PEDRETTI'S

Occupational Therapy

PRACTICE SKILLS FOR PHYSICAL DYSFUNCTION

PEDRETTI'S
Occupational Therapy

PRACTICE SKILLS FOR PHYSICAL DYSFUNCTION

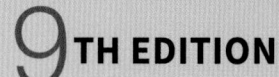

9TH EDITION

Heidi McHugh Pendleton,
PhD, OTR/L, FAOTA

Professor Emerita
Department of Occupational Therapy
San Jose State University
San Jose, California

Winifred Schultz-Krohn,
PhD, OTR/L, BCP, SWC, FAOTA

Professor Emerita
Department of Occupational Therapy
San Jose State University
San Jose, California

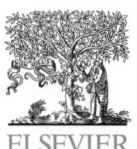

ELSEVIER

Elsevier
3251 Riverport Lane
St. Louis, Missouri 63043

PEDRETTI'S OCCUPATIONAL THERAPY: PRACTICE SKILLS FOR PHYSICAL
DYSFUNCTION, NINTH EDITION   ISBN 978-0-323-79255-4

Notice

Practitioners and researchers must always rely on their own experience and knowledge in evaluating and using any information, methods, compounds or experiments described herein. Because of rapid advances in the medical sciences, in particular, independent verification of diagnoses and drug dosages should be made. To the fullest extent of the law, no responsibility is assumed by Elsevier, authors, editors or contributors for any injury and/or damage to persons or property as a matter of products liability, negligence or otherwise, or from any use or operation of any methods, products, instructions, or ideas contained in the material herein.

Previous edition copyrighted 2018
International Standard Book Number 978-0-323-79255-4

Senior Content Strategist: Lauren Willis
Senior Content Development Manager: Lisa P. Newton
Senior Content Development Specialist: Tina Kaemmerer
Publishing Services Manager: Julie Eddy
Senior Project Manager: Jodi Willard
Design Direction: Brian Salisbury

Printed in India

Last digit is the print number: 9 8 7 6 5 4 3 2 1

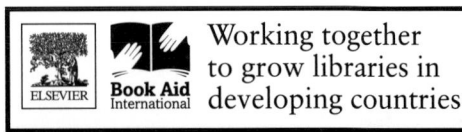

Working together to grow libraries in developing countries

www.elsevier.com • www.bookaid.org

CONTRIBUTORS

Michelle R. Abrams, OT, CHT
Occupational Therapist, Certified Hand
    Therapist
Department of Occupational Therapy
Mayo Clinic
Phoenix, Arizona

**Luis de Leon Arabit, OTD, MS, OTR/L,
BCN, BCPR, C/NDT, PAM, FAOTA**
Assistant Professor
Department of Occupational Therapy
San Jose State University
San Jose, California

**Cesar Cruz Arada, OTD, MHS, OTR/L,
PAM, SWC**
Academic Fieldwork Coordinator–Lecturer
Department of Occupational Therapy
San Jose State University
San Jose, California

Michal S. Atkins, MA, OTR/L
Instructor, Occupational Therapy
Department of Occupational and
    Recreation Therapy
Rancho Los Amigos National Rehabilitation
    Center
Downey, California

**Jennifer Bashar, OTD, OTR/L, BCPR,
CBIST**
Occupational Therapy Instructor
Department of Occupational and Recreation
    Therapy
Rancho Los Amigos National Rehabilitation
    Center
Downey, California

Jane Baumgarten, OTR/L
Instructor, Clinical Occupational Therapy
Division of Occupational Science and
    Occupational Therapy
University of Southern California
Los Angeles, California

Deborah J. Bolding, PhD, OTR/L, FAOTA
Associate Professor, Occupational Therapy
Department of Occupational Therapy
San Jose State University
San Jose, California

Brent Braveman, OTR, PhD, FAOTA
Director
Department of Rehabilitation Services
The University of Texas MD Anderson
    Cancer Center
Houston, Texas

Megan C. Chang, PhD, OTR/L, FAOTA
Professor
Occupational Therapy
Department of Occupational Therapy
San Jose State University
San Jose, California

Nancy Chee, OTD, OTR/L, CHT
Hand Therapist
Department of Physical Medicine and
    Rehabilitation–Hand Therapy
California Pacific Medical Center
San Francisco, California;
Adjunct Assistant Professor
Department of Occupational Therapy
Samuel Merritt University
Oakland, California

Janice Kishi Chow, PhD, DOT, OTR/L
Occupational Therapist
Physical Medicine and Rehabilitation Service
Veterans Affairs Palo Alto Health Care System
Palo Alto, California

Brenna Craig, MSOT, OTR/L
Occupational Therapist
Home Health (Pediatric Early Intervention
    and Neuro-rehabilitation)
San Jose, California

Elin Schold Davis, OTR/L, CDRS, FAOTA
Manager
Workforce Capacity and Engagement
American Occupational Therapy Association
North Bethesda, Maryland

Sharon Dekelboum, OTR/L, ATP
Occupational Therapist
Physical Medicine and Rehabilitation Service
Veterans Affairs Palo Alto Health Care System
Palo Alto, California

Elizabeth DePoy, PhD, MSW, BS
Professor
Social Work and Disability Studies
University of Maine
Orono, Maine

Lisa Deshaies, OTR/L, CHT
Clinical Specialist
Outpatient Therapy Services
Rancho Los Amigos National Rehabilitation
    Center
Downey, California;
Adjunct Clinical Faculty
Division of Occupational Science and
    Occupational Therapy
University of Southern California
Los Angeles, California

Heidi A. Dombish, MS, OTR/L
Occupational Therapist
Acute Inpatient Rehabilitation
Rancho Los Amigos National Rehabilitation
    Center
Downey, California;
Adjunct Instructor of Clinical Occupational
    Therapy
Division of Occupational Science and
    Occupational Therapy
University of Southern California
Los Angeles, California

Honor Duderstadt-Galloway, BS, OTR/L
Occupational Therapist II
Department of Occupational and
    Recreation Therapy
Rancho Los Amigos National Rehabilitation
    Center
Downey, California

Fiona Dunbar, OTR/L, MSOT, MALD
Occupational Therapist, Inpatient Acute
    Rehab
Department of Pediatric Rehabilitation
UCSF Benioff Children's Hospital Oakland
Oakland, California

Joyce M. Engel, PhD, OT
Professor
Department of Occupational Science and
    Technology
University of Wisconsin
Milwaukee, Wisconsin

Daniel Geller, EdD, MPH, MSOT
Assistant Professor
Programs in Occupational Therapy
Department of Rehabilitation and
    Regenerative Medicine
Vagelos College of Physicians and Surgeons
Columbia University
New York, New York

Alison Hewitt George, MS, OTR/L
Lecturer, Occupational Therapy
Department of Occupational Therapy
San Jose State University
San Jose, California

Glen Gillen, EdD, OTR, FAOTA
Professor, Regenerative and Rehabilitation
    Medicine (Occupational Therapy)
Columbia University Medical Center
Programs in Occupational Therapy
Columbia University
New York, New York

Lynn Gitlow, PhD, OTR/L, ATP
Lecturer, Occupational Therapy
Ithaca College
Ithaca, New York

Monica Godinez-Becerril, MA, OTR/L
Occupational Therapist II
Department of Occupational and
  Recreation Therapy
Rancho Los Amigos National Rehabilitation
  Center
Downey, California

Denise Haruko Ha, OTR/L
Occupational Therapist II
Occupational Therapy Work
  Rehabilitation
Rancho Los Amigos National Rehabilitation
  Center
Downey, California

Agnes Haruko Hirai, MA, OTR/L
Assistant Rehab Manager, Occupational
  Therapy
Rehabilitation Services
Los Angeles General Medical Center
Los Angeles, California

Jennifer Kaye Hughes, OTR, MOT
Senior Occupational Therapist
Rehabilitation;
Clinical Informatics Specialist
IS Shared Services
The University of Texas MD Anderson
  Cancer Center
Houston, Texas

**Cynthia Clare Ivy, MEd, OTD, OTR/L,
CHT**
Clinical Professor
Department of Occupational Therapy
Northern Arizona University
Phoenix, Arizona

**Vicki Kaskutas, BS, MHS, OTD, OTR/L,
FAOTA**
Associate Professor, Retired
Program in Occupational Therapy
Washington University School of Medicine
St. Louis, Missouri

Jean S. Koketsu, OTD, MS, OTR/L
Occupational Therapist
Rehabilitation
On Lok PACE;
Lecturer, Occupational Therapy
Department of Occupational Therapy
San Jose State University
San Jose, California

**Barbara L. Kornblau, JD, OTR/L,
FAOTA, DASPE, CCM, CDMS, CPE**
Principal
Barbara L. Kornblau Consulting
Washington DC;
Founder and Chief Executive Officer
Coalition for Disability Health Equity;
Program Director, Occupational Therapy
Professor, Occupational Therapy
Department of Physical and Occupational
  Therapy
Idaho State University
Pocatello, Idaho

Mark Kovic, OTD, OTR/L, FAOTA
Associate Director and Professor
Occupational Therapy
Department of Physical and Occupational
  Therapy
Midwestern University
Downers Grove, Illinois

**Sheama Krishnagiri, PhD, OTR/L,
FAOTA**
Associate Professor
Department of Brain Health
University of Nevada Las Vegas
Las Vegas, Nevada

Dawn Kurakazu, OTD, OTR/L
Occupational Therapy Instructor
Department of Rehabilitation Medicine
Los Angeles General Medical Center
Los Angeles, California

**Donna Lashgari, DHSc, OTR/L,
CHT Retired**
Lecturer/Guest Lecturer
Department of Occupational Therapy
San Jose State University
San Jose, California

Sonia Lawson, PhD, OTR/L, FAOTA
Associate Professor
Department of Occupational Therapy and
  Occupational Science
Towson University
Towson, Maryland

Katrina M. Long, EdD, MS, OTR/L
Assistant Professor, Occupational Therapy
Department of Occupational Therapy
San Jose State University
San Jose, California;
Research Affiliate
Biobehavioral Sciences
Teachers College, Columbia University
New York, New York

Cara Masselink, PhD, OTRL, ATP
Assistant Professor
Department of Occupational Therapy
Western Michigan University
Grand Rapids, Michigan

Rose McAndrew, OTD, OTR/L, CHT
Assistant Professor
Occupational Therapy Assistant Program
St. Louis Community College
St. Louis, Missouri

**Rochelle McLaughlin, MS, OTR/L,
MBSR**
Adjunct Faculty
Department of Occupational Therapy
San Jose State University
San Jose, California

Lynne F. Murphy, EdD, OTR/L
Associate Professor
Department of Occupational Therapy
East Carolina University
Greenville, North Carolina

Jennifer Nicholson, MOT, OTR/L
Senior Occupational Therapist
Department of Rehabilitation Services
The University of Texas MD Anderson
  Cancer Center
Houston, Texas

Annemarie E. Orr, MA, OTD
Director of Human Performance
Human Performance Program
Naval Special Warfare Center
San Diego, California;
Assistant Professor, Physical Medicine and
  Rehabilitation
Uniformed Services University of Health
  Sciences
Bethesda, Maryland

**Debra S. Ouellette, MS, OTR/L, BCPR,
SCLV, FNAP**
Clinical Director
Outpatient Neurological Rehabilitation
Casa Colina Hospital and Centers for
  Healthcare
Pomona, California

Jill J. Page, OTR/L, CEAS
Co-Owner, CapacityLAB
Birmingham, Alabama

Karen Parecki, OTR/L, MS, ATP
Occupational Therapist
Physical Medicine and Rehabilitation
  Service
Veterans Affairs Palo Alto Health Care System
Palo Alto, California

Heidi McHugh Pendleton, PhD, OTR/L, FAOTA
Professor Emerita
Department of Occupational Therapy
San Jose State University
San Jose, California

Barb Phillips-Meltzer, MS, OTD, OTR/L
Owner, Chief Executive Officer
Ergonomics
Ergo Life Solutions
El Segundo, California

Michael A. Pizzi, PhD, OTR/L, FAOTA
Wellness Lifestyle Coach
Associate Professor
Department of Occupational Therapy
Dominican College
Orangeburg, New York

Samia Husam Rafeedie, OTD, OTR/L, BCPR, CBIS, CEAS, FAOTA
Associate Professor of Clinical Occupational Therapy
Professional Program Director
Health and Safety Director
Chan Division of Occupational Science and Occupational Therapy
University of Southern California
Los Angeles, California

Pamela Roberts, PhD, OTR/L, SCFES, FAOTA, CPHQ, FNAP, FACRM
Executive Director and Professor
Physical Medicine and Rehabilitation
Cedars-Sinai Health System;
Executive Director
Office of Chief Medical Officer
Medical Affairs
Cedars-Sinai Health System;
Co-Director, Division of Informatics
Biomedical Sciences
Cedars-Sinai Health System;
Senior Director of Quality, Outcomes, and Research
Quality and Research
California Rehabilitation Institute
Los Angeles, California

Michelle Rodriguez, MA, OTR/L
Occupational Therapist
Rehabilitation
On Lok Lifeways
San Jose, California

†Kelly McGaughey Roseberry, DPT, BS
Adjunct Professor
Department of Occupational Therapy
University of Southern Maine
Lewiston, Maine;
Adjunct Professor
Department of Physical Therapy
Shenandoah University
Winchester, Virginia

Robert J.T. Russow, OTD, OTR/L
Assistant Professor of Clinical Occupational Therapy
Chan Division of Occupational Science and Occupational Therapy
University of Southern California
Los Angeles, California

Winifred Schultz-Krohn, PhD, OTR/L, BCP, SWC, FAOTA
Professor Emerita
Department of Occupational Therapy
San Jose State University
San Jose, California

Deborah A. Schwartz, OTD, OTR/L, CHT
Product and Educational Specialist
Physical Rehabilitation
Orfit Industries America
Leonia, New Jersey

Tim Shurtleff, BA, MA, OTD, OTR/L
Instructor, Retired
Program in Occupational Therapy
Washington University School of Medicine
St. Louis, Missouri

Ashley Uyeshiro Simon, OTD, OTR/L
Associate Professor of Clinical Occupational Therapy
Chan Division of Occupational Science and Occupational Therapy
University of Southern California
Los Angeles, California

Jerilyn (Gigi) Smith, PhD, OTR/L, FAOTA
Chair and Professor, Occupational Therapy
Graduate and Undergraduate Coordinator/Advisor
Department of Occupational Therapy
San Jose State University
San Jose, California

Shohei Takatani, MS, OTR/L, HTC
Occupational Therapist, Clinical Specialist
Rehabilitation Services
Stanford Health Care
Stanford, California

Graham Teaford, OTD, MS, OTR/L
Lecturer
Occupational Therapy
Department of Occupational Therapy
San Jose State University;
Occupational Therapist
On Lok
San Jose, California

Michelle Tipton-Burton, MS, OTR/L, CBIS
Lecturer
Department of Occupational Therapy
San Jose State University;
Occupational Therapist
Rehabilitation Case Manager
Private Practice
San Jose, California

Susan Martin Touchinsky, OTR/L, SCDCM, CDRS
Owner
OT Driver Rehabilitation
Adaptive Mobility Services, LLC
Orwigsburg, Pennsylvania

J. Martin Walsh, OTRL, CHT
Executive Director
Hand Therapy Certification Commission
Sacramento, California

Jacqueline Reese Walter, PhD, OTR/L, CHT
Associate Professor
Department of Occupational Therapy
Jacksonville University
Jacksonville, Florida

Mary Warren, PhD, SCLV, FAOTA
Associate Professor Emerita
Department of Occupational Therapy
University of Alabama at Birmingham
Birmingham, Alabama

Kristin Winston, PhD
Program Director and Associate Professor
Master of Science in Occupational Therapy
University of New England
Portland, Maine

Stephanie Yang, MA, OTR/L
Occupational Therapist
Department of Occupational and Recreation Therapy
Rancho Los Amigos National Rehabilitation Center
Downey, California

†Deceased.

We are honored to dedicate this ninth edition of *Pedretti's Occupational Therapy: Practice Skills for Physical Dysfunction* to Lorraine Williams Pedretti. Lorraine Williams Pedretti was selected by the American Occupational Therapy Association as one of the 100 Influential People in the field of Occupational Therapy as part of the professional Centennial Celebration. Her thoughtfulness, love of her profession, and dedication to the education of her students provided the impetus to embark on the daunting task of writing and editing an original textbook (and ensuing editions) for evaluation and treatment of adults with physical disabilities. As academic colleagues of Professor Pedretti, we were inspired by her example and challenged to accept the responsibility to continue in her footsteps to contribute to the advancement of the profession. It is our hope that our efforts have honored her example and lived up to her faith in us.

We would also like to dedicate this edition to occupational therapy students (past, present, and future), who are the future of our wonderful profession: may you find the happiness and fulfillment that we have as proud occupational therapists.

It was a great honor to continue the editorship of the ninth edition of *Pedretti's Occupational Therapy: Practice Skills for Physical Dysfunction*. To continue to follow in the footsteps of the inimitable Lorraine Pedretti is at once an awesome responsibility and a rewarding journey. The opportunity to work with the authors, each a leading expert in his or her field, continues to be an unparalleled experience of the exceptional ability of stellar occupational therapists to organize their time and unselfishly devote their scholarship to the education of future generations of the profession.

Since the publication of the eighth edition, there have been changes within the profession and within the clinical practice of occupational therapy for clients with physical dysfunction. Many of those changes served to shape the approach we took to the new edition and are reflected within the context of each of the chapters. Our mission and intention was to embrace these changes and continue to honor the primacy of occupation that has been the foundation of this textbook for the past several editions.

The ninth and latest edition is framed and guided by the Occupational Therapy Practice Framework: Domain and Process—4 (OTPF-4), designed to describe the focus and dynamic process of the profession. Key to the OTPF-4 is its view of the overarching goal of occupational therapy; that is, engagement in occupation to support participation in life. This conceptualization of the importance of occupation is emphasized throughout the text. The concepts of process and practice, evaluation and intervention, performance skills and patterns, contexts and activity demands, client factors, and intervention applications are all thoroughly illustrated throughout.

To honor the centrality of the client to occupational therapy practice, the chapters begin with case studies, which are then threaded throughout, guiding the reader through the information and relating the content to the specific case descriptions. Thus, the reader is able to experience the clinical reasoning and decision-making skills of the expert clinicians who authored the chapters. Authors of individual chapters were asked to follow the initial presentation of their case studies by crafting several probative or "critical thinking" questions that would pique the readers' curiosity, further motivating their attention to and questioning of the chapter content and consequently facilitating the learning process. Direct answers to these critical thinking questions are provided either within or at the end of each of the chapters.

This textbook, written for an intended audience of occupational therapy graduate students and as a reference for practicing occupational therapists, has always been acknowledged for its practical application and focus on practice. Theory and evidence-based content are presented in each chapter and then applied using case descriptions as a foundation for practice. Occupational therapy's role in health and wellness, as well as prevention, is addressed throughout the text. Similarly, occupational therapy's commitment to the importance of considering cultural and ethnic diversity is reflected in every chapter.

The ninth edition continues to feature the OT Practice Notes and the Ethical Considerations boxes that are highlighted throughout many of the chapters. The information contained in these boxes (pulled from the chapter content) conveys ideas that are relevant to students' future practice areas and thoughts about some of the possible ethical dilemmas and decisions with which they might be confronted.

During the process of editing this book, including the stages of envisioning and designing the content and format, selecting the authors, and reading and giving input to their work, we were guided by our commitment to honoring the occupational welfare of our clients, particularly adults with physical disabilities, through excellent preparation of their future occupational therapists. To that end we sought preeminent authors, those who not only had recognition for expertise in their topic area, but who also embraced the primary importance of occupation to their practice and scholarship. Our goal was to engender excitement in the reader for occupational therapy in the area of physical dysfunction while providing cutting-edge information and promoting models of best practice. Our extensive and rewarding clinical and academic careers in the profession of occupational therapy and our experiences with hardworking and inspiring clients and students served as the inspiration for our best efforts, which we trust are evident in this book.

Heidi McHugh Pendleton
Winifred Schultz-Krohn

ACKNOWLEDGMENTS

We would like to thank the authors, past and present, for their exceptional contributions and willingness to continue the tradition of excellence that has come to be associated with the Pedretti book. The impressive list of authors for the ninth edition continues the Pedretti reputation for including nationally and internationally known experts in their topic areas and disciplines. We are fortunate to feature contributions from new authors, and included among them are administrators, educators, researchers, and master clinicians.

We would also like to acknowledge the superb contribution of the dedicated editors and staff at Elsevier. We are especially grateful to Lauren Willis, Senior Content Strategist, and Tina Kaemmerer, Senior Content Development Specialist, who patiently and painstakingly mentored us through the long and arduous editing process. They are simply outstanding! Our thanks go to Jodi Willard, Senior Project Manager, who, with exceptional attention to detail, made sure that the final product reflected the efforts of all involved.

To those publishers and vendors who permitted us to use material from their publications, we extend our sincere gratitude. Photographers and artists, and the clients and models who posed for photographs, are gratefully acknowledged. We are grateful to the contributors who were particularly generous in finding just the right photographs to capture the importance of occupation to participation in life—we thank you!

Finally, we would like to extend heartfelt appreciation to our colleagues, friends, and families, without whose help and support this accomplishment could not have been achieved. Special expressions of *thank you* go to the faculty and staff at San José State University, who could be counted upon for their support and good wishes during this process.

Heidi McHugh Pendleton extends her gratitude to her husband, Forrest Pendleton (for immeasurable love and support, without which this endeavor could never have succeeded) and to her sisters, Deirdre McHugh and Kathleen McHugh (for a lifetime of support). Her love and appreciation go to all of her nieces, nephews, and stepson, including Dar, Jim, Nicky, Elizabeth, Jimmy D, Megan, Kelsey, Jamie, Jessica, and Katie—their love and enthusiasm make everything possible.

Winifred Schultz-Krohn extends a huge thank you to her always supportive, ever-patient husband, Kermit Krohn. His tireless love made the project possible. She is also very grateful for the support and encouragement received from her brother Tom Schultz and his wife Barb Fraser; her niece Sarah; her sister Donna Friedrich and her husband Don; her nephews Brian and Andrew; Andrew's wife Kirsten; her grandnephew Zachary; and her sister Nancy Yamasaki and her husband Bryan.

The co-editors would like to thank each other—great friends at the beginning of the process—as we were able to be there for each other, make our own unique contributions, and ultimately sustain our friendship throughout the process, emerging even better friends in the joy of our accomplishment.

CONTENTS

---

†Deceased.

1

The Occupational Therapy Practice Framework and the Practice of Occupational Therapy for People With Physical Disabilities

Heidi McHugh Pendleton and Winifred Schultz-Krohn

LEARNING OBJECTIVES

After studying this chapter, the student or practitioner will be able to do the following:

1. Briefly describe the evolution of the Occupational Therapy Practice Framework (OTPF), from the original OTPF through the OTPF-4.
2. Describe the need for the OTPF-4 in the practice of occupational therapy (OT) for persons with physical disabilities.
3. Describe the fit between the OTPF-4 and the *International Classification of Functioning, Disability, and Health* (ICF), and explain how they inform and enhance the

occupational therapist's (OT's) understanding of physical disability.

4. Describe the elements of the OTPF-4, including domain and process and their relationship to each other.
5. List and describe the components that make up the OT domain and give examples of each.
6. List and describe the components that make up the OT process and give examples of each.
7. Briefly describe the OT intervention levels, and give an example of each as it might be used in a physical disability practice setting.

CHAPTER OUTLINE

KEY TERMS

Activities
Client factors
Contexts
Domain
Environment
Evaluation
International Classification of Functioning, Disability, and Health (ICF)
Intervention

Occupational justice
"The Occupational Therapy Practice Framework: Domain and Process," fourth edition (OTPF-4)
Occupations
Performance patterns
Performance skills
Process
Targeted outcomes

THREADED CASE STUDY

Kent and Keri, Part 1

Kent (who identifies with the pronouns he, him, his) is a highly skilled and very competent OT with more than 25 years of clinical experience. He works in a large rehabilitation center with adult clients who have physical disabilities. He currently is the supervising OT on the spinal cord injury (SCI) unit. Through his reading of OT publications,[5,13,19,31] attendance at conferences and workshops, and interactions with his OT staff and interning OT students, he has become increasingly knowledgeable about the Occupational Therapy Practice Framework (OTPF) and its current version, the OTPF-4. When the OTPF was first published in 2002, he initially was annoyed that, among the many challenges to his professional time and efforts, he would have to learn, yet again, a new "language" to provide competent interventions and that even before he had mastered the first three models, a fourth, updated, edition had appeared. He couldn't help thinking, "Why fix something that isn't broken?" He reluctantly acknowledged the necessity for the change. Now, however, he is impressed by what he has learned so far, and he is convinced that it will be beneficial to delve into and integrate the OTPF-4 into his clinical practice.

Throughout his practice, Kent found it helpful to relate new or novel OT information he is learning to the relevant circumstances that either he or one of his clients is experiencing; in this way he considers the impact the new information might have on either his own life or that of his client.

Kent has decided that, as he works on learning the OTPF-4 and any updates, changes, additions, or eliminations, he will keep in mind one of his recently admitted clients, Keri. Keri is a single 25-year-old woman (preferring the pronouns she, her, hers) who lives alone in her own apartment and works as an administrative assistant for a busy law office. Keri incurred a cervical SCI and now has C6 functional quadriplegia/tetraplegia that necessitates use of a wheelchair for mobility. By keeping Keri in mind, Kent expects not only to learn the changes and updates to the OTPF-4 but also to reinforce his new knowledge by putting it to immediate use in his practice.

Critical Thinking Questions

As you read through the chapter, keep in mind the challenges that learning the OTPF-4 and integrating it into his practice will pose for Kent. Think of strategies you might recommend or use yourself to learn and integrate the information into your practice. In addition, consider the objectives for the chapter, outlined previously, and also these questions:

1. Why was there a need for the OTPF and its subsequent three versions, and how do they fill that need?
2. How might the specific information presented about the OTPF-4 apply to Kent or Keri?
3. Are there tools that Kent and other seasoned OT practitioners, students, and novice OT practitioners can use to help them learn the OTPF initially or learn the changes brought about by the fourth edition of the OTPF and integrate this vital information into their practice?

THE OCCUPATIONAL THERAPY PRACTICE FRAMEWORK: DOMAIN AND PROCESS, FOURTH EDITION (OTPF-4)—OVERVIEW

Many changes have occurred in the practice of occupational therapy (OT) for persons with physical disabilities since the publication of the previous edition of *Occupational Therapy: Practice Skills for Physical Dysfunction* in 2018. OT practice settings are increasingly moving away from traditional healthcare environments, such as the hospital and rehabilitation center, and have made significant strides moving more toward the home and community milieus. With the pandemic of 2020, occupational therapy practitioners were challenged to provide intervention via online services such as videoconferencing tools (e.g., Zoom) and delve extensively into the realm of telehealth (See Chapter 52). The provision of OT service has become progressively more client centered, and the concept of occupation is increasingly and proudly named as both the preferred intervention and the desired outcome of the services. Clinicians, researchers, and scholars have sought to implement evidence-based practice by learning more about the benefits of occupation not only to remediate problems after the onset of physical disability but also to anticipate and prevent physical disability and promote wellness. Not surprisingly, economic concerns have severely shortened the amount of time allotted for OT services, thus necessitating more deliberate and resourceful decisions about how these services can be delivered most effectively.

In response to these changes and many other practice advances, came a change, or ongoing evolution, in the language that OTs use to describe what they do and how they do it. This change, in turn, resulted in the document "The Occupational Therapy Practice Framework: Domain and Process," initially published in 2002 by the American Occupational Therapy Association (AOTA) in the *American Journal of Occupational Therapy* (AJOT).[2] (The model set forth in the initial document is commonly referred to as the Occupational Therapy Practice Framework [OTPF] or just the Framework.) As mentioned at the beginning of this chapter, with the fourth edition came the recommendation to call it simply, the OTPF.

The OTPF is a tool developed by the OT profession to more clearly articulate and enhance the understanding of what OT practitioners do (occupational therapy domain) and how they do it (occupational therapy process). The intended beneficiaries of all four editions of the OTPF were envisioned as including not only OT practitioners (an internal audience of OTs and occupational therapy assistants [OTAs]), but also the recipients of OT services (referred to as clients, including the individual, family members, the community, groups, and populations), other healthcare professionals, and those providing reimbursement for OT services (an external audience).

The first version of the Framework was put into practice, and its relevance and efficacy were assessed; this evaluation resulted in the OTPF-2,[3] which was published in the AJOT in 2008, and subsequently the OTPF-3, which was published in the AJOT in 2014.[4] The same rigorous examination was applied to produce the current version, "The Occupational Therapy Practice Framework: Domain and Process," fourth edition (OTPF-4), which appears in the August 2020 AJOT.[5]

The OTPF-4 is an important document that every OT practitioner should have and consult frequently. It can be downloaded from the AOTA website (http://www.aota.org) by selecting AJOT (under Publications & News at the top of the homepage) and then the August 2020 issue; a PDF copy of this document can be downloaded and printed for convenience to members of AOTA. Another helpful tool for learning the OTPF is the introductory article by Youngstrom[31] titled "The Occupational Therapy Practice Framework: The Evolution of Our Professional Language," which appeared in the November/December 2002 issue of the AJOT.

It is not the intention of this chapter to supplant the comprehensive OTPF-4 document but, rather, to describe the model and increase the reader's understanding of the OTPF-4 and its relationship to the practice of occupational therapy with adults with physical disabilities. To achieve this, the chapter begins with a discussion of the history of the OTPF, followed by sections describing the need for the OTPF and the fit between the OTPF and the World Health Organization's (WHO) *International Classification of Functioning, Disability, and Health* (ICF).[30] Next, a detailed description of the OTPF-4 is presented, with emphasis on explicating the domain of occupational therapy through examples from the case study and introducing the OT process (discussed in depth in Chapter 3) in the transactional application of the OTPF-4 when working with individuals with physical dysfunction. The types of OT intervention proposed by the OTPF-4 are examined and illustrated by examples typically used in physical disabilities practice settings. The chapter concludes with suggestions and strategies for learning the OTPF and an overview of how the latest version—the OTPF-4—is integrated as a unifying thread throughout the remaining chapters in the book.

Evolution of the Occupational Therapy Practice Framework

In 1999 the AOTA's Commission on Practice (COP) was charged with reviewing the "Uniform Terminology for Occupational Therapy," third edition (UT-III), a document that had been published by the association 5 years earlier.[5] Under the leadership of its chair, Mary Jane Youngstrom, the COP sought feedback from numerous OT practitioners, scholars, and leaders in the profession about the continued suitability of the UT-III to determine whether to update the document or to rescind it. Previous editions of the UT, in 1979 and 1989, had been similarly reviewed and updated to reflect changes and the evolving progress of the profession. The reviewers found that the UT-III, although considered a valuable tool for OTs, lacked clarity for both consumers and professionals in associated fields about what OTs do and how they do it. Furthermore, they found that the UT-III did not adequately describe or emphasize OT's focus on occupation, the foundation of the profession.[13] Given the feedback from the review, COP determined that a new document was needed, one that would preserve the intent of the UT-III (outlining and naming the constructs of the profession) while providing increased clarity about what OTs and OTAs do and how they do it. Additionally, it was determined that the new document would refocus attention on the primacy of occupation as the cornerstone of the profession and desired intervention outcomes, in addition to showing the process OTs use to help their clients achieve their occupational goals.

Need for the Occupational Therapy Practice Framework

The original OTPF and the revised versions (OTPF-2, 3, and now 4) make it clear that the profession's central focus and actions are grounded in the concept of occupation. Although some of what OTs do could be construed by clients and other healthcare professionals as similar to or even duplication of the treatment efforts of other disciplines, formally delineating occupation as the overarching goal of all that OT does, and clearly documenting supportive goals intended to achieve that main goal, establish the profession's unique contribution to client intervention.

This is not to say that before the OTPF, OT practitioners did not recognize or focus on occupation or occupational goals with their clients—most did.[14,15,19,23] However, in the physical disabilities practice setting, with the reductionistic, bottom-up approach and pervasive influence of the medical model, occupation was seldom mentioned or linked to what was being done in OT. A premium seemed to be placed on "medical speak," and it was difficult, if not impossible, to document occupational performance or occupational goals using the types of documentation characteristic of physical disabilities practice settings. Kent, the OT from the case study, still occasionally experiences the medical team members' heightened interest when the OT report focuses on muscle grades and sensory status and, in comparison, their quizzical, glazed-over looks when the clients' difficulties resuming homemaking, leisure, or other home and community skills are described. The OTPF-4 provides a means of communicating to healthcare professionals who are not OTs that engagement in occupation should be the primary outcome of all intervention.

The OTPF-4 provides a language and structure that communicates occupation more meaningfully. It empowers OTs to restructure evaluation, progress, and other documentation forms to reflect the primacy of occupation in what OT does, and it shows the interaction of all the aspects that contribute to supporting or constraining the client's participation. Thus, by clearly showing and articulating the comprehensive nature of OT's domain of practice to clients, healthcare professionals, and other interested parties, OTs enlist support and demand for their services and, most importantly, ensure that clients receive the unique and important services that OT provides. Equally important, the OTPF-4 positions the client as a collaborator with the OT at every step of the process, thereby empowering the individual as a change agent and reframing the image of the client as a passive recipient of services.[13]

Fit Between the OTPF-4 and the *International Classification of Functioning, Disability, and Health* (ICF)

There appears to be an excellent fit between the OTPF (all editions) and the ICF. About the same time the UT-III was being studied for continued suitability for contemporary language and practice, the WHO was revising its language and classification model. The result, the *International Classification of Functioning, Disability, and Health*, contributes to the understanding of the complexity of having a physical disability.[30]

The ICF "moved away from being a 'consequences of disease' classification to become a 'components of health' classification,"[30] progressing from impairment, disability, and handicap to body functions and structures, activities, and participation. In the ICF, *body structures* refers to the anatomic parts of the body, and *body functions* refers to a person's physiological and psychological functions. Also considered in this model is the impact of environmental and personal factors as they relate to functioning. The ICF adopted a universal model that considers health along a continuum that shows the potential for everyone to have a disability. The WHO perceived this as a radical shift—from emphasizing people's disabilities to focusing on their level of health.

The ICF also provides support and reinforcement for OT to specifically address activity and activity limitations encountered by people with disabilities.[30] In addition, it describes the importance of participation in life situations, or *domains,* including (1) learning and applying knowledge; (2) general tasks and task demands; (3) communication; (4) movement; (5) self-care; (6) domestic life areas; (7) interpersonal interactions; (8) major life areas associated with work, school, and family life; and (9) community, social, and civic life. All of these domains are historically familiar areas of concern and intervention for the OT profession. Although a physical disability may compromise a person's ability to reach up to brush his or her hair, the ICF redirects the service provider to also consider activity limitations that may result in restricted participation in desired life situations, such as sports or parenting. A problem with a person's bodily structure, such as paralysis or a missing limb, is recognized as a potentially limiting factor, but that is not the focus of intervention.

OT practitioners think that intervention provided for people with physical disabilities should extend beyond a focus on recovery of physical skills and address the person's engagement, or active participation, in occupations. This viewpoint is the cornerstone of the OTPF-4 and previous versions. Such active participation in occupation is interdependent on the client's psychological and social well-being, which must be simultaneously addressed through the OT intervention. This orientation is congruent with the emphasis reflected in the ICF.

In many instances the language of the UT-III was different from that used and understood by the external audience of other healthcare professionals. Similarly, the terminology of the previous WHO classification frequently differed from that used by the audience with which the organization was trying to communicate (e.g., healthcare professionals and other service providers). The goals of the new WHO classifications, the ICF, are to increase communication and understanding about the experience of having a disability and unify services. In a similar manner, the original OTPF, and now the updated OTPF-4, was designed to increase others' knowledge and understanding of the OT profession and, where appropriate, to incorporate the language of the ICF, as will be seen in the following discussion of the OT domain and process.

Detailed information on the ICF can be found in the document referenced in this chapter,[30] or an overview of the document can be downloaded from http://www.who.int.

A helpful resource for learning the ICF is the Beginners Guide to the ICF, which also can be accessed at the website http://www.who.int. Additional and annually updated documents on the ICF also are available at this website.

THE OTPF-4: DESCRIPTION

The OTPF-4 is composed of two interrelated parts, the domain and the process. The domain articulates the focus and factors addressed by the profession and where the profession has an established body of knowledge and expertise, and the process describes how occupational therapy does what it does (evaluation, intervention, and outcomes)—in other words, how the domain is put into practice by providing client-centered care focused on engagement in occupations. Central to both parts is the essential concept of occupation. The definition of occupation used by the developers of the original Framework is:

Activities of everyday life, named, organized, and given value and meaning by individuals and a culture. Occupation is everything people do to occupy themselves, including looking after themselves, enjoying life, and contributing to the social and economic fabric of their communities.[2,19]

The next two revised Frameworks (OTPF-2 and OTPF-3), rather than adopting a single definition, used several definitions found in the OT literature[3,4,16,22,27] (OTPF-3, pp. S5–S6). The committee charged with producing the OTPF-3 ultimately suggested that an array of selected definitions of the term *occupation*, offered by the scholars of the profession, would add to an understanding of this core concept (see OTPF-3, pp. S5–S6).[4] For the OTPF-4, a singular definition of occupation was adopted, which is: "Everyday personalized activities that people do as individuals, in families, and with communities to occupy time and bring meaning and purpose to life. Occupations can involve the execution of multiple activities for completion and can result in various outcomes. The broad range of occupations is categorized as activities of daily living, instrumental activities of daily living, health management, rest and sleep, education, work, play, leisure, and social participation" (see Appendix A, pp. 79).[5] The term *occupation* is differentiated from *activities* in the OTPF. Activities is defined as "actions designed and selected to support the development of performance skills and performance patterns to enhance occupational engagement" (see Appendix A pp. 74).[5]

In adopting the essence of this definition, the developers of the OTPF-4 characterized the profession's focus on occupation in a dynamic and action-oriented form, in which they echoed the words of the OTPF-3, articulated as "achieving health, well-being and participation in life through engagement in occupation"[4,5] (OTPF-3, p. S2 and OTPF-4, p. 5). This phrase links the two parts of the Framework, providing the unifying theme or focus of the OT domain and the overarching target outcome of the OT process—an inextricable linkage between domain and process that the authors of both the OTPF-3 and the OTPF-4 describe as "transactional."[4,5]

The Occupational Therapy Domain

The domain of occupational therapy encompasses the gamut of what OTs do, along with the primary concern and focus of the profession's efforts. Everything that occupational therapy does or is concerned about, as depicted in the domain of the OTPF-4, is directed at supporting the client's engagement in meaningful occupation that ultimately affects the health, well-being, and life satisfaction of that individual.

The current five broad areas that constitute the OT domain are occupations, client factors, performance skills, performance patterns, and context. These categories, which are dynamically interrelated, represent the practice domain of the occupational therapy profession. The OTPF stipulates that there is no hierarchy of categories within the domain of occupational therapy practice. The developers of the OTPF-3 pointed out that there is a complex interplay among all of these areas or aspects of the domain, that no single part is more critical than another, and that all aspects are viewed as influencing engagement in occupations. This concept was reinforced with the fourth edition of the OTPF. Furthermore, the success of the OT process (evaluation, intervention, and targeted outcomes) is incumbent on the OT's expert knowledge of all aspects of the domain. The expert practice of OT requires the therapeutic use of self, clinical reasoning (knowledge of theory and evidence), and skills in activity analysis and activity demands to create the overview that guides each step of the process.

Occupations

OTs frequently use the terms *occupation* and *activity* interchangeably. In the Framework, the term *occupation*

encompasses the term *activity*. **Occupations** may be characterized as being meaningful and goal directed but not necessarily considered by the individual to be of central importance to her or his life. Similarly, occupations also may be viewed as (1) activities in which the client engages, (2) activities that have the added qualitative criteria of giving meaning to the person's life and contributing to his or her identity, and (3) activities in which the individual looks forward to engaging. For example, Keri, Kent's client with quadriplegia, regards herself as an excellent and dedicated clothes and accessories shopper; holidays and celebrations always include her engagement in her treasured occupation of shopping. Kent, on the other hand, regards the activity of shopping for clothes as important only to keep himself clothed and maintain social acceptance. Kent avoids the activity whenever possible. Each engages in this activity to support participation in life but with a qualitatively different attitude and level of enthusiasm. In the OTPF-4, both of these closely related terms are used to recognize that individual clients determine the occupations he or she regards as meaningful and those that are simply necessary or are activities that support the person's participation in life. For Kent, shopping is a necessary occupation or activity, but for Keri, it is a favorite occupation.

The occupation category of the domain includes nine comprehensive types of human activities or occupations. Each is outlined in the following discussion; a list of typical activities included in each type is provided; and examples from the physical disability perspective, as provided by Keri's circumstances, are presented.

THREADED CASE STUDY

Kent and Keri, Part 2

Perusing the list of activities of daily living (ADLs) in Table 1 of the OTPF, Kent noted that virtually every category, with the exception of eating (which involves the ability to keep and manipulate food in the mouth and the ability to swallow), would be a concern for his client, Keri, because of the nature and extent of her SCI disability. When Kent discussed this list, Keri viewed practically all as necessary activities but personally valued feeding, sexual activity, and personal hygiene and grooming as being extremely important for her satisfactory participation in life. Keri was a little surprised to learn that sexual activity was included. "So this is occupational therapy? Maybe I'll wait awhile before I talk about this topic, but it's good to know I'm expected to be interested."

For the present, Keri's attention turned to activities of immediate interest, including those tasks associated with the personal hygiene and grooming category and its detailed description:

Obtaining and using supplies, removing body hair (use of razors, tweezers, lotions, etc.), applying and removing cosmetics, washing, drying, combing, styling, brushing and trimming hair; caring for nails (hands and

feet), caring for skin, ears, eyes, and nose, applying deodorant, cleaning mouth, brushing and flossing teeth; or removing, cleaning, and reinserting dental orthotics and prosthetics.[5] (OTPF, p. S30)

The numerous details reminded her of how important all these grooming activities were to her, and they indicated the scope of the daily activities she would like to address in OT. Of particular concern to Keri were the grooming activities of shaping her eyebrows and styling her hair; these were bodily care activities she regarded as very personal. In fact, she was reluctant to let anyone do these for her. Although under similar circumstances Kent might have gladly deferred these two ADLs, it was clear that Keri prioritized them as personally meaningful occupational goals.

In studying the list of ADLs, Kent noted that, just like personal hygiene and grooming, each ADL item listed had a similarly helpful definition and detailed list of examples in the tables throughout the OTPF-4 document. He remembered reading that these lists were provided to give a few examples, that they were not to be considered exhaustive, and in fact that there was an expectation that

(Continued)

Kent and Keri, Part 2

the lists would be modified and expanded on as the OTPF became more familiar and integrated into practice.

ADLs (also referred to as personal activities of daily living [PADLs] or *basic activities of daily living* [BADLs]) are activities that have to do with accomplishing one's own personal body care. The body care activities included in the ADL category are bathing/showering, toileting and toileting hygiene, dressing, eating and swallowing, feeding, functional mobility, personal hygiene and grooming, and sexual activity.

Instrumental activities of daily living (IADLs) are "activities to support daily life within the home and community"[5] (OTPF, p. S30). The specific IADLs included in the domain are care of others (including selecting and supervising caregivers), care of pets, childrearing, communication management, driving and community mobility, financial management, home establishment and management, meal preparation and cleanup, religious and spiritual expression, safety and emergency maintenance, and shopping.

Knowing that the IADL shopping was certain to be a priority occupation for Keri, Kent made a note of the full description of shopping from the corresponding lists of IADLs in the OTPF-4. Shopping is described there as "Preparing shopping lists (grocery and other); selecting, purchasing, and transporting items; selecting method of payment and completing payment transactions; managing internet shopping and related use of electronic devices such as computers, cell phones, and tablets"[5] (OTPF, p. S31). This is not as detailed as some descriptions, but it is a good start for looking at the related activities that would have to be addressed if Kent and Keri were to collaborate on Keri's resumption of engagement in shopping. Kent also noted that the occupation category of driving and community mobility included both driving and the use of public transportation, another IADL that would be important to explore with Keri as she contemplates returning to paid work. In fact, the entire list of IADLs held numerous concerns to be addressed in OT.

Health management is an occupational domain that addresses "[a]ctivities related to developing, managing, and maintaining health and wellness routines, including self-management, with the goal of improving or maintaining health to support participation in other occupations" (OTPF, p. S32). This is an important area for Kent to address with Keri considering the health management concerns when an individual has sustained a C6 SCI. This area of occupation includes social and emotional health promotion and maintenance, symptom and condition management, communication with the healthcare system, medication management, physical activity, nutrition management, and personal care management.[5]

Rest and sleep, recognized as an occupation in the OTPF-4, includes "activities related to obtaining restorative rest and sleep to support healthy, active engagement in other occupations"[5] (OTPF, p. S32). The component activities constituting rest and sleep include rest, sleep preparation, and sleep participation (see Chapter 13 for an expanded discussion of this important occupation). Keri's sleep occupations will be significantly changed as a result of her diagnosis. To name just two of the concerns OT will have to address, she will need to be repositioned frequently during the night for skin precautions and equipment will have to be set up to manage her bladder function while she sleeps.

Education is an occupation that includes "activities needed for learning and participating in the environment"[5] (OTPF, p. S33). Specific education activity subcategories include formal education participation, informal personal educational needs or interests exploration (beyond formal education), and informal personal

education participation. Table 2 of the OTPF includes more details about the specific activities in each of these subcategories.

Work includes activities associated with both paid work and volunteer efforts (see Chapter 14). Specific categories of activities and concerns related to the occupation of work include employment interests and pursuits, employment seeking and acquisition, job performance, retirement preparation and adjustment, volunteer exploration, and volunteer participation[5] (OTPF, pp. S33–S34).

Activities associated with the occupation play are described as "[a]ctivities that are intrinsically motivated, internally controlled, and freely chosen and that may include suspension of reality (e.g., fantasy; Skard & Bundy, 2008), exploration, humor, risk taking, contests, and celebrations (Eberle, 2014; Sutton-Smith, 2009). Play is a complex and multidimensional phenomenon that is shaped by sociocultural factors."[20] Considered under this area of occupation are play exploration and play participation[5] (OTPF, p. S34).

Leisure is defined as "nonobligatory activity that is intrinsically motivated and engaged in during discretionary time, that is, time not committed to obligatory occupations such as work, self-care, or sleep."[5] Leisure exploration and leisure participation are the major categories of activity in leisure occupations[5] (OTPF, p. S34) (see Chapter 16). Keri shared with Kent her interests in spending leisure time listening to music, traveling, antiquing, swimming, playing bridge, and reading books. As Kent was studying the description of leisure, it occurred to him that for Keri, shopping might be characterized as a leisure occupation in addition to an IADL. It probably would depend on the circumstances or context in which she engaged in the activity of shopping, he thought—another parameter of the OTPF domain.

Social participation is another occupation that encompasses the "interweaving of occupations to support desired engagement in community and family activities as well as those involving peers and friends[7]; also, involvement in a subset of activities that involve social situations with others[1] and that support social interdependence.[7] Social participation can occur in person or through remote technologies, such as telephone calls, computer interaction, and video conferencing"[4] (OTPF, p. S21). The occupation of social participation, as stated in the OTPF, views this as the activities that involve social interaction with others, including family, friends, peers, and community members, and that support social interdependence.[6,18] The occupation of social participation further encompasses engaging in activities that result in successful interaction at the community, family, and peer/friend levels. (Just as for previously discussed occupations, see the OTPF, Table 2, for definitions and more detailed information about the breadth of activities that constitutes OT's involvement in work, play, leisure, and social participation.)

Like Kent, readers currently learning the OTPF could benefit from studying the expanded lists to broaden their understanding of the OT domain. As Kent studied these sections of Table 2, he found it helpful to make note of the content of each one that included specific activities that would be relevant to Keri when engaging in the various occupations. For example, Kent considered the range of job skills and work routines necessary for Keri to return to the paid position as an administrative assistant. Kent also made a list of similar concerns involved in resumption of Keri's preferred play and leisure occupations, including swimming, reading, and board games. Kent was reminded of the importance of considering the activities that can support or constrain Keri's continued social participation in her community as a Girl Scout leader, in her family as the oldest daughter, and with her treasured circle of friends.

Performance Skills and Performance Patterns

Remember that throughout the OTPF document, there is no correct or incorrect order in which to study or follow the areas of the domain—there is no hierarchy: "All aspects of the occupational therapy domain transact to support engagement, participation, and health (OTPF-4, p. S7).[5] With this in mind, the next main areas of the domain to consider are performance skills and performance patterns. Both are related to the client's performance capabilities in the areas of occupation previously described, and they can be viewed as the actions and behaviors observed by the OT as the client engages in occupations.

The category of performance skills includes three components of concern: motor skills, process skills, and social interaction skills. The client's successful engagement in occupation or occupational performance depends on his or her having or achieving adequate ability in performance skills.[15] In the OTPF, performance skills are defined as "observable, goal-directed actions that result in a client's quality of performing desired occupations" (OTPF, p. S43).[5] Briefly, **performance skills** are the abilities clients demonstrate in the actions they perform. Problems in any of the three areas of performance skills are the focus for formulating short-term goals or objectives to reach the long-term goal of addressing participation in occupation. The OTPF provides an example of performance skills for persons and for groups. In this portion of the OTPF, the term "group" refers to a collective of members, not the intervention strategy.

Motor skills consist of actions or behaviors a client uses to move and physically interact with tasks, objects, contexts, and environments, including planning, sequencing, and executing new and novel movements. In Table 7 of the OTPF, motor skills are defined as "skills that represent small, observable actions related to moving oneself and interacting with tangible task objects … in the context of performing a personally and ecologically relevant daily life task.[15] Examples of motor skills include coordinating body movements to complete a job task, anticipating or adjusting posture and body position in response to environmental circumstances, such as obstacles and manipulating keys or a lock to open a door.

Kent observed Keri as she played a game of bridge with friends one afternoon in the OT clinic. Observing her performance skills, particularly her motor skills, Kent noted that Keri looped one elbow around the upright of her wheelchair, leaned her trunk toward the table, reached her other arm toward the cardholder, and successfully grasped a card, using tenodesis grasp, after three unsuccessful attempts. Kent perceived this as indicating that Keri felt the need to calibrate her attempts and endure or persist (see Chapter 38).

The OTPF defines process skills as "small, observable actions related to selecting, interacting with, and using tangible objects; … carrying out individual actions and steps; and preventing problems of occupational performance from occurring or reoccurring in the context of performing a personally or ecologically relevant daily life task."[15] Simply stated, process skills are observable actions taken to manage and modify the occupational task; for example, using knowledge, attending to and discerning solutions to problems, and organizing the task, including choosing appropriate tools and methods for performing the task.

Kent also observed Keri's process skills as she set up her cardholder so that her cards were not visible to her opponents (selecting and gathering proper equipment and arranging the space), perused her cards, paused, rearranged them using her tenodesis hand splint/orthotic device (attending to the task, using knowledge of the rules of bridge, and selection of proper equipment), and then stated her bid (demonstrating discernment, choosing, and problem solving).

Social interaction skills, the third category of performance skills, are "small, observable actions related to communicating and interacting with others in the context of engaging in personally and ecologically relevant daily life tasks that involve social interaction with others."[15] Such skills could include asking for information, expressing emotion, and interacting with or relating to others in a manner that supports engagement in the occupation at hand.

During the card game, Kent was able to observe a wide array of examples of Keri's social interaction skills. He saw Keri furrowing her brow; squinting her eyes shut in a thoughtful, cogitating manner; pursing her lips; and showing neither happiness nor despair on her face as she studied her cards in the cardholder (expressing affect consistent with the activity of card playing and thus demonstrating or displaying appropriate emotions and cognitive skill in determining her next strategy). As she reached for the cards, the holder moved out of her reach; she turned and asked the friend next to her to push it back, cautioning her in a smiling and light manner, "Don't you dare look!" (demonstrating her ability to multitask—asking for assistance and simultaneously using socially acceptable teasing behavior [social interaction skills] that enlists an opponent's cooperation in preserving the secrecy of her cards, thus conveying or disclosing the image of a savvy card player). Her observable performance skills supported Keri's continued inclusion with friends in a favorite leisure occupation.

Each of these particular motor skills, process skills, and social interaction skills categories has detailed lists of representative skills annotated with definitions, descriptions, and examples (see OTPF, Table 7).[5]

Performance patterns are the "habits, routines, roles, and rituals that may be associated with different lifestyles and used in the process of engaging in occupations or activities" (OTPF, p. 41).[5] Examples of habits listed in Table 6 of the OTPF include automatically putting car keys in the same place and spontaneously looking both ways before crossing the street.[5] Routines reflect the "patterns of behavior that are observable, regular, repetitive, and that provide structure for daily life. They can be satisfying, promoting, or damaging. Routines require delimited time commitment and are embedded in cultural and ecological contexts"[5] (OTPF, p. S41). Routines show how the individual configures or sequences occupations throughout daily life. Habits typically contribute (positively or negatively) to a person's occupational routines, and both are established with repetition over time. *Roles* refers to how the person's "identity is shaped by culture and context that may be further conceptualized and defined by the client"[5] (OTPF, p. S41). Rituals are described as "symbolic actions with spiritual, cultural, or social meaning, contributing to the client's identity and reinforcing values and beliefs. Rituals have a strong affective component and represent a collection of events"[5] (OTPF, p. S41). Table 6 of the OTPF outlines definitions and examples of performance patterns for groups and populations.[5]

Performance patterns for the individual and the ways these can support (or, by inference, hinder) occupational performance are further illustrated in Part 3 of the Kent and Keri case study.

THREADED CASE STUDY

Kent and Keri, Part 3

Some might view Keri's engagement in the occupation of paid work as an example of the role of worker. Inherent in this role are accepted norms that customarily include regular attendance, timely adherence to schedules, and acceptance of responsibility for completing assignments. Keri's work role is consistent with the sets of behaviors that would be expected of an administrative assistant at a busy law firm, including arriving at work on time, handling e-mail and other correspondence in a professional manner, managing the office budget and payroll according to accepted audit practices, and interacting with her supervisors, co-workers, and supervisees in a fair and respectful manner, to name just a few. To honor her stellar work performance, a ritual that evolved as part of Keri's work role experience at the law office is the annual Holiday Shopping Day. Keri and her three administrative assistant colleagues are given the Friday before the holiday off with pay. The law firm arranges transportation for all administrative assistants and transports them to the downtown shopping district, where they are given a generous gift card, lunch at a downtown restaurant, an afternoon of shopping, and transportation back home at the end of the day.

Keri's workday routine involves waking at 6:30 am; showering, grooming, and dressing; driving to work, with a stop for breakfast on the way; and arriving at her workplace early (at 7:45 am) for an 8:00 am expected work start. A habit that Keri regards as beneficial to her workday routine is her scrupulous use of her phone to record appointments; contact information, including phone numbers; and additions to her things-to-do list. Another habit she thinks contributes to the success of her workday routine is selecting her clothes the night before to save time in the morning, thus ensuring a punctual arrival at work. A habit that negatively affects her daily work routine is hitting the snooze button on her cell phone. Both Kent and Keri recognize that although Keri may resume her work occupation or worker role, her SCI has substantially altered her ability to carry out expected behaviors and her customary habits and routines; she will have to develop the ability to establish new and expanded habits and routines. Successful integration of these new habits and routines will undoubtedly determine the continuation of Keri's participation in the highly anticipated and beloved Holiday Shopping Day ritual.

Keri's occupational performance, performance skills, and patterns will be significantly influenced by the next two main areas of the domain to be discussed: contexts and client factors.

Contexts, as described in OTPF-4, includes both environmental and personal factors. Each will be discussed in relation to Keri's occupational engagement. Contexts are regarded as the variety of interrelated conditions, circumstances, or events that surround and influence the client and in which the client's daily life occupations take place. Contexts can either support or constrain health, well-being, and participation in life through engagement in occupation.

The OTPF states that "*environmental factors* are aspects of the physical, social, and attitudinal surroundings in which people live and conduct their lives" (OTPF-4, p. 36).[5] The **environment** includes the natural and the human-made factors, including the environmental modifications made by people and characteristics of the human populations within the environment. The environment addresses not only the physical aspects but also products and technology, supports and relationships, attitudes, services, systems, and policies (Table 4).[5] Personal factors, another part of Contexts, describes the "background of the person's life and living and consists of the unique features of the person that are not part of a health condition or health state" (Table 5, p. S40).[5] *Personal factors* include age, gender identity, sexual orientation, socioeconomic status, and educational status; it can also include group membership (e.g., volunteers, employees) and population membership (e.g., members of society).[5]

Each of these contexts, as they pertain to Keri's specific circumstances, will significantly affect her future engagement in occupation. Keri's physical environment includes aspects that will support her engagement in occupation, including an accessible work site, a reliable and accessible system of public transportation in her neighborhood, and a well-appointed downtown area of stores, shops, and restaurants within wheelchair distance. Aspects of her physical environment that may interfere with resumption of occupations include Keri's second floor apartment and small bathroom, which are inaccessible to a wheelchair. Supportive aspects of Keri's personal context are her college education in business and the fact that she has unemployment insurance, which will supplement her sick leave and continue her health coverage. From a social environment perspective, Keri is supported by both her family and her friends; additionally, her employer and co-workers are anxious to have her come back to the law firm. The attitudinal environment—those values, customs, and beliefs—includes the presence of the Americans with Disabilities Act (ADA), which acknowledges the job essentials at the law firm can be performed by Keri. This knowledge motivates Keri to resume engagement in previous levels of occupation for full participation in all environments and contexts and, ultimately, occupations of her life.[7]

Given the difficulty that resuming Keri's shopping occupation may present, Kent suggested the possibility of using online shopping for some items. Although interested, Keri indicated that her preference was to shop "in the real world" with her colleagues and friends. Keri's ultimate decisions no doubt will be influenced by the changes she experiences and adjusts to, such as the increased amounts of time required to accomplish basic daily routines that, in turn, support her engagement in preferred occupations.

Client Factors

OTPF-4 describes **client factors** in a manner similar to the ICF.[5,23] There are three sections in this portion of the OTPF-4: values, beliefs, and spirituality; body functions; and body structures. These three categories of client factors are regarded as residing within the client, and they may affect or influence the performance of occupations.[5] Client factors may be affected by performance skills, performance patterns, and contexts; in addition, they may have a cyclical/reciprocal relationship with and profound effect on the client's ability in those areas and, ultimately, satisfactory performance of occupations.

The client factor category of values, beliefs, and spirituality is described as encompassing the client's perceptions, motivations, and related meaning that influence or are influenced by engagement in occupations.[4] Table 9 of the OTPF describes values as beliefs and commitments, derived from culture, about what is good, right, and important to do (e.g., commitment to family), whereas beliefs are described as cognitive content held as true by the client (e.g., hard work pays off).[5] The third aspect, spirituality, is described as "a deep experience of meaning brought about by engaging in occupations" (OTPF, p. S 51).[5] For example, Keri's values, including her strong work ethic and her beliefs and spirituality, provide her the reassurance that her SCI was part of a higher power's plan and she will be given the strength to cope and succeed.[26]

The body structure category refers to the integrity of the actual body part, such as the integrity of the eye for vision (see Chapter 24) or the integrity of a limb (see Chapter 44). When the integrity of the body structure is compromised, this can affect function or require alternative approaches to engagement in activities, such as enlarged print for persons with macular degeneration or the use of a prosthesis for a person who sustained a below-elbow amputation. It is unlikely that this category of the domain would apply to Keri because the integrity of her body structures is not necessarily compromised by her diagnosis. Should she develop a pressure sore, a possible complication of SCI in which the integrity of a body structure (i.e., the skin) is compromised, her ability to engage in occupation could become significantly limited, requiring alternative approaches, such as positioning devices and adaptive equipment to compensate for the need to stay off the pressure sore.

The body function category of client factors refers to the physiological and psychological functions of the body. It includes a variety of systems, such as mental functions, sensory functions, and neuromusculoskeletal and movement-related functions. This category of body functions includes muscle function, which in turn includes muscle strength. A distinction is made between body functions and performance skills. As was described earlier, performance skills are observed as the client engages in an occupation or activity. The category of body function refers to the available ability of the client's body to function. For example, a client may have the available neuromuscular function (client factor of body function; specifically, muscle strength) to hold a comb and bring the comb to the top of the head, and also the strength to pull the comb through the hair, but when you ask the client to comb his hair (an activity), you observe that he has difficulty with manipulating the comb in his hand (motor skill of manipulation) and with using the comb smoothly to comb his hair (motor skill of flow). In the OTPF, these motor skills are considered performance skills.

In Keri's case, the absence of functioning muscles in her hands necessitates the use of a functional hand splint to access her phone or a credit card when engaged in her shopping occupation. To use a wrist-driven flexor hinge (i.e., tenodesis) hand splint to hold her phone, she must have adequate body function; in this case, fair or better muscle strength in her radial wrist

extensors. However, Keri also must have adequate performance skills, including the motor skills to exert enough force to adequately hold her phone while accessing information or when selecting a credit card.

The mental functions group includes emotional, cognitive, and perceptual abilities. This group also includes the experience of self and body image (see Chapters 6, 25, and 26). A client such as Keri, who has sustained a physically disabling injury, may have an altered self-concept, lowered self-esteem, depression, anxiety, decreased coping skills, and other problems with emotional functions after the injury[24,25] (see Chapter 6). Sensory functions and pain also are included in the body functions category (see Chapters 23 and 28).

Neuromuscular and movement-related functions refer to the available strength range of motion and movement (see Chapters 19 through 22); however, they do not refer to the client's application of these factors to activities or occupations, as was seen in the example of Keri accessing her credit card as part of engaging in the occupation of shopping. The body functions category also refers to the ability of the cardiovascular, respiratory, digestive, metabolic, and genitourinary systems to function to support client participation. These are further described in both the OTPF and the ICF. Table 9 in the OTPF presents a more detailed description of each function included in this category.[5]

THE OCCUPATIONAL THERAPY PROCESS

As mentioned, the OTPF consists of two parts, the domain and the process. From a very general perspective, the domain describes the scope of practice or answers the question, "What does an OT do?" The process describes the methods of providing OT services, or answers the question, "How does an OT provide occupational therapy services?"

The process is outlined briefly here for continuity; the reader is referred to Chapter 3 for a more in-depth discussion. The primary focus of the OTPF process is **evaluation** of the client's occupational abilities and needs to determine and provide services (**intervention**) that foster and support occupational performance (**targeted outcomes**). Throughout the process the focus is on occupation; the evaluation begins with determining the client's occupational profile, the analysis of occupational performance, and synthesis of the evaluation process along with the client's occupational history. Preferred intervention methods are occupation based, and the overall outcome of the process is achievement of the client's health, well-being, and participation in life through engagement in occupation. Throughout each step of the process, therapists are guided by the knowledge and skills learned and perfected over the course of their career, including the skills associated with clinical reasoning, therapeutic use of self, activity analysis, and activity demands.[9,11-12,24,29]

Interventions also vary, depending on the client, whether person, groups, or populations. In the practice of occupational therapy with adults with physical disabilities, the term *client*, at the person or individual level, may vary, depending on the treatment setting or environment. In a hospital or rehabilitation center, the person might be referred to as a *patient*, whereas in a community college post-stroke program, the person receiving occupational therapy may be referred to as a *student*. The term *client* or *consumer* might best describe the person who receives OT intervention at a center for independent living, where the individual typically lives in the community and seeks intervention for a specific, self-identified problem or issue.

Skills That Inform and Guide the Occupational Therapy Process

As mentioned previously, the therapist is guided in the OT process by the knowledge and skills acquired during the course of the therapist's career; these skills include professional reasoning, therapeutic use of self, activity analysis, and activity demands.

Professional reasoning is described as the process that enables occupational therapy practitioners to identify the demands, skills and meanings of activities/occupations and understand "the interrelationships of the domain . . . that support client-centered interventions and outcomes" (OTPF-4, p. S21).[5] OTs rely on the expertise and knowledge they have developed throughout their careers, including understanding of theory, research interpretation, and clinical skills.

The OTPF describes the therapeutic use of self as "an integral part of the occupational therapy process . . . in which occupational therapy practitioners develop and manage their therapeutic relationship with clients by using professional reasoning, empathy, and a client-centered, collaborative approach to service delivery" (OTPF-4, p. S20).[5] The professional literature describes an OT who is successful in the therapeutic use of self as having the qualities or attributes of showing empathy (including sensitivity to the client's disability, age, gender, religion, socioeconomic status, education, and cultural background); being self-reflective and self-aware; being able to communicate effectively using active listening; and consistently keeping a client-centered perspective, which in turn engenders an atmosphere of trust.[8-9,11-12,24,29]

The focus of the OT process supports the therapeutic use of self by the OT. When the therapist uses a client-centered approach and begins the process with an evaluation that seeks information about the client's occupational history and occupational preferences, the client sees the therapist as being interested in what the client does (occupational performance), who the client is (contexts, and client factors such as values, beliefs, and spirituality), and what occupations give meaning to the client's life. (Part 4 of the Kent and Keri case study, presented later in the chapter, describes how Kent demonstrates therapeutic use of self in each step of the therapeutic process.)

The analysis of occupational performance is a critical part of the overall evaluation process and examines the "client's ability to effectively complete desired occupations" (OTPF-4, p. S22).[5] The analysis considers the importance of the occupation or activity to the client as paramount, bearing in mind the client's goals, interests, and abilities and the demands of the activity itself on body structures, body functions, performance skills, and performance patterns. Activity analysis and activity demands are inextricably linked; activity demands focus on what is required to engage in the activity or occupation. For the OT, this skill requires a knowledge of several aspects that must be addressed for a client to perform a specific activity, including the activity's relevance and importance to the client, the objects used and their properties, space demands, social demands, sequencing and timing, required actions and performance skills, required body functions, and required body structures. Table 11 of the OTPF-4 document provides a comprehensive list of definitions and examples for a clearer understanding of each of these categories.[5]

Consider Keri's keen interest in resuming the occupation of shopping in the "real world" instead of online clothing purchases. The materials or tools needed are a phone with a payment app or credit card holder. The space demands are the accessibility of the store or shopping mall and the dressing room for Keri to try on the clothes before making a purchase. The social demands include paying for the items before leaving the store. The sequence and timing process includes being able to make a selection, go to the register, potentially wait in line, place the clothing on the counter, pay for the item, and then leave the store. The required actions refer to the performance skills necessary to engage in this activity, such as the coordination needed to try on clothing, the process skills needed to select one sweater or blouse from a large array of possible choices, and the social interaction skills needed to ask for assistance or directions if needed.

These performance skills are not viewed in isolation, but rather are seen as Keri engages in the occupation of clothes shopping. The required body functions and structures refer to the basic client factors necessary to perform the activity of shopping. The act of shopping requires a level of cognition or judgment because inherent in the activity of shopping is having the opportunity to make a choice among available items. Keri's ability to engage in the activity demand of making a choice of purchases indicates that she has an adequate level of cognition for shopping.

Using his skills of professional reasoning, therapeutic use of self, and expert knowledge of activity analysis and activity demands, Kent continually assesses the interplay of Keri's strengths and abilities and her occupational goals to select the interventions that will most effectively achieve these goals. These interventions are described next.

Types of Occupational Therapy Intervention

Table 1.1 shows the types of OT intervention typically used in physical disability practice and their relationship to the domain of occupational therapy. The general categories of intervention are presented in the OTPF, Table 12: Occupations and Activities, Interventions to Support Occupations (previously referred to as preparatory activities), Education and Training, Advocacy, Group Intervention, Virtual Intervention.[5] These categories of intervention are not designed or organized in a hierarchy but provide a range of options to support the client's occupational engagement. The OT reflects on the client's goal of engagement in preferred, self-selected occupations and then collaborates with the client in selecting the type or types of intervention that would best help the client achieve each occupational goal.

Since the inception of the OTPF (continued in the OTPF-2 and OTPF-3), the traditional concept of "intervention levels" has been dismissed in favor of viewing interventions as types, with no one type considered more important than another;

TABLE 1.1	Types of OT Intervention Typically Used in Physical Disability Practice
Intervention	**Description**
Occupations and Activities	Occupations and activities selected as interventions for specific clients are designed to meet therapeutic goals and address the underlying needs of the client's mind, body, and spirit. To use occupations and activities therapeutically, the practitioner considers activity demands and client factors in relation to the client's therapeutic goals and contexts.
Occupations	Broad and specific daily life events that are personalized and meaningful to the client.
Activities	Components of occupations that are objective and separate from the client's engagement or contexts. Activities as interventions are selected and designed to support the development of performance skills and performance patterns and to enhance occupational engagement.
Interventions to Support Occupations	Methods and tasks that prepare the client for occupational performance are used as part of a treatment session in preparation for or concurrently with occupations and activities or provided to a client as a home-based engagement to support daily occupational performance. Includes PAMs and mechanical modalities; Orthotics and Prosthetics; Assistive technology and Environmental modification; Wheeled mobility; and Self-regulation,
Education and Training	
Education	Imparting of knowledge and information about occupation, health, well-being, and participation that enables the client to acquire helpful behaviors, habits, and routines.
Training	Facilitation of acquisition of concrete skills for meeting specific goals in a real-life, applied situation. Differentiated from education by its goal of enhanced performance as opposed to enhanced understanding.
Advocacy	Efforts directed toward promoting occupational justice and empowering clients to seek and obtain resources to support health, well-being, and occupational participation. Can be advocacy efforts by the practitioner on behalf of the client or self-advocacy efforts undertaken by the client.
Group Intervention	Use of distinct knowledge of the dynamics of group and social interaction and leadership techniques to facilitate learning and skill acquisition across the life span. Groups are used as a method of service delivery.
Virtual Intervention	Use of simulated, real-time, and near-time technologies for service delivery absent of physical contact such as telehealth or mHealth.

From the American Occupational Therapy Association: Occupational therapy practice framework: domain & process, ed 4, *Am J Occup Ther* 74(Suppl 2):S1–S87, 2020.

rather, each type has a potential contribution to make in facilitating the ultimate goal of achieving health, well-being, and participation in life through engagement in occupation.

OT PRACTICE NOTES

Throughout the OT process, the therapist should make sure the client understands that they will select the outcomes together, based on the client's choice, and they will collaborate in planning the intervention. This lays the foundation for a relationship based on caring and trust.

Occupations and Activities

In the first version of the OTPF (2002), the occupations and activities category of OT intervention was adapted from the section "Treatment Continuum in the Context of Occupational Performance" (Chapter 1) in the fifth edition of this textbook. In the OTPF-4, this category is defined as "interventions for specific clients, designed to meet therapeutic goals and address the underlying needs of the mind, body, and spirit. To use occupations and activities therapeutically, the practitioner considers activity demands and client factors in relation to the client's therapeutic goals and contexts"[5] (OTPF-4, p. S59). Specific activities considered to be representative of the occupations and activities category are further separated into two types, including occupation and activity, that will each be discussed here.

THREADED CASE STUDY

Kent and Keri, Part 4

Kent did not originally regard therapeutic use of self as an integral, identified component of the OT process. However, through his study of the previous versions and current iteration of the OTPF, he has come to value it highly and use it in his practice. Clients respond well to Kent's caring and gentle approach. He enjoys the personal and interactive aspects of the therapeutic relationship, shows genuine interest in his clients' histories, and actively listens to their responses. He makes it a practice to introduce himself and explain his role to his clients as the first step in the OT process. This practice allows Kent to reinforce the primacy of the client's occupational participation and to associate and integrate the information about the client when providing occupational therapy services.

Kent practiced therapeutic use of self throughout the OT process with Keri. He brought to the process his 25 years of experience, continued education, and knowledge of SCI, in addition to his well-developed professional reasoning skills and his experiences in providing successful—and not-so-successful—OT intervention for numerous clients. Kent's college roommate and subsequent best friend has a physical disability, and this has served to increase Kent's understanding of, and inform his attitudes and beliefs about, the experience of having a disability. His close and loving relationships with his sisters, wife, and teenage daughters have provided him with an increased awareness of women's concerns and issues and have caused him to consider how disability might be experienced differently by clients. All of these aspects of Kent's personal and professional repertoire supported his ability to include therapeutic use of self, activity analysis, and professional reasoning as effective therapeutic skills that continually informed his actions throughout Keri's OT process.

The OTPF describes occupations (as interventions) as "Broad and specific daily life events that are personalized and meaningful to the client"[5] (OTPF-4, p. S59). For Keri, an example might entail a clothes shopping trip using public transportation or independently completing a typical morning of office skills at the law firm.

Activities (as interventions) are "selected and designed to support the development of performance skills and performance patterns to enhance occupational engagement" (OTPF-4, p. S59).[5] Examples from Table 12 of the OTPF include selecting and manipulating clothing fasteners before engaging in dressing.

After reading the descriptions of occupations and activities as interventions, Kent now thinks that occupation-based intervention would promote engagement in all areas of occupation, including ADLs, IADLs, rest and sleep, education, work, play, leisure, and social participation. Most of the OT intervention for Keri was occupation based. To reach her targeted goal of resuming her favorite leisure occupation of clothes shopping, Kent and Keri took a trip to a nearby department store, where Keri looked for a blouse that buttoned up the front. Keri perused the racks, inspecting the blouses on display; asked for help from a salesperson; tried on blouses in the dressing room; made her selection; and paid for her purchase—all parts of a typical shopping excursion in a customary shopping environment. When necessary, Kent suggested ways Keri could perform some of the more difficult shopping activities with less effort, such as negotiating her wheelchair into the dressing room from a narrow hallway, and transporting the blouses on her lap without having them slide to the ground.

The purpose of activity as intervention in the OTPF and the examples provided helped Kent reframe or slightly reconfigure his view of the relationship between an activity and an occupation during intervention. He was providing activity intervention when he had Keri practice what she would encounter as part of the occupation of clothes shopping. In the OT clinic, before the shopping trip, Keri and Kent collaborated on developing her ability to perform the activities of accessing her credit card from her wallet or a payment app on her phone, using a button hook to button her sweater, and lifting clothes on hangers out of a closet. Some of the shopping activities she performed while buying her blouse were learned as part of other occupation-based interventions, such as wheelchair mobility and dressing. When using activity as intervention, the OT practitioner is concerned primarily with assessing and remediating deficits in performance skills and performance patterns.

Interventions to Support Occupations

These are the interventions used to prepare the client before engaging in the occupation or activity or simultaneously when engaging in the occupation or activity. This includes both preparatory methods and tasks.

Preparatory methods used in occupational therapy may include exercise, facilitation and inhibition techniques, positioning, sensory stimulation, selected physical agent modalities, and provision of orthotic devices, such as braces and splints. *Preparatory tasks* involve active participation of the client and

sometimes comprise engagements that use various materials to simulate activities or components of occupations. Preparatory tasks themselves may not hold inherent meaning, relevance, or perceived utility as standalone entities.

OT services for persons with physical disabilities often introduce these preparatory methods, devices, and tasks during the acute stages of illness or injury. When using these methods, the OT is likely to be most concerned with assessing and remediating problems with client factors such as body structures and body functions. It is important for the therapist to plan the progression of this type of intervention so that the selected methods are used as preparation for occupation or activity and are directed toward the overarching goal of achieving health, well-being, and participation in life through engagement in occupation.

Kent reflected that in preparing for Keri's occupation intervention of clothes shopping, he used several other interventions that would be considered preparatory methods. For example, he and Keri looked at her options for grasping items and decided on a tenodesis hand splint, using orthotics as an intervention. To use the splint more effectively, she needed increased wrist extensor strength, and to push her wheelchair or to reach for and lift hangers with clothes, she needed stronger shoulder muscles; therefore, the preparatory intervention of exercise was chosen to facilitate Keri's ultimate engagement in purposeful occupations and activities.

Education and Training

The OTPF-4 describes *education* as "imparting knowledge and information about occupation, health, well-being, and participation that enables the client to acquire helpful behaviors, habits, and routines" (OTPF-4, p. S61).[5]

Kent considered this definition, thinking of instances when he provided education as intervention. Most recently, with Keri, he responded to her concerns about returning to her job as an administrative assistant. She was having misgivings about the amount of physical work and energy involved; the modest salary she received, which barely covered her preinjury expenses; and the additional expenses she would have for personal and household assistance. Using his years of knowledge and experience, Kent provided an education-focused intervention to inform Keri about her options. He explained the services offered by vocational rehabilitation and described the possibilities and opportunities for further education to support her work goal of becoming an attorney—a job position, he pointed out, that held the potential for higher pay and one that could be less physically demanding than her administrative assistant position. Kent also provided Keri with information about her rights to employment accommodations under the ADA (see Chapter 15). He informed her about the similar circumstances with his former clients, describing the various scenarios and outcomes of each (being mindful to preserve the former clients' anonymity and privacy). He also drew on his wealth of experience to discuss the many resources available to facilitate such options. Keri was already preparing to resume her job (an occupational goal she prioritized) and was actively participating in OT by engaging in occupations and activities that involved her actual work occupations and supporting activities. The education intervention made her aware of her options but did not involve any actual performance of an activity.

Kent could use the same intervention process to educate Keri's vocational counselor and the law firm where Keri works.

In the OTPF-4, *training* is distinguished from education; it is described as "facilitation of the acquisition of concrete skills for meeting specific goals in a real-life, applied situation. In this case skills refers to measurable components of function that enable mastery. Training is further differentiated from education by its goal of enhanced performance as opposed to enhanced understanding, although these goals often go hand in hand"[5] (OTPF-4, p. S61). Examples of training include interventions such as teaching a personal care attendant ways to help a client with ADLs.

Kent considered that he provided training when he taught Keri how to complete her administrative assistant duties by showing her how to access files, operate her environmental controls system, and dictate notes using voice recognition software. Kent anticipates training Keri in how to manage her bladder (empty her leg bag), perform regular weight shifts, and access the cafeteria at work—all skills that are part of Keri's personal care in the work setting that she wants to master before returning to full-time employment.

Advocacy

The intervention type identified as advocacy is provided when efforts are "directed toward promoting occupational justice (access to occupation) and empowering clients to seek and obtain resources to support health, well-being, and occupational participation" (OTPF-4, p. S61).[5] Kent worked with Keri and her work supervisor to advocate to the law firm partners for reasonable accommodations to support Keri's continued employment. After a year of Keri's successful job performance and her newly learned abilities to continually self-advocate, Kent and Keri were invited to the state bar association conference to advocate for similar collaborations on behalf of other employees with disabilities.

Group Intervention

Group intervention is described as functional groups, activity groups, task groups, social groups, and other groups used in healthcare settings within the community or within organizations that allow clients to explore and develop skills for participation, including basic social interaction skills and tools for self-regulation, goal setting, and positive choice making[5] (OTPF-4, p. S62).

In reflecting on Keri's OT process, Kent concluded that perhaps one of the most important interventions for Keri was the Home and Community Skills classes offered by the OT department during her rehabilitation stay. This eight-session experiential group class, led by Kent and several of his OT colleagues, introduced topics such as managing friendships, negotiating occupations in the environment (e.g., going to movie theaters, hair salons, or grocery stores), asking for assistance, dating, childrearing, and using public transportation, to name but a few. Former clients who had achieved their goal of health, well-being, and participation in life through engagement in occupation were invited as peer experts to provide the lived experience for the discussions facilitated by the therapists. In addition to talking about issues (as an OT intervention), Kent made sure

that each client had follow-up opportunities for "doing" the occupations and activities.

A year or so after her SCI, Keri was invited to return to the Home and Community Skills group and share her experiences of returning to work, seeking accessible housing, and beginning a new intimate relationship. Kent facilitated the discussion. He used his professional reasoning skills and knowledge of these topics, along with activity analysis and activity demands, to ask Keri strategic questions, to make sure the discussion included specific details, and to point out alternative solutions that others in the class might have found more applicable.

Kent carefully studied the OTPF domain, process, and types of interventions and reinforced his learning by applying this knowledge to his own circumstances and those of his client Keri. However, Kent still feels the need for additional suggestions or strategies for learning the Framework more thoroughly. The next section explores these strategies.

STRATEGIES FOR LEARNING THE OTPF-4

The most effective first step in learning the OTPF-4 would be to obtain and thoroughly read the published document, making notations as points arise, drawing diagrams for increased understanding, writing questions or observations in the margins, and consulting tables, figures, and the glossary, when directed to do so, to reinforce or clarify information.[5,8] The OTPF-4 is a comprehensive conceptualization of the profession, and it requires a substantial investment of time and commitment to study and integrate it into practice before a therapist will feel comfortable using it. Box 1.1 provides an abbreviated list of the core terminology and concepts of the OTPF-4; this can serve as a quick reference or can be used to jog the reader's memory in learning to use the OTPF-4.

More experienced OTs who are accustomed to using the previous iterations of the OTPF will find it helpful to consult the Preface in the OTPF-4 (pp. S1–S4), where changes and major revisions to the OTPF are listed and discussed.[5]

Several pioneering authors[7,10,17,25,26,28] have written helpful articles demonstrating application of the Framework for the AJOT's various Special Interest Section (SIS) quarterlies or OT Practice articles.[17] Writing for the *Home and Community Health SIS Quarterly*, Siebert[28] encouraged practitioners to realize that it is important to use the OTPF "as a tool to communicate practice, to support practice patterns that facilitate engagement in occupation, and to reflect on and refine our practice." She also pointed out the dominant role that context plays in home and community practice by providing continuity to the client, noting how firmly the Framework supports this concept. She expressed her belief that the OTPF's focus on occupation, in addition to beginning the process with the client's occupational profile, ensures that the results of OT intervention will matter to the client.[28]

Coppola,[10] writing for the *Gerontology SIS Quarterly*, described how the Framework can be applied to geriatric practice and explained that the evaluation is one of occupational therapy's most powerful means of informing others (including clients and colleagues) what OT is and what OT does. She provided a working draft of an Occupational Therapy Evaluation Summary form, which was developed to be incorporated into

BOX 1.1   Quick Guide to the Occupational Therapy Practice Framework

Achieving Health, Well-Being, and Participation in Life Through Engagement in Occupation: The OT's Unique Contribution, the Overarching Theme of the Domain, and the Overarching Outcome of the Process

Occupational therapists (OTs) use their knowledge and expertise in the therapeutic use of self and in activity analysis and activity demands (space demands, social demands, sequencing, and timing), in addition to critical thinking skills, to guide their actions throughout each step of the occupational therapy (OT) process. Clients (persons, groups, populations: Table 1 of OTPF-4) contribute their life experiences, knowledge, and expertise to the process in collaboration with the OT.[10,21]

The OTPF-4 is composed of two primary interrelated parts: domain and process. These major elements are enhanced and supported by additional parts of the OTPF.

Domain: What (OTs) do—no single aspect is considered more critical than another.

- *Performance of occupations* (activities of daily living [ADLs], instrumental activities of daily living [IADLs], health management, rest and sleep, education, work, play, leisure, and social participation: Table 2 of the OTPF-4).
- *Contexts* (Environmental factors: Table 4 of the OTPF-4, Personal factors: Table 5 of the OTPF-4).
- *Performance patterns* (habits, routines, roles, and rituals: Table 6 of the OTPF-4).
- *Performance skills* (motor skills, process skills, and social interaction skills: For persons—Table 7 of the OTPF-4, for groups—Table 8 of the OTPF-4).
- *Client factors* (values, beliefs and spirituality, body functions, and body structures: Table 9 of the OTPF-4).

Process: How OTs provide their services—collaborative process between client and OT.

- *Evaluation* (occupational profile and analysis of occupational performance).
- *Intervention* (preferred term rather than *treatment*—includes intervention plan, intervention implementation, and intervention review).
- *Targeted outcomes* (all goals aimed at the overarching goal of achieving health, well-being, and participation in life through engagement in occupation).

Client: Recipient of OT services (*client* is the preferred term, but the term used varies by practice setting—could be *patient, student, consumer, employee, employer,* and so on)

- *Individual* (broad view of client—could be the actual person with a disability or an individual providing support for the client, such as a family member, caregiver, teacher, or employer, who also may help or be served indirectly).
- *Groups* (collection of individuals having shared characteristics and/or common or shared purpose).
- *Populations* (within a community).
- *Client-centered approach*—an approach to the evaluation of the need for and provision of an intervention with emphasis on the client and his or her goals.
- *Occupation versus activity*—Activities are characterized as meaningful and goal directed but not of central importance to the life of the individual.

Occupations are viewed as activities that give meaning to the person's life and contribute to his or her identity; they are also the activities in which the individual looks forward to engaging.

Engagement: Includes both the subjective (emotional or psychological) and objective (physically observable) aspects of performance.

Types of Intervention
Occupations and Activities

- *Occupations*—client-directed daily life activities that match and support or address identified participation goals.
- *Activities*—actions that support the development of performance skills and patterns to enhance occupational engagement; client learns and practices parts or portions of occupations.

Interventions to Support Occupations

- *Preparatory methods*—modalities, devices, and techniques to prepare client for occupational performance; includes splints, assistive technology and environmental modifications, and wheelchair mobility.
- *Preparatory tasks*—actions to target specific client factors or performance skills.

Education and Training

- *Education*—OT imparts knowledge and information about occupation, health, well-being, and participation that enable the client to acquire helpful behaviors, habits, and routines, which may or may not require application at the time of the intervention session.
- *Training*—facilitation of acquisition of concrete skills for meeting specific goals in a real-life, applied situation. Differentiated from education by its goal of enhanced performance as opposed to enhanced understanding.

Advocacy

- *Advocacy*—promotes occupational justice and empowers clients to obtain resources for full participation in occupation. Can be advocacy efforts by the practitioner on behalf of the client or self-advocacy efforts undertaken by the client.

Group Interventions

- *Group interventions*—use of distinct knowledge and leadership techniques to facilitate learning and skill acquisition across the lifespan through the dynamics of group and social interaction. Groups also may be used as a method of service delivery.

Virtual Interventions

- *Virtual interventions*—use of simulated, real-time, and near-time technologies for service delivery absent of physical contact such as telehealth or mHealth.

---

the Framework and to highlight occupation in a visual way into her practice in a geriatric clinic. This summary form is unconstrained by the more traditional documentation forms that seem to bury occupation under diagnostic and clinical terminology.[10]

Similarly, Boss[7] offered readers of the *Technology SIS Quarterly* his reflections on how the Framework can be operationalized in an assistive technology setting. Addressing each of the categories of the domain, he offered examples of how assistive technology supports engagement in occupation (allowing completion of an activity or occupation) and how the use of assistive technology (personal device care and device use) can be an occupation in and of itself. He concluded his article by pointing out that "assistive technologies are all about supporting the client's participation in the contexts of their choice and are therefore part of the core of occupational therapy."[7]

Although the previously cited articles refer to use of the original OTPF, they thoroughly demonstrate how creatively the Framework, now referred to as simply the OTPF, can be applied to the array of OT practice settings. Another strategy for facilitating the reader's education in the OTPF-4 is the format of the chapters in this book, as described next.

THE OTPF-4: ITS USE IN THIS BOOK

In keeping with the OTPF-4's central focus on the client and the importance of contexts and participation in occupation, each chapter begins with a case study and then integrates the information presented into the consideration of that client and those circumstances, similar to Kent's and Keri's experiences as described and threaded throughout this chapter. As the particular content information is presented, the reader frequently is asked to refer back to the case study and consider how the information applies to the specifics of the client portrayed. The probative questions asked at the conclusion of Part 1 of the case study are answered throughout the text or addressed at the end of the chapter.

SUMMARY

"Occupational Therapy Practice Framework: Domain and Process," the first article on this model, was published in 2002 by the AOTA. The subsequent editions, OTPF-2, OTPF-3, and the current version, OTPF-4, were developed by the OT profession for two purposes: to reassert occupational therapy's focus on occupation and to clearly articulate and enhance understanding of the domain of occupational therapy (what OT practitioners do) and the process of occupational therapy (how they do it) for both internal audiences (members of the profession) and external audiences (clients, healthcare professionals, and interested others). The overarching goal of OTPF-4 is "achieving health, well-being, and participation in life through engagement in occupation"[5]—this emphasizes the primacy of occupation, regarding it as both the theme of the domain and the outcome of the process.

The domain comprises five categories that constitute the scope of occupational therapy: occupations, client factors, performance skills, performance patterns, and contexts. The OT process involves three interactive phases of OT services—evaluation, intervention, and outcomes—that develop in a collaborative and nonlinear manner. The types of OT intervention included in the OTPF-4 and typically used in physical disabilities practice settings include occupations and activities (including occupation-based activity and purposeful activity); interventions to support occupations (including modalities, devices, and techniques to prepare the client for occupational performance, orthotics and prosthetics, assistive technology and environmental modifications, and wheeled mobility, including seating and positioning); education and training; advocacy (by the practitioner and also by the client as self-advocacy); group intervention; and virtual interventions.[5]

In addition to studying the chapter, readers are encouraged to explore the OTPF-4 in its entirety and to reinforce their learning by applying it to their own life experiences and those of their clients, meaning both the clients in the case studies presented throughout this book and those they encounter in real life in the clinic.

REVIEW QUESTIONS

1. Briefly describe the evolution of the Occupational Therapy Practice Framework, including the OTPF-4.
2. Describe the need for the OTPF-4 in the practice of OT for persons with physical disabilities.
3. Describe the fit between the OTPF-4 and the ICF and explain how they inform and enhance the OT's understanding of physical disability.
4. List and describe the components that make up the OT domain, and give examples of each.
5. List and describe the components that make up the OT process, and give examples of each.
6. Briefly describe the OT intervention levels, and give an example of each as it might be used in a physical disability practice setting.

REFERENCES

1. American Occupational Therapy Association: Uniform terminology for occupational therapy, ed 3, *Am J Occup Ther* 48:1047, 1994.
2. American Occupational Therapy Association: *Occupational therapy practice framework: domain and process, Am J Occup Ther* 56(6):609, 2002.
3. American Occupational Therapy Association: Occupational therapy practice framework: domain and process, ed 2, *Am J Occup Ther* 62(6):625–683, 2008.
4. American Occupational Therapy Association: Occupational therapy practice framework: domain and process, ed 3, *Am J Occup Ther* 68(Suppl 1):S1–S48, 2014.
5. American Occupational Therapy Association: Occupational therapy practice framework: domain and process, ed 4, *Am J Occup Ther* 74(Suppl 2):S1–S48, 2020.
6. Bedell GM: Measurement of social participation. In Anderson V, Beauchamp MH, editors: *Developmental social neuroscience and childhood brain insult: theory and practice*, New York, 2012, Guilford Press, pp 184–204.
7. Boss J: The occupational therapy practice framework and assistive technology: an introduction, *Technol Special Interest Section Quarterly* 13(2):1–3, 2003.
8. Boyt Schell BA, et al: Glossary. In Boyt Schell BA, Gillen G, Scaffa M, editors: *Willard and Spackman's occupational therapy*, ed 12, Philadelphia, 2014, Lippincott Williams & Wilkins, p 607.

9. Cara E: Methods and interpersonal strategies. In Cara E, MacRae A, editors: *Psychosocial occupational therapy: a clinical practice*, Clifton Park, NY, 2005, Thomson/Delmar Learning, p 359.

10. Coppola S: An introduction to practice with older adults using the occupational therapy practice framework: domain and process, *Gerontol Special Interest Section Quarterly* 26(1):1–4, 2003.

11. Crabtree JL, et al: Cultural proficiency in rehabilitation: an introduction. In Royeen M, Crabtree JL, editors: *Culture in rehabilitation: from competency to proficiency*, Upper Saddle River, NJ, 2006, Pearson/Prentice Hall, p 1.

12. Crawford K, et al: *Therapeutic use of self in occupational therapy, unpublished master's project*, San Jose, CA, 2004, San Jose State University.

13. Delany JV, Squires E: From UT-III to the framework: making the language work, *OT Practice* 20, May 10, 2004.

14. Dunn W: *Best practice occupational therapy: in community service with children and families*, Thorofare, NJ, 2000, Slack.

15. Fisher AG, Marterella A: *Powerful practice: A model for authentic occupational therapy*, Fort Collins, CO, 2019, Center for Innovative OT Solutions.

16. Gutman SA, et al: Revision of the occupational therapy practice framework, *Am J Occup Ther* 61:119–126, 2007.

17. Hunt L, et al: Putting the occupational therapy practice framework into practice: enlightening one therapist at a time, *OT Practice* 12:18–22, 2007.

18. Khetani MA, Coster W: Social participation. In BA Boyt Schell & G Gillen, editors: *Willard and Spackman's occupational therapy*, ed 13, Wolters Kluwer.

19. Law M, et al: Core concepts of occupational therapy. In Townsend E, editor: *Enabling occupation: an occupational therapy perspective*, Ottawa, ONT, 1997, CAOT, p 29.

20. Lynch A, Moore A: Play as an occupation in occupational therapy. *Br J Occup Ther* 2016, 79(9) 519–520, 2006. DOI: 10.1177/0308022616664540.

21. Magasi S, Hammel J: Social support and social network mobilization in older African American women who have experienced strokes, *Disabilities Studies Quarterly* 24(4), 2004. http://dsq-sds.org/article/view/878/1053.

22. Nelson DL: Critiquing the logic of the domain section of the occupational therapy practice framework: domain and process, *Am J Occup Ther* 60:511–523, 2006.

23. Parham LD, Fazio LS, editors: *Play in occupational therapy for children*, St Louis, 1997, Mosby.

24. Peloquin S: The therapeutic relationship: manifestations and challenges in occupational therapy. In Crepeau EB, Cohn ES, Schell BAB, editors: *Willard and Spackman's occupational therapy*, ed 10, Philadelphia, 2003, Lippincott Williams & Wilkins, p 157.

25. Pendleton HMH, Schultz-Krohn W: Psychosocial issues in physical disability. In Cara E, MacRae A, editors: *Psychosocial occupational therapy: a clinical practice*, ed 3, Clifton Park, NY, 2013, Delmar/Cengage Learning, p 501.

26. Puchalski C, et al: Improving the quality of spiritual care as a dimension of palliative care: the report of the Consensus Conference, *J Palliat Med* 12(10):885–904, 2009. https://doi.org/10.1089/jpm.2009.0142.

27. Roley SS, Delany J: Improving the occupational therapy practice framework: domain and process: the updated version of the framework reflects changes in the profession, *OT Practice*, February 2, 2009.

28. Siebert C: Communicating home and community expertise: the occupational therapy practice framework, *Home Community Special Interest Section Quarterly* 10(2), 2003.

29. Taylor RR, Van Puymbrouck L: Therapeutic use of self: applying the intentional relationship model in group therapy. In O'Brien JC, Soloman JW, editors: *Occupational analysis and group process*, St Louis, 2013, Elsevier, pp 36–52.

30. World Health Organization: *International classification of functioning, disability, and health*, Geneva, 2001, WHO.

31. Youngstrom MJ: The occupational therapy practice framework: the evolution of our professional language, *Am J Occup Ther* 56:607, 2002.

SUGGESTED READINGS

Christiansen CH, Baum CM, editors: *Occupational therapy: enabling function and well-being*, Thorofare, NJ, 1997, Slack.

Law M: *Evidence-based rehabilitation: a guide to practice*, Thorofare, NJ, 2002, Slack.

Law M, et al: *Occupation-based practice: fostering performance and participation*, Thorofare, NJ, 2002, Slack.

Youngstrom MJ: Introduction to the occupational therapy practice framework: domain and process, AOTA continuing education article, *OT Practice* September: CE1-7, 2002.

History and Practice Trends in Physical Dysfunction Intervention

Deborah J. Bolding[a]

LEARNING OBJECTIVES

After studying this chapter, the reader will be able to do the following:

1. Trace the ideas, values, beliefs, and people that influenced the development of occupational therapy for persons with illness and physical disabilities in the United States (U.S.).

2. Consider the development of occupational therapy within the larger context of U.S. and global scientific, cultural, social, economic, political, and legislative forces.

3. Explore changes in the practice of occupational therapy over the decades.

CHAPTER OUTLINE

KEY TERMS

Arts and crafts movement
Diversional therapy
Moral treatment
Occupational Therapy Practice Framework
Postmodern philosophy

Pragmatism movement
Progressive Era
Social model of disability
Tuberculosis

This chapter will examine some of the people, ideas, events, and movements that influenced the early practice of occupational therapy for persons with medical conditions and physical disabilities. It surveys the expanding role of occupational therapists through subsequent decades, the transformation of practitioners from technicians to professionals, and the subsequent growth and changes in the profession in the areas of injury, illness, health, and wellness. The eminent occupational therapy historian, Kathleen Barker Schwartz, stated that the purpose of history is to "elucidate connections in the hope that we can learn from our rich past and feel more related to it."[65] It is hoped that readers of this chapter will develop an affinity to the values of occupational therapy that have been consistent over the 100 plus years of the profession and the changes in response to advances in medicine and within the larger context of U.S. and global scientific, cultural, social, economic, political, and legislative forces. To facilitate the reader's understanding of the evolving nature of occupational therapy (OT) practice, three case studies are presented, each of which is illustrative of an important era in occupational therapy history. Of note, occupational therapy developed in the United States and other Western countries, and the movements and philosophical ideas discussed in this chapter reflect the history of the profession. Readers are encouraged to explore other important cross-cultural perspectives on occupational therapy that are shaping the future of occupational therapy globally, such as those expressed by Rafeedie and Russow (see Chapter 6) and the review article and references by Mahoney and Kiraly-Alvarez (2019).[46]

[a]The author acknowledges the contributions of Kathleen Barker Schwartz, EdD, Emeritus Professor, San José State University, as the author of earlier editions of this chapter and for some of the content of the current edition of this chapter. Any omissions or errors are those of this author.

FOUNDATIONS OF OCCUPATIONAL THERAPY

Occupational therapy emerged in response to societal and healthcare changes in the United States and the world in the early part of the 20th century. Individuals with illness and injury until this period were often cared for at home or in institutions. Reasons for this were to protect the community from communicable diseases, because the physical environment was not accessible to persons with disabilities, or because of ignorance, fear, and stigma or outward signs of social unacceptability which resulted in discrimination. For example, cities in the United States in the 1880s and 1890s had laws prohibiting public appearances by people who were "diseased, maimed, deformed."[67] These perspectives began to change with advances in medicine and surgery that created new medical models of care, and by progressive reformers who wanted to help persons with disability reclaim their place in the community and the workplace.[82]

The Progressive Era (1890s–1920s)

The Progressive Era, spanning the period from the 1890s to the 1920s, was a time of social activism and reform in the United States. Cities were undergoing rapid industrialization. The majority population was shifting from rural to urban as a result of an agrarian depression, and there was also an influx of immigrants from other countries. These changes resulted in urban conditions of poverty, slums, hunger, homelessness, and exploitation of labor. Cholera, tuberculosis, smallpox, diphtheria, measles, and polio were only some of the communicable diseases which were rampant and resulted in chronic health conditions for city inhabitants. Reformists called for legislation to prevent child labor, protect workers, and provide accident insurance for injured workers and their families; penal reform; women's suffrage; and expanded charitable services for the poor. Through membership in clubs and charitable organizations, women gained leadership abilities and spearheaded many of the social reform initiatives.[56] The settlement house movement was one of the important ways in which women were leaders in creating change.

Settlement houses, first developed in Great Britain, were established in the United States to address social problems resulting from poverty, unsanitary living conditions, and exploitation. Members of more privileged White families, in particular young women, "settled" in immigrant and impoverished communities to help organize education about hygiene, health, work skills, and language and to develop daycare, recreational, vocational, and social activities. Settlers often became advocates for social reform and made contributions to areas such as education, public health, legal aid, housing, and parks.[29] The settlement houses played key roles in many U.S. cities, although they were later criticized because of volunteers' conscious attempts to teach White, middle-class, and religious values and reports of prejudice or ethnic stereotyping.[29]

Hull House, founded in Chicago by Jane Addams and Ellen Starr Gates in 1889, is a settlement house of particular importance to occupational therapy history. The Chicago School of Civics and Philanthropy, established at Hull House in 1908, created early courses to teach attendants and nurses about the efficacy of using occupations and amusements with patients with mental illness.[59] An occupational therapy founder, Eleanor Clarke Slagle, was a student in one of the courses, and was later recruited by the school and the Illinois Society for Mental Hygiene to develop an occupational center for people with mental and orthopedic disabilities in 1915. The workshop taught skills such as furniture making, sewing, rug weaving, toy-making, and other crafts often referred to as occupations at the time. Proceeds from sales of the work went to the clients, who would otherwise have been unemployable.[61] Before and during this period a philosophy of humane treatment of those with disabilities was simultaneously emerging, as will be discussed in the next section.

Moral Treatment Movement

The moral treatment movement for persons with mental and physical illnesses emerged from humanistic philosophy originating in late 18th-century Europe and was promoted by physician Philippe Pinel of France and philanthropist Samuel Tuke of England. This movement represented a shift in thinking from a pessimistic viewpoint that labeled the mentally ill as subhuman and incurable to an optimistic one that viewed the mentally ill as capable of reason when treated humanely. Strengths of the moral treatment movement were its respect for human life, belief in the unity of mind and body, and the recognition that health and well-being were affected by physical and social environments.[45,66]

The movement emphasized a homelike atmosphere for hospitals and asylums where patients could be cared for "with respect and kind treatment upon all circumstances, and in most cases manual labor, attendance at religious worship on Sunday, the establishment of regular habits of self-control, [and] diversion of the mind from morbid trains of thought."[45] Engagement in occupations was key to the program and included music, exercise, art, agriculture, carpentry, painting, and manual crafts.[66]

Both private and public asylums were created based on the moral treatment model. Private institutions were typically for middle- and upper-class clients. Patients in public institutions were often classified by class, sex, degree of illness, behavior, and ability to pay for services. For example, men engaged more in agriculture, carpentry, and other physical tasks, whereas women performed domestic chores and crafts. The "curable" clients engaged in reading, writing, music, and other educational and cultural pursuits, whereas "incurables" engaged in manual pursuits.[52]

Although the moral treatment movement reported early success with patients, public institutions became overwhelmed with chronic patients, overcrowding, and communicable diseases and were challenged to provide the humane treatment that was their initial goal.[9] Moral treatment was also limited by its narrow focus on the values of the dominant culture of the place and era (often based on Protestant beliefs), which did not meet the needs of many immigrants.[45] By the end of the 19th century, advances in surgical and medical treatments served to decrease the influence of moral treatment in hospitals. Psychiatric institutions, however, continued to retain elements of moral treatment, including the use of occupations as treatment.[9,45,52]

One positive outcome of the moral treatment movement was the recognition that occupation, or the "proper use of time in some helpful and gratifying activity," was considered fundamental to care for psychiatric patients at the turn of the century.[48] Coinciding with this belief in the fundamental need for meaningful occupation was resistance to what were considered the dehumanizing effects of the industrial revolution, as will be discussed in the next section.

Arts and Crafts Movement (1895–1920)

The **arts and crafts movement** developed in Europe and the United States as a reaction to the mass-produced goods created by the Industrial Revolution. The movement represented a longing, primarily among the socially advantaged, for a return to the use of natural materials and processes and simple designs.[42] Arts and crafts societies were established with the belief that "true work fixes attention, develops ability, and enriches the life; it strengthens the mind, forms the will, and inures to patience and endurance."[80]

Members of the arts and crafts movement developed programs for persons with physical and mental disabilities to develop discipline and improve worker roles.[64] A strong proponent for the use of arts and crafts in patient care was Dr. Herbert Hall, an occupational therapy founder who in 1904 developed a treatment program he called the "work cure."[5] Although best known for working with neurasthenia (chronic fatigue) patients, he set up training programs for women to teach crafts in schools, sanatoriums, and hospitals, and created industries to help people with physical disabilities such as cardiac disease and arthritis become self-supporting.[5] George Barton, another occupational therapy founder, credited the application of the principles from the arts and crafts movement with helping him regain function after contracting tuberculosis and also later when he developed paralysis of his left side.[64]

The therapeutic value of handicrafts was their ability to provide occupations that stimulated "mental activity and muscular exercise at the same time."[36] Handicrafts could be graded for the desired physical and mental effects. During World War I, occupational therapy "reconstruction aides" successfully used crafts for the physical and mental restoration of disabled servicemen.[56] Another example is the treatment for persons with tuberculosis, in which occupational therapists started with a graduated approach that began with bedside crafts and habit training and proceeded to occupations related to shop work and ultimately actual work.[38] The use of arts and crafts for restoration also fit into the pragmatism philosophers' view that persons needed to be challenged and engaged to live up to their potential, as discussed in the next section.

Pragmatism Movement (1870s–1940s)

Pragmatism was an important philosophy during the early 20th century, with proponents arguing that it was through doing or actions, being confronted with obstacles, making choices, and experiencing that an individual's potential was realized. John Dewey, a psychologist, educator, and philosopher, stressed the importance of people learning by doing.[77] He postulated that learning occurs in the context of one's past experiences, the environment in which the event takes place, and one's level of engagement.[32] Susan Tracy and Eleanor Clarke Slagle, early occupational therapists, cite the influence of John Dewey on their work.[11,49] They and other occupational therapists similarly recognized the importance of assessing clients' values, experiences, and context to help establish more effective intervention plans and programs.

Another pragmatist philosopher, William James, thought habits were created by repetition of meaningful actions. When a habit is created, the person can complete an activity with decreased cognitive load, allowing them to focus on more important tasks.[33] Eleanor Clarke Slagle applied the principle of habit training to help psychiatric patients develop more organized behaviors. Clients followed an organized schedule during the day, and activities were chosen to help patients take their minds off their illness and focus on their productive pursuits.[9,53]

The first occupational therapists (primarily nurses, social workers, and craft teachers) and their supporters thought that occupations, which at that time were primarily arts and crafts, aided in both the physical and psychological recovery of their patients. They demonstrated the value of their ideas to patients and physician allies, and the profession began to spread to an increasing number of settings, as discussed in the next section.

Medical and Scientific Models of Healthcare

Until the 20th century, hospitals in the United States were established primarily to isolate people with contagious diseases (e.g., smallpox or leprosy) and to care for poor, homeless, chronically ill, disabled, those with mental illnesses that might be dangerous to the community, and the dying.[57] As people began immigrating to cities in the United States and Canada from rural areas or other countries, they often lacked family and financial support for home care and increasingly turned to hospital care.[23,63] At about the same time, Frederick Taylor, a prominent engineer, introduced his theory of scientific management. He proposed that rationality, efficiency, and systematic observation could be applied to industrial management and all other areas of life, including teaching, preaching, and medicine.[74] Progressive reformers of the period supported his ideas and urged hospitals to adopt a more scientific approach to medicine and hospital operations.

Medical care in hospitals was also becoming safer and more effective because of advances in medicine, surgery, and infection control. Hospital administrators ran the business, seeking governmental and community support and offering amenities such as hot meals and semi-private rooms to attract middle-class patients, with physicians supervising all aspects of patient care.[41,63] Occupational therapists worked in hospitals under the direction of physicians who prescribed therapy just as they would medication.[64] Dunton, a physician himself, supported this arrangement, saying, "The occupational therapist, therefore, has the same relation to the physician as the nurse, that is, she [sic] is a technical assistant."[18]

The founders of occupational therapy were attracted to the idea of a scientific approach to treatment, and by 1920 were calling for the profession to promote the notion of the "science" of occupation by calling for "the advancement of occupation as a therapeutic measure, the study of the effects of occupation upon the human being, and the dissemination of scientific knowledge on this subject."[15] Barton[7] was particularly taken with Taylor's time and motion studies and thought these might provide a model for occupational therapy research. Similarly, Slagle urged research in occupational therapy to validate its efficacy, and Dunton advocated that practitioners should be educated to engage in systematic inquiry in order to further the profession's goals.[19,70]

Although the founders advocated a scientific approach, there is little evidence to suggest that occupational therapy practice during this period was informed by systematic observation. One exception was the Department of Occupational Therapy at Walter Reed Hospital in Washington, D.C., under the direction of psychologist Bird T. Baldwin.[66] Occupational therapy "reconstruction aides" were assigned to the orthopedic ward, where methods of systematically recording range of motion and muscle strength were established. Activities (typically arts and crafts) were selected based on motion analysis, including joint position, muscle action, and muscle strengthening. Methods of adapting tools were suggested, and splints were fabricated to provide support during the recovery process. Treatment with this systematic approach was narrowly focused but was applied within the context of what Baldwin called "functional restoration," in which the occupational therapist's purpose was to "help each patient find himself and function again as a complete man [sic] physically, socially, educationally, and economically."[66]

Treating Persons With Illness and Injury in the Early Years of the Profession

In the first part of the 20th century, craft teachers were commonly employed to work with patients in mental hospitals, although the practice was not common for medical facilities.[20] Susan Tracy, a nurse and occupational therapy founder, observed that surgical patients seemed happier when occupied and that activities helped restore strength and range of motion to joints and addressed other physiological problems.[36] Other occupational therapy advocates recognized that the mind of the sick person, especially during the prolonged hospitalization, caused worry, confusion, and negative thinking that affected one's spirit.[28,36]

In 1906, Tracy developed an invalid occupations course for nurses on a continuum from acute care to convalescence and return to work.[54] She thought that nurses, because of their medical training, were best suited to teach occupations in the sickroom or hospital shop, although she also supported the use of craft instructors with the convalescent patient.[54] Her book, *Studies in Invalid Occupations*, provided comprehensive suggestions for working with patients who could only use one hand, were without vision, were confused, or had other physical or cognitive conditions.[79] The book also described strategies for working in a variety of settings, including the homes of those who were socially and economically disadvantaged.[42] Nine additional courses of occupational therapy were created by nurses and social service workers between 1908 and 1916.[60] The new profession recruited educated young women, often from nursing, social work, and teachers of arts and crafts.[56] Practitioners and supporters corresponded through informal networks until 1917, when the National Society for the Promotion of Occupational Therapy (NSPOT) was established.

William Rush Dunton, a psychiatrist in charge of patient occupations at Sheppard and Enoch Pratt Hospital in Maryland, and George Barton, a strong supporter of occupational therapy because of personal illness and injury—which he thought responded positively to occupation—arranged the inaugural meeting of NSPOT to incorporate the new society. Eleanor Clarke Slagle, who directed the occupational therapy program at the Phipps Clinic at Johns Hopkins Hospital and had established the Henry B. Favill School of Occupations in Chicago, was an invitee. Also attending the organizational meeting were Susan Cox Johnson, Director of Occupations for the Department of Public Charities in New York City; Thomas Kidner, an architect and Vocational Secretary of the Canadian Military Hospital Commission, and Isabel Gladwin Newton as secretary. Susan Tracy was invited but unable to attend the first meeting.[59] Dr. Edward Hall, who is also considered a founder of the profession, was purposely not invited by George Barton who planned the founding meeting. The first annual meeting of association was held a few months later (September 1917) in New York City, with 26 attendees.[59]

The NSPOT organizers were cognizant that the United States was being drawn into World War I, and thought occupational therapists (or reconstruction aides, as they were called by the military) could provide a valuable service to their country and the war wounded. Only days after the OT inaugural meeting, the United States entered WWI. Mirroring rehabilitation programs developed in England for injured soldiers, training programs were established and over 200 occupational therapy "reconstruction aides" served in the army.[20] During and after the war, teams of occupational therapists, physical therapists, and vocational educators helped injured soldiers return to work (Fig. 2.1).[27] It was during this period that occupational therapy training programs increased requirements for medical knowledge and the ability to work with persons with physical disabilities.

During the period after WWI and before WWII, American occupational therapists worked in a variety of nonmilitary medical settings with people with diagnoses that included tuberculosis, blindness, polio, industrial accident cases, heart disease (often secondary to rheumatic fever), and orthopedic injuries.[30,41] While on bedrest and convalescing, patients would work on handicrafts, such as knitting or basket weaving. These were often described as "diversional" therapy, to direct patients' attention from their illness, prevent depression, and make use of their limited abilities.[51] In the second stage of recovery, patients engaged in occupations to strengthen the body and mind. Examples included knitting, weaving, ceramics, or gardening. Finally, patients engaged in occupations that would prepare them for return to work, such as manual crafts or carpentry, or to a sheltered workshop or agricultural or industrial colonies.[31,66] As occupational therapy treatment became more "scientific," the use of arts and crafts was more commonly prescribed by physicians to increase endurance, coordination, dexterity, muscle power, strength, range of motion, and functional results.[69]

The Rehabilitation Model

The rehabilitation model of care gained strength after World War II. A large number of returning soldiers had injuries that required

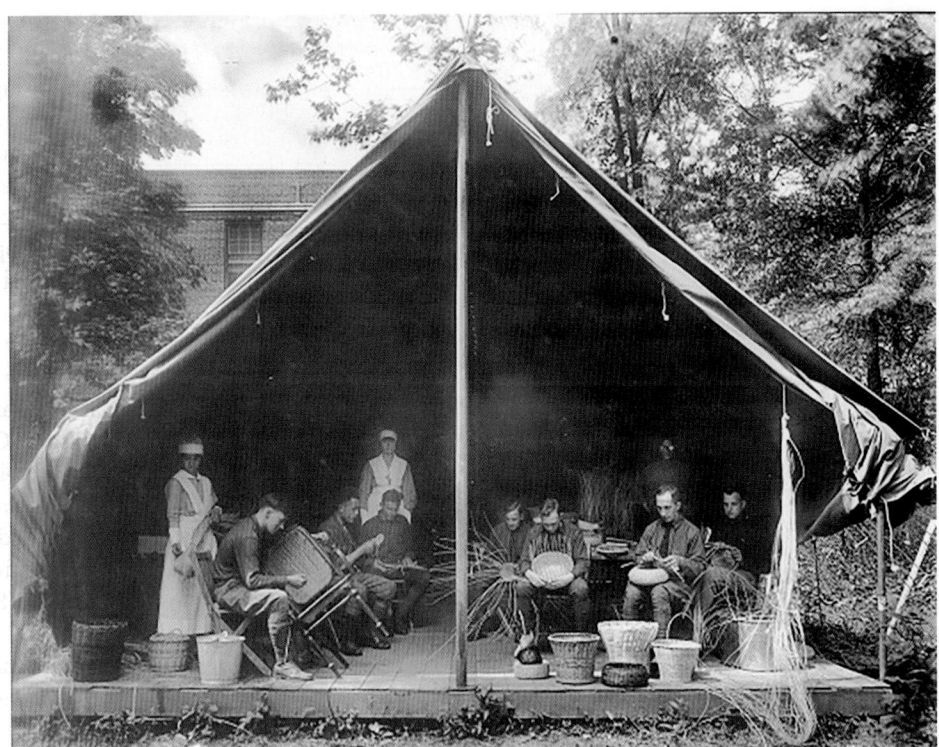

Fig. 2.1 Occupational therapy basketry and chair caning workshop, U.S. General Hospital #38, Eastview, N.Y. Circa 1919. (Courtesy of the Archive of the American Occupational Therapy Association, Inc.)

THREADED CASE STUDY

1920s

The case study of Mary is illustrative of the type of occupational therapy that was being offered during this early era.

Because of her tuberculosis, Mary was admitted to a sanitarium, isolated from her husband, young daughter, parents, and siblings to protect them from the incurable, infectious disease. At first, she was on strict bed rest, although her bed was moved outside when weather permitted so that she would benefit from the fresh air. She looked forward to visits from the occupational therapist, who came to her bedside every other day and brought a basket of activities (knitting, sewing, drawing) from which to choose. These activities helped her pass the long days, did not tax her endurance, and kept her from worrying too much about her future. As she gained strength, she was encouraged to go for short walks in the garden. She visited the occupational therapy room, which offered a range of activities, including weaving and pottery. The occupational therapist helped her choose activities that both were engaging and helped her regain endurance after weeks in bed. As her disease went into remission, she had a period of "conditioning" and then began livelihood training in stenography.[31]

Mary was fortunate. During the late 19th and early 20th century, tuberculosis, or "consumption," was the leading cause of death (1 in 7) in the United States and feared throughout the world (Fig. 2.2). Most patients were advised to rest, eat well, and exercise outdoors, but few recovered and many patients who survived had recurrent bouts of illness that limited activities throughout their lives. The disease affected poor city-dwellers the most because of crowded living conditions and the inability to pay for treatment. Persons with the disease were stigmatized and had to worry about being evicted from their dwellings because of fear of the highly contagious disease.

The discovery of effective medications in the 1940s helped control the spread of tuberculosis and helped patients recover. The United States now has the lowest worldwide rate of tuberculosis in the world (approximately 9000 reported cases in 2019), and approximately 13 million people have latent tuberculosis.[12] However, it is estimated that one third of the world's population carries the latent disease,[85] and some strains of the disease have become drug resistant. For stories of survivors and people living with the disease today, visit https://www.cdc.gov/tb/topic/basics/personalstories.htm.

care and training to help them return to productive lives. The Veterans Administration hospital system developed departments of physical medicine and rehabilitation to bring together all the services needed to care for the soldiers. As this model proved successful, it was implemented in the private sector for persons with polio, stroke, multiple sclerosis, spinal cord injury, head injury, arthritis, and other chronic conditions. Howard Rusk, MD, a physiatrist and prominent voice in the development of rehabilitation medicine, asserted that trained personnel were needed to

deliver services to the more than 5 million people in the United States who had a chronic disability.[37] He cited occupational therapy as one of the essential rehabilitation services. In response to the growing demand for rehabilitation services, Congress passed the Hill-Burton Act in 1946 to provide federal aid for the construction of rehabilitation centers. A proviso of the legislation was that rehabilitation centers had to include four integrated services: medical (including occupational therapy and physical therapy), psychological, social, and vocational.

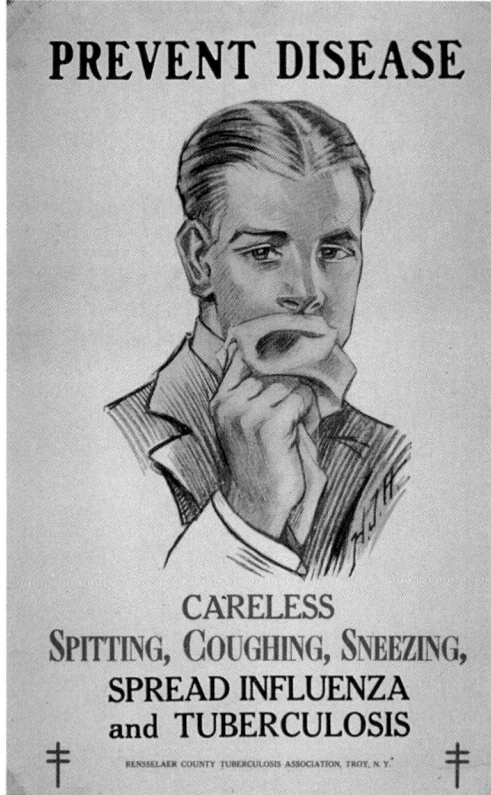

PREVENT DISEASE

CARELESS
SPITTING, COUGHING, SNEEZING,
SPREAD INFLUENZA
and TUBERCULOSIS

RENSSELAER COUNTY TUBERCULOSIS ASSOCIATION, TROY, N.Y.

Fig. 2.2 Rensselaer County Tuberculosis Association Poster. (From National Institutes of Health, National Library of Medicine, https://profiles.nlm.nih.gov/101584655X5.)

Close ties with the American Hospital Association and the American Medical Association benefited the profession in its early years; and during and after World War II, the occupational therapy profession was aided by their association with physical medicine and rehabilitation.[37] However, as physiatrists attempted to exert more control over the education and leadership of the profession, occupational therapy leaders resisted these attempts. Leaders recognized that occupational therapists worked in a variety of settings and with many medical specialties, and they did not want to limit the practice settings.[4,81] During this period, therapists began to seek greater autonomy from physician referrals and to focus more on community, rather than hospital-based care.[50]

Although occupational therapy was not subsumed under the physical medicine framework, therapists continued to specialize in particular kinds of medical knowledge and technological skills. Claire Spackman, who along with Helen Willard wrote the most influential textbook on occupational therapy of the time, argued that therapists must become skilled in carrying out new treatments based on improved techniques. According to Spackman, occupational therapists serving people with disability needed to be skilled in teaching activities of daily living, work simplification, and training in the use of upper extremity prostheses. But foremost, she asserted, "Occupational therapy treats the patient by the use of constructive activity in a simulated, normal living and/or working situation."[71]

THREADED CASE STUDY

1970s

Jacob, a 67-year-old man who recently had a cerebrovascular accident (stoke), was admitted to a 30-bed rehabilitation unit for persons with stroke, spinal cord injury, head injury, and other neurological and orthopedic conditions. It was expected that his stay at the rehabilitation center would last 4 to 5 weeks and he would participate in therapy (physical, occupational, and speech) for a minimum of 3 hours each day. After his initial evaluation, the occupational therapist talked with Jacob about his schedule for the first week. Treatment in the mornings would consist of activities related to hygiene, toileting, dressing, and bathing. Later in the day, they would work on regaining function in his paralyzed right arm. This would consist of neurodevelopmental treatment activities (such as weight-bearing and the use of reflex-inhibiting postures) to decrease tone in the arm. Weak muscles would be facilitated (e.g., tapping, quick stretch) and strengthened by exercises (e.g., stacking cones or sliding his arm on the tabletop) as well as using the hand during functional activities. Jacob made a cutting board that could be used in the kitchen with one hand by hammering two stainless steel nails into a cutting board, and adding suction cup feet. While working in the shop, Jacob observed patients with spinal cord injuries make their own transfer boards by sanding the wood smooth and then applying a finish to the wood. Some of Jacob's therapy sessions were with the occupational therapist; however, a number of the sessions were with the occupational therapy assistant who worked closely with supervision from the occupational therapist.

Before discharge, many patients on the rehabilitation unit would become independent with basic self-care, but in Jacob's case, he still required some assistance for safety when transferring to a toilet, tub, or car and for bathing. His occupational therapist suggested to the rehabilitation team that he be referred for home health occupational therapy, a service that was relatively new in this region of the country. This occupational therapy service would help Jacob work on skills in his home environment, and as he improved, he could transition to outpatient therapy.

Occupational therapists often used their shops to create assistive devices for their patients. Fred Sammons, an occupational therapist who earned his degree using the G.I. Bill benefits after WWII, created a company that sold assistive devices to therapy clinics. In the early days, clinics had to stock items because delivery time could take several weeks. For more about Fred Sammons, visit https://www.aotf.org/About-AOTF/Staff/fred-sammons. Today, patients are often directed to the internet to purchase their own equipment, although some custom items are still fabricated by therapists. The advent of three-dimensional printing has created exciting new possibilities for therapists to provide assistive devices, and proponents of universal design have helped make some everyday items more usable by persons with physical limitations. For more information about universal design, see http://universaldesign.ie/What-is-Universal-Design/.

Expansion and Specialization

Special education programs were established to train restoration aides during World War I, but occupational therapy leaders in the 1920s recognized the need for stronger educational standards. By 1930, educational programs were required to be 18 months long, with 9 months of classroom and technical work, and 9 months of hospital practice under supervision.[4] By the end of that decade, a college degree was required. At the request of the American Occupational Therapy Association (AOTA; created when NSPOT changed its name in 1921), the American Medical Association was asked to take over inspection of training programs to ensure they met minimum standards.[14,59]

In the period before and after World War II, occupational therapists continued to expand their practice in the area of physical disabilities. A shortage of trained occupational therapists during and after World War II led to the development of the aide role, and in 1958 the first certified occupational therapy assistant (COTA) programs were established.[16] Although the first COTA educational programs were established for training assistants to work in mental health settings, programs for training COTAs to work in general practice and nursing home care were developed soon afterward.[16]

As occupational therapy expanded into new practice areas, therapists in rehabilitation and outpatient centers began to focus on restoring self-care skills, creating self-help devices, the use of technology, orthotics, prosthetics, neuromuscular facilitation, therapeutic use of self, prevocational evaluation, and work simplification.[50,72] One paper of the era described the purpose of occupational therapy as the following: to increase endurance; to improve coordination, dexterity, muscle power, strength, and range of motion; to relieve tightness of fascial planes; and to obtain best functional results.[69] The occupational therapy assistant's role in general practice was to help patients develop and maintain skills for daily living and working.

The "typical" practitioner also changed somewhat in the post–World War II era. During the early years of the profession, the profession was exclusively young White women, most often from middle or upper classes and single. There were no males or people of color who were therapists. Concerns related to gender, racial, and cultural diversity began to be discussed during World War II, with AOTA considering whether schools should admit males, Blacks, persons with disabilities, and older (up to age 35) students.[10] Males began to enter the profession in larger numbers in the 1950s and 1960s; however, only 10% of therapists in the present day identify as males.[1] The first two Black therapists, Ruth Denard and Naomi Wright, graduated from occupational therapy school in 1946; only a small number of schools accepted Black applicants at that time.[10] It was not until the 1980s that AOTA began actively studying minority recruitment and retention for the profession.[10] Currently, Whites still represent the largest group (83.7%), followed by Asian/Pacific Islanders (5.8%), Latinx (3.9%), Blacks (3.0%), Multiethnic persons (1.8%), and American Indian/Alaskan Native, (0.3%),[1] and efforts to recruit people of color into the profession have been largely unsuccessful. There are many factors at play: many career choices are based on personal relationships, and high school and college students have few role models; lack of preparation in the sciences; poor performance of minority students on standardized tests,[83] and institutional racism have limited access to healthcare and healthcare and educational institutions, as well as more basic resources.[34] This lack of diversity within the profession has consequences for patient and client outcomes and professional development. For example, therapists may not fully understand contextual factors that are important to their patients without a broad understanding of culture that can be developed in a rich community of practice.

There was global interest in occupational therapy in the 1920s and beyond. Canadian programs developed in the same period as American clinics and expanded during World War I.[23] England, Germany, Switzerland, and Italy all reportedly had programs in the 1930s, although the therapy was oriented more toward mental health conditions.[6,22] The World Federation of Occupational Therapists held an organizational meeting in England in 1951, and the association started in 1952 with 10 member associations from the following countries: Australia, Canada, Denmark, India, Israel, New Zealand, South Africa, Sweden, United Kingdom (England and Scotland), and the United States. Today there are 106 regional and individual country member organizations. The organization is the global voice for practice, and supports a "quality of practice that is relevant and sensitive to context and culture."[84] This organization is also committed to occupational justice, advocating actions to counter injustice caused by social problems, poverty, economic restrictions, disease, discrimination, and other causes.

Theory-Practice Gap

Traditional arts and crafts treatment approaches were not suited to rehabilitation settings, and by the 1960s, self-care and social skills activities were becoming the norm for treatment (Fig. 2.3).[75] Dr. Frank Krusen, a leader in physical medicine and rehabilitation, stated that "while the average occupational therapist is more concerned with the liberal arts than with the science; nevertheless, the scientific approach is essential to your further advancement." He suggested that therapists focus more on kinetic occupational therapy and better education and research to strengthen the field.[40]

Occupational therapists working in hospitals and rehabilitation centers were under pressure to decrease the length of inpatient hospital stays, demonstrate positive outcomes for their interventions, and increase productivity. The value of arts and crafts was limited under these conditions, and patients themselves often did not understand the purpose or value of arts and crafts. Therapists began to disassociate themselves from the "basket weaver" image and the arts and crafts activities associated with diversional therapy, which were not reimbursable by insurance companies and Medicare.[47,58]

Changes in practice set the stage for conflict between occupational therapists who used exercises, neurodevelopmental treatment approaches, and modalities (e.g., biofeedback, electrical stimulation) and practitioners who thought all occupational therapy treatment should be "purposeful."[11,21,75] Critics asserted that some occupational therapists were becoming reductionist in their practice, and treating symptoms rather than the person.[68] Scholars such as Gill brought the perspective of the social model of disability rights to the discussion about occupational therapy practice. Gill urged occupational therapists to examine their practice and make sure that treatment did not focus solely on the individual's physical condition, but also their needs, values, interests, and the limitations in reaching their goals because of a discrimination and lack of opportunities.[25]

A study by Pendleton supported Gill's concerns. Pendleton found that occupational therapists were much less likely to provide training in independent living skills than physical remediation. She defined independent living skills as "those specific abilities broadly associated with home management and social/community problem solving." Pendleton recommended that if occupational therapists were not able to provide sufficient

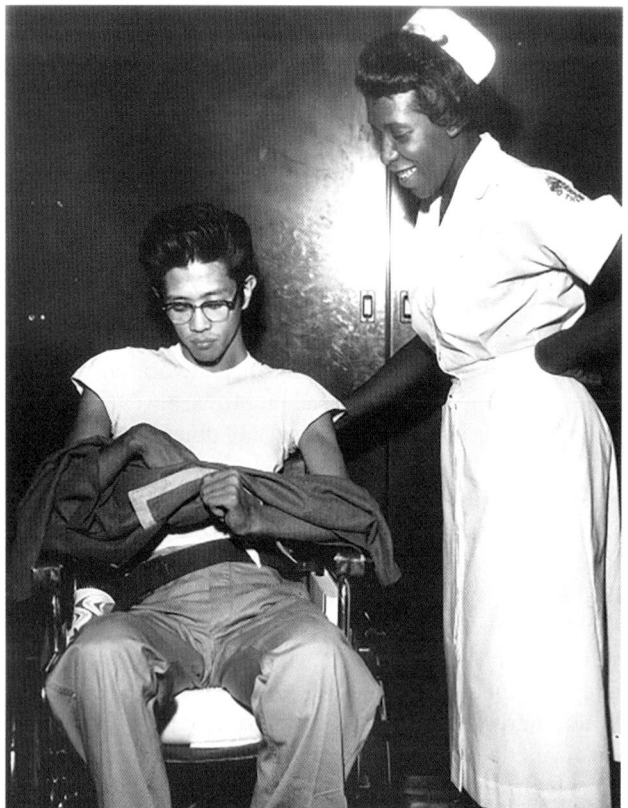

Fig. 2.3 Dorothy (Dottie) Wilson, OTR, at Rancho Los Amigos Hospital, circa late 1950s or early 1960s. Rancho Los Amigos Hospital was one of the preeminent rehabilitation centers established on the West Coast in response to the Hill-Burton Act of 1946. Occupational therapists worked with patients with spinal cord injury on activities of daily living, such as eating, dressing, hygiene, and bathing, and underlying motor function such as strengthening, endurance, and coordination. Patients also worked on community living skills. In the next decade, therapists would begin to incorporate more technology, such as environmental control devices (electronic assistive technology that enables persons with disabilities to control functions such as nurse call lights, lighting, heat, telephone) and personal computers, but these devices were primitive and expensive in comparison to today. (Courtesy of the Archive of the American Occupational Therapy Association, Inc.)

independent living skills training in inpatient rehabilitation centers, they should shift their treatment to community-based programs. Pendleton viewed independent living skills as the essence of occupational therapy and urged therapists to make it one of their priorities.[55]

It was during this same period that occupational therapy theorists were critically examining and questioning practice, developing the first occupation-based theories, and exploring the interrelationship of theory with practice.[13] There was a transition from empirical to more scientific approaches,[43] with the process including a "narrowing of the range of empirical content and the broadening of the range of rational theory."[62] Reilly's occupational behavior theory reflected the founders' philosophy that participation in meaningful occupations directly enhanced one's sense of well-being and promoted healthy role functioning.[13]

The *Uniform Terminology*, created by AOTA in 1979, helped occupational therapists conceptualize how occupations, adjunctive therapies, and multiple frameworks and theories might coexist in practice. The document incorporated performance areas (activities of daily living, work, play, or leisure), and performance components (activities, modalities, techniques).[17] For example, a patient who had a cerebrovascular accident might have a deficit in a performance area (dressing), and the patient's goals and intervention plan might include regaining function, as well as working on underlying strength, tone, or balance issues. The Occupational Therapy Practice Framework, which succeeded the *Uniform Terminology* in 2002, further clarified that although occupational therapists use everyday occupations to enhance or enable participation, therapists might also work on underlying motor and process and social skills, as well as body functions.[2]

The theory-practice gap also highlighted the need for more research about occupations, and occupational science was born as an academic discipline. As described by Yerxa,[87] the context for the development of occupational science was the increasing number of people with chronic impairments, the public policy debates about the rights of people with disabilities, efforts to show efficacy and cost-effectiveness across health professions, and greater acceptance of qualitative research methods. As an applied science, researchers and practitioners began to be able to translate knowledge about occupation as a guide for practice.[86] Scholarship that focuses on the disability experience can add to the profession's body of knowledge, increase our understanding of disability from the individual's perspective, help us develop more effective and meaningful interventions, and to be better advocates for social change. One school of thought that has influenced occupational therapy development in this area is postmodern philosophy, which will be discussed in the next section.

Postmodern Philosophy

Postmodern philosophy is a movement that developed in the 1940s and grew stronger through the late 20th century. It was characterized by subjectivism and a suspicion of reason and meaning. Medical and scientific research and practice were criticized for relying too heavily on technology and science, and ignoring the voices of disabled individuals, minority groups, and others.[24] Postmodern healthcare, it was suggested, should be concerned with values as well as evidence; health as well as healthcare; evaluation of services with respect to appropriateness and necessity; concern with patients' satisfaction and experience of care; commitment of continual quality assurance; and empowerment of patients.[24] Occupation-based theories developed within these broader views of the person (client); their values, motivations, occupations; and their physical and socioeconomic environments.

Postmodern philosophy also influenced the growth of identity politics in the United States, including disability rights activism which resulted in legislative changes in the United States such as the Rehabilitation Act of 1973, the Individuals with Disabilities Education Act of 1973 (IDEA), and the Americans with Disabilities Act of 1990. Despite legislation, however, people with disabilities continued to experience marginalization and financial inequity.[44,66] Although occupational therapists were allies in legislative efforts, disability scholars argued that the implicit assumption underlying rehabilitation and occupational therapy was that disability was undesirable. This reflected a societal perspective

THREADED CASE STUDY

2020s

Mara K. is a 26-year-old woman who sustained a T4 ASIA A spinal cord injury 1 year earlier. She is enrolled in a Parenting Self-Management Program that meets online weekly for 4 weeks. There are 10 other parents in the group. Topics include baby care techniques for persons using wheelchairs; parenting toddlers and school age children; safety and emergency planning; talking with children about disability; managing pain, fatigue, and other physical concerns; planning family outings and travel; and community resources. Group sessions are planned and facilitated by the occupational therapist in partnership with a lay leader who is a parent and who has a spinal cord injury. Guest speakers include other parents with disabilities, representatives from community agencies and schools, and others as requested by the group. Participants establish personal goals that they would like to explore during the month-long class. Participants are encouraged to share resources (as with other self-help groups).

This is the first time this center has offered the program. The therapist who developed the group heard about a similar program at a conference, explored the evidence for such a program, gathered input and support from other team members and administrators (including parents, for whom the group was targeted), and determined the best way to implement the program in their setting. The therapist is collecting outcome information related to participant satisfaction, goal attainment, and parental self-efficacy. These data will help determine what changes, if any, might be needed for future classes. One plan for the group is to transition to being led by a parent or parents with a spinal cord injury, with the occupational therapist acting as a resource for the group.

that impairment is a negative state that must be reduced or eliminated. Reduction of a client's disability would lessen social and or economic burden.[39] Disability rights advocates, using the social model of disability, say that people are disabled by physical structures and attitudinal and social barriers, not by their impairment.[26] Kielhofner[39] urged occupational therapists to rethink their concepts and approaches to disabilities, to consider how people experience impairment, how impairments change over time, and how therapists can better understand and support clients and their families.[39] An example of how this postmodern thinking influenced occupational therapy practice can be seen in the following case study circa 2020.

A focus on the therapeutic relationship is one way to ensure that clients' diverse needs are addressed, as was seen in the 2020 Case Study. As reported by Taylor and colleagues,[77] "Most therapists considered therapeutic use of self as the most important skill in occupational therapy practice and a critical element of clinical reasoning. By focusing on the client-therapist relationship, the practitioner is more likely to understand the client's experience as an individual with a disability and thus to work jointly with them to formulate an intervention plan that centers on the client's goals." When an effective therapeutic relationship is formed, practice is much more likely to be client-centered.[76]

USING HISTORY TO UNDERSTAND TODAY'S PRACTICE

During the latter part of the 20th century and into the 21st century, occupational therapists began to consider health as not just as the absence of disease but also risk factors, including exposure to health threats, genetic factors, and social and economic conditions. They began to work in community settings to promote healthy occupations and habits.[8,35] Baum and Law[8] suggested that therapists needed an understanding of community-based organizations (e.g., public health departments, housing services) to be able to work in teams markedly different from "traditional" settings.[8] An example of how this might work is the CAPABLE model for functionally impaired community-dwelling older adults.[73] This program integrated occupational therapy home visits and treatment with nursing, who addressed pain, depression, polypharmacy, and primary care provider communication. The program also included a handy person for simple repairs and home modifications to promote safety. The CAPABLE program has demonstrated a number of positive outcomes for participants, including increased independence with activities of daily living, improved walking, a reduction in depressive symptoms, and a decrease in home hazards, all while keeping costs relatively low.

A knowledge of history can provide a context from which to understand current challenges to physical disabilities practice. As this history has demonstrated, early treatment in occupational therapy was based on belief in the importance of occupation, habit training, knowledge of crafts, and the application of crafts therapeutically to improve clients' mental and physical condition. As scientific knowledge and technology advanced, occupational therapy defined a role for itself within the rehabilitation model. This closer relationship with medicine helped the profession gain credibility. As medical knowledge increased, specialty areas within occupational therapy began to emerge, such as the areas of spinal cord injury, burn rehabilitation, and hand therapy. However, the scientific reductionism of the medical model placed occupational therapy at odds with occupational therapy's more holistic view of practice, empowerment of clients, the growth of community-based and wellness models of care, the social model of disability, and postmodern analysis of justice and equity in healthcare.

The American Occupational Therapy Association's current definition of occupational therapy, published online, is the following: "Occupational therapy is the only profession that helps people across the lifespan to do the things they want and need to do through the therapeutic use of daily activities (occupations). Occupational therapy practitioners enable people of all ages to live life to its fullest by helping them promote health, and prevent—or live better with—injury, illness, or disability."[3] The description of occupational therapy continues: "Occupational therapy practitioners have a holistic perspective, in which the focus is on adapting the environment and/or task to fit the person, and the person is an integral part of the therapy team. It is an evidence-based practice deeply rooted in science."[3] Over the decades, the common conditions that occupational therapists might treat have changed (e.g., tuberculosis, polio, head injury, cancer, heart disease, human immunodeficiency virus, COVID-19), the settings have changed (e.g., hospital, long-term care, home, hospice, wellness centers, community centers), and other contextual factors have evolved. However, occupational therapists continue to view clients and their roles through a humanistic, holistic lens that defines its goals by what is important to the client.

■ REVIEW QUESTIONS

1. What were the primary contributions of moral treatment, the arts and crafts movement, and pragmatist philosophy to the early practice of occupational therapy? Are these same contributions part of practice today?
2. Explain why you think the early founders of OT emphasized the need for research.
3. Discuss the pros and cons of occupational therapy's alliance with physicians' organizations and the medical model.
4. Occupational therapists were divided about the use of modalities and treatments that were not "occupation-based." How was this issue resolved by the professional community?
5. Analyze how the social model of disability influenced occupational therapy practice.
6. Occupational therapy practitioners are described as having a "holistic perspective." Describe what that means to you.
7. Consider ways in which increasing globalization will affect the future practice of occupational therapy.

For additional practice questions for this chapter, please visit eBooks.Health.Elsevier.com.

REFERENCES

1. American Occupational Therapy Association: *2019 Workforce and salary survey.* Bethesda, MD, 2020a, American Occupational Therapy Association.
2. American Occupational Therapy Association: Occupational therapy practice framework: domain and process, 4th ed, *Am J Occup Ther* 74(Suppl 2):1–87, 2020b.
3. American Occupational Therapy Association: *What is occupational therapy?* 2021. https://www.aota.org/Conference-Events/OTMonth/what-is-OT.aspx.
4. Anderson LT, Reed KL: *The history of occupational therapy: the first century,* Thorofare, NJ, 2017, SLACK, Inc.
5. Anthony SH: Dr. Herbert J. Hall: Originator of honest work for occupational therapy 1904–1923 (Part 1), *Occup Ther Health Care* 19(3):3–19, 2005.
6. Armstrong-Jones R: Occupational therapy, *Br Med J* 2(3844):486, 1934.
7. Barton GE: *The movies and the microscope,* Bethesda, MD, American Occupation Therapy Foundation, Wilma West Library, 1920.
8. Baum C, Law M: Community health: a responsibility, an opportunity, and a fit for occupational therapy, *Am J Occup Ther* 52(1):7–10, 1998.
9. Bing RK: Occupational therapy revisited: A paraphrastic journey, *Am J Occup Ther* 35(8):498–518, 1981.
10. Black RM: Occupational therapy's dance with diversity, *Am J Occup Ther* 56(2):140–148, 2002.
11. Breines E: The issue is: an attempt to define purposeful activity, *Am J Occup Ther* 38(8):543–544, 1984.
12. Centers for Disease Control and Prevention. Tuberculosis data and statistics. https://www.cdc.gov/tb/statistics/default.htm.
13. Cole MB, Tufano R: *Applied theories in occupational therapy,* Thorofare, NJ, 2020, SLACK Incorporated.
14. Colman W: Structuring education: development of the first educational standards in occupational therapy, 1917–1930, *Am J Occup Ther* 46(7):653–660, 1992.
15. Constitution of the National Society for the Promotion of Occupational Therapy (1917). Baltimore, MD, Sheppard Pratt Hospital Press.
16. Cottrell RPF: COTA education and professional development: a historical review, *Am J Occup Ther* 54(4):407–412, 2000.
17. Dunn W, McGourty L: Application of uniform terminology to practice, *Am J Occup Ther* 43(12):817–831, 1989.
18. Dunton WR: *Prescribing occupational therapy,* Springfield, IL, 1928, Charles C. Thomas.
19. Dunton WR: The three "R's" of occupational therapy, *Occup Ther Rehabilitation* 7:345–348, 1928.
20. Dunton WR: History and development of occupational therapy. In Willard H, Spackman C, editors: *Principles of occupational therapy,* Philadelphia, 1947, J. B. Lippincott Company, pp 1–9.
21. English C, Kasch M, Silverman P, Walker S: On the role of the occupational therapist in physical disabilities, *Am J Occup Ther* 36(3):200–202, 1982.
22. Franks RM: Occupational therapy in Europe, *Can J Occup Ther,* 1933. https://doi.org/10.1177/000841743300100104.
23. Friedland J: *Restoring the spirit: the beginnings of occupational therapy in Canada, 1980–1930,* Montreal, Canada, 2011, McGill-Queen's University Press.
24. Gergen KJ: Toward a postmodern psychology. In Kvale S, editor: *Psychology and postmodernism,* Newbury Park, CA, 1992, SAGE Publications, pp 17–28.
25. Gill C: A new social perspective on disability and its implications for rehabilitation, *Occup Ther Health Care* 4:49–55, 1987.
26. Goering S: Rethinking disability: the social model of disability and chronic disease, *Curr Rev Musculoskelet Med* 8(2):134–138, 2015.
27. Gutman SA: Influence of the U.S. military and occupational therapy reconstruction aides in World War I on the development of occupational therapy, *Am J Occup Ther* 49(3):256–262, 1995.
28. Hall HJ: Remunerative occupations for the handicapped, *Mod Hospital* 8(6):383–386, 1917.
29. Hansan, J.E. (2011). Settlement houses: An introduction. VCU Libraries Social Welfare History Project. https://socialwelfare.library.vcu.edu/settlement-houses/settlement-houses/.
30. Harmon M: The history of the New Jersey Occupational Therapy Association, *Occup Ther Rehabilitation* 17(1):49–54, 1938.
31. Heaton TG: Occupational therapy for the tuberculous: Motives and methods, *Can J Occup Ther* 4:54–61, 1937.
32. Hickman LA: John Dewey: his life and work. In Hickman LA, Neubert S, Reich K, editors: *John Dewey between pragmatism and constructivism,* New York, 2009, Fordham University Press.
33. Ikiugu MN, Nissen RM: Pragmatic foundations: instrumentalism and transactionalism in occupational therapy. In Taff SD, editor: *Philosophy and occupational therapy: informing education, research, and practice,* Thorofare, NJ, 2021, SLACK Incorporated.
34. Institute of Medicine: *Unequal treatment: confronting racial and ethnic disparities in healthcare,* Washington, DC, 2009, National Academies Press.
35. Johnson JA: Wellness: its myths, realities, and potential for occupational therapy, *Occup Ther Health Care* 2(2):117–138, 1985.
36. Johnson SC: Instruction in handcrafts and design for hospital patients, *Mod Hospital* 15(1):69–72, 1920.
37. Kevorkian CG, Bartels M, Franklin DJ: To believe in humanity and in rehabilitation: Howard A. Rusk, MD, and the birth of rehabilitation medicine, *Phys Med Rehabilitation* 5:247–254, 2013.
38. Kidner TB: Planning for occupational therapy, *Mod Hospital* 21:414–428, 1923.
39. Kielhofner G: Rethinking disability and what to do about it: disability studies and its implications for occupational therapy, *Am J Occup Ther* 59:487–496, 2005.

40. Krusen FH: Relationships between occupational therapy and physical medicine and rehabilitation, *Can J Occup Ther* 21(1):3–9, 1954.

41. LeVesconte HP: Expanding fields of occupational therapy, *Can J Occup Ther* 3:4–12, 1935.

42. Levine RE: The influence of the arts-and-crafts movement on the professional status of occupational therapy, *Am J Occup Ther* 41(4):248–254, 1987.

43. Llorens LA, Gillette NP: The challenge for research in a practice profession, *Am J Occup Ther* 39(3):143–145, 1985.

44. Longmore P: *Why I burned my book and other essays on disability*, Philadelphia, 2003, Temple University Press.

45. Luchins AS: Moral treatment in asylums and general hospitals in 19th-century America, *J Psychol* 123(6):585–607, 1989.

46. Mahoney WJ, Kiraly-Alvarez AF: Challenging the status quo: infusing non-Western ideas into occupational therapy education and practice, *Open J Occup Ther* 7(3):1–10, 2019. https://doi.org/10.15453/2168-6408.1592.

47. Mead S, Harell A: Failures in functional occupational therapy, *Arch Phys Med rehabilitation* 31(12):753–756, 1950.

48. Meyer A: The philosophy of occupational therapy, *Arch Occup Ther* 1(1):1–10, 1922.

49. Morrison R: Pragmatist epistemology and Jane Addams: Fundamental concepts for the social paradigm of occupational therapy, *Occup Ther Int* 23:295–304, 2016.

50. Mosey AC: Involvement in the rehabilitation movement – 1942–1960, *Am J Occup Ther* 25(5):234–236, 1971.

51. Osthoff H: Occupational therapy and poliomyelitis, *Can J Occup Ther* 17(4):151–153, 1939.

52. Peloquin SM: Moral treatment: contexts considered, *Am J Occup Ther* 43(8):537–544, 1989.

53. Peloquin SM: Occupational therapy service: individual and collective understandings of the founders, Part 1, *Am J Occup Ther* 45(4):352–360, 1991.

54. Peloquin SM: Occupational therapy service: Individual and collective understandings of the founders, Part 2, *Am J Occup Ther* 45(8):733–744, 1991.

55. Pendleton HM: Occupational therapists current use of independent living skills training for adult inpatients who are physically disabled, *Occup Ther Health Care* 6:93–108, 1990.

56. Quiroga VAM: *Occupational therapy: the first 30 years*, Bethesda, MD, 1995, American Occupational Therapy Association.

57. Ransom JE: The beginnings of hospitals in the United State, *Bull History Med* 13(5):514–539, 1943.

58. Reed KL: Tools of practice: heritage or baggage? *Am J Occup Ther* 40:597–605, 1986.

59. Reed KL: Identification of the people and critique of the ideas in Meyer's philosophy of occupational therapy, *Occup Ther Ment Health* 33(2):107–128, 2017. https://doi.org/10.1080/016421 2X.2017.1280445.

60. Reed KL: The pioneer schools of occupation: reflections for current practice, *Occup Ther Health Care* 32(3):251–274, 2018. https://doi.org/10.1080/07380577.2018.1493760.

61. Reed KL: Henry B. Favill and the School of Occupations: origins of occupational therapy practice and education, *Occup Ther Health Care* 33(2):159–180, 2019. https://doi.org/10.1080/073805 77.2018.1553087.

62. Reilly M: An occupational therapy curriculum for 1965, *Am J Occup Ther* 12(6):293–299, 1958.

63. Risse GB: *Mending bodies, saving souls: a history of hospitals*, Oxford, UK, 1999, Oxford University Press.

64. Schemm RL: Bridging conflicting ideologies: the origins of American and British occupational therapy, *Am J Occup Ther* 48(11):1082–1088, 1994.

65. Schwartz KB: Reclaiming our heritage: connecting the founding vision to the centennial vision, *Am J Occup Ther* 63:681–690, 2009. https://doi.org/10.5014/ajot.63.6.681.

66. Schwartz KB: History and practice trends in physical dysfunction intervention. In Pendleton HM, Schultz-Krohn W, editors: *Pedretti's Occupational Therapy*, St Louis, 2018, Elsevier, pp 16–23.

67. Schweik SM: *The ugly laws: disability in public*, New York, NY, 2009, New York University Press.

68. Shannon PD: The derailment of occupational therapy, *Am J Occup Ther* 31(4):229–234, 1977.

69. Shields CD, Oelhafen WR, Sheehan HR: The role of occupational therapy in the physical medicine management of physical disabilities, *South Med J* 45(5):395–400, 1952.

70. Slagle EC: Training aides for mental patients, *Arch Occup Ther* 1(1):11–18, 1922.

71. Spackman CS: A history of the practice of occupational therapy for restoration of physical function: 1917–1967, *Am J Occup Ther* 22:67–71, 1968.

72. Strickland LR: Directions for the future—occupational therapy practice then and now, 1949–the present, *Am J Occup Ther* 45(2): 105–107, 1991.

73. Szanton SL, Gitlin LN: Meeting the health care financing imperative through focusing on function: the CAPABLE studies, *Public Policy Aging* 26(3):106–110, 2016. https://doi.org/10.1093/ppar/prw014.

74. Taylor F: *The principles of scientific management*, New York, 1911, Harper.

75. Taylor E, Manguno J: Use of treatment activities in occupational therapy, *Am J Occup Ther* 45(4):317–322, 1991.

76. Taylor R, Lee SW, Kielhofner G, Ketkar M: Therapeutic use of self: a nationwide survey of practitioners' attitudes and experiences, *Am J Occup Ther* 63:198–207, 2009.

77. Thayer HS: *Meaning and action: a critical history of pragmatism*. Indianapolis, IN, 1981, Hackett Publishing Company.

79. Tracy SE: *Studies in invalid occupation: a manual for nurses and attendants*, Boston, MA, 1910, Whitcomb and Barrows.

80. Triggs, OL: *Chapters in the history of the arts and crafts movement*. Bohemia Guild of the Industrial Arts League, 1902. https://archive.org/stream/chaptersinhistor00trigrich?ref=ol.

81. West WL: Ten milestone issues in AOTA history, *Am J Occup Ther* 46(12):1066–1074, 1992.

82. Wiebe R: *The search for order, 1877–1920*, New York, 1967, Hill and Wang, A division of Farrar, Strauss and Giroux..

83. Wilbur, KL: (2016). Race matters: occupational therapy as a career choice by high school students of color. Tacoma, WA, University of Washington, 2016. https://digitalcommons.tacoma.uw.edu.

84. World Federation of Occupational Therapists. Practice development. 2021. https://www.wfot.org/programmes/practice.

85. World Health Organization (WHO). *Global tuberculosis report*, 2022. https://www.who.int/teams/global-tuberculosis-programme/tb-reports/global-tuberculosis-report-2022.

86. Wright-St. Claire VA, Hocking C: Occupational science. In Boyt Schell BA, Gillen G, editors: *Willard and Spackman's Occupational therapy*, Philadelphia, 2019, Wolters Kluwer, pp 123–139.

87. Yerxa EJ: Occupational science: a renaissance of service to humankind through knowledge, *Occup Ther Int* 7(2):87–98, 2000.

3

Application of the Occupational Therapy Practice Framework to Physical Dysfunction

Winifred Schultz-Krohn and Heidi McHugh Pendleton

LEARNING OBJECTIVES

After studying this chapter, the student or practitioner will be able to do the following:

1. Identify and describe the major functions of the occupational therapy (OT) process.
2. Describe how clinical reasoning adjusts to consider various factors that may be present in the intervention context.
3. Identify how theories, models of practice, and frames of reference can inform and support OT intervention.
4. Identify appropriate delegation of responsibility among the various levels of OT practitioners.
5. Discuss ways in which OT practitioners may effectively collaborate with members of other professions involved in client care.
6. Recognize ethical dilemmas that may occur frequently in OT practice, and identify ways in which these may be addressed and managed.
7. Describe the various practice settings for OT practice in the arena of physical disabilities.
8. Discuss the types of services typically provided in the various practice settings.
9. Identify ways in which different practice settings affect the occupational performance of persons receiving occupational therapy services.
10. Identify the environmental attributes that afford the most realistic projections of how the client will perform in the absence of the therapist.
11. Identify environmental and temporal aspects of at least three practice settings.
12. Describe ways in which the therapist can alter environmental and temporal features to obtain more accurate measures of performance.

CHAPTER OUTLINE

KEY TERMS

Acute care
Acute rehabilitation
Clinical reasoning
Community-based settings
Conditional reasoning
Ethical dilemmas
Ethics
Evaluation
Frame of reference (FOR)
Inpatient settings
Interactive reasoning
Intervention plan

Narrative reasoning
Occupational therapist (OT)
Occupational therapy aide
Occupational therapy assistant (OTA)
Occupational therapy practitioners
Practice setting
Pragmatic reasoning
Procedural reasoning
Referral
Screening
Skilled nursing facility (SNF)
Subacute rehabilitation

THREADED CASE STUDY

Serena, Part 1

Serena is an occupational therapy student who began her first fieldwork internship 2 weeks ago. Serena prefers use of the pronouns she/her/hers during social interactions. She felt fortunate to be assigned a site that provides a wide array of services. Serena's site is a community hospital that provides a continuum of care, from emergency services and critical care (intensive care unit [ICU]) to outpatient rehabilitation services. Her internship includes providing occupational therapy (OT) intervention in a variety of settings. Her clinical instructor (CI) requested that Serena review the process of developing an intervention plan and be prepared to differentiate the roles of occupational therapy in the various settings.

Critical Thinking Questions
1. What process should be used to develop an intervention plan?
2. How do theories, models of practice, and frames of reference guide an intervention plan?
3. What forms of clinical reasoning are used when providing OT services?

This chapter is divided into two sections. The first section introduces the occupational therapy process, summarizing the functions of evaluation, intervention, and outcomes described in the "Occupational Therapy Practice Framework," fourth edition (OTPF-4).[11] The chapter acquaints the reader with the complexity and creativity of clinical reasoning within the context of the contemporary clinical environment. The complementary roles of different OT practitioners are described, as are the relationships between the occupational therapist and other healthcare professionals involved in the care of the client with physical dysfunction. Common ethical dilemmas are introduced, and ways to analyze these are presented.

The second section describes various practice settings in which OT services are provided for individuals who have physical disabilities. In addition, the typical services provided in each setting are discussed.

SECTION 1: THE OCCUPATIONAL THERAPY PROCESS

Winifred Schultz-Krohn and Heidi McHugh Pendleton

THE STEPS OF THE OCCUPATIONAL THERAPY PROCESS

The OTPF-4 discusses both the domain and the process of the occupational therapy profession.[11,91] The domain is described in Chapter 1, and the reader should be familiar with the domain before reading about the process of occupational therapy.

The OT process, as described by the OTPF-4, is part of the framework in which services are focused on "achieving health, well-being, and participation in life through engagement in occupation" (OTPF-4, p. S5). The OT process should be conceptualized as an iterative process typically initiated by a referral (Fig. 3.1). The referral may be generated by another professional or by the client seeking services. The profession of occupational therapy identifies the "client" as "persons, groups, and populations" (OTPF-4, p. S2).[7] For intervention services delivered to groups and populations, the initiation of services (referral) may occur through a collaborative discussion, needs assessment, or request by an organization or agency. Following the referral, an evaluation is conducted to identify the client's occupational needs. The intervention is developed based on the evaluation results. The targeted outcome of intervention "should ultimately be reflected in the clients' ability to engage in their desired occupations" (OTPF-4, p. S26).[7] The steps of evaluation, intervention, and outcome should not be viewed in a linear fashion, but instead should be seen as a circular or spiraling process in which the parts are mutually influential (see Fig. 3.1).

Referral

The physician or another legally qualified professional often requests occupational therapy services for the client. The referral may be oral, but a written record is often a necessity. Persons, groups, and/or populations may also seek occupational

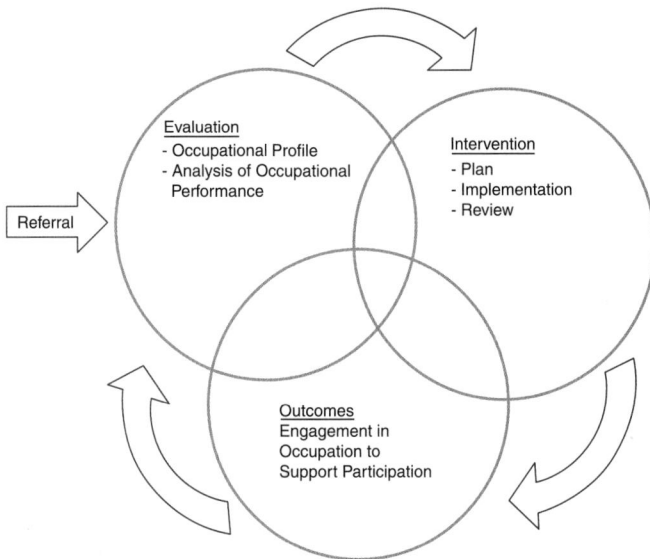

Fig. 3.1 Intervention process.

therapy services without a formal referral from another party. Guidelines for referral vary, and in some situations OT services may require a physician's referral before the initiation of services. The occupational therapist is responsible for responding to the referral. Although clients may seek OT services without first obtaining a referral, the occupational therapist may need a referral before the initiation of intervention services. State regulatory boards and licensing requirements should be reviewed before initiation of services to determine whether a referral for service is necessary.

Screening

The OT determines whether further evaluation is warranted and if OT services would be helpful to this client. The therapist may perform a screening independently or as a member of the healthcare team. Screening procedures are generally brief and do not cover all areas of occupation. A formal screening is not always conducted with the client; however, during the review of the client's record before the evaluation, the OT considers the client's diagnosis and physical condition, the reason for the referral, and information from other professionals. The therapist synthesizes this information before initiating an evaluation. In some settings, the screening process flows directly into the evaluation of the client in a seamless manner. This requires the OT to assess and view multiple influential factors through the lens of how the client would like to engage in occupations.

Evaluation

Evaluation refers to "the process of obtaining and interpreting data necessary to understand the person, system, or situation" and "requires synthesis of all data obtained, analytic interpretation of that data, reflective clinical reasoning, and consideration of occupational performance and contextual factors."[46] Assessment refers to "specific tool, instrument, or systematic interaction" used during the evaluation process.[46] Three parts of the evaluation process have been identified: the generation

of an occupational profile, the analysis of occupational performance, and the synthesis of the evaluation process (OTPF-4, p. S16).[7] The assessments chosen, if necessary, help further analyze the occupational performance. The OT then synthesizes the data from all sources while considering the client's values, priorities, occupational performance strengths and weaknesses, along with contextual factors. Goals and desired outcomes of the OT intervention services are identified during the evaluation process.

The evaluation is directed by the occupational therapist who makes initial contact with the client. The evaluation process begins with developing an occupational profile that reviews the client's occupational history and describes the client's current needs and priorities (OTPF-4, p. S16).[3,11,43] This portion of the evaluation process includes the client's previous roles and the contexts for occupational performance. For example, Serena has been assigned to develop an occupational profile for a 56-year-old, who identifies as male, and recently had a tumor removed from his right cerebral hemisphere, resulting in dense left hemiplegia. He has been married to his wife for 27 years and reports that he never cooks. On further exploration during the development of the occupational profile, the man reports that one of his most treasured occupations is being able to grill, and he discusses the importance of grilling over charcoal versus using a gas grill. Although Serena may have initially ignored the need to work on cooking skills with this client, she now understands the occupational significance of grilling and, from the client's perspective, the difference between grilling and cooking! The occupational profile allows the OT to understand the client's occupational history, current needs, and priorities, and it also identifies which occupations or activities are successfully completed and those that are problematic for the client.

The occupational profile is most often initiated with an interview with the client and significant others in the client's life and by a thorough review of available records.[11] Interviews may be completed using a formal instrument or informal tools. Although the occupational profile is used to focus subsequent intervention, this profile is often revised throughout the course of intervention to meet changing client needs. The Occupational Profile Template provides a structure to collect this information through a series of questions.[7] These questions provide an example of how the occupational therapy student, Serena, initiates the occupational profile of one of her clients, Nora.

1. *Why is the client seeking service, and what are the client's current concerns relative to engaging in occupations and in daily life activities?* This requires consideration of the individual and significant others in the client's life. In some settings the client may be identified as a group or population and not as an individual. Serena's client, Nora, is a 28-year-old, who identifies as female, and sustained a traumatic brain injury (TBI), resulting in memory deficits and slight difficulties with coordination. She is a wife and the mother to two young children. During the evaluation process, Serena considers not only Nora's occupational needs, but also the needs of Nora's family and her roles as a family member.

2. *In what occupations does the client feel successful, and what barriers are affecting the client's success?* This requires an understanding of which occupations are successfully completed by the client. Nora has the physical ability to drive, yet she also has severe memory problems and difficulty remembering the routes for driving her children to school and various activities.

3. *What is the client's occupational history?* Nora has a college degree and is a registered nurse. She worked full time as a nurse in a skilled nursing facility (SNF) before the birth of her first child and since has worked on a per-diem basis, primarily on weekends when her husband is able to care for the children. Before her TBI, she was employed by an agency to provide per-diem work at a variety of different SNFs within 50 miles of her home. Nora was also an avid runner and ran trails but expressed concern about running on poorly marked trails with her memory issues.

4. *What are the client's values and interests?* This includes the level of engagement in various occupations and activities, along with the value attributed to those occupations by the client. Although before her traumatic brain injury Nora was responsible for most of the housecleaning tasks, she did not highly value these duties. She was also responsible for meal preparation, and she says that she enjoys cooking. She places a much higher value on being able to drive her children to school and various after-school activities. She was working on a per-diem basis before her TBI.

5. *What are the client's patterns of engagement in occupations, and how have they changed over time? What are the client's daily life roles?* (Patterns can support or hinder occupational performance.) During the evaluation session, Nora explains that she has always been very active in the community and with her family. If anyone was sick, Nora was the person to provide support. Nora reveals to Serena that she has concerns about others needing to care for her; Nora has never been the one to receive care and support. Serena considers this marked change in a sense of self that Nora is experiencing after her TBI.

6. *What aspects of the client's environmental and personal factors (contexts) influence engagement in occupations and desired outcomes?* Some contexts may be supportive, whereas others present challenges or prohibit occupational performance. Nora's parents expect her to be the primary caregiver for her children, and when her husband attempts to support Nora, her parents interfere. Her home is a single story and does not present a barrier, but her children are very active.

7. *What are the client's priorities and targeted outcomes?* These may be identified as occupational performance, role competence, adaptation to the circumstance, health and wellness, prevention, or quality-of-life issues. For Nora, the need to drive safely to resume responsibility for fostering community participation for her children was a primary outcome. This reflects her interest in occupational performance. She was not interested in having her parents or her husband assume these roles. Additionally, she is interested in resuming her role as a per-diem registered nurse.

After the occupational profile has been developed, the OT identifies the necessary additional information to be collected, including areas to be evaluated and what assessment instruments should be used before the analysis of occupational performance. The OT may delegate parts of the evaluation, such as the administration of selected assessment tools, to the occupational therapy assistant (OTA).[10] OTAs contribute to the evaluation process by providing information and data collected to the OT. The interpretation of data is the responsibility of the OT. This requires the OT to direct the evaluation by completing an occupational profile, interpreting the data collected from the profile, and then analyzing the client's occupational performance before selecting additional assessment tools. The selection of additional information beyond the occupational profile should answer the following questions:

1. What additional data are needed to understand the client's occupational needs, including contextual supports and challenges (both environmental and personal)?
2. What is the best (most efficient and accurate) way to collect these data?
3. How will this information support the intervention plan?
4. How will this information influence potential outcomes?

The ability of the client to successfully plan, initiate, and complete various occupations is then evaluated. The occupations chosen are based on the occupational profile. The OT then analyzes the data to determine the client's specific strengths and weaknesses that have an impact on occupational performance. The impact of contextual factors on occupational performance is included in the analysis of data. This can be easily seen when a client who depends on a wheelchair for all mobility is faced with several stairs to enter an office building to conduct business. The client has functional mobility skills but is prohibited from participating because of an environmental factor that restricts access. The analysis includes integrating data regarding the activity demands, the client's previous and current occupational patterns, and the client factors that support or prohibit occupational performance. Data about specific client factors may be helpful in developing an intervention plan but should be performed after the occupational profile is completed and an analysis of occupational performance has been initiated. The information generated from the profile and analysis will allow more careful selection of necessary assessment tools to collect further data. The OT also considers if the client would benefit from a referral to other professionals.

THREADED CASE STUDY

Serena, Part 2

Although Serena is able to competently perform a manual muscle test and range-of-motion assessment, these assessments would not be necessary for all clients. Serena must first develop the client's occupational profile as a guide and then select the most appropriate assessment instruments to complete her evaluation of the client's occupational performance. After she has completed these steps, Serena will be able to identify more clearly what additional information is needed to plan and implement intervention services.

Intervention Process[11]

The intervention process consists of three interconnected parts driven by the collaborative efforts among the client(s) and occupational therapy practitioners. These three parts of intervention planning, intervention implementation, and intervention review are all focused on facilitating "engagement in occupation related to health, well-being, and achievement of established goals."[11]

Intervention Planning

In collaboration with the client, the occupational therapy practitioners (OT and OTA) develop an intervention plan using the approaches or strategies to enhance the client's ability to participate in occupational performance.[3,11,43] Although the OT is responsible for the plan, the OTA contributes to the plan and supports the development of the intervention plan based on the client's needs and priorities.[10] The strategies selected should be linked to the intended outcomes of service.[11] These approaches or strategies answer the question, "What type of intervention will be provided to meet the client's goals?" There are several types of interventions that can be used to support the client.[11] The type of intervention is selected to meet the client's goals and with consideration of the client; specifically, whether the client receiving the OT services a person, group, or population. During the planning process, an intervention may be selected that directly addresses *occupations or activities*. Serena considers interventions related to driving for her client, Nora, as an example of an intervention focused on occupational performance. Interventions may also *support occupations*, such as the use of orthotics, physical agent modalities, or assistive technology. Serena considers how Nora's memory affects driving and plans for the use of voice-activated directions to support the occupation of driving. *Education and training* are another type of OT intervention provided. As Serena develops the intervention plan, she consults with her fieldwork educator, a certified driving rehabilitation specialist, who will provide training for Nora. Intervention services can also take the form of *advocacy*. Serena considers Nora's interest in returning to work and the potential accommodations that may be necessary for this to occur. In the intervention plan, Serena includes working with Nora on self-advocacy skills to request accommodations at her worksite. Interventions also include *group* and *virtual*. As Serena further develops the intervention plan, she considers the "return to work" support group in the community for persons who sustained TBI. This group is included in the collaborative planning process between Serena and Nora.

The intervention planning process includes not only the types of interventions to be used but also the approaches and strategies.[3,11] Examples of each form of intervention approach or strategy are provided with selected literature to support this form of occupational therapy intervention.[3,11]

1. *Create or promote healthy occupational engagement (health promotion)*. A disabling condition is not assumed; rather, OT services are provided to enhance and enrich occupational pursuits. This approach may be used to help clients who are transitioning in roles or to foster occupational performance across contexts. An example would be using narratives to promote a healthy transition from the role of a worker to retirement.[33] As workers described what they anticipated in retirement, they linked "past, present, and future." This process of anticipating changes and making choices was considered to be an important factor in "understanding how people adapt to life changes."[49]

2. *Establish or restore a skill or ability*. This strategy is aimed at improving a client's skills or abilities, thus allowing greater participation in occupations. Evidence of the effectiveness of OT services provides this form of intervention, as demonstrated by several investigators. Walker et al.[88] investigated the effectiveness of OT services in restoring skills for activities of daily living (ADLs) and instrumental activities of daily living (IADLs) in clients who had sustained a cerebrovascular accident (CVA) but who had not received inpatient rehabilitation services. Using a randomized controlled trial, these researchers demonstrated that clients who received OT services had significantly better ADLs and IADLs performances compared to clients who had not received these services. Rogers and associates[76] demonstrated that performance of ADLs can be significantly improved when clients are provided with systematic training by OT practitioners.

3. *Maintain current functional abilities*. This approach recognizes that many clients are faced with degenerative disorders, and OT services should actively address the need to maintain occupational engagement.[22,36] Intervention may focus on the activity demands, performance patterns, or context for occupational performance. For example, an individual in the early stage of Parkinson disease is still able to complete many self-care activities but should develop the habits that will maintain these skills as motor function continues to deteriorate. Maintenance also includes clients who have a chronic, nonprogressive disorder; these individuals need to maintain physical conditioning to meet activity and environmental demands.

4. *Modify, adapt, or compensate*. This approach focuses on modifying the environment, the activity demands, or the client's performance patterns to support participation in occupations. Instruction and use of energy conservation techniques for clients who have dyspnea (shortness of breath or difficulty breathing) as a result of chronic obstructive pulmonary disease (COPD) is an example of this approach.[64] The use of electronic aids to daily living (EADLs) is another example of how the activity can be modified to promote participation. When clients who had an acquired brain injury were provided with training in the use of EADLs, they reported a sense of mastery.[34] Even if a client's previous abilities cannot be restored, using this adaptive or compensatory approach can promote participation in occupations.

5. *Prevention*. A prevention approach can be used for clients who have no identified disabling condition or circumstance. This approach focuses on developing the performance skills and patterns that support continued occupational performance, and it provides intervention that anticipates potential hazards or challenges to occupational performance. Contextual issues are also addressed using this approach, and environmental barriers would be similarly considered.

An example of services representing a preventive approach would be instructing a client who has compromised standing balance in fall prevention techniques and asking the family to remove loose throw rugs from the home to prevent falls.[27] Clark et al.[24] demonstrated the beneficial effects of preventive OT services in the investigation of well, elderly adults. Adults who received preventive OT displayed far fewer health and functional problems compared to adults who did not receive these services.

Through collaboration with the client and significant others, the OT can develop an intervention plan that identifies not only the specific focus of the goal, but also the explicit content of the goal. For example, Serena's client, Nora, who sustained a TBI, indicated that she wanted to be able to return to driving her children to various community-based activities. Services for Nora would focus on two approaches: restoring the skills needed to engage in this occupation of driving her children to community activities and adapting the performance by avoiding community activities that necessitate driving during heavy traffic periods in the morning and late afternoon.

Specific driving skills would be improved using strategies to enhance reaction time, problem solving, and attention to potential safety risks. Because of Nora's diminished memory and difficulty with processing complex information, the occupation of driving her children to community activities should be modified. Nora could select community activities that are close to her children's school and home, thereby decreasing the length of time she is driving her children. Through the use of a programmable guidance system in her car she is able to follow the specific directions to the various community activities. If these intervention approaches are unsuccessful, the OT may explore alternatives to driving with Nora, such as bicycling or walking with her children to nearby community activities or carpooling with another parent, who assumes the actual driving role, while Nora contributes by providing snacks or gas money. Such alternatives could provide a safer solution and still meet the need for Nora to be involved in the occupation of driving or transporting her children to their community activities.

The OT is responsible for the plan and collaborates with the OTA to determine which parts of the intervention plan will be implemented by the OTA.[28] The plan includes client-centered goals and methods for reaching them using the previously mentioned approaches or strategies. The values and goals of the client are primary; those of the therapist are secondary.[11] Cultural, social, and environmental factors are incorporated into the plan, which must identify the scope and frequency of the intervention and the anticipated date of completion. The outcomes of the intervention must be written at the time the intervention plan is developed. Discharge planning is initiated during the intervention planning process. This is accomplished by developing clear outcomes and targeted time frames for the completion of goals.

Developing clear and measurable goals is a very important step in the planning process. Long-term goals or terminal behaviors must reflect a change in occupational performance. For a client to receive authentic OT services, the program must focus on "supporting health and participation in life through engagement in occupation."[11] This outcome may be achieved by several means, such as improved occupational performance, role competence, adaptation, prevention, and quality of life or by fostering health and wellness.[3] Outcomes may also focus on occupational justice to afford individuals, groups, and populations the opportunity for occupational engagement. Short-term goals or behavioral objectives reflect the incremental steps that must be taken to achieve this outcome. An example would be the long-term goal for Nora's return to driving. Several short-term steps would be necessary before meeting this terminal behavior or long-term goal. An intervention plan may address bilateral coordination and speed of reaction before having Nora return to driving. Several authors have provided detailed descriptions of the critical parts of a well-written goal.[50] Table 3.1 serves as a brief guide for the development of goals and objectives. (See Chapter 8 for additional details about goals and documentation.)

TABLE 3.1 ABCDE Format for Writing Goals

A—Actor	Begin the goal with a statement such as, "Nora will." Name the client as the performer of the action for the goal.
B—Behavior	The occupation, activity, task, or skill to be performed by the client. If this is an outcome or terminal goal, the behavior must reflect occupational performance. Short-term goals or behavioral objectives are often steps to reaching a long-term goal or outcome. A short-term goal or objective may identify a client factor or performance skill as the targeted behavior. An outcome behavior for Nora, the client in the case study, would be the ability to drive a car, whereas a short-term behavior would be to enter the car and fasten a seat belt.
C—Condition	The situations for the performance of the stated behavior include social and physical environmental situations for the behavior. Examples of conditions included in a goal are the equipment used, social setting, and training necessary for the stated behavior. For Nora, driving a car with an automatic transmission is a far different condition than driving a car with a manual transmission.
D—Degree	The measure applied to the behavior and the criteria for how well the behavior is performed. These may include repetitions, duration, or the amount of the activity completed. A client may be expected to complete only a small portion of an activity as a short-term goal, but the long-term goal would address the targeted occupation. The amount of support provided serves as a measure of degree of behavioral performance. This would include whether the client required minimal assistance, verbal prompts, or performed the task independently. The criteria must be appropriate for the behavior. Safely driving 50% of the time is an inappropriate criterion; using a percentage to indicate that Nora will independently fasten her seat belt 100% of the time provides an appropriate criterion for the behaviour.
E—Expected Time Frame	When is the goal to be met, the time period that is anticipated to meet the goal as stated.

Adapted from Kettenbach G: *Writing SOAP notes*, ed 3, Philadelphia, 2004, FA Davis.

Intervention Implementation

The intervention plan is implemented by the OT practitioners. The OT may assign to the OTA specific responsibilities in the delivery of the intervention plan. Nonetheless, the OT retains the responsibility to direct, monitor, and supervise the intervention and must ensure that relevant and necessary interventions are provided in an appropriate and safe manner and that documentation is accurate and complete.[10] The method used to provide interventions could include therapeutic use of self, therapeutic use of occupations and activities, preparatory interventions to support occupations, group interventions, education and training, use of virtual interventions, or advocacy.[3,11] (See Chapter 1 for a more detailed description of these methods of providing intervention.) These methods answer the question, "How will intervention strategies be provided?" The intervention plan would identify which approach or strategy would be used in combination with the method of intervention. During the actual implementation of intervention services, a clinician may seamlessly shift between different methods, depending on the needs of the client.

OT PRACTICE NOTES

Implementation of the intervention plan does not occur in isolation; rather, it requires the OT to continuously review the effectiveness of the services delivered by monitoring the client's response to intervention. At the beginning of each intervention session, the OT should answer the following questions:
1. What is the primary focus of intervention for this session?
2. How will this service meet the client's goals and needs?

Implementation of services should also include helping the client anticipate needs and solutions. A method developed by Schultz-Krohn,[83] known as anticipatory problem solving, provides a structure for this process. This method was developed from client-centered models, such as the model of human occupation[46] and the person-environment-occupation model[56,59] (these are described later in the chapter). The method was designed to empower the client to anticipate potential challenges and develop solutions before encountering the challenges. The key elements of the anticipatory problem-solving process are:
1. The client and clinician identify the occupation or activity to be performed.
2. The specific features of the environment that are required for occupational/activity performance are identified. This includes contextual and environmental factors in addition to the necessary equipment to engage in the occupation/activity.
3. The OT and client identify potential safety risks or challenges to engagement in the occupation/activity that are located in the environment or with the objects required.
4. The OT and client develop a solution for these risks or challenges.

Remember that Nora would like to be able to drive her children to after-school activities. As she regains her abilities to drive, anticipatory problem-solving strategies are used to prepare her for potential environmental challenges. The process follows these steps:
1. Nora and the OT have identified the occupation of Nora driving her children to after-school music lessons as the focus for intervention.
2. Nora's car has an automatic transmission. The route she typically has taken to drive her children from school to the music lessons includes a busy street with four lanes, but no highway driving is required. She needs to make one left-hand turn on this street, but there is a left-turn light. The travel time typically is 10 minutes.
3. Nora reports that traveling on the one busy street can be a challenge because many drivers exceed the speed limit on this road and drive erratically. This is the quickest route to the music lessons, and because she is very familiar with it, it provides less challenge to her memory. Nora's husband also reports that this road often has construction, presenting an additional challenge.
4. Instead of changing her route, Nora develops a solution by allocating an additional 5 minutes to transport her children to lessons; this allows her to feel less pressure when drivers are exceeding the speed limit. Strategies to address the erratic drivers encountered on this road include frequent checks of her side mirrors and moving to the left lane two intersections before the left-hand turn light. In addition, an alternative route has been mapped out for Nora to use when road construction presents a challenge.

This process provides a brief illustration of how anticipatory problem-solving methods can be used during intervention implementation. The method can be equally applied to other activities. For example, for bathing, a client may anticipate the potential hazard of a slippery surface and make appropriate plans before getting in the bathtub. The foundation of this process is to engage the client in developing solutions for everyday challenges encountered when engaging in occupations/activities. The client is actively involved in identifying not only the occupation/activity but also potential challenges or risks encountered, and in generating solutions for those challenges or risks.

Included in the intervention implementation process is ongoing monitoring of the client's response to the services provided. As services are initiated, the OT monitors the client's progression on a continuous basis and modifies the intervention methods used as needed to support the client's health and participation in life.

Intervention Review

The OT practitioner evaluates the intervention plan on a regular basis to determine whether there is sufficient progress toward meeting the client's goals.[11] The OT and OTA[2] collaborate on the effectiveness of the intervention plan, but the OT is responsible for determining the need for continuing, modifying, or discontinuing occupational therapy services and referring to other services as appropriate.[11] The review may include a reevaluation of the client's status to determine what changes have occurred since the previous evaluation. This reevaluation also offers an opportunity to determine whether the intervention provided is focused on the outcomes articulated in the plan.

Outcomes

Working in collaboration with the client, the client's family, and the intervention team, the OT and OTA identify the intended outcome of the intervention. The OTPF-4 clearly states that the outcome of OT services is multifaceted, including improved occupational performance, quality of life, enhanced role competence, and the well-being of client/caregivers, to name only a few potential outcomes.[11] These outcomes can be measured in several ways. Outcomes may be written to reflect a client's improved occupational performance; a change in the client's response to an occupational challenge; effective role performance; habits and routines that foster health, wellness, or the prevention or lessening of further disability; and client satisfaction in the services provided. Client satisfaction can include overall quality-of-life outcomes that often incorporate several of the previously mentioned outcomes. Caregiver confidence may serve as an outcome measure, along with prevention of loss of occupational engagement for caregivers. For groups or populations, outcomes are often designed to address gains in health and wellness, prevention, and quality of life.[3,11]

Although the overarching outcome of OT intervention is achieving "health, well-being, and participation in life through engagement in occupation,"[11] this goal can be achieved through several types of outcomes. The decision on whether the selected outcomes have been successfully met is made collaboratively with the members of the intervention team, including the client. The outcomes may require periodic revisions because of changes in the client's status. When the client has reached the established goals or achieved the maximum benefit from OT services, the OT formally discontinues service and creates a discontinuation plan that documents follow-up recommendations and arrangements. Final documentation includes a record of any change in the client's status from first evaluation through the end of services.

Fig. 3.1 shows the interrelationship of the various parts of the intervention process. This process is not completed in a linear fashion, but instead requires constant monitoring, and each section informs the other parts of the process. The outcome generated during the planning step should direct an OT to select intervention methods best suited to reach the desired client goals. During the intervention process, it may become apparent that the desired outcome is not realistic, necessitating revision of the client's goals and outcome of services.

CLINICAL REASONING IN THE INTERVENTION PROCESS

Since 1986 the American Occupational Therapy Association (AOTA) has funded a series of investigations to examine how occupational therapists think and reason in their work with clients.[39] Clinical reasoning can be defined informally as the process used by OT practitioners to understand the client's occupational needs and make decisions about intervention services and also as a means to think about the interactions of multiple factors that influence occupational engagement. There are several forms of clinical reasoning, and authors do not consistently use the same term for specific forms of clinical reasoning.

The term "professional reasoning" also has been used by authors to capture the broad practice settings of OT because clinical reasoning is often associated with medical settings.[81] The AOTA Standards for Continuing Competence uses the term "critical reasoning" to refer to the approach used by OT practitioners to make judgments and decisions.[5] This chapter uses the term clinical reasoning to focus on the relationship between the OT practitioner and the client.

The chapter includes information from authors discussing both professional and critical reasoning skills. Fleming[37] identified three "tracks" of clinical reasoning used by the expert clinician to organize and process data: procedural, interactive, and conditional. Yet another dimension of clinical reasoning, identified as narrative reasoning, has been discussed in the literature by Mattingly.[62] The fifth form of clinical reasoning, pragmatic reasoning, describes the practical issues and contextual factors that must be addressed.[66,80] This section describes how the five basic forms of clinical reasoning, discussed in the current literature, can be applied to practice.

Procedural reasoning is concerned with getting things done, with what "has to happen next." This reasoning process is closely related to the medical form of problem solving. The emphasis is often placed on client factors and body functions and structures when this form of reasoning is used. A connection between the problems identified and the interventions provided is sought using this form of reasoning, and this can be seen in the "critical pathways" developed in some hospitals. A critical pathway is a form of decision-making tree that is based on a series of yes/no questions that can direct client intervention. For example, a client who had total hip replacement surgery would receive intervention that follows a predicted or anticipated trajectory of recovery.

Critical pathways are often developed to support best practice when there is substantial information about a client's course of recovery from a surgical procedure or medical treatment. Procedural reasoning would be used to develop critical pathways and is driven by the client's diagnosis and the potential outcomes anticipated for individuals with this diagnosis. This form of clinical reasoning is influenced by the current evidence regarding the client's condition and the selected intervention.[60] An OT should review the literature on an ongoing basis to provide effective and appropriate intervention services.[63] Using this knowledge to develop and implement intervention reflects procedural reasoning in practice.

This form of clinical reasoning supports evidence-based practice. Schaaf[79] describes the process of engaging in data-driven decision making, in which OT practitioners not only effectively use the current evidence to make decisions about selecting interventions but also use the current evidence to determine appropriate outcome data. This approach connects the process of developing the occupational profile, selecting intervention methods, and determining not only the appropriate outcomes but also the data that best represent the outcomes of OT services.

Interactive reasoning is concerned with the interchanges between the client and therapist. The therapist uses this form of reasoning to engage with, to understand, and to motivate the client. Understanding the disability from the client's point of view is fundamental to this type of reasoning. This form of reasoning is used during the evaluation to detect the important information provided by the client and to further explore the client's occupational needs. During intervention, this form of reasoning is used to understand how the client is responding to the intervention selected and whether the intervention is effective in meeting the client's goals. The therapeutic use of self fits well with this form of clinical reasoning as the therapist uses personal skills and attributes to engage the client in the intervention process.

Conditional reasoning is concerned with the contexts in which interventions occur, the contexts in which the client performs occupations, and the ways in which various factors might affect the outcomes and direction of therapy. Using a "what if?" or conditional approach, the therapist imagines possible scenarios for the client. The therapist engages in conditional reasoning to integrate the client's current status with the hoped-for future. Intervention is often revised on a moment-to-moment basis to proceed to an outcome that will allow the client to participate in various contexts. Although an intervention is designed and implemented to foster occupational pursuits, conditional reasoning is not singularly focused on reaching the outcome. Conditional reasoning recognizes that the process of intervention often necessitates a reappraisal of outcomes. This reappraisal should be encouraged to help the client refine goals and outcomes.

Narrative reasoning uses story making or storytelling as a way to understand the client's experience. The client's explanation or description of life and the disability experience reveals themes that permeate the client's understanding and that will affect the enactment and outcomes of therapeutic intervention. In this sense, narrative reasoning is phenomenological. Therapists also use narrative reasoning to plan the intervention session to create a story line of what will happen for the client as a result of therapy. Here the therapist draws on both interactive and conditional reasoning, using the client's words and metaphors to project possible futures for the client.

The therapeutic use of self is critical when using this form of clinical reasoning. Providing an opportunity for the client to share the meaning of the disability experience helps the OT practitioners formulate plans and project future occupational performance. This is where the context and occupational performance intersect. A person may be able to engage in an activity with modifications, but those modifications may be unacceptable within the client's cultural and social context. For example, an individual who was an avid motorcyclist before a stroke now has impaired balance and is unable to operate the clutch and hand controls necessary to drive a motorcycle safely. Although automatic motorcycles are now available with three wheels, this client refuses the option, considering this to be not part of the motorcycle culture.

Pragmatic reasoning extends beyond the interaction of the client and therapist. This form of reasoning integrates several variables, including the demands of the intervention setting, the therapist's competence, the client's social and financial resources, and the client's potential discharge environment. Pragmatic reasoning recognizes the constraints faced by the therapist from forces beyond the client-therapist relationship. For example, a hospital that provides inpatient services may not have the resources for a therapist to make a home visit before a client's discharge. A therapist working solely through a home health agency will not have full access to clinic equipment when working in the client's home. These challenges to providing intervention would be considered when an intervention plan is developed using pragmatic reasoning.

Experienced master clinicians engage in all forms of reasoning to develop and modify their plans and actions during all phases of the OT process. Some of the questions a therapist might consider with each form of clinical reasoning are listed in Box 3.1.

BOX 3.1 Questions to Engage in Clinical Reasoning

Procedural Questions
What is the diagnosis?
What prognosis, complications, and other factors are associated with this diagnosis?
What is the general protocol for assessment and intervention with this diagnosis?
What interventions (adjunctive methods, enabling activities, purposeful activities) might be employed?
What evidence supports the use of specific interventions to foster occupational performance?

Interactive Questions
Who is the client?
What are the client's goals, concerns, interests, and values?
How does the client view his or her occupational performance status?
How does the illness or disability fit into the client's performance patterns?
How might I engage this client?
How can we communicate?

Conditional Questions
What contexts has the client identified as important in his or her life?
What future(s) can be imagined for the client?
What events could or would shape the future?
How can I engage the client to imagine, believe in, and work toward a future?

Narrative Reasoning
What does the change in occupational performance mean to this client?
How is this change positioned within the client's life history?
How does the client experience the disabling condition?
What vision do I, as the client's therapist, hold for him or her in the future?
What "unfolding story" will bring this vision to fruition?

Pragmatic Reasoning
What organizational supports and constraints must be incorporated into the provision of services?
What physical environmental factors must be considered when designing an intervention plan?
What are my knowledge and skill levels as a therapist?

CLINICAL REASONING IN CONTEXT

Pressures for cost containment and reduction of unnecessary services require therapists to balance the needs of the client and the practical realities of healthcare reimbursement and documentation. Thus, on first meeting the client, the therapist will want to know the anticipated or required date of discharge, in addition to the scope of services that will be reimbursed and those that are likely to be denied. Simultaneously, the therapist is formulating an occupational profile with the client, evaluating the client's occupational performance, engaging the client in identifying outcomes and goals, and determining which interventions would best meet the desired outcomes. The OT also considers the contextual factors that will influence occupational performance. Further, the therapist is alert to requirements for documentation and the particular Current Procedural Terminology (CPT) codes that may apply. The OT must document services accurately and effectively so that reimbursement will not be challenged and the client's needs may be adequately addressed. (See Chapter 8 for a more detailed discussion of documentation.)

From the first meeting with the client, the therapist is guided by the client's goals and preferences. Client-centered service delivery requires client (or family) involvement and collaboration at all stages of the intervention process.[11] Effectively engaging the client and family demands cultural sensitivity and an ability to communicate with people of diverse backgrounds.[19,87,89,90] In some cultures the idea of participating equally in decision making with a health professional may be unknown. Being asked by a therapist to make decisions may feel quite unfamiliar and uncomfortable to the client. Thus, the therapist must support the client's ability to collaborate, adjust to the client's point of view, and find other ways to ensure that the intervention plan, including intended outcomes, is acceptable to the client and significant others in the client's life. Understanding the influence of culture on the client's occupational performance and performance patterns is fundamental to the provision of services.[19] The OT should answer the following questions to foster cultural competence in the provision of services:

1. *What do I know about the client's culture and beliefs about health?* This represents the basic knowledge of cultural health practices and beliefs. Conclusions or judgments should not be formed about why these practices are present.
2. *Does the client agree with these beliefs?* Although a client may affiliate with a specific cultural group, the OT must investigate to determine whether the cultural beliefs about health and the client's beliefs about health are similar.
3. *How will these beliefs influence the intervention and outcomes of services provided?* The OT must acknowledge and respond to the influences of cultural beliefs and practices within the intervention plan. To design a plan that conflicts with cultural beliefs would not only be counterproductive to client-centered services, but also would be disrespectful of the client's belief system. If a client, in deference to the authority of the OT, follows an intervention that conflicts with cultural practices, the client may risk losing the support of and affiliation with that cultural group.

4. *How can the intervention plan support culturally endorsed occupations, roles, and responsibilities to promote the client's engagement in occupation?* The OT must consider the important occupations from a cultural perspective. Evening meals may include specific behaviors that have strong cultural symbols for one client, but another client may view an evening meal as merely taking in food with no prescribed rituals.

CLIENT-CENTERED PRACTICE

- Involving clients in identifying their own goals and in making decisions about their own care and intervention is highly valued by leaders in the OT profession[38,71,82] and is endorsed by the AOTA in its policy and practice guidelines. Client-centered practice begins when the therapist first meets the client. Therapists using an occupation-based assessment tool, such as the Canadian Occupational Performance Measure (COPM),[54] initiate assessment by asking clients to identify and choose goals early in the evaluation process. This process can be fostered when the therapist is aware of potential biases that could influence the development of goals.[78] Regardless of the individual's disability status or perceived limitations in cognitive functioning, every client should be invited to participate in evaluation and intervention decisions. Client-centered practice is guided by these concepts[5]:
  - The language used reflects the client as a person with occupational interests. The client is offered choices and is supported in directing the OT process. This requires the occupational therapist to provide information about the client's condition and the evidence available about the various types of intervention.
  - Intervention is provided in a flexible and accessible manner to meet the client's needs.
  - Intervention is contextually appropriate and relevant.
  - There is clear respect for differences and diversity in the OT process.

Although client-centered practice is most often conceptualized as the OT practitioner working with a person and those significant in that person's life, the OTPF-4 describes "clients" as persons, groups, and/or populations.[11] However, even when providing OT services to organizations or populations, the OT practitioner is expected to apply the same values of client-centered practice and enlist the client, whether an organization or population, in identifying goals and selecting outcomes.

THEORIES, MODELS OF PRACTICE, AND FRAMES OF REFERENCE

The profession of occupational therapy acknowledges the need for theories, models of practice, and frames of reference to advance the profession, demonstrate evidence-based intervention, and more clearly view occupation.[51] Theories, models of practice, and frames of reference offer the OT practitioner a means to understand and interpret information so as to develop an effective intervention plan. These terms require definition and understanding before application to practice.

Theory

The term *theory* refers to the process of understanding phenomena, including articulating concepts that describe and define phenomena and the relationships between observed events across situations or settings. A theory is tested across settings for confirmation of concepts and relationships. Although a theory may be generated by one profession, it is often applied across professions if it becomes an accepted method of understanding phenomena. According to Reed,[73] theory attempts to:

- Define and explain relationships between concepts or ideas related to the phenomenon of interest (e.g., occupational performance and occupation).
- Explain how these relationships can predict behavior or events.
- Suggest ways that the phenomenon can be changed or controlled.

A clear example of a theory that meets these expectations and is well known is germ theory.[17] Widely accepted and tested, germ theory states that microorganisms produce infections. Before the relationship between these microorganisms and infections was understood, physicians would perform an autopsy and then go to an adjacent room to deliver a baby—without washing their hands between the two events. The number and severity of infections after childbirth declined dramatically when germ theory became accepted and then functionally applied to practice (a frame of reference) through the use of proper handwashing procedures. From an OT perspective, theories provide the profession with a means to examine occupation and occupational performance and to understand the relationship between engagement in occupations and participation in context.[45] The main purpose of a theory is to understand the specific phenomenon. Mary Reilly's theory of occupational behavior was designed to explain the importance of occupation and the relationship between occupation and health.[74,75] Her theory served as a foundation for several models of practice within the profession of occupational therapy.

Model of Practice

Model of practice refers to the application of a theory to OT practice. This process is achieved through several means, such as the development of specific assessments and articulation of principles to guide intervention. Models of practice are not intervention protocols, but instead serve as a means to view occupation through the lens of theory, with the focus on the client's occupational performance. Models of practice often serve as a mechanism to engage in further testing of the theory.[45] Some authors refer to models of practice as conceptual models,[21] whereas other authors include models of practice in the discussion of professional theories.[26] In the profession of occupational therapy, several models of practice exist, but the commonality of all of them is the focus on occupation. The main purpose of a model of practice is to facilitate the analysis of the occupational profile and to consider potential outcomes with selected interventions. Models should be applicable across settings and client groups, rather than designed primarily for a specific diagnostic group. Using a very colloquial expression, a model of practice requires the practitioner to "put on the OT eyeglasses" to bring into focus the client's needs and abilities, various contextual issues, and engagement in occupation. Three of these models of practice are briefly described here. The reader is encouraged to seek additional information from the materials used in this brief description.

Model of Human Occupation

In the model of human occupation (MOHO),[50] the engagement in occupation is understood as the product of three interrelated subsystems: volitional, habituation, and performance capacity. These subsystems cannot be reduced to a linear process; they are linked to produce occupational performance.

- The *volitional subsystem* refers to the client's values, interests, and personal causation. A client may clearly identify values and interests to an OT practitioner, but then express a sense of incompetence to engage in a desired occupation. Volition is the client's thoughts and feelings, including occupational choices.
- The *habituation subsystem* refers to the habits and roles that are often critical to a sense of self. Colloquial phrases expressed by a client, such as, "I don't feel like myself," often speak of a distortion of habit or role experienced in life. A client faced with a disabling condition often experiences a severe disruption in roles and habits. The sense of self can deteriorate when roles such as driving to work, driving to go shopping, or driving friends to enjoy a picnic are eliminated because of a disabling condition.
- The *performance capacity subsystem* reflects the client's lived experience of the body. This does not refer to the muscle strength or range of motion available, but rather to the client's previous experience, changes, and expectations of performance capacity. The colloquial phrase "Once you've ridden a bicycle, you never forget" captures a portion of this concept and requires the therapist to consider the client's experience of successes or failures in using the body to engage in occupations.

Ecology of Human Performance

The ecology of human performance (EHP)[31] was not designed to be used exclusively within the occupational therapy profession; rather, it was intended to serve as a mechanism for understanding human performance across professions. An important concept expressed in EHP is the interaction of the person, the task (activity demands), and the context. Occupational performance is intertwined with, and the product of, the interaction of these three variables. EHP is a client-centered model in which each person is viewed as unique and complex, having his or her own past experiences, skills, needs, and attributes. The task is understood as the objective and observable behaviors to accomplish a goal. The context includes the person's age, stage of life, and health status from a perspective of the cultural and societal meanings of each. Context also addresses the physical, social, and cultural factors that influence performance. EHP recognizes that these three factors influence each other and that the person and task are inextricably linked with the context. Performance is the product of the person engaged in a task within a context.

A significant contribution of this model is the equal importance placed on each variable in producing occupational performance. Instead of focusing only on improving the client's skills, intervention using this model can assume several forms. Five intervention strategies are described, reflecting a close similarity to the OTPF-3.[32]

1. *Establish/restore.* Although focused on improving the person's abilities and skills, the intervention includes the context for performance.
2. *Alter.* Intervention is designed to alter the contextual factors to foster occupational performance; an example would be home modifications to allow wheelchair access.
3. *Adapt/modify.* The task or context is adapted or modified to support performance, such as using a reacher to obtain objects or elastic shoelaces to eliminate the need to tie shoelaces.
4. *Prevent.* Intervention may address the person, the context, or the task to prevent potential problems. Examples would be teaching the client back safety techniques to prevent back injuries; removing rugs in an environment to reduce the risk of falls as a contextual prevention method; and turning down the water temperature for a client with sensory problems to reduce the risk of burns when bathing.
5. *Create.* Intervention addresses all three variables of the person, task, and context and is designed to develop or create opportunities for occupational performance.

Person-Environment-Occupation Model

The person-environment-occupation (PEO) model[55,56] shares characteristics of the EHP model; occupational performance is seen as the intersection of the person, environment, and occupation. This is a client-centered approach, but equal emphasis is placed on the environment and the occupation when the intervention is designed. PEO defines the person as a dynamic and changing being with skills and abilities to meet roles over the course of time. The environment includes the physical, social, cultural, and institutional factors that influence occupational performance. Occupations include self-care and productive and leisure pursuits. PEO further differentiates the progression from an activity, a small portion of a task, a task that is a clear step toward an occupation, and the occupation itself, which often evolves over time. An example would be the activity of safely handling a knife. This is a small portion of the task of making a peanut butter and jelly sandwich, and the task of making a sandwich is seen as a part of the occupation of meal preparation. Occupational performance is the result of the person, environment, and occupation interacting in a dynamic manner.

Frame of Reference

The purpose of a frame of reference (FOR) is to help the OT practitioner link theory to intervention strategies and to apply clinical reasoning to the chosen intervention methods.[50,65] An FOR tends to have a more narrow view of how to approach occupational performance compared to models of practice. The intervention strategies described within various FORs are not meant to be used as a protocol, but rather offer the practitioner a way to structure intervention and think about intervention progressions. The practitioner must always engage in the various forms of clinical reasoning to question the efficacy of the intervention in meeting the client's goals and outcomes.

A frame of reference should be well fitted to meeting the client's goals and hoped-for outcomes. The concept of "one size fits all" definitely does not apply to the use of an FOR to guide intervention; that is why there is a need for multiple FORs to meet varied client goals and outcomes. A practitioner may blend intervention strategies from several FORs to meet the client's needs effectively. As an example, a client may be able to recover precise coordination and control of both arms after a TBI if the OT practitioner combines a biomechanical FOR and a sensorimotor FOR, but the client may have persistent memory deficits, requiring the use of strategies from a rehabilitative FOR. The following brief descriptions are not meant to be an exhaustive review of all possible FORs that can be used in occupational therapy. Examples are provided to illustrate how an FOR can be used to guide the intervention process.

Biomechanical Frame of Reference

The understanding of kinematics and kinesiology serves as the foundation for the biomechanical FOR.[73] The practitioner views the limitations in occupational performance from a biomechanical perspective, analyzing the movement required to engage in the occupation. Based on principles of physics, the force, leverage, and torque required to perform a task or activity are assessed. These also serve as the basis for intervention. A client may be unable to open a jar of peanut butter or jelly because of limitations in grip strength or the range of motion available for the hands to hold the jar. A biomechanical approach would focus intervention on addressing these basic client factors to improve occupational performance. Although intervention may take the form of exercises, splinting, or other orthopedic approaches, the outcome must reflect engagement in occupation.[48]

Rehabilitation Frame of Reference

The rehabilitation FOR focuses on the client's ability to return to the fullest possible physical, mental, social, vocational, and economic functioning. The emphasis is placed on the client's abilities and using the current abilities, coupled with technology or equipment, to accomplish occupational performance. Compensatory intervention strategies are often used. An example would be teaching one-handed dressing techniques to an individual who no longer has functional use of one hand because of a CVA. The focus of intervention is often engagement in occupation through alternative means. (For additional examples of intervention strategies supported by the rehabilitation FOR, see Chapters 10, 11, and 17.) Returning to the example of making a peanut butter and jelly sandwich, instead of having the client work on strengthening the hands to finally open the jar, the OT practitioner would suggest using a device to stabilize the jar and a gripper to help accomplish the task using the client's current abilities. Regardless of the technology or equipment available, the practitioner must always link the intervention to the client's occupational performance.

Sensorimotor Frame of Reference

Several FORs are included in the sensorimotor category, such as proprioceptive neuromuscular facilitation (PNF) and neurodevelopmental treatment (NDT) (see Chapter 32 for additional information). These approaches have a common foundation: they view a client who has sustained a central nervous system (CNS) insult to the upper motor neurons as having poorly regulated control of the lower motor neurons. To recapture control of the lower motor neurons, various techniques are used to promote reorganization of the sensory and motor cortices of the brain. The specific techniques vary, but the basic premise is that when the client receives systematic sensory information, his or her brain will reorganize and motor function will return.

Meeting the Client's Needs

As mentioned previously, the occupational therapist relies on theories, models of practice, and FORs to interpret and integrate evaluation data to meet the client's identified outcomes. These elements are used in conjunction with clinical reasoning to develop an intervention plan and critically review the success of the plan. For example, the therapist would use procedural reasoning to select a theory, model, or FOR that has proven successful with clients who have a similar diagnosis. Interactive reasoning is used to assess whether the chosen model or FOR is meeting the client's needs. As a therapist applies theories, models, or FORs to meet the client's needs, a series of professional questions should be posed:

1. Does the theory, model of practice, or FOR help me understand and interpret the evaluation data as I consider the client's expressed needs?
2. Does the theory, model of practice, or FOR provide a good fit for the type of intervention that will meet the client's needs?
3. What evidence is available that the theory, model of practice, or FOR can efficiently produce the results requested by the client?
4. What are my skills, as an OT in delivering intervention using this theory, model of practice, or FOR?

These questions should be posed throughout the intervention process as a review of the effectiveness of services provided. Although the OT is responsible for interpreting and integrating evaluation data, collaborating with the client to develop the intervention plan, and engaging in ongoing review of the effectiveness of intervention, the OTA contributes to the evaluation and intervention process. Additionally, it is important for the OT and OTA to engage in continuing professional development to improve the occupational therapy services to all clients.[8]

TEAMWORK WITHIN THE OCCUPATIONAL THERAPY PROFESSION

The OT profession recognizes and certifies two levels of practitioners: the occupational therapist (OT) and the occupational therapy assistant (OTA).[2,3] The AOTA has provided many documents to guide practice and to clarify the relationship between the two levels of practitioner.[6,10] The OT operates as an autonomous practitioner with the ability to provide OT services independently, whereas the OTA "must receive supervision from an occupational therapist to deliver occupational therapy services."[10] There should be a collaborative relationship between the OT and OTA to deliver cost-effective services to meet the client's goals.[28] Even though OTs are considered able to independently provide OT services, they should seek supervision and mentoring to foster professional growth. The OT who is managing a case or providing services to clients should use the following points as a guide:

- Services are to be provided by personnel who have demonstrated service competency. Some states require advanced training and proficiency in specified arenas of practice. For example, advanced certification in dysphagia (difficulty swallowing) and physical agent modalities is required in California for an OT to provide those services.
- In the interest of rendering the best care at the least cost, the OT may delegate tasks to OTAs and, in some specific instances, to aides or other personnel, provided these individuals have the competencies to render such services. This requires the OT to establish the level of competence required and assess the ability of the OTA, aides, or other personnel to perform those duties.
- The OT retains final responsibility for all aspects of care, including documentation.

Occupational Therapist and Occupational Therapy Assistant Relationship

To work effectively with OTAs, the OT must understand the role of the practitioner trained at the technical level.[10] It is common for OTs to alternately overestimate and underestimate the capabilities of OTAs.[28] In overestimating the training and abilities of OTAs, OTs might assume that the OTA is trained to provide all services identical to those of the OT but perhaps at a lesser pace and level and with a smaller caseload. In underestimating the OTA, the OT might assume that the OTA is capable of performing only concrete and repetitive tasks under the strictest supervision.[10]

The appropriate role of the OTA is complementary to that of the OT. Employed effectively, the OTA can provide occupational therapy services under supervision that ranges from close to general. The AOTA has identified critical factors that must be considered in the delegation of delivery of OT services.[10] These factors include the severity and complexity of the client's condition and needs, the competency of the person to whom the services would be delegated, the type of intervention selected to meet the identified outcomes, and the requirements of the practice setting. Working together with several OTAs, the OT will be able to manage a larger caseload and will have the option of introducing more advanced and specialized services because the role of the OTA is often to provide routine services. Many variations in the use of OTAs exist across settings. Some services the supervising OT may delegate to the service-competent OTA include:

1. Administering selected screening instruments or assessments, such as range-of-motion (ROM) tests, interviews, questionnaires, ADL evaluations, and other assessments that follow a defined protocol.[6]

2. Collaborating with the OT and client to develop portions of the intervention plan (e.g., planning for dressing training or for kitchen safety training).[6]

3. Implementing interventions supervised by the OT in the areas of ADLs, work, leisure, and play. With appropriate training and supervision, the OTA can implement interventions related to other areas of occupational performance.[6] As determined by the OT, an OTA can also implement interventions for which he or she has demonstrated competence. An example would be intervention related to the client factors of strength or ROM.

4. As assigned by the OT, assisting with the transition to the next service setting; for example, by making arrangements with or educating family members or contacting community providers to address the client's needs.

5. Contributing to documentation, record keeping, resource management, quality assurance, selection and procurement of supplies and equipment, and other aspects of service management.

6. Under the supervision of the OT, educating the client, family, or community about OT services.

Occupational Therapy Aides

The OT may also extend the reach of services by employing aides.[10] Under AOTA guidelines, the **occupational therapy aide** may work only under the direction and close supervision of an OT practitioner (OT or OTA) and may provide only supportive services: "Aides do not provide skilled occupational therapy services."[10] Aides may perform only specific, selected, delegated tasks. Although the OTA may direct and supervise the aide, the OT is ultimately responsible for the actions of the aide. Tasks that might be delegated to an aide include transporting clients, setting up equipment, preparing supplies, and performing simple and routine client services for which the aide has been trained. Individual jurisdictions and healthcare regulatory bodies may restrict aides from providing client care services; reimbursement also may be denied for some services provided by aides. Where permitted, the OT may delegate routine tasks to aides to increase productivity.[6]

Teamwork With Other Professionals

Many healthcare workers collaborate in the care of individuals with physical disabilities. Depending on the setting, the OT may work with physical therapists (PTs), speech and language pathologists (SLPs), activity therapists, recreational therapists, nurses, vocational counselors, psychologists, social workers, spiritual leaders, orthotists, prosthetists, rehabilitation engineers, vendors of durable medical equipment, and physicians from many different specialties.

Relationships among and expectations of various healthcare providers are often determined by the context of care or the setting. For example, in some situations home care services are coordinated by a nurse. In a hospital or rehabilitation setting using a medical model, the physician most often directs the client care program. Some rehabilitation facilities use a team approach to assessment and intervention, which reduces duplication of services and increases communication and collaboration. Several individuals from different professions may together perform a single evaluation. For example, the OT may be the lead member of the team in some settings or may be the director of rehabilitation services. In a team, members adjust scheduling and expectations to collaborate with one another to promote effective client care.

Many factors affect relationships among professionals across disciplines: the intervention setting, reimbursement restrictions, licensure laws and other jurisdictional elements, and the training and experience of the individuals involved. Relationships develop over time, based on experience and interaction and sometimes on personality. Even when formal jurisdictional boundaries may appear to limit roles for OT, informal patterns often develop at variance with the prescribed rules. For example, although in some states a physician's referral may be required to initiate OT service, the physicians may expect the OT to initiate the referral and actually perform a cursory screening before the physician becomes involved. Some physicians rely on OT staff to identify clients who are most likely to benefit from OT service, and they generate referrals upon the recommendation of the OT.

Another example in which interdisciplinary boundaries may be at variance with actual practice is in the relationships among the rehabilitation specialists of OT, PT, and SLP. By formal definition, each discipline has a designated scope of practice, with some areas of overlap and occasional dispute. The scope of OT practice is described in the domain section of the OTPF-4 and in the AOTA document "Scope of Practice."[4] Nonetheless, it is common for practitioners to share skills and caseloads across disciplines and to train each other to provide less complex aspects of each discipline's care. Two terms used to describe this are *cross training* and *multiskilling*.

Cross training is the training of a single rehabilitation worker to provide services that would ordinarily be rendered by several different professions. Multiskilling is sometimes used synonymously with cross training but may also mean the acquisition by a single healthcare worker of many different skills.

Arguments have been made for and against cross training and multiskilling.[25,38,70,90] The consumer may benefit by having fewer healthcare providers and better integration of services, and involving fewer providers may reduce costs. Disadvantages cited include the prospect of erosion of professional identity, possible risk to consumers of harm at the hands of less skilled providers, and ceding the control of individual professions to outside parties, such as insurers and advocates of competing professions.

ETHICS

Although the study of **ethics** in an OT curriculum may be addressed as a separate course or topic, practitioners encounter **ethical dilemmas** with surprising frequency. In an ethics survey conducted by Kyler for the AOTA,[52] practitioner respondents ranked the following as the five most frequently occurring ethics issues they confront in practice:

1. Cost-containment policies that jeopardize client care
2. Inaccurate or inappropriate documentation

3. Improper or inadequate supervision
4. Provision of treatment to individuals who do not need it
5. Violation of client confidentiality by colleagues

Additional concerns were related to conflict with colleagues, lack of access to OT for some consumers, and discriminatory practice.[52] The study found 20% of practitioners reported that they faced ethical dilemmas daily, 31% weekly, and 32% at least monthly. New OT practitioners are often faced with ethical dilemmas of navigating differing values of various team members related to client choice along with feelings of being undervalued and unsupported.[44]

The AOTA has provided several documents to assist OT practitioners in analyzing and resolving ethical questions, including the "Occupational Therapy Code of Ethics and Ethics Standards"[2]; the "Core Values and Attitudes of Occupational Therapy Practice"[1]; the "Standards for Continuing Competence"[5]; and the "Scope of Practice."[4] These documents provide a basis for resolving ethical issues; practitioners may find additional resources and support if they approach institutional ethics committees and review boards for guidance. Kyler[52] also suggests that OT practitioners act to formalize resolutions for recurring questions by engaging with peers and others to analyze and consider courses of action.

ETHICAL CONSIDERATIONS

One process of ethical decision making in clinical practice follows these steps:
1. Gather sufficient data about the problem.
2. Clearly articulate the problem, including the action and consequences.
3. Analyze the problem using theoretical constructs and principles.
4. Explore practical options.
5. Select and implement an action plan to address the problem.
6. Evaluate the effectiveness of the process and outcome.

Adapted from Doherty RF, Purtilo RB: *Ethical dimensions in the health professions*, ed 6, St. Louis, 2016, Elsevier.

Lohman et al.[59] expanded the discussion of ethical practice to include the public policy arena. Instead of OT practitioners considering ethical practice only from the perspective of service delivery to an individual, these researchers recommended that the practitioner consider the need to influence public policy to better serve all clients.

OT practitioners should anticipate that in clinical practice they will frequently encounter ethical distress (defined as the subjective experience of discomfort originating in a conflict between ethical principles). Many approaches for resolving this may be useful. For example, a plan of action for addressing ethical distress and resolving ethical dilemmas may involve the following:

1. Reviewing AOTA guidelines[2,10]
2. Seeking guidance from institutional ethics and review boards
3. Approaching and engaging colleagues, peers, and the community to identify and debate ethical questions and formalize resolutions

SUMMARY: SECTION 1

The OT process begins with referral and ends with discontinuation of service. Although discrete stages can be named and described as evaluation, intervention, and outcomes, the process is more spiraling and circular than stepwise. The processes of evaluation, intervention, and outcomes influence and interact with one another. This may look confusing to the novice, but it is actually a hallmark of clinical reasoning.

Different types of clinical reasoning are simultaneously used to make decisions about the form and type of service provided. While logically analyzing how to proceed through the steps of therapy using procedural reasoning, the therapist also considers how best to interact with the client. Further, the therapist creates scenarios of possible future situations. The expert clinician seeks to uncover how the client understands the disability and uses a narrative or story-making approach to capture the client's imagination of how therapy will be of benefit in pursuing occupational engagement. This process is also influenced by the pragmatic reasoning that draws attention to the demands of the current healthcare arena.

The OT profession endorses client-centered practice, engaging the client in all stages of decision making, beginning with assessment. To achieve this ideal, clinical reality requires that the OT approach every client as a coparticipant, whom the OT assists in identifying and prioritizing goals and in considering and selecting intervention approaches.

The OT and OTA have specific responsibilities and areas of emphasis within the OT process. The OT is the manager and director of the process, who delegates specific tasks and steps to the qualified OTA. Aides also may be employed to extend the reach of OT services.

Effective practice typically involves interactions with members of other professions. This requires that the OT practitioner consider the intervention setting, the scope of practice of other professions, the applicable jurisdictions and healthcare regulations, and other factors that affect the individual situation (e.g., culture, personality, history).

Ethical questions arise with increasing frequency in modern healthcare. The AOTA provides guidelines and other resources to help resolve these. In addition, practitioners are urged to consider institutional and local resources and to take an active role in identifying and resolving ethical concerns.

SECTION 2: PRACTICE SETTINGS FOR PHYSICAL DISABILITIES
Winifred Schultz-Krohn

Individuals who have a physical disability receive OT services in a variety of settings. These may include acute care hospitals, acute inpatient rehabilitation, subacute rehabilitation, outpatient clinics, skilled nursing facilities, assisted living units, home health, day treatment, community care programs, and work sites. Regardless of the physical setting in which services are delivered, the OT should always focus on enhancing occupational performance to support participation across contexts.

The OT practitioner needs to be mindful of the supports and constraints encountered in the various practice settings.

The term **practice setting** refers to the environment in which OT intervention occurs, an environment that includes the physical facility or structure, along with the social, economic, cultural, and political situations that encompass it. Several factors influence the delivery of OT service within a specific practice setting, including (1) government regulations, (2) the economic realities of reimbursement rules, (3) the workplace pressures of critical pathways and other clinical protocols, (4) the range of services considered customary and reasonable, and (5) the traditions and culture staff members have developed over time.

Physical aspects, such as the building itself, the temperature and humidity of the air, the colors and materials used, the layout of the space, and the furnishings and lighting, also play a role. Practitioners must always be aware that context influences client performance in evaluation and intervention. The practice setting also influences the type of intervention available.[69] Limitations on the length of stay (LOS) and the number of visits require the OT practitioner to carefully examine interventions that can produce outcomes within the allotted time. Each practice setting has unique physical, social, and cultural circumstances that influence the individual's ability to engage in occupations or activities. These environmental features are important to consider when projecting how the client will perform in another setting. For example, individuals who are in control in their home environment may abdicate control for even simple decisions in an acute care hospital, giving the erroneous impression of being passive and indecisive.[18]

The following section describes the typical practice settings in which OT services are provided for individuals with physical disabilities. Table 3.2 provides a comparison of the approaches used in the various settings, the length of time services are provided, and the frequency of services. Notice that although the typical client conditions do not substantially change across settings, the approaches change to meet the client's needs. Suggestions are given for modifications of the therapeutic environment and clinical approach.

TABLE 3.2	Comparison of Practice Settings			
Practice Setting	**Length of Time Services Are Provided**	**Examples of Client Conditions Needing OT Services**	**Examples of Typical OT Approaches Used in the Setting**	**Frequency of Services**
Acute care hospitalization	Days to 1 or 2 weeks	Acute injuries and illnesses, exacerbations of chronic conditions	Restore ability or skill, modify the activity or context, prevent further disability with an emphasis on discharge setting	Daily
Acute rehabilitation	Weeks	Neurological, orthopedic, cardiac, and general medical conditions	Restore ability or skill, modify the activity or context, prevent further disability with emphasis on occupational performance	Daily, 3 hours a day
Subacute rehabilitation	Weeks to months	Neurological, orthopedic, cardiac, and general medical conditions	Restore ability or skill, modify the activity or context, prevent further disability with emphasis on occupational performance	Daily to weekly
Skilled nursing facilities	Months to years	Neurological, orthopedic, cardiac, and general medical conditions	Restore ability or skill, modify the activity or context, prevent further disability, preserve current skills	Daily, weekly, monthly consultation
Home- and community-based settings	Weeks to months	Neurological, orthopedic, cardiac, and general medical conditions	Restore ability or skill, modify the activity or context, prevent further disability with emphasis on occupational performance	Daily to weekly
Residential care and assisted living units	Months to years	Neurological, orthopedic, cardiac, and general medical conditions	Restore ability or skill, modify the activity or context, prevent further disability, preserve current skills, promote health	Weekly, monthly consultation
Home healthcare	Weeks to months	Neurological, orthopedic, cardiac, and general medical conditions	Restore ability or skill, modify the activity or context, prevent further disability	Weekly
Outpatient	Weeks to months	Neurological, orthopedic, cardiac, and general medical conditions	Restore ability or skill, modify the activity or context, prevent further disability with emphasis on occupational performance	Weekly
Day treatment	Months to years	Neurological, orthopedic, cardiac, and general medical conditions	Restore ability or skill, modify the activity or context, prevent further disability, preserve current skills, promote health	Daily, weekly
Work site	Weeks to months	Neurological, orthopedic, cardiac, and general medical conditions	Restore ability or skill, modify the activity or context, prevent further disability with emphasis on occupational performance	Weekly, monthly consultation

CONTINUUM OF HEALTHCARE

The variety of settings forms a continuum of care, albeit not always in a sequential fashion, for the client who has a physical disability. People with physical disabilities who are referred to OT services may enter the healthcare system at any point on the continuum and do not necessarily follow a direct progression through the various settings described here. A client in an acute care hospital might be referred for bed mobility, transfers, and self-care retraining. Depending on the severity of the condition and the potential to improve, the client may be transferred to a rehabilitation or day treatment program for additional services. A home health or outpatient therapist may see the same individual to address unresolved problems and modify the home environment to maximize occupational performance.

A client planning on returning to work may benefit from such OT services as an assessment and recommendations about modifications to the work environment or job tasks (see Chapter 14). Evidence has demonstrated the effectiveness of OT services in helping individuals return to work after they have experienced a disabling condition.[61] Some hospitals offer a range of healthcare services, from an emergency department and acute care or an intensive care unit (ICU) to inpatient and outpatient rehabilitation services. Other settings may offer only outpatient rehabilitation services.

Inpatient Settings

Settings in which the client receives nursing and other healthcare services while staying overnight are classified as **inpatient settings**.

Acute Care Inpatient Setting

Clients in an **acute care** inpatient setting typically have either a new medical condition (e.g., heart attack, burn, CVA, or TBI) that led to hospitalization or an exacerbation of a chronic condition (e.g., multiple sclerosis). An acute decline in a chronically progressive condition abruptly confronts the client with a long-term prognosis of increasing disability. The client may require life support because of the severity of the condition. Terminally ill clients who have managed to remain in their own home with support from a hospice program may require acute hospitalization for pain management, placement, or imminent death; in such cases, a client's hospice goals should be clearly stated and respected by the hospital staff. The client may also elect to die at home with hospice care. (For additional information on hospice care, see the section Skilled Nursing Facilities later in this chapter.)

Acute hospitalization, especially when unplanned, results in a sudden change in the client's environmental supports and context or contexts. Previous social roles may be abandoned when the person is hospitalized. External stressors (e.g., financial issues or disruption of career and educational pursuits) must be considered when services are provided in an acute care setting. An individual who felt in control of his or her life becomes controlled by the circumstances requiring the hospitalization.

Three general roles have been identified for the occupational therapist working in the acute care setting: education, initiation

THREADED CASE STUDY

Serena, Part 3

Nora, Serena's client in the case study, experienced a sudden change in her ability to control her environment and exercise her roles as wife and mother. When the TBI occurred, she was admitted through the emergency department and hospitalized in an ICU to stabilize her condition. Both a nasogastric (NG) tube and a catheter were inserted. On Nora's second day in the ICU, the OT evaluated her ability to manage oral secretions and swallow her own saliva. She would continue to receive most of her nutrition through the NG tube but was cleared to begin to eat thick liquids, such as nectar. When her vital signs stabilized on day 3, she was transferred to an acute rehabilitation setting for continued therapy services.

of the rehabilitation process, and consultation.[15] Education may address safety precautions and activity analysis. Rehabilitation services may be initiated for clients who will be transferred to a rehabilitation facility. Consultation focuses on the discharge environment and the client's needs after leaving the acute care hospital. An experienced occupational therapist, equipped with a knowledge of available resources in the hospital and community, can offer a better coordinated and more efficient intervention plan to promote the client's progress toward anticipated outcomes. For example, a therapist who determines that a client living alone at discharge would be unable to prepare meals should contact the social worker, who would help arrange for the delivery of meals to the home. Another example is a therapist who evaluates a client scheduled for imminent discharge and finds that the client is impulsive, lacks insight into the consequences of actions, and is confused when performing self-care tasks with potential safety risks. In this instance, the therapist expresses these concerns to the discharge coordinator or the physician. The social worker might be consulted about available family support, or discharge may be delayed until it can be determined whether appropriate environmental supports are available for the client.

Acute hospitalization is frequently stressful and frustrating for clients. Away from home while ill and subjected to multiple tests and examinations, in addition to interrupted sleep, clients are in a socially compromised environment. They may experience sleep deprivation and overstimulation because of the frequency of procedures or interventions. Some clients, after 2 or 3 days in the ICU, may display marked difficulties with orientation, appearing confused, agitated, and disorganized.[70] This has been referred to as "ICU psychosis," and clients may experience hallucinations in addition to anxiety and confusion. The client's history should be reviewed to determine whether he or she had had previous episodes of disorientation and confusion, or whether these conditions have been produced by the disorienting effects of hospitalization in an ICU. Concerns about whether the client will be able to return home after hospitalization, who will help with care, or who is helping care for dependent loved ones may add to a client's feelings of stress.

Acute hospitalization involves many physical environmental factors that present a challenge to clients. Often clients have several monitors in place or tubes inserted (e.g., oxygen saturation monitors, cardiac monitors, arterial lines, and catheters) that may compromise engagement in occupations.[47] The arrangement of hospital room and extra equipment can further affect the client's occupational performance. The absence of carpeting and the presence of a slippery floor surface may prove challenging for clients during a transfer and when walking. The incidence of falls in the geriatric population is higher in acute care hospitals than in either the community or skilled nursing facilities.[23]

Providing OT intervention services in an acute care setting may be challenging for therapists because it is often necessary to perform assessments in a client's room rather than in more natural environments designed for ADLs. As mentioned, performance of various activities may be affected by catheters, feeding tubes, or monitors. Likewise, client performance in some self-care activities may be artificially enhanced by a lack of the extraneous stimuli found in the home and by the physical attributes of hospital equipment. For example, a client whose home includes three very active cats, several throw rugs on a slippery floor, a very soft bed several feet from the bathroom, and a tiny bathroom faces far more challenges getting up in the middle of the night to use the toilet compared to the same activity performed in the hospital. The hospital has no throw rugs or active cats as obstacles, and often the bathroom is adapted to support safety and performance in toileting.

To partially replicate the home environment during the intervention session, the therapist might position the client's bed flat, eliminate the bed rails, and lower the bed. Most hospitals would not allow further challenges, such as bringing a cat into the room or scattering throw rugs on the floor as an obstacle for the client. Using clinical experience and judgment, along with information provided by the client about the home environment, the therapist must be able to anticipate the client's performance at home. However, referral to a home health occupational therapist is also advisable to assess occupational performance and accessibility in the client's home.

The acute care hospital also presents the occupational therapist with unique economic, social, and physical challenges. Medical intervention is directed toward promoting medical stability and providing for safe, expedient discharge. It is not unusual for the individual in acute care to receive OT services for the first time on the day of discharge. During this single visit, the therapist must communicate the role of occupational therapy, establish an occupational profile, and assist the client in identifying problems and assets in the discharge environment. The client and the family frequently look to the therapist to identify what the client will need at home. The therapist, in collaboration with the client and family, must develop intervention priorities by identifying issues and concerns after discharge from the acute care setting. The intervention plan may include purchase of durable medical equipment and referral for further intervention to inpatient rehabilitation, a skilled nursing facility, an outpatient clinic, or home health therapy providers. By contacting other members of the healthcare team and communicating concerns, the occupational therapist can facilitate implementation of the recommendations.

Inpatient Rehabilitation Setting

Clients may be admitted to an inpatient rehabilitation unit when they are able to tolerate several hours (usually 3) of therapy per day and are deemed capable of benefiting from rehabilitation services. Rehabilitation settings may be classified as acute or subacute (discussed later). Clients are generally medically stable in this setting and require less acute medical care compared to services provided in an acute care hospital. Pain, which may be present and can affect the client's performance, should be addressed in this setting. Performance of ADLs reflects the client's adaptation to pain, and the energy expended to perform self-care tasks should be considered. (See Chapter 28 for a further discussion of pain.)

During Nora's acute rehabilitation hospitalization, she received OT services twice a day, along with daily services from a speech and language pathologist and a physical therapist. These services were coordinated to support the outcomes she and her OT had selected. As is common during acute rehabilitation hospitalization, Nora was expected to dress in her typical street clothing and eat meals at a table in a dining area. This environmental feature of the acute rehabilitation setting provides a social element that is not present in the acute care hospital.

Acute Rehabilitation

When clients are medically stable and able to tolerate 3 hours of combined therapy services for 5 to 6 days a week, they may be transferred to an acute inpatient rehabilitation setting. Clients may still require some level of acute medical care in this setting. The LOS in **acute rehabilitation** settings generally ranges from 1 to 3 weeks, but it varies according to the client's needs. The usual discharge plan from acute rehabilitation is to a lesser level of care (e.g., residential care or the client's home with assistance, such as a home health aide or personal care attendant).

The process of adjusting to disability may have just begun by the time the client enters acute rehabilitation. As the client begins to participate in areas of occupation, deficits and strengths become more defined. An improvement in the client's function from the onset of the disabling condition may have occurred. Within a rehabilitation center, many clients form new social relationships with individuals who have similar disabilities. The advantages of these relationships are emotional support and encouragement from the progress of others. In rehabilitation, interventions focus on resuming the roles and occupations deemed important to the client's life. For example, an adolescent will reestablish social roles with peers; a parent will resume childcare responsibilities.

Although bedrooms in acute inpatient rehabilitation settings are similar to those found in acute care hospitals, clients are often encouraged to personalize their room by having family and friends bring in pictures, comforters, and other items from home. In this setting, clients are expected to wear street clothes during the day rather than pajamas. The clothing that clients most often select is easy-to-don leisure wear. However, the OT practitioner must consider the range of clothing the client will be expected to wear to resume occupational roles upon discharge, and the practitioner must include training with appropriate clothing.

Simulated living environments, family rooms, kitchens, bathrooms, and laundry facilities can be found at most rehabilitation centers. These environments may be inaccurate replicas of the client's home. For example, at home, laundry machines may be side-by-side and top-loading versions rather than coin-operated and front-loading machines. Kitchens may be wheelchair accessible in the rehabilitation center but inaccessible in the home. Clutter, noise, and types of appliances encountered in the rehabilitation setting often vary from the client's natural environment.

Access to the community is not generally evaluated during the acute rehabilitation hospitalization. Some urban facilities are able to integrate community training more smoothly because stores, restaurants, and theaters are located near the hospital. Although the community surrounding the hospital may differ from the client's neighborhood, this offers an opportunity to experience a more natural environment.

The culture of rehabilitation facilities focuses on the client's performance and goal attainment. The client's own culture may be compromised in the process of rehabilitation unless the team is sensitive to and incorporates the client's perspective into the intervention plan.[19] For example, some cultures view hospital settings as a place for respite and passive client involvement. Engaging clients in ADLs can be in direct conflict with the client's and family's expectations. When cultural perspectives clash, unrealistic goals may result. As in any setting, achieving planned outcomes requires clear communication and the identification of goals that are relevant and meaningful to the client.[78]

Upon completion of the acute inpatient rehabilitation program, some clients return home and receive home health services. Unfortunately, not all clients eligible to receive home health services are referred for these services.[67] The occupational therapist should actively participate in discharge planning for clients to ensure that they receive the necessary services when discharged from the acute rehabilitation setting. Upon discharge from the acute rehabilitation facility, some clients are referred to a subacute rehabilitation setting for continued services. There are several similarities between the acute and subacute rehabilitation settings. The primary differences found in subacute settings are discussed in the next section.

Subacute Rehabilitation

Subacute rehabilitation facilities are found in skilled nursing facilities and other facilities that do not provide acute medical care. This setting is also known as a short-term skilled nursing facility. The equipment available to the occupational therapist for intervention and evaluation in the subacute setting may be comparable to that found in the acute rehabilitation facility. The focus of intervention continues to be restoring functional abilities; however, because of the slower rate of change, the occupational therapist must also consider the need to adapt or modify the environment or the task demands to promote occupational performance. LOS in the subacute setting varies; stays may last a week to several months. Clients are usually discharged to a lesser level of care when they leave a subacute rehabilitation setting.

The pace of intervention services varies, and engaging in 3 hours of therapy per day is not mandatory. The client's endurance influences the frequency and duration of therapy. A client may continue to make steady gains, but at a slower pace than was seen during the acute inpatient rehabilitation stay.

Because many subacute rehabilitation programs are located in skilled nursing facilities, the client may have roommates who are convalescing rather than actively participating in rehabilitation services. This presents as an additional variable to be considered in the intervention plan because the social context does not always support participation in the rehabilitation services provided at the setting. Staff members may be more oriented to the skilled nursing care services and may not allocate comparable effort to the rehabilitation goals of independence.

Skilled Nursing Facilities

A skilled nursing facility (SNF) is an institution that meets Medicare or Medicaid criteria for skilled nursing care, including rehabilitation services. Although subacute and short-term rehabilitation programs may be housed in SNFs, OT services are also provided to individuals who are not in a subacute rehabilitation program; these services are known as long-term skilled programs. Many residents (the preferred consumer label for people who live in long-term care settings) will stay in an SNF for the remainder of their lives; others will be discharged home.[14] Goals should be directed toward independence and meaningful occupational pursuits, and they may include fostering engagement in occupations through environmental modifications and adaptations. An example would be reading materials and playing cards with enlarged print to foster leisure pursuits for clients with macular degeneration.

Hospice services may be included in the SNF setting if appropriate.[87] Hospice care requires the physician to document that the client "probably has 6 months or fewer to live."[86] The services provided do not focus on rehabilitation, but instead address palliative care and environmental modifications. OT services for hospice clients should address access to the environment and participation in occupation through support and modifications. For example, OT services could address participation in leisure pursuits as a hospice client creates a memory book for significant others.

The physical and social environments in SNFs may impede the natural performance of ADLs. Clients often receive assistance with self-care tasks to expedite task completion, but this assistance is not focused on fostering engagement in occupational performance.[77] An investigation conducted in SNFs demonstrated that even clients who were severely cognitively impaired benefited from intervention focused on fostering the client's participation in ADLs. Additionally, the investigators found that not only did clients increase participation in self-care tasks, but disruptive behavior also declined.

Clients in an SNF have a wide range of both disabling conditions and severity of the conditions. Observing residents who are severely and permanently disabled may lead newly disabled individuals to form negative expectations of their own prognosis and performance. Younger adults placed in SNFs may feel isolated and abandoned, which can adversely affect performance.

Friends are less likely to visit in this environment. Family and friends may expect less of the individual than they would in other settings. Maintaining connections with friends from the community may require the client to actively pursue these relationships. A therapist who facilitates identification of realistic and meaningful expectations and goals with the resident can promote a more positive outlook and outcome. A strong family commitment can support outside relationships by providing transportation to various community gatherings.

Community-Based Settings

Community-based settings often afford the occupational therapist access to the client's natural physical, social, and cultural environments. Services provided in community settings can foster not only skill acquisition and habit formation but also engagement in occupations in natural environments. Community-based settings may include a residential aspect, but the client is not hospitalized. Clients also reside in their homes when receiving community-based services.

Home-Based and Community-Based Settings

An alternative to an acute inpatient rehabilitation program for clients with traumatic injuries (e.g., head injuries or spinal cord injuries) is a home-based and community-based therapy program. This type of program provides intensive rehabilitation in the client's own home and community. The client receives comprehensive rehabilitation services and acquires functional skills in daily activities in the normal environments of home, school, work site, and community. This enhances the likelihood of a successful and functional outcome. Nora, for example, may benefit more from working on tasks in her home and community than in a clinic or an acute rehabilitation setting.

In home-based and community-based settings, the client is performing in her natural physical, social, and cultural environment. Scheduling is within the client's control, and intervention sessions vary in length and frequency, depending on the goals. An all-morning session to work with the client as she moves through her daily routine (e.g., bathing and dressing her child, going grocery shopping, and performing various household chores) would be possible.

OT PRACTICE NOTES

The occupational therapist must be able to adapt the intervention to the natural social and cultural aspects present in the home. Attempts to alter the natural social and cultural order are ill advised because things are likely to return to their natural state after the session ends and the therapist has left.

When practice is necessary for goal attainment, a rehabilitation technician or therapy aide may be charged with carrying out specific and limited programs established by the therapist. The technician who spends many hours with the client can provide insight when the program is not succeeding because it interferes with the natural context of the client's lifestyle. Adjusting intervention strategies to adapt to these lifestyle differences will ensure better clinical outcomes.

Intermediate Care Facilities (Residential Care)

Generally, residential facilities more closely resemble home situations; clients may reside there on a permanent or transitional basis, depending on their prognosis.[64] Similarities in the age of residents, their disability status, and even diagnoses are common. Although clients do not require ongoing intensive medical care, the facilities are staffed with care providers 24 hours a day because of the clients' need for safety and supervision. OT services may not be available on a daily basis, and rehabilitation technicians may implement the unskilled portions of the intervention plans addressing ADLs, select IADLs, and leisure. Often clients require ongoing assistance for portions of these tasks, and personal care attendants or health aides complete portions of the activity or task. The therapist can identify key performance issues in this context. Difficulties with evening self-care, follow-through with safety guidelines, problem solving, schedules, and client performance are reviewed and discussed with the OT. Modifications in the intervention plan can be more easily tailored to promote independence under such close supervision.

Assisted Living Unit or Residence

An assisted living unit (ALU) provides health services in a cooperative living setting. A client may live in an apartment or a cottage where one or more meals are provided on a daily basis; medication management is provided as needed; and 24-hour support is available. These settings usually have age restrictions: commonly, residents must be older than 55 years of age or, if a couple is involved, one person must be older than age 55. The client generally does not plan or anticipate a move to another type of setting and is often expected to own or rent the living space in the ALU. Because of the age restriction in most ALUs, social and environmental support is present to enable a person to live in their own space. For example, apartments or cottages may be equipped with safety railings in the bathroom and walk-in closets for ease of accessibility.

In this setting, OT services are provided to foster and enhance the habits and routines necessary to remain housed in this environment, which often includes personal care skills such as dressing, grooming, hygiene, and simple home care tasks. Some household tasks may be partially assumed by the services provided in the assisted living setting. For example, an ALU may provide a service of laundering towels and bed linen, but the individual is responsible for the care of his or her own clothing. Some ALU settings provide all meals, whereas others provide only one meal, and the individual will need simple meal preparation skills to live in that setting. It is important for the OT to determine what services are available at the ALU before designing an intervention plan with the client. An important occupational pursuit for those in this setting would be leisure activities. Environmental supports such as magnifiers for reading, enlarged print playing cards, and a universal remote to access the television may provide opportunities for leisure activities in this setting.

Home Health

Home healthcare provides services within the client's home and affords the most natural context for intervention.[16] The desired outcome for services provided within the home could include supported completion of ADLs or IADLs such as bathing, dressing, and meal preparation. The client, returning home from the hospital, begins to resume life roles at home. Stark et al.[84] provided guidelines to foster the decision-making process for providing home modifications; these guidelines cover both intrinsic and extrinsic factors. The intrinsic factors included the client's willingness to accept changes to the home and his or her ability to maintain any home modification, in addition to the esthetics of the proposed modifications. Extrinsic factors included financial resources, the type of home structure, and the typical weather conditions encountered. This approach allows the OT to focus intervention on supporting occupational participation in the home environment.[85]

A visiting therapist is a guest in the client's home and is subject to certain social rules associated with guests. For example, the family may practice the custom of removing street shoes within the home, and the therapist should respect and comply with this practice. The client and family establish daily schedules for meals, waking, and sleeping. Appointments should support the family's routines and not interfere with daily schedules. For example, if the client is accustomed to eating a larger meal during the middle of the day and a very small evening meal, an intervention to address meal preparation skills should be scheduled to support this routine.

Self-care, homemaking, and cooking tasks evaluated in the context of the home clearly identify the challenges that the client meets daily. The familiar clothing, furniture, appliances, and utensils used in everyday life are present and promote orientation and task performance. However, moving furniture to make things more accessible and safe for the client or modifying equipment to be used within the home may challenge the client's orientation skills and increase confusion. Caring for and feeding pets, answering the door safely, and determining a grocery list for the week are potential issues to be addressed within the home setting. Self-care tasks such as bathing can be addressed within the natural environment, and when appropriate modifications to the home are made, the client's dependence on others may decrease.[35]

Social and family support, or lack thereof, is readily evident to the home health therapist. Individuals who appeared alone and unsupported while hospitalized may have a network of friends and family members who lend support at home. Conversely, individuals who had frequent visitors in the hospital may be abandoned when the realities of disability reach the home setting.

The client who receives home health services typically requires assistance for some aspects of his or her ADLs. Nearly 19% of all family caregivers are employed full time outside the home.[13] These caregivers are available for only part of the client's day and will be concerned primarily with the safety of the client during their absence.

Stress is common among caregivers. Respite care, which temporarily places the client under the care and supervision of an alternative caregiver for a few hours and up to several days, can provide necessary relief for a caregiver.[13] Caring for a person with a disability in one's home is not an easy task. Box 3.2

BOX 3.2 Concerns in Caring for a Person With Disability in One's Home

Amount and Type of Care Needed
Long-term versus temporary care; intensive supervision or assistance versus minimal needs; help available to the caregiver; alternative solutions; and personal feelings about the client and the type of care required (intimate assistance versus household tasks).

Impact on the Household
Effect on spouses, children, and others living in the home; possible involvement of family in making decisions.

Environmental Concerns
Need for and possibility of adapting the home, expenses of adaptations.

Work and Finance
Options for family medical leave; ability and need to quit work; and benefits available.

Adapted from Visiting Nurses Association of America: *Caregiver's handbook: a complete guide to home medical care*, New York, 1997, DK Publishing.

identifies practical concerns that arise when a client is cared for in the home. A study by Dooley and Hinojosa[29] found that when individualized OT recommendations were provided for home modifications, caregiver approaches, and community-based resources for clients who had Alzheimer's disease, caregivers reported a decrease in a sense of burden and an improved quality of life.[29]

When viewing the client's home environment, the therapist can make recommendations for environmental adaptations, see them implemented, and modify those changes as needed to best meet the client's needs.[45] Physical changes to the home, including moving furniture, dishes, or bathing supplies, should not be undertaken without the permission of the client and are best considered through a team approach to support the collaboration between professionals and client.[72] If the client is in the home of a family member or friend, the permission of the homeowner must also be sought.

The client and family are in control of the home environment. Clinicians who fail to ask permission before adapting the environment will rapidly alienate their clients. A throw rug, viewed by the therapist as a tripping hazard, may be a precious memoir from the client's childhood home. In seeking the permission of the client and family and providing options, the therapist opens communication. An adhesive mat placed beneath the throw rug will provide a safer surface on which to walk. Another possible solution is to hang the rug as a wall tapestry, where it will be more visually prominent and less prone to damage.

Healthcare workers in the home occasionally encounter ethical dilemmas, typically involving safety.[68] The therapist must determine the best method for resolving issues of safety hazards. Fire and health hazards must be discussed and corrected when the safety of the client or adjacent households is in jeopardy. By broaching the subject diplomatically and directly, the therapist can address most hazards and provide acceptable solutions. Inclusion of the client, family, and other team members in the process of problem identification and solution generation is strongly recommended.

When Nora returned home after her acute rehabilitation hospitalization, Serena arranged for her to receive OT services through a home health agency. Nora, Serena, and the home health OT identified concerns with meal preparation, laundry, and playing with the children as important occupations to be addressed. Serena was not able to make a home visit before Nora's discharge from the acute rehabilitation program, but she was able to coordinate continued services through the home health agency. The home health OT worked with Nora on strategies to improve her safety in meal preparation, helped her to simplify her laundry and cleaning routines, and provided suggestions for leisure activities in which Nora could engage with her children in the home.

Outpatient Settings

Outpatient OT service is provided in hospitals and freestanding clinics to clients who reside elsewhere. Clients receiving services in this setting are medically stable and able to tolerate a few hours of therapy and travel to an outpatient clinic. Although many clients are adjusting to a new disability, some individuals with long-standing disability may be referred for reevaluations of functional status and equipment-related issues. The frequency of services provided in this setting varies substantially; some clients receive services several times a week, and other clients are seen once every few months. The frequency of service is determined by the client's needs and the services offered at the outpatient clinic.

Clients exert more control over outpatient therapy schedules compared to inpatient therapy schedules. Transportation issues and pressing family matters necessitate that clinics offer a variety of times from which a client may choose. Otherwise, the client may select a different clinic or choose to forgo therapy.

To evaluate a client's performance of ADLs or IADLs in an outpatient setting, the therapist must extrapolate how task performance would occur at home.[77] Engaging in self-care tasks in an outpatient clinic may be awkward for the client. Individuals who have been assisted with bathing and dressing before coming to the clinic may resist working on these same tasks during therapy. The more contrived and inappropriate a task and context seem to a client, the less likely he or she is to perform well and benefit from services addressing those needs.

The physical design and equipment in outpatient clinics vary to meet the intervention needs of specific disabilities. Clinics with hand therapy programs, for example, will have treatment tables for activities and areas for splint fabrication. A clinic designed to address industrial work is often equipped with specialized equipment which simulates work tasks. Although less frequent, outpatient clinics may have complete kitchens with cooking equipment and therapeutic apartments with bathing facilities, living rooms, and bedrooms.

The social context found in outpatient programs is quite distinctive. The client has begun to resume life in the home and community and may be newly aware of problems not previously foreseen or acknowledged. If the therapist is viewed as an ally in resolving problems and promoting a smooth transition to the home, the client or family members may easily disclose concerns. However, if the client and family fear that the client will be removed from the home because of an inability to manage there, they may actively hide concerns from the therapist. In the former case, the client and family view themselves as being in control of the situation. In the latter, control and power are assumed to belong to the healthcare professional. An outpatient therapist must be skilled in empowering the client. Soliciting the client's opinion and listening for unspoken needs are two methods of increasing the client's sense of control.[43] Providing choices for intervention does much to motivate clients and improve performance in desired tasks.

Day Treatment

Day treatment programs are becoming more popular as a community-based intervention setting. Programs vary, but the underlying philosophy is to provide an intensive interdisciplinary intervention for clients who do not need to be hospitalized.[40] Clients receiving day treatment typically live at home but frequently require support and assistance for ADLs or IADLs. Most programs offer a team approach. Professionals from all disciplines are engaged cooperatively, sharing their expertise to meet the client's individual goals. Clients may seek services from a day treatment program to further recover functional skills after an acute injury or illness such as a TBI or CVA, and clients with a progressively deteriorating disorder such as Parkinson's disease or Alzheimer's disease may benefit from a day treatment program to foster continued participation in occupations through environmental modifications and adaptations.

Many day treatment programs are designed without the time constraints often seen in outpatient programs. Lengthy community outings and home and work site intervention sessions may be used as methods of attaining goals. In a day treatment setting, the occupational therapist may have the best opportunity to evaluate and provide intervention for clients in all their natural environments.

Work Site Therapy Settings

Industrial rehabilitation can be conducted in the context of the employee's place of work. Work site therapy programs are designed to address an employee's therapy needs related to a work injury. The injured worker receives intervention to foster the occupational performance necessary in the workplace, which may include work hardening, back safety, energy conservation, and work simplification techniques. This approach places the client back into the work role. Prevention of further injury occurs in a more natural context when employees are treated at the work site.

Providing OT services to individuals at their place of work helps them make the transition from the patient role to the role of worker. The therapist providing service at the work site must avoid compromising the worker's status.[42] The employer and peers view the employee as a worker rather than as a client. Maintaining confidentiality can be challenging because co-workers' curiosity is often aroused by the unfamiliar face of the therapist in the workplace. The therapist should remember never to answer queries that would compromise client-therapist confidentiality. Unsolicited requests from co-workers for medical advice and work site modifications are best referred to that employee's healthcare provider or manager.

In the work setting, the therapist interacts not only with the client but also with the employer and often the insurance company. By encouraging the injured employee to communicate his or her needs for work modification and how productivity might be maintained, the therapist paves the way for a successful transition to work. The therapist strives to balance the needs of both the employee and employer while promoting resolution of work-related issues that would interfere with a smooth transition to productive work. Scheduling of therapy visits to the workplace should meet the needs of both the employee and employer. Work site visits should be scheduled in a manner that minimizes interference with the natural flow of work.

The financial impact of work modifications will concern the employer. Employers do not have unlimited resources for modifying work environments. Only reasonable and necessary work modifications should be considered. Suggestions for work modifications that have an associated cost should be discussed with the employer. The therapist can suggest work modifications but must also consider the impact of these modifications on co-workers using the same equipment. As a general rule, modifications that affect workers other than the employee must be discussed with management before they are presented to the employee as possible options.

In a traditional clinic setting, a secretary with a repetitive motion injury of her wrist may receive various modalities to control her symptoms of pain and edema and may be educated about techniques for protecting joints and tendons while performing various movements. When the secretary receives OT services in her work environment, additional benefits often occur. Joint and tendon protection techniques are applied at work while the client performs day-to-day work tasks. Because the client's injury occurred at work, this type of injury could be exacerbated or prevented at work. (See Chapters 14 and 15 for more information on the role of the OT in providing services to workers and in work settings.)

TELEMEDICINE AND TELEHEALTH

Telemedicine is the use of "electronic information and communications technologies to provide and support healthcare when distance separates the participants."[41] This approach can be effectively used to meet the needs of clients who live in rural settings, where it can be difficult to receive the needed OT services.[30] AOTA has published a document discussing the use of telemedicine for both evaluation and intervention, along with the ethical considerations when using this approach.[9]

Telemedicine also has been used as a method to monitor and modify a client's home exercise program.[53,58] Cason[20] clearly discussed the important role of occupational therapy in telehealth to promote access for populations. This focus allows far more individuals to receive OT services. Linder et al.[58] investigated the use of telemedicine to improve motor outcomes after a stroke, in addition to improving the quality of life and reducing depression for individuals who had a stroke. They used a randomized controlled trial with 99 participants to compare two intervention approaches. One group received telemedicine focused on monitoring and modifying the home exercise program, and the other group received similar telemedicine coupled with robot-assisted rehabilitation to foster hand use. All participants significantly improved in motor skills and quality-of-life measures and reduced depressive symptoms. This investigation demonstrated that significant improvements were made using telemedicine to modify and monitor home exercise, but it did not demonstrate any superiority of coupling robotics with telemedicine to produce better outcomes than telemedicine alone.

Asano et al.[12] investigated the use of teleconferencing to help individuals diagnosed with multiple sclerosis manage symptoms of fatigue. The occupational therapist used weekly conference calls with small groups of four to seven participants to address a variety of topics, including self-management strategies related to fatigue and energy conservation techniques. Of the 81 participants in the investigation, more than 75% indicated that they had made gains in their goals and approximately 50% said they had achieved their goal of managing fatigue.

SUMMARY: SECTION 2

Practice settings, the environment in which intervention occurs, have temporal, social, cultural, and physical contextual dimensions that affect both the therapist and the person receiving therapy services. Knowing the features of each practice setting and anticipating how the context will affect occupational performance prepares the therapist to best meet the client's needs. The continuum of care must be considered as the OT develops the intervention plan with the client in a specific intervention setting. A skilled therapist collaborates with the client to develop meaningful and attainable goals and then clearly communicates those goals from one setting to the next to foster meaningful outcomes. Evidence-based interventions and quality outcome measures should be used throughout the provision of OT services.[57] Sensitivity to the unique needs of each individual in each practice setting is critical.

REVIEW QUESTIONS

1. What are the major functions of the OT process?
2. How are the various forms of clinical reasoning used to guide the OT process?
3. How do theories, models of practice, and frames of reference inform and support OT intervention?
4. What is the appropriate delegation of responsibility among the various levels of OT practitioners (OT and OTA)?
5. What services may be assigned to the OT aide? What are the limits and why?

6. How should OT practitioners effectively collaborate with members of other professions involved in client care?

7. What are some of the ethical dilemmas that occur frequently in OT practice, and how can these be addressed and managed?

8. What are the various practice settings for OT services in the arena of physical disabilities?

9. What types of services are typically provided in the various practice settings?

For additional practice questions for this chapter, please visit eBooks.Health.Elsevier.com.

REFERENCES

1. American Occupational Therapy Association: Core values and attitudes of occupational therapy practice, *Am J Occup Ther* 47:1083, 1993.
2. American Occupational Therapy Association: Occupational therapy code of ethics and ethics standards, *Am J Occup Ther* 64(Suppl):S17–S26, 2010.
3. American Occupational Therapy Association: Occupational therapy practice framework: domain and process, ed 3, *Am J Occup Ther* 68(Suppl 1):S1–S48, 2014. http://doi.org/10.5014/ajot.2014.682006.
4. American Occupational Therapy Association: Scope of Practice, *Am J Occup Ther* 68:S34–S40, 2014. https://doi.org/10.5014/ajot.2014.686S04.
5. American Occupational Therapy Association: Standards for continuing competence, *Am J Occup Ther* 69(Suppl 3):1–3, 2015. http://doi.org/10.5014/ajot.2015.696S16.
6. American Occupational Therapy Association: Standards of practice for occupational therapy, *Am J Occup Ther* 69(Suppl. 3), 1–6, 2015. https://doi.org/10.5014/ajot.2015.696S06.
7. American Occupational Therapy Association: AOTA occupational profile template, *Am J Occup Ther* 71(Suppl. 2): 7112420030p1, 2017. https://doi.org/10.5014/ajot.2017.716S12.
8. American Occupational Therapy Association: Continuing professional development in occupational therapy, *Am J Occup Ther* 71,(Suppl 2):1–5, 2017. https://doi.org/10.5014/ajot.2017.716S13.
9. American Occupational Therapy Association: Telehealth in occupational therapy, *Am J Occup Ther* 72(Suppl. 2):1–18, 2018. https://doi.org/10.5014/ajot.2018.72S219.
10. American Occupational Therapy Association: Guidelines for supervision, roles, and responsibilities during the delivery of occupational therapy services, *Am J Occup Ther* 74(Suppl. 3):1–6, 2020.
11. American Occupational Therapy Association: Occupational therapy practice framework: domain and process (4th ed.), *Am J Occup Ther* 74(Suppl. 2):1–87, 2020. https://doi.org/10.5014/ajot.2020.74S2001.
12. Asano M, Preissner K, Duffy R, et al: Goals set after completing a teleconference-delivered program for managing multiple sclerosis fatigue, *Am J Occup Ther* 69:1–8, 2015. http://doi.org/10.5014/ajot.2015.015370.
13. Atchison B: Occupational therapy in home health: rapid changes need proactive planning, *Am J Occup Ther* 51:406, 1997.
14. Bausell RK, et al: *How to evaluate and select a nursing home*, Beverly, MA, 1988, Addison-Wesley, pp 264–277.
15. Belice PJ, McGovern-Denk M: Reframing occupational therapy in acute care, *OT Pract* April 29:21, 2002.
16. Benthall D: Out of the physician's office and into the home: Exploring OT's role on a home-based primary care team, *OT Pract* 22(3):8–13, 2016.
17. Black JG: *Microbiology: principles and applications*, ed 3, Upper Saddle River, NJ, 1996, Prentice Hall, pp 9–25.
18. Blau SP, Shimberg EF: *How to get out of the hospital alive: a guide to patient power*. New York, 1997, Macmillan.
19. Bonder B, et al: *Culture in clinical care*, Thorofare, NJ, 2002, Slack.
20. Cason J: Telehealth and occupational therapy: integral to the triple aim of health care reform, *Am J Occup Ther* 69:1–8, 2015. doi:10.5014/ajot.2015.692003.
21. Burke JP: Philosophical basis of human occupation. In Kramer P, Hinojosa J, Royeen CB, editors: *Perspectives in human occupation*, Baltimore, 2003, Lippincott Williams & Wilkins, pp 32–44.
22. Chan SCC: Chronic obstructive pulmonary disease and engagement in occupation, *Am J Occup Ther* 58:408, 2004.
23. Chu LW, Pei CK, Chiu A, et al: Risk factors for falls in hospitalized older medical patients, *J Gerontol A Biol Sci Med Sci* 54:M38, 1999.
24. Clark F, et al: Occupational therapy for independent-living older adults: a randomized controlled trial, *JAMA* 278:1321, 1999.
25. Collins AL: Multiskilling: a survey of occupational therapy practitioners' attitudes, *Am J Occup Ther* 51:749, 1997.
26. Crepeau EB, Schell BAB, Cohn ES: Theory and practice in occupational therapy. In Crepeau EB, Cohn ES, Schell BAB, editors: *Willard and Spackman's occupational therapy*, ed 11, Baltimore, 2009, Lippincott Williams & Wilkins, pp 428–434.
27. Cumming RG, Thomas M, Szonyi G, et al: Home visits by an occupational therapist for assessment and modification of environmental hazards: a randomized trial of falls prevention, *J Am Geriatr Soc* 47:1397, 1999.
28. Diamant R, Pitonyak JS, Corsilles-Sy C, James AB: Examining intraprofessional competencies for occupational therapist and occupational therapy assistant collaboration, *Occup Ther Health Care* 32(4):325–340, 2018. http://doi.10.1080/07380577.2018.1465211.
29. Dooley NR, Hinojosa J: Improving quality of life for persons with Alzheimer's disease and their family caregivers: brief occupational therapy intervention, *Am J Occup Ther* 58:561, 2004.
30. Dreyer NC, Dreyer KA, Shaw DK, Wittman PP: Efficacy of telemedicine in occupational therapy: a pilot study, *J Allied Health* 30:39–42, 2001.
31. Dunn W, Brown C, McGuigan A: The ecology of human performance: a framework for considering the effect of context, *Am J Occup Ther* 48:595, 1994.
32. Dunn W, Brown C, Youngstrom MJ: Ecological model of occupation. In Kramer P, Hinojosa J, Royeen CB, editors: *Perspectives in human occupation*, Baltimore, 2003, Lippincott Williams & Wilkins, pp 222–263.
33. Eagers J, Franklin RC, Broome K, Yau MK: The experiences of work: Retirees' perspectives and the relationship to the role of occupational therapy in the work-to-retirement transition process, *Work* 64:341–354, 2019.
34. Erikson A, et al: A training apartment with electronic aids to daily living: lived experiences of persons with brain damage, *Am J Occup Ther* 58:261, 2004.

35. Fänge A, Iwarsson S: Changes in ADL dependence and aspects of usability following housing adaptation: a longitudinal perspective, *Am J Occup Ther* 59:296, 2005.

36. Finlayson M: Concerns about the future among older adults with multiple sclerosis, *Am J Occup Ther* 58:54, 2004.

37. Fleming MH: The therapist with the three-track mind *Am J Occup Ther* 45:1007, 1991.

38. Foto M: Multiskilling: who, how, when, and why? *Am J Occup Ther* 50:7, 1996.

39. Gillette NP, Mattingly C: Clinical reasoning in occupational therapy, *Am J Occup Ther* 41:399, 1987.

40. Gilliand E: The day treatment program: meeting rehabilitation needs for SCI in the changing climate of health care reform, *SCI Nurs* 13:6, 1996.

41. Grigsby J, Sanders JH: Telemedicine: where it is and where it's going, *Ann Intern Med* 129:123–127, 1998.

42. Hajfey WJ, Abrams DL: Employment outcomes for participants in a brain injury reentry program: preliminary findings, *J Head Trauma Rehabil* 6:24, 1991.

43. Hazelwood T, Baker A, Murray CM, Stanley M: New graduate occupational therapists' narratives of ethical tensions encountered in practice, *Australian Occup Ther J* 66:283–291, 2019.

44. Head J, Patterson V: Performance context and its role in treatment planning, *Am J Occup Ther* 51:453, 1997.

45. Hinojosa J, Kramer P: Occupation as a goal. In Hinojosa J, Kramer P, Royeen CB, editors: *Perspectives in human occupation*, ed 2, Philadelphia, PA, 2017, FA Davis, pp 2017.

46. Hinojosa J, Kramer P, Crist P: Evaluation: where do we begin? In Hinojosa J, Kramer P, editors: *Evaluation in occupational therapy: Obtaining and interpreting data*, ed 4, Bethesda, MD, 2014, AOTA Press, pp 1–18.

47. Hogan-Kelley D: Occupational therapy frames of reference for treatment in the ICU February *OT Practice*, February 7:15, 2005.

48. James AB: Biomechanical frame of reference. In Crepeau EB, Cohn ES, Schell BAB, editors: *Willard and Spackman's occupational therapy*, ed 10, Baltimore, 2003, Lippincott Williams & Wilkins, pp 240–242.

49. Jonsson H, Kielhofner G, Borell L: Anticipating retirement: the formation of narratives concerning an occupational transition, *Am J Occup Ther* 51:49, 1997.

50. Kettenbach G: *Writing SOAP notes*, ed 2, Philadelphia, 2004, FA Davis.

51. Kielhofner G: Motives, patterns, and performance of occupation: basic concepts. In Kielhofner G, editor: *Model of human occupation*, ed 3, Baltimore, 2002, Lippincott Williams & Wilkins, pp 13–27.

52. Kyler P: Issues in ethics for occupational therapy, *OT Pract* 3:37, 1998.

53. Laver KE, Schoene D, Crotty M, et al: Telerehabilitation services for stroke, *Cochrane Database Syst* Rev(12):CD010255, 2013. https://doi.10.1002/14651858.CD010255.pub2.

54. Law M, et al: *Canadian occupational performance measure*, ed 2, Toronto, 1994, Canadian Association of Occupational Therapists.

55. Law M, et al: Theoretical contexts for the practice of occupational therapy. In Christensen C, Baum C, editors: *Enabling function and well-being*, ed 2, Thorofare, NJ, 1997, Slack.

56. Law M, Cooper B, Stewart D, et al: The person-environment-occupation model: a transactive approach to occupational performance, *Can J Occup Ther* 63:9–23, 1996.

57. Leland NE, Crum K, Phipps S, et al: Advancing the value and quality of occupational therapy in health service delivery, *Am J Occup Ther* 69(1):1–7, 2015. http://doi.org/10.5014/ajot.2015.691001.

58. Linder SM, Rosenfeldt AB, Bay RC, et al: Improving quality of life and depression after stroke through telerehabilitation, *Am J Occup Ther* 69, 2015. http://doi.org/10.5014/ajot.2015.014498.

59. Lohman H, Gabriel L, Furlong B: The bridge from ethics to public policy: implications for occupational therapy practitioners, *Am J Occup Ther* 58:109–112, 2004.

60. Lou JQ, Durando P: Asking clinical questions and searching for the evidence. In Law M, MacDermid J, editors: *Evidence-based rehabilitation: a guide to practice*, ed 2, Thorofare, NJ, 2008, Slack, pp 95–117.

61. Macedo AM, Oakley SP, Panayi GS, Kirkham BW: Functional and work outcomes improve in patients with rheumatoid arthritis who receive targeted, comprehensive occupational therapy *Arthritis Rheum* 61(11):1522–1530, 2009.

62. Mattingly C: The narrative nature of clinical reasoning, *Am J Occup Ther* 45:998, 1991.

63. McCluskey A, Home S, Thompson L: Becoming an evidence-based practitioner. In Law M, MacDermid J, editors: *Evidence-based rehabilitation: a guide to practice*, ed 2, Thorofare, NJ, 2008, Slack, pp 35–60.

64. Migliore A: Case report: improving dyspnea management in three adults with chronic obstructive pulmonary disease *Am J Occup Ther* 58:639–646, 2004.

65. Mosey AC: *Three frames of reference for mental health*, Thorofare, NJ, 1970, Slack.

66. Neistadt ME: Teaching clinical reasoning as a thinking frame, *Am J Occup Ther* 52:221, 1998.

67. Neufeld S, Lysack C: Allocation of rehabilitation services: who gets a home evaluation, *Am J Occup Ther* 58:630, 2004.

68. Opacich KJ: Moral tensions and obligations of occupational therapy practitioners providing home care, *Am J Occup Ther* 51:430, 1997.

69. Park S, Fisher AG, Velozo CA: Using the assessment of motor and process skills to compare occupational performance between clinic and home setting, *Am J Occup Ther* 48:697, 1994.

70. Pew Health Professions Commission: *Health professions education for the future: schools in service to the nation*, San Francisco, 1993, The Commission.

71. Pollock N: Client-centered assessment, *Am J Occup Ther* 47:298, 1993.

72. Pynoos J, et al: A team approach for home modifications, *OT Pract April* 8:15, 2002.

73. Reed KL: Theory and frame of reference. In Neistadt ME, Crepeau EB, editors: *Willard and Spackman's occupational therapy*, Philadelphia, 1998, Lippincott, pp 521–524.

74. Reilly M: Occupational therapy can be one of the great ideas of 20th century medicine, *Am J Occup Ther* 16:1, 1962.

75. Reilly M: The educational process, *Am J Occup Ther* 23:299, 1969.

76. Rogers JC, Holm MB, Burgio LD, et al: Improving morning care routines of nursing home residents with dementia, *J Am Geriatr Soc* 47:1049, 1999.

77. Rogers JC, Holm MB, Stone RG: Evaluation of daily living tasks: the home care advantage, *Am J Occup Ther* 51:410, 1997.

78. Rosa SA, Hasselkus BR: Finding common ground with patients: the centrality of compatibility, *Am J Occup Ther* 59:198, 2005.

79. Schaaf RC: The issue is: creating evidence for practice using data-driven decision making, *Am J Occup Ther* 69(2):1–6, 2015. http://doi.org/10.5014/ajot.2015.010561.

80. Schell BA, Cervero RM: Clinical reasoning in occupational therapy: an integrative review, *Am J Occup Ther* 47:605, 1993.

81. Schell BAB, Schell JW: *Clinical and professional reasoning n occupational therapy*, Baltimore, 2008, Lippincott Williams & Wilkins.

82. Schlaff C: From dependency to self-advocacy: redefining disability, *Am J Occup Ther* 47:943, 1993.

83. Schultz-Krohn WA: ADLs and IADLs within school-based practice. In Swinth Y, editor: *Occupational therapy in school-based practice*, Bethesda, MD, 2004. Online course: Elective Sessions (Lesson 10) at http://www.aota.org.

84. Stark SL, Somerville E, Keglovits M, et al: Clinical reasoning guideline for home modification interventions, *Am J Occup Ther* 69:1–8, 2015. https://doi.org/10.5014/ajot.2015.014266.

85. Steultjens EM, Dekker J, Bouter LM, et al: Evidence of the efficacy of occupational therapy in different conditions: an overview of systematic reviews, *Clin Rehabil* 19:247–254, 2005.

86. Trump SM: Occupational therapy and hospice: a natural fit, *OT Pract Novemb* 5:7, 2001.

87. Velde BP, Wittman PP: Helping occupational therapy students and faculty develop cultural competence, *Occup Ther Health Care* 13:23, 2001.

88. Walker MF, Gladman JR, Lincoln NB, et al: Occupational therapy for stroke patients not admitted to hospital: a randomised controlled trial, *Lancet* 354:278, 1999.

89. Wells SA, Black RM: *Cultural competency for health professionals*, Bethesda, 2000, American Occupational Therapy Association.

90. Yerxa EJ: Who is the keeper of occupational therapy's practice and knowledge? *Am J Occup Ther* 49:295, 1995.

91. Youngstrom MJ: From the guest editor: The Occupational Therapy Practice Framework: the revolution of our professional language, *Am J Occup Ther* 56:607, 2002.

SUGGESTED READINGS

Heron E: *Tending lives: nurses on the medical front pulse*, New York, 1998, Ballantine.

Visiting Nurses Association of America: *Caregiver's handbook: a complete guide to home medical care*, New York, 1997, DK Publishing.

4

Evidence-Based Practice for Occupational Therapy

Lynn Gitlow and Elizabeth DePoy

LEARNING OBJECTIVES

After studying this chapter, the student or practitioner will be able to do the following:

1. Distinguish among diverse models of evidence-based practice.
2. Define systematic occupational therapy practice (SOTP).
3. List, in sequence, the five steps of SOTP and detail the content and processes of each step.
4. Compare SOTP with the occupational therapy (OT) process as articulated in the Occupational Therapy Practice Framework.

CHAPTER OUTLINE

KEY TERMS

Abductive reasoning
Action processes
Deductive reasoning
Evidence
Evidence-based practice (EBP)
Goals
Inductive reasoning
Need statement

Objectives
Outcome objectives
Problem mapping
Problem statement
Process objectives
Specificity
Systematic occupational therapy practice (SOTP)
Thinking processes

In this chapter we present, discuss, and apply systematic occupational therapy practice (SOTP), a model that critically synthesizes and builds on evidence-based approaches to professional practice. The importance of systematically grounded practice has become well established within occupational therapy (OT) and the broader healthcare arena. The need for empirical analysis of the problems and needs that OT practitioners address is emphasized at local, national, and international levels, as reflected by numerous initiatives from the American Occupational Therapy Association (AOTA), the National Board for Certification in Occupational Therapy (NBCOT), and the American Occupational Therapy Foundation (AOTF). Box 4.1 lists some of the current initiatives.

Educators, scholars, and practitioners discuss and encourage the use of theoretically grounded and supported OT interventions and the development of solid evidence of successful outcomes of interventions.[1,23,30] We assert that current and ongoing systematic OT practice is needed in all professional domains (persons, groups, populations, and environmental changes) if OT is to remain a sustainable and respected field that will continue to flourish in the competitive environment of value-based service and fiscal healthcare-related surveillance and scarcity.

Systematic OT practice involves the creative integration of research-based techniques into all elements of OT practice.[29,33] This chapter provides a framework that will help readers understand and learn the research-based systematic thinking and action processes necessary to conduct all or part of the sequence of SOTP. The chapter begins with a discussion and analysis of current models of evidence-based practice (EBP). We then define systematic OT practice and proceed through the presentation and application of our model. As you will see, SOTP is valuable in all arenas of OT.

THREADED CASE STUDY

Maria, Part 1

Maria, an occupational therapist (OT) who uses the pronouns she/her/hers, receives a referral to treat a client who has been diagnosed with carpal tunnel syndrome. The referral states, "Client needs to improve hand strength in order to increase independence in ADLs [activities of daily living]."

Critical Thinking Questions

Think about how to answer the following questions as you proceed through this chapter.

1. How do you clarify the occupational therapy (OT) problem, and what is needed to resolve all or part of it? What evidence do you need to support your decision?
2. What factors do you need to consider in systematically examining your professional activity and interventions, and what evidence do you need?
3. How do you establish the extent to which you have determined the need and resolved the problem? What evidence do you need?

MODELS OF EVIDENCE-BASED PRACTICE

Many models of EBP have been presented in the literature. Practice models that integrate multiple methods of inquiry into all domains of professional practice have been called evidence-based medicine,[9,24,30] evidence-based practice,[8] evidence-based rehabilitation,[21] data-driven decision making,[27] research informed practice, outcomes research,[10] and so on. Because of the expansive literature on EBP approaches, it is beyond the scope of a single chapter to review all the work in its entirety. Therefore, we have chosen to present important definitions that have been advanced in the literature and to discuss their variations. This discussion provides a rationale for systematic OT practice, our model for the critical application and use of evidence-based approaches relevant to and consistent with OT practice. At this point you may be asking, "Why create another model if there are so many?" Our approach synthesizes and builds on the elements of other models such that it is used critically and consistent with the values, knowledge, and skills of OT practice. Different from other models that distinguish between research and practice, the SOTP is a comprehensive organizational framework that does not differentiate between systematic OT practice and inquiry and thus transcends frequent views that the use of systematically developed knowledge in practice is "tedious and impractical."[5] In other words, following the integrative steps of SOTP throughout the full sequence of professional activity leads not only to sound practice but, reciprocally, to the continuing creation of OT knowledge.

Table 4.1 presents diverse approaches to evidence- and inquiry-based practice. As you read these descriptions, you will notice that each approach identifies different sources as credible evidence in three categories: client generated, professionally generated, or scientifically grounded. By *client generated*, we mean that information put forth by the client is considered as part of the evidence base for professional interaction. Professionally generated refers to the provider's education and experience as a valued source of knowledge for use. Scientifically grounded means that the evidence was developed by diverse rigorous methods of inquiry.[26,28] As Table 4.1 shows, not all models may value all three sources.

ETHICAL CONSIDERATIONS

Consistent with OT ethics, philosophy, values, and theory, we subscribe to the principle that it is our ethical obligation as professionals[4,22] to collaborate with clients regarding all aspects of their service need, provision, risk, and outcome. Therefore, we not only support the value of evidence generated by the client, the practitioner, and science, but we also encourage critical use of diverse sets of evidence as viable and purposive.

THE SYSTEMATIC OCCUPATIONAL THERAPY PRACTICE MODEL—SOTP

Building on and synthesizing the excellent work in EBP, we have defined systematic OT practice as the seamless integration of critical, analytic, scientific thinking, and action processes throughout all phases and domains of OT practice. Let's look at this definition more closely.

Although thought and action are intertwined processes, for educational purposes we distinguish between them. In systematic inquiry, it is essential for the thinking sequence and its rationale to be presented clearly. Similarly within the practice arena, thinking processes comprise the reasoning sequence and logic that OT practitioners use to conceptualize intervention and specify desired outcomes, even if the practitioner does not conceptualize and express practice rationale in similar terms. Thinking processes involve the selection of a theoretical framework on which the OT practitioner grounds and plans the steps necessary to assess problems, evaluate intervention, specify desired outcomes, and plan a strategy to determine and systematically demonstrate the degree to which client-centered outcomes were met for an individual receiving

TABLE 4.1   Approaches to Evidence- and Inquiry-Based Practice

Author	Description	CREDIBLE EVIDENCE		
		Client Generated	Scientifically Grounded	Professionally Generated
Sackett et al.[28]	Evidence-based medicine is the conscientious, explicit, and judicious use of current best evidence in making decisions about the care of individual patients. The practice of evidence-based medicine means integrating individual clinical expertise with the best available clinical evidence from systematic research		X	X
Institute of Medicine[16]	To the greatest extent possible, the decisions that shape the health and healthcare of Americans will be grounded on a reliable evidence base, will account appropriately for individual variation in patient needs, and will support the generation of new insights on clinical effectiveness. Evidence is generally considered to be information from clinical experience that has met some established test of validity, and the appropriate standard is determined according to the requirements of the intervention and clinical circumstance	X	X	X
Law[19]	Evidence-based rehabilitation is a subset of EBP that consists of four concepts: 1. *Awareness:* Being aware of the existence and strength of evidence in one's field 2. *Consultation:* Collaborating with the client and other healthcare professionals to determine the client's relevant problems and their clinical solutions 3. *Judgment:* Being able to apply best evidence to the individual with whom one is working 4. *Creativity:* Emphasizes that EBP is not a "cookie cutter" approach, but rather the combination of art and science	X	X	X
Tomlin and Dougherty[35]	"Evidence Informed Practice (EIP) , . . . the everyday practice of a profession's practitioners, should draw upon all sources of information: the published literature and one's own outcome studies, the practitioner's own experience, peer experience and expertise, and evidence internal to the intervention process, including client values and preferences"	X	X	X
Kielhofner, Hammel, Helfrich, et al.[18]	Investigation that provides evidence about the effects of services Identifying the client's need Creating the best possible services to address those needs Generating evidence about the nature of specific services and their impact Accumulating and evaluating a body of evidence about specific OT services	X	X	X

OT services. Sometimes we are not fully aware of our thought processes, but they are there nonetheless and are the foundation of systematic OT practice, as we will see later in this chapter.

Action processes are the specific behaviors involved in implementing thinking processes.[12] Action processes are behavioral steps. In systematic OT practice, these steps are founded on logical inquiry such that any claim is supported with empirically derived information from a variety of sources.

Although SOTP is not research in itself, it is the organized application of research to the conceptualization, enactment, and investigation of the process and outcome of intervention and reciprocally the use of practice-generated knowledge to build on the repository of OT knowledge. Thus, SOTP

stimulates research and can be used as an organizing framework in which research questions are posed and answered. OT and healthcare researchers, educators, and practitioners have identified many arenas in which EBP is valuable. One of the AOTA's Vision 2025 guideposts, which builds on the Centennial Vision, states that a tenet of OT is that it "is evidence based, client centered, and cost-effective."[3] Synonyms for evidence include terms such as data, documentation, indication, sign, proof, authentication, report, and confirmation. In some models of EBP, the highest evidence in the hierarchy of credibility is considered to be data generated by positivist, true-experimental inquiries, the methods most frequently used in clinical trials. This perspective is reflected in the AOTA's use of standards of evidence based on those described by Sackett et al.[27] However, other OTs and authors suggest that a broader range of methods can generate useful evidence.[15,21,36]

In this chapter and in SOTP, we define evidence as information used to support a claim. This expansive definition allows for the identification and acceptance of a broad scope of evidence as the basis for decision making in practice, as long as the evidence is identified and used within the systematic thinking and action processes that we discuss in detail here.

Within the OT profession, practitioners can use the information obtained from SOTP not only to improve the processes and outcomes of their practices but also to engage in informed thinking when choosing among possible interventions and simultaneously to contribute to the overall knowledge base of our profession. Although the importance of using evidence to inform practice has been emphasized in the OT literature and scholarship, a study of practitioners' use of EBP for informing intervention revealed that only a minority of the practitioners surveyed used EBP when planning interventions.[7] SOTP systematically guides practitioners in determining which interventions will be effective at producing desired outcomes, which interventions must be improved, and what kinds of new knowledge need development. Additionally, having credible evidence to support the interventions OT practitioners use to produce desirable outcomes provides concrete feedback to the consumer.[32,34] Furthermore, by systematically evaluating interventions, OT practitioners can develop evidence for advancing clinical practices in the profession.

Pressures and demands on health practitioners from external sources render SOTP even more critical to adopt as a professional framework, for three reasons:

- First, both the location and the time allowed for service delivery are in flux. Long-term hospital stays and treatments in acute care settings have been replaced by community-based treatment, and the length of time for delivery of treatment is decreasing as third-party payers demand more efficient and cost-effective healthcare. SOTP guides the practitioner in balancing the multiple factors involved in practicing within a value-based, fiscally driven, technologically advanced healthcare environment.
- Second, by systematically examining the processes and outcomes of current practice, OT practitioners can provide an evidentiary basis for clinical thinking and action, which then can be presented to consumers, other professionals, insurers, and policy makers.

- Third, systematic inquiry transcends professional boundaries through shared language and theory. Within the context of physical rehabilitation, for example, the systematic foundation of the World Health Organization (WHO) *International Classification of Functioning, Disability and Health* (ICF)[34] is consistent with the current Occupational Therapy Practice Framework (OTPF-4)[22] and provides a common forum and language for cross-disciplinary communication.

As we proceed through SOTP, keep in mind that the skills and knowledge you already have are largely relevant to this conceptual approach. Let's now turn to the philosophical foundation and steps of the model.

Theoretical and Logical Foundations of SOTP

SOTP is grounded in logic and the systematic thinking that undergirds all research thinking processes. Inductive, abductive, and deductive reasoning methods form the basis for these thinking processes. Moreover, the three major research design traditions—naturalistic, experimental, and mixed methods inquiry—are based on these logic structures.[12] Therefore, OT practitioners must understand them and use them to guide their thinking and action and to support claims about the process and outcomes of OT intervention.

Inductive reasoning is a thinking process in which a person begins with seemingly unrelated data and then links these data by discovering relationships and principles within the data set. In inductive systematic approaches, the data may take many forms. Inductive reasoning leads us to select naturalistic strategies, those in which theory is derived from gathered evidence rather than tested by scientific experimentation. Among the methods used in naturalistic design are interview, observation, and textual analysis.[12] Data are collected, and themes that emerge from repeated examination of the data are named, defined, and placed in a taxonomic and then theoretical context.

Abduction, a term introduced by Charles Peirce[25] in 1957, currently is used by researchers and logicians to refer to an iterative process in naturalistic inquiry. This process involves the development of new theoretical propositions that can best account for a set of observations that cannot be accounted for or explained by a previous proposition or theoretical framework. The new theoretical proposition becomes validated and modified as part of the research process.

What distinguishes abduction from induction is that in inductive reasoning, an attempt is made to fit the data to a theoretical framework or to generate a set of identified and well-defined concepts that emerge from the data. In abductive reasoning, the data are analyzed for their own patterns and concepts, which in some cases may relate to available theories and in other cases may not.

Deductive reasoning begins with a theory and reduces the theory to its parts, which are then verified or falsified within a degree of certainty through examination. Deductive reasoning provides the foundation for experimental-type research, in which theories or parts are stated in measurable terms and standardized measurement forms the basis of all inquiry. Strategies used in deductive traditions include sampling, measurement, and statistical analysis. Because the rules of logic guide thinking, one can easily follow thinking processes and identify the basis on which guesses, claims, decisions, and pronouncements are made and verified.

Approaches that combine abduction and/or induction with deduction constitute mixed-methods research, in which techniques and strategies from both the naturalistic and experimental-type traditions are used. We place data analytics within the mixed-methods tradition as this large and increasingly health-relevant set of methods used, strategies, and logic structures from both experimental-type and naturalistic designs.

Complementarity With Contemporary Practice Models

Although it may seem difficult at first to engage in the formal, logical thinking processes that provide the foundation for research, we do it every day. Consider the ways the decision-making skills used in OT practice mirror the logical thinking processes that form the foundation of SOTP. Box 4.2 presents the steps of SOTP, and Table 4.2 illustrates the relationship between the OT process/clinical decision making and systematic thinking processes.

Sequence of SOTP

Our model of SOTP has five steps (see Box 4.2). The process begins with a conceptualization of the problem to be addressed. But what exactly is a problem?

Statement of the Problem

Although we often see problems as entities existing outside ourselves, problems are contextually embedded in personal and cultural values. A problem is a value judgment about what is undesirable or in need of modification. Therefore, a problem statement is defined as a specific claim of what is not desired or

TABLE 4.2   Relationship Between SOTP and the OT Process

SOTP	OT Process/Clinical Decision Making
Initial problem statement	Referral to OT
Need statement	Systematic assessment of client/occupational profile and analysis of occupational performance
Goals and objectives	Intervention goals and objectives
Reflexive intervention	Regular practice and progress monitoring and revision of intervention in response
Outcome assessment	Final assessment of client's progress

of what should be changed. Although it seems simple to specify a problem, we often see problems stated in terms of a preferred solution; this error limits our options in analyzing problem components and solutions. Moreover, in systematic OT practice, problem statements must be derived from credible, systematically generated knowledge, including scholarly literature and inquiry, client reports and data, and other sources discussed later in the chapter.

THREADED CASE STUDY

Maria, Part 2

Remember that the referral Maria received specified the client's problem as "needs to improve hand strength in order to increase independence in ADLs." This problem, stated as a preferred need, suggests only one solution: to increase hand strength. However, through systematic analysis and problem solving, together with the client, Maria expands her analysis of the problem to "limited hand strength does not allow the client to participate in work or self-care occupations"; this allows Maria to generate additional potential solutions. For example, the client may take the following measures: increase hand strength, look for alternative work, focus on use of adaptive equipment to compensate for reduced strength, adapt the environment, and so forth. By expanding a problem statement, the OT practitioner moves beyond the obvious primary difficulty or impairment and a singular solution and can capture the breadth of the problem, as revealed by systematically derived evidence from the literature, the client, or others.

If the OT practitioner proceeds merely from the problem statement in the referral, he or she may miss the essence of the client's problem and thus may select inappropriate and ineffective interventions to achieve the most positive outcomes. The OTPF-4 provides a guide for defining problems in OT by using a client-centered approach. Therefore, in SOTP it is critical to include the client and other diverse sources of knowledge, beyond the practitioner's guesses or referral orders, to formulate the problem statement.

There are many ways to identify problems. Problem mapping is a method in which the OT practitioner expands a problem statement beyond its initial conceptualization by asking two questions repeatedly: "What caused the problem?" and "What are the consequences of the problem?"[3] As with other professionals,

BOX 4.2   Steps in SOTP

1. Identification and clarification of the problem to be addressed by the intervention
2. Understanding of need—what is needed to resolve all or part of the problem?
3. Setting of goals and objectives to address the need
4. Reflexive intervention to achieve the goals and objectives
5. Outcome assessment

OTs do not address all aspects of the problem statement but can visualize how our expertise fits in integrated healthcare.

Problem mapping helps us operationalize the OTPF in that it provides a thinking process to locate impairment and individual function (1) within several broad contexts (cultural, personal, temporal, and virtual), (2) within diverse environments, and (3) as influenced by social and physical factors.[22] As we see in the example that follows, the problem areas for OT intervention are delimited by the scope of our professional activity.

In the following clinical example, we apply the problem mapping method to the statement, "Jane, who identifies as female, has impaired short-term memory resulting from a traumatic brain injury sustained in an automobile accident caused by a drunk driver." To conduct problem mapping, we first need to conceptualize the problem as a river. Articulating the original statement of the problem is analogous to stepping into the river and picking up one rock. As we look upstream, we see what shapes (and therefore causes) the problem; as we look downstream, we see the problem's ripples, or consequences. How does this mapping technique work?

Look at the problem map in Fig. 4.1. Each box above the initial problem contains a possible answer to the question of what caused the problem. Once we have determined the first-level causes of

the problem, we ask, "What caused the cause of the problem?" and so on, until we reach cultural and social value statements, both of which are specified as contexts for OT practice in the OTPF-3. Keep in mind that the evidence used to identify causes and consequences must be generated from credible, identifiable sources, including client, professional, and scientific sources.

Below the initial problem statement, we repeatedly ask the question, "What is the consequence of the problem?" As with the upstream map, this question about the consequences of consequences is repeated until we reach the effect of the problem on ourselves. At this point, you may be asking "Why?" The reason is, problems are values and thus are in the eye of the beholder. The problem map expands the problem statement from documented cultural, social, and environmental causes to personal effect, and it suggests many different sites or targets for intervention.

As you might imagine from the clinical example of Jane's situation, many causes and consequences of problems are not within the scope of OT practice and thus cannot be resolved by OT intervention. Many OT practitioners will likely expand their efforts into political action or other areas at some point in their careers; however, others will continue primarily to look for clinical interventions that can improve the occupational performance of individuals. Given the focus of this text, the emphasis

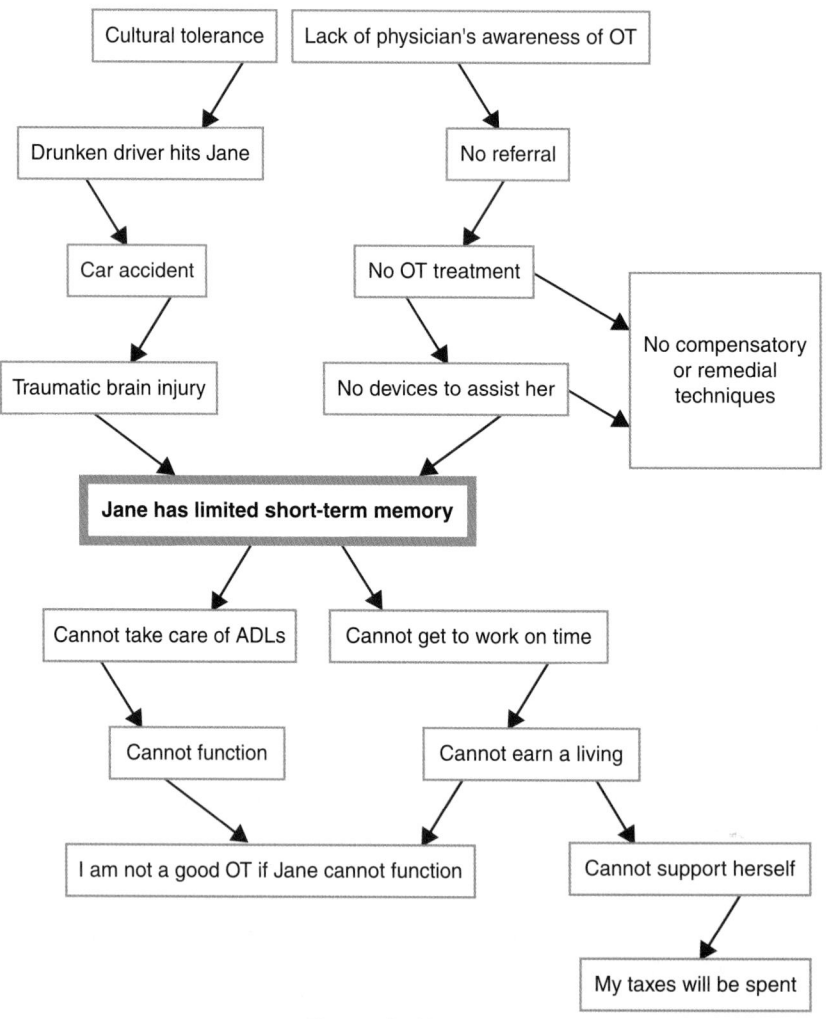

Fig. 4.1 Problem map.

in this chapter is on clinical interventions rather than other roles OTs might assume.

Jane's problem map suggests numerous points of intervention for clinical OT; for example, in cognitive remediation, compensatory training, and provision of assistive devices and services, such as assistive technology (AT). Because our focus is on clinical practice, in Jane's case, an area of occupational performance is considered—developing vocationally related strategies that will enable Jane to return to work. The OT practitioner could also make a referral to a social service agency for Jane, who might be eligible for Social Security disability income; in this way, the OT practitioner would indirectly intervene (through referral to another professional on the team) at the level of Jane's inability to support herself financially. In addition, as we look at the expanded problem, the OT practitioner may want to intervene on the macro level by advocating for stricter legislation and cultural "zero tolerance" of drunk driving, perhaps by educating adolescents and young adults. These areas of practice are beyond the scope of this chapter, but they allow us to see the expansiveness of problems and how mapping can assist occupational therapists to identify diverse areas for OT to target or address through collaboration.

Consider the initial problem statement focusing on Jane's impaired short-term memory. This is not a problem that can be resolved by an OT practitioner as it is stated. Therefore, the occupational therapist, in collaboration with the client, must reconceptualize and restate the problem so that the occupational therapist can intervene using meaningful and systematic methods within the OT professional scope of practice.[2] Problem mapping or other logical, evidence-based problem identification techniques help the OT practitioner to examine and analyze problems beyond their initial presentation and to identify the strength of the evidence by which problems are analyzed. In SOTP, problem analysis and a careful statement of the part of the problem to be addressed are critical if the rest of the steps are to be implemented. Including in the process, evidence from the client's perspective is essential in our model. Clarifying the problem will help the therapist ascertain what is needed to resolve the part of the problem that will be addressed. Now let's move to the next step of SOTP, ascertaining need.

Ascertaining Need

After problem mapping, the next step is ascertaining need. In this step, the practitioner must clarify exactly what is needed to resolve the part of the problem that has been targeted for change.

A distinction must be made between *problem* and *need*. As discussed earlier, a problem is a value statement about what is not desired. For a problem to be relevant to OT practitioners, it must concern improvement or maintenance of occupational performance. Thus, the problem area on the map that the OT practitioner would target for resolution would be delimited and guided by the professional and theoretical domains of OT concern. A need statement is a systematic, evidence-based claim, linked to all or part of a problem, that specifies what conditions and actions are necessary to resolve the part of the problem to be addressed. The identification of need involves collecting and analyzing diverse sets of information (e.g., assessment data and the information from the client interview) to form an occupational profile to ascertain what is necessary to resolve a problem.

At this needs assessment stage of the SOTP sequence, the occupational therapist already may have information on which to formulate need, or he or she may collect data in a systematic fashion to clearly delimit and identify need. A need statement should include four specifics: (1) who is the target of the problem (this strategy identifies the client or recipient of OT service), (2) what changes are desired, (3) what degree of change is desired in each specified area of change, and (4) how it will be recognized that the change has occurred. The need statement must be based on systematically derived data already contained in credible resources (e.g., the relevant practice and research literature or documentation, and professional education, knowledge, and experience) or as revealed by the client in a needs assessment activity. Can you see that the need statement uses systematic, research-based processes to define the next steps: specifying goals and objectives, determining the intervention, and specifying the evaluative criteria to determine the extent to which and how the desired outcomes of an intervention have been met?

Let's return to the example from our problem statement. As already mentioned, the problem as stated (impaired short-term memory) is not a problem an OT practitioner can resolve. Yet it is common for referrals for OT intervention to identify problems such as this one. Thus the use of a problem map or similar problem analysis strategy is not only a reasonable thinking tool, it is also essential if we are to define the nature of our interventions more clearly and thereby document the unique contributions and outcomes of OT both within and outside of our field. In Jane's case, therefore, the OT practitioner chose to reason about the causes and consequences of the problem to identify whether an area existed in which Jane would require OT intervention. By mapping the problem, the therapist found that OT did indeed have a critical role to play in Jane's treatment. The occupational therapist's problem statement then changed its focus to Jane's ability to engage in meaningful occupational performance is impaired because she is unable to manage her time and arrive at work on time as a result of her impaired short-term memory.

Given this problem statement, the therapist decided to conduct a research-based needs assessment to determine what was necessary to resolve the targeted part of the problem, to set goals and objectives to guide the selection of an intervention, and to determine what processes and outcome should be expected.

Using a systematic approach to data collection, the OT practitioner used mixed-method techniques, including an interview and systematic observation of Jane, to ascertain Jane's desires and skills. The OT practitioner also administered a standardized cognitive assessment and an occupational performance assessment. In this instance the OT practitioner is integrating qualitative and quantitative inquiry strategies to document a complete understanding of need and to provide the empirical basis for clinical decisions, in addition to expected outcomes.

One of the tools the OT practitioner can use to collect data is the Canadian Occupational Performance Measure (COPM). This criterion-referenced measure is used to identify client-perceived problems in daily functioning in the areas of self-care, productivity, and leisure. By means of a semistructured interview format, the COPM may be used to assess the performance skills and patterns the client identifies as interfering with his or her ability to function in a particular area. The data from the COPM are credible, rigorous, outcome based, and accepted as evidence in the research world.[20]

Systematic assessment revealed that Jane identified returning to her job as a saleswoman in a boutique as her most important goal. Additionally, the results of the COPM interview revealed that Jane was not satisfied with her ability to manage her time or her ability to be punctual and that she perceived these two issues as the greatest barriers to achieving her desired goal of returning to work. She recognized that her difficulties with short-term memory would affect her ability to do other work-related tasks, but she reported being most immediately concerned about time management and promptness.

Standardized testing indicated that Jane's short-term memory was impaired but that her capacity to respond well to external cues remained intact. Additionally, Jane's performance on the Wisconsin Card Sorting Test (WCST), another systematically derived and validated instrument used routinely in OT practice revealed that she was able to solve problems and that she demonstrated abstract reasoning. (The WCST is a standardized cognitive assessment of executive function that was developed to assess problem solving, abstract reasoning, and the ability to shift cognitive strategies.[14]) The results of standardized testing also suggested that Jane was able to learn new behaviors with specific, well-structured practice in the environment in which she would function. The WCST also provided an assessment of cognitive flexibility, and those data were extrapolated to suggest that Jane would be able to learn new skills in a structured environment, but that the number of variables and complexity of her work setting should also be considered.

With this empirically generated information, the therapist and Jane had a sound and credible basis for deciding that the OT intervention would be directed to the need to find and teach Jane compensatory strategies for time management and promptness, and thus would address the original problem statement through resolving a significant consequence of short-term memory impairment.

In addition, Jane had indicated in her occupational profile that she was married and that her husband would be supportive in helping her get to work. Based on this information, generated from the naturalistic part of the needs assessment, the therapist and Jane decided to include Jane's husband in the intervention, and to work first in Jane's home environment and then transfer her treatment to the work environment.

Can you see from this example how SOTP both provides the guidance and the documentation for clinical decisions and suggests future steps in the intervention and outcome assessment processes? Anyone who observes the intervention process can easily see the rationale for decisions and actions. Credible, evidence-based knowledge is structured in a manner that provides a clear reasoning trail.

The desired outcomes are implicit in the need statement, which provides a basis for formulating ascertainable outcomes of an intervention. According to the literature on closed head injury and professional wisdom,[17] what is needed in Jane's situation is contextually based OT intervention in the home and in the workplace to assist her with time management and promptness, as a skill to facilitate her return to work. The evidence for

targeting this intervention and for the goals and objectives to follow is clear and specified, as is the desired outcome.

The following case example features George, another OT practitioner, and considers a different type of need statement that illustrates why OT practice requires systematic inquiry.

CASE STUDY

George

George, an OT practitioner who identifies as male and uses the pronouns he, him, his, is asked by an employer to address a problem involving several computer operators whose ability to perform their jobs has been impaired or lost as a result of neck pain. After constructing a problem map based on literature about causes and consequences of neck pain, George formulates a need statement based on two areas that he thinks will address the problem: instruction in proper body mechanics and instruction in a regularly scheduled upper body stretching routine. A literature review provided him with empirical evidence on which to base his intervention. He begins his intervention by teaching proper body mechanics and upper body stretching techniques to the computer operators, but the problem is not resolved. The computer operators continue to be unable to do their jobs, and their complaints of neck pain continue. George's intervention has not successfully resolved the problem for which he was hired.

What was missing from George's reasoning? He based his problem map on empirical literature and educated but narrowly preconceived guesses without fully assessing the situation. Had he conducted a systematic needs assessment that included interviewing, testing, and observing the workers, he might have found that the monitors were too high for the operators and the chair heights were not adjustable. Thus, the intervention of body mechanics instruction and upper body stretching that may have been viable in another situation did not address the specific needs that George failed to identify. Had he used systematic thinking and action to ascertain need, rather than guessing and then jumping from the problem to the intervention, George would quickly have identified the appropriate target areas.

In needs assessment, many systematic approaches can be useful in identifying and documenting needs, including but not limited to formal research strategies, well-conducted a priori studies, and mixed methods of information gathering and analysis. For individual clinical problems, strategies such as single case design are extremely useful for guiding and testing the efficacy of intervention decisions with a client.[12] For program development, the therapist may want to use "group" (also called nomothetic) approaches, such as survey, interview, or standardized testing strategies, to obtain needed information on which to support a needs claim. Naturalistic inquiry or mixed-method thinking and action strategies may be valuable to ascertain the perspectives of client groups about whose problems and needs the therapist knows little. Many excellent research texts are available from which to build research knowledge (see the Suggested Readings at the end of this chapter).

The next step in the process of systematic OT practice is translating the needs into goals and objectives.

Goals and Objectives

Goals and objectives are two words with which OT practitioners are familiar because these concepts are used to structure treatment. In SOTP, goals and objectives emerge from the need statement and are essential not only for structuring intervention but also for specifying how the process and outcome of intervention will be examined and supported. Can you see how the SOTP and practice are seamless?

Definitions of the two terms are helpful. **Goals** are statements developed by clients and relevant others identifying the client's desired outcome of the service—what would the client like to be able to do or be.[6] In other words, a goal is a vision statement about future desires that is delimited by the need that it addresses. **Objectives** are statements about how to reach a goal and how to determine whether all or part of the goal has been reached. The objective sets up the systematic approach to attaining the goal and determining its empirical measurement or assessment.[13]

There are two basic types of objectives: process and outcome. **Process objectives** define concrete steps necessary to attain a goal. Process objectives are interventions or services that will be provided or structured by the OT practitioner.[11] **Outcome objectives** define the criteria that must be met to determine that all or part of the goal has been reached; outcome objectives further specify how these criteria will be demonstrated. Ultimately, assessing the attainment of outcome objectives focuses on ascertaining the extent to which the desired change has taken place following and/or as a result of participation in the OT process.

To develop goal and objective statements in our model, the therapist examines the need carefully, including the evidence supporting the need statement. Then, the therapist and the client formulate conceptual goal and objective statements that guide and imply how the process and outcomes of intervention will be assessed. Goals are overall conceptual statements about what is desired; objectives are statements that are operationalized (i.e., stated in terms of how they will be measured or known). Both are based on systematically generated knowledge from the needs assessment.[11]

Let's now return to Jane to illustrate goals and objectives. From the problem and need statements, the OT practitioner determined that an overall goal for Jane's intervention was to develop, teach, and have Jane learn compensatory strategies for promptness and time management so she could improve her performance in these areas and return to work. Based on the evidence given in the needs assessment, the OT intervention was to be carried out at first in Jane's home, with her husband participating; after this, a transition would be made to the workplace.

A critical element of goal setting in SOTP is **specificity**. The following example uses the treatment goal discussed previously as the basis for writing specific goal and objective statements.

Goal: Jane will improve her promptness so as to be able to get to work on time (performance), to her satisfaction. The process (P) and outcome (O) objectives to be used to attain this goal are:

1. Jane will be presented with assistive technology supports and services and repositories of assistive devices from which to select those she thinks will be most useful for her to achieve the goal. (P)
2. Given a choice of a variety of assistive devices (e.g., smart watches, notification apps, and clocks), Jane will choose one or more devices to use as an external cue provider for promptness. (P)

3. Jane will select one daily activity at home for which she needs an external promptness cue. (P)
4. With assistance from the OT practitioner, Jane and her husband will configure the device to cue Jane to attend to this daily event. (P)
5. Jane's husband will monitor her promptness (O) and provide feedback to Jane and the therapist regarding the effectiveness of the assistive device in meeting the goal. (P)
6. Once Jane has demonstrated that she can promptly attend to her schedule at home (O), she will begin to use the promptness cue to arrive at work. (P)
7. Once Jane has demonstrated that she can arrive at work on time (O), the therapist will work with Jane at the work site so that she can use the device to attend promptly to her work schedule, to her and her employer's satisfaction. (P)
8. Using the most effective strategy and devices, Jane will improve her promptness and satisfaction with her performance at work. (O)

As you can see by reading this goal and its related objectives, in SOTP, objectives are very directive conceptual statements designed to address the articulated broad goal statements based on an empirical understanding of need. As we will see in the following sections, Reflexive Intervention and Outcome Assessment, stating the goals and objectives as demonstrated in this chapter determines what will be formatively monitored and examined to ascertain treatment success.

Reflexive Intervention

Extrapolating from naturalistic methods of inquiry, DePoy and Gilson[11] chose the term *reflexive intervention* to highlight the fact that systematic thinking does not stop during the implementation of interventions. Therefore, we have integrated this term into our model to remind the practitioner that as practice proceeds, the occupational therapist monitors the professional activity and makes decisions based on feedback from the actual intervention itself, as well as on examination of the therapeutic use of self and other influences on the intervention process. We use the term reflexive intervention to refer to the thinking and action strategies that occur during the intervention phase of OT practice. In reflexive intervention, the occupational therapist systematically monitors the client, the collaboration, the professional practice, setting-based resources, the therapeutic use of self, and other internal and external influences that affect the practice process and outcome. That is not to say that practice wisdom and intuition do not occur or are not used as evidence. They do occur, and in SOTP the occupational therapist makes it a point to be well aware of the pluralistic evidentiary basis from which he or she is making decisions, to carefully look at all practice to obtain clarity about what was done, and to consider feedback from engaging in practice. An important point to be made here is that occupational therapists and other concerned parties cannot know anything about the success of the intervention if we do not know and articulate what we actually did.

Process assessment, the systematic monitoring of process objectives (denoted in the objective list by "P"), occurs throughout the reflexive intervention phase to provide the evidence on which to describe intervention and the context in which the intervention occurs. It also yields the evidence on which decisions are made about the need for intervention or programmatic change. Knowing what outcomes occurred without knowing what was done to influence and/or cause them limits our knowledge base and our ability to communicate the benefits of OT practice to those outside of the profession. Thus, reflexive intervention is critical to the growth of OT knowledge, theory, and practice strategies. Let's return to Jane to illustrate.

As we mentioned previously, the COPM is an excellent measure for documenting performance that is meaningful to the client. In process assessment, the COPM can be used to document changes in occupational performance and to illustrate the benefits of OT to Jane and other diverse audiences. Using this tool to collect data at multiple points during intervention can support the intervention "as is," or it can help the therapist reconceptualize the intervention. The occupational therapist might also have tracked and documented Jane's promptness over the course of her treatment to determine whether revisions in the intervention were necessary. Moreover, documentation is an excellent way to show Jane and others that Jane has improved while participating in OT. Similar strategies could be used to examine and document time management and other areas that Jane and the occupational therapist were addressing. The OTPF provides excellent guidance on reflexive intervention.

Outcome Assessment

Outcome assessment is a set of thinking and action processes conducted to ascertain and document what occurs following and/or as a result of the client being voluntarily or involuntarily

exposed to a purposive intervention process and to assess the worth of an intervention. (In the objective list shown earlier, outcome objectives were identified with an "O.") These objectives can be assessed by using quantitative, naturalistic techniques, and mixed methods, and by applying systematic inquiry to examine the extent to which objectives have been attained. To brush up on inquiry, we suggest that you consult one of the many excellent research method texts, some of which we list at the end of this chapter.

To perform an outcome assessment of Jane's intervention, the OT selected a pre-post test design using the COPM and the other documentation noted in the discussion on reflexive intervention. Although Jane's performance was measured multiple times, only the change from beginning to end was used for outcome assessment. As you can see, all OTs already do outcome assessment. The trick is to realize that you do it and to purposefully select methods that are credible and useful. We suggest that you choose strategies that use mixed-method approaches. Box 4.3 shows how each objective was assessed in Jane's case.

OT PRACTICE NOTES

SOTP in Professional Practice

An occupational therapist should deliberately perform each of the steps of SOTP and find a personal style for using evidence in professional practice. SOTP not only serves as a valuable approach in direct intervention, it also provides the foundation for knowledge building and intervention development in all professional domains.

BOX 4.3   **Putting It All Together**

Goal, Objectives, Evidence, and Success Criteria

Goal: Jane will improve her promptness so as to be able to get to work on time (performance), to her satisfaction.
1. **(P)** Jane will be supplied with repositories and assistive devices from which to select those that she thinks will be most useful for her to achieve the goal.
   Criterion for success: Completion of activity
   Evidence: Notes of each session documenting progress toward goal
2. **(P)** Given a variety of assistive devices (e.g., smart watches, notification apps, and clocks), Jane will choose a device to use as an external cue provider for promptness (O).
   Criterion for success: Selection of device
   Evidence: Notes of each session documenting progress toward goal
3. **(P)** Jane will select one activity at home for which she needs an external promptness cue.
   Criterion for success: Selection of activity
   Evidence: Notes of each session documenting progress toward goal
4. **(P)** With assistance from the occupational therapist, Jane and her husband will configure the device to cue Jane to attend to this daily event.
   Criterion for success: Demonstration that Jane and her husband have completed the objective
   Evidence: Progress notes indicating mastery of task
5. **(P)** Jane's husband will monitor her promptness (O) and provide feedback to Jane and the therapist regarding the effectiveness of the assistive device in meeting the goal.
   Criterion for success: Daily record of Jane's promptness, supplied to her each evening after dinner
   Evidence: Husband's recorded time charts

6. **(O)** Jane will demonstrate that she can promptly attend to her schedule at home.
   Criterion for success: Daily record of Jane's promptness at home
   Evidence: Husband's recorded time charts
7. **(P)** Once Jane has demonstrated that she can promptly attend to her schedule at home, she will begin to use the promptness cue to arrive at work.
   Criterion for success: Daily record of Jane's use of cues
   Evidence: Client self-report
8. **(O)** Jane will regularly arrive at work on time.
   Criterion for success: Daily record of Jane's promptness at work
   Evidence: Client's documented arrival time
9. **(P)** Once Jane has demonstrated that she can arrive at work on time, the therapist will work with Jane at the work site so that she can use the device to attend promptly to her work schedule to her and her employer's satisfaction.
   Criterion for success: Occupational therapist will meet Jane at work daily for 1 week to support use of device
   Evidence: OT notes
10. **(O)** Using the most effective strategy and devices, Jane will improve her promptness sufficient to work and sufficient for her satisfaction.
    Criterion for success: Significant improvement in Jane's promptness
    Evidence: COPM score on this item, compared with COPM score on pretest on this item

COPM, Canadian Occupational Performance Measure; O, outcome objective; P, process objective.

SUMMARY

In this chapter we presented SOTP, a practice approach in which systematic thinking and action are essential tools in OT practice. Our model begins with a clear problem statement that guides all the remaining steps. Naturalistic, experimental and mixed-method research traditions are applied to clinical decision making to guide the subsequent steps of identifying and documenting need, positing goals and objectives, reflexive intervention, and outcome assessment.

Reexamine Table 4.2 now in light of the need statement. The links among problem, needs, goals and objectives, process, and outcome have been clearly illustrated. Each step of SOTP emerges from and is anchored in the previous step. Moreover, systematic thinking and action provide the specificity and credible evidence supporting the extent to which the intervention resolved the part of the problem that was identified as falling within the OT domain.

REVIEW QUESTIONS

1. List three reasons OT practitioners need to use SOTP to demonstrate the efficacy of OT to external audiences.
2. Name and describe each of the steps of SOTP.
3. Compare the steps of SOTP to the steps of the OT process.
4. Using a potential OT client as a case study, select a problem and develop a problem map.
5. Suggest strategies to ascertain the need based on your problem statement.
6. Identify a need for your client based on your problem statement.
7. What is the difference between a goal and an objective, and what is their relationship?
8. How do goals and objectives relate to need?
9. How do goals and objectives relate to a problem?
10. Identify goals for your client.
11. What are the two types of objectives described in this chapter, and what are the differences between them?
12. Based on your goals for your client, identify at least two process objectives and two outcome objectives.
13. Explain how you will know that your objectives have been met.
14. Choose at least two interventions to achieve the goals and objectives you established in question 12.
15. Identify what questions you will ask and how you will answer them in reflexive intervention.
16. Discuss how you will use reflexive intervention and outcome assessment data to contribute to OT knowledge.

For additional practice questions for this chapter, please visit eBooks.Health.Elsevier.com.

REFERENCES

1. 2018 Accreditation Council for Occupational Therapy Education (ACOTE®) Standards and Interpretive Guide (effective July 31, 2020) December 2019 Interpretive Guide Version. https://www.aota.org/~/media/Corporate/Files/EducationCareers/Accredit/StandardsReview/2018-ACOTE-Standards-Interpretive-Guide.pdf.
2. American Occupational Therapy Association: EBP Project 1 CAP guidelines evidence exchange. https://www.aota.org/Practice/Researchers.aspx.
3. American Occupational Therapy Association: Evidence based resource directory. http://www.aota.org/practice/researchers/ebp-resource-directory.aspx.
4. American Occupational Therapy Association: OT practice guidelines. https://www.aota.org/Practice/Researchers/practice-guidelines.aspx.
5. American Occupational Therapy Association: Vision 2025, *Am J Occup Ther* 71(3):7103420010, 2017. https://doi.org/10.5014/ajot.2017.713002.
6. American Occupational Therapy Foundation: Implementation Research grant. https://www.aotf.org/Grants/Implementation-Research-Grant.
7. Bloom M, Fischer J, Orme JG: *Evaluating practice: guidelines for the accountable professional*, ed 6, Boston, 2009, Pearson.
8. Brownson RC, et al: *Evidence-Based Public Health*, ed 3, Oxford, UK, 2018, Oxford University Press.
9. Cochrane. www.cochrane.org.
10. Coster WJ: Making the best match: selecting outcome measures for clinical trials and outcome studies, *Am J Occup Ther* 67:162–170, 2013.
11. DePoy E, Gilson S: *Social work research and evaluation: examined practice for action*, Los Angeles, 2017, Sage.
12. DePoy E, Gitlin L: *Introduction to research: understanding and applying multiple strategies*, ed 7, St Louis, 2020, Mosby. https://doi.org/10.5014/ajot.2013.006015.
13. Fitzpatrick JL, Sanders JR, Worthen BR: *Program evaluation: alternative approaches and practical guidelines*, ed 4, Boston, 2011, Allyn & Bacon.
14. Heaton RK, et al: *Wisconsin card sorting test professional manual*, Lutz, FL, 1993, Psychological Assessment Resources (PAR).
15. Hinojosa J: The evidence-based paradox, *Am J Occup Ther* 67:e18–e23, 2013. http://doi.org/10.5014/ajot.2013.005587.
16. Institute of Medicine 2008: Evidence-Based Medicine and the Changing Nature of Health Care. *IOM Annual Meeting Summary*, Washington, DC, 2007, The National Academies Press. https://doi.org/10.17226/12041.
17. Johnstone B, et al, editors: *Rehabilitation of neuropsychological disorders: a practical guide for rehabilitation professionals and family members*, ed 2, Brighton, NY, 2009, Psychology Press.
18. Kielhofner G, et al: Studying practice and its outcomes: a conceptual approach, *Am J Occup Ther* 58:15–23, 2004.
19. Law MC, MacDermid J, editors: *Evidence-based rehabilitation: a guide to practice*, ed 3, Thorofare, NJ, 2013, Slack.
20. Law MC, et al: *The Canadian Occupational Performance Measure*, Ottawa, ONT, 1998, Canadian Association of Occupational Therapists.
21. MacDermid J, Law MC: Evaluating the evidence. In Law MC, editor: *Evidence-based rehabilitation: a guide to practice*, ed 3, Thorofare, NJ, 2013, Slack, pp 175–186.

22. Occupational Therapy Code of Ethics (2015). *Am J Occup Ther* 2015;69(Supplement_3):1–8. https://doi.org/10.5014/ajot.2015.696S03

23. Occupational Therapy Practice Framework: Domain and Process—Fourth Edition, *Am J Occupational Ther* 74(Supplement_2):1–87, 2020. https://doi.org/10.5014/ajot.2020.74S2001.

24. OTseeker. http://www.otseeker.com/About/Welcome.aspx#:~:text=OTseeker%20is%20a%20database%20that%20contains%20abstracts%20of,to%20inform%20their%20practice%20by%20quickly%20locating%20it.

25. Peirce CS: *Essays in the philosophy of science*, Indianapolis, IN, 1957, Bobbs-Merrill.

26. Risjord M: Genes, neurons, and nurses: new directions for nursing's philosophy of science, *Nurs Philos* 15(4):231–237, 2014. https://doi.org/10.1111/nup.12069.

27. Sackett DL, Richardson WS, Rosenberg WM, et al: *Evidence-based medicine: how to practice and teach EBM*, ed 2, New York, 2000, Churchill Livingstone.

28. Sackett DL, Rosenberg WM, Gray JA, et al: Evidence based medicine: what it is and what it isn't, *Br Med J* 312(7023):71–72, 1996.

29. Samuelsson K, Wressle E: Turning evidence into practice: barriers to research use among occupational therapists, *British Journal of Occupational Therapy* 78:175–181, 2015. https://doi-org.ezproxy.ithaca.edu/10.1177/0308022615569511.

30. Schaaf R: Creating evidence for practice using data-driven decision making, *Am J Occup Ther* 69(2):1–6, 2015. https://doi.org/10.5014/ajot.2015.010561.

31. Scope of Practice. *Am J Occup Ther* 68(Supplement_3):S34–S40, 2014. https://doi.org/10.5014/ajot.2014.686S04.

32. Sudsawad P: Creating outcomes research for evidence-based practices. In Taylor R, editor: *Kielhofner's Research in occupational therapy: methods of inquiry for enhancing practice,* ed 2, Philadelphia, 2017, FA Davis.

33. Tickle-Degnan L: Communicating evidence to clients, managers, and funders. In Law MC, editor: *Evidence-based rehabilitation: a guide to practice,* ed 3, Thorofare, NJ, 2013, Slack.

34. Tomlin G, Borgetto B: Research Pyramid: a new evidence-based practice model for occupational therapy, *Am J Occup Ther* 65:189–196, 2011.

35. Tomlin GS, Dougherty D: Decision-making and sources of evidence in occupational therapy and other health professions. evidence-informed practice/Entscheidungsfindung und evidenzquellen in der ergotherapie und weiteren gesundheitsberufen. Evidenzinformierte praxis, *International Journal of Health Professions (Warsaw, Poland)* 1(1):13–19, 2014. Walter de Gruyter GmbH. https://doi.org/10.2478/ijhp-2014-0001.

36. World Health Organization: International classification of functioning, disability and health, Geneva. https://www.who.int/classifications/documents/2018ICFUpdates.pdf?ua=1.

SUGGESTED READINGS

Babbie E, Wagner WE, Zaino JS: *Adventures in social research*, ed 13, Los Angeles, CA, 2018, Sage.

Coley SM, Scheinberg CA: *Proposal writing*, ed 5, Thousand Oaks, CA, 2017, Sage.

Creswell J: *Research Design: Qualitative, Quantitative, and Mixed Methods Approaches*, ed 5, Los Angeles, CA, 2018, Sage.

Denzin NK, Lincoln YS: *Handbook of qualitative research*, ed 5, Thousand Oaks, CA, 2018, Sage.

Fetterman DM: *Ethnography step-by-step*, ed 4, Thousand Oaks, CA, 2020, Sage.

Gambrill E: *Critical thinking in clinical practice: improving the quality of judgments and decisions*, ed 3, Hoboken, NJ, 2012, Wiley.

Grinnell RM: *Social work research and evaluation*, Itasca, IL, 2019, Peacock.

McNiff J: *Action research*, Los Angeles, CA, 2017, Sage.

Patton MQ: *Qualitative research and evaluation methods: integrating theory and practice*, ed 4, Thousand Oaks, CA, 2014, Sage.

Royse D, et al: *Program evaluation: an introduction to an evidence-based approach*, ed 6, Boston, MA, 2016, Cengage.

Yin R: *Case study research: design and methods*, ed 6, Los Angeles, CA, 2018, Sage.

5

Health Promotion, Well-Being, and Quality of Life for People With Physical Disabilities

Michael A. Pizzi

LEARNING OBJECTIVES

After studying this chapter, the student or practitioner will be able to do the following:

1. Discuss historical influences on occupational therapy's (OT's) role in health promotion and well-being.
2. Define key health promotion and prevention constructs and terminology.
3. Describe the impact of *Healthy People 2030* on OT practice.
4. Identify strategies for integrating health promotion into physical disability practice.
5. Develop a holistic client- and occupation-centered health promotion perspective for physical disability practice.
6. Develop health promotion interventions based on the OTPF-4 and supported by theory.

CHAPTER OUTLINE

KEY TERMS

Client-centered care (client-centered practice)
Empowerment
Enablement
Environment-Health-Occupation-Wellness (EHOW) Model
Health promotion
Health protection
Moral treatment
Occupational justice
Pizzi Health and Wellness Assessment (PHWA)
PRECEDE-PROCEED model

Prevention
Primary prevention
Quality of life
Risk factors
Secondary conditions
Secondary prevention
Tertiary prevention
Transtheoretical model
Well-being
Wellness

Achieving health, well-being, and participation in life through engagement in occupation is the overarching statement that describes the domain and process of occupational therapy in its fullest sense. This statement acknowledges the profession's belief that active engagement in occupation promotes, facilitates, supports, and maintains health and participation (p. 5).[2]

THREADED CASE STUDY

Jean, Part 1

Jean is a 49-year-old woman who identifies as female (prefers use of the pronouns she/her/hers) and has three grown children, two of whom live away from home. The one living at home has a 2-year-old child. She has been married for 27 years. Jean developed gestational diabetes with her first-born child and has been insulin dependent for most of her married life. Jean is knowledgeable about diet, the need for exercise and activity, and insulin regulation; however, she does not manage her health condition well despite this knowledge. She is active in her community, works part-time as a cashier to supplement her husband's income, and enjoys bowling, playing cards with friends every Friday night, crocheting, and maintaining her home.

Jean developed symptoms later confirmed to be a minor stroke, a transient ischemic attack (TIA). She lost sensation in her fingertips and in both lower extremities. As a result, she developed altered dynamic balance and grasp in both hands. She has coped with diabetic neuropathies for several years and is now faced with beginning signs of glaucoma. She has had a weakened cardiac status secondary to her diabetes despite her being active much of her life. The TIA was a result of poor health management, and she now has difficulties with her leisure participation, paid work, and home maintenance. Jean is overweight and has smoked a pack of cigarettes per day since she was 18 years old. Her husband also smokes regularly.

Critical Thinking Questions

1. How would you evaluate this client from a health promotion perspective?
2. In addition to standard occupational therapy services, what health promotion interventions might you use with this client and/or her family?
3. What theoretical perspective can best be used to support your interventions?

The value a society places on the health and welfare of its people can be measured by its level of commitment to policies and funding for healthcare. The wisdom of a society also can be measured by its commitment to prevention and health promotion. The profession of occupational therapy's (OTs) involvement in health promotion and prevention activities, as well as with policy development, is described. A review of health promotion principles and a description of health promotion–focused evaluation and intervention for individuals with physical disabilities is detailed in this chapter. A case study, threaded throughout, helps readers to integrate the principles and practice of health promotion and prevention for people with physical disabilities.

HISTORICAL INFLUENCES AND CONSIDERATIONS

Development of a Profession

Many descriptions of the development of occupational therapy as a profession either start with or include a discussion of moral treatment.[39,64,65,69] Moral treatment was defined as a "humane approach to the insane" that included occupation-based intervention that emphasized self-discipline, hard work, and learning self-control while developing "good habits."[97] The values and beliefs of the founders of occupational therapy in the United States were consistent with and influenced by the values and beliefs of the mental hygiene movement, the arts and crafts movement, the settlement house movement, and the actions of other social activists and reformers in the United States at that time.[12,13,41] These idealistic individuals and groups influenced the social injustice of their time and are viewed as helping to promote health, well-being, quality of life, and social participation.[69] The backgrounds and contributions of the founders of occupational therapy in the United States are well documented.[a] Therefore, the rest of this discussion focuses on (1) a summary of key events for involvement in health promotion and policy development in the United States and (2) recent international developments that may influence practice in the United States in the coming decades.

Milestones in Occupational Therapy Health Promotion Interventions

Leaders within the field of occupational therapy have been encouraging the profession's increased attention to health promotion for many decades. As early as the 1960s, leaders[b] articulated their vision of the role of occupational therapy in prevention and health promotion. Themes included (1) concerns of emphasis on cure or the saving of life versus the provision of services to maximize the quality of a saved life or the prevention of the illness or injury, (2) the match of occupational therapy values and principles with those of public health, (3) the untapped potential and responsibility for occupational therapy to contribute to the well-being of society, (4) the need to build and redefine the knowledge base of the profession, and (5) the responsibility to conduct research to determine effectiveness of community-based health promotion and prevention initiatives. Finn continued to encourage this involvement through an Eleanor Clarke Slagle Lecture[27] and subsequent work.[25,26]

Through the years the American Occupational Therapy Association (AOTA) has developed a series of statements and employed other means to focus attention on health promotion. In 1979, "Role of the Occupational Therapist in the Promotion of Health and the Prevention of Disabilities," the first official document related to health promotion and prevention, was published.[1] This document has been revised and republished several times since then, the latest being 2020 with a name change to "Occupational Therapy in the Promotion of Health and Well-Being" made in 2013.[5] In 1986, the AOTA supported this role by devoting an entire issue of its journal, the *American Journal of Occupational Therapy (AJOT)*, to health promotion.[94] Another special issue of AJOT on health, well-being, and quality of life, reflecting the profession's move toward prevention and wellness, was published in 2017, with an emphasis on evidence-based practice and research.[53]

Besides encouraging occupational therapy's role in health promotion within the profession, the AOTA also promoted it to external audiences. The AOTA was a participant in the Healthy People 2000 Consortium.[2,88] The consortium, together with 22 expert groups and numerous state and national governmental agencies and services, worked cooperatively to set the nation's health agenda for the next decade. Both this document and its current version, *Healthy People 2030*,[89,90] include targeted health

[a] References 9, 12–14, 38, 43, 64, 65, 76.

[b] References 23–25, 66–68, 73, 92–96.

goals for individuals with disabilities. *Healthy People 2030*[89,90] was released in 2020 identifying the goals for the next decade. The overarching goals of *Healthy People 2030* include:

- Attain healthy, thriving lives and well-being, free of preventable disease, disability, injury, and premature death.
- Eliminate health disparities, achieve health equity, and attain health literacy to improve the health and well-being of all.
- Create social, physical, and economic environments that promote attaining full potential for health and well-being for all.
- Promote healthy development, healthy behaviors, and well-being across all life stages.
- Engage leadership, key constituents, and the public across multiple sectors to take action and design policies that improve the health and well-being of all.

A review of the current version at https://healthypeople.gov can assist occupational therapists (OTs) in the development of new intervention strategies to address the documented unmet health needs of U.S. residents, both with and without disabilities. In 2007, the AOTA selected six focus areas for the profession to emphasize in the decade leading to its centennial in 2017. Health and wellness is one of these six areas; the others include children and youth;[17] productive aging; mental health; work and industry; and rehabilitation, disability, and participation.[3]

An additional AOTA official document, *The Role of Occupational Therapy in Disaster Preparedness, Response, and Recovery*,[4] is another helpful prevention and action tool for occupational therapy practitioners to meet the disaster preparedness needs of individuals with disabilities and to assist employers in preparing for mass casualties resulting from extreme weather, mass transportation accidents, or terrorist activities. COVID-19, caused by infection with coronavirus (called SARS-CoV-2) and appearing in the United States in 2020, also can be considered a natural disaster requiring occupational therapy health promotion and prevention interventions. As will be discussed later in this chapter, prevention is part of a comprehensive health promotion strategy.

Lifestyle Redesign Programs

The development of the Lifestyle Redesign programs by faculty at the University of Southern California (USC), Mrs. T. H. Chan, Division of Occupational Science and Occupational Therapy, is a significant contribution in health promotion occupational therapy practice.[86,87] The outcome of the first of these programs for well elderly was published in a landmark article in the *Journal of the American Medical Association*.[19] The intervention protocol that evolved for the Well Elderly Study was eventually named "Lifestyle Redesign."[44] Results of this Lifestyle Redesign program indicated that "preventive occupational therapy greatly enhances the health and quality of life of independent-living adults" (p. xi).[44] Other Lifestyle Redesign programs have since been developed for individuals both with and without disabilities.[87] These include Lifestyle Redesign programs addressing weight, pain, headache, and diabetes management, as well as ergonomics among others. The occupational therapy faculty at the University of Southern California designed an interdisciplinary program with physical therapy entitled *Optimal Living with MS* to support a wide variety of groups using life coaching and lifestyle risk assessment.[87]

International Trends

An international discussion started by Wilcock and Townsend has shaped the future of occupational therapy's involvement in health promotion and prevention worldwide. Wilcock and Townsend called attention to the potential for occupational therapists and occupational therapy assistants to combat social and occupational injustice.[8,82,97,98] The idea of occupational justice first emerged in Australia and Canada. Occupational justice is "the promotion of social and economic change to increase individual, community, and political awareness, resources, and equitable opportunities for diverse occupational opportunities which enable people to meet their potential and experience well-being" (p. 257).[97] The World Federation of Occupational Therapists (WFOT) also is active in the call for the profession's involvement in promoting occupational justice by encouraging occupational therapists' contributions to the eradication of occupational deprivation.[79] Occupational Justice is now a major principle for OT practice in the AOTA document Occupational Therapy Practice Framework-4.

The WFOT continues to advocate for occupational therapy to address broad societal concerns that affect health and well-being. In 2012, the WFOT approved the document *Environmental Sustainability, Sustainable Practice within Occupational Therapy*,[99] which encourages the profession "to re-evaluate practice models and expand clinical reasoning about occupational performance to include sustainable practice."

Ethical Considerations

The profession of occupational therapy has the potential to be able to assess societal issues that affect the daily occupational rights and function of marginalized individuals, groups, and communities. Through education, political advocacy, and activism, occupational therapists can draw attention to the inequities that exist.

As occupational therapy practitioners gain additional working knowledge of the political process, they can advocate for both the prevention of disability and the promotion of health and prevention of secondary conditions for individuals with disabilities who have been marginalized. In preparation for this advocacy, occupational therapy practitioners should familiarize themselves with the goals, especially the second overarching goal, "Achieve health equity, eliminate disparities, and improve the health of all groups" (p. 3), and other data available in *Healthy People 2030*[89,90] concerning reducing disparities and improving quality of life for individuals with disabilities.

One possible action occupational therapy practitioners can take is increasing their awareness of current history-making efforts that can be joined and supported. The independent living movement, which is working to combat these disparities and social injustice for individuals with disabilities, is one such example. However, if an occupational therapy practitioner singularly embraces the rehabilitation paradigm, he or she may not feel comfortable with either the principles of the independent living movement or its political agenda. Integrating a proactive approach to health that includes health promotion, wellness, and rehabilitation can significantly affect the quality of life of people with disabilities and their loved ones.[54,58]

The rehabilitation paradigm is one clearly used by occupational therapy practitioners. Wellness and health promotion strategies can easily be introduced into any practice area. An example of this is to work with a client after a stroke who is obese on healthy nutrition and activity levels, identifying positive environmental supports, and helping to develop routines that promote health and well-being. Working from a client-centered versus expert-centered perspective permits more control for the client for positive independent living. "As new approaches are developed in Medicare and in private insurance, occupational therapy's role may move from being considered a rehabilitation service to being an essential component of any well-designed, effective, and efficient health care system. Areas in which occupational therapy practitioners may be involved with healthy and frail community-dwelling older adults include several fully supported by the evidence" (p. 382).[7] An important milestone in international efforts to ensure independent living and other equal rights for individuals with disabilities was the adoption in 2006 of the United Nations Convention on the Rights of Persons with Disabilities. The United States did not sign this convention until 2009, at which time 142 other countries had signed.[84,85]

Occupational therapy practitioners need to look beyond the immediate rehabilitation goals to be truly client centered in their practice.[82] This includes advocacy for equal access and rights for all people, marginalized or not, with or without physical disabilities. In a sense, this discussion has come full circle, with the opportunity to emulate the original founders of the profession by becoming social activists.

HEALTH PROMOTION PRINCIPLES AND PRACTICE

Health is a constant interplay of a variety of factors. Important determinants of health status include biology and genetics, individual behavior, social factors, policymaking, and health services.[6,89,90] Public health professionals evaluate the health status of a population by examining birth and death rates, incidence and prevalence of disease, injury and disability, use of health care services, life expectancy, quality of life, and other factors. Leading health indicators for the U.S. population were established during the development of *Healthy People 2020* in an effort to set priorities and focus the national health promotion agenda. The leading health indicators were revised in the *Healthy People 2030* to serve as the foundation for the strategic planning process and include:[89,90]

- Access to health services
- Clinical preventive services
- Environmental quality
- Injury and violence
- Maternal, infant, and child health
- Mental health, including suicide prevention
- Nutrition, physical activity, and obesity
- Oral health
- Reproductive and sexual health
- Social determinants
- Substance abuse
- Tobacco

Health promotion is defined by the World Health Organization (WHO) as:

The process of enabling people to increase control over, and to improve, their health. To reach a state of complete physical mental and social well-being, an individual or group must be able to identify and to realize aspirations, to satisfy needs, and to change or cope with the environment. Health is, therefore, seen as a resource for everyday life, not the objective of living (1).[100]

Health promotion encompasses both health protection and prevention of disease. Health protection strategies are targeted at populations and include control of infectious diseases, immunizations, protection from occupational hazards, and governmental standards for the regulation of clean air and water, sanitation, and food and drug safety, among other things.[21] Prevention refers to "anticipatory action taken to reduce the possibility of an event or condition from occurring or developing, or to minimize the damage that may result from the event or condition if it does occur" (p. 81).[47] Prevention strategies can be categorized using three levels: primary, secondary, and tertiary. Primary prevention focuses on healthy individuals to decrease vulnerability or susceptibility to disease or dysfunction. Primary prevention strategies include good nutrition, regular physical activity, adequate housing, recreation and working conditions, periodic physical examinations, and seatbelt laws. Secondary prevention focuses on persons at risk or in the early stages of disease with the goal of arresting the disease progression and preventing complications and disability. Secondary prevention strategies include early detection and intervention, as well as screening for chronic diseases such as cancer, coronary artery disease, and diabetes. Tertiary prevention focuses on persons with disease or disability and attempts to prevent further complications, minimize the effects of the condition, and promote social opportunity. Tertiary prevention strategies include rehabilitation services and the removal of architectural and attitudinal barriers to social participation.[22,32,74]

Health promotion and prevention approaches attempt to reduce risk factors and enhance protective or resiliency factors. Risk factors are human characteristics or behaviors, circumstances, or conditions that increase the likelihood or predispose an individual or community to manifest certain health problems. Risk factors include not only physical conditions such as hypertension and behaviors such as smoking but also social, economic, and environmental conditions such as poverty, homelessness, exposure to radiation, and pollution.[22,74] Research indicates that "it is usually the accumulation of risk rather than the presence of any single risk factor that affects outcomes, and that multiple risks usually have multiplicative rather than merely additive effects" (p. 512).[21] Protective or resiliency factors are human characteristics or behaviors, circumstances, or conditions that decrease susceptibility or increase an individual's or community's resistance to illness, dysfunction, or injury. Protective factors include not only an individual's genetic profile, personality, and health behaviors, but also peer and family relationships, social norms, and social support.[21,74]

MODELS FOR HEALTH PROMOTION PRACTICE

In the health promotion field there are a number of individual, interpersonal, and community models and theories of health behavior change.[70,71] Three models will be presented here briefly to help the practitioner better conceptualize health promotion interventions. One model, the **transtheoretical model**, also known as the stages of change model, was designed to facilitate individual health behavior change and is therefore extremely relevant to occupational therapy practitioners. The second model, PRECEDE-PROCEED, is an approach to planning that facilitates the design, implementation, and evaluation of health promotion interventions.[29] A third model, the **Environment-Health-Occupation-Wellness (EHOW) Model**, was developed by the author. That model is an OT health- and wellness-specific model, with well-being and quality of life, not occupational performance, being the outcomes of OT services.[59]

Transtheoretical Model

The transtheoretical model (TTM) is based on the premise that change occurs in stages. The model consists of six stages: precontemplation, contemplation, preparation, action, maintenance, and termination. Precontemplation is the stage in which the person has no intention of taking action to modify health behaviors. This may be due to lack of knowledge, previous failed attempts at changing health behavior, or simply a lack of motivation. The contemplation stage is characterized by intention to modify behaviors within the next 6 months, but with some ambivalence regarding the costs and benefits of doing so. The preparation stage is an indication that the person is ready to take action in the very near future (30 days or less) and has demonstrated some initiative to plan the change strategies such as reading a self-help book, joining a health club, or talking to a physician. Action refers to specific overt manifestations of lifestyle modification. The duration of this stage is a minimum of 6 months. After 6 months of sustained health behavior change, a person is considered to be in the maintenance stage. The goal of this stage is to prevent relapse into previous unhealthy behaviors. Termination is the stage at which a person is no longer tempted and has a sense of self-efficacy that permits the person to maintain healthy behaviors even in stressful, high-risk situations. True termination may be unrealistic for most behavioral changes, and lifelong maintenance may be the appropriate goal for the majority of people.[63]

According to the TTM, change occurs through "covert and overt activities that people use to progress through the stages" (p. 103).[63] These activities or processes of change include consciousness raising, dramatic relief, self-reevaluation, environmental reevaluation, self-liberation, helping relationships, counter-conditioning, contingency or reinforcement management, stimulus control, and social liberation. The developers of the TTM discovered that each of these processes is more or less effective during different stages of change. For example, consciousness raising is critical in the precontemplation stage for the person to progress to the contemplation stage. Contingency management and stimulus control strategies are most useful in the maintenance stage to prevent relapse.[63]

PRECEDE-PROCEED Model

The **PRECEDE-PROCEED model** is used for planning interventions and consists of nine steps (Box 5.1). The PRECEDE portion

---

BOX 5.1   Steps of the PRECEDE-PROCEED Model

PRECEDE
Step 1: Social Assessment
Step 2: Epidemiologic Assessment
Step 3: Behavioral and Environmental Assessment
Step 4: Educational and Ecological Assessment
Step 5: Administrative and Policy Assessment

PROCEED
Step 6: Implementation
Step 7: Process Evaluation
Step 8: Impact Evaluation
Step 9: Outcome evaluation

From Green LW, Kreuter MW: *Health promotion planning: an educational and ecological approach*, ed 3, Mountain View, CA, 1999, Mayfield.

---

of the model is based on the assumption that health behaviors are the result of a complex interaction of multiple factors.[30,31] In the PRECEDE framework, these factors are identified and specific objectives are developed for a population. The PROCEED portion of the model consists of policy development, intervention implementation, and evaluation. The first five steps represent a comprehensive needs assessment that evaluates a number of social, epidemiologic, behavioral, environmental, educational, ecologic, administrative, and policy issues that might affect the development, implementation, and ultimate success of a health promotion intervention. After all of these factors are considered, the intervention is developed and implemented. The final three steps represent a comprehensive evaluation of the intervention, including process, impact, and outcome measures.[31]

PRECEDE-PROCEED has been used to plan, implement, and evaluate health promotion interventions in school, work, health care, and community settings. It has been used to address a number of health issues, including smoking cessation, HIV prevention, seatbelt use, driving under the influence of alcohol, nutrition, exercise and fitness, blood pressure control, stress management,[31] and depression and pain among individuals with rheumatoid arthritis.[45] Typically, interventions designed using the PRECEDE-PROCEED model address multiple risk factors and health behaviors and use multiple intervention strategies.

Environment-Health-Occupation-Wellness Model

An OT clinical model focused on well-being and quality of life as the outcomes of interventions is the Environment-Health-Occupation-Wellness Model (EHOW) (Fig. 5.1). This model proposes that the interaction between one's health; the cultural, social, or physical environment in which occupation is engaged; and participation in occupation yields the level of one's well-being and quality of life. Most recently, the EHOW model was used as the basis for older adults residing in a skilled nursing facility, with emphasis on how leisure can be used as a therapeutic modality and be a health-promoting occupation (https://www.otinsnf.com/).[36]

The EHOW model emphasizes participation over performance. For example, if a person can make minimal to no progress (a person at the end of life, a child with severely involved

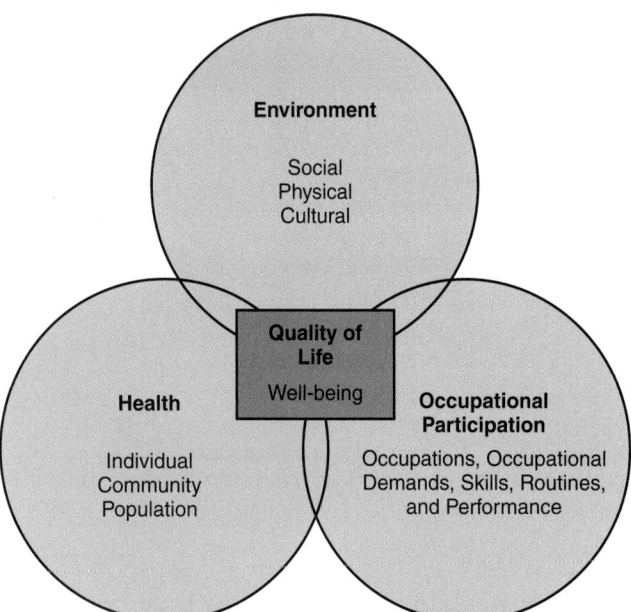

Fig. 5.1 Environment-Health-Occupation-Wellness (EHOW) Model. (Courtesy Michael Pizzi PhD, OTR/L, FAOTA © 2017.)

motor challenges) yet continue to participate in meaningful occupation, they are still engaging in that occupation, but not necessarily performing that occupation. The following assumptions support the EHOW model[59]:

- Individuals, communities, and populations strive to optimize their health, well-being, and quality of life.
- Health, environments, and occupational participation have a dynamic influence on quality of life and well-being.
- Health behavior change can occur when clients become aware of a need for such change.
- Participation in daily activities that are meaningful promotes a positive health trajectory for daily living.
- Health is a resource used daily to pursue and participate in important and meaningful activity in life.[100]
- Use of time for an individual, community, or population in meaningful, culturally relevant, and socially appropriate daily activities can be health promoting.

OCCUPATIONAL THERAPY INVOLVEMENT IN HEALTH PROMOTION AND PREVENTION

According to population health measures, persons with disabilities (PWDs) experience health disparities in comparison to individuals without disabilities. Persons with disabilities are more likely to have high blood pressure, use tobacco, be overweight, and experience psychological distress. They are also less likely to get the health care they need, have an annual dental visit, engage in fitness activities, and participate in health screenings.[84] The *Healthy People 2030* goals cited previously in the area of disability and health apply to disabled and nondisabled individuals and communities. The objectives in *Healthy People 2030* address both individuals with disabilities and the environments in which they function, because it is recognized

that disability is the result of the interaction between individual limitations and barriers in the environment.[85,89,90]

In the *Occupational Therapy Practice Framework: Domain and Process–4*,[6] AOTA describes health promotion and prevention as appropriate intervention approaches for the profession. "Health promotion is equally and essentially concerned with creating the conditions necessary for health at individual, structural, social, and environmental levels through an understanding of the determinants of health: peace, shelter, education, food, income, a stable ecosystem, sustainable resources, social justice, and equity" (p. 441).[83] AOTA embraces the WHO definition of well-being as "the process of enabling people to increase control over, and to improve, their health."[100] Occupational therapist Ann Wilcock[98] (2006, as cited in the OTPF-4[6]) stated,

Following an occupation-based health promotion approach to well-being embraces a belief that the potential range of what people can do, be, and strive to become is the primary concern, and that health is a by-product. A varied and full occupational lifestyle will coincidentally maintain and improve health and well-being if it enables people to be creative and adventurous physically, mentally, and socially (p. 315).[6]

The OTPF-4, more than any previous AOTA Practice Framework document, focuses on health, well-being, and quality of life.

Health promotion programming can assist individuals, families, and communities reach a state of wellness in their lives.[75] **Wellness** has been described as the "perception of and responsibility for psychological and physical well-being as these contribute to overall satisfaction with one's life situation" (p. 1243).[11] occupational therapy practitioners facilitate wellness through holistic and client-centered health promotion practice.

Occupational therapy involvement in health promotion and prevention can assume a variety of forms. For example, primary prevention could include providing education to workers regarding their personal risk factors for injury on the job (e.g., poor body mechanics) or altering the environment to reduce the incidence of workplace accidents. Secondary prevention strategies in occupational therapy practice include joint protection, energy conservation, and work simplification techniques. Fall prevention programs and home safety evaluations for frail elderly clients are other examples of secondary prevention. occupational therapy practitioners are already experts in tertiary prevention, because they provide services to maximize function and minimize barriers to occupational performance.[32,75] It is important that occupational therapy practitioners begin to engage in primary and secondary prevention to build the evidence for occupational therapy in health and wellness. One population that could benefit from all three levels of prevention is military personnel.[20] As the Patient Protection and Affordable Care Act enables an increase in occupational therapy services, telehealth occupational therapy services in all areas of health promotion and prevention can also be enabled.[15,16] Telehealth services have been used more than ever as a health prevention tool to access medical and therapy services given the onset of COVID-19, because it limits large crowds in waiting rooms and schools.

Health Promotion and Occupational Participation

Health promotion interventions assist in enabling people with disabilities to more fully engage and participate in society. According to Hills,[33] there are three "pillars and related assumptions" of health promotion: (1) the primacy of people, (2) empowerment, and (3) enablement. All three of these constructs, especially the primacy of people, focus on what the profession of occupational therapy calls **client-centered care** or client-centered practice. Client-centered practice can be defined as: An "approach to service that incorporates respect for and partnership with clients as active participants in the therapy process. This approach emphasizes clients' knowledge and experience, strengths, capacity for choice, and overall autonomy" (p. 1230).[11] It is this client-centered approach that is health promoting for individuals with physical disabilities. The respect for and involvement in decision-making, particularly in occupational participation, is a foundational similarity in both health promotion and occupational therapy. Occupational therapists facilitate meaning and assist people in seeing a hopeful future through occupational engagement and enablement of participation. This focus will help foster optimal health and well-being for people with disabilities. There is increasing occupational therapy evidence for client-centered care and client-centered practice. Pizzi[55] was one of the first occupational therapists to demonstrate the effectiveness and validity of client-centered care and people at the end of life, a population needing preventive occupations to diminish the psychological impact of the dying process and enable the physical body to optimally participate in meaningful occupation until death.

Empowerment speaks to the development of autonomy and self-control. Occupational therapists are skilled at creating contexts and occupation-based interventions that support and facilitate the feeling of being empowered. "To increase control over and to improve one's health, one must not only be empowered to do so but also able to do so. To be able, one must possess the requisite skills, resources and knowledge" (p. 232)."[32] People with impairments and disabilities and those at risk for impairment and disability can be knowledgeable about the need to change health behaviors that undermine the promotion of healthy living (e.g., smoking); however, they may be lacking skills and resources to achieve optimal well-being. "The fundamental assumption underlying the notion of **enablement** is that people have capacity to identify their own needs, to solve their own problems and to generally know what is best for them" (p. 232).[32]

To effectively promote health and well-being, occupational therapists should embrace the belief that people are capable of identifying needs and are able to problem-solve life challenges. Implementing client-centered approaches versus expert-centered approaches (those approaches that come from therapists without inclusion of clients or their caregivers) will empower people with disabilities to view themselves as valued and contributing members of society.

Powers provided a glimpse into the lived experiences of people with disabilities and their perceptions of health and well-being.[62] She believes there is need to develop more models of health and wellness that specifically address the needs of people with disabilities. There are models currently used, such as some discussed earlier, that do enhance the knowledge of health professionals regarding people with disabilities. Health and illness can and do coexist on a daily basis for people with physical impairments and disabilities:

> *Living healthy and well is not something new for people with disabilities. Currently, a stereotype exists that suggests people with disabilities are "sick" or are "perpetual patients" who cannot be considered "healthy" or "well." However, for years people with disabilities have used strategies to maintain health and wellness, created supportive relationships, and accessed needed resources from various service systems. It is from these resourceful people that health professionals need to be willing to continue learning about issues related to health, wellness and long-term disability (p. 73).[62]*

Secondary Conditions and People With Disabilities

Secondary conditions can be defined as "those physical, medical, cognitive, emotional, or psychosocial consequences to which persons with disabilities are more susceptible by virtue of an underlying impairment, including adverse outcomes in health, wellness, participation, and quality of life" (p. 162).[33] The term *secondary conditions* expanded the term *comorbidity*, which is a term often used in medical settings.

However, the term *secondary condition* adds three dimensions not fully captured by the term *comorbidity*. It includes (1) nonmedical events (e.g., isolation), (2) conditions that affect the general population (e.g., obesity, with higher prevalence among people with disabilities), and (3) problems that arise any time during the life span (e.g., inaccessible mammography). Children and adults with disabilities can experience secondary conditions any time during their life span.[18] Childhood obesity, with its concomitant impact on social, physical, and mental health, is an example of a secondary condition that is often overlooked by occupational therapists. There has been considerable research in this area, including development of an occupation-based assessment and intervention programs.[b] Obesity and healthy weight management occupational therapy goes beyond exploring performance issues of children, and incorporates performance and participation while also focusing on a child's health and well-being.

Occupational therapy practitioners can aid in the prevention of secondary conditions through increasing client awareness and patient education about health, healthy habits and routines, and strategies to offset increasing secondary conditions or other disability. In view of the increased rates of disability among youth, it is particularly important to target activities and services

---

> **OT PRACTICE NOTES**
>
> It behooves occupational therapy practitioners to make a paradigm shift and transition from defining oneself as a rehabilitation specialist to a specialist in occupation, health promotion, and well-being using occupation to facilitate healthy living. Through listening to the narratives of people with disabilities and engaging in client-centered evaluation and interventions, occupational therapists and occupational therapy assistants can enable people with disabilities and chronic illnesses to maximize quality of life and participation in society.[49,59]

---

[b] References 40, 50–52, 56, 57, 60, 61.

that address all aspects of health and well-being, including promoting health, preventing secondary conditions, and removing environmental barriers, as well as providing access to medical care.[49] For an older person with a disability, it is important to target worsening coexisting conditions that may intensify and thus threaten general well-being. For example, declining vision combined with declining hearing can greatly impair mobility, nutrition, and fitness, conditions that may intensify and thus threaten general well-being.[84]

Hough thinks that a paradigm shift from disability prevention to prevention of secondary conditions is needed.[34] After the inability to prevent primary disability, "it is within the environment that the negative effects of secondary conditions could be ameliorated and even prevented" (pp. 187–188).[34] Public health agencies often focus efforts toward primary prevention, and secondary conditions need to be of equal concern. The emphasis on policy change and education of health professionals on health promotion for people with disabilities can help foster interventions toward self-management of one's disability.

Stuifbergen et al. emphasized the need for health practitioners to integrate health promotion strategies in neurorehabilitation for people with stroke.[81] Krahn emphasized the need to encourage self-responsibility for health to promote health and well-being while living with a disability,[39] whereas Rimmer[72] has viewed health promotion as a means to maintain functional independence by preventing secondary conditions. "People with disabilities have increased health concerns and susceptibility to secondary conditions. Having a long-term condition increases the need for health promotion that can be medical, physical, social, emotional, or societal."[83]

The development of secondary conditions and occupational impairments can be directly related to one's mental health. Psychosocial aspects of physical disabilities are as important to identify and help ameliorate as the physical barriers to occupational participation.

People who have activity limitations report having had more days of pain, depression, anxiety, and sleeplessness and fewer days of vitality during the previous month than people not reporting activity limitations. Increased emotional distress, however, does not arise directly from the person's limitations. The distress is likely to stem from encounters with environmental barriers that reduce the individual's ability to participate in life activities and that undermine physical and emotional health.[85]

Exploration of a person's disability, in the context of one's life situations, and the physical and emotional impacts of that disability on participation exemplifies OT practice committed to optimizing quality of life. Quality of life (QOL) is an outcome of occupational therapy as defined by the framework. It is "a person's dynamic appraisal of his or her life satisfactions (perceptions of progress toward one's goals), self-concept (the composite of beliefs and feelings about oneself), health and functioning (including health status, self-care capabilities, role competence), and socioeconomic factors (e.g., vocation, education, income)" (p. 82).[6]

Stuifbergen and Rogers interviewed 20 individuals with MS who shared their stories about health promotion, QOL, and factors that affected these areas of health.[80] They identified six

life domains related to QOL, including family (most frequently identified domain), functioning to maintain independence, spirituality, work, socioeconomic security, and self-actualization. Six broad themes also emerged related to health-promoting behaviors. These included exercise or physical activity, nutritional strategies, lifestyle adjustment, maintaining a positive attitude, health responsibility behaviors, and seeking and receiving interpersonal support.[47] Occupational therapy practitioners play a key role in helping people actualize QOL through interventions that include these themes. Physical disability does not translate to being unable to participate and experience a good QOL. The paradigm shift to promoting health, well-being, and wellness is necessary to optimize QOL.

Creating links among occupation, occupational participation, and health in ways that are understandable to the general public, other health professionals, policymakers, and society must be occupational therapy's mission. The profession must continue to strategize how occupational therapy becomes the leader, and not the follower, in the promotion of health, well-being, and QOL. There also must be a shift from performance to participation in daily life, with evidence supporting the link between participation and a person's health status. A paradigm shift is imperative to reorganize the profession and make a dramatic, if not revolutionary, shift.[52]

Evaluation: Emphasizing the Promotion of Health and Well-Being

Evaluation of people with disabilities must include the life story or narrative of the person as elicited through careful obtaining of an occupational history. This occupational profile is coupled with physical, sensorimotor, social, psychological, and emotional assessments to create a holistic view of the person. The most important element in evaluation is incorporating the client's perspectives of health and well-being, as well as his or her values, beliefs, and contexts of living experiences. Client-centered care promotes healthy views of living for the client and the family system, from the beginning of occupational therapy intervention through discharge.

The Pizzi Health and Wellness Assessment (PHWA)[48,59,78] was created for adults and is a subjective, occupation-focused, and client-centered assessment tool. It measures, both qualitatively and quantitatively, self-perceptions of a person's health and well-being in six different categories. It is an assessment that is not focused on the disability but instead emphasizes one's abilities and current self-perceived levels of health and well-being, not performance, that support or are barriers to occupational participation. Collaboratively, the client and therapist work on strategies that the client identifies as health promoting for each area, as well as using the clinical reasoning of the therapist to problem-solve health issues related to occupational participation. A systems perspective was used during its development, with the TTM noted above as the underlying theoretical framework. The EHOW model also can be used to support health promotion and prevention interventions. Thus, it is a useful assessment and research tool for clients as well as caregivers of people with disabilities. For example, a caregiver may report additional burden achieving occupational balance of roles and occupations, as well as the caregiving responsibilities. The caregiver could benefit from occupational therapy intervention to address identified needs based on responses from the PHWA. The assessment is available by contacting the author at phwa58@gmail.com.

Table 5.1 shows a number of assessments from a variety of disciplines that may be helpful to occupational therapists as they consider how to enhance their health promotion interventions with people with disabilities.[35] The purpose of this table is to encourage practitioners to seek resources outside of the discipline that may increase options to facilitate the end goal

of enhanced participation in occupations. Inclusion of a tool in this table should not be considered an endorsement of the tool. Readers are encouraged to critically examine assessment tools in terms of reliability, validity, sensitivity, and practicability, as well as possible training or certification required before use. Similar tables and lists of assessments that are more commonly used and known by occupational therapy practitioners exist that include assessments developed both within and external to the field.[10,18] These compilations include numerous additional assessments, which, along with other resources, should be reviewed and considered before an assessment being selected for a specific client or client group. Assessments, when chosen appropriately and used competently, can be an important tool in implementing client-centered care.[42,46] Table 5.2 offers additional guidance and considerations for the selection of an assessment.[75]

Intervention

For people with disabilities, health promotion interventions are designed to optimize health status. One focus of these interventions is to help prevent secondary conditions from occurring and thus help people with disabilities maintain a level of well-being that allows them to engage in meaningful life roles. The framework identifies six areas of focus for intervention: (1) areas of occupation, (2) performance skills, (3) performance patterns,

TABLE 5.1 A Selection of Assessments for Use in Health Promotion Physical Disabilities Practice

Assessment Type	Examples
Adjustment scales	Profile of Adaptation to Live
	Social Support Questionnaire
Other well-being scales	Perceived Well-Being Scale
Arthritis	Arthritis McMaster-Toronto Arthritis Patient Reference Disability Questionnaire (MACTAR)
	Health Assessment Questionnaire (HAQ)
	Arthritis Impact Measurement Scales (AIMS)
Back pain	Disability Questionnaire
Cancer	Karnofsky Performance Status Measure (KPS)
	Functional Living Index: Cancer
COPD	American Thoracic Society Respiratory Questionnaire and Grade of Breathlessness Scale
Depression	Beck Depression Inventory
Diabetes	DCCT Questionnaire
Family scales	Caregiver Time-Tradeoff Scale
	Family Hardiness Inventory
Hardiness scales	Hardiness Scale
Health risks appraisals	The Healthier People Network Risk Appraisal
	1999 Youth Risk Behavior Survey
HIV/AIDS	AIDS Health Assessment Questionnaire
Heart	New York Heart Association Functional Classification (NYHA)
Life satisfaction scales	Kansas Family Life Satisfaction Index
	Index of Life Satisfaction
Multiple sclerosis	Expanded Disability Status Scale
Neurological head injury	Modified Sickness Impact Profile
Orthopedic	Musculoskeletal Outcomes Data Evaluation and Management System (MO-DEMS)
Pain	MOS Pain Measures
Quality of life	Overall Life Status

COPD, Chronic obstructive pulmonary disease; HIV/AIDS, human immunodeficiency virus/acquired immunodeficiency syndrome.
Data from Hyner GC, Peterson KW, Travis JW, et al., editors: Society of prospective medicine handbook of health assessment tools, Stoughton, WI, 1999, Wellness Associates Publications.

TABLE 5.2 Organizing the Search for Assessment Evidence to Discuss With Different Decision Makers

Decision Maker	Decision Maker's Use of Evidence	Question That Guides the Search for Evidence
Client and family members	To make informed decisions related to choosing assessment procedures	Is goal attainment scaling a reliable and valid method for assessing personally meaningful goal achievement among 75-year-old men with Parkinson's disease?
Manager	To decide which assessment procedures should be supported and provided by the organization	What are the most reliable and valid methods for assessing personally meaningful goal achievement among persons with Parkinson's disease?
Funder	To determine whether or not assessment procedures will effectively document important attributes of clients and their responses to rehabilitation	Same question as for manager

From Tickle-Degnen L: Communicating evidence to clients, managers, and funders. In Law M, editor: Evidence-based rehabilitation: a guide to practice, Thorofare, NJ, 2002, Slack, p. 225.

THREADED CASE STUDY

Jean, Part 2

For Jean, the PHWA could be used to evaluate the following:

- Occupational habits, routines, and patterns that may be barriers to general health (e.g., smoking, eating habits).
- Balance in daily life activity and barriers to fuller participation in occupation.
- Stress and psychosocial areas that may exacerbate cardiac insufficiency, increase smoking and eating problems, and create insulin imbalance (use stress and depression scales to help assess these areas).
- Physical versus sedentary activity levels and reasons for these activity patterns.
- Risk factors for development of secondary conditions related to her physical function and past medical history.
- Contexts for occupation, including the current support system at work and at home. Caregiver assessment, especially level of support for Jean, can be crucial for health promotion programming.
- The PHWA will also identify Jean's altered leisure participation and reveal her maladaptive health management routines and habits.

(4) context(s) or physical environment, (5) activity demands, and (6) client factors.[6] All of these areas affect each other, and, in turn, affect occupational performance and participation.

Interventions to promote health and well-being are implemented with consideration of all of these areas. Five approaches to intervention are listed in the framework. Although they all can relate to health promotion, the framework specifically links create and promote approaches to health promotion. As indicated earlier, the approaches can be used with people with occupational impairments and disability. The updated OTPF-4 includes health management, which is defined by the framework as "activities related to developing, managing, and maintaining health and wellness routines, including self-management, with the goal of improving or maintaining health to support participation in other occupations" (p. 32).[6] It includes social and emotional health promotion and maintenance, symptom and condition management, communication with the healthcare system, medication management, physical activity, nutrition management, and personal care device management.

As stated earlier, a paradigm shift for therapists' therapeutic reasoning is needed to understand that health, wellness, and disability can be co-mingled and interventions to promote healthy living with a disability are vital for a person with disability. Although the intervention approach of create or promote is most closely related to health promotion, the other four approaches (i.e., establish/restore, maintain, modify, and prevent)[6] are all related to the creation of healthy lifestyles and well-being. They also should be considered as potential approaches for the restoration and promotion of health for individuals with disabilities.

Often, such work is more successful when performed by a multidisciplinary team. An excellent example of a multidisciplinary

THREADED CASE STUDY

Jean, Part 3

The Jean case example illustrates how a health promotion approach for a person with disability can be implemented. In addition to standard occupational therapy services, a health promotion approach might be appropriate with this client or her family. Potential health promotion interventions are described next.

If Jean's occupational habits, routines, and patterns are maladaptive and are barriers to healthy living, patient education around developing healthy habits (including how her habits can result in further medical complications) should be implemented. This includes developing a health management routine that will prevent further illness and secondary conditions.

An imbalance in occupations and occupational performance can contribute to the exacerbation of stress, cause cardiac issues, and affect insulin production. Increasing awareness of the need for balance in daily life, including balance of work, play, rest, sleep, and leisure, can assist Jean in creating a new structure for her daily living and optimize her quality of life. This new structure will include health maintenance and resumption of favored leisure occupations.

Stress, depression, and other psychosocial factors can exacerbate preexisting conditions and lead to inactivity, poor self-esteem, and eventually poorer health. Client-centered care that incorporates meaningful and interesting occupation relevant to the person can help offset psychosocial conditions. Areas of concern could be feelings of worthlessness or ineffectiveness because one cannot occupationally engage in meaningful life activity. Jean may experience these issues because of her limited (and potentially limiting) medical condition. Exploring the impacts of stress, depression, and other factors on occupational performance and creating new occupational strategies for Jean can improve occupational performance and lead to Jean developing a future that includes "preventive occupations"—in this case, preventing further or future depression and managing her stress.

After assessing activity levels, occupational interventions that promote a healthier heart, decrease smoking and overeating, and improve general mental and physical fitness are primary in Jean's case. Once Jean is aware of her abilities and develops a knowledge based on her real and perceived levels of activity, the occupational therapy practitioner can help her modify and adapt her lifestyle to incorporate activity that optimizes mental and physical health. Health management strategies also should be implemented. It is important for Jean to optimize health for both present and future occupational performance in multiple contexts.

Interventions must include measures to prevent the development of secondary conditions. For example, Jean has developed the warning sign (TIA) of potential future stroke. Preventive occupations can include increasing walks outdoors by 5 minutes each week to reach a daily target of 30 minutes maximum, working with an occupational therapy practitioner to help decrease smoking and overeating habits, or developing a stress management program. These health promotion program ideas can be habituated in the acute care and home care settings and followed through by Jean and her loved ones.

Caregiver support is critical for implementing and following through with a health promotion program. In Jean's case, she requires strong support to help her recognize and prevent future health problems (e.g., reminders, environmental and verbal cues, ongoing education). She also will need support with smoking cessation, developing healthy eating (and cooking) habits, and increasing optimism for a healthy and bright future.

program that uses interprofessional perspectives discussed above is the MS Care Center at New York University's Langone Medical Center.[37]

SUMMARY

Readers were introduced to health promotion, well-being, and wellness terminology within the context of physical disability practice. An introduction to the power of symbols, important constructs such as occupational justice, and principles and practice of health promotion help support best practice. Although practitioners have long promoted optimal health for clients of all ages, there has been little discussion about theoretical foundations for evaluation and intervention in health promotion. The framework is a helpful guide to assist practitioners in bridging gaps in service delivery and integrating health promotion into everyday practice. Through the framework, AOTA emphasizes occupational engagement and participation in life as the means to health and wellness, quality of life, and well-being. Occupational therapy practitioners create and promote healthy living by careful attention to the physical, psychosocial, spiritual, social, and emotional abilities and challenges that support, or are barriers to, occupational performance. Holistic evaluation and goal planning using a client-centered approach should include health promotion goals that are co-developed between the client and the practitioner.

Engagement in occupation to support participation in context is a key focus of the framework. A health promotion approach enhances awareness of barriers to health and wellness, and strategies are developed to optimize health and well-being, as well as prevent future health problems. Risk factors are considered, and interventions are implemented to support participation while creating a new lifestyle that is meaningful to the client. Client factors, although important to address to optimize occupational performance, are integrated into a top-down approach to care when providing a health promotion program. In the case example, Jean can engage in a physical activity program designed to improve her cardiac status while she develops strategies to control the pain and discomfort, which are the secondary complications of her diabetes, as she works to decrease or cease smoking. If Jean decreases or stops smoking, she also will have a positive impact on the overall health of her family, especially her grandchildren, by decreasing or removing the health risks of secondary smoke exposure.

As practitioners learn more about health promotion, prevention, and wellness, they will be better equipped to promote healthy living within the context of a person's lifestyle. Client-centered and occupation-centered care that includes health promotion and focuses on the whole person living with disability can be occupational therapy's unique contribution to humanity.

REVIEW QUESTIONS

1. Describe the historical relationship between social activism and occupational justice for individuals with disabilities.
2. Identify an objective from *Healthy People 2030* to support a new health promotion program you want to develop for your client group.
3. Describe the determinants of health as identified in *Healthy People 2030* and discuss how occupational therapy can address these determinants.
4. Identify the levels of prevention, and give examples of potential occupational therapy interventions at each level.
5. Choose a health behavior of interest, and describe the stages of change associated with that health behavior using the transtheoretical model.
6. Discuss how occupational therapists and occupational therapy assistants can facilitate resiliency for their clients with disabilities.
7. How would health promotion approaches fit within the Occupational Therapy Practice Framework?
8. Develop a clinical case and explain the case using the EHOW model. How might this be different than using the TTM or other OT models/frames of reference to support interventions?

For additional practice questions for this chapter, please visit eBooks.Health.Elsevier.com.

REFERENCES

1. American Occupational Therapy Association: Association official position paper: role of the occupational therapist in the promotion of health and the prevention of disabilities, *Am J Occup Ther* 26:59, 1979.
2. American Occupational Therapy Association: Year 2000 health consortium meets, *OT Week*:9, 1989.
3. American Occupational Therapy Association: *April 2007 RA meeting highlights.* https://www.aota.org/governance/ra/pastmeetings/highlights/40465.aspx.
4. American Occupational Therapy Association: The role of occupational therapy in disaster preparedness, response, and recovery, *Am J Occup Ther* 65(Suppl):S11–S25, 2011. https://doi.org/10.5014/ajot.2011.65 S11.
5. American Occupational Therapy Association: Occupational therapy in the promotion of health and well-being, *Am J Occup Ther* 74(3):1–14, 2020. https://doi.org/10.5014/ajot.2020.743003.
6. American Occupational Therapy Association: Occupational therapy practice framework: domain and process, Fourth Edition, *Am J Occup Ther* 74(Supplement_2):1–87, 2020. https://doi.org/10.5014/ajot.2020.74S2001.
7. Arbesman M, Lieberman D, Metzler CA: Using evidence to promote the distinct value of occupational therapy, *Am J Occup Ther* 68:381–385, 2014.
8. Arnold MJ, Rybski D: Occupational justice. Scaffa ME, et al., editors: *Occupational therapy in the promotion of health and wellness*, Philadelphia, 2010, FA Davis, pp 135–156.

9. Bing RK: Point of departure (a play about founding the profession), *Am J Occup Ther* 46:27, 1992.

10. Boop C, Appendix A: Assessments: listed alphabetically by title. In Crepeau EB, et al., *Willard and Spackman's occupational therapy*, ed 10, Philadelphia, 2003, Lippincott Williams & Wilkins, pp 981.

11. Boyt Schell BA, Gillen G, Scaffa ME: Glossary. In Boyt Schell BA, et al: *Willard and Spackman's occupational therapy*, ed 12., Philadelphia, 2014, Lippincott Williams & Wilkins, pp 1229–1243.

12. Breines EB: *Origins and adaptations*, Lebanon, NJ, 1986, Geri-Rehab. [(preface, pp ix–xii; Chapters 2 and 8)]

13. Breines EB: *From clay to computers*, Philadelphia, 1995, FA Davis.

14. Brunyate RW: After fifty years, what stature do we hold? *Am J Occup Ther* 21:262, 1967.

15. Cason J: Telehealth opportunities in occupational therapy through the Affordable Care Act, *Am J Occup Ther* 66:131–136, 2012.

16. Cason J: Telehealth and occupational therapy: integral to the triple aim of healthcare reform, *Am J Occup Ther* 69:1–8, 2015.

17. Centers for Disease Control and Prevention. *Disability and health related conditions.* https://www.cdc.gov/ncbddd/disabilityandhealth/relatedconditions.html; 2020.

18. Christiansen C, Baum C: Index of Assessments. In Christiansen C, Baum C, editors: *Occupational therapy: enabling function and well-being*, ed 2., Thorofare, NJ, 1997, Slack, pp 607.

19. Clark F, Azen SP, Carlson JJ, et al: Occupational therapy for independent-living older adults: a randomized controlled trial, *J Am Med Assoc* 278:1312, 1997.

20. Cogan AM: Supporting our military families: a case for a larger role for occupational therapy in prevention and mental healthcare, *Am J Occup Ther* 68:478–483, 2014.

21. Durlak JA: Common risk and protective factors in successful prevention programs, *Am J Orthopsychiatry* 68:512, 1998.

22. Edelman CL, Mandle CL: *Health promotion throughout the lifespan*, ed 5, St Louis, 2002, Mosby.

23. Fidler G: Introductory overview. In Fidler G, Velde B, editors: *Activities: reality and symbols*, Thorofare, NJ, 1999, Slack, pp 1.

24. Fidler G, Velde B: *Activities: reality and symbols*, Thorofare, NJ, 1999, Slack.

25. Fine S: Symbolization: making meaning for self and society. In Fidler G, Velde B, editors: *Activities: reality and symbols*, Thorofare, NJ, 1999, Slack, pp 11.

26. Finn G: The occupational therapist in prevention programs, *Am J Occup Ther* 26:59, 1972.

27. Finn G: Update of Eleanor Clarke Slagle Lecture: The occupational therapist in prevention programs, *Am J Occup Ther* 31:658, 1977.

28. Reference deleted in proofs.

29. Glanz K, Rimer BK, Lewis FM: *Health behavior and health education: theory, research and practice*, ed 3, San Francisco, 2002, Jossey-Bass.

30. Green LW, Kreuter MW: *Health promotion planning: an educational and environmental approach*, ed 2, Mountain View, CA, 1991, Mayfield.

31. Green LW, Kreuter MW: *Health promotion planning: an educational and ecological approach*, ed 3, Mountain View, CA, 1999, Mayfield.

32. Harlowe D: Occupational therapy for prevention of injury and physical dysfunction. In Pedretti LW, Early MB, editors: *Occupational therapy practice skills for physical dysfunction*, ed 5, St Louis, 2001, Mosby, pp 69–82.

33. Hills MD: Perspectives on learning and practicing health promotion in hospitals: nursing students' stories. In Young L, Hayes V, editors: *Transforming health promotion practice: concepts, issues, and applications*, Philadelphia, 2002, FA Davis, pp 229.

34. Hough J: Disability and health: a national public health agenda. In Simeonsson RJ, Bailey DB, editors: *Issues in disability and health: the role of secondary conditions and quality of life*, Chapel Hill, 1999, North Carolina Office on Disability and Health, pp 161.

35. Hyner GC, et al: *Society of Prospective Medicine handbook of health assessment tools*, Stoughton, WI, 1999, Wellness Associates Publications.

36. Janssen S., Hauck E., Miller S.: Leisure as a therapeutic modality. https://www.otinsnf.com, 2020.

37. Kalina JT: The role of occupational therapy in a multiple sclerosis center, *OT Practice.* 14:9, 2009.

38. Kielhofner G: The development of occupational therapy knowledge. In Kielhofner G, editor: *Conceptual foundations of occupational therapy*, ed 3. Philadelphia, 2004, FA Davis, pp 27.

39. Krahn G. *Institute on Disability and Development. Changing concepts in health, wellness and disability.* Proceedings of Changing Concepts of Health and Disability: State of the Science Conference and Policy Forum 2003. Portland OR: Oregon Health and Science University; 2003.

40. Kuo F, Pizzi M, Chang W-P, Fredrick A, Koning S: An exploratory study on the clinical utility of the Pizzi Healthy Weight Management Assessment (PHWMA) among Burmese high school students, *Amer J Occup Ther* (70):1–9, 2016. https://doi.org/10.5014/ajot.2016.021659.

41. Larson E, Wood W, Clark F: Occupational science: building the science and the practice of occupation through an academic discipline. In Crepeau EB, et al., editors: *Willard and Spackman's occupational therapy*, ed 10, Philadelphia, 2003, Lippincott Williams & Wilkins, pp 15.

42. Law M: *Evidence-based rehabilitation*, Thorofare, NJ, 2002, Slack.

43. Licht S: The founding and the founders of the American Occupational Therapy Association, *Am J Occup Ther* 21:269, 1967.

44. Mandel DR, et al: *Lifestyle Redesign: implementing the well-elderly program*, Bethesda, MD, 1999, American Occupational Therapy Association.

45. Oh H, Seo W: Decreasing pain and depression in a health promotion program for people with rheumatoid arthritis, *J Nurs Scholarsh* 35:127–132, 2003.

46. Ottenbacher KJ, Christiansen C:, ed 2. C: Occupational performance assessment. In Christiansen C, Baum C, editors: *Occupational therapy: enabling function and well-being*, ed 2, Thorofare, NJ, 1997, Slack.

47. Pickett G, Hanlon JJ: *Public health: administration and practice*, St Louis, 1990, Mosby.

48. Pizzi M: The Pizzi Holistic Wellness Assessment, *Occup Ther Health Care* 13:51, 2001.

49. Pizzi M: Health promotion for people with disabilities. In Scaffa M, Reitz SM, Pizzi M, editors: *Occupational therapy in the promotion of health and wellness*, Philadelphia, 2010, FA Davis, pp 376–396.

50. Pizzi M, editor: Editorial: Special issue on obesity and the role of occupational therapy. *Occup Therap in Health Care* 27(2):75–77, 2013.

51. Pizzi M. Obesity, health and quality of life: A conversation to further the vision in occupational therapy Occup Therap in Health Care 27(2):78–83, 2013.

52. Pizzi M: *Childhood obesity institute*, Chicago IL, April 9, 2016, Presentation at the AOTA 2016 annual conference.

53. Pizzi MA: editor: Special issue on health, well-being, and quality of life. *Am J Occup Ther* 2017; 71(4):7104170010. https://doi.org/10.5014/ajot.2017.028456.

54. Pizzi MA: Promoting disability awareness and occupational and social justice through a community-based arts and education not for profit organization. [Presentation at the Medical Anthropology at the Intersections conference, Yale University, September 27] 2009.

55. Pizzi MA: Promoting health and well-being at the end of life through client-centered care, *Scand J Occup Ther* 22:442–449, 2015.

56. Pizzi MA: Editorial: Promoting health, well-being, and quality of life for children who are overweight or obese and their families, *Am J Occup Ther* 70:1–6, 2016. https://doi.org/10.5014/ajot.2016.705001.

57. Pizzi M, Orloff S: Childhood obesity: emerging practice in occupational therapy, *New Zealand J Occup Ther* 61(1):29–38, 2015.

58. Pizzi MA, Renwick R: Quality of life and health promotion. In Scaffa ME, Reitz SM, Pizzi MA, editors: *Occupational therapy in the promotion of health and wellness*, Philadelphia, 2010, FA Davis, pp 122–134.

59. Pizzi MA, Richards LG: Promoting health, well-being, and quality of life in occupational therapy: a commitment to a paradigm shift for the next 100 years, *Am J Occup Ther* 71(4):1–5, 2017. 7104170010p1-7104170010p5

60. Pizzi M, Vroman KE: Childhood obesity: effects on children's participation, mental health, and psychosocial development, *Occup Therap in Health Care* 27(2):99–112, 2013.

61. Pizzi M, Vroman KG, Lau C, Gill SV, Bazyk S, Suarez-Balcazar Y, Orloff S: Occupational therapy and the childhood obesity epidemic: research, theory and practice. *J Occup Ther, Schools & Early Intervention* 7(2):87–105, 2014.

62. Powers L: *Health and wellness among persons with disabilities.* Proceedings of Changing Concepts of Health and Disability: State of the Science Conference and Policy Forum 2003; Portland, OR: Oregon Health and Science University; 2003.

63. Prochaska JO, Redding CA, Evers KE: The transtheoretical model and stages of change. In Glanz K, Rimer BK, Lewis FM, editors: *Health behavior and health education: theory, research and practice*, ed 3, San Francisco, 2002, Jossey-Bass, pp 99.

64. Punwar AJ: The development of occupational therapy. In Punwar AJ, Peloquin SM, editors: *Occupational therapy: principles and practice*, Baltimore, 2000, Lippincott Williams & Wilkins, pp 21.

65. Reed K: The beginnings of occupational therapy. In Hopkins H, Smith H, editors: *Willard and Spackman's occupational therapy*, ed 8, Philadelphia, 1993, Lippincott Williams & Wilkins, pp 26.

66. Reilly M: Occupational therapy can be one of the great ideas of the 20th century medicine, *Am J Occup Ther* 16:1, 1962.

67. Reitz SM: A historical review of occupational therapy's role in preventive health and wellness, *Am J Occup Ther* 46:50, 1992.

68. Reitz SM: Functional ethics. In Sladyk K, Ryan SE, editors: *Ryan's occupational therapy assistant: principles, practice issues, and techniques*, ed 4, Thorofare, NJ, 2005, Slack.

69. Reitz SM: Historical and philosophical perspectives of occupational therapy's role in health promotion. In Scaffa ME, Reitz SM, Pizzi MA, editors: *Occupational therapy in the promotion of health and wellness*, Philadelphia, 2010, FA Davis, pp 1–21.

70. Reitz SM, Scaffa ME, Pizzi MA: Occupational therapy conceptual models for health promotion practice. In Scaffa ME, Reitz SM, Pizzi MA, editors: *Occupational therapy in the promotion of health and wellness*, Philadelphia, 2010, FA Davis, pp 22–45.

71. Reitz SM, Scaffa ME, Campbell RM, Rhynders PA: Health behavior frameworks for health promotion practice. In Scaffa ME, Reitz SM, Pizzi MA, editors: *Occupational therapy in the promotion of health and wellness*, Philadelphia, 2010, FA Davis, pp 46–69.

72. Rimmer JH: Health promotion for people with disabilities: the emerging paradigm shift from disability prevention to prevention of secondary conditions, *Phys Ther* 79:495, 1999.

73. Rybski D, Arnold MJ: *Broadening the concepts of community and occupation: perspectives in a global society*, Park City, UT, [October 17] 2003, [Paper presented at the Society for the Study of Occupation: USA Second Annual Research Conference].

74. Scaffa ME: *Occupational therapy in community-based practice settings*, Philadelphia, 2001, FA Davis.

75. Scaffa ME, Reitz SM, Pizzi MA: *Occupational therapy in the promotion of health and wellness*, Philadelphia, 2010, FA Davis.

76. Schwartz KB: The history of occupational therapy. In Crepeau EB, Cohn ES, Schell BA, editors: *Willard and Spackman's occupational therapy*, ed 10, Philadelphia, 2003, Lippincott Williams & Wilkins, pp 5.

77. Reference deleted in proofs.

78. Serwe KM, Walmsley, ALE, Pizzi MA: Reliability and responsiveness of the Pizzi Health and Wellness Assessment, *Annals of International Occup Ther* 3(1):7–13, 2019.

79. Sinclair K. *Message to the AOTA Representative Assembly from the WFOT President.* [Department of Rehabilitation Sciences, Hong Kong Polytechnic University, May] 2004.

80. Stuifbergen AK, Rogers S: Health promotion: an essential component of rehabilitation for persons with chronic disabling conditions, *ANS Adv Nurs Sci* 19:1–20, 1997.

81. Stuifbergen AK, Gordon D, Clark AP: Health promotion: a complementary strategy for stroke rehabilitation, *Topics Stroke Rehabil.* 5:11–18, 1998.

82. Townsend E: Enabling occupation in the 21st century: making good intentions a reality, *Aust Occup Ther J* 46:147, 1999.

83. Trentham B, Cockburn L: Participatory action research: creating new knowledge and opportunities for occupational engagement. In Kronenberg F, Simo Algado S, Pollard N, editors: *Occupational therapy without borders: learning from the spirit of survivors*, London, 2005, Elsevier, pp 440–453.

84. United Nations. *Convention and optional protocol signatures and ratifications.* https://www.un.org/development/desa/disabilities/resources/handbook-for-parliamentarians-on-the-convention-on-the-rights-of-persons-with-disabilities/chapter-four-becoming-a-party-to-the-convention-and-the-optional-protocol.html#:~:text=The%20Convention%20and%20the%20Optional%20Protocol%20both%20provide,the%20State%20becomes%20legally%20bound%20by%20the%20treaty.

85. United Nations. *Convention on the Rights of Persons with Disabilities.* https://www.un.org/development/desa/disabilities/convention-on-the-rights-of-persons-with-disabilities/convention-on-the-rights-of-persons-with-disabilities-2.html.

86. University of Southern California: *Department of Occupational Science and Occupational Therapy. Occupational science and the making of community, Fourteenth Annual Occupational Science Symposium*, Los Angeles, January 26, 2002, Davidson Center.

87. University of Southern California: Chan Division of Occupational Science and Occupational Therapy. *Patient*

care—about the USC occupational therapy practice. http://chan.usc.edu/patient-care/faculty-practice.

88. US Department of Health and Human Services: *US Public Health Service. Healthy people 2000: national health promotion and disease prevention objectives. [conference edition],* Washington, D.C., 1990, US Government Printing Office.

89. US Department of Health and Human Services. *Healthy people 2030: about healthy people.* https://health.gov/our-work/healthy-people-2030.

90. US Department of Health and Human Services. *Healthy people 2030: framework.* https://www.healthypeople.gov/2020/About-Healthy-People/Development-Healthy-People-2030/Framework.

91. Reference deleted in proofs.

92. West WL: The occupational therapist's changing responsibility to the community, *Am J Occup Ther* 21:312, 1967.

93. West WL: The growing importance of prevention, *Am J Occup Ther* 23:226, 1969.

94. White V: Special issue on health promotion, *Am J Occup Ther* 40:743–748, 1986.

95. Wiemer R: Some concepts of prevention as an aspect of community health, *Am J Occup Ther* 26:1, 1972.

96. Wiemer R, West W: Occupational therapy in community healthcare, *Am J Occup Ther* 24:323, 1970.

97. Wilcock AA: *An occupational perspective of health.* Slack: Thorofare, NJ; 1998.

98. Wilcock AA, Townsend E: Occupational terminology interactive dialogue: occupational justice, *J Occup Sci.* 7:84, 2000.

99. World Federation of Occupational Therapists. Position statement—environmental sustainability, sustainable practice within occupational therapy.

100. World Health Organization: *The Ottawa Charter for Health Promotion*, First International Conference on Health Promotion, Ottawa. http://www.euro.who.int/AboutWHO/Policy/20010827_2#.

6

The Lived Experience of Disability: The Intersection of Disability Perspectives and Occupational Justice

Samia Husam Rafeedie and Robert J.T. Russow

LEARNING OBJECTIVES

After studying this chapter, the student or practitioner will be able to do the following:

1. Identify the environmental factors and personal factors that have an impact on participation and engagement in occupation, as defined by the Occupational Therapy Practice Framework-4.
2. Describe the complex construction of a disability identity and why people with disabilities may or may not disclose that identity in a clinical setting.
3. Describe how stigma, spread, and negative attitudes toward people with disabilities have impacted the care and services received by people with disabilities.
4. Identify ways in which the medical model and social model fall short of meeting the needs of people living with disabilities.
5. Apply concepts of occupational justice to occupational therapy practice, with a focus on maximizing capabilities.
6. Describe the impact of a social justice framework and contemporary models of practice on the role of OT practitioners when working with the disability community.

CHAPTER OUTLINE

KEY TERMS

Ableism
Capabilities approach
Capabilities, Opportunities, Resources and Environments (CORE) approach
Disclosure
Environmental factors
Neurodiversity

Occupational justice
Occupational rights
Personal factors
Social justice
Spread
Stigma

Occupational therapy (OT) practitioners have a long and rich history of working with clients who have different abilities, whether the differences are congenital or acquired. The profession has defined its work through the *Framework* (American Occupational Therapy Association [AOTA], 1979), which was originally a document developed in response to a federal requirement to develop a uniform reporting system. This document gradually morphed into the *Uniform Terminology for Occupational Therapy* (AOTA, 1989), and it was not until 1994 that the AOTA included contextual aspects of performance into the document. With revisions every 5 years, clients were defined as persons, groups, and populations in 2012; and finally, with the 2020 revisions of the *Occupational Therapy Practice Framework v.4 (OTPF-4)*, a *community* has been defined as a "collection of populations that is changeable and diverse and includes various people, groups, networks, and organizations."[6,77,90] The reader of the OTPF-4 is reminded that it is "important to consider the community or communities with which a client identifies throughout the occupational therapy process."[6] The disability community draws attention to the complexities of occupational therapy practitioners having their historical place in the

medical model as rehabilitation practitioners while attempting to embrace the social model of disability (see Chapter 2 for more about the social model of disability, disability rights, and the independent living movement).

Occupational therapy has been criticized by the disability community for unintentionally extending the perspective of the medical community into the realm of rehabilitation, in that disabled people need to be fixed and that they are not "normal." Abberley[1] concluded that, "[Occupational therapy], despite what may be the best intentions on the part of its practitioners, serves to perpetuate the process of disablement of impaired people" (p. 222). Through experiences in the classroom during occupational therapy educational programs, these dominating medical views of disabilities are reinforced, even when learning activities are not planned with this intention.

The late Gary Kielhofner[47] reported that disability rights scholars[10,29,35,49] "further argue that rehabilitation's traditional beliefs and perspectives misconstrue disability and can result in unnecessary negative consequences for disabled persons" (p. 488). He challenged the field to consider two questions: What is the cause of the disability, and what should be done

THREADED CASE STUDY

Katie, Part 1

Katie is a graduate student in an occupational therapy program and ready to embark on her second semester of school. This semester she is taking the physical dysfunctions course and has heard about the 24-hour wheelchair assignment from students who have taken the course in the past. Students, faculty, and staff on campus are accustomed to seeing the occupational therapy students using wheelchairs across campus, in the dining halls, loading the wheelchairs in and out of their vehicles in the parking garage, or requesting that the lift on the university tram be lowered so they can access the shuttle to get to another part of campus. The reputation of the assignment has moved through generations of students, and Katie was anxious to see how the experience would shape the minds and hearts of her peers and future colleagues.

Katie needs to use a wheelchair. She spent the majority of her life moving from point A to point B without the use of an assistive device; however, a recent hip fracture after a fall on wet pavement means that Katie needs this wheelchair for energy conservation, safety, and a way to get around campus efficiently. Katie was diagnosed with osteogenesis imperfecta, or "brittle bone disease" as a baby. The condition is hereditary, and her parents knew she was at risk, because Katie's father has the same diagnosis. The 24-hour wheelchair assignment was timely, as she progressed in her rehabilitation and learned how to manage the environmental barriers associated with using a wheelchair on campus.

In fact, Katie grew to learn that the 24-hour wheelchair assignment had those very same intentions and objectives for the students taking the physical dysfunctions course—that environmental barriers would be identified and analyzed, that students would learn to recognize issues related to access such as buildings without ramps or pneumatic switches for opening doors, that the lack of curb cuts will limit safe access onto a sidewalk, and that people will stare when they see someone moving around campus in a different way. Disability simulations have a long history of existing in occupational therapy programs and curricula across the United States, from blindfolding students to simulate "being blind" and tying one arm behind their backs to simulate "having hemiplegia." This was an opportunity for students to become more sensitive to a person's feelings, when functional skills are negatively affected by a medical condition, or when a person's independence is compromised. Katie felt

excited about the potential for this assignment and anticipated a positive outcome from her peers, who could benefit from this experience to gain empathy in preparation for working as future clinicians.

Each student was to "sign out" a generic, attendant-propelled wheelchair that was not custom-fit or available with the necessary leg rests or seat cushions. They would borrow the wheelchair and then return it after 24 hours of "living life" and experiencing the environmental barriers, outward societal stigmas, and physical challenges associated with this new way of moving. Several students lived in a graduate apartment complex on the university's main campus, and Katie saw those students hoisting their wheelchairs out of their trunks and contemplating how they would get the wheelchairs up the stairs, since the elevator in the building was rarely working. She overheard one student call the university and demand that the elevator be repaired immediately. She saw another student put the wheelchair back in the trunk and walk up the stairs, not willing to inconvenience herself or her evening plans. Back at school, she saw students from the course park their wheelchairs in the hallway outside of the bathroom, and then walk into the space to use the bathroom and wash their hands before returning to the hallway to sit in their wheelchairs again. She overheard others complaining about sore arms, sore bottoms, and discomfort as people stared at them using their chairs at the grocery store, at the library, and at the restaurant. One classmate even described an argument they had with the university tram driver. The driver refused to "waste time" lowering the lift, because he knew that the students were "just faking it" and they could get up and walk onto the tram. Katie felt discouraged and confused.

Critical Thinking Questions
1. How could an assignment with so much good intention be sending the wrong message?
2. How can this assignment be modified so that stigmas and stereotypes are not reinforced with a negative experience by the students?
3. How can occupational justice and social justice frameworks address what Katie is feeling towards the assignment, her identity as a disabled person, and a future occupational therapist?

about the disability? According to the literature and history of the occupational therapy profession, the answer to the first question followed the traditional medical model by defining disability as a personal deficiency or deviation from normal development.[47,52,60,78,96] This is echoed in the occupational therapy paradigm shift away from occupation, reflecting that of reductionism and focusing on neurological, kinesiological, and the intrapsychic workings of the human body, as seen in the 1980s and 1990s.[46] Measuring range of motion, manual muscle strength, cognition, and other quantitative outcomes became more important than engaging in a meaningful occupation because that is what was needed to keep in step with the medical professionals with whom occupational therapy practitioners worked. These measurements were essential in proving to the medical team that occupational therapy was beneficial in making progress and documenting improvements to help a client get back to normal or to the previous level of functioning and "fix the problem." Oliver[67] described normalization as a popular ideology and wrote that a normal state of existence was far more desirable than having an impairment or disability.

With respect to what should be done about disability,[47] occupational therapy, among other rehabilitation disciplines, developed a response. The response was to create solutions and find strategies that supported those with disabilities to, "ameliorate or minimize the impact of impairments and their consequences while encouraging the person with impairments to be as independent and normal as possible."[47] This perspective negatively reinforced the identity of the disabled person and further reinforced the oppression felt by disabled people. In the OTPF-4, identity falls within personal factors and oppression falls within environmental factors, both important areas for occupational therapy practitioners to consider during the occupational therapy process.

CONTEXT: ENVIRONMENTAL FACTORS AND PERSONAL FACTORS SUPPORTING OCCUPATION

According to the OTPF-4, context is the term used to describe the environmental and personal factors that are specific to each client, whether that client is a person, group, or population. The context also "affects clients' access to occupations and the quality of and satisfaction with performance."[6] It is important for an occupational therapy practitioner to consider the contexts in which occupations take place, or where they could potentially take place, as part of an occupation-based, top-down approach to evaluation and intervention.

PERSONAL FACTORS

Personal factors are "the unique features of a person that are not part of a health condition or health state and that constitute the particular background of the person's life and living."[6] Personal factors should be viewed as neither positive nor negative, but rather as a reflection of who the client is as a person. They have an impact on function and disability and are, at times, described as basic demographic information such as chronological age, sexual orientation/preference/identity, gender identity, race, ethnicity, cultural identity, socioeconomic status, life experiences, lifestyle, professional identity, and fitness status, to name a few.[6] There are clear connections between personal factors and one's identity, particularly one who identifies as disabled or having a disability.

Disability Identity

Identity is a complex construction developed to make sense of the internal and external realities surrounding a person. Internal realities are defined by the way people view themselves from within, and external realities are defined by the way people view themselves based on societal perspectives. What complicates this aspect of identity construction further is that this process is trying to reconcile the internal and external realities simultaneously.[27] Siebers saw identity as a tool for helping navigate through the social world.[82] As people become inserted into the social world, interactions with others continue to develop that identity. Self-narrative, then, is a tool for navigating the complexities of self and world.[72] Stories have power in their ability to define reality for a person, and the societal accumulation of these stories, in the context of disability, helps define what is and is not a life worth living.[33]

Development of Disability Identity

Narrative plays an essential role in the development of disability identity. One model of disability identity development has been proposed by Forber-Pratt and Zape based on their interviews with persons with disabilities.[27] The authors conceptualized four different statuses that an individual might identify with during their lived experience with disability. These are not stages to be moved through in a linear fashion, but rather statuses that may be moved through in any order or even experienced concurrently. These statuses are identified as *acceptance, relationship, adoption, and engagement.*

Acceptance status consists of the individual accepting their own disability. This may happen earlier or later in life in relation to the occurrence of the disability, or it may never be achieved. This includes acceptance by both the individual and family and friends. Often, conflict can arise by family or friends being slower to accept the disability compared to the person's acceptance. *Relationship status* focuses on the social support created by the person, especially in relationships with other persons with disabilities. Forber-Pratt and Zape found that some study participants were able to connect immediately with others who had similar disabilities, whereas some needed warming up time to enrich their network.[27] There appears to be power in connecting to others in similar circumstances. Thinking in terms of disability identity and community, there is comfort in being understood and supported during times of need. The proliferation of online communities is evidence of this desire to connect, even if it is in a virtual context.

When persons' focus moves beyond individual relationships to disability culture as a whole, they may be working toward attainment of *adoption status.* They begin to "adopt" the values of the disability community and engage in a broader manner. Identity develops as they consciously or unconsciously explore how they relate to those broader values and determine which of them to "adopt." This includes becoming familiar with the formal and informal rules of what it means to have a disability. There is also an emerging focus on advocacy, more specifically, people may be more cautious in applying this strategy and weighing the consequences of potential retaliation versus being successful in their advocacy efforts. *Engagement status* is when a person with a disability shifts beyond taking on characteristics of disability culture and moves to a role model position to give back to the community. This could involve leadership in disability organizations, mentorship, public speaking, and even leading by example. As part of that mentorship, a person might help individuals who are currently in other statuses.[27]

It would seem that there is a progression to these statuses—a widening of scope from the individual to close relationships to community and then to leadership within the community—which might make the distinction of statuses and stages more of a semantic one than a practical one. Individuals experiencing these statuses, however, may identify with more than one at the same time, move fluidly between them, and also do not necessarily have to experience all of them to have a strong disability identity.[27]

Disclosure of Identity

Disability, at least in part, is shaped by social forces and influences manners of relating. **Disclosure** of impairment information, a relational tool, has historically been central to the disability experience and the shaping of disability identity.[25] Significant physical disability was often much more apparent and overt than invisible disabilities, giving the latter group more freedom with regard to how much to disclose and with whom to disclose. Changing technology and societal structures, including more frequent digital communication and a normalization of remote work, has served to minimize some of the overt visibility for a person with disabilities.

Different methods of disclosure reflect different disability self-images. Evans describes three methods for disclosure as *confessional disclosure, pragmatic disclosure,* and *validating disclosure* and what those methods reveal about an individual's self-image.[25] An individual with feelings of guilt or shame related to their disability may practice *confessional disclosure* when something arises that requires them to discuss their disability. Often, this disclosure is used as a reason to ask for help, not when advocating for certain rights (e.g., obtaining an accommodation), but rather as a justification. These feelings of guilt may also lead a person to not ask for help, which can further exacerbate a situation. Confessional disclosure also can be used for a different type of justification, such as poor performance at work, which can be a frequent source of shame for those who have centered their identity around their professional selves.[25]

Pragmatic disclosure is centered around individuals clearly communicating their needs in a given context. Those with disabilities or their family/allies may suggest ways in which an environment can be adjusted to better suit those needs, whether that be related to the built environment or any other barriers in the social or structural environment. Pragmatic disclosure also can be associated with legal requirements for access to curriculum at a public school or access to the entry of a public building.

There might be additional difficulty in advocating for needs in more complex environments, such as information systems or within the policies of a larger corporation, but building flexibility into these facets of a person's life creates many pragmatic benefits. In an ideal situation, these disclosures would help facilitate communication between relevant parties that would ultimately result in improved participation and clear expectations, such as between family members, student-teacher relationships, and employer-employee relationships.[25]

If a person discloses information with the intention of highlighting the validity of their difference, they are practicing *validating disclosure*. One benefit of this approach is that it serves "to invite dialogue, identify allies, or to signal one's identification with a disability community."[25] When a disability is not apparent, validating disclosures can be a discerning tool for finding allies who can then help with processing situations and information. These types of disclosures can be seen as a "declaration" that the difference they are living with is an equally valid expression of life—something that could be disorienting to existing societal assumptions of disability.[25]

ENVIRONMENTAL FACTORS

According to Kielhofner, "Disability scholars point out that the rehabilitation focus on impairment can also reinforce the idea that impairments are the essential characteristics of disability and that persons are disabled because they are lacking in some functional capacity such as moving, seeing, hearing, or thinking."[47] This harmful notion further strengthens the idea that society imposes onto people with disabilities in that impairment is an individual's problem, not a problem with the environment or society. The focus on the individual's limitations obscures the deeper concerns inherent in the social, political, and economic environments in which we live and function.[53,73]

Environmental factors are defined as "aspects of the physical, social, and attitudinal surroundings in which people live and conduct their lives."[6] They include the natural environment and human-made changes to the environment; products and technology; support and relationships; attitudes; and services, systems, and policies. Each of these environmental factors becomes critical when working with a person who has a disability. *Support and relationships* are critical facets of the environmental factors considered by a clinician. Support can be provided by people or animals and can be provided in a physical or emotional sense in the home, school, or work environment where daily occupations take place. The *natural environment and human-made changes to the environment* include animate or inanimate elements in the natural or physical environment, including those elements that have been modified or adapted to meet the needs of a client. This is one of the basic tenets of occupational therapy, to modify an object or adapt a space to promote engagement in a task or participation at the highest level of independence.

Products and technology are either natural or human-made pieces of equipment or technology that are created, produced, or manufactured to support the needs of a person. Bickenbach,[11] a disability rights law and policy maker who has drawn on Irving Zola's work, reminds us that the "special needs" approach to disability is inevitably shortsighted. If the mismatches between impairments and the social, attitudinal, architectural, medical, economic, and political environment are viewed as merely a problem facing the individual with a disability, we are ignoring that disability is an essential feature of the human condition. It is not whether a disability will occur, but when; not so much which one, but how many and in what combination. The entire population is at risk for the impairments associated with chronic illness and disability. As people live longer, the incidence of disability increases. Viewing disability as an abnormality does not provide a realistic picture of the human experience. Bickenbach, in his discussion of disability as a human rights issue, underlined the fact that disability is a constant and fundamental part of the human experience and that no individual has a perfect set of abilities for all contexts; there are no fixed boundaries dividing all the variations in human abilities. Our usual description of contrast between ability and disability is, in fact, a continuum of functionality in various settings.[11]

This perspective affects occupational therapy's role in the realm of assistive technology and modification of the environment to enhance individual performance of occupational behavior. Our literature is overflowing with discussions about assistive technology (see Chapter 17) and environmental modifications; applications with various diagnostic classifications, methods for training in the use of assistive technology, the usefulness of providing a specialized device to enhance performance, and home modifications. The concept of universal design (the way the environment may be designed to support individual differences) is not as prominent in our professional literature. This idea includes the built environment, information technology, and consumer products, in addition to a host of commercial and social transactions, usable by all people, to the greatest extent possible, without the need for adaptation or specialized design. The concept is this: if devices (e.g., buildings, computers, educational services) are designed with the needs of people with disabilities in mind, they will be more usable for all users, regardless of whether they have disabilities.

Disability is just one of many characteristics that an individual might have that should influence the design of our environments. An example of universal design is ramped entries, which are required by federal law (Americans with Disabilities Act Accessibility Guidelines [ADAAG]) in public buildings (including transportation services, such as airports and train stations) and designed for those who use wheelchairs. As that design requirement has become increasingly implemented, the use of wheeled luggage by all travelers, in addition to parents pushing children in strollers and delivery staff with rolling carts, has become commonplace. Just imagine the impact on home modification if new housing construction design regulations included the legal requirement for one entrance easily adaptable and a bathroom door wide enough for wheelchair access (see Chapter 15).

Activists in the independent living movement have influenced the personal computer and digital device industry to integrate a multitude of individual preferences, from the size and type of the font to the ease with which adaptive technologies such as speech recognition and alternative keyboards interact with operating systems. In another example of successful advocacy, standards were issued under the Rehabilitation Act in 2000 to address access to electronic and information technology for people with physical, sensory, or cognitive disabilities (see the website http://www.access-board.gov/guidelines-and-standards/communications-and-it/about-the-section-508-standards). Universal design in instruction is becoming evident as educators are increasingly trained to include multiple modalities of visual, auditory, and tactile systems to address the needs of people with wide differences in the ability to see, hear, speak, move, read, write, understand English, attend, organize, engage, and remember.[15]

Some argue that universal design principles could make assistive technology unnecessary in many situations involving an impairment. A can opener that has been designed for one-handed use by anyone busy preparing multiple steps in a recipe will also be usable by the cook who has hemiparesis caused by a cerebrovascular accident (CVA). Universally designed devices and aids may be one remedy for the stigmatization attached to special equipment. As Daarragh et al.[19] pointed out, there is a trade off with the potential usefulness of a device and the concerns about social acceptability and aesthetics. Beatrice Wright, a social psychologist, studied and wrote for many years about society's reactions to people with disability.[94] She used the term spread to describe how the presence of disability or an atypical physique serves as a stimulus to inferences, assumptions, or expectations about the person who has a disability. For example, a person who is blind may be shouted at, as though lack of vision also indicates impaired hearing; or a person with cerebral palsy and a speech impairment may be assumed to be intellectually challenged. An extreme manifestation of spread is the belief that an individual's life must be a tragedy because he or she has a disability, and this is experienced through various methods from movies and television shows to social media and personal interactions.

Attitudes include "observable evidence of customs, practices, ideologies, values, norms, factual beliefs, and religious beliefs held by people other than the client."[6] Negative attitudes toward those with disabilities have been described by researchers in the disability community and must be a priority for occupational therapy practitioners because they will shape the relationships developed between practitioners and clients, and they also affect a person's emotional and psychological contributions to the therapeutic process.

Attitudes Toward Disability

Goffman defined stigma as "an attribute that is deeply discrediting" (p. 3),[32] not because of anything inherent to that attribute, but because of contextual factors. Goffman's theoretical work shaped conceptualizations of the performative nature of disability and stigma: acting out the expectations others place on an individual in different social contexts, even when those expectations fail to align with that individual's actual self.

Goffman's work has since been critiqued and expanded upon as the theoretical models of disability have come into existence and a broader lexicon has been adopted by disability scholars. Similarly, the use of stigma as a concept for

THREADED CASE STUDY

Katie, Part 2

Katie decided to meet with her professor, because she was worried that this assignment was more of a hassle and inconvenience to her peers, the managers of the university apartment housing, and even the tram driver. She worried that her friends were not experiencing the eye-opening and educational opportunity of this assignment, but rather, that it was turning into a nuisance, a dreaded experience, and ultimately changing their emotions to those of feeling pity for people with disabilities and for those who actually use wheelchairs in their day-to-day lives. Katie described to her professor that students (who do not actually have limitations in participating in occupation or a medical diagnosis that warrants using a wheelchair) are only experiencing 24 hours of inconvenience and frustrations and not truly getting a sense of what a person's life is like when overcoming these initial feelings and "barriers." People living with disabilities learn how to navigate a campus, open heavy doors from a seated position, adjust the leg rests, acquire a seat cushion, and learn how to talk to someone who is staring at them. People who use wheelchairs develop their own ways of adapting, living, and demonstrating resilience. What her peers were experiencing was not truly reflective of what it is like to be her for one day, and the assignment was feeling increasingly more like an insult to her. Katie asked her professor, "How could the students know what it is like to be me, by pretending to use a wheelchair for one day and then getting up, and stepping back into their able-bodied worlds, as if it never happened?"

Each student was required to complete the 24-hour wheelchair assignment experience by writing a one-page reflection upon returning the wheelchair. The reflections mirrored Katie's fears, that students would get out of those chairs and simply walk to their cars as if nothing happened and that they were merely inconvenienced for 24 hours. They simply completed something they had to do for class and crossed that item off the list of homework due that week. Student reflections included comments like, "I'm so glad I don't have to use a wheelchair. It is so hard. I can't stand when people stare at me;" and "I hope nobody in my family ever has to live life like that;" and "I got out of that wheelchair and just

thanked God that wasn't my life." Katie's professor could see that the intention of the assignment was skewed, and the students were certainly receiving "the wrong message." Katie and her professor knew that the assignment had to change; and that something had to be done so that the very lessons that were intended in the assignment could still be addressed, but students would not literally walk away from the assignment experiencing only the negative outcomes of a "day in the life."

Katie and her professor consulted with Ann, an expert in the fields of disability studies and occupational therapy. That expert was known for her disability rights advocacy because she had a disability, and expressed concerns she long held related to class activities such as the 24-hour wheelchair assignment and how they were implemented in occupational therapy programs. Ann summarized that there were, indeed, educational benefits of simulation and role-play in a professional program curriculum; however, they needed to be implemented carefully and thoughtfully.

Ann told Katie and her professor that role-playing is used in healthcare curricula to teach students about the literature, history, or even the technical procedures used in practice. Simulations are also used in areas such as assertiveness and social skills training as a way to get the students to become interested and involved in a safe environment, where mistakes can be made and corrected by the educator, without endangering a patient. It is generally understood that simulations and role-playing can create the very challenges that practitioners experience in a real clinical setting and that there are benefits to creating these experiences in the safety of a classroom. They have to be implemented carefully, however, so as to not reinforce the negative stigmas or perceptions of society onto people with disabilities. The consultation left Katie and her professor with much to consider. They could now also recognize that simulations and role-playing could be problematic if the experience is not carefully implemented and if reflection and discussion are not part of the process.

---

understanding negative societal attitudes toward persons with disabilities has been expanded. Stigma has three main qualities: fear, stereotyping, and social control.[18] Fear represents the affective facet of stigma—when a person fears having to use a wheelchair, for example, that is the effect of stigma on their emotions. Stereotyping represents the cognitive facet of stigma. In the previous example of using a wheelchair, when people think that using a wheelchair means they will be unable to do anything for themselves (false stereotype), that is the effect of stigma on their thoughts. Barriers resulting from attitudes toward persons with disabilities arise from stereotypes, fear, and insufficient knowledge,[13] leading to the third quality of stigma: social control. Social control represents the behavioral facet of stigma. Continuing the example of wheelchair users, when there are insufficient curb cutouts and other physical barriers or when a person does not hire persons with disabilities for jobs they are qualified for, those are the effects of stigma on behaviors.

The process of stigmatization occurs in four stages.[51] The first stage is that difference is distinguished and named, or labeled. This is followed by stage two, in which a connection is made between that difference and something that is undesirable. Stage three is when the person with an undesirable difference is categorized, creating a separation; and in the last stage, that

separation creates discrimination and differences in health and life outcomes.[51] These stages parallel the concepts of ableism and disablism, which bookend the process of stigmatization. Ableism creates the false truth that people without disabilities are superior through an assumption of normalcy.[13] Assuming that such a thing as "normal" exists, it follows that there must be abnormal that can then be distinguished (as in stage 1 above). Once abnormal, or different, has been defined and identified as something undesirable, action can be taken against individuals in these categories (as in stage 4). This exclusionary process is known as disablism.[13]

Different types of stigma can result from exclusionary policies and attitudes: enacted stigma, anticipated stigma, internalized stigma, and perceived community stigma.[21,22,85] Enacted stigma is the actual experience of discrimination as a result of the "undesirable" difference. Anticipated stigma is when people believe there will be some form of discrimination in the future as a result of their difference. Internalized stigma is when people with disabilities begin to accept those negative characterizations of their difference as inherent to them. Finally, perceived community stigma "refers to a person's perceptions of the *severity* of stigmatizing attitudes that exist in the community."[85] These forms of stigma have consequences for different domains in the life of a person with a disability.

Consequences of Stigmatization

Stereotyping and stigma are powerful tools for shaping what a society defines as "ideal." Several studies on attitudes toward persons with disabilities suggest an inverse relationship between social distance and disability severity. That is, the more severe the disability, the greater social distance (maintaining friendships versus dating or marriage) a person without disabilities would choose.[42,55,57] In one study, respondents were more willing to have a relationship with a person with physical disabilities over intellectual or psychological disabilities.[57] In another study, females were more willing than males to have a relationship with a person with disabilities.[42] Some of the reasons given for not wanting to have a more intimate relationship with a person with disabilities include the relationship being too much work, awkwardness interacting with a person with disabilities, the person being too sick or ill, and a fear over perceived lack of sexual satisfaction.[55]

In terms of affective consequences for persons with disabilities, research has found that stigma is connected to lower self-esteem, decreased social support, and increased depressive symptoms.[85] Gill[31] labeled the erosion of self-esteem by continued stigmatization "internalized oppression." These psychological effects were primarily the result of the interplay between perceived community stigma and internalized stigma. The more severely a person perceives stigmatizing attitudes to be in a community, the more a person appears to accept these negative stereotypes as part of their identity. In addition to the psychological effect, behaviorally, persons who experience continued stigmatization may have a decrease in medication adherence and a decrease in physician trust.[85]

Stigma in Rehabilitation

Medicine and rehabilitation have both been accused of using structures and policies to create distance between the practitioner and their client.[56] Within institutions such as hospitals and skilled nursing facilities, these structures and policies are commonplace. Ritual task performance, especially when time is limited, creates the possibility that practitioners could treat their client like a homogenous item on an assembly line. Tasks such as taking blood pressure, drawing blood, bringing and setting up meals at established times, and emptying bedpans or urinals are all examples of tasks that could become depersonalized.

Another institutional policy that depersonalizes care is when professionals are regularly moved to different units. For those institutions that employ such a policy, deeper connection is much more difficult because of the lack of consistency. In addition, clients continue to be faced with new strangers performing intimate tasks. This lack of familiarity can also lead to clients being labeled "difficult" or "noncompliant." These clients might be in extreme pain, for example, but because they do not conform to the "deferential norm," they are seen as "difficult."[56]

"Noncompliance" or "nonadherence" to medical or rehabilitative recommendations is not an intrinsic failure on the part of the client. It is a failure of the client-therapist relationship; the client has goals and plans that are different from what the medical or rehabilitation practitioner has determined are important; and the professional has failed to facilitate meaningful conversation to bridge the divide.[75] When a client is labeled as "unmotivated," it just means the practitioner has discovered something not intrinsically valuable to the client. Whatever the practitioner expected and valued does not have the same importance to the client, and the practitioner needs to reconnect with more skill and empathy.

At their core, all of these policies and practices are limiting intimacy; avoiding intimacy encourages sympathy and pity rather than empathy. Visit any hospital and listen to the common refrain of, "Oh that poor person with [name a health condition] and their family. . . ." That phrase ultimately belies a deeper truth, that pity is just "stigma clothed as compassion."[33] Labels and language have power; understanding how that power manifests in the context of disability is important in reassigning power within the therapeutic relationship.

Use of Language

Language is one tool by which the powerful group remains in control[33,97] and has historical power with implications for persons with a disability. During World War I, the phrase "shell shock" was coined to describe certain mental health symptoms associated with the war and was predominantly used when describing the symptoms for officers. Common soldiers were persecuted minorities at the time (Irish and Jewish soldiers), and the word "hysteria" was used to describe their mental health symptoms.[33] Those soldiers who were said to have hysteria were much less likely to receive treatment compared to the officers with "shell shock." The function of a label is to perpetuate the connection between disability and abnormality or wrongness.[97] That association between a label such as "crazy" or "noncompliant" and wrongness allows people to dismiss the labeled person and their behavior without looking deeper. Another problem with labels, as with categories or even diagnoses, is that they become broad categories with certain expectations that miss individual differences and subtleties unique to the experience of the person with disabilities.[97]

Language, as seen in the previous example of soldiers during World War I, can communicate a message beyond the literal meaning of the words used.[97] Choosing to use active versus passive verbs dramatically changes the connotation underlying a statement. When using passive verbs, such as "being confined to a wheelchair," the person is controlled by the action of the verb. Using active verbs, on the other hand, the person is in control and performs the action, such as "using a wheelchair." Another associational meaning in language choice is the difference in using "to be" as compared to "to have." By saying someone "is a father," one implies equivalence between the subject and the label of "father" as opposed to saying someone "has children," which implies the subject possesses that quality. A similar separation is achieved with the use of prepositions in person-first language, for example, with the phrase "person *with* disabilities."[97]

Opponents of person-first language argue that this separation and distancing between a person and the person's disabilities in fact weakens the political power of the disability rights movement. For some, there is political power in categorization and pride in labeling oneself.[97] In addition, changing language avoids acknowledging the offensive associations and the discomfort with those terms. "Mentally handicapped" became "special needs," which then became "learning disabled" or having an "intellectual disability."[56] The goal in changing language used to describe disability is to change the perceptions, or stigma, associated with the disability. However, one concern with this strategy is that people will simply transfer the negative connotations or hostility to the new term, rather than having the hostility be transparent as with "mentally handicapped." Stigma will be hidden behind the new, "sterilized" language.[13]

Terminological modification can help change attitudes, especially if they maintain an essence of the reality of the condition.[13,97] One example of this is the term "neurodiversity," which was created to bring a more positive connotation to autism. Autism was once highly stigmatized, but increased awareness has led to a more flexible understanding of personhood and acceptance within society.[33] The term neurodiversity connotes that autism is one of many neurological states that are unique and valuable. Pairing with "neurotypical," a point society determines as normal thought and behavior, these terms recognize the social construction of language and normalcy, as opposed to using "normal," which implies a universal truth or value.[33]

Social Media and Attitudes Toward Disability

Historically, disability studies focused on critiques of traditional media, such as film and television, when examining portrayals of disability. Despite the emergence of new media, with new methods of communication and connection, many common stereotypes have persisted. One stereotype, elucidated by Black and Pretes,[12] is the person with a disability as pitiable and pathetic, a stereotype strategically deployed for charity drives, as a tool for creating sympathy from a nondisabled viewer. Typically, this stereotype might have been seen during a telethon to raise money, most famously demonstrated by the Jerry Lewis telethon for muscular dystrophy broadcast every Labor Day holiday for over 40 years in the United States.

With social media, new forms of pity-generating images took shape, a phenomenon that came to be known as "inspiration porn." Stella Young, a disability activist described inspiration porn as "an image of a person with a disability, often a kid, doing something completely ordinary—such as playing, or talking or running, or drawing a picture, or hitting a tennis ball—carrying a caption such as 'your excuse is invalid' or 'before you quit, try. . . .' Inspiration porn shames people with disabilities. It says that if we fail to be happy, to smile and to live lives that make those around us feel good, it's because we are not trying hard enough. . . . Let me be clear about the intent of this inspiration porn; it's there so that non-disabled people can put their worries into perspective."[95] Pity is easier, or more palatable, for a nondisabled person; it is also disguised, when the person with a disability is also inspiring.[36] In viewing inspiration porn, the nondisabled viewer does not feel as bad about pitying the person with a disability, and a subconscious desire to save them results in the generation of money and other forms of support for whatever charity or internet group is behind the image or story. Inspiration porn further reinforces another dangerous stereotype: connecting disability to suffering and death.[12,36]

These stereotypes frame "cure" as the ultimate objective for people with a disability, that their disability is a problem to be fixed, and that life with a disability is not a life worth living.

Although social media provided a platform for the proliferation of inspiration porn and other forms of ableist stereotypes, it also created opportunities for disability activists to push back through cultivation of their own online content. Memes emerged pushing back against the success of hoaxes using sick children as the foundation of money-generating content. The hoax would often involve images and stories of children with disabilities being shared through social media and a call to donate money or "like" the image or fan page. Many of these images went viral and only later would people find out the story or image was fictional. In one response from disability activists, a meme was created featuring an image of a doctor talking to a parent of a sick child with the caption "I'm sorry we didn't get enough likes in time. Your little boy is going to die."[36] Social media also enabled persons with disabilities to resist through online activism.

The Netflix show *Daredevil*, an adaptation of a popular Marvel comic book series, featured a protagonist who was blind; however, the show initially debuted on the streaming service without audio description, which would have allowed blind comic book fans to participate along with sighted individuals. After organized activism and advocacy through social media and other channels from blind individuals and the Accessible Netflix Project, Netflix released audio descriptions for *Daredevil* in 2015[23] and has since expanded the service to include hundreds of other titles.[61]

Another example of advocacy through social media took place in Montreal, Canada, where disability activists used different digital channels to advocate for improved public transportation and increased accessibility in both the physical aspects of travel and in online communities in which the public transportation company would communicate with the public.[68] Through the sharing of personal stories and the gathering of individuals who share similar perspectives, a community was created in which people could connect and be empowered to advocate for themselves and others.

Social media have helped to develop disability communities, especially among people who are not geographically connected, bringing together groups of people around the globe.[76] Aside from joining interest groups, individuals can share information about themselves and their group identity through the various hashtags they use. One common hashtag used by individuals with an amputation who enjoyed exercise was "#amputeefitness." This hashtag, combined with others such as "#fitfam" helped create in-group connections and served to connect individuals with amputations to a broader fitness community, expanding on what is seen as the "ideal" body.[58]

One innovative program used Pinterest to create new forms of expression for people with aphasia, helping build community through mediated face-to-face interactions.[3] Pinterest provided a way for these members of an older generation to connect with younger family members when the persons with aphasia were no longer able to do so verbally. Individuals used Pinterest to curate significant images as a means of introducing themselves and their passions, order food from restaurants, and control a conversation, expressing themselves in novel ways, as depicted in the following example:

Myra is an over-50 black stroke survivor; the stroke affected her vocal cords, which no longer allows her to make a sound. Myra used her Pinterest page to introduce herself to me and the international visitors through her curated images and captions. Of her 30 pins, the first 10 were about SCALE activities, her family, her dog, but the other 20 pins were about her love of Westerns, both films and TV shows, with several pins about the actor Rory Calhoun, who starred in film Westerns in the 1950s and 1960s. What was so powerful about her Pinterest introduction was that if we had interacted with Myra verbally, it is unlikely that we would have learned about her interest in Westerns. In a verbal conversation, we might have only learned the information in the first 10 pins. This image-based curation on Pinterest of what interested Myra gave everyone meeting her in-depth information and a glimpse into her real passions.[3]

Social media allow for many of the same stereotypes surrounding disability to be perpetuated, but it also offers more avenues for persons with disabilities to resist stereotypes, change the narrative, and form communities with similar people around the globe. The importance of services available to those with disabilities, the systems that are structured in our communities, and the policies that affect everything from healthcare delivery to payment must not be overlooked.

Services, Systems, and Policies

The final environmental factor described in the OTPF-4, *services, systems, and policies,* must not be overlooked, because they are the "benefits, structured programs, and regulations for operations provided by institutions in various sectors of society designed to meet the needs of persons, groups, and populations."[6] A brief historical overview of examples of environmental factors follows as an attempt to situate the reader to the many ways that *services, systems, and policies* were intended to support the disability community.

The independent living movement, which achieved public recognition in the early 1970s, is a political social justice, civil rights challenge to prior disability policy, practice, and research.[20] It is aligned with other minority groups (e.g., race, gender, ethnicity) in a call for equality in the dominant society. The independent living movement is a civil rights movement founded on the idea that the difficulties of having a disability are primarily based on the myths, fears, and stereotypes established in society.[81] This movement seeks to modify the convention of habilitating the isolated individual with disability through social and environmental changes.[81] A major political achievement was the passage of the Americans with Disabilities Act (ADA), which was signed into law in 1990, and the enactment of the ADA Amendments Act of 2008 (and subsequent partial amendments in 2010 and 2011) (see Chapters 2 and 15). The ADA's broad definition of disability emphasizes that perhaps the most significant factor people with various disabilities have in common is the experience of disability-based discrimination.[38,43] This civil rights movement has had its share of detractors,

including representatives of the healthcare industry, but it has sustained expansive momentum.[45]

In 2001, the World Health Organization (WHO) restructured its classification of health and health-related domains (*the International Classification of Functioning, Disability and Health* [ICF]) that describes body functions and structures, activities, and participation. The domains are classified from body, individual, and societal perspectives. The ICF also includes a list of environmental factors because the individual performs within a context. The aim of the ICF classification is to provide a unified and standard language and framework to describe changes in body function and structure, what a person with a health condition can do in a standard environment (the person's level of capacity), and what the person actually does in their usual environment (the person's level of performance). The text produced with the language depends on the users, their creativity, and their scientific orientation. This text is a companion to the WHO's *International Classification of Disease, Tenth Revision* (ICD-10).[91] For healthcare providers, including occupational therapy practitioners, the ICF challenges mainstream ideas on how health and disability are understood.

The ICF stresses health and functioning, rather than disability. Abandoned is the notion that disability begins at the point at which health ends. The ICF is a tool for measuring the act of functioning, without regard for the etiology of the impairment. This radical shift emphasizes the person's level of health, not the individual disability.[92] Fougeyrollas and Beauregard[28] pointed out that the revised ICF is more aligned with social ecology's theoretical description of disability and distances itself from reductionist social theory by emphasizing the role of environmental factors. It is also more in accord with the disability rights movement (see Chapter 2).

Health, as defined by the WHO, is a state of physical, mental, and social well-being. It is the capacity of individuals to function optimally within their environment or the adaptation of the persons to their environment or setting.[28] The ICF measures biological changes in body function or structure, but places equal emphasis on the contextual domains of personal and environmental factors. This is a shift from an exclusive view of disability from the medical model (i.e., directly caused by disease, trauma, or other health conditions that require individual treatment by professionals) to a paradigm that allows for integration of a social model, in which disability is not an attribute of an individual but rather a complex collection of conditions, many of which are created by environmental factors, as defined by the OTPF-4. The social model requires social action, and it is the collective responsibility of society at large to make the environmental modifications necessary for the full participation of people with disabilities in all areas of social life.[91] According to the WHO, neither the medical model nor the social model provides a complete picture of disability, although both are partially useful. The complex phenomenon called *disability* can be viewed at the level of a person's body and also primarily viewed at the social level.

The social justice movement successfully entered the international arena on May 3, 2008, with the United Nations Convention on the Rights of Persons with Disabilities (CRPD). The CRPD treaty obligates the United Nations (UN) member nations that sign it to provide equal access to healthcare and related services for people with disabilities; it represents the first legally binding international instrument that specifically protects the rights of persons with disabilities. The UN has estimated that 1 billion people (residing in 1 in 4 households) have at least one disabling condition.[30] The CRPD is also the first treaty in which nongovernmental organizations were present during negotiations and could offer interventions. People with disabilities participated as members of organizations for persons with disabilities, delegations from many countries, and UN organizations. Partly because of this inclusive process, the CRPD has received wide support, and as of 2016, it had been ratified by 157 countries, excluding the United States of America.[30]

The core principles of the CRPD are respect for human dignity, nondiscrimination, full participation, social inclusion, equality of opportunity, and accessibility.[84] The American Occupational Therapy Association (AOTA) is in full agreement with this focus, and this complements the WHO's perspective on health.[93] The WHO highlights the fact that a person's health can be influenced by the inability to participate in daily life occupations, and this can be caused by contextual barriers and by impairments in the human body. The OTPF-4 emphasizes the application of context to occupational justice and also identifies it as an outcome of occupational therapy practice.[6] Nilsson and Townsend[62] define occupational justice as "a justice that recognizes occupational rights to inclusive participation in everyday occupations for all persons in society, regardless of age, ability, sex, social class, or other differences."[6]

Occupational therapy practitioners must consider respect, fairness, impartiality, and equitable opportunities when addressing the contexts of their clients.[4,6] The relationship between occupation, justice, and client-centered practice is increasingly a focus of the profession and the approach to evaluation and intervention.[5,14] The necessity and power of occupation in the everyday lives of all humans is acknowledged. Health is supported and maintained when individuals are able to engage in their valued occupations. Occupation always occurs within the context of interrelated conditions that will affect client performance.[5,14] Occupational therapy practitioners must recognize that aspects of occupational justice and injustice, as well as the environmental and personal contexts of disability, are inextricably intertwined in the lived experience of those with disability.[8] This must be taken into consideration when collaborating with clients to facilitate engagement in occupation.[8] A critical lens also must be used when evaluating theories and models, because the development of those models is not void of their time in history or the context in which they were developed (i.e., Western or global North perspectives).

OCCUPATIONAL JUSTICE

According to Bailliard,[7] "Occupational scientists have a role to play in promoting justice" (p. 13). With the complex understanding of occupation within the sociocultural, economic, and political contexts, occupational scientists are experts at studying the impact of occupation on health and well-being. The role of occupational justice in occupational science should be explored for a better understanding on how occupational therapy practitioners can further engage with people who have disabilities to maximize their capabilities and occupational possibilities.

According to Hocking,[44] "occupational justice is taken to be an aspect, subset, derivative, or complementary to social justice" (p. 29). Wilcock and Hocking[87] define occupational justice as equitable or fair opportunities and resources "to do, be, belong and become what people have the potential to be and the absence of avoidable harm" (p. 414).[87] There are three foundational ideas supporting occupational justice. The first describes the need for humans to engage in occupations as a determinant of health, in ways that are agreeable to their culture and belief systems and support sustaining well-being. The second highlights that occupation is immersed in the environmental and personal contexts, as described earlier, and includes many structural factors such as the economy, various policies, and cultural values. According to Stadnyk et al.,[83] these factors are also considered determinants of occupation. The third foundational idea behind occupational justice is focused on engagement in occupation and how that can improve the lives of people who are in vulnerable situations.[44] Therefore, according to Hocking,[44] occupational justice "is concerned with enabling, mediating and advocating for environments in which all people's opportunities to engage in occupation are just, health-promoting and meaningful" (p. 33).

Occupational justice will look different, based on the culture, time, and place because different people have different occupational patterns, standards, and performances.[44] As Wilcock and Townsend[88] point out, some established occupational patterns and structures might be inherently inequitable or unfair, leading to occupational injustice. Hocking[44] defines an occupational injustice as "patterns of occupation so deficient as to seriously retard children's development, result in substantive health issues, or shorten people's lifespan" (p. 33). Human potential is wasted and various burdens are experienced, particularly of health, social unrest, and social discontent, threatening a sense of safety, according to Christiansen and Townsend.[17]

Five forms of "cause and effect" of occupational injustice are described in the literature: *occupational deprivation, occupational imbalance, occupational alienation, occupational marginalization,* and *occupational apartheid.* A brief description of each, according to Hocking,[44] follows; however, the reader is directed to the greater library of literature in occupational science for a more in-depth discussion of occupational injustice. *Occupational deprivation* is when a person's meaningful occupations are being negatively affected by an external barrier. An *occupational imbalance* occurs when people think they are overoccupied or underoccupied, like being overworked with too many responsibilities at work, or the complete opposite in not having enough meaningful occupation in which to engage. *Occupational alienation* is described as incompatibility with specific occupations that are associated with a place or situation in which it seems that even basic needs and wants are impossible to achieve, such as medical treatment or shelter. Occupational alienation may manifest as more aggressive occupations that could be associated with civil unrest. An example of this is the recent civil unrest experienced across the United States after the murder of George Floyd, an unarmed Black man who was killed by a White police officer in the summer of 2020. These occupations associated with civil unrest resulted in protesting, looting, and unrest across the country.[50] Another example of a response to occupational alienation is the work of *Not Dead Yet: The Resistance*, a national grassroots disability rights group that opposes legalization of assisted suicide as a deadly form of discrimination through media and public education campaigns to bring attention to their cause.[64] Other organizations to be considered include the AIDS Coalition to Unleash Power (ACT UP), which is a group working to end the acquired immunodeficiency syndrome (AIDS) pandemic through direct action, medical research, and advocacy to change legislation and public policies.[2] Another current example is the advocacy implemented in the state of California in the United States to shift COVID-19 vaccine prioritization to those living with chronic and serious health conditions such as heart, lung, or kidney disease; diabetes; cancer; or disabilities to be eligible for the vaccine at the same time that it was being offered to essential workers in March 2020.[16] *Occupational marginalization* occurs when people are discriminated against, such that they are systematically denied opportunities and resources to participate in everyday occupations, except for those that are less valued in a given society. Finally, *occupational apartheid* is defined as the systematic segregation of groups of people who are intentionally denied access to basic occupations such as quality education and paid employment based on prejudice.[44,87] These social conditions are not natural, and as Hocking[44] describes, they "give rise to occupational injustice [and] can be changed" (p. 33).

Social Justice

Although there are several definitions and variations of the concept of social justice, the commonalities among them are equal rights, equal opportunity, and equal treatment. Hocking reports that when a social justice lens is used, it is accepted that some inequities are created by societies rather than the forces of nature or the will of a higher power. Hocking also reports that societies can do something to change the inequities, such as amending the social arrangements to make a situation more equitable.[44] She argues, "in accepting that proposition, we are conceding that social institutions—politics, the economy, religion, schools, and the family—have a real-world impact on people's material circumstances."[44]

According to the literature, debates regarding the outcomes and processes of working toward social justice exist, with two main ideas prevailing in the discussion. The first is that a "just society is one in which people are treated equitably"[44] and the second is that "all citizens should receive a fair share of societal resources."[44] This leads to the question of where health fits into the discussion and whether it falls under the social justice umbrella. Although there are researchers who claim that health is not part of social justice,[44,74] Sen[79] insisted that "health is a

fundamental capability for functioning in society that ought to be protected."[44] He argued that when someone is in ill health, it further disadvantages a socially disadvantaged individual or group and becomes a barrier to realizing human rights and participation in society. Because societies have the power to protect, nurture, and restore people's capability to be healthy through fair distribution of the determinants of health, health disparities are considered an issue of justice.[44]

It has been established in the occupational therapy profession's literature that occupations are health-promoting and that engaging in meaningful occupations positively affects a person's health and well-being.[26,48,70] Occupational scientists and practitioners alike view occupation as a right; and inequities experienced by people who want to engage in meaningful occupations can be harmful. According to Hocking,[44] "occupational justice can be directly linked to human rights through the United Nations' (1948) Universal Declaration of Human Rights" (p. 34). Various occupations such as slavery, unfavorable work conditions, work without reimbursement, and not being able to vote or participate in leisure and recreation are all considered violations of human rights. Stadnyk et al.[83] reported four areas in which people have an occupational right in which to participate in a variety of occupations that bolster health, development, and inclusion; making choices and sharing decision-making power for everyday tasks; experiencing meaning; and receiving fair privileges from engagement in occupation.

Occupational rights have been defined as "the right of all people to engage in meaningful occupations that contribute positively to their own well-being and the well-being of their communities."[37] A violation of occupational rights, as a result of unfair and inequitable social conditions, constitutes an occupational injustice.[37] In fact, the World Federation of Occupational Therapy (WFOT) revised its position statement on occupational therapy and human rights in 2019, declaring that, "Occupational justice requires occupational rights for all."[90] the WFOT further clarified that occupational justice is "the fulfillment of the right for all people to engage in the occupations they need to survive, define as meaningful, and contribute positively to their own well-being and the well-being of their communities."[90]

Hammell and Iwama[41] further support this notion in that "human rights are associated with occupational rights" (p. 386) and that the true impairments are not associated with the physical limitations, but may actually be a consequence of "environmental barriers and inequity of opportunity."[40] As an example, consider the basic occupational therapy evaluation that includes assessments in self-care, functional mobility, manual muscle testing, range-of-motion testing, safety and cognition, and a vision screen completed by an occupational therapy practitioner before discharge from an acute care setting. The clinician has not seen the client's home or physical environment where the client will need to ascend two flights of stairs before getting into his or her apartment, nor addressed the social isolation and lack of community supports the person was experiencing before the hospitalization, and the fact that the client will likely not be able to return to work and earn a sustainable salary has not made it into the occupational therapy intervention plan of care.

THREADED CASE STUDY

Katie, Part 3

Consulting with disability community experts and reading more about disability studies, social justice, and occupational justice, Katie and her professor knew how they wanted to proceed in making changes to the original class activity. After discussing the 24-hour wheelchair assignment and outcomes with Ann, Katie's professor came to the realization that occupational therapy education must move beyond the traditional medical, rehabilitation, and functional models of disability. It became clear that the occupational justice lens should be more explicit, and in an overarching way, exposure and consideration of the social justice perspective must be included in the course.

Ann stressed the importance of occupational therapy educational programs needing to aggressively and intentionally prepare new practitioners to intervene against the social, political, and economic barriers to participation. Occupational therapy research, intervention development, and occupational therapy curricula need to be infused with the disability studies perspective, as well as a social justice framework if this critical work is to be accomplished during the training students receive in occupational therapy education programs.

This means that faculty members with disabilities need to be hired, students with disabilities should be recruited, people with disabilities should be consultants while developing or redesigning educational programs, and people with disabilities should be teaching in the classrooms and experiential learning laboratories.

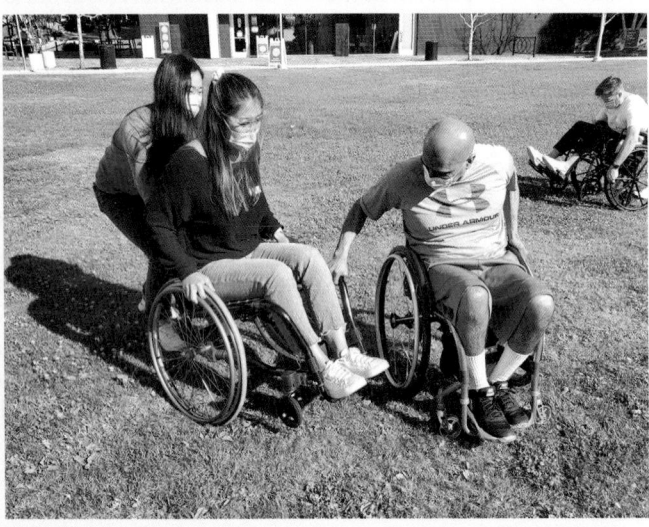

Community mentor and invited guest speaker, Juan, teaches students how to perform a wheelie.

Katie and her professor came up with the following options to incorporate into the physical dysfunctions course, with support from other faculty and administrative personnel in their occupational therapy department. The 24-hour wheelchair assignment would be replaced with a combination of the following learning activities. Students would be assigned to read a novel or autobiography (such as Golem Girl by Riva Lehrer) about a disabled person's lived experience, or to watch a documentary about disability rights (i.e., When Billy Broke His Head, Crip Camp). Students would write about their experiences with reading the book or viewing the documentary, how their perspectives were affected, and how those perspectives may affect their future practice through examining their own biases. People with disabilities would also be invited into their classrooms and learning laboratory spaces to teach content related to how activities of daily living are completed, how wheelchairs are used inside and outside of the classroom, and how a person lives life to its fullest, regardless of ability or disability.

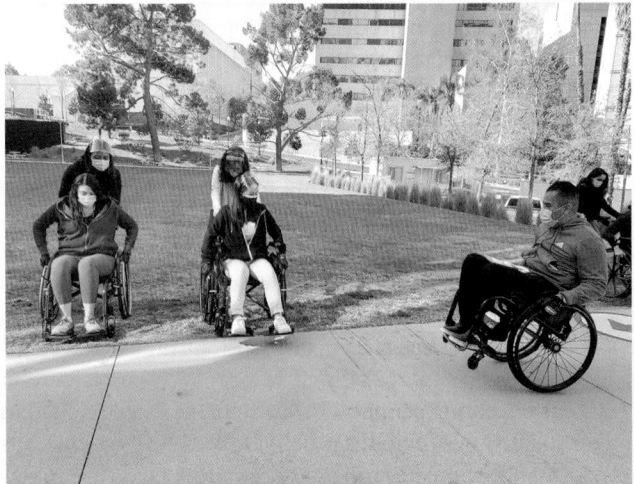

Community mentor and invited guest speaker, Lee, teaches students how to perform a wheelie to manage transitions from grass to concrete.

Simulations that occur in the classroom will be informed by the disability studies perspective, and perhaps the department could even hire people with disabilities to serve as standardized patients so that students can learn the technical skills, while still interacting with a disabled person in a safe classroom space, where mistakes can be made and professional growth can occur.

Katie also offered to talk to her peers about her personal experiences with the assignment and the suggestions discussed with her professor. Katie truly believed that the real experts of disability are those who live life every day and overcome the barriers and stigmas encountered in society. Occupational therapy practitioners have much to learn from their clients, in addition to their classroom experiences. The social justice and occupational justice perspectives felt like a breath of fresh air to Katie, and she was so grateful to have a professor who was open and willing to learn, grow, and change.

IMPLICATIONS FOR OCCUPATIONAL THERAPY PRACTITIONERS

It has long been tradition for occupational therapy, practitioners to assess the intersection of a person and the diagnosis or impairments, the occupation or task attempted, and the environment or context in which the person lives, works, or plays. Much of what clinicians do in the Western culture is grounded in traditional medical settings in which services are reimbursed by third-party payers, and practice is constrained by the context

and payment that follow. Kielhofner[47] describes additional challenges in healthcare, reporting that "reimbursement for rehabilitation services, including occupational therapy, is consistently tied to the aims of increasing an individual's likelihood of being an accountable, productive societal member or of reducing costs associated with necessary care" (p. 489).

Using occupation as a therapeutic modality, occupational therapy practitioners have a long history of evaluating and intervening with their clients from a traditional medical-rehabilitation lens, aiming to "remediate the individual, rather than target their interventions at the oppressive nature of social structures."[71] According to Barton,[9] the way in which a disability is defined is important because the language that is used to describe those who do things differently also influences expectations and interactions they will have with other people, including healthcare providers. Within this medical-rehabilitation perspective, disability, just like poor health, takes into account problems with the mind or body and is viewed as a problem that needs to be medically cured so that a person can function within a society in a "normal" way. By default, people are considered disabled on the basis that they are not able to function as "normal" people would.[34] According to Njelesani and colleagues, the concept of client-centered practice is actually guided by "prevailing social values and beliefs about what are 'normal' occupational possibilities" (p. 252).[63] For these reasons, it is critical for occupational therapy practitioners to examine their own biases and the framework in which they will situate their clinical interactions.

Consider Models With a Social Justice Framework

Hammell[40] describes the categorization of occupations according to dominant models that inform current occupational therapy practices as "simplistic, individualistic and inapplicable to collectivistic occupations, exclusionary, value laden, culturally specific to urban Western contexts, ethnocentric, ableist, class bound, artificially restrictive, potentially culturally unsafe, and devoid of contextual relevance" (p. 212). These models also portray the environment as something peripheral to and separate from the people who are functioning within the environment.[40] Njelesani and colleagues[63] also describe the challenges of categorizing occupations, and particularly those that are labeled as leisure because these kinds of classifications may reflect moral judgments. Even the long coveted Canadian Occupational Performance Measure (COPM) assessment is guilty of organizing what people need to do, want to do, or are expected to do into three neatly arranged categories of self-care, productivity, and leisure.

Rather than viewing a disability as an individual deficit remedied by experts in the medical field, a social justice lens encourages helping professions to explore other models and frameworks that examine the social, political, cultural, and economic factors that define disability and help determine personal and collective responses to difference.

Capabilities Approach

It is important for occupational therapy and occupational science to consider different models or approaches when working with people who have disabilities. Occupational equity is a phrase described by Hammell[40] as freedom to fully and fairly "access occupational opportunities necessary to fulfill occupational needs and rights for health and well-being" (p. 391) and should be available to all people, regardless of their differences. There is a clear connection between occupational equity and occupational rights, informed by existing literature on human capabilities.[40] A more critical perspective of occupation is emerging through the lens of the capabilities approach, originally developed by Amartya Sen in 1979 and further adapted by Nussbaum in 2000. In fact, this approach has been substantially refined over the last two decades by various authors across

many disciplines. It appeals to interdisciplinary scholars and students alike, although originally intended to answer questions related to social justice, economics, social sciences, and public affairs, in addition to the study of welfare states reform and issues related to the global South or North.

The capabilities approach links development, quality of life, and freedom for human beings with key ideas about capabilities, functioning, agency, human diversity, and public participation in generating valued capabilities.[86] In its simplest form, the capabilities approach "refers to what people are actually able to be and do, rather than to what resources they have access to. It focuses on developing people's capability to choose a life that they have reason to value."[84] Walker argues that freedom and capabilities go hand-in-hand, and to develop capabilities, one must have the freedom to do so. The approach highlights the ability that people should have to make meaningful choices from a range of options and have the freedom to choose a life that is valued.

The core concepts of the approach involve "functioning" and "capabilities." Functioning is defined as "the various things a person may value doing or being"[79]; whereas capability refers to the "freedom to promote or achieve valuable functionings."[86] Capability is a combination of functionings that a person can choose and achieve.[86] This approach highlights the realities in a person's life—do people have the freedom to achieve the things they find meaningful and have real opportunities to accomplish the occupations they value? Sen argues that "what people can positively achieve is influenced by economic opportunities, political liberties, social powers, and the enabling conditions of good health, basic education, and the encouragement and cultivation of initiatives."[79] If people live in communities or situations in which there is poverty, social deprivation, or neglect of public services, can people actually develop real alternatives and choices that can substantially change their lives?[86]

Human diversity is central to this approach, as Sen describes: "Human diversity is no secondary compilation to be ignored, or to be introduced later on; it is a fundamental aspect of our interest in equality" (1992, p. xi). This approach highlights the importance of interrelationships between practitioners and the disability community, and critically addresses perspectives that are "brought to the table." The lives of men, able-bodied people, heteronormative people, people of power, or people from any one racial majority cannot serve as the norm, or point of comparison, for occupational therapy practitioners performing clinical evaluations and interventions while working with persons who have disabilities.

Through this approach, people's capability to do the things they have reason to value is protected and promoted.[7] There is a focus on quality of life, in terms of what people are "actually capable of doing or becoming in the real world."[7,65] This approach was created for those clinicians who "seek to address inequalities of occupational opportunity and inequities in participation."[40] There are disagreements among scholars regarding this approach and its interpretations and applicability; however, it has been recently evaluated for its application to occupational therapy.

Because functionings are considered "states of being," they include things such as shelter, education, mental health, and nourishment. Functionings also include "doings," such as traveling, caregiving, work, and family gatherings. According to Bailliard,[7] the obvious parallels between doings and occupation indicate that the capabilities approach is compatible with the fundamental priorities of occupational science. The capabilities approach takes into consideration both internal and external conditions of evaluating a situation. Nussbaum[66] describes the internal capacities as being personality traits, emotional capacities, and states of health and fitness; and the external conditions are the political, cultural, social, economic, and historical environments that can restrict the expression of those capacities. Bailliard reports that "capabilities for functioning are interdependent and cannot be conceptualized as separate from the environments in which they develop" (p. 5).[7]

Sen[80] made a connection between individual and environmental factors, which basically come together to have actual capabilities for functioning. The minimum threshold of capability cannot be attained without environmental conditions that support the individual factors to develop basic capacities. This minimum threshold "cannot be obtained without careful consideration of the skills necessary to convert those resources or services into real and desirable beings and doings.[7] Conversion skills will be different among individuals, groups, and populations; therefore, "efforts to promote justice must both design favorable environmental conditions to enhance capabilities and consider whether those conditions can be effectively converted into desired functionings."[7] In other words, the environment must be considered, in addition to the person's abilities, to turn opportunities into personal action. If an entire gym is built in someone's home, the person's health is not going to improve unless the person demonstrates the motivation to use the gym and works toward changing their lifestyle. For that person to work toward physical fitness and good health, both things have to happen: the person needs a way to exercise and the person has to be motivated to work out. Moving beyond the individual, the capabilities model points out that the capability thresholds should be established by each society through "full participatory public deliberation."[7] Sen[80] claims that justice is the opportunity and freedom to choose the functionings that one values.

In fact, the capabilities approach elevates the "doings" and the "beings" as key factors of social justice. The philosophical work of this approach "has embraced the nuance of justice work and concludes that the pathway to justice is to enhance or support human capabilities to achieve desired and valued functioning."[7] According to Mitra,[59] the capability approach does offer a new and useful perspective on disability by focusing on two levels of the problem, as well as a framework for understanding the possible causes of disability. The focus of the model is to highlight the interaction among the individual's personal characteristics, available resources, and the environment. It moves away from the traditional perspectives of the disability being "within the person" and points to the impairment as being within the economic environment. Assessing a person's physical limitations in an acute care setting will not be a comprehensive or thorough approach, unless the person's home, or physical environment, and economic resources have also been addressed and resolved before discharge. This is not often a reality that can be achieved in the increasingly short-term hospitalizations experienced by people with disabilities in the United States' healthcare systems.

Capabilities, Opportunities, Resources, and Environments Approach

Another approach developed within the occupational therapy profession that can be considered in light of this discussion is the Capabilities, Opportunities, Resources, and Environments (CORE) approach. It provides a mechanism for occupational therapy practitioners to view their practice through an inclusive lens while enacting inclusive, occupation-centered services to their clients.[70] The CORE approach was first developed in an Australian context from a synthesis of multidisciplinary social inclusion and exclusion research, as well as Pereira's own research on poverty, disability, and social exclusion.[70] Put simply, this approach provides a mechanism for occupational therapy practitioners to "view practice through an inclusive lens, and *do* inclusive occupational therapy through applying reflexive questions."[70] Complimentary to the capabilities approach by Sen described previously, the CORE approach also enhances a client's capabilities, social inclusion, and well-being.[69]

The four key elements of social inclusion in this approach are a focus on capabilities, a focus on opportunities, resources to enable those capabilities, and environments that support social inclusion. The author of this approach cites Sen,[79] describing capabilities "as the opportunities and freedoms to live a life that we have reason to value so that human beings are able to do and be."[70] For people to achieve meaningful and valuable "functionings," they need to have real opportunities to do so with the freedom to access or discover the possibilities. Therefore, this approach brings capabilities and opportunities together, as this enhances "the scope and potential of occupational fulfillment in practice."[70] Resources are described as not only the things that are needed or wanted to participate in occupations, but the perspective on resources extends to include "personal, social, cultural, emotional, material, physical, spiritual, and/or technological resources."[70] Finally, environments are necessary, because occupations occur in contexts in which facilitators and barriers can be identified and addressed.

CORE elements and guiding questions are presented by Pereira and colleagues[69] for practical "how to" questions that serve as a framework for occupational therapy practitioners to consider when applying a person-centered, strengths-based, and occupation-based approach through the CORE approach lens. The authors believe this approach "promotes the goals, aspirations and occupational potential of the people with whom they [occupational therapy practitioners] work, as well as understanding and respecting their values."[70] The authors also think that this approach can support practitioners in working toward interventions that highlight true occupation-based practice that enhances human life and occupational justice.[70]

Practical "how to" questions that can facilitate the implementation of the CORE approach are offered by its authors. Under *capabilities*, questions regarding what is valued most in life should be asked, in addition to what the client would like to do and be. Inquiries into what the client needs to be able to do should be made, and a consideration of how social inclusion can be achieved is necessary. With regard to *opportunities*, the practitioner should ask themselves how a plan can be created with the client receiving services that will make it possible for them to do and be, and how best can the practitioner advocate for those occupational opportunities. When addressing *resources*, the practitioner should ask what personal, social, cultural, emotional, material, physical, spiritual, and/or technological resources are available to facilitate capabilities and how to best mobilize those resources. Finally, under the component of *environment*, the practitioner should consider how the environment can be designed, modified, or enriched to maximize social inclusion while supporting diverse identities, aspirations, and abilities.[69]

Opportunities for Reflection in Practice

When working with a person who has a disability, interventions should reflect real opportunities to develop capabilities that are based on what a person finds meaningful, not what society pushes onto them as normal, or even possible. A heightened sense of awareness of the relevance of justice issues related to everyday occupations should inform practice, from the mundane self-care tasks to extreme circumstances of hunger, ethnic violence, civil unrest, pandemics, and war.[7] Bailliard argues that "issues of justice occurring in everyday practice should be emphasized and participation in occupation can be reconceptualized as unavoidably affected by social institutions and systems of power" (p. 14).[7] However, Hammell[39] insists that "occupational therapists remain preoccupied with assessing and addressing individual dysfunctions and have directed little attention to assessing and challenging inequitable environmental constraints on people's occupational opportunities" (p. 78). That critical aspect of occupational therapy services cannot be ignored.

A client's perspectives on what they need to do, want to do, or are expected to do are highly influenced by social values and beliefs about occupations that are "normal" and socially expected. Njelesani and colleagues suggest "that therapists abandon efforts to be client-centered, as client-centered practice has benefits for all parties involved; what this paper supports is for occupational therapy practitioners to be reflexive and think critically about implicit values of "normal" embedded in daily practice and whether there could be any harm related to how these values influence their practice" (p. 254).[63] They continue with the fact that occupational therapy needs critical reflexivity to examine the assumptions and ideologies underlying human activity; how knowledge is produced and reproduced when participating in occupations, who controls the knowledge production, how the occupation is chosen, and what are the social, cultural, and political contexts of occupations. A clinician, who is practicing through a client-centered approach, may unintentionally be facilitating "normal" ways of doing certain occupations and, at the same time, marginalizing those who are different or simply doing things differently.[63]

How can clinicians incorporate this type of reflexivity into their practice? Njelesani et al.[63] recommend the reflection of the following questions when working with clients through a client-centered lens: (1) What assumptions underpin preferences toward some occupations and not to others? (2) Whose interests do preferred or "normal" occupations serve? What are the effects, feasibility, or practicality of a range of alternative occupational possibilities? (3) Is there the possibility that there can be harm in supporting occupations that seem to be "normal?" What is missed when a clinician neglects to reflect upon other occupational possibilities? (4) Is there a discussion with a client about limitations that may be encountered while trying to be "normal?"

Can the clinician support a discussion focusing on the positive value of considering a range of achievable and practical occupational possibilities? More consideration must be given to a client's unique sets of needs, capabilities, and resources to enable them to try out different occupational possibilities in all categories of occupation across the lifespan, not just the ones that have been normalized by Western society. In addition to this support and advocacy at the individual level, occupational therapy providers must also work to shift perspectives of state and national organizations, associations, and various practice contexts in which decisions are made regarding policy that can broaden the visioning of a wider range of occupational possibilities. Njelesani et al. conclude with this: "Engaging in critical reflexivity can help therapists, together with clients, embrace individual differences and envision possibilities for occupations that would be missed altogether in the pursuit of "normal." Being client-centered involves opening up discussion with clients and their families regarding the positive value of alternative occupational possibilities that are available in the world" (p. 258).[63]

Connection to Resources

An occupational therapy practitioner can serve as a resource for persons with disabilities, especially during rehabilitation, when the experience might be new and the rights and opportunities unfamiliar. Something as basic as helping people with disabilities understand their rights, not just in the sense of filing legal claims, but rights in daily life, can help them advocate for themselves. That empowerment translates into improved self-image and participation.[24] This awareness of rights should also include helping persons with disabilities understand avenues to complain in a hospital or other institutional setting, as this is often a tool to "get things done" that many hospital patients either do not feel empowered to do or do not have the institutional knowledge required to complete.[37]

Another important way occupational therapy practitioners can connect persons with disabilities to resources is through facilitating peer mentorship and social connection. Therapists can facilitate events and spaces for people with disabilities to come together.[27] There are many different realms for this social connection to occur, including sports, arts, and advocacy, provided that the person has interests in those areas.[31] These social opportunities can be important for providing practical information—sharing details peer-to-peer that a person might not hear from staff—as well as facilitating positive group identification. A final resource that is critical as a "bridge" to participation for persons with disabilities is having access to reliable and affordable transportation. Leaving an institutional setting, whether after a short or long stay, can be shocking depending on the suitability of the environment a person is returning to, so it is important to have resources in place to allow for community mobility.

Building Disability Identity

During rehabilitation, occupational therapy practitioners often focus on interventions that remediate an impairment and restore function over managing the long-term consequences of an acquired disability such as cerebrovascular accident (CVA). Even though some function is likely to be regained with time and treatment, rehabilitation professionals spend a disproportionate amount of time on biomechanical approaches to disability. Instead, some of the time could be spent managing the impact of the disability and the environment over time.[89] There are programs that are built upon ideas of building self-efficacy and using social learning with peers who are having (or have had) the same experience. This can include persons with disabilities as group leaders and facilitators who can model behaviors and share resources. Programs such as this can improve a patient's participation in different spheres of their life including home, work, and community.[89]

Building on ideas of self-efficacy and self-management of disability, stigma resistance is a central skill for persons with disabilities. One author even went so far as to imagine stigma resistance as an ADL.[31] One of the first ways an occupational therapy practitioner can affect a person with disabilities in the therapeutic process is in being a guide to expanding the person's view of disability.[31] An occupational therapy practitioner is often a key member of the interdisciplinary team in traditional rehabilitation settings, and can set the tone for how disability is framed. As mentioned earlier, this skill is not about telling the person what to think, as people have their own pace for understanding and adapting to disability; but rather, the occupational therapy practitioner can help celebrate new ways of doing things—"normal" functioning is no longer the gold standard. People and their families may be slow to accept this new perspective and may not be fully accepting of their disability.[27] Instead of labeling that person as "lacking insight," a therapist should be respectful of the power of self-narrative, as part of the rehabilitation process. Therapists can skillfully relate to the current narrative a person is creating for themselves, rather than insisting on an intervention or dialogue that is not relevant to that story.[72] For this to be effective, rehabilitation personnel also need to be trained in areas of disability history and theoretical models, disability rights, and other elements of disability culture

(see Chapter 2). Occupational therapy practitioners can collaborate with members of the disability community and invite them to facilitate trainings for staff who have not had this type of education, especially education that involves persons with disabilities leading or playing a key role in those sessions.

Another practical skill that can be applied by occupational therapy practitioners in the therapeutic context is role playing. This can be useful to help brainstorm ways for persons with disabilities to recognize stigmatizing behavior and manage responses. There are two main forms of stigma resistance: deflections and challenges, which can then both be further subdivided into strategies that align with either the medical or social model (Table 6.1). Deflections can be a tool to "smooth the social interaction while preserving both the self and the existing social order."[54] This strategy does not address the underlying structures that perpetuate stigma, but does attempt to minimize the consequences of stigmatizing behavior. Examples of medical deflections include behavioral or physical remediation of impairment. Social deflections include apologizing, passing, or avoiding situations or in which disability is likely to be more stigmatized. Passing is the attempt to present oneself as "normal" by managing or minimizing the stigmatizing aspect of oneself.[32]

Challenges encompass activism toward changing the social structure in which the stigma continues to thrive. Challenges "place the burden of embarrassment, discomfort, and inconvenience on those people and institutions that enact stigmatization."[54] Medical challenges are a way of explaining why certain things occur by situating the problem within the person's body; for example, explaining that a consequence of Parkinson's disease can be walking slower to an impatient caregiver. Social challenges are those that fully embody the activist movements and include educating people about laws and rights of persons with disabilities, actively addressing problematic stigmatizing behaviors, and advocating for change to unjust systems and policies. Although social challenges are most in line with the activism paralleling the disability rights movement, all four of these response forms might have utility in different practical situations. Often, social responses fail to address the embodied reality of disability. Physical, behavioral, and medical interventions do not have to be pushed upon the person as an attempt to fix a flawed body, but instead may be actively chosen by the person as a form of empowerment, especially if it is part of them enacting their rights within the medical system.[54]

TABLE 6.1 Summary of Forms of Stigma Resistance		
Type of Stigma Resistance	Examples That Align With the Medical Model of Disability	Examples That Align With the Social Model of Disability
Deflection	Behavioral modification Medical modification Physical modification	Apologizing Passing Avoiding
Challenge	Education about disability Informing of reason for behavior	Education about society/laws Calling out behavior as unacceptable Advocating for policy or system to be changed

Adapted from Manago B, Davis JL, Goar C: Discourse in action: parents' use of medical and social models to resist disability stigma. *Soc Sci Med* 184;169–177, 2017.

SUMMARY

Maximize capabilities or maximize independence? This is a question that all occupational therapy practitioners should ask themselves when considering a framework or model of practice to implement with a client who has a disability. The medical model sets the stage for the occupational therapy profession to think in reductionistic ways about people and their limitations. The social model of disability asked the occupational therapy profession to consider that *different* is neither positive or negative, and that the limitations being assessed are only one small part of a client's story that does not always need to be fixed.

What needs to be fixed are the attitudes that healthcare providers and members of society embrace about those who do things differently, those who look different, and those who are interdependent on systems and services that are critical to *being* and *functioning*. A critical lens must be used to analyze the profession's theories, beliefs, and ideals on what occupations matter, because everyone has a right to choose what matters to them.

Human beings want to *be*, and they want to *do*. Human beings are occupational beings who have a right to participate in the meaningful occupations they think are of value to them; and those occupations do not necessarily fit into the story of the Western culture or the founders of the profession.

That being said, a social justice perspective is at the heart of the discussion where occupational justice intersects with disability rights. It encourages occupational therapy practitioners to consider other models and frameworks, like the capabilities approach or the CORE approach, to critically examine the social, political, cultural, and economic factors that define disability. This will allow practitioners to capitalize on capabilities and move away from the focus on limitations; and it will also support a new personal and collective response to difference.

REVIEW QUESTIONS

1. What are the environmental and personal factors that affect participation and engagement in occupation? How can those factors be included in the occupational therapy evaluation and intervention processes?
2. What are some of the challenges faced by people with disabilities when constructing their personal disability identity?
3. How do stigma, spread, and negative attitudes toward people with disabilities influence the social context of disability and access to healthcare?
4. In what ways does the International Classification of Functioning, Disability, and Health (ICF) promote a biopsychosocial model of disability? What are the ways in which the medical model and social model fall short of meeting the needs of people living with disabilities?
5. How can concepts from an occupational justice perspective be applied to occupational therapy practice?
6. What is the impact of a social justice framework and contemporary models practice on the role of occupational therapy practitioners when working with the disability community?

For additional practice questions for this chapter, please visit eBooks.Health.Elsevier.com.

ACKNOWLEDGMENTS

The authors wish to acknowledge several important colleagues who have contributed to the development of this chapter. We thank Sandra Burnett for her exemplary work in previous editions, in addition to her consultation and collegiality as the chapter moved in a different direction. We also extend our gratitude to Heidi Pendleton for her contributions to previous iterations of the chapter and her openness to embracing new perspectives that inform the study of occupational therapy. Thank you both for initiating this critical discussion by bringing disability studies and occupational therapy together in one chapter.

Thank you to Kiara Ota, OTD, OTR/L; Creig Smith, OTD, OTR/L; and Erika Julyann Tolentino, OTRP, OTS, for contributing to the literature review and reference lists in preparation for submission. We greatly appreciate the consultation with Rebecca Aldrich, PhD, OTR/L, and her expertise in the area of occupational science and occupational justice. And lastly, a final heartfelt thank you to the late Ann Neville-Jan, PhD, OTR/L, FAOTA, our colleague and dear friend, who influenced generations of occupational therapy students, clinicians, and researchers with her unwavering desire to promote the power of occupation, whether it was by choosing her favorite shoes to wear or critically analyzing an injustice that would never stand in her way. We are forever grateful for her role in our lives, personally and professionally.

REFERENCES

1. Abberley P: Disabling ideology in health and welfare – the case of occupational therapy, *Disability and Society* 10:221–232, 1995.
2. AIDS Coalition to Unleash Power (ACT UP). (2021, May 21). In *Wikipedia*. https://en.wikipedia.org/wiki/ACT_UP
3. Alper M, Haller B: Social media use and mediated sociality among individuals with communication disabilities in the digital age. In Ellis K, Kent M, editors: *Disability and Social Media: Global perspectives*, New York, 2017, Routledge, pp 133–145.
4. American Occupational Therapy Association: Occupational therapy code of ethics (2015), *American Journal of Occupational Therapy* 69(Suppl. 3):1–8, 2015. https://doi.org/10.5014/ajot.2015.696S03.

5. American Occupational Therapy Association: Occupational therapy practice framework: domain and process, ed 3, *American Journal of Occupational Therapy* 68(Suppl 1):S1–S48, 2014.

6. American Occupational Therapy Association: Occupational therapy practice framework: Domain and process (4th ed.), *American Journal of Occupational Therapy* 74(Suppl. 2):1–87, 2020. https://doi.org/10.5014/ajot.2020.74S2001.

7. Bailliard A: Justice, difference, and the capability to function, *Journal of Occupational Science* 23(1):3–16, 2016. https://doi.org/10.1080/14427591.2017.1294016.

8. Bailliard AL, Dallman AR, Carroll A, Lee BD, Szendrey S: Doing occupational justice: a central dimension of everyday occupational therapy practice, *Canadian Journal of Occupational Therapy* 87(2):144–152, 2020. https://doi.org/10.1177/000841741989893.

9. Barton L: Disability, physical education and sport: some critical observations and questions, *Disability and Youth Sport*:39–50, 2009.

10. Behler GT Jr: Disability simulations as a teaching tool: some ethical issues and implications, *Journal on Postsecondary Education and Disability* 10(2):3–8, 1993.

11. Bickenbach JE: Disability human rights, law, and policy. In Albrecht GL, Seelman KD, Bury M, editors: *Handbook of disability studies*, Thousand Oaks, CA, 2001, Sage.

12. Black RS, Pretes L: Victims and victors: representation of physical disability on the silver screen, *Research and Practice for Persons with Severe Disabilities* 32(1):66–83, 2007.

13. Bolt D: Introduction: Perspectives from historical, cultural, and educational studies. In Bolt D, editor: *Changing social attitudes toward disability: perspectives from historical, cultural and educational studies*, New York, 2014, Routledge, pp 1–11.

14. Braveman B, Bass-Haugen JD: Social justice and health disparities: an evolving discourse in occupational therapy research and intervention, *Am J Occup Ther* 63:7–12, 2009.

15. Burgstahler S: Universal design of instruction. In Cory R, editor: *Beyond compliance: an information package on the inclusion of people with disabilities in postsecondary education*, Syracuse, NY, 2003, Center on Human Policy, Syracuse University.

16. Calmatters.org. (February 12, 2021). *California shifts vaccine priorities again: people with health conditions are eligible next month.* https://calmatters.org/health/coronavirus/2021/02/california-shifts-priorities-vaccine-chronic-conditions/.

17. Christiansen CH, Townsend EA, editors: *Introduction to occupation: the art and science of living*, 2nd ed., Upper Saddle River, NJ, 2010, Pearson Education.

18. Coleman LM: Stigma: an enigma demystified. In Davis LJ, editor: *The Disability Studies Reader (2, 141–152)*, New York, 2006, Routledge.

19. Darragh AR, et al: "Tears in my eyes 'cause somebody finally understood": client perceptions of practitioners following brain injury, *Am J Occup Ther* 55:191, 2001.

20. DeJong G: Defining and implementing the independent living concept. In Crewe NM, Zola IK, editors: *Independent living for physically disabled people, San Francisco*, 1983, Jossey-Bass.

21. Earnshaw VA, Chaudoir SR: From conceptualizing to measuring HIV stigma: a review of HIV stigma mechanism measures, *AIDS and Behavior* 13(6):1160–1177, 2009.

22. Earnshaw VA, Smith LR, Chaudoir SR, Amico KR, Copenhaver MM: HIV stigma mechanisms and well-being among PLWH: a test of the HIV stigma framework, *AIDS and Behavior* 17(5):1785–1795, 2013.

23. Ellis K: #Social conversations: disability representation and audio description on Marvel's *Daredevil*. In Ellis K, Kent M, editors: *Disability and social media: global perspectives*, New York, 2017, Routledge, pp 146–160.

24. Engle DM, Munger FW: *Rights of inclusion: law and identity in the life stories of Americans with disabilities*, Chicago, 2003, University of Chicago Press.

25. Evans HD: 'Trial by fire': forms of impairment disclosure and implications for disability identity, *Disability & Society* 34(5):726–746, 2019. https://doi.org/10.1080/09687599.2019.1580187.

26. Fisher A: Occupation-centred, occupation-based, occupation-focused: same, same or different? *Scandinavian Journal of Occupational Therapy* 20(3):162–173, 2013. https://doi.org/10.3109/11038128.2012.754492.

27. Forber-Pratt AJ, Zape M: Disability identity development model: voices from the ADA-generation, *Disability and Health Journal* 10:350–355, 2017.

28. Fougeyrollas P, Beauregard L: An interactive person-environment social creation. In Albrecht GL, Seelman KD, Bury M, editors: *Handbook of disability studies*, Thousand Oaks, CA, 2001, Sage.

29. French S: Simulation exercises in disability awareness training: a critique, *Disability, Handicap & Society* 7(3):257–266, 1992.

30. Geiger BF: Establishing a disability-inclusive agenda for sustainable development in 2015 and beyond, *Glob Health Promot* 22:64–69, 2014.

31. Gill CJ, Mukherjee S, Garland-Thomson R, Mukherjee D: Disability stigma in rehabilitation, *PM&R* 8:997–1003, 2016.

32. Goffman E: *Stigma: notes on the management of spoiled identity*, New Jersey, 1963, Prentice Hall.

33. Grinker RR: Autism, "stigma," disability: a shifting historical terrain, *Current Anthropology* 61(21):S55–S67, 2020.

34. Haegele JA, Hodge S: Disability discourse: overview and critiques of the medical and social models, *Quest* 68(2):193–206, 2016. https://doi.org/10.1080/00336297.2016.1143849.

35. Hallenbeck CE: The trouble with simulation, *AHSSPPE Bulletin* 2(3), 1984.

36. Haller B, Preston J: Confirming normalcy: 'inspiration porn' and the construction of the disabled subject? In Ellis K, Kent M, editors: *Disability and social media: global perspectives*, New York, 2017, Routledge, pp 41–56.

37. Hammel J, Magasi S, Heinemann A, Whiteneck G, Bogner J, Rodriguez E: What does participation mean? An insider perspective from people with disabilities, *Disability and Rehabilitation* 30(19):1445–1460, 2008.

38. Hammel J, Magasi S, Heinemann A, et al: Environmental barriers and supports to everyday participation: a qualitative insider perspective from people with disabilities, *Arch Phys Med Rehabil* 96:578–588, 2015.

39. Hammell KW: Quality of life, participation and occupational rights: a capabilities perspective, *Australian Occupational Therapy Journal* 62:78–85, 2015. https://doi.org/10.1111/1440-1630.12183.

40. Hammell KW: Action on the social determinants of health: advancing occupational equity and occupational rights, *Cadernos Brasileiros de Terapia Ocupacional* 28(1):378–400, 2020. https://doi.org/10.4322/2526-8910.ctoARF2052.

41. Hammell KW, Iwama MK: Well-being and occupational rights: an imperative for critical occupational therapy, *Scandinavian Journal of Occupational Therapy* 19:385–394, 2012.

42. Hergenrather K, Rhodes S: Exploring undergraduate student attitudes toward persons with disabilities: application of the disability social relationship scale, *Rehabilitation Counseling Bulletin* 50(2):66–75, 2007.

43. Hill E, Goldstein D: The ADA, disability and identity, *JAMA* 313:2227–2228, 2015.

44. Hocking C: Occupational justice as social justice: the moral claim for inclusion, *Journal of Occupational Science* 24(1):29–42, 2017. https://doi.org/10.1080/14427591.2017.1294016.

45. Johnson M: *Make them go away: Clint Eastwood, Christopher Reeve and the case against disability rights*, Louisville, KY, 2003, Advocado Press.

46. Kielhofner G: *Conceptual foundations of occupational therapy*, Philadelphia, 1997, F.A. Davis.

47. Kielhofner G: Rethinking disability and what to do about it: disability studies and its implications for occupational therapy, *American Journal of Occupational Therapy* 59:487–496, 2005.

48. Kielhofner G: Emergence of the contemporary paradigm: a return to occupation. In Kielhofner G, editor: *Conceptual foundations of occupational therapy practice*, Philadelphia, PA, 2009, F.A. Davis Company, pp 41–55.

49. Kiger G: Disability simulations: logical, methodological and ethical issues, *Disability, Handicap & Society* 7(1):71–78, 1992.

50. Lavalley R, Johnson KR: Occupation, injustice, and anti-black racism in the united states of America, *Journal of Occupational Science*, 29:487–499, 2020. https://doi.org/10.1080/14427591.2020.1810111.

51. Link BG, Phelan JC: Conceptualizing stigma, *Annual Review of Sociology* 27:363–385, 2001.

52. Linton S: Disability studies/not disability studies. In Linton S, editor: *Claiming disability: knowledge and identity*, New York, 1998, University Press, pp 132–156.

53. Longmore PK, Goldberger D: The league of the physically handicapper and the Great Depression: a case study in the new disability history [electronic version], *Journal of American history* 87(3):888–922, 2000.

54. Manago B, Davis JL, Goar C: Discourse in action: parents' use of medical and social models to resist disability stigma, *Social Science & Medicine* 184:169–177, 2017.

55. Marini I, Chan R, Feist A, Flores-Torres L: Student attitudes toward intimacy with persons who are wheelchair users, *Rehabilitation Education* (25):15–26, 2011.

56. Marks D: Dimensions of oppression: theorising the embodied subject, *Disability & Society* 14(5):611–626, 1999. https://doi.org/10.1080/09687599925975.

57. Miller E, Chen R, Glover-Graf NM, Kranz P: Willingness to engage in personal relationships with persons with disabilities: examining category and severity of disability, *Rehabilitation Counseling Bulletin* 52(4):211–224, 2009.

58. Mitchell FR, Santarossa S, Ramawickrama IL, Rankin EF, Yaciuk JA, McMahon ER, van Wyk PM: An evaluation of social media images portrayal of disability discourse: #amputeefitness, *European Journal of Adapted Physical Activity* 12(11):1–15, 2019.

59. Mitra S: The capability approach and disability, *Journal of Disability Policy Studies* 4(16):236–247, 2006.

60. Nagi SZ: Disability concepts revisited: implications for prevention. In Pope A, Tarlou A, editors: *Disability in America: toward a national agenda for prevention*, Washington, D.C., 1991, National Academy Press, pp 309–327.

61. Netflix (n.d.). *Audio description for TV shows and movies.* https://help.netflix.com/en/node/25079.

62. Nilsson I, Townsend E: Occupational justice: bridging theory and practice, *Scandinavian Journal of Occupational Therapy* 17(1):57–63; 2010.

63. Njelesani J, Teachman G, Durocher E, Hamdani Y, Phelan S: Thinking critically about client-centred practice and occupational possibilities across the lifespan, *Scandinavian Journal of Occupational Therapy* 22:252–259, 2015.

64. Not Dead Yet: The Resistance (2020). https://notdeadyet.org/ndys-non-violent-direct-action.

65. Nussbaum MC: *Women and human development*, New York, NY, 2000, Cambridge University Press.

66. Nussbaum MC: *Creating capabilities: The human development approach*, Cambridge, MA, 2011, Harvard University Press.

67. Oliver M: Capitalism, disability, and ideology: a materialist critique of the normalization principle. In Flynn RJ, Raymond AL, editors: *A quarter century of normalization and social role valorization: evolution and impact*, 1999, Internet publication. http://www.independentliving.org/docs3/Oliver99.pdf.

68. Parent L, Veilleux ME: *Transport mésadapté*: exploring online disability activism in Montréal. In Ellis K, Kent M, editors: *Disability and social media: global perspectives*, New York, 2017, Routledge, pp 89–100.

69. Pereira RB: Towards inclusive occupational therapy: introducing the CORE approach for inclusive and occupation-focused practice, *Australian Occupational Therapy Journal* 64(6):429–435, 2017. https://doi.org/10.1111/1440-1630.12394.

70. Pereira RB, Whiteford G, Hyett N, Weekes G, Di Tommaso A, Naismith J: Capabilities, Opportunities, Resources, and Environments (CORE): using the CORE approach for inclusive, occupation-centered practice, *Australian Occupational Therapy Journal* 67:162–171, 2020.

71. Pitts, D. & Rafeedie, S. (2004). *Disability simulations in one occupational therapy curriculum: a pedagogical practice in need of a critique.* Unpublished manuscript.

72. Polkinghorne D: *Narrative knowing and the human sciences*, Albany, New York, 1988, SUNY Press.

73. Raman S, Levi SJ: Concepts of disablement in documents guiding physical therapy practice, *Disability and Rehabilitation*, 24(15):790–797, 2002.

74. Rawls J: In Kelly E, editor: *Justice as fairness: a restatement*, Cambridge, MA, 2001, Harvard University Press.

75. Roush SE, Sharby N: Disability reconsidered: the paradox of physical therapy, *Advances in Disability Research* 91(12):1715–1727, 2011.

76. Ryan S, Julian G: Personal reflections on the #107days campaign: Transformative, subversive or accidental? In Ellis K, Kent M, editors: *Disability and social media: global perspectives*, New York, 2017, Routledge, pp 25–40.

77. Scaffa, M: Occupational therapy interventions for groups, communities, and populations. In BAB Schell & G Gillen, editors: *Willard and Spackman's occupational therapy*, 13th ed, Philadelphia, 2019, Wolters Kluwer.

78. Scotch RK: *From good will to civil rights: transforming federal disability policy*, 2nd ed., Philadelphia, 2001, Temple University Press.

79. Sen A: *Development as Freedom*, New York, 1999, Alfred A. Knopf.

80. Sen A: *The idea of justice*, Cambridge, MA, 2009, Harvard University Press.

81. Shapiro JP: *No pity: people with disabilities forging a new civil rights movement*, New York, 1993, Times Books.

82. Siebers T: *Disability Theory*, Ann Arbor, MI, 2008, The University of Michigan Press.

83. Stadnyk R, Townsend E, Wilcock A: Occupational justice. In Christiansen CH, Townsend EA, editors: *Introduction to occupation: the art and science of living* 2nd ed., Upper Saddle River, NJ, 2010, Pearson Education, pp 329–358.

84. Stein MA, Stein PJS, Weiss D, Lang R: Healthcare and the UN disability rights convention, *Lancet* 374:1796–1798, 2009.

85. Turan B, Budhwani H, Fazeli PL, Browning WR, Raper JL, Mugavero MJ, Turan JM: How does stigma affect people living with HIV? The mediating roles of internalized and anticipated HIV stigma in the effects of perceived community stigma on health and psychosocial outcomes, *AIDS and Behavior* 21:283–291, 2017.

86. Walker M: Amartya Sen's capability approach and education, *Educational Action Research* 13(1):103–110, 2005.

87. Wilcock AA, Hocking C: *An occupational perspective of health*, 3rd ed., NJ: Slack, 2015, Thorofare.

88. Wilcock A, Townsend E: Occupational terminology interactive dialogue, *Journal of Occupational Science* 7(2):84–86, 2000. https://doi.org/10.1080/14427591.2000.9686470.

89. Wolf TJ, Baum CM, Lee D, Hammel J: The development of the improving participation after stroke self-management program (IPASS): an exploratory randomized clinical study, *Topics in Stroke Rehabilitation* 23(4):284–292, 2016.

90. World Federation of Occupational Therapists (WFOT): *Position Statement: Occupational therapy and human rights*, 2019, World Federation of Occupational Therapists.

91. World Health Organization: International classification of functioning, disability and health (ICF). 2001. http://www.who.int/icf/icftemplate.cfm.

92. World Health Organization: Towards a common language for functioning, disability and health. 2002. http://www.who.int/icf/beginners/bg.pdf.

93. World Health Organization: *International classification of functioning, disability and health: ICF*, Geneva, 2008, WHO Press.

94. Wright B: *Physical disability: a psychological approach, ed 2*. In *New York*, 1983, Harper & Row.

95. Young S: *We're not here for your inspiration*, Australia, 2012, July 2, *ABC News*. https://www.abc.net.au/news/2012-07-03/young-inspiration-porn/4107006.

96. Zola IK: Medicine as an institution of social control, *Sociological Review* 20:487–503, 1972.

97. Zola IK: Self, identity and the naming question: reflections on the language of disability, *Social Science and Medicine* 36(2):167–173, 1993.

Implementation of Occupational Therapy Services

Megan C. Chang and Winifred Schultz-Krohn

LEARNING OBJECTIVES

After studying this chapter, the student or practitioner will be able to do the following:

1. Identify the unique characteristics of implementation science.
2. Differentiate implementation science from evidence-based practice.
3. Discuss purposes and outcome goals for teaching in occupational therapy.
4. Analyze how teaching strategies will differ depending on the characteristics of the client, task, and context.
5. Apply current knowledge about factors that influence motivation and active participation to the implementation of occupational therapy services.
6. Provide appropriate instruction, feedback, and practice tailored to individual tasks and client goals.
7. Promote transfer of learning to real-life situations through effective teaching strategies.
8. Implement occupational therapy interventions designed to promote self-monitoring and strategy development.

CHAPTER OUTLINE

KEY TERMS

Blocked practice
Conation
Contextual interference
Declarative learning
Extrinsic feedback
Evidence-based practice
Implementation Science
Intrinsic feedback

Metacognition
Procedural learning
Random practice
Somatosensory instruction
Strategies
Transfer of learning
Verbal instruction
Visual instruction

IMPLEMENTATION STRATEGIES IN OCCUPATIONAL THERAPY

Occupational therapists spend much of their time with clients teaching a variety of activities. At the core of the profession is the concept of working with clients to achieve the client's occupational goals.[2] Effectiveness in instructing clients depends on several factors, including the therapist's ability to use and implement evidence-based practice, organize the environment and the instructional methods to meet the learning needs of the client, while including family members, friends, and other caregivers. This chapter discusses the steps of implementing evidence through the use of implementation science and then describes the occupational therapy process of working with clients who have physical disabilities. It also presents the reasons occupational therapists teach activities, the phases and types of learning, and principles of teaching and learning with this population.

IMPLEMENTATION SCIENCE AND OCCUPATIONAL THERAPY

The term *implementation science* is the process of systematically applying the results of research to practice.[4,5,41] Five steps outlined for implementation science are described by Rapport and associates[41] as *diffusion, dissemination, implementation, adoption,* and *sustainability.*

Diffusion, as the first step, is the spread of information and knowledge throughout practice areas using informal channels of communication. An investigation at a local hospital found that occupational therapists who actively engage their clients in problem solving to remove potential safety hazards at home had fewer falls once discharged from the hospital. This approach was compared to other methods of providing instructional materials and information on how to prevent falls within the home after hospital discharge. The information about using this collaborative problem-solving approach spreads throughout the hospital and surrounding community, but the evidence is not distributed in a planned or organized manner.

The next step is *dissemination.* The same hospital recognizes the benefit for their clients, and the occupational therapists continue to collect data to publish a paper and present the data at a national conference. This next step in the process of implementation science, dissemination, reflects the organized manner of distributing the evidence to targeted audiences.

The third step in the process is the *implementation* of research results into the daily practice of occupational therapists. In this example, how occupational therapists structure their intervention services to systematically include using this collaborative problem-solving strategy to reduce falls in the home would reflect the implementation step. This would require administrative support to fund this process as part of the occupational therapy services delivered to clients.

The next step is *adoption* and reflects how the practice of collaborative problem solving with clients becomes widespread throughout the regional hospitals and beyond. The adoption of the collaborative problem-solving approach initiated by a few occupational therapists in a single hospital now becomes a model of practice to avoid falls once clients are discharged to home.

THREADED CASE STUDY

Li, Part 1

Li is a 67-year-old retired high school science teacher who identifies as male (prefers use of the pronouns he/him/his). Li was hit by a car as he walked across a city street. Before his accident, Li was active in a variety of volunteer activities that included teaching English as a second language at an adult education program, working as a docent at the local botanical gardens, and leading nature hikes in a nearby county park. He also was an amateur watercolor artist who had recently begun to receive recognition for his landscape paintings.

On referral to occupational therapy, he was nonambulatory because of a fracture of the right pelvis and right femur. He also had fractures of his right clavicle and humerus and multiple fractures of his dominant right forearm and hand. He had a severe concussion and experienced dizziness and impaired balance, memory loss, and episodes of confusion.

In the initial occupational therapy evaluation, Li stated his desire to return to his volunteer activities and his painting. He understood that the healing and rehabilitation process would take time, and his immediate concern was to regain physical capacity so that he could be more independent in his self-care. His wife attended his occupational therapy sessions and was committed to assisting him in his recovery.

Critical Thinking Questions
1. What does Li need to learn?
2. What strategies should Li's therapist use to facilitate his learning?
3. What should Li learn first?

The final phase of implementation science is called *sustainability* and reflects the need to monitor not only the outcome of the service provided but also the ability for this practice to occur in the real world of a busy inpatient hospital. To support the sustainability of the collaborative problem-solving approach, the occupational therapists from the original hospital developed guided questions that can be used to gather information from clients before discharge. Additional systematic questions were developed that foster collaborative problem solving so environmental changes are made in the home that not only reduce the risk of falling but are endorsed by the client. The reason the suggested questions were developed was to support the sustainability of this approach.

Implementation science is closely linked to evidence-based practice (see Chapter 4) and has emerged as a systematic means to translate evidence into everyday practice.[30] Evidence-based practice has been advocated by the occupational therapy profession for many years, but the implementation of evidence into practice remains difficult, and occupational therapy practitioners often face many challenges in interpreting research results that support practice.[27] Evidence-based practice is to provide a foundation for best practice, and implementation science provides an approach to infuse evidence into the practice.[27] This dedication to using the best available evidence to implement services is considered an important feature of ethical behavior, as discussed in the Code of Ethics.[1]

The Occupational Therapy Practice Framework 4th edition (OTPF-4)[2] describes the process used when providing occupational therapy services. The implementation of services clearly includes education and training as important forms of occupational therapy intervention. Training and education are differentiated in occupational therapy implementation of services. The focus of occupational therapy intervention using education with clients is to provide "knowledge and information about occupation, health, well-being, and participation" (S61). When an occupational therapist provides training, the focus is on "enhanced performance" as the outcome. The occupational therapist often seamlessly blends interventions addressing education and training together, but the outcomes are not the same. The outcome of the services provided for education are understanding and knowledge, whereas the outcomes for training are improved performance and skills needed for occupational engagement.

The following examples illustrate both training and education when implementing occupational therapy services:

1. *To help clients regain skills lost as a result of illness or injury.* Clients may need to learn new strategies to perform daily occupations such as eating and dressing. They may also need to relearn basic performance skills, such as the ability to maintain sitting or standing balance, reaching, or grasping. In the case of Li, his head injury affected both short- and long-term memory, impairing his ability to perform self-care skills. One of the first goals of his OT program was to relearn hygiene and grooming skills so that he could regain independence in this aspect of self-care. This goal requires both education and training. The occupational therapist, using implementation science, would search for strategies that can improve Li's ability to complete grooming and hygiene tasks and enhance both short- and long-term memory skills. The application of evidence-based practices to support client success is coupled with careful examination of the client's desired outcomes.[20]

2. *To develop alternative or compensatory strategies for performing valued occupations.* Clients may need to be taught new ways to perform familiar activities. Alternative or compensatory strategies also can be taught to prevent injury and increase safety. These strategies may be temporary, as in the case of an individual who needs to learn hip precautions after hip replacement surgery, or permanent, as in the case of an individual who needs to learn to use a tenodesis grasp after a complete spinal cord injury at the C6 level. In some cases, adaptive equipment may be needed to achieve independence, and instruction in the use of adaptive equipment must be included in the teaching of compensatory strategies. Li's occupational therapist instructed him in adaptive dressing and bathing techniques so that he could maintain independence in these activities while his fractures healed. Implementation science supports the professional reasoning used by the occupational therapist in determining why alternative or compensatory strategies would be preferred to address Li's dressing and bathing skills instead of working on regaining previous skills.[33] An example can be seen with the use of a bath chair as a safety precaution to avoid a fall in the bathtub while bathing.

3. *To develop new performance skills to support role performance in the context of a disabling condition.* In some cases clients will need to learn new skills to enable participation in daily occupations. Propelling a wheelchair, operating a prosthetic device, and managing a bowel and bladder program are examples of new skills that clients with specific disabilities must learn. These new skills require both education and training. The education part provides the client with the knowledge of why the new skill should be acquired. This approach requires careful consideration of the client's social, cultural, economic, and environmental contextual factors.[2] The training is focused on creating an efficient means of engaging in the new skill. Implementation science is focused on how evidence can be effectively applied to support the client's preferred outcomes.[37] Li's therapist worked with him to develop a reminder system to compensate for his memory loss. He learned to record and keep important information with him in his phone so that he could easily access phone numbers, appointments, and other needed information.

4. *To provide therapeutic challenges that will help to improve performance skills to support participation in areas of occupation.* Therapists may teach clients activities that provide physical and/or cognitive challenges to facilitate the rehabilitation process. Activities such as board games and crafts can be used to improve strength, dexterity, postural control, and problem-solving and sequencing skills, among others. Clients may need to be instructed in the rules or procedures of the activity and also in how to position or organize themselves to engage in the activity. To improve dexterity in Li's injured right arm after the cast was removed, and also to improve his attention and task orientation, his occupational therapist worked with Li on repotting orchids. This activity addressed Li's deficits in both motor and process skills and supported his return to participation in his valued occupation of gardening.

5. *To instruct family members or caregivers in activities that will enhance the client's independence and/or safety in daily occupations.* If the client is not able to learn to perform an activity using compensatory and/or adaptive strategies, it is necessary to teach family members or caregivers how to assist or supervise the client in the activity. Many self-care and home activities may require assistance or supervision to ensure safety. Environmental modifications may need to be made to ensure the safety of the client and the caregiver and to facilitate maximal independence for the client. Li's wife was instructed on how to help him with wheelchair transfers. She was also instructed on how to cue him to use his reminder notebook at home.

PHASES OF LEARNING

Learning is a process that requires both education and training[2] and generally proceeds through three phases. Not all clients are able to progress through all three phases. This requires careful consideration of supports that may be needed for client safety in daily occupations. These three phases of learning are known as *acquisition, retention,* and *transfer* phases. The acquisition phase occurs during initial instruction and education along with practice. This phase is often characterized by numerous errors of performance as the learner develops strategies and schemata for how to successfully complete the task. The retention phase is demonstrated during subsequent sessions, when the learner demonstrates recall or retention of the task in a similar situation. The transfer phase focuses on generalization of skill that is seen when the learner is able to spontaneously perform the task in different environments, such as the client who is able to correctly apply safety precautions after a total hip replacement at home after learning the precautions in the hospital.

LEARNING CAPACITIES

Dynamic assessment is one approach used to determine an individual's capacity to benefit from education and training. In this assessment framework an interactive process is used by which the therapist uses feedback, encouragement, and guidance to facilitate an individual's optimal performance using a test-teach-retest format.[46] Dynamic assessment provides therapists the opportunity to observe learning and change within various environments while considering the client's culture, beliefs, and values, which can help guide intervention.

Not all clients are able to transfer skills learned in one environment to another setting. Clients who cannot transfer learning will need environmental modifications, supervision, and/or cueing to engage successfully in the activity being taught. Therefore, the therapist needs to determine each client's capacity for retaining and transferring knowledge so that therapist and client can establish appropriate goals and use appropriate teaching methods. For example, electronic devices can provide cues and prompts to support skill performance across environments.

Li's occupational therapist (OT) used education to inform both Li and his wife about safe transfers on and off the toilet early in his rehabilitation program. After providing initial instruction, the OT asked him to demonstrate a transfer. The OT then provided additional instruction to address unsafe techniques observed. After providing revised instruction, the OT had Li demonstrate the transfer to determine if he was incorporating the feedback. These skills were then practiced to promote training of the safe transfer skills. This education-training process was repeated during each session until the OT was confident that Li was able to consistently use safe technique in the hospital.

Transfer of knowledge can be evaluated by changing one or more attributes of the task and observing whether the client is still able to perform the task. For instance, a therapist who has been teaching upper body dressing can change the type of garment used in the task, the location or orientation of the garment relative to the client, or the client's positioning. A client who is not able to perform the task with one or more attributes changed may not be capable of transferring new skills. In Li's case, he used safe transfer skills within his hospital room and the inpatient therapy clinic, demonstrating transfer of the skill across two environmental contexts.

OT PRACTICE NOTES

Learning capacities can change dramatically in some clients because of spontaneous recovery from neurological insults, so therapists should frequently reassess clients to determine whether teaching methods and goals need to be adjusted.

PROCEDURAL AND DECLARATIVE LEARNING

Therapists teach tasks in which learning occurs both consciously and unconsciously. Knowledge is demonstrated in different ways for the two types of tasks. Procedural learning occurs for tasks that are typically performed automatically, such as many motor and perceptual skills (see Chapter 33 for additional details). Procedural knowledge is developed through repeated practice in a variety of environmental settings. For instance, an individual learns to maneuver a wheelchair through a process of procedural learning while gradually developing a movement schema for the activity.[39] Verbal instruction alone is of little value. Rather, the procedures for performing this activity are learned through opportunities to experiment with different combinations of arm or arm and leg movements in a variety of directions, speeds, surfaces, and around various obstacles. Learning is demonstrated through efficiency of performance; therefore, individuals who have limitations in cognition or language can still demonstrate procedural knowledge.

Declarative learning creates knowledge that can be cognitively recalled. Learning a multistep activity, such as dressing self or performing a transfer, is often facilitated if the client can verbalize the steps of the task while completing it. Learning also can be demonstrated by verbally describing (declaring) the steps involved in completing the activity. Through repetition of an activity, declarative knowledge can become procedural, as the movement becomes more automatic and requires less cognitive attention. Mental rehearsal is an effective technique for enhancing declarative learning. During mental rehearsal the individual practices the activity sequence by reviewing it mentally or by verbalizing the process. This method can be used effectively with clients who, because of weakness or fatigue, are limited in their ability to physically practice an activity. However, because of the cognitive requirements, clients with significant cognitive or language deficits may not be able to express declarative knowledge.

Li described the similarities and differences between his bathroom at home and the hospital room bathroom. The occupational therapist created an environment similar to his home setting to assess Li's procedural knowledge and transfer of skills from the hospital training to home environment.

STRATEGIES FOR IMPLEMENTING OCCUPATIONAL THERAPY SERVICE

The process of implementing occupational therapy services involves a sequence of clinical reasoning decisions. Regardless of the characteristics of the client and the activity, basic learning principles can be applied when providing services.

The principles listed in Box 7.1 identify the strategies for implementing occupational therapy services. Before initiating an activity, the occupational therapist must be aware of the

BOX 7.1   Strategies for Implementing Occupational Therapy Services

- Identify an activity that has meaning or value to the client and/or family.
- Choose an instructional mode that is compatible with the client's cognition and the characteristics of the task to be taught.
- Organize the learning environment.
- Provide reinforcement and grading of activities.
- Structure feedback and practice schedules.
- Help the client develop self-awareness and self-monitoring skills.

client's cognitive capacity, valued occupations of the client and family, the attributes of the task being taught, and the personal and environment contexts for the activity.[2] The therapist gathers information during the initial assessment to create an accurate occupational profile from which to develop the intervention plan, the choice of activities, and the method of teaching to support the client. Effective intervention requires appropriate evidence-based application of these principles to each client's unique situation. This is where implementation science becomes critical.[33,41] The use of effective interventions must be considered within the context of personal and environmental contexts.

Two examples of teaching methods used during intervention include occupational gradation and goal-directed training. Occupational gradation is a method of systematically adjusting or altering the properties of the task performance, the person, the object, and the environment to optimally support the individual's engagement in the occupation. It includes the interaction of these various elements in occupational performance, such as donning shoes and then instructing how to don shoes using a long-handled shoe horn to avoid hip flexion. Occupational gradation incorporates principles of motor learning, motor control, personal factors, environmental factors, and properties of tasks and objects. Meaningfulness of the task, client goals, and ability to incorporate the task into daily life are also key considerations.[39] The goal-directed training approach uses client-selected goals to create active problem-solving opportunities for the client. Intervention is focused on the task to be achieved, rather than on impairments that may limit performance. This approach is based on the dynamic systems models of motor control and motor learning and the ecological occupation-based models of intervention. Progress is measured through incremental steps using goal attainment scaling.[29]

Each of these approaches combines occupation-centered activities and active engagement of the client, with application of specific motor learning and teaching techniques tailored to the cognitive and motor abilities of the client. Professional reasoning assists the therapist in determining the appropriate configuration of goals, activities, and teaching methods for each individual. The principles of teaching and learning in occupational therapy are further discussed in the following sections.

Identify a Meaningful Occupation, Activity, or Task

When conducting a client-centered assessment, the therapist explores which occupations have the greatest value and importance to the client. Engagement in these occupations can serve both as outcomes of intervention and as activities used in the intervention process. The client will be motivated to be an active partner in the therapy process if the activities are perceived to be meaningful.[47] If the client does not have the capability to engage in the occupation itself, performance skills and activities that contribute to participation in the occupation are often addressed in the intervention. The therapist collaborates with the client to develop or improve skills that contribute to the client's ability to engage in valued occupations. Doing so helps the client ascribe meaning to the activities and facilitates optimal participation.

Li's occupational therapist learned of his skill as a painter during the initial interview with Li and his wife. The therapist was able to use Li's motivation to return to this valued occupation to guide the choice of drawing and painting activities to improve function in his injured arm. The therapist also was able to explain to Li how his participation in other therapeutic activities to improve strength, range of motion, and endurance would contribute to his ability to resume his occupation of painting, in addition to independence in daily living skills. The therapist's attention to Li's interests and values created trust that led to a productive learning partnership.[12]

Choose Instructional Mode Compatible With Client's Cognition

Many people consider education and specifically teaching skills as synonymous with verbal instruction, but occupational therapists us several forms of education and training approaches.

Verbal instruction is an effective means of conveying information in many situations. It is an efficient method for instructing groups, such as in back safety classes, during training in hip precautions after hip replacement surgery, and through instruction in body mechanics and ergonomic principles for employee groups. Verbal instruction also can be used effectively when instructing individual clients. Verbal cues can be used to provide reinforcement or to give information about the next step in the sequence or the quality of performance. Verbal cues can be an effective method to provide feedback in the early and middle stages when training new skills; however, it should be phased out as soon as possible so that the client does not become dependent on verbal cues to complete the task. Family members and caregivers can be instructed on how to provide appropriate verbal cues if the client is unable to recall a task sequence independently. Li's wife was present during instruction on transfer techniques, and the therapist taught her brief verbal cues she could use to remind Li of key steps of the safe transfer process.

Visual instruction is effective for clients who have cognitive and/or attention deficits and difficulty processing verbal language and also for tasks that are too complex to describe verbally. The therapist demonstrates discrete steps of the activity, and the client observes the therapist and then follows the therapist's demonstration. The therapist may need to repeat the demonstration for the client to accurately reproduce the task. Other forms of visual instruction include drawings, photographs, or short video clips of the performance that can be used to remind a client and/or caregiver about the task sequence or desired performance outcome. Visual instruction can effectively be paired with verbal instruction, but therapists must avoid overwhelming the client with combined verbal and visual input.

Somatosensory instruction involves the use of tactile, proprioceptive, and kinesthetic cues to help guide the speed and direction of a movement. Manual guidance is a form of somatosensory instruction that is especially effective for procedural learning, such as the process of weight shifting and postural adjustment involved in coming from sit to stand. Hand-over-hand assistance is effective in teaching activities to clients who have cognitive and/or sensory processing deficits; the therapist guides the client's hands in completion of a task.

Forward and backward chaining represents another method of instruction. The therapist can also break the task into steps, demonstrating one step at a time and continuing to the next step as the client completes the previous step. This strategy then links or "chains" each of the steps together to help train the task performance. The steps can be taught in a forward progression or in reverse order.

When the steps are taught in a forward progression, known as *forward chaining*, the therapist demonstrates the first step of the task, works with the client to achieve mastery of this step, and then teaches the second step connected or chained to the first step. This process of forward chaining can be used with a variety of tasks, such as donning a front closing shirt in which the client places one arm in the sleeve and receives support for the remainder of the task. As the client gains mastery of the first step (placing one arm in the shirt sleeve), the second step of swinging the shirt around the back of the neck is taught and client mastery is met before moving to the third step. In this approach the task is broken into incremental steps and taught in a forward progression until the client has mastered the task performance.

The process of training can also occur in a backward manner, known as *backward chaining*, in which the full task is broken into discrete steps and the client is first taught the last step in performance. This allows a sense of task completion and may motivate a client to participate in the task. The therapist would assist or complete the first few steps of the task and have the client complete the final step of the task. An example can be seen with the task of preparing a salad in which ingredients need to be selected, washed, cut, and combined and then applying a salad dressing. In this sequence of steps, the therapist would have the client apply the preferred salad dressing as the first step mastered. The next session would ask the client to both combine the salad ingredients and apply the salad dressing.

Li's therapist used all instructional modes. Verbal instruction was most effective for reteaching self-care skills; verbal cueing was used to orient Li to the task sequence during the acquisition phase of learning. Visual instruction was used to teach many of the therapeutic activities the therapist used to enhance upper extremity function. Somatosensory instruction was effective for balance retraining during safe toilet transfers to avoid weight bearing on the fractured lower extremity. Backward chaining was used in which the therapist prepared the canvas and secured it to his easel, paints were arranged, and brushes selected before Li began painting.

Structure the Learning Environment

Choosing the appropriate environment in which to instruct a client is critical to teaching success. If a client is confused or easily distracted, a quiet environment with minimal visual distraction is often needed when teaching of a task is begun. As the client becomes more proficient in the skill being taught, visual and auditory distractions need to be introduced so the environment more closely resembles the one in which the client will eventually engage in the activity. For instance, a therapist working with a client on self-feeding may initially conduct the intervention in the client's room. As the client becomes more

proficient and confident, the therapist may move the intervention to the facility's dining room, where multiple distractions are present. In addition to providing challenges to the client's attention, the dining room provides opportunities for social interaction, which may act as a motivator for the client to further improve self-feeding skills.

Similarly, clients need opportunities to practice new skills in a variety of environments so that they are proficient in meeting environmental challenges. A client who is learning how to control a wheelchair needs to practice both outdoors and indoors on a variety of surfaces. A client who is working on refining grasp and dexterity needs experience in manipulating objects of a variety of sizes, shapes, and weights while engaging in functional tasks with a variety of demands similar to those that will be encountered in the client's daily activities.

Li's therapist determined that his initial confusion necessitated a quiet, minimally stimulating environment for initiation of teaching in self-care skills. As Li's confusion cleared, he was able to work in the therapy clinic on activities to improve balance for transfers and upper extremity control for dressing and hygiene tasks, and later he worked in the kitchen and garden areas on more demanding and varied skills.

Provide Reinforcement and Grading of Activities

The concept of reinforcement comes from operant conditioning theory, which states that behaviors that are rewarded or reinforced tend to be repeated.[21] Many types of reinforcement may be used. For some clients, social reinforcement such as a smile or verbal encouragement creates motivation to continue. Other clients may require more tangible rewards, such as rest periods, snacks, favorite activities, and so on. Still other clients are motivated by visible indications of their progress. Use of a graph or chart to demonstrate daily improvement in performance skills or client factors such as grip strength, sitting tolerance, or range of motion can help a client to engage more actively in the therapy process. These are examples of extrinsic reinforcement.

Many clients are motivated by completion of a task—for example, preparing a snack and then eating it or dressing themselves independently so they can visit with friends. Completion of the task provides intrinsic reinforcement, seen in the individual's satisfaction in his or her ability to participate in desirable activities as a result of completing the task. An activity that is motivating and meaningful to the client can increase active participation and improve intervention outcomes. As occupational therapists, the focus of services should address occupational performance. Clients engaged in meaningful and/or purposeful occupations demonstrated greater time engaged in the task, better attention to task performance, greater functional gains, and expressed higher levels of satisfaction.[3,8,14,35]

Visual imagery, in which the client is asked to imagine seeing the movement of the extremity to achieve the intended task, is often used. The use of visual imagery has been promoted as an avenue to enhance the effectiveness of exercise, but results have been inconclusive. A randomized controlled trial (RCT) provided one group of clients with daily exercise and additional visual imagery, and the control group received only exercise. Both groups improved, and no statistical significant difference in outcomes was demonstrated between the two groups.[34] In another RCT, intervention compared the use of imagery to observation with an additional control group of individuals.[49] Both treatment groups, using imagery and observation, improved over the control group, but there was no difference in outcomes between the two treatment groups.

In addition to structuring the type of reinforcement, the therapist needs to carefully grade the challenges of the activity, so the client can experience success and mastery during the process of learning the activity. If the client has too much difficulty completing a task, social reinforcement or inherent meaningfulness of the activity will not be enough to override frustration or fatigue. Therefore, therapists must analyze the activity and determine how to grade the activity to meet the learning and reinforcement needs of the individual client. This includes deciding on the most appropriate mode of instruction (as described in the previous section), what type of reinforcement will facilitate intrinsic motivation, and how best to structure feedback and practice schedules; these decisions are discussed in the next section.

Li's therapist knew that his strong desire to return to his occupation of leading nature hikes would motivate him to improve his balance and standing tolerance. The therapist explained how a variety of activities involving challenges to Li's sitting and standing balance would help him regain his ability to engage in activity, such as gardening, painting, and hiking. Li participated actively in these tasks, and he generated ideas for additional tasks that could be incorporated into his OT program; he also practiced outside of the therapy environment. His intrinsic motivation to return to preferred occupations was incorporated into intervention across various environments.

Structure Feedback and Practice

Feedback is information about a response[38] that can provide knowledge about the quality of the learner's performance or the results of the performance. Intrinsic feedback is generated by an individual's sensory systems. An individual learning to hit a golf ball uses visual and somatosensory feedback to evaluate performance. The visual system is used to align the head of the golf club and the golfer's body in correct orientation to the ball. Kinesthetic and proprioceptive inputs inform the golfer about joint position and the location of body segments in space; this allows the golfer to make the necessary postural adjustments and upper extremity movements to bring the club head into contact with the ball while using appropriate speed and force.

Extrinsic feedback is information from an outside source. The trajectory of the golf ball, the distance of the drive, and the location of the ball on the fairway all provide extrinsic feedback about the results of the golfer's actions. An observer can provide extrinsic feedback about task performance by giving the golfer information such as, "Your stance was too wide," "You did not follow through far enough on the swing," or "Your head position was good." For clients whose sensory recognition or processing abilities have been impaired, extrinsic feedback from a therapist or technological device can provide useful supplementary information to facilitate learning during the acquisition phase. Technological feedback mechanisms include biofeedback systems, virtual reality, and gaming technology,[22] and digital displays of kinetic or cardiovascular data on exercise equipment. These feedback systems can allow manipulation of practice conditions and often provide more immediate and consistent feedback than can be obtained from a therapist.

Although extrinsic feedback may be helpful early in the learning process, clients will achieve greater independence and efficiency in activities by developing the ability to continue learning through intrinsic rather than extrinsic feedback. In fact, extrinsic feedback may not produce optimal learning and may create dependency, with deterioration in performance if the feedback is removed.[23] Therefore, extrinsic feedback must be gradually decreased if the client's goal is independent performance in a variety of performance contexts.

Practice is a powerful component of the occupational therapy process. The ways in which a therapist structures practice conditions can influence a client's success in retention and transfer of learning. Several aspects of practice are discussed in the following paragraphs.

Li experienced mild sensory loss in his right arm as part of his injury. When his cast was removed and active rehabilitation commenced, he benefited from extrinsic verbal cues and somatosensory feedback provided by his therapist about the quality of his movement. As his upper extremity function improved, the therapist gradually decreased the amount of extrinsic feedback provided. Li learned to use intrinsic feedback to adjust the timing, speed, and direction of his movements while engaged in a variety of functional activities designed to improve strength, range of motion, and dexterity. Participation in practice sessions that included varied task challenges helped him learn strategies that could be transferred to many activities.

Contextual Interference

Contextual interference refers to factors in the learning environment that increase the difficulty of initial learning. Limiting extrinsic feedback provided about the results of performance is one example of contextual interference. A therapist who is attempting to limit extrinsic feedback will minimize the amount of verbal feedback about performance and/or the amount of manual guidance provided during the task. Performance during the acquisition phase may be poorer with high contextual interference; retention and generalization are more effective. This may occur because a high level of contextual interference forces the learner to rely on intrinsic feedback and to adapt motor and cognitive strategies to complete the task, resulting in more effective learning.[16]

Blocked and Random Practice Schedules

Blocked and random practice schedules are examples of low and high contextual interference, respectively. During blocked practice, clients practice one task until they master it. This is followed by practice of a second task until it is also mastered. In random practice, clients attempt multiple tasks or variations of a task before they have mastered any one of the tasks. A random practice schedule may be used to teach wheelchair transfer skills. The client practices each of several transfers during the course of a single session. For example, the client will practice moving between the wheelchair and a therapy mat, between the wheelchair and a chair, and between a toilet and the wheelchair. A random practice schedule for improving postural stability might include having the client stand on a variety of unstable surfaces, such as an equilibrium board, a balance beam, or a foam cushion, while playing a game of catch. These types of practice schedules may slow the initial acquisition of skills but are better for long-term retention of these skills[10] and for transfer of the learning to another context or task.[13] This is because random practice engages deeper cognitive processing than blocked practice. As a result, the stronger motor memory formed facilitates retention, particularly for more complex motor tasks.[18,36]

Whole Versus Part Practice

Breaking a task into its component parts for teaching purposes is useful only if the task can naturally be divided into discrete, recognizable units.[50] This is so because continuous skills (or whole task performance) are easier to remember than discrete responses.[43] For example, once a person has learned to ride a bicycle, this motor skill will be retained even without practicing for many years. Continuous skills should be taught in their entirety rather than in segments. For example, the activity of making vegetable soup includes several discrete tasks, including chopping vegetables, measuring ingredients, assembling the ingredients in the soup pot, and cooking the ingredients. During one session, the therapist could teach a client to chop the vegetables; the other components of the task could be taught in subsequent sessions. However, for the activity of making a pot of coffee, the task components (measuring the water, pouring it into the coffeemaker, measuring the coffee, putting the coffee into the coffeemaker, turning on the coffeemaker) need to be completed in a specific order. Teaching any of these task components in isolation would not result in meaningful learning or independent activity performance. For best retention and generalization, making coffee should be taught as a complete task, rather than having the client practice a different portion of the task during each therapy session.

To facilitate the learning process, the therapist may provide demonstration, verbal cueing, or manual guidance as needed for selected aspects of the task. This way the client experiences completion of the task on each trial, and the therapist gradually gives less assistance as practice sessions continue.

Cognitive Strategies

A growing body of literature supports the efficacy of cognitive strategies in helping individuals to learn motor skills. Cognitive strategies are goal-directed, consciously controlled processes that support motor learning and include conation, memory, problem solving, mental imagery, perception, and metacognition.[32] Cognitive strategies can be general or specific. Metacognition refers to the client's ability to examine knowledge acquisition or think about the thinking process. Conation refers to the coupling of thinking and action.[11,15] The effort expended by a client to engage and complete a task is a reflection of conation. General strategies are used in a variety of situations, and specific strategies are used for a particular task. An RCT compared the use of exercises to exercises combined with functional cognitive

therapy to reduce chronic neck pain.[17] Clients had significantly better outcomes in reduction of chronic neck pain when exercises were coupled with functional cognitive strategies to foster stress relief and relaxation. Evidence from a variety of studies suggests that cognitive strategies can assist individuals with stroke to transfer skills to different environments.[24,25,32,48] Cognitive strategies can be used in conjunction with practice in variable contexts to facilitate learning of motor and functional performance skills.

Based on the meta-analysis study provided by Park et al.,[35] the use of occupation-based cognitive rehabilitation for clients with traumatic brain injury (TBI) improved activities of daily living (ADLs) and mental functions in addition to psychosocial functions. Li was very motivated to regain control of his dominant arm to return to his treasured occupation of watercolor painting. Following the study suggestion,[35] Li's therapist asked him to review the systematic steps needed to prepare the watercolor canvas before painting. He explained the process and the need for the canvas to be prepared approximately 1 day before painting. The occupational therapist engaged Li in problem-solving strategies to consider where to position the canvas to dry in anticipation of returning to the canvas the next day to begin painting. He spent far more time and energy engaged in preparing his canvas before engaging in watercolor painting compared to rote exercises. This reflects the use of occupations to regain function.

Practice under variable contexts enhances transfer of learning. Optimal retention and transfer of motor skills occur when the practice context is natural rather than simulated.[26,31] This may reflect the fact that the enriched natural environment provides more sources of feedback and information about performance than the more impoverished simulated environment. However, transfer of learning is better when the demands of the practice environment more closely resemble the demands of the environment in which the client will eventually be expected to perform.[51] Therefore, teaching kitchen skills in a client's own home or in a kitchen environment that is very similar to the client's kitchen will result in better task performance when the client engages in the task at home.

Client factors may also influence outcomes related to the practice context. A meta-analysis of the effects of context found that treatment effects were much greater for populations with neurological impairments than for those without neurological impairment.[23] Errorless learning, also known as systematic instruction, is an intervention paradigm based on the principle that learning will occur more quickly and efficiently if the learner does not engage in trial and error throughout the learning process. This learning strategy has been used effectively with individuals who have cognitive or memory deficits as a result of acquired brain injury or dementia,[40] but it has also been effective in facilitating learning of a practical skill (fitting a prosthetic limb) during the rehabilitation process.[9]

One aspect of the practice context that has received little research attention is the role of the social environment in task learning. The importance of the social context of occupational performance and of the occupation of social participation is endorsed by the Occupational Therapy Practice Framework: Domain and Process, 3rd edition (OTPF-3).[2] Working with other clients in a group promotes socialization, cooperation, and competition, which can increase clients' motivation. Acquisition of skills is enhanced through observation of others who are learning a task. Additionally, group intervention can promote the development of problem-solving skills and can create a bridge between the supervised therapy environment and the unsupervised home environment.[7]

Help Client Develop Self-Awareness and Self-Monitoring Skills

To maximize the retention and transfer of learning, clients must develop the ability to self-monitor, so they are not dependent on extrinsic feedback and reinforcement. The knowledge and regulation of personal cognitive processes and capacities is known as *metacognition*.[19] It includes awareness of personal strengths and limitations and the ability to evaluate task difficulty, to plan ahead, to choose appropriate strategies, and to shift strategies in response to environmental cues. Although metacognition is typically discussed in relation to improving cognitive skills, self-awareness and monitoring of relevant performance skills may be equally important prerequisites to developing effective motor, interpersonal, and coping strategies. Specifically, an intervention directed toward helping clients develop enhanced awareness of body kinematics and alignment may be an important component of motor learning.[6] Self-review of performance and guided planning for tackling the challenges of future tasks are key factors in the therapeutic process and are critical prerequisites to a person's ability to generate and apply appropriate strategies.

Strategies are organized plans or sets of rules that guide action in a variety of situations.[42] Motor strategies include the repertoire of kinematic linkages and schemata that underlie the performance of skilled, efficient movement. The process of stepping to the side when one is abruptly jostled is a motor strategy for the maintenance of standing balance.[44] Cognitive strategies include the variety of tactics used to facilitate processing, storage, retrieval, and manipulation of information. Using a mnemonic device to remember a phone number is a cognitive strategy. Interpersonal strategies help in social interactions with other individuals. A person who uses direct eye contact and greets another by name when being introduced is using an interpersonal strategy. Coping strategies allow people to adapt constructively to stress. Coping strategies can include deep breathing, exercise, or relaxation activities.

Strategies provide individuals with foundational skills that can be adapted to the changing demands of occupational tasks within a variety of contexts. Thus, learning is more likely to be transferred to new situations when opportunities arise to develop foundational strategies.[45] Individuals develop strategies through a process of encountering problems, implementing solutions, and monitoring the effects of these solutions. Occupational therapists use activities to help clients develop useful strategies by presenting task challenges within a safe environment that provide opportunities to try out different solutions.[42]

As Li was nearing discharge from occupational therapy services, the therapist worked with him to develop strategies to facilitate his occupational performance. Although his memory was improved, recall of names and numbers was still poor, so the cognitive strategy of using a notebook for recording important information was continued. In addition, to cope with persistent mild deficits in balance, Li and his therapist developed a motor strategy of keeping a sturdy table nearby when he stood to talk to visitors at the botanical gardens. This strategy provided a support that he could lean on or hold onto if needed, and it was a strategy that also could be used in other situations.

FACTORS THAT INFLUENCE THE LEARNING PROCESS

The ultimate goal of learning is to create strategies and skills that individuals can apply flexibly in a variety of contexts and occupations. As this chapter has presented, occupational therapists have many methods available to them to help their clients achieve this goal. The concepts discussed in this chapter that facilitate transfer of learning to other environments are listed in Box 7.2.

THREADED CASE STUDY

Li, Part 2

In the case of Li, the therapist used the information gathered in the initial assessment process to determine what should be taught to Li and his wife and in what order various tasks, activities, and occupations would be presented. The intervention began with hygiene tasks because these could be accomplished in a sitting position and because of Li's stated desire to perform these tasks independently. Transfer skills and adapted activity of daily living (ADL) techniques were important within the occupational therapy services provided so that Li could maximize his mobility, safety, and functional independence in a wheelchair while his lower extremity fractures healed.

As Li's healing progressed, his therapist was able to begin teaching tasks to improve postural stability and upper extremity strength and coordination. Occupations taught during this phase included ADLs and instrumental ADLs (IADLs), in addition to activities designed to improve motor skills. As Li's performance skills improved, the therapist was able to introduce more complex tasks and occupations that further challenged his motor and process skills and prepared him to return to his valued occupations of painting, hiking, and teaching.

As Li's discharge from therapy neared, the therapist changed to focus on teaching cognitive and motor strategies that Li could use to help compensate for residual deficits in balance and memory. Throughout the intervention process the therapist reassessed Li's functional status to adjust teaching strategies to support Li's current cognitive and motor skills and to the specific demands of the task and environment.

BOX 7.2   Factors That Support Transfer of Learning

- Active participation
- Occupationally embedded instruction
- Intrinsic feedback
- Contextual interference
- Random practice schedules
- Naturalistic contexts
- Whole task practice
- Strategy development

SUMMARY

Occupational therapists teach activities for a variety of reasons. They reteach familiar activities, teach alternative or compensatory strategies of performing valued activities, teach new performance skills to support role performance, teach therapeutic challenges to improve performance skills to support occupational participation, and teach caregivers and/or family members to facilitate the client's independence and safety in the home environment.

Occupational therapists use a variety of teaching strategies to promote skill acquisition, skill retention, and transfer of learning. Procedural and declarative learning represent unconscious and conscious learning processes, respectively.

Occupational therapists maximize the learning process by (1) identifying activities that have meaning or value to the client/family, (2) providing instruction tailored to the needs of the individual and the task, (3) structuring the environment to facilitate learning, (4) providing reinforcement and grading of activities to establish intrinsic motivation, (5) structuring feedback and practice to facilitate acquisition, retention, and transfer of learning, and (6) helping clients develop self-awareness and self-monitoring skills.

REVIEW QUESTIONS

1. What is the difference between acquisition, retention, and transfer of learning? Apply these terms to describe the learning stages in a client you have observed.
2. When are declarative learning and procedural learning processes used? How will OT services differ if declarative or procedural processes are used?
3. What are the reasons therapists use education and training? Give an example of desired outcomes for each of the reasons presented in the chapter.
4. In which situations is extrinsic feedback valuable to the therapeutic process? What are some advantages and disadvantages of providing extrinsic feedback to clients?
5. How does contextual interference contribute to transfer of learning? Think of an example of how contextual interference can be incorporated into an OT session.
6. Differentiate between random and blocked practice schedules. In which situations would each of these practice schedules be chosen?
7. Provide examples of how a therapist might structure whole practice versus part practice. In which situations might each of these types of practice be appropriate?
8. In which ways can occupational therapists enhance the variability of practice contexts? Give practical examples of how occupational therapists working in inpatient settings can provide treatment in natural contexts.
9. How can occupational therapists help clients develop metacognitive skills? Why are these skills important in the learning process?
10. What strategies can be used during occupational therapy services to foster self-awareness and self-motivation?

For additional practice questions for this chapter, please visit eBooks.Health.Elsevier.com.

REFERENCES

1. American Occupational Therapy Association (AOTA): AOTA 2020 Occupational Therapy Code of Ethics, Am J Occup Ther 74(Suppl 3): 1–13, 2020. https://doi.org/10.5014/ajot.2020.74S3006/.
2. American Occupational Therapy Association: Occupational therapy practice framework: Domain and process (4th ed.), *American Journal of Occupational Therapy* 74(Suppl. 2):1–87, 2020. https://doi.org/10.5014/ajot.2020.74S2001.
3. Arya KN, Verma R, Garg RK, Sharma VP, Agarwal M, Aggarwal GG: Meaningful task-specific training (MTST) for stroke rehabilitation: a randomized controlled trial, *Topics in Stroke Rehabilitation* 19(3):193–211, 2012. https://doi.org/10.1310/tsr1903-193.
4. Bauer MS, Kirchner J: Implementation science: what is it and why should I care? *Psychiatry Res* 283:112376, 2020. https://doi.org/10.1016/j.psychres.2019.04.025.
5. Bauer MS, Damschroder L, Hagedorn H, Smith J, Kilbourne AM: An introduction to implementation science for the non-specialist, *BMC Psychol* 3(1):32, 2015. https://doi.org/10.1186/s40359-015-0089-9.
6. Carr JH, Shepherd RB: *Neurological rehabilitation: optimizing motor performance*, Oxford, England, 1998, Butterworth-Heinemann.
7. Carr JH, Shepherd RB: *Stroke rehabilitation: guidelines for exercise and training to optimize motor skill*, London, 2003, Butterworth-Heinemann.
8. Celinder D, Peoples H: Stroke patients' experiences with Wii Sports® during inpatient rehabilitation, *Scandinavian Journal of Occupational Therapy* 19(5):457–463, 2012. https://doi.org/10.3109/11038128.2012.655307.
9. Donaghey CL, McMillan TM, O'Neill B: Errorless learning is superior to trial and error when learning a practical skill in rehabilitation: a randomized controlled trial, *Clin Rehabil* 24:195–201, 2010.

10. Ferguson JM, Trombly CA: The effect of added-purpose and meaningful occupation on motor learning, *Am J Occup Ther* 51:508–515, 1997.

11. Gerdes KE, Stromwall LK: Conation: a missing link in the strengths perspective, *Social Work* 53:233–242, 2008.

12. Guidetti S, Tham K: Therapeutic strategies used by occupational therapists in self-care training: a qualitative study, *Occup Ther Int* 9:257–276, 2002.

13. Giuffrida CG, Demery JA, Reyes LR, et al: Functional skill learning in men with traumatic brain injury, *Am J Occup Ther* 63:398–407, 2009.

14. Gustafsson L, McKenna K: Is there a role for meaningful activity in stroke rehabilitation? *Topics in Stroke Rehabilitation* 17(2):108–118, 2010. https://doi.org/10.1310/tsr1702-108.

15. Hill BD, Aita SL: The positive side of effort: a review of the impact of motivation and engagement on neuropsychological performance, *Applied Neuropsychology: Adult* 25(4):312–317, 2018. https://doi.org/10.1080/23279095.2018.1458502.

16. Jarus T: Motor learning and occupational therapy: the organization of practice, *Am J Occup Ther* 48:810–816, 1994.

17. Javdaneh N, Letafatkar A, Shojaedin S, Hadadnezhad M: Scapular exercise combined with cognitive functional therapy is more effective at reducing chronic neck pain and kinesiophobia than scapular exercise alone: a randomized controlled trial, *Clinical Rehabilitation* 34:1485–1496, 2020. https://doi.org/10.1177/0269215520941910.

18. Kantak SS, Winstein C: Learning-performance distinction and memory processes for motor skills: a focused review and perspective, *Behav Brain Res* 228:219–231, 2011.

19. Katz N, Hartman-Maier A: Metacognition: the relationships of awareness and executive functions to occupational performance. In Katz N, editor: *Cognition and occupation in rehabilitation: cognitive models for intervention in occupational therapy*, Bethesda, MD, 1998, American Occupational Therapy Association.

20. Kirchner JE, Smith JL, Powell BJ, Waltz TJ, Proctor EK: Getting a clinical innovation into practice: an introduction to implementation science. *Psychiatry Research* 283:112467, 2020. https://doi.org/10.1016/j.psychres.2019.06.042.

21. Kupferman I: Learning and memory. In Kandel ER, Schwartz JH, Jessell TM, editors: *Principles of neuroscience* ed 3, New York, 1991, Elsevier.

22. Levin MF, Weiss PL, Keshner EA: Emergence of virtual reality as a tool for upper limb rehabilitation: incorporation of motor control and motor learning principles, *Phys Ther* 95:415–425, 2015.

23. Lin K-C, Wu C-Y, Tickle-Degnen L, Coster W: Enhancing occupational performance through occupationally embedded exercise: a meta-analytic review, *Occup Ther J Res* 17:25–47, 1997.

24. Liu KP, Chan CC, Lee TM, Hui-Chan CW: Mental imagery for promoting relearning for people after stroke: a randomized controlled trial, *Arch Phys Med Rehabil* 85:1403–1408, 2004.

25. Liu KP, Chan CCH, Wong RSM, et al: A randomized controlled trial of mental imagery augments generalization of learning in acute poststroke patients, *Stroke* 40:2222–2225, 2009.

26. Ma H, Trombly CA, Robinson-Podolski C: The effect of context on skill acquisition and transfer, *Am J Occup Ther* 53:138–144, 1999.

27. Marr D: Centennial topics: fostering full implementation of evidence-based practice, *American Journal of Occupational Therapy*, 71, 2017.

28. Reference deleted in proofs.

29. Mastos M, Miller K, Eliasson AC, Imms C: Goal-directed training: linking theories of treatment to clinical practice for improved functional activities in daily life, *Clin Rehabil* 21:47–55, 2007.

30. Mathieson A, Grande G, Luker K: Strategies, facilitators and barriers to implementation of evidence-based practice in community nursing: a systematic mixed-studies review and qualitative synthesis, *Primary Health Care Research & Development* 20(e6):1–11, 2018. https://doi.org/10.1017/S1463423618000488.

31. Mathiowetz V, Haugen JB: Motor behavior research: implications for therapeutic approaches to central nervous system dysfunction, *Am J Occup Ther* 48:733–745, 1994.

32. McEwen SE, Huijbregts MPJ, Ryan JD, Polatajko HJ: Cognitive strategy used to enhance motor skill acquisition post-stroke: a critical review, *Brain Inj* 23:263–277, 2009.

33. McNett M, Tucker S, Melnyk BM: Implementation science: a critical strategy necessary to advance and sustain evidence-based practice, *Worldviews on Evidence-Based Nursing* 16(3):174–175, 2019. https://doi.org/10.1111/wvn.12368.

34. Özcan Ö, Karaali H, Ilgin D, Gündüz ÖS, Kara B: Effectiveness of motor imagery training on functionality and quality of life in chronic neck pain: a randomized controlled trial, *Exercise Therapy and Rehabilitation* 6(1):1–9, 2019.

35. Park HY, Maitra K, Martinez KM: The Effect of Occupation-based cognitive rehabilitation for traumatic brain injury: A meta-analysis of randomized controlled trials, *Occupational Therapy International*, 22:104–116, 2015.

36. Pauwels L, Swinnen SP, Beets IAM: Contextual interference in complex bimanual skill learning leads to better skill persistence, *PLoS ONE* 9(6):e100906, 2014. https://doi.org/10.1371/journal.pone.0100906.

37. Peters DH, Adam T, Alonge O, Agyepong I, Tran N: Implementation research: What it is and how to do it, *British Medical Journal* 347:f6753, 2013. https://doi.org/10.1136/bmj.f6753.

38. Poole J: Application of motor learning principles in occupational therapy, *Am J Occup Ther* 45:53–57, 1991.

39. Poole J, Burtner PA, Stockman G: The Framework of Occupational Gradation (FOG) to treat upper extremity impairments in persons with central nervous system impairments, *Occup Ther Health Care* 23:40–59, 2009.

40. Powell LE, et al: Systematic instruction for individuals with acquired brain injury: results of a randomised controlled trial, *Neuropsychol Rehabil* 22:85–112, 2012.

41. Rapport F, Clay-Williams R, Churruca K, Shih P, Hogden A, Braithwaite J: The struggle of translating science into action: foundational concepts of implementation science, *Journal of Evaluation in Clinical Practice* 24:117–126, 2018. https://doi.org/10.1111/jep.12741.

42. Sabari J: Activity-based intervention in stroke rehabilitation. In Gillen G, Burkhardt A, editors: *Stroke rehabilitation: a function-based approach* ed 2, St Louis, 2004, Mosby.

43. Schmidt RA: *Motor performance and learning: principles for practitioners*, Champaign, IL, 1992, Human Kinetics.

44. Shumway-Cook A, Woollacott M: *Motor control: theory and practical applications,* ed 3. Baltimore, 2007, Williams & Wilkins.

45. Singer RN, Cauraugh JH: The generalizability effect of learning strategies for categories of psychomotor skills, *Quest* 37:103–119, 1985.

46. Toglia J, Cermak SA: Dynamic assessment and prediction of learning potential in clients with unilateral neglect, *Am J Occup Ther* 63:569–579, 2009.

47. Trombly CA: Occupation: purposefulness and meaningfulness as therapeutic mechanisms: 1995 Eleanor Clark Slagle Lecture, *Am J Occup Ther* 49:960–972, 1995.

48. Walker MF, et al: The DRESS trial: a feasibility randomized controlled trial of a neuropsychological approach to dressing therapy for stroke inpatients, *Clin Rehabil* 26(8):675–685, 2011.

49. Williams SE: Comparing movement imagery and action observation as techniques to increase imagery ability, *Psychology of Sport and Exercise*, 44:99–106, 2019.

50. Winstein CJ: Designing practice for motor learning clinical implications. In Lister MJ, editor: *Contemporary management of motor control problems: proceedings of the II STEP conference*, Alexandria, VA, 1991, Foundation for Physical Therapy.

51. Zimmerer-Branum S, Nelson DL: Occupationally embedded exercise versus rote exercise: a choice between occupational forms by elderly nursing home residents, *Am J Occup Ther* 49:397–402, 1995.

8

Documentation of Occupational Therapy Services

Jerilyn (Gigi) Smith

LEARNING OBJECTIVES

After studying this chapter, the student or practitioner will be able to do the following:

1. Identify five purposes of documentation.
2. Describe the basic technical points that should be adhered to when writing in the medical record.
3. Explain why only approved abbreviations should be used in occupational therapy documentation.
4. Describe the acceptable method of correcting an error in the medical record.
5. Explain why occupational therapy documentation should reflect the terminology outlined in the Occupational Therapy Practice Framework (OTPF).
6. Describe the components of a well-written progress note.
7. Briefly summarize the content of the initial evaluation.
8. Define assessments as they apply to the OT process.
9. Describe the purpose of the intervention plan.
10. Explain why establishment of goals should be a collaborative effort between the client and the therapist.
11. Explain the meaning of client-centered goal.
12. Describe the purpose of progress reports.
13. Explain what is meant by a skilled intervention.
14. List the components of a SOAP note and give an example of each component of the note.
15. Identify the purpose of the discharge report.
16. Explain how professional reasoning is used in the documentation of occupational therapy services.
17. Describe two ways to ensure that confidentiality in documentation is maintained (refer to the American Occupational Therapy Association Code of Ethics and the regulations established by the Health Insurance Portability and Accountability Act [HIPAA]).

CHAPTER OUTLINE

KEY TERMS

Assessments
Checklist notes
Client record
Conditions supporting outcomes
Confidentiality
Discharge report
Documentation
Ethical practice
Evaluation

Evaluation report
Expected outcome behavior
Health Insurance Portability and Accountability Act (HIPAA)
Initial evaluation report
Intervention plan
Legal document
Long-term goal
Measurable expectation of performance
Medical record

THREADED CASE STUDY

Jane, Part 1

Jane (who prefers use of the pronouns she/her/hers) just started her first job as an occupational therapist (OT) at a skilled nursing facility. This week she completed two initial evaluations, and she has seen four clients for therapy each day. Jane knows the importance of accurate documentation, and she wants to make sure she includes data that will communicate the necessary information for reimbursement. She also knows that documentation is essential to demonstrate the value of occupational therapy. However, she has never worked in this practice setting and is worried about what terminology to use and how to document effectively to guarantee reimbursement.

Professional Thinking Questions

As you read this chapter, reflect on the following questions as they pertain to the case study.
1. What specific skills must Jane use in deciding how she will document the evaluation process?
2. What information is important to include in the SOAP note for reimbursement? Will the practice setting have an influence on what is included in the note?
3. How might federal regulations (HIPAA) and the principles put forth in the Occupational Therapy Code of Ethics influence how Jane communicates the results of the OT evaluation and the intervention program?

Documentation is an essential component of occupational therapy practice. It is the primary method of communication that is used to convey what was done with the client. Documentation supplements the practitioner's memory and creates a longitudinal record to enhance the continuity of care for the client. It demonstrates to others the value of OT intervention, and it provides validation of services to substantiate reimbursement. Documentation also serves as a means for collecting data that can later be used to support evidence-based clinical research.

PURPOSES OF DOCUMENTATION

Documentation is a permanent record of what occurred with the client. It is also a legal document and as such must follow the guidelines that will enable it to withstand a legal investigation. Reimbursement depends on accurate, well-written documentation that provides the necessary information to justify the need for and value of OT services.

The American Occupational Therapy Association (AOTA) has identified these purposes of documentation[1]:

- To communicate information about the client from the OT perspective
- To articulate the rationale for provision of OT services and the relationship of those services to the client's outcomes
- To create a chronological record of the client's status, the OT services provided to the client, the client's response to OT interventions, and client outcomes
- To provide justification for skilled occupational therapy services and reimbursement

Clear, concise, accurate, and objective information is essential to communicate the OT process to others. The clinical record should provide sufficient data to support the need for OT intervention and must reflect the OT practitioner's **clinical reasoning** and professional reasoning.

Documentation is required whenever OT services are performed. This includes a record of what occurred during direct client care, in addition to supportive documentation required to justify the need for OT intervention.

OT PRACTICE NOTES

Examples of Documentation

Documentation is an ongoing process that continues throughout the client's therapy program. For example, the OT will document screening reports, **initial evaluation reports**, reevaluation reports, progress notes, discharge summaries, other medical record entries (e.g., interdisciplinary care plans, provider telephone orders), intervention and equipment authorization requests, letters and reports to families and other healthcare professionals, and outcomes data.

BEST PRACTICES

Regardless of where documentation takes place, several basic technical points are important to adhere to when writing in the medical record. Box 8.1 lists the fundamental elements of documentation as set forth by the AOTA.[1] Proper grammar, correct spelling and syntax, and well-written sentences are essential components of any professional correspondence. Keeping lists of commonly used terms and using a handheld spell-check device are two strategies that can help the practitioner with spelling difficulties. Poor grammar or inaccurate spelling can lead the reader to question the skills of the therapist. If documentation is handwritten, legibility is important to ensure that misinterpretation does not occur.

Only approved abbreviations are to be used in the medical record. All clinical sites should have a printed list of acceptable abbreviations that can be used at the site. It is important to

BOX 8.1   AOTA's Fundamental Elements of Documentation

The following elements should be present in all documentation.

1. Client's full name, date of birth, and case number (if applicable) on each page.
2. Date.
3. Identification of type of documentation (e.g., evaluation report, progress note).
4. Occupational therapy practitioner's professional signature with a minimum of first name or initial, last name, and professional designation.
5. When applicable on notes or reports, the signature of the recorder directly at the end of the note and the signature.
6. Countersignature and credential by an OT on documentation written by students and occupational therapy assistant as required by the payer source, state regulations, or the employer.
7. Acceptable terminology defined within the boundaries of the setting.
8. Abbreviation usage as acceptable within the boundaries of the setting.
9. All errors corrected by drawing a single line through an error and initialing the correction.
10. Adherence to professional standards of technology when OT services are documented with electronic claims or records.
11. Compliance with confidentiality requirements.
12. Compliance with agency and state and federal regulations and guidelines for storage and disposal of records.
13. Documentation should reflect the professional clinical reasoning and expertise of an OT practitioner and the nature of OT services delivered in a safe and effective manner. Clear rationale for the purpose, value, and need for skilled OT services is provided. The client's diagnosis or prognosis should not be the sole rationale for OT services.

Modified from the American Occupational Therapy Association: Guidelines for documentation of occupational therapy, *Am J Occup Ther* 72 (Suppl 2):1–7, 2018.

obtain this list and to use it as a reference when documenting. Examples of abbreviations commonly used in clinical practice are listed in Box 8.2. Misinterpretation of the intended meaning can occur when unfamiliar abbreviations or casual language unsuitable for therapeutic context is used. Language particular to a profession (slang or jargon) should never be used in the client record.

All entries made in the medical record must be signed with the therapist's legal name. Your professional credentials should follow your signature. Do not leave blank spaces at the end of an intervention note. Instead, draw a single line that extends from the last word to the signature. This prevents additional information from being added after the entry has been completed.

One of the greatest challenges for students and new therapists is writing notes that are concise yet comprehensive and include all the relevant information necessary to meet the goals of documentation as described earlier. Most third-party payers do not reimburse for time spent on documentation, so efficiency becomes essential. Although it is particularly important to accurately describe what occurred in the therapy session, care must be taken to keep this information to the point, relevant, and specific to established goals identified in the intervention plan. A common error is to describe each event that occurred in the intervention session in a step-by-step format. This is far too time-consuming and in fact does not meet the objectives of good documentation. Rather, short statements should be used that clearly and objectively convey necessary information to the reader. Abbreviations that have been approved by and are appropriate for the practice setting can be used to save time and space. Customized forms and checklists that include information relevant to the practice setting help streamline documentation and reduce time spent on narrative writing.

OT practitioners have an obligation to present information (verbally, in writing, or electronically) that is clear and at a level of linguistic clarity that the recipient of the information can understand.

ETHICAL CONSIDERATIONS

Principle 5 of the AOTA's Code of Ethics[2] addresses the OT practitioner's duty to provide comprehensive, accurate, and objective information when representing the profession. Principle 5 states that OT personnel shall "implicitly promise to be truthful and not deceptive."[2] This pertains to all types of communication, including documentation. To maintain ethical standards when documenting, therapists must be truthful and accurate in all that they report about the client.

Documentation must be written by the therapist providing the intervention. It is never acceptable to write a note for another therapist; in fact, it is considered fraudulent to do so. It is best practice to complete documentation as soon after the therapy session as possible. The longer the interval between evaluation or intervention and completion of the written record, the greater the chance that details or other important information will be forgotten. Although documenting at the time of service delivery is ideal, it is not always possible. At these times, it may be beneficial for the therapist to carry a notepad or clipboard to record data that can later be included in the official write-up.

Altering, substituting, or deleting information from the client's record should never take place. Changes made to the original documentation could be used to support allegations of tampering with the medical record, even when this was not the intent of the writer. However, at times, corrections must be made. These might include errors in spelling, mistakenly writing in the wrong medical record, or inadvertently omitting information or assessment results. Several principles should be followed to avoid questioning of the validity of the corrected information. Nothing should be deleted or removed from the record. Never use correction fluid when correcting an entry in the client's record. An acceptable method of correcting an error in the documentation is to draw a single line through the word or words, initial and date the entry, and indicate that this was an "error." Do not try to obliterate the sentence or word because this may appear to be an attempt to prevent others from knowing what was originally written. Late entries to the medical record cannot be backdated. If it is necessary to enter information that is out of sequence (e.g., a note that the therapist forgot to write), it must be entered into the medical record as a "late entry" and be identified as such. Words or sentences cannot be squeezed into existing text "after the fact." Attempts to do this

BOX 8.2   Abbreviations Commonly Used in Clinical Documentation

abd	abduction	post	posterior
Add	adduction	Pt, pt	patient
ADLs	activities of daily living	PTA	prior to admission
Ⓐ	assistance	PWB	partial weight bearing
AE	above elbow	q	every
AFO	ankle-foot orthosis	qd	every day
AK	above knee	qh	every hour
AM	morning	qid	four times a day
ant	anterior	qn	every night
A/P	anterior-posterior	Ⓡ	right
AROM	active range of motion	RCF	residential care facility
Assist	Assistance, assistive	re:	regarding
Ⓑ	bilateral	rehab	rehabilitation
BE	below elbow	reps	repetitions
BM	bowel movement	R/O	rule out
BP	blood pressure	ROM	range of motion
c̄	with	RR	respiratory rate
CHF	congestive heart failure	RROM	resistive range of motion
CHI	closed head injury	Rx	prescription
C/O	complains of	s̄	without
D/C	discontinue or discharge	SNF	skilled nursing facility
dept	department	SOB	short of breath
DNR	do not resuscitate	S/P	status post
DOB	date of birth	S/S	signs and symptoms
DOE	dyspnea on exertion	STM	short-term memory
Dx	diagnosis	Sx	symptoms
ECF	extended care facility	TDWB	touch down weight bearing
eval	evaluation	TTWB	toe touch weight bearing
ext	extension	t.o.	telephone order
F/U	follow up	Tx	treatment
flex	flexion	UE	upper extremity
FWB	full weight bearing	VC	vital capacity
fx	fracture	v.o.	verbal orders
HOB	head of bed	WBAT	weight bearing as tolerated
HOH	hand over hand	w/c	wheelchair
LE	lower extremity	WFL	within functional limits
LOS	length of stay	WNL	within normal limits
NWB	non-weight bearing	y.o.	year old
OOB	out of bed	<–>	to and from
PO	by mouth	–>	to; progressing toward
PMH	past medical history	@	at
PM	afternoon	1°	primary
prn	as needed	2°	secondary; due to

From Gateley C, Borcherding S: *Documentation manual for occupational therapy: writing SOAP notes*, ed 4, Thorofare, NJ, 2017, Slack.

may be interpreted as adding missing information to support something that occurred after the original documentation was completed. Although it is acceptable to make immediate corrections in the medical record, the medical record itself should never be altered.[7]

Corrections in an electronic medical record (EMR) are managed differently from paper-based documentation corrections. Each facility or organization has its own protocol for correcting errors in the medical record. Therapists must take the initiative to learn the site-specific guidelines for making corrections in the medical chart.

ETHICAL CONSIDERATIONS

OT notes can be the best defense against a denial of reimbursement of services or a lawsuit. Although no fraudulent intent may be present, it could be suspected if the content of a claim is ever called into question.

Do not leave blank spaces on evaluation and preprinted forms. If it is not appropriate to complete a section, N/A can be inserted to indicate that the particular area was not addressed. If sections are left blank, others reading the chart may think these areas were overlooked.

Documentation should incorporate the terminology outlined in the *Occupational Therapy Practice Framework*, fourth edition (OTPF-4).[3] One of the purposes of the OTPF-4 is to assist therapists in communicating to other professionals, consumers of services, and third-party payers the unique focus of occupational therapy on occupation and daily life activities. Documentation should reflect the impact of occupational therapy on supporting function and performance in daily life activities and those factors that support well-being, participation, and health (performance skills, performance patterns, client factors, and context) through engagement in occupation during the evaluation and intervention process.[3] Many practice settings that follow the medical model, such as hospitals, use the term *patient* to describe the recipient of services. Other settings may prefer the term *resident*. Although these are acceptable, the OTPF-4 advocates use of the term *client*. *Client* encompasses not only the individual receiving therapy, but also others who are involved in the person's life (e.g., a spouse, parent, child, caregiver, employer), in addition to larger groups, such as organizations or communities. The OTPF-4 provides terminology that can be used at each stage of the therapy process. This is explained in further detail when the various parts of the therapy evaluation, intervention, and discharge processes are described.[3]

CLINICAL/PROFESSIONAL REASONING SKILLS

Occupational therapists must use clinical or professional reasoning throughout the OT process. The more contemporary term professional reasoning is used by some authors to more closely align with language used in OT practices outside of medical settings, such as educational and community settings. However, the term *clinical reasoning* is still widely used by OTs, especially those working in physical disability practice settings. Professional reasoning is also defined in the OTPF-4 as "enabling

practitioners to identify the multiple demands, required skills, and potential meanings of the activities and occupations, and to gain a deeper understanding of the interrelationships among aspects of the domain that affect performance and that support client-centered interventions and outcomes" (p. 23).[3] For the purpose of this chapter, the term *professional reasoning* will be used to refer to the comprehensive types of thinking and judgment used by OTs in making client-related decisions. Professional reasoning also includes determining how to appropriately document information obtained during the evaluation, intervention, and discharge process. Clinical/professional reasoning is used to plan, direct, perform, and reflect upon client care.[10] Documentation must demonstrate that professional reasoning was used in the decision-making process during all aspects of the client's therapy program.

Professional reasoning comprises many different aspects of reasoning: scientific, diagnostic, procedural, narrative, pragmatic, ethical, interactive, and conditional.[11] *Scientific reasoning* is used to help the therapist understand the client's impairments, disabilities, and performance contexts and to determine how these might influence occupational performance. Scientific reasoning guides the therapist's choice of interventions that will most benefit the client. *Diagnostic reasoning* is specifically concerned with clinical problem identification related to the client's condition. *Procedural reasoning* is used when the therapist considers and uses intervention routines for identified conditions that are typically used for clients in that particular setting. *Narrative reasoning* guides the therapist in evaluating the personal meaning that occupational performance limitations might have for the client. This involves an appreciation of the client's culture as a basis for understanding the client narrative. *Pragmatic reasoning* is used when the therapist addresses the practical realities associated with delivery of therapy services while looking at the context or contexts within which the client must perform their desired occupations. The therapist's personal situation, such as clinical competencies, preferences for particular therapy techniques, commitment to the profession, and comfort level in working with certain clients or conditions, is a part of the pragmatic reasoning process.[10] *Ethical reasoning* is the process by which the therapist considers what should be done, taking into consideration all interested parties' needs and wishes when they develop the intervention plan[10] For OT practitioners, keeping these points in mind and using professional reasoning skills in determining what and how to document will enhance client care and facilitate reimbursement for therapy services.

Professional Reasoning in Documentation

Choosing appropriate assessments based on an understanding of the client's diagnosis and the occupations that might be affected involves professional reasoning. Skilled observations, theoretical knowledge, and professional reasoning are used to identify, analyze, interpret, and document components of occupational performance that may contribute to the client's engagement in occupation. OTs demonstrate professional reasoning when they include information in their documentation that demonstrates synthesis of information from the occupational

BOX 8.3   **Examples of Professional Reasoning in Documentation**

- Because of Mr. Page's change in affect after a total hip replacement, the Geriatric Depression Scale will be administered and the client's primary physician will be contacted.
- Using neurodevelopmental techniques (NDT), including facilitation at the hips, the client is now able to independently stand at the sink with good balance for 2 minutes to brush his teeth.
- A home assessment is recommended to determine what adaptive equipment is necessary to allow the client to independently and safely complete activities of daily living (ADL) tasks.
- The client's difficulty with problem solving, task initiation, and task progression impedes ability to independently prepare a simple meal.
- A resting hand splint was fabricated for the client because of the emergence of spasticity, poor passive positioning of the upper extremity, and a high risk for development of contractures.
- Mrs. Rogers requires maximal assistance to complete upper/lower body dressing because of poor sitting balance, right neglect, and apraxia.

profile; interpretation of objective and subjective data to identify facilitators and barriers to client performance; collaboration with the client to establish goals; and a clear understanding of the demands, skills, and meaning of the activities used in intervention to reach established goals.[3,10] Professional reasoning skills are also used to analyze client responses and make decisions about modifications to improve outcomes. Terminology used in documentation should reflect the unique skilled services that the OT uses to address client factors, performance skills, performance patterns, context and environment, and activity demands as they relate to the client's performance (Box 8.3) provides some examples of professional reasoning.

OT PRACTICE NOTES

Concise, clear, accurate documentation that keeps the target audience in mind will ensure that the appropriate information is conveyed to other healthcare professionals and will meet the criteria for reimbursement.

LEGAL LIABILITY

The medical record is a legal document. All written and computerized therapy documentation must be able to pass a legal review. The AOTA Ethics Commission enforces the Standard of Conduct, which states that documentation done for reimbursement purposes must be in accordance with all applicable laws, guidelines, and regulations.[10] The medical record may be the most important document in a malpractice suit because it outlines the type and amount of care or services that were given.[7] The therapist must know what information is necessary to include in the client record to reduce the risk for malpractice in a legal proceeding. All information must be accurate and based on firsthand knowledge of care. Deductions and assumptions are to be avoided; judgmental statements do not belong in the therapy notes. The therapist instead should describe the action, behavior, or signs and symptoms that are observed. As described earlier, it is considered fraudulent to alter the medical record in any way.

The False Claim Act is a federal law that makes it a crime to knowingly make a false record or a claim for services provided through insurance or otherwise that are funded in full or in part by the U.S. Government or any state healthcare system. [6,12] Examples of documentation fraud include misrepresentation of services rendered, diagnosis, place of service, date of service, and/or provider to justify reimbursement; falsifying plans of treatment, and medical records to justify payment; billing for goods and services never delivered or rendered; billing for more services than provided; medical documentation not consistent with the service billed; and improper coding practices (e.g., misuse of CPT codes).[5,6,12]

INITIAL EVALUATION

The initial evaluation report is a very important document in the OT process. It is the foundation upon which all other components of the client's program is based. including long- and short-term goals, the intervention plan, progress notes, and therapy recommendations. Evaluation is the process of obtaining and interpreting objective and subjective data necessary for understanding the individual, system, or situation. It includes planning for and documenting the evaluation process, results, and recommendations, including the need for intervention.[3] The OTPF-4 stresses that the evaluation process should focus on identifying what the client wants and needs to do, in addition to identifying factors that function as supports for or barriers to performance. The client's involvement in this process is essential for guiding the therapist in choosing the appropriate tools to assess these areas. The OT takes into account the performance skills, performance patterns, context and environment, activity and occupational demands, in addition to the client factors required for the client to successfully engage in occupation. This information must be articulated and supported by assessments in the initial evaluation write-up. For reimbursement purposes, it is particularly important to include measurable, evidence-based, objective data in the evaluation whenever possible.

A clear, accurately written account of the client's current status, in addition to a description of their prior status, is essential to justify the need for OT services. This initial report also provides necessary information to establish a baseline against which reevaluation data and progress notes can be compared to demonstrate the efficacy of therapy intervention. The evaluation must clearly "paint a clinical picture" of the client's current functional status, strengths, impairments, and need for skilled occupational therapy services.

The occupational profile is a key component of the evaluation process. The occupational profile includes information about the client's occupational history and experiences, patterns of daily living, interests, values, and needs. The client provides information as to their concerns relative to engaging in occupation, as well as what client factors they think support engagement in desired occupations and which aspects are barriers to engagement.[3] Information obtained from the occupational profile is essential in guiding the therapist to make clinically sound decisions about appropriate assessments, interventions, and goals (which are made in collaboration with the client).

Assessments are the tools, instruments, and interactions used during the evaluation process.[3,4] Assessments comprise standardized and nonstandardized tests and can include written tests or performance checklists. Interviews and skilled observations are examples of assessments frequently used in the evaluation process. The specific assessments used are determined by the needs of the client and the practice setting in which the client is being seen. Assessments should be chosen that evaluate the client's occupational needs, challenges, and concerns. Clinical reasoning skills are used to decide which assessments are appropriate and which areas should be evaluated. It is not necessary to evaluate every occupation and all performance skills for every individual. For example, it is not appropriate to assess a client's ability to cook a meal if he or she lives in a setting in which meals are provided. Results of the assessment should be clearly identifiable and stated in measurable terminology that is standardized to the practice setting. Table 8.1 shows an example of terminology that can be used to describe the level of assistance required during the performance of a functional task.

The occupational therapist initiates and directs the evaluation process. The occupational therapist assistant contributes to this process by performing assessments identified by the occupational therapy as well as providing written and verbal reports about assessment results. The occupational therapist then interprets the information and integrates it into the evaluation.[5]

The AOTA has outlined the recommended components of professional documentation used in occupational therapy in the text *Guidelines for Documentation of Occupational Therapy*,[1] which provides suggestions for what information should be included in screening reports, evaluation and reevaluation reports, intervention plans, progress reports, transition plans, and discharge reports.

Screening Report

The **screening report** is an initial brief assessment to determine the client's need for further OT evaluation or for referral to another service. Suggested content includes:

1. *Client information:* Name/agency; date of birth; gender; applicable medical, educational, and developmental diagnosis; precautions; and contraindications
2. *Referral information:* Date and source of referral; services requested; reason for referral; funding source; and anticipated length of service
3. *Brief occupational profile:* Client's reason for seeking OT services; current areas of occupation that are successful and areas that are problematic; contexts that support or hinder occupations; medical, educational, and work history; occupational history; client's priorities; and targeted outcomes
4. *Assessments used and results:* Types of assessments used and results (e.g., interviews, record reviews, observations)
5. *Recommendations:* Professional judgments regarding appropriateness of need for complete OT evaluation

Evaluation Report

The **evaluation report** should contain the following information:
1. *Client information:* Name/agency; date of birth; gender; applicable medical, educational, and developmental diagnosis; precautions; and contraindications

TABLE 8.1 Levels of Assistance

Assistance Level	Description
Independent	• Client is completely independent. • No physical or verbal assistance is required to complete the task. • Task is completed safely.
Modified independence	• Client is completely independent with task but may require additional time or adaptive equipment.
Supervised	• Client requires supervision to safely complete task. • A verbal cue may be required for safety.
Contact guard/standby assistance	• Hands-on contact guard assistance is necessary for client to safely complete the task, or caregiver must be within arm's length for safety.
Minimum assistance	• Client requires up to 25% physical or verbal assistance from one person to safely complete the task.
Moderate assistance	• Client requires 26% to 50% physical or verbal assistance from one person to safely complete the task.
Maximal assistance	• Client requires 51% to 75% physical or verbal assistance from one person to safely complete the task.
Dependent	• Client requires more than 75% assistance to complete the task.
	• *NOTE:* For all levels it is important to state whether the assistance provided is physical or verbal assistance.

2. *Referral information:* Date and source of referral; services requested; reason for referral; funding source; and anticipated length of service
3. *Occupational profile:* Client's reason for seeking OT services; current areas of occupation that are successful and areas that are problematic; contexts that support or hinder occupations; medical, educational, and work history; occupational history; client's priorities; and targeted outcomes
4. *Assessments:* Types of assessments used and results (e.g., interviews, record reviews, observations, standardized or nonstandardized assessments)
5. *Analysis of occupational performance:* Description and judgment about performance skills; performance patterns; contextual or environmental aspects or features of activities; client factors that facilitate or inhibit performance; and confidence in test results
6. *Summary and analysis:* Interpretation and summary of data as they relate to the occupational profile and referring concerns
7. *Recommendation:* Judgment regarding appropriateness of OT services or other services

INTERVENTION PLAN

On completion of the assessment, the intervention plan is established. Information obtained from the occupational profile and the various tools used to assess the client is analyzed, and a problem list is generated. Problem statements should include a description of the underlying factor (performance skill, performance pattern, client factor, contextual or environmental limitation, activity demand) and its impact on the related area of occupation. Based on the client's specific problems, an intervention plan is developed. The therapist must use theoretical knowledge and professional reasoning skills to develop long- and short-term goals in collaboration with the client, to decide upon intervention approaches, and to determine the interventions to be used to achieve stated goals. Recommendations and referrals to other professionals or agencies are also included in the plan.[1] The intervention plan is formulated on the basis of selected theories, frames of reference, practice models, and best available evidence. It is directed by the client's goals, values, beliefs, and occupational needs.[3]

Establishment of the intervention plan is a collaborative effort between the therapist and the client or, if the client is unable, the client's family or caregivers. Although the OT has primary responsibility for development of the intervention plan and goal setting, the occupational therapy assistant (OTA) may contribute to the process. The OTA collaborates with the occupational therapist to select, implement, and make modifications to the interventions consistent with demonstrated competence levels and client goals and provides documentation in the client's record.[5]

Intervention Goals

Intervention goals are established based on identified problems. Goals must be measurable and directly related to the client's ability to engage in desired occupations. The overarching goal of interventions provided by the OT practitioner in collaboration with the client is "to facilitate engagement in occupation related to health, well-being, and achievement of established goals" (p. 27).[3] This must be kept in mind at all times when long- and short-term goals are developed. The OTPF-4 further identifies the outcome of OT intervention "may be traced to improvement in areas of the domain, such as performance skills and client factors, but should ultimately be reflected in clients' ability to engage in their desired occupations. Outcomes targeted in occupational therapy can be summarized as occupational performance, prevention, health and wellness, quality of life, participation, role competence, well-being, and occupational justice" (p. 30).[3] Documentation that uses this terminology and speaks to these areas will support the unique focus that occupational therapy contributes to the client's care plan and the rehabilitation process.

The AOTA defines intervention goals as "measurable and meaningful occupation-based long-term and short-term goals directly related to the client's ability and need to engage in desired occupations and to the justification of the need for skilled occupational therapy intervention to meet the goals."[1] Writing goals that are clear, realistic, measurable, and appropriate for the client is an essential part of the therapeutic process that will lead to desired outcomes. Goals are written as a part of the evaluation and are critical factors in justifying the need for therapeutic intervention. As the client's status changes throughout the course of treatment, goals are upgraded or downgraded to guide further intervention. Reimbursement requirements and the setting in which the therapist works often direct the specific wording of the goal.

The client's intervention plan contains both short- and long-term goals. Some therapists prefer to use the term *objective* in place of *short-term goal*. Short-term goals, or objectives, are written for specific time periods (e.g., 1 or 2 weeks) within the overall course of the client's therapy program. They are periodically updated as the client progresses or in accordance with the guidelines of the practice setting or payer requirements. Short-term goals are the steps that lead to accomplishment of the long-term goal, which is also called the *discharge goal* in some settings. The long-term goal is generally considered to be the overall goal of the intervention and is broader in nature than the short-term goal. For example, the client's long-term goal may be to become independent with dressing. One short-term goal to accomplish this might be that the client will be able to independently put on and take off a simple pullover shirt without fasteners. When this short-term goal has been achieved, a subsequent goal might be for the client to be able to dress independently in a shirt with buttons. Eventually, lower extremity dressing would be added as an objective, then socks, shoes, and outerwear, until the long-term goal of independent dressing is achieved.

Establishing objective, occupation-based, client-centered goals that focus on engagement in occupations and activities to support participation in life is central to the philosophy of occupational therapy. Skillful goal writing requires practice and careful consideration of the desired outcome of therapy intervention. Client-centered goals are written to reflect what the client will accomplish or do, *not* what the therapist will do, and are written in collaboration with the client. The goal must reflect the outcome, not the technique or intervention used to achieve the outcome. *The client will be taught energy conservation techniques to use during dressing* is an example of a poorly written goal that focuses on the process, rather than the outcome, of therapy. The correct way to write the goal would be: *The client will independently use three energy conservation techniques during dressing.*

Goals must be objective and *measurable* and must include a *time frame*. The time frame may be written in a separate section of the evaluation form. A well-written goal clearly identifies the expected outcome behavior using concrete terms that describe a specific functional task, action, behavior, or activity (e.g., The client will put on pants); a measurable expectation of performance (e.g., independently); and the conditions (or circumstances) supporting outcomes listed (e.g., using a dressing stick). Examples of measurable expectations of performance include levels of assistance, degrees of motion, number of repetitions, and length of time. Examples of conditions include use of assistive devices, adaptive aids, the location where performance takes place (e.g., edge of the bed), and additional time necessary to complete the activity. The following goal has all the necessary components: *Mr. B will feed himself* (expected outcome behavior) *with moderate verbal cues* (measurable expectation of performance) *while sitting in a quiet environment* (condition). Table 8.2 shows examples of short- and long-term goals.

SMART

A strategy that may assist the therapist in writing goals is a framework called SMART goals (Table 8.3). SMART stands for **s**pecific, **m**easurable, **a**chievable, **r**elevant, and **t**ime based. Each element of the SMART framework works together to create a goal that is carefully planned, clearly presented, and measurable.

- Make your goals specific and addressed toward the identified problem.
- Have a clear, measurable target to aim for. Define the evidence that will demonstrate that progress is being made.
- Make sure that it is reasonable that the client be able to achieve this goal in the identified time frame.
- Long- and short-term goals should align with each other and be relevant to the client's occupational needs.
- The goal is time-based: Short- and long-term goals have a designated realistic end-date.

Once the short- and long-term goals have been established, the therapist, in collaboration with the client, chooses appropriate interventions that will lead to goal attainment. The intervention plan consists of skilled interventions that the therapist will provide throughout the client's therapy program. Interventions are chosen that involve the therapeutic use of occupations or activities (occupation-based activity, purposeful activity, preparatory methods) in consultation with the client/caregiver.[3] Examples of OT interventions are activities of daily living (ADLs) training; instrumental activities of daily living (IADLs) training; therapeutic activities; therapeutic exercises; splint/orthotic fabrication, modification, and application; neuromuscular retraining; cognitive-perceptual training, community reintegration training, client/caregiver training; and discharge planning. The OTPF-4 outlines various approaches that may guide the intervention process (Table 8.4).

TABLE 8.2 Examples of Short- and Long-Term Goals

Short-Term Goal[a]	Long-Term Goal[b]
Client will transfer wheelchair <–> (from wheelchair onto and off of) toilet with a raised seat and handrails with minimal physical assistance.	Client will safely and independently transfer to a nonmodified toilet using a walker.
Client will brush teeth with moderate physical and verbal assistance while seated at the sink.	Client will complete morning hygiene and grooming routine independently after task setup using assistive devices while seated at the sink.
Client will don socks with minimal assistance using a sock aid while seated in a regular chair with armrests.	Client will independently complete lower body dressing without assistive devices while seated at the edge of the bed.

[a]Short-term goals are to be completed in 2 weeks.
[b]Long-term goals are to be completed in 4 weeks.

TABLE 8.3 Differentiating SMART and Not-SMART Goals

Not a SMART Goal	SMART Goal
Improve swallow with liquids using chin tuck	Client will safely swallow 250 mL of water from an open cup using a chin tuck strategy with two or three verbal cues, as evidenced by no throat clearing or cough after swallow by the end of four visits.
Client will transfer with less assistance	Client will safely transfer from the wheelchair to the toilet using a stand-pivot technique with minimal verbal cues for sequencing of task and contact guard for hand placement by the end of six visits.

TABLE 8.4 OT Intervention Approaches

Intervention Approach	Designed to . . .
Create, promote (health promotion)	Provide enriched contextual and activity experiences to enhance performance for persons in the natural contexts of life. It does not assume that a disability is present or that there is anything specific that would interfere with performance. An example of this approach might be to develop a falls prevention program for either an individual client or for older adults at a senior center.
Establish, restore (remediation, restoration)	Change client variables to develop a skill or ability that has not yet been developed or to restore a skill or ability that has been impaired. An example of this approach might be to collaborate with a client who has had a traumatic brain injury (TBI) to establish a new routine and strategies that will allow them to complete work duties on time.
Maintain	Provide the supports that will allow the client to maintain performance capabilities. Without continued maintenance intervention, client performance would decline and/or occupational needs would not be met, affecting the individual's health and quality of life. An example of this might be to maintain safe and independent access to the dining hall for individuals with low vision living in an independent living center by recommending lighting and environmental contrasts.
Modify (compensation, adaptation)	Find ways to revise the current context or activity demands to support performance. This includes using compensatory techniques, enhancing some features to provide cues, or reducing features to reduce distractibility. An example of this approach is to simplify the steps of an activity so that an individual with cognitive impairment can successfully complete the a.m. self-care routine.
Prevent (disability prevention)	Prevent the occurrence or development of barriers to performance in context. This approach is directed toward clients with or without a disability who are at risk for occupational performance problems. An example of this would be to design a series of group activities for individuals living in a senior apartment complex to prevent social isolation.

Adapted from the American Occupational Therapy Association: Occupational therapy practice framework: domain and process, fourth edition, *Am J Occup Ther* 74(Suppl 2):1–87, 2020.[3]

These approaches are based on theory and best practice evidence. It is expected that the intervention plan will be modified according to the client's needs, priorities, and responses to the interventions. Modifications to the intervention plan must be documented in the client's record in the weekly or monthly progress reports.

PROGRESS REPORTS

Progress toward goal attainment is an expected criterion for reimbursement of OT services in most practice settings. Documentation that demonstrates progression toward goal achievement is critical to support the need for ongoing therapy. The purposes of the progress report are to document the client's improvement, describe the skilled interventions provided, and update goals. Progress reports may be written daily or weekly, depending on the requirements of the work site and the payer source. Various reporting formats are used to document client progress. The most prevalent formats used in physical disabilities settings are SOAP notes, checklist notes, and narrative notes.

Regardless of the format used, progress reports should identify the following key elements of the intervention session: the client outcome (using measurable terminology from the OTPF); the skilled interventions provided by the OT; and progress that resulted from the OT intervention. Skilled interventions are those that require the expertise, knowledge, clinical judgment, decision making, and abilities of an OT. Skilled therapy services have a level of inherent complexity such that they can be performed safely and/or effectively only by or under the general supervision of a qualified therapist.[9] Skilled services include evaluation; determination of effective goals and services in collaboration with the client, the client's caregivers, and other medical professionals; analysis and modification of functional activities and tasks; determination that the modified task obtains optimum performance through tests and measurements; client/caregiver training; and periodic reevaluation of the client's status, with corresponding adjustment of the OT program. Box 8.4 shows examples of terminology that reflect the provision of skilled services.

Documentation of skilled services includes a description of the type and complexity of the skilled intervention and reflects the therapeutic rationale underlying the choice of the intervention. Reimbursement for clinical services provided depends on documentation that demonstrates the professional reasoning that underlies the intervention. The progress note must identify the skilled intervention provided and indicate the progress made toward established goals. Comparison statements are an excellent way to convey this information. Current status information is compared with baseline evaluation findings to clearly identify progress: *Client now requires minimal assistance to regain sitting posture in a regular chair with armrests during lower body dressing (last week required moderate assistance).* Documentation that includes functional assessment scores from validated tests and measurements to demonstrate client progress provides strong justification for reimbursement of therapy services. A statement explaining why additional therapy services are needed substantiates the need for ongoing therapy: *Occupational therapy*

BOX 8.4   Terminology Used in the Provision of OT Services

Skilled Terminology
Assess
Analyze
Interpret
Modify
Facilitate
Inhibit
Instruct in:
    compensatory strategies
    hemiplegic dressing
    techniques
    safety
    adaptive equipment
Fabricate
Design
Adapt
Environmental modifications
Determine
Establish

Unskilled Terminology
Maintain
Help
Watch
Observe
Practice
Monitor

---

services are required for facilitation of balance and postural corrections to improve independence and safety with lower body dressing. Goals are modified and updated on the basis of the client's progress: *Client will don pants independently, without loss of balance, while seated on the edge of the bed.* Upgrading of the client's goals can consist of reducing the amount of assistance required to complete the task, increasing the complexity of the task, or introducing a new component to the activity. This is an ongoing process, and meticulous documentation is necessary to demonstrate the need for continued OT services. If a client is not making progress toward stated goals, a clear explanation of the reasons for this must be included in the progress note, with a modification of the existing goal and intervention approach.

SOAP Progress Note

The format for the SOAP note was introduced by Dr. Lawrence Weed in 1970 as a method of charting in the problem-oriented medical record (POMR).[13] In the POMR, which focuses on a client's problems instead of on his or her diagnosis, a numbered problem list is developed that becomes an important part of the medical record. Each member of the healthcare team writes a SOAP note to address problems on the list that are specific to his or her area of expertise. The POMR is constantly modified and updated throughout the client's stay. The SOAP progress note is one of the most frequently used formats for documenting a patient's status. Each letter in the acronym SOAP stands for the name of a section of the note:

S—Subjective
O—Objective
A—Assessment
P—Plan

The *Subjective* (**S**) part of the note is the section in which the therapist includes subjective information reported by the client that gives one's perspective on the client's condition or treatment.[8] Information provided by the family or caregivers also can be included here. Many types of statements can be included in the subjective section of the SOAP note. Any information the client gives the therapist about their current condition that is relevant to treatment (e.g., complaints of pain or fatigue; statements about feelings, attitudes, or concerns; and goals or plans) is appropriate to include in this section.[8] A client's subjective response to treatment is recorded in this section. Direct quotes can be used when appropriate. Family, caregivers, and others involved in the client's care also can provide valuable information. For example, nursing may report that the client was unable to feed themselves at breakfast, or a family member may supply information on the client's normal routine before hospitalization. If the client is nonverbal, gestures, facial expressions, and other types of nonverbal responses are appropriate to include. This information can be used to demonstrate improvement, support the benefit of chosen interventions, document the client's response, and show client compliance. However, discretion must be used when deciding what information to include. A common error in the "S" section is to list everything that the client says during the intervention session. Rather, summarize the pertinent statements in a concise manner. Using careful, effective communication skills during client treatment sessions will enhance the therapist's ability to gather relevant subjective information about the client's attitudes and concerns that can be used to ensure proper intervention.[8] The Subjective section should include only relevant information that will support the therapist's decision regarding which interventions should be used and which goals are appropriate for this client. The therapist should avoid statements that can be misinterpreted or that can jeopardize reimbursement. Subjective statements that do not relate to information in the other parts of the note are not useful and should not be included.[8] Negative quotes from the client that do not relate to the intervention session are not necessary or beneficial to include. If there is nothing relevant to report in the Subjective section, it is permissible to not include a statement. In this case, write a circle with a line through it (ϕ) to indicate that you have intentionally left the section blank.

In the *Objective* (**O**) section of the SOAP note, the therapist documents the objective results of assessments, tests, and measurements performed, in addition to objective observations.[8] Data that are recorded in the *Objective* section are measurable, quantifiable, or observable. Only factual information may be included. Results of standardized and nonstandardized tests are documented in this part of the note. Measurable performance of functional tasks (ADLs, IADLs), range-of-motion (ROM) measurements, muscle grades, results of sensory evaluations, and tone assessments are examples of appropriate information for this section of the SOAP note. It is important that the therapist not interpret or analyze data in the *Objective* section.

Rather, statements should include only concise, specific, objective recordings of the client's performance. Simply listing the activities that the client engaged in is not sufficient. The emphasis is on the results of the interventions, not on the interventions themselves. Information in the *Objective* section can be organized chronologically, discussing the results of each treatment event in the order it occurred during the session, or categorically. Information that is organized categorically should follow the categories outlined in the OTPF-4: performance skills, performance patterns, context, and client factors. Four steps to guide you when writing good observations for the O section are[9]:

1. Begin with a statement about the length, setting, and purpose of the treatment session.
2. Provide a brief overview of the key deficits that affect the client's performance.
3. Provide a summary of what you observed.
4. Be professional, concise, and specific.

Table 8.5 presents examples of documentation that can be used in the *Objective* section.

In the *Assessment* (**A**) section of the SOAP note, the therapist draws from the subjective and objective findings and interprets the data to establish the most appropriate therapy program. In this section, impairments and functional deficits are analyzed and prioritized to determine what impact they have on the client's occupational performance and ability to engage in meaningful occupation. Only information that was included in the *Subjective* or *Objective* section is discussed in the *Assessment* section. Professional reasoning is required to analyze the information and develop the intervention plan. The *Assessment* portion of the SOAP note is where the therapist demonstrates their ability to summarize relevant assessment findings, synthesize the information, analyze its impact on occupational performance, and use it to formulate the intervention plan. It requires keen observation, professional reasoning, and judgment skills, in addition to an ability to identify relevant factors that inhibit or facilitate performance. The *Assessment* section should end with a statement justifying the need for continued therapy services: *Client would benefit from activities that encourage trunk rotation and forward lean to facilitate transfers and lower body dressing.*[8] Insight and skill in completing the *Assessment* section improves with clinical experience.

In the *Plan* (**P**) section of the SOAP note, the OT practitioner outlines the intervention plan. As the client achieves the short-term goals, the plan is revised and new short-term goals are established. Documentation reflects the client's updated goals, in addition to any modifications to the frequency of therapy. Suggestions for additional interventions are also included in this section. This information will guide subsequent treatment sessions. Fig. 8.1 shows an example of a progress note using the SOAP format.

Narrative Notes

The **narrative note** is another format used to document daily client performance. One way to organize the narrative note is to categorize the information into the following subsections: problem, program, results/progress, and plan. The *problem* being

TABLE 8.5　Examples of Categories and Documentation for Objective Section of SOAP Note

Category	Objective Documentation
Activities of daily living (ADLs) task performance	Note how each of the performance skills and client factors affects completion of ADLs tasks. Use objective measurements, such as levels of assistance and setup needed, adaptive equipment required, amount of time required to complete the task, quality of task performance, or specialized techniques used. Include client response to the intervention.
Posture and balance	Note whether balance was static or dynamic during the task or activity the client was involved in doing. Note whether the client leans in one direction, has rotated posture, or has even or uneven weight distribution. Indicate what cues or assistance was necessary to maintain or restore balance and how the client responded to this feedback. Indicate if the client was sitting or standing.
Coordination	Include hand dominance, type of prehension used, ability to grasp and maintain grasp, reach and purposeful release, object manipulation, and gross versus fine motor ability. Indicate purposeful activity client was engaged in as you describe these areas.
Swelling or edema	Give volumetric measurements if possible, pitting or nonpitting type, or measure using a soft tape measure if appropriate.
Movement patterns in affected upper extremities	Note tone, rigidity, spasticity, tremors, synergy patterns, facilitation required to elicit or inhibit movement or positioning of upper extremities.
Ability to follow directions	Note type and amount of instruction required and ability to follow one-, two-, or three-step directions. Be specific.
Cognitive status	Report on ability to initiate tasks, verbal responses to questions, approach to the task, ability to stay on task, sequencing, orientation, judgment, and problem solving. Use measurable terminology such as amount/type of assistance to do these things during the completion of an activity or task.
Neurological factors	Note perseveration, sensory losses (specific), motor deficits, praxis, spasticity, flaccidity, rigidity, neglect, bilateral integration, and tremors. Describe in objective terms.
Functional mobility	Note amount and type of assistance, need for special techniques or assistive devices required for the client to complete all types of mobility.
Psychosocial factors	Objectively describe the client's overall mood, affect, and ability to engage with others. Also note family support, response to changes in body image, and ability to make realistic discharge decisions. State in objective terms; do not interpret the behavior in this section. Use measures (e.g., number of times the client engaged with others during the session) whenever possible.

S: Client states that "it takes too much energy to dress each day and my hands are too stiff to manage buttons and ties anyways." Client's family reports that client no longer seems interested in self-care activities.

O: Client became SOB with seated self-care task (dressing) after 5 minutes of activity. Client required minimal assistance for upper body dressing, moderate assistance to don pants, and maximal assistance to don shoes (last week she required maximal assistance with all tasks). Client had moderate difficulty with buttons (last week she was unable to button blouse). Client was unable to tie shoes. BUE shoulder strength is 3+/5 (was 3/5).

A: Client is improving in her ability to complete her self-care tasks. COPD still interferes with ADL independence. She may benefit from adaptive equipment for lower body dressing.

P: Continue ADL training: assess for independence with adaptive equipment (dressing stick, long-handled shoe horn, and elastic shoe laces). Instruct client in energy-conservation techniques during ADL task completion. Instruct client in AROM exercises before beginning morning ADL tasks.

Fig 8.1 SOAP (**s**ubjective, **o**bjective, **a**ssessment, **p**lan) note.

addressed in the treatment intervention should be clearly identified. The impact on occupational performance and the underlying impairment is stated (e.g., *Unable to put on socks due to poor sitting balance and postural instability*). The intervention or intervention modality is identified in the *program* section. The *results*, including progress, are documented in measurable, objective terminology. Barriers to progress are included in this section. The plan for future intervention is outlined in the *plan* section. The need to modify goals and the rationale for this would be included here. In some practice settings, the narrative note is written directly in the medical chart. Occupational therapy may have a designated area in the medical chart in which the therapist can write notes, or all clinicians involved with the client may document in a single comprehensive interdisciplinary note. The date and often the beginning and ending times of the therapy session must be included in the note. The therapist's signature follows the last word of the note. Fig. 8.2 shows an example of a narrative note using this format.

A narrative format also may be used to write any type of information the therapist wishes to convey to the other team members. For example, the therapist may document that the evaluation was initiated or that the client was unable to attend therapy because of illness. Documentation of communication between team members regarding the client's program may be expressed in a narrative format.

Descriptive Notes

At times a short descriptive note is useful to relay important information about the client. Although it is preferable to keep

Problem:	Client was seen for 60 minutes. IADL task: light meal preparation.
Results:	Client was able to assemble necessary items to prepare a simple sandwich with minimal verbal cues, which were necessary because of unfamiliarity with clinic kitchen. Minimal verbal assistance was necessary for task initiation and progression from one step to the next. Although physical assistance was not required, client demonstrated mild coordination deficits resulting in difficulty opening jars, manipulating knife, and opening packages. Endurance was good for this activity — client was able to stand for 30 minutes without rest.
Plan:	Therapeutic exercise and activities will be performed to improve coordination. Instruct client in strategies for improving task initiation. Progressive IADL assessment — hot meal preparation.

Fig. 8.2 Narrative progress report.

notes as objective as possible, it is sometimes appropriate to include subjective information. Judgmental comments, negative statements, comments about other staff members, and information not directly related to the client's intervention program do not belong in the official medical record. Unobserved behaviors that are included in the client record should be recorded as such and a clear explanation provided as to who provided the information to the therapist.

Progress Checklists or Flow Sheets

Checklists or flow sheets can be used to document daily performance in a concise, efficient manner. High productivity demands in many settings, in addition to lack of reimbursement for documentation, have made this type of documentation a useful option. Flow sheets typically have a table or graph format, which the therapist uses to record measurements at regular intervals, usually after each session. Advantages of using a flow sheet or a checklist to document daily performance on specific tasks include improved clarity and organization of data; reduction in the quantity of data that needs to be recorded after each session; improved focus on interventions that are specific to the client's goals; and ease in clearly identifying the client's functional status and progress. A disadvantage of using this format for documentation is that often there is not sufficient space for the therapist to include subjective statements to explain client performance, document the therapist's interpretation of objective information, or describe the client's response to the intervention. The checklist provides a description of what the client did based on a level of assistance or an objective measurement, but it does not provide information on the quality of how the task was accomplished or modifications that were made to facilitate successful completion of the task. Whenever possible, this information should be included in a narrative format on a separate note sheet. Information from the daily checklist or flow sheet is used to write a weekly progress note and discharge reports.

Discharge Reports

Discharge reports are written at the conclusion of the therapy program. A comparison statement of occupational performance from initial evaluation to discharge is documented to demonstrate progress. Emphasis should be placed on the progress the client has made in engaging in occupations. A summary of the skilled interventions provided to the client is also included. Discharge recommendations (e.g., home programs, therapy follow-up, and referral to other programs) are made to facilitate a smooth transition from therapy. Clients are discharged from therapy when they have achieved established goals, have received maximal benefit from OT services, do not desire to continue services,[4] or have exceeded reimbursement allowances. The discharge summary should clearly demonstrate the efficacy of OT services and is often used to obtain information for outcome studies.

ELECTRONIC DOCUMENTATION

Many healthcare facilities and other healthcare providers have adopted electronic health records (EHR) to standardize the collection of client data, improve coordination of care, improve productivity, and facilitate reporting of quality measures. Electronic documentation can be used to record all aspects of the OT process, from the evaluation report to the discharge report. Reporting forms can be accessed on the computer, and the results of the initial evaluation and the discharge report can be typed directly onto the forms. This guarantees legibility and ensures that no areas are left uncompleted.

Electronic evaluation forms and progress notes are formatted to meet the needs of the facility and include information required for reimbursement (Fig. 8.3). Therapists often are able to choose responses from a pull-down menu, thereby reducing the time spent in deciding on the appropriate terminology to use. Space also is usually available to include narrative information. Because all healthcare providers enter information in a common database, members of the team are able to quickly access information about the patient by reviewing relevant sections on the computerized medical chart. One of the problems or inconveniences that may occur with electronic documentation is the accessibility of computers. Therapists must allow time to locate a computer that is not in use so that they can enter data. However, many clinical sites are now using handheld devices, which alleviates this obstacle. Additionally, some electronic forms are very restrictive in terms of what information the therapist may enter. This may make it difficult for the therapist to adequately document the session. Information entered solely from a pull-down menu may not give a clear picture of what occurred with the client. The use of electronic clinical documentation should not compromise the quality of the content in documentation. Software that allows for ease of use, the ability to customize the documentation record to meet the individual needs of the practice setting, and the ability to allow for custom entries in narrative form to clarify information enhances the quality of electronic documentation.[14] In general, electronic documentation and billing can be an asset in the therapy setting.

```
DATE:                                                                              PAGE 1
TIME:                            NURSING ASSESSMENT
                                 O.T. PROGRESS REPORT

Client :                                                          Age/Sex :
Account :                                                         Unit # :
Admit Date :                                                      Location :
Status : ADM IN                                                   Room/Bed :
Attending :
```

Diagnosis :
Precautions :
Onset Date :   Equipment :

	INITIAL STATUS	STATUS WEEK
FUNCTIONAL SKILLS	Date :	From : To :
Eating :	.	:
Grooming :	.	:
Sponge Bathing UB/LB :	.	:
Showering :	.	:
Toileting :	.	:
Dressing UB :	.	:
Dressing LB :	.	:
Kitchen/Homemaking :	.	:
Bed/Chair Transfers :	.	:
Toilet Transfer :	.	:
Tub/Shower Transfer :	.	:

Pain :   Pain Scale : (1-10)   /10
Pain Location :   Quality of Pain:
Effects of pain on ADLs :
 Pain Comment :

CURRENT SHORT-TERM GOALS
1 :   MET :
2 :   :
3 :   :

Current Problems :
1 :   4 :
2 :   5 :
3 :   6 :

NEW SHORT-TERM GOALS
1 :
2 :
3 :

COMMENTS :   Conferred with OT for Treatment Plan Adjustment:
:
:
:
:
:

                                EDUCATED
Client Instructed :   Parent/Significant Other Instructed :   Translator Used :
Instruction Given On :
                     :

Fig. 8.3 Computerized documentation form.

FORMATS FOR DOCUMENTATION OF OCCUPATIONAL THERAPY SERVICES

Many different written formats can be used to document OT services. The content of the form used is usually determined by the requirements of the third-party payer reimbursing the service and the unique needs of the practice setting. As stated previously, documentation must contain the information necessary to justify the need for OT services, demonstrate the provision of skilled therapeutic interventions, and show client progress

DATE: TIME:	NURSING ASSESSMENT O.T. PROGRESS REPORT	PAGE 2

Client : Account : Admit Date : Status : ADM IN Attending :	Age/Sex : Unit # : Location : Room/Bed :

                :

Mode of Instruction :

    Fact Sheet/Handout Title :

Instruction comment :
Understanding Validated By :
MD aware of current status via conference notes (SNU)

Occurred Date : Monogram : Initials : Name :	Occurred Time : Nurse Type :

Fig. 8.3 Cont'd

toward identified goals. OT documentation should address all of these components to ensure reimbursement and to convey accurate information about the client's performance.

Primary reimbursement systems for OT services in the physical disabilities setting include Medicare, Medicaid, various health maintenance organizations (HMOs), and preferred provider organizations (PPOs). Each of these organizations requires specific information that must be included in the documentation for reimbursement to occur. Individual facilities (e.g., hospitals, clinics, home health agencies, skilled nursing facilities) often design documentation forms to meet their specific needs and to ensure that the information necessary for reimbursement is included. Billing systems may also influence the type of documentation format that is used in a particular setting.

Medicare is a major payer source in the older adult (geriatric) physical disability setting. Medicare is a national insurance program and as such has set national standards for documentation. This government agency has put forth detailed guidelines stating expectations for what information must be included in the medical record to justify the need for OT services. Intermediaries will reimburse OT services only if all of the requirements established by the Medicare guidelines and regulations have been met. The 2019 Medicare Benefit Policy Manual[9] describes the key words and phrases medical reviewers are looking for when they review a claim for payment. Medicare requires that specific information be clearly documented for each part of the therapy process for therapy services to be reimbursed. Many other payers of therapy services in adult rehabilitation follow Medicare's guidelines when establishing documentation policies for reimbursement. A thorough and up-to-date understanding of these requirements is critical for ensuring reimbursement for services provided. The therapist working with Medicare clients must become familiar with these guidelines and regulations to prevent denial of services. Detailed information can be found at the

Medicare website (https://www.medicare.gov). It is important to keep up to date on current Medicare regulations to ensure that documentation is sufficient and includes all the components required for reimbursement. The AOTA (http://www.aota.org) maintains current information on Medicare reimbursement coverage on its website.

The Centers for Medicare and Medicaid Services (CMS)[9] has identified the required documentation for reimbursement of both inpatient and outpatient therapy services. An initial evaluation and plan of care that demonstrate the need for services is completed by the occupational therapist. It is important to include a statement of the client's prior level of function and the change in function that precipitated the OT referral. Objective tests and measurements are used to establish baseline status. Results from assessments that support the need for therapeutic intervention are included in the evaluation report. This information serves as the basis for short- and long-term goals. The therapist must be able to concisely present data that clearly demonstrate the need for occupational therapy. A recent change in function (a decline or an improvement) is required to justify therapy services. The plan of treatment includes functional, measurable goals based on assessment results). Goals cannot address issues that do not have supporting baseline data. The plan of treatment is the skilled intervention that the therapist will provide and must include the frequency, intensity, and duration of the requested services. Medicare defines skilled therapy to be those services that require the skills of a qualified therapist and must be reasonable and necessary for the treatment of the patient's illness or injury.[9] The inherent complexity of the service provided is such that it can only be performed safely and/or effectively by, or under the supervision of, a qualified occupational therapy practitioner. This requires the expertise, knowledge, clinical judgment, decision-making skill, and abilities of an OT practitioner that others cannot provide independently.

Documentation must explicitly include the services provided that require these specialized skills, knowledge, and judgement to ensure the safety of the client and the effectiveness of the program. In addition, a therapist's skills may be documented, for example, by the clinician's descriptions of the skilled treatment, the changes made to the treatment as a result of a clinician's assessment of the patient's needs on a particular treatment day or changes because of progress the clinician judged sufficient to modify the treatment toward the next more complex or difficult task. Skilled intervention also may be required for safety reasons. For example, a client with a cardiac condition might require the skill of a therapist to instruct him or her on how to safely complete an activity that might otherwise be done independently. Or the skill of a therapist might be required for a client learning compensatory swallowing techniques to perform cervical auscultation (examination with a stethoscope) and identify changes in voice and breathing that might signal aspiration. After the client is judged safe for independent use of these compensatory techniques, the skill of a therapist is no longer required to feed the client or check what was consumed.

The Occupational Therapy Practice Framework (OTPF)[3] provides the foundation for documenting all aspects of the occupational therapy process and should be used to highlight the unique contributions of occupational therapy. Fig. 8.4 shows an example of an OT evaluation report and initial intervention plan that incorporates the language of the OTPF.

CONFIDENTIALITY AND DOCUMENTATION

Maintaining confidentiality in documentation is the responsibility of the OT. Confidentiality, which is a part of principle 3 (Autonomy) of the AOTA 2020 Code of Ethics,[2,11] addresses the issue of privacy and confidentiality in all forms of communication, including documentation. Furthermore, the Enforcement Procedures for the Code of Ethics addresses standards of conduct for occupational therapy personnel:

Occupational therapy personnel shall maintain the confidentiality of all verbal, written, electronic, augmentative, and nonverbal communications, in compliance with applicable laws, including all aspects of privacy laws and exceptions thereto (e.g., Health Insurance Portability and Accountability Act [HIPAA] and the Family Educational Rights and Privacy Act [FERPA]); and maintain privacy and truthfulness in the delivery of occupational therapy services, whether in person or virtually.[2,11]

Similarly, Fremgen,[7] addressing the rules of medical law and ethics, explained that patients "have the right to have their personal privacy respected and their medical records handled with confidentiality. No information, test results, patient histories, or even the fact that the person is a patient, can be transmitted to another person without the patient's consent."

AOTA's Occupational Therapy Code of Ethics provides additional guidance regarding confidentiality issues[2,11]:

Information that is confidential must remain confidential. This information cannot be shared verbally, electronically, or in writing without appropriate consent. Information must be shared on a need-to-know basis only with those having primary responsibilities for decision making.

5.1 All occupational therapy personnel shall respect the confidential nature of information gained in any occupational therapy interaction. The only exceptions are when a practitioner or staff member believes that an individual is in serious, foreseeable, or imminent harm. In this instance, laws and regulations require disclosure to appropriate authorities without consent.

5.2 Occupational therapy personnel shall respect the client's and colleagues' right to privacy.

5.3 Occupational therapy personnel shall maintain the confidentiality of all verbal, written, and electronic, augmentative, and nonverbal communications (as required by HIPAA).[2] Ethical practice demands that the therapist understand what is meant by confidential information and is knowledgeable about how to maintain client confidentiality. Information about clients, including their names, diagnoses, and intervention programs, cannot be discussed outside of the treatment environment. Client charts should not be removed from the facility. Reports containing personal information (name, Social Security number, medical diagnosis) cannot be left out in plain view where others can read the information. Therapists, students, and staff cannot discuss clients in public areas where others may overhear the conversation.

Federal laws have been enacted to protect the consumer against breaches of confidentiality. The privacy sections of the HIPAA clearly outline the expectations of healthcare professionals in issues of confidentiality. HIPAA was enacted in 1996 and consisted of a series of provisions that required the Department of Health and Human Services to adhere to national standards for electronic transmission of healthcare information. The law also required that healthcare providers adopt privacy and security standards by which to protect confidential medical information of patients. Beginning in April 2003, healthcare providers were required to adhere to the privacy standards mandated by HIPAA. Individually identifiable health information, also known as protected health information (PHI), is federally protected under HIPAA regulations. PHI is health information that relates to a past, present, or future physical or mental health condition. The HIPAA rule limits the use and disclosure of PHI to the minimum necessary to perform the intended purpose. It also gives patients the right to access their medical records. This regulation protects the medical records of clients, whether the information is written or electronic (computer) or is verbally communicated. Violations of the HIPAA rules are subject to criminal or civil sanctions.[7,11]

The law requires that all staff members be trained in HIPAA policies and procedures and that they understand the implications specific to their work setting. In addition to the client confidentiality procedures explained earlier, safeguards must now be adhered to for compliance with HIPAA regulations. The therapist has a responsibility to protect confidential information from unauthorized access, use, or disclosure. This includes information documented in the medical record. Papers, reports, and forms containing PHI should not be disposed of in the regular trash. Instead, they must be shredded. Never leave medical records or

Occupational Therapy Initial Assessment

Name: _____ DOB: _____ Start of Service Date: _____

HICN: _____ Onset: _____

Medical Dx/ICD-9 # _____Treatment Dx/ICD-9# _____

Past Medical History:_____

Occupational Profile:

Areas of Occupation:

ADL Status	dep	max	mod	min	sup	indep	comments:
Self-feeding							
Hygiene/grooming							
UB bathing							
UB dressing							
LB dressing							
Wet tub/shower							
Toilet transfer							
Toileting skills							
Functional mobility:							
Personal device care							

IADL Status							
Kitchen survival skills							
Meal preparation							
Shopping							
Laundry							
Light housekeeping							
Community mobility							
Financial mgmt							
Care of others							

Work/Leisure/social participation

Fig. 8.4 OT evaluation report and initial intervention plan.

Vocational:
Avocational:
Leisure participation:
Social participation:

Client Factors:

Functional cognition	
Perceptual status	
Memory	
Vision/hearing	
Pain	
ROM: RUE: LUE:	
Motor control: RUE: LUE:	
Strength: RUE: LUE:	
Muscle tone	
Coordination/bilateral integration	
Body system function	

Performance Skills: Patient/family goals:

Posture Sit: Stand:	
Mobility	
Endurance/effort	

Short-term goals:	Long-term goals:
OT intervention plan:	Frequency/duration:

_____   _____

Therapist's Signature   Date

Fig. 8.4 Cont'd

ETHICAL CONSIDERATIONS

Special safety measures, such as personal identification and user verification codes for access to records, as well as having dedicated computers for client records, should be established to unauthorized individuals from accessing client information.

THREADED CASE STUDY

Jane, Part 2

Reflect on the questions posed in Part 1 of this case study. Jane, the OT beginning her first job at the skilled nursing facility, must use professional (previously referred to as clinical) reasoning skills at all stages of the therapy process, including the documentation of services delivered. The evaluation, the intervention plan, and short-term and long-term goals are written using sound reasoning to decide which assessments are appropriate to administer, how to use best practice evidence to develop interventions, and how to best collaborate with the client (taking into account the client's goals, priorities, and desires) throughout the process. Evidence of this comprehensive approach must be reflected in the documentation provided by Jane. It is essential that OT notes also indicate the skilled service or skilled intervention that was provided for reimbursement purposes. The format used for recording this information, and also the terminology used, may be specific to the practice setting. Federal (i.e., HIPAA) privacy mandates and the Occupational Therapy Code of Ethics must be adhered to at all times for all methods of documentation, whether written, verbal, or electronically generated.

portions of records (i.e., therapy notes) unattended in public view. Information (written, verbal, or electronic) cannot be shared with the client's family members unless permission has been provided in writing by the client.

If documentation is done electronically, special care must be taken to prevent unauthorized individuals from accessing client information. Log-in pass codes cannot be shared among staff members, and therapists must take care to ensure privacy when entering information.

SUMMARY

Documentation is a necessary part of the OT process. Occupational therapy practitioners have a responsibility to the client, to the employer, and to the profession to develop the skills that will allow them to accurately document the therapy process. Well-written documentation promotes the profession by providing proof of the value of OT intervention. It can provide valuable information for outcome research and evidence-based practice. It is a professional expectation that OTs will keep current on documentation requirements for their practice area and will acquire the skills necessary to accurately document the OT process.

REVIEW QUESTIONS

1. What are four purposes of documentation in OT practice?
2. What key elements should be reflected in OT documentation?
3. What are three technical points that the therapist must be aware of when writing in the medical record? Why is it important to adhere to these when documenting OT services?
4. Why is it considered best practice to complete documentations as soon after the therapy session as possible?
5. Why is it unacceptable to alter or delete information from the client's record once it has been written by the therapist?
6. Why should occupational therapy documentation reflect the terminology outlined in the Occupational Therapy Practice Framework (OTPF-4)?
7. How is professional reasoning used during documentation of occupational therapy services?
8. What type of professional reasoning is used when the OT considers the personal meaning that involvement in a particular activity might have for the client? Give an example.
9. What are three examples of documentation fraud?
10. Why is it important to collaborate with the client in the development of goals?
11. What is the role of the occupational therapy assistant in the assessment process?

12. How is an assessment different from an evaluation in the occupational therapy process?
13. How does the therapist use professional reasoning skills in the development of the intervention plan?
14. What are the components of a SMART goal?
15. Explain why the goal must reflect the outcome of services, not the technique or intervention used to achieve the outcome.
16. Why is it necessary to identify the skilled intervention provided in the occupational therapy progress note?
17. What is an example of documenting "skilled services" in a client progress note?
18. What does the "A" refer to in the SOAP note? Give an example of a statement that would be appropriate to include in the "A" section of a SOAP note.
19. When would a descriptive note be the most appropriate type of note for the OT to use?
20. List two benefits and two possible drawbacks of electronic documentation to document the outcome of a therapy session.
21. What is one way to ensure that confidentiality is maintained during the documentation of occupational therapy services?

For additional practice questions for this chapter, please visit eBooks.Health.Elsevier.com.

REFERENCES

1. American Occupational Therapy Association: Standards of practice for occupational therapy, *Am J Occup Ther* 69(Suppl 3): 1–6, 2015.
2. American Occupational Therapy Association: Guidelines for documentation of occupational therapy, *Am J Occup Ther* 72(Suppl 2):1–7, 2018.
3. American Occupational Therapy Association: AOTA 2020 Occupational Therapy Code of Ethics, *Am J Occup Ther* 74(Suppl 3):1–13, 2020a.
4. American Occupational Therapy Association: Guidelines for supervision, roles and responsibilities during the delivery of occupational therapy services, *Am J Occup Ther* 74(Suppl 3):1–6, 2020b.
5. American Occupational Therapy Association: Occupational Therapy Practice Framework: domain and process, fourth edition, *Am J Occup Ther* 74(Suppl 2):1–87, 2020c.
6. US Department of Justice, US Department of Health and Human Services: *Health care fraud and abuse control program FY 2020*, 2021. https://oig.hhs.gov/publications/docs/hcfac/FY2020-hcfac.pdf.
7. Fremgen B: *Medical law and ethics*, ed 6, Upper Saddle River, NJ, 2020, Pearson Education.
8. Gateley CA, Borcherding S: *Documentation manual for occupational therapy: writing SOAP notes*, ed 4, Thorofare, NJ, 2017, Slack.
9. Medicare Benefit Policy Manual: Covered medical and other health services, 2019. https://www.hhs.gov/guidance/sites/default/files/hhs-guidance-documents/38399_bp102c15_0.pdf.
10. Schell BAB: Professional reasoning in practice. In Schell BAB, Gillen G, editors: *Willard and Spackman's occupational therapy* ed 13, Baltimore, MD, 2018, Wolters Kluwer Health.
11. Scott JB, Reitz SM: *Practical applications for the Occupational Therapy Code of Ethics*, Bethesda, MD, 2015, American Occupational Therapy Association.
12. Total Health Care. False Claims Act. 2020. Retrieved from: https://thcmi.com/false-claimsact/#:~:text=The%20False%20Claim%20Act%20is,or%20otherwise%2C%20which%20is%20funded.
13. Weed LL: *Medical records, medical education and patient care*, Chicago, 1971, Year Book Medical Publishers.
14. Weiner M: Forced Inefficiencies of the Electronic Health Record, *J Gen Intern Med* 34:2299–2301, 2019. https://doi.org/10.1007/s11606-019-05281-3.

9

Infection Control and Safety Issues in the Clinic

Alison Hewitt George

LEARNING OBJECTIVES

After studying this chapter, the student or practitioner will be able to do the following:

1. Recognize the role of occupational therapy personnel in maintaining safety and preventing accidents.
2. Identify recommendations for safety in the clinic.
3. Describe the purposes of special medical equipment.
4. Identify precautions that should be taken when treating clients who require special equipment.
5. Describe the difference between Standard Precautions and Transmission-Based Precautions.
6. Identify Standard Precautions for infection control and explain the importance of following them with all clients.
7. Describe proper techniques of hand hygiene.
8. Recognize the importance for all healthcare workers of understanding and following standard procedures used in client care to prevent the transmission of infectious agents.
9. Identify proper procedures for handling client injuries.
10. Describe the guidelines for handling various emergency situations.

CHAPTER OUTLINE

KEY TERMS

Arterial monitoring line
Autoclave
Cardiopulmonary resuscitation (CPR)
Catheter
Centers for Disease Control and Prevention (CDC)
COVID-19
Dyspnea control postures
Endotracheal tube (ET)
Feeding pump
Fowler's position
Healthcare-associated infection (HIA)
Hyperalimentation

Intravenous (IV) feeding
Intravenous (IV) lines
Isolation systems
Nasogastric (NG) tube
Nosocomial infection
Occupational Safety and Health Administration (OSHA)
Pathogens
Personal Protective Equipment (PPE)
Standard Precautions
Total parenteral nutrition (TPN)
Tracheostomy
Transmission-Based Precautions

Donna, Part 1

Donna (prefers use of the pronouns she/her/hers) is a registered occupational therapist (OT) hired as director of Occupational Therapy (OT) Services in a recently opened community hospital. This 300-bed general acute care hospital provides inpatient and outpatient services for individuals with a wide range of medical needs, including cardiac problems, brain injury, neurological and orthopedic problems, and needs in oncology, obstetrics, and gynecology. OT services are provided in acute care, skilled nursing, acute rehabilitation, and outpatient units.

As director of OT Services, Donna must establish policies and procedures pertaining to client safety, infection control, medical emergencies, and precautions with special equipment. Donna must develop written guidelines and must identify and/or develop training requirements to ensure adequate orientation and preparation of OT personnel.

Critical Thinking Questions

In preparing these policies and procedures, Donna must consider the following:

1. What general safety procedures and infection control standards should be followed to maintain a safe clinic environment?
2. What items of specialized medical equipment are occupational therapy personnel likely to encounter in their interventions with clients, and what precautions should be taken when treating a client who requires special equipment?
3. What are the basic guidelines and/or procedures to be applied in emergency situations?
4. What resources are available to healthcare providers that offer up-to-date information pertaining to safety procedures and infection control?

As you read through the chapter, keep in mind these questions and any other concerns confronting Donna in developing protocols, policies, and procedures for the safety of clients and OT personnel.

ETHICAL CONSIDERATIONS

Occupational therapists (OTs) have an ethical obligation to refrain from causing harm, injury, or wrongdoing to recipients of service and to not to impose risks of harm even if the potential risk is without malicious or harmful intent (p. 3, 2020 Code of Ethics)[1] to recipients of OT services. To meet these ethical obligations to clients and to provide a physical context that supports clients' engagement in meaningful occupations, occupational therapists need to be educated in proper safety procedures, infection control standards, and emergency interventions.

The current (2020) version of the OT Framework, the "Occupational Therapy Practice Framework: Domain and Process," fourth edition[2] (OTPF-4), describes the occupational therapy (OT) process as the client-centered delivery of services facilitated by a collaboration between the client and the OT practitioner. This collaboration can occur in a variety of settings (e.g., hospitals, schools, community settings, and home). Environmental factors within these settings can enable or restrict participation and engagement in meaningful occupations. These environmental factors include: the natural and human-made changes to the physical environment; products and technology; support and relationships; attitudes; and services, systems, and policies."[2] Therefore, the setting, or environmental context, in which OT intervention occurs plays a significant role in the delivery of services in terms of supporting or inhibiting the client's performance.

Medical technology and cost control pressures have made it necessary for rehabilitation professionals to treat seriously ill clients early in their illness and for shorter periods. In the hospital setting it is not unusual for occupational therapists (OTs) to work with clients using interventions that include specialized medical equipment, such as catheters, intravenous (IV) lines, monitoring devices, and ventilators. These circumstances increase the potential for injuries to clients. In addition to ethical obligations to provide safe and proper intervention, OT personnel can be held legally liable for negligence if a client is injured because staff failed to follow proper procedures or standards of care.[6]

This chapter reviews specific safety precautions for use with a variety of clients. It identifies precautions to consider when encountering equipment commonly used with clients. Guidelines for handling various emergency situations are reviewed. It is important to note that the chapter is only an overview and cannot substitute for training in specific procedures used in many facilities. In addition to following these procedures, it is incumbent upon the occupational therapist to teach clients and their families applicable techniques that can be followed at home.

SAFETY RECOMMENDATIONS FOR THE CLINIC

Prevention of accidents and subsequent injuries begins with consistent application of basic safety precautions for the clinic[16,17]:

1. Hand hygiene (hand-washing or the use of alcohol-based hand rubs) should be performed before and after treating each client to reduce cross-contamination.
2. Make sure space is adequate to maneuver equipment. Avoid placing clients where equipment or passing personnel may bump them. Keep the area free from clutter.
3. Do not attempt to transfer clients in congested areas or in areas where your view or movement is blocked.
4. Routinely check equipment to ensure that it is working properly.
5. Make sure that the furniture and equipment in the clinic are stable. When not using items, store them out of the way of the treatment area.
6. Keep the floor free of cords, scatter rugs, litter, and spills. Ensure that the floors are not highly polished because polished floors may be very slippery.
7. Do not leave clients unattended. Follow federal guidelines for the proper use of restraint equipment (e.g., bed rails, belts, vests) to protect clients when they are not closely observed.
8. Have the treatment area and supplies ready before the client arrives.
9. Allow only properly trained personnel to provide client care.
10. Follow the manufacturer's and the facility's procedures for handling and storing potentially hazardous material. Make sure that such materials are marked and stored in a place

that is in clear view. Do not store such items above shoulder height.

11. Clearly label emergency exits and evacuation routes.
12. Have emergency equipment, such as fire extinguishers and first aid kits, readily available.

PRECAUTIONS WITH SPECIAL EQUIPMENT

Newly hired OT personnel need orientation and education regarding the types of medical equipment they are likely to encounter when treating clients. Before providing any intervention to a client at bedside, the OT should carefully review the medical chart to determine whether any specific instructions regarding movement precautions, positioning, or handling should be followed. For example, a client may need to follow a turning schedule and may be limited in the length of time allowed to remain in one position. Certain joint movements may be contraindicated, or special bed and wheelchair positioning requirements may need to be followed, such as with clients recovering from a burn injury, spinal cord injury, stroke, hip replacement surgery, and so forth. Special handling techniques may be required when working with clients who have catheters, feeding tubes, IV lines, or special monitors.[7] The various chapters throughout this book that address specific diagnoses will identify necessary precautions and handling recommendations.

Hospital Beds

OT personnel must be educated in the proper use of hospital beds to ensure client safety. The most commonly used hospital bed is electrically powered, but some are adjusted manually (cranked) or by hydraulic methods. All hospital beds are designed to make it easier to support the client and to change a client's position. Other, more specialized beds are needed for management of more complicated or more traumatic cases. Whatever type is used, the bed should be positioned so that the client is easily accessed and the therapist can use good body mechanics during mobility activities (see Chapter 11).

Most standard electrically adjustable beds are adjusted by means of electrical controls attached to the head or the foot of the bed or to a special cord that allows the client to operate the controls. The controls are marked according to their function and can be operated with the hand or foot. The entire bed can be raised and lowered, or upper and lower sections of the bed can be elevated or lowered to meet the client's needs. When the upper portion is raised 45 to 60 degrees, the client's position is referred to as **Fowler's position**.[5] This commonly used position facilitates lung expansion, improves breathing, and decreases cardiac workload (as compared with supine lying). However, an important precaution for the OT to observe and address is that in this position, the client may slide down in the bed, which increases shearing forces on tissues of the back.[22]

Side rails are attached to most beds as a protective measure. Some rails are lifted upward to engage the locking mechanism, whereas others are moved toward the upper portion of the bed until the locking mechanism is engaged. If a side rail is used for client security, the OT should be sure the rail is locked securely before leaving the client. The rail should be checked to ensure

that it does not compress, stretch, or otherwise interfere with any IV or other tubing.

Ventilators

Ventilators (respirators) move gas or air into the client's lungs and are used to maintain adequate air exchange when normal respiration is decreased. Current ventilator systems are complex, computer-driven devices that mix air under pressure with variable oxygen concentrations to provide inspiration and expiration. Ventilation can be invasive or noninvasive. Noninvasive ventilation systems use a face mask, nasal cannula, or mouth piece to introduce positive pressure ventilation to the client.[19] Invasive ventilation delivers oxygen to the client via a tracheostomy or endotracheal tube (ETT). The tracheostomy is a tube placed in a surgically made opening into the trachea (windpipe) at the base of the neck. The ventilator is attached to the tracheostomy for providing respiratory support. The ETT is an airway catheter inserted via the nose or mouth into the trachea.[24] Insertion of a tracheostomy or ETT will prevent verbal communication by the client. It is important to use alternative methods (message boards, hand signals, picture boards) to facilitate communication. When the ETT is removed, the client may complain of a sore throat and may have a distorted voice for a short period. For both invasive and noninvasive ventilator systems, it is important to avoid disturbing, bending, kinking, or occluding the tubing or accidentally disconnecting the ventilator tube from the delivery systems (e.g., face masks, the ETT, tracheostomy). The client who uses a ventilator may participate in various bedside activities, including sitting and ambulation. Make sure the tubing is sufficiently long to allow the activity to be performed.[10] A client using a ventilator may have a lower tolerance for activities and should be monitored for signs of respiratory distress, such as an increase in the breathing rate, bluish color to the mouth, lips, or fingernails, grunting with exhalation or change in body position (e.g., leaning forward to take deeper breaths).[23]

Monitors

Various monitors are used to observe the physiological state of clients who need special care. Therapeutic activities can be performed by clients who are being monitored, provided that care is taken to prevent disruption of the equipment. Many monitors have auditory and visual signals that are activated by a change in the client's condition or position or by a change in the function of the equipment. It may be necessary for a nurse to evaluate and correct the cause of the alarm unless the OT has received special instruction.

The cardiac monitor provides a continuous check on the function of the client's heart, including electrical functioning.[15] Acceptable or safe ranges for the three physiological indicators (heart rate, blood pressure, and respiration rate) can be set in the unit. An alarm is activated when the upper or lower limits of the ranges are exceeded or if the unit malfunctions. A monitoring screen provides a graphic and digital display of the values so that healthcare staff can observe the client's responses to treatment.

The pulmonary artery catheter (PAC) (e.g., Swan-Ganz catheter) is a long, plastic IV tube that is inserted into a large vein (e.g., subclavian, femoral, or jugular) and then threaded through the right side of the heart into the pulmonary artery. It provides accurate and continuous measurements of pulmonary artery pressures and will detect subtle changes in the client's cardiovascular system, including responses to medications, stress, and activity.[5] Activities, including OT interventions, can be performed with the PAC in place, providing they do not interfere with the location of insertion of the catheter. For example, if the catheter was inserted into the subclavian vein, elbow flexion should be avoided and shoulder motions restricted.

The intracranial pressure (ICP) monitor measures pressure exerted against the skull by brain tissue, blood, or cerebrospinal fluid (CSF). It is used to monitor ICP in clients with a closed head injury, cerebral hemorrhage, brain tumor, or overproduction of CSF.[15] Some of the complications associated with this device are infection, hemorrhage, and seizures. Three methods commonly used to monitor ICP are the intraventricular catheter, the subdural screw, or the epidural sensor. All methods involve placement of a catheter and sensor through a hole drilled in the skull. Physical activities should be limited when these devices are in place.[13] Activities that would cause a rapid increase in ICP, such as straining or isometric exercises, should be avoided. Positions to avoid include neck flexion, hip flexion greater than 90 degrees, and the prone position. Care must be taken to avoid disturbing the device and connected catheter tubing. Bed positioning for clients involves keeping the neck in neutral position and elevating the head of the bed to 30 degrees, but this should always be confirmed with the nurse or the physician.[9]

The **arterial monitoring line** (A line) is a catheter that is inserted into an artery to continuously and accurately measure blood pressure or to obtain blood samples without repeated needle punctures.[5] OT intervention can be provided with an A line in place, but care should be taken to avoid disturbing the catheter and inserted needle.

Feeding Devices

Special feeding devices may be necessary to provide nutrition for clients who are unable to ingest, chew, or swallow food. Some of the more commonly seen devices are the **nasogastric (NG) tube**, the gastric tube, and **intravenous (IV) feedings**.

The NG tube is a plastic tube that is inserted through a nostril and terminates in the client's stomach. The tube may cause the client to have a sore throat or an increased gag reflex. Feeding training can be initiated while the NG tube is in place. However, care should be taken because the tube may desensitize the swallow mechanism.[5] Caution should be used when moving the client's head and neck, especially in forward flexion, to avoid dislodging the tube.

The gastric tube (G tube) is a plastic tube inserted through an incision in the client's abdomen directly into the stomach.[5] Care should be taken so that the tube is not disturbed or removed during intervention activities.

Intravenous feeding, **total parenteral nutrition (TPN)**, or **hyperalimentation** devices permit infusion of the large amounts of nutrients needed to promote tissue growth. A hyperalimentation device is used when a client is unable to eat or absorb nutrients through the gastrointestinal tract.[5] A catheter

is passed into a large vein (typically the subclavian vein) that empties directly into the heart. The catheter may be connected to a semipermanently fixed cannula or sutured at the point of insertion. The OT should carefully observe the various connections to be certain they are secure before and after intervention. A disrupted or loose connection may result in the development of an air embolus, which could be life-threatening.[5]

The system usually includes a specialized **feeding pump**, which will administer fluids and nutrients at a preselected, constant flow rate. An audible alarm will be activated if the system becomes imbalanced or when the fluid source is empty.[5] Intervention activities can be performed as long as the tubing is not disrupted, disconnected, or occluded and as long as undue stress to the infusion site is prevented. Motions of the shoulder on the side of the infusion site may be restricted, especially abduction and flexion.

Most **intravenous (IV) lines** are inserted into superficial veins. Various sizes and types of needles or catheters are used, depending on the purpose of the IV therapy, the infusion site, the need for prolonged therapy, and site availability. Care should be taken during intervention to prevent any disruption, disconnection, or occlusion of the tubing. The infusion site should remain dry, the needle should remain secure and immobile in the vein, and no restraint should be placed above the infusion site.[5] For example, a blood pressure cuff should not be applied above the infusion site. The total system should be observed to ensure that it is functioning properly when intervention begins and ends. If the infusion site is in the antecubital area, the elbow should not be flexed. The client who ambulates with an IV line in place should be instructed to grasp the IV support pole so that the infusion site will be at heart level. If the infusion site is allowed to hang lower, blood flow may be affected. Similar procedures to maintain the infusion site in proper position should be followed when the client is treated while in bed or at a treatment table. Activities involving elevation of the infusion site above the level of the heart for a prolonged period should be avoided.[5] Problems related to the IV system should be reported to nursing personnel. Simple procedures, such as straightening the tubing or removing an object that is occluding the tubing, may be performed by the properly trained therapist.

Catheters

A urinary catheter is used to remove urine from the bladder when the client is unable to satisfactorily control retention or release. Urine is drained through plastic tubing into a collection bag, bottle, or urinal. Any form of trauma, disease, condition, or disorder affecting neuromuscular control of the bladder sphincter may necessitate the use of a urinary catheter. The catheter may be used temporarily or for the remainder of the client's life.[15]

A urinary catheter can be applied internally (indwelling catheter) or externally. Female clients require an indwelling catheter inserted through the urethra and into the bladder. In addition to indwelling catheters, males may use an external catheter. A condom catheter is applied over the shaft of the penis and is held in place by an adhesive applied to the skin or by a padded strap or tape encircling the proximal shaft of the penis. The condom is connected to a drainage tube and a urine collection bag.[5]

When clients with urinary catheters are receiving OT intervention, several precautions are important. Disruption or stretching of the drainage tube should be prevented, and no tension should be placed on the tubing or the catheter. The urine collection bag must not be placed above the level of the bladder for longer than a few minutes to avoid backflow of urine into the bladder or kidneys (with an indwelling catheter) or soiling of the client (with an external catheter). The bag should not be placed in the client's lap when the client is being transported. The production, color, and odor of the urine should be observed. The following observations should be reported to a physician or nurse: foul-smelling, cloudy, dark, or bloody urine or a reduction in the flow or production of urine. The collection bag must be emptied when it is full.[5]

Infection is a major complication for persons using catheters, especially for those using indwelling catheters. Everyone involved with the client should maintain cleanliness during treatment. The tubing should be replaced or reconnected only by those properly trained. Treatment settings in which clients with catheters are routinely treated have specific protocols for catheter care.[5]

Two types of internal catheters that are frequently used are the Foley catheter and the suprapubic catheter. The Foley catheter is a type of indwelling catheter that is held in place in the bladder by a small balloon inflated with air, water, or sterile saline solution. For removal of the catheter, the balloon is deflated and the catheter is withdrawn. The suprapubic catheter is inserted directly into the bladder through incisions in the lower abdomen and the bladder. The catheter may be held in place by adhesive tape, but care should be taken to avoid its removal, especially during self-care activities.[5] Catheter application and bladder management are activities of daily living (ADLs) that are frequently taught to clients as part of a comprehensive OT intervention program (see Chapters 10 and 37 for examples).

INFECTION CONTROL

Currently worldwide we are experiencing a pandemic caused by the coronavirus disease 19 (COVID-19). In late December 2019, a cluster of novel human pneumonia cases, which would later be attributed to COVID-19, were reported in Wuhan, China, and then rapidly spread throughout the world.[11] The highly contagious virus spreads primarily through airborne transmission (coughing, sneezing). Transmission can also occur through the contact of hands with contaminated surfaces that are then transferred to mucosa of the eyes, nose, and mouth. As of April 7, 2021, the World Health Organization (WHO) reports over 2.8 million deaths resulting from COVID-19 (updates to worldwide statistics can be found at the WHO Coronavirus Dashboard at covid19.who.int).[26] In the United States (US), as of March 1, 2021, over 550,000 individuals have died from this disease.[3]

Early in 2020, the US experienced a severe shortage of personal protective equipment (PPE) needed by essential healthcare workers providing services to infected populations while fighting the COVID-19 pandemic. The significant lack of proper PPE such as protective face masks, gowns, eye wear/shields, and gloves led to higher rates of infectious transmission of the virus to healthcare workers, which in turn reduced the quality and quantity of care available to infected individuals as well as contributing to further viral transmission.[4,20] As of April 7, 2021, according to the CDC, there have been more than 460,000 confirmed COVID-19 cases among healthcare workers in the US, leading to at least 1529 deaths.[3] The devastating effects of the shortage of PPE during this pandemic illustrates the importance of providing adequate and appropriate PPE for healthcare workers in infectious disease prevention and control.[4] It is vital to ensure that all essential healthcare workers are adequately protected for more effective containment of infectious diseases such as COVID-19.

In healthcare settings, consistent infection control procedures are used to prevent the spread of disease and infection among clients, healthcare workers, and others. They are designed to interrupt or establish barriers to the infection cycle. In 1996 the Centers for Disease Control and Prevention (CDC) published "Guidelines for Isolation Precautions in Hospitals."[21] This document described Universal Precautions (UP), which were established to protect healthcare workers and the clients they served from infectious agents, such as the human immunodeficiency virus (HIV), and diseases, such as acquired immunodeficiency syndrome (AIDS), hepatitis B, and hepatitis C. UP placed an emphasis on preventing the transmission of pathogens (infectious microorganisms) through contact with blood and bodily fluids.[21] The CDC revised and developed additional guidelines for a system of isolation, called body substance isolation (BSI), which focused on isolating moist and potentially infectious body substances (blood, feces, urine, sputum, saliva, wound drainage, and other body fluids) from all patients. These guidelines recommended the use of Standard Precautions, which synthesized the primary features of BSI and UP. Standard Precautions apply to blood, all bodily secretions and fluids, mucous membranes, and nonintact skin (Box 9.1 and Fig. 9.1).[21]

The most recent revision by the CDC, the "2007 Guideline for Isolation Precautions Preventing Transmission of Infectious Agents in Healthcare Settings,"[21] updated July 2019, recommends the use of two tiers of precautions to prevent transmission of infectious agents: Standard Precautions and Transmission-Based Precautions. The document states,

Standard Precautions are intended to be applied to the care of all patients in all healthcare settings, regardless of the suspected or confirmed presence of an infectious agent. Implementation of Standard Precautions constitutes the primary strategy for the prevention of healthcare-associated transmission of infectious agents among patients and healthcare personnel (p. 68).[21]

Standard Precautions include hand hygiene, use of protective clothing (e.g., gloves, gowns, masks, eye protection, or face shield, depending on anticipated exposure), and safe injection practices. A new strategy of infection control that has been added to Standard Precaution is Respiratory Hygiene/Cough Etiquette. This strategy is targeted at reducing the spread of undiagnosed respiratory infections and includes covering sneezes and coughs directing into one's elbow crease, use of masks, hand hygiene, and social distancing (of more than 3 feet).[21] Specific recommendations for each area of the Standard Precautions are detailed in the CDC guidelines. Key features of these recommendations are summarized in Box 9.1 and Table 9.1.

BOX 9.1 Summary of Standard Precautions

1. Use extreme care to prevent injuries caused by sharp instruments.
2. Cover minor, nondraining, noninfected skin lesions with an adhesive bandage.
3. Report infected or draining lesions and weeping dermatitis to your supervisor.
4. Avoid personal habits (e.g., nail biting) that increase the potential for oral mucous membrane contact with body surfaces.
5. Perform procedures involving body substances carefully to minimize splatters.
6. Cover environmental surfaces with moisture-proof barriers whenever splattering with body substances is possible.
7. Wash hands regularly, whether or not gloves are worn.
8. Avoid unnecessary use of protective clothing. Use alternative barriers whenever possible.
9. Wear gloves to touch the mucous membranes or the nonintact skin of any client, and whenever direct contact with body substances is anticipated.
10. Wear protective clothing (e.g., gown, mask, and goggles) when splashing of body substances is anticipated.
11. Ensure that the hospital has procedures for care, cleaning, and disinfection of environmental surfaces and equipment.
12. Handle and process soiled linens in a manner that minimizes the transfer of microorganisms to other patients and environments.
13. Handle used patient care equipment appropriately to prevent transfer of infectious microorganisms. Ensure that reusable equipment is thoroughly and appropriately cleaned.

Transmission-Based Precautions are additional standards that are implemented with clients who are known to be infected with infectious agents and require additional control measures to effectively prevent transmission. The most recent standards of the CDC also reflect current trends in the transition of healthcare delivery from primarily acute hospital settings to other settings (e.g., long-term care, home care). These recommendations "can be applied in all healthcare settings using common principles of infection control practice, yet can be modified to reflect setting-specific needs."[16] Additionally, the term **nosocomial infection** (i.e., hospital-acquired infection) has been replaced by **healthcare-associated infection (HIA)** "to reflect the changing patterns in healthcare delivery and difficulty in determining the geographic site of exposure to an infectious agent and/or acquisition of infection."[21]

The **Occupational Safety and Health Administration (OSHA)** issues regulations to protect the employees of healthcare facilities. All healthcare settings must do the following to comply with federal regulations[17]:

1. Educate employees on methods of transmission and on prevention of hepatitis B, HIV, and other infections.
2. Provide safe and adequate protective equipment and teach employees where the equipment is located and how to use it.
3. Teach employees about work practices used to prevent occupational transmission of disease, including, but not limited to, Standard Precautions, proper handling of client specimens and linens, proper cleaning of body fluid spills (Fig. 9.2), and proper waste disposal.
4. Provide proper containers for the disposal of waste and sharp items and teach employees the color-coding system used to distinguish infectious waste.
5. Post warning labels and biohazard signs (Fig. 9.3).

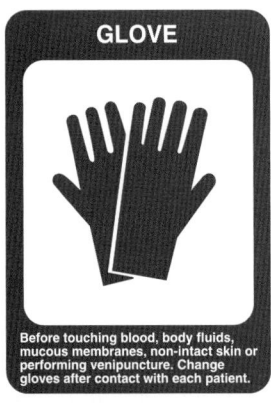

GLOVE

Before touching blood, body fluids, mucous membranes, non-intact skin or performing venipuncture. Change gloves after contact with each patient.

WASH

Wash hands immediately after gloves are removed. Wash hands and other skin surfaces immediately if contaminated with blood or other body fluids.

GOWN/APRON

For procedures likely to generate splashes of blood or other body fluids.

MASK/EYEWEAR

Masks and protective eyewear or face shields for procedures likely to generate splashes of blood or other body fluids.

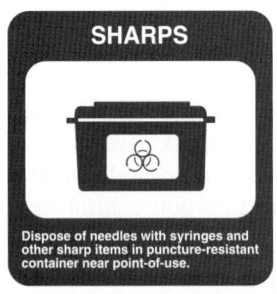

SHARPS

Dispose of needles with syringes and other sharp items in puncture-resistant container near point-of-use.

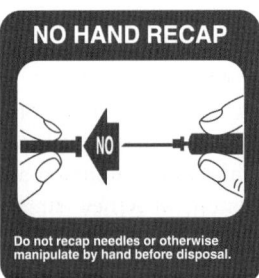

NO HAND RECAP

Do not recap needles or otherwise manipulate by hand before disposal.

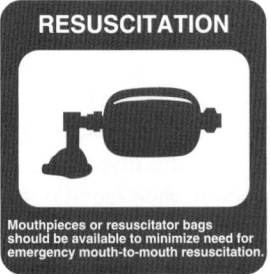

RESUSCITATION

Mouthpieces or resuscitator bags should be available to minimize need for emergency mouth-to-mouth resuscitation.

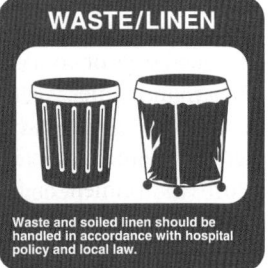

WASTE/LINEN

Waste and soiled linen should be handled in accordance with hospital policy and local law.

Universal Precautions apply to blood, visibly bloody fluid, semen, vaginal secretions, tissues and to cerebrospinal, synovial, pleural, peritoneal, pericardial and amniotic fluids.

Fig. 9.1 Universal blood and body fluid precautions. (Courtesy Brevis, Salt Lake City, UT.)

TABLE 9.1   Recommendations for Application of Standard Precautions in All Healthcare Settings

Component	Recommendations
Hand hygiene	After touching blood, body fluids, secretions, excretions, contaminated items; immediately after removing gloves; between patient contacts
Personal Protective Equipment (PPE)	
Gloves	For touching blood, body fluids, secretions, excretions, contaminated items; for touching mucous membranes and nonintact skin
Gown	During procedures and patient care activities when contact of clothing/exposed skin with blood/body fluids, secretions, and excretions is anticipated
Mask, eye protection (goggles), face shield	During procedures and patient care activities likely to generate splashes or sprays of blood, body fluids, secretions, especially suctioning, endotracheal intubation
Soiled patient care equipment	Handle in a manner that prevents transfer of microorganisms to others and to the environment; wear gloves if visibly contaminated; perform hand hygiene
Environmental control	Develop procedures for routine care, cleaning, and disinfection of environmental surfaces, especially frequently touched surfaces in patient care areas
Textiles and laundry	Handle in a manner that prevents transfer of microorganisms to others and to the environment
Needles and other sharps	Do not recap, bend, break, or hand-manipulate used needles; if recapping is required, use a one-handed scoop technique only; use safety features when available; place used sharps in puncture-resistant container
Patient resuscitation	Use mouthpiece, resuscitation bag, or other ventilation devices to prevent contact with mouth and oral secretions
Patient placement	Prioritize for single-patient room if patient is at increased risk of transmission, is likely to contaminate the environment, does not maintain appropriate hygiene, or is at increased risk for acquiring infection or developing adverse outcomes following infection
Respiratory hygiene/cough etiquette (source containment of infectious respiratory secretions in symptomatic patients, beginning at initial point of encounter [e.g., triage and reception areas in emergency departments and physician offices])	Instruct symptomatic persons to cover mouth/nose when sneezing/coughing; use tissues and dispose of in no-touch receptacle; perform hand hygiene after soiling of hands with respiratory secretions; wear surgical mask if tolerated or maintain spatial separation greater than 3 feet if possible

From Healthcare Infection Control Practices Advisory Committee: 2007 guideline for isolation precautions: preventing transmission of infectious agents in healthcare settings, updated July 2023. https://www.cdc.gov/infectioncontrol/pdf/guidelines/Isolation-guidelines-H.pdf.

6. Offer the hepatitis B vaccine to employees who are at substantial risk of occupational exposure to the hepatitis B virus.
7. Provide education and follow-up care to employees who are exposed to communicable disease.

OSHA has also outlined the responsibilities of healthcare employees. These responsibilities include the following[17]:

1. Use protective equipment and clothing provided by the facility whenever the employee contacts or anticipates contact with body fluids.
2. Dispose of waste in proper containers, applying knowledge and understanding of the handling of infectious waste and using color-coded bags or containers.
3. Dispose of sharp instruments and needles in proper containers without attempting to recap, bend, break, or otherwise manipulate them before disposal.
4. Keep the work environment and the client care area clean.
5. Wash hands immediately after removing gloves and at any other times mandated by the hospital or agency policy.
6. Immediately report any exposures, such as needle sticks or blood splashes, or any personal illnesses to the immediate

supervisor and receive instruction about any further follow-up action.[17]

Although it is impossible to eliminate all pathogens from an area or object, the likelihood of infection can be greatly reduced. The largest source of preventable client infection is contamination from the hands of healthcare workers. Hand hygiene (Fig. 9.4) and the use of gloves are the most effective barriers to the infection cycle.[25] The use of gloves does not eliminate the need for hand hygiene and vice versa. Latex gloves provide the best protection from infectious materials. However, many individuals have latex allergies, so nonlatex gloves can be used as an alternative. The World Health Organization (WHO) recommends the use of alcohol-based hand rubs as the most effective way to ensure optimal hand hygiene.[25]

Alcohol-based hand rubs have the advantage of eliminating the majority of germs, are fast acting, cause minimal skin irritation, are available at the point of care and do not require any particular infrastructure (clean water supply, washbasin, soap, hand towel).[25]

In the clinic, general cleanliness and proper control of heat, light, and air are important for infection control. Spills should

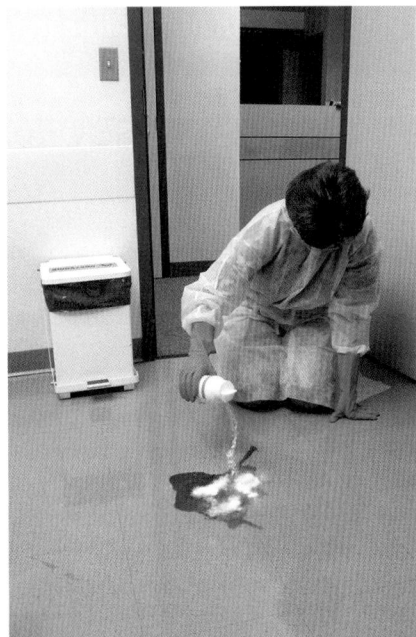

Fig. 9.2 Spills of body fluids must be cleaned up by a gloved employee using paper towels, which should then be placed in an infectious waste container. Afterward a solution of 5.25% sodium hypochlorite (household bleach) diluted 1:10 should be used to disinfect the area. (From Niedzwiecki B: *Kinn's the medical assistant*, ed 14, St Louis, 2020, Elsevier.)

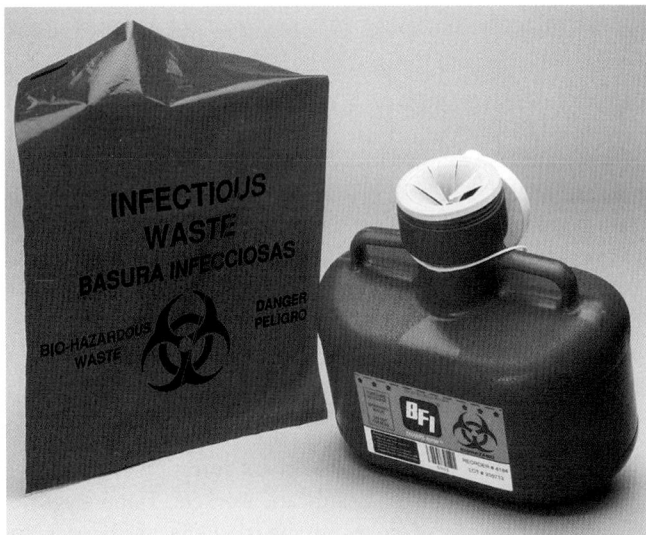

Fig. 9.3 Biohazard label. (From Niedzwiecki B: *Kinn's the medical assistant*, ed 14, St Louis, 2020, Elsevier.)

be cleaned up promptly. Work areas and equipment should be kept free from contamination.

To decontaminate is to "remove, inactivate, or destroy blood-borne pathogens on a surface or item to the point where they are no longer capable of transmitting infectious particles and the surface or item is rendered safe for handling, use, or disposal" (p. 1).[17] Items to be sterilized or decontaminated should first be cleaned thoroughly to remove any residual matter. Sterilization is used to destroy all forms of microbial life,

including highly resistant bacterial spores. An **autoclave** is used to sterilize items by steam under pressure. Ethylene oxide, dry heat, and immersion in chemical disinfectants are other methods of sterilization.[5]

A variety of disinfectants may be used to clean environmental surfaces and reusable instruments. When liquid disinfectants and cleaning agents are used, gloves should be worn to protect the skin from repeated or prolonged contact. The CDC, local health department, or hospital infection control department can provide information about the best product and method to use.

Instruments and equipment used to treat a client should be cleaned or disposed of according to institutional or agency policies and procedures. Contaminated reusable equipment should be placed carefully in a container, labeled, and returned to the appropriate department for sterilization. Contaminated disposable items should be placed carefully in a container, labeled, and discarded.[17]

Contaminated or soiled linen should be disposed of with minimal handling, sorting, and movement. It can be bagged in an appropriate bag and labeled before transport to the laundry, or the bag can be color coded to indicate the type or condition of linen it contains. Other contaminated items, such as toys, magazines, personal hygiene articles, dishes, and eating utensils, should be disposed of or disinfected. They should not be used by others until they have been disinfected.

OT PRACTICE NOTES

Therapists should routinely clean and disinfect personal items such as pens, keys, cell phones, and clipboards because these objects are touched frequently and may become contaminated. If white coats or scrubs are worn, these should be cleaned regularly as well.

Isolation Systems

Isolation systems are designed to protect a person or an object from becoming contaminated or infected by transmissible pathogens. Various isolation procedures are used in different institutions. It is important for all healthcare workers to understand and follow the isolation approach used in their facilities so protection can be ensured. As mentioned, the CDC established Transmission-Based Precautions to be used for patients documented to have or suspected of being infected with highly transmissible or epidemiologically important pathogens: "Transmission-Based Precautions are used when the route(s) of transmission is (are) not completely interrupted using Standard Precautions alone" (p. 69).[21] Three types of Transmission-Based Precautions may be used, singly or in combination, to control infectious transmission: contact precautions, droplet precautions, and airborne precautions. The CDC provides specific recommendations for each infection control measure. In addition, Appendix A of the 2007 guidelines provides a comprehensive list of the types of precautions (e.g., standard, contact, airborne, droplet) recommended for selected infections and conditions.[21]

When Transmission-Based Precautions are needed, a client is usually isolated from other clients and the hospital environment

How to handrub?
WITH ALCOHOL-BASED FORMULATION

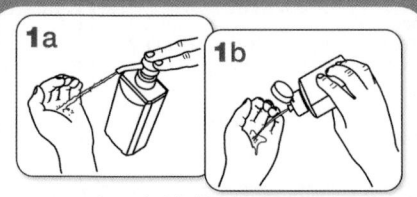

Apply a palmful of the product in a cupped hand and cover all surfaces.

How to handwash?
WITH SOAP AND WATER

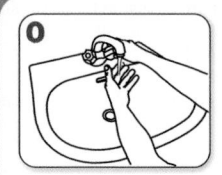

Wet hands with water

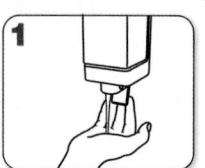

apply enough soap to cover all hand surfaces.

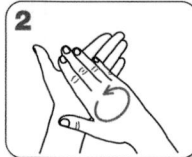

Rub hands palm to palm

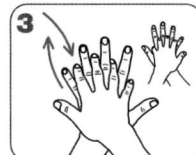

right palm over left dorsum with interlaced fingers and vice versa

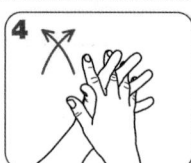

palm to palm with fingers interlaced

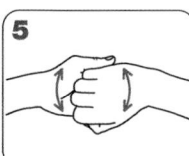

backs of fingers to opposing palms with fingers interlocked

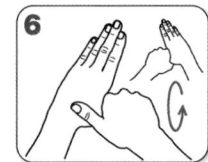

rotational rubbing of left thumb clasped in right palm and vice versa

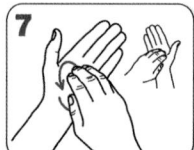

rotational rubbing, backwards and forwards with clasped fingers of right hand in left palm and vice versa

Design: mondofragilis network

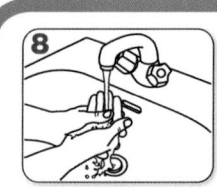

rinse hands with water

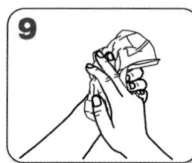

dry thoroughly with a single use towel

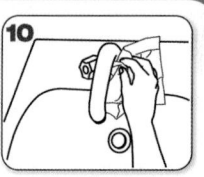

use towel to turn off faucet

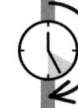

20-30 sec

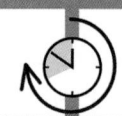

40-60 sec

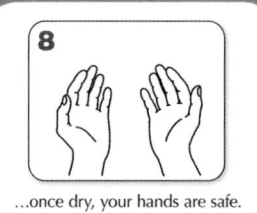

...once dry, your hands are safe.

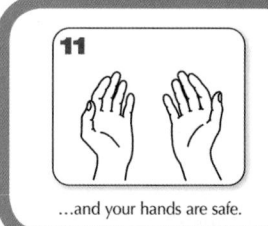

...and your hands are safe.

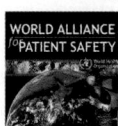

WORLD ALLIANCE for PATIENT SAFETY

WHO acknowledges the Hôpitaux Universitaires de Genève (HUG), in particular the members of the Infection Control Programme, for their active participation in developing this material.

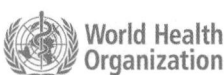

World Health Organization

October 2006, version 1.

Fig. 9.4 Guidelines on hand hygiene with hand rubs or hand-washing. (From PAHO/WHO, 2020. https://www.paho.org/en/documents/infographic-clean-your-hands.)

STRICT ISOLATION

VISITORS: REPORT TO NURSES' STATION BEFORE ENTERING ROOM
1. Masks are indicated for all persons entering the room.
2. Gowns are indicated for all persons entering the room.
3. Gloves are indicated for all persons entering the room.
4. HANDS MUST BE WASHED AFTER TOUCHING THE PATIENT OR POTENTIALLY CONTAMINATED ARTICLES AND BEFORE TAKING CARE OF ANOTHER PATIENT.
5. Articles contaminated with infective material should be discarded or bagged and labeled before being sent for decontamination and reprocessing.

A

RESPIRATORY ISOLATION

VISITORS: REPORT TO NURSES' STATION BEFORE ENTERING ROOM
1. Masks are indicated for those who come close to the patient.
2. Gowns are not indicated.
3. Gloves are not indicated.
4. HANDS MUST BE WASHED AFTER TOUCHING THE PATIENT OR POTENTIALLY CONTAMINATED ARTICLES AND BEFORE TAKING CARE OF ANOTHER PATIENT.
5. Articles contaminated with infective material should be discarded or bagged and labeled before being sent for decontamination and reprocessing.

B

Fig. 9.5 A, Strict isolation procedures sign. The card will be color-coded yellow and will be placed on or next to the door of the client's room. B, Respiratory isolation procedures sign. The card will be color-coded blue and will be placed on or next to the door of the client's room.

because that client has a transmissible disease. Isolation involves placing the client in a room alone or with one or more clients with the same disease to reduce the possibility of transmitting the disease to others. Specific infection control techniques must be followed by all who enter the client's room.[21] These requirements are based on the type of infectious organism and common routes of transmission (i.e., airborne, direct or indirect physical contact, and droplets). Specific instructions are listed on a color-coded card and are placed on or next to the door of the client's room. Strict isolation and respiratory isolation procedures are shown in Fig. 9.5. Personal protective equipment (PPE), including gown, mask, cap, and gloves, may be required. The specific sequence for donning and the safe removal of PPE can be found in Fig. 9.6A and 9.6B. When leaving the client, the caregiver must also dispose of the protective clothing in an appropriately designated area or container for storage, washing, decontamination, or disposal. Examples of diseases that require Transmission-Based Precautions are COVID-19, tuberculosis, severe acute respiratory syndrome (SARS), *Clostridioides difficile* (C. diff) infection, chickenpox, measles, and meningitis.[21]

Occasionally a client's condition (e.g., burns, systemic infection) makes him or her more susceptible to infection. This client may be placed in protective isolation. In this approach, persons entering the client's room may have to wear protective clothing to prevent the transmission of pathogens to the client.

Healthcare-associated infections continue to be a significant problem in a variety of healthcare delivery settings.[21] It is critical that OT personnel be given proper education and training in

infection control standards to prevent the spread of unnecessary infections.

INCIDENTS AND EMERGENCIES

Occupational therapists should be able to respond to a variety of medical emergencies and to recognize when it is better to get assistance from the most qualified individual available, such as a physician, emergency medical technician, or nurse. Securing such assistance should be relatively easy in a hospital but may require an extended period before response if the OT intervention is conducted in a client's home or an outpatient clinic. It is a good idea to keep emergency telephone numbers readily available.

ETHICAL CONSIDERATIONS

In most cases it is best to call for assistance before initiating emergency care unless delay is life-threatening to the client.

All OT practitioners should be certified in **cardiopulmonary resuscitation (CPR)** and should have received basic first aid training. Training and certification can be obtained through organizations such as the American Heart Association (http://www.americanheart.org) and the American Red Cross (http://www.redcross.org).

Consistently following safety measures will prevent many accidents. However, the therapist should always be alert to the

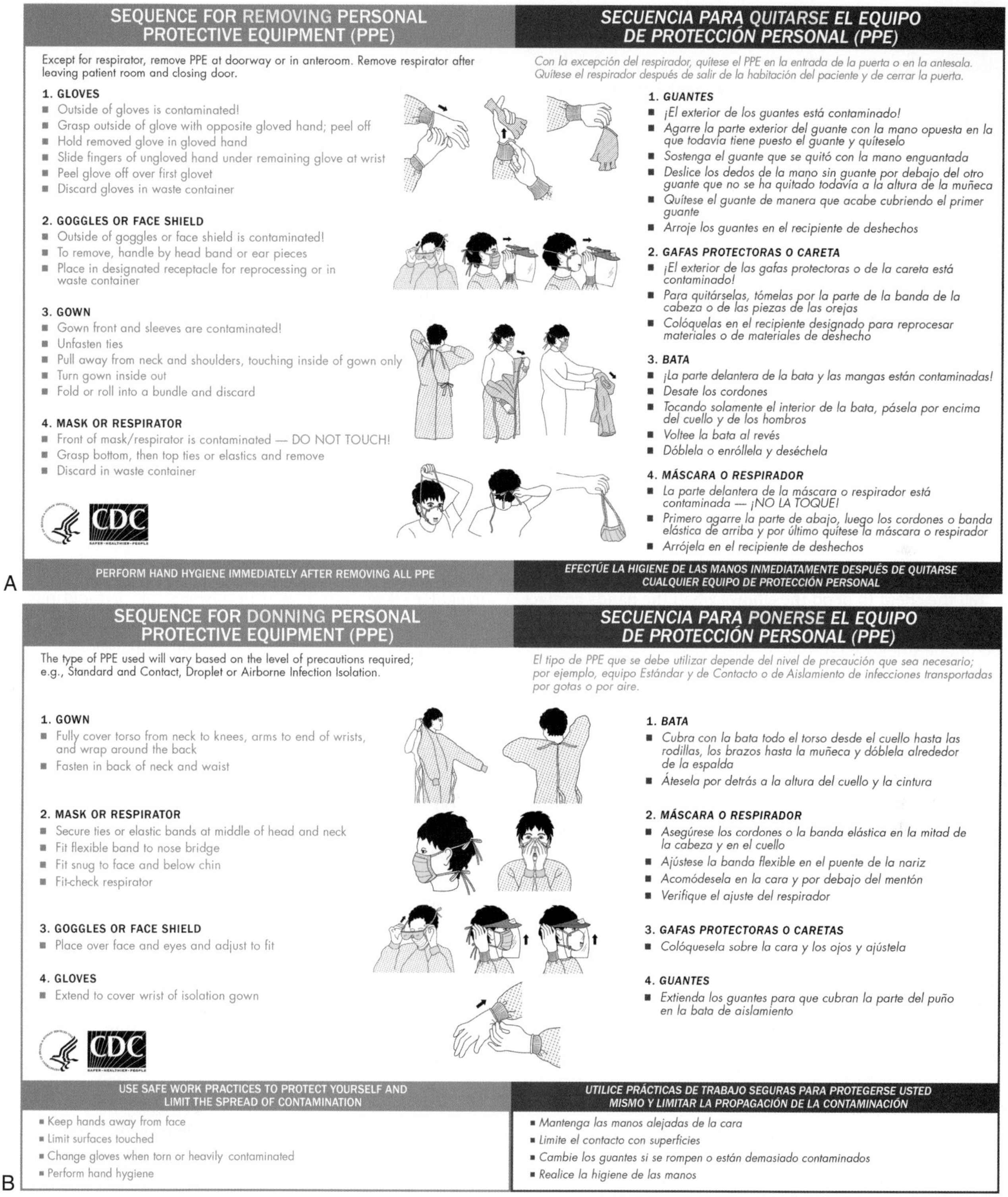

SEQUENCE FOR REMOVING PERSONAL PROTECTIVE EQUIPMENT (PPE)

Except for respirator, remove PPE at doorway or in anteroom. Remove respirator after leaving patient room and closing door.

1. GLOVES
- Outside of gloves is contaminated!
- Grasp outside of glove with opposite gloved hand; peel off
- Hold removed glove in gloved hand
- Slide fingers of ungloved hand under remaining glove at wrist
- Peel glove off over first glove
- Discard gloves in waste container

2. GOGGLES OR FACE SHIELD
- Outside of goggles or face shield is contaminated!
- To remove, handle by head band or ear pieces
- Place in designated receptacle for reprocessing or in waste container

3. GOWN
- Gown front and sleeves are contaminated!
- Unfasten ties
- Pull away from neck and shoulders, touching inside of gown only
- Turn gown inside out
- Fold or roll into a bundle and discard

4. MASK OR RESPIRATOR
- Front of mask/respirator is contaminated — DO NOT TOUCH!
- Grasp bottom, then top ties or elastics and remove
- Discard in waste container

PERFORM HAND HYGIENE IMMEDIATELY AFTER REMOVING ALL PPE

SECUENCIA PARA QUITARSE EL EQUIPO DE PROTECCIÓN PERSONAL (PPE)

Con la excepción del respirador, quítese el PPE en la entrada de la puerta o en la antesala. Quítese el respirador después de salir de la habitación del paciente y de cerrar la puerta.

1. GUANTES
- ¡El exterior de los guantes está contaminado!
- Agarre la parte exterior del guante con la mano opuesta en la que todavía tiene puesto el guante y quíteselo
- Sostenga el guante que se quitó con la mano enguantada
- Deslice los dedos de la mano sin guante por debajo del otro guante que no se ha quitado todavía a la altura de la muñeca
- Quítese el guante de manera que acabe cubriendo el primer guante
- Arroje los guantes en el recipiente de deshechos

2. GAFAS PROTECTORAS O CARETA
- ¡El exterior de las gafas protectoras o de la careta está contaminado!
- Para quitárselas, tómelas por la parte de la banda de la cabeza o de las piezas de las orejas
- Colóquelas en el recipiente designado para reprocesar materiales o de materiales de deshecho

3. BATA
- ¡La parte delantera de la bata y las mangas están contaminadas!
- Desate los cordones
- Tocando solamente el interior de la bata, pásela por encima del cuello y de los hombros
- Voltee la bata al revés
- Dóblela o enróllela y deséchela

4. MÁSCARA O RESPIRADOR
- La parte delantera de la máscara o respirador está contaminada — ¡NO LA TOQUE!
- Primero agarre la parte de abajo, luego los cordones o banda elástica de arriba y por último quítese la máscara o respirador
- Arrójela en el recipiente de deshechos

EFECTÚE LA HIGIENE DE LAS MANOS INMEDIATAMENTE DESPUÉS DE QUITARSE CUALQUIER EQUIPO DE PROTECCIÓN PERSONAL

A

SEQUENCE FOR DONNING PERSONAL PROTECTIVE EQUIPMENT (PPE)

The type of PPE used will vary based on the level of precautions required; e.g., Standard and Contact, Droplet or Airborne Infection Isolation.

1. GOWN
- Fully cover torso from neck to knees, arms to end of wrists, and wrap around the back
- Fasten in back of neck and waist

2. MASK OR RESPIRATOR
- Secure ties or elastic bands at middle of head and neck
- Fit flexible band to nose bridge
- Fit snug to face and below chin
- Fit-check respirator

3. GOGGLES OR FACE SHIELD
- Place over face and eyes and adjust to fit

4. GLOVES
- Extend to cover wrist of isolation gown

USE SAFE WORK PRACTICES TO PROTECT YOURSELF AND LIMIT THE SPREAD OF CONTAMINATION
- Keep hands away from face
- Limit surfaces touched
- Change gloves when torn or heavily contaminated
- Perform hand hygiene

SECUENCIA PARA PONERSE EL EQUIPO DE PROTECCIÓN PERSONAL (PPE)

El tipo de PPE que se debe utilizar depende del nivel de precaución que sea necesario; por ejemplo, equipo Estándar y de Contacto o de Aislamiento de infecciones transportadas por gotas o por aire.

1. BATA
- Cubra con la bata todo el torso desde el cuello hasta las rodillas, los brazos hasta la muñeca y dóblela alrededor de la espalda
- Átesela por detrás a la altura del cuello y la cintura

2. MÁSCARA O RESPIRADOR
- Asegúrese los cordones o la banda elástica en la mitad de la cabeza y en el cuello
- Ajústese la banda flexible en el puente de la nariz
- Acomódesela en la cara y por debajo del mentón
- Verifique el ajuste del respirador

3. GAFAS PROTECTORAS O CARETAS
- Colóquesela sobre la cara y los ojos y ajústela

4. GUANTES
- Extienda los guantes para que cubran la parte del puño en la bata de aislamiento

UTILICE PRÁCTICAS DE TRABAJO SEGURAS PARA PROTEGERSE USTED MISMO Y LIMITAR LA PROPAGACIÓN DE LA CONTAMINACIÓN
- Mantenga las manos alejadas de la cara
- Limite el contacto con superficies
- Cambie los guantes si se rompen o están demasiado contaminados
- Realice la higiene de las manos

B

Fig. 9.6 A, Sequence for putting on PPE. B, Sequence for removing PPE. (From PPE sequence. Centers for Disease Control and Prevention. Accessed June 11, 2022. https://www.cdc.gov/hai/pdfs/ppe/ppe-sequence.pdf.)

possibility of an injury and should expect the unexpected to happen. Most institutions have specific policies and procedures to follow. In general, the therapist should do the following when an injury to a client occurs:

1. Ask for help. Do not leave the client alone. Prevent further injury to the client and provide emergency care.

2. When the emergency is over, document the incident according to the institution's policy. Do not discuss the incident with the client or significant others or express information to anyone that might indicate negligence.

3. Notify the supervisor of the incident and file the incident report with the appropriate person within the organization.

Falls

The risk of falling is always present when functional mobility is addressed with clients. The OT can reduce the risk of falling by carefully preparing the environment before initiating intervention. This includes use of a gait belt, as needed, during mobility activities; clearing the environment of potential hazards; and having a wheelchair or chair nearby to pull into position for clients who might be prone to falling. The therapist can prevent injuries from falls by remaining alert and reacting quickly when clients lose their balance. Proper guarding techniques must be practiced. In many instances it is wise to resist the natural impulse to keep the client upright. Instead, the therapist can carefully assist the client to the floor or onto a firm object.

If a client begins to fall forward, the following procedure should be used: Restrain the client by firmly holding the gait belt. Push forward against the pelvis and pull back on the shoulder or anterior chest. Help the client stand erect once it is determined that no injury has occurred. The client may briefly lean against you for support. If the client is falling too far forward to be kept upright, guide the client to reach for the floor slowly. Slow the momentum by gently pulling back on the gait belt and the client's shoulder. Step forward as the client moves toward the floor. Tell the client to bend the elbows when the hands contact the floor to help cushion the fall. The client's head should be turned to one side to avoid injury to the face.

If the client begins to fall backward, the following procedure should be used: Rotate your body so one side is turned toward the client's back and widen your stance. Push forward on the client's pelvis and allow the client to lean against your body. Then, assist the client to stand erect. If the client falls too far backward, to stay upright, continue to rotate your body until it is turned toward the client's back and widen your stance. Instruct the client to briefly lean against your body or to sit on your thigh. You may need to lower the client into a sitting position on the floor using the gait belt and good body mechanics.

Burns

In general, only minor, first-degree burns are likely to accidentally occur in occupational therapy. These can be treated with basic first aid procedures. Skilled personnel should be contacted for immediate care if the burn has any charred or missing skin or shows blistering. The following steps should be taken for first-degree burns in which the skin is only reddened[8]:

1. Rinse or soak the burned area in cold (not iced) water.
2. Cover with a clean or sterile dressing.
3. Do not apply any cream, ointment, or butter to the burn because this will mask the appearance and may lead to infection or a delay in healing.
4. Report the incident so that the injury can be evaluated by a physician.

Bleeding

A laceration may result in minor or serious bleeding. The objectives of first aid treatment are to prevent contamination of the wound and to control bleeding. The following steps should be taken to stop the bleeding[12]:

1. Wash your hands and put on protective gloves. Continue to wear protective gloves while treating the wound.
2. Remove any clothing or debris on the wound. Do not attempt to remove large or deeply embedded objects.
3. Place a clean towel or a sterile dressing over the wound and apply direct pressure to the wound. If no dressing is available, use your gloved hand.
4. Elevate the wound above the level of the client's heart to reduce blood flow to the area.
5. Help the client to lie down if possible. The client needs to remain quiet and to avoid using the extremity.
6. Do not apply a tourniquet unless you have been trained to do so.
7. Get medical help as soon as possible.

Shock

Clients may experience shock as a result of excessive bleeding, sepsis, and respiratory distress; as a reaction to the change from a supine to an upright position; or as a response to excessive heat or anaphylaxis (severe allergic reaction). Shock causes a drop in blood pressure and inefficient cardiac output, resulting in inadequate perfusion of organs and tissues. Signs and symptoms of shock include pale, moist, and cool skin; shallow and irregular breathing; dilated pupils; a weak or rapid pulse; dizziness or nausea; and an altered level of consciousness.[8] Shock should not be confused with fainting, which would result in a slower pulse, paleness, and perspiration. Clients who faint generally will recover promptly if allowed to lie flat. If a client exhibits symptoms of shock, the following actions should be taken[8]:

1. Get medical assistance as soon as possible because shock can be life-threatening.
2. Try to determine the cause of shock and correct it if possible. Monitor the client's blood pressure, breathing, and pulse rate.
3. Place the person in a supine position, with the head slightly lower than the legs. If head and chest injuries are present or if respiration is impaired, it may be necessary to keep the head and chest slightly elevated.
4. Do not add heat, but prevent loss of body heat if necessary by applying a cool compress to the client's forehead and covering the client with a light blanket.
5. Do not allow exertion. Keep the client quiet until emergency medical help arrives.

Seizures

Seizures may be caused by a specific disorder, brain injury, or medication. The OT should be able to recognize a seizure and should take appropriate action to keep the client from getting hurt. A client having a seizure will usually become rigid for a few seconds and then will begin to convulse with an all-over jerking motion. The client may turn blue and may stop breathing for up to 50 to 70 seconds.[8] A client's sphincter control may be lost during or at the conclusion of the seizure, so the client may void urine or feces involuntarily. When a client shows signs of entering a seizure, the following steps should be taken[8]:

1. Place the person in a safe location and position him or her away from anything that might cause injury. Do not attempt to restrain or restrict the convulsions.

2. Loosen clothing around the person's neck to assist in keeping the client's airway open.
3. Do not insert any objects into the person's mouth; this can cause injury.
4. Remove sharp objects (glasses, furniture, and other objects) from around the person to prevent injury.
5. When the convulsions subside, roll the person onto his or her side to maintain an open airway and to prevent the person from aspirating any secretions.
6. After the convulsions cease, have the client rest. He or she may experience confusion for a period of time. It may be helpful to cover the client with a blanket or screen to provide privacy.
7. Get medical help.[8]

Insulin-Related Illnesses

Many clients seen in occupational therapy have insulin-related episodes. These episodes can occur as the result of severely inadequate insulin levels (hyperglycemia, or a high blood glucose level) or from excessive insulin (hypoglycemia, or a low blood glucose level).[8] It is very important for the OT to be able to differentiate between the conditions of hypoglycemia (insulin reaction) and hyperglycemia (ketoacidosis), which can lead to diabetic coma (Table 9.2). Both conditions can result in loss of consciousness, but medical intervention for each condition is very different.

An insulin reaction (also called insulin shock) can be caused by too much systemic insulin, the intake of too little food or sugar, or too much physical activity. If the client is conscious, some form of sugar (e.g., candy, orange juice) should be provided. If the client is unconscious, glucose may have to be provided intravenously. The client should rest, and all physical activity should be stopped. This condition is not as serious as ketoacidosis, but the client should be given the opportunity to return to a normal state as soon as possible.[8]

Hyperglycemia can develop when a person with diabetes fails to take enough insulin or deviates significantly from a prescribed diet. Ketoacidosis and dehydration occur and can lead to a diabetic coma and eventual death if not treated. This should be considered a medical emergency requiring prompt action, including assistance from qualified personnel.[8] The client should not be given any form of sugar. Usually, an injection of insulin is needed, followed by IV fluids and salt. A nurse or physician should provide care as quickly as possible. Table 9.2 explains how to differentiate the symptoms of hyperglycemia and hypoglycemia.

Respiratory Distress

Dyspnea control postures may be used to reduce breathlessness in clients in respiratory distress. The client must be responsive and must have an unobstructed airway.[14] The high Fowler's position (Fig. 9.7A) may be used for clients in bed. The head of the bed should be in an upright position at a 90-degree angle. If available, a footboard should be used to support the client's feet. The orthopneic position (see Fig. 9.7B) may be used for clients who are sitting or standing. In either case the client bends forward slightly at the waist and supports the upper body by leaning the forearms on a table or counter. Pursed-lip breathing (i.e., a breathing pattern of inhaling through the nose and slowly exhaling through pursed lips) can help decrease dyspnea and the respiratory rate[14] (see Chapter 45 for additional suggestions).

Choking and Cardiac Arrest

All healthcare practitioners should be trained to treat clients who are choking or suffering from cardiac arrest. Cardiopulmonary resuscitation (CPR) is a series of potentially lifesaving actions that increase an individual's chance of surviving cardiac arrest.[18] Basic Life Support (BLS) certification involves instruction in recognizing a cardiac arrest, activating the emergency response system, performing specific CPR techniques, and using an automatic external defibrillator (AED). In addition, training in recognizing and providing intervention when an individual is choking is provided. The American Heart Association (AHA) regularly publishes recommended standards for the performance of CPR and emergency cardiovascular care. The 2020 AHA Guidelines for Cardiopulmonary Resuscitation (CPR) and Emergency Cardiovascular Care (ECC) advise initiating chest compressions first, followed by establishing the airway and then breathing (or C-A-B).[18] Specific certification training courses are offered by both the AHA and the American Red Cross. The following information is presented as a reminder of the basic techniques and is not meant to be substituted for training.

The urgency of choking cannot be overemphasized. Immediate recognition and proper action are essential (Fig. 9.8). When assisting a conscious adult or a child who is older than 1 year, the following steps should be taken[18]:

1. Ask the client, "Are you choking?" If the client can speak or cough effectively, do not interfere with the client's own attempts to expel the object.
2. If the client is unable to speak, cough, or breathe, check the mouth and remove any visible foreign object.
3. If the client is unable to speak or cough, position yourself behind the client. Clasp your hands over the client's abdomen, slightly above the umbilicus but below the diaphragm.
4. Use the closed fist of one hand, covered by your other hand, to give 3 or 4 abrupt thrusts against the person's abdomen by compressing the abdomen in and up forcefully

TABLE 9.2 Warning Signs and Symptoms of Insulin-Related Illnesses		
	Insulin Reaction (Insulin Shock)	**Ketoacidosis (Diabetic Coma)**
Onset	Sudden	Gradual
Skin	Moist, pale	Dry, flushed
Behavior	Excited, agitated	Drowsy
Breath odor	Normal	Fruity
Breathing	Normal to shallow	Deep, labored
Tongue	Moist	Dry
Vomiting	Absent	Present
Hunger	Present	Absent
Thirst	Absent	Present

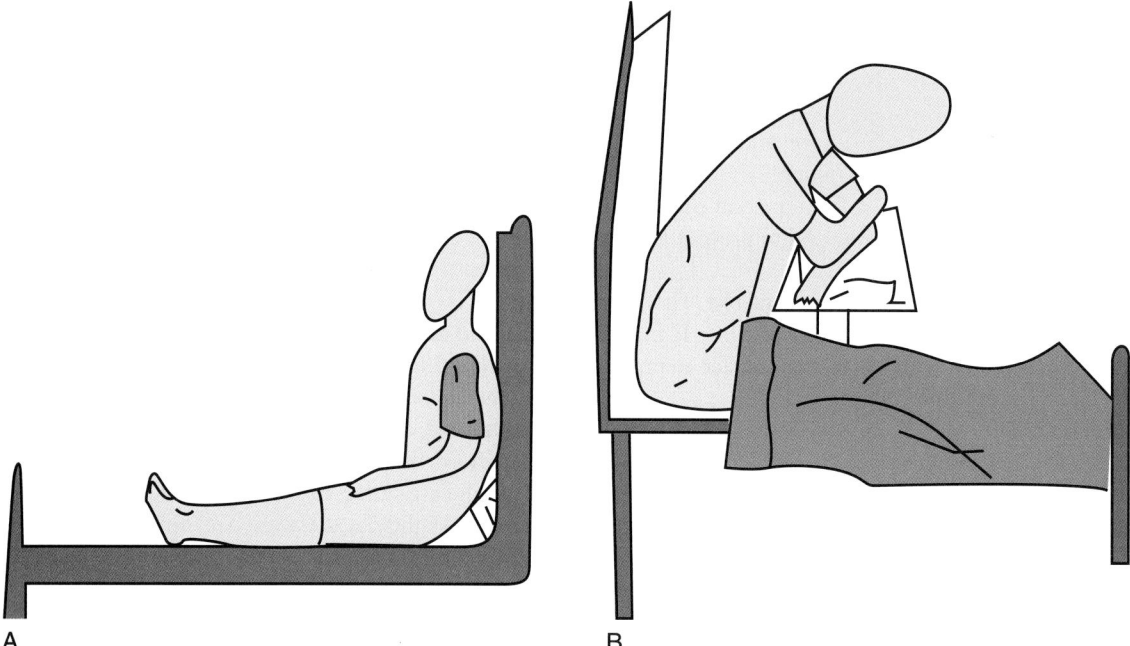

Fig. 9.7 A, High Fowler's position. B, Orthopneic position.

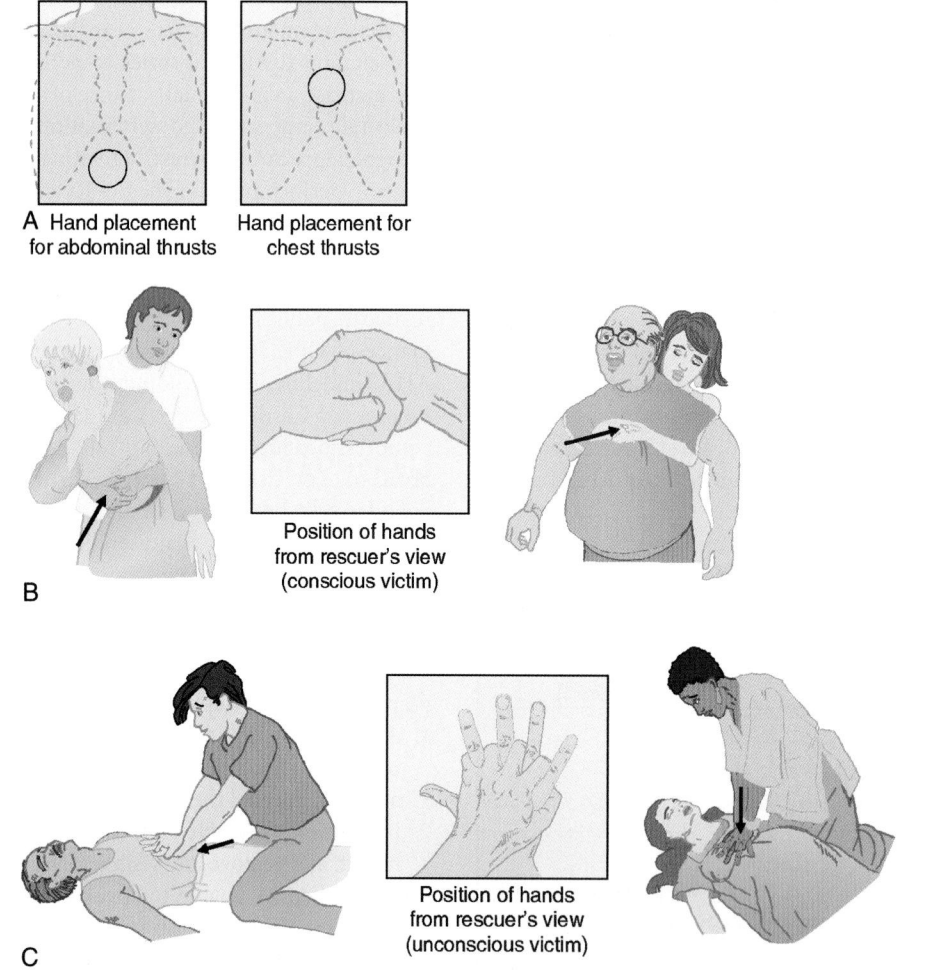

Fig. 9.8 Abdominal thrust maneuver (also known as the Heimlich maneuver) used for removal of foreign bodies blocking the upper airway. A, Hand placement. B, Maneuver for conscious victims. C, Maneuver for unconscious victims. (From Black JM, Hawks JH: *Medical-surgical nursing: clinical management for positive outcomes,* ed 8, St Louis, 2009, Saunders.)

(this technique is also known as the Heimlich maneuver). Continue to apply the thrusts until the obstruction becomes dislodged or is relieved or the person becomes unconscious. It is no longer recommended that a rescuer perform a finger sweep to remove the object.

5. Seek medical assistance.

When assisting an adult or a child who is older than 1 year who appears to be unconscious, the following steps should be taken[18]:

1. Ensure that it is safe for you to intervene (no hazards or risky environmental conditions).

2. Activate the emergency response system (call for help, or call 9-1-1). Get an AED (defibrillator), if available. If two persons are available, one should call for help and get the AED while the other individual initiates CPR.

3. Attempt to awaken or rouse the individual.

4. If the individual is unresponsive, place the person in a supine position on a firm surface. Look for no breathing or only gasping and check for a pulse, limiting the time to do this to no more than 10 seconds.

5. If there is no normal breathing or pulse, initiate chest compressions. Kneel next to the client and place the heel of one hand on the inferior portion of the sternum superior to the xiphoid process (approximately in line with the nipples). Put your other hand over your first hand with your fingers interlaced. Position your shoulders directly over the client's sternum, keep your elbows extended, and press down firmly, depressing the sternum at least 2 inches with each compression; avoid excessive depths (greater than 2.4 inches). Relax after each compression, allowing the chest to fully recoil after each compression, but do not remove your hands from the sternum. The relaxation and compression phases should be equal in duration. Compressions should be applied at a rate of 100 to 120 per minute.

6. If you are not trained in CPR, continue to perform only chest compressions until help arrives or the victim awakens ("hands only" CPR).

7. If you are trained in CPR, perform 30 chest compressions, then open the victim's airway using the head-tilt, chin-lift method.

8. Check for respiration by observing the chest or abdomen for movement, listen for sounds of breathing, and feel for breath by placing your cheek close to the person's mouth. If no sign of breath is present, the client is not breathing and you should initiate breathing techniques.

9. Pinch the client's nose closed and maintain the head tilt to open the airway. Place your mouth over the client's mouth and form a seal with your lips. Perform two full breaths. Your breaths should be strong enough to make the victim's chest rise. Some persons prefer to place a clean cloth over the client's lips before initiating mouth-to-mouth respirations. If available, a plastic CPR device can be used to decrease contact between the caregiver's mouth and the client's mouth and any saliva or vomitus.

10. Evaluate for circulation by palpating the carotid artery for a pulse. Sometimes it can be difficult to locate a pulse, so also observe the client for signs of life—breathing, movement, consciousness. If no pulse or signs of consciousness are noted, you must return to performing external chest compressions.

11. If you are performing CPR procedures without assistance, you should repeat 30 chest compressions, followed by 2 breaths. Continue this sequence (30 compressions/2 rescue breaths) until qualified help arrives, the victim shows obvious signs of life (e.g., moving or breathing), or you are physically unable to continue. Limit the interruption of chest compressions to less than 10 seconds. In all instances the client will require hospitalization and evaluation by a physician.

12. If you have access to an AED, continue to perform CPR until you can attach the chest pads and turn on the machine. If you are alone and you observed the victim collapse, put the AED on immediately. If you did not observe the collapse, attach the AED after approximately 1 minute of CPR. The AED will analyze the victim's heart for rhythm and will provide a shock if necessary. The AED provides auditory instructions for operation. After placement of the chest pads, it will analyze the victim's heart for rhythm and will direct the rescuer to provide a shock or to continue CPR.

NOTE: Extreme care must be taken when attempting to open the airway of a person who may have experienced a cervical spine injury. In such cases use the chin lift, but avoid the head tilt. If the technique does not open the airway, the head should be tilted slowly and gently until the airway is open.

As mentioned, these procedures are appropriate to use for adults and for children 1 year of age or older. CPR is contraindicated if clients have clearly expressed their desire for "do not resuscitate" (DNR). This information should be clearly documented in the medical chart. A pamphlet or booklet containing diagrams and instructions for CPR techniques can be obtained from most local offices of the AHA or from a variety of websites.[18]

THREADED CASE STUDY

Donna, Part 2

To adequately prepare the OT clinic as a safe environment for clients and staff, clear policies and procedures pertaining to client safety, medical emergencies, infection control, and precautions with special equipment need to be developed and implemented. In the case study presented at the beginning of this chapter, Donna, the director of OT Services, is responsible for developing such policies and procedures. It should be mandatory for all OT personnel to become certified in CPR and first aid. Employee manuals can be produced that orient staff to general safety procedures and infection control standards. Furthermore, in-service education should be developed for newly hired personnel that familiarizes them with the types of specialized medical equipment that OT personnel are likely to encounter in their interventions with clients.

Many resources are available that can assist Donna in establishing these policies and procedures. The Centers for Disease Control and Prevention (http://www.cdc.gov), the Occupational Safety and Health Administration (http://www.OSHA.gov), and the National Institutes of Health (http://www.nih.gov) are government organizations that provide up-to-date information pertaining to health standards, infection control, medical research, and workplace safety. Information on first aid, choking, and CPR can be obtained from most local offices of the AHA and from the American National Red Cross. In addition, information on emergency procedures may be found on a variety of websites.

SUMMARY

All OT personnel have a legal and professional obligation to promote safety for self, the client, visitors, and others. The OT should be prepared to react to emergency situations quickly, decisively, and calmly. The consistent use of safe practices helps reduce accidents for both clients and workers and reduces the length and cost of treatment.

REVIEW QUESTIONS

1. Why is it important to teach the client and significant others guidelines for handling various emergency situations?
2. Describe at least four behaviors that you can adopt to improve client safety.
3. Why is it important to review a client's chart before initiating an intervention?
4. What types of activities are appropriate when providing an intervention to a client who is ventilator dependent? What precautions must be taken during such activities?
5. Define the following: IV line, A line, NG tube, TPN or hyperalimentation, and catheter.
6. Describe Standard Precautions.
7. Why is it important to follow Standard Precautions with all clients?
8. Demonstrate the proper technique for hand-washing.
9. How should you respond to a client emergency?
10. Distinguish between an insulin reaction and ketoacidosis (diabetic coma). What is the appropriate medical intervention for each condition?
11. Describe how you would help a client who is falling forward and one who is falling backward.
12. Which emergency situations might require getting advanced medical assistance, and which situations could a therapist handle alone?

For additional practice questions for this chapter, please visit eBooks.Health.Elsevier.com.

REFERENCES

1. American Occupational Therapy Association: AOTA 2020 code of ethics, *Am J Occup Ther* 74(Suppl 3):1–13, 2020. https://doi.org/10.5014/ajot.2020.74S3006.
2. American Occupational Therapy Association: Occupational therapy practice framework: domain and process, ed. 4, *Am J Occup Ther.* 74 (Suppl 2):1–87, 2020. https://doi.org/10.5014/ajot.2020.74S2001.
3. Centers for Disease Control and Infection: COVID data tracker (2021). https://covid.cdc.gov/covid-data-tracker/#datatracker-home.
4. Cohen J, Van der Meulen Rodgers Y: Contributing factors to personal protective equipment shortages during the COVID-19 pandemic, *Preventive Medicine* 141:106263, 2020. https://doi.org/10.1016/j.ypmed.2020.106263.
5. Cooper K, Gosnell K, editors: *Foundations of adult health nursing,* ed 8, St Louis, 2018, Mosby.
6. Ekelman Ranke BA, Moriarty MP: An overview of professional liability in occupational therapy, *Am J Occup Ther* 51:671–680, 1997.
7. Fairchild SL, O'Shea RK, Washington R: *Pierson and Fairchild's principles and techniques of client care,* ed 6, St Louis, 2017, Elsevier.
8. Frazier MS, Drzymkowski JW: *Essentials of human diseases and conditions,* ed 5, St Louis, 2015, Saunders.
9. Gaspari C, Lafayette S, Cavalcanti D, et al: Safety and feasibility of out-of-bed mobilization for patients with external ventricular drains in a neurosurgical intensive care unit, *Journal of Acute Care Therapy* 9:171–178, 2018. https://doi.org/10.1097/JAT.0000000000000085.
10. Hinkel JL, Cheever KH: *Brunner and Suddarth's textbook of medical-surgical nursing,* ed 14 Philadelphia, 2017, Lippincott Williams & Wilkins.
11. Liu Y-C, Kuo R-L, Shih S-R: COVID-19: The first documented coronavirus pandemic in history, *Biomedical Journal* 43:328–333, 2020. https://doi.org/10.1016/j.bj.2020.04.007.
12. Mayo Clinic Staff: Severe bleeding: first aid. (2020), Mayo Clinic. https://www.mayoclinic.org/first-aid/first-aid-severe-bleeding/basics/art-20056661.
13. MedlinePlus (2021): Intracranial pressure monitoring. US National Library of Medicine, National Institutes of Health: https://medlineplus.gov/ency/article/003411.htm.
14. Migliore A: Management of dyspnea: guidelines for practice for adults with chronic obstructive pulmonary disease, *OT Health Care* 18:1–8, 2004.
15. *Mosby's dictionary of medicine: nursing & health professions,* ed 10, St Louis, 2016, Elsevier.
16. Occupational Safety and Health Administration: Hospital e-tool: healthcare wide hazards, slips/trips/falls. https://www.osha.gov/SLTC/etools/hospital/hazards/slips/slips.htm.
17. Occupational Safety and Health Administration: Bloodborne pathogens. https://www.osha.gov/SLTC/etools/hospital/hazards/bbp/bbp.html.
18. Panchal AR, Bartos JA, Cabañas JG, et al: Part 3: Adult basic and advanced life support: 2020 American Heart Association Guidelines for Cardiopulmonary Resuscitation and Emergency Cardiovascular Care., *Circulation* 142(16 Suppl 2):S366–S468, 2020. https://doi.org/10.1161/CIR.0000000000000916.
19. Popat B, Jones A: Invasive and non-invasive mechanical ventilation, *Medicine (Abingdon)* 40(6):298–304, 2012.
20. Rutgers University. Health care workers most at risk for COVID-19: A new study finds nurses have the highest prevalence of infection. *ScienceDaily*, 16 November 2020. https://www.sciencedaily.com/releases/2020/11/201116125608.htm.
21. Siegel JD, Rhinehart E, Jackson M, Chiarello L, the Healthcare Infection Control Practices Advisory Committee: 2007 guideline for isolation precautions: preventing transmission of infectious agents in healthcare settings, US Department of Health and Human Services, Centers for Disease Control

(Updated July 2023). https://www.cdc.gov/infectioncontrol/pdf/guidelines/isolation-guidelines-H.pdf.

22. Sussman C, Bates-Jensen B: *Wound care: a collaborative practice manual for health professionals*, ed 4, Philadelphia, 2013, Lippincott Williams & Wilkins.

23. University of Rochester Medical Center (2021). Signs of respiratory distress. Health Encyclopedia. https://www.urmc.rochester.edu/encyclopedia/content.aspx?contenttypeid=85&contentid=P01326.

24. Walter J, Corbridge T, Singer B: Invasive mechanical ventilation. *Southern Medical Journal*, 111(12):746–753, 2018. https://doi.org/10.14423/SMJ.0000000000000905.

25. World Health Organization: *WHO guidelines on hand hygiene in healthcare,* Geneva. Switzerland, 2009, World Health Organization.

26. World Health Organization: *WHO coronavirus (COVID-19) dashboard*, 2021, World Health Organization. https://covid19.who.int/.

10

Activities of Daily Living

Jean S. Koketsu and Michelle Rodriguez

LEARNING OBJECTIVES

After studying this chapter, the student or practitioner will be able to do the following:

1. Describe activities of daily living (ADLs) and instrumental activities of daily living (IADLs), and explain how ADLs and IADLs relate to the current Occupational Therapy Practice Framework (OTPF-4).
2. Explain why it is important to consider environmental and personal factors when performing ADL and IADL assessments and training. Give examples of specific environmental and personal factors that a person, group, or population may have that can affect ADLs and IADLs.
3. Describe a client-centered approach to evaluation, and explain why it is an important consideration in ADL and IADL training.
4. Explain the general procedures for ADL and IADL assessments.
5. Explain how to record levels of independence and summarize the results of an ADL/IADL evaluation.
6. Explain the purpose of performing a home safety assessment and when it may be indicated.

7. Give at least five examples of client factors that may have limitations that can affect performance in occupations and how each can affect an ADL and IADL (e.g., if someone has shoulder range-of-motion limitations, they may have difficulty putting on a shirt [ADL] and reaching for object on a shelf when cooking a meal [IADL]).
8. Give examples of how difficulties in performance skills (motor skills, process skills, and social interaction skills) can affect specific ADL and IADL abilities.
9. Discuss considerations for selecting adaptive equipment for performance of ADLs and IADLs. Describe at least five pieces of adaptive equipment that may be used to increase independence and the conditions for which each device may be indicated.
10. Describe, perform, and teach specific ADL techniques for individuals with limited range of motion (ROM) and strength, incoordination, paraplegia, tetraplegia, low vision, and if a very large size.

CHAPTER OUTLINE

KEY TERMS

Activities of daily living (ADLs)

Adaptive equipment and techniques

Client-centered approach

Cultural humility

Home Safety Assessment

Instrumental activities of daily living (IADLs)

Occupational profile

THREADED CASE STUDY

Anna, Part 1

Anna is a 29-year-old woman (prefers use of the pronouns she/her/hers) who has been diagnosed with a T4 spinal cord injury (SCI) from a car accident. She has complete sensory and motor loss below the level of injury. Anna is currently in an inpatient rehabilitation program. Before her injury, Anna lived in a recently purchased one-story house with two bedrooms and one bathroom with her husband and 2-year-old daughter. In addition to caring for her daughter, Anna spent much of her time performing household chores, such as cooking, laundry, and grocery shopping. Anna also took care of her family's finances and enjoyed leading a Bible study group with her friends. Anna dropped their daughter off at a daycare center while she worked part-time as a bookkeeper at her church. Her husband picked up their daughter after spending a full day at his job as an auto mechanic. The family depended on Anna's part-time income to pay some of the bills. Anna's mother, Martha, has been caring for her granddaughter since Anna's accident. Martha agreed to temporarily live with Anna and her husband and granddaughter after Anna's discharge home until Anna can independently take care of her child.

Anna currently requires minimal assistance with basic transfers, bed mobility, and lower body dressing because of decreased endurance, pain in her back, and decreased trunk control. She requires minimal assistance with verbal cues for proper techniques for weight shifts in her wheelchair and skin checks to ensure skin integrity. Anna reports that she has been overwhelmed with all the new things she has had to learn. She requires moderate assistance with bowel and bladder care and showering/bathing tasks. She is independent with wheelchair

mobility on indoor flat surfaces but requires standby assistance to propel in tight areas and corners and while propelling up ramps because of fatigue, decreased trunk control, and reduced upper body strength. She is independent with seated-level activities, such as hygiene and grooming at the sink and light kitchen tasks in the rehabilitation unit's kitchen.

Anna and her husband are concerned about the amount of assistance she may require when discharged from the rehabilitation program. They want to eventually grow their family and have concerns about sexual functioning, intimacy, and fertility. Their home is not wheelchair accessible. Although they appreciate Martha and her offer to live with them after Anna's discharge home from the hospital, they prefer that Martha does not have to live with them long term.

Anna wants to be independent in taking care of herself, her daughter, her household, and her husband. She wants to drive again, return to her Bible study classes, and resume her part-time job. She is not sure how she can resume the occupations she considers important to fulfilling her roles as a wife, mother, homemaker, worker, and active community member.

Critical Thinking Questions

1. What ADL and IADL tasks will Anna need to master to be more independent and to return home safely with her family?

2. What is the role of occupational therapy in helping Anna to return home safely and to eventually reach her goals of independence?

3. With all the occupational performance areas that need to be addressed, how can an occupational therapist prioritize which areas to address?

The American Occupational Therapy Association (AOTA), the U.S. national professional organization for occupational therapy practitioners, presents its current intervention guidelines in the "Occupational Therapy Practice Framework: Domain and Process," fourth edition (OTPF-4), an official document intended for both internal and external audiences (AOTA, 2020).[12] This chapter describes both the aspects of the domain and the process of occupational therapy in regard to activities of daily living (ADLs) and instrumental activities of daily living (IADLs). It also focuses on specific intervention strategies for assisting clients to optimize occupational functioning.

According to the OTPF-4, ADLs and IADLs are considered two of nine broad categories of occupation in which clients

engage.[12] ADLs and IADLs include, but are not limited to, routine tasks of personal care, functional mobility, communication, home management, and community mobility.[28] Evaluation and training in the performance of these important life tasks have long been important aspects of assessments and treatments in virtually every type of health and wellness practice area. Loss of ability to care for personal needs and to participate in daily activities to fulfill important life roles can be life-changing and devastating.

In the broadest sense, service delivery in the areas of occupation begins with the occupational therapist (OT) receiving a referral for service, performing an evaluation, forming and instituting an intervention plan, and assessing the outcome of the process.[12] Occupational therapists develop an occupational profile, a summary of a client's occupational history and experiences, patterns of daily living, interests, values, needs, and relevant contexts, with the purpose of understanding what is currently important and meaningful to the client.[12] Keeping information from a client's occupational profile in mind, an OT practitioner (OT practitioners include the occupational therapist and the occupational therapy assistant who works under the supervision of the occupational therapist; in this chapter OT practitioner is referring to the occupational therapist) will usually analyze a client's occupational performance during evaluation and treatment to inform what interventions to implement. As treatment commences, outcomes are looked at to assess progress and includes transitions in continuums of care and eventual discharge from services.[12]

The process is not strictly linear and is dynamic, which allows OT practitioners, along with the clients, to reflect and change plans as needed.[12] The OT practitioner and client collaborate to identify which occupation, such as ADLs and IADLs, the client wants or needs to participate in to optimize health and wellness. The need to learn new methods, use assistive devices to perform daily tasks, or modify the environment may be temporary or permanent, depending on the particular dysfunction, the environment, the prognosis for recovery, and a multitude of other factors.

DEFINITIONS OF ACTIVITIES OF DAILY LIVING AND INSTRUMENTAL ACTIVITIES OF DAILY LIVING

Daily living activities can be separated into two areas: activities of daily living (ADLs) (also called personal activities of daily living [PADLs] and basic activities of daily living [BADLs]) and instrumental activities of daily living (IADLs). ADLs require basic skills and focus on activities involved in taking care of one's own body. ADLs include self-care tasks such as bathing and showering, toileting and toilet hygiene, dressing, eating and swallowing, feeding, functional mobility (e.g., transfers and bed mobility), personal hygiene and grooming, and sexual activity.[12]

IADLs require a more advanced level of skills in all performance areas and includes activities performed in the home or community.[12] IADLs generally require use of executive functions,[51] social skills, and more complex environmental interactions than ADLs. IADL tasks include care of others and of pets and animals, childrearing, communication management, community mobility (e.g., driving and use of public transportation), and financial management; Anna, the client in our case study, has reported most of these as areas to be addressed. Other IADLs include home establishment and management, a category that includes housecleaning and meal preparation and cleanup, which are two IADLs that Anna was responsible for in her home. Religious and spiritual expression occupations (e.g., Anna's ability to lead and participate in her Bible study), and safety and emergency maintenance (e.g., Anna's ability to appropriately notify authorities in case of emergencies), and shopping are other important IADLs (Box 10.1).

BOX 10.1 OTPF-4 Categories for ADLs and IADLs

Activities of Daily Living (ADLs)
- Bathing and showering
- Toileting and toilet hygiene
- Dressing
- Eating and swallowing
- Feeding
- Functional mobility
- Personal hygiene and grooming
- Sexual activity

Instrumental Activities of Daily Living (IADLs)
- Care of others (including choosing and supervising caregivers)
- Care of pets and animals
- Childrearing
- Communication management
- Driving and community mobility
- Financial management
- Home establishment and management
- Meal preparation and cleanup
- Religious and spiritual activities and expression
- Safety and emergency maintenance
- Shopping

For a more examples, refer to the OTPF-4.

CONSIDERATIONS IN ADL AND IADL OCCUPATIONAL ANALYSIS AND TRAINING

The overall goal of any ADL and IADL training program is for the client and family to learn to adapt to life changes or situations and to participate as fully as possible in occupations that are meaningful to them. The following sections present important areas the occupational therapist must consider when analyzing ADLs and IADLs. Each area is defined in relation to an ADL or IADL evaluation and intervention plan.

Definition of "Client"

According to the OTPF-4, the term clients refers to persons, groups, and populations who receive occupational therapy services.[12] "Persons" include the actual person receiving services (e.g., Anna) and those involved in the client's care (e.g., Anna's husband and immediate family). "Groups" refers to collectives of individuals (e.g., Anna's church community) who may receive general consultation or referral by an occupational therapist on accessibility. "Populations" refers to larger collectives of people who live in similar locales, such as cities or states, or who share similar concerns; for example, refugees, survivors of particular natural or manmade disasters, or people with paraplegia who live in the United States, such as Anna. Most of the intervention strategies in this chapter relate to providing such intervention to persons or individuals as clients (e.g., Anna), although it is acknowledged that occupational therapists also provide services to groups and populations in the areas of ADLs and IADLs.

Client Factors

Client factors are specific abilities, characteristics, or beliefs that reside within the client to influence performance in occupations.[12]

This aspect of occupational therapy's domain includes (1) values, beliefs, and spirituality; (2) body functions; and (3) body structures.[12] Numerous questions can be investigated to different ends in the category of values, beliefs, and spirituality. Using Anna's case as an example: does her belief in her potential to improve or her ideas about her purpose in life influence her performance? OT practitioners' comfort level with the topic and self-reflection in the area may help them be more client-centered and may enhance their therapeutic use of self with a client such as Anna.[117] Other general categories include body functions and structures (Box 10.2). Does Anna have the strength, range of motion (ROM), coordination, sensation, balance, and cognitive functions to participate in occupations? How is Anna coping emotionally?

Client factors can be assessed to determine the potential for remediation or the possible need for adaptive equipment or other modifications. In Anna's case, it would be important to know whether the spinal cord injury (SCI) is complete and whether

she has potential for muscle return to determine an appropriate approach to treatment. Cardiovascular system functioning is another area of pertinence. Is Anna's blood pressure stable enough for her to perform ADLs, or does she have orthostatic hypotension? Anna's cognitive functions (e.g., memory, attention, and problem solving) are also important to assess in relation to ADLs and IADLs. Performance of ADLs and IADLs are occupations in which clients are directly confronted with what they can and cannot do as they had done previously; therefore, it is important to be alert to emotional functioning. The occupational therapist questions, "Is Anna requiring cues to perform her weight shifts and skin checks because she has a memory deficit? Or is she having difficulty learning new techniques and strategies because of issues surrounding coping with the disability?" Specific assessments to identify and measure client factors contribute information that influences ADL and IADL performance.

Sleep and Rest

Adequate sleep and rest are essential to optimal functioning in occupations for all people but particularly for clients in the hospital setting or those who are medically or otherwise compromised (see Chapter 13). Individuals who are hospitalized are particularly at risk of poor sleep, which can affect how a client may function while in a hospital. As cited in Young et al.,[129] research has shown that approximately 50% of individuals admitted to general medical units complain of sleep disruption.[44,71] In a later study, Young et al. found that 50% to 70% of people with chronic pain complained of poor sleep, which suggested poorer pain tolerance.[129] A prospective study on sleep-related breathing disorder (SRBD) and rehabilitation outcomes of stroke patients showed poorer functional recovery rates during a hospital rehabilitation stay.[30] Research has shown that electronic alerting sounds, staff conversations, and voice paging can be particularly disruptive to sleep while a client is in the hospital.[24] Researchers posit that sleep disturbance may be a modifiable predictor of rehabilitation outcomes and suggest that improving sleep/wake patterns during rehabilitation may result in better functional recovery among older adults.[4] Education in good sleep hygiene, optimal sleep/wake patterns, and advocacy for optimal sleep environments in hospital settings can go far to help clients such as Anna, who are treated by occupational therapists in that setting. An occupational therapist working with Anna can expect better outcomes from interventions for ADLs and IADLs if Anna gets adequate sleep and rest.

Performance Skills

The OTPF-4 describes performance skills as "goal-directed actions and consist of motor skills, process skills, and social interaction skills."[12] Whereas client factors reside within a person, performance skills are observable and demonstrable. Examples of motor skills may be Anna's ability to maintain balance while performing the ADL of transferring to a low, soft surface or her ability to bend down and reach for a pot from a low cupboard when preparing to cook. A client who has difficulty sequencing the steps involved in taking a shower or cooking an egg may demonstrate difficulty with a process skill. Examples of social interaction skills may include initiating conversations in

---

BOX 10.2 Client Factors

Examples of Values, Beliefs, and Spirituality

Values: Honesty, fairness, inclusion, and commitment

Beliefs (thoughts held as true): "Practice makes perfect"; trials are punishment for previous wrongs

Spirituality: Purpose and meaning of life

Examples of Body Functions

- *Specific mental functions (affective, cognitive, perceptual):* Emotional regulation, anxiety, executive functions (e.g., organization and time management), attention, memory, and discrimination of sensation, awareness of own identity
- *Global mental functions:* Alertness, orientation to person, temperament/personality, energy, and quality of sleep
- *Sensory functions:* Vision, hearing, vestibular (perception of body position and movement), taste, smell, proprioception, touch, pain, temperature, pressure
- *Neuromusculoskeletal and movement-related functions:* Joint mobility and stability, muscle strength/tone/endurance, reflexes, involuntary/voluntary control (e.g., coordination, fine motor control, and eye movement), gait patterns
- *Cardiovascular, hematological, immunological, and respiratory functions:* Blood pressure, heart rate, respiratory rate/rhythm/depth, physical endurance, stamina, aerobic capacity*
- *Voice and speech functions:* Fluency of speech, rate of speech, alternative vocalization functions*
- *Digestive, metabolic, and endocrine functions:* Effect on bowel movements, continence, hormonal imbalance*
- *Genitourinary and reproductive functions:* Continence, ability to have intercourse or reproduce*
- *Skin and related structure functions (hair and nail function):* Wound healing, protection of the skin, nail care, and awareness of abnormalities

Body Structures*

- Includes structures of the nervous system, eyes, ears, voice/speech/swallow structures, cardiovascular, immunological, endocrine, respiratory, digestive, genitourinary, reproductive, movement structures

  For a more detailed list, refer to the OTPF-4.

---

* OT practitioners must be knowledgeable about these functions and structures as they relate to occupations, which include ADLs and IADLs, the focus of this chapter.

a support group or allowing a friend to finish asking a question before interrupting with a response.

Performance Patterns

Habits, routines, roles, and rituals are all performance patterns according to the OTPF-4.[12] All can be helpful or detrimental to occupational performance. The OTPF-4 describes habits as "specific, automatic behaviors."[12] An example of an ADL habit may be automatically placing a napkin on one's lap before starting to eat or placing the right leg into pant legs first, then the left leg.

Routines are "established sequences of occupations or activities that provide a structure for daily life."[12] An example this may be Anna's routine of waking up at the same time every day and completing toileting, showering, dressing, hygiene and grooming, and eating breakfast in the same sequence. With changes in medical or functional status, some clients must adjust their established routines. In the case of Anna, her ADL routine may have to be drastically altered to accommodate additional ADL tasks that she previously never had to perform, such as skin checks and weight shifts because her diagnosis of paraplegia places her at high risk for pressure ulcers.[46] Anna's IADL routine may have been to help her daughter get ready for the day by completing such activities as changing her diaper, getting her dressed and cleaned, making her breakfast, packing her lunch, and driving her to daycare.

Roles are sets of behaviors that are expected by society, shaped by culture and context with further refinement by a client.[12] Examples of roles might include the husband of a wife with severe rheumatoid arthritis or a college student who lives independently in an apartment with a roommate. Important roles for Anna are those of wife, mother, daughter, worker, and Bible study leader.

Rituals are "symbolic actions with spiritual, cultural, or social meaning" than can contribute to a client's identity and reinforce values and beliefs.[12] Examples of rituals that are in the realm of ADLs and IADLs include praying or saying grace before every meal or celebrating particular holidays with foods served only on that date that have special cultural meanings.

Understanding performance patterns described previously allows the OT practitioner to identify performance deficits, determine priorities in goal setting, and help the client reestablish continuity in daily living. For example, with her new functional status, Anna may not be able to perform all the previous morning IADL routines with her daughter. She may have to establish new routines with her daughter and learn to perform those activities differently. At least in the early stages of her recovery, others may have to assume occupations previously completed by Anna. She may need to redefine her own expectations to perform activities that she currently sees as her role in the family, an important undertaking for an occupational therapist to help facilitate.

Context: Environmental and Personal Factors

The OTPF-4 described *context* as a broad construct and is explained as *environmental factors* and *personal factors* that can influence participation in occupations. The terms *context* and *environment* are not used interchangeably in the OTPF-4.[12]

Environmental factors include the physical, social, and attitudinal backdrop to how and where people live. The natural and human-made environments and the objects in them, such as products and technology, social relationships, attitudes and systems, services, and policies available are included. A few of the human-made external environments for Anna are her home and its contents, her place of work, and her church. Larger natural context can include the climate in which Anna lives, road conditions, and natural disasters that may occur in her area. Also included are access and ability to use technology and the internet and sensory environments such as lighting.

The social environment includes people or even animals in a person's setting. Anna's social surroundings includes her spouse, her mother, her child, her Bible study group, neighbors, colleagues, and community members. Attitudes, which are observable customs, practices, and beliefs held by those around people are also included as environmental factors. Services, systems, and policies are other important environmental factors that can affect people. For Anna, this may include health benefits, transportation access, policies set at immediate, local, regional, and national levels.

Personal factors are the features of a person that make them unique and include demographic information and things such as cultural identification, social backgrounds, type of upbringing, socioeconomic status, and lifestyle. Included in personal factors are temperament and coping abilities. The ADL and IADL tasks and routines may differ based on any one of many of these factors. For example, a young adult woman may consider it important to regain the ability to shave her armpits if she is from a part of the world where this is the norm, whereas she may not care to do this if she were from a different part of the world.

Given Anna's circumstances regarding her context, questions abound regarding environmental and personal factors. Here are a few questions:

Environmental:
- Is her home accessible? Can Anna's family home be modified?
- Will Anna be alone at home at times?
- What is the terrain and typical weather patterns in her area?
- How does her community view people with disabilities? Will she continue to maintain her current social network of friends, or will she also need to develop others?
- Who will be her primary caregiver when she goes home, her mother or her husband? How long will Anna's mother live with her family?
- Personal:
- If her home needs modifications, can the family afford to make changes?
- Does Anna have the ability to emotionally manage all the life changes?

The client's answers to these questions strongly influence treatment priorities.

Culture and Cultural Humility

Culture is a way of living that includes what people consider important, beliefs, how people talk and communicate, behavioral norms that influence how a group of people operate, that is passed on from generation to generation and to others.[21] Culture is not inborn but is learned.[21] Culture is explained as a "kaleidoscope" and as encompassing a variety of elements such as language, values, and traditions.[50] Many think that culture is only about race and ethnicity, but it is a much broader concept and includes many other diversity factors such as gender identity, class, sexual orientation, abilities, whether one is a civilian or in the military, or even a healthcare provider, to name a few.[3]

Cultural humility is an idea and process considered a lifelong endeavor that acknowledges power differences between recipients and receivers of healthcare, acknowledges that people have biases, and emphasizes self-reflection of the healthcare provider.[3] An attitude of cultural humility for the occupational therapy practitioner is an important consideration with ADLs and IADLs as people vary vastly in terms of whether, when, how, with whom these occupations are performed. It is important that therapists acknowledge they have a worldview, that they have biases and power in the therapist-client relationships. For example, some people may consider that bathing daily is an imperative, whereas others may not. An OT practitioner with an agenda to have someone bathe daily when someone was not raised to think it necessary will not find success or respect. One culture may view bathing as a private event, whereas another may consider it a communal event. Another idea that may differ significantly based on culture is the construct of independence.

The AOTA position paper on the construct of independence supports the view that independence is "defined by the individual's culture, values, support systems, and ability to direct his or her life."[55] A thorough evaluation allows the OT practitioner to understand what activities are critical to each client; this aids the occupational therapist in reestablishing the client's sense of directing his or her own life. An example of differing cultural values frequently occurs when an occupational therapist raised in a more Westernized culture considers it important to foster independence in ADLs and IADLs, but a client from a different cultural view may not see independence in ADL tasks as highly valued. The OT practitioner may unfairly label the client as unmotivated. For the individual whose culture does not value ADLs or IADLs independence, the occupational therapist may focus primarily on teaching the client and family to adapt. The focus would be on family training and identifying the activities of highest value to the client and family.

With relation to power, occupational therapists work within what can be perceived to be complicated, hierarchical systems. Whereas some clients' cultures value self-determination, other clients' may place high value in the words and actions of their healthcare providers because providers occupy a position of knowledge and authority. This may lead to misunderstandings at best or to people receiving unnecessary and inappropriate interventions at worst. Whatever the scenario, it is important for OT practitioners to recognize where they fit in existing power structures and to hold themselves and their colleagues accountable to optimize care.

Occupational Justice

The term *occupational justice* was coined by Townsend in 2003 (OTPF-2, p. 630)[8] and describes the occupational therapist profession's concerns with the ability of all people, to be given the opportunity to engage in occupations, including the ADLs and IADLs that are important to them.[12] Bailliard et al. argue that occupational therapy is a justice-oriented profession and that practitioners in all settings can enact its principles.[17] They

espouse the "centrality of justice to everyday occupational therapy, and to encourage therapists to further infuse justice-related practices into therapy" (p. 45).[17] Many times, occupational therapists are the first to recognize the disparity in abilities to meet occupational needs because of social, economic, and other factors. Occupational therapists can assist in supporting social policies, actions, and laws that allow all people to engage in occupations that are important to them.[12]

Occupational therapists can incorporate occupational justice at the micro-, meso-, and macro-levels.[17] An example of applying this principle of occupational justice at the micro-level can be listening and validating client concerns. Another example at the micro-level is for occupational therapists to use interpreters when there are language barriers and to have written materials translated into appropriate languages when needed. A common situation for an occupational therapist is a client who needs a piece of adaptive equipment, such as a transfer bath bench, that is neither covered by insurance nor within the client's ability to purchase. At the meso-level, resourceful occupational therapists can help bridge this disparity and thus help all clients participate in ADLs and IADLs that are important to them by establishing or making contacts with equipment donor closets. At the macro-level, occupational therapists can advocate and be involved at population levels to ensure that policies regarding durable medical equipment (DME) are favorable to all people.

Public health crises, like the COVID-19 pandemic, can change lives at all levels of occupational functioning and thus raise many examples related to occupational justice. Mandated use of masks, recommendations for appropriate hygiene such as hand-washing, and changes in how one may enter business establishments are just a few examples of adjustments required. Occupational therapists may be involved at the micro-, meso-, and macro-levels for the self-care task of wearing a mask. At the micro-level, the occupational therapist may need to ensure that a client can use the mask appropriately based on their function: Does the client have access to an appropriate mask and information about current protocols? Can the client don and doff the mask? Can the client tolerate the mask? Is a different design of mask required? At the meso-level, occupational therapists may be involved in ensuring that groups of clients have access to appropriate masks and information in appropriate languages using communication channels that are effective. At the macro-level, occupational therapists may advocate in the policy realm to ensure that financial resources are available and initiatives support people having access to masks.

Finances

Financial resources available for potential expenses, such as assistant care, special equipment, and home modifications, are another important consideration for performance of ADLs and IADLs. For example, consider a client who is a new full-time wheelchair user and who can no longer stand to take showers, thus requiring significant assistance from a caregiver to perform the task. If the client has unlimited financial resources; owns his or her home; has an able-bodied, committed caregiver; wants to take showers daily; and is eager to fully remodel the home for accessibility, an occupational therapist experienced in home modifications may recommend a fully remodeled bathroom by a licensed contractor. Anna has fewer financial resources, but she has reliable caregivers, and she and her husband own their home. She also wants to shower regularly. In Anna's case, an occupational therapist may make recommendations for less costly modifications, such as removing the sliding glass door from the bathtub/shower and replacing it with a shower curtain, and obtaining a bath bench and other equipment.

EVALUATION OF ADLS AND IADLS

According to the OTPF-4, occupational therapy's overarching goal for both the domain and the process is "achieving health, well-being, and participation in life through engagement in occupation."[12] A comprehensive evaluation of occupational performance involves collaborating with the client to determine what the client wants and needs to do to support health and participation.[12] In the OTPF-4, occupations include ADLs, IADLs, health management, rest and sleep, education, work, play, leisure, and social participation. A comprehensive evaluation includes a thorough occupational profile and an analysis of occupational performance, including assessing client factors, performance skills, performance patterns, and contexts.[12]

As outlined by the OTPF-4, the process of delivering OT services to a client occurs by means of evaluation, intervention, and targeted outcomes. The process may seem linear but is actually dynamic, allowing the OT practitioner to continually assess the progress toward reaching goals.[12]

In a client-centered approach, the therapist collaborates with the client or the family/caregivers to understand what is "important and meaningful" to the client.[12] This approach centers the occupational therapy process on the client's priorities and fosters active participation toward the outcome. Evaluation consists of initially creating an occupational profile and analyzing occupational performance. An occupational profile is central to the client-centered approach because it describes the client's occupational history, patterns of daily living, interests, values, and needs.[12]

General Procedure

The focus of the occupational therapy evaluation is to discover what occupations are important for the client, to determine what a client can do, and to identify barriers, problems, and supports that affect the client's participation in those occupations.[12] The type of client information and data collected differs, based on the client's needs, the practice setting, and the frame of reference or practice models of the occupational therapist.[12] This textbook focuses on occupational therapists who treat adults with physical dysfunction; therefore, the general procedure described highlights areas that may be targeted in assessing that group.

The initial interview may serve as a screening device to help determine the need for further assessment or treatment. The therapist makes a determination of further need for assessment and occupational therapy intervention based on knowledge of the client, the dysfunction, and previous assessments. Not all clients who receive an OT referral will need intervention. However, the interview alone can lead to inaccurate assumptions about actual performance. Clients may overestimate or underestimate their abilities, may not understand the timelines for which they are being asked, or may simply misinterpret interview questions. For example, a client may report that they are independent with lower body dressing and forget to report that their spouse assists them with donning their socks every morning because of chronic low back pain. To have a more complete picture of a client's functional status and to determine need for services, observation of actual performance of ADLs is invaluable.

Clinical assessment of relevant client factors, such as ROM, strength, sensation, and cognition, may occur before the actual observations of ADLs or IADLs. In any physical disabilities settings, particularly in the hospital setting, or after any new surgery or procedure, it is essential that occupational therapists educate themselves about any medical precautions or contraindications by reading the medical chart or consulting with the medical staff. For example, the physician may still have bed-rest orders in place, a neck brace may be required before any out-of-bed activities, an extremity may have non–weight-bearing precautions, active range of motion to a joint may not be allowed, or a person may not be allowed to shower.

When the occupational therapist first met Anna shortly after her admission, she may have been seen in the intensive care unit, or she may have been on bed rest and awaiting surgery or some type of stabilization of her spine. The occupational therapist at that point may have interviewed Anna, gotten some background and her occupational history, and assessed her upper body ROM and also sensation. The occupational therapist would have gleaned information about Anna's cognition and emotional status based on those brief assessments: Is she alert, oriented (person, place, time)? Can she follow directions? Can she recall what she had for breakfast that morning? Does she initiate asking for help?

Ideally, the occupational therapist assesses the performance of activities in the environment and context in which they usually take place.[14] For example, a dressing assessment could be arranged early in the morning in the treatment facility, when the client is dressed by nursing personnel, or in the client's home. A self-feeding assessment should occur at regular meal hours. If this timing is not possible, the assessment may be conducted during regular treatment sessions in the occupational therapy clinic under simulated conditions. Requiring the client to perform routine self-maintenance tasks at irregular times in an artificial environment may contribute to a lack of carryover, especially for clients who have difficulty generalizing learning. With clients who have cognitive impairments, it is important to consider that facilitating simulated tasks in an artificial environment can also cause confusion and may not completely reflect a client's actual ability to complete the original, unsimulated task.

The therapist should initially select relatively simple and safe tasks from the ADL and IADL checklist/assessment form and then progress to more difficult and complex items. For example, with Anna, transfer training would likely start with transfers from her wheelchair to her bed and then progress to commode transfers, which are more difficult. Tasks that would be unsafe or that obviously cannot be performed should be omitted and the appropriate notation made in the occupational therapist's written assessment.

During the performance analysis, the therapist should observe the methods the client uses or attempts to use to accomplish the task and try to determine the causes of performance problems.

Common causes include weakness, spasticity, involuntary motion, perceptual deficits, cognitive deficits, and low endurance. If problems and their causes can be identified, the therapist has a good foundation for establishing training objectives, priorities, methods, and the need for assistive devices.

Other important aspects of this analysis that should not be overlooked are the client's need for privacy and dignity in the performance of personal ADLs and the occupational therapist's questions about them. The client's feelings and cultural attitudes about having one's body viewed, discussed, and touched should be respected. With safety in mind, privacy should be maintained for performance of basic ADLs such as toileting, grooming, bathing, and dressing tasks. For example, even if the occupational therapist needs to be an arm's length away (or closer) for safety while assessing a private ADL, dignity and a semblance of "privacy" could be provided by the therapist turning his or her gaze away, by closing the curtains, by making sure nobody else can see or hear the discussion, or by placing a small towel in a strategic location. Attempts by the therapist to honor a client's privacy as best able are usually highly appreciated and can go far to build trust in the development of the therapeutic relationship.

Even if the therapeutic relationship between the primary occupational therapist and client may be good, situations may arise in which it may be necessary to change therapists when more private ADLs are practiced. For example, Anna may be fine with working with a male occupational therapist during cooking tasks but may prefer a female occupational therapist when performing showering and dressing tasks or when questions arise about sexual function or fertility. Situations such as this are important to note because as the therapist interacts with the client during the performance of daily living tasks, they may elicit some of the client's attitudes and feelings about particular tasks, priorities in training, dependence and independence, and cultural, family, and personal values and customs regarding performance of ADLs.

Performance of ADLs and IADLs

An occupational performance analysis of ADLs and IADLs may include using a checklist as a guide for questioning and selecting specific activities to perform, as identified during the interview for the occupational profile. For example, in Anna's case the occupational therapist may select lower extremity dressing and basic transfers as two key activities to have Anna perform. The occupational therapist can then determine strategies to promote independence and provide caregiver instruction regarding how to provide Anna with the appropriate level of assistance.

Many types of ADL and IADL checklists and standardized tests are available. They cover similar categories and performance tasks. The use of a standardized test ensures a more objective assessment and provides a standard means of measurement. A standardized assessment tool can be used at a later time for reevaluation, and some assessments allow for comparison to a norm group. Both Asher[15] and Letts et al.[62] have developed resources on assessments that can be used for selecting appropriate tools for evaluation. The occupational therapist should review the literature periodically to learn about new assessments developed by occupational therapists and about those that have

been developed as interdisciplinary assessments. One example is the internationally recognized Assessment of Motor and Process Skills (AMPS), an OT-focused assessment of the quality of a person's ADL performance.[38–41,72] Another interdisciplinary assessment is the Functional Independence Measure (FIM).[38,106]

Recording the Results of the ADL Assessment

During the interview and performance analysis, the therapist makes appropriate notations on the checklists. If a standardized assessment is used, the standard terminology identified for that assessment is used to describe or measure performance. Nonstandardized tests may include separate checklists for self-care, home management, mobility, and home environment assessments. When describing levels of independence, occupational therapists often use terms such as *maximum, moderate*, and *minimal assistance*. These quantitative terms have little meaning to healthcare professionals unless they are clearly defined. It also should be specified whether the level of independence refers to a single activity, a category of activities (e.g., dressing), or all ADLs. The following general categories and their definitions are suggested.

1. **Independent**. Client can independently perform the activity without cueing, supervision, or assistance, with or without assistive devices, at normal or near normal speeds. Task is completed safely. If the client requires assistive devices or performs the activity at a slower than customary speed, the term *modified independence* may be used in some settings.
2. **Supervised**. Client requires general supervision (not hands on) and may require a verbal cue for safety. The occupational therapist feels comfortable being greater than an arm's length away at all times.
3. **Standby assistance (SBA)/contact guard assistance (CGA)**. Client requires caregiver or someone to provide hands-on guarding to perform a task safely. NOTE: Occupational therapists may tend to use the term standby assistance, whereas other disciplines may use contact guard assistance.
4. **Minimal assistance**. Client requires 25% physical or verbal assistance of one person to complete a task safely. (Client performs 75% or more of the task.)
5. **Moderate assistance**. Client requires 50% physical or verbal assistance of one person to complete a task safely. (Client performs 50% to 74% of the task.)
6. **Maximal assistance**. Client requires physical or verbal assistance for 51% to 75% of an activity by one person. (Client performs 25% to 49% of the task.) The helper is doing more than half the work or task, while client is performing less than half.
7. **Dependent**. Client requires more than 75% physical or verbal assistance. Client does less than 25% of the task. For example, they can only perform very few steps.

These definitions are broad and general, and they can be modified to suit the approach of the particular treatment setting.

As stated previously, the AOTA published a position paper on a definition of *independence* that differs from the relatively narrow definition noted earlier. Hinojosa stated, "Independence is a self-directed state of being characterized by an individual's ability to participate in necessary and preferred occupations in a satisfying manner, *irrespective of the amount or kind of external assistance desired or required."[55]* This means that an individual's independence is not related to whether an individual performs the activity or not or in a modified fashion or with assistance.

Information from the ADL assessment is summarized succinctly for inclusion in the client's permanent record so that other professionals involved in the care of the client can refer to it. Fig. 10.1 presents two forms related to the sample case

---

OCCUPATIONAL THERAPY DEPARTMENT
Activities of Daily Living Evaluation/Progress Form

Name: Mrs. Hayes   Age: 72   Onset Date: 2/3   Today's Date: 4/3

Medical Diagnosis: Lt. CVA   Treatment Diagnosis: dysphagia, mild right hemiparesis; ↓'d independence ADL/IADL

Past Medical History: Unremarkable per pt. report and chart

Precautions: Soft foods, thick liquids

Mode of Ambulation: Mod A 20' with FWW, primarily uses w/c   Hand Dominance: Right

Social / Home environment: Married 45 years, was primary caregiver to husband, lives in one-story house which they own; four adult children live out of area; has 24 hour caregivers to assist in home since CVA

Occupational Profile/Previous Level of Function: Prior to the CVA, pt. was I with ADL, IADL, volunteering at thrift store, going for walks with friends, paying bills, driving and caring for husband who has ↓'d vision and diabetes but who is otherwise ambulatory and cognitively intact. Pt. was a homemaker while she raised her four children and highly values her independence, community involvement and volunteering. Pt. enjoyed spending time with friends, potted gardening and entertaining her family including many grandchildren when they visit from out of town. Her goals are to be as independent as possible in her ADL/IADL, to be able to help her husband and to be able to enjoy previous leisure activities.

Grading key:	Abbreviations key:		Symbol key:
I = Independent S = Supervised SBA = Standby assistance Min A = Minimal assistance Mod A = Moderate assistance Max A = Maximum assistance D = Dependent N/A = Not applicable N/T = Not tested	ADL = activity of daily living AROM = active range of motion avg. = average bilat. = bilateral c/o = complains of CVA = cerebrovascular accident Executive Function Performance Test = EFPT FWW = front-wheeled walker HTN = hypertension lbs. = pounds LE = lower extremity min. = minutes DTL = dysphagia thickened liquids	PROM = passive range of motion Pt. = patient PT = physical therapist ther ex = therapeutic exercise UE = upper extremity w/c = wheelchair WFL = within functional limits WNL = within normal limits	↓ decrease ↑ increase ↔ to and from ' feet " inch 2° secondary to (due to)

Activities of Daily Living
Functional Mobility: Transfers/Ambulation

Date	4/3/11	5/3		Comments
Tub or shower transfer	Min A	S		Cues for safety, balance, set-up required of bath bench
Toilet transfer	S	I		
Wheelchair transfer	S	I		
Bed and chair transfer	S	I		
Car transfer	N/T	S		
Wheelchair management	SBA	I		Difficulty managing armrest and footrest.
Wheelchair mobility	I (indoor, flat surface)	I (outdoor, smooth surfaces, slight incline)		
Functional ambulation	Mod A 20' per PT report	Min A 20' per PT report		FWW 20'

A

Fig. 10.1 (A) ADL evaluation form.

Continued

Self feeding/Eating (swallowing)

Date	4/3/11	5/3		Comments
Butter bread	N/T	I		
Cut meat	Min A	I		Rocker knife
Eat with fork	I	I		
Eat with spoon	I	I		
Eat with chopsticks	N/T	N/A		
Drink with straw	N/T	I		Nectar DTL
Drink from cup (cold)	I	I		
Drink from mug (hot)	N/T	I		
Pour from pitcher	N/T	I		
Diet:				Soft Diet/Nectar DTL
Managing fluids	Min A	I		Written instructions provided
Managing foods	Min A	I		Written instructions provided
Follow through with swallow techniques	Dep	S		Poor follow-through of techniques

Undress

Date	4/3/11	5/3		Comments
Underwear	Mod A	I		Seated
Slip/Undershirt/Bra	Min A	I		Seated
Dress	N/A	N/A		Pt. reports, "I only wear pants."
Skirt	N/A	N/A		
Blouse/Shirt	N/T	I		Seated, slowed pace with buttons
Slacks/Jeans	Mod A	I		Seated
Panty hose/Tights	N/A	N/A		
Housecoat/Robe	N/T	I		
Jacket/Coat	I	I		
Belt/Suspenders	N/A	N/A		
Hat	N/A	N/A		
Sweater (cardigan)	N/T	I		
Sweater (pullover)	N/T	I		
Mittens/Gloves	N/A	N/A		
Glasses	I	I		
AFO/Prosthesis	N/A	N/A		
Shoes	Min A	I		Seated, slip-on, prefers Velcro to laces
Socks	Min A	I		Seated
Boots	N/A	N/A		

Fig. 10.1A cont'd

Dress

Date	4/3/11	5/3		Comments
Underwear	Mod A	I		
Slip/Undershirt/Bra	Min A	I		
Dress	N/A	N/A		
Skirt	N/A	N/A		
Blouse/Shirt	N/T	I		
Slacks/Jeans	Min A	I		Seated, stand to hike pants
Panty hose/Tights	N/A	N/A		
Housecoat/Robe	N/T	I		
Jacket/Coat	I	I		
Belt/Suspenders	N/A	N/A		
Hat	N/A	N/A		
Sweater (Cardigan)	N/T	I		
Sweater (Pullover)	N/T	I		
Mittens/Gloves	N/A	N/A		
Glasses	I	I		
AFO/Prosthesis	N/A	N/A		
Shoes	Min A	I		Seated, slip-on, prefers Velcro to laces
Socks	Min A	I		Seated
Boots	N/A	N/A		

Clothing Fasteners

Date	4/3/11	5/3		Comments
Button	Min A	I		Slowed pace with ½" diameter buttons
Snap	Min A	I		
Zipper	Min A	I		Uses large (1" x ¼") zipper pull on jacket
Hook and eye	N/T	I		Slowed pace (bra)
Untie shoes	Mod A	I		Pt. currently prefers Velcro or slip-on shoes
Velcro	Mod A	I		Seated: shoes

Fig. 10.1A cont'd

Continued

Hygiene and Grooming/Bathing/Toileting

Date	4/3/11	5/3		Comments
Blow/Wipe nose	I	I		
Wash face and hands	I	I		Seated
Showering/Bathing general status	Mod A	S (set-up only)		Seated on bath bench
Wash upper body	Min A	I		
Wash lower body	Mod A	I		Long-handled sponge, handheld shower hose
Shampoo hair	Min A	I		Seated
Brush teeth	I (seated)	I (standing)		Seated
Brush dentures	N/A	N/A		
Brush/comb hair	I	I (standing)		Seated
Curl hair	N/A	N/A		
Shave	N/A	N/A		
Apply makeup	N/T	I (seated)		Lipstick only
Clean fingernails	N/T	I		
Trim nails	N/T	SBA		Recommended nail file
Apply deodorant	N/A	N/A		
Initiate need to perform toileting task, bowel/bladder mgmt.	I	I		
Use toilet paper	I	I		
Use feminine hygiene products	N/A	N/A		
Personal Device Care (e.g., glasses, hearing aids, splints, etc.)	I	I		Glasses

Sexual Activity

Date	4/3/11	5/3		Comments
Able to have needs met	Dep	I		4/3 Pt. reports she and her husband have not had intercourse for 5 years due to her husband's erectile dysfunction. Couple sleeps in the same bed but husband is afraid to cuddle because he is afraid he will "hurt" her. 5/3 Couple instructed that cuddling will not injure pt.

Fig. 10.1A cont'd

IADL
Health Management and Maintenance

Date	4/3/11	5/3		Comments
Identify proper medication	Min A	S		Reading glasses required.
Open medicine bottle	Min A	S		Recommended non-child-proof and use of Dycem
Manipulate pills	SBA	SBA		Needs pill-organizer (at least 1" large pill holders)
Manage syringe	N/T	Min A		For husband's meds
Draw medication	N/T	Min A		For husband's meds
Follow medication routines	N/T	S		
Follow home exercise program/therapy program	Min A	S		Rt. UE home exercise program and with swallowing techniques
Arrange medical appointments	Dep	Min A		Uses large wall calendar

Communication Management

Date	4/3/11	5/3		Comments
Verbal	S	S		Dysarthria with slowed/slurred but understandable speech. Cues needed to slow down.
Initiate communication verbal or nonverbal	I	I		
Read	I	I		
Hold book	S (paperback)	I (book holder)		Reports fatigue with holding book.
Turn page	S	I		
Write	Mod A	SBA (1/4" letters); fair legibility		Poor legibility (1/2" letters)
Type/Use keyboard	N/A	N/A		Pt. "doesn't like" computers
Handle mail	N/T	S		
Use of call light	N/A	N/A		
Use home telephone	Mod A	I		
Use cell phone	N/T	S (answer phone only)		Recommended cell phone with larger buttons. Prior to CVA, pt. did not use often
Retrieve messages	N/A	N/A		
Use personal digital assistant	N/A	N/A		Pt. reports she does not like electronic gadgets though her children want her to use them to communicate.

Fig. 10.1A cont'd

Continued

Care of Others

Date	4/3/11	5/3		Comments
Care of pets	N/A	N/A		
Childrearing	N/A	N/A		
Caregiving for others:	Dep	Dep		Difficulty with assisting with husband's insulin due to poor coordination in hand

Financial Management

Date	4/3/11	5/3		Comments
Managing cash	Mod A	I		
Using checkbook	Mod A	S		
Paying bills	Mod A	S		
Other				

Religious Observance (To Participate in Chosen Belief Practices)

Date	4/3/11	5/3		Comments
Individually	I	I		To say "grace" before meals
Corporately	N/T	Dep		Pt. reports she goes to church twice a year during the holidays.

Safety and Emergency Maintenance

Date	4/3/11	5/3		Comments
Initiates getting help in emergency	S	I		
Recognizes safety hazards	S	I		
Awareness of deficits and limitations	S	I		Husband reports pt. doesn't always ask for help when she needs it (e.g., with transfers)

Fig. 10.1A cont'd

Rest and Sleep

Date	4/3/11	5/3		Comments Check here if there are no problems with sleep and rest.
# hours of sleep at night: # naps taken per day: Time in naps:	6 1 2 hours	7.5 1 45 min.		4/3 Pt. c/o discomfort in her bilat. LEs and waking at night with inability to fall asleep 2° "too much on my mind." Pt. reports difficulty with sleep prior to CVA. MD notified.
Wakes up rested to perform ADL/IADL	No	No, but "better" than before per pt.		5/3 Pt. following through with at least two sleep hygiene strategies a day per OT recommendations.
Emotions & energy level WFL in late afternoon (poor, fair, good) to perform occupations	Poor	Fair		"I have a hard time remembering things and concentrating." Recommended pt. see primary MD regarding sleep issues: Pt. agreed. 5/4 Overnight sleep study scheduled for 6/7.

Combined Performance Activities
Operate Objects in External Environment

Date	4/3/11	5/3		Comments
Light switches	I	I		w/c level
Doorbell	N/T	I		
Door locks/Handles	Dep	S (adapted key holder)		Difficulty turning key 2° hand weakness.
Faucets	I	I		Lever style
Shades/Curtains	N/T	S		
Open/Close window	N/T	Dep		Windows throughout house are difficult to open. Husband to call children to fix.
Hang up garment	N/T	N/A		

Community Mobility

Date	4/3/11	5/3		Comments
Driving	Dep	Dep		
Walking	Mod A	Min A 20'		5/3 Uses w/c in community
Bicycle	Dep	Dep		
Powered mobility	N/A	N/A		
Public transportation				
Bus	NT	NT		
Train or light rail, other	NT	NT		
Taxi cab	NT	NT		
Paratransit	NT	NT		

Fig. 10.1A cont'd

Continued

Summary of Evaluation Results (Client Factors)
Perceptual/Cognitive/Emotional Regulation

Date	4/3/11		5/3				Comments
Intact = IN Impaired = IM	IN	IM	IN	IM	IN	IM	☐ Check here if perceptual, cognitive status are grossly intact
Follows directions	√		√				
Orientation (person, place, time)	√		√				
Topographical orientation	√						
Memory		√	√		√		
Attention span		√			√		Min A to attend for 15 min during ADL eval.
Problem solving		√			√		4/3 Min A with cooking tasks 5/3 SBA with cooking tasks
Sequencing of task	√		√				
Visual spatial	√		√				
Left/right discrimination	√		√				
Motor planning	√		√				
Emotional regulation and coping		√			√		4/3 Min cues/encouragement required when pt. frustrated with fine motor tasks. 5/3 Only occasional cues for 45 min session

Functional Range of Motion

Date	4/3/11				5/3								Comments
Intact = IN Impaired = IM	L		R		L		R		L		R		☑ Check here if AROM or PROM is WNL for all functional tasks below (Circle AROM, PROM or both)
	IN	IM	IN	IM	IN	IM	IN	IM	IN	IM	IN	IM	
Comb Hair													
Feed Self													
Fasten Buttons													
Pull up back of pants													
Zip Zipper													
Tie shoes													
Reach shelf													
Put on socks													

Sensation

Date	4/3/11				5/3								Comments
Intact = IN Impaired = IM	L		R		L		R		L		R		☑ Check here if sensation is WNL for UE
	IN	IM	IN	IM	IN	IM	IN	IM	IN	IM	IN	IM	
Light Touch													
Pain (Location)													
Temperature													
Proprioception													
Stereognosis													
Other													

Fig. 10.1A cont'd

Vision (Sensory and Perceptual)

Date	4/3/11				5/3								Comments
Intact = IN Impaired = IM	L IN	L IM	R IN	R IM	L IN	L IM	R IN	R IM	L IN	L IM	R IN	R IM	☑ Check here if vision is grossly intact ☑ Needs corrective lenses
Visual fields													
Visual attention (e.g., "neglect")													
Visual acuity (near)													
Visual acuity (far)													
Visual tracking													

Strength: Indicate Muscle Grade as Appropriate

Date	4/3/11		5/3				Comments
Left = L or Right = R	L	R	L	R	L	R	☑ Check here if strength is grossly WFL for UE, head/neck
Head/Neck							
Shoulder flexion							
Shoulder extension							
Elbow flexion							
Elbow extension							
Supination							
Pronation							
Wrist extension	WNL	WFL	WNL	WNL			
Gross grasp	WNL	WNL	WNL	WNL			
Grip strength	35 lb	25 lb	37 lb	27 lb			Jamar Dynamometer avg. of 3 measurements
Muscle tone	WNL	WNL	WNL	WNL			

Coordination/Endurance

Date	4/3/11				5/3								Comments
Left = L or Right = R	L IN	L IM	R IN	R IM	L IN	L IM	R IN	R IM	L IN	L IM	R IN	R IM	☑ Check here if UE fine and gross motor ability are WFL
Fine motor	√			√	√			√					Difficulty with buttons, dialing phone.
Gross U.E.	√		√		√		√						
General endurance (good, fair, poor)	Fair (for eval)												Pt. c/o "I'm tired" at end of eval. Pt. reports endurance declines as day progresses.

Fig. 10.1A cont'd

Continued

Performance Skills
Functional Balance

Date		4/3/11	5/3		Comments
Sitting	Static	I (w/c)	I		
	Dynamic	Min A	I		Edge of bed
Standing	Static	Min A	I		5/3 While stabilizing with one UE on counter.
	Dynamic	Mod A	Min A		
Walking	Even surfaces	Mod A (20' per PT report)	Min A per PT report for 50'		
	Uneven surfaces	N/T	Mod A per PT for 20'		
Stoop		N/T	Min A		
Carry objects		N/T	I (w/c) Mod A walking		
Open/ Close door					
Reach for objects off floor		Max A	Min A		

Fig. 10.1A cont'd

Occupational Therapy Initial Assessment

Name: _____ DOB: _____ Onset Date: _____ Today's Date: _____

Medical Dx: _____ Treatment Dx: _____

Past Medical History: _____

Precautions: _____

Occupational profile/previous level of function: _____

Areas of occupation: _____

ADL Status	Date:	Date:	Comments	I-ADL Status	Date:	Date:	Comments
Eating/Swallowing				Care of others/Child rearing			
Self feeding				Care of pets			
Hygiene/Grooming				Communication management (e.g., writing, phone, etc)			
UE dressing				Community mobility			
LE dressing				Financial management			
Bowel/Bladder management and toilet hygiene				Health mgmt and maintenance			
Bed mobility				Laundry			
Functional AMB/ transporting objects				Light housekeeping			
Transfers				Meal prep. and clean-up			
Bathing/Showering				Religious observance			
Personal device care				Safety and emergency maintenance			
Sexual activity				Shopping			

Key:
Independent — I
Supervised — S
Stand by assist — SBA
Minimum assist — Min
Moderate assist — Mod
Maximum assist — Max

B

Fig. 10.1 cont'd (B) OT initial assessment.

Rest & Sleep:	Date:	Date:	Comments	Functional Cognition	Date:	Date:	Comments
Poor: Feels unrested after night's sleep, fatigue during day affecting ADL due to poor sleep. Poorly educated in good sleep hygiene techniques. Fair: Sleep is adequate to perform ADL/IADL during day but could use more productive sleep. Fair knowledge and follow-through of good sleep hygiene techniques. Good: Feels well-rested after a night's sleep, demonstrates good knowledge of good sleep hygiene techniques with good follow-through.				☐ Check here if cognition is WNL for ADL/IADL			
Education (formal and informal):				Attention			
Work Employment/Volunteer:				Short-term memory:			
Leisure participation:				Long term memory:			
Social participation (community, family, peers):				Problem solving:			
				Safety awareness:			

Client Factors	Date:	Date:	Comments		Date:	Date:	Comments
ROM RUE: LUE: Other:				Strength RUE: LUE: Other:			
Sensation RUE: LUE: Other:				Muscle Tone RUE: LUE: Other:			
Fine coordination RUE: LUE: Other:				Selective muscle movement and control RUE: LUE: Other:			
LE function:				Endurance			
Hearing				Vision			

Performance Skills	Date:	Date:	Comments	Functional Cognition	Date:	Date:	Comments
Balance Static: Sit: Stand:				Sensory/Perceptual skill (position in space, body awareness, midline, neglect etc)			
Dynamic: Sit: Stand:				Emotional regulation (behavior, coping, etc)			

Fig. 10.1B cont'd

Continued

Pt/Family goals:

OT short term goals:

OT long term goals:

Rehab Potential: ☐ Poor   ☐ Fair   ☐ Good   ☐ Excellent
OT Intervention Plan: _____
_____
_____

Frequency/Duration:
Patient/Family in agreement with plan of treatment and goals: ☐ yes   ☐ no

Therapist's signature:	Date:	Re-eval Date:	Re-eval Date:
Physician's signature:	Date		

Adapted from Smith, J. (2006). Documentation of occupational therapy services. In H.M. Pendleton and Schultz-Krohn (Eds),
Pedretti's occupational therapy: Practice skills for physical dysfunction (6th ed, p. 127). St. Louis: Mosby Elsevier.

American Occupational Therapy Association. (2008). Occupational therapy practice framework: Domain and process (2nd ed).
American Journal of Occupational Therapy Association, 62, 625-683.

Fig. 10.1B cont'd

study for Mrs. Hayes, a 79-year-old woman who had had a cerebrovascular accident (CVA). Two evaluation forms are provided to illustrate Mrs. Hayes's progress: a detailed ADL assessment form (see Fig. 10.1A), and an abbreviated ADL form (Fig. 10.1B). The detailed form with Mrs. Hayes's information incorporated into it will help the novice OT practitioner appreciate the details of many ADLs and IADLs that may be taken for granted. Abbreviated forms or electronic templates are more likely to be used in actual practice. A third form, also frequently used, is a home management checklist (Fig. 10.2). When reviewing the forms just discussed, the reader should keep in mind that the assessment and progress summaries relate only to the ADL and IADL portions of the intervention program.

It must be noted that computerized documentation has become the standard for medical records.[61] The term *electronic health record* (EHR) is widely used in the United States. The EHR is a digitized/electronic version of a client's medical chart and is kept by the provider.[25] OT documentation is included in the EHR.

INSTRUMENTAL ACTIVITIES OF DAILY LIVING

Home Management Assessment

Home management tasks are assessed similarly to self-care tasks. First, the client should be interviewed to elicit a description of the home and of previous and current home management responsibilities. Tasks the client needs to perform when returning home, in addition to those that they would like to perform, should be determined during the interview. If the client has communication or cognitive deficits, reliable friends or family members may be enlisted to obtain relevant information. Clients also may be questioned about their ability to perform relevant tasks on the activities list. The assessment is more meaningful and accurate if the interview is followed by a performance assessment in the ADL kitchen or apartment of the treatment facility or, if possible, in the client's home. An example of a standardized assessment to evaluate the executive skills required to perform IADLs is the Executive Function Performance Test (EFPT).[20,51,79] Examples of specific IADL tasks

Occupational Therapy Department
Home Management Checklist

Name _____   Date _____

Address _____   Age _____

Roles _____

Diagnosis _____

Activity Precautions _____

Description of home

Owns home _____   Apartment _____   Board and care _____

    No. of rooms _____   Bathroom description _____

    No. of floors _____   _____

    Stairs _____   _____

    Elevator _____   _____

Will client be required to perform the following activities? If not, who will perform?
Identify with ** the I-ADLs most important to the client.

Activity	Yes/NO	Who will perform?	Activity	Yes/NO	Who will perform?
Meal prep			Laundry		
Serving			Child care		
Wash dishes			Housekeeping		
Shopping			Other:		

Key:

Independent- I
Supervised- S
Stand by Assist- SBA
Minimum Assist- Min
Moderate Assist- Mod
Maximum Assist- Max
Dependent- D
Not Applicable- N/A
Not Tested- NT

Meal preparation

Date				Remarks
Manage faucets				
Handle stove controls				
Open packages				
Carry items				
Open cans				
Open jars				
Handle milk carton				
Empty garbage				
Retrieve refrigerator items				
Reach cupboards				
Peel vegetables				
Cut safely				
Break eggs				
Use electric mixer				
Use toaster				
Use coffee maker				
Use microwave				
Manage oven				
Pour hot water				

Fig. 10.2 Home management checklist. (Courtesy Lorraine Pedretti, MS, OTR.)

Continued

Set up/clean up for meal preparation

Date				Remarks
Set table				
Carry items to table				
Load/empty dishwasher				
Wash dishes				
Wash pots and pans				
Wipe counters/stove				
Wring out dishcloth				

Cleaning activities

Date				Remarks
Pick up object from floor				
Wipe spills				
Make bed				
Use dust mop				
Dust high surfaces				
Dust low surfaces				
Mop floor				
Sweep				
Use dust pan				
Vacuum				
Clean tub and toilet				
Change sheets				
Carry pail of water				
Carry cleaning tools				

Laundry/cleaning activities

Date				Remarks
Do hand washing				
Wring out clothes				
Hang clothing				
Carry laundry to and from washer and dryer				
Manage controls on appliances				
Use washing machine				
Retrieve clothes from dryer				
Iron				

Heavy household activities

Date				Remarks
Clean stove and oven				
Clean refrigerator				
Shopping				
Put away groceries				
Wash windows				
Change light bulbs				
Wash bathtub & toilet				
Maintain smoke alarms				
Recycle/compost				

Fig. 10.2 cont'd

Miscellaneous household activities

Date				Remarks
Retrieve newspaper				
Retrieve mail				
Feed pet				
Manage pet waste				
Let pet in and out				
Reach thermostat				
Use scissors				
Water houseplants				

Shopping

Date				Remarks
Prepare shopping list				
Select appropriate items				
Finding items in store				
Initiates asking for help as needed in store				
Reaching for objects in store				
Pushing cart				
Manage money, ATM, checkbook at store				
Purchasing within budget				
Putting away groceries or purchased items				

Suggestions for home modification: _____

_____

_____

_____

_____

_____

_____

_____

_____

_____

Fig. 10.2 cont'd

to evaluate for home management can be found in the home management checklist (see Fig. 10.2).

The therapist should select tasks and exercise safety precautions consistent with the client's capabilities, limitations and interests. The initial tasks should be simple one- or two-step procedures that are not hazardous, such as wiping a dish, sponging a tabletop, and turning the water on and off. As the assessment progresses, tasks graded in complexity and involving safety precautions should be performed, such as making a sandwich and a cup of coffee and vacuuming the carpet. For example, with Anna, initial tasks may include making a sandwich and using

the microwave because using a manual wheelchair in her own home is new for her and requires working from a seated versus a standing position. As Anna performs these simple tasks using her wheelchair, the occupational therapist will be able to observe and make suggestions about modification to her kitchen, reorganization, safety techniques, or methods to transport items and simplify tasks.

Individuals may live independently or share home management responsibilities with others. In some homes, it is necessary for a role reversal to occur after the onset of a physical disability. In Anna's case, she has stated she would like to participate in previous home management activities and eventually return to work. Anna's occupational therapist will collaborate with her on home tasks to be completed by her so that interventions can be prioritized. Until Anna can perform the tasks more independently, Anna's mother or husband may be available to perform some of these tasks with direction from Anna.

If a client will be home alone, several basic ADL and IADL skills are needed for safety and independence. Lysack et al.[66] studied 122 African American women from urban areas who previously had lived alone who had a primary rehabilitation condition, such as a CVA or hip replacement. The researchers looked at FIM scores 3 and 6 months after discharge from a hospital. In telephone interviews they found that independence in five ADLs (eating, grooming, toileting, dressing, bathing) was significantly related to live-alone status. In the same study,

9 of 10 IADLs were significantly related to live-alone status at 6 months after discharge, and four items (phone use, taking medications, managing finances, food preparation) were highly significant.[66]

The data suggest that investment in improved functional outcome is worthwhile, and higher functional performance is related to live-alone status. Findings such as these underscore the importance of OT intervention as it is in the domain of practice to focus on occupations and areas such as ADLs and IADLs.[12] The occupational therapist can assess the potential for remaining at home alone through the activities of the home management assessment. An evaluation such as the EFPT can be used to assist in determining whether a person is safe to remain at home or to help determine how much assistance is required for some IADL tasks.[20,51] Children with a permanent disability also need to be considered

CASE STUDY

Mrs. Hayes

Mrs. Hayes is a 79-year-old woman (prefers use of the pronouns she/her/hers) who incurred a cerebral thrombosis, which resulted in a left CVA 2 months ago. She lives in a modest home with her husband of 45 years. Mrs. Hayes was active before the CVA, volunteering 10 hours a week at a local thrift store with her friends and caring for her husband, who has diabetes and poor vision. Mrs. Hayes was independent with all of the indoor home management activities and paid the bills for herself and her husband using checks. Mrs. Hayes enjoyed gardening with potted plants.

After the CVA, Mrs. Hayes spent 3 weeks in the acute inpatient rehabilitation unit. While she was in the rehabilitation facility, the occupational therapist performed a home safety assessment (see the following section, Home Safety Assessment). Following through with the occupational therapist's recommendations, Mrs. Hayes's family made simple home modifications to increase her safety and independence when she came home.

The CVA resulted in an ataxic gait, mild dysarthria (slurred speech), dysphagia (swallowing deficit), and mild right hemiparesis (weakness). Mrs. Hayes was referred to outpatient occupational therapy for evaluation and training in ADLs and IADLs and for treatment of dysphagia.

The initial evaluation started with an interview with the client and her husband to create an occupational profile. Mrs. Hayes expressed concern about how she and her husband would manage because her four adult children lived 5 hours away. Her children hired caregivers who are with the couple in shifts for 8 hours a day. Mrs. Hayes and her husband want to be on their own again and do not want to be a financial burden on their children.

Based on the priorities and problems identified by the client and her husband, the occupational performance analysis included the use of the EFPT and an ADLs performance evaluation.[20,51] The initial performance evaluation was completed during the first 1-hour session, and the EFPT was completed during the second visit.

During the initial evaluation, Mrs. Hayes became restless after 15 minutes, but with minimal redirection she continued to attend to the tasks. She also demonstrated decreased frustration tolerance and required minimal encouragement to continue with fine motor tasks, which were difficult for her. The results of the initial evaluation showed that Mrs. Hayes was independent with eating, basic hygiene, and grooming while seated and with toileting tasks. Mrs. Hayes required supervision with transfers from her wheelchair to the bed and toilet but minimal assistance to transfer onto the bath bench because of occasional loss of balance, setup, and cues for safety. She required minimal to moderate assist for dressing and bathing. She required minimal assistance with upper body dressing and bathing and moderate assistance for lower body dressing. She has difficulty with handwriting, using the phone, and handling keys. She requires moderate

assistance to walk 20 feet using a quad cane but is independent with manual wheelchair mobility on indoor flat surfaces. Her visual fields are intact and she has no visual-spatial deficit. Her left upper extremity (UE) strength and active range of motion (AROM) are within normal limits (WNL). Her right UE strength is WNL proximally, but testing by use of a dynamometer demonstrates mild weakness in her hand. Right UE AROM is WNL. Her muscle tone in her bilateral UEs is WNL. Her right hand coordination is mildly impaired, as demonstrated with moderate difficulty pushing buttons on the phone and putting on socks. She is able to stand while holding on to a stable surface but cannot use her hands for a task while standing because of mild balance impairments.

Results of the EFPT demonstrated significant deficits in organization of cooking and bill-paying tasks, requiring moderate assistance to complete both. The EFPT results indicated that Mrs. Hayes required minimal assistance with medication management and phone management.

A swallow assessment demonstrated moderately impaired tongue coordination and minimal delay with a swallow. Mrs. Hayes has already modified her diet by selecting very soft foods and slightly thickened liquids.

Mrs. Hayes tolerated the full OT evaluation but reported, "I'm tired," at the end of the session. She reported diminished endurance since the CVA, especially toward the end of the day. She admitted that in the later afternoon hours, "I have a hard time remembering things and concentrating." When queried about her sleep, Mrs. Hayes reported that she had difficulty falling asleep and that she wakes up in the middle of the night and cannot fall back asleep because of "too much on my mind" and discomfort in her legs. She reported having sleep difficulties before the CVA and stated that her husband complains that she snores loudly.

Mrs. Hayes is motivated and has the potential to prepare simple hot meals and perform basic self-care independently, except for showering, for which she may require supervision. Mrs. Hayes would like to be as independent as possible in her ADLs and IADLs. She acknowledges that her right hand has gotten stronger, but she reports frustration that it is taking longer than she expected. She would like to eventually resume her leisure activities.

Progress Report

Mrs. Hayes has attended occupational therapy two times a week for 6 weeks. She is generally cooperative and motivated, although periodically becomes discouraged as she continues to have an ataxic gait and requires use of the manual wheelchair for independent mobility. Treatment has focused on lower extremity (LE) dressing, tub transfers, oral-motor exercises to improve swallowing, instruction in sleep hygiene techniques, and simple meal preparation. Because

Mrs. Hayes

the caregiver drives Mrs. Hayes and her husband to the occupational therapy appointments, the occupational therapist has also trained the caregiver in how to assist the client to be more independent in her ADLs.

Mrs. Hayes has made significant progress in the treatment program, progressing from requiring moderate assistance with LE dressing to being independent while seated. She has improved from chair-level grooming to standing with one-hand stabilization while using the other hand to brush her hair and teeth. Progress has been made from requiring minimal assistance with bathing to requiring supervision only with bathing on a shower bench. Initially requiring supervision with bed to wheelchair transfers, she is now independent. From requiring minimal assistance with transfers onto the shower bench, she now requires supervision, mainly for setup of the environment. From moderate difficulty with use of the phone, she has progressed to using the phone independently; from requiring moderate assistance with bill-paying activities and medication management, she has progressed to the supervised level. From being dependent with oral-motor exercises, she has progressed to supervised. Mrs. Hayes is now independent in cold meal preparation after initially requiring moderate assistance. Mrs. Hayes reports some improvement in her sleep at night and states that she is following through with two sleep hygiene strategies, but she says that she still has difficulties and does not wake up refreshed.

Mrs. Hayes continues to require a soft diet and slightly thickened liquids because of swallowing difficulties. She consistently follows through with the use of safety techniques for swallowing and is safe and independent to do so. She continues to have impaired hand function but is learning compensatory techniques to adapt her method of performing various ADLs. To continue working on Mrs. Hayes' right hand strength and coordination, the occupational therapist worked with Mrs. Hayes to develop regular gardening activities, initially with

the help of her husband or caregiver, to increase strength and coordination (e.g., sowing seeds in small containers, pinching dead leaves off plants, filling the watering can and watering plants, etc.).

The occupational therapist, in consultation with Mrs. Hayes, has coordinated treatment and goals with the physical therapist (PT) and social worker. Mrs. Hayes also has been referred to her primary physician, who referred her to a physician specializing in sleep medicine. The sleep specialist evaluated Mrs. Hayes and scheduled her for an overnight sleep study in 4 weeks. (See Chapter 13 for more information on the occupation of sleep and rest.)

Mrs. Hayes and her husband are pleased with her increased independence. With input provided by the occupational therapist, the family will reduce the hours needed for a hired caregiver to 4 hours a day. The hired caregiver will assist Mrs. Hayes with bathing, meals, driving to appointments, shopping, and housekeeping. Occupational therapy will now focus on hot meal preparation, bed making, and exploration of future community mobility options, along with continuing to work toward improvement of oral-motor and hand function and improving sleep hygiene techniques.

Critical Thinking Questions

1. What deficits is Mrs. Hayes experiencing, and what compensatory strategies can she be taught to improve her ADLs and IADLs?
2. What role does the occupational therapist have in helping Mrs. Hayes meet her goals for ADLs and IADLs?
3. With all the areas that Mrs. Hayes needs to work on with the occupational therapist, how can the occupational therapist prioritize the goals that are most important for Mrs. Hayes to accomplish so that she can continue to live in her home safely with her husband?

---

for assessment and training for IADL skills because they will develop and mature, and have a growing need for independence.

Home Safety Assessment

The AOTA Representative Assembly's position paper on complex environmental modifications asserts that evaluation and provision of complex adaptations to environments where people complete daily occupations is within the scope of practice of OT practitioners.[82] One of the most important places where people complete many life occupations is the home.[28] To help with the transition from a treatment facility to home, or to optimize performance in a dwelling in which a client already lives, a home safety assessment may be performed, in which the occupational therapist goes to the home. A home safety assessment can serve several purposes; it allows the occupational therapist to assess the home for safety and accessibility, and it also provides a way for the occupational therapist to assess client functioning at home and to perform some caregiver training. The home assessment provides the family with a list of modifications and DME (Box 10.3) and strategies to maximize safety and independence in the home to prevent falls.[110,111] It also helps the occupational therapist understand clients' environmental and personal factors that can affect ADLs and IADLs. Insufficient or incorrect information about the home can lead to costly mistakes in terms of safety, independence, and finances, so a home assessment can be useful. In a randomized controlled study, researchers demonstrated that even one home visit with an occupational therapist

BOX 10.3 Durable Medical Equipment

- Equipment that can withstand repeated use ("durable" and long-lasting)
- Primarily and customarily used to serve a medical purpose
- Generally not useful to a person in the absence of an illness or injury
- Appropriate for use in the home

DME that occupational therapists in the United States customarily recommend includes hospital beds, commodes, bath equipment, and client lifts (for transfers). Other professionals may recommend DME in the realm of their expertise, such as walkers, medication infusion pumps, and blood glucose monitors

DME, Durable medical equipment.
From the US Social Security Administration: Program operations manual system (POMS) website. https://secure.ssa.gov/poms.nsf/lnx/0600610200; and the Medicare: Durable medical equipment (DME) coverage. http://www.medicare.gov/coverage/durable-medical-equipment-coverage.html.

after a hip fracture, while the client was still at the hospital, increased adherence to recommendations and reduced hospital readmission 30 days after discharge home.[64]

Regardless of the setting, from the initial meeting with a client or caregivers, the occupational therapist must have an idea about the home environment to which the client will return. For example, the occupational therapist treating Anna or Mrs. Hayes should know from early on whether the client lives in a second story apartment without an elevator or in a one-story house. When the client's discharge from the treatment facility is imminent, a home assessment may be carried out to facilitate the client's maximal independence and safety in the living environment. Other professionals also make home modification recommendations, but they are often provided by occupational therapists.[80,90] Stark et al.[96] found that home modification interventions by occupational therapists have demonstrated greater efficacy in reducing falls and improving function in older adults than interventions delivered by other professionals. In a later study, Stark et al. found that OT practitioners can deliver home modifications with high fidelity, at relatively reasonable cost, with interventions being maintained for 12 months to older adults in the community.[99]

The AOTA document "Research Opportunities Tables on Home Modifications" points future researchers toward areas that can be studied further, and it acknowledges the strong evidence that occupational therapists make important contributions in this area.[11]

Generalist occupational therapists who work with clients with physical dysfunction regularly provide recommendations, but occupational therapists can also specialize in this practice area and obtain advanced training.[82] Occupational therapists who make larger recommendations must have the training to do so. For example, an occupational therapist who has not had advanced training or experience in home modification, or without consultation with a licensed contractor, should not recommend that Anna's family make large structural changes to their home. The Occupational Therapy code of Ethics and Ethics Standards (2020) regarding advanced practice must be followed.[10]

Before performing a home assessment, occupational therapists must recognize that they will be assessing someone else's space. Chase and Christianson[26] pointed out that the "choices regarding the home belong to clients and may be highly significant to them" (p.6). In addition, these researchers noted that the home is not just the sum of its physical characteristics; emotional components also are a part of it.[26] It is important that occupational therapists be mindful of this throughout the home assessment process and that they use a client-centered approach; studies have shown greater adherence to recommendations with this method.[112]

It should be noted that not all clients seen by an occupational therapist in a facility need or receive a home safety assessment. These clients may be those who are ambulating, those who are at a higher functional level, and those who live out of the area. A home safety assessment is performed when a client demonstrates a change from previous level of functioning that can present safety or accessibility issues.

Preparing to Return Home

If the client is in a facility with plans to return home, the home assessment should be performed when the client's mobility status has been stabilized and is close to what is expected at discharge. Collaboration with the PT about a client's ambulatory status and potential is essential to determine the necessity and timing of home assessment. For example, if the PT reports that a client will be primarily walking at discharge, recommendations for home modifications may be very different from those for a client whose primary mode of mobility will be a wheelchair.

Ideally, the occupational and physical therapists perform the home assessment together. During the home visit, the client and essential caregivers and family members should be present. However, if it is not feasible to take the client, a wheelchair and other necessary equipment may be taken. Budget, time factors, and reimbursement issues may not allow two professionals to go to the client' home or may prohibit a home visit altogether.

In some situations, some clients are allowed a trial of a few hours at home before discharge (a visit that must be approved by the insurance company). Much of the information can be obtained by interviewing the client and family members after a client's trial home visit. The family member or caregiver may be instructed to complete the home safety checklist (audit) during the trial home visit and provide photographs or sketches of the rooms and their arrangements. Problems encountered by the client during a trial home visit should be discussed and the necessary recommendations for their solution made.

The client and a family member should be interviewed before the home assessment to determine the client's and family's expectations and the roles the client will assume in the home and community. The family's values or those of their culture regarding people with disabilities may influence role expectations and whether independence will be encouraged. Willingness to make modifications in the home also must be determined. The purposes and procedure of the home assessment should be clearly explained to the client and caregivers before the actual visit.

Understandably, the first-time home (which may be at the home assessment) after an illness or injury can be emotional for everyone concerned. Before the occupational therapist performs a home assessment, especially with the client present, it is important that they know whether the home being evaluated is new for the client or whether drastic home changes have already had to be made. For example, if Anna had lived in a second story apartment before her accident, her family may have had to move to a first story home. Or, if Anna's mother was going to move into her home to help care for her daughter and granddaughter, rooms may have been switched, furniture moved, belongings displaced. Knowing this ahead of time can help the occupational therapist and other rehabilitation team members be ready to provide emotional support to the client as needed.

If the client is present during the home visit, sufficient time should be scheduled so that they can demonstrate required functional mobility skills, such as selected self-care and home management tasks in the dwelling. During the assessment, the client should use the mobility aid and any assistive devices that they are accustomed to using or expected to use. As examples, Anna and Mrs. Hayes would be asked to propel their manual wheelchairs throughout the home to determine what access issues they will encounter. The therapist should bring a tape measure to measure the width of doorways, the height of stairs, the height of the bed, and other dimensions. With permission, the occupational therapist can take photos during the assessment and refer to them later to assist with problem-solving placement of safety equipment, adaptive devices, and home modifications.

The therapist can take the required measurements while surveying the general arrangement of rooms, furniture, and appliances. Fig. 10.3 provides a format for documenting critical

Home Evaluation Checklist

Name _____   Date _____

Address _____

Roles _____

Diagnosis _____

Number of people who live in the home _____

Current mobility status   ☐ independent   ☐ needs assist   ☐ dependent

Mobility Device used in home: ☐ ambulatory, no device   ☐ walker   ☐ cane

    ☐ power wheelchair   ☐ manual wheelchair

Exterior

Home located on: _____

Type of house   ☐ owns home   ☐ mobile home

    ☐ apartment   ☐ board and care

Number of floors   ☐ one story   ☐ split level   ☐ two story

Driveway surface   ☐ inclined   ☐ smooth

    ☐ level   ☐ rough

Is the DRIVEWAY negotiable
with current mobility device?   ☐ yes   ☐ no

Is the GARAGE accessible?   ☐ yes   ☐ no

Entrance

Accessible entrances   ☐ front   ☐ side   ☐ back

Steps   Number_____

    Height of each_____

    Width_____

    Depth_____

Are there HANDRAILS?   ☐ yes   ☐ no

If yes, where are they located?   ☐ left   ☐ right

HANDRAIL height from step surface? _____

If no, how much room is available for HANDRAILS? _____

Are landings negotiable?   ☐ yes   ☐ no

Briefly describe any problems with LANDINGS:

_____

_____

_____

Fig. 10.3 Home safety assessment checklist. (Adapted from Ralph K Davies Medical Center: Occupational/physical therapy home safety assessment form, San Francisco, 1993; and Alta Bates Hospital: Occupational therapy home safety assessment form, Albany, CA, 1993.)

Continued

Ramps

☐ yes ☐ no

☐ front ☐ back

Height _____

Width _____

Length_____

Are there HANDRAILS? ☐ yes ☐ no

If yes, where are they located? ☐ left ☐ right Height _____

Condition of current ramp _____

If no ramp, how much room is available for one? _____

Given 1" rise:12" length ratio for ramp, how long should the ramp be? _____

Porch

Width _____

Length_____

Level at threshold? ☐ yes ☐ no

Lighting available at porch? ☐ yes ☐ no

Door

Width_____

Threshold height _____

Negotiable? ☐ yes ☐ no

☐ swing in

☐ swing out

☐ sliding

Do door locks work? ☐ yes ☐ no

Can door lock be reached with use of current mobility device and can it be safely locked and unlocked considering current status? ☐ yes ☐ no

Type of door knob? ☐ lever ☐ round

Interior

Living Room
Is furniture arranged for safe maneuverability with current mobility status? ☐ yes ☐ no

Height of frequently used furniture/chair? _____

Type of floor covering: _____

Able to control TV, phone, lights from seat in living room? ☐ yes ☐ no

Comments _____

_____

Fig. 10.3 cont'd

Hallways

Can current mobility device be maneuvered in hallway? ☐ yes ☐ no

Hall width _____

Is it adequate for current mobility status? ☐ yes ☐ no

Door width _____

Is it adequate for current mobility status? ☐ yes ☐ no

Sharp turns? ☐ yes ☐ no

Steps? ☐ yes ☐ no   Number _____

Are there HANDRAILS? ☐ yes ☐ no

If yes, where are they located? ☐ left ☐ right   Height _____

Lighting: Is switch within reach with current mobility status? ☐ yes ☐ no

Bedroom

☐ single ☐ shared

Is there room for current mobility device? ☐ yes ☐ no

Type of floor covering? _____

Door:

Width _____

Threshold height _____

Negotiable? ☐ yes ☐ no

☐ swing in ☐ swing out

Bed:

☐ twin ☐ double ☐ queen

☐ king ☐ hospital bed

Overall height _____

Safe and accessible with current mobility status? ☐ yes ☐ no

Would hospital bed fit into room if needed? ☐ yes ☐ no

Able to control TV, phone, lights from bed? ☐ yes ☐ no

Clothing:

Are drawers accessible with current mobility status? ☐ yes ☐ no

Able to reach all items in closet (higher and lower)? ☐ yes ☐ no

Is there adequate lighting in closet? ☐ yes ☐ no

Comments: _____

Fig. 10.3 cont'd

Continued

Bathroom   ☐ private   ☐ shared

Door:

Width _____

Swings   ☐ in   ☐ out

Will door close with current mobility device inside?   ☐ yes   ☐ no

Threshold height _____

Negotiable?   ☐ yes   ☐ no

Tub/Shower   ☐ tub/shower combination   ☐ shower stall   ☐ tub only

Height, floor to rim _____

Height, inside bottom to rim _____

Width and length inside   Width _____   Depth _____

Glass doors?   ☐ yes   ☐ no

☐ sliding   ☐ swing   ☐ in   ☐ out

Width of doors _____

Handheld shower?   ☐ yes   ☐ no

Type of faucet controls   ☐ 2 levers   ☐ single lever   ☐ round

If seated, will user be able to reach faucets?   ☐ yes   ☐ no

Is tub/shower accessible safely with current mobility status?   ☐ yes   ☐ no

The following equipment is currently being used for bathing in the home   ☐ shower seat   ☐ transfer tub bench   ☐ 3 in1 commode

☐ shower/commode tub slider system   ☐ power tub lift

☐ shower commode chair

Is there room for the caregiver to assist?   ☐ yes   ☐ no

Sink:

Height _____   ☐ open (no cabinets)

Faucet type _____   ☐ closed (cabinets below)

Able to reach and use faucet and sink with current mobility status?   ☐ yes   ☐ no

Height of mirror _____

Appropriate height to sit?   ☐ yes   ☐ no

Can shelf be reached with current mobility status?   ☐ yes   ☐ no

Are hot water pipes insulated?   ☐ yes   ☐ no

Type of faucet controls   ☐ 2 levers   ☐ single lever   ☐ round

Electrical outlets within reach from seated or standing position   ☐ yes   ☐ no

Comments on clutter/organization? _____

_____

Fig. 10.3 cont'd

Toilet:

Height from floor_____

Location of toilet paper_____

Distance from toilet to side wall L _____   R _____

Grab bars: ☐ yes ☐ no

Location _____

Comments: _____

The following equipment is
currently being used for toileting ☐ raised toilet seat ☐ toilet safety rails ☐ 3 in1 commode
☐ grab bars ☐ bidet

Kitchen

Door:

Width_____

Threshold height_____

Negotiable? ☐ yes ☐ no

Stove:

Height_____

Location of controls ☐ front ☐ rear

Able to reach and operate
controls/burners with current
mobility status? ☐ yes ☐ no

Oven:

Height from floor to door hinge and door handle _____

Location of oven_____

Is there a nearby surface to rest
hot foods on when removed
from oven? ☐ yes ☐ no

Microwave Oven:

Height from floor to door hinge and door handle _____

Location of microwave oven _____

Is there a nearby surface to rest
hot foods on when removed
from microwave oven? ☐ yes ☐ no

Sink:

Will w/c fit underneath? ☐ yes ☐ no

Type of faucet controls ☐ 2 levers ☐ single lever ☐ round

Can faucet be reached while
seated? ☐ yes ☐ no

Are hot water pipes insulated? ☐ yes ☐ no

Fig. 10.3 cont'd

Continued

Cupboards:

Height of counters? _____

Accessible from seated position
or with current mobility status?   ☐ yes   ☐ no

Is there under-the-counter knee
space for a work area?   ☐ yes   ☐ no

Refrigerator:

Type: ☐ side by side   ☐ freezer on top   ☐ freezer on bottom

Hinges on   ☐ left   ☐ right

Able to reach all shelves in the
refrigerator?   ☐ yes   ☐ no

Able to reach all shelves in the
freezer?   ☐ yes   ☐ no

Switches/outlets:

Able to reach with current
mobility status?   ☐ yes   ☐ no

Lighting:

Adequate in work areas of
kitchen?   ☐ yes   ☐ no

Kitchen table:

Height from floor _____

Will w/c fit under table?   ☐ yes   ☐ no

Comments: _____

Laundry

Door:

Width _____

Threshold height _____

Negotiable?   ☐ yes   ☐ no

Steps: ☐ yes   ☐ no

Number _____

Height _____

Width _____

Are there HANDRAILS?   ☐ yes   ☐ no

If yes, where are they located?   ☐ left   ☐ right   Height _____

Washer: ☐ Top load   ☐ Front load

Can user reach controls and
inside to retrieve clothing?   ☐ yes   ☐ no

Dryer: ☐ Top load   ☐ Front load

Can user reach controls and
inside to retrieve clothing?   ☐ yes   ☐ no

Comments: _____

Fig. 10.3 cont'd

Safety

Throw rugs ☐ yes ☐ no

Location _____

Is client and/or family willing to remove? ☐ yes ☐ no

Water Temperature

Is water temperature set at 120 degrees Fahrenheit? ☐ yes ☐ no

Phone

Type ☐ programmable ☐ cordless ☐ mobile
☐ attached to base

Within reach of chair? ☐ yes ☐ no

Within reach of bed? ☐ yes ☐ no

Able to retrieve phone, dial and hear caller? ☐ yes ☐ no

Emergency phone numbers posted and programmed into phone? ☐ yes ☐ no

Location _____

Mailbox

Able to reach and empty? ☐ yes ☐ no

Location _____

Doorbell

Able to identify visitors? ☐ yes ☐ no

Able to hear doorbell? ☐ yes ☐ no

Thermostat

Able to reach and read controls? ☐ yes ☐ no

Location _____

Electric outlets/switches

Height of outlets? _____

Electrical extension cord hazards? ☐ yes ☐ no

Drapes/Curtains/Blinds

Able to open with current mobility status? ☐ yes ☐ no

Windows/Doors

Able to open with current mobility status? ☐ yes ☐ no

Fig. 10.3 cont'd

Continued

Imperfect floor/floor covering? ☐ yes ☐ no

Location _____

Sharp-edged furniture? ☐ yes ☐ no

Location _____

Fire extinguisher ☐ yes ☐ no

Location _____

Smoke detector ☐ yes ☐ no

Location _____

Client hears and understands
meaning of smoke detector? ☐ yes ☐ no

Guns present: ☐ yes ☐ no

Locked? ☐ yes ☐ no

Comments on condition of house:

Cleanliness: _____

Disrepair: _____

Clutter issues: _____

Health issues:_____

Equipment present: ☐ shower seat   ☐ transfer tub bench   ☐ 3 in1 commode

                      ☐ shower/commode tub slider system   ☐ power tub lift

                      ☐ raised toilet seat   ☐ toilet safety rails   ☐ grab bars installed

                      ☐ tub safety rail   ☐ shower commode chair   ☐ lift recliner chair

                      ☐ hospital bed with rails   ☐ stair glide

Other equipment/Status of equipment (e.g., borrowed, in disrepair, etc): _____

_____

Problem list: _____

_____

_____

Recommendations for modifications: _____

_____

_____

Equipment recommendations: _____

_____

_____

Patient/Family willing to make modifications: ☐ yes ☐ no

Patient/Family able to make modifications: ☐ yes ☐ no

Cost constraints: _____

Referrals needed: _____

Comments: _____

Fig. 10.3 cont'd

measurements. It may be helpful to sketch the size and arrangement of rooms for later reference and to attach these sketches to the home assessment checklist.

Next, the client demonstrates functional mobility skills and essential self-care and home management tasks. The client's ability to use the entrance to the home and to transfer to and from an automobile, if it is to be used, should be included in the home assessment.

During the performance assessment, the therapist should observe safety factors, ease of mobility and performance, and limitations imposed by the environment. If the client needs assistance for transfers and other activities, the caregiver should be instructed in the methods that are appropriate. The client also may be instructed in methods to improve maneuverability and to simplify the performance of tasks in a small space.

Access to the bathroom and maneuvering with a wheelchair or walker are common problems. Frequently, a bedside commode is recommended until a bathroom can be made accessible or modified to allow independence with toileting (Fig. 10.4). Shower seats can be used in the tub if a client can transfer over the edge of the tub and also may be used in a shower. A transfer tub bench (Fig. 10.5) is recommended for individuals who cannot safely or independently step over the edge of the tub, but glass doors need to be removed and replaced with a shower curtain. Installation of a handheld shower hose increases access to the water and also eliminates risky turns and standing while bathing.

The Americans with Disabilities Act (ADA) established standards for accessible design, which can be used as general guidelines and are available at the ADA's website (https://www.ada.gov).[109] Not all modifications recommended should necessarily meet the ADA guidelines because the home will be modified to suit the individual and to compensate for the person's situation. As Thompson (2019) points out, there are no specific rules that should govern the heights at which personal grab bars are placed and that optimal heights should consider the

person who needs it.[105] The ADA guidelines are meant to apply to public areas and to meet the needs of people with a variety of disabilities (see Chapter 15). The ADA standards may serve as a resource, but they should not be the only guidelines the occupational therapist uses when making recommendations.[28] The occupational therapist should recommend that the family use only licensed contractors who are aware of building code requirements in their area.

Christenson and Lorentzen suggested the optimal reach zone (OZR) as a more realistic criterion for recommendations.[28] According to the OZR method, items should be placed in a zone that is 20 to 44 inches above the floor and a maximum depth of 20 inches.[125] No specific rule can accommodate every person, but ideal heights have been determined for some items that require vision, reach, or grasp; for example, clothing rods, thermostats, electric switches, and door handles should be placed between 27.3 and 45.5 inches from the ground.[28,125]

In a study by Cummings et al., the most common home safety recommendations were to remove mats and throw rugs (48%), to change footwear (24%), and to use a nonslip bathmat (21%).[35] Other recommendations included changing behaviors, such as using a commode, keeping a light on at night, or motion detecting nightlights.[35] In their small study of older adults in an independent living community, Van Oss et al., found that items rated most useful included nonslip bath strips, a suction-bottom foot scrubber, a tub seat, a bath mat for outside the tub, a reacher, a magnified mirror, a pill bottle magnifier, a raised toilet seat, and a jar gripper.[112] Box 10.4 presents additional common recommendations for home safety and access, and Box 10.5 shows a list of supplies to take on a home safety assessment.

When the home assessment is completed, the therapist writes a report summarizing the information on the form and describes the client's performance in the home. The report should conclude with a summary of the environmental barriers and the functional limitations the client encountered. Recommendations should include additional safety equipment

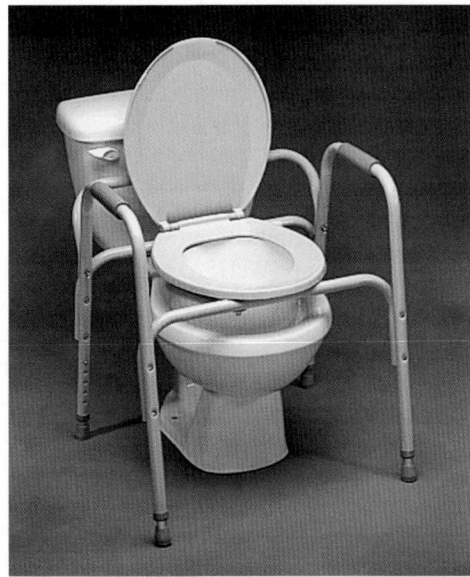

Fig. 10.4 Three-in-one commode. (Courtesy North Coast Medical, Gilroy, CA.)

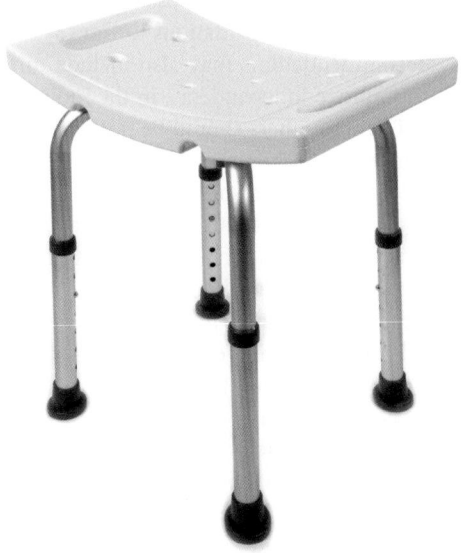

Fig. 10.5 Adjustable bath and shower safety chair. (iStock.com/Chiyacat. ID: 1189207031.)

BOX 10.4   Common Home Recommendations

1. Installation of a ramp or railings at the entrance to the home
2. Removal of throw rugs, clutter, and exposed electrical wires
3. Removal of door thresholds (if not level) and doorjambs
4. Installation of safety grab bars around the toilet and bathtub
5. Rearrangement or removal of furniture to accommodate a wheelchair or other assistive devices
6. Rearrangement of kitchen and other storage for access
7. Lowering of clothes rods in closets

BOX 10.5   Supplies to Take on a Home Safety Assessment

- Measuring tape—use heavy duty (at least 30 ft long) or infrared distance measurer[16]
- Paper and pen for notations and sketches
- Digital device for notations, to take pictures, video (explicit permission must be obtained and documented)
- Home safety assessment checklist
- Light meter[16]
- Maps or GPS
- Important emergency phone numbers (e.g., nursing station, your supervisor, and healthcare provider)
- Any durable medical equipment you think the client may need (e.g., wheelchair, walker, commode, and bath bench)
- Tool kit for quick fixes
- Cell/mobile phone

Other Considerations

- Urinal, as appropriate
- Blood pressure cuff, stethoscope, gloves, pulse oximeter, thermometer
- Infection control personal protective equipment (PPE), as required per policies: Appropriate masks, goggles/shields, disposable gown, hand sanitizer, biohazard trash bag. Training in donning and doffing (https://www.cdc.gov/) (see Chapter 9).

---

and assistive devices needed and possible modifications that could be made, with recommendations to work with a licensed contractor. Recommendations may also include further functional goals to improve independence in the individual's home environment. Team members should be notified about the client's performance in the home and accessibility problems so that they can practice skills or be made aware of issues before discharge. For example, the occupational therapist may report to the PT that a client such as Mrs. Hayes will eventually need to negotiate a step down into the living room to be more independent. The occupational therapist may report to the psychologist that Anna had a difficult time emotionally handling her visit home with her new functional status.

The occupational therapist should carefully review all recommendations with the client and family. The family should receive a written report with the recommendations clearly written. This review should be done with tact and diplomacy in a way that gives the client and family options and the freedom to decline them or consider alternative possibilities. Family finances may limit the implementation of needed changes. The

social worker, case manager, and/or insurance company may be involved in working out funding for needed equipment and alterations, and the client should be made aware of this service when cost is discussed. Sprague noted that determination of a household's available resources and obtaining further funding, if needed, are among the most important activities in the home modification process.[93] The occupational therapist may assist in helping to justify and prioritize projects for funding. Sprague provided ideas and a detailed list of possible funding sources in the United States for home modifications.[93] The therapist should include recommendations regarding the feasibility of the client's discharge to the home environment or of the client remaining in or managing the home alone. If there is a question regarding the client's ability to return home safely and independently, the home assessment summary should include the additional functional skills the client needs to return home. If the occupational therapist thinks that the home is not safe to live in or if there is imminent danger, appropriate parties should be notified immediately and steps taken to ensure the safety of the client.

If a home safety assessment is not possible before discharge, an environmental audit, which consists of checklists with potential hazards, can be performed.[96,97] The rehabilitation team along with the client and family members should identify the most serious concerns and develop a plan to address them. Fig. 10.6 shows a home safety checklist (audit) that can be completed by the client or the client's family. Family members or caregivers could take pictures and measurements of the home or draw floor plans. Another option if a home safety assessment is not possible before discharge is to refer this task to an occupational therapist in a home health agency who can regularly provide skilled assessment and services in the home. Occupational therapists who work in outpatient settings can also ensure follow-through of previous and their own safety recommendations.

Assessments

Stark et al. discuss the importance of choosing the right assessment instruments and/or audits based on the needs of the people.[97] Their chapter shows a chart of examples of environmental assessments that have been developed for specific populations (p. 34).[97] An example of a frequently used housing audit with older adults is the Home Falls and Accidents Screening Tool (Home FAST).[69,116] Other assessments developed for use with older adults are the Safety Assessment of Function and the Environment for Rehabilitation (SAFER),[78] the Westmead Home Safety Assessment (WeHSA),[31,32] and, for adults, the Housing Enabler.[56] However, researchers found that commonly used assessments do not address environmental features specific to individuals with vision loss.[18] Another assessment that can be used with older adults is the In-Home Occupational Performance Evaluation, a valid and reliable self-report and performance-based assessment of activity performance in the home, which can be used to examine the person-environment fit.[96] For more information on standardized assessments, see Letts et al.,[62] Anemaet et al.,[13] and Stark et al.[96,98] Recently, a Japanese version of the WeHSA was developed by Hasegawa and Kamimura (2018) to be more applicable to older adults and

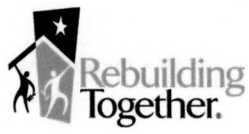

Safe AT HOME
Checklist

Created in partnership with the Administration on Aging and the
American Occupational Therapy Association

Rebuilding Together
1899 L Street NW, Suite 1000
Washington, DC 20036
800-473-4229
www. rebuildingtogether.org

Rebuilding Together has long recognized that greater attention must be given our elderly population, so they may age-in-place and safely in their homes. We have also built lasting national partnerships with Area Agencies on Aging, AARP, American Occupational Therapy Association, National Association of Home Builders, National Council on Aging, and others.

Use this list to identify home safety, fall hazards and accessibility issues for the homeowner and family members. Home safety, fall prevention and accessibility modification interventions on the reverse side of this page can help prioritize your work. Underline or use a highlighter to note. problems and add comments.

1. EXTERIOR ENTRANCES AND EXITS
- ☐ Note condition of walk and drive surface; existence of curb cuts
- ☐ Note handrail condition, right and left sides
- ☐ Note light level for driveway, walk, porch
- ☐ Check door threshold height
- ☐ Note ability to use knob, lock, key, mailbox, peephole, and package shelf
- ☐ Do door and window locks work easily?
- ☐ Are the house numbers visible from the street?
- ☐ Are bushes and shrubs trimmed to allow safe access?
- ☐ Is there a working door bell?

2. INTERIOR DOORS, STAIRS, HALLS
- ☐ Note height of door threshold, knob and hinge types; clear width door opening; determine direction that door swings
- ☐ Note presence of floor level changes
- ☐ Note hall width, adequate for walker/wheelchair
- ☐ Determine stair flight run: straight or curved
- ☐ Note stair rails: condition, right and left side
- ☐ Examine stairway light level
- ☐ Note floor surface texture and contrast
- ☐ Note if clutter on stairway

3. BATHROOM
- ☐ Are sink basin and tub faucets, shower control and drain plugs manageable?
- ☐ Are hot water pipes covered?
- ☐ Is mirror height appropriate, sit and stand?
- ☐ Note ability reach shelf above, below sink basin
- ☐ Note ability to step in and out of the bath and shower
- ☐ Can resident use bath bench in tub or shower?
- ☐ Note toilet height; ability to reach paper; flush; come from sit to stand posture
- ☐ Is space available for caregiver to assist?

4. KITCHEN
- ☐ Note overall light level, task lighting
- ☐ Note sink and counter heights
- ☐ Note wall and floor storage shelf heights
- ☐ Are under sink hot water pipes covered?
- ☐ Is there under counter knee space?
- ☐ Is there a nearby surface to rest hot foods on when removed from oven?
- ☐ Note stove condition and control location (rear or front)
- ☐ Is there adequate counter space to safely prepare meals?

5. LIVING, DINING, BEDROOM
- ☐ Chair, sofa, bed heights allow sitting or standing?
- ☐ Do rugs have non-slip pad or rug tape?
- ☐ Chair available with arm rests?
- ☐ Able to turn on light, radio, TV, place a phone call from bed, chair, and sofa?

6. LAUNDRY
- ☐ Able to hand-wash and hang clothes to dry?
- ☐ Able to safely access washer/dryer?

7. BASEMENT
- ☐ Are the basement stairs stable and welllit?
- ☐ Is there any storage of combustible materials?

8. TELEPHONE AND DOOR
- ☐ Phone jack location near bed, sofa, chair?
- ☐ Able to get phone, dial, hear caller?
- ☐ Able to identify visitors, hear doorbell?
- ☐ Able to reach and empty mailbox?
- ☐ Wears neck/wrist device to obtain emergency help?
- ☐ Is there an answering machine?
- ☐ Is there a wireless phone system?

9. STORAGE SPACE
- ☐ Able to reach closet rods and hooks, open bureau drawers?
- ☐ Is there a light inside the closet?

10. WINDOWS
- ☐ Opening mechanism at 42 inches from floor?
- ☐ Lock accessible, easy to operate?
- ☐ Sill height above floor level?
- ☐ Are storm windows functional?

11. ELECTRIC OUTLETS AND CONTROLS
- ☐ Sufficient outlets?
- ☐ Are there ground fault outlets in kitchen and bathroom?
- ☐ Light switch at the entrance to each room
- ☐ Outlet height, wall locations
- ☐ Low vision/sound warnings available?
- ☐ Extension cord hazard?
- ☐ Are there any uncovered outlets or switches?

12. HEAT, LIGHT, VENTILATION, SMOKE, CARBON MONOXIDE, WATER TEMP CONTROL
- ☐ Are there smoke/CO alarms and a fire extinguisher?
- ☐ Are thermostat displays easily accessible and readable?
- ☐ Note rooms where poor light level exists
- ☐ Able to open windows; slide patio doors?
- ☐ Able to open drapes or curtains?
- ☐ Note last service date for heating/cooling system
- ☐ Observe temperature setting of the water heater

COMMENTS:

_____

_____

_____

_____

_____

_____

Fig. 10.6 Safe at Home Checklist. (Rebuilding Together. Created in partnership with the Administration on Aging and the American Occupational Therapy Association). https://www.aota.org/~/media/Corporate/Files/Practice/Aging/rebuilding-together/RT-Aging-in-Place-Safe-at-Home-Checklist.pdf

Continued

HELP PREVENT FALLS-SAVE A LIFE

> **Safety enhancements, fall prevention and accessibility modification interventions that can help prioritize your work.**

1. EXTERIOR ENTRANCES AND EXITS
- ☐ Increase lighting at entry area
- ☐ Install stair rails on both sides
- ☐ Install door lever handles; double-bolt lock
- ☐ Install beveled, no step, no trip threshold
- ☐ Remove screen or storm door if needed
- ☐ Create surface to place packages when opening door
- ☐ Install peephole on exterior door
- ☐ Repair holes, uneven joints on walkway
- ☐ Provide non-slip finish to walkway surface
- ☐ Add ramp as needed
- ☐ Trim bushes and shrubs to provide clear view from doors and windows
- ☐ Trim low hanging branches

2. INTERIOR DOORS, HALLS, STAIRS
- ☐ Create clear pathways between rooms
- ☐ Apply color contrast or texture change at top and bottom stair edges
- ☐ Install door lever handle
- ☐ Install swing-clear hinges to widen doorway. Minimum width: 32 inches
- ☐ Install beveled thresholds (max 1/2 inch)
- ☐ Replace or add non-slip surface on steps
- ☐ Repair or install stair handrails on both sides

3. BATHROOM
- ☐ Install swing-clear hinges to widen doorway. Minimum width: 32 inches
- ☐ Install secure grab bars at toilet, bath and shower
- ☐ Install adjustable-height, handheld shower head
- ☐ Install non-slip strips in bath/shower
- ☐ Secure floor bathmat with non-slip, double-sided rug tape
- ☐ Adapt flush handle or install flush sensor
- ☐ Adapt or relocate toilet paper dispenser
- ☐ Round counter corners to provide safety
- ☐ Insulate hot water pipes if exposed
- ☐ Create sitting knee clearance at basin by removing vanity door and shelves underneath
- ☐ Install mirror for sitting or standing view
- ☐ Install good-quality non-glare lighting
- ☐ Install shower with no threshold if bathing abilities are severely limited
- ☐ Elevate toilet height by adding under seat riser, portable seat, or raising toilet at the base

4. KITCHEN
- ☐ Increase task lighting at sink, stove, etc.
- ☐ Install D-type cupboard door handles
- ☐ Install adjustable shelving to increase access to upper cabinets
- ☐ Increase access to under counter storage space by installing pull-out units
- ☐ Insulate hot water pipes if exposed
- ☐ Install hot-proof surface near oven
- ☐ Install switches and outlets at front of counter
- ☐ Install pressure-balanced, temperature-regulated, lever faucets
- ☐ Expand counter surface
- ☐ Create sitting knee clearance under work sites by removing doors or shelves
- ☐ Improve color contrast of cabinet and counters surface edges for those with low vision
- ☐ Add tactile and color-contrasted controls for those with low vision
- ☐ Provide sturdy step stool with hand rail
- ☐ Clean or install new range hood

5. LIVING, DINING, BEDROOM
- ☐ Widen or clear pathways within each room by rearranging furniture
- ☐ Secure throw and area rug edges with double-sided tape
- ☐ Improve access to and from chairs and beds by inserting risers under furniture legs
- ☐ Use side bed rail or chairs with armrests
- ☐ Enlarge lamp switch or install touch-control lamp at bedside
- ☐ Install adjustable closet rods, shelving, and light source for better storage access
- ☐ Install vertical pole adjacent to chair and sofa
- ☐ Raise furniture to appropriate height using leg extender products
- ☐ Install uniform level floor surfaces using wood, tile, or low-pile rugs
- ☐ Install telephone jack near bed and favorite chair

6. LAUNDRY
- ☐ Build a counter for sorting and folding clothes
- ☐ Adjust clothesline to convenient height
- ☐ Relocate laundry appliances
- ☐ Clean dryer vent or replace with metallic hose

7. BASEMENT
- ☐ Identify and eliminate sources of water in basement (usually gutters our plumbing)
- ☐ Add additional lighting as needed
- ☐ Remove combustible materials and hazardous waste
- ☐ Clear pathway to utilities

8. TELEPHONE AND DOOR
- ☐ Install wireless phone system near bed, sofa, and chair
- ☐ Install peephole at convenient height
- ☐ Install flashing light or sound amplifier to indicate ringing doorbell for those with visual or hearing problems
- ☐ Install mailbox at accessible height

9. STORAGE SPACE
- ☐ Install lights inside closet
- ☐ Install adjustable closet rods and shelves
- ☐ Install bi-fold or pocket doors

10. WINDOWS
- ☐ Install handles and locks that are easy to grip, placed at appropriate heights
- ☐ Replace windows or storms that are not functional

11. ELECTRICAL OUTLETS AND CONTROLS
- ☐ Install light fixtures or outlet for lamps
- ☐ Install switches at top and bottom of stairs
- ☐ Install ground fault outlets in kitchen and bathroom
- ☐ Install wireless light switches where needed

12. HEAT, AIR, LIGHT, SMOKE, CARBON MONOXIDE, WATER TEMP CONTROLS
- ☐ Install smoke/CO alarms, fire extinguishers
- ☐ Replace thermostat with easy to read programmable type
- ☐ Order service for heating/AC system
- ☐ Install compact florescent lightswhere appropriate
- ☐ Reduce hot water temperature to 120 degrees

COMMENTS:

_____

_____

_____

_____

_____

_____

_____

_____

_____

_____

_____

_____

Fig. 10.6 cont'd

their homes in Japan, where 49 of the original 72 items in the original version of the assessment were found to have fair to good or excellent reliability and validity.[52]

Financial Management

If the client is to resume management of money and financial matters independently, a cognitive and perceptual assessment that accurately tests these skills should be implemented. Because some persons with physical disabilities have concurrent involvement of cognition and perception, the level of impairment should be determined. The occupational therapist evaluates the methods and routines the client typically implements for financial management. For example, one client may pay each bill as it arrives by writing a check, whereas another client may pay bills once a month online. The skills needed for each are different and require different levels of organization. As with any other performance area, the occupational therapist will break down the activity into small tasks and focus treatment on building skills for each component of the task. Caregivers may require training if the role of financial manager is new and must be assumed. In the case of Mrs. Hayes, she is having cognitive deficits and handwriting difficulties. She may need to teach her husband how to manage bill paying, or they may choose to work together. The client may be capable of handling only small amounts of money or may need retraining in activities that require money management, such as shopping, balancing a checkbook, or making a budget. If a physical limitation is involved, the therapist may introduce adaptive writing devices or practice skills, such as handling coins or bills, taking a wallet out of the pocket, and calculating appropriate tips for service provided. If a client uses a smartphone or mobile device, digital payments may be an advisable option with careful consideration of a client's motor, process, and social interaction skills and activity demands in specific contexts. When a client experiences significant changes in ability to manage finances independently, occupational therapists must be vigilant for signs of financial abuse and report to relevant parties. A social worker should be notified if a client is cognitively unable to manage finances and has no reliable support and therefore is at risk of financial abuse.

Community Mobility

The OTPF-4 classifies community mobility as an IADL and includes the use of public or private transportation such as walking, driving, riding the bus, taking a taxi, riding a train, and traveling by airplane or any number of other transportation systems.[12] Wesselhoff et al., found that people who have had a stroke may experience a significant decrease in community mobility, which affects independence.[122] Occupational therapists with advanced training and experience can specialize in the area of adaptive driving (see Chapter 11), but occupational therapists in all areas of practice need to address community mobility. The ability to maneuver in the community opens up doors for access to many other occupations.[100,101] Lack of access can close the door, preventing many people from participating in all the other occupations, such as work, education, play, leisure, and social participation. A study by Metz found that mobility in the

community can contribute to positive health outcomes physically, psychologically, socially, and with overall life satisfaction.[73]

The occupational therapist evaluates the client's potential to participate in the community under circumstances in which some type of community mobility is required. Zahoransky categorized community mobility in these ways[130]:

- Walking with or without the use of an ambulation aid, such as a cane or walker. A study by Lynott and Figueiredo[65] found that walking is second to driving a private automobile as the preferred way for older adults to be mobile in the community.
- Using wheeled mobility devices (e.g., bicycle, motorcycle)
- Using a powered device (e.g., power wheelchair or scooter)
- Riding as a passenger, with a family member, friend, or caregiver as primary transport
- Driving oneself in a vehicle that may or may not be adapted (see Chapter 11)
- Using public transportation (e.g., taxi, bus, van, subway, airplane, or other transit system)

The occupational therapist must assess the client's physical, perceptual, cognitive, functional, and social capabilities to be independent and safe with community mobility. The occupational therapist should be familiar with the environment in which the client lives and accesses the community, and the therapist also should be aware of available resources, such as special parking placards and how to obtain them, adaptive driving programs, and types of transportation available.[130]

Examples of physical capabilities to be considered are whether the client has the endurance to be safely mobile in the community and whether they can safely use assistive devices (e.g., a walker, cane, crutch, or wheelchair) and perform transfers needed to go beyond the home environment. Wheelchair mobility skills include managing uneven pavement, curbs, and inclines and crossing the street. Other functional skills the occupational therapist must evaluate that influence community mobility are handling money, carrying objects in a wheelchair or with other assistive devices, and managing toileting in a public restroom.

Cognitive skills include geographic and topographic orientation, reading a schedule and a map or knowing how to get directions, and problem solving or obtaining help if an issue arises.

If the disability is new, the client may need to develop new social skills or relearn old skills with modifications. Assertive or confident behaviors, such as requesting an accessible table at a restaurant, obtaining assistance with unreachable items in the grocery store, becoming comfortable with a new body image in the community, and asking for help when needed, can be daunting for a person who is newly disabled.

Visuo-spatial skills are critical to safety in judging distance such as stepping down from a curb, driving a car, and maneuvering a wheelchair on a narrow sidewalk. The visual-spatial skills are identified during an evaluation and considered in relation to the cognitive, physical, and functional deficits the client exhibits. Some individuals have awareness of their deficits and compensate well. Others are not aware of the deficits or have difficulty with devising or remembering compensatory strategies and therefore will require greater supervision with community mobility than others.

The occupational therapist should also assess the client's community environment, such as security, terrain, availability of curb cutouts, travel distance, location of bus and train stations, duration of traffic lights, and availability of help if needed. For Anna, her place of worship is important, so this could be an area that should be assessed. Accessibility of worship space is not mandatory according to the ADA, but inclusion is a basic part of worship in synagogues, temples, mosques, churches.[89] Shamberg and Kidd provided a useful checklist in their article for basic worship space accessibility that would be helpful for Anna and others in her church.[89]

Accessibility of public transportation should be considered. Some communities have door-to-door cab and van services, which have certain restrictions or set protocols. Some of these restrictions include the need to arrange transportation a week in advance, the ability to get out the front door and to the curb independently, and the ability to transfer independently into the vehicle. If clients are to use a public bus, they must learn how to use the electric lifts or be aware that buses can lower for access and they need to know how to ask for help to lock a wheelchair into place. Because not all bus stops are wheelchair accessible, the neighboring bus stops should be surveyed. Since 2017 ridehailing services, which require use of smartphones to use taxi-type services have proliferated and are more commonly used by younger people with higher income and those living in more dense, metropolitan areas.[123] It is important for the occupational therapist to consider whether the recommended transportation mechanism is appropriate based on comfort, affordability, and accessibility to those services.

HEALTH MANAGEMENT

Health management and maintenance include the client's ability to develop, manage, and maintain routines to promote health and wellness.[12] The client's abilities in the practical aspects of health management must be assessed, including the ability to maintain fitness and an adequate nutrition and fluid intake, avoid unhealthy behaviors, obtain adequate sleep, handle medications, implement public health recommendations, and know when to call a healthcare provider and how to make a medical appointment. The evaluation of the client's ability to perform these activities may be completed by the occupational therapist but will probably include other team members, such as a nurse, primary care provider, dietician (for proper nutrition and hydration), or social worker. Caregivers and family members may also need to be involved in this area. Sanders and Van Oss found in their study of 149 community-living older adults that 51% of the sample required some type of social support to take medications.[85,112] Most of the help involved verbal reminders and assistance with picking up or arranging for refills.[112] The information provided by the occupational therapist's evaluation of the client's cognition, visual perception, and physical abilities can greatly enhance the skilled nurse's ability to use appropriate interventions and strategies when teaching medication management to the client. Assessment tools such as the In-Home Medication Management Performance Evaluation (HOME-Rx), developed by Somerville et al. have been found to be a valid and reliable performance-based tool for occupational therapists to measure an older adult's medication management ability, which can guide treatment planning and improve performance in this area.[92]

The occupational therapy assessment can be helpful in determining which aspects of the task need to be modified for the client to be independent. For example, the occupational therapist can work jointly with a nurse to ensure that a client with hemiplegia and diabetes can manage insulin shots. The occupational therapy evaluation considers the client's cognitive and perceptual abilities to make judgments about drawing the insulin out of the bottle, measuring the insulin, and injecting the insulin. Physical concerns include how to stabilize the insulin bottle, accurately see the measurement, and handle the syringe with one hand. Another example might involve determining the best strategies for a client using eye drops to open the container and measure and dispense the correct amount of medication into the eye. Sanders and Van Oss found that 91% in their study of older adults used timing of activities to remember to take medications.[85] Of the participants, 71% planned medications around mealtimes and 52% around wake or bedtimes.[85] Because the occupational therapist usually questions clients about their ADLs and IADLs routines, the connection of commonly performed activities with timing of the taking of medication can be a valuable strategy for some clients. The researchers also found that 64% of the older adults in their study embedded medication use around breakfast, 40% around morning hygiene, and 33% around evening hygiene. Weekly routines (e.g., loading pillboxes on Sundays) and monthly routines were also used to help with medications. Interestingly, it was noted that although physicians recommended that their clients use charts to track medication usage, fewer than 10% did so.[85,112]

The occupational therapist may evaluate and train the client in other skills that affect health management. Examples include using the phone, finding the appropriate phone numbers, and providing the needed information to make a medical appointment. During public health crises like the COVID-19 pandemic, an occupational therapist may consider a client's ability to access information about local public health mandates, to don appropriate protective equipment like face masks, and to obtain basic needs such as food or medicine if business operations change.

Because she has paraplegia, Anna's new health management and maintenance routine may include performing regular skin checks and weight shifts to prevent decubiti (pressure sores) from developing. An occupational therapist can help Anna obtain necessary adaptive aids and devise strategies to ensure good skin health. Considering that many lifestyle factors can affect skin integrity, OT practitioners are well suited to assist clients such as Anna in this area.[46]

Health maintenance is an issue for the client and the entire healthcare team. The occupational therapist plays an important role because of the scope of the ADL and IADL assessments, which may identify and help resolve problems related to health maintenance.

ADL AND IADL TRAINING

If it is determined after an assessment that ADL and IADL training are to be initiated, it is important to establish appropriate short- and long-term goals, based on the assessment and on the client's priorities and potential for independence.

The occupational therapist should estimate which ADL and IADL tasks are possible and which are not within the client's potential to achieve. The therapist should explore with the client the use of alternative methods of performing the activities, environmental modifications to support safety and independence, and the use of any assistive devices that may be helpful.

The ADL and IADL training program may begin with simple tasks and gradually increase in complexity.

Methods of Teaching ADLs

The occupational therapist must tailor methods of teaching the client to perform daily living tasks to suit each client's learning ability. The client who is alert and grasps instructions quickly may be able to perform an entire process after a brief demonstration and oral instruction. Clients who have perceptual problems, poor memory, and difficulty following instructions of any kind need a more concrete, step-by-step approach in which the amount of assistance is gradually reduced as success is achieved. For these clients it may be important to break down the activity into small steps and progress through them slowly. A demonstration of the task or step by the therapist in the same plane and in the same manner in which the client is expected to perform it can be helpful. Accompanying the demonstration with oral instructions may or may not be helpful, depending on the client's receptive language skills and ability to process and integrate two modes of sensory information simultaneously.

Evidence suggests that a variety of interventions may be effective in helping people with cognitive deficits after a CVA and that a focus on use of "authentic occupations" in the clinic were more effective than contrived cognitive activities.[47] A review of the literature by Gillen et al.[48] showed some correlation in the use of "gesture training" on measures of functional independence in ADLs for people with apraxia as described by Smania et al.[91]; cognitive strategy training, such as internal rehearsal, verbalizing actions while executing ADLs, and external cueing, may also help. In general, the review suggested that the literature supports a performance focus and use of strategy training techniques and compensatory techniques as being effective in treating clients with CVA-related cognitive impairment.[48]

Physical cueing, such as passive movement of the part through the desired pattern to achieve a step or a task, and gentle manual guidance through the task are helpful tactile and kinesthetic modes of instruction. These techniques can augment or replace demonstration and oral instruction, depending on the client's best avenues of learning. It is necessary to perform a step or complete a task repeatedly to achieve skill and speed and to have a task that is currently declarative learning (consciously knowing what to do) become automatic/procedural learning (unconsciously knowing how to do it). Tasks may be repeated several times during the same training session if time

and the client's physical and emotional tolerance allow, or they may be repeated daily until the desired retention or level of skill is achieved.

Other methods of teaching include forward and backward chaining. As Batra and Batra[19] pointed out, forward chaining is a concept first described by B. F. Skinner in relation to operant conditioning (reinforcement or punishment to change behavior). In this technique, tasks ("chains") are broken down into serial steps and then taught from first step to last step. In backward chaining, the task is taught in reverse chronological order. Forward or backward chaining can be used to teach ADLs skills. An example of forward chaining for the ADL of putting on a sock may be having a client practicing holding a sock open, then the occupational therapist finishing the rest of the task if the client gets stuck. After that step has been mastered, the client may place the sock over the toes and, eventually, pull up the whole sock. In backward chaining, the therapist assists the client until the last step of the process is reached. The client then performs this last step independently. In the sock example, when training starts, the therapist helps the client perform the early steps of keeping the sock open, putting on the toes, and then the foot, and then the heel of the sock. The client then pulls up the sock past the ankle and masters that step. The process continues, with the therapist offering less and less assistance and the client performing successive steps of the task, from last to first ("backward"), until the client can perform the whole task from start to finish. In their small study of children in India who had intellectual disabilities, Batra and Batra found that forward and backward chaining techniques were equally effective for ADLs training (putting on socks or tying shoelaces).[19] Most likely, occupational therapists use both methods, sometimes in the same session.

Before beginning training in any ADL, the occupational therapist must prepare by providing adequate space and arranging equipment, materials, and furniture for maximal safety and convenience; this serves as an example to the client of using work simplification and energy conservation techniques. The OT practitioner should be familiar with the task to be performed and any special methods or assistive devices that will be used in its performance. The occupational therapist should be able to perform (or should know how to perform) the task as skillfully as they expect the client to perform it. After preparation, the activity is presented to the client, usually in one or more of the modes of guidance, demonstration, and oral instruction described earlier. The occupational therapist ensures the appropriate environmental setup for success and safety. For example, a chair with arms or a safely locked wheelchair may be provided to start. The client's feet are placed flat on the floor (or, if a wheelchair is used, on the footplates). Personal care items are located within safe reaching distance when the client is initially learning an activity. The client then performs the activity either along with the occupational therapist or immediately after being shown, with the required amount of supervision and assistance. Performance is modified and corrected as needed, and the process is repeated to ensure learning.

Because other staff or family members are frequently reinforcing the newly learned skills, staff and family training is critical to reinforce learning and ensure that the client carries over the skills from previous treatment sessions. The therapist should check performance in progress and later arrange to check on the adequacy of performance and carryover of learning with the client, the nursing personnel, the caregiver, or the supervising family members.

Recording Progress in ADL Performance

The ADL checklists used to record performance on the initial assessment usually have one or more spaces for recording changes in abilities and the results of reassessment during the training process. The sample checklist shown earlier in this chapter (see Fig. 10.1) is designed and completed for illustration purposes using Mrs. Hayes' information. If a standardized assessment is used during the initial evaluation, it should be used in the reevaluation process to objectively measure the level of progress the client has attained.

Progress is usually summarized for inclusion in the medical record. The progress record should summarize skilled services provided by treating occupational therapists, changes in the client's abilities and current level of independence and should also estimate the client's potential for further independence, attitude, motivation for ADL training, and future goals for the ADL program. The information about the client's level of assistance needed for ADLs and IADLs will help with the discharge planning. For example, if clients continue to require moderate assistance with self-care, they may need to hire a personal care attendant, or the occupational therapist may justify ongoing treatment if the client has potential for further independence.

Assistive Technology and Adaptive Equipment

The terms *assistive technology, adaptive equipment*, and *assistive devices* are generally used interchangeably throughout the profession. An assistive technology (AT) device is defined in the Assistive Technology Act of 2004 as "any item, piece of equipment, or product system whether acquired commercially off the shelf, modified, or customized that is used to increase, maintain, or improve functional capabilities of individuals with disabilities."[105,107] When considering the aging global population and noncommunicable diseases, the World Health Organization approximates over 2 billion people will require at least one assistive device by 2030.[124]

Adaptive equipment is used to compensate for a physical limitation, to promote safety, and to prevent injury. Electronic aids to daily living (EADLs) provide a bridge between an individual with limited function and an electrical device such as a door operator,[102] even devices used to manage chronic conditions (e.g., blood pressure monitors).[128] Physical limitations necessitating the use of these aids may include a loss of muscle strength, loss of ROM, incoordination, or sensory loss. An example of using adaptive equipment to improve safety is the use of a bed or door alarm to alert a caregiver that a client with impaired cognition and poor balance is getting out of bed or wandering. The use of adaptive equipment to prevent joint injury is indicated for the person with rheumatoid arthritis (e.g., an eating utensil with a built-up handle). Occupational

therapists in general practice assess the need for and recommend adaptive equipment and technology on a regular basis. Occupational therapists can also specialize in this area and obtain further education and certifications, such as Assistive Technology Professional (ATP), a credential granted by the Rehab Engineering and Assistive Technology Society of North America (RESNA) (https://www.resna.org).[81]

Before recommending a piece of adaptive equipment, the OT practitioner must complete a thorough assessment to determine the client's functional problems and the causes of the problems. The OT practitioner may also consider other solutions first, before settling on adaptive equipment as the solution, which at first may seem like a quick and easy fix. Some practical solutions would be to avoid the cause of the problem, use a compensatory technique or alternative method, get assistance from another person, or modify the environment. Typical of these considerations is the case of Mr. Rojas (discussed in the case study that follows). The environment was adapted, wheelchair positioning and setup were adapted, and compensatory strategies were used, instead of just the provision of adaptive equipment.

Other factors to consider in the selection of adaptive equipment are whether the disability is short or long term, the client's tolerance for gadgets, the client's feelings about the device, and the cost and upkeep of the equipment.

Offering good suggestions and sound advice on improving engagement in occupations is within the domain of occupational therapy and is an important responsibility; however, these good qualities, in and of themselves, may not actually mean use of the strategies provided by the therapist. In a study of 154 community-dwelling, functionally vulnerable adults over 70 years old, Chee looked at modifiable factors that can influence the use of adaptive strategies.[27] These adaptive strategies, offered mainly by occupational therapists and physical therapists, comprised environmental strategies (assistive technology, home modifications) or behavioral strategies (energy conservation, performance techniques). The researcher looked at sociodemographic information, functional status, perceived importance of learning new strategies, and degree of readiness to change or adapt to functional decline. "Readiness" was defined as the extent to which a study participant acknowledged a functional deficit and demonstrated or showed a willingness to change or modify the environment. The study's findings concurred with those of other studies; that is, that individuals with a higher stage of "readiness" are more likely to use home environmental adaptations than those who are not ready. Chee suggested that environmental strategy adherence could be improved by enhancing the readiness of older adults through education, problem solving, and more opportunities to practice. The study targeted older adults, but the results suggested that an intervention process–related variable (e.g., readiness) may affect the acceptability of therapeutic strategies offered by therapists to other clinical populations. Another finding was that living arrangements of the participants significantly predicted adherence to behavioral strategies offered. Participants who lived alone demonstrated higher use of prescribed behavioral strategies than those who lived with others.[27]

CASE STUDY

Mr. Rojas

Mr. Rojas is 75 years old and lives in a nursing home. The occupational therapist received a referral for a self-feeding assessment because he has recently lost weight, and the nursing aides have reported that he needs assistance with eating. The nurse mentioned that he thought Mr. Rojas needed a utensil with a built-up handle to feed himself.

The occupational therapy assessment included an interview with Mr. Rojas, observation of him eating lunch in his usual location (in his room with the use of an over-bed table while seated in his wheelchair), physical assessment (including strength, ROM, sensation, and coordination), and gross cognitive and perceptual assessments. Mr. Rojas stated that he would like to be able to feed himself because he likes to eat his food when it is hot, and he likes to be as independent as possible. The results indicated that Mr. Rojas had problems with sitting properly in his wheelchair. The over-bed table was too high and limited his ability to reach the plate. His strength, ROM, coordination, and sensation were within normal limits, except that bilateral shoulder flexors and abductors were F− (3−/5). Mr. Rojas' cognition and perception were adequate to relearn simple self-care tasks.

Treatment involved working on wheelchair positioning, lowering the over-bed table, and then teaching the client how to use a compensatory technique of elbow propping to bring his hand to his mouth during eating. The occupational therapy assessment did not indicate a need for adaptive equipment at this time; instead, the environment was adapted, wheelchair positioning modified, and a compensatory method taught.

If the results of the assessment had indicated that Mr. Rojas had a weak grasp or hand incoordination, a utensil with a built-up handle and plate guard might have been used to promote independence with self-feeding. In either case, a treating occupational therapist would summarize findings to the referring party and complete any necessary training with nursing staff to update Mr. Rojas' care plan.

SPECIFIC ADL AND IADL TECHNIQUES

In many instances specific techniques to solve specific ADL problems are not possible. Sometimes the occupational therapist has to explore a variety of methods or assistive devices to reach a solution. It is occasionally necessary for the therapist to design a special device, method, orthotic, or piece of equipment to make a particular activity possible for the client to perform. Many of the assistive devices available today were first conceived of and made by occupational therapists and clients. Special methods used to perform specific activities also evolved through the trial-and-error approaches of therapists and their clients. Clients often have good suggestions for therapists because they live with the limitation and are confronted regularly with the need to adapt the performance of daily tasks.

The purpose of the following summary of techniques is to give the reader some ideas about how to solve ADL and IADL problems for specific classifications of dysfunction. The focus is on compensatory strategies involving changing the method in which an activity is performed, changing the environment, or using an assistive device. If the client has the potential for improvement of specific deficits, treatment that includes remediation and restoration should be considered. For example, if a client has hand weakness as a result of a fracture of his hand, the therapist may offer alternative methods and adaptive equipment to manage until strength improves, but hand strengthening also should be a component of the treatment program, assuming there are no contraindications. Ideally, every suggestion provided should be actually tried with a client before recommendations are made.

In the following chapter sections, recommended techniques are summarized for individuals with these physical deficits:

- Limited ROM or strength
- Incoordination
- Hemiplegia or use of only one UE
- Paraplegia
- Quadriplegia
- Low vision (low vision is addressed in Chapter 24)
- Exceptionally large size body (bariatric population)
- These ADLs and IADLs are addressed for each of the physical deficits previously listed:
- Dressing activities
- Feeding activities (eating and swallowing are addressed in Chapter 27)
- Personal hygiene and grooming activities
- Communication management and environmental adaptations
- Functional mobility (transfers and wheelchair mobility are addressed in Chapter 11)
- Home management, meal preparation, and cleanup activities

ADLs for the Person With Limited Range of Motion or Strength

The major problem for persons with limited joint ROM is compensating for the lack of reach and joint excursion through such means as environmental adaptation and assistive devices. Individuals who lack muscle strength may require some of the same devices or techniques to compensate and to conserve energy. Some adaptations and devices are outlined here.[9,84]

Lower Extremity Dressing Activities

1. Use one of many commercially available dressing sticks with a plastic-coated coat hook on one end and a small hook on the other for pushing and pulling garments (e.g., underwear, pants) off and on the feet and legs.
2. To put on socks, use one of many different commercially available models of sock aides (Fig. 10.7). To take off socks, use a reacher (Fig. 10.8).
3. Eliminate the need to bend to tie shoelaces or to use finger joints in this fine motor activity by using elastic shoelaces or other adapted shoe fasteners (e.g., Velcro-fastened shoes or secure slip-on shoes).
4. Use reachers (see Fig. 10.8) to pick up socks and shoes, arrange clothes, remove clothes from hangers, pick up objects on the floor, and put on and take off pants.

Upper Extremity Dressing Activities

1. Use front-opening garments that are one size larger than needed and made of fabrics that have some stretch.
2. Use dressing sticks to push a shirt or blouse over the head.
3. Use larger buttons or zippers with a loop on the pull-tab.
4. Replace buttons, snaps, and hooks and eyes with Velcro or zippers (clients who cannot manage traditional fastenings).

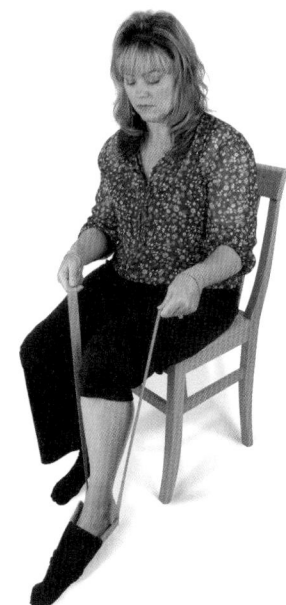

Fig. 10.7 Easy-Pull Sock Aid. (Courtesy North Coast Medical, Gilroy, CA.)

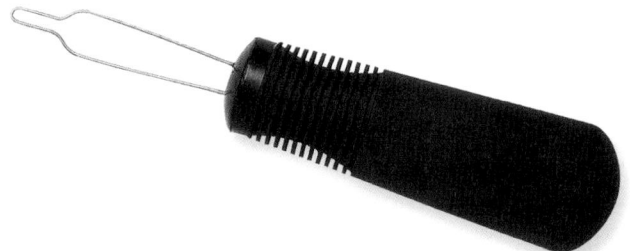

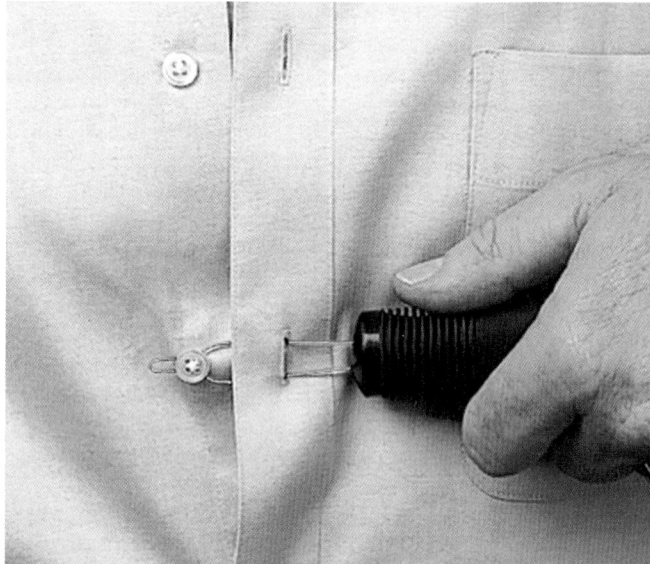

Fig. 10.9 Buttonhook with built-up handle. (Courtesy North Coast Medical, Gilroy, CA.)

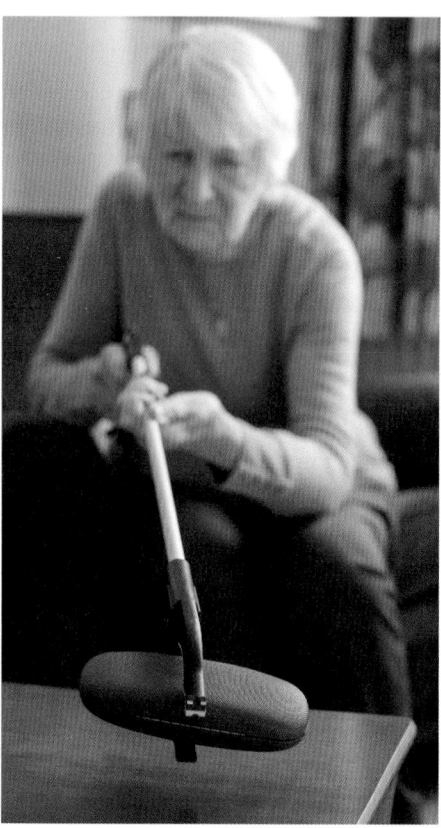

Fig. 10.8 Extended-handle reacher. (iStock.com/Daisy-Daisy. ID: 9414-20734).

5. Use one of several types of commercially available button-hooks (Fig. 10.9) if finger ROM or strength is limited or unavailable.
6. A front opening or Velcro replacements for the usual hook-and-eye fasteners may make it easier to put on and remove a bra. Slipover, stretchable bras (which may be called sleep bras or comfort bras) or a bra-slip combination also may

eliminate the need to manage fastenings. Regular bras may be fastened in front at waist level, then slipped around to the back and the arms put into the straps, which are then worked up over the shoulders. Bra band extenders may be suggested. An ambulatory person with narrow hips, good balance, and leg ROM but poor UE ROM may find it easier to put on a bra by clasping the bra, putting the bra on the floor, stepping into it, and pulling it up over the hips onto the chest.
7. Quilted vests with armhole openings that are large (but not so large they get caught on things) are easier to put on and take off than jackets for those with shoulder ROM limitations.

Feeding Activities
1. Use built-up handles on eating utensils that can accommodate limited grasp or prehension (grip or pinch pattern) (Fig. 10.10).
2. Elongated or specially curved handles on spoons and forks may be needed to reach the mouth. A swivel spoon or spoon-fork combination can compensate for limited forearm supination (see Fig. 10.10).
3. Long plastic straws and straw clips on glasses or cups can be used if neck, elbow, or shoulder ROM limits hand-to-mouth motion or if grasp is inadequate to hold the cup or glass.
4. Universal cuffs (Fig. 10.11) or utensil holders can be used if grasp is very limited and built-up handles are not sufficient. Notice that the utensil sleeve is placed so that the tool to be used is put in the palm of the hand, not on the top of the hand.

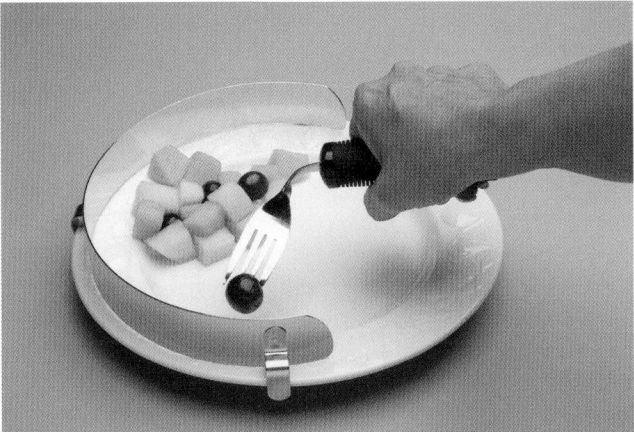

Fig. 10.10 Fork with built-up handle and swivel. (Courtesy North Coast Medical, Gilroy, CA.)

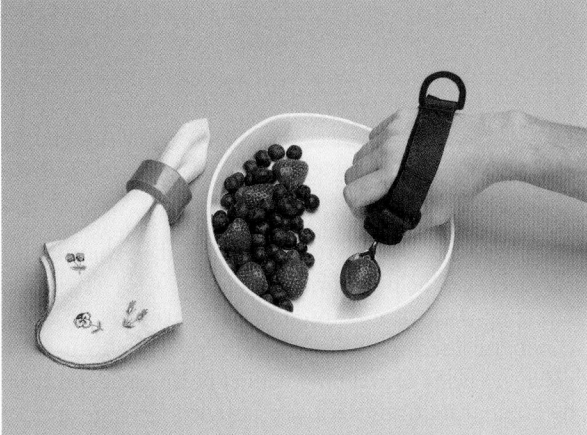

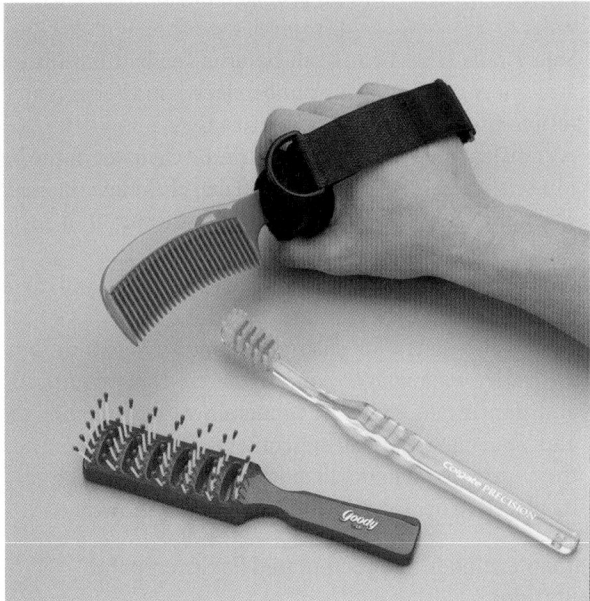

Fig. 10.11 Universal cuff. (Courtesy North Coast Medical, Gilroy, CA.)

5. Plate guards or scoop dishes may be useful to prevent food from slipping off the plate (see Fig. 10.10).
6. Cups with nose cutouts may be useful to persons who have limited neck ROM or who may be wearing a neck brace (Fig. 10.12).

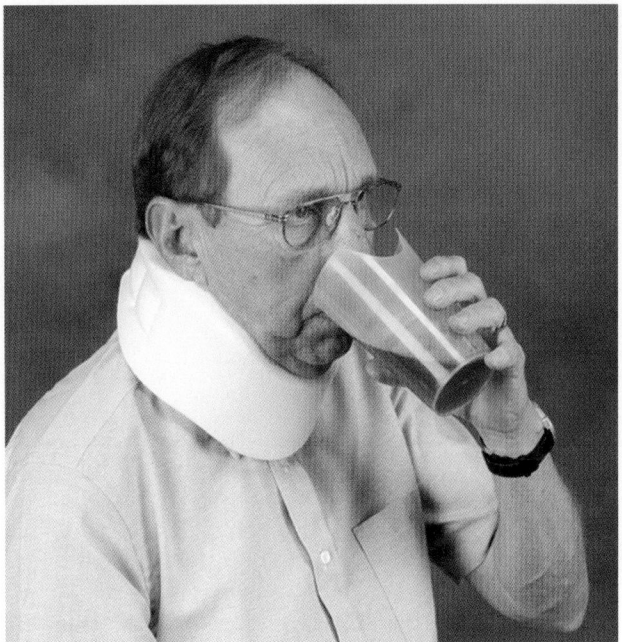

Fig. 10.12 Nose cutout tumbler. (Courtesy North Coast Medical, Gilroy, CA.)

Personal Hygiene and Grooming Activities

1. A handheld flexible shower hose for bathing and shampooing hair can eliminate the need to stand in the shower and offers the user control of the direction of the spray. The handle can be built up or adapted for limited grasp.
2. A long-handled bath brush or sponge with a soap holder (Fig. 10.13) or a long cloth scrubber can allow the user to reach the legs, feet, and back. A wash mitt (Fig. 10.14) and soap on a rope can aid limited grasp. For the economically minded, bar soap can be placed in a cutoff leg of light-colored pantyhose and tied to the bath chair to eliminate the need to bend to pick up soap. If reach is limited to wash the hair, a soft rubber brush with extended handle or specially designed long-handled adaptive aid can be used to shampoo the hair.
3. A wall-mounted hair dryer or one on a stand may be helpful. This device is useful for clients with limited ROM, UE weakness, incoordination, or hemiplegia. The dryer is mounted (wall or stand) to allow the user to manage the hair with one arm or to position himself or herself to compensate for limited ROM.[37]
4. Long handles on a comb, brush, toothbrush, lipstick, mascara brush, and safety or electric razor may be useful for clients with limited hand-to-head or hand-to-face movements. Extensions may be constructed from inexpensive wooden dowels or lengths of various diameter polyvinyl chloride (PVC) pipe found in hardware stores. The handles can be built up or adapted for limited grasp.
5. Pump deodorant, hair spray, and spray powder or perfume can extend the reach by the distance the material sprays.
6. Electric toothbrushes and a Water-Pik may be easier to manage than a standard toothbrush; each may need to be adapted for limited grasp.
7. A short reacher (or kitchen tongs) can extend reach for using toilet paper. Several types of toilet aids are available

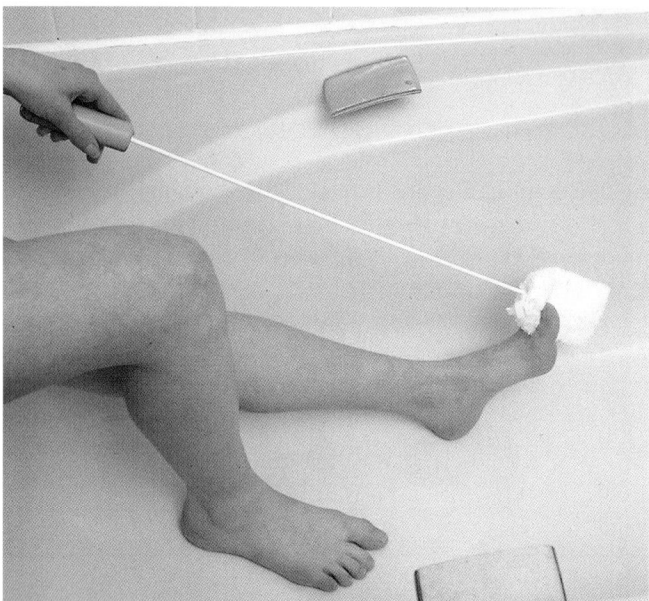

Fig. 10.13 Long-handled brush. (Courtesy Patterson Medical, Warrenville, IL.)

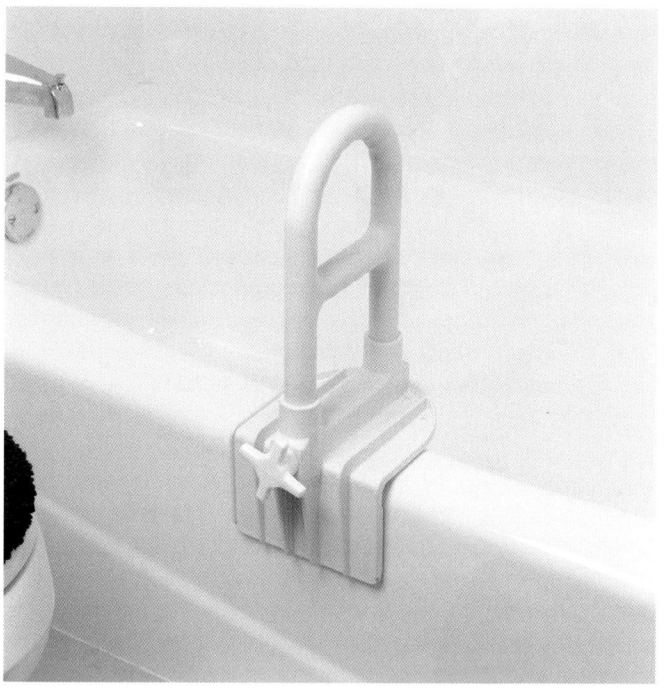

Fig. 10.15 Tub safety rail. (Courtesy North Coast Medical, Gilroy, CA.)

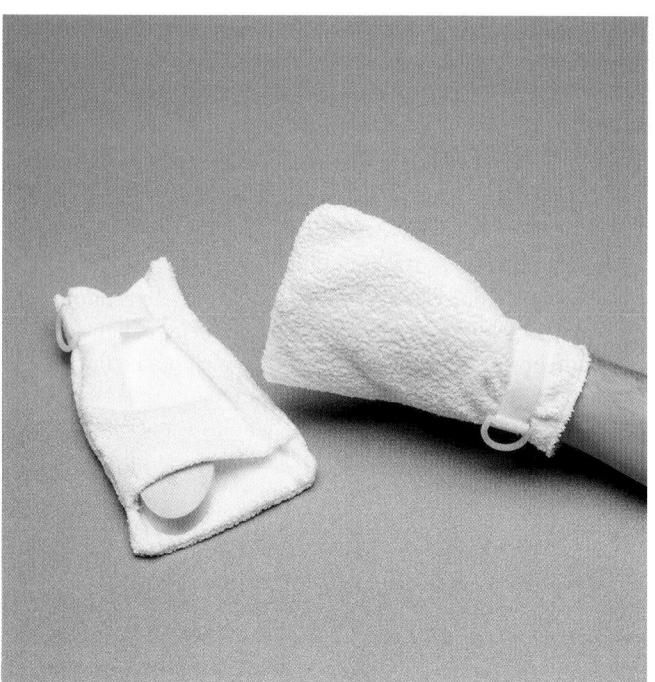

Fig. 10.14 Bath mitt. (Courtesy North Coast Medical, Gilroy, CA.)

in catalogs that sell assistive devices. Bidets can be used to help with perineal cleansing; more expensive products, such as the Toto Washlet, can help wash (variable temperature settings) and dry the area while providing a warm seat. Squeeze bottles with water may be sufficient for some who have limited ROM to reach their backside to wipe. Products such as the One-Drop Powerful Deodorizer can be a portable way for those with weak pinch strength to get rid of offensive odors.

8. If the shoulder cannot be raised enough to allow removal of hair from the underarms with a razor or wax, an epilator hair removal system (e.g., Epilady rechargeable hair remover) can help perform this task.

9. Dressing sticks can be used to pull garments up after the client has used the toilet. An alternative is to use a long piece of elastic or webbing with clips on each end that can be hung around the neck and fastened to pants or panties, preventing them from slipping to the floor during use of the toilet.

10. Safety rails (Fig. 10.15) can be used for bathtub transfers, and safety mats or strips can be placed on the bathtub bottom to prevent slipping.

11. A transfer tub bench, shower stool, or chair set in the bathtub or shower stall (see Fig. 10.5) can eliminate the need to sit on the bathtub bottom or stand to shower, thus increasing safety.

12. Grab bars can be installed to prevent falls and to ease transfers.

13. Pump dispensers for shampoo, conditioners, and lotions are easier to manage than containers that require lifting and pouring of contents. If containers that require lifting and pouring are used, the contents should be transferred from larger containers to smaller ones, and objects should be placed in an accessible location in the shower.

Communication Management and Environmental Adaptations

1. Extended built-up or lever handles on faucets can accommodate limited grasp.

2. Telephones should be placed within easy reach, or cordless phones can be used and kept with the client. A speakerphone or headset may be necessary. Phones with large push buttons or voice-activated phones may be helpful if individual finger movements are difficult or not possible. Mobile phones

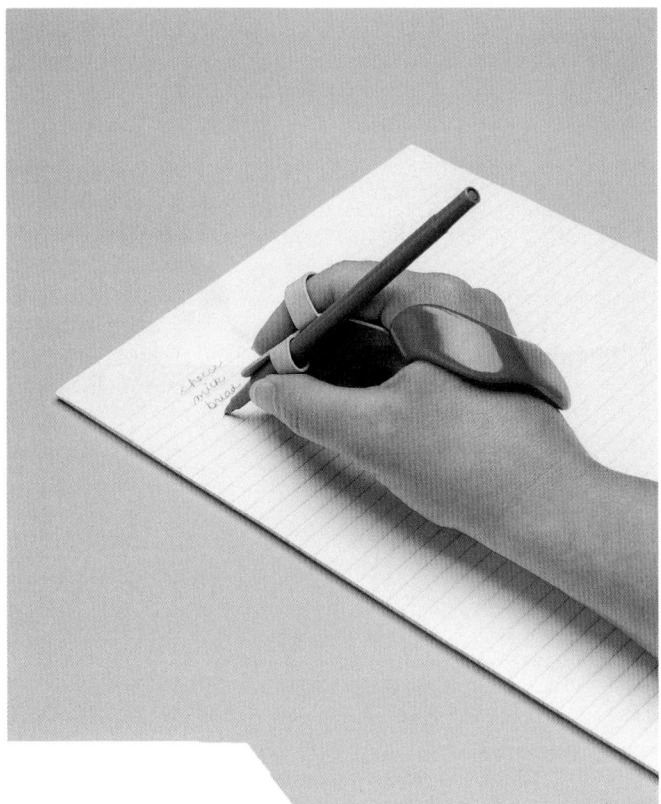

Fig. 10.16 Wanchik writer. (Courtesy North Coast Medical, Gilroy, CA.)

paired with Bluetooth devices can be used for hands-free, voice-activated answering and calling.

3. Built-up pens and pencils can be used to accommodate limited grasp and prehension. A Wanchik writer (Fig. 10.16) and several other commercially available or custom-fabricated writing aids also can be used.

4. Personal computers, word processors, voice recognition computer software, book holders, and electronic books can facilitate communication for those with limited or painful joints.

5. Lever-type doorknob extensions (Fig. 10.17), commercially available lever-style doorknobs, adapted car door openers, doors with push-button combination locks, and adapted key holders can compensate for hand ROM and strength limitations.

Functional Mobility

The individual who has limited ROM and may have some generalized weakness, but no significant muscle weakness, may benefit from the following assistive devices.

1. Platform crutches can prevent stress on hand or finger joints and can accommodate limited grasp. Confer with the PT about this option because platform crutches may increase the weight and size of the walking aid and may actually be a detriment to the client's gait or may increase pressure on the shoulder.

2. Enlarged grips on crutches, canes, and walkers can accommodate limited grasp. Confer with the PT about this option.

3. A raised toilet seat can be used if hip and knee motion is limited.

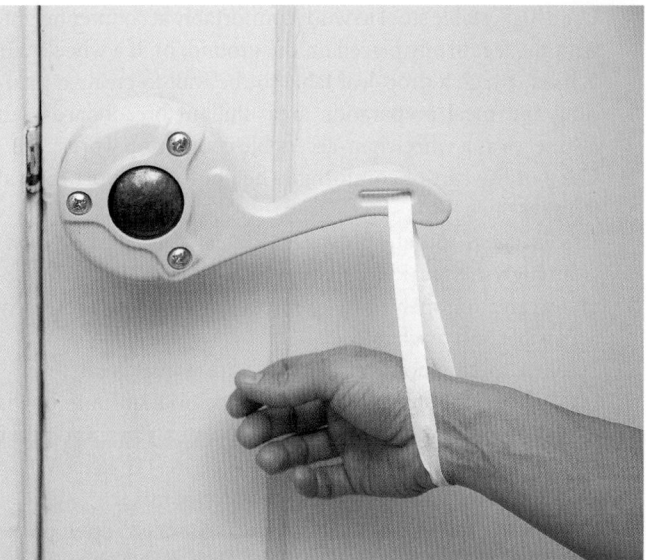

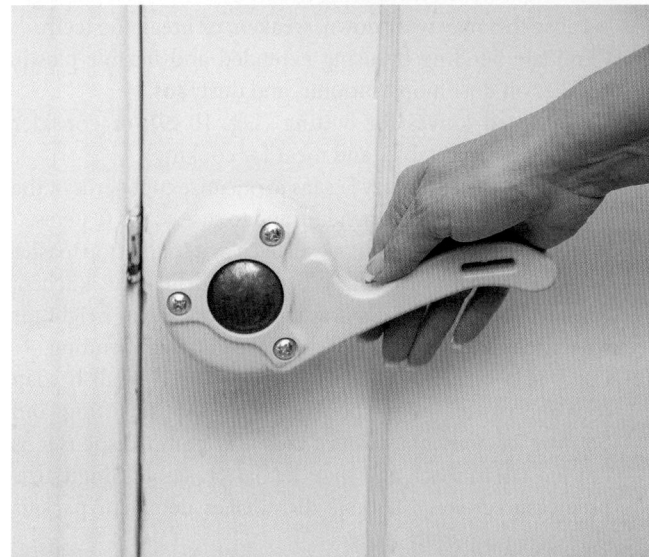

Fig. 10.17 Doorknob extension. (Courtesy North Coast Medical, Gilroy, CA.)

4. A walker with padded grips and forearm troughs can be used if marked hand, forearm, or elbow joint limitations are present. Confer with the PT about this option.

5. A walker or crutch bag, tray, or basket can facilitate the carrying of objects.

Home Management, Meal Preparation, and Cleanup Activities

Home management activities can be facilitated by a wide variety of environmental adaptations, assistive devices, management, energy conservation methods, and work simplification techniques.[29,127] The principles of joint protection are essential for those with rheumatoid arthritis and other inflammatory joint conditions (see Chapter 39). The following are suggestions to facilitate home management for persons with limited ROM.[60]

1. Store frequently used items on the first shelves of cabinets, just above and below counters or on counters where possible. Eliminate unnecessary items.

2. Use a high, stable stool to work comfortably at counter height, with the feet firmly placed on the ground; or, if a wheelchair is used, attach a drop-leaf table to the wall to create a planning and meal preparation area. Pullout breadboards can also serve as a wheelchair-accessible countertop workspace.

3. Use a utility cart of comfortable height to transport several items at once.

4. Use reachers to get lightweight items (e.g., a cereal box) from high shelves. Place frequently used items in the refrigerator and on shelves in cabinets where items are easily accessible and reachable.

5. Stabilize mixing bowls and dishes with nonslip mats.

6. Use lightweight utensils, such as plastic or aluminum bowls and aluminum pots. Use lightweight plates, cups, and other serving containers.

7. Use an electric can opener and an electric mixer.

8. Use electric scissors or adapted loop scissors to open packages (Fig. 10.18). Avoid using the teeth to rip open packages because this may wear down, weaken, or break the teeth.

9. Eliminate bending by using extended and flexible plastic handles on dust mops, brooms, and dustpans.

10. Use adapted knives for cutting (Fig. 10.19), or consider using precut vegetables and meat for cooking.

11. Use pullout shelves or lazy Susans to organize cupboards or the refrigerator to eliminate bending and to ease access to items.

12. Eliminate bending by using a wall oven or a countertop toaster oven or microwave oven. When remodeling the kitchen, consider elevating the dishwasher to a convenient height for wheelchair use or for those who have difficulty bending.

13. Use pump dispensers for dish soap instead of dish soap containers with pour spouts, which require lifting and pouring of contents. Ensure that the pump dispenser is not too tall to reach and that the base is stable. Single-use, premeasured, water-soluble dishwasher detergent packets eliminate numerous steps.

14. Use a piece of Dycem or other nonslip material (e.g., a piece of puffy shelf liner, a thick rubber band around a jar lid, or jar openers) to open containers. Keep these handy in multiple locations.

15. Eliminate leaning and bending by using a top-loading automatic washer and elevated dryer. Alternatively, mount front-loading washers and dryers on an elevated platform. Wheelchair users or people of shorter stature can benefit from front-loading appliances. Use a reacher or other extended tool (e.g., tongs or even a small bamboo rake) to remove clothes from the washer or dryer. Place smaller items in net bags for ease of retrieval from the machines.

16. Use an adjustable ironing board to make it possible to sit while ironing, or eliminate ironing by choosing permanent press clothing or wrinkle-free material.

17. For child care, elevate the playpen and diaper table and use a bathinette (portable folding baby bathtub) or a plastic tub on the kitchen counter for bathing to reduce the amount of bending and reaching by the ambulatory parent. The crib mattress can be in a raised position until the child is 3 or 4 months of age.

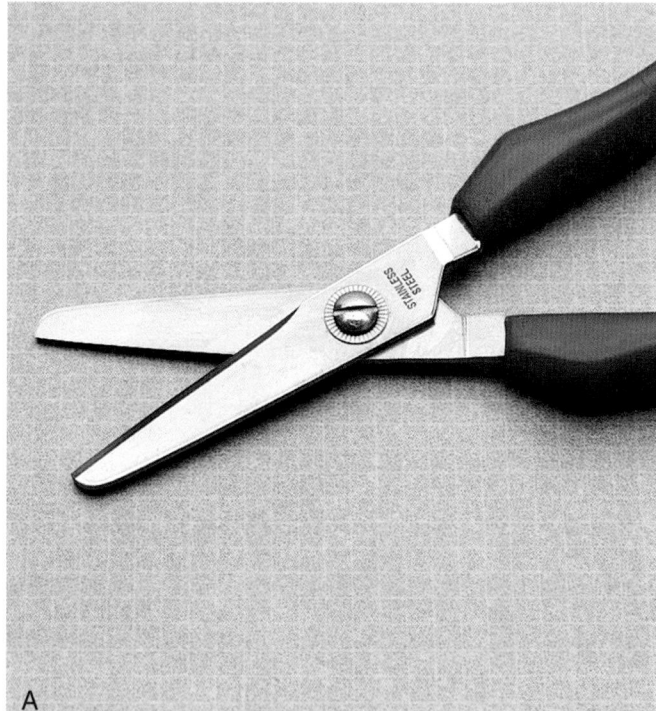

A

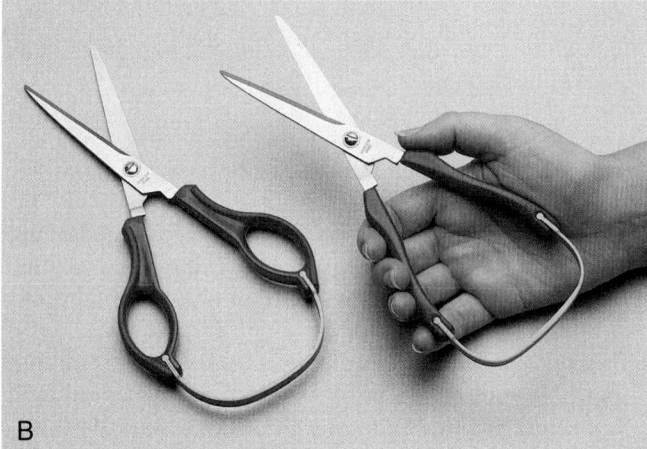

B

Fig. 10.18 (A) Round-tip scissors. (B) Loop scissors. (Courtesy North Coast Medical, Gilroy, CA.)

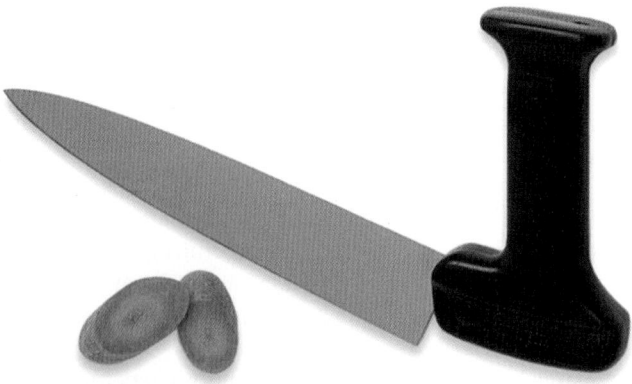

Fig. 10.19 Swedish steak knife. (Courtesy North Coast Medical, Gilroy, CA.)

18. Use slightly larger and looser fitting garments with Velcro fastenings on children.
19. Use a reacher to pick up items from the floor. For individuals without hand function, investigate the Cripper, a reaching device designed for people with quadriplegia who have use of wrist extensors, elbow flexors, and shoulder musculature (Fig. 10.20).
20. Use a lightweight comforter instead of a top sheet and blanket to increase the ease of making the bed.[60]

ADLs for the Person With Incoordination

Incoordination in the form of tremors, ataxia, and athetoid or choreiform movements can be caused by a variety of central nervous system (CNS) disorders, such as Parkinson's disease, multiple sclerosis, cerebral palsy, Friedreich's ataxia, Huntington's disease, and head injuries. Major problems that may be encountered in ADL performance are safety and adequate stability of gait, body parts, and objects to complete the tasks.

Fatigue, stress, emotional factors, fear, and environmental factors may influence the severity of uncoordinated movement.[60] The client must be taught appropriate fatigue management techniques, along with appropriate work pacing and safety methods to prevent the fatigue and apprehension that could increase incoordination and affect performance (see Chapter 35).[60] Occupational therapists should be aware of the sensory environment in which occupations take place. Evidence has shown that auditory stimuli that require semantic processing (e.g., weather forecast) may distract attention from the primary task and cause a decline in performance in people with mild to moderate Parkinson's disease.[67]

Stabilizing the trunk and arm reduces some of the incoordination and may allow the individual to improve occupational performance.[47] Propping the elbow on a counter or tabletop, pivoting from the elbow, and moving only the forearm, wrist, and hand in the activity can help provide some stability to the arm when in use. When muscle weakness is not a major deficit for the individual with incoordination, device weight can affect a client's ability to stabilize objects. Use of weights on the wrists by those with intention tremors caused by static brain lesions has been found to provide some functional improvement in self-feeding.[70] A Velcro-fastened weight can be attached to the

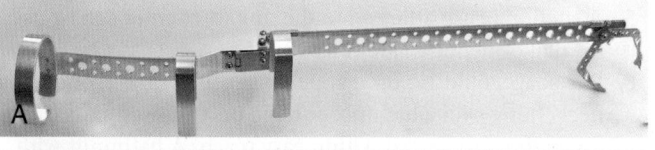
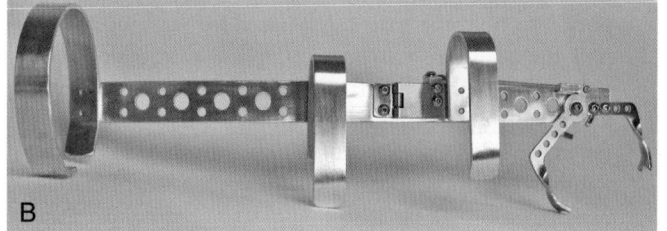

Fig. 10.20 Crippers. (A) Original Lightweight Cripper. (B) Shorty Lightweight Cripper. (Courtesy Quadtools, Camino, CA.)

client's arm or to the back of the client's hand to reduce ataxia, or the device being used (e.g., eating utensils, pens, and cups) can be weighted. On the other hand, a lightweight eating utensil appears to help smooth arm movements for people with Parkinson's disease. [67,68]

Dressing Activities

To prevent falls, the client should attempt to dress while sitting on a sturdy surface (e.g., a chair with arms and a back) with the feet planted firmly on floor, or in a wheelchair with the wheels locked. The following adaptations can reduce dressing difficulties.

1. Front-opening garments that fit loosely can facilitate the process of putting on and removing garments.
2. Large buttons, Velcro closures, and zippers with loops on the tab are fasteners that are easier to open and close. Clothing with magnetic closures or clasps should be considered carefully because some clients may have implanted devices, like deep brain stimulators or pacemakers, that can be accidentally turned off when in close proximity to magnets.[7,95] A buttonhook with a large, weighted handle may be helpful.
3. Elastic shoelaces, Velcro fasteners, other adapted shoe closures, and slip-on shoes eliminate the need for bow tying.
4. Slacks with elastic tops for women or Velcro closures for men are easier to manage than slacks with hooks, buttons, and zippers.
5. Bras with a front opening or Velcro replacements for the usual hook-and-eye fasteners may be easier to put on and take off. A slipover, stretch bra or bra-slip combination also may eliminate the need to manage bra fastenings. Regular bras may be fastened in front at waist level, then slipped around to the back and the arms put into the straps, which are then worked up over the shoulders.
6. When hand function or dexterity is impaired or absent, clip-on ties can be used, as can claspless necklaces that slip over the head and stretchable beaded bracelets.

Feeding Activities

Feeding can be a challenge for clients with problems of incoordination. Lack of control during eating is not only frustrating but also can cause embarrassment and social rejection. As mentioned previously, some evidence indicates that the use of weights on the wrist may increase functional ability in feeding.[70] It is important to make eating safe, pleasurable, and as neat as possible. Some suggestions for achieving this goal are as follows.

1. Use plate stabilizers, such as nonskid mats (Dycem), suction bases, or even damp dishtowels.
2. Use a plate guard or scoop dish to prevent food being pushed off the plate. The plate guard can be clipped to any ordinary dinner plate, so the client can use it when away from home (Fig. 10.21).
3. Prevent spills during the plate-to-mouth excursion by using weighted or swivel utensils for stability. A plate platform, like the Meal Lifter (https://www.meallifter.com), also may be used to reduce the distance from plate to mouth.
4. Weighted cuffs may be placed on the forearm or a glove with weights can be placed on the back of the hand, to reduce involuntary movement. Some clients, like those with Parkinson's disease, may demonstrate smoother arm movements when using lightweight utensils.[68]

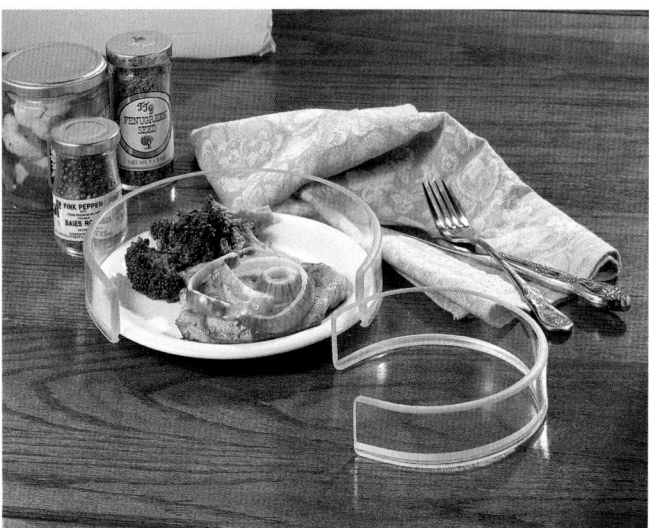

Fig. 10.21 Plate guard. (Courtesy Patterson Medical, Warrenville, IL.)

5. Use long plastic straws with a straw clip on a glass, or use a cup with a weighted bottom to eliminate the need to carry the glass or cup to the mouth, thus avoiding spills. Plastic cups with covers, one or two handles, and spouts may be used for the same purpose (Fig. 10.22). Having more than one cup designed for different drinks at a meal promotes independence and saves time and effort for the individual and caregivers.
6. Use a resistance or friction feeder (similar to a mobile arm support) to help control patterns of involuntary movement during the feeding activities of adults with cerebral palsy and athetosis. These devices may help many clients with severe incoordination to achieve some degree of independence in feeding. The device is available in adaptive equipment catalogs and is listed as a Friction Feeder MAS (Mobile Arm Support) Kit (see Chapter 31).
7. Use a mechanical self-feeding device that turns the plate, scoops the food, and brings it to the mouth. Several models are available.
8. If possible, eliminate distractions in the environment where self-feeding is taking place (e.g., turn off television during breakfast). For people with Parkinson's disease, research suggests that eliminating sound helps facilitate fast, forceful and efficient task performance.[67] If removal of sound is not possible and the client has adequate selective attention skills, people with mild-moderate Parkinson's disease may demonstrate improved performance by consciously ignoring auditory stimuli and focusing their attention to the functional task at hand.[67]

Personal Hygiene and Grooming Activities

Stabilization and handling of toilet articles may be achieved by having the client use the following measures.

1. Articles such as a razor, lipstick, or toothbrush may be attached to a cord if frequent dropping is a problem. An electric toothbrush may be more easily managed than a manual one. It is important to check the weight, operating mechanisms, and other properties of recommended devices to determine whether the client can manage safely.

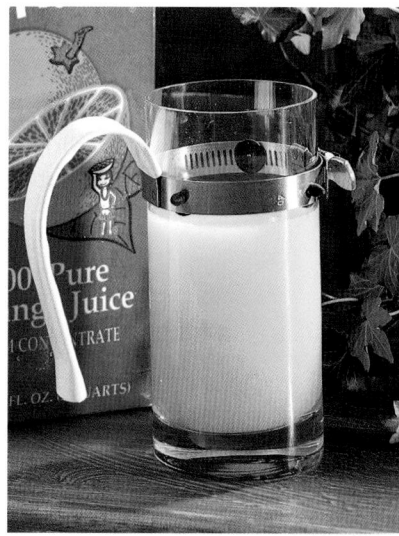
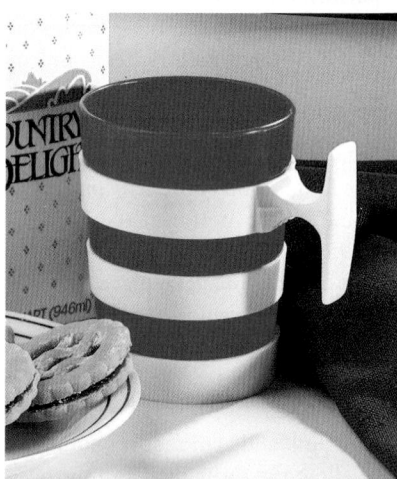

Fig. 10.22 Cup adaptors. (Courtesy Patterson Medical, Warrenville, IL.)

2. Weighted wrist cuffs may be helpful for some during the finer hygiene activities, such as hair care, shaving, and applying makeup.
3. A wall-mounted (or stand-mounted) hair dryer (described earlier for clients with limited ROM) also can be useful for clients with incoordination.[37]
4. An electric razor offers more stability and safety than a blade razor. A strap around the razor and hand can prevent dropping.
5. A suction brush attached to the sink or counter can be used for nail or denture care (Fig. 10.23).
6. Bar soap could be on a rope. It can be worn around the neck, hung over a bathtub, or hung on a shower fixture during bathing to keep it within easy reach. A bath mitt with a pocket to hold the soap can be used for washing to eliminate the need for frequent soaping and rinsing and wringing a washcloth. A leg from a pair of light-colored panty hose (which can stretch for use) with a bar of soap in the toe may be tied over a faucet or on a bath chair to keep soap within reach. Liquid soap with a soft nylon scrubber may be used to minimize the handling of soap. Bath gloves can be worn, and liquid soap that is not too slippery can be applied to eliminate the dropping of soap bars and washcloths.

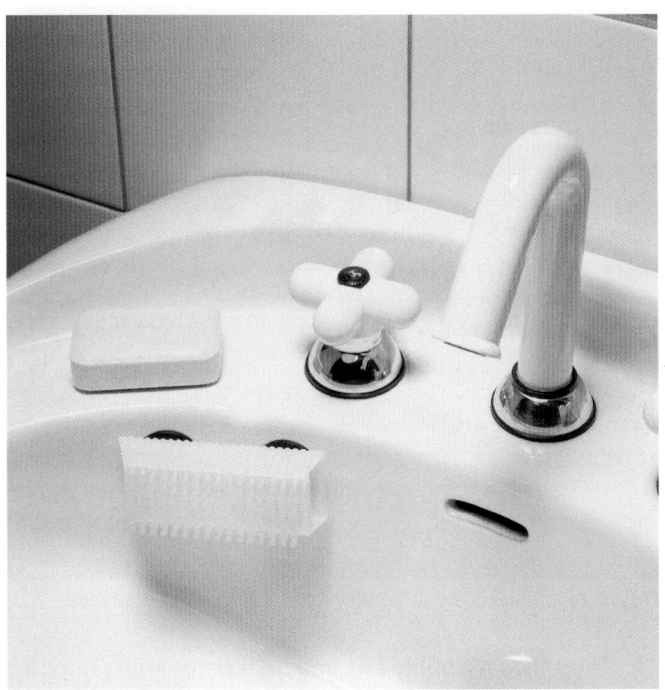

Fig. 10.23 Suction denture brush. (Courtesy North Coast Medical, Gilroy, CA.)

7. An emery board or small piece of wood with fine sandpaper glued to it can be fastened to the tabletop for filing nails. A nail clipper can be stabilized in the same manner.
8. Large solid deodorants are preferable to sprays.
9. Sanitary pads that stick to undergarments may be easier to manage than tampons.
10. Nonskid mats should be used inside and outside the bathtub during bathing. Their suction bases should be fastened securely to the floor and bathtub before use. Safety grab bars should be installed on the wall next to the bathtub, or one could be fastened to the edge of the bathtub. A bathtub seat or shower chair or bench with backrest could be used. Sponge bathing while seated at a bathroom sink may be substituted for bathing or showering several times a week.

Communication Management and Environmental Adaptations

1. Doorknobs may be managed more easily if replaced or adapted with lever-type handles or covered with rubber or friction tape (see Fig. 10.17).
2. Large-button phones, speakerphones, or using a headset as a telephone receiver may be helpful. Operator assistance services for dialing may be implemented. Alternatives to the phone may also include Voice Over Internet Protocol (VOIP) services such as Google Hangouts that allow people to initiate phone calls on their computer.[1]
3. Mobile phones or smartphones should be selected based on need for larger key pads and voice dialing capabilities. Understand what accessibility options are available for common smartphone models and specialized phones.
4. Writing may be managed by using a weighted, enlarged pencil or pen. A personal computer with a keyboard guard is a helpful aid to communication. A computer mouse may frequently be substituted for the keyboard. A voice recognition program may be used with a personal computer to minimize use of the keyboard or mouse. Most computers have "accessibility" features as a choice on the control panels. These features allow for adjustments such as reducing the sensitivity of the keys to eliminate redundancy of keystrokes and reducing the sensitivity of the mouse. The My Computer My Way website by AbilityNet (https://mcmw.abilitynet.org.uk/) provides free resources and factsheets to guide adjustment of computers and other devices.
5. Keys may be managed by placing them on an adapted key holder that is rigid and offers more leverage for turning the key. Inserting the key into the keyhole may be difficult, however, unless the incoordination is relatively mild. Locks for cars and homes can be modified with keypads or electronic door openers.
6. Extended lever-type faucets are easier to manage than knobs that turn and push-pull spigots. To prevent burns during bathing and kitchen activities, the person with incoordination should turn the cold water on first and add hot water gradually. The thermostat on the water heater can be turned down to a safe level or shower heads and tub spigots replaced with models that have a built-in shutoff valve to prevent scalding.
7. Lamps that can be turned on and off with a wall switch, a signal-type device, by motion, or by touch can eliminate the need to turn a small switch. Lights can also be programmed to turn on at specific times of the day if a timer is attached. Smart lights use Wi-Fi or Bluetooth technology and can be controlled by a smartphone or a Wi-Fi-enabled smart speaker (e.g., Amazon Echo Dot).

Functional Mobility

Clients with problems of incoordination may use a variety of adaptive aids, depending on the type and severity of incoordination. Clients with degenerative diseases sometimes need help recognizing the need for and accepting mobility and ambulation aids; the occupational therapist must consult with the PT about devices for gait. The following suggestions can improve stability and mobility for clients with incoordination.

1. Instead of lifting objects, slide them on floors or counters.
2. Use suitable ambulation aids (e.g., cane, crutches, or walker) based on suggestions by a physical therapist.
3. Use a utility cart, preferably a heavy, sturdy cart that has good treads on the wheels to increase friction with the ground.
4. Remove doorsills or thresholds, throw rugs, and thick carpeting.
5. Install railings on indoor and outdoor staircases.
6. Substitute ramps for stairs wherever possible.
7. Use a bed transfer handle (or railing) to assist with bed mobility and transfers.
8. Use a wheelchair for indoors or outdoors if upright ambulation is deemed unsafe. Either the occupational therapist or physical therapist may assist in accurate selection, depending on the facility.

Home Management, Meal Preparation, and Cleanup Activities

It is important for the occupational therapist to carefully assess performance of homemaking activities to determine which activities can be done safely (with or without modification) and which require another person's assistance. Major considerations include, but are not limited to, stabilization, handling and moving objects, and use of tools. Potential problems need to be addressed to prevent spills, accidents, and injuries such as cuts, burns, bruises, electric shock, and falls. The following are suggestions for performing home management tasks safely.[49]

1. Use a wheelchair and wheelchair lapboard, even if ambulation is possible with devices. The wheelchair saves energy and increases stability if balance and gait are unsteady. Some people with UE incoordination who do not want a lap tray find it safer to place a plastic tray on their lap (when stationary) while performing tasks with their hands.
2. If possible, use convenience and prepared foods to eliminate as many processes as possible (e.g., peeling, chopping, slicing, and mixing). Prewashed salads may help eliminate multiple meal preparation steps.
3. Use easy-open containers, or store foods in plastic containers once the original container has been opened. A jar opener is also useful.
4. Use heavy utensils, mixing bowls, and pots and pans to increase stability.
5. Use nonskid mats on work surfaces.
6. Consider using electrical appliances such as crock pots, indoor plate grills, electric fry pans, an electric water heater, toaster ovens, and microwave or countertop convection ovens because they can be safer than using a range-top stove. Safe cleanup of the appliances needs to be strongly considered because appliances such as crock pots are very heavy. Automatic shutoff devices would be safer.
7. Use a blender and stand mixer because they are safer than handheld mixers and easier than mixing with a spoon or whisk. Cleanup needs to be considered because blenders and stand mixers may be heavy or difficult to clean or may have sharp parts.
8. If possible, adjust the work heights of counters, the sink, and the range to minimize leaning, bending, reaching, and lifting, whether the client is standing or using a wheelchair.
9. Use long oven mitts, which are safer than potholders.
10. Use pots, pans, casserole dishes, and appliances with two handles because they may be easier to manage than those with one handle.
11. Use an adapted cutting board with side rails (Fig. 10.24) to stabilize meats and vegetables while cutting. The bottom of the board should have suction cups, should be covered with stair tread, or the board should be placed on a nonskid mat to prevent slipping during use.
12. Consider weight of dinnerware. Heavy dinnerware may be easier to handle because it offers stability and control to the distal part of the UE. On the other hand, unbreakable dinnerware may be more practical if dropping and breakage are problems.

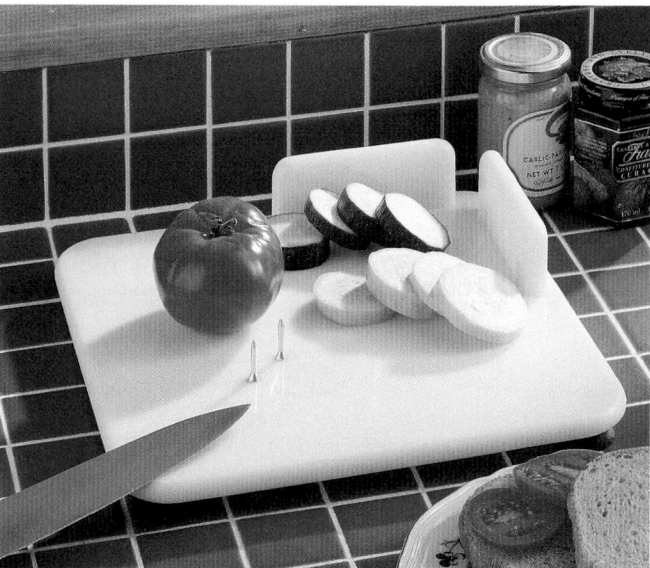

Fig. 10.24 Cutting board. (Courtesy Patterson Medical, Warrenville, IL.)

13. Cover the sink, utility cart, and countertops with protective rubber mats or mesh matting to stabilize items.
14. Use a serrated knife for cutting and chopping because it can be easier to control.
15. Use a steamer basket or deep-fry basket for preparing boiled or fried foods to eliminate the need to carry and drain pots containing hot liquids.
16. Use tongs to turn foods during cooking and to serve foods because tongs may offer more control and stability than a fork, spatula, chopsticks, or serving spoon.
17. Use blunt-ended loop scissors to open packages.
18. Vacuum with a heavy, upright cleaner, which may be easier for the ambulatory client. The wheelchair user may be able to manage a lightweight tank-type vacuum cleaner or electric broom.
19. Use dust mitts for dusting. Consider eliminating breakable knickknacks, unstable lamps, and other objects to minimize the dusting required.
20. Eliminate ironing by using permanent press fabrics or a timed dryer or by assigning this task to other members of the household. Lower the ironing board so that the task can be accomplished from a seated position.
21. Use a front-loading washer, a laundry cart on wheels, and premeasured detergents, bleaches, and fabric softeners.
22. Sit when working with an infant and use foam rubber bath aids, an infant bath seat, and a wide, padded dressing table with Velcro safety straps to achieve enough stability for bathing, dressing, and diapering an infant. Some childcare tasks may not be possible if the incoordination is severe.
23. Use disposable diapers with tape or Velcro fasteners because they are easier to manage than cloth diapers and pins and also require less frequent changing.
24. Do not feed the infant with a spoon or fork unless the incoordination is very mild or does not affect the upper extremities. This task may need to be performed by another household member.

25. Children's clothing should be large, loose, and made of non-slip stretch fabrics and have Velcro fastenings.
26. Use front infant carriers or strollers for carrying.

ADLs for the Person With Hemiplegia or Use of Only One Upper Extremity

Suggestions for performing daily living skills apply to persons with hemiplegia secondary to brain injury and also to those with conditions such as unilateral UE amputation, fractures, rotator cuff injuries, adhesive capsulitis, burns, and peripheral neuropathic conditions that can result in the dysfunction of one UE.

The client with hemiplegia as a result of conditions such as CVA, brain injury, or other conditions that affect the brain may have greater difficulty learning and performing one-handed skills than do those with orthopedic or lower motor neuron dysfunction and may need specialized methods of teaching. The client with normal perception and cognition and the use of only one UE may learn the techniques quickly and easily.

In a client with hemiplegia as a result of brain injury, the trunk and leg may be involved, and static or dynamic balance difficulties may exist in both seated and standing positions. Sensory, visual, perceptual, cognitive, and speech disorders may be present in a mild to severe degree. These disorders may profoundly affect the ability to learn and retain information and to carry over techniques into functional tasks, especially if inattention or neglect of one side of the body is present. Any type of apraxia (e.g., difficulty with motor planning, using objects), which is sometimes seen in this group of clients, can also have a profound effect on the potential for relearning different ways to perform once familiar tasks. These clients need to be assessed for sensory, perceptual, and cognitive deficits to determine the potential for ADL performance and to establish appropriate teaching methods to facilitate learning.

The following sections present primarily adaptive techniques rather than restorative techniques. However, it is important to incorporate the UE with hemiplegia to assist in returning function to the extremity. Waddell et al. conducted a study of 15 clients in an inpatient rehabilitation facility each of whom had incurred a CVA and consequently had UE paresis.[118] These individuals were provided high-repetition, task-specific training in the affected extremity. The researchers found that the clients' UE function had improved enough to allow an occupational therapist to devise a treatment plan that provided both adaptive strategies and an intensive focus on restorative strategies.[118]

Research also has shown promise of improved function in the affected extremity with constraint-induced movement therapy (CIMT); the unaffected UE is purposefully constrained to force the client to use the affected UE, when applied in original and modified forms. Hayner et al. found that constraint of the unaffected extremity, in combination with "intrusive cueing" of bilateral use of UEs, may lead to improvement in motor function of the affected extremity.[53]

Major problems for the individual who is newly one-handed, either permanently or temporarily, include reduction of work speed and dexterity, difficulty stabilizing objects in tasks that require both hands, and learning to use the normally nondominant hand to perform tasks that the dominant hand had previously performed. Occupational therapists have an important role in helping such individuals use adaptive strategies to perform occupations in ways that maximize safety and independence.

Dressing Activities

General setup. The following one-handed dressing techniques can facilitate dressing for persons who can use only one UE. The list below summarizes the general setup.

- Begin by using a sturdy chair or wheelchair and progress to more difficult surfaces (e.g., higher, lower, softer, or more unstable—yet safe—surfaces).
- Keep clothing within easy reach, and keep adaptive equipment set up and within reach.
- Support the feet (or foot) on floor or some other sturdy surface.
- Usually, maintain the body in the upright and midline positions, depending on the task.
- The therapist is usually positioned on the affected side, or in the client's midline, or in front of the client.

A general rule for putting on clothing is to begin with the affected arm or leg; start with the unaffected extremity when removing clothing. Additionally, compensatory techniques are preferable to using unnecessary devices. Assistive devices should be used minimally for dressing and other ADLs. A reacher may be helpful for securing articles and assisting in some dressing activities.

Shirts. Any of the three following methods can be used to manage front-opening shirts. The first method also can be used for jackets, robes, sweaters, and front-opening dresses.

Method 1. This method also works well with individuals who have decreased shoulder ROM or pain in the shoulders.

Donning a shirt

1. Grasp the shirt collar with the stronger hand and shake out any twists (Fig. 10.25A).
2. Position the shirt on the lap with the inside up and the collar toward the chest (see Fig. 10.25B).
3. Position the sleeve opening on the affected side so that the opening is as large as possible and close to the affected hand, which is resting on the lap (see Fig. 10.25C).
4. Using the stronger hand, place the affected hand in the sleeve opening and work the sleeve over the elbow by pulling on the garment. Make sure the affected hand is visible through the sleeve before proceeding to the next step (see Fig. 10.25D1–D2).
5. Put the stronger arm into its sleeve and raise the arm to slide or shake the sleeve into position past the elbow (see Fig. 10.25E).
6. With the stronger hand, gather the shirt up the middle of the back from hem to collar and raise the shirt over the head (see Fig. 10.25F).
7. Lean forward, duck the head, and pass the shirt over and behind the head (see Fig. 10.25G).
8. With the stronger hand, adjust the shirt by leaning forward and working the shirt down past both shoulders. Reach in

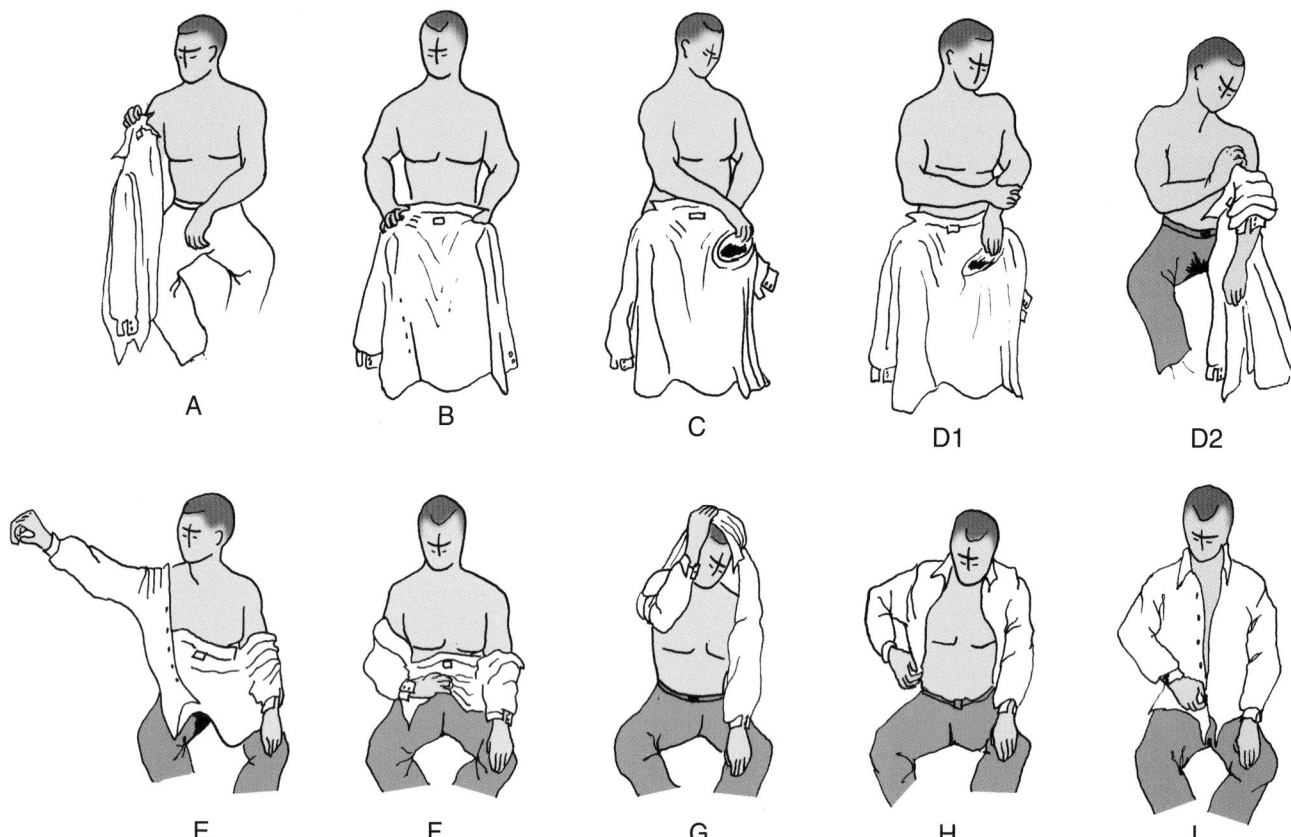

Fig. 10.25 Steps in donning a shirt—method 1. (Courtesy Christine Shaw, Metro Health Center for Rehabilitation, Metro Health Medical Center, Cleveland, OH.)

back and pull the shirttail down (see Fig. 10.25H). Adjust the shirt so that it is smooth, any wrinkles have been removed, and the sleeve is properly positioned on the shoulders and arms. (A person with hemiplegia may not have the sensation, cognition, or vision to realize that a shirt needs adjustment.)

9. Line up the two sides of the shirt front for buttoning and begin with the bottom button (see Fig. 10.25I). Button the sleeve cuff of the affected arm. The sleeve cuff of the stronger arm may be pre-buttoned if the cuff opening is large. A button may be sewn on with elastic thread or sewn onto a small tab of elastic and fastened inside the shirt cuff (commercially available button extenders can be found in the adaptive equipment catalogs). A small button attached to a crocheted loop of elastic thread is another option. Slip the button on the loop through the buttonhole in the garment so that the elastic loop is inside. Stretch the elastic loop to fit around the original cuff button. This simple device can be transferred to each garment and positioned before the shirt is put on. The loop stretches to accommodate the width of the hand as it is pushed through the end of the sleeve.

Removing a shirt

1. Unbutton the shirt.
2. Lean forward.
3. With the stronger hand, grasp the collar, or gather up the material in back from collar to hem.

4. Lean forward, duck the head, and pull the shirt over the head.
5. Remove the sleeve from the stronger arm first, then from the affected arm.

Method 2. Clients who get their shirts twisted or have trouble sliding the sleeve down onto the stronger arm can use method 2.

Donning a shirt

1. Position the shirt as described in method 1, steps 1 to 3.
2. With the stronger hand, place the involved hand into the sleeve opening and work the sleeve onto the hand and forearm, but do not pull it all the way up over the elbow.
3. With the stronger arm, reach for the shirt from behind and wrap the shirt around the back. Put the stronger arm into the sleeve, and bring the arm out to the side (about 180 degrees of abduction) to get the shirt on. Tension on the fabric from the stronger arm to the wrist of the affected arm will bring the sleeve into position.
4. Lower the arm and work the sleeve on the affected arm up over the elbow.
5. Continue as in steps 6 through 9 of method 1.

Removing a shirt (one sleeve off at a time)

1. Unbutton the shirt.
2. With the stronger hand, push the shirt off the shoulders, first on the affected side and then on the stronger side.
3. Pull off the cuff of the stronger side with the stronger hand.

4. Work the sleeve off by alternately shrugging the shoulder, shaking the arm, and working the sleeve off the stronger arm.
5. Lean forward, bring the shirt around the back (toward affected side), and pull the sleeve off the affected arm.

Method 3

Donning a shirt

1. Position the shirt and work it onto the arm as described in method 1, steps 1 to 4.
2. Pull the sleeve on the affected arm up to the shoulder (Fig. 10.26A). The affected hand should be visible through the sleeve before the next step is done.
3. With the stronger hand, grasp the tip of the collar on the stronger side, lean forward, and bring the arm over and behind the head, to wrap the shirt around to the stronger side (see Fig. 10.26B).
4. Put the stronger arm into the sleeve opening, directing the arm up and out (see Fig. 10.26C).
5. Adjust the shirt and button it as described in method 1, steps 8 and 9.

Removing a shirt. The shirt may be removed using the procedure described for method 2.

Variation—donning a pullover shirt

1. Position the shirt on the lap, with the bottom of the shirt toward the chest and the label and front of the shirt facing down.
2. With the stronger hand, gather the bottom edge of the back of the shirt up to the sleeve on the affected side.
3. Position the sleeve opening so that it is as large as possible, and use the stronger hand to place the affected hand into the sleeve opening. While sitting upright, pull the shirt sleeve up onto the weaker arm past the elbow. Or, bend forward at the hips so that gravity can assist in placing the arm into the sleeve until the hand emerges from the cuff. Then, sit up and pull the sleeve onto the weaker arm past the elbow.
4. Insert the stronger arm into the sleeve.
5. Adjust shirt on the affected side up and onto the shoulder.
6. Gather the shirt back with the stronger hand, lean forward, duck the head, and pass the shirt over the head.
7. Adjust the shirt. Make sure it is adjusted properly on the shoulders and in the front and back.

Variation—removing a pullover shirt

1. Gather up the shirt with the stronger hand, starting at the top back.
2. Lean forward, duck the head, and pull the gathered back fabric over the head.
3. Remove the shirt from the stronger arm and then from the affected arm.

Trousers/pants. Trousers may be managed by one of the following methods, which may be adapted for shorts and women's panties. For some people, a well-constructed button fly front opening may be easier to manage than a zipper. Velcro may be used to replace buttons and zippers. Trousers should be worn in a size slightly larger than that worn previously and should have a wide opening at the ankles. They should be put on after the socks have been put on, but before the shoes are put on. If the client is dressing in a wheelchair, the feet should be placed flat on the floor, not on the footrests of the wheelchair.

Method 1

Donning trousers

1. Sit in a sturdy armchair or in a locked wheelchair (Fig. 10.27A).
2. Position the stronger leg in front of the midline of the body with the knee flexed to 90 degrees. Using the stronger hand, reach forward and grasp ankle of affected leg or sock around ankle (see Fig. 10. 27B1). Lift the affected leg over the stronger leg to crossed position (see Fig. 10. 27B2).
3. Slip the trousers up the affected leg to a point at which the foot is completely inside the trouser leg (see Fig. 10.27C). Do not pull the trousers above the knee, or it will be difficult to insert the stronger leg.
4. Uncross the affected leg by grasping the ankle (or the portion of sock around the ankle) (see Fig. 10.27D). Do not allow the affected leg to just drop because this can cause injury.
5. Insert the stronger leg and work the trousers up onto the hips as far as possible (see Fig. 10).
6. To prevent the trousers from dropping while pulling them over the hips, place the affected hand in the pocket or place one finger of the affected hand into a belt loop (this is an optional technique). If able to do so safely, stand and pull the trousers over the hips (see Fig. 10.27F1–F2). This step may take more time and effort, but it is a tip that may prove useful for some.
7. If standing balance is good, remain standing to pull up zipper or to button (see Fig. 10.27F3). Sit down to button front (see Fig. 10.27G).

Removing trousers

1. Unfasten trousers and work them down the hips as far as possible while seated.
2. Stand, letting the trousers drop past the hips, or work them down past the hips.
3. Remove the trousers from the stronger leg first.
4. Sit and cross the affected leg over the stronger leg, remove the trousers, and uncross the leg.

Method 2. Method 2 is used in three situations: (1) for a client sitting in a wheelchair with the brakes locked, the footrests swung away, the feet on the ground, and the wheelchair anti-tips in place; (2) for a client sitting in a sturdy, straight-backed

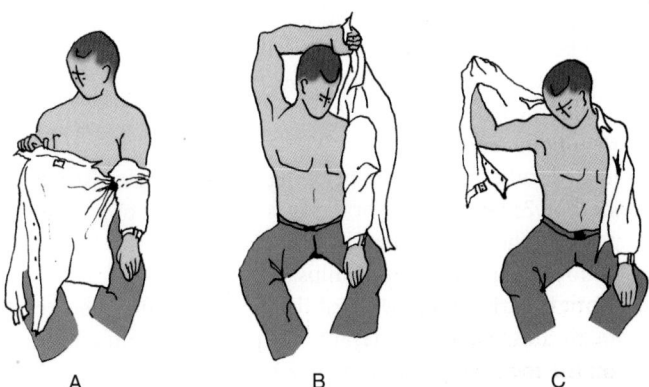

Fig. 10.26 Steps in putting on a shirt—method 3. (Courtesy Christine Shaw, Metro Health Center for Rehabilitation, Metro Health Medical Center, Cleveland, OH.)

A   B   C

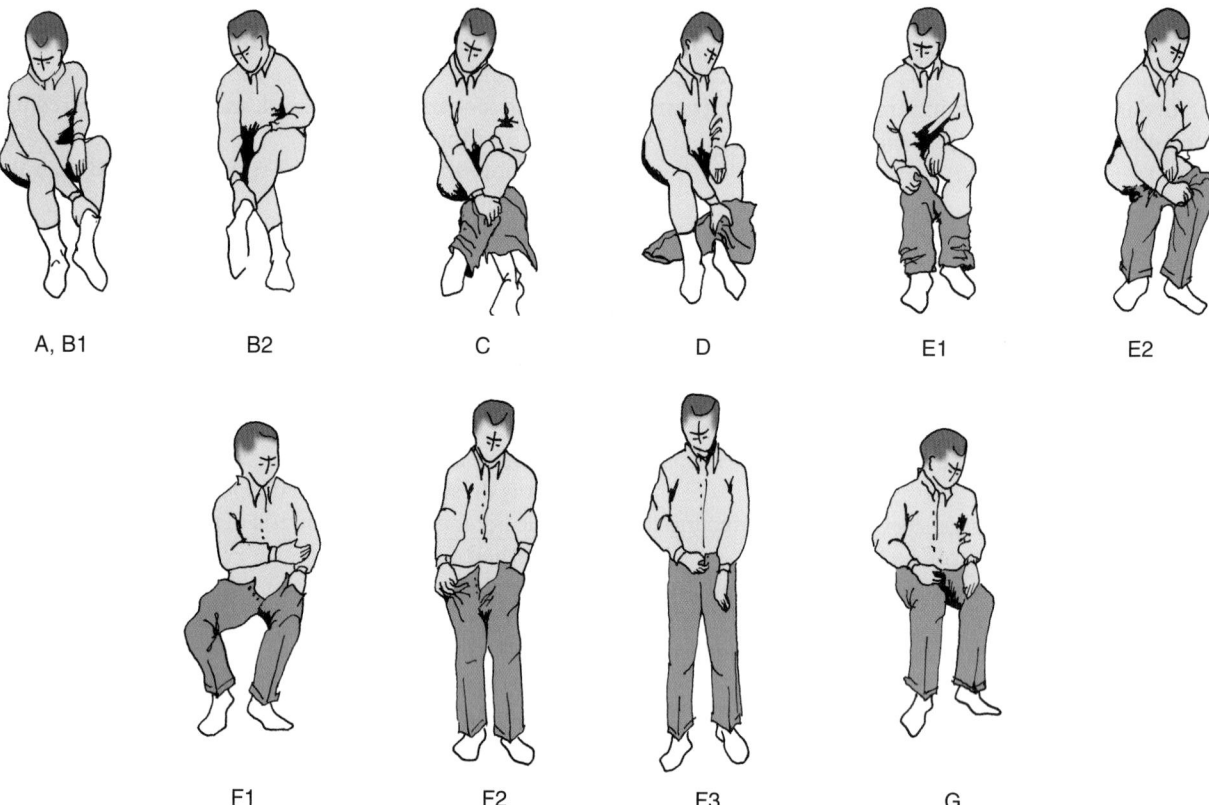

Fig. 10.27 Steps in putting on trousers—method 1. (Courtesy Christine Shaw, Metro Health Center for Rehabilitation, Metro Health Medical Center, Cleveland, OH.)

armchair that is positioned with the chair back against the wall; and (3) for a client who cannot stand independently. This method is not recommended for clients who cannot safely extend (bridge) the hips up; those who have severe sensory or perceptual deficits in the affected extremity; those with poor safety judgment and impulsivity control; or those who have a tendency to tip the wheelchair backward.

Donning trousers/pants
1. Position the trousers on the legs as in method 1, steps 1 through 5.
2. Elevate the hips by leaning back against the chair and pushing down against the floor with the stronger leg. As the hips are raised, work the trousers over them with the stronger hand.
3. Lower the hips back into the chair and fasten the trousers.

Removing trousers
1. Unfasten the trousers and work them down on the hips as far as possible while sitting.
2. Lean back against the chair, push down against the floor with the stronger leg to elevate the hips, and use the stronger arm to work the trousers down past the hips.
3. Proceed as in method 1, steps 3 and 4.

Method 3. Method 3 is used for clients in a recumbent position. It is more difficult to perform than the seated methods. If possible, the head of the bed should be raised to a semi-reclining position for partial sitting.

Donning trousers
1. Using the stronger hand, place the affected leg in a bent position and cross it over the stronger leg, which may be partially bent to prevent the affected leg from slipping.
2. Position the trousers and work them onto the affected leg first, up to the knee. Then uncross the leg.
3. Insert the stronger leg and work the trousers up onto the hips as far as possible.
4. This step may be easier if the bed is flat. With the stronger leg bent, press down with the foot and shoulder to elevate the hips from the bed. With the stronger arm, pull the trousers over the hips, or work the trousers up over the hips by rolling from side to side. If bridging (hips off the bed) is difficult or not possible, the bed should be positioned flat, both knees can be bent, and the client can roll from side to side to hike the pants up over the hips.
5. Fasten the trousers.

Removing trousers
1. In bed, hike the hips by bridging (see Putting on trousers, method 3, step 4). Or, if bridging is not possible or is difficult, position the bed flat, bend the knees, and roll side to side to remove the pants from the hips.
2. Work the trousers down past the hips by bending the knees and rolling side to side; remove the pants first from the stronger leg and then from the affected leg.

Bra

Donning a bra

1. Tuck one end of the bra into the pants, girdle, or skirt waistband and wrap the other end around the waist (wrapping toward the affected side may be easiest). Hook the bra in front at waist level and slip the fastener section around to the back (at waistline level).
2. Place the affected arm through its shoulder strap; then place the stronger arm through the other strap.
3. Work the straps up over the shoulders. Pull the strap on the affected side up over the shoulder with the stronger arm. Put the stronger arm through its strap and work the strap up over the shoulder by directing the arm up and out and pulling with the hand.
4. Use the stronger hand to adjust the breasts in the bra cups.

It is helpful if the bra has elastic straps and is made of stretch fabric. If there is some function in the affected hand, a fabric loop may be sewn to the back of the bra near the fasteners. The affected thumb may be slipped through the loop to stabilize the bra while the stronger hand fastens it. All-stretch bras, pre-fastened or without fasteners, may be put on by adapting method 1 for pullover shirts, described previously. For clients with some gross arm function, front-opening bras may be adapted with a loop for the affected hand.

Removing a bra

1. Slip the straps down off the shoulders, stronger side first.
2. Work the straps down over the arms and off the hands.
3. Slip the bra around to the front with the stronger arm.
4. Unfasten the bra and remove it.

Necktie

Putting on a necktie.

Clip-on neckties are convenient. If a conventional tie is used, the following method is recommended.

1. Place the collar of the shirt in the "up" position. Bring the necktie around the neck and adjust it so that the smaller end is at the desired length when the tie is completed.
2. Fasten the small end to the shirt front with a tie clasp or spring-clip clothespin.
3. Loop the long end of the tie around the short end (one complete loop) and bring it up the middle of the V at the neck. Then bring the tip down through the loop at the front and adjust the tie, using the ring and little fingers to hold the tie end, and the thumb and forefingers to slide the knot up tightly.

Removing a necktie

1. Pull the knot at the front of the neck until the small end slips up enough for the tie to be slipped over the head.
2. The tie may be hung up in this state. To put it on again, slip it over the head, position it around the upturned collar, and tighten the knot as described in step 3 of the preceding section.

Socks or stockings

Donning socks or stockings

1. Sit in a straight-backed armchair or in a wheelchair with the brakes locked, the feet on the floor, and the footrests swung away.
2. With the stronger leg directly in front of the midline of the body, cross the affected leg over the stronger leg.

3. Open the top of the stocking by inserting the thumb and first two fingers near the cuff and spreading the fingers apart.
4. Work the stocking onto the foot before pulling it over the heel. Care should be taken to eliminate wrinkles.
5. Work the stocking up over the leg. Shift the weight from side to side to adjust the stocking around the thigh.
6. Thigh-high stockings with an elastic band at the top are often an acceptable substitute for pantyhose, especially for the individual who is nonambulatory.
7. Pantyhose may be put on and taken off as one would for a pair of slacks, except that the legs are gathered up one at a time before the feet are placed into the leg holes.

Removing socks or stockings

1. Work the socks or stockings down as far as possible with the stronger arm.
2. Cross the affected leg over the stronger one as described in step 2 of the preceding section.
3. Remove the sock or stocking from the affected leg. A dressing stick may be required by some clients to push the sock or stocking off the heel and off the foot.
4. Lift the stronger leg to a comfortable height or to seat level and remove the sock or stocking from the foot.

Shoes. If possible, select supportive slip-on shoes to eliminate lacing and tying. If an individual uses an ankle-foot orthosis (AFO) or short leg brace, shoes with fasteners are usually needed.

1. Use elastic laces and leave the shoes tied.
2. Use adapted shoe fasteners.
3. Use one-handed shoe-tying techniques (Fig. 10.28).
4. It is possible to learn to tie a standard bow with one hand, but this requires excellent visual, perceptual, and motor planning skills, along with much practice.

Ankle-foot orthosis. The individual with hemiplegia who lacks adequate ankle dorsiflexion to walk safely and efficiently frequently uses an AFO, which may be recommended by a PT, prescribed by a physician, and made by an orthotist. The following methods are two techniques that may be used. The shoe needs to be half to one size bigger than usual.

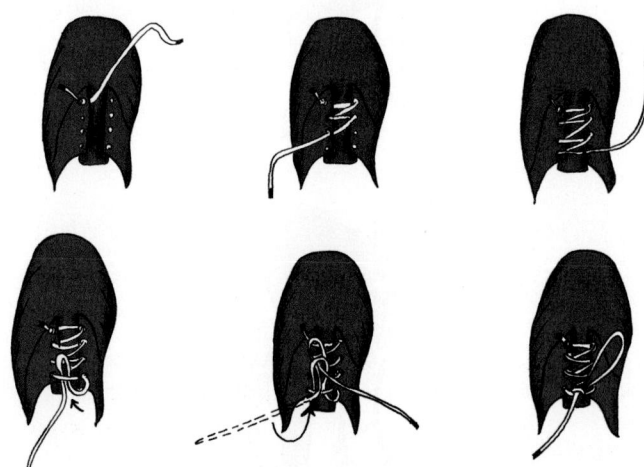

Fig. 10.28 Method for tying shoelaces with one hand. (Courtesy Christine Shaw, Metro Health Center for Rehabilitation, Metro Health Medical Center, Cleveland, OH.)

Donning an ankle-foot orthosis
Method 1

1. Sit in a straight-backed armchair or in a wheelchair with the brakes locked and the feet on the floor. Loosen the fasteners on the shoe, and pull back the tongue to allow the AFO to fit into the shoe. Place the AFO into the shoe (Fig. 10.29A).
2. Place the AFO and the shoe on the floor between the legs (but closer to the affected leg), facing up (see Fig. 10.29B).
3. With the stronger hand, lift the affected leg behind the knee and place the toes into the shoe (see Fig. 10.29C).
4. Reach down with the stronger hand and lift the AFO by the calf piece. Simultaneously, use the unaffected foot against the affected heel to keep the shoe and AFO together. The heel will not be pushed into the shoe at this point (see Fig. 10.29D).
5. If leg strength is not sufficient, use the stronger hand to apply pressure directly downward on the affected knee, pushing the heel into the shoe (see Fig. 10.29E). To prevent injury, especially with clients who have poor sensation, make sure the client does not jam the heel into the AFO.
6. Fasten the Velcro calf strap, and then fasten the shoes (see Fig. 10.29F). The affected leg may be placed on a footstool to assist with reaching shoe fasteners.
7. To fasten the shoes, the client may use one-handed bow-tying techniques, elastic shoelaces, or other commercially available shoe fasteners; alternatively, Velcro-fastened shoes may be used.

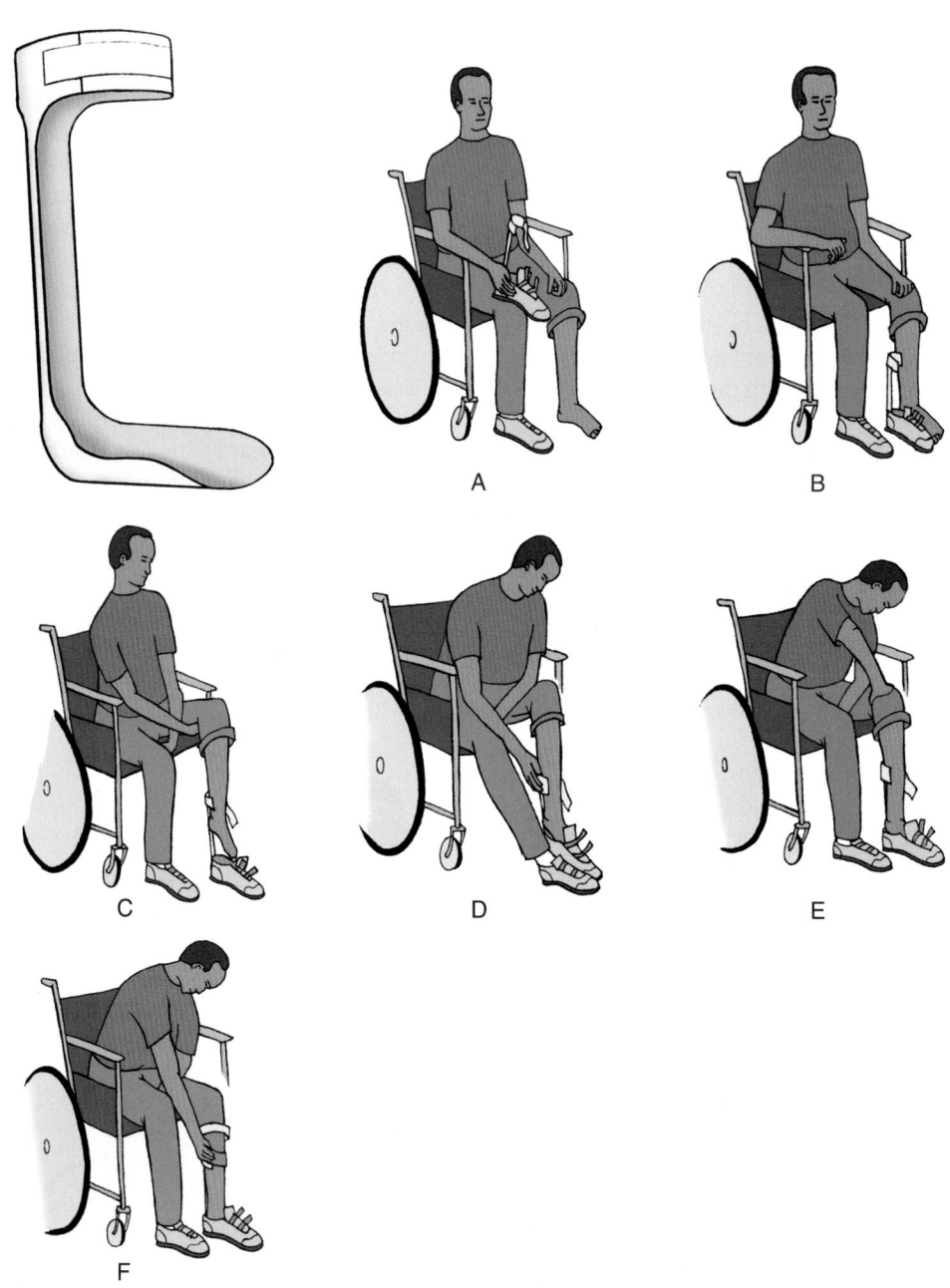

Fig. 10.29 Steps in donning an ankle-foot orthosis (AFO).

Method 2.   Steps 1 and 2 are the same as the positioning required for putting on trousers.

1. Sit in a sturdy armchair or in a locked wheelchair.
2. Position the stronger leg in front of the midline of the body with knee flexed to 90 degrees. Using the stronger hand, reach forward and grasp the ankle of the affected leg (or the sock around the ankle). Lift the affected leg over the stronger leg to crossed position.
3. Loosen the fasteners of the shoe and pull back the tongue to allow the AFO to fit into the shoe; unfasten the Velcro fastener on the AFO. Place the AFO in the shoe.
4. Using the stronger hand, hold the heel of the shoe and work the shoe over the toes of the affected foot and leg. Once the toes are in the shoe, work the top part of the AFO around the calf.
5. Pull the heel of the shoe onto the foot with the stronger hand, or place the foot on the floor, put pressure on the knee, and push the heel down into the shoe.
6. Fasten the Velcro calf strap on the AFO and then fasten the shoes.

Removing an ankle-foot orthosis
Variation 1
1. While seated as for putting on an AFO, cross the affected leg over the stronger leg.
2. Unfasten the straps of the AFO and the fasteners of the shoe with the stronger hand.
3. Push down on the calf part of the AFO until the shoe is off the foot.

Variation 2
1. Unfasten the straps of the AFO and the fasteners of the shoe with the stronger hand.
2. Straighten the affected leg by putting the stronger foot behind the heel of the shoe on the affected leg and pushing the affected leg forward.
3. Push down on the AFO upright with the stronger hand, and at the same time, push forward on the heel of the AFO shoe with the stronger foot.

Feeding Activities

A primary problem for individuals with only one functional hand is inability or difficulty using one hand to stabilize an object while using that same hand to perform another task. An example in feeding is a person with one functional hand trying to cut food, such as meat, using a knife while stabilizing the food at the same time. This problem can be resolved by the use of a rocker knife (Fig. 10.30) for cutting meat and other foods. This knife cuts with a rocking motion rather than a back-and-forth slicing action. Use of a rocking motion with a standard table knife or a sharp paring knife may be adequate to cut tender meats and soft foods. If such a knife is used, the client is taught to hold the knife handle between the thumb and the third, fourth, and fifth fingers, and the index finger is extended along the top of the knife blade. The knife point is placed in the food in a vertical position, and then the blade is brought down to cut the food. The rocking motion, using wrist flexion and extension, is continued until the food is cut. To stabilize a plate or bowl, a product such as foam-padded shelf liner or Dycem can be placed under it. There are many other

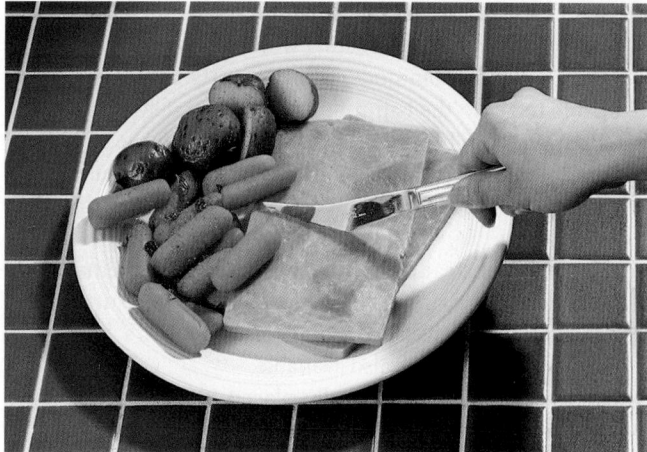

Fig. 10.30 Rocker knife. (Courtesy Patterson Medical, Warrenville, IL.)

adaptive devices, such as a plate guard (see Fig. 10.21), that the person who eats with only one fully functional hand can use.

Another feeding issue that may arise is opening packages such as yogurt containers, drink bottles, and milk cartons, in addition to containers such as margarine tubs and ketchup holders. These tasks require practice, and the less functional hand should be incorporated into the task, if appropriate.

Personal Hygiene and Grooming Activities

Clients with the use of one hand or one side of the body can accomplish personal hygiene and grooming activities by using assistive devices and alternative methods. The following are suggestions for achieving hygiene and grooming with one hand.

1. Use an electric razor rather than a razor with a blade.
2. Use a shower seat in the shower stall or a transfer tub bench in a bathtub-shower combination. Other helpful devices include a bath mat, wash mitt, long-handled bath sponge, safety rails on the bathtub or wall, soap on a rope or a suction soap holder, and a suction brush for fingernail care.
3. Take a sponge bath while sitting at the lavatory using the wash mitt, suction brush, and suction soap holder. The stronger forearm and hand may be washed by placing a soaped washcloth on the thigh and rubbing the hand and forearm on the cloth.
4. Consider an easily accomplished hairstyle. Or, use a wall-mounted hair dryer, which frees the stronger UE to hold a brush or comb to style the hair during blow-drying.[28]
5. As described previously for clients with incoordination, an emery board or small piece of wood with fine sandpaper glued to it can be fastened to the tabletop for filing nails, and a nail clipper can be stabilized in the same manner. For toenails, a large nail file can be used. If circulatory issues or diminished sensation is a problem, a podiatrist may need to be consulted or should perform this important (but often neglected) ADL.
6. Use a suction denture brush (see Fig. 10.23) for care of dentures. The suction fingernail brush may also serve this purpose.

Toileting

Clients with the use of one hand or one side of the body can accomplish toileting activities by using assistive devices and alternative methods. The following are suggestions for achieving independent and safe toileting with one hand.

1. Use a bedside commode with or without drop arms if unable to get to the bathroom quickly or safely (Fig. 10.31). Commodes can be placed over the toilet, with use of a splash guard (looks like a bucket without the bottom). Toilet safety frames and raised toilet seats can also facilitate safe transfers for toileting.
2. Use a urinal instead of transferring to the toilet. Female- and male-designed urinals are available, but female urinals are not always effective, depending on the client's body size. Spill-proof urinals are also available.
3. Grab bars can be strategically placed to assist with sit-to-stand or stand-to-sit movements.
4. Place toilet paper on the unaffected side.
5. Bidets or specialty toilets with wash, dry, and other features can be useful to optimize and facilitate cleansing.
6. Incontinence supplies may need to be considered, especially for community outings.

Communication Management and Environmental Adaptations

1. The primary problem with writing is stabilization of the paper or tablet. This problem can be overcome by using a clipboard, paperweight, or nonskid surface (e.g., Dycem) or by taping the paper to the writing surface. In some instances,

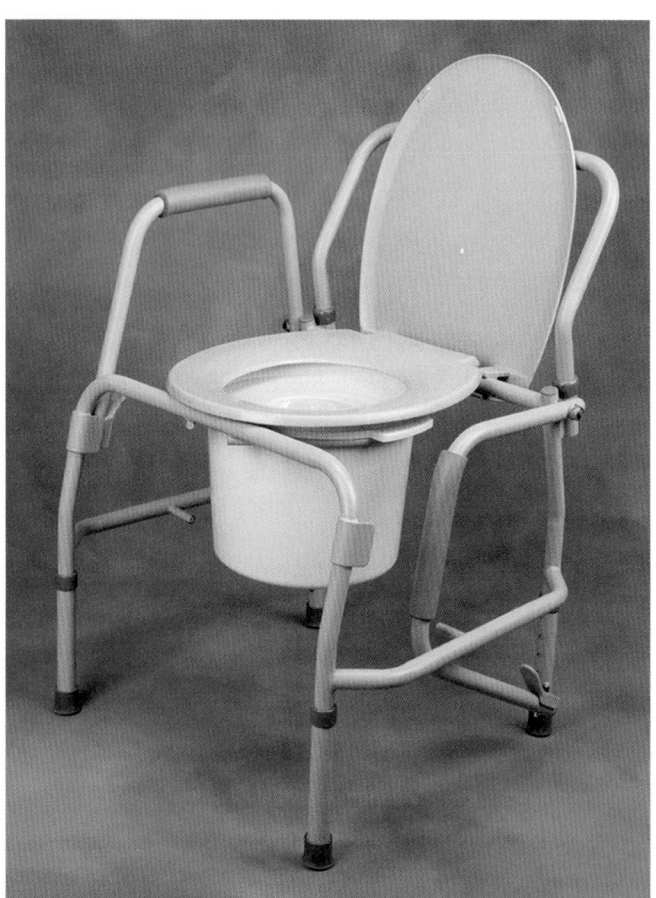

Fig. 10.31 Drop-arm commode. (Courtesy North Coast Medical, Gilroy, CA.)

the affected arm may be positioned on the tabletop to stabilize the paper.
2. If dominance must be shifted to the nondominant extremity, writing practice may be necessary to improve speed and coordination. Single-handed keyboards, onscreen keyboards, and voice control features on computers, tablets, and smartphones can help enable clients to compose messages as well.[2] One-handed writing and keyboarding instruction manuals are available.
3. Book holders may be used to stabilize a book while reading or holding copy for typing and writing practice. A soft pillow placed on the lap easily stabilizes a book while the client is seated in a chair. Clients who enjoy reading may want to consider an e-reader (e.g., Kindle), which allows touch page turning and options to increase the font size to the reader's preference.
4. Dialing numbers on a telephone with one hand requires several motions, including lifting the receiver to listen for the dial tone, setting it down, pressing the keys, and lifting the receiver to the ear. A speakerphone or headset can also leave the hands free to take messages. For writing while using the telephone, a stand or shoulder telephone receiver holder can be used for classic older model receivers. One-touch or voice-activated dialing using preprogrammed phone numbers eliminates or reduces the need to press as many keys, simplifies sequencing, and may help compensate for memory deficits. As previously described in the section on incoordination, VOIP services may be used to make calls from an internet-enabled computer.

Functional Mobility

Principles of transfer techniques for clients with hemiplegia are described in Chapter 11.

Home Management, Meal Preparation, and Cleanup Activities

Many assistive devices are available to facilitate home management and meal activities. Various factors determine how many home management and meal activities can realistically be performed, which methods can be used, and how many assistive devices can be managed. These factors include whether the client is disabled by the loss of function of one arm and hand, as in amputation or a peripheral neuropathic condition, or whether both arm and leg are affected, along with possible sensory, visual, perceptual, and cognitive dysfunctions, as in hemiplegia. The following are some suggestions for home management and meal activities for the client with the use of one hand.[60]

1. Stabilizing items is a major problem for the one-handed homemaker. Stabilize foods for cutting and peeling by using a cutting board with two stainless steel or aluminum nails in it. A raised corner on the board stabilizes bread for making sandwiches or spreading butter. Suction cups or a rubber mat under the board will keep it from slipping. A nonskid surface or rubber feet may be glued to the bottom of the board.

2. Use nonskid mats or pads, wet dishcloths, or suction devices to keep pots, bowls, and dishes from turning or sliding during food preparation.

3. To open a jar, stabilize it between the knees or in a partially opened drawer while leaning against the drawer. Break the air seal by sliding a pop bottle opener under the lid until the air is released, then use a Zim jar opener (Fig. 10.32).

4. Open boxes, sealed paper, and plastic bags by stabilizing between the knees or in a drawer as just described and cut open with household shears. Special box and bag openers are also available from ADL equipment vendors.

5. Crack an egg by holding it firmly in the palm of the hand. Hit it in the center against the edge of the bowl. Then, using the thumb and index finger, push the top half of the shell up and use the ring and little fingers to push the lower half down. Separate whites from yolks by using an egg separator, funnel, or large slotted spoon.

6. Eliminate the need to stabilize the standard grater by using a grater with suction feet, or use an electric countertop food processor instead.

7. Stabilize pots on the counter or range for mixing or stirring by using a pan holder with suction feet (Fig. 10.33).

8. Eliminate the need to use hand-cranked or electric can openers, which necessitate the use of two hands, by using a one-handed electric can opener.

9. Use a utility cart to transfer items from one place to another. For some clients, a cart that is weighted or constructed of wood may be used as a minimal support during ambulation.

10. Transfer clothes to and from the washer or dryer by using a clothes carrier on wheels.

11. Use electrical appliances (e.g., lightweight electrical hand mixer, immersion blender, traditional blender, and food processor) that can be managed with one hand and that save time and energy. Safety factors and judgment need to be evaluated carefully when electrical appliances are considered.

12. Floor care becomes a greater problem if, in addition to one arm, ambulation and balance are affected. For clients with involvement of only one arm, a standard dust mop, carpet sweeper, or upright vacuum cleaner should present no problem. A self-wringing mop may be used if the mop handle is stabilized under the arm and the wringing lever operated with the stronger arm. Clients with balance and ambulation problems may manage some floor care from a sitting position. Dust mopping or using a carpet sweeper may be possible if gait and balance are fairly good without the aid of a cane. Some people may benefit from a programmable robotic vacuum cleaner (Roomba) or floor scrubber (Braava) from iRobot (http://store.irobot.com/home/index.jsp). However, careful consideration must be used for these devices because they can also be a safety or tripping hazard if they do not return to the docking station.[60]

These are just a few of the possibilities for solving homemaking problems for one-handed individuals. The occupational therapist must evaluate each client to determine how the dysfunction affects the performance of homemaking activities. One-handed techniques take more time and may be difficult for some clients to master. Activities should be paced to accommodate the client's physical endurance and tolerance for one-handed performance and use of special devices. Fatigue management techniques should be used. New techniques and devices should be introduced on a graded basis as the client masters first one technique and device and then another. Family members need to be oriented to the client's skills, special methods used, and schedule. The therapist, with the family and client, may facilitate the planning of homemaking responsibilities to be shared by other family members, in addition to the supervision of the client, if that is needed. If special equipment and assistive devices are needed for IADLs, it is advisable for the client to practice using the devices in the clinic if possible. The therapist can then train the client and demonstrate use of the equipment to a family member before these items are purchased and used

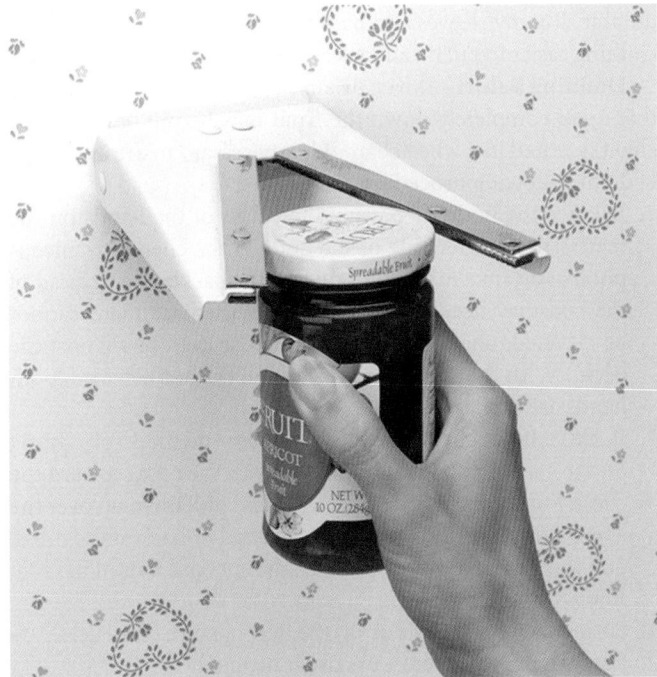

Fig. 10.32 Zim jar opener. (Courtesy ZIM Manufacturing, Chicago, IL.)

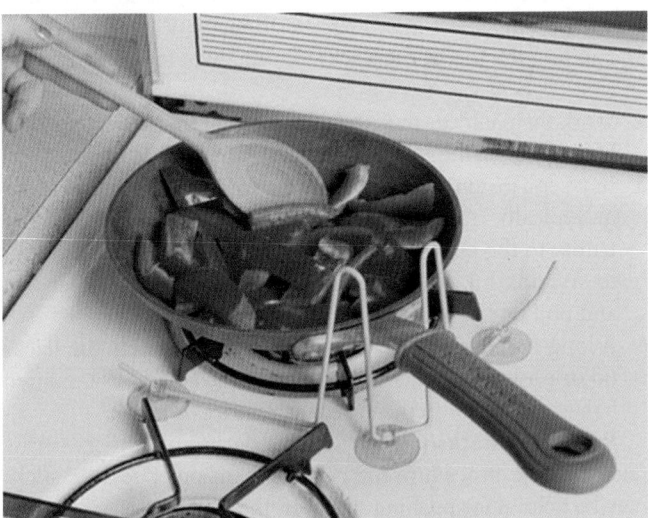

Fig. 10.33 Pan stabilizer. (Courtesy SP Ableware–Maddak, Inc., Wayne, NJ.)

at home. After training, the occupational therapist should provide the client with sources for replacing items independently, such as a consumer catalog of adaptive equipment or websites.

ADLs for the Person With Paraplegia

Clients who use a wheelchair for mobility need to find ways to perform ADLs from a seated position, to transport objects, and to adapt to an environment designed for standing and walking. Given normal function in the upper extremities and otherwise good health, the wheelchair user can probably perform ADLs independently. The client should have a stable spine or use an appropriate orthotic or stabilization device, and the healthcare provider should clearly identify mobility precautions.

Dressing Activities

It is recommended that clients who must use wheelchairs put on clothing in this order: stockings or socks, undergarments, braces (if worn), slacks, shoes, and then shirt or dress. Underwear may be eliminated because it is an extra step, has the potential to contribute to skin breakdown, and results in greater difficulty for toileting. During the initial rehabilitation, the client with paraplegia will likely begin dressing training in bed; as his or her strength, endurance, and balance improve, the client will progress to dressing in the wheelchair. The ability to dress in the wheelchair simplifies toileting by eliminating the need to go back to bed to manage clothing.

Slacks/pants

Putting on slacks/pants. Slacks are easier to fasten if they button or zip in front. If braces are worn, zippers in side seams may be helpful. Wide-bottom slacks of stretch fabric are recommended. The following steps comprise the procedure for putting on shorts, slacks, and underwear.

1. Use side rails, a trapeze, or other adaptive technique to pull up to a sitting position, with the back supported by pillows or the headboard of the bed. If side rails or a trapeze is not required, the client props up on the elbows in a semi-reclined position and generates momentum by alternately pushing with one elbow and then the other until the elbow comes up high enough for the client to prop the hands on the bed.[58]
2. Sit on the bed and reach forward to the feet, or sit on the bed and pull the knees into flexed position.
3. Holding the top of the slacks, flip the pant legs down to the feet.
4. Work the pant legs over the feet, and pull the slacks up to the hips. Crossing the ankles may help get the slacks over the heels.
5. In a semi-reclining position, using rotation and momentum by typically transferring momentum from the arms to the trunk, to the pelvis, and then to the lower extremities,[58] roll to one side, hike up the slacks, and then roll to the other side and pull up the pant leg.
6. A long-handled reacher may be helpful for pulling the slacks up or positioning them on the feet if the client has impaired balance or ROM in the lower extremities or trunk.

Removing slacks/pants. Remove slacks and underwear by reversing the procedure for putting them on. Dressing sticks may be helpful for pushing slacks off the feet.

Socks or stockings. Soft stretch socks or stockings are recommended. Pantyhose that are slightly larger may be useful. Elastic garters or stockings with elastic tops should be avoided because of potential skin breakdown. Dressing sticks or a stocking device may be helpful to some clients.

Donning socks or stockings

1. Put on socks or stockings while sitting up in bed with the legs extended (long-sitting).
2. While propped up when long-sitting with the legs initially extended, pull one leg into flexion with one hand and cross the leg over onto the other extended leg.
3. Use the other hand to slip the sock or stocking over the foot, and pull on the sock or stocking. To prevent pressure skin breakdown, make sure there are no wrinkles or creases in the socks.

Removing socks or stockings. Remove socks or stockings by flexing the leg as described for putting them on, and then push the sock or stocking down over the heel. A dressing stick may be needed to push the sock or stocking off the heel and toe and to retrieve the sock. This is a good time to perform a skin check on the feet and lower legs to detect any skin breakdown or red areas.

Slips and skirts. Slips and skirts slightly larger than usually worn are recommended. A-line, wraparound, and full skirts are easier to manage and may drape better on a person seated in a wheelchair than narrow skirts, which can ride up.

Putting on slips and skirts

1. Sit on the bed, slip the garment over the head, and let it drop to the waist.
2. In a semi-reclining position, roll from hip to hip and pull the garment down over the hips and thighs.

Removing slips and skirts

1. In a sitting or semi-reclining position, unfasten the garment.
2. Roll from hip to hip, pulling the garment up to waist level.
3. Pull the garment off over the head.

Shirts. Fabrics should be wrinkle resistant, smooth, and durable. Roomy sleeves and backs and full shirts may make this clothing easier to put on and take off than closely fitted garments.

Donning a shirt. Shirts, pajamas, jackets, robes, and dresses that open completely down the front may be put on while the client is seated in a wheelchair. If it is necessary to dress while in bed, the following procedure can be used.

1. Balance the body by putting the palms of the hands on the mattress on either side of the body. If the client's balance is poor, assistance may be needed, or the backboard or head of the bed may need to be elevated. (If the backboard cannot be elevated, one or two pillows may be used to support the back.) With the backboard or head of the bed elevated, both hands are available.
2. If difficulty occurs with the customary methods of putting on the garment, open it on the lap with the collar toward the chest. Put the arms into the sleeves and pull them up over the elbows. Then, holding on to the shirttail or back of the dress, pull the garment over the head, adjust it, and button it.

Removing a shirt

1. Sitting in a wheelchair or on the bed, open the fasteners.
2. Remove the garment in the usual manner.

3. If the usual manner is not feasible, grasp the collar with one hand while balancing with the other hand. Gather up the material from collar to hem.
4. Lean forward, duck the head, and pull the shirt over the head.
5. Remove the arms from the sleeves, first the supporting arm and then the working arm.

Shoes

Donning shoes. If an individual has sensory loss and is at risk for injury during transfers, shoes should be put on in bed.

Variation 1

1. Sit on the bed, on the edge of the bed (requires good balance, high skill), or in a wheelchair for back support. Pull one knee at a time into the flexed position with the hands.
2. While supporting the leg in the flexed position with one hand, use the free hand to put on the shoe.

Variation 2

1. Sit on the edge of the bed or in a wheelchair for back support.
2. Cross one leg over the other and slip the shoe onto the foot.
3. If sitting in a wheelchair, put the foot on the floor or footrest and press down on the knee to push the foot into the shoe.

Removing shoes

1. Flex or cross the leg as described for the appropriate variation.
2. For variation 1: Remove the shoe with one hand while supporting the flexed leg with the other hand.
3. For variation 2: Remove the shoe from the crossed leg with one hand while maintaining balance with the other hand, if necessary.

Feeding Activities

Eating activities should present no problem for the person who uses a wheelchair but has good to normal arm function. Wheelchairs with desk-style armrests and footrests that fit under tabletops are recommended so that the client can sit close to the table. Footrests on the wheelchair may be detachable or fixed but need to function within the client's environment for maximum independence.

Personal Hygiene and Grooming Activities

Facial and oral hygiene and arm and upper body care should present no problem. Reachers may be helpful for getting towels, washcloths, makeup, deodorant, and shaving supplies from storage areas. Special equipment is needed for tub baths and showers. (Transfer techniques for the toilet and bathtub are discussed in Chapter 11.) The following are suggestions for facilitating safety and independence during bathing activities.

1. Use a handheld shower hose and keep a finger over the spray to determine sudden temperature changes in the water. Make sure the water heater is set at a safe temperature (120°F [49°C]) to prevent scald burns.[108]
2. Use a long-handled bath brush with a soap insert for ease in reaching all parts of the body.
3. Use soap bars attached to a cord around the neck or use liquid soap.
4. Use a padded shower chair or padded transfer tub bench. Consider a commode cutout if the bowel program is performed in the shower.

5. Increase safety during transfers by installing grab bars on the wall near the bathtub or shower and on the bathtub to provide a balance point during transfers and when bending to wash the legs and buttocks.
6. Fit a bathtub or shower floor with a nonskid mat or adhesive material.
7. Remove doors on the bathtub and replace with a shower curtain to increase safety and ease of transfers.

Skin integrity and hygiene. Because sensory loss increases the risk of skin breakdown, regular skin checks and weight shifts should be considered a normal part of the ADL routine. Clients should be instructed in the following procedures.

1. Checking for potential areas of skin breakdown and signs of developing skin problems, and practicing methods to maintain good skin integrity.
2. How and when to perform proper weight shifts while up in the wheelchair and how to position oneself in bed to prevent skin breakdown.
3. Performing skin checks and complying with the recommended frequency. The client can use a long-handled mirror (Fig. 10.34) to see areas that are otherwise difficult to observe.
4. Maintaining all equipment to ensure that disrepair is not contributing to skin breakdown. For example, a tear in a padded tub bench could tear the skin on the buttocks, resulting in skin breakdown.

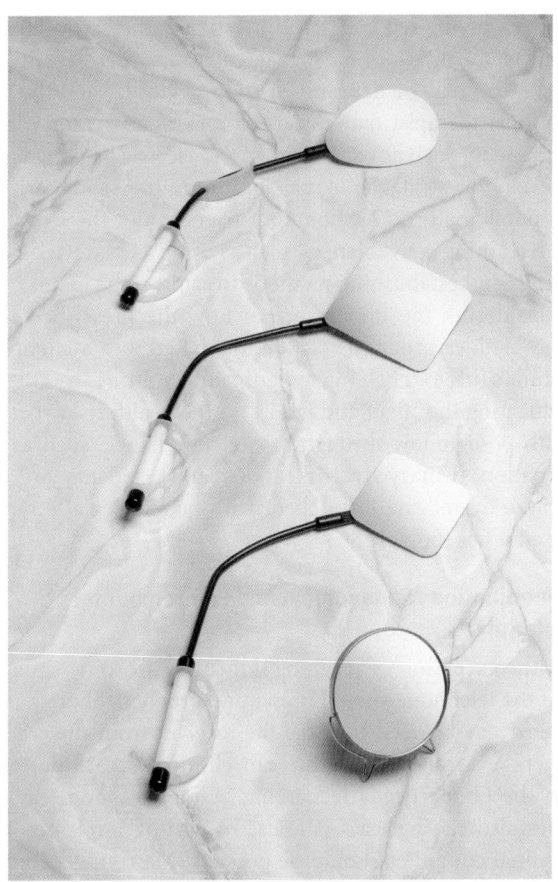

Fig. 10.34 Long-handled mirrors. (Courtesy North Coast Medical, Gilroy, CA.)

Bowel and bladder management. The physician customarily is responsible for prescribing the bowel and bladder program, but the occupational therapist and other team members can provide valuable insight into adaptations and routines that may be ideal or most suitable.[94] For example, an occupational therapist, along with nursing staff members, may be involved in instructing the client about digital stimulation or the use of intermittent catheterization for elimination. Helping the client establish a routine for this ADL is important because ineffective bowel and bladder management may lead to significant limitations in other activities, if the client is experiencing accidents or infections. Significant time and close monitoring may be required to perform this crucial ADL, which can affect many aspects of life, including sleep. An interdisciplinary approach is critical for health maintenance in bowel and bladder care. The following are some areas in which an occupational therapist may be helpful.

1. Determining the optimal DME for performing a task (e.g., a padded commode, padded raised toilet seat, or padded roll-in-shower chair) and practicing transfers on and off toileting surfaces.
2. Assisting the interdisciplinary team in determining a client's readiness and cognitive/physical/emotional capacity to learn and perform the required skills.[94]
3. Determining the appropriate adaptive equipment and/or techniques for performing tasks such as inserting a suppository or an adaptive digital stimulator for bowel management, and emptying leg bags and inserting catheters for bladder management. Clothing management and perineal hygiene tasks also may be determined and practiced,[94] and the occupational therapist may make recommendations for adaptive equipment such as pants holders and electric bag openers.
4. Developing strategies to manage intermittent catheterization in public bathrooms, homes of friends, and the workplace; determining conveniences, such as using a waist pack to hold items; and establishing methods to sanitize the hands.[57,94]
5. Considering the importance of how the prescribed bowel and bladder programs can be integrated into a client's and family's life, and helping to figure out a routine.[94]
6. Educating the client and family on the health risks that arise with poor follow-through or noncompliance, such as constipation, urinary tract infections, and accidents and autonomic dysreflexia for a client with quadriplegia/tetraplegia or a higher thoracic SCI.[94]

Communication Management and Environmental Adaptations

With the exception of reaching difficulties in some situations, use of the telephone should present no problem. Short-handled reachers may be used to grasp the receiver from the cradle or charger. A cordless telephone can eliminate reaching, except when the phone needs recharging. A mobile phone or smart phones also can be used. The use of writing implements and a personal computer should be possible. Managing doors may present some difficulties. If the door opens toward the person, it can be opened using the following procedure (Fig. 10.35).

1. If the doorknob or handle is on the right, approach the door from the right and turn the doorknob or pull the handle with the left hand.
2. Open the door as far as possible and move the wheelchair close enough so that it helps keep the door open.
3. Holding the door open with the left hand, turn the wheelchair with the right hand and wheel through the door.
4. Start closing the door when halfway through.

If the door is very heavy and opens out or away from the person, the following procedure is recommended.

1. Back up to the door so that the knob can be turned or the handle operated with the right hand.
2. Open the door and back through it so that the large drive (rear) wheels keep it open.
3. Also use the left elbow to keep the door open.
4. Propel backward with the right hand.

Functional Mobility

Principles of transfer techniques are discussed in Chapter 11.

Home Management, Meal Preparation, and Cleanup Activities

When homemaking activities are performed from a wheelchair, the major problems are work heights, adequate space for maneuverability, access to storage areas, and transport of supplies, equipment, and materials from place to place. If funds are available for kitchen remodeling, recommendations include lowering the counters to a comfortable height for wheelchair use and opening the space under the counters and the range. Such extensive adaptation is often not feasible for many people. The following are some suggestions for homemaking activities.[60]

1. Remove cabinet doors to eliminate the need to maneuver around them for opening and closing. Frequently used items should be stored toward the front of easy to reach cabinets above and below the counter surfaces.
2. If entrance and inside doors are not wide enough, make doors slightly wider by removing the strips along the doorjambs. Offset hinges can replace standard door hinges and increase the doorjamb width by 2 inches (Fig. 10.36).
3. Use a wheelchair cushion to increase the user's height so that standard-height counters may be used. This recommendation may or may not work for some because changing cushions takes energy and/or may have consequences for skin care or safety.
4. Detachable, desk-style armrests allow wheelchair users to get closer to counters and tables than is possible with detachable (or fixed) full-length armrests. Swing-away detachable footrests should be removed to allow the client to get closer to counters and tables and also to stand at counters if possible.
5. Transport items safely and easily with a wheelchair lapboard. The lapboard may also serve as a work surface for writing, preparing food, or drying dishes (Fig. 10.37). It protects the lap from injury from hot pans and prevents utensils from falling into the lap. Use silicone pads as nonslip surfaces and to prevent burning.

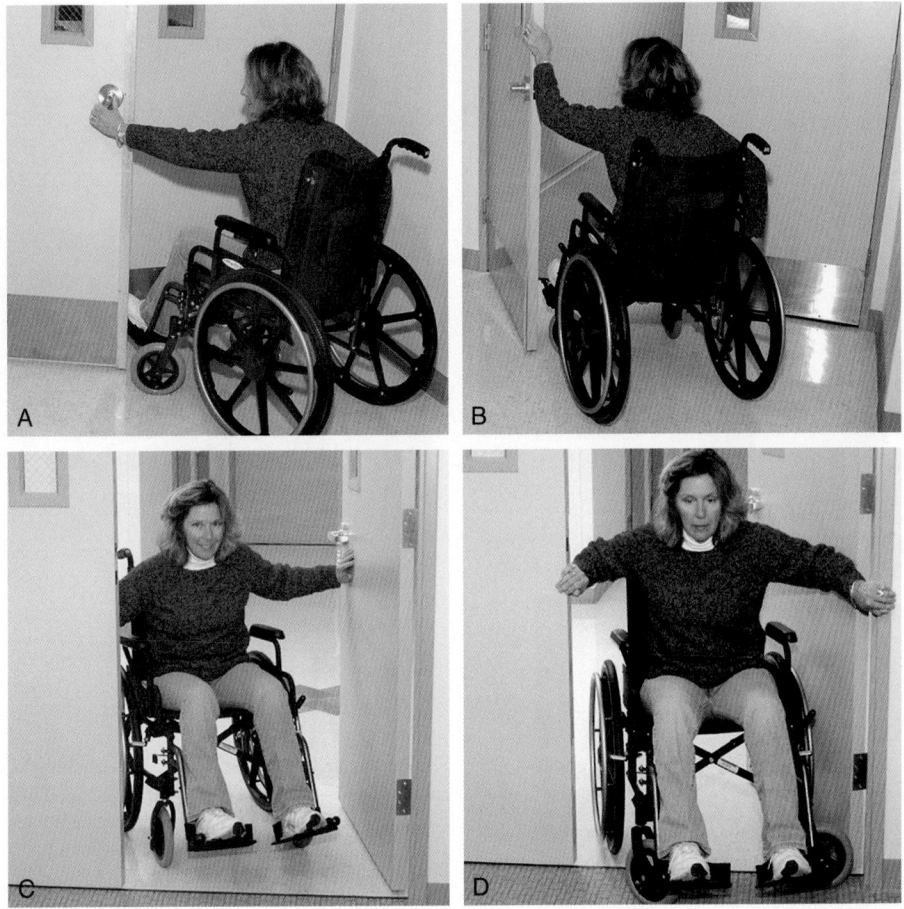

Fig. 10.35 Independent navigation through an open door with the door opening toward the client. (A) As the door is pulled open, the wheelchair is angled and ready to pivot. (B) The client turns and begins to move the wheelchair through the doorway. (C) The client pulls on the door frame with one hand and pushes the door farther open with the other. (D) The client then quickly propels the wheelchair through the doorway. If the door closes before the client is all the way through, the client allows the door to bump against the wheelchair (first moving his or her hand out of the way) and then applies an additional push to the door. (From Fairchild SL: Pierson and Fairchild's principles and techniques of patient care, ed 5, St Louis, 2013, Saunders.)

6. Fasten a drop-leaf board to a bare wall, or install a slide-out board under a counter to provide a work surface that is a comfortable height in a kitchen that is otherwise standard. When not in use, the drop-leaf board can be securely fastened to the wall to increase accessibility to the kitchen space.

7. Place a cutting board on an open drawer to set up a workstation. The drawer should be stable when pulled out and should be at a height that allows the wheelchair user to roll under it and reach with a comfortable arm position.

8. Fit cabinets with custom or prefabricated pullout shelves for ease in reaching back spaces.

9. Pull-down cupboards can be installed for reaching stored items.[28]

10. A commercially available wooden or plastic round turntable, commonly known as a Lazy Susan, can be used to store items for easy access by just rotating the device.

11. Cook tops that are open underneath to accommodate wheelchairs and front-panel stove controls are easier to access.[28]

12. Tilted or angled mirrors over the range can allow cooks to see the contents of pots.

13. A small electric toaster oven with a microwave oven or a microwave convection oven can be substituted for the range if the range is not safely manageable.

14. Ovens that have doors that swing sideways (instead of the standard doors that open down) can make it safer to put items into an oven and take them out.[28]

15. Use front-loading washers and dryers. Use a reacher for items that are difficult to access in the washer and dryer.

16. Vacuum carpets with a carpet sweeper or tank-type cleaner that rolls easily and is lightweight or self-propelled. A retractable cord may prevent the cord from tangling in the wheels. Robotic vacuum cleaners may also be considered, but safety should be a concern, if it gets stuck and can be tripped on.

17. Sweep and mop floors with lightweight swivel head cleaners that allow easier reach.

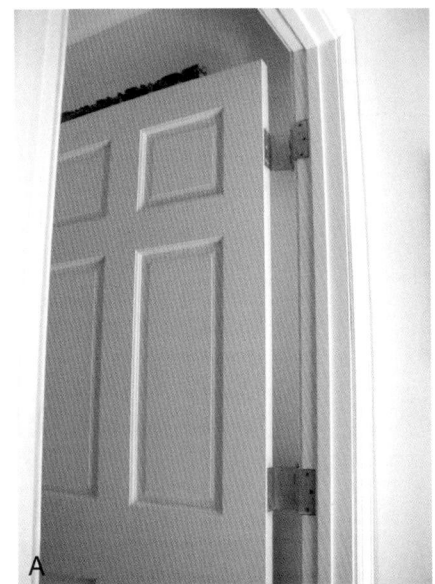

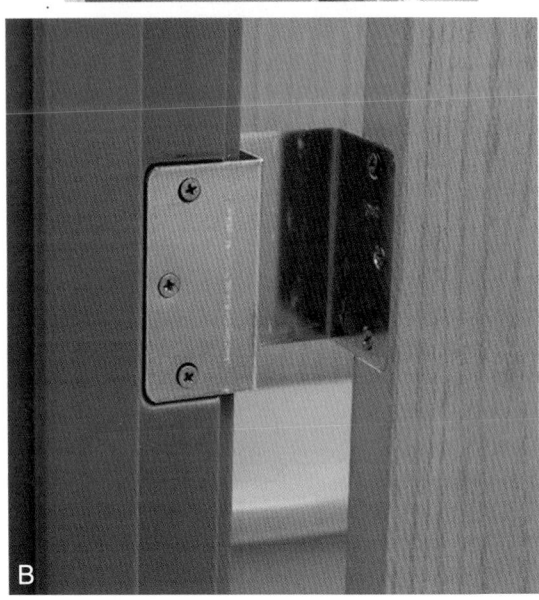

Fig. 10.36 (A) Offset door hinges allow for a wider doorway for wheelchair users. (B) Close-up of offset hinges. (A courtesy How to Adapt: www.howtoadapt.com; B courtesy Brigs Healthcare, West Des Moines, IA.)

ADLs for the Person With Quadriplegia/Tetraplegia

For an overview of expected functional outcomes for ADLs and IADLs for each level of SCI, refer to the detailed tables in Chapter 37. Expected outcomes depend in part on whether a complete or incomplete injury occurred. Persons with C1-4 injuries will require assistance for all ADLs except communication and mobility, if appropriate equipment is available. A person with a C5 injury will require considerable special equipment and assistance. (Externally powered orthotics and arm braces or mobile arm supports are recommended for C3, C4, and C5 levels of muscle function (see Chapters 31 and 37. Individuals with muscle function from C6 can be relatively independent

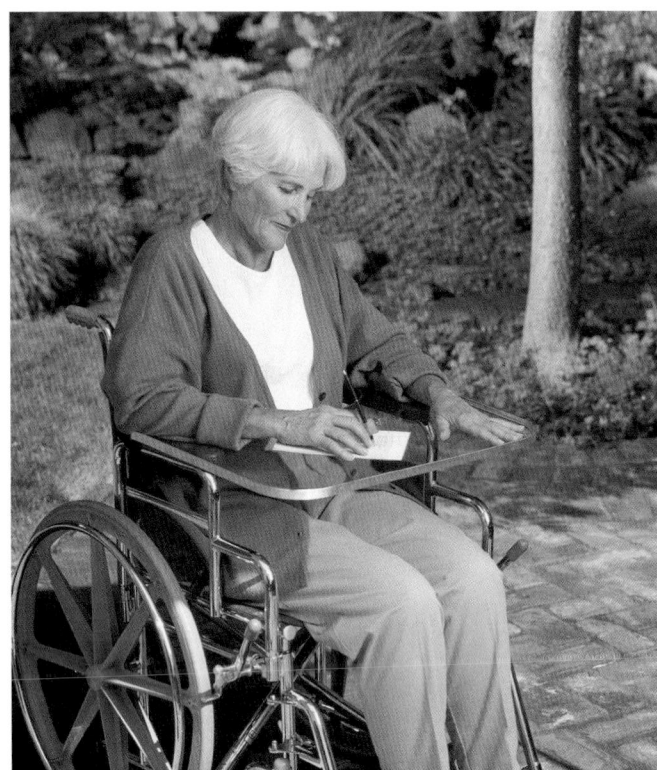

Fig. 10.37 Wheelchair with lapboard. (Courtesy North Coast Medical, Gilroy, CA.)

with adaptations and assistive devices and may benefit from the use of a wrist-driven flexor hinge hand splint (also known as a tenodesis hand splint).

It is important to consider that some people, such as those with high-level quadriplegia/tetraplegia (e.g., C1-4 injury), may be physically dependent in performing an ADL or IADL but independent in directing others to assist in those areas. It is within the purview of the occupational therapist to ensure that such clients can independently direct others, such as personal care attendants, in ADLs and IADLs as needed.[12]

Dressing Activities

Training in dressing can be commenced when the spine is stable and precautions, if present, are followed. The minimum criteria for UE dressing are:
1. Fair to good muscle strength in the deltoids, upper and middle trapezii, shoulder rotators, rhomboids, biceps, supinators, and radial wrist extensors.
2. ROM of 0 degrees to 90 degrees in shoulder flexion and abduction, 0 degrees to 80 degrees in shoulder internal rotation, 0 degrees to 30 degrees in external rotation, and 15 degrees to 140 degrees in elbow flexion.
3. Sitting balance in bed or wheelchair, which may be achieved with the assistance of bed rails, an electric hospital bed, or a wheelchair safety belt.
4. Finger prehension achieved with adequate tenodesis grasp or wrist-driven flexor hinge orthosis.

Additional criteria for dressing the lower extremities are:

1. Fair to good muscle strength in the pectoralis major and minor, serratus anterior, and rhomboid major and minor.
2. ROM of 0 degrees to 120 degrees in knee flexion, 0 degrees to 110 degrees in hip flexion, and 0 degrees to 80 degrees in hip external rotation.
3. Body control for transfer from bed to wheelchair with minimal assistance.
4. Ability to roll from side to side, turn from supine position to prone position and back, and balance in side-lying.
5. Vital capacity must be greater than 50%.

Dressing is contraindicated if any of the following factors are present[17,68]:

1. Unstable spine at the site of injury
2. Pressure sores or a tendency for skin breakdown during rolling, scooting, and transferring
3. Uncontrollable muscle spasms in the legs
4. Less than 50% vital capacity

Sequence of dressing. The recommended sequence for training to dress is to put on slacks while still in bed, then transfer to a wheelchair and put on shirt, socks, and shoes.[84] Some clients may want to put on their socks before their pants because socks may help the feet slip through the pant legs more easily. They may also want to put on their shoes in bed, after putting on their slacks, to prevent injury during the transfer.

Expected proficiency. Clients with spinal cord lesions at C7 and below can achieve independence with dressing for both the upper and lower extremities. Clients with lesions at C6 can also achieve independence with dressing, but LE dressing may be difficult or impractical in terms of time and energy for these clients. Clients with lesions at C5 to C6 can achieve independence in UE dressing, with some exceptions. It is difficult or impossible for these clients to put on a bra, tuck a shirt or blouse into a waistband, or fasten buttons on shirt fronts and cuffs. Factors such as age, physical proportions, coordination, secondary medical conditions, and motivation affect the degree of proficiency in dressing skills that any client can achieve.[22] Many people with various injuries, including quadriplegia/tetraplegia, now post educational videos on platforms such as YouTube to share how they perform ADLs such as dressing. However, it is important for the information to be vetted by more experienced therapists and sources to ensure that the techniques are appropriate.

Types of clothing. Clothing should be loose and have front openings. Slacks need to be a size larger than usually worn to accommodate the urine collection device or leg braces if worn. Wraparound skirts and incontinence pads are helpful for women. The fasteners that are easiest to manage are zippers and Velcro closures. Because the client with quadriplegia often uses the thumb as a hook to manage clothing, loops attached to zipper pulls, undershorts, and even the back of the shoes can be helpful. Belt loops sewn onto the waistbands of slacks with reinforced stitching are used for pulling. Bras should have stretchy straps and no wires. Front-opening bra styles can be adapted by fastening loops and adding Velcro closures; back-opening styles can have loops added at each side of the fastening. Underwear may be eliminated because it is an extra step, has the potential to contribute to skin breakdown, and results in greater difficulty in toileting.

Shoes can be half to one size larger than normally worn to accommodate edema and spasticity and to prevent pressure sores and even autonomic dysreflexia. Shoe fasteners can be adapted with Velcro, elastic shoelaces, large buckles, or flip-back tongue closures. Some people use shoes with zippers and looped draw cords with adjustable stoppers. Loose woolen or cotton socks without elastic cuffs should be used initially. Nylon socks, which tend to stick to the skin, may be used as skill is gained. If neckties are used, the clip-on type or a regular tie that has been pre-knotted and can be slipped over the head may be manageable for some clients.

Slacks/pants

Donning slacks (SCI level C6-7). Setup—pants, socks, shoes, and adaptive devices (if needed) can be placed in the wheelchair, which is placed next to the bed the night before for easier access when the client gets dressed in the morning.

Method 1 (no assistive device)

1. Long-sit on the bed with the bed rails up and, if needed, the head of the bed elevated (if using a full electric bed).
2. Position the slacks at the foot of the bed with the pant legs over the end of the bed and front of pants side up.[84]
3. Sit up and lift one knee at a time by hooking the right hand under the right knee to pull the leg into flexion; put pants over the right foot by using patting motions of the palms while keeping bent at the waist.
4. Return the right leg to extension or semi-extended position and repeat the procedure with the left hand and left knee. Work the slacks up the legs, using patting and sliding motions with the palms of the hands. Vernon uses fingerless weight-lifting gloves to help grip the pants.[113-115] Ellis showed how he used rubber wristbands on his wrists to give traction for pants to grip.[36]
5. Return to the sitting position and repeat this procedure, pulling and patting on the slacks up to thigh level. Remain long-sitting, lean on the left elbow, and pull the slacks over the right buttock; reverse the process for the other side.
6. Alternatively, flatten the bed (if it is raised up) remain in the supine position and roll side to side while using bed rails for support; place free arm behind the back and hook the thumb in the waistband, belt loop, or pocket, and pull the slacks up over the hips. Repeated as often as necessary to get the slacks over the buttock.
7. Using the palms of the hands in pushing and smoothing motions, straighten the slack legs.
8. In the supine position, fasten the slacks by hooking the thumb in the loop on zipper pull, patting the Velcro closed, or using hand splints and buttonhooks for buttons or a zipper pull.[22,84]

YouTube videos demonstrating this technique have been posted by individuals who have been injured, such as Beau Vernon and Mason Ellis.[36,113-115]

Method 2—assistive device

1. Follow steps 1 and 2 in method 1.
2. If unable to maintain the leg in flexion by holding it with one arm or through advantageous use of spasticity, use a dressing band. This device is a piece of elasticized webbing that has been sewn into a figure-8 pattern, with a small loop and a

large loop. The small loop is hooked around the foot, and the large loop is anchored over the knee. The band is measured for the individual client so that its length is appropriate to maintain the desired amount of knee flexion. Once the slacks are in place, the knee loop is pushed off the knee and the dressing band is removed from the foot with a dressing stick.

3. Work the slacks up the legs, using patting and sliding motions with the palms of the hands. While still long-sitting, with the pants to midcalf height, insert the dressing stick into a front belt loop. Grip the dressing stick by slipping its loop over the wrist. Pull on the dressing stick while extending the trunk, returning to the supine position. Return to the sitting position and repeat this procedure, pulling on the dressing sticks and maneuvering the slacks up to thigh level.

4. Follow steps 5 to 8 in method 1.

Variation. Substitute the following for step 2: Sit up and lift one knee at a time by hooking the right hand under the right knee to pull the leg into flexion, then cross the foot over the opposite leg (which is extended) above the knee. This position frees the foot so that the slacks can be placed more easily, and it requires less trunk balance. Continue with all other steps.

Removing slacks/pants (SCI level C6-7)

1. Lying supine in the bed (a flat bed is easier than if the head of the bed is up) with the bed rails up, unfasten the belt and fasteners.

2. Placing the thumbs in the belt loops, waistband, or pockets, work the slacks past the hips by stabilizing the arms in shoulder extension and scooting the body toward the head of the bed.

3. Use the arms as described in step 2 and roll from side to side to get the slacks past the buttocks.

4. Coming to a sitting position and alternately pulling the legs into flexion, push the slacks down the legs.

5. Slacks can be pushed off over the feet with a dressing stick or by hooking the thumbs in the waistband.

Front-opening and pullover garments (SCI level C5-7). Front-opening and pullover garments include blouses, jackets, vests, sweaters, skirts, and front-opening dresses.[22,84] UE dressing is frequently performed in the wheelchair for greater trunk stability.

Donning front-opening or pullover garments (SCI level C5-7)

1. Position the garment across the thighs with the back facing up and the neck toward the knees.

2. Place both arms under the back of the garment and in the armholes.

3. Push the sleeves up onto the arms, past the elbows.

4. Using a wrist extension grip, hook the thumbs under the garment back and gather up the material from the neck to the hem.

5. To pass the garment over the head, adduct and externally rotate the shoulders and flex the elbows while flexing the head forward.

6. When the garment is over the head, relax the shoulders and wrists and remove the hands from the back of the garment. Most of the material will be gathered up at the neck, across the shoulders, and under the arms.

7. To work the garment down over the body, shrug the shoulders, lean forward, and use elbow flexion and wrist extension. Use the wheelchair arms for balance if necessary. Additional maneuvers to accomplish this task are to hook the wrists into the sleeves and pull the material free from the underarms, or lean forward, reach back, and slide the hand against the material to help pull the garment down.

8. If hand function is inadequate, the garment can be buttoned from bottom to top with the aid of a buttonhook and a wrist-driven flexor hinge splint.

Removing front-opening or pullover garments (SCI level C5-7)

1. Sit in the wheelchair and wear wrist-driven flexor hinge splints. Unfasten the buttons (if any) while wearing orthotics and using a buttonhook. Remove the splints for the remaining steps.

2. For pullover garments, hook the thumb in back of the neckline, extend the wrist, and pull the garment over the head while turning the head toward the side of the raised arm. Maintain balance by resting against the opposite wheelchair armrest or pushing on the thigh with an extended arm.[113-115]

3. For stretchy front-opening clothing, hook the thumb in the opposite armhole and push the sleeve down the arm. Elevation and depression of the shoulders with trunk rotation can be used to get the garment to slip down the arms as far as possible.

4. Hold one cuff with the opposite thumb while the elbow is flexed to pull the arm out of the sleeve.

See Beau Vernon's progression as he took his t-shirt off in his wheelchair by himself for the first time, then, later after practice.[113]

Bra (back opening)

Putting on a bra (SCI level C5-7). The bra is adapted and has loop extenders attached on both the right and left sides of the fasteners. The bra is around the trunk and fastened in the front first, then it is twisted around into the correct position. The arms are placed in the straps last.

1. Place the bra across the lap with the shoulder straps toward the knees and the inside of cups, which are facing up.

2. Using a right-to-left procedure, hold the end of the bra closest to the right side with the hand or a reacher and pass the bra around the back from right to left side. Lean against the bra at the back to hold it in place while hooking the thumb of the left hand in a loop attached near the bra fastener. Hook the right thumb in a similar loop on the right side, and fasten the bra in front at waist level.

3. Next, use thumbs to grasp bra and use wrist extension, elbow flexion, shoulder adduction, and internal rotation, to rotate the bra around the body so that the front of the bra is in the front of the body.

4. While leaning on one forearm, hook the opposite thumb in the front end of the strap and pull the strap over the shoulder; repeat procedure on the other side.[22,84]

Variation (similar to putting on shirt) (SCI C6-C7). For C6-7, this technique may be easier than that described previously, unless the client has very large breasts or broad shoulders, which may make it difficult to put head and shoulders through straps that are pre-clasped.

1. Bra is back closure–type with hook and eye. Seated in wheelchair, place bra on lap with shoulder straps at knees with inside of cups of bra facing breasts. Using tenodesis grasp, with each hand holding each side of back strap, clasp bra straps together.
2. Once clasped, put arms through straps (like a pullover shirt). If one arm has limited range of motion or is painful, put that arm in first, and bring strap up to elbow by bending at hips and/raising elbows up. Place other arm into other shoulder strap past elbow.
3. Put head through by looping thumbs into back of strap and lift up enough for head to fit through. Bend head forward into bra so that bra is now around the body.
4. Use thumbs and wrists to place breasts into cups and to straighten shoulder straps.[74] See Milz demonstrate this technique[74] at https://www.youtube.com/watch?v=3LxhO3ISZ60.

Removing a bra
1. Hook the thumb under the opposite bra strap, and push the strap down over the shoulder while elevating shoulder.
2. Pull the arm out of the strap and repeat the procedure for other arm.
3. Push the bra down to waist level and turn it around as described previously to bring the fasteners to the front.
4. Unfasten the bra by hooking the thumbs into the adapted loops near the fasteners.

Alternatives for a back-opening bra are (1) a front-opening bra with loops for using a wrist extension grip or (2) a stretchable bra that has no fasteners (e.g., sports bra that is not tight) and can be put on like a pullover shirt.

Socks
Putting on socks (SCI level C6-7)
Method 1
1. Sit in a wheelchair (or on the bed if balance is adequate) in cross-legged position with one ankle crossed over the opposite knee.
2. Pull the sock over the foot using wrist extension and patting movements with the palm of the hand.[22] To prevent pressure areas, check to make sure there are no creases or thickened areas on the socks.

Method 2
1. Sitting in a wheelchair with the seat belt fastened, hook one arm at the elbow around the push handle of the wheelchair, which allows for improved stability at the truck while reaching forward.
2. Position the foot on a stool, chair, or stable open drawer to elevate it enough to reach easily. Unhook the arm from the push handle once stable.
3. Pull the sock over the foot using wrist extension and patting movements with the palm of the hand.[22] To prevent pressure areas, check to make sure there are no creases or thickened areas on the socks.

Method 3 (using an adaptive device)
1. Use a sock aid (see Fig. 10.7) to assist in putting on socks while seated in a wheelchair. Powder sock aide (to reduce friction) and put the sock on the aide, using the thumbs and the palms of the hands to smooth out the sock.
2. With the cord loops of the sock aide around the wrist or thumb, throw the aide beyond the foot.
3. Maneuver the aide over the toes by pulling the cords, using elbow flexion. Insert the foot as far as possible into the aide.
4. To remove the aide from the sock after the foot has been inserted, move the heel forward off the wheelchair's footrest. Use wrist extension (of the free hand) behind the knee and continue pulling the cords of the aide until it is removed and the sock is in place on the foot. Use the palms to smooth the sock with patting and stroking motions.[22] Two loops can be sewn on either side of the top of the sock so that the thumbs can be hooked into the loops and the socks pulled on.

Removing socks (SCI level C6-7)
Method 1 (no adaptive device)
1. While long-sitting in the bed and with the hips flexed forward, slide the hands into the sock with the wrist extended, gradually working the sock off the feet and toes.
2. If seated in a wheelchair, hook the thumb in the sock and use wrist extension to slide it off.

Method 2 (using an adaptive device). While sitting in a wheelchair or long-sitting in the bed with the hips flexed forward, use a dressing stick with a coated end or a long-handled shoehorn to push the sock down over the heel. Cross the legs if needed.

Shoes
Putting on shoes (SCI level C6-7)
1. Use the same position as for putting on socks.
2. Use the thumbs or, if needed, a long-handled dressing stick and insert the aid into the tongue of the shoe. Place the shoe opening over the toes. Remove the dressing aid from the shoe and dangle the shoe on the toes.
3. Place the palm of the hand on the sole of the shoe and pull the shoe toward the heel of the foot. One hand is used to stabilize the leg while the other hand pushes against the sole of the shoe to work the shoe onto the foot. Use the palms and sides of the hand to push the shoe on.
4. With the feet flat on the floor or on a wheelchair footrest and the knees flexed 90 degrees, place a long-handled shoehorn (if needed) in the heel of the shoe and press down on the flexed knee until the heel is in the shoe. Fasten the shoe.

Removing shoes (SCI level C6-7)
1. Sitting in a wheelchair with the legs crossed as described previously, unfasten the shoes.
2. Use a shoehorn or dressing stick, if needed, to push on the heel counter of the shoe, dislodging it from the heel. The shoe will drop, or it can be pushed to the floor with the dressing stick.

Feeding Activities

Feeding may be assisted by a variety of devices, depending on the level of the client's muscle function. Someone with a C1-4 injury will likely need assistance to eat unless an electrical self-feeding device is used. These devices allow independence because the client uses head movement to hit a switch that turns the plate and then brings the spoon down to the plate and back up to mouth level.

An injury at C5 may require mobile arm supports or externally powered splints and braces. A wrist splint and a universal cuff (see Fig. 10.11) may be used together if a wrist-driven flexor hinge splint is not used. The universal cuff holds the eating utensil, and the splint stabilizes the wrist. A nonskid mat and a plate with a plate guard may adequately stabilize the plate for pushing and picking up food (C5-7).

A regular or swivel spoon-fork combination with a universal cuff can be used when there is minimal muscle function (C5). A long plastic straw with a straw clip to stabilize it in the cup or glass eliminates the need for picking up cups. A bilateral or unilateral clip-type holder on a glass or cup makes it possible for many individuals with hand and arm weakness to manage liquids without a straw.

Built-up utensils may be useful for those with some functional grasp or tenodesis grasp. Food may be cut with an adapted knife if arm strength is adequate to manage the device. Food also may be cut with a sharp knife if a wrist-driven flexor hinge splint is used.

Personal Hygiene and Grooming

1. Use a padded shower seat or padded transfer tub bench and transfer board for transfers (SCI level C1-7).
2. Extend reach by using a long-handled bath sponge with a loop handle or a built-up handle (SCI level C6-7).
3. Eliminate the need to grasp a washcloth by using bath mitts or bath gloves (SCI level C5-7).
4. Hold a toothbrush with a universal cuff (SCI level C5-7).
5. Use a wall-mounted hair dryer. Use a universal cuff to hold a brush or comb for hair styling while using the mounted hair dryer[28] (SCI level C5-7) (Fig. 10.38).
6. Use a clip-type holder for an electric razor (SCI level C5-7).

7. Individuals with quadriplegia can use suppository inserters to manage bowel care independently (SCI level C6-7).
8. Use a skin inspection mirror with a long stem and looped handle (see Fig. 10.34) for independent skin inspection. Devices and methods selected must be adapted to the degree of weakness of each client (SCI level C6-7).
9. Adapted leg bag clamps for emptying catheter leg bags are also available for individuals with limited hand function. Elastic leg bag straps may be replaced with Velcro straps (SCI level C5-7).
10. If the client is unable to reach the leg bag clamp, or does not have hand function to do so, commercially available manual, electric, and wireless leg bag systems allow people to empty the leg bag with the pull of a cord, or a push of a button (SCI level C1-7).[33,34]

Communication Management and Environmental Adaptations

1. For nondigital book or magazine: Turn pages in with an electric page turner, mouth stick (Fig. 10.39), or head wand if hand and arm function is inadequate (SCI level C4-5).
2. For keyboarding, writing, and painting, insert a pen, pencil, typing stick, or paintbrush into a universal cuff that has been positioned with the opening on the ulnar side of the palm (Fig. 10.40) (SCI level C5-7).
3. Touch telephone keys with the universal cuff and a pencil positioned with the eraser down (SCI level C5-7). The receiver may need to be positioned for listening. For clients with no arm function, a speakerphone can be used, along with a mouth stick to push the button, or voice activation to initiate a call. Set any frequently used numbers for speed-dial. An operator can also assist with dialing (SCI level C1-5).
4. Mobile phones allow many functions with voice activation including calling out, Web searches, calendar programs, and

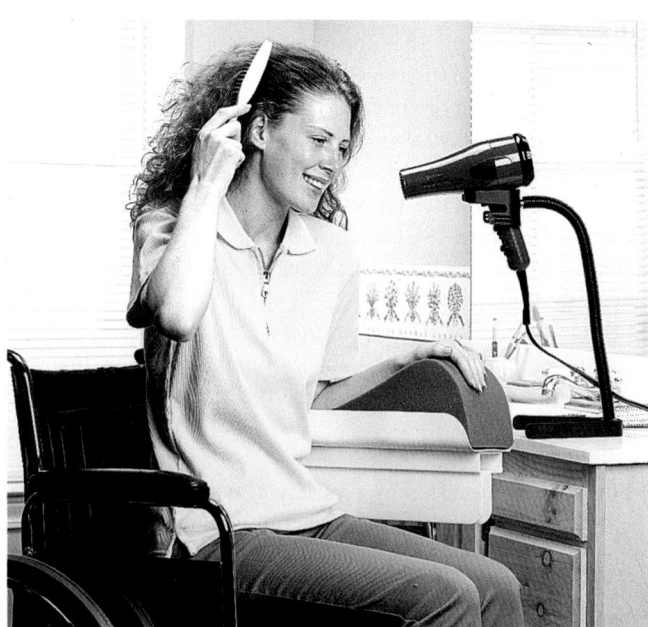

Fig. 10.38 Hair dryer holder. (Courtesy Patterson Medical, Warrenville, IL.)

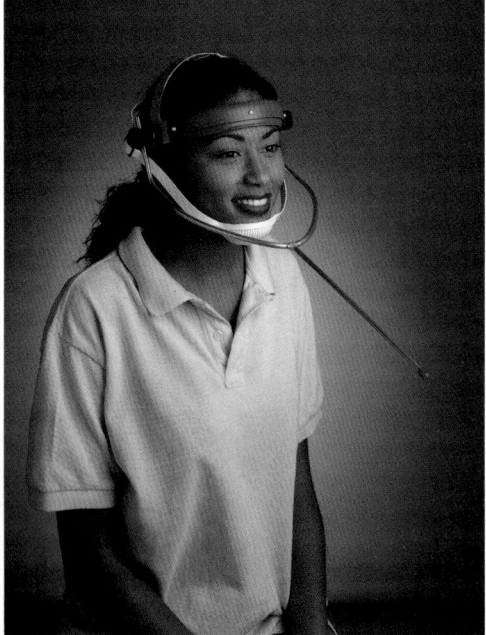

Fig. 10.39 Mouth wand. (Courtesy Patterson Medical, Warrenville, IL.)

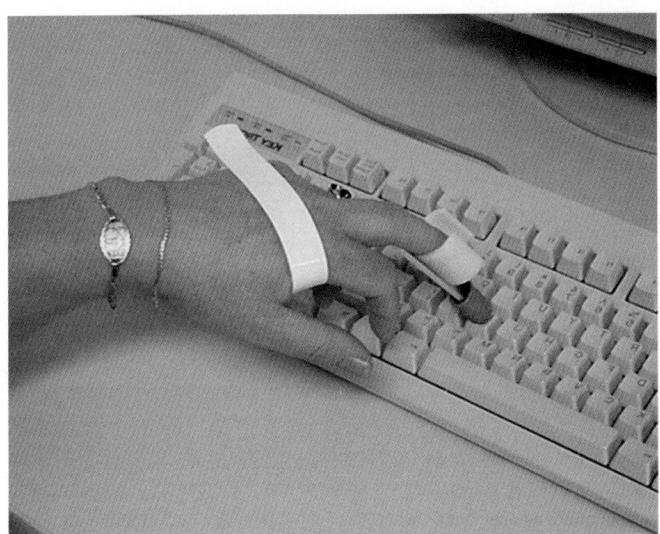

Fig. 10.40 Typing with a keyboard aid. (Courtesy Patterson Medical, Warrenville, IL.)

directories, to name a few. A touch-screen phone with multiple functions can eliminate the need for multiple devices to organize information (SCI level C1-7).

5. Use personal computers or smart phones. A computer mouse, hands-free mouse, or voice recognition program may be substituted for use of the keyboard. A variety of different mouse and keyboard designs and sizes are available (SCI level C1-7).

6. Clients with hand weakness can use built-up pencils and pens or special pencil holders. The Wanchik writer (see Fig. 10.16) is an effective adaptive writing device (SCI level C5-7).

7. Sophisticated electronic communication devices operated by mouth, pneumatic controls, and head controls are available for clients with no function in the upper extremities. Other communication devices are available that rely on eye blinks and gazes (SCI level C1-5).

8. MP3 (a digital audio recording format) players are capable of playing digitally available music and podcasts and can be used with a universal cuff and a pencil positioned with the eraser down or other adapted pointer to press buttons (SCI level C5-7).

9. Environmental controls allow easy operation from a panel designed to run multiple devices, such as televisions, radios, lights, telephones, intercoms, and hospital beds (see Chapter 17) (SCI level C1-7).

Functional Mobility

The principles of wheelchair transfer techniques for the individual with quadriplegia are discussed in Chapter 11. Mobility depends on the degree of weakness. Electric wheelchairs operated by hand, chin, head, or pneumatic controls have greatly increased the mobility of individuals with severe UE and LE weakness. Vans fitted with wheelchair lifts and stabilizing devices provide transportation for these clients, allowing them to pursue community, vocational, educational, and leisure activities with the help of an assistant. In addition, adaptations for hand controls have made it possible for many clients with function of at least the C6 level to drive independently.

Home Management, Meal Preparation, and Cleanup Activities

Clients with muscle function of C6 or better may be independent for light homemaking with appropriate devices, adaptations, and safety awareness. Many of the suggestions for wheelchair maneuverability and environmental adaptation for a person with paraplegia also apply here. In addition, clients with UE weakness need to use lightweight equipment and special devices. A classic book that is still available, *The Mealtime Manual for People with Disability and the Aging*, compiled by Klinger,[60] contains many helpful specific suggestions that apply to homemakers with weak upper extremities. Specialty suppliers for cooking devices to make meal preparation and cooking easier and more efficient are an excellent source for new ideas. The kitchen and home sections of general national and international stores are other good resources for ideas and products. As mentioned, many people with various disabilities post themselves online performing ADLs and IADLs.

1. Use extended lever-type faucets for easier reach and control or motion sensor faucets (SCI level C5-7).
2. To eliminate the need for grasp and release, use pump bottles for cleaners and soaps or motion sensor dispensers (SCI level C5-7).
3. For cooking utensils, use universal cuff adaptations, a tenodesis splint, or adapted long-handled utensils (SCI level C5-7).
4. For opening cans, use one-touch can openers.
5. For opening jars, use electric jar openers.
6. To wash dishes, use a combination soap dispenser/sponge.
7. To wash and rinse lettuce, use a salad spinner with a push-button center.

ADLs for the Person With Low Vision

Many people with or without physical disabilities also have low vision as a result of advancing age or age-related eye diseases, or as a complication of diabetes.[63] Occupational therapists specialize in the area of vision rehabilitation itself. However, occupational therapists who work with clients with physical disabilities frequently see individuals with visual impairment; therefore, it is important for occupational therapists to be knowledgeable about this condition so they can help promote independence in occupations.[86,87,119]

Low vision is defined as a visual impairment that cannot be corrected by regular eyeglasses or other corrective lenses, or by surgery or medication, and that negatively affects the performance of daily occupations.[63,75,76] Research indicates that for older people, low vision is a greater threat to independence than hearing loss.[23,63] With respect to practice guidelines for older adults with low vision, a systematic review of literature from 2010 to 2016 highlights the efficacy of low vision rehabilitation to improve performance of ADLs and IADLs, as well as reading for occupational performance and leisure.[59] In reviewing this literature, Kaldenberg and Smallfield emphasize that available evidence strongly supports routine use of multicomponent low vision intervention to improve ADLs and IADL performance.[59]

Visual changes are considered part of a comprehensive OT evaluation. Evaluation of the person with low vision should initially involve understanding the specific condition that has caused the low vision, such as whether visual acuity is affected or whether a specific field of vision is impaired. (For more information on visual loss in the aging, see Chapter 47). The type of visual loss, along with any other physical or cognitive deficits, influences treatment and adaptive equipment choices. Providing low vision devices is not sufficient in itself to optimize performance in ADLs and IADLs. OT literature in older adults with low vision has shown that multiple components are crucial, such as education, use of low vision devices, problem-solving strategies, and community resources.[63]

In addition to assistive technology, adaptive equipment, and environmental modifications, reorganization and task restructuring may be needed. Weisser-Pike and Kaldenberg provided a framework of intervention strategies that the occupational therapist can consider when addressing functional activities for the person with low vision.[120] Box 10.6 presents the modified

---

BOX 10.6 Framework for Low Vision Interventions

Use of Corrective Lenses
Have client wear glasses for activities as needed. Some people use multiple pairs of glasses, depending on the task performed (e.g., writing, reading, use of the computer, or driving). Ask about the client's most recent eye examination to make sure they have the most recent prescription.

Adequate Lighting
Examples include adding light that shines from behind the client onto the work area, avoiding glare and shadows on writing areas, and using natural light behind the work area.

Good Ergonomic Positioning
Examples include raising reading material within the field of vision and moving closer to an object, such as the television or a person. Ideal positions include upright, midline, comfortable postures.

Increase Contrast Enhancement
Examples include using black ink on white or yellow paper in an easy-to-read font (e.g., Times New Roman or Arial) if providing printed materials. Mark edges of doorways or stairs with contrasting strip.

Simplification of Environment
An example is using a pill organizer, which can eliminate many pill bottles that create clutter and require numerous steps to manage.

Resize Written Materials
Examples include larger print, larger television, and larger label on pill bottles. For people with peripheral vision loss, enlargement of print may be contraindicated. Provide resources for large print materials.

Provide Sensory Substitutes
Use tactile or auditory cues, such as rubber bands on doorknobs and on frozen meals, to indicate how many minutes an item should be cooked; also, talking books and TV ears.

Restructure Routines
Use the time of day when vision is the best to perform difficult activities; use pill organizer.

Visual Skills/Referrals
Refer to vision specialist or low-vision rehab specialist.

Data from Weisser-Pike O, Kaldenberg J: Occupational therapy approaches to facilitate productive aging for individuals with low vision, *OT Practice* 15:CE1–CE8, 2010.

---

version of this framework, which has nine categories, and provides some examples for each category. The occupational therapist may use this model in combination with interventions under the specific functional activity.[120]

Adequate training and selection of the appropriate intervention and adaptive equipment are essential. Allow the client to touch and explore the piece of adaptive equipment before beginning practical teaching, break the steps down into small chunks of information, have the client practice a few days before doing the functional activity with the adaptive equipment, and request a return demonstration after the client has practiced.[54]

The modifications described in the following sections are appropriate for all people with low vision for performing ADLs.

Dressing Activities

1. Light the closet to improve acuity. Hang matching outfits together on the same hanger.
2. Place a safety pin on the label of the backs of shirts, pants, and dresses so that clothing is oriented correctly when worn.
3. Pin socks together before placing them in the washer and dryer so they stay matched.

Feeding Activities

1. Provide high contrast. Ensure that plates contrast with the table surface or place mats. Avoid patterned tablecloths.
2. Arrange food on the plate in a clockwise fashion and orient the person with low vision to the arrangement.

Personal Hygiene and Grooming Activities

1. Reduce clutter in bathroom drawers and cabinets.
2. Use an electric razor.
3. Use magnified mirrors. A front-facing camera can be used to take a photo in the absence of a magnified mirror.[88]
4. Use a high-contrast bath mat in the bathtub.
5. Install high-contrast grab bars in the shower.
6. Use a high-contrast bath chair in the bathtub.
7. Train the client and other caregivers to keep supplies organized by replacing and storing them in the same location.

Communication Management and Environmental Adaptations

1. Use talking watches or clocks to tell time.
2. Use a talking scale to determine weight.
3. Use a large-print magnification screen on the computer.
4. Use large-print books, menus, and pharmacy labels.[103] If the client has a smartphone, use a camera app to take pictures and zoom in on small text on menus, documents, or other objects.[88]
5. Use high-contrast doorknobs. Paint the doorframe a color that contrasts highly with the door to improve ease of identifying the door.
6. Use speakerphones, preprogrammed phone numbers, or a phone with large print and high-contrast numbers. Identify phone buttons with contrasting tape or a Velcro dot to teach the client how to turn the phone on and the correct buttons to push. Use a mobile phone with voice recognition

commands. Enable sound on mobile phones and smartphones to provide auditory feedback when buttons have been pushed.[1] Understand phone accessibility features and use when appropriate.

7. Use writing guides to write letters, checks, or signatures.

8. To read, use books on tape, talking books, electronic books, digital books (e.g., Kindle), or a tablet (e.g., iPad). Screens can be magnified, and some of the devices have "reading" capability so the reader can listen to a story or newspaper article. Software is available, such as the JAWS screen reader, which reads aloud information on a computer screen.

9. To promote verbal communication, provide specific information when giving directions, avoid gestures, and offer to read educational materials out loud.[103]

10. When ending a conversation or leaving the room, notify the client and offer to help guide him or her out of a room because novel environments may be difficult.[103]

11. Do not have clients with low vision "guess" your identity by your voice (e.g., "Do you remember me?"). Clearly introduce yourself.

Lighting and magnifiers

1. Improve lighting by aiming light at the work area, not into the eyes.

2. Reduce glare by having adjustable blinds, sheer curtains, or tinted windows. Wearing dark glasses indoors may also reduce glare.[103]

3. Maximize contrast by providing a work surface that is in contrast to the task. For example, serve a meal on a white plate if the table is dark. Paint a white edge on a dark step. Replace white wall switches with black to contrast with the wall.

4. Simplify figure-ground perception by clearing pathways and eliminating clutter.

5. Work in natural light by placing a chair by a window with the back toward the window.

6. Use magnifiers with lights. These come in a variety of sizes and degrees of magnification. Specialists in low vision can determine the appropriate degree of magnification needed. Some magnifiers are portable, others are attached to stands to do needlework or fine work, and others are sheets of plastic used to magnify an entire page of print.[49]

Functional Mobility

1. Mobility is eased with the clearing of pathways and the minimizing of clutter and furniture. Furniture can be used as guides for going from one place to another.

2. Lighting in hallways and entryways is also needed.

3. The person with low vision needs to optimize visual scanning abilities by learning to turn and position the head frequently when mobile or participating in an activity.[126]

4. Use scan courses (paths), which consist of letters and numbers that are placed systematically along a hallway to encourage those with peripheral vision loss to use visual search and scanning patterns (also see Chapter 24).[103]

5. The OT practitioner may need to refer a client with severe vision loss to an orientation and mobility specialist who is specifically trained in teaching mobility in the community, such as human guide techniques, use of a white cane, and use of service animals by people with low vision or those who are legally blind.

Home Management, Meal Preparation, and Cleanup Activities

Various devices are available to compensate for low vision while managing the home. Organization and consistency are critical to the safe and efficient performance of home management tasks. Family members need to remember to replace items where they were found and to refrain from reorganizing them without the assistance of the person with low vision. Suggestions include the following.[60]

1. For safety, cleaning supplies should be kept in a separate location from the food supplies.

2. Eliminate extra hazardous cleaning supplies and replace them with one multipurpose cleanser. Place this cleaning agent in a uniquely shaped bottle or in a specific location.

3. Mark appliance controls with high-contrast tape or paint to identify start and stop buttons or positions. Place Velcro tabs to mark frequently used positions on dials (e.g., on the 350°F position for the stove or for the wash-and-wear cycle on the washer or dryer).

4. Label cans by using rubber bands to attach index cards with bold, dark print to each can. When the can is used, the card may be placed into a stack to create a shopping list.

5. Indicate the number of minutes needed for microwave cooking by placing rubber bands on the items. Two rubber bands would indicate that the item should be cooked for 2 minutes. Assistance will be needed for the initial setup.

6. Use a liquid level indicator to determine when hot liquid reaches 1 inch from top of a cup or container.

7. Use cutting guides or specially designed knives to cut meat or bread.[49]

8. Audio-record reminder lists or grocery lists. A client with decreased memory may also benefit from a motion-activated voice player. This device may be placed in the home and used to remind the client to complete important tasks whenever they trigger the motion sensor.

9. Discourage the wearing of long, flowing gowns with flowing sleeves (e.g., kimono style) while performing cooking tasks at the stove.

Medication management

1. Use a medication organizer to organize pills.

2. For diabetic management, many products are available for individualized evaluation of the client (e.g., syringe magnifiers, talking or large-print glucometers, and a device to count the insulin dosages).

3. Use talking scales to evaluate weight.

Money management

1. Use a consistent method of folding money to identify denominations, as in the following example:

$1	Keep flat
$5	Fold in square half
$10	Fold lengthwise
$20	Fold in half and then lengthwise

2. Keep different denominations in different sections of the wallet. Learn to recognize coins by size and type of edge (smooth or rough).[125]

3. For clients who want to avoid using credit cards for online purchases, consider payment systems such as PayPal and Google Wallet.[6] At stores that have compatible point-of-sale terminals, tap-to-pay options on mobile devices (e.g., Apple Pay) can eliminate the need to swipe a credit card, enter a pin on a keypad, and have a digital record of how much is spent.[6]

Leisure

1. Use low vision playing cards with large letters and symbols.

2. Search for resources in the community for activities aimed at people with low vision.[86,87] See Chapters 16 and 47.

ADLs for the Person of Large Size/Body Mass

The terms *morbidly obese* and *bariatrics* both have been used to describe the population that is exceptionally large. Morbidly obese is defined as a body mass index (BMI) of 40 or greater. Because the word "morbid" is a term that may be misconstrued, the preferred terms are "class III obesity" or "severe obesity."[121] A person who is considered to be class III is not considered to have a disability, because many people in this category of obesity can function well, but occupational therapists often see people who are of a large size, so consideration needs to be made.[121]

The following are levels of obesity based on BMI.[121]:

- Overweight: BMI 25.0 to 29.9 kg/m²
- Class I Obesity: BMI 30.0 to 34.9 kg/m²
- Class II Obesity: BMI 35.0 to 39.9 kg/m²
- Class III Obesity: BMI ≥40.0 kg/m²

Bariatrics is defined as the medical investigation, prevention, and treatment of obesity with interventions such as diet, nutrition, exercise, behavior modification, lifestyle changes, surgical alternatives, and appropriate medications. It is an area of practice that is continuing to expand.[9,42,43]

Individuals who are exceptionally large may experience difficulty performing ADLs and IADLs.[5,83,104] They may have difficulty with ADLs and IADLs because of limitations in reach, strength, pain, and endurance. They may also experience neuropathies that require increased safety awareness to prevent skin breakdown. People of larger size also experience negative biases in many areas, including healthcare (https://www.obesityaction.org/).[77] As with all clients, a comprehensive evaluation should include primary and secondary medical problems that result in additional functional deficits.

Adaptive techniques, adaptive equipment, and home modifications may allow for increased independence and safety. When recommending adaptive equipment and DME, the occupational therapist must consider the size and durability of equipment. For example, the standard molded sock aid may not fit around the client's calf, whereas softer fabric or flexible plastic sock aids likely will accommodate larger calf sizes.[42,43]

The standard DME issued may have maximal weight limits for safe use. As examples, bath chairs, hospital beds, wheelchairs, or transfer (sliding) boards may accommodate only individuals up to 250 pounds. Issuing adaptive equipment and DME that are inadequate for a client's weight may put the client at risk of injury.

Dressing Activities

Provide resources for clothing available in larger sizes that may help the client feel more comfortable in the community and help with self-esteem. Some manufacturers have designed exercise clothing, swimsuits, and work attire in larger sizes. Many resources can be found on the Internet that offer larger sizes.

Lower extremity dressing activities

1. Use dressing sticks with a Neoprene-covered coat hook on one end and a small hook on the other for pushing and pulling garments off and on the feet and legs.

2. For socks, use a large, flexible, commercially available sock aid (see Fig. 10.7). The rigid sock aids available may not fit around larger calves.

3. Compensate for the need to bend to tie shoelaces by using elastic shoelaces or other adapted shoe fasteners, such as Velcro-fastened shoes or secure slip-on shoes. Edema is frequently a problem with this population and should be taken into account when shoes are selected.

4. Use reachers (see Fig. 10.8) for picking up socks and shoes, arranging clothes, removing clothes from hangers, picking up objects on the floor, and putting on pants, to avoid bending or unsafe reaching.

Upper extremity dressing activities

1. Use front-opening or pullover garments that are one size larger than needed and are made of fabrics that have some stretch.

2. Use dressing sticks to push a shirt or blouse over the head and reach around shoulders. Some exceptionally large individuals are not able to touch the shoulder with the opposite hand because of the girth of the trunk.

Personal Hygiene and Grooming Activities

Bathing

1. A handheld flexible shower hose for bathing and shampooing the hair can eliminate the need to stand in the shower and offers the user control of the direction of the spray.

2. A long-handled bath brush or sponge with a soap holder (see Fig. 10.13) or long cloth scrubber can allow the user to reach the legs, feet, and back. If the standard long-handled bath brush/sponge is not long enough, add an extension with PVC pipe and a bend about one third of the distance from the handle to improve reach.

3. Safety rails that can accommodate the larger individual's weight (see Fig. 10.15) can be used for bathtub transfers, and safety mats or strips can be placed on the bathtub bottom to prevent slipping.

4. A transfer tub bench or a shower stool (see Fig. 10.5) set in the bathtub or shower stall can eliminate the need to stand to shower, thus increasing safety and conserving energy. The bench should be built to accommodate the user's weight. The larger equipment may not be easily obtainable and may need to be special ordered. It is usually more functional to remove the back on the shower equipment to allow for increased sitting surface and room for the posterior buttocks to shift back on the seat and allow the user to lean back as legs are lifted into the shower or over the edge of the tub. The user must have adequate sitting balance before removing the back of the bench or stool.

5. Evaluate issues with water spillage from the tub or shower when using a transfer tub bench. Tub benches typically have three panels on it where the client sits on two of the panels that are inside the tub. A shower curtain is tucked in between the panel that is inside the tub and the panel that is outside so that water does not spill out onto the floor. A person of larger size who uses a transfer tub bench that fits into the standard tub may need to plan ahead to manage water over-flow because the width of the hips may cover the area on the bench originally designed for placement of the shower curtain. Water on the floor can lead to a fall and create extra cleanup. Extra towels may be required when setting up the shower.

6. Grab bars can be installed to prevent falls and ease transfers and should accommodate appropriate weight limits. A licensed contractor must securely mount these into the studs of the wall. The suction grab bars commercially available would not be safe for this population because the amount of pull and weight would cause the suction to release from the wall.

7. Use a hair dryer to thoroughly dry the skin in hard-to-reach areas (e.g., buttocks, crotch, and abdominal folds) to prevent rashes and fungal infections in the folds.

Grooming

1. Use a long-handled mirror for regular skin checks of the feet to detect skin breakdown.

2. Over-the-counter spray products, such as deodorant, hair spray, and spray powder, can compensate for limited reach because the user does not need to make direct skin contact with the product. The spray can be aimed in the general direction (e.g., the underarms) to provide adequate coverage.

Toileting

1. Use toilet paper holders/extenders for toilet hygiene because reach is often difficult for optimal hygiene. Several types of toilet aids are available in catalogs that sell assistive devices.

2. Use a bidet mounted on the toilet for toilet hygiene. Select one on which the controls are not mounted to the seat and likely to be covered by the user's wide hips. Many options are available, ranging from one as simple as a pump with a hand-held spray to deluxe models that include front and rear wash, warm-air drying, and water pressure control. The deluxe models may not accommodate rails place on it in the future.

3. Dressing sticks can be used to pull garments up after using the toilet.

4. Bedside commodes made for larger people can be used over the toilet, but only if there is enough room on the sides. The commode also may be used at the bedside. The commode should be built to accommodate the user's weight. The sitting surfaces should be smooth to prevent skin tears or pressure areas. Because body size may push the large person forward, the standard hole size is not in the correct location for toileting. The commode hole should be larger than that for a standard commode to allow space to reach for toilet hygiene and proper alignment for elimination. If the user is not able to stand and pivot to the commode, drop-arm commodes are available for the bariatric population (Fig. 10.41).

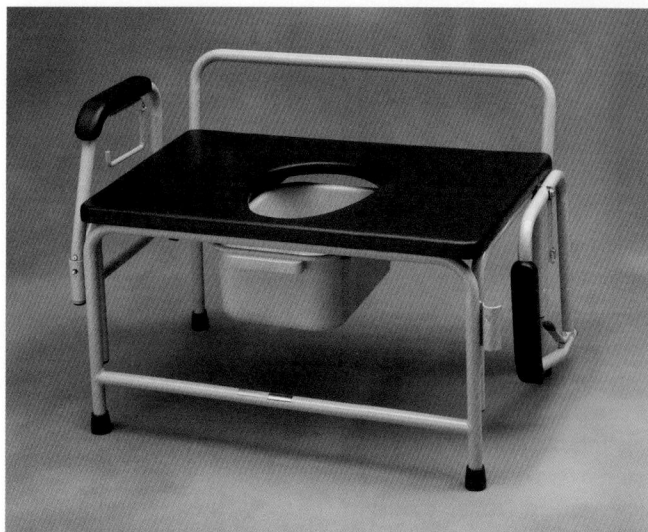

Fig. 10.41 Bariatric commode. (Courtesy North Coast Medical, Gilroy, CA.)

5. Adapt male urinals with a PVC pipe handle to allow for independent use. This allows the client to use one hand to hold the urinal and the other hand to lift abdominal folds to place the urinal.

6. Some people of very large size who may have lost weight in a shorter time may have large extra skin folds on the legs that may get caught on commodes, so it is important to be aware of this.

Functional Mobility

1. Set up furniture at an appropriate height by raising it on blocks to elevate it or by shortening leg rests to lower it. Multiple sitting surfaces allow the large individual to alter sitting pressures during the day; elevate lower extremities, which may be prone to edema; and provide alternatives to staying in bed. Several manufacturers make electrical lifts for furniture or chairs that accommodate individuals weighing up to 1000 lb.

2. A glider/office chair that is operated by the feet can facilitate transportation if LE endurance is limited. It should be built to accommodate the user's weight, and the user should be able to demonstrate a safe sit-to-stand technique because the chair is mobile and without brakes to secure it during transfers.

3. Encourage the use of mobility aids for safety that may have been issued by a PT. A PT can assess whether a four-wheeled walker with a seat may improve mobility and function because the seat can be used as a fatigue management method to carry items when moving from room to room. The user can sit on the four-wheeled walker seat to conserve energy while cooking, brushing teeth, shaving, and washing.

4. For the client of larger size with limited functional mobility, a manual wheelchair is generally not functional because it is too wide for most doorways in the home. If the client is discharged home with a wheelchair that has a seat width greater than 24 inches (at the seat), the user is likely to use it in only one room because doorways in most homes are too narrow

to accommodate such a large wheelchair. The occupational therapist and team should consider alternatives if a bariatric wheelchair is needed but access is limited.

5. If an electric hospital bed is required, weight limits and size should be checked to ensure it can accommodate the client's weight and size.

Home Management, Meal Preparation, and Cleanup Activities

The person of larger size may be unable to reach faucet handles, reach into lower cabinets or a clothes dryer, be safe on step stools, or carry heavy items with proper body mechanics because of abdomen size, limited endurance, and limited reaching and bending.[42] Home management activities can be facilitated by a wide variety of environmental adaptations, assistive devices, and fatigue management techniques.[42] The following are suggestions to facilitate home management for the exceptionally large individual.

1. Store frequently used items on the first shelves of cabinets, just above and below counters, or on counters where possible. Eliminate unnecessary items.
2. If the individual is unable to reach faucet handles, add an extension onto the handle.
3. Use a high, stable stool to work comfortably at counter height, with the feet firmly placed on the ground; or, if a wheelchair is used, attach a drop-leaf table to the wall for a planning and meal preparation area.
4. Use a utility cart of comfortable height or a four-wheeled walker to transport several items at once.
5. Use reachers to get lightweight items (e.g., a cereal box) from high shelves. Place frequently used items on shelves in cabinets and in the refrigerator where the items are easily accessible and reachable.
6. Eliminate bending by using extended and flexible plastic handles on dust mops, brooms, and dustpans. Sit to do cleaning and move the chair as needed.
7. Use pullout shelves or lazy Susans to organize cupboards to eliminate bending and to ease access to items.
8. Eliminate bending by using a wall oven, countertop broiler, microwave oven, and convection oven.
9. Use a metal kitchen spatula to pull out and push in oven racks. There also are commercially available tools for this purpose.

10. Eliminate leaning and bending by using a top-loading (or tall front-loading) automatic washer and elevated dryer. Wheelchair users or people of shorter stature can benefit from front-loading appliances. Use a reacher or other extended tool to obtain clothes from the washer or dryer.
11. Use an adjustable ironing board to make it possible to sit while ironing, or eliminate ironing with the use of permanently pressed clothing.[5,42,43,104]

Community Mobility

Special mention will be made of community mobility regarding a person of very large size because many ADL are performed in the community as well. Occupational therapy practitioners can participate to help advocate for more inclusive social and physical environments in clinics and healthcare settings such as having sturdy armless chairs in waiting rooms, having bathroom facilities that can accommodate them, having blood pressure cuffs and hospital gowns available in larger sizes.[77]

THREADED CASE STUDY

Anna, Part 2

At the beginning of this chapter, Anna's case introduced questions regarding ADLs and IADLs participation. Anna identified many ADLs and IADLs that she wanted to engage in as independently as possible, such as self-care, child-rearing, spiritual activities, sexual function and fertility, community mobility, financial management, home management, meal preparation and cleanup, and shopping. All of these areas are in the domain of occupational therapy and can be addressed while Anna is in the inpatient setting and further along in the continuum of care, which might include outpatient, home, and community settings. The topic of sexual function and fertility were not addressed in this chapter. However, it is an important ADL that occupational therapists can and should discuss with clients such as Anna (also see Chapter 12).[45] With the many areas that must be addressed, an occupational therapist, along with the client, family, and rehabilitation team, must prioritize which areas to address at each stage. Before discharge home, a home safety assessment is indicated for safety and accessibility, as is an assessment for appropriate DME such as a wheelchair and padded bath bench. Other equipment and adaptive techniques in ADLs and IADLs also may be recommended to foster Anna's independence and return to her roles as wife, mother, worker, and active community member.

SUMMARY

Occupational therapists routinely assess performance in ADLs and IADLs to determine a client's level of functional independence. Interviews and performance analysis are used to carry out the assessment. Occupational therapists also assess and take into consideration the client factors, performance skills, and patterns and contexts when they evaluate and establish the treatment goals.

The results of the assessment and ongoing progress are recorded on one of the many available ADL checklists or with a standardized assessment, the content of which is summarized for the permanent medical record (see Chapter 8 for further

information on documentation). Intervention is client centered and directed at training in independent living skills or at teaching a caregiver to assist the client with ADLs and IADLs, if it is their goal to do so. During the therapy process, the OT practitioner exhibits professional behaviors that are mindful of cultural factors and cultural humility and focuses on occupation-based treatment.[12] The occupational therapist can include in the intervention plan compensatory strategies, home modification, adaptive equipment, DME, work simplification, and energy conserving or fatigue management techniques to improve ADLs and IADLs performance.

REVIEW QUESTIONS

1. Define ADLs and IADLs. List three classifications of tasks that may be considered in each category.
2. What is the role of occupational therapy in restoring ADLs and IADLs independence?
3. List at least three activities considered self-care skills, three functional mobility skills, three functional communication skills, and three home management or meal preparation and cleanup skills.
4. List three factors the occupational therapist must consider before commencing ADLs performance assessment and training. Describe how each could limit or affect ADLs performance.
5. What is the ultimate goal of the ADLs and IADLs training program?
6. Discuss the concept of maximal independence as defined in the text.
7. List the general steps in the procedure for ADLs assessment.
8. Describe how the occupational therapist can use the ADLs checklist.
9. What is the purpose of the home safety assessment?
10. What areas of the home are assessed in a home assessment?
11. How does the occupational therapist, with the client, select ADLs and IADLs training objectives after an assessment?
12. Describe three approaches to teaching ADLs skills to a client with perception or memory deficits.
13. List the important factors to include in an ADLs or IADLs progress report.
14. Describe the levels of independence as defined in the text.
15. Give an example of a health management issue.
16. Give three examples of adaptations that may be helpful for the person with low vision.

For additional practice questions for this chapter, please visit eBooks.Health.Elsevier.com.

REFERENCES

1. AbilityNet. (2019). Telephones and mobile phones. https://abilitynet.org.uk/factsheets/telephones-and-mobile-phones#simple-table-of-contents-11
2. AbilityNet. (2020). Stroke and computing. https://abilitynet.org.uk/factsheets/stroke-and-computing
3. Agner J: Moving from cultural competence to cultural humility in occupational therapy: A paradigm shift, *Am J Occup Ther* 74, 7404347010, 2020. https://doi.org/10.5014/ajot.2020.038067.
4. Alessi CA, Martin JL, Webber AP, et al: More daytime sleeping predicts less functional recovery among older people undergoing inpatient post–acute rehabilitation, *Sleep* 31:1291–1300, 2008.
5. Alley DE, Chang VW: The changing relationship of obesity and disability, 1988–2004, *JAMA* 298:2020–2027, 2007.
6. American Federation for the Blind. (n.d.). Accessible payment systems for people with visual impairments. https://www.afb.org/blindness-and-low-vision/using-technology/online-shopping-and-banking-accessibility-people-visual-2
7. American Heart Association. (2016). Devices that may interfere with ICDs and pacemakers. https://www.heart.org/en/health-topics/arrhythmia/prevention--treatment-of-arrhythmia/devices-that-may-interfere-with-icds-and-pacemakers
8. American Occupational Therapy Association: Occupational therapy practice framework: domain and process, ed 2, *Am J Occup Ther* 62:630, 2008.
9. American Occupational Therapy Association: AOTA official documents: obesity and occupational therapy, *Am J Occup Ther* 67(Suppl 6):S39–S46, 2013.
10. American Occupational Therapy Association: Occupational therapy code of ethics and ethics standards, *Am J Occup Ther* 74(Supplement_3), 7413410005p1–7413410005p13, 2020. https://doi.org/10.5014/ajot.2020.74S3006.
11. American Occupational Therapy Association: Research opportunities in the area of home modifications, *Am J Occup Ther* 69:1–2, 2015. https://doi.org/10.5014/ajot.2015.693001.
12. American Occupational Therapy Association: Occupational therapy practice framework: Domain and process (4th ed.), *Am J Occupl Ther* 74(Suppl. 2), 7412410010, 2020. https://doi.org/10.5014/ajot.2020.
13. Anemaet WK, Moffa-Trotter ME: *Home rehabilitation: guide to clinical practice*, St Louis, 2000, Mosby.
14. Arilotta C: Performance in areas of occupation: the impact of the environment, *Phys Disabil Special* 26:1–3, 2003.
15. Asher IE:: *Asher's occupational therapy assessment tools: an annotated index*, ed 4, Bethesda, MD, 2014, American Occupational Therapy Association.
16. Bachner S: Completing the home modification evaluation process. In Christenson M, Chase C, editors: *Occupational therapy and home modification: promoting safety and supporting participation*, Bethesda, MD, 2012, American Occupational Therapy Association.
17. Bailliard AL, Dallman AR, Carroll A, Lee BD, Szendrey S: Doing occupational justice: A central dimension of everyday occupational therapy practice, *Canadian J Occup Ther* 87(2):144–152, 2020. https://doi.org/10.1177/0008417419898930.
18. Barstow BA, Bennett DK, Vogtle LK: Perspectives on home safety: do home safety assessments address the concerns of clients with vision loss? *Am J Occup Ther* 65:635–642, 2011. https://doi.org/10.5014/ajot.2011.001909.
19. Batra M, Batra V: Comparison between forward chaining and backward chaining techniques in children with mental retardation, *Ind J Occup Ther* 37:57–63, 2005.
20. Baum CM, Tabor Connor L, Morrison T, et al: Reliability, validity, and clinical utility of the executive function performance test: a measure of executive function in a sample of people with stroke, *Am J Occup Ther* 62:446–455, 2008. https://doi.org/10.5014/ajot.62.4.446.
21. Black RM, Wells SA: *Culture and occupation: A model of empowerment in occupational therapy*, , 2007, AOTA Press.
22. Bromley I: *Tetraplegia and paraplegia: a guide for physiotherapists*, ed 6, London, 2006, Churchill Livingstone Elsevier.
23. Burmedi D, Becker S, Heyl V, et al: Behavioral consequences of age-related low vision, *Vis Impair Res* 4:15–45, 2002. http://doi.org/10.1076/vimr.4.1.15.15633.
24. Buxton OM, Ellenbogen JM, Wang W, et al: Sleep disruption due to hospital noises: a prospective evaluation, *Ann Intern Med* 157:170–179, 2012.

25. Centers for Medicare and Medicaid Services. Electronic health records. https://www.cms.gov/medicare/e-health/ehealthrecords/index.html?redirect=/ehealthrecords/.

26. Chase C, Christenson M: Recognizing the meaning of home. In Christenson M, Chase C, editors: *Occupational therapy and home modification: promoting safety and supporting participation*, Bethesda, MD, 2011, American Occupational Therapy Association, pp 6.

27. Chee YK: Modifiable factors on use of adaptive strategies among functionally vulnerable older adults, *Aging International* 38:364–379, 2013. https://doi.org/10.1007/s12126-013-9188-1.

28. Christenson M, Lorentzen L: Proposing solutions. In Christenson M, Chase C, editors: *Occupational therapy and home modification: promoting safety and supporting participation*, Bethesda, MD, 2011, American Occupational Therapy Association, pp 69–78.

29. Christiansen CH, Matuska KM: *Ways of living: adaptive strategies for special needs*, ed 3, Bethesda, MD, 2004, American Occupational Therapy Association.

30. Cherkassky T, Oksenberg A, Froom P, King H: Sleep-related breathing disorders and rehabilitation outcome of stroke patients: a prospective study, *Am J Phys Med Rehabil* 82:452–455, 2003.

31. Clemson L: *Home fall hazards and the Westmead Home Safety Assessment*, West Brunswick, Australia, 1997, Coordinates Publications.

32. Clemson L, Fitzgerald MH, Heard R: Content validity of an assessment tool to identify home fall hazards: The Westmead Home Safety Assessment, *British J Occup Ther* 62(4):171–179, 1999.

33. Collie, Z. (2018, October 18). *How a quadriplegic drains his own pee bag*. [Video]. YouTube. https://www.youtube.com/watch?v=A4UqJ__0d10&t=222s

34. Collie, Z. (2019, September 22). *Freedom Flow (Wireless Leg Bag Emptier)*. [Video]. https://www.youtube.com/watch?v=7U8hiR3VMIo

35. Cummings RG, Thomas M, Szonyi G, et al: Adherence to occupational therapist recommendations for home modifications for falls prevention, *Am J Occup Ther* 55:641–648, 2001. https://doi.org/10.5014/ajot.55.6.641.

36. Ellis, M. (2016, June 7). *Head To Toe - Dressing | Quadriplegic(C5,C6,C7)*. [Video]. YouTube. https://www.youtube.com/watch?v=5SAl1yMECXc

37. Feldmeier DM, Poole JL: The position-adjustable hair dryer, *Am J Occup Ther* 41:246, 1987.

38. Fioravanti AM, Pettit SM, Bordignon CM, et al: Comparing the responsiveness of the Assessment of Motor and Process Skills and the Functional Independence Measure, *Can J Occup Ther* 79:167–174, 2012. https://doi.org/10.2182/cjot.2012.79.3.6.

39. Fisher AG: *Assessment of motor and process skills*, ed 3, Fort Collins, CO, 1999, Three Star Press.

40. Fisher AG: Assessment of Motor and Process Skills, ed 6 *Development, standardization, and administration manual*, vol 1, Fort Collins, CO, 2006, Three Star Press.

41. Fisher AG: Assessment of motor and process skills, ed 6 *User manual*, vol 2, Fort Collins, CO, 2006, Three Star Press.

42. Foti D: Caring for the person of size, *OT Practice* 9:9–14, 2005.

43. Foti D, Littrell E: Bariatric care: practical problem solving and interventions, *Phys Disab Special Interest Sect Quart* 27:1–3, 2004.

44. Frighetto L, Marra C, Bandali S, et al: Failure of physician documentation of sleep complaints in hospitalized patients, *West J Med* 169:146–149, 2004.

45. Fritz HA, Dillaway H, Lysack CL: "Don't think paralysis takes away your womanhood": sexual intimacy after spinal cord injury, *Am J Occup Ther* 69:02260030p1–6902260030p10, 2015. https://doi.org/10.5014/ajot.2015.015040.

46. Ghaisas S, Payatak EA, Blanche E, et al: Lifestyle changes and pressure ulcer prevention in adults with spinal cord injury in the Pressure Ulcer Prevention Study lifestyle intervention, *Am J Occup Ther* 69:1–10, 2015. https://doi.org/10.5014/ajot.2015.012021.

47. Gillen G: Case report: improving activities of daily living performance in an adult with ataxia, *Am J Occup Ther* 54:89–96, 2000.

48. Gillen G, Nilsen DM, Attridge J, et al: Effectiveness of interventions to improve occupational performance of people with cognitive impairments after stroke: an evidence-based review, *Am J Occup Ther* 69, 2015. https://doi.org/10.5014/ajot.2015.012138.

49. Girdler S, Packer T, Boldy D: The impact of age-related vision loss, *OTJR: Occup, Partic Health* 28:P110–P120, 2008.

50. Gupta J: Exploring culture. In Wells SA, Black RM, Gupta J, editors: *Culture & occupation: Effectiveness for occupational therapy practice, education and research*, ed 3, Bethesda, MD, 2016, AOTA Press, pp 3–21.

51. Hahn B, Baum C, Moore J, et al: Brief report: development of additional tasks for the Executive Function Performance Test, *Am J Occup Ther* 68:e241–e246, 2014. https://doi.org/10.5014/ajot.2014.008565.

52. Hasegawa A, Kamimura T: Development of the Japanese version of the Westmead Home Safety Assessment for the elderly in Japan, *Hong Kong J Occup Ther* 31(1):14–21, 2018. https://doi.org/10.1177/1569186118764065.

53. Hayner K, Gibson G, Giles GM: Comparison of constraint-induced movement therapy and bilateral treatment of equal intensity in people with chronic upper-extremity dysfunction after cerebrovascular accident, *Am J Occup Ther* 64:528–539, 2010. https://doi.org/10.5014/ajot.2010.08027.

54. Herget M: New aids for low vision diabetics, *Am J Nurs* 89:1319–1322, 1989.

55. Hinojosa J: Position paper: broadening the construct of independence, *Am J Occup Ther* 56:660, 2002.

56. Iwarsson S, Isacsson A: Development of a novel instrument for occupational therapy assessment of the physical environment in the home: a methodologic study on "the Enabler, " *OTJR: Occup, Participation Health* 16:227–244, 1996.

57. Jennings J, Laredo R: Beyond expectations: innovative strategies for bowel and bladder management after spinal cord injury, *Paper presented at the 2009 Congress on Spinal Cord Medicine and Rehabilitation*, September, 2009. Dallas, TX.

58. Johansson C, Chinworth SA: *Mobility in context: principles of patient care skills*, Philadelphia, 2012, FA Davis.

59. Kaldenberg J, Smallfield S: Practice Guidelines—Occupational therapy practice guidelines for older adults with low vision, *Am J Occup Ther* 74, 7402397010, 2020. https://doi.org/10.5014/ajot.2020.742003.

60. Klinger JL: *Mealtime manual for people with disabilities and the aging*, Thorofare, NJ, 1997, Slack.

61. Kurfuerst S: The transition to electronic documentation: managing the change, *AOTA's Admin Manag SIS Quarty* 26:1–3, 2010.

62. Letts L, Law M, Rigby B, et al: Person-environment assessments in occupational therapy, *Am J Occup Ther* 48:608, 1994.

63. Liu C-J, Brost MA, Horton VE, et al: Occupational therapy interventions to improve performance of daily activities at home

for older adults with low vision: a systematic review, *Am J Occup Ther* 67:279–287, 2013.

64. Lockwood KJ, Harding KE, Boyd JN, Taylor NF: Home visits by occupational therapists improve adherence to recommendations: Process evaluation of a randomised controlled trial, *Aust Occup Therp J* 67(4):287–296, 2020. https://doi-org.libaccess.sjlibrary.org/10.1111/1440-1630.12651.

65. Lynott J, Figueiredo C: *How the travel patterns of older adults are changing: highlights from the 2009 National Household Travel Survey, AARP Public Policy Institute.* http://assets.aarp.org/rgcenter/ppi/liv-com/fs218-transportation.pdf.

66. Lysack CL, MacNeill SE, Lichtenberg PA: The functional performance of elderly urban African-American women who return home to live alone after medical rehabilitation, *Am J Occup Ther* 55:433–440, 2001.

67. Ma HI, Hwang WJ, Lin KC: The effects of two different auditory stimuli on functional arm movement in persons with Parkinson's disease: A dual-task paradigm, *Clin Rehabil* 23(3):229–237, 2009. https://doi.org/10.1177/0269215508098896.

68. Ma HI, Hwang WJ, Tsai PL, Hsu YW: The effect of eating utensil weight on functional arm movement in people with Parkinson's disease: A controlled clinical trial, *Clin rehabil* 23(12):1086–1092, 2009. https://doi.org/10.1177/0269215509342334.

69. Mackenzie L, Byles J, Higgenbotham N: Reliability of the Home Falls and Accidents Screening Tool (Home FAST) for identifying older people at increased risk of falls, *Disabil Rehabil* 24:266–274, 2002.

70. McGruder J, Cors D, Tiernan AM, Tomlin G: Weighted wrist cuffs for tremor reduction during eating in adults with static brain lesions, *Am J Occup Ther* 57:507–516, 2003.

71. Meissner HH, Riemer A, Santiago SM, Stein M: Failure of physician documentation of sleep complaints in hospitalized patients, *West J Med* 169:146–149, 1998.

72. Merritt BK: Validity of using the Assessment of Motor and Process Skills to determine the need for assistance, *Am J Occup Ther* 65:643–650, 2011. https://doi.org/10.5014/ajot.2011.000547.

73. Metz D: Mobility of older people and their quality of life, *Transport Policy* 7:149–152, 2000. https://doi.org/10.1016/S0967-070X(00)00004-4.

74. Milz. (2019, March 21). *Quadriplegic: How I put on my bra with limited hand function.* [Video]. YouTube. https://www.youtube.com/watch?v=3LxhO3ISZ60

75. National Eye Institute: (2010). nei.nih.gov.

76. National Eye Institute: Living with low vision: what you should know. (2013). nei.nih.gov.

77. Obesity Action Coalition. (n.d.). Understanding obesity stigma: An education resource provided by the Obesity Action Coalition. Public Educational Resources: Brochures/Guides. https://www.obesityaction.org/get-educated/public-resources/brochures-guides/

78. Oliver R, Blathwayt J, Brackely C, Tamaki T: Development of the Safety Assessment of Function and the Environment for Rehabilitation (SAFER) tool, *Can J Occup Ther* 60:78–82, 1993.

79. Rand D, Lee Ben-Haim K, Malka R, Portnoy S: Development of Internet-based tasks for the Executive Function Performance Test, *Am J Occup Therap* 72, 7202205060, 2018. https://doi.org/10.5014/ajot.2018.023598.

80. Rashcko B: *Housing interiors for the disabled and elderly*, New York, 1982, Van Nostrand Reinhold.

81. Rehab Engineering and Assistive Technology Society of North America (RESNA). resna.org.

82. Renda M, Shamberg S, Young D: Complex environmental modifications, *Am J Occup Ther* 69, 6913410010p1–691341, 2015.

83. Reynolds SL, Saito Y, Crimmins EM: The impact of obesity on active life expectancy in older American men and women, *Gerontology* 45:438–444, 2005.

84. Runge M: Self-dressing techniques for clients with spinal cord injury, *Am J Occup Ther* 21:367, 1967.

85. Sanders MJ, Van Oss T: Using daily routines to promote medication adherence in older adults, *Am J Occup Ther* 67:91–99, 2013.

86. Scheiman M: *Understanding and managing vision deficits: a guide for occupational therapists*, ed 3, Thorofare, NJ, 2011, Slack.

87. Scheiman M, Scheiman M, Whittaker SG: *Low vision rehabilitation: a practical guide for occupational therapists*, Thorofare, NJ, 2007, Slack.

88. Scope. (2019). Phone accessibility features. https://www.scope.org.uk/advice-and-support/phone-accessibility-features-for-mobile-android-iphone/#:~:text=these%20to%20work.-,Finding%20phone%20accessibility%20features,features%20on%20and%20off%20individually.

89. Shamberg S, Kidd A: Making places of worship more accessible, *OT Practice* 15:18–20, 2010.

90. Siebert C, Smallfield S, Stark S, et al: *Occupational therapy practice guidelines for home modifications*, Bethesda, MD, 2014, AOTA.

91. Smania N, Agliotti SM, Girardi F, et al: Rehabilitation of limb apraxia improves daily life activities in patients with stroke, *Neurology* 67:2050–2052, 2006. https://doi.org/10.1212/01.wnl.0000247279.63483.1f.

92. Somerville E, Massey K, Keglovits M, Vouri S, Hu Y-L, Carr D, Stark S: Scoring, clinical utility, and psychometric properties of the In-Home Medication Management Performance Evaluation (HOME–Rx), *Am J Occup Ther* 73, 7302205060, 2019. https://doi.org/10.5014/ajot.2019.029793.

93. Sprague D: Sources and management of funding for home modifications. In Christenson M, Chase C, editors: *Occupational therapy and home modification: promoting safety and supporting participation*, Bethesda, MD, 2011, American Occupational Therapy Association, pp 105–112.

94. Staats Z: The role of occupational therapy in bowel and bladder management in clients with spinal cord injury and disease, *AOTA's Phys Disabil SIS Quart* 37:1–4, 2014.

95. Stanford Health Care. (n.d). The deep brain stimulator. https://stanfordhealthcare.org/medical-treatments/d/deep-brain-stimulation/devices.html

96. Stark SL, Somerville EK, Morris JC: In-Home Occupational Performance Evaluation (I–HOPE), *Am J Occup Ther* 64:580–589, 2010. https://doi.org/10.5014/ajot.2010.08065.

97. Stark S, Somerville E, Russell–Thomas D: Choosing assessments. In Christenson M, Chase C, editors: *Occupational therapy and home modification: promoting safety and supporting participation*, Bethesda, MD, 2011, American Occupational Therapy Association.

98. Stark S, Somerville E, Keglovits M, et al: Clinical reasoning guideline for home modification interventions, *Am J Occup Ther* 69(2), 6902290030p1–6902290030p8, 2015.

99. Stark S, Somerville E, Conte J, Keglovits M, Hu Y-L, Carpenter C, Hollingsworth H, Yan Y: Feasibility trial of tailored home modifications: Process outcomes, *Am J Occup Ther* 72, 7201205020, 2018. https://doi.org/10.5014/ajot.2018.021774.

100. Stav WB: Updated systematic review on older adult community mobility and driver licensing policies, *Am J Occup Ther* 68:681–689, 2014. https://doi.org/10.5014/ajot.2014.011510.

101. Stav WB, Lieberman D: From the desk of the editor, *Am J Occup Ther* 62:127–129, 2008. https://doi.org/10.5014/ajot.62.2.127.

102. Steggles E, Leslis J: Electronic aids to daily living, *AOTA's Home Commun Health SIS Quart* 8:1, 2001.

103. Sternberg K: Low vision strategies for the non–low–vision specialist, *AOTA's Phys Disabil SIS Quart* 36:1–4, 2013.

104. Sturn R, Ringel JS, Andreyeva T: Increasing obesity rates and disability trends, *Health Aff* 23:199–205, 2004.

105. Thompson MR: Around the house: grab bars, *PN* 73(4):43–45, 2019, April. https://search-ebscohost-com.libaccess.sjlibrary.org/login.aspx?direct=true&db=ccm&AN=135343257&site=ehost-live&scope=site.

106. Uniform Data System for Medical Rehabilitation: Functional Independence Measure (FIM), Buffalo, NY, 1993, State University of New York at Buffalo.

107. US Assistive Technology Act of 2004. Public Law 108-364. https://www.govinfo.gov>details>PLAW-108publ364.

108. US Department of Consumer Product Safety Commission: CPSC safety alert: avoiding tap water scalds. Doc #5098 009611 032012. https://www.cpsc.gov.

109. US Department of Justice: Civil Rights Division: ADA standards for accessible design. http://www.ada.gov/2010ADAstandards_index.htm.

110. US Department of Medicare. Durable medical equipment (DME) coverage. http://www.medicare.gov/coverage/durable-medical-equipment-coverage.html.

111. US Social Security Administration. Program operations manual system (POMS). https://secure.ssa.gov/poms.nsf/lnx/0600610200.

112. Van Oss T, Rivers M, Macri C, Heighton B: Bathroom safety: environmental modifications to enhance bathing and aging in place in the elderly, *OT Practice* 17:14–16, 2012.

113. Vernon B.: Dressing techniques C5-C6. (2014). https://www.youtube.com/watch?v=V0FbWlhN2u8.

114. Vernon, B. (2014, April 16). *Beau Vernon getting dressed c5-6 quadriplegic.* [Video]. YouTube https://www.youtube.com/watch?v=V0FbWlhN2u8

115. Vernon, B. (2014, April 22). *Quadriplegic taking t-shirt on and off C5-6.* [Video]. YouTube. https://www.youtube.com/watch?v=g7HNchv09UE

116. Vu TV, Mackenzie L: The inter-rater and test-retest reliability of the Home Falls and Accidents Screening Tool, *Aust Occup Ther J* 59(3):235–242, 2012. https://doi.org/10.1111/j.1440-1630.2012.01012.x.

117. Waite A: Have faith: How spirituality is a regular part of occupational therapy practice, *OT Practice* 19:13–16, 2014.

118. Waddell KJ, Birkenmeier RL, Moore JL, et al: Feasibility of high-repetition, task-specific training for individuals with upper-extremity paresis, *Am J Occup Ther* 88:444–453, 2014.

119. Warren M: *The Brain Injury Visual Assessment Battery for Adults: test manual,* Hoover, AL, 2008, visAbilities Rehab Services.

120. Weisser-Pike O, Kaldenberg J: Occupational therapy approaches to facilitate productive aging for individual with low vision, *OT Practice* 15:CE1–CE8, 2010.

121. Welcome, A. (2019, February 26). What is morbid obesity? Not what you might think. https://obesitymedicine.org/what-is-obesity/

122. Wesselhoff S, Hanke TA, Evans CC: Community mobility after stroke: a systematic review, *Topics in Stroke Rehabilitation* 25(3):224–238, 2018. https://doi-org.libaccess.sjlibrary.org/10.1080/10749357.2017.1419617.

123. Wigginton Conway M, Salon D, King DA: Trends in taxi use and the advent of ridehailing, 1995-2017: Evidence from the U.S. National Household Travel Survey, *Urban Science* 2(79):1–23, 2018. https://doi.org/10.3390/urbansci2030079.

124. World Health Organization. (2018, May 18). *Assistive technology.* https://www.who.int/news-room/fact-sheets/detail/assistive-technology#:~:text=With%20an%20ageing%20global%20population,have%20access%20to%20assistive%20products

125. Wylde M, Baron-Robbins A, Clark S: *Building for a lifetime: the design and construction of fully accessible homes,* Newtown, CT, 1994, Taunton Press.

126. Yano E.: Working with the older adult with low vision: home health OT interventions. Paper presented at the Kaiser Permanente Medical Center Home Health Department, Hayward, CA, 1998.

127. Yasuda YL, Leiberman D: *Adults with rheumatoid arthritis: practice guidelines series,* Bethesda, MD, 2001, American Occupational Therapy Association.

128. Young D: Technology for managing high blood pressure at home, *OT Practice* 10(3):5–6, 2013.

129. Young J, Bourgeois JA, Hilty DM, Hardin KA: Sleep in hospitalized medical patients, Part 1. Factors affecting sleep, *J Hosp Med* 3:473–482, 2008.

130. Zahoransky M: Community mobility: it's not just driving anymore, *AOTA's Home Commun Health SIS Quart* 16:1–3, 2009.

11

Mobility[a]

Luis de Leon Arabit, Cesar Cruz Arada, Michelle Tipton-Burton, Elin Schold Davis, and Susan Martin Touchinsky

LEARNING OBJECTIVES

After studying this chapter, the student or practitioner will be able to do the following:

1. Define functional ambulation.
2. Discuss the roles of physical and occupational therapists and other caregivers in functional ambulation.
3. Identify safety issues in functional ambulation.
4. Recognize basic lower extremity orthotics and ambulation aids.
5. Develop goals and plans that can help ambulatory clients resume occupational roles.
6. Identify the components necessary to perform a wheelchair evaluation.
7. Explain the process of wheelchair measurement and prescription completion.
8. Identify wheelchair safety considerations for drivers and passengers.
9. Follow guidelines for proper body mechanics.
10. Apply principles of proper body positioning.
11. Identify the steps necessary for performing various transfer techniques.
12. Identify considerations necessary to determine the appropriate transfer method based on the client's clinical presentation.
13. Identify different transportation systems and contexts and the treatment implications each system presents.
14. Discuss and distinguish the roles between the occupational therapy practitioner in general practice and the specialized service provider in driving rehabilitation.
15. Identify the performance skills and client factors that should be considered when determining the intervention plan that includes referral to a driver rehabilitation specialist.
16. Discuss the value of driving within this society and how loss of license or mobility affects participation in occupation.
17. Develop awareness of the complexities involved in a driver referral and evaluation.
18. Develop an awareness and understanding of driving rehabilitation terminology and program service distinctions when selecting or referring to a program for establishing goals, exploring options with patients, hope, and awareness.
19. Discuss why driver competency assessment is a specialty practice area requiring advanced training, a driving test, driving risk assessment, comprehensive driving evaluation, and includes in car performance that is regulated by state regulatory procedures, and professional practice and ethical considerations.

CHAPTER OUTLINE

---

[a] The authors gratefully acknowledge past contributions from Susan M. Lillie and Ana Verran.

KEY TERMS

Ambulation aids	Gait training
Americans with Disabilities Act (ADA)	Medical necessity
Body mechanics	Older drivers
Community mobility	On-road assessment
Driver rehabilitation	Paratransit
Driver training	Pelvic tilt
Driving	Positioning mass
Driving cessation	Primary controls
Driving rehabilitation	Private transportation
Driving retirement	Rehabilitation technology supplier
Driving simulation	Secondary controls
Durable medical equipment (DME)	Skin breakdown
Fixed-route system	Stair ambulation
Functional ambulation	Vital capacity
Gait belt	

Walking, climbing stairs, traveling within one's neighborhood, using public transportation, using an elevator or escalator, and driving a car are so customary that most people would not consider these to be complex mobility activities. The basic capacities to move within the environment, to reach objects of interest, to explore one's surroundings, and to come and go at will appear natural and easy. For persons with disabilities, however, mobility is rarely taken for granted or thought of as automatic. A disability may prevent a person from using legs to walk or hands to operate controls of motor vehicles and other mobility devices/aids. Cardiopulmonary and medical conditions may limit aerobic capacity or endurance, requiring the person to take frequent rests and to curtail walking to cover only the most basic of needs, such as toileting. Deficits in motor coordination, vision, flexibility, sensation, and strength may create serious difficulties with activities that require a combination of mobility (e.g., walking or moving in the environment) and stability (e.g., holding the hands steady when carrying a cup of coffee or a watering can).

Occupational therapy (OT) practitioners assist persons with mobility restrictions to achieve maximum access to environments and objects of interest to them to perform necessary occupations of daily life. Typically, OT practitioners (OTPs) provide remediation and compensatory training as part of intervention services. During this process, occupational therapists collaborate with clients to perform a task analysis of valued occupations and the environments most often used by clients. Therapists should consider future changes that can be anticipated based on an individual's medical history, prognosis, and developmental status.

This chapter guides the OT practitioner in evaluation and intervention for persons with mobility restrictions. Three main topics are explored. The first section addresses functional ambulation, which combines the act of walking within one's immediate environment (e.g., home, workplace) with other activities chosen by the individual. Feeding pets, preparing a meal and carrying it to a table, and doing simple housework are tasks that may involve functional ambulation. Mobility aids such as walkers, canes, and crutches may be used during the occupation of functional ambulation. Also included in this section is stair ambulation.

The second section is focused on wheelchairs and their selection, measurement, fitting, and use. For many persons with disabilities, mobility becomes possible only with a wheelchair and specific positioning devices. Consequently, individual evaluation is needed to select and fit this essential piece of personal medical equipment. Proper training in ergonomic principles supports the person who is dependent on the use of a wheelchair, for many years of safe and comfortable mobility. Safe and efficient transfer techniques based on the individual's status are introduced in this chapter. Attention also is given to the body mechanics required to safely assist an individual in transfers and mobility.

The third section covers community mobility, which for many in the United States is synonymous with driving. Increased advocacy by and for persons with disabilities has improved access and has yielded an increasing range of options for adapting motor vehicles to meet individual needs. Public transportation also has become increasingly accessible. Driving is a complex activity that requires multiple cognitive and perceptual skills. Evaluation of individuals with medical conditions and physical limitations is thus important for the safety of the person with the disabling condition and the public at large.

Mobility is an area of occupational therapy practice that requires close coordination with other healthcare providers, particularly physical therapists (PTs) and providers of **durable medical equipment (DME)**. Improving and maintaining the functional and community mobility of persons with disabilities can be one of the most gratifying practice areas. Clients experience tremendous empowerment when they are able to access and explore wider and more varied environments.

SECTION 1: FUNCTIONAL AMBULATION

Luis de Leon Arabit and Cesar Cruz Arada, with contributions from Deborah Bolding

THREADED CASE STUDY

Pyia, Part 1

Pyia is 75 years old and identifies as female (prefers use of the pronouns she/her/hers). Pyia was treated for breast cancer 8 years earlier. She developed spinal metastases, with an onset of acute, bilateral lower extremity (LE) weakness and loss of sensation. For 2 days Pyia felt "unsteady" when walking and had one fall. She was unable to walk by the time of admission to the hospital. Pyia underwent a laminectomy and decompression of the spinal cord, with debulking of the tumor, followed by CyberKnife treatment.

Pyia was hospitalized for 1 day before surgery and for 4 days after surgery. Postoperatively she learned to ambulate 50 feet with a front-wheeled walker and minimal assistance and to get on and off a commode chair. Pyia required an ankle-foot orthosis (AFO) for her left foot because of weakness. Pyia was discharged from the hospital with plans to stay with her daughter and had a rental wheelchair for community mobility. A referral for home-based occupational and physical therapy was made through a home care agency.

An occupational profile provided the following information about Pyia. Pyia was widowed and lived alone in a three-bedroom house with three steps by which to enter the home. At the age of 62, Pyia retired from retail sales. She was independent in driving, was active in church, and attended occasional programs at the local senior citizens' center. Pyia volunteered 3 hours per week at a thrift shop that benefits the local children's hospital. She has two close friends with whom she would go to lunch each Tuesday. Pyia has three children, two sons who live in other states and a daughter who lives in the same town. She has two grandchildren, ages 10 and 13, who live nearby. Two or three times per year, Pyia would fly to visit the rest of her children.

An important part of Pyia's life for the past few years has been going to her daughter's home one or two afternoons per week to help watch the grandchildren after school or drive them to activities. Pyia would also help her daughter with laundry and dinner preparation.

After 3 weeks at her daughter's home, Pyia was asked to identify problematic areas of occupational performance, what areas are successfully performed, and what other goals she wanted to address during occupational therapy sessions. Pyia reported being happy to be able to walk better but felt endurance was still a problem. She used the walker independently in the home but still needed assistance for **stair ambulation**. The PT thought that Pyia would soon be independent with stair ambulation and may be able to transition to using a cane because her LE strength, especially in her left leg, had improved. Pyia was able to walk to the bathroom and use the toilet independently and was independently able to dress upper and lower body. Pyia's daughter helped her transfer into and out of the tub for safety reasons. Pyia used a shower chair inside the tub for bathing. She was able to prepare a simple breakfast and lunch but needed a rest period each morning and afternoon.

Pyia felt like a burden to her daughter and son-in-law. Pyia felt guilty that her daughter had taken a week off from work to be with her after her hospitalization. Additionally, her son-in-law continued to help her 2 weeks after discharge. She was happy to be able to take care of herself during the day but would also like to be able to help with household chores. Pyia had to rely on family and friends to drive her to doctor and therapy appointments while transitioning to outpatient care. Pyia wanted to return home but recognized the need to be ready and prepared. Her friends brought lunch to her daughter's home once a week, and she was grateful for their support and the support she received from her pastor and church.

Critical Thinking Questions

1. How did Pyia's needs, goals, and occupational roles change during the course of her illness and recuperation?
2. Where would you start your intervention plan, considering her current goals?
3. What are Pyia's safety issues and how would you address them?

The Occupational Therapy Practice Framework (2020) defines functional mobility as "moving from one position or place to another (during performance of everyday activities), such as in-bed mobility, wheelchair mobility, and transfers (e.g., wheelchair, bed, car, shower, tub, toilet, chair, floor); includes functional ambulation and transportation of objects." The definition of functional mobility in the Occupational Therapy Practice Framework (OTPF) clearly includes **functional ambulation** within the domain of occupational therapy practice. Functional ambulation is the term used to describe how a person walks while achieving a goal, such as carrying a plate to the table or carrying a bag of groceries from the car to the house. Functional ambulation training is applicable for all individuals with safety or functional impairments and for a variety of

diagnoses, such as lower extremity (LE) amputation, cerebrovascular accident (CVA), brain trauma or tumor, neurological disease, spinal cord injury (SCI), orthopedic injury, and total hip or knee replacement. Older adults and persons with neurological conditions are at higher risk for falls, and as such, training is important and key to prevent any foreseeable injuries. Intervention goals should focus on the ability of individuals to engage in occupations and to promote wellness and safety during performance of those occupations.

Because occupational therapists are experts in rehabilitating and restoring occupations after disease or trauma, it is essential that the occupation of functional ambulation be addressed in OT intervention plans. Functional ambulation is often a key component for the client to engage in desired occupations. For example, a client would need skilled occupational therapy intervention to address functional ambulation at home so the client is able to safely walk from the bedroom to the bathroom to use the toilet. In a similar manner, a client who wishes to engage in the occupation of meal preparation would need training to safely ambulate to and within the kitchen. In addition, the occupational therapist must also pay close attention to environmental hazards as well as the terrain and various floor surfaces as part of safe functional ambulation during the performance of activities of daily living (ADLs) and instrumental activities of daily living (IADLs).

Occupational therapy practitioners provide skilled interventions to support clients with a variety of problems that result in limitations in functional ambulation. Functional ambulation problems may be considered temporary or permanent in nature. As an example, a middle-aged client involved in a motor vehicle accident who sustained a spinal cord compression injury with a spinal fracture may require a wheelchair or a pair of crutches initially for a few weeks until the vertebrae have healed and the client has regained enough sensation and strength to ambulate. An older person who suffered a fall resulting in a hip fracture may require the use of a front-wheel walker for several weeks or months until the fracture has healed, and the client is able to bear weight on the operated hip. The therapist must carefully consider other factors, such as the client's condition or nature of the disability, the energy required to perform ambulation, and the client's occupational roles, habits, and routines.

Evaluation of ambulation, **gait training** (treatments used to improve walking and ameliorate deviations from normal gait), and recommendations for LE bracing and **ambulation aids** are included in the professional role and scope of practice of the physical therapist (PT). The PT makes recommendations to be followed by the client, families, hospital staff, or other caregivers. The occupational therapist works closely with PT colleagues to determine when clients may be ready to advance to the next levels of functional performance. For example, the occupational therapist may begin having a client ambulate to the bathroom for toileting instead of using a bedside commode. The PT often collaborates with the occupational therapist to recommend techniques, mobility equipment, or specific cues to improve safety during ambulation. Mutual respect and good communication between all professionals help coordinate care and maximize client outcomes. For example, the need for coordinated care can be seen in practice when a client with Parkinson's disease ambulated well with the PT in the morning immediately after taking medication but has difficulty walking to the refrigerator to select items for preparing lunch with the occupational therapist a few hours later when the effects of medication are waning. Holistic, client-centered care, with strong interprofessional communication and collaboration, will help meet the client's identified goals.

The following section introduces the occupational therapist to the basics of functional ambulation, ambulatory aids (e.g., crutches, canes, walkers, and braces) and stair ambulation to assist the client with ADLs and IADLs. It is not meant as a substitute for close collaboration with a physical therapist. A basic introduction will also be provided to fall prevention and safety.

BASICS OF AMBULATION

Normal walking is a method of using two legs, alternately, to provide support and propulsion. The terms *gait* and *walking* are often used interchangeably, but gait more accurately describes the style of walking.[220] The "normal" gait pattern of walking includes body support alternating on each leg (stance phase), advancement of the swinging leg to allow it to assume a supporting role (swing phase), balance, and power to move the legs and trunk. Normal gait is achieved without difficulty and with minimal energy consumption. During normal walking the person has more time in the stance phase compared to the swing phase.

Descriptors of the events of walking include loading response, midstance, terminal stance and pre-swing, and mid-swing and terminal swing; the duration of the complete cycle is called cycle time. Cadence is the average step rate. Stride length is the distance between two placements of the same foot. Various diseases may shorten a person's stride length. Walking base is the distance between the line of the two feet. It may be wider than normal for people with balance deficits.[219]

Abnormal gait is seen with disruption to the complex interaction between neuromuscular and structural elements of the body. It may result from problems with the brain, spinal cord, nerves, muscles, joints, or skeleton or from pain. Problems may include weakness, paralysis, ataxia, spasticity, loss of sensation, and inability to bear weight through the limb or pelvis. Deficits may include decreased velocity, decreased weight bearing, increased swing time of the affected leg, an abnormal base of support, and balance problems. Functional deficits may include loss of mobility, decreased safety (increased fall risk), and insufficient endurance.[177] Problems with vision and the vestibular system affect how clients move around their homes. Reduced sensation in extremities exposes clients to injury and safety risks. Low endurance affects distance covered and pacing during occupation-based functional ambulation.

When the client is engaged in various occupations, the occupational therapist should reinforce gait training recommendations developed by the PT.

Functional ambulation can be negatively affected by client sensory, kinesthetic, and activity tolerance deficits. The occupational therapist should note client deficit areas during the evaluation and collaborate with the client to address these areas on the intervention plan. This may include training with new skills, adaptive devices and compensatory strategies, and environmental modifications.

Orthotics

The occupational therapist should be familiar with basic LE orthotics, including the reason for using braces or orthotics, often recommended by the PT. The occupational therapist will often teach clients to put on the LE orthotics as part of dressing training.

Orthotics, or braces, are used to provide support, protection, and stability for a joint, to prevent or correct deformity, or to replace lost function. They should be comfortable, easy to apply, and lightweight, if possible. They can be prefabricated products or custom-molded to meet the client's specifications. The more joints of the LE that require orthotic support, the higher the energy cost of ambulation for the client.

Orthotics are named by the part of the body that is supported. A supramalleolar orthosis, or supramalleolar ankle-foot orthosis (AFO), is made of plastic and fits into a shoe. It provides medial-lateral stability at the ankle, provides rear foot alignment during gait, supports midfoot laxity, and can control pronation/supination positions of the forefoot. An AFO is usually made of plastic; it inserts into a shoe and extends up the back of the lower leg. It is sometimes called a foot drop splint because it is used in cases of central or peripheral nerve lesions, which cause weakness of ankle dorsiflexors. An AFO may consist of one piece or may be hinged to permit ankle dorsiflexion. A knee-ankle-foot orthosis (KAFO) may be recommended for clients with knee weakness or hyperextension or with foot problems. The KAFO might be used with clients diagnosed with paraplegia, cerebral palsy, or spina bifida (myelomeningocele). For clients with spinal cord lesions or spina bifida involving the hip muscles, a hip-knee-ankle-foot orthosis (HKAFO) might be used. A reciprocating gait orthosis (RGO) is a type of HKAFO that may be used to help advance the hip in the presence of weak hip flexors. High energy costs are associated with use of HKAFOs during ambulation, and clients' upper extremities are used for support on walkers and crutches. This makes functional ambulation tasks extremely challenging for these clients, and it may be more energy efficient and safer to perform some tasks while seated in a chair or wheelchair.

When cost is an issue or access to AFO is not possible, the occupational therapist can collaborate with the PT to secure low-cost alternatives to help with functional ambulation. For example, an ankle dorsiflexion assist device can be fabricated supporting the ankle joint at 90 degrees of dorsiflexion during the swing phase, thus preventing dragging of the toes. A band is strapped around the client's calf and another strap, attached from the anterior shin area, extends down to the front of the foot. This anterior strap is then attached to another band that encircles the metatarsal area of the foot or is attached to the top of the shoe keeping the ankle at 90 degrees of dorsiflexion. This device provides ankle dorsiflexors during functional ambulation.

Walking Aids

Ambulation aids may be used to compensate for deficits in balance and strength, to decrease pain, to decrease weight bearing on involved joints and help with fracture healing, or in the absence of a LE. Walking aids are generally classified as canes, crutches, and walkers. All three help support part of the body weight through the arm or arms during gait. They are also used as sensory cues for balance and enhance stability by increasing the base of support.

A single-point cane may be used with clients who have minor balance problems to widen the base of support or provide sensory feedback through the upper extremity (UE) about position. For clients with a painful hip or knee, a cane is most often used on the contralateral side to reduce loading on the painful joint. The cane is advanced during the swing phase of the leg with the painful hip or knee. Variations of cane designs include quad canes and hemiwalkers, which are heavier and bulkier than single-point canes but provide greater stability. A quad cane provides additional stability with the distal end of the cane having four "feet" instead of a single point. The hemiwalker is used for clients with hemiplegia and provides great stability compared to the single-point or quad cane. The client uses the stronger (less involved) side UE on this device and uses the hemiwalker like a cane.

Axillary crutches transmit forces in a horizontal plane because two points of attachment exist: one at the hand and the other higher on the arm. Clients should be cautioned not to lean on crutches at the axilla because this may cause damage to blood vessels or nerves. The lever between the axilla and the hand is long, and enough horizontal force can be generated to permit walking when one leg has restricted weight-bearing capacity or when both legs are straight and have limited weight-bearing capacity. Crutches are suitable for short-term use, such as for a fractured leg.

Forearm crutches are also called Lofstrand or Canadian crutches. The points of contact are on the hand and forearm. Forearm crutches are lighter than the axillary type, and the lever arm is shorter. For most people mobility is easier with forearm crutches than with the axillary type, and forearm crutches are useful for active people with leg weakness. All crutches require good upper body strength.

Walkers are more stable than canes or crutches. With a standard walker without wheels, the pick-up style walker is moved first; the client takes a short step with each foot to the stable walker and then moves the walker slightly forward again. This type of walking can be slow. Depending on factors such as balance and control of pace, a client may use a front-wheeled walker instead of a standard walker. Most clients who need a walker are able to use a front-wheeled walker, which has two wheels on the front, making it lighter and easier to advance. Another variation is a walker with four wheels, along with a braking system. Some walkers have seats so that clients can rest when they become fatigued. Walkers require the use of both arms but do not require as much upper body strength or balance as crutches. Forearm platforms can be added to forearm crutches or walkers when clients are unable to bear weight through their hands or wrists, perhaps because of fracture or arthritis. For example, the client in the case study, Pyia, is currently using a walker that supplies substantial support during ambulation but requires additional energy to use compared with a cane. The PT may recommend a cane as Pyia progresses, but a walker may still be necessary in some situations within the home environment.

Ambulation Techniques

Basic ambulation techniques recommended by the PT vary from client to client, depending on the individual's goals, strengths, and weaknesses and may be more complex than the descriptions provided previously. The occupational therapist reinforces the PT's recommendations and incorporates them into functional ambulation activities while performing ADLS and IADLs.

During functional ambulation on a level surface, the occupational therapist is positioned slightly behind and to one side of the client. The therapist is typically positioned on the client's weaker side, but consult with the PT and consider the goals of the activity. The occupational therapist moves in tandem with the client when providing support during ambulation. The occupational therapist's outermost LE moves with the ambulation aid, and the occupational therapist's inside foot moves forward with the client's LE. Of course, some clients who are independent with basic ambulation and may need guarding or assistance only when practicing new activities, such as transporting hot foods, mopping a floor, or reaching into a dryer.

Safety

OT PRACTICE NOTES

Safety for Functional Ambulation

1. Know the client (e.g., current status, orthotics and aids, precautions, any history of falls).
2. Always guard and stay on the weaker/more-involved side (if there is asymmetry of strength or balance based on condition of the client) while maintaining a wide base of support.
3. Use appropriate footwear.
4. Always observe proper body mechanics
5. Monitor physiological responses.
6. Use a **gait belt** to direct and guide the client's center of mass back over the client's base of support. Do not use the client's clothes or UE to guide the client.
7. Think ahead and try to anticipate potential problems.
8. Never leave the client unattended, position yourself appropriately at all times
9. Assess the environment. Clear potential environmental hazards and suggest modifications when appropriate to facilitate safety.

Safety is a concern and is of the utmost priority and importance for clients during functional ambulation. Before beginning an evaluation of ADLs or IADLs, the occupational therapist should review the client's medical record, especially the current status, medical history, and any precautions. Does the client currently use any assistive device or have a history of falls? Does the client need to use an oxygen tank? If so, does the oxygen level need to be increased during activity? In the hospital setting it may be useful to be aware of the client's laboratory values such as hematocrit level, if available, to help predict the client's tolerance to sustained activity. The occupational therapist should review PT notes and confer with the PT as needed about gait techniques, aids, orthotics, and ambulatory status. For example, it is important to always guard and stay on the client's weaker side and encourage the client to maintain a wide base of support during functional ambulation. To prepare the client for functional ambulation, the therapist and the client should have safe and appropriate footwear. Soft-soled shoes or shoes with a slippery sole should be avoided, and slippers or shoes without an enclosed heel support can compromise safety and stability for the client.

Another key to safe and successful engagement with ADLs/IADLs is modifying the session to match the client's physical endurance level, including the distance the client can safely ambulate. It is very important for the therapist to anticipate and plan ahead for the activity. The therapist should have a wheelchair, a chair, or a stool readily available for use at appropriate intervals or as necessary in case of client fatigue. The area should be free of potential safety hazards, such as throw rugs or other objects and clutter on the floor. In certain cases, however, as with a client with unilateral neglect, hemianopsia, or visual or perceptual deficits, the therapist may want to challenge the client within safety boundaries to manage a complex environment.

The client's physiological responses should be monitored during the activity. The therapist should be aware of the client's precautions and should respond appropriately. Physiological responses may include a change in breathing patterns, perspiration, reddened or pale skin, a change in mental status, nausea, pain, dizziness, and decreased responsiveness. These changes may require termination of the activity to allow the client a period of rest, monitoring, and observation. Recall that Pyia continues to experience limited endurance and was easily fatigued. Activities that require prolonged and sustained standing or walking may be too challenging for Pyia at this time.

Elderly clients who use assistive devices for ambulation before hospitalization are particularly at risk for loss of ADL and IADL function after hospitalization. A history of use of assistive devices may be a marker for decreased ability to recover.[126] It may be necessary to provide older persons with intensive therapy to improve and restore function.

Falls represent a major problem for older persons. Studies suggest that one-fourth of persons aged 65 to 79 and half of those older than 80 fall every year.[64] Falls result from many factors, including both intrinsic (e.g., health, existence of balance disorders) and external, or environmental, factors. Home hazards include poor lighting, poor visual contrast with changes in floor surfaces, inadequate bathroom grab rails, inadequate stair rails, exposed electrical cords, items on the floors, and throw rugs. Elderly people with health problems such as cardiac disease, stroke, and degenerative neurological conditions have an even greater risk of falling.[115,176] Occupational therapists may visit the client's home while the client is hospitalized or may work through home health agencies, fall prevention programs, or senior citizen centers to help evaluate homes for potential hazards.[153] All reasonable efforts should be made to decrease the risk of falls.

Occupational therapists must consistently observe proper body mechanics during functional ambulation with a client. If a client loses balance or stumbles, the therapist will have better control of the client if supporting the client's trunk while using a gait belt. If a client begins to lose balance or fall, the therapist should use their own legs to support or lower the client to the floor instead of pulling or twisting with the upper body to avoid possible back injuries. For a client who feels faint or develops sudden leg weakness, the therapist lowers the client onto the therapist's flexed leg using a gait belt, as if onto a chair, and then down to the floor.

Use of Gait Belts

A gait belt (Fig. 11.1) is a safety device used with clients during functional mobility such as transfers from bed toward the wheelchair, wheelchair to car, into a shower or tub, onto a toilet, or from a chair to stand and use a walker. The purpose of the gait belt is to direct and guide the client's center of mass during

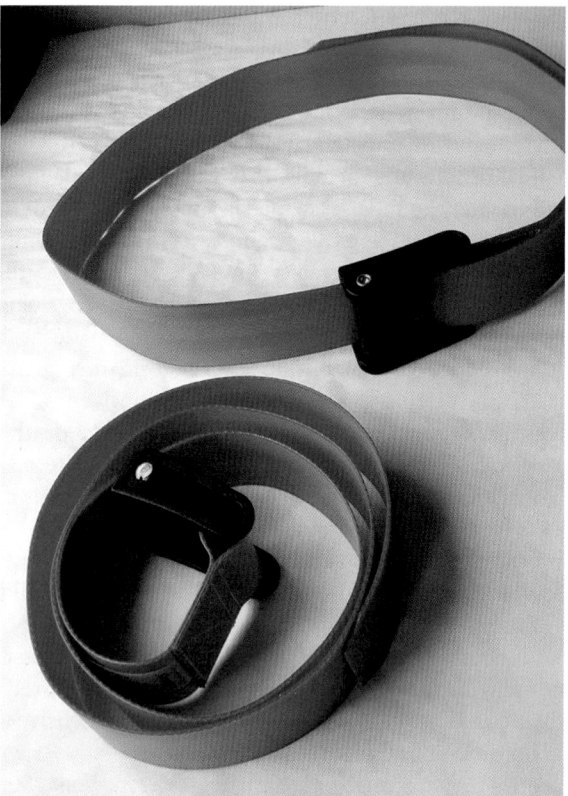

Fig. 11.1 Gait belt.

functional mobility, control descent in the event of a fall, and reduce the chances of grabbing the client's garments or upper extremities. The gait belt is securely fastened around the client's waist above the pelvis to assist in facilitating the client to move safely and perform functional mobility while engaging in desired occupations. Once fastened, the gait belt may need to be adjusted in tightness when the client changes position, such as coming up from sitting to a standing position. During functional ambulation, the therapist holds on to the gait belt from the back of the client in an underhand fashion for a more secure and stronger grip. The use of a gait belt is found to be helpful in reducing the risk of falling and the risk of fall-related injury.[211] Gait belts are a necessity to safely assist clients during functional mobility and to help support therapists in preventing incidence of falls during therapy sessions, which can cause bodily harm to the client. In the event of a fall, a gait belt also can be used to control a client's descent toward a lower surface.[97]

Most institutions provide training to their employees regarding proper body mechanics in the mobility of clients and in the use of gait belts. It is important to check in with the facility/institution regarding policies and procedures in the use of gait belts.

> ### OT PRACTICE NOTES
>
> All clients who are at risk for falling and who are alone for significant periods of time should be connected to a lifeline-type phone system by which help can be summoned in the event of a fall or other emergency. Local hospitals or senior citizen centers will have further information about lifeline services.

Communication among clients and healthcare providers is an important in every healthcare setting. In the hospital setting, call lights or a call system are used by clients to initiate communication with healthcare providers. In a study regarding call light use and inpatient falls in acute care settings, Tzeng and Yin[202] found that the key in reducing injurious fall rates is to encourage clients to use the call light. Therapists working in healthcare settings must ensure that after every therapy session (regardless of whether the client is at a high risk for fall) the hospital call light is placed within reach of the client in the event the client needs assistance. The occupational therapist needs to evaluate if the client can remember/understand how to use the call light or if an adaptive input is required for operation. The call system must be accessible and functional, and the occupational therapist needs to ensure that the device can be activated by the client. Incorporating this simple procedure in practice by therapists can help reduce the incidence of falls in hospital settings.

FUNCTIONAL AMBULATION ACTIVITIES

> ### OT PRACTICE NOTES
>
> The therapist must develop a good working relationship with the equipment supplier and reimbursement sources to facilitate payment of the most appropriate mobility system for the client. The therapist must have the oral and written documentation skills needed to clearly communicate the medical necessity, appropriateness, and cost-effectiveness of each item throughout the assessment and recommendation process.

In the occupational therapy process, functional ambulation is integrated into the performance of ADLs and IADLs. Clients with a history of previous falls are at risk for another fall during functional ambulation. It is important to assess the client's cognitive awareness and motor, sensory and vestibular skills as factors affecting performance at home. Functional ambulation activities are customized to each client, thereby helping the client perform valued roles and activities. Safe and independent functional mobility at home is an important factor for all clients and particularly an older adult's well-being. Older Americans overwhelmingly express a desire to age in place and receive care at home rather than in institutional settings. Recognizing these preferences and the potential for home-based care to reduce care delivery costs system-wide, policies have begun to prioritize noninstitutional care settings.[117] "All of these drivers of change point to a shift in the delivery system toward clinically appropriate care in the community, with the home as a central node."[1] Beyond ADLs and IADLs, functional ambulation during a client's engagement in work, play, or leisure activities is incorporated into a comprehensive client occupational therapy plan of care. The following occupational areas are commonly desired outcomes the occupational therapist addresses with clients.

Kitchen Ambulation

Moving around the kitchen during meal preparation, including setup and clean up involves dynamic and varied tasks. This includes opening/closing cupboards/drawers, reaching for and returning items into a refrigerator, and use of appliances such as a microwave, stove, oven, toaster, and dishwasher. The occupational therapist suggests strategies to the client to maintain balance while using arms and hands in meal preparation tasks. For example, items can be stored at a level between the client's shoulder and knee height in the refrigerator, kitchen cabinets, and drawers to facilitate easy reach or use adaptive equipment such as a reacher. Items stored overhead or below the height of the client's knee place the client at greater risk of a fall when attempting to retrieve these items. Attaching the reacher to a walker with Velcro allows the client easy access. During kitchen activities, a client can be encouraged to place one hand on to the ambulation device or stable furniture while the other hand is engaged in the activity. This approach provides additional stability for the client. Cooking food may require standing with or without support from an ambulation device to stir, cut, pour, and move items from a counter to the stove area. The occupational therapist should collaborate with the client to focus on sliding items on the countertop instead of picking items up and attempting to carry the item from one location to another within the kitchen. Retrieving fallen objects from the floor is another task that must be addressed during the occupational therapy session. Clients may be able to pick up items from the floor by kicking or pushing the item close to a counter, where they can hold on to the counter while bending to pick up the item. If they have had a total hip replacement and have hip flexion precautions, they can position the affected leg behind them, being careful not to internally rotate the hip, while they reach down to the floor.

Transporting items such as food, plates, and eating utensils during functional ambulation invites creative problem solving on the part of the OT, particularly when the client is using an ambulation aid (Figs. 11.2 and 11.3). The occupational therapist

may have a client practice carrying a glass of water or a plate of food or other items while moving around the kitchen. Baskets attached to a walker, rolling kitchen carts, or sliding the item on the countertops may be appropriate in these situations. Walker trays and walker bags or pouches are alternatives to walker baskets. Clients must clearly desire the equipment or adaptations, and care should be taken not to provide unwanted or unnecessary equipment. Collaboration with clients and their family is necessary when prioritizing goals and tasks. A client who does not live alone may prefer to share jobs with other family members; that is, the client may do the cooking while a family member sets and clears the table. Although Pyia was able to prepare a simple meal, she still experiences fatigue after doing so and is unable to fully assist her daughter in meal preparation. Suggestions regarding adaptations and energy conservation techniques may support Pyia's goal of being able to help with this activity while still living with her daughter.

Bathroom Ambulation

Toileting is a necessary task related to bodily functions. Once a client is ready to progress from using a bedpan, urinal, and/or bedside commode, functional ambulation to the bathroom commences with or without ambulation devices. Safety precautions are followed, such as LE weight-bearing restrictions as necessary to access the toilet and sink. Similarly, this applies when a client transitions from bathing bedside to showering/bathing in the bathroom stall or bathtub.

Trip-and-fall hazards along the path from the bed to the toilet are assessed. For example, removal of rugs, clearing pathways, and ensuring ample lighting is available reduces fall risks. The texture of the floor is critically assessed for safety (e.g., smooth floor compared to dense carpeting); transition thresholds may exist between the room and the bathroom requiring specific consideration during the occupational therapy session. Care should be

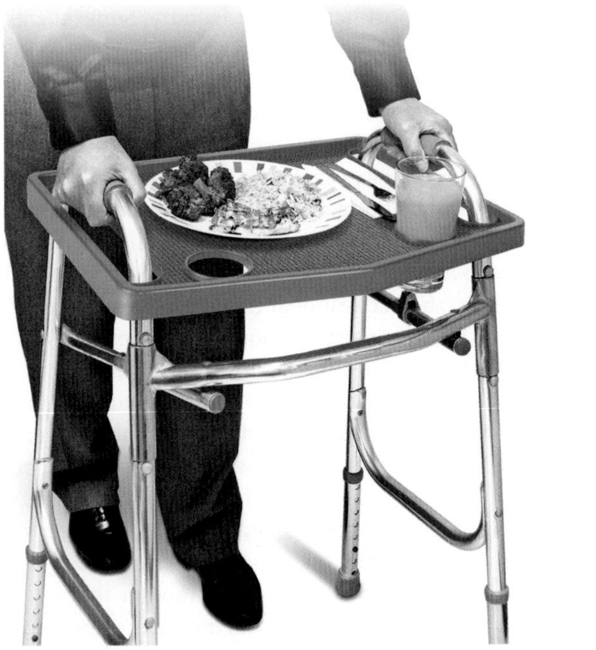

Fig. 11.2 Functional ambulation with an active walker and serving tray. (©2016 Problem Solvers.)

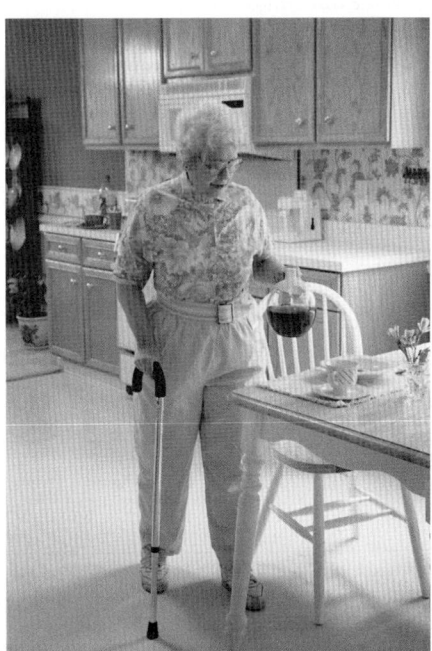

Fig. 11.3 Functional ambulation with a straight cane.

taken during activities in the bathroom because of the many fall risks associated with water and hard surfaces. Well-lit bathroom paths and task areas are necessary. Lighting strips can be added to the edge where the wall meets the floor. Spills on the floor are slipping hazards, and loose bathmats are tripping hazards. Nonslip surfaces or mats should be used on tub and shower floors. Clients must be informed about these dangers, including the need to create an environment promoting independence and safety. This includes use of bathroom adaptive devices, equipment, and environmental modifications in facilitating bathroom ambulation. Falls in the bathroom are a common cause of injury in the home. Having the client approach the sink and stand as close as possible when engaged in tasks of personal hygiene and grooming reduces the risk of falls. If the walker has a walker basket, the client can position the walker at the side of the sink and, while holding on to the walker with one hand, can place the other hand on the sink or countertop for support. The client can then turn to face the sink. Alternatively, by using a walker bag instead of a walker basket, the client can position the walker closer to the sink.

The importance of helping the client become as independent as possible in toileting cannot be overemphasized. People who are unsure about their abilities to safely use a toilet in friends' or families' homes, in restaurants, in the mall, or at gas stations may become homebound as a result. When safe to do so, practice toileting in a variety of community settings, with and without equipment such as commodes or raised toilet seats and grab bars. One limiting factor may be postoperative precautions; a tall client who has had a total hip replacement may not be able to sit safely on a regular-height toilet while observing the postsurgical precaution of no hip flexion greater than 90 degrees. A shorter client may be able to sit successfully on a toilet of regular height without difficulty. Collaboration is needed with the PT to address LE strength and balance when a client is unable to get up and down from the toilet without assistance or if the task is done with extreme difficulty.

When the client is ambulating to a tub or shower, make sure the equipment and supplies are in position for the client to use. When using a *shower stall/walk in shower* with a low rim, clients use the same technique used to go up a curb or step with their walking aid, provided it fits into the shower. If the walking aid does not fit within the shower stall, the therapist can evaluate the client's ability to safely step into the shower without the equipment. An alternative is to have the client walk as close as possible to the stall where a shower chair is strategically positioned; the client then turns around and sits on the shower chair using grab bars as needed and then "steps" into the shower from a seated position. A client who has non–weight-bearing precautions on a leg will not be able to step into a shower without walking aids and a tub bench seat. *Bathtub:* When a client uses a walker, the client positions the side of the walker beside the tub and steps into the tub, typically with the use of grab bars and a tub seat or bench. A tub bench must be used for clients who are non–weight-bearing or unable to step into a tub. Pyia is able to negotiate her daughter's home and to use the toilet but still requires assistance to transfer into and out of the tub. These skills will have to be addressed before Pyia can return to her own home.

Grab bars are important safety items for clients in the shower and tub. The therapist should practice shower or tub transfers under trial conditions before practicing an actual shower or bath. Practicing transfer into and out of shower and tub allows identification of best locations where grab bars need to be installed. Collaboration with clients is often necessary in the types and location of grab bars just like in any home modifications. Some older persons have become accustomed to taking sponge baths because of a fear of falling in the bathroom. The therapist should determine whether the client is satisfied with this system or would like to work toward independent showering.

Home Establishment and Management Ambulation

The ability to live alone is closely tied to the ability to perform IADLs.[124] Safety and independent performance of this occupation allows clients to age in place. Home establishment and management activities include cleaning, laundry, household maintenance, and transportation. Cleaning includes tidying; vacuuming, sweeping, and mopping floors; dusting; and making beds. It also includes sorting trash, replacing trash bags, and carrying them to the garbage bins. Clients may support their balance with one hand holding on to a counter or a sturdy piece of furniture while cleaning floors if they are not stable or dependent on a walking aid. Lightweight duster-style sweepers, which come with dry or wet replaceable pads, are easy to handle and use. When making the bed, the client can use the walking aid or the bed for support and stability while straightening and pulling up sheets and bedcovers. The client then moves around the bed to the other side to repeat the process. Some clients find that carrying items in a small fanny pack or shoulder bag slung over the neck is an easy way to transport small items such as cell phones, bottled water, and books. Moving clothes to or from a laundry room may present a challenge for people with mobility impairments, particularly if they use a walking aid. Rolling carts may be useful to transport items to the laundry. Some clients carry items over the front of their walkers, in a bag attached to the walker, or in a bag that they hold while walking with crutches or a cane. Whichever method is safe for the client is acceptable. It is important that the clothes do not shift while the client is carrying them; the shift can challenge the client's balance.

In establishing and managing a home, personal and household possessions and environments are maintained. Assessing the ability to move around different areas of the home is essential. Similarly, the occupational therapist assesses the ability to ambulate while maintaining household appliances, outdoor equipment, and vehicles. Through use of the occupational profile, the client should identify the most valued home management activity before the functional activity is begun. Sometimes the client has goals that are not safe for the client to perform. For example, the client who has had a mild stroke who wants to climb a ladder and trim tree branches with a power saw may need to be persuaded by the OT practitioner to wait until balance and strength have improved. Although this is a valued activity, it may be incompatible with the client's functional abilities at the time. Gardening is an area in which the occupational therapist and the PT may collaborate to work toward the client's goals. The client learns how to maneuver over uneven surfaces, get up and down from the ground, carry tools and other equipment, and dispose of clippings and weeds. The occupational therapist may also suggest use of environmental modifications such as using a gardening stool or gardening using a raised garden bed to eliminate the need to get down and back up from the ground.

Clients should learn how to get up and down from the floor or ground during therapy sessions. It may be a functional activity with the occupational therapist when clients want to sit within the tub instead of using a tub seat or bench, reach objects stored under a bed or in a lower section of a cabinet or cupboard, or sit on the floor to play with their children or grandchildren.

The client's habits and familiarity of their personal spaces can be beneficial and integrated in the occupational therapy plan of care. Therapists should listen to clients about the techniques they have developed to be independent and safe. Some clients with fall risks manage to walk to the bathroom from their bed every night without putting on braces and/or using equipment. They will say things such as, "I lean against the wall as I walk," or "There is a couch there, and I brace myself on the back." If the technique is safe and if the client has not had falls, the routine may not need modification.

Stair Ambulation

Stair ambulation or stair climbing is another important aspect of functional mobility that is essential to independent mobility in homes and in community settings.[107] The inability to use stairs to access multistory facilities may create a social disadvantage for persons with disabilities, those with cardiovascular and musculoskeletal conditions, as well as older adults. Regular stairs create an architectural barrier for persons with disabilities to the point that it could prevent them from leaving/entering and becoming mobile within their own homes. Some people with disabilities have relied on the use of ramps as a means to access their homes and community buildings, and others resort to various equipment such as stair climbers (Fig. 11.4)[225] to manage stairs and steps.

The inability to manage stair ambulation also increases the risk for injury for older adults. Starzell et al.[188] identified several

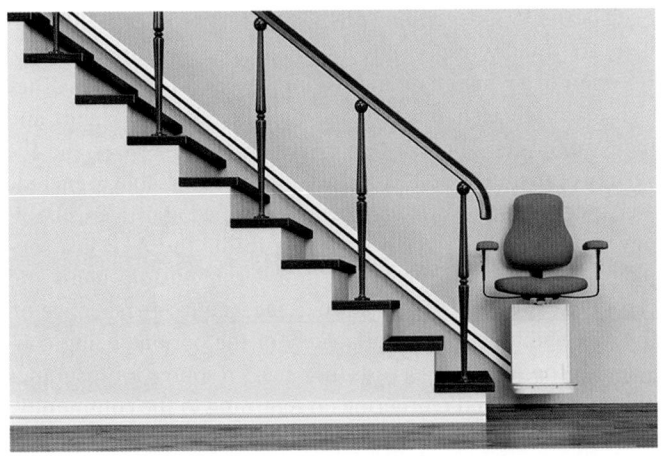

Fig. 11.4 Stair climber.

age-related impairments associated with difficulty and safety on stairs, including poor vision, somatosensory loss, cardiovascular demands, musculoskeletal limitations, joint disease and surgery, reduced cognition, and neurological disorders. For some older adults stair ambulation is a necessity tied to their physical living situation. For example, an older adult who recently had hip replacement surgery and is scheduled to return home would need stair ambulation training to learn how to navigate stairs to access the second story apartment unit.

Functional ambulation is classified under functional mobility in the OTPF.[28] Stair ambulation or stair climbing may be considered as part of functional ambulation or may be seen as gait training. The American Occupational Therapy Association (AOTA)[29,30] suggests checking your specific state licensure laws to see if there is any language related to gait assessment/training. In addition, the AOTA also asserts that language in practice acts tend to be quite broad so there may not be language specific to gait training. Checking with the licensure board within your state is highly recommended as they have the ultimate authoritative decision about what is or is not covered in a profession's scope of practice.

However, occupational therapy practitioners have a role in the evaluation and intervention of skills related to stair ambulation. These include but are not limited to visuoperceptual skills, spatial relations, balance reactions, safety awareness, cognition, and sensorimotor skills. It is critical that occupational therapy practitioners share and discuss these important client findings with physical therapy colleagues as part of interdisciplinary communication to assess and determine client readiness and endurance level before attempting stair ambulation/climbing with the client.

A general safety practice in stair ambulation training is to start with the client ascending stairs by leading with the stronger/less-affected LE and when descending stairs by leading with the weaker/more-affected LE. Ascending stairs with the stronger leg is needed to propel and lift the client upward, while the weaker leg follows. The stairs are not ascended using a reciprocal motion but by leading with the stronger leg and then having both feet on the same step and then again leading with the stronger leg. This pattern is used instead of a reciprocal stair climbing pattern. Descending stairs leading with the weaker leg allows the client to bear weight on the stronger leg as they lower the weaker leg to the step. Again, this approach has the client place both feet on the step and descend placing the weaker leg on the lower step and then following with the stronger leg instead of using a reciprocal pattern to descend stairs. Some therapists like to direct and cue their clients by saying "go up with the good and go down with the bad." It is always advisable that handrails are present on both sides for support and as a safety precaution. When the client is ascending stairs, the therapist is positioned posteriorly and laterally toward the client's weaker/affected side. When the client is descending stairs, the therapist is positioned in front of the client, anteriorly and lateral toward the weaker/affected side. Recall that Pyia had three steps to enter her home. It is important to follow the stair ambulation strategies and to work collaboratively with the physical therapist to improve the client's overall mobility and safety in this area.

SECTION 1 SUMMARY

Functional ambulation is typically incorporated during ADLs, IADLs, health management, work, play, leisure, and social participation. Occupational therapists and physical therapists have an opportunity to collaborate to support the client's function, with the physical therapist providing gait training, exercises, and ambulation aid recommendations, and the occupational therapist reinforcing training and integrating it during purposeful activities.

THREADED CASE STUDY

Pyia, Part 2

With Pyia's condition, her roles as homemaker, caregiver, grandmother, mother, and volunteer have changed. Her role became more passive as others became her caregivers. Initially, Pyia was very concerned about her disease, whether and how long it would last, and if there would ever be a chance for her to walk again. After surgery, Pyia's goals were to be able to walk and to go to her daughter's home. Once this was achieved, she began to experience loss about change in roles and planning for the future: taking care of herself during the day, resuming homemaking activities, planning a return to her own home, visiting with friends, and becoming more independent in the community.

Pyia is home alone during the day. She would like to be more active with homemaking, both to help her daughter and to prepare for the return to her own home. The therapist could begin practice with laundry and light house cleaning tasks. Pyia is already able to complete basic meal preparation. The therapist could help assess safety in Pyia's home, make recommendations for equipment or modifications, and refer the family for lifeline services. Pyia might arrange transportation services for the disabled through the county or could have a driver's evaluation to determine whether she could start driving again. She would need to get into and out of the car safely and be able to put her walker and other items in the car independently.

SECTION 2: WHEELCHAIR ASSESSMENT AND TRANSFERS

Michelle Tipton-Burton[b]

WHEELCHAIRS

A wheelchair can be the primary means of mobility for someone with a permanent or progressive disability, such as cerebral palsy, brain injury, SCI, multiple sclerosis, or muscular dystrophy. Someone with a short-term illness or orthopedic problem may need it as a temporary means of mobility. In addition to mobility, the wheelchair can substantially influence total body positioning, skin integrity, overall function, and the general well-being of the client. Regardless of the diagnosis or the client's condition, the occupational therapist must understand the complexity of wheelchair technology; available options and modifications; the evaluation and measuring process; the use, care, and cost of the wheelchair; and the process by which this equipment is funded.

[b] The authors wish to acknowledge previous work by Carol Adler.

THREADED CASE STUDY

William, Part 1

William is a 17-year-old patient (prefers use of the pronouns he/his/him) who sustained a C6 spinal cord injury (SCI) after a diving accident approximately 2 weeks ago. Sensation and motor function are absent below the level of the lesion. He is medically stable, is receiving rehabilitation services, and has been referred for a wheelchair assessment. William has a halo vest for stabilization and is able to tolerate sitting upright for 1 hour before he complains of getting dizzy. He still asks the rehabilitation therapists, nurses, and his physician when he will be able to move his legs. He has been told that because he has had no return of function during the past 2 weeks, it is unlikely that he will have significant changes in his current level of motor and sensory function.

On discharge from the inpatient rehabilitation unit, William will be returning to his home, where he lives with his parents and younger brother. The home is two stories, and William's bedroom is located on the second floor. A bathroom is located on the first floor.

Before his injury William was very physically active and was on the track and field team at his high school. He was also an avid hiker and often would go camping with his family and friends. William is a high school senior and received early acceptance to a university located within 2 hours of his home. He was very excited about attending this university because of the track and field program, in addition to his interest in becoming a marine biologist. Although William's friends have come to visit him, his girlfriend of 2 years has not visited.

Critical Thinking Questions

1. How would you anticipate that William would respond to being fitted for a wheelchair? What emotional responses may be evoked in William by this experience? How could you minimize his potential distress?
2. What decisions could William make regarding selection of the wheelchair?
3. Considering William's needs across several contexts, what type of wheelchair would you recommend?
4. What client factors must be considered when a wheelchair is selected for William?

Wheelchairs have evolved considerably in recent years, and significant advances have been made in powered and manual wheelchair technology by manufacturers and service providers. Products are constantly changing. Many improvements are the result of user and therapist recommendations. Durable medical equipment reimbursement (DME benefit) has also changed, and clients' benefits should be explored before initiating a wheelchair assessment.

OTs and PTs, depending on their respective roles at the facilities, are usually responsible for evaluation, measurement, and selection of a wheelchair and seating system for the client. They also teach wheelchair safety and mobility skills to clients and their caregivers. The constant evolution of technology and the variety of manufacturers' products make it advisable to include an experienced, knowledgeable, and certified assistive technology provider (ATP) on the ordering team. The ATP is a supplier of DME who is proficient in ordering custom items and can offer an objective and a broad mechanical perspective on the availability and appropriateness of the options being considered. The ATP will serve as the client's resource for insurance billing, repairs, and reordering on returning to the community.

Whether the client requires a noncustom rental wheelchair for temporary use or a custom wheelchair for use over many years, an individualized prescription clearly outlining the specific features of the wheelchair is needed to ensure optimal performance, safety, mobility, and enhancement of function. A wheelchair that has been prescribed by an inexperienced or nonclinical person is potentially hazardous and can cause undue financial harm to the client. Once a wheelchair has been purchased, the DME benefit has been used, and therefore another wheelchair may not be purchased. Typically, payer sources do not authorize another wheelchair for at least 5 years unless there has been a significant change in physical status. An ill-fitting wheelchair can, in fact, contribute to unnecessary fatigue, skin breakdown, and trunk or extremity deformity, and it can inhibit function.[158] A wheelchair is an extension of the client's body and should facilitate rather than inhibit good alignment, mobility, and, most importantly, function.

WHEELCHAIR ASSESSMENT

The therapist has considerable responsibility in recommending the wheelchair appropriate to meet immediate and long-term needs. When evaluating for a wheelchair, the therapist must know the client and have a broad perspective on the client's clinical, functional, and environmental needs. Careful assessment of physical status must include the specific diagnosis, the prognosis, and current and future problems (e.g., age, spasticity, loss of range of motion [ROM], muscle weakness, reduced endurance) that may affect wheelchair use. Additional client factors to be considered in assessment of wheelchair use are sensation, cognitive function, and visual and perceptual skills. Functional use of the wheelchair in a variety of environments must be considered, along with how the wheelchair will be transported. For instance, if a power wheelchair is being considered, there must be a means of transporting the patient and the wheelchair safely.[164-166] Collaboration with representatives of other disciplines treating the client is important. Box 11.1 lists questions to consider before making specific recommendations.

Before the final prescription is prepared, the collected information must be analyzed to understand the advantages and disadvantages of recommendations based on the client's condition and how to provide an optimally effective mobility system.

To ensure that payment for the wheelchair is authorized, therapists should have an in-depth awareness of the client's insurance DME benefits and should provide documentation with thorough justification of the medical necessity of the wheelchair and any additional modifications. Therapists must explain clearly why particular features of a wheelchair are being recommended. They must be aware of standard versus "up-charge" items, the cost of each item, and the effects of these items on the end product.

WHEELCHAIR ORDERING CONSIDERATIONS

Before selecting a specific manufacturer and the wheelchair's specifications, the therapist should carefully analyze the following sequence of evaluation considerations.[6,158,217]

Propelling the Wheelchair

The wheelchair may be propelled in a variety of ways, depending on the physical capacities of the user. If the client is capable of self-propulsion by using his or her arms on the rear wheels of the wheelchair, sufficient and symmetric grasp, arm strength, and physical endurance may be assumed to be present to maneuver the chair independently over varied terrain throughout the day.[217-219] An assortment of push rims are available to facilitate self-propelling, depending on the user's arm and grip strength. A client with hemiplegia may propel a wheelchair using the extremities on the unaffected side for maneuvering. A client with tetraplegia may have functional use of only one arm and may be able to propel a one-arm drive wheelchair, or a power chair may be more appropriate. Although William, the 17-year-old introduced in the beginning of this section, who sustained a C6 SCI, has functional strength in both biceps,

---

BOX 11.1 Questions to Ask Before Making Specific Recommendations for a Wheelchair

- Who will pay for the wheelchair?
- Who will determine the preferred durable medical equipment (DME) provider: the insurance company, the client, or the therapist?
- What is the specific disability?
- What is the prognosis?
- Is range of motion limited?
- Is strength or endurance limited?
- How will the client propel the chair?
- How old is the client?
- How long is the client expected to use the wheelchair?
- What was the client's lifestyle, and how has it changed?
- Is the client active or sedentary?
- How will the dimensions of the chair affect the client's ability to transfer to various surfaces?
- What is the maneuverability of the wheelchair in the client's home or in the community (e.g., entrances and egress, door width, turning radius in bathroom and hallways, floor surfaces)?

- What is the ratio of indoor to outdoor activities?
- Where will the wheelchair be primarily used—in the home, at school, at work, or in the community?
- Which mode of transportation will be used? Now and in the future? driver or passenger? If in the role of driver, will the client be driving a van from the wheelchair? How will it be loaded and unloaded from the car? If in the role of passenger, what are the needs for support to load/unload and secure? (and some, are in both roles . . . are options and choices required?
- Which special needs (e.g., work heights, available assistance, accessibility of toilet facilities, parking facilities) are recognized in the work or school environment?
- Does the client participate in indoor or outdoor sports activities?
- How will the wheelchair affect the client psychologically?
- Can accessories and custom modifications be medically justified, or are they luxury items?
- What resources does the client have for equipment maintenance (e.g., self, family, caregivers)?

energy expenditure and potential injury in the future must be considered if he is to use only a manual wheelchair.

If independence in mobility is desired, a power wheelchair should be considered for those who have minimal or no use of the upper extremities, limited endurance, or shoulder dysfunction. Power chairs are also preferred in situations involving inaccessible outdoor terrain.[217-219] Power wheelchairs have a wide variety of features and can be programmed; driven by foot, arm, head, or neck; or pneumatically controlled (sip and puff), or even controlled by eye gaze or tongue driven.[108] Given current sophisticated technology, assuming intact cognition and perception, even a person with the most severe physical limitations is capable of independently driving a power wheelchair.

If the chair is to be propelled by the caregiver, consideration must be given to ease of maneuverability, lifting, and handling, in addition to the positioning and mobility needs of the client.

Regardless of the method of propulsion, serious consideration must be given to the effect the chair has on the client's current and future mobility and positioning needs. In addition, lifestyle and the home environment; available resources, such as the ability to maintain the chair; transportation options; and available reimbursement sources are major determining factors.

Although William is physically fit, his upper body strength has been compromised by the SCI. If he is interested in engaging in outdoor activities, he may lack the physical strength to propel a manual wheelchair on uneven terrain. A powered wheelchair seemed an appropriate option for William, but the occupational therapist also considered his previous occupations of camping and hiking when selecting a wheelchair that could potentially be used in outdoor terrain.

Rental Versus Purchase

The therapist should estimate how long the client will need the chair and whether the chair should be rented or purchased; this will affect the type of chair being considered. This decision is based on several clinical and functional issues. A rental chair is appropriate for short-term or temporary use, such as when the client's clinical picture, functional status, or body size is changing. Rental chairs may be necessary when the permanent wheelchair is being repaired. A rental wheelchair also may be useful when the prognosis and expected outcome are unclear or when the client has difficulty accepting the idea of using a wheelchair and needs to experience it initially as a temporary piece of equipment. Often the eventual functional outcome is unknown. In this case a chair can be rented for several months until a reevaluation determines whether a permanent chair will be necessary.[6]

A permanent wheelchair is indicated for the full-time user and for the client with a need for a wheelchair over a long period. It may be indicated when custom features are required or when body size is changing, such as in the growing child.[6]

Frame Style

Once the method of propulsion and the permanence of the chair have been determined, several wheelchair frame styles are available for consideration. The frame style must be selected before specific dimensions and brand names can be determined. The therapist needs to be aware of the various features, the advantages and disadvantages of each, and the effects of these features on the client in every aspect of the client's life, from both short-term and long-term perspectives.

William is still in emotional shock that he no longer has motor control of his legs and hands. These variables must be considered when William is approached about wheelchair selection. Although a power wheelchair seemed the most appropriate choice for William, the therapist was concerned about the appearance of the wheelchair. The therapist actively engaged William in making choices regarding the type, model, and options available on various wheelchairs.

WHEELCHAIR SELECTION

The questions in the following sections regarding client needs should be considered carefully before the specific type of chair is determined.[6]

Manual Versus Electric/Power Wheelchairs

Manual Wheelchair (Fig. 11.5A)

- Does the user have sufficient strength and endurance to propel the chair at home and in the community over varied terrain?
- Does manual mobility enhance functional independence and cardiovascular conditioning of the wheelchair user?
- Will the caregiver be propelling the chair at any time?
- What will be the long-term effects of the propulsion choice?

Power Chairs

Power chair controls come in several designs and allow for varying degrees of customization and programming. Most power chair users drive using a joystick control mounted on the armrest. For those without UE function, several other types of controls are available, such as head controls, chin drives, and breath controls (sip and puff). Technology is available to accommodate a client with only eye or tongue movement that can be used to operate a power wheelchair (see Fig. 11.5B).

- Does the user demonstrate insufficient endurance and functional ability to propel a manual wheelchair independently?
- Does the user demonstrate progressive functional loss, making powered mobility an energy-conserving option?
- Is powered mobility needed to enhance independence at school, at work, and in the community?
- Does the user demonstrate cognitive, visual, and perceptual ability to safely operate a power-driven system?
- Does the user or caregiver demonstrate responsibility for care and maintenance of equipment?
- Is a van available for transportation?
- Is the user's home accessible for use of a power wheelchair?
- Has the user been educated regarding rear, mid, and front wheel drive systems, and has the client been guided objectively in making the appropriate selection?

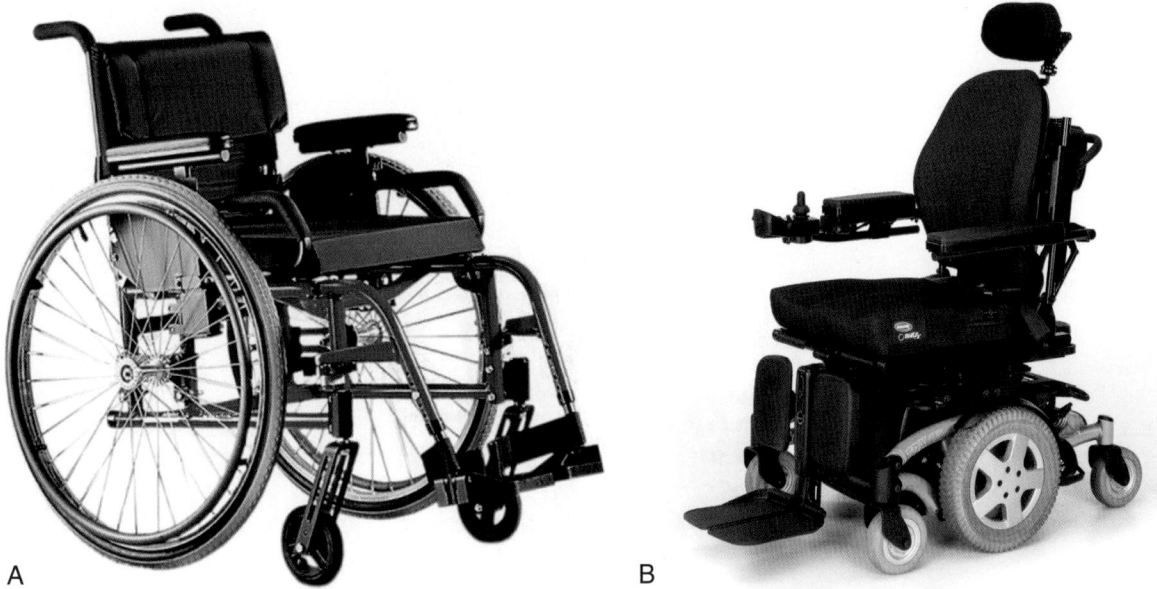

Fig. 11.5 Manual versus electric wheelchair. (A) Rigid-frame chair with swing-away footrests. (B) Power-driven wheelchair with hand control. (A Courtesy Quickie Designs, Phoenix, AZ. B Courtesy Invacare, Elyria, OH.)

Manual Recline Versus Power Recline Versus Tilt-in-Space Wheelchairs

Reclining chairs allow the wheelchair back to recline and the angle of the client's hip flexion increases with a reclining chair. A tilt-in-space wheelchair maintains the client's sitting position with 90 degrees of hip flexion while tipping backward to reduce the forces of gravity.

Manual Recline Wheelchair (Fig. 11.6A)

- Is the client unable to sit upright because of hip contractures, poor balance, or fatigue?
- Is a caregiver available to assist with weight shifts and position changes?
- Is relative ease of maintenance a concern?
- Is cost a consideration?

Power Recline Versus Tilt-in-Space (Fig. 11.6B–C)

- Does the client have the potential to operate the controls independently?
- Are independent weight shifts and position changes indicated for skin care and increased sitting tolerance?
- Does the user demonstrate safe and independent use of controls?
- Are resources available for care and maintenance of the equipment?
- Does the user have significant spasticity that is facilitated by hip and knee extension during the recline phase?
- Does the user have hip or knee contractures that prohibit the ability to recline fully?
- Will a power recline or tilt-in-space decrease or make more efficient use of caregiver time?
- Will a power recline or tilt-in-space feature on the wheelchair reduce the need for transfers to the bed for catheterizations and rest periods throughout the day?

- Will the client require quick position changes in the event of hypotension and/or dysreflexia?
- Has a reimbursement source been identified for this add-on feature?

Folding Versus Rigid Manual Wheelchairs
Folding Wheelchairs (Fig. 11.7A)

- Is the folding frame needed for transport, storage, or home accessibility?
- Which footrest style is necessary for transfers, desk clearance, and other daily living skills? (Elevating footrests are available only on folding frames.)
- Is the client or caregiver able to lift, load, and fit the chair into necessary vehicles?

Equipment suppliers should have a variety of brands available and be knowledgeable about each. Frame weight can range from approximately 28 to 50 lb, depending on size and accessories. Frame adjustments and custom options vary with the model.

Rigid Wheelchairs (Fig. 11.7B)

- Does the user or caregiver have the UE function and balance needed to load and unload the nonfolding frame from a vehicle if driving independently?
- Will the user benefit from the improved energy efficiency and performance of a rigid frame?

Footrest options are limited, and the frame is lighter (20–35 lb). Features include an adjustable seat angle, rear axle, caster mount, and back height. Efficient frame design maximizes performance. Options are available for frame material composition, frame colors, and aesthetics. These chairs are usually custom ordered; availability and expertise are generally limited to custom rehabilitation technology suppliers.

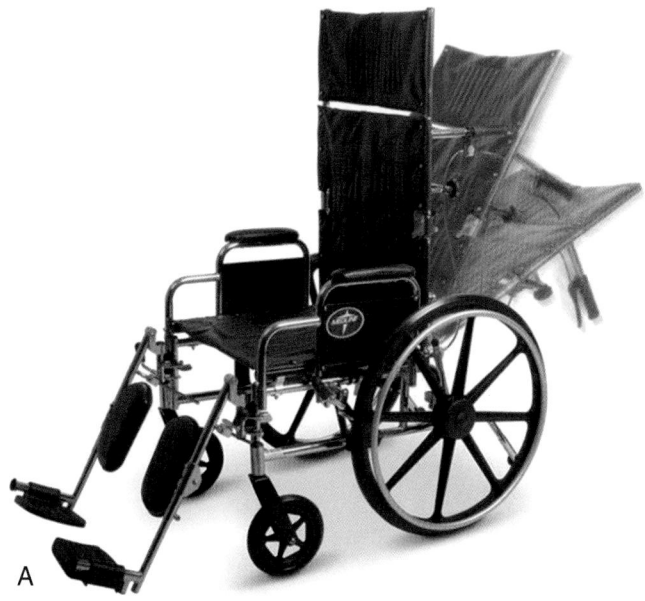

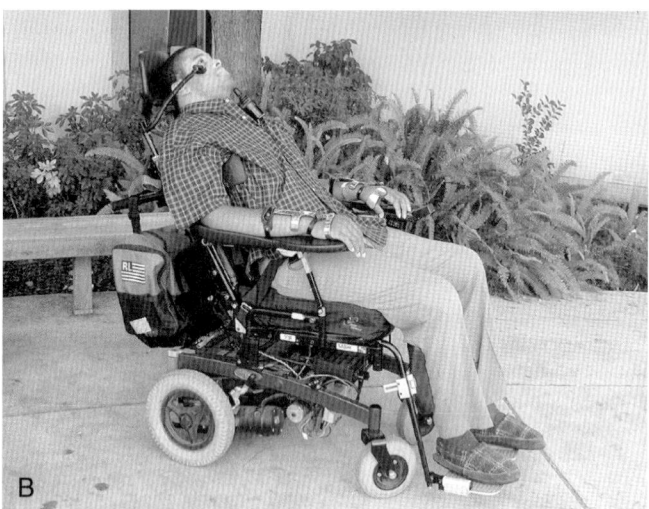

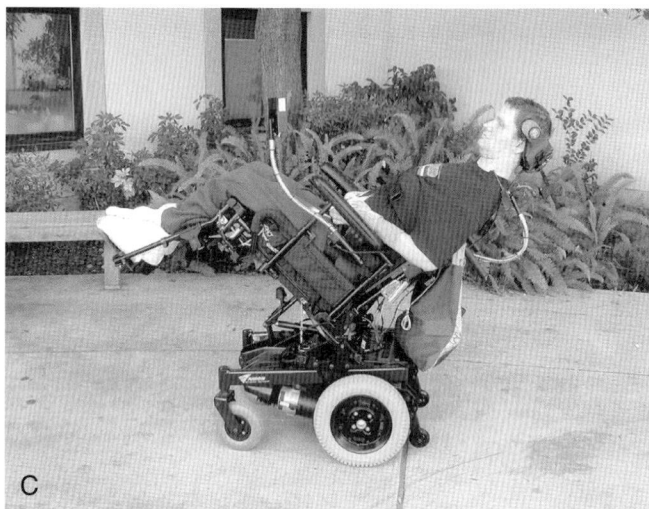

Fig. 11.6 Manual recline versus power recline wheelchair. (A) Reclining back on folding frame. (B) Low-shear power recline with collar mount chin control on electric wheelchair. (C) Tilt system with head control on electric wheelchair. (A Courtesy Medline Industries, Inc., 2016. B and C Courtesy Luis Gonzalez.)

Lightweight (Folding or Nonfolding) Versus Standard-Weight (Folding) Wheelchairs

Lightweight Wheelchairs: Under 35 Pounds (see Fig. 11.7A)

- Does the user have the trunk balance and equilibrium necessary to handle a lighter frame weight?
- Does the lighter weight enhance mobility by reducing the user's fatigue?
- Will the user's ability to propel the chair or handle parts be enhanced by a lighter weight frame?
- Are custom features (e.g., adjustable height back, seat angle, axle mount) necessary?

Standard-Weight Wheelchairs: More Than 35 Pounds (Fig. 11.8)

- Does the user need the stability of a standard-weight chair?
- Does the user have the ability to propel a standard-weight chair?

- Can the caregiver manage the increased weight when loading the wheelchair and fitting into a vehicle?
- Will the increased weight of parts be unimportant during daily living skills?

Custom options are limited, and these wheelchairs are usually less expensive (except for the heavy-duty models required for users weighing more than 250 lb).

Standard Available Features Versus Custom, Top-of-the-Line Models

The price range, durability, and warranty within a specific manufacturer's model line must be considered.

Standard Available Features

- Is the chair required only for part-time use?
- Does the user have a limited life expectancy?

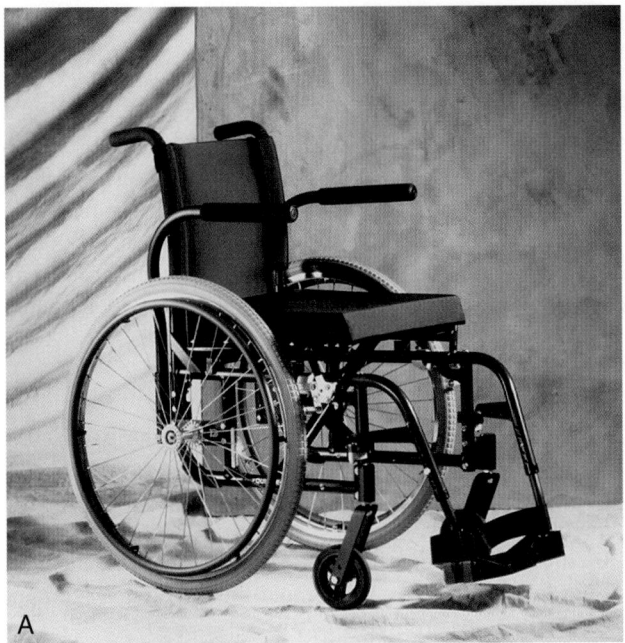

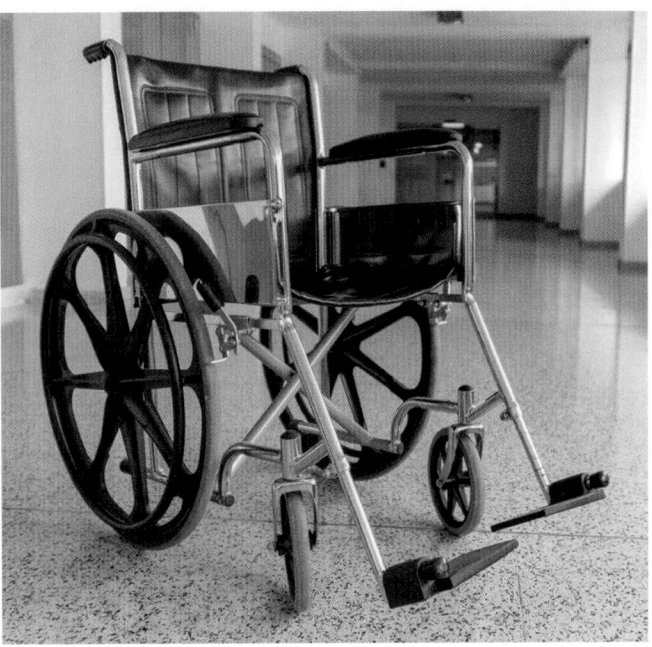

Fig. 11.8 Standard folding frame (>35 lb) with swing-away footrests. (Courtesy iStock.com.)

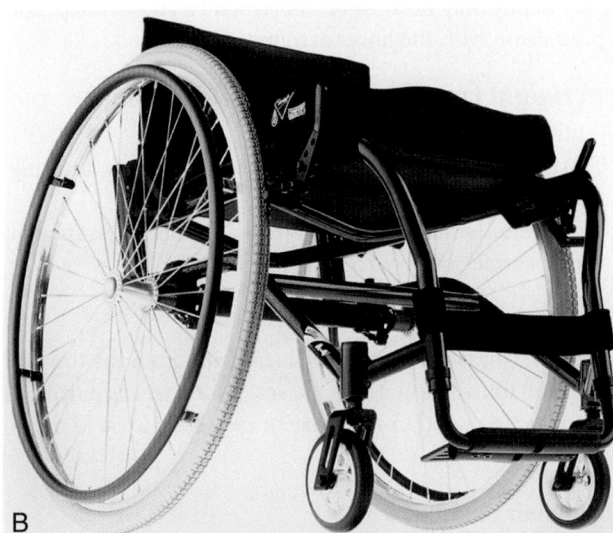

Fig. 11.7 Folding versus rigid wheelchair. (A) Lightweight folding frame with swing-away footrests. (B) Rigid aluminum frame with tapered front end and solid foot cradle. (A Courtesy Quickie Designs, Phoenix, AZ. B Courtesy Invacare, Elyria, OH.)

- Is the chair needed as a second or transportation chair, used only 10% to 20% of the time?
- Will the chair be primarily for indoor or sedentary use?
- Is the user dependent on caregivers for propulsion?
- Will the chair be propelled only by the caregiver?
- Are custom features or specifications not necessary?
- Is substantial durability unimportant?

For standard wheelchairs, a limited warranty is available on the frame. These chairs may be indicated because of reimbursement limitations. Limited sizes, options, and adjustability are available. These cost considerably less than custom wheelchairs.

Custom and Top-of-the-Line Models
- Will the client be a full-time user?
- Is long-term use of the wheelchair a likely prognosis?

- Will this be the primary wheelchair?
- Is the user active indoors and outdoors?
- Will this frame style improve the prognosis for independent mobility?
- Is the user a growing adolescent, or does the client have a progressive disorder requiring later modification of the chair?
- Are custom features, specifications, or positioning devices required?

Top-of-the-line wheelchair frames usually have a lifelong warranty on the frame. A variety of specifications, options, and adjustments are available. Many manufacturers will work with therapists and providers to solve a specific fitting problem. Experience is essential in ordering top-of-the-line and custom equipment.

WHEELCHAIR MEASUREMENT PROCEDURES

The client is measured in the style of chair and with the seat cushion that most closely resembles those being ordered. If the client will wear a brace or body jacket or will need any additional devices in the chair, these should be in place during the measurement. Observation skills are important during this process. Measurements alone should not be used. The therapist should visually assess and monitor the client's entire body position throughout the measurement process.[6,217–219]

Seat Width (Fig. 11.9, A)
Objectives
1. To distribute the client's weight over the widest possible surface.
2. To keep the overall width of the chair as narrow as possible.

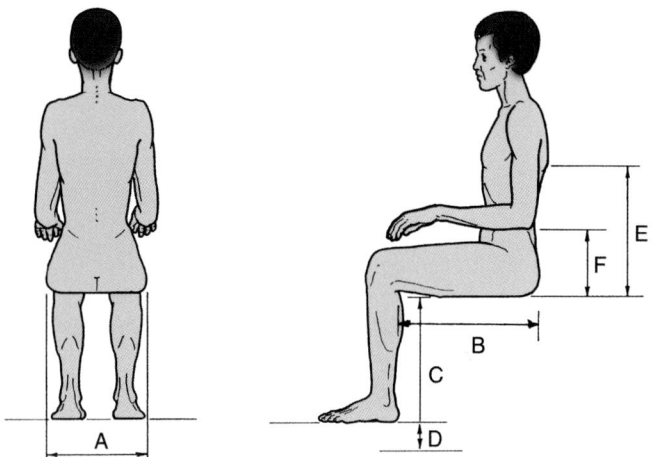

Fig. 11.9 Measurements for wheelchairs. *A*, Seat width. *B*, Seat depth. *C*, Seat height from floor. *D*, Footrest clearance. *E*, Back height. *F*, Armrest height. (Adapted from Wilson A, McFarland SR: *Wheelchairs: a prescription guide*, Charlottesville, VA, 1986, Rehabilitation Press.)

Measurements

Measure the individual across the widest part of the thighs or hips while the client is sitting in a chair comparable to the anticipated wheelchair.

Wheelchair Clearance

Add ½ to 1 inch on each side of the hip or thigh measurement taken. Consider how an increase in the overall width of the chair will affect accessibility.

Checking clearance. Place the flat palm of the hand between the client's hip or thigh and the wheelchair skirt and armrest. The wheelchair skirt is attached to the armrests in many models, and clearance should be sufficient between the user's thigh and the skirt to avoid rubbing or pressure.

Considerations

- User's potential weight gain or loss (i.e., male [tendency for abdominal weight gain] and female [tendency for weight gain in hips and buttocks])
- Accessibility of varied environments
- Overall width of wheelchair. Camber, axle mounting position, rim style, and wheel style can also affect overall wheelchair width.

Seat Depth (Fig. 11.9, B)
Objective

The objective is to distribute the body weight along the sitting surface by bearing weight along the entire length of the thigh to just behind the knee. This approach is necessary to help prevent pressure sores on the buttocks and the lower back and to attain optimal muscle tone normalization to assist in prevention of pressure sores throughout the body.

Measurements

Measure from the base of the back (the posterior buttocks region touching the chair back) to the inside of the bent knee; the seat edge clearance needs to be 1 to 2 inches less than this measurement.

Checking clearance. Check clearance behind the knees to prevent contact of the front edge of the seat upholstery with the popliteal space. (Consider front angle of leg rest or foot cradle.)

Considerations

- Braces or back inserts may push the client forward.
- Postural changes may occur throughout the day from fatigue or spasticity.
- Thigh length discrepancy: the depth of the seat may be different for each leg.
- If considering a power recliner, assume that the client will slide forward slightly throughout the day and make depth adjustments accordingly.
- Seat depth may need to be shortened to allow independent propulsion with the lower extremities.

Seat Height From Floor and Foot Adjustment
Objectives

1. To support the client's body while maintaining the thighs parallel to the floor (Fig. 11.9, C).
2. To elevate the foot plates to provide ground clearance over varied surfaces and curb cuts (Fig. 11.9, D).

Measurements

The seat height is determined by measuring from the top of the wheelchair frame supporting the seat (the post supporting the seat) to the floor, and from the client's popliteal fossa to the bottom of the heel.

Wheelchair Clearance

The client's thighs are kept parallel to the floor, so the body weight is distributed evenly along the entire depth of the seat. The lowest point of the foot plates must clear the floor by at least 2 inches.

Checking clearance. Slip fingers under the client's thighs at the front edge of the seat upholstery. Note that a custom seat height may be needed to obtain footrest clearance. One inch of increased seat height raises the foot plate 1 inch.

Considerations

If the knees are too high, increased pressure at the ischial tuberosities puts the client at risk for skin breakdown and pelvic deformity. This position also impedes the client's ability to maneuver the wheelchair using the lower extremities.

Posterior pelvic tilt makes it difficult to shift weight forward as needed to propel the wheelchair, especially with uphill grades.

Sitting too high off the ground can impair the client's center of gravity, seat height for transfers, and visibility if the client is driving a van from the wheelchair.

Back Height (Fig. 11.9, E)
Objective
Back support consistent with physical and functional needs must be provided. The chair back should be low enough for maximal function and high enough for maximal support.

Measurements
For full trunk support for the client, the back must be of sufficient height. Full support height is obtained by measuring from the top of the seat frame on the wheelchair (seat post) to the top of the user's shoulders. For minimum trunk support, the top of the back upholstery is below the inferior angle of the client's scapulae; this should permit free arm movement, should not irritate the skin or scapulae, and should provide good total body alignment.

Checking back height. Ensure that the client is not being pushed forward because the back of the chair is too high or is not leaning backward over the top of the upholstery because the back is too low.

Considerations
- Adjustable-height backs (usually offer a 4-inch range)
- Adjustable upholstery
- Lumbar support or another commercially available or custom back insert to prevent kyphosis, scoliosis, or other long-term trunk deformity

Armrest Height (Fig. 11.9, F)
Objectives
1. To maintain posture and balance.
2. To provide support and alignment for upper extremities.
3. To allow change in position by pushing down on armrests.

Measurements
With the client in a comfortable position, measure from the wheelchair seat frame (seat post) to the bottom of the user's bent elbow.

Wheelchair Clearance
The height of the top of the armrest should be 1 inch higher than the height from the seat post to the user's elbow.

Checking armrest height. The client's posture should look appropriately aligned. The shoulders should not slouch forward or be subluxed or forced into elevation when the client is in a relaxed sitting posture, with flexed elbows resting slightly forward on armrests.

Considerations
- Armrests may have other uses, such as increasing functional reach or holding a cushion in place.
- Certain styles of armrests can increase the overall width of the chair.

- Are armrests necessary?
- Is the client able to remove and replace the armrest from the chair independently?
- Review all measurements against standards for a particular model of chair.
- Manufacturers have lists of the standard dimensions available and the costs of custom modifications.

PEDIATRIC WHEELCHAIRS
The goals of pediatric wheelchair ordering, as with all wheelchair ordering, should be to obtain a proper fit and to facilitate optimal function. Rarely does a standard wheelchair meet the fitting requirements of a child. The selection of size is variable; therefore, custom seating systems specific to the pediatric population are available. A secondary goal is to consider a chair that will accommodate the child's growth.

For children younger than 5 years of age, a decision must be made about whether to use a stroller base or a standard wheelchair base. Considerations include the child's ability to propel the chair relative to the child's developmental level and the parents' preference for a stroller or a wheelchair.

Many variables must be considered when a wheelchair frame is customized. An experienced ATP or the wheelchair manufacturer should be consulted to ensure that a custom request will be filled successfully.

BARIATRIC WHEELCHAIRS
According to the latest data from the National Center for Health Statistics, more than 30% of American adults 20 years of age or older (more than 60 million people) and more than 16% of children and adolescents aged 2 to 19 years are obese.[62] The average wheelchair is rated to hold up to 250 lb, and most bariatric wheelchairs can accommodate 500 pounds. It is imperative that the therapist order a wheelchair that not only meets the client's functional needs but also will safely accommodate the client's weight. Using a wheelchair for clients who exceed the weight limit has potential safety issues, such as skin breakdown and the risk of the wheelchair bending or buckling, which may cause injury to the client. Bariatric wheelchairs feature heavy-duty frames, reinforced padded upholstery, and heavy-duty wheels. An experienced DME supplier should be able to guide the therapist and the client to the most appropriate and safe wheelchair.

ADDITIONAL CONSIDERATIONS
A wheelchair evaluation is not complete until the seat cushion, the back support, and any other positioning devices—in addition to the integration of those parts—have been carefully thought out, regardless of the diagnosis. The therapist must appreciate the effect that optimal body alignment has on skin integrity, tone normalization, overall functional ability, and general well-being (Fig. 11.10).[6]

Consider William's potential need for a wheelchair seat cushion that will distribute weight evenly and avoid excessive pressure on his ischial tuberosities while sitting. He lacks sensory

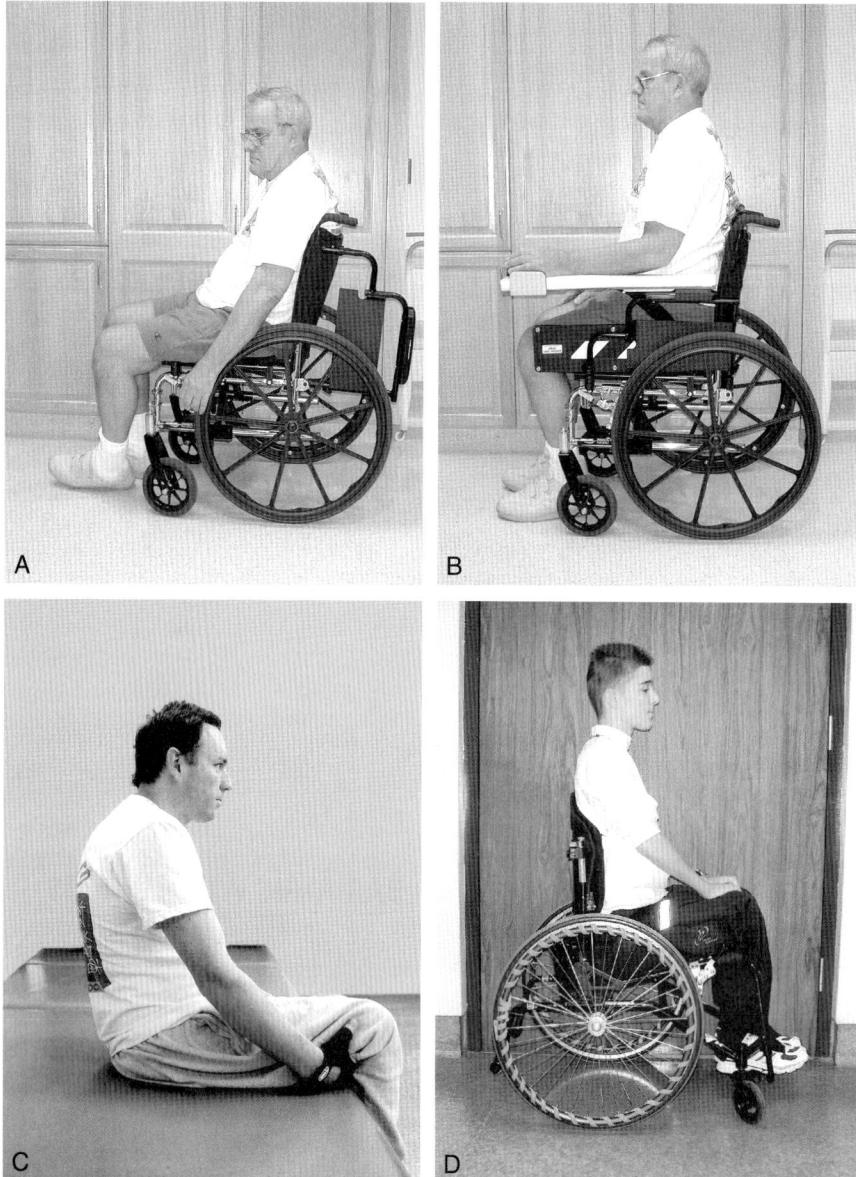

Fig. 11.10 (A) Client who had a stroke, seated in wheelchair. Poor positioning results in kyphotic thoracic spine, posterior pelvic tilt, and unsupported affected side. (B) Same client now seated in wheelchair with appropriate positioning devices. Seat and back inserts facilitate upright midline position with neutral pelvic tilt and equal weight bearing throughout. (C) Client who sustained a spinal cord injury, sitting with back poorly supported; this results in posterior pelvic tilt, kyphotic thoracic spine, and absence of lumbar curve. (D) Client seated with rigid back support and pressure-relief seat cushion, resulting in erect thoracic spine, lumbar curve, and anterior tilted pelvis.

awareness in the buttocks region, and that places him at risk for developing decubitus ulcers. He should develop sitting tolerance that extends beyond the current 1-hour period to help him pursue his educational goals of attending college. An appropriate seat cushion that distributes weight evenly will help William remain seated for a longer period. He will also need to develop the habit of shifting his weight while seated. This can be done by having William position his arm around the upright posts of the wheelchair back and pulling his body slightly to one side and then repeating the process on the other side. This shifting of the body from side to side reduces the risk of developing decubitus ulcers.

The following seven sections present the goals of a comprehensive seating and positioning assessment.

Goals for Wheelchair Assessment
Prevention of Deformity

Providing a symmetric base of support preserves proper skeletal alignment and discourages spinal curvature and other body deformities.

Tone Normalization

With proper body alignment, in addition to bilateral weight bearing and adaptive devices as needed, tone normalization can be maximized.

Pressure Management

Pressure sores can be caused by improper alignment and an inappropriate sitting surface. The proper seat cushion can provide comfort, assist in trunk and pelvic alignment, and create a surface that minimizes pressure, heat, moisture, and shearing—the primary causes of skin breakdown.

Promotion of Function

Pelvic and trunk stability is necessary to free the upper extremities for participation in all functional activities, including wheelchair mobility and daily living skills.

Maximum Sitting Tolerance

Wheelchair sitting tolerance will increase as support, comfort, and symmetric weight bearing are provided.

Optimal Respiratory Function

Support in an erect, well-aligned position can decrease compression of the diaphragm, thus increasing vital capacity.

Provision for Proper Body Alignment

Good body alignment is necessary for prevention of deformity, normalization of tone, and promotion of movement. The client should be able to propel the wheelchair and to move around within the wheelchair. Positioning starts with the pelvis, then progresses to the trunk and finally to the head. If the pelvis is not properly positioned, the trunk and head will not be aligned in a neutral and midline position. Spending time addressing the trunk and head positions, rather than starting at the pelvis, will often address the symptoms, but not the root problem.

A wide variety of seating and positioning equipment is available for all levels of disability. Custom modifications are continually being designed to meet a variety of client needs. In addition, technology in this area is ever growing, as is interest in wheelchair technology as a professional specialty. However, the skill of clinicians in this field ranges from extensive to negligible. Although it is an integral aspect of any wheelchair evaluation, the scope of seating and positioning equipment is much greater than can be addressed in this chapter. The Suggested Readings list at the end of this chapter provides additional resources.

Considerations for Transportation

Considering how the individual will use the wheelchair during transportation outside of the home and into the community must also be considered. Ideally, the individual should always transfer from the wheelchair into a vehicle's seat and seatbelt system. If the individual is unable to transfer from the wheelchair into a seat, then additional considerations must be made, including the height, weight, and size of the chair; space for maneuvering the wheelchair within the vehicle; and the total applied weight to the vehicle once the individual and the chair have been secured. Loading of the wheelchair by a lift, ramp, or other mode must also be considered.

Accessories

Once the measurements and the need for additional positioning devices have been determined, a wide variety of accessories are available to meet a client's individual needs. It is extremely important for the therapist to understand the function of each accessory and how an accessory interacts with the complete design and function of the chair and with seating and positioning equipment.[6,217-219]

Armrests come in fixed, flip-back, detachable, desk, standard, reclining, adjustable height, and tubular styles. The fixed armrest is a continuous part of the frame and is not detachable. It limits proximity to table, counter, and desk surfaces and prohibits side transfers. Flip-back, detachable desk, and standard-length arms are removable and allow side-approach transfers. Reclining arms are attached to the back post and recline with the back of the chair. Tubular arms are available on lightweight frames.

Footrests may be fixed, swing-away detachable, solid cradle, and elevating. Fixed footrests are attached to the wheelchair frame and are not removable. These footrests prevent the person from getting close to counters and may make some types of transfers more difficult. Swing-away detachable footrests can be moved to the side of the chair or removed entirely. This allows a closer approach to bed, bathtub, and counters, and, when the footrests are removed, reduces the overall wheelchair length and weight for easy loading into a car. Detachable footrests lock into place on the chair with a locking device.[217] A solid cradle footrest is found on rigid, lightweight chairs and is not removable. Elevating leg rests are available for clients with such conditions as LE edema, blood pressure changes, and orthopedic problems.

Foot plates may have heel loops and toe straps to aid in securing the foot to the foot plate.[217] The angle of the foot plate itself can be fixed or adjustable, raising or lowering toes relative to heels. A calf strap can be used on a solid cradle or when additional support behind the calf is necessary. Other accessories can include seatbelts, various brake styles, brake extensions, anti-tip devices, caster locks, arm supports, and head supports.

PREPARING THE JUSTIFICATION/ PRESCRIPTION

Once specific measurements and the need for modifications and accessories have been determined, the wheelchair prescription must be completed. It should be concise and specific so that everything requested can be accurately interpreted by the DME supplier, who will be submitting a sales contract for payment authorization. Before-and-after pictures can be helpful to illustrate medical necessity. The requirements for payment authorization from a particular reimbursement source must be known, so that medical necessity can be demonstrated. The therapist must be aware of the cost of every item being requested and must provide a reason and justification for each item. Payment may be denied if clear reasons are not given to substantiate the necessity for every item and modification requested.

Before the wheelchair is delivered to the client, the therapist should check the chair against the specific prescription and ensure that all specifications and accessories are correct. When a custom chair has been ordered, the client should be fitted by the ordering therapist to ensure that the chair fits and that it provides all the elements expected when the prescription was generated.

Often there are many adjustments that need to be made to ensure that the patient is properly positioned, supported, and, most importantly, symmetrically aligned to participate in wheelchair propulsion and functional activities. Even the smallest misalignment of the body can affect the client's ability to operate the wheelchair or, most importantly, could cause future skin

WHEELCHAIR SAFETY

Wheelchair parts tend to loosen over time and should be inspected and tightened on a regular basis. Elements of safety for the wheelchair user and the caregiver are as follows:

1. Brakes should be locked during all transfers.
2. The client should never bear weight or stand on the foot plates, which are placed in the "up" position during most transfers.
3. In most transfers it is an advantage to have footrests removed or swung away if possible.
4. If a caregiver is pushing the chair, the caregiver should be sure that the client's elbows are not protruding from the armrests and that the client's hands are not on the hand rims. If approaching from behind to assist in moving the wheelchair, the caregiver should inform the client of this intent and should check the position of the client's feet and arms before proceeding.
   - To push the client up a ramp, the caregiver should move in a normal, forward direction.
   - If the ramp is negotiated independently, the client should lean slightly forward while propelling the wheelchair up the incline.[218]
   - To push the client down a ramp, the caretaker should tilt the wheelchair slightly backward by pushing down on the anti-tippers with one foot to a tilt of approximately 30 degrees. Then the caregiver should ease the wheelchair down the ramp in a forward direction, while maintaining the chair in its balance position. The caregiver should keep knees slightly bent and the back straight.[218] The caregiver may also move down the ramp backward while the client maintains some control of the large wheels to prevent rapid backward motion. This approach is useful if the grade of the ramp is relatively steep. Ramps with only a slight grade can be managed in a forward direction if the caregiver maintains control of the wheelchair by grasping the hand grips with the wheelchair slightly tipped backward, and the client again maintains some control of the big wheels to prevent rapid forward motion.

   - If the ramp is negotiated independently, the client should move down the ramp facing forward, while leaning backward slightly and maintaining control of speed by grasping the hand rims. The client can descend a steep grade by traversing the ramp slightly back and forth to slow the chair. Push gloves may be helpful to reduce the effects of friction.[218]

5. A caregiver can manage ascending curbs by approaching them forward, tipping the wheelchair back, and pushing the foot down on the anti-tipper levers, thus lifting the front casters onto the curb and pushing forward. The large wheels then are in contact with the curb and roll on with ease as the chair is lifted slightly onto the curb.
6. The curb should be descended using a backward approach. A caregiver can move self and the chair around as the curb is approached and can pull the wheelchair to the edge of the curb. Standing below the curb, the caregiver can guide the large wheels off the curb by slowly pulling the wheelchair backward until it begins to descend. After the large wheels are safely on the street surface, the caregiver can tilt the chair back to clear the casters, move backward, lower the casters to the street surface, and turn around.[218]

With good strength and coordination, many clients can learn to manage curbs independently. To ascend and descend a curb, the client must have good bilateral grip, arm strength, and balance. To ascend the curb, the client tilts the chair onto the rear wheels and pushes forward until the front wheels hang over the curb, then lowers them gently. The client then leans forward and forcefully pushes forward on the hand rims to bring the rear wheels up on the pavement. To descend a curb, the client should lean forward and push slowly backward until the rear and then the front wheels roll down the curb.[53]

The ability to lift the front casters off the ground and balance on the rear wheels ("pop a wheelie") is a beneficial skill that expands the client's independence in the community with curb management and in rural settings with movement over grassy, sandy, or rough terrain. The chair will have to be properly adjusted so that the axle is not too far forward, which makes the wheelchair tip over backward too easily. Clients who have good grip and arm strength, and balance usually can master this skill and perform safely. The technique involves being able to tilt the chair on the rear wheels, balance the chair on the rear wheels, and move and turn the chair on the rear wheels. Wheelies make it possible to wheel up or down (jump) curbs. The client should not attempt to perform these maneuvers without instruction and training in the proper techniques, which are beyond the scope of this chapter. Specific instructions on teaching these skills can be found in the sources cited at the end of the chapter.[53]

TRANSFER BASICS

Transferring is the movement of a client from one surface to another. This process includes the sequence of events that must occur both before and after the move, such as the pretransfer sequence of bed mobility and the post-transfer phase of wheelchair positioning. If it is assumed that a client has some physical or cognitive limitations, it will be necessary for the therapist to assist in or supervise a transfer. Many therapists are unsure of the transfer type and technique to use or feel perplexed when a particular technique does not succeed with the client. Each client, therapist, and situation is different. This chapter does not include an outline of all techniques but presents the basic techniques with generalized principles. Each transfer must be adapted for the particular client and his or her needs. If there is a team involved, it is best to discuss with the physical therapist the most appropriate and safe transfer technique for the client. Discussion in this chapter includes directions for some transfer techniques that are most commonly used in practice. These techniques include the stand pivot, the bent pivot, and one person– and two person–dependent transfers.

Preliminary Concepts

The therapist must be aware of the following concepts when selecting and carrying out transfer techniques to ensure the safety of both the client and the therapist:

1. The client's status, especially physical, cognitive, perceptual, and behavioral abilities and limitations
2. The therapist's own physical abilities and limitations and ability to communicate clear, sequential instructions to the client (and if necessary to the long-term caregiver of the client)
3. The use of correct moving and lifting techniques

Guidelines for Using Proper Body Mechanics

The therapist should be aware of the following principles of basic body mechanics[7]:

1. Get close to the client or move the client close to you.
2. Position your body to face the client (face head on).
3. Bend the knees; use your legs, not your back.
4. Keep a neutral spine (not a bent or arched back).
5. Keep a wide base of support.
6. Keep your heels down.
7. Do not tackle more than you can handle; ask for help.
8. Do not combine movements. Avoid rotating at the same time as bending forward or backward.

The therapist should consider the following questions before performing a transfer:

1. What medical precautions affect the client's mobility or method of transfer?
2. Can the transfer be performed safely by one person or is assistance required?
3. Has enough time been allotted for safe execution of a transfer? Are you in a hurry?
4. Does the client understand what is going to happen? If not, does the client demonstrate fear or confusion? Are you prepared for this limitation?
5. Is the equipment (wheelchair, bed) that the client is being transferred to and from in good working order and in a locked position? Is it the appropriate size and type?
6. What is the height of the bed (or surface) in relation to the wheelchair? Can the heights be adjusted so that they are similar? (Transferring downhill is easier than uphill.)
7. Has all equipment been placed in the correct position?

8. Have all unnecessary bedding and equipment (e.g., footrests, armrests) been moved out of the way so that you are working without obstruction?
9. Is the client dressed properly in case you need to use a waistband to assist? If not, do you need a transfer belt or other assistance?
10. What are the other components of the transfer, such as leg management and bed mobility?

The therapist should be familiar with as many types of transfers as possible so that each situation can be resolved as it arises. It is also important to consult other team members, such as the physical therapist, to discuss the client's condition and the appropriate technique. It is best to start with basic, even-level transfers (e.g., mat table to wheelchair) and then progress to more complex transfers (e.g., toilet and car) because these have more variables and are more challenging.

Many classifications of transfers exist, based on the extent of the therapist's participation. Classifications range from dependent, in which the client is unable to participate and the therapist moves the client, to independent, in which the client moves independently while the therapist merely supervises, observes, or provides input for appropriate technique related to the client's disabling condition.

Before attempting to move a client, the therapist must understand the biomechanics of movement and the effect the client's center of positioning mass has on transfers.

Principles of Body Positioning
Pelvic Tilt

Generally, after the acute onset of a disability or prolonged time spent in bed, clients assume a posterior pelvic tilt (i.e., a slouched position with lumbar flexion). In turn, this posture moves the center of mass back toward the buttocks. The therapist may need to verbally cue or manually assist the client into a neutral or slightly anterior pelvic tilt position to move the center of mass forward over the center of the client's body and over the feet in preparation for the transfer.[175]

Trunk Alignment

It may be observed that the client's trunk alignment is shifted to the right or the left side. If the therapist assists in moving the client while the client's weight is shifted to one side, this movement could throw the client and the therapist off balance. The client may need verbal cues or physical assistance to come to and maintain a midline trunk position before and during the transfer.

Weight Shifting

Transfer is initiated by shifting the client's weight forward, thus removing weight from the buttocks. This movement allows the client to stand, partially stand, or be pivoted by the therapist. This step must be performed regardless of the type of transfer.

Lower Extremity Positioning

The client's feet must be placed firmly on the floor with the ankles stabilized and with the knees aligned at 90 degrees of flexion over the feet. This position allows the weight to be shifted easily onto and over the feet. The heels should be pointing toward the surface to which the client is transferring. The client should be barefoot or should have shoes on to prevent slipping out of position. Shoes with proper ankle support are beneficial for patients who have weakness or instability in the ankles or feet. The feet can easily pivot in this position, and the risk of twisting or injuring an ankle or a knee is minimized.

Upper Extremity Positioning

The client's arms must be in a safe position or in a position to assist in the transfer. If one or both of the upper extremities are nonfunctional, the arms should be placed in a safe position that will not be in the way during the transfer (e.g., in the client's lap). If the client has partial or full movement, motor control, or strength, the client can assist in the transfer by reaching toward the surface to be reached or by pushing off from the surface to be left. The decision to request the client to use the arms during the transfer is based on the therapist's prior knowledge of the client's motor function. The client should be encouraged to not reach or grab for the therapist during the transfer because this could throw both the therapist and the client off balance.

Preparing Equipment and Client for Transfer

The transfer process includes setting up the environment, positioning the wheelchair, and helping the client into a pretransfer position. The following four sections present a general overview of these steps.

Positioning the Wheelchair

1. Place the wheelchair at approximately a 0- to 30-degree angle to the surface to which the client is transferring. **The angle depends on the type of transfer and the client's level of assist.**
2. Lock the brakes on the wheelchair and the bed.
3. Place both of the client's feet firmly on the floor, hip width apart, with the knees over the feet.
4. Remove the wheelchair armrest closest to the bed.
5. Remove the wheelchair pelvic seatbelt.
6. Remove the wheelchair chest belt and trunk or lateral supports if present.

Bed Mobility in Preparation for Transfer
Rolling the Client Who Has Hemiplegia

1. Before rolling the client, you may need to put your hand under the client's scapula on the weaker side and gently mobilize it forward (into protraction) to prevent the client from rolling onto the shoulder, potentially causing pain and injury.
2. Assist the client in clasping the strong hand around the wrist of the weak arm, and lift the upper extremities upward toward the ceiling.
3. Assist the client in flexing knees.
4. You may assist the client to roll onto the side by moving first the arms toward the side, then the legs, and finally by placing one of your hands at the scapular area and the other hand at the hip, guiding the roll.

Side-Lying to Sit Up at the Edge of the Bed

1. Bring the client's feet off the edge of the bed.
2. Stabilize the client's lower extremities with your knees.
3. Shift the client's body to an upright sitting position.
4. Place the client's hands on the bed at each side of the body to help maintain balance.

Scooting to the Edge of the Bed

When working with a client who has sustained a stroke or a traumatic brain injury (TBI), the therapist should "walk" the client's hips toward the edge of the bed. Shift the client's weight to the less affected or unaffected side, position your hand behind the opposite buttock, and guide the client forward. Then shift the client's weight to the more affected side and repeat the procedure if necessary. Move forward until the client's feet are flat on the floor.

In the case of an individual with an SCI, grasp the client's legs from behind the knees and gently pull the client forward, placing the client's feet firmly on the floor and making sure that the ankles are in a neutral position.

TRANSFER TECHNIQUES

Stand Pivot Transfers

The standing pivot transfer requires the client to be able to come to a standing position and pivot on both feet. It is most commonly used with clients who have hemiplegia, hemiparesis, or general loss of strength or balance. If the client has significant hemiparesis, stand pivot transfers encourage the less affected or the unaffected side to accommodate most of the body weight and may put the more affected limb (ankle) at risk while pivoting.

Transfer From Wheelchair to Bed or to Mat Table

1. Facilitate the client's scoot to the edge of the surface and put the client's feet flat on the floor. The client's heels should be pointed toward the surface to which the client is transferring. The feet should not be perpendicular to the transfer surface, but the heel should be angled toward the surface.
2. Stand on the client's affected side with your hands on the client's scapulae or around the client's trunk, waist, or hips. Stabilize the client's involved foot and knee with your own foot and knee. Provide assistance by guiding the client forward as the buttocks are lifted up from the present surface and toward the transfer surface (Fig. 11.11A).
3. The client may reach toward the surface to which the client is transferring or may push off the surface from which the client is transferring (Fig. 11.11B).
4. Guide the client toward the transfer surface and gently help the client down to a sitting position (Fig. 11.11C).

Variations: Stand Pivot and/or Stand/Step Transfer

A stand pivot and/or stand/step transfer is generally used when a client can take small steps toward the surface goal and not just pivot toward the transfer surface (Fig. 11.11D–F). The therapist's intervention may range from physical assistance to accommodation for potential loss of balance to facilitation of near

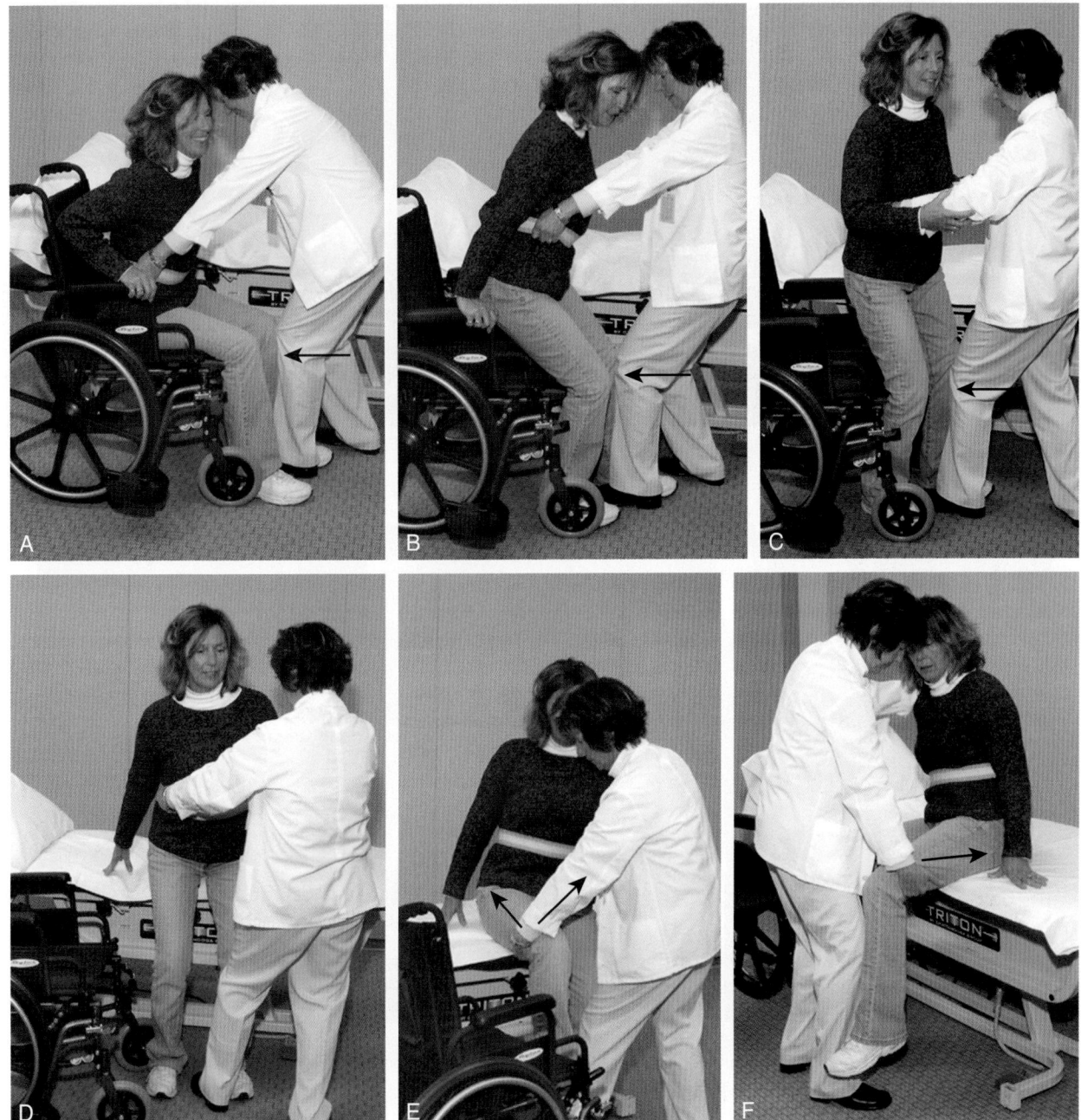

Fig. 11.11 Standing pivot transfer—wheelchair to bed, assisted. (A–C) Therapist stands on client's affected side and stabilizes client's foot and knee. He or she assists by guiding client forward and initiates lifting the buttocks up. (D) Client reaches toward transfer surface. (E–F) Therapist guides the client toward transfer surface. (Courtesy Luis Gonzalez.)

normal movement, equal weight bearing, and maintenance of appropriate posture for clients with hemiplegia or hemiparesis. If a client demonstrates impaired cognition or a behavior deficit, including impulsiveness and poor safety judgment, the therapist may need to provide verbal cues or physical guidance.

Sliding Board Transfers

Sliding board transfers are best used with those who cannot adequately bear weight on the lower extremities and who have paralysis, weakness, or poor endurance in their upper extremities. If the client is going to assist the caregiver in this transfer,

the client should have good UE strength. This transfer is most often used with persons who have LE amputations, individuals with spinal cord injuries, and bariatric clients.

Method (Fig. 11.12)

1. Position and set up the wheelchair as previously outlined.
2. Lift the leg closer to the transfer surface and place the board under this leg, at midthigh between the buttocks and the knee, angled toward the opposite hip. The board must be firmly under the thigh and firmly on the surface to which the client is transferring.

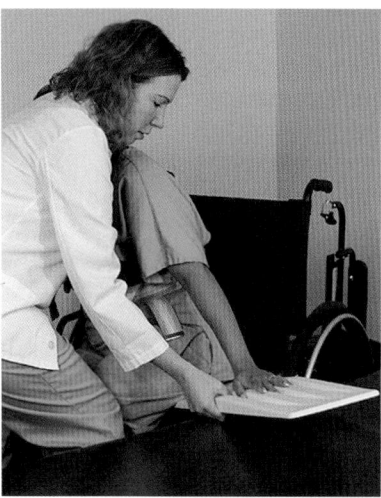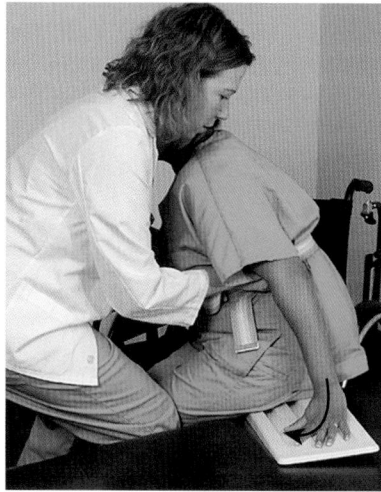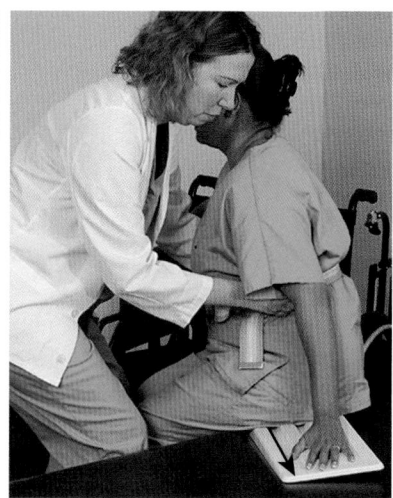

Fig. 11.12 Positioning sliding board. Lift leg closest to transfer surface. Place board midthigh between buttocks and knee, angled toward opposite hip. (Courtesy Luis Gonzalez.)

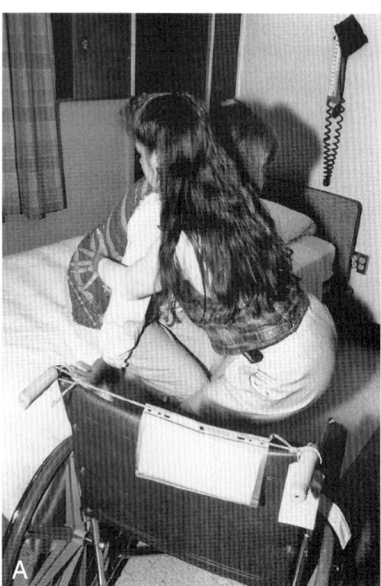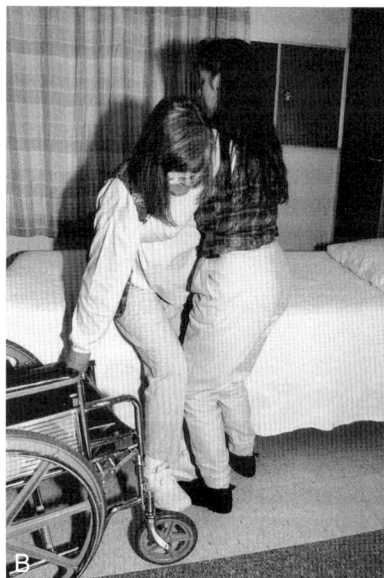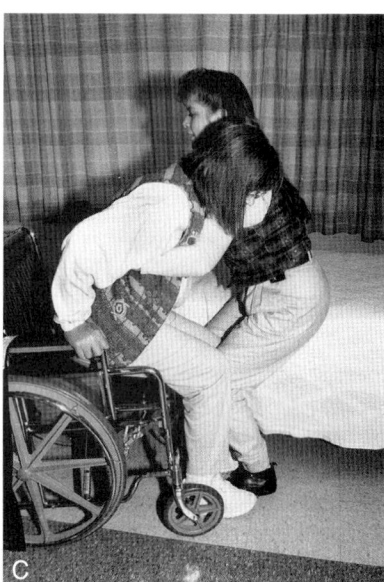

Fig. 11.13 Bent pivot transfer—bed to wheelchair. (A) Therapist grasps client around trunk and assists in shifting client's weight forward over feet. (B) Client reaches toward wheelchair. (C) Therapist assists client down toward sitting position. (Courtesy Luis Gonzalez.)

3. Block the client's knees with your own knees.
4. Instruct the client to place one hand toward the edge of the board and the other hand on the wheelchair seat.
5. Instruct the client to lean forward and slightly away from the transferring surface.
6. The client should transfer upper body weight in the direction opposite to which the client is going. The client should use both arms to lift or slide the buttocks along the board.
7. Assist the client where needed to shift weight and support the trunk while moving to the intended surface.

Bent Pivot Transfer: Bed to Wheelchair

The bent pivot transfer is used when the client cannot initiate or maintain a standing position. A therapist often prefers to keep a client in the bent knee position to maintain equal weight bearing, provide optimal trunk and LE support, and perform a safer and easier therapist-assisted transfer.

Procedure

1. Assist the client to scoot to the edge of the bed until both of the client's feet are flat on the floor. Grasp the client around the waist, trunk, or hips, or even under the buttocks, if a moderate or maximal amount of assistance is required.
2. Facilitate the client's trunk into a midline position.
3. Shift the weight forward from the buttocks toward and over the client's feet (Fig. 11.13A).
4. Have the client reach toward the surface he or she is transferring to or push from the surface he or she is transferring from (Fig. 11.13B).
5. Provide assistance by guiding and pivoting the client around toward the transfer surface (Fig. 11.13C).

Depending on the amount of assistance required, the pivoting portion can be done in two or three steps, with the therapist repositioning himself or herself and the client's lower extremities between steps. The therapist has a variety of choices regarding where to hold or grasp the client during the bent pivot transfer, depending on the weight and height of the client in relation to the therapist and the client's ability to assist in the transfer. Variations include using both hands and arms at the waist or trunk, or one or both hands under the buttocks. The therapist never grasps under the client's weak arm or grasps the weak arm; such an action could cause significant injury because of weak musculature and poor stability around the shoulder girdle. The choice is made with consideration of proper body mechanics. Trial and error in technique is advised to allow for optimal facilitation of client independence and safety, and the therapist's proper body mechanics.

Dependent Transfers

The dependent transfer is designed for use with the client who has minimal to no functional ability. If this transfer is performed incorrectly, it is potentially hazardous for therapist and client. This transfer should be practiced with able-bodied persons and should be used first with the client only when another person is available to assist.[7]

The purpose of the dependent transfer is to move the client from surface to surface. The requirements are that the client must be cooperative and willing to follow instructions and the therapist must be keenly aware of correct body mechanics and his or her own physical limitations. With heavy clients it is always best to use the two-person transfer, or at least to have a second person available to spot the transfer.

One Person–Dependent Sliding Board Transfer (Fig. 11.14)

The procedure for transferring the client from wheelchair to bed is as follows:

1. Set up the wheelchair and bed as described previously.
2. Position the client's feet together on the floor, directly under the knees, and swing the outside footrest away. Grasp the client's legs from behind the knees and pull the client slightly forward in the wheelchair, so the buttocks will clear the large wheel when the transfer is made (Fig. 11.14A).
3. Place a sliding board under the client's inside thigh, midway between the buttocks and the knee, to form a bridge from the bed to the wheelchair. The sliding board is angled toward the client's opposite hip.
4. Stabilize the client's feet by placing your feet laterally around the client's feet.
5. Stabilize the client's knees by placing your own knees firmly against the anterolateral aspect of the client's knees (Fig. 11.14B).
6. Facilitate the client's lean over the knees by guiding the client forward from the shoulders. The client's head and trunk should lean opposite the direction of the transfer. The client's hands can rest on the lap.
7. Reach under the client's outside arm and grasp the waistband of the trousers, a transfer belt positioned around the client's waist, or under the client's buttock. On the other

side, reach over the client's back and grasp the waistband, transfer belt, or under the buttock (Fig. 11.14C).
8. After your arms are positioned correctly, lock them to stabilize the client's trunk. Keep your knees slightly bent and brace them firmly against the client's knees.
9. Gently rock with the client to gain some momentum and prepare to move after the count of three. Count to three aloud with the client. On three, holding your knees tightly against the client's knees, transfer the client's weight over the client's feet. You must keep your back straight and your knees bent to maintain good body mechanics (Fig. 11.14D).
10. Pivot with the client and move onto the sliding board (Fig. 11.14E). Reposition yourself and the client's feet and repeat the pivot until the client is firmly seated on the bed surface, perpendicular to the edge of the mattress and as far back as possible. This step usually can be achieved in two or three stages (Fig. 11.14F).
11. You can secure the client onto the bed by easing him or her against the back of an elevated bed or onto the mattress in a side-lying position and then lifting the legs onto the bed.

The one person–dependent sliding board transfer can be adapted to move the client to other surfaces. It should be attempted only when therapist and client feel secure with the wheelchair-to-bed transfer.

Two Person–Dependent Transfers (Fig. 11.15)

Bent Pivot: With or Without a Sliding Board, Bed to Wheelchair. A bent pivot transfer is used to allow increased therapist interaction and support. It provides the therapist with greater control of the client's trunk and buttocks during the transfer. It is often used with neurologically involved clients because trunk flexion and equal weight bearing are often desirable with this diagnosis. The steps in this two-person procedure are as follows:

1. Set up the wheelchair and bed as described previously.
2. One therapist assumes a position in front of the client and the other in back.
3. The therapist in front assists in walking the client's hips forward until the feet are flat on the floor.
4. The same therapist stabilizes the client's knees and feet by placing the therapist's knees and feet lateral to each of those of the client.
5. The therapist in back positions self squarely behind the client's buttocks, grasping the client's waistband or transfer belt, grasping the sides of the client's pants, or placing his or her hands under the buttocks. Maintain proper body mechanics (Fig. 11.15A).
6. The therapist in front moves the client's trunk into a midline position, grasps the client around the back of the shoulders, waist, or hips, and guides the client to lean forward and shift weight forward, over the feet and off the buttocks. The client's head and trunk should lean in the direction opposite the transfer. The client's hands can rest on the lap (Fig. 11.15B).
7. As the therapist in front shifts the client's weight forward, the therapist in back shifts the client's buttocks in the direction of the transfer. This can be done in two or three steps, making sure the client's buttocks land on a safe, solid surface. The

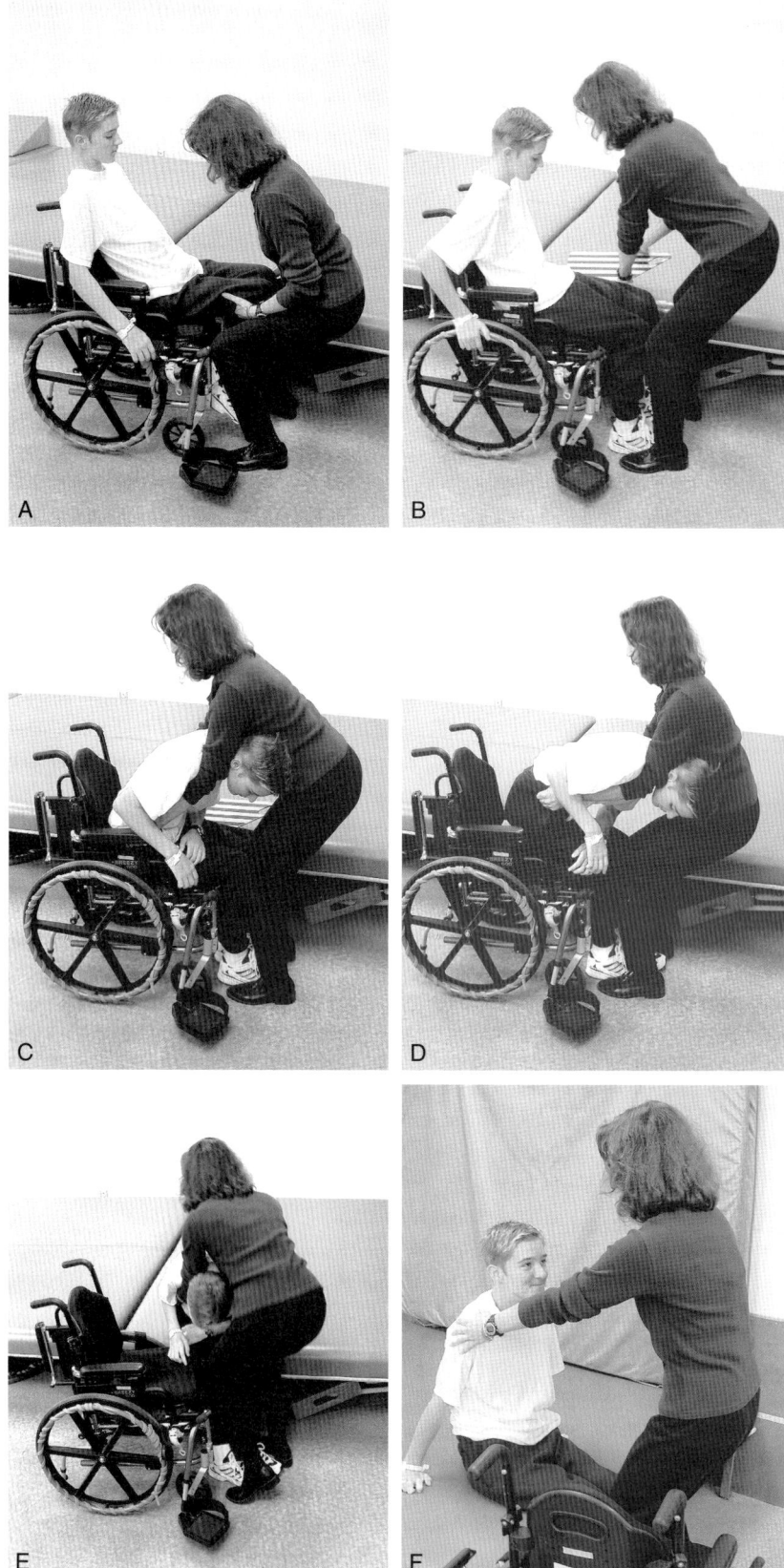

Fig. 11.14 One person–dependent sliding board transfer. (A) Therapist positions wheelchair and client and pulls client forward in chair. (B) Therapist stabilizes client's knees and feet after placing sliding board. (C) Therapist grasps client's pants at lowest point of buttocks. (D) Therapist rocks with client and shifts client's weight over client's feet, making sure client's back remains straight. (E) Therapist pivots with client and moves client onto sliding board. (F) Client is stabilized on the bed. (Courtesy Luis Gonzales.)

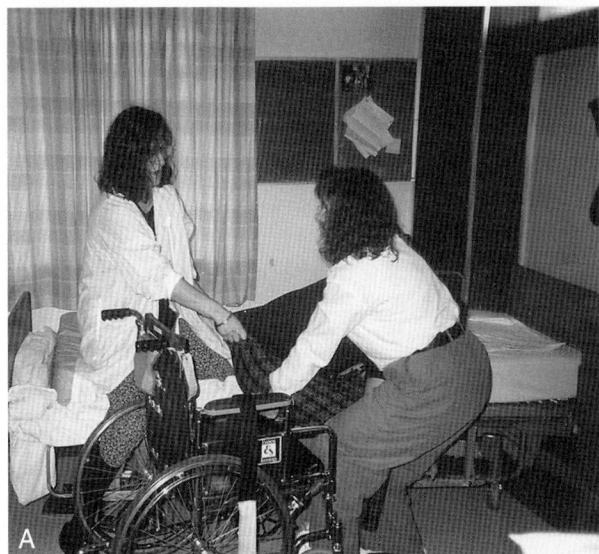
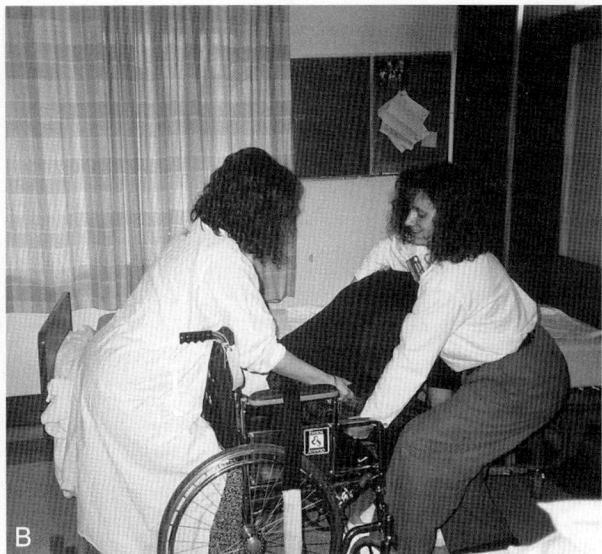
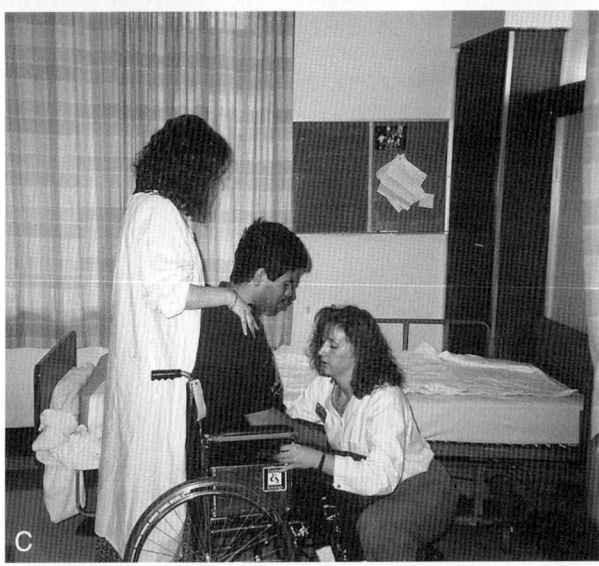

FIG 11.15 Two person–dependent transfer: bed to wheelchair. (A) One therapist positions self in front of client, blocking feet and knees. The therapist in back positions self behind client's buttocks and assists by lifting. (B) Person in front rocks client forward and unweights buttocks as the back therapist shifts buttocks toward wheelchair. (C) Both therapists position client in upright, midline position in wheelchair. Seatbelt is secured, and positioning devices are added. (Courtesy Luis Gonzales.)

therapists reposition themselves and the client to maintain safe and proper body mechanics (Fig. 11.15C).

8. The therapists should be sure they coordinate the time of the transfer with the client and one another by counting to three aloud and instructing the team to initiate the transfer on three.

9. Transfer or gait belts may be used to offer a place to grasp while assisting the client in a transfer. The belt is placed securely around the waist and often is used instead of the client's waistband. The belt should not be allowed to slide up the client's trunk because leverage will be compromised.

Mechanical Lift Transfers (Fig. 11.16)

Some clients, because of body size, degree of disability, or the health and well-being of the caregiver, require the use of a mechanical lift. A variety of mechanical lifting devices can be used to transfer clients of any weight (see Fig. 11.16). A properly trained caregiver, even one who is considerably smaller than the client, can learn to use the mechanical lift safely and independently.[218] The client's physical size, the environment in which the lift will be used, and the uses to which the lift will be put must be considered to order the appropriate mechanical lift. The client and caregiver should demonstrate safe use of the lift for the therapist before the therapist prescribes it.

Transfers to Household Surfaces
Sofa or Chair (Fig. 11.17)

Wheelchair to sofa and wheelchair to chair transfers are similar to wheelchair to bed transfers; however, a few unique concerns should be assessed. Transfers to surfaces that are variable are described as complex transfers. The therapist and the client need to be aware that the chair may be light and not as stable as a bed or wheelchair. When transferring to the chair, the client must be instructed to reach for the seat of the chair. The client should not reach for the armrest or the back of the chair because this action may cause the chair to tip over. When moving from a chair to the wheelchair, the client should use a hand to push off from the seat of the chair as he or she begins to stand. Standing from a chair is often more difficult if the chair is low or the seat cushions are soft. Dense cushions may be added to increase height and provide a firm surface to which to transfer.

Toilet and Bedside Commode

In general, wheelchair to toilet and wheelchair to bedside commode transfers are difficult because of the confined space in most bathrooms, the height of the toilet, and the instability and lack of support of a toilet seat. The therapist and client should attempt to position the wheelchair next to or at an appropriate angle to the toilet or commode. The therapist should check the space around the toilet and wheelchair to ensure that no obstacles are present. Adaptive devices such as grab bars and raised toilet seats can be added to a regular toilet to enhance the client's independence during this transfer. Raised toilet seats that are poorly secured to toilets and may be unsafe for some clients. The client can use these devices for support during transfers and to maintain a level surface to which to transfer.

Bathtub

The occupational therapist should be cautious when assessing or teaching bathtub transfers because the bathtub is considered one of the most hazardous areas of the home. Transfers from the wheelchair to the bottom of the bathtub are extremely difficult and are used with clients who have good bilateral strength and motor control of the upper extremities (e.g., clients with paraplegia and LE amputation). A commercially produced bath bench or bath chair or a well-secured straight-back chair is commonly used by therapists for seated bathing. Therefore, whether a standing pivot, bent pivot, or sliding board transfer is performed, the technique is similar to a wheelchair to chair transfer. However, the transfer may be complicated by the confined space, the slick bathtub surfaces, and the bathtub wall between the wheelchair and the bathtub seat.

If a standing pivot transfer is used, it is recommended that the locked wheelchair be placed at a 45-degree angle to the bathtub if possible. The client should stand, pivot, sit on the bathtub chair, and then place the lower extremities into the bathtub.

If a bent pivot or sliding board transfer is used, the wheelchair is placed next to the bathtub with the armrest removed. The transfer tub bench may be used and removes the need for a sliding board. This approach allows the wheelchair to be placed right next to the bench, which permits safe and easy transfer of the buttocks to the seat. Then the lower extremities can be assisted into the bathtub.

In general, the client may exit by first placing one foot securely outside the bathtub on a nonskid floor surface and then performing a standing or seated transfer back to the wheelchair. Often the client's buttocks may be bare; therefore, a pillowcase may be placed over the sliding board, or a SafetySure Transfer Sling (The Wright Stuff [http://www.thewright-stuff.com/]). (Fig. 11.18) may be used for safe transfers for bathing.

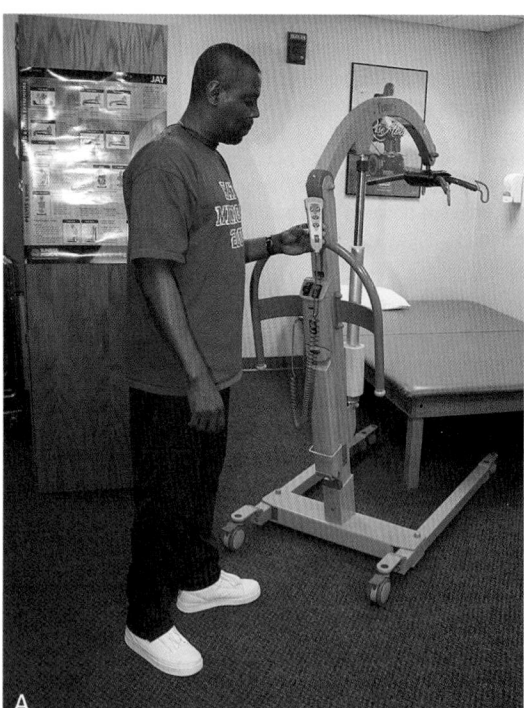
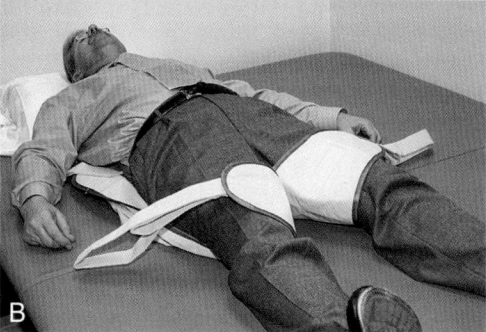
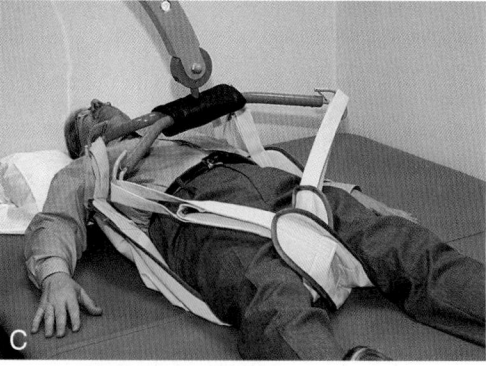

FIG 11.16 (A) Traditional boom-style mechanical lift. (B) Sling attachments should be exposed with the outside seams of the sling directed away from the patient. (C) Position the lift perpendicularly to the patient, close to the bed, and with the spreader bar over the chest; attach the chains or web straps to the spreader bar.

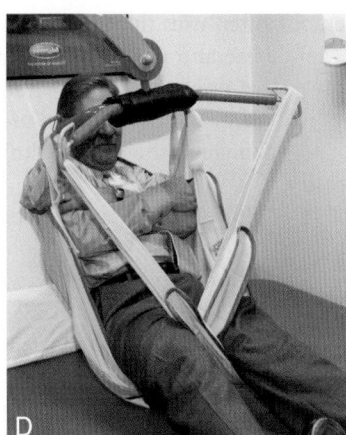
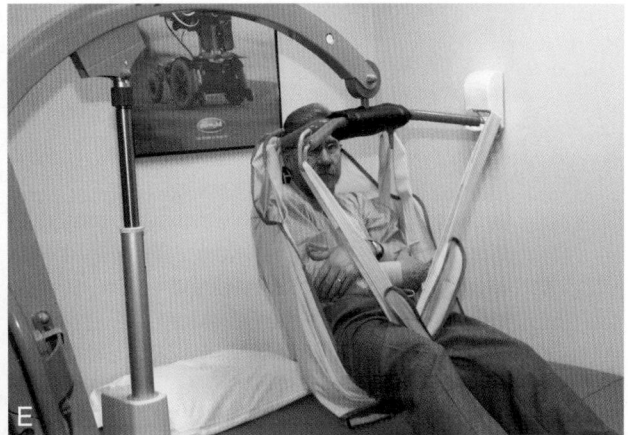
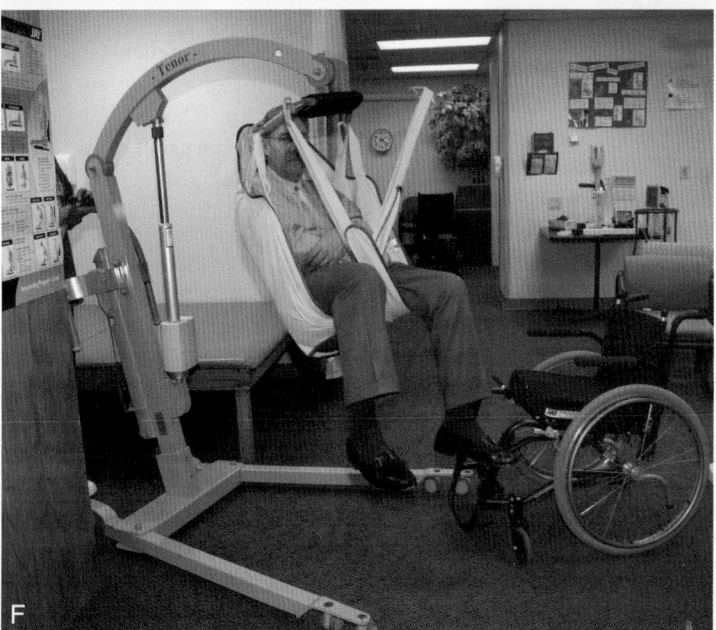
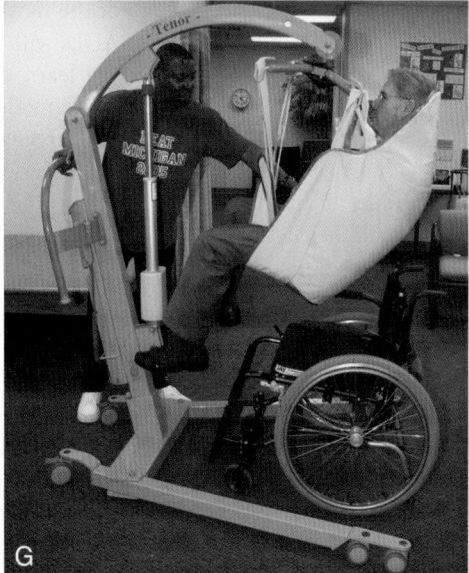
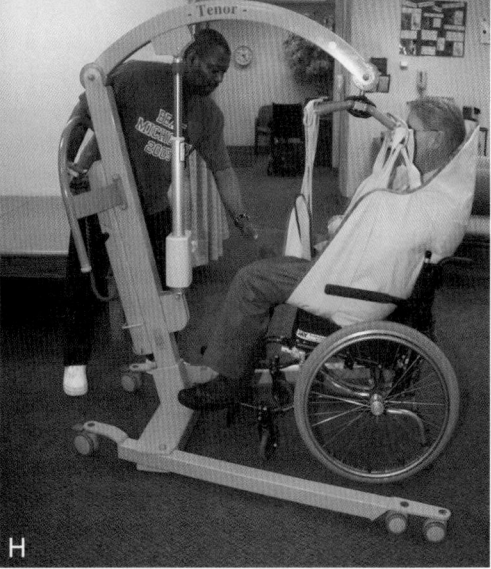

FIG 11.16 cont'd (D–E) Fold the patient's arms over the abdomen and elevate the body. Elevate the patient until the buttocks clear the surface of the bed. (F–H) The patient's knees can be allowed to flex or can be kept extended. Carefully move the lift away from the side of the bed and then turn the patient to face the support column. Transport the patient to the wheelchair and lower into the chair.[93] (From Fairchild S: *Pierson and Fairchild's principles and techniques of patient care*, ed 5, St Louis, 2013, Saunders.)

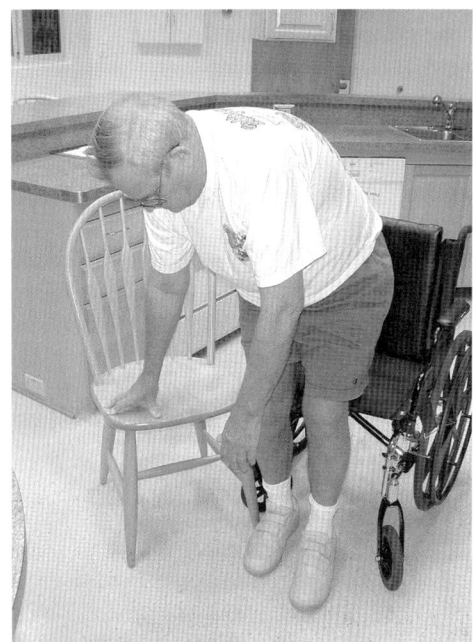

Fig. 11.17 Client who sustained a stroke in midtransfer reaches for seat of chair, pivots, and lowers body to sitting. (Courtesy Luis Gonzales.)

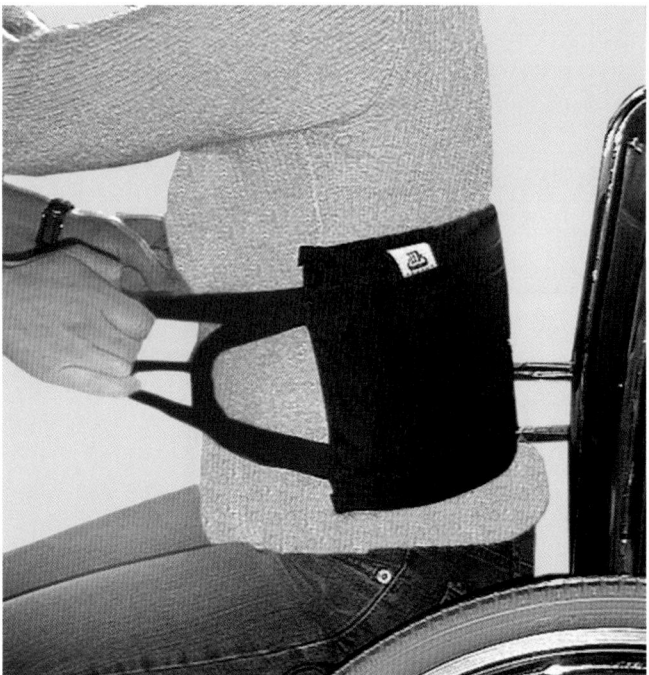

Fig. 11.18 SafetySure Transfer Sling fastened around the client's waist and lower back for support. (Courtesy Scan Medical, North Billerica, MA.)

Car Transfers

A car transfer is often the most challenging for therapists because it involves trial-and-error methods to develop a technique that is safe and easy for the client and caregiver to carry out. The therapist often uses the client's existing transfer technique. The client's size and degree of disability, in addition to the vehicle style (two door or four door), must be considered. These factors will affect the client's level of independence and may necessitate a change in the usual technique to allow a safe and easy transfer.

In general, it is difficult to get a wheelchair close enough to touch the car seat, especially with four-door vehicles. The following are some additional considerations when making wheelchair to car transfers:

1. Car seats are often much lower than the standard wheelchair seat height, which makes the uneven transfer much more difficult, especially from the car seat to the wheelchair. Sport utility vehicles (SUVs) and trucks are especially challenging because of the increased height.
2. Occasionally clients have orthopedic injuries that necessitate the use of a brace, such as a halo body jacket or an LE cast or splint. The therapist often must alter the technique (e.g., recline the car seat) to accommodate these devices.
3. The therapist may suggest the use of an extra-long sliding board for this transfer to compensate for the large gap between transfer surfaces.
4. Because uphill transfers are difficult and the level of assistance may increase for this transfer, the therapist may choose a two person–assist instead of a one person–assist transfer to ensure a safe and smooth technique.
5. The therapist may have to practice transfers in both the front and back seats to determine which car position would be safest for the client.

SECTION 2 SUMMARY

A wheelchair that fits well and can be managed safely and easily by its user and caregiver is one of the most important factors in the client's ability to perform ADLs with maximal independence.[216] All wheelchair users must learn the capabilities and limitations of the wheelchair and safe methods of performing all self-care and mobility skills. If a caregiver is available, that individual needs to be thoroughly familiar with safe and correct techniques of handling the wheelchair, the positioning equipment, and the client.

Transfer skills are among the most important activities that must be mastered by the wheelchair user. The ability to transfer increases the possibility of mobility and travel. However, transfers can be hazardous. Safe methods must be learned and followed.[218] Several basic transfer techniques are outlined in this chapter. Additional methods and more detailed training and instructions are available, as discussed previously.

Many wheelchair users with exceptional abilities have developed unique methods of wheelchair management. Although such innovative approaches may work well for the person who has devised and mastered them, they cannot be considered basic procedures that everyone can learn.

SECTION 3: DRIVING AND COMMUNITY MOBILITY

Elin Schold Davis and Susan Martin Touchinsky

THREADED CASE STUDY

Jacqueline, Part 1

Jacqueline (prefers use of the pronouns she/her/hers) is a 67-year-old retired teacher referred to outpatient occupational therapy by her rheumatologist. She describes increased difficulty in her ADLs because of painful arthritis in her neck, hands, back, hips, knees, and ankles. While establishing an occupational profile for Jacqueline, her occupational therapist, Sergio, an occupational therapist in general practice, asks Jacqueline if she drives. Jacqueline's husband, a retired accountant who has diabetes, peripheral neuropathies in his legs, and diabetic retinopathy, ceased driving in the past year. This brought about a major change in Jacqueline's role. Whereas Jacqueline had previously been a passenger and navigator, she has now assumed the primary role for transportation and driving, including assisting her husband with his wheelchair and car transfers. Jacqueline is 5 feet, 6 inches tall and weighs 138 lb. Her husband is 6 feet tall and weighs 220 lb. The family vehicle is a 20-year-old sedan, which is meticulously maintained.

The occupational therapist, Sergio, reviews Jacqueline's chart and notes she is in good health other than the limitations imposed by the arthritis. During the IADL evaluation, Sergio carefully observes Jacqueline's occupational performance in the kitchen and notes that she is able to plan and problem solve easily. Her primary deficits are in motor areas. Larger grip kitchen utensils are recommended to facilitate meal preparation. Because Jacqueline has emphasized the importance of being the caregiver and driver for her husband, Sergio decides to observe how her deficits affect her ability to support her husband's vehicle transfers and management of his mobility device. Sergio observes that Jacqueline has difficulties loading her husband's manual wheelchair into the car, managing the key in the car door, and manipulating the hand lever to open the door. Jacqueline tells Sergio that she does not mind driving, but she does not drive at all on days when she is experiencing a lot of pain or fatigue.

During therapy sessions, Jacqueline reports that she feels fatigued from driving so much. She mentions that she drives herself and her husband to all doctor appointments, to the pharmacy for medicines, and to church. When Sergio asks about her preferred occupations, she states that she rarely participates in her hobby of scrapbooking anymore because of fatigue and lack of time. She is worried about what the future will bring in terms of transportation because their two adult children live out of state, more than 500 miles away.

Critical Thinking Questions

1. What tests and measures has the occupational therapist used to consider Jacqueline's driving risk and potential?
2. What areas of Jacqueline's community mobility are appropriate for OT intervention in general practice?
3. Upon analysis of the occupation of driving relative to her diagnosis, what client factors and performance skills indicate the need for further intervention and a referral to a driver rehabilitation specialist?
4. What adaptations or recommendations can Jacqueline and her therapist consider to improve mobility for her and her husband, especially on days when she is not feeling up to driving?

Community mobility is an essential occupation that supports a range of occupations, habits, routines, roles, and rituals.[18,50] As highlighted in the OTPF-4,[28] the occupation of driving and community mobility (D&CM) includes not just the task of operating a vehicle, but the "planning and moving around in the community using public or private transportation, such as driving, walking, bicycling, or accessing and riding in buses, taxi cabs, ride shares, or other transportation systems" (p. 31). Driving is especially critical in our industrialized nation and will have an impact on the engagement and health of patients. Thus, it is imperative that all OT practitioners include considerations for engagement in D&CM as part of the evaluation and plan of care.[26] While the role of the OT practitioner in general practice differs from that of a driver rehabilitation specialist, both are important for supporting and optimizing the health and engagement of patients.

The potential for engagement in areas of occupation and community mobility are closely linked.[60] OTs understand that community mobility is critical for accomplishing necessary activities and enabling individuals to maintain social connectedness.[223] In the United States, community mobility, and the subset of driving in particular, is often seen as an important part of independence.[88] Conversely, limitations in community mobility and loss of a driver's license can negatively affect autonomy and feelings of well-being. Lack of transportation to engage in occupations such as grocery shopping, going to medical appointments, and attending religious and/or recreational events can result in diminished social participation.[98,101] Transportation problems are often cited as a primary barrier among individuals with disabilities.[200,220] In addition, older adults faced with driving cessation risk depression[161] and entry into long-term care[97] and have increased self-perceptions of disability.[113]

ROLE OF OCCUPATIONAL THERAPY

The OT practitioner is ideally suited to identify when community mobility occupations require assessment and intervention.[26,132] OT practitioners understand the interplay between engagement in occupation, the existence or lack of mobility options, and physical and mental health. Knowledge in this area makes the profession relevant to clients, the community, and public and private entities.[16] Occupational therapists develop treatment plans by analyzing the interplay of client factors, performance skills and patterns, and the contexts and environments involved in community mobility (Fig. 11.19).[28] Within

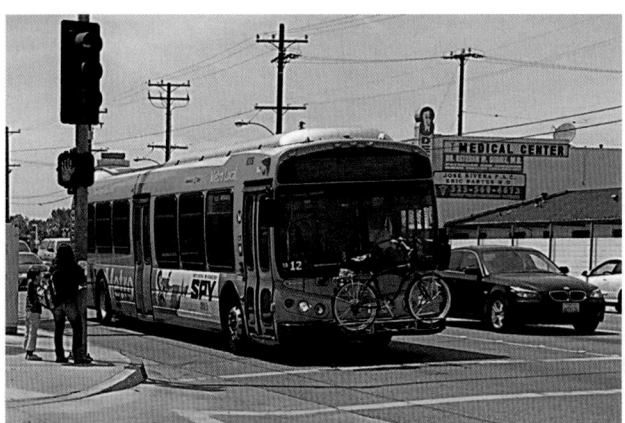

Fig. 11.19 Occupational therapists must take a comprehensive view of community mobility throughout the lifespan. Community mobility in this context includes pedestrian, bicycling, public transportation, and driver issues.

this framework, OT practitioners consider the community mobility needs of clients with varying disabilities at all stages of life. Service recipients could be as diverse as a toddler with cerebral palsy, an adolescent with autism spectrum disorder, a young adult with an SCI, an adult who has suffered a stroke, and a senior citizen with dementia.[16]

OT services in general practice are directly related to a client's mobility concerns and the occupations in which they engage. OT practitioners can address various aspects of passenger safety, walking, biking, and use of mass transit. Interventions may also involve pre-driver readiness in preparation to acquire a first driver's license, assessment of experienced drivers with age-related changes that interfere with driving, and exploration of alternative transportation options for those people who must temporarily or permanently discontinue driving.[16] Although clients are often individual persons, organizations or populations may also benefit from occupational therapy services.[16,50] Examples of services that might be provided to organizations include modification of the paratransit eligibility evaluation for a transit company seeking to increase ridership of disabled persons and training of drivers and bus aides for a school system seeking to improve the safety of student passengers with special needs. Services to populations may include collaboration with municipal planning organizations to promote roadway design, bike lanes, and pedestrian paths to support older drivers and persons using other modes of transportation.[16]

Historical Context

Understanding that aspects of driving rehabilitation fall within specialty practice, the responsibility to address the IADLs of driving and community mobility has evolved to a responsibility of medical practitioners concerned with an individual's IADLs.[160] Driver rehabilitation practices are founded on the commitment that adaptation of the physical vehicle or driving environment can be redesigned or modified to make the personal vehicle accessible to any disabled driver wishing to drive. Multiple disciplines from rehab engineering to vehicle designers to occupational therapy professionals have collaborated to define the field of driver rehabilitation and led to formation of the Association for Driver Rehabilitation Specialists (ADED) in 1977.[33] The organization, a multidisciplinary trade association, includes members from both medical and nonmedical professions. ADED offers members resources and education, a code of ethics[36] and best practice guidelines.[37,38] Since 1995, ADED has offered an examination based certification in driver rehabilitation to a variety of individuals with both medical and nonmedical backgrounds, including but not limited to counseling, criminal justice/law enforcement, education, exercise physiology, health and physical education, kinesiotherapy, nursing, occupational therapy, physical therapy, social work, special education, speech language pathology, therapeutic recreational therapy, and vocational rehabilitation.[35]

Expansion of the driver rehabilitation field prompted trade and government agencies to address safety issues related to vehicle modifications and the practice of driver rehabilitation. In 1997 the National Mobility Equipment Dealers Association (NMEDA), a national organization to promote and support

individual members engaged in the modification of transportation for people with disabilities, established their Quality Assurance Program (QAP). This is an accreditation program to promote quality, safety, and reliability within the mobility industry.[141,148] The National Highway Traffic Safety Administration (NHTSA), a federal agency charged with saving lives, preventing injuries, and reducing the economic costs related to traffic accidents, is involved in overseeing vehicle safety related to vehicle modifications for people with disabilities.[140]

For some, using the physical vehicle is not the primary concern. The concept that anyone can drive with the proper modifications has evolved to reflect broader practitioner responsibilities. Practitioners are asked to provide opinions regarding delicensing (or canceling a driver's license) and consider that a potential negative outcome of driving rehabilitation services is driving cessation.

As medical practitioners and decision makers sought evidence-based measures for addressing medically related changes that placed driving competence at risk, research efforts have diligently sought to clarify uncertainty surrounding testing (or selecting the right test) and driving licensing decisions. As delicensing and driving cessation gained recognition as both a community and healthcare issue, the need for addressing and expanding transportation alternatives for the aging American population became recognized, and the NHTSA developed a plan to address the needs of older drivers.[137,207] The agency funded research and developed educational materials to increase awareness of the transportation needs of older drivers. A seminal document that described the controversial complexities around delicensing an older driver with diminishing abilities was the first edition, published in 2001, of the American Medical Association's (AMA) *Physician's Guide to Assessing and Counseling Older Drivers*.[63] This was created in collaboration with the NHTSA to help physicians address the public health issue of older adult driver safety. This document firmly established that concerns for driving safety were within the realm and scope of medical practice. This document has been updated and the title changed to the *Clinician's Guide to Assessing and Counseling Older Drivers* to reflect the multidisciplinary responsibilities to address driving.[160] To increase the quality and availability of service providers dealing with senior driving, the NHTSA has promoted partnerships with professional organizations serving the older population. The agency recognized the role of OT practitioners in driving and community mobility of older adults and acknowledges that OT practitioners in general practice, who frequently encounter seniors with medical conditions, are in a position to screen for changes that may affect the capacity to operate a vehicle and refer at-risk individuals for additional services. This screening for risk (discussed later in this chapter) can be considered an important step between medical practice or general rehabilitation and a referral to the specialist in driving rehabilitation. The NHTSA also recognized that OT practitioners with a specialty in driver rehabilitation have acquired an advanced skill set to offer driving-related services and interventions beyond what can be expected at the level of general or entry level practice.[143] The *Clinician's Guide*, now into its fourth edition, supports the growing need for medical professionals to address driving risk. This guide has been published by the American Geriatric Society, and because its development was funded through NHTSA,[160] it is available for download at no cost (https://geriatricscareonline.org/ProductAbstract/clinicians-guide-to-assessing-and-counseling-older-drivers-4th-edition/B047).

In 2003 the AOTA received funding from the NHTSA for an Older Driver Initiative (ODI) to expand occupational therapy's role in driving and driving safety. Awareness initiatives and practice resources were developed to raise awareness of senior driving issues, needs, and opportunities.[16] The ODI resulted in various continuing education materials, development of resources available on both AOTA and partner websites. AOTA's annual Older Driver Safety Awareness Week encouraged a wide range of programs to use social media platforms to make resources known. The ODI encouraged partnering with other providers and stakeholders in older driver safety. CarFit is a collaborative educational program developed and coordinated through a partnership between AOTA, AARP, and AAA. The CarFit program was based on crash data analysis suggesting that seniors are at greater risk for injury in lower-speed crashes and that these injuries could be reduced or prevented by the proper and consistent use of the vehicle provided safety devices (Fig. 11.20). The premise is to offer safety education to seniors with occupational therapy expanding the conversation by building awareness of aftermarket solutions for attaining the safest fit when needs exceed the solutions offered by the original equipment manufacturer's (OEM's) features of the vehicle.[10] For example, if the seat base does not bring a short-statured person's line of sight above the obstruction of the dashboard, a simple cushion may add the inch or two needed to allow that driver full view of the road environment.[9,10,193] The Gaps and Pathways Project, launched by the AOTA in 2011, was funded through a cooperative agreement with the NHTSA. The intent of the Gaps and Pathways Project was to provide guidance to OT practitioners to effectively address the IADLs of driving with all clients, either through direct service or through referral pathways.[179]

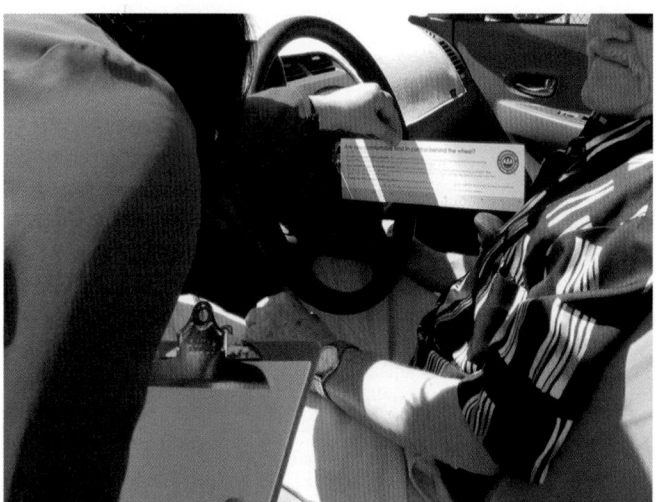

Fig. 11.20 Participation in CarFit events provides the OT generalist with experience in evaluating the fit between an older adult and his or her vehicle.

One of the outcomes of the Gaps and Pathways Project was a special issue of *Occupational Therapy in Health Care*,[66a] which presented resources and papers to guide practitioners in promoting client participation in driving and other forms of community mobility.[25]

The Centennial Vision endorsed by the AOTA board of directors in 2003 has served as a road map for the profession,[15,32] prompting practitioners to identify opportunities to expand occupational therapy practice. An initial focus on opportunities for meeting the needs of senior drivers led to recognition of community mobility and older drivers as an emerging practice niche.[28,51] The future challenges occupational therapists within all practice settings to evolve to address driving and community mobility throughout the life span in a comprehensive way that considers needs at the levels of prevention, planning, transition, and driving rehabilitation.[16,132] The Centennial Vision's strategy of linking education, research, and practice has been implemented by increased scholarly research in the area of driving and community mobility. Several evidence-based literature reviews related to driving and community mobility for older adults have been published in the *American Journal of Occupational Therapy*.[14,66,103] The AOTA continues to develop resources to support OT practitioners in the area of driving and community mobility[21] and to expand clinically applicable programs such as OT-DRIVE toolkit (available at https://www.aota.org/practice/clinical-topics/driving-community-mobility/driving--community-mobility-toolkit-for-professionals).

DRIVING

Driving is cited numerous times as the basis for personal independence, employment, and aging in place.[63,132,141] A driver's license has deep social and cultural contexts; it serves as a rite of passage for the teenager and provides the adult with an ability to pursue employment and recreational opportunities. The social impact of an aging population (20% of the U.S. population will be 65 or older in 2030[94]) has brought the issues of maintaining independence and quality of life, especially as they pertain to driving, to the forefront of public attention.

Generalist and Specialist Roles

The World Federation of Occupational Therapy 2019[222] Position Statement related to driving and community mobility asserts, "The scope of occupational therapy practice enables occupational therapists, with or without specialized training in driver rehabilitation, to develop functional, safe and realistic client centered outcomes in driving and community mobility." All OT practitioners, in general and specialized practice settings, have the professional skills and training necessary to address questions, concerns, and needs in the areas of driving and community mobility.[16,50] All OT practitioners can be expected to identify client risks and strengths, support participation in the community, and strive to optimize independence in community mobility through skilled occupational therapy intervention thereby reducing driving disability (or over restriction), crashes, injuries, and fatalities. To optimally meet driving and community mobility needs, occupational therapy services are provided along a continuum.[44,71a] The depth at which the individual practitioner addresses community mobility issues with clients depends on their level of expertise and education.[158,178] In general practice, community mobility to maximize occupational engagement is focused on driving and community mobility risk as a driver, passenger, pedestrian, transit user, or individual aspiring to drive. For the experienced driver who wants to resume driving, the first step is identification of driving

risk through a specific assessment process that serves to identify possible actions and prompt individualized interventions that may include referrals. Box 11.2 lists driving considerations.

When focused on the IADL of driving, the committed driving rehabilitation provider addresses a driver's fitness to drive through the administration of a comprehensive driving evaluation with the option of a performance on road component and subsequent driver rehabilitation training.[65]

BOX 11.2 Normalizing Conversations of Driving and Community Mobility Needs Across the Lifespan

- **Children's mobility roles:** May include crawling, walking, biking, navigating the (home) environment, exploring and learning, and transport as passengers.
  - Medically at-risk status because of factors of size, stature, disability, or behavior
  - Mobility needs are at the role of passenger. Needs may include car seat, with specialized car seats for addressing positioning, securement, and elopement. Safe transport in family vehicles, school bus, and transit options. Safe securement of equipment: walker, mobility devices, wheelchair.
  - Family/support system may require education, awareness of options, access to family transport vehicles (that may require modification), training in transfers, or consideration of the capacity and needs of all support and transportation providers involved. These may include parents, grandparents, paraprofessionals, etc.
  - **Specialist role:** Specialized or modified seating systems and vehicle modifications, family transport vehicles that may be modified to provide the means to transport individuals, mobility equipment/supplies.
- **Youth, nondriver mobility roles:** May include walking, biking, navigating the home and community environment, observer of driving or driving readiness.
  - Medically at risk because of factors of attention deficit–hyperactivity disorder (attention disorders), congenital diagnosis (cerebral palsy, spina bifida, amputation, etc.), knowledge and emerging skills that include situational awareness.
  - Mobility roles and needs: passenger role may include car seats, education for parents and grandparents or ride providers, securement in vehicle, school bus, and transit; unloading/loading and securement of mobility device (walker, mobility devices, wheelchair), strategies to address issues of passenger elopement affecting safety during transportation.
  - Future driver: Role with expectations? Preparation? Early family awareness may include the purchase of a family vehicle that would eventually be a candidate for adaptation for the new novice driver. Involvement of the family/support system must begin early, often years before the driving evaluation.
  - **Specialist role:** Mentor generalist with potential driver's level of independence, using IADL engagement to guide readiness and support transition.
- **Youth/adult nondriver mobility roles when of driving age, with special consideration for the individual with the goal or hope to drive.** Roles here may include walking, biking, motorized mobility, transit (private or public), observant passenger, driving readiness.
  - Intervention and readiness to expand access, offer choice flexibility, spontaneity, employment options.
  - Medically at risk. Explore reasons behind not driving? Yet? Medical diagnosis. Assumptions or actual? Attention? Learning? "Disability."
  - Mobility roles: Passenger, potential as driver include navigating the environment, knowledge, emerging skills, and situational awareness.
  - Goals may include transition from passenger to driver, The novice driver learning to drive (learners permit, rules of the road, state driver licensing,

etc.) in addition to driving rehabilitation needs and potential to manage equipment/walker, mobility devices, etc.
  - Considering the specialist role for the aspiring driver: Might this individual drive with/from equipment? Transport or drive while seated in a wheelchair? Offer hope and a pathway? Engage the specialist role early to build awareness and readiness, and for some offer early evaluation to build awareness of options for training, equipment, and associated costs. Select OT-DRS with driving instructor credentials and training required in your state to teach the novice driver/"disabled driver" to drive.
  - The nondriver is a novice driver, and all steps toward driving must include the required training and interventions toward state approved driver licensing.
  - Family/support systems need to understand the importance of driving rehabilitation perspective in driver training, the possibility of focusing on a family transport vehicle (family as driver, flexible and available personal transportation for family), as well as transfers, equipment management.
  - **Specialist role:** Access to a specialist in driving rehabilitation is required when an injury or illness may be affecting engagement in the occupation of driving. This may be for adults learning to drive or returning to driving. Interventions include comprehensive driving evaluation, driver rehabilitation training, and/or adaptive equipment training.
- **Adult experienced drivers (distinguish loss of skill from novice nondriver/learner)** experiencing loss where the role of driving is at risk. Driving is a role in addition to possibly walking, biking, motorized mobility, rideshare, paratransit, public transit, and increased dependence on family support for transportation. The goals at this level are to preserve mobility, prevent driving disability.
  - Medically at risk may include any identified impediments to safe operation of a vehicle, or driving. Outcome of interventions address current driving status, temporary and or long-term restrictions. Particular attention to conditions that affect attention, learning, and the subskills of vision, physical abilities, and cognition.
  - Evaluation at the level of general practice may involve a driving risk assessment as an appropriate intervention that considers medical status, diagnosis or progressive conditions placing a driving future at risk.
  - Mobility roles take into consideration the importance of driving, ability to manage mobility equipment/walker, mobility devices, role as caregiver and capacity to manage expectations and demands for mobility related equipment, transfers, etc.
  - **Specialist role:** Access to a specialist in driving rehabilitation is required when the need for more advanced evaluation and intervention is indicated. Justifications for this level of intervention, often by referral, include evaluation of the potential to return to driving with or without equipment, training, and equipment prescription, training to drive with adaptive equipment and/or vehicle modification.
  - Family/support systems may advocate for their loved one's role of driver, or the focus may be on the family securing a transport vehicle with training and equipment to safely transport the client as a passenger.

Generalist: Driving Risk Assessment

It is the role of the occupational therapist in general practice to make the connection between medically related changes and their potential impact on the IADL of driving.[11,65] A driving risk assessment offers a framework for the clinician to consider the data, the results of assessments that measure impairments and strengths in the critical areas to driving, vision, cognition, and physical function. With the OT DRIVE as a guiding framework, all OTs should assess how a client's performance skills and client factors affect community engagement. Through a driving risk assessment, the OT practitioners provides a data-driven report, offers targeted interventions to address deficits, and makes referrals to specialists when indicated. While the components of an individualized driving risk assessment will vary based on an individual's stage of recovery and reason for referral, in general it includes review of medical history, occupational profile, assessment of client factors, and performance skills that include vision, cognition, and motor assessments and observation of an IADL.[11,44,72]

Occupational Profile

A review of the available medical records and a client interview are necessary to establish an occupational profile that identifies the importance of driving and the contexts and environments in which driving or community mobility access are performed.

The medical record will contain valuable information related to driving abilities, including whether a client's medical condition is acute, chronic, or progressive; the client's medication regimen; the presence of symptoms (e.g., pain and fatigue); and the client's communication status.[11,77] Clients should be asked about driving frequency; whether they drive with passengers; whether they have experienced driving problems, such as seeing clearly, turning the steering wheel, confusing the pedals, getting lost, committing driving infractions, or having near misses; and whether family members or friends have expressed concern about their driving ability.[105] License status and the availability of a suitable vehicle should also be established. It is also helpful to determine what, if any, other alternative modes of transportation have been used. Without this information it is very difficult to project the client's future needs for driver rehabilitation, adaptive driving equipment, or a modified vehicle.

The information-gathering process should focus on establishing what the client and family goals for driving and community mobility/family transport. Is the goal to be able to conduct errands and get to medical appointments? Does the client want to be able to commute to work? Does he or she want to drive on surface streets or freeways or both? Can the family transport the client with or in their mobility equipment? A client-centered focus is necessary to understand the client and family perspective, guide assessment, and help therapists plan interventions that are contextually appropriate. The Canadian Occupational Performance Measure can be used to help adult clients identify and prioritize goals important to them and to make decisions about their care.[106] If driving is not an option at the time of assessment, addressing alternative transportation needs would be appropriate, to optimize mobility during recovery or as a long-term alternative.

Jacqueline was concerned that she was the primary driver for her husband and lacked a backup transportation plan. Based on her identified priority, Sergio's immediate intervention was to provide information about alternative public and para-transit transportation options that offered the support required by both Jacqueline and her husband.

Analysis of Occupational Performance

Once the goal of driving has been identified through the occupational profile, an analysis of occupational performance is conducted to more specifically identify the client's assets or problems through observation, measurement, and inquiry about supporting and limiting factors. OT generalists are not equipped to observe a client's performance on road or in the driving context; however, occupational therapy practitioners are skilled at making inferences about "other IADLs," including driving performance risk based on how well the client performs on other complex IADLs. Emerging evidence suggests that the Assessment of Motor and Process Skills,[96] a standardized assessment to observe IADL performance, can be used to understand driving risk and potential.[72]

There are any assessments are available that address contexts, environments, and client factors that influence performance skills and patterns in driving. Some of these screening tools are appropriately used by a generalist; other, more complex tests are more appropriate for use by a specialist in driving rehabilitation. The reader is referred to Driving and Community Mobility: Occupational Therapy Strategies Across the Lifespan[132] for an extensive list of various tests. This section describes a few assessments that are commonly used or are recognized for their usefulness in predicting fitness to drive.

Driver Safety Screens Administered by Healthcare Professionals

Driver safety screening tools allow OTs to obtain data about a client and identify areas of concern for additional evaluation and intervention. Driver safety screening tools supplement observations of risk obtained during IADL performance and offer additional data or evidence to justify the need for a next or more advanced service, including the comprehensive driving evaluation with an OT driving rehabilitation specialist (OT-DRS). The Assessment of Driving Related Skills (ADReS)[63] is a screening test battery, originally developed by the AMA with support from the NHTSA, to assist physicians and healthcare professionals in preventing motor vehicle crashes in older adults. It screens aspects of vision, cognition, and motor function, three areas that have been identified as necessary for safe driving. The ADReS does not predict crash risk, although some of its components have documented associations with crash risk.[105] A limitation of this test is its poor sensitivity because it tends to recommend intervention even for people who do not demonstrate a lack of fitness to drive.[129] The test battery is available in the fourth edition of the Clinician's Guide to Assessing and Counseling Older Drivers, which can be accessed at no cost on the NHTSA website.

Self-Administered or Family/Caregiver-Administered Driver Screens

Self-screening measures intended for client self-administration outside of a clinical setting are developed to increase self-awareness about "changes associated with driving" or driving risk. These activities may be less threatening for some clients than more formal assessments, but they may offer little benefit for cognitively impaired persons who lack insight.[86] These types of assessment tools may contribute to the assessment process when completed in conjunction with a clinical assessment. An example of a self-screening tool is the SAFER Driving found in *The Enhanced Driving Decisions Workbook*.[86] This self-assessment is free and available online: https://www.drivesmartbc.ca/older-drivers/self-help-enhanced-driving-decisions-workbook

The Fitness-to-Drive Screening Measure is a Web-based tool designed for caregivers and/or family members of older drivers to identify at-risk older drivers. Caregivers and family members who have driven with the driver in the past 3 months rate the driver's difficulties with 54 driving skills. A rating profile classifying the driver into at-risk, routine, or accomplished driver categories is generated, and recommendations based on the category are provided.[203] The recommendations can be used to begin a conversation about fitness to drive and to identify the need for further intervention.

Clinical Assessments Related to Specific Client Factors

OTP generalists may administer a variety of tests as part of a driving risk assessment. The tests supplement observations of driving risk gleaned from observations of IADL performance. Screening results inform decisions for improving function in a specific area, to establish a basis for advising clients of the need for a temporary hold on driving or driving cessation, and to provide evidence of the need to refer to an OT-DRS for a comprehensive driving evaluation.

Vision: Acuity, Eye-Motor Skills, Visual Fields, and Contrast Sensitivity

Vision provides most of the sensory input related to driving.[182] Not surprisingly, uncorrectable vision deficits are a leading cause of driving cessation.[110] Visual conditions that are substantial concerns for driving include cataracts, glaucoma, macular degeneration, diabetic retinopathy, diplopia, and strabismus, and visual field cut. Specialists may have access to an instrument such as the Optec Functional Vision Analyzer[191] to test skills such as visual acuity, depth perception, color perception and recognition, phorias, and eye teaming. However, there are many tests that can be performed by either generalists or specialists with minimal equipment or by using mobile phone or tablet apps. Clients should be referred to a vision care practitioner to maximize visual skills before a referral to an OT-DRS is initiated.[50] Vision care specialist interventions, such as a corrective lens prescription, prisms, and eye occlusion or surgery, can have a significant impact on safe driving potential. Because standards for licensing vary among the various states, OTs should be aware of the requirements in their particular area to appropriately educate clients.

Visual acuity, typically tested using a Snellen wall chart, is the most widely tested skill among driver licensing agencies. Acuity can affect the ability to read signage if it is worse than 20/30,[151] but it does not appear to be related to crash risk unless it is worse than 20/70.[63] Most state driver licensing agencies have established a far acuity standard of 20/40 with both eyes for initial licensing and for some renewals. Clients with acuity worse than 20/40 or who do not meet their state vision standards should be referred to a vision care specialist for further assessment.

Screening of ocular range of movement and ocular alignment (pursuits, saccades, phorias, and tropias) is also valuable because these functions can impact on the ability to efficiently scan the road for hazards.[157,192] Visual field testing identifies the range of the traffic environment a person can see. Peripheral vision is particularly important for detecting cues such as a signal light blinking on a car in the next lane. Visual field deficits have been linked to crash risk, but there is currently no conclusive evidence about the visual field range that is adequate for driving.[63] Eye movements can serve as a compensatory strategy to increase the visual environment that can be seen.[151] However, the difficulty of accomplishing this successfully is increased in a fast-paced driving environment. There is evidence that educational programs improve a client's awareness of visual deficits; however, they do not appear to result in lowered crash risk.[110] Training to compensate for visual skill deficits in a protected environment using a driving simulator may be appropriate before initiating an actual driving assessment.[110]

The useful field of view (UFOV) can be conceptualized as the spatial area from which a person can quickly extract visual information without head or eye movement.[205] It requires identification and localization of targets, and it is not the same as the visual sensory field. Age-related issues can cause a slowed speed of processing and UFOV size can be reduced by poor vision and difficulty in dividing attention and ignoring distraction (Fig. 11.21).[87] Driving demands efficient processing speed and selective and divided attention. For instance, quick processing speed is necessary for a driver to recognize when a child's ball has rolled into the street. Selective attention is needed to attend to urgent stimuli (the person in the crosswalk) without being distracted by unimportant ones (a family walking on the sidewalk). Divided attention, or task shifting, is required to focus on the multiple relevant stimuli that are encountered in a complex driving environment (e.g., viewing traffic to the front and sides of the vehicle when changing lanes).[63] The UFOV test is a computerized measure of visual processing speed, divided attention, and selective attention. Test takers are assigned to five crash risk categories based on results from the assessment. The test has been widely used in research related to crash risk in older drivers. There is moderate evidence that it correlates with crash outcomes and fitness to drive.[20] Although the UFOV test is becoming more widely used, it is still not consistently used by DRSs[69] and may not be available to a generalist.

Contrast sensitivity, the perception of contrast between visual stimuli,[63] is an important visual function that is not currently used as a measure for driver licensing. It has been found to be a valid predictor of crash risk among older drivers.[76] Testing is

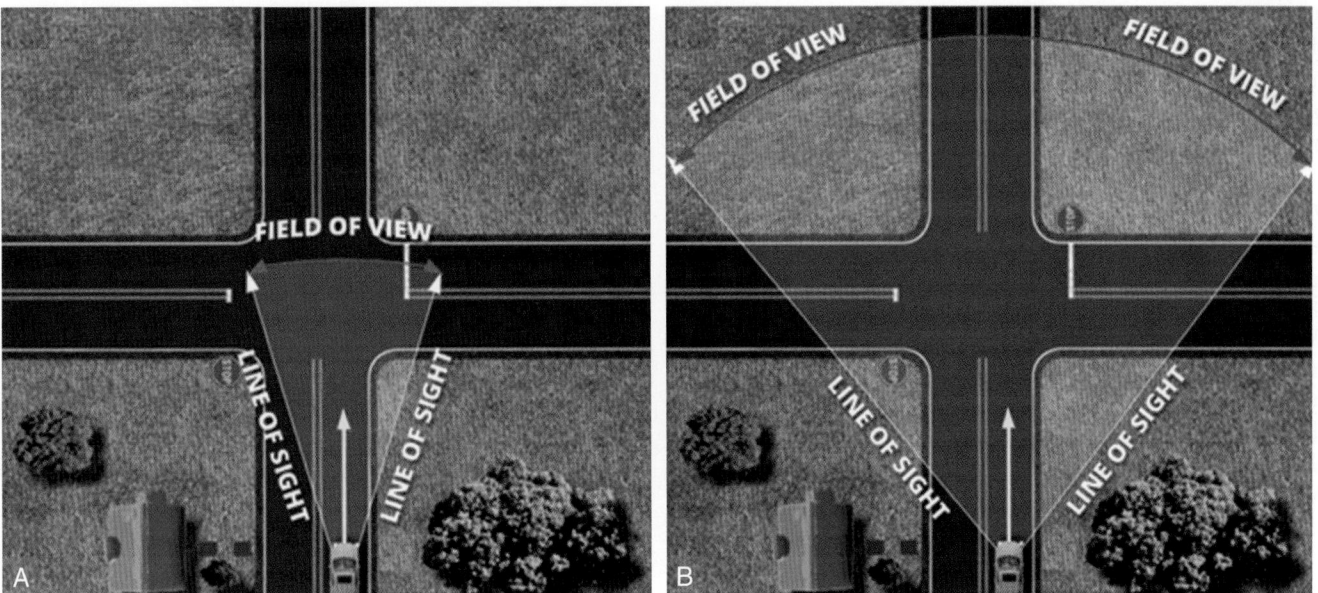

Fig. 11.21 The useful field of view of a 76-year-old (A) is smaller than that of a 16-year-old (B). Reduction of the useful field of view can prevent the individual from seeing things that are a safety risk to driving. (Courtesy American Automobile Association, Heathrow, FL.)

accomplished using a Pelli Robson Contrast Sensitivity Chart,[159] which presents lines of letters with progressively less contrast relative to the chart's background color, is one example of a contrast sensitivity test. Deficits in this function are common in cataracts and glaucoma. OT-DRS will consider contrast to identify the lighting conditions under which a client will drive because low-light conditions such as fog, dawn, and dusk exacerbate deficits in contrast sensitivity.

Visual perception. Although visual skills, visual perceptual processing skills, and cognition are typically evaluated individually, in the dynamic and complex driving context they work synergistically and must be used quickly. The Motor-Free Visual Perception Test is a widely used standardized test that measures various aspects of perception without requiring a motor response. The most recent version includes norms for ages 4 to 80 years.[54] Research results linking it to fitness to drive have been inconsistent, with some showing a link and others no relationship.[20] In relation to driving, visual closure, which is the ability to complete a figure when only fragments are presented, might be needed for tasks such as anticipating where lane markers would continue when they are divided by an intersection or for recognizing a stop sign that is partially occluded by a branch.

The Clock Drawing Test is widely used with geriatric populations to discriminate healthy individuals from those who have dementia.[63] There are several versions and various procedures for scoring it.[128] In the Freund Clock Drawing form that is used in the ADReS, the person is asked to draw a circular analog clock on a blank sheet of paper with the numbers and hands arranged to read 10 minutes after 11. Scoring is based on correct completion of seven different elements, not time for completion.[63] This seemingly simple measure involves visual spatial skills, language, selective attention, long- and short-term memory, abstract thinking, and executive functioning. The visual spatial demands appear to be significant in identifying fitness

to drive, given that visual spatial skills have the highest level of prediction in the driving performance of older adults.[163]

Cognition: Attention, Processing Speed, Memory, and Executive Function

A significant part of what is required to drive safely occurs "between the ears." Cognitive factors in driving include the ability to focus and sustain attention on single and multiple stimuli, the speed with which traffic information is perceived, and many aspects of memory.[199] There is clear evidence that executive functioning is critical to on-road performance.[20] There are many tests of executive function with varying levels of ability to predict safe driving.

The Brief Cognitive Assessment Test is a multifactorial test for executive function, attentional capacity, and working memory that predicts participation in instrumental and basic activities of daily living.[126,127,130] The Assessment of Motor and Process Skills (AMPS) is an occupational therapy standardized assessment tool that reviews motor and processing functions—planning, organization, initiation, sequencing, adaptation—of individuals engaged in ADLs and IADLs.[73] The Weekly Calendar Planning Activity (WCPA) is an occupation based performance test that is useful for identifying difficulties in executive function and higher level cognitive skills. It may be used for a individuals between the age of 12 to 90.[198,221]

The Trail Making Tests (TMTs) Parts A and B are paper-and-pencil assessments of overall cognitive function measuring selective and divided attention, mental flexibility, visual scanning, sequencing, and visual memory. Part A involves connecting scattered numbers in order, and Part B requires alternately connecting numbers and letters in sequential order. Poor performance on Part B has been significantly correlated with poor driving performance. Part B is one of the components of the ADReS and is scored by the time needed to correctly connect the letters and numbers. Completing Part B in over 3 minutes signals a need for intervention, including consideration for referral to a specialist.[63] Use of this test by the generalist should be coordinated with the OT-DRS. This test has specific requirements on how frequently it may be repeated.

There are several assessments from the field of neuropsychology that test memory, orientation, attention, calculation, recall, language, and visual-spatial perception. These include the St. Louis University Mental Status Exam, the Mini-Mental State Examination, the Short Blessed Test, the Montreal Cognitive Assessment, and the Brief Cognitive Assessment Test. Driving requires intact working memory, attentional capacity, executive function, and processing speed. Practitioners should consider these factors when selecting the best cognitive test to use with clients. Many of these tests have documented correlation with ADLs and IADLs performance safety.[126] Lower scores on these assessments are associated with increase driving risk and may warrant referral to an OT-DRS.[132]

Motor Skills: Strength, Range of Motion, Sensation, and Balance

Strength, ROM, sensation, and balance are important to many driving-related tasks. Paralysis, incoordination, tremors, amputations, limitations in static and dynamic balance, fatigue, and slowing of reaction time can affect performance of driving tasks such as loading and unloading a mobility device, entering and exiting a vehicle, turning a key in an ignition, and operating the primary and secondary controls. Both OTP generalist and OT-DRSs are trained in evaluation of client factors such as strength, ROM, and sensation using well-established testing protocols. The OTP generalist can use clinical reasoning and task analysis to anticipate the impact of identified limitations on driving. For example, when a client demonstrates restriction in cervical ROM, that same client may have difficulty turning the head to see blind spots or check cross traffic. Decreased cervical ROM has been linked to an increased risk of a motor vehicle crash. When deficits are identified, the generalist should determine whether it is possible to remediate skills, either through OT intervention or through treatment by other professionals and consider referral to an OT-DRS for possible adaptive driving equipment.

The OT-DRS will have an in-depth understanding of how motor skills relate to driving. The assessment information will be used by the specialist to determine when it is appropriate to use adaptations and vehicle modifications to compensate for deficits. Technological advances have made it possible to compensate for motor deficits in many instances. In addition to aftermarket equipment, matching client abilities with vehicle characteristics and equipment features, particularly when high-tech equipment is required, is critical to driving safety and is the purview of the specialist.

In terms of usefulness for predicting driving safety, some research has demonstrated a link between the Rapid Pace Walk (RPW) test and fitness to drive.[20,63] This test asks clients to walk 10 ft, turn around, and return to the starting point as fast as possible, using a mobility device if necessary. The RPW test, which is another component of the ADReS, measures LE mobility,

trunk stability, and balance. The Toe Tap Test simulates the LE mobility for alternately pressing gas and brake pedals with a foot. To observe potential deficits in proprioception, the test can be performed with the eyes closed. Scores have not been shown to be predictive of at-fault crashes in older drivers, but the test has face validity as a measure of one's ability to move the leg/foot quickly from the accelerator to the brake.[186] Brake reaction time is typically measured as the length of time between the stimulus to the time the brake pedal is depressed. It increases with age[132] and is affected by surprise, urgency, and critical situations. Although shown not to be predictive of crashes,[20] brake reaction time does have face validity and may be an effective tool for observing psychomotor performance.[132] Despite the preceding list of tests and their correlation to driving risk, it is the clinician's responsibility to weigh test scores and observe functional performance with the integration of solid clinical judgment when making conclusions about driving risk, potential, and recommendations. This expert analysis is what places occupational therapy in the role of using the aforementioned tools to ethically address the needs of the individuals we serve.

Driving Simulators

Interactive driving simulators use computer-based technology that provides virtual scenarios of driving situations. Ranging in cost and size, they enable observation of performance and the assessment of discrete driving performance components in a safe environment coupled with the ability to change the scenarios to reflect factors that simulate various traffic situations, daytime or nighttime driving, and weather (e.g., sunshine, rain, fog). Driving simulators can provide an effective way to initiate a stationary assessment of components and to train a client in preparatory components of driving skills in controlled situations, but it must be clearly understood and distinguished that the interactive driving simulator is not a replacement for the actual on road experience and is not to be considered to replace the need for an on-road assessment with an OT-DRS.[190] Factors that raise the appeal of simulators include the capability to replicate features of driving conditions, and then repeat these environments and conditions for data comparison after treatment. The question of whether they can predict driving behavior in real-life situations remains. These devices may not accurately represent the reality of driving because they do not drive like an actual car, and the depictions of driving situations may not be perceived as realistic. Promising evidence lies more in the assessment of critical vehicle control components such as "foot to pedal" reaction time or delayed initiation of movement for a driver with Parkinson's disease.

Currently there is a limited amount of evidence that driving simulators can be used to comprehensively determine driving fitness.[20] One key limitation that must be appreciated by clinicians is the phenomenon described as simulator sickness. The problem is similar to motion sickness and is sometimes experienced when the ocular, motor, and kinesthetic systems receive sensory input of movement in the absence of true motion.[132] Client factors such as recent head injury, concussion, seizure, or vertigo; being female; and being over age 70 appear to contribute to simulator sickness.[132] Other concerns include unfamiliarity with the technology, inconsistent standardization between simulators, inconsistent outcome metrics measured by simulators, and anxiety. Extensive clinician training is required to ensure the proper use and delivery of simulation technology. Therefore, driving simulators should not be the sole determinant of fitness to drive, with added caution when analyzing the data generated through simulation as a component of the older adult driving evaluation.[190]

Applying the Driving Risk Assessment

The OT practitioner in general practice should incorporate questions about driving and community mobility during the development of the occupational profile and consider activity demands when performing an initial IADLs evaluation.[8] The observation of performance skills during the IADL assessment, in combination with specific tests and measures, enables a determination of the client's strengths and whether his or her impairments have the potential to affect driving.[71a] Applying resources, such as the Generalist Resource to Integrating Driving (GRID)[41,43] or the Occupational Therapy-Driver Off-Road Assessment (OT-DORA), will support the OT generalist understanding of performance skill patterns for driving.

In general, the OT practitioner uses driving risk assessment to determine an individual's level of driving risk and potential to return to driving. Clients with low risk are often provided with education and referred back to their physician for readiness to return to driving. Clients with risk and potential are likely referred to the OT-DRS for an on-road assessment to determine fitness to drive. Those with high risk and who have maximized recovery are considered for driving retirement. Addressing driving risk is not equivalent to determining fitness to drive. Although in practice the OT practitioner may use similar ADLs and IADLs to help anticipate engagement potential (i.e., using performance during meal preparation to help anticipate needs for discharge to home), it is important to distinguish that the driving risk assessment is not a review of engagement in the actual occupation of driving. Therefore, the driving risk assessment is only used to anticipate risk and potential and not to determine fitness to drive. This is an important distinction for two reasons. First, this means the OT practitioner in general practice has not seen the client drive and therefore may not say they are "safe to drive." Second, this means it is not the responsibility of the OT practitioner in general practice to carry the burden of whether someone is safe to drive. Instead, the driving risk assessment becomes a screening tool to understand level of risk and potential and help facilitate conversations and appropriate referrals.

Furthermore, based on the state of recovery, the OT practitioner must consider the opportunity to initiate treatments that may improve driving capabilities.[112] The driving risk assessment allows the OT practitioner to expand beyond basic ADLs and consider additional deficits that may benefit from OT interventions. Examples may be applying therapeutic intervention to improve processing speed, scanning, and task shifting. If at any point a client presents with risk, the OT practitioner may recommend a temporary hold on driving. This is often recommended for clients with acute medical conditions based on the evidence.[105]

Additionally, if it is determined that a client must eliminate complex IADLs (e.g., cooking or financial management) because of a progressive condition, such as moderate to severe dementia, the generalist, in conjunction with the referring physician, may appropriately recommend driving retirement and focus intervention efforts on exploration of transportation alternatives.[132] Recommendations for driving retirement require the collaboration of the medical team with the OT practitioner providing evidence to guide recommendations in collaboration with the referring physician and other team members. Decisions regarding driving retirement can have a profound impact on an individual's health and therefore should not be made based on one test, during one day, or be made by one person.

To improve seating and positioning in the vehicle and prepare for the occupation of driving, OT practitioner in general practice can assist clients in choosing simple aids that do not directly affect vehicle control (e.g., a key holder or a handle that attaches to the door latch to assist with entering and exiting a vehicle). As with all adaptive equipment, the OT practitioner must consider the potential effect of any recommended piece of equipment.[132] OT practitioners in general practice may NOT recommend adaptive equipment that affects the **primary controls** of the vehicle (starting, stopping, steering).

Finally, and perhaps most importantly the OTP generalist helps to facilitate the timing of appropriate referrals to the specialists. The OTP generalist has a unique and thorough understanding of the client's recovery and performance skills. This understanding is pivotal for helping to identify the appropriate point in recovery to refer to an OT-DRS and other resources. A diagram outlining the decision making process is depicted in Fig. 11.22.

Spectrum of Driver Service Programs

There are a variety of resources and programs available, and understanding the distinct differences is imperative to generating appropriate referrals. *The Spectrum of Driver Services: Right Services for the Right People at the Right Time* is a document developed as part of the AOTA Gaps and Pathways project funded by NHTSA.[118] Through this project AOTA enlisted the collaboration of the Association for Driver Rehabilitation Specialists to describe service categories and add clarity for providers and the public seeking driving services. This chart helps to differentiate the role of various programs and the outcome that may be expected from that level of provider. Driver rehabilitation programs provide a wide range of services related to driving and community mobility for individuals with disabilities, medical conditions, or age-related changes. These programs offer driving skills assessment, education and training, and instruction in the use of driving adaptations and compensatory techniques. Identifying the program that is best for a particular person can be challenging for consumers and referral sources. The *Spectrum of Driver Services Table*, approved in 2013, describes three broad categories of driving program services: community-based education programs; medically based assessment, education, and referral programs; and specialized evaluation and training programs.[39]

Community-based education programs include driver safety programs having specific credentials (e.g., AARP and AAA

Occupational Therapy Process
for Driving and Community Mobility

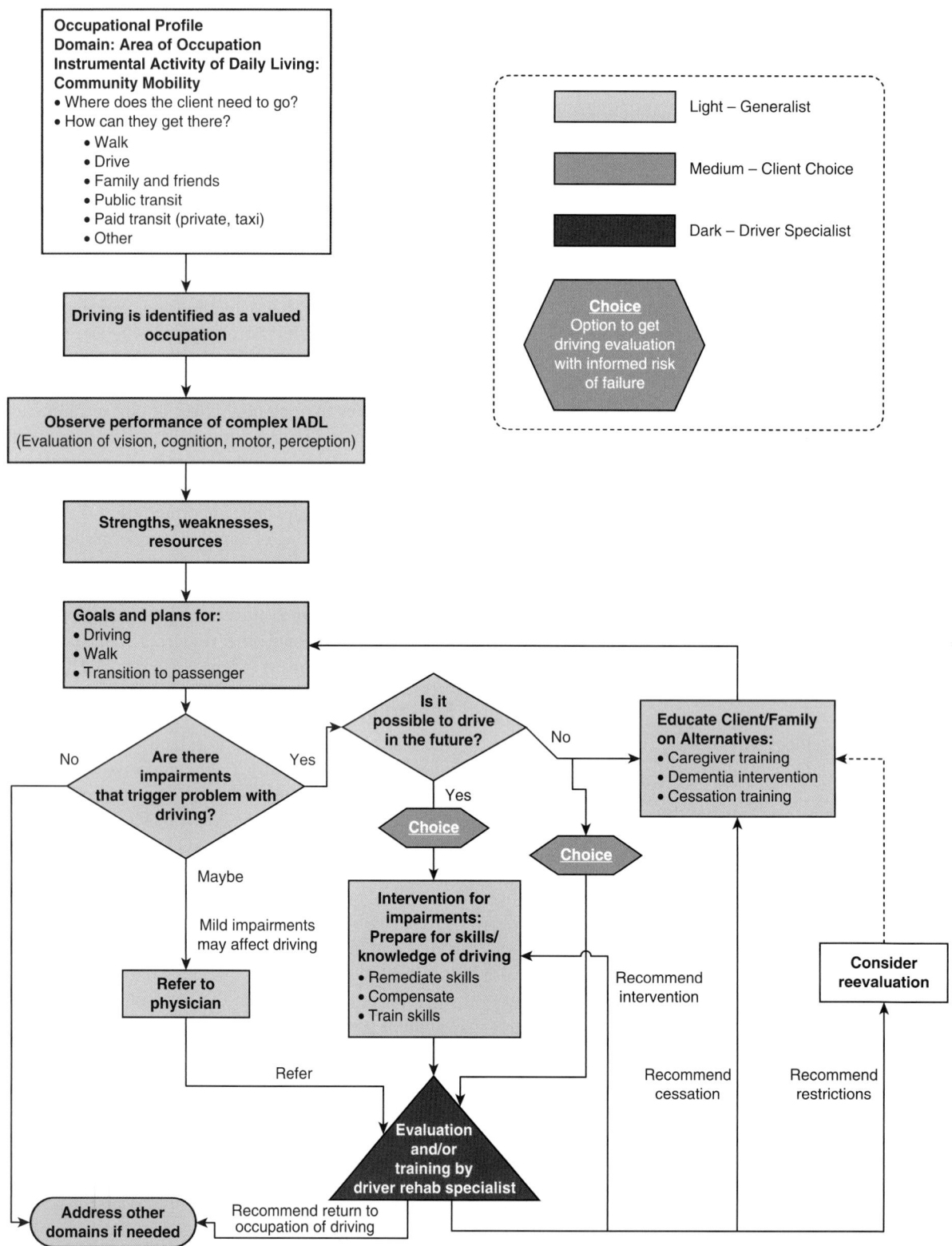

Fig. 11.22 This algorithm illustrates the decision-making process for effective referral to and delivery of driving-related services. (From Dickerson AE, Reistetter T, Schold Davis E, Monahan M: Evaluating driving as a valued instrumental activity of daily living, *Am J Occup Ther* 65:64–75, 2011.)

driver improvement programs) and driving schools. Driver safety programs offer classroom or computer-based refresher courses for licensed drivers. Driving schools employ licensed driving instructors to teach, train, and refresh driving skills for novice or relocated drivers. These schools focus on well individuals rather than people who have medical or age-related conditions that might interfere with driving. Driving schools typically provide services to enhance driving skills and to assist in acquisition of a driver's license or permit.[39]

Medically based assessment, education, and referral programs offer driver risk screens and IADL evaluations. Programs offering driver screening are typically staffed by healthcare professionals with knowledge of medical conditions, assessment tools, and intervention processes. They understand the limits and value of the assessment tools used as a measure of driving risk and potential fitness to drive and can counsel consumers regarding the risks associated with medical conditions and make referrals when indicated.[39]

Programs offering clinical IADL evaluations or driving risk assessment employ OT practitioners (either generalists or a driver rehabilitation specialists) or another healthcare professional with expertise in IADLs who has knowledge of medical conditions and their implications for community mobility, including driving. Clinical IADL evaluators interpret risks associated with changes in vision, cognition, or sensory motor functions caused by acute or chronic conditions; they also facilitate remediation of deficits, develop individualized transportation plans, and discuss resources for vehicle adaptations. They refer to driver rehabilitation specialists when appropriate, discuss driving cessation, and follow professional ethics on referrals to other resources or to the driver licensing authority.[39]

Specialized driver rehabilitation programs employ individuals with advanced or specialized training (DRS and CDRS) and offer evaluation and training programs; they also administer comprehensive driving evaluations that include clinical and on-road components to establish fitness to drive.[49] The driving rehabilitation programs are broadly described in three levels, distinguished primarily by the complexity of evaluations, types of equipment used, and expertise of the provider. Basic programs offer comprehensive driving evaluations and training for individuals who can independently transfer and drive using standard primary driving controls (e.g., a standard steering wheel and standard gas and brake pedals). Low-tech programs offer comprehensive evaluation and training services with or without the use of adaptive equipment. At this level of service, the adaptations for primary control are typically mechanical (e.g., a mechanical gas/brake hand control, pedal extensions, and left foot accelerator). Wireless or remote access to secondary controls (e.g., turn signal, horn) may be used.[39]

High-tech driver rehabilitation programs offer all the services available through basic and low-tech programs; however, they also have high-tech equipment for primary control (e.g., powered hand controls, remote steering, and joystick driving controls) and devices such as powered transmission shifters, remote panels, and switch arrays for secondary control. They can address the needs of drivers able to transfer to an unmodified vehicle seat, those who require a transfer seat base to facilitate a transfer, and those who cannot transfer and must drive while seated in a wheelchair. Service providers in this category can recommend vehicle structural modifications (e.g., ramps or lifts) that allow people in wheelchairs access to the vehicle's interior and to the driving position.[116]

Jacqueline's OTP generalist, Sergio, noticed that she demonstrated some difficulties with motor skills when performing kitchen tasks. Because Jacqueline planned to continue to drive as her primary way of getting around, Sergio was concerned that she might have problems gripping the steering wheel, turning her head to check traffic, and applying the brakes quickly. Sergio designed a home exercise program to address these areas of limitation and recommended that Jacqueline undergo a comprehensive driving evaluation with an OT-DRS.

ETHICAL CONSIDERATIONS

Principle 1. Beneficence of the AOTA Code of Ethics states, "Occupational therapy personnel shall demonstrate a concern for the well-being and safety of persons." In Jacqueline's case, supporting her with identification of alternative modes of transportation is essential for both her and her husband's well-being.

Principle C-46 of the ADED's Code of Ethics states that, "Driver rehabilitation specialists use only assessment techniques that they are qualified and competent to use. They do not misuse assessment results or interpretations."

The OT practitioner should readily consult with the local OT-DRS for support in guiding discussion about driving. By applying the OT DRIVE model, completing a driving risk assessment including IADL assessment, and applying focused interventions, OTP generalist optimizes engagement in the occupation of driving and facilitate appropriate referrals.

Role of the Specialist

While the OTP generalist considers risk and potential, it is the role of the OT-DRS to determine a client's fitness to drive in the context of a medical condition or injury. Driving presents a greater possibility of personal and public harm than does any other ADL or IADL; therefore, OT practitioners offering comprehensive driver evaluation services should, at a minimum, have advanced specialty education including formal hands-on training in a driver rehabilitation vehicle, expanded liability coverage, knowledge of the state's licensing regulatory processes, and specialized driver rehabilitation equipment. Individuals specializing in the field of driver rehabilitation, after gaining experience, may choose to obtain advanced credentials that may include a certification in driver rehabilitation from ADED.[14]

Occupational Therapist Driver Rehabilitation Specialist Training

Advanced Education

While training may vary, it is imperative that the OT practitioner interested in becoming a Driver Rehabilitation Specialist select advanced training that includes both education and hands-on experience in a driver rehabilitation vehicle with another trained OT-DRS. Learning to work, cue, and operate defensively in a moving vehicle requires training and skill. It is imperative that the OT-DRS complete hands-on training in this new treatment environment to ensure the safest experience for themselves, their clients, and all others on the road.

Driver Rehabilitation Vehicle

The OT-DRS uses a driver rehabilitation vehicle that is outfitted with specialized equipment such as an instructor brake and eye check mirror. The driver rehabilitation vehicle is the OT-DRS treatment environment and therefore must be equipped to help keep both the driver and specialist safe. In addition to careful maintenance, many driver rehabilitation programs perform daily checks to ensure the vehicles are in optimal condition.

Advanced Liability Insurance and Coverage

In many cases the driver rehabilitation vehicle is considered a non-traditional treatment environment. As such, many traditional occupational therapy liability coverage programs will not include the evaluation and treatment completed in a moving vehicle. Therefore, it is essential that the OT-DRS research and obtain appropriate liability coverage for themselves, the driver rehabilitation vehicle, and their drivers.

State-Specific Regulatory Considerations

Within the United States, each state has its own licensing processes and procedures. Therefore, it is essential that the OT-DRS has a working knowledge and understanding of their state's regulatory process to ensure compliance. In some states OT practitioners specializing in driving must also be certified driver instructors (CDIs) and/or a driving school to perform on-road assessments and provide driver training.[16,132] The OT-DRS who works with novice drivers also often has advanced training in driver education principles and/or partners with local driving instructors who provided novice driver instruction. It is also the responsibility of the OT-DRS to understand their state's specific licensing regulations, work within their state's requirements, and appropriately support communication of medical concerns per their state's licensing and medical reporting processes. Finally, the OT-DRS must also understand and support any licensing processes related to the application of adaptive equipment (Fig. 11.23).

Specialty Training and Certification

Currently there are two ways by which OT practitioners can designate themselves as offering advanced or specialized services in driver rehabilitation. The first is the Driving and Community Mobility Micro Credential, which is available to occupational therapists (Ots) and occupational therapy assistants (OTAs) through the AOTA. The Driving and Community Mobility Micro Credential Badge is awarded after completing a series of courses addressing topics such as the ethical and professional obligations related to driving, the impact of low vision on driving and community mobility, community mobility interventions for those with functional cognitive, screening and evaluation of driving risk, and interventions for driving and community mobility for older adults. These micro credential badges are recognized as quality markers and communicate expertise to consumers and professionals outside the profession.

The second alternative is the Certified Driver Rehabilitation Specialist (CDRS) who obtains a certification in driver

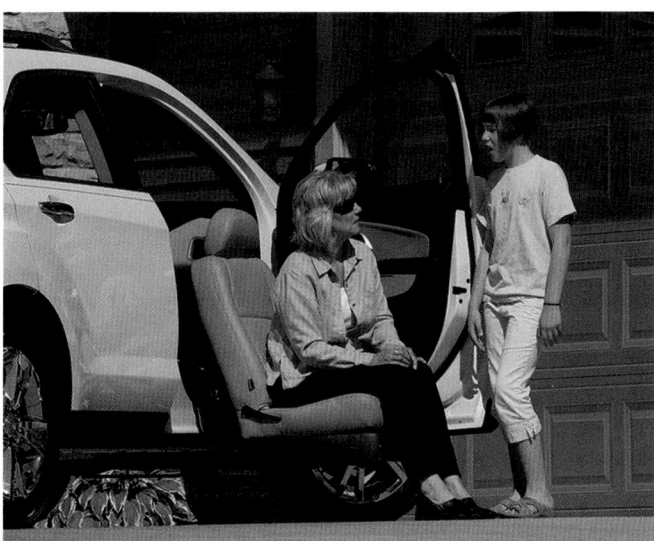

Fig. 11.23 Bruno's Valet Plus aids vehicle entry by modifying activity demands for caregiver and client. (Courtesy Bruno Independent Living Aids, Oconomowoc, WI.)

rehabilitation, available through the ADED. The CDRS represents a varied group of individuals from various disciplines who have met the required educational backgrounds. An individual is eligible to apply for the CDRS examination after practicing in the field of driver rehabilitation for an extensive number of hours (often over 1000 hours) based on training and educational background.[34]

Occupational Therapy Assistants

OTAs are a valuable asset to driving rehabilitation. The OT/OTA roles and responsibilities are identified by the AOTA,[27] and the suggested model indicates that the OTA can complete delegated portions of the evaluation process and collaborate on the intervention planning and implementation. The OT and OTA work together to provide services to meet the client's occupational needs, including community mobility and driving. To provide competent occupational therapy services addressing community mobility and driving, both the OT and OTA must comply with supervisor requirements and specific state licensure laws.

Completion of clinic-based standardized testing, vehicle entry/exit and lift safety training, transfer training, and driver rehabilitation training are just some of the ways the OTA-DRS can contribute to a driver rehabilitation program. The OTA must work under the supervision of and in partnership with the OT-DRS.[27] Expanded roles are possible when intervention protocols are developed, documented, and followed, again under the OT-DRS's supervision. For example, OTAs can be used to administer specific assessments to measure performance skills, such as the Motor Free Visual Perceptual Test, the Brief Cognitive Assessment Tool (BCAT), or Weekly Calendar Planning Activity, provide interventions using a driver simulator, and with appropriate advanced training, provide driver rehabilitation, including adaptive equipment training. Clear treatment protocols facilitate supervision by enhancing communication among colleagues.

It is important to understand that some OTAs choose to leave the profession and operate as a DRS or CDRS on their own. In this capacity, the OTA is no longer supervised by an OT and therefore not operating within the scope and ethics of the OT/OTA relationship. In these situations, the OTA no longer operates under the OTA state license.

Best Practice Standards for Driving Programs

Practice guidelines for driving and community mobility for older adults, which use an evidence-based perspective have been developed by AOTA. The guidelines emphasize the expertise of occupational therapists in general practice in understanding the occupations of driving and community mobility. These guidelines are helpful for OT practitioners, program developers, administrators, legislators, third-party payers, educators, and others to understand the contribution of occupational therapy in serving the needs of the older adult population.[189] An additional resource, *Driving and Community Mobility: Occupational Therapy Strategies Across the Lifespan*,[132] serves as an excellent guide.

In addition to the occupational therapy–based resources referenced previously, for the OT-DRS, *Best Practices Guidelines for the Delivery of Driver Rehabilitation Services* was initially published by the ADED in 2004 and continues to be revised. The document is intended for any individual providing rehabilitation services to persons with various disabilities or age-related impairments that affect driving. Guidelines for assessment, behind-the-wheel (BTW) training, and intervention are discussed, as are the recommended procedures for documentation, completion of a prescription for equipment, and conducting a final fitting.[37]

Comprehensive Driving Evaluation

Distinguish Testing From Therapeutic Evaluation and Intervention

Driving test	Outcome is pass/fail usually based solely on operational and tactical driving skills. It does not factor in judgment. Consistency is important and criteria developed to measure the minimum knowledge and skill set of the entry level novice driver. Not developed to measure medically related change. *Example:* State-administered (novice) driver's test, test offered by a driving school or driver safety program.
Driving screen	A screen that involves administration of tests to measure client factors and performance skills correlated to driving, usually performed in a medical setting/clinic. Moderate to severe impairment in vision and cognition flag driving risk. Physical impairments should flag referral to driver rehabilitation. *Example:* Driving risk assessment completed by the occupational therapist in general practice.
Comprehensive driving evaluation	Completed by the specialist in driving rehabilitation and includes clinical assessment, on-road assessment, and outcome discussion. The outcome generates a plan that may include intervention by driver rehabilitation that includes training, adaptive equipment, and/or vehicle modification. The outcome of cessation must prompt intervention or referral to preserve mobility as a nondriver.

Driver rehabilitation specialists provide a comprehensive driver evaluation that may include completion of clinical assessments, on-road assessment (also known as behind-the-wheel assessment) and outcome discussion. Similar to the OT practitioner, the OT-DRS completes clinical assessments of vision, motor skills, and cognition to help prepare for an understanding of anticipated driving performance.[49] As highlighted in the Evidenced Based Consensus Statements, "In the hands of a general practice occupational therapist, screening/assessment tools serve as criteria for referral and action. In the hands of the driver rehabilitation specialist, the same tools can contribute to a decision for fitness to drive."[190] While similar assessment tools may be used by the occupational therapist in general practice, the OT-DRS provides the expertise that will impact next steps.[70] A systematic review of the research on screening and assessment tools used to determine fitness to drive revealed that although some measures were better able to discriminate the skills and abilities necessary for driving, no measure, by itself, was sufficient to predict fitness to drive.[71]

During clinical assessment, the OT-DRS completes an occupational profile and then uses clinical reasoning to select and administer assessments specific to the requirements involved in driving, including those for vision, cognition, motor performance, reaction time, and coordination, knowledge of traffic rules, and a behind-the-wheel BTW) assessment of skill.[16,49,70] Many individuals will then progress to the on-road assessment where the OT-DRS will have the client drive the driver rehabilitation vehicle in a variety of traffic environments. The specialist will use a fixed driving route, which is a pre-planned route set up with specific driving maneuvers, or a geographic drive, which is often based in the client's community and uses established driving routes, or a combination of both. The OT-DRSs then uses their clinical reasoning and training, along with systematic analysis of the driver's ability using Michon's driving behaviors.[133a] Michon's driving behaviors address three levels.[68a] First is the strategic level where the driver creates a general plan for the destination, route, and driving conditions. Next is the tactical level where the driver is operating the vehicle and the last is the control level where the driver is avoiding collisions. The OT-DRS synthesizes the information to consider the pattern of performance between the clinical testing and on-road performance to hold an outcome discussion. Outcome discussions may range from recommendations on fitness to drive, additional driver rehabilitation training, or driving retirement. The completed comprehensive driving evaluation is then shared with the referring physician for discussion and consideration.

Driver Rehabilitation: Client Training

Driver training offered by **driver rehabilitation** providers for clients will vary, depending on the person's driving experience and the need to use adaptive vehicle controls. A young person with a disability who has never driven may have training needs related both "learning to drive" as a novice driver and approaches to compensate for limitations imposed by the disability. Individuals with driving experience who have perceptual impairments or older adults with age-related declines may benefit from driver rehabilitation training to relearn specific driving behaviors or implement compensatory skills to obtain consistent driving performance. Some clients require training in their own vehicle equipped with unique modifications. Depending on each state's requirements and the individual client's needs, driver training may occur before or after the vehicle has been modified. It is the role of the OT-DRS to carefully consider the individual's cognitive capacity for learning and carryover before initiating driver rehabilitation training.

Interventions: Adaptive Driving Equipment and Vehicle Modifications

The OT-DRS will use the comprehensive driving evaluation results to determine interventions that may include the need for adaptive equipment. For those who have experienced a change in motor skills, adaptive driving equipment may be the solution that would put them back behind the wheel. There are a range of adaptive driving equipment options, including hand controls, left foot accelerators, steering devices, and more. Adaptive driving equipment is often categorized into low technology and high technology categories. Both require that the OT-DRS offer training sessions for the client to establish new motor patterns for controlling the vehicle consistently and safely. Selection and training of adaptive driving equipment requires the skills of a specialist.

Although some clinics may have driving simulators with adaptive equipment options available, it is important that application of this equipment occurs in collaboration with an OT-DRS to ensure correct identification of equipment and establishment of motor patterns. Simulators are a resource for assessment and intervention but do not replace the on-road evaluation and training.

The legality of driving with adaptive equipment varies and is established by each state's driver's licensing agency. OT practitioners who think their clients may benefit from adaptive equipment should consult with their local OT-DRS and work to support timing of referrals and to facilitate the adaptive driving equipment process. In general, the OT-DRS completes the comprehensive driving evaluation, helps to match the driver with the best adaptive driving equipment, provides necessary training, facilitates completion of any state licensing requirements (i.e., relicensing with appropriate permissions to use equipment), generates the adaptive equipment prescription, helps to identify mobility vendors, and then completes a final fitting with the client and the modified vehicle.

Final Fittings

Final fittings, completed by the OT-DRS are an important aspect of adaptive driving and vehicle modification process. When adaptive equipment is recommended, this fitting ensures that the equipment is positioned and adjusted to meet the client's functional needs.[37] The final fitting for the client's equipment typically occurs at the mobility vendor occurs and often includes the OT-DRS. This is the first time that the client, adaptations, and selected vehicle have interfaced. Adjustment are frequently needed to meet functional goals and to have the adaptations perform as envisioned.[132] A short drive with the client in the vehicle is often completed to ensure adjustments are adequate for function given the dynamic forces involved in driving. It is important for the OT-DRS to consider liability coverage before initiating a ride with the client in the vehicle.

Vehicle Modifications

In addition to adaptive driving equipment, the OT-DRS will also consider the client's current vehicle and the need for additional vehicle modifications. The vehicle type, size, height of seat, space of trunk, weight capacity, etc., must all be considered. Client factors, adaptive equipment features, and vehicle modifications must match appropriately before an expectation of safe and independent driving can be met. The OTP generalist can play an important role by advising clients and their families that vehicle choices will have implications and by recommending that they consult with a specialist before making a vehicle purchase. Vehicle modifiers and funders may have requirements for the age, mileage, make, and model of a vehicle. It may not be feasible to install costly modifications in an old vehicle.[132]

Vehicle modifications are selected to support ease of ingress/egress and management of mobility devices. Examples of vehicle modifications may include the addition of a ramp, transfer seat, lift, or securement system. Vehicle modifications for drivers should include collaboration with the OT-DRS. Vehicle modifications for the passenger may be completed with the support of a trained OT practitioner (Fig. 11.23). Partnering with the local, qualified vendor for vehicle modifications is essential to ensure proper installation and integration of equipment. The vehicle's safety system is set up to work with the vehicle's seating system; therefore, whenever possible, being seated in the vehicle's original seating system is prioritized over transportation in a mobility device. If an individual is being transported in his or her mobility device, proper securement is required. Securement includes both device securement and the addition of seatbelt securements (Fig. 11.24). A wheelchair seatbelt does not replace the need for a vehicle safety belt.

It is the role of the OT-DRS to provide choice and options when supporting the selection of the mobility vendor. The NMEDA is a nonprofit trade association for mobility vendors and certifying body for the QAP. Vendors who are members of this program are committed to following established safety guidelines for adaptive equipment installation.

Learn more about becoming an OT-DRS, adaptive equipment, and vehicle modifications by accessing continuing education through Adaptive Mobility Services, American Occupational Therapy Association (AOTA), Association of Driver Rehabilitation Specialists (ADED), and National Mobility Equipment Dealers Association (NMEDA).

Adaptive Equipment and Risks of Online Buying

Practitioners and clients must understand that adaptive driving equipment requires the establishment of new motor patterns. In many cases an individual must change 25 to 35 years of engrained driving habits. Purchasing adaptive driving equipment online without proper evaluation, training, use of qualified installers, and understanding of state-specific licensing laws may place the client at great risk. If practitioners are implicated as recommending, there is professional liability risk as well. As a precaution, practitioners should be careful to describe the purpose, but not the device that could be construed as recommending.

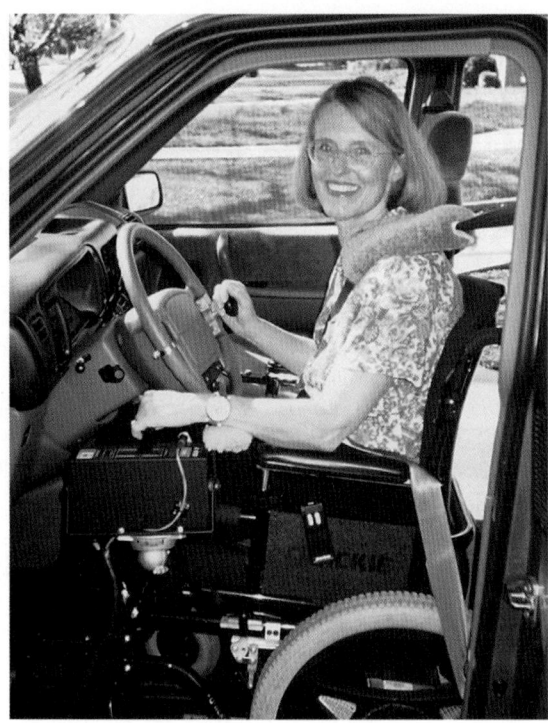

Fig. 11.24 This client was experiencing difficulties driving and at work because progression of her multiple sclerosis exceeded the activity demands of pushing a manual wheelchair. Driving from a power wheelchair and using an electronic gas-brake hand control decreased the activity demands on her upper extremities, enabling her to drive safely and work full time as a teacher.

Example

Wrong: I think you should see a specialist in driving rehabilitation for hand controls.

Risk: The client has a product name and proceeds to purchase "hand controls" online and claim they were recommended. Risk exacerbated if involved in a crash.

Correct: I think you should see a specialist in driving rehabilitation to explore the best equipment that would allow you to operate a car following your leg amputation.

Risk: None. Your message focused on the why and where and not the what.

Driver Licensing Assistance

Each state's driver licensing administration will have their own established rules, laws, and regulations around first-time licensure, licensure needed for driving with adaptive equipment, and medical reporting.[1] The OT-DRS working with a novice driver will understand and support the individual through the first-time driver licensing process for the state. For adaptive equipment, many states require the individual to obtain an updated license with "permission" or "restrictions" applied to the license providing permission to drive with the prescribed adaptive equipment. While some states may allow licensed individuals to have adaptive equipment installed into their vehicle before updating their license, many OT-DRS will encourage clients to update their license before having adaptive equipment installed.

This ensures the individual is licensed to use the adaptive equipment before investing in the equipment.

Regarding medical reporting, state laws often determine when and who is responsible for medical reporting. Clients who present with a medical concern should be assessed for driving risk by the OT practitioner and then discussed with the medical team. Collaborating with the OT-DRS can be helpful when there are concerns about safety, reporting, and need for driving retirement.

It is the role and responsibility of the OT-DRS to be well versed in their state's driver licensing laws and procedures.[89] Occupational therapists must be knowledgeable about the licensing procedures, requirements, and reporting laws in their state; understand how they may affect the client's ability to begin or return to driving and participation in their valued occupations; and share this information with their clients.[180]

Driving Retirement

Driving is the most complex IADL, requiring visual, cognitive, and sensory-motor skills be in peak condition. With increasing age, the older adult may experience functional declines brought about by medical conditions common in aging and safe driving may no longer be realistic.[89] Driving retirement is the term first used by the AMA to refer to the transition from driver to nondriver.[63]

Driving retirement is a process. Recommendations for transition from the driver's seat to the passenger's seat should not be based on one test or one session or be made by one provider. Recommendations for driving retirement should be based on a pattern of changes, often identified in more than one test, made over more than one session, and involve at a minimum the occupational therapist and referring doctor. Furthermore, the opportunity for recovery, rehabilitation, remediation, and adaptation must be considered. Individuals recommended for driving retirement have a medical condition or impairment that will either not improve or will progress. Examples include vision loss from macular degeneration, changes in cognitive capacity due to Alzheimer's disease or other dementia syndrome, or significant motor control loss. Consulting with an OT-DRS is often helpful for confirming the plan toward driving retirement.

Occupational therapists should approach this very emotional topic with compassion. The Hartford Center for Mature Market Excellence has created several free publications related to older adult driving.[194] *We Need to Talk: Family Conversations with Older Drivers* is their guidebook of practical information to help families and caregivers initiate productive and caring conversations about driving safely. It is available at http://www.thehartford.com/mature-market-excellence/publications-on-aging. The AARP has produced a free, three-module, online seminar with videos, printable worksheets, practice activities, and an interactive review based on the Hartford materials. The seminar is available at http://www.aarp.org/home-garden/transportation/we_need_to_talk/.

Adaptive Mobility offers practitioners and families a strategy called the "Three R's of Driving Retirement." This strategy outlines removing access to the vehicle, replacing all community mobility needs with a scheduled routine, and remembering to integrate leisure and fun activities as part of the driving retirement process. Training video available at https://youtu.be/WFIZXDYF8D8.

Whenever possible, the discussion of driving retirement should be initiated well before the need arises for driving cessation so that the client can begin exploring available resources for alternative transportation within the structure of his or her home and community. Making a "plan" for driving retirement helps to normalize the process so that it feels similar to planning for financial retirement or retirement from gainful employment. Discussions of this subject should include transportation alternatives and barriers to participation, such as finances, limited service destinations, and reluctance to rely on family and friends.[156]

Technology-based resources that can ease the transition from driver to passenger are becoming increasingly obtainable and should be discussed with the client facing driving retirement. Many goods and services can be procured on the worldwide Web. Home delivery of groceries and medications has become more common. As they gradually become more accepted by society, app-based transit services (e.g., Uber, Sidecar, and Lyft) have the potential to foster independence in the community and facilitate engagement in occupations. Finally, self-driving vehicles, which have been in development for over a decade, have the potential to transform community mobility. Client factors and performance skills must be carefully considered when matching resources with clients. Individuals with dementia syndrome may not be appropriate for using shared rides and may benefit from being with a trusted family member or friend for community integration.

Although the subject is sensitive, when deficits that preclude driving safely are demonstrated, it is imperative that the occupational therapist make the recommendation for the client to refrain from driving. If the client's medical condition is one with potential for functional improvement, the recommendation should be that the client refrain from driving until the deficit has been remediated. However, if additional functional decline is anticipated, retirement from driving should be clearly recommended. If possible, the client's family or another individual within the support system should be included in the discussion. Recommendations should be provided to the client both verbally and in writing. All aspects of the assessment and recommendations should be clearly documented in the medical report. Additionally, the client's physician should be informed in writing of the assessment results and recommendations made by the OT.

Individuals being considered for driving retirement may choose to participate in a comprehensive driving evaluation with an OT-DRS. The OT-DRS can provide an objective review of performance skills as well as observation of the task of driving. For many families, being provided with this option helps to lessen their own burden with the driving retirement decision. Completing a comprehensive driving evaluation helps to give this highly valued occupation the objective data, weight, and consideration it deserves.

INTERVENTION IMPLICATIONS FOR VARIOUS DISABILITIES

Many different types of disabilities affect driving ability. Occupational therapists can apply their knowledge of the various conditions to understand the client factors that might be affected and to anticipate how disease progression could influence the need for driving equipment over the course of time. A discussion of the driving issues related to some commonly seen disabilities is presented in the following section.

Wheelchairs and Driving

People with many different types of disabilities use wheelchairs to move about in the community. It is important to keep clients informed about how their wheelchair choices will affect their ability and safety as passengers and drivers. Whether moving in a personal vehicle or public transportation, as a passenger or driver, there are several considerations when it comes to wheelchairs. Loading, unloading, ingress, egress, weight, size, maneuverability, and securement options must all be considered and will be affected by the client's mode of transportation.[99]

For the driver or passenger transferring from a wheelchair into a vehicle seat, the ability to load and unload the wheelchair must be considered. Drivers using a rigid wheelchair may find disassembling the chair to be the easiest method. But the repetition of this task can be exhausting and difficult on joins over time. This type of loading requires good trunk motor skills, sitting balance, and upper body strength. Adding an electric lift to the trunk of a small SUV or van may be an option as well, but the size of the trunk and chair must be considered (Fig. 11.25). If the lift user is also the driver, the individual must be able to manage closing the trunk, navigate from the back of the trunk, and transfer into the driver's seat. Car toppers may be another option for individuals using a folding wheelchair. Once transferred out of the chair and into the vehicle seat the operator can consider an option that uses a remote to open the box located on top of the car, lower down a hook, and then lift the chair up on top of the car and into the box. Wheelchair lift equipment options continue to evolve and change. Mobility equipment vendors are skilled at matching wheelchair loading options with the specific vehicles. If the wheelchair user will be a driver, coordinating with the OT-DRS is essential.

Passengers or drivers entering into the vehicle in their wheelchair or power mobility device, will likely use a vehicle with remote entry, a ramp, and the ability for the vehicle to lower (Fig. 11.26). Vehicle options for this type of entry are usually minivans, vans, or some larger SUVs, although vehicle types and options continue to evolve. Ramps may be applied either to the side passenger door or through the rear of the vehicle. The height of the individual sitting in the chair, along with the weight of the chair and person, dimensions of the chair, and maneuverability must be carefully considered. Many vehicles have weight restrictions, as well as limits on seated height space and maneuverability. The chair also must be secured to ensure it does not shift while in transport. Once in the vehicle, sitting in an original vehicle seat, with that seat's designed safety system is priority. This may mean the addition of a remote-controlled transfer

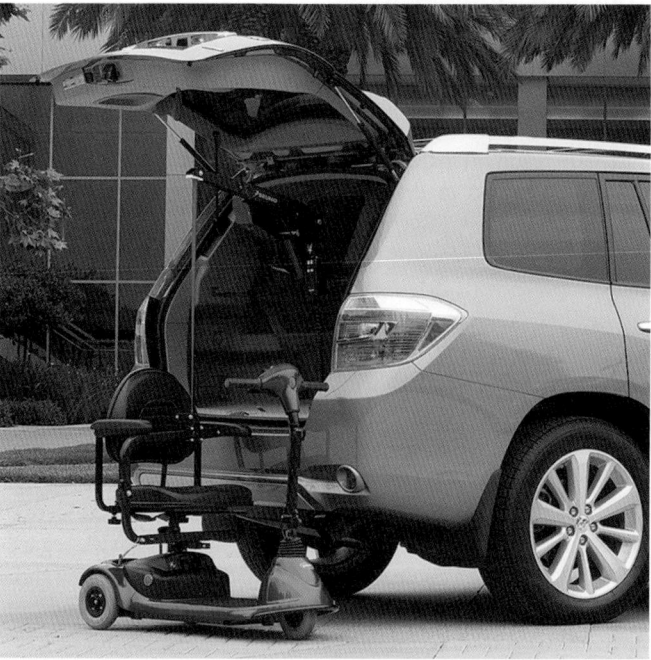

Fig. 11.25 Bruno's Curb-Sider lifts and stows a scooter or power wheelchair inside a minivan by the push of a button on a handheld pendant. (Courtesy Bruno Independent Living Aids, Oconomowoc, WI.)

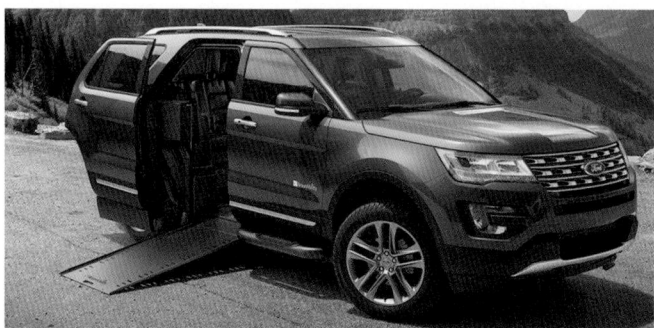

Fig. 11.26 The BraunAbility MXV is a wheelchair-accessible SUV that might be an appropriate alternative to a minivan for some clients. (Courtesy Braun, Winamac, IN.)

seat. Working closely with your mobility vendor for passengers and an OT-DRS for drivers will be essential to ensure the proper combination of options is selected to support safety.

Drivers who will be driving from their seat must be carefully assessed to ensure safety. Individuals who will be driving from their mobility device partner with both the OT-DRS and mobility vendor to ensure proper seating and positioning and wheelchair securement is achieved. The individual's wheelchair seatbelt does not replace the need for a vehicle seatbelt system.

Client education about the safety risk involved in driving from a wheelchair is necessary. It is generally accepted that the hierarchy of safe seating for a driver begins with the OEM driver's seat, which is designed to withstand crash forces. The OEM seat is followed by an aftermarket powered seat base. Driving from a wheelchair is next, with a power wheelchair considered safer than a manual wheelchair, even when both are WC19 compliant. The heavier weight of the power wheelchair allows it to withstand forces at the higher speeds typical in many driving situations. Proper securement of the wheelchair in the vehicle is critical to safety in either case.[99] Guidelines for using a wheelchair tiedown and occupant restraint system (WTORS) for this purpose were discussed earlier in this chapter. For safety reasons, it is not possible to drive from a scooter.

Spinal Cord Injury

Many people with an SCI have a goal to resume driving or become independent drivers. (NOTE: If not a licensed driver before, the client's driver rehabilitation program would begin at the level of novice driver). Driving-related interventions for clients with SCI requires critical thinking early on in a rehabilitation program. Mild or undiagnosed TBI is common among people with an SCI.[125] It is important to remain alert to possible signs of TBI so that intervention services addressing the future demands of driving can be planned. Because there is evidence that transfers can increase the risk for upper limb injury in people with an SCI,[152] the client's efficiency and technique during transfers into and out of a vehicle should be carefully assessed. If limiting transfers is necessary to preserve upper limb function, the client may need to consider driving from a wheelchair.

The functional outcomes and equipment needed for driving with an SCI depend on a number of factors, explored carefully through the clinical portion of the comprehensive driving evaluation. Particularly critical are the identification of which key muscle groups are functioning and whether the injury is complete or incomplete. A significant percentage of SCIs are incomplete,[149] which allows varying levels of motor and/or sensory function below the level of the lesion that can facilitate task performance. Steering devices may be needed to accommodate hand and UE impairments (Fig. 11.27). Upper torso supports or chest straps may be required in addition to a diagonal seatbelt to maintain an upright position during a sharp or fast turn. LE spasms in some people may necessitate the use of pedal blockers to prevent accidental activation of the brake and gas pedals.

In practice, even some people with a C5 SCI can drive safely from a wheelchair in a lowered floor minivan with a ramp. A high-tech, one-arm driving system in which the steering, gas,

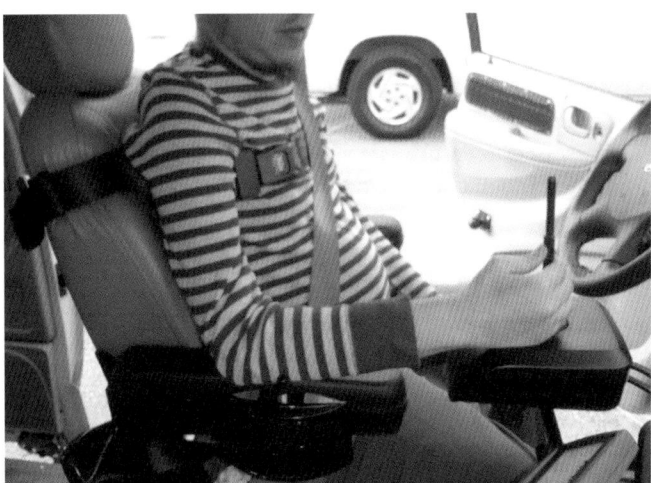

Fig. 11.27 This client with muscular dystrophy required a joystick system to operate the primary controls for driving. Evaluations and training requirements for clients using high-tech systems are more complicated and time intensive.[78]

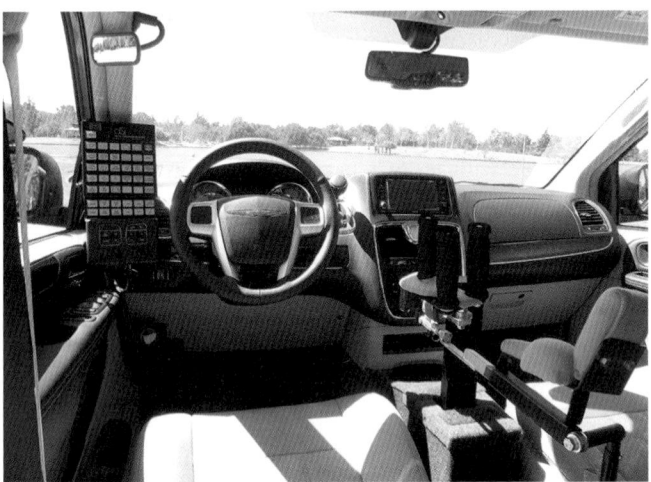

Fig. 11.28 Some people with severe disabilities can drive if matched with the right technology. This variation of the Scott Driving system allows the steering, gas, and brake to be operated with a single arm.[81] (Courtesy Driving Systems, Van Nuys, CA.)

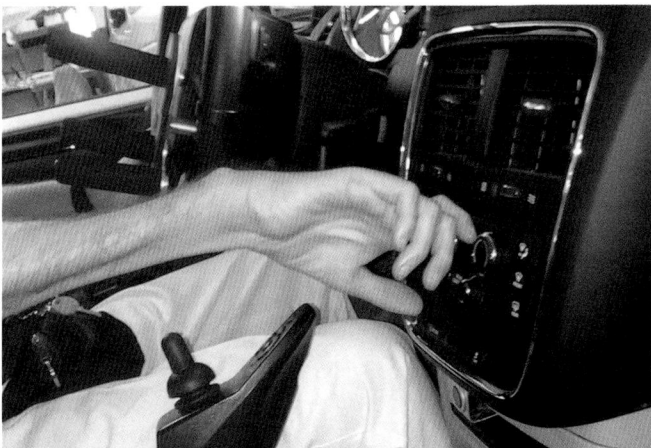

Fig. 11.29 A follow-up fitting determined that this client with tetraplegia from a spinal cord injury required extension modifications to operate the dials on the dashboard.[79,80]

Traumatic Brain Injury

Diffuse and local damage from TBI can cause physical and visual deficits; impairments in aspects of cognition such as attention, processing speed, language function, and memory; and visuo-spatial and visuo-motor limitations. Moderate and severe TBI can result in paresis, plegia, and post-traumatic seizures that affect fitness to drive.[102] However, even mild TBI, which accounts for most TBIs,[61] can lead to concentration and attention difficulties, irritability, and executive functioning challenges that interfere with driving performance.[67,68] Although research studies have not consistently identified the risk for crashes after a TBI, there is evidence that even mild cognitive difficulties can lead to increased risk while driving.[52] Despite this, between 40% and 80% of people with moderate to severe injuries return to driving after injury, many without evaluations for driving competency.[67,68]

These findings suggest that clinicians should be concerned about fitness to drive in any client with a history of TBI, regardless of its severity. People with mild TBIs may experience a short hospitalization and may be discharged before their symptoms have fully resolved. Occupational therapists in an acute care setting may be called upon to provide advice about whether it is safe to return to driving. Based on the time for resolution of symptoms from mild TBI, some facilities have developed clinical protocols identifying the timing for safe return to driving.[42] Clinicians in a facility without such established protocols should administer a driving screen to identify whether referral to a specialist for more in-depth evaluation and BTW assessments is warranted. Generalists should be aware of their state's laws for reporting loss of consciousness or seizure disorders to the state's Department of Motor Vehicles.

Cognitive and perceptual impairments are common problems post-TBI that can interfere with driving safety. OTP generalists should be familiar with the evidence-based guidelines for practice with TBI clients using key concepts from the OTPF.[102] Additionally, the AOTA's "Critically Appraised Topics and Papers" series reviews current evidence for interventions related to cognitive impairments and skills, vision and visual

and brakes are operated with a lever modified with a tri-pin is needed (Fig. 11.28). Individuals with C6 tetraplegia typically require a modified van and sensitized steering and hand controls for driving (Fig. 11.29). Some are able to transfer into the driver's seat if it is modified with a powered seat base, which moves up/down and forward/back and rotates to facilitate transfers. People with C7-8 injuries and paraplegia typically have sufficient upper limb function to use mechanical hand controls and can usually transfer into the driver's seat of a car. However, full hand function is not present in low-level tetraplegia SCI, and there may be balance limitations because of varying degrees of trunk musculature paralysis. These two factors can make dismantling and loading/unloading a manual wheelchair from a car difficult and time-consuming and should be considered when evaluating the feasibility of driving from a car.

processing, psychosocial, behavioral, and/or emotional impairments, and skills.[24]

It is important to establish whether driving or a return to driving is a goal for a client with a TBI. Family members and other caregivers often have valuable insight into a client's ability to return to driving[162] and should be included in the conversation about driving potential, provided the client agrees. The timing of consultations, driver risk assessments, and referrals to on-road driving programs should be carefully considered. Clients whose functional return has stabilized require less adaptive equipment than those who are newly injured. A referral made too early can use up limited therapy visits from an insurance provider or tax the financial resources of the individual or family. Exploration of driving potential becomes appropriate when the client has insight about personal physical and cognitive limitations and when improvement in the ability to demonstrate new learning, divided attention, and incorporate good judgment into decision making is consistently observed. Consultation with the OT-DRS can identify the important performance skills that can be included in inpatient, outpatient, day treatment, or community intervention programs before the actual referral. The OT-DRS can render a valuable service, even if driving is not a realistic goal, by providing information about transportation alternatives.

Cerebrovascular Accident

A CVA can have varying effects on function, depending on the anatomical location and extent of brain damage. Deficits that can interfere with driving include hemiparesis or hemiplegia, visual limitations, problems with memory and concentration, slowed reactions, spasms, speech and reading difficulties, and other consequences.[144] Scores on the Functional Independence Measures and Disabilities of the Arm, Shoulder and Hand (DASH) questionnaire in inpatient and outpatient rehabilitation may be helpful in developing treatment goals for clients who want to resume driving. Low scores on these measures have been linked to a lower likelihood of return to driving at 6 months.[40] Driving screens are a valuable service that an OTP generalist can provide to identify people who are at risk for unsafe driving following a stroke. Many stroke survivors do not receive professional advice or a formal evaluation on which to base a decision to resume driving.[105] The NHTSA has produced a series of short videos to show how different medical conditions can affect driving abilities.[136] The educational video about stroke, available as part of the NHTSA video tool kit on the agency's website, can be an important tool for educating clients with stroke about the driving risks resulting from their functional deficits[139]: https://www.nhtsa.gov/search?q=stroke%20video%20toolkit#gsc.tab=0&gsc.q=stroke%20video%20toolkit&gsc.page=1.

Hemianopia is a common occurrence after a CVA.[156] Visual field loss is of concern because it has the potential to affect driving safety.[63] Visual neglect often occurs in conjunction with visual field loss and can result in lack of attention to the more involved side. In these cases, driving is usually contraindicated.[132] However, there is evidence that people with hemianopia or quadrantanopia with no spatial neglect may demonstrate safe driving.[90] Occupational therapists in general practice should carefully screen these clients, refer to a vision care specialist for formal assessment, and consider the need for referral for a comprehensive driving evaluation. Most states have both visual acuity and visual field requirements and a deficit of this nature could prohibit driving.[63]

Equipment used for driving after a CVA will depend on the individual's functional impairments. If the person cannot steer with both hands, a steering aid may be needed to assist with turning. When there is paralysis of the right leg, modification of the vehicle with a left foot accelerator might be appropriate, if the person is able to operate it reliably. Extra mirrors may be necessary to compensate for visual deficits. Individuals who may require adaptive equipment should be referred to a medical provider for a comprehensive driving evaluation.

Arthritis

Arthritis is the most prevalent disease of people over 65 years of age. The pain, fatigue, ROM deficits, and diminished strength and reaction time caused by arthritic conditions can negatively affect driving performance.[212] Depending on the location of joint involvement, arthritis can limit specific driving skills. For example, involvement of the cervical spine can impair head turning and the ability to check traffic to the side and rear of a vehicle. Clients report difficulties in turning a key, operating the switches for the secondary controls, entering and exiting a vehicle, managing seatbelts, and operating gas and brake pedals. Loading and unloading mobility devices can also prove to be problematic. Occupational therapists should be aware that side effects from medications used to treat pain associated with arthritis also have the potential to affect reaction time and alertness for driving.

The NHTSA video tool kit, previously referenced, can assist OTP generalists in educating clients and their families about the driving problems associated with arthritis. Exercise programs to improve strength and ROM and instruction in proper body mechanics and energy conservation also may be warranted. Some clients will benefit from adaptations such as key turners and simple devices to facilitate getting into and out of a car. Identifying vehicle design features that facilitate comfort and safety for drivers with arthritis may also be helpful. The website MyCarDoesWhat.org offers a wealth of information on safety features and their functions presented by each vehicle make and model. OT practitioners need to appreciate that all levels of equipment affect how a driver interfaces with a vehicle and must be ready to refer clients to an OT-DRS for a comprehensive evaluation when a client's needs exceed simple aids. Examples of adaptations to compensate for ROM and strength limitations include steering using a modified position for a steering wheel (Fig. 11.30).

Medically At-Risk Older Drivers

The question is: How much risk is too much? In 2018 there were more than 45 million licensed drivers aged 65 or older and 83% of those aged 70 or older hold an active driver's license in the United States. Licensed drivers will account for approximately 75% of this group.[63] Driving in this age group is often viewed negatively by the public, but age alone is not an ethical

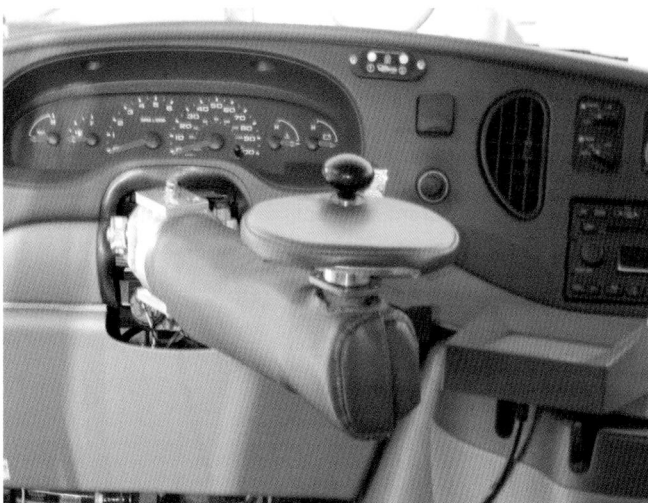

Fig. 11.30 A steering wheel that can be placed in a horizontal position can enable steering for clients who lack upward range to reach a traditional wheel. (Courtesy Drive-Master, Fairfield, NJ.)

or accurate determinant of one's fitness to drive.[109,114] Evidence indicates that older drivers, as a cohort, do not engage in risky behaviors such as speeding, not wearing a seatbelt, and drinking and driving, and they often self-regulate their driving by using strategies such as not driving at night or forgoing left turns.[63] The concern is that for many, age increases the likelihood that they will experience the type of medical conditions that can impair driving abilities and increase crash risk.[132] Even with self-regulation, the rate of crashes per mile driven starts to increase after age 65.[63] Another factor is that seniors are more susceptible to injury because of fragility and do not survive crashes as well as younger people. Their risk of being involved in a fatal car crash begins to increase at ages 70 to 84 and is highest for drivers 85 or older.[108,109] Functional declines brought on by polypharmacy also have been shown to be associated with an increased risk of motor vehicle crashes. This is significant because more than 40% of persons aged 65 or older use five or more medications per week.[114,120,139] Considered all together, these issues are the reason that older adult driving is a pressing public health concern.

Driving is often the preferred transportation for older adults[46,139,187] and how many remain connected to goods, services, and leisure activities. Loss of driving privileges can be the cause of social isolation with a very harmful effect on engagement outside of the home. Because current estimates project that most older adults will outlive their ability to drive (men by 6 years and women by 10 years),[63] OT practitioners must be diligent in helping those with the goal of "aging in place or in community" to remain drivers as long as it is safe to do so. When driving is no longer feasible, the focus shifts to community mobility, in which practitioners have an important role in identifying transportation alternatives.

The OT practitioner provides an important role in supporting older drivers in making early decisions about driving and community mobility. Driving status should be explored routinely when the occupational therapist is establishing occupational profiles. Medical records should be carefully reviewed to identify health issues and medications with the potential to

impair driving. Observation of a client's performance on complex IADL tasks, a routine part of the OT generalist's intervention, provides valuable information about whether the client is likely to encounter problems in driving; it is a key factor in helping generalists identify when a client requires referral to a specialist.[111,132]

When clients demonstrate a lack of insight into how their health issues and driving interact, many of the tools discussed earlier in this chapter (e.g., Enhanced Driving Decisions Workbook, and the Fitness to Drive Screening Measure) are useful for assisting them to gain self-awareness. Education through the CarFit program, https://www.Car-Fit.org, a collaboration between AOTA, AAA, and AARP, provides an opportunity for clinicians and clients to understand the in-car environment, the challenges that may be faced from ingress to managing controls to achieving the safest seating position and how to ascertain fit with the vehicle. The program also provides a platform to increase the public's awareness of the role of occupational therapy in older driver safety, the role of adaptation and driver support, and a means to identify clients who would benefit from referral to a specialist. OT practitioners working with clients who have progressive diseases, when driving cessation is an eventual outcome, need to introduce local transportation options well in advance of the need to cease driving, to allow for productive preparation for eventual driving retirement. To facilitate referrals for clients requiring comprehensive driver evaluation services, OTP generalists should be aware of the various driver rehabilitation programs available in their particular area.

PUBLIC TRANSPORTATION

Impact of the Americans with Disabilities Act

Public transportation refers to services operated by public agencies or supported by public funds that are available to anyone for any trip purpose.[213] Public transportation involves the use of buses, trolleys and light rail, subways, commuter trains, streetcars, cable cars, vanpool services, paratransit services, ferries and water taxis, and monorails and tramways.[31] Title II of the Americans with Disabilities Act (ADA) of 1990[4] prohibits discrimination on the basis of disability by all public entities that provide transportation at the local and state levels. Title III extends coverage to private entities that provide public transportation services.[4] The ADA has jurisdiction over most modes of transportation, including buses, trains, and ships but transportation that is specifically covered through other laws is excluded. For example, discrimination on the basis of disability in air travel is prohibited by the Air Carrier Access Act of 1986 (ACAA).[5]

The ADA's public transportation requirements for vehicles, facilities, and service were meant to create integration so that people with disabilities could travel to desired activities and do so in a nonsegregated way.[83] The law established accessibility guidelines for buses, trains, and light rail systems and specified the need for wheelchair lifts and ramps.[205] ADA guidelines also provide for priority seating, handrails to facilitate interior circulation, public address systems to announce stops, stop request controls, clearly marked destination and route signs, and various other features intended to ease navigation by persons with disabilities. Major improvements in transit systems across the United States have resulted from this legislation.[95]

Fixed-Route and Demand-Response Systems

Public transportation includes both fixed-route and demand-response systems of service delivery. Fixed-route systems use defined routes with predetermined stops and run on a published schedule.[213] Trains, city buses, and shuttles are types of fixed-route transportation. Demand-response transit refers to transportation service delivery in which rides are generated by calling a transit operator who then dispatches a vehicle to pick up passengers and transport them to their destination. The vehicles do not operate over a fixed route or on a fixed schedule. They may be dispatched to pick up several passengers at different points before taking them to their respective destinations.[209]

Fixed-route transportation creates links to home, work, schools, recreation areas, and other important destinations. The fixed-route system does not have a process for qualification and is open to anyone. It is an important transportation alternative for many segments of the population because it costs less and offers greater autonomy and flexibility than demand-response systems. In some locations the use of fixed-route transit by people with disabilities is two to six times higher than ADA paratransit ridership.[193] Older nondrivers also rely on public transit significantly, using it for 9% of their trips.[2] Public transit appears to be important to people born between 1983 and 2000 who appear less focused on using cars for transportation than older generations and seem to use alternative transportation methods, including public transportation, more extensively.[82]

The ADA requires public transit agencies that provide fixed-route service to offer a type of demand-response service called "complementary paratransit" to people unable to use the fixed-route service because of a disability. The individuals are entitled to the complementary service as a civil right and the service characteristics that must be provided are defined by the law.[84] Some communities offer demand-response transit referred to as "call-a-ride services" in addition to ADA complementary paratransit. These services may be offered in place of ADA complementary paratransit in locations where there is no fixed-route service.[83] Call-a-ride systems may be open to the general public or may be limited to people who participate in specific social service programs. The services such systems offer can vary from community to community.[84]

The people entitled to use complementary ADA paratransit include those with physical or mental impairments who cannot board and ride accessible fixed-route transit systems, those in areas where the fixed-route system lacks accessible vehicles, and those who have specific impairments that prevent them from getting to and from a stop. Eligibility may be conditional if the person can use fixed-route transit for some trips and not others. Examples of situations that might prevent an individual from using a fixed-route service for some trips include weather conditions for a person with temperature sensitivity, presence of a variable medical condition, and environmental barriers at certain locations.[84,215]

Complementary paratransit service considered equivalent to the fixed route must be provided within three-fourths of a mile of a bus route or rail station, at the same hours and days, for no more than twice the regular fixed-route fare. The ADA further requires that paratransit rides be provided if requested at any time during the previous day. Trip times can be negotiated but must not be more than 1 hour before or after the requested departure. Personal care attendants can ride for free.[119]

Transit authorities are required to have a process for determining paratransit eligibility.[74,121] An application is usually needed to qualify. Some transit authorities also ask for supporting documentation, an in-person interview, and/or an in-person assessment of the applicant's ability to use fixed-route service.[215] The in-person assessment is conducted either in a real setting or using a transit simulator. The focus of the in-person assessment is to determine whether the person can perform the tasks involved in using public transportation, not on the presence of a disability.[74]

Intervention Implications for Fixed-Route Transit

Trepidation about traveling alone can make an older adult or a person with a disability reluctant to use the fixed-route system, even when it is a viable transportation alternative.[50,154,213] To achieve increased ridership, occupational therapists must match the task demands of the local fixed-transit environment with client factors and performance skills.[215] If possible, the client's proficiency and destination points, management of mobility, skill in boarding and exiting the vehicle, and the actual time of travel as a fixed-transit user should be evaluated in the setting in which the bus or rail services will be used. Factors such as the ability to efficiently get to a bus stop, the safety of bus stops at origin and destination points, skills in boarding and exiting the bus, including the management of any mobility devices, and whether the time at which travel will occur is optimal for the client should be addressed.

If barriers to successful use of fixed transit are identified,[152] a focused intervention plan may be necessary to remediate or compensate for limited skills. Strengthening, balance, and endurance programs to increase ambulation or efficiency in using a mobility device[214] can be addressed in the clinic. Occupational therapists recommending a scooter or wheelchair should determine whether the device's weight and dimensions will allow it to fit and be safely transported on a bus's lift. Guidelines require buses to have lifts with a minimum design load of 600 lb and the lift platform to accommodate a wheelchair measuring 30 inches by 48 inches.[208] Lower footrests tend to make a wheelchair functionally longer. The length may make the wheelchair incompatible with some transit lifts and complicate maneuverability within the bus or light rail system. Clients should know where securement devices should be placed on their wheelchair and if their wheelchair is fit for traveling in. WC19 is an industry standard ensuring a wheelchair is safe to be seated in during vehicle transport. Bus drivers receive training to become proficient in using securement devices but in practice may not know how to work them properly.[73]

Skills such as reading a schedule can be practiced in the clinic. Trip-planning tools found on transit authority websites and those available through smart phone apps from third-party developers are useful resources. Clients who do not use computers or smart phones can be shown how to obtain travel information by dialing 511 on their phone. The Federal Communications Commission has designated this number as the single travel information telephone number available to states and local jurisdictions across the country.[206]

The natural environment poses limitations that cannot always be anticipated or duplicated in a clinic setting. Many clients benefit from participation in real-life sessions to develop the competence and confidence to use fixed-route transit independently. Community outings provide opportunities for skill practice and discussion of problems. Some transit systems offer individualized training programs, known as travel training, to assist persons who cannot negotiate the fixed-route system to travel safely and independently to a regularly visited destination such as work or school. Occupational therapists who are part of an Individualized Educational Plan (IEP) team should consider the need for travel training when they plan for a child's post-secondary transition needs.[201] This needs to be incorporated into the Individualized Transition Plan (ITP) for the student. Occupational therapists have the academic competencies to provide travel training.[132] Additional education in this area is available through Easter Seals Project Action, a national technical assistance program for community transportation.[83,84] Some transit authorities offer travel instruction geared specifically to older adults. In some cases, a senior is paired with an experienced bus user who will accompany them on a test ride to a destination of their choosing.[122]

Intervention Implications for Paratransit

OT practitioners can play a critical role in helping clients determine whether paratransit service best meets their community transportation needs. OT practitioners must become familiar with the policies of the local transit company and clearly understand their clients' passenger assistance level. The ADA allows transit companies to determine whether door-to-door or curb-to-curb service will be provided. In door-to-door service, the driver offers help from the door at the origin point of the trip and comparable assistance to the door at the destination point. In curb-to-curb service, help is not provided until the person reaches the curb. Guidance provided by the federal Department of Transportation to transit agencies has clarified that transit agencies with curb-to-curb service must still provide assistance to riders who need it because of a disability; however, door-to-door service may be provided only as needed, not necessarily for all rides.[75] The OT practitioner should prepare the client to advocate for door-to-door service if the person's functional limitations require it.

Because Jacqueline had reported that she was sometimes unable to drive because of arthritic flare-ups, her therapist, Sergio. used the opportunity to talk in greater depth about her transportation needs. Jacqueline had never heard of paratransit, but after Sergio explained how it operated and what the qualification process to use it would involve, Jacqueline decided it would be an option worth trying. However, because she was still concerned about her husband's blood sugar level if the ride caused them to be way from home for an extended time, Sergio recommended that she pack appropriate diabetic snacks to avoid low blood sugar problems during the trip. After Jacqueline had established paratransit eligibility for herself and her husband, she expressed relief that she had found an effective transportation safety net.

The costs to taxpayers or the transit system of providing a paratransit trip are significantly higher than for a fixed-transit trip—often 10 times higher.[56] The high expense of providing paratransit service has caused some transit providers to implement a stringent eligibility certification process as a way to contain costs.[55] Occupational therapists have a potential role in all aspects of eligibility certification.[215] To ensure appropriate categorization of disability, assistance can be provided during the application process. Clients can be encouraged to accurately report all significant disabling conditions that interfere with using fixed-route service. Assistance during the interview process could involve educating the person to provide necessary documentation of problems and helping the client articulate the difficulties encountered when using fixed-route service. During this process, the occupational therapist should also identify potential benchmarks of recovery that would allow the client more independence in using transportation options. Occupational therapy services are also needed by transit authorities to determine whether a person's wheelchair conforms to the common wheelchair ADA requirements, to prescreen an applicant for balance and motor capabilities, and to assess the person's skills during an actual transit trip.

OT interventions may include orientation to the local system, training in making a reservation, and education related to service limitations. Paratransit ridership combines the trips of several individuals to meet the capacity of the vehicles; consequently, travel often takes longer than private transportation. In some cases, it can exceed fixed-route timelines. Long trips can pose a hardship for those whose medical conditions or symptoms include urinary urgency and frequency, pain with prolonged immobility, insensate skin, or decreased endurance. OT intervention in such cases may call for cushioning and positioning devices to decrease discomfort and fatigue during the trip. Clients who are reluctant to travel alone can gain confidence in their abilities when accompanied by an occupational therapist on a trip to a destination and back.

PRIVATE TRANSPORTATION

Private transportation refers to vehicles that are privately owned, either individually or by a group, and are used for the benefit of those individuals.[71a,150] When individuals' goal is to "drive," they are most likely referring to "private transportation." It is imperative that the rehabilitation team understands the role of driving rehabilitation and the bridge this practice provides toward the goal of operating a private vehicle. This is accomplished through the application of strategies, adaptive devices, and/or modifications of the vehicle itself. The primary advantages of private transportation are the on-demand,

24-hour availability of origin-to-destination travel, the flexibility to modify travel plans, and the strong sense of control over one's life. Individuals in rural areas that are not served by fixed-transit routes may have limited to no acceptable alternatives and be highly motivated to explore all options to use private transportation. The perception and barrier to full information and awareness may actually prohibit potential candidates from using private transportation options. Nondrivers may also choose to continue to own and maintain their vehicles, bridging the driver gap by hiring drivers.

Supplemental Transportation Programs for Seniors

The aging of America has resulted in a focused effort to develop supplemental transportation programs (STPs) for seniors.[46] The primary purpose of these programs is to support the gap in transportation service for older adults, particularly those over age 85, who may not be driving. STPs are found in many geographic regions, sponsored by a wide variety of private organizations, places of worship, government agencies, and even public transportation authorities. Some STPs have their own vehicles, purchased through public funding. Others, such as volunteer driver programs, rely on the vehicles of their volunteer drivers. Eligibility criteria are established by the sponsor organization, and the services provided can vary significantly. Depending on the program, door-to-door, door-through-door, escort, and assistance at the destination services might be offered. Service

destinations may be affected by who sponsors a program. In some cases, an organization may offer transportation only for a specific purpose, such as to attend religious services or to participate in a hot lunch program. Some STPs do not restrict the types of trips that can be taken and provide very flexible service, allowing for multiple stops during a single outing.

Intervention Implications for Supplemental Transportation Programs for Seniors

Occupational therapists should be aware of the factors (availability, accessibility, acceptability, affordability, and adaptability) that have been identified as facilitating senior-friendly transportation services.[47] Knowledge of the resources available for locating programs in a particular community is helpful in matching services to a client's particular needs (Box 11.3). The Eldercare locator (https://eldercare.acl.gov/Public/Index.aspx) is a public service of the Federal Administration on Aging that connects users to information and assistance resources, including transportation services, for older adults at the state and community level. The interactive maps on the AAA's Senior Driving website provide additional resources for finding STPs. The nonprofit Independent Transportation Network of America (ITNAmerica), offers a searchable national database and toll-free telephone number at which callers can obtain information about the transportation alternatives available in their geographic areas.[110]

BOX 11.3   Resources for Driving Safety Programs

AARP
http://www.aarp.org (search under driver safety resources)
- Contains We Need to Talk online seminar about driving retirement, information about driver safety education classes, brain games, and various tools, including interactive **driving simulations** and a link to the University of Florida's Fitness to Drive Screening Tool.

Beverly Foundation
http://www.beverlyfoundation.org/map/stps
- Provides an interactive map with a city and state listing of volunteer transportation providers. The Beverly Foundation dissolved in 2014 but made arrangements for the map to be maintained by the National Volunteer Transportation Center.

ITN Rides in Sight Hotline
1-800-60-RIDES
- A free service uses ITN America's database of senior transportation options to identify local availability for callers.

National Mobility Equipment Dealers Association
http://www.nmeda.org
- Trade association for manufacturers of equipment and vehicle modifiers. Has a quality assurance program.

National Highway Traffic Safety Administration (NHTSA)
http://www.nhtsa.gov (search under driving safety)
- The Older Driver subsection contains a video toolkit on medical conditions, a link to the Physician's Guide to Assessing and Counseling Older Drivers, and driver fitness medical guidelines. Parents Central has information about

child safety, including selecting the right car seat, a database of installation locations, and information to promote seatbelt use. Information about Safe Routes to Schools programs and pedestrian safety workshops for youth and older adults is provided under the Pedestrian subsection. The Bicycles subsection has materials and videos related to bicycling safety for youth and adults.

Resources: Transportation in Wheelchairs
- Wheelchair Transportation Safety: https://wc-transportation-safety.umtri.umich.edu/
  - Contains information and educational materials about safe transportation of people who use wheelchairs as a seat in a motor vehicle.
- Rehabilitation Engineering Research Center on Wheelchair Transportation Safety (https://www.rercwts.org/)

Safe Kids Worldwide National Child Passenger Safety Certification
https://cert.safekids.org/
- Contains information for becoming a child passenger safety technician, certified to provide one-on-one personalized instruction on how to properly install a child's safety seat. Practitioners working with infants and young children should consider working closely with a child safety seat technician or to seek out this education to integrate into practice.

U.S. Administration On Aging Eldercare Locator
https://eldercare.acl.gov/Public/Index.aspx and 1-800-677-1116
- The Eldercare Locator is a public service of the U.S. Administration on aging. 33333The site connects users to information and assistance resources, including transportation services, for older adults at the state and community levels.

Taxis and Ride-Sharing Services

Taxi service is a significant source of transportation for people with disabilities affecting mobility, vision, thinking and other mental processes. Easter Seals Project Action (mentioned earlier), a government-funded program to assist the disability community and transportation industry to achieve the goal of accessible community transportation, reports that as many as 10% of taxi service customers are people with disabilities.[85] Taxi services are mandated to comply with ADA requirements as private companies that provide demand-response type services. Companies do not have to purchase accessible sedan-type automobiles; however, if a new vehicle type other than a sedan is purchased, it must meet ADA accessibility requirements for transportation vehicles. Service cannot be denied to a person who uses a service animal or to a person who is able to transfer from a wheelchair to a vehicle seat if the wheelchair can be stowed in the cab or the trunk. Additionally, personnel must be trained. Dispatchers must know how to operate communications equipment, such as a Telecommunications Display Device (TDD), and have sufficient knowledge about various disabilities to dispatch an appropriate vehicle. Training in the correct operation of lifts and securement devices is required for drivers.

Ride-sharing services, primarily Uber, Sidecar, Lyft and specialty services such as GoGoGrandparent (https://get.gogograndparent.com/gogostart?utm_source=bing&utm_medium=cpc&utm_campaign=267706219&utm_content=79237331078215&utm_term=keyword=gogograndparent%20transportation&msclkid=706a55cdd8a91531cb3330ceb781df91) offer additional options within the transportation industry.[123,184,210] These businesses use smart phone apps and the smart phone's GPS function to identify a user's location and connect the person to a ride in the personal vehicle of the nearest available driver. Payment transactions can be cashless when completed using the smart phone app. Proponents of ride-sharing services proclaim their convenience, environmental benefits, and potential savings in fuel and parking costs. Ride-sharing services have faced criticism from disability rights advocates because they lack accessible vehicles for people who use wheelchairs and they sometimes discriminate against people who use service animals.[131,166,167] In 2013 California became the first state to regulate ride-sharing services and mandated that ride-sharing companies provide incentives to attract accessible vehicles to their fleets, report annually on the demand for them, and ensure accessibility accommodations for their apps and websites.[55]

Interventions for Taxi and Ride-Sharing Services

For some clients, practicing in the clinic using the computer, tablet, or smart phone apps to arrange for taxi and ride-sharing services may be helpful. A client who uses a wheelchair should be trained in the procedure for correctly securing it in a vehicle and should be able to communicate these steps to another person. Clients who believe they have been denied transportation services or have been treated unfairly should know where to seek information about legal requirements. The ADA National Network, funded by the National Institute on Disability and Rehabilitation Research, provides informal guidance on the ADA to meet the needs of business, government, and individuals at local, regional, and national levels. Inquiries can be submitted to the 10 regional centers comprising the network, either online (https://adata.org/), by email, or by calling a toll-free number (1-800-949-4232). Specialists can answer most questions immediately, and, if necessary, will research complex questions. Referrals to local resources for disability issues not addressed by the ADA are also provided.[3]

TRAVELING AS A PASSENGER

General Considerations

In the United States, motor vehicle crashes are a source of significant medical and work costs. They are a leading cause of death among people ages 1 to 54 years. Seatbelts reduce serious crash-related injuries and deaths by half, but not everyone wears them.

Seatbelts are designed to be used in conjunction with air bags to provide optimal protection. Without the seatbelt, occupants can be thrown into the rapidly inflating front air bag, which could result in significant injury or death. Passengers need to wear both a lap and shoulder belt to best distribute crash forces. The chances of living through a collision are three to four times higher when both belts are worn. The shoulder belt should be placed across the middle of the chest and away from the neck, and the lap belt should be adjusted to fit low on the pelvis, across the hips and below the stomach. The shoulder belt should never be worn behind the back or under an arm. Special consideration should be explored for individuals managing a physical illness, treatment, or disability that may interfere with the proper fitting of the seatbelt. An example is the chemo port that runs across the clavicle or a colostomy bag that may interfere with the lap belt. There are adaptive aids and solutions, and those working with these clients need to be informed.

Intervention for Passengers

Seatbelts play a significant role seatbelts in reducing injuries and fatalities in a car crash and should be used by all clients. Occupational therapists should be aware of the populations with lower seatbelt use (i.e., teens, adults aged 18–34, people living in rural areas, and men[59]), and the occupational therapist should be ready to provide information about seatbelt effectiveness and how to wear them properly.

CarFit is a program collaboratively developed by AAA, AARP, and AOTA, launched in 2006 and expanded to Australia, New Zealand, and Canada. Training and information can be found at https://www.car-fit.org/. The focus of CarFit is to support and educate both active drivers and aging driver to stay on the road safely. Questions may arise after the CarFit educational session that would warrant therapeutic services offered by an OT practitioner or a driver rehabilitation program.

Safety in entering and exiting a vehicle, stowing any mobility device, and securing the seatbelt are all part of mobility and must be carefully assessed. Training family and personal care attendants may be warranted. Occupational therapists not primarily responsible for teaching transfers should work in conjunction with physical therapists to maximize safety during the process. OTP generalists can make recommendations for low-tech equipment to facilitate entering and exiting the vehicle and twisting in a seat. Cushions, either commercially available or custom made, can aid in positioning and maximizing comfort and should be considered when pain and joint limitations are present, or the short statured driver can no longer bring their line of sight above the obstruction of the dashboard. Jacqueline, the client described in the case study, may benefit from the use of a specialized motorized passenger seat to help her husband transfer under his own power reducing the repetitive stress demands that cause pain for Jacqueline, and potentially exacerbate her arthritis. These motorized seats move outside the car and rotate, easing the physical demands created by assisted car transfers (see Fig. 11.23).

Traveling While Riding in a Wheelchair

In most cases sitting in a motor vehicle seat offers the highest level of protection for a person riding in a vehicle. Cars, vans, and SUVs are designed with seats and belt restraint systems that work in conjunction with air bags to prevent occupant ejection and minimize the potential for contact with the vehicle interior. For various reasons people who use wheelchairs may find that they have to ride in their wheelchair when traveling in a motor vehicle. However, wheelchairs are not typically designed for this purpose. Protecting vehicle occupants who use a wheelchair as a seat requires attention to the position of the wheelchair in the vehicle, the structure of the wheelchair itself, and the systems for securing the wheelchair to the vehicle and restraining the occupant in the wheelchair.

Occupied wheelchairs should face forward during transport. A sideways orientation is the least safe for enduring a frontal crash, which produces the most serious injuries. Wheelchairs that meet standard WC19 of the American National Standards Institute/Rehabilitation Engineering Society of North America (ANSI/RESNA) are recommended by safety experts. However, not every wheelchair will meet this standard. A WC19-compliant wheelchair (also known as a wheelchair with the transit option) has a frame and transit components that have been sled-impact tested to determine how they will respond in a crash. The chair also has four securement points, specific securement point geometry, a clear path of travel for proper placement of vehicle-mounted occupant safety belts, and anchor points for an optional wheelchair-anchored pelvic safety belt.[164] Wheelchairs that meet this standard are labeled to show that they comply.

Wheelchair tiedown and occupant restraint systems (WTORS) should meet standard J2249 of the Society of Automotive Engineers (SAE), which ensures that these systems have undergone dynamic strength testing conducted on an impact sled.[165,204] The wheelchair tiedown portion of the system secures the wheelchair to the vehicle. It consists of two front straps and two rear straps, all four of which are needed for safe transport. If an individual is traveling in a personal vehicle, an SAE J2249 docking system can be recommended in place of the straps.[164] Adaptor hardware is attached to the wheelchair frame so it can engage with a docking device installed on the vehicle's floor. The occupant restraint part of WTORS keeps the wheelchair occupant safely in the seat. The postural support belts of a wheelchair cannot do this effectively. Occupant restraint can be provided either by the vehicle manufacturer's three-point restraint or by an upper and lower torso occupant restraint provided by the WTORS manufacturer.[185] All parts of the WTORS must be used to safely transport a person in a wheelchair.

Interventions for Passengers Traveling in Wheelchairs

Passenger evaluations, which can significantly improve the safety of a rider, are too often overlooked as a focus of OT intervention. Determining whether a client can safely and efficiently transfer to a vehicle seat or should ride in the wheelchair is an important first step in addressing passenger transportation safety. Riding in the vehicle's seat with the vehicle's securement system should always be prioritized; however, if the client cannot transfer, the occupational therapist should advocate for a WC19 wheelchair by providing justification and documentation of need to third-party payers. Collaboration with physical therapy may be needed if the occupational therapist is not directly responsible for ordering the wheelchair. OT-DRS should recommend that SAE J2249–compliant WTORS be installed by vehicle manufacturers or accredited members of NMEDA.[98] The website of the Rehabilitation and Engineering Research Center on Wheelchair Transportation Safety (https://www.rerc-wts.org/) provides valuable resource information about WC19-compliant wheelchairs and other issues of transportation safety for occupants of motor vehicles who remain seated in their wheelchair. Installation of additional seatbelts with the securement system also must be considered. The individual's wheelchair seatbelt does not replace the need for a vehicle securement system including a seatbelt.

OT practitioners working in a school setting must consider that their responsibility for students who use wheelchairs extends to their safe transportation to and from school.[166] Educating transporters in the safe loading of a wheelchair onto a lift (passenger facing away from the vehicle and wheel locks applied) and in deciding whether an individual with a power wheelchair can safely drive onto a lift is warranted. Additional opportunities exist for school-based therapists to work with transporters in developing a bus evacuation plan for disabled students.[183]

Child Passengers

Children are at significant risk when traveling in a motor vehicle. The leading cause of death among those ages 3 to 14 years is car crashes.[168] Fortunately, several steps can be taken to mitigate risk. Safety seats have been shown to reduce fatal injuries by 71% for infants and 54% for toddlers. The safety seat should be selected according to the child's age, height, and weight and should be positioned in the back seat of a vehicle. The NHTSA recommends a four-step progression from rear-facing car seats, to forward-facing car seats, to booster seats, to seatbelts. Children are ready to use seatbelts in the back seat when they are tall enough to sit without slouching and are able to keep their back against the vehicle seat, naturally bend their knees over the edge of the seat, and keep their feet flat on the floor. The NHTSA advises that children remain in the back seat at least until age 12.

Incorrect installation of car seats can jeopardize the safe transport of a child in a motor vehicle. Most parents think that they are putting their children in car seats correctly and installing the car seats in the right way; however, NHTSA research has shown that 7 of 10 children are improperly restrained.[181] Typical mistakes include using the wrong harness slot, improper harness retainer/chest clip position, loose car seat installation, loose harness strap, and improper seatbelt placement. The confusion is understandable because there are different installation instructions for every vehicle and car seat.

Intervention for Child Passengers

Parents may need help in selecting and installing a car seat that is appropriate for their child's needs. The NHTSA's Parent Central website (http://www.safercar.gov/parents/index.htm) offers information about various car seat types, in addition to tools for finding an appropriate seat based on the child's age and size. The site allows parents to register the car seat so that they can be notified if there is a safety recall.[147] Occupational therapists can also refer families to a SeatCheck program for assistance in installing the car seat provided by the NHTSA. SeatCheck is a national campaign to promote proper securement of children in motor vehicles. The program's website (http://www.seatcheck.org) and live chat options at this site identify local inspection stations where trained and certified child safety technicians provide a free installation check (https://www.nhtsa.gov/equipment/car-seats-and-booster-seats#installation-help-inspection). The website also contains tips and tools for keeping children safe in a motor vehicle, a listing of safety seat manufacturers, and a seat recall list.

Occupational therapists may want to take a more active role in child safety seat inspection by providing this service themselves. Safe Kids Worldwide, a global organization dedicated to preventing injuries in children, offers a Child Passenger Safety Technician certification course that provides specialized training in this area.[171] The certification course combines classroom instruction, hands-on activities, and skills assessments with car seats and vehicles. It concludes with a checkup event in which new technicians teach caregivers how to properly install and use car seats and booster seats.

Safe transport of infants and children with medical needs or disabilities is another practice area that should not be overlooked. Car seats should not be modified unless the person performing the modification is certified to do so. Inappropriate recommendations for car seat adaptations can have life-threatening implications.[45]

Assessment for children and teenagers must take into account future physical growth. For example, a 6-year-old riding in a van seated in a wheelchair may no longer fit in the vehicle by age 15 because of increased height. Also, activity demands associated with caregiving will be greater for a 15-year-old than for a 6-year-old. Alternative mechanical or power lifts or adaptations may become necessary for children or adults when their body size becomes unmanageable (and therefore unsafe) for their caregiver. Growth, development and aging affect the choice of equipment that will meet the individual's needs at a given age.

PEDESTRIANS AND CYCLISTS

General Considerations for Pedestrians

Regardless of transportation preferences, many Americans rely on their role as a pedestrian, either by walking or using a wheelchair or other mobility device. Although walking is an important means for getting around and has health, environmental, and economic benefits, it also involves risk. In 2020 alone, traffic accidents in the United States resulted in 6721 pedestrian deaths.[104] Awareness of the factors that cause risk for various age groups is necessary to plan effective OT interventions that allow clients to engage in community mobility as a pedestrian.

Older adults are one of the population groups most at risk for pedestrian injury. Decreased visual acuity, reduced reaction time, and slower walking speed contribute to the risk.[136] Nonfatal injuries from walking due to falls, especially while attempting to navigate curbs, are common.[135] Due to greater physical frailty, older adult pedestrians are less likely to survive a collision with a motorized vehicle than are younger pedestrians.

Children are also at significant risk for injury when walking. In 2019, 17% of children killed in a car crash were pedestrian.[135] Young children may not have fully developed judgment of speed and distance or use of peripheral vision, which can make crossing the street by themselves unsafe. Safety experts suggest that children aged 10 or younger should not cross the street without an accompanying adult.[173] A child's experiential basis for judging traffic situations is small. Emotions such as excitement may overwhelm their regard for safety. Older children have a more mature sensory processing skills, but the brain areas that control impulses and weigh the long-term consequences of actions are not fully mature.[175]

Adolescents and young adults become increasingly mobile as they strive to gain independence. Teens have both the highest death rate and the highest nonfatal pedestrian injury rate of any group of children.[169] The problem appears to be distractions while walking brought about by listening to music, texting, and talking on cell phones.[169] Walking while intoxicated is connected to very significant risk because of impaired judgment and diminished appreciation of hazards. More than one-third of the pedestrians killed in crashes were intoxicated.

Intervention for Pedestrian Safety

Mitigation of walking risk begins with pedestrian education. Some basic rules apply to all pedestrians and are fundamental to walking safety. These include walking on the sidewalk or facing traffic when there is no crosswalk, and crossing at intersections whenever possible, looking left, right, and left again before crossing the street. Additional recommendations are to increase visibility by wearing light-colored or reflective clothing, avoiding alcohol and distractions such as cell phones and headsets, and carrying identification.

The NHTSA and the Federal Highway Administration (FHWA) have developed a one-stop shop website (http://www.nhtsa.gov/pedestrians) with tips and resources for pedestrian safety that can be incorporated into OT interventions for people at various ages and developmental levels. The site includes links to the NHTSA's *Child Pedestrian Safety Curriculum* for students in kindergarten through the 5th grade and to the *Pedestrian Safety Workshop: A Focus on Older Adults.* There are additional links to the FHWA's *Pedestrian Safer Journey* series of videos about walking safety for children ages 5 to 18, checklists for conducting environmental audits, educational materials to teach parents about walking safety, and guides for community pedestrian safety advocates.

Individual assessment of skills to determine a person's potential to move about safely and independently as a pedestrian should be conducted. Impairments in vision, cognition, and motor skills caused by medical conditions and aging can potentially affect walking speed and endurance, management of uneven terrain, stepping up and down curbs, wayfinding, accurately estimating the time for street crossing, and recognizing and reacting appropriately to hazards. If assessments show that walking independently would be unsafe, OT practitioners have an obligation to advise the client and family of the risks involved.

When pedestrian skill acquisition or remediation appears feasible, skills should be practiced within a natural context as much as possible.[132] Real-life settings are valuable for reviewing the basic rules of safe walking, showing clients how to effectively visually scan for traffic hazards, and for practice in managing mobility devices outdoors. In many clinical settings there are opportunities to improve pedestrian skills. Tasks such as reading a map and selecting an ideal route to a destination do not have to occur on the streets to be practiced. The clinic also can be an ideal setting for educating families with children about pedestrian risks and helping parents develop strategies for modeling safe pedestrian behaviors.

According to the Centers for Disease Control and Prevention (CDC), many Americans view walking and biking in their communities as unsafe because of the presence of environmental barriers and absence of sidewalks, crosswalks, and bicycle paths.[57] Crashes between pedestrians and motor vehicles commonly involve people attempting to navigate environments designed primarily for use by cars.[224] In contrast, "walkable" communities are those in which it is easy and safe to walk to goods and services. These communities encourage pedestrian activities, expand options for transportation, and have safe streets that serve people with different ranges of mobility.[174] Occupational therapists can be helpful in improving the walkability of a neighborhood and intervention in this area requires a change in focus from serving individuals to serving communities. The FHWA's *A Resident's Guide for Creating Safe and Walkable Communities*[174] is a useful resource for practitioners interested in influencing neighborhood walkability. In addition to providing a section on assessing environmental problem areas, the guide discusses ways to take action, the various government agencies responsible for maintaining roads, the engineering improvements and law enforcement strategies needed to lower pedestrian risk.[174]

Safe Routes to School (SRTS) is a national and international movement to create safe, convenient, and fun opportunities for children to bicycle and walk to and from schools through its "Walking School Bus" and "Bike Train" programs.[133,170] The website for this organization offers free tools and resources for establishing SRTS programs and ideas for integrating SRTS considerations into community planning.[142] SRTS allows occupational therapists to address issues of childhood obesity with individual pediatric clients, and it also offers a platform for occupational therapists to serve the community by providing input for the design of roadways, bike lanes, and pedestrian paths that foster mobility for people of various ages and abilities.

General Considerations for Cyclists

Bicycling can be a means of exercise, recreation, conducting personal errands, or commuting to work or school. According to the National Survey of Pedestrian and Bicyclist Attitudes and Behaviors, 18% of the population aged 16 or older rode a bicycle at least once during the summer of 2012.[155] Like walking, bicycling has many health benefits. Yet bicycling is not without risk. In the United States, bicyclists are at greater risk for injury and fatality from crashes than occupants of motor vehicles, even though bicycle trips represent only a small portion of all trips taken.[58] Most bicycling deaths occur at night and in urban areas.[145] In 2010, roughly half of the cyclists killed or injured in the United States were children and adolescents under the age of 20. Annually 26,000 of the bicycle-related injuries to this age group have been traumatic brain injuries.[60] Alcohol use also appears to be a significant risk factor to safe bicycle riding. One in four bicycle riders killed in a crash had an illegal blood alcohol level.[145]

Bicycles are considered vehicles, and bicyclists are considered operators of vehicles in all 50 states.[145] Bicycle riders consequently have the same rights and are subject to the same rules as other motorists when they operate in traffic. There is no federal law requiring bicycle helmets; however, close to half of the states have laws mandating that children wear helmets. Additionally, some areas have local ordinances related to helmet use.[48] The League of American Bicyclists, an organization dedicated to creating a more bicycle-friendly America, is an excellent resource for information about the rules of the road and bike riding laws in the various states.[195,196]

Intervention for Cycling Safety

Bicycling requires clients to simultaneously pedal, balance, look around, and make decisions about whether it is safe to proceed. OT practitioners should determine whether a client has these skills before recommending bicycling. Interventions to improve subskills such as strength, ROM, coordination, and balance may be needed before bicycling can become a realistic goal.

Knowledge of a client's physical and cognitive functioning allows occupational therapists to provide guidance in selecting the contexts in which bicycling can safely occur. Not every person will be able to bike ride in all environments. Heavy city traffic conditions may be too fast moving for some people who can ride effectively in their familiar residential neighborhood. Off-road conditions may prove too physically challenging for some clients who can ride easily on paved roads.

Most clients will benefit from classes to ensure they can ride confidently, safely, and legally. The bicycle safety education classes shown to be the most effective in preventing crashes are those that involve lectures to teach rules and include several hours of supervised riding to practice their application in dynamic situations.[91] The League of American Cyclists offers online lessons with interactive components and videos, in addition to local education classes for all experience levels taught by certified instructors.[197,198] The FHWA's *Bicycle Safer Journey*, a series of three free educational videos for those ages 5 to 18, can be used to introduce safe bicycling skills or augment a comprehensive biking curriculum.[92] The NHTSA's *Bike Safe–Bike Smart*[134] and *Ride Smart–It's Time to Start*[146] videos use a peer-to-peer approach to teach bicycle safety to children from elementary to high school. A safety video targeting adult bicycle riders is also available on the NHTSA website.

Use of appropriate bicycling equipment should be encouraged. Knowledge of the client's functional abilities is valuable for selecting an appropriate bicycle. Occupational therapists should familiarize themselves with the many design options available for various abilities. These range from hand-pedaled bikes to recumbent bikes to adult tricycles. Bicycle helmet use during every ride should be encouraged for clients of all ages. These helmets are the single most effective safety device to reduce head injury and death from bicycle crashes.[172] An instructional video for correctly fitting a bicycle helmet is available from the NHTSA at the following website: https://www.nhtsa.gov/bicycles.

Occupational therapists can make a significant impact on reducing the number and extent of bicycling injuries by advocating to increase bicycle safety on a community level. Advocacy efforts in the community could focus on bringing about engineering changes to alter the infrastructure affecting the operation and movement of traffic and pedestrians or involve education to motivate behavioral change among various groups. Advocacy might also entail efforts to enforce laws and regulations or encouragement to promote bicycling in a community.[174]

ETHICAL CONSIDERATIONS

Occupational therapists in this practice area must seek out advanced education and have the knowledge and skill to support their selected evaluation tools and process of analysis to withstand what may seem at times to be significant challenges to their decision making. A novice driver with significant cognitive and perceptual impairments, for example, may press to curtail or even skip the assessment process prematurely because of time and financial considerations. Pressure to sway the therapist's opinion before completion of an assessment may come from biased third-party payers; even family members may strongly attempt to influence the outcomes of the assessment in a direction that is not supported by performance observations. Collaboration with other healthcare members is essential. Decisions, especially regarding driving retirement, should be made with data and support from the referring physician and other members of the client's healthcare team. Although the occupational therapist may lead conversations about safety with regard to engagement in the occupation of driving, expertise from the other healthcare providers must be included.

IN-VEHICLE ASSESSMENTS

THREADED CASE STUDY

Jacqueline, Part 2

After completing her driving risk assessment in outpatient, the OT, Sergio, referred Jacqueline for a comprehensive driving evaluation with the OT-DRS. Jacqueline was initially concerned that the driving evaluation would result in her losing her license and was hesitant about participating. Sergio took the time to communicate the intent of the evaluation. After Jacqueline realized that the purpose was to help her drive safely for as long as possible, she readily agreed to a referral to the low-tech driving program at the hospital.

The specialist completed the comprehensive driving evaluation with Jacqueline, including an on-road assessment. The OT-DRS observed how Jacqueline's hand limitations affected turning the key in the ignition and gripping the steering wheel. Jacqueline received an adaptive key holder and tried a simple steering wheel wrap to build up the steering wheel diameter. The OT-DRS also discussed wheelchair loading options for Jacqueline to consider when loading her husband's wheelchair. They explored the pros and cons of a car-top carrier versus internal wheelchair lift, but Jacqueline decided to wait to purchase it because of financial considerations. The specialist then worked with Jacqueline on strategies for tipping the wheelchair into the trunk of the car and reinforced proper body mechanics.

During the on-road assessment, Jacqueline had a near miss with a vehicle in her blind spot while changing lanes. Jacqueline had difficulty turning her neck to complete a full head check of the environment. The OT-DRS and Jacqueline

tried both a wide-angle interior rearview mirror and blind spot mirrors on the car's exterior mirrors. Education was provided and after practicing Jacqueline was thrilled she had increased visibility and confidence in viewing traffic and completing blind spot checks. The OT-DRS also found that she sat too low in the driver's seat, where her field of view out the windshield was obstructed by the dashboard. Jacqueline's seat was adjusted, and a cushion with securement was used to raise her eye level to the recommended 3 inches of unobstructed view above the dashboard/top of the steering wheel.

The OT-DRS also talked with Jacqueline about the future. Her current vehicle, while in good shape, is 20 years old. If she were to consider a newer vehicle, there are several technology updates that would benefit Jacqueline. The specialist shared information about blind spot warning lights, increased visibility with newer side view and rear-view mirrors, and the benefits of rear avoidance systems. They also discussed potential for financial support because her husband is a veteran. The OT-DRS encouraged Jacqueline to talk to her husband's counselor about vehicle options because his benefits may provide support for a vehicle that allows for his transport, such as a minivan with a remote entry, ramp, and wheelchair securement. Many dealers offer substantial discounts if modifications are ordered through manufacturer mobility programs at the time of new vehicle purchase. The OT-DRS provided Jacqueline with information and support to help her make considerations for the future.

SECTION 3 SUMMARY

Community mobility, whether it occurs while accessing a school bus, driving one's own vehicle, or riding in the local senior transport van, is a pivotal IADL. All forms of community mobility have the ability to enable engagement in necessary and meaningful occupations and are thus the concern of OT practitioners, whether they are generalists or specialists in the practice area. Individual evaluation, with consideration of valued occupational roles and the transportation systems available to a person, provides a foundation for determining the necessary level of intervention. Evidence-based research should be used to support practice, but without losing sight of the importance of driving and community mobility for facilitating social participation and involvement in other occupations throughout the lifespan. OT practitioners are encouraged to provide driving and community mobility services that will be widely recognized and valued by consumers, communities, and organizations.

THREADED CASE STUDY

Jacqueline, Part 3

Jacqueline's generalist OT and her OT driver rehabilitation specialist both played important roles in meeting her needs in driving and community mobility. Her generalist OT, Sergio, first identified problem areas in community mobility as he formulated Jacqueline's occupational profile. He assisted Jacqueline in successfully applying for paratransit services, to be used as backup transportation when pain from her arthritis prevented her from driving. After evaluating Jacqueline's performance capabilities, he also designed a home exercise program to improve her limited neck ROM and grip strength. Because these deficit areas could negatively affect Jacqueline's performance behind the wheel, Sergio discussed the benefits of a comprehensive driving evaluation with her. Sergio used his knowledge of local driver rehabilitation programs to determine that Jacqueline's needs could be met through the low-tech program at her hospital. The OT-DRS prescribed equipment to help Jacqueline compensate for the physical limitations to driving imposed by the arthritis. The OT-DRS provided Jacqueline with training in adaptive techniques for vehicle entry/exit, car transfers, wheelchair loading, and driving performance. In this program, Jacqueline was helped to think about a future transportation plan, if she needed to retire from driving. Jacqueline's quality of life was greatly improved through therapeutic intervention in several aspects of community mobility. She reported satisfaction and described herself as pleased with the outcomes achieved with the help of both occupational therapists.

REVIEW QUESTIONS

1. Define functional ambulation. List three ADLs or IADLs in which functional ambulation may occur.
2. Who provides gait training?
3. What is the role of the OT practitioner in functional ambulation?
4. How do OT and PT practitioners collaborate in functional ambulation?
5. List and describe safety issues for functional ambulation.
6. Name five basic ambulation aids in order of most supportive to least supportive.
7. Discuss why great care should be taken during functional ambulation within the bathroom.
8. List at least three diagnoses for which functional ambulation may be appropriate as part of occupational therapy services.
9. What purpose does a task analysis serve in preparation for functional ambulation?
10. What suggestions could be made regarding carrying items during functional ambulation when an ambulation aid is used?
11. What is the objective in measuring seat width?
12. What is the danger of having a wheelchair seat that is too deep?
13. What is the minimal distance for safety from the floor to the bottom of the wheelchair step plate?
14. List three types of wheelchair frames and the general uses of each.
15. Describe three types of wheelchair propulsion systems and tell when each would be used.
16. What are the advantages of detachable desk arms and swing-away footrests?
17. Discuss the factors for consideration before wheelchair selection.
18. Name and discuss the rationale for at least three general wheelchair safety principles.
19. Describe or demonstrate how to descend a curb in a wheelchair with the help of an assistant.
20. Describe or demonstrate how to descend a ramp in a wheelchair with the help of an assistant.
21. List four safety principles for correct moving and lifting technique during wheelchair transfers.
22. Describe or demonstrate the basic standing pivot transfer from a bed to a wheelchair.
23. Describe or demonstrate the wheelchair-to-bed transfer using a sliding board.
24. Describe the correct placement of a sliding board before a transfer.
25. In what circumstances would you use a sliding board transfer technique?
26. List the requirements for client and therapist to perform the dependent transfer safely and correctly.
27. List two potential problems and solutions that can occur with the wheelchair-to-car transfer.
28. When is the mechanical lift transfer most appropriate?
29. How is community mobility defined?
30. What unique qualifications do therapists have that enable them to address community mobility issues?

31. What are the primary advantages and disadvantages of public and private transportation?
32. What are the basic components for protecting passengers seated in a wheelchair within motor vehicles?
33. What are three resources for educating clients about safe pedestrian behavior?
34. Describe the role of the OT generalist and specialist in driving rehabilitation.
35. Name four ways the OTA may be used in a driver evaluation program.
36. Describe the decision-making process for assessment, referral, and training of clients with driving related needs.

37. What are the three categories of driving program services?
38. Why are older driver issues of particular interest?
39. What additional credentials can therapists obtain in the field of driver rehabilitation?
40. What is the function of driver training?
41. Why is a follow-up evaluation necessary when adaptive equipment is prescribed?
42. What legal issues must be considered by a driver rehabilitation therapist?
43. Where can the interested therapist go for additional information on this area of practice?

For additional practice questions for this chapter, please visit eBooks.Health.Elsevier.com.

REFERENCES

1. AAA Foundation for Traffic Safety: Driver licensing policies, practices, and noteworthy programs database. (2015). https://aaafoundation.org/.
2. AARP Public Policy Institute: Fact sheet 218: how the travel patterns of older adults are changing—highlights from the 2009 National Household Travel Survey. (2011). https://www.aarp.org/ppi/about-ppi/.
3. ADA National Network: ADA National Network: information, guidance, and training on the Americans with Disabilities Act. (nd). https://adata.org/.
4. ADA National Network: Information, guidance, and training on the Americans with Disabilities Act: What is the Americans with Disabilities Act (ADA)? (nd): https://adata.org/.
5. ADA National Network: Overview of disability rights laws: Air Carrier Access Act (ACAA). (nd). https://adata.org/factsheet/ADA-overview.
6. Adler C: *Wheelchairs and seat cushions: a comprehensive guide for evaluation and ordering.* In *Occupational Therapy Department,* San Jose, CA, 1987, Santa Clara Valley Medical Center.
7. Adler C, Musik D, Tipton-Burton M: *Body mechanics and transfers: multidisciplinary cross training manual,* San Jose, CA, 1994, Santa Clara Valley Medical Center.
8. Alexander H: On the road: Are we prepared to keep older drivers safe? [AOTA], *Physical Disabilities SIS Quarterly* 33:1–3, 2010.
9. American Association of Retired Persons, American Automobile Association, and the American Occupational Therapy Association: Frequently asked questions—CarFit. (2015). https://car-fit.org/faq.
10. American Automobile Association (AAA): Find the right vehicle for you: smart features for older drivers. (2011). https://www.ace.aaa.com/publications/auto/car-guide/how-to-choose-a-car.html.
11. American Automobile Association (AAA): Medical conditions and medications can affect safe driving. (2020). https://mwg.aaa.com/via/car/medications-and-driving.
12. Reference deleted in proofs.
13. Reference deleted in proofs.
14. American Occupational Therapy Association: *Occupational therapy practice guidelines for driving and community mobility for older adults,* Bethesda, MD, 2006, The Association.
15. American Occupational Therapy Association: The centennial vision: a call to action. (2006). http://www.otcentennial.org/100-events/2006.

16. American Occupational Therapy Association: Driving and community mobility, *Am J Occup Ther* 64:S112–S124, 2010.
17. Reference deleted in proofs.
18. American Occupational Therapy Association: The occupational therapy role in driving and community mobility across the life span. (2022). https://www.aota.org/practice/clinical-topics/driving-community-mobility.
19. Reference deleted in proofs.
20. American Occupational Therapy Association: Critically appraised topics: clinical and performance-based assessments (vision, cognition, physical function) and performance-based assessments (behind the wheel/simulated and on the road) for determining driving safety/competence and driving cessation. (2013). http://www.aota.org//media/Corporate/Files/Secure/Practice/CCL/OD/Driving%20Assessments.pdf.
21. American Occupational Therapy Association: Critically appraised topics: interventions to address cognitive and visual function, motor function, driving skills, self-regulation/self-awareness, and the role of passengers and family involvement in driving ability, performance, and safety. (2013). http://www.aota.org/-/media/Corporate/Files/Secure/Practice/CCL/OD/Driving-Person.pdf.
22. Reference deleted in proofs.
23. Reference deleted in proofs.
24. American Occupational Therapy Association: Evidence based practice: traumatic brain injury. (2015). http://www.aota.org/Practice/Rehabilitation-Disability/Evidence-Based#TBI.
25. American Occupational Therapy Association: Older driver safety: AOTA and NHTSA collaborative agreement. (2015). http://www.aota.org/Practice/Productive-Aging/Driving/gaps-and-pathways.aspx.
26. American Occupational Therapy Association: Driving and community mobility, *Am J Occup Ther* 70(Suppl. 2), 7012410050, 2016. https://doi.org/10.5014/ajot.2016.706S04.
27. American Occupational Therapy Association: Guidelines for supervision, roles, and responsibilities during the delivery of occupational therapy services, *Am J Occup Ther* 74(Suppl. 3), 7413410020, 2020. https://doi.org/10.5014/ajot.2020.74S3004.
28. American Occupational Therapy Association: Occupational therapy practice framework: Domain and process (4th ed.), *Am J Occup Ther* 74(Suppl. 2), 7412410010, 2020. https://doi.org/10.5014/ajot.2020.74S2001.
29. American Occupational Therapy Association: Occupational therapy scope of practice, *Am J Occup Ther* 75(Suppl. 3), 7513410030, 2021. https://doi.org/10.5014/ajot.2021.75S3005.

30. American Occupational Therapy Association. (2021) Scope of Practice Q & A: Gait assessment for fall risks https://www.aota.org/Practice/Manage/Scope-of-Practice-QA/gait.aspx

31. American Public Transportation Association (APTA): Public transportation benefits. (2015). http://www.apta.com/mediacenter/ptbenefits/Pages/default.aspx.

32. Amini D, et al: : The centennial vision in physical disabilities practice, [AOTA], *Phys Disab SIS Quart* 31:1–4, 2008.

33. Association for Driver Rehabilitation Specialists (ADED): ADED history. (nd). http://www.aded.net/?page=130.

34. Association for Driver Rehabilitation Specialists (ADED): CDRS certification: driver rehabilitation specialist certification exam. (nd). http://www.aded.net/?page=215.

35. Association for Driver Rehabilitation Specialists (ADED): Learn about: CDRS. (nd). http://www.aded.net/?page=210.

36. Association for Driver Rehabilitation Specialists (ADED): Code of ethics/standards of practice. (2003). http://c.ymcdn.com/sites/www.aded.net/resource/resmgr/P&P_Current/803-Code_of_Ethics_Standards.pdf.

37. Association for Driver Rehabilitation Specialists (ADED): Best practices for the delivery of driver rehabilitation services. (2009). https://c.ymcdn.com/sites/aded.site-ym.com/resource/resmgr/Docs/ADED_Best_Practices_2009_Edi.pdf.

38. Association for Driver Rehabilitation Specialists (ADED): Publications and links: disabilities and driving fact sheets. (2013). http://www.aded.net/?page=510.

39. Association for Driver Rehabilitation Specialists and the American Occupational Therapy Association: Spectrum of driver services: right services for the right people at the right time. (2014). https://www.aota.org/-/media/Corporate/Files/Practice/Aging/Spectrum-of-Driving-Services-2014.pdf.

40. Aufman EL, Blanco MD, Carr DB, Lang CE: Predictors of return to driving after stroke, *Am J Phys Med Rehabil* 92: 627–634, 2013.

41. Babulal G, Dickerson AE: Driving and Transportation: Aging Drivers. Occupational Therapy with Aging Adults, ed 2, editors: Karen Frank Barney & Margaret Perkinson, 2024.

42. Baker A, Bruce C, Unsworth C: Fitness to drive decisions for acute care and ADHD, *OT Practice* 19:7–10, 2014.

43. Barney KF, Perkinson M: ed *Occupational Therapy with Aging Adults*, ed 2, St Louis, 2016, Elsevier.

44. Berlly M, Lillie SM: Long term disability: the physical and functional impact on driving, 2000 Association for Driver Rehabilitation Professionals Annual Conference, Symposium at the Meeting of the Association for Driver Rehabilitation Professionals, San Jose, CA. (2000).

45. Berres S: Keeping kids safe: passenger restraint systems, *OT Practice* 8:13–17, 2003.

46. Beverly Foundation: Fact sheet 3: STPs in America. (2008). http://beverlyfoundation.org/wp-content/uploads/Fact-Sheet-3-STPs-in-America.pdf.

47. Beverly Foundation: Fact sheet 4: The 5 A's of senior friendly transportation. (2008). http://beverlyfoundation.org/wp-content/uploads/Fact-Sheet-5-the-5-as.pdf.

48. Bicycle Helmet Safety Institute: Helmet laws for bicycle riders. (2015). http://www.helmets.org/mandator.htm.

49. Bouman J, Pellerito JM: Preparing for the on-road evaluation. In Pellerito J, editor: *Driver rehabilitation and community mobility: principles and practice*, St Louis, 2005, Elsevier/Mosby, pp 239–253.

50. Brachtesende A: Ready to go? *OT Practice*:14–25, 2003.

51. Brachtesende A: New markets emerge from society's need,, *OT Practice* 23:17–19, 2005.

52. Brain Injury Association of America: Driving after brain injury: issues, obstacles, and possibilities. (2007). http://www.biausa.org/_literature_43315/driving_after_brain_injury.

53. Bromley I: *Tetraplegia and paraplegia: a guide for physiotherapists*, ed 3, London, 1985, Churchill Livingstone.

54. Calarusso RP, Hammill DD: *Motor-free visual perceptual test*, ed 4, Los Angeles, 2015, Western Psychological Services.

55. California Public Utilities Commission: CPUC establishes rules for transportation network companies (Docket #: R 12-12-011). (2013). http://docs.cpuc.ca.gov/publisheddocs/published/g000/m077/k132/77132276.pdf.

56. Center for Urban Transportation Research, University of South Florida: Creative ways to manage paratransit costs (BD 549 RPWO 28). (2008). http://www.nctr.usf.edu/pdf/77606.pdf.

57. Centers for Disease Control and Prevention (CDC): Healthy places. (2012). http://www.cdc.gov/healthyplaces/healthtopics/injury.htm.

58. Centers for Disease Control and Prevention (CDC): Home and recreational safety: bicycle-related injuries. (2013). http://www.cdc.gov/HomeandRecreationalSafety/Bicycle/.

59. Centers for Disease Control and Prevention (CDC): Injury prevention and control: motor vehicle safety—seat belts: get the facts. (2014). http://www.cdc.gov/motorvehiclesafety/seatbelts/facts.html.

60. Centers for Disease Control and Prevention (CDC): Gateway to health communication and social marketing practice: head injuries and bicycle safety. (2015). http://www.cdc.gov/healthcommunication/toolstemplates/entertainmented/tips/headinjuries.html.

61. Centers for Disease Control and Prevention (CDC): Traumatic brain injury in the United States: fact sheet. (2015). http://www.cdc.gov/traumaticbraininjury/get_the_facts.html.

62. Centers for Disease Control and Prevention/National Center for Health Statistics: *Prevalence of obesity in the United States, 2009–2010, NCHS data brief no 82*, Hyattsville, MD, 2012, National Center for Health Statistics.

63. Centers for Disease Control Transportation Safety (Last reviewed in November 2021) https://www.cdc.gov/transportationsafety/older_adult_drivers/index.html#:~:text=In%202018%2C%20there%20were%20more,a%2060%25%20increase%20since%202000.&text=Driving%20helps%20older%20adults%20stay,crash%20increases%20as%20people%20age.

64. Cesari M: Prevalence and risk factors for falling in an older community-dwelling population, *J Gerontol* 57:722, 2002.

65. Chaudhary NK, Ledingham KA, Eby DW, Molnar LJ: Evaluating older drivers' skills (DOT HS 811 773). (2013). http://www.nhtsa.gov/staticfiles/nti/pdf/811773.pdf.

66. Christopher and Dana Reeve Foundation Paralysis Resource Center: Prevalence of paralysis. (2014). http://www.christopherreeve.org/site/c.mtKZKgMWKwG/b.5184255/k.6D74/Prevalence_of_Paralysis.htm.

66a. Classen S, Monahan M, Auten B, Yarney A: Evidence-based review of interventions for medically at-risk older drivers, *Am J Occup Ther* 68:e107–e114, 2014. https://doi.org/10.5014/ajot.2014.010975.

67. Clay OJ, Wadley VG, Edwards JD, et al: : Cumulative meta-analysis of the relationship between useful field of view and

driving performance in older adults: current and future implications, *Optom Vis Sci* 82:724–731, 2005.

68. Defense Centers of Excellence for Psychological Health and Traumatic Brain Injury: Driving following traumatic brain injury: clinical recommendations. (2009). http://www.dcoe.mil/content/navigation/documents/Driving%20Following%20Traumatic%20Brain%20Injury%20-%20Clinical%20Recommendations.pdf.

68a. Devos H, Hawley CA, Conn AM, Marshall SC, Akinwuntan AE. Driving after stroke. In Platz T, editor: *Clinical Pathways in Stroke Rehabilitation,* pp 243–260, 2021. https://doi.org/10.1007/978-3-030-58505-1_13.

69. Di Stefano M, Macdonald W: On-the road evaluation of driving performance. In Pellerito J, editor: *Driver rehabilitation and community mobility: principles and practice*, St Louis, 2005, Elsevier/Mosby, pp 255–308.

70. Dickerson AE: Driving assessment tools used by driver rehabilitation specialists: survey of use and implications for practice, *Am J Occup Ther* 67:564–573, 2013.

71. Dickerson AE, Bedard M: Decision tool for clients with medical issues: a framework for identifying driving risk and potential to return to driving, *Occup Ther Health Care* 28:194–202, 2014.

71a. Dickerson A, Schold Davis E: Checklist of community mobility skills: Connecting clients to transportation options. OT Practice, Sept 21, 2020. https://www.aota.org/publications/ot-practice/ot-practice-issues/2020/transportation-checklist.

72. Dickerson AE, Brown Meuel D, Ridenour CD, Cooper K: Assessment tools predicting fitness to drive in older adults: a systematic review, *Am J Occup Ther* 68:670–680, 2014.

73. Dickerson AE, Reistetter T, Davis Schold, Monahan E: M: Evaluating driving as a valued instrumental activity of daily living, *Am J Occup Ther* 65:64–75, 2011.

74. Disability Rights California: Transportation rights for people with disabilities under the Americans with Disabilities Act. (nd). http://www.disabilityrightsca.org/pubs/541001.htm.

75. Disability Rights Education and Defense Fund: Topic guides on ADA transportation: topic guide 3: eligibility for ADA paratransit. (nd). http://dredf.org/ADAtg/elig.shtml.

76. Disability Rights Education and Defense Fund: Topic guides on ADA transportation: topic guide 5: origin to destination service in ADA paratransit. (nd). http://dredf.org/ADAtg/O-D.shtml.

77. Dobbs BM: Medical conditions and driving: a scientific review of the literature (1960–2000) (DOT HS 809 690). (2005). http://www.nhtsa.gov/people/injury/research/Medical_Condition_Driving/pages/TRD.html.

78. Driving Systems: Joysteer. (2008). http://www.drivingsystems.com/joysteerdrivingsystem.html.

79. Driving Systems: Paravan space drive. (2008). http://www.drivingsystems.com/paravanspacedrive.html.

80. Drive Master: Modified steering systems. (2015). http://www.drivemastermobility.com/steering.htm.

81. Driving Systems: Scott driving system. (2008). http://www.drivingsystems.com/ScottSystem.html.

82. Dutzik T, Ingliss J, Baxandall P: Millennials in motion: changing travel habits of young Americans and the implications for public policy. (2014). http://www.uspirg.org/sites/pirg/files/reports/Millennials%20in%20Motion%20USPIRG.pdf.

83. Easter Seals Project Action: Ask Project Action: ADA complementary paratransit. (nd). https://www.projectaction.com/our-services/training-on-americans-with-disabilities-act-requirements/.

84. Easter Seals Project Action: Introduction to travel training. (nd). https://www.projectaction.com/certification-programs/travel-trainer-certification/.

85. Easter Seals Project Action and the American Public Transportation Association (APTA). ADA essentials for transit board members: fundamentals of the Americans with Disabilities Act and transit public policy. (2010). http://www.fhwa.dot.gov/livability/cia/index.cfm.

86. Easter Seals Project Action and the Taxicab, Limousine and Paratransit Association. The Americans with Disabilities Act and you: frequently asked questions on taxicab service. (2015). http://www.tlpa.org/news/adanotice.pdf.

87. Eby DW: Older driver self-screening and functional assessment. In Senior Mobility Awareness Symposium: Science, Policy, and Practice (PowerPoint presentation). (2012). https://secure.hosting.vt.edu/www.apps.vtti.vt.edu/PDFs/smas-2012/Eby.pdf.

88. Edwards JD, Ross LA, Wadley VG, et al: : The useful field of view test: normative data for older adults, *Arch Clin Neuropsychol* 21:275–286, 2006.

89. Eisenhandler SA: The asphalt identikit: old age and the driver's license, *Int J Aging Hum Dev* 30:1–14, 1990.

90. Electronic Mobility Solutions (EMC): AEVIT 2.0 gas/brake and steering systems. (2015). http://www.emc-digi.com/explore.cfm/aevitgasbrakesteer/?s=1001408.

91. Elgin J, McGwin G, Wood JM: Evaluation of on-road driving in people with hemianopia and quadrantanopia, *Am J Occup Ther* 64:268–278, 2010.

92. Ellis J: Bicycle safety education for children from a developmental and learning perspective (DOT HS 811 880). (2014). http://www.nhtsa.gov/staticfiles/nti/bicycles/pdf/Bicycle_Safety_Education_For_Children-811880.pdf.

93. Fairchild SL, Kuchler O'Shea R, Washington RD: Principles and techniques of patient care *Assistive devices, patterns, and activities*, 6, St. Louis, MO, 2018, Elsevier, pp 211–260.

94. Federal Highway Administration: Bicycle Safer Journey: skills for safe bicycling for ages 5 to 18. (2015). http://www.pedbikeinfo.org/bicyclesaferjourney/.

95. Federal Interagency Forum on Aging Related Statistics: Older Americans 2012: key indicators of well-being. (2012). http://www.agingstats.gov/agingstatsdotnet/Main_Site/Data/2012_Documents/Docs/EntireChartbook.pdf.

96. Federal Transit Administration: Highlights of the Federal Transit Administration's impact on public transportation in the United States. (nd). http://www.fta.dot.gov/documents/FtaImpactBook_Web.pdf.

97. Fisher G, Jones KB: *Assessment of motor and process skills*, ed 7, Fort Collins, CO, 2010, Three Star Press.

98. Freeman EE, Gange SJ, Munoz B, West SK: Driving status and risk of entry into long term care in older adults, *Am J Public Health* 96:1254–1259, 2006.

99. Fuhrman S, Buning ME, Karg PE: Wheelchair transportation: ensuring safe community mobility, *OT Practice* 13:10–14, 2008.

100. Reference deleted in proofs.

101. Glantz C, Curry MK: Professional development and certification: what's in it for me? *OT Practice* 13:21–22, 2008.

102. Glass TA, Leon CM, Marottoli RA, Berkman LF: Population based study of social and productive activities as predictors of survival among elderly Americans, *Br Med J* 319(7208):478–483, 1999.

103. Golisz K: *Occupational therapy practice guidelines for adults with traumatic brain injury*, Bethesda, MD, 2009, AOTA Press.

104. Governor's Highway Safety Administration (2020) (https://www.ghsa.org/resources/Pedestrians21#:~:text=An%20analysis%20of%20data%20reported,from%206%2C412%20fatalities%20in%202019.)

105. Green M: How long does it take to stop?": methodological analysis of driver perception–brake times, *Transportation Human Factors* 2:195–216, 2000.

106. Hegberg A: An older driver rehabilitation primer for occupational therapy professionals. (2007). http://www.aota.org/-/media/Corporate/Files/Practice/Aging/Driving/Brochures-and-Fact-Sheets/AMAPrimerLowRes.pdf.

107. Hinman MR, O'Connell JK, Arnold LA, et al: Functional predictors of stair-climbing ability in older adults, *MOJ Gerontol Ger* 1(5):115–118, 2017. https://doi.org/10.15406/mojgg.2017.01.00025.

108. Huo X, Ghovanloo M: Using unconstrained tongue motion as an alternative control surface for wheeled mobility, *IEEE Trans Biomed Eng* 56:1719–1726, 2009.

109. Insurance Institute for Highway Safety, Highway Loss Data Institute: Older drivers. (2019). https://www.iihs.org/topics/older-drivers#age-and-driving-ability

110. ITN America: Senior transportation: helping seniors keep their independence. (2012). http://www.itnamerica.org/.

111. Iverson DJ, Gronseth GS, Reger MA, et al: Quality Standards Subcommittee of the American Academy of Neurology: Practice parameter update: evaluation and management of driving risk in dementia: report of Quality Standards Subcommittee of the American Academy of Neurology, *Neurology* 74(16):1316–1324, 2010.

112. Justiss MD: Occupational therapy interventions to promote driving and community mobility for older adults with low vision: a systematic review, *Am J Occup Ther* 67:296–302, 2013.

113. Kartje P: Approaching, evaluating, and counseling the older driver, *OT Practice* 11:11–15, 2006.

114. Kelley-Moore JA, Shumacher JG, Kahana E, et al: : When do older adults become "disabled"? Social and health antecedents of perceived disability in a panel study of the oldest old, *Am J Public Health* 47:126–141, 2006.

115. Korner-Bitensky N, Bitensky J, Sofer S, et al: : Driving evaluation practices of clinicians working in the United States and Canada, *Am J Occup Ther* 60:428–434, 2006.

116. Lamb SE, Ferrucci L, Volapato S, et al: : Risk factors for falling in home-dwelling older women with stroke: the Women's Health and Aging Study, *Stroke* 34:494, 2003.

117. Reference deleted in proofs.

118. Lane A, Green E, Dickerson AE, Schold Davis E, et al: Driver Rehabilitation Programs: Defining Program Models, Services, and Expertise, *Occupational therapy in health care* 28:177–187, 2014. https://doi.org/10.3109/07380577.2014.903582.

119. Law M, Baptiste S, Carswell A, McColl MA: *Canadian Occupational Performance Measure*, ed 5, Ottawa, ON, Canada, 2014, CAOT Publications.

120. Legal Information Institute (nd): 49 CFR 37.125: ADA paratransit eligibility: process. (nd). https://www.law.cornell.edu/cfr/text/49/37.125.

121. Legal Information Institute: 49 CFR 37.131: Service criteria for complementary paratransit. (2006). https://www.law.cornell.edu/cfr/text/49/37.131.

122. Lococo KH, Staplin L: Polypharmacy and older drivers: identifying strategies to study drug usage and driving functioning among older drivers (DOT HS 810 681). (2006). http://www.nhtsa.gov/people/injury/olddrive/polypharmacy/images/Polypharmacy.pdf.

123. Los Angeles County Metropolitan Transit Authority: Tips for seniors: On the Move Riders' Club. (nd). http://www.metro.net/riding/senior-tips/.

124. Lyft: How Lyft works. (2015). https://www.lyft.com/.

125. Lysack CL, Neufeld S, Mast BT, et al: : After rehabilitation: an 18-month follow-up of elderly inner-city women, *Am J Occup Ther* 57:298, 2003.

126. Macchiocchi S, Seel RT, Thompson N, et al: : Spinal cord injury and co-occurring traumatic brain injury: assessment and incidence, *Arch Phys Med Rehabil* 89:1350–1357, 2008.

127. MacDougall EE, Mansbach WE, Mace RA, Clark KM: The Brief Cognitive Assessment Tool (BCAT): Cross-validation in a Community Dwelling Older Adult Sample, *Int Psychogeriatrics* 27(2):243–250, 2015. https://doi.org/10.1017/S1041610214001458.

128. Mahoney JE: Use of an ambulation assistive device predicts functional decline associated with hospitalization, *J Gerontol* 54:83, 1999.

129. Manos PJ, Wu R: The ten point clock test: a quick screen and grading method for cognitive impairment in medical and surgical patients, *Int J Psychiatry Med* 24:229–244, 1994.

130. Mansbach WE, Mace RA: Predicting functional dependence in mild cognitive impairment: differential contributions of memory and executive functions, *The Gerontologist* 59(5):925–935, 2019. https://doi.org/10.1093/geront/gny097.

131. McCarthy DP, Mann WC: Sensitivity and specificity of the Assessment of Driving-Related Skills older driver screening tool, *Top Geriatr Rehabil* 22:139–152, 2006.

132. McGuire MJ, Davis ES: *Driving and community mobility: occupational therapy strategies across the life span*, Bethesda, MD, 2012, American Occupational Therapy Association.

133. Meronek T: Disabled Americans fight for transport rights. *Aljazeera* [Doha, Qatar]. (2014). http://www.aljazeera.com/humanrights/2014/03/disabled-americans-fight-transport-rights-201436104326992795.html.

133a. Michon J: A critical view of driver behavior models: what do we know, what should we do?. In Evans L, Schwing RC, editors: *Human behaviour and traffic safety*, Boston, 1985, Springer, pp 485–524.

134. National Center for Safe Routes to School. Connecting the trip to school with (2015). http://www.saferoutesinfo.org/.

135. National Center for Statistics and Analysis (2021, May) Pedestrians: 2019 data (Traffic Safety Facts. Report No. DOT HS 813 079). National Highway Traffic Safety Administration. U.S. Department of Transportation National Highway Traffic Safety Administration. 1200 New Jersey Avenue SE, Washington, DC 20590

136. National Council on Disability (nd): Workforce infrastructure in support of people with disabilities: matching human resources to service needs. http://www.ncd.gov/publications/2010/Jan202010.

137. National Highway Traffic Administration Bike Safe–Bike Smart (25MB and 146MB, WMV format). (2015). http://www.nhtsa.gov/Driving+Safety/Bicycles/Bike+Safe+-+Bike+Smart+(25MB+and+146MB,+WMV+format).

138. Reference deleted in proofs.

139. National Highway Traffic Safety Administration: Older driver traffic safety plan. (nd). https://www.nhtsa.gov/search?q=stroke%20video%20toolkit#gsc.tab=0&gsc.q=stroke%20video%20toolkit&gsc.page=1

140. National Highway Traffic Safety Administration: Parents Central: find the right car seat to fit your child. (nd). http://www.safercar.gov/cpsApp/crs/index.htm.

141. National Highway Traffic Safety Administration: Video toolkit on medical conditions in older drivers. (nd). http://www.nhtsa.gov/Driving+Safety/Older+Drivers/Video+Toolkit+On+Medical+Conditions.

142. National Highway Traffic Safety Administration: Specific needs. (1997). http://www.safercar.gov/Vehicle+Shoppers/Air+Bags/Specific+Needs.

143. National Highway Traffic Safety Administration: Safe Routes to School: overview. (2002). http://www.nhtsa.gov/people/injury/pedbimot/bike/Safe-Routes-2002/overview.html#3Collaboration.

144. National Highway Traffic Safety Administration: Driver rehabilitation: a growing niche, *OT Practice Magazine* 9:13–18, 2004.

145. National Highway Traffic Safety Administration: Safety in numbers newsletter: Halloween pedestrian safety. (2014). http://www.nhtsa.gov/nhtsa/Safety1nNum3ers/october2014/S1N_Halloween_Drunk_Peds_Oct_2014.pdf.

146. National Highway Traffic Safety Administration: Safety in numbers: preventing two-wheeled tragedies—the mistakes we all make. (2014). http://www.nhtsa.gov/nhtsa/Safety1nNum3ers/july2014/S1N_Bicycles_812047.pdf.

147. National Highway Traffic Safety Administration: Ride smart: it's time to start. (2015). http://www.nhtsa.gov/Driving+Safety/Bicycles/Ride+Smart+-+It's+Time+to+Start.

148. National Mobility Equipment Dealers Association: About NMEDA. (2015). http://www.nmeda.com/about/.

149. National Mobility Equipment Dealers Association: Adaptive vehicle steering aids: From reduced effort to foot steering. (2015). http://www.nmeda.com/nmeda-blog/adapted-vehicle-steering-aids-from-reduced-effort-to-foot-steering/.

150. National Spinal Cord Injury Statistical Center: Spinal cord injury (SCI) facts and figures at a glance. (2014). https://www.nscisc.uab.edu/PublicDocuments/fact_figures_docs/Facts%202014.pdf.

151. Office of the Assistant Secretary for Research and Technology/Bureau of Transportation Statistics: Dictionary. (nd). http://www.rita.dot.gov/bts/dictionary/list.xml?search=private+transportation&letter=&=Go.

152. Owsley C, McGwin G, Jr: Vision and driving, *Vis Res* 50:2348–2361, 2010.

153. Paralyzed Veterans of America Consortium for Spinal Cord Medicine: Preservation of upper limb function following spinal cord injury: a clinical practice guideline for health-care professionals, *J Spinal Cord Med* 28:434–470, 2005.

154. Pardessus V: Benefits of home visits for falls and autonomy in the elderly, *Am J Phys Med Rehabil* 81:247, 2002.

155. Peck MD: Barriers to using fixed-route public transit for older adults (MTI Report 09-16). (2010). http://transweb.sjsu.edu/MTIportal/research/publications/documents/2402_09-16.pdf.

156. Pedestrian and Bicycle Information Center: Who's walking and bicycling? (2015). http://www.pedbikeinfo.org/data/factsheet_general.cfm.

157. Peli E: Field expansion for homonymous hemianopia by optically induced peripheral exotropia, *Optom Vis Sci* 77:453–464, 2000.

158. Pezenik D, Itoh M, Lee M: Wheelchair prescription. In Ruskin AP, editor: *Current therapy in physiatry*, Philadelphia, 1984, Saunders.

159. Pierce S: The occupational therapist's roadmap to safety for seniors, [AOTA], *Gerontology SIS Quarterly* 26:1–2, 2003.

160. Pomidor A: *Clinician's Guide to Assessing and Counseling Older Drivers*, ed 4, New York, 2019, The American Geriatrics Society.

161. Purwanto D, Mardiyanto R, Arai K: Electric wheelchair control with gaze direction and eye blinking, *Artificial Life and Robotics* 14:397–400, 2009.

162. Ragland DR, Satariano WA, MacLeod KE: Driving cessation and increased depressive symptoms, *J Gerontol A Biol Sci Med Sci* 60:399–403, 2005.

163. Rappaport LJ, Hanks RA, Bryer RC: Barriers to driving and community integration after traumatic brain injury, *J Head Trauma Rehabil* 21:34–44, 2006.

164. Rehabilitation Engineering Research Center on Wheelchair Transportation Safety (RERCWTS): Best practices for using a wheelchair as a seat in a motor vehicle. (2008). http://www.rercwts.org/RERC_WTS2_KT/RERC_WTS2_KT_Stand/WC19_Docs/BestPractices.pdf.

165. Rehabilitation Engineering Research Center on Wheelchair Transportation Safety (RERC WTS): Wheelchair transportation safety: frequently asked questions. (2009). http://www.rercwts.org/RERC_WTS2_FAQ/RERC_WTS_FAQ.html#WTS_FAQ_Answer_A1_anchor.

166. Rehabilitation Engineering Research Center on Wheelchair Transportation Safety (RERCWTS): Wheelchair tiedown and occupant restraints. (2010). http://www.rercwts.pitt.edu/RERC_WTS2_FAQ/RERC_WTS2_FAQ_refdocs.html.

167. Rosenbloom S: Transportation patterns and problems of people with disabilities. In Field MJ, Jette AM, editors: The future of disability in America, 2007. http://www.ncbi.nlm.nih.gov/books/NBK11420.

168. Rosenthal BM: Texas disability advocates sue Uber and Lyft. (2014). http://www.chron.com/news/houston-texas/article/Texas-advocates-file-32-disabilities-act-lawsuits-5644400.php.

169. Safe Kids USA: Child passenger safety: kids can live with it! (2007). https://www.safekids.org/sites/default/files/documents/CPS-Kids-Can-With-Live-It_0.pdf.

170. Safe Kids Worldwide: Pedestrian safety. (nd). http://www.safekids.org/walkingsafelytips.

171. Safe Kids Worldwide: Bike. (2014). http://www.safekids.org/bike.

172. Safe Kids Worldwide: Teens on the move. (2014). http://www.safekids.org/sites/default/files/documents/ResearchReports/skw_pedestrian_study_2014_final.pdf.

173. Safe Kids Worldwide: National child passenger safety certification. (2015). http://cert.safekids.org/.

174. Safe Routes to School National Partnership. What is Safe Routes to School? (2015). http://saferoutespartnership.org/about/history/what-is-safe-routes-to-school.

175. Sandt L, Thomas L, Langford K, Nabors D: *A resident's guide to creating safe and walkable communities (FH WA-SA-07-016)*, Washington DC, 2008, Federal Highway Administration.

176. Santa Clara Valley Medical Center: *Physical Therapy Department: Lifting and moving techniques*, San Jose, CA, 1985, The Center.

177. Schaafsma JD, Giladi N, Balash Y, et al: : Gait dynamics in Parkinson's disease: relationship to Parkinsonian features, falls and response to levodopa, *J Neurol Sci* 212:47, 2003.

178. Schewbel DC, Davis AL, O'Neal EE: Child pedestrian injuries: a review of behavioral risks and preventative strategies, *Am J Lifestyle Med* 6:292–302, 2012. https://doi.org/10.1177/0885066611404876.

179. Schold Davis E: Defining OT roles in driving, *OT Practice* 8:15–18, 2003.

180. Schold Davis E, Dickerson AE: The Gaps and Pathways Project: meeting the driving and community mobility needs of OT clients, *OT Practice* 17:9–19, 2012.

181. Scott JB: Legal and professional ethics in driver rehabilitation. In Pellerito J, editor: *Driver rehabilitation and community mobility: principles and practice*, St Louis, 2006, Elsevier/Mosby, pp 465–485.

182. SeatCheck (nd): SeatCheck frequently asked questions. http://www.seatcheck.org/news_fact_sheets_faq.html.

183. Shinar D, Shieber F: Visual requirements for safety and mobility of older drivers, Human Factors, *J Human Factors Ergon Soc* 33:507–519, 1991.

184. Shutrump SE, Manary M, Buning ME: Safe transportation for students who use wheelchairs on the school bus, *OT Practice* 13:8–12, 2008.

185. Sidecar: Shared rides are here. And here. And here. (2015). https://www.side.cr/.

186. Society of Automotive Engineers: J2249 Guidelines: wheelchair tiedown and occupant restraint systems. (1999). http://www.rercwts.org/RERC_WTS2_KT/RERC_WTS2_KT_Stand/SAE_Restraints_RefDocs/J2249Guide_4_SAE2249.pdf.

187. Staplin L, Lococo KH, Gish KW, Decina LE: Maryland pilot older driver study, vol 2, (DOT HS 809 583). (2003). http://icsw.nhtsa.gov/people/injury/olddrive/modeldriver/.

188. Startzell JK, Owens DA, Mulfinger LM, et al: Stair negotiation in older people: A review, *J Am Geriatric Soc* 48(5):567–580, 2000.

189. Stav W: Differentiating yourself in the market as a specialist, *OT Practice* 13:21–22, 2008.

190. Stav WB: Consensus Statements on Occupational Therapy Education and Professional Development Related to Driving and Community Mobility, *Occup Ther Health Care* 28(2):169–175, 2014. https://doi.org/10.3109/07380577.2014.904536.

191. Stav WB, Lieberman D: From the desk of the editor, *Am J Occup Ther* 62:127–129, 2008.

192. StereoOptical: Vision screeners. (2015). http://www.stereooptical.com/category/vision-screeners/.

193. Thatcher R, Ferris C, Chia D, et al: Strategy guide to enable and promote the use of fixed route transit by people with disabilities (163). (2013). http://onlinepubs.trb.org/onlinepubs/tcrp/tcrp_rpt_163.pdf.

194. Thate M, Gulden B, Lefebrve J, Springer E: CarFit: Finding the right fit for the older driver, [AOTA], *Gerontol SIS Quart* 34:1–3, 2011.

195. The Hartford Financial Services Group: The Hartford publications on aging: home and car safety guide. (2015). http://www.thehartford.com/mature-market-excellence/publications-on-aging.

196. The League of American Bicyclists: Rules of the road. (2013). http://bikeleague.org/content/rules-road-0.

197. The League of American Bicyclists: State bike laws. (2013). http://bikeleague.org/StateBikeLaws.

198. The League of American Bicyclists: Take a class. (2013). http://bikeleague.org/content/take-class.

199. Toglia J, Berg C: Performance-based measure of executive function: comparison of community and at-risk youth, *Am J Occup Ther* 67(5):515–523, 2013. https://doi.org/10.5014/ajot.2013.008482. PMID: 23968789

200. TransAnalytics Health and Safety Services: (2014). http://drivinghealth.com/dhi-background.html.

201. Trautman T: Will Uber serve customers with disabilities? (2014). http://nextcity.org/daily/entry/wheelchair-users-ride-share-uber-lyft.

202. Tzeng HM, Yin CY: Relationship between call light use and response time and inpatient falls in acute care settings, *J Clin Nurs* 18(23):3333–3341, 2009.

203. Uber (nd): Your ride, on demand: transportation in minutes with the Uber app. https://www.uber.com.

204. University of Florida Institute for Mobility, Activity and Participation: Fitness-to-Drive Screening Measure. (2013). http://fitnesstodrive.phhp.ufl.edu/.

205. University of Michigan Transportation Research Institute (nd): Wheelchair and wheelchair tiedown/restraint testing at UMTRI. http://www.rercwts.pitt.edu/RERC_WTS2_KT/RERC_WTS2_KT_Stand/WC19_Docs/C_WTORS_CrashTesting@UMTRI07.pdf.

206. US Department of Education: Building the legacy of IDEA 2004. (2009). http://idea.ed.gov/explore/view/p/,root,dynamic,QaCorner,12.

207. US Department of Transportation/Federal Transit Administration: Part 38—Accessibility specifications for transportation vehicles. (1998). http://www.fta.dot.gov/12876_3905.html.

208. US Department of Transportation/Federal Transit Administration: Demand response service explained. (2013). http://www.fta.dot.gov/documents/Demand_Response_Fact_Sheet_Final_with_NEZ_edits_02-13-13.pptx.

209. US Department of Transportation/Federal Highway Administration: 511—America's traveler information telephone number. (2015). http://www.fhwa.dot.gov/trafficinfo/511.htm.

210. US Government Accountability Office: ADA paratransit service: demand has increased but little is known about compliance (GAO-13-17). (2012). http://www.gao.gov/assets/660/650079.pdf.

211. Venema DM, Skinner AM, Nailon R, Conley D, High R, Jones KJ: Patient and system factors associated with unassisted and injurious falls in hospitals: an observational study, *BMC geriatrics* 19(1):348, 2019. https://doi.org/10.1186/s12877-019-1368-8.

212. Visual Awareness Research Group: What is UFOV? (2015). http://www.visualawareness.com/Pages/whatis.html.

213. Vrkljan BH, Cranney A, Worswick J, et al: : Supporting safe driving with arthritis: developing a driving toolkit for clinical practice and consumer use, *Am J Occup Ther* 64:259–267, 2010.

214. Wacker RR, Roberto KA: Transportation. In Wacker RR, Roberto KA, editors: *Community resources for older adults: programs and services in an era of change* ed 4, Thousand Oaks, CA, 2014, Sage Publications, pp 282–307.

215. Walker KA, Morgan KA, Morris CL, et al: : Development of a community mobility skills course for people who use mobility devices, *Am J Occup Ther* 64:547–554, 2010.

216. Welch P: Transportation options for people with disabilities, *OT Practice* 12:10–15, 2007.

217. Wheelchair prescription: *measuring the client (booklet 1)*, Camarillo, CA, 1979, Everest & Jennings.

218. Wheelchair prescription: *wheelchair selection (booklet 2)*, Camarillo, CA, 1979, Everest & Jennings.

219. Wheelchair prescription: *safety and handling (booklet 3)*, Camarillo, CA, 1983, Everest & Jennings.

220. Whittle MW: *Gait analysis: an introduction*, Oxford, 2002, Mosby.

221. Williamson Weiner N, Toglia J, Berg C: Weekly Calendar Planning Activity (WCPA): a performance-based assessment of executive function piloted with at-risk adolescents. Published 1 November 2012. Psychology, Medicine. The American journal of occupational therapy: official publication of the American Occupational Therapy Association.

222. World Federation of Occupational Therapists. (2019). Position Statement: Occupational Therapy in Driving and Community Mobility. https://www.scribd.com/document/458506082/WFOT-Position-Statement-Occupational-Therapy-in-Driving-and-Community-Mobility-2019-1

223. World Health Organization: Make walking safe: a brief overview of pedestrian safety around the world (WHO/NMH/VIP13.02). (2013). http://who.int/violence_injury_prevention/publications/road_traffic/make_walking_safe.pdf.

224. Zahoransky M: Community mobility: it's not just driving anymore, [AOTA], *Home Commun Health SIS Quart* 16:1–3, 2009.

225. Zonzini website: (Photo) https://www.zonzini.us/2020/05/06/choosing-a-stair-climber-for-disabled-people-wheelchair/

SUGGESTED READINGS

Adler C: Equipment considerations. In Whiteneck G, editor: *Treatment of high quadriplegia*, New York, 1988, Demos Publications.

Bergen A, Presperin J, Tallman T: *Positioning for function* Valhalla, NY, 1990, Valhalla Rehabilitation Publications.

Davies PM: *Steps to follow: a guide to the treatment of adult hemiplegia* New York, 1985, Springer-Verlag.

Ford JR, Duckworth B: *Physical management for the quadriplegic client* Philadelphia, 1974, FA Davis.

Gee ZL, Passarella PM: *Nursing care of the stroke client: a therapeutic approach* Pittsburgh, Pa, 1985, AREN Publications.

Hill JP: *Spinal cord injury: a guide to functional outcomes in occupational therapy* Rockville, Md, 1986, Aspen.

Paralyzed Veterans of America: *Outcomes following traumatic spinal cord injury: clinical practice guidelines for health-care professionals. Paper presented at the Consortium for Spinal Cord Medicine* Washington, DC, 1999, Paralyzed Veterans of America.

Hill JP, editor: *Spinal cord injury: a guide to functional outcomes in occupational therapy,* Rockville, Md., 1986, Aspen. Paralyzed Veterans of America: *Outcomes following traumatic spinal cord injury: clinical practice guidelines for health-care professionals. Paper presented at the Consortium for Spinal Cord Medicine,* Washington, DC, 1999, Paralyzed Veterans of America.

12

Sexuality and Physical Dysfunction

Michelle Tipton-Burton, Fiona Dunbar, and Brenna Craig[a]

LEARNING OBJECTIVES

After studying this chapter, the student or practitioner will be able to do the following:

1. Justify sexuality as a concern of the occupational therapist.
2. List at least five possible reactions of the person with physical disability to their sexuality.
3. List some attitudes and assumptions that the able-bodied population may make about the sexuality of people with physical disability.
4. Discuss how sexuality and sensuality are related to self-esteem and a sense of attractiveness.
5. Define sexual harassment and describe how to handle a situation in which clients harass staff members.
6. Describe the effects that such items as mobility aids and splints can have on sexuality.
7. List signs of potential sexual abuse of adults.
8. List at least two intervention goals designed to improve sexual functioning.
9. Discuss ways in which the occupational therapist can provide a safe environment for discussing sexual issues.
10. Describe how sexual values can be communicated.
11. List at least five effects that physical dysfunction can have on sexual functioning, in addition to possible solutions for each.
12. Discuss the potential hazards of birth control.
13. List the potential complications of pregnancy and childbirth for a woman with disability.
14. Discuss methods of sex education.
15. Define PLISSIT and Ex-PLISSIT.

---

[a]The authors would like to acknowledge contributions from Gordon Umphred Burton and Winifred Schultz-Krohn to previous editions of this chapter.

KEY TERMS

Autonomic dysreflexia

Emasculation

Erogenous

New body

PLISSIT

Reflexogenic erection

Self-perception

Sensuality

Sexual abuse

Sexual harassment

Sexual history

Sexual values

Sexuality

Sexually transmitted infection (STI)

Vaginal atrophy

THREADED CASE STUDY

Shivani, Part 1

Shivani has cerebral palsy and identifies as female (prefers use of the pronouns she/her/hers). She is 29 years old and has been married for 2 years. She would like to have a child but has some barriers to overcome with the occupation of reproduction. To start with, as she was growing up, she was never taught by her therapists or anyone else to enjoy her body. Also, she has never had a role model who has cerebral palsy give birth to and raise a child. For 2 years she has been trying to relax and enjoy sexual activities with her spouse. This has been complicated by the fact that several people sexually molested her as she grew up, including her physician and a caretaker. Shivani has also found that sex is uncomfortable for her when she is lying on her back with her husband on top of her, but this is the only position she is aware of for sexual intercourse. She feels like a failure as a partner and a woman, and in her culture, she feels that she should not discuss this topic with anyone.

Critical Thinking Questions
1. Can Shivani enjoy having sex, get pregnant, and raise a child?
2. Do issues such as sexual positioning, enjoyment of the body, and abuse have anything to do with occupational therapy?
3. How would you approach this situation with Shivani and her partner?

BOX 12.1   Factors Related to Sexuality and Sensuality

- Quality of life
- Role delineation
- Cultural aspects
- Impulse control
- Energy conservation
- Muscle weakness
- Hypertonicity and hypotonicity
- Appreciation of body
- Psychosocial issues
- Range of motion
- Joint protection
- Motor control
- Cognition
- Increased or decreased sensation

This chapter is a brief, general overview and introduction to the topic of sexuality. As a disclaimer, the points of view portrayed in this chapter are mostly a cisgender and heteronormative perspective. However, the author acknowledges that all individuals experience, define, and practice sexuality differently, and that there is a broad spectrum of gender and sexual identities and ways of expressing and engaging in sexual activity. Nevertheless, occupational therapists (OTs) need to be prepared to work with clients, their partners, and family members from all backgrounds and be open to their differences.

Sensuality and sexuality are important aspects of activities of daily living (ADLs) and directly relate to the quality of each person's life.[2] As an ADL, sexual activity is in the domain of occupational therapy (OT).[82] Occupational therapists work with clients in all areas related to sensuality and sexuality (Box 12.1). Sexuality is an integral part of the human experience and is important for self-esteem, self-concept, well-being, and overall quality of life. It includes emotions, feelings, and hopes for the future. Individuals express sexuality in different ways.

Sexual expression is not only the sexual act of intercourse; it may include talking, touching, hugging, kissing, or fantasizing.

Engagement in sexual activities does not always take priority when individuals are coping with many other problems and deficits related to their disabling condition (Fig. 12.1).

Physical limitations may cause clients to question their physical attractiveness, sexual desire, arousal, and/or general ability to experience sexual pleasure. With the onset of physical disability, clients undergo a significant change in how they perceive the world and how others perceive them. This transformation significantly affects clients' perception of the commonly held roles and practices of the able-bodied population.[12,74,89]

Individuals with disabilities have a broad range of sexual expression and orientation, just as with individuals without disabilities. Healthcare providers and individuals without disabilities often incorrectly assume that individuals with disability are sexually inactive, or the healthcare provider neglects to consider the issue of sexuality. Adults with physical disabilities reported far lower levels of sexual activity and satisfaction compared to nondisabled adults.[58] A longitudinal investigation found that those who identified as male with disabilities had a similar number of sexual partners when compared to males without physical disabilities.[39] This investigation did reveal that those who identified as female with physical disabilities had significantly fewer sexual partners when compared to males, regardless of disability status.

There is a growing body of information in the medical and scientific literature about sexuality in individuals with

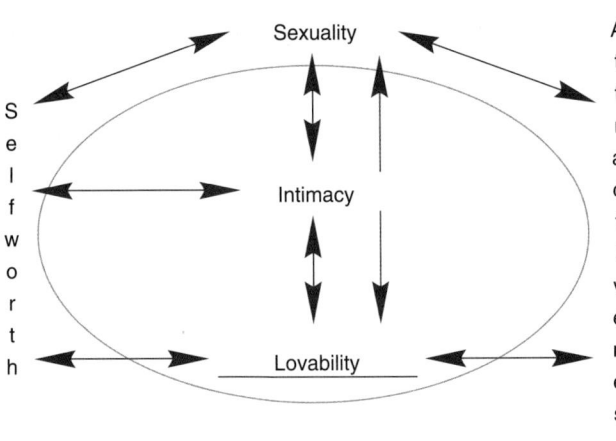

Fig. 12.1 Sexuality and disability.

disabilities. Even with the new literature available discussing sexuality for those who have disabilities, the translation of this evidence into practice has been slow.[62] In particular, women with disabilities are poorly understood.[25] For example, an investigation interviewed over 80 women with physical disabilities and the women reported that their healthcare provider never asked about their sexual function and presumed that they were sexually inactive.[40] The women had great difficulty locating information about sexual intimacy, and healthcare providers did not offer support in this area. Several women indicated that pressing medical concerns took a priority over attention to their sexuality. These incorrect assumptions by healthcare providers often negatively influence how healthcare providers perceive and treat sexuality in individuals with disabilities.[1,66] The result of this general lack of attention of healthcare providers to sexuality is that individuals with disabilities may not receive adequate and/or appropriate healthcare, including screening, education, and/or treatment for sexual problems or reproductive health.[1] This includes identifying physicians and other healthcare professionals who are knowledgeable about the disability.[13]

For individuals with disabilities, the associated features of the disabling condition may significantly influence the assessment of the client's sexuality. For example, incontinence, pain, spasticity, medications, cognition, and many other associated features may have a significant impact on sexual functioning. Many healthcare professionals may not recognize the ways in which the disabling condition may affect sexuality and intimacy. Therefore OTs must not only receive training in sexuality, but they also must be educated about how disabling conditions influence sexual functioning and how best to create a welcoming environment in which a client may feel more comfortable discussing sexual needs. Additionally, OTs must recognize the sexual health risks for various groups of people, such as those who identify as LGBTQ+, the elderly, and those with socioeconomic background issues who may have unique health and sexuality concerns.

The individual with a disability may be regarded by people without disabilities as asexual, or hyposexual, an object of pity, and unattractive.[6,45,54] Being perceived as unattractive and possibly unlovable can cause clients to think that they can never be intimate with anyone. Holding this belief can lead the client and related others to a sense of despair. McCabe and Taleporos[60] found that "people with more severe physical impairments experienced significantly lower levels of sexual esteem and sexual satisfaction and significantly higher levels of sexual depression than people who had mild impairments or who did not report having a physical impairment."

Low and Zubir[54] and Kettl and colleagues[43] found that females with acquired spinal cord injuries (SCIs) reported feeling less attractive after they acquired the disability, even though SCI is a disability with little observable physical change in body appearance. Slocum and associates[78] noted that women who had sustained an SCI were very unsatisfied with the sexual counseling they received, although sexuality remained an important aspect of their identities after the SCI. These studies showed a major decrease in the self-perception of attractiveness.[54] Another study found that with the advent of a disability, males felt a loss of their sense of masculinity and sensed a threat to the male role.[71]

These are just a few examples of the feelings and perceptions that affect the sensuality and sexuality of the person who has a physical disability. To provide comprehensive rehabilitation with the client, the OT and other health professionals must address self-perception, beliefs, and needs related to sexuality. This chapter examines issues related to sexuality and sensuality in individuals with physical disability.

REACTIONS TO SEXUALITY AND DISABILITY

The many obstacles encountered by people with a disability should not interfere with the expression of sensuous and sexual needs. As an informed professional, each therapist can help the adult client eliminate unnecessary obstacles, overcome anxieties, and appreciate personal uniqueness. The expression of sexuality or sensuality is a sign of self-confidence, self-validation, and a sense of being lovable.[55] When people acquire a disability or are born with a disability, they can feel less positive about themselves and less lovable or unattractive to others.[24,70,71] Sexuality can symbolize how a person is dealing with the world. If a person feels inadequate as a sexual, sensual, and lovable human being, the motivation to pursue other avenues of life can be affected.[87] When people have a negative self-image, their approach to other challenges in their lives may also be negatively affected. Coping with life's problems thus becomes much more difficult. Because sexuality can be seen as a barometer of how one feels about oneself, it is productive for the therapist to help the client feel as positive as possible about his or her physical and personal qualities. A healthy attitude toward one's sexuality enhances motivation for all aspects of therapy. The therapist must try to help the client adjust self-perceptions enough to function positively in life.

Sexuality has been found to be a predictor of marital or relationship satisfaction, adjustment to physical disability, social interaction, and success of vocational training. In society, people are often judged by their physical attractiveness.[74] In Western civilization, physical intimacy is closely associated with love. Therefore, if a person perceives themselves as incapable of expressing sensuality or sexuality, it is possible that they feel incapable of loving and being loved. The majority of people who have had a stroke "reported a marked decline in all measured sexual functions."[28,44] Without the capability to love and be loved, a sense of isolation and being valueless may ensue.[8,54,65,70] Adaptive devices such as splints, wheelchairs, and communication aids can be a detriment to a person's self-perceived attractiveness and sexuality. For example, it may be hard to perceive oneself as sexual when an indwelling catheter is present or when splints are worn. By discussing the effects of these devices on social interaction, the client can get some ideas about how to handle difficult situations when they arise.[3,52,65,91]

OT intervention should include goals that facilitate an increase in self-esteem and enable the client to feel lovable.[72,87] The therapist's role is to foster feelings of self-worth and a positive body image to help the client engage in occupations and to minimize feelings of worthlessness and hopelessness.[8,26,54,70,74] Feeling lovable engenders a sense of self-worth, attractiveness, sensuality, sexuality, and being capable of intimacy.[46,48] Achieving this goal enhances the development of a healthy and realistic life balance in which the client engages in occupations.

Whether sex is still possible is a concern that arises after the onset of physical disability. This concern is often set aside in the immediacy of coping with the adjustment to hospital life and activities that make up the daily routine. However, the concern is not forgotten. A common complaint from people with disabilities about members of the healthcare team is that the staff members do not readily bring up the subject of sexuality, and it is not an integral part of the rehabilitation process, treatment plan, or medical appointment.[25] Individuals with disabilities think that if their sensuality and sexuality are often negated, a significant facet of their personhood is negated. This lack of acceptance causes people with a disability to lose the feeling that they are being treated as a whole person. Currently, no single healthcare profession has been designated to address issues concerning the physiological and psychosocial changes related to sexuality after an injury or illness; rather, interdisciplinary team approaches are often used.

However, when a single discipline is not designated, the subject may be left unaddressed.[89] Often individuals with disabilities have an increased dependence on an able-bodied partner, which can result in a decrease in the couple's sex life.[22] One possible explanation is that the able-bodied partner is less inclined to be aroused when having just bathed the partner or assisted the partner with toileting. It is often difficult to transition from caregiver to intimate partner. The therapist must be sensitive to the possibility of these perceptions and help clients deal appropriately with the feelings they evoke.

The client's sense of masculinity or femininity may be threatened by the disability.[56,71,76] Men who have recently acquired a disability report that they feel emasculated.[71,76] Feelings of emasculation can be reinforced by physical limitations, as Western culture stereotypically associates masculinity with physical and emotional strength, which translates into power and social status. For example, relying on one's own physical strength may no longer be possible, engaging in physical activities such as sports or even basic ADLs may not be possible without adaptations, and the need to use a wheelchair and ask for assistance can engender feelings of dependency.

A man with a disability may react to feelings of dependency and emasculation[71] by flirting or making sexual comments to prove his masculinity. The client may attempt to flirt, making sexually inappropriate gestures or comments to a therapist.

Women experience many of the same feelings but may interpret and react to them in a different way.[6] Although many women with physical disabilities may be just as sexually active as women without disabilities,[13,25] some women with disabilities report feeling unattractive and undesirable. This can lead to despair if a woman feels that she cannot achieve some of her major goals in life. Thus the female client may flirt to see whether she is still attractive to others.

The therapist must realize that clients may be seeking confirmation of their sexuality. The therapist should not be surprised by flirtations or sexual advances from clients. The OT practitioner should deal with these behaviors and set therapeutic boundaries in a positive and professional manner, but therapists should never allow themselves to be harassed. All of the therapist's interactions should be directed toward creating an environment that promotes the client's self-esteem, positive and appropriate sexuality, and adjustment to disability.

ETHICAL CONSIDERATIONS

When responding to the client, the therapist should be alert to the client's current sexuality issues to avoid doing further damage to the client's sense of self. If the therapist rejects or makes the client feel uncomfortable, the client may hesitate to attempt similar interactions in which these behaviors are more socially appropriate. If the therapist rejects the client, the client may assume that if someone who is familiar with people who have disabilities is rejecting, then a person who is unfamiliar with them would not be likely to be accepting, either.

Inappropriate sexual advances, sexual harassment, and exploitation of either the therapist or the client cannot be permitted.[61,81] Behavior is considered harassment when it causes the therapist to feel threatened, intimidated, or treated as a sexual object. If sexual harassment is allowed, it can be damaging to the client and to staff morale.[31] The therapist should provide direct feedback, explaining that they feel offended and that the behavior is inappropriate and must stop. All staff members should be informed of the situation, and they should develop and implement a plan to modify the client's behavior if it persists.

Care of Minors

It is important to consider the education for minors who have yet to go through puberty and those who have not had sexual education thus far. Parents and healthcare workers can often minimize the need for sexual education after a catastrophic injury or illness, which prevents education that could offer safe and healthy decisions. Minors with physical and/or cognitive impairment should be provided with sex education,[41,47] similar to their peers, but modified depending on the individual's learning abilities.[75] Unaddressed sexual issues can cause distress, low self-esteem, and conflict with present and future relationships. Younger people may need more guidance for self-confidence. It is just as important to inform minors about safe sex practices to minimize the risk of contracting sexually transmitted infections (STIs) and contraceptives to prevent unwanted pregnancies. Sexual exploration is common during puberty, and it is appropriate for individuals to engage in self-stimulation; healthcare providers, along with parents of minors, may need to establish rules for privacy. It is also prudent that care providers and family be aware of sexual advances and inappropriate behaviors that the minor may display and/or be protected against.

LGBTQIA+ and Health

It is important for the therapist to have an understanding of terminology (Box 12.2) related to the Lesbian Gay Bisexual Transgender Queer/Questioning, Intersex, and Asexual (LGBTQIA+) Community as well as a basic knowledge of medical interventions (gender-affirming care, hormone therapy) unique to this group and guidelines for practice consideration.

Another consideration is to ensure you are using your client's preferred pronouns; if you do not know them, it is important to ask. It is also important to use appropriate language and to include this language in your documentation.[68]

The main focus for OTs to be aware of when working with clients who identify as a sexual and gender minority (SGM) is creating a welcoming and nonjudgmental communication and providing the prevalent health concerns of this specific population. SGM clients report not disclosing their sexual and/or gender identity or related health concerns to healthcare professionals because of fear or past experiences of being judged, disrespected, and harassed. These individuals also express not feeling welcomed or properly represented in most medical facilities, either simply through intake forms not offering options for their preferred pronouns or gender, or healthcare professionals misgendering or making assumptions about their lifestyles and health.[50] Therefore it is imperative that OTs are aware of their own attitudes, knowledge, and preparedness when working with SGM clients to create a therapeutic relationship that would best serve these clients in need.

OTs understanding the health risks related to this population is essential to provide effective and quality healthcare interventions. Health risks for people who identify with the LGBTQIA+

BOX 12.2 Key Terms and Definitions for LGBTQIA+ Clients

The following are key terms, as defined by the National LGBT Health Education Center (2016) and Coalition of Occupational Therapy Advocates for Diversity (COTAD), for OTs to be aware of when treating LGBTQIA+ clients:

- *Asexual:* An umbrella term or identity that describes individuals who experienced little or no sexual attraction to others and/or lack of interest in sexual relationships and/or behaviors; may have romantic relationships, but they would not have the interest in adding a sexual component to the relationship.
- *Bisexual:* A sexual orientation that describes people who are emotionally and sexually attracted to people of their own gender and people of other genders.
- *Cisgender:* A term used to describe people whose gender identity aligns with those typically associated with the sex assigned to the person at birth.
- *Gay:* A sexual orientation that describes people who are emotionally and sexually attracted to people of their own gender; used regardless of gender identity, but is more commonly used to describe men.
- *Gender:* Sex; the behavioral, cultural, or psychological traits typically associated with a person's sex.
- *Gender dysphoria:* Clinically significant distress caused when people's assigned birth gender is not the same as the one with which they identify.
- *Gender expression:* External appearance of one's gender identity, usually expressed through behavior, clothing, haircut, or voice, and which may or may not conform socially defined behaviors and characteristics typically associated with being either masculine or feminine.
- *Gender identity:* One's innermost concept of self as male, female, a blend of both, or neither; how individuals perceive themselves and what they call themselves; can be the same or different from their sex assigned at birth.
- *Gender transition:* Process by which some people strive to more closely align their internal knowledge of gender with its outward appearance; some socially transition by dressing, using names and pronouns and/or being socially recognized as another gender; others undergo physical transitions by modifying their bodies through medical interventions.
- *Genderqueer/Nonbinary:* Individuals who identify their gender as falling outside the binary constructs of male and female.

- *Heteronormativity:* The assumption that everyone is heterosexual, and that heterosexuality is superior to all other sexualities.
- *Heterosexual (straight):* A sexual orientation that describes a person's emotional, romantic, and sexual attraction to people of the sex opposite to their own.
- *Homosexual:* A sexual orientation that describes a person's emotional, romantic, and sexual attraction to people of the same sex as their own.
- *Intersex:* A term for a combination of chromosomes, hormones, sex organs, or genitals that differs from the male/female binary. For example, a person might be born appearing to be female on the outside but having mostly male-typical anatomy on the inside.
- *Lesbian:* A sexual orientation that describes a woman who is emotionally and sexually attracted to other women.
- *Pansexual (pan):* Someone who is emotionally, physically, spiritually, and sexually attracted to all gender identities.
- *Fluidity (or gender fluid):* A gender identity that may shift or change over time.
- *Demisexual:* A term or identity that represents an individual who has little or no sexual attraction to another individual, unless there is romantic connection/involvement; mostly considered to be under the umbrella of asexuality, though some view it separately.
- *Queer:* An umbrella term used by some to describe those who view their sexual orientation or gender identity as outside of societal norms; sometimes seen as more fluid and inclusive than traditional categories for sexual orientation and gender identity; others view it as a derogatory term because of historical use.
- *Questioning:* Describes individuals who are unsure about or are exploring their own sexual orientation and/or gender identity.
- *Sexual orientation:* A person's sense of identity, referring to a person's emotional, romantic, or sexual attraction to another individual; divided into three categories: heterosexual, bisexual, homosexual.
- *Transgender (trans):* Describes a person whose gender identity and assigned sex at birth do not align; umbrella term to include gender identities outside of male and female.

population depend on a multitude of factors (e.g., age, socio-economic status, ethnicity), but generally include depression, anxiety, suicide ideation and/or attempts, bullying and/or feeling unsafe in public areas, acquired disability as a result of emotional or physical harm, mental health issues, substance abuse and related health concerns, unsafe sex and related health risks such as autoimmune diseases, partner abuse, cardiovascular issues related to hormonal medications for transitioning, surgical recovery and care after transition surgery, eating disorders, and overall poor physical health such as obesity and asthma.[38,50,53,59,67] This population also may be less likely to have caregiver support, safe living situations, and/or finances to cover medical expenses compared to those outside of this group.[53] LGBTQIA+ individuals are also less likely to have access to healthcare services because of financial barriers from employment discrimination and a general lack of cultural awareness education among healthcare providers, including OTs (https://www.salus.edu/News/News-Stories/But-What-Does-the-Q-Stand-For.aspx).

When addressing sexuality and intimacy with this population, consider clients' preference and comfort level with a specific gender of OT and their desired privacy while being treated. Transgender patients might also have additional modification devices or practices that promote their sexual identity, such as male transgender individuals wearing chest binders or elastic wraps and a phallic prosthesis; female transgender individuals may tuck genitals and wear garments that mimic soft tissue or a bra.

Therapeutic Communication

Conversations about sexuality can be opportunities for discussing personal feelings and perceptions. Before initiating a conversation about sexuality, the OT practitioner should ask the client for permission to discuss topics that some may find uncomfortable. Beginning with open-ended, nonthreatening questions can help the client feel more comfortable and assist the therapist in obtaining important information. One way to approach a discussion of intimate matters would be to ask the female client how she will perform breast self-examination with her disability. A way to introduce the subject to a male client would be to ask if he has noticed any physical changes in his body or how he will perform self-examination of the testicles. If the treatment facility does not have information about these examinations, the client can obtain them from the American Cancer Society or the local Planned Parenthood Association. Each of these activities falls into the domain of health maintenance and may not have been discussed by other health team members either because of lack of knowledge or the team member's own discomfort in discussing sexuality with clients. This interaction can set the stage for discussion of other personal matters; it also impresses upon the client the necessity for concern about personal health and reaffirms the client's sexual identity.

Clients may feel safe asking the OT about sexual matters related to their disabilities because the therapist deals with other intimate activities, such as bathing, dressing, and toileting. It is also important to discuss sexual hygiene as an ADL. The trust built up in the relationship encourages this communication.

The therapist should be prepared with accurate information and resources. The therapist does not need to know everything or be a sex expert but should ensure that the client gets the necessary information or appropriate referral.[55]

The OT is the most appropriate professional to solve some problems, such as the motor performance needed for sexual activity.[15] For example, discussing positioning to reduce pain or hypertonicity or to enable the client to more comfortably engage in sexual relations will help the client deal with problems before they occur.[18,49,65]

In the case study, Shivani, who has hypertonicity, particularly in the hip adductors, experiences discomfort in a sexual position in which she abducts her legs during intercourse with her husband. She and her husband have not explored other positions, but instead have reduced the number of times they have intercourse during the month. Shivani's sense of failure and feelings of diminished worth as a wife may have further affected the intimacy of her marriage.

Approaches to intervention can include individual, partner, or group sessions. The format in which the information is presented can also vary and depends on the client's status physically, cognitively, and emotionally. It is important to provide the information in a way that can be best understood and when the individual is ready to assimilate it. Information can be presented in many ways and may include diverse media such as videos, pamphlets, or booklets. Varied media may be used to address the unique learning style and need of the individual.[10]

During all aspects of the rehabilitation process, the therapist, staff members, and the client's sexual partner should work on communication with the client. The therapist can facilitate this process simply by giving the client permission to discuss feelings and potential problems, especially sexual problems, and initiate the discussion through open-ended questions. The client needs to learn how to accurately communicate sexual needs, desires, and position options to a partner, either verbally or nonverbally, to have a mutually satisfactory sexual relationship.[23,43] Each client will have unique problems or issues that are related to the nature of the disability. An example is a client with Parkinson's disease in whom the lack of facial expression impedes the nonverbal communication of intimacy. The client can be taught to communicate feelings verbally that were previously conveyed with facial expressions.

> ### OT PRACTICE NOTES
> Discussion of sexuality is a way to explore feelings of dependency, identity, attractiveness, and unattractiveness.[43,51] Communication must be established about the client's feelings of sexual role changes. If a client's perceived roles are threatened, this situation should be dealt with as early as possible during intervention. If it is not, the effects could persist throughout the client's life and impinge on occupations important to the client.

VALUES CLARIFICATION

The **sexual values** of the client, the partner, and the therapist must be examined for the therapist to interact with the client in the most effective and positive manner.[6,21,56,65,74] Many professional schools do not train healthcare workers on the subject of sexuality and disability.[6,30,76,83]

In-service training can be arranged to help staff members become aware of the sexual needs of people with disability.[27,43] Books, articles, videos, training packets, and internet resources are available for professional education.[11,19,21,76] Sensitivity training for staff members is imperative in creating an atmosphere of openness to discussing issues of sexuality. The Sexual Attitude Reassessment Seminar (SARS)[32] uses lectures, media, and small group discussions to help participants explore their knowledge and beliefs about sexuality. This seminar also describes sexual problems, how they develop, and how education and therapy can help with their clients. At the very least, it is helpful for therapists to participate in in-service classes and to role-play situations so as to improve their knowledge and comfort in dealing with questions about sexuality from patients and families.

Unless the staff members are educated about the significance of sexuality and related issues, they may have negative feelings about dealing with these matters.[6,11,83,90] If the therapist is not aware of the thoughts and feelings of all of the individuals involved, the therapist could make incorrect assumptions that have negative results.[18] One of the most direct ways of gaining information is by taking a sexual history.[18,76,79] The purpose of a sexual history is to learn how a person thinks and feels about sex and bodily functions and to discover the needs of those concerned.[18,51,76] According to some researchers, individuals with a disabling condition may have had a sexual dysfunction before they acquired the physical disability. Taking the sexual history can help identify such a problem.[52]

SEXUAL HISTORY

When taking a sexual history, the therapist should create an environment that ensures confidentiality and encourages comfort and self-expression. Early in the intervention process, the therapist should ask about the client's concerns regarding contraception, safe sex, sexual orientation, gender, masturbation, sexual health, aging, menopause, and physical changes.

Box 12.3 lists some questions that could be asked. All questions should not be asked at the same time, nor would all questions be asked of every client.

After taking the sexual history, the therapist can often ascertain whether guilt or discomfort is connected with the sex act, body parts, or sexual alternatives (e.g., masturbation, oral sex, sexual positions, or sexual devices). For example, some clients report feelings of guilt or fear in relation to having sex after a heart attack or a stroke—fear that sex can cause a stroke, or guilt that it may have caused the first episode. Another fear is that the partner will not accept the presence of catheters, adaptive equipment, or scars. Performance is often an issue. Able-bodied individuals and those with disabilities ask questions about the sexual ability of the person with disabilities.

The therapist can provide appropriate and accurate information by (1) directing the client to other professionals; (2) providing references, websites, and books that discuss the subject; (3) showing movies; or (4) suggesting role models. The therapist

BOX 12.3 Questions to Ask in a Sexual History

- How did you first find out about sexuality?
- When and how did you first learn about heterosexuality and homosexuality?
- Who furnished you with information about sexuality when you were young?
- Were you ready for the information when you first heard about sexuality?
- How important is sexuality at this time in your life?
- How would you describe your sexual activities at this time?
- How do you feel sexuality expresses your feelings and meets your needs and those of others?
- If you could change aspects of your current sexual situation, what would you change and how would you change it?
- What concerns do you have about birth control, disease control, and sexual safety?
- What physical, medical, or drug-related concerns do you have relating to your sexuality?
- Have you ever been pressured, threatened, or forced into a sexual situation?
- Which sexual practices have you engaged in, in the past (e.g., oral, anal, and genital)?
- Do you consider certain sexual activities "kinky"? How do you feel about participating in such activities?
- How important do you think sexuality will be in your future?
- What concerns do you have about your sexuality?
- Are there questions or concerns that you have regarding this interview?

THREADED CASE STUDY

Shivani, Part 2

The following questions may have been able to elicit important responses from Shivani.

1. *How important is sexuality at this time in your life?*
   Shivani's answer would reveal that she does not feel that sexuality is important to her, but that it is to her spouse and also for having a child.
2. *How would you describe your sexual activities at this time?*
   The OT would find out that sex is uncomfortable for Shivani; the OT would also learn how Shivani views sexual activities—whether sexual activity is a meaningful activity to her, or more of a responsibility.
3. *If you could change aspects of your current sexual situation, what would you change and how would you change it?*
   Shivani may say that she is uncomfortable during sex because she had been molested previously and that sex is physically uncomfortable for her now, which makes her feel like a failure. The therapist may not want to pursue the discussion about the sexual molestation and the psychological counseling aspects, but may ask for a referral to a psychiatric professional. The physical discomfort may be then addressed. Positions could be found to make intercourse more comfortable, helping Shivani to feel less like a failure as a partner.

must be tactful and remember that the client may be questioning her or his own values and previous notions about sexuality.

Personal care issues (e.g., toileting, personal hygiene, menstrual hygiene, bathing, and birth control) can evoke reflection on values about sex and body image.

Self-care issues, particularly personal hygiene and sexuality, usually are not emphasized during acute illness and rehabilitation. Discussing such issues once or twice is not sufficient. The circumstances and environment in which these issues are discussed should also be considered. The therapist must create an environment that allows personal discussions. A personal conversation cannot take place in a crowded therapy room, during a rushed and impersonal treatment session, or with a therapist with whom a good personal rapport does not exist. Building rapport is a problem in healthcare facilities in which therapists are frequently rotated or work on a per diem basis.

A discussion of feelings will also help clients explore their new body, or adapt to ongoing degeneration of the body if there is a progressive disability. These conversations may take place while other therapeutic activities are in progress so that billing insurers for time is not a barrier.

SEXUAL ABUSE

The sexual abuse of adults with disabilities is a significant problem.[3,80,83,90] Clients should be made aware of the possibility of exploitation, especially when they use the internet for social networking and online dating. Others have reported that medical staff members took inappropriate liberties with them and that personal care attendants, on whom they depended, demanded sexual favors. Clients can and should report such abuse to their state's Adult Protective Services agency. The therapist also must report cases of suspected sexual abuse. The client may be reluctant to report abuse because of a concern that it will not be possible to get another aide or that, during the time it takes to hire another aide, essential assistance will not be available. These are major problems for a person who is dependent on others for care. However, therapists must discuss with clients the need for mandatory reporting, to reduce their reluctance to report. In addition, the therapist should provide emotional support throughout this reporting process and/or provide a mental health referral to assist the client once an abuse report has been made.

Therapists may not suspect caregivers, medical staff members, aides, transportation assistants, or volunteers of sexual abuse, but the therapist should be alert to signs of possible abuse even from these sources. Some individuals are sexual predators who prey on adults and children with disabilities. They may be drawn to the health fields with this motive.[3] The therapist must always be alert for signs of potential abuse, such as clients usually being upset after interacting with a specific person, the client being reluctant to be left alone with a particular caregiver, caregivers taking the client off alone for no apparent reason, excessive touching in a sensual manner by caregivers, the client being agitated when around a particular individual, and the client being overly compliant with a specific individual.

The therapy session should help clients develop a sense of personal ownership of their body. However, this goal is sometimes overlooked when the OT is working with adults and children. For example, children who believe that they do not have the right to say "no" to being touched, who cannot physically resist unwanted touching, and who may not be able to communicate that unwanted touching or frank abuse has taken place, are in jeopardy of being victimized.[3]

The therapist should ask permission before touching the client; the therapist should touch with respect and maintain the client's sense of dignity. If the therapist does not ask permission

to touch a client, the client can lose the sense of control over being touched by others. The therapist should guard against communicating this notion to clients and should educate clients about their personal rights regarding others touching them.

Naming body parts and body processes is a good way of helping clients take charge of their bodies. Once the body parts and processes have been named, using correct terminology rather than slang, the possibility exists for the client to communicate and to relate in an appropriate manner.[3,17,63,79] The use of the proper terms has the effect of helping the client view the body in a more positive way, whereas slang tends to communicate negative images.[79]

EFFECTS OF PHYSICAL DYSFUNCTION

Specific physical problems that may create difficulties in sexual performance for people with disabilities and their partners and suggestions for management of the problems are outlined next and summarized in Table 12.1.

Hypertonia

Hypertonia can increase when muscles are quickly stretched. To prevent quick stretching of muscles involved in a movement pattern, motion should be performed slowly. It is advisable to incorporate rotation into the movement to break up the tone. Slow rocking can be used to inhibit hypertonic musculature. Gentle shaking or slow stroking (massage) can also be inhibitory. Heat or cold can be used to inhibit tone. Clients with hypertonia should review options for different positions in which to have sexual intercourse. Alternative ways of dealing with personal hygiene (e.g., toileting, inserting tampons, gynecologic examinations, and birth control) may also need to be explored in relation to hypertonicity.

Shivani's OT discussed strategies that could be used to relax the hypertonicity in her legs, such as gently rocking her legs side to side while she was seated. Although initially presented as a means to reduce the hypertonicity affecting Shivani's sitting balance when toileting and for personal hygiene during menstruation, this technique also was suggested as a means to relax her legs before intercourse.

Hypotonia

Clients with low muscle tone (hypotonia) need physical support during sexual activity. Pillows, wedges, or bolsters may be used to support body parts, allowing for endurance and protecting the body from overstretching and fatigue. Sexual positions that

TABLE 12.1   Possible Effects of Selected Conditions on Sexual Functioning

Symptoms / Diagnosis	Anxiety/ Fear	Contractures	Cultural Barriers	Decreased Libido	Depression	Impotence	Incontinence	Limited ROM	Loss of mobility	Low Endurance	Medication	Paralysis/ Spasticity	Poor Body Image	Tremor	Catheter/ Ostomy
Amputation	X	X	X		X				X				X		
Arthritis	X	X	X	X	X			X	X	X	X		X		
Burns	X	X	X		X			X	X	X		X	X		
Cardiac disease	X		X	X	X	X	X		X	X	X		X		
Cerebral palsy	X	X	X		X			X	X	X		X	X	X	X
Cerebrovascular accident	X	X	X	X	X	X	X	X	X	X	X	X	X	X	X
Diabetes	X	X	X	X	X	X			X	X			X	X	
Hand injury	X	X	X		X			X	X			X	X		
Head injury	X	X	X	X	X	X	X	X	X	X	X	X	X	X	X
Musculoskeletal injury	X	X	X		X		X	X	X	X	X	X	X	X	
Spinal cord injury	X	X	X		X	X	X	X	X	X	X	X	X	X	X

allow support of the joints involved should be explored. The client and her or his partner should also explore their attitudes about the positions.

Ataxia, Decreased Coordination, Balance, and Apraxia

These conditions may have an impact on safe transfers and transitioning from various positions as well as movement with sexual activity and specific intended movements and positions. Clients with these difficulties may require assistance with safe positioning,

Low Endurance and Stamina

Prolonged sexual activity can be challenging because of low physical endurance. Some techniques for dealing with low endurance apply the principles of work simplification to sexual activity; for example, using timing to engage in sex when the client has the most energy and assuming positions in which sexual performance uses less energy.

Range of Motion and Contractures

Limited mobility and contractures prohibit many movement patterns and limit the number of positions for sex. Activity analysis must be done to find positions that allow sexual activity. This system often requires creative problem solving on the part of the client, the partner, and the responsible professional counselor.

Joint Degeneration

Conditions such as arthritis can cause pain, damage to the joints, and contractures. Avoiding stress and repetitive weight bearing on the joints can reduce joint damage. Activity analysis is needed to reduce joint stress and excessive weight bearing on the joints. It is necessary to find a position that takes weight and stress off the knees or hips, such as the one in Fig. 12.2. This position is sometimes referred to as the missionary position. A position with substantial hip abduction may not be acceptable for the client, in which case a side-lying position may be more comfortable. If hip abduction is limited, the woman should avoid positions such as those shown in Fig. 12.2 (also see Figs. 12.5 and 12.9, presented later in the chapter).

After Shivani's OT introduced the technique of slow rocking, Shivani asked about other positions that would be more

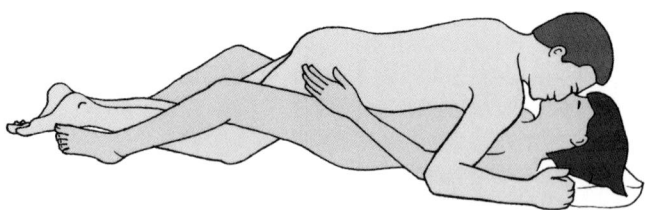

Fig. 12.2 This position places pressure on a female's bladder and requires hip abduction but little energy expenditure for her. An excellent discussion of these alternatives can be found in the journal *Sexuality and Disability* 12:1, 1994.

comfortable during intercourse. The OT discussed the possibility of using side-lying intercourse.

Pain and Pain Management

Pain limits the enjoyment of sexual activities.[35] Usually, at some time of day, pain is diminished and energy is at its highest. Sexual activities can be scheduled for such times. Many people find that sexual activity is possible after pain medication has taken effect. However, pain medications can also interfere with sexual functioning. These medications can interfere with alertness, sexual desire, and arousal. Another alternative can be the use of physical agents (heat and ice) and manual therapy (massage/soft tissue and joint mobilization) to be used before sexual activity and/or potential options incorporated into foreplay. Communication between partners is especially important when pain is involved. An unaffected partner who does not understand the negative effects of pain and/or the negative effects of pain medications may believe that the affected partner is not interested in sex and/or is not considering her or his personal needs. A referral to a psychotherapist who understands the effects of pain or to a pain specialist can help address emotional and physical aspects of this problem. The OT can help the client think of acceptable ways of meeting the partner's and the client's own sexual needs without causing pain. Masturbation and mutual masturbation with sexual fantasy are possible ways of meeting sexual needs in these circumstances. In this way, the partners are interacting and neither person feels isolated.

Loss of Sensation

The loss of sensation can affect the sexual relationship in several ways. The lack of erogenous sensation in the affected area can block proper warning that an area is being abraded (e.g., the vagina is not being sufficiently lubricated) or damaged (e.g., the bladder or even bones if the partner is on top and being too forceful). A lack of sensation may be a sign of disruption of the reflex loop responsible for sensation and erections in the male and sensation and lubrication in the female. Altered sensation also presents an increased risk of injury with sexual activities; it is important to be aware of this precaution. Having decreased sensation or impairment with vision, hearing, taste, and smell may affect sexual arousal and function as well.[31]

Cognitive Impairments and Behavioral Changes

Disabilities such as traumatic brain injury (TBI), multiple sclerosis (MS), and cerebrovascular accident (CVA) may affect sexual relationships and sex drive. Clients may have difficulties with impulsivity, poor initiation, attention/concentration, multitasking, memory, social communication, decreased awareness, and executive functions, such as problem solving and reasoning, all of which can affect relationships and successful sexual interactions.[9,73]

Emotional Factors

Depression and anxiety adversely affect sexual desire and arousal, and new onset of a disability has a high incidence of depression. For example, depression is seen in 11% to 61% of those with TBI or a spinal cord injury (SCI).[14,57]

Aging and Sexuality

With aging, changes take place that can affect sexuality. In women, menopause and the resulting hormonal changes cause vaginal atrophy, decreased lubrication, pain, an increased need for direct stimulation, and slower reactions to sexual stimulation. In men, greater stimulation may be needed to develop and maintain an erection, and the recovery time between erections may be greater. Men may also experience a shrinkage of their penis as their testosterone levels decrease with age. Both men and women can experience emotional changes involving their sexual desire or libido as they age. Partners can be informed of ways to increase direct stimulation and can be helped to understand that it is the quality, not the quantity, of sexual activity that is important in the relationship. In addition, many couples over time develop maladaptive sexual patterns. One common pattern is that any type of sexual or affectionate expression always culminates in sexual intercourse. Unfortunately, any type of sexual dysfunction that arises can lead to a significant decrease in expressions of affection or any sexual touching or communication for these individuals and their partners. Clients and their partners should be educated on the importance of intimacy, sexual and nonsexual touching, and other ways of expressing affection. The client should be made aware of the maturation process and its normal effect on sexuality so that the disability is not blamed for all problems.

Isolation

The environment is composed of objects, persons, and events. All activities involve an interaction between the person and environment. Some of the objects with which people with disabilities interact are wheelchairs, braces, canes, crutches, and splints. These objects are all hard, cold, and angular. They can communicate a hard exterior and a fragile interior and can convey the notion that no softness exists, that it is not safe to hug, and that a person in a wheelchair or in braces or on crutches can get hurt or toppled if touched. As a result of these ideas, individuals with a disability may feel isolated by the appliances or equipment they need to successfully interact with the world around them.

Some people tend to withdraw from the objects around the client. This may reinforce the client's notion of a lack of sensuousness and increase the client's sense of isolation. Clients often feel isolated and different from the "normal" population.[21] This phenomenon is more common among clients who have been out of the healthcare facility for a period of time. In the early phases of the disability, the therapist and the client can role-play about how to deal with a new partner or how to explain the equipment used, such as a catheter. This approach may help ease the client's anxieties and fears and increase their comfort with such issues. At the same time, the therapist should be communicating that sex may be a possibility in the future. It should be pointed out to clients that at no time in human history have people with disabilities not existed in society, that they are a part of society, and that it is not "abnormal" to have a disability. All people who live long enough eventually acquire a disability, to a greater or lesser extent.

Medication

An average of 4.5 million people in the United States experience various side effects from prescription medications.[5] Potential side effects of medication are impotence, delayed sexual response, or other problems. Diuretics and antihypertensives can cause erectile dysfunction, decreased desire, and changes in orgasm. Tranquilizers, selective serotonin reuptake inhibitors (SSRIs), and antidepressants can contribute to changes in sexual desire, arousal, and orgasm in some individuals.[77] Side effects of medication should be discussed with the prescriber and the pharmacist to see whether medications can be altered or changed. If they cannot be, acknowledging that the problem is a side effect of a needed medication can be helpful to the client. Clients should be strongly discouraged from stopping their medications on their own, without first discussing the implications with their prescriber.

Street drugs also have sexual side effects and adversely affect sexual functioning at every level of the sexual response cycle. For example, methamphetamines and cocaine may have the sexual side effect of decreased interest in sex and difficulty reaching orgasm. Marijuana and alcohol can cause difficulty in obtaining and sustaining erections. Occupational therapists do not condone the use of street drugs, but it is important for the OT to consider that such drugs may be part of a client's life, and providing education on these side effects is critical.

Performance Anxiety

At times of emotional stress, regardless of his age, a male client may have difficulty obtaining and maintaining an erection. Even one or two instances of difficulty with an erection can lead to increased anxiety and create a cycle of erectile dysfunction and even avoidance of sex. Another problem that can arise is premature ejaculation, which can in turn lead to performance anxiety. It can be helpful for the client and his partner to take the emphasis off erection and genital intercourse and focus on sensuality and making each other feel good. A massage or nondemand touching are techniques that can be helpful with performance anxiety. More specifically, with premature ejaculation there are very useful techniques the patient and his partner can be taught to manage the issue. If these approaches do not work and it has been determined that the problem is not physical or related to medications, a sex therapist or psychotherapist trained in sexuality may be needed to help the couple deal with the problem.

Skin Care

The person with a disability should be informed that positioning modifications might be needed to protect the skin, prevent skin breakdown, and increase pleasure. If a sexual position causes repeated rubbing on the skin, this friction can cause abrasions and result in skin damage. The therapist and client can discuss the use of various positions, and lubrication agents are important in preventing skin breakdown or issues related to decreased sensation. Pressure on bony prominences or pressure exerted in a specific area by a partner can also cause problems with skin irritation and must be avoided.

Lubrication

Stimulating natural lubrication in female clients is important. It may be overlooked in a woman with paralysis because she may not be able to feel the stimulation or lack of natural lubrication. Stimulation to cause reflexive lubrication should occur even when the woman does not feel it. Without proper lubrication, damage may occur without the woman being aware of the problem. If needed, artificial water-based lubricants should be used. The individual should be warned that only water-based lubricants are appropriate because petroleum-based lubricants can cause irritation and can attack the integrity of latex condoms, causing condom failure. This is a major concern because the female partner is more likely than the male to become infected with the human immunodeficiency virus (HIV) in any given heterosexual encounter.

Erection

Many men regard the ability to achieve an erection as one of the most significant signs of masculinity.[51] If awareness of sensory stimulation to the penis is blocked by the sensory loss associated with paralysis and if the male client does not try to stimulate a reflexogenic erection, he may believe that he is unable to obtain an erection. This is not necessarily true, and the client may go through much needless anguish. The client should be encouraged to explore his body.

Rubbing the penis, the thighs, or the anus can be effective ways to evoke a reflexogenic erection. Even rubbing the big toe has been reported by some men with quadriplegia to stimulate an erection. If the normal reflex arc is interrupted, it is usually not possible to achieve an erection, and alternative methods must be explored.

Alternative methods can be forms of sex that do not require an erect penis, such as using a vibrator or oral or digital sex. If the client feels that penile intercourse is the only acceptable method, other possibilities exist.[16] Injections or penile suppositories that stimulate erections can be used, but this practice may have adverse reactions or lead to problems if the client does not have good judgment or lacks hand dexterity. Penile vacuum devices are available that are very easy to use and result in erections firm enough for penetration. The use of a vibrator or massager against the penis to help produce ejaculate is sometimes effective and is one of the less invasive techniques.[79] Prescription medications are readily available for men with erectile dysfunction (i.e., sildenafil, vardenafil, tadalafil).

Fertility

Some disabilities may directly affect an individual's ability to biologically become a parent. For example, women who sustain an SCI or a TBI may experience a disruption in their menstrual cycle. This pause may last as long as 6 months or even a few years depending on the injury. However, a woman's ability to have children is not usually affected once menstruation resumes.

It should be noted that depending on the disability, women may be subject to certain pregnancy-related complications, and those should be discussed with a physician before considering pregnancy. Men with catastrophic injuries or illnesses (e.g., SCI) also experience difficulty with fertility. Typically, the reason for this is the inability to ejaculate during intercourse. Men who wish to father a child do have options, and a fertility specialist should be consulted.

Birth Control

Client should consult their healthcare provider when weighing the pros and cons of various methods of birth control. People with disabilities must consider a number of factors when planning birth control.[15,16,33,49,63] Because most disabling conditions do not impair fertility (especially for women), it is important for clients to be aware of birth control and potential complications of the use of birth control.

Adequate hand function is needed to successfully apply a condom. An applicator can be adapted in some cases, but someone with good hand dexterity must assemble the device beforehand. Diaphragms are not very feasible for people who have poor hand function, unless the partner does have hand function and both parties feel comfortable about inserting the diaphragm as part of foreplay. Insertable contraception options require functional use of the hands.

Using birth control pills can increase the risk of thrombosis, especially when the client is paralyzed or has impaired mobility. If the client has decreased sensation, the intrauterine device (IUD) can result in complications from bleeding, cramping, puncturing of the uterus, or infection. The use of spermicides requires good control of the hands or the assistance of the partner who has normal hand function. The use of nonoxynol-9 has been suspected to increase the risk of HIV transmission and should be avoided.[64] The injectable type of birth control may allow for easy use but has many of the same side effects as the pill. In using any method of birth control, the client must always be concerned with reducing the chance of infection and practicing safe sex.

Adaptive Aids

Adaptive aids may be necessary, especially if the client lacks hand function. One aid is a vibrator for foreplay or masturbation.[29] Special devices have been adapted for men and women.[18,49,63] Pillows may be used for positioning, and other equipment may be used for clients who have special needs. The therapist must prepare the client for the concept of using sexual aids before suggesting the option to the client. For example, the therapist can suggest that the client privately explore the sensation that the vibrator produces in the lower extremities. The client might discover the possible use of the vibrator for sexual stimulation or at least, when told how it can be used, may be more open to the idea of using a vibrator as a sexual aid.

There are many specially designed adaptive devices and tools available to enhance the sexual experience and facilitate access to a quality sex life for people with disabilities. The following are a sample of potential adaptive options:

- The IntimateRider Chair assists with sexual activity positioning and mobility. The small seat glide provides a fluid motion facilitated through minimal movement of the upper torso to mimic a pelvic thrust. A seat cushion or positioning support strap also can be applied.

- The Strapper Harness is a leather harness with a short smooth surface pubic plate to ensure no covering or irritation to the clitoris where a dildo can be attached.
- The Body Bouncer is made with a spring activated seat where slight momentum shifts allow the seated partner 8 to 9 inches of thrusting motion.
- Love bumper is a soft foam positioning pillow with an opening that can be used with a vibrator and dildo.
- The Thigh Sling is made of leather and positioned around the neck with adjustable padded loops for thigh straps. The design allows the person to maintain the pelvis in an open and elevated position, requiring little to no motor control during sexual activity.
- The Liberator Shapes are positioning devices with pillows and cushions in a variety of shapes and sizes to assist with necessary motions during various sexual activities.
- The Encore Deluxe Powered/Manual Vacuum Erection Device uses an external vacuum system to help with impotence and allows users to maintain erections for up to 30 minutes.

Safe Sex

Safe sex is an important aspect of sexual and overall health that needs to be addressed to minimize STIs, including the acquired immunodeficiency syndrome (AIDS), as well as unplanned pregnancies.[33] Clients need to be advised that this is a crucial issue. If there is sensory impairment in and around the genital area, the person might not be aware of an abrasion or infection. Any genital irritation or infection allows easy entrance of STD pathogens. The person with disability must be informed of the increased risk of HIV and STDs so that extra care can be taken.

Hygiene

Catheter care is a concern, especially when hand function is impaired. Questions may be raised about how or if a person with an indwelling catheter can have sex. Sex is possible for both men and women, but some precautions should be taken. If the catheter becomes kinked or closed off (which will definitely happen in the case of a catheterized man having vaginal intercourse), pressure should not be placed on the bladder. The bladder should be fully voided before sexual activity. Urine flow should be restricted for as short a time as possible, and no longer than 30 minutes. Damage to the bladder and kidneys could result if these precautions are not followed. The client should not drink fluids for at least 2 hours before sex to prevent the bladder from filling during this time. Sexual positions that avoid placing pressure on the bladder should be used, such as those shown in Figs. 12.3 to 12.10. Many of the same positions can be used if the client uses a stoma appliance.

Women who have various disabling conditions have reported irregular menstrual periods and deterioration of their neurological condition during menstruation.[88] Hygiene issues may occur for several reasons. Lack of education, poor hand function, and poor sensation are conditions that may contribute to menses complications. Information about toxic shock syndrome should

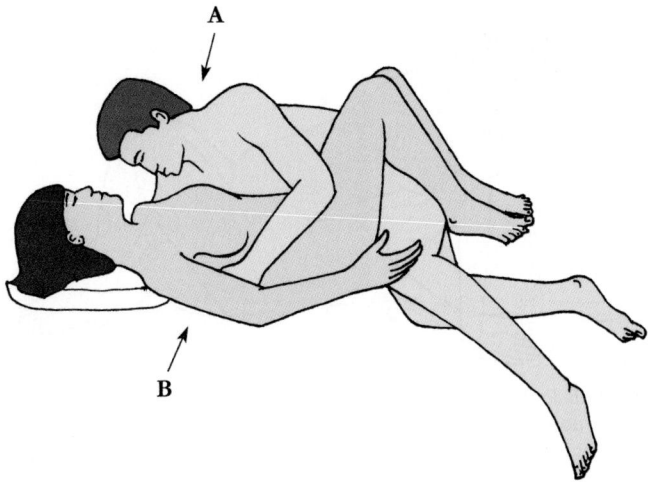

Fig. 12.3 Vaginal entry of partner B requires no hip abduction, and hip flexion tightness would not impede performance. Energy requirements for both partners are minimal, and bladder pressure, catheter safety, and stoma appliance safety should not be an issue for partner B. This position also may be recommended if partner B has back pain or is paralyzed, especially if a rolled-up towel is used to support the lumbar spine.

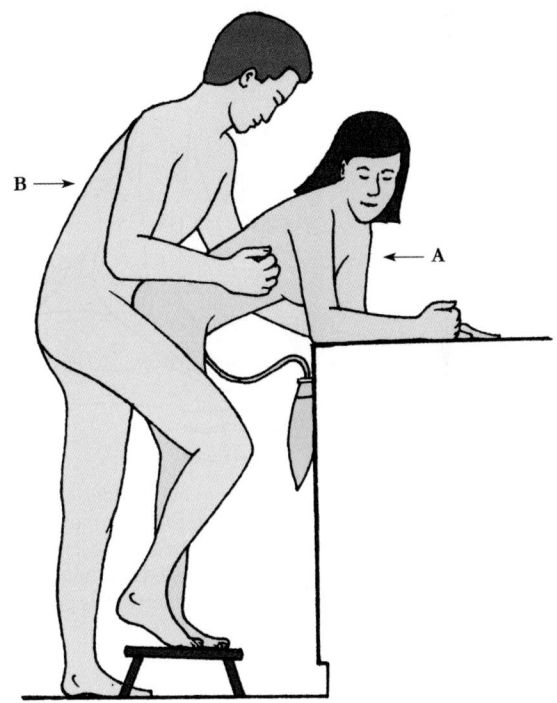

Fig. 12.4 Partner A needs little hip abduction but good strength. Partner B may feel less strain on his back. Hip, knee, or ankle joint degeneration would preclude this position for either partner.

be given to clients who may not feel or be aware of infection. A sanitary napkin or pad requires less fine motor skill and is less dependent on intact sensation than a tampon. Although the client's preferences must be considered, the therapist is responsible for educating a woman about the pros and cons of using either sanitary pads or tampons, menstruation cups, or specialized underwear during menstruation. Menopause complications may be increased, but this area may need further research.

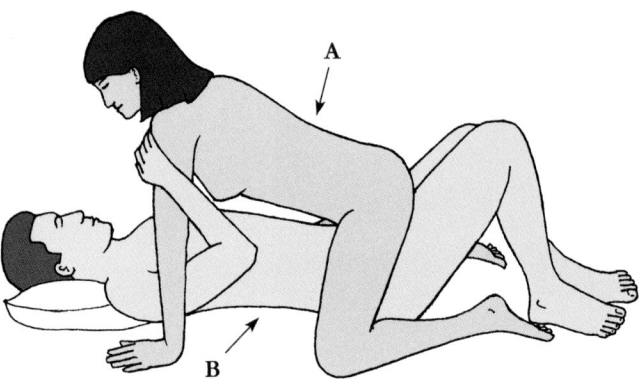

Fig. 12.5 Partner A must have hip abduction, balance, and endurance in this position, but pressure is kept off the bladder and stoma. If a catheter is used, it would be unrestricted. Back pain may be avoided by keeping the trunk vertical. Partner B's hip flexors could be contracted. If low back pain is a problem, the legs should be flexed and a rolled-up towel placed under the lower back. If a stoma appliance is used, this position would prevent interference. If low endurance is a problem, this position can be used effectively for partner B.

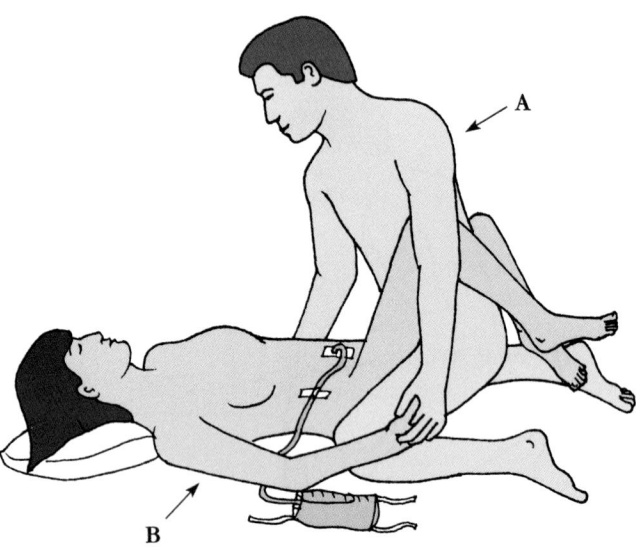

Fig 12.6 This position keeps pressure off the bladder, lessens the chance of tubing becoming bent, reduces pressure on the back (especially if a small rolled-up towel is used under the lower back), and does not require partner B to use much energy. The legs do not need to be as high as shown, but if the hip flexors are contracted, this position may be comfortable.

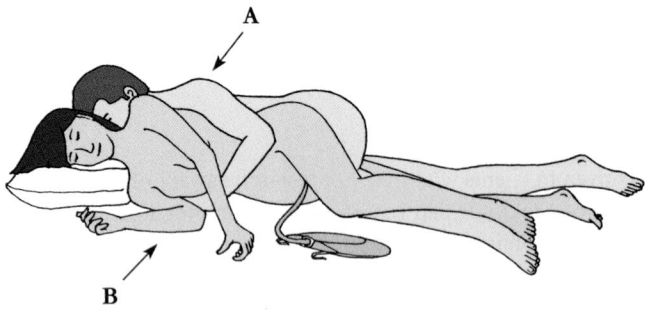

Fig 12.7 Partner B need not expend much energy in this position, and both partners may avoid swayback. Either partner may have hemiparesis. Partner B will not need hip abduction, and pressure on the stoma bag may be avoided.

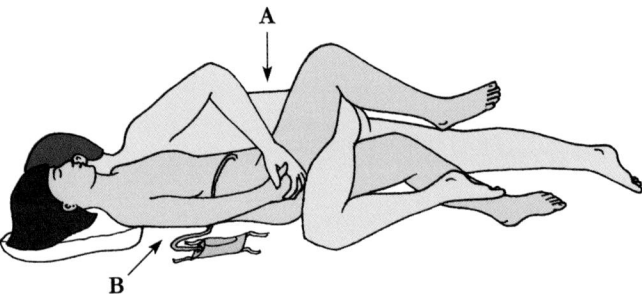

Fig. 12.8 This position can be used if either partner has hemiparesis, or if low endurance is a problem. Partner A may avoid swayback in this position.

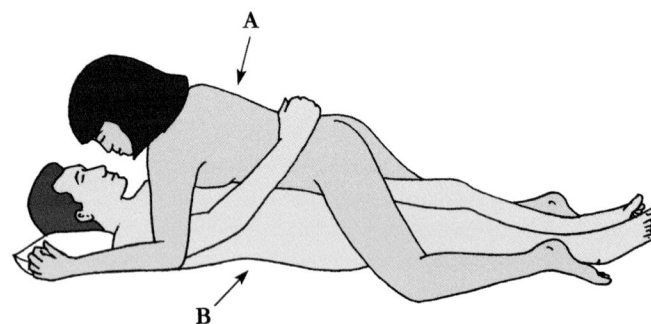

Fig 12.9 Partner B may be paralyzed or have limited range of motion. His back may need a rolled-up towel for support, and he must be concerned with pressure on his bladder.

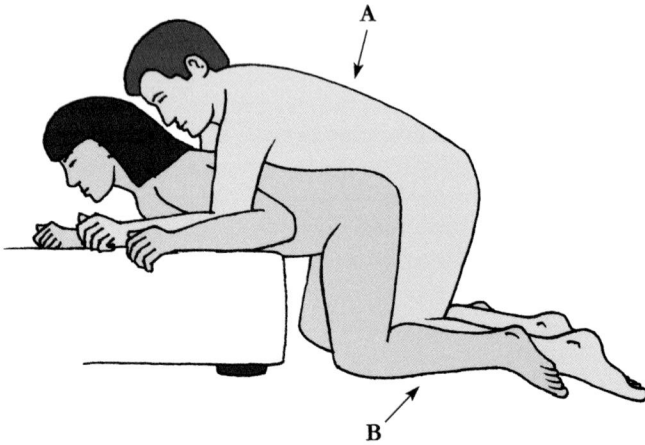

Fig. 12.10 Rear vaginal entry of partner B, who does not need much energy because support is provided by a low-level bed or cushioned footstool and little or no abduction of the hips is required. Flexion tightness of the hips does not affect performance. Because of the weight on partner B's knees, hips, and back, in addition to the inevitable repetitive movement at the hips, this would not be a good position for individuals with back, hip, or knee joint degeneration.

A person with an impairment of bowel or bladder function may have an occasional episode of incontinence during sexual activities. If the client and the therapist discuss this possibility and how to deal with it, some embarrassment can be averted when the episode occurs. The client and the therapist can role-play to explore various scenarios, such as, "You are planning intimacy with a new partner. How will you explain your catheter and appliances to the person?" These may be awkward conversations for the therapist and the client, but dealing with these issues beforehand is usually easier than waiting for the situation to arise. Such topics must be approached with caution and discretion.

Pregnancy, Delivery, and Childcare

Before becoming pregnant, women must weigh the risks and benefits of pregnancy, childbirth, and childcare. Complications of pregnancy may affect the client's function and mobility. These complications include the potential for respiratory or kidney problems, the effect of the increased body weight on transfers, an increased possibility of autonomic dysreflexia, and the need for increased bladder and bowel care; all of these should be considered when pregnancy is contemplated.[86] Labor and delivery can present some special problems, such as a lack of awareness of the beginning of labor contractions. Induction of labor may be contraindicated if a person has an SCI at T6 or above and the medical staff members are not trained to deal with the respiratory problems or dysreflexia that can result. After delivery, the parent with disability will need to have modifications made to the wheelchair. The client may need consultations to achieve an optimal level of function in the parenting role.[33]

Using Shivani as an example, the therapist may help her find information about pregnancy. Introducing her to sites appropriate for an online search or encouraging her to contact Planned Parenthood or United Cerebral Palsy can help her locate the information she needs to make informed decisions. She also could ask these agencies for a list of healthcare providers who have experience with women who were pregnant and had cerebral palsy.

The therapist may then simulate situations during the first year after birth. These may include how to transport an infant, change diapers and dress the child at different stages, play with the child, bathe the child, and deal with parenting despite mobility impairments, just to name a few possible scenarios.

SEXUAL SURROGATES

A sexual surrogate is someone trained to work with individuals to help them deal with sexual dysfunction or to explore their sexuality. Typically, a surrogate works with a therapist and a client. A sexual surrogate engages in sexual behaviors with the client, often using specific techniques that have been shown to be effective. The goal is to allow the client to explore aspects of sexual response, sexual feelings, and sexual techniques in a safe environment with a professional who is trained to provide feedback and offer advice.[42] The main goal of the interaction is education.

METHODS OF EDUCATION

The following techniques or approaches have been used effectively to deal with the emotional aspects of sex education for people with disability.

Repeat Information

Mentioning sexual issues just once is not enough for anyone. Whether the individual has a disability or not, most people need

to hear information more than once to fully understand the complexity of sexual function. This fact is especially true for people who are in crisis or who are in the process of adjustment to a disabling condition. Too much information, or more than is asked for, should not be offered at one time. Whenever possible, the therapist should try to say something positive in every conversation. Holding out hope for the restoration of function or alternative function is important. The therapist should not assume that the client understands all of the information. To verify that the client understands the information, the therapist should invite the client to ask questions and to paraphrase what was said.

Help the Client Discover the "New" Body

With any disability, the client's body image and perception of the body are altered. In effect, the client has a new body and must find altered ways of moving, interpreting sensations, and performing ADLs. A large part of the therapeutic experience is directed toward helping the client discover how to use this new body as effectively as possible. The therapist can facilitate this discovery of the new body by creating situations that encourage awareness of the body through the input of sensation and function.[52] The client alone or with the sexual partner can accomplish this awareness through exercises that encourage exploration of the body. Exercises such as the gentle tapping or rubbing of a specific area can be developed to see if sensation exists or if the stimulation causes a change in muscle tone. Many people with a disability such as paralysis report that they have experienced nongenital orgasms[15] by stimulating other new erogenous areas, often in the area just above where sensation starts to appear. The therapist may suggest ways to use this sensation or change in tone in ADLs or may ask the client to think of ways this change in tone could be used, such as triggering reflex leg extension to help with putting on pants. This discussion stimulates problem solving by the client.

PLISSIT, Ex-PLISSIT, and Recognition Models

The acronym PLISSIT, which was originally developed in 1976 by Jack Annon, stands for *p*ermission, *l*imited *i*nformation, *s*pecific *s*uggestions, and *i*ntensive *t*herapy. The Extended PLISSIT (Ex-PLISSIT) was introduced to the medical community to address permission at each stage of the process. PLISSIT is a progressive approach to guide the therapist in helping the client deal with sexual information.[4] The extended PLISSIT model was developed in the 2000s, which added the reflection and review process at each step of the process to encourage clinicians to reflect with clients and family members at each stage[85] (Fig. 12.11). The Ex-PLISSIT model also emphasizes the role of permission giving at each and every stage of the conversation between healthcare professionals and the client; thus, each stage has a foundation of permission-giving. *Permission* refers to allowing the client to feel new feelings and experiment with new thoughts or ideas regarding sexual functioning. *Limited information* refers to explaining what effect the disability can have on sexual functioning. An explanation with great detail is not usually necessary early in the counseling process. The next level of information is providing specific suggestions. It may be in the therapist's domain to give *specific suggestions* on

The Extended PLISSIT Model

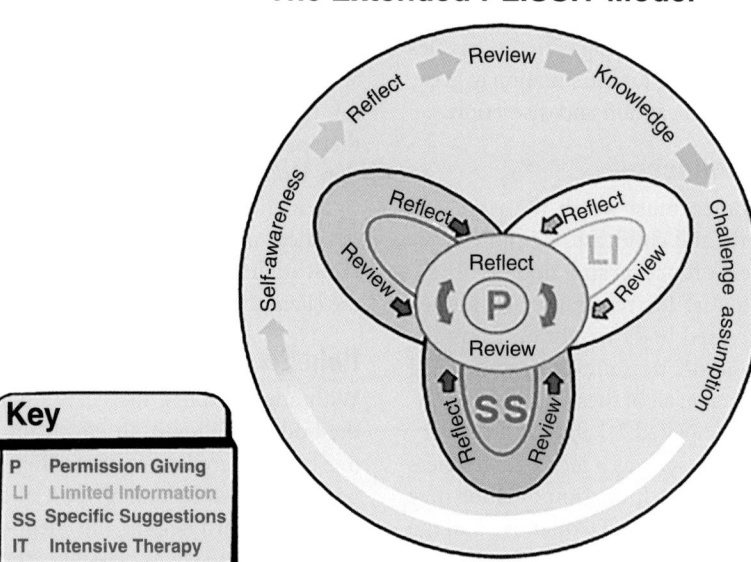

Fig. 12.11 The Ex-PLISSIT model is an extension of Annon's original PLISSIT model. (Reproduced from Davis S, Taylor B: From PLISSIT to Ex-PLISSIT. In David S, editor: *Rehabilitation: the use of theories and models in practice,* Edinburgh, 2006, Churchill Livingstone.)

dealing with specific problems that relate to the disability, such as positioning.

This is the highest level of input the average occupational therapist should attempt without advanced education and training in sexual counseling. *Intensive therapy* should be reserved for the rare client who has an abnormal coping pattern in dealing with sexuality. An extensive counseling background is needed to provide intensive therapy; therefore referral to a trained sex therapist is required in these situations.

An alternative framework to the Ex-PLISSIT is the Recognition Model.[20] This model was developed to address some of the limitations noted with the Ex-PLISSIT model. The Ex-PLISSIT model assumes that a team member or several team members will address the issue of sexuality using the steps outlined previously. Unfortunately, this does not consistently occur. The responsibility was often placed on the individual service user to request information instead of the service provider offering an opportunity to discuss issues related to sexuality. The Recognition Model uses a team approach whereby each team member has the responsibility to introduce the topic of sexuality as part of the rehabilitation process. A five-stage process has been outlined in which the first stage clearly recognizes the service user, client, or patient as a "sexual being with sexual needs and desires (p. 294)."[20] The second stage is that of providing sensitive, permission-giving strategies. This stage is focused on providing opportunities for conversations. Within the Recognition Model, there is the understanding that some team members, for various reasons, may not be able to provide this information. That is where specific team members can be identified to support the client. During this stage, printed materials can be provided to support the conversations about sexuality. The third stage involves exploration of sexuality and may include the

occupational therapist in considering how to manage spasticity or pain, or being unable to independently undress. This stage also includes experts in sexual health. The fourth stage identifies what issues fit within the team's expertise and boundaries. This includes the analysis of the activity and development of an intervention plan with client-centered goals. The fifth stage of the Recognition Model specifies the team make a referral to fully serve the client if the client's needs cannot be met with the team's level of skill and expertise. Key to the Recognition Model is the recognition of the client's sexuality and acknowledgement of the client as a sexual being.

Perform Activity Analysis

To assess the client's positioning needs, the therapist must analyze the demands of the particular activity. This analysis entails looking at the physical, psychological, social, cultural, and cognitive aspects of the client's functioning. Activity analysis should be implemented, using an objective and professional perspective. The therapist must realize that the sex act itself, if one exists, is only a small part of the act of making love and should be treated as just one more ADL that must be analyzed and with which the client needs professional assistance. The therapist must also remember that not all partners had sexual intercourse on a daily, weekly, or even yearly basis before the onset of the disability. The therapist's values and biases should not be imposed on the client. Same-sex partners, multiple partners, masturbation, or a preference for no sexual activities are some client practices that could evoke bias.

Provide Basic Sex Education

Some clients need basic sex education if they did not have the information before the onset of disability (Box 12.4). Some

BOX 12.4   The Sexual Response Cycle

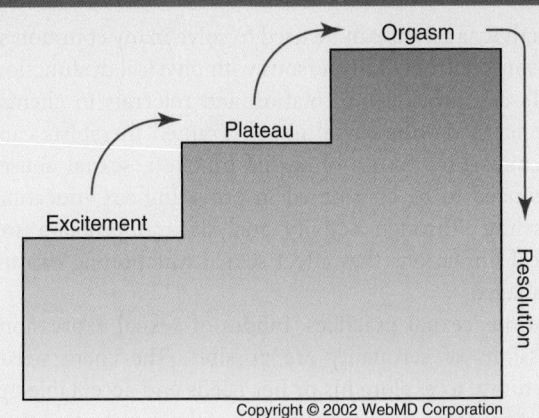

Copyright © 2002 WebMD Corporation

The sexual response cycle has four phases: excitement, plateau, orgasm, and resolution. Both men and women experience these phases, although the timing usually is different. For example, it is unlikely that both partners will reach orgasm at the same time. In addition, the intensity of the response and the time spent in each phase varies from person to person. Understanding these differences may help partners better understand one another's bodies and responses and thus enhance the sexual experience.

Phase 1: Excitement
General characteristics of the excitement phase, which can last a few minutes to several hours, include the following:
- Muscle tension increases.
- Heart rate quickens, and breathing is accelerated.
- Skin may become flushed (blotches of redness appear on the chest and back).
- Nipples become hardened or erect.
- Blood flow to the genitals increases, resulting in swelling of the woman's clitoris and labia minora (inner lips) and erection of the man's penis.
- Vaginal lubrication begins.
- The woman's breasts become fuller, and the vaginal walls begin to swell.
- The man's testicles swell, his scrotum tightens, and he begins secreting a lubricating liquid.

Phase 2: Plateau
General characteristics of the plateau phase, which extends to the brink of orgasm, include the following:
- The changes begun in phase 1 are intensified.
- The vagina continues to swell from increased blood flow, and the vaginal walls turn a dark purple.
- The woman's clitoris becomes highly sensitive (may even be painful to touch) and retracts under the clitoral hood to avoid direct stimulation from the penis.
- The man's testicles are withdrawn up into the scrotum.
- Breathing, heart rate, and blood pressure continue to increase.
- Muscle spasms may begin in the feet, face, and hands.
- Muscle tension increases.

Phase 3: Orgasm
The orgasm is the climax of the sexual response cycle. It is the shortest of the phases and generally lasts only a few seconds. General characteristics of this phase include the following:
- Involuntary muscle contractions begin.
- Blood pressure, heart rate, and breathing are at their highest rates, with a rapid intake of oxygen.
- Muscles in the feet spasm.
- There is a sudden, forceful release of sexual tension.
- In women, the muscles of the vagina contract, and the uterus undergoes rhythmic contractions.
- In men, rhythmic contractions of the muscles at the base of the penis result in the ejaculation of semen.
- A rash, or "sex flush," may appear over the entire body.

Phase 4: Resolution
During resolution, the body slowly returns to its normal level of functioning, and swollen and erect body parts return to their previous size and color. This phase is marked by a general sense of well-being, enhanced intimacy and, often, fatigue. Some women are capable of a rapid return to the orgasm phase with further sexual stimulation and may experience multiple orgasms. Men need recovery time after orgasm, called a *refractory period*, during which they cannot reach orgasm again. The duration of the refractory period varies among men and usually lengthens with advancing age.

Data from Kaplan HS: *The new sex therapy: active treatment of sexual dysfunctions*, New York, 1974, Routledge; and Masters WH, Johnson VE: *Human sexual response*, Boston, 1966, Little, Brown.

---

clients may not have been informed because of the disability, or they may be misinformed about sexual practices.[3,15,54,64] Research has shown that people with hearing impairments have substantially less information about sex than do those without hearing impairments.[84] In one study of adolescents with congenital disabilities, it was found that they were misinformed or not informed about sexual issues and that they relied on health professionals and parents to keep them informed.[7] Women who had not had sex before age 18 years may be less inclined to have sex later if they are not given sexual information.[23,29,54]

If the OT is not the one to educate the client or the client's partner, the therapist should anticipate the need for information and have resources available for the client to acquire the information. It is not advisable to recommend only books about sexuality and people with disabilities. Such books are useful, but their focus on the disability may be discouraging to some. Books written for the able bodied, such as *The Hite Report: A Nationwide Study of Female Sexuality*,[36] *The Hite Report on Male Sexuality*,[37] and *How to Satisfy a Woman Every Time*,[34] can be helpful. These books will not only give clients an understanding of sex, but they will also show clients that they are normal, while minimizing the focus on the disability.

Excellent books written for individuals with disabilities also can be recommended. Some of these are *Choices: A Guide to Sexual Counseling with the Physically Disabled*,[63] *Reproductive Issues for Persons with Physical Disabilities*,[33] *The Sensuous Wheeler*,[69] *Sexuality and the Person with Traumatic Brain Injury*,[31] *Sex and Back Pain*,[35] *Sexuality and Disabilities*,[56] *Sexual Function in People with Disability and Chronic Illness*,[76] and *Enabling Romance*.[49]

SUMMARY

This chapter began with the case of Shivani and examined some of the possible needs of people with disabilities that affect the ADLs of sexuality. This topic is a powerful one that the OT must deal with in a professional and sensitive manner. We have seen that Shivani can engage in sexual activity, become pregnant, and be a good parent. She may need assistance with finding the better positions to have sex, and she may learn to enjoy her body and sex even though she was sexually abused. All of these issues may be within the role of the OT and should be dealt with to improve the quality of life for the client.

OTs are concerned with the sexuality of their clients because sexuality is related to self-esteem, it influences the adjustment to disability, and it is an activity of daily living. As with other ADLs, a physical dysfunction can necessitate some changes in the performance of sexual activities. Education, counseling, and activity analysis can be used to solve many common sexual problems confronted by persons with physical dysfunction.

OTs can provide information and referrals to clients who are concerned with sexual issues. Trained therapists can provide counseling. Issues of sexual function, sexual abuse, and values need to be considered in providing sex education and counseling. Through activity analysis and problem solving, physical limitations that affect sexual functioning can usually be managed.

Various sexual practices, modes of sexual expression, and expressions of sensuality are possible. The client needs the opportunity to explore his or her needs and acceptable options to meet those needs. The OT is one of the members of the rehabilitation team who has something to offer the client in the area of rehabilitation and sexuality and sensuality.

REVIEW QUESTIONS

1. List at least five areas related to sensuality or sexuality that are usually the concerns of the OT.
2. What are some common attitudes of the able-bodied population about the sexuality of persons with physical dysfunction?
3. How do these attitudes affect disabled persons' perception of themselves and attitudes toward their own sexuality?
4. How is sexuality related to self-esteem and a sense of attractiveness?
5. Describe some typical questions for taking a sexual history. How can these questions be used to clarify values about sexuality?
6. How do mobility aids and assistive devices affect sexual functioning? How can this concern be managed?
7. What are some signs of potential sexual abuse of adults?
8. What are some suggestions for dealing with the following physical symptoms during sexual activity: hypertonia, low endurance, joint degeneration, and loss of sensation?
9. List some medications that may cause sexual dysfunction.
10. Discuss some issues and precautions relative to birth control for the woman with a physical disability.
11. How is a catheter managed during sexual activity?
12. What are some potential problems in pregnancy, delivery, and childcare?
13. Discuss some techniques for educating a person about sexual issues.

REFERENCES

1. Aloni R, Katz S: *Sexual difficulties after traumatic brain injury and ways to deal with it*, Springfield, IL, 2003, Charles C Thomas, pp 9–19.
2. American Occupational Therapy Association: Occupational therapy practice framework: Domain and process (4th ed.), *American Journal of Occupational Therapy* 74(Suppl. 2):1–87, 2020. https://doi.org/10.5014/ajot.2020.74S2001.
3. Andrews AB, Veronen LJ: Sexual assault and people with disabilities, *J Soc Work Hum Sex* 8:137–159, 1993.
4. Annon JS: *The behavioral treatment of sexual problems (vols 1 and 2)*, Honolulu, 1974, Enabling Systems.
5. Barry P: Prescription drug side effects. *AARP Bulletin*, Sept 1, 2011, https://www.aarp.org/health/drugs-supplements/info-09-2011/prescription-drug-side-effects.html.
6. Becker H, Stuifbergen A, Tinkle M: Reproductive healthcare experiences of women with physical disabilities: a qualitative study, *Arch Phys Med Rehabil* 78(12 Suppl 5):S26, 1997.
7. Berman H, Harris D, Enright R, et al: Sexuality and the adolescent with a physical disability: understandings and misunderstandings, *Issues Compr Pediatr Nurs* 22:183, 1999.
8. Blum RW: Sexual health contraceptive needs of adolescents with chronic conditions, *Arch Pediatr Adolesc Med* 151:330–337, 1997.
9. Bombardier CH, Ehde DM, Stoelb B, Molton IR: The relationship of age-related factors to psychological functioning among people with disabilities, *Phys Med Rehabil Clin N Am* 21:281–297, 2010.
10. Booth S, Kendall M, Fronek P, Miller D, Geraghty T: Training the interdisciplinary team in sexuality rehabilitation following spinal cord injury: a needs assessment, *Sex Disabil* 21:249–261, 2003.
11. Boyle PS: Training in sexuality and disability: preparing social workers to provide services to individuals with disabilities, *J Soc Work Hum Sex* 8:45, 1993.
12. Braithwaite DO: From majority to minority: an analysis of cultural change from able-bodied to disabled, *Int J Intercult Relat* 14:465, 1990.
13. Center for Research on Women with Disabilities: National Study of Women with Physical Disabilities. (2003). http://www.bcm.tmc.edu/crowd/national_study/MAJORFIN.htm.
14. Chevalier Z, Kennedy P, Sherlock O: Spinal cord injury, coping and psychological adjustment: a literature review, *Spinal Cord* 47:778–782, 2009.

15. Choquet M, Du Pasquier Fediaevsky L, Manfredi R: National Institute of Health and Medical Research (INSERM), Unit 169, Villejuif, France: Sexual behavior among adolescents reporting chronic conditions: a French national survey *J Adolesc Health*, 20:62–67, 1997.

16. Cole SS, Cole TM: Sexuality, disability, and reproductive issues for persons with disabilities. In Haseltine FP, Cole SS, Gray DB, editors: *Reproductive issues for persons with physical disabilities*, Baltimore, 1993, Paul H Brooks.

17. Cole SS, Cole TM: Sexuality, disability, and reproductive issues through the lifespan, *Sex Disabil* 11:189, 1993.

18. Cole TM: Gathering a sex history from a physically disabled adult, *Sex Disabil* 9:29–37, 1991.

19. Cornelius DA: *Who cares? A handbook on sex education and counseling services for disabled people*, Baltimore, 1982, University Park Press.

20. Couldrick L, Sadlo G, Cross V: Proposing a new sexual health model of practice for disability teams: the Recognition Model, *International Journal of Therapy and Rehabilitation* 17:290–298, 2010. https://doi.org/10.12968/ijtr.2010.17.6.48152.

21. Ducharme S, Gill KM: Sexual values, training, and professional roles, *J Head Trauma Rehabil* 5:38–45, 1990.

22. Edwards DF, Baum CM: Caregivers' burden across stages of dementia, *OT Practice* 2:13, 1990.

23. Ferreiro-Velasco ME, Barca-Buyo A, Salvador de la Barrera S, et al: Sexual issues in a sample of women with spinal cord injury, *Spinal Cord* 43(1):51–55, 2005.

24. Fisher TL, Laud PW, Byfield M, et al: Sexual health after spinal cord injury: a longitudinal study, *Arch Phys Med Rehabil* 83:1043, 2002.

25. Fritz HA, Dillaway H, Lysack CL: "Don't think paralysis takes away your womanhood": sexual intimacy after spinal cord injury, *Am J Occup Ther* 69(2):1–10, 2015. http://doi.org/10.5014/ajot.2015.015040.

26. Froehlich J: Occupational therapy interventions with survivors of sexual abuse, *Occup Ther Health Care* 8:1, 1992.

27. Gender AR: An overview of the nurse's role in dealing with sexuality, *Sex Disabil* 10:71, 1992.

28. Giaquinto S, Buzzelli S, Di Francesco L, Nolfe G: Evaluation of sexual changes after stroke, *J Clin Psychiatry* 64:302, 2003.

29. Goldstein H, Runyon C: An occupational therapy educational module to increase sensitivity about geriatric sexuality, *Phys Occup Ther Geriatr* 11:57, 1993.

30. Greydanus DE, Rimsza ME, Newhouse PA: Adolescent sexuality and disability, *Adolesc Med* 13:223, 2002.

31. Griffith E, Lemberg S: *Sexuality and the person with traumatic brain injury: a guide for families*. Philadelphia, 1993, FA Davis.

32. Halstead LS, Halstead MG, Salhoot JT, Stock DD, Sparks RW: Sexual attitudes, behavior and satisfaction for able-bodied and disabled participants attending workshops in human sexuality, *Arch Phys Med Rehabil* 59:497–501, 1978.

33. Haseltine FP, Cole SS, Gray DB: *Reproductive issues for persons with physical disabilities*, Baltimore, 1993, Paul H Brooks.

34. Hayden N: *How to satisfy a woman every time*, New York, 1982, Bibli O'Phile.

35. Hebert L: *Sex and back pain*, Bloomington, MN, 1987, Educational Opportunities.

36. Hite S: *The Hite Report: a nationwide study of female sexuality*, New York, 1991, Seven Stories Press.

37. Hite S: *The Hite report on male sexuality*, New York, 1981, Knopf.

38. Institute of Medicine (IOM): *The Health of Lesbian, Gay, Bisexual, and Transgender (LGBT) People: Building a foundation for better understanding*, 2011, National Academies Press (US). https://www.ncbi.nlm.nih.gov/books/NBK64801/.

39. Kahn NF, Suchindran CM, Halpern CT: Sexual partner accumulation from adolescence to early adulthood in populations with physical disabilities in the U.S, *Journal of Adolescent Health* 68:991–998, 2021. https://doi.org/10.1016/j.jadohealth.2020.08.020.

40. Kalpakjian CZ, Kreschmer JM, Slavin MD, Kisala PA, Quint EH, Chiaravalloti ND, Jenkins N, Bushnik T, Amtmann D, Tulsky DS, Madrid R, Parten R, Evitts M, Grawi CL: Reproductive health in women with physical disability: a conceptual framework for the development of new Patient-Reported Outcome Measures, *Journal of Women's Health* 29:1427–1436, 2020. https://doi.org/10.1089/jwh.2019.8174.

41. Kaufman M: *Easy for you to say: Q & As for teens living with chronic illness or disability*, Richmond Hill, ON, Canada, 1995, Firefly Books.

42. Kaufman M, Silverberg C, Odette F: *The ultimate guide to sex and disability: for all of us who live with disabilities, chronic pain, and illness*, San Francisco, 2003, Cleis Press.

43. Kettl P, Zarefoss S, Jacoby K, et al: Female sexuality after spinal cord injury, *Sex Disabil* 9:287, 1991.

44. Korpelainen JT, Nieminen P, Myllylä VV: Sexual functioning among stroke patients and their spouses, *Stroke* 30:715, 1999.

45. Krause JS, Crewe NM: Chronological age, time since injury, and time of measurement: effect on adjustment after spinal cord injury, *Arch Phys Med Rehabil* 72:91, 1991.

46. Kreuter M: Partner relationships, sexuality and quality of life in persons with spinal cord injury and traumatic brain injury, *Spinal Cord* 1998(36):252–261, 1997.

47. Kriegsman K: Taking charge: teenagers talk about life and physical disabilities, 1992, Woodbine House.

48. Kroll, K. (2001). *Enabling romance: a guide to love, sex, and relationships for the disabled (and the people who care about them)*. No Limits Communication.

49. Kroll K, Klein EL: *Enabling romance*, New York, 1992, Harmony Books.

50. Kuzma EK, Pardee M, Darling-Fisher CS: Lesbian, gay, bisexual, and transgender health: creating safe spaces and caring for patients with cultural humility, *Journal of the American Association of Nurse Practitioners* 31(3):167–174, 2019. https://doi.org/10.1097/JXX.0000000000000131.

51. Lefebvre KA: Sexual assessment planning, *J Head Trauma Rehabil* 5:25, 1990.

52. Lemon MA: Sexual counseling and spinal cord injury, *Sex Disabil* 11:73, 1993.

53. Lim FA, Brown DV Jr, Kim SMJ: Addressing health care disparities in the lesbian, gay, bisexual, and transgender population: a review of best practices. AJN, *The American Journal of Nursing* 114(6):24–34, 2014.

54. Low WY, Zubir TN: Sexual issues of the disabled: implications for public health education, *Asia Pac J Public Health* 12(Suppl):S78, 2000.

55. Lynch C, Fortune T: Applying an occupational lens to thinking about and addressing sexuality, *Sexuality and Disability* 37:145–159, 2019. https://doi.org/10.1007/s11195-019-09566-7.

56. Mackelprang R, Valentine D: *Sexuality and disabilities: a guide for human service practitioners*, Binghamton, NY, 1993, Haworth Press.

57. Maller JJ, et al: Traumatic brain injury, major depression, and diffusion tensor imaging: making connections, *Brain Res Rev* 64:213–240, 2010.

58. Mamali FC, Chapman M, Lehane CM, Dammeyer J: A national survey on intimate relationships, sexual activity, and sexual satisfaction among adults with physical and mental disabilities, *Sexuality and Disability* 38:469–489, 2020. https://doi.org/10.1007/s11195-020-09645-0.

59. Mayer K, Bradford J, Makadon H, Stall R, Goldhammer H, Landers S: Sexual and gender minority health: What we know and what needs to be done, *American Journal of Public Health* 98(6):989–995, 2008. https://doi.org/10.2105/AJPH.2007.127811.

60. McCabe MP, Taleporos G: Sexual esteem, sexual satisfaction, and sexual behavior among people with physical disability, *Arch Sex Behav* 32:359, 2003.

61. McComas J, Hébert C, Giacomin C, Kaplan D, Dulberg C: Experiences of students and practicing physical therapists with inappropriate patient sexual behavior, *Phys Ther* 73:762–769, 1993.

62. Morozowski M, Roughley RA: The journey of sexuality after spinal cord injury: implications for allied health professionals, *Canadian Journal of Human Sexuality* 29:354–365, 2020. https://doi.org/10.3138/cjhs.2020-0024.

63. Neistadt ME, Freda M: *Choices: a guide to sexual counseling with physically disabled adults*, Malabar, FL, 1987, Krieger.

64. Neufeld JA, et al: Adolescent sexuality and disability, *Phys Med Rehabil Clin North Am* 13:857, 2002.

65. Nosek M, et al: Psychological and psychosocial disorders: sexuality issues for women with physical disabilities, *Rehabil Res Development Progress Reports* 34:244, 1997.

66. Olkin R: *What psychotherapists should know about disability*, New York, 1999, Guilford Press, pp 226–237.

67. Price-Feeney M, Ybarra ML, Mitchell KJ: Health indicators of lesbian, gay, bisexual, and other sexual minority (LGB+) youth living in rural communities, *The Journal of Pediatrics* 205:236–243, 2019. https://doi.org/10.1016/j.jpeds.2018.09.059.

68. Primary care protocol for Transgender Patient care: *Center of excellence for transgender health*. University of California, San Francisco, April 2011, Department of Family and Community Medicine.

69. Rabin BJ: *The sensuous wheeler*, Long Beach, CA, 1980, Barry J Rabin.

70. Rintala D, Howland CA, Nosek MA, et al: Dating issues for women with physical disabilities, *Sex Disabil* 15:219, 1997.

71. Romeo AJ, Wanlass R, Arenas S: A profile of psychosexual functioning in males following spinal cord injury, *Sex Disabil* 11:269, 1993.

72. Rose N, Hughes C: Addressing sex in occupational therapy: a constructed autoethnography, *American Journal of Occupational Therapy* 72:1–6, 2018. https://doi.org/10.5014/ajot.2018.026005.

73. Sandel ME, Delmonico RL, Kotch MJ: Sexuality, intimacy and reproduction following traumatic brain injury. In Zasler N, Katz D, Zafonte R, editors: *Brain injury medicine* ed 2, New York, 2013, Demos Medical Publishing.

74. Sandowski C: Responding to the sexual concerns of persons with disabilities, *J Soc Work Hum Sex* 8:29, 1993.

75. Schmidt EK, Hand BN, Havercamp S, Sommerich C, Weaver L, Darragh A: Sex education practices for people with intellectual and developmental disabilities: A qualitative study, *American Journal of Occupational Therapy* 75:7503180060, 2021.

76. Sipski M, Alexander C: *Sexual function in people with disability and chronic illness*, Gaithersburg, MD, 1997, Aspen.

77. Sipski ML, Alexander CJ: *Sexual function in people with disability and chronic illness: a health professional's guide*, New York, 1997, Aspen.

78. Slocum C, Halloran M, Unser C: A primary care provider's guide to clinical needs of women with spinal cord injury, *Topics in Spinal Cord Injury Rehabilitation* 26:166–171, 2020. https://doi.org/10.46292/sci2603-166.

79. Smith M: Pediatric sexuality: promoting normal sexual development in children, *Nurse Pract* 18:37, 1993.

80. Sobsey D, Randall W, Parrila RK: Gender differences in abused children with and without disabilities, *Child Abuse Negl* 21:707, 1997.

81. Stockard S: Caring for the sexually aggressive patient: you don't have to blush and bear it, *Nursing* 21:72, 1991.

82. Summerville P, McKenna K: Sexuality education and counselling for individuals with a spinal cord injury: implications for occupational therapy, *Br J Occup Ther* 61:275–279, 1998.

83. Suris JC, Resnick MD, Cassuto N, Blum RW: Sexual behavior of adolescents with chronic disease and disability, *J Adolesc Health* 19:124, 1996.

84. Swartz DB: A comparative study of sex knowledge among hearing and deaf college freshmen, *Sex Disabil* 11:129, 1993.

85. Taylor B, Davis S: The extended PLISSIT model for addressing the sexual wellbeing of individuals with an acquired disability or chronic illness, *Sexuality and Disability* 25(3):135–139, 2007. https://doi.org/10.1007/s11195-007-9044-x.

86. Verduyn WH: Spinal cord injured women, pregnancy, and delivery, *Sex Disabil* 11:229–234, 1993.

87. Walker B, Otte K, Lemond K, Hess P, Kaizer K, Faulkner T, Christy D: Development of the Occupational Performance Inventory of Sexuality and Intimacy (OPISI): Phase One, *The Open Journal of Occupational Therapy* 8(2):1–18, 2020. https://doi.org/10.15453/2168-6408.1694.

88. Weppner DM, Brownscheidle CM: The evaluation of the healthcare needs of women with disabilities, *Prim Care Update Ob Gyns* 5:210, 1998.

89. Yim SY, et al: Quality of marital life in Korean spinal cord injured patients, *Spinal Cord* 36:826, 1998.

90. Young ME, Nosek MA, Howland C, Chanpong G, Rintala DH: Prevalence of abuse of women with physical disabilities, *Arch Phys Med Rehabil* 78(12 Suppl 5):S34, 1997.

91. Zani B: Male and female patterns in the discovery of sexuality during adolescence, *J Adolesc* 14:163, 1991.

SUGGESTED READINGS

Amador MJ, Lynn CM, Brackett NL: *A guide and resource directory to male fertility following spinal cord injury/dysfunction*, 2000, Miami Project to Cure Paralysis.

Gregory MF: *Sexual adjustment: a guide for the spinal cord injured*, Bloomington, IL, 1993, Accent on Living.

Greydanus DE: *Caring for your adolescent: the complete and authoritative guide*, New York, 2003, Bantam Books.

Karp G: *Disability and the art of kissing*, San Rafael, CA, 2006, Life on Wheels Press.

Kaufman M, Silverberg C, Odette F: *The ultimate guide to sex and disability*, San Francisco, 2003, Cleis Press.

Kempton W, Caparulo F: *Sex education for persons with disabilities that hinder learning: a teacher's guide*, Santa Barbara, CA, 1989, James Stanfield.

Leyson JF: *Sexual rehabilitation of the spinal-cord-injured patient*, Totowa, NJ, 1991, Humana Press.

Mackelprang R, Valentine D: *Sexuality and disabilities: a guide for human service practitioners*, Binghamton, NY, 1993, Haworth Press.

Sandowski C: Sexual concern when illness or disability strikes, Springfield, IL, 1989, Charles C Thomas. In *Resources for people with disabilities and chronic conditions*, ed 2, Lexington, KY, 1993, Resources for Rehabilitation.

Shortridge J, Steele-Clapp L, Lamin J: Sexuality and disability: a SIECUS annotated bibliography of available print materials, *Sex Disabil* 11:159, 1993.

Sipski M, Alexander C: *Sexual function in people with disability and chronic illness*, Gaithersburg, MD, 1997, Aspen.

Sobsey D, Gray S, editors: *Disability, sexuality, and abuse*, Baltimore, 1991, Paul H Brooks.

RESOURCES

Sexuality Reborn

Video available for purchase from the Kessler Medical Rehabilitation Research and Education Center

https://www.kflearn.org/courses/sexuality-reborn

Through the Looking Glass

2198 Sixth Street, Suite 100, Berkeley, CA 94710-2204

http://lookingglass.org

American Association of Sexuality Educators, Counselors and Therapists

435 North Michigan Avenue, Suite 1717, Chicago, IL 60611

https://www.aasect.org/

Association for Sexual Adjustment in Disability

PO Box 3579, Downey, CA 90292

Sex Information and Education Council of the United States (SIECUS)

130 West 42nd Street, Suite 2500, New York, NY 10036

https://siecus.org/

Sexuality and Disability Training Center—University of Michigan Medical Center

Department of Physical Medicine and Rehabilitation

1500 East Medical Center Drive, Ann Arbor, MI 48109

https://www.uofmhealth.org/conditions-treatments/sexual-health

The Task Force on Sexuality and Disability of the American Congress of Rehabilitation Medicine

11654 Plaza America Drive, Suite 535

Reston, VA 20190-4700

https://acrm.org/about/committees-groups/evidence-and-practice/

13

Sleep and Rest

Jean S. Koketsu

LEARNING OBJECTIVES

After studying this chapter, the student or practitioner will be able to do the following:

1. Describe sleep architecture in the young adult population.
2. Describe how sleep architecture changes across the life span.
3. Describe the difference between sleep and rest.
4. Describe at least five negative consequences of poor sleep and rest in daily occupations.
5. Name at least seven techniques to promote good sleep hygiene techniques that will optimize conditions to facilitate sleep.
6. Describe the role of the occupational therapy practitioner in sleep and rest.

CHAPTER OUTLINE

KEY TERMS

Circadian rhythm
Comorbid insomnia
Excessive daytime sleepiness (EDS)
Homeostasis
Hypnogram
Insomnia
Non–rapid eye movement (NREM) sleep

Polysomnography (PSG)
Rapid eye movement (REM) sleep
Rest
Sleep
Sleep architecture
Sleep hygiene

THREADED CASE STUDY

Mrs. Tanaka, Part 1

Mrs. Tanaka (prefers use of the pronouns she/her/hers), a 63-year-old first-grade teacher born and raised in California, was diagnosed with left ischemic cerebro-vascular accident (CVA) and right hemiplegia. She was admitted to the in-client rehabilitation unit that specializes in clients with neurological injuries or events. She is married and lives with her husband of 40 years in a single-story house, to which she will return. Mrs. Tanaka has two adult children and three grandchildren. Her 65-year-old husband is in good health and will be her caregiver upon discharge.

Before the CVA, Mrs. Tanaka enjoyed working as a teacher and taking care of her grandchildren. Her status at evaluation consisted of the following: She had right hemiplegia with severe sensory and perceptual motor deficits. Her right arm was edematous, her muscles were hypotonic and dependent for movement. She was able to follow one-step verbal/gestural cues with moderate assistance. She required maximum assistance for bed mobility, dressing, hygiene, and grooming because of distractibility and impairments in trunk control, balance, awareness of her right side, and endurance. She was totally dependent for bathing, basic transfers, all instrumental activities of daily living (IADLs), and community mobility. Mrs. Tanaka tolerated 15 minutes of the team evaluation before falling asleep. The prior hospital did not note any sleep disturbance.

The occupational therapist (OT) scheduled an appointment to see Mrs. Tanaka in the morning to work on activities of daily living (ADLs), such as bed mobility,

transfers, dressing, and hygiene activities. The nursing staff noted that the client had a "rough night" and slept for only 2 to 3 hours. Her hospital roommate complained to the occupational therapist that Mrs. Tanaka snores loudly and stated that she wanted to change rooms because of this. Throughout the day, Mrs. Tanaka was unable to participate in all therapies because of her sleepiness. As the first week of her rehabilitation stay progressed, she continued to have difficulty participating in therapies because of her sleepiness.

Mrs. Tanaka, her family, and the rehabilitation team are concerned about her inability to get restful sleep at night and to stay awake during the day, so as to fully benefit from therapies and to reach her rehabilitation goals before returning home.

This chapter addresses sleep and rest, two occupational performance areas within the domain of OT practice.

Critical Thinking Questions

1. What is the role of the occupational therapist in addressing Mrs. Tanaka's sleep disturbance?
2. What are sleep and rest, and why do occupational therapists need to address these areas of occupation?
3. What can an occupational therapist do to help with Mrs. Tanaka's sleep difficulty?

To help guide occupational therapists in their practice, the American Occupational Therapy Association (AOTA), the national organization representing occupational therapy in the United States, has established the Occupational Therapy Practice Framework (OTPF) (2020).[15] The OTPF is reviewed every 5 years and is considered an evolving document. The original OTPF (2002) identified seven performance areas in which humans engage; in this first edition, sleep and rest were organized under the category Activities of Daily Living (ADLs).[10] The second edition (OTPF-2 [2008]) contained several revisions, and one change was reclassification of sleep and rest as its own category of occupation.[11] In the 2014 OTPF-3, sleep and rest remained its own separate category of occupation among seven other categories and the OTPF-4, kept rest and sleep as one of nine major occupations in which humans engage.[13,15]

In 1922 Adolf Meyer,[128] considered one of the founders of occupational therapy, wrote that the "big four" areas in life that need to be balanced and in rhythm, even under difficult circumstances, were work, play, rest, and sleep. Many years later the OTPF-2 stated, "Unlike any other area of occupation, all people rest as a result of engaging in occupations and engage in sleep for multiple hours per day throughout their life span" (OTPF-2, p. 665).[11] Another reason cited in the OTPF-2 for categorizing sleep and rest as its own occupation was "[s]leep significantly affects all other areas of occupation" (OTPF-2, p. 665).[11] In 2007, Jonsson had suggested that providing sleep prominence in the Framework as an area of occupation promoted the consideration of lifestyle choices as an important aspect of participation and health (OTPF-2, p. 665).[11,102] As mentioned, the OTPF-4 continues to present sleep and rest prominently as an occupation.[15]

Because sleep and rest are considered an occupation in its domain of practice, it is appropriate for an occupational therapist to address sleep and rest when treating Mrs. Tanaka.

HISTORY OF SLEEP AND REST IN OCCUPATIONAL THERAPY

From the earliest published writings in occupational therapy, sleep was considered to be important. In October 1921, while presenting a paper at the Fifth Annual Meeting of the National Society for the Promotion of Occupational Therapy (now known as the American Occupational Therapy Association), Adolf Meyer stated:

There are many other rhythms that we must be attuned to: the larger rhythms of night and day, of sleep and waking hours, or hunger and its gratification, and finally the big four—work and play and rest and sleep, which our organism must be able to balance in all this actual doing, actual practice, a program of wholesome living as the basis of wholesome feeling and thinking and fancy and interests.[128]

Even though the founders of occupational therapy considered sleep and rest important for a healthy balance in life, this area was forgotten in the OT literature, and in OT practice for decades.

Green suggested that occupational therapy has paid little attention to the area of sleep because influential scholars in the field have omitted sleep definitions from classifications of occupations.[79] Green also noted that occupational scientists are uncertain about whether sleep is considered an occupation. In his research, Green found evidence in the occupational science literature on sleep with respect to time use and of occupational therapists giving advice on sleep. However, he noted, "Coverage has been neither consistent nor comprehensive and it is unclear why sleep has been considered by so few writers."[79]

Howell and Pierce suggested that Meyer's ideas about the importance of the occupations of sleep and rest were not embraced or further developed in occupational therapy because of the culture's overemphasis on productivity in industry, business, home management, and even leisure.[94] The authors think that the Protestant work ethic, the Industrial Revolution, and the Victorian era all played a role in shaping current Western views on restorative occupations. They pointed out that Meyer's message was ignored in Western society because "it is generally believed that valuable time is wasted while sleeping, time that could be spent more productively."[94]

In a review of OT textbooks published since 1990, Green found that information on sleep was limited.[79] He pointed out, however, that Yasuda[205] and Hammond and Jefferson[87] addressed the topic more thoroughly in chapters on fibromyalgia and rheumatoid arthritis, respectively. Melvin and Jenson[125] and Melvin and Ferrell[126] also emphasized the importance of sleep for adults with rheumatological diseases and fibromyalgia with chapters devoted to fatigue management, sleep retraining, positioning, lifestyle changes and bedding.

More recent major textbooks used by occupational therapy students and practitioners have included chapters on the topic of sleep and rest.[112,114,176] Similarly, Green and Westcomb edited a book on sleep in which the perspectives of various disciplines, including occupational therapy, were represented.[81] In 2015 Green and Brown edited a book focused on sleep that was intended specifically for occupational therapists.[80]

The AOTA has produced the document "Blueprint for Entry-Level Education," which identifies key content areas that should be included in occupational therapy students' course of study.[12] The topic of sleep and rest was included on the list of occupation-centered factors that should be included in entry-level curriculum content.

In 2013, in an opinion piece in the *British Journal of Occupational Therapy*, Fung et al.[71] proposed that "sleep (and wakefulness) should be routinely assessed and addressed as part of standard occupational therapy practice." They recommended more sleep and wakefulness education in OT curriculums; more education on sleep itself and on assessments, interventions, and tools pertaining to it, and more attendance by occupational therapists at professional development workshops held by experts in the field.[71] Tester and Foss also encouraged occupational therapists to perform routine screening on sleep.[185] O'Donoghue and McKay studied the impact of obstructive sleep apnea (OSA) on occupations in Ireland and agreed that interventions by occupational therapists can have a significant impact on the lives of people with sleep disorders.[150]

It should be considered that occupational therapists may be so busy helping clients in areas of occupations when the client is awake that focusing on the area of sleep may be given lower priority. For example, the areas an occupational therapist needs to address with Mrs. Tanaka are numerous and can be overwhelming for a novice practitioner, or even for an experienced OT, given the time pressures for clients to meet functional and other occupational goals. Data have shown that in-client rehabilitation stays have shortened for clients with a cerebrovascular accident (CVA), whereas acuity levels have risen, as evidenced by lower Functional Independence Measure (FIM) scores on admission and discharge.[78] Pressures for Mrs. Tanaka to meet her goals quickly are high.

Because sleep and rest are now identified as a category of occupation in itself; major occupational therapy textbooks cover the topic more thoroughly; and the AOTA blueprint supports sleep education and the interest of international OT researchers, it is anticipated that educational programs will cover the occupation of sleep and rest more thoroughly in their curriculums and that practicing therapists will advance their knowledge in this area.

Occupational Therapy's Definition of Sleep and Rest

Sleep

OT definitions of sleep and rest are fluid (or fluctuating), changing as more research is dedicated to this understudied occupation. The OTPF-4 does not give a definition of sleep, but rather describes the activities surrounding sleep preparation and participation.[15] The OTPF-4 describes sleep in relation to other occupations and to its role in supporting "healthy, active engagement in other occupations" (p. 46).[15] Sleep and rest are described separately in the OTPF-4 because they are distinct from each other.[15]

It should be pointed out that people are not unconscious during sleep, as previous editions of the OTPF (second edition) described that consciousness could be completely lost during sleep.[11] Mahowald, a sleep researcher, has stated, "There is now overwhelming evidence that the primary states of being (wakefulness, non–rapid eye movement [NREM] sleep and rapid eye movement [REM] sleep) are not mutually exclusive, but may become admixed or may oscillate rapidly, resulting in numerous clinical phenomena" (p. 159).[120] Coren, a psychologist and author on sleep, pointed out that at some level, our vision, hearing, and sense of touch are still functioning to some extent when we are asleep.[48]

Human sleep is not just the opposite of wakefulness, or wakefulness the opposite of sleep.[121] It appears that consciousness is not completely lost during sleep.

Rest

According to the OTPF-4, rest includes identifying a need to rest and relax, decreasing involvement in taxing (physically, mentally, or socially) activities, and participating in relaxation or other activities that restore energy, calm, and renewed engagement.[15]

Nurit and Michal compared how the literature of the various fields that interact with occupational therapy conceptualize rest.[148] Psychology (Maslow), they pointed out, considers rest a basic human need, whereas the nursing profession differentiates between physical and mental rest.[123,148] Various religions and philosophies view rest as important for restoration and focus. The researchers concluded that although the various fields may have different concepts of rest, they all concur with occupational therapy that rest is important for a healthy, balanced life.

Nurit and Michal also reviewed debates surrounding the concept of bed rest in medicine. They noted that, historically, rest was highly recommended; however, they also pointed to research that has shown that clients on bed rest, compared to clients in ambulatory groups, may experience detrimental effects to their health.[6,32,148]

This chapter focuses on the general concept of rest, rather than the idea of physician-ordered bed rest (i.e., not allowing a client out of bed for medical or safety reasons).

Sleep and Rest

The OTPF-4 explains that the concepts of both sleep and rest include "activities related to obtaining restorative rest and sleep to support healthy active engagement in other occupations" (p. 46).[15] Instead of categorizing the occupations into what she called "adopted cultural categories" of work, play, leisure, and self-care, Pierce[161] described the categories of occupation based on how the individual experiences them. She described three categories of occupation as *pleasurable*, which includes play and leisure; *productive*, which includes work; and *restorative* types of occupations, which include sleep, self-care, and quiet activities.[160,161] Among the pleasurable, productive, and restorative occupations, Howell and Pierce considered restorative occupations the least recognized.[94] In 2003, Pierce stated, "In our clients, the need for improvements in the restorative quality of their occupational patterns can be critical. Without adequate restoration, productivity and pleasure also remain low" (p. 98).[161]

NEED TO ADDRESS SLEEP IN OCCUPATIONAL THERAPY

It is important to emphasize that a founding figure of the OT profession, Adolf Meyer, regarded sleep as one of the four main areas that determine whether humans can function (in addition to work, rest, and play). It is also noteworthy that the OTPF considers sleep a major human occupation.[15] Perhaps an even more compelling reason that occupational therapists should address sleep is because it is an occupation in which every human being across the age span engages in or should engage in. Of the nine occupations listed in the OTPF-4, sleep and rest is the only one that cannot be performed by someone else or by an alternative means. The environment and actions surrounding sleep can be adapted, but the act of sleeping itself is the only occupation that cannot be adapted for an individual to function optimally, let alone survive. As Dahl bluntly stated, "Sleep is not some biological luxury. Sleep is essential for basic survival, occurring in every species of living creature that has ever been studied. Animals deprived of sleep die" (p. 33).[53]

As this chapter illustrates, sleep (or the lack thereof) affects almost every client population with whom OT practitioners work and within virtually every setting.

NEED TO ADDRESS REST IN OCCUPATIONAL THERAPY

As mentioned previously, in the OTPF-4, rest, along with sleep, is considered one of the primary occupations in the purview of occupational therapy in which people engage.[15] However, rest should not be confused with sleep. According to Dahl, "Sleep is not simply rest. Mere rest does not create the restorative state

of having slept" (p. 32).[53] If a client such as Mrs. Tanaka "rests" during the day but does not sleep, she will still suffer the loss of sleep and therefore of all its unique restorative benefits.

Howell and Pierce discussed the importance of rest in addition to sleep for physical, cognitive, and mental restoration.[94] They noted the uniqueness of individuals in deciding which occupations are restorative, and how one person may consider a particular activity to be relaxing and calming, whereas another may not. The authors also pointed out that occupations that are highly restorative tend to have strong routines of a simple and even repetitive nature, and they are often considered pleasurable and have personal meaning to the individual based on tradition and history with the occupation.[94]

Edlund, an expert on rest, body clocks, and sleep, described four different forms of active rest that are needed in addition to sleep: physical rest, mental rest, social rest, and spiritual rest. He stated, "Rest is not useless but a major pathway to our renewal, our survival" (p. 3). His book, *The Power of Rest: Why Sleep Alone Is Not Enough: A 30-Day Plan to Reset Your Body*, provides information on how a person can obtain those types of rest efficiently.[65]

SLEEP AND REST AND OCCUPATIONAL JUSTICE

Occupational justice describes the occupational therapy profession's concerns with the ability of all people, "regardless of age, ability, gender, social class or other differences" to be given the opportunity to engage in occupations.[147] Occupational justice describes concerns that OT practitioners have about the ethical, moral, and civic aspects of clients' environments and contexts.[15] Sleep is an occupation that is optimized by a safe setting and environment, especially for someone with a physical or mental disability. In a 2014 point-in-time survey of communities across the United States, 49,933 homeless veterans (8.6% of the total) were identified.[134] Significantly, 54% of these homeless veterans were found to have a mental or physical disability.

Homeless veterans tend to be male (91%), single (98%), live in a city (76%), and have a mental and/or physical disability (54%). Black veterans are substantially overrepresented among homeless veterans, accounting for 39% of the total homeless veteran population, but only 11% of the total veteran population.[134]

Sleep researchers Dement and Pelayo stated, "It is a deplorable fact that in the inner portions of our large cities, we have begun to see large numbers of individuals who are homeless and who do not have a comfortable, safe place to sleep" (p. 16).[59] Occupational therapists work with many people in society who may not statistically be considered homeless, but these people may live (and sleep) in substandard environments. Even other species attempt to find safe places to sleep.

HISTORY OF SLEEP IN SOCIETY AND CULTURAL INFLUENCES

Howell and Pierce stated that one of the most significant forces to shape our current view of occupations is the Protestant work ethic, which evolved during the Protestant Reformation of the 1500 s.[94] The values of honesty, thrift, and hard work were embraced during this time in Europe. Leisure (often associated with pleasurable, "nonproductive" activities such as sleep and rest) was considered a potential temptation into sin and thus to be avoided, similar to the belief in the adage "idle hands are the devil's workshop."[94]

In 1996, Coren[48] pointed out that the invention of the light bulb by Thomas Edison had a powerful influence over sleep and served to transform society, making shift work possible throughout the night. Before the introduction of the modern tungsten filament light bulb in 1913 (an inexpensive and long-lasting bulb), the average person slept 9 hours a night, as was documented by a 1910 study. The new light bulb served to "free" working people from working in darkness; but, ironically, it may have simultaneously served to reduce the hours of sleep for future generations.[48]

The National Commission on Sleep Disorders Research, mandated by the U.S. Congress, concluded in the 1990s that the "root cause of pervasive sleep deprivation and unidentified sleep problems is the continued low level of public and professional awareness due to failure to give sleep topics adequate attention in the educational system."[59] In 2015, Dement and Pelayo pointed out that international surveys conducted since the 1800s show that people in industrialized nations are sleeping less than they did a century ago.[59] These researchers referred to studies in Japan, where surveys were conducted annually; they noted that these surveys showed an overall reduction in the daily amount of sleep of 1½ hours since 1920.[59]

In a poll conducted in 2009 by the U.S. National Sleep Foundation (NSF), 1000 telephone interviews were conducted among a random sample of Americans in the continental United States.[140] Respondents were at least 18 years of age and a head of the household. They were asked how many hours of sleep they needed to function at their best during the day. On average, respondents reported needing 7 hours and 24 minutes to function at their best. However, they reported getting an average of 6 hours and 40 minutes of sleep on a typical workday or weekday, almost 2½ hours less than people had reported in 1910.[140] The 2014 NSF poll found that of 1103 adults polled who were parents of or had parental responsibility for a child aged 6 to 17 in their household, more than 90% thought that sleep was either very or extremely important for their own mood, health, and performance, in addition to the mood, health, and performance of their children.[142] Although the parents thought that getting enough sleep was important, they acknowledged that their children were not getting enough, especially as the children got older.[142] In 2018, the NSF polled 1010 respondents about their effectiveness at getting things done, and 65% thought that sleep contributed to next day effectiveness.[143] Though they acknowledged sleep's importance, when asked what activities were important to them, sleep was not prioritized over other activities. Of the respondents, 10% chose sleep, compared with 35% who chose physical fitness and nutrition, 27% who chose work, 17% who selected hobbies and personal interests, and 9% chose social life.[143]

These statistics point to the existence of a culture-wide "sleep debt," and deprioritization of sleep, a point of relevance for occupational therapists, whose overarching goal, according to the OTPF-4, is "achieving health, well-being, and participation in life through engagement in occupation" (p. 4).[15]

Mrs. Tanaka, whose primary cultural influence is Western, has her own beliefs and values about sleep. Therefore, it is of utmost importance to identify Mrs. Tanaka's and her family's beliefs about sleep. Is sleep considered important or a waste of time?

Cultures of Sleep Practices

Sleep behavior among Western industrial societies is distinctive to that culture. In a comparative analysis of sleep among industrialized Western society and indigenous cultures, Worthman and Melby pointed out several uniquely Western sleep practices, including the following[202]:

1. Solitary sleep from early infancy, supported by cultural norms and beliefs about the risk of an overlying need for infant independence or autonomy and the need for sexual decorum
2. Consolidation of sleep into a single long bout
3. Distinct bedtimes enforced in childhood and reinforced by highly scheduled daytime hours for work or school and mechanized devices for waking
4. Housing design and construction that provide remarkably sequestered, quiet, controlled environments for sleep in visually and acoustically isolated spaces

In contrast, non-Western sleepers habitually engage in co-sleep in shared beds or spaces. In 2012, Steger[180] reported that in some cultures, it would be "simply unthinkable" to leave a baby or toddler to sleep alone in a room. Steger found that mothers in Japan are convinced that it is important to convey a sense of security and belonging to their children by sleeping with them, not firmly putting children to bed alone in a room and letting them cry themselves to sleep.[180]

Steger pointed out that in monophasic sleep cultures (one long bout of night sleep), only "marginal social groups" (e.g., children or sick people) or night shift workers are allowed to sleep during the day. A "siesta culture," as described by Steger, supports biphasic sleep in which there is a predetermined time for night and midday sleep. Social life quiets down during the night and early afternoon. A "napping culture" (polyphasic sleep) occurs when there are often irregular sleep times during the day in addition to the regulated nighttime sleep. However, there are many other sleep cultures within those three basic types.[180]

Compared to Western cultures, other cultures may have more fluid sleep schedules and more fluid sleep/wake states, and may fall asleep and remain asleep in more sensorially dynamic settings.[202] As mentioned, Western sleep areas, by design, provide minimal sensory stimulation[186] (i.e., protection from the elements, minimal contact with others, climate control, and negligible noise, movement, or light). Compared to this, sleepers in other cultures may sleep exposed to the elements and co-sleep, and may be accustomed to sounds, movement, and light. For example, the Ache (Paraguay), Hiwi (southern Venezuela), Efe (Zaire), and !Kung (northwest Botswana) use fire as light, heat, and protection at night and therefore may need to tend the fire and awaken frequently to monitor it.[202]

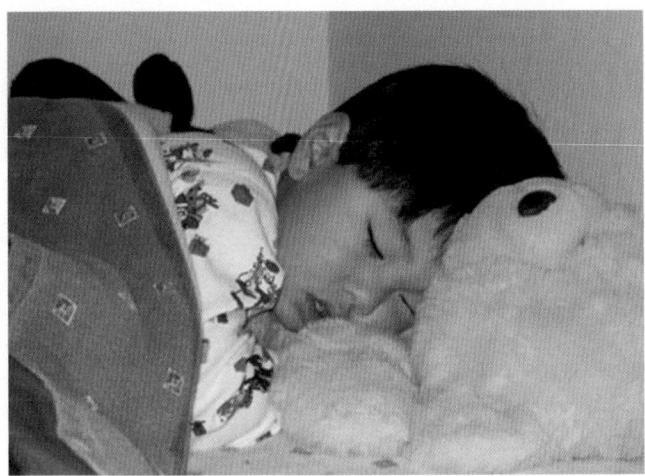

Fig. 13.1 This 3½-year-old boy uses a teddy bear as a sleep aid, for comfort and a sense of security. It is considered socially acceptable at this young age, but it would not be so as he moves into the teen years and adulthood. (Courtesy Jean S. Koketsu.)

Humans universally sleep in a recumbent position (unless ill or during infancy) but can differ widely in terms of accessories (e.g., bedding).[202] For example, "foragers" (e.g., Ache, Efe, !Kung) who inhabit tropical or mild climates and move regularly do not sleep on platforms but directly on the ground.[202] !Kung sleep on skin, a blanket (or nothing) over conforming sandy ground. Efe sleep on thin layers of leaves or between logs. Hiwi use hammocks. According to Worthman and Melby, none of the groups listed regularly use pillowing material or coverings, whereas Westerners use an abundance of these.[202] The minimal use of bedding by the groups listed may have to do with available technology and resources, but it may also have to do with avoidance of pests such as fleas, bedbugs, lice, or mites, which thrive in bedding material.[202]

Human beings have a tremendous diversity in sleep patterns and sleep developmental histories based on cultural background and upbringing.[202] Steger suggested that four major sources of the emotional security required for relaxing and peaceful sleep shape sleep practices around the world[180]:

1. Stability of the physical sleep environment/sleeping place
2. The presence of trusted people
3. Recurring rituals or routines
4. Social acceptance of certain sleep behavior (Fig. 13.1)

It is important for occupational therapists to be aware of a client's sleep history and culture so they can set realistic and meaningful goals for the client in the area of sleep. The OTPF-4 acknowledges that client engagement in occupations within cultural contexts influence how the occupation is organized.[15]

The occupational therapist treating Mrs. Tanaka should find out what her typical sleep habits were prior to the stroke. Did she sleep in her bed alone or with her husband? What time did she normally go to bed and wake up? Did she usually take naps? What habits or routines did she have before going to sleep or upon waking up? Did she experience interruptions during sleep, such as getting up to go to the bathroom? What kind of bed did she sleep on? What are her sheet and pillow preferences? Was

there noise in the room where she slept? What are comfortable light and temperature levels for her?

Brief History of Sleep Medicine

Sleep medicine as a medical specialty is relatively new. William C. Dement, a pioneer in sleep medicine himself, considers Nathaniel Kleitman, a physiologist who started studying sleep in the 1920s, as the first to devote his professional life to the study of sleep.[57-59] Kleitman and Aserinsky first described rapid eye movement (REM) sleep in the early 1950s, and overnight electroencephalograms (EEGs) were first reported in the late 1950s by Dement and Kleitman.[56] In 1965, sleep apnea was identified in Europe, and in 1970, Dement founded the first sleep disorders center at Stanford University Hospital. The 1970s saw a proliferation of sleep disorder clinics. Since that time, sleep medicine has become a specialty in medicine; scholarly journals focusing on sleep were launched; national and international organizations that focused on sleep research and education were founded; and a congressional commission focused on sleep was mandated.

Dement and Pelayo[59] reported that there was no scholarly discipline that was the "best candidate to assume responsibility for the education of the public about sleep." They found that traditional academic organizations of colleges and universities viewed psychology and biology departments as the "obvious homes" of the topic. Fung et al.[71] argued that "occupational therapists should be equipped with a subset of skills to assess and address sleep in practice." In these researchers' view, occupational therapy seemed to be an "obvious home," or at least a good home, for this discipline.

The OTPF-4 highlights the importance of how engagement and participation in an occupation (e.g., sleep) occur in contexts, which includes environmental and personal environments, which must be considered in the process of helping people with occupational concerns.[15] Sociologists, Williams, Meadows, and Arbor, made note of the "medicalization" of sleep issues (i.e., the "cultural framing of sleep problems as medical matters") and described how popular culture and media can play a role in defining and highlighting sleep concerns and opinions about sleep.[197]

This chapter addresses sleep definitions and problems sometimes more from a medical perspective. However, the complex and varied dimensions of sleep must be considered; occupational therapists cannot just "medicalize" the issue.

Definition of Sleep According to Sleep Medicine
Behavioral Definition

According to Carskadon and Dement, the two defining characteristics of sleep are (1) being a reversible behavioral state and (2) demonstrating perceptual disengagement from and unresponsiveness to the environment.[40] The perceptual disengagement is compared to the waking state in which humans are conscious or aware of various sights, sounds, and smells in the world.[59] For example, Dement and Pelayo pointed out that even if the eyelids are taped open, we stop seeing when we fall asleep.[59] However, this perceptual disengagement is not unconscious and is still considered an active process. Reversibility, the other essential defining characteristic quality of sleep, means that a person could be taken out of that state relatively easily based on the stage of sleep in which they are. Other sleeplike states, such as coma, anesthesia, and hibernation, are differentiated from normal sleep because of the difference in reversibility.[59]

Dement and Pelayo considered sleep a restorative process, with "sleep and wakefulness occur(ring) as complementary phases in the daily cycle of existence."[59] Sleep is usually characterized by closed eyes, postural recumbence (lying down), and behavioral quiescence.[40] Other sleep behaviors also may occur, such as sleep talking and sleepwalking.[40]

Scientists have described several discrete stages of sleep based on brain wave patterns and eye and muscle activity. The two major types of sleep are NREM (pronounced *non-rem*) and REM sleep.[40] The two states (NREM and REM) exist in virtually all mammals and birds and are as distinct from each other as sleep is from the waking state.[59]

The American Academy of Sleep Medicine (AASM) characterizes the sleep stages as stage N1 (NREM 1), stage N2 (NREM 2), stage N3 (NREM 3), and stage R (REM).[97] It should be noted that from 1968 to 2007, NREM sleep was divided into four stages (stages 1–4); at that point, stages 3 and 4 were combined into one (N3, or slow-wave sleep [SWS]), according to the AASM.[59] NREM sleep accounts for 75% to 80% of total sleep time in young adults. The stages are defined by brain wave patterns from an EEG. The EEG pattern in NREM sleep is synchronous and shows wave forms called spindles and K complexes, in addition to high-voltage slow waves (Fig. 13.2). Carskadon and Dement gave a shorthand definition of NREM as a relatively inactive state yet actively regulating the brain in a movable body.[40]

REM sleep accounts for approximately 20% to 25% of total sleep time in young adults and is defined by EEG activation, muscle atonia or paralysis, and occasional bursts of rapid eye movements.[40] The eye movements are binocularly synchronous and rapid, although drifting movements may be seen.[59] REM sleep is associated with dreaming.[59] This is based on vivid dream recall

reported after approximately 80% of arousals from this state of sleep.[58] Spinal motor neurons are inhibited by brainstem mechanisms that suppress postural motor tonus during REM sleep. It is thought that the body is paralyzed during REM sleep to protect dreaming individuals from physically acting out dream content and injuring themselves or others, although brief, minor position shifts or limb movements occur. Carskadon and Dement's short definition of REM sleep is an activated brain in a paralyzed body.[40]

Evidence from human beings and other species suggests that mammals have only minimal ability to thermoregulate during REM.[40] The poor ability to respond to temperature extremes during REM suggests that problems with temperature regulation may be worse later during the night, when REM sleep tends to predominate; these are important considerations for OT practitioners working with people with thermoregulation problems. Interestingly, Carskadon and Dement pointed out that sweating or shivering during sleep under ambient temperature extremes occurs in NREM sleep and is limited during REM sleep.[40]

Sleep Architecture
Polysomnography

A **polysomnograph (PSG)** is a continuous recording of specific physiological variables during sleep. It is typically performed at night during a sleep study in a sleep clinic. The PSG quantifies sleep; the AASM recommends measuring brain waves (by EEG), eye movements (by electrooculogram [EOG]), chin and leg muscle movements (via electromyogram [EMG]), airflow, oxygen saturation, and body positions.[97] The AASM also recommends that in addition, the PSG record respiratory, arousal (wake-up), cardiac (e.g., heart rate), movement, and behavioral events.[97]

The sleep stages are charted on a diagram, called a **hypnogram** (histogram, or graphical representation of sleep), made from the data collected from the PSG. The chart resembles a city skyline and is referred to as **sleep architecture** by sleep experts (Fig. 13.3). A client's sleep architecture describes the details of an individual's sleep after an overnight recording of EEG, EOG, and EMG. The histogram shows the following[56]:

- Time needed to fall asleep (sleep latency)
- Sequence of sleep stages
- Time spent in each stage of sleep
- Total sleep time
- Number and length of nighttime wakenings

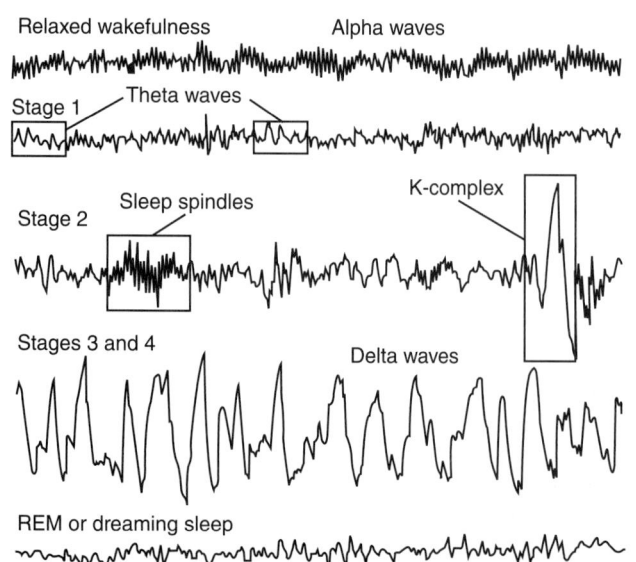

Fig. 13.2 Brain waves recorded on an electroencephalogram (EEG) to identify stages of sleep. (From Epstein LJ, Mardon S: *Harvard Medical School guide to a good night's sleep*, New York, 2007, McGraw-Hill.)

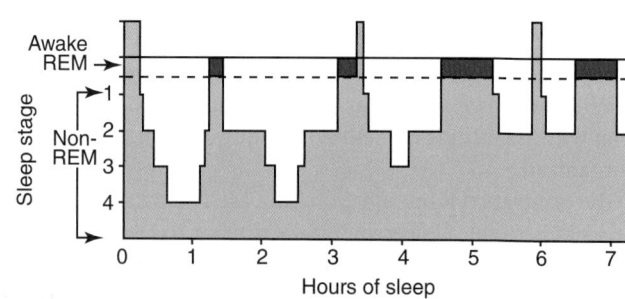

Fig. 13.3 Sleep architecture. The tracing on this hypnogram, which resembles a skyline, illustrates a typical night's sleep. A hypnogram charts the sleep stages during an overnight sleep study. (From Epstein LJ, Mardon S: *Harvard Medical School guide to a good night's sleep*, New York, 2007, McGraw-Hill.)

Actigraphy

Actigraphy is another way sleep is measured. It is increasingly used in research and in the clinical care of clients with sleep issues and is a recommended for use to evaluate sleep disorders under certain guidelines.[175] The client wears a motion sensor on the wrist, and the sensor continuously monitors movement.[59] The data can be downloaded immediately, or the sensor can be worn for a specified period. Actigraphy is more convenient and less expensive than a PSG.[59] In recent years smart phone apps and sleep management systems have been developed to track sleep.

Progression of Normal Sleep

Normal young adults first enter sleep through NREM sleep, and REM sleep occurs 80 to 100 minutes afterward. Throughout the night, in approximately 90-minute periods, cycles of NREM and REM sleep alternate, usually with progressively increasing periods of REM sleep.[40] Box 13.1 lists the general stages of sleep and describes the bodily functions that occur during these stages.[a]

Sleep Across the Age Span

Research shows that age is the strongest and most consistent factor that affects sleep stages (Fig. 13.4).[40,152] The biggest difference in sleep stages is seen in newborns, who enter from wake to sleep through the REM phase first for the first year of life (Fig. 13.5). Infants also cycle between REM and NREM, but they cycle through the phases in 50 to 60 minutes instead of the approximately 90 minutes seen in adults. At birth, active (REM) sleep accounts for approximately 50% of total sleep and declines over the first 2 years to approximately 20% to 25%.[40] Infants do not seem to have fully developed and recognizable NREM sleep until they are 2 to 6 months old.[40] Stage N3, also known as deep or SWS, is maximized in young children but decreases markedly with age in quantity and quality (Fig. 13.6). That may explain why children may be very difficult to arouse when they are in SWS in the first cycle, whereas an older adult may be easier to awaken in that phase.

Adolescence. Contrary to popular belief, teenagers require more sleep than adults. As cited by Carskadon[39] and Carskadon et al.,[41] evidence shows that teenagers need at least 9 to 9¼ hours of sleep a night to maintain optimal alertness. Teenagers also have been shown to have a phase delay in the circadian timing system, which means that their biological clocks alert them to stay up late and sleep in later (e.g., sleep from midnight to 9 am).[41] The quantitative change in SWS may best be seen across adolescence; SWS decreases by nearly 40% during the teen years, even while nocturnal sleep remains constant.[40] These are important considerations in occupational therapy practice in terms of clients' scheduling and optimal performance of occupations.

Adulthood and aging. From ages 20 to 60, sleep patterns do not change as rapidly as during childhood. However, there are consistent trends that occur in sleep patterns, such as decreased

---

[a] References 40, 59, 66, 88, 91, and 174.

BOX 13.1   Stages of NREM and REM Sleep

Non–Rapid Eye Movement (NREM) Sleep
Stage N1 (1–7 Minutes)
Stage N1 is considered transitional wakefulness to sleep onset or to rapid eye movement (REM) sleep. The body temperature begins to drop, muscles start to relax, and the eyes may move slowly from side to side. An electroencephalogram (EEG) shows brain waves slowed to 4–7 cycles per second *(theta waves)*. A person in this phase can be easily wakened by tapping him or her or softly calling the individual's name (low arousal threshold). However, everyone experiences stage N1 differently. If awakened in this stage, one person may say he or she was asleep, whereas another may only say that he or she was drowsy. A common sign of severely disrupted sleep is an increased amount and percentage of sleep in this phase.

Stage N2 (About 10–30 Minutes)
Stage N2 follows stage N1. The eyes are not moving much, and the heart rate and breathing are slower than when the person is awake. This is the first stage of established sleep. Brain waves are irregular; the EEG shows intermediate-sized brain waves with brief bursts of fast sleep spindles, or K-complexes, that occur about every 2 minutes. Generally, a more intense stimulus is required to arouse a person in this stage (higher arousal threshold). In the later phases of this stage, the EEG shows high-voltage slow wave activity. Overall, this stage may account for half the night.

Stage N3 (About 20–40 Minutes in the First Cycle)
Stage N3 sleep is also called *delta sleep* or *slow wave sleep* (it formerly was called stage 3 and stage 4 sleep). Breathing slows and becomes more regular, and the blood pressure and pulse fall to 20% to 30% of the waking state. The EEG shows high-amplitude slow waves. Stage N3 accounts for approximately 10%–15% of total sleep time, but it may be undetectable in older adults, especially men.

Rapid Eye Movement (REM) Sleep
Stage R (About 1–5 Minutes in the First Cycle, Increases up to 30 Minutes)
The body temperature, blood pressure, heart rate, and respiratory rate all increase and are often irregular. The clitoris or penis may become erect. The EEG shows a dramatic decline in amplitude, which resembles the waking state. Thermoregulation is severely inhibited. Motor neurons also are inhibited, which means major muscles are paralyzed, except the diaphragm and the ocular muscles.

NOTE: See Fig. 13.1 for brain wave patterns during sleep. Slow wave sleep (SWS) is considered the most restorative phase for physiological repair, whereas REM sleep is thought to be necessary for memory consolidation.

---

sleep efficiency, decreased time in restorative deep sleep, and easier arousal during the deep sleep phase (Table 13.1). After age 60, the sleep trends of adulthood continue.[66] A hallmark of aging is an increased percentage of time in stage N1 (NREM sleep) and a decreased percentage of time in N3 (deep, SWS), particularly in men. Sleep efficiency also decreases as a person ages. Sleep efficiency is measured by dividing the actual time a person is asleep by the amount of time he or she is in bed. Sleep efficiency at approximately age 45 is 86%, and it declines to 79% for those over age 70. Brief arousals are also more common in the elderly. In addition, older adults may have an advanced sleep phase, meaning that they may get sleepy in the early evening and tend to awaken early in the morning.[40]

Carskadon and Dement reported that possibly the most notable finding about sleep in older adults is the profound

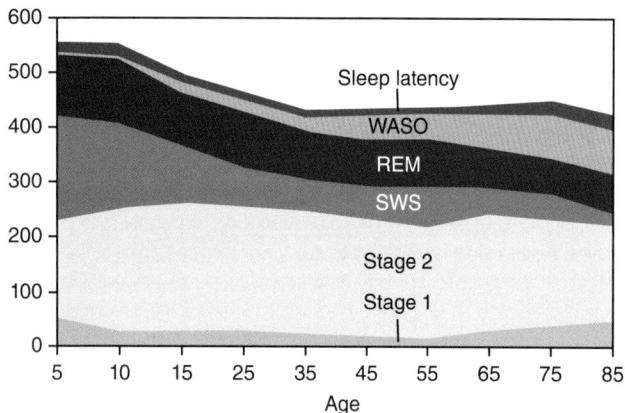

Fig. 13.4 Time is measured in minutes, and the values recorded, in terms of age, are sleep latency (the time it takes to fall asleep), wake time after sleep onset *(WASO)*, rapid eye movement *(REM)*, slow wave sleep *(SWS)*, and stage 1 and stage 2 sleep. Note that as we age, it takes longer to fall asleep (sleep latency increases), the time spent in deep sleep decreases, and the time spent in stages 1 and 2 increases. Also note that SWS decreases markedly during adolescence. As we age, night awakenings (WASO) also increase. (From Ohayon M, Carskadon MA, Guilleminault C, Vitiello MV: Meta analysis of quantitative sleep parameters from childhood to old age in healthy individuals: developing normative sleep values across the human lifespan, *Sleep* 27:1255–1273, 2004.)

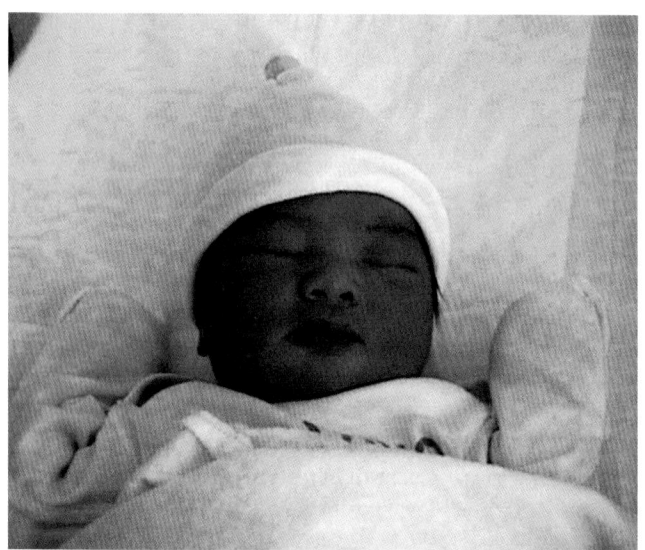

Fig. 13.5 Newborns enter REM sleep first for the first year of life and cycle through rapid eye movement and non–rapid eye movement sleep within 50–60 minutes, instead of the 90 minutes seen in adults. (Courtesy Jean S. Koketsu.)

increase in interindividual variability, which precludes generalizations such as those made for young adults.[40]

Circadian Rhythm, Homeostasis, and Allostasis

The timing of human sleep is regulated by two systems in the body: the circadian biological clock and sleep/wake homeostasis.

Circadian rhythms are approximately 24-hour cycles of behavior and physiology that are generated by biological clocks (pacemakers or oscillators).[130] The internal biological clock regulates the timing and periods of sleepiness and wakefulness,

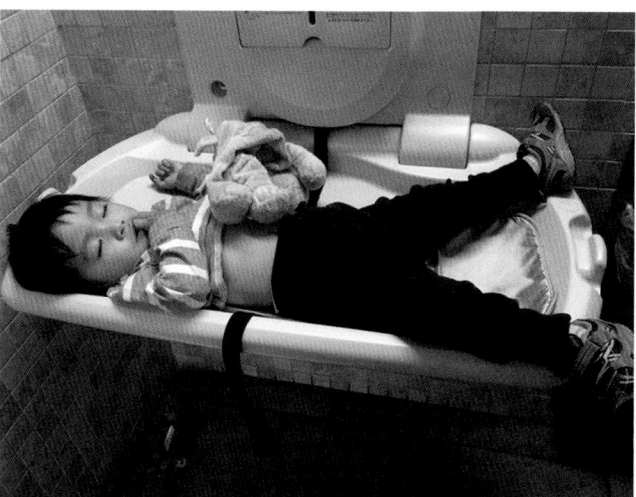

Fig. 13.6 A 22-month-old child has no social qualms about falling asleep anywhere, even on a public diaper-changing table. Young children's deep sleep is maximized, so they may be very difficult to arouse from stage N3 sleep. (Courtesy Windy Chou.)

TABLE 13.1	**Sleep Changes With Aging**				
	Age 20	**Age 40**	**Age 60**	**Age 70**	**Age 80**
Sleep latency	16 min	17 min	18 min	18.5 min	19 min
Total sleep time	7.5 hr	7 hr	6.2 hr	6 hr	5.8 hr
Time in stage 2 sleep	47%	52%	53%	55%	57%
Time in deep sleep	20%	15%	10%	9%	7.5%
Time in REM sleep	22%	21%	20%	19%	17%
Sleep efficiency	95%	88%	84%	82%	79%

Data from Epstein LJ, Mardon S: *Harvard Medical School guide to a good night's sleep*, New York, 2007, McGraw-Hill, p 43; and Ohayan M, Carskadon MA, Guilleminault C, Vitiello MV: Meta analysis of quantitative sleep parameters from childhood to old age in healthy individuals: developing normative sleep values across the human life span, *Sleep* 27:1255–1273, 2004.

temperature, blood pressure, and the release of hormones throughout the 24-hour day without need of outside cues for the clock to persist. However, environmental stimuli known as *zeitgebers*, or "time cues," help synchronize the internal clock to the 24-hour day. Light is the most dominant zeitgeber for most species[130]; bright light has the ability to shift circadian rhythms. Blind people who may not have a conscious perception of light can still entrain to the 24-hour day because human eyes have irradiance detectors that can sense light despite the inability to produce a visual image.[158] The receptors may remain intact in many people with blindness, which allows entrainment as usual. However, people without eyes (or the receptors) often have difficulty with entrainment and may have circadian rhythm problems.[158]

The master circadian (24-hour) clock, which is located in the suprachiasmatic nucleus in the hypothalamus of the brain, dictates when we feel sleepy and when we feel most awake. Melatonin, a naturally occurring hormone, is inhibited by light. It is secreted by the pineal gland at night, which induces

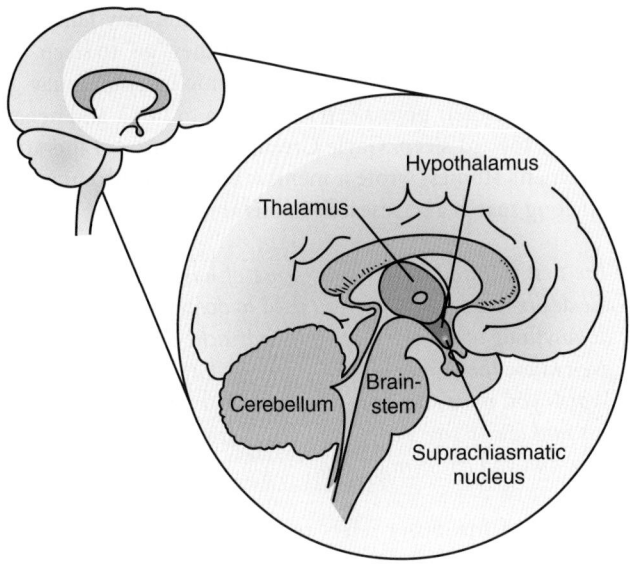

Fig. 13.7 The sleep/wake control center is located in the suprachias-matic nucleus in the hypothalamus. This "pacemaker" regulates the cir-cadian rhythm of sleep and wakefulness. (From Epstein LJ, Mardon S: *Harvard Medical School guide to a good night's sleep,* New York, 2007, McGraw-Hill.)

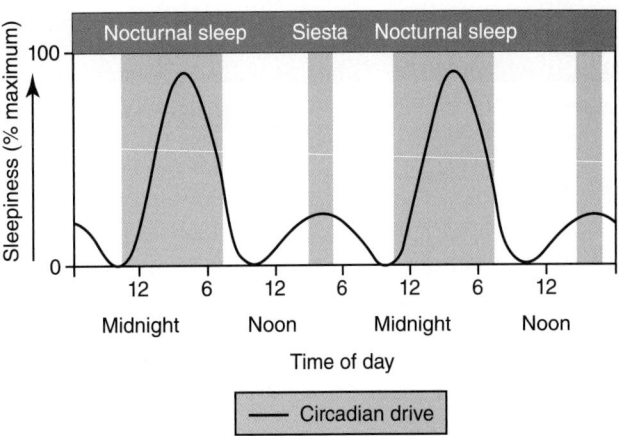

Fig. 13.8 The circadian rhythm of sleep and wakefulness has two peaks of sleepiness during the 24-hour day. These peak times of sleepiness are between midnight and dawn (higher peak) and in the afternoon after the typical lunchtime. (From Epstein LJ, Mardon S: *Harvard Medical School guide to a good night's sleep,* New York, 2007, McGraw-Hill.)

sleep and has the ability to synchronize circadian rhythms (Fig. 13.7).[166,167]

The circadian rhythm for sleep and wakefulness is bimodal; the strongest desire to sleep occurs between midnight and dawn and in the midafternoon (Fig. 13.8).[66,131] This explains why people have the most difficult time staying awake between 2 and 4 in the morning and why they feel most sleepy in the afternoon after lunch. A person who is sleep deprived will feel sleepier during the afternoon dip in the circadian rhythm than if he or she had sufficient sleep. On the other hand, if a person is sleep deprived and has been awake for a long time, he or she may have difficulty falling asleep during the clock "alerting" times. This may explain the quandary of the world traveler who has flown through many time zones and wants to sleep but is unable to do so because the biological clock is telling the body to stay awake.[166]

All phases of normal sleep are considered to be under homeo-static control (homeostasis), or the tendency to maintain equi-librium. The longer a person is awake or deprived of certain sleep stages, the greater will be the drive to obtain that lost sleep or stage.[188] Stated differently, as soon as a person awakens, the sleep debt starts to accumulate. This sleep/wake homeostasis creates a drive that balances sleep and wakefulness.[25] Studies have shown that adenosine, a by-product of energy metabolism, increases in concentration with increased neural activity and is released during wakefulness.[25] The adenosine may promote sleepiness by inhibiting wakefulness-promoting neurons.[25] Caffeine and other stimulants counteract the effects of adenosine by serving as antagonists at their receptors.

A third, less understood mechanism, the allostatic process, is another factor involved in controlling the sleep/wake cycle.[158] Allostasis achieves stability of a system through many or variable physiological or behavioral changes, and it can be controlled by external forces such as social or ecological cues. Those mechanisms can override the circadian or homeostatic propensity for sleep, if

necessary.[158] Social factors may include work, family, and societal structure.[158] Examples of ecological factors include habitat, light, food, warmth, shelter, and the presence of young; these are drivers that can determine the timing and duration of sleep and whether sleep actually occurs because of other pressing needs.[158] As cited by Czeisler et al., humans can override the signals of the circadian and sleep/wake system short term if they have very urgent matters to which they must attend.[52] The invention of artificial light and the alarm clock contributed to human beings' need (or desire) to override the biological clock, simply because they can or because of societal and cultural pressures to do so.

What is considered adequate sleep?. Determining what is considered adequate sleep varies widely based on age, genetics, and many other factors. Table 13.2 presents the recommenda-tions of the National Sleep Foundation for determining how much sleep an individual needs.[92]

SLEEP DISORDERS

Many sleep disorders have been researched and identified by sleep medicine researchers. Only the more common sleep dis-orders are reviewed here.

Insomnia

In general, insomnia is defined as repeated difficulty with initi-ating sleep or maintaining sleep, awakening earlier than desired, or having poor-quality sleep that is not restorative despite ade-quate opportunities for sleep.[64,173] *The International Classification of Sleep Disorders,* third edition (ICSD-3), is the authorita-tive clinical text for the diagnosis of sleep disorders; the text was updated in 2014.[8] The American Psychiatric Association also described "sleep-wake disorders" in the *Diagnostic and Statistical Manual of Mental Disorders,* fifth edition (DSMV).[186] Insomnia is the most common sleep disorder and in isolation affects 30% to 50% of the general population; 9% to 15% of those report impairment in daily activities as a result.[64]

Insomnia is primarily diagnosed by clinical evaluation (by a physician) with a thorough sleep history and detailed medical,

TABLE 13.2   How Much Sleep Do You Need?

Age	Sleep Needs (Hours)
Newborns (0–3 months)	14–17
Infants (4–11 mo)	12–15
Toddlers (1–2 yr)	11–14
Preschoolers (3–5 yr)	10–13
School-age children (6–13 yr)	9–11
Teens (14–17)	8–10
Young adults (18–25)	7–9
Adults (26–64)	7–9
Older adults (65+)	7–8

Data from the National Sleep Foundation. http://sleepfoundation.org/how-sleep-works/how-much-sleep-do-we-really-need. To view the full research report, visit SleepHealthJournal.org.

substance, and psychiatric history.[173] A diagnosis of insomnia requires an associated daytime dysfunction in addition to appropriate insomnia symptoms.[173] Because occupational therapists well understand occupations and the process of assessing function, they can provide valuable information to the treatment team on occupational performance in relation to sleep issues.[71] Treatment for insomnia may include:

- Initially, at least one behavioral intervention is tried, such as stimulus control therapy or relaxation therapy, or a combination of cognitive therapy, stimulus control therapy, and sleep restriction therapy, with or without relaxation therapy. Cognitive-behavioral therapy (CBT) for insomnia (CBT-I) is a combination of cognitive therapy with behavioral treatments (e.g., stimulus control, sleep restriction). Trained occupational therapists can use these therapies, but they are traditionally offered by other mental health professionals.
- Adherence to good sleep hygiene is recommended, but there is insufficient evidence to indicate that sleep hygiene alone is effective in the treatment of chronic insomnia. It is agreed that sleep hygiene education should be used in combination with other therapies. Occupational therapists can certainly provide education and training in this area.[173]

Table 13.3 presents more detailed information on possible treatments for chronic insomnia. Advanced training in CBT-I is required if it is used because there are contraindications for its use, and it could be dangerous for some people if not prescribed appropriately. Occupational therapists also may be trained in CBT-I, and research has shown that occupational therapists can effectively use CBT-I.[63] It is the recommended treatment for people with chronic insomnia.[164]

Risk factors for insomnia include advancing age; female; psychiatric, medical, or substance abuse problems; shift work; and possibly unemployment and lower socioeconomic status.[173] Individuals with comorbid medical and psychiatric conditions are at particularly increased risk; the insomnia rates in clients with psychiatric and chronic pain disorders are as high as 50% to 75%.[27,149,183]

The consequences of insomnia are impaired cognition, fatigue or tiredness, depressed mood or irritability, and impaired work or school performance.[114,149,153] Dement and

Pelayo described how a person with insomnia may talk about "trying" to go to sleep, whereas others say they "go" to sleep, and effort is not required.[59] People with chronic insomnia may get worse because their poor sleep leads them to think and behave negatively toward sleep. Gayle Greene, a professor of literature and women's studies, wrote a memoir about her insomnia and her lifelong search and research in this area.

> *The first thing to lose is your sense of humor. The next is the desire to do the things you used to do, then the desire to do anything at all. Parts of your body ache that you do not even know the names of, and your eyes forget how to focus. Words you once knew are not there anymore, and there is less and less to say. People you once cared about fall by the way, and you let them go, too.*[79]

Comorbid insomnia refers to clients who have a medical or psychiatric diagnosis but also have symptoms of insomnia. Treatment begins by addressing the comorbid condition, such as treatment of major depression or pain.[173] Previously it was assumed that treating the condition would eliminate the insomnia, but it is now apparent that numerous psychological and behavioral factors develop that perpetuate the insomnia problem (Box 13.2).[173] As Khurshid points out, "Insomnia is a disorder unto itself that needs independent clinical attention" (p. 28), and that focus on treatment should be not only on the primary diagnosis, because treating the insomnia has been shown to improve in psychiatric disorders.[109] Thus, treatment should also include treatment of insomnia separately. A meta-analysis was conducted and found that CBT-I had positive effects on the treatment decreasing insomnia symptoms in comorbid insomnia.[203]

Insomnia can be severe; it is a pervasive condition and should not be taken lightly. Most people who do not have chronic insomnia may have had the occasional sleepless night and may feel they can relate to a person whose insomnia is chronic. However, the occupational therapist working with a client with insomnia should show sensitivity and should not assume that he or she fully understands the situation; the therapist also must be able to recognize the need to refer the client to a specialist, if necessary.

Obstructive Sleep Apnea

OSA can be a serious medical condition. It has been shown to affect 3% to 7% of men and 2% to 5% of women in the adult general population.[163] Untreated OSA impairs daytime functioning and can diminish the quality of life, accelerate multiple health risks, compromise public safety, and result in increased healthcare spending.[18] Despite increasing awareness by both the public and clinicians, OSA remains considerably underdiagnosed and undertreated.[18] The most common terminal events induced by OSA are heart attack, CVA, and accidents.[59] OSA is twice as common in men as in women before age 50, but the prevalence in the sexes equalizes with age.[90]

OSA is one of several sleep-related breathing disorders (SRBDs) that healthcare providers treat. In OSA the upper airway narrows and normal ventilation becomes impaired during sleep.[107] This causes the person to stop breathing and then awaken (though not usually fully wake up) throughout

TABLE 13.3 Summary of Interventions for Chronic Insomnia

Intervention	Treatment Type	Description
CBT-I	Multicomponent	CBT-I combines one or more of the cognitive therapy strategies with education about sleep regulation plus stimulus control instructions and sleep restriction therapy. CBT-I also often includes sleep hygiene education, relaxation training, and other counterarousal methods. Treatment progresses using information typically gathered with sleep diaries completed by the patient throughout the course of treatment (typically 4–8 sessions).
BTIs	Multicomponent	BTIs include abbreviated versions of CBT-I (typically 1–4 sessions) emphasizing the behavioral components. BTIs typically consist of education about sleep regulation, factors that influence sleep, and behaviors that promote or interfere with sleep, along with a tailored behavioral prescription based on stimulus control and sleep restriction therapy and on information typically derived from a pretreatment sleep diary. Some therapies include brief relaxation or cognitive therapy elements.
Stimulus control	Single-component	A set of instructions designed to (1) extinguish the association between the bed/bedroom and wakefulness to restore the association of bed/bedroom with sleep, and (2) establish a consistent wake-time. Stimulus control instructions: (1) go to bed only when sleepy, (2) get out of bed when unable to sleep, (3) use the bed/bedroom for sleep and sex only (e.g., no reading or watching television in bed), (4) wake up at the same time every morning, and (5) refrain from daytime napping.
Sleep restriction therapy	Single-component	A method designed to enhance sleep drive and consolidate sleep by limiting time in bed equal to the patient's sleep duration, typically estimated from daily diaries. Time in bed is initially limited to the average sleep duration and is subsequently increased or decreased based on sleep efficiency thresholds until sufficient sleep duration and overall sleep satisfaction are achieved.
Relaxation therapy	Single-component	Structured exercises designed to reduce somatic tension (e.g., abdominal breathing, progressive muscle relaxation, autogenic training) and cognitive arousal (e.g., guided imagery training, meditation) that may perpetuate sleep problems.
Cognitive therapy	Single-component	A set of strategies including structured psychoeducation, Socratic questioning, use of thought records, and behavioral experiments designed to identify and modify unhelpful beliefs about sleep that may support sleep-disruptive habits and/or raise performance anxiety about sleeping.
Sleep hygiene	Single-component	A set of general recommendations about lifestyle (e.g., diet, exercise, substance use) and environmental factors (e.g., light, noise, temperature) that may promote or interfere with sleep. Sleep hygiene may include some education about what constitutes "normal" sleep and changes in sleep patterns with aging.
Biofeedback	Single-component	A variant of relaxation training that employs a device capable of monitoring and providing ongoing feedback on some aspect of the patient's physiology. This technique has most commonly employed continuous monitoring of frontalis electromyography activity to assess the overall level of muscle tension. Typically, the biofeedback device produces an ongoing auditory tone to train the patient to relax by learning how to alter the auditory feedback tone in the desired direction (e.g., reduced muscle tension).
Paradoxical intention	Single-component	The patient is instructed to remain awake as long as possible after getting into bed. The patient is instructed to purposefully engage in the feared activity (staying awake) to reduce performance anxiety and conscious intent to sleep that confound associated goal-directed behavior (falling asleep). This method alleviates both the patient's excessive focus on sleep and anxiety over not sleeping; as a result, sleep becomes less difficult to initiate.
Intensive sleep retraining	Single-component	This newly described treatment is designed to markedly enhance homeostatic sleep drive to reduce both sleep onset difficulties and sleep misperception. After a night wherein the patient limits time in bed to no more than 5 hours, the treatment includes a 24-hour laboratory protocol in which the patient is given an opportunity to fall asleep every 30 minutes in sleep-conducive conditions. If sleep occurs, then the patient is awakened after 3 minutes and remains awake until the subsequent 30-minute trial. For each sleep opportunity, the patient is given feedback as to whether or not sleep occurred.
Mindfulness	Multicomponent or single-component	Mindfulness approaches are used as a form of meditation emphasizing a nonjudgmental state of heightened or complete awareness of one's thoughts, emotions, or experiences on a moment-to-moment basis. Mindfulness therapies are typically administered in a group format. Structured exercises teach momentary awareness, self-acceptance, and muted reactivity. Home practice of mindfulness exercises is required. When applied to people with insomnia, standard mindfulness is often combined with other insomnia therapies such as stimulus control, sleep restriction therapy, and sleep hygiene (described previously).

Multicomponent treatment is a combination of approaches, and single-component treatment is delivered in isolation.
The American Academy of Sleep Medicine commissioned a task force of experts to conduct an evidence review of treatment for chronic insomnia. Provision of interventions requires advanced training. See original article for risks and benefits.
BTIs, Brief therapies for insomnia, *CBT-I*, cognitive-behavioral therapy for insomnia.
From Edinger JD, Arnedt JT, Bertisch SM, et al: Behavioral and psychological treatments for chronic insomnia disorder in adults: an American Academy of Sleep Medicine systematic review, meta-analysis, and GRADE assessment. *J Clin Sleep Med* 17(2):263–298, 2021.

the night, sometimes hundreds of times. Apnea is defined as a complete cessation of airflow for a minimum of 10 seconds, regardless of whether there is oxygen desaturation or fragmented sleep. Hypopnea (shallow breathing) is defined as air flow decreased by 30% or more with oxygen desaturation of 3% to 4%.[85] The apnea/hypopnea index (AHI) is the frequency of abnormal breathing events per hour of sleep.[59] An AHI of

40 means that a person experiences complete or partial air flow blockage 40 times an hour.[85] Snoring and daytime sleepiness are prevalent symptoms of OSA (Box 13.3),[18] and recent research has shown that nocturia (waking one or more times a night to urinate) is comparable to snoring as a screening tool for OSA.[165,169] This constant awakening throughout the night can lead to severe daytime sleepiness and fatigue and higher rates of depression.[152,154] Furthermore, the decrease in oxygen levels throughout the night can cause an increase in blood pressure and can lead to cardiovascular disease.[59,100]

No treatment modalities are universally accepted or used by all clients with OSA; however, evidence indicates that several modalities can improve alertness or quality of life.[18] Currently, OSA is typically treated with a positive airway pressure (PAP) device that provides continuous positive airway pressure (CPAP, pronounced "C-pap") (Fig. 13.9), bilevel PAP (BPAP), or auto-titrating PAP (APAP).[18] The client is fitted with a mask, from which a hose attaches to a generator that provides (for CPAP) a continuous flow of pressurized air through the nose to keep the airway open while the client sleeps. A variety of masks are available (Fig. 13.10), but the three general types are the nasal mask,

---

BOX 13.2 Common Comorbid Disorders, Conditions, and Symptoms Seen With Insomnia

Neurological	Stroke, dementia, Parkinson's disease, seizure disorders, headache disorders, traumatic brain injury, peripheral neuropathy, chronic pain disorders, neuromuscular disorders
Cardiovascular	Angina, congestive heart failure, dyspnea, dysrhythmias
Pulmonary	Chronic obstructive pulmonary disease, emphysema, asthma, laryngospasm
Digestive	Reflux, peptic ulcer disease, cholelithiasis, colitis, irritable bowel syndrome
Genitourinary	Incontinence, benign prostatic hypertrophy, nocturia, enuresis, interstitial cystitis
Endocrine	Hypothyroidism, hyperthyroidism, diabetes mellitus
Musculoskeletal	Rheumatoid arthritis, osteoarthritis, fibromyalgia, Sjögren's syndrome, kyphosis
Reproductive	Pregnancy, menopause, menstrual cycle variations
Sleep disorders	Obstructive sleep apnea, central sleep apnea, restless legs syndrome, periodic limb movement disorder, circadian rhythm sleep disorders, parasomnias
Other	Allergies; rhinitis; sinusitis; bruxism; alcohol and other substance use, dependence, or withdrawal; cancer[115]; pain from any source[115]

From Schutte-Rodin S, Broch L, Buysse D, et al: Clinical guideline for the evaluation and management of chronic insomnia in adults, *J Clin Sleep Med* 4:492, 2008.

BOX 13.3 Symptoms of Obstructive Sleep Apnea

- Snoring
- Witnessed apnea
- Excessive daytime sleepiness
- Morning headache
- Dry throat in the morning
- Depressive symptoms
- Erectile dysfunction
- Insomnia
- Impaired vigilance and memory

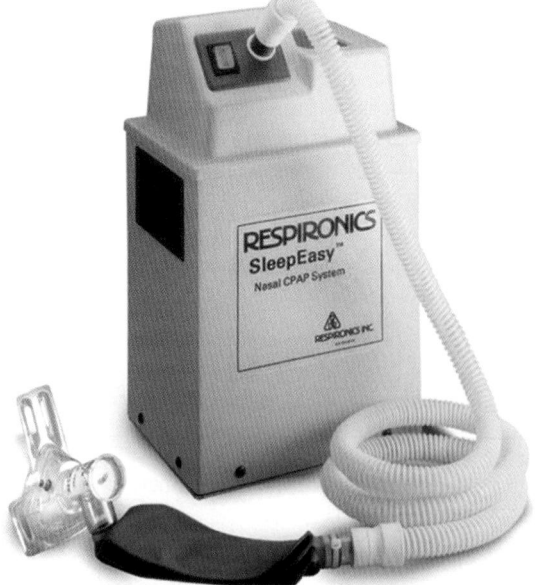 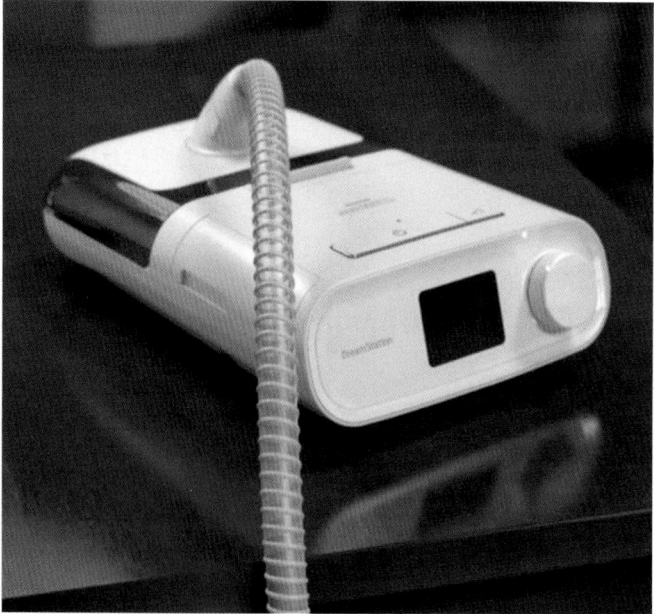

Fig. 13.9 Continuous positive airway pressure (CPAP) machines have dramatically decreased in size since they were first introduced. *Left,* The SleepEasy system (1985). *Right,* The DreamStation system (2016). (Courtesy Philips Respironics, Murrysville, PA.)

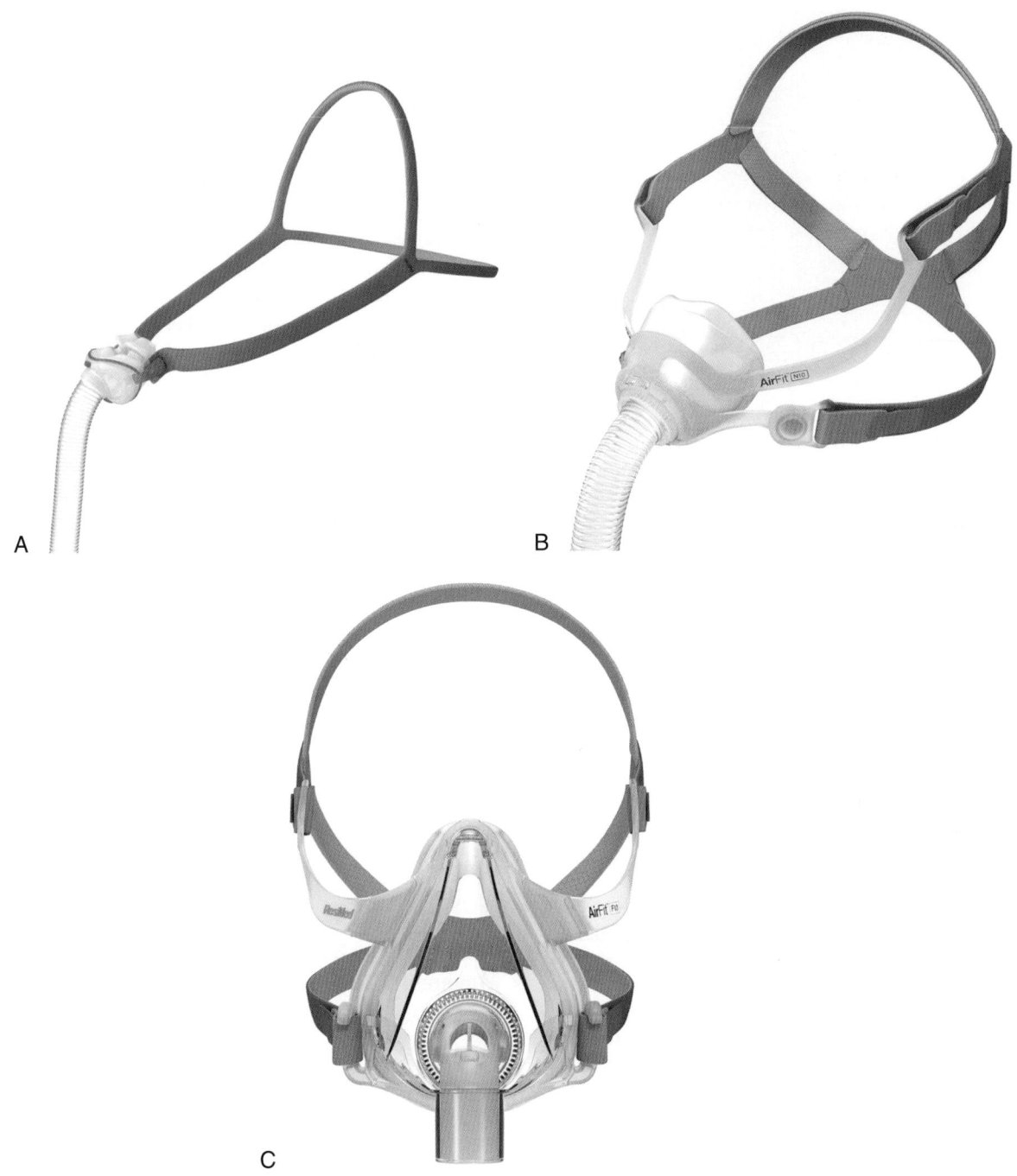

Fig. 13.10 Sample of available CPAP masks and headgear. Three general types of masks are used for adults. (A) A nasal pillow mask, for which prongs are inserted into the nostrils (AirFit P10. Airfit is a trademark of ResMed.). (B) A nasal mask (AirFit N10). (C) A full face mask (AirFit F10). (D) Pediatric mask (the Pixi). (Courtesy ResMed, San Diego, CA.)

nasal pillow, and full-face mask (Fig. 13.11). CPAP has proved to be effective and is a standard for use in OSA.[116] It can be critical for reducing blood pressure in some clients and has been found to eliminate apneas, improve sleep quality, reduce EDS, and improve quality of life.[54,92] However, many people do not follow the recommendations for proper use of a CPAP; 29% to 93% of clients do not adhere to the therapeutic recommendation when adherence is defined as using the CPAP for more than 4 hours a night.[157]

Internationally, adherence also has been shown to be poor. Researchers in Tianjin, China, found adherence to CPAP therapy to be about 50%; many clients did not follow through, abandoned use of the device, or did not even purchase it in the first place.[191] Swedish researchers described nonadherence as occurring for a variety of reasons, such as dry throat, difficulty adjusting the mask, mask leakage, disturbing noise, difficulty changing sleep positions with the mask on, dry eyes, and difficulty traveling with the device.[31] Other barriers to CPAP adherence include negative attitudes toward the CPAP machine, insufficient support from healthcare personnel and family, feelings of shame about the need for CPAP, reduced freedom, a

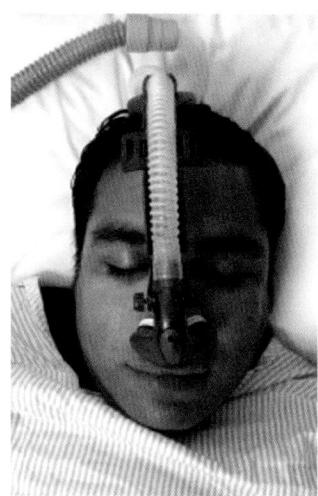

Fig 13.11 Patient with continuous positive airway pressure (CPAP) device. Patient is wearing nasal pillows (positive pressure only through nose). (From Goldman L, Schafer AI: *Goldman-Cecil medicine*, ed 25, Philadelphia, 2016, Elsevier.)

desire to avoid lifelong treatment, claustrophobic thoughts, and anxiety about the technology itself.[31]

Other primary treatments for OSA include oral appliances or dental devices provided by dentists trained in this specialty, in addition to surgery to open the airway.[18,90] Oral appliance application is relatively simple and reversible and may be used for snoring and mild OSA.[59] Examples of dental appliances include molds for the teeth to move the lower jaw forward or a tongue retainer that pulls the tongue forward.[59] Surgical procedures may include removal of nasal polyps, tonsils, or redundant palatal tissue; advancement of the mandible (cutting of the bone of upper and lower jaw and pulling structures forward), and tracheostomy.[59] Weight reduction, topical nasal corticosteroid use, and positional therapies[18,132] are all within the guidelines of the AASM as possible treatments for OSA. Positional therapy, which involves sleeping in the nonsupine position and using pillows, is most useful (i.e., normalizes the AHI) for clients who have less severe OSA, are less obese, and are younger.[132] A pilot study showed that use of trained "peer buddies" who were successful in CPAP use increased adherence to CPAP therapy in a group of veterans newly diagnosed with OSA.[157]

If left untreated, OSA can have severe adverse effects on a client's functioning throughout the day. When a person is chronically sleep deprived, daytime function is affected by slowed thought processes, forgetfulness, slowed responses, and difficulty concentrating.[192] Clients who had sustained a CVA and had been treated in a hospital rehabilitation program were found to have a comorbid SRBD that predicted a poorer outcome in the functional recovery rate.[42] Researchers suspect that two processes contribute to decreased cognitive functioning in clients with OSA: nocturnal hypoxia (decreased oxygen to the brain) and fragmented sleep. Furthermore, as a group, OSA clients' risk of motor vehicle accidents is increased twofold. Research also has shown that sleep-disordered breathing precedes stroke and may contribute to its development.[105]

A small, qualitative study in Ireland looked at how occupations were affected in nine people diagnosed with OSA. The six

men and three women participants were interviewed, and an overarching theme emerged: sleep apnea is a life-changing condition.[150] Five subthemes representing the life-altering aspects of OSA also became apparent: occupational participation, psychological well-being, relationships, executive functioning, and treatment. Participants reported inability to fully enjoy and partake in daily life, being forced into early retirement, having worries about the future, having relational/social difficulties, memory/executive function problems, and the need to use a CPAP (described as an "albatross" that must be lugged around until death) because of OSA.[150]

Considering the functional and cognitive impairments that can result from OSA, it is important for occupational therapists to ask clients about their sleep when evaluating those who may have a secondary diagnosis of OSA or symptoms that indicate an SRBD and referral to a physician. Functional-cognitive impairments may affect follow-through on home programs, safety, and ability to meet goals, and they can diminish the quality of life.

Since the mid-1990s it has been known that 60% to 70% of all stroke clients exhibit sleep-disordered breathing (SDB) as defined by an AHI of 10 episodes per hour.[26] As cited by Alessi et al.,[5] studies of older adults admitted to rehabilitation hospitals after a stroke showed that sleep apnea is commonplace,[105] is associated with lower admission functional levels, and results in poorer outcomes.[105,194]

Could it be that Mrs. Tanaka has a history of an undiagnosed SRBD? Or is the sleep disturbance the result of the CVA and location of the brain insult? Or is poor sleep hygiene in the hospital the biggest contributor to Mrs. Tanaka's sleep problems? It is critical for the occupational therapist treating Mrs. Tanaka to keep the physician informed about the client's sleepiness during treatment and her loud snoring, both of which can be indicators of OSA.

Restless Legs Syndrome and Periodic Limb Movement Disorder

Restless legs syndrome (RLS), also known as Willis-Ekbom disease,[37] is a common disease that affects a person's ability to fall asleep and stay asleep.[7,20] RLS affects 10% of adults in the United States, and the prevalence increases with age. The International Restless Legs Syndrome Study Group's guidelines for diagnosis of the disease are the following five criteria[7]:

- An *urge to move the legs* is usually but not always accompanied by or felt to be caused by uncomfortable sensations (e.g., creepy-crawly) in the legs.
- The urge to move the legs and any unpleasant sensations begin or *worsen during periods of rest or inactivity*, such as lying down or sitting.
- The urge to move the legs and any accompanying unpleasant sensations are *partially or totally relieved by movement*, such as walking, getting up, or stretching, at least as long as the activity continues.
- The urge to move the legs and any accompanying unpleasant sensations during rest or inactivity only occur or are *worse in the evening or night* rather than during the day.
- The occurrence of the previously listed features is *not due to other medical or behavior problems* (e.g., muscle pain, leg

edema, arthritis, leg cramps, positional problems, or foot tapping behaviors).

The clinical significance of this disorder is determined by issues or impairments in social, occupational, educational or other areas of functioning and by their impact on sleep, energy and vitality, daily activities, behavior, and cognition or mood,[7] all of which are in the realm of occupational therapy.[15]

Many clients with comorbid conditions associated with RLS are treated by occupational therapists as in-clients or out-clients and in-home health, nursing home, and other settings (Fig. 13.12). RLS symptoms can occur anytime in the day during prolonged immobilization (e.g., a long car drive), but they typically occur in the evening, with increasing symptoms until bedtime. The urge to move the legs results in insomnia, the effects of which can be detrimental to occupational performance.

Some think that RLS is related to dopamine deficiency, whereas other hypotheses focus on brain iron deficiency. Current nonpharmacological treatment includes encouraging alerting (mentally challenging) activities, which have been found to relieve RLS symptoms, and avoiding caffeine, alcohol, and nicotine.[20] Because occupational therapists focus on occupation and wellness, these are certainly areas in which practitioners can provide treatment.

Periodic limb movement disorder (PLMD) is frequently confused with RLS, but it is a different condition, although the two can coexist. PLMD affects up to 34% of clients over 60 years of age, and the prevalence increases with age. PLMD can be definitively diagnosed only with an EMG and a sleep study/ PSG. In this disorder, a client has periodic episodes of repetitive and stereotyped movements of the limbs (arms or legs), which the client cannot control, during sleep. This results in client arousals or awakenings during sleep, which the client often does not recognize. The creepy-crawly sensations present in RLS do not exist in PLMD. When PLMD is severe, clients experience excessive sleepiness, which can affect daytime functioning.[21]

Narcolepsy

Narcolepsy is a neurological sleep disorder characterized by **excessive daytime sleepiness (EDS)**, cataplexy, sleep paralysis, and hypnagogic hallucinations; it is most likely an autoimmune disease.[57,59] Cataplexy, sleep paralysis, and hypnagogic hallucinations are abnormal manifestations of REM sleep into wakefulness.[19] The excessive sleepiness is not relieved by adequate time sleeping.[19] Cataplexy, which affects 60% to 100% of individuals with narcolepsy,[19] manifests when a person has a sudden loss of postural and muscle tone during an emotional

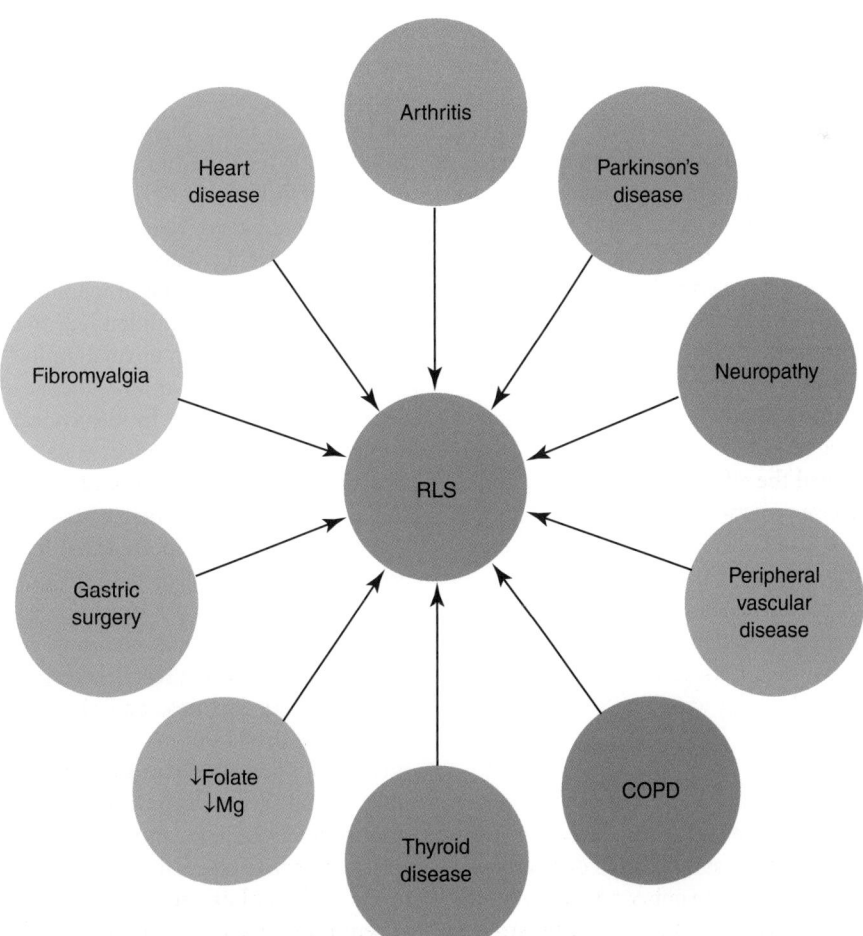

Fig. 13.12 Comorbid conditions associated with late-onset (after 45 years of age) secondary restless legs syndrome (RLS). Occupational therapists treat many of these clients in their practice. *COPD*, Chronic obstructive pulmonary disease; *Mg*, magnesium. (From Avidon A: Restless legs syndrome and periodic limb movements in sleep. In Kryger MH, editor: *Atlas of clinical sleep medicine*, Philadelphia, 2010, Saunders Elsevier.)[20]

event such as laughter, joking, anger, excitation, startle, fear, and even sex.[19,57,59] The person is still conscious when the cataplexy occurs, and his or her breathing is normal.[19] People with this disorder have disturbed and fragmented nocturnal sleep. Sleep paralysis occurs at the start or end of sleep and is demonstrated by the fact that a person cannot move for a few seconds or minutes.[19,57,59] Hypnagogic hallucinations are characterized by vivid, dreamlike experiences that occur at the onset or end of sleep; they are generally frightful and visual but can be tactile or auditory.[19] The goal of therapeutic approaches is to control the narcoleptic symptoms, maintain wakefulness and alertness during the day, and allow the client to have full participation in life.[57,59] Good sleep hygiene, instruction in anticipation of attacks, behavioral treatments, and support groups may be important.[5]

Parkinson's Disease and Alzheimer's Disease

Alzheimer's disease (AD) and Parkinson's disease (PD) are not sleep disorders, but they are the two most common neurodegenerative disorders in our society.[170] Sleep disturbances are commonly reported in both PD and AD,[170] especially insomnia, hypersomnia, and excessive daytime napping.[170] The most commonly seen neurodegenerative disorder in a sleep disorders clinic is PD.[21]

Sleep problems are common in all forms of PD.[21,187] Among clients with PD, 60% to 90% have sleep complaints. A majority of clients with PD have sleep complaints that adversely affect sleep, including excessive sleepiness, insomnia, nightmares, and other sleep disorders. As the severity of the disease increases, sleep complaints also increase. Foster[69] and Dixon et al.[61] pointed out that people with PD are referred to occupational therapy when significant physical disabilities are present, so clients referred to an occupational therapist may already have severe sleep complaints.[61] Gregory et al.[84] found that the chronically disturbed sleep of a person with PD can also adversely affect the coping ability and sleep quality of the person's caregivers. Improved sleep hygiene is an important treatment that can be provided to this population, in addition to training in safe bed mobility, transfer training, and adaptive equipment (e.g., bedside commode) for safety in toileting tasks.[84,187]

Nascimento et al.[50] studied the effects of a multimodal mild to moderate physical exercise program on 35 people diagnosed with AD and 42 subjects with PD in Brazil. Examples of exercises included calisthenics, resistive, balance, and aerobic exercises performed over a 6-month period by both PD and AD clients. The results showed a reduction in IADL deficits and attenuation of sleep disturbance in both groups.[50]

Consequences of Poor Sleep
Sleepiness

The seemingly obvious but not so obvious consequence of sleep debt is sleepiness or drowsiness. Behavioral signs of sleepiness include yawning; ptosis (drooping of the upper eyelid); reduced activity; lapses in attention; head nodding,[168] with decreased animation; and head-drop, accompanied by sudden jerking up with a startle, which may indicate a "microsleep."[59] Dement and Pelayo[59] suggested that the "real essence" of the onset of

sleepiness is the awareness that remaining alert and attentive takes effort. Besides the embarrassment that may be caused by those behaviors in a public place, there are serious consequences to sleepiness.

The terms *sleepiness, fatigue,* and *somnolence* are sometimes used interchangeably. However, sleepiness should be distinguished from fatigue. Sleepiness is a sleep state that is characterized by the tendency to fall asleep, whereas fatigue is the exhaustion that occurs after exertion.[77] As cited by Bushnik et al.,[33] another definition of fatigue is "the awareness of a decreased capacity for physical and/or mental activity due to an imbalance in the availability, utilization and/or restoration of resources needed to perform activity."[3] Although many people, including sleep experts, use the word *somnolence* and *sleepiness* interchangeably, Gooneratne et al.[76] stated that the terms should not be considered the same. Somnolence is an impaired neurological state that can lead to lethargy or coma, whereas sleepiness is a tendency to fall asleep.

Roehr et al.[168] described sleepiness as a physiological need state, much like hunger or thirst. The body's desire to sleep cannot be met by resting, eating, taking a cold shower, or exercising. It can only be met by sleep. Researchers have quantified sleepiness by how readily subjects fall asleep, by subjects rating how likely they are to fall asleep in certain situations, and by subjects rating themselves on how they feel at the moment. The Multiple Sleep Latency Test (MSLT) is considered the standard method for quantifying sleepiness and is performed by trained sleep technologists.[59,168,179] With this test, subjects are placed in a dark room on a bed. The amount of time it takes the subject to fall asleep is measured every 2 hours during the waking hours on several occasions. Severely sleep-deprived individuals fall asleep instantly (zero sleep latency). Generally, many clinicians consider an average latency of 5 to 8 minutes to be consistent with EDS, a chronic state of inability to stay awake during the day that occurs when unintended; 10 to 12 minutes or longer is considered to be within normal limits.[43]

Research has shown that those who are the most sleep deprived, as evidenced by behavioral measures, are the least accurate in rating their sleepiness. Roehr et al.[168] speculated that adaptation to the chronic sleepiness state occurs, such that some people actually forget what complete alertness feels like. The researchers also reported that for those with mild to moderate sleepiness, subjective complaints of sleepiness and even its behavioral indicators can be masked by a number of factors, such as motivation, environment, posture, activity, light, and food intake. The researchers reported, "Heavy meals, warm rooms, boring lectures, and the monotony of long-distance automobile driving unmask physiological sleepiness when it is present, but they do not cause it."[168] However, for those with significant and severe sleep debt, the ability to override sleepiness diminishes. Even in the most exciting environment, microsleeps (brief episode of sleep, usually NREM)[59] can occur, in addition to the likelihood of sleep onset. An example would be a person falling asleep while watching a live basketball game.

A healthy individual becoming sleepy while watching a sporting event is a relatively benign problem, if it is isolated. However, research has found that sleepiness can be a detriment to functioning. One study found that excessive sleepiness in the older adult without dementia or depression was associated with self-reports of moderate impairments in activities such as housework, sports, activities in the morning or evening, and keeping pace with others.[77] This study showed strong associations between having a number of medical conditions and reporting excessive sleepiness.

Other studies have shown that activities and positioning may affect sleepiness. One study showed that sleep latency increased by 6 minutes when the subject was sitting up rather than lying down. Sleep latency also has been shown to increase by 6 minutes when subjects went for a 5-minute walk before taking the MSLT.[28,29]

Instead of investigating behaviors (of purposefully not getting enough sleep), one group of researchers examined the clinical and PSG predictors of the natural history of EDS in a random population sample. Seven and a half years after the initial data were collected from 1741 individuals (known as the Penn State Adult Cohort), 1395 of them provided follow-up data. Obesity and weight gain were found to play a key role in the development and chronicity of EDS, and weight loss was associated with its remission.[68]

Many well-known disasters have been attributed to workers who were sleep deprived, including the *Exxon Valdez* oil spill (1989), the Three-Mile Island nuclear meltdown (1979), and the *Challenger* space shuttle explosion (1986).[48,56,209]

Countermeasures, or techniques and behaviors used to counteract the drive to fall asleep, are frequently used by sleepy drivers to try to stay awake. The National Sleep Foundation's 2012 poll found that pilots and train operators use caffeine more than controls to stay awake and alert on the job.[142] Staffan's small study in Sweden[178] used social media to find subjects to investigate the kinds of countermeasures used by people to avoid falling asleep while driving. The more common countermeasures included changing seat position, pulling off the road to get fresh air, increasing the fan speed, decreasing the temperature, turning on loud music, and opening windows, among others. Staffan suggested a mismatch between what researchers suggested (short naps) and how people actually behave when sleepy on the road. The research (sponsored by Volvo) suggested the possibility that cars of the future could be designed to include seats that automatically changed position, and systems that could change the temperature in the car or announce to the driver that he or she should get a cup of coffee.[178] Researchers have been studying and developing self-driving cars, also known as autonomous cars and driverless cars have been have been researched since the mid-1980s.[23] Spurred on by challenges in 2004, 2005, and 2007 by the U.S. Defense Advanced Research Projects Agency to develop self-driving cars, advances have developed in this endeavor, though much still needs to be done for safe products to be available to the general public.[23]

These findings have implications for occupational therapists who work with sleepy clients in setting goals and creating treatment plans.

For Mrs. Tanaka, if medical or psychiatric conditions or medication problems are ruled out, occupational therapists can help ensure the client gets adequate sleep at night. If Mrs. Tanaka's

sleep problem includes a shifted circadian rhythm, light exposure during treatment and between therapies during the day may help shift her circadian pattern so that she sleeps at night, not during the day. Treatment in an upright posture in a bright room may help keep her alert longer during treatment so that she can participate in therapy during the day.

Drowsy Driving

The AAA Foundation for Traffic Safety sampled 3511 respondents in the United States, ages 16 and older, on their driving attitudes and behaviors.[2] Approximately 96% of the drivers considered drowsy driving as very or extremely dangerous, and over 97% of drivers disapprove of driving while drowsy. Although it is considered dangerous and there is social disapproval of drowsy driving behaviors, about 24% of respondents admitted driving while sleepy, so much so that their eyes were difficult to keep open, at least one time in 30 days.[2]

A March 2011 report by the U.S. National Highway Traffic Safety Administration (NHTSA) found that drowsy driving was reportedly involved in 2.2% to 2.6% of fatal car crashes annually from 2005 to 2009.[137] However, in 2014, a study conducted by the AAA Foundation for Traffic Safety found that the numbers were much higher than reported by the NHTSA.[1] The AAA foundation study focused on the 14,268 crashes that occurred from 2009 to 2013 in which a vehicle was towed. The study found that a drowsy driver was involved in 7% of crashes in which a person received treatment for injuries sustained in a crash; 13% of crashes in which a person was hospitalized; and 21% of crashes in which a person was killed. If these proportions are applied to all reported crashes nationwide, results suggest that an average of 328,000 crashes annually, including 109,000 crashes that result in injuries and 6,400 fatal crashes, involve a drowsy driver.[1]

In an earlier study, the NHTSA looked at data collected annually from 1991 to 2007 on fatal single-vehicle crashes in which the car ran off the road.[136] The most influential factor in the occurrence of these fatal crashes was sleepiness. The NHTSA reported that a sleepy driver's odds of being involved in a run-off-the-road crash are more than three times higher than those for a driver who is not sleepy. In comparison, the odds of a driver with alcohol in his system (blood alcohol concentration = 0.01 + grams per deciliter) being in a similar crash are almost two times higher than those for a sober driver. Currently, of the 50 states in the United States, only New Jersey (Maggie's Law, passed in 2003) and Arkansas (SB 874, passed in 2013) consider falling asleep at the wheel and fatigued driving a criminal offense in a fatal crash if the driver is found not to have slept in 24 consecutive hours.[13] As of this writing, six other states have "Drowsy Driving Awareness Days" or weeks or have enacted laws to post road signs about the dangers of drowsy driving.[135]

Drowsy driving is a serious international concern. According to data from Australia and from England, Finland, and other European nations, all of which have more consistent crash reporting procedures than the United States, drowsy driving accounts for 10% to 30% of all crashes.[139]

The NSF has reported the following groups as most at risk of being involved in a fall-asleep crash[142]:

- Young people, especially males under 26
- Shift workers and people with long work hours
- Commercial drivers, especially long-haul drivers
- People with undiagnosed or untreated disorders (for individuals with untreated OSA, the risk of falling asleep at the wheel is up to seven times higher)
- Business travelers who drive many hours or are jet lagged

Most drowsy driving crashes happen between midnight and 6:00 am or in the midafternoon during the circadian dip. They typically occur when a driver is alone; they tend to involve a single vehicle running off the road and often hitting a stationary object; and, as opposed to alcohol-related driving, there may not be any evidence of the driver braking or taking evasive maneuvers.[144]

Regarding occupational therapy recommendations in terms of drowsy driving, the safest option is for people to not drive while drowsy and to obtain adequate sleep. Countermeasures to combat drowsy driving such as rolling down the window, turning up the volume on the radio, and singing do little to increase alertness while driving.

The American Academy of Sleep Medicine[9] makes these recommendations:

- Get a full night of 7 to 8 hours of sleep before driving
- Avoid driving late at night
- Avoid driving alone
- For long trips, share driving duties with another passenger
- Pull over at a rest stop and take a nap
- Use caffeine for a short-term boost
- Take a short nap after consuming caffeine to maximize the effect
- Arrange for someone to give you a ride home after working a late shift

Shift Work

Research results suggesting that shift work can be deleterious to people's health are well documented. As previously mentioned, the invention of artificial light and the Industrial Revolution changed the work world so that people could now work around the clock. The prevalence of shift work sleep disorder that results in insomnia is estimated to be about 10% of the night and rotating shift worker population.[167]

Neuromuscular Disorders and Sleep

Individuals with neuromuscular disorders are considered in a "state of vulnerability" during sleep because normal REM-related changes, such as atonia and other changes in ventilation, are magnified as a result of muscle weakness. Sleep disturbance also can be related to spasticity, poor secretion clearance, sphincter dysfunction, inability to turn, pain, and any associated or secondary autonomic dysfunction. These factors can impair sleep and decrease daytime functioning.[76] Individuals who rely on accessory muscles to breathe (e.g., those with quadriplegia/tetraplegia) are also in a vulnerable state during sleep. Indeed, research has shown that individuals with a spinal cord injury (SCI) have a two to five times greater prevalence of SDB than that seen in the general population.[171] Researchers suggest that all clients with SCI undergo full PSG studies to better

detect sleep-disordered breathing because many such cases may go undetected with a limited sleep study recording.[171] Sleep disturbance also is a common consequence of traumatic brain injury,[156] and individuals with this condition are another group of clients that occupational therapists treat.[33,62,198]

Other Consequences of Sleep Deprivation

Young et al.[206] noted that sleep deprivation can result in a multitude of negative physical and psychological consequences, even when the person is healthy. These negative consequences include but are not limited to hypertension,[73,151] decreased postural control,[67] possible obesity, and diabetes[73,75,111] and decreased insulin sensitivity (seen in a group of nondiabetic White males).[200] Inadequate sleep can also result in greater likelihood of falls.[181] In older adults the consequences of poor sleep are significant; they can include overall poorer health, physical function, and cognitive function and increased mortality.[16]

Sleep Considerations in the Hospital Setting

As mentioned previously, inadequate sleep can have serious consequences in and of itself. Acute hospitalization combined with inadequate sleep can further hinder recovery. Studies have shown that approximately half of clients admitted to general medical wards complain of sleep disruption. Young et al.[206] found that clients who were hospitalized had difficulty initiating and maintaining sleep and complained of early awakening and nonrestorative sleep.[206] Hospital sounds have been found to disrupt sleep even in healthy individuals.[34] Buxton et al. studied the effects of typical sounds present in hospital settings on 12 healthy young subjects.[34] They found that electronic sounds designed to alert medical staff were more arousing than other sounds and that even brief frequent noises can increase heart rates, which is especially important to consider in critical care settings. These researchers stressed that their study was conducted on young, healthy subjects and that many hospital clients are older, have decreased quality and quantity of deep sleep, and would be less able to tolerate the noises present in hospital settings.[34] They concluded that "protecting sleep from acoustic assault in hospital settings is a key goal in advancing the quality of care for in-client medicine."[34]

Hardin reported that for more than 30 years (now 40+ years), sleep abnormalities have been documented in clients in the intensive care unit (ICU).[88] Current research continues to show that ICU sounds and lights interrupt sleep and that earplugs, eye masks, and oral melatonin improve sleep quality in healthy subjects.[95] Environmental noises and client care activities account for about 30% of awakenings in ICU clients.[72] The noise levels in ICUs are found to be especially high.[129]

Although noise in the hospital is a concern, a study by Freedman et al.[70] suggested that nursing care activities, such as taking vital signs and giving sponge baths, may actually contribute more to client awakening than the environmental conditions. Bartick et al.[24] reported similar results in their study, which found that hospital staff was the factor most responsible for sleep disruption in clients and that behavioral interventions for hospital staff members can actually reduce the use of sedatives. A qualitative study by Hopper et al.[93] of nurses and physicians working in an ICU found multiple environmental barriers to sleep; in addition, the study found that attitudinal barriers also may contribute to sleep disruption in the ICU. Attitudinal barriers included staff uncertainty about the significance of sleep, the tensions of providing protocol-driven care versus allowing the client to sleep, and lack of consensus about interventions.[93]

The cause of sleep disturbances in the hospital or institutional setting is multifactorial and can be related to a client's medical illness, medical treatments, and the environment.[206] Clients treated in a traditional rehabilitation setting may also have a higher likelihood of sleep disturbance. In one study[122] of 31 consecutively admitted clients, diagnosed with a closed head injury (CHI), who were admitted to a brain injury unit, 68% had sleep/wake cycle disturbance. Those with the aberrations in nighttime sleep had longer stays in both the acute and rehabilitation settings—an important consideration in an era of concern over high healthcare costs.[122]

Taking account of these factors, it is important to consider Mrs. Tanaka's sleep patterns at the facility or unit before admission to the rehabilitation hospital or unit. Was Mrs. Tanaka in the ICU? How long was she there before admission to the rehabilitation unit? Was her sleep disturbed in that setting?

To Nap or Not to Nap?

According to the NSF, napping can be categorized in three ways[145]:

- *Planned napping:* Also known as preparatory napping, planned napping involves taking a nap before one becomes sleepy. This type of nap is used when a person knows that a later bedtime than usual is planned for that day.
- *Emergency napping:* This type of nap occurs when a person suddenly realizes that sleep is imminent and that the activity he or she is engaged in will not be possible very shortly. This type of napping can be used to help a drowsy driver or a worker who is operating dangerous machinery.
- *Habitual napping:* This type of nap is taken at the same time every day and is frequently done by children or by adults who require an afternoon nap.

The research has been mixed on whether it's a good idea for a person to nap during the day.[89] The primary concerns are that napping fragments sleep and that consolidated nighttime sleep may be disrupted as a result. A study by Alessi et al.[5] suggested that sleep disruption is common and severe among older persons receiving in-client post-acute rehabilitation and that excessive daytime napping was associated with less functional recovery for up to 3 months after admission. As cited by Woods et al.,[201] other studies have shown that naps longer than 1½ hours in the afternoon can be associated with increased falls and hip fractures,[22] more night awakenings, and higher mortality.[182] In their study of nursing home residents with moderate to severe dementia, Woods et al.[201] found that excessive daytime naps may be linked to elevated evening cortisol levels, indicative of circadian rhythm dysregulation (phase delay).

In a large population-based study of middle- to older-aged cohorts of British citizens, associations were found between daytime napping and an increased risk of mortality from all causes and respiratory diseases.[119] Another study, conducted in China, suggested an association between frequent napping and a higher prevalence of type 2 diabetes in the older population.[117]

On the other hand, some researchers are finding benefits to napping and thus recommending short naps, and other researchers have found that daytime naps do not necessarily hinder night sleep. In their study of 100 community-dwelling older adults with typical age-related health issues, Dautovich et al.[55] found that naps do not hinder consolidated night sleep. A study by Payne et al.[159] added to a growing body of evidence suggesting that even a short daytime nap can be enough to produce marked memory advantages, and that these benefits can be selective for emotionally salient and adaptive information. A study of clients with myasthenia gravis found that naps longer than 5 minutes can mitigate symptoms of fatigue.[108] A still limited but growing body of literature suggests that a daily afternoon nap may be a safe and effective means of increasing 24-hour sleep and improving waking functions.[36] The NSF considers that good naps may have psychological benefits and can be a "pleasant luxury, a mini-vacation. It can provide an easy way to get some relaxation and rejuvenation."[145] Box 13.4 presents tips on napping.

The debate over whether naps are beneficial continues. Current research seems to indicate that shorter daytime naps (e.g., 20–30 minutes) may be beneficial, but overly extended daytime naps (1½–2 hours) may actually have negative health effects.[89] More research needs to be done in this area; the OT practitioner should keep up to date on current research and not simply rely on commonly held beliefs. For example, caregivers who work in nursing homes frequently view napping during the day as good for residents with dementia. However, they may not be aware of the potentially negative consequences of extended naps.[201]

Nocturia

Nocturia is defined as waking one or more times to void (urinate) at night. It is the most common lower urinary tract symptom.[30] Booth and McMillan[30] cited prevalence studies[98,172] indicating that nocturia increases in both sexes with age. The most significant consequence of nocturia is sleep disturbance, with evidence of fatigue during the day affecting energy and activity.[17] Zeitzer et al.[208] examined the sleep and toileting patterns of 147 community-dwelling older men and women with insomnia and found that more than half of all reported awakenings

---

BOX 13.4   How to Take a Good Nap

- Keep the nap short. A 20- to 30-minute nap may be ideal, but even a few minutes has benefits. A longer nap may lead to post-sleep grogginess ("sleep inertia").
- Find a dark, quiet, cool place. Do not waste a lot of time getting to sleep. Dimming the light and reducing noise help most people fall asleep faster.
- Plan a nap in the afternoon instead of napping haphazardly.
- Time caffeine intake so that it does not coincide with the nap.
- Do not feel guilty about taking a nap. A good, well-timed nap can actually help increase productivity.

Modified from the Harvard Health Letter: How to take a good nap, Boston, 2009, Harvard Medical School Publications.

were associated with nocturia. The need for more trips to the toilet was associated with decreased feelings of being rested and decreased sleep efficiency; thus, nocturia compounds the negative impact of insomnia.[208]

Obayashi et al.[149] reported similar results from their large-scale study of general community-dwelling older adults in Japan. They found an association between nocturnal voiding frequency and poor objective sleep quality (lower sleep efficiency, longer duration of wakefulness after sleep onset, and shorter duration of sleep latency). Other studies have shown an association between the risk of falls and nocturia, and that caregivers and other sleeping partners also are at risk of falls during the night and day because of fatigue resulting from sleep disruption.[17]

In an editorial on the study by Obayashi et al.,[149] Mehra[124] pointed out that nocturia is also highly prevalent in the non-older adult population, citing a study[49] that showed that in a U.S. sample, 31% reported voiding more than once a night, and 14% reported voiding two or more times a night. Mehra suggested that more research should be done on ways interventions could influence nocturia so as to improve sleep health.[124]

When evaluating a client's ADL status, occupational therapists should always ask the client about his or her voiding habits at night. The frequency of voiding can alert the OT practitioner to sleep disturbances or other issues. Information on voiding habits also can help the occupational therapist determine whether the client is using safe toileting practices, and whether he or she needs durable medical equipment (DME; e.g., bedside commode), adaptive equipment, routines, splint/orthotic schedules, a safe environmental setup, or possibly referral to the client's physician to address problems in this area.

Hunjan and Twiss[96] suggested that OT practitioners embrace the practice of helping clients with urinary incontinence in general, not just nocturia. They offered behavioral strategies that can be explored, including evaluating schedules; implementing timed, scheduled, or prompted voids; seeking assistance as needed; modifying the diet (with the help of a dietitian); and managing fluids and medications (in consultation with the physician or healthcare provider)—all of which may also help with nocturia.[96] Cunningham and Valasek[51] did preliminary research on three women regarding treatment of urinary symptoms and found reduced symptom severity and positive life impacts and agree that occupational therapists should be included on primary healthcare teams to support effective treatments of urinary issues.

OCCUPATIONAL THERAPY AND SLEEP

In current practice, a sleep disturbance may not be the primary reason a client seeks occupational therapy services. However, because it has been established that insufficient sleep can impair or negatively affect all occupations, this is clearly an important area to consider in occupational therapy treatment in all practice settings.

Occupational therapists work in many settings, including hospitals, long-term care and skilled nursing facilities, home health, out-client rehabilitation clinics, psychiatric facilities, community health programs, schools, and academia.[14] OT

practitioners in all practice settings can be educated about the occupations of sleep and rest; they therefore can potentially have a significant positive impact on the general health of society.

OCCUPATIONAL THERAPY EVALUATION

It is important to obtain a thorough occupational profile of the client during the evaluation, including the client's history and experiences, patterns, interests, values, and needs.[15] The profile also should include questions about the client's sleep and rest patterns, routines, and habits. The Occupational Profile of Sleep[162] can be used to collect more specific information on sleep. A thorough medical history and information on whether the client has a history of sleep disorders or difficulties are other elements of the profile. A standardized, valid measure, such as the Epworth Sleepiness Scale (ESS)[133] (Fig. 13.13), originally designed to measure sleepiness but is now widely used for screening for OSA, or the Pittsburgh Sleep Quality Index (PSQI),[35] can be used to collect initial and later outcome information on sleep. Screening tools such as the Berlin questionnaire,[146] STOP-BANG questionnaire (SBQ),[46] STOP questionnaire,[47] and ESS[133] are widely used for OSA screening, but the findings on diagnostic accuracy are controversial, so a meta-analysis investigated and compared the summary sensitivity, specificity, and diagnostic odds[44] and found that the SBQ compared with the others was a more accurate tool for detecting mild, moderate, and severe OSA. Chiu and team[44] suggest that sleep specialists should use the SBQ to conduct patient interviews for the early diagnosis of OSA in clinical settings, especially if resources are lacking and testing by PSG is unavailable or not possible. This writer suggests that the SBQ be used for regularly screening people for OSA, a common diagnosis for people seen by OT. This writer combined the SBQ with Pierce and Summers Occupational Profile of Sleep[162] and with Carney et al.'s[38] Consensus Sleep Diary to be an effective sleep screen to use with older adults and anticipates that it could be used with other adult populations (Fig. 13.14).[113]

Fung et al.[71] found the Functional Outcome of Sleep Questionnaire[193] to be well suited to helping occupational therapists understand the impact of sleep on function and daily occupational performance. They also suggested use of the Daily Cognitive-Communication and Sleep Profile,[193] another self-reporting instrument that investigates sleep/wake disturbances in terms of cognition, communication, and mood.

A unique way to collect information on clients' pre-sleep routines is to have people draw pictures of their pre-sleep routine. In a qualitative study Koketsu[113] had 16 typical adult sleepers draw pictures of their pre-sleep routines, then interviewed people about the sleep routine. The drawings were found to be a useful method for people to describe pre-sleep routines and a way to dig deeper in describing routines during the interview.[113]

OCCUPATIONAL THERAPY INTERVENTION FOR SLEEP AND REST

Leland et al.[118] conducted a scoping review/systematic summary of the literature on sleep interventions and identified four

---

Epworth Sleepiness Scale

Using the following scale, circle the *most appropriate number* for each situation.

0 = Would doze *less than once a month*
1 = *Slight* chance of dozing
2 = *Moderate* chance of dozing
3 = *High* chance of dozing

Situation		Chance of Dozing		
Sitting and reading	0	1	2	3
Watching TV	0	1	2	3
Sitting, inactive in a public place (in a theater or in a meeting)	0	1	2	3
As a passenger in a car for an hour without a break	0	1	2	3
Lying down to rest in the afternoon (when circumstances permit)	0	1	2	3
Sitting and talking to someone	0	1	2	3
Sitting quietly after a lunch without alcohol	0	1	2	3
In a car, while stopped for a few minutes in the traffic	0	1	2	3

Add the 8 numbers you have circled   Total _____

Fig. 13.13 The Epworth Sleepiness Scale has been validated in clinical settings and can be used by occupational therapists to collect information for referring a client to a physician. A score of 10 or higher indicates excessive daytime sleepiness. A score of 6 is the norm. However, clients with insomnia can have scores in the normal range. A score of 12 to 24 may indicate a severe abnormality. (Modified from Johns MW: A new method for measuring daytime sleepiness: the Epworth Sleepiness Scale, *Sleep* 14:540–545, 1991.)

intervention areas in which OT practitioners can help clients with sleep: (1) cognitive behavioral therapy for insomnia, (2) physical activity, (3) multicomponent interventions, and (4) other intervention strategies that improve sleep and fall within OT's scope of practice. Physical activity included a variety of activities, such as stretching, resistance training, yoga, tai chi, Qigong, dancing, and running. Examples of multicomponent interventions included sleep restriction/compression, sleep hygiene, relaxation techniques, and bright lights. Other interventions included strategies such as earplugs, eye masks, light therapy, music, and headphones to help with sleep. With all these interventions, the emphasis was on consistent focus on modifying existing habits and routines, and participation in activity that followed adherence to sleep restriction/compression.[118] Fung et al.[71] suggested that occupational therapists can provide education and interventions such as awareness of pain, energy levels, sleepiness, fatigue, and stress levels, in addition to environmental recommendations and strategies to pace activities (also see Chapter 51).[71]

According to the OTPF-4,[15] the types of OT intervention include therapeutic use of occupations and activities, interventions to support occupations, education and training, advocacy, and group and virtual interventions. All of these interventions can be used for treating clients in the occupations of sleep and rest. They are reviewed after the discussions of the therapeutic use of self and consultation.

Therapeutic Use of Self

The therapeutic use of self is a therapeutic agent (not necessarily an "intervention") that should be integral to the practice of occupational therapy and interwoven in all interactions with clients.[15] Therapeutic use of self allows OT practitioners to develop and manage their relationships with clients by using narrative and professional reasoning, empathy, and a client-centered and collaborative focus.[15] With therapeutic use of self, the OT practitioner can demonstrate caring and concern for the client or caregivers about the amount and quality of their rest and sleep. Sleep medicine is a relatively new discipline, so many physicians do not ask their clients about their sleep or do not recognize the signs of sleep disorders or issues.[66] Therefore, because of occupational therapy's attention to occupations, routines, and life balance, the OT practitioner may be the first to ask a client or caregiver about sleep concerns.

The OT practitioner can practice "mindful empathy," a mode of observing the client's emotions, needs, and motives while remaining objective.[184] For example, instead of judging a client for canceling appointments or not fully participating in treatment, the occupational therapist should actively listen to the client and reassess the situation; this approach could reveal a sleep-deprived client.

Therapeutic use of self also means that OT practitioners must be more knowledgeable and have competency in the areas of sleep and rest so as to help clients optimize their sleep and rest patterns. Becoming knowledgeable about sleep and sleep disorders can help the OT practitioner recognize any problems that may indicate severe sleep disturbance so the client can be referred to a physician or sleep specialist.

OT practitioners can also model good sleep practices, so that they are alert, safe, and functioning at their best when working with clients. In addition, occupational therapists need to examine their own values about sleep and rest because attitudinal barriers on the part of the healthcare staff may affect the sleep of clients.[93] For example, do you consider sleep and rest a waste of time? Is a person lazy if he or she requires a nap during the afternoon?

Developing cultural competency is a "central skill" for using oneself therapeutically.[184] As previously mentioned, recognizing

Koketsu OT Sleep Profile

Name:_____   Date: _____

Client Record #: _____   Date of Birth: _____

Diagnosis: _____

Precautions/Allergies: _____

Level of function for ADL: _____   Level of function for IADL: _____

Medications (include over the counter, herbal supplements)

Medication Name   **Dosage**   **Time taken**

If you take sleep medications, is it a goal of yours to eventually stop it? (Notify PCP)

Client's (or caregiver) Sleep Concerns /Effects on function (If "none," state here):

When did this issue start? _____   Any mind racing? _____

How high of a priority is sleep to you?

Naps (frequency, time of day, length, wake refreshed?):

Sleep pattern on weekend:

New stresses in life:

<u>**AWAKE ROUTINE**</u>

Morning routine (times and what you do):

Other activities in bedroom besides sleep:

Exercise regularly: yes no **Type:** _____   **Time of day?** _____

Meals (time and foods):

Fig. 13.14 Koketsu Occupational Therapy Sleep Profile. (From Koketsu, J: *Pre-sleep routines of adult normal sleepers.* 2018. [Occupational Therapy Doctorate Capstone Projects, 34]. https://encompass. eku.edu/otdcapstones/34.)

How much control do you have over timing of meals and types of food?

Caffeine intake: Yes No **How much?** _____ **Time of day?**_____

Drink alcoholic beverages? Yes No **How much?**_____ **Time of day?** _____

Smoke? Yes No **How much?** ____**Are you around smoke on a regular basis?** Yes No

Evening routine from dinner to bedtime (times and what you do):

SLEEP ENVIRONMENT

Location of sleep (do not assume on bed):_____

Bed size: king, queen, full, twin **Bedding type (mattress)/condition/age:**_____

Do you like your bed? If not, why not? _____

Equipment used at night: w/c commode oxygen PAP Cath Other:

Linens type and texture: _____

Type of pajamas or night clothes:_____

Temperature: _____ **Light level:** _____ **Noise level:** _____

Bed sharers: partner, children, pets other: _____

Number of people who sleep in same space_____ **Who are they?**_____

Do the others in same bedroom negatively affect sleep? Yes No **If yes, how?**_____

Sleep environment (Is it dark, quiet, cool, comfortable, safe?):

SLEEP PATTERNS: STOP-BANG[47]

Snore loudly	**Yes**	**No**
Tired, fatigued, sleepy during day?	**Yes**	**No**
Observed apnea?	**Yes**	**No**
Pressure (Hypertension)?	**Yes**	**No**
BMI >35 mg/m2?	**Yes**	**No**
Age >50 years	**Yes**	**No**
Neck circumference > 16"?	**Yes**	**No**
Gender: male?	**Yes**	**No**

Fig. 13.14 Cont'd   *(Continued)*

High risk of OSA: yes 5–8, Intermediate risk of OSA Yes 3–4, Low risk of OSA: Yes 0–2

*Do you move around in your sleep a lot?

*Do you move your legs, have the urge to move them, or have pain? _____

*Do you have nightmares regularly?   _____

*Above questions may indicate possible sleep disorders (PLMD, parasomnias, RLS)

Any changes in sleep due to menstruating, pregnancy, or menopause: _____

Core Items from the Consensus Sleep Diary[38]

Today's Date			
What time did you get into the bed?			
What time did you try to go to sleep?			
How long did it take you to fall asleep?			
*How many times did you wake up, not counting your final awakening?			
In total, how long did these awakening last?			
What time was your final awakening?			
What time did you get out of bed for the day?			
How would you rate the quality of your sleep?	☐ Very poor ☐ Poor ☐ Fair ☐ Good ☐ Very good	☐ Very poor ☐ Poor ☐ Fair ☐ Good ☐ Very good	☐ Very poor ☐ Poor ☐ Fair ☐ Good ☐ Very good
Medication and dose (including over-the-counter and herbal)			

The Consensus Sleep Diary was designed for people to fill out information over a period of time sleep over a period of time (1–2 weeks). This writer found this tool be a useful to collect information on sleep for the initial meeting and thereafter, especially for those who refuse to fill out a sleep diary or are unable to do so. *Particularly for people with physical disabilities, for the question on number of awakening, note reason (e.g., voiding, cathing, bed positioning, orthotics)

Fig. 13.14 Cont'd

and appreciating diversity in sleep and rest are important because others' definitions, patterns, practices, and environments may completely differ from our own. The concept of cultural humility is an idea considered a lifelong process that acknowledges power differences between recipients and receivers of healthcare and also acknowledges that people have biases and emphasizes self-reflection of the healthcare provider.[4] An attitude of cultural humility for the occupational therapy practitioner is an important consideration with sleep and rest as people vary vastly in terms of whether, when, how, with whom sleep and rest are performed. It is crucial that therapists acknowledge they have a worldview, that they have biases and power in the therapist-client relationships that can have an impact on care.[4]

Mrs. Tanaka's views about and experiences with sleep, in addition to her sleep habits and patterns of sleep, are all important considerations in her treatment. For example, if Mrs. Tanaka's family reports that she always used a night-light to sleep and was afraid of the dark, the OT practitioner should not impose complete darkness in her room at night as a sleep hygiene technique (see Chapter 51).

Consultation

Infused throughout the OTPF is the role of the occupational therapist providing consultation as a method of service delivery versus being considered a separate intervention.[15] Consultation takes place when practitioners provide services to clients indirectly on their behalf, such as within multidisciplinary teams or community agencies.[15] Occupational therapists can provide consultation in institutional settings where a 24-hour operational schedule is in place. Typical delivery of service addressing sleep and rest could include consulting with the treatment team and staff about providing an optimal sleep environment for clients at night. Or, the OT consultant might discuss with the team the necessity of middle-of-the-night, nonurgent blood pressure readings, sponge baths, and blood draws, and recommend they be avoided. Providing training to night-shift aides, nurses, orderlies, and caregivers in bed mobility, bed positioning, transfer techniques, and body mechanics is another common form that OT consultation can take.

The occupational therapist also can act as a consultant in worksite settings, meeting with managers and administrators about the importance of sleep for optimal functioning and safety. The OT consultant can encourage balance in life for a more productive and safer workforce. West points out that consultation services may be particularly useful in settings that employ shift workers (e.g., hospitals, factories, airlines), providers of driver education, the military, and emergency relief programs.[195]

Driving rehabilitation specialists and certified driving rehabilitation specialists (CDRSs), many who are OT practitioners trained in driving and community mobility and OT generalists, can educate clients and the public about the dangers of drowsy driving. Occupational therapists who are specialists in adaptive driving and evaluation of disabled or at-risk individuals are usually the most up to date about regulations and information on driving, and they can act as consultants to other OT practitioners and healthcare professionals. The CDRS also can counsel clients on driving training or driver retirement when appropriate. See Chapter 11, Section 3 for more information on the occupational therapist's role in driving.

OCCUPATIONAL THERAPY INTERVENTIONS IN VARIOUS PRACTICE SETTINGS

Therapeutic Use of Occupations and Activities

Occupational therapy offers an abundance of therapeutic occupations and activities that can focus on helping the client have a healthy lifestyle balance and well-planned routines to ensure adequate rest and sleep.[15] An activity configuration or pie chart can be used with the client to review occupations that are important to the client and to assess how time is spent and the portion of time allocated to each of the occupations.

Woods et al.[201] stated that nursing home staff or caregivers can alter daytime napping behavior to prevent prolonged napping in residents. The researchers suggested increasing physical activity and activity programs to increase engagement with the environment. Interventions that maintain a more normal sleep/wake cycle may help the person with dementia maintain a more normative cortisol diurnal rhythm. Increased daytime activities may decrease excessive daytime napping and mitigate sleep dysregulation.

Activities of Daily Living

Schedules. Consider optimal times for ADL training; for example, if the client is a "night owl," do not schedule training in showering and dressing for 7 am. Try to schedule certain ADLs at "customary" times, especially for clients with cognitive impairment (e.g., work on dressing in the morning rather than at 1:30 pm), so that they become accustomed to a routine. Consult with other team members or family members and ensure that clients are getting sleep and rest. Keep track of sleep by using a sleep chart or diary. Schedule regular daytime naps (in bed, if possible; not in a wheelchair or recliner) or rest breaks if needed. Keep the medical team informed about the client's alertness during therapies.

Dressing. If dressing is considered a usual habit for a client, dissuade the use of pajamas during the day and have clients dress in "street" clothes. Encourage pajamas or "usual" sleeping clothes at night while the client is on a rehabilitation unit or recovering from illness or injury at home. However, it is important to note that some clients regularly wear housecoats during the day. Some cultures may also deem it necessary to wear pajamas because the client is still considered "sick."

Hygiene and grooming. If a client normally shaves or wears makeup during the day, encourage this as part of the morning/daytime routine, if it is important to the client. Ensure that the client and caregiver have a routine for activities to get ready for the day and to go to sleep at night.

Bed positioning, bed mobility, the bed, and bedding.

- *Bed positioning.* Train the client and caregivers in bed positioning to ensure comfort and optimal functioning. Are there enough pillows? Does the head of the bed need to be elevated? Does an extremity need to be elevated? Are there other precautions that need to be followed while the client is in bed (e.g., total hip, logroll)? As previously mentioned, "positional therapy" was recommended as a practice guideline for medical professionals in the treatment of OSA. This type of positioning entails keeping clients in a nonsupine position, which has been found to be useful as a secondary therapy (to PAP therapy) for people with OSA.[132]

- *Bed mobility.* Train the client and caregivers in bed mobility techniques for safety. Assist in determining the optimal bed for the client to use to facilitate sleep, with consideration for skin protection, breathing, and mobility and transfer status at the forefront. Ensure that the client has easy access to a call light, and make or request adaptations to the call light if needed. Provide adaptive equipment for safe bed mobility, such as a transfer handle, bed rails, loops on bed rails, and a trapeze, as indicated.

- *Bed.* Consider the type of bed required for safety and independence in bed mobility, transfers and even to support relationships. Factors to consider include size; height for safe transfers; height if the client tends to fall out of bed (lower bed may be safer); whether the client co-sleeps; mattress materials (some absorb and retain heat, which can be an issue for people with thermoregulation problems, such as those with severe burns or quadriplegia/tetraplegia, or women going through menopause); whether a mechanical bed (semi-electric or full-electric) is required; whether the bed helps protect the skin, requiring fewer turns at night; and how the client with mobility problems can maneuver on a particular type of mattress. For example, some clients may find it more difficult to position themselves on a foam mattress than on a spring mattress. Consider that some people do not sleep in beds at all: Some may sleep on the floor, in recliner chairs, in hammocks, or on the couch.

- *Bedding.* If the client is going to be away from home, consider whether a special quilt or blanket from home may assist him or her to sleep, or whether particular textures for sheets may be more suitable during sleep for skin protection or comfort. The 2012 National Sleep Foundation Bedroom Poll[141] of 1500 Americans between the ages of 25 and 55 found that 92% of people said that a good mattress was important for good sleep; 91% identified pillows; and 85% mentioned bedding; and 78% said that sheets with a fresh scent helped them become enthusiastic about going to sleep.[141]

OT practitioners are well versed in bed positioning, mobility, and the use of DME, in addition to environmental setup; therefore, occupational therapists are a natural fit when it comes to addressing these areas for sleep and rest concerns.

Transfers. Train the client, caregivers, and family members in safe techniques for transferring onto a commode or other surfaces where transfers may occur at night. Consider DME that may make transfers safer, such as transfer handles, as appropriate, and only as necessary.

Toileting. Consider the most appropriate times for catheterization, voiding, and a bowel program to optimize rest and sleep. Ensure that any equipment (e.g., commode, urinal) is readily available by the bedside or in the toileting area. Help the client and caregivers choose incontinence products, such as seat and bed protectors, disposable underwear ("pull-up" style), diapers, and so on. Discuss with the medical team, the client, and the caregivers the optimal toileting techniques to encourage sleep at night for all concerned and for safety. For example, if transfers are difficult for a male client, with the physician's approval a condom catheter initially can be used at night for urination rather than a commode.

Showering and bathing. Consider the optimal time for a bath or shower to encourage sleep at night or wakefulness during the day to participate in therapies or daytime activities. Perhaps a morning shower would "wake up" a client. Or, the optimal time

for a client to take a shower or bath may be at night, to help with sleep. The shower increases the core temperature, which then decreases to the optimal body temperature for sleep. Safety should be the primary consideration in determining showering and bathing times.

Eating and meals. Work on feeding activities. Encourage the client to eat meals with the rest of the family in the family dining area, as appropriate, to ensure that daily rhythms are reinstated to help distinguish day from night. Avoid allowing the client to eat in bed, even the hospital bed, if possible. The appropriate dietary and fluid intakes and their timing should be discussed with the dietitian and physician.

Instrumental Activities of Daily Living

IADLs call for more advanced skills than basic ADLs and generally require use of executive functions.[86]

Homemaking, bed making, and laundry. The 2012 National Sleep Foundation Bedroom Poll of 1500 Americans between the ages of 25 and 55 found that nearly 9 in 10 (88%) made their beds at least a few days a week[141]; 7 in 10 (71%) made their beds every day or almost every day. Respondents living in the Northeast, women, older respondents, and those married or partnered were more likely to make their beds every day or every other day. Those who made their beds every day or almost every day were more likely than those who did so less often, or not at all, to say that they got a good night's sleep every day or almost every day (44% versus 37%).[141] These are interesting statistics to consider because bed making as an IADL is under the domain of occupational therapy and should not be forgotten. The same poll found that 53% of respondents rated sleeping on sheets with a fresh scent an important contributor to their sleep experience. More research is needed to determine whether fresh-smelling sheets actually help people sleep better, but it is an important consideration for an OT practitioner when working on laundry tasks with clients or when considering sleep environments in industrial or home settings. See Chapter 10 for more information on ADLs and IADLs.

Community mobility. If clients are no longer deemed safe to drive because of sleep disorders, OT practitioners can train them in community mobility and alternative transit (see Chapter 11, Section 3).

Home Safety Assessment

As appropriate, perform a home evaluation to ensure that the home is safe for transfers, toileting, and ambulation at night and to determine any equipment needs (see Chapter 10). Suggestions can be made for bed placement, and night-lights and call bells can be set up as needed. Lighting and security are also important to facilitate sleep. Blackout curtains are frequently recommended, but sufficient lighting for safety in mobility is also important, as is a clean, uncluttered sleeping area. Confer with a physical therapist about optimal ambulation devices the client can use at night. According to Solet, an OT and sleep researcher at Harvard Medical School, the optimal sleep environment is quiet, dark, cool, comfortable, and clean.[177] She recommended that the occupational therapist help adapt and organize the sleep environment. Because the body temperature drops as part of the sleep cycle, a cooler bedroom is more conducive to sleep.[177] Solet also noted that clean environments are especially important to consider for people with allergies.[177]

Healthcare environment. Check with the nursing staff before making changes to the environment, especially in the acute hospital setting. To encourage sleep, turn off lights, encourage a quiet room, turn off the TV, and close the door fully if needed and if safe. Consider whether the client may be overstimulated if too many items are posted on the wall. However, keep in mind that photos of loved ones and personal blankets and objects may provide comfort and a sense of security to a person in the hospital. For safety, make sure the floor is clear of clutter and obstructions. Make sure the temperature in the room is comfortable for the client to sleep. Extra blankets may be needed for clients who tend to get cold. Make sure call lights, water (if allowed), and a phone are accessible to the client before leaving the room. Bed rails should be up unless the medical team states that they may be down.

Leisure Activities, Social Participation, and Restorative Activities

Try to schedule treatments outdoors so that the client is exposed to light because it is the strongest zeitgeber (time cue) and can help reset the biological clock if it is off kilter. Collaborate with the client and family to make sure activities selected are interesting and important for the client. Clients sometimes sleep during the day because they're bored. Encourage participation in activity groups, therapeutic recreation groups, and community events if it helps the client sleep at night. Make suggestions for and encourage quiet restful evening activities. As mentioned previously, Howell and Pierce[94] have pointed out that occupations that are highly restorative tend to have strong routines of a simple and repetitive nature, are often considered pleasurable, and have personal meaning to the individual. West[195] has suggested relaxing activities such as reading, stretching, meditating, or praying before bedtime. Use of sleep preparatory activities such as visual imagery and massage also can be used.[195] Some evidence suggests that aromatherapy with essential oils such as lavender and chamomile may have some promise in helping induce a state of mind that assists with sleep.[196] However, continued research is needed to find evidence of its effects on sleep architecture by polysomnography.[196]

Interventions to Support Occupations

Instruction and training in good sleep hygiene strategies can be considered preparatory activities to facilitate sleep. Occupational therapy practitioners also have many interventions that can support or hinder sleep, so they need to be considered carefully.

Orthotics, prosthetics, exercise schedule, and pain. Consider client sleep when giving orthotic (splinting) schedule instructions. Ensure proper fit for comfort so that the client can sleep. Make sure the orthotic schedule does not interfere with sleep or that the continuous passive motion (CPM) machine, typically used with clients who require a total knee replacement, does not keep the client awake all night. Collaborate with physical therapy about CPM use. Ensure people who use prosthetic devices can don and doff independently and have a regular routine and placement of devices before bedtime. Make

sure exercises are performed at a time that will optimize sleep at night. Consider the client's pain levels and consult with the medical staff and physicians. Talk to the client about whether he or she is unable to sleep at night because of pain, edema, or immobility.

Sleep hygiene. Sleep hygiene refers to activities involving lifestyle choices and environmental factors that can lead to healthy sleep. "Hygiene" does not just imply cleanliness, but generally stands for everyday habits to promote good health; "sleep hygiene" emphasizes proper habits to promote healthy sleep.[59] Sleep specialists provide sleep hygiene education with the intent of providing information about lifestyles and environments that either interfere with or promote sleep. OT practitioners can also provide sleep hygiene information to support healthy, active engagement in other areas of occupation (Box 13.5).[15]

According to Dement and Pelayo,[59] general guidelines for sleep hygiene are:

1. Create an optimal environment for sleep.
2. Reinforce predictability.
3. Avoid substances that negatively affect the sleep/wake cycle.
4. Follow good general health practices, which favor optimal sleep.

Box 13.6 provides more specific examples for each of these four categories.[59]

BOX 13.5   Important Considerations in Sleep Preparation and Participation (OTPF-4)

Preparation of Oneself
- Developing routines that prepare one for comfortable sleep, such as grooming, undressing/dressing, reading, listening to music to fall asleep, saying goodnight to others, meditation or prayers
- Determining the time of day and length of time desired for sleeping or the time needed to wake
- Establishing patterns that support growth and health (patterns are personally and culturally determined)

Preparation of the Environment
- Making the bed or space in which to sleep
- Providing for warmth/coolness and protection
- Setting an alarm clock
- Securing the home (e.g., locking doors, closing windows or curtains)
- Turning off electronics or lights
- Setting up sleep-supporting equipment (e.g., CPAP, positioning devices, etc.)

Participation in Actual Sleep
- Stopping all activities so as to ensure the onset of sleep, napping, and dreaming
- Sustaining a sleep state without disruption
- Ensuring nighttime care of toileting needs or hydration
- Negotiating needs of others in the social environment
- Interacting with those who share the sleeping space (e.g., children or partners)
- Nighttime caregiving (e.g., breastfeeding)
- Participating in activities to monitor the comfort and safety of others (e.g., the family) while sleeping

Data from the American Occupational Therapy Association: *Occupational therapy practice framework: domain and process* (4th ed.). *Am J Occup Ther* 74(Suppl 2):7412410010, 2020. https://doi.org/10.5014/ajot.2020.74S2001.

BOX 13.6 General Recommendations for Sleep

1. Create an optimal environment for sleep.
   - Remember that the only activities that should occur in bed are sleep and sex (avoid reading, watching TV, texting, tweeting, or using other media or computer devices in bed).[112]
   - In the hour before bedtime, turn off electronics. Research has shown that blue light from a television, personal computer, or tablet screen can interfere with sleep.[74] Culture and generational differences should be considered. Kaji and Shigeta[104] found that Japanese teenagers considered their mobile device a "teddy bear" that provided reassurance that they could connect to friends if needed.[180]
   - Prepare a quiet environment for sleep or use "white noise" to foster sleep.[112]
   - Ensure that the environment is dark, quiet, comfortable, cool,[74] and clean.[176]
2. Reinforce predictability (and activity).
   - Develop a regular sleep/wake cycle. Use an alarm clock if needed.[59]
   - Develop a relaxing routine before bedtime.
   - Avoid mentally stimulating or arousing activities before bedtime.[106]
   - Keep a sleep diary, which is considered the gold standard for subjective sleep assessment.[34] Sleep diaries are currently not standardized. However, insomnia experts, with feedback from potential users, have created a Consensus Sleep Diary, which is considered a living document.[38] In addition, the National Sleep Foundation (NSF) has created the NSF Official Sleep Diary.[138]
   - If a person cannot fall asleep within a reasonable amount of time (e.g., 15 minutes) while in bed, he or she should leave the bed, go to another room, or perform another activity until the individual feels sleepy. Mindfulness-based activities (e.g., mental body scanning, deep breathing) may be considered for those who cannot readily hop out of bed.[103]
3. Avoid substances that negatively affect the sleep/wake cycle.
   - Do not use alcohol to fall asleep. Alcohol can make snoring and obstructive sleep apnea (OSA) worse. Evidence exists that three to five glasses of alcohol in the evening can cause arousal when the effects of the alcohol wear off.[56,59]
   - Do not use caffeine before sleep. Caffeine has a half-life of 3.5 to 5 hours, depending on a person's age, activity level, or body chemistry; this means that it could remain in the body for many hours after ingesting it.[56,127] Keep in mind that besides coffee, some teas, soft drinks, and chocolate also contain caffeine.[56,127]
   - Avoid medicines that will keep a person awake at night. Confer with a prescriber about medications taken at night, timing of when the medications are taken, particularly those that affect sleep occupations (eg, diuretics taken at night).[206]
4. Follow good general health practices (e.g., exercise, diet, timing of meals), which favor optimal sleep.
   - Exercise daily, but do not do vigorous exercise in the 2 hours before bedtime.[74] Research has shown that participation in an exercise training program can have positive effects on sleep quality in middle-aged and older adults.[204]
   - Avoid going to bed with a full stomach; try to finish dinner at least 2 hours before bedtime.[74]
   - Avoid spicy foods and heavy eating in the evening, but do not go to bed when hungry.[59]
   - Limit liquids at night. Talk to a healthcare provider about this.

Education and Training

In the healthcare setting, the occupational therapist can educate and empower the client and family to set a strict visitation schedule, if necessary, to dissuade visitors from arriving at night or during scheduled rest times, which may interrupt rest and sleep. OT practitioners can help empower caregivers to limit visits to short periods, or they can help with the enforcement of visitation rules. The occupational therapist can educate caregivers about sleep and make sure they realize how important it is for them to get their own rest and sleep.

Some institutions require doors in rooms to be open at night despite the lights and noise. Education can be provided to staff about how best to facilitate sleep in these settings. Young et al.[207] suggested several strategies, including offering earplugs and eye masks, encouraging regular nocturnal sleep time, and discouraging long daytime naps. Other suggestions included encouraging the medical staff to minimize nighttime bathing, dressing changes of wounds, or other medical procedures and to avoid discussing emotionally charged topics with the client at night.[207]

OT practitioners can also train people in pain awareness and management, energy levels (work simplification techniques), sleepiness and fatigue, time management, and cognitive behavioral techniques.[71]

OT instructors can educate their students about the consequences of sleep deprivation; as college and graduate students, they are a group known to be at risk for erratic sleep behaviors and significant sleep debt. If afternoon classes are scheduled, more "active" class activities may be required to fend off sleepiness for instructors and students during the circadian clock's "sleepiness" times. During short breaks for longer classes, instructors can encourage students to stand up, stretch, or walk around instead of remaining in their chairs to check their mobile devices. Occupational therapy and occupational science educators can coordinate assignment due dates and spread them out to encourage balance for the instructor and students and to ensure proper sleep for both.

Green et al.[82] noted that many clients complain of lack of information about the management of insomnia. Occupational therapists can provide education to the sleep-deprived public in community practice settings.

Advocacy

OT practitioners can provide services in the form of advocacy to their clients.[15] The OTPF-4 defines clients as persons, groups, or populations.[15] Advocacy as an OT service involves more than just education; it includes follow-up and an assertive voice and action to ensure that people's needs are met. Advocacy is defined as an "act of pleading, supporting, recommending; active espousal."[60]

For occupational therapists, advocacy can take any of the following forms:

- *Persons (includes those involved in care of the client):* Simply asking clients about their rest and sleep is the first step in advocacy. If the assessment indicates problems with sleep and rest, notify the primary care provider. If indicated, recommend to the primary care provider that a sleep specialist be consulted. Inform the treatment team of poor function resulting from inadequate sleep. Encourage families and friends to abide by hospital visitation rules if the client lives (temporarily or permanently) in a facility. Advocate for appropriate environments for adequate rest and sleep. Through detailed documentation or calls to vendors, advocate for timeliness for delivery of appropriate DME and adaptive equipment to maximize sleep; examples include a hospital bed, mattress with skin protection, diapers, pads, urinal, and appropriate pillows. Ensure follow-through with adequate client positioning by nursing staff and caregivers; talk to the treatment team about adequate pain control to maximize sleep.

- *Groups:* Advocate for appropriate sleep and nap environments in any number of settings. For example, in day health-care centers for frail older adults or dementia activity centers where seniors may stay all day, promote the creation of nap or rest areas. Options for reclining and lounging should be provided, in addition to just dining-type chairs. Ensure that workers, injured or not, have appropriate sleep and rest to perform their jobs. Advocate for students in OT educational settings to have adequate sleep and rest.

- *Oneself and the role of the OT profession:* Educate others on the role of occupational therapy in sleep. Advocate for more involvement of occupational therapists in IADLs, leisure, and rest activities, not just basic ADLs, so that clients will have meaningful activity to engage in during the daytime to avoid prolonged napping because of boredom. In an evidence-based review of the literature on OT intervention for people who had had a CVA, Wolf et al. found an overemphasis on ADLs, with less attention paid to other areas of occupation, such as leisure, social participation, rest and sleep, and work and productivity.[199] As the authors noted, "In general, regardless of diagnosis, occupational therapy is too focused on ADL performance, which limits practitioners' role in the other areas of occupation that are meaningful to clients" (p. 8).[199]

- *Populations:* Occupational therapy practitioners can be involved in informing the population about the dangers of drowsy driving. Many organizations such as the American Sleep Association (https://www.sleepassociation.org/), the National Sleep Foundation (https://www.sleepfoundation.org/), and the American Academy of Sleep Medicine (https://aasm.org/), and Centers for Disease Control (https://www.cdc.gov/) have information on sleep and drowsy driving. Advocacy also can be conducted on school start times. School times for high school students in metropolitan Minneapolis were shifted to match adolescent circadian rhythms (i.e., later school start times), and a subsequent study[189] found statistically significant improvements in graduation rates, rates of continuous enrollment, tardiness, and attendance. OT practitioners can be involved in future research in this area or in political advocacy.

In addition to individual client treatment, the topics of sleep and rest lend themselves well to group occupational therapy sessions, as is discussed in the next section. Marilyn B. Cole's book, *Group Dynamics in Occupational Therapy: The Theoretical Basis and Practice Application of Group Intervention*, fourth edition (2012), offers the beginning occupational therapy student or novice group leader a helpful seven-step format for leading groups. Experienced group leaders can also benefit from this book.

Group Interventions

Occupational therapists should develop cognitive strategies to help manage negative, anxiety-producing thoughts and concerns.[106] These strategies can be used successfully in both group and individual interventions.[83] Examples of negative, anxiety-producing thoughts are, "I'll never sleep again," or "I won't be able to function tomorrow." Occupational therapists can consider training in CBT-I. CBT-I usually focuses on consolidating sleep with sleep restriction, using stimulus control techniques so that people equate the bed with sleep, altering dysfunctional beliefs and attitudes about sleep, and educating clients about healthier sleep hygiene practices.[155] Research has supported the use of CBT-I in groups as a nonpharmacological treatment for sleep disturbance.[99]

In a 2013 article in *OT Practice*, a magazine published by the AOTA, Gentry and Loveland[74] discussed how an occupational therapist and a recreational therapist co-led a 10-week sleep hygiene therapy group for military veterans. The group sessions were attended by 20 to 25 members and lasted 90 minutes. The leaders led discussions on topics such as the nature of sleep, sleep-related problems. and nightmares because many members had post-traumatic stress disorder (PTSD). The group leaders reported that participants felt healthier and more engaged in daily life after attending the group sessions.[74]

Gentry and Loveland also provided suggestions for documentation and the use of Current Procedural Terminology (CPT) codes when billing for sleep-related services in the United States. CPT codes are maintained by the American Medical Association and are important for billing purposes in the United States.[74]

Determining When to Refer a Client to a Physician or Sleep Specialist

Refer the client to a physician or sleep specialist if he or she complains of any of the following conditions[66]:

- Has trouble initiating sleep or getting restful sleep for more than a month or two
- Does not feel rested despite getting the usual amount of sleep or more sleep than he or she is accustomed to getting to feel rested
- Falls asleep at inappropriate times, even though he or she is getting 7½ to 8 hours of sleep
- Has been told that he or she snores loudly or gasps and has periods of not breathing that disrupt a bed partner or roommate
- Has to sleep in a different room because a bed partner claims the client's snoring is too disruptive
- Follows good sleep hygiene habits but still has difficulty sleeping
- Other reasons to refer a client to a physician or sleep specialist are:
  - Caregivers complain that the client is awake all night and sleeps all day.
  - A cognitively impaired client is not able to report clearly his or her sleep habits but has obviously declined in occupational performance areas (e.g., ADLs, mobility) and you suspect poor sleep.
  - The client falls asleep regularly during your treatment in the daytime.

If appropriate, have the client fill out a sleepiness scale, such as the ESS (see Fig. 13.13), which has been validated in clinical settings.[101] A score of 10 or higher indicates EDS; a score of 6 is the norm.[209] Present the data to the client's physician, and notify him or her of the client's deficits in occupational performance or other symptoms resulting from sleep deprivation.

SUMMARY

Historically, occupational therapists and occupational scientists have been interested in the importance of helping clients maintain a healthy, balanced lifestyle.[45] Included in that balance should be adequate sleep and rest, two "restorative" occupations.[161] According to the OTPF-4 the category of sleep and rest is considered a major occupation that is in the domain of occupational therapy practice; accordingly, addressing this area in all practice settings is appropriate.[15]

Occupational therapists have not traditionally treated clients whose diagnosis or problem has been primarily a sleep disorder. However, the sleep medicine literature abounds with information about the deleterious effects of sleep deprivation, including the effects on the at-risk clients occupational therapists treat daily in physical disability and other practice settings. Although occupational therapy has not focused research or practice on rest and sleep, sleep medicine research affirms what OT practitioners have known all along: Humans need to sleep, and they need to rest. Otherwise, occupational performance declines, negatively affecting a person's quality of life and health.

However, compelling evidence suggests that occupational therapists could and should put more emphasis, research, and practice into helping clients who have sleep difficulties. A study in Scotland of 38 healthcare professionals (including 19 occupational therapists) who took a 3-day course on sleep in people with Parkinson's disease showed that cognitive-behavioral sleep management can be successfully transferred to healthcare professionals who were not sleep specialists.[84] Clients who were seen by the healthcare professionals who took the course reported reduced anxiety over sleep problems, better ability to manage sleep, and more of a sense of control over sleep.[84]

Solet points out that there are 10 influences on sleep: exercise activity levels, sleep schedule, bed partner/pets, caffeine/alcohol/medications, psychological state, age/sex/genetics, cultural norms/social context/"lifestyle," light/circadian drive, sleep environment, and sleep debt.[176,177] The only area that occupational therapists cannot influence from that list is age/sex/genetics.

An emerging body of research shows that purpose in life is linked with a variety of healthy behaviors, positive health outcomes, longevity, and a lower incidence of sleep disturbances.[110] In a nationally representative sample of U.S. adults over age 50, Kim et al.[110] found that purpose showed an independent association with sleep disturbances, even after adjusting for psychological distress such as anxiety and depression. This finding may suggest that purpose is important for good sleep above and beyond the absence of negative psychological factors. Further research is needed, but interventions to enhance purpose in life could be an approach for reducing sleep disturbances.[110]

Another important client factor, spirituality, is not considered the same as religion; the OTPF-4 describes it as deeper experiences of meaning that are experienced through engagement in occupations that involve values, beliefs, and reflection and is evolving.[15] Waite offered ideas on how OT practitioners can incorporate spirituality into practice.[190]

OT practitioners are in the front lines of those working closely with clients who must cope with life-altering events. They help people face the realities of needing to change or alter their life course. Occupational therapy practice emphasizes the occupational nature of humans' drive to achieve a healthful, productive, and satisfying (meaningful) life; thus, OT practitioners are primed to help people find meaning through occupation, even when their lives have been drastically altered.[15]

Reflecting on the case of Mrs. Tanaka, it is evident that OT practitioners can help make a difference in her rehabilitation outcomes by focusing on her sleep disturbance, once medical issues have been ruled out. A multitude of reasons may explain Mrs. Tanaka's sleep disturbance. The exact location of her brain injury may help the medical team determine whether the disturbance is organic, but further study may also reveal a sleep disorder. An OT practitioner who is educated and attuned to Mrs. Tanaka's sleep and rest needs can help her reach her rehabilitation goals and improve her quality of life.

REVIEW QUESTIONS

1. What is sleep architecture?
2. How does sleep architecture change as we age?
3. What is REM sleep, and how does it differ from NREM sleep?
4. Why should OT practitioners address sleep in their practice?
5. What is the difference between sleep and rest?
6. Where does the area of sleep and rest fit into the OTPF-4?
7. What is sleep hygiene?
8. What is the Multiple Sleep Latency Test? What is the Epworth Sleepiness Scale?
9. When is it appropriate to refer a client to a physician or sleep specialist?
10. How can an occupational therapist help improve a client's sleep hygiene in a hospital setting?
11. Name at least five consequences of inadequate sleep.
12. What is obstructive sleep apnea, and what are some signs and symptoms of the disorder?

For additional practice questions for this chapter, please visit eBooks.Health.Elsevier.com.

REFERENCES

1. AAA Foundation for Traffic Safety: AAA prevalence of motor vehicle crashes involving drowsy drivers, United States, 2009–2013. <https://www.aaafoundation.org/prevalence-motor-vehicle-crashes-involving-drowsy-drivers-us-2009-2013>, 2014.
2. AAA Foundation for Traffic Safety. (2020, June). 2019 *Traffic Safety Culture Index*. https://aaafoundation.org/wp-content/uploads/2020/06/2019-Traffic-Safety-Culture-Index.pdf.
3. Aaronson LS, Teel CS, Cassmeyer V, et al: Defining and measuring fatigue, *J Nurs Scholarsh* 31:45–50, 1999.
4. Agner J: The Issue Is—Moving from cultural competence to cultural humility in occupational therapy: a paradigm shift, *Am J Occup Ther* 74(4), 2020. https://doi.org/10.5014/ajot.2020.038067. 7404347010
5. Alessi CA, Martin JL, Webber AP, et al: More daytime sleeping predicts less functional recover among older people undergoing in client post-acute rehabilitation, *Sleep* 31:1291–1300, 2008.
6. Allen C., Glasziou P., Del Mar C: Bed rest: A potentially harmful treatment needing more careful evaluation, *Lancet* 354(9186):1229–1233, 1999.
7. Allen RP, Picchietti DL, Garcia Borreguereo D, et al: Restless legs syndrome/Willis-Ekbom disease diagnostic criteria: updated International Restless Legs Syndrome Study Group (IRLSSG) consensus criteria—history, rationale, description, and significance, *Sleep Med* 15:860–873, 2014. https://doi.org/10.1016/j.sleep.2014.03.025.
8. American Academy of Sleep Medicine: The international classification of sleep disorders—third edition (*ICSD-3*). <http://www.aasmnet.org/library/default.aspx?id=9>, 2014.
9. American Academy of Sleep Medicine. (2020). *Sleep education: Drowsy driving*. http://sleepeducation.org/sleep-topics/drowsy-driving.
10. American Occupational Therapy Association: Occupational therapy practice framework: domain and process, *Am J Occup Ther* 56:609–639, 2002.
11. American Occupational Therapy Association: Occupational therapy practice framework: domain and process, ed 2, *Am J Occup Ther* 62:625–683, 2008.
12. American Occupational Therapy Association: Blueprint for entry level education, *Am J Occup Ther* 64:186–203, 2010.
13. American Occupational Therapy Association: Occupational therapy practice framework: domain and process, ed 3, *Am J Occup Ther* 68(Suppl 1):S1–S48, 2014. https://doi.org/10.5014/ajot.2014.682006.
14. American Occupational Therapy Association: Surveying the profession: the 2015 AOTA Salary & Workforce Survey, OT Practice 20:7–11, 2015. <http://www.aota.org/education-careers/advance-career/salary-workforce-survey.aspx>.
15. American Occupational Therapy Association: Occupational therapy practice framework: Domain and process (4th ed.), *Am J Occup Ther* 74(Suppl. 2), 2020. https://doi.org/10.5014/ajot.2020.74S2001. 7412410010
16. Ancoli-Israel S: Sleep and its disorders in aging populations, *Sleep Med* 10:S7–S11, 2009.
17. Asplund R: Nocturia: consequences for sleep and daytime activities and associated risks, *Eur Urol Suppl* 3:24–32, 2005.
18. Aurora RN, Collop NA, Jacobowitz O, et al: Quality measures for the care of adult clients with obstructive sleep apnea, *J Clin Sleep Med* 11:357–383, 2015.
19. Avidan AY: Neurologic disorders: narcolepsy and idiopathic hypersomnia. In Kryger HM, editor: *Atlas of clinical sleep medicine*, Philadelphia, 2010, Saunders/Elsevier, pp 107–114.
20. Avidan AY: Restless legs syndrome and periodic limb movements in sleep. In Kryger MH, editor: *Atlas of clinical sleep medicine* ed 5, Philadelphia, 2010, Saunders/Elsevier, pp 115–124.
21. Avidan AY: Sleep in Parkinson's disease. In Kryger MH, editor: *Atlas of clinical sleep medicine* ed 5, Philadelphia, 2010, Saunders/Elsevier, pp 131–134.
22. Avidan AY, Fries BE, James ML, et al: Insomnia and hypnotic use, recorded in the minimum data set, as predictors of falls and hip fractures in Michigan nursing homes, *J Am Geriatr Soc* 53:955–962, 2005.
23. Badue C, Guidolini R, Vivacqua Carneiro R, Azevedo P, Cardoso VB, Forechi A, Jesus L, Berriel R, Paixão TM, Mutz F, de Paula Veronese L, Oliveira-Santos T, De Souza AF: Self-driving cars: A survey, *Exp Syst App* 165(1):1–27, 2020. https://doi.org/10.1016/j.eswa.2020.113816.
24. Bartick MC, Thai X, Schmidt T, et al: Brief report: Decrease in as-needed sedative use by limiting nighttime sleep disruptions from hospital staff, *J Hosp Med* 15(3):E20–E24, 2009. https://doi.org/10.1002/jhm.549.
25. Basheer R, Strecker RE, Thakkar MM, McCarley RW: Adenosine and sleep–wake regulation, *Prog Neurobiol* 73:379–396, 2004.
26. Bassetti C, Aldrich M, Chervin R, Quint D: Sleep apnea in the acute phase of TIA and stroke, *Neurology* 47:1167–1173, 1996.
27. Benca R, Ancoli-Israel S, Moldofsky H: Special considerations in insomnia diagnosis and management: depressed, elderly, and chronic pain populations, *J Clin Psychiatry* 65:S26–S35, 2004.
28. Bonnet MH, Arand DL: Sleepiness as measured by the MSLT varies as a function of preceding activity, *Sleep* 21:477–484, 1998.
29. Bonnet MH, Arand DL: Arousal components which differentiate the MWT from the MSLT, *Sleep* 24:441–447, 2001.
30. Booth J, McMillan L: The impact of nocturia on older people: implications for nursing practice, *Br J Nurs* 18:592–596, 2009.
31. Broström A, Nilsen P, Johansson P, et al: Putative facilitators and barriers for adherence to CPAP treatment in clients with obstructive sleep apnea syndrome: a qualitative content analysis, *Sleep Med* 11:126–130, 2010.
32. Browse NL: *The physiology and pathology of bed rest*, Springfield, IL, 1965, Thomas.
33. Bushnik T, Englander J, Katznelson L: Fatigue after TBI: association with neuroendocrine abnormalities, *Brain Inj* 21:559–566, 2007.
34. Buxton OM, Ellenbogn JM, Wang W, et al: Sleep disruption due to hospital noises: a prospective evaluation, *Ann Intern Med* 157:170–179, 2012.
35. Buysse DJ, Reynolds CF 3rd, Monk TH, et al: The Pittsburgh Sleep Quality Index (PSQI): a new instrument for psychiatric research and practice, *Psychiatry Res* 28:193–213, 1989.
36. Campbell SS, Stanchina MD, Schlang JR, Murphy PJ: Effects of a month-long napping regimen in older individuals, *J Am Geriatr Soc* 59:224–232, 2011. https://doi.org/10.1111/j.1532-5415.2010.03264.x.
37. Carmona Toro BE: New treatment options for the management of restless leg syndrome, *J Neurosci Nurs* 46:227–233, 2014.
38. Carney CE, Buysse DJ, Ancoli-Israel S, Edinger JD, Krystal AD, Lichstein KL, Morin CM: The Consensus Sleep Diary: Standardizing prospective sleep self-monitoring, *Sleep* 35(2):287–302, 2012. https://doi.org/10.5665/sleep.1642.
39. Carskadon MA: Factors influencing sleep patterns of adolescents. In Carskadon MA, editor: *Adolescent sleep patterns: biological, social, and psychological influences*, Cambridge, UK, 2002, Cambridge University Press, pp 4–26.

40. Carskadon MA, Dement WC: Normal human sleep: an overview. In Kryger MH, Roth T, Dement WC, editors: *Principles and practice of sleep medicine* ed 5, St Louis, 2011, Elsevier/Saunders, pp 16–26.

41. Carskadon M, Orav EJ, Dement WC: Evolution of sleep and daytime sleepiness in adolescents. In Guilleminault C, Lugaresi E, editors: *Sleep/wake disorders: natural history, epidemiology, and long-term evolution*, New York, 1983, Raven Press, pp 201–216.

42. Cherkassky T, Oksenberg A, Froom P, King H: Sleep-related breathing disorders and rehabilitation outcome of stroke clients: a prospective study, *Am J Phys Med Rehabil* 82:452–455, 2003.

43. Chervin RD: Use of clinical tools and tests in sleep medicine. In Kryger MH, Roth T, Dement WC, editors: *Principles and practice of sleep medicine* ed 4, Philadelphia, 2004, Elsevier/Saunders, pp 602–614.

44. Chiu HY, Chen PY, Chuang LP, Chen NH, Tu YK, Hsieh YJ, Wang YC, Guilleminault C: Diagnostic accuracy of the Berlin questionnaire, STOP-BANG, STOP, and Epworth Sleepiness Scale in detecting obstructive sleep apnea: A bivariate meta-analysis, *Sleep Medicine Reviews* 36:57–70, 2017. https://doi.org/10.1016/j.smrv.2016.10.004.

45. Christiansen CH, Matuska KM: Lifestyle balance: a review of concepts and research, *J Occup Sci* 13:49–61, 2006.

46. Chung F, Abdullah HR, Liao P: STOP-Bang questionnaire: A practical approach to screen for obstructive sleep apnea, *Chest* 149:631–638, 2016.

47. Chung F, Yegneswaran B, Liao P, Chung SA, Vairavanathan S, Islam S, et al: STOP questionnaire: A tool to screen patients for obstructive sleep apnea, *Anesthesiology* 108:812–821, 2008.

48. Coren S: *Sleep thieves: an eye opening exploration into the science and mysteries of sleep*, New York, 1996, The Free Press.

49. Coyne KS, Zhou Z, Bhattacharyya SK, et al: The prevalence of nocturia and its effect on health-related quality of life and sleep in a community sample in the USA, *BJU Int* 92:948–954, 2003.

50. Crispim Nascimento CM, Ayan C, Cancela JM, et al: Effect of a multimodal exercise program on sleep disturbances and instrumental activities of daily living performance on Parkinson's and Alzheimer's disease clients, *Geriatr Gerontol Int* 14:259–266, 2014. https://doi.org/10.1111/ggi.12082.

51. Cunningham R, Valasek S: Case Report: Occupational therapy interventions for urinary dysfunction in primary care: A case series, *Am J Occup Ther* 73, 2019. https://doi.org/10.5014/ajot.2019.038356. 7305185040

52. Czeisler CA, Buxton OM, Singh Khalsa SB: The human circadian timing system and sleep/wake regulation. In Kryger MH, Roth T, Dement WC, editors: *Principles and practice of sleep medicine* ed 4, Philadelphia, 2004, Elsevier/Saunders, pp 375–394.

53. Dahl RE: The consequences of insufficient sleep for adolescents: links between sleep and emotional regulation. In Wahlstrom KL, editor: *Adolescent sleep needs and school starting times*, Bloomington, IN, 1999, Phi Delta Kappa Educational Foundation.

54. D'Ambrosio C, Bowman T, Mohsenin V: Quality of life in clients with obstructive sleep apnea: Effect of nasal continuous airway pressure: a prospective study, *Chest* 115:23–29, 1999.

55. Dautovich ND, McCrae CS, Rowe M: Subjective and objective napping and sleep in older adults: are evening naps "bad" for nighttime sleep? *J Am Geriatr Soc* 56:1681–1686, 2008. https://doi.org/10.1111/j.1532-5415.2008.01822.x.

56. Dement W, Kleitman N: The relation of eye movements during sleep to dream activity: an objective method for the study of dreaming, *J Exp Psychol* 53:339–346, 1957.

57. Dement WC: *The promise of sleep*, New York, 1999, Delacort Press/Random House.

58. Dement WC: History of sleep physiology and medicine. In Kryger MH, Roth T, Dement WC, editors: *Principles and practice of sleep medicine* ed 4, Philadelphia, 2004, Elsevier/Saunders, pp 1–12.

59. Dement WC, Pelayo R: *Dement's sleep and dreams*, Palo Alto, CA, 2015, William C Dement.

60. Dictionary.com: Advocacy. <http://dictionary.reference.com/browse/advocacy>, nd.

61. Dixon L, Duncan D, Johnson P, et al: Occupational therapy for clients with Parkinson's disease, *Cochrane Database Syst Rev*(3), 2007. https://doi.org/10.1002/14651858.CD002813.pub2. CD002813

62. Duclos C, Beauregard M-P, Bottari C, et al: The impact of poor sleep on cognition and activities of daily living after traumatic brain injury: a review, *Aust Occup Ther J* 62:2–12, 2015.

63. Eakman AM, Schmid AA, Henry KL, Rolle NR, Schelly C, Pott CE, Burns JE: Restoring effective sleep tranquility (REST): A feasibility and pilot study, *British J Occup Ther* 80(6):350–360, 2017. https://doi.org/10.1177/0308022617691538.

64. Edinger JD, Means MK: Overview of insomnia: definitions, epidemiology, differential diagnosis, and assessment. In Kryger MH, Roth T, Dement WC, editors: *Principles and practice of sleep medicine* ed 4, Philadelphia, 2004, Elsevier/Saunders, pp 702–713.

65. Edlund M: *The power of rest: why sleep alone is not enough—a 30-day plan to reset your body*. NY, 2010, Harper Collins.

66. Epstein LJ, Mardon S: *Harvard Medical School guide to a good night's sleep*. New York, 2007, McGraw Hill.

67. Fabbri M, Martoni M, Esposito MJ, et al: Postural control after a night without sleep, *Neuropsychologia* 44:2520–2525, 2006.

68. Fernandez-Mendoza J, Vgontzas AN, Kritikou I, et al: Natural history of excessive daytime sleepiness: role of obesity, weight loss, depression, and sleep propensity, *Sleep* 38:351–360, 2015. https://doi.org/10.5665/sleep.4488.

69. Foster ER: Instrumental activities of daily living performance among people with Parkinson's disease without dementia, *Am J Occup Ther* 68:353–362, 2014. https://doi.org/10.5014/ajot.2014.010330.

70. Freedman NS, Kotzer N, Schwab RJ: Client perception of sleep quality and etiology of sleep disruption in the intensive care unit, *Am J Respir Crit Care Med* 159:1155–1162, 1999.

71. Fung C, Wiseman-Hakes C, Colantonio A, et al: Time to wake up: bridging the gap between theory and practice for sleep in occupational therapy, *Br J Occup Ther* 76:384–386, 2013.

72. Gabor JY, Cooper AB, Crombach SA, et al: Contribution of the intensive care unit environment to sleep disruption in mechanically ventilated clients and healthy subjects, *Am J Respir Crit Care Med* 167:708–715, 2003.

73. Gangwisch JE, Hemysfield SB, Boden-Albala B, et al: Short sleep duration as a risk factor for hypertension: analyses of first National Health and Nutrition Examination Survey, *Hypertension* 47:833–839, 2006.

74. Gentry T, Loveland J: Sleep: essential to living life to its fullest, *OT Practice* 18:9–14, 2013.

75. George C: Diabetes mellitus. In Kryger MH, editor: *Atlas of clinical sleep medicine*, Philadelphia, 2010, Saunders/Elsevier, pp 240.

76. George CFP, Guilleminault C: Sleep and neuromuscular diseases. In Kryger MH, Roth T, Dement WC, editors: *Principles and practice of sleep medicine* ed 4, Philadelphia, 2004, Elsevier/Saunders, pp 831–838.

77. Gooneratne NS, Weaver TE, Cater JR, et al: Functional outcomes of excessive daytime sleepiness in older adults, *J Am Geriatr Soc* 51:642–649, 2003.

78. Granger CV, Markello SJ, Graham JE, et al: The uniform data system for medical rehabilitation: report of clients with stroke discharged from comprehensive medical programs in 2000–2007, *Am J Phys Med Rehabil* 88(12):961–972, 2009. https://doi.org/10.1097/PHM.0b013e3181c1ec38.

79. Green A: Sleep, occupation and the passage of time, *Br J Occup Ther* 71:343, 2008.

80. Green A, Brown C, editors: *An occupational therapist's guide to sleep and sleep problems*, London, 2015, Jessica Kingsley Publishers.

81. Green A, Westcomb A, editors: *Sleep: multi-professional perspectives*, Philadelphia, 2012, Jessica Kingsley Publishers.

82. Green A, Hicks J, Wilson S: The experience of poor sleep and its consequences: a qualitative study involving people referred for cognitive-behavioral management of chronic insomnia, *Br J Occup Ther* 71:196–204, 2008.

83. Green A, Hicks J, Weekes R, Wilson S: A cognitive-behavioral group intervention for people with chronic insomnia: an initial evaluation, *Br J Occup Ther* 68:518–522, 2005.

84. Gregory P, Morgan K, Lynall A: Improving sleep management in people with Parkinson's, *Br J Community Nurs* 17:14–20, 2012.

85. Guilleminault C, Bassiri A: Clinical features and evaluation of obstructive sleep apnea–hypopnea syndrome and upper airway resistance syndrome. In Kryger MH, Roth T, Dement WC, editors: *Principles and practice of sleep medicine* ed 4, Philadelphia, 2004, Elsevier/Saunders, pp 1043–1052.

86. Hahn B, Baum C, Moore J, et al: Brief report: development of additional tasks for the Executive Function Performance Test, *Am J Occup Ther* 68:e241–e246, 2014. https://doi.org/10.5014/ajot.2014.008565.

87. Hammond A, Jefferson P: Rheumatoid arthritis. In Turner A, Foster M, Johnson SE, editors: *Occupational therapy and physical dysfunction: principles, skills and practice* ed 5, Edinburgh, 2002, Churchill Livingstone, pp 543–564.

88. Hardin KA: Sleep in the ICU, *Chest* 136:284–294, 2009.

89. Harvard Health Letter: Napping may not be such a no-no. <http://www.health.harvard.edu/newsletter_article/napping-may-not-be-such-a-no-no>, 2009.

90. Hayes D Jr, Phillips B: Sleep apnea. In Kryger MH, editor: *Atlas of clinical sleep medicine*, Philadelphia, 2010, Saunders/Elsevier, pp 167–196.

91. Heller C: Temperature, thermoregulation, and sleep. In Kryger MH, Roth T, Dement WC, editors: *Principles and practice of sleep medicine* ed 4, Philadelphia, 2004, Elsevier/Saunders, pp 292–300.

92. Hirshkowitz M, Whiton K, Albert SM, et al: National Sleep Foundation's sleep time duration recommendations: Methodology and results summary, *Sleep Health* 1(1):40–43, 2015. https://doi.org/10.1016/j.sleh.2014.12.010.

93. Hopper K, Fried TR, Pisani MA: Health care worker attitudes and identified barriers to client sleep in the medical intensive care unit, *Heart Lung* 44:95–99, 2015.

94. Howell D, Pierce D: Exploring the forgotten restorative dimension of occupation: quilting and quilt use, *J Occup Sci* 7:68–72, 2000.

95. Huang H-W, Zheng B-L, Jiang L, et al: Effect of oral melatonin and wearing earplugs and eye masks on nocturnal sleep in healthy subjects in a simulated intensive care unit environment: which might be a more promising strategy for ICU sleep deprivation? *Crit Care* 19:124, 2015. https://doi.org/10.1186/s13054-015-0842-8.

96. Hunjan R, Twiss KL: Urgent interventions: promoting occupational engagement for clients with urinary incontinence, *OT Practice* 18:8–12, 2013.

97. Iber C, Ancoli-Israel S, Chesson AL, Quan SF: *The AASM manual for the scoring of sleep and associated events: rules, terminology and technical specifications*, Westchester, IL, 2007, The American Academy of Sleep Medicine (AASM).

98. Jackson S: Lower urinary tract symptoms and nocturia in men and women: prevalence, etiology and diagnosis, *BJU Int* 84(Suppl 1):5–8, 1999.

99. Jansson M, Linton SJ: Cognitive-behavioral group therapy as an early intervention for insomnia: a randomized controlled trial, *J Occup Rehabil* 15:177–190, 2005.

100. Javaheri S: Cardiovascular disorders. In Kryger MH, editor: *Atlas of clinical sleep medicine*, Philadelphia, 2010, Saunders/Elsevier, pp 216–227.

101. Johns MW: Sleepiness in different situations measured by the Epworth Sleepiness Scale, *Sleep* 17:703–710, 1994.

102. Jonsson H.: Towards a new direction in the conceptualization and categorization of occupation, Wilma West Lecture, Occupational Science Symposium, Los Angeles, 2007, University of Southern California, Occupational Science and Occupational Therapy.

103. Kabat-Zinn J: *Full catastrophe living: using the wisdom of your body and mind to face stress. In pain, and illness*, NY, 1991, Dell Publishing.

104. Kaji M, Shigeta M: *Knick-knacks for sleeping (nemuri komono) in contemporary Japan, Unpublished manuscript for the workshop New Directions in the Social and Cultural Study of Sleep. In Vienna*, , June 7–9, 2007, University of Vienna.

105. Kaneko Y, Hajek VE, Zivanovic V, et al: Relationship of sleep apnea to functional capacity and length of hospitalization following stroke, *Sleep* 26:293–297, 2003.

106. Kannenberg K: Practice perks: addressing sleep, *OT Practice* 14(15):5–6, 2009.

107. Kapur VK, Auckley DH, Chowdhuri S, Kuhlmann DC, Mehra R, Ramar K, Harrod CG: Clinical practice guideline for diagnostic testing for adult obstructive sleep apnea: an American Academy of Sleep Medicine clinical practice guideline, *J Clin Sleep Med* 13(3):479–504, 2017. https://doi.org/10.5664/jcsm.6506.

108. Kassardjian CD, Murray BJ, Kokokyi S, et al: Effects of napping on neuromuscular fatigue in myasthenia gravis, *Muscle Nerve* 48:816–818, 2013.

109. Khurshid KA: Comorbid insomnia and psychiatric disorders: An update, *Innov Clin Neurosci* 15(3-4):28–32, 2018.

110. Kim ES, Hershner SD, Strecher VJ: Purpose in life and incidence of sleep disturbances, *J Behav Med* 38:590–597, 2014. https://doi.org/10.1007/s10865-015-9635-4.

111. Knutson KL, Spiegel K, Penev P, Van Cauter E: The metabolic consequences of sleep deprivation, *Sleep Med Rev* 11:163–178, 2007.

112. Koketsu J: Rest and sleep. In Pendleton HM, Schultz-Krohn W, editors: *Pedretti's occupational therapy: practice skills for physical dysfunction* ed 7, St Louis, 2013, Mosby/Elsevier, pp 313–336.

113. Koketsu, J. (2018). *Pre-sleep routines of adult normal sleepers*. [Occupational Therapy Doctorate Capstone Projects, 34]. https://encompass.eku.edu/otdcapstones/34

114. Koketsu JS: Rest and sleep. In Pendleton HM, Schultz-Krohn W, editors: *Pedretti's occupational therapy: Practice skills for physical dysfunction* 8th ed., 2018, Elsevier, pp 305–335.

115. Kryger M, Roth T: Insomnia. In Kryger MH, editor: *Atlas of clinical sleep medicine*, Philadelphia, 2010, Saunders/Elsevier, pp 98–106.

116. Kushida CA, Littner MR, Hirshkowitz M, et al: Practice parameters for the use of continuous and bilevel positive airway pressure devices to treat adult clients with sleep-related breathing disorders, *Sleep* 29:375–380, 2006.

117. Lam KB, Jiang CQ, Thomas GN, et al: Napping is associated with increased risk of type 2 diabetes: the Guangzhou Biobank Cohort Study, *Sleep* 33:402–407, 2010.

118. Leland NE, Marcione N, Schepens Niemiec SL, et al: What is occupational therapy's role in addressing sleep problems among older adults? *OTJR (Thorofare N J)* 34:141–149, 2014.

119. Leng Y, Wainwright NWJ, Cappuccio FP, et al: Daytime napping and the risk of all-cause and cause-specific mortality: a 13-year follow-up of a British population, *Am J Epidemiol* 179:1115–1124, 2014. https://doi.org/10.1093/aje/kwu036.

120. Mahowald M: What state dissociation can teach us about consciousness and the function of sleep, *Sleep Med* 10:159–160, 2009.

121. Mahowald MW, Schenck CH: Evolving concepts of human state dissociation, *Arch Ital Biol* 139:269–300, 2001.

122. Makley MJ, English JB, Drubach DA, et al: Prevalence of sleep disturbance in closed head injury clients in a rehabilitation unit, *Neurorehabil Neural Repair* 22:341–347, 2008.

123. Maslow AH: *Motivation and personality*, New York, 1954, Harper & Row.

124. Mehra R: Nocturnal voiding: yet another sleep disruptor in the elderly (editorial), *Sleep Med* 16:557–558, 2015.

125. Melvin J, Jenson G: *Rheumatologic rehabilitation series: Assessment and management*, Volume 1, 1998, American Occupational Therapy Association.

126. Melvin JL, Ferrell KM: *Rheumatologic rehabilitation series: Adult rheumatic diseases*, Volume 2, 2000, The American Occupational Therapy Association.

127. Mendelson W: Pharmacology. In Kryger MH, editor: *Atlas of clinical sleep*, Philadelphia, 2010, Saunders/Elsevier, pp 69–79.

128. Meyer A: The philosophy of occupational therapy, *Arch Occup Ther* 1:1–10, 1922.

129. Meyer T, Eveloff S, Bauer M: Adverse environmental conditions in the respiratory and medical ICU settings, *Chest* 105:1211–1216, 1994.

130. Mistlberger RE, Rusak B: Circadian rhythms in mammals: formal properties and environmental influences. In Kryger MH, Roth T, Dement WC, editors: *Principles and practice of sleep medicine* ed 4, Philadelphia, 2004, Elsevier/Saunders, pp 321–334.

131. Mitler MM, Miller JC: Methods of testing for sleepiness, *Behav Med* 21:171–183, 1996.

132. Morgenthaler TI, Kapen S, Lee-Chiong T, et al: Practice parameters for the medical therapy of obstructive sleep apnea, *Sleep* 29:1031–1035, 2006.

133. Murray W, Johns A: New method for measuring daytime sleepiness: The Epworth Sleepiness Scale, *Sleep* 14(6):540–545, 1991. https://doi.org/10.1093/sleep/14.6.540.

134. National Alliance to End Homelessness: Fact sheet: veteran homelessness. <http://www.endhomelessness.org/library/entry/fact-sheet-veteran-homelessness>, 2015.

135. National Conference of State Legislatures: Summaries of current drowsy driving laws. <http://www.ncsl.org/research/transportation/summaries-of-current-drowsy-driving-laws.aspx>, 2014.

136. National Highway Traffic Safety Administration: *Factors related to fatal single-vehicle run-off-road crashes*, Washington DC, 2009, US Department of Transportation, p 23. <http://www-nrd.nhtsa.dot.gov/Pubs/811232.pdf>.

137. National Highway Traffic Safety Administration: *Traffic safety facts: a brief statistical summary—drowsy driving*, Washington DC, 2012, US Department of Transportation. <http://www-nrd.nhtsa.dot.gov/pubs/811449.pdf>.

138. National Sleep Foundation: *NSF Official Sleep Diary*. <http://sleepfoundation.org/content/nsf-official-sleep-diary>, nd.

139. National Sleep Foundation: *National Sleep Foundation Drowsy Driving Prevention Week*, n.d. https://www.thensf.org/drowsy-driving-prevention/.

140. National Sleep Foundation: *2009 Sleep in America Poll*, Washington, DC, 2009, The Foundation.

141. National Sleep Foundation: 2012 bedroom poll: summary of findings, 2012. https://www.thensf.org/wp-content/uploads/2021/03/2012-NSF-bedroom-poll.pdf.

142. National Sleep Foundation: *2014 Sleep in America Poll: sleep in the modern family*, Washington, DC, 2014, The Foundation. <http://www.sleepfoundation.org/sleep-polls-data/sleep-in-america-poll/2014-sleep-in-the-modern-family>.

143. National Sleep Foundation. (2018). Sleep in America® Poll 2018: Sleep & effectiveness are linked, but few plan their sleep. https://doi.org/10.1016/j.sleh.2018.02.007.

144. National Sleep Foundation. 2019 Drowsy Driving Prevention Week® Key Messages. https://live-drowsydriving.pantheonsite.io/wp-content/uploads/2019/10/DDPW-2019-Key-Messages-and-Talking-Points-rev-10-31-91.pdf.

145. National Sleep Foundation. (2020, July 28). *Napping*. https://www.sleepfoundation.org/articles/napping.

146. Netzer NC, Stoohs RA, Netzer CM, Clark K, Strohl KP: Using the Berlin Questionnaire to identify patients at risk for the sleep apnea syndrome, *Ann Internal Med* 131, 485–449, 1999. https://doi.org/10.7326/0003-4819-131-7-199910050-00002.

147. Nilsson I, Townsend E: Occupational justice: bridging theory and practice, *Scand J Occup Ther* 17:57–63, 2010. https://doi.org/10.3109/11038120903287182.

148. Nurit W, Michal AB: Rest: a qualitative exploration of the phenomenon, *Occup Ther Int* 10:227–238, 2003.

149. Obayashi K, Saeki K, Kurumatani N: Quantitative association between nocturnal voiding frequency and objective sleep quality in the general elderly population: the HEIJO-KYO cohort, *Sleep Med* 16:577–582, 2015. https://doi.org/10.1016/j.sleep.2015.01.021.

150. O'Donoghue N, McKay EA: Exploring the impact of sleep apnea on daily life and occupational engagement, *Br J Occup Ther* 75:509–516, 2012.

151. Ogawa Y, Kanbayashi T, Saito Y, et al: Total sleep deprivation elevates blood pressure through arterial baroreflex resetting: a study with microneurographic technique, *Sleep* 26:986–989, 2003.

152. Ohayon M, Carskadon MA, Guilleminault C, Vitiello MV: Meta analysis of quantitative sleep parameters from childhood to old age in healthy individuals: developing normative sleep values across the human life span, *Sleep* 27:1255–1273, 2004.

153. Ohayon MM: Epidemiology of insomnia: what we know and what we still need to learn, *Sleep Med Rev* 6:97–111, 2002.

154. Ohayon MM: The effects of breathing-related sleep disorders on mood disturbances in the general population, *J Clin Psychiatry* 64:1195–2000, 2003.

155. Ong JC: *Mindfulness-based therapy for insomnia*, , 2017, American Psychological Association.

156. Orff HJ, Ayalon L, Drummond SP: Traumatic brain injury and sleep disturbance: a review of current research (abstract), *J Head Trauma Rehabil* 24:155–165, 2009.

157. Parthasarathy S, Wendel C, Haynes PL, et al: A pilot study of CPAP adherence promotion by peer buddies with sleep apnea, *J Clin Sleep Med* 13:543–550, 2013.

158. Paterson LM: The science of sleep: what is it, what makes it happen and why do we do it?. In Green A, Westcombe A, editors: *Sleep: multi-professional perspectives*, Philadelphia, 2012, Jessica Kingsley Publishers.

159. Payne JD, Kensinger EA, Walmsley E, et al: Napping and the selective consolidation of negative aspects of scenes, American Psychological Association, *Emotion* 15:176–186, 2015. https://doi.org/10.1037/a0038683.

160. Pierce D: Untangling occupation and activity, *Am J Occup Ther* 55:138–146, 2001.

161. Pierce D: *Occupation by design: building therapeutic power*, Philadelphia, 2003, FA Davis.

162. Pierce D, Summers K: Rest and sleep. In Brown C, Stoffel VC, editors: *Occupational therapy in mental health: A vision for participation*, Philadelphia, 2011, F. A. Davis, pp 736–758.

163. Punjabi NM: The epidemiology of adult obstructive sleep apnea, *Proc Am Thorac Soc* 5:136–143, 2008.

164. Qaseem A, Kansagara D, Forciea MA, Cooke M, Denberg TD: Management of chronic insomnia disorder in adults: A clinical practice guideline from the American College of Physicians, *Ann Internal Med* 165:125–133, 2016. https://doi.org/10.7326/M15-2175.

165. Raheem OA, Orosco RK, Davidson TM, Lakin C: Clinical predictors of nocturia in the sleep apnea population, *Urol Ann* 6:31–35, 2014. https://doi.org/10.4103/0974-7796.127019.

166. Reid KJ, Zee PC: Circadian rhythm sleep disorders. In Kryger MH, editor: *Atlas of clinical sleep medicine*, Philadelphia, 2010, Saunders/Elsevier, pp 91–97.

167. Reid KJ, Zee PC, Buxton O: Circadian rhythms regulation. In Kryger MH, editor: *Atlas of clinical sleep medicine*, Philadelphia, 2010, Saunders/Elsevier, pp 25–27.

168. Roehr T, Carskadon MA, Dement WC, Roth T: Daytime sleepiness and alertness. In Kryger MH, Roth T, Dement WC, editors: *Principles and practice of sleep medicine* ed 4, Philadelphia, 2004, Elsevier/Saunders, pp 39–50.

169. Romero E, Krakow B, Haynes P, Ulibarri V: Nocturia and snoring: predictive symptoms for obstructive sleep apnea, *Sleep Breath* 14:337–343, 2010.

170. Rothman SM, Mattson MP: Sleep disturbances in Alzheimer's and Parkinson's diseases, *Neuromolecular Med* 14:194–204, 2012.

171. Sankari A, Bascom A, Oomman S, Safwan Badr M: Sleep disordered breathing in chronic spinal cord injury, *J Clin Sleep Med* 10:65–72, 2014. https://doi.org/10.5664/jcsm.3362.

172. Schatzl G, Temml C, Schmidbauer J, et al: Cross sectional study of nocturia in both sexes: analysis of a voluntary health screening project, *Urology* 56:71–75, 2000.

173. Schutte-Rodin S, Broch L, Buysse D, et al: Clinical guideline for the evaluation and management of chronic insomnia in adults, *J Clin Sleep Med* 4:487–504, 2008.

174. Siegel JM: REM sleep. In Kryger MH, Roth T, Dement WC, editors: *Principles and practice of sleep medicine* ed 4, Philadelphia, 2004, Elsevier/Saunders, pp 10–35.

175. Smith MT, McCrae CS, Cheung J, Martin JL, Harrod CG, Heald JL, Carden KA: Use of actigraphy for the evaluation of sleep disorders and circadian rhythm sleep-wake disorders: An American Academy of Sleep Medicine clinical practice guideline, *J Clin Sleep Med* 14(7):1231–1237, 2018. https://doi.org/10.5664/jcsm.7230.

176. Solet JM: Sleep and rest. In Schell BAB, Gillen G, Scaffa ME, editors: *Willard and Spackman's occupational therapy* ed 12, Philadelphia, 2014, Lippincott Williams & Wilkins, pp 714–730.

177. Solet JM: Sleep and rest. In Schell BAB, Gillen G, editors: *Willard and Spackman's occupational therapy* 13th ed, 2019, Wolters Kluver, pp 828–846.

178. Staffan D: Countermeasure drowsiness by design: using common behavior, *Work* 41:5062–5067, 2012. https://doi.org/10.3233/WOR-2012-0798-5062.

179. Standards of Practice Committee of American Academy of Sleep Medicine: Practice parameters for clinical use of the Multiple Sleep Latency test and the Maintenance of Wakefulness test, *Sleep* 28:113–121, 2005.

180. Steger B: Cultures of sleep. In Green A, Westcombe A, editors: *Sleep: multiprofessional perspectives*, Philadelphia, 2012, Jessica Kingsley Publishers.

181. St George RJ, Delbaere K, Williams P, Lord SR:: Sleep quality and falls in older people living in self-and assisted-care villages, *Gerontology* 55:162–168, 2008.

182. Stone KL, Blackwell T, Cummings SR, et al: Rest-activity rhythms predict risk of mortality in older women, *Sleep* 29:160, 2006.

183. Taylor D, Mallory LH, Lichstein KL, et al: Comorbidity of chronic insomnia with medical problems, *Sleep* 30:213–218, 2007.

184. Taylor RR: *The intentional relationship: Occupational therapy and use of self*, 2nd ed., 2020, F. A. Davis.

185. Tester NJ, Foss JJ: The Issue Is—Sleep as an occupational need, *Am J Occup Ther* 72, 2018. https://doi.org/10.5014/ajot.2018.020651. 7201347010

186. Thorpy M: International Classification of Sleep Disorders. In Chokroverty S, editor: *Sleep Disorders Medicine*, New York, NY, 2017, Springer. https://doi.org/10.1007/978-1-4939-6578-6_27.

187. Trotti LM, Bliwise DL: *Treatment of the sleep disorders associated with Parkinson's disease*, *Neurotherapy* 11:68–77, 2014. https://doi.org/10.1007/s13311-013-0236-z.

188. Turek FW, Dugovic C, Laposky AD: Master circadian clock: master circadian rhythm. In Kryger MH, Roth T, Dement WC, editors: *Principles and practice of sleep medicine* ed 4, Philadelphia, 2004, Elsevier/Saunders, pp 318–320.

189. Wahlstrom KL: Accommodating the sleep patterns within current educational structures: an uncharted path. In Carskadon MA, editor: *Adolescent sleep patterns: biological, social, and psychological influences*, NY, 2002, Cambridge University Press, pp 172–197.

190. Waite A: Have faith: how spirituality is a regular part of occupational therapy practice, *OT Practice* 19:13–16, 2014.

191. Wang Y, Gao W, Sun M, Chen B: Adherence to CPAP in clients with obstructive sleep apnea in a Chinese population, *Respir Care* 57:238–243, 2012.

192. Weaver TE, George CFP: Cognition and performance in clients with obstructive sleep apnea. In Kryger MH, Roth T, Dement WC, editors: *Principles and practice of sleep medicine* ed 4, Philadelphia, 2004, Elsevier Saunders, pp 1023–1042.

193. Weaver TE, Laizner AM, Evans LK, et al: An instrument to measure functional status outcomes for disorders of excessive sleepiness, *Sleep* 20:835–843, 1997.

194. Wessendorf TE, et al: Sleep-disordered breathing among clients with first-ever stroke, *J Neurol* 247:41–47, 2000.

195. West L: Sleep: an emerging practice area? *OT Practice* 14(8): 9–10, 2009.
196. Wheatley D: Medicinal plants for insomnia: a review of their pharmacology, efficacy and tolerability, *J Psychopharmacol* 19:414–421, 2005.
197. Williams S, Meadows R, Arber S: The sociology of sleep. In Cappuccio FP, Miller MA, Lockley SW, editors: *Sleep health, and society: from aetiology to public health*, Oxford, UK, 2010, Oxford University Press, pp 275–299.
198. Wiseman-Hakes C, Colantonio A, Gargaro J: Sleep and wake disorders following traumatic brain injury: a critical review of the literature, *Crit Rev Phys Rehabil Med* 21:317–374, 2009.
199. Wolf TJ, Chuh A, Floyd T, et al: Effectiveness of occupation-based interventions to improve areas of occupation and social participation after stroke: an evidence-based review, *Am J Occup Ther* 69:1–11, 2014. https://doi.org/10.5014/ajot.2015.012195.
200. Wong PM, Manuck SB, DiNardo MM, et al: Shorter sleep duration is associated with decreased insulin sensitivity in healthy white men, *Sleep* 38:223–231, 2015.
201. Woods DL, Kim H, Yefimova M: To nap or not to nap: excessive daytime napping is associated with elevated evening cortisol in nursing home residents with dementia, *Biol Res Nurs* 15:185–190, 2011. https://doi.org/10.1177/109980041142086.
202. Worthman CM, Melby MK: Toward a comparative developmental ecology of human sleep. In Carskadon MA, editor: *Adolescent sleep patterns: biological, social, and psychological influences*, New York, 2003, Cambridge University Press.
203. Wu JQ, Appleman ER, Salazar RD, Ong JC: Cognitive Behavioral Therapy for Insomnia Comorbid With Psychiatric and Medical Conditions: A Meta-analysis, *JAMA Intern Med* 175(9):1461–1472, 2015. https://doi.org/10.1001/jamainternmed.2015.3006.
204. Yang P-Y, Ho K-H, Chen H-C, Chien M-Y: Exercise training improves sleep quality in middle-aged and older adults with sleep problems: a systematic review, *J Physiother* 58:157–163, 2012.
205. Yasuda YL: Rheumatoid arthritis, osteoarthritis and fibromyalgia. In Radomski MV, Trombly Latham CA, editors: *Occupational therapy for physical dysfunction* ed 6, Philadelphia, 2008, Wolvers Kluver/Lippincott Williams & Wilkins, pp 1214–1241.
206. Young JS, Bourgeois JA, Hilty DM, Hardin K: Sleep in hospitalized medical patients. Part 1. Factors affecting sleep, *J Hosp Med* 2:473–482, 2008.
207. Young JS, Bourgeois JA, Hilty DM, Hardin K: Sleep in hospitalized medical patients. Part 2. Behavioral and pharmacological management of sleep disturbance, *J Hosp Med* 4:50–59, 2009.
208. Zeitzer JM, Bliwise DL, Hernandez B, et al: Nocturia compounds nocturnal wakefulness in older individuals with insomnia, *J Clin Sleep Med* 9:259–262, 2013.
209. Zupancic M, Swanson L, Arnedt T, Chervin R: Impact, presentation and diagnosis. In Kryger MH, editor: *Atlas of clinical sleep medicine*, Philadelphia, 2010, Saunders/Elsevier, pp 85–90.

OTHER RESOURCES

American Academy of Sleep Medicine: http://www.aasmnet.org
The American Board of Sleep Medicine: http://www.absm.org
The American Sleep Association: http://www.sleepassociation.org
National Sleep Foundation: http://www.sleepfoundation.org
Sleep Research Society: http://www.sleepresearchsociety.org
Edinger JD, Arnedt JT, Bertisch SM, et al: Behavioral and psychological treatments for chronic insomnia disorder in adults: an American Academy of Sleep Medicine systematic review, meta-analysis, and GRADE assessment, *J Clin Sleep Med* 17(2):263–298, 2021.

Work Evaluation and Work Programs*

Denise Haruko Ha, Jill J. Page, and Barb Phillips-Meltzer

LEARNING OBJECTIVES

After studying this chapter, the student or practitioner will be able to do the following:

1. Understand the role of occupational therapy in the development of work programs.
2. Describe the different types of work evaluation and work programs that are currently being practiced.
3. Identify the components of a work rehabilitation program.
4. Understand the difference between work hardening and work conditioning.
5. Identify the aspects of a well-designed functional capacity evaluation.
6. Explain the importance of reliability and validity in the context of evaluation.
7. Understand the differences between job demands analysis, ergonomic evaluation/hazard identification, and worksite evaluation.
8. Discuss the application of job demands analysis.
9. Discuss basic ergonomic interventions.
10. Describe the components of worker wellness programs.
11. Describe school-to-work transition services.
12. Describe the purpose of a work readiness program.
13. Identify various community-based work programs.

CHAPTER OUTLINE

*The authors would like to acknowledge the significant and outstanding contributions of Christine M. Wietlisbach to this and the previous two editions.

KEY TERMS

Ergonomic evaluation
Ergonomics
Essential tasks
Functional capacity evaluation
General vocational evaluation
Job demands analysis
Primary prevention
Secondary prevention
Specific vocational evaluation

System theory
Tertiary prevention
Vocational evaluation
Work conditioning
Work hardening
Work readiness program
Work rehabilitation
Work-related musculoskeletal disorders
Worksite evaluations

THREADED CASE STUDY

Joe, Susan, and Henry, Part 1

Joe is a 26-year-old man (prefers use of the pronouns he/him/his) who worked two jobs to support himself and his daughter, who lived with his ex-wife. He worked as a janitor during the day at a hotel and spa, and cleaned offices at night. Because of a motor vehicle accident, he sustained a T11 spinal cord injury resulting in complete paralysis of his legs. This injury affected his mobility, strength, and effort, impeding his ability to return to janitorial work. He would not be able to effectively carry out the essential functions of the job from a wheelchair. Fortunately, the hotel and spa thought Joe was a good worker and offered him an alternative job as a laundry attendant, as long as he met the physical demands of the job. Joe was referred to occupational therapy by his physician.

Susan is a 34 year-old woman (prefers use of the pronouns she/her/hers) who works in the accounting department for a large corporation. She was asked to telecommute during the COVID-19 pandemic. Susan's telecommuting work environment is less than ideal. Susan, her husband and her 8-month-old baby were relocated to her in-law's home, with all three of them sleeping in her husband's old bedroom. Her father-in-law set up an "office" for her in the basement, using an old chair from his office and a folding table. The basement had poor air circulation and there was a mildew smell. Susan is having difficulty with completing work assignments due to pain in her neck, arms, upper and lower back as well as headaches. Susan contacted her Human Resources Department who suggested that she meet with the occupational therapist consultant.

Henry (prefers use of the pronouns he/him/his) is a 42-year-old father and husband who has been supporting his family by working as a roofer for the past 15 years. On one of his work assignments he fell off the roof and sustained a traumatic brain injury and a couple of lower extremity fractures. As a result, his motor and praxis skills, sensory-perceptual skills, cognitive skills, emotional regulation skills, and communication and social skills have been affected. He has been receiving workers' compensation for 2 years. Henry now feels ready to return to some type of work but does not know what he can do. He has sufficient insight to know that he cannot return to roofing but would like to do something with his life.

Critical Thinking Questions

As you read through the following information on occupational therapy work evaluation and intervention, keep in mind the circumstances of Joe, Susan, and Henry to determine which services each may benefit from most.

1. What type of evaluation and services could occupational therapy offer to assist Joe, his physician, and the employer?
2. What services can the occupational therapy consultant offer to Susan to help her improve her work environment and help remedy her physical and emotional discomfort?
3. What work-related occupational therapy services can help Henry discover what type of work he can do at this point?

One of the most significant occupations in which adults engage is work. A stable job provides the means to fulfill the most basic physiological and safety requirements that humans need to survive and thrive: food and water, a safe place to sleep, and the security of knowing that these resources will continue to be available. For many, belonging and esteem needs are also met at the workplace. Anything that prevents an adult from participating in the occupation of work will have significant consequences for that individual's health and well-being. According to the Office of Disability Employment Policy of the U.S. Department of Labor, in 2020, 21.0% of the labor force consisted of people with disabilities (up from 17.1% in 2014). The unemployment rate for those with disabilities was 16.5% (which interestingly was an increase from 12.5% in 2014—a discrepancy that should be researched further).[99] Occupational therapy practitioners play a key role in helping workers maintain their employment despite the symptoms they experience; they also facilitate an individual's entry or reentry into the workforce.

HISTORY OF OCCUPATIONAL THERAPY INVOLVEMENT IN WORK PROGRAMS

The therapeutic use of work has always been a core tenet of occupational therapy, since the inception of the profession.[38] Work programs have their roots in efforts to help those with mental illness during the moral treatment movement, which started in Europe in the late 18th and early 19th centuries.[1] In 1801, Philippe Pinel, one of the founders of moral treatment, introduced work treatment in the Bicentre Asylum for the Insane. He suggested that "prescribed physical exercises and manual occupations should be employed in all mental hospitals. . . . Rigorously executed manual labor is the best method of securing good morale. . . . The return of convalescent patients to their previous interests, to industriousness and perseverance have always been for me the best omen of a final recovery."[78] Later in the 1800s, several psychiatric settings instituted productive activity programs.

In 1914, George Barton, one of the founding fathers of the occupational therapy profession, who was disabled by tuberculosis and a foot amputation, established the Consolation House in New York.[86] This program enabled convalescents to use occupations to return to productive living.[86] Barton stated, "The purpose of work was to divert the mind, exercise the body, and relieve the monotony and boredom of illness."[81]

In 1915, Eleanor Clarke Slagle, another founder of the occupational therapy profession, was hired to create a program for persons with mental or physical disabilities that would enable them to work and become self-sufficient.[86] The program was located at Hull House, a settlement house in Chicago, and was funded by philanthropic contributions. The participants involved in the program produced goods such as baskets, needlework, toys, rugs, and cabinets while developing manual skills and receiving wages for their work.

The early leaders of occupational therapy identified the importance of work when defining the profession's focus and purpose. Adolph Meyer, a psychiatrist who emigrated from Germany at the time and was an early proponent of moral treatment, observed that healthy living involved a "blending of work and pleasure."[63] Dr. Herbert Hall helped establish a medical workshop at Massachusetts General Hospital in Boston, where clients were involved in "work cure."[36] In this workshop clients produced marketable goods and received a share of the profits. The focus of treatment in these curative workshops was to restore the impaired body part to as normal function as possible, with the goal of returning the client to work.

While this curative workshop movement was transpiring on the East Coast, similar programs were developing elsewhere in the United States. For example, at the Los Angeles County Poor Farm, now recognized as Rancho Los Amigos National Rehabilitation Center in Downey, California, "all inmates were requested to do an amount of work that was commensurate with their physical strength and mental capacity, which was determined by the admitting doctor."[33] Inmates used woodworking machinery to build a large amount of furniture, which was used at the farm. Commodes, bedside tables, wheelchair tables, park benches, cabinets, and other items were built in the shops. In later years, when there was a true occupational therapy department, patients made Navajo-type rugs, rag or braided rugs, brushes, shawls, pottery, pictures, baskets, and leatherwork (Fig. 14.1A). Patients took special occupational therapy classes "which were designed to enable those who are crippled, blinded, or otherwise handicapped to make themselves useful" by producing articles that could be used at the County Farm or sold to employees or the California Crafts and Industries Society in Los Angeles (see Fig. 14.1B).[33]

In the early 1900s the medical profession did not seem to consider vocational readiness programs to be important. The focus of care for persons with physical illnesses was primarily palliative and involved immobilization and bed rest. This attitude shifted after World War I, with the need to rehabilitate the large number of injured soldiers to help them become functional and gain employment.

The U.S. Federal Board for Vocational Education (FBVE) was created after adoption of the Vocational Education Act of 1917.[48] In 1918 the Division of Orthopaedic Surgery in the Medical Department of the Army organized a reconstruction program for disabled soldiers.[77] One of the founders of occupational

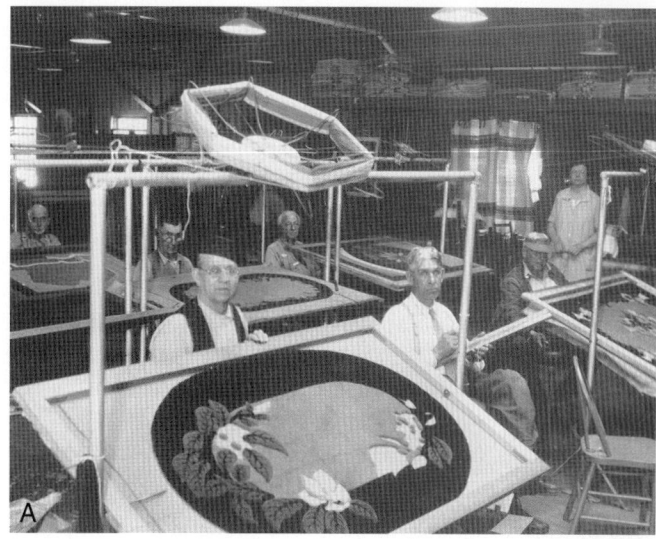

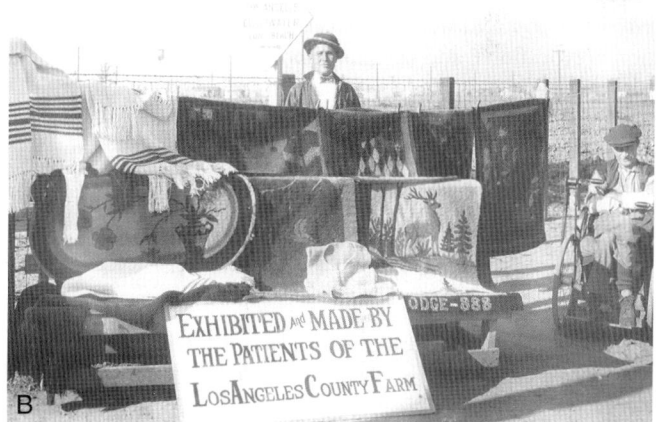

Fig. 14.1 A, Patients at work weaving rugs in the occupational therapy shop at the Los Angeles (LA) County Poor Farm. B, Patients with a display of their products made at the LA County Poor Farm. (From Fliedner CA: Occupational therapy: for the body and the mind. In Rodgers GM, editor: Centennial Rancho Los Amigos Medical Center 1888-1988, Downey, CA, 1990, Rancho Los Amigos Medical Center.)

therapy, Thomas Kidner, served as an advisor. This program led to the development of reconstruction aides, who were the precursors to occupational and physical therapists. Treatment involved both handicrafts and vocational education. The reconstruction aides used work activities to return the injured soldiers to military duty or civilian life to the highest degree possible.

In 1920, Congress passed the Civilian Rehabilitation Act of 1920 (Smith-Fess Act, Public Law 66-236). This law provided funds for vocational guidance and training, work adjustment, prostheses, and placement services.[48] If therapy was part of a medical treatment program, the law provided payment for occupational therapy services; however, it did not provide payment for physician services. Physicians either provided free services or received payment through state or volunteer contributions. This limited the use of occupational therapy services in vocational rehabilitation to the states that received supplemented federal program funds to support services such as the curative workshops.

The Social Security Act of 1935 defined rehabilitation as "the rendering of a person disabled fit to engage in a remunerative occupation."[56] This was the first attempt to provide vocational rehabilitation to the physically handicapped in the community.

In 1937, industrial therapy, called employment therapy, was born.[61] The occupational therapist used activities as treatment modalities. It was common for patients to have work assignments in the hospital that matched their experience, aptitude, and interest. Sheltered work environments within the hospital were used, including the hospital laundry, barber shop, and carpenter shop.

The term *prevocational* started appearing in the literature by the late 1930s. It referred to the use of crafts to develop skills readily transferable to industry.[100] Prevocational therapy prepared patients for the work role. Occupational therapists worked as directors, work evaluators, and prevocational therapists in work programs. In the 1940s, prevocational programs and work evaluation were accepted as part of the practice of occupational therapy. Patients in acute care facilities who were physically disabled were transferred to outpatient or rehabilitation prevocational and vocational programs.

World War II brought more opportunities for occupational therapists to become involved in work programs. With the advancement of medicine and pharmacology, many injured soldiers survived their wounds. Federal funding for rehabilitating disabled veterans increased as the government discharged the disabled soldiers. This led to an increase in the development of work programs designed to evaluate and rehabilitate injured veterans.[20]

In 1943, the Barden-LaFollette Act (Public Law 78-113) modified the original provisions of the Civilian Rehabilitation Act of 1920.[48] This new law, called the Vocational Rehabilitation Act, covered many medical services, including occupational therapy and vocational guidance. Services were expanded to those with physical and mental limitations. This law also created the Office of Vocational Rehabilitation, a state and federally funded agency that is still in existence today and provides job training and placement services to people with disabilities. Industrial therapy continued in various settings as a form of vocational rehabilitation.

During the 1950s, many occupational therapists thought that work evaluation belonged to a newly established profession, vocational rehabilitation, rather than to occupational therapy.[61] Occupational therapy involvement declined, and vocational counselors, vocational evaluators, and work adjusters were primarily the leaders in this field. There were, however, still a few occupational therapists who remained active in work programming.

A high point in the development of prevocational exploration and training techniques in the field of occupational therapy occurred in 1960.[48] Rosenberg and Wellerson published an article on development of the TOWER (Testing, Orientation, and Work Evaluation in Rehabilitation) system in New York.[82] The TOWER system was one of the first work sample programs to use real job samples in a simulated work environment. In 1959, Lilian S. Wegg gave the Eleanor Clarke Slagle Lecture on "Essentials of Work Evaluation," based on her experiences at the May T. Morrison Center for Rehabilitation in San Francisco. Wegg promoted the need for both sound testing procedures and training programs.[100] Florence S. Cromwell, a past president of the American Occupational Therapy Association (AOTA), established norms for disabled populations on certain prevocational tests while evaluating the performance of adults with cerebral palsy at the United Cerebral Palsy Organization.[20,48] Cromwell continued to be an important advocate of occupational therapy–based work-related therapy in the ensuing decades.

Occupational behavioral theory, which emerged in the mid-1960s and early 1970s, offered a return to the profession's concern for occupation. Mary Reilly, an early proponent of occupational behavior theory and a 1962 Eleanor Clark Slagle lecturer, thought that productive activity as treatment was the unique contribution of occupational therapy.[48] Occupational behavior theory advocated that persons can achieve healthy living only through a balance of work, rest, and play.

The increasing number of industries in the late 1970s and early 1980s introduced a whole new arena for occupational therapists: industrial rehabilitation and work hardening.[48] Work hardening used actual work tasks in a simulated, structured work environment, generally in community-based settings.[1,87] Occupational therapists used their knowledge of neuromuscular characteristics, including range of motion (ROM) and endurance, along with task analysis skills and knowledge of the psychosocial aspects of work, in evaluating, planning, and implementing a work-hardening program.

In 1989, the Commission on Accreditation of Rehabilitation Facilities (CARF) developed work-hardening standards requiring an interdisciplinary approach.[19] The interdisciplinary team consisted of occupational therapists, physical therapists, psychologists, and vocational specialists.

The Americans with Disabilities Act of 1990 (ADA; Public Law 101-336) was important legislation that addressed the civil rights needs of those with disabilities and simultaneously opened major markets for occupational therapists.[48] Occupational therapists were involved in providing both work training for persons with disabilities and assistance to employers in meeting the requirements of the ADA. This legislation continues to have important implications for work practice.[26] (See Chapter 15 for more information on the ADA.)

Also in 1990 the National AgrAbility Project (http://www.agrability.org) was established through the 1990 Farm Bill (PL 101). This opened up opportunities for occupational therapy practitioners to help farmers, ranchers, and other agricultural workers with disabilities safely return to work. AgrAbility funds occupational therapy practitioners' site visits to evaluate and identify what is needed for a farmer or rancher to return to work. If assistive technology or other workplace modifications are needed, various funding sources (e.g., the state's vocational rehabilitation office) usually support some or all of the recommendations that need to be implemented.

In 1992, the AOTA published a document that defined work as "all productive activities and included life roles such as homemaker, employee, volunteer, student, or hobbyist."[2] This document was replaced in 2000 by "Occupational Therapy Services in Facilitating Work Performance."[3] This statement asserted that "occupational therapists and occupational therapy assistants contribute to the delivery of services for the promotion and management of productive occupations as well as the prevention and treatment of work-related disability." Subsequent to a third revision in 2011,[4] in 2017 this document was again revised by AOTA and entitled Occupational Therapy Services in Facilitating Work Participation and Performance.[6]

In 2002, the Occupational Safety and Health Administration (OSHA) unveiled a comprehensive approach to ergonomics to reduce the incidence of musculoskeletal disorders (MSDs) in the workplace. This four-pronged, comprehensive approach includes guidelines, enforcement, outreach and assistance, and a national advisory committee on ergonomics.

Occupational therapists have traditionally consulted and continue to consult with employers and employees on making recommendations about equipment, posture, and body mechanics to prevent injuries. Ergonomic intervention continues to be an area of many opportunities for occupational therapists who have received additional training and education in the area of ergonomics.[92]

ROLE OF THE OCCUPATIONAL THERAPIST IN WORK PROGRAMS

Occupational therapists (OTs) and occupational therapy assistants (OTAs) play an important role in helping individuals participate in all aspects of work. According to the "Occupational Therapy Practice Framework: Domain and Process," fourth edition (OTPF-4), work is an area of occupation that is defined by Christiansen et al. as "labor or exertion related to the development, production, delivery, or management of objects or services; benefits may be financial or nonfinancial (e.g. social connectedness, contributions to society, adding structure and routine to daily life)" OTPF-4, p. S20).[7] Work is further described in the OTPF-4 as "employment interests and pursuits, employment seeking and acquisition, job performance and maintenance, retirement preparation and adjustment, volunteer exploration, and volunteer participation" (OTPF-4, p. S20).[7]

Entry-level occupational therapy practitioners have obtained the education and training to address clients' work participation goals. When work-related services are provided, the characteristics of the worker, the worker's tasks, environments, and contexts are examined. Additional training and certifications, however, are available and beneficial for specializing in ergonomics, functional or work capacity evaluations, and job analysis. Occupational therapy practitioners provide client-centered services to "to promote health and wellness, prevent injury, and maximize work performance and participation for clients who experience challenges in attaining, maintaining, or resuming work because of disease, disability or injury."[7] The following roles can be fulfilled by occupational therapy practitioners: "independent contractor or business owner; consultant; industrial rehabilitation specialist; ergonomist; health and safety specialist; therapist or consultant employed within an institution, hospital, or facility; and vocational rehabilitation specialist."[7] Work-related services are provided in a variety of settings, including,

but not limited to, acute care and rehabilitation facilities, industrial and business environments, mental health centers, schools, vocational programs, and community settings. The occupational therapy process involves "evaluation, intervention planning" implementation, and review; and outcome monitoring."[7] This chapter describes the range of work evaluations and interventions in which occupational therapists are involved in assisting people in actively participating in meaningful work roles.

WORK REHABILITATION

The Occupational Therapy Intervention Process Model (OTIPM) described by Fisher et al. builds a persuasive case for how well occupational therapists' training and philosophy of care can benefit the injured worker.[30] Therapeutic rapport integrated with information assemblage and functional performance analysis leads to the appropriate selection of intervention based on the injured worker's needs and insures the best possible outcome.[30] **Work rehabilitation** includes functional capacity evaluation (FCE), vocational evaluation, job demands analysis (JDA), worksite evaluation/fitness for duty testing, pre-employment screening, work hardening/conditioning, onsite rehabilitation, modified/transitional employment, education, ergonomics, wellness, health promotion, and preventive services. Occupational therapists are integral in providing these services, and this area of practice provides a tangible way for therapists to experience the tremendous reward of seeing lives changed through their efforts. The AOTA has developed a Work and Industry Special Interest Section for those who are involved in or wish to know more about this area of specialization.

FUNCTIONAL CAPACITY EVALUATION

A **functional capacity evaluation** is an objective assessment of an individual's ability to perform work-related activity.[b][3] These functionally based tests have been used since the early 1970s to assist in making return-to-work decisions and were primarily performed by occupational and physical therapists.[45] Today, however, the results of such an evaluation can be used in many different ways, and the evaluation is performed by a multitude of disciplines. Occupational therapists are remarkably qualified to conduct FCEs because of their education and background in task analysis.[3,4] An FCE can be used to set goals for rehabilitation and readiness for return to work, assess residual work capacity, determine disability status, and screen for physical compatibility before hiring a new employee and case closure.[73,74]

ETHICAL CONSIDERATIONS

The FCE is a tremendous tool in the course of rehabilitation that allows a therapist to have objective findings for making thoughtful and appropriate recommendations regarding initiation, continuation, or cessation of treatment, or for referring the client to another service. Great care must be taken to ensure that the results are not derived lightly because of the enormous impact that such results can have on a person's life.[51,55]

---

[b] References 30,34,45,46,53,55,74.

An FCE usually consists of a review of medical records, an interview, musculoskeletal screening, evaluation of physical performance, formation of recommendations, and generation of a report.[51] Evaluation of physical performance usually takes the form of assessing the client's physiology, both cardiovascular and muscular endurance, during the course of strength, static, and dynamic tasks. The report usually contains information regarding the overall level of work, tolerance for work over the course of a day, individual task scores, job match information, level of client participation (cooperative or self-limited), and interventions for consideration.[51,55]

> ## OT PRACTICE NOTES
>
> The referral source for an FCE can and does vary. Physicians, attorneys, case managers, insurance carriers, and other therapists are the primary sources for FCE referrals. Some states, institutions, and insurance carriers require a physician's prescription for an FCE; therefore, it is important to be aware of each state's practice act, employer, and insurance carrier guidelines for accepting referrals. Reimbursement also varies with geographic location.

A wide variety of FCEs are currently used in practice today, both commercially available systems and evaluations developed by individual therapists or clinics (Fig. 14.2).

FCEs can be (1) all inclusive when looking at case closure or settlement; (2) job specific when making a match between a person's abilities and the job description, such as "cashier at XYZ store" or a broader occupational title such as "cashier"; or (3) injury specific, such as an upper extremity evaluation after bilateral carpal tunnel release. Joe, the 26-year-old man with T11 paraplegia, could benefit from a job-specific FCE to determine whether he can meet the physical demands of the alternative job as a laundry attendant. Using Fisher's terminology during the assessment of performance skills in an initial evaluation phase as "Effective" or "Ineffective" provides a broad categorical range that can be further detailed with *Dictionary of Occupational Titles terminology.*[30]

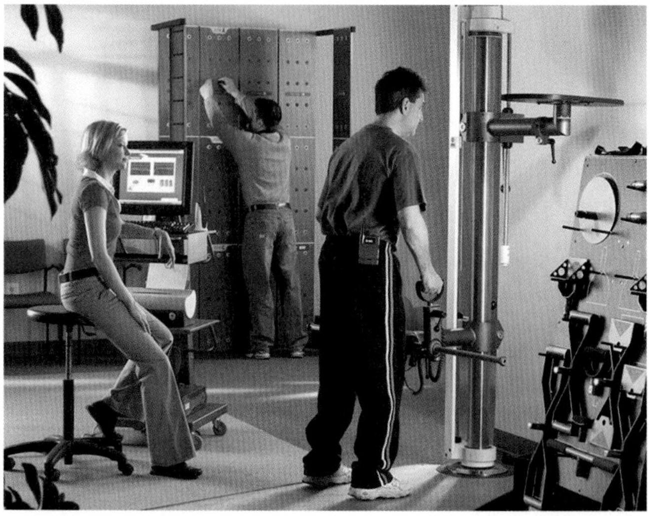

A well-designed FCE is comprehensive, standardized, practical, objective, reliable, and valid.[51,55,83]

A comprehensive FCE will include all of the physical demands of work as defined by the *Dictionary of Occupational Titles* (DOT), published by the U.S. Department of Labor and last revised in 1991 (Box 14.1).[96] The main focus of Joe's FCE will be on the physical demands of work that he can still reasonably do from the wheelchair, such as lifting, carrying, pushing, pulling, balancing, reaching, handling, fingering, feeling, talking, hearing, and seeing.

It is also important for the individual being tested to understand the correlation between the test items and the functions of the job. The application of meaningful activity can improve individuals' cooperation during testing and encourage maximum effort. For example, an individual who performs secretarial duties may have difficulty understanding the need to test her ability to climb ladders if she does not actually perform this function during the course of her job.[7,75] An FCE needs to be practical in terms of length of testing, cost, space, and report generation.[55,71]

Standardization in FCEs means having a procedure manual, task definitions and instructions, a scoring methodology, and equipment requirements and set-up.[53,55,73] This type of structure helps ensure that individuals are being assessed in a fair and consistent manner, and it demonstrates the effort to minimize observer bias. Verbal instructions are critical in establishing rapport between the evaluator and the individual being tested. During the initial interview, the tone is set for the course of the evaluation, and the individual's trust in the evaluator is implicit in maximizing cooperation and effort during the evaluation.[55] Objectivity is not limited to weights, distances, heights, or some other numerical quantity; subjective measures can be made objective with operational definitions. Objectivity during the course of an FCE does not exclude clinical judgment and decision making, but it does require the measure to be as free as possible of examiner bias.[83] This includes physical performance, in addition to client cooperation during testing. Objectivity is accomplished through standardization of the testing protocol and a structured scoring methodology.

Fig. 14.2 The EvalTech Functional Testing System, an example of a functional capacity evaluation system. (Courtesy BTE, Hanover, MD.)

> ## BOX 14.1   Twenty Physical Demands of Work
>
> - Lifting
> - Standing
> - Walking
> - Sitting
> - Carrying
> - Pushing
> - Pulling
> - Climbing
> - Balancing
> - Stooping
> - Kneeling
> - Crouching
> - Crawling
> - Reaching
> - Handling
> - Fingering
> - Feeling
> - Talking
> - Hearing
> - Seeing
>
> Data from US Department of Labor, Employment and Training Administration: *Revised dictionary of occupational titles*, vols I and II, ed 4, Washington, DC, 1991, US Government Printing Office.

The most important aspects of an FCE are reliability and validity of the testing protocol. Two types of reliability are deemed important in an FCE: interrater and test-retest reliability.[53] Interrater reliability in an FCE means consistency; if two therapists administer the same test to the same client, will they get the same results.[51] King and Barrett state that "test-retest reliability or intra-rater reliability refers to the stability of a score derived from one administration of an FCE to another when administered by the same rater."[51] Being able to establish reliability is the first step in determining the validity or accuracy of the results.[83] If there is not agreement between evaluators, it is difficult to determine whose results are correct.[51] Once reliability has been proved, validity can be assessed. The term *validity* is used in many ways, often with significance placed on issues surrounding sincerity of effort. In scientific terms validity means accuracy; in other words, does the FCE provide results that truly describe how the client can perform at work?[55,83]

There are several types of validity, with content, criterion (both concurrent and predictive), and construct validity having the most impact on the results of an FCE.[51,55] Content validity is the easiest to establish in an FCE because this measure refers to whether the evaluation tests the physical demands of work, as defined by a panel of experts, by job analysis, or by a recognized document, such as the DOT.[53,55,73,96]

Criterion validity refers to whether conclusions can be drawn from the measures taken, and in an FCE this refers to whether a person can actually perform at the level demonstrated during testing.[51,53,55] Criterion validity is often determined by comparing the methodology in question with a gold standard—another instrument that has been proved to be reliable and valid.[51,53,55] This is difficult to do in an FCE because there are a limited number of available assessments with proven reliability and validity to compare against and because other methods, such as comparing the person's tested ability with the actual work level, can be seriously flawed.[53,55,60] Criterion validity includes concurrent and predictive validity.

Concurrent validity refers to the ability of a test to measure existing abilities, and in an FCE this would be demonstrated by the test's ability to determine which clients can perform at a given level and which clients cannot perform at a given level.[51,53,55]

Predictive validity is indicated by the test's capacity to predict future ability and has great value in an FCE by determining who can safely return to work and remain without injury.[51,55,62] The first FCE to be studied for validity and published in peer-reviewed literature was developed by the occupational therapist Susan Smith and has served as an important contribution to the knowledge base.[89] Without reliability and validity, a referral source cannot know whether the results of the evaluation would vary if the individual were tested by another therapist or whether the results are accurate.[51,53,55]

VOCATIONAL EVALUATIONS

Work evaluations, or vocational evaluations, are "a comprehensive process that systematically uses work, real or simulated, as the focal point for vocational assessment and exploration to assist individuals in their vocational development."[28] According to CARF, the following factors are addressed in the traditional vocational evaluation model: physical and psychomotor capacities; intellectual capacities; emotional stability; interests, attitudes, and knowledge of occupational information; aptitudes and achievements (vocational and educational); work skills and work tolerances; work habits; work-related capabilities; and job-seeking skills.[41] These assessments can last from 3 to 10 consecutive days, depending on the goals of the assessment. Vocational evaluators generally conduct these types of assessments in private vocational agencies; however, some occupational therapists also have been involved in conducting these evaluations in public and private medical or nonmedical settings. Vocational rehabilitation, worker's compensation, and long-term disability carriers pay for these services, but most medical plans do not.

Standardized work samples, such as the Valpar Component Work Sample System or the Jewish Employment Vocational Services, are used to assess specific skills in the areas of data or other job-related topics (Fig. 14.3).[42] Dexterity tests, such as the Bennett Hand Tool (Fig. 14.4), Crawford Small Parts, and Purdue Pegboard, are used to evaluate motor skills.[41,42] When no standardized work samples are available to assess the specific skills needed for a particular occupation, specially designed

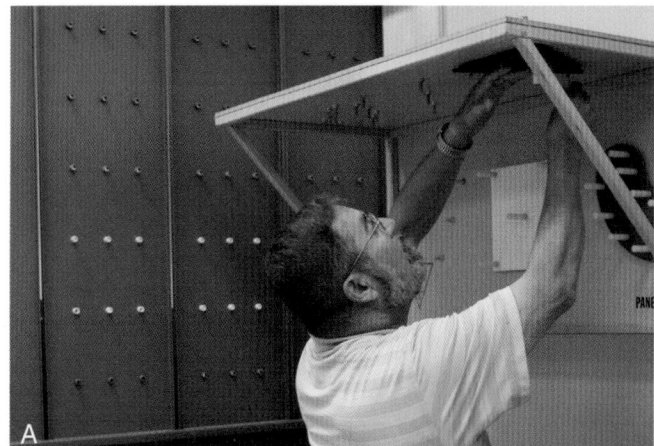
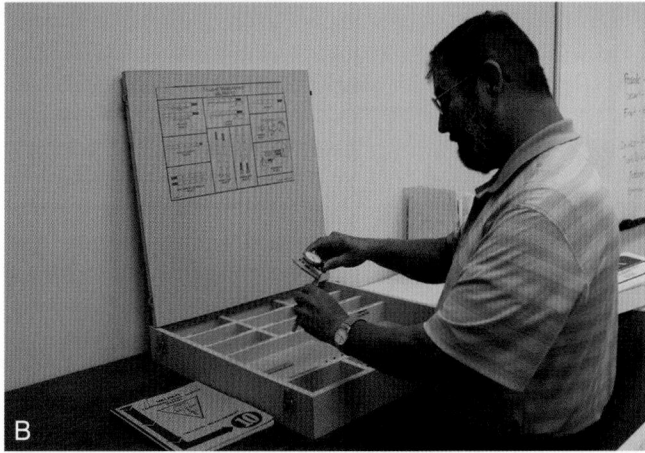

Fig. 14.3 (A) Valpar 9 Total Body Range of Motion work sample, which is used to evaluate functional abilities such as standing, bending, crouching, reaching, and gross manipulation and handling. (B) The Valpar 10 Tri-Level Measurement is used to evaluate a person's ability to follow a multistep sequence to inspect metal parts with various jigs and tools.

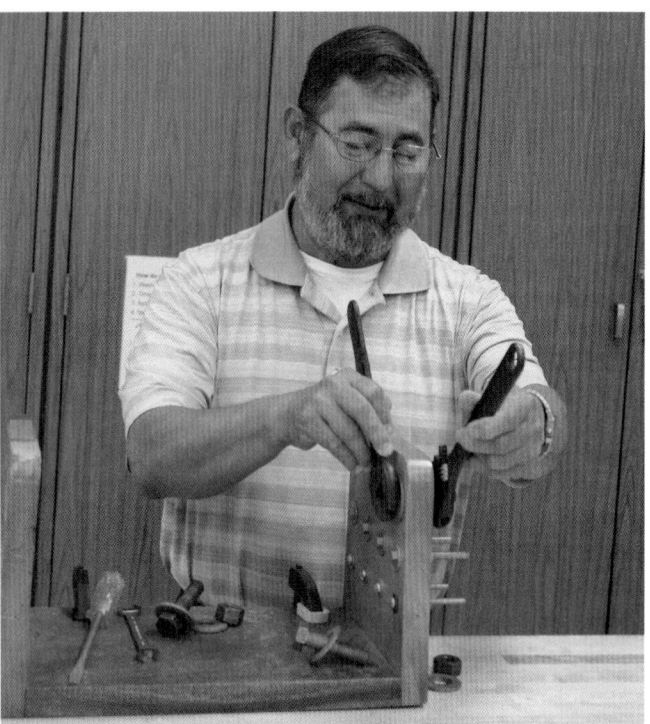

Fig. 14.4 The Bennett Hand Tool is a dexterity test to assess a person's ability to use hand tools.

situational assessments are also used to create real-life work situations that are related to actual work tasks that would be conducted on particular jobs.[42] For example, persons who are interested in working as floral arrangers could have their motor skills evaluated to see whether they have the coordination, energy, and strength and effort to grip and manipulate tools to cut the stems of flowers and plants and arrange them in floral containers. Individuals also can be evaluated in real worksites and perform actual job tasks that one would perform on the job.[42]

ETHICAL CONSIDERATIONS

The tasks need to take clients' safety into account and not jeopardize their health or put them at risk for injury by allowing them to perform in an unsafe manner or push beyond their maximum level of performance.[55]

There are generally two different types of vocational evaluation: a general vocational evaluation and a specific vocational evaluation. A general vocational evaluation is a comprehensive assessment to evaluate a person's potential to do any type of work. For an individuals who have never worked, do not have a job to return to, or cannot return to the previous job because of a disability, this type of evaluation is beneficial in determining their aptitudes, abilities, and interests to explore all reasonable options for work. For example, Henry, the roofer who experienced a traumatic brain injury from a fall while working, could benefit most from a general vocational evaluation to explore other options for employment. A general vocational evaluation could help identify other vocational interests and abilities by exploring a person's cognitive and motor skills and physical and

mental tolerances that could be applied to a different occupation. A specific vocational evaluation assesses a person's readiness to return to a particular occupation. For a person who has suffered a stroke and wants to return to work as a general office clerk, a specifically tailored vocational evaluation to assess the person's ability to return to this particular type of work can be done. Clerical work samples and specially designed situational assessments that gauge the person's ability to multitask, pay attention to detail, file, answer a telephone, and take messages can be incorporated as an integral component of the vocational evaluation.

JOB DEMANDS ANALYSIS

Assessing the physical demands of a job by JDA is often beneficial in the rehabilitation process inasmuch as recommendations for initiation or return to work require objective information about both the client's abilities and the job itself. Contextual assessment is an important part of evaluation of work-related demands that can include motor skills, process skills, and social interaction skills.[30] A well-written job description that includes the essential tasks of the job, physical requirements, cognitive aptitudes, educational requirements, equipment operated, and environmental exposure assists in selecting suitable candidates for employment, setting compensation packages, and making appropriate return-to-work decisions after an injury.[12,92]

A JDA should not be confused with ergonomic evaluations or identification and abatement of hazards. A job demands analysis seeks to define the actual demands of the job, whereas ergonomic evaluations and hazard assessment focus more on work practice and risk for injury secondary to postural or manual material-handling extremes or excesses.[8,12] Certainly these areas can overlap, but it is important to be clear about the differences and the reasons behind the request for information and to use suitable methods for each.[8,12]

Approaches to a JDA include questionnaires, interviews, observations, and formal measurement.[8,12] It is common to interview incumbents or supervisors about the job requirements.[75] Such an informal approach often leads to narrative descriptions with little functional information and questionable accuracy of demand estimates.[41,64,75] As with other types of assessment, it is important to have an objective process for analyzing the demands of the job and standardized evaluations help to provide objective information about the job demands.[90]

In the context of attempting to make return-to-work decisions based on matching the results of an FCE with the job description, many FCEs include a JDA component.[55] However, these are often subjective interviews with the client and can lack accuracy regarding the physical demands.

The occupational therapist who was working with Joe contacted the employer and conducted a JDA to obtain a complete picture of the job demands and requirements of the laundry attendant position. The occupational therapist spoke to the supervisor and to other employees while they were performing the actual job at the worksite. Being able to actually observe the job being done in the real work environment allowed the occupational therapist to gather the information needed to adequately assess Joe's ability to carry out the essential functions of this job.

A standardized classification system is crucial to ensure consistency in terminology and among professionals. The Dictionary of Occupational Titles (DOT) defines occupations in the United States, in addition to the physical demands of work (Tables 14.1 to 14.3).[96] It provides definitions of the overall level of work, strength demands, and frequency of the physical demands.[96,97] Many countries around the world use the DOT as their primary reference for generic occupational descriptions.

The DOT was last revised in 1991. In the early 1990s the U.S. government made the decision not to revise the DOT again; instead, it created a new format for classifying occupations.[29] The intent was to create a more generic classification system, or framework, for defining work. The American Institutes of Research (AIR) was awarded a contract for this purpose by the Utah Department of Employment Security, acting on behalf of the U.S. Department of Labor. AIR developed O*NET, an online, searchable database for information about occupations. Although the format includes an enormous amount of data, its definitions can make it difficult for rehabilitation professionals to use in a qualitative fashion.[72] O*NET is not intended to take the place of the DOT, but rather to provide a more structured approach for "career exploration."[72] It is recommended that both the DOT and O*NET be consulted when obtaining occupational information.[29]

In terms of recent legislation that has had an impact on employment law, both the ADA and the Equal Employment Opportunities Commission (EEOC) have defined **essential tasks** as being the reason that a job exists.[9,11,27] The ADA further defines essential tasks as those that are highly specialized (i.e., the reason the incumbent was hired to perform the job), and for which a limited number of people are available at the job site to perform the tasks.[9] During the course of a JDA, it is important to distinguish between tasks that are essential and those that are

---

TABLE 14.1 Definitions for Overall Level of Work

Level of Work	Definition
Sedentary	Exerting up to 10 lb of force occasionally or a negligible amount of force frequently to lift, carry, push, pull, or otherwise move objects, including the human body. Sedentary work involves sitting most of the time but may involve walking or standing for brief periods. Jobs are sedentary if walking and standing are required only occasionally but all other sedentary criteria are met.
Light	Exerting up to 20 lb of force occasionally, up to 10 lb of force frequently, or a negligible amount of force constantly to move objects. Physical demand requirements are in excess of those for sedentary work. Even though the weight lifted may be only a negligible amount, a job should be rated light work (1) when it requires a significant degree of walking or standing, (2) when it requires sitting most of the time but entails pushing or pulling arm or leg controls, or (3) when the job requires working at a production rate pace entailing constant pushing or pulling of material even though the weight of the material is negligible. NOTE: The constant stress and strain of maintaining a production rate pace, especially in an industrial setting, can be and is physically demanding on a worker even though the amount of force exerted is negligible.
Medium	Exerting 20–50 lb of force occasionally, 10–25 lb of force frequently, or greater than negligible and up to 10 lb of force constantly to move objects. Physical demand requirements are in excess of those for light work.
Heavy	Exerting 50–100 lb of force occasionally, 25–50 lb of force frequently, or 10–20 lb of force constantly to move objects. Physical demand requirements are in excess of those for medium work.
Very heavy	Exerting force in excess of 100 lb of force occasionally, in excess of 50 lb of force frequently, or in excess of 20 lb of force constantly to move objects. Physical demand requirements are in excess of those for heavy work.

Data compiled from the US Department of Labor, Employment and Training Administration: *Revised dictionary of occupational titles*, vols I and II, ed 4, Washington, DC, 1991, US Government Printing Office; and the US Department of Labor, Employment and Training Administration: *The revised handbook for analyzing jobs*, Indianapolis, IN, 1991, JIST Works.

TABLE 14.2 Definitions of Physical Demand Frequencies

Physical Demand Frequency	Definition
Never	Activity or condition does not exist
Occasionally	Up to 1/3 of the day
Frequently	1/3 to 2/3 of the day
Constantly	2/3 to full day

Data compiled from the US Department of Labor, Employment and Training Administration: *Revised dictionary of occupational titles*, vols I and II, ed 4, Washington, DC, 1991, US Government Printing Office; and US Department of Labor, Employment and Training Administration: *The revised handbook for analyzing jobs*, Indianapolis, IN, 1991, JIST Works.

TABLE 14.3 Strength Demands of Work

Strength Rating	Occasional (Up to 1/3 of the Day)	Frequent (1/3 to 2/3 of the Day)	Constant (Over 2/3 of the Day)
Sedentary	10 lb	Negligible	Negligible
Light	20 lb	10 lb	Negligible
Medium	20–50 lb	10–25 lb	10 lb
Heavy	50–100 lb	25–50 lb	10–20 lb
Very heavy	Over 100 lb	50–100 lb	20–50 lb

Data from the US Department of Labor, Employment and Training Administration: *Revised dictionary of occupational titles*, vols I and II, ed 4, Washington, DC, 1991, US Government Printing Office.

not. This can be challenging because it is a nontraditional way for both the employee and the employer to look at the job. It is important that both hiring and return-to-work decisions be based on job descriptions that define the essential tasks to be congruent with both the ADA and language.

OT PRACTICE NOTES

In preparation for an observational JDA, an interview can be conducted on the telephone to glean initial information about the job to allow adequate research on the job title and equipment. Advance preparation also aids in selecting the personal protective equipment that needs to be worn while performing the analysis.

Jobs are composed of the tasks that are performed, the physical demands that make up the tasks, and the frequency with which the physical demands are performed, including weights handled, forces exerted, and distances both ambulated and reached.[8,30] The frequency of each physical demand must be weighted appropriately for the given duration of each task because there is often a significant difference in the amount of time spent on each task during the workday. For example, the job of "loader" in ABC warehouse is composed of two tasks: (1) loading crates with boxes and (2) wrapping the crate with packing tape when loaded. The loader completes 48 cycles of loading and taping in an 8-hour shift, with loading the crate taking approximately 80% of the work shift. The boxes weigh 10 lb each. To correctly assess the overall level of work, the amount of weight lifted must be determined, in addition to the frequency of the manual materials handling.

Task 1 is composed of the physical demands of lifting, carrying, stooping, walking, reaching, handling, and standing. Task 2 is composed of walking, reaching, handling, fingering, and standing. To correctly sum the amount of the physical demands for the job of loader, one must determine how much time is spent on each physical demand within each task and then account for the proportion of the time that the task is performed during the workday. This type of assessment can be performed manually or through the use of various software protocols available in the marketplace.

Whatever methods are selected, clinicians should strive to provide an accurate picture of the job and its requirements, with an emphasis on functional demands, for easier application in the rehabilitation continuum.

ETHICAL CONSIDERATIONS

Whatever methods are selected, clinicians should strive to provide an accurate picture of the job and its requirements, with an emphasis on functional demands, for easier application in the rehabilitation continuum.

WORK HARDENING/WORK CONDITIONING

The idea of using work for rehabilitation is at the very core of occupational therapy. In the 1970s the idea of occupational rehabilitation developed from the necessity of improving strategies to control work-related injuries.[c] Work hardening was first illustrated conceptually by Leonard Matheson, a psychologist at Rancho Los Amigos, who worked very closely with Dempster, an occupational therapist, in developing his material.[46,52,71] The goal then, and remains, the rehabilitation of injured workers, maximization of their function, and returning them to work as quickly and safely as possible. The delivery system for this type of rehabilitation has evolved over time from a lengthy, hospital-based program, to structured interdisciplinary programs in outpatient settings, to the more progressive partnership between outpatient intervention and transitional work, in addition to rehabilitation occurring at the workplace in company-sponsored clinics. In the 1980s, CARF developed guidelines for work-hardening programs and offered certification for a fee through adherence to their guidelines and periodic surveys.[29,46,52,73] In 1991, a committee of the American Physical Therapy Association (APTA) developed another set of principles for clinics that wanted to follow recognized standards but did not desire to undertake the CARF accreditation process.[20,46,52]

Work hardening refers to formal, multidisciplinary programs for rehabilitating an injured worker.[1,22,50,54,71] The disciplines represented on the team can often include occupational and physical therapists and assistants, psychologists, vocational evaluators and counselors, licensed professional counselors, addiction counselors, exercise physiologists, and dieticians.[22,50,54] The programs typically range from 4 to 8 weeks and consist of an entry and exit evaluation (usually an FCE or a derivative thereof), a job site evaluation, graded activity, both work simulation and strength and cardiovascular conditioning, education, and individualized goal setting and program modification, with the goal of return to work at either full or modified duty.[22,50,54] Actual equipment from the job is preferred during the work simulation to maximize cooperation of the worker and more closely replicate the actual demands of the job.[46] Work conditioning is more often defined as physical conditioning alone, which covers strength, aerobic fitness, flexibility, coordination, and endurance and generally involves a single discipline.[1,22,46,48,50] Job simulation may also occur during work conditioning. Both approaches involve evaluation of the worker to establish a baseline from which to plan treatment and measure progress.

Motivational issues are a constant concern and are often thought to be at the forefront of unsuccessful return to work.[88] Maladaptive behavior regarding return to work can develop in an injured worker as a result of depression, financial issues, family pressures, and feelings of being manipulated by the "system."[88] This can lead to employer mistrust, interest in litigation, and a need to exaggerate symptoms. Fraud on the part of the injured worker is also an issue.[88] Employer indifference is a concern and can have a remarkable impact on a worker's attitude toward returning to the job.[88] Surveys of attitudes among employers have indicated that activity on the part of the

---

[c] References 20,46,50,53,54,73.

employer can affect costs; as many as 90% of respondents indicated that how well the employee perceived that he or she was treated at the time of the injury was associated with decreased costs as a result of the injury.[88]

OT PRACTICE NOTES

It is essential for the therapist to recommend that the employer be involved with the employee after the injury; the employer should be encouraged to investigate injury claims that are worthy of investigation, to call to inquire about how the employee is feeling, and to consider modified duty and transitional work options to promote a successful return to work.

Ensuring a positive outcome for the injured worker requires early intervention and a customized plan of treatment to address the various areas affected by the injury, including both physical and psychosocial.[88] Therapeutic use of self to establish rapport and build trust is a key component of how OT intervention is beneficial in caring for the injured worker.[93] Incorporation of a multidisciplinary team allows the patient to have the benefit of many areas of expertise working toward his or her common good. Intervening and initiating the rehabilitation program as soon as possible after the injury dramatically increase the chance for successful return to work. Based on a study of 5620 worker's compensation beneficiaries, there was a 47% return-to-work rate in workers referred to rehabilitation within the first 3 months after injury, with a cost savings of 71%. When referred during months 4 through 6, the rates dropped to 33% for return to work and 61% for cost savings. For those referred beyond 12 months after injury, only 18% returned to work and cost savings dropped to 51%.[88]

Outcome measurement, both for the individual and overall program success can be impactful in practice.[88] Documentation of Return to Work (RTW) and Stay at Work metrics for the individual are important for case resolution. Documentation of the same for the injured worker population is key in supporting the value of the treatment platform and refinement of care planning to develop more effective future outcomes.

Transitional work and modified duty programs involve a combination or a progression of acute rehabilitation and return to work at a level consistent with the individual's current ability, with the goal of returning to work at full duty or maximizing the individual's work capacity. An example of transitional duty would have a worker performing work-conditioning activities under supervision in an outpatient clinic from 8 to 10 a.m., going to the worksite and performing the less physically demanding portions of his job from 11 am to 1 pm, breaking for lunch, and then returning to the "lighter" duties of the job for the duration of the shift. More regular duty activities are added under supervision as the worker's skill and strength improve, with eventual return to full duty. This type of structure provides a much better environment for the worker to be involved in the work culture and allows co-workers and supervisors to participate in job modification and overall recovery of the injured worker.[88] Modified duty follows a similar path but typically does not include the clinical portion of the day. There are challenges to return to work at less

than full duty, however; some employers do not want workers to return to the site unless they are at "100%." It is imperative to demonstrate the benefit to the company and the employee, both economically and psychologically, of early transitional return to the long-term success of returning the employee to the workforce.

Work rehabilitation programs will continue to evolve as the tides of economy, industry needs, and legislation change. Occupational therapists play a key role in directing the changes that lie ahead.

FITNESS FOR DUTY TESTING

A frequent use of functional testing includes assessing a person's ability to meet certain physical requirements before being hired for a job; hence the term "fitness for duty."[76] Some pre-employment testing may consist of isometric strength testing, ROM testing, or actual measurement of a person's ability to perform selected tasks from the job description. These types of testing may be known by a variety of names: Post Offer Employment Testing (POET), Post Offer Screening (POS), Pre Employment Testing (PET), Post Offer Physical (POP), and Essential Function Testing (EFT), among others. This type of testing can be an integral part of a company's comprehensive injury prevention and management strategy.[76]

OT PRACTICE NOTES

Occupational therapists are excellent candidates for assisting companies with expansion of plans to more effectively manage employee injuries because of their task analysis training and holistic approach.

When a company is looking at the overall impact of an employee injury bottom line, it goes much further than simply the cost associated with the injury itself. It extends beyond the medical costs to include the employee's compensation, benefit package payments, training of replacement personnel, replacement personnel wages, and overtime payment for existing personnel if they are needed for coverage. This does not include the indirect costs of diminished productivity during the period when coverage is being arranged. The total impact can be quite staggering. The cost of developing an employment screening process is significant; however, the cost savings to the company can be dramatic.[76]

The EEOC's *Uniform Guidelines on Employee Selection Procedures* sets forth guidelines for the structure and function of human resource departments within companies and businesses. The guidelines also address how an organization can select and manage employees and places strong emphasis on the necessity of policies and procedures being job related.[27,76] The EEOC also mandates that an employer's selection process not have an adverse impact on any group of people and must not discriminate on the basis of race, color, religion, gender, or national origin, as established by Title VII of the Civil Rights Act of 1964.[27,76] Meeting these criteria requires that the selection procedures demonstrate validation, be of business necessity, and be a bona fide occupational requirement.[27,76]

To be compliant with the ADA, pre-employment screening must be based on an accurate job description, test only the essential functions (although not every function need be assessed), and have high face validity, often referred to as content validity (i.e., it tests what the examiner really wants to know), or closely mirror the aspects of the job for which the person is being tested.[9,76] Dynamic testing (actually replicating physical tasks from the job) is recommended; it can be conducted onsite at the company or off-site, and it needs to use equipment from the job as it is available.[76] It is vital that companies take the time to thoroughly develop their screening process to be able to defend why the screening was considered necessary, maintain awareness and vigilance in the development phase of good test design, and be prepared to explain and demonstrate the applicability of the screening to the job in question.[76]

Pre-employment testing can also occur at several points in the hiring process; however, many healthcare providers and legal experts recommend conducting such testing after an offer of employment has been extended.[37,57] With post-offer screening (POS), the most advantageous progression is to interview the applicant and determine whether the person is an acceptable candidate for employment.[76] A conditional offer is extended to the applicant based on the applicant's ability to meet a variety of conditions, such as passing a drug screen, acceptable background check, and physical testing. A problem with pre-offer testing is that Title 29 of the Code of Federal Regulations specifically states that medical examination is permissible "after making an offer of employment to a job applicant."[17] Monitoring blood pressure or the heart rate or inquiring about medical history is considered to be part of a medical examination and is precluded in pre-offer testing.[76]

Anything that a therapist does in the way of evaluating an applicant might be deemed medical simply because an occupational therapist is a medical professional. It is also important to look critically at any testing that is considered to be general strength testing because it has been found to be a poor predictor of potential for injury.[24,67,76] Normative databases also are of little use in making hiring decisions because, according to both the ADA and the EEOC, it does not matter whether the applicant falls into the 5th percentile or the 95th percentile; the only thing of importance is whether the applicant can perform the tasks of the job.[9,27]

If the applicant passes the screening, he or she is hired and begins working. If the applicant does not pass, the employer must assess whether the applicant has a disability as defined under the ADA (see Chapter 15).[9] If the applicant does, the employer must determine whether reasonable accommodation can be offered to the applicant so that the individual may be able to perform the job. Reasonable accommodation means providing accommodation in such a way that the employer is not placed under undue financial strain for the accommodation to be implemented. If the company can and does offer accommodation to the applicant, the hiring process is completed and the employment begins. If the company cannot offer reasonable accommodation or if the applicant does not have a disability yet fails the screening, the employer can choose to rescind the offer of employment, examine opportunities for alternative placement elsewhere in the company, or offer remediation of some type and allow the applicant to retest if certain criteria are met.[76] For example, if a nondisabled applicant does not pass the lifting portion of a POS and otherwise meets the employment criteria, the company might elect to allow the applicant 2 weeks to improve strength with the goal of returning for a retest screen in an attempt to pass the lifting portion.

Suppose Henry (the roofer in the case study) had difficulty balancing on one leg as a result of an early childhood accident but that this balance problem was not something that was readily apparent. If a POS had been conducted on Henry before he was hired at the roofing company, and balance was a component of testing for working as a roofer, his difficulty could have been detected and Henry could have been denied the job or offered alternative placement. Either way Henry would have been protected from a fall that would radically change his life.

A company does not have to test applicants for every job. Typically, it is suggested that a company survey all of its injuries and determine where the majority of injuries are occurring and if they are occurring within the first 6 months of hiring. If so, this company is a good candidate for implementing a physical screen as part of the hiring process. Once it has been determined which jobs are going to be selected for testing, the physical demands of the job must be evaluated. This can be done by survey, questionnaire, or observation (either direct or video).[11] The job description must include information that is functional in terms of physical demands, describe the essential tasks of the job, and be presented in such language that one can test for an individual's ability to perform them.[11] In the case of a company requesting that existing job descriptions be used for development of the screen, it is extremely important to document that the company provided the job descriptions and that the therapist does not assume any liability for errors in their accuracy.

Physical demand items can then be selected for testing during screening based on either the difficulty or the frequency of the item. It is not necessary to test all of the physical demands for each job. For instance, a job might include carrying 10 lb a distance of 10 feet twice a day and lifting 40 lb from pallet height to waist height 200 times per day. Testing the ability to lift 40 lb would be a better selection for testing because if the applicant is able to lift 40 lb from pallet height to waist height, it is likely that he or she will also be able to carry 10 lb a distance of 10 feet. It is important to select a method of testing the tasks that is reliable and valid and demonstrates job applicability, whether choosing from a standardized battery of physical demand tests or developing job-specific tasks to improve the applicant's understanding of the relevance of the task and defensibility of hiring decisions.[27,76]

After tasks have been selected, implementation can begin. It is suggested that a statistically significant sample of incumbents be tested to ensure that the correct demands have been selected and that the minimum requirements for each demand have been set appropriately. Once pilot testing has been completed, the screening can be administered consistently to all applicants for a given job. It is also recommended that the screening process be monitored to ensure that fair and nondiscriminatory selection of applicants is occurring and that modifications in the screening process can occur as needed.[76]

ETHICAL CONSIDERATIONS

It is imperative for the clinician to encourage companies to have written policies regarding the screening process, including how to handle screening failures.[76] It is also important to extricate the therapist from the hiring process in that all communications come from the employer, so the therapist is allowed to maintain objectivity and third-party distance from the course of action.[76] Continuing documentation and follow-up help establish a definitive paper trail demonstrating the business necessity for implementing a pre-employment screening process, the steps taken to select and analyze the job and tasks to be tested, the implementation phase, ongoing quality assurance to monitor any changes in the job and reflect subsequent changes in the screening and the actions taken to handle screening failures, reasonable accommodation, and avoidance of adverse impact.[76]

WORKSITE EVALUATIONS

Worksite evaluations are on-the-job assessments to determine whether an individual can return to work after the onset of a disability or whether a person can benefit from reasonable accommodations to maintain employment.[50,92] For example, a person who worked at a manufacturing company as a machine operator has a stroke, and the employer is willing to take this person back as long as the physical and cognitive demands of the job can be met. An occupational therapist can go to the worksite to evaluate the person's ability to safely and adequately operate the machinery and carry out the essential functions of the job. Consider another example. A person who previously worked as an office clerk without any difficulty is now experiencing extreme fatigue, pain, and muscle weakness with repetitive tasks as a result of post-polio syndrome. This person could benefit from a worksite evaluation to identify reasonable accommodations to allow continued working at this job while minimizing the employee's symptoms. Several factors are assessed at the worksite with the worker present: the essential functions of the job, the functional assets and limitations of the worker, and the physical environment of the workplace.[58]

A worksite evaluation is usually conducted after a job analysis has been done. Larger companies may already have information on job analyses done on specific jobs. If a job analysis has not been done, the occupational therapist can conduct a job analysis if the employer is willing, or a job description could be obtained from the employer before going out to the worksite. If there is no written job description, a phone call to the supervisor/manager of the worker should be made to obtain verbal information regarding the essential functions of the job and the physical and cognitive requirements for the job. After this information has been obtained, the occupational therapist schedules a time with the employer and the worker to meet at the worksite. This is exactly what happened with Joe as he prepared to switch from the job of janitor to laundry attendant at the hotel and spa. After the occupational therapist conducted the job analysis, Joe met with both the occupational therapist and the employer at the worksite for the worksite evaluation.

When the occupational therapist meets the employer and worker at the worksite, the occupational therapist assesses the work, the worker, and the workplace.[52] The evaluation begins with an analysis of the essential functions that may require

accommodation.[92] The occupational therapist should have an idea of what these functions are, based on the information obtained, before going to the worksite. The desired outcome of the work tasks should be emphasized, not just the process of performing the essential function.[92] The occupational therapist should find out certain details, such as how the outcome will be affected if a particular task is done incorrectly, in a different sequence, or omitted; whether there are quotas, standards, or time constraints that must be met[77]; and whether the frequency with which a task is done will affect the outcome.

Activity analysis is a useful tool for evaluating a person at the worksite.[16] It can be used to address all areas, including motor, sensory, cognitive, perceptual, emotional and behavioral, cultural, and social. When assessing a person's ability to carry out the essential functions of the job, the occupational therapist has expertise in breaking down the tasks and determining the parts of the task with which the worker is having difficulty or may have difficulty over the course of a workday. The occupational therapist can suggest accommodations to allow the worker to carry out the essential functions of the job.

The final step in the worksite evaluation is to assess the work environment. The environment outside the immediate work area should be evaluated (parking if driving or access to public transportation; access into the building, break room, and restroom), as well as the workstation itself. All work areas that the worker may use need to be investigated to identify obstacles and solutions to increase accessibility. The location and placement of machines, supplies, and equipment that the worker needs to access should be assessed, as well as other environmental factors such as lighting, temperature, and noise level.

Taking photographs or video recordings at the worksite can be very useful; however, permission must be obtained from both the employer and the worker to do so. The occupational therapist should also bring a tape measure to measure the height of work surfaces, width of doorways, and other factors, depending on the person's needs. Drawing a layout of the work area to scale on graph paper is also very helpful, especially when the worker is in a wheelchair. Critical measurements can be recorded on the diagram.

The outcome of the worksite evaluation is to determine whether the person can safely and adequately carry out the essential functions of the job with or without any reasonable accommodations. Ergonomic principles (addressed in the following section) should be considered and applied when recommending reasonable accommodations. The process of identifying reasonable accommodations requires cooperation between the person with the disability, the employer, and the occupational therapist.[77] Each person has valuable insights and information to contribute to the process of identifying the best accommodations. The Job Accommodation Network (JAN) is a service provided by the Office of Disability Employment Policy (ODEP), an agency of the U.S. Department of Labor, and is the best resource for assisting employers and disabled workers in making reasonable accommodations (http://askjan.org).[84] JAN's website points out that most job accommodations are not usually expensive. According to JAN, more than half of all accommodations cost nothing. JAN offers one-on-one guidance on workplace accommodations, the ADA, and self-employment options for people with disabilities. JAN consultants can be contacted both over the phone and online. JAN's toll-free number is (800) 526-7234.

The occupational therapist analyzes the need for modification of the equipment that the worker is using or modification of the workplace to help the person perform with greater efficiency, effectiveness, and safety.[1]

After the worksite evaluation has been completed, a report is prepared and sent to the qualified employee, the referring party, and the employer. The problem areas that relate to the essential job functions should be listed clearly, in addition to the accommodations necessary to solve them. If training is necessary to use a recommended accommodation, sources for the training should be identified. If commercially available equipment is recommended, exact model numbers, local sources, and approximate expenses should be provided.[94] If custom equipment needs to be fabricated, sources, cost estimates, and the amount of time required to fabricate the equipment also should be included. The report should summarize the findings of the evaluation and the accommodations that were recommended.

After Joe's worksite evaluation, it was determined that he could safely and dependably carry out the essential functions of the job from his wheelchair. Just one accommodation was recommended and implemented. Because it gets very hot in the laundry room and Joe is sensitive to the heat, the employer agreed to purchase additional fans to ventilate the room better, and to allow the door to the laundry room to be propped open. The employer agreed to schedule Joe's shift in the evening or early morning, when it was cooler, so that he would not have to work in the heat of the day.

The occupational therapy practitioner thus evaluates the worker, the work, the workplace, and the relationship among them. Therapeutic intervention is used when deficits in performance are found. The occupational therapist can modify the way that the worker performs the work or modify the work environment to allow the worker to perform optimally.

ERGONOMICS

For full engagement in the occupation of work, the demands of the job and the environment must fit with the employee's physical, mental, and psychosocial makeup. Any mismatch between the demands of the job, the context, or individual client factors will interfere with performance and could lead to poor worker productivity, stress, or injury.

Occupational therapists use the science of **ergonomics** to assist clients in the occupation of work. The goal of ergonomics is to improve the health, safety, and efficiency of both the worker and the workplace.[68] The term *ergonomics* is derived from the Greek words *ergos*, meaning "work," and *nomos*, meaning "laws"—hence the laws of work.[23] The Polish educator and scientist Wojciech Jastrzebowski (1799–1882) introduced the term *ergonomics* in the literature about 150 years ago.[22] However, the concept of ergonomics—that there is some connection between physical well-being and the type of work performed—is as old as humanity itself: "From the very first tools of the Stone Age, humans have tried to find better ways of

working, taking advantage of human talents and making up for human shortcomings."[60]

Often, work settings and processes are designed to satisfy space and budget limitations as well as the demands of productivity and aesthetics. When these designs fail to take into account the people who will be using the work settings and procedures, injury and inefficiency can result. Matching individual employees' abilities with the context and activity demands of a job can significantly improve workplace productivity as well as worker safety and morale.[47]

The principles of ergonomics help address a variety of work-related concerns. Common issues include work-related injury or stress, the disabled and aging workforces, tool and equipment design, architectural design, and accessibility. **Primary prevention** is when an ergonomic intervention is applied proactively, preventing problems before they occur. **Secondary prevention** emphasizes identification and intervention in the early, reversible stages of injury. **Tertiary prevention** occurs after a worker suffers nonreversible injury, illness, or disease. Many occupational therapists use ergonomic principles as part of their comprehensive rehabilitation or wellness client-centered programs. Some occupational therapists choose to specialize and become professional ergonomists.

With regard to ergonomic services, the occupational therapist's client base may include the individual worker, workers in the context of employee groups, and/or the employer itself. The ideal environment for ergonomic services is at the client's place of work. Occupational therapists providing ergonomic services must become skilled in navigating what can be an unfamiliar business world with its unique lingo, social norms, and culture. Occupational therapists providing ergonomic services share a similar focus with occupational therapists in all areas of practice, that is, a focus on marketing and sale of the product (wellness), cost-effectiveness, definable outcomes, and client satisfaction.

Occupational therapists are not the only professionals suited to specialize in the field of ergonomics. It is not unusual to see ergonomists who have been academically trained in industrial hygiene, engineering, safety, business administration, human resources, medicine, physical/occupational rehabilitation, psychology, architecture, epidemiology, or computer science.[21] Ergonomic equipment sales representatives commonly perform ergonomic assessments at the time that they deliver or install equipment. For the occupational therapist, the road to becoming a professional ergonomist can take many paths. Table 14.4 outlines a variety of methods for acquiring advanced knowledge and certification in the field of ergonomics.

The holistic nature of their training provides a unique advantage for occupational therapists working in the field of ergonomics. The occupational therapist understands the complexity of achieving a perfect fit between individual workers, their jobs, job contexts, and social parameters.

Looking at worker performance by the interactions of all aspects of the domain of occupational therapy is known as **system theory**. Rannell Dahl, MS, OTR, explains that the "components of work systems are workers, job tasks, tools and equipment, work environments, and organizational structure, and the interactions among these components."[21] Dahl offers an excellent schematic of this concept of the ergonomics work system (Fig. 14.5).

TABLE 14.4 Education and Training Opportunities in Ergonomics

Name	Type	Certification or Certificate
1. Board of Certification in Professional Ergonomics (BCPE) International Ergonomics Association Endorsement based on ISO/IEC 17024 standard for certifying bodies (http://www.bcpe.org)	National Board Certification	CPE: Certified Professional Ergonomist AEP: Associate Ergonomics Professional
2. Oxford Research Institute (ORI) (https://www.oxfordresearch.org/)	National Board Certification	CIE: Certified Industrial Ergonomist CAE: Certified Associate Ergonomist
3. Worksite International, Inc. (https://www.worksiteinternational.com)	Private Business Certificate	COESp: Certified Office Ergonomics Specialist (using the Worksite International System of Ergonomic Evaluations) CASp: Certified Chair Assessment Specialist
4. Matheson's Ergonomic Evaluation Certification Program (http://www.roymatheson.com)	Private Business Certificate	CEES: Certified Ergonomic Evaluation Specialist
5. The Back School of Atlanta (http://www.backschoolofatlanta.com)	Private Business Certificate	CEAS I, II, III: Certified Ergonomic Assessment Specialist
6. OCCUPRO (https://www.occupro.net)	Private Business Certificate	COEE: Certified Office Ergonomic Evaluator
7. Humanscale (https://www.humanscale.com/)	Private Business Certificate	COEE-Certified Office Ergonomics Evaluator

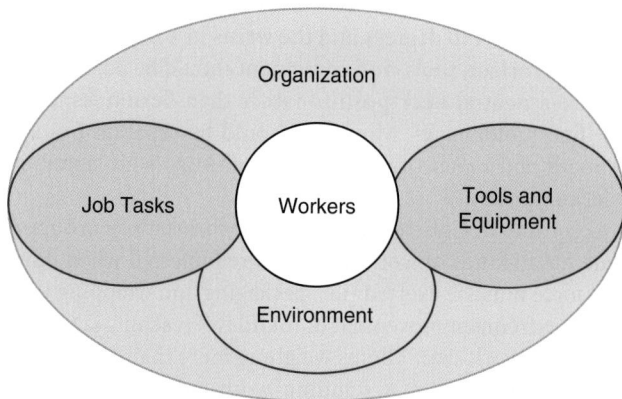

Fig. 14.5 Dahl's ergonomics work system. (From Dahl R: Ergonomics. In Kornblau B, Jacobs K, editors: Work: principles and practice, Bethesda, MD, 2000, American Occupational Therapy Association.)

In his groundbreaking text *Conceptual Aspects of Human Factors*, David Meister explained that in [ergonomics], the system concept is the belief that human performance in work can be meaningfully conceptualized only in terms of organized wholes. He emphasized the fundamental Gestalt ideas that "the whole is more than the sum of its parts, that the parts cannot be understood if isolated from the whole, and that the parts are dynamically interrelated or interdependent."[62] Occupational therapists understand that one can conceive of worker performance only in terms of the interaction among performance skills, performance patterns, context, activity demands, and client factors (Box 14.2). The *Occupational Therapy Practice Framework: Domain and Process* (supports this concept: "Engagement in occupation as the focus of occupational therapy intervention involves addressing both subjective (emotional and psychological [skills and abilities]) and objective (physically observable) aspects of performance. Occupational therapy practitioners understand engagement from this holistic perspective and

BOX 14.2 Anthropometry

Anthropometry is the study of people in terms of their physical dimensions. It includes the measurement of human body characteristics such as size, breadth, girth, and distance between anatomical points. It also includes segment masses, centers of gravity of body segments, and ranges of motion, which are used for biomechanical analysis of work and postures. Standard anthropometric tables are available to assist designers of work areas, work surfaces, chairs, and equipment. The tables outline the average dimensions of adult men and women in the 5th, 50th, and 95th percentiles of the population. Ideally, designs should "fit" a wide range of persons between the 5th percentile (smallest people) and the 95th percentile (largest people). Retail merchandise labeled "ergonomic" is based on these anthropometric dimensions. In practice, however, few designs meet the needs of such a wide range of people, which explains why expensive equipment labeled "ergonomic" does not always produce the desired results. Professional ergonomic intervention seeks to create a better "fit" for the individual user as demonstrated in the sketch below showing measurement ratios relevant to the occupation being performed by the individual rather than specific measurements used by a wide range of individuals of average dimensions.

An example of ergonomic chair design offering adjustable features that can be adapted to the individual is presented in Fig. 14.8.

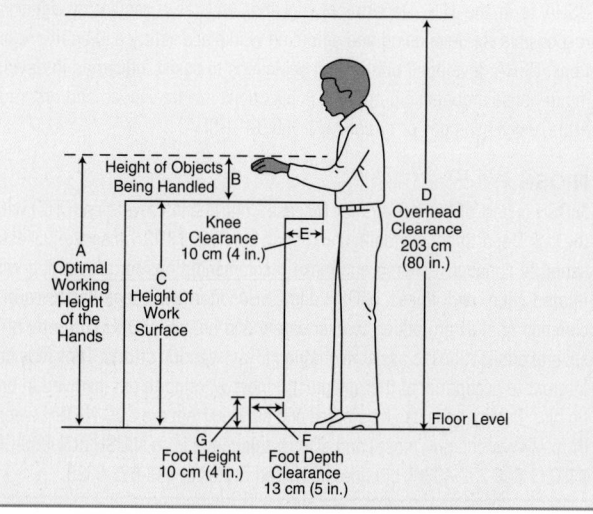

Image reproduced with permission from Eastman Kodak Company. Adapted from Alf Nachemson, 1975.

address all aspects of performance when providing interventions" (OTPF-3 p. 628).[5]

The system theory supports the importance of independent aspects of the domain of occupational therapy. The quality of the work system can suffer if there are deficiencies or deviations in performance skills, performance patterns, context, activity demands, or individual client factors. Dahl explains that each component of the ergonomics work system (see Fig. 14.5) "has its own set of characteristics that affect the performance of the work system"[21] as a whole. The ergonomic practitioner modifies and strengthens certain aspects of the system with the goal of enhancing the overall quality of the work system interactions (i.e., improving the fit between the worker and his or her job).

Ergonomic Design Principles

Although it is beyond the scope of this chapter to review the complete array of ergonomic design considerations, the following is a discussion of selected ergonomic design principles. Many resources are available for occupational therapists interested in learning more about the science of ergonomics. The authors of this chapter direct you to the references listed at the end of the chapter. Additionally, readers may be interested in the ergonomics information available through OSHA (https://www.osha.gov) and National Institute for Occupational Safety and Health (NIOSH) (http://www.cdc.gov/niosh/) (Box 14.3).

When discussing ergonomic design it is important to understand that it is the relationship between the worker and work equipment, tools, or processes that needs to be addressed, not any specific characteristic on either side. This can be confusing to an employer who orders expensive ergonomic tools and equipment for workers and is disappointed when the workers continue to suffer work-related injuries and illnesses. A tool or piece of equipment is never in itself ergonomic; rather, it is the fit between a particular piece of equipment, tool, or process and the intended user of that equipment, tool, or process that creates a proper ergonomic solution.[47] For Susan, there were several factors affecting her comfort in the temporary work environment; she was using equipment that did not fit her size, and she was working in the basement of her in-law's home. Also contributing was the fact that her husband lost his job and they had to leave their home, moving in with her in-laws.

Workstations

There are three major types of workstations: seated, standing, and combination sit/stand. The type of task being performed dictates the best choice. Seated workstations are best for fine motor assembly, writing, and computer tasks when all required items can be supplied and handled within comfortable arm's reach in the seated workspace.[18] Items handled at a seated workstation should not require hands to work more than 6 inches (15 cm) above the workspace, and the items handled should not weigh more than 10 lb (4.5 kg).[18] For this reason, the height of the work surface should be above elbow height for precision work. For computer keyboard and mouse operation, the ideal height of the desk is at or just below elbow height, placing elbow flexion at 90 to 110 degrees and the wrists in a neutral position. The work surface, tools, and equipment should be positioned to produce a neutral neck posture rather than flexion, especially with fine motor tasks. Monitors should be separate from the keyboard and mouse, rather than attached as with laptop and tablet computers.

According to Cohen et al., standing workstations are appropriate for all kinds of work tasks but are preferred when downward force must be exerted (i.e., packaging and wrapping tasks) and when frequent movement or multilevel reaching is required around the work area.[18] Items weighing more than 10 lb (4.5 kg) should be handled at a standing workstation. Work surface heights for heavy work should be 4 to 6 inches (10–15 cm) below elbow height. For computer workstations, the desktop height should be a little higher, positioning the elbows in 90 to 110 degrees of flexion and wrists in a neutral position. As with a seated workstation, the work surface, tools, and equipment should be positioned to produce a neutral neck posture.

The combination sit/stand workstation is best for jobs consisting of multiple tasks, some that are best done sitting and some that are best done standing,[23] or to allow for postural changes throughout the day. For computer operators who perform light duty tasks from a seated position, having the option to stand and change their posture is essential to the maintenance of a healthy work environment. Equipment and tools should be adjustable to account for subtle postural changes that occur when transitioning between seated and standing positions. Fig. 14.6 shows the recommended dimensions for both a seated and a standing workstation.

Seating

If seating is required, the design of the chair is of utmost importance for worker comfort and safety. Poor seating leads to poor working posture. The result can be fatigue, musculoskeletal

---

BOX 14.3 OSHA and NIOSH

The Occupational Safety and Health Act of 1970 created both the National Institute for Occupational Safety and Health (NIOSH) and the Occupational Safety and Health Administration (OSHA). Although NIOSH and OSHA were created by the same act of Congress, they are two distinct agencies with separate responsibilities.

OSHA

OSHA is in the U.S. Department of Labor and, as a regulatory agency, is responsible for developing and enforcing workplace safety and health regulations. OSHA developed publication guidelines to assist industries in developing in-house ergonomic programs. Publications can be viewed and ordered at http://www.osha.gov or by calling 1-800-321-OSHA.

NIOSH

NIOSH is part of the Centers for Disease Control and Prevention (CDC) within the U.S. Department of Health and Human Services. NIOSH is an agency established to conduct research and make recommendations for preventing work-related injury and illness. NIOSH and OSHA often work together toward the common goal of protecting worker safety and health. NIOSH currently offers several publications to assist in ergonomic intervention efforts. They may be of interest to occupational therapy practitioners wanting to get involved in ergonomics. Publications can be viewed and ordered from the CDC-NIOSH website (http://www.cdc.gov/niosh) and also by telephone from NIOSH at 1-800-CDC-INFO (1-800-232-4636); outside the United States at 513-533-8328.

Seated work

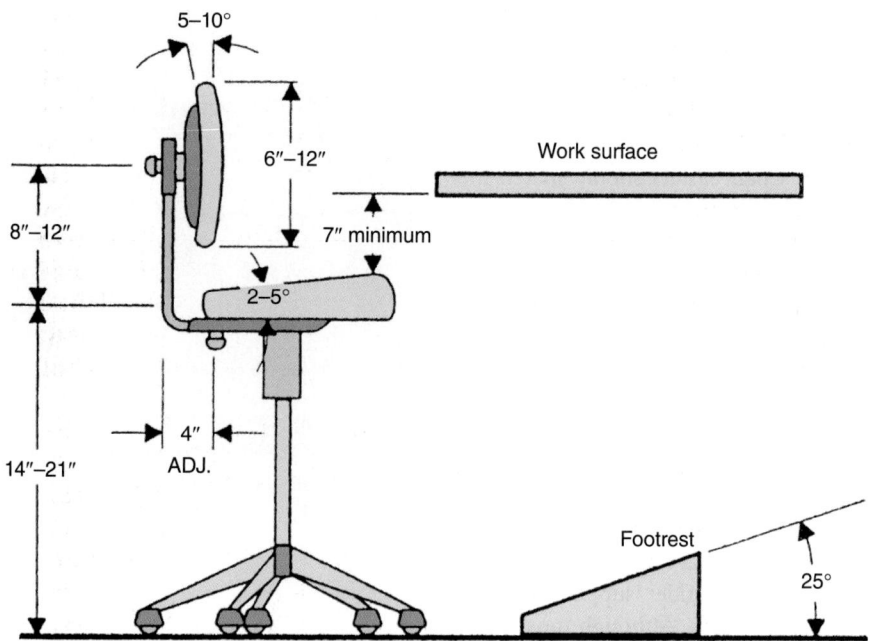

Optimal work surface height varies with work performed:
Precision work = 31–37 inches
Reading/writing = 28–31 inches
Typing/light assembly = 21–28 inches
Seat and back rest heights should be adjustable as noted in chair requirements

A

Standing work

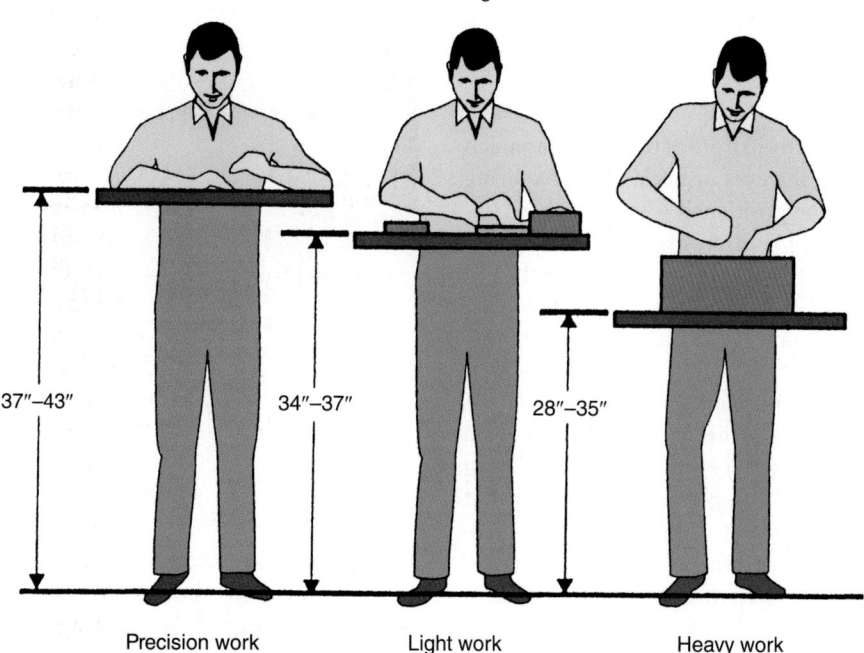

Precision work   Light work   Heavy work

Workbench heights should be:
Above elbow height for precision work
Just below elbow height for light work
4–6 inches below elbow height for heavy work

B

Fig. 14.6 Recommended dimensions of workstations. (A) Seated work. (B) Standing work. (From Cohen AL, Gjessing CC, Fine LJ, et al: Elements of ergonomics programs: a primer based on workplace evaluations of musculoskeletal disorders, Washington, DC, 1997, US Government Printing Office.)

injury, back injury, and/or poor work performance. Although chair preference is highly variable, there are some basic characteristics to consider. Chairs should be easily adjustable for seat height, armrest and backrest position, and seat pan depth and tilt adjustment. Appropriate lumbar support is important. Seats upholstered in woven fabric are cooler and more comfortable in warmer work environments.[25] Chair casters should match the flooring (i.e., hard floor versus carpet casters). A seat pan that is too deep or a chair that is too high will press into the back of the leg and compromise lower extremity circulation. Sitting in a chair without foot support will also cause pressure on the back of the legs. When the worker is at a seated workstation, both feet should be supported on the floor or a footrest (Fig. 14.7). Choosing a seat pan with a front-edge "waterfall" design will also decrease pressure on the back of the legs. Seats that are too high or too deep can put stress on the lower back. Armrests are an area of controversy but should generally be provided when the work task requires the arms to be held away from the body.[44] It can be challenging to find a chair that offers armrests positioned optimally for forearm and shoulder support, without applying pressure on bony prominences. Although most ergonomic chairs have armrests, they tend to be positioned poorly for upper extremity support. For fully adjustable armrests, highe-end chair manufacturers such as Bodybilt (https://bodybilt.com/), Steelcase (https://www.steelcase.com/), RFM Seating (http://rfmseating.com/), and Herman Miller (https://www.hermanmiller.com/) offer adjustable armrests with options. Fig. 14.8 illustrates the recommended chair characteristics for generalized seated workstations. Fig. 14.9 illustrates a seated position for computer users.

Visual Factors

Tasks should be located as directly in front of the worker as much as possible without straining the eyes or neck. Tasks requiring close-range viewing should be positioned 6 to 10 inches (15–25 cm) above the work surface, and if possible at an angle to reduce the need to bend the neck over the work. Minimum and maximum viewing distances depend on the size of the object being viewed and any prescription eyewear the worker is using. Workers can be encouraged to speak with their eye doctors to optimize their eye-wear for specific work tasks.

Inadequate lighting can lead to headaches, blurry vision, eyestrain, burning, itchy, and watery or dry eyes. Lighting should be adequate for the worker to perform the job task, but not so bright that it causes discomfort. Three basic lighting factors need to be considered for performance of work: quantity, contrast, and glare. General work environment illumination is typically provided by sunlight and light fixtures. The color and finish of the workstation walls and equipment, as well as the arrangement of the lighting sources, should all be designed to avoid reflective glare on the job task (Fig. 14.10).[69] Monitor(s) should be positioned perpendicular to the light source if natural light is available, or parallel to the light source for overhead florescent lighting. If overhead lighting is too bright, the use of light diffusers is helpful. Other options include removing one light bulb from the overhead light fixture, or using desktop task lighting instead of overhead lighting.[69]

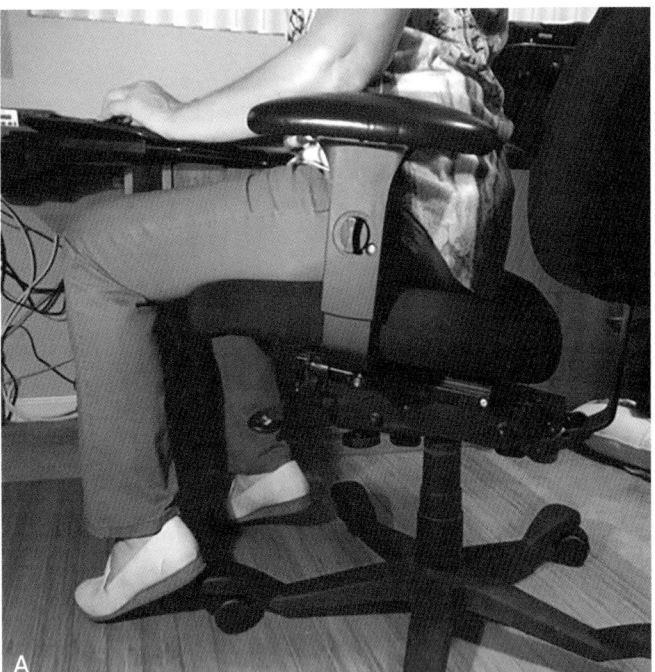

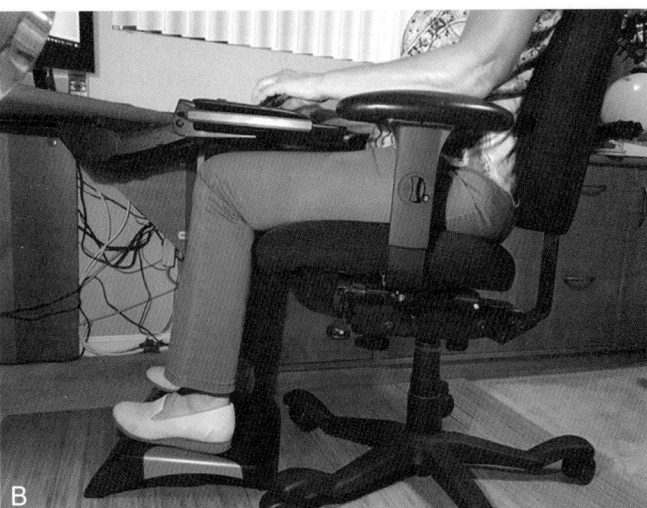

Fig. 14.7 (A) Before: chair is too high. No lower extremity, back or arm support. Pressure on the back of the thighs. (B) After: footrest in place. Sitting back in the chair with lower extremities, back and arms supported. Pressure relieved from the back of the thighs.

Tools

Tools should be designed to protect the worker from hand vibration, extreme temperatures, and soft tissue compression. "A properly designed tool handle should isolate the hand from contact with the tool surface, enhance tool control and stability, and serve to increase the mechanical advantage while reducing the amount of required exertion."[18] The length of the tool handle must be designed to avoid unnecessary pressure on the palm of the hand. Handles of scissors and pliers should be spring-loaded to avoid trauma to the back and sides of the hands.

Tool design should minimize muscular effort and awkward posturing of the upper extremity. Whenever possible, opt for battery operated or electric power tools to minimize the physical

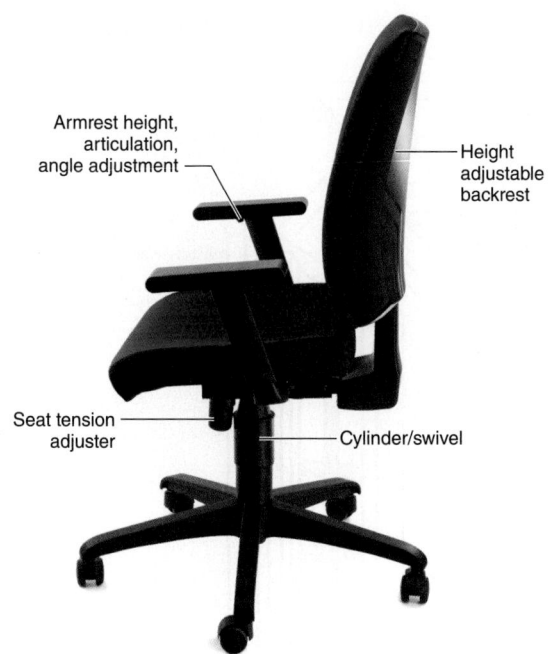

Fig. 14.8 Recommended chair characteristics: height-adjustable backrest, lumbar support, backrest depth adjustment, seat height, seat rotation and height cylinder, seat tilt (seat depth adjustment not shown), armrest width, seat tilt tension, armrest height and arm pad adjustability. (From iStock.com/shutterman99. ID: 625524830.)

effort required. Choose tool shapes that allow the wrist to stay neutral and the elbow to stay flexed and close to the body during use. The shape of the tool will depend on the job task and work surface (Fig. 14.11). Suspension systems and counterweights should be designed for use with heavy hand tools.

Whole-body vibration can cause back pain and performance problems when the workstation vibrates, as in the case of long-distance truck drivers and in production industries using high-powered drills or saws in the work area.[14] Hand-arm vibration has been linked to vascular compromise, peripheral nerve damage, muscular fatigue, bone cysts, and central nervous system disturbances.[35] The effects of hand tool vibration should be minimized as much as possible. Use antivibration tools at low speeds when available. Ensure that tool handles and gloves fit the workers' hands. Train workers to grip tool handles as lightly as possible and allow the tool to do all the work instead of the worker adding force behind the tool. Encourage frequent rest breaks and educate workers that smoking increases the risk for vibration-related hand problems.[21,35]

Materials Handling

Back injury is a common occurrence for jobs requiring materials handling, including lifting, pushing, pulling, bending, and twisting. The heavier the material, the more risk for injury. Back

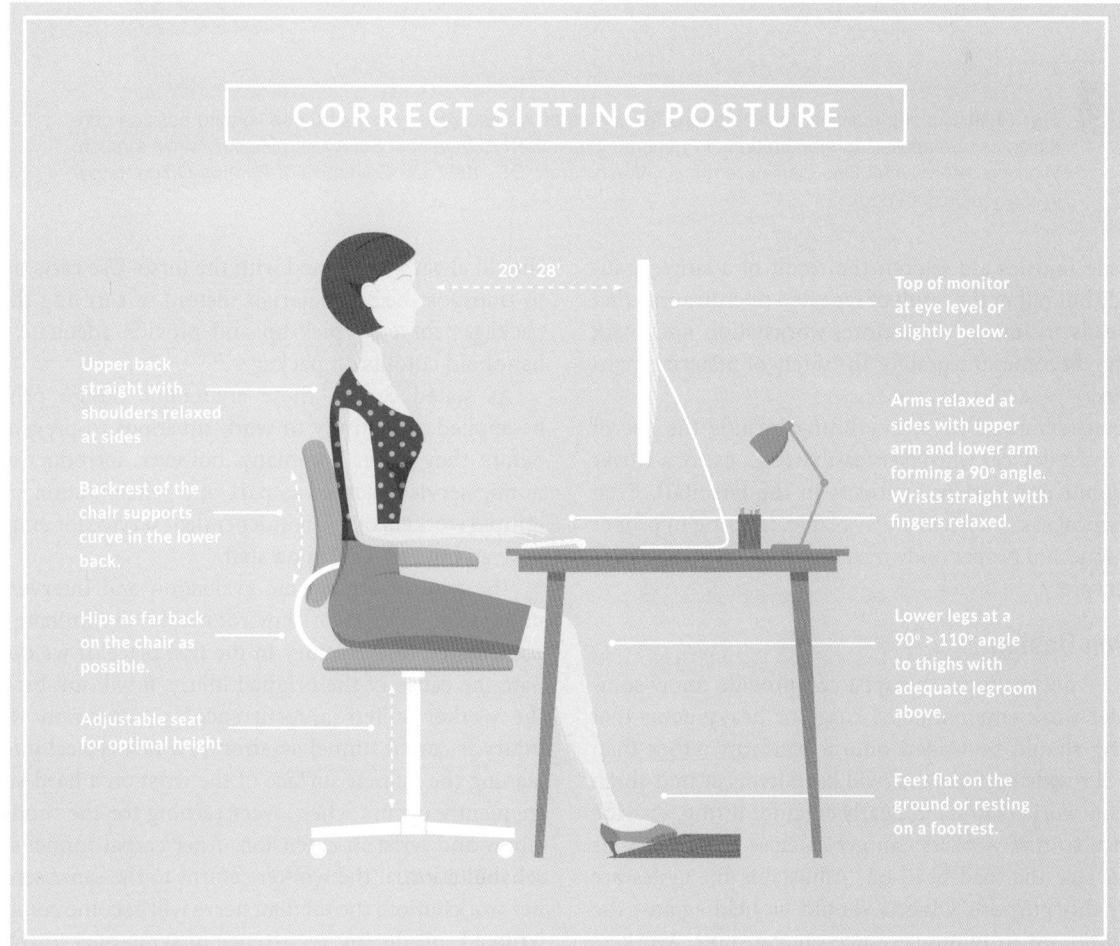

Fig. 14.9 Correct seating position for ergonomic computer workstation. (iStock.com/wetcake.).

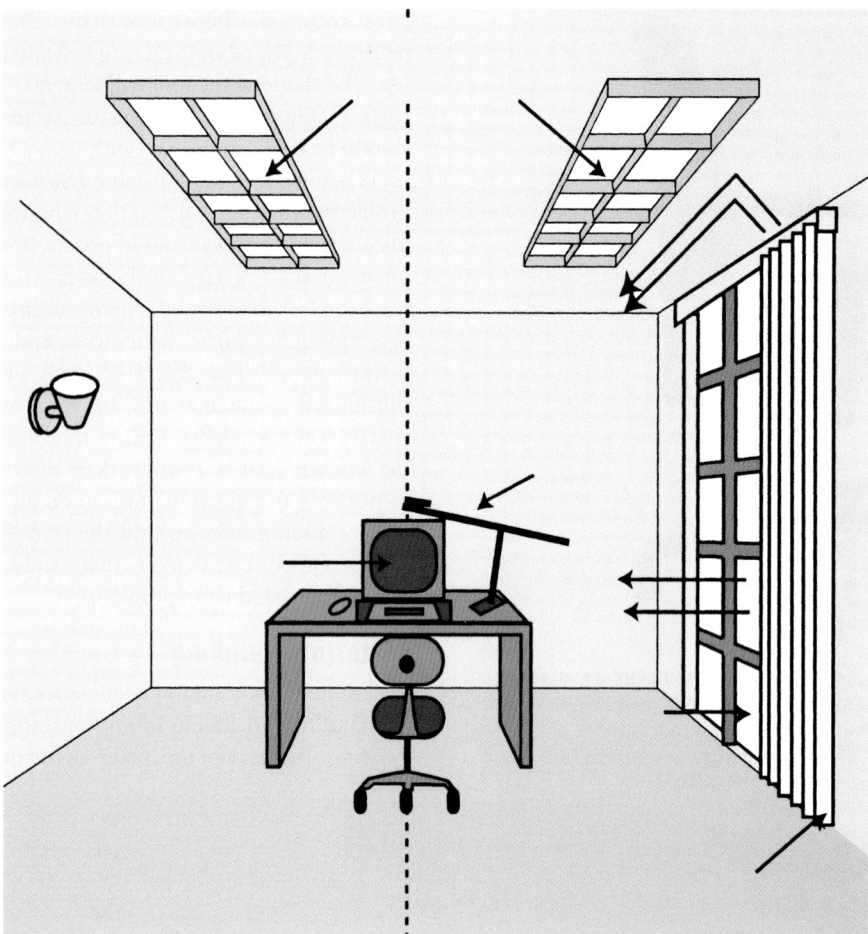

Fig. 14.10 Lighting position considerations for computer workstations. Most of these lighting position principles can be applied to workstations in general. (From the Occupational Safety and Health Administration: Working safely with video display terminals, Washington, DC, 1997, US Government Printing Office. http://www.google.com/books.)

and soft tissue injuries are seldom the result of a single traumatic episode but rather the result of repeated microtrauma that ultimately leads to injury.[39] Therefore, workstation and work process design becomes integral for the safety of materials handling workers.

Design considerations for heavy lifting include the use of mechanical assist devices whenever feasible (e.g., use of a Hoyer lift for immobile and bariatric patients in the hospital). Even when mechanical assist devices are available, training in proper lifting technique and proper body mechanics is essential to promote worker safety.

Workstation Design

The perceptive occupational therapist can provide many solutions for safer work environments. Large or heavy items that require lifting should be loaded onto a platform rather than on the floor. Provide surfaces that will keep items at mid-thigh height to allow workers to stand nearly erect for lifting. Provide foot clearance so that workers can get as close to the item as possible and face the load head-on. Adjustable lift tables are excellent for this purpose. Objects should be held against the torso during the lift to minimize force on the spine. Workers should never twist their torsos to lift or place an object and feet

should always be aligned with the torso. Use carts or conveyors to transport heavy materials instead of carrying them. Orient packages for easy pick-up and provide adequate handles or handhold cutouts on packages.[21]

As stated earlier, these ergonomic design principles can be applied proactively to work situations to prevent problems before they arise. For many, however, introduction to ergonomic services comes as part of a rehabilitation program for injured workers or as an independent service for employers who have an injured worker on staff.

The goal of ergonomic evaluation and intervention in an injured employee's work environment is to eliminate factors that contributed to the injury in the first place. If we do not eliminate the cause of the original injury, it will not be long before the worker suffers a recurrence.[47] A common work-related injury is carpal tunnel syndrome, which typically results from leaning the palmar surface of the wrist on a hard surface. This frequently occurs when over-reaching for the mouse with the elbow and wrist in extension. After carpal tunnel surgery and rehabilitation, if the worker returns to the same setup of his or her workstation, the median nerve will become compressed and irritated, producing recurrence of symptoms to the area. It is essential that the workstation is adjusted so that the employee

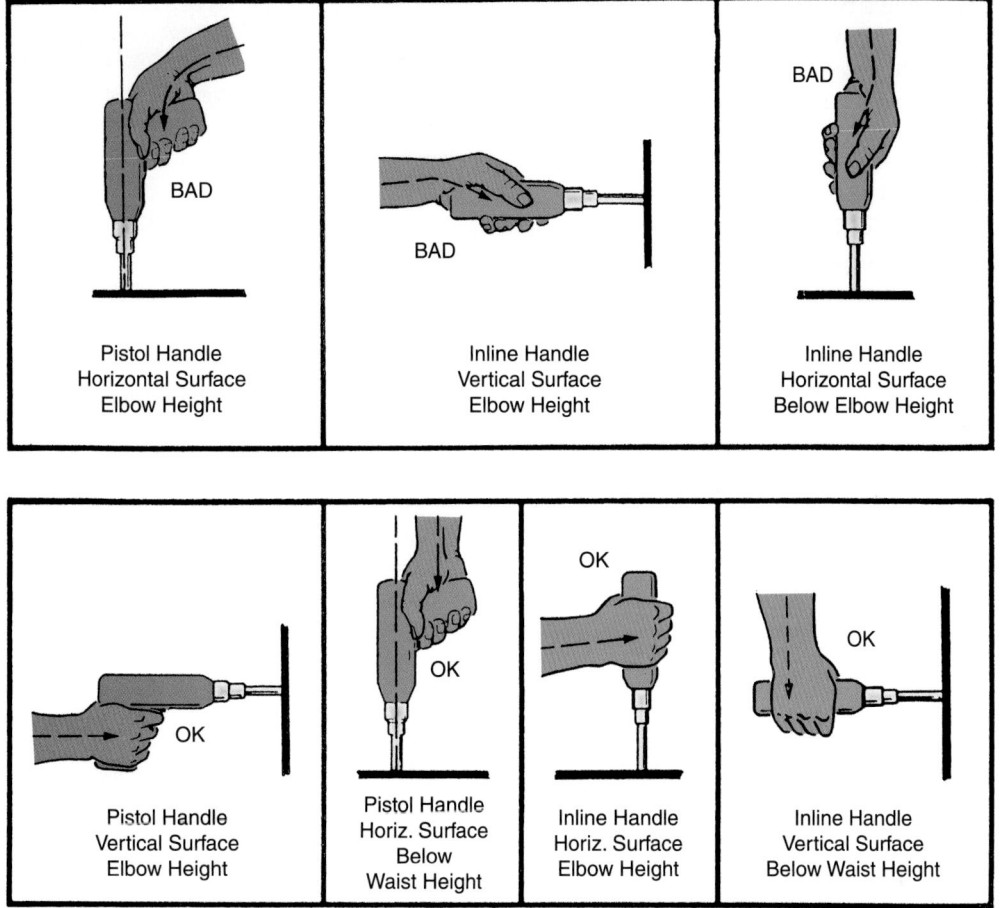

Fig. 14.11 Hand tool design and wrist posture. (From Armstrong T: An ergonomic guide to carpal tunnel syndrome, Akron, OH, 1983, American Industrial Hygiene Association.)

can obtain distributed support through the forearm on an appropriate armrest, to relieve any pressure on the volar surface of the wrist (Fig. 14.12).

Ergonomic Evaluation

The ergonomic evaluation is an important assessment and intervention tool when used as part of a comprehensive rehabilitation or injury prevention program. This tool can be used along the entire continuum of prevention services. Ergonomic evaluation can be performed during workstation and work methods planning to assist in efforts to prevent worker injury. Ergonomic evaluation also can be performed for workers in whom symptoms of a work-related musculoskeletal disorder (WMSD) develop and for workers who come to therapy for rehabilitation and are ready to return to work, the goal being to prevent reinjury. Finally, an ergonomic assessment can be useful in modifying a job in preparation for a disabled worker's return to work with the goal of preventing further injury related to the disability.

The ergonomic evaluation should begin with the occupational therapist scheduling a time to meet with both the worker(s) to be assessed and the direct supervisor of the work area. The evaluation should be scheduled during the normal work hours of the worker(s). The goal is to obtain the best understanding of

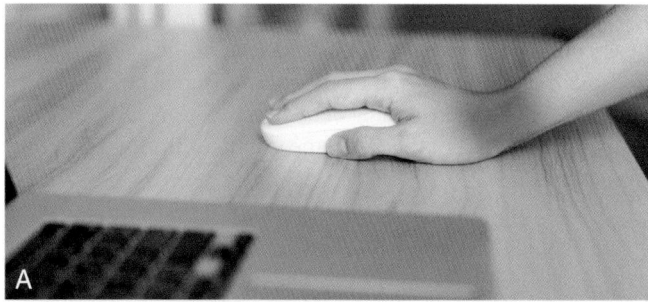

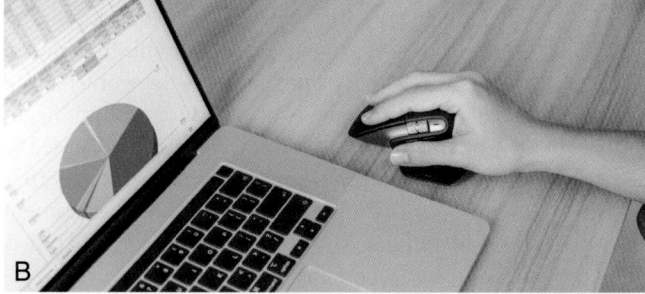

Fig. 14.12 Carpal tunnel risk factors (A), leaning weight of arm on the mouse rest, platform too low. Not using armrest of the chair. Carpal tunnel risk factor remediated (B). Using the armrest of the chair to support upper arm, elevated mouse platform to bring forearm and wrist to neutral position. (From iStock.com/Panuwat Dangsungnoen. ID: 1438845702 and 1438845704.)

what actually occurs during a typical work shift, so the conditions should be closely approximated. It is extremely important that the actual worker(s) be present. The purpose of the evaluation is to look at the fit between the specific worker(s) and the specific job methods, equipment, and context. If any element is missing, the evaluation is of little or even no value.[47]

Ideally, the occupational therapist evaluator will arrive at the worksite and meet first with the direct supervisor of the work area to be evaluated. The supervisor will be asked to give an overview of the circumstances leading up to the request for ergonomic evaluation. The occupational therapist will want to know what kinds of injuries are occurring in the work area(s), when the problem started, and how many employees have been affected. The supervisor will be able to review how the organization has handled the problem to date. Frequently, the supervisor will also describe what sorts of psychosocial and environmental influences may be affecting the situation. This brief encounter with the supervisor will give an observant occupational therapist evaluator a good feel for the organization's management culture and organizational priorities.

After the supervisor interview, the occupational therapist evaluator will want to see the work area and meet the employees. The supervisor may give the evaluator a brief tour of the work area and describe the job tasks and methods that occur there, and describe any areas that he or she believes is contributing to worker injury. This part of the evaluation will give the evaluator an understanding of how management views the situation. Next, the evaluator will meet with the workers.

Once alone with the worker(s) it is important to establish a level of trust. The evaluator will explain to the workers(s) why the organization has asked for an ergonomic evaluation. It should be explained that the purpose of the evaluation is to make the job safer and more comfortable for them. The worker(s) should be encouraged to give the evaluator a tour of the work area and to explain their job tasks. If there are any discrepancies between management's understanding of the job situation and the workers' understanding of the same, the evaluator must seek definitive clarification.

Finally, the worker(s) should be observed performing the job as normally as possible. The evaluator will explain that he or she will be watching and perhaps videotaping, taking photographs, or taking notes. The evaluator should assure the worker(s) that the information that is being recorded will be used to develop strategies to make the job tasks safer and more comfortable to perform. The evaluator must stress that he or she wants the workers(s) to do the job just like any other day. The evaluator will not begin analysis of the work methods until several minutes has elapsed to allow the workers time to fall into a more normal work pattern.

The ergonomic workstation and work methods assessment should focus on identifying known risk factors for MSD. It is often very useful to videotape the work area and work methods performed (Box 14.4). Recording the worker(s) performing their job tasks will allow the evaluator to return to one's office to further analyze the data. If the evaluator plans to photograph or videotape any work areas or methods, signed permission should be obtained from the company and the worker before going to the site or conducting the evaluation.

BOX 14.4 Protocol for Videotaping Jobs for Ergonomic Evaluation

The following is a guide for preparing a videotape and related task information to facilitate job analysis and assessment of risk factors for **work-related musculoskeletal disorders**.

Materials Needed
- Video software through electronic device
- Clipboard, pens, paper, blank checklists
- Stopwatch, strain gauge (optional) for weighing objects

Videotaping Procedures
1. To verify the accuracy of the video camera to record in real time, videotape a worker or job with a stopwatch running in the field of view for at least 1 minute. Playback of the tape should correspond to the elapsed time on the stopwatch.
2. Announce the name of the job on the voice channel of the video camera before taping any job. Restrict running time comments to the facts. Make no editorial comments.
3. Tape each job long enough to observe all aspects of the task. Tape 5 to 10 minutes for all jobs, including at least 10 complete cycles. Fewer cycles may be needed if all aspects of the job are recorded at least 3 to 4 times.
4. Hold the camera still with a tripod if available. Do not walk unless absolutely necessary.
5. Begin taping each task with a whole-body shot of the worker. Include the seat/chair and the surface that the worker is standing on. Hold this shot for 2 to 3 cycles and then zoom in on the hands/arms or other body parts that may be under stress because of the job task.
6. It is best to tape several workers to determine whether workers of varying body size adopt different postures or are affected in other ways. If possible, try to tape the best- and worst-case situations in terms of worker fit to the job. The following suspected upper body problems suggest focusing on the parts indicated:
   - Wrist problems/complaints
   - Hands/wrists/forearms
   - Elbow problems/complaints
   - Arms/elbows
   - Shoulder problems/complaints
   - Arms/shoulders

   For back and lower limb problems, the focus would be on movements of the trunk of the body and the leg, knee, and foot areas under stress as a result of task loads or other requirements.
7. Tape from whatever angles are needed to capture the body part(s) under stress.
8. Briefly tape the jobs performed before and after the one under actual study to see how the targeted job fits into the total department process.
9. For each taped task, obtain the following information to the maximum extent possible:
   - Whether the task is continuous or sporadic
   - Whether the worker performs the work for the entire shift or whether there is rotation with other workers
   - Measures of work surface heights and chair heights and whether adjustable
   - Weight, size, and shape of handles and textures for tools in use; indications of vibration in power tool use
   - Use of hand wear
   - Weight of objects lifted, pushed, pulled, or carried
   - Nature of the environment in which the work is performed (too cold or too hot?)

From Cohen AL, Gjessing CC, Fine LJ, et al: *Elements of ergonomics programs: a primer based on workplace evaluations of musculoskeletal disorders*, Washington, DC, 1997, US Government Printing Office.

It is helpful to develop a prescreening questionnaire and an ergonomic checklist to assist with expediting the performance of the onsite evaluation. The checklist should include the most common ergonomic risk factors and be tailored to the specific needs and conditions of the workplace that the occupational therapist intends to evaluate. Fig. 14.13 is an example of a typical ergonomic risk factor identification checklist. Fig. 14.14 is an example of a checklist for computer workstation evaluation. Fig. 14.15 is a typical hand tool risk factor checklist.

Risk factors to look for include the following:

1. *Forceful exertions:* Heavy lifting, pushing, pulling, twisting, gripping, or pinching.
2. *Repetition:* Performing the same motion or series of motions continually or frequently for an extended period.
3. *Awkward or static posturing:* Positions that place stress on the body such as reaching, kneeling, squatting, leaning over a surface, using tools or a keyboard with the wrists bent, twisting the torso or the neck.
4. *Contact stress:* Pressing or leaning the body part against hard or sharp surfaces.
5. *Vibration:* For example, from power tools or sitting in a truck cab all day while driving.
6. *Temperature:* Working in cold temperatures or handling cold tools or products. Temperatures that are too warm lead to fatigue and poor productivity.

Once the workstation and work methods risk factors have been identified and the worker(s) have had a chance to familiarize themselves with the occupational therapist, focus should turn to the psychosocial aspects of the job. Frequently, these factors will surface during the evaluation process without any prompting whatsoever. Factors such as workload and productivity stressors, quality of the relationship between the worker(s) and other co-workers and the supervisor, genuine job task enjoyment, and overall health and fitness cannot be overlooked. Work-related musculoskeletal injury is never the result of any one factor; rather, it is the accumulation of a variety of risk factors and situations that ultimately result in injury. Occupational therapists evaluate the entire occupational profile to determine what components are contributing to the system as a whole.

Finally, it is important to ask the workers for their perspective on problem areas or risk factors in their work area. If their perspective matches what has been identified in the ergonomic evaluation of the work area and work methods, the workers should be encouraged to share their ideas for correcting the problem. Although the occupational therapist is the expert in workstation and work methods analysis, the onsite workers know their job best. The workers have likely spent hours formulating and discussing how they would change things if ever given the chance. Make sure to ask them. Often, one will find a wealth of knowledge and many useful ideas for reducing or eliminating risk factors. It is, however, the occupational therapist's ultimate responsibility to ensure that the changes implemented will serve to reduce and prevent injury. If possible, it is important to consult with union representatives, human resources and the safety department for a well-rounded perspective on the workplace culture.

Following the onsite evaluation, the occupational therapist returns to the office to analyze the data and prepare a report. The report will be shared with whoever requested the ergonomic evaluation. (Always check before sharing the results with the worker because an employer may have budget constraints or other plans.) The report should contain an introduction explaining the background and purpose of the ergonomic evaluation, a description of the actual work area, risk factors, and work methods assessment. Most importantly, the report should include the evaluator's findings with comprehensive directives to implement the recommendations, as well as resources for purchasing any equipment or services. Job tasks found to contain several risk factors for the development of work-related musculoskeletal disorder (WSMD) have the greatest risk for injury and should be prioritized by the company. Recommendations will focus on ways to eliminate or reduce risk factors.

New Trends in Ergonomics
Open Office Design

Before the onset of the COVID-19 pandemic one of the newest trends in office ergonomics was the shift from cubicles to open office designs. High-tech companies, especially, were removing walls and eliminating organized seating arrangements, with the intention of promoting informal collaboration among workers. Many of these offices provided adjustable workstations and adjustable equipment, making it easier to obtain safe (for the time) and comfortable work postures for the staff, including those who job share or multiple shift workers. The open space allows for more light, more air flow, and illusion of fewer restrictions. However, obstacles include noisy environments where workers may wear headphones to help focus their attention, and glare from various lighting options. In open environments, it is very difficult for workers to personalize their space. They are often limited to a single surface prohibiting the display of personal items. Tethers of wires can restrict movement when the desk height is adjustable, making it more difficult to alternate between sitting and standing positions. Some offices have general seating and standing workstations where workers select a temporary station for the day, much like a coffee shop or library. At the end of the shift, worker clear the desk where they were working and places their belongings into a locker. With generalized open design concepts, there is no personalization of workstation equipment (chairs or desks). Here, the occupational therapist is more likely to provide emotional or psychological support for the stress of not having a "home-base" at work, rather than the physical equipment itself. Small things that make workers feel comfortable and reduce stress, have a great impact on their quality of work life. Being able to post photographs of a child or a favorite pet, or use a favorite coffee mug, can contribute to positive feelings and reduce stress. Restrictions in the ability to personalize a workspace can inadvertently contribute to worker injury or illness (Fig. 14.16). It will be interesting to see how the "open office design" fares long term once the pandemic is over.

General Ergonomic Risk Analysis Checklist

Check the box if your answer is "yes" to the question. A "yes" response indicates that an ergonomic risk factor that requires further analysis may be present.

Manual Material Handling
❏   Is there lifting of loads, tools, or parts?
❏   Is there lowering of loads, tools, or parts?
❏   Is there overhead reaching for loads, tools, or parts?
❏   Is there bending at the waist to handle loads, tools, or parts?
❏   Is there twisting at the waist to handle loads, tools, or parts?

Physical Energy Demands
❏   Do tools and parts weigh more than 10 lbs?
❏   Is reaching greater than 20 inches?
❏   Is bending, stooping, or squatting a primary task activity?
❏   Is lifting or lowering loads a primary task activity?
❏   Is walking or carrying loads a primary task activity?
❏   Is stair or ladder climbing with loads a primary task activity?
❏   Is pushing or pulling loads a primary task activity?
❏   Is reaching overhead a primary task activity?
❏   Do any of the above tasks require five or more complete work cycles to be done within a minute?
❏   Do workers complain that rest breaks and fatigue allowances are insufficient?

Other Musculoskeletal Demands
❏   Do manual jobs require frequent, repetitive motions?
❏   Do work postures require frequent bending of the neck, shoulder, elbow, wrist, or finger joints?
❏   For seated work, do reaches for tools and materials exceed 15 inches from the worker's position?
❏   Is the worker unable to change his or her position often?
❏   Does the work involve forceful, quick, or sudden motions?
❏   Does the work involve shock or rapid buildup of forces?
❏   Is finger-pinch gripping used?
❏   Do job postures involve sustained muscle contraction of any limb?

Computer Workstation
❏   Do operators use computer workstations for more than 4 hours a day?
❏   Are there complaints of discomfort from those working at these stations?
❏   Is the chair or desk nonadjustable?
❏   Is the display monitor, keyboard, or document holder nonadjustable?
❏   Does lighting cause glare or make the monitor screen hard to read?
❏   Is the room temperature too hot or too cold?
❏   Is there irritating vibration or noise?

Environment
❏   Is the temperature too hot or too cold?
❏   Are the worker's hands exposed to temperatures less than 70° F?
❏   Is the workplace poorly lit?
❏   Is there glare?
❏   Is there excessive noise that is annoying, distracting, or producing hearing loss?
❏   Is there upper extremity or whole body vibration?
❏   Is air circulation too high or too low?

General Workplace
❏   Are walkways uneven, slippery, or obstructed?
❏   Is housekeeping poor?
❏   Is there inadequate clearance or accessibility for performing tasks?
❏   Are stairs cluttered or lacking railings?
❏   Is proper footwear worn?

Tools
❏   Is the handle too small or too large?
❏   Does the handle shape cause the operator to bend the wrist in order to use the tool?
❏   Is the tool hard to access?
❏   Does the tool weigh more than 9 pounds?
❏   Does the tool vibrate excessively?
❏   Does the tool cause excessive kickback to the operator?
❏   Does the tool become too hot or too cold?

Gloves
❏   Do the gloves require the worker to use more force when performing job tasks?
❏   Do the gloves provide inadequate protection?
❏   Do the gloves present a hazard of catch points on the tool or in the workplace?

Administration
❏   Is there little worker control over the work process?
❏   Is the task highly repetitive and monotonous?
❏   Does the job involve critical tasks with high accountability and little or no tolerance for error?
❏   Are work hours and breaks poorly organized?

Fig. 14.13 General ergonomic risk analysis checklist. (From Cohen AL, Gjessing CC, Fine LJ, et al: Elements of ergonomics programs: a primer based on workplace evaluations of musculoskeletal disorders, Washington, DC, 1997, US Government Printing Office.)

Risk Analysis Checklist for Computer-User Workstations

"No" responses indicate potential problem areas which should receive further investigation.

1. Does the workstation ensure proper worker posture, such as

   - horizontal thighs? ☐ Yes ☐ No
   - vertical lower legs? ☐ Yes ☐ No
   - feet flat on floor or footrest? ☐ Yes ☐ No
   - neutral wrists? ☐ Yes ☐ No

2. Does the chair

   - adjust easily? ☐ Yes ☐ No
   - have a padded seat with a rounded front? ☐ Yes ☐ No
   - have an adjustable backrest? ☐ Yes ☐ No
   - provide lumbar support? ☐ Yes ☐ No
   - have casters? ☐ Yes ☐ No

3. Are the height and tilt of the work surface on which the keyboard is located adjustable? ☐ Yes ☐ No

4. Is the keyboard detachable? ☐ Yes ☐ No

5. Do keying actions require minimal force? ☐ Yes ☐ No

6. Is there an adjustable document holder? ☐ Yes ☐ No

7. Are arm rests provided where needed? ☐ Yes ☐ No

8. Are glare and reflections avoided? ☐ Yes ☐ No

9. Does the monitor have brightness and contrast controls? ☐ Yes ☐ No

10. Do the operators judge the distance between eyes and work to be satisfactory for their viewing needs? ☐ Yes ☐ No

11. Is there sufficient space for knees and feet? ☐ Yes ☐ No

12. Can the workstation be used for either right- or left-handed activity? ☐ Yes ☐ No

13. Are adequate rest breaks provided for task demands? ☐ Yes ☐ No

14. Are high stroke rates avoided by

    - job rotation? ☐ Yes ☐ No
    - self-pacing? ☐ Yes ☐ No
    - adjusting the job to the skill of the worker? ☐ Yes ☐ No

15. Are employees trained in

    - proper postures? ☐ Yes ☐ No
    - proper work methods? ☐ Yes ☐ No
    - when and how to adjust their workstations? ☐ Yes ☐ No
    - how to seek assistance for their concerns? ☐ Yes ☐ No

Fig. 14.14 Risk analysis checklist for computer workstations. (From Cohen AL, Gjessing CC, Fine LJ, et al: Elements of ergonomics programs: a primer based on workplace evaluations of musculoskeletal disorders, Washington, DC, 1997, US Government Printing Office.)

Handtool Risk Factor Checklist

"No" responses indicate potential problem areas which should receive further investigation.

1. Are tools selected to limit or minimize

   - exposure to excessive vibration? ☐ Yes ☐ No
   - use of excessive force? ☐ Yes ☐ No
   - bending or twisting the wrist? ☐ Yes ☐ No
   - finger pinch grip? ☐ Yes ☐ No
   - problems associated with trigger finger? ☐ Yes ☐ No

2. Are tools powered where necessary and feasible? ☐ Yes ☐ No

3. Are tools evenly balanced? ☐ Yes ☐ No

4. Are heavy tools suspended or counterbalanced in ways to facilitate use? ☐ Yes ☐ No

5. Does the tool allow adequate visibility of the work? ☐ Yes ☐ No

6. Does the tool grip/handle prevent slipping during use? ☐ Yes ☐ No

7. Are tools equipped with handles of textured, non-conductive material? ☐ Yes ☐ No

8. Are different handle sizes available to fit a wide range of hand sizes? ☐ Yes ☐ No

9. Is the tool handle designed not to dig in the palm of the hand? ☐ Yes ☐ No

10. Can the tool be used safely with gloves? ☐ Yes ☐ No

11. Can the tool be used by either hand? ☐ Yes ☐ No

12. Is there a preventive maintenance program to keep tools operating as designed? ☐ Yes ☐ No

13. Have employees been trained

   - in the proper use of tools? ☐ Yes ☐ No
   - when and how to report problems with tools? ☐ Yes ☐ No
   - in proper tool maintenance? ☐ Yes ☐ No

Fig. 14.15 Hand tool risk factor checklist. (From Cohen AL, Gjessing CC, Fine LJ, et al: Elements of ergonomics programs: a primer based on workplace evaluations of musculoskeletal disorders, Washington, DC, 1997, US Government Printing Office.)

Working From Home

Before the year 2020, working from home (WFH) was an evolving concept, with many employees working distributed hours between home and the office. With the onset of the COVID-19 global pandemic, WFH quickly became the new world standard.[32] Advances in technology catapulted workers from almost every industry into WFH. Some companies provided equipment for their staff to establish an office space at home, some provided stipends for the workers to purchase equipment, and some expected workers to find their own accommodations.

Remote assessments offer the occupational therapist a unique opportunity to view both the client's home and work environment simultaneously. Awkward postures and the blurring of work/life balance create a new set of ergonomic challenges in

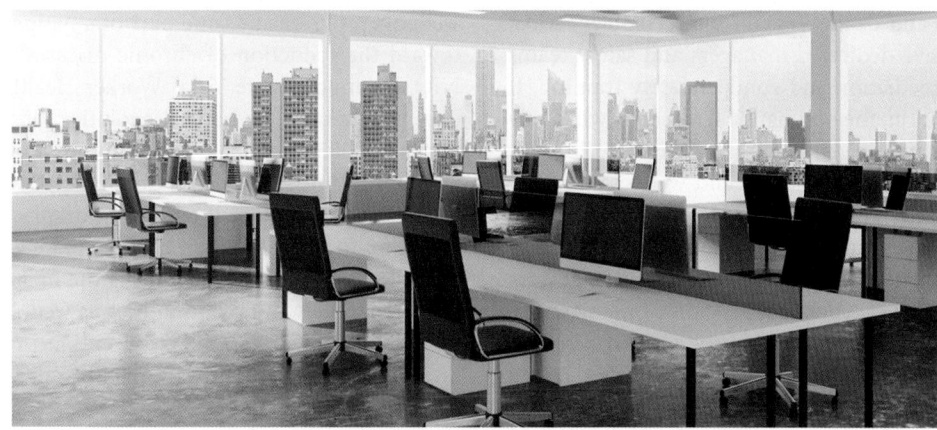

Fig. 14.16 Open office space. (iStock.com/imaginima. ID: 1127657173.)

which occupational therapists can intervene. Many people WFH are using temporary equipment that does not provide adequate support or adjustability. By directing the worker to locate items within their home to provide postural support, the occupational therapist empowers the worker to make the necessary changes to prevent injury or further discomfort.

There are many opportunities for the ergonomist providing services for WFH. Clients may have limited space and find themselves working with makeshift offices or in the family's social center like the kitchen, dining, or living room, posing distractions that are atypical for a workday. For others, WFH creates social isolation that can lead to sadness or depression. Still, other complications may result from lack of mobility. In an office setting, there are natural posture breaks built in throughout the workday, such as walking to use the bathroom, attend meetings, or make copies on a copy machine, etc. Conducting all business from one location significantly limits one's mobility. Workers may experience new discomfort or lower extremity edema related to longer periods of static work. Occupational therapists can assist with helping workers separate work from leisure time, assisting children with home schooling, incorporating physical activity, and organizing workspaces.[32]

Because Susan developed pain symptoms while telecommuting during COVID-19, the occupational therapy consultant interviewed her using video software in her home office before observing her work. Susan shared that her husband lost his job 2 months earlier and they had to move back to their home state and live with her in-laws. Susan's father-in-law set up an "office" for her to work in the musty basement. During the remote evaluation, Susan was observed working in awkward positions. The chair she was borrowing was unstable, tilting backward if she leaned on the backrest. The armrests were too low and the makeshift desk was too high, producing pressure on the underside of her forearms. She used a 24-inch monitor and a tablet computer, both of which were too low on the desktop surface. Susan had to lean in while looking down to see the screens. She often found herself sitting on her crossed leg on the chair seat to obtain more stability.

The following changes were made during Susan's assessment: the lock function on the chair was enabled so the chair would not rock backward. The seat was elevated and a book was placed on the floor as a temporary footrest. The armrests of the chair were elevated to the height of the table to provide support to her forearms. Both the monitor and the tablet were elevated on temporary "risers" (boxes) to bring the screens up to eye-level. They were brought closer to reduce the need for Susan to lean in to see the text clearly. In addition, the occupational therapist affirmed the feelings that Susan was having and made some suggestions to improve the basement environment; finding a way to open the windows, getting a fan to circulate the air and an oil diffuser. She was also encouraged to speak with her husband and his family about options to relocate her workstation and look into remediating the musty smell in the basement. A report was written and the following equipment recommendations were made: footrest, monitor risers and her own chair (so she could return her father-in-law's chair). The employer was in agreement and made the purchases for Susan. A follow-up appointment was scheduled for once the recommendations were implemented.

INJURY PREVENTION AND WORKER WELLNESS PROGRAMS

Worksite evaluations and ergonomic interventions can be important aspects of comprehensive injury prevention and worker wellness programs.[31] The Department of Labor was established in the early 1900s, to protect workers from becoming injured while on the job. Surprisingly, it was not until 1970 that the federal government legally mandated organizations to protect workers' safety.[59] Injury prevention programs focus on the reduction of exposure to risk factors (tools equipment and physical space) within the work environment itself. These proactive processes are geared to reduce hazards leading to injuries, illness, and fatalities. Successful injury prevention programs are onsite and have the cooperation of upper management, union representatives, and line-staff. There has been at least a 60% drop in workplace deaths and reported occupational injuries in the five decades since the Occupational Safety and Health Act was signed into law; however, the number of preventable work-related injuries and deaths remain unacceptable.[70] Most large organizations have dedicated managers and safety teams to address hazard remediation and conduct safety training. If holding an onsite position, the occupational therapist will likely be part of the occupational health and safety team. Duties may include encouraging a climate of safety and wellness through hazard recognition and remediation, and worker empowerment. The team may collaborate with health and safety representatives, union representatives, human resources, and engineers to implement solutions that reduce risks.[49] Some organizations will hire an occupational therapist as a consultant to control the severity and incidence of work-related muscular injuries, rather than hire them into a full-time position. Either way, there are many opportunities to make a positive impact on the health and safety of workers in the workplace.

Worker Wellness

Global chronic medical conditions are reaching crisis levels, holding significant public health concerns because of illness, mortality, and the burden of healthcare costs.[31] The World Health Organization (WHO) defines health as "A state of complete physical, mental and social well-being, and not merely the absence of disease." In 1958, the WHO reported that a healthy population is the most relevant and important basic resource of any society.[32] Modifiable chronic conditions have essential characteristics that can be altered to reduce risk and improve overall health and well-being. Some modifiable chronic physical conditions include diabetes, cardiovascular disease, tobacco use, obesity, hypertension, hypercholesterolemia, and inactivity. Depression, anxiety, and stress disorders are also considered modifiable chronic conditions.[31] Of adults in the United States, 6 in 10 have one chronic condition and 4 in 10 adults have two or more chronic conditions. "Chronic conditions are the leading causes of death and disability and the leading drivers in the nation's $3.5 trillion in annual healthcare costs."[65]

In an effort to improve global health by reducing chronic conditions, several consecutive and correlated health policies have been enacted. Every 10 years since 1980, the U.S. Department of Health and Human Services released initiatives with national disease prevention and health promotion objectives. The Healthy People initiatives lead the nation with their social determinants of health and shared vision for a healthier nation.[95] The U.S. Chamber of Commerce generates initiatives specifically supporting the Healthy Workforce.[98] The WHO developed a global model for action, including a "Five Keys to a Healthy Workplace" with resources in 13 languages.[32] There are parallel interests held by private and corporate business owners to sustain a healthy workforce to keep medical costs and lost productivity to a minimum. For successful health and wellness programming, employers recognize that they must manage the health behaviors of their staff.

The American workforce is a microcosm of society, and workers present with most of the chronic health issues that are evident within society. Addressing wellness in the workplace translates to wellness in the community, wellness in society, and ultimately wellness for the world. With the passage of the Patient Protection and Affordable Care Act in 2014, worksite wellness programs became part of a national strategy working toward the reduction of chronic diseases.[10] In June 2011, the NIOSH launched the Total Worker Health (TWH) Program. This program is the natural evolution of NIOSH efforts that began in 2003 with the creation of the Steps to a Healthier U.S. Workforce Initiative.[79] The exciting paradigm shift with the TWH program is that it expands workplace injury prevention programs to include worker health and well-being outside of the workplace. The TWH program is the first worker initiative to include families and communities as well. TWH programs are designed to integrate injury prevention programs with health promotion programs to ultimately advance worker safety, health, and well-being.[49]

More than 60% of Americans obtain health insurance through their place of employment; thus, workplace wellness programs are uniquely positioned to respond to the varied health needs of their workers.[10] The WHO defines a healthy workplace as one in which workers and managers collaborate to protect and promote the health, safety, and well-being of all workers.[32] These policies provide exciting and ideal opportunities for occupational therapists to address the physical and psychosocial work contexts, including culture, personal health resources, and community participation within the work environment.

Occupational Therapy Role in Workplace Wellness

The principles of preventing injury or illness and promoting a healthy society are deeply embedded in the roots of occupational therapy. Our training in the total integration of our clients' physical, mental, psychological, social, and environmental schema allows us to be key players by assisting employees and employers to create healthy workers and healthy workplaces. Presently, many occupational therapists are either including wellness into their treatment plans, or focusing their practices specifically on wellness promotion and disease prevention.

Successful wellness programs should be comprehensive, tailored to the population, and embraced by the recipients. For the workplace, this includes upper management, union representatives, and the employees. It is very important to have the support of management because they carry the financial burden as well as implementation responsibility of the wellness plans. The culture of the business is also very important to consider, although this may be difficult to formally assess. An organization that proposes regular work hours, but in which the managers stay late every day, creates a conflict for the worker who must leave on time to pick up a child from daycare. A company that provides healthy cafeteria choices but brings donuts to staff meetings is sending mixed messages to their workers. When developing or running an onsite program, a consultant occupational therapist who may be viewed as an outsider, or may not be present and visible at all times, must have strong allies within the workforce. Recruiting management and front-line workers is vital for the successful monitoring and implementation of wellness programming. It is also essential for the workers to contribute to the program and feel they are part of the organization's commitment to safety and wellness.[70]

The benefits of wellness programming are manifold. By keeping employees healthy and reducing health-care expenditures, evidence suggests that work site wellness programs are cost-effective for the employer. Baicker et al. calculated an average return on investment to be $3.27 for every $1 spent on worksite wellness programs. In addition to improving worker health, wellness programs create a sense of community, improve morale, improve productivity, and improve worker retention. Worker absenteeism and "presenteeism" (in which a worker is present but not productive) are also reduced through integrated wellness programming.[10a]

An example of this is the situation with Lisa, a young woman (prefers use of the pronouns she/her/hers) who returned to work from maternity leave about 3 months before requesting an ergonomic evaluation. Lisa was having wrist and neck pain. The occupational therapist visited her and after the evaluation, recommended some changes to her workstation including elevating her monitors and bringing her mouse and keyboard closer to avoid overreaching for the desktop accessories. After a month, Lisa requested a follow-up because her pain had not improved. The occupational therapist spent more time observing Lisa work, and noticed that her cubicle walls were becoming covered with photos of her new baby. The occupational therapist recommended a different ergonomic keyboard and recommended Lisa take more frequent posture breaks throughout the day. She also spent time talking with Lisa about her baby and possible posture changes she could use while caring for him. After 2 more weeks, Lisa's discomfort still had not improved. The occupational therapist took Lisa into a private room where Lisa burst into tears. She had gone through fertility treatments to conceive and was so happy being a new mom that being at work was the last place she wanted to be. All of her anxiety about being away from her baby was adding to the stress she was holding in her body and contributing to her discomfort. The occupational therapist spent time listening to Lisa as she finally felt the freedom to express her feelings. The occupational therapist helped her problem-solve with conversations she could have with her family to see what options she had other than working full time. Not surprisingly, Lisa's productivity at work was far less than before her maternity leave. Just because workers are physically present does not mean that they will be optimally productive; thus—presenteeism.

The TWH program provides opportunities for occupational therapists to broaden their scope by leading and coordinating efforts under the umbrella of the TWH.[49] Occupational therapists can expand their role within more comprehensive workplace wellness programs. "The TWH™ strategy encompasses many areas relevant to occupational therapy practice, especially the holistic approach acknowledging that factors inside and outside of work have an effect on the worker and families."[49] It is the occupational therapist who is naturally aligned to address worker's interests in meaningful occupations and to address the multidimensional aspects of the worker, workplace, and organization.

The occupational therapist hired to develop or implement wellness programming may be doing it as part of another program. Some organizations are more receptive to ergonomic programs, where there are tangible costs associated with the purchase of ergonomic equipment, and data can be collected measuring the effects of the program. Employee morale and satisfaction are more difficult to capture and measure. An occupational therapist working onsite as part of a team will have the insider advantage when developing a culture of health and wellness. For many though, working as a consultant is the only option.

Although policies are in place promoting health and wellness programs, there is little consistency between organizations. A climate of wellness can be as informal as providing fliers suggesting stretch breaks, or as expansive as programs involving several different departments. The perceptive occupational therapist hired to develop or implement wellness programming should embrace collaboration with insurance companies and community wellness organizations (Weight Watchers, American Heart Association, American Diabetes Association, etc.) rather than beginning anew. Many employee health insurance companies offer incentive programs. Those who maintain a healthy weight and body mass index, have regular doctor's visits, or participate in health challenges, can earn rewards or have financial incentives deposited into personal health savings accounts. "In companies with a strong culture of health, employees are three times as likely to report taking action to improve their health. Employee health and well-being are critical to overall job satisfaction and for many, are more important than salary or benefits."[10]

TRANSITION SERVICES FROM SCHOOL TO WORK

Occupational therapy practitioners can make a valuable contribution to students with disabilities who are transitioning from school to the community. The 1997 amendments to the Individuals with Disabilities Education Act (IDEA) of 1990 specified that transition planning is to be part of the Individualized Education Program (IEP). Representatives from community agencies that provide postschool services, such as state-sponsored vocational rehabilitation, must join the education team. Related services, such as occupational therapy, are formal contributors to the transition planning for students who need these types of services.[91] Transition services are defined by the IDEA as "a coordinated set of activities for a student designed within an outcome-oriented process, which promotes movement from school to post-school activities, includes postsecondary education, vocational training, integrated employment (including supported employment), continuing and adult education, adult services, independent living, or community participation."[91] Occupational therapy's unique focus on occupational performance can be a strong asset to the transition team.

The three main roles that an occupational therapist will participate in are transition-related evaluation, service planning, and service implementation. The occupational therapist contributes vital information about students' performance abilities and needs in any of the transition domains: domestic, vocational, school, recreational, and community.[91]

Transition-Related Evaluation

Effective transition-related evaluation primarily uses nonstandardized interviews, situational observation, and activity analysis approaches. These approaches are top-down, which means that they first consider what the student wants or needs to do and secondarily identify the occupational performance issues that are causing difficulties.[1] The transition team helps the student identify a positive, shared vision for the future. This can include living alone or with others in the community, attending postsecondary schools or training programs, working in a paid or volunteer job, using community services, and participating in activities of interest. The occupational therapist and other members of the team work together to identify the student's present interests and abilities within the context in which performance is expected or needed. The evaluation process also allows the team to identify areas in which the student is likely to need ongoing support and resources to achieve his or her vision and goals for the future.

Service Planning

In a collaborative transition team, the team members collectively share information and write down the student's goals.[93] The team members do not record discipline-specific goals that focus on remediating the student's underlying deficits. The occupational therapist, for example, does not need to write specific goals addressing cognitive, motor, or psychosocial skills. Instead, two or more group members work together to write the goals and work collaboratively with the student to accomplish the goals. A student with limited movement in her arms and hands may have the goal of being able to complete written assignments. The occupational therapist may take the lead in evaluating the effectiveness of using alternative writing methods such as assistive technology. Recommendations are made to the student and the team. If the team supports the recommendations, the team would assign responsibility for obtaining the equipment and also provide training to the student and other team members. Rainforth and York-Barr define collaboration as "an interactive process in which persons with varied life perspectives and experiences join together in a spirit of willingness to share resources, responsibility, and regards in creating inclusive and effective educational programs and environments for students with unique learning needs."[80]

Program Implementation

The occupational therapist provides services in collaboration with the student and his or her teachers, parents, employers, co-workers, and others as necessary to address the student's goals in the domestic, vocational, school, recreation, and community areas. Occupational therapy personnel (including the occupational therapist and the OTA) deliver transition services in the student's natural environments. Therefore, occupational therapy may provide intervention in the student's school, workplace, home, or any other relevant setting in the community. Collaborative problem solving with others involved in the student's environment is essential to help the student use alternative methods to complete the necessary activities. For example, an occupational therapist may introduce and train the teacher in using assistive technology to help a student be able to access the computer at school to do written assignments. The occupational therapy practitioner may provide direct or consultative

services to help minimize discrepancies in the student's abilities and the demands of any environment. Evaluating whether the student reaches his or her goals should be the outcome measure to evaluate the effectiveness of occupational therapy services.

WORK READINESS PROGRAMS

Many times people who have survived a major accident or illness cannot return to their prior employment and need to explore other options for employment. For example, Henry can no longer meet the job demands of a roofer. Henry may really want to return to some type of meaningful work but needs guidance and direction to explore what his present abilities and work skills are so that he can set some realistic vocational goals.

A work readiness program is designed to help individuals who desire to work identify vocational options that match their interests, skills, and abilities. At Rancho Los Amigos National Rehabilitation Center in Downey, California, an occupational therapist developed and implemented an ongoing work readiness program as part of the Occupational Therapy Vocational Services. This is an 8-week program that meets two times a week for 2 hours. It consists of people with various diagnoses (e.g., stroke, traumatic brain injury, and spinal cord injury) who meet as a group. Topics addressed include work habits, goals, interests, work skills, vocational exploration, job hunting strategies, and community resources. Instruction, group discussion, and hands-on exploration of work skills by standardized work samples and situational assessments are used to help people explore their readiness to work and discover their potential for pursuing training for a different occupation. Field trips to a real business in the community are sometimes conducted to allow participants to practice actual work tasks in the community. For example, one field trip may be to a hardware store to practice dusting shelves, reorganizing and moving misplaced merchandise in the aisles and to practice visual scanning, dynamic standing balance, reaching, and bending.

Each person's program is individualized to address specific goals and interests. For example, Henry may be interested in working with a computer. He would be given the opportunity to do different work-related tasks using a computer so that he could see whether he has an aptitude for this type of work. If Henry was not familiar with the types of jobs that a person could do with a computer, he would learn how to do vocational research by using various reference books in the library or on the internet.

A work readiness program can help people identify specific goals to pursue and develop a plan to help them work toward their goals. This program can help persons prepare for returning to work, but it does not provide a job for the participant. At the completion of the program, if a person demonstrates readiness to work, that person can be referred to the state's department of rehabilitation for assistance in job training and job placement. After completing a work readiness program, the occupational therapist can provide valuable information on a person's skills, aptitudes, and interests to assist the rehabilitation counselor in developing a feasible plan for the worker. While Henry was attending the work readiness program, he identified the goal of becoming a computer support technician. Based on the vocational testing and research that he did during the program, this was determined to be a reasonable goal for him to pursue. He was referred to his state's department of rehabilitation for job training and job placement in his new career.

WORK ACTIVITY GROUPS

Occupational therapists can develop and implement work-related functional activity groups for people with physical disabilities to build the strength and stamina, hand dexterity, standing balance and endurance to engage in productive activities. At Rancho Los Amigos National Rehabilitation Center, the Rancho Works occupational therapy program was developed for people who desire to return to work after sustaining a stroke, brain injury, spinal cord injury, amputations as a result of diabetes or who have been diagnosed with any other neurologic illnesses. By engaging in various activities, such as woodworking, basic carpentry, ceramics, card making, sewing, and jewelry making, people can improve their motor, process, and social interaction skills while producing tangible products. Participants can also learn adaptive strategies to use tools and complete tasks using one hand after a stroke or can practice using the affected hand as an active assist to complete a bimanual task. Clients manufacture handcrafted gift items which are sold in the hospital gift shop operated by paid workers who have completed the vocational program. This program gives individuals the opportunity to build the appropriate work habits and skills to work at the Rancho Works Café and Gift Shop to acquire customer service, cashiering, cleaning, and food service skills or to prepare for other work in the community. Clients gain confidence and self-esteem while developing new work skills and interests by participating in this program with the goal of being able to transition to work out in the community.

COMMUNITY-BASED SERVICES

Historically, work-related programs took place within medical model clinics, such as rehabilitation programs or settings designed for work intervention, as opposed to the site where the worker actually performed his or her role.[87] Today work programs are increasingly being located in the community in which the participant resides or within the work setting itself.[87] This trend toward increased community practice is probably due to changes in the field of occupational therapy and external forces influencing the practice. Current thinking in occupational therapy recognizes that "occupational dysfunction is multidimensional, resulting from the interplay of biological, psychological, and ecological factors."[87] Decreasing reimbursement in medical model settings has resulted in occupational therapists exploring other options for reimbursement in the community.

Funding for most community-based programs is derived from grants or contracts through local, state, or the federal government and also from foundations. Grants are funds that are awarded for a specific purpose and a specific period, usually for research or a service project, "based on a submission of a creative original proposal."[87] Contracts also provide funding

for research or service projects; however, the funding agency defines the scope of the project and requests bids from competing organizations in the community. The majority of funding for community-based programs comes from foundations; "foundations are operated by philanthropic families, corporations, or community agencies that have reserved significant amounts of money for the purpose of supporting charitable organizations and programs to address specific community needs."[87] Many associations and civic groups, such as the United Way, American Head Injury Foundation, Kiwanis Club, and others, provide funding for community projects related to specific areas of interest. It is important to note that community-based programs should develop a broad financial base with multiple funding sources for programs to "survive and thrive" in the long run.

Community Rehabilitation Programs

There are almost 600 community rehabilitation programs (CRPs) with federal contracts under the Javits-Wagner-O'Day (JWOD) program, according to Source America (formerly NISH, the National Industries for the Severely Handicapped). These community-based nonprofit organizations train and employ individuals with severe disabilities (primarily developmental disabilities and blindness) and provide quality goods and services to the federal government. The CRPs subcontract work from various industries to allow individuals with severe disabilities the opportunity to be productive, earn a competitive wage, and contribute to society. (See the Source America website [http://www.sourceamerica.org] for more details.) These programs receive most of their funding from regional centers or the Office of Vocational Rehabilitation. Although most of these programs are run by individuals who are not OT professionals, this is an area that some occupational therapists may want to explore for future involvement. There is a great need for these types of programs for individuals with other severe, chronic disabilities (e.g., brain and spinal cord injuries), but creative funding needs to be obtained to support them.

Homeless Shelter Programs

Emerging in the 1980s, another practice area for occupational therapists is working with persons who are homeless. Because of the increasing number of persons experiencing homelessness, Congress enacted the Stewart McKinney Homeless Assistance Act of 1987 (Public Law 100-77).[40] This act was designed to meet the needs of those who are homeless by providing funds for emergency shelters, food, healthcare, housing, education, job training, and other community services. The act funded a Department of Labor project to plan, implement, and evaluate the effectiveness of a comprehensive spectrum of employment, training, and other support services to help persons who are homeless to locate and sustain employment. Based on the Job Training for the Homeless Demonstration Program (JTHDP), which consisted of 63 organizations across the United States that provided comprehensive services for persons who were homeless from September, 1988, to November, 1995, the Department of Labor created a best practices guide.[87] Box 14.5 lists the findings of the JTHDP, which recommended that a sponsoring

---

BOX 14.5   Core Services to Aid Underserved Community Members

The Job Training for the Homeless Demonstration Program has defined the following as necessary services to aid the underserved members of a community:
- Case management and counseling
- Evaluation and employability development planning
- Job training services (e.g., remedial education, basic skills training, literacy instruction, job search assistance, job counseling, vocational and occupational skills training, and on-the-job training)
- Job development and placement services
- Postplacement follow-up and support services (e.g., additional job placement services, training after placement, self-help support groups, mentoring)
- Housing services (e.g., emergency housing assistance, evaluation of housing needs, referrals to appropriate housing alternatives)
- Other support services (e.g., child care, transportation, chemical dependence evaluation, counseling, and referral to outpatient or inpatient treatment as appropriate)
- Mental health evaluation, counseling, and referral to treatment
- Other healthcare services
- Clothing
- Life skills training

From Herzberg GL, et al: Work and the underserved: homelessness and work. In Kornblau BL, Jacobs K, editors: *Work: principles and practice*, Bethesda, MD, 2000, American Occupational Therapy Association.

---

agency provide the core services or that the agency develop linkages with other local human service providers to assist persons who are homeless in obtaining and sustaining employment.

Occupational therapists have the skills to design and implement programs that incorporate the JTHDP recommendations for best practices. Client-centered job readiness and job training programs can and have been developed for community service agencies to address the concerns of persons who are homeless. This population desires intervention services that are "sensitive, respectful, and responsive to their self-identified needs."[15]

Occupational therapy practitioners work with those who are homeless and with agencies providing services for people who are homeless to build skills for accessing resources, solving problems by identifying strengths and assets, and learning to critically analyze situations for win-win situations for employers and the persons who are homeless.

WELFARE-TO-WORK PROGRAMS

Congress passed the Personal Responsibility and Work Opportunity Reconciliation Act (Public Law 104-193) in 1996 to move people from welfare to work.[15] It required welfare recipients to find work after receiving 2 years of public assistance. The Balanced Budget Act of 1997 (Public Law 105-33) provided funds for welfare-to-work grants. These grants are for training long-term recipients of welfare or public assistance to enter the job market in unsubsidized jobs. People who are most difficult to place because of multiple barriers to work,

such as low academic skills, poor work history, or those who need substance abuse treatment, are the target of these grants. A substantial percentage of welfare recipients have learning problems, mental health and substance use disorders, and issues of domestic violence that interfere with their sustained employability.[87]

Welfare-to-work programs are another innovative practice area for occupational therapists. Therapists who are interested in entering this area of practice must find out which agencies within the local or state communities control the welfare-to-work funds. Occupational therapists can subcontract with these agencies and collaborate with them. This information can be accessed from the National Governors Association (NGA) Center for Best Practices welfare reform website.[66] Private foundations that are involved in the welfare-to-work programs also may be a source of entry for occupational therapists.

There are many barriers that a person receiving welfare must face to enter into competitive employment. Lack of transportation, lack of childcare, problems with domestic violence, illiteracy, lack of housing, substance abuse, and medical needs can interfere with a welfare recipient's ability to obtain and retain a job.[15] Successful welfare-to-work programs attempt to break these barriers down. For example, programs combine basic education and job development, provide refurbished cars for transportation to work, and provide one-on-one mentoring for improving self-sufficiency. Transitioning welfare recipients to the workplace presents a challenging practice area for occupational therapists to use their creativity to design and deliver effective services to help clients set goals, explore vocational options, and introduce them to different community resources to achieve successful and continued employment.[40,87]

Ticket to Work

The Ticket to Work and Work Incentives Improvement Act was enacted in December, 1999. This law created a voluntary program for recipients of Supplemental Security Income (SSI) and Social Security Disability Insurance (SSDI) to receive job-related support services and encourage beneficiaries to return to work and pursue their employment goals.[94] Those who have tickets can go to any Employment Network (EN), an organizational entity (state or local, public or private) that has contracted with the Social Security Administration (SSA) to coordinate and deliver employment services, vocational rehabilitation services, and/or other support services under the Ticket to Work Program. Interested individuals can contact the Ticket to Work Help Line at 1-866-968-7842 (V)/866-833-2967 (TTY) to verify eligibility and find out how the program works. The Ticket to Work Program can also be contacted via the website http://www.yourtickettowork.com or https://www.ssa.gov/work. The Ticket to Work Program creates opportunities for occupational therapists to serve on advisory panels, work as program managers, or provide employment support services.[87,94] Those who are interested in learning how this program will affect their Social Security benefits can register for free Work Incentive Seminar Events (WISE) at https://www.ssa.gov/work/.

Volunteerism

Some people may not be able to return to competitive employment due to the nature or extent of their disability, but they still may be interested in participating in some type of productive activity in the community. Occupational therapy practitioners can help people identify the type of work activities they can successfully do by practicing different skills that may be done by a volunteer at a hospital, school, community center, or any place of interest. Simulated clerical tasks, such as making photocopies, collating and stapling papers, making and receiving phone calls, and data entry, can be practiced. Customer service skills, hospitality and greeting skills, and providing directions and information can be practiced. Helping people identify their strengths will give them more confidence to advocate for themselves when applying and interviewing for a volunteer position. Additionally, occupational therapy practitioners can offer practical assistance to individuals in locating a suitable volunteer site in their local community by educating them on locating the various resources available on the internet, such as the websites https://www.volunteermatch.org and https://www.idealist.org.

THE AGING WORKER

As occupational therapists, we can also offer an increasing emphasis on special programs to accommodate older workers. The Bureau of Labor Statistics[13,14] projects that by year 2026, 30.2% of the total labor force will be between the ages of 65 to 74 and 10% of the working population will be 75 or older.[85] People 60 years and over are the fastest-growing segment of the population and their numbers are expected to triple by the year 2100.[43] The population of older workers is increasing, whereas the population of younger workers between 25 and 44 is decreasing.[85] It is predicted that there will be a shortage of younger workers to replace the baby boomers when they retire, thereby creating a gap in the labor market. One proposal to fill this gap would be to employ more people with disabilities.[85] Occupational therapists can work with human resource managers to educate and provide resources for workplace accommodations. The Society for Human Resource Management has recently partnered with the Office of Disability Employment Policy (ODEP).[85] This collaboration reveals that human resource professionals are seeking support and services for hiring and accommodating workers with disabilities.

In the United States alone, older people will account for roughly 20% of the population by 2030.[43] Not only are people living longer, but life expectancies are predicted to continue to increase. Many in the baby boomer generation (those born between 1946 and 1964) continue to be gainfully employed well into their 70s and beyond. In a study by the Equality and Human Rights commission, 10% of men and 7% of women between the ages of 50 and 75 planned to set up their own businesses after retiring from mainstream employment. Throughout their lives, baby boomers have pushed social boundaries.[43] As a group, they are healthier, are better educated, and have greater expectations than previous generations. They have taken control of work-life balance opportunities and redefined what was historically considered a typical retirement age. With factors such as rising cost of living expenses, medical expenses, and adult children who continue to live at home, our growing economic demands as a society drives the need for many seniors to work for as long as possible.[43]

No matter how physically or mentally fit one is, biological changes can make work productivity more challenging as one ages. For most, the aging process involves some level of decline in physical, sensory, and potentially cognitive capacity. Conversely, the pace of the modern office with younger co-workers and rapidly evolving technology only compounds challenges for the aging worker. Although no one can argue that the invention and application of technology holds incredible benefits, for the older worker some of these challenges can be daunting (see Chapter 47).

Occupational therapists working with older workers recognize the value of purposeful, meaningful occupation and recognize the importance of helping our clients be able to work for as long as they desire. By embracing the potential challenges that they face, we can provide a proactive approach to adaptation that allows them to adjust in ways that will promote ongoing employment. For the worker who wants to make a vocational shift, we can assist by exploring alternative vocational or leisure options for the future (see Chapter 16).

For older workers with visual changes, there are options to enlarge the font or change the contrast on monitor screens. Task lighting, proper eyewear and organization systems help for desktop paperwork activities. For workers who have motor or orthopedic changes, a variety of adaptive equipment can be very helpful in the workplace. For specific technology modifications, please refer to Chapter 17. Other barriers for the older worker can include stress related to fast-paced cultures, difficulty taking supervision from less experienced managers, the physical demands of the environment and job security. Fear of losing a job can lead to occupational imbalance that could contribute to poor health. Focusing on the strengths of older workers as valued contributors to the work environment should be top priority for the occupational therapist in this role.

Baby boomers represent one of the largest percentages of the working population.[85] As the baby boomers age, employers may need to be sensitive to workers for whom multiple disabilities develop that eventually may have an impact on their job performance. Changes in the workplace offer new opportunities for occupational therapists to help aging workers stay employed with their functional limitations. As older workers retire, occupational therapists can help individuals plan for their retirement and explore ways to remain active in the community by participation in leisure pursuits or volunteer activities. Occupational therapists can help older individuals identify their strengths and abilities and provide community resources to allow meaningful participation in valued occupations.

THREADED CASE STUDY

Joe, Susan, and Henry, Part 2

Reflecting back on the introductory case scenarios, the reader sees opportunities for the application of these comprehensive work-related occupational therapy interventions. For example, Joe's occupational therapist could conduct a job demands analysis of the laundry attendant position and a worksite evaluation at the hotel and spa where he worked before his spinal cord injury. Then the occupational therapist would determine whether Joe could successfully carry out the essential functions of that alternative job. The occupational therapist could recommend any modifications that needed to be done to make the work area wheelchair accessible. An FCE may be helpful to determine whether Joe could carry out any of the specific physical demands of the job on an occasional or frequent basis. Based on the results, the occupational therapist could then make recommendations to the physician and the employer for any reasonable accommodations that may be necessary for Joe to successfully return to work, in addition to informing them of any concerns regarding Joe's ability to safely meet the physical demands of the job.

Susan can benefit from occupational therapy consultation services provided by her employer. A remote interview and work assessment of Susan's home office would be helpful to identify problematic postures and work positions contributing to her pain and eliminate these factors through modifying the environment or the task. Education of proper positioning to eliminate risk factors is key. The occupational therapist could teach Susan how to "lock" the chair so it does not rock backward and direct Susan to elevate her chair and place a temporary riser under her feet (book or box). Susan can also elevate the armrests of the chair to bring her forearms up to the height of the desktop surface.

In addition, the monitors should be elevated to promote a neutral neck and upright posture.

The expertise and knowledge of psychosocial skills an occupational therapist brings to each interaction can be extremely beneficial in a situation in which the client is upset. In this case, because of the COVID-19 pandemic, Susan was displaced from her home and work location, her husband lost his job, and her family was living in her husband's childhood home. There are many things that the occupational therapist can assist with in helping Susan to problem solve her options and help her regain control of a situation that feels out of her control. In this case, the work equipment and set up are equally important as the psychosocial components of this evaluation. (See Chapter 15 for latest legislation on "Long COVID," which may now qualify as a disability under the ADA).

Finally, contemplate the third scenario, which involves Henry. Henry needs the assistance of an occupational therapy practitioner to help him discover what type of work that he would best be suited for, while taking into consideration his present physical and cognitive abilities and limitations. He could also benefit from a comprehensive vocational evaluation to assess his cognitive and physical abilities, work habits, work skills, and work tolerances, in addition to interests and attitudes, to determine whether he could return to any other type of work. Another alternative would be for Henry to participate in a work readiness program. The same areas assessed during a vocational evaluation would be addressed in the work readiness program; however, Henry could also benefit from a discussion on work-related topics and could receive peer interaction and feedback on his work performance, work habits, and attitudes.

SUMMARY

This chapter has provided an overview of the varying types of work programs in which occupational therapists are currently practicing; it also has identified and discussed areas for further involvement. There are tremendous opportunities for occupational therapists and certified occupational therapy assistants to expand their role and involvement in hospitals, schools, industrial settings, and the community in general in the area of work rehabilitation. Occupational therapy practitioners are challenged to take a proactive approach in advocating the need for and benefit of these types of work-related programs in all communities, to help restore the occupation of work and the worker role in many people's lives. Training in occupational performance, problem identification, intervention planning, implementation and outcomes makes the area of work evaluation and rehabilitation, including ergonomics, injury prevention, and wellness programming, ideally suited for occupational therapy practitioners.

REVIEW QUESTIONS

1. How has involvement of occupational therapy in work programs evolved over the years?
2. What is the role of occupational therapy in work programs?
3. Describe the difference between an FCE and a vocational evaluation.
4. What components are usually included in an FCE report?
5. Describe the difference between work hardening and work conditioning.
6. List the common applications of the results of a JDA.
7. What interventions are used to determine whether someone is capable of returning to a specific occupation after an injury?
8. Discuss the ergonomic design considerations for workstations, seating, visualizing job tasks, tools, and materials handling.
9. What are some common soft tissue injuries that can occur when an employee sits in a chair that is too high for long periods?
10. Describe why occupational therapists are good candidates for assisting companies in the development of workplace wellness programs.
11. Name and describe some innovative types of work programs in which occupational therapists can be involved in the community.

For additional practice questions for this chapter, please visit eBooks.Health.Elsevier.com.

REFERENCES

1. American Occupational Therapy Association: Work hardening guidelines, *Am J Occup Ther* 40(12):841, 1986.
2. American Occupational Therapy Association: Occupational therapy services in work practice, *Am J Occup Ther* 46(12):1086, 1992.
3. American Occupational Therapy Association: Statement: occupational therapy services in facilitating work performance, *Am J Occup Ther* 54(6):626–628, 2000.
4. American Occupational Therapy Association: Statement: occupational therapy services in facilitating work performance, *Am J Occup Ther* 65(6):S55–S64, 2011.
5. American Occupational Therapy Association: Occupational therapy practice framework: domain and process, ed 3, *Am J Occup Ther* 68(2):S20–S21, 2014.
6. American Occupational Therapy Association: Statement: occupational therapy services in facilitating work participation and performance, *Am J Occup Ther* 71(6):S2, 2017.
7. American Occupational Therapy Association: Occupational therapy practice framework: domain and process, ed 4, *Am J Occup Ther*:74, 2020. https://doi.org/10.5014/ajot.2020.74S2001.
8. American Occupational Therapy Association (2020). Retrieved September 24, 2020, from https://www.aota.org/about-occupational-therapy/professionals/wi/work-rehab.aspx
9. Americans with Disabilities Act: *Technical assistance manual*, Washington, DC, 1992, Equal Employment Opportunity Commission.
10. Anderko L, Roffenbender JS, Goetzel RZ, et al: Promoting prevention through the affordable care act: Workplace wellness, *Prevention chronic disease* 9:120092, 2012. https://doi.org/10.5888/pcd9.120092.
10a. Baicker K, Cutler D, Song Z: Workplace wellness programs can generate savings, February 2010, *Health Affairs: E-Health in the Developing World*, 29(2), https://doi.org/10.1377/hlthaff.2009.0626.
11. Baum CM, Law M: Occupational therapy practice: focusing on occupational performance, *Am J Occup Ther* 51(4):277, 1997.
12. Bohr PC: Work analysis. In King PM, editor: *Sourcebook of occupational rehabilitation*, New York, 1998, Plenum Press.
13. Bureau of Labor Statistics. TED: The economics daily. 2008. http://www.bls.gov/opub/ted/2008/dec/wk1/art02.htm.
14. Bureau of Labor Statistics: Persons with a disability: labor force characteristics – 2014. http://www.bls.gov/.
15. Callahan SR: *Understanding health-status barriers that hinder the transition from welfare to work*, Washington, DC, 1999, National Governors Association Center for Best Practices, Health Policy Status Division.
16. Canelon MF: An on-site job evaluation performed via activity analysis, *Am J Occup Ther* 51(2):144, 1997.
17. Code of Federal Regulations, Title 29, Vol 4. Revised as of July 1, 2003. Part 1630: Regulations to implement the equal employment provisions of the Americans with Disabilities Act. Section 1630.14, Washington, DC.
18. Cohen AL, Gjessing CC, Fine LJ, et al: *Elements of ergonomics programs: a primer based on workplace evaluations of musculoskeletal disorders*, Washington, DC, 1997, US Government Printing Office.
19. Commission on Accreditation of Rehabilitation Facilities: *Standards manual for organizations serving people with disabilities*, Tucson, AZ, 1989, CARF.
20. Cromwell FS: Work-related programming in occupational therapy: its roots course and prognosis, *Occup Ther Healthcare* 2(4):9, 1985.
21. Dahl R: Ergonomics. In Kornblau B, Jacobs K, editors: *Work: principles and practice*, Bethesda, MD, 2000, American Occupational Therapy Association.
22. Darphin LE: Work-hardening and work-conditioning perspectives. In Isernhagen SJ, editor: *The comprehensive guide to work injury management*, Gaithersburg, FL, 1995, Aspen.
23. Davis H, Rodgers S: Using this book for ergonomics in industry: introduction. In: Eggleton E, editor: *Rodgers S, technical editor, Ergonomic design for people at work*, vol 1, New York, 1983, Van Nostrand Reinhold.
24. Deuker JA, Ritchie SM, Knox TJ, Rose SJ: Isokinetic trunk testing and employment, *J Occup Med* 36(1):42, 1994.
25. Eggleton E, editor: *Rodgers S, technical editor: Ergonomic design for people at work*, vol 1, New York, 1983, Van Nostrand Reinhold.
26. Ellexon M: *What every rehab professional in the USA should know about the ADA*, Miami, 1992, ADA Consultants.
27. Equal Employment Opportunity Commission: *Uniform guidelines on employee selection procedures*, Washington, DC, 1978, EEOC.
28. Eser G: *Overview of vocational evaluation*, Las Vegas, 1983, Stout University Training Workshop.
29. Field JE, Field TF: *COJ 2000 with an O*NETTM 98 Crosswalk*, Athens, GA, 1999, Elliot & Fitzpatrick.
30. Fisher AG, Marterella A: *Powerful practice: A model for authentic occupational therapy*, Fort Collins, 2019, Center for Innovative OT Solutions.
31. Fisher MA, Ma Z: Multiple chronic conditions: Diabetes associated with comorbidity and share risk factors using CDC WEAT and SAS analytic tools, *Journal of Primary Care and Community Health*, 2013. https://journals.sagepub.com/doi/full/10.1177/2150131913503347.
32. Fletcher, T. (2020, April 6) *Why the ergonomics of working from home are so important*. https://www.evoluted.net/thinktank/agency-life/
33. Fliedner CA: Occupational therapy: for the body and the mind. In Rodgers GM, editor: *Centennial Rancho Los Amigos Medical Center 1888–1988*, Downey, CA, 1990, Rancho Los Amigos Medical Center.
34. Gibson L, Strong J: A conceptual framework of functional capacity evaluation for occupational therapy in work rehabilitation, *Aust Occup Ther J* 50(2):64–71, 2003.
35. Grubbs R, Hamilton A, editors: *Criteria for a recommended standard: occupational exposure to hand-arm vibration*, Washington DC, 1989, US Government Printing Office.
36. Hall H, Buck M: *The work of our hands*, New York, 1919, Moffat Yard.
37. Harbin G, Olson J: Post-offer, pre-placement testing in industry, *Am J Ind Med* 47(4):296–307, 2005.
38. Harvey-Krefting L: The concept of work in occupational therapy: a historical review, *Am J Occup Ther* 39(5):301, 1985.
39. Hepper E, et al: Back school. In Kirkaldy-Willis WH, Burton CV, editors: *Managing low back pain,* ed 3, New York, 1992, Churchill Livingstone.
40. Herzberg GL, et al: Work and the underserved: homelessness and work. In Kornblau BK, Jacobs K, editors: *Work: principles and practice*, Bethesda, MD, 2000, American Occupational Therapy Association.
41. Holmes D: The role of the occupational therapist–work evaluator, *Am J Occup Ther* 39(5):308, 1985.

42. Homan NM, Armstrong TJ: Evaluation of three methodologies for assessing work activity during computer use, *Am Ind Hyg Assoc J* 64(1):48–55, 2003.

43. Hunt LA, Wolverson CE: *Work and the older person: increasing longevity and well-being,* Thorofare, NJ, 2015, SLACK.

44. *IBM ergonomics handbook,* New York, 2000, IBM.

45. Isernhagen SJ: Advancements in functional capacity evaluation. In D'Orazio BP, editor: *Back pain rehabilitation,* Boston, 1993, Butterworth.

46. Jacobs K: Preparing for return to work. In Trombly K, editor: *Occupational therapy for physical dysfunction,* ed 4, Baltimore, 1995, Williams & Wilkins.

47. Jacobs K: *Ergonomics for Therapists,* 3rd Edition, St. Louis, MO, 2008, Mosby Elsevier.

48. Jacobs K, Baker NA: The history of work-related therapy in occupational therapy. In Kornblau BL, Jacobs K, editors: *Work: principles and practice,* Bethesda, MD, 2000, American Occupational Therapy Association.

49. Jagers L: Total Worker Health™: An opportunity for integrated occupational therapy practice, *Work & Industry Special Interest Section Quarterly* 3(29):1–4, 2015.

50. King PM: Work hardening and work conditioning. In King PM, editor: *Sourcebook of occupational rehabilitation,* New York, 1998, Plenum Press.

51. King PM, Barrett T: A critical review of functional capacity evaluations, *Phys Ther* 78(8):852, 1998.

52. Kornblau B: The occupational therapist and vocational evaluation, *Work Programs Special Interest Section Newsletter* 10:1, 1996.

53. Lechner D, Roth D, Stratton K: Functional capacity evaluation in work disability, *Work* 1:37, 1991.

54. Lechner DE: Work hardening and work conditioning interventions: do they affect disability? *Phys Ther* 74(5):102, 1994.

55. Lechner DE: Functional capacity evaluation. In King PM, editor: *Sourcebook of occupational rehabilitation,* New York, 1998, Plenum Press.

56. Legislative Committee, National Rehabilitation Association: Meeting the nation's needs by the expansion of the program of vocational rehabilitation of physically handicapped persons, *Occup Ther Rehabil* 16(3):186, 1937.

57. Littleton M: Cost-effectiveness of prework screening program for the University of Illinois at Chicago physical plant, *Work* 21(3):243–250, 2003.

58. MacFarlane B: Job modification, *Work Special Interest Section Newsletter* 2(1):1, 1988.

59. MacLaury, J. (1981, Mar). *The job safety law of 1970: its passage was perilous.* Retrieved from: https://dol.gov/general/aboutdol/history/osha

60. MacLeod D: *The ergonomics manual: guidebook for managers, supervisors, and ergonomic team members,* Minneapolis, 1990, Comprehensive Loss Management.

61. Marshall EM: Looking back, *Am J Occup Ther* 39(5):297, 1985.

62. Meister D: *Conceptual aspects of human factors,* Baltimore, 1989, Johns Hopkins Press.

63. Meyer A: The philosophy of occupational therapy, *Am J Occup Ther* 31(10):639, 1977.

64. Mikkelson S, Vilstrup I, Funch Lassen C, et al: Validity of questionnaire self-reports on computer, mouse and keyboard usage during a four week period, *Occup Environ Med* 64(8): 541–547, 2007.

65. National Center for Chronic Disease Prevention and Health Promotion, *Chronic diseases in America*: Center for disease control. Retrieved from: https://www.cdc.gov/chronicdisease/resources/infographic/chronic-diseases.htm

66. National Governors Association Center for Best Practices. Welfare reform. http://www.nga.org/portal/site/nga/menuitem.1b7ae943ae381e6cfcdcbeeb501010a0/?vgnextoid=4bb8aa9c00ee1010VgnVCM1000001a01010aRCRD&vgnextfmt=print.

67. Newton M, Waddell G: Trunk strength testing with iso-machines. I. Review of a decade of scientific evidence, *Spine* 18(7):801, 1993.

68. O'Callaghan J: Primary prevention and ergonomics: the role of rehabilitation specialists in preventing occupational injury. In Rothman J, Levine R, editors: *Prevention practice: strategies for physical therapy and occupational therapy,* Philadelphia, 1992, Saunders.

69. Occupational Safety and Health Administration: *Working safely with video display terminals,* Washington, DC, 1997, US Government Printing Office.

70. Occupational Safety and Health Administration: *Injury and illness prevention programs [White paper],* 2012, OSHA. https://www.osha.gov/sites/default/files/OSHAwhite-paper-january2012sm.pdf.

71. Ogden-Niemeyer L, Jacobs K: Definition and history of work hardening. In Ogden-Niemeyer L, Jacobs K, editors: *Work hardening state of the art,* Thorofare, NJ, 1989, Slack.

72. O*NET. O*NET online. http://online.onetcenter.org/.

73. Owens LA, Buchholz RL: Functional capacity assessment, worker evaluation strategies, and the disability management process. In Shrey DE, Lacerte M, editors: *Principles and practices of disability management in industry,* Winter Park, FL, 1995, GR Press.

74. Page J: Functional capacity evaluation: making the right decision, *RehabPro* 9(4):34–35, 2001.

75. Patterson C: A historical perspective of work practice services. In Pratt J, Jacobs K, editors: *Work practice: international perspectives,* Boston, 1997, Butterworth.

76. Perry L: Preemployment and preplacement testing. In King PM, editor: *Sourcebook of occupational rehabilitation,* New York, 1998, Plenum Press.

77. Peterson W, Perr A: Home and worksite accommodations. In Galvin JC, Scherer J, editors: *Evaluating, selecting and using appropriate assistive technology,* Gaithersburg, MD, 1996, Aspen.

78. Pinel P: *A treatise on insanity,* New York, 1962, Hafner.

79. Punnett L, Cavallari JM, Henning RA, et al: Defining 'integration' for total worker health: a new proposal, *Ann Work Expo Health* Apr;64(3):223–235, 2020. https://academic.oup.com/annweh/article/64/3/223/5719338.

80. Rainforth B, York-Barr J: *Collaborative teams for students with severe disabilities: integrating therapy and educational services,* ed 2, Baltimore, 1997, Brookes.

81. Reed K: The beginnings of occupational therapy. In Hopkins HL, Smith HD, editors: *Willard and Spackman's occupational therapy,* Philadelphia, 1993, Lippincott.

82. Rosenberg B, Wellerson T: A structured pre-vocational program, *Am J Occup Ther* 14:57, 1960.

83. Rothstein J, Echternach J: *Primer on measurement: an introductory guide to measurement issues featuring the APTA's standards for tests and measurements in physical therapy practice,* Alexandria, VA, 1993, American Physical Therapy Association.

84. Ryan DJ: *Job search handbook for people with disabilities,* Indianapolis, IN, 2000, Job Information Seeking and Training (JIST) Publishing.

85. Sabata D, Endicott S: Workplace changes: seizing opportunities for persons with disabilities in the workplace: work programs special interest section, *Q Am Occup Ther Assoc* 21:2, 2007.

86. Sabonis-Chafee B: *Occupational therapy: introductory concepts*, St Louis, 1989, Mosby.

87. Scaffa ME, et al: Future directions in community-based practice. In Scaffa ME, editor: *Occupational therapy in community-based practice settings*, Philadelphia, 2001, FA Davis.

88. Shrey DE: Worksite disability management and industrial rehabilitation: an overview. In Shrey DE, Lacerte M, editors: *Principles and practices of disability management in industry*, Winter Park, FL, 1995, GR Press.

89. Smith SL, Cunningham S, Weinberg R: The predictive validity of the functional capacities evaluation, *Am J Occup Ther* 40:564, 1986.

90. Soer R, van der Schans CP, Groothoff JW, Geertzen JH, Reneman MF: Towards consensus in operational definitions in functional capacity evaluation: A Delphi survey, *Journal of Occupational Rehabilitation* 18(4):389–400, 2008.

91. Spencer K: Transition from school to adult life. In Kornblau B, Jacobs K, editors: *Work: principles and practice*, Bethesda, MD, 2000, American Occupational Therapy Association.

92. Symons J, Veran A: Conducting worksite evaluations to identify reasonable accommodations. In Hamil J, editor: *Integrating assistive technology into your practice (AOTA online course)*, Bethesda, MD, 2000, American Occupational Therapy Association.

93. Taylor RR, Van Puymbroeck L: Therapeutic use of self: Applying the intentional relationship model in group therapy. In O'Brien JC, Solomon JW JW, editors: *Occupational analysis and group process*, St. Louis, 2013, Elsevier, pp 36–52.

94. The Work Site: Ticket to work fact sheet. http://www.ssa.gov.

95. U.S. Department of Health and Human Services, *Healthy People, 2030*. Office of disease prevention and health promotion. Retrieved from: https://healthypeople.gov.

96. US Department of Labor: *Employment and Training Administration: Revised dictionary of occupational titles (vol I and II)*, ed 4, Washington, DC, 1991, US Government Printing Office.

97. US Department of Labor: *Employment and Training Administration: The revised handbook for analyzing jobs*, Indianapolis, IN, 1991, Job Information Seeking and Training (JIST).

98. U.S. Department of Labor, Immigration and Employee Benefits Division, U.S. Chamber of commerce, Healthy Workforce *2010 and Beyond*. https://www.uschamber.com/assets/archived/images/documents/files/HealthyWorkforce2010FINALElectronicVersion111709.pdf.

99. Wegg LS: The essentials of work evaluation, *Am J Occup Ther* 14:65, 1960.

100. World Health Organization: *Healthy workplaces: a model for action for employers, workers, policy-makers and practitioners*, 2010, https://iris.who.int/bitstream/handle/10665/44307/9789241599313_eng.pdf?sequence=1&isAllowed=y.

15

Americans With Disabilities Act and Related Laws That Promote Participation in Work, Leisure, and Activities of Daily Living

Barbara L. Kornblau

LEARNING OBJECTIVES

After studying this chapter, the student or practitioner will be able to do the following:

1. Explain how the Americans with Disabilities Act (ADA) defines disability and how that definition may apply to clients seen by occupational therapists (OTs) as a tool to increase professional advocacy and client participation.
2. Compare and contrast definitions of discrimination and discuss how they may apply to clients served by occupational therapy and lead to increased participation of our clients in everyday life.
3. Recognize and define specific terms used in the ADA, Fair Housing Act, and Air Carrier Access Act and how they can lead to increased independence and participation.
4. Discuss the roles that occupational therapy can play in advocating for clients under the ADA, Fair Housing Act, and Air Carrier Access Act and how advocacy can lead to increased participation and independence in employment, community life, housing, and travel.
5. Discuss the roles that occupational therapy can play in consulting with employers, places of public accommodation, airline carriers, and landlords to improve clients' participation, independence, and integration into community life.
6. Explain the process used to determine "essential job functions" and how occupational therapy can use this information to help clients maintain their employment, and/or promote return to work following an accident, injury, or illness.
7. Analyze "reasonable accommodations" as an intervention strategy in occupational therapy and explain the decision-making process involved in making reasonable accommodations in employment, places of public accommodations, housing, and community living.
8. Outline the process for removing physical and other barriers to access in places of public accommodation and the steps necessary to perform an accessibility audit.
9. Prepare and train employers, co-workers, supervisors, airline employees, and those who work with the public to treat individuals with disabilities with dignity and respect.

CHAPTER OUTLINE

KEY TERMS

Accessibility audit
Auxiliary aids
Direct threat
Discrimination
Essential job functions
Individual with a disability

Major life activities
Places of public accommodation
Qualified individual or person with a disability
Reasonable accommodations
Undue hardship

INTRODUCTION

Readers may see this chapter and ask, "Why is this chapter in a textbook on physical dysfunction?" Here is the answer: Some years ago, one of the author's students, who was out on fieldwork, went to do a home assessment with a client awaiting discharge from an inpatient rehabilitation unit. As part of the assessment, she told her supervising OTR (Registered Occupational Therapist) that the client—like Carlotta in the Threaded Case Study—would need to install grab bars in her bathroom, so she could be safe and independent in bathing. The client, a participant in the conversation, told the fieldwork student and the supervising OTR there was no way her landlord would allow her to put grab bars in HIS apartment building.

The supervising OTR shifted the conversation to discussing possible alternative living arrangements for the client. My former student spoke up. "The landlord has to let her put in the grab bars that she needs," she said. "She has to pay for them and pay to install them, but he must let her do this under the Fair Housing Act." The student explained a few more things about the Fair Housing Act that she learned in her occupational therapy program, and with this information, the client was able to pay a contractor to install the grab bars and return home to live independently.

The purpose of this chapter is to get readers thinking about policies that function as tools for independent living and community integration and the importance of educating our clients about policies that contribute to independence and advocating for them. Applying the knowledge acquired in this chapter can mean the difference between one's clients returning to/entering employment versus remaining dependent on government benefits and absent independence, living independently or in an institutional setting, and/or maintaining a place in everyday community activities or finding themselves excluded from community life.

AMERICANS WITH DISABILITIES ACT

To understand the protection the ADA affords Carlotta and the roles it provides for occupational therapists and occupational therapy assistants (OTAs), one must first have a basic understanding of the ADA, its definitions, and how the courts have interpreted the law. Congress passed the ADA in 1990 in an effort to reduce discrimination against individuals with disabilities and promote their inclusion in the mainstream of society. The law's antidiscrimination provisions cover employment, certain state and local government services, public accommodations, communications, and public transportation. This chapter

THREADED CASE STUDY

Carlotta, Part 1

Carlotta is a 50-year-old woman (prefers she, her, hers) with severe rheumatoid arthritis. Since her most recent exacerbation, she finds she must use a wheelchair for mobility. She has always prided herself on her independence and does not want to rely on her children or husband for assistance. She loves going to the movies, shopping, and traveling. Carlotta works as a Spanish teacher at a local high school.

She comes to the occupational therapist (OT) concerned about several things. How will she be able to participate in her work and leisure occupations from her wheelchair when some places (and people) in the community, including her classroom, are not wheelchair friendly or accessible? How will she manage airplane travel from a wheelchair? How can she independently participate in activities of daily living (ADLs) from a wheelchair when her landlord of 12 years will not allow her to make the changes needed in her apartment?

This chapter addresses Carlotta's concerns by expanding the concept of occupational therapy (OT) interventions to include advocacy as a key concept of intervention. As we address the occupations significant to Carlotta, we will look at three important laws for guidance and support in promoting occupational performance; we also will look to these laws to support our intervention plan. These laws are:

- The Americans with Disabilities Act (ADA),[81] including the Americans with Disabilities Act Amendments (ADAA)[82] and the 2010 ADA Standards for Accessible Design[113]
- The Air Carrier Access Act[78]
- The Fair Housing Act[95]

Each law provides an avenue for OT intervention that promotes the greater good for many individuals with disabilities. Each law also provides specific supports for our efforts to promote our client's desire to increase and improve her participation at work, at home, and in the community.

Carlotta's evaluation shows that as a person with a chronic disability, she is a very sophisticated player.[80] Over almost 25 years of living with arthritis, she has acquired many adaptive devices and adaptive behaviors (e.g., reachers, jar openers, bathtub benches, joint protection techniques, work simplification) to make her life easier, facilitate independent participation, and prevent further damage to the joints of her hands. She requires the assistance of others for some tasks.

Her occupational profile shows that her job as a Spanish teacher at the large private school where she has worked for 18 years is very important to her.[80] She believes that she can do her job but will have some difficulty navigating the classroom in her wheelchair because of the presence of multiple levels. Her classroom is the former orchestra classroom. She also expresses concerns about continuing her weekly excursions to the movies. How can she navigate the old theater in town in which the old upstairs balcony was turned into a separate screen theater with a one-flight walk up? Before she began to use a wheelchair herself, she saw wheelchair users at the local shopping mall struggling to get in the door, and she thinks that this will present a barrier to her shopping or, as she puts it, "retail therapy." How will she manage at the airport and aboard airplanes in her quest to find the perfect bed and breakfast (another hobby)? Finally, from her experience as an individual with a disability, she knows that she will need more adaptations in her bathroom to participate in activities of daily living. She is particularly concerned because her landlord has already told her she cannot widen the bathroom door or install grab bars in the bathtub. She is interested in finding alternatives so that she can take care of herself and not have to move. She also expressed concern about her difficulty carrying out a home aquatics program prescribed by her previous occupational therapist. She now requires assistance to get into the pool at her apartment complex, but the complex's rules do not allow guests on weekends.

Disability laws heavily influence the facilitation of participation in work, leisure, and the community. Ignoring disability laws can promote ineffective intervention plans.[80] To move forward with an intervention plan, Carlotta's occupational therapists first must understand both the disability laws that affect the areas of concern to their client and the ways these laws can provide a basis for intervention.

explores Title I (employment), Title II (state and local government services), and Title III (public accommodations) and how they affect OT practice.

Title I: Employment

Before the ADA became law, the Rehabilitation Act of 1973 prohibited discrimination against qualified individuals with disabilities in employment by three categories of employers: (1) the federal government, (2) employers who contract with the federal government to provide goods and service, and (3) employers who were recipients or beneficiaries of federal funding.[105]

Congress extended that protection by expanding it to private employers who are not dependent on federal funding by passing the ADA in 1990. Because one of Carlotta's concerns is her work and whether she can continue to participate in her work from a wheelchair, knowledge of Title I of the ADA can provide a foundation for OT intervention.

Title I of the ADA prohibits discrimination against individuals with disabilities in employment with private, nongovernment employers who have 15 or more employees. In a nutshell, the prohibition against discrimination in Title I states[74]:

No covered entity shall discriminate against a qualified individual on the basis of disability in regard to job application procedures, the hiring, advancement, or discharge of employees, employee compensation, job training, and other terms, conditions, and privileges of employment.

To understand this statement, one must understand the terms used by answering the following questions:
- Who is considered "an individual with a disability" under the ADA?
- What is a "qualified individual with a disability" under the ADA?
- What is considered "discrimination" under the ADA?

The ADA refers to "individuals with disabilities," as opposed to "disabled individuals" to give voice to politically correct terminology that stresses the individual first, not the disability. It defines the phrase individual with a disability broadly under three umbrella categories, which are considered in the court cases discussed in the next section.

Changes in the ADA

When Congress passed the original ADA, it intended to create an inclusive society in which people with disabilities would work, engage in everyday community activities, and benefit from state and local benefits and services side by side and on the same basis as people without disabilities.[81] Looking back, on the 30th anniversary of the ADA, we see that individuals with disabilities have achieved success in gaining access to participation in the community and in government benefits and services.

Employment under Title I had proved to be the biggest disappointment with the ADA. Greeted with great fanfare by the disability community, the courts took a civil rights bill intended to provide employment rights for people with disabilities and decimated its intent. Though originally given a broad mandate by Congress and intended to cover all who fit within the

definition of "individual with a disability," the Supreme Court and lower courts chipped away at these protections and narrowed the definition of "individuals with a disability."

Ruling on three cases in one day, the Supreme Court severely restricted protection for individuals with disabilities in the employment arena.[79] For example, the Court ruled that individuals were not considered persons with disabilities if they used ameliorative measures to reduce the impact of their disabling condition.[102] The lower courts interpreted this to mean that someone with diabetes, who took insulin, was not considered a person with a disability.[94]

In *McClure v. General Motors Corp.*, 75 Fed. Appx. 983 (5th Cir. 2003), the court held that Mr. McClure's fascioscapulohumeral muscular dystrophy, which prevented him from lifting his arms above his shoulders and required him to use an accommodation to perform his job as a mechanic, did not make him a person with a disability. The court stated, "But the evidence [of limitations from his fascioscapulohumeral muscular dystrophy] does not show that these differences rise to the level of severe restrictions."[99] Like Carlotta, Mr. McClure had many adaptive devices that "ameliorated the effects"[99] of his disability and its impact on everyday activities.

The lower courts also interpreted the Supreme Court's restrictions as imposing significant restrictions on individuals with intellectual disabilities. As presented in *Littleton v. Wal-Mart*,[98] Mr. Littleton had an intellectual disability and, with the assistance of a job coach, went for an interview with Wal-Mart for a shopping cart attendant position. Although arrangements were made in advance for the job coach to attend the interview, when they arrived, Wal-Mart's personnel would not allow the job coach to attend the interview. Mr. Littleton did not get the job. The court acknowledged that Mr. Littleton had an intellectual disability, which it referred to as "mental retardation," a term now considered offensive. In denying Mr. Littleton a trial and declaring that he was not an individual with a disability, the court said in its opinion, "He has pointed to no evidence which would create a genuine issue of material fact regarding whether he was substantially limited in the major life activity of learning because of his mental retardation [now referred to as intellectual disability]."[98] The Supreme Court refused to hear Mr. Littleton's appeal (128 S.Ct. 302 [2007]).

The Court also said that episodic conditions, such as epilepsy, did not qualify as a disability. For example, in *Todd v. Academy Corp.*,[109] the court found that Mr. Todd was not an individual with a disability because the effects of his seizures were not substantial, since they lasted "only" 10 to 15 seconds and did not occur frequently enough.[109] In another case, *EEOC v. Sara Lee*,[93] the court held that the employee was not entitled to a reasonable accommodation from the employer because the employee took medications for seizures and therefore was not a person with a disability.[93]

The Supreme Court further limited the rights of people with disabilities when it reviewed what it means to be "substantially limited in a major life activity" in the case of *Williams v. Toyota Motor Mfg.* Mrs. Williams had carpal tunnel syndrome and myotendinitis. The Court declared that people with disabilities had to have multiple limitations in their everyday activities to be considered a person with a disability; one limitation was not enough.[115]

As a result of these decisions, the ADA faded into a hollow promise for people with disabilities in employment. Its definitions were meaningless. Its safeguards no longer provided protection for people with any disability. Veterans returning from the wars in Iraq and Afghanistan with limb loss feared that employers could discriminate against them and that the courts would not stand behind them because of the mitigating effect of their prostheses. Carlotta could have found herself without the ADA's protection because her wheelchair and adaptive aids mitigated the impact of her arthritis.

The disability advocacy community lobbied Congress to change the law to restore Congress' original intent to ensure that people with disabilities could work and not face unnecessary discrimination. These efforts led to the passage of the ADA Amendments Act (ADAAA), which specifically rejected the Supreme Court's decisions and broadened the definitions portion of the ADA to return the law to its original intent: a broad scope of protection under the ADA.[74] It also extended all of its changes to the Rehabilitation Act of 1973.[82]

The first definition states that with reference to individuals, disability means "(i) A physical or mental impairment that substantially limits one or more of the major life activities of such individual."[41] A physical or mental impairment includes "any physiological disorder or condition, cosmetic disfigurement or anatomical loss affecting one or more of the following body systems: neurological, musculoskeletal, special sense organs, respiratory (including speech organs), cardiovascular, reproductive, digestive, genitourinary, hemic and lymphatic, skin, and endocrine."[44] The revised definition of physical or mental impairment included most of the traditional medical diagnoses seen by occupational therapists in the individuals they treat; including, for example, individuals with multiple sclerosis, spinal cord injury, cerebrovascular accident (CVA), cerebral palsy, and arthritis—Carlotta's condition—which affects the musculoskeletal system. Mental or psychological impairments included "any mental or psychological disorder, such as an intellectual disability [formerly termed 'mental retardation'], organic brain syndrome, emotional or mental illness, and specific learning disabilities."[45]

The ADAAA broadened the meaning of the phrase "substantially limits" based on Congress' finding that the former regulation that defined "substantially limited" to mean "significantly restricted" was inconsistent with Congressional intent because the standard was too high.[81,83] The ADAAA specified that the term "substantially limits" be interpreted consistently with the findings and purposes of the ADAAA enacted in 2008.[84]

The implementing regulations incorporated the policies that Congress outlined in the ADAAA into a series of rules to help define "substantially limiting." The closest one to an actual definition states[48]:

An impairment is a disability within the meaning of this section if it substantially limits the ability of an individual to perform a major life activity as compared to most people in the general population. An impairment need not prevent,

or significantly or severely restrict, the individual from performing a major life activity in order to be considered substantially limiting. Nonetheless, not every impairment will constitute a disability within the meaning of this section.

The remaining rules explained how to interpret this general rule. As Congress intended, the rule was to be interpreted "broadly in favor of expansive coverage"[48] so that people such as Carlotta were covered by the ADA. Furthermore, the ADAAA required that lawsuits brought under the ADA focus on whether employers "complied with their obligations and whether discrimination has occurred, not whether an individual's impairment substantially limits a major life activity."[48] Accordingly, the threshold issue of whether an impairment "substantially limits" a major life activity should not demand extensive analysis.[48]

At the same time, the regulations say that the "determination of whether an impairment substantially limits a major life activity requires an individualized assessment."[47] This is an area in which occupational therapists can provide consultation. If Carlotta must prove that she is an individual with a disability, the occupational therapist can help provide the individualized assessment of her disability and specify the major life activities limited by her arthritis. The regulations reiterate that the standard used for this assessment is lower than the previous "substantially limited" standard.[47]

The regulations also say that the "comparison of an individual's performance of a major life activity to the performance of the same major life activity by most people in the general population usually will not require scientific, medical, or statistical analysis."[49] However, an individual with a disability, such as Carlotta, could present "scientific, medical, or statistical evidence" to show the comparison, which could include evidence from an occupational therapy therapist and an occupational therapy assessment.[49]

The other rules governing "substantially limited" incorporated the specific concerns that Congress expressed in the law to address the problems created by the Supreme Court cases: mitigating measure, an impairment that is episodic or in remission, and an impairment in only one major life activity. Under the ADAAA, the ameliorative effects of mitigating measures would no longer play a role in the determination of whether an impairment substantially limited a major life activity.[50] Congress specified examples of mitigating measures, several of which fall under the umbrella of occupational therapy intervention, as follows[84]:

1. "Medication, medical supplies, equipment, or appliances, low-vision devices (which do not include ordinary eyeglasses or contact lenses), prosthetics including limbs and devices, hearing aids and cochlear implants or other implantable hearing devices, mobility devices, or oxygen therapy equipment and supplies"
2. "Use of assistive technology"
3. "Reasonable accommodations or auxiliary aids or services"
4. "Learned behavioral or adaptive neurological modifications"

An episodic impairment or one that is in remission is considered a disability "if it would substantially limit a major life activity when active."[51] An impairment need limit only one major life activity to be considered a substantially limiting impairment.[52] For Carlotta, this means that *none* of the following circumstances—her use of assistive technology, a limitation only in walking, and remission of her arthritis—would prevent her from qualifying as substantially limited or a person with a disability.

Major life activities include many areas of occupation and functions related to ADLs, including "but . . . not limited to, caring for oneself, performing manual tasks, seeing, hearing, eating, sleeping, walking, standing, sitting, reaching, lifting, bending, speaking, breathing, learning, reading, concentrating, thinking, communicating, interacting with others, and working."[46] Another category of major life activities includes "operation of a major bodily function, including functions of the immune system, special sense organs and skin; normal cell growth; and digestive, genitourinary, bowel, bladder, neurological, brain, respiratory, circulatory, cardiovascular, endocrine, hemic, lymphatic, musculoskeletal, and reproductive functions. The operation of a major bodily function includes the operation of an individual organ within a body system."[46]

Sometimes, when determining whether a person is limited in a major life activity, one may want to look at the condition under which individuals perform the activities, the manner in which they perform them, and/or how long it takes individuals to perform them.[48] However, the regulations give examples of certain disabilities that one could easily conclude will substantially limit at least the major life activity indicated in Box 15.1.

The OT evaluation provides the information the court will want to use to make a determination whether an individual is substantially limited in major life activities. Occupational therapists may find themselves assisting employers, attorneys, and others by providing this information, if requested.

The OT evaluation of Carlotta shows that she has arthritis, which substantially limits the major life activity of walking. Carlotta's arthritis also substantially limits her musculoskeletal function. She has difficulty participating in or is unable to

participate in a variety of tasks related to everyday living. In light of these limitations, she probably falls under the first definition of disability.

The second definition of an individual with a disability under the ADA includes someone who has a record of having had such an impairment, as described in the first definition.[42] This category includes individuals with a history of a disabling condition, such as a person who had multiple sclerosis that is now in remission or a person who has been cured of hepatitis C.

The third definition of an individual with a disability includes situations in which a person is regarded as having a substantially limiting impairment that is a perception of a disability based on myths, misperceptions, fears, and stereotypes.[43] For example, suppose a morbidly obese individual, Sue, seeks a promotion to a position that requires frequent trips out of town. The person empowered to decide whether Sue gets that promotion assumes that Sue will have difficulty managing the traveling because of her size. The manager is concerned that Sue will struggle with walking through the airports, breathing, and other nonsedentary aspects of her job. Sue has had a perfect attendance record and has always received excellent performance appraisals. The manager bases his failure to promote Sue on his assumptions about her supposed difficulty walking, breathing, and completing nonsedentary tasks, and these assumptions are simply not true. The manager regards Sue as being an individual with a substantially limiting impairment.

Individuals Not Covered by the ADA

The ADA provides protection against disability discrimination only for those who meet the criteria outlined earlier. This means that individuals with temporary impairments, such as a broken leg or a knee replacement that is likely or expected to heal normally, will not find that the ADA protects them. Individuals who have impairments that are not substantially limiting, such as a visual limitation correctable with eyeglasses, will not find benefits under the ADA.

Furthermore, the ADA enumerates specific exclusions in its definition of disability. For example, it does not provide protection for individuals who fall into one of the following categories: transvestites, homosexuals, pedophiles, exhibitionists, voyeurs, and gender disorders not caused by physical impairments.[63] The ADA further excludes from its protection illegal drug users, compulsive gamblers, kleptomaniacs, pyromaniacs, and alcoholics whose alcohol use prevents them from performing their jobs as well as people with substance use disorders resulting from their current illegal use of drugs.[64] The ADA does provide protection against discrimination based on disability for recovering illegal drug users, as long as they participate in a rehabilitation program.

Qualified Individual With a Disability

Title I of the ADA does not protect all individuals with disabilities. It protects only those who are a qualified individual or person with a disability. The ADA specifies that "the term 'qualified,' with respect to an individual with a disability, means that the individual satisfies the requisite skill, experience, education, and other job-related requirements of the employment

---

BOX 15.1 Impairments That Substantially Limit Major Life Activities

- Deafness substantially limits hearing.
- Blindness substantially limits seeing.
- An intellectual disability (formerly termed mental retardation) substantially limits brain function.
- Partially or completely missing limbs or mobility impairments requiring the use of a wheelchair substantially limit musculoskeletal function.
- Autism substantially limits brain function.
- Cancer substantially limits normal cell growth.
- Cerebral palsy substantially limits brain function.
- Diabetes substantially limits endocrine function.
- Epilepsy substantially limits neurological function.
- Human immunodeficiency virus (HIV) infection substantially limits immune function.
- Multiple sclerosis substantially limits neurological function.
- Muscular dystrophy substantially limits neurological function.
- Major depressive disorder, bipolar disorder, posttraumatic stress disorder, obsessive compulsive disorder, and schizophrenia substantially limit brain function.

Adapted from 29 CFR §1630.2 (j)(3)(i-iii).

position such individual holds or desires and, with or without reasonable accommodation, can perform the essential functions of such position."[53] The first inquiry in deciding whether an individual with a disability meets the basic job requirements looks at the individual's amount of experience, level of education, and skills necessary to perform the job. Carlotta meets these requirements because the school hired her as a qualified teacher more than 18 years ago; therefore, she meets the basic education, skills, and experience requirement. The next inquiry is whether the individual can perform the essential functions of the job.

Essential Job Functions

The ADA defines essential job functions as job duties fundamental to the position that the individual holds or desires to hold, as opposed to functions that are marginal functions.[54] Essential functions are those that the individual who holds the position must be able to perform with or without the assistance of a reasonable accommodation. One may consider a function essential because the position exists to perform the particular function. These essential functions are usually obvious. For example, a typist must type and a proofreader must proofread.

A function is essential because of the limited number of employees available who can share the particular function. For example, because there are only three Spanish teachers at Carlotta's school, Carlotta must collaborate with the other two Spanish teachers to write and direct the annual Spanish language pageant. If the school employed 20 Spanish teachers, it could divide responsibilities so that Carlotta did not have to participate in the annual Spanish language pageant.

An essential function is also one in which the function is so specialized that the employer hires the person in the position for his or her particular expertise or ability to perform that function. For example, the position of brain surgeon is a highly specialized one, and the person in this position is hired to perform highly technical surgery.

Whether a function is an essential function is determined on a case-by-case basis. Specific evidence will support whether a particular function is essential. The Equal Employment Opportunity Commission (EEOC), the federal agency that enforces Title I's provisions, and the courts look at seven factors[55] as evidence of whether a function is essential (Box 15.2).

In some situations, essential functions are obvious. For example, the essential functions of a receptionist's position may include answering telephones, taking messages, and greeting and announcing visitors. Typing may be a marginal function for a receptionist in a very busy office where the receptionist has

not had to type anything at all over the last 6 months. Essential job functions are determined on a case-by-case basis by looking at the facts of each situation. Occupational therapists can help determine essential job functions by looking at the job description, by conducting focus groups with employees, and by performing a job analysis as discussed in Chapter 14.

In determining essential job functions, the focus must be on the outcome or job tasks that employers expect employees to perform. The definition of essential job functions focuses on the concept of job duties or expected outcomes, not the physical demands required to perform a job duty. In other words, an essential function is a task that one must perform to perform the job, not a physical function. Essential functions are not bending, lifting, walking, climbing, or other physical demands. For example, being a mail clerk for a large corporation includes delivering mail as one of the essential functions. The essential function is not walking and carrying the mail, but rather the outcome of delivering the mail. A mail clerk who is not able to carry the mail could push the mail on a cart to accomplish the same result or outcome. Essential functions are what you do, not how you do it.

The job description, job analysis, and discussions with Carlotta about her job show that as a teacher, Carlotta must perform several essential functions, including grading papers and tests and recording their results, discussing student progress with parents, preparing lesson plans, motivating students, and maintaining order in the classroom. (Note that these essential functions are all specific job tasks and not physical functions, such as "hand manipulation skills for writing" or "walking around the classroom.") The OT evaluation shows that Carlotta is able to perform these functions for her position as a Spanish teacher. However, she may have difficulty maneuvering around the classroom to the desks of the individual students because of steps and multiple levels in the former band classroom in which she currently teaches Spanish. Carlotta will also have difficulty writing on the blackboard from a wheelchair. The key to facilitating Carlotta's continued participation in the workplace lies in making reasonable accommodations.

Reasonable Accommodations

The ADA defines reasonable accommodations as any change in the work environment or in the way that work is customarily performed that enables an individual with a disability to enjoy equal employment opportunity.[56] Not all employees are entitled to reasonable accommodation. Employers need to make reasonable accommodations only for employees with disabilities who are qualified (Box 15.3).

Reasonable accommodations include three subcategories. First, reasonable accommodations include modifications or adjustments in the job application process that enable consideration of a qualified applicant with a disability for employment in a position that the person wants.[57] This would include reading a job application to an individual with dyslexia or modifying the way a preplacement screening is performed to accommodate an individual with one hand. If Carlotta were to apply for another position, her potential employer would need to provide her with an accessible entrance to the human resources department so that she could obtain a job application.

BOX 15.2 Seven Factors That Determine Essential Job Functions

- The employer's judgment of which functions are essential
- Written job descriptions prepared before the hiring process begins
- The amount of time spent performing the job function
- The consequences of not requiring the performance of a particular function
- The terms of the collective bargaining agreement
- The work experience of previous employees who held the job
- The current work experience of incumbents in similar positions

The potential employer would also have to allow her to use a larger pen for filling out an application because she uses the larger pen to prevent joint changes in her hand. As an alternative, the potential employer can provide someone to assist her in filling out the application.

The modifications and adaptations that occupational therapists most typically provide fall under the umbrella of the second category of reasonable accommodations. The second category includes modifications or adjustments to the work environment or to the manner or circumstances in which the position is customarily performed to enable an individual with a disability who is qualified to perform the essential functions of that position.[58] Occupational therapists have traditionally been involved in this area by modifying job sites, including raising or lowering work heights, making a jig, or having the individual with a disability use a piece of equipment (e.g., a cart) to move objects rather than carrying them.

OT PRACTICE NOTES

Occupational therapists may help human resources personnel to understand how disabling conditions, and the limitations in performance skills and client factors that accompany them, can affect the hiring process. In addition, occupational therapists can suggest appropriate, reasonable accommodations available for the application and interview process, which can prevent unintentional discrimination.

Carlotta's continued participation in her work environment will require reasonable accommodations in her intervention plan in the form of changes in the way the work is performed. For example, Carlotta's employer could reasonably accommodate her by moving her to a different classroom, one that is on a single level and that does not have steps or risers; this would provide Carlotta physical access to the students at their desks. Carlotta could also benefit from a laptop computer with a projector that has a liquid crystal display (LCD), which will eliminate the need for her to write on the board—an impossible task from wheelchair level. (See Chapter 14 for a more detailed discussion of job modifications.)

Occupational therapists and OTAs working on the development of reasonable accommodations should note that employers must provide an effective reasonable accommodation—this means one that works, not the most expensive accommodation or the specific accommodation the employee wants. Although the employee suggests the specific type of accommodation, ultimately the employer gets to select the accommodation used. If a shoebox with some rubber bands wrapped around it works as well as the high-tech computerized gadget that the employee requests, the employer need only provide the shoebox with the strategically placed rubber bands.

The third category of reasonable accommodations includes modifications or adjustments that enable employees with a disability to enjoy equal benefits and privileges of employment as other similarly situated employees without disabilities enjoy.[59] For example, suppose the language department at Carlotta's school customarily holds an annual international fair for all the students and their families at the school. The teachers compete by class for the best food, costumes, and projects. The teacher of the winning class wins prizes supplied by the Parent-Teacher Association (PTA). Under the ADA, the school would be required to hold the fair at an accessible location so that Carlotta could participate. This would also apply to the school's annual holiday party and all other school functions for employees. Occupational therapists can improve awareness on the part of employers, assist them in making reasonable accommodations, and help sensitize them to the needs of individuals with disabilities in these situations.

According to the ADA, reasonable accommodations may include physical changes to make facilities accessible, in addition to other nonenvironmental changes. Depending on the individual circumstances, reasonable accommodations can include job restructuring; part-time or modified work schedules; reassignment to a vacant position; acquisition or modification of equipment or devices (e.g., Carlotta's laptop computer and LCD projector); appropriate adjustment or modification of examinations, training materials, or policies; provision of qualified readers or interpreters; and other similar accommodations for individuals with disabilities.[57,58]

For example, an individual who needs to begin kidney dialysis may find that leaving work early 3 days a week reasonably accommodates his needs. Allowing a cashier with fatigue from multiple sclerosis to sit instead of stand while working may reasonably accommodate her needs. Because of their knowledge of the limitations of impairments and how to adapt the work environment to the individual, occupational therapists can suggest and/or design many of these accommodations while working with the client. Carlotta has a good understanding of much of what she needs to reasonably accommodate her work needs, and her intervention plan should incorporate her insights and suggestions.

The most efficient way for employers to identify the reasonable accommodations that an individual employee may need is to initiate an informal, interactive process with the qualified individual with a disability in need of the accommodation.[85] Employers will find that individuals with a disability are often in the best position to determine which reasonable accommodations they may need to enable job performance. Occupational therapists may participate in this effort when the parties need additional expertise to make these accommodations. The EEOC recognizes the expertise of occupational therapists in helping employers and individuals with disabilities make reasonable accommodations.[91]

The ADA provides an exception to the employer's requirement to provide reasonable accommodations for qualified individuals with disabilities. Employers need not provide reasonable accommodations when provision of the accommodation would cause an undue hardship to the employer. **Undue hardship** refers to any accommodation that would be unduly costly, extensive, substantial, or disruptive or that would fundamentally alter the nature or operation of the business.[60] For example, it would probably be an undue hardship for the school to fix Carlotta's classroom by ripping out the floor in the old band room to remove the risers and level the floor because this would eliminate the use of a very needed classroom for an extended period and might represent a significant expense. The alternative, to swap classrooms with another teacher, would be more cost-effective and less disruptive.

Determination of whether an accommodation presents an undue hardship to the employer involves looking at whether the proposed action requires significant difficulty or expense when the following factors are considered[61]:

- Nature and cost of the accommodation needed in light of tax credits and deductions and/or outside funding
- Overall financial resources of the facility, the number of people employed at the facility, and the effect on expenses and resources
- Overall financial resources, overall size of the business, and the number, type, and location of facilities
- Composition, structure, and functions of the workforce
- Impact of the accommodation on operation of the facility, including impact on the ability of other employees to perform their duties and impact on the facility's ability to conduct business

According to the Job Accommodations Network,[96] a federally funded program that has provided technical assistance in making accommodations for more than 25 years, data show that more than 56% of all accommodations cost nothing, and the remaining have a typical cost of $500, a cost that has remained consistent over time. The network's statistics also show that employers experience financial gains from the decreased costs of training new employees, a decrease in insurance costs, and an increase in worker productivity.

Discrimination Under the ADA

The ADA does not give one specific definition of discrimination. Instead, it specifies at least nine categories of activities considered discriminatory.

Limiting, classifying, or segregating. The first prohibited activity includes limiting, classifying, or segregating the employee because of his or her disability.[65] For example, if Carlotta's school were to require all employees who use wheelchairs for mobility to work in one wing of the first floor, it would be segregating the employees with disabilities. This section also forbids employers from asking any questions about an applicant's workers' compensation history during the interview or on the employment application because employers can use this information to limit or classify individuals because of their disability.

Poor disability etiquette can lead to limiting, classifying, and segregating individuals with disabilities in the workplace. The way co-workers treat people with disabilities and the language they use to refer to individuals with disabilities can also make people feel bad or left out of the workplace culture. One method employers may use to avoid limiting, classifying, or segregating employees because of their disabilities is to sensitize supervisors and other employees to working with individuals with disabilities. Nondisabled individuals who lack familiarity in socializing with individuals with disabilities may not know how to shake hands with a person who does not have a right hand. They may shout at a person who is deaf, instead of speaking clearly and facing the person with the hearing impairment.

OT PRACTICE NOTES

Occupational therapists can assist employers in providing sensitivity training experiences similar to those used in some OT program classrooms to develop an understanding of the disability experience. Giving co-workers time in a wheelchair or with a blindfold during planned activities can help them experience functional limitations, if only for a brief time, that may encourage the development of some sensitivity to how it feels to have limitations in performance and participation. Using lay language, free of confusing jargon during this kind of training, makes it easier to get the message across to co-workers unfamiliar with OT lingo.

OTs can work with supervisors and co-workers on basic disability etiquette tips, such as using politically correct terminology in which, as mentioned earlier, the person comes before the disability. For example, using the phrase "a person who had a stroke" is better than calling someone a "stroke patient" or "stroke victim" because the word *victim* has negative connotations. Using the phrase "wheelchair user" is more appropriate than "wheelchair bound" because no one is physically bound to the wheelchair, as a book is bound to its binding. Box 15.4 gives more tips on disability etiquette, and Box 15.5 presents tips on conducting the interview process that might help occupational therapists in consulting with employers on how to interview people with disabilities.

Contractual relationships that discriminate. The second prohibited activity includes participating in a contractual or other relationship that results in discrimination against qualified applicants or employees because of their disability.[66] This provision applies to collective bargaining agreements, contracts with employment agencies, and other contracts. For example, suppose Carlotta's employer contracted with an outside

BOX 15.4 **Disability Etiquette Do's and Don'ts**

- Do try to treat an individual with disabilities as you would treat any other person.
- Don't raise your voice at someone because he or she is in a wheelchair or has a visual or hearing impairment.
- Do address the person, not the wheelchair, interpreter, or guide.
- Don't trap yourself into thinking, "If I were disabled, how would I feel?"
- Do refer to an individual with a disability as "an individual with a disability."
- Don't refer to an individual with a disability as "the quadriplegic" or "Mary is a diabetic or epileptic."
- Do cleanse your vocabulary of offensive, outdated terms, such as wheelchair bound or stroke "victim" or as "afflicted with . . ." or "suffering from . . ."
- Don't refer to able-bodied persons as "normal."
- Do avoid generalizations such as "People with epilepsy are unpredictable" or "People with learning disabilities are not very intelligent."
- Don't apologize for comments such as "Let's take a walk" to an individual in a wheelchair or "Do you see my point?" to a person with a visual impairment.
- Do avoid statements such as "I admire your courage" or "You've done so much for a person in a wheelchair."
- Don't use outdated terminology such as "handicapped," "crippled," "retarded," "lame," "the disabled," or "the handicapped."
- Do provide assistance only in the manner requested.
- Don't take hold of an individual's wheelchair or push his or her wheelchair unless asked to do so.
- Do put yourself on the same level as the individual in a wheelchair as soon as possible by sitting down during the conversation or interview.
- Don't turn away when conversing with an individual with a hearing impairment.
- Do speak directly to the person, not the interpreter.
- Don't complete the sentences of an individual with communication impairments.
- Do rid your thinking of stereotypes about disabilities.
- Don't perpetuate another person's insensitivity to an individual with a disability.

Courtesy Barbara L. Kornblau, ADA Consultants.

BOX 15.5 **Interview Do's and Don'ts**

- Don't make notes about an individual's physical or mental condition.
- Do discuss reasonable accommodations when possible. The interviewee is an expert on accommodating his or her disability.
- Don't rely on body language as a measure during the interview process. Lack of eye contact or a mild grip handshake may be caused by an applicant's disability, not his or her lack of confidence.
- Do remember that individuals with disabilities may make poor interviewees if judged against many "traditional" interviewing standards.
- Don't try to put yourself in the applicant's place and ask yourself, "Could I do this job if I were disabled?"
- Do offer an applicant a job based on his or her abilities, not disabilities.
- Don't job stereotype.
- Do remember that communications skills are often an inaccurate measure of the intelligence, ability, or confidence of an individual with a speech or hearing problem.
- Don't patronize the applicant with a disability with your own body language.

Courtesy Barbara L. Kornblau, ADA Consultants.

workplace.[62] However, the direct threat must pose a significant risk for substantial harm to the health or safety of the individual or others that employers or others cannot eliminate or reduce to less than a significant risk by reasonable accommodation. Employers must consider the duration of the risk, the nature and severity of the potential harm, the likelihood that the potential harm will occur, and the imminence of the potential harm.[62]

For example, suppose Carlotta wanted to swap classrooms with a teacher whose classroom is on the second floor of the school, which has three stories and an elevator. The headmaster could not refuse to allow Carlotta to use this second-floor classroom because he fears that Carlotta, as a wheelchair user, would pose a direct threat in the event of a fire. The chance of a fire occurring is small; therefore, little likelihood exists that any harm will occur. Moreover, the school could develop an emergency plan in advance that would further lower the risk.

Employers must base the determination that an individual poses a direct threat on an individualized assessment of the person's present ability to safely perform the essential functions of the job. Employers must base the assessment on a reasonable medical judgment that relies on the most current medical knowledge and/or on the best available objective evidence.[62]

The regulations suggest that employers seek opinions from professionals who have expertise in the disability involved or direct knowledge of the individual with the disability. The EEOC recognizes that documentation of direct threat can come from occupational therapists "who have expertise in the disability involved and/or direct knowledge of the individual with a disability."[91] Often a reasonable accommodation can reduce the risk. For example, say that a teenager with epilepsy has a seizure every time the buzzer goes off on the fryer while he is working at the local fast-food restaurant. The occupational therapist could suggest that the employer could reasonably accommodate him by changing the buzzer to a bell.

Discrimination based on association with an individual with a disability. The fourth prohibited activity includes excluding or otherwise denying an equal job or benefits to a qualified individual because of a disability identified in an individual with

company to provide continuing education courses at her school. The continuing education company would have to comply with the ADA by offering reasonable accommodations when needed, such as allowing Carlotta to tape sessions or providing her with a note taker if she is unable to take notes during the classes. The occupational therapist could work with the continuing education provider to help develop other reasonable accommodations for Carlotta and other individuals with disabilities.

Using standards, criteria, and methods of administration that discriminate. The third prohibited activity includes the use of standards, criteria, or methods of administration that are not job related and consistent with business necessity and that have the effect of discrimination based on the disability.[67] For example, an employer could not require that Carlotta have a driver's license for promotion to chair of the Spanish Department if driving is not an essential function of the position.

Employers may use a direct threat standard to exclude from employment individuals whose disabilities pose a direct threat to the health and safety of themselves or others in the

whom the qualified individual is known to have a family, business, social, or other relationship or association.[68] For example, an employer could not refuse to hire Carlotta's husband because Carlotta has arthritis and is in a wheelchair and the employer is worried that Carlotta's husband may have excessive absences because of Carlotta's condition. In fact, this principle prohibits the employer from asking any questions that may reveal information about his wife's disability.

Failing to make a reasonable accommodation. The fifth prohibited activity includes failing to make a reasonable accommodation after a request for a particular accommodation for a known disability of a qualified individual or denying someone employment to avoid providing a reasonable accommodation, unless the employer can show that the accommodation would impose undue hardship on operation of the business.[69] As discussed previously, the occupational therapist can play a major role in assisting employers to determine reasonable accommodations. Carlotta's intervention plan includes her need for the following reasonable accommodations: a laptop computer with an LCD projector and a one-level classroom. Carlotta must request the specific accommodations that she wants. As part of the intervention plan, the occupational therapist may prepare a report for the school as documentation, explaining Carlotta's need for the particular accommodations, for submission with Carlotta's accommodation request. The occupational therapist may meet with the school's staff members to help them understand the needed accommodations. Should Carlotta's school fail to make the reasonable accommodations she requests, it would violate this provision of the ADA.

The employer must know that a prospective or actual employee is an individual with a disability before its obligation to make accommodations arises. Courts have found that an employer cannot discriminate based on disability if it does not know about the disability (*Morisky v. Broward County*).[101] Vague statements about one's limitations or past are not sufficient to put the employer on notice of a disability.[101] Disabilities such as multiple sclerosis, arthritis, learning disabilities, and mental health disorders may not be as obvious to an employer as the disability of a person in a wheelchair. To obtain reasonable accommodations for these hidden disabilities, employees or potential employees must disclose their disability to the employer. Occupational therapists can work with clients as employees or potential employees in determining whether to disclose the disability, when to disclose it, and how to disclose it.

Employment tests that screen out individuals with disabilities. The sixth prohibited activity involves using employment tests that tend to screen out individuals with disabilities on the basis of their disability, unless the test is shown to be job related for the position in question and is consistent with business necessity.[70] The EEOC considers a test job related if it measures a legitimate qualification for the specific job in question.[91] A test is not consistent with business necessity if it excludes an individual with a disability because of the disability and is not related to the essential functions of the job.[91] For example, under this section of Title I, the private school where Carlotta works could not give a written, 12th grade–level reading test to an individual with a known learning disability who applies for a janitorial

position. The janitorial position requires reading labels, which are on a fourth-grade reading level. The 12th grade–level test would screen out the applicant based on her disability and is neither job related nor consistent with business necessity.

Administering tests to measure physical attributes, not skills or aptitudes. The seventh prohibited activity involves failing to administer tests in a manner to ensure that when administered to a job applicant or employee with a disability that impairs sensory, manual, or speaking skills, the test results accurately reflect the skill, aptitude, or whatever other factor of the applicant or employee that the test purports to measure rather than the sensory, manual, or speaking skills, except when such skills are the factors that the test purports to measure.[71] For example, in *Stutts v. Freeman*,[108] an individual with dyslexia was denied a heavy equipment job because he could not pass the written test required to enter a training program. The standard that he pass a written test had the effect of discriminating against the plaintiff as a result of his disability because the test was not meant to test the applicant's ability to read and write but rather his knowledge of heavy equipment operation. Had the employer administered the test orally, the potential employer would have focused on evaluation of the applicant's qualifications for the job, not his ability to read the material.

Retaliating against individuals who file discrimination claims. The eighth prohibited activity prevents employers from retaliating against individuals who file claims for discrimination under Title I.[72] Before an applicant can file a lawsuit in court under Title I, he or she must file a complaint with the EEOC. This section prohibits an employer from firing, demoting, or otherwise retaliating against an employee who files a charge of discrimination with the EEOC or otherwise pursues his or her rights under this law.

Conducting preemployment medical examinations or inquiries. The ninth and final prohibited activity prevents employers from conducting preemployment medical examinations of an applicant or employee or inquiring into whether the applicant is an individual with a disability or the nature and extent of the person's disability, before the employer extends an offer of employment to the applicant.[73] Under the ADA, a medical examination means a "procedure or test that seeks information about an individual's physical or mental impairments or health."[92] The EEOC considers a variety of factors in deciding whether a test is a medical examination. These factors include, among others, whether the test is administered or the results interpreted by a healthcare professional or someone trained by a healthcare professional; whether the test is designed to reveal an impairment; and whether the test measures the applicant's performance of a task or his or her physiologic responses to performing the task.[92]

Preplacement Screenings and Functional Capacity Assessments

The preplacement screenings and functional capacity assessments provision of Title I affects the way occupational therapists do business. Occupational therapists are often involved in preplacement screenings and functional capacity evaluations, which are sometimes considered under the category of fitness-for-duty examinations. Employers often hire occupational therapists to perform these tests (see Chapter 14). The ADA regulations outline the types of testing that employers (or those acting on their behalf) may perform and the stages at which they may perform them.

The hiring process involves two relevant stages. The first stage, the pre-offer, occurs during the interview process, before an employer extends an offer of employment to an applicant or candidate. The second stage, the post-offer, occurs after the employer has made a hiring decision and extends an offer of employment to the applicant or candidate. We often speak of this offer of employment as a conditional offer of employment because it is subject to withdrawal under certain circumstances, which this chapter addresses later.

During the pre-offer stage, an employer may conduct only a simple agility test. Employers and occupational therapists acting on their behalf may not conduct medical examinations or inquiries, preemployment physical examinations, preplacement screening, or functional capacity assessments during the pre-offer stage. An agility test is a simple test that looks at a person's physical agility. It is not a medical test. Agility tests do not involve medical examinations, physicians, or medical diagnoses. Employers may request clearance from the applicant's physician before administering an agility test.[91] The classic agility test for police recruits shows them running through tires, scaling a wall, and climbing ropes. Another example of a permissible agility test would include an employer asking an applicant to carry a piece of wallboard from one end of the construction site to the other.

Although employers may conduct these agility tests, the ADA rules govern their use. If an employer chooses to use an agility test, he or she must give the test to all similarly situated applicants or employees. If the agility test screens out individuals with disabilities, the employer must show that the test is job related, consistent with business necessity, and that the applicant could not perform the job with a reasonable accommodation.

During the post-offer stage, employers or those acting on their behalf may conduct agility tests, medical examinations and inquiries, preemployment physicals, preplacement screenings, and functional capacity assessments. If the employer chooses to give medical examinations, once a conditional offer of employment has been made, he or she must give the examination to all employees entering the same job category. The ADA does not require that a medical examination satisfy the job-related and consistent-with-business-necessity standards. However, if the employer withdraws a conditional offer of employment because of the results of the medical examination, he or she must be able to show (1) the reasons for the exclusion are job related and consistent with necessity, or the person is being excluded to avoid a direct threat to health or safety, and (2) no reasonable accommodation was available that would enable this person to perform the essential functions without a significant risk to health or safety or the accommodation would cause an undue hardship.

As mentioned earlier, during the post-offer stage, employers and occupational therapists acting on their behalf may perform preplacement screenings and functional capacity assessments. Both are subject to the same requirements as medical examinations. In other words, although the tests need not comply with the job-related and business-necessity requirements,

should the tests screen out individuals with disabilities, job related and business necessity become the required standard to meet. Reality dictates then that to comply with the ADA, the preplacement screening must be job related and test only the essential functions of the job. For example, assessing Carlotta's hand strength as part of the interview process for hiring her as a Spanish teacher would violate this provision of the ADA because hand strength is not job related and not related to an essential job function.

Employers and those acting on their behalf must keep the results of all medical examinations and inquiries confidential, with some limited exceptions. These exceptions include work restrictions information, insurance purposes, government investigations of ADA complaints, and state workers' compensation and second injury funds, which are funds set up by some states to encourage employers to hire individuals with previous workers' compensation–related or other injuries.

This prohibition against inquiries into medical and disability-related information also extends to job applications and interviews. Employers cannot ask questions about a person's disability or questions that will lead to information about a person's disability during the job interview process. Box 15.6 shows examples of questions employers may not ask during the interview process.

Occupational therapists can assist human resources professionals in the proper way to inquire into an individual's ability to perform the essential functions of a position without asking prohibited questions. Employers must base their interview questions on specific job functions, information that occupational therapists gather from the job analysis (described in more detail in Chapter 14). Ideally, the interviewer should have a job description prepared from the occupational therapist's job analysis and ask interviewees questions about the match between their skills and abilities and the job's essential functions.

Role of the Occupational Therapist

Occupational therapists can work with individuals with disabilities, as part of their intervention plan, to identify needed

---

BOX 15.6 Questions Not Permitted Under the ADA

- How did you become disabled?
- Are you in good health?
- Have you recovered from your prior disability?
- How much can you lift?
- How far can you walk?
- Have you been in a wheelchair your whole life?
- Do you have a driver's license? (if the job does not require driving or if a reasonable accommodation cannot eliminate the driving)
- Does your wife, husband, child, or roommate have a disability?
- Who takes care of your disabled husband (or wife or child)?
- Have you ever been injured in an accident?
- Have you ever filed a claim for worker's compensation?
- How were you burned?
- Do you have any physical conditions that would prevent you from doing your job?
- Do you have a good back?
- Have you ever been hospitalized?

accommodations that will enable participation in the workplace; they also can help the individual plan a strategy to obtain those accommodations from the employer. Occupational therapists can help their clients understand their right to reasonable accommodations under Title I of the ADA. This includes the requirement to request the specific accommodations needed and to furnish documentation of the need, which the occupational therapists can prepare for the client to provide to the employer. Occupational therapists may find themselves advocating for the accommodations to their client's employer.[86]

For example, as described earlier, Carlotta's occupational therapist can play a major role in her employer's provision of the accommodations she needs. Carlotta and her occupational therapist identified the accommodations she needs as part of her occupational profile and intervention plan. If the employer refuses to provide the accommodations after Carlotta provides the occupational therapist's documentation and if Carlotta eventually files a lawsuit, the occupational therapist may find himself or herself testifying in court about Carlotta's need for the accommodations.

Occupational therapists can also provide consultation services for employers who want to avoid litigation and who seek advice on making reasonable accommodations for their employees with disabilities. If Carlotta's employer were proactive, he or she may have contacted an occupational therapist for advice on how to accommodate Carlotta.

This kind of consultation, in which the client is the employer, not the individual with a disability, usually begins with a job analysis (see Chapter 14) to see what the job requires. The therapist compares this information with the individual's limitations and tries to develop accommodations to enable performance. This accommodation development stage cannot proceed without input from the person with the disability.

For example, the author was hired by a hospital to look at whether a nurse affected by some post-polio weakness and arthritis could use a scooter (wheelchair substitute–type scooter) as her requested accommodation to cut down on the number of steps she took during the day. The nurse had filed a charge of discrimination with the EEOC, and the hospital's attorney suggested hiring an occupational therapist to see whether the requested accommodations were reasonable, so that a full-blown lawsuit could be avoided if possible. The head nurse could not imagine a nurse using a scooter. The author performed a job analysis and determined that the scooter was a reasonable accommodation. Convincing the head nurse that the scooter was reasonable took more work in the form of sensitivity training (an area in which occupational therapists also make major contributions).

Suppose Carlotta decided she did not want to return to her teaching position because she wanted a career change from classroom teaching. An occupational therapist might suggest that Carlotta look for jobs with potential employers who are federal government contractors. Federal government contractors must develop affirmative action plans to recruit, hire, promote, and retain people with disabilities, with a workplace goal of 7%.[114] This recent workplace mandate also requires employers to evaluate their hiring practices and adjust them to achieve this goal.[114] In theory, this means that as a person with a disability,

Carlotta would have preference in hiring if she applied for a job with a company that contracts with the federal government, as long as she is qualified for the position.

If Carlotta were out of work for a period of time and needed to transition from disability benefits to employment, many work incentive programs exist to help ease her transition. Occupational therapists can learn more about the return-to-work incentive programs designed for people with disabilities from the Social Security Administration's *Red Book: A Guide to Work Incentives*.[107]

Title II: State and Local Government Services

Title II of the ADA prohibits state and local government entities, and those with whom they contract, from denying a qualified individual with a disability participation in or the benefits of services, programs, or activities provided to individuals without disabilities.[23] Title II's antidiscrimination protection in the employment of individuals with disabilities by state governments has been limited by cases decided by the U.S. Supreme Court. Individual state employees can no longer bring lawsuits for monetary damage in federal court when a state discriminates in its employment practices based on the disability.[89]

Title II's other requirements look similar to those of Title III, described in detail later for nongovernment entities. However, Title II goes further in its requirement for state and local government services than for privately owned entities in one particular concept: Title II requires that government agencies give qualified individuals with disabilities equal opportunity to participate in or benefit from the state or local government aid, benefits, or services.[24] This requires providing more access than in Title III's requirements to provide what is readily achievable, as described later in this chapter. Providing equal opportunity to state and local government services requires taking specific measures that allow access to equal services. These may include making facilities physically accessible, making policy changes, providing reasonable accommodations in the form of auxiliary aids and services, providing accessibility in public transportation, and supplying communication aids, such as 911 services for people with hearing impairments. It may include other accommodations described more fully under Title III later in this chapter. Occupational therapists can help state and local governments make some of the needed changes, as will be discussed further in this chapter.

Title II and Title III were amended through the rule-making process, and new regulations took effect March 15, 2011.[110-112] Most of the changes apply to both Title II and Title III. Several are specific to Title II. In particular, residential housing programs and detention and correctional facilities run by state and local governments must now comply with the applicable design requirements listed in the new 2010 Standards for Accessible Design, commonly called the 2010 Standards.[111,113]

Title III: Public Accommodations

Title III of the ADA prohibits discrimination against individuals with disabilities in places of public accommodation (PPAs). This description may seem slightly misleading because, despite its name, this section of the ADA covers privately owned entities that own or lease to others, places that effect commerce. In

TABLE 15.1   Places of Public Accommodation Under Title III

Category	Examples
Places of lodging	Hotels, motels
Establishments serving food or drink	Restaurants, bars
Places of exhibition or entertainment	Movie theaters, stadiums
Places of public gathering	Convention centers
Sales or rental establishments	Bakeries, shopping malls
Service establishments	Laundromats, funeral homes, physician's offices
Public transportation terminals	Train stations
Places of public display or collection	Museums, libraries
Places of recreation	Parks, zoos, amusement parks
Places of education	Preschools, private schools, colleges
Social service establishments	Daycare centers, senior centers
Places of exercise or recreation	Health clubs, bowling alleys, golf courses

other words, PPAs are privately owned entities where business of some kind is transacted or affected. The term PPA covers 12 broad categories enumerated in the ADA (Table 15.1).[25] The U.S. Department of Justice, the federal government agency charged with overseeing and enforcing Title III, reports that more than 5 million PPAs exist in the United States.[85]

The "super rule," which forms the basis for Title III, prohibits discrimination as follows:

> *No individual shall be discriminated against on the basis of disability in the full and equal enjoyment of the goods, services, facilities, privileges, advantages, or accommodations of any place of public accommodation by any private entity who owns, leases (or leases to), or operates a place of public accommodation.*[26]

Under Title III, PPAs must remove barriers to access, and if the PPA cannot remove the barriers, it must provide an alternative or reasonable accommodation to enable access to the goods and services it provides. Many think of the barriers that Title III addresses as architectural barriers or barriers in the physical environment, such as steps and curbs, that limit physical access to a place a person desires to go. However, although many view the requirements of Title III as a quasi–building code, removing barriers to access as described in the ADA refers to more than mere access through removal of physical barriers. It also refers to access caused by attitudinal barriers and rules and to policies based on myths, misperceptions, and fears about individuals with disabilities that act as barriers to their access to PPAs.

For example, before the ADA became law, some banks refused to allow individuals who are blind to have safe deposit boxes. The rationale behind this policy was that because individuals who are blind cannot see what is in their safe deposit boxes, how can they remove things that they need from the box? Only the safe deposit box holder can go into the viewing booth.

Based on misperceptions, banks believed themselves at risk for accusations of theft from the boxes, and consequently, they disallowed individuals who were blind from benefiting from the services they provided to individuals who were not blind. This practice discriminated against individuals with visual impairments. The ADA prohibits these practices and seeks to break down these kinds of barriers.

To further its mission of breaking down physical and attitudinal barriers, Title III specifies three broad principles that provide the foundation for its philosophy of inclusion of individuals with disabilities in society. First, PPAs must provide individuals with disabilities an equal opportunity to participate in or benefit from the goods and services offered.[27] Furthermore, PPAs must give individuals with disabilities an equal opportunity to benefit from the goods and services that they offer.[27] Finally, PPAs must provide the benefits in the most integrated setting possible.[27,28]

PPAs can violate Title III's mandates against discrimination by doing the following, among other things.

- Refusing to admit an individual with a disability merely because he or she has a disability.[27] For example, a restaurant cannot refuse to admit and/or serve an individual with cerebral palsy because he or she drools.

- Failing to provide goods and services to individuals with disabilities in the most integrated setting appropriate to the individual's needs.[28] For example, a professional or college football team cannot segregate all wheelchair users in a "handicapped" section in the end zone. It must allow wheelchair users to sit with family members and disperse wheelchair seating throughout the stadium.

- Using eligibility criteria that screen out or tend to screen out individuals with disabilities from full and equal enjoyment of goods and services.[30] For example, retail stores located in a busy tourist area require that individuals using credit cards show a driver's license as proof of identification as a way of cutting down on the use of stolen credit cards. However, this practice screens out individuals with visual impairments or other disabilities who do not qualify for driver's licenses. The retail stores would have to accept state identification cards in place of a driver's license from individuals with disabilities who do not qualify for driver's licenses.

- Failing to make reasonable modifications in policies, practices, or procedures when the modifications are necessary to offer goods, services, or facilities to individuals with disabilities.[31] The example given earlier about bank policies for safe deposit boxes and individuals who are blind is a good illustration of a policy that discriminates on the basis of disability. As another example, Great Grocery Store has a policy by which cashiers must place all checks in a specific column in the cash drawer. Carlotta's occupational therapist recommended that she use large-print checks because she can write more legibly with larger print. She attempts to give the cashier a large-print check. The cashier refuses to take the check because it does not fit in the cash drawer column for checks. She also tells Carlotta that their policy is to accept large-print checks only from blind people. Great Grocery Store must modify its policies and accept Carlotta's check.

- Failing to take steps to ensure that individuals with disabilities are not excluded or denied services, segregated, or otherwise treated differently from individuals without disabilities because of the absence of auxiliary aids and services.[33] Auxiliary aids as used in the ADA include devices that occupational therapists usually refer to as adaptive equipment or assistive technology. According to the regulations, auxiliary aids and services include, among other things, qualified interpreters on site or through video remote interpreting (VRI) real-time computer-aided transcription services, assistive listening devices, closed captioned decoders on televisions, Braille materials, taped texts, and "acquisition or modification of equipment or devices."[33]

For example, suppose Carlotta stays at a restored historic hotel in her quest for the perfect bed and breakfast. She finds that she can use the bathing facilities in her room only if she has a tub bench. The hotel would have to provide her with a bathtub bench as an auxiliary aid so that it will not exclude or deny her bathing services.

Two exceptions exist to the auxiliary aid provision requirement. The PPA need not provide an auxiliary aid that fundamentally alters the nature of the goods and services offered, or one that causes an undue burden.[33] An undue burden means that provision of the auxiliary aid would cause significant difficulty or expense. The impact on the PPA varies, depending on such elements as the size of the business and its budget. A major corporation should expect to spend more money on auxiliary aids and services than a neighborhood "mom and pop" operation. A fundamental alteration in the nature of the goods and services offered would occur, for example, if an individual with a visual impairment requested management to raise the lights in a bar in which the lights are customarily turned down low to create a particular ambiance or atmosphere.

- The PPA need not provide personal devices and services such as individually prescribed devices (e.g., eyeglasses) or services of a personal nature (e.g., eating, toileting, or dressing).[37] However, it would probably be a reasonable auxiliary service should Carlotta request that the restaurant cut her meat in the kitchen before serving her steak if weakness in her hands prevents her from performing this task.

- Failing to furnish auxiliary aids and services when necessary to ensure effective communication, unless an undue burden or fundamental alteration would result.[33] For example, Bob is deaf and needs a sign language interpreter to converse with others. When seeking counseling services at a private mental health clinic, he requests a sign language interpreter to enable him to communicate with the mental health therapist. The mental health clinic must provide the sign language interpreter unless it is an undue burden.

- Refusing to remove architectural and structural communication barriers in existing facilities when this is readily achievable.[34] Readily achievable means removal of barriers that can easily be accomplished and carried out without much difficulty or expense.[34] The ADA regulations provide 21 examples of steps PPAs can take to remove barriers (Box 15.7).

- The ADA regulations recognize that not all changes are immediately readily achievable. In concert with input from members of the disability community, the Justice

---

BOX 15.7 Examples of Ways to Remove Barriers

- Installing ramps
- Making curb cuts in sidewalks and entrances
- Repositioning shelves
- Rearranging tables, chairs, vending machines, display racks, and other furniture
- Repositioning telephones
- Adding raised markings on elevator control buttons
- Installing flashing alarm lights
- Widening doors
- Installing offset hinges to widen doorways
- Eliminating a turnstile or providing an alternative accessible path
- Installing accessible door hardware
- Installing grab bars in toilet stalls
- Rearranging toilet partitions to increase maneuvering space
- Insulating lavatory pipes under sinks to prevent burns
- Installing a raised toilet seat
- Installing a full-length bathroom mirror
- Repositioning the paper towel dispenser in a bathroom
- Creating designated accessible parking spaces
- Installing an accessible paper cup dispenser at an existing inaccessible water fountain
- Removing high-pile, low-density carpeting
- Installing vehicle hand controls

Department set forth four priorities in the ADA regulations that PPAs should follow to comply with the barrier removal requirements (Box 15.8).[33]

- Refusing to provide access to goods and services through alternative, readily achievable measures when removal of barriers is not readily achievable.[36] The ADA regulations give three examples of alternatives to removal of barriers, including, for instance, providing curb service or home delivery for an inaccessible restaurant, retrieving merchandise from inaccessible shelves or racks in the grocery store, and relocating activities to accessible locations.[36] For example, in pursuit of her movie hobby, Carlotta wants to see the latest popular art film. A multiscreen cinema is showing the film, but the particular theater the film is being shown in requires climbing a flight of steps. The theater must rotate the films to provide Carlotta access to the film that she wants to see.[36]

- Failing to provide equivalent transportation services and to purchase accessible vehicles in certain circumstances.[38] For example, Robby Rat's Fantasy Garden, a large amusement park, provides trams to take people to their cars in its enormous parking lots. On one of her trips, Carlotta takes her grandchildren to the Fantasy Garden. The Fantasy Garden must provide accessible transportation from the parking lot to the entry gates for Carlotta.

- Failing to maintain the accessible features of facilities and equipment so it is readily accessible and usable by people with disabilities.[29] For example, Streams Department Store must maintain its accessible ramped entrance into the store. This means shoveling snow in the winter and raking leaves in the fall so that Carlotta has access into the store on her trips to the city.

Priority 1: Access Into a Place of Public Accommodation
First, the place of public accommodation (PPA) should try to provide access to and into the PPA from public sidewalks, parking, or public transportation. In other words, provide a way for individuals with disabilities to get into the building. For example, this includes, among other things as may prove necessary in individual circumstances, installing a ramp to the entrance, widening entrances, and providing accessible parking spaces.[34] Under this provision, the PPA is responsible for making sure that Carlotta can get from her parking space into the lobby of the movie theater.

Priority 2: Access to Areas Where Goods and Services Are Made Available
The second priority the PPA should focus on is providing access to areas of public accommodation where it makes goods and services available to the public. This step answers the following question: Now that individuals with disabilities can enter through our door, how do we get them to the actual part of the PPA where we provide the goods and services? This can include changes such as adjusting the layout of display racks, providing Braille and raised-character signage, widening doorways, providing visual alarms, and installing ramps.[33] The movie theater, under this section, would want to make sure Carlotta could get to the snack bar to purchase her popcorn and into the theater to watch the movie.

Priority 3: Access to Restrooms
The third priority for access is access to the restroom facilities. This may include modifications such as removing obstructing furniture or vending machines, widening doorways, installing ramps, providing accessible signage, widening toilet stalls, lowering paper towel dispensers and mirrors, and installing grab bars, usable faucet handles, and soap dispensers, to name a few. The movie theater would provide Carlotta access to the restrooms under this provision.[33]

Priority 4: Access to Goods and Services
The fourth and final priority for access is access to the goods, services, facilities, privileges, advantages, or accommodations offered at the PPA. This includes access to the actual goods or services that the PPA provides.[34] For Carlotta, the PPA needs to consider whether a place exists for her to sit in the movie theater so that she can watch the movie she wants to see. Can they remove seats to provide her a place to sit where she can sit with her family? Can they disperse the seats in the theater so that they do not have to segregate all of the wheelchair users in the back or front of the theater?

- Failing to design and construct new facilities and, when undertaking alterations, alter existing facilities in accordance with the ADA Accessibility Guidelines issued by the Architectural and Transportation Barriers Compliance Board and incorporated in the final Department of Justice Title III regulations or the 2010 Standards, depending on the date of completion of the new or altered facilities.[35,39,40,113] This is where the "building code" flavor of the ADA comes in. Specific requirements dictate how builders should design and decorate buildings to provide access. The 2010 ADA Standards for Accessible Design (2010 Standards) requirements are available online at (http://www.ada.gov/regs2010/2010ADAStandards/2010ADAStandards_prt.pdf).

Government agencies periodically update the accessibility guidelines and related standards. For example, the 2010

Standards allow PPAs to ask individuals to remove their service animal if it is out of control and the handler is not able to get it under control or if it is not housebroken.[32] The 2010 Standards also adopt a two-tiered approach to mobility devices by distinguishing wheelchairs and "other power-driven mobility devices," to include mobility devices used by individuals with disabilities, but not necessarily developed for that purpose, such as a Segway PT.[112] Wounded soldiers returning from war often use adapted Segway PTs for mobility. The new rules allow access for these alternative mobility devices. Another change in the 2010 Standards provides that places of lodging must allow individuals to make reservations for accessible guest rooms during the same hours and in the same manner as people without disabilities.[112]

Keep in mind that some state regulations differ from the 2010 Standards requirements. For example, Florida requires accessible parking spaces to have a 12-foot width (144 inches) and a 5-foot access aisle,[103] whereas the 2010 Standards require a width of 8 feet (96 inches) with a 5-foot access aisle.[76] The ADA regulations advise PPAs to follow the rule that provides the most access to individuals with disabilities.

Sometimes standards developed by government agencies exist only as recommended guidelines. For example, Carlotta may find it difficult to transfer from her wheelchair to an examination table for her annual Pap smear or to access mammography equipment from her wheelchair. Other wheelchair users may not have access to weight scales or other diagnostic equipment in their healthcare providers' offices. To address these needs, Section 4203 of the Patient Protection and Affordable Care Act established Section 510 of the Rehabilitation Act.[77] This new section required the Architectural and Transportation Barriers Compliance Board (also known as the U.S. Access Board), in consultation with the U.S. Food and Drug Administration (FDA), to develop accessibility standards for medical diagnostic equipment.

The Architectural and Transportation Barriers Compliance Board (Access Board) published a "Notice of Proposed Rulemaking" in 2012 as a first step in developing accessibility standards for medical diagnostic equipment (MDE) that would "allow independent entry to, use of, and exit from the equipment by individuals with disabilities to the maximum extent possible."[104] The MDE Advisory Committee included medical device manufacturers; healthcare providers, including an OT; standards-setting organizations; organizations representing individuals with disabilities; federal agencies; and other stakeholders and submitted its report to the U.S. Access Board with recommended standards at the end of 2013.[99,100] The Access Board issued its final standards in 2017 as recommended or voluntary standards.

As of this writing, these standards are recommendations only and are not required, but politics and advocacy could change their status to "required" in the future. However, occupational therapists should consider these standards when advising clients with disabilities about access needs in medical settings. These standards are also important for occupational therapists advising clients who seek OT consultation services for assistance in meeting their Title II and Title III access obligations in connection with the provision of medical services.

Role of the Occupational Therapist

Even though Congress passed the ADA more than 25 years ago, many examples point to a pervasive lack of compliance with access requirements.[88,97] Occupational therapists are in a unique position to promote Title III's access and inclusion mandates. With our knowledge of performance in occupations, performance skills, performance patterns, activity analysis, and client factors, we have the skills to look at how the physical environment can affect performance.[80] We know how to make adaptations in the environment, the task, or the person to enable performance despite the limitations an individual may have in performance skills. This knowledge base equips occupational therapists to act as consultants, helping PPAs comply with Title III's access requirement, by looking at limitations to accessibility and making recommendations to PPAs to improve access, both physical and nonphysical (including attitudes, policies, and procedures).

Occupational therapists may find themselves working from two angles in providing access intervention. Their clients may include individuals with disabilities, such as Carlotta, who seek to increase their participation in the community by increasing their access and inclusion. Alternatively, occupational therapists may find that their clients include proactive PPAs seeking to make their goods and services accessible to individuals with disabilities to avoid lawsuits and/or do the right thing.

When the individual with a disability is the client, the occupational therapist should perform an occupational profile that delves into the client's interests in the community, as was done with Carlotta.[80] The occupational therapist works with the client to determine what the barriers are to the client's participation in the community activities of his or her choice. In Carlotta's case, we know that movies and going to the mall are important to her. Part of our intervention plan will include problem-solving the changes

that Carlotta needs to be able to participate in these occupations, explaining her right to accommodations under Title III, and suggesting ways to advocate to the PPA for the needed changes. If the PPA fails to make changes to provide access for Carlotta, she can file an administrative complaint with the Department of Justice in Washington (https://www.ada.gov/t3compfm.htm) or immediately file a lawsuit. The occupational therapist may serve as a witness in Title III litigation, should it come to that.

When the PPA is the client, the occupational therapist should look at the goods and services the PPA offers, the policies and procedures it uses (especially customer service–related

---

OT PRACTICE NOTES

Consulting With Places of Public Accommodation

- Advise businesses that offer public accommodations, such as restaurants, movie theaters, hospitals, medical clinics, and hotels, how to make their facilities accessible to individuals with disabilities.
- Ensure that places of public accommodation are accessible to individuals with disabilities and make recommendations to remove architectural and other barriers.
- Assist in the acquisition of auxiliary aids to allow individuals with disabilities to have an equal opportunity to participate in or benefit from programs offered.
- Prevent lawsuits by performing accessibility audits and making recommendations for increased access and barrier removal on a proactive basis.
- Locate and/or acquire auxiliary aids and services for places of public accommodation.
- Train employees in how to make people with disabilities feel welcome in their facilities, how to use the auxiliary aids, and how to provide auxiliary services to individuals with disabilities.

OT PRACTICE NOTES

Consulting With Employers

- Analyze jobs to determine essential job functions and possible accommodations that one can easily make for a specific job.
- Develop or rewrite job descriptions based on job analysis that include specific descriptions of essential job functions.
- Modify job sites to make reasonable accommodations for individual employees with disabilities.
- Suggest specific devices and adaptive equipment that allow the employer to hire an individual with a disability who, with the assistance of the device, can now perform the essential functions of a given job.
- Sensitize co-workers and supervisors to interacting, supervising, and working effectively with individuals with disabilities.
- Train supervisors to develop reasonable accommodations for injured workers returning to the job, including workers' compensation claimants.
- Ensure that job sites are accessible to individuals with disabilities and make recommendations to remove architectural barriers when inaccessible features are found or to allow employees to work remotely when feasible.
- Propose post-offer, job-related employee screenings and/or evaluations for positions associated with high risk for injury.
- Perform an individualized assessment of a worker's present ability to safely perform the essential functions of the job to determine whether the worker with a disability poses a direct threat to the health and safety of himself or herself or others.
- Save businesses money by promoting cost-effective reasonable accommodations during the complaint or mediation process to avoid costly litigation.

OT PRACTICE NOTES

Advocating for Employees With Disabilities

- Analyze physical functions to determine, for the employee, whether he or she can perform the essential functions of a given job with or without reasonable accommodations.
- Suggest specific reasonable accommodations, such as adaptive equipment, auxiliary aids, modifications to the worksite, or working remotely to enable the prospective or returning employee to perform the essential functions of his or her job.
- Obtain adaptive devices or auxiliary aids to facilitate performance in the workplace and in the community.
- Develop strategies to prepare the prospective employee to suggest reasonable accommodations to human resources personnel during the interview and hiring process.
- Teach adolescents with disabilities entering the job market for the first time how to manage the application, hiring, and interview processes.
- Expand access to public accommodations in the mainstream of independent living, such as theaters, conference centers, hotels, and restaurants, through focusing on mobility in the community; identification of equipment, aids, and services; and advocacy to obtain them.
- Provide information to clients so they can develop a basic understanding of their rights under the ADA.

policies), and the physical access offered, in the ADA-delineated priority order. Just as an employment-related ADA consultation with an employer usually begins with a job analysis, an access consultation with a PPA begins with an accessibility audit. An accessibility audit is a review of the access and inclusion practices of a PPA from a physical and policy perspective. The accessibility audit looks at the 2010 Standards requirements, the types of modifications the PPA can make to increase access, and the readily achievable changes the PPA can make according to the priorities set in Title III. Fig. 15.1 presents an accessibility audit that includes examination of physical and nonphysical barriers to access according to the 2010 Standards and follows the priorities specified in Title III. Occupational therapists can also provide consultation services for employers.

How to Do an Accessibility Audit Under the ADA

A. Remember, Title III, Public Accommodations, is not limited to the physical accessibility of a building. Title III includes meaningful access and equal participation in all programs and services offered by the public accommodation.

1. Making something accessible is worthless if you do not identify its location. For example, public accommodations must include accessible signage to assist individuals in locating accessible bathrooms and building entrances.

B. Title III sets forth the following priorities for accessibility:

1. **Access to and into the place of public accommodation** from public sidewalks, parking, or public transportation. This includes installing a ramp to the entrance, widening entrances, and providing accessible parking spaces.

2. **Access to those areas of public accommodation where goods and services are made available to the public.** This includes adjusting the layout of display racks, providing Brailled and raised character signage, widening doorways, providing visual alarms, and installing ramps.

3. **Access to restroom facilities.** This includes removing obstructing furniture or vending machines, widening doorways, installing ramps, providing accessible signage, widening toilet stalls, lowering paper towel dispensers and mirrors, and installing grab bars.

4. **Access to the goods, services, facilities, privileges, advantages, or accommodations offered at the place of public accommodation.** This includes access to the actual goods or services themselves.

C. **The Accessibility Audit should follow the priorities set forth in Title III.**

STEP ONE: According to the first priority, look at the access to and into the place of public accommodation from public sidewalks, parking, or public transportation:

		YES	NO
1.	Are parking spaces 96 inches wide with an adjacent access aisle of 60 inches?	_____	_____
2.	Is one in every eight parking spaces served by a 96-inch access aisle marked "van accessible"?	_____	_____
3.	How many parking spaces are designated for individuals with disabilities? _____ (_____% of spaces) (compare with chart at ADAAG § 4.1.2(5)(a); 10% of total number provided for outpatient units or facilities should be accessible.)	_____	_____
4.	If covered parking is provided, is the ceiling at least 114 inches high to allow access to high-top vans?	_____	_____
5.	Are all curb ramps (curb cuts) from the parking spaces at a gradient of 1:20 with a textured, non-slip surface?	_____	_____

Fig. 15.1 How to do an accessibility audit to check for compliance with ADA requirements.[113] (Courtesy Barbara L. Kornblau, ADA Consultants, 1992, 2002, 2011.)

6. Are parking area and building separated by a street? _____ _____

7. Are the accessible parking spaces located on the shortest accessible route of travel from the parking area to the accessible building entrance? _____ _____

8. Is the surface of the accessible route smooth (no sand, gravel, or utility hole covers)? _____ _____

9. Are all ramps along the accessible route at a gradient of at least 1:12 (1:16 - 1:20 preferred)? _____ _____

10. Do ramps have 5-foot level landings at the bottom and top that are as wide as the ramp itself? _____ _____

11. Do all ramps have handrails with top handrail, non-slip, gripping surfaces mounted between 34 inches and 38 inches above the ramp surface? _____ _____

12. Is the accessible route walkway at least 48 inches wide? _____ _____

13. Is the accessible route marked with appropriate signage? _____ _____

14. Is there a passenger loading and unloading zone? _____ _____

15. The accessible entrance is located _____
    _____ _____ _____

16. Is the accessible door marked with appropriate signage? _____ _____

17. Is the entrance door a minimum of 32 inches wide? _____ _____

18. Is the door automatic? _____ _____

19. Is the door-opening mechanism set to less than _____ pounds of pressure (as measured by a push then pull scale, although no specific requirements are set for exterior doors at this time)? _____ _____

20. If there are two doors in series at the entrance, do the doors open in the same direction or away from the space between the two doors and is the space at least 48 inches plus the width of any door opening into the space? _____ _____

21. Is there an alternative to a revolving door? _____ _____

22. Is door hardware shaped so as to require one hand to open and not to require tight grasping, tight pinching, or twisting of the wrist to operate? _____ _____

23. Are thresholds less than ½ inch high? _____ _____

24. If the primary entrance has steps, is there a proper sign directing patrons to the accessible entrance? _____ _____

Fig. 15.1 Cont'd

(Continued)

STEP TWO: Look at access to those areas of public accommodation where goods and services are made available to the public. This includes adjusting the layout of display racks, providing Brailled and raised character signage, widening doorways, providing visual alarms, and installing ramps.

A. List all areas in the facility where goods, services, and programs are provided to the public. (Remember, this includes areas in places that are not normally considered places of public accommodations, but parts of those facilities where members of the public would go, i.e., the showroom of a factory not open to the general public but where outside buyers and salespersons might go.)

B. Are all areas where goods, services, and programs are located accessible?
(This section should be repeated for all goods, services, and programs offered at the location.)

Goods/Service/Program and Location

Fig. 15.1 Cont'd

		YES	NO
1.	Is the width of the pathway to the area, including corridors and aisles, at least 32 inches of usable space?	_____	_____
2.	Is the pathway free of protruding telephones, water fountains, or other items?	_____	_____
3.	Is the pathway flooring covered with high-density, low-pile (½ inch) carpeting, non-slip tile, or vinyl?	_____	_____
4.	Are doorways at least 32 inches wide?	_____	_____
5.	If there are steps along the pathway, is the area also served by an elevator?	_____	_____
6.	Are steps covered with non-slip surfaces, provided with adequate lighting, and designed with curved nosings and sloped risers?	_____	_____
7.	Do all stairways have handrails positioned at both sides of the stairs with top handrail, non-slip, gripping surfaces mounted between 34 inches and 38 inches above the stair nosing?	_____	_____
8.	Do the handrails extend 12 inches beyond the top riser and 12 inches plus the width of one thread beyond the bottom riser?	_____	_____
9.	Are thresholds at ½ inch high or less for interior doors?	_____	_____
10.	Is the door-opening mechanism set to 5 pounds of pressure or less?	_____	_____
11.	Is door hardware shaped so as to require one hand to open and not to require tight grasping, tight pinching, or twisting of the wrist to operate?	_____	_____
12.	If doorways have two independently operated door leaves, is one leaf at least 32 inches wide?	_____	_____
13.	If there are two doors in series along the pathway, do the doors open in the same direction or away from the space between the two doors and is the space at least 48 inches plus the width of any door opening into the space?	_____	_____
14.	Are elevator call buttons centered at 42 inches above the floor and at least ¾ inch in diameter?	_____	_____
15.	Do objects mounted below the elevator call button protrude more than 4 inches into the elevator lobby?	_____	_____
16.	Are visible and audible signals provided at each elevator entrance to indicate which car is answering the call and the direction the car is going (once for up and twice for down)?	_____	_____

Fig. 15.1 Cont'd

(Continued)

17.   Are raised and Braille characters at least 2 inches high, provided on both jambs of the elevators, and centered 60 inches above the floor?   _____ _____

18.   Are elevators provided with an automatic reopening device?   _____ _____

19.   Is the minimum amount of time the elevators remain open in response to a call at least 3 seconds?   _____ _____

20.   Are control buttons inside the elevator designated by Braille and raised letters?   _____ _____

21.   Are floor buttons 54 inches or less above the floor for a side wheelchair approach and 48 inches or less for a front approach?   _____ _____

22.   If public telephones are provided, are they on an accessible floor at an accessible location?   _____ _____

23.   Is at least one telephone mounted so that its operable parts are no more than 54 inches or less above the floor for a side wheelchair approach and 48 inches or less for a front approach?   _____ _____

24.   Is there a clear floor or ground space of at least 30 inches by 48 inches under the telephone absent bases, enclosures, fixed seats, and protruding objects of more than 4 inches?   _____ _____

25.   Is at least one telephone equipped with an amplifier for individuals with hearing impairments and located near an electrical outlet for portable TTDs?   _____ _____

26.   Is the telephone cord at least 29 inches long?   _____ _____

27.   Is at least one text telephone provided?   _____ _____

28.   Where are the accessible telephones located?   _____ _____

29.   Are accessible telephones marked with appropriate signage?   _____ _____

30.   Are water fountains mounted so that spouts are no higher than 36 inches from the floor?   _____ _____

31.   Are fire alarms and other warning signals provided in both a visual and audible manner?   _____ _____

32.   Are room numbers, directional signs, emergency directions, and other signs and markings indicated in large, block letters and numerals, using contrasting colors so they can be read by individuals with visual impairments?   _____ _____

33.   Are signs provided in raised and Braille letters and numbers?   _____ _____

Fig. 15.1 Cont'd

If the answer to any of the above questions is no, what reasonable accommodations may be made to allow access to the area where the goods, services, and programs are provided?

_____

_____

_____

STEP THREE: Look at access to restroom facilities.

		YES	NO
1.	Where are the accessible restrooms located? _____ _____	_____	_____
2.	Is the accessible restroom designated with appropriate signage?	_____	_____
3.	Is the restroom on an accessible pathway?	_____	_____
4.	Can one use the restroom without going up or down steps?	_____	_____
5.	Is the width of the pathway to the restrooms, including corridors, and aisles, at least 32 inches of usable space?	_____	_____
6.	Is the pathway to the restrooms free of protruding telephones, water fountains, or other items?	_____	_____
7.	Is the pathway flooring to the restrooms covered with high-density, low-pile (½ inch) carpeting, non-slip tile, or vinyl?	_____	_____
8.	Are the doorways to the restrooms at least 32 inches wide?	_____	_____
9.	Do doorways to the restrooms require 5 pounds or less of pressure to open?	_____	_____
10.	Is the entrance to the toilet stall at least 32 inches wide?	_____	_____
11.	Is the top of the seat of the accessible toilet between 17 inches and 19 inches from the floor?	_____	_____
12.	Does the toilet paper dispenser allow for the continuous flow of toilet paper without delivery control?	_____	_____
13.	Does the toilet stall have a minimum depth of 56 inches where toilets are wall mounted and 59 inches where toilets are floor mounted?	_____	_____
14.	Is at least one stall a minimum of 36 inches wide with an outwardly opening, self-closing door?	_____	_____

Fig. 15.1 Cont'd

(Continued)

15. Are there a minimum of two grab bars at least 36 inches long in the accessible toilet stall with one grab bar mounted behind the toilet? _____ _____

16. Are grab bars between 33 inches and 36 inches from the floor? _____ _____

17. Are urinal rims at a maximum of 17 inches from the floor? _____ _____

18. Is there a clear space in front of the urinal of 30 inches by 48 inches to allow a front approach? _____ _____

19. Are soap dispensers, paper towel dispensers, hand dryer, and feminine product dispensers within 48 inches of the floor? _____ _____

20. Are mirrors mounted so that the bottom edge is within 40 inches of the floor? _____ _____

21. Are sinks mounted so that the rim or counter surface is within 34 inches of the floor and a 29-inch clearance space is provided from the floor to the bottom of the apron? _____ _____

22. Is there a clear space in front of the sink of 30 inches by 48 inches to allow a front approach? _____ _____

23. Are hot water pipes insulated or configured to avoid contact? _____ _____

24. Are sink faucets lever-operated, push-type, electronically controlled, or otherwise operable with one hand without requiring tight grasping, pinching, or twisting of the wrist? _____ _____

25. Do self-closing faucets remain open for at least 10 seconds? _____ _____

STEP FOUR: Look at access to the goods, services, facilities, privileges, advantages, or accommodations offered at the place of public accommodation.

This step answers the question, "Can people use or take advantage of the goods, services, facilities, or programs provided at the place of public accommodation?"

Look back at the goods, services, facilities, or programs identified in **STEP TWO** and determine whether they are usable. **For example:**

YES   NO

1. Are printed materials provided in alternative formats where needed? _____ _____

2. Are items in racks or on walls within reach? _____ _____

3. Are special listening devices provided for individuals with hearing impairments in theaters, conference centers, and concert halls? _____ _____

Fig. 15.1 Cont'd

4.   Can individuals in wheelchairs reach the microfilm
       machines at the library?   _____ _____

5.   Is there an integrated location for individuals in
       wheelchairs to sit at the football stadium without having to
       transfer out of one's chair?   _____ _____

6.   Can individuals with disabilities reach the items on the
       grocery store shelves?   _____ _____

STEP FIVE: If STEPS ONE through FOUR identify goods, services, facilities, or programs that are not usable by individuals with disabilities, can an accommodation be made to enable the individual to take advantage of the goods, services, facilities, or programs?

Are there policies that need to be changed to enable participation by individuals with disabilities?

Fig. 15.1 Cont'd

AIR CARRIER ACCESS ACT

Carlotta's occupational profile shows that travel is a meaningful occupation for her. To pursue that occupation now that she uses a wheelchair for mobility, she will need to know what to expect while traveling and how she can advocate for herself. The key is the Air Carrier Access Act of 1986 (ACAA). The ACAA, as amended,[78] prohibits discrimination against qualified individuals with physical or mental impairments in air transportation by foreign and domestic air carriers. The ACAA applies only to air carriers that provide regularly scheduled services for hire to the public. As with the ADA and Fair Housing Act, the ACAA lists specific actions that it considers discriminatory.

Discrimination Prohibited Under the ACAA

Airline carriers may not refuse to transport qualified individuals with disabilities on the basis of their disability.[3] The definitions of disability are similar to the definitions found in the ADA. A qualified individual with a disability in the airline travel context means that he or she seeks to purchase or has a ticket to fly. The ACAA would protect Carlotta because she has arthritis and an airline ticket. By federal statute, carriers may exclude anyone from a flight if carrying the person would pose a direct threat to the health and safety of others.[4] This parallels the direct threat criteria under the ADA. If the airline carrier excludes persons with disabilities on safety grounds, the carrier must provide a written explanation of the decision within 10 days of the refusal, including the specific basis for the refusal.[6]

Airline carriers may not deny transportation to a qualified individual with a disability "because the person's disability results in appearance or involuntary behavior that may offend, annoy, or inconvenience crewmembers or other passengers."[5] Airline carriers cannot limit the number of people with disabilities they will allow on flights as a means of refusing transportation based on disability.[2] The ACAA prohibits airlines from requiring a person with a disability to accept special services, such as preboarding, if the passenger does not request them.[1] Similarly, air carriers cannot segregate passengers with disabilities, even if separate or different services are available to them.[8]

Under the ACAA, airline carriers cannot require qualified individuals with a disability to provide advance notice of their intention to travel or of their disability as a condition of receiving transportation or of receiving services or required accommodations.[7] Carlotta would not have to notify the airline in advance that she planned to fly. A limited exception to this rule exists, however. An airline carrier may require up to 48 hours' notice for certain specific accommodations that require advance preparation. These include, for example, 48 hours advance notice and check-in 1 hour before other passengers, if the passenger intends to use their own ventilator, respirator, or CPAP machine.[8] There are some items the ACAA states the airline may provide, but are not *required* to provide that include, for example, provision of an on-board wheelchair on an aircraft with more than 60 seats that does not have an accessible lavatory, and an electrical hook-up for inflight respirators or ventilators.[8]

Airlines cannot exclude a passenger with disabilities from a particular seat, or require him or her to sit in a certain seat, except to comply with safety regulations established by the Federal Aviation Administration (FAA), such as exit row seating, which requires that passengers have specific abilities to open the exit door in case of an emergency.[15] Airlines must accommodate passenger seat assignments if they are required, based on the person's disability, and requested 24 hours in advance. For example, if Carlotta traveled with a service animal that assisted her in tasks such as pulling her wheelchair and picking up items from the floor, the carrier would have to assign them to a bulkhead seat or another seat that could accommodate the service animal.[14]

Airline carriers may not require a person with a disability to travel with an attendant except in certain limited circumstances.[9] Such limited circumstances include, among others, those in which a person with an impairment in mobility is unable to assist in his or her own evacuation and in which a person with a mental disability cannot understand or respond to the crew's safety instructions.[9] If the person with a disability and the carrier disagree about whether the individual's circumstances meet the ACAA's criteria, the carrier may require the attendant but may not charge for the attendant's transportation cost.[9]

Airline Carriers' Obligations

Airline carriers must provide assistance in boarding and deplaning by providing personnel, ground wheelchairs, boarding wheelchairs, and ramps or mechanical lifts.[16] If entry-level boarding is unavailable, airlines must provide boarding assistance through lifts or ramps.[17] Exceptions exist for certain small airplanes and low-volume airports. Occupational therapists should review with Carlotta how to explain to airline personnel the safest way to transfer her. Carlotta should also know that the carrier cannot leave her unattended in a ground or boarding wheelchair for more than 30 minutes if she cannot independently operate that wheelchair.[18] The carrier must also accept her wheelchair as carry-on baggage if a place exists to store it on the plane or as gate-checked baggage, which the airline returns to her as soon as possible and as close to the airplane door as possible if she wishes—and the airline cannot count assistive devices, such as a ventilator, toward the airline's limit on luggage.[20] Carlotta can also choose to have her wheelchair delivered to her in the baggage claim area.[20]

The ACAA requires airlines to provide other assistance to individuals with disabilities as outlined in Box 15.9.[19] Carriers cannot charge for providing these services.[10] However, they can charge for the use of more than one seat "if the passenger's size or condition (e.g., use of a stretcher) causes him or her to occupy the space of more than one seat."[10]

Wide-bodied aircraft must have accessible lavatories, and those with 100 seats or more must have priority space for storing wheelchairs in the cabins.[12,13] This information may help Carlotta select her flights based on the services that the plane provides. In addition to services and access on the airplanes themselves, airlines must make sure that their terminals are accessible.[11]

BOX 15.9   Services Airlines Must Provide if Requested

- Assistance moving to and from seats during boarding and deplaning
- Assistance in preparation for eating, such as opening cartons (but not assistance in eating)
- Assistance to and from the lavatory if the aircraft has an on-board wheelchair (but no assistance in the lavatory)
- Assistance moving to and from the lavatory for a semiambulatory person, not involving lifting or carrying
- Assistance loading and retrieving carry-on items, including mobility aids stored on board

If Carlotta does have a service animal, the airline must allow her to bring her service animal with her on the airplane. The ACAA "defines a service animal as a dog that is individually trained to do work or perform tasks for the benefit of a person with a disability."[a] Rules promulgated in 2020 no longer consider emotional support animals to be service animals, so if Carlotta has an emotional support animal, she cannot bring it with her on a commercial airline flight.[a]

The ACAA requires airline carriers to train their employees in awareness and appropriate response to persons with a disability, "including persons with physical, sensory, mental, and emotional disabilities, including how to distinguish among the differing abilities of individuals with a disability."[21] This could provide opportunities for advocating for a particular client such as Carlotta or to provide consultation services to the airline staff in the form of sensitivity training and disability awareness.

Each airline must designate a complaint resolution official at each airport that it serves to receive and make efforts to resolve complaints. If it cannot resolve the complaint, it must give the passenger a written summary of the problem and outline the steps that the carrier will take to solve it. It must also notify the passenger of his or her right to pursue the complaint with the U.S. Department of Transportation (DOT).[22] Information about filing a complaint with the DOT is available online at https://www.transportation.gov/airconsumer/complaints-alleging-discriminatory-treatment-against-disabled-travelers.

The DOT takes the ACAA very seriously. In February 2011, one airline agreed to a $2 million settlement with the DOT for failing to provide adequate and prompt enplaning and deplaning wheelchair assistance to passengers with disabilities, failing to provide dispositive responses to written complaints alleging ACAA violations, and failing to properly categorize and accurately report its disability-related complaints.[75]

Role of the Occupational Therapist

Occupational therapists can work with their clients to help them understand what their needs will be for air travel and also to

---

[a]U.S. Department of Transportation. (December 2, 2020). U.S. Department of Transportation announces final rule on traveling by air with service animals (https://www.transportation.gov/briefing-room/us-department-transportation-announces-final-rule-traveling-air-service-animals).

help them develop a strategy to follow for meeting their needs. They can also play a key role in informing clients of the rights to which they are entitled in air travel and how to advocate for those rights for themselves.

ETHICAL CONSIDERATIONS

As occupational therapists we are in a unique position to facilitate an understanding of disabilities and the impact they have on everyday activities and functions. Occupational therapists can use this knowledge to work directly with airlines as consultants and conduct the training mandated by law to promote a culture of sensitivity and awareness.

FAIR HOUSING ACT

Congress passed the Fair Housing Amendments Act of 1988 to add "handicaps" (hereafter referred to as individuals with disabilities, a more politically correct term with the same legal meaning[90]) to the list of those protected against discrimination in housing. Before passage of the Fair Housing Act Amendments, the Fair Housing Act (FHA) prohibited discrimination based only on race, color, religion, sex, familial status, or national origin.[95]

Generally, the FHA prohibits discrimination in the sale, rental, or advertising of housing dwellings, in the provision of brokerage services, or in other residential real estate–related transactions, such as the provision of mortgage loans. The FHA covers private housing, housing that receives federal government assistance, and state and local government housing. Some exceptions exist to the FHA. For example, the FHA does not apply to owner-occupied apartment buildings with four or fewer units, or to private homes when the owner owns fewer than three single-family homes and is not in the business of selling or renting dwellings.

The FHA uses the same definition of individuals with disabilities as the ADA. Discrimination means denying or making a sale or rental unavailable because of the disability of a buyer or renter, the disability of an intended resident, or the disability of any person associated with a person with a disability. Landlords may not inquire whether a person applying to buy or rent housing is an individual with a disability, and they cannot charge a higher price or provide different services because a renter or purchaser of a dwelling unit is an individual with a disability.

Passage of the Fair Housing Act Amendments gave individuals with disabilities certain additional rights to use and enjoy their dwellings. These additional rights play a significant role in promoting independent living and participation for individuals with disabilities. Under the FHA, it is illegal to refuse to permit reasonable modification of existing premises occupied or to be occupied by individuals with disabilities if the proposed modification is necessary to allow the person with the disability full use and enjoyment of the dwelling. However, unlike the ADA, which requires businesses to pay for modifications that provide access, the FHA does not require landlords to pay for modifications; it requires only that the landlord allow the tenant to make modifications, at the expense of the person with a disability who needs them.

The landlord may condition permission for modification on the renter's agreeing to restore the interior to its condition before the modification, if this is reasonable. If the renter plans to make a modification in the dwelling, the landlord may not increase a security deposit. The landlord may, however, condition permission for modification on provision of a reasonable description of the proposed modification and assurances that the work will be properly performed by licensed professionals with permits, in addition to other stipulations.

The FHA also makes it illegal for any person to refuse to make reasonable accommodations in rules, policies, practices, or services, when needed, to afford a person with a disability equal opportunity to use and enjoy a dwelling unit, including public and common use areas. For example, an apartment building management company would have to make an exception to a "no pets" policy so that an individual with a spinal cord injury could keep a service dog. Another often-disputed example involves parking. A person with a disability may need an assigned parking space close to his or her apartment in a development that prides itself on unassigned parking. It would be a reasonable accommodation to modify the parking policy to allow assignment of a parking space to the person with the disability.

Research shows that interventions based on home assessments, such as providing bath benches and recommending grab bars, help prevent falls in the home and encourage safe and independent participation in everyday home life.[87,106] Carlotta's intervention plan would include a home assessment. Applying the provisions of the FHA to Carlotta's case affords her some assistance in her quest for independent participation. First, the landlord would have to allow Carlotta to install the grab bars that her occupational therapist recommended for her bathtub, as long as this was done in a workmanlike manner with permits and all necessary requirements. The landlord would probably have to allow Carlotta to widen her bathroom door, as the occupational therapist recommended, so that Carlotta could wheel her wheelchair into the bathroom. With these modifications and others developed by the occupational therapist in collaboration with Carlotta, Carlotta can independently participate in her ADLs.

The second issue for Carlotta involves her need for assistance to carry out her aquatics home program. To do this, she must be able to use the pool, an amenity to which she is entitled, as are all residents of the apartment complex. Carlotta has no access to the pool unless her friend can help her get into and out of the pool each day. The landlord would probably have to modify the "no guests in the pool on weekends" policy to allow Carlotta access to and use of the pool on weekends.

What if the landlord does not want to allow Carlotta to make these accommodations? Even the most wonderful suggestions for accommodation made by the occupational therapist and/or OTA are worthless if the client cannot use them. Because the success of the occupational therapist intervention plan may rest on provision of these accommodations, the OT and/or OTA should steer Carlotta to the website for the U.S. Department of Housing and Urban Development (HUD) (https://www.hud.gov/program_offices/fair_housing_equal_opp/online-complaint) where Carlotta can find information on how to file an administrative complaint to encourage the landlord to allow her to make the needed accommodations. Remember, under the FHA the landlord is not responsible for making the accommodations but must allow the tenant to make needed reasonable accommodations. HUD staff members will contact the landlord and/or property management company, mediate the situation by encouraging them to follow the law, and try to resolve the issues without the need for filing a lawsuit.

Occupational therapists and OTAs will also find the FHA helpful in other, very commonly encountered situations. For example, occupational therapists who make home visits to patients' and clients' homes before hospital discharge will appreciate the support of the FHA. During these home visits, occupational therapists customarily evaluate the individual's ability to function in the home as independently as possible. This assessment includes making recommendations about adaptive equipment and other modifications to the home to promote independent participation. The FHA gives the therapist's recommendations clout should the landlord refuse to allow the modifications to the dwelling unit. Clients in need of grab bars and other accommodations in their homes have an alternative route to take should the landlord say "no" to the accommodations needed.

ADVOCACY AS INTERVENTION

Occupational therapists promote participation in work, leisure, and ADLs (see Chapters 10, 14, and 16). As shown earlier,

sometimes barriers to participation exist despite the efforts of occupational therapists and their clients. For example, the client may successfully transfer from the wheelchair to the toilet and bath bench in the clinic but cannot get into the bathroom at home if the landlord will not allow modifications to the apartment. Carlotta can do her job from a wheelchair, but the headmaster will not transfer her to an accessible classroom.

To promote participation in these instances, the occupational therapist may have to include advocacy as an intervention strategy. The occupational therapist may need to act as an advocate, or he or she may have to guide the client through a self-advocacy process.

ETHICAL CONSIDERATIONS

Eight Rules of Advocacy

- Know the basics of how the laws help your patients/clients.
- Read the regulations or summaries of them on websites of disability advocacy organizations, such as the Centers for Independent Living (CIL). (You can find your local CIL listed at https://www.ilru.org/projects/cil-net/cil-center-and-association-directory.)
- Believe that you or your client has a right to what you seek.
- Organize yourself, document your efforts, get everything in writing, and keep copies of all correspondence.
- Start with the source of the problem.
- Be specific; tell them exactly what you want.
- File a complaint with the administrative agency that oversees the matter.
- Follow through.

SUMMARY

The ADA, ACAA, and FHA exist to provide individuals with disabilities certain rights. These laws, in concert with OT intervention, have the potential to open many avenues to participation for individuals with disabilities. By familiarizing themselves with these laws and sharing that information with clients, occupational therapists can play a major role in ensuring that those whom they serve have more opportunities to participate in work, leisure, and ADLs.

With the assistance of the ADA, ACAA, and FHA, Carlotta should be able to continue in her job as a teacher with the reasonable accommodations provided by her employer under Title I of the ADA. Carlotta can continue traveling by airplane to find the perfect bed and breakfast with accommodations provided to her under the ACAA. She can continue shopping and going to movies with the protection afforded her under Title III of the ADA. The FHA will provide the legal tools Carlotta needs to stay in her current apartment and care for herself independently, with cooperation from her landlord for the accommodations she needs.

ADDENDUM: GUIDANCE ON "LONG COVID" AS A DISABILITY UNDER THE AMERICANS WITH DISABILITIES ACT

Months after this chapter was completed for this, the 9th edition, it became apparent that one of the many repercussions of the global COVID-19 pandemic would be resulting long-term disability for many of those who survived the disease. This potential for long-term disability would undoubtedly need to be addressed by the ADA and, not surprisingly, these issues are being studied and will be considered under the ADA. The argument for inclusion shows the following thinking.

The passage of the Patient Protection and Affordable Care Act (ACA) included Section 1557, the antidiscrimination provisions, which prohibits discrimination "on the basis of race, color, national origin, sex, age, or disability in health programs or activities that receive Federal financial assistance or are administered by an Executive agency or any entity established under Title I of the ACA."[1]

In July 2021, the U.S. Department of Health and Human Services, Office of Civil Rights, and the U.S. Department of Justice, Civil Rights Division, Disability Rights Section, issued its "Guidance on 'Long COVID' as a Disability Under the ADA, Section 504, and Section 1557."[2] The Guidance provides specific criteria, including symptoms of long COVID that may include[3]:

- Tiredness or fatigue
- Difficulty thinking or concentrating (sometimes called "brain fog")
- Shortness of breath or difficulty breathing
- Headache
- Dizziness on standing
- Fast-beating or pounding heart (known as heart palpitations)
- Chest pain
- Cough
- Joint or muscle pain
- Depression or anxiety
- Fever
- Loss of taste or smell

The Guidance further provides that if "long COVID" limits one or more major life activities, it is a disability under the ADA, Section 504 of the Rehabilitation Act, and Section 1557.[4] The Guidance also explains that long COVID is not *always* a disability. To determine whether or not it is a disability, "[A]n individualized assessment is necessary to determine whether a person's long COVID condition or any of its symptoms substantially limits a major life activity."[5] OTs can play a key role in this assessment for clients, attorneys, and employers.

REVIEW QUESTIONS

1. Study the ADA definition of disability and explain how that definition may apply to clients seen by OTs and used as a tool to increase professional advocacy and client participation.
2. Compare and contrast definitions of discrimination provided throughout the chapter and discuss how they may apply to clients served by occupational therapy and lead to increased participation of our clients in everyday life.
3. Discuss the roles that occupational therapy can play in advocating for clients under the ADA, Fair Housing Act, and Air Carrier Access Act and how advocacy can lead to increased participation and independence in employment, community life, housing, and travel.
4. Discuss the roles that occupational therapy can play in consulting with employers, places of public accommodation, airline carriers, and landlords to improve clients' participation, independence, and integration into community life.
5. Explain the process used to determine "essential job functions" and how occupational therapy can use this information to help clients maintain their employment, and/or promote return to work following an accident, injury, or illness.
6. Analyze "reasonable accommodations" as an intervention strategy in occupational therapy and explain the decision-making process involved in making reasonable accommodations in employment, places of public accommodations, housing, and community living.
7. Using the How to Do an Accessibility Audit Under the ADA (Fig. 15.1) conduct a practice audit of a business or community service such as a movie theater, concert hall, gymnasium, senior center, or library. Share your observations with a colleague or service provider.

For additional practice questions for this chapter, please visit eBooks.Health.Elsevier.com.

REFERENCES
1. 14 CFR § 382.11(a)(2) (as amended at 75 FR 44887, July 30, 2010).
2. 14 CFR § 382.17 (2009).
3. 14 CFR § 382.19(a) (2009).
4. 14 CFR § 382.19(c)(1) (2009).
5. 14 CFR § 382.19(b) (2009).
6. 14 CFR § 382.19(d) (2009).
7. 14 CFR § 382.27(a) as amended (2020).
8. 14 CFR §§ 382.27(b)(c) as amended (2020).
9. 14 CFR §§ 382.29(a)-(c) (2011).
10. 14 CFR § 382.31 (as amended at 78 FR 67914, Nov. 12, 2013).
11. 14 CFR § 382.51 (as amended at 74 FR 11471, Mar. 18, 2009; 75 FR 44887, July 30, 2010).
12. 14 CFR § 382.63 (2009).
13. 14 CFR § 382.67 (as amended at 78 FR 67923, Nov. 12, 2013.
14. 14 CFR § 382.81(c) (2009).
15. 14 CFR § 382.87(a) (2009).
16. 14 CFR § 382.95(a) (2009).
17. 14 CFR § 382.95(b) (2009).
18. 14 CFR § 382.103 (2009).
19. 14 CFR § 382.111 (as amended at 75 FR 44887, July 30, 2010).
20. 14 CFR § 382.121-131 (2009).
21. 14 CFR § 382.141(a)(2) (2009).
22. 14 CFR § 382.151-155 (as amended at 75 FR 44887, July 30, 2010).
23. 28 CFR § 35.130 (1991).
24. 28 CFR § 35.130(a) (2010).
25. 28 CFR § 36.104 (1991).
26. 28 CFR § 36.201(a) (2010).
27. 28 CFR §§ 36.202(a)-(c) (2010).
28. 28 CFR § 36.203(a)(b) (2010).
29. 28 CFR § 36.211(a) (as amended by AG Order No. 3181-2010, 75 FR 56251, Sept. 15, 2010).
30. 28 CFR § 36.301(a) (1991).
31. 28 CFR § 36.302(a) (as amended by 76 FR 13287, Mar. 11, 2011; AG Order 3702-2016, 81 FR 53243, Aug. 11, 2016).
32. 28 CFR § 36.302(c) (2010). (as amended by 76 FR 13287, Mar. 11, 2011; AG Order 3702-2016, 81 FR 53243, Aug. 11, 2016).
33. 28 CFR §§ 36.303(a)(b)(c) (as amended by AG Order 3779-2016, 81 FR 87378, Dec. 2, 2016).
34. 28 CFR §§ 36.304(a)-(c) (as amended by AG Order No. 3181-2010, 75 FR 56254, Sept. 15, 2010; AG Order No. 3332-2012, 77 FR 30179, May 21, 2012).

35. 28 CFR §§ 36.304(d) (2010). (as amended by AG Order No. 3181-2010, 75 FR 56254, Sept. 15, 2010; AG Order No. 3332-2012, 77 FR 30179, May 21, 2012).
36. 28 CFR §§ 36.305(a)-(c) (1991).
37. 28 CFR § 36.307 (1991).
38. 28 CFR § 36.310 (1991).
39. 28 CFR § 36.401 (1991).
40. 28 CFR § 36.406(a)(5) (2010).
41. 29 CFR § 1630.2(g)(1) (2011).
42. 29 CFR § 1630.2(g)(2) (2011).
43. 29 CFR § 1630.2(g)(3) (2011).
44. 29 CFR § 1630.2(h)(1) (2011).
45. 29 CFR § 1630.2(h)(2) (2011).
46. 29 CFR § 1630.2(i)(1)(i) (2011).
47. 29 CFR § 1630.2(j)(iv) (2011).
48. 29 CFR §§ 1630.2(j)(2)(i)-(iii) (2011).
49. 29 CFR § 1630.2(j)(1)(v) (2011).
50. 29 CFR § 1630.2(j)(1)(vi) (2011).
51. 29 CFR § 1630.2(j)(1)(vii) (2011).
52. 29 CFR § 1630.2(j)(1)(viii) (2011).
53. 29 CF § 1630.2(m) (2011).
54. 29 CFR § 1630.2(n)(1) (2011).
55. 29 CFR § 1630.2(n)(3) (2011).
56. 29 CFR § 1630.2(o) (2011).
57. 29 CFR § 1630.2(o)(1)(i) (2011).
58. 29 CFR § 1630.2(o)(1)(ii) (2011).
59. 29 CFR § 1630.2(o)(1)(iii) (2011).
60. 29 CFR § 1630.2(p) (2011).
61. 29 CFR § 1630.2(p)(2)(i)-(v) (2011).
62. 29 CFR § 1630.2(r) (2011).
63. 29 CFR § 1630.3(d)(1) (2011).
64. 29 CFR §§ 1630.3(d)(2)(3) (2011).
65. 29 CFR § 1630.5 (2011).
66. 29 CFR § 1630.6 (2011).
67. 29 CFR § 1630.7 (2011).
68. 29 CFR § 1630.8 (2011).
69. 29 CFR § 1630.9 (2011).
70. 29 CFR § 1630.10 (2011).
71. 29 CFR § 1630.11 (2011).
72. 29 CFR § 1630.12 (2011).
73. 29 CFR § 1630.1 4 (2011).
74. 42 USC 12112(a).
75. 2011-2-10 Consent Order (Delta Air Lines, Inc): Violations of 14 CFR Part 382 and 49 USC §§ 41310, 41702,41705 and 41712. http://www.regulations.gov/#!documentDetail;D=DOT-OST-2011-0003-0007.
76. ADAAG § 4.6.3.
77. Affordable Care Act (Public Law 111-148, 124 Stat L 119 (2010).
78. Air Carrier Access Act, as amended 14 CFR § 382.1 *et. seq.* (2020).
79. *Albertsons, Inc, v Kirkingburg, 527 U.S. 555,* (1999); *Murphy v United Parcel Service, Inc,* 527 US 516, (1999); *Sutton v United Air Lines, Inc,* 527 U.S. 472, (1999).
80. American Occupational Therapy Association Commission on Practice. Occupational therapy practice framework: domain and process, fourth edition, *American Journal of Occupational Therapy,* 74(Suppl 2):1–87, 2020. https://doi.org/10.5014/ajot.2020.74S2001.
81. Americans with Disabilities Act, codified at 29 CFR § 1630 et seq and 28 CFR § 36.101 et seq (1991).
82. Americans with Disabilities Act Amendments (ADAA), Pub L No 110-325 (2008).
83. ADAAA § 2(a)(8).
84. ADAAA § 4(a).
85. Americans with Disabilities Act Title III Regulations. 2017. https://www.ada.gov/regs2010/titleIII_2010/titleIII_2010_regulations.htm.
86. Appendix to Part 1630—Interpretive Guidance on Title I of the Americans With Disabilities Act 29 CFR § 1630 (1992). Section on the interactive process following a request for reasonable accommodations was not affected by ADAA.
87. Bakker R: Elderdesign: home modifications for enhanced safety and self-care, *Care Manage J* 1(1):47–54, 1999.
88. Berry S: Top 10 ADA access violations. *Disability Smart Solutions,* 2014. https://disabilitysmartsolutions.com/top-10-ada-access-violations.
89. *Board of Trustees of the University of Alabama v Garrett,* 531 US 356 (2001).
90. *Bragdon v Abbott,* 524 US 624, 631 (1998).
91. Equal Employment Opportunity Commission (EEOC): *A technical assistance manual on the employment provisions (Title I) of the Americans with Disabilities Act,* Washington, DC, 1992, US Government Printing Office.
92. Equal Employment Opportunity Commission (EEOC): Notice concerning The Americans With Disabilities Act (ADA) Amendments Act of 2008. https://www.eeoc.gov/statutes/notice-concerning-americans-disabilities-act-ada-amendments-act-2008; Equal Employment Opportunity Commission (EEOC): Enforcement guidance on disability-related inquiries and medical examinations of employees under the ADA. http://www.eeoc.gov/policy/docs/guidance-inquiries.html, 2000.
93. *Equal Employment Opportunity Commission v Sara Lee,* 237 F.3d 349 (4th Cir 2001).
94. *Equal Employment Opportunity Commission and Landers v Wal-Mart Stores, Inc,* 2001. US Dist LEXIS 23027 (WDNY 2001).
95. Fair Housing Act, 42 USC § 3601 *et. seq.* (1989).
96. Job Accommodation Network. Costs and benefits of accommodation. October 21, 2020. https://askjan.org/topics/costs.cfm.
97. Lilker S: New LSHA boss refuses to comply with ADA wheelchair requirements, *Columbia County Observer.* January 11, 2010. https://www.columbiacountyobserver.com/master_files/LSHA/LSHA_Stories/10_0111_ADA-compliance---little-better-but-not%20much.html.
98. *Littleton v Wal-Mart Stores, Inc,* No. 05-12770 (11th Cir May 11, 2007) unpublished opinion available at https://casetext.com/case/littleton-v-wal-mart; cert. denied 128 S.Ct. 302 (2007).
99. *McClure v General Motors Corp,* 75 Fed Appx 983 (5th Cir 2003).
100. Medical Diagnostic Equipment Accessibility Standards Advisory Committee: Advancing equal access to diagnostic services: recommendations on standards for the design of medical diagnostic equipment for adults with disabilities. https://www.regulations.gov/document?D=ATBCB-2013-0009-0001, December 6, 2013.
101. *Morisky v Broward County,* 80 F.3d 445, 447 (11th Cir 1996).
102. *Murphy v United Parcel Service, Inc,* 527 US 516, (1999).
103. Parking spaces for persons who have disabilities. Fl Stat § 553.5041.
104. Proposed accessibility standards for medical diagnostic equipment, 36 CFR Part 1195 (2012). https://www.regulations.gov/document?D=ATBCB-2012-0003-0001.
105. Rehabilitation Act of 1973, 29 USC 791 §§ 501, 503, 504.

106. Rogers J: The occupational therapy home assessment: the home as a therapeutic environment, *J Home Health Care Pract* 2:73, 1989.

107. Social Security Administration: The red book: a guide to work incentives. SSA Publication 64-030. http://ssa.gov/redbook/, January, 2020.

108. *Stutts v Freeman*, 694 F.2d 666 (11th Cir 1983).

109. *Todd v Academy Corp*, 57 F. Supp 2d 448 (SD Tex 1999).

110. US Department of Justice: Fact sheet: adoption of the 2010 Standards for Accessible Design. Retrieved January 6, 2011. http://www.ada.gov/regs2010/factsheets/2010_Standards_factsheet.html, August 3, 2010.

111. US Department of Justice: Fact sheet: highlights of the final rule to amend the Department of Justice's regulation implementing Title II of the ADA. http://www.ada.gov/regs2010/factsheets/title2_factsheet.html, October 7, 2010.

112. US Department of Justice: Fact sheet: highlights of the final rule to amend the Department of Justice's regulation implementing Title III of the ADA. http://www.ada.gov/regs2010/factsheets/title3_factsheet.html, May 26, 2011. Retrieved January 24, 2021.

113. US Department of Justice: 2010 ADA Standards for Accessible Design. http://www.ada.gov/regs2010/2010ADAStandards/2010ADAStandards_prt.pdf, September 15, 2010.

114. US Department of Labor, Office of Federal Compliance Programs: Section 503. https://www.dol.gov/agencies/ofccp/section-503, 2021; US Department of Labor, Office of Federal Compliance Programs, Federal Contract Compliance Manual, 1G13 Utilization Goal Analysis for Individuals with Disabilities. https://www.dol.gov/general/topic/disability/ada.

115. *Williams v Toyota Motor Mfg*, 534 US 184 (2002).

REFERENCES FOR ADDENDUM: GUIDANCE FOR "LONG COVID" AS A DISABILITY UNDER THE AMERICANS WITH DISABILITIES ACT

1. U.S. Department of Health and Human Services, Office of Civil Rights. (2017, May 18). *Section 1557: Frequently Asked Questions.* https://www.hhs.gov/civil-rights/for-individuals/section-1557/1557faqs/index.html.

2. *Guidance on "Long COVID" as a Disability Under the ADA, Section 504, and Section 1557* (2021, July 26). https://www.hhs.gov/civil-rights/for-providers/civil-rights-covid19/guidance-long-covid-disability/index.html.

3. *Guidance on "Long COVID" as a Disability Under the ADA, Section 504, and Section 1557* at 3.

4. *Guidance on "Long COVID" as a Disability Under the ADA, Section 504, and Section 1557* at 2.

5. *Guidance on "Long COVID" as a Disability Under the ADA, Section 504, and Section 1557* at 4.

16

Leisure Occupations[a]

Megan C. Chang and Sheama Krishnagiri

LEARNING OBJECTIVES

After studying this chapter, the student or practitioner will be able to do the following:
1. Discuss the benefits of leisure for adults.
2. Describe the key areas in which humor can be used.
3. Understand the different leisure needs of people in different stages of life.
4. Use the Occupational Profile and other appropriate assessments to evaluate factors and needs for clients to engage in leisure.
5. Identify specific strategies to promote leisure activity for people with disabilities.

CHAPTER OUTLINE

KEY TERMS

Humor
Leisure
Leisure exploration

Leisure participation
Modeling
Play

THREADED CASE STUDY

Jeri, Part 1

Before she was involved in a traffic accident, Jeri, a 29-year-old newly married woman (prefers the pronouns she/her/hers), lived a full and happy life. She was employed as an interior designer; spent time with her husband, friends, and family; and participated in leisure occupations. She particularly enjoyed going hiking with friends, playing video games, scrapbooking, and playing with and caring for her dogs. As Jeri was driving home from running errands one evening, a drunk driver hit her car. It rolled over, and she was trapped inside. She was taken by paramedics to the local hospital, where she was found to have a traumatic brain injury, a broken wrist, and a broken leg. Jeri was transported to the regional brain trauma center for rehabilitation. She recovered over a period of months and returned home.

Jeri continues rehabilitation as an outpatient for residual problems from her brain injury and for continuing problems using her dominant hand because of the wrist fracture. Jeri receives occupational therapy twice weekly and is demonstrating significant improvement; she has progressed from needing maximum assistance for activities of daily living (ADLs) to minimum assistance. Jeri has no apparent cognitive deficits, she uses a walker to ambulate, and she still needs a family member or aide at home on a full-time basis because she has poor balance, which impairs her safety when moving around in her environment. The occupational therapist (OT) is ready to discharge Jeri because her ADL goals have been met. However, during the intervention review before discharge, Jeri tells her OT that she spends most of her days hanging out at home, watching TV, that she feels lonely and disengaged from her friends, and that she will miss occupational therapy because it is her only activity outside the home.

Critical Thinking Questions
1. Is Jeri ready to be discharged from occupational therapy?
2. Why is Jeri dissatisfied with her current lifestyle?
3. What intervention could the OT provide to improve Jeri's quality of life?

---

[a]The authors acknowledge the outstanding work of Dr. Marti Southam in previous editions of this text. The present chapter is built on her foundational work.

Participating in meaningful leisure occupations is vital to a healthy, balanced lifestyle.[10,78,79,85] As one of nine categories of occupation in the domain of occupational therapy, leisure is defined in the *Occupational Therapy Practice Framework* (fourth edition [AOTA, OTPF-4]) as "a nonobligatory activity that is intrinsically motivated and engaged in during discretionary time, that is, time not committed to obligatory occupations such as work, self-care, or sleep" (AOTA, OTPF-4, p. S50).[7] Key phrases in the definition are that these activities are intrinsically motivated and that they are not obligatory. In other words, people participate in leisure occupations that they choose and enjoy. For instance, for some people cooking may be a chore, whereas for others it is a pleasure.

Leisure time may be spent in a variety of ways indicative of an individual's unique interests. Examples of leisure occupations are reading, playing games, participating in sports, doing arts and crafts, engaging in outdoor activities (biking, hiking, fishing), cooking, taking a yoga class, exercising at the gym, going to concerts, watching movies, and so on. Because of the uniqueness of individuals, this list is as long as there are people who participate in leisure occupations.

LEISURE AND LIFE SATISFACTION FOR PEOPLE WITH PHYSICAL DISABILITIES

When adults sustain injuries (e.g., traumatic brain injury, stroke, spinal cord injury, carpal tunnel syndrome), have health conditions (e.g., multiple sclerosis, Parkinson's disease, arthritis, Alzheimer's disease), undergo life transitions (e.g., empty nest syndrome, menopause, retirement), or experience natural disasters (e.g., hurricanes, earthquakes, pandemics) that disrupt normal habits and routines, they face devastating losses. Loss of work, social activities, and meaningful leisure activities may contribute to depression, and the self must be redefined.[65,105]

Occupational therapists are skilled in collaborating with people with physical disabilities to assist them in resuming a full life.[103] It has been suggested that one method of measuring whether a person is fully engaged in life is to consider the individual's participation in leisure activities.[16,86] This is especially important because research indicates that the perception of leisure satisfaction by adults with physical disabilities is the most significant predictor of life satisfaction.[55,73] Reduced risk for dementia has been shown when participating in leisure over time.[4] Depressive symptoms also have been shown to diminish when the number and variety of pleasant activities increase.[45,60,91,98] Dance-based approach has shown significant improvements in quality of life, executive functioning, and psychological well-being,[5,30,31,73] whereas other studies have demonstrated benefits of music listening on reducing pain, enhancing cognitive recovery, or improving mood.[14,94] Leisure participation in older adults is associated with fewer depressive symptoms as well as increases in ADL and IADL.[58] Studies with adults who have developmental and intellectual disabilities indicate an association between participation in leisure and an improved sense of well-being,[67] as well as increased quality of life.[37] Engaging in familiar or novel leisure activities provides

a receptive environment for opportunities for socializing and making friends, in which people with physical disabilities have a chance to demonstrate their occupational skills to others who might not otherwise view those with a disability as capable or as a candidate for friendship.[88] Subsequent studies of people with multiple sclerosis, stroke, and Parkinson's disease have demonstrated similar findings about social participation.[3,25,43]

OT PRACTICE NOTES

Benefits of Leisure Activities
Participation in leisure activities can offer many psychosocial and physical benefits.

Psychosocial Benefits
- Increased sense of self-worth
- Practice in adaptive behavior and coping skills
- Improved emotional well-being
- Adjustment to living arrangements
- Improved quality of life
- Release of hostility and aggression
- Shared control of self and environment
- Experience of choice
- Increased socialization
- Development of leadership
- Increased attention span
- Increased tolerance of groups and other people
- Experience of intellectual stimulation
- Decreased life stress

Physical Benefits
- Increased circulation
- Promotion of gross, fine, bilateral, and eye-hand coordination
- Provision of vestibular stimulation
- Provision of sensory stimulation
- Promotion of motor planning
- Improvement or maintenance of perceptual abilities
- Maintenance or improvement of adaptive and coping skills
- Increased strength, range of motion, and physical tolerance
- Improved balance
- Improved activities of daily living (ADLs) and instrumental activities of daily living (IADLs) function
- Provision of opportunity to grade activities

OT PRACTICE NOTES

The Therapist's Role in Encouraging Leisure Activities
If therapists provide interventions aimed only at physical rehabilitation (e.g., strengthening, range-of-motion exercises) and improving performance in activities of daily living and instrumental activities of daily living, the recovering individual may never experience the opportunity of resuming old leisure interests or developing new ones. Leisure skills are integral to rekindling one's inner spirit and redefining one's identity, self-worth, and self-efficacy.

Leisure also has been shown to contribute to individual development, well-being, happiness,[70,74] and quality of life,[57] as well as to provide a significant mechanism for coping.[7] Unfortunately, studies indicate that most leisure activities are abandoned after the onset of a physical disorder such as rheumatoid arthritis or stroke.[86,117] Adults with physical disabilities seem to relinquish activities that are purely for enjoyment, especially community-based social activities, and focus their effort and time on ADLs and work.[86,90]

The emphasis on the physical model of recovery is most likely due to healthcare professionals who deliver treatment with a focus on mobility and independence in ADLs and also the fact that rehabilitation outcome measures are commonly based on these factors.[86] Occupational therapists recognize that people often experience difficulty adapting their interests and activities by themselves after a physical or neurological disorder, and yet leisure can influence one's life in many diverse and meaningful ways that contribute to one's growth, advancement, or maturity.[28]

Leisure comes in different forms and function; it can be sedentary (e.g., reading and listening to music) or active (such as dancing, bowling, bike riding). Taking dance as an example, Hackney et al. examined the effectiveness of an adapted Tango program to improve balance, mobility, and quality of life in older adults with visual impairment.[53] Thirty-two individuals participated in this study (mean age = 79.3, age range 51–95 years). The Tango intervention consists of 20 classes of 90 minutes for 12 weeks. Each class started with upbeat music for 15 minutes standing warm-ups to increase postural alignment, ROM, and entrainment to rhythmic beats. New steps were then introduced weekly, and previously learned steps were repeated. Every fifth class was a review, so no new steps were introduced. Dance steps were progressed by increasing its rhythmic complexity, balance challenge, and number of steps combined. Unlike the traditional ballroom style, participants were asked to hold the elbows facing one another and maintain their forearms parallel to the floor. This study shows that this adapted dance Tango intervention, a multimodal exercise program, significantly improved endurance, cognitive dual-tasking, and vision-related quality of life.[53] It is worth noting that similar adapted Tango programs have been implemented with other conditions, such as Parkinson's disease[75] and individuals with chronic stroke.[53] Findings from these studies also showed an improvement in balance and walking velocity and cadence. Participants in these studies expressed enjoyment and interest in continuing in the dance program.[49–51,75] These studies affirm the need for occupational therapists to address the leisure area of occupation to encourage clients to engage in their leisure interests to enhance physical well-being and social participation.

On a different form of leisure, some clients may prefer sedentary activities. If so, therapists must follow their clients' preferences to support their occupational pursuits and use research evidence to support their decision. One of the pieces of recent research evidence demonstrates how listening to music supports one's leisure pursuit and psychological well-being. Baylan et al. conducted a pilot randomized controlled trial (RCT) to evaluate the feasibility and acceptability of incorporating brief mindfulness training into an 8-week music listening intervention on clients with ischemic stroke in the acute phase (less than 14 days after a stroke).[13] There were three study groups: (1) music listening with brief mindfulness training (mindful-music group);

(2) music listening alone; and (3) audiobook. All 72 participants were asked to choose their preferred music or audiobooks from any genre and required to keep a daily record of listening. Participants in the mindful-music group were introduced to the concept of mindfulness at the first visit and given a recording that included mindfulness exercise (5-minute Body Scan) to complete daily before music listening. Results showed that not only were most of the participants (94%) compliant with the intervention protocol but also the adherence and retention rates were high (above 80% for all three groups). Interestingly, compared to the mindful-music group, the music and audiobook groups were more likely to engage in daily music listening, and the audiobook group was more likely to continue audiobook listening compared to the other groups. The mindful-music group more frequently referred to listening aiding relaxation, emotional regulation, and attentional control, although there was no statistically significant difference in engaging relaxation, mindfulness, or meditation-based leisure activities among the three groups. Participants in the music or audiobook groups often expressed that listening to music or audiobooks was enjoyable and uplifting. As the authors noted, there may be sampling bias that participants who were vulnerable to mood disorders may choose not to participate in the study. Thus, the depression scores for all groups were within the normal range at baseline, and there was no significant change after the intervention. Yet, it is apparent that the medication usage for antidepressants in the mindful-music group was decreased by 20%, whereas the music group remained about the same and the audiobook group was increased about 7%.[13] This pilot RCT study suggested that mindful music listening is feasible and acceptable after a stroke. Moreover, when clients enjoy the leisure activities, they may continue such engagement and that may enhance or maintain their physical and/or psychological well-being. Therefore, occupational therapists need to inquire regarding clients' interest and values and tailor those preferences in the intervention plan.

There are times that adults with physical disabilities may give up leisure activities because they are not aware of ways to adapt valued activities to enable them to participate in those activities again, or they may not know how to explore new hobbies or crafts that they might enjoy. Occupational therapists have an important role in helping people both discover and plan engagement in leisure occupations so that they can participate in activities that bring joy to life.[17,81,93,105] Engagement in "serious leisure" (a term used in the literature to indicate fulfilling leisure activities that engage the individual's special skills, knowledge, and experience) has been associated with positive effects on affect,[55,72] quality of life,[57] and mood.[34] Additionally, it can serve as a mechanism for upholding identity and for helping the individual remain engaged in a fulfilling and meaningful life with the disability.[43,46,56,57]

One way to ensure that the occupational therapist allocates appropriate focus on this key aspect of life is to place oneself in the client's shoes and/or ask the client questions such as what the client's day to day life is like. What do they miss doing that they previously loved to do for fun and relaxation? What do they wish to do now for fun and relaxation? A second method is for the occupational therapist to make it a habit to gather a detailed "leisure profile" as part of the occupational profile during evaluation.[8] This action serves to not only connect with the individual but also allows a glimpse into the individual's inner spirit. Further, the leisure profile can serve as a beginning list of activities to draw from in choosing meaningful activities for therapy. In other words, one can use the individual's preferred activities to meet the therapeutic goals. A thorough occupational analysis, with appropriate grading and adaptation to the individual's abilities and context, makes this possible. Leisure occupations, therefore, can be both the means and the ends of occupational therapy.[27]

BENEFITS OF PLAY AND LAUGHTER IN LEISURE OCCUPATIONS

When talking about participating in leisure occupations, people often use the word *play*: play golf, play the piano, play sports, play cards, play board games, and so on. Other types of leisure occupations involve being creative, such as dressing uniquely, preparing original recipes, writing poetry, and such.[115] **Play** allows adults to escape the reality of everyday life and immerse themselves in a world of carefree spontaneity that provides meaning to their existence and sometimes an avenue for self-expression.[20] Play suggests fun, and fun is often accompanied by laughter.

Many physical health benefits of laughter have been demonstrated through numerous research studies. For example, immune cells increase and stress hormones decrease, thereby possibly preventing illness or aiding recovery.[15,89,104] Some people experience relief from pain and a sense of well-being after hearty laughter.[1,33,64] Laughter also benefits people psychologically and psychosocially.[36,92,100,113,115] Laughing together facilitates bonding, reduces anxiety, and improves coping[47,66]—all important factors in a therapeutic alliance between the occupational therapist and the client (Box 16.1).

Facilitating psychosocial and physical adaptations is integral to occupational therapy; given the current healthcare climate of high productivity and short hospital and rehabilitation stays, it is imperative that occupational therapists be able to quickly form a therapeutic alliance with their clients. **Humor** and laughter are natural ways that therapists and clients connect. Recent studies have found that all of the occupational therapists who were interviewed or surveyed agreed that humor has a place in occupational therapy.[62,69,100]

In a national, cross-sectional, randomized survey of 283 occupational therapists that examined their attitudes and use of humor in interacting with adult clients with physical disabilities, humor was classified into four key areas: building relationships, helping clients cope with adversity, promoting clients' physical health, and facilitating compliance with treatment.[100] Although therapists reported positive attitudes about humor in all four of these areas, most were actually using humor only to build relationships and to help clients cope. The majority of therapists in Southam's study reported feeling more comfortable using spontaneous humor with clients as part of the therapeutic use of self rather than using planned humor as a therapeutic intervention.[100]

People who are disabled may need to learn ways to adapt to their new circumstances. Humor is a skill that can be learned

---

BOX 16.1 Health Benefits of Laughter

Physical Health Benefits of Laughter[36,92]

- Stress hormones decrease (e.g., cortisol and noradrenaline).[15]
- Immune functions increase (e.g., immunoglobulin A and natural killer cells).[15,104]
- Muscle tension relaxes.
- Blood pressure drops, and cardiovascular functions improve; blood flow increases to aid healing.
- Respiratory airways are cleared (through laughing and coughing).
- Pain relief may be attained after hearty laughter and may last for several hours as a result of release of opioids and endorphins.[89]
- "Feel good" hormones (e.g., beta-endorphins and serotonin) are released.

Psychological and Psychosocial Health Benefits of Laughter[64,92,100]

- Facilitates bonding—laughter occurs more often with others than when alone
- Improves ability to cope with problems[1]
- Increases well-being and promotes hope and optimism[66]
- Diverts negative thoughts—it is hard to maintain destructive thoughts when laughing[33]
- "Saves face" in embarrassing situations
- Facilitates mental clarity, creativity, and brainstorming because the two brain hemispheres communicate better during humor, and the limbic system is aroused[66]
- Adds vibrancy to facial tone and sparkle to the eyes

---

and may provide the client with the ability to manage concerns related to his or her health and life situations. Within a larger relational context, humor may be modeled by occupational therapists to teach coping skills. Based on his Social Learning Theory, Bandura described four essential factors for **modeling** to be an effective intervention.[11] These four factors include attention, retention, reproduction, and motivation. These are necessary in any form of observational learning and modeling behaviors. During the intervention, therapists must first make sure the client must have an adequate attention span that allows him or her to focus on the modeled behavior. Second, the client must be able to cognitively form and retain a mental image of the behavior. Third, the client must be able to recall the image and then produce the behavior. Therapists then need to document the frequency and duration as well as the client's responses and feedback. Last, and perhaps most important, the client must have the motivation to engage in the behavior. It is important for therapists to adopt leisure activities their clients choose; the clients view these occupations as meaningful to them and therefore will be more motivated to engage in it repeatedly.

ETHICAL CONSIDERATIONS

Establishment of trust through the bond of a therapeutic relationship may provide the encouragement clients need to try new behavior, such as humor and laughter.[54]

The intimacy that humor presumes may provide the client with a sense of connection with the therapist. This connection, which occurs on conscious and unconscious levels, has many benefits for clients. When the therapist is able to demonstrate professionalism and empathy with a touch of humor, a client may feel less alone and more cared for as an individual.[100] An improved sense of equality with the healthcare provider may occur that could increase the client's active involvement in her or his treatment.[2,36]

Although laughter has been shown to be beneficial, there are times when humor may not be a good choice and must be used with caution or avoided altogether. Seizures and cataleptic or narcoleptic attacks may follow a laughter episode in a small number of people.[44] In addition, because laughing increases abdominal and thoracic pressure, people with recent abdominal surgery, upper body fractures, acute asthma, or "preexisting arterial hypertension and cerebral vascular fragility" should not be encouraged to laugh.[44]

ETHICAL CONSIDERATIONS

Occupational therapists need to be aware that humor can have destructive elements and may be used intentionally or unintentionally to hurt a person. Following the "AT&T principle" (appropriate, timely, and tasteful) can help OTs determine the proper use of humor.[97] As Klein pointed out, this principle means that the therapist must be attuned to the patient's humor style, culture, and current status (physical, emotional, and cognitive) before introducing humor and facilitating laughter.[62]

Leisure exploration is defined in the OTPF-4 as "identifying interests, skills, opportunities, and leisure activities," and leisure participation is "planning and participating in leisure activities; maintaining a balance of leisure activities with other occupations; and obtaining, using, and maintaining equipment and supplies."[7] In exploring leisure options with the client, the occupational therapist must evaluate the appropriateness of an occupation with respect to the client's age and gender, the cultural fit, and the meaning of the occupation to the specific individual. These concerns are addressed in the next section.

MEANINGFUL LEISURE OCCUPATIONS: AGE, CULTURAL ISSUES, AND GENDER

Clients choose the leisure occupations they want to pursue.[7,103] Choices may be based on past experiences or on a desire to explore something new. As people move through the developmental stages of adulthood, the occupation of leisure may vary in intensity and time allotted. The continuity theory of aging suggests that personality plays a major role in adjustment to aging. Because personality does not radically change throughout life, preferences, lifestyle, and activities remain relatively the same in individuals who age successfully.[9,21,82,107,108]

Age and Leisure

It is crucial that occupational therapists have knowledge of the typical progression through adulthood, the common life-stage choices of leisure activities, and the ways physical disabilities can disrupt participation in leisure activities. Armed with this information, OTs are able to discover gaps in developmental stages and to assist clients in the mastery of valued and meaningful occupations.[38]

Early Adulthood (20 to 40 Years)

Young adults are typically healthy, active, working, and engaged in relationships. Erikson's sixth stage of psychosocial development, intimacy versus isolation, describes young adulthood as a time in life when people know who they are and are ready to form intimate relationships with others.[84] Inability to make commitments on an intimate level may lead to isolation. Levinson (as cited in Papalia et al.) views this age period as a time of becoming independent from parents, choosing and beginning a career, and imagining one's dream future.[84]

Young adults are often involved in career training and education, decision about life roles and establishing social and intimate relationships that encompass family, work, and leisure activities.[77] According to the U.S. Bureau of Labor Statistics, over 95% of people aged 15 and older engaged in some sort of leisure activity, such as exercising, watching TV, or socializing.[111] Other examples of leisure activities in which young adults engage may include social and family group activities, sports (e.g., basketball, off-road biking), exercise (e.g., Zumba and yoga), travel, computer games, social networking on the internet, hobbies and crafts (e.g., scrapbooking), outdoor activities, dancing, dating, and sex. In addition, the popularity of outdoor adventure sports continues to grow at a rapid pace. Many outdoor adventure sports are fully accessible, even if the individual has limited arm movement. These include paragliding, flying a sailplane, hang gliding, sky diving, surfing, white water rafting, and zip lining (Fig. 16.1).[112] Accidents or physical disorders that affect an individual's areas of occupation, performance skills, and body functions can severely impede progress through the normal activities of young adulthood and may delay the development of age-related roles such as spouse, parent, employer/employee, social participant, participator in leisure occupations,

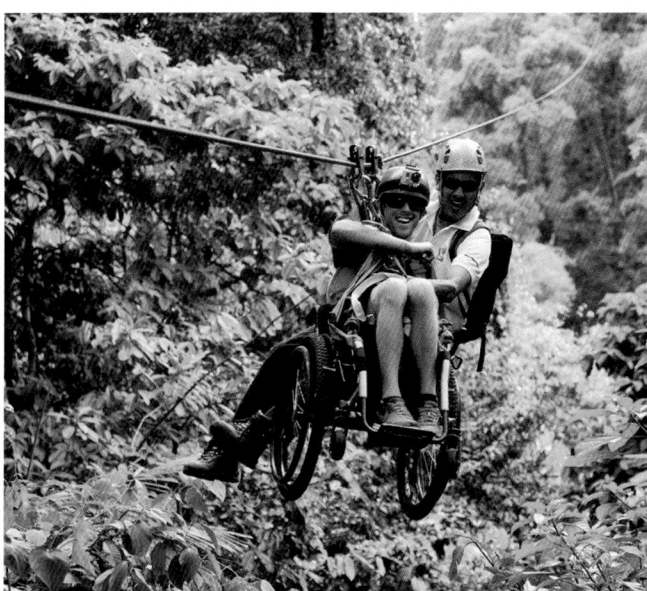

Fig. 16.1 Wheelchair user zip lining in Costa Rica. (From Vogel B: Outdoor recreation: you can do it, *New Mobility* 26(263):32–42, 2015.)

and sexual being. Individuals at the beginning stage of adulthood who sustain an irreversible injury may need to redefine themselves to successfully navigate the aging process. Leisure problems may include social isolation and changes in relationships, lack of ability to perform favorite sports, difficulty traveling, and decreased knowledge of how to creatively express the self.[48,52,53,105] A sense of incompetence may ensue that could lead to depression.

Middle Adulthood (40 to 65 Years)

People in this age group are typically immersed in work and family life. They have usually developed expertise in their chosen field of employment and may have risen to supervisory levels. Financial independence is attained as people purchase homes and cars and build a nest egg. Some adults in this age group experience a midlife review of self and career and may change careers or retire. This is the stage of generativity versus stagnation (Erikson's seventh stage of psychosocial development) in which the person enjoys developing the skills and talents of younger people (e.g., serving as a sports coach or work mentor).[84] Lack of generativity may lead to stagnation in life, disappointment, and burnout.

Examples of leisure activities typical of this age group are friend and family activities, sports (e.g., golf, bowling, coaching [Fig. 16.2]), card games, internet surfing, socializing and shopping, travel, pet care, gardening, movies, attending plays and concerts, boating, fishing, reading, television, bike riding, dating, and sexual activity with a spouse or partner.

Disruption caused by a physical disability can impair the individual's ability to engage in cherished leisure occupations. Spouses or significant others are called on to be caregivers, and the relationship may undergo changes. Leisure occupations such as travel and fishing may be put aside for the more immediate concerns of learning to cope with self-care, rehabilitation exercises, and therapeutic equipment.[96,117] Friend relationships often change as well. For example, if two men had a friendship based on golfing every Saturday and one of them experiences a stroke and needs to use a wheelchair, either they will have to be proactive and figure out a way to

enjoy each other's company in a new way (e.g., playing golf with adapted equipment or trying out a new activity that they both enjoy), or they may drift apart. Finally, changes caused by life transitions such as menopause and empty nest syndrome are ameliorated many times by engagement in leisure occupations. For example, a qualitative study of women experiencing menopause indicated that leisure activities not only gave the women a sense of familiarity, security, and continuity, but also provided them opportunities to develop new interests and to focus on themselves.[87]

Late Adulthood (65 Years or Older)

Occupational roles typically go through transformations during this age span. Some changes seen in older adults include a shift of emphasis from parent to grandparent and from worker to retiree or volunteer. As time spent in work/career/parenting diminishes, free time increases, and leisure occupations come into full bloom. The interests and activities that were put aside during career attainment now can be given full rein. Erikson's last stage of psychosocial development (stage 8, ego integrity versus despair) is described as the time when people review their lives and hopefully accept the life cycle as being complete and satisfying.[84] The "use it or lose it" principle is particularly important as people age. If activity levels are not maintained, strength, coordination, and skills may deteriorate rapidly.[84] Some aspects of aging considered fairly normal include diminishing hearing and eyesight, arthritis, and decreased sensory abilities, in addition to general aches and pains (see Chapter 47).

Examples of leisure activities in which older adults engage are dining with or cooking for friends and family, social activities, card games, bingo (Fig. 16.3), travel, sports (e.g., golf, or attending games or watching them on TV), walking, exercise

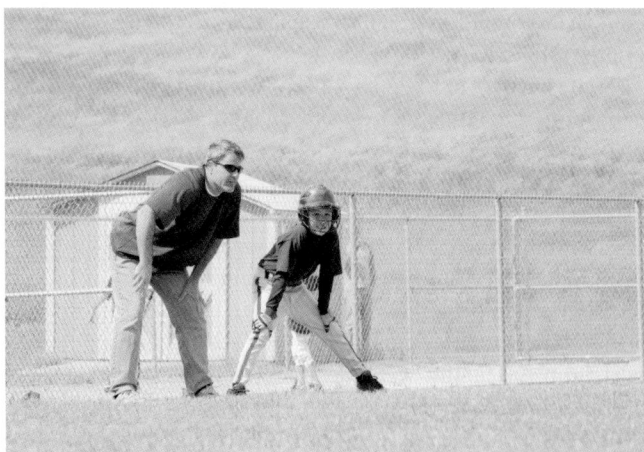

Fig. 16.2 Middle-aged man coaching a baseball player at third base. (Courtesy iStock.com.)

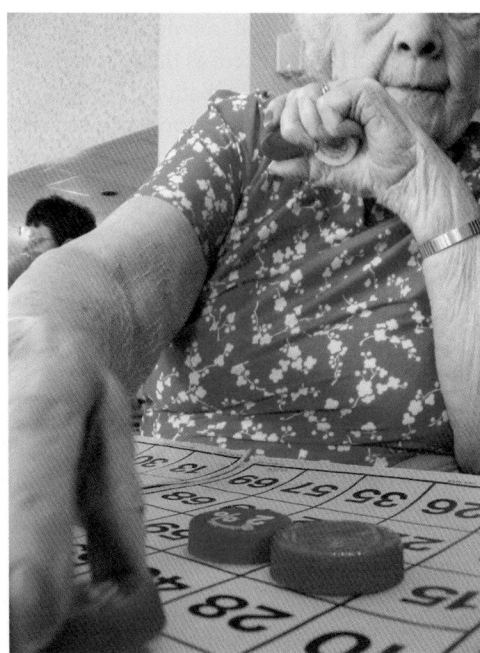

Fig. 16.3 Older adult woman participating in bingo tournament. (Courtesy iStock.com.)

at the gym, swimming, boating, sexual activity with a spouse or partner, reading, television, pet care, gardening, and hobbies (e.g., crafts, genealogy, collecting, birding).[19,65]

If a physically disabling event or disease progression occurs, spouses or significant others may be called on to assist their partners in performing ADLs, including leisure. This can be problematic because the caregiver also may be advanced in age and may not be well suited to provide the care needed.[77] Consequently, leisure activities may be forgotten except for sedentary activities, such as watching television.[117]

For some in late adulthood, isolation and depression could set in and diminish the person's quality of life. A quantitative study of 383 retirees indicated that leisure plays a significant role in achieving a high level of life satisfaction, which the authors propose is equivalent to successful adaptation to retirement.[82] In a study of 324 older Swedes living in the community, Silverstein and Parker discovered that people who increased participation in leisure activities reported being more satisfied with life.[97] The researchers stated, "The results suggest that maximizing activity participation is an adaptive strategy taken by older adults to compensate for social and physical deficits in later life."[97] Mental acuity also may be strengthened or preserved by engaging in novel activities. Engagement with life is vital to successful aging.[65,99]

Culture and Leisure

Because of the increasing diversity of the U.S. populace, occupational therapists must know how culture affects the choices and performance of leisure activities for clients. The client's choice for leisure activities is driven by their self-construct composed of cognition, emotion, and motivation,[78] which is influenced by the culture of their beliefs.[76] Every culture recognizes some aspects of independence and interdependence,[113] and every client and family may value these aspects at a different level. As therapists, we need to understand that everyone has some elements of both independence and interdependence,[41] and clients may not have the same preferences as their family members.

Thus, depending on where occupational therapy is delivered, therapists should make themselves familiar with leisure activities related to the culture of their clients and attend to their desires, goals, and needs to find a best solution for the clients and their families.

Leisure Occupations Related to Culture

Games and leisure occupations instruct, inspire, and reflect the values and beliefs of the parent cultures. For people who immigrate to a new country (e.g., Hispanics to the United States), leisure activities can be used to maintain connections with their heritage. Other possible uses of leisure that aid community integration are to gain pleasure from the new environment and people and learn their language and customs.[61] Watching television, reading, and attending adult education school are some of the ways newcomers use leisure to improve their conversational skills and to understand cultural features.[6,71,101] Depending on the interest of the client involved, occupational therapists may offer leisure occupations that reflect the client's traditional background, thus fostering security in a new country, or provide

leisure experiences of the new country to increase learning, comfort, and integration. Keeping the leisure interventions client centered is the critical element for a successful outcome. Table 16.1 presents ideas for leisure resources.

Leisure-Time Physical Activity by Gender, Age, and Racial/ Ethnic Groups

Physical inactivity has been associated with various health risks, such as obesity; cardiovascular disease, including stroke; diabetes; some cancers; and premature mortality.[26] Occupational therapists can help clients live a healthy lifestyle by encouraging them to participate in some type of leisure-time occupation that involves physical exercise at least several times a week. Some examples of leisure occupations that provide physical exercise but that could be more attractive alternatives to some people are dancing, swimming, boating, bowling, golfing, gardening, and yoga.

To discover national leisure-time physical activity (LTPA), researchers at the Centers for Disease Control and Prevention conducted a multipurpose, cross-sectional healthy survey of U.S. civilian noninstitutionalized population using a stratified multistage sample of U.S. households.[18] The data were collected from 2010 to 2015, and a total of 155,134 respondents aged 18 to 64 completed the survey from 50 states and the District of Columbia.[18] The interview questions inquired about current leisure-time behavior. Specifically, they asked about frequency and duration of muscle-strengthening activities (e.g., lifting weights), light or moderate-intensity physical activity (e.g., cause only light sweating or a slight to moderate increase in breathing or heart rate) and vigorous-intensity physical activity (cause heavy sweating or large increases in breathing or heart rate). Results showed that nationally, only 22.9% of U.S. adults aged 18 to 64 met the guidelines for both aerobic and muscle-strengthening activities during LTPA in 2010 to 2015. Fourteen states and the District of Columbia had significantly higher percentage of adults meeting the LTPA guidelines than the national average. Thirteen states were significantly lower than national average, and most of those are in the Southeast regions, such as Florida, Georgia, Arkansas, etc. Nationally, the percentage of men meeting the LTPA guidelines is higher than women (men: 27.2%; women: 18.7%), although it varies by states.[18] Other studies discovered that women in all cultures engaged in the least amount of physical activity.[39,83,110]

Some barriers to LTPA have been identified. Although many people of different cultures and ages think that movement (e.g., exercise, gardening, walking) yields positive benefits, such as improved health and appearance, they do not engage in physical activities because of "self-consciousness and lack of discipline, interest, company, enjoyment and knowledge."[32] Additional barriers to activity were identified, such as lack of transportation, prohibitive cost, and perceived lack of safety.[65] Social issues, such as gender roles for activity and poor support from the family, were identified by minority women. As barriers to activity, these women additionally reported problems with language, isolation in the community, and lack of childcare because of lack of relatives in the area. In planning interventions, occupational therapists can collaborate with

TABLE 16.1 Resources on Leisure Occupations for Individuals With Disabilities

Media	Titles
Examples of internet resources	*National Center on Health, Physical Activity and Disability* (http://www.nchpad.org/Directories/Programs) *Disabled Sports USA* (moveunitedsport.org/): Provides links to technology available for some disabled sports.
	Adaptive Sports
	Access Sport America (http://www.accessportamerica.org) *Outdoors for All* (http://www.outdoorsforall.org/) *PE Central: Adapted Physical Education Websites* (http://pecentral.org/adapted/adaptedsites.html) *Professional Association of Therapeutic Horsemanship International* (http://www.pathintl.org/)
	Video Games
	Video games accessibility (http://www.ablegamers.com): Provides reviews of games and hardware for accessibility, as well as a forum for discussion of issues.
	Animal Therapy
	Animal Assisted Therapy (AAT) (http://www.petpartners.org/) and *Canine Companions for Independence* (http://www.cci.org) A national nonprofit that enhances the lives of people with disabilities by providing highly trained assistance dogs and ongoing support to ensure quality partnerships.
	Gardening
	Christopher and Dana Reeve Foundation (https://www.christopherreeve.org/living-with-paralysis/health/staying-active/gardening-from-a-wheelchair) and *University of Florida Gardening Solutions* (https://gardeningsolutions.ifas.ufl.edu/): Provides tips for tools, raised garden beds, garden design, planting, watering, etc.
Books	J.A. Decker: *Making the moments count: leisure activities for caregiving relationships* (1997)[29] C. Kenney: *Have crutch, will travel* (2002)[59] J.L. Klinger: *Meal preparation and training: the healthcare professional's guide* (1997)[63] L.H. Meyer: *Lifelong leisure skills and lifestyles for persons with developmental disabilities* (1994)[80] R. Steadward et al.: *Adapted physical activity* (2003)[102]
Journals	*Adapted Physical Activity Quarterly* *Leisure Sciences* *Journal of Leisure Research* *Leisure Studies*
Magazines specifically for individuals with disabilities	*New Mobility Magazine* (http://www.newmobility.com): Serves people with disabilities by providing information, humor, and inspiration to unite the disabled community. *Sports N Spokes*: (https://sportsnspokes.com/): Sports N Spokes is an online sports and recreation online media source for people living with spinal cord injury and disease, spina bifida, MS, and amputations. *Ability Magazine* (http:...www.abilitymagazine.com): Provides information on new technologies, travel and leisure, and employment opportunities. *Audacity Magazine* (http://www.audacitymagazine.com/): A lifestyle magazine that examines issues of the able-minded individual with a disability, ranging from fashion, sports, and dating to cooking, money, hobbies, and advice.

OT PRACTICE NOTES

Barriers to Leisure Participation

Incurring any type of disability or health condition may result in barriers to leisure engagement, such as the following:[16,40]

- Perception of constraint, inability to problem solve and adapt around constraint
- Loss of interest, motivation
- Lack of facilities/support, lack of physical access
- Reduced ability/limited tolerance of activity (e.g., low vision, endurance)
- Lack of time
- Attitude of others (caregivers may not value leisure)
- Attitudes of fellow participants (awkwardness displayed by able bodied)
- Challenging behaviors (e.g., in those with neurological disability)
- Communication issues (e.g., in those with cognitive deficits)
- Increased expense (as a result of adaptations, career support, equipment)

clients to address these problems, find community resources, and develop strategies to improve participation in leisure-time physical activities.

LEISURE OCCUPATIONS: EVALUATION AND INTERVENTION

The OTPF-4 focuses on a client-centered approach, and as the first step in the therapy process, the OTPF-4 requires the OT to work collaboratively with the client and family/caregivers to develop an occupational profile.[7] The profile includes the client's occupational history, past and current interests, performance, and values. Knowledge of the problems and goals the client and family/caregivers consider important gives the therapist a basis for a meaningful intervention plan. Evaluation includes formal

TABLE 16.2 Standardized and Nonstandardized Leisure Assessments and Descriptions Used by OTs

Assessment	Descriptions
Activity Card Sort[12] (standardized)	Picture cards of adults performing various activities, which include 20 instrumental activities, 17 social activities, 17 high physical demand leisure activities, and 35 low physical demand leisure activities. Client sorts them into piles, depending on his or her interest level. Provides a "retained activity level" score indicating engagement levels of performance of past and current activities, which guides the clinician to further examine the reason and develop intervention plans.
Canadian Occupational Performance Measure[68] (standardized)	Interview conducted before and after interventions to describe problems, level of satisfaction in performing activities, and level of perceived performance abilities in areas of self-care, productivity, and leisure. Available in multiple languages. The English version is available in both digital and paper versions.
Leisure Attitude Scale—Short Version for adolescents and young adults (LAS-SV)[106] (standardized)	Measures leisure attitudes using 18 self-report items, comprising three subscales, that address cognitive, affective, and behavioral components of attitude. Rated on a 5-point Likert scale from 1 (strongly disagree; very unfavorable or negative attitude) to 5 (strongly agree; favorable or positive attitude).
Leisure Satisfaction Scale (LSS—Short Form)[109] (Standardized)	Measures whether personal needs are met through leisure activities. Scale of 24 items scored on a 5-point Likert scale from 1 (almost never true for me) to 5 (almost always true for me). Higher scores indicate greater satisfaction.
Nottingham Leisure Questionnaire (shortened version)[35,114] (Standardized)	Outcome measure for leisure participation in patients who received physical rehabilitation. Questionnaire of 30 items scores on a 3-point Likert scale (regularly, occasionally, never).
Physical Activity Scale for the Elderly (PASE)[116] (Standardized)	A 10-item self-report physical activity assessment that includes leisure, household, and occupational activities during the previous 7-day period on community-dwelling older adults aged 65 years or older. Available in other languages, such as Chinese, Italian, etc.
Physical Activity Scale for Individuals with Physical Disabilities (PASIPD)[116] (Standardized)	Modification of the PASE specifically for individuals with physical disabilities; 13 items consist of leisure, household, and occupational activity components.
Quality of Life Scale[22,23,42,117] (Standardized)	Perceived quality of life measured by given conceptual domains: material and physical well-being; relationships with other people; social, community and civic activities; personal development and fulfillment; and recreation. This 16-item instrument is available in several other languages and has been used in patients with cardiac disease, chronic obstructive pulmonary disease, diabetes fibromyalgia, gastrointestinal disorders, rheumatic diseases, and spinal cord injury. Rated on a 7-point Likert scale of "very satisfied" to "very dissatisfied."
Occupational Profile (AOTA Template)[8] (nonstandardized, use with clinical observation)	Interview with the client (and family/caregivers if appropriate), along with observations to gather information about demographics, language, health status, and social and medical history. Questions address why the client needs OT services, what his or her concerns are, the client's occupational history (e.g., values, meanings associated with life experiences), and the client's priorities.
Modified Interest Checklist (https://moho-irm.uic.edu) (nonstandardized)	Checklist of 68 activity items that assesses the client's level of interest (casual, strong, or no interest). Includes many leisure-time activities. Available in multiple languages.
Role Checklist Version 2[95]: Quality of Performance (Role Checklist V2: QP)[95] (https://moho-irm.uic.edu/)	Interview to discover past, present, and future occupational roles (including leisure roles) and their value to the client. Available in multiple languages. Nonstandardized.

and informal assessments, conducted initially and over the course of the therapy process, to guide the therapist in providing an individualized intervention program that meets the client's expressed needs and desires.[7] Examples of possible assessments that address the leisure area of occupation and a description of each are presented in Table 16.2.

Intervention: Where There's a Will, There's a Way

Based on information gathered during the evaluation process, an intervention plan incorporating leisure occupations is developed; this plan must be one that the client and family/caregivers view as important to improving quality of life. Clients (including family members or caregivers, as necessary) and therapists develop goals and plan interventions together,

thus ensuring that the client is motivated to engage in therapy sessions to the best of his or her ability.[7] In occupational therapy, leisure occupations can be both a means and an end. As a means of intervention, the client is provided with the therapeutic use of leisure that is motivating because it is chosen and fun. Leisure as an end is seen when the client voluntarily engages in leisure occupations after therapy intervention stops.[7] As stated by Taylor and McGruder, when developing discharge plans that include leisure, the therapist should consider "attributes of novelty and challenge, meaningful use of time, and identity construction," which are imperative to the continued growth, adaptation, and quality of life of clients.[105] Occupational therapists may offer a variety of leisure activities that are delivered to individuals or groups, depending on the relevance to the client's interests, abilities, and activity demands. In the case of Andrew (see the following case study), individual activities need to be mastered before group activity can be considered.

CASE STUDY

Andrew

Andrew, a 22-year-old man (prefers the pronouns he/him/his) with a spinal cord injury (paraplegia), has an avid interest in playing wheelchair basketball. To prepare him for this sport, the occupational therapist (OT) works with him individually to order the correct wheelchair; strengthen his upper extremities; develop skill in dribbling, catching, and throwing the ball; making baskets from the wheelchair; finding appropriate sports apparel (e.g., to hide his leg bag; shirts that can stay down in back when he is reaching for the basket; push cuffs or golf gloves to protect his hands); and learning how to get back into the wheelchair when he falls out on the court. Referral is then made to a recreational therapist, who helps Andrew incorporate these basic skills into an existing team of players. By developing his individual skills before entering the group activity, his potential to successfully participate in his leisure activity of choice is increased.

Balloon volleyball is a fun and social activity. For example, in a long-term care facility, residents with appropriate cognitive and motor skills can be organized into two teams, seated and facing each other. A real or simulated volleyball net is erected between the two teams, and a balloon is hit back and forth. Music adds to the enjoyable atmosphere. This game can meet several OT goals, such as improving eye pursuit, upper extremity range of motion, socialization, and cognition (keeping track of the score). In addition, because joking and laughing often occur, physical, social, and psychological benefits may be gained (see Box 16.1). The therapist must ensure that clients are interested in participating and that each person is safe, with wheelchairs locked and, if necessary, seat belts attached. Cardiac patients may not be appropriate to include because of the upper extremity workout and increased respiration, heart rate, and blood pressure that could occur.

Adapting the Activity for Success

Occupational therapists are uniquely qualified to adapt the activity, including the equipment, the environment, or the nature of the activity, to make leisure occupations accessible to clients. By participating in leisure occupations that are meaningful, clients are able to continue to make positive adaptations that lead to greater life satisfaction. Table 16.3 describes some leisure occupations and possible adaptations.

Level of Functioning

Occupational therapists view the client as a whole person with myriad dimensions (e.g., physical, cognitive, spiritual, psychological). Leisure occupations are self-enhancers that add joy and pleasure to life. For effective implementation, activities must be analyzed according to the individual's level of functioning (e.g., performance skills, performance patterns, client factors, activity demands, and context). Examples of clients by level of function, along with leisure occupations that are meaningful to the individual, are presented in the case studies of Tina, John, and Miguel.

TABLE 16.3 Examples of Adapted Leisure Occupations

Leisure Occupation	Possible Adaptations	
Gardening	Raised beds for flower or vegetable gardens that are accessible from a chair or wheelchair. Nonskid surface under pots to prevent sliding during potting.	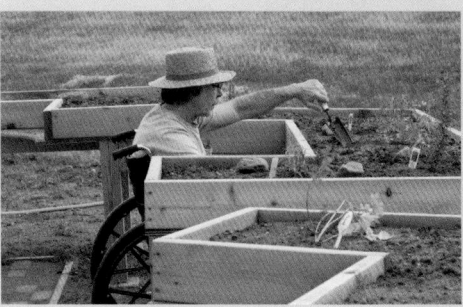

(Courtesy iStock.com.)

(Continued)

TABLE 16.3 Examples of Adapted Leisure Occupations—cont'd

Leisure Occupation	Possible Adaptations	
Bowling	Wheelchair specially designed for bowling, on which the wheels are set under the chair for ease of bowling action. Bowling ball can be made with handles for people with arthritis or hand dexterity problems.	 (Cpl. David Bessey, Public domain, via Wikimedia Commons)
Golf	Adapted golf clubs (e.g., constructed to be used from a seated or wheelchair position or to be used one handed), lower extremity prosthetics specially made for golf.	 (Courtesy David B Windsor, PGA, Georgia State Golf Association Adaptive Golf; Adaptive Golf Academy and Adaptive Golf Association.)
Playing cards	Card shuffler, card holder, large-print or Braille cards	 (Courtesy iStock.com.)
Computer activities or internet surfing	Large monitor screen, large-print font, voice-activated controls or software (e.g., Dragon NaturallySpeaking).	 (Courtesy iStock.com.)
Cooking	Energy conservation techniques, sliding instead of lifting heavy pots, nonskid surface to prevent slippage, rocker knife, perching stool.	 (Courtesy iStock.com.)

TABLE 16.3	Examples of Adapted Leisure Occupations—cont'd	
Leisure Occupation	**Possible Adaptations**	
Pets	Canine companions to manage daily tasks (e.g., open drawers and doors, acknowledge phone ringing, obtain objects) and to provide love and licks. Therapy dogs to visit clients in hospitals, skilled nursing facilities, and homes to bring joy and opportunities for touch. Pets such as fish, cats, dogs, and others provide companionship and may promote motivation for engagement in caring activities.	(Courtesy iStock.com.)
Bike riding	Handcycles for those with lower extremity weakness or paralysis. These bikes are propelled and controlled by arm strength and coordination.	
Swimming	Hydraulic lifts are used to lower people with disabilities into pools for accessibility. Arm bands and flotation belts are adaptations used for those who cannot tread water to float.	(Copyright © iStock.com/kali9. ID: 53123736.)
Ping pong	Wheelchairs with a third wheel to prevent tipping and few adapted rules based on level of disability are the typical adaptations needed for Para-table-tennis, a Paralympic sport	(Copyright © iStock.com/South_agency. ID: 911723688.)
Reading	Audible books, electronic readers	(Copyright © iStock.com/Gaysorn Eamsumang. ID: 1434779765.)

CASE STUDIES

Adapting and Grading Leisure Occupations for Clients

Tina, John, and Miguel

Tina

Level of Function: Maximum Assistance Needed

Tina, a 41-year-old mother of two (prefers the pronouns she/her/hers), had a severe stroke that left her unable to smoothly coordinate movement. She enjoys listening to tapes of her son playing the guitar.

Leisure Occupation

Occupational therapy assessment revealed that when Tina was positioned correctly, her left hand could be guided to hit a large-button switch (Fig. 16.4). Stephanie, the occupational therapist, connected the button switch to a tape player, which held a tape of her son's recent musical accomplishments. Her family members were instructed in how to assist Tina so that they could all participate in a valued leisure activity together.

John

Level of Function: Moderate Assistance Needed

John, a 50-year-old man (prefers the pronouns he/him/his), suffered a traumatic brain injury 3 years earlier. He demonstrates poor dynamic balance, short-term memory deficits, and weakness on his right side. He uses a three-wheeled walker for ambulation. John lives with his wife and is independent in the majority of activities of daily living. His passion is bowling.

Leisure Occupation

After assessing his satisfaction and perceived bowling performance using the Canadian Occupational Performance Measure (COPM),[68] DeShawn, John's occupational therapist, accompanied John, his wife, and their adult son to the bowling alley. DeShawn called ahead to make sure the bowling alley was accessible and had accommodations for people with disabilities. The lanes were set up with gutter bumpers and a bowling ball ramp. Using a gait belt and moderate assistance, John was able to place a lightweight ball on the ramp, set up his shot, release the ball, and knock down some of the pins. When he, his wife, and his son saw that bowling was possible again, they set up a family night once a week to resume a cherished fun activity.

Miguel

Level of Function: Independent

Miguel, a 25-year-old single man (prefers the pronouns he/him/his), was in a skiing accident 5 years earlier and incurred a spinal cord injury that resulted in paraplegia. He progressed through rehabilitation and is independent in activities of daily living (ADLs) and instrumental activities of daily living (IADLs). He uses a power wheelchair, drives, and has a job as a police dispatcher. Miguel has come to occupational therapy to upgrade his wheelchair and discuss leisure occupations. He reports that his free time is boring and he wants to return to a sport.

Leisure Occupation

Wheelchair sports abound in variety. Miguel's occupational therapist, Eric, began by helping Miguel explore the many options for people who want to participate as a wheelchair athlete, including basketball, mountaineering, hunting, rugby (the fastest-growing wheelchair sport), weightlifting, racing (including handcycle racing), tennis, javelin throwing, and snow skiing. When Miguel indicated that he might be interested in resuming his previously loved leisure occupation of camping, Eric showed him how to locate helpful resources, such as magazines, journals, websites, catalogs, and other related publications. For example, in an article in the *British Journal of Occupational Therapy*, Butler, 1997, reviewed sports wheelchairs, and that article also provided information on the chairs' suitability for use on camping trails.[24]

Miguel was further directed to *New Mobility*, a magazine written for and by people with physical disabilities, which had an excellent article on accessible campgrounds and suggestions for making a trip successful. Eric also recommended other magazines, such as *Adapted Physical Activity Quarterly* and *Sports N Spokes*, so that Miguel could read about others' experiences and stories and broaden his ideas of equipment and gadgets for wheelchair users. Eric was thrilled to hear from Miguel a few months later that he had indeed gone camping (Fig. 16.5) and that it was a "super experience!"

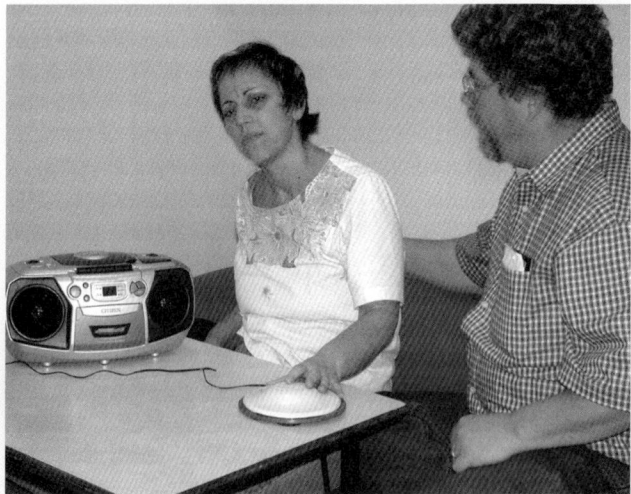

Fig. 16.4 Tina, with her husband, Scott, using a large-button device to turn on a tape player so she can listen to her son playing the guitar.

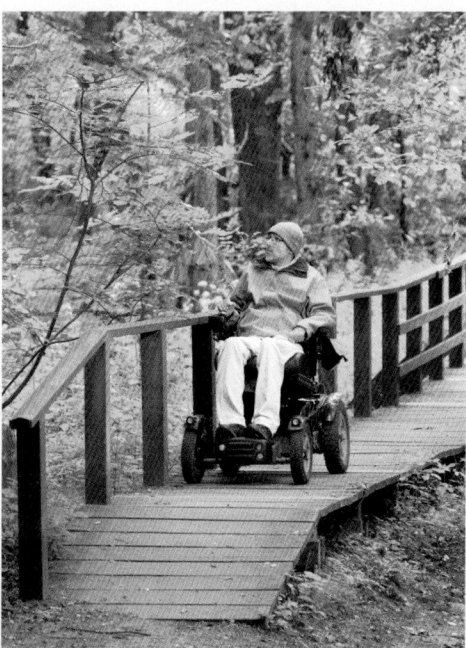

Fig. 16.5 Miguel, in his power wheelchair, is able to enjoy the experience of forests and camping. (Courtesy iStock.com.)

THREADED CASE STUDY

Jeri, Part 2

Reconsider the questions posed about Jeri, a 29-year-old newly married woman whose case study opened the chapter.

1. Is Jeri really ready to be discharged from occupational therapy?

Probably not. Although the occupational therapist has done a thorough job of teaching Jeri how to be competent in ADLs, we now know that there is more to life for occupational therapists to consider than just instructing clients in personal care techniques. OT assessments of Jeri's leisure attitudes, interests, skills, and abilities need to be undertaken and a further intervention plan developed that addresses her quality of life, as well as physical and emotional well-being issues. To ensure that as an occupational therapist you have considered Jeri's life as an individual and not just her activities of daily living, revisit the occupational profile with her and consistently inquire about her daily routines and what she is doing for fun and to relax. Maintaining that connection with the client as a human and a person, and not just as someone with physical rehabilitation goals, will remind the therapist of the larger picture of Jeri's life and what makes her spirits soar.

2. Why is Jeri dissatisfied with her current lifestyle?

Jeri is leading a restricted life, compared with her life before the accident. She has lost many of the activities that brought joy to her life. She is unable to do scrapbooking because she still lacks the fine motor coordination in her dominant hand to manipulate scissors and small decorative paper pieces. She wants to drive again and misses working as an interior designer, playing video games with friends, meeting friends for lunch, and playing with the dogs. Her husband treats her as though she will break and is unsure whether she is capable of caring for the dogs again. Jeri is no longer engaging in leisure activities that reaffirm her age-related competencies.

3. What interventions could the OT provide to improve Jeri's quality of life?

To improve Jeri's ability to resume her cherished hobby of scrapbooking, the occupational therapist could provide fine motor activities that incorporate scrapbooking materials. Manipulation of materials can be improved by gluing small pieces of paper onto sturdy cards to make them easier to hold and using adapted scissors for cutting. A home visit to adapt and set up materials, tools, and access for Jeri to work on the craft would be helpful. Assisting Jeri in problem-solving various ways of playing with the dog outside and how she can physically accomplish caring for the dogs would be needed. Use of two hiking sticks to assist with balance and choosing flat trails to restart this outdoor nature activity with one or two people would probably bring joy to her. A pre-driving assessment and perhaps driver training may help Jeri resume her outside activities, or the assessment may determine that driving is not advisable at this time. If Jeri is unable to drive, the occupational therapist may determine that an intervention aimed at accessing and using public transportation may be the first step in increasing community independence.

A collaborative session with Jeri's husband can be set up to talk through his concerns and to instruct him in the use of adaptive equipment and other means of assisting her in resuming former life roles, such as hiking with friends and playing with the dog. Jeri, her husband, and the occupational therapist could discuss Jeri's missed social roles and need for emotional expression. The occupational therapist can explore what element within the stated leisure activities brings her joy and suggest other leisure, play, and craft activities that she can try. They may set mutual goals that encourage Jeri and her husband to invite friends and family over for a few hours for socializing. She may also be interested in joining a brain injury support group that the OT department runs to provide her with needed peer interaction; her husband may wish to be included in a support group for families. Sexual and sensual expression may be brought up in this meeting, and the occupational therapist could offer suggestions regarding communication of perceived changes, use of touch, and positions to enhance intimacy. The occupational therapist may also indicate referrals, as necessary. All of these leisure-related accomplishments will help reestablish 29-year-old Jeri's perception of herself as a whole human being.

SUMMARY

Occupational therapists assist clients in attaining life satisfaction through a variety of occupations that are meaningful to the individual. Engaging and reengaging in leisure occupations, which may include social interactions, movement, playfulness, and pleasure, are important aspects of a balanced lifestyle. Realizing that lack of leisure activities may lead to isolation and depression and detrimentally affect an individual's recovery and joy in life, occupational therapists need to include leisure evaluation, intervention planning, and implementation for people with physical disabilities. Consideration of the client's age, gender, culture, interests, and environment is paramount when investigating or implementing leisure so that the intervention is client centered. A skilled occupational therapist can facilitate participation in meaningful leisure occupations that may lead to improved psychological and physical well-being, social relationships, and quality of life.

REVIEW QUESTIONS

1. What can the absence of a meaningful leisure occupation lead to for people with a physical disability?
2. List five psychosocial benefits and five physical benefits of leisure activities.
3. Why is the client's cultural background important when considering leisure occupations?
4. How will you modify the leisure occupation that is identified by the client based on his or her cultural background and contextual factors?
5. When should humor and laughter be used with caution?
6. What four factors are essential for modeling behavior to be an effective intervention?
7. Why is it important for the client to be involved in setting his or her own goals?

For additional practice questions for this chapter, please visit eBooks.Health.Elsevier.com.

REFERENCES

1. Abel MH: Humor, stress, and coping strategies, *Humor* 15:365, 2002.

2. Adams P (with Mylander M): Gesundheit! Rochester, VT, 1998, Healing Arts Press.

3. Ahn S-N, Hwang S: An investigation of factors influencing the participation of stroke survivors in social and leisure activities, *Phys Ther Rehabilitation Sci* 7:67–71, 2018.

4. Akbaraly TN, Portet F, Fustinoni S, Dartigues JF, Artero S, Rouaud O, Touchon J, Ritchie K, Berr C: Leisure activities and the risk of dementia in the elderly: results from the Three-City study, *Neurology* 73:854–861, 2009.

5. Allen JL, McKay JL, Sawers A, Hackney ME, Ting LH: Increased neuromuscular consistency in gait and balance after partnered, dance-based rehabilitation in Parkinson's disease, *J Neurophysiol* 118:363–373, 2017.

6. Allison MT, Geiger CW: Nature of leisure activities among the Chinese-American elderly, *Leisure Sci* 15:309, 1993.

7. American Occupational Therapy Association: Occupational therapy practice framework: domain and process, ed 4, *Am J Occup Ther* 74(Suppl_2), 2020. https://doi.org/10.5014/ajot.2020.74S2001.

8. American Occupational Therapy Association. Occupational Profile Template. https://www.aota.org/~/media/Corporate/Files/Practice/Manage/Documentation/AOTA-Occupational-Profile-Template.pdf.

9. Atchley RC: *Social forces and aging: an introduction to social gerontology*, ed 10, Belmont, CA, 2004, Wadsworth.

10. Backman CI: Occupational balance: exploring the relationships among daily occupations and their influence on well-being, *Can J Occup Ther* 71:202, 2004.

11. Bandura A: *Social foundations of thought and action: a social cognitive theory*, Englewood Cliffs, NJ, 1986, Prentice-Hall.

12. Baum CM, Edwards D, editors: *Activity card sort* ed 2, St Louis, 2008, Washington University.

13. Baylan S, Haig C, MacDonald M, Stiles C, Easto J, Thomson M, Cullen B, Quinn TJ, Stott D, Mercer SW, Broomfield NM, Murray H, Evans JJ: Measuring the effects of listening for leisure on outcome after stroke (MELLO): a pilot randomized controlled trial of mindful music listening, *Int J Stroke* 16: 149–158, 2020.

14. Baylan S, Swann-Price R, Peryer G, Quinn T: The effects of music listening interventions on cognition and mood post-stroke: a systematic review, *Expert Review of Neurotherapeutics* 16:1241–1249, 2016.

15. Bennett MP, Zeller JM, Rosenberg L, McCann J: The effect of mirthful laughter on stress and natural killer cell activity, *Altern Ther Health Med* 9(2):38–45, 2003.

16. Bhogal SK, Teasell RW, Foley NC, Speechley MR: Community reintegration after stroke, *Top Stroke Rehabil* 10:107, 2003.

17. Blacker D, Broadhurst L, Teixeira L: The role of occupational therapy in leisure adaptation with complex neurological disability: a discussion using two case study examples, *NeuroRehabilitation* 23:313, 2008.

18. Blackwell, DL, & Clarke, TC: State variation in meeting the 2008 Federal Guidelines for both aerobic and muscle-strengthening activities through leisure-time physical activity among adults aged 18–64: United States, 2010–2015. National Health Statistics Reports, 112, 2018. National Center for Health Statistics. Retrieved from: https://www.cdc.gov/nchs/data/nhsr/nhsr112.pdf.

19. Bjorkland C, Gard G, Lilja M, Erlandsson L-K: Temporal patterns of daily occupations among older adults in Northern Sweden, *J Occup Sci* 21:143–160, 2014. https://doi.org/10.1080/14427591.2013.790666.

20. Blanche E: The expression of creativity through occupation, *J Occup Sci* 14:21–29, 2007. https://doi.org/10.1080/14427591.2007.9686580.

21. Brown CA, McGuire FA, Voelkl J: The link between successful aging and serious leisure, *Int J Aging Hum Dev* 66:73, 2008.

22. Burckhardt C, Anderson KL: The Quality of Life Scale (QOLS): reliability, validity, and utilization, *Health Qual Life Outcomes* 1:60, 2003.

23. Burckhardt C, Archenholtz B, Bjelle A: Measuring the quality of life of women with rheumatoid arthritis or systemic lupus erythematosus: a Swedish version of the Quality of Life Scale (QoLS), *Scand J Rheumatol* 21:190, 1992.

24. Butler B: Overview of sports wheelchairs, *Br J Occup Ther* 4:66, 1997.

25. Cahill M, Connolly D, Stapleton T: Exploring occupational adaptation through the lives of women with multiple sclerosis, *Br J Occup Ther* 73:106–115, 2010. https://doi.org/10.4276/030802210X12682330090415.

26. Centers for Disease Control and Prevention: State indicator report on physical activity. 2014. http://www.cdc.gov/physicalactivity/downloads/pa_state_indicator_report_2014.pdf.

27. Chen S-W, Chippendale T: Leisure as an end, not just a means, in occupational therapy intervention, *Am J Occup Ther* 72:1–5, 2018.

28. Creighton-Smith BA, Cook M, Edginton C: Leisure, ethics, and spirituality, *Ann Leisure Res* 20:546–562, 2017.

29. Decker JA: *Making the moments count: leisure activities for caregiving relationships*, Baltimore, MD, 1997, Johns Hopkins University Press.

30. Delabary MS, Komeroski IG, Monteiro EP, Costa RR, Haas AN: Effects of dance practice on functional mobility, motor symptoms and quality of life in people with Parkinson's disease: a systematic review with meta-analysis, *Aging Clin Exp Res* 30:727–735, 2018.

31. de Natale ER, Paulus KS, Aiello E, Sanna B, Manca A, Sotgiu G, Leali PT, Deriu F: Dance therapy improves motor and cognitive functions in patients with Parkinson's disease, *NeuroRehabilitation* 40:141–144, 2017.

32. Dergance JM, et al: Barriers to and benefits of leisure-time physical activity in the elderly: differences across cultures, *J Am Geriatr Soc* 51:863, 2003.

33. Dilley DS: Effects of humor on chronic pain and its relationship to stress and mood in a chronic pain population, doctoral dissertation, 2006, Alliant International University, Available through Dissertation Abstracts International. www.proquest.com/products-services/dissertations-Abstract-International.html.

34. Dorstyn D, Roberts R, Kneebone I, Kennedy P, Lieu C: Systematic review of leisure therapy and its effectiveness in managing functional outcomes in stroke rehabilitation, *Top Stroke Rehabil* 21(1):40–51, 2014. https://doi.org/10.1310/tscir2001-40.

35. Drummond AER, Park CJ, Gladman JRF, Logan PA: Development and validation of the Nottingham Leisure Questionnaire (NLQ), *Clin Rehabil* 15:647–656, 2001.

36. du Pré A: *Humor and the healing arts: a multimethod analysis of humor use in healthcare*, Mahwah, NJ, 1998, Lawrence Erlbaum Associates.

37. Duvdevany I, Arar E: Leisure activities, friendships, and quality of life of persons with intellectual disability: foster homes vs. community residential settings, *Int J Rehabilitation Res* 27:289–296, 2004. https://doi.org/10.1097/00004356-200412000-00006.

38. Erlandsson L-K, Christiansen CH: The complexity and patterns of human occupations. In Christiansen CH, Baum CM, Bass JD, editors: *Occupational therapy: performance, participation, and well-being*, 2015, Slack, pp 113–127.

39. Eyler AE, et al: Correlates of physical activity among women from diverse racial/ethnic groups, *J Womens Health Gend Based Med* 11:239, 2002.

40. Fenech A: The benefits and barriers to leisure occupations, *NeuroRehabilitation* 23:295, 2008.

41. Fiske A, Kitayama S, Markus H, Nisbett R: The cultural matrix of social psychology 4th ed. In Gilbert DT, Fiske ST, Lindzey G, editors: *The handbook of social psychology*, Vol. 2, 1998, Wiley, pp 915–981.

42. Flanagan J: A research approach to improving our quality of life, *Am Psychologist* 33(2):138, 1978.

43. Foster ER, Golden L, Duncan RP, Earhart GM: Community-based Argentine tango dance program is associated with increased activity participation among individuals with Parkinson's disease, *Arch Phys Med Rehabil* 94:240–249, 2013. https://doi.org/10.1016/j.apmr.2012.07.028.

44. Fry W: The physiologic effects of humor, mirth, and laughter, *JAMA* 267:1857, 1992.

45. Fullagar S: Leisure practices as counter-depressants: emotion-work and emotion-play within women's recovery from depression, *Leisure Sci* 30:35, 2008.

46. Genoe MR, Dupuis SL: "I'm just like I always was": a phenomenological exploration of leisure, identity and dementia, *Leisure* 35:423–452, 2011.

47. Godfrey JR: Toward optimal health: the experts discuss therapeutic humor, *J Women's Health (Larchmt)* 13:474, 2004.

48. Guo L, Lee Y: Examining the role of leisure in the process of coping with stress in adult women with rheumatoid arthritis, *Annu Ther Recreat* 18:100, 2010.

49. Hackney ME, Earhart GM: Effects of dance on movement control in Parkinson's disease: a comparison of Argentine tango and American ballroom, *J Rehabilitation Med* 41:475–481, 2009.

50. Hackney ME, Earhart GM: Effects of dance on gait and balance in Parkinson disease: a comparison of partnered and non-partnered dance movement, *Neurorehabilitation Neural Repair* 24:384–392, 2010.

51. Hackney ME, Hall CD, Echt KV, Wolf SL: Application of adapted tango as therapeutic intervention for patients with chronic stroke, *J Geriatric Phys Ther* 35:206–217, 2012.

52. Hackney ME, Hall CD, Echt KV, Wolf SL: Dancing for balance: feasibility and efficacy in oldest-old adults with visual impairment, *Nurs Res* 62:138–143, 2013.

53. Hackney ME, Hall CD, Echt KV, Wolf SL: Multimodal exercise benefits mobility in older adults with visual impairment: a preliminary study, *J Aging Phys Act* 23:630–639, 2015.

54. Hampes WP: The relationship between humor and trust, *Humor* 12:253, 1999.

55. Heo J, Lee Y, McCormick B, Pedersen PM: Daily experience of serious leisure, flow and subjective well-being of older adults, *Leis Stud* 29:207, 2010.

56. Hunt L, Nikopoulou-Smyrni P, Reynolds F: "It gave me something big in my life to wonder and think about which took over the space … and not MS": managing well-being in multiple

57. sclerosis through art-making, *Disabil Rehabil* 36:1139–1147, 2014. https://doi.org/10.3109/09638288.2013.833303.

57. Iwasaki Y: Leisure and quality of life in an international and multicultural context: what are major pathways linking leisure to quality of life? *Soc Indic Res* 82:233–264, 2007.

58. Janke MC, Payne LL, Van Puymbroeck M: The role of informal and formal leisure activities in the disablement process, *Int J Aging Hum Dev* 67:231–257, 2008. https://doi.org/10.2190/AG.67.3.c.

59. Kenney C: *Have crutch, will travel*, Denver, CO, 2002, Tell Tale Publishing.

60. Kiepe MS, Stöckigt B, Keil T: Effect of dance therapy and ballroom dances on physical and mental illness: a systematic review, *The Arts in Psychotherapy* 39:404–411, 2012.

61. Kim E, Kleiber DA, Kropf N: Leisure activity, ethnic preservation, and cultural integration of older Korean Americans, *J Gerontol Soc Work* 36:107–129, 2002.

62. Klein A: *The healing power of humor*, Los Angeles, Calif, 1989, Jeremy P Tarcher.

63. Klinger JL: *Meal preparation and training: the healthcare professional's guide*, Thorofare, NJ, 1997, Slack.

64. Kolkmeier LG: Play and laughter: moving toward harmony. In Dossey BM, editor: *Holistic health promotion: a guide for practice*, Rockville, MD, 1989, Aspen Press.

65. Krishnagiri S, Fuller E, Ruda L, Diwan S: Occupational engagement and health in older South Asian immigrants, *J Occup Sci* 20(1):87–102, 2013. https://doi.org/10.1080/14427591.2012.735614.

66. Kuiper NA, Martin RA: Laughter and stress in daily life: relation to positive and negative affect, *Motiv Emot* 22(2):133–153, 1998.

67. Kuykendall L, Tay L, Ng V: Leisure engagement and subjective well-being: a meta-analysis, *Psychological Bull* 141:364–403, 2015. https://doi.org/10.1037/a0038508.

68. Law M, Baptiste S, Carswell A, et al: *Canadian Occupational Performance Measure*, ed 5, Toronto, 2014, Canadian Association of Occupational Therapy.

69. Leber DA, Vanoli EG: Therapeutic use of humor: occupational therapy clinicians' perceptions and practices, *Am J Occup Ther* 55:221–226, 2001.

70. Lee KJ, Cho S, Kim EK, Hwang S: Do more leisure time and leisure repertoire make us happier? An investigation of the curvilinear relationships, *J Happiness Stud* 21:1727–1747, 2020.

71. Lee M-Y, Sheared V: Socialization and immigrant students' learning in adult education programs, *N Directions Adult Continuing Educ* 96:27–36, 2002.

72. Letts L, Edwards M, Berenyi J, et al: Using occupations to improve quality of life, health and wellness, and client and caregiver satisfaction for people with Alzheimer's disease and related dementias, *Am J Occup Ther* 65:497–504, 2011.

73. Lewis C, Annett L, Davenport S, Hall AA, Lovatt P: Mood changes following social dance sessions in people with Parkinson's disease, *J Health Psychol* 21:483–492, 2016.

74. Liu H, Da S: The relationships between leisure and happiness: A graphic elicitation method, *Leisure Stud* 39:111–130, 2020.

75. Lötzke D, Ostermann T, Büssing A: Argentine tango in Parkinson disease – a systematic review and meta-analysis, *BMC Neurol* 15:226, 2015.

76. Markus H, Kitayama S: Culture and the self: implications for cognition, emotion, and motivation, *Psychological Rev* 98:224–253, 1991.

77. Martin P: Family leisure experiences and leisure adjustments made with a person with Alzheimer's, *Top Geriatr Rehabil* 22:309, 2006.

78. Matuska K, Barrett K: Occupations of adulthood. In Christiansen CH, Baum CM, Bass JD, editors: *Occupational therapy: performance, participation, and well-being*, 2015, Slack, pp 113–127.

79. Matuska KM, Christiansen CH: A proposed model of lifestyle balance, *J Occup Sci* 15:9, 2008.

80. Meyer LH, Schleien SJ: *Lifelong leisure skills and lifestyles for persons with developmental disabilities*, Baltimore, MD, 1994, Brookes.

81. Mitchell EJ, Veitch C, Passey M: Efficacy of leisure intervention groups in rehabilitation of people with an acquired brain injury, *Disabil & Rehabil* 36(17):1474–1482, 2014. https://doi.org/10.310 9/09638288.2013.845259.

82. Nimrod G: Retiree's leisure: activities, benefits, and their contribution to life satisfaction, *Leis Stud* 26:65, 2007.

83. Outley CW, McKenzie S: Older African American women: an examination of the intersections of an adult play group and life satisfaction, *Act Adapt Aging* 31:19–36, 2007.

84. Papalia DE, editor: *Human development* ed 9, New York, 2004, McGraw-Hill.

85. Parham LD, Fazio LS: *Play in occupational therapy for children*, ed 2, St Louis, 2007, Mosby.

86. Parker CJ, Gladman JR, Drummond AE: The role of leisure in stroke rehabilitation, *Disabil Rehabil* 19:1, 1997.

87. Parry D, Shaw SM: The role of leisure in women's experiences of menopause and mid-life, *Leisure Sci* 21:205, 1999.

88. Pendleton HM: Establishment and sustainment of friendship of women with physical disability: the role of participation in occupation, doctoral dissertation, Los Angeles, 1998, University of Southern California. Available through Dissertation Publishing, University of Michigan. www.proquest.com/ products-services/dissertations-Abstract-International.html.

89. Pert C: *Molecules of emotion: why you feel the way you feel*, New York, 1997, Scribner.

90. Ponsford JL, et al: Longitudinal follow-up of patients with traumatic brain injury: outcome at two, five, and ten years post-injury, *J Neurotrauma* 31:64–77, 2014. https://doi.org/10.1089/ neu.2013.2997.

91. Riley J: Weaving an enhanced sense of self and collective sense of self through creative textile making, *J Occup Sci* 15:63, 2008.

92. Robinson VM: *Humor and the health professions: the therapeutic use of humor in healthcare*, ed 2, Thorofare, NJ, 1991, Slack.

93. Sander AM, Clark A, Pappadis MR: What is community integration anyway? Defining meaning following traumatic brain injury, *J Head Trauma Rehabil* 25:121–127, 2010.

94. Särkämö T, Tervaniemi M, Laitinen S, Forsblom A, Soinila S, Mikkonen M, Autti T, Silvennoinen HM, Erkkilä J, Laine M, Peretz I, Hietanen M: Music listening enhances cognitive recovery and mood after middle cerebral artery stroke, *Brain* 131:866–876, 2008.

95. Scott PJ, McFadden R, Yates K, Baker S, McSoley S: The Role Checklist V2: QP: establishment of reliability and validation of electronic administration, *Br J Occup Ther* 77:96–102, 2014.

96. Shannon CS: Breast cancer treatment: the effect on and therapeutic role of leisure, *Am J Recreat Ther* 4:25, 2005.

97. Silverstein M, Parker MG: Leisure activities and quality of life among the oldest old in Sweden, *Res Aging* 24:528, 2002.

98. Soh S-E, Morris ME, McGinley JL: Determinants of health-related quality of life in Parkinson's disease: a systematic review, *Parkinsonism Relat Disord* 17:1–9, 2011.

99. Son JS, Kerstetter DL, Yarnal C, Baker BL: Promoting older women's health and well-being through social leisure environments: what we have learned from the Red Hat Society, *J Women Aging* 19:89, 2007.

100. Southam M: Therapeutic humor: attitudes and actions by occupational therapists in adult physical disabilities settings, *Occup Ther Health Care* 17:23, 2003.

101. Sparks B: A sociocultural approach to planning programs for immigrant learners, *Adult Learn* 13:22–25, 2001.

102. Steadward R, Wheeler GD, Watkinson EJ: *Adapted physical activity*, Alberta, CA, 2003, University of Alberta Press.

103. Suto M: Leisure in occupational therapy, *Can J Occup Ther* 65:271, 1998.

104. Takahashi K, et al: The elevation of natural killer cell activity induced by laughter in a crossover designed study, *Int J Mol Med* 8:645, 2001.

105. Taylor LPS, McGruder JE: The meaning of sea kayaking for persons with spinal cord injuries, *Am J Occup Ther* 50:39, 1996.

106. Teixeira A, Freire T: The Leisure Attitude Scale: psychometrics properties of a short version for adolescents and young adults, *Leisure* 37:57–67, 2013.

107. Trenberth L: The role, nature and purpose of leisure and its contribution to individual development and well-being, *Br J Guid Couns* 33:1, 2005.

108. Trenberth L, Dewe P: An exploration of the role of leisure in coping with work related stress using sequential tree analysis, *Br J Guid Couns* 33:101, 2005.

109. Trottier AN, Brown GT, Hobson SJG, Miller W: Reliability and validity of the Leisure Satisfaction Scale (LSS-short form) and the Adolescent Leisure Interest Profile (ALIP), *Occup Ther Int* 9(2):131–144, 2002.

110. Umeda M, Kim Y: Gender differences in the prevalence of chronic pain and leisure time physical activity among US adults: a NHANES study, *Int J Environ Res Public Health* 16:988–999, 2019.

111. United States Bureau of Labor Statistics. American time use survey summary. 2022. Retrieved from: https://www.bls.gov/ news.release/atus.nr0.htm.

112. Vogel B: Outdoor recreation: you can do it, *N Mobil* 26:32–42, 2015.

113. Walker GJ, Deng J, Dieser RB: Culture, self-construal, and leisure therapy and practice, *J Leisure Res* 37:77–99, 2005.

114. Walker MF, Leonardi-Bee J, Bath P, et al: Individual patient data meta-analysis of randomized controlled trials of community occupational therapy for stroke patients, *Stroke* 35:2226–2232, 2004.

115. Warren B, editor: *Using the creative arts in therapy and healthcare: a practical introduction* ed 3, New York, NY, 2008, Routledge/Taylor & Francis Group.

116. Washburn RA, Zhu W, McAuley E, Frogley M, Figoni SF: The Physical Activity Scale for individuals with physical disabilities: development and evaluation, *Arch Phys Med Rehabil* 83: 193–200, 2002.

117. Wikström I, Isacsson Å, Jacobsson LT: Leisure activities in rheumatoid arthritis: change after disease onset and associated factors, *Br J Occup Ther* 64:87, 2001.

17

Assistive Technology

Cara Masselink

LEARNING OBJECTIVES

After studying this chapter, the student or practitioner will be able to do the following:
1. Define and describe assistive technology.
2. Compare and contrast therapeutic technology and occupation-enabling technology.
3. Describe the purpose of device access, speech generating devices, and electronic aids to daily living, providing examples and relating to occupational performance.
4. Describe the occupational therapist (OT) role in augmentative communication.
5. Evaluate for positioning and access for commercial and disability-specific device use.
6. Match appropriate assistive technology to a person's unique abilities, occupations, and environments.

CHAPTER OUTLINE

KEY TERMS

Access method
Assistive technology
Bridge
Dedicated device
Direct access

Dynamic display
Equipment abandonment
Indirect access
Letter of medical necessity
Occupation-enabling technology

Proportional control
Switched control
Synthesized speech
Therapeutic technology

Word acceleration techniques
Word prediction
Word completion

WHAT IS ASSISTIVE TECHNOLOGY?

The Technology Act of 1988 defined assistive technology devices as "any item, piece of equipment, or product systems, whether acquired commercially off the shelf, modified, or customized, that is used to increase, maintain, or improve functional capabilities of individuals with disabilities."[21] This definition, although written almost 35 years ago, has stood the test of time as broad enough to encompass the breadth of devices that enable people with a variety of disabilities to improve their independence with daily tasks.

The Technology Act of 1988 further defined assistive technology services, describing "any service that directly assists an individual with a disability in the selection, acquisition, or use of an assistive technology device." The accompanying process in the legislation described evaluation through integration of the equipment in the person's preexisting routines,[21] closely imitating the occupational therapy (OT) process of evaluation,

intervention, and outcomes.[4] Although other professions are also involved in assistive technology practice, the emphasis of occupational therapy on analyzing the person, environment, and occupation, as well as understanding the interactions between each, make our profession a key player in matching a person with appropriate assistive technology devices.[4]

Various proposed typologies for assistive technology equipment exist, based on a variety of factors that often range from two to four categories.[20] Pragmatically, OTs use technology in practice for two reasons: (1) to remediate body functions or performance skills to promote independent occupational performance without equipment and (2) to compensate for chronic deviations in occupational performance, facilitating engagement and participation with equipment. Therefore, the categories of assistive technology described in this chapter include, respectively, therapeutic technologies and occupation-enabling technologies (OETs).

THREADED CASE STUDY

Gianna, Part 1

Gianna, who is 26 years old (identifies as female using the pronouns she/her/hers), has completed her undergraduate degree and wants to apply to law school. Her path to the legal profession is challenged by a complete spinal cord injury at the C4 level, which she sustained 12 years previously in an automobile accident that killed her parents. She no longer is dependent on a ventilator and is able to breathe without mechanical assistance. Gianna is bright, articulate, and exceptionally popular in her rural community. She recently received a new wheelchair with sip-and-puff controls, which allows her mobility in her home and community, and she would now like to attend law school. Ultimately, Gianna would like to specialize in disability rights to support the civil rights of others with profound disabilities. She believes that her insider perspective on the issues might make her arguments more compelling when disabled workers are seeking reasonable accommodations.

The admissions office at the nearby university where Gianna wants to apply for law school suggested that Gianna may have a difficult time completing the required work. As a law student, she will have to research legal precedence in case law and write briefs. She can get into the library, which meets many of the requirements of the Americans with Disabilities Act (ADA), but will need to be able to navigate the legal records, take notes on her findings, and write formal responses to legal challenges. The admissions counselor thinks that Gianna, who has no movement below her neck, may find that the challenge of the legal profession exceeds her capabilities. Gianna does have full-time attendant care, and the attendant would be allowed to sit with Gianna in the classroom and act as a note taker for her. The school also provides lecture notes to disabled students within 3 days of a class session, if requested.

However, because Gianna's attendant must constantly monitor Gianna's physical needs, the ability of the attendant to focus on the lecture content may be impaired. In addition, because the attendant does not have the interest or background in coursework addressing issues related to the law, her ability to identify and record the important content during the lecture is limited. Finally, because of the required hours and hourly wage, Gianna is often faced with attendants quitting after 6 months or so. The new attendant would not have a complete background to help in interpreting the material Gianna is studying.

In her home life Gianna would like to be able to adjust the lights in the room, the room temperature, and the music playing (she prefers to study with music in the background) without interrupting her attendant. She knows that she will always be dependent on others for bathing, dressing, meal preparation, and many other aspects of her activities of daily living. However, she thinks that if she were able to make fewer demands on her attendants, they might be able to remain in her employ longer.

Gianna is seeking an assistive technology consultation to explore technological aids that could help her reach her life goals.

Critical Thinking Questions

1. Which of Gianna's areas of occupation might be improved through the application of assistive technology?
2. What might the occupational therapist (OT) ask, observe, and assess in the evaluation?
3. What positioning considerations and access methods might the OT trial with Gianna?
4. What occupation-enabling technology will the OT trial with Gianna?

THERAPEUTIC AND OCCUPATION-ENABLING TECHNOLOGIES

It is important to note that whether or not a technology is considered an "assistive technology" depends on the application; what is a convenience for some people may be an assistive technology for another.

Therapeutic Technology

Merriam-Webster[13] defines therapeutic as "relating to the treatment of disease or disorders by remedial agents or methods." When applied to this chapter, therapeutic technology refers to the technology that occupational therapists use in treatment to facilitate the remediation of deficits. Using therapeutic technology in occupational therapy intervention aims to progress the person to perform the desired occupation without technology or adaptive equipment—fully independently.

There are two main types of therapeutic technology. First, physical agent modalities and mechanical modalities, defined by AOTA OTPF-4 as an "intervention to support occupation" (p. 59).[4] These are addressed further in Chapter 29. The second type uses technology systems to remediate; this category is often identified as virtual reality, and equipment ranges from commercial gaming to rehabilitation-specific systems. Virtual reality systems are able to engage the individual in a state of immersion. Nonimmersive virtual reality occurs with computer games or gaming systems with handheld controllers.[11] The level of immersion increases on a continuum to increase the virtual experience with head-mounted displays and body tracking sensors emulating natural movement.[11]

Exercises are a common way to remediate range-of-motion or strength deficits. However, using therapeutic technology, the client engages in a concrete task and is motivated to produce many repetitions of movement because of the enjoyable nature of the task and/or rewards with participation.[7] Lange et al.[11] proposed that when using virtual reality in treatment, the OT must fit the game to the user's needs, matching the desired body function or performance skill from current status to the client's end-goal and also to the client's preferences and interests. Furthermore, the OT must gather objective data with the task, provide feedback, and adapt the environment to facilitate performance improvement.[11] When these techniques have done their job, the client will have improved intrinsic function.

Occupation-Enabling Technology

Occupation-enabling technology (OET) is equipment or technology that aids in the performance of an occupation. Assistive technologies and environmental modifications are described as "interventions that support occupation,"[4] as well as "products and technology"[4] that OTs consider as a part of the person's context. Consistent with the definition of assistive technology devices and therapeutic technology, OET can be commercial, disability-specific, or even custom-designed products. An individual would likely benefit from OET when clinical reasoning predicts that presented deficits cannot be remediated. In a successful match of the person and appropriate OET, the OET is regularly and consistently used outside of occupational therapy sessions for safe, efficient, and satisfactory occupational participation.

Products that can be used as OET are limited only by our imaginations and resources, in relation to the individual's needs. Technological advances contributed to the plethora of commercial options available that enable occupational tasks. Furthermore, creating custom equipment, through partnering with a rehabilitation engineer or using three-dimensional (3-D) printing plans from a maker website, can result in unique products that meet individual needs. Although the opportunities for OET are endless, this chapter will focus on the use of devices to support occupational performance, specifically phones, tablets, and computers.

The differences between therapeutic technology and OET have clinical implications for practice (Table 17.1).

The OT Process for Device-Based OET

Device-based OET supports many occupations within the domain of occupational therapy (Table 17.2). The three main categories of OET that will be discussed in this chapter include device (phone, tablet, and computer) access, speech generating devices (SGDs, sometimes also referred to as augmentative and alternative communication [AAC]), and electronic aids to daily living (EADLs). However, OTs start with the occupational problem the person is experiencing, not the equipment (see Table 17.2). Sometimes, after hearing an expressed problem, the OT may try a remediation approach before fitting or matching a person with OET. Other times, the OT concludes, based on the therapist's clinical reasoning and the client's perception, that an adaptation approach should be taken first. Often this occurs within an OT encounter, in an outpatient, home health, or other setting. However, if the person has complex needs, a referral to a specialized assistive technology department may be necessary.

Matching a Person With OET: Interview-Observe-Assess-Trial-Train (IOATT) Evaluation Process

Matching an individual with appropriate equipment relies on solid foundations of occupational therapy practice. Whether the process is implemented in one evaluation session or across 3 months of weekly occupational therapy sessions, matching OET to achieve optimal outcomes must blend occupational therapy practice with technology-specific knowledge. The process can be summarized to interview-observe-assess-trial-train (IOATT), consistent with a top-down occupational therapy evaluation process.[4] However, the process quickly moves into intervention in the "trial" portion, addressing the person's positioning and access (how the person will use the device), and then "trialing" different equipment to improve navigating the display and selecting icons, entering text, and doing other essential tasks as needed to fulfill the individual's needs (Fig. 17.1). The last step in the IOATT process is "train." As we will talk about later, setup and training are necessary to ensure that the recommended equipment, when received, meets the person's needs.

The approach starts with an interview to understand the client's desired occupations, performance patterns, perceptions, specific client factors that affect occupations, as well as to identify the client's specific goals. Use of the AOTA Occupational Profile Template[5] or the Canadian Occupational Performance Measure[12] to frame this conversation will enhance systematic data collection. In addition to specific information about preferred occupations and the environmental context, the OT must ask about the client's associated current technology and any prospective changes, such as device type, and even brand names and models. These details are necessary to ensure that the software and hardware setup for the trials will interface with the individual's current equipment. Furthermore, inquiring about

TABLE 17.1 Comparison of Therapeutic Technology and Occupation-Enabling Technology

	Therapeutic Technology	Occupation-Enabling Technology
Intervention Approach	Remediate/Establish	Adapt/Compensate
Setting of equipment use	Clinical sessions	In home and community environments during everyday occupations
OT role	OT sets up the equipment, selecting games to fit with the person's: 1. Interests and preferences 2. Current abilities as well as the abilities needed to meet end goal OT must adjust game as needed to continue challenging person's improving abilities OT will gather objective data to measure progression and for documentation	Interview client about occupation Observe client performing desired occupation or equivalent occupation Assess the individual's physical, cognitive, and psychosocial status Trial occupation-enabling technology to determine optimal setup that will enable client to participate in the occupation Support person in funding, setup, and training of the equipment to facilitate occupational performance in the home environment
Optimal outcome	Client to perform desired occupation without equipment or technology	Client to perform desired occupation with equipment or technology
Example intervention activity and goal	Activity: Laptop with a USB adaptor and switch system setup to be activated by right thumb and pointer finger in pincer grasp motion. Switch will be placed at midline; client will activate switch to feed fish in computer game. Goal: "Client will independently button a cardigan with large buttons ×2 using dominant (affected) right hand in 8 weeks."	Activity: Client will trial voice recognition software for typing an email. Goal: "Client will check the accuracy of an independently entered, four-sentence email to client's mother using alternative text entry method as appropriate with no errors in less than 4 minutes in 4 weeks."

TABLE 17.2 Occupational Problems, the OT Domain, and OET

Reported Occupational Problem (Examples)	OT Domain Area[4]	OET Category
Unable to write, spell, or type accurately or efficiently enough to complete assignments, communicate with health professionals, and/or do work tasks	IADLs (communication management) Health Management Education/Work Play/Leisure Social Participation	Device access
Difficulty reading (paying attention, listening and comprehending, or fluency)	Education/Work	Device Access
Unable to call outside contact in case of emergency	IADLs (safety and emergency maintenance, communication management)	Device Access
Ordering food for home delivery, if unable to go out into the community	IADLs (shopping)	Device Access
Expressing verbal speech	Social Participation IADLs (communication management)	Speech Generating Device
Too slow on speech device (software or app) to keep up with the conversation	Social Participation	Speech Generating Device
Unable to physically control TV, lights, fans, thermostat, or door lock either at the source or remotely	Rest and Sleep	Electronic Aid to Daily Living
Caregivers need access to locked front door when individual is in bed	IADLs (safety and emergency maintenance)	Electronic Aid to Daily Living

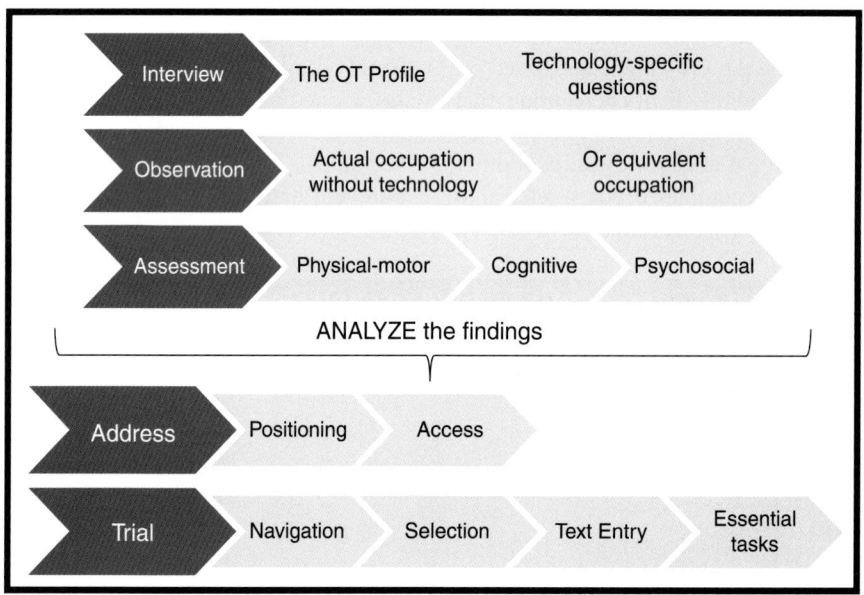

Fig. 17.1 The IOATT evaluation and intervention process.

how the person uses the technology, how they want to use the technology, and what the technology means to the person, is important to understand the client's perspective.

Next, the assessment relates to the analysis of occupational performance,[3,4] in which the OT observes and assesses occupational performance and pertinent body functions and performance. Ideally, the observation would occur in the person's natural setting; pragmatically, the OT may choose an equivalent task that would allow them to gather the same or similar data, but with tools found in the clinic. If the client lacks the necessary body functions to participate, setting up an activity that will

allow the OT to observe the client's strengths and weaknesses related to the occupation is also appropriate. For example, if you are seeing the client to improve text entry because of spelling and handwriting concerns, an observation activity may be watching the client write a shopping list, type an email, or complete a color-by-number. When writing a shopping list, the OT receives valuable information about composing written work, legibility, grasp patterns, fine motor coordination, and position during tabletop tasks. Typing an email will provide an opportunity to observe the person's text entry method at baseline, including spelling, if he or she needs visual attention to the keyboard while typing, hand-eye coordination, bilateral upper extremity use, and cognitive ability to navigate the computer. A color-by-number lends insight into the client's hand-eye coordination, following directions, and sequencing. In each of these activities, the goal is to identify the client's specific strengths and weaknesses, which will guide the process into the assessment portion of the process.

The assessment aims to objectively measure the person's abilities for occupational performance.[4] Gathering more specific details about the individual is a critical part of the occupational therapy process, typically in order to support the need for occupational therapy treatment. For OET, this information combines with the interview and observation to inform the occupational therapist in two additional ways: (1) selecting appropriate trial equipment and (2) justifying (in documentation) the need for, and fit of, the final recommended OET equipment. Common assessments for OET are the same as those used in a typical occupational therapy process, including but not limited to vision screens and assessment of visual perceptual skills, range of motion and muscle strength or muscle tone, cognition, fine motor coordination, posture, and sensation. The occupational therapist must use clinical reasoning to select the appropriate assessment tools to examine the individual's needs.

In the interview, observation, and assessment periods, the occupational therapist gathers information specific to the person's desired occupational goals. The synthesis of this information will determine the individual's baseline status, as well as areas of strengths and weaknesses. The next steps, trialing and training, should be approached as the occupational therapy intervention, with the goal to improve the client's "health, well-being, and participation."[4]

Matching a Person With OET: IOATT Trial

Synthesis of the information from the interview, observation, and assessment provides the basis for the trials. Moderate to complex SGD and EADL software runs on phone, tablet, or computer operating systems; therefore, the procedure to trialing phones, tablets, and computers for occupational performance will be the focus of this section. Variations will be explained in the equipment-specific sections.

Examining the individual's position and determining the optimal access method, or the way the person interacts with the device, is a critical starting point to device use. Trunk stability supports upper extremity mobility; therefore, addressing any postural instabilities in the person's position will support more efficient and accurate upper extremity function. A neutral sitting posture is often perceived as the gold standard for seated occupational performance, with 90-degree flexion of the elbow, hip, and knee angles. This remains true; however, it can be difficult to maintain for a period of time. Therefore, the OT needs to examine closely the person's needs and balance the neutral sitting posture with alternative appropriate positions, such as prone, tall kneeling, or standing for ambulatory people (Box 17.1). Additional equipment may be needed to adapt the device's position when the person moves to an alternative position. Nonambulatory people, or those with low muscle tone, strength, or endurance, may benefit from additional secondary supports such as appropriate arm rests or forearm supports, mobile arm supports, a lumbar

support, and well-placed foot supports, which can facilitate security when in a seated position. Finally, when the individual is a wheelchair user or in an alternative position, a mount or device support should be considered to provide a consistent position from which the person can use the device. Mounts can be secured to the wheelchair, tabletop, or even a body part in some cases to stabilize the position of the device for use, as well as to keep the device safe from falling or being thrown.

BOX 17.1 Positioning Checklist

For device use over a period of time (e.g., during work/school tasks):

____ 1. Can the person achieve the reference neutral seating posture of 90-90-90? Can the person's feet rest flat on the floor or footrests?

If not, we need to work with the person's optimal position and examine equipment fit.

Look at the pelvis first. Is the chair depth sufficient for the person's hip to knee length? The person's thighs should be supported by the chair with a 0- to 2-inch gap behind the knee when the person is sitting with the back against the chair back.

Look at the person's trunk. Is the back height sufficient for the person's trunk? For tabletop work, the back height should reach about three fourths of the way up the person's back, stopping at about the lower scapula. This may be different for wheelchair users, as other occupations (not just tabletop tasks) need to be considered.

Look at the person's feet. Do the feet sit flat on the floor when the knees are at 90 degrees flexion? If the person's feet are dangling, support with an appropriate height stool that supports the feet in neutral.

Look at the person's elbows. Can the person access the keyboard at 90 degrees and sustain that posture? If not, the patient may need chair arms, with articulating or mobile arm rests positioned supportively to achieve and sustain that position.

Look at the person's workstation. Is the device positioned appropriately to support the person's posture? The top to middle of the display should be at the person's eye level and 20 to 24 inches away from the person. If not, it may need to be elevated. A wired or wireless keyboard may help to separate the display from the device, if needed, to obtain the optimal display position.

____ 2. Is the person able to sustain the posture for the necessary period of time to participate in the occupation?

If not, does the person have sensory processing needs? The person may need different equipment (e.g., Move 'N' Sit, therapy ball) or alternative positioning (e.g., prone, tall kneeling) that supports the need for sensory input to support attention.

If not, does the person have the strength and endurance to maintain the posture? If not, may need to try secondary supports to sustain the position over a period of time. Some people even benefit from working in a reclined or tilted position.

Intermittent device use throughout the day (e.g., phones, SGDs):

____ 3. Can the person carry and set up the device, safely, without risk of dropping, throwing, or forgetting?

If not, consider a wearable harness, pocket in clothing, carrying bag, or wearable device holder. This may work for lighter weight, smaller devices.

If not, consider a mount. The mount may secure the device to a specific surface, such as tabletop, that the person frequents throughout the day. Or, a mount may be affixed to a wheelchair. The mount needs to position the device to provide a consistent, secure, and stable surface when the person moves to use it but cannot occlude vision for other occupations.

There are two main types of access methods: direct and indirect access. An access method is the way a person interacts with a device. Direct access is when the person can activate to any icon desired, without additional steps. With indirect access, the person must navigate through nested functions within the display to activate the intended icon. This requires memory of what actions are needed to navigate to the display or icon. Think of when you navigate to a single subfolder on a computer located within several subfolders. To access a specific subfolder, the user needs to open the folder, then subsequent subfolders, until the intended icon is activated. In indirect access, software directs the highlighting of groups of icons on the display, which the user selects when the desired icon is present in the group. This sequence is repeated until the user may select the desired icon directly.

Direct access is the most intuitive type of access. When we use a smartphone, touching icons with our fingers to select apps or move pages, or when we type on a keyboard with our fingers, we are directly accessing these devices. The most common type of direct access is with our hands. However, when a person experiences motor planning deficits, the person's hands often are unable to access a device accurately and efficiently. Adaptations to the task can improve accuracy and efficiency.

Adapting access methods may require hardware and/or software. *Hardware* is physical objects; a keyboard or monitor is considered hardware. *Software* tells the device what to do. Common types of software are applications (apps) or computer programs. Built-in software is software that comes with the device, like accessibility options in the system settings. Add-on software is software purchased for the device and may be related to accessing the device or may be occupation-specific. Direct access for devices may be adapted using hardware such as stylus or typing splints, or through different computer mice (also hardware) that can be controlled by the person's mouth, head, eyes, an arm, or foot (Box 17.2). Given the level of Gianna's spinal cord injury, the use of eye gaze and speech-to-text software to access devices is important to consider when she needs

---

BOX 17.2 Access Checklist

_____ 1. Can the person navigate the device—that is, can the person find and touch (or move the mouse pointer onto) the desired icon?

If not, is it a vision issue—can the person see it? Modify the display to enlarge icons, spread out icons, or change contrast. Enabling auditory feedback with system settings, add-on zoom software, or screen-reading software may also improve function.

If not, is it a cognitive issue—does the person understand the direction or the content? Simplify the directions and the display. Remove unnecessary icons, decrease the number of words, or color code.

If not, is it a mobility or motor planning issue—does the person try but cannot reach, miss the icon, or tremor too greatly to accurately move his or her arm?

Try potential control options for upper extremities, such as an access method that allows the person to anchor the forearm to the tabletop (e.g., trackball mouse), or hardware that guides motor movement (e.g., keyguard, disability-specific joystick).

An access method that uses **proportional control** (i.e., controls movement in any direction with one piece of equipment, such as a joystick) is more efficient and intuitive over **switched control** (i.e., pairs one direction of movement with one activation so that multiple activations are needed to move in various directions, such as mouse keys). Although switched control may be needed to adapt for significant motor planning difficulties.

May be paired with software to slow mouse pointer movement or change touch sensitivity.

Try one- or two-switch scanning. This requires hardware, a switch, and (depending on the device) an adaptor, and built-in software settings or add-on software that will program the timing and switch scanning pattern.

Try potential control options for the person's head and neck, such as a chin or mouth-controlled joystick, or a head-tracking mouse. If those do not work, eye gaze may be trialed. Typically, lower-level access methods need to be ruled out before trialing eye gaze systems.

_____ 2. Can the person select the desired icon? Can they execute the selection actions of single click, double click, right click, click and drag? Or, on a touchscreen, single tap, double tap, tap-hold, flick, and drag and drop, among other device-specific gestures?

If not, does the person need a selection method because the one with the navigation method will not work for them? Or, are their movements too slow, or does the mouse move under the person's hand when they try to select?

Try changing the software settings for mouse pointer or touchscreen sensitivity. A hold or increasing the firmness needed to select may increase accuracy and decrease unintended selections.

Try selection with a switch, to separate selection from the mouse pointer movements. To do this, use a compatible adaptor with the device (e.g., Swifty USB Switch Interface[15]), plug in an appropriate switch, and plug the adaptor into the computer. Once installed, it will work as a mouse click.

Try dwell software, with built-in device settings or add-on software. This software presents different selection methods, allows for the person to activate the desired selection, and then applies it the next time the person "dwells" the mouse pointer in a small (definable) area.

_____ 3. Can the person enter intelligible text? When asked to type, do they touch-type or hunt-and-peck? (NOTE: For EADLs, entering text is not often necessary.)

Do they have the potential to touch-type? If so, try learning-to-type programs. There are even programs for one-handed typing.

Try alternative hardware (e.g., keyboard with keyguard) that may guide digit movements to the appropriate key.

Try an onscreen keyboard, especially if the person has a reliable navigation and selection method. Many built-in onscreen keyboards have **word acceleration techniques** such as **word prediction** (the software predicts the next word given the context of the sentence) and **word completion** (the software will insert the completed word into the text when selected). Onscreen keyboards often work great for short periods of text and are very reliable.

Try voice recognition software. For longer periods of text, voice recognition software is the optimal method to efficiently enter text, as long as the person has a consistent voice. Otherwise, voice recognition software can be frustrating, and in certain software systems, can be unreliable. Voice recognition software will not spell a word wrong, but can put the wrong word in. Proofreading skills are necessary, and training can improve accuracy!

_____ 4. If the person cannot spell or talk, a symbol-based system, like that often found in communication apps and software, is necessary to support the person's communication of medical-based wants and needs. Many of the access methods described here work with communication software, including touch access, mice controlled by different body parts, one- and two-switch scanning, and even eye gaze.

to generate written assignments for school. Software may also adapt access methods, with mouse or touch modifications that change the sensitivity of how the device accepts input, or screen-reading software that navigates the computer display for a person who is blind, or dwell software for selection that activates a mouse click based on "dwelling" the mouse pointer in a target area for a set period of time. Furthermore, voice access has progressed with technological advances and is quite functional for directly accessing text entry. However, functionality differs within voice recognition programs for navigating and selecting functions, and add-on software is generally better than built-in software to support voice navigation. Due to the disparities in software, attempting, or "trialing," all tasks the person needs to do is important to ensure the person has full functionality and control of the device.

When assessing device access, whether direct or indirect, there are three main tasks a person must be able to do in the following order: (1) navigate to where the person needs to go on the device, (2) select icons and/or text (in all quadrants of the device screen), and (3) enter text. During these tasks, the OT needs to think both about the person doing the specific task, as well as the cumulation of doing all the necessary tasks with the device in the home, work, or school environment, to ensure that all of the technology will work effectively in various settings. For example, it may be feasible that the client uses typing splints to type, but if he or she cannot control the mouse with the typing splints donned and needs to navigate to a new webpage, the typing splints become barriers without a compatible mouse. In this case, a solution might be to find a mouse the individual can control well and type using an onscreen keyboard.

Software programs aimed at objectively capturing the person's performance with various access methods exist. Koester Performance Research (KPR)[9] assessment software examines computer accessibility and may be used with different access methods to compare user efficacy and accuracy. Some of the software programs can even adjust software settings based on assessment results to optimize access. Scanning Wizard by KPR[10] is a free website that assesses switch fit and provides ways to optimize switch access for device or SGD access. Using these objective measurements can help when collaborating with the client to make decisions for equipment recommendations, as well as justify the person's need for the equipment to a funding source.

Device trials. The majority of tasks on a device can be accomplished by navigating, selecting, and entering text. However, difficulties in reading, spelling, and taking notes also may be adapted using a device.

Text-to-speech software. Auditory books are common adaptations when a person has trouble reading print, but text-to-speech (TTS) software can read aloud digital print, providing a multimodal reading platform with visual and auditory feedback. Implementing TTS can support reading comprehension and vocabulary.[16,19] TTS software options range from simple to complex. Simple options, which may be enabled through built-in software settings or web extensions, read aloud highlighted digital text on demand. As TTS increases

in complexity, features are added, such as the ability of the software to highlight words while reading, modify the speech rate, and also include note-taking or comprehension supplements (e.g., dictionary). At greatest complexity, TTS programs convert scanned images of book pages or worksheets into digital text (providing the user complete control to read any document), include study tools, mask lines or paragraphs to direct visual attention, and further modify the text for vision impairments.

Difficulty spelling can be debilitating, but software can help through the access method for text entry, or alternative software that addresses spelling and comprehension apart from typing. For example, voice recognition software eliminates the need to spell words, as accurate spelling is used during the transcription process from the software's dictionary. However, the software may put the wrong word in the text. Therefore, close proofreading to ensure accuracy is required. Apart from the access method, built-in options in word processing software programs such as spellcheck can identify any misspelled words in its dictionary and propose modifications. Add-on software, such as Grammarly,[8] reviews grammar as the person is typing and suggests improvements, which can be selected and inserted into the text. However, reading corrections may not provide enough support for someone with a concurrent reading disability. Therefore, add-on software, such as WordQ 5,[17] uses (modifiable) speech output to read aloud lists of words, using word prediction and word completion. Some TTS software programs have word processing capabilities and can also provide word prediction and completion with speech output for words, sentences, and highlighted content.

Notes are often taken for studying purposes, but also in vocational roles such as administrative assistant, sales, or customer service positions. When approaching trials for note-taking, first consider if voice recordings, written text, or both, are needed for the outcome to be successful. Asking a student "How do you study?" can provide insight into the student's preferred method of learning. Note-taking by hand can be limited; however, using a digital notebook allows notes to be imported to the computer, increasing accessibility. Typed notes are often used as well and are easily searchable when key words are used. However, the demands for typing efficiently during a meeting or phone call are great. Both built-in and add-on options exist for adapting note-taking. Onscreen keyboards or spelling software with word lists may speed up typing long words. Voice recording software or apps can be helpful, but they should possess a "bookmark" option so that the person can easily return to important spots in the recording. Voice recordings may later be turned to text through a transcription service or app, although the text should be proofread to ensure accuracy. Additionally, it is important to note that although transcriptions of lectures or meetings may be helpful, the person still needs to identify priorities in the transcribed document and summarize them to be useful. Finally, add-on software programs that record auditory synchronously with text entry allow the user to easily return after the lecture or meeting to fill in the notes. This may increase accuracy and enable studying by repetition to improve learning (if that is the desired outcome). However, video recordings of lectures and meetings may require a lot of digital space.

Finally, many occupational tasks, especially those that are vocational in nature, require the use of specific software for full participation. For example, OTs use electronic medical records to document client visits, and faculty and students use virtual platforms to transmit course documents and assignments. These specific software programs, and even different web browsers (e.g., Apple's Safari,[5] Microsoft's Edge[14]), present varying levels of accessibility. The compatibility of the software with different accessibility hardware and software may change with software updates. Therefore, when the individual uses specific software for occupations, the OT should trial the recommended equipment with the software before pursuing purchase.

Speech generating devices. Speech therapists typically lead the process to match a person with an appropriate SGD (sometimes referred to as augmentative and alternative communication [AAC] devices) however, occupational therapists provide valuable input on the positioning and access of the person needing the device, especially when upper extremity compromises, mobility impairments, vision problems, or sensory processing concerns are present.[22] SGDs are one of the only device-based OETs that most medical insurances cover, as they are classified as "durable medical equipment,"[6] although the coverage extends only to **dedicated devices**, or those that are locked into the communication software at delivery. It is important to note that many funding sources require a physical or occupational therapy evaluation accompanies the SGD request. Customizing the documentation to demonstrate occupational therapy's distinct value in the OET matching process will provide further proof of the individual's ability to functionally use the device, thereby improving the potential that the funding source will cover the equipment for the individual.

A wide range of SGDs exist. Simple SGDs often consist of one to two switches, or a grid of 4 to 32 icons, that allow for the voice recording of messages that play upon activation. Complex SGDs consist of a communication software or app and a device. Currently, many communication software programs, and even SGDs, run on a commercial operating system. An *operating system* is the software that tells a device how to work (e.g., ChromeOS, MacOS, iOS, Android, Windows). Because many of the communication software systems run on commercial operating systems, many commercial devices are used as the basis for SGDs; although, to comply with the funding source rules, they are delivered locked into the communication software or app. Complex SGDs have **dynamic displays** that change when icons are activated, use **synthesized speech** (a computer-generated voice), and possess a range of vocabularies that meet the needs of initial communicators (that represent language as symbols and speak whole phrases upon activation) to emerging communicators (that represent language and symbols and text and require the user to link together nouns, verbs, and other words to create messages to speak) to text-based communicators which, if given an appropriate access method, communicate their own unique messages from spelling and stored phrases.

The commercial devices that are employed for SGDs use access methods in similar ways to those used in phones, tablets, and computers because, in essence, that is what they are. However, some access methods are easier to use on an SGD because of the grid-based format with simple interface and specific settings created directly for people with disabilities in mind. For example, the organized grid-based format and larger targets increase the simplicity when navigating using one- and two-switch scanning systems and eye gaze, and switch and dwell selection methods are often built in, making these features easier to program. Additionally, some SGDs use a propriety device design with a commercial operating system. By doing this, they can build in switch ports and eye gaze systems so that the device is one integrated and seamless system.

Addressing positioning and determining optimal access methods for SGDs follows the same process as that of devices described previously with one major difference: the occupational therapist will likely collaborate with the speech therapist on the communication software and vocabulary appropriate for the person. Furthermore, occupational therapist interaction with the SGD does not end at recommendation if the person is receiving OT services. A person's SGD should be integrated into occupational therapy treatment and used to elicit participation and engagement in occupations, as the end goal of OET is competence using the device for occupational participation in daily living activities.

Electronic aids to daily living. EADLs are a unique category of equipment that provides the user with control over home features such as opening and closing, or locking and unlocking, doors, lights (plug-in and hardwired), television and entertainment system control, temperature regulation, caregiver and family call, bed control, and even home appliances. There are two main categories of EADLs: single-purpose and multipurpose. *Single-purpose EADLs* provide control over one task, whereas *multipurpose EADLs* provide control over two or more tasks. Both commercial and disability-specific systems may work for a person's needs, depending on the occupational goal, or goals. Commercial systems use more recent technology but may be unstable after device updates, and customer support may be limited. Disability-specific systems often have built-in alternative access methods, similar to dedicated SGDs, and the impact of updates are considered in the software design. Whether the person needs a single-purpose or multipurpose system, the same positioning and access method assessment needs to occur to determine how the individual will interact with the EADL.

EADLs range from simple to complex; simple EADLs are often single-purpose, and more complex are often multipurpose. However, more distinctions between the two categories exist. EADLs must communicate with accessories in the environment. Simple, single-purpose EADLs often communicate in one way, whereas multipurpose, complex EADLs may communicate in a variety of ways. There are four main ways that EADLs communicate: direct, through house wiring, infrared (IR), and radio frequency (RF). Direct, or wired, communication occurs when the device and accessory are connected through wires, often receiving power when plugged into the wall. For example, the Ablenet Powerlink 4[1] is a simple EADL that gets power when connected to a wall plug. The Powerlink 4 makes the power on/off of simple appliances (e.g., fan, blender, radio) switch controlled by plugging the appliance into the Powerlink 4 and the switch into the Powerlink 4. House wiring is an older communication method and not often used anymore, but an example of this is X10 technology. X10 connected on/off for plug-in devices to remote control. IR is known as "line of sight" communication and is often used in remote controls to communicate with paired televisions. If the remote control uses IR communication, putting a barrier (such as your hand) over the end of the remote control, will stop it from working. EADLs that communicate by IR may possess a dictionary of IR commands, like a universal remote does, and apply selected codes to actions or may "learn" IR codes from an existing remote control so they can be programmed into remote control software. Finally, RF is the quickest growing technology category, containing both Bluetooth and Wi-Fi communication methods. RF can be found in many garage door openers, and Bluetooth communication pairs many phones with wireless earphones and other accessories. However, Bluetooth has a limited distance for connectivity, which can be reduced by barriers in the physical environment, such as walls. Wi-Fi can cover a greater distance, and even may be communicated with outside of the home. Because of this, devices that use Wi-Fi as a communication method are quickly growing in popularity.

Many occupational therapists are familiar with smart home technology and may assume this is a perfect option for the individual; however, when planning EADL trials, the OT must start by assessing a reliable access method, then ensure that the access method can interface with the EADL. The EADL may be a phone with an app, a smart speaker, or a disability-specific device. It is important to read carefully through the entire setup and installation instructions of commercial devices. These instructions will provide imperative information on specifically what is needed to set up the equipment and how the equipment works. For many commercial smart home devices, such as the Amazon Echo devices and smart lights, access to a phone or tablet-based app is needed for setup and installation and, in some cases, even for continued customization and use of the equipment.[2] Furthermore, sometimes a **bridge**, or piece of hardware to interface between two incompatible communication methods, is needed. For example, some smart blinds (providing remote shade control through windows) only communicate in RF, so a bridge is needed to interpret the signals from a Wi-Fi smarthub.

Equipment recommendation and equipment abandonment. The occupational therapist has interviewed, observed, and assessed the individual. The therapist has analyzed the information and setup activities in which the client participated in approximately three equipment trials or trial activities. During this time, the occupational therapist observed the person navigating, selecting, and entering text on one or many devices. The results of the trials were discussed with the person and the

person's support system, and together the team has come to a decision: the final equipment recommendation, including all of the equipment needed for the person to participate in the desired occupation at the person's greatest potential.

If the comprehensive approach was followed, the occupational therapist and the individual should have enough information to make an informed decision. If not, equipment abandonment may occur. **Equipment abandonment** is when an equipment is recommended, but upon approval and ordering, the equipment sits unused, generally stashed away in a closet. Discussing the four qualities of equipment abandonment in the concluding discussion may help reduce the potential of this occurring. First, is the device easy to use? Is the interface intuitive, and is it light enough to carry or easy enough to take on and off the mount? Determine who will install the equipment. Second, does the person like the look of the device? Can the person picture himself or herself using the device during daily tasks? Third, is the device sturdy enough to be present during the person's daily activities? If there are any questions about this, what is the warranty? (Disability-specific equipment tends to be more durable than commercial equipment and has better customer service, although this varies). Last, does the person have a diagnosis that is progressive or may change over time, and will the device fit the person's changing needs? We can often pursue different access accessories if the person's needs change in the future; however, it takes time, money, and effort to get accustomed to a whole new device.

Now what? The occupational therapist needs to write up the information in a **letter of medical necessity**, a specific occupational therapy document with the purpose of justifying the need for the equipment. In contrast to occupational therapy documents that serve to justify need for services, this document provides a summary of the client's interview, observation, and assessment and then describes the equipment trialed and the person's performance in the occupation. This document is entered into the individual's record but also may be given to the funding source, such as medical insurance or vocational rehabilitation services, or the person's family to pursue private funding.

Matching a Person With OET: IOATT Training

Once the person has the equipment, installation and setup, or customization of the equipment to the person's unique needs, must occur. The adaptations programmed during the trial need application to the person's own equipment. As equipment use occurs, modifications to settings and other issues may need addressing, as fluctuations in abilities because of fatigue, temperature changes, or other factors will arise that were not observed during the evaluation. Additionally, some equipment, such as voice recognition software, or SGDs, need further training to maximize occupational performance. Incorporation of this training into occupational therapy treatment allows the therapist to ensure that the individual achieves optimal independence; but also, this follow-through will improve clinical reasoning skills for future OET processes.

THREADED CASE STUDY

Gianna, Part 2

Gianna has difficulty in her current areas of occupational performance in instrumental activities of daily living (IADLs), education, and social participation, which might be addressed through assistive technology, specifically occupation-enabling technology because of the length of time that has passed since her injury and the deficits in body functions and performance skills that still remain. Gianna's ability to write letters to her friends and socially communicate on social media would benefit from the same technologies (primarily mobility [addressed in Chapter 11] and device access) that will allow her to pursue her education. Additionally, providing her with a means to make contact in the event of an emergency may enable further independence.

Furthermore, the occupational therapist asked about Gianna's goals, observed occupational participation, and assessed Gianna's vision, cognition, psychosocial status, and physical-motor abilities in preparation for device trials. The occupational therapist observed her posture in the power wheelchair, but it did not need direct intervention at this time because no problems were present. Gianna's verbal communication skills are excellent, so she will not need a speech generating device. Because this is an area of strength, the occupational therapist observes that this may be a viable access method for longer periods of text. Alternatively, a mouth-controlled joystick or a head tracking mouse are other access methods the occupational therapist considered.

For device access, Gianna will need to use a computer for school and a phone for emergency contact. Gianna currently uses a power wheelchair with sip-and-puff controls, so access through the power wheelchair electronics to a computer mouse and a phone by Bluetooth or television control by infrared may be possible. However, control through her power wheelchair would limit her participation to when she is in her wheelchair. After a trial, Gianna decides that because she does not have a history of bedrest due to pressure injuries or other comorbidities, computer access through her sip-and-puff wheelchair electronics would work well. She further trials the onscreen keyboard, which works for short periods of text entry, and voice recognition software for longer periods of text entry. Gianna demonstrates excellent potential for using these three adaptions for schoolwork.

Gianna decides that she will likely need to use a smartphone while in bed for calling in the event of emergencies, but the smartphone would need to be accessible by voice. Therefore, the occupational therapist and Gianna find a smartphone option that will allow for voice calling in the event of an emergency and a mount that will stabilize the phone so that it is visible and accessible by voice at her bedside. Gianna will also be able to use this phone setup when she is up in her power wheelchair with a voice-controlled Bluetooth headset for privacy.

Through the use of an EADL, Gianna can gain control over her immediate environment. The smartphone pairs with the Alexa app and an Amazon Echo Show, as well as appropriate accessories, to control the temperature of her home, the radio, and/or television; control the lighting; and open doors as desired. Gianna's uncle enjoys tinkering with technology and has smart home technology at his house; he has committed to setting up this technology for his niece.

Through the application of appropriate assistive technology, it will become possible for Gianna to have more control over her life in terms of both her immediate surroundings and her future occupations. Gianna will be able to access online resources, write papers for college, and ultimately, if she has the cognitive skills, become a successful lawyer. Her assistive technology does not guarantee that Gianna will succeed, but it does give her the same opportunities to succeed or fail as her peers in law school who do not currently have functional limitations.

SUMMARY

Matching a person with appropriate OET maximizes function with occupations in the presence of chronic or progressive injuries and disabilities. The occupational therapist plays a key role in this process as experts of occupation and the disability process. Advocating for the equipment needs of the person results in outcomes with impact far greater than the immediate occupational process. When the person's needs reach outside of the occupational therapist's current knowledge, the person may benefit from consulting an expert in assistive technology through the Rehabilitation Engineering and Assistive Technology Society of North America.[18] Remaining up to date on current technology requires attention and effort; however, it is a worthwhile undertaking in the path to becoming an expert practitioner.

REVIEW QUESTIONS

1. Compare and contrast therapeutic and occupation-enabling technology.
2. In what way do devices using universal design assist individuals with disabilities? Why are they not considered assistive technologies?
3. Why might a person with a disability not require any assistive technology for the completion of some tasks?
4. In pediatric applications, complex EADL devices might not be considered appropriate. What sort of EADL might be used with a very young child?
5. Some EADL devices allow control of the features of devices in the environment. Discuss the benefit of providing such control. What additional load does this place on the user?

6. SGD devices can be used to provide alternative or augmentative communication. Discuss the difference between these two strategies. Might an SGD device be a rehabilitation technology in some applications?
7. Describe how positioning can support effective communication using a SGD or AAC.
8. Discuss the difference between direct and indirect access of technology devices for communication. How might each of these be important in an educational setting? What are the dominant demands of each type of communication?
9. Explain the steps in the IOATT method and when to introduce OET to support a client's occupational performance.

10. If an individual is able to use a physical keyboard but can only use one hand, what keyboard options might help him or her with text production?

11. Consider the keypad providing control for a microwave oven. How might the keypad present difficulty to an individual who is blind? How might it be modified by an OT to improve its usability?

12. Word prediction and word completion are often touted as means to improve typing speed, yet research suggests that they do not improve speed. What advantage might these technologies offer to improve productivity for a person with a disability?

13. Abbreviation expansion is generally considered a means of typing long words and phrases with only a few keystrokes, although this requires the user to remember the abbreviation. How else can this technology be used for individuals with learning disabilities in ways that do not require memorization of keystroke sequences?

14. Integrated control systems allow a single control device to serve as the interface for a range of assistive technologies. What are the advantages of integrated control systems? Why might an integrated control system not be desirable for an individual user?

REFERENCES

1. Ablenet, Inc: Powerlink 4 (North America), n.d. https://www.ablenetinc.com/powerlink-4-north-america/.
2. Amazon: *Amazon Echo and Alexa Devices*, n.d. https://amzn.to/3y0NQw5.
3. American Occupational Therapy Association: AOTA Occupational Profile Template, 2020. https://www.aota.org/-/media/Corporate/Files/Practice/Manage/Documentation/AOTA-Occupational-Profile-Template.pdf.
4. American Occupational Therapy Association: Occupational therapy practice framework: Domain and process (4th ed), *American Journal of Occupational Therapy* 74(Suppl. 2):1–87, 2020.
5. Apple: *Safari*, 2021. https://www.apple.com/safari/.
6. Centers for Medicare and Medicaid: *Speech Generating Devices*, November 6, 2014. https://www.cms.gov/medicare-coverage-database/details/medicare-coverage-document-details.aspx?MCDId=26.
7. Choi JY, Yi S-H, Ao L, Tang X, Shim D, Yoo B, Park ES, Rha D-W: Virtual reality rehabilitation in children with brain injury: a randomized controlled trial, *Developmental Medicine & Child Neurology* 63(4):480–487, 2021. https://doi.org/10.1111/dmcn.14762.
8. Grammarly, 2021. https://bit.ly/3hcymiA.
9. Koester Performance Research: *Koester Performance Research*, 2019. https://kpronline.com
10. Koester Performance Research: *KPR Scanning Wizard*, 2016. https://scanningwizard.com/#/account-overview.
11. Lange B, Koenig S, Chang C-Y, McConnell E, Suma E, Bolas M, Rizzo A: Designing informed game-based rehabilitation tasks leveraging advances in virtual reality. *Disability and Rehabilitation,* 34(22):1863–1870, 2012. https://doi.org/10.3109/09638288.2012.670029.
12. Law M, Baptiste S, Carswell A, McColl M, Polatajko H, Pollock N: *Canadian occupational performance measure*, 4th ed., Ottawa, CAOT Publications ACE, 2005.
13. Merriam-Webster: *Definition of Therapeutic*, nd. https://www.merriam-webster.com/dictionary/therapeutic.
14. Microsoft: *Microsoft Edge*, 2021. https://www.microsoft.com/en-us/edge.
15. Origin Instruments: *Swifty USB Switch Interface*, 2020. https://orin.com/access/swifty/.
16. Park HJ, Takahashi K, Roberts KD, Delise D: Effects of the text-to-speech software use on the reading proficiency of high school struggling readers, *Assistive Technology* 29(3):146–152, 2017. https://doi.org/10.1080/10400435.2016.1171808.
17. Quillsoft: *WordQ5*, nd. https://www.quillsoft.ca/wordq5.
18. Rehabilitation Engineering and Assistive Technology Society of North America: *RESNA*, 2021. https://www.resna.org.
19. Scammacca NK, Roberts G, Vaughn S, Stuebing KK: A meta-analysis of interventions for struggling readers in grades 4–12: 1980–2011, *Journal of Learning Disabilities* 48(4):369–390, 2015. https://doi.org/10.1177/0022219413504995.
20. Smith RO: Technology and occupation: past, present, and the next 100 years of theory and practice, *American Journal of Occupational Therapy*, 71(6):1–15, 2017.
21. Technology-Related Assistance for Individuals With Disabilities Act of 1988, 29 U.S.C. § 2201, 1988. Retrieved from the Government Publishing Office website https://www.gpo.gov/fdsys/pkg/STATUTE-102/pdf/STATUTE-102-Pg1044.pdf.
22. Trujillo C, Del Monte B, Conatser M, Norris G, Malmgren T, Westcott C, Moritz K: Establishing OT's distinct value in AAC evaluations for children with disabilities, *The American Journal of Occupational Therapy* 74(4_Supplement_1):7411520480p1, 2020. https://doi.org/10.5014/ajot.2020.74S1-PO4202.

18

Performance Skills: Definitions and Evaluation in the Context of the Occupational Therapy Practice Framework

Winifred Schultz-Krohn and Mark Kovic

LEARNING OBJECTIVES

After studying this chapter, the student or practitioner will be able to do the following:

1. Explain the difference between a performance skill and a client factor.
2. Develop an understanding of client-centered, occupation-based performance.
3. Relate how improvements in performance skills may affect habits, roles, and routines.
4. Define impairment, strategy, and function.
5. Identify principles that may affect client outcomes.
6. Explain how a skilled intervention with clients facilitates cortical reorganization.

CHAPTER OUTLINE

KEY TERMS

Adaptive plasticity
Client factor
Contrived
Control parameter
Cortical reorganization
Function

Impairment
Motor control theory
Neuroplasticity
Occupational performance
Occupational therapy practitioner (OTP)
Performance skill

Plateau
Strategy
Task-oriented approach (TOA)

CURRENT OCCUPATIONAL THERAPY PRACTICE FRAMEWORK

The current version of the *"Occupational Therapy Practice Framework: Domain and Process,"* fourth edition (OTPF-4), was published in 2020. The revisions in this document were designed both to guide occupational therapy (OT) practice and to convey to others the domain and process of the profession.[2] The OTPF-4 is meant to be an "ever-evolving document," and the current revisions were offered to "build on a set of values that the profession has held since 1917"[2] (OTPF-4, p. S4). The OTPF-4 serves as a guide for the occupational therapy practitioner (OTP), which means both the OT and OTA use this document in practice. This chapter reviews the roles of performance skills and client factors as applied to a client case presentation and addresses how these elements relate to any client throughout the lifespan. It also describes how neuroscientific research supports an occupation-based approach to facilitate changes in the central nervous system (CNS) that directly correlate with improvements in occupational performance and client-centered outcomes.

THREADED CASE STUDY

John, Part 1

John is a 50-year-old construction worker who identifies as male and uses the pronouns he/him/his. John has been out of work for a year following a cerebrovascular accident (CVA). He has taken on a new role, keeping the house clean while his wife continues to work full time. He lives with his wife and two children, ages 10 and 15.

John sustained a right middle cerebral artery (MCA) CVA. The resultant client factor deficits from this CVA include mild impairment in his left lower extremity and moderate impairment in his left upper extremity, with greater impairment in distal motor control compared to proximal motor control. His available movement patterns in his left upper limb include lifting his shoulder and bending his elbow to position his hand so that it is better able to pick up items, but he is only able to use a gross grasp and has limited precision for release of objects with his left hand. He presents with a left visual field deficit and decreased sustained attention to tasks regardless of environment. He requires occasional indirect verbal cues to attend to tasks and activities. He benefits from the use of strategies to compensate for his deficits. He is currently able to complete all basic self-care activities, with occasional to minimal physical assistance required. Much of the physical assistance required is for starting the activity and the quality of performance. He is medically stable and taking antiseizure medications. He is right-hand dominant.

John lives in a one-story ranch home without any steps inside the house. He is currently walking with the use of a large-based quad cane. He and his family live in an urban setting with access to public transport. He has numerous friends and family members who live nearby. His children participate in several after-school activities, and this requires a parent to pick them up and bring them home. His wife has been picking up the children over the past year because her work is near the children's school.

John wants to improve his home management skills and continue to maintain his role as a homemaker in support of his wife. He has prioritized the following occupations with his occupational therapy (OT) practitioner: being able to complete his morning routine, take his medications, and manage the home. He is currently unable to do stovetop cooking activities, and he has difficulty vacuuming the carpet and sweeping the floors in the house. He is unable to perform shaving activities as he did before the CVA. Previously John had used a safety razor with his right hand while holding part of his face with his left hand to allow the safety razor to glide smoothly over the skin, without cuts or nicks. Since the CVA, John has used an electric razor, which he holds in his right hand; however, he does not like the poor results, and he often has razor irritation after shaving. He is unable to use his left hand to assist in the shaving process.

Critical Thinking Questions

1. What performance skills would potentially negatively affect John's ability to engage in desired occupations?
2. Given John's stated concerns, what additional occupations may be compromised?
3. What evidence is available to support services designed to improve John's occupational performance?

Role of Performance Skills and Client Factors in Occupational Performance

Occupational performance is the engagement in meaningful and purposeful activities that relate to habits, routines, and roles. Performance skills, as defined in the OTPF-4, are "observable, goal-directed actions" (S13).[2] These actions are further differentiated into three distinct skills: *motor skills*, meaning goal-directed movement. *Process skills* refers to how objects needed for the occupation are organized, the timing related to the occupational performance, and the use of space for occupational performance. The final performance skill is referred to as *social interaction*. This includes the "verbal and nonverbal skills to communicate, including initiating and terminating" (S13). Active client engagement in occupation-based evaluation and intervention can facilitate changes in performance skills and performance patterns, and this may influence habits, roles, routines and, ultimately, occupational performance. The term *client*, using the case illustration, refers to an individual, John. The OTPF-4 clearly articulates that performance skills occur with persons and groups. Considering the task of shaving, John's grasp on the razor and movement reflects the motor skills; the organizational flow of shaving including the speed and direction would be examples of the process skills.

Client factors, within the occupational therapy profession, are the "specific capacities, characteristics, or beliefs that reside within the person, group, or population" (S15).[2] Client factors include values, beliefs, and spirituality within a person, group, or population. John values being a contributing member of his family, although in a different capacity after his CVA. His stated goals include not only self-care but also helping with household chores. Applying client factors beyond the person, a group may hold a belief that household chores should be a collaborative effort that includes all members of the household or may hold a belief that only adults within the household are responsible for household chores. A population may value interdependence far more than independence. The term *spirituality* is referring to the meaning of the occupation, not religiosity. A person, group, or population may find meaning in cherished occupations, and this is often closely related to values and beliefs. Client factors also refer to body functions and body structures. These client factors are generally not applied to groups or populations and follow the World Health Organization (WHO) Classification (2008).[31] Body functions refer to the physiological and psychological functions of the body, whereas body structures refer to the anatomic parts of the body.

The importance of client-centered interactions in selecting specific occupations that will help clients progress through their course of occupational therapy (OT) is a concept endorsed by the American Occupational Therapy Association (AOTA)[2] and several leaders in the OT profession.[10,12,19,29] There are several variations of how this process may occur; however, regardless of whether the Assessment of Motor and Process Skills (AMPS),[10] the occupational functioning model,[29] or the task-oriented approach (TOA)[21] is used, the message is similar: analysis of client performance provides the OT practitioner with a means of understanding what is observed.

These authors follow a common thread, consistent with the World Health Organization's current International Statistical Classification of Diseases and Health Problems (ICD-11), 11th revision,[31] along with the previous International Classification of Functioning, Disability and Health,[32] that performance analysis is important. This analysis may be formal or informal. Yet, one particular caution is to make sure that during any informal analysis, the intended outcome is specifically identified. This allows the OT practitioner to anchor what was expected with what is actually performed and observed. Thus, the focus remains on the tasks and corresponding performance skill, rather than on the client factor serving as the key determining variable in the OT process.

Occupation-Based Approaches and Neuroscientific Evidence

Connecting occupation-based approaches to the neuroscientific realm provides a framework to consider these concepts as they relate to learning. Learning, as defined in this context, occurs as a result of neuroplasticity produced by new neuronal connections and axonal sprouting that occurs within the central nervous system through multisensory input.[6,14,27] Application of this concept may be seen with clients who have sustained upper motor neuron (UMN) injuries. Evidence exists demonstrating that axonal sprouting occurs after a stroke and contributes to the recovery of function.[6] Axonal sprouting adjacent to the damaged CNS after a stroke is known as reactive sprouting and has been attributed to the limited recovery that spontaneously occurs after the stroke. Axonal sprouting that occurs over a longer distance is known as reparative and, coupled with reactive sprouting, accounts for the functional changes. Current trends in occupational therapy to ameliorate upper extremity hemiparesis as a result of UMN lesions are varied, yet research indicates that a potentially beneficial way to achieve a successful client-centered outcome is to include those interventions that address how the client interacts with the task and the environment. This particular approach, focused on how the client engages in functional tasks within an appropriate environment, may direct cortical changes and facilitate neuromuscular recovery. Consequently, this type of approach may improve completion of activities of daily living (ADLs) through improvements in performance skills[13] via engagement in occupational performance-based activities. Occupational performance, as such, often arises from a person performing a particular task in a particular environment. This dynamic interaction among the individual, the task, and the environment is consistent with the foundational framework provided by the **task-oriented approach (TOA)**.[21] From an occupational therapy perspective, the TOA is client-centered and individualized and addresses performance of functional tasks meaningful to the client.[1] A single-blind randomized crossover trial demonstrated significant improvement in arm function with greater gains in the client's self-identified skills using the Canadian Occupational Performance Measure. The TOA is one of a variety of approaches to evaluation and intervention that incorporates an underlying understanding of a variety of concepts. Among these is the ecologic approach to the performance of functional tasks (and purposeful movements). This approach emphasizes the interaction among the person, environment, and

task performance.[21] Within this approach, the term "task" is not equivalent to "occupation."[10] Although several definitions of the term *occupation* have been offered, the elements that distinguish occupations from tasks include the specific meaning to the occupational performance and the occupational performance within a context or environment.[9] A task is often a small portion of an occupation, such as the task of cutting with a knife and fork within the occupation of self-feeding. The performance skill in this task may be grasping the fork. Yet, an appreciation for the task-oriented approach (TOA) can be seen with understanding the potential impact the task has upon occupational engagement. The OT practitioner may then apply motor learning concepts, adapt, modify, or otherwise facilitate successful completion of an occupation-based goal.

Application of the TOA directs OT practitioners to address the performance skill[13] deficits that their clients experience while simultaneously incorporating current understanding of neuroscience concepts. Both the process and outcome are important with regard to this approach. The net result of this approach is that the client may benefit from improved ADLs performance. Ultimately, this may support habits and routines and eventually facilitate return to desired, client-centered roles.

A new model of intervention builds on the TOA and serves to promote recovery of function, particularly upper extremity control, following a CVA called the Accelerated Skill Acquisition Program (ASAP).[20] The ASAP uses principles of motor learning and provides a systematic approach that addresses four components: building capacity, skill acquisition, motivation enhancement, and autonomy support. These components articulate well with the OTPF-4.[2] Capacity building is focused on the foundational movement needed for the task completion, including practice of the smaller motor elements needed for a task.[20] Skill acquisition, as the name implies, is focused on collaborative assessment of what motor skills are needed to complete the task, including having the client anticipate potential challenges. Motivational enhancement is blended with creating incremental goals that are selected by the client. Autonomy support refers to the continuous involvement of the client in evaluating performance and setting new goals. This process clearly supports a client-centered approach.

Assessment of Performance Skills and Client Factors

The OTPF-4 identifies client factors and performance skills as separate elements and describes how they impact and are affected by client interaction with task and the environment in the process of performance of ADLs.[2] Fisher[10] provided a background to the process of how to formally and informally assess performance skills and patterns in relation to occupations. She stated that to understand how the client factors affect occupational performance, it is important to thoroughly determine how these components affect performance skills during occupational performance. Thus, it could be inferred that any attempt to assess this relationship without an appreciation and understanding for this dynamic process may lead to potentially "misdirected" conclusions. There will be a mismatch between client need and OT practitioner choice of intervention. In other

TABLE 18.1 Performance Skills in the OTPF-4

Performance Skills	Definition
Motor skills	Skills observed as a person interacts with and moves task objects and self around the environment
Process skills	Skills observed as a person selects and uses tools and materials, carries out actions and steps, and modifies performance when problems are encountered
Social interaction skills	Skills observed during a social exchange

Adapted from American Occupational Therapy Association: Occupational therapy practice framework: Domain and process (4th ed.), *American Journal of Occupational Therapy* 74(Suppl. 2): 1–87, 2020. https://doi.org/10.5014/ajot.2020.74S2001.

words, the OT practitioner may make clinical decisions that are not in the best interests of the client and will not reflect best practice.

Table 18.1 lists the performance skills from the OTPF-4.

In what way could the OT practitioner evaluate John to identify what assets and deficits this client may be able to use?

It is necessary to understand current client abilities relative to specified task performance. This can be understood with measurement of particular client factors such as John's left upper limb active range of motion (AROM) and strength. As discussed in the chapter, it is important to have an understanding of particular deficit areas before the initiation of occupational therapy services. This should then be combined with observation of John participating in certain activities. The activities may occur in a structured or unstructured manner. They could include performance of his morning routine. This may include dressing, brushing his teeth, or shaving. The OT practitioner would observe what specific strategies are used. If John turned his body to the side to position his left arm across his lap to then place his left arm into the sleeve of a shirt, it is likely that this particular strategy maximizes his performance skill. The evaluation process would be a combination of the client factor measurement with the occupational performance and would most likely reflect what John is able to do for these ADLs.

Client factors related to body and structure function are important as they inform the OT process and ultimately contribute to understanding of how these functions (or lack thereof) contribute to the evaluation process and development of an intervention plan. Additionally, values, beliefs, and spirituality are included as client factors in the OTPF-4.[2] Within the OTPF-4,[2] client factors are differentiated at the person, organization, and population level; this chapter will primarily address client factors applied to the level of the person. Some of the specific client factors identified at the level of the person are: neuromusculoskeletal functions related to strength, muscle tone, motor reflexes, and voluntary and/or involuntary movement. Global and specific mental functions are important client factors that support incorporation of the input from one's interaction with a task within an environment. These mental functions, collectively termed cognition, are required for a person to make sense of sensorimotor input from the environment. These functions

are important to overall functional ability. Also, the degree to which the central nervous system is intact following damage or a lesion will affect a client's occupational performance.

As it relates to upper motor neuron (UMN) cortical lesions, these client factors may result in peripheral soft tissue changes, hypertonia, spasticity, and changes in range of motion. Any combination of these changes will likely have an impact on how a client participates in a particular task. These client factors remain relevant and supportive in their role in the overall OT process. In other words, they are a means to understanding an end that focuses on performance skills because these skills support performance of occupations.

Client factors differ from performance skills in that they represent the responses to system control. Client factors often can be measured and quantified—strength, range of motion, visual acuity, muscle tone, attention. Client factors represent bodily functions and what the body "does," rather than what the person does. This distinction is made clear by Fisher[10] in that client factors are the actual body structures and basic body functions aligning with the WHO International Classification of Functioning, Disability and Health.[32] Additionally, client factors represent what a person can use to perform a particular task. Thus, client factors facilitate performance skills but merely assessing available client factors is not predictive of occupational performance.[2]

Performance skills include the motor, process, and communication/social interaction skills required to perform specific tasks (i.e., ADLs, instrumental ADLs [IADLs], work). Fisher[10] described performance skills as "small units of action [that] are always goal-directed because they are enacted in the context of carrying out and completing a daily life task." Therefore, performance skills are not assessed in the absence of occupational performance but must be assessed *while* the client is engaged in an occupation. For example, John would like to be able to complete a dinner that includes cooking on the stove, specifically cooking pasta and spaghetti sauce. Although assessment of specific body functions may reveal limited isolated active range of motion (AROM) of his left arm, making it difficult to hold the handle of the sauce pan while stirring the sauce with a spoon in his right hand, during the actual task performance the OT practitioner would also notice the difficulties with positioning his body appropriately to the stove and poor pacing of the actions that are in the performance skill category of motor and process skills. Motor and process skills are required in adequate and appropriate amounts to interact with an object in the environment during performance of a task in an accurate and efficient manner. This process can be quite dynamic and complex, and understanding this interaction informs and directs the OT evaluation and intervention. The ability to judge and respond to task demands is an aspect of the cognitive performance skills linked to overall occupational performance. Returning to the example of John cooking pasta and spaghetti sauce for dinner would require him to sequence the task appropriately by starting spaghetti sauce, then placing the water on the stove for the pasta, and as the sauce simmers, adding the pasta to the boiling water. These aspects of the task may require reaching, manipulation, and calibration. All of these are motor performance skills. He would need to time all these events appropriately for dinner to avoid serving cold pasta with overcooked sauce. He needs to endure and pace his performance. With John's difficulties in attention (a client factor), an OT practitioner may assume the complex task of cooking spaghetti and sauce would be a challenge. Without observing the actual performance, the therapist may have suggested a checklist as an intervention method and not understand how the motor and process performance skills interact with cognitive skills during the occupation of meal preparation. Thus, a person presents with specific deficits (client factors) that have an impact on performance skills, which relates to occupational performance. Significant changes/impairments with these client factors may sufficiently affect a client's performance patterns and skills and eventually (adversely) affect occupational roles. The analysis of the occupational performance requires consideration of the strategies currently available to the client and intervention considers options to modify the environment, the task, and the client's performance skills. Research indicates that the TOA is more likely to affect and positively influence outcomes when compared to treatment that addresses only client factors.[1,23] Neuroscientific research is pointing toward the possibility that the central nervous system is organized in such a way that tasks can be addressed through interaction with the environment rather than specific muscle groups meant to perform specific tasks. This is consistent with the TOA. Thus, understanding a client's roles and routines will guide an OT practitioner's ability to address performance skills as they relate to occupational performance. In summary, performance skills are required for interaction with task, object, and environment.[25]

How would John benefit most from occupational therapy intervention with a focus on performance skills to support improvements in client chosen activities?

John is motivated to improve his self-care and home management skills at home. He is able to complete his morning routine and self-care activities with limited physical assistance from another person. He has a supportive family who provides assistance as needed. He stated that he wants to be able to improve his ability to complete his morning routine, self-care activities, and home management. If the OT practitioner were to focus on prioritizing these activities, it would be possible to determine the best way to address reacquisition of these abilities. Although there are multiple control parameters (a control parameter refers to the motor element that influences performance) that influence successful task completion, it is likely that in any particular activity, at least one key parameter may be the most limiting factor to successful task completion. For example, with the shaving activity; John's impaired movement in his left hand compromises bilateral task performance and serves as the control parameter. This impairment, as described in the case illustration, comes from the inability to have sufficient distal control. It is important to observe the actual performance of the shaving activity when possible to avoid any contrived situations. Merely having John use a safety razor with the cover in place to simulate the act of shaving would not accurately replicate the actual performance of shaving. In this instance, it needs to be determined if focusing on how the performance skill of bilateral control can be achieved will improve shaving or if the task needs to be adapted to maximize independence. The OT practitioner

can validate these approaches by observing John with the actual task of shaving. This same approach may be taken with each activity to be addressed.

Motor Control Theory

Interaction among the task, person, and environment represents important aspects of motor control. Motor control theory (i.e., the ability to make dynamic changes/responses of body and limb to complete a purposeful activity[27]) has undergone much development in recent years. This development has expanded our knowledge base, answered some questions, introduced other questions, and has permitted a further appreciation of the complexity of cortical function as it relates to motor performance.

A variety of sources indicates that multisensory input will provide the nervous system with input that will ultimately lead to improved quality of movement performance, result in decreased error, and support more efficient movement patterns.[7,23,24] These multiple sensory inputs to learning (or relearning) will attempt to work together to contribute to understanding interaction with the environment whether they are intact or not intact. When one sensory input (or system) is impaired, others may need to compensate. When one part of a system is impaired, the performance pattern is affected. For example, if a person presents with impaired ability to perform dynamic distal (hand and finger) movements because of decreased motor control, then he or she may move the proximal upper limb in such a manner as to compensate for this impairment. The net result of this compensatory movement may present as "shoulder hiking" and may include other movements such as lateral trunk flexion or even shortening of the lever arm (i.e., elbow flexion) to control degrees of freedom.[26]

John "hikes" (abnormally elevates) his left shoulder as movement is initiated with his left arm as he attempts to reach for objects such as his razor or toothbrush. Doing so allows him to be able to move his left arm to a position where he can then access these items. John is aware that his pattern of reaching for objects with his left hand was more effective before the CVA. The OT practitioner may ask John to reach for these items with his right hand for comparison (recall that John is right-hand dominant). This serves as an informal task analysis. If the position of the items and how John interacts with the objects in the environment is changed, it also can be analyzed as to how this may affect the strategy, given available skills.

It is possible that this inefficient movement pattern could then be repeated and eventually develop into a new adapted or maladapted pattern. However, unless this process is properly analyzed, the client is more likely to "learn" and repeatedly use this inefficient movement pattern to accomplish a task. Poor and ineffective patterns may emerge, overuse syndromes may occur, and the net result is potentially poor self-efficacy and extra energy expenditure with occupational performance.

Repetition alone as part of a neuromuscular rehabilitation approach is insufficient to create and reinforce cortical reorganization.[3,6,15,26] This statement is neither novel nor groundbreaking in meaning, yet its intent is shared by multiple researchers in a variety of arenas from basic neuroscience to the field of occupational therapy.[3,15,16,22] It is a well-established hallmark of occupational therapy to work with the client to develop an occupational profile and to engage the client in meaningful and purposeful activities. Additionally, intense task-oriented training of the sensorimotor cortex is thought to lead to cortical reorganization. Bayona et al.[3] found that rehabilitation outcomes have greater success when the tasks are meaningful to the patient. Volpe et al.[30] shared this same conclusion.

Yet, client-centered, therapist-driven, task-oriented approaches may not directly translate to anecdotal or clinically measurable/significant before and after changes. Motor learning concepts[29] indicate that the degree to which a task is learned is positively correlated with the "depth" of the "well" in which it is kept. In other words, the more ingrained a task is to a person, the more challenging it may be to change or alter the movement or behavior. The key point at which that transition occurs also may be influenced by control parameters.

Control parameter is a motor control term that could be anything that shifts a motor behavior from one manner of performance to another type of performance. Control parameters can be internal to the person (strength, vision—for example, John's left visual field deficit) or external (location of an object, lighting). Consider the task of washing your back, the length of your arm, size of your back, established habits from training, all serve as control parameters—do you attempt to wash your left scapular area with your right hand or left? When the control parameter is a client factor, this may be an appropriate instance in which the OT practitioner may attempt to address/remediate the client factor.[21] This approach to the OT process, often termed a "bottom-up" approach, assumes that addressing the underlying client factors will foster improved occupational performance. Yet, doing so may not translate to the client's improved performance skills or occupational performance. In fact, it is likely that the further the intervention is from the actual occupational activity or performance, the less likely there will be a positive correlation between these two items. Ultimately, the degree to which the client factor is impaired will have an impact on the end result and how there is compensatory or adaptive interventions by the OT practitioner and the client. These concepts could be at least part of the explanation as to why there have been improvements measured in clinical outcome measures in some well-developed studies in this arena, but that there are limited long-term improvements. Consequently, it may be challenging to overcome (sometimes poorly) practiced performance skills and patterns. Return to the example of John cooking dinner. He has a left visual field cut that compromises his ability to obtain visual information, and when the pot with pasta (located on the left side of the stove) begins to boil over, John is not receiving that visual input. He could be trained to visually scan the environment to compensate for the visual field cut, and it would be most appropriate to provide this training within a natural environment and with preferred occupations.

Fundamentals of experience-driven neuroplasticity include the adaptive capacity of the central nervous system to make fundamental changes and alterations on the cellular and eventually the systems level that can then lead to new learned/adapted behaviors. There are key critical "signals" that can facilitate such recovery.[6,13] Additionally, the brain continually reorganizes itself, with or without damage.[13,16] This process of learning will occur spontaneously without any explicit learning or formal rehabilitation. Lack of skilled therapeutic intervention may lead to maladaptive behavioral responses. It is the skilled learning that occurs through the use of strategies and adaptation to facilitate this adaptive response. This has been shown to occur with the use of the TOA and task-specific techniques.[5] Focus on the performance skill in therapy allows the opportunity for skilled learning to occur. A person may present with compensatory movements or adaptations to control parameters such as decreased agonist strength. The TOA, with a focus on the person interacting with the task in the environment, can address this limiting performance client factor (compensation), in part, by guiding the performance skill via skilled management of the dynamic interaction of these items.[5] Compensatory behavioral changes are a regular part of this process.[16]

John has been attempting to move his left arm as much as possible since the CVA. He tells family and caregivers frequently that he wants to do as much as possible for himself. He is motivated to make improvements. When he attempts to complete self-care activities on his own, he does not make adjustments in the environment. He interacts with objects with poorly coordinated movement patterns. His performance skills are relative to how he uses objects. The OT practitioner can maximize the quality of the performance skills with a focus on how John brushes his teeth or shaves. This would then serve as the foundation for how to modify the task or the environment.

Kleim and Jones[15] identify 10 principles that fit this process: (1) use it or lose it, (2) use it and improve it, (3) specificity, (4) repetition matters, (5) intensity matters, (6) time matters, (7) salience matters, (8) age matters, (9) transference, and (10) interference. These principles come from basic and applied neuroscience research concepts that have shown evidence that they can affect outcomes. These principles can support evaluation and treatment.

Effective evaluation of the client who presents with upper limb hemiparesis as has been described in this chapter should then include an understanding of the specific impairments (client factors) that have an impact on the performance of occupation-based, client-centered tasks. Although addressing specific client factors may be a part of treatment, this may not necessarily reflect changes in occupational performance. A client may need to improve bicep strength in order to complete a hand-to-mouth pattern, yet improving the bicep strength to a point at which the strength is sufficient to facilitate the movement does not guarantee that the task can be completed successfully. Thus, the focus should be on the performance skills and patterns. Observation of the client strategy with use of remaining abilities as it relates to overall function is an important part of the evaluation process. This should occur with respect for current understanding of how skilled interventions by the OT practitioner may direct learning/relearning and lead to neuroplastic cortical changes. These changes in performance skills can lead to improvements in occupational performance.

Comprehensive evaluation with respect for the TOA requires a thorough assessment of impairment, strategy, and function.

As stated earlier in this chapter, the specific impairments are those that result as a consequence of the UMN lesion. These impairments may include but are not limited to: weakness (of the agonist), decreased coordination, decreased in-hand manipulation, inability to manage agonist and agonist efficiently, impaired/absent sensation, proprioception, impaired vision, and decreased overall cognitive ability. These impairments may be measured with traditional assessment approaches used by OT practitioners: manual muscle testing, range of motion testing, sensation testing, vision testing, strength (grip) testing via a dynamometer (for example), coordination testing via the Nine-Hole Peg Test (for example), and so on. The appropriate standardized test may be, in part, determined by the site/setting. The benefit of these assessments is that they provide a pretest foundation from which to measure progress. Yet, these client factors remain relevant in so much as they affect occupational performance via performance skills. Thus, it is important for the OT practitioner to have an appreciation of the strategies and performance patterns used by the client.

John has less than 5 lb of grip strength in his left hand as measured by the dynamometer. He has impaired sensation on his left hand. He does not visually attend to the environment in his left peripheral visual field. These are client factors. John grasps objects such as eating utensils with insufficient strength and has difficulties when he attempts to use his left hand to hold a fork while cutting foods with the knife in his right hand. He is unable to judge the water temperature from a faucet on his left hand before shaving. He does not always attend to the left side of his environment when he is attempting to cook. These are performance skills. He requires assistance and verbal cues to complete his morning routine with good quality. This is occupational performance.

Ultimately, it is the occupational performance that arises from performance skills and patterns supported by clinical observations and leads to clinical decisions for "best practice." The benefit from use of the TOA with respect for current neuroscientific concepts such as cortical neuroplasticity is that the OT practitioner addresses a client's needs from a top-down approach rather than from a bottom-up approach. The top-down approach directs the OT practitioner to work with the client from the view of actual occupational performance. Fisher[10] describes these approaches along with the benefits and potential pitfalls of each of these approaches. It is possible to complete the impairment-based measurements and progress to function or to start with functional performance and to use these observations to guide assessment and treatment, yet caution is suggested when a "motor behavior perspective"[11] is solely used.

John has decreased strength and range of motion throughout his left upper limb. This impairment is observable and measurable. Sole measurement of these items is insufficient to create a client-centered occupation-based treatment plan. It might be possible to measure these client factors. Improvement with strength or range of motion may not reflect improvements with John being able to raise his left arm to apply shaving cream to his face. It is important to understand the deficits as they relate to real performance of some client-identified, clinician-driven approach.

Neuroscience Research Related to Practice

Recent research relating neuroscientific concepts from the animal model (rodent and primate) to the human model provide evidence of the potential benefits of provision of skilled learning opportunities to direct cortical reorganization.[6,14,22,23,25] Cortical reorganization is the concept that the adult brain has a neuroplastic ability to alter or modify its synaptic connections in the context of performance of a skilled activity—whether the brain and central nervous system are intact or not intact. Nudo and Milliken[22] and Nudo et al.[23] completed groundbreaking research demonstrating that through skilled learning principles, it is possible to create topographical cortical map changes that directly correspond to specific "pellet retrieval" (distal forelimb) tasks after induced focal cortical lesions in these particular representative areas in squirrel monkeys. Task-specific training can lead to increased cortical representation of the trained areas along with a decreased representation of the previously postinfarct compensatory areas. The net result of performance skill in these primates was improved quality of movement. Most of the "improved performance patterns" occurred via observation of and interpretation of behavior by the researcher before and after intervention assessment. This demonstrates the ability of the cortical region to reorganize when demands are placed on it to function. Of course there are limits to the process of reorganization, particularly if large sections of the cortex are damaged.

Animal (primate) model research in this area has provided invaluable information, yet these conclusions have resulted from specific, focally induced lesions[26] with clear boundaries as to the lesioned area. In many instances with animal models, the adjacent tissue is undamaged.[26] In humans, research has demonstrated that peri-infarct (cortical) reorganization may occur. Additionally, in humans, the "edges" of the lesioned area are not always clear.[25] Aside from the clinical implications of these variances, other potential issues may arise from more complex cortical damage. These may include medical complexity, family/caregiver support, comorbidity, cultural expectations, or other client-specific variables. These challenges have not been the focus of nor have they been addressed in the animal model.

What would be the best fit for treatment interventions for John, given the current evidence available and understanding of neuroscience to facilitate occupational performance? Current research indicates that it may be most beneficial to observe how John participates in particular daily activities. This allows the OT practitioner to understand what repeated behaviors are used and where new strategies may be effective in assisting John in his desired occupational outcomes. In doing so, it may be possible to better fit treatment to his needs. This allows the possibility to focus on activities of interest to John and use concepts related to the task-oriented approach (TOA). This approach is both client-centered and occupation-based. The specific treatment activities will focus on matching the client performance patterns.

Data from both animal and human models lead to the likelihood that client-centered, client-specific intervention plans and approaches may be best practice. This, of course, may introduce challenges in how to implement such approaches into the current standard of care. Regardless, the distinction between animal and human models will likely continue to be a topic of discussion. This discussion is relevant when we attempt to consider what defines the aforementioned "best practice." Birkenmeier et al.[4] attempted to address this translation from neuroscientific concepts to animal model research to clinical research implementation. Their description of how they made these decisions is one of the most comprehensive presentations of this issue. Lang and Birkenmeier[18] collaborated on a resource book that aligns animal model research with a parallel human model treatment regimen. These examples are comprehensive and include dozens of examples. Additionally, there are suggestions to guide the OT practitioner to upgrade and downgrade (modify) specific interventions.[18]

Research sponsored Northstar Neuroscience Phase III Clinical Trial[17] has taken these neuroplastic concepts and knowledge from animal models and applied them to a treatment protocol based on occupational therapy concepts of client-centeredness. This randomized controlled trial included nearly 150 subjects in close to 20 sites. The study intended to investigate the potential benefits of sub-threshold cortical stimulation in combination with "skilled" (already defined in this chapter) learning via a therapy protocol grounded in the TOA.

Similar investigations have identified possible potential benefits from sub-threshold (i.e., non-evoked action potentials) cortical stimulation to support synaptic connections, dendritic density, and to facilitate overall cortical reorganization.[25] Although the exact dosage of the stimulation and whether specific cortical stimulation to the region responsible for post-lesion upper limb (distal) control or another approach such as transcranial magnetic stimulation (TMS) remains unclear at this time, this area holds potential future benefits.[25]

The treatment protocol for the Northstar Neuroscience Phase III Clinical Trial[17] study incorporated the approach of evaluation (and corresponding intervention) of *impairment*, *strategy*, and *function* in the realm of the TOA. The impairment corresponds to the client factor. The strategy corresponds to how the person attempts to perform a task as it relates to occupation, given specific impairments. Function corresponds to how the impairment and corresponding strategy relates to performance skills and patterns. Ultimately, subjects in this clinical trial were evaluated and treated with this framework. The research therapists evaluated and treated the subjects with a focus on performance skills. This focus arose from client-centered occupation-based tasks determined by each participant with the Canadian Occupational Performance Measure (COPM).[19] Clients' self-perceived changes in the performance patterns for ADLs were measured by the COPM. Other assessments used as outcome measures included the Fugl-Meyer[11] and Arm Motor Ability Test.[16] The latter two are well-established and validated clinical measures and were primary outcome measures for this particular study and are focused on limb movement (Fugl-Meyer) and contrived activity performance (Arm Motor Ability Test). Clients demonstrated improvements in COPM outcome measures but significant changes were not noted in the other two measures. The evaluation of the clients occurred according to the principles outlined by the TOA. The treating therapists were trained and followed standardized

procedures to focus with the client on the client-centered goals. Once an individual improved on a client factor or performance skill, the treating therapist reviewed how that change affected the performance pattern and what this represented in the occupational performance. The changes in performance skills with participants in this study—addressed through client-centered functional activities focused on the use of strategies related to task performance—corresponded to changes in client factors. This treatment approach and protocol is consistent with neuroscience concepts of skilled learning supporting cortical changes that may lead to changes (improvements) in occupational performance, performance patterns, habits, routines, and roles. A portion of this protocol included evaluation and understanding of the impact of client factors on performance skills. Consistent with this chapter, caution was heeded as to how the client factor was a means to understanding its relevance to performance skills and overall occupational performance.

Muscle strength, range of motion, sensation, and a variety of other client factors are necessary to engage in functional activities and therefore important to measure in a quantifiable manner. An adequate amount of strength, for example, is necessary to grip an eating utensil or sufficient active range of motion is necessary to complete a hand-to-mouth pattern. Yet, the key with this protocol was that neuroplastic concepts were used to link client factors to performance skills to facilitate adaptive plasticity. Isolated work on the client factors of muscle strength or range of motion was not part of the protocol.

Adaptive plasticity (the innate ability of the central nervous system to adapt or modify behavioral responses after exposure to a challenge to the system) implies that by addressing the performance skill, direct change toward improved quality of occupational performance will occur. As defined, the performance skill occurs in the process of engaging in the occupation and cannot be separated from the occupation.

The examples provided in this chapter reflect neuroscientific knowledge as it relates to how OT practitioners work with the neurologically impaired client, and these same fundamental concepts can guide clinical interventions with a variety of other clients across the lifespan.

Although the approach discussed in this chapter may relate to any client, a few other examples have been provided for consideration. This list is not exhaustive. In this chapter, the focus is on adults. For example, a client who has cancer, chronic obstructive pulmonary disease (COPD), total knee replacement (TKR), or Parkinson's disease may benefit from the approach discussed in this chapter. The condition will inform the OT practitioner as to etiology, clinical and medical presentations, prognosis, and other valuable information. The client factors affected by any condition, such as the ones previously listed, may have an impact on performance skills. This may affect performance patterns. Ultimately, this leads to the possibility that habits, routines, and roles may be affected. Observation and assessment of performance skills may still guide the OT practitioner to a client-centered occupation-based intervention.

The older client with the TKR may present with decreased bilateral upper extremity strength, not as a result of the TKR but due to deconditioning from diminished activity secondary

THREADED CASE STUDY

John, Part 2

John has sustained a right MCA CVA. This condition informs the OT practitioner that it is likely that he has left upper limb motor impairment. Additionally, there may be other consequences from the CVA. John may have decreased attention and decreased visual attention to the left side. Yet, it remains important to be aware that John is also a parent and a housekeeper. He wants to return to these roles. Thus, mere measurement of the specific client factors that have resulted from the CVA will not explicitly return him to these roles and routines.

to knee problems. This decreased bilateral upper extremity strength will limit the ability to efficiently use a walker for functional mobility around the home. This client may also have a history of cognitive impairments that affect the ability to learn new concepts. The OT practitioner may need to consider these items to develop a client-centered intervention plan. Relating this example to the framework provided in this chapter, the OT practitioner will likely assess upper limb strength and range of motion. Part of the OT intervention may even include exercises and activities that may improve these client factors. Yet, this does not mean that in doing so, the client will improve the performance skill of (for example) a morning routine. Nor does it imply that engaging a client with a purposeful activity will translate to improved occupational performance. How a task is practiced in the clinic may not translate to the home environment. Thus, the formal or informal occupational profile and analysis will provide the foundation from which the OT practitioner may link the current status to desired outcomes.

Best Practice Occupational Therapy Service

It is important to bring this discussion back to clients who have acquired neurological deficits in order to identify how this particular group of clients can best be treated by OT practitioners. As occupational therapy practice for the adult neurological practice moves further from an "expert opinion" approach to one grounded in evidence (whether that evidence supports or refutes traditional practice approaches), there is much more to be learned to determine "best practice." There have been attempts to identify both current trends and task-specific training to identify what defines "best practice." In support of this comment, Carter et al.[8] describe that much of the effort in rehabilitation research is going toward the direction of "motor restoration." Additionally, they state that the quality of the research is more rigorous than it has ever been in the past. There is no doubt that these efforts will continue and may involve other novel means to address these deficits such as post-stroke bilateral upper limb training interventions.[28]

When it comes to measuring performance and improvements in clients with neurological insults, it may be that previous outcome measures used to identify improvements are insufficient at this point in time. For example, some standardized and validated measures that address ADLs do so with contrived ADLs. Contrived activities are those that are artificially created in an attempt to recreate real scenarios. Although there are potential

benefits gained from using a standardized ADL assessment as a common, consistent approach to measuring performance and conveying performance information that is clearly recognized because of the standardization process, if this standardization lacks the fundamental elements of the task or is too "contrived," it may affect performance and the corresponding measurement of performance. An example of a contrived situation would be having a client "spread" butter on bread by having the client use a knife on a plate in the spreading motion without the actual bread or butter. In this example, the client may possess the motor control needed for the task but in the actual task (real-world experience) of spreading butter on the bread the client may fail to notice that all the butter is located on one corner of the bread or may use excessive force and tear the bread. These observations would not be possible using a contrived activity but would be immediately noticed if the client was given an actual piece of bread and butter. Wu et al.[33] describe that real performance of activities results in different and better results than imagined or contrived activities. Additionally, there is a variety of means to measure performance, including time to complete portions of a task, time to complete the entire task, and subjective observations of quality of performance. Further research may advance newer ways to measure performance skills and occupational performance. This does not mean that we, as OT practitioners, should not attempt to incorporate current trends, concepts, measures/assessments, and techniques.

There are other considerations to make with the impact of how we intervene with clients such as John. Timing, dosage, and method of delivery are important variables to control for in clinical studies, and these variables should also be considered in clinical practice. Although evidence-based practice is expected, using data from an investigation that did not attempt to control these factors needs to be considered with some caution.[8] Given the competition for space in the cortex after UMN damage,[22] it is necessary for OT practitioners to respond immediately and effectively to client needs. This clinical reasoning process may affect how performance plateaus are determined in clinical practice.

Plateau is a term that is all too common in the realm of current rehabilitation practice with persons with upper limb hemiparesis, as well as other conditions across the lifespan. Page et al.[24] suggest that the way in which therapists frame the upper limb hemiparetic population may need to be reconsidered. They state that what defines: (1) "motor recovery plateau," (2) "ability to recover motor function," and (3) when to "use different modalities" may need to be reconsidered. Traditional expectations of most (motor) recovery occurring in 6 to 12 months often guides insurance and is tied into clinical practice. This chapter identifies the reasons as to why this may not necessarily be the case. Immediately after a CVA some clients may be able to participate in a rehabilitative approach designed to foster self-care skills, whereas other clients may be far too ill. The timing, intensity (dosage), and method of delivery for these two clients will most likely vary, but a similar functional outcome may ultimately be met. Hubbard et al.[13] summarize principles that should be considered for incorporation of task-specific interventions. These suggestions may serve as a guide for "best practice" while addressing the potential for improvements in performance skills. They suggest that such training/intervention should "be relevant to the patient/client and to the context; be randomly assigned; be repetitive and involve massed practice; aim towards reconstruction of the whole task; and be reinforced with positive and timely feedback."[15] They further conclude that, although as noted in this chapter, there is much evidence pointing toward the benefit of task-oriented or task-specific training techniques, common practice approaches are grounded in accepted practice or custom and may be beneficial at specific points in time. An appreciation for this conclusion and the current state of neuroscience as it relates to this population can serve to transform clinical practice. Given the complexity of human beings, it may ultimately prove that what emerges as best practice may incorporate a multifactorial approach to guide client-centered evaluation and treatment, maximize outcomes, and facilitate client habits, routines, and roles.

SUMMARY

It is possible to address client-centered, occupation-based needs with a focus on performance skills. Neuroscientific research indicates that this approach can be applied with the use of certain methods, such as the TOA. The TOA emphasizes a dynamic interaction between the person, the task, and the environment. OT practitioners are educated and trained to address control parameters and complete performance analyses to maximize overall occupational performance.

REVIEW QUESTIONS

1. What are the advantages of using real situations when assessing clients rather than contrived situations?
2. What are the advantages of using contrived situations when assessing clients instead of real situations?
3. What does the term *plateau* mean in reference to clients who have sustained neurological insults?
4. What is the difference between a client factor and a performance skill?
5. Using the task of brushing your teeth as part of your morning routine, identify two client factors and two performance skills that influence the way you engage in this task.
6. What does the term *control parameter* mean with regard to working with clients who have sustained neurological insults?
7. Explain the term *neuroplasticity*.
8. Explain the term *cortical reorganization*.
9. How do the meanings of the terms *neuroplasticity* and *cortical reorganization* support occupation-based interventions?
10. Explain how the TOA was used with the case of John.

For additional practice questions for this chapter, please visit eBooks.Health.Elsevier.com.

REFERENCES

1. Almhdawi KA, Mathiowetz VG, White M, delMas RC: Efficacy of occupational therapy task-oriented approach in upper extremity post-stroke rehabilitation, *Occupational Therapy International* 23:444–456, 2016. https://doi.org/10.1002/oti.1447.
2. American Occupational Therapy Association: Occupational therapy practice framework: Domain and process (4th ed.), *American Journal of Occupational Therapy* 74(Suppl. 2):1–87, 2020. https://doi.org/10.5014/ajot.2020.74S2001.
3. Bayona NA, Bitensky J, Salter K, Teasell R: The role of task-specific training in rehabilitation therapies, *Top Stroke Rehabil* 12:58–65, 2005.
4. Birkenmeier RL, Prager EM, Lang CE: Translating animal doses of task-specific training to people with chronic stroke in 1-hour therapy sessions: a proof-of-concept study, *Neurorehabil Neural Repair* 24(7):620–635, 2010.
5. Bondoc S, Booth J, Budde G, Caruso K, DeSousa M, Earl B, Hammerton K, Humphreys J: Mirror therapy and task-oriented training for people with a paretic upper extremity, *American Journal of Occupational Therapy* 72(2):1–8, 2018. https://doi.org/10.5014/ajot.2018.025064.
6. Carmichael ST, Kathirvelu B, Schweppe CA, Nie EH: Molecular, cellular and functional events in axonal sprouting after stroke, *Experimental Neurology* 287:384–394, 2017. https://doi.org/10.1016/j.expneurol.2016.02.007.
7. Carr J, Shepherd R: The adaptive system: plasticity and recovery. In Carr J, Shepherd R, editors: *Neurological rehabilitation: optimizing motor performance*, ed 2, London, 2010, Churchill Livingstone, pp 3–14.
8. Carter AR, Connor LT, Dromerick AW: Rehabilitation after stroke: current state of the science, *Curr Neurol Neurosci Rep* 10:158–166, 2010.
9. Dickie V: What is occupation? In Crepeau EB, Cohn ES, Schell BAB, editors: *Willard and Spackman's occupational therapy*, ed 11, Philadelphia, 2009, Lippincott Williams & Wilkins, pp 15–21.
10. Fisher A: Overview of performance skills and client factors. In Pendleton H, Schultz-Krohn W, editors: *Pedretti's occupational therapy for physical dysfunction*, ed 6, St Louis, 2006, Elsevier/Mosby, pp 372–402.
11. Fugl-Meyer AR, Jääskö L, Leyman I, Olsson S, Steglind S: The post-stroke hemiplegic patient. I. A method for evaluation of physical performance, *Scand J Rehabil Med* 7:13–31, 1975.
12. Gillen G: *Stroke rehabilitation: a function-based approach*, ed 3, St Louis, 2011, Elsevier/Mosby.
13. Hubbard IJ, Parsons MW, Neilson C, Carey LM: Task-specific training: evidence for and translation to clinical practice, *Occup Ther Int* 16(3–4):175–189, 2009.

14. Joy MT, Carmichael ST: Encouraging an excitable brain state: mechanisms of brain repair in stroke, *Nature Reviews Neuroscience* 22:38–53, 2021. https://doi.org/10.1038/s41583-020-00396-7.

15. Kleim JA, Jones TA: Principles of experience-dependent neural plasticity: implications for rehabilitation after brain damage, *J Speech Lang Hear Res* 51:S225–S239, 2008.

16. Kopp B, Kunkel A, Flor H, et al: The Arm Motor Ability Test: reliability, validity, and sensitivity to change of an instrument for assessing disabilities in activities of daily living, *Arch Phys Med Rehabil* 78:615–620, 1997.

17. Kovic M, Stoykov ME: A multi-site study for cortical stimulation and occupational therapy. Poster session presented at the Fifteenth Congress for the World Federation of Occupational Therapists, May, 2010, Santiago, Chile.

18. Lang CE, Birkenmeier RL: *Upper-extremity task-specific training after stroke or disability: a manual for occupational therapy and physical therapy*, Bethesda, MD, 2014, AOTA Press.

19. Law M, et al: *Canadian Occupational Performance Measures*, ed 3, Ottawa, ON, 1998, CAOT.

20. Lewthwaite R, et al: Accelerating stroke recovery: body structures and functions, activities, participation, and quality of life outcomes from a large rehabilitation trial. *Neurorehab Neural Repair* 32(2) 150–165, 2018.

21. Mathiowetz V: Task-oriented approach to stroke rehabilitation. In Gillen G, editor: *Stroke rehabilitation: a function-based approach*, ed 3, St Louis, 2011, Elsevier/Mosby, pp 80–99.

22. Nudo RJ, Milliken GW: Reorganization of movement representations in primary motor cortex following focal ischemic infarcts in adult squirrel monkeys, *J Neurophysiol* 75:2144–2149, 1996.

23. Nudo RJ, Milliken GW, Jenkins WM, Merzenich MM: Use-dependent alterations of movement representations in primary motor cortex of adult squirrel monkeys, *J Neurosci* 16:785–807, 1996.

24. Page SJ, Gater DR, Bach Y, Rita P: Reconsidering the motor recovery plateau in stroke rehabilitation, *Arch Phys Med Rehabil* 85:1377–1381, 2004.

25. Plow EB, Carey JR, Nudo RJ, Pascual-Leone A: Invasive cortical stimulation to promote recovery of function after stroke: a critical appraisal, *Stroke* 40:1926–1931, 2009.

26. Rossini PM, Calautti C, Pauri F, Baron J-C: Post-stroke plastic reorganisation in the adult brain, *Lancet Neurol* 2:493–502, 2003.

27. Shumway-Cook A, Woollacott MH: *Motor control: translating research into clinical practice*, ed 3, Philadelphia, 2007, Lippincott Williams & Wilkins.

28. Stoykov ME, Corcos DM: A review of bilateral training for upper extremity hemiparesis, *Occup Ther Int* 16:190–203, 2009.

29. Trombly CA: Occupation: purposefulness and meaningfulness as therapeutic mechanisms, *Am J Occup Ther* 49:960–972, 1995.

30. Volpe BT, et al: Intensive sensorimotor arm training mediated by therapist or robot improves hemiparesis in patients with chronic stroke, *Neurorehabil Neural Repair* 22:305–310, 2008.

31. World Health Organization: *International statistical classification of diseases and related health problems (ICD)* 11th Revision, 2022. https://www.who.int/classifications/classification-of-diseases.

32. World Health Organization: *International classification of functioning, disability and health: ICF*, Geneva, 2008, WHO Press.

33. Wu C-Y, Trombly CA, Lin K-C, Tickle-Degnen L: A kinematic study of contextual effects on reaching performance in persons with and without stroke: influences of object availability, *Arch Phys Med Rehabil* 81:95–101, 2000.

SUGGESTED READINGS

Hebb DO: *The organization of behavior: a neuropsychological theory*, New York, 1949, Wiley.

Muellbacher W, et al: Improving hand function in chronic stroke, *Arch Neurol* 59:1278–1282, 2002.

World Health Organization: *International statistical classification of diseases and related health problems (ICD)* 11th Revision, 2022. https://www.who.int/classifications/classification-of-diseases.

Wu C, Trombly CA, Lin K, Tickle-Degnen L: Effects of object affordances on reaching performance in persons with and without cerebrovascular accident, *Am J Occup Ther* 52:447–456, 1998.

19

Evaluation of Motor Control

Winifred Schultz-Krohn[a]

After studying this chapter, the student or practitioner will be able to do the following:

1. Differentiate between upper and lower motor neuron pathological conditions.
2. State the principles of neuroplasticity and explain to clients the potential for recovery after a neurological injury or cerebrovascular disorder.
3. Describe four types of rigidity and the ways each affects movement.
4. Clinically differentiate between spinal and cerebral hypertonia.
5. Rate hypertonia on the Modified Ashworth Scale or the mild-moderate-severe scale.
6. Name standardized assessments designed to evaluate function after a cerebrovascular accident.
7. List the components of the postural mechanism.
8. Describe at least four types of cerebellar disorders.
9. List and describe at least four extrapyramidal disorders.
10. Choose a coordination assessment that objectively assesses function.
11. Name three current medical or surgical treatment options for the management of spasticity.
12. List at least three conservative occupational therapy interventions for spasticity.
13. Describe a conservative, evidence-based, client-centered occupational therapy program for treating Parkinson's disease.

CHAPTER OUTLINE

[a] With contributions from Linda Anderson Preston.

KEY TERMS

Clonus
Coordination
Decerebrate rigidity
Decorticate rigidity
Flaccidity
Hypertonicity
Hypertonus

Hypotonus
Intrathecal baclofen pump
Motor control
Movement disorders
Nerve blocks
Neuroplasticity
Paresis

Plegia
Postural mechanism
Rigidity
Serial casting
Spasticity
Spinal hypertonia

Motor control is the ability of the central nervous system (CNS) to direct or regulate the musculoskeletal system in purposeful activity.[90] The components necessary for motor control include normal muscle tone, normal postural tone and postural mechanisms, selective movement, and coordination. Complex neurological systems (i.e., the cerebral cortex, basal ganglia, and cerebellum) collaborate to make motor control possible. A neurological insult, such as a cerebrovascular accident (CVA) (stroke), brain injury, or disease such as multiple sclerosis or Parkinson's disease, affects motor control. Functional recovery depends on the initial amount of neurological damage, prompt access to medical treatment to

(hopefully) limit the extent of neurological damage, the nature of the neurological damage, whether it is static or progressive, and therapeutic intervention that can facilitate motor recovery.

Plasticity is an important concept in neurological rehabilitation because it helps explain why recovery is possible after a brain injury or lesion. The term *plasticity* simply means the ability to change. Neuroplasticity is defined as the capacity for anatomic and electrophysiological changes in the CNS. Neuroplasticity, seen as dendritic and axonal sprouting, has occurred not only directly adjacent to the site of the lesion but in more remote brain regions to support functional recovery.[22]

THREADED CASE STUDY

Daniel, Part 1

Daniel is a 54-year-old salesman who is right-hand dominant (he identifies as male and uses the pronouns of he/his/him). Daniel had an embolic cerebrovascular accident (CVA) 2 months ago that weakened the right side of his body. He has just completed 3 weeks of inpatient rehabilitation services that included occupational therapy, and he is starting outpatient occupational therapy today. His 76-year-old mother must drive him to therapy, and he finds this quite frustrating because he values his independence. His goal is to start his car ignition with his right hand and eventually resume driving. His vision and visual fields were not compromised by the CVA, as assessed by an ophthalmologist and the inpatient occupational therapist. Daniel is concerned about the future, and he wants to return to full-time employment. The occupational therapist knows that the ability to return to work after a stroke varies substantially, and each year many individuals surviving a stroke are left permanently disabled.[8,49] Additionally, those who do return to work after a stroke are often working part-time instead of full-time.[92]

One of the best predictors of the ability to return to work is independence in activities of daily living (ADLs).[49]

Daniel's right upper extremity (RUE) shows hypertonia in a flexion synergy, with moderate spasticity in his shoulder internal rotators, elbow flexors, forearm pronators, wrist and finger flexors, and thumb adductors. Daniel does not have active range of motion (ROM) of the right shoulder external rotation or right forearm supination. His active finger extension on his right hand is emerging and is a 2− on the strength grade scale. He is currently at stage 4 of the Modified Brunnstrom Motor Recovery Scale (Table 19.1 and Figs. 19.1 to 19.5). He has only 1 lb of lateral pinch strength in his right hand. His ROM losses and impairments, coupled with RUE spasticity, prevent him from starting his car ignition with his right hand. He needs occupational therapy (OT) rehabilitation services to regain the performance skills of holding a steering wheel, releasing a steering wheel, and turning on the ignition with his right hand.

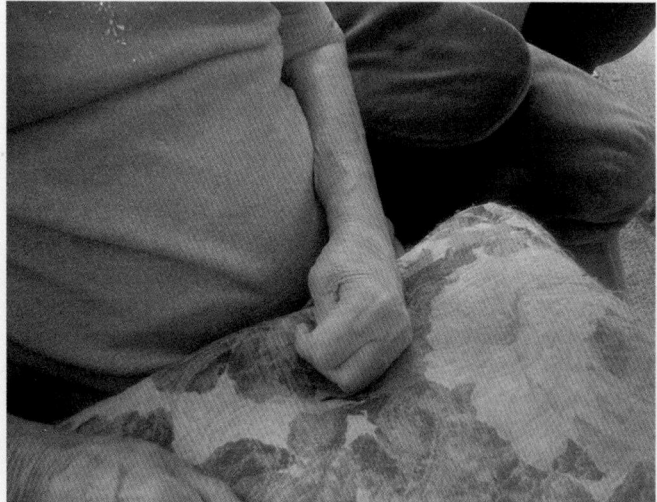

Fig. 19.1 Modified Brunnstrom stage 1 in female patient.

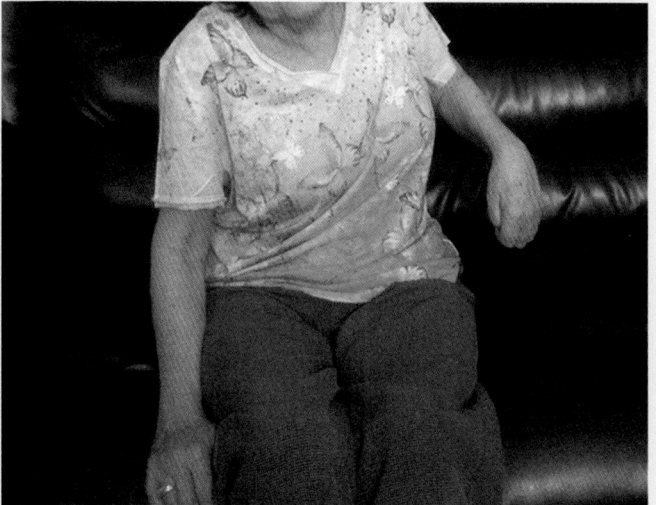

Fig. 19.2 Modified Brunnstrom stage 2 in female patient.

(Continued)

THREADED CASE STUDY—cont'd

Daniel, Part 1

Critical Thinking Questions

1. What performance skills or standardized assessments would you select as part of your initial evaluation to assess Daniel's motor function?

2. What activities or intervention would you plan for Daniel to reduce the spasticity in his right arm?

3. What home exercises or activity program would you prescribe to help him reach his goals of using his right hand to insert the key into the car ignition and then drive with both hands on the steering wheel?

TABLE 19.1   Modified Brunnstrom Stages of Motor Recovery[a]

Stage	Modified Brunnstrom Motor Recovery of Arm and Hand	Interdisciplinary Spasticity Management Options
0	Flaccidity with no active movement.	• Prevent contractures with PROM and consider splinting. • Functional electrical stimulation.
1	Spasticity developing. Trace muscle contraction in elbow flexors and scapular retractors (see Fig. 19.1).	• Same as stage 0.
2	Weak synergistic movement of scapular retractors, scapular elevators, elbow flexors, and forearm pronators. Promote active movement in gravity-reduced planes. Eccentric, side-lying, and supine exercises are good ways to start facilitating movement. Functional electric stimulation may speed up motor recovery. Clients tend to use trunk lateral flexion to substitute for weak shoulder/scapular muscles (see Fig. 19.2).	• Prevent contractures with PROM and consider splinting. Risk for shoulder, elbow, forearm, and finger flexion contractures. • Blocks[b] and surgery generally are not indicated at this stage.
3	Spasticity increasing. Synergy patterns and their components can be performed voluntarily to almost full ROM. Gross grasp is developing; however, there is no active finger release. Lateral pinch is possible via thumb adduction tone and flexor pollicis longus tone. Synergy pattern may be useful for carrying objects (e.g., envelopes with lateral pinch, or grocery bags in client's affected hand with finger flexion tone). Clients in this stage also tend to substitute with trunk lateral flexion to make up for shoulder weakness (see Fig. 19.3).	• *Acute:* Client is a good candidate for nerve or motor point blocks to prevent contractures. Recovery may be facilitated by unmasking movement in antagonists if spastic agonists are weakened by blocks. See text for OT treatment suggestions. • *Chronic:* After all conservative measures have failed, orthopedic surgery may be performed to release contractures so as to improve hygiene in the hand and ease UE dressing.
4	Spasticity declining, movement combinations from synergies are now possible. Elbow extension and wrist and finger extension are emerging but are not to full range. Occupational therapy should incorporate functional tasks that promote extension of the elbow, wrist, fingers, and thumb (see Fig. 19.4).	• *Acute:* Client is a good to excellent nerve block candidate. Better chance of gaining motor control of antagonists with blocks to the spastic agonists. • *Chronic:* Ongoing blocks three or four times per year if the risk-to-benefit ratio for orthopedic surgery is not acceptable to client. Orthopedic surgery options include procedures to gain function and to ameliorate contractures.
5	Synergies are no longer dominant. Finger extension is full range. Isolated finger extension is possible. Three-jaw chuck pinch and tip pinches are possible, but motor control is only fair. Emergence of intrinsic function. Occupational therapy should focus on purposeful fine motor activities (see Fig. 19.5).	• Client is an excellent candidate for fine-tuning motor control via blocks (e.g., neuromuscular blocks to the extrinsic flexor pollicis longus supports the goal of improved intrinsic motor control of the thumb by allowing action of the opponens pollicis, abductor pollicis brevis, and flexor pollicis brevis to be unmasked). It should be noted that reducing hypertonia does not always result in improved dexterity.[33]
6	Isolated joint movements are performed with ease. Intrinsic function is normal. All types of prehension are possible with normal motor control.	• Client is not a candidate for blocks or surgery. Discharge from occupational therapy if all goals have been met.

[a]These stages may be used as a guideline for OT intervention and interdisciplinary spasticity management in clients with hemiplegia or hemiparesis. NOTE: Upper extremity recovery is variable owing to varying degrees of paralysis. Some clients may never progress through all the stages.
[b]The term *blocks* refers to chemical denervation with botulinum toxin type A or type B; neurolysis; or motor point blocks with phenol or alcohol.
CVA, Cerebrovascular accident; *PROM*, passive range of motion; *ROM*, range of motion; *UE*, upper extremity.
Adapted from Brunnstrom S: *Movement therapy in hemiplegia*, Philadelphia, 1970, Lippincott Williams & Wilkins.

THREADED CASE STUDY—cont'd

Daniel, Part 1

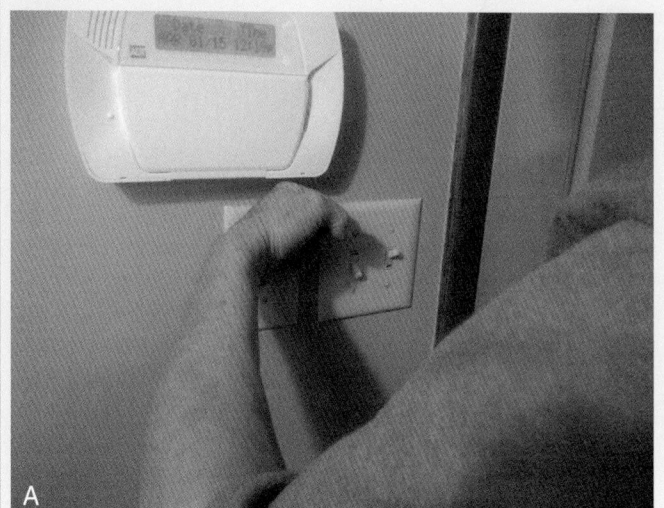
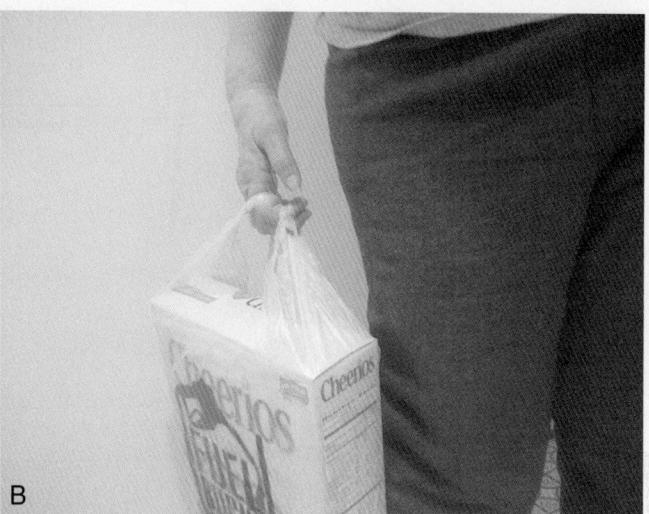

Fig. 19.3 Modified Brunnstrom stage 3.

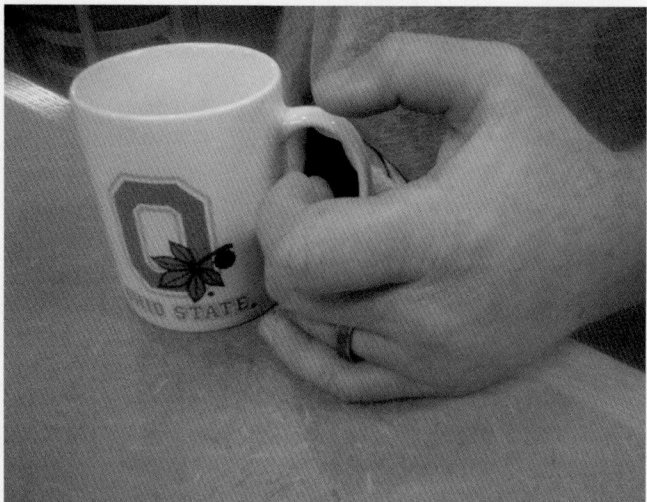
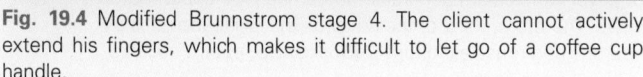
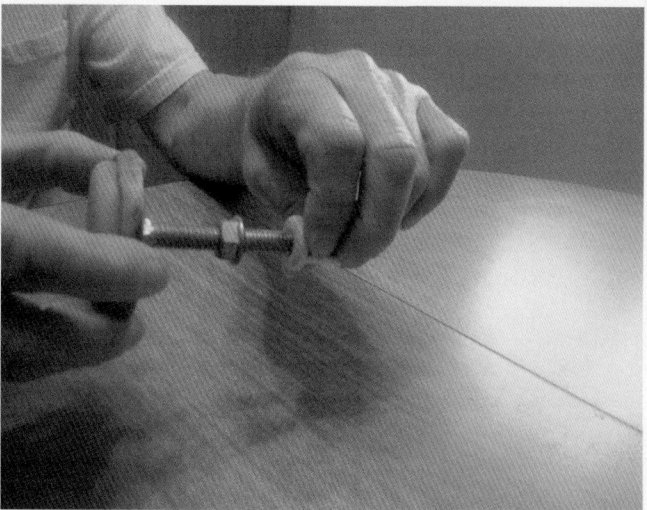

Fig. 19.4 Modified Brunnstrom stage 4. The client cannot actively extend his fingers, which makes it difficult to let go of a coffee cup handle.

Fig 19.5 Modified Brunnstrom stage 5. The client is able to use a three-jaw chuck pinch to loosen the nut on the screw.

In some instances, the CNS is able to reorganize and adapt to functional demands after injury. Motor relearning can occur through the use of existing neural pathways (unmasking) or through the development of new neural connections (neural sprouting) (Fig. 19.6). With unmasking, it is thought that seldom-used (secondary) pathways become more active after the primary pathway has been injured. Adjacent nerves take over the functions of damaged nerves.[25] With sprouting, dendrites from one nerve form a new attachment or synapse with another. Axonal sprouting also occurs and allows for flexible synaptic connections to be formed. Neural sprouting is thought to be the primary process for neuroplasticity, leading to improvement in function.[57]

Observing movements during occupational performance is a way to assess motor control. Then, after occupational performance has been evaluated, it may be necessary to evaluate the specific components that underlie motor control. These components include muscle tone, postural tone and the postural mechanism, reflexes, selective movement, and coordination.

THE UPPER MOTOR NEURON AND LOWER MOTOR NEURON SYSTEMS

This chapter focuses on the functional effects of lesions in the upper motor neuron (UMN) system. The UMNs originate in the cerebral hemispheres, cerebellum, and brainstem and influence the intention, accuracy, and smoothness of movements. UMN "signs" often seen after damage has occurred include hyperreflexia, a positive Babinski's sign, and spasticity.[32] These "signs" of UMN damage are seen when the UMN can no longer efficiently

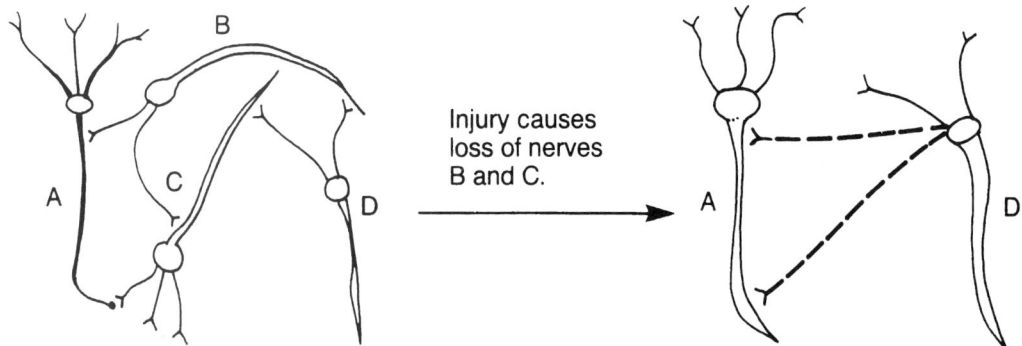

Fig. 19.6 Sprouting theory of nerve cell replacement. Injury causes loss of nerves B and C. New dendrite connections "sprout" from nerve D to reestablish contact with nerve A. (From DeBoskey DS, et al: *Educating families of the head injured*, Rockville, MD, 1991, Aspen.)

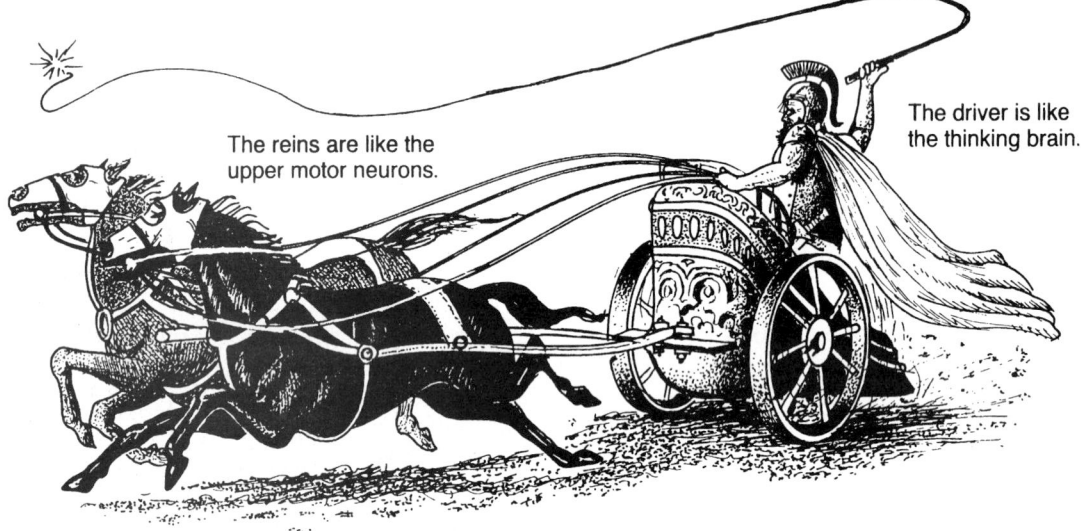

Fig 19.7 The control of movement works much as does a chariot driver with a team of horses. Remember, the upper motor neuron system facilitates or inhibits the lower motor neuron system. Therefore, think of the driver as the brain, the reins as the upper motor neurons, and the horses as the lower motor neurons and muscles. (From DeBoskey DS, et al: *Educating families of the head injured*, Rockville, MD, 1991, Aspen.)

and accurately influence the lower motor neuron (LMN). Weakness, paralysis, and fatigue often accompany UMN syndrome. Individuals who sustain a CVA or traumatic brain injury (TBI) often have resultant UMN dysfunction.

The lower motor neuron system (LMNS) includes the anterior horn cells of the spinal cord, the nuclei and axons of the cranial nerves, and the peripheral nerves, both efferent and afferent portions. LMN dysfunction results in diminished or absent deep tendon reflexes and muscle weakness, atrophy, or flaccidity. An example of an LMN disease is Guillain-Barré syndrome. Individuals who have sustained a spinal cord injury can show both UMN and LMN signs if the anterior horn cells have been damaged. The findings of electromyography and nerve conduction studies are abnormal with LMN dysfunction.[4] Fig. 19.7 illustrates the influence of the UMNS on the LMNS.[24]

OT PRACTICE NOTES

These questions may help guide evaluation of motor control dysfunction:
1. Is the client having difficulty with sitting or standing balance?
2. Is trunk control adequate to perform the activity?
3. Do changes in body position affect muscle tone (e.g., more hypertonia when standing than supine, more hypertonia when walking than standing)?
4. Are primitive reflexes evoked during performance?
5. Is spasticity limiting antagonist movement?
6. Are spatial or temporal sequencing problems interfering with coordinated movement?
7. Does weakness prohibit antigravity activity?
8. Is tremor present?
9. Is incoordination apparent (i.e., overshooting or undershooting the target)? Are there extraneous movements?

CLIENT-CENTERED PERFORMANCE INTERVIEWS TO DETECT PROBLEM AREAS IN MOTOR CONTROL

The occupational therapist faces the challenge of maximizing the client's ability to return to purposeful and meaningful occupation in his or her physical, cultural, and social environment. Therefore, evaluating functional performance is primary in helping clients set realistic goals. A simple method of goal setting is to ask the client to name the top two or three things he or she would like to be able to resume doing. The Canadian Occupational Performance Measure (COPM), an assessment tool, is a more structured interview that ensures client-centered therapy.[63] It helps prioritize the client's functional activity goals in the areas of self-care, leisure, and productivity.

Two other noteworthy, client-centered, quality-of-life surveys frequently are used in interdisciplinary settings with clients who have been diagnosed with a CVA. The Stroke Impact Scale (SIS) version 3.0 contains 59 items grouped into 8 domains that include items addressing strength, hand function, activities of daily living (ADLs), instrumental activities of daily living (IADLs), mobility, communication, emotion, memory, thinking, and social participation.[27] The Stroke Specific Quality of Life Scale consists of 49 items divided into 12 domains: energy, family roles, language, mobility, mood, personality, self-care, social roles, thinking, upper extremity (UE) function, vision, and work/productivity.[94] Both scales are scored on a 5-point Likert scale.

The occupational therapist (OT) can observe the client for motor control dysfunction during assessment of ADLs and IADLs and productive and leisure activities. The therapist must observe how problems in motor control affect occupational performance while considering the client's sensation, perception, cognition, and medical status.

STANDARDIZED ACTIVITIES OF DAILY LIVING ASSESSMENTS FOR MOTOR CONTROL

Many standardized ADL tests are available for assessing occupational performance and are useful for observing motor control. The Test d'Évaluation des Membres Supérieurs de Personnes Âgées (TEMPA) is a UE functional activity performance test developed to help therapists distinguish between "normal and pathologic[al] aging in upper extremity performance."[26] Test items include picking up and moving a jar, writing on an envelope, tying a scarf, and handling coins, among others.

Several assessments have been designed to assess function after a CVA. These can be used to observe for motor control problems.

1. The Graded Wolf Motor Function Test[72] (GWMFT) was developed to measure functional gains after a hemiparetic event from a CVA or TBI. This test was based on the Wolf Motor Function Test.[14] It is called "graded" because there are two levels of difficulty for each task; level A is more advanced, and level B is easier. Gorman investigated the interreliability and intrareliability of the GWMFT with a sample of eight physical therapists and three subjects (Gorman IG: Personal communication, June 2004).

Intrarater and interrater reliability was .935 on the timing scores. Intrarater reliability was .897, and interrater reliability was .879 on the functional ability scores. This is a very useful test that can be used with a wide variety of clients with hemiparesis who have varying degrees of motor recovery. More research is needed to confirm the validity and reliability of this test.

2. The Wolf Motor Function Test (WMFT) has been and continues to be widely used to quantify the motor abilities of clients with chronic and persistent high levels of UE dysfunction after a CVA or TBI.[1,95,96] It has an interrater reliability range of .95 to .97 (Fig. 19.8).

3. The Functional Test for the Hemiplegic/Paretic Upper Extremity[95] assesses the client's ability to use the involved arm for purposeful tasks. This test provides objective documentation of functional improvement and includes tasks ranging from those that involve basic stabilization to more difficult tasks requiring fine manipulation and proximal stabilization. Examples include holding a pouch, stabilizing a jar, wringing a rag, hooking and zipping a zipper, folding a sheet, and putting in a light bulb overhead.[95]

4. The Fugl-Meyer Assessment[58] (FMA) is based on the natural progression of neurological recovery after a CVA. Low scores on the FMA have been closely correlated with the presence of severe spasticity. Fugl-Meyer and colleagues developed a quantitative assessment of motor function after a stroke by measuring such parameters as range of motion (ROM), pain, sensation, and balance.[41] Scores on the FMA correlate with ADL performance, and this tool is widely used to document UE recovery after a CVA.[1,53,85,96]

5. The Arm Motor Ability Test[61] (AMAT) is a functional assessment of UE function. Cutting meat, making a sandwich, opening a jar, and putting on a T-shirt are some of the tasks included in this test. It has high interrater and test-retest reliability.

6. The Motricity Index[23] (MI) is a valid and reliable test of motor impairment that can be performed quickly. The test assesses the client's ability to pinch a cube with the index finger and thumb, in addition to elbow flexion, shoulder abduction, ankle dorsiflexion, knee extension, and hip flexion.

7. The Assessment of Motor and Process Skills (AMPS)[12] is a standardized test that assesses the quality of performance in ADLs, in addition to motor and process skills in ADLs and IADLs. The test was created by occupational therapists. Although this test is not diagnosis specific, it has been widely used with clients who have had a CVA. Occupational therapy (OT) practitioners can become certified in the use of this test by completing a 5-day training course.[12]

As mentioned, after observing functional performance, the OT usually finds it necessary to assess the performance components that underlie motor control: muscle tone (normal/abnormal), the postural mechanism, muscle tone assessment/reflexes, sensation, and coordination.

MUSCLE TONE

Muscle tone is the resistance felt by the examiner while passively moving a client's limb.[87] It is dependent on the integrity of peripheral and CNS mechanisms and the properties of muscle. It should be high enough to resist gravity, yet low enough to allow movement. The tension is determined partly by mechanical factors (e.g., the connective tissue and viscoelastic properties of muscle) and partly by the degree of motor unit activity. When passively stretched, normal muscle offers a small amount of involuntary resistance.

Normal muscle tone relies on normal function of the cerebellum, motor cortex, basal ganglia, midbrain, vestibular system, spinal cord, and neuromuscular system (including the mechanical-elastic features of the muscle and connective tissues) and on a normally functioning stretch reflex. The stretch reflex is mediated by the muscle spindle, a sophisticated sensory receptor that continuously reports sensory information from muscles to the CNS.

WOLF MOTOR FUNCTION TEST
DATA COLLECTION FORM

Subject's Name: _____   Date: _____

Test (check one):   Pre-treatment _____   Post-treatment _____   Follow-up _____

Arm tested (check one):   More-affected _____   Less-affected _____

Task	Time	Functional Ability	Comment
1. Forearm to table (side)		0 1 2 3 4 5	
2. Forearm to box (side)		0 1 2 3 4 5	
3. Extend elbow (side)		0 1 2 3 4 5	
4. Extend elbow (weight)		0 1 2 3 4 5	
5. Hand to table (front)		0 1 2 3 4 5	
6. Hand to box (front)		0 1 2 3 4 5	
7. Weight to box		_____lbs.	
8. Reach and retrieve		0 1 2 3 4 5	
9. Lift can		0 1 2 3 4 5	
10. Lift pencil		0 1 2 3 4 5	
11. Lift paper clip		0 1 2 3 4 5	
12. Stack checkers		0 1 2 3 4 5	
13. Flip cards		0 1 2 3 4 5	
14. Grip strength		_____kgs.	
15. Turn key in lock		0 1 2 3 4 5	
16. Fold towel		0 1 2 3 4 5	
17. Lift basket		0 1 2 3 4 5	

A

Fig. 19.8 Wolf Motor Function Test score sheet (A) and functional ability scale (B). (From Taub E, Morris DM, Crago J: *Wolf Motor Function Test [WMFT] manual,* revised 2011, University of Alabama at Birmingham CI Therapy Research Group. http://www.uab.edu/citherapy/.)

FUNCTIONAL ABILITY SCALE

0 – Does not attempt with upper extremity (UE) being tested.

1 – UE being tested does not participate functionally; however, attempt is made to use the UE. In unilateral tasks the UE not being tested may be used to move the UE being tested.

2 – Does, but requires assistance of the UE not being tested for minor readjustments or change of position, or requires more than two attempts to complete, or accomplishes very slowly. In bilateral tasks the UE being tested may serve only as a helper.

3 – Does, but movement is influenced to some degree by synergy or is performed slowly or with effort.

4 – Does; movement is close to normal,* but slightly slower; may lack precision, fine coordination or fluidity.

5 – Does; movement appears to be normal.*

*For the determination of normal, the less-involved UE can be utilized as an available index for comparison, with pre-morbid UE dominance taken into consideration.

B

Fig. 19.8, cont'd

Normal muscle tone varies from one individual to another. Within the range considered normal, the degree of normal tone depends on such factors as age, gender, and occupation. Normal muscle tone is characterized by a number of factors:

1. Effective coactivation (stabilization) at axial and proximal joints
2. Ability to move against gravity and resistance
3. Ability to maintain the position of the limb that has been passively positioned by the therapist and then the support from the therapist is removed
4. Balanced tone between agonistic and antagonistic muscles
5. Ease of ability to shift from stability to mobility and to reverse as needed
6. Ability to use muscles in groups or selectively with normal timing and coordination
7. Resilience or slight resistance in response to passive movement

Hypertonicity (increased tone) interferes with the performance of normal selective movement because it affects the timing and smoothness of agonist and antagonist muscle groups (see Chapters 32, 33, and 34). Normalization of muscle tone and amelioration of paresis (incomplete paralysis/weakness) are desirable when striving for selective motor control. Some function can be achieved even though tone may not be normal. Plegia is defined as complete paralysis.

ABNORMAL MUSCLE TONE

Abnormal muscle tone usually is described with the terms *flaccidity, hypotonus, hypertonus, spasticity,* and *rigidity.* To plan the appropriate intervention, the OT practitioner must recognize the differences among these tone states and must be able to identify these states during the clinical assessment.

Flaccidity

Flaccidity refers to the absence of tone. Deep tendon reflexes (DTRs) and active movement are absent. Flaccidity can result from spinal or cerebral shock immediately after a spinal or cerebral insult. With traumatic UMN lesions of cerebral or spinal origin, flaccidity usually is present initially and then often, but not always, changes to hypertonicity within a few weeks, depending on the location and amount of brain damage.

Flaccidity also can result from LMN dysfunction, such as peripheral nerve injury or disruption of the reflex arc at the alpha motor neuron level. The muscles feel soft and offer no resistance to passive movement. If the flaccid limb is moved passively, it will feel heavy. If moved to a given position and released, the limb will drop because the muscles are unable to resist the pull of gravity.[4]

Hypotonus

Hypotonus is considered by many to be a decrease in normal muscle tone (i.e., low tone). DTRs are diminished or absent. Van der Meche and Van der Gijn[90] suggested that hypotonus could be an erroneous clinical concept. They performed electromyographic (EMG) analysis on the quadriceps muscles in "hypotonic" clients (e.g., those with peripheral neuropathy, cerebral infarction, and other diagnoses) and in relaxed normal subjects in a lower leg free-fall test. They concluded that if a client's limb feels hypotonic or flaccid, this is the result of weakness, not of long-latency stretch reflexes.

Hypertonus

Hypertonus is increased muscle tone. Hypertonicity can occur when a lesion is present in the premotor cortex, the basal ganglia, or descending pathways. UMNs tend to have an inhibitory influence on LMNs. Damage to the UMNS has the effect of increasing stimulation of the LMNs, with resultant increased alpha motor activity. Any neurological condition that damages and compromises the function of the UMN pathways can directly or indirectly facilitate alpha motor neuron activity, which may result in hypertonicity. Other spinal or brainstem reflexes may become hyperactive, which leads to hypertonic patterns, such as flexor withdrawal or the dominance of primitive reflexes during movement activities.[32]

Hypertonicity often occurs in a synergistic neuromuscular pattern, particularly when seen after a CVA or TBI. Synergies are defined as patterned movement characterized by co-contraction of flexors or extensors. A typical synergy seen in the UE after a CVA or TBI is a *flexion synergy*. The flexion synergy is shoulder adduction; internal rotation; elbow flexion; forearm pronation; wrist, finger, and thumb flexion; and thumb adduction. In contrast, an extension synergy is seen in the lower extremity.

For the client who has sustained damage to the UMNs, the energy cost of moving against hypertonicity is considerable. It takes a great deal of effort for clients with moderate to severe hypertonicity to move against this force. Antagonist power may be insufficient to overcome the spastic agonist muscle groups. Daniel, in the case study, had problems overcoming the pull of his spastic finger flexors with his weak finger extensors. Even clients with mild hypertonicity report frustration during functional activities. Loss of reciprocal inhibition is noted between spastic agonists and antagonists.[4] Clients are unable to rapidly and efficiently coordinate the activity between agonist and antagonist groups of muscles. The client with a UMN lesion will have dysfunction in spatial and temporal timing of movement. This makes his or her movements uncoordinated. This frustration, coupled with the fatigue, decreased dexterity, and paresis associated with UMNs, can influence therapy participation. Furthermore, the architecture of hypertonic muscles changes over time. The muscles lose their ability to lengthen and shorten because of viscoelastic changes that result from the hypertonia.[82]

Not everyone recovers full UE motor function after a CVA or TBI. Table 19.1 can help the OT practitioner to explain the stages of motor recovery to families, and to clarify that not all clients will progress through all seven stages. The table can be used for preparation for discharge, allowing the therapist to explain to the client and family that the client has reached a plateau in motor recovery.

Hypertonicity can increase as a result of painful or noxious stimuli. These stimuli often can be reduced with appropriate medical care. Stimuli that can increase tone include pressure sores, ingrown toenails, tight elastic straps on a urine collection leg bag, tight clothing, an obstructed catheter, a urinary tract infection, and fecal impaction. Other triggering factors include fear, anxiety, environmental temperature extremes, heterotopic ossification, and sensory overload. These triggering factors are seen in both cerebral and spinal hypertonicity; however, they are more pronounced in spinal hypertonia. Therapeutic

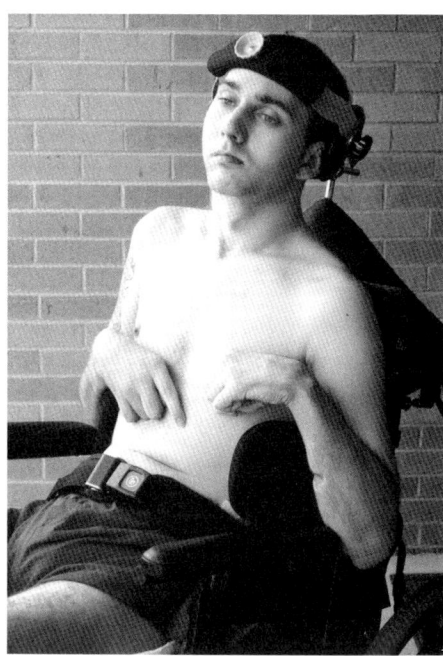

Fig. 19.9 A client with dystonia in his right index finger (extension). His left wrist shows severe hypertonicity. Tone abnormalities are the result of a traumatic brain injury.

intervention should be designed to reduce, eliminate, or cope with the various external factors.[72]

Clients with hypertonicity often have difficulty initiating movement, especially rapid movement. Although hypertonic muscles appear to be able to resist substantial external force (as in manual muscle testing), they do not function as normal, strong muscles. Through the mechanism of reciprocal inhibition, hypertonic muscles inhibit the activity of their antagonists and thus can mask potentially good or normal function of antagonists.[74] Four types of hypertonia are described in the following sections: cerebral hypertonia, spinal hypertonia, spasticity, and rigidity.

Cerebral Hypertonia

Cerebral hypertonia is caused by TBI, stroke, anoxia, neoplasms (brain tumors), metabolic disorders, cerebral palsy, and diseases of the brain. In multiple sclerosis, hypertonia is produced from both spinal and cerebral lesions. With cerebral hypertonia, muscle tone fluctuates continuously in response to extrinsic and intrinsic factors. Cerebral hypertonia usually occurs in definite patterns of flexion or extension, causing the limb to frequently assume and remain in a specific position (Fig. 19.9). Typically, these patterns occur in the antigravity muscles of the upper and lower extremities (e.g., flexors of the upper extremities, extensors of the lower extremities).

The dominance of primitive reflexes and associated reactions alters postural tone. When an individual is supine, muscle tone is less than when the individual is sitting or standing. Tone is highest during ambulation. Thus, attention to postural tone is important when positioning a client for splinting or casting. A cast or splint fabricated on a client in a supine position may not fit when the client is sitting up because of the influence of gravity and posture on increasing muscle tone.[82]

Spinal Hypertonia

Spinal hypertonia results from injuries and diseases of the spinal cord. In slow-onset spinal disease (e.g., spinal stenosis, tumor), there is no period of spinal shock. With a traumatic spinal cord injury, spinal shock occurs and is characterized by initial flaccidity. Over time (weeks or months), the flaccidity diminishes and hypertonia develops. The affected extremities first develop flexor and adductor tone. Over time, extensor tone develops and becomes predominant in the lower extremities. Spinal hypertonia can lead to muscle spasms severe enough to cause an individual to fall out of a wheelchair, off a gurney, or out of bed. The degree of hypertonicity in incomplete spinal lesions varies, depending on the degree of damage to the spinal cord. Tone tends to be more severe in individuals with incomplete spinal cord lesions than in those with complete lesions.[82]

Spasticity

According to Nance and colleagues,[74] the most commonly cited definition of spasticity is from the American Academy of Neurology: "Spasticity is a motor disorder that is characterized by a velocity dependent increase in tonic stretch reflexes (muscle tone) with exaggerated tendon jerks, resulting from hyperexcitability of the stretch reflex, as one component of the upper motor neuron syndrome."[7]

Spasticity has two characteristics:
- *Velocity dependence:* The stretch reflex is elicited only by the examiner's rapid passive stretch.
- *Clasp-knife phenomenon:* When the examiner takes the extremity through a quick passive stretch, a sudden catch or resistance is felt, followed by a release of the resistance. What actually happens is that the initial high resistance felt by the therapist is due to spasticity and then the hypertonia is suddenly inhibited, allowing the extremity to be moved through the full passive ROM.

One of the main CNS tracts involved in the pathophysiology of spasticity is the corticospinal tract. It is a major motor tract that originates from many areas in the cerebral cortex, including the cells of the prefrontal region, the cingulate gyrus, and the postcentral gyrus of the parietal lobe.[32]

Clonus. Clonus is a specific type of spasticity. This condition often is present in clients with moderate to severe spasticity. Clonus is characterized by repetitive contractions in the antagonist muscles in response to rapid stretch. Recurrent bursts of Ia afferent activity result in a cyclical oscillation of phasic stretch reflexes. Clonus is seen most commonly in the finger flexors and ankle plantar flexors. The occurrence of clonus can interfere with participation in purposeful activity, transfers, and mobility. Therapists should educate clients and their families in how to use weight-bearing actively because this usually stops the clonus. Therapists and physicians record clonus by counting the number of beats elicited after a quick stretch to an extremity, such as a quick stretch of the ankle plantar flexors or finger flexors. A 3-beat clonus can be rated as mild and is less likely to interfere with ADLs than a clonus of 10 beats or more. Clonus may be elicited during quick stretch tone evaluation or may become apparent during assessment of occupation (e.g., grasping, ambulation, pushing the involved foot into a shoe). If

clonus greatly interferes with ADLs, the client may be referred to a physiatrist or neurologist for oral medication, Botox[16] injection, Myobloc[73] injection, or phenol motor point block.[82]

Daniel is going to have a Botox injection in his flexor carpi ulnaris and ring finger flexor digitorum profundus to help reduce the spasticity in these muscles; this will help him work on finger and wrist extension ROM and strength.

Rigidity

Rigidity is a simultaneous increase in muscle tone of agonist and antagonist muscles (i.e., muscles on both sides of the joint). Both groups of muscles contract steadily, leading to increased resistance to passive movement in any direction and throughout the ROM. Rigidity is seen in disorders such as Parkinson's disease, TBI, some degenerative diseases, encephalitis, and tumors and also after poisoning with certain toxins and carbon monoxide. Rigidity also is seen in conjunction with spasticity in individuals with stroke and TBI. Rigidity is not velocity dependent (i.e., the tendon reflexes are not exaggerated, and no catch is felt on quick stretch).[2]

Rigidity is evaluated during muscle tone evaluation and can be rated as mild, moderate, or severe. Four types of rigidity are commonly seen:
- Lead pipe rigidity
- Cogwheel rigidity
- Decorticate rigidity
- Decerebrate rigidity

Both lead pipe and cogwheel rigidity can occur in Parkinson's disease. In lead pipe rigidity, constant resistance is felt throughout the ROM when the part is moved slowly and passively in any direction, not unilaterally, as in spasticity. This rigidity feels similar to the bending of solder or a lead pipe (thus its name). In cogwheel rigidity, a rhythmic give in resistance occurs throughout the ROM, much like the feeling of turning a cogwheel. It is thought that cogwheel rigidity is lead pipe rigidity with concomitant tremor, which results in the stopping and starting of resistance to passive movement.[70] DTRs are often normal or are only mildly increased in clients with Parkinson's rigidity.

Decerebrate and decorticate rigidity can occur after severe TBI with diffuse cerebral damage or anoxia. These abnormal postures occur immediately after injury and can last a few days or weeks if recovery occurs or can persist indefinitely if there is little or no recovery.

Decerebrate rigidity results from lesions in the bilateral hemispheres of the diencephalon and midbrain. It appears as rigid extension posturing of all limbs and the neck. Bilateral cortical lesions can result in decorticate rigidity, which appears as flexion rigidity in the upper extremities and as extension rigidity in the lower extremities. Supine positioning increases the abnormal tone, and with either type of rigidity, it may be extremely difficult to position clients in a sitting position.

MUSCLE TONE ASSESSMENT

Objective assessment of muscle tone in the client with cerebral spasticity is difficult because the tone fluctuates continuously in response to extrinsic and intrinsic factors. The postural reflex mechanism, the position of the body and head in space, the position of the head in relation to the body, synergies, the presence of primitive reflexes, and associated reactions all influence the degree and distribution of abnormal muscle tone.[86]

Guidelines for Muscle Tone Assessment

The following steps describe correct procedures for assessing muscle tone.

1. It is helpful to rate spasticity and hypertonia with the client in the same position, preferably at the same time of day, to enhance reliability because the body and head position influence hypertonia. The client's UE muscle tone usually is evaluated with the client sitting on a mat table when possible. Remember that the client's trunk posture (e.g., seated, bearing weight symmetrically rather than slumped or leaning to one side) will affect the results of the tone evaluation. Tone fluctuates from hour to hour and from day to day because of intrinsic and extrinsic factors that influence it. This fluctuation makes accurate measurement difficult, particularly for cerebral hypertonia. Nevertheless, rating tone is still worthwhile, especially in the managed care environment, in which objective measures of progress are needed to justify the continuation of therapy.

2. Securely hold the client's limb proximal and distal to the joint to be tested and move the joint slowly through its range to determine the free and easy ROM available. Note the presence and location of pain. If there is no active movement and if the limb feels heavy, record that the limb is flaccid or "0" in strength. If the limb has some active movement and no evidence of increased tone, the affected muscle or muscle group may be labeled "paretic" instead of "hypotonic." The paretic antagonist muscle can then be graded in strength (usually the strength grade will fall between 1 and 4−). Grading the paretic antagonist muscles provides more objective clinical information than merely labeling the muscles as hypotonic. Strength-grading antagonists can help the occupational therapist triage candidates for phenol block and botulinum toxin injection who have the potential to improve function; for example, a client with an elbow extension strength grade of 2− (in the presence of elbow flexor tone) would be a better block candidate than a client with a triceps strength grade of 0. The injection temporarily diminishes the hypertonicity of the spastic muscle group restricting freedom of movement and provides a greater opportunity to strengthen the opposing muscle group.

3. Hold the limb on the lateral aspects to avoid giving tactile stimulation to the belly of the muscle being tested.

4. Clinical assessment of spasticity involves holding the client's limb as just described and moving it rapidly through its full range while the client is relaxed. The easiest scale to use is the mild/moderate/severe scale. Some physicians find goniometric measurement of the location of the first tone helpful before and after long-acting nerve block. Record the findings for various muscle groups (see the tone rating scales in the next section).

5. Clinical assessment of rigidity involves moving the limb slowly during the range, noting the location of first resistance to movement in degrees; label it mild, moderate, or severe.

> ### OT PRACTICE NOTES
>
> It is important to note the client's overall posture during evaluation of muscle tone. Is the client's posture symmetric, with equal weight bearing on both hips (if sitting) or on both feet (if standing)? Note how the client moves in general. Is the head aligned or tilted to one side? Is one shoulder elevated? Does the client have a forward head posture? Is the trunk rotated or elongated on one side and shortened on the other? Such postural deviations affect the client's ability to move the limbs functionally. Current intervention focuses heavily on quality of movement, achieving as normal motor control as possible during occupation.

BOX 19.1   Ashworth Scale

0 = No increase in muscle tone
1 = Slight increase in muscle tone; "catch" when limb moved
2 = More marked increase in muscle tone, but limb easily flexed
3 = Considerable increase in muscle tone; passive movement difficult
4 = Limb rigid in flexion or extension

From Ashworth B: Preliminary trial of carisoprodol in multiple sclerosis, *Practitioner* 192:540–542, 1964.

Manual Rating Scales for Spasticity and Hypertonicity

Ashworth Scale

The Ashworth Scale[9] (Box 19.1) and the Modified Ashworth Scale[6,15] (MAS) are the two scales most widely used to manually rate spasticity. The literature reflects some controversy over the validity and reliability of these scales. Fleuren and associates[38] studied 30 clients with elbow flexion spasticity, correlating the Ashworth Scale with EMG studies, and concluded that the Ashworth Scale is not a reliable measure of spasticity.[38] Pandyan colleagues noted that the Ashworth Scale and the MAS should be used as an ordinal scale of resistance to passive movement, but that they are not valid for assessing spasticity.[76,77]

Four studies have demonstrated that the MAS is a reliable scale for the assessment of spasticity[47,48]; four other studies have reported that it is not reliable.[5,13,37]

Therapists familiar with the Ashworth Scale or the MAS can help physicians evaluate candidates for neurosurgical procedures. For example, some of the selection criteria for implantation of the Synchromed Intrathecal Baclofen Pump[69] are based on the occurrence of a point reduction, on either of the aforementioned scales, after administration of a test dose of medication; a 2-point reduction is required in spinal spasticity, and a 1-point reduction is required in cerebral spasticity.

Tardieu Scale

Both the Modified Tardieu Scale (MTS)[17] and the Tardieu Scale[50] measure spasticity.[39] The Tardieu Scale is written in French and has been shown to have excellent test-retest and interrater reliability, when used with inertial sensors, in assessing elbow flexor tone in patients with a CVA.[78] The MTS had an interrater reliability coefficient of .7 and was shown to be more reliable than the MAS.[45]

BOX 19.2   Mild/Moderate/Severe Spasticity Scale

Mild: Stretch reflex (palpable catch) occurs at the muscle's end range (i.e., the muscle is in a lengthened position).
Moderate: Stretch reflex (palpable catch) occurs in midrange.
Severe: Stretch reflex (palpable catch) occurs when the muscle is in a shortened range.

Farber S: *Neurorehabilitation: a multisensory approach,* Philadelphia, 1982, Saunders.

BOX 19.3   Preston's Hypertonicity or Rigidity Scale

0	No abnormal tone is detected during slow, passive movement.
1 (mild)	First tone or resistance is felt when the muscle is in a lengthened position during slow, passive movement.
2 (moderate)	First tone or resistance is felt in the midrange of the muscle during slow, passive movement.
3 (severe)	First tone or resistance occurs when the muscle is in a shortened range during slow, passive movement.

Mild/Moderate/Severe Spasticity Scale

Some therapists and physicians find a mild/moderate/severe scale easier to use than the scales just discussed. The scale in Box 19.2 is suggested as a guide for estimating the degree of spasticity.[35] The scale in Box 19.3 is suggested as a guide for estimating the extent of hypertonia.[80]

Mechanical and Computer Rating Systems for Spasticity and Hypertonicity

Mechanically determined parameters for assessing hypertonia may be more reliable than the manual methods. McCrea and colleagues[66] concluded that using a linear spring-damper model to assess the hypertonic elbow was reliable and valid. This model is not widely used in clinical practice, nor even in research practice, because of time constraints and difficulty accessing certain muscle groups (e.g., it is easier to set up and measure elbow hypertonia than hip hypertonia with a mechanical tone rating device).

Leonard and associates[64] investigated the construct validity of the Myotonometer (Neurogenic Technologies, Missoula, Montana), a computerized electronic device with a probe (resembling an ultrasound transducer) that is placed on top of the skin over the muscle belly. Measurements were taken over the biceps brachii at rest and during maximum voluntary muscle contraction. They revealed a significant difference between affected and unaffected extremities in subjects with UMN spasticity. The authors concluded that the Myotonometer could provide objective data about the tone reduction efficacy of various tone-reducing procedures.

Clearly, more research is needed in the areas of manual, mechanical, and computer rating systems for the assessment

of hypertonia. Identification of a uniformly acceptable, reliable, and valid measure of spasticity continues to confound clinicians.

Range-of-Motion Assessment in Evaluation of Tone

Assessment of passive ROM (PROM) supplements and often correlates with tone assessment. For example, if a client with an acute CVA (1 month after onset) has a wrist ROM measurement of 20 degrees extension (normal, 70 degrees) and if orthopedic causes have been ruled out (e.g., arthritis, fixed contracture), the therapist should assess the tone in the wrist flexors and the extrinsic finger flexors. Spasticity of any of these muscles can inhibit full wrist extension. Assessment of PROM can reveal possible signs of joint changes (e.g., subluxation, dislocation, and contracture) resulting from chronic hypertonia, such as proximal interphalangeal joints (PIPs) of the hands. Some physicians find PROM measurements useful for documenting the location of the first tone, or resting position, before and after Botox[16] or Myobloc[73] injections.

Other Considerations in Tone Assessment

Changes in bone or other peripheral structures can lead to ROM limitations. For example, heterotopic ossification can limit joint ROM. Heterotopic ossification is the formation of new bone in soft tissue or joints, which can lead to pain and/or joint contracture. Heterotopic ossification can occur in individuals with TBI and spinal cord injury, along with severe spasticity, or with other types of severe injuries. Conversely, the presence of fixed contractures may be incorrectly labeled as hypertonia. Physiatrists and other physician specialists can aid in the diagnosis of contractures through the use of diagnostic short-term nerve blocks, EMG, and/or radiographs.[82]

Assessing Movement and Control

Along with the assessment of muscle tone, the occupational therapist performs an assessment of UE movement and control. The therapist identifies where and how much the client's motor control is dominated by synergies, and where selective, isolated movement is present. The degree to which abnormal tone interferes with selective control is identified. Also, identifying in which direction of movement spasticity occurs and how it affects function helps in determining the need for intervention.

Manual muscle testing usually is not appropriate for clients who show moderate to severe spasticity or rigidity because the relative tone and strength of the muscles are not normal, and movement is not voluntary or selective. Tone and strength are influenced by the position of the head and body in space and by abnormal contraction, deficits in tactile and proprioceptive sensation, and impaired reciprocal inhibition. However, if hypertonia is mild and selective movements are possible, it is helpful to grade the strength of the antagonists to measure progress objectively.[82]

Sensation

The sensibility tests recommended for clients with CNS damage include static two-point discrimination, kinesthesia, proprioception, pain, and light touch using the Semmes-Weinstein monofilament test.[5] The therapist can assess light touch more accurately with the Semmes-Weinstein monofilaments because they provide better pressure control than a cotton ball (see Chapter 23 for the procedures for administering these sensory tests). If a client has a significant sensory impairment (i.e., is unable to detect deep pressure or pain), the therapist must instruct the individual to watch his or her limb to help compensate for the sensory loss. Sensory impairment is one of the main reasons clients do not automatically use their neurologically impaired hand during ADL tasks. Another reason is unilateral neglect, also known as hemi-inattention.

Medical Assessment of Muscle Tone

Physiatrists, orthopedic surgeons, and neurologists are some of the physicians who may specialize in assessment of muscle tone. They may use static or dynamic surface or percutaneous (needle) EMG. Multiple channels are used in dynamic EMG to evaluate the hypertonicity of many contributing muscles. EMG helps the physician determine abnormal, excessive electrical activity in muscles. EMG can help physiatrists and neurologists plan and implement short- and long-acting nerve blocks to treat hypertonia.[82]

NORMAL POSTURAL MECHANISM

The normal postural mechanism is composed of automatic movements that provide an appropriate level of stability and mobility. These automatic reactions develop in the early years of life and allow for trunk control and mobility, head control, midline orientation of self, weight bearing and weight shifting in all directions, dynamic balance, and controlled voluntary limb movement. Components of the normal postural mechanism include normal postural tone and control, integration of primitive reflexes and mass movement patterns, righting reactions, equilibrium and protective reactions, and selective movement.

In clients with UMNS damage, the normal postural mechanism has been disrupted. Abnormal tone and synergistic patterns of movement dominate clients' movements, and these clients have impaired balance and stability. Movements are slow and uncoordinated. Therapists must assess the extent of damage to the postural mechanism in clients with CNS trauma or disease.

Normal postural tone allows automatic and continuous postural adjustment to movement. Postural control is the ability to control "the body's position in space for the dual purposes of stability and orientation."[4] It is important to assess the automatic righting, equilibrium, and protective reactions, which are part of the postural mechanism, in clients with CNS trauma or disease.

Righting Reactions

Righting reactions direct the head to an upright position. They help a person assume a standing position. Automatic reactions maintain and restore the normal position of the head in space and the normal relationship of the head to the trunk, in addition to the normal alignment of the trunk and limbs. Without effective righting reactions, the client will have difficulty getting up from the floor, getting out of bed, sitting up, and kneeling.[4]

Equilibrium Reactions

Equilibrium reactions help the individual sustain or keep an upright position. According to Ryerson,[86] they are the "first line of defense against falling." Equilibrium reactions, which are elicited by stimulation of the labyrinths in the inner ear, are used to maintain and regain balance in all activities. These reactions ensure sufficient postural alignment when the body's center of gravity is altered by a change in the supporting surface. Without equilibrium reactions, the client will have difficulty maintaining and recovering balance in all positions and activities.

Protective Reactions

Protective reactions are the second line of defense against falling if the equilibrium reactions cannot correct a balance perturbation. They consist of protective extension of the arms and hands, which is used to protect the head and face when an individual is falling. Stepping and hopping are examples of lower extremity protective reactions. Without protective reactions, the client may fall or may be reluctant to bear weight on the affected side during normal bilateral activities.[85]

Assessment of Righting, Equilibrium, and Protective Reactions and Balance

Formal testing of the righting, equilibrium, and protective reactions may be difficult because of the cognitive and physical limitations of the client or time constraints of the therapist. The therapist can evaluate righting reactions, however, during transfers and ADLs. Equilibrium and protective reactions can be observed when the client shifts farther out of midline than necessary during functional activities, such as lower extremity dressing.

Postural stability is also known as balance. Balance depends on normal equilibrium and protective reactions. Balance is the ability to maintain the center of mass over the base of support.[88] Balance involves the complex interaction of many systems, including the vestibular, proprioceptive, and visual systems, in addition to motor modulation from the cerebellum, basal ganglia, and cerebral cortex. Occupational and physical therapists must also observe the client's ankle, hip, and step strategies and note areas of breakdown in the kinetic chain.

When assessing a client with CNS dysfunction, the therapist should assess the client's static and dynamic balance before leaving the client unattended on a mat table, in a wheelchair, or during ambulatory ADLs. Dynamic balance involves maintaining balance while moving, and static balance involves maintaining equilibrium while stationary.

The Physical Performance Test assesses physical function during activity. Seven of the nine items in this assessment involve static and dynamic balance.[93] The test takes only 10 minutes to complete.[84] Fig. 19.10 shows the test form and test protocol. Four other noteworthy balance assessments are the Tinetti Balance Test of the Performance-Oriented Assessment of Mobility Problems[89] and the Berg Balance Scale.[11] The Berg Balance Scale is a good assessment for lower functioning

PHYSICAL PERFORMANCE TEST SCORING SHEET

	Time*	Physical Performance Test Scoring	
Score			
1. Write a sentence (Whales live in the blue ocean.)	_____ sec	≤10 sec = 4 10.5-15 sec = 3 15.5-20 sec = 2 >20 sec = 1 unable = 0	_____
2. Simulated eating	_____ sec	≤10 sec = 4 10.5-15 sec = 3 15.5-20 sec = 2 >20 sec = 1 unable = 0	_____
3. Lift a book and put it on a shelf	_____ sec	≤2 sec = 4 2.5-4 sec = 3 4.5-6 sec = 2 >6 sec = 1 unable = 0	_____
4. Put on and remove a jacket	_____ sec	≤10 sec = 4 10.5-15 sec = 3 15.5-20 sec = 2 >20 sec = 1 unable = 0	_____
5. Pick up penny from floor	_____ sec	≤2 sec = 4 2.5-4 sec = 3 4.5-6 sec = 2 >6 sec = 1 unable = 0	_____
6. Turn 360°	discontinuous steps continuous steps unsteady (grabs, staggers) steady	0 2 0 2	_____
7. 50-foot walk test	_____ sec	≤15 sec = 4 15.5-20 sec = 3 20.5-25 sec = 2 >25 sec = 1 unable = 0	_____
8. Climb one flight of stairs	_____ sec	≤5 sec = 4 5.5-10 sec = 3 10.5-15 sec = 2 >15 sec = 1 unable = 0	_____
9. Climb stairs†		Number of flights of stairs up and down (maximum 4)	_____

TOTAL SCORE (maximum 36 for nine-item, 28 for seven-item)

_____ nine-item
_____ seven-item

*For timed measurements, round to nearest 0.5 second.
†Omit for seven-item scoring.

Fig. 19.10 Physical performance test scoring sheet. (From Reuben DB, Siu AL: An objective measure of physical function of elderly outpatients: the Physical Performance Test, *J Am Geriatr Soc* 38:1105–1112, 1990.)

clients (e.g., those who are less ambulatory). Shumway-Cook and Woollacott[87] developed the Dynamic Gait Index (DGI) to assess balance with changes in task demands in ambulatory patients. It has been widely used with ambulatory clients who have been diagnosed with vestibular disorders, CVA, multiple sclerosis, or Parkinson's disease and in the geriatric population. It is a reliable and valid test.[29] The Functional Gait Assessment (FGA) is another reliable and valid balance assessment.[98]

Primitive Reflexes

Dominance of primitive reflex movement patterns can interfere with the client's occupational performance. Difficulties that may be encountered are described in the following sections. Observation of these motor behaviors is a way of evaluating for the presence of primitive reflexes.

Brainstem-Level Reflexes

Asymmetric tonic neck reflex. The asymmetric tonic neck reflex (ATNR) is tested with the client positioned supine or sitting.
- *Stimulus:* Actively or passively turn the client's head 90 degrees to one side.
  Response: An increase in the extensor tone of both extremities (upper and lower) on the face side, and an increase in the flexor tone of both extremities (upper and lower) on the skull side.[44]

Symmetric tonic neck reflex. The symmetric tonic neck reflex (STNR) is tested with the client positioned sitting or quadruped.
- *Stimulus 1:* Flex the client's head and bring the chin toward the chest.
  Response: Flexion of the upper extremities and extension of the lower extremities.
- *Stimulus 2:* Extend the client's head.
  Response: Extension of the upper extremities and flexion of the lower extremities.[60]

Tonic labyrinthine reflex. The tonic labyrinthine reflex (TLR) can be tested with the client supine with his or her head in midposition.
- *Stimulus:* The test position.
  Response: An increase in extension tone or extension of the extremities.

The TLR also can be tested with the client prone with the head in midposition.
- *Stimulus:* The test position.
  Response: An increase in flexor tone or flexion of the extremities.

Positive supporting reaction. The positive supporting reaction is caused by pressure on the ball of the foot.
- *Stimulus:* Pressure on the ball of the foot.
  Response: Rigid extension of the lower extremities due to co-contraction of the flexors and extensors of the knee and hip joints. The practitioner may also see internal rotation of the hip, ankle plantar flexion, and foot inversion.[60]

Spinal-Level Reflexes

Spinal reflexes can occur after a UMN lesion. They appear because of lack of integration with higher centers. Some examples of exaggerated spinal reflexes are hyperactive DTRs, Babinski's sign, and the flexor withdrawal, crossed extension, and grasp reflexes.[54]

Crossed extension reflex. The crossed extension reflex causes increased extensor tone in one leg when the other leg is flexed. Therefore, if the client with hemiplegia who is influenced by this reflex flexes the unaffected leg for walking, a strong extensor hypertonicity occurs in the affected leg and interferes with the normal pattern of ambulation.

Flexor withdrawal reflex. The client with a flexor withdrawal reflex shows flexion of the ankle, knee, and hip when the sole of the foot is touched (swiped heel to ball of foot). This reflex clearly interferes with gait pattern and transfers.

Grasp reflex. The client with a grasp reflex will not be able to release objects placed in the hand, even if active finger extension is present. The flexor withdrawal, crossed extension, and grasp reflexes are rarely seen in isolation.[60]

Trunk Control Assessment

Collin and Wade[23] designed a quick and easily administered test of trunk control that is valid and reliable in clients with a diagnosis of CVA. It involves four timed tests: (1) rolling to the weak side, (2) rolling to the sound side, (3) moving from supine to sitting, and (4) sitting on the side of the bed with the feet off the floor for 30 seconds.

To accurately assess trunk control, the therapist must evaluate strength and control in four muscle groups: the trunk flexors, the extensors, the lateral flexors, and the rotators. For all the tests, the client should be sitting upright on a mat table with the feet supported. Remember that the client should not be left unattended on the mat table until the therapist determines that he or she has adequate trunk control and sitting balance. The procedures described in the following sections are condensed from Gillen's *Stroke Rehabilitation: A Function-Based Approach*.[42]

Trunk Flexors

The examiner asks the client to sit upright, to slowly move his or her shoulders behind the hips (eccentric control), and to hold the end-range posture (isometric control) (Fig. 19.11A). The client then is asked to move forward (concentric control) to resume the initial upright posture (see Fig. 19.11B).

The examiner should observe for evidence of unilateral weakness, potential for falls, and symmetry of weight shift. A functional test for trunk flexor control is to observe the client move from supine to sitting.

Trunk Extensors

Test 1. The client sits in a position of spinal flexion with a posterior pelvic tilt and moves into trunk extension while simultaneously moving the pelvis into neutral or into a slight anterior tilt. This test assesses concentric trunk extensor control, which is a prerequisite for lower extremity dressing and forward reach (Fig. 19.12A).

Test 2. The client is seated in an upright posture. The examiner asks the client to maintain an erect spine and lean forward. This test evaluates eccentric trunk extensor control (see Fig. 19.12B).

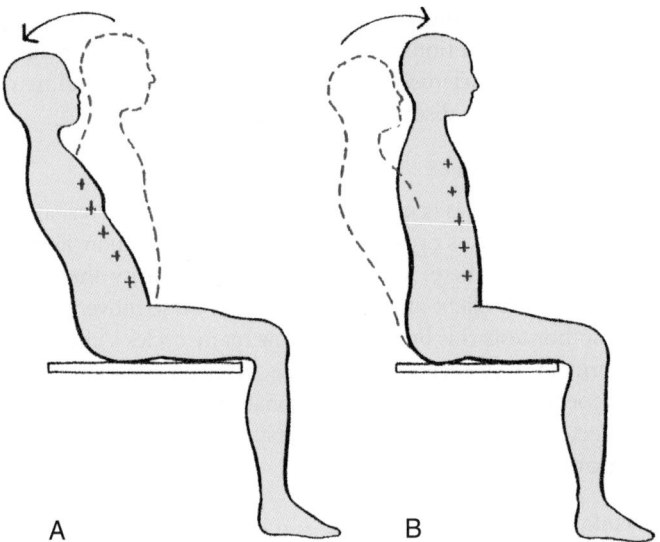

Fig. 19.11 Trunk flexor control. The *dotted lines* indicate the trunk's starting position; the *solid lines* indicate the trunk's final position. The *arrows* indicate the direction of movement, and the *plus symbols* indicate the muscle groups primarily responsible for control of the pattern. Skeletal muscle activity occurs on both sides of the trunk (reciprocal innervation). (From Gillen G, Nilsen D: *Stroke rehabilitation: a function-based approach*, ed 5, St Louis, 2021, Elsevier.)

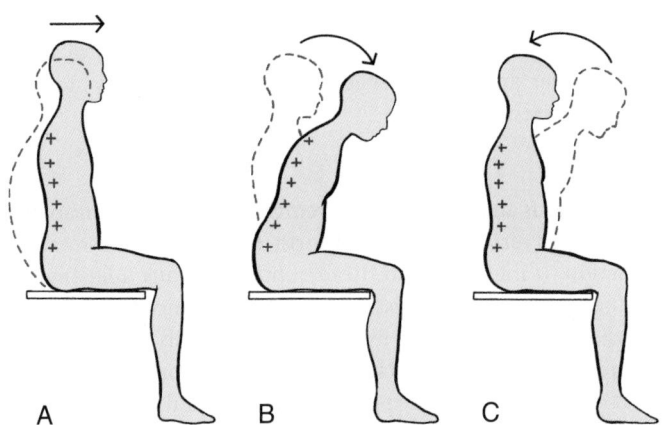

Fig. 19.12 Trunk extensor control. The *dotted lines* indicate the trunk's starting position; the *solid lines* indicate the trunk's final position. The *arrows* indicate the direction of movement, and the *plus symbols* indicate the muscle groups primarily responsible for control of the pattern. Skeletal muscle activity occurs on both sides of the trunk (reciprocal innervation). (From Gillen G, Nilsen D: *Stroke rehabilitation: a function-based approach*, ed 5, St Louis, 2021, Elsevier.)

For both trunk extensor tests, the examiner should observe for signs of unilateral weakness and note end-range control.

Test 3. The client is asked to move his or her shoulders back to assume a seated, aligned, upright position. The trunk extensors are contracting concentrically (see Fig. 19.12C).

Lateral Flexors

The client sits in an upright posture. The pelvis is stationary, and the upper trunk laterally flexes toward the mat table. Fig. 19.13 shows eccentric contraction of the left side and muscle shortening of the right side. The client is asked to return to

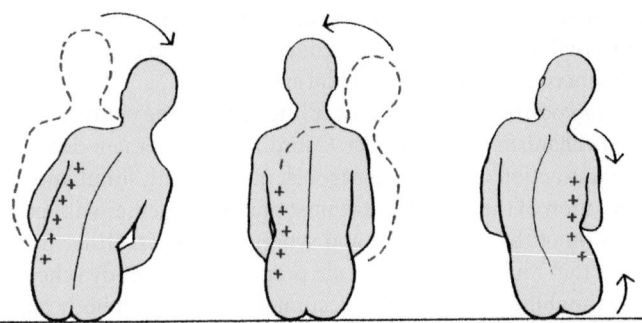

Fig. 19.13 Lateral flexor control. The *dotted lines* indicate the trunk's starting position; the *solid lines* indicate the trunk's final position. The *arrows* indicate the direction of movement, and the *plus symbols* indicate the muscle groups primarily responsible for control of the pattern. Skeletal muscle activity occurs on both sides of the trunk (reciprocal innervation). (From Gillen G, Nilsen D: *Stroke rehabilitation: a function-based approach*, ed 5, St Louis, 2021, Elsevier.)

the original test position (concentric control of the left side) (see Fig. 19.13).

Fig. 19.13 shows assessment of trunk and pelvis lateral flexion, in which movement is initiated from the lower trunk and pelvis. The end position is one of trunk elongation on the weight-bearing side and shortening on the non–weight-bearing side, which involves concentric contraction of the right side.

Lateral flexion is needed for fall prevention when a client is reaching to the side (e.g., shutting a car door).[35]

Trunk Rotation

The primary muscles responsible for rotation are the obliques. When a person rotates the trunk to the left, the right external and the left internal obliques are recruited. Rotational control is a prerequisite for UE dressing and reaching across the midline. Three movement patterns are evaluated:

1. The client sits upright with the pelvis in a neutral, stable position. The client reaches with his or her right arm, across the body, in the direction of the floor. This motion helps in assessment of concurrent flexion and rotation. The motion tests concentric control of the obliques and the back extensors (particularly the thoracic region). Both sides need to be tested.
2. The second movement pattern involves trunk extension with rotation. The upper trunk remains stable, and the lower trunk and pelvis moved forward on one side (i.e., shifting forward). Again, both sides are tested.
3. The client is positioned supine for the third movement. Farber[35] described this as the client initiating a "segmental roll by lifting the shoulders from the support surface and toward the opposite side of the body. This pattern is controlled by a concentric contraction of the abdominals (obliques)."

COORDINATION

Coordination is the ability to produce accurate, controlled movement. Characteristics of coordinated movement include smoothness, rhythm, appropriate speed, refinement to the minimum number of muscle groups needed, and appropriate muscle tension, postural tone, and equilibrium. Coordination of muscle action is under the control of the cerebellum and is influenced by the extrapyramidal system.

For coordinated movement, all elements of the neuromuscular mechanism must be intact. Coordinated movement depends on contraction of the correct agonist muscles with simultaneous relaxation of the correct antagonist muscles, together with contraction of the joint fixator and synergist muscles. Other functions that must be intact include proprioception, body scheme, and the ability to judge space accurately and to direct body parts through space, with correct timing, to the desired target.

INCOORDINATION

Many types of lesions can produce disturbances in coordination. Disturbances in coordination often stem from cerebellar and extrapyramidal disorders. Noncerebellar causes include diseases and injuries of muscles and peripheral nerves, lesions of the posterior columns of the spinal cord, and lesions of the frontal and postcentral cerebral cortex.[31]

Cerebellar Disorders

Cerebellar dysfunction can cause incoordination that may affect any body region and cause a variety of clinical symptoms. For example, the client may have postural difficulties that include slouching or leaning positions (caused by bilateral lesions) or spinal curvature (caused by unilateral lesions) and wide-based standing. Eye movements, both voluntary and reflexive, may be affected, as may the resting position of the eye.[70] One interesting fact about the cerebellum is that lesions or disease in one cerebellar hemisphere show signs of impairment on the same side of the body (ipsilateral).[3] Common signs of cerebellar dysfunction that the therapist may encounter include ataxia, dysdiadochokinesis, dysmetria, dyssynergia or asynergia, nystagmus, and dysarthria.

Ataxia

Ataxia is manifested as delayed initiation of movement responses, errors in range and force of movement, and errors in the rate and regularity of movement. Poor coordination is noted between the agonist and antagonist muscle groups. This results in jerky, poorly controlled movements. When a client with ataxia reaches for an object, the movement lacks an organized acceleration upon initiating the reach and deacceleration when approaching the object with additional jerkiness while reaching for the object. The client with gait ataxia has a staggering, wide-based gait with reduced or no arm swing. The person is unable to tandem walk (heel to toe); step length may be uneven; and the client may have a tendency to fall.[33] The client with cerebellar dysfunction isolated to one cerebellar hemisphere will have a tendency to fall on the side of the lesion or dysfunction because of the ipsilateral (same side) influence of the cerebellum on the lower motor neurons.

Many ataxias are hereditary and are classified by chromosomal location and type of inheritance: autosomal dominant, in which the affected client inherits a normal gene from one parent and a faulty gene from the other parent; or autosomal recessive,

in which both parents pass on the faulty gene. Ataxia also can be acquired. Conditions that can cause acquired ataxia include stroke, multiple sclerosis, tumors, alcoholism, peripheral neuropathy, metabolic disorders, and vitamin deficiencies.[75]

Dysdiadochokinesis

Dysdiadochokinesis is an inability to perform rapid alternating movements, such as pronation and supination or elbow flexion and extension. There is a breakup and irregularity that happens when the client attempts to perform these movements.[33] This author tests this by counting how many cycles a client can perform in a 10-second time frame. A cycle consists of one full repetition of supination and pronation. It is best to test the unaffected (or lesser affected) side first. The affected side is then compared with the unaffected side.[79]

Dysmetria

Dysmetria is an inability to estimate the ROM necessary to reach the target of movement. The target is missed. The two types of dysmetria are hypermetria, in which the limb overshoots the target, and hypometria, in which the limb undershoots the target.

Dyssynergia or Asynergia

Literally, dyssynergia is a decomposition of movement in which voluntary movements are broken up into their component parts and appear jerky. Dyssynergia is one of the main clinical signs of cerebellar dysfunction or lesions involving pathways to and from the cerebellum.[33]

Nystagmus

Nystagmus is an involuntary movement of the eyeballs in an up-and-down (vertical), back-and-forth (horizontal), or rotating direction. It interferes with head control and fine adjustments required for balance. Nystagmus can be induced by specific procedures, but induced nystagmus is typically brief in neurotypical clients (e.g., nystagmus is observed for a few seconds after quickly spinning the person around several times and then stopping the motion). Nystagmus also can occur as a result of vestibular system, brainstem, or cerebellar lesions or dysfunction.[3] When nystagmus occurs after a CNS lesion or dysfunction, it is typically sustained for a longer time and with a larger excursion or movement range of the eyeball in the socket. This can significantly disrupt an individual's functional performance.

Dysarthria

Dysarthria is explosive or slurred speech caused by incoordination of the speech mechanism. The client's speech may also vary in pitch or may seem nasal and tremulous, or both.[25]

Extrapyramidal Disorders

Extrapyramidal disorders are characterized by hypokinesia (small movement) or hyperkinesia (exaggerated movement). Hypokinesia examples are discussed first. Parkinson's disease is characterized by hypokinesia, bradykinesia (slow movement), cogwheel and lead pipe rigidity, a decrease in or loss of postural mechanisms, and a resting, pill-rolling tremor.[34]

Parkinson's plus is the name given to a group of movement disorders that have signs of Parkinson's disease with concomitant neurological deficits. Progressive supranuclear palsy (PSP) is an example of a Parkinson's plus disorder. Clients affected with PSP have loss of vertical ocular gaze, balance dysfunction, rigidity of the neck and trunk muscles, dementia, and usually absence of tremor. The life expectancy is shorter than in Parkinson's disease; death often occurs within 6 to 10 years.[46]

Chorea

Chorea is characterized by irregular, purposeless, quick movements. They are not movements that occur in a regular pattern, such as the alternating movement seen with clonus, nor is chorea as quick as clonus. The jerky movements randomly flow from one muscle to another. Chorea usually stems from disorders in the caudate nucleus.[33] These movements may occur during sleep.[25] Two diagnoses often present with chorea: tardive dyskinesia (TD) and Huntington's disease. TD is a drug-induced disorder, often associated with neuroleptic drug use. Occupational therapists may see clients who have TD in psychiatric settings. It also can occur as a side effect of certain medications for Parkinson's disease. Huntington's disease is an inherited, autosomal dominant disease. Clients with Huntington's disease have chorea that compromises functional movement (e.g., walking) or tasks that require fine coordination of movements. As the disease progresses, rigidity develops.

Athetoid Movements

Athetoid movements are continuous, slow, writhing, arrhythmic movements that primarily affect the distal portions of the extremities. These movements are not present during sleep. Adult athetosis can occur after cerebral anoxia and with Wilson's disease. Movement patterns include alternating extension and flexion of the arm, supination and pronation of the forearm, and flexion and extension of the fingers. Athetosis that occurs with chorea is called *choreoathetosis*.

Dystonia

Dystonia results in sustained muscle contraction of the extremities (e.g., hyperextension or hyperflexion of the wrist and fingers), often with concurrent torsion of the spine and associated twisting of the trunk.[33] Dystonic movements are often continuous and often seen in conjunction with spasticity. The client in Fig. 19.14 sustained a TBI, and his right wrist and fingers show dystonia. Dystonia can be primary or secondary, the latter occurring with other CNS disorders (e.g., hypoxic brain injury, tumor). Segmental dystonia involves two or more adjacent body parts. Generalized and multifocal types of dystonia also exist. Focal dystonia involves only one limb, as is seen in writer's cramp, musician's cramp, and spasmodic torticollis.[31]

Ballism

Ballism is a rare symptom produced by continuous, abrupt contractions of the axial and proximal musculature of the extremity. Ballism causes the limb to fly out suddenly, with a much greater amplitude than chorea. It occurs on one side of the body

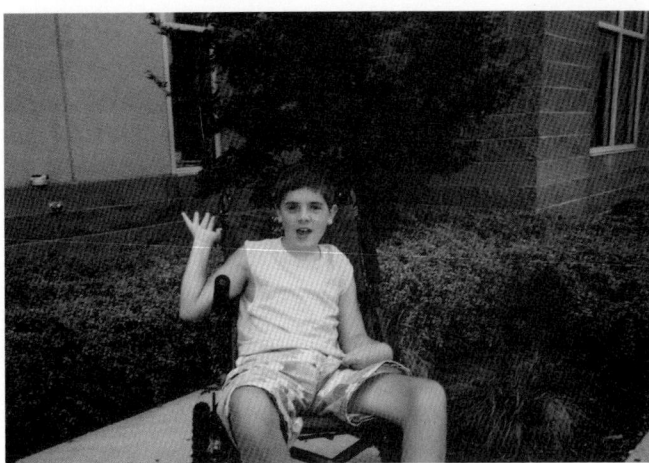

Fig. 19.14 A client with right upper extremity dystonic posturing of the wrist and finger extensors. His left wrist shows severe hypotonicity. Tone abnormalities are the result of a traumatic brain injury.

(hemiballism) and is caused by lesions of the opposite subthalamic nucleus.

Tremor

Tremors stem from alternating contractions of opposing muscle groups. They are rhythmic oscillatory movements. There are three common types of tremors:

1. *Action tremor*, formerly known as intention tremor associated with cerebellar disease, occurs during voluntary, intentional movement. It is intensified at the termination of the movement and is often seen in multiple sclerosis. The client with action tremor may have trouble performing tasks that require accuracy and precision of limb placement (e.g., drinking from a cup, inserting a key into a lock).
2. *Resting tremor* occurs at rest and subsides when voluntary movement is attempted. It occurs as a result of damage to or disease of the basal ganglia and is seen in Parkinson's disease.[33]
3. *Essential familial tremor* is inherited as an autosomal dominant trait. It is most visible when the client is carrying out a fine precision task, such as writing or pouring liquids. The pathophysiology is not known. This is the most common movement disorder.[31]

ASSESSMENT OF COORDINATION

Medical Assessment of Coordination

Incoordination consists of errors in rate, rhythm, range, direction, and force of movement. Therefore, observation is an important element of the clinical examination. The neurological examination for incoordination may include the nose-finger-nose test; the finger-nose test; the heel-knee test; the knee pat (pronation-supination), hand pat, and foot pat tests; finger wiggling; and drawing a spiral. Such tests can reveal dysmetria, dyssynergia, dysdiadochokinesis, tremors, and ataxia. Usually the neurologist or the physiatrist performs these examinations. Magnetic resonance imaging (MRI) and computed tomography (CT) scans also may be ordered. Infrequently EMG is used to better characterize the frequency and pattern of the tremor.

For example, the rate of the resting tremor often seen in a client with Parkinson's disease is 3 to 5 per second. A faster or slower tremor effectively rules out this condition.

Occupational Therapy Assessment of Coordination

Selected activities and specific performance tests can reveal the effects of incoordination on function. The occupational therapist can observe for coordination difficulties during ADL assessment by observing the client write, open containers, or button a garment. The therapist should observe for irregularity in the speed of movement. Movement during the performance of various activities may appear irregular and jerky and may overreach the mark. The following general guidelines and questions can be used when evaluating incoordination.

1. Assess muscle tone and joint mobility first in a sitting position.
2. Observe for ataxia, proximal to distal, during functional UE movement. Are movements away from or toward the body more difficult for the client?
3. Stabilize joints proximally to distally during the functional task and note differences in client performance compared with performance without stabilization. (Stabilization can be attained by splinting, holding the wrist stable with the other hand, or stabilizing the affected body part against a wall.) Weighted cuffs may be applied to the extremity during task performance to determine whether weighting or resistance reduces the tremor. Note the amount of resistance provided. Observe whether the cuff weights make the coordination worse because sometimes the use of weights increases tremor.
4. Observe for tremor. Are the head and speech affected by the tremor?
5. How do the client's ataxia and coordination problems affect participation in occupation?

Perform an occupational profile, in addition to a performance patterns interview, to ask about the client's roles, routines, goals, and environment to determine which activities are important for the client.

Standardized functional assessments for a CVA (e.g., the WMFT), mentioned earlier, may be useful for measuring the efficacy of OT intervention for impaired coordination.[14] Additional instruments such as the Bennett Hand Tool Dexterity Test,[10] Jebsen Taylor Hand Test,[56] Minnesota Manual Dexterity Test,[71] Nine Hole Peg Test,[65] and the Purdue Pegboard[83] may be helpful in assessing a client's coordination.

OCCUPATIONAL THERAPY INTERVENTION

Intervention for Hypertonicity and Spasticity

It is very important to assess how UMN deficits such as hypertonicity, paresis, fatigue, and decreased dexterity affect occupational performance. Intervention should address not only the impact hypertonicity has on function but how these other deficits compromise a client's performance.[31]

Before treating hypertonia, the therapist and physician need to closely evaluate the function of the tone. Hypertonicity can have beneficial effects, such as aiding in standing and transfers, maintaining muscle bulk, and preventing deep vein thrombosis,

osteoporosis, and edema. Intervention is necessary when spasticity interferes with ADLs, gait, sleep, or wheelchair positioning, or when it causes severe pain and limits hygiene (e.g., the client is unable to wash the hand or axilla) or leads to contractures or decubitus ulcers. Hypertonicity or spasticity may be treated with conservative therapeutic interventions, pharmacologic agents, or surgery.[31,82]

Conservative Treatment Approaches

Weight bearing.   For hypertonicity reduction and paresis remediation in the UE, therapists have been using weight-bearing skills and activities for many years with clients who have UMN lesions, but evidence of treatment efficacy has not been fully established.

Brouwer and Ambury[18] concluded that corticospinal facilitation of motor units occurred during UE weight bearing. They thought that afferent input from weight bearing increased motor cortical excitability. Chakerain and Larson[20] studied the effects of UE weight bearing on hand opening and prehension in children with spastic cerebral palsy. Computer calculations of clients' hand surface area were performed. An increase in surface area was noted after weight bearing, along with an increase in the maturity of movement components needed for prehension. McIlroy and Maki[68] demonstrated that if the affected arm is used when weight bearing, postural responses occur throughout the weight-bearing extremity and during other perturbations of posture.

Despite the fact that few well-controlled studies document how and why weight bearing works physiologically, it certainly is a requirement for improving functional performance. Seated clients who reach to the floor to pick up an object need UE postural support to prevent them from falling. Standing clients who reach into a high cabinet need UE weight bearing to facilitate balance.[42]

Traditional Sensorimotor Approaches

Proprioceptive neuromuscular facilitation has been shown to be effective in gaining motor control for clients with a variety of diagnoses (see Chapter 32).[86] The Neuro-Developmental Treatment (NDT) Association[52] has stated that therapists who follow an NDT approach:

- Perform an in-depth analysis of the intricacies of movement and of how the details relate to the whole to allow for functional movement in a wide variety of environments.
- Believe that control of movement is based on a complex interaction of many body systems, which are plastic and adaptable, and on the tasks presented and the environments in which the tasks are performed. Therefore, function can be altered by changing one or more of these elements.
- Implement an understanding of the development of atypical movement, in addition to the compensations, to help minimize the impact of CNS pathology and prevent the emergence of contractures and deformities, which contribute to the functional problems.

Another OT objective is to have the client manage muscle tone to engage in and complete basic ADLs (BADLs) and IADLs. Positioning and movement in patterns opposite to hypertonic or synergistic patterns are important to expand the motor repertoire and develop movement that is as close to normal as possible. At times it is appropriate to facilitate synergistic movements in the client with chronic disease, or if the client does not recover beyond stage 3 of the Modified Brunnstrom's Stages of Motor Recovery (see Table 19.1 and Fig. 19.3). The synergy patterns can be facilitated to improve lateral pinch or elbow flexion function. The client should also be taught how to incorporate the affected UE as much as possible into BADLs and IADLs. (See Chapter 10 for a more detailed review of traditional treatment strategies.)

Even when motor control is adequate for participation in occupation, the sensory, cognitive, and perceptual abilities of the client may affect the achievement of functional goals. Perceptual dysfunction may alter the client's abilities, requiring the therapist to focus on perceptual training concurrently.

Casting. In some cases, unilateral hypertonicity is severe enough to necessitate serial inhibitive casting or splinting. Casting in inhibitive postures has been shown to be effective in tone reduction.[44] The beneficial effect of casting on hypertonia and UE contractures has been well documented in the literature.[13,32]

Casting in inhibitive postures is effective because it provides neutral warmth, maintained pressure, and constant joint positioning with static lengthening of muscle. Serial casting is most successful when a contracture has been present for less than 6 months. The cast may be bivalved (cut in half) and worn as a splint. This helps protect the skin and allows the therapist to work with the extremity out of the cast. However, many clinicians think that a nonbivalved cast is more effective and actually causes less skin breakdown. A dropout cast, which can be used as part of the serial casting process, includes a cutout area, allowing movement of the joint in the desired direction. For example, for an elbow with flexor hypertonicity, the dorsal upper arm portion of a long arm cast can be cut out to allow the triceps to be facilitated to extend the arm.

Serial casting should stop when the desired position has been achieved and tone is manageable with the last cast or splint. If no evidence of increased PROM is seen after two or three casts have been removed, serial casting must stop; however, the last cast should be kept, bivalved, and used as a "retainer" splint to prevent additional contractures, similar to retainer use in orthodontics.

Many innovations have occurred in commercially available spasticity reduction splints that are used to place the wrist and hand in inhibitive postures. The client and the family need to be educated on continuing to incorporate the extremity in occupation and on bearing weight on the extremity as much as possible to retain the ROM gains achieved during casting.[43,82]

Physical Agent Modalities

Physical agent modalities, such as cold, superficial heat, ultrasound, and neuromuscular electrical stimulation, can be used as preparation for or in conjunction with purposeful activity and muscle reeducation, provided the OT practitioner has the appropriate training and meets the license criteria for his or her state or country. Ultrasound can help inhibit or reduce hypertonicity temporarily and can increase tendon and muscle extensibility. It is helpful to provide concurrent stretch during the ultrasound procedure. Even though neuromuscular electrical

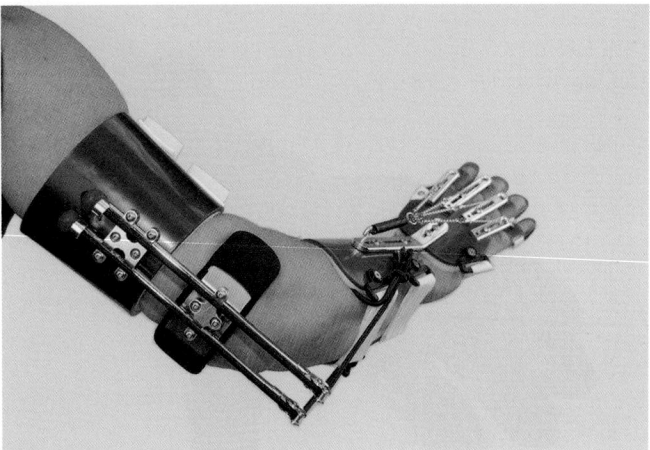

Fig. 19.15 SaeboReach dynamic orthosis. (Courtesy Saebo, Charlotte, NC.)

stimulation has been shown to strengthen paretic muscles,[19,51] more research needs to be done. Quandt and Hummel[84] reached this conclusion after completing a comprehensive review on the effect of functional electrical stimulation on hand motor recovery after a CVA.

Distal-to-Proximal Approach

The Functional Tone Management (FTM) Arm Training Program (Saebo, Charlotte, North Carolina) was developed to address the weaknesses of therapeutic interventions currently applied to the neurologically impaired upper extremity and hand. The occupational therapists who founded Saebo theorized that because grasp and release capabilities are pivotal to reintegrating the upper extremity into daily activities, a paradigm shift for UE neurological rehabilitation was needed. Although traditional therapeutic interventions such as Bobath-based (NDT) programs are based on a proximal-to-distal recovery pattern, Saebo developed the FTM Arm Training Program on the basis of a distal activation model, which focused on the key point of early initiation of upper extremity movements that incorporate grasp and release. To incorporate the hand into the FTM Arm Training Program, Saebo developed a dynamic orthosis for the hand and elbow, called the SaeboReach (Fig. 19.15).

The SaeboReach orthosis assists an individual with hypertonia in the hand to place the hand in an open, functional position. This positioning is accomplished by means of a fixed wrist support and a finger and thumb spring system of variable strength. Once the hand is open, the client can begin to retrain the finger flexors for improved motor control of the hand. While wearing the SaeboReach, the client relearns to produce a graded muscle contraction of the finger flexors to grasp an object. The finger and thumb spring system, coupled with the client's own efforts to relax muscle activation, allows the hand to open enough for the object held in the hand to be released while assisting the elbow extensors.

The SaeboGlove's lightweight, low-profile design assists with finger and thumb extension in clients with neurological or orthopedic problems. The SaeboGlove positions the wrist and fingers into extension in preparation for functional activities. The client grasps an object by voluntarily flexing the fingers. The

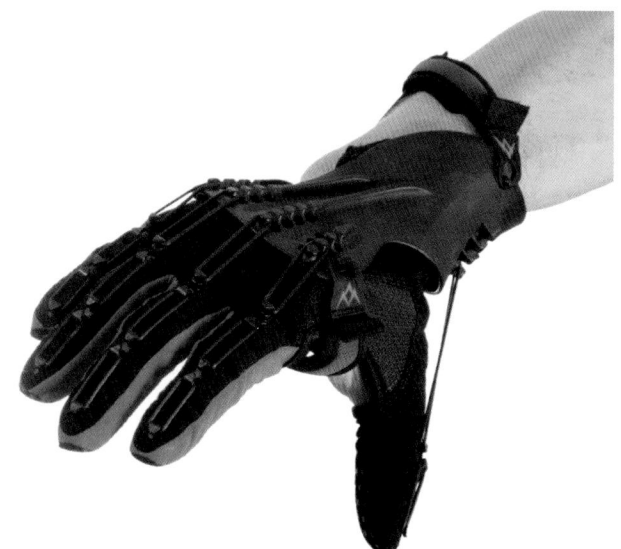

Fig. 19.16 SaeboGlove. (Courtesy Saebo, Charlotte, NC.)

extension system assists with reopening of the hand to release the object (Fig. 19.16).

Once the client is comfortable using the SaeboReach, the FTM Arm Training Program can begin. The FTM program combines high-repetition grasp and release with task-specific arm training drills to progress the client toward a functional goal. A body of research supports the FTM Arm Training Program; however, this program does not require the wrist or finger extension typically needed for participation in a constraint-induced program. Clinically observed improvements with use of the SaeboFlex (hand and wrist splint only) for 1 hour per day, 5 days per week, were improved scores on the Fugl-Meyer Assessment and the Box and Blocks test.[97] Another study of the SaeboFlex involving eight clients found that seven of the eight showed improved test scores on the upper limb Motricity Index after using the SaeboFlex for 12 weeks.[89] Most recently the SaeboGlove has been combined with virtual reality and demonstrated improvements in UE function for individuals who sustained a stroke.[5]

Surgical Methods

Surgery to control hypertonicity is an option. Dynamic EMG can help orthopedic surgeons plan surgery. Orthopedic surgical intervention can improve function or release contractures. Examples of upper extremity functional surgery include lengthening of the biceps tendon to reduce elbow flexion and to gain elbow extension, thumb-in-palm release, and transfer of the flexor carpi ulnaris tendon to the extensor carpi radialis longus or brevis tendon to reduce the deforming force of wrist flexion while simultaneously augmenting wrist extension. An example of a contracture release procedure is the flexor digitorum superficialis-to-profundus transfer to gain length in the extrinsic finger flexors.[59]

Therapists will encounter clients with severe spasticity who have undergone a neurosurgical procedure called intrathecal baclofen pump (ITB) implantation. This procedure enables baclofen, a spasticity-reducing medication, to enter the body at the spinal level, preventing the centrally mediated side effects

of oral baclofen. The ITB dispenses the baclofen directly into the intrathecal (subarachnoid) space via a catheter attached to a subcutaneous implantable pump in the abdomen. The client must undergo a lumbar puncture test dose of intrathecal baclofen to determine candidacy before pump implantation. A 2-point lower limb spasticity reduction on the Ashworth Scale or MAS is needed for spinal spasticity, and a 1-point reduction is required for cerebral spasticity.[69]

The ITB has been shown to be very effective in reducing severe spinal spasticity and spasticity associated with multiple sclerosis, and it is also effective for cerebral spasticity. For additional details on medical and surgical treatments and their relation to occupational therapy, see Preston and Hecht's *Spasticity Management: Rehabilitation Strategies.*[82]

Pharmacological Agents

Pharmacological agents prescribed and administered by physicians include oral medications, short-term nerve blocks, and long-term blocks.

Clients with severe hypertonicity accompanied by severe pain may need evaluation to determine the cause of the pain. Drug therapy and other pain management techniques may be part of the treatment approach. The four commonly used oral medications for spasticity of UMN origin are baclofen, dantrolene sodium, tizanidine, and diazepam. These medications are generally well tolerated, but a common side effect is drowsiness. Dantrolene sodium acts at the skeletal muscle. It is preferred in cerebral spasticity because it is less apt to cause sedation, but it can cause weakness and liver damage. Tizanidine HCl is labeled for spasticity reduction in multiple sclerosis and spinal cord injury. Its side effects may include hypotension, sedation, and visual hallucinations. Side effects of diazepam include drowsiness, fatigue, and possible dependency. Neither diazepam nor baclofen can be discontinued suddenly because doing so may cause seizures.

No matter which drug is used, it is crucial for the OT practitioner to alert the medical staff to any side effects that may interfere with the client's overall function.[74,82]

Nerve blocks and motor point blocks consist of injections of a chemical agent to diminish or obliterate tone. Short- and long-term blocks may be used. Short-term blocks are injections of an anesthetic (e.g., bupivacaine) to temporarily reduce pain and muscle tone. Short-term blocks help the physician differentiate between hypertonus and contracture. Short-term blocks last 1 to 7 hours, depending on which anesthetic is used.[81]

Long-term blocks, which usually consist of injections of phenol or botulinum toxin (Botox) generally last several months. Botox lasts for 2 to 5 months with spastic hypertonia and has been shown to diminish the negative effects of cervical dystonia for 12 to 16 weeks. Phenol blocks last 2 to 8 months, depending on whether the motor points (2 to 3 months) or the motor branch (8 months) is injected.[21,42]

Hsu et al.[53] studied a 52-year-old client who had spastic hypertonia after a CVA. Botulinum toxin type A was injected into the elbow, wrist, and finger flexors; this treatment was combined with a 4-week program of modified constraint-induced movement therapy (CIMT) and a 5-month home exercise program. (CIMT involves constraining the sound arm to encourage use of the affected arm.) The client made functional progress, as evidenced by improved scores on the Motor Activity Log, Wolf Motor Function Test, Action Research Arm Test, and Fugl-Meyer Assessment of Motor Recovery.

Treatment of Rigidity

Decerebrate and decorticate rigidity can increase and decrease during the day for a client. When rigidity is increasing, it is recommended that the client be transferred to a wheelchair or a reclining chair because rigidity decreases in sitting. Rigidity increases during episodes of agitation.[60] Parkinson's rigidity diminishes temporarily when the client is provided with heat, massage, stretching, and ROM exercises. Rocking back and forth before standing can aid in the transition from sitting to standing and diminish the rigidity seen in clients who have Parkinson's disease. The Lee Silverman Voice Training BIG (LSVT BIG) program (described later in the chapter) involves exercises geared toward ameliorating rigidity and enhancing large movements. The focus of the LSVT-BIG is to diminish the slowness (bradykinesia) and limited range of movement (hypokinesia) observed in clients with Parkinson's disease. (See Chapter 36 for further discussion of Parkinson's disease and additional treatment strategies.)

Treatment of Flaccidity

Flaccidity stemming from UMN dysfunction (e.g., a client recovering from spinal or cerebral shock caused by acute CNS insult or injury) is treated with facilitation techniques such as weight bearing, high-frequency vibration, tapping, quick stretch, bed positioning with weight on the flaccid side most of the time, and functional neuromuscular electrical stimulation. Splinting of the hand and wrist may be indicated for support. Therapists should closely supervise splinting because contractures can result from excessive splint wear. PROM exercises also are indicated. The arm can be passively positioned as normally as possible during ADL tasks to provide sensory and proprioceptive feedback. For example, when the client is eating, have him or her place the affected arm on the dining room table, resting on top of a piece of Dycem.[28] Client and family education on proper positioning and joint protection is important to prevent overlengthening of soft tissues and trauma (e.g., the arm falls off the client's lap and bumps the wheel of the wheelchair).

Treatment of Incoordination

Treatment of incoordination is challenging. Activities graded on the basis of motor learning and control may be helpful for attaining proximal stability and then mobility. Therapy directed toward the modulation of reflexes and abnormal synergy patterns and the enhancement of postural control mechanisms, such as the righting and equilibrium reactions, can help improve coordination. Weight bearing, joint approximation, placing and holding techniques, and fixed points of stability (having the client stabilize the elbow or wrist on the tabletop) can be helpful.

It is critical that the therapist encourage the client to use his or her vision to help direct upper extremity movements. The therapist should begin with small ranges of movement and

gradually increase them as the client progresses. Initially work is done in the plane and direction of movement that are easiest for the client; it then progresses toward more difficult areas. Some of the involuntary movements of cerebellar or extrapyramidal origin, particularly primary movement disorders, are difficult to manage or change. Therapists have greater influence over movement disorders associated with TBI, stroke, and the first three stages of Parkinson's disease.

LSVT BIG, mentioned earlier, is an intensive, evidence-based treatment protocol for clients with all stages of Parkinson's disease. The LSVT BIG protocol consists of 16 visits (four times per week for 4 weeks). It is delivered by occupational and/or physical therapists who have completed the LSVT BIG Training and Certification Workshop. The focus of the program is to address both the motor and sensory impairments related to Parkinson's disease by training larger amplitude movements and translating these movements into everyday functional activities.

Three studies have shown the efficacy of LSVT BIG in improving function in clients with Parkinson's disease. Ebersbach et al.[30] studied 60 clients with Parkinson's disease and randomly assigned them to three groups: home exercise, Nordic walking, or LSVT BIG (individual 1-hour treatment sessions, 4 days per week, for 4 weeks). The main outcome measure rated before and after treatment was the motor score of the United Parkinson's Disease Rating Scale (UPDRS). The clients in the LSVT BIG group showed a significant 5-point improvement on the UPDRS motor score, whereas the other two groups experienced mild deterioration.[30] Another study revealed that clients with Parkinson's disease who underwent 16 sessions of LSVT BIG had generalized transference of higher amplitude during reach and also demonstrated improved gait speed.[36] In both studies the clients were evaluated by blinded raters after treatment. A case series reported positive improvements in gait, balance, and bed mobility in three clients with Parkinson's disease.[55] Fox et al.[40] provide the reader with an overview of the rationale for the LSVT protocols, in addition to a description, summary of efficacy data, and discussion of limitations and future research directions. A systematic review of the literature and meta-analysis completed by McDonnell et al.[67] identified clear advantages of using the LSVT-BIG to enhance motor control for individuals who have Parkinson's disease.

Methods and devices to compensate for incoordination may be necessary to make BADLs and IADLs safer, more achievable, and more satisfying. The OT practitioner must obtain a thorough occupational profile to make appropriate activity and equipment choices and to determine adaptive strategies the client can carry over to the home environment. The physician may decide to use pharmacological agents or surgical intervention to try to damp tremor or other involuntary movement patterns.

Surgical Intervention for Movement Disorders

Neurosurgical interventions for movement disorders may include stereotactic thalamotomy to reduce ballistic movement, essential tremor (multiple sclerosis), resting tremor (Parkinson's disease), and athetosis. Surgical treatment for dystonia may include ramisectomy, stereotactic thalamotomy, or ITB implantation.[31] Deep brain stimulation has been effective in tremor reduction in essential tremor and Parkinson's disease.[34]

Because of the current managed care system, occupational therapists are receiving more referrals than ever before from primary care physicians. Occupational therapists who have a basic knowledge of medical and surgical options for ameliorating motor control problems can play a triage role in suggesting referral to physician specialists.

REHABILITATION ROBOTICS

Rehabilitation robotics is an exciting interdisciplinary field in which OT practitioners can participate. Recent rehabilitation robotics conventions have organized this field into three tracts: gerotechnology (user group characteristic), biorobotics (source of design inspiration), and neurorobotics (harness neurorecovery or neuron connectivity).[62]

Researchers at the Massachusetts Institute of Technology (MIT) invented the MIT-Manus, a device that robotically assists arms with paresis for clients who have had a CVA. The MIT study involved 96 clients, who were an average of 2 weeks post-CVA. Shoulder and elbow function improved twice as much in the experimental group (the group that used the MIT-Manus) as in the control group (the group that received conventional therapy).[91]

More information on the role of robotics in rehabilitation is available in the article by Krebs et al.[62] listed in the references.

THREADED CASE STUDY

Daniel, Part 2

1. What performance skills or standardized assessments would you select to evaluate Daniel's motor function?

Rating Daniel's muscle tone on a mild-moderate-severe scale is a low-tech, quick way to rate the hypertonia throughout his treatment and to observe the influence it has on his movement over time. Spasticity often peaks at 3 months post-CVA and then starts to decline. This varies from client to client, depending on the level of brain damage. Active and passive range of motion (AROM and PROM) are also indicated for his shoulder through his fingers. PROM is needed to make sure he does not have any contractures that inhibit his ability to reach the steering wheel. AROM is needed to see whether he has the active range to reach the steering wheel, grasp it, and release it. Sensibility testing (e.g., kinesthesia and Semmes-Weinstein monofilaments) would be useful. It is important to know whether Daniel can feel his hand position on the steering wheel. The Wolf Motor Function Test[14] or the Graded Wolf Motor Function Test[72] could be used initially and then once a month thereafter to monitor his functional progress.

2. What activities or intervention would you plan for Daniel to reduce the hypertonia in his right arm?

Weight bearing on a mat table or a kitchen counter with his right fingers, wrist, and elbow extended would serve as a good method of stretching Daniel's extrinsic finger flexors, wrist flexors, and elbow flexors. He can participate in activity with his left hand, such as putting away dishes or folding laundry one-handed.

The OT practitioner should consider fabricating a custom resting hand splint/orthotic that stretches his extrinsic finger flexors and wrist flexors. Wearing the splint/orthosis 7 hours at night is preferable so that it does not inhibit use of the affected extremity during the day.

Modality-certified OT practitioners can use ultrasound with concurrent stretch to lengthen tendons and muscles that have become shortened because of hypertonia/spasticity. In-clinic functional electrical stimulation can be used to strengthen antagonists to the spastic muscles (i.e., triceps, wrist extensors, extrinsic finger extensors, and extensor pollicis longus to obtain thumb extension). If Daniel has good results in the clinic, a home functional electrical stimulation unit can be ordered with a physician's prescription.

3. What home exercise or activity program would you prescribe for Daniel to help him reach his goals of starting the ignition of his car and driving with his RUE?

Daniel should perform passive and active stretching in any plane of motion that is needed for him to reach the steering wheel and also to turn on the ignition. This would include scapular protraction, shoulder flexion, elbow extension, forearm supination, wrist extension, finger flexion and extension, and lateral pinch. Throwing a ball forward can help him work out of the flexion synergy and speed up the release of his fingers. The hammer and inverted hammer exercises will help him gain ROM, motor control, and strength in his supinator muscles (biceps and supinator) (Figs. 19.17 and 19.18).

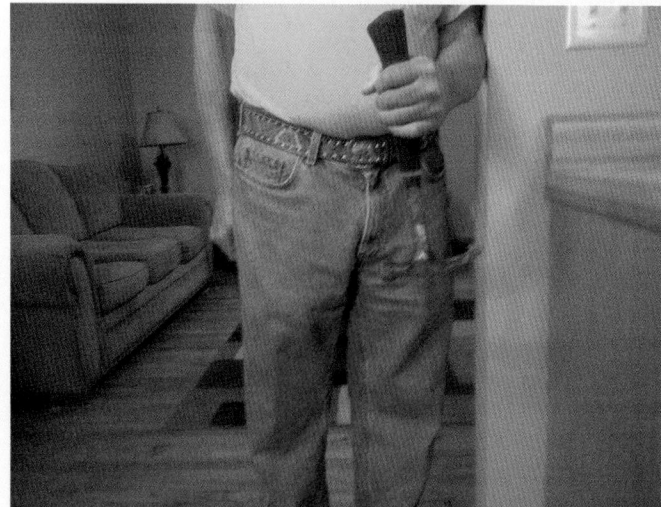

Fig. 19.17 Starting position for the inverted hammer exercise to strengthen the supinator muscles.

Daniel, Part 2

He needs both supination and lateral pinch to turn the key in the ignition. He can use therapy putty to help him acquire the strength to hold on to the car key. Home functional electrical stimulation units can be used to strengthen the triceps and the extensors of the fingers, wrist, and thumb.

Daniel reached his goals of driving and returning to work full duty as a salesperson 4 months after his CVA (Fig. 19.19).

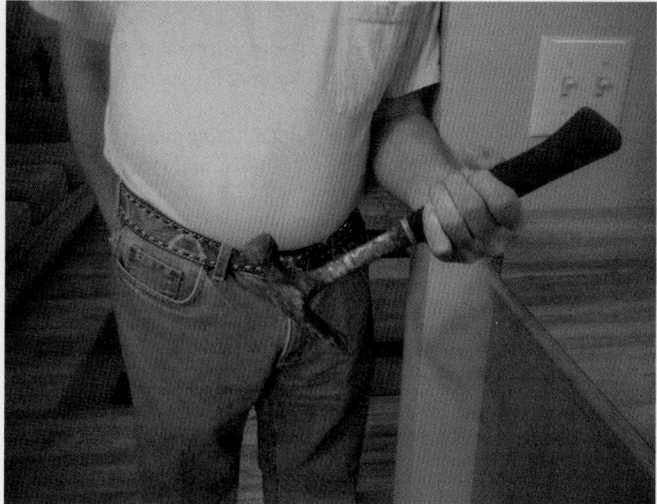

Fig. 19.18 Ending position for the inverted hammer exercise to strengthen the supinator muscles. The therapist can put a cuff weight on the hammer when the client can do the exercise easily to full range.

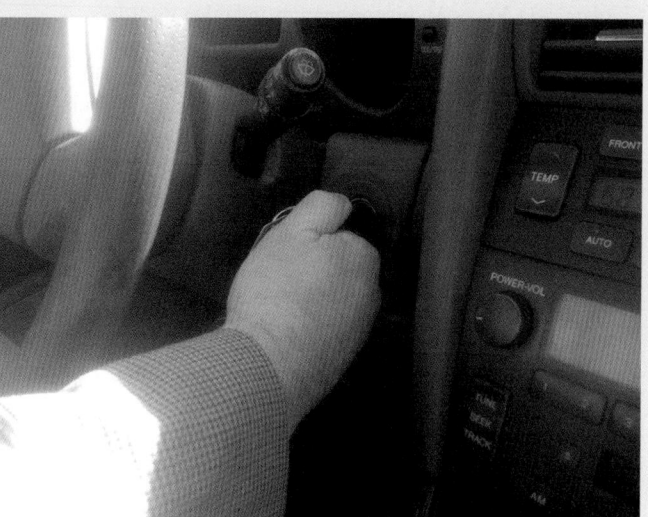

Fig. 19.19 Daniel's last day of therapy, driving himself to work.

SUMMARY

From reading Daniel's case study, we can see how abnormal elements of motor control affect the quality of movement and the ability to perform in areas of occupation. The occupational therapist assesses muscle tone, UE recovery, and coordination using standardized tests and observation of movement during occupational performance. The results of the motor control assessment can help the client and the therapist collaborate on appropriate intervention. Ameliorating motor control problems can be a rewarding experience for the client and the therapist.

REVIEW QUESTIONS

1. What is neuroplasticity?
2. Describe the circumstances in which a physician would recommend a long-term nerve block or a motor point block for a person with spastic wrist and finger flexors.
3. Describe the characteristics of rigidity.
4. Explain the major difference between spasticity and hypertonia.
5. Demonstrate how to perform an upper extremity muscle tone evaluation.
6. What is the name of the certification program that focuses on helping clients with Parkinson's disease take bigger steps and reach higher in ADLs?
7. What are equilibrium reactions?
8. Compare chorea and athetosis.
9. What is ataxia?
10. What is the most common type of tremor?

REFERENCES

1. Abo M, et al: Randomized, multicenter, comparative study of NEURO versus CIMT in poststroke patients with upper limb hemiparesis: the NEURO-VERIFY study, *Int J Stroke* 9:607–612, 2014. https://doi.org/10.1111/ijs.12100.
2. Adams RD, Victor M: Abnormalities of movement and posture caused by disease of the basal ganglia. In Ropper AH, Samuels MA, editors: *Principles of neurology* ed 9, New York, 2009, McGraw-Hill.
3. Adams RD, Victor M: Incoordination and other disorders of cerebellar function. In Ropper AH, Samuels MA, editors: *Principles of neurology* ed 9, New York, 2009, McGraw-Hill.
4. Adams RD, Victor M: Motor paralysis. In Ropper AH, Samuels MA, editors: *Principles of neurology* ed 9, New York, 2009, McGraw-Hill.
5. Adams RJ, Ellington AL, Armstead K, Sheffield K, Patrie JT, Diamond PT: Upper extremity function assessment using a glove orthosis and virtual reality system, *OTJR: Occup Ther J Res* 39:81–89, 2019. https://doi.org/10.1177/1539449219829862.
6. Allison SC, Abraham LD, Petersen CL: Reliability of the Modified Ashworth Scale in the assessment of plantar-flexor muscle spasticity in patients with traumatic brain injury, *Int J Rehabil Res* 19:67–78, 1996.
7. American Academy of Neurology: Assessment: the clinical usefulness of botulinum toxin A in treating neurological disorders—report of the Therapeutics and Technology Assessment Subcommittee, *Neurology* 40:1332–1336, 1990.
8. Ashley KD, Lee LT, Heaton K: Return to work among stroke survivors, *Workplace Health & Safety* 67:87–94, 2019. https://doi.org/10.1177/2165079918812483.
9. Ashworth B: Preliminary trial of carisoprodol in multiple sclerosis, *Practitioner* 192:540–542, 1964.
10. Bennett Hand Tool Test. Lafayette Instruments, Lafayette, IN. http://lafayetteevaluation.com.
11. Berg KO, Wood-Dauphine S, Williams JI, Gayton D: Measuring balance in the elderly: preliminary development of an instrument, *Physiother Can* 41:304–311, 1989.
12. Bernspång B, Fisher AG: Differences between persons with right or left cerebral vascular accident on the Assessment of Motor and Process Skills, *Arch Phys Med Rehabil* 76:1114–1151, 1995.
13. Blackburn M, van Vliet P, Mockett SP: Reliability of measurements obtained with the Modified Ashworth Scale in the lower extremities of people with stroke, *Phys Ther* 82:25–34, 2002.
14. Blanton S, Wolf S: An application of upper-extremity constraint-induced movement therapy in a patient with subacute stroke, *Phys Ther* 79:847–853, 1999.
15. Bohannon RW, Smith MB: Interrater reliability of a Modified Ashworth Scale of muscle spasticity, *Phys Ther* 67:206–207, 1987.
16. Botox package insert. Allergan Pharmaceuticals, Irvine, CA. http://www.allergan.com.
17. Boyd R, Graham H: Objective measurement of clinical findings in the use of botulinum toxin type A for the management of children with cerebral palsy, *Eur J Neurol* 6:S23–S36, 1999.
18. Brouwer BJ, Ambury P: Upper extremity weight-bearing effect on corticospinal excitability following stroke, *Arch Phys Med Rehabil* 75:861–866, 1994.
19. Carmick J: Clinical use of neuromuscular electrical stimulation for children with cerebral palsy, part 2: upper extremity, *Phys Ther* 73:514–522, 1993.
20. Chakerian DL, Larson MA: Effects of upper-extremity weight-bearing on hand-opening and prehension patterns in children with cerebral palsy, *Dev Med Child Neurol* 35:216–229, 1993.
21. Chironna RL, Hecht JS: Subscapularis motor point block for the painful hemiplegic shoulder, *Arch Phys Med Rehabil* 71:428–429, 1990.
22. Coleman ER, Moudgal R, Lang K, Hyacinth HI, Awosika OO, Kissela BM, Feng W: Early rehabilitation after stroke: a narrative review, *Curr Atheroscler Rep* 19(12):59, 2017. https://doi.org/10.1007/s11883-017-0686-6.
23. Collin C, Wade D: Assessing motor impairment after a stroke: a pilot reliability study, *J Neurol Neurosurg Psychiatry* 53:576–579, 1990.
24. DeBoskey DS, Hecht JS, Calub CJ: *Educating families of the head injured: a guide to medical, cognitive, and social issues*, Gaithersburg, MD, 1991, Aspen.
25. deGroot J, editor: *Correlative neuroanatomy* ed 21, Norwalk, CT, 1991, Appleton & Lange.
26. Desrosiers J, Hébert R, Bravo G, Dutil E: Upper extremity performance test for the elderly (TEMPA): normative data and correlates with sensorimotor parameters, *Arch Phys Med Rehabil* 76:1125–1129, 1995.
27. Duncan PW, et al.: Rasch analysis of a new stroke-specific outcome scale: the Stroke Impact Scale, *Arch Phys Med Rehabil* 84:950–963, 2003.
28. Dycem package insert. Patterson Medical. https://dycem.com/products/.
29. Dye DC, Eakman AM, Bolton KM: Assessing the validity of the Dynamic Gait Index in a balance disorders clinic: an application of Rasch analysis, *Phys Ther* 93:809–818, 2013.
30. Ebersbach G, Ebersbach A, Edler D, et al: Comparing exercise in Parkinson's disease: the Berlin LSVT/BIG Study, *Mov Disord* 25:1902–1908, 2010. https://doi.org/10.1002/mds.23212.
31. Elovic E, Bogey R: Spasticity and movement disorders. In DeLisa JA, Gans BM, editors: *Physical medicine & rehabilitation: principles and practice* ed 4, Philadelphia, 2004, Lippincott Raven.
32. Elovic EP, Eisenberg ME, Jasey NN: Spasticity and muscle overactivity as components of the upper motor neuron syndrome ed 5. In: Frontera WR, editor: *DeLisa's physical medicine and rehabilitation principles and practice*, vol I and II, Philadelphia, 2010, Lippincott Williams & Wilkins, pp 1319–1344.
33. Fahn S: Involuntary movements. In Rowland LP, Pedley TA, editors: *Merritt's neurology* ed 12, Philadelphia, 2010, Lippincott Williams & Wilkins.
34. Fahn S, Przedborski S: Parkinson disease. In Rowland LP, Pedley TA, editors: *Merritt's neurology* ed 12, Philadelphia, 2010, Lippincott Williams & Wilkins.
35. Farber S: *Neurorehabilitation: a multisensory approach*, Philadelphia, 1982, Saunders.
36. Farley BG, Koshland GF: Training BIG to move faster: the application of the speed amplitude relation as a rehabilitation strategy for people with Parkinson's disease, *Exp Brain Res* 167:462–467, 2005.
37. Farrell JF, Hoffman HB, Snyder JL, et al: Orthotic aided training of the paretic limb in chronic stroke: results of a phase 1 trial, *NeuroRehabilitation* 22:99–103, 2007.
38. Fleuren JM, Voerman GE, Erren-Wolters CV, et al: Stop using the Ashworth Scale for the assessment of spasticity, *J Neurol Neurosurg Psychiatry* 81:46–52, 2010.
39. Fosang AL, Galea MP, McCoy AT, et al: Measures of muscle and joint performance in lower limbs of children with cerebral palsy, *Dev Med Child Neurol* 45:664–670, 2003.

40. Fox C, Ebersbach G, Ramig L, Sapir S: Behavioral treatment programs for speech and body movement in Parkinson disease, *Parkinsons Dis*, 2012. https://doi.org/10.1155/2012/391946. Epub 2012 Mar 15.

41. Fugl-Meyer AR, Jääskö L, Leyman I, et al: The post-stroke hemiplegic patient 1. A method for evaluation of physical performance, *Scand J Rehabil Med* 7:13–31, 1975.

42. Gillen G: Trunk control: supporting functional independence. In Gillen G, editor: *Stroke rehabilitation: a function-based approach* ed 4, St Louis, 2015, Elsevier/Mosby.

43. Goga-Eppenstein PG, Hill JP, Yasukawa A: *Casting protocols of the upper and lower extremities*, Chicago, 1999, Aspen.

44. Goldberg C, VanSant A: Normal motor development. In Tecklin JS, editor: *Pediatric physical therapy* ed 3, Philadelphia, 1999, Lippincott Williams & Wilkins.

45. Gracies JM, Marosszeky JE, Renton R, et al: Short-term effects of dynamic Lycra splints on upper limb in hemiplegic patients, *Arch Phys Med Rehabil* 81:1547–1555, 2000.

46. Green P: Parkinson's plus syndrome. In Rowland LP, Pedley TA, editors: *Merritt's neurology* ed 12, Philadelphia, 2010, Lippincott Williams & Wilkins.

47. Gregson JM, Leathley MJ, Moore AP, et al: Reliability of measurements of muscle tone and muscle power in stroke patients, *Age Ageing* 29:223–228, 2000.

48. Gregson JM, Leathley MJ, Moore AP, et al: Reliability of the Tone Assessment Scale and the Modified Ashworth Scale as clinical tools for assessing poststroke spasticity, *Arch Phys Med Rehabil* 80:1013–1016, 1999.

49. Hackett ML, Glozier N, Jan S, Lindley R: Returning to paid employment after stroke: the Psychosocial Outcomes in StrokE (POISE) cohort study, *PLoS ONE* 7(7):e41795, 2012. https://doi.org/10.1371/journal.pone.0041795.

50. Held JP, Pierrot-Deseilligny E: *Reeducation motrice des affections neurologiques*, Paris, 1969, Bailliere.

51. Hill J: The effects of casting on upper extremity motor disorders after brain injury, *Am J Occup Ther* 48:219–224, 1994.

52. Howle JM: *Neurodevelopmental treatment approach: theoretical foundations and principles of clinical practice*, Laguna Beach, California, 2002, Neuro-Developmental Treatment Association.

53. Hsu C-W, et al: Application of combined botulinum toxin type A and modified constraint-induced movement therapy for an individual with chronic upper extremity spasticity after stroke, *Phys Ther* 86:1387, 2006.

54. Jain SS, Kirshblum SC: Movement disorders, including tremors. In DeLisa JA, editor: *Rehabilitation medicine: principles and practice* ed 2, Philadelphia, 1993, Lippincott.

55. Janssens J, Malfroid K, Nyffeler T, et al: Application of LSVT BIG intervention to address gait, balance, bed mobility, and dexterity in people with Parkinson disease: a case series, *Phys Ther* 94:1014–1023, 2014.

56. Jebsen RH, Taylor N, Trieschmann RB, et al: An objective and standardized test of hand function, *Arch Phys Med Rehabil* 50:311–319, 1969.

57. Joshi Y, Grando Sória M, Quadrato G, et al: The MDM4/MDM2-p53-IGF1 axis controls axonal regeneration, sprouting and functional recovery after CNS injury, *Brain* 138:1843–1862, 2015.

58. Katz RT, Rovai GP, Brait C, Rymer WZ: Objective quantification of spastic hypertonia: correlation with clinical findings, *Arch Phys Med Rehabil* 73:339–347, 1992.

59. Keenan ME, Matzon JL: Upper extremity dysfunction after stroke or brain injury. In: Wolfe S.W.Hotchkiss RN, Pederson WC, Kozin SH, editors: *Green's operative hand surgery*, vol I, Philadelphia, 2010, Elsevier/Churchill Livingstone.

60. Kohlmeyer K: Evaluation of performance skills and client factors. In Crepaeau EB, Cohn ES, Boyt–Shell BA, editors: *Willard and Spackman's occupational therapy* ed 10, Philadelphia, 2003, Lippincott Williams & Wilkins.

61. Kopp B, Kunkel A, Flor H, et al: The Arm Motor Ability Test: reliability, validity, and sensitivity to change of an instrument for assessing disabilities in activities of daily living, *Arch Phys Med Rehabil* 78:615–620, 1997.

62. Krebs HI, et al: Rehabilitation robotics ed 5. In: Frontera WR, editor: *DeLisa's physical medicine and rehabilitation: principles and practice*, vol I and II, Philadelphia, 2010, Lippincott Williams & Wilkins, pp 2187–2198.

63. Law M, et al: *Canadian Occupational Performance Measure*, ed 3, Ottawa, ON, 1998, Canadian Association of Occupational Therapists.

64. Leonard CT, Stephens JU, Stroppel SL: Assessing the spastic condition of individuals with upper motoneuron involvement: validity of the myotonometer, *Arch Phys Med Rehabil* 82:1416–1420, 2001.

65. Mathiowetz V, Weber K, Kashman N, Volland G: Adult norms for the Nine Hole Peg Test of finger dexterity, *Occup Ther J Res* 5:24–38, 1985.

66. McCrea PH, Eng JJ, Hodgson AJ: Linear spring-damper model of the hypertonic elbow: reliability and validity, *J Neurosci Methods* 128:121–128, 2003.

67. McDonnell MN, Rischbieth B, Schammer TT, Seaforth C, Shaw AJ, Phillips AC: Lee Silverman Voice Treatment (LSVT)-BIG to improve motor function in people with Parkinson's disease: A systematic review and meta-analysis, *Clinical Rehabilitation* 32:607–618, 2018. https://doi.org/10.1177/0269215517734385.

68. McIlroy WE, Maki BE: Early activation of arm muscles follows external perturbation of upright stance, *Neurosci Lett* 184:177–180, 1995.

69. Medtronic ITB. Therapy. Clinical reference guide. Medtronic Neurological, Minneapolis, MN. http://www.medtronic.com.

70. Melnick ME: Clients with cerebellar dysfunction. In Umphred DA, editor: *Neurological rehabilitation* ed 5, St Louis, 2007, Elsevier/Mosby.

71. Minnesota Manual Dexterity Test. https://www.prohealthcareproducts.com/blog/minnesota-dexterity-test-guide-and-instructions/.

72. Morris D.M., et al: Graded Wolf Motor Function Test, University of Alabama at Birmingham, revised May 6, 2002.

73. Myobloc. Solstice Neurosciences, Louisville, KY. http://www.solsticeneuro.com/.

74. Nance PW, Ethans K: *Spasticity management*. In *Physical medicine and rehabilitation*, ed 4, Philadelphia, 2010, Elsevier/Saunders.

75. National Institute of Neurological Disorders and Stroke (NINDS): Information page: ataxias and cerebellar or spinocerebellar degeneration. https://www.ninds.nih.gov/health-information/disorders/ataxia-and-cerebellar-or-spinocerebellar-degeneration?search-term=ataxia.

76. Pandyan AD, Johnson GR, Price CIM, et al: A review of the properties and limitations of the Ashworth and Modified Ashworth Scales as measures of spasticity, *Clin Rehabil* 13:373–383, 1999.

77. Pandyan AD, Price CIM, Rodgers H, et al: Biomechanical examination of a commonly used measure of spasticity, *Clin Biomech (Bristol, Avon)* 16:859–865, 2001.

78. Paulis WD, Horemans HD, Brouwer BS, Stam HJ: Excellent test-retest and inter-rater reliability for Tardieu Scale measurements

with inertial sensors in elbow flexors of stroke patients, *Gait Posture* 33:185–189, 2011.

79. Preston LA: Effects of botulinum toxin type B on shoulder pain, master's thesis, Nashville TN, 2003, Belmont University.

80. Preston LA: Motor control. In Pendleton HM, Schultz-Krohn W, editors: *Pedretti's occupational therapy practice skills for physical dysfunction* ed 7, St Louis, 2013, Elsevier/Mosby, pp 461–488.

81. Preston LA: OT's role in enhancing nerve blocks for spasticity, *OT Practice* 3:29–35, 1998.

82. Preston LA, Hecht JS: *Spasticity management: rehabilitation strategies*, Bethesda, MD, 1999, American Occupational Therapy Association.

83. Purdue Pegboard. Science Research Associates, Chicago. http://www.mheducation.com/.

84. Quandt F, Hummel F: The influence of functional electrical stimulation on hand motor recovery in stroke patients; a review, *Exp Transl Stroke Med* 6:1–11, 2014. https://doi.org/10.1186/2040-7378-6-9.

85. Rickards T, et al: Diffusion tensor imaging study of the response to constraint-induced movement therapy of children with hemiparetic cerebral palsy and adults with chronic stroke, *Arch Phys Med Rehabil* 95:506–514, 2014.

86. Ryerson SD: Hemiplegia. In Umphred DA, editor: *Neurological rehabilitation* ed 5, St Louis, 2007, Elsevier/Mosby.

87. Shumway-Cook A, Woollacott MH: Constraints on motor control: an overview of neurological impairments. In Shumway-Cook A, Woollacott MH, editors: *Motor control: translating research into clinical practice* ed 3, Philadelphia, 2007, Lippincott Williams & Wilkins.

88. Shumway-Cook A, Woollacott MH: Development of postural control. In Shumway-Cook A, Woollacott MH, editors: *Motor control: translating research into clinical practice* ed 3, Philadelphia, 2007, Lippincott Williams & Wilkins, pp 76.

89. Stuck RA, Marshall LM, Sivakumar R: Feasibility of SaeboFlex upper limb training in acute stroke rehabilitation: a clinical case series, *Occup Ther Int* 21:108–114, 2014. https://doi.org/10.1002/oti.1369.

90. Van der Meche F, van Gijn J: Hypotonia: an erroneous clinical concept? *Brain* 109(Pt 6):1169–1178, 1986.

91. Volpe BT, Krebs HI, Hogan N: Is robot–aided sensorimotor training in stroke rehabilitation a realistic option? *Curr Opin Neurol* 14:745–752, 2001.

92. Vyas MV, de Oliveira C, Laporte A, Kapral MK: The association between stroke, integrated stroke systems, and the employability and productivity of Canadian stroke survivors, *Neuroepidemiology* 53:209–219, 2019. https://doi.org/10.1159/000502010.

93. Whitney SL, Poole JL, Cass SP: A review of balance instruments for older adults, *Am J Occup Ther* 52:666–671, 1998.

94. Williams LS, et al: Development of a stroke-specific quality of life scale, *Stroke* 30:1362–1369, 1999.

95. Wilson DJ, Baker LL, Craddock JA: Functional Test for the Hemiplegic/Paretic Upper Extremity, Downey, CA, 1984, Los Amigos Research and Education Institute.

96. Wolf SL, et al: The EXCITE trial: attributes of the Wolf Motor Function Test in patients with subacute stroke, *Neurorehabil Neural Repair* 19:194–205, 2005. https://pubmed.ncbi.nlm.nih.gov/16093410/l.

97. Woo Y, et al: Kinematics variations after spring-assisted orthosis training in persons with stroke, *Prosthet Orthot Int* 37:311–316, 2013. https://doi.org/10.1177/0309364612461050.

98. Wrisley DM, Marchetti GF, Kuharsky DK, Whitney SL: Reliability, internal consistency, and validity of data obtained with the Functional Gait Assessment, *Phys Ther* 84:906–918, 2004.

SUGGESTED READINGS

Amyotrophic lateral sclerosis, 1998–2015. January 19, 2015. Mayo Foundation for Medical Education and Research. http://www.mayoclinic.org.

Bell-Krotoski JA, Fess EE, Figarola JH, Hiltz D: Threshold detection and Semmes-Weinstein monofilaments, *J Hand Ther* 8:155–162, 1995.

Brunnstrom S: *Movement therapy in hemiplegia*, Philadelphia, 1970, Lippincott Williams & Wilkins.

Cramer SC: Neural repair and plasticity ed 5. In: Frontera WR, editor: *DeLisa's physical medicine and rehabilitation principles and practice*, vol I and II, Philadelphia, 2010, Lippincott Williams & Wilkins, pp 2155–2172.

Gorman SL: Contemporary issues and theories of motor control, motor learning, and neuroplasticity: assessment of movement and posture. In Umphred DA, editor: *Neurological rehabilitation* ed 5, St Louis, 2007, Elsevier/Mosby.

Hecht JS: Subscapular nerve block in the painful hemiplegic shoulder, *Arch Phys Med Rehabil* 73:1036–1039, 1992.

Hines AE, Crago PE, Billian C: Functional electrical stimulation for the reduction of spasticity in the hemiplegic hand, *Biomed Sci Instrum* 29:259–266, 1993.

Hoffman HB, Blakey GL: New design of dynamic orthoses for neurological conditions, *Neuro Rehabilitation* 28:55–61, 2011. https://doi.org/10.3233/NRE-2011-0632.

Pandyan AD, Price CI, Barnes MP, Johnson GR: A biomechanical investigation into the validity of the Modified Ashworth Scale as a measure of elbow spasticity, *Clin Rehabil* 17:290–293, 2003.

Reuben DB, Siu AL: An objective measure of physical function of elderly outpatients, *J Am Geriatr Soc* 38:1105–1112, 1990.

Shumway-Cook A, Woollacott MH: Clinical management of the patient with a mobility disorder. In Shumway-Cook A, Woollacott MH, editors: *Motor control: translating research into clinical practice* ed 3, Philadelphia, 2007, Lippincott Williams & Wilkins.

Shumway-Cook A, Woollacott MH: Physiological basis of motor learning and recovery of function. In Shumway-Cook A, Woollacott MH, editors: *Motor control: translating research into clinical practice* ed 3, Philadelphia, 2007, Lippincott Williams & Wilkins, pp 84.

St John K, Stephenson J: *PNF I: the functional approach to proprioceptive neuromuscular facilitation*, Steamboat Springs, CO, 2002, The Institute of Physical Art.

Tinetti ME: Performance oriented assessment of mobility problems in elderly patients, *J Am Geriatr Soc* 34:119–126, 1986.

20

Occupation-Based Functional Motion Assessment

Alison Hewitt George[a]

LEARNING OBJECTIVES

After studying this chapter, the student or practitioner[b] will be able to do the following:

1. Define occupation-based functional motion assessment.
2. Explain why it is desirable to assess motor function through observation of engagement in occupation and activity performance.
3. State two circumstances under which assessment of performance skills is indicated.
4. Define individual activity analysis, or "dynamic performance analysis."
5. Explain why it is not possible to do an accurate objective activity analysis.
6. List at least three questions that can guide the clinical observation and clinical reasoning of the occupational

therapy (OT) practitioner while conducting an occupation-based functional motion assessment.

7. List factors other than range of motion (ROM), strength, and motor control that can affect motor performance.
8. Discuss how information gained from the occupation-based functional motion assessment differs from that gained during assessment of specific client factors.
9. State the minimum level of strength required throughout the lower extremities for normal stance and positioning.
10. Compare levels of muscle strength and associated endurance in the upper extremities.
11. List occupations that can be used to access functional motion in the upper extremities and in the lower extremities.

CHAPTER OUTLINE

KEY TERMS

Functional motion assessment
Individual activity analysis

Objective activity analysis
Occupation-based functional motion assessment

THREADED CASE STUDY

Raymond, Part 1

Raymond (prefers use of the pronouns he/him/his) is a 60-year-old foreman of several lineman crews of the telephone company. He has been with the company for more than 40 years; although he could have moved into a more administrative

position over the years, he has always enjoyed working out in the field, being a mentor to the younger workers, and dealing with emergencies. He is known throughout his neighborhood as the person to call when help is needed with

(Continued)

---

[a] The author wishes to acknowledge Amy Phillips Killingsworth for her work on previous editions of this chapter.

[b] In this chapter, the term *occupational therapy practitioner* refers to occupational therapists (OTs) or occupational therapy assistants (OTAs) as defined in the current version (2020) of the OT Framework, the *Occupational Therapy Practice Framework: Domain and Process*, fourth edition (OTPF-4).[2] Throughout the chapter, distinctions will be made regarding which practitioner, when appropriate, depending on the job responsibilities of each in the evaluation process as defined in three important documents published by the American Occupational Therapy Association (AOTA): the Standards of Practice for Occupational Therapy (2021)[4]; the Guidelines for Supervision, Roles, and Responsibilities During the Delivery of Occupational Therapy Services (2020)[1]; and the Scope of Practice for Occupational Therapy (2021).[3] In general, the OT is responsible for all aspects of the evaluation process, and the OTA contributes to the process under the supervision of the OT.

Raymond, Part 1

home repair tasks, whether it is carpentry, plumbing, or electrical work. He is a member of a championship senior softball team and plays most weekends during the season, sometimes traveling out of town to participate in tournaments. He does quite a bit of volunteering through the outreach program at his church, participating in such activities as collecting, preparing, and delivering food to home-bound elderly and driving new immigrants to various appointments. He shares household duties with his wife and enjoys cooking for her.

Raymond was first diagnosed with rheumatoid arthritis 10 years ago, when he began experiencing pain and stiffness in his shoulders, hips, and knees. His symptoms were managed with medication and, except for occasional exacerbations, he was able to fully engage in those occupations that were meaningful to him. In the last 6 months he has experienced an exacerbation of his symptoms. The pain in his shoulders, hips, and knees has increased, and he also has begun experiencing pain in his wrist and hands. His wife began to notice Raymond's change in mood as he became increasingly reluctant to engage in occupations in which he always took the lead, such as helping his neighbors with home projects, preparing food in his church outreach program, and participating in the softball games.

Because he could not do things the way he used to, he did not want to do them at all. He stated that he did not want people seeing him fumbling as he attempted to hold tools or cooking utensils because his grip was so weak, nor did he want to let his teammates down because of the decreased power in his batting swing and speed in running the bases. At work he found himself giving more verbal instructions to his crew rather than demonstrating techniques, as he had always done before, at times speaking in a gruff, impatient tone, which was surprising to his fellow workers. His frustration with the increased amount of time it was taking him to complete activities of daily living (ADLs), such as shaving,

buttoning his shirt, and putting on the boots he was required to wear at work, was making him irritable. The fatigue he was experiencing at the end of the day "just from trying to move my body around" was also adding to the depression of this client. This previously outgoing person was withdrawing and becoming increasingly more socially isolated.

The occupational therapist (OT) to whom he was referred began anticipating the needs of this client based on the profile she developed. Evaluating this client as he engaged in occupations in specific contexts would provide the best information for determining intervention strategies that would be most helpful, such as adaptive equipment and joint protection techniques. Getting information underlying those client factors (muscle strength, range of motion [ROM]) contributing to his decrease in function was critical. Arrangements were made to assess the client in his home and to make a job site visit. By observing the client perform occupation-based tasks and motions at work and home, the OT could obtain important information concerning his ROM, strength, and endurance and could assess his motor control.

Critical Thinking Questions
1. What is the advantage of administering an occupation-based functional motion assessment versus more specific assessments, such as joint measurement and manual muscle testing?
2. What information about the client's muscle strength and joint ROM can be determined through the occupation-based functional motion assessment? What cannot be determined?
3. What is the value of administering the occupation-based functional motion assessment in different environmental contexts?

Many physical disabilities cause limitations in motor performance skills and client factors, including joint range of motion (ROM), muscle strength, and endurance or control of voluntary movement (gross and fine motor control). These physical impairments in body functions and motor skills result in movement limitations that can cause slight to substantial deficits in performance of areas of occupation and prevent pursuit of self-care, work, leisure, and educational and social activities. The occupation-based functional motion assessment is a way of assessing the ROM, strength, and motor control available for task performance by observing the client during performance of everyday occupations (activities of daily living [ADLs], instrumental activities of daily living [IADLs], education, work, social participation, leisure activities, and rest and sleep) in varied contexts and environments.[2]

Because the primary responsibility of the occupational therapist (OT) is to assess occupational performance, identify performance problems, and plan intervention strategies that will improve the client's ability to fully engage in occupations, sensorimotor limitations first should be assessed through observation of functional activities. When improvement of performance skills is a goal of the intervention program, assessment of performance skills, occupation demands, and client factors in a variety of environmental contexts (e.g., home, workplace, or school) may be indicated to make an objective assessment of

physical limitations and gains (see Chapters 19, 21, and 22 for additional information.)

Mental functions, including cognitive and perceptual abilities, such as motivation or the ability to sequence complex movement patterns, interpret incoming stimuli, and exhibit coping and behavioral regulation, can also affect motor function. These client factors must be considered in any performance evaluation (see Chapters 25 and 26) for additional information. However, this chapter is limited to consideration of motor function (i.e., ROM, strength, motor control) during the occupation-based functional motion assessment.

OT PRACTICE NOTES

Except for a few diagnoses, specific assessments of ROM, muscle strength,[5] and motor control are seldom necessary. For example, performing a full ROM assessment or manual muscle test is time-consuming, can be tiring to the client, and may duplicate other services, whereas assessing these factors while the client is engaging in occupation yields the most comprehensive picture of the client's actual abilities and limitations.

CLINICAL OBSERVATION

It is possible to administer a gross assessment of joint mobility and muscle strength by having the client perform those motions associated with functional tasks (i.e., a functional motion assessment). The OT practitioner could observe as the client reaches overhead, as would happen when putting dishes away in an overhead cupboard, or taking a step to the side, as when stepping into a bathtub.[11] This will give the practitioner some basic, although nonspecific, information about those factors that affect function.

OT practitioners (the OT in collaboration with the OTA) analyze the occupations of a client to assess the quality of that client's effectiveness in valued occupations, to identify the impact of contextual factors on performance, and to "determine the impact of personal factors (including health condition) on current performance."[6] With occupational analysis, client factors such as muscle strength, ROM, and motor control can be observed during the performance of ordinary ADLs, IADLs, work, and leisure tasks.[4] For example, while assessing ADLs, the therapist can observe for performance difficulties and movement patterns that may signal limited ROM, muscle weakness, muscle imbalance, poor endurance, limited motor control, and compensatory motions used for function.

An occupation-based functional motion assessment has an advantage over the functional motion assessment because, although the client will perform motions as described previously, there is the added resistance to body structures that will occur as the result of using equipment such as a sliding door, manipulating objects such as cards, or resisting fatigue and having endurance during repetitive activities such as folding clothes or bouncing a ball. Also, because the client is performing these tasks in environments and contexts that are meaningful, the client's full participation and engagement in the task may be heightened.

Essentially, when observing a client perform selected tasks, the occupational therapist is doing an individual activity analysis or "dynamic performance analysis"[11] to diagnose the occupational performance problems of that client. Because people perform the same task in a variety of ways and because there are so many variables in task performance, it is not possible to do an objective activity analysis, one that can be applied universally, and describe the sensorimotor requirements of the myriad of ADLs. The purpose of observation is to understand the client's occupational performance problems in the context of the interaction between the person, the task, and the environment.[6] This type of screening will serve the occupational therapist well in deciding a course of intervention for Raymond, who because of the current exacerbation status of his disease, is not a candidate for more specific muscle strength assessment (see Chapter 22). While observing Raymond in his home as he performs the functional tasks described later in this chapter, the therapist will not only be able to assess available ROM but also make some determination of the client's muscle strength, endurance, and coordination.

The therapist's scientific knowledge of the particular dysfunction and an analysis of the ways in which activities are generally performed (activity demands) influence the assessment of performance problems and aid in the development of plans to remediate those problems. Analyzing the client while engaged in a specific occupation parallels activity analysis but also allows

the practitioner to gain additional knowledge of the client's unique way of performing that occupation.[6]

The following are questions to guide the clinical observation and clinical reasoning processes:

1. Does the client have adequate ROM to perform the task?
   a. Where are the joint limitations?
   b. What are some possible causes of the limitations?
   c. Are there true ROM limitations, or are apparent limitations actually caused by decreased muscle strength?
2. Does the client have enough strength to perform the task?
   a. In which muscle groups is there apparent weakness?
   b. If strength appears inadequate to perform a task because the client cannot complete the ROM, is there truly muscle weakness, or is there actually limited ROM?
3. Does the client have enough motor control to perform the task?
   a. Is the movement smooth and rhythmic?
   b. Is movement slow and difficult (e.g., as seen in spasticity and rigidity)?
   c. Are there extraneous movements when the client performs the task (e.g., tremors, athetoid, or choreiform movements)?

The observing OT practitioner must also consider the client's understanding of the instructions and perception of task importance, in addition to the possibility of sensory, perceptual, and cognitive deficits. An analysis of the results of the occupation-based functional motion assessment may indicate that formal assessment of performance skills or body functions is needed. For example, such an assessment may be needed to differentiate muscle weakness from limited ROM or to quantify (with a muscle grade) muscle weakness in specific muscle groups.

Assessing ROM, strength, and motor control by observing the client perform functional activities can aid in selecting meaningful intervention goals relative to improving occupational performance. The therapist can ask the client about his or her ability to perform the tasks of daily living but should also observe the client performing such activities as dressing, walking, standing, and sitting to make an accurate assessment.[7] Having the client perform ADLs in addition to other tasks associated with his or her habits and routines while interacting in varied environmental contexts can also add to the depth of information concerning the client's ROM and muscle strength. The occupational therapist delivering OT services to Raymond has determined that doing both a home visit and job site visit will enhance understanding of the demands on this client. Observation of Raymond interacting with materials, equipment, tools, and products in these environments will provide information about those critical motions and complex motor patterns required for him to fully engage in those occupations most meaningful to him. Completion of the tasks by Raymond in the timely manner required in these contexts will also give information about the client's endurance, thus giving more information about his muscle strength.

Joint ROM, manual muscle testing, and motor control assessments (see Chapters 21, 22, and 19) will give the therapist specific information about the function of the musculoskeletal, neurophysiological, and sensorimotor systems. Although the tests require minimum to maximum active output by the client, the therapist will not be able to determine the client's ability to integrate these systems to perform specific goal-directed tasks based on the results of these assessments. Rather, the therapist will have information about movements of a specific limb or a combination of limbs. Under carefully controlled conditions, the therapist will know about the flexibility of the components of the joint and the strength of muscles to create movements such as flexion, abduction, and external rotation. However, the client's motor performance capabilities are not measured by these assessments. For example, the manual muscle test cannot measure muscle endurance (number of times the muscle can contract at its maximum level and resist fatigue), motor control (smooth rhythmic interaction of muscle function), or the client's ability to use the muscles for functional activities.[7]

OT PRACTICE NOTES

While observing a client performing functional activities, it would be most helpful if a therapist could also estimate the client's existing ROM, muscle strength, and motor control.

At his job site Raymond had difficulty stepping up into his truck (the cab of which was somewhat elevated because of the oversize tires), not having enough ROM during flexion of the hip and knee flexion. The OT also observed that if the truck was parked near a curb or if Raymond could step first on a box and then onto the step of the truck, thus requiring less flexion ROM, he had less difficulty. However, in both instances he lacked sufficient strength in hip and knee extension to launch himself into the truck without compensating with his upper extremities.

OCCUPATION-BASED FUNCTIONAL MOTION ASSESSMENT

The activities listed in the following sections for the occupation-based functional motion assessment are suggested as a general starting place for the student or beginning practitioner (within the guidelines of the roles and responsibilities of the OT or the OTA). Only upper and lower extremity activities are included. Movements of the face, mouth, neck, and spine are beyond the scope of this chapter. Many more motions and tasks could be suggested in each category. The reader is referred to *Joint Motion, Muscle Length and Function Assessment: A Research-Based Practical Guide*, by Clarkson,[7] for a comprehensive and detailed discussion of musculoskeletal assessment and its functional application.

Lower Extremity

Because of the somewhat stereotypical movements of the lower extremity, the arrangement of the large muscle groups, and the nature of the overall functions of weight bearing and ambulation, assumptions can be made about muscle strength during functional activities. For example, to assume a normal stance pattern, ambulate without any compensatory gait patterns, or position the lower extremities (without the assistance of the upper extremities) during dressing, a minimum of fair plus (F+) muscle strength is required in the musculature of the hips, knees, ankles, and feet. If muscle strength in the lower extremities is only fair (F) throughout the lower extremity, ambulation without aids will not be possible.[5] Good to normal muscle strength is required for the endurance to perform the small postural adjustments needed for maintained standing, repetitive movement patterns inherent in walking, and the lifting, maneuvering, and balancing on the lower limbs that usually occur during dressing.[5]

Hip Complex

The hip joints support the body weight. Each joint acts as a fulcrum when a person is standing on one leg. Hip movement makes it possible to move the body closer to or farther from the ground, bring the foot closer to the trunk, and position the lower limb in space.[7]

During functional activities, lumbar-pelvic movements accompany hip movement, which extends the functional capabilities of the hip joint. The hip is capable of flexion, extension, adduction, abduction, and internal and external rotation.[7]

Flexion and extension. Full flexion and extension are required for many ADLs and IADLs. Standing requires full hip extension. Squatting, bending to tie a shoelace with the foot on the ground, and toenail care done with the foot on the edge of a chair all require full or nearly full hip flexion. Other activities that require moderate to full flexion and extension are donning pantyhose or socks, bathing the feet in a bathtub, ascending and descending stairs or a step stool, sitting and rising in a standard chair, and riding a stationary bicycle.[7]

Abduction and adduction. Most ordinary ADLs and IADLs do not require full ranges of abduction and adduction. The main function of the hip abductors is to keep the pelvis level when one foot is off the ground. For ADLs, hip abduction may be used when stepping sideways into a shower or bathtub, donning trousers when sitting, squatting to pick up an object, sitting with the foot across the opposite thigh, getting on a bicycle, or, as in the case of Raymond, shifting weight from one foot to the other as he steps out when swinging the bat.[7,8]

Hip adduction brings the foot across the front of the body. An individual uses this motion when kicking a ball, moving an object on the floor with the foot, or crossing one thigh over the other for donning or removing shoes and socks.[7]

Internal and external rotation. Internal rotation occurs when a person is pivoting medially on one foot. When a person is sitting, there is internal rotation when the person reaches to the lateral side of the foot for washing or donning socks. Internal rotators are active in walking.[7]

External rotation with hip flexion and abduction brings the foot across the opposite thigh for donning shoes or socks or examining the sole of the foot.[7,8]

Knee

The knee joint supports the body weight. With the foot fixed on the ground, knee flexion lowers the body toward the ground and knee extension raises the body. If the foot is off the ground, as in sitting, the knee and hip are used to orient the foot in space.[7]

ADLs that require moderate to full ranges of knee flexion and extension are coming to standing and walking, squatting to lift an object from the floor, crossing the ankle of one foot over the thigh of the opposite leg, sitting down and rising from a chair, and dressing the feet.

Ankle and Foot

The foot is a flexible base of support when a person is on rough terrain. It functions as a rigid lever during terminal stance in the walking pattern. It absorbs shock when transmitting forces between the ground and the leg. The foot and ankle function to elevate the body from the ground when the foot is fixed. Dorsiflexion and plantar flexion occur at the ankle joint. Foot inversion and eversion occur at the subtalar joint.[7]

Plantar flexion and dorsiflexion. Full plantar flexion is used when a person is rising on the toes to reach upward to a high shelf. Some plantar flexion is used to depress the accelerator in an automobile or the control pedal on a sewing machine and when donning socks or shoes. Full range of dorsiflexion is needed to descend stairs. Dorsiflexion is used in such activities as positioning the foot to cut the toenails or tying shoelaces.[7] During walking the ankle moves from dorsiflexion to a neutral position and then into plantar flexion as a person strides.

Inversion and eversion. Inversion and eversion function to provide flexibility when an individual is walking on uneven ground. Inversion is used when the foot is crossed over the opposite thigh and the sole is inspected.[7]

THREADED CASE STUDY

Raymond, Part 2

In administering an occupation-based functional motion assessment at Raymond's home, the occupational therapist was able to observe that in his attempt to don his shoes and socks, Raymond was unable to abduct and externally rotate his hip sufficiently, in combination with full flexion of the knee, to place the ankle of one foot over the opposite thigh.

Upper Extremity

By simply observing a client engaging in functional activities, the therapist cannot make general assumptions as easily about muscle strength in the upper extremities as in the lower extremities. There are three reasons why this is the case: (1) the variety of ways in which the upper extremity can be positioned to complete any given task (i.e., there is not one right way to do the task), (2) the complexity of motor patterns possible requiring gross motor and fine motor skill, and (3) the dependency of the distal joints and musculature on the more proximal joints for positioning.

If several people are observed donning shirts, it will be apparent that different techniques are used by each. One person may lift the arm out to the side, increasing shoulder abduction as the shirt is drawn onto the arm. Another person might prefer to dress with the arm more in front of the body, thus positioning the humerus in flexion. A third person might hyperextend the humerus as the shirt is pulled on. The difficulty, of course, is determining exactly how much ROM and muscle strength are minimally required at all of the joints involved when so many options are available to perform one task.

In the first two examples of donning a shirt, the musculature of the shoulder complex would certainly have to create more tension than if the humerus were in the adducted position. It would be inappropriate for the therapist to instruct the client on how to don the shirt if the therapist's goal was to attain some information regarding the client's level of independence in dressing and secondarily to make assumptions about ROM and muscle strength.

When observing a client perform occupation-based tasks and motions with the upper extremities, it is important to remember that even when it is not obvious or readily apparent, the muscles of the shoulder complex are contracting with varying degrees of tension. They may have to contract with enough force to position the hand in space and maintain it there, such as when a person is combing his or her hair. At other times the humerus must be held close to the body to provide a stable base from which the forearm, wrist, and hand can maneuver, such as when hitting the keys on a keyboard, cutting food with a knife, or writing. It would be an inaccurate assumption that the extremity is just hanging passively at the side, when in fact, the static contractions around the proximal joints make it possible for the musculature of the distal extremity to work effectively. Conversely, the shoulder complex may have to be a moving unit, as opposed to a positioning one, such as when moving groceries from a countertop to shelves in a kitchen cabinet.

General guidelines exist for assessing strength for function in the upper extremities. With good to normal endurance, the client with good (G) to normal (N) muscle strength throughout the upper extremity will be able to perform all ordinary ADLs and IADLs, work, play, and enjoy leisure and social participation occupations without undue fatigue.[5] The client with fair plus (F+) muscle strength usually will have low endurance and will fatigue more easily than a client with G to N strength. The client will be able to perform many basic ADLs and IADLs independently but may need frequent rest periods. Work, play, and some social participation occupations may prove to be too strenuous, as in the case of Raymond attempting to hit a ball with force.

The client with muscle grades of fair (F) will be able to move parts against gravity and perform light tasks that require little or no resistance.[5] Low endurance is a significant problem and will limit the amount of activity that can be done. The client with low endurance probably will be able to eat finger foods and perform light hygiene if given the time and rest periods needed to reach the goals.

Poor (P) strength is considered below functional range, but the client with poor strength will be able to perform some ADLs with mechanical assistance and can maintain ROM independently when the range of motion is completed in gravity-eliminated planes or movement (see Chapter 31).

Clients with muscle grades of trace (T) and zero (0) will be completely dependent and unable to perform ADLs without externally powered devices. Some activities will be possible with special controls on equipment. Examples include power wheelchairs and electronic communication devices, such as voice recognition computers or environmental control systems (see Chapter 17).

Individuals use a variety of motor patterns when performing a functional task, and no one way is the right way to perform the task. These facts make it impossible for the therapist to predetermine the level of muscle strength, amount of ROM, and degree of motor control needed in the upper extremity to perform any given task. Individual styles of moving, numerous possibilities for compensatory movements when faced with loss of joint flexibility, poor endurance, lack of motor control, impaired sensation, and pain are all factors that may affect the client's ability to generate tension in a muscle or muscle group and sustain muscle activity. The pain Raymond experiences in his hands may be the primary cause of his inability to manipulate objects such as the buttons on his shirt.

Shoulder Complex

The shoulder complex is the most mobile joint complex in the body. Its function is to move the arm in space and position the hand for function.[9] The shoulder complex is composed of the acromioclavicular, sternoclavicular, scapulothoracic, and glenohumeral joints and the muscles, ligaments, and other structures that move and support these joints.[9,10] In the performance of functional activities, scapular, clavicular, and trunk motions normally accompany glenohumeral motion. These associated movements increase the range of glenohumeral motion for function. The shoulder complex functions in a coordinated manner that is accomplished through scapulothoracic and glenohumeral movement. This coordinated function is called scapulohumeral rhythm.[9,10] Thus, movements at the shoulder are actually combinations of several joint motions and are dependent on scapulohumeral rhythm in the performance of any given activity.[7]

Shoulder flexion and abduction with scapula upward rotation (overhead movements). Activities such as placing an object (e.g., book, box, or cup) on an overhead shelf or reaching overhead to pull on a light cord require these movements.

Shoulder extension and adduction with scapula downward rotation. Activities such as reaching back for toilet hygiene, Raymond swinging his arm backward when preparing to pitch the softball, reaching backward to put an arm through the sleeve of a coat, and pulling open a refrigerator door require these movements.[7]

Horizontal adduction and abduction. These movements allow the arm to be moved around the body. Reaching the opposite axilla or opposite ear for hygiene activities, opening and closing a sliding door, combing the hair on the opposite side of the head, fastening a necklace at the back of the neck and reaching the upper back while bathing are some activities that use horizontal adduction and abduction.[7]

Internal and external rotation. Some degree of either internal or external rotation accompanies every glenohumeral motion. The ROM varies in various positions of the arm. Full range of external rotation is required for reaching the back of the head for combing or washing the hair. External rotation is often associated with supination when the elbow is extended, as when rotating a doorknob in a clockwise direction.[7]

Internal rotation is used when buttoning a shirt, eating, and drinking from a cup. Full range of internal rotation with scapu-

lothoracic motion is used to reach into a back pocket, fasten a bra, put a belt through the belt loops on trousers, or do toilet hygiene. Internal rotation is often associated with forearm pronation, as when putting a pillow behind the low back, turning a screwdriver to unfasten a screw, rotating a doorknob in a counterclockwise direction, and pouring water from a vessel.[7]

Extension and adduction. Extension and adduction are used to return the arm to the side of the body from shoulder flexion and abduction, as after reaching overhead. These motions are also used when quick movement or force is required, as when an individual is closing a vertically oriented window, crutch walking, or pushing off to rise from an armchair, or when stabilizing the humerus to the lateral trunk, as when carrying a basket of laundry.[7]

Flexion and adduction. Flexion and adduction are used in activities that require reaching the same side of the body, such as washing the cheek or ear and combing the hair on the same side. Slight shoulder flexion with adduction is used for hand-to-mouth activities and putting on an earring back.

Elbow and Forearm

Elbow and forearm movements serve to place the hand for function.[9] Elbow flexion moves the hand toward the body, and elbow extension moves the hand away from the body. Forearm pronation or supination usually accompanies elbow flexion and extension. Pronation and supination position the hand precisely for the requirements of the given activity. The elbow and forearm support skilled and forceful movements of the hand that are used during performance of ADLs and work activities.[7]

Full or nearly full range of elbow flexion, usually with some humeral flexion and forearm supination, is used to bring food to the mouth, shave the face or underarms, hold a telephone receiver, place an earring on the ear, and reach the neck level of a back zipper.

Full range of elbow extension, usually with forearm pronation, is used when an individual is reaching to the feet to tie shoes, throwing a ball overhand, and using the arms to push off from a chair. Many other ADLs and IADLs require less than full range of these movements.[7]

Wrist and Hand

The wrist controls the length-tension relations of the extrinsic muscles of the hand. It positions the hand relative to the forearm for touch, grasp, or manipulation of objects.[8] Wrist extension and ulnar deviation are most important in performance of ADLs.[7] It is possible to perform some ADLs when there is a loss of wrist ROM by using compensatory movements of the proximal joints.

The primary functions of the hand are to grasp and manipulate objects and to discriminate sensory information about objects in the environment. The arches of the hand make it possible to adapt the hand to the shape of the object being manipulated.[12]

Power grip and precision grip are the basis of all hand activities. Power grip is used when force is required for grasping, such as holding a hammer handle, a full glass, or the handle of a purse or suitcase. Precision grip is used when an object is pinched and when it is being manipulated between the thumb and one or more fingers. Precision grip is used for holding a pencil, moving checkers or chess pieces, turning a key, threading a needle, and opening the cap of a medicine bottle.[12]

The occupational therapist observed Raymond in his home as he was preparing to make homemade soup. She noted that Raymond easily accessed ingredients that were on the first two shelves of above-counter cabinets but displayed quite a bit of facial grimacing and two attempts reaching overhead to the top shelf. He was observed being able to fully open his fingers but not able to make a tight fist. When chopping vegetables, he was able to manage the less resistive ones, such as tomatoes and celery, but could not exert enough force to cut through the carrots. Although he could carry an empty pot to the sink without difficulty, he was not able to stabilize his wrists to carry a full pot of water to the stove. At his job site the occupational therapist again noted Raymond having difficulty holding some of the heavier tools in position and exerting appropriate force, such as with the large wire cutters.

THREADED CASE STUDY

Raymond, Part 3

Because of the difficulty Raymond experienced when donning his socks and shoes, getting in and out of his truck, reaching overhead, and manipulating and applying needed force to kitchen and work tools, the occupational therapist has determined that ROM and muscle testing assessments should be administered to some of this client's specific joints and muscles.

After the occupation-based functional motion assessment, the next step in the OT process would be for the OT to plan the intervention. See Chapter 39 (Arthritis) for some ideas for interventions that could be implemented to return Raymond to participation in his customary rounds of occupation. Also, refer back to the beginning of this chapter and reflect on the three probative questions posed at the end of Raymond's case study; be able to describe the advantages of using the occupation-based functional motion assessment, the amount and type of information that was gleaned regarding Raymond from this assessment, and the value to the OT of conducting this assessment in both the home and work contexts and environments.

SUMMARY

Many physical disabilities cause deficits in ROM, strength, and motor control that limit occupational performance. The occupational therapy practitioner (i.e., the OT or the OTA under the supervision of the OT) is primarily responsible for assessing occupational performance, identifying performance problems, and planning intervention that will improve the client's occupational performance.

Because people perform the same activity in a variety of ways, the level of ROM, strength, or motor control needed to do a task is variable. Assessment of physical limitations can be made through observation of a client's performance while engaged in a variety of occupations. Therefore, as in the case of Raymond, the therapist must observe the client performing selected tasks in the person-task-environment interaction.[6]

While assessing the client's ability to perform ADLs, IADLs, work, or leisure occupations, the therapist should observe for sensorimotor problems. An analysis of the results of observation may indicate that an assessment of specific body factors or performance skills is needed.

Questions to guide clinical observation and clinical reasoning and suggested activities to assess function of the upper and lower extremities were outlined in this chapter.

REVIEW QUESTIONS

1. Compare and contrast functional motion assessment with occupation-based task and motion assessment.
2. In occupation-based practice, how are sensorimotor functions first assessed?
3. What is meant by individual activity analysis?
4. Why is it not possible to do an objective activity analysis?
5. List three major questions that can guide the clinical observation and clinical reasoning of the OT practitioner when doing an occupation-based functional motion assessment.
6. Which factors, other than strength, ROM, and motor control, can affect the functional task-motion assessment?
7. How is the information gained from assessment of specific body factors different from that gained in an occupation-based functional motion assessment?
8. What is the minimum level of strength required throughout the lower extremities for normal stance and positioning?
9. List some activities or occupations that can be used to assess general function in the lower extremities: hip, knee, ankle, and foot.
10. Compare levels of muscle strength with endurance in the upper extremities.
11. List some activities that can be used to assess general function in the upper extremities: shoulder complex, elbow and forearm, and wrist and hand.

For additional practice questions for this chapter, please visit eBooks.Health.Elsevier.com.

REFERENCES

1. American Occupational Therapy Association: Guidelines for supervision, roles, and responsibilities during the delivery of occupational therapy services, *Am J Occup Ther* 74(Suppl 3):1–6, 2020. https://doi.org/10.5014/ajot.2020.74S3004.
2. American Occupational Therapy Association: Occupational therapy practice framework: domain and process, ed 4, *Am J Occup Ther* 74(Suppl 2):1–87, 2020. https://doi.org/10.5014/ajot.2020.74S2001.
3. American Occupational Therapy Association: Occupational therapy scope of practice, *Am J Occup Ther* 75(Suppl 3): 7513410020, 2021. https://doi.org/10.5014/ajot.2021.75S3005.
4. American Occupational Therapy Association: Standards of practice for occupational therapy. 75(Suppl 3):7513410030, 2021. https://doi.org/10.5014/ajot.2021.75S3004.
5. Avers D, Brown M: *Daniels and Worthingham's muscle testing: techniques of manual examination and performance testing*, ed 10, St Louis, 2018, Elsevier.
6. Boyt Schell BA, Gillen G, Crepeau EB, Scaffa ME: Analyzing occupations and activity. In Boyt Schell BA, Gillen G, editors: *Willard and Spackman's occupational therapy* ed 13, Philadelphia, 2018, Lippincott Williams & Wilkins.
7. Clarkson HM: *Joint motion, muscle length, and function assessment: a research-based practical guide*, 2 ed. Philadelphia, 2020, Wolters Kluwer.
8. Dadio G, Nolan J: *Clinical pathways: An occupational therapy assessment for range of motion & manual muscle strength*, Philadelphia, 2019, Wolters Kluwer.
9. Lippert L: *Clinical kinesiology and anatomy*, ed 6, Philadelphia, 2017, FA Davis.
10. Muscolino JE: *Kinesiology: the skeletal system and muscle function*, ed 3, St Louis, 2017, Elsevier.
11. Polatajko HJ, Mandich A, Martini R: Dynamic performance analysis: a framework for understanding occupational performance, *Am J Occup Ther* 54:65–72, 2000.
12. Provident I, et al: Wrist and hand. In Houglum P, Bertoti D, editors: *Brunnstrom's clinical kinesiology* ed 6, Philadelphia, 2012, FA Davis.

21

Joint Range of Motion[a]

Tim Shurtleff, Vicki Kaskutas, and Rose McAndrew

LEARNING OBJECTIVES

After studying this chapter, the student or practitioner will be able to do the following:

1. Define active, passive, and functional range of motion (ROM).
2. List the purposes of measuring ROM.
3. Name two methods used to screen for ROM limitations.
4. Name disabilities for which joint measurement is often an assessment tool.
5. Describe how ROM measurements are used to select intervention goals and methods.
6. Describe how to establish ROM norms for clients with unilateral involvement.
7. Describe what the therapist should do before actually measuring the joints with the goniometer.
8. Describe proper positioning of the therapist and methods to support limbs.
9. List precautions for and contraindications to joint measurement.
10. List and describe the steps in the joint measurement procedure in correct order.
11. Describe how to record results of the joint measurement.
12. Measure all the joints of a typical practice subject by using the 180-degree method and correct procedure.
13. Describe at least three intervention strategies that can be used to increase ROM.

CHAPTER OUTLINE

---

[a]The authors would like to acknowledge previous contributions from Amy Phillips Killingsworth, Lorraine Williams Pedretti, and Heidi McHugh Pendleton.

KEY TERMS

Active range of motion

End-feel

Functional range of motion

Goniometer

Joint measurement

Palpation

Passive range of motion

Range of motion

THREADED CASE STUDY

Evelyn, Part 1

Evelyn is an 83-year-old who identifies as a woman (prefers use of the pronouns she/her/hers). She sustained a Colles fracture when she fell on her outstretched, nondominant left hand in an attempt to break her fall after tripping on a doorstop as she exited a building. The fracture was reduced, and Evelyn was placed in a hand-to-below-elbow cast for 6 weeks. On removal of the cast, Evelyn's wrist and hand appeared swollen. She complained of pain and stiffness in the carpometacarpal and metacarpal joints of her thumb and the metacarpophalangeal and proximal interphalangeal joints of her fingers. She was unable to make a fist or oppose her thumb to her fingers.

Evelyn is a widow; her two grown children live nearby. Before her injury she was independent in all ADLs and the majority of IADLs. She used public transportation to move around her community, although her children and friends usually drove her to appointments. Evelyn volunteered at the local hospital weekly in its telecare program and called elderly, home-bound persons. She is an accomplished seamstress, makes all of her own clothing, and attends a weekly sewing class, primarily for the camaraderie of the other students, although she states, "There is always something new to learn." She also enjoys baking for her family, gardening, and generally engaging in tasks that contribute to the upkeep of her home. She attends church regularly and enjoys dining out with friends and family members.

Since her injury, her ability to participate in occupations that are meaningful to her has been curtailed. She requires moderate to maximal assistance to hold a utensil in her left hand while cutting food with her right, wash and style her hair, put on jewelry, bathe the right side of her body, transfer out of the bathtub, and engage in home maintenance tasks (e.g., changing bed linen). At her volunteer work site, she is unable to hold the telephone with her left hand while writing with her right hand and because of privacy issues does not want to use the speaker phone feature. When cooking, she has difficulty stabilizing bowls, pots, and pans with her left hand while manipulating a cooking utensil with her right. Evelyn is experiencing a great deal of frustration with her loss of independence and inability to fully engage in occupations that got her out in the community and facilitated interaction with others.

In reviewing Evelyn's occupational profile, the occupational therapist must focus on client factors that are interfering with function. Loss of range of motion (ROM) in her left upper extremity, especially the inability to flex the fingers to make a fist and oppose the thumb to the fingers, which is required for fine motor activities, is prohibiting the client from fully engaging in the physical, social, personal, cultural, and spiritual contexts that bring meaning to her life. Before determining intervention goals and strategies, the therapist must assess her ROM limitations to establish a baseline for treatment. While reading and studying this chapter, keep in mind Evelyn's ROM limitations and the restrictions that they impose on her engagement in occupation.

Critical Thinking Questions

1. Why should the occupational therapist proceed with caution when assessing the ROM limitations of this client?
2. What is the appropriate sequencing of joint measurement assessment for this client? What methods should be applied first?
3. What is the advantage of joint measurement in evidence-based practice?

Joint range of motion (ROM) is the amount of movement that is possible at a joint.[3,15] It is the arc of motion at a joint within a specific plane. When the joint is moved by the muscles that act on the joint, it is called active range of motion (AROM). When the joint is moved by an outside force such as the therapist, it is called passive range of motion (PROM).[3] In normal individuals, PROM is slightly greater than AROM because of the slight elasticity of soft tissue.[3,10] The additional PROM that is available at the end of normal AROM helps protect joint structures because it allows the joint to give and absorb extrinsic forces. If PROM is significantly greater than AROM for the same joint motion, it is likely that muscle weakness is present.[13]

Decreased ROM can cause limited function and interfere with performance in areas of occupation. Limitations in ROM may occur as a result of injury to or disease in the joint or the surrounding joint tissue structures, joint trauma, or joint immobilization. These limitations may restrict the client's ability to perform successfully in chosen day-to-day occupations. Inflexibility at a joint may adversely affect both speed and strength of movement. A client who constantly has to work to overcome the resistance of an inflexible joint will probably demonstrate decreased endurance and fatigue during activity. The functional motion test (see Chapter 20), screening tests, and measurement of joint ROM with a goniometer can all be used to assess ROM.

RANGE OF MOTION AND THE OCCUPATIONAL THERAPY PRACTICE FRAMEWORK, VERSION 4

The Occupational Therapy Practice Framework (OTPF) version 4 does not specifically mention ROM testing, because it is an enabling physical component of participating in occupation, which is the primary focus of occupational therapy. However, many of the areas of emphasis of the OTPF can be seen to support the testing of ROM in the process of evaluating a client's capability, or of their limitations in the performance of their desired activities and occupations. To illustrate the importance of ROM testing in the context of the occupation focus of the OTPF, the following sections and references are provided with page numbers noted in parentheses.

- Motor skills[2] *is one of the observable and measurable subsets of the category of performance skills* (also listed under Domain in Exhibit 1 [p. 7], and detailed in Table 7 [p. 42]): These are defined as to how a person effectively "moves self, positions the body, obtains, and holds objects" to enable occupation. Measurement of a client's ROM quantifies how much a client can "move self" and "position the body" and whether they can "obtain and hold objects" to perform tasks, activities, and occupations. Measurement of ROM enables an occupational therapist to understand baseline limitations in movement and forms a basis to develop interventions to increase ROM or to compensate for limited ROM depending on the cause of the ROM limitation, all in the interest of improving occupational performance. ROM measurement is also a means of measuring progress and the effectiveness of interventions. Although ROM does not independently predict success at occupational performance, improving ROM can be a source of feedback and encouragement to a client to continue with interventions developed with an OT.

- *Performance skills are observable in the context of activities* (p. 13): ROM is a critical component of the performance of many activities that require movement of the body, even the most basic ADLs. For example, without sufficient shoulder flexion ROM, it is difficult to don a shirt without assistance or devices. Limited finger/thumb ROM makes it difficult to grasp items with which to perform everyday activities that add up to complex occupations. Toileting requires shoulder extension and rotation and sufficient elbow, wrist, and finger ROM to achieve and maintain hygiene. An occupational therapist may decide to measure the ROM of component movements to determine where and how to focus treatment to improve the performance of these and many other basic and necessary tasks.
- "The practitioner analyzes the client's challenges in performance and generates a hypothesis about gaps between current and effective performance" (p. 14): ROM limitation is often one of the underlying reasons for the gaps identified. Measuring and documenting those limitations provides useful information in the evaluation and treatment planning process, as well as the measurement of progress toward effective performance.
- *"Client factors are specific capacities, . . . affected by . . . disability"* (p. 15): ROM limitations are often outcomes from disease, injury, and congenital or developmental disabilities.
- *Evaluation (Exhibit 2—Evaluation* (p. 16): One component of the occupational profile is the answer to the question: "How are the client's performance patterns supporting or limiting occupational performance and engagement?" Motor skills, including ROM, are some of those performance patterns referenced here.
- *Analysis of occupational performance* (p. 23): "Selecting specific assessments . . . relevant to occupations . . . effectiveness of performance skills and performance patterns." One of the specific assessments that is often employed to provide a starting point to understand performance limitations is ROM screening, which can lead to specific measurement of those movements that show limitations. Interpretation of those assessments, including ROM, helps to identify supports and limitations.
- *Intervention:* Of the intervention approaches listed in the OTPF (p. 24), "establish or restore, maintain, modify, or prevent" may benefit from ROM data to develop a treatment plan and to measure progress in these enabling skills toward improved occupational performance.
- *Direct services* (p. 18): Working with a client to improve ROM may fit into the category of "person-level direct service delivery."

- *Occupation and activity analysis* (pp. 19, 23): "Occupational therapy practitioners analyze the demands of an occupation or activity to understand the performance patterns, performance skills, and client factors that are required to perform it."[2] Understanding the ROM required to perform activities that are components of occupation can be a valuable input to understanding how gaps in a person's ROM compared to the ROM activity demands affect a person's ability to perform. This becomes part of the basis of an intervention plan to improve ROM or find compensatory methods or equipment support performance of the activities. Additionally, the OTPF section describing the Analysis of Occupational Performance (pp. 22–23) states that this process includes "selecting and using specific assessments to measure client factors (including ROM) that influence performance skills and performance patterns."
- *Evaluation: Screening and measurement activities* (p. 21): Most practitioners have their favorite initial screens. Many of them include a basic screen of ROM. These screens determine if detailed measurement of specific joint ROM is needed to provide sufficient information to develop an effective intervention strategy. This chapter specifies that *standardized or structured ROM screening and measurement methods* are needed so practitioners can have interrater and intrarater reliability by communicating and documenting limitations in a standardized way. This is especially important when multiple OT practitioners and OT assistants use evaluation data about a single client, which is the case in many treatment settings.
- *Occupations* (Table 2, pp. 30–34): This table defines and details categories of occupation. Reading through the listing provides too many examples to list of activities to support occupations.
- *Examples of occupations* (Table 3, p. 35): Includes many activities that would benefit from an activity analysis being performed (with ROM of needed movement), would provide a comparison baseline with which to compare the client's ROM to determine gaps that might affect performance.
- *Motor skills and performance skills for persons* (Table 7, p. 43): Positions self—ROM is an essential component of skills to position the body (e.g., stabilize, align, position, reach, bend, grip, manipulate). Examples of effective and ineffective performance of these skills are given in the table. Similar examples are given for "moving self and objects."

The listed items are some of the many references in the OTPF in which ROM might be relevant and indicate that screening/measurement of ROM might be helpful for an occupational therapist as part of the evaluation of a client's limitations. ROM screening and measurement can be used in the context of an activity analysis within that occupational profile to develop an effective treatment plan. Although the specific terms of ROM, AROM, or PROM might not be mentioned in the OTPF, ROM is relevant and critically important in the occupational performance of many desired client tasks and necessitate occupational therapy practitioners to possess the knowledge and skills to assess this client factor. The procedures and skills in this chapter are intended to provide a consistent foundation for occupational therapy practitioners (both therapists and assistants) to screen and measure ROM, both active and passive, and do it in a way that is precise and consistent to ensure intrarater and interrater reliability creating valid and useful data to support OT intervention.

OT PRACTICE NOTES

The primary concern of the occupational therapist using the skills described in this chapter is to determine whether ROM is adequate for the client to engage in meaningful occupations.

Methods used to screen limitations in ROM involve the observation of AROM and PROM. To screen for AROM, the therapist asks the client to perform all the active movements that occur at the joint.[3] To screen for PROM, the therapist moves the joint passively through all of its motions to estimate ROM, detect limitations, and observe the quality of movement, end-feel, and the presence of pain.[3] The therapist can then decide at which joints precise ROM measurement is indicated.

JOINT MEASUREMENT

The joints of the body need to move fluidly to perform the activities and occupations that are meaningful to people, such as driving, parenting, working, playing, studying, and social participation. Reaching overhead to shampoo hair, squatting to pick up a child, and operating the foot pedals in an automobile require movements of the joints of the body. A wide array of client factors influence joint motion, such as aging, obesity, developmental conditions, injuries and illnesses, and chronic health conditions. Body structures that affect joint ROM include the bones and joints, ligaments and cartilage, muscles and tendons, skin and fat, and the nervous system. The ability of the muscles that are performing the movement to generate tension is important, as is the ability of the muscles on the opposite side of the joint to stretch to allow movement. Restricted ROM may result from skin contracture caused by adhesions or scar tissue; arthritis, fractures, burns, and hand trauma; displacement of fibrocartilage or the presence of other foreign bodies in the joint; bony obstruction or destruction; and soft tissue contractures, such as tendon, muscle, or ligament shortening. Limited ROM may be secondary to spasticity, muscle weakness, pain, and edema.[8,13] For example, for full knee extension ROM to occur, the muscles that straighten the knee must have adequate contractibility and the muscles that flex the knee must be long enough to stretch across the backside of the knee. Lifestyle, environmental, and occupational factors can also affect joint mobility. Goniometry is an evaluation tool used to assess ROM of the joints of the body.

ROM measurements can help the therapist identify treatment goals, intervention methods, and preventive activities to restore, compensate, modify, and prevent limitations and enhance occupational performance. ROM measurement is useful to identify limitations that interfere with function or may produce deformity, additional motion needed to increase functional capacity or reduce deformity, the need for orthoses and assistive devices,

and progression of treatment. The use of formal joint measurement will assist in determining the efficacy of intervention and may also serve as evidence in assisting the client to see the outcome of the intervention through quantifiable data.

Tables documenting ranges for normal ROM measurements exist in the literature.[4] These may be useful guides; however, ROM varies from one person to another. It is important to avoid making assumptions about identified ROM limitations when comparing to normative values; the client may be able to function remarkably well with the ROM limitations, although the client may need more ROM than is considered "normal" to perform an especially meaningful activity. The occupational history and client interview will help identify baseline ROM. If one extremity is impaired, the analogous uninvolved part also can be a useful guide.[4,5] The presence of joint and other structural limitations from previous health conditions and the immediate illness or injury should be considered. Joints should not be forced when resistance is met on PROM. Pain may limit ROM, and crepitus (grinding, crackling sound or feeling) may be heard or felt with movement in some conditions. Therefore, before beginning joint measurement procedures, the therapist must explain what will be done and ask if the client is experiencing any joint pain and, if so, where it is located and how severe it is. To not cause undue pain, the occupational therapist further explains to the client the importance of indicating any changes in pain throughout the procedure.

Planes and Axes of Movement

It is important to understand the planes and axes of movement. Motion occurs in three cardinal planes, two of which are vertical, the frontal (coronal) and sagittal planes, and one that is horizontal, the transverse plane (Figs. 21.1 to 21.4). The planes of movement do not change even if the position of the body changes, that is, supination/pronation is always in the transverse plane even if the elbow is straight or bent to 90 degrees. The axes, which are perpendicular to the joint, are the pivot point for the joints. The frontal (coronal) plane divides the body into anterior (front) and posterior (back) portions.

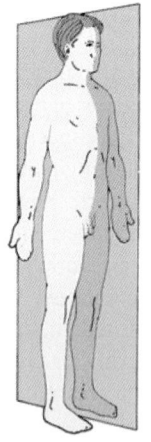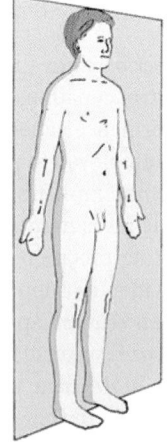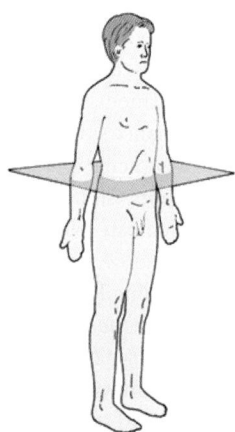

Sagittal plane   Frontal plane   Transverse plane

Fig. 21.1 Sagittal, frontal, and transverse planes. (From Cameron MH, Monroe L: *Physical rehabilitation for the physical therapist assistant*, St Louis, 2011, Saunders.)

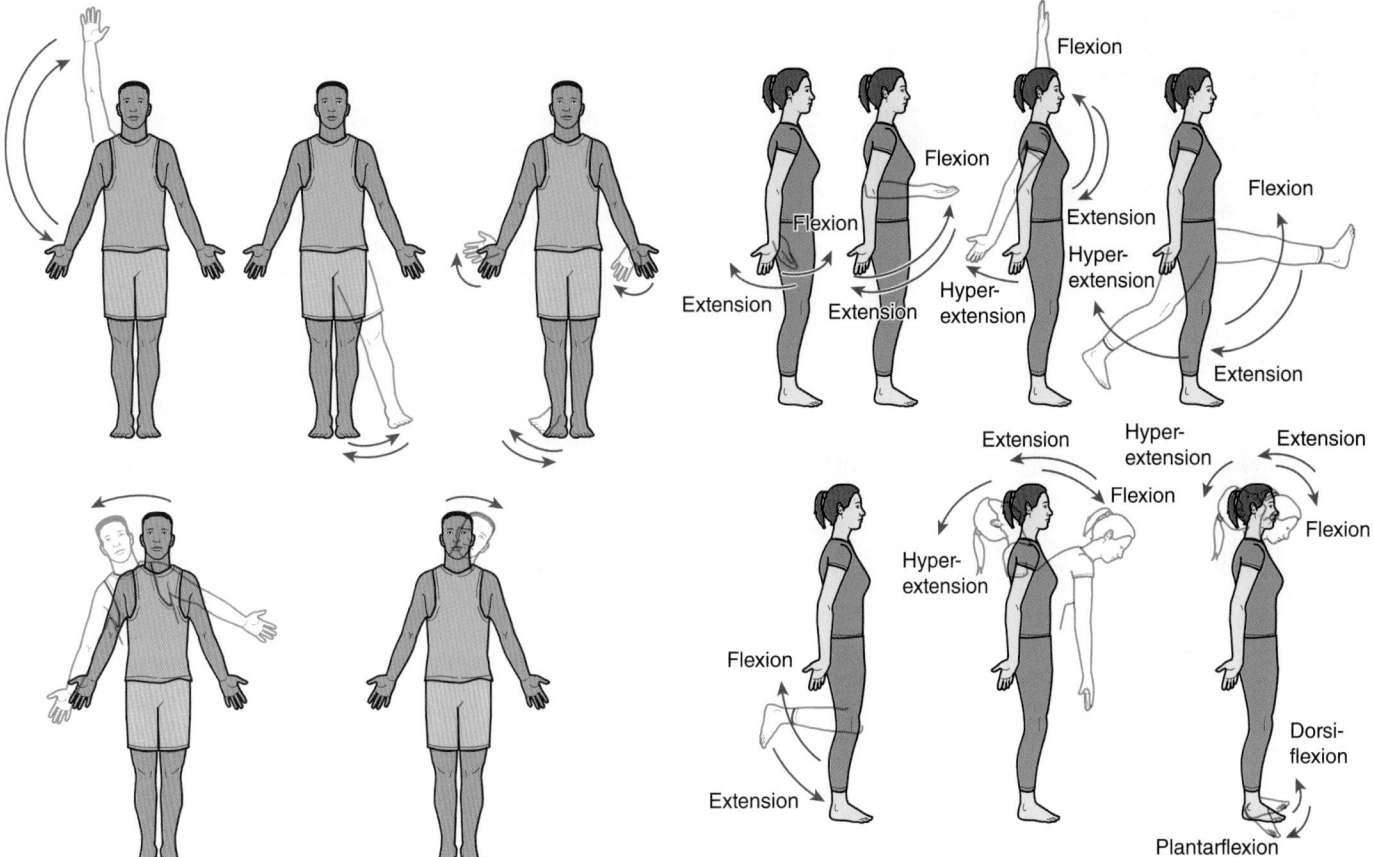

Fig. 21.2 Motions that occur in the frontal plane include abduction, adduction, and spine lateral flexion to the right and left (side-bending).

Fig. 21.3 The sagittal plane divides the body into right and left portions, whether it is through the center of the entire body (spine) or through an extremity (upper or lower extremity). Motions that occur in the sagittal plane are flexion and extension.

PRINCIPLES AND PROCEDURES IN JOINT MEASUREMENT

Before measuring PROM, the therapist should be familiar with normal end-feel, average normal PROM ranges, joint structure, and function, safe handling methods, and bony landmarks related to each joint and joint axis.[4,5,11] The therapist should be skilled in correct positioning and stabilization for measurements, palpation, alignment and reading of the goniometer, and accurate recording of measurements.[10] For the most reliable measurements, it is best that the same therapist assesses and reassesses the client at the same time of day with the same instrument and the same measurement protocol.[3] Because that is not always feasible, when there are alternative measurement protocols and tools, the specific protocol used for measurement must be described with the measurement data to ensure test-retest and interrater reliability.

Visual Observation

The joint to be measured should be exposed, and the therapist should observe the joint and adjacent areas.[4] The therapist asks the client to move the part through the available ROM actively and independently, if muscle strength is adequate, and observes the movement.[4] The therapist should look for compensatory motions, posture, muscle contours, skin color and condition, and skin creases and compare the joint with the noninjured part, if possible.[4] The therapist should then move the part through its range to the tolerance of the client to see and feel how the joint moves and to estimate PROM.

Palpation

Feeling the bony landmarks and soft tissue around the joint is an essential skill gained with practice and experience. The pads of the index and middle fingers are used for palpation. The thumb is sometimes used. The therapist's fingernails should not contact the client's skin. Pressure is applied gently but firmly enough to detect underlying muscle, tendons, or bony structures. For joint measurement, the therapist must palpate to locate bony landmarks for placement of the goniometer.[3]

Positioning of Therapist and Support of Limbs

The therapist's position varies, depending on the joints being measured. When measuring finger or wrist joints, the therapist may sit next to or opposite the client. If sitting next to the client, the therapist should measure the wrist and finger joints on that side and then move to the other side to measure the joints on the client's opposite side. This procedure makes the client more comfortable (eliminating the need to stretch across the midline)

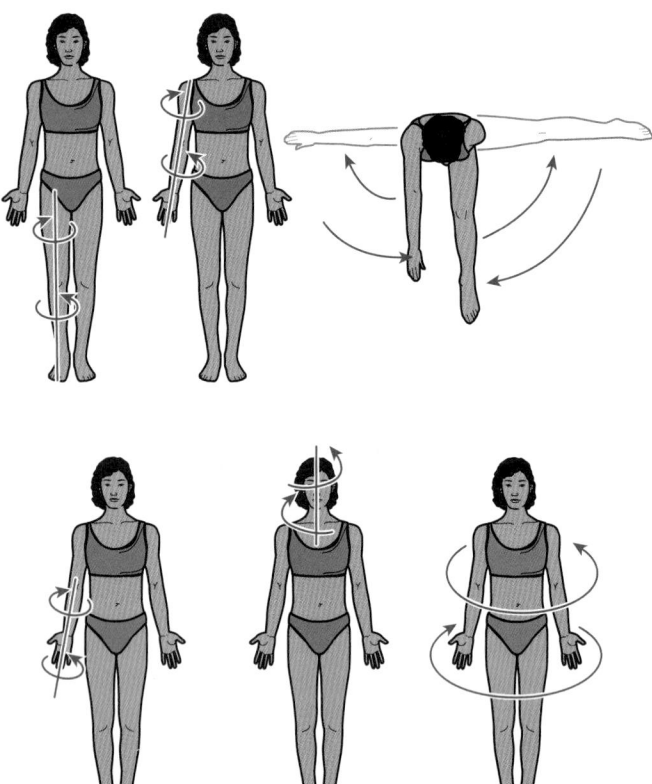

Joint measurement must always be done carefully. The following situations call for extreme caution[3,10]:

1. The client has joint inflammation or an infection.
2. The client is taking either medication for pain or muscle relaxants.
3. The client has osteoporosis, osteoarthritis or rheumatoid arthritis, hypermobility, or subluxation of a joint.
4. The client has hemophilia.
5. The client has a hematoma.
6. The client has just sustained an injury to soft tissue.
7. The client has a newly united fracture.
8. The client has undergone prolonged immobilization.
9. Bony ankyloses or excessive osteophyte formation around joint surfaces is suspected.
10. The client has carcinoma of the bone or any fragile bone condition (e.g., osteogenesis imperfecta—brittle bone disease).

End-Feel

PROM is normally limited by the structure and health of the joint and surrounding soft tissues. Thus, ligaments, the joint capsule, muscle, and tendon tension, contact of joint surfaces, and soft tissue approximation may limit the end of a particular ROM. Each of these structures has a different end-feel as the therapist moves the joint passively through its ROM. End-feel is the resistance to further joint motion because of stretching of soft tissue, ligamentous and joint capsule limitations, approximation of soft tissue, and contact of bone on bone. End-feel is normal when full PROM is achieved, and the motion is limited by normal anatomic structures. Abnormal end-feel occurs when PROM is increased or decreased or when PROM is normal but structures other than normal anatomy stop the PROM.[3]

End-feel is normally classified as hard, soft, or firm. An example of hard end-feel is bone contacting bone when the elbow is passively extended, and the olecranon process comes into contact with the olecranon fossa. Soft end-feel can be detected on elbow flexion when there is soft tissue apposition of the forearm with the elbow flexor muscles of the upper arm. A firm end-feel has a firm or springy sensation that has some give, as when the ankle is dorsiflexed with the knee in extension and PROM is limited by tension in the gastrocnemius muscle.[3]

In pathologic states, end-feel is abnormal when PROM is increased or decreased significantly from the standards listed in Table 21.1 (later in chapter) or when PROM is normal but movement is stopped by structures other than normal anatomy.[3] For example, elbow flexion may have a hard end-feel because of a bony osteophyte or surgically implanted plate, or the end-feel may be firmer than normal as a result of excessively large muscle bulk. Practice and sensitivity are required for the therapist to detect different end-feels and to distinguish normal from abnormal.[3,10] The normal end-feel for each joint and directions for joint measurement are described in the following sections.

Two-Joint Muscles

Many of the deep muscles that move a joint cross only one joint; however, the more superficial muscles usually cross two or more joints. When a one-joint muscle contracts, it moves the one joint

Fig. 21.4 The transverse (horizontal) plane divides the body into upper and lower portions: motion occurs around a vertical axis in the transverse plane, whether it is rotation to the right and left (spine), internal and external rotation (shoulder and hip), or pronation and supination (forearm).

and ensures more accurate placement of the goniometer. When measuring the larger joints of the upper or lower extremity, the therapist may stand next to the client on the side being measured. The client may be seated or lying down. The therapist needs to use good body mechanics when reaching, lifting, and moving heavy limbs. The therapist should use a broad base of support and stand with the head upright while keeping the back straight. The feet should be shoulder width apart, with the knees slightly flexed. The therapist's stance should be in line with the direction of movement. The therapist should be positioned close to the client when lifting the limb. The limb should be supported at its center of gravity, approximately where the upper and middle thirds of the segment meet. To ensure patient comfort, the therapist's hands should be in a relaxed broad grasp that conforms to the contours of the part without pinching or allowing fingers to dig into the body part. The therapist can provide additional support by resting the part on his or her forearm.[4]

Precautions and Contraindications

In some instances, measuring joint ROM is contraindicated or should be undertaken with extreme caution. It is contraindicated if there is a joint dislocation or unhealed fracture, immediately after surgery on any soft tissue structures surrounding joints, in the presence of myositis ossificans, or when ectopic ossification is a possibility.[3]

that it acts at; subsequently this muscle is stretched when the joint is moved into the opposite direction. A muscle that crosses two or more joints is not long enough to allow for full stretch when both joints that it crosses are simultaneously moved into the opposite direction of muscle contraction. A two-joint muscle feels taut when it is at its full length over both joints that it crosses and before it reaches the limits of the normal PROM of both joints.[7] Positioning is of utmost importance as PROM at one joint may be affected by the position of the other joint because of passive insufficiency.[3] For example, the extrinsic finger flexor muscles cross anterior to the wrist and finger joints, so they have insufficient length to allow for simultaneous extension of the wrist and fingers. When joints crossed by two-joint muscles are being measured, it is necessary to place the other joint (the one not being measured) in a neutral or relaxed position to place the two-joint muscle in slack. In the finger flexor example, the wrist should be placed in a neutral position when measuring finger extension PROM to prevent passive insufficiency of the extrinsic finger flexor from restricting finger extension PROM. Similarly, when hip flexion is being measured, the knee should be flexed to place the hamstrings in the slackened position,[3] and when knee flexion is measured, the hip should be flexed to relax the rectus femoris, which crosses both the hip and knee joints. Avoiding passive insufficiency ensures that the measurement of a joint actually measures only the limits of the joint and not unintended limits of the muscles.

METHODS OF JOINT MEASUREMENT

There are two systems for measuring joint ROM, the 180-degree and the 360-degree systems. Both systems use a goniometer, a protractor with two arms (movable and stationary), to measure ROM. The goniometer is superimposed on the body in the plane in which the motion is to occur. The axis of the goniometer is placed on the moving joint and the two arms are placed on the body parts that form the joint. When measuring the elbow joint, the axis is at the elbow, the stationary arm is on the proximal upper extremity, and the movable arm is on the forearm. In the 360-degree system the protractor is a full circle, whereas the protractor is a half-circle in the 180-degree system. Either system can be used to measure the moving elbow joint with results easily transposed between systems. This chapter focuses on the 180-degree system; however, the 360-degree system is briefly discussed.

The 360-Degree System

In this system, movements occurring in the coronal and sagittal planes are related to the full circle. When the body is in the anatomic position, the circle is superimposed on it in the same plane in which the motion is to occur, with the goniometer axis placed on the joint center in line with the axis of movement. "The 0-degree (360-degree) position will be overhead and the 180-degree position will be toward the feet."[5] Thus, for example, shoulder flexion and abduction are movements that proceed toward 0 degrees, and shoulder adduction and extension proceed toward 360 degrees. The average normal ROM for shoulder flexion is 170 degrees in the 180 degree system (outlined below). Therefore, in the 360-degree system, the movement would start

at 180 degrees and progress toward 0 to 10 degrees. The ROM recorded would be 10 degrees. On the other hand, shoulder extension that has a normal ROM of 60 degrees would begin at 180 degrees and progress toward 360 to 240 degrees, and 240 degrees would be the ROM recorded.[5] The total ROM of extension to flexion would be 240 to 10 degrees—that is, 230 degrees.[5,6]

The 180-Degree System

A more common method of joint measurement is the 180-degree system. In the 180-degree system of joint measurement, 0 degrees is the starting position for all joint motions. For most motions, the anatomic position is the starting, or 0-degree, position (Fig. 21.5). All joint motions begin at 0 degrees and increase toward 180 degrees.[3,5,10] Some motions cannot be related to the full circle. In these instances, a 0-degree starting position is designated (as anatomic or neutral position) and the movements are measured as increases from 0 degree. These motions occur in a horizontal plane around a vertical axis. They are forearm pronation and supination as well as hip and shoulder internal rotation (IR) and external rotation (ER).

The exceptions to the rule that the anatomic position defines the 0 point of all measurements of joint movement are illustrated by forearm pronation/supination. The anatomic position always includes shoulder ER and elbow extension, which make it very difficult to isolate supination and pronation in this position. In the anatomic position the palms face forward, with the forearms at maximum supination, requiring some shoulder ER to reach this position. This is not 0 for pronation/supination or shoulder rotation. The 0-degree position or starting point of movement for forearms and shoulder occurs when the palms

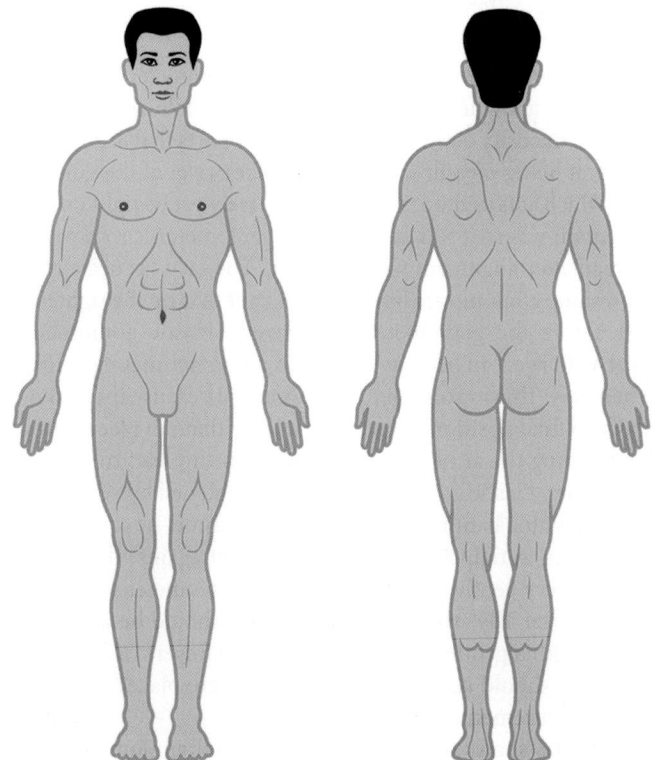

Fig. 21.5 For most motions, the anatomic position is the starting or 0-degree position. (From GettyImages.com.)

face the thigh, thumbs forward. This exception to the 0 point for supination/pronation and shoulder IR/ER has everything else in the standard anatomic position, but the palm is facing the thigh with thumbs facing forward. This position is a variation on the traditional anatomic position and is called the 0 position, or the neutral position.

Goniometers

Usually made of metal or plastic, goniometers come in several sizes and types and are available from medical and rehabilitation equipment companies.[6,11,12] The word *goniometer* is derived from the Greek *gonia*, which means angle, and *metron*, which means measure.[9,14] Thus, goniometer literally means "to measure angles." The universal goniometer consists of a body attached to a stationary (proximal) bar and a movable (distal) bar.[3,10] The stationary bar is attached to the body of the goniometer. The body is a half-circle or a full-circle protractor printed with a scale of degrees from 0 to 180 for the half-circle and 0 to 360 for the full-circle goniometer.[3,4] The movable bar is attached at the center, or axis, of the protractor and has a line or pointer on the protractor. As the movable bar rotates around the axis, the dial points to the number of degrees on the protractor scale.

In many goniometers, two scales of figures are printed on the full or half circle. Each starts at 0 degree and progresses toward 180 degrees, but in opposite directions, often printed in black in one direction and in red in the other. Because the starting position in the 180-degree system is always 0 degree and increases toward 180 degrees, the outer row of figures is read if the bony segments being measured are end to end, as in elbow flexion. The inner row of figures is read if the bony segments being measured are alongside one another in anatomic position, as in shoulder flexion. The scale to read is the one that reads 0 in the anatomically neutral position.

To ensure accuracy, it is best to use a goniometer that is long enough to allow for the stationary and movable arms to align over the majority of the length of the body parts that articulate at the joint being measured. The grommet or rivet of the goniometer, which acts as the axis, must move freely yet be tight enough to remain where it was set when the goniometer is removed to be read after alignment with the joint.[4] For easy, accurate readings, some goniometers have a locking nut that can be tightened just before the goniometer is removed.[5] Plastic goniometers wear with age, can become loose, and are sometimes even loose when new. This makes them difficult to use because they do not stay in a final position to be read. Holding them in place to read by pinching the arms to immobilize them can lead to slippage and errors. Plastic goniometers may be tightened by very gently tapping with a hammer on the rivet or grommet or squeezing it with pliers to tighten the rivet or grommet against the plastic. Do this very gently because a too-tight goniometer is also difficult to use. The arms of the goniometer should be able to be moved with a gentle force applied with the fingers of one hand. The arms should stay in the position they are placed in during joint measurement.

Fig. 21.6 shows several types and styles of goniometers. The first five (Figs. 21.6A–E) are full-circle goniometers and may

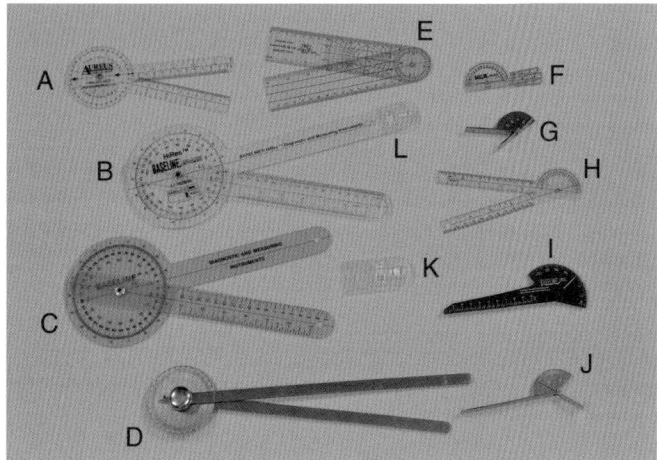

Fig. 21.6 Types and styles of goniometers.

have calibrations for both the 360-degree and the 180-degree systems printed on their face. Figs. 21.6B–D have longer arms and are usually best for use on the large joints of the body. Figs. 21.6B–C are the same size but note that one is shaded plastic and one is clear. They function the same and shading or clear may be more visible in some situations (as noted in the following images). Figs. 21.6F and 21.6H have half-circle protractors used for the 180-degree system. Fig. 21.6F is simply an inexpensive 6-inch goniometer, like Fig. 21.6H, that has been cut to more easily measure the small joints of the hand and digits. The movable arms in Figs. 21.6F and 21.6H have an extension that crosses the axis and allows one to read either scale regardless of whether the convexity of the half circle is directed toward or away from the direction of motion. Thus, the evaluator does not have to reverse the goniometer and thereby obscure the scale to read it. Figs. 21.6G, Fig. 21.6I, and 21.6J are special finger and hand goniometers. Figs. 21.6G and 21.6J have arms that are short and flattened. They are designed to lie flat over the finger joints and adjacent dorsal surfaces rather than on their lateral aspects, as is done for most of the larger joint motions. It is also designed to be used on the hand and digits, but the protractor itself rotates and the flat side follows the dorsal surface of the joints of the hand rather than the arm rotating on the stationary protractor. Figs. 21.6E and 21.6H are best for smaller joints as shown throughout this chapter, but they can also be used for larger joints if a large goniometer is not available. These small plastic goniometers are inexpensive and easy to carry in a pocket.

Note that one of the larger goniometers (Fig. 21.6L) has a set of spirit levels (bubble levels) on the end of the stationary bar. These enable correct vertical and horizontal orientation of the stationary bar and protractor for movements that are compared to the level line of the world when a patient is in anatomic or neutral position (e.g., forearm pronation and supination, IR, and ER of the shoulder when measured in abduction). Fig. 21.6K is a spirit level that can be slipped over the end of a large (12-inch) goniometer like Fig. 21.6C and removed when not needed.

Other types of goniometers are available. Some are inclinometers, which have a fluid indicator that responds to gravity and provides the reading after the motion is completed; they must be read while they are on the body part.[5] Others can be attached to two body segments and have dials that register ROM electronically with digital output, but are normally used only in research settings. There are special goniometers for cervical and spine ROM measurements and for forearm rotation.[11] A tape measure or metric scale also may be used on some joints by measuring the distance between two segments, for example, the distance between the chin and chest when measuring cervical flexion, extension, and rotation, the distance between the center of the tips of two fingers for finger flexion or abduction, and the distance between the tip of the thumb and the tip of the little finger for opposition.[3]

RECORDING MEASUREMENTS

The 180-Degree System

When using the 180-degree system, the evaluator should record the number of degrees at the starting position and the number of degrees at the final position after the joint has passed through the maximally possible arc of motion.[10] Normal ROM always starts at 0 degrees in anatomic or neutral positions and increases toward 180 degrees. When it is not possible to start the motion at 0 degrees because of limitation of motion, ROM is recorded by writing the number of degrees at the starting position followed by the number of degrees at the final position.[3] For example, elbow ROM limitations can be noted as follows:

- Normal: 0 to 140 degrees
- Extension limitation: 15 to 140 degrees
- Flexion limitation: 0 to 110 degrees
- Flexion and extension limitation: 15 to 110 degrees

Abnormal hyperextension of the elbow may be recorded by indicating the number of degrees of hyperextension below the 0-degree starting position with a minus sign, followed by the 0-degree position and then the number of degrees at the final position.[10] This may be noted as follows:

- Normal: 0 to 140 degrees
- Abnormal hyperextension: −20 to 0 to 140 degrees. A potential problem with this numbering system is that it works for an elbow but does not work well for joints such as the shoulders, hips, and metacarpals that naturally move past 0 without indicating a potentially pathological excess ROM, which is written with the negative number.

An alternative that avoids this problem is the three-number system. The three-number system is most useful with joints that can move in either direction past their neutral position, with 0 being the typical anatomic position; however, it can be used with any joint. Negative numbers are never used to avoid the confusion cited earlier. The three numbers represent total motion of a joint, with the first number denoting the amount of motion that occurs when the extremity moves beyond the expected anatomic position (extension or hyperextension in the sagittal plane, and toward the body in the frontal or horizontal planes), the second number representing whether neutral (anatomic position) was achieved or not, and the third number denoting the amount of motion achieved as joint moves in opposite direction from anatomic position (flexion in the sagittal plan, and away from body in frontal and horizontal planes). Normal ROM of the shoulder in the sagittal plane is to extend to 60 degrees, to swing neutral (0 degrees or anatomic position), and flex to 170 degrees. In the three-number system the measurement is recorded as 60/0/170. The total amount of motion in the sagittal plane at the shoulder joint is the amount of hyperextension plus the amount of flexion (60 + 170), for a total of 220 degrees. Normal elbow ROM is from 0 degrees extension to 135 to 150 degrees of flexion. A client with elbow flexion to 140 degrees and extension to 0 degrees is reported as 0/0/140 in the three-number system. Their elbow is capable of moving through 140 degrees of motion (0 + 140 = 140). If this client could hyperextend the elbow 15 degrees past neutral, the measurement is recorded as 15/0/140. The client's elbow is capable of moving 155 degrees of motion (15 + 140 = 155). If this client lacks 15 degrees of elbow extension (unable to achieve 0/neutral/anatomic position), the measurement is recorded as 0/15/150. The elbow moves through 135 degrees of motion (150–15 = 135 degrees), but the starting position is in 15 degrees of elbow flexion. ROM in any joint and plane can be reported in this manner, with the motion toward the body always reported first: adduction, IR, ulnar deviation, pronation, and inversion. The OT practitioner should always state the motion in each position of the three-number system.

Because there are alternative methods of recording ROM, the evaluator is advised to learn and adopt the particular method commonly and consistently used by the healthcare facility and professional peers with whom one works to limit any misunderstanding of AROM or PROM notation and to ensure interrater reliability in remeasuring and interpretation.

A sample form for recording ROM measurements is shown in Fig. 21.7. Average normal ROM for each joint motion is listed on the form and in Table 21.1 (later in chapter). When recording ROM, there are rare instances in which it is clinically important to measure every joint on the form. Every space on the form should be filled in with numbers for those joints tested. If the joint was not tested, "NT" should be entered in the space or some sections lined through to avoid confusion in the future.[3]

When joint measurements are performed in more than one position (e.g., as in alternative shoulder IR and ER positions), the evaluating occupational therapist should document the position in which the measurement was taken. The therapist should also note the position of the joint at the point pain or discomfort is experienced by the client, the appearance of protective muscle spasm, and whether AROM or PROM or both was being measured. Record the points (degrees of ROM) where tightness started, progressed to discomfort, and then became felt as pain and any deviations from recommended testing procedures or positions.[10] This becomes important information to document recovery from injury over time or as a result of therapist intervention.

JOINT RANGE MEASUREMENTS

Client's name _____ Chart no. _____

Date of birth _____ Age _____ Sex _____

Diagnosis _____ Date of onset _____

Disability _____

LEFT					RIGHT		
3	2	1	**SPINE**		1	2	3
			Cervical spine				
			Flexion	0-45			
			Extension	0-45			
			Lateral flexion	0-45			
			Rotation	0-60			
			Thoracic and lumbar spine				
			Flexion	0-80			
			Extension	0-30			
			Lateral flexion	0-40			
			Rotation	0-45			
			SHOULDER				
			Flexion	0 to 170			
			Extension	0 to 60			
			Abduction	0 to 170			
			Horizontal abduction	0-40			
			Horizontal adduction	0-130			
			Internal rotation	0 to 70			
			External rotation	0 to 90			
			ELBOW AND FOREARM				
			Flexion	0 to 135-150			
			Supination	0 to 80-90			
			Pronation	0 to 80-90			
			WRIST				
			Flexion	0 to 80			
			Extension	0 to 70			
			Ulnar deviation	0 to 30			
			Radial deviation	0 to 20			
			THUMB				
			MP flexion	0 to 50			
			IP flexion	0 to 80-90			
			Abduction	0 to 50			
			FINGERS				
			MP flexion	0 to 90			
			MP hyperextension	0 to 15-45			
			PIP flexion	0 to 110			
			DIP flexion	0 to 80			
			Abduction	0 to 25			
			HIP				
			Flexion	0 to 120			
			Extension	0 to 30			
			Abduction	0 to 40			
			Adduction	0 to 35			
			Internal rotation	0 to 45			
			External rotation	0 to 45			
			KNEE				
			Flexion	0 to 135			
			ANKLE AND FOOT				
			Plantar flexion	0 to 50			
			Dorsiflexion	0 to 15			
			Inversion	0 to 35			
			Eversion	0 to 20			

Fig. 21.7 Form for recording joint ROM measurement.

Results of Assessment as the Basis for Planning Intervention

After joint measurement, the therapist should analyze the results in relation to the client's life role requirements. The therapist's first concern should be to correct ROM that is below functional limits. Many ordinary activities of daily living (ADLs) do not require the maximum ROM listed in the tables. Functional range of motion refers to the amount of joint range necessary to perform essential ADLs and instrumental activities of daily living (IADLs) without the use of special equipment. The first concern of intervention is to attempt to increase to functional levels any ROM that is limiting performance of self-care and home maintenance tasks, if deemed reasonable based on body structure impairments the client experiences.[8] For example, severe limitation of elbow flexion affects eating and oral hygiene. Therefore, it is important to increase elbow flexion to nearly full ROM for function. Likewise, severe limitation of forearm pronation affects eating, washing the body, telephoning, caring for children, and dressing. Because sitting comfortably requires hip ROM of at least 0 to 100 degrees, a first goal might be to increase flexion to 100 degrees if it is limited. Of course, if additional ROM can be gained, the therapist should plan the progression of intervention to increase ROM to the normal range.

Some limitations in ROM may be permanent. The role of the therapist in such cases is to work with the client to develop methods to compensate for the loss of ROM. Possibilities include assistive devices, such as a long-handled comb, brush, shoehorn, and device to apply socks or stockings, or adapted methods of performing a particular skill. (See Chapter 10 for further suggestions for ADL techniques in those with limited ROM.)

In many conditions, such as burns and arthritis, loss of ROM can be anticipated with clients. The goal of intervention is to prevent joint limitation with orthoses, positioning, exercise, activity, and application of the principles of joint protection.

Limited ROM, its causes, and the prognosis for increasing ROM will suggest intervention approaches. Some of the specific methods used to increase ROM are discussed elsewhere in this text (see Chapters 29 and 39). Such methods include stretching exercises, resistive activity and exercise, strengthening of antagonistic muscle groups, activities that require active motion of the affected joints through the full available ROM, splints, and positioning. To increase ROM, the physician may perform surgery or manipulate the part while the client is under anesthesia. The OT, PT, or certified hand therapist may use joint mobilization techniques such as manual stretching with heat and massage.[8] Some surgeries (e.g., rotator cuff repair) require long periods of restriction of AROM while the surgery site (tendon grafts to bone) heals. During these periods (often 6–8 weeks) a shoulder can develop persistent or even permanent loss of ROM during this period if it is not moved passively to its limits. During this precaution period it is often the role of the therapist (OT or PT) to passively move the shoulder on a regular treatment schedule in all planes to the point of tolerance as specified by the surgeon. This will maintain joint mobility while the patient observes surgical precautions of no AROM in physician-specified planes that would pull on the grafts and damage the repairs. Monitoring PROM during these treatments provides data about progress or maintenance of joint ROM or helps identify problems to communicate to the surgeon.

PROCEDURE FOR MEASURING PASSIVE RANGE OF MOTION

Average normal maximum ROM for each joint motion is listed in Table 21.1 and before each of the following procedures used for measurement. The reader should keep in mind that ROM may vary considerably among individuals, and these tables contain averages of maximum ROM. Normal ROM is affected by age, sex, injury, and other factors, such as lifestyle and occupation.[10] Therefore, the client in the illustrations may not always demonstrate the average maximum ROM listed for the particular motion.

In the illustrations, the goniometer is shown in such a way that the reader can most easily see its positioning. Therefore, the occupational therapist in the pictures may not always be in the optimum position for body mechanics during the measurement. For the purposes of clear illustration, the therapist may be shown off to one side and may have only one hand, rather than both hands, on the instrument and the joint. For many of the motions the occupational therapist would typically be in front of the client, or the therapist's hands may obscure the goniometer. For this reason, do not assume that the pictures indicate the *correct* position for the therapist during measurement and do not assume you must follow the picture precisely. How the therapist holds the goniometer and supports the body part being measured in practice is determined by several factors such as the position of the client, amount of muscle weakness, presence or absence of joint pain, and whether AROM or PROM is being measured. Both the therapist and the client should be positioned based on the judgment of the therapist and the feedback from the client for the greatest comfort, correct placement of the goniometer, and adequate stabilization of the body part being tested, to ensure the desired motion in the correct plane is measured accurately.

General Procedure: 180-Degree Method of Measurement[3,10]

1. The client should be comfortable and relaxed in the appropriate position (described later) for the joint measurement.
2. Uncover the joint to be measured.
3. Explain and demonstrate to the client what you are going to do, why, and how you expect him or her to cooperate.
4. If there is unilateral involvement, assess PROM on the analogous limb to establish normal ROM for the client.
5. Establish and palpate bony landmarks, which will be used to align the axis and arms of the goniometer.
6. Stabilize joints proximal to the joint being measured.
7. Ensure that when measuring joints that are operated by two-joint muscles (e.g., finger flexors, extensors, and rectus

TABLE 21.1   Average Normal Range of Motion (180-Degree Method)

Joint	Range of Motion (Degrees)	Associated Girdle Motion	Joint	Range of Motion (Degrees)
Cervical Spine			**Thumb**	
Flexion	0 to 45		DIP flexion	0 to 80–90
Extension	0 to 45		MP flexion	0 to 50
Lateral flexion	0 to 45		Palmar abduction	Neutral to 50
Rotation	0 to 60		Radial abduction	Neutral to 50
Thoracic and Lumbar Spine			Opposition	Thumb pad to touch pad of little finger
Flexion	0 to 80		**Fingers**	
Extension	0 to 30		MP flexion	0 to 90
Lateral flexion	0 to 40		MP hyperextension	0 to 15–45
Rotation	0 to 45		PIP flexion	0 to 110
Shoulder			DIP flexion	0 to 80
Flexion	0 to 170	Abduction, lateral tilt, slight elevation, slight upward rotation	Abduction	0 to 25
Extension	0 to 60	Depression, adduction, upward tilt	**Hip**	
Abduction	0 to 170	Upward rotation, elevation	Flexion	0 to 120 (bent knee)
Adduction	0	Depression, adduction, downward rotation	Extension	0 to 30
Horizontal abduction	0 to 40	Adduction, reduction of lateral tilt	Abduction	0 to 40
Horizontal adduction	0 to 180	Abduction, lateral tilt	Adduction	0 to 35
Internal rotation		Abduction, lateral tilt	Internal rotation	0 to 45
Arm in abduction	0 to 70		External rotation	0 to 45
Arm in adduction	0 to 40		**Knee**	
External rotation		Adduction, reduction of lateral tilt	Flexion	0 to 135
Arm in abduction	0 to 90		**Ankle and Foot**	
Arm in adduction	0 to 60		Plantar flexion	0 to 50
Elbow			Dorsiflexion	0 to 15
Flexion	0 to 135–140		Inversion	0 to 35
Extension	0		Eversion	0 to 20
Forearm				
Pronation	0 to 80–90			
Supination	0 to 80–90			
Wrist				
Flexion	0 to 80			
Extension	0 to 70			
Ulnar deviation (adduction)	0 to 30			
Radial deviation (abduction)	0 to 20			

DIP, Distal interphalangeal; *MP*, metacarpophalangeal; *PIP*, proximal interphalangeal.

Data from American Academy of Orthopaedic Surgeons: *Joint motion: method of measuring and recording*, Chicago, IL, 1965, The Academy; and Esch D, Lepley M: *Evaluation of joint motion: methods of measurement and recording*, Minneapolis, MN, 1974, University of Minnesota Press.

femoris), the other joint is positioned to put those muscles in a relaxed (shortened) state avoiding passive insufficiency, which will limit ROM of the joint you are measuring.

8. Move the part passively through ROM to assess joint mobility and end-feel.

9. Return the part to the starting position.

10. To measure the starting position, place the goniometer just over the surface of the joint and in the plane of movement. Place the axis of the goniometer over the axis of the joint by using the designated bony prominence or anatomic landmark. With some joints that are embedded in soft tissue (such as the glenohumeral joint) the therapist must visualize the center based on knowledge of skeletal anatomy and adjacent surface landmarks (e.g., two fingers inferior to the acromion is a good approximation of the placement of the glenoid fossa and humeral head which are the true joint center). Place the stationary bar on or parallel to the longitudinal axis of the proximal part (e.g., the trunk) or along the stationary/proximal bone and place the movable bar on or parallel to the longitudinal axis of the distal or moving bone. Keep the plane of the goniometer aligned with the correct plane of movement of the joint.

11. Record the number of degrees at the starting position and follow the movement or remove (or back off) the goniometer until maximum ROM is achieved. It is acceptable but not necessary to hold the goniometer in place and follow the joint through the arc of ROM. Measurements at each end of ROM are sufficient.

12. To measure PROM, hold the part securely above and below the joint being measured and gently move the joint through ROM. Do not force the joint. Watch for signs of pain and discomfort. Note that PROM also may be measured by asking the client to move actively through ROM. Note the degree of AROM. From the final AROM position the therapist then moves the joint passively through the final few degrees to a normal stop or to the point at which the client indicates movement becomes painful and then measures PROM. There is no need to force a joint past a normal maximum ROM even if it is not painful (remember that there also may be sensory damage and pain may not be felt, even if it will go further or joint or soft tissue damage may result).

13. Reposition the goniometer and record the number of degrees at the final position. It is often necessary to stabilize the joint in its maximum PROM position with one hand, with furniture or with an assistant in difficult cases. Learning to operate the goniometer with the other hand alone becomes a very useful skill in PROM measurement.

14. Remove the goniometer and gently place the part in the resting position.

15. Record the reading at the final position and make any notes on the evaluation form about which of the alternative measurement methods you might have used or variations from standard procedure that were necessary because of client condition or position.

Understanding the Goniometry Measurement Figures

The figures in this chapter help guide the correct client and goniometer positioning for AROM and PROM. When an alternative method for taking measurements is used in clinical practice, additional descriptions and figures are provided.

MOTION SCREEN

It is almost never necessary to measure the ROM of all joints of the body. Most injuries, disabilities, and health conditions affect only part of the body. The first step to measuring ROM is to conduct a quick screen of the motions of the major joints of the body. This gives the therapist a first look at movement ability and limitations. It also gives the therapist early information about which motions the therapist might want to measure and document in detail. Some movements might be observed as "Within Normal Limits" (WNL) or "Within Functional Limits" (WFL). In this case they need no further measurement because they are not limited enough to impair ADL, IADL, or other important occupations. There are many varieties and sequences of motion screens with different levels of completeness. A new therapist in a treatment facility would be advised to confer with colleagues to see what they use as a screen so they can be consistent in the way their screens are documented and to ensure test-retest reliability for monitoring a patient's progress in treatment notes. The motion screen (unnumbered table) provides an illustrated example of one way to do a screen:

1. The therapist stands in front of the client to model each movement and performs each movement and asks the client in layman language to perform it. Because they are facing each other, the therapist should perform movements on the opposite side (mirror image) from what the client is asked to do so the client is not confused by the left-right instructions compared to what they see as the therapist models each movement.

2. The screen is ideally performed standing, but if a client cannot stand unaided, it can be modified to be done from a sitting position.

3. Because some movements are mirror images, some are only illustrated with a left or right movement when both are requested in the screen.

4. Motion screen sequence:

A. Starting Position
"Stand straight looking forward; look at me."

B. Cervical Flexion
"Look down, bend your neck so your chin is close to your chest."

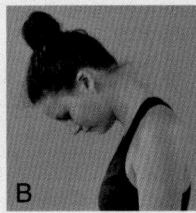

C. Cervical Extension
"Look up, bend your head back as far as you can."

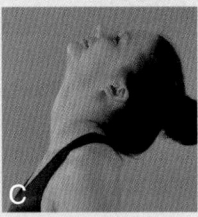

D. Cervical Horizontal Rotation
"Turn your head to the right as far as you can. Now turn your head to look to the left."

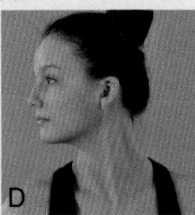

E. Thoracolumbar Lateral Flexion
"Bend your body as far as you can to the left. Now bend to the right."

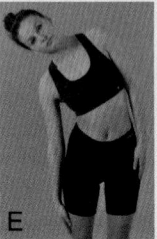

F. Thoracolumbar Horizontal Rotation
"Twist your body to the right as far as you can. Now twist to the left."

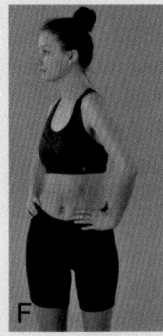

G. Thoracolumbar Flexion
"Bend over and touch your toes or the floor."

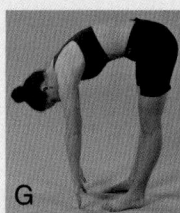

H. Shoulder Flexion With Elbow Extension
"Raise both arms as high and straight as you can."

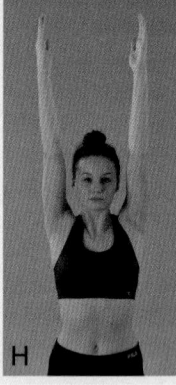

I. Shoulder External/Lateral Rotation
"Touch the back of your head with both hands."

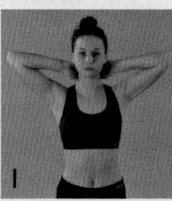

J. Shoulder Internal/Medial Rotation
"Touch your back with both hands."

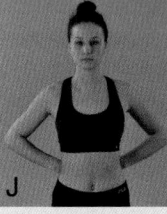

K. Elbow Flexion
"Bend your elbows up and touch your chin or shoulders."

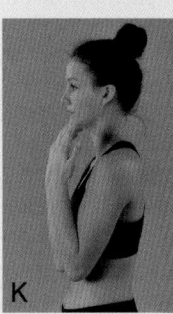

(Continued)

L. Elbow Extension
"Straighten your elbows down with palms forward."

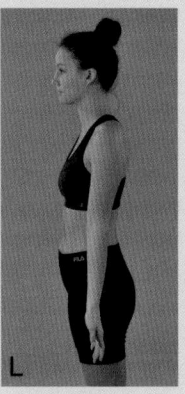

M. Hip and Knee Flexion While Balancing and Weight Bearing
"Squat down like this." (Therapist should stand near client to assist with balance.)

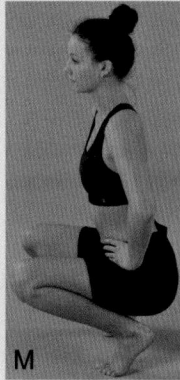

N. Alternative Methods for Hip and Knee Flexion
Alternative Method 1 (Top):
"Lift your right knee as high as you can while standing. Now your left knee. You can hold onto a chair if you need to." (Therapist should stand near client for balance assistance.)
Or
Alternative Method 2 (Bottom):
"Sit down and pick up each knee as high as you can."

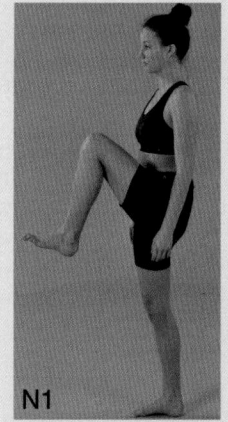

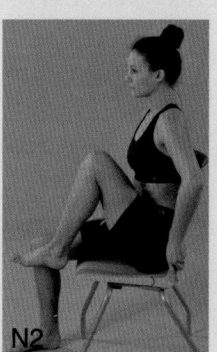

O. Dorsiflexion
"While sitting, point your foot up."

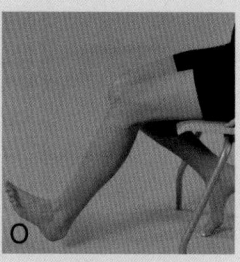

P. Plantar Flexion
"Now point your foot down."

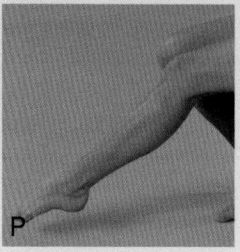

The following movements can be done in either a sitting or standing position.

Q. Wrist Extension
"Bend your elbows so both hands are out in front of you. Lift your hands at the wrist, like this."

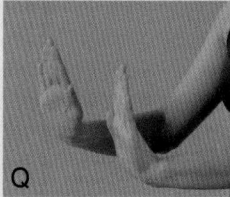

R. Wrist Flexion
"Now bend your wrists down."

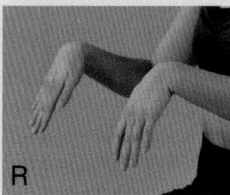

S. Composite Digit Flexion
"Make a fist with both hands, thumbs on top."

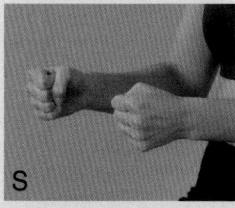

T. Composite Digit Extension
"Open both hands and spread your fingers."

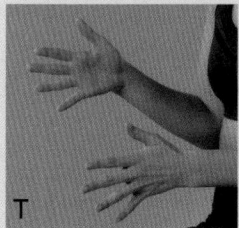

(Continued)

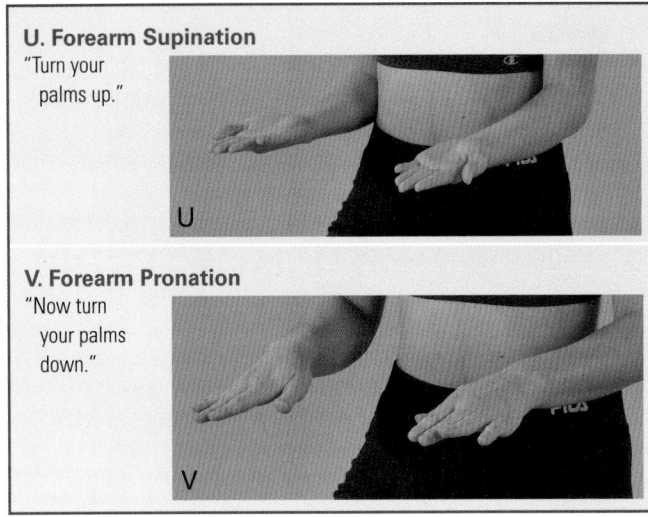

U. Forearm Supination
"Turn your palms up."

V. Forearm Pronation
"Now turn your palms down."

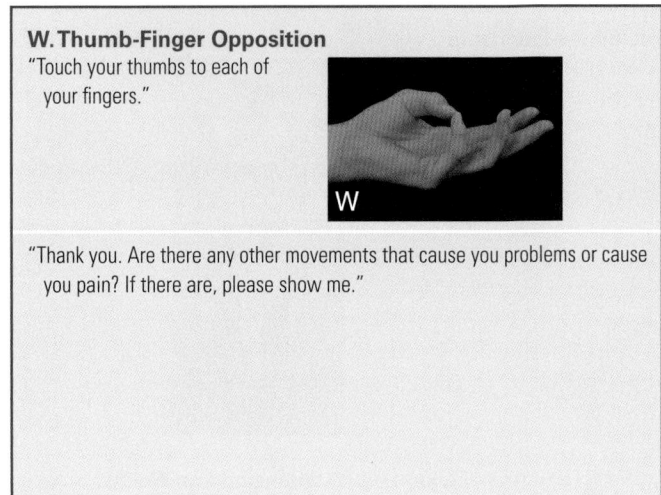

W. Thumb-Finger Opposition
"Touch your thumbs to each of your fingers."

"Thank you. Are there any other movements that cause you problems or cause you pain? If there are, please show me."

The following sections demonstrate specific directions for joint measurement using the 180-degree system (see Fig. 21.7).

SPINE

Cervical Spine

Measurements of neck movements are the least accurate because the neck has few bony landmarks and much soft tissue overlying the bony segments. It is also composed of a series of joints and therefore does not have only one axis.[4] Radiographic examination is the best means to make an accurate measurement of the specific joints.[12] However, general measurements may be taken with a tape measure to record the distance between the chin and chest for flexion and extension, between the chin and shoulder for neck rotation, and between the mastoid process and shoulder for lateral flexion.[3]

Approximate estimates of cervical flexion, extension, rotation, and lateral flexion may be made with the goniometer or by estimating the number of degrees of motion by using a fixed landmark and axis (e.g., midline on posterior aspect of head compared to the horizontal line from C7 to acromion or vertically down spine as proximal base of movement). Then the arc of motion is measured between those two lines.[1,4]

Cervical Flexion

- 0 to 45 degrees (Fig. 21.8)
  Neutral Position of the Client
- Sitting or standing erect, with the head vertical
  Measurement. The client is asked to flex the neck so that the chin moves toward the chest. If a goniometer is used (see Fig. 21.8A), the axis is placed over the angle of the jaw. The stationary bar is held horizontal to align with the starting motion of the mandible. The movable bar follows the mandible toward the point of the chin.

As an alternative method, the movable arm of the goniometer can be aligned with a tongue depressor, which the client is holding between the teeth. As the client performs neck flexion,

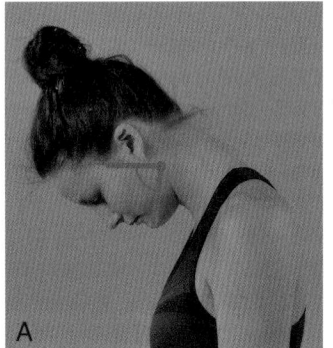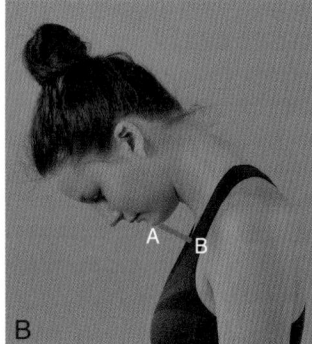

Fig. 21.8 (A) Axis, landmarks, arc. (B) Chin to sternal notch.

the movable bar of the goniometer is adjusted downward to align with the new position of the tongue depressor.[4,10]

In another alternative method, the number of degrees of motion may be estimated, or the therapist may measure the number of inches or centimeters from the bone at the tip of the chin to the sternal notch (see Fig. 21.8B).[1,3,10] Recognize that when the head is flexed forward, soft tissue may bunch up around the chin. The bony tip of the chin must be found by palpation to measure this distance.

Cervical Extension

- 0 to 45 degrees (Fig. 21.9)
  Neutral Position of the Client
- Sitting or standing erect, with the head vertical
  Measurement. The client is asked to extend the neck as though looking at the ceiling so that the back of the head approaches the thoracic spine. The number of degrees of motion may be estimated, or the number of inches or centimeters from the chin to the sternal notch may be measured.[3] If a goniometer is used, the axis is placed over the angle of the jaw and the stationary bar is held horizontal corresponding with a theoretically level mandible. The therapist grasps the corner of the protractor and steadies his or her arm against the client's shoulder to stabilize and avoid substitution by extending the thoracic spine. The client can hold a tongue depressor in the teeth. The movable

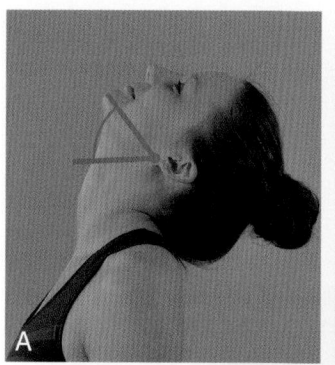
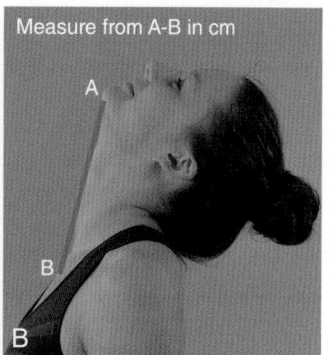

Measure from A-B in cm

A

B

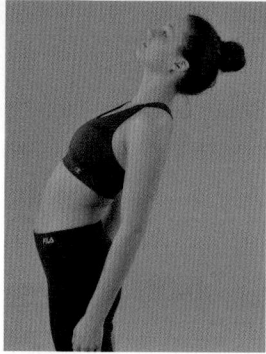

Fig. 21.9 (A) Axis, landmarks, arc. (B) AROM. (C) Substitution.

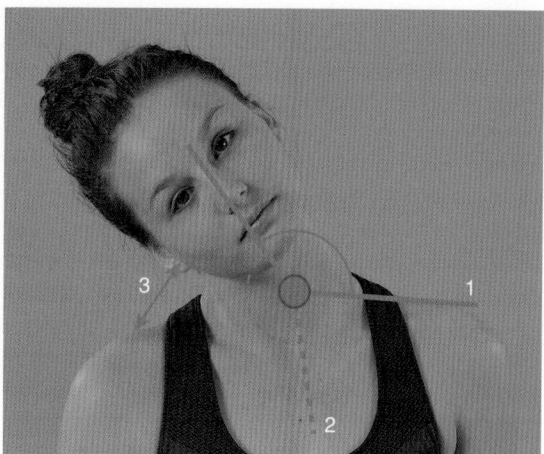

Fig. 21.10 Alternative methods.

bar of the goniometer is moved upward to align with the mandible or the tongue depressor as the client extends the neck. It is important to document which method is used to ensure reliable measurements over time or between therapists.[4,10]

Substitution. If cervical extension is inadequate, a client may attempt to achieve additional extension by extending the thoracic and lumbar spine (see Fig. 21.9C). Although this may enable the client to look upward, it does not actually increase cervical extension by changing the angle of the head to the trunk.

Cervical Lateral Flexion

- 0 to 45 degrees
  Neutral Position of the Client
- Sitting or standing erect, with the head vertical
  Position of the Client
- Sitting or standing erect
  Measurement. The client is asked to flex the neck laterally without rotation by moving the ear toward the shoulder. The number of degrees of motion may be estimated. If a goniometer is used, the axis is typically placed over the spinous process of C7 (the seventh cervical vertebra) if measured on the posterior neck, or with the axis pointed toward the larynx if measured from the anterior side. The stationary bar may be over the shoulder toward the acromion if that yields a starting position of 0 degrees (Fig. 21.10, labeled *1*) or parallel to the floor if the trunk is vertical so that the motion begins at 90 degrees. Or it may be aligned with the thoracic vertebra or sternal notch (see Fig. 21.10, labeled *2*) if the client is not in a vertical position. On the posterior side, the movable bar is aligned with the midline of the external occipital protuberance or the midline of the forehead between the eyes if measured anteriorly, as in Fig. 21.10.

As an alternative method (see Fig. 21.10, labeled *3*), the therapist may measure the number of inches or centimeters between the mastoid process and the acromion process of the shoulder. Given these alternatives, and because there is no single standard method of measuring this movement, it is critical that the measurement method and landmarks be described in the notes to ensure reliability in repeat measurement.

Cervical Horizontal Rotation

- 0 to 60 degrees
  Neutral Position of the Client
- Sitting or standing erect, with the head vertical, facing forward
- Lying supine or seated
  Measurement

Sitting/Standing. The client is asked to rotate the head right or left without rotating the trunk. The therapist can provide stabilization to reduce shoulder movement occurring because of trunk rotation.

As a screen, the amount of rotation may be estimated in degrees from the neutral position,[1] or from a therapist position above the head with client in a seated position, a goniometer can be used. The goniometer will be set at 90 degrees with the axis placed over the vertex in the center of the top of the head, aligned with C1, as close as the therapist may estimate the axis of rotation of the head on the entire cervical spine. The stationary bar can be held in one of three positions. (1) It can be held steady on the sagittal plane relative to the trunk. (2) If the client is sitting, the stationary bar can be aligned with the frontal plane of the trunk in line with the acromion process on the side being tested. (3) If the client is lying supine with both shoulders on a firm horizontal surface, the goniometer can be held parallel to the table or floor or vertically. In any of these positions, the movable bar is aligned with the tip of the nose on the sagittal plane of the head to follow the rotation in the horizontal plane as the head rotates on the neck relative to the shoulders. The deviation from the 0 point, regardless of how it is found, is the horizontal rotation of the head on the cervical spine (this method is not illustrated in a photograph).[4,10]

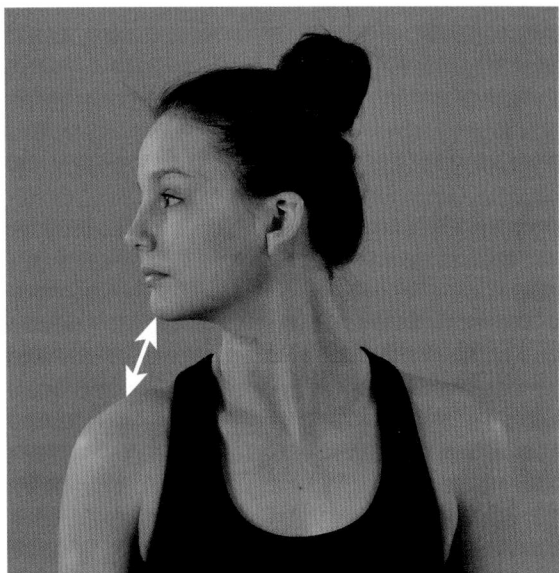

Fig. 21.11 Measurement of the distance from the tip of the chin to the acromion process with neck rotated.

Alternative Method. A tape measure also may be used to measure the distance from the tip of the chin to the acromion process of the shoulder. The measure is taken first in the anatomic position with the face forward aligned with the sagittal plane of the trunk, and the deviation is measured again after the head has been rotated in the horizontal plane on the cervical spine. The difference in measurement between the two positions is the amount of rotation (Fig. 21.11).[3]

Thoracic and Lumbar Spine

Thoracolumbar Flexion

- 0 to 80 degrees and 4 inches
  Neutral Position of the Client
- Standing erect, facing forward
  Measurement. Spinal flexion is a combination of several joints and is difficult to measure with a goniometer because the axis of movement varies along the thoracolumbar spine providing no single point of flexion on which to anchor a goniometer. However, the combined movement can be measured with a goniometer using two reference points for the movable bar, the greater trochanter of the femur at the hip and the acromion process at the shoulder. Both points can be palpated. The stationary bar can be aligned with the greater trochanter and the lateral epicondyle of the femur at the knee. This method is illustrated in Fig. 21.12A and B (using the *red lines* drawn on the photograph).

  Alternative Methods. Four alternative methods of estimating the range of spinal flexion are as follows:

1. Measuring trunk forward flexion in relation to the longitudinal axis of the body (the therapist must hold the pelvis stable with the hands and observe any change in the client's normal lordosis), recording the level of the fingertips along the front of the client's leg.
2. Measuring the number of inches or centimeters between the client's fingertips and the floor, and
3. Measuring the length of the spine from the seventh cervical vertebra to the first sacral vertebra when the client is erect

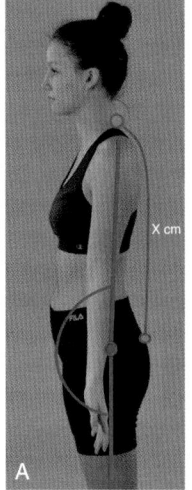
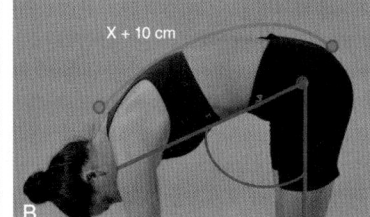

Fig. 21.12 (A) Beginning measure. (B) Ending measure.

and again after the client has flexed the spine. This measurement method is illustrated with the blue lines in Figs. 21.12A and B).[3,10] The third alternative method Fig. 21.12B may be the most accurate.[1] In a normal adult, the average increase in length in forward flexion of the spine is 4 inches (approximately 10 cm).[3]

As long as the method of aligning the stationary bar is described so a follow-up measure can be replicated with interrater and intrarater reliability, any of these methods are acceptable.

Thoracolumbar Extension

- 0 to 30 degrees (Fig. 21.13)
  Neutral Position of the Client
- Standing erect, facing forward, level pelvis (same neutral position as thorocolumbar flexion depicted in Fig. 21.12A)
  Measurement. The client is asked to bend backward while maintaining stability of the pelvis. If necessary, the therapist can stabilize the pelvis to maintain a neutral pelvis by holding their pelvis between the anterior superior iliac spines and the iliac crests from the front. If freestanding, the client will likely thrust the pelvis in an anterior direction while tilting the pelvis anteriorly (as in Fig. 21.9C) to keep center of gravity over the base of support to not fall. Another method of stabilizing would be to place the client's pelvis against a table or desk before leaning back to secure a neutral pelvis. In any of these alternative methods, the range of extension is measured as the arc illustrated in Fig. 21.13 or estimated in degrees from a neutral pelvis by using the superior iliac crest as the pivotal point in relation to the spinous process of C7. If the client is freestanding and the pelvis naturally tilts anteriorly with thoracolumbar extension to maintain the center of gravity over the base of support, the stationary bar of the goniometer must still be aligned with the pelvis instead of being held vertical relative to the earth as it would be for a neutral stabilized pelvis. This is depicted as a *dotted line* at a right angle to the line between the anterior superior iliac spine (ASIC) and the posterior superior iliac spine (PSIC) as depicted in Fig. 21.13A.

  Alternative method.

  Fig. 21.13B shows the same starting position that is used for thoracic flexion above (using the blue lines). The measurement points are also the same. Extension will shorten the measurement

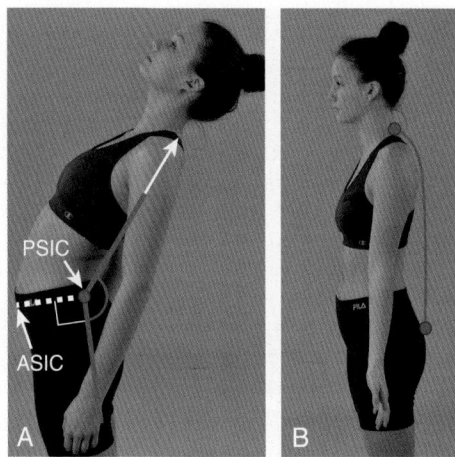

Fig. 21.13 Thoracolumbar extension, starting position (A) and ending position with substitution (B). Note that thoracolumbar extension has the same starting position as thoracolumbar flexion with the same measurement points. The measurement will shorten with thoracolumbar extension.

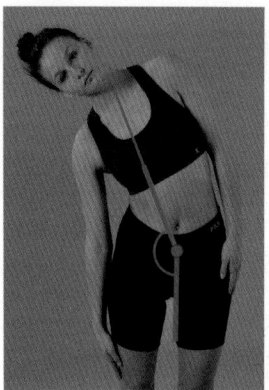

Fig. 21.14 Thoracic lateral flexion ending measure. The beginning measurement is not shown.

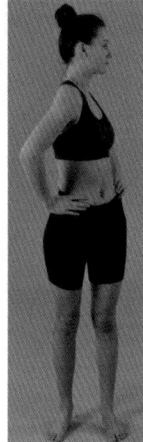

Fig. 21.15 Trunk and pelvic rotation without stabilization.

during thoracolumbar extension. The *difference* between the measurements in anatomic position and in extension is recorded as the amount of extension. This method should be documented specifically in notes to ensure reliability with repeated measurements.

Alternative Position. With the client in the prone position, the client's hands are placed at shoulder level on the treatment table. The pelvis is stabilized with a strap (a long gait belt around the table will work) or by an assistant. The client extends the elbows to raise the trunk from the table into thoracolumbar extension. A perpendicular measurement can be taken of the distance between the suprasternal notch and the supporting surface at the end of the ROM,[3] or a goniometer can be used, with the stationary bar held horizontal (aligned with the stabilized pelvis), the axis at the iliac crest, and the movable bar points toward C7. In all methods above, the arc being measured is the deviation from the vertical line of a theoretically neutral pelvis as shown in the AROM picture in Fig. 21.13A.

Thoracolumbar Lateral Flexion

- 0 to 40 degrees
  Neutral Position of the Client
- Standing erect, facing forward
  Measurement. Several methods may be used to estimate the range of lateral flexion of the trunk. A straight edge or yardstick may be held in place during the motion and be used to estimate the number of degrees of lateral inclination of the trunk with respect to the vertical position.

Measuring Using Goniometer. A long-arm goniometer (Fig. 21.14) can be used on the dorsal or ventral surface of the trunk. Placing the axis on the mid-pubic bone (as in the photograph) or at the sacroiliac joint, hold the stationary bar perpendicular to the floor and the movable bar aligned with the larynx (or with C7).[1,10]

Alternative Methods. Other methods include estimating the angle of the spinous process of C7 in relation to a vertical line from the sacroiliac joint of the pelvis; measuring the distance of the fingertips from the knee joint in lateral flexion; and measuring the distance between the tip of the third finger and the floor.[3] Because there are several measurement method options, it is important to describe the method used in any treatment

notes to ensure test-retest reliability so this movement is measured again in a comparable manner.

Thoracolumbar Rotation

- 0 to 45 degrees (Fig. 21.15)
  Neutral Position of the Client
- Standing erect, facing forward, or sitting
  Measurement. Because of the distance from the hips to the shoulders, this is a measurement that can be best approximated only in standing. It is also difficult for a client to isolate thoracolumbar rotation from pelvic rotation at the hips, as illustrated in Fig. 21.15. The client is asked to rotate the upper part of the trunk while maintaining a neutral position of the pelvis as much as possible. Because these movements are difficult to isolate, the therapist might visually align the stationary bar of the goniometer with a line between the left and right anterior superior iliac spine to represent the sagittal plane and ignore any rotation of the pelvis on the hips. This motion is recorded in degrees by aligning the movable bar with a line between the shoulders, or using the center of the crown of the head, which is held at 90 degrees to the shoulders.

Alternative Method. Using the same goniometer placement, trunk rotation also can be measured in the sitting position. The seated position will stabilize the pelvis from moving with trunk rotation and may provide a simpler, more accurate and replicable measurement.

It is important to specify the position of the client in notation to ensure clarity for interpretation or for follow-up measurement.

UPPER EXTREMITY[1–3,5,10,12]

Shoulder

Glenohumeral Joint Movement Versus Total Shoulder Movement

It should be noted that scapula movement accompanies total shoulder movement. The range of shoulder motion is highly dependent on scapula mobility, which adds flexibility and wide ranges of motion to the shoulder. Although it is difficult to measure scapula movement directly with the goniometer, the evaluator should assess scapula mobility by observation of active motion or passive movement before proceeding with additional shoulder joint measurements. Scapular ROM can be noted as full or restricted.[3] If scapular motion is restricted, as when the musculature is in a state of spasticity or contracture, and the shoulder joint is moved into extreme ROMs (e.g., above 90 degrees of flexion or abduction), pain at the end of ROM stops AROM or indicates to the therapist to stop PROM measurement or glenohumeral joint damage can result.

Isolating glenohumeral joint movement. Approximately two-thirds of shoulder flexion and abduction comes from movement of the humerus in the glenohumeral joint, and one-third of total shoulder movement comes from scapular movement. This is referred to as "scapular rhythm." The measurement methods below and the ROMs shown in the text and in the table (see Table 21.1) are for total shoulder movement. However, in some cases (e.g., when treating a patient after a shoulder replacement or rotator cuff repair) it may be desirable to measure glenohumeral joint movement without scapular movement because the ROM of the humerus relative to the scapula is what is important and targeted in treatment. In that situation, the hand of the therapist can be laid on the scapula with the distal palm (the metacarpophalangeal joints of digits 2–4) on the spine of the scapula and the fingers over the acromion. In that position, the therapist can feel when the angle of the scapula begins to move (rotate for abduction or retract for flexion) and can stop the client at that point to measure isolated glenohumeral joint movement using the same axis and goniometer arm positions as described in movements in Fig. 21.16A–D. This method is also applicable to isolate and measure internal and external rotation of the humerus relative to the scapula when measured in a position of abduction of the shoulder (see figures with shoulder internal rotation and external rotation).

Shoulder Flexion

- 0 to 170 degrees (see Figs. 21.16A–D)
  Position of the Client
- Seated or supine with the humerus adducted in neutral rotation
  Axis, Landmarks, and Arc/Position of the Goniometer. At the beginning point of this movement is the 0 position (anatomic position variation with the palm facing the thigh, leading with the thumb). This position rotates the head of the humerus, allowing maximum flexion ROM by limiting restriction in the

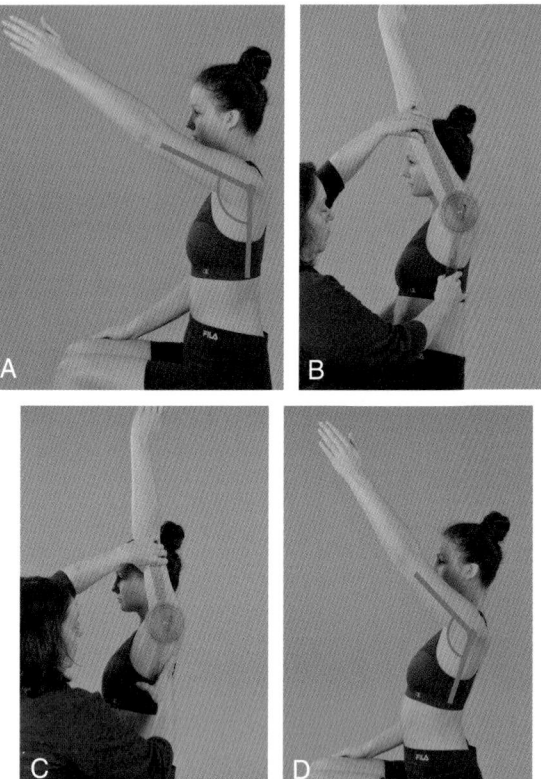

Fig. 21.16 (A) Axis, landmarks, arc. (B) AROM. (C) PROM. (D) Substitution.

glenohumeral joint. The goniometer axis is placed over the center of the humeral head, just distal to the acromion process on the lateral aspect of the humerus. The stationary bar is parallel to the trunk, and the movable bar is parallel to the humerus, aligned with the sagittal plane. If the landmarks are found before the movement into flexion, note that when the shoulder is flexed, the shape of the deltoid muscle mass changes as the shoulder flexes. The point on the skin where the initial axis is found in the 0 position moves upward and backward to the posterior surface of the shoulder and is no longer the axis of movement of the glenohumeral joint in flexion. Thus, to take a measurement of the final position, the therapist uses knowledge of the skeletal structures for placement of the goniometer on the lateral surface of the shoulder joint and aligns it by visualizing the skeleton along with palpating the axis through the center of the humeral head, slightly superior to the crease formed by the distal end of the deltoid mass and approximately two fingers below the acromion. The acromion can be palpated as it forms a hollow between the proximal deltoid attachments when the shoulder is in flexion or abduction.

Fig. 21.16A shows the landmarks for ideal placement of the axis and arms of the goniometer. In Fig. 21.16B, the client holds the limb herself in her own maximum flexed position and the therapist's hand lightly holds the goniometer in place, with the axis aligned with the joint center and the stationary and movable arms on the proximal and distal parts. In Fig. 21.16C (PROM) the therapist holds the movable limb firmly with the left hand while also holding the moving arm of the goniometer aligned with the humerus. This is done simultaneously while stabilizing the trunk with the right hand to offset pressure of moving the limb toward maximum flexion and pushing the humerus to the shoulder's firm end-feel. The therapist's right hand stabilizes the stationary arm of the goniometer against the client's trunk, as seen in Fig. 21.16C, to maintain correct goniometer alignment.

End-Feel

- Firm[3]

Common Substitution. Sometimes a client has limitations of shoulder movement. Most clients want to please their therapist or may not even realize that they have learned to use compensatory movements to "get the job done" so they can perform their ADLs, IADLs, or other occupations, even with limited ROM. In such a case as in Fig. 21.16D, the individual may still be able to reach a top shelf but has substituted thoracolumbar extension for limited shoulder flexion to be able to elevate the arm and hand to reach the target. However, the client's shoulder AROM has not actually increased. In this illustration the arc of the model's shoulder flexion AROM is identical to that in the axis and landmark picture above (see Fig. 21.16A) where the thoracic spine is held in a neutral anatomic position. The stationary bar follows a vertical line. The evaluator must be careful to watch for substitutions and align the goniometer with the correct landmarks, that is, follow the thoracic spine, regardless of the angle of the spine, and not be tempted to follow a vertical line and incorrectly add ROM when there is no more than before.

Shoulder Extension

- 0 to 60 degrees (Fig. 21.17A–D)
  Neutral Position of the Client
- Seated or prone, with no obstruction behind the humerus and the humerus in neutral rotation, held parallel to the spine in the 0 position

Position of the Goniometer. The axis for measuring shoulder extension is the same as for shoulder flexion, but the axis point appears to remain the same for the starting and final positions. Movement should be accompanied by only a slight upward tilt of the scapula. Excessive scapular motion should be avoided so only glenohumeral joint ROM is measured. Angular changes of the scapula can be seen if the shoulder is exposed but can also be palpated if a hand is laid on the scapula from behind with the palm over the spine of the scapula and the fingers over the acromion. During PROM the therapist must hold the goniometer while maximizing PROM (see Fig. 21.17C), illustrated by the therapist lifting upward at the elbow in Fig. 21.17C. Stabilization method depends on whether the therapist wants to isolate glenohumeral joint movement or measure total shoulder movement (glenohumeral joint with scapular elevation).

End-Feel

- Firm[3]

Substitution. Just as with flexion, a substitution for limited extension of the glenohumeral joint may be accomplished by a client by excess anterior flexion of the trunk with no difference in actual extension of the glenohumeral joint or total shoulder ROM. If the client substitutes as in 21.17D, the therapist can either stabilize the trunk and scapula with a firm hand on the anterior shoulder over the acromion or allow the substitution but compensate in measurement by aligning the stationary bar with the upper trunk/thoracic spine with the movable bar still

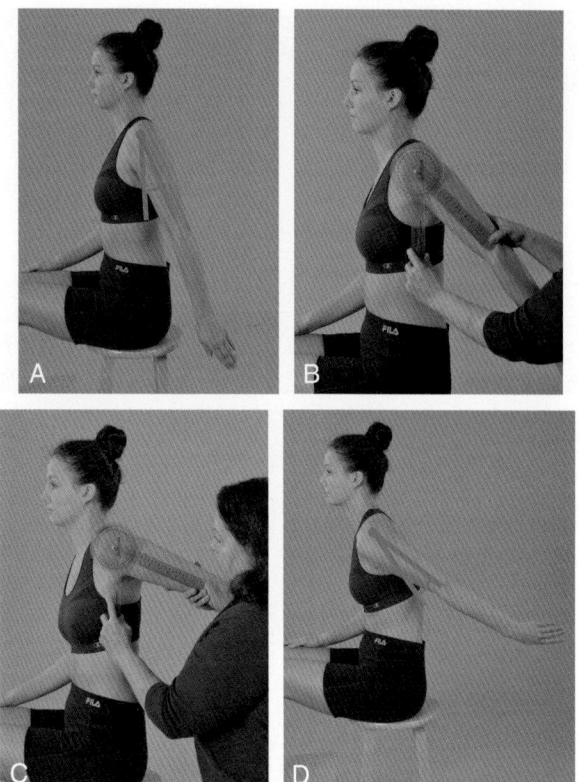

Fig. 21.17 (A) Axis, landmarks, arc. (B) AROM. (C) PROM. (D) Substitution.

aligned with the humerus, yielding the same shoulder extension measurement as in Fig. 21.17A.

Shoulder Abduction

- 0 to 170 degrees (Fig. 21.18A–D)
  Neutral Position of the Client
- Seated or lying supine, with the humerus in adduction and external rotation, with the thumb pointing upward, in the direction of abduction.

Position of the Goniometer. Measure on the posterior surface. The axis is below the acromion process on the posterior surface of the shoulder in line with the joint center at the head of the humerus. The therapist can visualize the joint center based on knowledge of skeletal anatomy (or approximate its position two fingers width directly below the acromion process). The stationary bar is held parallel to the trunk, and the movable bar is parallel to the humerus, pointing at the lateral epicondyle of the elbow. For PROM measurement, those positions do not change, but the therapist must find a way to hold the goniometer in position while also pushing the limb to maximum PROM. In Fig. 21.18C, note that the therapist holds the goniometer in position with the left thumb and index finger while using the palm and digits 3 to 5 to push the humerus to maximum PROM abduction.

End-Feel

- Firm[3]

Substitution. If a client cannot abduct to an ideal or desired level, he or she will likely substitute by leaning the trunk away from the limb thinking they are changing the angle of the joint itself when they are only raising the hand to accomplish the task at hand. This does not change the maximum AROM angle of the

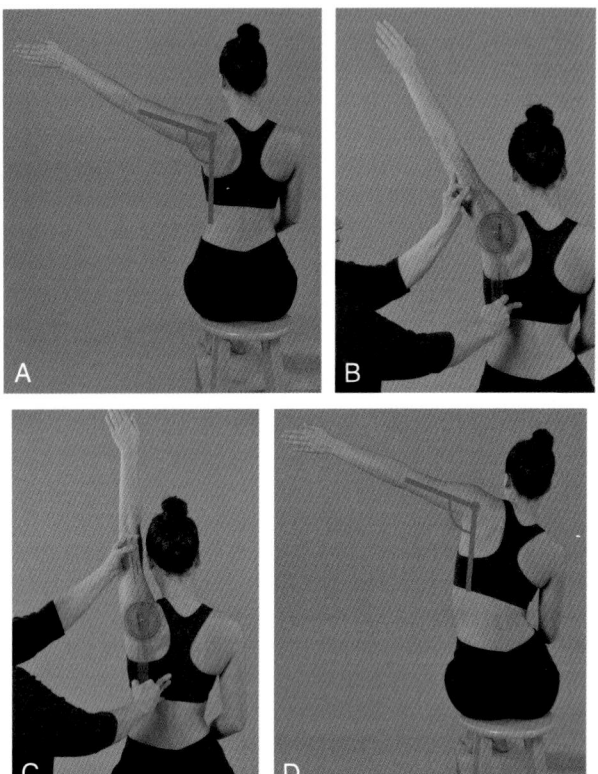

Fig. 21.18 (A) Axis, landmarks, arc. (B) AROM. (C) PROM. (D) Substitution.

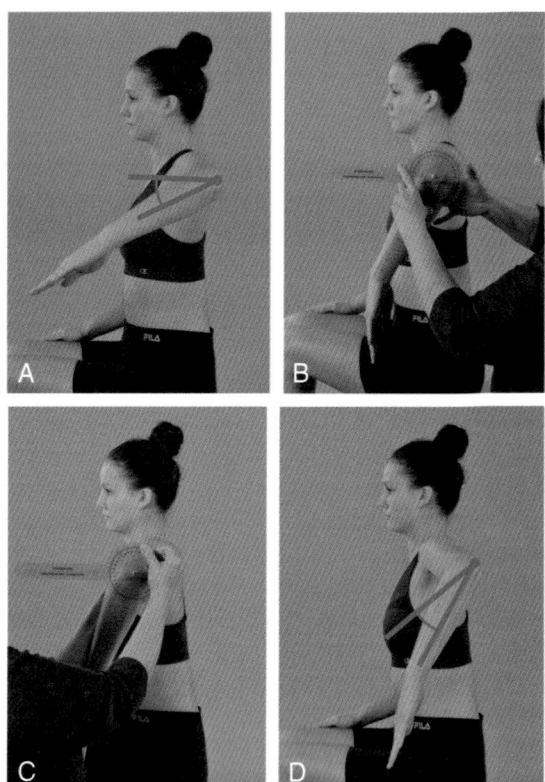

Fig. 21.19 (A) Axis, landmarks, arc. (B) AROM. (C) PROM. (D) Substitution.

shoulder. When measuring ROM, the therapist follows the same landmarks and should still produce the same measurement as in Fig. 21.18A, which shows landmarks and axis.

Shoulder Internal Rotation (Shoulder Abducted)

- 0 to 70 degrees (Fig. 21.19A–D)

Neutral Position of the Client. The following position is used if there is no danger of posterior dislocation and if abduction to 90 degrees is possible and not painful for the client.

Neutral/0 Position

- In seated or standing position, with the humerus abducted to 90 degrees and the elbow flexed to 90 degrees, with the forearm in pronation, parallel to the floor

Position of the Goniometer. The axis is on the olecranon process of the elbow because it is the humerus that actually rotates in the glenohumeral joint for this movement. The stationary bar is held in a horizontal position, and the movable bar is parallel to the forearm, aligned with the ulna. For maximum precision, this is a measurement in which the goniometer illustrated previously with the spirit level (bubble level) could be useful. The therapist could also sight along the stationary bar to a horizontal line in the room (e.g., a table, a line on the wall, or piece of furniture, or the joint between the wall and floor to ensure a horizontal stationary bar).

End-Feel

- Firm[3]

Substitution. In Fig. 21.19D the client is substituting for inadequate IR of the glenohumeral joint with excessive elevation of the scapula, which gives the illusion of increased IR of

the humerus in the glenohumeral joint, and it does cause the forearm to point more downward. Although the scapula is not visible in the picture (see Fig. 21.19D), the stationary bar is still positioned perpendicular to the scapula just as it is while held horizontal in Fig. 21.19A relative to a neutral scapula and should yield the same AROM measurement of rotation of the humerus in the glenohumeral joint.

Shoulder Internal Rotation (Adducted—Alternative position)

- 0 to 40 degrees

The following position (no picture) is used if abduction cannot be achieved. Neutral (0) rotation is when seated or standing with the humerus adducted against the trunk, the elbow flexed at 90 degrees, and the forearm at the midposition and perpendicular to the body (projected forward into the sagittal plane).[3]

Position of the Goniometer. The axis is on the olecranon process below the elbow, the stationary bar is horizontal and pointed forward into the sagittal plane. The movable bar is parallel to the forearm, follows the arc of movement, and moves in a horizontal plane. This position has a limitation in that maximum IR ROM may not be achieved because the forearm's maximum arc in IR stops at the abdomen.

Shoulder External Rotation (Abducted)

- 0 to 90 degrees (Fig. 21.20A–D)

Neutral Position of the Client. Starting in the same position as in Fig. 21.19A when measuring IR, this position is used if

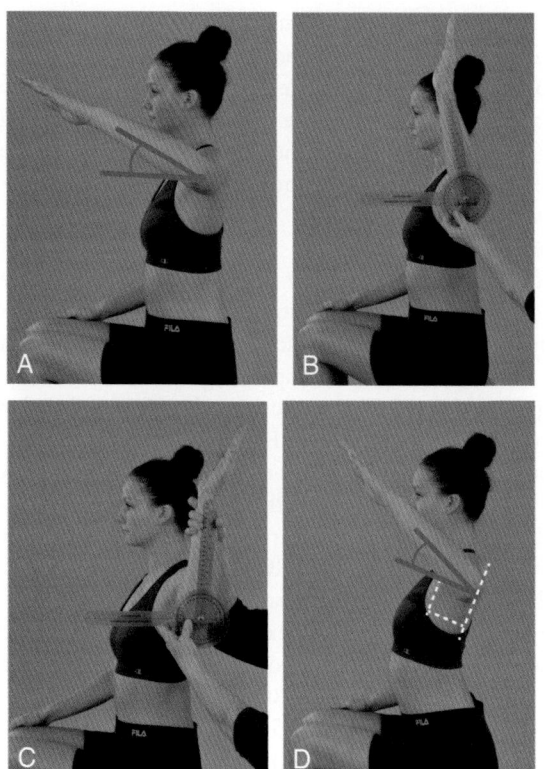

Fig. 21.20 (A) Axis, landmarks, arc. (B) AROM. (C) PROM. (D) Substitution.

there is no danger of anterior dislocation of the humerus[3] or discomfort. Seated or supine with the humerus abducted, the elbow is flexed to 90 degrees and the forearm pronated.

Position of the Goniometer. The axis is the same as previously described with IR. The axis is on the olecranon process of the elbow, and the stationary bar is horizontal in neutral, parallel to the forearm (which points forward in the sagittal plane) at the beginning of the movement. The movable bar follows the forearm in a vertical arc in the sagittal plane to the end of ROM. Specifics for measuring this movement are analogous to measuring IR.

Substitution. When ER is limited, a client will often substitute thoracic extension to enable the hand to go higher. Actual ER of the shoulder does not change as indicated by the *dotted line* parallel to the upper thoracic vertebrae and the *right-angle symbol* in Fig. 21.20D showing that the stationary bar is still perpendicular to the trunk. The client may develop this substitution to reach higher or might lean back to throw a ball higher and farther with some elevation rather than only being able to throw close and to the ground because of limited ER of the shoulder.

Shoulder External Rotation (Adducted—Alternative Position)

- 0 to 60 degrees

Neutral Position of the Client. This position is the same as the alternative position to measure IR. The following position is used if abduction to 90 degrees is not possible or is painful.

In seated or standing position, the humerus is adducted, with the elbow held at the mid-lateral trunk with the elbow flexed to 90 degrees; the elbow is in midposition, perpendicular to the trunk; and the forearm is in neutral rotation (thumb up).

Position of the Goniometer. The axis is aligned with and below the olecranon process of the elbow. In neutral/0, the stationary bar and movable bar are parallel to the forearm (which points forward in the sagittal plane) in 0 rotation/starting position. The movable bar follows the forearm in a lateral arc toward the abdomen in the horizontal plane to the end of AROM or PROM. There is no interference with the trunk in ER, but in this position the abdomen may restrict maximum IR. Because the head of the humerus is in a different position in the glenohumeral joint, there also may be a difference in measurement between the adducted position and the abducted position for ER measurement. The position of measurement must be noted to ensure consistency with follow-up measurements.

End-Feel

- Firm[3]

Shoulder Horizontal Adduction

- 0 to 130 degrees

Neutral Position of the Client. Seated erect with the shoulder to be tested abducted to 90 degrees, the elbow extended, and the palm facing down. The therapist may support the arm in abduction.[3]

Position of the Goniometer. The axis is over the acromion process. The stationary bar is parallel to the line between the left and right acromion, over the shoulder toward the neck, and the movable bar is parallel to the humerus on the superior aspect. The arm is rotated forward toward the opposite shoulder, past the anterior midline as far as possible in a horizontal plane.

End-Feel

- Firm or soft[3]

Shoulder Horizontal Abduction

- 0 to 40 degrees

Neutral Position of the Client and Goniometer. Same positions and goniometer placements as for horizontal adduction. The arm rotates in the horizontal plane in a posterior direction to end range while the shoulder is abducted.

End Feel

- Firm or soft[3]

Elbow

Elbow Flexion/Extension

- 0 to 135-150 degrees (Fig. 21.21)

Neutral Position of the Client

- Standing, sitting, or supine with the humerus adducted (at side), in neutral rotation, the elbow in anatomic position (extension), and the forearm supinated

Position of the Goniometer. The axis is placed over the lateral epicondyle of the humerus at the end of the elbow crease. The stationary bar is parallel to the midline of the humerus or aimed

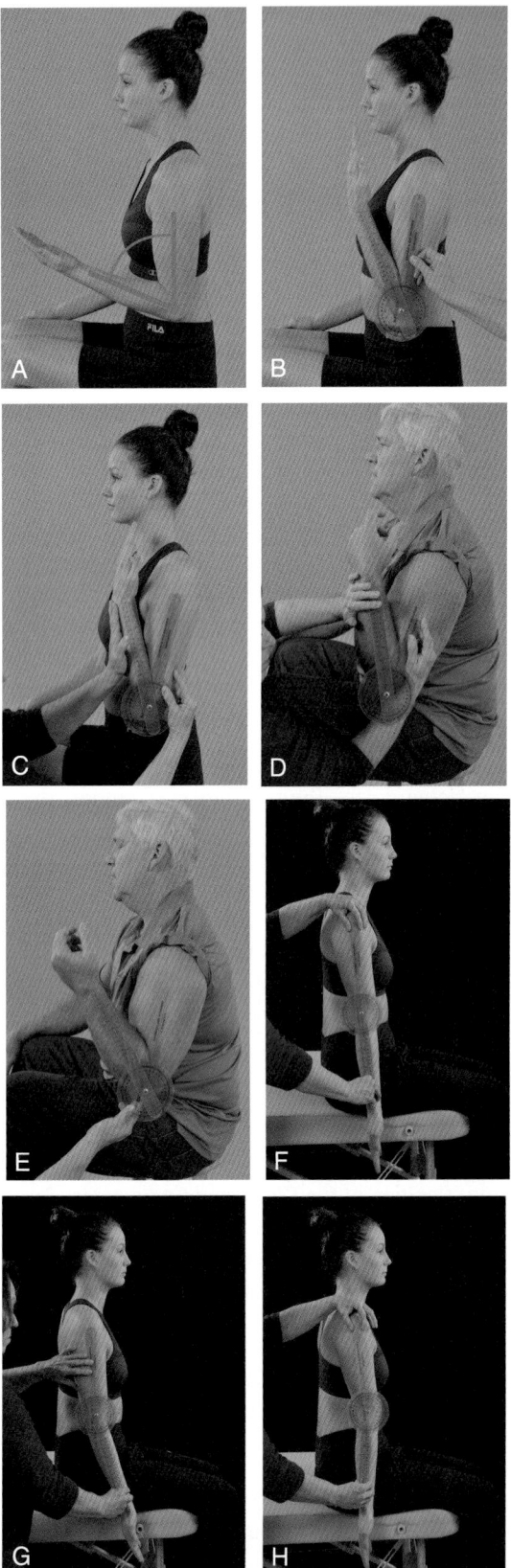

at the head of the humerus, and the movable bar is parallel to the radius. After the movement has been completed, the position of the elbow crease changes in relation to the lateral epicondyle because of the rise of the muscle bulk during the motion. The axis of the goniometer should be repositioned so that it is aligned with the lateral epicondyle.

End-Feel
- Soft, hard, or firm: flexion

Elbow Extension. Hard or firm: extension and hyperextension.[3] End-feel for flexion of some joints (elbow and knee) may depend on relaxed flexor muscle mass compared to the bulk of those muscles in flexion. Compare Figs. 21.21B and E (AROM) to Figs. C and D (PROM) to illustrate the effect of flexed muscle mass on AROM vs. PROM. In Figs. 21.21B and E, during active flexion, the muscle mass of the elbow flexors bulk up to flex the elbow and thus limit flexion with a firm end-feel. In Figs. 21.21C and D (passive range measurement), the elbow flexors are relaxed, allowing additional PROM flexion with a soft end-feel.

Elbow extension typically starts at 0 for neutral extension (see Fig. 21.21F). The elbow extends to a hard stop when the olecranon impacts the olecranon fossa. However, many people vary with their typical elbow ROM and some cannot quite get their elbow to neutral (21.21G), whereas some may hyperextend a few degrees (21.21H). In such cases the measurement of ROM of elbow extension will use the same landmarks as noted earlier. The three-number notation system described previously is useful in this instance to avoid confusion about the meaning of negative numbers when measuring elbow flexion and extension, especially when hyperextension or limited extension occur.

Forearm

Forearm Supination
- 0 to 80 to 90 degrees (Fig. 21.22A–C)
Neutral Position of the Client
- Seated or standing with the humerus fully adducted, with the elbow flexed to 90 degrees, and the forearm in midposition (thumb up)

Position of the Goniometer. The arc to be measured is indicated in Fig. 21.22A. The axis is at the ulnar border of the volar aspect of the wrist, just proximal to the ulnar styloid. The movable bar is resting against the volar aspect of the wrist, and the stationary bar is vertical, perpendicular to the floor (see Fig. 21.22B). After the forearm is supinated, the goniometer should be repositioned so that the movable bar rests on a tangent across the middle of the curved center of the distal forearm, across the flexor tendons at the midpoint of the wrist between radial and ulnar styloids.

Substitution. The most common substitution for this movement is to slightly flex and adduct the shoulder, allowing the forearm to only appear more supinated relative to the vertical line, but this does not actually change the ROM angle of forearm rotation measured at the wrist relative to the humerus (see Fig. 21.22C).

Fig. 21.21 (A) Axis, landmarks, arc. (B) AROM. (C) PROM. (D) PROM limited by large muscle mass. (E) AROM limited by large muscle mass. (F) AROM neutral extension. (G) Elbow AROM showing limited extension. (H) Elbow PROM showing slight hyperextension.

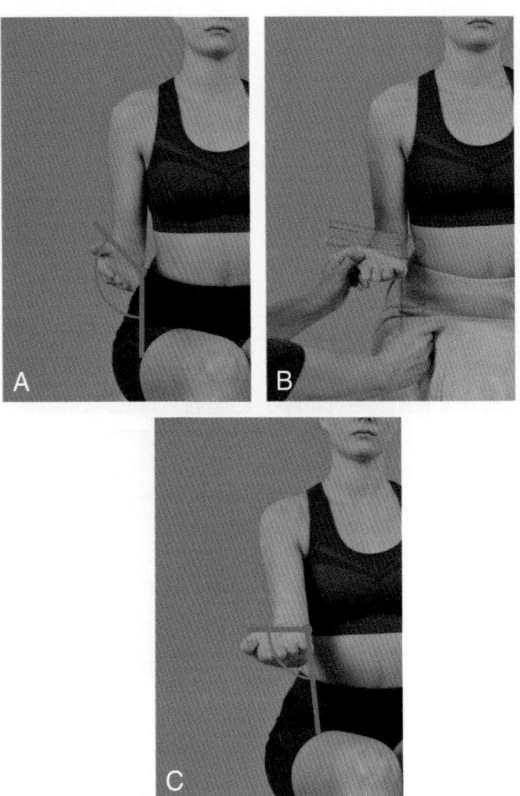

Fig. 21.22 (A) Axis, landmarks, arc. (B) AROM. (C) Substitution.

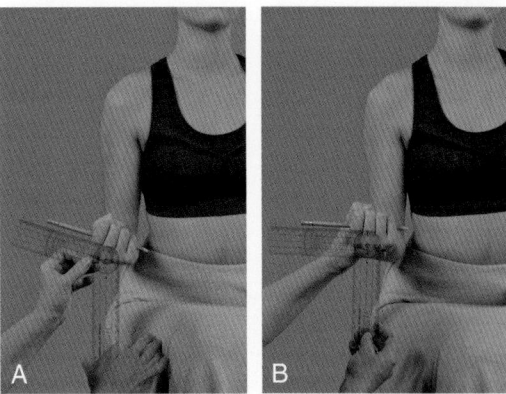

Fig. 21.23 (A) AROM. (B) PROM.

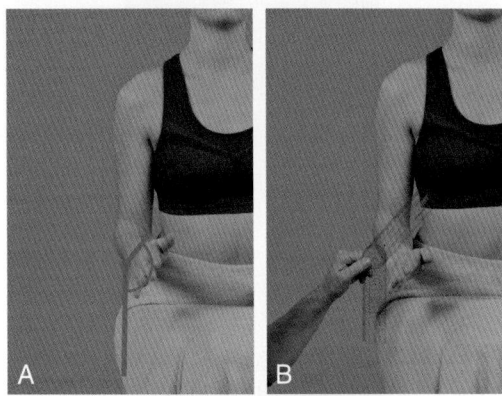

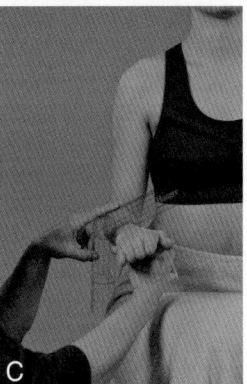

Fig. 21.24 (A) Axis, landmarks, arc. (B) AROM. (C) PROM.

Forearm Supination (Alternative Method)

- 0 to 80-90 degrees (Fig. 21.23A–B)
  Neutral Position of the Client. Seated or standing with the humerus adducted, the elbow at 90 degrees, and the forearm in midposition (thumb up). In neutral position, place a pen or pencil in the client's hand. Client will rotate the forearm and pencil toward horizontal or beyond.
  Position of the Goniometer. The axis is over the head of the third metacarpal. The stationary bar is perpendicular to the floor. The movable bar is held parallel to the pencil.
  End-Feel
- Firm[3]

Forearm Pronation

- 0 to 80 to 90 degrees (Fig. 21.24)
  Neutral Position of the Client
- Seated or standing with the humerus adducted, the elbow at 90 degrees, and the forearm in midposition (thumb up).
  Position of the Goniometer. The axis is at the ulnar border of the dorsal aspect of the wrist, just proximal to the ulnar styloid. Place the goniometer so that the movable bar rests squarely across the center of the dorsum of the distal end of the forearm between the styloids. The stationary bar is held perpendicular to the floor with the forearm fully pronated for AROM (see Fig. 21.24B) and PROM (see Fig. 21.24C).

Forearm Pronation (Alternative Method)

- 0 to 80 to 90 degrees (Fig. 21.25)
  Neutral Position of the Client. Same as alternative method to measure supination. A pencil can be used to measure pronation. The client is seated or standing with the humerus adducted to neutral, elbow at 90 degrees, and the forearm in midposition. A pencil is placed in the hand. In neutral position (0 degrees) the pencil will be vertical, perpendicular to the floor.
  Position of the Goniometer. When the forearm is rotated into pronation, the axis of the goniometer is over the head of the third metacarpal, the stationary bar is perpendicular to the floor, and the movable bar is parallel to the pencil.

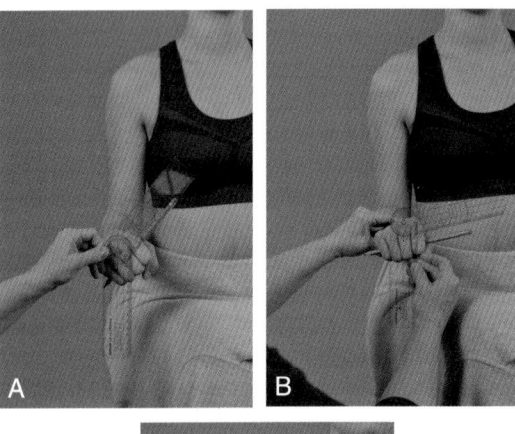

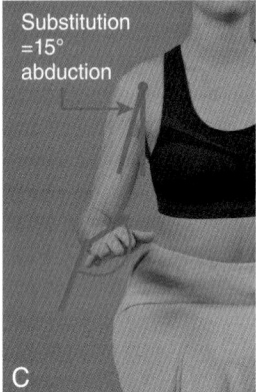

Fig. 21.25 (A) AROM. (B) PROM. (C) Substitution.

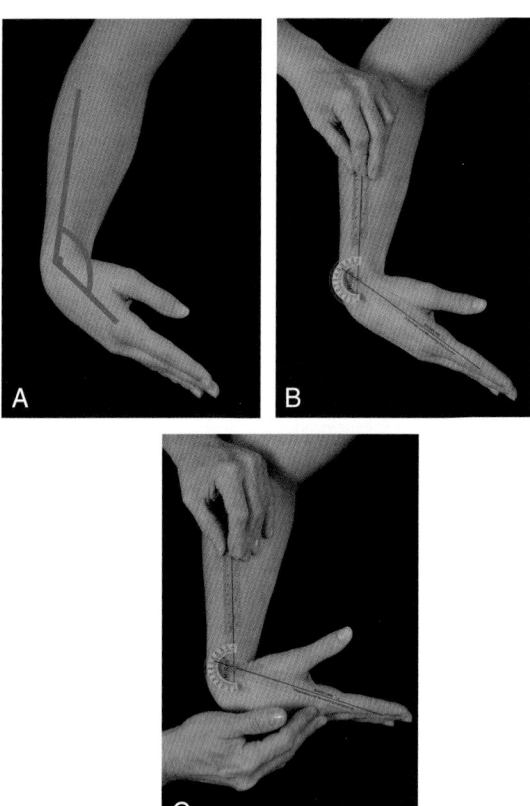

Fig. 21.26 (A) Axis, landmarks, arc. (B) AROM. (C) PROM.

End-Feel

- Hard to firm[3]

Substitution. The most common substitution when ROM of forearm pronation is limited is to achieve the desired position of the forearm/hand by substituting shoulder abduction for a limit in pronation (see Fig. 21.25C). This turns the wrist/hand flatter relative to the horizontal surfaces but does not change the rotation angle of the forearm relative to the humerus. To avoid this substitution during measurement, instruct the client verbally (or stabilize manually) so the humerus remains in adduction, (i.e., vertical or aligned with the trunk, with the elbow held close to the lateral trunk).

Wrist

Wrist Flexion

- 0 to 80 degrees (Fig. 21.26)

Neutral Position of the Client. Seated with the forearm in midposition and the hand and forearm resting on a table on the ulnar border with the wrist aligned with the forearm. The fingers are relaxed or extended to avoid passive insufficiency from tight extensors, which would limit wrist ROM in flexion.

Position of the Goniometer. The wrist is typically measured with the forearm in midposition, with the axis on the lateral aspect of the wrist just distal to the radial styloid in the anatomic snuffbox. The stationary bar is parallel to the radius, and the movable bar is parallel to the metacarpal of the index finger. This measurement also could be taken with the elbow partially flexed and the forearm resting on something (e.g., pillow, rolled

towel, or bolster) that elevates the hand enough to clear the table and enables full ROM of the wrist while avoiding interference with the fingers on the table.[3]

End-Feel

- Firm[3]

Wrist Extension

- 0 to 70 degrees (Fig. 21.27)

Neutral Position of the Client and Goniometer. The positions for the client and goniometer are the same as for wrist flexion, except that the wrist is extended and fingers should be relaxed in flexion instead of extended, to avoid passive insufficiency from tight flexors, which would limit wrist ROM in extension.

End-Feel

- Firm or hard[3]

Measurement Error. Fig. 21.27D demonstrates a measurement error. Measuring passive wrist extension ROM with the fingers extended may result in inaccurate measurement of wrist extension PROM because the finger flexors may become passively insufficient, limiting the amount of wrist extension.

Wrist Radial Deviation

- 0 to 20 degrees (Fig. 21.28)

Neutral Position of the Client. Seated with the forearm pronated, the wrist at neutral (straight), the fingers relaxed in extension, and the palm of the hand resting flat on the table surface.

Position of the Goniometer. Neutral (0 degrees) is a straight wrist and goniometer. The axis is on the dorsum of the wrist at the base of the third metacarpal, in a hollow that can be palpated

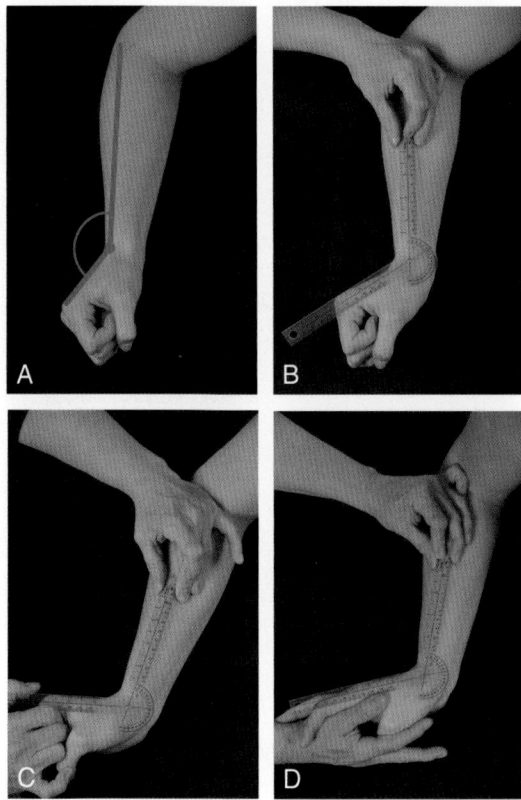

Fig. 21.27 (A) Axis, landmarks, arc. (B) AROM. (C) PROM. (D) Measurement error, passive insufficiency.

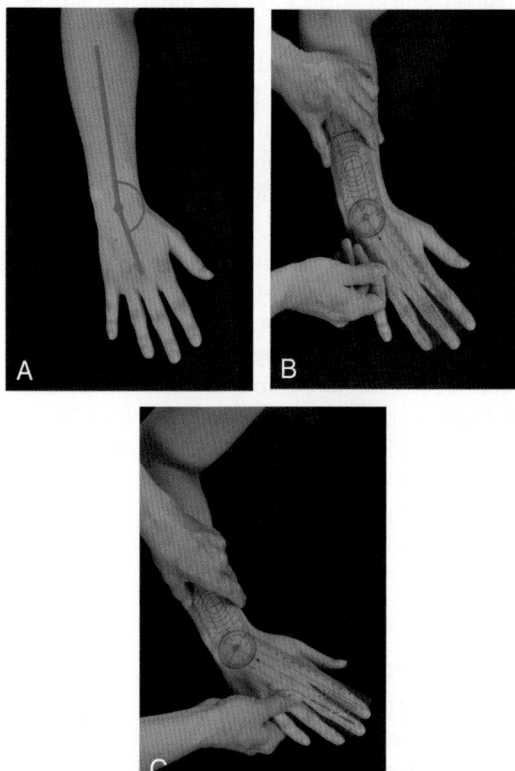

Fig. 21.28 (A) Axis, landmarks, arc. (B) AROM. (C) PROM.

over the capitate bone. The movable bar is parallel to the third metacarpal aligned with the third MCP joint, and the stationary bar follows the midline of the dorsal aspect of the forearm.

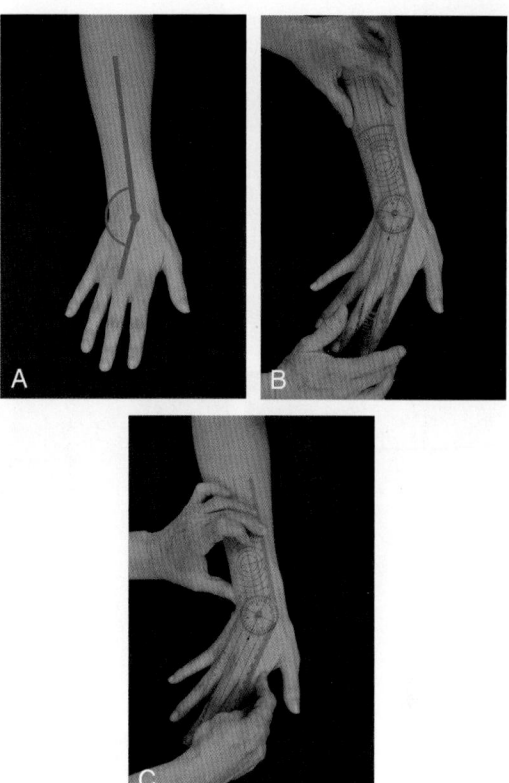

Fig. 21.29 (A) Axis, landmarks, arc. (B) Partial AROM. (C) PROM.

End-Feel
- Firm[3]

Substitution. A common substitution for limited radial deviation is to abduct the shoulder and pronate the forearm and flex the wrist slightly, which turns the wrist/hand relative to the trunk but does not change wrist radial deviation AROM measurement relative to the forearm.

Wrist Ulnar Deviation
- 0 to 30 degrees (Fig. 21.29)

Position of the Client and Goniometer. Same client position and goniometer placement as for radial deviation. Wrist deviates toward the ulnar side.

End-Feel
- Firm or hard[3]

Fingers
Metacarpophalangeal (MP or MCP) Flexion
- 0 to 90 degrees

The joint center viewed from the side is as indicated in Fig. 21.30A. The actual axis is on the lateral side of the MP joint, but only the second digit (index finger) and the fifth digit (small finger) can be measured, as in Fig. 21.30B, on the side of the joint. So, the most common method of measuring MP joints is to place a small goniometer (cut to 3 inches long) on the dorsal surface of the MP joint, as in Fig. 21.30C, on the dorsum of both the hand and proximal phalanx. Specialized goniometers are also illustrated that simplify dorsal ROM measurement. PROM is illustrated in Figs. 21.30D–E using a specialized goniometer. The MPs of digits 2 to 5 can all be measured in this manner.

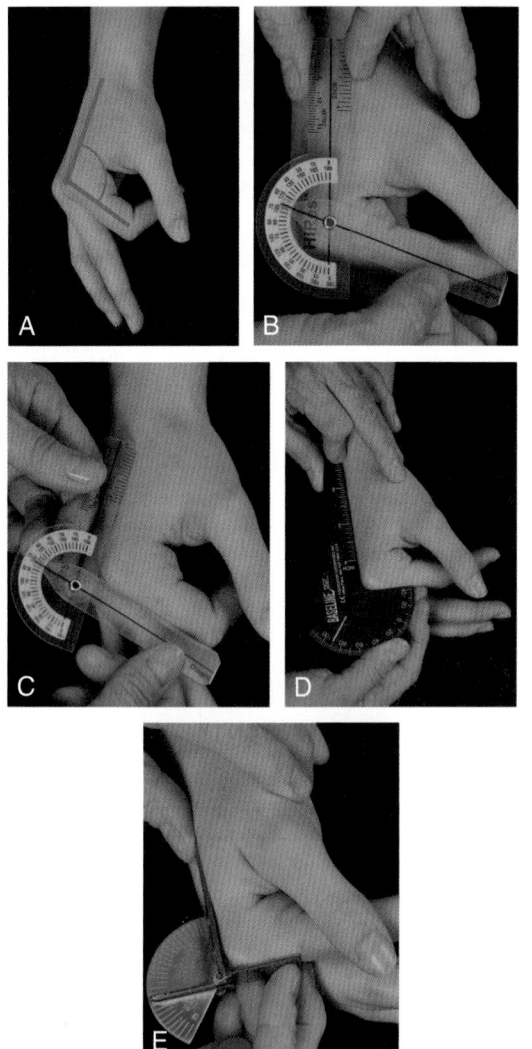

Fig. 21.30 (A) Axis, landmarks, arc. (B) Lateral AROM. (C) Dorsal AROM. (D–E) Dorsal PROM with specialized goniometers.

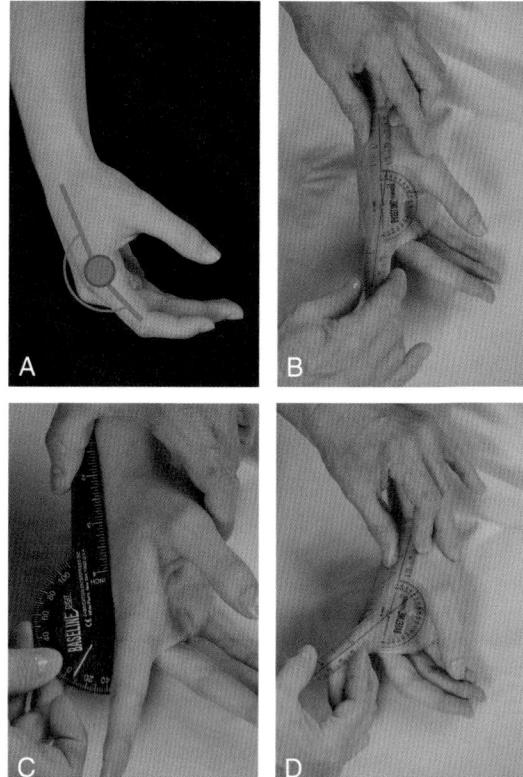

Fig. 21.31 (A) Axis, landmarks, arc. (B–C) AROM. (D) PROM.

Neutral Position of the Client. Seated with the elbow flexed, the forearm in midposition, the wrist at 0-degree neutral position, the proximal and distal IP joints relaxed to avoid passive insufficiency and the forearm and hand supported on a firm surface on the ulnar border.

Position of the Goniometer
- *Method 1* (see Fig. 21.30C): The axis is centered on the dorsal aspect of the metacarpophalangeal (MP) joint. The stationary bar lies on the dorsal surface of the hand, following the metacarpal for the MP joint being measured, and the movable bar lies on the dorsal surface of the proximal phalanx.
- *Method 2* (see Fig. 21.30D–E): Use the specialized finger goniometers on the dorsal surfaces.

End-Feel
- Hard or firm[3]

Metacarpophalangeal Extension/Hyperextension
- 0 to 45 degrees

Neutral Position of the Client. Seated with the forearm in midposition, the wrist at 0-degree neutral position, the interphalangeal joints relaxed or in flexion, and the forearm and hand

supported on a firm surface on the ulnar border. Regardless of which way the protractor is turned on the goniometer, the extension angle being measured is illustrated in Fig. 21.31A.

Position of the Goniometer. The axis is over the lateral aspect of the MP joint of the index finger. The stationary bar is parallel to the metacarpal, and the movable bar is parallel to the proximal phalanx. The small finger's MP joint may be measured similarly. ROM of the long and ring fingers can be estimated by comparison or specialized finger goniometers can be used on the dorsal surface of the hand and fingers.

An alternative is to place the goniometer on the volar aspect of the hand. With use of the edge of a shortened goniometer (a 6-inch goniometer can be cut to more easily measure the small joints of the hand), the axis is aligned over the MP joint being measured, the stationary bar is parallel to the metacarpal, and the movable bar is parallel to the proximal phalanx. As another alternative, these joints can be measured using specialized goniometers (illustrated in Fig. 21.31C and previously in 21.30D–E).

End-Feel
- Firm[3]

Metacarpophalangeal Abduction
- 0 to 25 degrees (Fig. 21.32)

Neutral Position of the Client. Seated with the forearm pronated, the wrist at 0-degree neutral deviation, the fingers straight, and the hand resting on a firm surface.

Position of the Goniometer. The axis is centered over the MP joint being measured. The stationary bar is over the corresponding metacarpal, and the movable bar is over the proximal phalanx. The arc of the abduction angle is measured as the

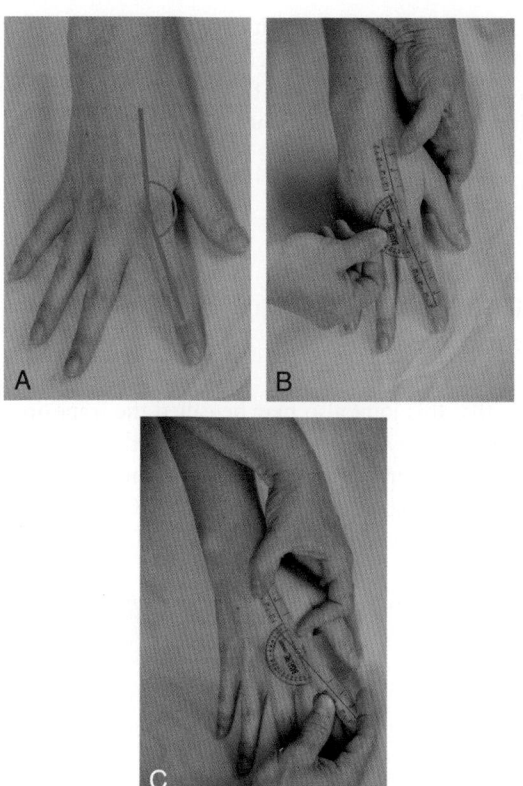

Fig. 21.32 (A) Axis, landmarks, arc. (B) AROM. (C) PROM.

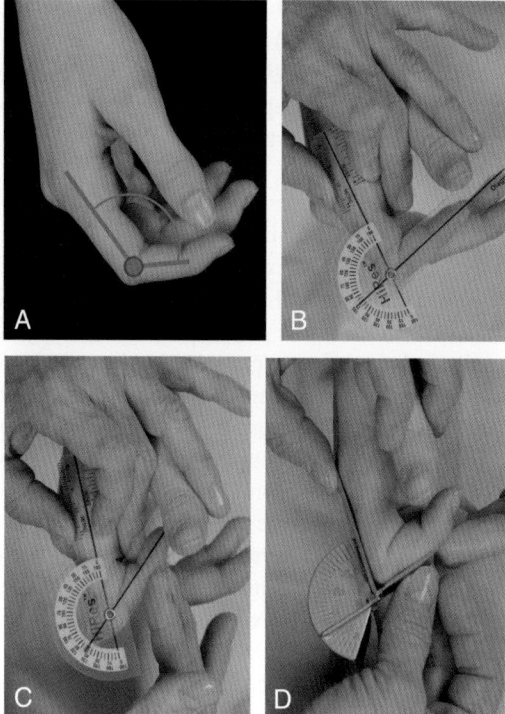

Fig. 21.33 (A) Axis, landmarks, arc. (B) AROM. (C) PROM. (D) PROM with specialized goniometer.

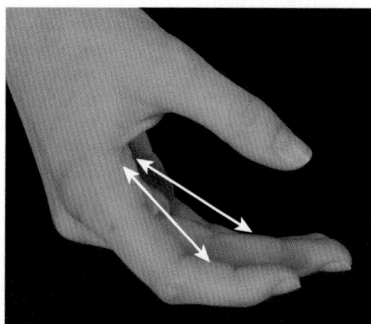

Fig. 21.34 Alternative method.

deviation from 0 (0 = straight MP) for the MP joint/finger being measured. Measurements can be taken in both radial and ulnar directions for each finger.

End-Feel

- Firm[3]

Proximal Interphalangeal (PIP) Flexion/Extension

(Fingers: second through fifth digits)

- 0 to 110 degrees (Fig. 21.33)

Neutral Position of the Client. Seated with the forearm in midposition, the wrist at 0-degree neutral position or relaxed and slightly extended, with the forearm and hand supported on a firm surface on the ulnar border.

Position of the Goniometer

- *Goniometry Method 1:* The axis is centered on the lateral surface of the proximal interphalangeal (PIP) joint being measured. The stationary bar is placed along the lateral side of the proximal phalanx, and the movable bar follows the middle phalanx (see Figs. 21.33A–C).
- *Method 2:* Using a shortened goniometer or a specialized dorsal goniometer (see Fig. 21.33D), place the stationary bar on the lateral aspect or dorsum of the proximal (first) phalanx and the movable bar on the lateral aspect or dorsum of the middle (second) phalanx. When the stationary and movable bars of the goniometer are so aligned, the axis will fall into alignment with the joint center. For the index finger (digit 2) and the small finger (digit 5), the lateral measurement method presents few problems. However, digits 3 and 4 are easier to measure using the dorsal method shown in

Fig. 21.33D because there is not enough room to get a shortened goniometer between the fingers. The dorsal method illustrated in Fig. 21.33D, PROM, is equally valid on digits 2 to 5 and is often the only method used for all of the fingers (digits 2 to 5).

PIP extension is typically close to 0 and without significant and painful hyperextension is usually not measured with straight fingers. However, problematic hyperextension can be measured in the same manner as flexion with the same landmarks and stationary and movable bar positions.

Proximal Interphalangeal Flexion (Alternative Method). This joint also can be measured with a ruler. The IP and MP joints of the fingers are flexed toward the palm (Fig. 21.34). A ruler is used to measure from the midpoint of the middle phalanx of each finger to the distal palmar crease.[3]

End-Feel

- Usually hard; may be soft or firm depending on the health of the surrounding tissues.[3]

Distal Interphalangeal Flexion (DIP)

- 0 to 80 degrees (Fig. 21.35)

Neutral Position of the Client. Seated with the forearm in midposition, the wrist at 0-degree neutral slight extension, and the forearm and hand supported on the ulnar border on a firm surface.

Position of the Goniometer. A shortened goniometer is best to measure DIP flexion because a longer goniometer impacts the palm at maximum DIP flexion or interferes between the fingers. The axis is on the dorsal surface of the DIP joint. The stationary bar is over the middle phalanx, and the movable bar lies over the distal phalanx (see Fig. 21.35B). Alternative methods are to use a specialized goniometer on the dorsum of the DIP (see Fig. 21.35C). A standard long goniometer can be used as in Fig. 21.35D on the sides of the index and small fingers, but this becomes difficult with the second and third fingers as the palm interferes with the length of the goniometer.

MP, PIP, and DIP Composite Flexion (Alternative Method). Some clients may have very limited flexion of all of the finger joints. In this case, isolating flexion of each digit and each joint can have limited value. Alternatively, composite finger flexion can be measured if the client flexes all three finger joints (MP, PIP, and DIP) toward the palm (Fig. 21.36). A measurement is then taken with a ruler from the tip of the middle finger to the distal palmar crease. Progress toward 0 can be tracked during the course of treatment using this method. When the measurement is 0, the client has full composite flexion. If digits 2 to 5 all have similar flexion, this will yield a general composite measurement of finger flexion for the hand. Individual digit composite flexion also can be measured independently for each

finger if the situation warrants it (e.g., to monitor recovery from a single digit injury or surgery). Specific description of the measurement method is needed in therapist notes to ensure understanding and reliability of repeat measurement.

End-Feel

- Soft or firm[3]

Thumb

Thumb Carpometacarpal (CMC) Extension (AKA Radial Abduction)

- 0 to 50 degrees (Fig. 21.37)

Note that this joint also may be called the trapeziometacarpal (TMC) joint by hand surgeons or hand therapists because it is the joint between the trapezium (one of the carpal bones) and the first metacarpal. It is the first of five CMC joints between the wrist and the hand and operates differently from the other CMC

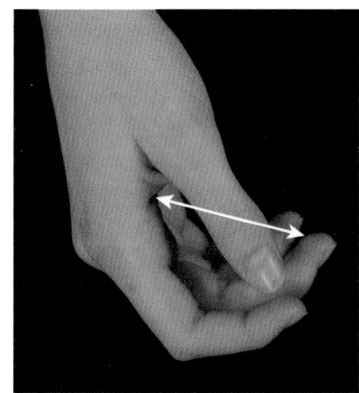

Fig. 21.36 Alternative method.

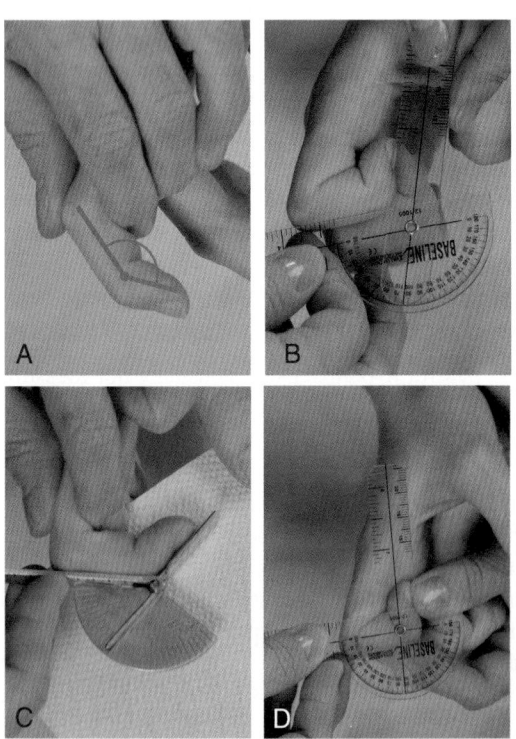

Fig. 21.35 (A) Axis, landmarks, arc. (B) AROM dorsal. (C) AROM. (D) PROM lateral.

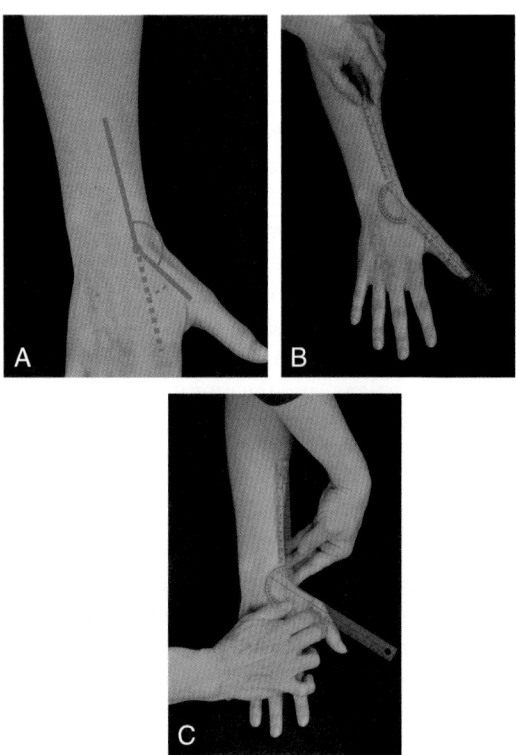

Fig. 21.37 (A) Axis, landmarks, arc. (B) AROM. (C) PROM.

joints. It is a unique and very mobile joint allowing more thumb flexibility than the other CMC joints provide to the metacarpals of the fingers. This joint enables the opposable thumb.

Neutral Position of the Client. Seated with the forearm pronated, wrist neutral, and the hand facing palm down, resting flat on a firm surface. The starting point is the thumb held as close to the first metacarpal as possible. Note that this starting position of the first metacarpal and the radius is 25 to 30 degrees but is considered a theoretical neutral position, and for measurement purposes, neutral/0 is parallel to the radius or first metacarpal.

Position of the Goniometer. The axis is over the dorsal surface of the thumb carpometacarpal (CMC or TMC) joint at the base of the thumb metacarpal, in the anatomic snuffbox. The stationary bar is parallel to the radius, and the movable bar is aligned with the thumb metacarpal extended in the same plane as the palm (frontal plane).

Thumb CMC extension (AKA Radial Abduction) (Alternative Method)

- 0 to 50 degrees

Position of the Client and Goniometer. The client is positioned the same as described in the first method. The axis is over the CMC joint at the base of the thumb metacarpal. The difference is that the stationary bar is parallel to the second metacarpal (index finger), which is in line with the radius, and the movable bar is parallel to the first metacarpal of the thumb (see *dotted line* on Fig. 21.37A). If both bars are parallel to the bones described, the axis will be correctly positioned automatically and the measurement will be correct.

End-Feel
- Firm[3]

CMC Abduction (Palmar Abduction)

- 0 to 50 degrees from radius (Fig. 21.38).

Similar to CMC extension, the thumb cannot reach a true 0 position relative to the radius with the wrist in neutral, instead measuring 25 to 30 degrees from first metacarpal and radius.

Position of the Client. Seated with the forearm in neutral, at 0-degree pronation/supination, the wrist flexion and extension are neutral. The forearm and hand are resting on the ulnar border. The thumb is rotated in a plane toward a right angle from the palm of the hand toward its maximum abduction, in the sagittal plane.

Position of the Goniometer. The axis is at the junction of the thumb and index finger metacarpals (in the anatomic snuffbox, the hollow that can be seen or palpated at the lateral base of the thumb). The stationary bar is over the radius and the movable bar is parallel to the thumb metacarpal as illustrated in Fig. 21.38A.

CMC Palmar Abduction (Alternative Method)

Maximum is 50 degrees from second metacarpal.

Neutral Position of the Client. The client is positioned in the same way as described in the first method with the same 0 position limitations described above.

Placement of the Goniometer. The axis is at the junction of the thumb and index finger metacarpals in the anatomic

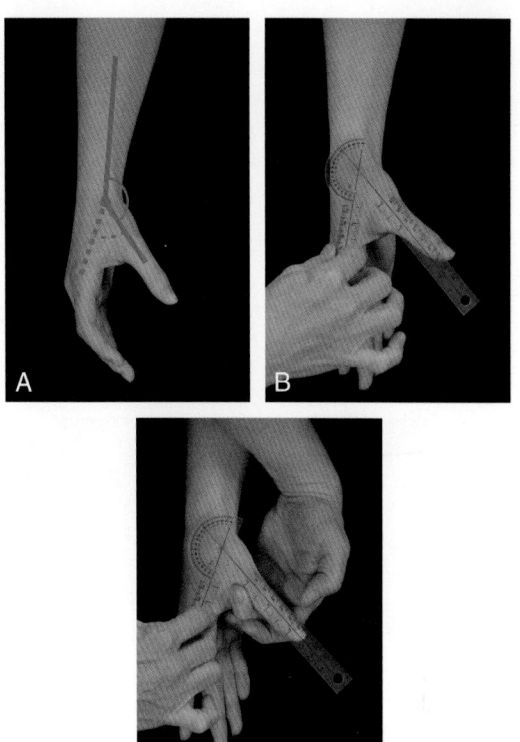

Fig. 21.38 (A) Axis, landmarks, arc. (B) AROM. (C) PROM.

snuffbox. The stationary bar is parallel to the metacarpal of the index finger and the movable bar follows the thumb metacarpal as illustrated in Fig. 21.38A with the *dotted lines* and Fig. 21.38B–C. The method of measurement must be specified in treatment notes.

End-Feel
- Firm[3]

Thumb Metacarpophalangeal (MP or MCP) Flexion

- 0 to 50 degrees (Fig. 21.39)

Neutral Position of the Client. Seated with the elbow flexed, the forearm in 45 degrees of supination, the wrist at neutral deviation, the MP and interphalangeal joints relaxed in extension, and the hand and forearm supported on a firm surface.

Position of the Goniometer. The axis is parallel to the dorsal surface of the MP joint. The stationary bar is over the thumb metacarpal, and the movable bar is over the proximal phalanx.

Alternative Method. A small goniometer can be used on the palmar side of the thumb MP (no picture).

End-Feel
- Hard or firm[3]

Thumb Interphalangeal (IP) Flexion

- 0 to 80 to 90 degrees (Fig. 21.40)

Position of the Client. Same as described for thumb MP flexion.

Position of the Goniometer. The axis is on the dorsal surface of the interphalangeal joint. The stationary bar is over the proximal phalanx, and the movable bar is over the distal phalanx.

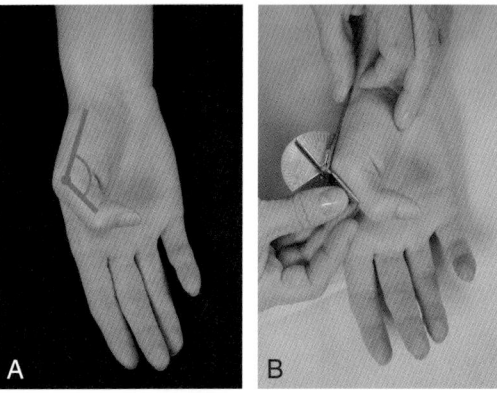

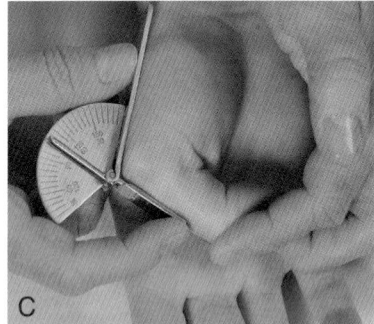

Fig. 21.39 (A) Axis, landmarks, arc. (B) AROM. (C) PROM.

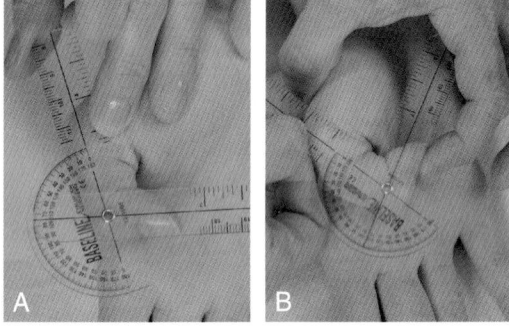

Fig. 21.40 (A) AROM. (B) PROM.

This joint also can be measured with a specialized or standard goniometer on the dorsal surface of the IP joint. Describe the measurement method in the clinical notes to ensure reliability of repeat measurements.

Opposition (Thumb to the Fifth Finger)

Opposition is a function of several joints between the thumb and fingers that could be measured individually with a goniometer, but that method provides only limited information about a deficit in total opposition. Deficits in opposition (composite of all joints involved) may be recorded by measuring the distance between the centers of the pads of the thumb and the fifth finger with a ruler (Fig. 21.41). Distance is 0 (no deficit) if the thumb can touch the small finger. Most goniometers have a ruler

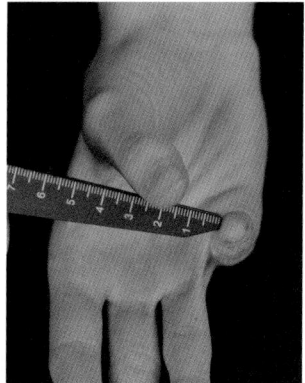

Fig. 21.41 AROM.

printed on one of the long arms that can be used to measure the gap if the thumb cannot touch the small finger. Progress can be monitored as the gap shrinks to 0.

End-Feel

- Soft or firm[3]

LOWER EXTREMITY

Principles from measuring the upper extremity can be easily applied to the lower extremity.[3,5,6,10] We present one hip and one knee measurement in this chapter as examples of this application of general principles and refer readers to many other texts for details that may be needed to measure ROM of lower extremity joints and movements.

Hip

Hip Flexion

- 0 to 120 degrees (Fig. 21.42)

   Neutral Position of the Client. Supine, lying with the hip and knee in 0-degree extension and rotation (femur straight in neutral, flexion at hip into sagittal plane).

   Position of the Goniometer. The axis is found by palpating the lateral aspect of the hip for the greater trochanter of the femur. The stationary bar is centered over the middle of the lateral aspect of the pelvis at the greater trochanter (which can be palpated), parallel to the trunk and to the horizontal surface on which the client is lying. The movable bar is parallel to the long axis of the femur on the midline of the lateral aspect of the thigh, aiming at the lateral epicondyle of the knee joint. The knee is flexed during the motion to relax the knee flexors and avoid passive insufficiency of the hamstrings, which cross both the hip and the knee and would limit hip flexion.

   End-Feel

- Soft[3]

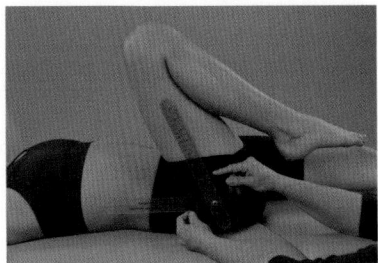

Fig. 21.42 AROM.

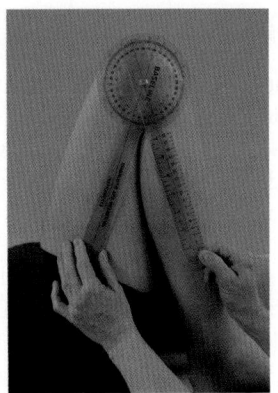

Fig. 21.43 AROM.

Knee

Knee Flexion

- 0 to 135 degrees (Fig. 21.43)

Position of the Client. Neutral position: The client should be supine, lying with the knees and hips flexed and the hip in 0-degree (neutral) rotation (flat on the table). To measure knee flexion with the client in the supine position, the hip must be flexed, relaxing the rectus femoris, which crosses the hip and the knee, avoiding passive insufficiency of this hip flexor at the knee and enabling maximal ROM in knee flexion. Knee flexion measured with the client in the prone position will likely show less ROM because of passive insufficiency from the rectus femoris across the hip being on stretch from lying on a flat surface in prone.

Position of the Goniometer. With the client in the supine position, the axis is centered on the lateral aspect of the knee joint at the lateral epicondyle of the femur (see Fig. 21.43). The stationary bar is on the lateral aspect of the thigh, parallel to the longitudinal axis of the femur, aimed at the greater trochanter. The movable bar is parallel to the longitudinal axis of the fibula, aligned with the lateral malleolus, on the lateral aspect of the ankle.

End-Feel

- Soft[3]

THREADED CASE STUDY

Evelyn, Part 2

At the beginning of the chapter, Evelyn's case study was introduced. She is an active 83-year-old woman with a rich occupational life who sustained a Colles fracture (of her distal radius) in her left nondominant upper extremity. She recently had her cast removed and was experiencing residual problems (including joint ROM deficits). Readers were asked to consider three questions while studying the chapter:

1. Why should the therapist proceed with caution when assessing the ROM limitations of this client?

    The therapist should proceed with caution with all clients. In the case of Evelyn, heightened caution is necessary during joint measurement because of the edema, pain, and stiffness that she is experiencing in the thumb and fingers of her recently injured left wrist. Failure to proceed with caution during measurement of ROM could exacerbate each of these symptoms.

2. What is the appropriate sequencing of joint measurement assessment for this client—that is, what methods should be applied first?

It is important for the therapist to first have Evelyn actively move her joints through all available pain-free (or with tolerable pain) ROM throughout both her left affected upper extremity and her unaffected right upper extremity (for comparison purposes). Next, the therapist should passively move Evelyn's affected joints through the available pain-free (tolerable) PROM, note the end-feel, and estimate the ROM in those joints. Finally, the therapist measures the affected joints with a goniometer by following the specific sequential directions for measuring each of the joints.

3. What is the advantage of joint measurement in evidence-based practice?

    An advantage of joint measurement in evidence-based practice is that the client's ROM baselines are recorded, and the effectiveness of interventions can be determined or substantiated on the basis of the results of follow-up joint measurements. Once these outcome data are collected by the therapist (along with standardized data, i.e., similar data from other clients), a body of evidence regarding effectiveness of intervention is compiled, which in turn can be used to select effective treatment of future clients with similar problems.

SUMMARY

Joint measurement is used to evaluate ROM in persons whose physical dysfunction affects joint mobility. Measurements of ROM are used in setting intervention goals, selecting intervention methods, and making objective assessments of progress that allow the therapist to select the intervention methods most likely to target the affected joints. The OTPF-4 provides many considerations for assessment, intervention planning, and treatment implementation. Measurement of ROM is a source of data to determine specific and measurable degrees of joint mobility limitations and to monitor progress that might enable a client to better perform activities that contribute to improved occupational performance.

Before measuring ROM, the therapist should know of any precautions or contraindications concerning the client's condition that may determine how extensive the joint measurement procedure can be. For example, after surgery, the surgeon will usually provide relevant precautions if needed, but surgery is not the only condition for which precautions and contraindications

might be indicated. Joint or tissue inflammation are additional considerations and the occupational therapist should also know the principles of joint measurement. The procedure for measuring joint ROM involves correct positioning of the client and therapist, exposure of the joints to be measured, palpation, appropriate stabilization and handling, protection of body parts, and correct placement of the goniometer at the beginning and end of the ROM. To support the efficacy of intervention strategies and modalities, the therapist must also consider which method of reporting will best serve as evidence of effective intervention and ensure interrater and intrarater reliability and note the method used in treatment notes.

Directions and illustrations for measuring all of the major joint motions in the neck, trunk, and upper and lower extremities are included in this chapter. The content is designed for development of the fundamental techniques of joint measurement. The reader is referred to the references for more comprehensive treatment of the topic.[3,9,10]

REVIEW QUESTIONS

1. Describe general rules for positioning the goniometer when measuring joint ROM.
2. With which conditions is joint measurement likely to be used?
3. List and discuss four purposes of joint measurement.
4. Is formal joint measurement necessary for every client? If not, how may ROMs be assessed?
5. What is the benefit of conducting precise joint measurement with a goniometer?
6. What is meant by palpation? Why and how is palpation done?
7. What should the therapist look for when observing joints and joint motions?
8. List at least five precautions during or contraindications to joint measurement.
9. What is meant by end-feel?
10. When measuring a joint crossed by a two-joint muscle, how should the occupational therapy practitioner position the joint not being measured?
11. List the steps in the procedure for joint measurement.
12. How is joint ROM measurement recorded on the evaluation form?
13. List the average normal ROM for elbow flexion, shoulder flexion, finger MP flexion, hip flexion, knee flexion, and ankle dorsiflexion.
14. Describe how to read the goniometer when using the 180-degree system of joint measurement.
15. What is meant by functional ROM?
16. List three intervention methods that could be used to increase ROM.

EXERCISES

1. Measure all of the upper extremity joint motions of a normal client. Record the findings on the form in Fig. 21.7.
2. Repeat the first exercise, but the client should play the role of someone with several joint limitations.
3. Observe the joint motions used in ordinary ADLs/IADLs (e.g., self-care and home management). Estimate the functional ROMs for the following joint motions: shoulder flexion, ER, IR, and abduction; elbow flexion; wrist extension; hip flexion and extension; knee flexion; and ankle plantar flexion.

REFERENCES

1. American Academy of Orthopaedic Surgeons: *Joint motion: method of measuring and recording*, Chicago, IL, 1965, The Academy.

2. American Occupational Therapy Association: Occupational therapy practice framework: Domain and process (4th ed.), *American Journal of Occupational Therapy* 74(Suppl. 2), 7412410010, 2020. https://doi.org/10.5014/ajot.2020.74S2001.

3. Baruch Center of Physical Medicine: *The technique of goniometry* (unpublished manuscript), Richmond, VA, Medical College of Virginia.

4. Clarkson HM: *Musculoskeletal assessment, joint range of motion and manual muscle strength*, ed 2, Philadelphia, PA, 2000, Lippincott Williams & Wilkins.

5. Cole T: Measurement of musculoskeletal function: goniometry. In Kottke FJ, Stillwell GK, Lehmann JF, editors: *Krusen's handbook of physical medicine and rehabilitation* ed 3, Philadelphia, PA, 1982, Saunders.

6. Esch D, Lepley M: In *Evaluation of joint motion: methods of measurement and recording*, Minneapolis, MN, 1974, University of Minnesota Press.

7. Hurt SP: Considerations of muscle function and their application to disability evaluation and treatment: joint measurement, reprinted from Am J Occup Ther 1:69, 1947; 2:13, 1948.

8. Kendall FP, Kendall McCreary E, Geise Provance P, et al: *Muscles, testing and function*, ed 5, Baltimore, MD, 2005, Williams & Wilkins.

9. Killingsworth A: *Basic physical disability procedures*, San Jose, CA, 1987, Maple Press.

10. Latella D, Meriano C: *Occupational therapy manual for evaluation of range of motion and muscle strength*, Clifton, NY, 2003, Delmar Thomson Learning.

11. Norkin CC, White DJ: In *Measurement of joint motion: a guide to goniometry*, ed 3, Philadelphia, PA, 2003, FA Davis.

12. Patterson Medical, Sammons Preston: Professional Rehabilitation Catalog, 2011, Warrenville, IL.

13. Rancho Los Amigos Hospital: *How to measure range of motion of the upper extremities* (unpublished manuscript), Rancho Los Amigos, CA, The Hospital.

14. Venes D, Thomas CL: *Taber's cyclopedic medical dictionary*, ed 21, Philadelphia, PA, 2011, FA Davis.

22

Evaluation of Muscle Strength

Vicki Kaskutas and Rose McAndrew[a]

LEARNING OBJECTIVES

After studying this chapter, the student or practitioner will be able to do the following:

1. Describe screening tests for muscle strength assessment.
2. Identify what is measured by the manual muscle test (MMT).
3. List diagnoses for which the MMT is appropriate and those for which it is not appropriate, with the rationale for each.
4. List the steps of the MMT procedure in correct order.
5. Describe the limitations of the MMT.
6. Define muscle grades by name, letter, and number.
7. Administer an MMT, using the directions in this chapter, on a normal practice subject.
8. Describe how results of the muscle strength assessment are used in intervention planning.

CHAPTER OUTLINE

---

[a]The authors would like to acknowledge the significant contributions of Amy Phillips Killingsworth and Lorraine Williams Pedretti to previous editions of this chapter.

KEY TERMS

Against gravity
Gravity-minimized
Manual muscle test
Muscle endurance

Muscle grades
Resistance
Screening tests
Substitutions

THREADED CASE STUDY

Sharon

After a week of experiencing increasing numbness and weakness in her extremities and shortness of breath, Sharon, a 32-year-old who identifies as a woman (prefers use of the pronouns she/her/hers), was admitted to an intensive care unit (ICU) at a local hospital with acute respiratory distress, generalized musculoskeletal weakness, decreased sensory processing, and difficulty swallowing. Sharon complained of pain and tenderness in her muscles and was very agitated and fearful. She was diagnosed as being in the acute phase of Guillain-Barré syndrome (GBS) and was placed on a ventilator.[11] The occupational therapy (OT) practitioner fitted her with resting splints to support Sharon's weakened hands and minimize muscle belly tenderness. When Sharon was moved from the ICU to the acute rehabilitation unit, as the symptoms of GBS began to plateau, the therapist was able to greatly reduce her fear by adapting an environmental system that gave Sharon more control of her environmental context, allowing her to operate her call button, room lights, bed, and television.[20]

Sharon is a senior editor for a monthly food magazine. She has two children, ages 2 and 6. She has been married for 8 years; her husband is a sales representative for a computer company. They live in a two-story townhouse in an urban community. Sharon primarily works at home, going into the magazine's office once or twice a week. However, once a month, during the week the magazine is being published, her life "becomes a bit crazy," and she may go into the office 5 days. She feels fortunate that she is able to employ a housekeeper/childcare person. In addition to caring for her home and family, Sharon is an avid photographer, exercises at a gym three times per week, and enjoys hiking and camping. She is a regular volunteer at her eldest child's school. She and her husband enjoy an active social life.

Six months after onset, Sharon is now being seen as an outpatient by an occupational therapist. Her GBS is in the recovery phase, with remyelination and axonal regeneration resulting in a generalized increase in muscle strength.[11] Sharon continues to be unable to fully engage in occupations that are meaningful to her, primarily because of residual weakness in her distal extremities and moderate limitation in endurance. She usually uses a wheelchair for mobility in the community, but she uses a walker in her home. She has an aide that comes in the morning to assist her with bathing and personal grooming and to drive her to her outpatient appointments. She states that "Although I can do things for myself, it takes so long that I end up being tired before my day even begins. I need help to safely shave my underarms and legs. Styling my hair can be exhausting." Sharon has also indicated that she cannot complete home maintenance tasks such as meal preparation (chopping food items, managing pots and pans) and grocery shopping without assistance. She is unable to fully provide for the care and supervision of her children, especially the 2-year-old, nor can she access the second story of her home on a regular basis. Regarding health maintenance, Sharon needs assistance managing medication bottles and performing exercises; however, she is capable of instructing caregivers in methods to manage her health needs. She is limited in her ability to participate in outdoor and community occupations, which formerly brought her a great deal of satisfaction. She has recently been able to resume some of her job responsibilities at home on a limited basis with a voice-activated computer and is "grateful my employer still wants me and has been willing to make accommodations." She indicated that with all the progress she has made, she and her husband are trying to be realistic but are feeling more and more hopeful about her making a full recovery.

In reviewing the previous occupational profile, the therapist must focus on client factors that are interfering with body function, namely, decreased muscle strength and endurance. Maintaining her arms at and above shoulder level without taking several rest breaks when vigorously brushing her back teeth, for example, remains a problem. Another problem is applying enough force to open jars or perform fine motor activities, such as manipulating coins. These deficits are prohibiting the client from fully engaging in occupations for participation in the physical, social, personal, cultural, and spiritual contexts that bring meaning to her life.

Critical Thinking Questions

1. At what stage in this client's recovery should the occupational therapist first administer a muscle strength assessment?
2. Several methods are available for assessing muscle strength; what are they? What information regarding the client's status could be gained from each of these methods?
3. What is the relationship between MMT and graded activity with this client?

Many physical disabilities cause muscle weakness. Slight to substantial limitations in occupational performance, such as bringing food to one's mouth, lifting a child, removing items from a grocery store shelf, and getting into and out of bed, can result from loss of strength, depending on the degree of weakness and whether the weakness is permanent or temporary.

If improvement is expected, the occupational therapist must assess the current muscle weakness and plan an intervention that will enable graded demands of occupational performance with increased strength.

MUSCLE STRENGTH

Muscle strength is defined as "the amount of force generated by muscle contraction," muscle contraction is the "process of development of tension in muscle tissue" (http://www.online-medical-dictionary.org). Muscle strength is a body function, specifically a muscle function, within the client factor domain according to the Occupational Therapy Practice Framework 4 (OTPF-4).[14] Muscle strength influences several motor skills identified within the performance skills domain of the OTPF, specifically stabilizing, reaching, bending, gripping, moving, lifting, walking, and transporting. Muscle strength is an underpinning of many of the occupations within occupational therapy's domain, such as work participation, home establishment and management, activities of daily living, instrumental activities of daily living, leisure, and play. Muscular strength depends on a wide array of anatomic, physiological, neurological, sensory, motivational, cognitive, environmental, occupational, and habitual factors. Muscle weakness can restrict or prevent performance of a wide array of performance skills and occupations within occupational therapy's domain. Muscle strength can be assessed by observing the client perform daily activities (see Chapter 20), screening tests, and manual muscle testing, when indicated.

OT practitioners must understand the components and function of the muscular system and its interaction with other systems of the body before performing MMT. To ensure that it is safe to evaluate muscle strength, any health conditions, injuries, and/or illnesses that the client may have should be known, and the OT practitioner must understand the effect that these condition(s) may have on the muscular system and contraindications to strength testing. Several factors should be screened and/or understood before assessing muscle strength, and the therapist must weigh the risks of strength testing with the benefits. Factors that may preclude a reliable and accurate assessment of strength should be considered, and muscle strength grades should never be reported unless the therapist can attest that the strength assessment is a true measure of strength and not a measure of other interfering factors such as pain, fatigue, motivation, cognition, or environmental conditions. This chapter assumes that the reader has this level of knowledge and clinical reasoning before participating in strength assessment.

CAUSES OF MUSCLE WEAKNESS

Muscle strength varies greatly among individuals based upon their:
- Stature/size
- Muscle fiber composition
- Occupations/activities
- Age
- Sex
- Routines
- Roles
- Motivation
- Health
- Injuries and illnesses

Athletes will likely demonstrate better strength than sedentary workers who do not pursue occupations involving physical effort. Those who have lived with neuromuscular conditions for an extended period, such as brachial plexus injuries or peripheral neuropathies, have diminished strength. As a result, there is a wide variation in the range of what is considered to be "normal" muscle strength. There are many health-related causes for decreased muscle strength.

1. Health conditions affecting the muscle tissue can result in decreased strength, including injuries (muscle strain, tear, laceration, tendinitis, and myositis), muscle length disorders (excessive tightness, length, or spasms), and a wide range of muscular dystrophies.
2. The muscular system requires messages from the nervous system to contract; therefore. strength can be affected because of conditions affecting the nervous system (brain, spinal cord, peripheral nervous system), whether due to disease, illness, or injury. This includes conditions such as stroke, traumatic brain injury, anoxia, amyotrophic lateral sclerosis, multiple sclerosis, tumor, cancer, spinal cord injury, peripheral nerve laceration or impingement, peripheral neuropathy, and nerve disease. The nerve supply to muscle(s) can be damaged from bone fracture, osteoarthritis, or herniation of an intervertebral disc, which can result in decreased strength.
3. Autoimmune disorders and infectious disease often affect the muscular system, resulting in decreased strength. This includes syndromes such as myasthenia gravis, Guillain-Barré syndrome, rheumatoid arthritis, and systemic lupus erythematosus.
4. Endocrine and metabolic disorders can have an impact on muscular function, such as Cushing syndrome, hyperthyroidism hormonal, and diabetes mellitus.
5. Inflammatory conditions, toxins, nutrition, and vitamin deficiencies may have an impact on muscle strength.
6. Medical interventions can affect muscle strength as a result of surgery, immobilization, and medications. Clients who have been hospitalized for an extended period can lose a significant amount of strength. Fatigue and disuse can affect strength.

Various other factors that can affect the amount of strength demonstrated during MMT. These may or may not represent an actual muscle strength deficit, but they need to be considered during testing and when interpreting the results. This includes factors within the client (e.g., pain, cognition, motivation, and affect), physical environmental factors (e.g., temperature, noise, privacy, and distractions), and OT practitioner–related factors (e.g., therapeutic relationship, instructions provided, and handling techniques).

METHODS TO EVALUATE MUSCLE STRENGTH

Information regarding a client's muscle strength can be ascertained by several different methods. For many clients seen in occupational therapy, it is important to evaluate strength before implementing other evaluations or interventions. Depending on the specific needs, the OT practitioner should choose the most appropriate method of those listed in the following section to evaluate strength. The OT practitioner should not assume a level of occupational performance based on strength. For example, a client with normal strength may be unable to perform the job essentials because of other factors, whereas a client with strength deficits may perform meaningful daily activities independently.

Screening tests are useful for observing areas of strength and weakness and for determining which areas require specific MMT.[6,10,12,19] Screening tests can help the therapist avoid unnecessary testing or duplication of services.[12] These tests are not as precise as MMT, and their purpose is to make a general evaluation of muscle strength and to determine areas of weakness, performance limitations, and the need for more precise testing. Screening may be accomplished by the following means:

1. Examination of the medical record for results of previous muscle testing or daily activity performance
2. Observing the client's movements while entering the clinic, moving about the hospital room, or getting in or out of a chair
3. Observing the client perform functional activities, such as removing an article of clothing and shaking hands with the therapist.[6,12,13]
4. Performing an occupation-based functional motion assessment, as described in Chapter 20.
5. Performing a gross check of bilateral muscle groups.[13] The client is comfortably seated in a sturdy chair or wheelchair and the OT practitioner asks the client to move both upper extremities through active range of motion. The OT practitioner applies pressure to both extremities at mid-range of selected motions to obtain a gross estimation of strength.

In the case of Sharon, who during the acute stage of her illness had very limited muscle strength, the OT practitioner would be able to observe changes by observing this client as she moved around her bed in an attempt to position herself. Initially she might require maximal assistance for bed repositioning or for food intake. The therapist will notice a gradual increase in automatic movements of the limbs as Sharon raises her arms to her forehead to brush back her hair with her forearm, cups her hands around the water glass being held by her husband as she sips through a straw, bends and straightens her legs in an attempt to get comfortable, or momentarily lifts her trunk away from the surface of the bed. Observation of these spontaneous movements as Sharon begins to engage within the context of her environment can serve as preliminary and informal screening of this client's muscle strength.

MANUAL MUSCLE TESTING

Manual muscle testing (MMT) measures the maximal contraction of a specific muscle or muscle group.[6,7] MMT is used to determine the amount of muscle power and to record gains and losses in strength. Criteria used to measure strength include evidence of muscle contraction, amount of ROM through which the joint passes when the muscle contracts, and amount of external pressure the muscle or muscle group can resist during contraction. Gravity is considered a form of resistance.[6,7,13]

This chapter presents MMT of muscle groups because this level of testing yields the type of data needed for most occupational therapy clinical settings. A muscle can be tested individually if a more precise measure is needed. This chapter presents several common tests of the strength of individual muscles to help the reader envision the differences in testing procedures and discrete actions when testing individual muscles versus groups of muscles that perform a specific action. Readers requiring further details on group MMT are referred to Daniels and Worthingham,[10] Hislop and Montgomery,[12,13] and the Rancho Muscle Testing Guide.[21] Details about specific MMT are available in Kendall and McCreary[15] and Cole et al.[8]

Purposes

The purposes of MMT are to determine the amount of muscle power available, to discern how muscle weakness is limiting performance in meaningful occupations, to prevent deformities that can result from imbalances of strength, to determine the need for assistive devices as compensatory measures, to aid in the selection of occupations within the client's capabilities, to establish a baseline and guide intervention, and to evaluate the effectiveness of intervention strategies and modalities.[16] MMT of individual muscles can be essential for diagnosis of some neuromuscular conditions, such as peripheral nerve lesions and spinal cord injury. In peripheral nerve or nerve root lesions, the pattern of muscle weakness may help determine which nerve or nerve roots are involved, whether the involvement is partial or complete, and progression over time. Careful evaluation can help determine the level(s) of spinal cord involvement and can provide an indication of whether the cord damage is complete or incomplete.[15] Along with sensory evaluation, MMT can therefore be an important diagnostic aid in neuromuscular conditions.

Individual Differences

The age, sex, body type, and lifestyle of the client; the muscle size and type and speed of contraction; the effect of previous training for the testing situation; joint position during the muscle contraction; previous training effects; and time of day, temperature, and fatigue all can affect muscle strength.[6,7] Occupations also influence the amount of pressure that a particular client can withstand during strength testing.[9,10,12–15] Strength tends to decline with age, and the amount of pressure the same muscle group will tolerate varies considerably from an 85-year-old to a 25-year-old.[7,15] When an individual has one side affected, such as a nerve injury, to establish an individual client's "normal" strength is recommended to test the unaffected extremity first. Evaluating strength on the unaffected extremity provides a comparison when testing the affected extremity. Learning about the activities, occupations, and tasks regularly performed in daily life can give the therapist a general idea of an individual's strength, however assumptions should be avoided. For example, an individual who regularly plays football for leisure or is employed as a construction worker is likely to have strength that is in the higher range of "normal." Conversely, the strength of a financial consultant, with a slight build, should not be assumed because that individual may regularly practice taekwondo.

Limitations

When done correctly, MMT measures the strength of a muscle or group of muscles. Although information about quality of movements (speed, smoothness, rhythm, and abnormal movements such as tremors),[19] muscle tone (resistance to passive movement), and motor performance (the use of muscles for functional activities)[8] may be gathered while assessing active and passive ROM, these are not directly measured during MMT. Assessment of muscle endurance involves assessment of ability to repetitively contract and resist fatigue,[6] which are not measured during MMT. In fact, the therapist should limit the number of times that the muscle is maximally contracted during MMT to ensure that strength (and not muscle endurance or fatigue resistance) is being measured.

Contraindications and Precautions

MMT is contraindicated when the client has inflammation or pain in the region to be tested; a dislocation or unhealed fracture; recent surgery, particularly of musculoskeletal structures; myositis ossificans; or bone carcinoma or any fragile bone condition.[7,16] Because weak muscles fatigue easily, MMT should not be performed when the client is tired or especially fatigued for two reasons: the results will not accurately reflect strength and negative ramifications can result when excessive force is applied to muscles that are compromised. Special precautions must be taken when resisted movement could aggravate the client's condition, as might occur with arthritis, osteoporosis, subluxation or hypermobility of a joint, hemophilia or any type of cardiovascular risk or disease, abdominal surgery or an abdominal hernia, and fatigue that exacerbates the client's condition.[6,7] Until recently, MMT was not performed with clients with muscle spasticity, otherwise known as hypertonicity; however, recent literature notes that MMT can result in accurate results in clients with mild spasticity. Critics of MMT in clients with hypertonicity suggest that primitive reflexes and gross synergistic movement patterns make it extremely difficult for the client to isolate joint motion, which is demanded in MMT procedures.[2,3,6,7,17] Refer to Chapters 19, 33, and 34 for detailed information about hypertonicity and MMT in clients with upper motor neuron disorders.

Unlike the PROM assessment discussed in Chapter 21, MMT requires the client's complete involvement in the testing procedure. MMT should not be compromised as a result of cognitive and language barriers or the client's inability to perform the motor skills required for the test.[13] Screening of clients' ability to understand and follow directions and their willingness and ability to expend maximal effort should be ascertained before MMT. If the OT practitioner suspects that the results of MMT may be compromised, MMT should not be performed. Likewise, if the therapist has any reason to believe that results of MMT that was administered do not accurately measure muscle strength, the results should not be recorded in the client's record.

The Role of Joint Range of Motion

The amount of motion through which a muscle group can move the body part is the first criterion used to evaluate MMT. As a result, it is common to perform MMT after evaluating range of motion (ROM) (Chapter 21). The amount of ROM actively performed when the client contracts the muscle group (AROM), is compared to the amount of ROM that the OT practitioner can passively move the client's body part through (PROM). It is important to note that PROM deficits do not affect assignment of muscle strength grades. Despite a PROM limitation, muscle strength within the available AROM may be normal. ROM in the direction of the muscle being tested should be screened before assessing strength; if AROM is within functional limits, further ROM evaluation is not necessary because PROM also will be within functional limits. However, if AROM is limited, the therapist must take the joint through PROM to identify the available amount of joint mobility before assigning a muscle grade.

Let's consider a client with joint contracture resulting from old fracture with passive and active right elbow flexion ROM of 120 degrees. Strength is not the factor limiting AROM, so the OT practitioner proceeds with the next step of MMT, placing the joint in mid-range and applying pressure. It is important to record the PROM limitation along with the muscle grade noted when pressure is applied.[10] Comparing the client's right elbow ROM with measurements of the left elbow ROM has more validity and meaning than comparing to published elbow ROM norms. Conversely, if the client's PROM for elbow flexion is 160 degrees and AROM is only 120 degrees, pressure would not be applied because the muscle group is capable only of moving the joint through partial ROM against gravity, and therapist would proceed with testing elbow flexion in a gravity-minimized plane, explained in detail in the next section. When assessing Sharon's muscle strength during the recovery phase of her illness, the OT practitioner most likely will find less active than passive ROM because of deficits in muscle strength. As remyelination and axonal regeneration occur, the discrepancy between active and passive ROM will likely decrease and strength will begin to recover.

The Role of Gravity

Gravity is a form of resistance that the muscular system must overcome to move the body through ROM. Movement against gravity is one criterion used to assess muscle strength.[15] Movement of a body part against gravity in a vertical plane (i.e., away from the floor or toward the ceiling) through the joint's full available PROM signifies a certain level of muscle strength. If a client is not able to perform a movement against gravity (plane that is vertical), the effect of gravity on the body part is minimized to determine the amount of movement possible. This involves placing the body part in a position that allows motion to occur in a horizontal plane (i.e., parallel to the floor). This position has been referred to as the gravity-eliminated, gravity-minimized, or gravity-lessened test position.[10,15,17,19] Because the effect of gravity cannot be completely eliminated, gravity-minimized or gravity-lessened are more accurate terms to describe this alternative position. The term *gravity-minimized*[10,15] is used in this chapter.

When the body part being moved has a substantial mass (and hence weight), the effect of gravity on muscle power must be considered when muscle testing. Such is the case when moving the trunk or head, lifting an entire extremity at the hip or shoulder, and performing knee, elbow, ankle, and wrist movements. In these cases, motion must occur in the vertical plane to account for gravity's effect, and when strength is inadequate to move the body part in the vertical plane, the body must be repositioned to measure movement in the horizontal or gravity-minimized plane. It is of lesser importance to position body with the motion occurring against gravity (in the vertical plane) when the moving body part is light-weight, such as the fingers, toes, and when rotating the forearm.[10,15] Therefore, when assessing strength of the muscle group that moves the forearm, fingers, or toes, testing can occur in either the horizontal or vertical plane. For some actions, positioning in the against-gravity or gravity-minimized position is not be feasible. For example, when testing scapula depression, the against-gravity position would require the client to assume an inverted position. In individual cases, positioning for movement in the correct plane may not be possible because of confinement to bed, generalized weakness, trunk instability, immobilization devices, medical devices, and precautions. In these instances, the OT practitioner must adapt the positioning to the client's needs and use clinical judgment in modifying the grading. Such modifications in positioning and grading should be noted by the therapist when documenting the results of the muscle test.

For consistency in procedure and grading, gravity-minimized positions and against-gravity positions are used in the manual muscle tests for all motions described later, except in cases in which the positioning is not feasible or would be awkward or uncomfortable for the client. Modifications in positioning and grading have been cited with the individual tests.

Application of Pressure

Application of pressure by the therapist is an additional external force that is used when assessing muscle strength. The amount of pressure a group of muscles performing an action can tolerate depends on a wide range of factors. Larger muscles have greater strength[7,10]; this relates to the diameter or cross-section of the fibers that make up a muscle. The number of muscles responsible for an action (the agonists) also affects the strength of an action. For example, the three muscles primarily responsible for wrist flexion are larger, have more power, and can withstand more pressure than the one muscle that adducts each finger. As a result, the OT practitioner must consider the size and relative power of the muscles and modify the amount of pressure applied accordingly. The amount of pressure that can be applied to grade a particular muscle group varies among individual clients.[9,10,12–15]

There are many other principles that must be followed during application of pressure. Pressure is applied opposite to the direction of the action being tested and should be applied directly opposite to the line of pull of the muscle or muscle group being tested. This means that the pressure is applied completely perpendicular to the long axis of the bony structure that is moving (Fig. 22.1). Application of pressure in this manner allows for all of the therapist's force to be applied to "un-rotate" the joint, and not to compress or distract the joint. Pressure is normally applied as distal as possible on the body part that is moving (avoiding crossing the next joint), which

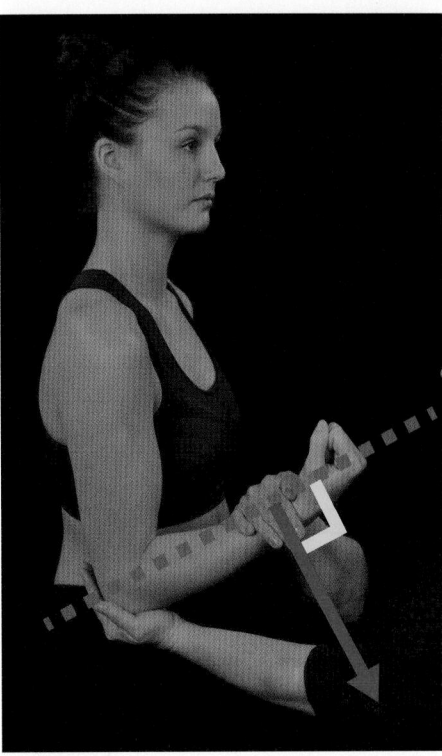

Fig. 22.1 Application of pressure during MMT. *Red arrow* denotes pressure application by OT, *blue dotted line* is the longitudinal axis of the moving body part. Note that pressure is applied perpendicular to the moving body part.

gives the therapist a mechanical advantage because of a longer moment arm. Applying pressure in a perpendicular manner to the moving body part and ensuring that pressure is applied as far distal as possible without crossing the next joint will increase the therapist's biomechanical advantage, resulting in the need to use less force when applying pressure. The therapist should tell the client when the pressure is going to be applied, which allows the client to "set" the muscle. Pressure should be applied gradually and be adjusted to the client's abilities.[12] The body part(s) proximal to the joint being tested should be well stabilized to ensure that pressure is directed only to the muscle group being tested. To prevent interference with muscle contraction, pressure should not be applied directly over the muscle belly or tendon of the muscles that are contracting. In some cases, all of these principles regarding pressure application cannot be observed at the same time. Therefore, the therapist considers the ramifications of breaking a principle, always erring on the side of safety.

The muscle test should not evoke pain, and pressure should be released immediately if pain or discomfort occurs.[10] After applying pressure, the therapist grades the muscle strength according to the standard definitions of muscle grades. This procedure is used for tests of strength of grades Fair+ (3+) and above. Pressure is not usually applied for tests of muscles from Fair (3) to Zero (0); however, slight pressure is applied to a muscle that has completed the full ROM in the gravity-minimized plane to determine whether the grade is Poor+. Fig. 22.2 shows a sample form for recording muscle grades.

MUSCLE EXAMINATION

Client's name _____ Chart no. _____

Date of birth_____ Name of institution_____

Date of onset_____ Attending physician_____ MD

Diagnosis:

LEFT   RIGHT

			Examiner's initials					
			Date					
			NECK	Flexors	Sternocleidomastoid			
				Extensor group				
			TRUNK	Flexors	Rectus abdominis			
				Rt. ext. obl. / Lt. int. obl. — Rotators	{ Lt. ext. obl. / Rt. int. obl.			
				Extensors	{ Thoracic group / Lumbar group			
				Pelvic elev.	Quadratus lumb.			
			HIP	Flexors	Iliopsoas			
				Extensors	Gluteus maximus			
				Abductors	Gluteus medius			
				Adductor group				
				External rotator group				
				Internal rotator group				
				Sartorius				
				Tensor fasciae latae				
			KNEE	Flexors	{ Biceps femoris / Inner hamstrings			
				Extensors	Quadriceps			
			ANKLE	Plantar flexors	{ Gastrocnemius / Soleus			
			FOOT	Invertors	{ Tibialis anterior / Tibialis posterior			
				Evertors	{ Peroneus brevis / Peroneus longus			
			TOES	MP flexors	Lumbricales			
				IP flexors (first)	Flex. digit. br.			
				IP flexors (second)	Flex. digit. l.			
				MP extensors	{ Ext. digit. l. / Ext. digit. br.			
			HALLUX	MP flexor	Flex. hall. br.			
				IP flexor	Flex. hall. l.			
				MP extensor	Ext. hall. br.			
				IP extensor	Ext. hall. l.			

Measurements:

Cannot walk   Date   Speech

Stands   Date   Swallowing

Walks unaided   Date   Diaphragm

Walks with apparatus   Date   Intercostals

KEY

5	N	Normal	Complete range of motion against gravity with full resistance.
4	G	Good*	Complete range of motion against gravity with some resistance.
3	F	Fair*	Complete range of motion against gravity.
2	P	Poor*	Complete range of motion with gravity eliminated.
1	T	Trace	Evidence of slight contractility. No joint motion.
0	0	Zero	No evidence of contractility.
S or SS			Spasm or severe spasm.
C or CC			Contracture or severe contracture.

*Muscle spasm or contracture may limit range of motion. A question mark should be placed after the grading of a movement that is incomplete from this cause.

Fig. 22.2 Sample form for recording the muscle examination. (Adapted from March of Dimes Birth Defects Foundation.)

LEFT | | | | | | | | | RIGHT

				Region	Movement	Muscle				
					Examiner's initials					
					Date					
				SCAPULA	Abductor	Serratus anterior				
					Elevator	Upper trapezius				
					Depressor	Lower trapezius				
					Adductors	Middle trapezius				
						Rhomboids				
				SHOULDER	Flexor	Anterior deltoid				
					Extensors	Latissimus dorsi				
						Teres major				
					Abductor	Middle deltoid				
					Horiz. abd.	Posterior deltoid				
					Horiz. add.	Pectoralis major				
					External rotator group					
					Internal rotator group					
				ELBOW	Flexors	Biceps brachii				
						Brachioradialis				
					Extensor	Triceps				
				FOREARM	Supinator group					
					Pronator group					
				WRIST	Flexors	Flex. carpi rad.				
						Flex. carpi uln.				
					Extensors	Ext. carpi rad. l. & br.				
						Ext. carpi uln.				
				FINGERS	MP flexors	Lumbricales				
					IP flexors (first)	Flex. digit. sub.				
					IP flexors (second)	Flex. digit. prof.				
					MP extensor	Ext. digit. com.				
					Adductors	Palmar interossei				
					Abductors	Dorsal interossei				
					Abductor digiti quinti					
					Opponens digiti quinti					
				THUMB	MP flexor	Flex. poll. br.				
					IP flexor	Flex. poll. l.				
					MP extensor	Ext. poll. br.				
					IP extensor	Ext. poll. l.				
					Abductors	Abd. poll. br.				
						Abd. poll. l.				
					Adductor pollicis					
					Opponens pollicis					
				FACE						

Additional data:

Fig. 22.2 cont'd

Because weak muscles fatigue easily, the results of MMT may not be accurate if the client is tired. There should be no more than three repetitions of the test movement because fatigue can result in grading errors if the muscle has low endurance.[7,8] Pain, swelling, or muscle spasm in the area being tested may also interfere with the testing procedure and accurate grading. Such problems should be recorded on the evaluation form.[19] When interpreting muscle testing results, the therapist must assess motivation, cooperation, and the effort put forth by the client.[10] Psychological, cognitive, and sensory difficulties encountered during MMT may render the results inaccurate; therefore, they should not be reported in the medical record.

Gravity-Minimized Position: Palpation of Muscle Contraction

If there is no visible movement when a muscle group is tested on a horizontal plane (gravity-minimized position), the therapist must ascertain if the muscle(s) is/are able to generate any tension, which is done by palpation. The therapist places fingertips (typically the index and long fingertips of one hand) over the muscle belly and/or tendon of the muscles that perform the action being tested and moves the body part into the target position several times while instructing the client to attempt to move the joint in the manner demonstrated. Palpating over the exact position of each muscle belly/tendon that performs is preferred, however placement over the general area of the muscle group performing the action is acceptable. The general area of palpation is common in all joints when moving out of anatomic positions. For example, because shoulder abduction occurs in the frontal (coronal) plane, the muscles performing abduction are palpable lateral to the glenohumeral joint (Fig. 22.3A). Similarly, knee flexion occurs in the sagittal plane, and the muscles that flex the knee lie posterior to the knee joint (muscle bellies are both superior and inferior to the knee), so that is where the OT practitioner palpates to assess if a muscle contraction is occurring (see Fig. 22.3B).

When palpating for contraction, it is important to tell the client that although the muscles can be too weak to physically move the joint, there can still be muscular activity that the OT practitioner can feel when the client attempts to perform the motion. The client should be given several opportunities to generate tension. It is also important for the OT practitioner to know the location of the target muscles and their tendinous attachments to discern from other muscles in the vicinity that may be attempting to substitute for the test action.

Substitutions

The OT practitioner must observe the client closely to ensure that the action they perform is the exact motion performed by the muscle group being tested. The brain thinks in terms of movement and not in terms of contraction of individual muscles.[10] Therefore, a muscle or muscle group may attempt to compensate for the function of a weaker muscle to accomplish a movement. These movements are called substitutions.[6,7,15] The therapist must provide careful instructions; provide correct positioning, stabilization, and palpation; and ensure that the

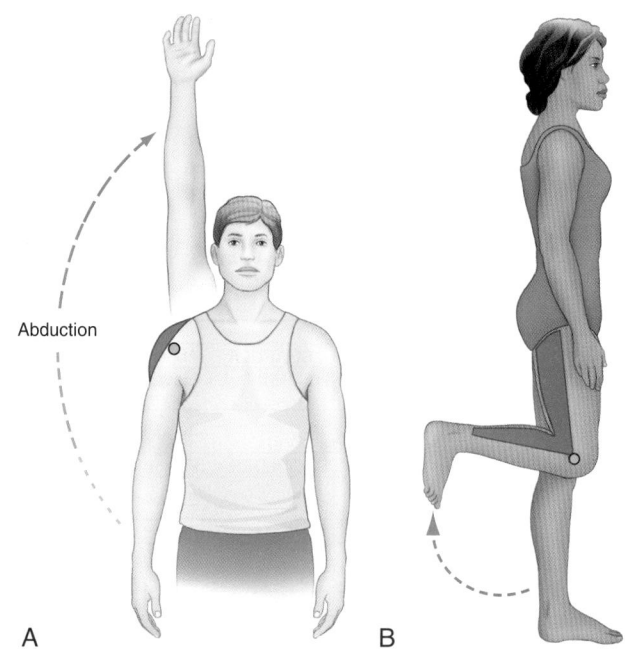

Fig. 22.3 (A) Abduction of the shoulder; *green dot* denotes general axis of motion, and *red shape* represents position of the shoulder abductor muscle group. (B) Flexion of the knee; *green dot* denotes general axis of motion, and *red shape* represents position of the knee flexor muscle group.

test motion occurs without extraneous movements. To prevent substitutions, the correct position of the body should be maintained and movement of the part performed without shifting the body or turning the part.[6,7,15] Undetected substitution movements can mask the client's problems, resulting in inaccurate treatment planning.[6] Palpation of the contractile tissue ensures that tension is being generated by the muscle under examination.[6,10] Palpation is used when the muscle grade is below Poor. The technique for muscle testing described in this chapter does not use palpation when testing grades normal, good, fair, or poor. The muscles that work in concert to perform a joint action often originate in different locations, making palpation of the contractile tissue impossible. For example, the muscle bellies of the elbow flexors lie in the anterior arm, lateral forearm, and deep anterior elbow joint. In addition, one of the OT practitioner's hands is stabilizing the proximal body part and the other is applying pressure to the moving body part, leaving no hand free for palpation. This chapter describes body and joint positioning in detail, placement of the body part in a specific position, and subtle movements clients may perform to help the OT practitioner identify substitutions. Detecting substitutions is a skill that OT practitioners gain with time and experience.

Knowledge and Skill of the Occupational Therapist

The safety, reliability, and validity of MMT depends on the knowledge, abilities, and skills of the OT practitioner. This begins with detailed understanding of the muscular system (muscle anatomy, innervation, origin, and insertion), kinesiology (muscle action and function, direction of muscle fibers, the role of muscles in fixation and substitution), and skeletal system (joints, motions, end-feels, and normal ROM). The therapist must be able to observe the contour of a muscle to determine if it is normal, atrophied, or hypertrophied. The OT practitioner must be able to detect abnormal movements, postures, and positions. Therapists must be able to position their body and the client's body and body part and apply stabilization and pressure adequately or must be able to instruct and closely supervise a proxy to help in performing these physical skills. The ability to locate and feel contracting muscles is required. The OT practitioner must know and be competent using consistent methods in the application of test procedures. Skilled observation of movement, careful and accurate palpation, correct positioning, consistency of procedure, and experience of the therapist are critical factors in accurate testing.[10,12-15] Knowledge and experience are necessary to detect substitutions and interpret strength grades with accuracy.[12-15]

It is necessary for the OT practitioner to acquire skill and experience in testing and grading the muscles of a wide range of typical individuals of all ages before to be able to determine how "normal" presents in the clinical setting. Although definitions of muscle grades are standardized, conducting MMT consists of both subjective and objective components. Subjective components relate to the OT practitioner's perception of how much pressure was applied, relative to their expectations based on experience of what is typical strength for a person of that size, age, history, etc. Objective factors primarily relate to the clients' ROM in a specific plane. Collectively, the objective and subjective components inform the therapist's clinical reasoning to assign a specific muscle grade. Because many factors affect muscle strength, experience is required to help therapists differentiate among strength grades.[19]

PRINCIPLES OF MANUAL MUSCLE TESTING

Preparation for Testing

After performing necessary screening tests, the client is positioned on a stable chair or table per directions outlined in specific testing procedures. If several tests are to be administered, they are sequenced to avoid frequent repositioning of the client.[12,13,21] Clothing is arranged or removed to avoid interference with motion, contraction, or application of pressure and to allow for observation of muscle contour (symmetry between sides, hypertrophy, or atrophy). The OT practitioners is positioned close to the client's body part being tested to minimize upward and outward reaching. This allows for support of a weakened extremity on the OT practitioner's body, decreases the amount of force the OT practitioner must generate when applying pressure, protects the OT practitioner's joint structures, and prevents overall fatigue.

Specific Procedure for Testing

To ensure accuracy and consistency, MMT must always be performed according to standardized procedures. If modifications are performed, they must be described and documented. The procedure for MMT of the extremities is described in Box 22.1. Scapular actions are not demonstrated in this chapter; however, muscles that move the scapula are being tested during shoulder

---

> ### BOX 22.1 Manual Muscle Test Procedure
>
> 1. **Body position:** The client is positioned in a stable position that allows for the muscle group to perform the action against gravity (vertical plane).
> 2. **Action:** After being shown the motion to be tested, the client actively performs the action against gravity through the maximal available range of motion.*
> 3. **Test position:** The joint is positioned midway through the available range of motion.
> 4. **Stabilize:** The OT practitioner stabilizes the body part just proximal to the joint that is moving.
> 5. **Pressure:** The OT practitioner applies pressure opposite to the direction of muscle contraction. NOTE: we use the word *pressure* and not *resistance*, because the therapist is not resisting the client's motion. We also do not use the term "break test," as the therapist is not attempting to apply enough pressure to overcome the client's effort.

* Depending on the results in step 2, the following procedures are followed:

a. If the client demonstrates active ROM through the available PROM, the OT practitioners positions the joint in mid-range (approximately 50% of full available PROM), stabilizes the body part proximal to the joint being tested (to isolate the muscle group, ensure the correct test motion, and prevent substitutions), and applies pressure perpendicular to the body part that moved to assume the test position in a direction that is opposite to the motion being tested. Pressure is applied as distal as possible on the moving body part without crossing the next joint. For example, when elbow flexion is tested, the therapist applies pressure over the distal volar forearm (just proximal to the wrist) in the direction of elbow extension. The client should be prepared to establish a maximal contraction when the OT practitioner applies pressure.[10,16]

b. If AROM is less than the available PROM, and no other reason for limited AROM is detected (e.g., joint contracture), the OT practitioner positions the client's body part in a manner that limits the effect of gravity (body part supported by the OT practitioner in a horizontal plane that is parallel to the ground) the client is asked to perform the action in the gravity-minimized (horizontal) plane. The OT practitioner will need to demonstrate the motion to the client by either performing the motion himself or herself or passively moving the client's through the motion.

   i. If the client performs the motion through full available PROM in the gravity-minimized plane, the body part is placed at mid-range and the therapist attempts to move the body part out of the test position using slight pressure.

   ii. If the client is unable to perform the motion through full available PROM, no pressure is applied.

   iii. If no motion is noted in the horizontal plane, the therapist palpates over the muscle belly and/or tendon of the muscles being tested and the OT practitioner demonstrates the action he or she wants the client to try to perform, positions the joint in midposition, and asks the client to attempt the motion while the OT practitioner palpates for muscle contraction.

MMT. Procedures for testing the face, neck, and trunk are documented elsewhere.[6,8,10,12-15]

Grading of Muscle Strength

The criteria for grading of muscle strength are listed in Table 22.1.[6,10,12,13,21] The highest grade that can be assigned is grade 5, or Normal. For a client to be assigned this muscle grade, the client must demonstrate full AROM against gravity and tolerate maximal pressure. If a muscle group is able to complete full range against gravity but is unable to withstand the maximal

TABLE 22.1 Muscle Grades

Grade (No.)	Grade (Name)		Gravity	AROM	Pressure
5	Normal	N	Against	Full	Maximal
4+	Good plus	G+	Against	Full	Moderate to maximal
4	Good	G	Against	Full	Moderate
4−	Good minus	G−	Against	Full	Minimal
3+	Fair plus	F+	Against	Full	Slight
3	Fair	F	Against	Full	None
3−	Fair minus	F−	Against	More than 50%	None
2+	Poor plus	P+	Against	Less than 50%	None
			Gravity minimized	Full	Slight
2	Poor	P	Gravity minimized	Full	None
2−	Poor minus	P−	Gravity minimized	Partial	None
1	Trace	T	Against or gravity minimized	No motion	Contract observed/felt
0	Zero	0	Against or gravity minimized	No motion	No movement

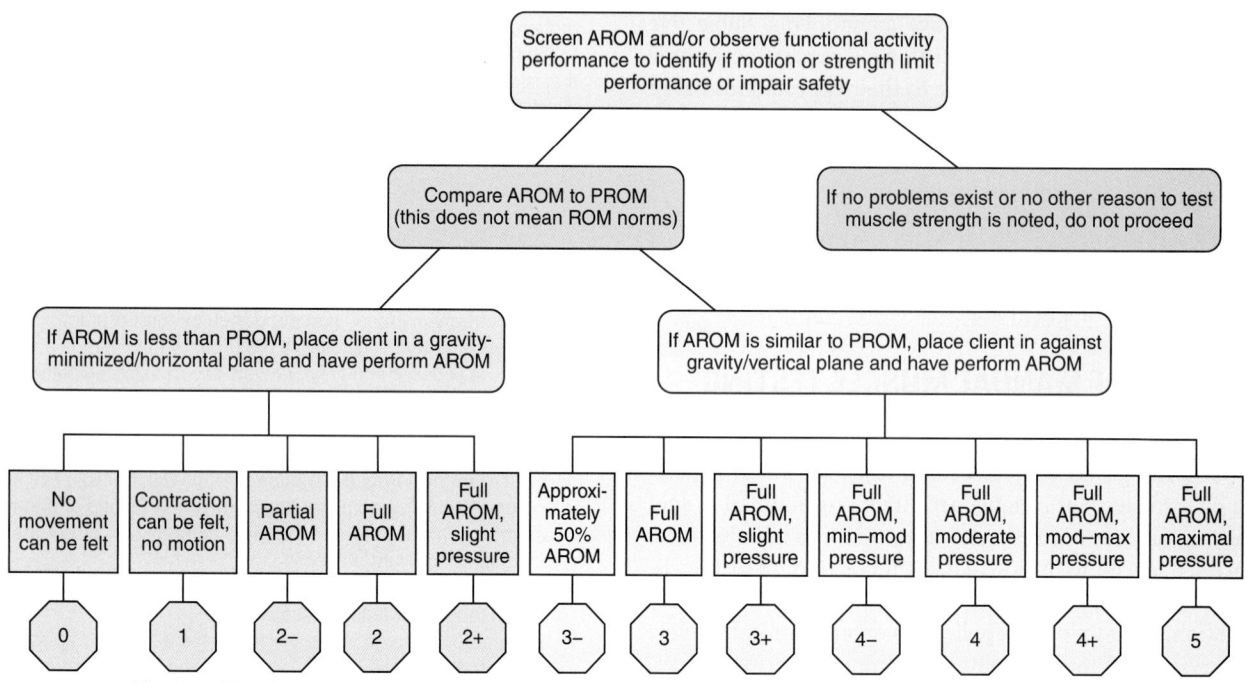

Fig. 22.4 Muscle testing decision tree. *AROM,* Active range of motion; *max,* maximum; *min,* minimum; *mod,* moderate; *PROM,* passive range of motion.

pressure, it is assigned a grade 4, Good. The therapist will assign a grade 4 when the muscle "yields" or "gives" when it is no longer to withstand maximal pressure. A muscle or muscle group is deemed a grade 3, Fair, if it can move through the full ROM against gravity but cannot tolerate additional pressure from the OT practitioner. The muscle group will easily yield if the therapist provides only slight pressure. If a muscle group is assigned a muscle grade of 2, Poor, the muscle group is able to complete full ROM in a gravity-minimized plane. If the muscle group is unable to move the body through any ROM in a gravity-minimized plane, but the therapist can feel tension or contraction in the muscle group upon palpation, the muscle is a grade 1, Trace.

The client does not need to be placed in a gravity-minimized plane to palpate the muscle contraction. When the therapist is unable to feel the contraction, the muscle is assigned a grade 0, Zero. The decision tree in Fig. 22.4 is a useful guide.

The purpose of using "plus" or "minus" designations with muscle grades is to "fine-grade" muscle strength. These designations are likely to be used by the experienced OT practitioner. Two OT practitioners testing the same individual may vary up to a half grade in their results, but there should not be a whole grade difference.[19] Practice among a work group of OT practitioners can standardize techniques and calibrate muscle grading to improve interrater reliability.

If tests of the forearm, fingers, and toes are performed against gravity rather than in the gravity-minimized plane, the standard definitions of muscle grades can be modified when muscle grades are recorded. Partial ROM against gravity is graded Poor (2), and full ROM against gravity is graded Fair (3).[10]

If the client cannot be placed in the correct position for the test, the OT practitioner must adapt the test and use clinical judgment in approximating strength grades.[19] In addition to correct positioning, test reliability and validity depends on careful stabilization, palpation of the muscles, and observation of movement.[10]

MANUAL MUSCLE TESTING OF THE UPPER EXTREMITY

The muscles performing each action, their innervation, and the specific procedures for testing are described in this section. The OT practitioner has positioned to allow for optimal viewing of client positioning, which may not be the most mechanically advantageous position for the OT practitioner. The evaluator should stand as close as possible to the body part that is being tested. Pressure should always be applied perpendicular to the distal body part, which may not always be demonstrated in the picture to maintain optimal viewing of the client's positioning.

Shoulder Flexion (Fig. 22.5)

Muscles[10,22]	Innervation[6,10,19,22]
Anterior deltoid	Axillary nerve, C5,6
Coracobrachialis	Musculocutaneous nerve, C5-7
Bicep brachii (short head)	Musculocutaneous, C5, C6
Pectoralis major (clavicular head)	Lateral and medial pectoral nerves, C5, C6

Procedure for Testing Grades Normal (5), Good (4), and Fair (3)

1. **Body position:** The client is seated on a supportive chair or mat; if trunk stability or balance is impaired, the trunk is externally supported. Shoulder is at side in neutrally rotated position. The therapist stands on the side being tested.
2. **Action:** While demonstrating movement from neutral to full shoulder flexion, the OT practitioner says, "move your arm like I am." Observe the client actively perform the movement. Allow client's scapula and clavicle to move along with the humerus (Fig. 22.5A).
3. **Test position:** If client performs through available PROM, place shoulder at 90 degrees of flexion and proceed. If not, follow procedure for testing grades Poor, Trace, and Zero.
4. **Stabilize:** Therapist stabilizes the scapula and clavicle by placing hand over superior shoulder girdle just proximal to glen-humeral joint. Client is stabilized in chair if needed.
5. **Pressure:** Tell the client, "don't let me move you." Apply pressure perpendicular to the distal humerus in downward fashion (toward shoulder extension), adjusting pressure to client's abilities (see Fig. 22.5B). If pressure maximal = Normal; moderate = Good, minimal = Good–, slight = Fair+, and no pressure = Fair.

Procedure for Testing Grades Poor (2), Trace (1), and Zero (0)

1. **Body position:** The client is side-lying on side that is not being tested. If the client cannot maintain the weight of the upper extremity against gravity, the therapist supports it[6,12] (see Fig. 22.5C). If the side-lying position is not feasible, the client may remain seated, and the test procedure is performed with grading modified.[10]
2. **Action:** Beginning in mid-position, move client's shoulder through partial flexion ROM twice while stating "move your arm like I did."

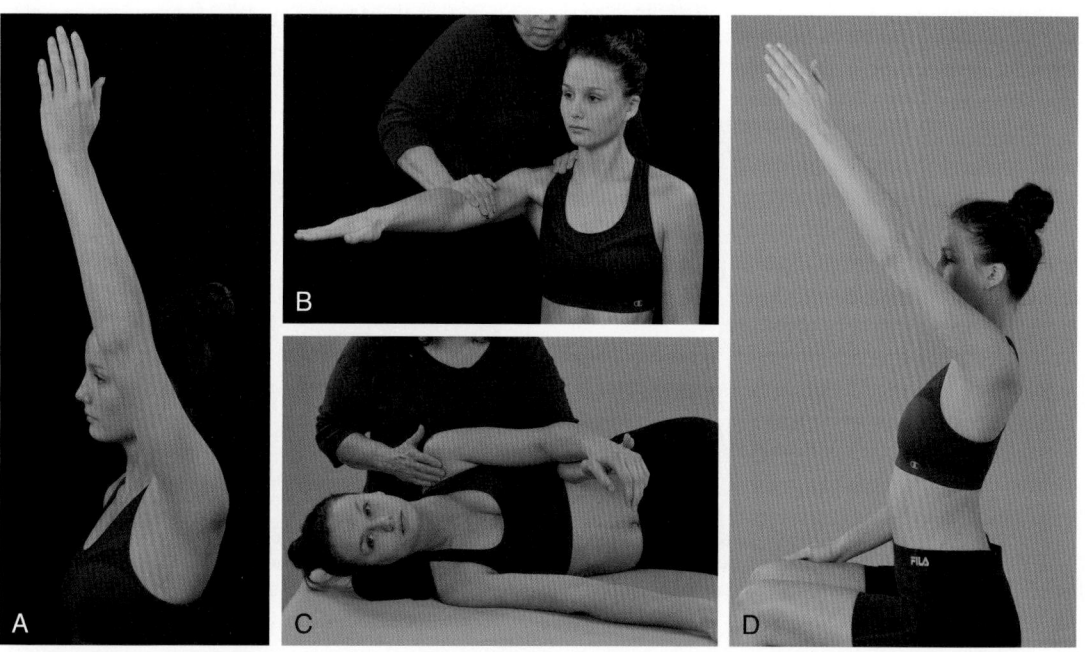

Fig. 22.5 (A) Shoulder flexion: action—muscle grades 3 and above. (B) Shoulder flexion: application of pressure. (C) Shoulder flexion: palpation—for muscle grades 2 and below. (D) Shoulder flexion: substitutions.

a. If client performs action through full ROM, place in 90 degrees of shoulder flexion and apply slight pressure perpendicular to the distal humerus toward shoulder extension.
   i. If tolerates pressure = Poor+.
   ii. No pressure = Poor.
b. If client performs through partial ROM, do not apply pressure = Poor–.
c. If client unable to perform motion, place in 90 degrees of shoulder flexion and state, "try to move your arm like I did." Palpate over anterior glenohumeral joint to feel for contraction in shoulder flexor muscle(s) (see Fig. 22.4).
   i. If muscle contraction palpable = Trace.
   ii. If no contraction palpable = Zero.

Substitution(s). Observe for flexion accompanied by horizontal adduction, external rotation, or scapula elevation.[10,16,21] Also, hyperextension (increased lumbar lordosis) of the trunk (see Fig. 22.5D)

NOTE: Arm elevation in the plane of the scapula, about halfway between shoulder flexion and abduction, is called *scaption*. This movement is used for function more commonly than shoulder flexion or abduction. Scaption is performed by the deltoid and supraspinatus muscles. It is tested in a way similar to that used for shoulder flexion, except the arm is in a position 30 to 45 degrees anterior to the frontal plane.[6,12]

Shoulder Extension (Figs. 22.6 to 22.11)

Muscles[4,10,14,19,22]	Innervation[6,10,19,22]
Latissimus dorsi	Thoracodorsal nerve, C6-8
Teres major	Lower subscapular nerve, C5-7
Posterior deltoid	Axillary nerve, C5,6
Infraspinatus	Suprascapular, C4-6
Teres minor	Axillary nerve, C5, 6
Triceps brachii (long head)	Radial nerve, C6-8
Pectoralis major (sternal head)	Lateral and medial pectoral nerve, C7, 8, T1

Procedure for Testing Grades Normal (5), Good (4), and Fair (3)

1. **Body position:** The client is sitting on chair without back or lying prone on mat. If trunk stability or balance is impaired, the trunk is externally supported. Shoulder is at side in neutral position.[6,7,12] The therapist stands behind the side being tested.
2. **Action:** While passively moving the client's shoulder from neutral to shoulder extension, the OT practitioner says, "move your arm like I did." Observe the client actively perform the movement.
3. **Test position:** If client performs through available PROM, place shoulder at 30 degrees extension and proceed (Figs. 22.6 and 22.7). If not, follow procedure for testing grades Poor, Trace, and Zero.
4. **Stabilize:** Therapist stabilizes scapula and clavicle by placing hand over superior shoulder girdle just proximal to glenohumeral joint. If sitting, client is stabilized in chair if needed.
5. **Pressure:** Tell the client, "don't let me move you." Apply pressure perpendicular to humerus at the distal humerus toward flexion, adjusting pressure to client's abilities (Figs. 22.8 and 22.9). If pressure maximal = Normal; moderate = Good, minimal = Good–, slight = Fair+, and no pressure = Fair.

Procedure for Testing Grades Poor (2), Trace (1), and Zero (0)

1. **Body position:** The client is placed side-lying on side that is not being tested. If the client cannot maintain the weight of the upper extremity against gravity, the therapist supports it[6,12] (Fig. 22.10). If the side-lying position is not feasible, the client may remain seated or in prone, and the test procedure is performed with the grading modified.[10]
2. **Action:** Beginning in mid-position, move client's shoulder through partial extension ROM twice while stating "move your arm like I did" (see Fig. 22.10).
   a. If client performs full ROM, place in 30 degrees of shoulder extension and apply slight pressure perpendicular to the distal humerus.
      i. If tolerates pressure = Poor+.
      ii. No pressure = Poor.

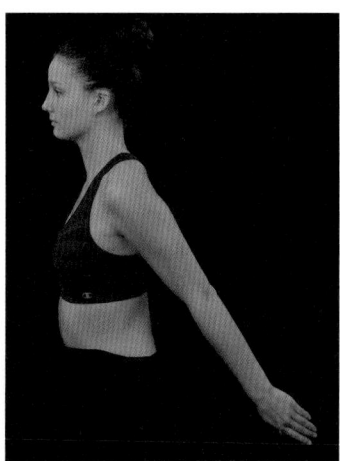

Fig. 22.6 Shoulder extension: action—muscle grades 3 and above.

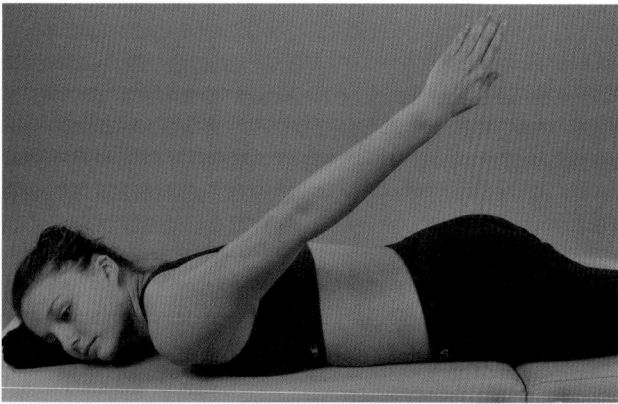

Fig. 22.7 Shoulder extension: alternate test position—muscle grades 3 and above.

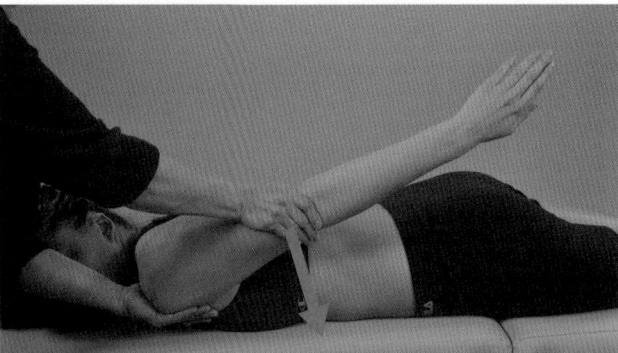

Fig. 22.8 Shoulder extension: application of pressure.

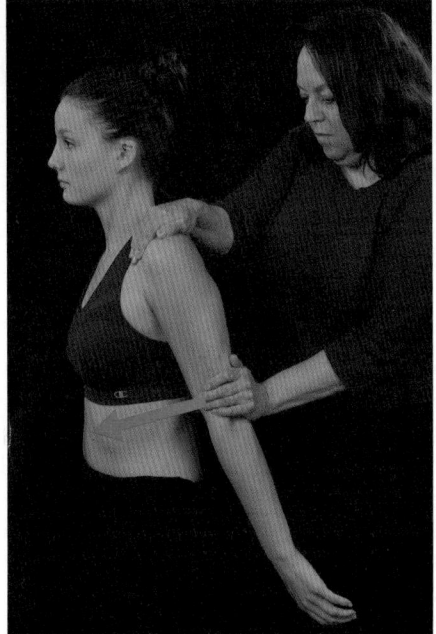

Fig. 22.9 Shoulder extension: application of pressure.

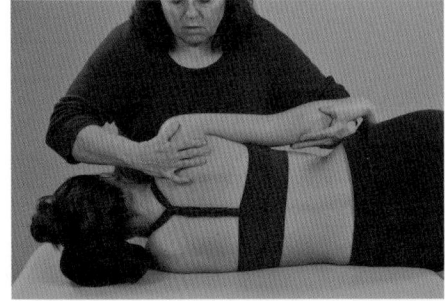

Fig. 22.10 Shoulder extension: positioning—for testing muscle grades 2 and below.

b. If patient performs through partial ROM, do not apply pressure = Poor–.
c. If client is unable to perform motion, place in 90 degrees of shoulder flexion and state, "try to move your arm like I did." Palpate over posterior glenohumeral joint to feel for contraction in shoulder extensor muscle(s).
   i. If muscle contraction palpable = Trace.
   ii. If no contraction palpable = Zero.

Substitutions. If sitting, trunk flexion or scapular anterior tilting (Fig. 22.11).

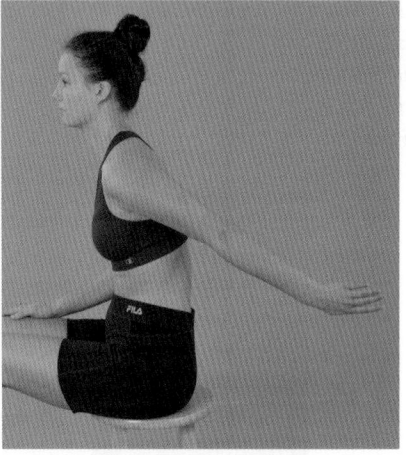

Fig. 22.11 Shoulder extension: substitution.

Shoulder Abduction (Figs. 22.12 to 22.14)

Muscles[10,15]	Innervation[1]
Middle deltoid	Axillary nerve, C5,6
Supraspinatus	Suprascapular nerve, C4, C5, C6

Procedure for Testing Grades Normal (5), Good (4), and Fair (3)

1. **Body position:** The client is seated on a supportive chair or mat; if trunk stability or balance is impaired, the trunk is externally supported. The therapist stands behind the client.[6,7,12]
2. **Action:** While demonstrating movement from neutral to full shoulder abduction, the therapist says, "move your arm like I am." Observe the client actively perform the movement. Allow client's scapula and clavicle to move along with the humerus (Fig. 22.12).
3. **Test position:** If client performs through available PROM, place shoulder at 90 degrees of abduction and proceed. If not, follow procedure for testing grades Poor, Trace, and Zero.
4. **Stabilize:** Therapist stabilizes scapula and clavicle by placing hand over superior shoulder girdle proximal to glenohumeral joint. Client is stabilized in chair if needed.
5. **Pressure:** Tell the client, "don't let me move you." Apply pressure perpendicular to the distal humerus in downward fashion toward adduction, adjusting pressure to client's abilities (Fig. 22.13). If pressure maximal = Normal; moderate = Good, minimal = Good–, slight = Fair+, and no pressure = Fair.

Procedure for Testing Grades Poor (2), Trace (1), and Zero (0)

1. **Body position:** The client is in the supine position, lying with the arm to be tested resting at the side of the body. The therapist stands on the side to be tested,[10,12] providing upper extremity support if needed.
2. **Action:** Beginning in mid-position, move client's shoulder through partial abduction ROM twice while stating "move your arm like I did" (Fig. 22.14).

a. If client performs full ROM, place in 90 degrees of shoulder abduction and apply slight pressure perpendicular to the distal humerus.
   i. If tolerates pressure = Poor+.
   ii. No pressure = Poor.

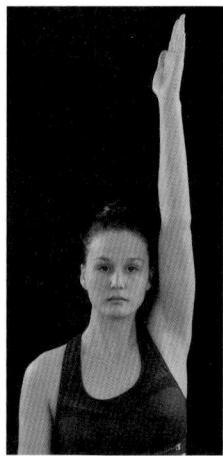

Fig. 22.12 Shoulder abduction: action—muscle grades 3 and above.

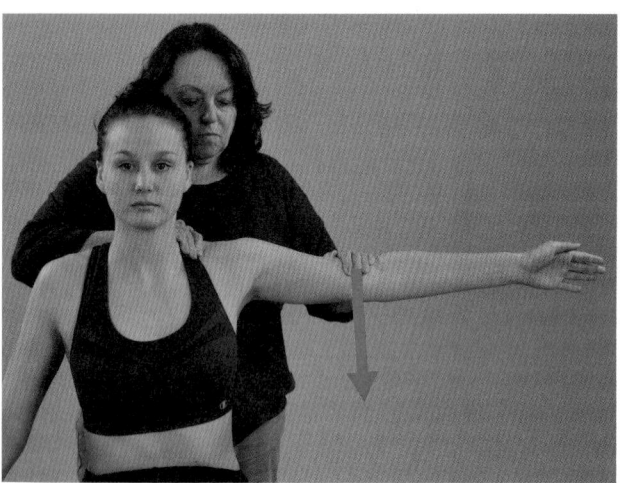

Fig. 22.13 Shoulder abduction: application of pressure.

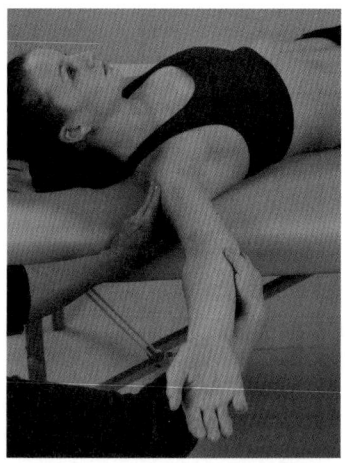

Fig. 22.14 Shoulder abduction: position and palpation—muscle grades 2 and below.

b. If client performs through partial ROM, do not apply pressure = Poor–.
c. If client unable to perform motion, place in 90 degrees of shoulder abduction and state, "try to move your arm like I did." Palpate superior to glenohumeral joint to feel for contraction in shoulder abductor muscle(s) (see Fig. 22.14).
   i. If muscle contraction palpable = Trace.
   ii. If no contraction palpable = Zero.

Substitutions. The long head of the biceps may attempt to substitute. Observe for elbow flexion and external rotation accompanying the movement.[12] The anterior and posterior heads of the deltoid can act together to effect abduction. The upper trapezius may attempt to assist. Observe for scapula elevation preceding movement.[7,16,21]

Shoulder External Rotation (Figs. 22.15 to 22.19)

Muscles[4,10,15]	Innervation[4,10,15]
Infraspinatus	Suprascapular nerve, C5,6
Teres minor	Axillary nerve, C5,6
Posterior deltoid	Axillary nerve, C5,6

Procedure for Testing Grades Normal (5), Good (4), and Fair (3)

1. **Body position:** The client is prone (or sitting), with the shoulder abducted to 90 degrees and the humerus in neutral rotation, elbow flexed to 90 degrees. The forearm is in neutral rotation, hanging over the edge of the table, perpendicular to the floor.[6–8,12] A rolled towel under distal humerus will elevate the humerus to full abduction and may increase comfort. The therapist stands in front of the supporting surface, toward the side to be tested.[10,15]
2. **Action:** The therapist demonstrates the movement from neutral to full shoulder external rotation. The therapist then says, "move your arm like I did" (Figs. 22.15 and 22.16).
3. **Test position:** If client performs through available PROM, place shoulder in mid-external rotation ROM (approximately 40 degrees) and proceed. If not, follow procedure for testing grades Poor, Trace, and Zero.

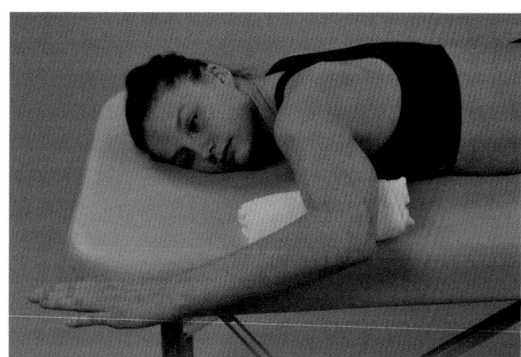

Fig. 22.15 Shoulder external rotation: test position—muscle grades 3 and above.

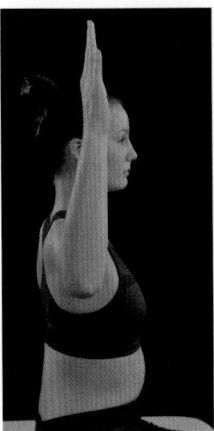

Fig. 22.16 Shoulder external rotation: alternate test position—muscle grades 3 and above.

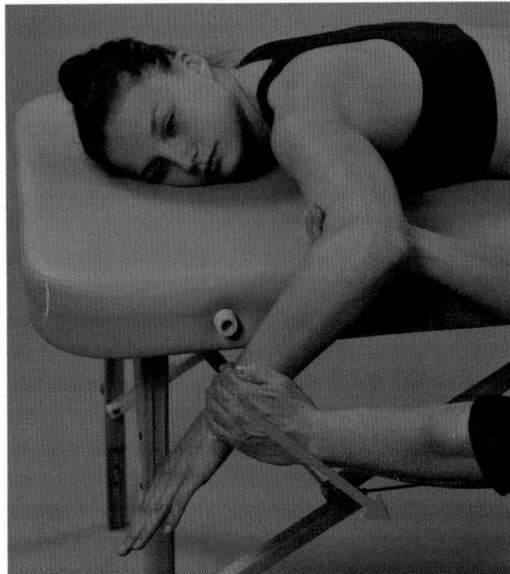

Fig. 22.17 Shoulder external rotation: application of pressure.

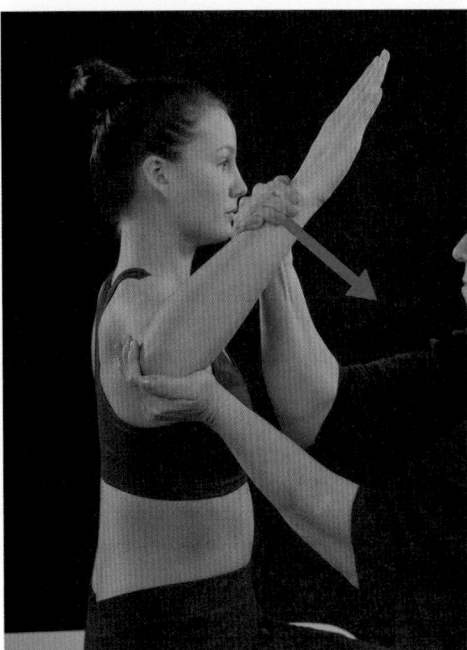

Fig. 22.18 Shoulder external rotation: application of pressure.

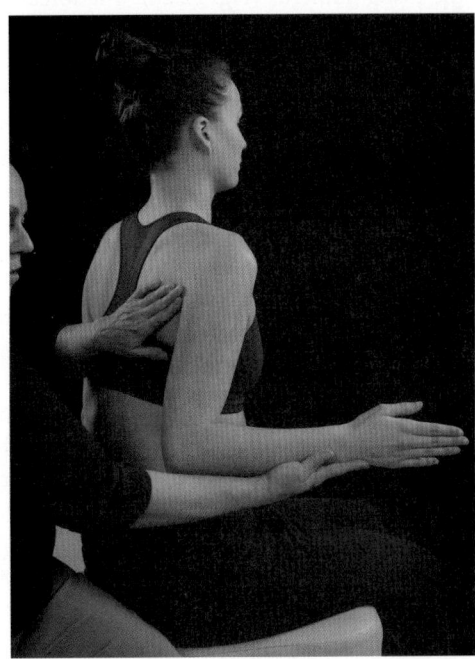

Fig. 22.19 Shoulder external rotation: position and palpation—muscle grades 2 and below.

4. **Stabilize:** The therapist provides stabilization at the distal end of the humerus by placing a hand under the distal humerus on supporting table.[7,15]

5. **Pressure:** The therapist tells the client, "don't let me move you." Apply pressure perpendicular to the distal end of the forearm toward the direction of internal rotation, adjusting pressure to the client's abilities. If pressure given is maximal = Normal; moderate = Good, minimal = Good−, slight = Fair+, and no pressure = Fair (Figs. 22.17 and 22.18).

Procedure for Testing Grades Poor (2), Trace (1), and Zero (0)

1. **Body position:** The client is seated, with arm adducted and in neutral rotation at the shoulder. The elbow is flexed to 90 degrees, with the forearm in neutral rotation. The therapist stands in front of the client toward the side to be tested.[6,7]

2. **Action:** Move client's shoulder through partial external rotation ROM twice while stating "move your arm like I did."

   a. If client performs full ROM, place in 40 degrees of external rotation and apply slight pressure to the distal forearm toward internal rotation.

   i. If tolerates pressure = Poor+.
   ii. No pressure = Poor.

   b. If client performs through partial ROM, do not apply pressure = Poor−.

   c. If client unable to perform motion, place in 40 degrees of external rotation and state, "try to move your arm like I did." Palpate over posterior shoulder and scapula to feel for contraction in external rotators (Fig. 22.19).

   i. If muscle contraction palpable = Trace.
   ii. If no contraction palpable = Zero.

   Substitutions. If the elbow is extended and the client supinates the forearm, the momentum could aid external rotation of the humerus. Scapular adduction can pull the humerus backward and into some external rotation. The therapist should observe for scapula adduction and initiation of movement with forearm supination.[16,21]

Shoulder Internal Rotation (Figs. 22.20 to 22.22)

Muscles[10,15,16]	Innervation[4,5,10]
Subscapularis	Subscapular nerve, C5-7
Pectoralis major	Medial and lateral pectoral nerves, C5-T1
Latissimus dorsi	Thoracodorsal nerve, C6-8
Teres major	Lower Subscapular nerve, C5-6
Anterior deltoid	Axillary nerve, C5-6

Procedure for Testing Grades Normal (5), Good (4), and Fair (3)

1. **Body position:** The client is prone, with the shoulder abducted to 90 degrees, the humerus in neutral rotation, and the elbow flexed to 90 degrees. A rolled towel may be placed under the distal humerus (Fig. 22.20). The forearm is perpendicular to the floor. The therapist stands on the side to be tested, just in front of the client's arm.[6-8,12]
2. **Action:** While demonstrating movement from neutral to full internal rotation, the therapist says, "move your arm like I am." Observe the client actively perform the movement (see Fig. 22.20).
3. **Test position:** If client performs through available PROM, place shoulder into mid-range of internal rotation (approximately 40 degrees) and proceed.
4. **Stabilize:** The therapist provides stabilization at the distal end of the humerus by placing a hand under the arm and on the supporting surface, as for external rotation.[6,7,10,15]
5. **Pressure:** The therapist tells the client, "don't let me move you," then applies pressure at the distal end of the volar surface of the forearm anteriorly toward external rotation, adjusting pressure to the client's abilities (Fig. 22.21).

Procedure for Testing Grades Poor (2), Trace (1), and Zero (0)

1. **Body position:** The client is seated, with the shoulder adducted and in neutral rotation, elbow flexed to 90 degrees with the forearm in neutral rotation. The therapist stands on the side to be tested[6,22] and supports forearm (Fig. 22.22).
2. **Action:** Beginning in mid-position, move client's shoulder through partial internal rotation ROM twice while stating "move your arm like I did."
   a. If client performs full ROM, place in mid-shoulder internal rotation (approximately 40 degrees) and apply slight pressure to distal forearm into internal rotation.
      i. If tolerates pressure = Poor+.
      ii. No pressure = Poor.
   b. If client performs through partial ROM, do not apply pressure = Poor−.
   c. If client unable to perform motion, place in mid-range of internal rotation (approximately 40 degrees) and state, "try to move your arm like I did." Palpate over anterior glenohumeral joint to feel for contraction in internal rotators (see Fig. 22.22).
      i. If muscle contraction palpable = Trace.
      ii. If no contraction palpable = Zero.

Substitutions. If the trunk is rotated, gravity will act on the humerus, rotating it internally.[6] The therapist should observe for trunk rotation. When the elbow is in extension, pronation of the forearm can substitute.[10,16,21]

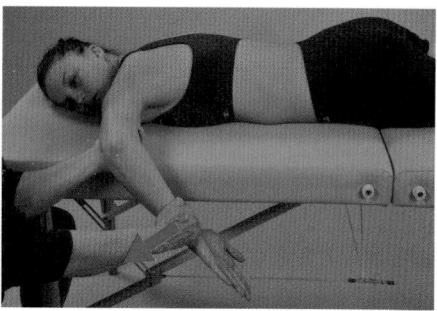

Fig. 22.21 Shoulder internal rotation: application of pressure.

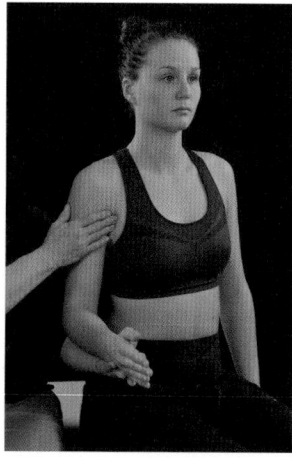

Fig. 22.22 Shoulder internal rotation: position and palpation—muscle grades 2 and below.

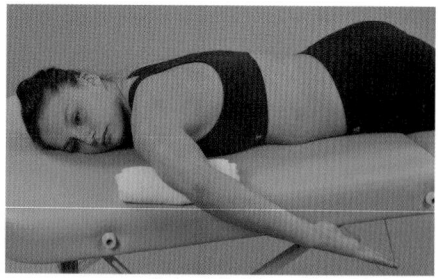

Fig. 22.20 Shoulder internal rotation: test position—muscle grades 3 and above.

Shoulder Horizontal Abduction (Figs. 22.23 to 22.26)

Muscles[4,10,16]	Innervation[10,13]
Posterior deltoid	Axillary nerve, C5, 6
Infraspinatus	Suprascapular nerve, C5, 6

Procedure for Testing Grades Normal (5), Good (4), and Fair (3)

1. **Body position:** The client is prone, with the upper extremity hanging over the edge of the mat, shoulder in approximately 90 degrees of scaption and neutral rotation, and elbow extended. The therapist stands on the side being tested[15,16] (Fig. 22.23).

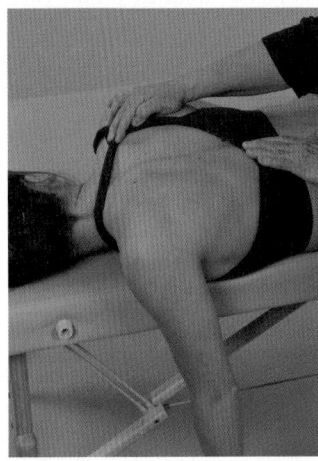

Fig. 22.23 Shoulder horizontal abduction: test position—muscle grades 3 and above.

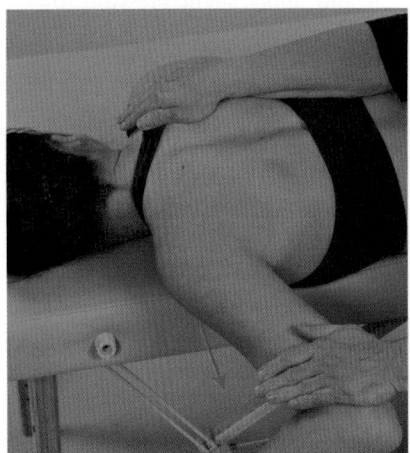

Fig. 22.24 Shoulder horizontal abduction: application of pressure.

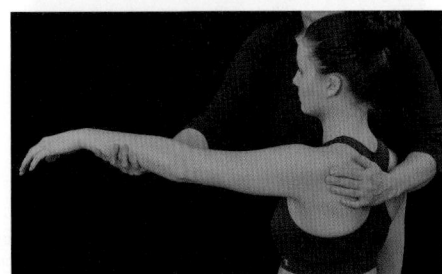

Fig. 22.25 Shoulder horizontal abduction: position and palpation for muscle grades 2 and below.

2. **Action:** The therapist moves the client's upper extremity from position above into full horizontal abduction and says, "move your arm like I did." Observe the client actively perform the movement (Fig. 22.24).

3. **Test position:** If client performs through available PROM, place shoulder into 90 degrees horizontal abduction (upper extremity will be parallel to the floor) and proceed. If not, follow procedure for testing grades Poor, Trace, and Zero.

4. **Stabilize:** The therapist provides stabilization over the scapula.[6,10] If needed, stabilization can move to the opposite scapula to keep client's trunk stable (see Fig. 22.24).

5. **Pressure:** Tell the client, "don't let me move you," then apply pressure over the distal humerus downward toward horizontal adduction. Be sure the table does not restrict motion (see Fig. 22.24).

Procedure for Testing Grades Poor (2), Trace (1), and Zero (0)

1. **Body position:** The client is seated, with the arm in 90-degree abduction and the palm down, supported on a high table or by the therapist[6,12] (Fig. 22.25). If a table is used to support the weight of the upper extremity, powder may be sprinkled on the surface or the limb can be placed on a rolling support (similar to a small skateboard) to reduce friction.

2. **Action:** Beginning in mid-position, move client's shoulder through partial horizontal abduction ROM twice while stating "move your arm like I did."
   a. If client performs full ROM, place in 90 degrees of horizontal abduction and apply slight pressure to distal humerus toward horizontal adduction.
      i. If tolerates pressure = Poor+.
      ii. No pressure = Poor.
   b. If client performs through partial ROM, do not apply pressure = Poor−.
   c. If client is unable to perform motion, place in 90 degrees of horizontal abduction and state, "try to move your arm

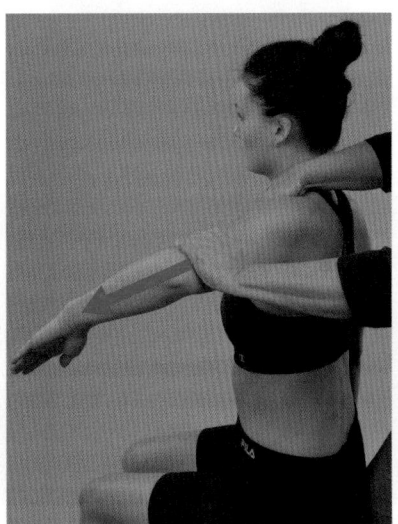

Fig. 22.26 Shoulder horizontal abduction: position, palpation, and pressure to posterior deltoid for muscle grades 2+.

like I did." Palpate over posterior glenohumeral joint to feel for contraction in horizontal abductors.

    i. If muscle contraction palpable = Trace.

    ii. If no contraction palpable = Zero.

Specific muscle testing. The posterior deltoid can be isolated by positioning the client in sitting, with the shoulder in 90 degrees abduction and approximately 35 degrees of internal rotation. The trunk is stabilized, and pressure is applied over the distal humerus toward horizontal adduction and flexion[4] (Fig. 22.26).

Substitutions. Latissimus dorsi and teres major may assist movement if the posterior deltoid is very weak. Movement will occur with more shoulder extension rather than at the horizontal level. Scapula adduction may produce slight horizontal abduction of the humerus, but trunk rotation and shoulder retraction would occur.[6,16,21] The long head of the triceps may substitute. Maintain some flexion at the elbow to prevent this.[12]

Shoulder Horizontal Adduction (Figs. 22.27 to 22.29)

Muscles[4,12–15]	Innervation[4,10,12,13]
Pectoralis major	Medial and lateral pectoral nerves, C5-T1
Anterior deltoid	Axillary nerve, C5, 6
Coracobrachialis	Musculocutaneous nerve, C6, 7
Biceps brachii (short head)	Musculocutaneous nerve, C5, 6

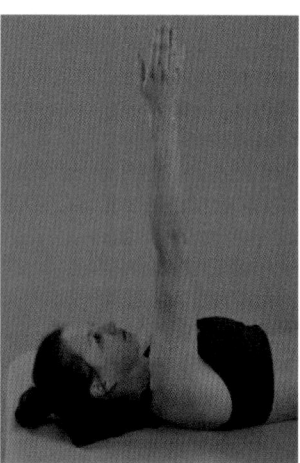

Fig. 22.27 Shoulder horizontal adduction: test position and action—muscle grades 3 and above.

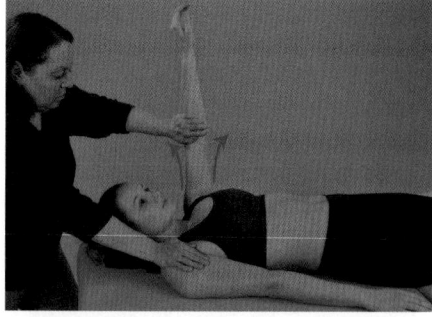

Fig. 22.28 Shoulder horizontal adduction: stabilizing and application of pressure.

Procedure for Testing Grades Normal (5), Good (4), and Fair (3)

1. **Body position:** The client is supine, with the shoulder abducted to 90 degrees, elbow flexed or extended. The therapist stands next to the client on the side being tested or behind the client's head.[4,6,7,10,12]

2. **Action:** The therapist moves the client into horizontal adduction and says, "move your arm like I did." Observe the client actively perform the movement (Fig. 22.27).

3. **Test position:** If client performs through available PROM, place shoulder into mid-horizontal adduction (approximately 80 degrees) (see Fig. 22.27) and proceed. If not, follow procedure for testing grades Poor, Trace, and Zero.

4. **Stabilize:** The therapist stabilizes the trunk by placing one hand over the anterior shoulder on the side opposite to that being tested to stabilize the trunk (Fig. 22.28).

5. **Pressure:** Tell the client, "don't let me move you," then apply pressure over the distal humerus in outward direction toward horizontal abduction (see Fig. 22.28).

Procedure for Testing Grades Poor (2), Trace (1), and Zero (0)

1. **Body position:** The client is seated with shoulder in 90 degrees of shoulder abduction with arm supported on high table[4,12,21] or by therapist (Fig. 22.29A). If a table is used to support the weight of the upper extremity, powder may be sprinkled on the surface or the limb can be placed on a rolling support (similar to a small skateboard) to reduce friction.

2. **Action:** Move client's shoulder into horizontal adduction twice while stating "move your arm like I did."

    a. If patient performs full ROM, place in slight horizontal adduction and apply slight pressure toward horizontal abduction.

        i. If tolerates pressure = Poor+.

        ii. No pressure = Poor.

    b. If patient performs through partial ROM, do not apply pressure = Poor–.

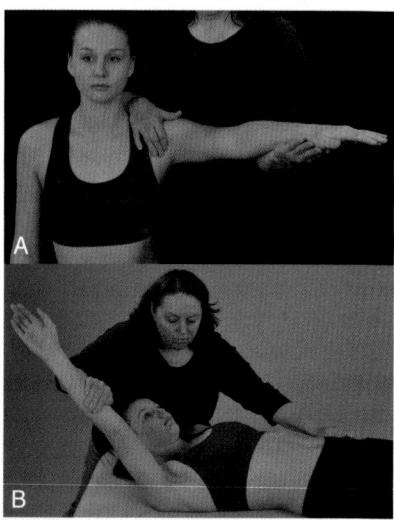

Fig. 22.29 (A) Shoulder horizontal adduction: position and palpation for muscle testing the clavicular portion grades 2 and below. (B) Shoulder horizontal adduction: position, palpation, and pressure to the sternal head of the pectoralis major—muscle grades 3 and above.

c. If client unable to perform motion, place shoulder in slight horizontal abduction and state, "try to move your arm like I did." Palpate over anterior shoulder girdle for muscle contraction (see Fig. 22.29A).
   i. If muscle contraction palpable = Trace.
   ii. If no contraction palpable = Zero.

Specific muscle testing. The sternal and clavicular heads of the pectoralis major can be tested individually. The described procedure tests the clavicular head (however, the thumb must point toward the opposite shoulder), whereas bringing the hand from the position demonstrated in Fig. 22.29B, toward the opposite hip (with the thumb pointing toward opposite hip) isolates the sternal head. Stabilization of the opposite hip is provided and pressure is toward horizontal abduction and abduction[15] (see Fig. 22.29B).

Substitutions. If the pectoralis major is not functioning, strength will be significantly weakened.[16] Contralateral trunk rotation can substitute if trunk is not adequately stabilized.[6]

Elbow Flexion (Figs. 22.30 to 22.32)

Muscles[10,12–14]	Innervation[12–14]
Biceps brachii	Musculocutaneous nerve, C5, 6
Brachialis	Musculocutaneous nerve, C5, 6
Brachioradialis	Radial nerve, C5-7
Pronator teres	Median nerve, C5, 6

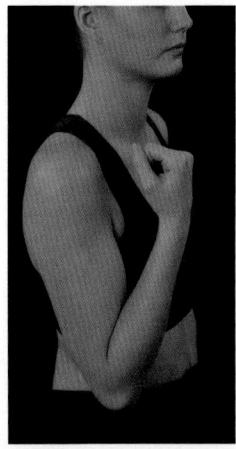

Fig. 22.30 Elbow flexion: action.

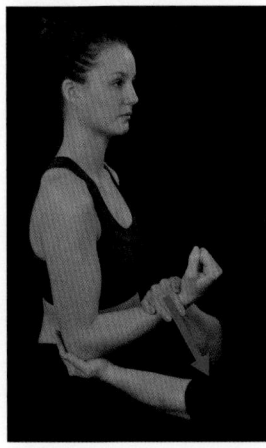

Fig. 22.31 Elbow flexion: application of pressure.

Procedure for Testing Grades Normal (5), Good (4), and Fair (3)

1. **Body position:** Client is seated on a supportive chair or mat; if trunk stability or balance is impaired, the trunk is externally supported. Shoulder and elbow in neutral. Therapist stands on side being tested.
2. **Action:** While demonstrating movement from neutral to full elbow flexion with forearm supinated, the therapist says, "move your arm like I am." Observe the client actively perform the movement (Fig. 22.30).
3. **Test position:** If client performs through available PROM, place elbow at 90 degrees of flexion with forearm supinated and proceeds. If not, follow procedure for testing grades Poor, Trace, and Zero.
4. **Stabilize:** The therapist provides stabilization under the elbow joint.
5. **Pressure:** Tell the client, "don't let me move you." Apply pressure over the distal volar forearm in downward fashion toward elbow extension, adjusting pressure to client's abilities (Fig. 22.31). If pressure maximal = Normal; moderate = Good, minimal = Good–, slight = Fair+, and no pressure = Fair.

Procedure for Testing Grades Poor (2), Trace (1), and Zero (0)

1. **Body position:** The client is sitting or supine with shoulder abducted to 90 degrees. The upper extremity can be supported on a high table with powder sprinkled on top to prevent friction. Therapist stands on side being tested and supports arm and forearm as needed (Fig. 22.32).
2. **Action:** Beginning in mid-position, move client's elbow through partial flexion ROM twice while stating "move your arm like I did."
   a. If client performs full ROM, place in 90 degrees of elbow flexion and apply slight pressure over distal volar wrist perpendicular to forearm.
      i. If tolerates pressure = Poor+.
      ii. No pressure = Poor.
   b. If client performs through partial ROM, do not apply pressure = Poor–.
   c. If client is unable to perform motion, place in 90 degrees of elbow flexion and state, "try to move your arm like I did." Palpate over anterior arm and forearm to feel for contraction in elbow flexor muscle(s).
      i. If muscle contraction palpable = Trace.
      ii. If no contraction palpable = Zero.

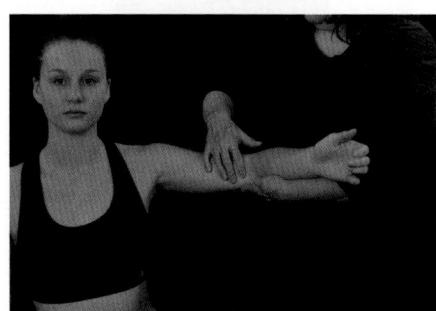

Fig. 22.32 Elbow flexion: body position, action, and palpation—muscle grades 2 and below.

Specific muscle testing. A supinated forearm position tests primarily the biceps brachii, whereas pronated position tests brachialis and pronator teres[16]; neutral forearm position tests brachioradialis.[10,12,13]

Substitution. Wrist and extrinsic finger flexors may assist elbow flexion, which will be preceded by finger and wrist flexion.[10,12,13,16]

Elbow Extension (Figs. 22.33 to 22.38)

Muscles[6,10,12]	Innervation[10,12–15]
Triceps	Radial nerve, C6-8
Anconeus	Radial nerve, C7,8, T1

Procedure for Testing Grades Normal (5), Good (4), and Fair (3)

1. **Body position:** The client is supine with shoulder in 90 degrees flexion, sitting with shoulder in full flexion, or prone with humerus abducted to 90 degrees. The elbow is flexed. The therapist stands next to the client, just behind the extremity to be tested.[7,15,21]
2. **Action:** While demonstrating movement from elbow flexion to full extension, the therapist says, "move your arm like I am." Observe the client actively perform the movement. (Figs. 22.33 and 22.34)

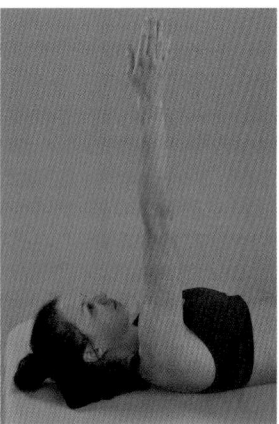

Fig. 22.33 Elbow extension: action.

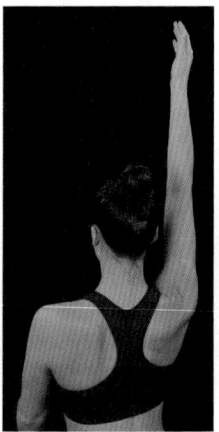

Fig. 22.34 Elbow extension: action—alternate action method.

3. **Test position:** If client performs through available PROM, place elbow in 45 degrees of flexion and proceeds. If not, follow procedure for testing grades Poor, Trace, and Zero.
4. **Stabilize:** The therapist provides stabilization at the humerus, avoiding the contracting fibers on posterior humerus.
5. **Pressure:** The therapist tells the client, "don't let me move you," then applies pressure at the distal end of the forearm into elbow flexion, adjusting pressure to the client's abilities (Fig. 22.35). The elbow should not be locked in full extension because this can cause joint injury.[6,10]

Procedure for Testing Grades Poor (2), Trace (1), and Zero (0)

1. **Body position:** The client is sitting with shoulder in 90 degrees flexion, scaption, or abduction.[7,10,12] Shoulder and forearm are in neutral rotation. The therapist supports the weight of the arm while standing next to the client's arm being tested (Fig. 22.36).[10]
2. **Action:** Beginning in mid-position, move client's shoulder through partial extension ROM twice while stating "move your arm like I did" (Fig. 22.37).
   a. If client performs full ROM, place in 90 degrees of elbow flexion and apply slight pressure perpendicular to the forearm.
      i. If tolerates pressure = Poor+.
      ii. No pressure = Poor.
   b. If client performs through partial ROM, do not apply pressure = Poor−.
   c. If client is unable to perform motion, place in 90 degrees of shoulder flexion and state, "try to move your arm like I did." Palpate just superior to the dorsal elbow over the tendon (Fig. 22.38) or over the mid-dorsal humerus over the muscle belly to feel for contraction in elbow extensor muscle(s).
      i. If muscle contraction palpable = Trace.
      ii. If no contraction palpable = Zero.

Substitutions. Extrinsic finger and wrist extensors may substitute for weak elbow extensors as their proximal attachment crosses the elbow joint in a posterior manner. Observe for the

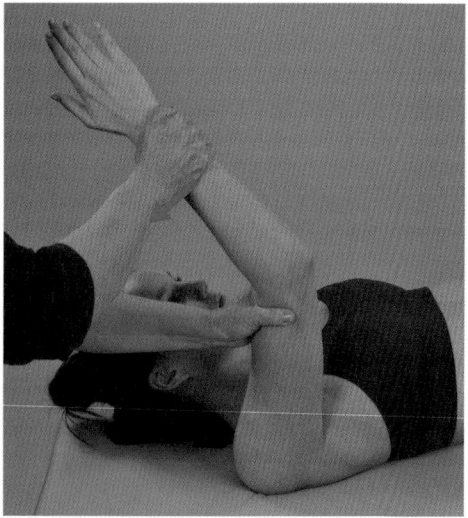

Fig. 22.35 Elbow extension: application of pressure.

presence of finger and wrist extension preceding elbow extension. When the client is upright, gravity and eccentric contraction of the biceps will affect elbow extension from the flexed position.[16] Scapula depression with shoulder external rotation aided by gravity may result in elbow extension.[6] The elbow will assume an extended position when a client who is sitting with the hand fixed on the bed or mat (closed chair) performs scapular protraction and contracts the shoulder flexors to move the proximal attachment. Once the elbow is "locked" in hyperextension, the client's body weight maintains elbow extension.

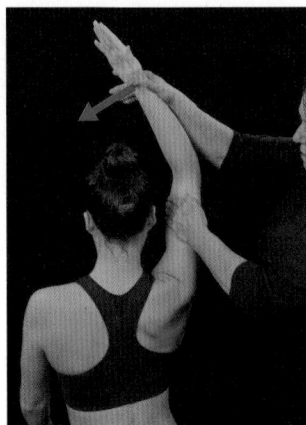

Fig. 22.36 Elbow extension: application of pressure.

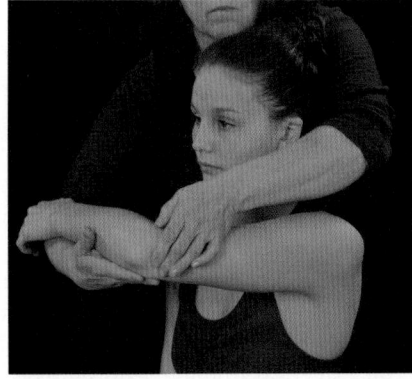

Fig. 22.37 Elbow extension: body position, action, and palpation—muscle grades 2 and below.

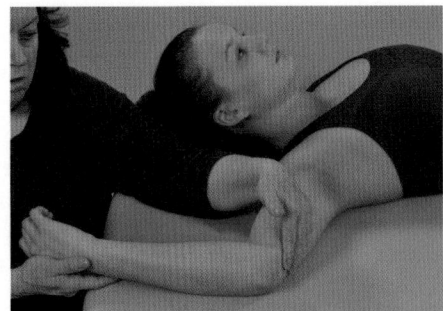

Fig. 22.38 Elbow extension: alternative body position, action, and palpation—muscle grades 2 and below.

Forearm Supination (Figs. 22.39 to 22.42)

Muscles[4,10,13]	Innervation[6,10,13]
Biceps brachii	Musculocutaneous nerve, C5, 6
Supinator	Radial nerve, C7-C8

Procedure for Testing Grades Normal (5), Good (4), and Fair (3)

1. **Body position:** The client is seated, with the humerus adducted, the elbow flexed to 90 degrees, and the forearm pronated. The therapist stands in front of the client or next to the client on the side to be tested.[6,7,10,12,13]
2. **Action:** While demonstrating movement from neutral to full forearm supination, the therapist says, "move your arm like I am." Observe the client actively perform the movement. (Fig. 22.39).
3. **Test position:** If client performs through available PROM, place forearm in neutral position and proceed. If not, follow procedure for testing grades Poor, Trace, and Zero.
4. **Stabilize:** If client is able to stabilize humerus next to side, therapist can use both hands to comfortably apply pressure to client. If not, therapist stabilizes humerus just proximal to elbow.[6,10]
5. **Pressure:** Tell the client, "don't let me move you." Therapist can "sandwich" the forearm between both hands on mid-forearm, applying pressure into pronation (Fig. 22.40). Therapist can also grasp around the dorsal aspect of the distal forearm with the fingers and heel of the hand, while turning the arm toward pronation. Adjust pressure to client's abilities (Fig. 22.41).

Procedure for Testing Grades Poor (2), Trace (1), and Zero (0)

1. **Body position:** The client is seated with shoulder and elbow flexed to 90 degrees and upper arm resting on table or supported by therapist (position demonstrated in Fig. 22.42). Can test lying supine with shoulder in neutral and elbow

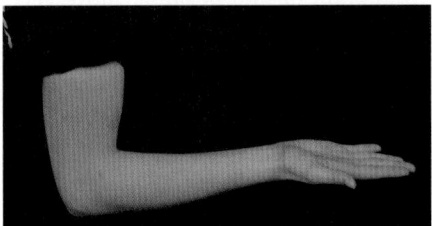

Fig. 22.39 Forearm supination: action.

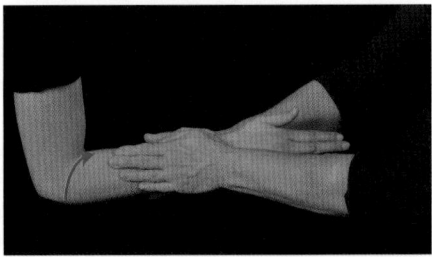

Fig. 22.40 Forearm supination: application of pressure.

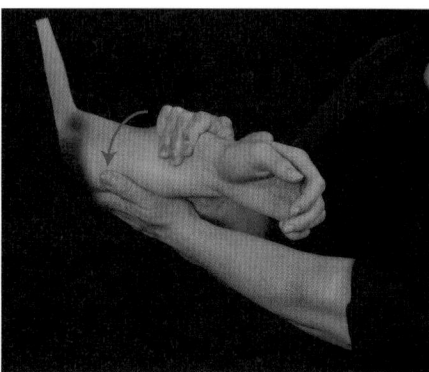

Fig. 22.41 Forearm supination: application of pressure—alternate method.

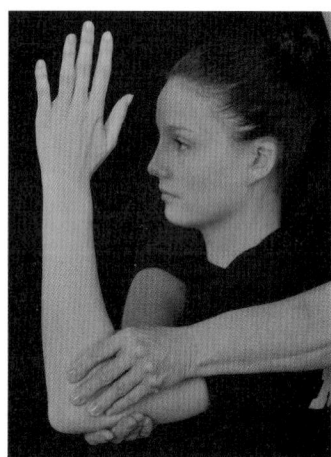

Fig. 22.42 Forearm supination: body position, action, and palpation—muscle grades 2 and below.

flexed to 90 degrees, or prone with shoulder in 90 degrees abduction and forearm lying over edge of table in a position perpendicular to the floor.[6,7,21] Therapist stands next to client on the side to be tested.

2. Action: Beginning in mid-position, move client's forearm into supination twice while stating "move your forearm like I did."
   a. If client performs full ROM, place in mid-position and apply slight pressure toward pronation.
      i. If tolerates pressure = Poor+.
      ii. No pressure = Poor.
   b. If client performs through partial ROM, do not apply pressure = Poor−.
   c. If client unable to perform motion, place forearm in mid-position and state, "try to move your forearm like I did." Palpate over anterior dorsal forearm just distal to lateral epicondyle to feel supinator contraction or over volar elbow for biceps brachii.
      i. If muscle contraction palpable = Trace.
      ii. If no contraction palpable = Zero.

Specific muscle testing. To test only the supinator muscle, the elbow and shoulder are fully flexed to make the biceps actively insufficient. In this position it is hard to tell if the

forearm is pronated or supinated, resulting in pressure applied into pronation. Therapist should orient to forearm position when elbow is flexed.

Substitutions. With the elbow flexed, external rotation and horizontal adduction of the humerus will effect forearm supination. With the elbow extended, shoulder external rotation will place the forearm in supination. The brachioradialis can bring the forearm from full pronation to mid-position. Wrist and thumb extensors, assisted by gravity, can initiate supination. The therapist should note any external rotation of the humerus, supination to midline only, and initiation of motion by wrist and thumb extension.[10,13,15,21]

Forearm Pronation (Figs. 22.43 to 22.46)

Muscles[4,12,13,16]	Innervation[12,15]
Pronator teres	Median nerve, C6,7
Pronator quadratus	Median nerve, C8, T1

Procedure for Testing Grades Normal (5), Good (4), and Fair (3)

1. **Body position:** The client is seated, with the shoulder and elbow flexed to 90 degrees, and the forearm supinated. The therapist stands beside client on the side to be tested.[6,7,10,13]
2. **Action:** While demonstrating movement from supination to full forearm pronation, the therapist says, "move your forearm like I am." Observe the client actively perform the movement (Fig. 22.43).
3. **Test position:** If client performs through available PROM, place forearm in neutral position and proceed. If not, follow procedure for testing grades Poor, Trace, and Zero.
4. **Stabilize:** If client is able to stabilize humerus next to side, therapist can use both hands to comfortably apply pressure to client. If not, therapist stabilizes humerus just proximal to elbow to prevent shoulder abduction.[6,7,10,15]
5. **Pressure:** Tell the client, "don't let me move you." Therapist can "sandwich" the forearm between both hands on midforearm, applying pressure toward supination (Fig. 22.44). Therapist can also grasp around the dorsal aspect of the distal forearm with the fingers and heel of the hand while turning the arm toward pronation (Fig. 22.45). Adjust pressure to client's abilities.

Procedure for Testing Grades Poor (2), Trace (1), and Zero (0)

1. **Body position:** The client is seated with shoulder and elbow flexed to 90 degrees and upper arm resting on table or supported by therapist. Can test with client in side-lying or supine with shoulder in neutral and elbow flexed to 90 degrees, or prone with shoulder in 90 degrees abduction and forearm lying over edge of table in a position perpendicular to the floor.[21] The therapist stands next to client on the side to be tested.
2. **Action:** Beginning in mid-position, move client's forearm into supination twice while stating "move your forearm like I did."

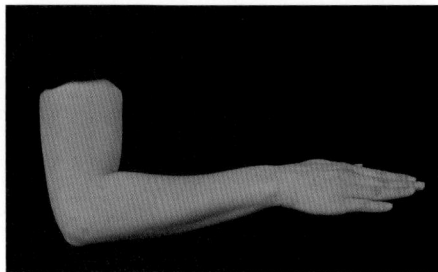

Fig. 22.43 Forearm pronation: action.

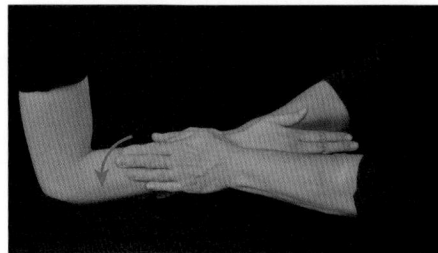

Fig. 22.44 Forearm pronation: application of pressure.

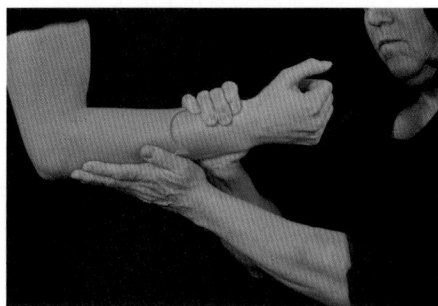

Fig. 22.45 Forearm pronation: application of pressure—alternate method.

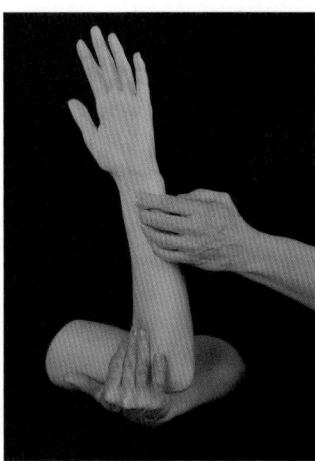

Fig. 22.46 Forearm pronation: body position, action, and palpation—muscle grades 2 and below.

a. If client performs full ROM, place in mid-position and apply slight pressure toward supination.
   i. If tolerates pressure = Poor+.
   ii. No pressure = Poor.
b. If client performs through partial ROM, do not apply pressure = Poor−.
c. If client is unable to perform motion, place forearm in mid-position and state, "try to move your forearm like I did." Palpate over anterior volar forearm just distal to elbow and the volar distal forearm for muscle contraction (Fig. 22.46).
   i. If muscle contraction palpable = Trace.
   ii. If no contraction palpable = Zero.

Specific muscle testing. To isolate the pronator quadratus only, the elbow is fully flexed to render the pronator teres actively insufficient.[4]

Substitutions. With the elbow flexed, internal rotation and abduction of the humerus will produce apparent forearm pronation. With the elbow extended, internal rotation can place the forearm in a pronated position. Brachioradialis can bring the fully supinated forearm to mid-position. Wrist flexion, aided by gravity, can effect pronation.[b]

Wrist Extension (Figs. 22.47 to 22.49)

Muscles[10,12,15]	Innervation[6,12]
Extensor carpi radialis longus	Radial nerve, C6, 7
Extensor carpi radialis brevis	Deep branch of radial nerve, C7, 8
Extensor carpi ulnaris	Posterior interosseous nerve off radial nerve, C7, 8

Procedure for Testing Grades Normal (5), Good (4), and Fair (3)

1. **Body position:** The client is seated or supine with the forearm resting on the supporting surface in pronation and the fingers and thumb relaxed. The therapist sits opposite to or next to the client on the side to be tested.[10,15]
2. **Action:** While demonstrating movement from neutral to full wrist extension, the therapist says, "move your wrist like I am" (Fig. 22.47). Observe the client actively perform the movement.
3. **Test position:** If client performs through available PROM, place the wrist in slight extension and proceed. If not, follow procedure for testing grades Poor, Trace, and Zero.
4. **Stabilize:** The therapist stabilizes over the volar or dorsal aspect of the distal forearm.[6,10,15]
5. **Pressure:** Tell the client, "don't let me move you." Apply pressure dorsally over distal metacarpals in perpendicular fashion toward flexion, adjusting pressure to client's abilities (Fig. 22.48). If pressure maximal = Normal; moderate = Good, minimal = Good−, slight = Fair+, and no pressure = Fair.

[b] References 6,7,10,12,13,16,21.

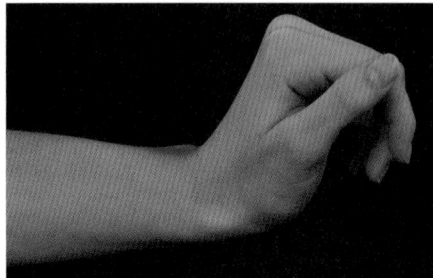

Fig. 22.47 Wrist extension: action.

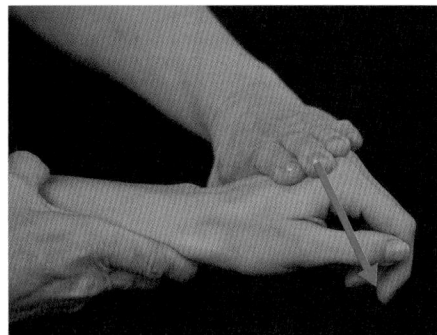

Fig. 22.48 Wrist extension: application of pressure.

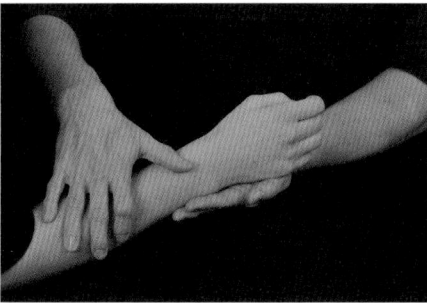

Fig. 22.49 Wrist extension: body position, action, and palpation—muscle grades 2 and below.

Procedure for Testing Grades Poor (2), Trace (1), and Zero (0)

1. **Body position:** Client is seated or supine with forearm resting in mid-position on its ulnar border[10,21] and fingers and thumb relaxed.
2. **Action:** Move client's wrist into extension twice while stating "move your wrist like I did."
   a. If client performs full ROM, place in slight wrist extension and apply slight pressure toward wrist flexion.
      i. If tolerates pressure = Poor+.
      ii. No pressure = Poor.
   b. If client performs through partial ROM, do not apply pressure = Poor−.
   c. If client unable to perform motion, place forearm in mid-position and state, "try to move your wrist like I did." Palpate over posterior dorsal forearm and dorsal wrist for muscle contraction (Fig. 22.49, lateral view).
      i. If muscle contraction palpable = Trace.
      ii. If no contraction palpable = Zero.

Specific muscle testing. Each wrist extensor muscle can be tested individually by combining wrist extension with radial deviation (extensor carpi radialis longus and brevis), or wrist

extension with ulnar deviation (extensor carpi ulnaris). Pressure is performed opposite to the action.

Substitution. The extensor digitorum and extensor pollicis longus can initiate wrist extension, but finger or thumb extension will precede wrist extension.[c]

Wrist Flexion (Figs. 22.50 to 22.52)

Muscles[10,13]	Innervation[5,10,13]
Flexor carpi ulnaris	Ulnar nerve, C7-T1
Palmaris longus	Median nerve, C7-T1
Flexor carpi radialis	Median nerve, C6-8

Procedure for Testing Grades Normal (5), Good (4), and Fair (3)

1. **Body position:** The client is seated or supine with the forearm resting in nearly full supination on the supporting surface, fingers and thumb relaxed. The therapist is seated opposite or next to the client on the side to be tested.[10,15]
2. **Action:** While demonstrating movement from neutral to full wrist flexion, the therapist says, "move your wrist like I am" (Fig. 22.50, lateral view). Observe the client actively perform the movement.
3. **Test position:** If client performs through available PROM, the therapist places the wrist in slight wrist and proceeds. If not, follow procedure for testing grades Poor, Trace, and Zero.
4. **Stabilize:** The therapist stabilizes the forearm[10,15]; therapist's hand under dorsal forearm increases client comfort.
5. **Pressure:** Tell the client, "don't let me move you." Therapist positions his or her hand over distal volar palm and applies pressure in a dorsal direct toward extension, adjusting pressure to client's abilities (Fig. 22.51). If pressure maximal = Normal; moderate = Good, minimal = Good−, slight = Fair+, and no pressure = Fair.

Procedure for Testing Grades Poor (2), Trace (1), and Zero (0)

1. **Body position:** Client is seated or supine with forearm resting in mid-position on its ulnar border,[10,21] and fingers and thumb relaxed.[10] The therapist sits opposite or next to the client on the side being tested.
2. **Action:** Move client's wrist into flexion twice while stating "move your wrist like I did."
   a. If client performs full ROM, place in slight wrist flexion and apply slight pressure toward wrist extension.
      i. If tolerates pressure = Poor+.
      ii. No pressure = Poor.
   b. If client performs through partial ROM, do not apply pressure = Poor−.
   c. If client is unable to perform motion, place forearm in mid-position and state, "try to move your wrist like I did."

---

[c]References 6,7,12,13,16,21.

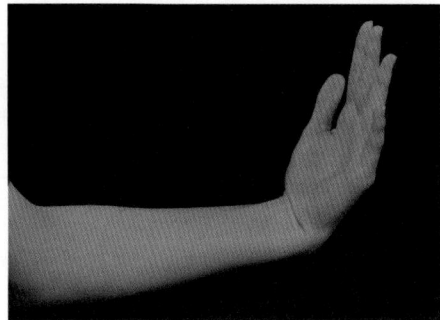

Fig. 22.50 Wrist flexion: action.

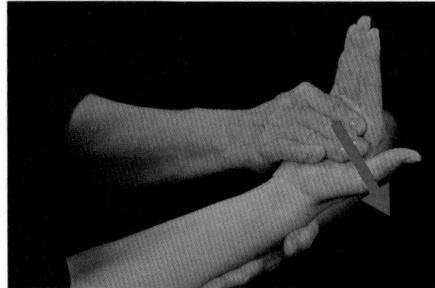

Fig. 22.51 Wrist flexion: application of pressure.

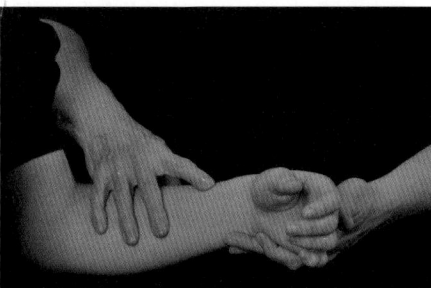

Fig. 22.52 Wrist flexion: body position, action, and palpation—muscle grades 2 and below.

Palpate over volar forearm and wrist for muscle contraction (Fig. 22.52, lateral view).

   i. If muscle contraction palpable = Trace.

   ii. If no contraction palpable = Zero.

Specific muscle testing. Each wrist flexor muscle can be tested individually by combining wrist flexion with radial deviation (flexor carpi radialis), or wrist flexion with ulnar deviation (flexor carpi ulnaris). The palmaris longus is tested by having the client oppose the thumb and small finger while flexing the wrist.[4] Pressure is applied to un-oppose (reposition) the thumb and extend the wrist.

Substitution. The extrinsic finger flexors can also assist wrist flexion, but the motion will be preceded by flexion of the fingers.[6,16,21]

Wrist Radial Deviation (Figs. 22.53 to 22.55)

Muscles[10,13]	Innervation[5,10,13]
Flexor carpi radialis	Median nerve, C6-8
Extensor carpi radialis longus	Radial nerve, C6, 7
Extensor carpi radialis brevis	Deep branch of radial nerve, C7, C8

Procedure for Testing Grades Normal (5), Good (4), and Fair (3)

1. **Body position:** The client is seated or supine with forearm in neutral rotation and wrist in slight extension and neutral deviation. Thumb will be pointing up. The therapist is seated or standing next to the client on the side to be tested.
2. **Action:** While demonstrating movement from neutral to full wrist radial deviation, the therapist says, "move your wrist like I am" (Fig. 22.53, lateral view). Observe the client actively perform the movement.
3. **Test position:** If client performs through available PROM, place the wrist in mid-radial deviation and proceed. If not, follow procedure for testing grades Poor, Trace, and Zero.
4. **Stabilize:** The therapist stabilizes the forearm, therapist's hand under dorsal ulnar forearm increases client comfort.
5. **Pressure:** Tell the client, "don't let me move you." Apply pressure radially over the distal second metacarpal or through the entire hand (not fingers) toward ulnar deviation, adjusting pressure to client's abilities (Fig. 22.54, lateral view). If pressure maximal = Normal; moderate = Good, minimal = Good–, slight = Fair+, and no pressure = Fair.

Procedure for Testing Grades Poor (2), Trace (1), and Zero (0)

1. **Body position:** Client is seated or supine with volar surface of forearm resting on table, bed, or supported by therapist. The therapist sits opposite or next to the client on the side being tested.
2. **Action:** Move client's wrist into radial deviation twice while stating "move your wrist like I did."
   a. If client performs full ROM, place in mid-radial deviation and apply slight pressure through distal second metacarpal or entire hand toward ulnar deviation.
      i. If tolerates pressure = Poor+.
      ii. No pressure = Poor.
   b. If client performs through partial ROM, do not apply pressure = Poor–.
   c. If client is unable to perform motion, place forearm in mid-position and state, "try to move your wrist like I did." Palpate over distal radial wrist for muscle contraction (Fig. 22.55).
      i. If muscle contraction palpable = Trace.
      ii. If no contraction palpable = Zero.

Substitution. The thumb extrinsic muscles (abductor and extensor pollicis longus) can radially deviate the wrist, but wrist motion will be preceded by thumb movement.

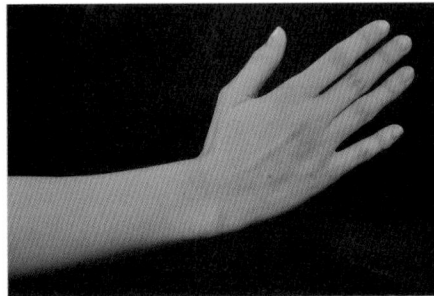

Fig. 22.53 Wrist radial deviation: action.

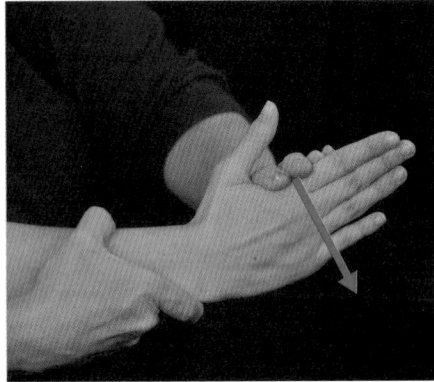

Fig. 22.54 Wrist radial deviation: application of pressure.

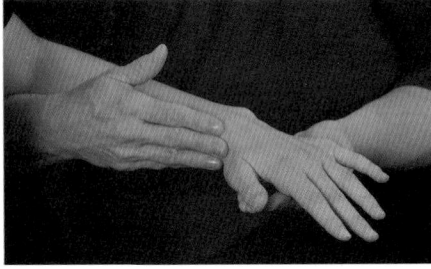

Fig. 22.55 Wrist radial deviation: body position, action, and palpation—muscle grades 2 and below.

Wrist Ulnar Deviation (Figs. 22.56 to 22.57)

Muscles[10,12,15]	Innervation[6,12]
Extensor carpi ulnaris	Posterior interosseous nerve of radial nerve, C7, 8
Flexor carpi ulnaris	Ulnar nerve, C7-T1

Procedure for Testing Grades Normal (5), Good (4), and Fair (3)

1. **Body position:** The client is seated or supine with forearm in neutral rotation and wrist in slight extension and neutral deviation. To get the action against gravity, the client's elbow and shoulder must be flexed. The therapist is seated or standing next to the client on the side to be tested.
2. **Action:** While demonstrating movement from neutral to full ulnar deviation, the therapist says, "move your wrist like I am." Observe the client actively perform the movement (Fig. 22.56A).
3. **Test position:** If client performs through available PROM, place the wrist in mid-ulnar deviation and proceed. If not, follow procedure for testing grades Poor, Trace, and Zero.
4. **Stabilize:** The therapist stabilizes the distal forearm, therapist's hand under the distal radial forearm.
5. **Pressure:** Tell the client, "don't let me move you." Apply pressure radially over distal fifth metacarpal or through the entire hand (not fingers) toward radial deviation, adjusting pressure to the client's abilities (see Fig. 22.56B). If pressure maximal = Normal; moderate = Good, minimal = Good–, slight = Fair+, and no pressure = Fair.

Procedure for Testing Grades Poor (2), Trace (1), and Zero (0)

1. **Body position:** Client is seated or supine with volar surface of forearm resting on table, bed, or supported by therapist. The therapist sits opposite or next to the client on the side being tested.
2. **Action:** Move client's wrist into ulnar deviation twice while stating "move your wrist like I did."

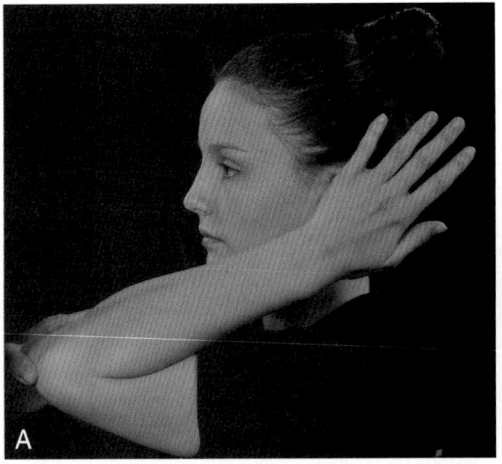
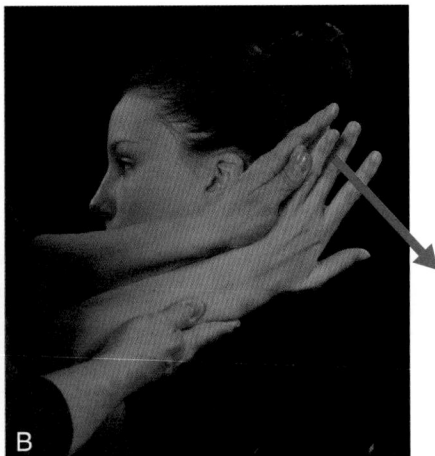

Fig. 22.56 (A) Wrist ulnar deviation: action. (B) Wrist ulnar deviation: application of pressure.

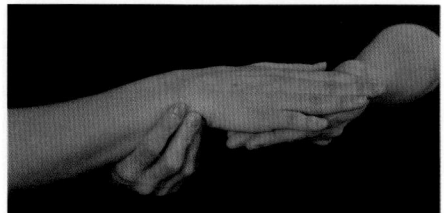

Fig. 22.57 Wrist ulnar deviation: body position, action, and palpation—muscle grades 2 and below.

a. If client performs full ROM, place in mid-ulnar deviation and apply slight pressure on ulnar border of hand (not fingers) toward radial deviation.
  i. If tolerates pressure = Poor+.
  ii. No pressure = Poor.
b. If client performs through partial ROM, do not apply pressure = Poor–.
c. If client is unable to perform motion, place wrist in mid-position and move toward ulnar deviation while stating "try to move your wrist like I did." Palpate over the ulnar wrist and distal forearm for muscle contraction (Fig. 22.57, lateral view).
  i. If muscle contraction palpable = Trace.
  ii. If no contraction palpable = Zero.

Metacarpophalangeal Flexion (Figs. 22.58 to 22.63)

Muscles[1,4,19,22]	Innervation[10,12,19]
Lumbricals 1 and 2 (index and long)	Median nerve, C8, T1
Lumbricals 3 and 4 (ring and small)	Ulnar nerve, C8, T1
Dorsal interossei (index, long, and ring)	Deep branch of ulnar nerve, C8, T1
Palmar interossei (index, ring, and small)	Deep branch of ulnar nerve, C8, T1
Flexor digitorum superficialis	Median nerve, C8, T1
Flexor digitorum profundus	Digit 2 and 3: Median nerve, C8, T1 Digit 4 and 5: Ulnar nerve, C8, T1
Flexor digiti minimi (small)	Ulnar nerve, C8, T1

Procedure for Testing Grades Normal (5), Good (4), and Fair (3)
1. **Body position:** The client is seated or supine with forearm fully supinated and wrist stabilized in neutral resting on a supporting surface.[8] The therapist sits next to the client on the side being tested.
2. **Action:** While demonstrating movement from neutral to full MP flexion, the therapist says, "move your finger(s) like I am" (Fig. 22.58). Observe the client actively perform the movement.
3. **Test position:** If client performs through available PROM, place the MP joint(s) in mid-flexion and proceeds (see Fig. 22.58). If not, follow procedure for testing grades Poor, Trace, and Zero.

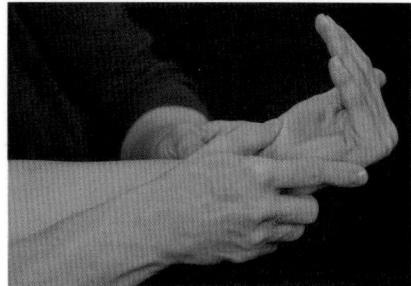

Fig. 22.58 Metacarpophalangeal flexion: action.

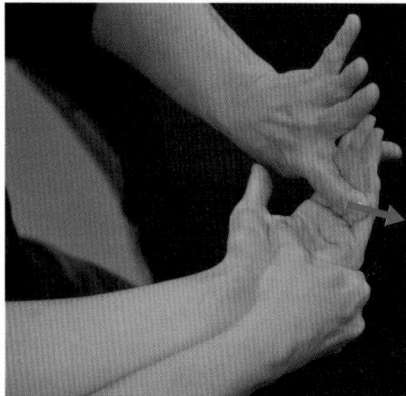

Fig. 22.59 Metacarpophalangeal flexion: application of pressure to all digits.

4. **Stabilize:** The therapist stabilizes the metacarpal of digit being tested. If digits 2 to 5 are tested simultaneously, metacarpals 2 to 5 are stabilized (Fig. 22.59).
5. **Pressure:** Tell the client, "don't let me move you." Apply pressure over the volar proximal phalange(s) toward MP extension, adjusting pressure to client's abilities. If pressure is maximal = Normal; moderate = Good, minimal = Good–, slight = Fair+, and no pressure = Fair. Fig. 22.59 depicts simultaneous testing of digits 2 to 5, with the intrinsic muscles that flex the MP joints targeted (as the IP joints are in extension), whereas Fig. 22.60 depicts index finger testing only, allowing the extrinsic finger flexors to assist as the PIP joint is flexed.

Procedure for Testing Grades Poor (2), Trace (1), and Zero (0)
1. **Body position:** Client's hand is resting on table or bed on the ulnar side of forearm and hand. The therapist is opposite or next to the client on the side being tested.
2. **Action:** Move client's MP joint(s) into flexion twice while stating "move your finger(s) like I did." Digits can be tested simultaneously or individually depending on the needs.
a. If client performs full ROM, place in mid–MP flexion and apply slight pressure toward MP extension.
  i. If tolerates pressure = Poor+.
  ii. No pressure = Poor.
b. If client performs through partial ROM, do not apply pressure = Poor–.

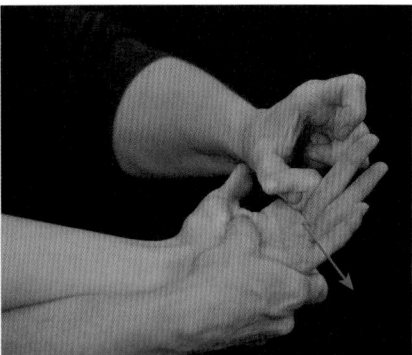

Fig. 22.60 Metacarpophalangeal flexion: application of pressure to index finger.

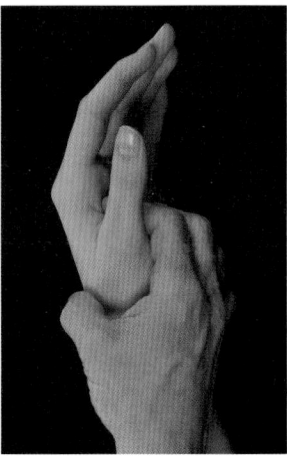

Fig. 22.61 Metacarpophalangeal flexion: body position, action, and palpation—muscle grades 2 and below. Palpation over volar surface of the palm.

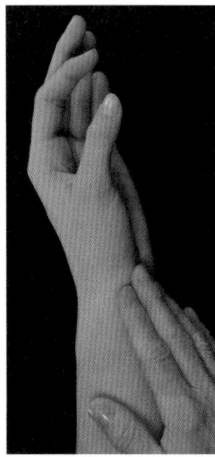

Fig. 22.62 Metacarpophalangeal flexion: body position, action, and palpation—muscle grades 2 and below. Alternate palpation method over volar surface of the wrist.

c. If client unable to perform motion, place MP joints in mid-position and state, "try to move your finger(s) like I did." Palpate over the volar palm for muscle contraction (Fig. 22.61, superior view); however, the intrinsics are very deep and contraction may not be

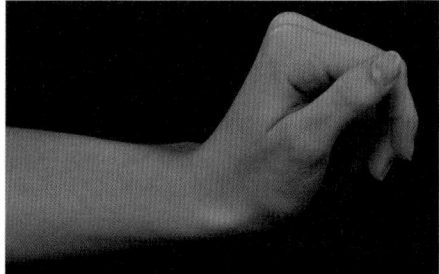

Fig. 22.63 Metacarpophalangeal flexion: substitution—tenodesis action.

palpable.[16,21] The first dorsal interossei is palpable over the distal web space. Contraction of the extrinsic finger flexors is palpable over the volar wrist (Fig. 22.62, superior view).

  i. If muscle contraction palpable = Trace.
  ii. If no contraction palpable = Zero.

Specific muscle testing. To isolate the intrinsic muscles that flex the MP joints, MP flexion must be performed with the IP joints in full extension because the intrinsics perform IP extension concomitantly with MP flexion. When testing the extrinsic finger flexor muscles, the IP joints are flexed along with the MP joints; however, the extrinsic flexors are best isolated by testing their actions at the PIP (flexor digitorum superficialis) and/or DIP joints (flexor digitorum profundus).[16,21] These tests are described in PIP and DIP sections.

Substitution. The joints of the fingers will move into a flexed position when the wrist is moved into extension; however, the motion is not due to active contraction of any muscles that flex the fingers. Because the extrinsic finger flexors pass volar to the wrist joint, they are of insufficient length to allow the fingers to stay extended when the wrist is actively or passively moved into extension; this is known as tenodesis, as insufficient tendon excursion pulls the fingers into flexion (Fig. 22.63). To prevent tenodesis action, the wrist should be stabilized while testing the muscles that flex the fingers so the client cannot actively extend the wrist.

Metacarpophalangeal Extension (Figs. 22.64 to 22.67)

Muscles[10,13]	Innervation[10,13,19]
Extensor digitorum (ED)	Radial nerve, C7, 8
Extensor indicis	Posterior interosseous nerve, C7, 8
Extensor digiti minimi (EDM)	Posterior interosseous nerve, C7, 8

Procedure for Testing Grades Normal (5), Good (4), and Fair (3)

1. **Body position:** The client is seated, with the forearm pronated and the wrist in neutral to slight extension and MP and IP joints relaxed in partial flexion.[7,10,12] The therapist sits opposite or next to the client on the side to be tested.
2. **Action:** While demonstrating movement from neutral to full MP extension, the therapist says, "move your finger(s) like

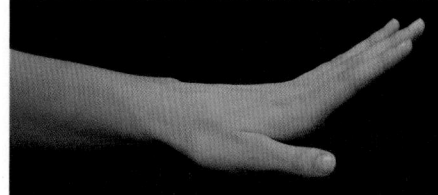

Fig. 22.64 Metacarpophalangeal extension: action.

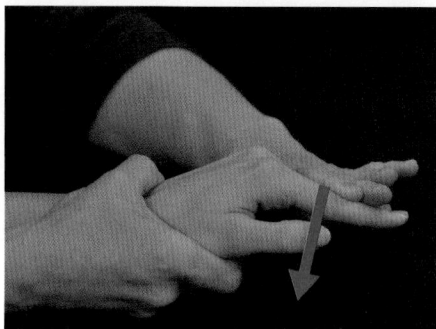

Fig. 22.65 Metacarpophalangeal extension: application of pressure.

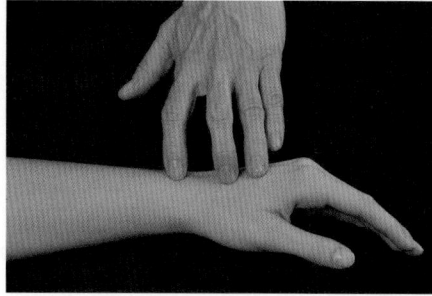

Fig. 22.66 Metacarpophalangeal extension: body position, action, and palpation—muscle grades 2 and below. Palpation of the individual tendons of the extensor digitorum.

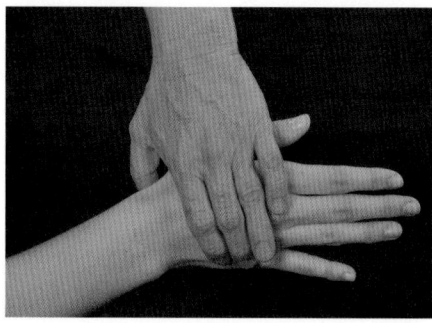

Fig. 22.67 Metacarpophalangeal extension: body position, action, and palpation—muscle grades 2 and below. Simultaneous palpation of all of the tendons of the extensor digitorum.

I am" (Fig. 22.64). Observe the client actively perform the movement.

3. **Test position:** If client performs through available PROM, place the MP joint in mid-extension and proceed. If not, follow procedure for testing grades Poor, Trace, and Zero.
4. **Stabilize:** The therapist stabilizes the wrist and metacarpals slightly above the supporting surface.[10,12–15] If testing fingers individually, the metacarpal corresponding to the finger being tested is stabilized.
5. **Pressure:** Tell the client, "don't let me move you." Provide pressure to each finger individually on the dorsum of the proximal phalanx toward MP flexion (Fig. 22.65).[6,10,15] Digits 2 to 5 can be tested simultaneously. If pressure maximal = Normal; moderate = Good, minimal = Good–, slight = Fair+, and no pressure = Fair.

Procedure for Testing Grades Poor (2), Trace (1), and Zero (0)

1. **Body position:** Client's hand is resting on table or bed on the ulnar side of forearm and hand.[10,12] The therapist is opposite or next to the client on the side being tested.
2. **Action:** Move client's fingers into MP extension twice while stating "move your fingers like I did." Digits can be tested simultaneously or individually depending on the needs.
   a. If client performs full ROM, place in mid–MP extension and apply slight pressure over distal proximal phalange(s) toward MP flexion
      i. If tolerates pressure = Poor+.
      ii. No pressure = Poor.
   b. If client performs through partial ROM, do not apply pressure = Poor–.

   c. If client is unable to perform motion, place MP joint in mid-position and state, "try to move your finger(s) like I did." Palpate the ED tendons where they course over the dorsum of the hand[6,7,10] (Fig. 22.66, superior view of hand resting on ulnar forearm, and Fig. 22.67, lateral view). In some individuals, the extensor digiti minimi tendon can be palpated or visualized just lateral to the ED tendon to the fifth finger. The extensor indicis tendon can be palpated or visualized just medial to the ED tendon to the first finger.[6] The intrinsic MP extensor muscles are small and deep, making palpation difficult for anything besides the first dorsal interrossei.
      i. If muscle contraction palpable = Trace.
      ii. If no contraction palpable = Zero.

Specific muscle testing. To isolate the extrinsic MP extensors, the IP joints should remain in some flexion[6,12] because the ED becomes actively insufficient if the IP joints are concurrently in IP extension.

Substitutions. With the wrist stabilized, no substitutions are possible. When the wrist is not stabilized, passive insufficiency of the ED can produce MP extension through tenodesis action.[d]

---

[d]References 6,7,10,13,16,21.

Proximal Interphalangeal Flexion, Second Through Fifth Fingers (Figs. 22.68 to 22.70)

Muscles[10,15]	Innervation[6,10,12]
Flexor digitorum superficialis (FDS)	Median nerve, C7, C8, T1
Flexor digitorum profundus (FDP)	Median and ulnar nerves, C8, T1

Procedure for Testing Grades Normal (5), Good (4), and Fair (3)

1. **Body position:** The client is seated, with the forearm supinated, wrist at neutral, fingers extended, and hand and forearm resting on the dorsal surface.[6,10,12] The therapist sits opposite or next to the client on the side being tested.
2. **Action:** While demonstrating movement from neutral to full PIP flexion, the therapist says, "move your finger like I am" (Fig. 22.68). Observe the client actively perform the movement.
3. **Test position:** If client performs through available PROM, place the PIP joint in mid-flexion and proceed. If not, follow procedure for testing grades Poor, Trace, and Zero (0).
4. **Stabilize:** The therapist stabilizes the MP joint and proximal phalanx of the finger being tested in extension.[6,7,10,15]
5. **Pressure:** Tell the client, "don't let me move you." Apply pressure over volar middle phalanx toward PIP extension,[6,10,15] adjusting pressure to client's abilities (Fig. 22.69). If pressure maximal = Normal; moderate = Good, minimal = Good−, slight = Fair+, and no pressure = Fair.

Procedure for Testing Grades Poor (2), Trace (1), and Zero (0)

1. **Body position:** The client is seated, with the forearm in neutral rotation and the wrist at neutral, resting on the ulnar border.[12,21] The therapist sits opposite or next to the client on the side to be tested.
2. **Action:** Move client's PIP joint into PIP flexion twice while stating "move your finger like I did."
   a. If client performs full ROM, place in mid–PIP flexion and apply slight pressure toward PIP extension.
      i. If tolerates pressure = Poor+.
      ii. No pressure = Poor.
      iii. If the test for grades poor and below is done with the forearm in full supination,
3. Partial ROM against gravity may be graded poor.[10]
   a. If client performs through partial ROM, do not apply pressure = Poor−.
   b. If client is unable to perform motion, place PIP joint in mid-position and state, "try to move your finger like I did." Palpate over the volar proximal phalanx and palm for muscle contraction (Fig. 22.70).
      i. If muscle contraction palpable = Trace.
      ii. If no contraction palpable = Zero.

Specific muscle testing. It is often important to isolate the flexor digitorum superficialis to ensure that it is intact and functioning. If DIP flexion precedes PIP flexion, the FDP is assisting with PIP flexion.[e] Stabilizing all of the fingers not being tested

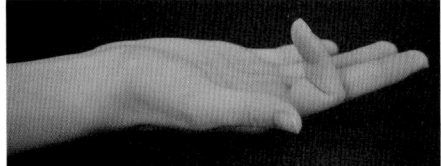
Fig. 22.68 Proximal interphalangeal flexion: action.

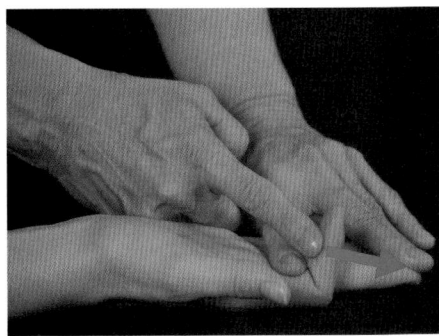
Fig. 22.69 Proximal interphalangeal flexion: application of pressure.

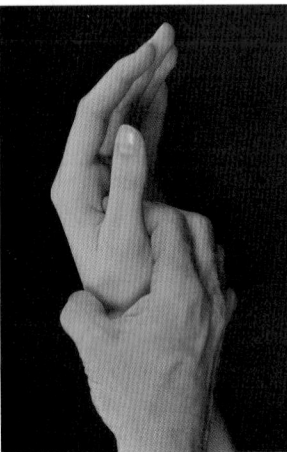
Fig. 22.70 Proximal interphalangeal flexion: body position, action, and palpation—muscle grades 2 and below. Simultaneous palpation of all of the tendons of the flexor digitorum superficialis.

in MP and IP extension prevents the FDP from flexing the PIP joint. Many individuals cannot isolate flexion of the small finger PIP joint even MP stabilization. To ensure that the FDP is inactive, the therapist may wiggle the DIP joint while applying pressure to the middle phalanx.[4,6,12,16,21]

Substitution. Active insufficiency of the extrinsic finger flexors can result in apparent finger flexion through partial ROM when the wrist is actively or passively extended because of tenodesis,[10,13,21] so the therapist should ensure this is not the mistaken for active finger flexion.

---

[e]References 7,12,13,16,18,21.

Distal Interphalangeal Flexion, Second Through Fifth Fingers (Figs. 22.71 to 22.74)

Muscle[10,13]	Innervation[10,13]
Flexor digitorum profundus (FDP)	Median and ulnar nerves, C8, T1

Procedure for Testing Grades Normal (5), Good (4), and Fair (3)

1. **Body position:** The client is seated, with the forearm supinated, wrist at neutral, fingers extended.[10] The therapist sits opposite or next to the client on the side being tested.[12]
2. **Action:** While demonstrating movement from neutral to full PIP flexion, the therapist says, "move your finger like I am" (Fig. 22.71). Observe the client actively perform the movement.
3. **Test position:** If client performs through available PROM, place the DIP joint in mid-flexion and proceed. If not, follow procedure for testing grades Poor, Trace, and Zero (0).
4. **Stabilize:** The therapist stabilizes the PIP joint and middle phalanx in extension on the finger being tested.[6,21]
5. **Pressure:** Tell the client, "don't let me move you." Apply pressure over volar distal phalanx toward DIP extension[6,7,10,15] adjusting pressure to client's abilities (Fig. 22.72). If pressure maximal = Normal; moderate = Good, minimal = Good−, slight = Fair+, and no pressure = Fair. Palpate.

Procedure for Testing Grades Poor (2), Trace (1), and Zero (0)

1. **Body position:** The client is seated, with the forearm in mid-position and the wrist at neutral, resting on the ulnar border.[12,21] The client is seated, with the forearm in mid-position and with the wrist at neutral, resting on the ulnar border.[12,21] The therapist sits opposite or next to the client on the side to be tested.
2. **Action:** Move client's DIP joint into flexion twice while stating "move your finger like I did."
   a. If client performs full ROM, place in mid–DIP flexion and apply slight pressure toward PIP extension.
      i. If tolerates pressure = Poor+.
      ii. No pressure = Poor.
      iii. If the test for grades poor and below is done with the forearm in full supination, partial ROM against gravity may be graded poor.[10]
   b. If client performs through partial ROM, do not apply pressure = Poor−.
   c. If client is unable to perform motion, place DIP joint in mid-position and state, "try to move your finger like I did." Palpate over the volar proximal surface of the middle phalanx[6,10,14] (Fig. 22.73) and palm for muscle contraction (Fig. 22.74).
      i. If muscle contraction palpable = Trace.
      ii. If no contraction palpable = Zero.

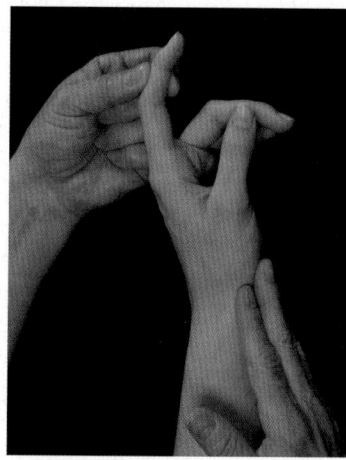

Fig. 22.73 Distal interphalangeal flexion: body position, action, and palpation—muscle grades 2 and below. Palpation of the flexor digitorum profundus tendon of the index finger.

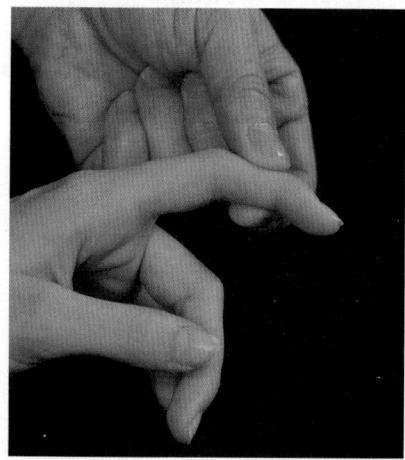

Fig. 22.71 Distal interphalangeal flexion: action.

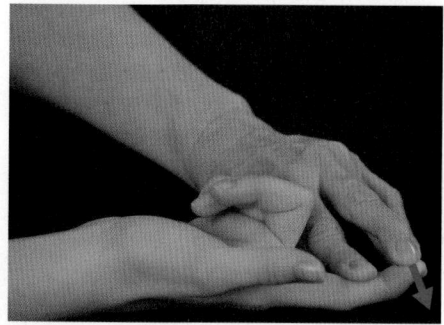

Fig. 22.72 Distal interphalangeal flexion: application of pressure.

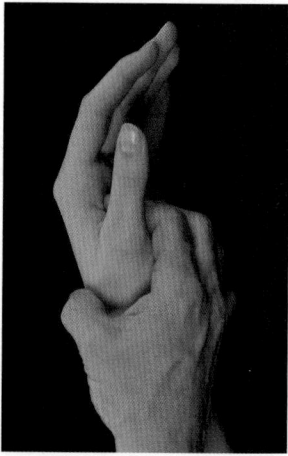

Fig. 22.74 Distal interphalangeal flexion: body position, action, and palpation—muscle grades 2 and below. Palpation of the flexor digitorum profundus tendons.

Substitutions. None are possible during the testing procedure if the wrist is well stabilized because the FDP is the only muscle that can act to flex the DIP joint when it is isolated. During normal hand function, however, wrist extension with tendon action of the finger flexors can produce partial flexion of the DIP joints.[10,16,21]

Finger Abduction (Figs. 22.75 to 22.78)

Muscles[10,12]	Innervation[10,12]
Dorsal interossei of the 2nd, 3rd, and 4th fingers	Ulnar nerve, C8, T1
Abductor digiti minimi (5th finger)	Deep branch of ulnar nerve, C8, T1

Procedure for Testing Grades Normal (5), Good (4), and Fair (3)

1. **Body position:** The client is seated or supine (Fig. 22.75). The forearm should be in midposition (with thumb pointing toward ceiling) for index and long fingers, and the hand positioned so ulnar aspect of ring and small fingers point toward ceiling (Fig. 22.76). Because the weight of the fingers is negligible and this testing position may be uncomfortable, it is acceptable to test in a position of comfort. The therapist is seated opposite or next to the client on the side to be tested.[10,13]

2. **Action:** While demonstrating movement from neutral to full finger abduction, the therapist says, "move your finger like I am." Observe client actively perform the movement of spreading the fingers apart (Fig. 22.77, lateral iew).

3. **Test position:** If client performs through available PROM, place the finger in mid-abduction and proceed. If not, follow procedure for testing grades Poor, Trace, and Zero.

4. **Stabilize:** The therapist stabilizes the wrist and metacarpals on the supporting surface.

5. **Pressure:** Tell the client, "don't let me move you." Apply pressure over lateral proximal phalanx (index and long fingers) and medial proximal phalanx (long, ring, and small fingers)[6,15] toward adduction, adjusting pressure to client's abilities (Fig. 22.78, lateral view). An alternative mode of applying pressure is to flick each finger toward adduction. If the finger rebounds, the grade is N (5).[12] Note that the long finger is the axis for the hand, so it abducts both radially and ulnarly. If pressure maximal = Normal; moderate = Good, minimal = Good−, slight = Fair+, and no pressure = Fair. If not tested against gravity, use professional judgment when grading. For example, partial ROM in the gravity-minimized position may be graded poor and full ROM graded fair.[10,13]

Procedure for Testing Grades Poor (2), Trace (1), and Zero (0)

1. **Body position:** The client is seated or supine with forearm pronated, wrist in neutral, and fingers extended and adducted. The therapist is seated opposite or next to the client on the side to be tested.[10,13]

2. **Action:** Move client's finger into abduction twice while stating "move your finger like I did."

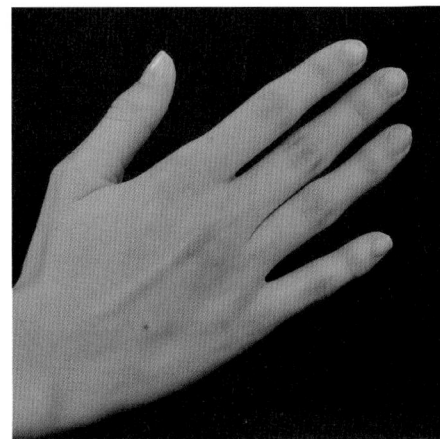

Fig. 22.75 Finger abduction: gravity-testing position for index and long fingers.

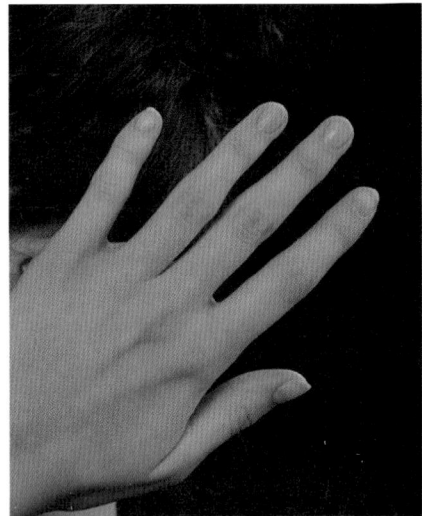

Fig. 22.76 Finger abduction: gravity-testing position for ring and small fingers.

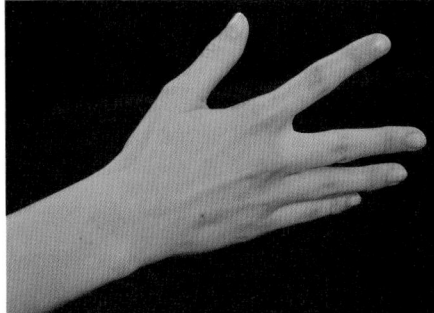

Fig. 22.77 Finger abduction: action—individual fingers (index finger).

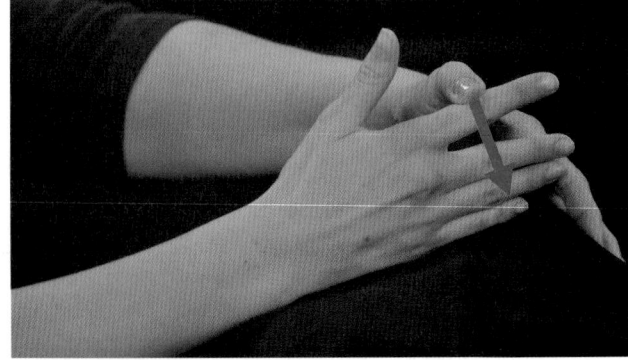

Fig. 22.78 Finger abduction: application of pressure to the index finger.

a. If patient performs full ROM, place in mid-MP abduction and apply slight pressure toward adduction.
  i. If tolerates pressure = Poor+.
  ii. No pressure = Poor.
b. If patient performs through partial ROM, do not apply pressure = Poor–.
c. If client is unable to perform motion, place MP joint in mid-abduction and state, "try to move your finger like I did." Palpate over lateral metacarpal for index and long fingers, and medial metacarpal for muscle contraction. Because the muscles for long and ring fingers are very small and deep, contraction may not be palpable.
  i. If muscle contraction palpable = Trace.
  ii. If no contraction palpable = Zero.

Substitutions. Extensor digitorum can assist weak or absent finger abduction, but abduction will be accompanied by MP extension.[6,16,21]

Finger Adduction (Figs. 22.79 to 22.82)

Muscles[10-15]	Innervation[10,13]
Palmar interossei, 2nd, 4th, and 5th fingers	Ulnar nerve, C8, T1

Procedure for Testing Grades Normal (5), Good (4), and Fair (3)

1. **Body position:** The client is seated or supine. Forearm is pronated and (shoulder in 90 degrees abduction) to test index finger (Fig. 22.79), and forearm is in mid-position to test ring and small fingers (Fig. 22.80). Because the digits are so light-weight, testing in any comfortable position is reasonable because the positions described may be awkward to assume and maintain. Wrist in neutral position and fingers extended and abducted.[10,13] The therapist is seated opposite or next to the client on the side to be tested.
2. **Action:** While demonstrating movement from neutral to full finger adduction, the therapist says, "move your finger like I am." Observe the client adducting the index, ring, and small fingers toward the middle finger (see Figs. 22.79 and 22.80).
3. **Test position:** If client performs through available PROM, place the finger in adduction and proceed. If not, follow procedure for testing grades Poor, Trace, and Zero.
4. **Stabilize:** The therapist stabilizes the wrist and metacarpals.[6]
5. **Pressure:** Tell the client, "don't let me move you." Apply pressure over medial proximal phalanx (index finger) (Fig. 22.81, lateral view) and lateral proximal phalanx (ring and small fingers) (Fig. 22.82, lateral view) toward abduction, adjusting pressure to client's abilities.[6,15] These muscles are very small, and pressure must be modified to accommodate their comparatively limited power. Fingers can be grasped at the distal phalanx and flicked in the direction of abduction. If the finger snaps back to the adducted position, the grade is Normal.[12] If pressure maximal = Normal; moderate = Good, minimal = Good–, slight = Fair+, and no pressure = Fair. If not tested against gravity, use professional judgment when grading. The therapist's judgment must be used in determining the degree of weakness.

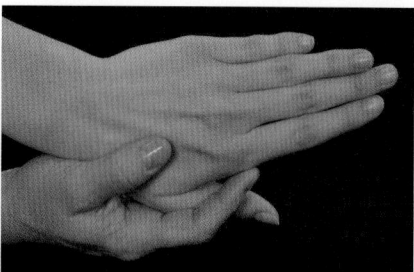

Fig. 22.79 Finger adduction: position and action—to test index and long fingers.

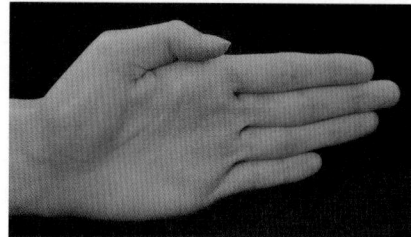

Fig. 22.80 Finger adduction: position and action—to test ring and small fingers.

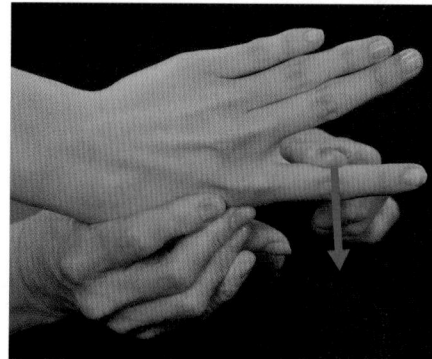

Fig. 22.81 Finger adduction: application of pressure—index finger.

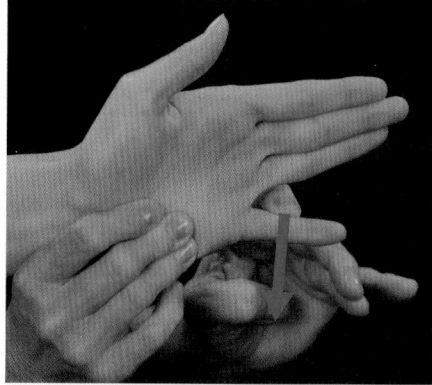

Fig. 22.82 Finger adduction: application of pressure—small finger.

Achievement of full ROM may be graded fair and partial ROM graded poor.[10,12]

Procedure for Testing Grades Poor (2), Trace (1), and Zero (0)

1. **Body position:** The client is seated or supine with forearm pronated, wrist in neutral, and fingers extended and

abducted. The therapist is seated opposite or next to the client on the side to be tested.[10,13]

2. **Action:** Move client's finger into adduction twice while stating "move your finger like I did."
   a. If patient performs full ROM, place in adduction and apply slight pressure toward abduction.
      i. If tolerates pressure = Poor+.
      ii. No pressure = Poor.
   b. If patient performs through partial ROM, do not apply pressure = Poor−.
   c. If client unable to perform motion, place MP joint in mid-abduction and state, "try to move your finger like I did." Because these muscles are very small and deep, contraction is not usually palpable.[6]
      i. If muscle contraction palpable = Trace.
      ii. If no contraction palpable = Zero.

   Substitutions. Flexor digitorum profundus and superficialis can substitute for weak adductors, but IP flexion will occur with finger adduction.[13,16,21]

Interphalangeal Extension (Figs. 22.83 to 22.85)

Muscles[10,13]	Innervation[10,13,19]
Lumbricals 1 and 2 (index and long)	Median nerve, C8, T1
Lumbricals 3 and 4 (ring and small)	Ulnar nerve, C8, T1
Dorsal interossei (index, long, and ring)	Deep branch of ulnar nerve, C8, T1
Palmar interossei (index, ring, and small)	Deep branch of ulnar nerve, C8, T1

Procedure for Testing Grades Normal (5), Good (4), and Fair (3)

1. **Body position:** The client is seated or supine with forearm pronated and wrist in mid-extension and neutral deviation. The therapist is seated or standing next to the client on the side to be tested.
2. **Action:** While demonstrating movement from neutral to full PIP and DIP extension, the therapist says, "move your finger like I am." Observe the client actively straighten both IP joints (Fig. 22.83).
3. **Test position:** If client performs through available PROM, place the IP joints in mid-extension and proceed. If not, follow procedure for testing grades Poor, Trace, and Zero.
4. **Stabilize:** The therapist stabilizes the proximal phalanx.

5. **Pressure:** Tell the client, "don't let me move you." Apply pressure over the dorsal middle (Fig. 22.84) and distal phalanx (Fig. 22.85) toward flexion, adjusting pressure to client's abilities. If pressure maximal = Normal; moderate = Good, minimal = Good−, slight = Fair+, and no pressure = Fair.

Procedure for Testing Grades Poor (2), Trace (1), and Zero (0)

1. **Body position:** The client is seated or supine with forearm in neutral rotation and wrist in mid-extension and neutral deviation. The therapist is seated or standing next to the client on the side to be tested.
2. **Action:** Move client's PIP and DIP joints into extension twice while stating "move your finger like I did."
   a. If patient performs full ROM, place in mid-extension and apply slight pressure toward flexion.
      i. If tolerates pressure = Poor+.
      ii. No pressure = Poor.

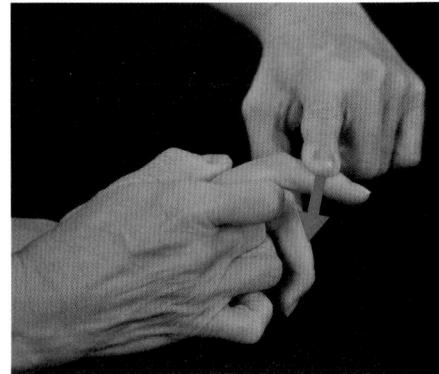

Fig. 22.84 Interphalangeal extension: application of pressure—middle phalanx.

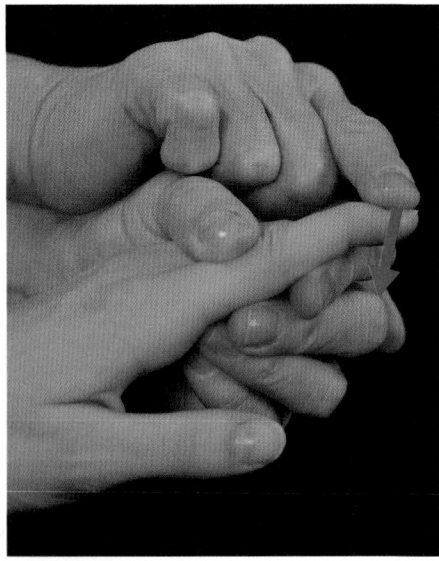

Fig. 22.85 Interphalangeal extension: application of pressure—distal phalanx.

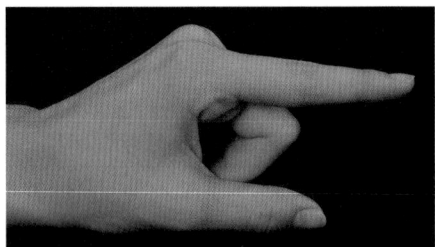

Fig. 22.83 Interphalangeal extension: action—to test the index finger.

b. If patient performs through partial ROM, do not apply pressure = Poor–.

c. If client unable to perform motion, place extension in mid-position and state, "try to move your finger like I did." Because the intrinsic hand muscles that perform IP extension are very small and deep, it may be difficult to palpate for muscle contraction.

   i. If muscle contraction palpable = Trace.

   ii. If no contraction palpable = Zero.

Substitution. Because the extensor digitorum inserts into the dorsal hood, if the wrist and MP joints are positioned in flexion (to prevent the ED from becoming actively insufficient), the ED can extend the IP joints. Passive tension in the ED can also result in finger extension at the MP and IP joints by tenodesis action. Positioning the wrist in extension when testing IP extension prevents this substitution from occurring.

Thumb Metacarpophalangeal Extension (Figs. 22.86 to 22.88)

Muscles[10,12–15]	Innervation[10,12–15]
Extensor pollicis brevis (EPB)	Radial nerve, C7, 8
Extensor pollicis longus (EPL)	Radial nerve, C7, 8

Procedure for Testing Grades Normal (5), Good (4), and Fair (3)

1. **Body position:** The client is seated or supine with forearm in mid-position, wrist in neutral, and hand and forearm resting on the ulnar border.[6,10,13] Because thumb extension occurs in the frontal plane (plane parallel to the hand), the thumb nail should face the ceiling to test against gravity. The therapist is seated or standing next to the client on the side to be tested. The thumb is flexed into the palm at the MP joint, and the IP joint is extended but relaxed.

2. **Action:** While demonstrating movement from neutral to full extension, the therapist says, "move your thumb like I am." Observe the client actively extend thumb MP joint (Fig. 22.86). It is difficult for many people to extend the MP joint without extending the IP joint simultaneously.

3. **Test position:** If client performs through available PROM, place the thumb in mid-extension and proceed. If not, follow procedure for testing grades Poor, Trace, and Zero.

4. **Stabilize:** The therapist stabilizes the first metacarpal and wrist in neutral.[6]

5. **Pressure:** Tell the client, "don't let me move you." Apply pressure over the dorsal surface of the proximal phalanx toward MP flexion,[6,10,12–15] adjusting pressure to client's abilities (Fig. 22.87). If pressure maximal = Normal; moderate = Good, minimal = Good–, slight = Fair+, and no pressure = Fair.

Procedure for Testing Grades Poor (2), Trace (1), and Zero (0)

1. **Body position:** Forearm is fully pronated and resting on the volar surface,[21] or forearm is supinated to about 70 degrees

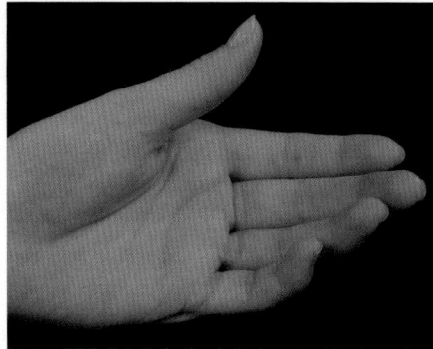
Fig. 22.86 Thumb metacarpophalangeal extension: action.

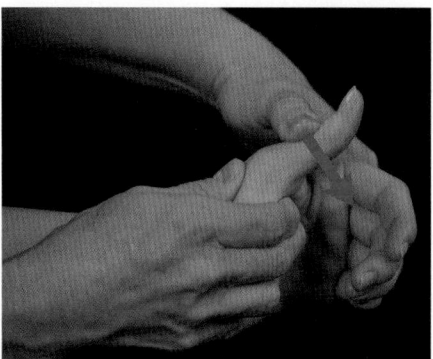
Fig. 22.87 Thumb metacarpophalangeal extension: application of pressure.

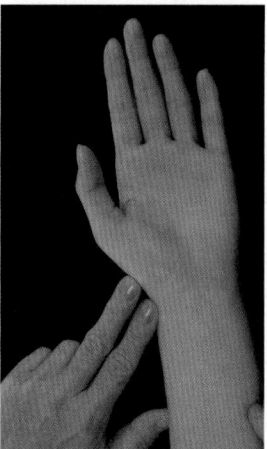
Fig. 22.88 Thumb metacarpophalangeal extension: body position, action, and palpation—muscle grades 2 and below.

resting on dorsal surface. The therapist sits opposite or next to the client on the side being tested, except that the therapist may stabilize the first metacarpal, holding the hand slightly above the supporting surface. The test may also be performed in the same manner as for grades normal to fair, with modified grading.[10]

2. **Action:** Move client's thumb MP into extension twice while stating "move your thumb like I did."
   a. If patient performs full ROM, place in mid-MP extension and apply slight pressure toward MP flexion.
      i. If tolerates pressure = Poor+.
      ii. No pressure = Poor.
      iii. If mid-position of the forearm was used, partial ROM is graded poor and full ROM is graded fair.[10,12]
   b. If patient performs through partial ROM, do not apply pressure = Poor–.
   c. If client unable to perform motion, place MP in mid-position and state, "try to move your thumb like I did." Palpate the extensor pollicis brevis tendon on the dorso-radial aspect of the base of the first metacarpal (Fig. 22.88, superior view). It lies just medial to the abductor pollicis longus tendon on the radial side of the anatomic snuffbox, which is the hollow space created between the EPL and EPB tendons when the thumb is fully extended and radially abducted.[4,6,7]
      i. If muscle contraction palpable = Trace.
      ii. If no contraction palpable = Zero.

Specific muscle testing. To isolate the extensor pollicis brevis, the thumb IP joint should be flexed or relaxed to prevent the extensor pollicis longus from acting.[6,7,13,16,21] It is difficult for many individuals to isolate this motion.

Thumb Interphalangeal Extension (Figs. 22.89 to 22.92)

Muscles[10,12–15]	Innervation[10,12–15]
Extensor pollicis longus (EPL)	Radial nerve, C7,8

Procedure for Testing Grades Normal (5), Good (4), and Fair (3)

1. **Body Position:** The client is seated or supine, forearm in mid-position, wrist at neutral, and hand and forearm resting on the ulnar border.[6,10,13] The thumb is adducted, the MP joint is extended or slightly flexed, and the IP is flexed.[6] The therapist sits opposite or next to the client on the side being tested. Because IP extension occurs in a plane parallel to the palm, the thumb nail should be facing the side.
2. **Action:** While demonstrating movement from neutral to full IP extension, the therapist says, "move your thumb like I am" (Fig. 22.89, lateral view). Observe the client actively perform the movement.
3. **Test position:** If client performs through available PROM, place the thumb in mid-extension and proceed. If not, follow procedure for testing grades Poor, Trace, and Zero.
4. **Stabilize:** The therapist stabilizes the wrist in neutral position, the first metacarpal, and the proximal phalanx of the thumb.[6]
5. **Pressure:** Tell the client, "don't let me move you." Apply pressure over dorsal distal phalanx toward flexion,[6,10,15] adjusting pressure to client's abilities (Fig. 22.90, lateral view). If pressure maximal = Normal; moderate = Good, minimal = Good–, slight = Fair+, and no pressure = Fair.

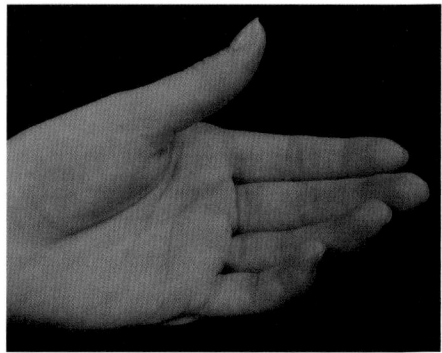

Fig. 22.89 Thumb interphalangeal extension: action.

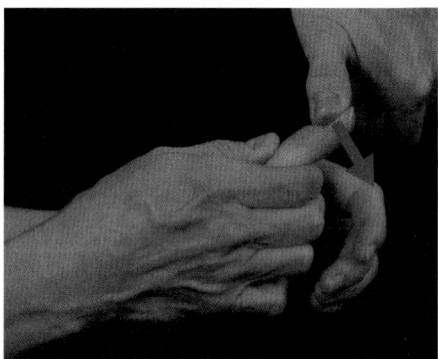

Fig. 22.90 Thumb interphalangeal extension: application of pressure.

Procedure for Testing Grades Poor (2), Trace (1), and Zero (0)

1. **Body position:** Forearm is fully pronated and resting on the volar surface,[21] or forearm is supinated to about 70 degrees resting on dorsal surface. The therapist may stabilize so that the client's hand is held slightly above the supporting surface. The thumb is adducted and IP joint is flexed. The therapist sits opposite or next to the client on the side being tested.
2. **Action:** Move client's thumb IP into extension twice while stating "move your thumb like I did."
   a. If patient performs full ROM, place in extension and apply slight pressure toward flexion.
      i. If tolerates pressure = Poor+.
      ii. No pressure = Poor.
      iii. If tested against gravity, partial ROM is graded Poor.[10]
   b. If patient performs through partial ROM, do not apply pressure = Poor–.
   c. If client unable to perform motion, place IP joint in mid-position and state, "try to move your thumb like I did." Palpate the EPL tendon on the dorsal surface of the hand medial to the EPB tendon, between the head of the first metacarpal and the base of the second on the ulnar side of the anatomic snuffbox[4,6,10] (Fig. 22.91, superior view). The EPL tendon also may be palpated over the dorsal proximal phalanx (Fig. 22.92, superior view)
      i. If muscle contraction palpable = Trace.
      ii. If no contraction palpable = Zero.

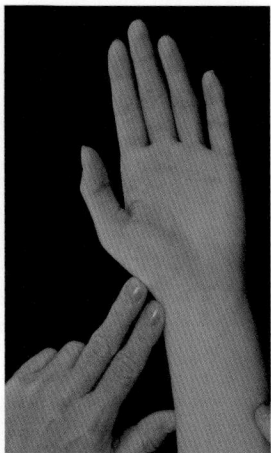

Fig. 22.91 Thumb interphalangeal extension: body position, action, and palpation of the extensor pollicis longus—muscle grades 2 and below.

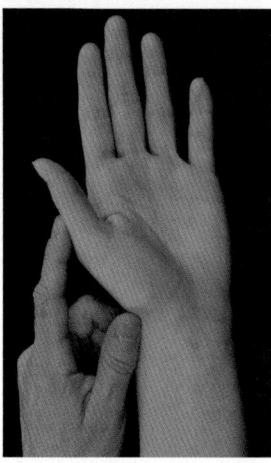

Fig. 22.92 Thumb interphalangeal extension: body position, action and alternate palpation of the extensor pollicis longus—muscle grades 2 and below.

Substitution. A quick contraction of the flexor pollicis longus followed by rapid release will cause the IP joint to rebound into extension.[6] IP flexion will precede IP extension.[7,14] The abductor pollicis brevis, the flexor pollicis brevis, the oblique fibers of the adductor pollicis, and the first palmar interosseous can extend the IP joint because of their insertions into the extensor expansion of the thumb.[15,21] Stabilization of the wrist in slight extension prevents thumb extension occurring from passive tension in the EPL with wrist flexion.

Thumb Metacarpophalangeal Flexion (Figs. 22.93 and 22.94)

Muscles[10,12–15]	Innervation[10,12–15]
Flexor pollicis brevis (FPB)	Median, C8, T1
Flexor pollicis longus (FPL)	Median nerve, C8, T1

Procedure for Testing Grades Normal (5), Good (4), and Fair (3)

1. **Body position:** The client is seated or supine. Thumb flexion occurs in the frontal plane (the plane parallel to the hand), so to perform this movement against gravity the client's shoulder is internally rotated and flexed to approximately 90 degrees (upper extremity must be parallel to the floor). The forearm will be fully pronated with the thumbnail facing the floor. The therapist is seated next to or opposite the client.[7,10,15]
2. **Action:** While demonstrating movement from neutral to full MP flexion, the therapist says, "move your thumb like I am." Observe the client actively perform the movement.
3. **Test position:** If client performs through available PROM, place the finger in mid-flexion and proceed. If not, follow procedure for testing grades Poor, Trace, and Zero.
4. **Stabilize:** The therapist stabilizes the wrist and first metacarpal.[12]
5. **Pressure**: Tell the client, "don't let me move you." Apply pressure over the volar surface of the proximal phalanx toward MP extension adjusting pressure to client's abilities[6,7,10,15] (Fig. 22.93, lateral view). If pressure maximal = Normal; moderate = Good, minimal = Good–, slight = Fair+, and no pressure = Fair.

Procedure for Testing Grades Poor (2), Trace (1), and Zero (0)

1. **Body position:** Client is seated with supinated forearm resting on table or in therapist's hand. The therapist sits opposite or next to the client on the side being tested.

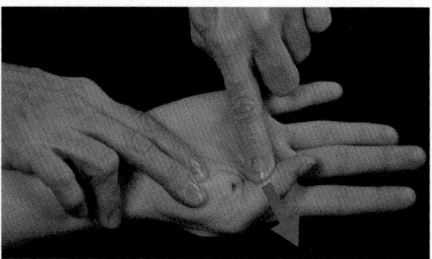

Fig. 22.93 Thumb metacarpophalangeal flexion: application of pressure.

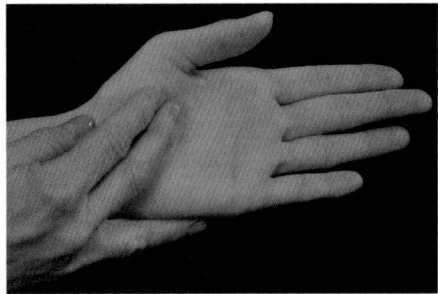

Fig. 22.94 Thumb metacarpophalangeal flexion: body position, action, and palpation—muscle grades 2 and below.

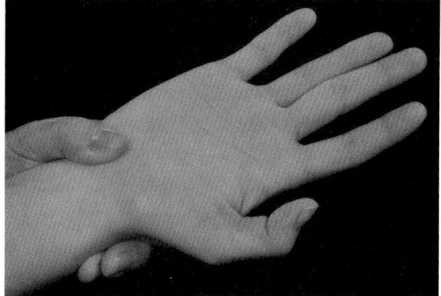

Fig. 22.95 Thumb interphalangeal flexion: action.

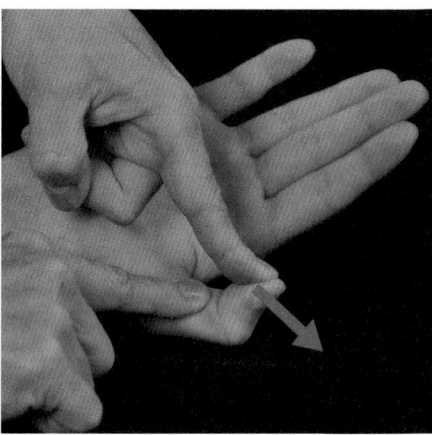

Fig. 22.96 Thumb interphalangeal flexion: application of pressure.

2. **Action:** Move client's MP into flexion twice while stating "move your thumb like I did."
   a. If patient performs full ROM, place in mid-flexion and apply slight pressure toward extension.
      i. If tolerates pressure = Poor+.
      ii. No pressure = Poor.
   b. If patient performs through partial ROM, do not apply pressure = Poor−.
   c. If client unable to perform motion, place MP in mid-position and state, "try to move your thumb like I did." Palpate the client over the middle of the palmar surface of the thenar eminence just medial to the abductor pollicis brevis muscle[6,10] (Fig. 22.94, superior view).
      i. If muscle contraction palpable = Trace.
      ii. If no contraction palpable = Zero.

Specific muscle testing. To test the integrity of the flexor pollicis brevis, ensure that the IP joint remains extended during MP flexion.[f] It may not be possible for some individuals to isolate flexion to the MP joint.

Substitution. Quick extension of the thumb is followed by a "rebound" to a flexed position if the first metacarpal and wrist are not stabilized.

Thumb Interphalangeal Flexion (Figs. 22.95 to 22.97)

Muscles[6,10,12]	Innervation[10,13]
Flexor pollicis longus (FPL)	Median nerve, C8, T1

Procedure for Testing Grades Normal (5), Good (4), and Fair (3)

1. **Body position:** The client is seated or supine. Thumb flexion occurs in the frontal plane (the plane parallel to the hand), so to perform this movement against gravity the client's shoulder is internally rotated and flexed to approximately 90 degrees (upper extremity must be parallel to the floor). The forearm will be fully pronated with the thumb nail facing the floor. The therapist is seated next to or opposite the client.[7,10,13]
2. **Action:** While demonstrating movement from neutral to full IP flexion, the therapist says, "move your thumb like I am" (Fig. 22.95, lateral view). Observe the client actively perform the movement.

[f]References 6,7,12,13,16,21.

3. **Test position:** If client performs through available PROM, place the thumb in mid-flexion and proceed. If not, follow procedure for testing grades Poor, Trace, and Zero.
4. **Stabilize:** The therapist stabilizes the wrist and first metacarpal.[12]
5. **Pressure:** Tell the client, "don't let me move you." Apply pressure over the volar surface of the distal phalanx toward MP extension adjusting pressure to client's abilities.[6,10,12,13] (Fig. 22.96, lateral view). If pressure maximal = Normal; moderate = Good, minimal = Good−, slight = Fair+, and no pressure = Fair.

Procedure for Testing Grades Poor (2), Trace (1), and Zero (0)

1. **Body position:** Forearm is fully pronated and resting on the volar surface[21] or forearm is supinated to about 70 degrees resting on dorsal surface. The IP joint is flexed. The therapist sits opposite or next to the client on the side being tested.
2. **Action:** Move client's thumb IP into extension twice while stating "move your thumb like I did."
   a. If patient performs full ROM, place in extension and apply slight pressure toward flexion.
      i. If tolerates pressure = Poor+.
      ii. No pressure = Poor.
   b. If patient performs through partial ROM, do not apply pressure = Poor−.
   c. If client is unable to perform motion, place IP in mid-position and state, "try to move your thumb like I did."

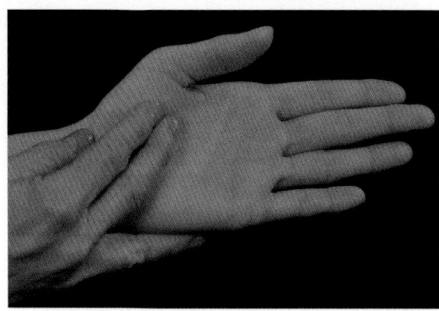

Fig. 22.97 Thumb interphala ngeal flexion: body position, action, and palpation—muscle grades 2 and below.

Palpate over the volar surface of the palmar surface of the proximal phalanx[6] (Fig. 22.97, superior view).
i. If muscle contraction palpable = Trace.
ii. If no contraction palpable = Zero.

Substitution. Quick extension of the thumb is followed by a "rebound" of the thumb IP joint into a flexed position if the proximal phalanx and metacarpal are not stabilized. The therapist should observe for IP extension preceding IP flexion.[g]

Thumb Palmar Abduction (Also Referred to as Abduction of the Carpometacarpal Joint) (Figs. 22.98 and 22.99)

Muscles[13,15]	Innervation[13,15]
Abductor pollicis brevis (APB)	Median nerve, C8, T1
Abductor pollicis longus (APL)	Posterior interosseous nerve C7, 8 continuation of deep branch of radial nerve

Procedure for Testing Grades Normal (5), Good (4), and Fair (3)

1. **Body position:** The client is seated or supine, forearm in supination, wrist at neutral, thumb relaxed in adduction against the volar aspect of the index finger. The therapist sits opposite or next to the client on the side to be tested.[6,7,10,12–15]
2. **Action:** Thumb abduction, also known as palmar abduction, is movement of the first metacarpal in a plane perpendicular to the palm.[6,15] While demonstrating movement from neutral to full abduction, the therapist says, "move your thumb like I am" (Fig. 22.98, lateral view). Observe the client actively perform the movement and note that movement is occuring at the carpal-metacarpal joint.
3. **Test position:** If client performs through available PROM, place the thumb in abduction and proceed. If not, follow procedure for testing grades Poor, Trace, and Zero.
4. **Stabilize:** The therapist stabilizes the wrist (and hand if needed).
5. **Pressure:** Tell the client, "don't let me move you." Apply pressure over the distal first metacarpal toward adduction (the palm),[6,15] adjusting pressure to client's abilities (Fig. 22.99A, lateral view). If pressure maximal = Normal; moderate = Good, minimal = Good–, slight = Fair+, and no pressure = Fair.

Procedure for Testing Grades Poor (2), Trace (1), and Zero (0)

1. **Body position:** Client is seated with the forearm and wrist in neutral, ulnar border of forearm and hand resting on table.[12,21] The therapist sits opposite or next to the client on the side being tested.
2. **Action:** Move client's thumb into abduction twice while stating "move your thumb like I did."
   a. If patient performs full ROM, place in abduction and apply slight pressure toward adduction.
      i. If tolerates pressure = Poor+.
      ii. No pressure = Poor.
   b. If patient performs through partial ROM, do not apply pressure = Poor–.
   c. If client is unable to perform motion, place in abduction and state, "try to move your thumb like I did." Palpate over volar radial wrist (Fig. 22.99B, lateral view) and superior surface of the thenar eminence for muscle contraction.
      i. If muscle contraction palpable = Trace.
      ii. If no contraction palpable = Zero.

Specific muscle testing. It is very difficult to test the abductor pollicis brevis and longus independently.

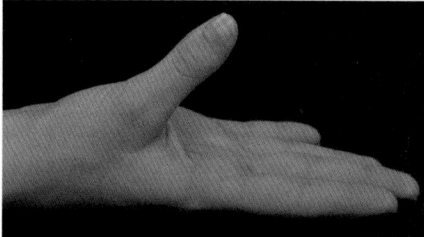

Fig. 22.98 Thumb palmar abduction: action.

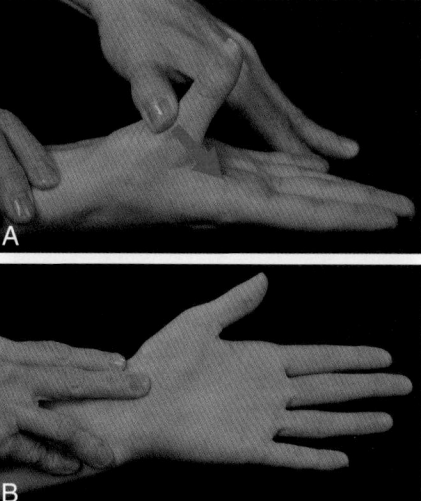

Fig. 22.99 (A) Thumb palmar abduction: application of pressure. (B) Thumb palmar abduction: body position, action, and palpation—muscle grades 2 and below.

gReferences 6,7,12,13,16,21.

Thumb Radial Abduction (Also Referred to as Extension of the Carpometacarpal Joint) (Figs. 22.100 to 22.102)

Muscles[12,15]	Innervation[12,15]
Extensor pollicis brevis (EPB)	Radial nerve, C7, 8
Extensor pollicis longus (EPL)	Radial nerve, C7, 8
Abductor pollicis longus (APL)	Radial nerve, C6-8

Procedure for Testing Grades Normal (5), Good (4), and Fair (3)

1. **Body position:** The client is seated or supine, forearm in neutral rotation, wrist at neutral, thumb adducted and slightly flexed across the palm. Hand and forearm are resting on the ulnar border.[15] The therapist sits opposite or next to the client on the side being tested.
2. **Action:** While demonstrating movement from neutral to full carpal-metacarpal extension, the therapist, says "move your thumb like I am." Observe the client perform the movement. The thumb should extend at the carpal-metacarpal joint, as well as the MP and IP joints (Fig. 22.100, lateral view).
3. **Test position:** If client performs through available PROM, place the finger in mid-abduction and proceed. If not, follow procedure for testing grades Poor, Trace, and Zero.
4. **Stabilize:** The therapist stabilizes the wrist and metacarpals of the fingers.[10,15]
5. **Pressure:** Tell the client, "don't let me move you." Apply pressure over distal, lateral surface of the first metacarpal toward flexion, adjusting pressure to client's abilities (Fig. 22.101, lateral view). If pressure maximal = Normal; moderate = Good, minimal = Good−, slight = Fair+, and no pressure = Fair.

Procedure for Testing Grades Poor (2), Trace (1), and Zero (0)

1. **Body position:** Client is seated with forearm in supination, dorsal surface of forearm resting on table.[10] The therapist sits opposite or next to the client on the side being tested.

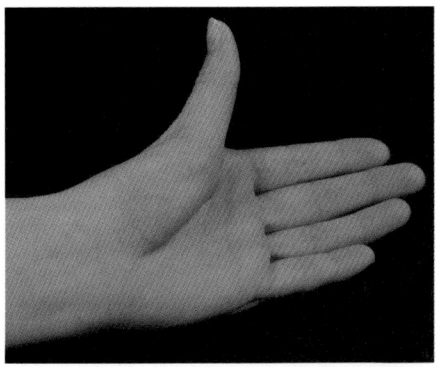

Fig. 22.100 Thumb radial abduction: action.

2. **Action:** Move client's first CMC into extension twice while stating "move your thumb like I did."
   a. If patient performs full ROM, place in extension and apply slight pressure toward flexion.
      i. If tolerates pressure = Poor+.
      ii. No pressure = Poor.
   b. If patient performs through partial ROM, do not apply pressure = Poor−.
   c. If client unable to perform motion, place CMC in extension and state, "try to move your thumb like I did." Palpate over dorsal lateral wrist for tension in the EPB, EPL, or APL. (Fig. 22.102, superior view).
      i. If muscle contraction palpable = Trace.
      ii. If no contraction palpable = Zero.

Specific muscle testing. Action in the EPB, EPL, and APL can be isolated by palpation and often visualization of the tendons in the lateral wrist.

Substitution. Stabilization of the wrist prevent radial deviation from CMC extension.

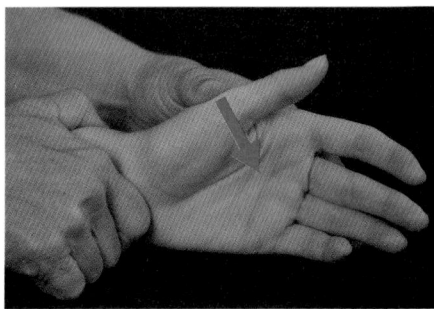

Fig. 22.101 Thumb radial abduction: application of pressure.

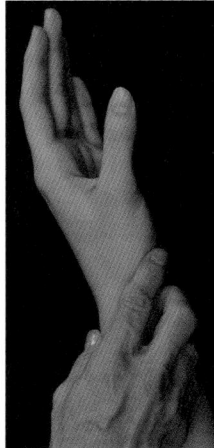

Fig. 22.102 Thumb radial abduction: body position, action, and palpation—muscle grades 2 and below.

Thumb Adduction (Figs. 22.103 to 22.105)

Muscles[10,12–15]	Innervation[10,12–15]
Adductor pollicis (AP)	Ulnar nerve, C8, T1

Procedure for Testing Grades Normal (5), Good (4), and Fair (3)

1. **Body position:** The client is seated or supine, forearm pronated, wrist at neutral, thumb relaxed and in palmar abduction.[10,13,21] The therapist is sitting opposite or next to the client on the side to be tested.
2. **Action:** While demonstrating movement from neutral to full adduction, the therapist says, "move your thumb like I am" (Fig. 22.103, lateral view). Observe the client adduct thumb into the palm.[10,12]
3. **Test position:** If client performs through available PROM, place the finger in mid-adduction and proceed. Space must be allowed between the first and second metacarpals for the

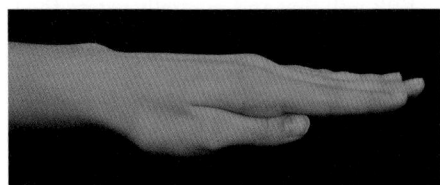

Fig. 22.103 Thumb adduction: action.

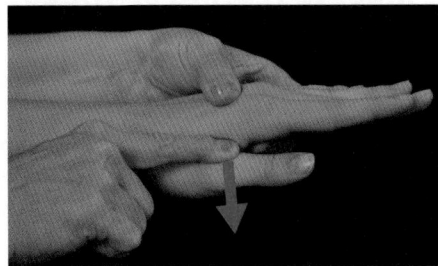

Fig. 22.104 Thumb adduction: application of pressure.

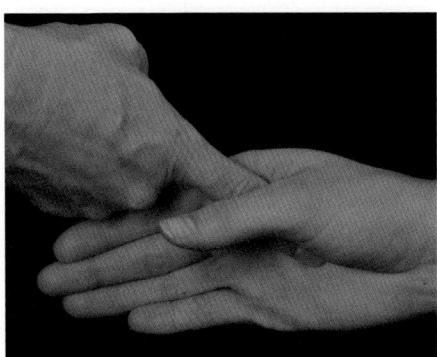

Fig. 22.105 Thumb adduction: body position, action, and palpation—muscle grades 2 and below.

therapist's finger. If not, follow procedure for testing grades Poor, Trace, and Zero.
4. **Stabilize:** The therapist stabilizes the wrist and metacarpals by grasping the hand around the ulnar side and supporting it slightly above the resting surface.[10,13]
5. **Pressure:** Tell the client, "don't let me move you." Apply pressure downward toward palmar abduction by placing finger between first and second metacarpals or grasping the first metacarpal head[10] (Fig. 22.104, lateral view). Adjust pressure to client's abilities. If pressure maximal = Normal; moderate = Good, minimal = Good–, slight = Fair+, and no pressure = Fair.

Procedure for Testing Grades Poor (2), Trace (1), and Zero (0)

1. **Body position:** Client is seated with the forearm and wrist in neutral, ulnar border of forearm and hand resting on table.[21] The therapist sits opposite or next to the client on the side being tested.
2. **Action:** Move client's thumb into adduction twice while stating "move your thumb like I did."
   a. If patient performs full ROM, place in adduction and apply slight pressure toward abduction.
      i. If tolerates pressure = Poor+.
      ii. No pressure = Poor.
   b. If patient performs through partial ROM, do not apply pressure = Poor–.
   c. If client unable to perform motion, place first CMC in mid-position and state, "try to move your thumb like I did." Palpate the AP on the palmar side of the thumb web space[6,16] (Fig. 22.105, lateral view).
      i. If muscle contraction palpable = Trace.
      ii. If no contraction palpable = Zero.
   Substitution. The FPL or EPL may substitute, but adduction will be preceded by thumb flexion or extension.[13,16,21]

Opposition of the Thumb to the Fifth Finger (Figs. 22.106 to 22.108)

Muscles[10,13]	Innervation[10,13]
Opponens pollicis	Median nerve, C8, T1
Opponens digiti minimi	Ulnar nerve, C8, T1

Procedure for Testing Grades Normal (5), Good (4), and Fair (3)

1. **Body position:** The client is seated or supine, with forearm supinated, wrist at neutral, thumb in palmar abduction, and fifth finger extended.[6,7,10,15] The therapist sits opposite or next to the client on the side to be tested.
2. **Action:** While demonstrating movement from open hand with small finger abducted and thumb extended, the therapist says, "touch your thumb to your small finger like I am." Observe the client opposing the thumb to touch the thumb pad to the pad of the fifth finger, which flexes and rotates toward the thumb (Fig. 22.106).[6,7]

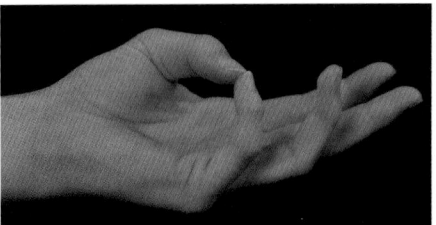

Fig. 22.106 Thumb opposition: action.

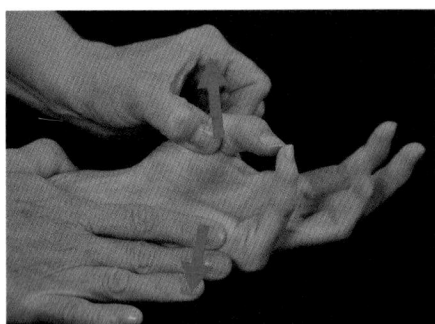

Fig. 22.107 Thumb opposition: application of pressure.

3. **Test position:** If client performs through available PROM, proceed with stabilization. If not, follow procedure for testing grades Poor, Trace, and Zero.
4. **Stabilize:** Rest forearm and wrist on table with padding to stabilize, as both of the therapist's hands must be free to apply pressure.
5. **Pressure:** Tell the client, "don't let me move you." Apply pressure at the distal ends of the first and fifth metacarpals toward reposition of these bones and flattening of the palm of the hand (Fig. 22.107).[10,12] Adjust pressure to client's abilities. If pressure maximal = Normal; moderate = Good, minimal = Good–, slight = Fair+, and no pressure = Fair.

Procedure for Testing Grades Poor (2), Trace (1), and Zero (0)

1. **Body position:** Client is seated with elbow flexed and resting on table, forearm and wrist in neutral and hand in open position. Therapist supports forearm and wrist if weak. The therapist sits opposite or next to the client on the side being tested.
2. **Action:** Touch client's thumb tip to the small finger-tip twice while stating "move your fingers like I did."
   a. If patient performs full ROM, leave in opposed position and apply slight pressure toward reposition.
      i. If tolerates pressure = Poor+.
      ii. No pressure = Poor.
   b. If patient performs through partial ROM, do not apply pressure = Poor–.
   c. If client unable to perform motion, touch client's thumb tip to small finger-tip and state, "try to move your fingers like I did." Palpate the thenar and hypothenar eminences of the palm[6,10,16] (Fig. 22.108, anterior view).
      i. If muscle contraction palpable = Trace.
      ii. If no contraction palpable = Zero.

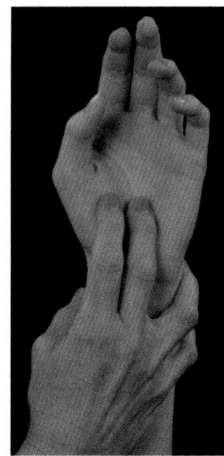

Fig. 22.108 Thumb opposition: body position, action, and palpation—muscle grades 2 and below.

Substitution. APB will assist with opposition by flexing and medially rotating the CMC joint, but the IP joint will extend. The FPB will flex and medially rotate the CMC joint, but the thumb will not move away from the palm of the hand. The FPL will flex and slightly rotate the CMC joint, but the thumb will not move away from the palm, and the IP joint will flex strongly.[16,21] The DIP joints of the thumb and little finger may flex to meet, giving the appearance of full opposition.[7,12]

MANUAL MUSCLE TESTING OF THE LOWER EXTREMITY

Muscle testing of lower extremity motions follows the same principles as the upper extremity. Because the distal lower extremity rotates in utero to allow humans to ambulate in a bipedal fashion, the muscles that flex the knee, ankle, and toes lie posterior to the knee joint, and the extensors lie anterior. Lower extremity muscle strength is traditionally measured by OT professionals by screening and not MMT; therefore, this chapter will present only a portion of the lower extremity motions.

Hip Flexion (Fig. 22.109)

Muscles[6,12,15]	Innervation[10,13]
Psoas major	Anterior rami off lumbar plexus, L1-L3
Iliacus	Femoral nerve, L2-L3
Sartorius	Sciatic nerve, L5-S2
Rectus femoris	Femoral nerve, L5-S2
Tensor fascia latae	Superior gluteal nerve, L5-S1

Procedure for Testing Grades Normal (5), Good (4), and Fair (3)

1. **Body position:** The client is sitting with hip in 90 degrees and knee relaxed (flexed to about 90 degrees).[12] Client should

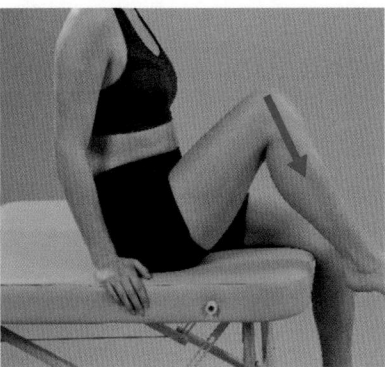

Fig. 22.109 Hip flexion: action.

rest hands on mat to stabilize body. The therapist stands next to the client on side being tested.[15]

2. **Action:** While demonstrating movement to full hip flexion, the therapist says, "move your leg like I am." Observe the client actively perform the movement (Fig. 22.109).

3. **Test position:** If client performs through available PROM, place the hip in enough flexion that it is off of the mat. Should be less flexion than pictured in Fig. 22.109. If not able to do motion, follow procedure for testing grades Poor, Trace, and Zero.

4. **Stabilize:** Client should rest stabilize body with both hands on the mat to maintain balance while pressure is applied. Therapist may stabilize trunk if client is unable to.

5. **Pressure:** Tell the client, "don't let me move you." Apply pressure at the distal femur, downward, toward hip extension,[12–15] adjusting pressure to client's abilities. OT practitioner is not pictured, but pressure should be applied where the tail of the *red arrow* begins, in the direction of the head (see Fig. 22.109). If pressure maximal = Normal; moderate = Good, minimal = Good–, slight = Fair+, and no pressure = Fair.

Procedure for Testing Grades Poor (2), Trace (1), and Zero (0)

1. **Body position:** Client is in a side-lying position on side opposite to hip being tested. The therapist stands in front of the client, supporting the weight of the lower extremity with the hip and knee in slightly flexed position.[10] The lower leg (not being tested) is flexed at the hip and knee to help maintain side-lying position.

2. **Action:** Move client's hip into flexion twice while stating "move your leg like I did."
   a. If patient performs full ROM, place in mid-flexion and apply slight pressure toward extension.
      i. If tolerates pressure = Poor+.
      ii. No pressure = Poor.
   b. If patient performs through partial ROM, do not apply pressure = Poor–.
   c. If client unable to perform motion, place hip in mid-position and state, "try to move your hip like I did." Palpate over the anterior hip joint and superior anterior thigh for muscle contraction.
      i. If muscle contraction palpable = Trace.
      ii. If no contraction palpable = Zero.

Hip Extension (Figs. 22.110 and 22.111)

Muscles[6,12,15]	Innervation[10,13]
Gluteus maximus	Inferior gluteal nerve, L5-S2
Semitendinosus	Sciatic nerve, L5-S2
Semimembranosus	Sciatic nerve, L5-S2
Biceps femoris (long head)	Sciatic nerve, L5-S2
Adductor magnus	Obturator, L2-L4

Procedure for Testing Grades Normal (5), Good (4), and Fair (3)

1. **Body position:** The client is prone, with the hip at neutral and the knee flexed to about 90 degrees[6,12] or extended.[12] The therapist stands next to the client on the opposite side.[15] Two pillows may be placed under the pelvis to flex the hips.[6,7]

2. **Action:** While demonstrating movement from neutral to full hip extension, the therapist says, "move your leg like I am." Observe the client actively perform the movement (Fig. 22.110).

3. **Test position:** If client performs through available PROM, place the hip in mid-extension and proceed. If not, follow procedure for testing grades Poor, Trace, and Zero.

4. **Stabilize:** The therapist stabilizes over the iliac crest on the side being tested.[10,12]

5. **Pressure:** Tell the client, "don't let me move you." Apply pressure at the distal end of the posterior aspect of the thigh, downward, toward flexion,[10,12–15] adjusting pressure to client's abilities (Fig. 22.111). If pressure maximal = Normal; moderate = Good, minimal = Good–, slight = Fair+, and no pressure = Fair.

Procedure for Testing Grades Poor (2), Trace (1), and Zero (0)

1. **Body position:** Client is in a side-lying position. The therapist stands in front of the client, supporting the upper leg in extension and slight abduction.[10] The lower extremity (to be tested) is flexed at the hip and knee.

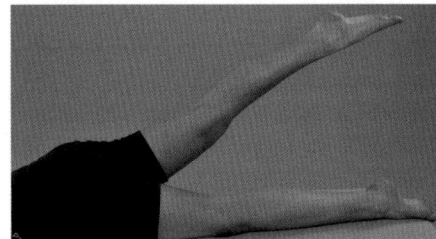

Fig. 22.110 Hip extension: action.

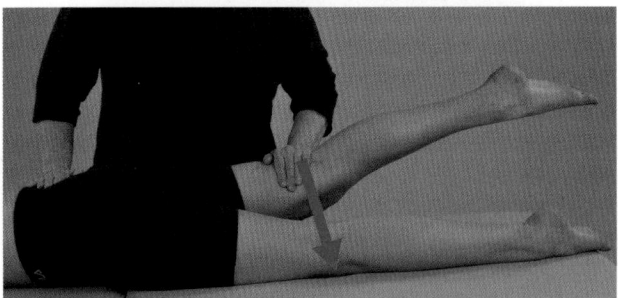

Fig. 22.111 Hip extension: application of pressure.

2. **Action:** Move client's hip into extension twice while stating "move your leg like I did."
   a. If patient performs full ROM, place in mid-extension and apply slight pressure toward flexion.
      i. If tolerates pressure = Poor+.
      ii. No pressure = Poor.
   b. If patient performs through partial ROM, do not apply pressure = Poor–.
   c. If client unable to perform motion, place hip in mid-position and state, "try to move your hip like I did." Palpate over the middle posterior surface of the buttock[16] and the posterior thigh for muscle contraction.
      i. If muscle contraction palpable = Trace.
      ii. If no contraction palpable = Zero.

Specific muscle testing. The gluteus maximus can be isolated by keeping the knee flexed while extending the hip to minimize action of the hamstring muscles on the hip.

Substitution. Elevation of the pelvis and extension of the lumbar spine can produce some hip extension. In the supine position, gravity and eccentric contraction of the hip flexors can return the flexed hip to extension.[16] Hip external rotation, abduction, or adduction may be used to substitute.[7]

Hip Abduction (Figs. 22.112 and 22.113)

Muscles[6,10,12]	Innervation[10,12–15]
Gluteus medius	Superior gluteal nerve, L4-S1
Gluteus minimus	Superior gluteal nerve, L4-S1
Tensor fasciae latae	Superior gluteal nerve, L4-S1
Sartorius	Femoral nerve, L2, l2

Procedure for Testing Grades Normal (5), Good (4), and Fair (3)

1. **Body Position:** The client assumes a side-lying position on the side not being tested with knee of bottom lower extremity flexed to stabilize client.[7] Lower extremity being tested is positioned with knee extended and hip extended slightly beyond the neutral position and slight forward rotation of the pelvis.[12] The therapist stands behind or in front of the client.[6,7,10,12–15]

2. **Action:** While demonstrating the movement from neutral to full hip abduction, the therapist says, "move your leg like I am." Observe the client actively perform the movement (Fig. 22.112).

3. **Test position:** Position the client's hip in mid-abduction.

4. **Stabilize:** Provide stabilization at the pelvis over the iliac crest.[10,15]

5. **Pressure:** Provide pressure just proximal to the knee in a downward direction, toward adduction (Fig. 22.113).[6,10,12]

Procedure for Testing Grades Poor (2), Trace (1), and Zero (0)

1. **Body position:** The client is supine, with both hips and knees in neutral. The therapist stands next to the client on the side that is being tested.[10] The therapist may use one hand to support at the ankle and slightly lift the test leg off the surface, being careful to avoid resisting or assisting the movement.[12]

2. **Action:** Move client's hip into abduction twice while stating "move your leg like I did."
   a. If patient performs full ROM, place in mid-abduction and apply slight pressure toward adduction.
      i. If tolerates pressure = Poor+.
      ii. No pressure = Poor.
   b. If patient performs through partial ROM, do not apply pressure = Poor–.
   c. If client is unable to perform motion, place hip in mid-position and state, "try to move your hip like I did." Palpate over the lateral hip, pelvis, and buttock[16] and palpate for muscle contraction.
      i. If muscle contraction palpable = Trace.

Substitution. Lateral muscles of the trunk may contract to bring the pelvis toward the thorax, effecting partial abduction at the hip.[10] If the hip is externally rotated, the hip flexors may assist in abduction.[6,7,10,16]

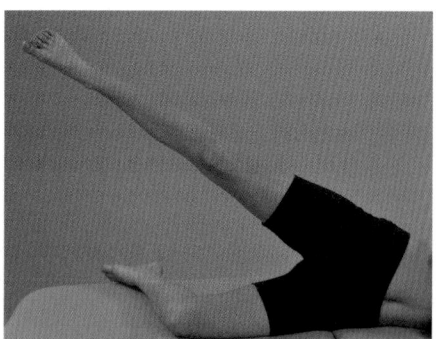

Fig. 22.112 Hip abduction: action.

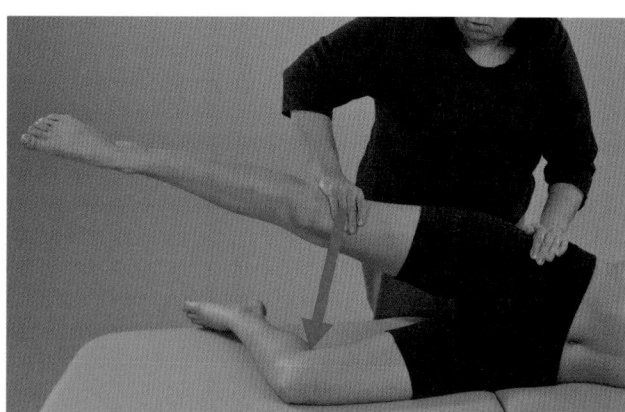

Fig. 22.113 Hip abduction: application of pressure.

Hip External Rotation (Figs. 22.114 and 22.115)

Muscles[10,12]	Innervation[10,12]
Quadratus femoris	Femoral nerve, L2-I4
Piriformis	Sacral plexus, S1, 2
Obturator internus	Sacral plexus, L5-S1
Obturator externus	Obturator nerve, L3,4
Gemellus superior	Obturator internus, I5, S1
Gemellus inferior	Obturator internus, I5, S1

Procedure for Testing Grades Normal (5), Good (4), and Fair (3)

1. **Body position:** The client is seated, with knees flexed over the edge of the table. A small pad or folded towel is placed

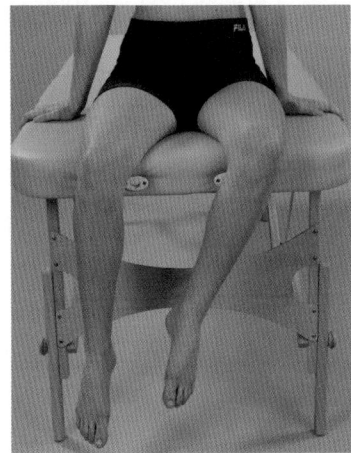

Fig. 22.114 Hip external rotation: action. (Note that the thigh is externally rotated despite the leg moving internally. Imagine this motion if the knee was extended instead of flexed.)

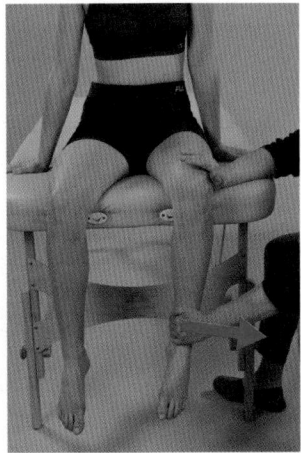

Fig. 22.115 Hip external rotation: application of pressure.

under the knee on the side to be tested. The therapist stands in front of the client toward the side to be tested.[6,10,12–15]

2. **Action:** While demonstrating movement from neutral to full external rotation, the therapist says, "move your leg like I am." Observe the client actively rotate the thigh outwardly—the foot will be move away from the midline (Fig. 22.114). Gravity may assist this motion once the client has passed the neutral position. Note that you are viewing the external rotation based upon the direction the thigh is rotating, not the direction the leg moved.

3. **Test position:** If client performs through available PROM, place the hip in mid-external rotation and proceed. If not, follow procedure for testing grades Poor, Trace, and Zero.

4. **Stabilize:** The therapist stabilizes the medial aspect of the knee on the side to be tested. The client may grasp the edge of the table to stabilize the trunk and pelvis.[6,10,15]

5. **Pressure:** Tell the client, "don't let me move you." Apply pressure over the distal leg (just proximal to the ankle joint) in medial direction toward internal rotation,[6,7,10,12–15] adjusting pressure to client's abilities. Because the long lever arm multiplies the force significantly, it is extremely important to apply pressure carefully and gradually; joint injury can occur if pressure is sudden and forceful (Fig. 22.115). Clients with knee instability should be tested in the supine position.[7,10] If pressure maximal = Normal; moderate = Good, minimal = Good–, slight = Fair+, and no pressure = Fair.

Procedure for Testing Grades Poor (2), Trace (1), and Zero (0)

1. **Body position:** The client is supine, with hips and knees extended; the hip to be tested is internally rotated. The therapist is standing next to the client on the opposite side.[10,12]

2. **Action:** Move client's hip into external rotation twice while stating "move your leg like I did." Observe the client actively rotate the thigh.[10]
   a. If patient performs full ROM, place in mid-external rotation and apply slight pressure toward internal rotation.
      i. If tolerates pressure = Poor+.
      ii. No pressure = Poor.
      iii. Muscles are graded poor if ROM in the gravity-minimized position can be achieved against slight pressure during the second half of the ROM.
   b. If client performs through partial ROM, do not apply pressure = Poor–.
   c. If client is unable to perform motion, place hip in mid-position and state, "try to move your leg like I did." These deep muscles are difficult or impossible to palpate.[6] Action of the external rotators may be detected by palpating deeply posterior to the greater trochanter of the femur.[10]
      i. If muscle contraction palpable = Trace.
      ii. If no contraction palpable = Zero.

   Substitution. The gluteus maximus may substitute for the deep external rotators when the hip is in extension. The sartorius may substitute, but external rotation will be accompanied by hip flexion, abduction, and knee flexion.[7,16]

Knee Extension (Figs. 22.116 and 22.117)

Muscles[10]	Innervation[10]
Rectus femoris	Femoral nerve, L2-4
Vastus intermedius	Femoral nerve, L2-l4
Vastus medialis	Femoral nerve, L2-l4
Vastus lateralis	Femoral nerve, L2-l4
Tensor fascia latae	Superior gluteal nerve, L4-s1

Procedure for Testing Grades Normal (5), Good (4), and Fair (3)

1. **Body position:** The client is seated, with knees flexed over the edge of the table and feet suspended off the floor. The client may lean backward slightly to release tension on the hamstrings and grasp the edge of the table for stability.[6,10,12] The therapist stands next to the client on the side to be tested.[6,12]

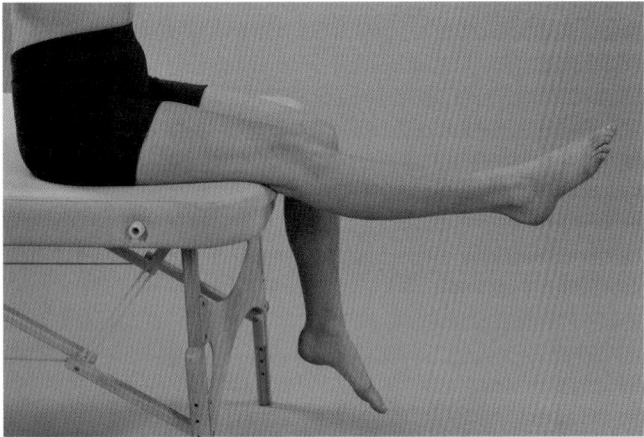

Fig. 22.116 Knee extension: action.

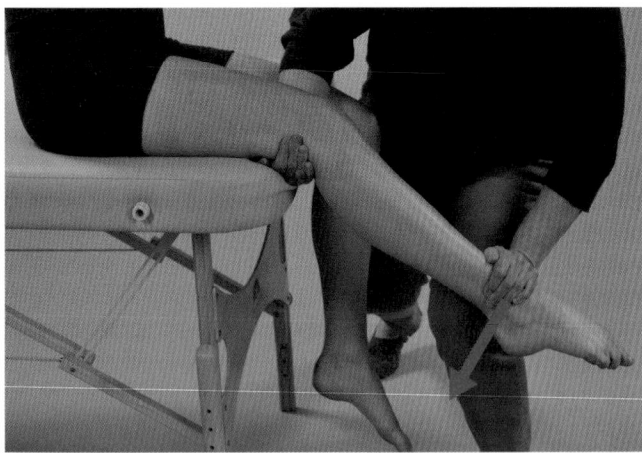

Fig. 22.117 Knee extension: application of pressure.

2. **Action:** While demonstrating movement from neutral to full extension, the therapist says, "move your leg like I am." Observe the client actively perform the movement (Fig. 22.116).
3. **Test position:** If client performs through available PROM, place the finger in mid-abduction and proceed. If not, follow procedure for testing grades Poor, Trace, and Zero.
4. **Stabilize:** The therapist stabilizes the thigh by placing one hand under the client's knee to cushion it from the edge of the table. The client may grasp the edge of the table.[7,10,12-15]
5. **Pressure:** Tell the client, "don't let me move you." Apply pressure on the anterior surface of the leg, just above the ankle, with downward pressure toward knee flexion,[6,10,15] adjusting pressure to client's abilities. Because applying pressure to a locked knee can cause joint injury,[10] ensure that the knee is tested in mid-extension and not at the end ROM of knee extension[7,10] (Fig. 22.117). If pressure maximal = Normal; moderate = Good, minimal = Good–, slight = Fair+, and no pressure = Fair.

Procedure for Testing Grades Poor (2), Trace (1), and Zero (0)

1. **Body position:** The client assumes a side-lying position on the side to be tested. The lower leg is positioned with the hip extended and the knee flexed to 90 degrees. The therapist stands behind the client.
2. **Action:** Move client's knee into extension twice while stating "move your leg like I did."
   a. If patient performs full ROM, place in mid–knee extension and apply slight pressure toward flexion.
      i. If tolerates pressure = Poor+.
      ii. No pressure = Poor.
   b. If patient performs through partial ROM, do not apply pressure = Poor–.
   c. If client is unable to perform motion, place knee in mid-position and state, "try to move your leg like I did." Palpate over the anterior aspect of the thigh.
      i. If muscle contraction palpable = Trace.
      ii. If no contraction palpable = Zero.

   Substitutions. Tensor fasciae latae may substitute for or assist weak quadriceps. In this case, hip internal rotation will accompany knee extension.[6,10,15] Observe for hip movement.

Ankle Dorsiflexion (Figs. 22.118 and 22.119)

Muscles[6,10,12]	Innervation[6,10,15]
Tibialis anterior	Peroneal nerve, L4-S1
Extensor digitorum longus	Deep fibular nerve, L5-S1
Peroneus (fibularis) tertius	Superficial fibular nerve, l5, S1, S2
Extensor hallucis longus	Deep fibular nerve, L5, S1

Procedure for Testing Grades Normal (5), Good (4), and Fair (3)

1. **Body position:** The client is seated, with the legs flexed at the knees, over the edge of the table. The therapist sits in front of the client, slightly to the side to be tested.[6,10,12-15]

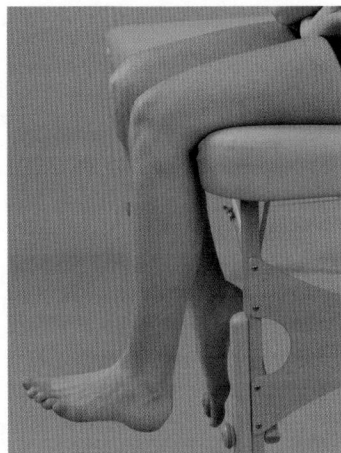

Fig. 22.118 Ankle dorsiflexion: action.

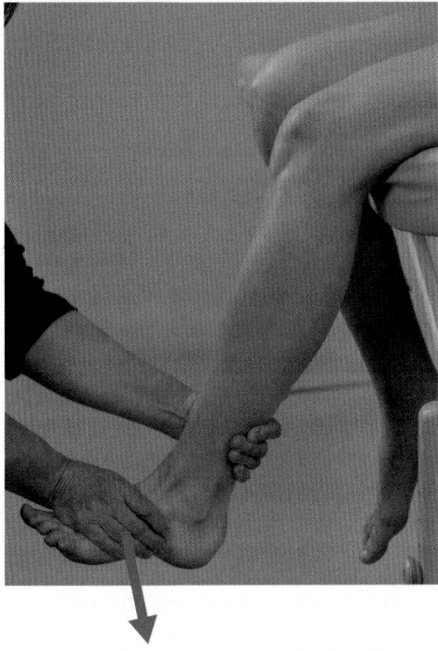

Fig. 22.119 Ankle dorsiflexion: application of pressure.

2. **Action:** While demonstrating movement from neutral to full dorsiflexion, the therapist says, "move your foot like I am." Observe the client actively perform the movement (Fig. 22.118).
3. **Test position:** If client performs through available PROM, place the finger in mid-abduction and proceed. If not, follow procedure for testing grades Poor, Trace, and Zero.
4. **Stabilize:** The therapist stabilizes the leg, just above the ankle. The client's heel can rest in the therapist's lap.[6,12]
5. **Pressure:** Tell the client, "don't let me move you." Apply pressure on the dorsal aspect of the foot (top of foot), toward plantar flexion (Fig. 22.119)[6,10,15] adjusting pressure to client's

abilities (see Fig. 22.119). If pressure maximal = Normal; moderate = Good, minimal = Good–, slight = Fair+, and no pressure = Fair.

Procedure for Testing Grades Poor (2), Trace (1), and Zero (0)

1. **Body position:** Client is positioned in a side-lying position.[7,10] The therapist stands or sits opposite or next to the client on the side being tested.
2. **Action:** Move client's ankle into dorsiflexion twice while stating "move your foot like I did."
   a. If patient performs full ROM, place in mid–ankle dorsiflexion and apply slight pressure toward plantarflexion (toward the floor).
      i. If tolerates pressure = Poor+.
      ii. No pressure = Poor.
   b. If patient performs through partial ROM, do not apply pressure = Poor–.
   c. If client unable to perform motion, place ankle in mid-dorsiflexion and state, "try to move your foot like I did." Palpate over the anterior medial aspect of the ankle joint[6,7,10] and the anterior surface of the leg, just lateral to the tibia.[16]
      i. If muscle contraction palpable = Trace.
      ii. If no contraction palpable = Zero.
      iii. If the against-gravity position is used, exercise clinical judgment to determine muscle grades. Partial ROM against gravity can be graded poor.[12] If the test is performed with the client in the supine position for these grades, standard definitions of muscle grades may be used.[10]

Specific muscle testing. To isolate the peroneus tertius, dorsiflexion should be combined with eversion, whereas the tibialis anterior is isolated with the foot in inversion and dorsiflexion. To prevent the extensor hallucis longus and extensor digitorum longus, do not allow the toes to extend.[7,10,12–16]

Foot Eversion (Figs. 22.120 and 22.121)

Muscles[10,15]	Innervation[10,15]
Peroneus longus	Peroneal nerve, L4-S1
Peroneus brevis	Superficial fibular nerve, L5-22
Peroneus tertius	Superficial fibular nerve, L5-22

Procedure for Testing Grades Normal (5), Good (4), and Fair (3)

1. **Body position:** The client assumes a side-lying position, with the lower leg flexed at the knee to keep it out of the way. The upper test leg is in hip extension with neutral rotation, knee extension, and ankle plantar flexion with foot inversion.[6]
2. **Action:** While demonstrating movement from neutral to full eversion, the therapist says, "move your foot like I am."

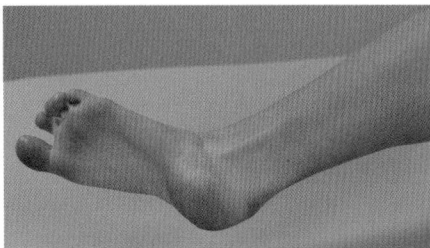

Fig. 22.120 Foot eversion: action.

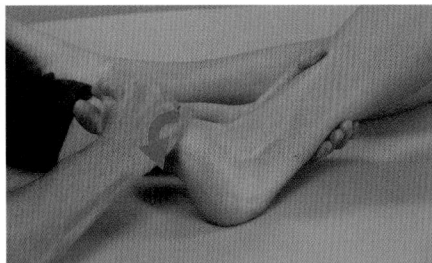

Fig. 22.121 Foot eversion: application of pressure.

Observe the client actively perform the movement. Eversion is normally accompanied by some degree of plantarflexion[15,16] (Fig. 22.120).

3. **Test position:** If client performs through available PROM, place the foot in eversion and proceed. If not, follow procedure for testing grades Poor, Trace, and Zero.

4. **Stabilize:** The therapist stabilizes the leg above the ankle in a medial or lateral manner.[6]

5. **Pressure:** Tell the client, "don't let me move you." Apply pressure against the lateral border and the plantar surface of the foot toward inversion and dorsiflexion,[6,15] adjusting pressure to client's abilities (Fig. 22.121). If pressure maximal = Normal; moderate = Good, minimal = Good–, slight = Fair+, and no pressure = Fair.

Procedure for Testing Grades Poor (2), Trace (1), and Zero (0)

1. **Body position:** The client is supine, hip extended and in neutral rotation.[10] The knee is extended, and the ankle is in mid-position.

2. **Action:** Move client's foot into eversion twice while stating "move your foot like I did."
   a. If patient performs full ROM, place in mid-eversion and apply slight pressure toward inversion.
      i. If tolerates pressure = Poor+.
      ii. No pressure = Poor.
   b. If patient performs through partial ROM, do not apply pressure = Poor–.

c. If client is unable to perform motion, place foot in mid-position and state, "try to move your foot like I did." Palpate over the upper half of the lateral aspect of the calf, ankle, and lateral border of the foot and over the base of the fifth metatarsal.[6,10,16]
   i. If muscle contraction palpable = Trace.
   ii. If no contraction palpable = Zero.

Specific muscle testing. To isolate the peroneus tertius, allow dorsiflexion along with eversion. To prevent the extensor hallucis longus from acting, do not allow the toes to extend.[7,10,12–16]

RESULTS OF ASSESSMENT AS A BASIS FOR INTERVENTION PLANNING

When planning intervention for maintenance or improvement of strength, the OT practitioner considers several factors in the clinical reasoning process before determining intervention priorities, goals, and modalities. Results of the muscle strength assessment will suggest the progression of the intervention program. What is the degree of weakness? Is it generalized or specific to one or more muscle groups? Are the muscle grades generally the same throughout, or is there significant disparity in muscle grades? If there is disparity, is there an imbalance of strength between the agonist and antagonist muscles that necessitates protection of the weaker muscles during OT intervention or when ADLs and IADLs are performed? When substantial imbalance between an agonist muscle and an antagonist muscle is noted, intervention goals may be directed toward strengthening the weaker group while maintaining the strength of the stronger group. Muscle imbalance may also suggest the need for an orthosis to protect the weaker muscles from overstretching while recovery is in progress. Examples of such orthoses are devices such as the bed footboard, used to prevent overstretching of the weakened ankle dorsiflexors, and the wrist cock-up splint, which can prevent overstretching of weakened wrist extensors.

Muscle grades will suggest the level of therapeutic activity or exercise that can help to maintain or improve strength. Is the weakness mild (G range), moderate (F to F+), or severe (P to 0)?[16] Muscles graded F+, for example, could be strengthened by active assisted exercise or light activity against gravity. Likewise, muscles graded P will require activity or exercise in the gravity-minimized plane, with little or no pressure, to increase strength. (See Chapter 29 for further discussion of appropriate exercise and activity for specific muscle grades.)

Endurance of the muscles (i.e., how many repetitions of the muscle contraction are possible before fatigue sets in) is an important consideration in intervention planning. A frequent goal of the therapeutic activity program is to increase endurance and strength. Because MMT does not measure endurance, the therapist should assess endurance by engaging the client in periods of exercise or activity graded in length to determine the length of time that the muscle group can be used in sustained activity. A correlation between strength and endurance is usually noted. Weaker muscles will tend to have less endurance than stronger ones. When selecting intervention modalities for increasing endurance, the therapist may elect not to tax the muscle to its maximal ability, but rather to emphasize repetitive action at less than the maximal contraction to increase endurance and prevent fatigue.[16]

Sensory loss, which often accompanies muscle weakness, complicates the ability of the client to perform in an activity program. If little or no tactile or proprioceptive feedback is obtained from motion, the impulse to move is decreased or lost, depending on the severity of sensory loss. Thus, the movement may appear weak and ineffective even when strength is adequate for performance of a specific activity. With some diagnoses, a sensory reeducation program (see Chapter 23) may be indicated to increase the client's sensory awareness and feedback received from the part. In other instances, the therapist may elect to teach compensation techniques to address the sensory loss. These techniques include the use of mirrors, video playback, and biofeedback, which can be used as adjuncts to the strengthening program.

Other important considerations in the therapist's clinical reasoning include the diagnosis and expected course of the disease. Is strength expected to increase, decrease, or remain about the same? If strength is expected to increase, what is the expected recovery period? What is the effect of exercise or activity on muscle function? Will too much activity delay the progress of recovery? If muscle power is expected to decrease, how rapid will the progression be? Are there factors to be avoided, such as vigorous activity or an exercise program that can accelerate the decrease in strength? If strength is declining, is special equipment practical and necessary? How much muscle power is needed to operate the equipment? How long will the client be able to operate a device before a decrease in muscle power makes it impracticable?[16] In the case of Sharon, the therapist must be aware of the change in muscle strength of this client. It is expected that muscle strength will return in a proximal-to-distal pathway, and it is critical to protect the intrinsic muscles of the hand against overexertion to ensure the possibility of full recovery. Frequent

OT PRACTICE NOTES

The therapist must consider the following questions: What is the client doing in each of the therapies? How long is each treatment session? Are the goals of all of the therapies similar and complementary, or are they divergent and conflicting? Is the client being over-fatigued in the total program? Are the various treatment sessions provided in rapid succession, or are they well spaced to meet the client's need for rest periods?

On the basis of these considerations and others pertinent to the specific client, the occupational therapist can select enabling and purposeful activities designed to maintain or increase strength, improve performance of ADLs, and enable the use of special equipment while protecting weak muscles from overstretching and overfatigue.

muscle testing of select muscle groups will serve as a means to monitor progression of the disease and to assist in the introduction of appropriate intervention strategies.[11,20]

The therapist should assess the effect of muscle weakness on the ability to perform ADLs; this can be observed during assessment. Which tasks are most difficult to perform because of muscle weakness? How does the client compensate for the weakness? Which tasks are most important for the client to be able to perform? Is special equipment necessary or desirable for the performance of some ADLs, such as mobile arm support for independence in eating (see Chapter 30)?

If the client is involved in a total rehabilitation program and is receiving several other healthcare services, the activity and exercise programs must be synchronized and balanced to meet the client's needs rather than the needs of the professionals, their schedules, and possibly their competition. The occupational therapist must be aware of the nature and extent of programs in which the client is engaged in physical therapy, recreation therapy, and any other services. Ideally, all members of the healthcare team should plan the exercise and activity programs together, to ensure that they complement one another.

SUMMARY

Many diseases and injuries result in muscle weakness. Screening tests can be used to assess the general level of strength available for the client to engage in ADLs, IADLs, and sleep and rest, educational, work, and leisure occupations. These tests can also help determine which clients and muscle groups might require MMT.

MMT evaluates the level of strength in a muscle or muscle group. It is used with clients who have motor unit (lower motor neuron) disorders and orthopedic conditions. It does not measure muscle endurance or coordination, and it cannot be used accurately in upper motor neuron disorders when spasticity and or patterned/synergistic motion is present or when selective motion is not present.

Accurate assessment of muscle strength depends on the knowledge, skill, and experience of the occupational therapist. Although there are standard definitions of muscle grades, clinical judgment is important in accurate evaluation.

Muscle test results are used to plan intervention strategies to improve occupational performance, compensate for muscle weakness, and increase strength. In some cases, muscle test results also can be used to track the expected course and progression of the disease or disorder, which can assist the OT practitioner when choosing intervention modalities and strategies, and when setting goals, as in the case of Sharon.

REVIEW QUESTIONS

1. List three general classifications of physical dysfunction in which muscle weakness is a primary symptom.
2. List at least three purposes for assessing muscle strength.
3. Discuss five considerations and their implications in intervention planning that are based on the results of muscle strength assessment.
4. Define endurance.
5. How can muscle weakness be differentiated from joint limitation?
6. If there is joint limitation, can muscle strength be measured accurately? How is strength recorded when available ROM is less than normal?
7. What does MMT measure?
8. What are the limitations of MMT?
9. When is MMT contraindicated?
10. What are the criteria for determining muscle grades?
11. In relation to the floor as a horizontal plane, describe or demonstrate what is meant by the terms "with gravity assisting," "with gravity minimized," "against gravity," and "against gravity and pressure."
12. List five factors that can influence the amount of pressure against which a muscle group can hold.
13. Define the muscle grades: N (5), F− (3−), F (3), P (2), P− (2−), T (1), and zero (0).
14. Explain what is meant by substitution.
15. How are substitutions most likely to be ruled out in the muscle testing procedure?
16. List the steps in the muscle testing procedure.
17. Is it always necessary to perform MMT to determine level of strength? If not, what alternatives may be used to make a general assessment of strength?
18. List the purposes of screening tests.

REFERENCES

1. Basmajian JF: *Muscles alive*, ed 4, Baltimore, 1978, Williams & Wilkins.
2. Bobath B: Adult hemiplegia: evaluation and treatment, ed 2, London, 1978, William Heinemann Medical Books.
3. Brunnstrom S: *Movement therapy in hemiplegia*, New York, 1970, Harper & Row.
4. Brunnstrom S: *Clinical kinesiology*, Philadelphia, 1972, FA Davis.
5. Chusid J: *Correlative neuroanatomy and functional neurology*, ed 19, Los Altos, CA, 1985, Lange Medical Publications.
6. Clarkson HM: *Musculoskeletal assessment*, ed 2, Philadelphia, 2000, Lippincott Williams & Wilkins.
7. Clarkson HM, Gilewich GB: *Musculoskeletal assessment*, Baltimore, 1989, Williams & Wilkins.
8. Cole JH, Furness AL, Twomey LT: *Muscles in action*, New York, 1988, Churchill Livingstone.
9. Crepeau EB, Cohn ES, Schell BA: *Willard and Spackman's occupational therapy*, ed 11, Philadelphia, 2008, Lippincott Williams & Wilkins.
10. Daniels L, Worthingham C: *Muscle testing*, ed 5, Philadelphia, 1986, WB Saunders.
11. Hallum A: Neuromuscular diseases. In Umphred DA, editor: *Neurological rehabilitation,* ed 5, St Louis, 2007, Mosby.
12. Hislop HJ, Montgomery J: *Daniels and Worthingham's muscle testing*, ed 6, Philadelphia, 1995, WB Saunders.
13. Hislop HJ, Montgomery J: *Daniels and Worthingham's muscle testing*, ed 8, St Louis, 2007, Saunders Elsevier.
14. American Occupational Therapy Association: Occupational therapy practice framework: domain and process, 4th edition, *Am J Occup Ther* 74: 7412410010p1–7412410010p87, 2020. .
15. Kendall FP, Kendall McCreary E, Provance PG, Rodgers M, Romani W: *Muscles – Testing and Function with Posture and Pain*, ed 5, Baltimore, MD, 2005, Lippincott Williams and Wilkins.
16. Killingsworth A: *Basic physical disability procedures*, San Jose, CA, 1987, Maple Press.
17. Landen B, Amizich A: Functional muscle examination and gait analysis, *J Am Phys Ther Assoc* 43:39, 1963.
18. Latella D, Meriano C: *Occupational therapy manual for evaluation of range of motion and muscle strength*, Clifton, NY, 2003, Thomson Delmar Learning.
19. Moore KL, Agur AR, Dalley AF: *Essential Clinical Anatomy with PrepU software*, ed 5, Baltimore, MD, 2014, Lippincott, Williams and Wilkins.
20. Pact V, Sirotkin-Roses M, Beatus J: *The muscle testing handbook*, Boston, MA, 1984, Little, Brown.
21. Pulaski KH: Adult neurological dysfunction. In Creapeau EB, Cohen ES, Schell BA, editors: *Willard and Spackman's occupational therapy*, ed 10, Philadelphia, 2003, Lippincott Williams & Wilkins.
22. Sieg KW, Adams SP: *Illustrated Essentials of Musculoskeletal Anatomy*, ed 4, Gainsville, FL, 2009, Megabooks, Inc.

23

Evaluation of Sensation and Intervention for Sensory Dysfunction

Michelle R. Abrams and Cynthia Clare Ivy

LEARNING OBJECTIVES

After studying this chapter, the student or practitioner will be able to do the following:

1. Describe how sensation is positioned within the current (2019) Occupational Therapy Practice Framework (OTPF-4).
2. Describe and compare the differences in sensory loss caused by a central nervous system dysfunction, a spinal segment, and a peripheral nerve injury and repair.
3. Perform a sensory evaluation on a client with peripheral nerve dysfunction.
4. Instruct a client in an appropriate intervention process for sensory reeducation; describe ways to upgrade the process and name the criteria that reflect a client's readiness to have the process upgraded.
5. Explain why lack of protective sensation puts people at risk for serious injury.
6. Identify whether a client is a candidate for compensatory strategies for sensory dysfunction, discriminative sensory reeducation, and/or cortical reorganization based on sensory evaluation findings.

CHAPTER OUTLINE

KEY TERMS

Allodynia
Chemoreceptors
Dermatome
Desensitization
Dexterity
Dysesthesia
Graded motor imagery
Habituation
Hyperalgesia
Hypersensitivity

Kinesthesia
Mechanoreceptors
Neuropathy
Neuroplasticity
Nociceptors
Paresthesia
Proprioception
Stereognosis
Thermoreceptors
Tinel's sign

THREADED CASE STUDY

Don, Part 1

Don is a 79-year-old, right hand–dominant gentleman (prefers use of the pronouns he/him/his) who sustained a spinal cord injury 45 years ago, with resultant incomplete paraplegia at the level of T12. He has relied solely on his bilateral upper extremities for his occupations because he has functioned independently from a wheelchair level since the injury. As stated in the Occupational Therapy Practice Framework (OTPF-4), "Occupations include things people need to, want to and are expected to do (p. 7)."[1] In Don's case, his occupations encompass tasks such as functional wheelchair mobility to independently maneuver through his daily activities, including self-care tasks, but he also enjoys playing tennis from a wheelchair level. In the course of his extensive arm use over the past 45 years, he has developed severe bilateral carpal tunnel syndrome. The sensory loss and increased pain in his hands associated with carpal tunnel syndrome are leading to difficulties

THREADED CASE STUDY—cont'd

Don, Part 1

with wheelchair mobility and his ability to complete basic and higher-level self-care tasks. During the occupational therapy (OT) initial evaluation, Don stated that the client factor that has had the greatest impact on his life is the sensory loss in his hands. This is leading to difficulty with the performance skill of wheelchair mobility, both as a means of transportation and as a means to engaging in recreational activities, because he now needs to use his vision to see how his hands are placed around the rim of the wheels for fear of them getting caught and injured in the spokes of the wheel. He believes that his wheelchair mobility signifies his level of independence and also provides for bilateral upper extremity exercise. He states that he typically chooses not to park in a "handicap" spot in order to allow others "who really need it" to park there and that he enjoys the extra exercise he feels he gains by parking farther away and using his arms to maneuver the wheelchair to get to his destination. Don believes that transitioning to a motorized wheelchair at this time would be a symbol of weakness and a loss of function. He and his OT practitioner will have to identify a client-centered approach that will allow him to improve his health and well-being and maintain his ideal engagement in occupations, including wheelchair tennis.

Don has recently undergone a right endoscopic carpal tunnel decompression, and his hand surgeon anticipates excellent sensory recovery. However, Don will need to work with his OT practitioner to learn strategies and make modifications to reduce weight bearing on his hands and repetitive strain to his palms at the area of the carpal tunnel during his recovery so as not to further irritate the median nerve as it passes through the carpal tunnel.

Critical Thinking Questions

1. What sensory tests would be most appropriate for Don?
2. Describe a sensory reeducation program that would be appropriate for Don in order for him to improve his functionality and safety with wheelchair mobility during wheelchair tennis.
3. What will you tell Don regarding typical sensory recovery after carpal tunnel release and the modifications that he will have to make to try to minimize weight bearing through his hands?

THREADED CASE STUDY

Mario, Part 1

Mario is an 84-year-old, right hand–dominant male (prefers use of the pronouns he/him/his) who sustained a circular saw injury, with resultant amputation of his right fourth (ring) finger and fifth (small) finger at the level of the fingertips, just distal to the distal interphalangeal (DIP) joints. He is an active senior who had been in the tile and granite profession and now enjoys woodworking, wine making, and dancing with his wife. He has osteoarthritis throughout many joints of his body, including his hands, hips, and knees, but is otherwise generally healthy. He has had prior hand surgeries, followed by hand occupational therapy for joint replacements in his fingers and also a thumb fracture. These surgical corrections and injuries grossly affected his function as a result of limitations in active range of motion (AROM) and functional strength, but they did not directly affect his sensation in his fingertips. Although Mario considered losing the tips of two fingers a relatively minor injury compared to the recovery required for joint replacements in his hand, he has come to realize the functional implications of sensory dysfunction. He not only has decreased sensation at the residual portion of his amputated digits, he also has hypersensitivity, along with phantom limb pain (PLP). Mario communicated that his leisure activities are the occupations that are the most affected by the amputation and resultant sensory dysfunction. He reports specific difficulty with tool use in both woodworking and

wine making. He also notices negative effects in his social participation because he has become less comfortable with driving, which he needs to do in order to go dancing with his wife; the sensory changes make it difficult to adequately and confidently grip the steering wheel. To sufficiently cover the residual portion of his fingers with soft tissue, surgical amputation was performed distal to the DIP joint of both his ring and small fingers. His hand surgeon expects full recovery in terms of AROM at those joints, but Mario will have sensory dysfunction at the residual distal ends of his ring and small fingers. The intervention plan for skilled occupational therapy services will address the client factor of sensory dysfunction while exploring resolutions to potential problems in performance skills related to his occupations of woodworking, winemaking, and driving his wife to go dancing.

Critical Thinking Questions

1. Why does sensation affect Mario's occupational roles?
2. How can an occupational therapist incorporate purposeful activity into Mario's treatment plan to enhance sensory perceptual skills?
3. What types of treatment interventions may you incorporate to improve the remapping of his brain to connect him with his fingers once again?

People who have not experienced sensory problems probably take for granted all that sensation contributes to their daily occupational performance. By comparison, people with sensory dysfunction are likely to be acutely aware of the lost picture that normal sensation provides. This chapter discusses the functional impact of somatosensory system dysfunction on occupational performance.

Sensation is explored in terms of touch, temperature, pain, proprioception (sense or awareness of body position and movement in space; for example, with loss of proprioception, the person experiences a lack of coordination with everyday tasks, such as buttoning), and stereognosis (the ability to

identify an item with the vision occluded). Techniques for sensory testing, desensitization, and sensory reeducation also are presented. This chapter offers cases illustrating sensory loss deficits and stimulates clinical reasoning that guides evaluation, intervention, and outcomes appropriate to various diagnoses. Additional information regarding upper extremity sensibility testing and reeducation may be found in Chapter 40 in this text.

Sensation, also called sensibility, is a body function, a component of the client factors that influence both the motor and processing aspects of performance skills.[1] Although there are several realms of sensibility or sensation in the body (e.g., the olfactory realm, the auditory realm, and even emotionality), this chapter is specific to cutaneous and proprioceptive sensation. Cutaneous refers to pain, temperature, and touch sensation where proprioceptive refers to sensation from the joints, skeletal muscles and tendons. According to the OTPF-4, the area of occupation that Don is limited in is the activity of daily living (ADL) of functional mobility because the lack of sensation in his first three digits affects his ability to grasp and maneuver the rims of his wheelchair.[1] Within the domain of occupation, this dysfunction will also affect his social participation. Client factors affected include body functions, such as mental functions, sensory functions, and pain resulting from the sensory loss. Body structures involved include the structure of the nervous system affected by sensory dysfunction. For this reason, sensation and sensory dysfunction may affect clients' performance in nearly all areas of occupation, including ADLs, instrumental activities of daily living (IADLs), education, work, play, leisure, and social participation. For people with carpal tunnel syndrome, as in Don's case, the sensory loss typically involves the volar surface of the thumb, index finger, long finger, and radial half of the ring finger. This distribution of sensory loss makes it difficult to pinch with a tip pinch or three-point pinch and to grasp objects with a lateral key pinch. It often forces people to oppose their thumb to the pad of their small finger instead. This would lead to difficulties for Don in maintaining a functional grasp and lateral pinch on his wheelchair rims.

All clients with sensory dysfunction, regardless of cause, should be evaluated to determine the occupational impact of the sensory loss.[12] The specific sensory tests and interventions may vary depending on the diagnosis and the prognosis for recovery. The battery of tests selected is contingent on whether the diagnosis defines the problem as either central nervous system (CNS) or peripheral nervous system (PNS) in origin. If CNS, it is important to determine whether the brain or the spinal cord is involved and, if PNS, whether it is a spinal nerve or named peripheral nerve.[12]

A person with CNS injury with brain involvement, with or without spinal cord injury, is more likely to have deficits in proprioception and stereognosis. Persons with CNS injury may also have difficulty processing sensory feedback, which would become evident during the evaluation and may require further testing (see Chapters 25 [perception] and 26 [cognition]). If there is an injury to a spinal nerve after it has exited the spinal cord, there may be a loss of all sensation at the dermatome at the level of injury, and if there is a CNS injury that only involves the spinal cord, there may be a loss of all sensation at the dermatome at the level of injury and below.

A person with PNS injury may have deficits in touch pressure awareness, including touch threshold and/or density, pain or temperature discrimination, or proprioceptive dysfunction. A client with a history of a cerebrovascular accident (CVA), which would be considered a previous CNS insult, who then sustains a wrist fracture (a PNS injury), should be evaluated for stereognosis as well as for pressure threshold and two-point discrimination because both the CNS and PNS systems are affected. Raynaud's phenomenon, brachial plexus injury, neuroma, severed nerve, and amputation are examples of other conditions that may lead to sensory dysfunction from the PNS. However,

radiculopathy, traumatic brain injury, neurodegenerative diseases, and CNS cancers or cancer treatments may lead to sensory dysfunction in the CNS.

Furthermore, it is useful to have the sensory test follow the motor examination, functional assessment, and interview with the client (see Chapters 19 and 20). These two preceding portions of the evaluation will allow greater information to determine where to begin sensory testing and the battery of sensory tests on which to focus. In Don's case, the occupational therapy (OT) interview allowed the therapist to focus on the distribution of the median and ulnar nerves of the hand. In Mario's case, the motor evaluation, which was normal, revealed that his functional deficits were due entirely to the sensory loss.

SOMATOTOPIC ARRANGEMENT

Sensory information is received and organized somatotopically in the primary somatosensory cortex of the brain.[7,18] The sensory homunculus (Fig. 23.1) is a diagram that shows the arrangement and proportions of cortical areas representing the surface of the body. Areas with large cortical representation indicate a high density of sensory receptors. As shown in Fig. 23.1, somatotopic arrangement is such that axons providing information from the index finger are situated closer to those from the thumb than to those from the foot. There is also a motor homunculus, or diagram, that follows roughly the same arrangements. Research studies have demonstrated the relevance of somatotopic arrangement to therapeutic strategies for normalizing impaired sensation.[28] These strategies are effective because of the brain's plasticity, or ability to adapt to new needs.

Referred sensations and PLP (pain felt in a part removed from its point of origin) in persons with amputations are

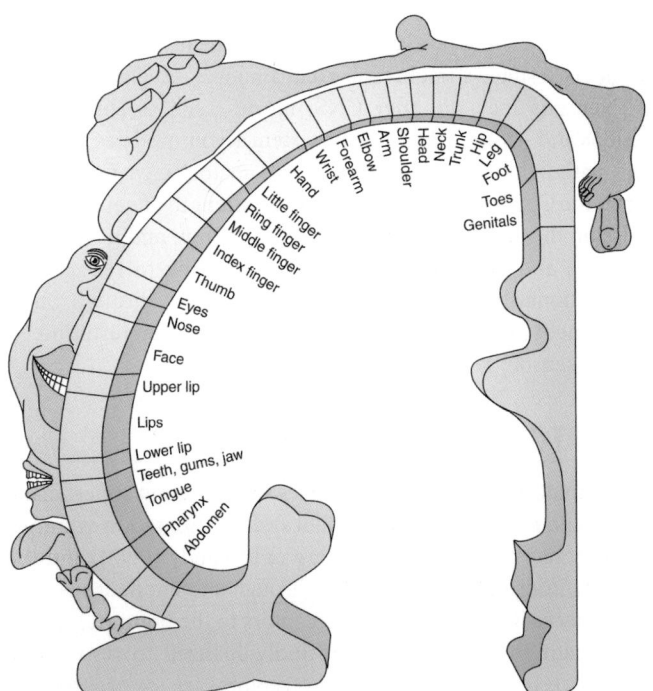

Fig. 23.1 Sensory homunculus. (From Banasik JL, Copstead LC: *Pathophysiology*, ed 6, St Louis, 2019, Elsevier.)

examples of cortical reorganization. Newer techniques, such as graded motor imagery, are being developed and used to address cortical reorganization at a clinical level. [27]

NEUROPLASTICITY

Our brain has the plasticity, called neuroplasticity (brain's ability to change, remodel, and reorganize for the purpose of better ability to adapt to new situations), to mechanically induce neuronal reorganization. Instances in which this occurs include the processes of habituation, learning, memory, and cellular recovery after an injury. Within the somatosensory cortex and other areas of the brain that interact with the somatosensory cortex, there is an inherent capacity for plasticity involving the complex firing of neurons and neurotransmitters.[43] Neuroplasticity involves changes in function or structure to the brain to adapt to external and/or internal factors.[56] Topographical reorganization of the cerebral cortex occurs after injury and can be influenced by sensory input and through learning and experience. This idea of a dynamic interplay between parts of the brain, including cognition, motor and sensory areas, was described as early as 1912[8] and in continued studies to the present time. [8,27,40,53,54] A concept of "occupational neuroplasticity" shows a relationship of changes in brain images related to specialized occupations with enhanced neural development in specific brain areas.[10] Some tenets of neuroplasticity are:

- Sensory perception is a dynamic process that is experienced by the CNS.[24,54]
- Receptor morphology is affected by hand use. The axiom, "Use it or lose it," is particularly applicable here. Immobilization or disuse (e.g., a casted fracture, a highly guarded injured upper extremity) contributes to retrogressive modifications in receptors. Conversely, promoting normal use may stimulate new receptors.[43]
- Because there is overlap of the receptive fields of various nerve fibers, a single stimulus will excite multiple receptors.[10]

Neurons may die after CNS injuries such as spinal cord lesions and strokes. The nervous system accommodates for injuries with behavioral, physiologic, and anatomic changes. Over time, the CNS can adapt by altering the strength of neural transmission through modifications in the structure and function of neurons and synapse.[10] It can be encouraging to realize that occupational therapists may facilitate recovery through functional activities and involvement in occupation resulting in somatosensory reeducation.

SOMATOSENSORY SYSTEM

The somatosensory system processes sensory input superficially (skin) and deeply (musculoskeletal system). Sensation is stimulated by receptors in the periphery of the body (PNS), and the sensory information then travels through afferent neurons, carrying nerve impulses from the receptors to the brain (CNS).

Somatosensory receptors are individualized to respond to specific types of input. These receptors are categorized as mechanoreceptors, chemoreceptors, and thermoreceptors. Mechanoreceptors respond to touch, pressure, stretch, and vibration and are stimulated by mechanical deformation. Chemoreceptors respond to cell injury or damage and are stimulated by substances (neuropeptides) that the injured cells release. Thermoreceptors respond to the stimulation of heating or cooling. Each of these three types of receptors has a subset called nociceptors, which sense pain when stimulated. Afferents, which are peripheral axons that carry information toward the brain, are categorized by the diameter of the axon. Axons with larger diameters transmit their information more quickly, in part because they are myelinated. In contrast to the axons with the larger diameter, pain is frequently carried on small-diameter, unmyelinated axons.[10]

Disturbances in somatosensation may be manifested as paresthesia, hyperalgesia, hypersensitivity, dysesthesia, or allodynia. Paresthesia is a tingling, electrical, or prickling sensation. Tapping the volar aspect of the wrist may elicit paresthesias in the distribution of the median nerve in a person who has carpal tunnel syndrome due to the compressive nature of the disease. When such tapping elicits paresthesia, it is referred to as Tinel's sign. Hyperalgesia is increased pain and may occur during nerve regeneration. Hypersensitivity is increased sensory pain. In our second case study Mario experienced hyperalgesia and hypersensitivity at his amputation sites after his surgery. Desensitization helps normalize the phenomenon of hypersensitivity. Dysesthesia is an unpleasant sensation that may be spontaneous or reactive to stimulation. Allodynia is pain caused by a stimulus that would not normally cause pain. An example of allodynia is observed when a person with complex regional pain syndrome (CRPS), formerly referred to as reflex sympathetic dystrophy (RSD), experiences pain with the mere movement of air wafting over the involved arm (Table 23.1).

A dermatome is the area of skin supplied by one spinal dorsal root and its spinal nerve. The affected dermatome correlates with the level of the spinal cord or spinal nerve lesion. However, some peripheral nerves have innervation patterns that differ from dermatome patterns. This is due to regrouping of sensory axons in the brachial plexus and in the lumbosacral plexus (Fig. 23.2). The clinical significance of such regrouping is that sensory assessment along a dermatomal pattern is more appropriate in clients with CNS lesions, not PNS lesions, unless the injury occurs at the level of the spinal nerve as it exits the spinal cord. Because of the central processing of sensory input, clients

TABLE 23.1 Disturbances in Somato-sensation

Sensory Disturbance	Description
Paresthesia	Tingling, electrical or prickling sensation
Hyperalgesia	Increased pain; often occurs during nerve regeneration
Hypersensitivity	Increased sensory pain
Dysesthesia	Unpleasant sensation that may be spontaneous or a reaction to stimulation
Allodynia	Pain caused by a stimulus that would not normally cause pain

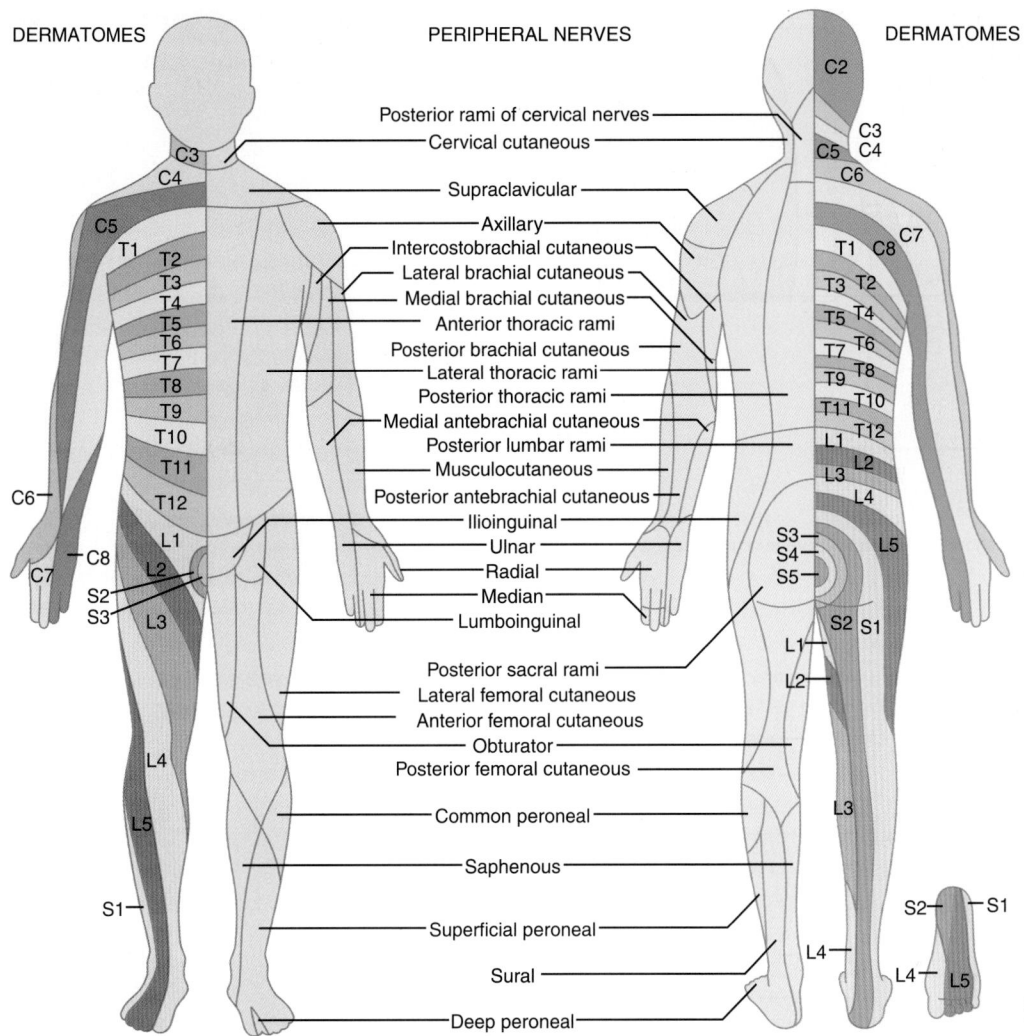

Fig. 23.2 Cutaneous sensory distribution and dermatomes. (From Lundy-Ekman L: *Neuroscience: fundamentals for rehabilitation*, ed 3, St Louis, 2007, Saunders.)

with some CNS lesions (e.g., CVA and multiple sclerosis) are more likely to have deficits in discriminatory sensation, as well as vibration, proprioception, and stereognosis. Clients with CNS dysfunction in the spinal cord and those with PNS lesions are more likely to experience deficits in pain, pressure threshold, and two-point discrimination. According to the American Spinal Injury Association (ASIA), persons with spinal cord injury are classified according to their "sensory level," which is the most caudal intact dermatome for both pinprick and light touch.[22,49] **Neuropathy** is defined as impairment of the PNS. Large sensory nerve fibers carry signals of vibration, light touch, and proprioception, whereas the smaller fibers, which are also often not myelinated, transmit messages of temperature and pain. Testing for light touch, proprioception, temperature, and pain will help discern whether small or large sensory nerve fibers are affected. This in turn, may help the therapist focus the intervention planning to the appropriate sensory stimuli.

Superficial Sensation

The upper and lower extremities have a higher density of large fiber cutaneous receptors with smaller receptor fields distally

than they do proximally.[20,21] Pain fibers, however, do not follow this pattern, and there are areas of increased density of pain fibers proximal to mechanoreceptors.[25,26] It is thought that there are approximately 3000 sensory nerve endings in a 1 cm² area on the pulp of the human finger (Fig. 23.3). This arrangement contributes to enhanced fingertip sensation, such as the ability to distinguish between one and two stimuli that are close together. The relevance of this in terms of daily occupations is that normal two-point discrimination enables a person to distinguish a dime from a penny without vision, as when one manipulates the coins in a pocket or wallet. Fig. 23.4 shows normal two-point discrimination values over various locations within the body.

Blisters, altered sweat patterns, calluses, shiny or dry skin, blanching of the skin, scars, and wounds are indicators of possible autonomic sensory problems and indicate the need to instruct the client in the use of compensatory techniques, such as vision, during daily occupations. In people with sensory problems, healing is slowed because of decreased vascularity because autonomic nerves also control the blood vessels. An absence of "wear" marks (e.g., calluses) or lack of dirt or grease

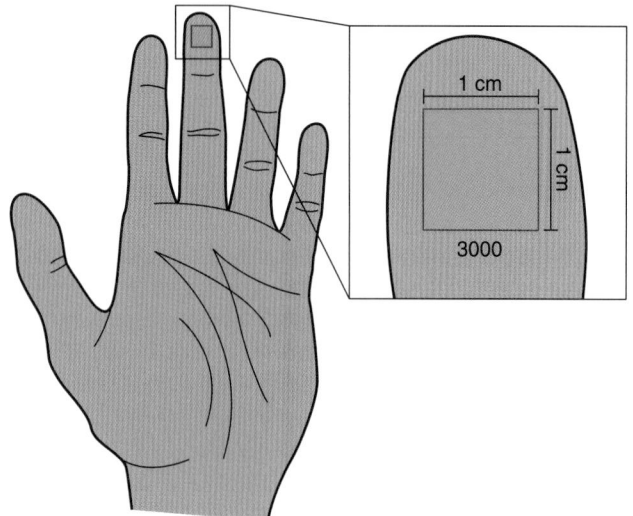

Fig. 23.3 Illustration showing sensory nerve endings in a 1 cm² area on the finger.

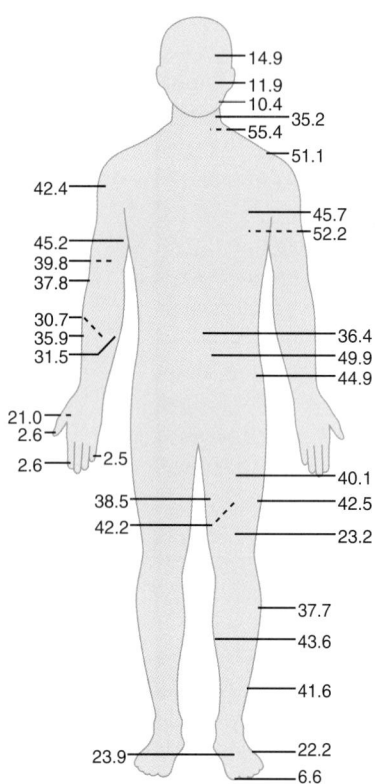

Fig. 23.4 Normal two-point discrimination values over different locations of the body. (From Lundy-Ekman L, Weyer A: *Neuroscience: fundamentals for rehabilitation,* ed 6, St Louis, 2023, Elsevier.)

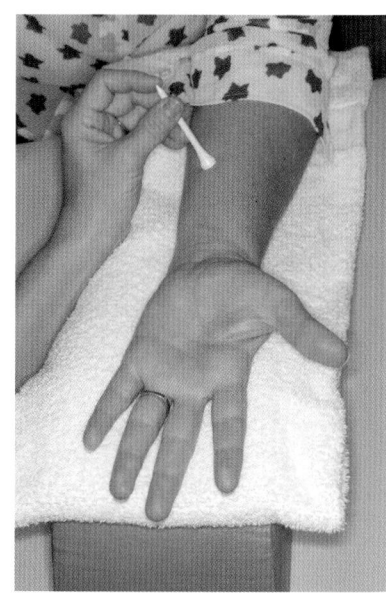

Fig. 23.5 The full forearm rests on a towel for sensory testing with a golf tee.

CRPS in clients with median nerve injury. Therefore, it is important to assess Don, the wheelchair user with bilateral carpal tunnel syndrome, for vasomotor function (e.g., blotching of the skin), sudomotor function (e.g., abnormal sweating), pilomotor changes (e.g., absence of goose bumps), and trophic changes (e.g., atrophy of finger pulp or hair growth) because all of these signs are indicators of CRPS.

Before sensory testing, the therapist must obtain a history through client interview and review of medical reports. The history should include client name, age, hand dominance, gender, occupation, date of injury, nature of injury, client description of the sensory problem and how sensation affects functional hand use, screening of motor function, and grip and pinch tests, if appropriate. In addition, any medications the client takes that may interfere with sensation should be noted. Some examples are gabapentin, an antiseizure medication that is sometimes used to treat nerve pain, and chemotherapy medications, which may sometimes induce peripheral neuropathy. Because pain is a sensation, a careful client description of pain should be obtained as a part of the history, including location, severity, aggravating factors, and elements of pain relief.

The most accurate sensory evaluation requires an environment free of background noise, high-quality instruments, consistent testing techniques, cooperative clients, and competent testers. It is important to support the client's hand fully, positioning it with a foam wedge or towels to prevent it from moving because movement could provide sensory information that interferes with the test being administered (Fig. 23.5). For all sensory testing, the client's vision should be occluded. This is accomplished by asking the client to keep the eyes closed or by occluding the area by other means, such as with a manila folder (Fig. 23.6). A hand grid worksheet may be used to record the findings (Fig. 23.7).

Sensory screening is a time-saving method to determine some parameters of the sensory loss experienced. With hand screening, specific sites can be used to reflect larger portions of the hand

stains on the hands of a mechanic, for example, may suggest that the hand is not being used. Nerve damage results in atrophy of soft tissue, which increases the tissue's susceptibility to injury because of the lack of protective padding.

Because upper extremity cutaneous sensory fibers and sympathetic nervous system fibers follow similar pathways, sympathetic phenomena may correlate with sensory function. In the upper extremity, the median nerve has more sympathetic fibers than the ulnar nerve, which may explain the increased risk for

innervated by the same peripheral nerve. For screening Don's median nerve function, test the thumb tip, index tip, and index proximal phalanx. For screening ulnar nerve function, test the distal and proximal ends of the small finger and the proximal ulnar aspect of the palm. For screening the radial nerve, test the dorsal part of the thumb web space (Fig. 23.8).[6] Screening also may be used for central nerves: for dermatome C5, test the anterior lateral arm; test C6 on the dorsum of the thumb at the distal phalanx; test C7 at the dorsal middle phalanx of the long finger; test C8 at the dorsal middle phalanx of the small finger; and test T1 on the anterior medial elbow (Fig. 23.9).

Pain Sensation

Pain is an unpleasant sensory and perceptual experience that is associated with either actual or potential cellular damage. The experience of pain is subjective and multidimensional.[16] Pain can be tested by pinching the digit firmly or by using a sharp point, as with a golf tee or the end of a partially unwound paper clip. Recent practices caution that one should avoid traditional use of a safety pin in testing pain sensation so as not to draw blood and risk compromising tissue. Intact pain sensation is indicative of available protective sensation. Sharp/dull testing, using both ends of a

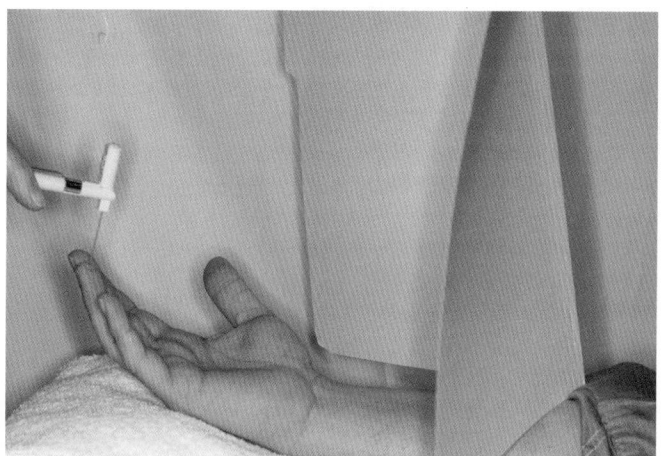

Fig. 23.6 Vision occlusion during sensory testing behind a manila folder.

golf tee, would be an alternative method to a safety pin to rule out a digital nerve laceration. This also could be accomplished by use of a paper clip opened to expose one end (Fig. 23.10).

Testing for pain sensation involves evaluating the client's perception of the type of pain. Note whether the pain is jabbing, tingling, sharp, deep, superficial, aching, dull, pounding, hot, or another descriptor that the client uses. This chapter focuses on sensation and sensory dysfunction and will describe specific testing for protective sensation. For detailed evaluation of pain, refer to Chapter 28.

Test for pain (protective sensation).

Purpose. Testing for pain is critical in the assessment of protective sensation and establishes a baseline for current function. Sensory testing for pain should be completed in clients with both PNS and CNS insult. Diminished or lack of protective sensation can lead to injury during daily activities, such as unknowingly sustaining a puncture wound while working with power tools. OT practitioners should also assess pain in the plantar foot, for example, in clients with peripheral neuropathy, to ensure that they can sense the presence of a sharp object in their shoes.

Procedure.
- Using a single-use golf tee or an opened paper clip, assess the amount of pressure required to elicit a pain response on the uninvolved hand or plantar foot. This is the amount of pressure that the examiner will use on the involved side.
- Alternate randomly between the sharp and dull sides of the golf tee or paper clip and ensure that each spot has at least one sharp and one dull application (see Figs. 23.5 and 23.10). Each application of pressure should last 1 to 1.5 seconds.
- Repeat five times total, using sharp or dull in random order.

Response.
- The client indicates "sharp" or "dull" after each application.

Scoring. Although evidence does not indicate a specific amount of trials for this type of sensory testing, anecdotally this scoring method provides a comprehensive picture of the client's current functional sensibility related to protective sensation.
- Intact protective sensation: Correct response to both sharp and dull on 5/5 trials

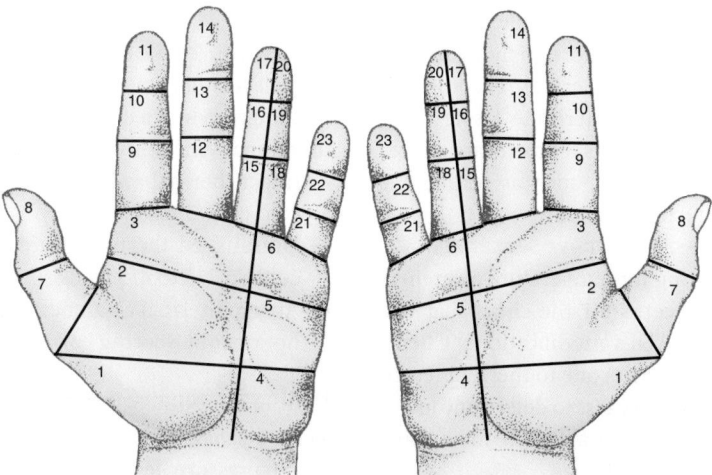

Fig. 23.7 Hand grid worksheet. (From Skirven T et al: *Rehabilitation of the hand and upper extremity*, ed 7, Philadelphia, 2021, Elsevier.)

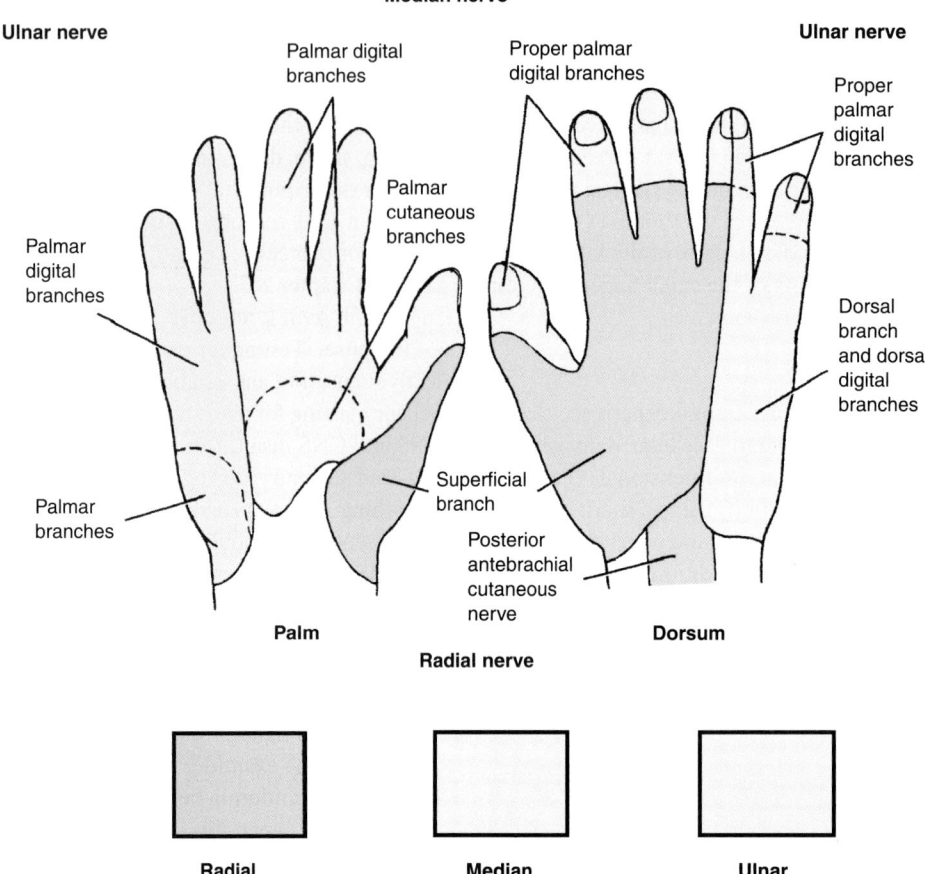

Fig. 23.8 Sensory distribution of the hand. (From Trumble TE, et al: *Principles of hand surgery and therapy*, ed 3, Philadelphia, 2017, Elsevier.)

- Diminished protective sensation: Correct response to sharp and dull on 1/5 to 4/5 trials
- Absent protective sensation: Inability to perceive being touched, scoring correctly on 0/5 trials
- Hyperalgesia: Heightened pain reaction to the stimulus

Temperature Awareness

Temperature awareness is another test for protective sensation. Thermal receptors detect warmth and cold. In the clinic, it is important to test temperature sensation before applying heat or cold modalities to avoid burn injuries. Thermal receptors are also critical for a person to be able to determine a safe water temperature for bathing. A client who lacks temperature awareness must learn compensatory strategies, such as testing the water temperature with an unaffected body part.

Test for temperature awareness (protective sensation).

Purpose. The purpose of testing for temperature awareness is to identify potential safety concerns for the client that will guide the therapist in suggesting ADLs modifications. Clients with burns or frostbite injury are more prone to thermal receptor dysfunction. Use this type of sensory test to determine likelihood of injury during occupations, such as not realizing that fingertips are burning while grilling food.

Procedure.

- Fill two test tubes or metal cylinders, one with hot water and the other with cold water.

- Examiner to test on self first to determine appropriate temperature level.
- Apply test tubes or metal cylinders filled with hot or cold water randomly to areas of the involved hand. Testing may follow dermatomal or peripheral nerve patterns. Test both the dorsal and volar surfaces.
- The client indicates "hot" or "cold" after each application.
- Repeat for five trials, randomly moving between hot and cold.

Scoring. While evidence does not indicate a specific amount of trials for this type of sensory testing, anecdotally, this scoring method provides a comprehensive picture of the client's current functional sensibility related to temperature awareness.

- Intact thermal awareness: Correct response to both hot and cold on 5/5 trials
- Diminished thermal awareness: Correct response to hot or cold on 1/5 to 4/5 trials
- Absent thermal awareness: Inability to discriminate between hot or cold, scoring correctly on 0/5 trials

Testing for Touch Sensation

Two-point discrimination. Two-point discrimination and touch pressure testing with monofilaments are two different tests examining various aspects of sensation. Two-point discrimination is a test for receptor density and is a good test to use for mapping improvement after nerve repair. One criticism

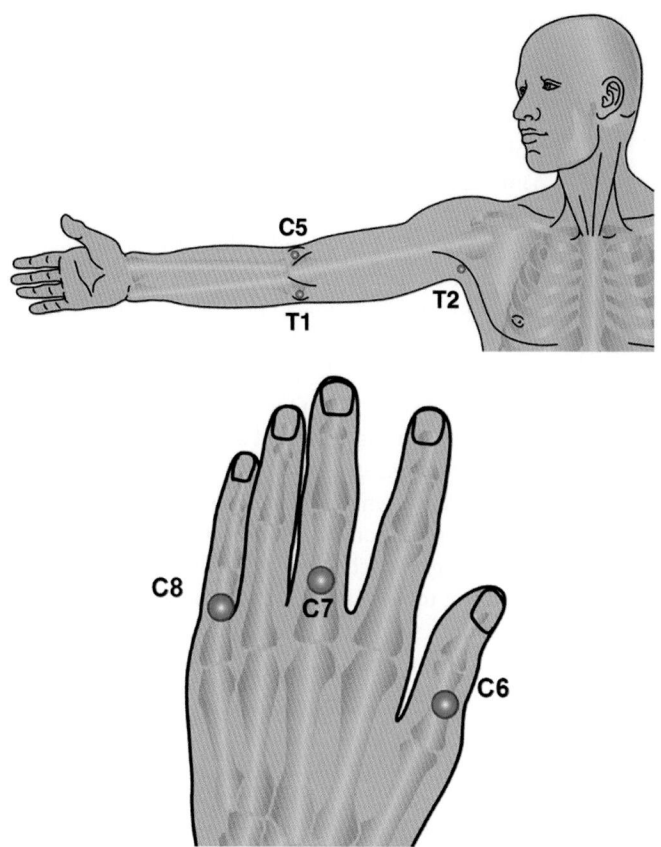

Fig. 23.9 Key sensory points (International Standards for the Classification of Spinal Cord Injury). (Adapted from Neurological Classification of Spinal Cord Injury. American Spinal Injury Association: International Standards for Neurological Classification of Spinal Cord Injury, Atlanta, GA. Revised 2011, Updated 2015. Courtesy American Spinal Injury Association, Richmond, VA.)

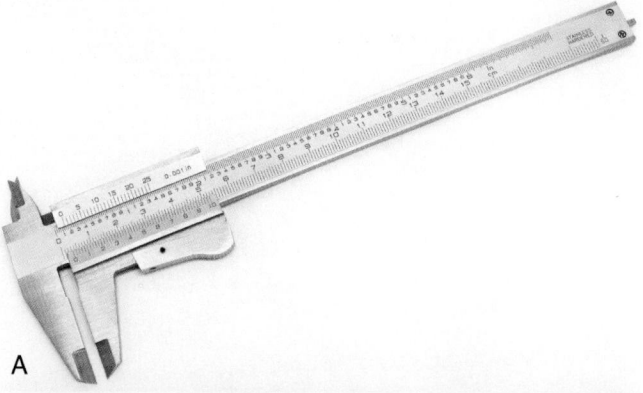

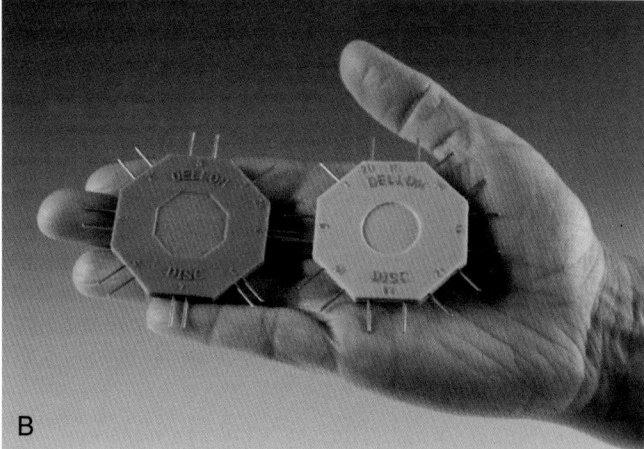

Fig. 23.11 The Boley gauge (A) and the Disk-Criminator (B) are used to test static and moving two-point discrimination. (A, iStock.com; B, courtesy Danmic Global, San Jose, CA.)

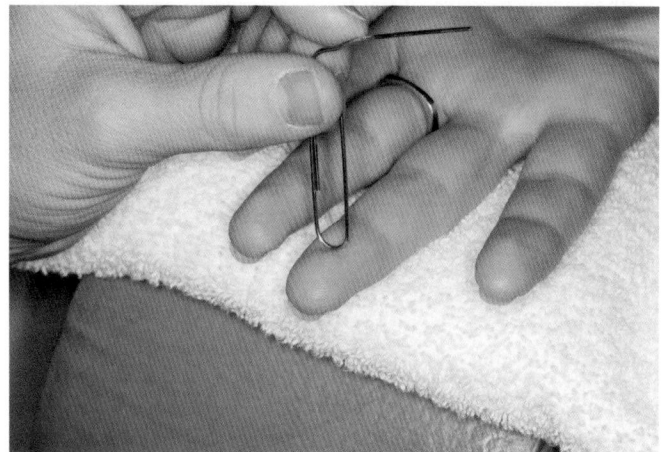

Fig. 23.10 Opened paper clip can be used for sharp/dull sensory testing on the hand.

concerns potential variability in the force of application during testing.[32] Nonetheless, good interrater reliability has been reported with the Disk-Criminator tool.[23]

Test for static two-point discrimination.

Purpose. OT practitioners should include sensory testing for two-point discrimination to assess area of receptor density at

the fingertips. This is especially important after digital and peripheral nerve injury and/or repair to establish a baseline and determine ongoing recovery. As in touch sensation (threshold), innervation density can also identify potential safety concerns. For example, a person with less innervation density will have decreased ability to perform fine motor tasks and will be less able to determine hot, cold, and sharp sensations.

Procedure.

- Use a device such as the Disk-Criminator or a Boley gauge with blunt testing ends (Fig. 23.11).
- Test only the volar tip of each finger because the fingertip is the primary area of the hand used for exploration of objects and the location of the majority of nerve endings.
- Begin with a distance of 6 mm between the testing points.
- Randomly test by depressing either a single point or two points spread to the testing distance on the radial and ulnar aspects of each finger. Apply testing points parallel to the longitudinal axis of the finger so that the adjacent digital nerve is not stimulated (Fig. 23.12).
- Apply pressure lightly; stop just when the skin begins to minimally deform.
- If the client is unable to accurately determine the difference between a single point and two points, widen the gauge by 1 mm. Continue widening the gauge until the client is able to accurately detect a single point versus two points or

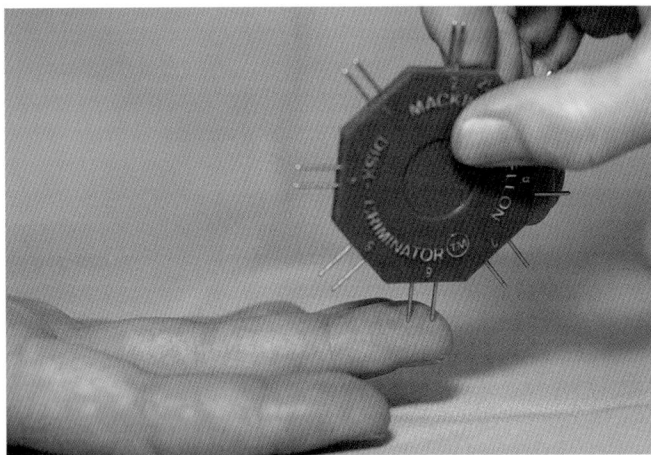

Fig. 23.12 Two-point discrimination testing.

demonstrates "protective sensation only" or an "anesthetic area" (see Scoring section later).

Response.
- The client will respond "One" or "Two" or "I don't know" after each application.

Scoring.
- The client responds accurately to 7 of 10 applications at that number of millimeters of distance between the two points.
- Norms are as follows[19]:
  - 1 to 5 mm: Normal static two-point discrimination
  - 6 to 10 mm: Fair static two-point discrimination
  - 11 to 15 mm: Poor static two-point discrimination
  - 1 point perceived: Protective sensation only
  - No points perceived: Anesthetic area

Test for moving two-point discrimination.

Purpose. Sensory testing for moving two-point discrimination should be completed with all digital and peripheral nerve injuries as the ability to sense moving discrimination returns before static discrimination and is therefore an objective indicator of recovery.

Procedure.
- Use a device such as the Disk-Criminator or a Boley gauge with blunt testing ends (see Fig. 23.11).
- Begin with a distance of 8 mm between points.
- Randomly select one or two points. Move slowly from proximal to distal on the distal phalanx, moving longitudinally along either the radial or the ulnar aspect of the fingertip so that the adjacent digital nerve is not stimulated (see Fig. 23.12). The pressure applied is just enough for the skin to be deformed.
- If the client responds *accurately*, decrease the distance between the points and repeat the sequence until you find the smallest distance that the client can perceive accurately.
- If the client responds *inaccurately*, increase the distance between the points and repeat the sequence until you find the smallest distance that the client can perceive accurately.

Response.
- The client responds "One," "Two," or "I don't know."

Scoring.
- The client responds accurately to 7 of 10 applications on any one given set distance on the gauge or tool.

- Score is indicated as either "normal" or "abnormal" based on the following normative data.
- Norms are as follows:
  - 2 to 4 mm (ages 4–60): Normal moving two-point discrimination[13,23]
  - 4 to 6 mm (ages 60 or older): Normal moving two-point discrimination[14]
  - *Note:* Lowest values are in second to third decades of life with increase in both stationary and moving two-point values beyond age 40, reaching a maximum in the seventh decade.

Touch Pressure

Light touch is perceived by receptors in the superficial skin. Pressure (or deeper touch) is perceived by receptors in the subcutaneous and deeper tissues. Light touch is important for fine discriminatory hand use, whereas deep pressure is important as a form of protective sensation. Touch pressure testing examines the spectrum from light touch to deep pressure. Touch pressure testing is a good test to use for clients with nerve compression, such as carpal tunnel syndrome. Many practitioners test two-point discrimination and the touch pressure of their hand therapy patients to gain a more objective clinical picture and track progress. Having intact light touch pressure awareness is an indicator of better sensation than having only intact deep touch pressure awareness. Light touch pressure awareness has to be intact for two-point discrimination to be testable because the two-point discrimination test uses light touch.

Touch pressure is tested with a set of 20 monofilaments, although most agree that the mini-kit with a set of 5 monofilaments is sufficient to gain objective data.[15] The Semmes-Weinstein monofilaments are often used in clinics, although there are various other brands of kits at this time.[45] These monofilaments are of varying thickness and are marked with numbers that represent a mathematical formula of the force required to bow them when applied perpendicularly. They are color coded to correspond to five threshold categories. Practitioners will frequently use an abbreviated set of five monofilaments, one for each of these categories, often referred to as the mini-kit. The five monofilaments used in the mini-kit are green (2.83), blue (3.61), purple (4.31), red (4.56 and 6.65), and untestable (6.65+).

Test for touch pressure.

Static touch pressure.

Purpose. Evaluating static light touch pressure is performed to gain a bottom threshold for which a stimulus is required to sense the presence of an object against the skin. This sensation is critical in tasks for safety when working with sharp objects or items that are extreme in either heat or cold. Touch pressure is required for tasks of fine motor coordination such as buttoning, zipping, or donning earrings. Static touch pressure should be assessed before assessing two-point discrimination, as touch pressure must be intact in order to sense the more detailed two-point stimulus.

Procedure (using mini kit).
- Begin with monofilament 2.83.
- Apply the monofilament for 1 to 1.5 seconds at the pressure needed to bow the monofilament (applied perpendicularly) (Fig. 23.13).

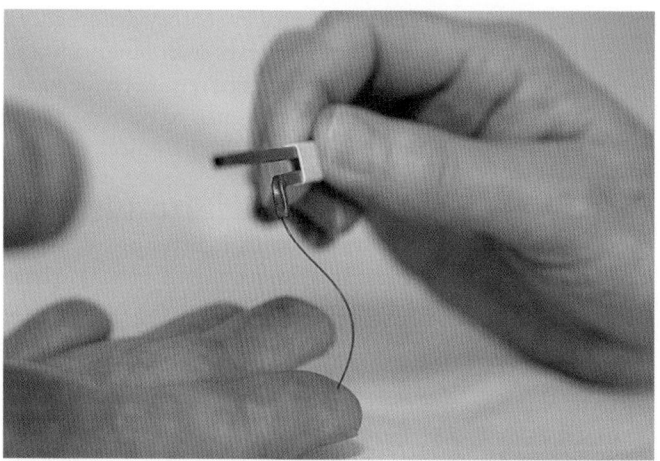

Fig. 23.13 Application of a touch pressure monofilament to the client's fingertip.

- Hold the pressure for 1 to 1.5 seconds.
- Lift the monofilament in 1 to 1.5 seconds.
- The proper amount of pressure is achieved when the filament bends.
- Repeat this three times in the same spot for monofilaments 2.83 and 3.61; monofilaments 4.31 and higher are applied only once.
- Randomly select areas of the hand to test and change the time interval between the application of monofilaments.
- If the client does not perceive the monofilament, proceed to the next (thicker) monofilament and repeat the sequence until you reach monofilament 6.65.
- If the client does perceive the monofilament, record this number on the hand grid and proceed to the next area of the hand.

    Response.
- The client says "Touch" when he or she feels the monofilament. The client does not need to localize or verbalize where the touch is felt on the hand.

    Scoring.
- The client responds to at least one of the three applications of the monofilament.
- Norms are as follows and include all 20 monofilaments in the full kit:
  - Green (1.65–2.83): Normal light touch
  - Blue (3.22–3.61): Diminished light touch
  - Purple (3.84–4.31): Diminished protective sensation
  - Red (4.56–6.65): Loss of protective sensation
- Untestable (6.65+): Inability to feel the largest monofilament

Moving Touch Pressure

Purpose. Moving touch pressure can be assessed by using the Ten Test.[46–48] In this method of screening, a client places a subjective value on his or her sensibility to light moving touch on their affected side and qualifies that number compared to the sensibility of that same touch on the contralateral, or unaffected, side. Assigning a number between 1 and 10 to describe the difference from their "normal" is often easier for clients than describing their sensation. This test can act as a quick screening

tool that yields measurable data. This sensibility test or screen can be completed at each visit to establish current status of recovery.

Procedure.
- The examiner lightly strokes an unaffected or "normal" area compared to the affected side. For example, stroke the small fingertip with normal sensation when evaluating sensory dysfunction in the index fingertip. The examiner can also stroke the contralateral side, as in touching the lateral upper arm on the left side when evaluating for sensory loss at the same location on the right arm.
- Stroke the unaffected area and tell the client that the sensation they are feeling is considered "normal," or a 10 of 10 on a scale of normalcy. The number 10 becomes the denominator in scoring.
- Next, stroke both the normal and abnormal areas *simultaneously* and *with equal pressure.*
- Ask the client to report how the affected side feels compared to the normal side. The client reports this by giving a numerical value from 1 to 10, with 10 being the best sensibility that can be appreciated. This value becomes the numerator in scoring.

Response. The client says a number between 1 and 10, with 10 being the best sensibility that can be appreciated (equal to the unaffected or "normal" area) and 1 being insensate.

Scoring.
- The client's given response becomes the numerator and the "normal" sensation of 10 becomes the denominator, so scores are indicated as a fraction or ratio with a range from 1/10 to 10/10.

Proprioception

Conscious proprioception derives from receptors found in muscles, tendons, and joints and is defined as awareness of joint position in space. It is through cerebral integration of information about touch and proprioception that objects can be identified by tactile cues and pressure. If proprioception is impaired, it may be difficult to gauge how much pressure to use when holding a paper cup.

Test for proprioception.

Purpose. Proprioception has been shown to diminish with age as the integrity of the end organs, such as muscle spindles, in the PNS slow, but proprioception also can be affected negatively by injury or insult to the CNS.[39]

Procedure.
- Hold the lateral and medial aspects of the body part to be examined, such as the elbow, wrist, or digit.
- Move the body part into flexion or extension (Fig. 23.14), being mindful not to touch the dorsal or volar aspect of the body so as not to give tactile cues to the direction that the body part is moving.
- Repeat three times at each testing joint, randomly moving into either flexion or extension.

Response.
- The client indicates whether the body part is being moved with "Up" and "Down" corresponding to the movements of flexion/extension and pronation/supination, depending on

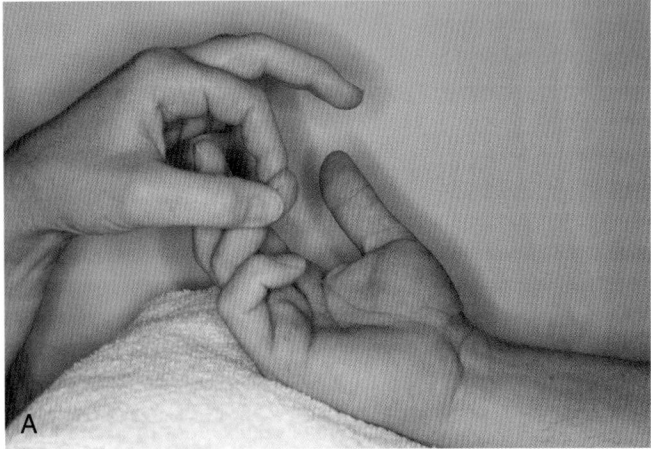

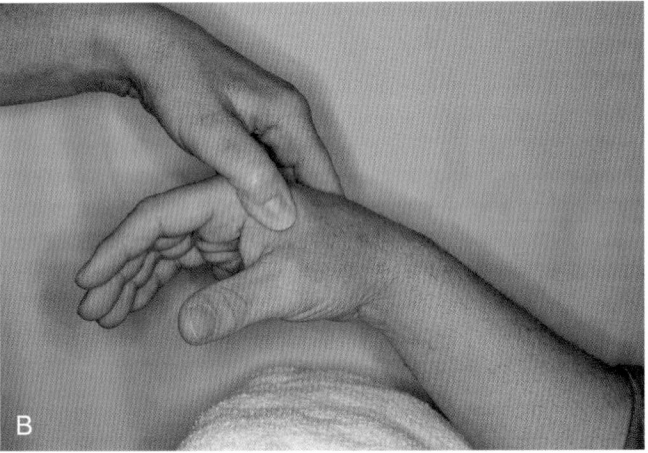

Fig. 23.14 Testing of proprioception of the finger (A) and the wrist (B).

the joint. "In" and "Out" may be used for ulnar/radial deviation, internal/external rotation, and inversion/eversion.

Scoring. While evidence does not indicate a specific amount of trials for this type of sensory testing, anecdotally this scoring method provides a comprehensive picture of the client's current functional sensibility related to proprioception.

- *Intact proprioception:* Correct response to both up and down movements on 3/3 trials
- *Diminished proprioception:* Correct response to up or down movements on 1/3 to 2/3 trials
- *Absent proprioception:* Inability to perceive movement of the body part, scoring correctly on 0/3 trials

The term kinesthesia is sometimes used interchangeably with the term *proprioception* but also can be defined as awareness of joint movement. Some therapists make a distinction between these two terms and test for kinesthesia by moving the unaffected limb into a certain posture and having the client copy the movement with the affected side while the eyes are closed.

Dexterity

Dexterity is the skill and ease in using the hands. Although dexterity is considered a motor function and therefore addressed in other chapter(s) in this textbook (see Chapters 20 and 40 as well as chapters covering individual diagnoses that affect dexterity),

fine motor dexterity is directly affected by sensory disturbances, especially in the median and ulnar nerves with innervation to the finger pads of the hands.[2] The fingertips rely on tactile input, with afferent fibers triggering sensory signals to distinguish the object's properties in order to manipulate the object with the appropriate fine motor dexterity.

The Dellon-Modified Moberg Pickup Test (DMMPUT) is a good test for dexterity for clients with injuries involving the median and/or ulnar nerves. This test requires the client to have the ability to participate motorically, so motor loss or weakness should be factored into the choice of this assessment. This test is based on the Moberg Pickup Test, which is a timed motor test of dexterity that does not require identification of objects.[2,3]

Dellon-Modified Moberg Pickup Test (DMMPUT).

Purpose. Pure sensory tests, such as the ones already addressed in this chapter, including those that measure for pain, temperature, and touch sensation, do not provide a picture of true hand function because hand function relies also on motor innervation and muscle activation. The Moberg Pickup Test was developed to fill the void in testing to quantify hand dexterity.[29] Advantages of the Moberg Pickup Test and Dellon-Modified Moberg Pickup Test include the use of relatively simple equipment and the ability to test both the dominant and nondominant hand independently.[2,3] In test 2, as described in the following text, clients repeat the test with vision occluded, thereby assessing sensory acuity at the fingertips in addition to dexterity.

Procedure.
- Begin with a group of 12 standardized items: Wing nut, large nut, hex nut, small square nut, screw, key, nickel, dime, washer, safety pin, paper clip, and nail.
- If the ulnar nerve is not involved, tape the ulnar two fingers to the client's palm if possible.
- Test 1
  - Place the 12 listed objects randomly on a table in front of the client, with the objects placed on the same side of the table as the hand being tested. Put the box for placement of the objects on the opposite side.
  - The client places the items one at a time into a box as quickly as possible (Fig. 23.15).
  - Repeat with client's other hand.
- Test 2 (initiate test 2 only if the client's motor deficits do not appear to be too severe during test 1)
  - With the client's vision occluded, the examiner places the items into the client's radial three digits one at a time
  - The examiner records the time that it takes to identify each item, with a maximum of 30 seconds for each item. The examiner also records any errors in recognition of items.
  - Each item is placed in the client's hand two times.

Response.
- *Test 1:* The client places the items in a box as quickly as possible with the radial three digits.
- *Test 2:* The client manipulates the objects with the radial three digits one at a time and attempts to identify them as quickly as possible. The client has 30 seconds to respond verbally with the name of the object.

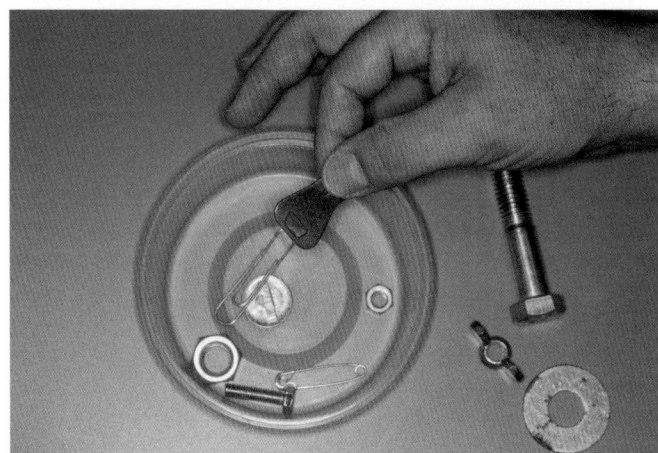
Fig. 23.15 The Dellon modification of the Moberg Pickup Test.

TABLE 23.2 Normative Data for Mean (SD) Moberg Pickup Test

	Male Subjects	Female Subjects
Group 1: Eyes open, dominant hand	11.5 (1.3)	10.6 (1.4)
Group 2: Eyes open, nondominant hand	11.9 (1.4)	11.3 (1.7)
Group 3: Eyes closed, dominant hand	22.1 (3.2)	20.3 (3.0)
Group 4: Eyes closed, nondominant hand	22.9 (3.4)	21.4 (3.6)

From Ng CL, Ho DD, Chow SP: The Moberg pickup test: results of testing with a standard protocol, *J Hand Ther* 12(4):309–312, 1999.

Scoring.
- *Test 1:* The time it takes to place all the items in the box. Normative data are found in Table 23.2.
- *Test 2:* The time it takes to identify all the items as well as the number of errors in recognition. Although normative data do not exist for the identification of objects, these scores can be used as a comparison for improvement on subsequent testing of the DMMPUT.

Stereognosis

Stereognosis is the use of both proprioceptive information and touch information to identify an item with the vision occluded. Without stereognosis, it is impossible to pick out a specific object such as a coin or a key from one's pocket, use a zipper that fastens behind you, or pick up a plate from a sink of sudsy water.
Test for stereognosis.
Purpose. Stereognosis is needed when identifying objects by touching or manipulating them with the fingertips. Thus, sensory dysfunction at the level of the median and ulnar nerves, which supply the volar aspect of the hand and thereby fingertips, can lead to deficits in stereognosis. Stereognosis testing provides information on functional sensibility and potential compensatory strategies. Use this test for patients with diagnoses such as severe carpal or cubital tunnel syndrome and with spinal cord injury to test their current abilities related to stereognosis.

Procedure.
- The examiner gathers 2 to 12 small objects that are known to the client and places them on the table.
- The client is asked to identify each object.
- The examiner then places the small objects in the hand to be tested one at a time with vision occluded.
- If a client is not able to perform in-hand manipulation, the examiner may provide assistance; this should be noted in the documentation.

Procedure and scoring is based on that described by Mulcahey and colleagues[31] and Tyler.[51]
Response.
- The client may manipulate the object and then is asked to name the object verbally.
- This test is not timed, although responses are expected within 2 to 3 seconds.
- If the client is not able to verbalize the response, pictures of the items may be used and they can point to the picture.
Scoring.
- Scoring is the number of correct responses divided by the number of objects tested.
- A modified scoring scale[31]:
  - 0 = absent
  - 1 = impaired, responses are delayed and/or inaccurate
  - 2 = intact, responses are correct and within approximately 3 seconds

Localization of Touch

Localization of touch is considered to be a test of functional sensation because there is a high correlation between this test and the test for two-point discrimination.[35] Localization of touch is an important test to perform after nerve repair because it helps determine the client's baseline and projected functional prognosis. This test can be done with a constant (static) touch or a moving touch. Localization of touch is higher order and processed in the cerebral cortex. Because it is considered to be a test of tactile discrimination that requires cortical processing, it is different from touch pressure testing.
Test for localization of touch.
Purpose. Localization of touch requires a higher processing in the cerebral cortex that is not required in solely recognizing touch pressure. This test is important in assessing nerve function after repair because the ability to localize touch pressure is appreciated following the ability to sense static or moving light touch. In the case that a client does not show higher level cortical processing dysfunction and is able to discriminate both localization in addition to static light touch, the examiner may have the client indicate localization as outlined in the procedure below during responses in the static light touch pressure test with the monofilaments.
Procedure.
- Apply the finest monofilament that the client can perceive to the center of a corresponding zone on the hand grid, according to the result of static touch pressure assessment using the mini-kit or full kit of monofilaments.
- Once the client feels a touch, have him or her open his or her eyes and use the index finger to point to the exact area where the stimulus was felt (see Fig. 23.6).

- Place a dot on the hand grid for a correct response.
- Place an arrow from the site of the actual stimulation to the identified site if the stimulus is identified incorrectly.
  Response.
- The client attempts to identify the exact location of a stimulus.
  Scoring.
- Correct identification of the area within 1 cm of actual placement indicates intact touch localization.

DESENSITIZATION

The existence or persistence of hypersensitivity will often limit use of the affected body part and may prevent sensory reeducation from proceeding, so it is important to address this problem early, if possible, as in the case of Mario, who will need to adjust to his amputated fingertips before regaining full functional hand use. Desensitization for hypersensitivity is a form of treatment that aims to elicit habituation and thereby reduce the client's hypersensitivity and improve function. Habituation is a decrease in a response after repeated benign stimuli. There is a reduction in the excitatory neurotransmitters released, and if the stimulation continues over a prolonged period, a permanent alteration will occur, consisting of a reduction in the number of synaptic connections.[9]

Desensitization uses graded stimulation with procedures and modalities that can be slightly aversive but tolerable[34] or applied around the area of pain but not directly over the pain and not aversive.[44] In an article on using a desensitization technique with CRPS, Packham suggests a technique called distant vibrotactile counter stimulation (DVCS), whereby no pain-evoking stimulus is applied but rather a comfortable light touch is used with a rabbit fur or plush microfleece and applied in a stroking motion for less than 1 minute, eight times per day. It is applied to an area with normal sensation that is anatomically related to the sensitized cutaneous branch hypothesized to underlie the painful area. The stimuli are upgraded to be slightly more noxious as the client's tolerance increases.[33] Lois Barber, an occupational therapist and pioneer in hand splinting and hand therapy, developed a desensitization approach that exposes the hypersensitive area to textures such as sandpaper, contact particles (e.g., rice), and vibration.[5] Treatment is performed for 10-minute intervals, three or four times a day. Clients can incorporate desensitization into their daily routine. For example, they may find that rubbing the hand on their textured shirt or denim pants is desensitizing and can be performed easily throughout the day.

SENSORY REEDUCATION

Stimulation and use of a body part affects the cortical map.[28] The passage of time, use of the involved hand, and training all help promote improved functional sensibility.[17] Children have greater capacity for neural regeneration and neuroplasticity than older people do. Sensory reeducation has been shown to improve the sensation of fingertip replantations even without repair of the nerves.[32] There are two categories of clients who may benefit from sensory reeducation: those who require

reeducation to compensate for the dangers associated with sensory loss and those who may need to effect change on nervous systems that are either hypersensitive or more dormant. These two groups are candidates for instruction in compensatory strategies for sensory loss and candidates for discriminative sensory reeducation.

Compensatory Strategies for Sensory Loss

People who lack protective sensation are at risk for serious injury because they cannot feel pinprick or hot or cold exposure. Blisters may develop after handling hot or cold objects with people not realizing this until they visually examine the hand or notice the stench of burning flesh. After a CVA a person with left hemiparesis and left neglect may inadvertently move the left hand on top of a stove burner during a cooking task. If the client lacks protective sensation, he or she will be burned without feeling the painful sensory stimulus of the hot stove. A person such as Don is at risk for getting fingers caught in the spokes of his wheelchair because of the lack of protective sensation in his first three digits. The same frequently happens to individuals with C6 quadriplegia. Protective sensation in the thumb, index finger, and long finger may be intact, whereas sensation in the ring and little fingers is absent. For example, a typical burn would occur to the little finger and the ulnar side of the hand while cooking or barbequing using the thumb and intact (sensory wise) thumb and radial fingers to turn food using a spatula, leaving the insensate ulnar fingers dangling above the hot stove or grill.

Callahan and Hunter identified the following instructions for compensatory strategies for sensory loss, which she refers to as protective sensory reeducation[11]:

- Protect from exposure to sharp items or to cold or heat.
- Try to soften the amount of force used when gripping an object.
- Use built-up handles on objects whenever possible to distribute gripping pressure over a greater surface area.
- Do not persist in an activity for prolonged periods. Instead, change the tool used and rotate the work task often.
- Visually examine the skin for edema, redness, warmth, blisters, cuts, or other wounds. This is important because tissue heals more slowly when a nerve injury has occurred.
- If there is tissue injury or damage, be very careful in treating and try to avoid infection.
- Maintain skin suppleness as much as possible by applying moisturizing agents.

Discriminative Sensory Reeducation

Clients are candidates for discriminative sensory training if they have intact protective sensation with recognition of at least 4.31 on the touch pressure monofilament test. A client such as Don, who is not able to localize the stimulus but can feel it is a candidate for discriminative sensory reeducation, as is a client with hypersensitivity, such as Mario. A client with a brain insult or nerve injury resulting in reduced discriminative sensation will be unable to fasten a bra in the back, manipulate a clasp on a necklace, or locate a wallet in a bag or pocket with the vision occluded. Discriminative sensory reeducation

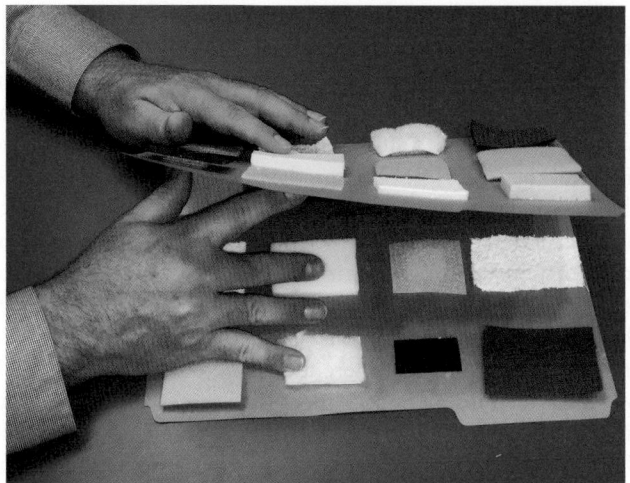

Fig. 23.16 Discriminative sensory reeducation using a sensory folder.

is graded by initially using grossly dissimilar objects, such as a spoon and a penny, and progressing over time to more similar objects, such as a dime and a penny. Another method of discriminative sensory reeducation is through the use of sensory folders which can be made with clinic materials. The same textures taken from items such as splinting materials are attached to both the outside and inside of file folders with the pattern of the textures differing from outside to inside. The client is instructed to place the affected hand inside the folder with eyes closed or vision occluded by external means. The client identifies a texture on the inside of the folder through touch with the affected fingertips and then attempts to localize the same texture on the outside of the folder with his unaffected hand (Fig. 23.16). When planning discriminative sensory reeducation intervention, it works best to identify short-term goals that are achievable and that will enhance function despite the sensory loss. If the client has motor involvement and cannot manually manipulate the stimulus, the stimulus can be moved over the hand instead. Discriminative sensory reeducation involves training in both localization and graded discrimination.

Localization

Localization of moving touch tends to return before localization of constant touch. Retraining is done for both. With the client's eyes closed, the eraser end of a pencil or the therapist's finger is used to touch the client's hand in the midline of one zone of the hand grid. This makes documentation easier and the intervention more accurate and consistent and minimizes afferent activity from adjacent areas of the skin. The stimulus is applied with either a moving or a constant touch. The client is told to open his or her eyes and point to the area that was touched. It has been shown that activity in the visual cortex is enhanced when touch of the hand is added to the visual stimulation, as long as the touch is provided on the same side as the visual stimulation.[52] If the answer was incorrect, the process is repeated. The steps are repeated again with the eyes closed. The full process is then repeated in a new area. As the client improves, the stimulus is changed to a lighter and smaller touch.

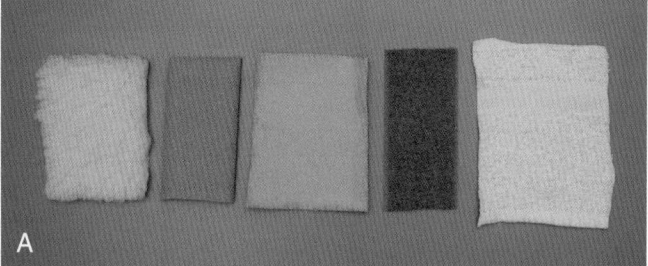

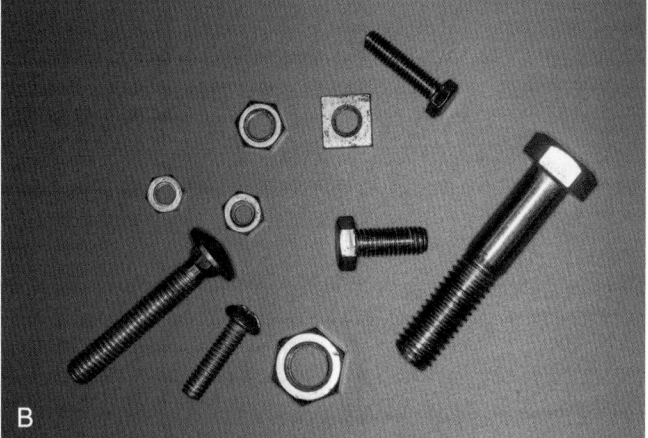

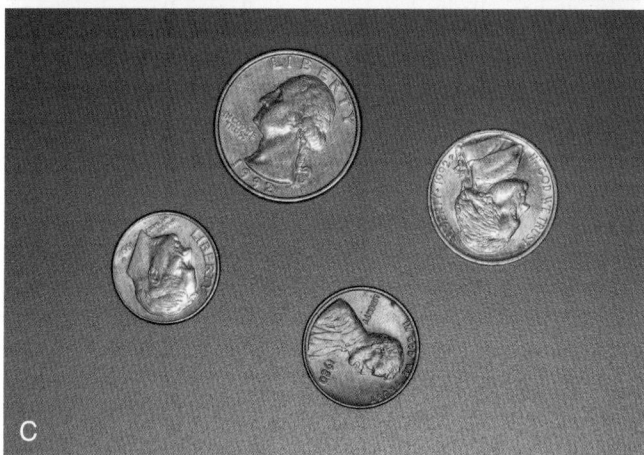

Fig. 23.17 Graded discrimination for sensory reeducation: textures (A), nuts and bolts (B), and coins (C).

Graded Discrimination

Stimulation is graded from that requiring gross discrimination to that requiring fine discrimination. Levels of difficulty in discrimination are represented by sequencing of the following three categories: (1) same or different, (2) how they are the same or different, and (3) identification of the material or object.

The stimulus is applied to the skin in an area corresponding to the hand grid. Either the hand or the stimulus is moved to provide input. As earlier, the eyes are closed, then opened, and then closed for the retraining steps. Various textures can be used, such as different grades of sandpaper or fabric or objects such as nuts and bolts or coins (Fig. 23.17). When using various textures as the stimulus, instruct the client to rub five different textures along the numb or hypersensitive areas for 2 minutes each, watching what he or she is doing for the first minute and then closing the eyes for the second minute.

Another version of discriminative training involves tracing a geometrical shape or a letter or number on the fingertip or small area of the hand. This can be accomplished with a fingertip, the end of an instrument such as a small dowel, or a pencil eraser. The client tries to identify the figure.

Difficulty is increased by adding the requirement of in-hand manipulation for motor stimulation if appropriate and by occluding the vision. Discriminative training may include identifying objects out of a box or embedded within therapeutic putty, retrieving and identifying items out of washable beads, or performing ADLs with the eyes closed. Progress can be determined by improvement in the number of accurate responses, better mapping of areas of localization, increased speed of completing motor tasks, better status of two-point discrimination, and improved level of function involving ADLs overall.

Cortical Reorganization

Occupational therapists can use graded motor imagery to affect cortical reorganization. Graded motor imagery is a treatment regimen that includes interventions such as mirror visual feedback, imagined hand movements, and laterality training.[30] In their studies, Ramachandran and Rogers-Ramachandran[37] speculated that PLP after amputation results from a disruption of the normal interaction between motor intention to move the limb and the absence of appropriate sensory or proprioceptive feedback to complete that motor task. The authors proposed that visual feedback may interrupt the pathologic cycle between the motor intention and sensibility. They developed a process by which a mirror could be used to superimpose an image of the normal limb on the location where the individual "felt" the phantom limb. Clinical observation and functional imaging studies were examined in subsequent research.[18] Based on these studies, Harris hypothesized that disorganized cortical representations may lead to the experience of peripheral pain or sensory disturbances based on a disconnect between motor intention and proprioceptive or visual feedback.[20]

Mirror therapy as an OT intervention technique is based on this research. In mirror therapy the client positions the hands on either side of a mirror so that the affected hand is placed in back of the mirror and the nonaffected hand is placed in front of it; all of the client's attention is focused on the image in the mirror (Fig. 23.18).[41,42] Mirror therapy may be incorporated into treatment of sensory dysfunction by placing the same textures or simple items (e.g., coins, beans, or foam pieces) in front of and behind the mirror. In addition, the client can retrain proprioception by viewing the noninvolved hand in the mirror while simultaneously moving both hands the same (flexion/extension, circumferential movements, touching each finger to the thumb, pronation/supination, radial/ulnar deviation, abduction/adduction of the digits). Studies using mirror therapy show favorable results in PLP after amputation and in patients who have had strokes.[50,55] The client (as in the case of Mario, who experiences PLP in his distal fingers) is then coached by the therapist to use both hands simultaneously to stimulate bilateral sensory receptors with attempts to affect cortical remapping. If pain in the affected hand precludes the client's ability to complete the task, then an imagined hand movement technique should be incorporated: the affected hand would not move beyond the limits of pain, but the unaffected hand would continue with the task and the client's attention would continue to focus on the mirror.

Reinersmann and associates[38] studied limb laterality recognition tasks for their effect on the lateralization of the somatosensory system of the cerebral cortex. The authors based their study of this use of the intervention on the assumption that cortical body representation becomes disrupted in disease states such as CRPS and PLP, resulting in a change in the client's body schema. They showed that there were delayed reaction times and higher error rates compared to healthy subjects, when the client was presented with pictures of right and left hands and asked to identify the laterality of the limb (Fig. 23.19).[38] After a 4-day training course, both the healthy subjects and the clients with CRPS and PLP improved in their reaction time in the laterality recognition task. From studies such as these, a

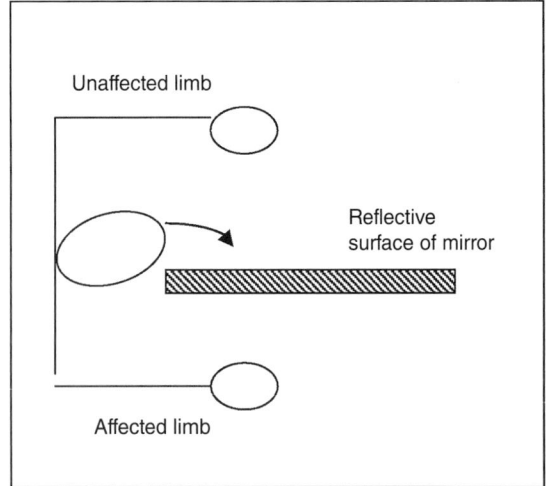
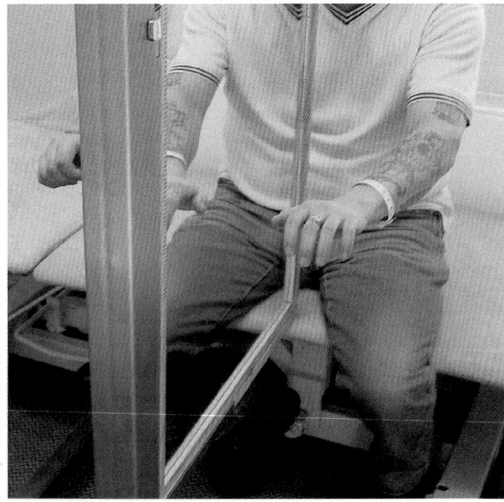

Fig. 23.18 Position of the mirror for upper limb mirror visual feedback therapy. (From McCabe C: Mirror visual feedback therapy: a practical approach, *J Hand Ther* 24:171–178, 2011.)

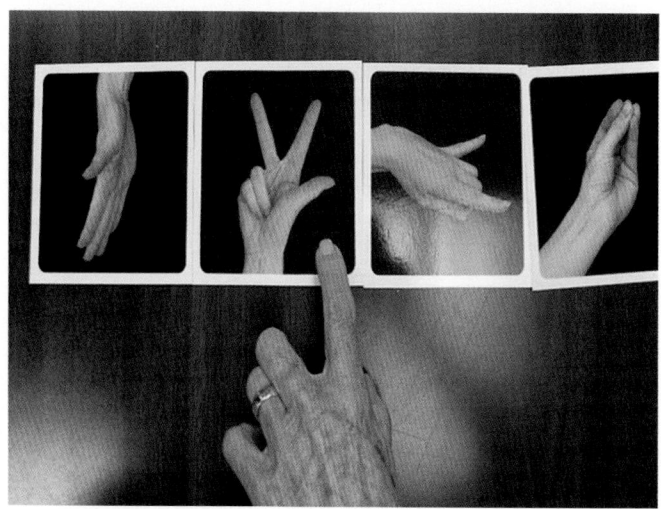

Fig. 23.19 The Recognise Hand Flash Cards (Noigroup Products; https://www.noigroup.com) are examples of laterality training cards. The pictures demonstrate different positions of the right and left hands. (From Priganc VW, Stralka SW: Graded motor imagery, *J Hand Ther* 24:164–169, 2011.)

connection can be drawn between the dysfunction in lateralization in the somatosensory cortex and various disease processes that affect sensation, such as CRPS and PLP. Because improvements in laterality recognition can be visualized through various treatments, as shown in these studies, this may indicate the possibility that laterality recognition training may lead to cortical reorganization.

Graded motor imagery is described as using a staged approach of 2 weeks each of laterality recognition, mental imagery (imagined hand movements), and mirror therapy. However, therapists have used any of the three stages independently.[4,36] The staged approach of graded motor imagery has been shown to be effective for long-standing CRPS.[30]

▌ SUMMARY

Now, using the information provided in this chapter regarding the evaluation of sensation and the determination of appropriate OT intervention for sensory dysfunction, review the application of this knowledge to the two case studies presented.

THREADED CASE STUDY

Don, Part 2

The most appropriate sensory tests for Don would be touch pressure, two-point discrimination, the Ten Test, and the Dellon modification of the Moberg Pickup Test. Assess for touch pressure first because light touch must be intact for two-point discrimination to be tested. The Dellon modification of the Moberg Pickup Test is particularly appropriate for Don because it tests sensory function of the digits that carpal tunnel syndrome is affecting. Those digits, including the thumb, index, long, and radial aspect of the ring finger, are generally used for fine motor coordination in picking up small objects such as medications and pinching the rim of his wheelchair. Don is a good candidate for discriminative sensory reeducation to stimulate neural recovery. To simulate grasping the rims of his wheelchair with a lateral pinch without the need for his vision to assist, Don could practice identifying objects out of a bowl of rice with his eyes opened and then eyes closed. He could also work to find and pinch marbles or small pegs out of therapeutic putty with the use of his vision and with his vision occluded. Tell Don that typical recovery after successful carpal tunnel release includes decreased hypersensitivity as the desensitization program progresses. The common progression of recovery as seen clinically is improved pain, followed by reduced tingling sensation, and then diminished numbness. Sensory disturbances after a carpal tunnel release may take several months to fully recover. The OT

practitioner should assess whether progress has been made and provide intervention if progress is delayed or if there is an unintended negative outcome, such as hypersensitivity. Progress should be assessed on each visit, although threshold testing may not demonstrate significant gains at each testing, especially when the mini-kit is used. In contrast, the Ten Test will provide a quick snapshot of their current subjective sensation and can often appreciate change at each visit.

Don should expect improving ability to feel and manipulate small objects as sensory recovery proceeds proximally to distally, with the fingertips being the last to recover. Deeper pressure will be felt before lighter pressure, and it will be easier to discern a nickel before he can discern a dime with his vision occluded; this will progress as two-point discrimination improves. Given Don's unique situation of using a wheelchair for all functional mobility, he must take special care to avoid weight bearing on his hands whenever possible so as not to further irritate the surgical site at the carpal tunnel. He may benefit from wearing a prefabricated wrist cock-up orthosis, which has a metal insert along the carpal tunnel and through the volar wrist to provide both support and a barrier during obligatory weight bearing for transfers, functional mobility, and recreational activities such as wheelchair tennis.

THREADED CASE STUDY

Mario, Part 2

In applying new knowledge of sensation to Mario's case, we note that several of his occupational leisure roles involve the use of significant tactile sensibility. This includes manipulating tools for woodworking to grade the pressure that he is applying with his grip, or the need to feel the texture of grapes in his fingertips during wine making. Sustaining a grasp on the steering wheel can be painful with the altered PLP in his residual digits, which causes Mario to choose not to drive to the dance hall and thereby eliminates one of his favorite occupations of dancing with his wife. An OT practitioner can incorporate purposeful activity into

Mario's intervention plan to enhance sensory perceptual skills by having Mario bring some of his tools for woodworking or wine making to therapy. The therapist can work with Mario to determine whether there are activity modifications or compensatory strategies that can be implemented to allow him maximal functional independence in these tasks. Types of interventions that may be incorporated to improve the remapping of Mario's brain to connect him with his partially amputated fingers once again include mirror therapy and laterality recognition cards.

REVIEW QUESTIONS

1. Describe how the PNS and the CNS are connected and ways in which sensory testing differs between the two.
2. Explain why the fingertips have enhanced sensation compared with more proximal body parts.
3. Name three signs that represent altered sympathetic nervous system status.
4. Explain how desensitization works.
5. What are the three categories of sensory reeducation and how do they differ?

For additional practice questions for this chapter, please visit eBooks.Health.Elsevier.com.

REFERENCES

1. American Occupational Therapy Association: Occupational therapy practice framework: domain and process, fourth edition, *Am J Occup Ther* 74(Supplement_2):1–87, 2020. https://doi.org/10.5014/ajot.2020.74S2001.
2. Amirjani N, Ashworth NL, Gordon T, Edwards DC, Chan KM: Normative values and the effects of age, gender, and handedness on the Moberg Pick-Up Test, *Muscle Nerve* 35(6):788–792, 2007. https://doi.org/10.1002/mus.20750.
3. Amirjani N, Ashworth NL, Olson JL, Morhart M, Chan KM: Discriminative validity and test-retest reliability of the Dellon-modified Moberg pick-up test in carpal tunnel syndrome patients, *J Peripheral Nerv Syst* 16(1):51–58, 2011. https://doi.org/10.1111/j.1529-8027.2011.00312.x.
4. Bakshi P, Chang W-P, Fisher TF, Andreae B: Client buy-in: an essential consideration for graded motor imagery in hand therapy, *J Hand Ther* 34(3): 348–350, 2021. https://doi.org/10.1016/j.jht.2020.03.014.
5. Barber L, Hunter JM, SL Mackin EJ, editors: *Rehabilitation of the Hand* ed 3, 1990, Mosby, pp 721–730.
6. Bell Krotoski JA: Flexor tendon and peripheral nerve repair, *Hand Surg* 7(1):83–100, 2002. https://doi.org/10.1142/s021881040200087x.
7. Borich MR, Brodie SM, Gray WA, Ionta S, Boyd LA: Understanding the role of the primary somatosensory cortex: opportunities for rehabilitation, *Neuropsychologia* 79(Pt B):246–255, 2015. https://doi.org/10.1016/j.neuropsychologia.2015.07.007.
8. Brown T, Sherrington C: On the instability of a cortical point, *Proc R Soc Lond* 85:250–277, 1912.
9. Burleigh-Jacobs A, Stehno-Bittel L, Lundy-Ekman L, editors: *Neuroscience: Fundamentals for Rehabilitation* ed 2, 2002, Saunders, pp 67–80.
10. Calford MB: Mechanisms for acute changes in sensory maps, *Adv Exp Med Biol* 508:451–460, 2002. https://doi.org/10.1007/978-1-4615-0713-0_51.
11. Callahan A, Hunter J: Sensibility testing: clinical methods. In *Rehabilitation of the hand*, 1984, Mosby, pp 407–431.
12. Dellon AL, Kallman CH: Evaluation of functional sensation in the hand, *J Hand Surg* 8(6):865–870, 1983.
13. Dellon ES, Mourey R, Dellon AL: Human pressure perception values for constant and moving one- and two-point discrimination, *Plast Reconstr Surg* 90(1):112–117, 1992. https://doi.org/10.1097/00006534-199207000-00017.
14. Desrosiers J, Hébert R, Bravo G, Dutil E: Hand sensibility of healthy older people, *J Am Geriatr Soc* 44(8):974–978, 1996. https://doi.org/10.1111/j.1532-5415.1996.tb01871.x.
15. Dros J, Wewerinke A, Bindels PJ, van Weert HC: Accuracy of monofilament testing to diagnose peripheral neuropathy: A systematic review, *Ann Fam Med* 7(6):555–558, 2009. https://doi.org/10.1370/afm.1016.
16. Engel JM, Jensen MP, Schwartz L: Coping with chronic pain associated with cerebral palsy, *Occup Ther Int* 13(4):224–233, 2006. https://doi.org/10.1002/oti.219.
17. Fess E, Mackin E, editors: *Rehabilitation of the Hand and Upper Extremity* ed 5, 2002, Mosby, pp 635–639.
18. Fink GR, Marshall JC, Halligan PW, et al: The neural consequences of conflict between intention and the senses, *Brain* 122(3):497–512, 1999. https://doi.org/10.1093/brain/122.3.497.
19. Harding-Forrester S, Feldman DE: Somatosensory maps. In: Vallar G.Coslett HB, editors: *Handbook of clinical neurology*, Vol 151, 2018, The Parietal Lobe. Elsevier, pp 73–102. https://doi.org/10.1016/B978-0-444-63622-5.00004-8.
20. Harris AJ: Cortical origin of pathological pain, *Lancet* 354(9188):1464–1466, 1999. https://doi.org/10.1016/S0140-6736(99)05003-5.
21. Johansson RS, Vallbo AB: Tactile sensibility in the human hand: relative and absolute densities of four types of mechanoreceptive units in glabrous skin, *J Physiol* 286:283–300, 1979.
22. Kirshblum S, Biering-Sørensen F, Betz R, et al: International standards for neurological classification of spinal cord injury: cases with classification challenges, *Top Spinal Cord Inj Rehabil* 20(2):81–89, 2014. https://doi.org/10.1310/sci2002-81.
23. Louis DS, Greene TL, Jacobson KE, Rasmussen C, Kolowich P, Goldstein SA: Evaluation of normal values for stationary and moving two-point discrimination in the hand, *J Hand Surg* 9(4):552–555, 1984. https://doi.org/10.1016/s0363-5023(84)80109-4.
24. Malaviya GN: Sensory perception in leprosy-neurophysiological correlates, *Int J Lepr Other Mycobact Dis* 71(2):119–124, 2003. https://doi.org/10.1489/1544-581x(2003)71<119:spilc>2.0.co;2.
25. Mancini F, Bauleo A, Cole J, et al: Whole-body mapping of spatial acuity for pain and touch, *Ann Neurol* 75(6):917–924, 2014. https://doi.org/10.1002/ana.24179.
26. Mancini F, Sambo CF, Ramirez JD, Bennett DLH, Haggard P, Iannetti GD: A fovea for pain at the fingertips, *Curr Biol* 23(6):496–500, 2013. https://doi.org/10.1016/j.cub.2013.02.008.
27. McCabe C: Mirror visual feedback therapy. a practical approach, *J Hand Ther* 24(2):170–179, 2011. https://doi.org/10.1016/j.jht.2010.08.003. quiz 179.
28. Merzenich MM, Jenkins WM: Reorganization of cortical representations of the hand following alterations of skin inputs induced by nerve injury, skin island transfers, and experience,

J Hand Ther 6(2):89–104, 1993. https://doi.org/10.1016/s0894-1130(12)80290-0.

29. Moberg E: Objective methods for determining the functional value of sensibility in the hand, *J Bone Jt Surg Br* 40-B(3):454–476, 1958.

30. Moseley LG: Graded motor imagery is effective for long-standing complex regional pain syndrome: a randomised controlled trial, *Pain* 108(1):192–198, 2004. https://doi.org/10.1016/j.pain.2004.01.006.

31. Mulcahey MJ, Kozin S, Merenda L, et al: Evaluation of the box and blocks test, stereognosis and item banks of activity and upper extremity function in youths with brachial plexus birth palsy, *J Pediatric Orthop* 32:S114–S1222, 2012. https://doi.org/10.1097/BPO.0b013e3182595423.

32. Novak CB: Evaluation of hand sensibility: a review, *J Hand Ther* 14(4):266–272, 2001. https://doi.org/10.1016/S0894-1130(01)80004-1.

33. Packham T, Holly J: Mechanism-specific rehabilitation management of complex regional pain syndrome: proposed recommendations from evidence synthesis, *J Hand Ther* 31(2):238–249, 2018.

34. Packham TL, Spicher CJ, MacDermid JC, Michlovitz S, Buckley DN: Somatosensory rehabilitation for allodynia in complex regional pain syndrome of the upper limb: a retrospective cohort study, *J Hand Ther* 31(1):10–19, 2018. https://doi.org/10.1016/j.jht.2017.02.007.

35. Periyasamy R, Manivannan M, Narayanamurthy VB: Correlation between two-point discrimination with other measures of sensory loss in diabetes mellitus patients, *Int J Diabetes Dev Ctries* 28(3):71–78, 2008.

36. Priganc VW, Stralka SW: Graded motor imagery, *J Hand Ther* 24(2):164–168, 2011. https://doi.org/10.1016/j.jht.2010.11.002.

37. Ramachandran VS, Rogers-Ramachandran D: Synaesthesia in phantom limbs induced with mirrors, *Proc Biol Sci* 263(1369):377–386, 1996. https://doi.org/10.1098/rspb.1996.0058.

38. Reinersmann A, Haarmeyer GS, Blankenburg M, et al: Left is where the L is right. Significantly delayed reaction time in limb laterality recognition in both CRPS and phantom limb pain patients, *Neurosci Lett* 486(3):240–245, 2010. https://doi.org/10.1016/j.neulet.2010.09.062.

39. Ribeiro F, Oliveira J: Factors influencing proprioception: what do they reveal? *Biomech Appl*, 2011. https://doi.org/10.5772/20335. Published online September 9.

40. Rosen K, Patel M, Lawrence C, Mooney B: Delivering telerehabilitation to COVID-19 inpatients: a retrospective chart review suggests it is a viable option. *HSS J* 16(Suppl 1):64–70. https://doi.org/10.1007/s11420-020-09774-4.

41. Rostami HR, Arefi A, Tabatabaei S: Effect of mirror therapy on hand function in patients with hand orthopaedic injuries: a randomized controlled trial, *Disabil Rehabil* 35(19):1647–1651, 2013. https://doi.org/10.3109/09638288.2012.751132.

42. Rothgangel A, Braun S, Winkens B, Beurskens A, Smeets R: Traditional and augmented reality mirror therapy for patients

with chronic phantom limb pain (PACT study): results of a three-group, multicentre single-blind randomized controlled trial, *Clin Rehabil* 32(12):1591–1608, 2018. https://doi.org/10.1177/0269215518785948.

43. Sharma N, Classen J, Cohen LG: Neural plasticity and its contribution to functional recovery. In *Handbook of Clinical Neurology*, Vol 110, 2013, Elsevier, pp 3–12. https://doi.org/10.1016/B978-0-444-52901-5.00001-0.

44. Skirvin T, Callahan A, Mackin E, editors: *Rehabilitation of the hand and upper extremity* ed 5, 2002, Mosby, pp 499–629.

45. Slater RA, Koren S, Ramot Y, Buchs A, Rapoport MJ: Interpreting the results of the Semmes-Weinstein monofilament test: accounting for false-positive answers in the international consensus on the diabetic foot protocol by a new model, *Diabetes Metab Res Rev* 30(1):77–80, 2014. https://doi.org/10.1002/dmrr.2465.

46. Strauch B, Lang A: The Ten Test revisited, *Plast Reconstr Surg* 112(2):593–594, 2003. https://doi.org/10.1097/01.PRS.0000070680.25190.E6.

47. Strauch B, Lang A, Ferder M, Keyes-Ford M, Freeman K, Newstein D: The Ten Test, *Plast Reconstr Surg* 99(4):1074–1078, 1997. https://doi.org/10.1097/00006534-199704000-00023.

48. Sun HH, Oswald TM, Sachanandani NS, Borschel GH: The "Ten Test": application and limitations in assessing sensory function in the paediatric hand, *J Plast Reconstr Aesthet Surg* 63(11):1849–1852, 2010. https://doi.org/10.1016/j.bjps.2009.11.052.

49. ten Donkelaar HJ, Broman J, van Domburg P: The somatosensory system. In ten Donkelaar HJ, editor: *Clinical neuroanatomy: brain circuitry and its disorders*, 2020, Springer International Publishing, pp 171–255. https://doi.org/10.1007/978-3-030-41878-6_4.

50. Thieme H, Morkisch N, Mehrholz J, et al: Mirror therapy for improving motor function after stroke, *Cochrane Database Syst Rev* 7:CD008449, 2018. https://doi.org/10.1002/14651858.CD008449.pub3.

51. Tyler NB: A stereognostic test for screening tactile sensation, *Am J Occup Ther* 26(5):256–260, 1972.

52. Wilson F: *The hand: how its use shapes the brain, language, and human culture*, 1998, Pantheon Books.

53. Wu H, Yan H, Yang Y, et al: Occupational neuroplasticity in the human brain: a critical review and meta-analysis of neuroimaging studies, *Front Hum Neurosci* 14:215, 2020. https://doi.org/10.3389/fnhum.2020.00215.

54. Wu JZ, Sinsel EW, Zhao KD, An K-N, Buczek FL: Analysis of the Constraint Joint Loading in the Thumb During Pipetting, *J Biomech Eng* 137(8):084501–084507, 2015. https://doi.org/10.1115/1.4030311.

55. Zeng W, Guo Y, Wu G, Liu X, Fang Q: Mirror therapy for motor function of the upper extremity in patients with stroke: A meta-analysis, *J Rehabil Med* 50(1):8–15, 2018. https://doi.org/10.2340/16501977-2287.

56. Zilles K: Neuronal plasticity as an adaptive property of the central nervous system, *Ann Anat* 174(5):383–391, 1992. https://doi.org/10.1016/s0940-9602(11)80255-4.

24

Evaluation and Treatment of Visual Deficits After Brain Injury

Mary Warren

LEARNING OBJECTIVES

After studying this chapter, the student or practitioner will be able to do the following:

1. Describe the role of vision in enabling the person to complete daily occupations.
2. Describe the components of the visual perceptual hierarchy as a framework for evaluation and intervention for vision impairment.
3. Describe the changes that may occur in visual acuity, visual field, oculomotor control, and visual attention after adult acquired brain injury.
4. Select appropriate assessments to screen visual acuity, visual field, oculomotor control, and visual attention in adults with acquired brain injury.
5. Describe how to use assessment results to establish an intervention plan.
6. Select appropriate interventions to enable adults with acquired brain injury to use their vision more efficiently and effectively to complete daily occupations.
7. Describe the occupational therapy role on the rehabilitation team when addressing visual impairment in the adult with acquired brain injury.

CHAPTER OUTLINE

KEY TERMS

Contrast sensitivity function
Convergence insufficiency
Diplopia
Hemianopia
Paralytic strabismus
Phoria
Tropia
Uncorrected refractive error
Visual acuity
Visual fields
Visual perceptual hierarchy
Visual scanning training
Visual spatial neglect
Yoked Prism Adaptation

Penny, Part 1

Penny Periwinkle, age 70 (identifies as female and prefers the use of the pronouns she/her/hers), sustained a right cerebrovascular accident (CVA) from a posterior cerebral artery occlusion. Penny also has a 5-year history of adult-onset type 2 diabetes. The stroke caused a left homonymous hemianopia, and possible hemiinattention. After diagnosing the hemianopia, Penny's ophthalmologist diagnosed the hemianopia and referred her to University Low Vision Rehabilitation Clinic because she stated that she was unable to read because of her vision loss. Penny is also a well-known local artist, famous for her detailed ink drawings of local architecture, and reported that she was no longer able to engage in this occupation. Penny has been married for 45 years. She has one son who lives several states away and no other family in the area. Her husband, Pot, sustained a severe stroke 5 years ago. Pot has right hemiplegia and global aphasia and requires assistance for all daily activities. Because of Pot's disability, Penny is responsible for all home management—cooking, cleaning, paying bills, shopping, and so on. As Pot's primary caregiver, Penny completes his self-care and medication management. Penny describes herself as fiercely independent and has refused to get outside help to care for Pot. She faces significant challenges continuing in her roles as homeowner, caregiver, and artist.

Critical Thinking Questions

1. How does Penny's left hemianopia limit her ability to complete her daily occupations?
2. Does Penny have hemiinattention in addition to a left hemianopia?
3. What intervention approaches will be the most effective to enable Penny to compensate for her vision impairment and participate in her daily occupations and roles?

ROLE OF VISION IN DAILY OCCUPATIONS

Vision is the primary way that the brain engages and learns from the world.[108] We use vision to identify resources that may help us complete our daily occupations and respond to threats from events occurring around us. We rely on vision because it offers certain attributes that enable us to rapidly assess and make decisions about our environment. Vision's attributes include:

- *Vision is our most far-reaching sensory system and takes us further into the environment than any of our other senses.* We can see *lightning* before we hear thunder; see a car careening toward us before we hear the squeal of the tires or smell the exhaust. By warning us of changes in our environment, vision enables us to *anticipate* developing situations, formulate a plan to handle them, and achieve a successful outcome. Thus, when an object is unexpectedly flung in our direction, we duck, or when we see the banana peel on the floor, we walk around it.
- *Vision rapidly conveys large amounts of detailed information.* Vision is a truly integrative sense in that it provides us with all of the information we need to identify the objects within our environment and size up situations. We can instantly recognize objects using vision but require more time to identify them by touch or by hearing a verbal description. Because we can rapidly get a complete picture using our visual system, we prefer to use vision when we quickly need to size up a situation and respond. This explains why we prefer to view images about the unfolding of significant events or prefer to watch sporting events instead of listening to the description of the competition.

- *Vision provides the processing speed that we need to adapt to dynamic environments.* We operate in two types of environments: static and dynamic. In static environments, we are the only object moving, which removes the temporal (e.g., timing) requirement for an activity. We can decide when to start and stop movement and how long to take to complete an activity. In contrast, dynamic environments contain objects moving independently of us. To successfully adapt to this environment, we must simultaneously monitor our own movement and that of the other moving objects. Only vision provides the processing speed that enables us to either interact with moving objects or avoid them.

These attributes are the reason we use vision as our primary interface with the world to guide how we respond to our surroundings. We rely on vision to "size up" situations. We say to ourselves, "He looks harmless," or "That looks delicious." We pepper our conversation with phrases that reflect the importance of vision in decision-making, such as, "I'll believe it when I see it," "I'll keep an eye out for it," or "I can see what you mean." We rely on vision for our social interactions, using it to detect and respond to the subtle gestures and facial expressions of our companions, and to understand the emotional nuance in conversations. Vision also plays an important role in our ability to safely navigate environments by warning us of upcoming obstacles like a curb or broken pavement. Our motor actions are also driven by what we see; for example, you are able to stick to your diet until you see the plate of donuts sitting on the table and find yourself reaching for one. The takeaway message is that "vision rules!" It is the primary way that we acquire information; it dominates our daily occupations, including recreational activities—consider life without Facebook and YouTube, watching or playing sports, completing crafts. Vision also enables us to participate in dynamic unpredictable activities such as driving. Research has shown that even mild vision impairment from brain injury can significantly disrupt a person's life, and significant visual impairment can be devastating.[32,59,81]

SHORT OVERVIEW OF VISUAL PROCESSING WITHIN THE BRAIN

For vision to be used for occupation, the raw material of vision (e.g., the pattern of light that falls on the retina) must be transformed into images that can be compared with visual memories and used to make decisions and respond to unfolding events. The visual processing journey encompasses many areas of the brain. Along the way visual input is sorted out, refined, and combined with other sensory input to provide a product that can be used to perceive and adapt to our surroundings and circumstances.[a] The process begins with the anterior structures of the eye—cornea, pupil, lens—that focus light rays onto the photoreceptor cells of the retina. The photoreceptor cells record the patterns of light and convey this visual input over the optic nerve and the optic tract to the lateral geniculate nucleus (LGN) in the thalamus[15,67,109] (Fig. 24.1). Each optic nerve carries visual

---

[a] References 4, 15, 67, 68, 71, 109.

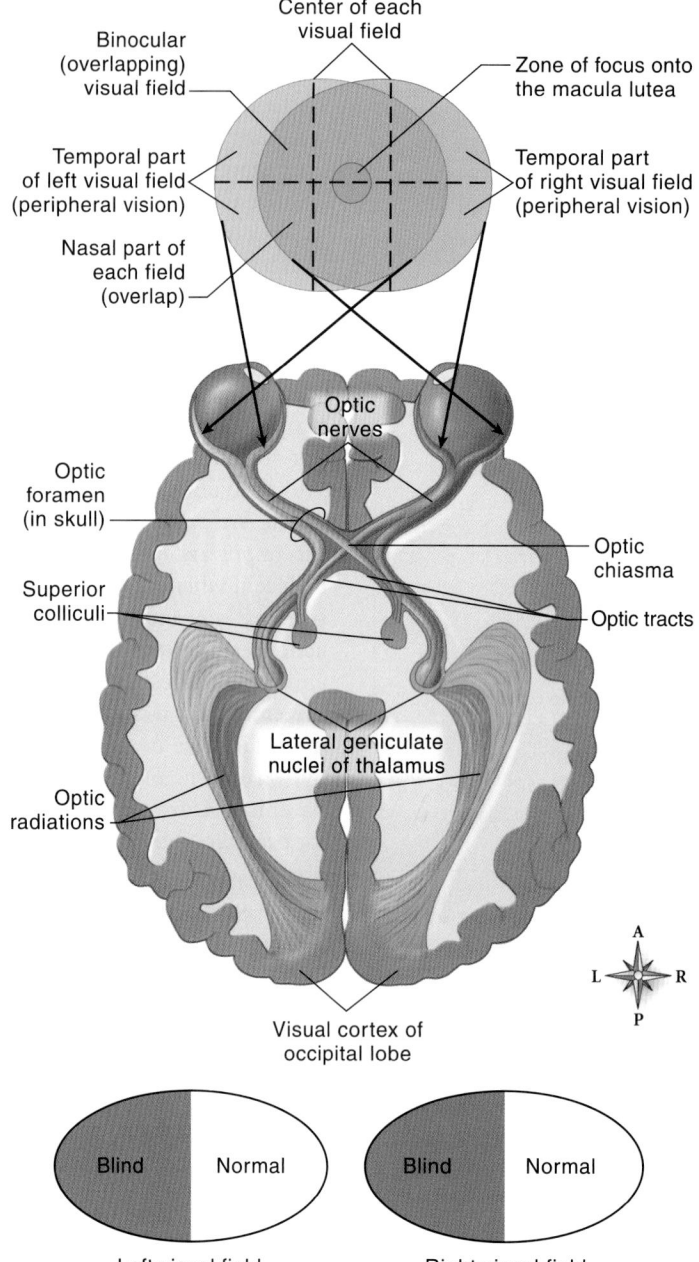

Fig. 24.1 The primary visual pathway conveying visual field information from the retina to the cortex. The *green-shaded* areas show the pathway conveying visual field information captured in the retina from the *left half* of the person's visual space to the occipital lobe in the right hemisphere. The *blue-shaded* areas show the pathway conveying visual field information from the *right half* of the person's visual space to the occipital lobe in the *left hemisphere*. Note that the nasal fibers of the optic nerves *cross over* at the optic chiasm to join the temporal fibers from the optic nerves to create the optic tract (comprising *green* and *blue* tracts). The optic tracts now carry a representation of the left side or right side of the visual field in both eyes that continues first to the lateral geniculate nucleus (LGN) in the thalamus and then onto the occipital cortex via geniculocalcarine tracts to the occipital lobes in the right or left hemisphere. Damage to the optic tract or geniculocalcarine tracts will create a right or left hemianopia depicted by *blue-shaded* area of the ovals at the bottom of the illustration. The top of the diagram shows how the visual fields of each eye overlap to provide a binocular visual field in the center of a person's vision. The far ends of the field retain their individual color to show how the far peripheral field can be seen by only one eye because the nose occludes the other eye's view. (From Patton K et al: *Anatomy & physiology*, ed 11, St Louis, 2022, Elsevier.)

input from just one eye until it reaches the optic chiasm. At this juncture, the nasal fibers of each optic nerve cross over and merge with the temporal fibers of the optic nerve in the opposite hemisphere. These newly merged fibers become the *optic tract* and, more importantly, now carry visual input from the *two eyes* as they continue on toward the LGN. The optic tracts deliver visual input from the same hemifield in each eye to the LGN. Thus, the right LGN receives images from the left half of the visual field in both eyes and the left LGN receives images from the right half of the visual field in both eyes.[67] After processing in the LGN, visual input representing half of the visual field in each eye travels over the large geniculocalcarine tracts (GCT: the optic radiations) in each hemisphere to the primary visual area of the occipital lobe (e.g., visual cortex).[67] Visual input from the left half of the visual field is conveyed over the GCT in the right hemisphere to the right occipital lobe, and input from the right half of the visual field is conveyed over the GCT in the left hemisphere to the left occipital lobe. *Penny's stroke occurred from an occlusion in the posterior cerebral artery feeding the right hemisphere of the brain. The stroke damaged the GCTs in the right hemisphere, causing Penny to develop a left homonymous hemianopia.*

The GCT terminate in the calcarine fissure of the occipital lobe. The calcarine fissure serves as the doorway to the cortical processing of visual input. The visual input that enters the cortex via the calcarine fissure is used to build and maintain a library of images in the posterior cortical areas of the brain. The prefrontal areas of the cortex will use this library to make decisions, direct actions, and achieve goals.[4,56] As visual input enters into the primary visual cortex, this area of the occipital lobes sorts through the incoming visual information, fine-tunes it, and then disperses the refined visual input to the posterior areas of temporal and parietal lobes.[4,53,56,132] The visual input sent to the posterior temporal lobe is combined with language and auditory input to identify and classify objects.[4,53,56] The purpose of this processing is to help answer the "what" question, as in "what am I looking at?" The visual input sent to the posterior areas of the parietal lobe is integrated with input from all of the other senses to create internal sensory maps that orient the body to space and time.[56,64,71,72,83] These sensory maps help answer the "where" question by tuning the brain into the location of features and objects that are important to completion of a goal.[56,64,71,74] The sensory maps are body-centered and dynamic, changing as the body moves through space.

The prefrontal cortex functions as the CEO of the brain using the library created by the posterior cortical areas to make decisions and formulate plans.[4,56,70] The frontal eye fields, located in the prefrontal cortex, direct voluntary visual search of the environment based on an expectation (memory) of where key visual information will be found.[4,70,98] For example, if you were looking for a light switch in a room, your frontal eye fields would direct your visual search toward the walls, because that is the most likely location of a light switch—you would not waste time searching the floor or the ceiling. Directing visual search based on the expected location of a key visual provides the visual processing speed needed to successfully engage in dynamic activities such as driving or walking down a busy street. The prefrontal

cortex also directs working visual (spatial) memory.[70,163,201] Working memory is the ability to hold more than one piece of information "on deck" in memory and ready for immediate recall to assist in completing a task.[70] *Working visual memory* is the specific ability to hold in mind a picture of an object and its location while completing a task.[70] An example of working visual memory would be holding in mind a picture of a specific brand of canned tomatoes along with its location in the aisle while shopping for the ingredients to make chili. It is "working" memory in the sense that once you accomplish the task, you discard the memory of the tomatoes and replace it with the next item on your list. We use working memory to sequence and stay on task while completing activities.

The brainstem and cerebellum also process visual information and contribute to the ability to use vision for daily activities.[98,169] The brainstem contains several important centers involved in visual processing. Brainstem centers direct the light (pupillary) reflex, the blink response, and the accommodation reflex.[98] The superior colliculi—located in the midbrain of the brainstem—monitor moving visual stimuli in the peripheral visual fields.[98] When motion is detected, the superior colliculi automatically initiate eye movement toward the location to identify the source of the movement. In performing this function, the superior colliculi serve as an early warning system to prevent us being caught off guard by intruders. The brainstem works with the cortex and cerebellum to control other visual functions, most notably executing eye movements and focusing.[98,169] The motor nuclei of cranial nerves (CNs) III, IV, and VI, which control the extraocular muscles and move the eyes, are located in the brainstem. The cortex uses eye movements to shift attention to objects in the environment and focus on critical details needed to complete a task.[98] The cerebellum adds synergy to eye movements to ensure that the eye lands precisely on the target so it can be clearly seen.[98] Finally, the brainstem houses the vestibular nerve nuclei and pathways that integrate vestibular input with eye movements to provide gaze stability during head and body movement.[98]

It is important to remember that the many brain areas that contribute to visual processing must work together to make sense of what is seen and use visual information to adapt.[b] Millions of long and short neural fibers (e.g., white matter pathways) tie the various cortical and subcortical structures together to form a complex network to produce effective and efficient visual processing.[4,51,67] Similar to a car, in which the fuel-injection system is as critical to performance as the starter, visual processing will not be completed efficiently unless all of its components are working together. Brain injury disrupts communication within the network and creates gaps in visual processing. The specific type of visual deficit that occurs after brain injury depends on the area(s) of the brain that were injured and whether the injury caused structural or pathway damage within the brain.[182] Moderate to severe brain injuries often cause structural damage to brain areas that recover more slowly.[182] In contrast, mild (concussive) injuries cause more shearing of the white matter

---

[b] References 4, 53, 67, 68, 71, 132.

pathways that connect the network together and may recover more quickly.[32,182]

FRAMEWORK FOR EVALUATION AND INTERVENTION

A Hierarchical Model of Visual Processing

The ability to use vision to adapt to the environment requires the integration of visual input within the brain to transform the raw data supplied by the retina into cognitive concepts (rules) that enable us to interpret and understand the visual world. Visual perceptual processing can be conceptualized as an organized hierarchy of visual processes and functions that interact with and subserve each other.[187] As Fig. 24.2 shows, the hierarchy consists of five visual processes: visual cognition (visuocognition), visual memory, pattern recognition, visual scanning, and visual attention. These perceptual processes are supported by three basic visual functions that form the foundation of the hierarchy: oculomotor control, visual fields, and visual acuity. Within the hierarchy, each process is supported by the one that precedes it and cannot properly function without the integration of the lower-level process. Thus, the ability to use vision for daily occupations results from the interaction of all of the processes within the hierarchy working together in a unified system. Although each perceptual process is discussed individually in this section, the reader should remember that they do not operate independently of one another.

The highest-order process in the hierarchy is *visual cognition*. Visual cognition is defined as the ability to interpret visual input (e.g., patterns) and integrate vision with other sensory information to identify, understand, and use objects to achieve goals. Visual cognition begins to develop in childhood as we combine vision with sensory input from the body to develop cognitive concepts (e.g., rules) for how space and objects operate.[108] Size constancy, which is the concept that an object is the same size whether it is near or far from us, is an example of a cognitive rule about space.[4] For example, if we see an adult person who is 12 inches tall, we assume that the adult must be several yards away because we know from interacting with adults in childhood that most adults are between 5 and 6 feet tall. We decide to move closer to the person, thinking that if we do so, the person will get larger. Visual cognition enables us to complete complex visual analysis and thus serves as a foundation for all of our academic endeavors and occupations.

Visual cognition cannot occur without the support of *visual memory*, the second process level in the hierarchy.[4] Mental manipulation of visual input requires the ability to create, retain, and recall memories of images to use for comparison during visual analysis. For example, to interpret the illustration in Fig. 24.3, one must be able to recall memories of the silhouettes of a goose and a hawk. Adults and older children can easily resolve this illusion, but a typical toddler lacks the stored memories of the shapes of these birds to identify them. Emotion is an important component of visual memory. We are more likely to attend to emotionally relevant objects, which increases the likelihood their images will be stored in memory.[4,50,70,108,132] It is

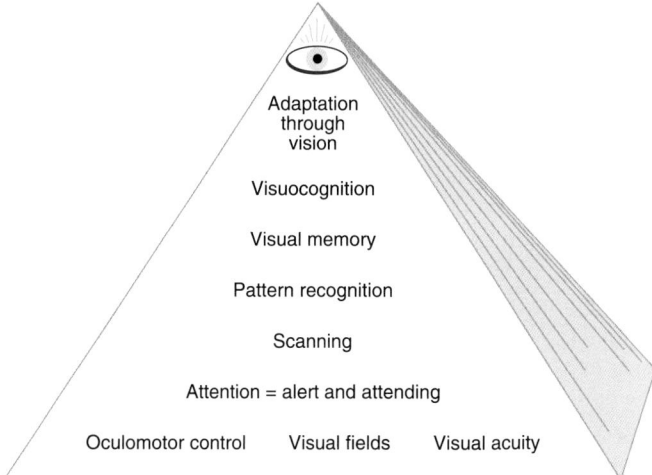

Fig. 24.2 Hierarchy of visual perceptual processing within the brain. (Courtesy Josephine C. Moore, PhD, OTR. From Warren M: A hierarchical model for evaluation and treatment of visual perceptual dysfunction in adult acquired brain injury, part I, *Am J Occup Ther* 47[1]:42–54, 1993.)

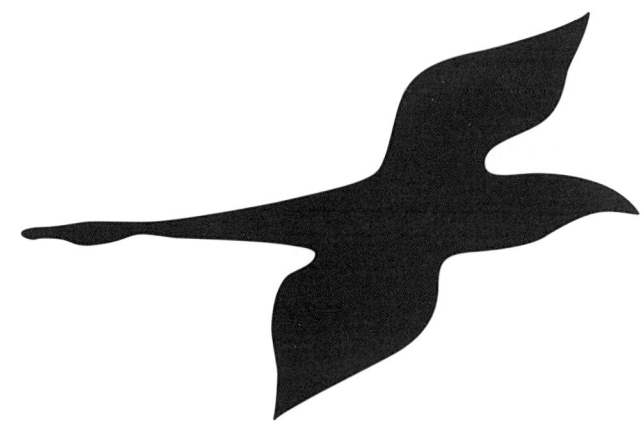

Fig. 24.3 Is this a goose or a hawk? (From Warren M: A hierarchical model for evaluation and treatment of visual perceptual dysfunction in adult acquired brain injury, part I, *Am J Occup Ther* 47[1]:42–54, 1993.)

easy to recall an image of your favorite food or your childhood pet and much more difficult to remember the face of the clerk who scanned your groceries last week.

To store and access images in memory, the person must recognize the pattern making up the image. *Pattern recognition*, which subserves visual memory in the hierarchy, involves identifying the salient features of an object and using these features to define and distinguish the object from its surroundings.[70,103] A salient feature is a noticeable feature that distinguishes a particular object from another. For example, the salient feature that differentiates an "E" from an "F" is the lower horizontal line on the "E." We develop pattern recognition through repetition; our ability to recognize patterns improves from having seen them before in meaningful contexts.[56,67] Children (and adults) spend hours viewing and deciphering patterns in order to develop a large library of images to assist with object recognition.[70] Generic memory, a subset of memory, consists of images that can be accessed by a broad range of sensory input.[70] They represent the common objects that we frequently encounter and use. An apple is an example of an everyday object that can be accessed through generic memory. To conjure up the image of an apple, I could show you an apple, have you close your eyes and put an apple in your hand to feel, release the scent of an apple, or place a slice of apple on your tongue. In each case you should be able to easily identify the object as an apple.

Pattern recognition can be accomplished only with the support of the next process in the hierarchy: organized and thorough scanning of the visual array. *Visual scanning* or search is accomplished through the use of saccadic eye movements. A saccade is a movement of the eye toward an object of interest in the environment.[98] The purpose of a saccade is to place the fovea, which is the retinal area with the greatest ability to see detail, precisely onto the targeted object so that it can be clearly seen and identified. When scanning a visual scene, the eyes selectively focus on the elements that are critical to accurately interpreting the array.[57,94,98,103,111] The person ignores unessential elements in the scene but scans the most important details several times to ensure accuracy.[57,94,98,111]

Visual scanning is actually the outward expression of visual attention. The saccadic eye movements observed when one is scanning reflect the engagement of visual attention as it is shifted from object to object.[c] Visual search occurs on two levels: an automatic, reflexive level largely controlled by the brainstem (through the superior colliculi) and a voluntary level driven by the prefrontal cortex.[70,71,98] On a reflexive level, visual attention (and therefore visual search) is automatically engaged by any novel object moving or suddenly appearing in the peripheral visual field, such as a flash of light.[71,98] The eyes move quickly to focus on and identify the object to protect us from unexpected intrusions in our environment. Voluntary visual search directed by the prefrontal areas of the cortex is completed for the explicit purpose of gathering the information needed to decide and formulate a plan.[70] Voluntary search is purposefully and consciously driven by a desire to locate certain objects in the environment, such as a misplaced set of keys, or to obtain specific information, such as where an exit is located.[57,71,94] Voluntary visual search is also completed in an organized, efficient, symmetric, and predictable pattern based on the qualities of the visual array and the goal.[57,94] For example, we execute a left to right and top to bottom scanning pattern when reading paragraphs of text written in English. Our search is guided by where we anticipate an object to be found in the environment, but it is also driven by the highly visible features of objects that "pop out" in the visual array.[4,57,103] A bright red stoplight at an intersection is an example of a feature that pops out and grabs ones' attention when driving down a roadway.

Visual attention, which subserves scanning in the hierarchy, is a critical prerequisite for visual cognitive processing. If and how a person attends to visual features determines whether the brain will use the visual input in making decisions. Persons who are unable to attend to visual images will not search for visual information and therefore will not complete pattern recognition or lay down a visual memory and, ultimately cannot use this visual input to make decisions. Likewise, persons who attend to

visual information in a random and incomplete fashion often miss important details needed to make an effective decision.[132]

The level and type of visual attention the brain engages depends on the type of visual analysis needed. For example, the type of attention needed to be aware that a chair is in the room is different from that needed to identify the style of the chair. The first instance requires a *global* awareness of the environment and the location of objects within it; the second requires *selective* visual attention to identify the features of the chair.[132] We must also be able to employ more than one type of visual attention at the same time. When crossing a crowded room to talk to a friend, we must monitor the other people and obstacles in the room to avoid collisions, while at the same time continue to focus on the location of our friend so we can successfully make contact. A large neural network that spans the brain is devoted to directing visual attention. The extensiveness of the network means that attention can be easily disrupted by brain injury, but it also increases the potential for recovery with intervention.[49,70,132]

Engagement of visual attention and the other higher-level processes in the hierarchy cannot occur unless the brain receives concise and accurate visual input from the environment.[187] Three primary visual functions ensure that the brain receives high-quality visual input: oculomotor control, visual field, and visual acuity. *Oculomotor control* ensures eye movements are executed quickly and accurately to locate visual information and keeps the desired target focused on the fovea to capture sharp detailed images. The visual fields register the entire visual scene and ensure that the brain receives complete visual information. Visual acuity ensures that details of the environment and tasks are captured, including color. Together these visual functions supply the accurate, complete, and detailed information needed for the cortex to direct attention, complete pattern recognition, lay down and access visual memory, and complete cognitive processing.[187]

Brain injury or disease can disrupt visual processing at any level within the hierarchy. Because of the unity of the hierarchy, if brain injury impairs a lower-level process or function, the processes above it will also be compromised.[187] When this happens, the client may appear to have a deficit in a higher-level process, even though the impairment actually occurred at a lower level in the hierarchy. Effective evaluation and intervention require an understanding of how brain injury affects the integration of vision at each process level and how the levels interact to enable visual perceptual processing.

Consider Penny, whose hemianopia prevents her from seeing objects in the left half of her visual field. Her vision loss on the left side will make it difficult for her to attend to and search for objects on the left side. Her failure to search for objects on the left limits her ability to locate items needed to complete daily activities. She is also missing the visual input needed to accurately map the left side of her environment, causing her to collide with objects on the left as she tries to navigate environments. During Penny's initial OT session, the occupational therapist (OT) observed that she was inattentive to the left side. The OT understood that the visual field deficit could disrupt the higher-level visual processes of attention and visual scanning

---

[c] References 70, 71, 94, 98, 103, 132.

and made a mental note to administer assessments that would help reveal just how Penny's attention to the left had changed and how it affected her occupational performance.

HOW VISION IMPAIRMENT AFFECTS OCCUPATIONAL PERFORMANCE

Visual impairment can occur from disease, trauma, and aging.[98,183] Older adults especially may experience a combination of causes.[139] *Penny sustained a hemianopia from the brain trauma caused by the stroke, but she also has diabetes, a disease that causes many vision-related impairments.*[91] Visual impairment can alter the quality and amount of visual input into the brain or alter how the brain processes and uses incoming visual input.[98] Either way, clients with brain injuries can experience a decrease in the ability to use vision to complete daily occupations. Changes are observed in vision-dependent activities, which are activities that can be successfully completed only using visual input.[110] Two of the most vision-dependent daily activities are reading printed material and driving—without vision it is impossible to read a printed book or drive a car. Many instrumental ADLS (IADLs; e.g., meal preparation, financial management, medication management) and some basic ADLS (e.g., applying make-up) also require good vision to successfully complete these activities. Persons with visual impairment must put more effort into seeing and may process visual information so slowly that they are unable to participate in dynamic activities such as driving or group activities such as playing a card game with friends. Persons with vision impairment are also prone to making errors because of insufficient or poor-quality visual input. They may misread a bill and pay the wrong amount, or step in front of an oncoming bicyclist because they did not see the bicyclist. Continuously making (even small) errors throughout the day can erode the person's self-efficacy and confidence. The person may even stop engaging in highly valued occupations because of fear and frustration.[59,100] In addition, because vision is needed most to successfully engage in dynamic environments, persons with vision impairment often avoid participation in community environments, which can lead to social isolation. The inability to complete valued activities and occupations can contribute to anxiety and depression in adults who, like Penny, acquire vision impairment after a lifetime of good vision.[22,150]

Visual impairment can potentially limit the client's participation in many vision-dependent daily activities inside and outside of the home.[188] *Recall, for example, that Penny reports difficulty completing reading, driving, home management, her art, and caring for Pot.* Yet, when vision impairment occurs with a brain injury, its effect on occupational performance is often attributed to other causes such as motor or cognitive impairment. This occurs because visual impairment is a *hidden disability.* Unlike a hemiplegia or slowness in responding, which can be easily observed following a stroke, clients display few outward signs that they have a significant visual impairment.[59] *Penny, despite the fact that she is missing 50% of her visual field because of hemianopia, looks just like a typical normally sighted older adult as she waits for her treatment session with the OT.*

THE OCCUPATIONAL THERAPY EVALUATION AND INTERVENTION PROCESS

Specific occupational therapy assessments and interventions for vision impairment will be described later in the chapter, but first it is important to consider the OT evaluation and intervention process. As stated earlier in the Occupational Therapy Practice Framework,[7] our profession believes that "achieving health, well-being, and participation in life [occurs] through engagement in occupation" (p S5). Although it is important for clients to become independent in their daily occupations, the ultimate goal of occupational therapy intervention is *participation*. Participation is driven by effort and a belief that one is capable of successfully completing an activity, and it is strongly influenced by personal expectations, current abilities, context, and environment. *Penny told her ophthalmologist that she could no longer paint, even though the ophthalmologist found that her visual acuity and thus her ability to see details and color was normal. Is Penny really incapable of engaging in this valued occupation or is the effort required to participate too great for her to derive any pleasure from painting or does she feel that she can no longer "measure up" to her previous high standard of performance? To answer these questions and determine why Penny will not paint requires the OT to consider all aspects of the OT domain, focusing on the interrelatedness among the client factors, performance skills, performance patterns, and context, both personal and environment context, that contribute and enable Penny to complete this occupation.*

An Overview of Evaluation

The OT evaluation has three purposes: (1) to identify limitations in occupation, (2) to link the occupational limitations to the presence of a visual impairment, and (3) to develop an appropriate intervention plan based on the results of the evaluation. If enabling the client to reengage in valued occupations is the primary goal of the OT intervention, it does not matter how much the client's vision deviates from an established performance norm but rather in how it interferes with occupational performance. A client's visual impairment requires intervention only when it interferes with performance of a necessary or desired daily occupation.

A team approach is required to provide effective intervention to a client with vision impairment.[61,63,115] The occupational therapist must collaborate with the ophthalmologist and/or optometrist to understand how vision has changed and determine the best intervention approach. Both of these eye doctors diagnose, manage, and treat visual impairment. As physicians, *ophthalmologists* are primarily responsible for diagnosing and treating the medical conditions that cause the visual impairment.[6] Board certified neuro-ophthalmologists treat the largest number of persons with visual impairment from brain injury. Consequently, they often serve as referral sources and consultants to OT practice. *Optometrists* are licensed healthcare providers who have a clinical doctorate of optometry and often use the credential of Optometry Doctorate (OD). Although they are not physicians, optometrists also diagnose and treat medical conditions causing vision loss and also provide most of the primary eye care in the United States.[10] Some optometrists specialize in neuro-rehabilitation and provide services to persons with vision impairment from brain injury.[9] *Because Penny's stroke affected only her vision, she made an appointment with her ophthalmologist when she noticed that her vision had changed. Her ophthalmologist referred her to a low vision rehabilitation program. The medical director of the low vision program was an optometrist who led the rehab team consisting of an occupational therapist with specialty certification in low vision (the credential, SCLV)[8] and a clinical social worker. Together this team addressed the limitations caused by Penny's vision loss.* Luckily, Penny's stroke caused limited neurological impairment, but many clients with brain injury experience significant deficits in multiple body functions that require comprehensive inpatient and outpatient rehabilitation. In an ideal medical rehabilitation program, an optometrist is a member of the rehabilitation team. The OD evaluates and diagnoses the client's vision impairment and provides the team with information on prognosis and medical/optical management.[63,115] Currently few optometrists are integrated into rehabilitation teams, and instead the client must be referred to an ophthalmologist or optometrist's private practice. Obtaining an outside referral can be a difficult and time-consuming process. The OT will be expected to provide evidence to the medical director or case manager that a visual impairment may be present and limiting the client's occupational performance. To advocate for referral, the occupational therapist must be able to administer basic visual assessments to screen for visual impairment.

Occupational therapists use a variety of assessments to screen visual performance. This chapter will use subtests from the Brain Injury Visual Assessment Battery for Adults (biVABA; http://www.visabilities.com) developed by the author to illustrate how to evaluate the client.[189] The biVABA was designed specifically as a tool to assist occupational therapists to develop effective intervention plans for adults with visual impairment caused by brain injury. The battery consists of 17 subtests that include commonly used assessments to screen basic visual function, along with tests designed specifically for occupational therapists. By definition, a screening assessment suggests that an impairment may exist but is not conclusive because the results do not provide enough information to diagnose the condition. Occupational therapists lack the professional qualifications to diagnose visual conditions; that is the role of the ophthalmologist or optometrist. However, occupational therapists are often the designated member of the rehabilitation team who screens for vision impairment. *If Penny's stroke had been more severe, causing hemiplegia and other impairment, she would have been taken to the emergency room and admitted for intensive rehabilitation. In this scenario, it is highly unlikely that an ophthalmologist would have been called in to evaluate and diagnose Penny's hemianopia before the rehabilitation team began providing therapy. Instead, if there was no ophthalmologist or optometrist on the rehabilitation team, the OT would screen Penny's vision during the initial evaluation using assessments described later in this chapter. When documenting the evaluation instead of using the diagnostic term left hemianopia, the OT would describe the behaviors that suggest a visual field deficit was present and report*

these findings to the rehabilitaion team. The team would then compare their observations of Penny's visual performance and determine the type of follow-up evaluation needed to address the suspected vision impairment.

An Overview of Intervention

Recovery from brain injury often spans months and years rather than days or weeks. Some vision impairment from brain injury, notably some forms of oculomotor impairment, can improve over time.[124] Other impairment, notably visual field deficits such as Penny's hemianopia, usually cause more permanent impairment.[31,139] Others, such as visual attention deficits, may recover slowly over several months.[116] Currently there is little research evidence to support the efficacy of interventions that aim to restore visual function to normal preinjury levels.[65,128,139,140,171] In addition, many proposed restorative interventions require significant amounts of therapy time that cannot feasibly be implemented within the very brief time allotted to rehabilitation.[90,140,170,171] For these reasons, rather than focusing on restoration of visual processing, the occupational therapy intervention should focus on enabling the client to use his or her *current* visual abilities to participate in valued activities and occupations. This approach aligns with the overarching goal of occupational therapy intervention as stated in the occupational therapy practice framework to promote the client's health and participation despite disability.[7] The approach is also consistent with research showing that neuroplasticity within the brain is stimulated when a person attempts to engage in meaningful tasks.[49]

Newer models of neocortical processing suggest that the brain uses past experience to create a context in which to evaluate incoming visual information and predict what is going to happen next.[16,76,77] For example, you see your mug of steaming coffee and based on your experience with drinking coffee you predict that the cup will feel warm when you pick it up. The brain continuously runs unconscious simulations such as the coffee example using previously learned information to predict what will happen next. These simulations keep you prepared to successfully respond to situations as they arise. It is important to remember that these predictive simulations are unlocked and activated by the physical environment. The OT Practice Framework[7] defines context as "the environmental and personal factors specific to each client . . . that influence engagement and participation in occupations" (S9). Contexts include environmental and personal factors. The physical environment includes "animate and inanimate elements of the natural or physical environment" (S36). We link environmental and personal factors together to construct a plausible hypothesis of what we will see next when we move our eyes or feel next when we move our bodies. For example, you are standing in the produce aisle of the grocery store (i.e., the physical environment) while shopping for ingredients for a pie, and you see something round and red. Based on the environmental factors, you predict it is the apples that you need for the pie and you walk over to see if you are correct. If what you see confirms that your prediction is correct, visual processing does not need to go any further; you just select the number of apples that you need and move on to the next item on your list. The critical takeaway message is that the ability to make an accurate prediction is predicated on the ability to accurately *see* the critical environmental features that trigger memory and unlock prediction. As stated earlier, vision is the primary way we acquire information about our world, and as such it dominates the interpretation of environment and context. Vision impairment then may reduce the accuracy, quality, and completeness of visual input into the brain, causing the person to miss the critical environment/task features needed to define the context and trigger prediction. As a result, the person may not be able to successfully participate in the activity or occupation.

Persons with vision impairment, whether it is from brain injury, age-related eye disease, or aging, are strongly influenced by the visual properties of the task and the environment. These properties include contrast, pattern, size, and illumination. The client's success in using their current visual capabilities to complete daily occupations depends on the OT's ability to create a visible and explicit environment that facilitates rather than inhibits performance. Because increasing visibility is the most important OT intervention for each type of vision impairment described in this chapter, the components of this intervention will be described here and then mentioned again in the sections on specific visual deficits.

Increase Contrast of Key Components of the Task and Environment

Key components are those features of a task or environment that guide completion of the desired occupation. Changing background color to contrast with an object can help the client see the object more clearly. The application of this technique can be as simple as using a black cup for milk and a white cup for coffee. In cases in which background color cannot be changed, such as on carpeted steps, color can be added to highlight critical features. For example, a line of bright orange duct tape can be applied to the edge of each step to distinguish between them. Adding contrast to an object also enables the client to locate a desired item more quickly. For example, adding a bright pink cover to a client's smartphone reduces the time and frustration spent in continually losing and searching for the device.[39,55]

Reduce or Eliminate Background Pattern in Environments and Objects

Patterned backgrounds have the effect of camouflaging visual details. Using solid colors on background surfaces such as bedspreads, place mats, dishes, countertops, rugs, towels, and furniture coverings increases the visibility of objects placed on them. Clutter also creates significant and distracting pattern in an environment, making it more difficult to locate needed items. Persons with visual processing deficits perform best in simple environments that contain only the objects needed for daily occupations.[55] Cluttered environments with haphazardly placed objects are challenging even for persons with normal visual processing. If possible, reduce the number of objects in a setting and arrange needed objects in an orderly fashion. Items that are used daily should be placed on accessible shelves in single rows. Rarely used items should be stored on upper and lower shelves or removed. Use commercially available organizing systems to store items together to create workstations. For example,

place all of the items used for grooming together in a basket. Reducing clutter and adding structure to an environment creates an explicit and predictable environment that places less demand on visual attention. Once the environment is organized and simplified, educate the client and family on the importance of maintaining the structure. Developing the habit of putting items back where they belong and maintaining organization reduces frustration and facilitates independence.

Enlarge Critical Features of Objects and Environments

Increasing the size of a feature or object makes it more visible. Enlarge the print on instructions, medications, calendars, and other items. The last line of print that the client can easily read on the reading acuity test card wearing eyeglasses provides a starting place; generally persons prefer to read 3 to 5 points greater than their minimum acuity.[97] Increase contrast along with size because it does little good to enlarge text if the print is faint. Black on white or white on black print is more visible than any other color combination. Modify the accessibility settings of digital devices to adjust the brightness and background color of the screen; enhance the size, color, and boldness of text, icons, and cursors. Many commonly used items are available with enlarged print, including calculators, clocks, watches, phones; health devices such as glucose monitors, blood pressure cuffs, and weight scales; and leisure items such as playing cards, games, and puzzles. These items can be purchased through specialty catalogs that carry low vision products and are also increasingly available in commercial stores.

Eliminate Vision-Dependent Steps in Tasks

If it is not possible to increase the visibility of a task component, consider eliminating the vision-dependent step from the occupation. For example, apply toothpaste directly onto the tongue rather than the toothbrush, voice dial phone numbers using the smartphone virtual assistant feature, and purchase prechopped vegetables. Train the client to use internet-connected virtual assistants (e.g., Apple Siri, Amazon Echo, Google Home) to perform tasks such as turning on lights; setting a timer; telling the time, temperature, and weather forecast; and ordering items.

Add Adequate, Good Quality Illumination

Increasing the intensity, amount, and quality of available light enables the client to see objects and environmental features more readily and reduces the need for high contrast between objects. For example, facial features can be identified more easily if a person's face is fully illuminated. Strategically place lighting to provide full, even illumination of the task without areas of surface shadow. The light should be positioned as close to the task surface as possible to obtain optimal brightness and illumination of the task[39] (Fig. 24.4).

Many persons with acquired brain injury experience photophobia—an abnormal sensitivity to light that is uncomfortable and often painful.[5,30,48,197] Light sensitivity is a common complaint of persons with vision impairment from traumatic brain injury (TBI); neurodegenerative diseases such as Parkinson's disease and multiple sclerosis; and age-related eye disease such as macular degeneration, diabetic retinopathy, and glaucoma.[48,197]

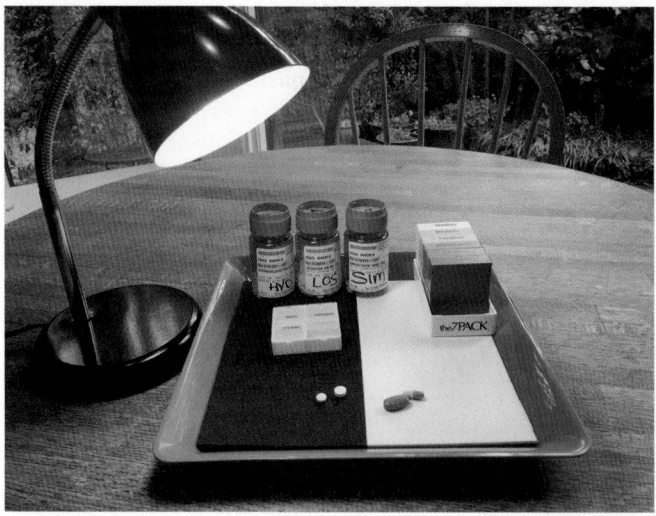

Fig. 24.4 Example of a medication workstation that provides a structured and organized location to complete medication management. The surface of the tray provides a high-contrast surface to identify pills, and a high intensity task lamp provides optimal illumination. (Courtesy Mary Warren, PhD.)

For these persons, light is often friend and foe. They need more illumination to see the details in the environment, while at the same time lighting often causes visual stress and uncomfortable side effects, including excessive blinking, tearing, eye pain, and headache. These side effects may cause a client to avoid or limit participation in environments where lighting cannot be controlled (e.g., virtually all community environments) or to take extreme measures to reduce light into the eye such as wearing dark sunglasses and wide-brimmed hats indoors, using thick drapes on windows, and turning off all of the lights within a room.

The challenge for the occupational therapist is to find lighting sources that provide adequate illumination without discomfort. Fluorescent lighting, which is commonly used because of its energy efficiency, is actually the least tolerated light source. Fluorescent lighting emits a short-wavelength, 50- to 60-Hz flicker that can be quite noxious to persons with photophobia associated with TBI and migraine.[5,48,197] Halogen and LED lights provide a well-tolerated source of bright illumination. However, all types of lighting should be considered, including fluorescent, because there is a wide variation among clients. Tinted eyeglass lenses or shields that fit over lenses and a wide-brimmed hat may reduce glare and ease discomfort in situations where lighting cannot be controlled, such as community use environments.[17,48,60,63] Changing the background on computer screens and smartphones from white to a darker color may also alleviate eyestrain. Filtering incoming light from windows using blinds and covering glossy surfaces such as countertops and floors with nonglare materials create more a comfortable environment.[39]

The OT must also help the client establish performance patterns that support occupational performance. Establishing routines such as shopping at off hours to avoid a crowded grocery store reduces both cognitive and visual stress. Establishing a habit of leaving the keys in a bowl by the door reduces the need for visual search; cleaning eyeglasses daily ensures a brighter image.

EVALUATION AND INTERVENTION FOR SPECIFIC VISUAL DEFICITS

The visual perceptual hierarchy provides the framework for the discussion of evaluation and intervention for specific visual impairments from brain injury. Many of the changes in visual processing after brain injury occur because of impairment in lower levels of the hierarchy. When lower-level processing is disrupted, the visual input into the brain can be limited, inconsistent, or of poor quality, which impairs the brain's ability to use vision for occupational performance. This section describes evaluation and intervention for impairments occurring within the first five levels of the hierarchy: visual acuity, oculomotor control, visual field, visual attention, and visual scanning.

Visual Acuity

Visual acuity is the ability to see visual details and color. In delivering these details, acuity contributes to the brain's ability to quickly identify objects. Good acuity therefore facilitates information processing and decision-making. For this reason, occupational therapists must know whether the client's acuity has been diminished from the brain injury or another cause and collaborate with the eye doctors to make sure the client is able to see as clearly as possible.

Acuity results from a multistep process that begins with the focusing of light onto the retina.[98,109] Light rays enter the eye through the pupil and are focused onto the retina by the anterior structures of the eye: the cornea, lens, and optic media (Fig. 24.5). The photoreceptor cells in the retina, acting like film in a camera, process the light and record a "picture" that is relayed to the rest of the brain via the optic nerve and pathway.[109] Although the concept is simple, the process is complex and involves many components. These components include the ability to focus light precisely onto the retinal cells and maintain a sharp focus for near and distant targets, the ability to allow just the right amount of light into the eye to enable the retina to capture a quality image, and the ability to transmit the image to other brain areas to interpret the image.[98,109] Any compromise of the structures involved in this process will cause images to blur and reduce acuity.

Visual acuity is measured by having the person identify progressively smaller optotypes (letters, numbers, or symbols) on a chart placed at a specified distance. In the United States, acuity level is commonly expressed as a Snellen equivalent fraction (e.g., 20/20).[62] The fraction represents a ratio of the test distance to size of the optotype. In layman's terms, a measurement of "20/20" means that standing at a distance of 20 feet, the viewer can see an optotype that a person with normal vision can see at 20 feet and 20/200 indicates that a person standing at a distance of 20 feet can see an optotype that a person with normal vision can identify at 200 feet. Visual acuity is associated with the ability to see high-contrast, black-on-white optotypes on a test chart. However, visual acuity actually represents a continuum of visual function ranging from the ability to detect high-contrast features on one end of the continuum to the ability to detect low-contrast features (e.g., beige on white) on the other end. Low-contrast acuity, also known as contrast sensitivity, is

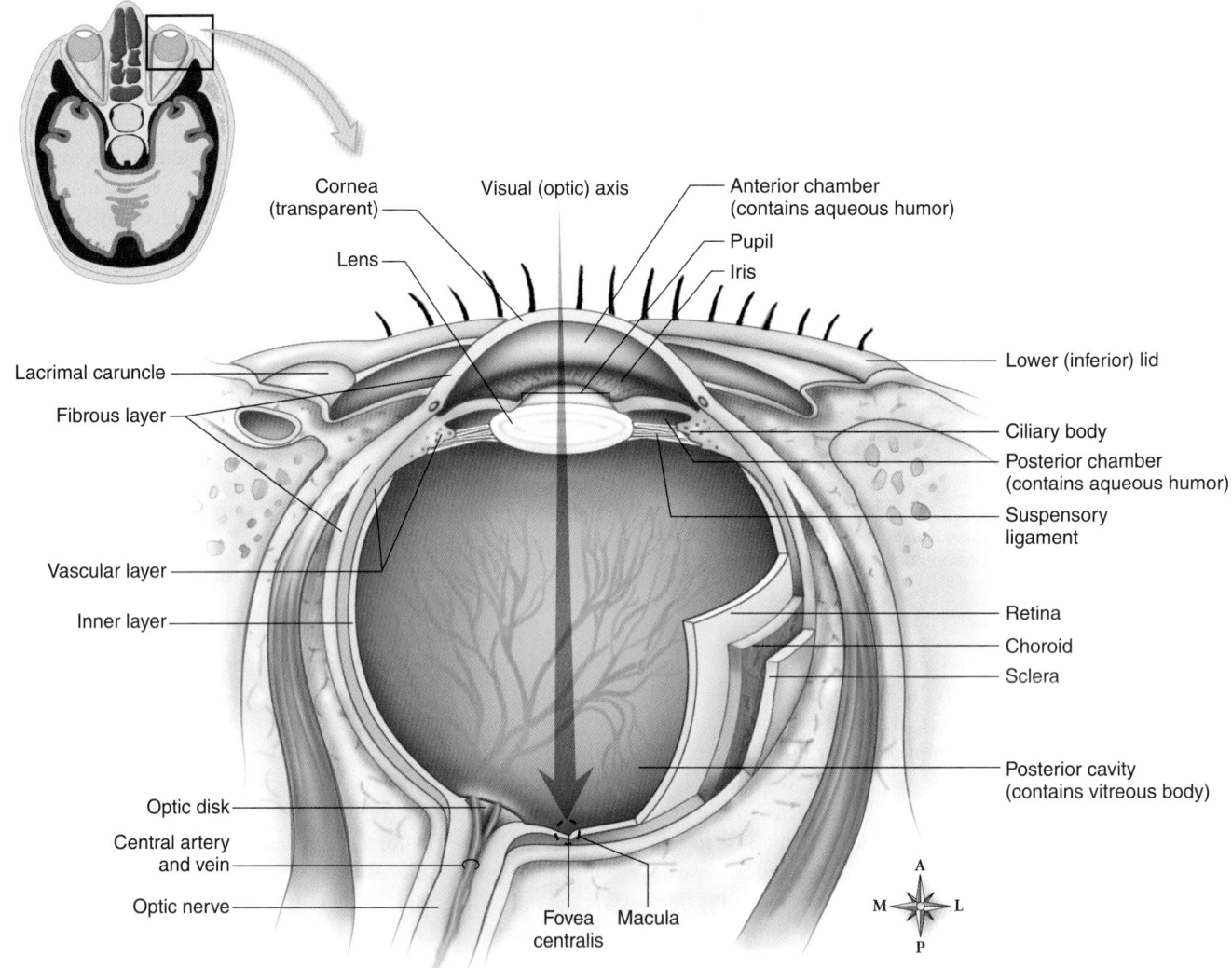

Fig. 24.5 The structures of the eyeball. Images pass through the transparent cornea, lens, and vitreous to focus on the photoreceptor cells of the retina. (From Patton K, Thibodeau GA: *The human body in health and disease*, ed 7, St Louis, 2018, Elsevier.)

the ability to detect the borders of objects as they decrease in contrast from their background.[120] Contrast sensitivity makes it possible to distinguish and identify faint features of objects, such as the curve of a concrete curb or the protrusion of the nose on the face. Because much of the environment is made up of low-contrast features, contrast sensitivity is a critical visual function for safely negotiating the environment. For example, contrast sensitivity is needed to see the depth in a single-color feature such as a step or detect the outline of a transparent substance such as water spilled on a floor. In poorly lit environments where carpets, walls, doors, doorframes, and furniture match in color, good contrast sensitivity may be needed to locate the exit or avoid a chair jutting out into the pathway. The human face is another frequently encountered low-contrast object. There is very little color difference between facial features; the nose is the same color as the forehead, cheeks, and chin. Very good contrast sensitivity is needed to identify the unique features of a human face and accurately distinguish one white-haired old

friend from another. Research has shown that persons with brain injury may experience impaired low-contrast acuity even when their high-contrast acuity is within normal limits.[52,120] Therefore, both forms of acuity (high and low contrast) must be measured to obtain an accurate assessment of acuity function.

Impaired Visual Acuity

There are many causes of impaired acuity, including congenital or acquired conditions, inherited or acquired imperfections in the eye structures, eye diseases that occur early or late in life, conditions that occur secondary to other diseases, neurological diseases, and brain injuries.[30,142] Among persons with acquired brain injury, blurred vision is the most commonly voiced cause of reduced acuity, and difficulty reading is the most common functional complaint.[30,37,74,142] Oculomotor impairment is a common cause of blurred vision because it diminishes the ability of the eye to focus at near distances.[35,74,169] To make it less confusing for the reader, the effect of oculomotor impairment on visual acuity will be covered in the next section of this chapter. This section will focus on acuity impairment from normal imperfections in the eye and damage to anterior eye structures, the retina, the optic nerves, the occipital lobes, and the posterior cortical processing areas of the brain.

Normal refractive errors. Although some people enjoy perfect visual acuity throughout their lifetimes, many of us are born with or acquire refractive errors that reduce our visual acuity.[112] Refractive errors affect how light rays are bent as they enter the eye and result from imperfections in the shape of cornea or eyeball or aging of the lens. Common refractive errors include hyperopia (far-sightedness), myopia (nearsightedness) astigmatism (uneven corneal surface), and presbyopia (loss of lens flexibility).[112] Ophthalmologists and optometrists are skilled at identifying and treating refractive errors with lenses or surgery. Fig. 24.6 describes the common refractive errors and the lens used to correct the error. In *myopia* the image of an object is focused on a point in front of the retina and is therefore blurred

when it reaches the retina. Myopia is corrected by placing a concave lens in front of the eye. In *hyperopia* the image comes into focus behind the retina, causing the image to remain out of focus on the retina. Hyperopia is corrected by placing a convex lens in front of the eye. In *astigmatism* light is focused differently by two meridians 90 degrees apart—images blur because both meridians cannot be simultaneously focused on the retina. A cornea that is shaped more like a spoon or is dimpled instead of smooth may cause astigmatism. Astigmatism is corrected by placing a cylindrical lens in front of the eye. *Presbyopia* occurs when the aging lens becomes more rigid and less capable of changing shape.[112] Adults with this condition frequently complain of difficulty reading small print. Presbyopia is corrected either by using reading glasses to magnify print or, if the person already wears eyeglasses, by adding a magnifying lens or "reading add" to the base of the lenses to create a bifocal. Although most refractive errors can be easily corrected with a trip to the eye doctor, uncorrected refractive error (URE) is a significant public health issue.

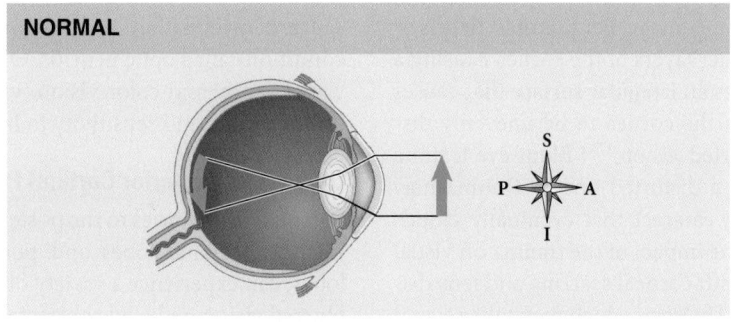
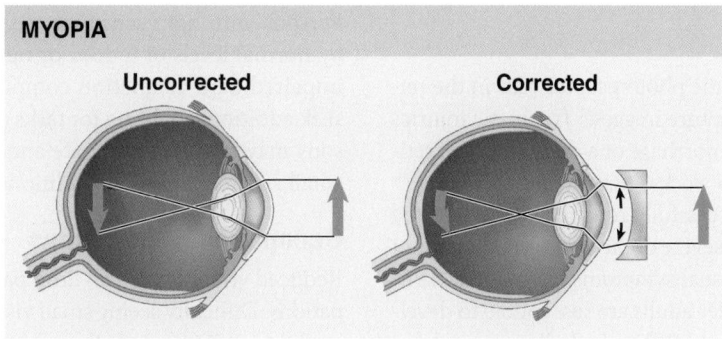
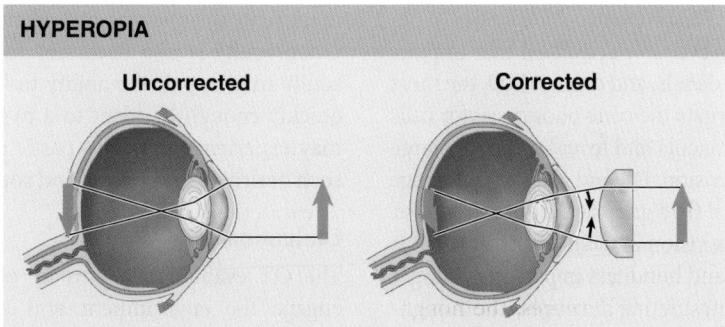

Fig. 24.6 Normal, myopic, and hyperopic optical refraction of light coming into the eye and the type of lens used to correct myopic and hyperopic optical refractive errors. (From Patton K, Thibodeau GA: *The human body in health and disease*, ed 7, St Louis, 2018, Elsevier.)

It has been estimated that over eight million Americans experience unnecessary vision impairment because of URE.[181] Older adults make up the largest number of Americans with correctable vision impairment. Although Medicare covers the cost of an annual eye examination, many older adults never receive an examination because of health reasons or limited access to eye doctors.[58,121] Other older adults cannot afford to update their eye glass prescription because Medicare does not cover the cost of eyeglasses. These barriers are more likely to affect older adults residing in nursing homes and assisted living facilities, where it is estimated that nearly a third of vision impairment can be corrected with glasses or surgery.[58,121]

Opacity or Irregularities in Anterior Eye Structures

Images entering the eye pass through four transparent mediums: the cornea, aqueous humor, crystalline lens, and vitreous humor. An opacity or irregularity in these structures will prevent light and images from properly reaching the photoreceptor cells in the retina. The eye's location in the head makes it vulnerable to injury during a traumatic head injury. Injury to the cornea and lens may result in opacities or irregularities that reduce the quality of the incoming image. For example, debris or shrapnel may penetrate the inner layers of the cornea causing a scar to develop. The scar creates an irregular surface that causes the light rays passing through the cornea to be unevenly dispersed, causing blurred, distorted vision.[37,74] Blunt eye trauma can displace the lens creating a distorted image. Trauma may also induce development of a cataract that eventually clouds the lens and blurs vision.[37,74] The impact of the trauma on visual acuity may be immediate, as with corneal scarring and lens displacement, or delayed, as with cataract, which may take several months to develop.

Damage to the Retina

Injury and disease can damage the photoreceptor cells in the retina, impairing their ability to capture images.[d] Traumatic injuries to the eye can cause a retinal hemorrhage or a detachment of retinal cells immediately or days to weeks after the initial trauma.[100] Retinal detachment may be successfully repaired when detected early. However, if the damage is severe or the trauma patient is not sufficiently aware to describe visual symptoms, permanent damage to the retina may occur. Older adults are susceptible to developing age-related eye diseases (ARED), including age-related macular degeneration (AMD), diabetic retinopathy (DR), and open-angle glaucoma (OAG).[183] Persons with these diseases experience *low vision*—a chronic, irreversible condition that impairs the ability to clearly see objects, details, and color. AMD, the most prevalent ARED, specifically targets the cone photoreceptor cells in the central visual field (e.g., macula and fovea) creating a large blind spot in the center of one's vision. DR and glaucoma damage the central and peripheral visual field and can lead to blindness. AMD is the leading cause of low vision in older adults, and DR is the leading cause of low vision and blindness in persons younger than 65.[91,183] Damage to the central retina diminishes both high- and low-contrast visual acuity, and an injury here impairs the

ability to accurately identify objects. It is not uncommon for an older adult referred to OT for intervention for stroke-related disability to also demonstrate reduced high- and low-contrast acuity from an age-related eye disease.[52,142] Too often the rehabilitation team either overlooks the vision loss from the eye disease or misinterprets it as impaired attention or cognition associated with the stroke.

Damage to the Optic Nerve

Trauma is the most common cause of optic nerve damage in brain injury.[12,158,182] Damage can occur from a penetrating injury to the nerve from a projectile or an optic canal fracture occurring with facial or blunt forehead fractures.[182] Severe closed head injuries can cause stretching or tearing of the optic nerves, resulting in significant and usually bilateral damage to the nerves.[158,182] Bilateral optic nerve injury can also result from compression of the nerves from intracranial swelling or hematoma.[158,182]

Two fairly common neurological diseases—glaucoma and optic neuritis—can damage the optic nerves. Persons who sustain significant damage to the eye can develop traumatic glaucoma that may reduce visual acuity.[119] Multiple sclerosis can cause demyelination and inflammation of the optic nerve, a condition called optic neuritis. Optic neuritis can cause reduced visual acuity and color vision, visual field deficit, orbital pain, dulled vision, and sensitivity to light.[41]

Damage to Posterior Cortical Processing

Persons with injuries to the posterior areas of the cortex, including the occipital lobes and posterior parietal and temporal lobes, can experience a variety of visual disturbances, including blurred vision, reduced contrast sensitivity, a perception of dark or dim vision, light sensitivity, and reduced dark adaptation.[e] Persons with light sensitivity (e.g., photophobia) are bothered by normal levels of indoor or outdoor lighting.[197] Persons with impaired dark adaptation complain of dark or dim vision and seek additional lighting for tasks and environments.[54] Some persons may be able to tolerate and see clearly only within a very small range of lighting conditions.[48]

Occupational Limitations

Reduced visual acuity can limit participation in many daily occupations. Difficulty seeing small visual details and color will impair reading, writing, and fine motor coordination. Occupations dependent on these skills include meal preparation, medication management, financial management, grooming, and shopping. Good acuity is also necessary to quickly identify objects. Poor acuity may impair the ability to locate landmarks and obstacles quickly enough to adapt to a dynamic environment. The client may experience difficulty participating in community activities such as driving, shopping, and social events.

Evaluation

The OT evaluation begins by observing the client's ability to engage the environment and complete daily activities. The OT may observe that the client does not notice small features

---

[d] References 12, 39, 74, 91, 100, 183.

[e] References 12, 48, 54, 74, 176, 182, 197.

of objects and may lean in very close to view an object, seek additional light to complete a task that involves reading or seeing small details, complain that colors seem faded, and is slow to locate and identify objects. Difficulty reading is the primary complaint of persons who experience reduced acuity after brain injury.[74,106,142] It is important to question the client about reading difficulties; common complaints include the print is too small or too faint to read, parts of words are missing, or the print is blurry. Clients with impaired contrast sensitivity may not recognize or may confuse acquaintances because they are unable to see faces clearly, they may demonstrate more difficulty completing tasks or walking in dimly lit surroundings and ask for additional lighting to complete tasks, they may experience difficulty reading faint print or accurately distinguishing shades of colors (e.g., red from pink), or they may misjudge depth in stairs and curbs.

A client who is struggling to see may miss items or perform so slowly on a timed assessment or one with small visual details that the resulting score suggests a significant impairment. Bertone et al.[23] tested the ability of educated, healthy, and normally sighted participants with artificially blurred vision to complete nonverbal neuropsychological tests commonly used to assess cognitive status in adults. They found that even a slight reduction in acuity from 20/20 to 20/40 resulted in poorer performance on certain nonverbal tests. This research study and others have shown that uncorrected visual impairment may mistakenly appear as cognitive impairment in adults,[23,85] increasing the risk that the client's acuity limitations are never diagnosed and addressed. Therefore it is important that high- and low-contrast acuity are the first screening assessments administered to the client.

Eye charts are used to measure high- and low-contrast acuity. High-contrast acuity is measured as distance acuity and near acuity using two different charts. Distance acuity charts measure acuity at a distance of 1 m or greater, and near acuity charts measure acuity at the typical reading distance of 40 cm (16 inches). Distance acuity charts require the person to identify single optotypes, such as a letter number or symbol. Although near acuity can be measured using single optotypes, requiring the person to read sentences provides the most accurate functional measurement of near acuity. Reading acuity charts contain sentences in progressively smaller sizes of print.

There are many types of acuity eye charts, but the same requirements and procedures are used to ensure that an accurate measurement is obtained. There are two requirements that must be met regardless of the chart used: (1) the chart face must be evenly and brightly illuminated and (2) the chart must be held at the correct distance from the client. Adequate chart illumination is important to ensure the maximum contrast of the optotypes. Because acuity is depicted as a fraction of distance over letter size (e.g., 20/20 or 20/200), the measurement is not accurate unless the viewing distance is precise. All test charts specify a distance at which they are to be used, and this must not be altered. The procedure for administering the test is described in Table 24.1.

Clients with brain injury may have deficits in cognition, language, and perception that interfere with the ability to provide an accurate and timely response in a testing situation.

TABLE 24.1 Procedure for Assessing High-Contrast Visual Acuity

Step	Description
1	The client must wear their glasses for the test if they habitually wear them either to see at a distance or to read. Bifocal users should view through the upper portion of the lens on the distant chart and the lower portion on the reading acuity chart.
2	Instruct the client to read the optotypes on the chart out loud, beginning with the largest line and continuing across and down the chart until the optotypes are too small to see. Although most clients should be able to easily see the top lines, beginning on the top line allows the client to practice reading the chart before the actual measurement is made.
3	If the client struggles but is able to identify the optotypes on each line, continue the test until the client accurately identifies fewer than half of the optotypes on a line.
4	Record the acuity level at the smallest line on which the client accurately identified the majority of the optotypes. The acuity level for each line will be printed on the chart.

Several modifications are permissible as long as the requirements are met for distance and lighting. Slowness in responding does not necessarily indicate that the client lacks the acuity to identify the optotype, so allow the client extra time to locate the optotype, process the image, and respond. If the client understands speech but is unable to speak, offer a choice—"is it this or is it that?" and ask the client to respond with a head nod. If the client has limited attention or scans slowly, cover all of the optotypes on a line except one and ask the client to identify the remaining optotype.

The most clinically useful high-contrast acuity chart is one that measures visual acuity as low as 20/1000 so that significant reductions in acuity can be identified. Because some conditions such as optic nerve damage or macular diseases can result in profound vision loss (less than 20/400 acuity), it is important to be able to measure acuity in the lower ranges so that appropriate referral and task modifications can be provided for the client. The Lea Numbers Chart for Vision Rehabilitation is a widely used standardized low-vision distance acuity chart that measures high-contrast visual acuity between 20/20 and 20/1000. The chart is manufactured by Good-Lite and is also included in the biVABA. Reading acuity charts typically measure a range between 20/20 and 20/400 Snellen acuity. Because these charts use sentences to measure acuity, the sentences must match the client's reading grade level and primary language in order to obtain an accurate measurement. The MNREAD Acuity Chart (http://legge.psych.umn.edu/mnread-acuity-charts) is a clinical and research instrument that measures reading acuity and also determines how print size influences maximum reading speed and critical print size. The chart consists of 10 short sentences written at a third-grade reading level and is available in several languages. The Warren Text Card (included in the biVABA) measures reading acuity between 20/400 and 20/20 visual acuity using short simple sentences. A Spanish version of the card is available.

Low-contrast acuity (e.g., **contrast sensitivity function**) also is measured by viewing optotypes printed on a chart held at a specified distance from the client. However, for this type of testing, the optotypes (letters, numbers, or symbols) remain the same size but diminish in contrast as the person proceeds down or across the chart. The client begins with the darkest optotype and proceeds through the chart until the optotype is too faint to be identified. As with high-contrast acuity testing, the test chart must be held at a specific distance and must be well illuminated to obtain an accurate measurement. There are many types of contrast sensitivity charts. The Mars Chart provides a comprehensive assessment of the client's ability to see contrast values between 100% and 1%, and scores can be used to classify the client as having normal, moderate, severe, or profound impairment in contrast sensitivity function.[11] The Lea Numbers Low Contrast Screener (part of the biVABA) was developed as a quick screening tool for the clinic and measures just five contrast values between 25% and 1.2% contrast. Clients who have difficulty identifying optotypes at these contrast values typically experience functional limitations in their daily activities. Dr. Lea Hyvarinen, the developer of the chart, provided a functional interpretation of the client's performance on the chart for the biVABA.

If you do not have a contrast sensitivity chart, you can get a sense of the client's limitations with a simple task analysis that compares the client's performance completing a task with low-contrast features with their performance completing a task with high-contrast features. For this task analysis, instruct the client to fill a black cup with black coffee or a white cup with milk to within half an inch of the rim (i.e., low-contrast task) and then repeat the task pouring black coffee into a white cup or milk into a black cup (i.e., high-contrast task). Observe the client and compare the ease and accuracy of their performance between the two contrast conditions.

Remember that the occupational therapist screens acuity to obtain a general understanding of how well the client is able to see and to determine if vision is limiting occupational performance. If a significant limitation in acuity is observed on the screening assessment, seek referral of the client to an ophthalmologist or optometrist. The eye doctor will determine the cause and prognosis of the impairment and whether acuity can be improved using lenses, surgery, or medications.

Intervention

The first step in intervention is to make sure that the client is wearing his or her glasses and that the glasses are clean and in good repair. Although every client should be wearing his or her corrective lenses, research has shown that persons are frequently admitted to rehabilitation floors without their glasses. Lotery et al.[101] found that over a quarter of persons who wore glasses and were receiving inpatient stroke rehabilitation did not have their eyeglasses with them in the hospital and among those who did, nearly a quarter of the eyeglasses were dirty, were scratched, or needed repair. Roche et al.[136] reported similar findings in a study of persons admitted onto an orthopedic floor: 25% of the patients did not have their glasses with them and, of those who did, 85% of the spectacles were dirty or in poor repair.

Seek a referral to an eye doctor if the acuity screening shows that the client has less than 20/20 acuity wearing his or her eyeglasses or if it has been more than 2 years since an older client's eyeglasses were last updated. In the Lotery et al. study, half of the participants benefitted from an updated eyeglasses refraction.[101] In another study, Park et al.[125] found that nearly half of the patients referred to optometry from an inpatient rehabilitation floor benefitted from updated refraction of their glasses. The participants in the study by Park et al. had been admitted to the rehabilitation floor with 27 different primary diagnoses, but nearly three quarters of the sample had a documented neurological condition in their medical history. If the acuity screening shows significant reduction in acuity (e.g., 20/60 or below) and the client is wearing a pair of recently updated glasses, seek a referral to a low-vision rehabilitation program for specialized assessment and intervention.

When screening shows that the client has reduced high-contrast or low-contrast acuity, the OT should modify the environment and tasks to increase the visibility of key features. Use the interventions described in the previous section to increase contrast, reduce pattern, enlarge features, provide good quality and even illumination, and provide a structured, predictable environment. There are also many resources available to assist persons with poor acuity. The services are generally free of charge. Advocacy organizations like the American Foundation for the Blind (www.afb.org) provide many resources. Examples of other available services include:

1. The National Library Service for the Blind and Print Disabled offers free recorded books, magazines, and music through its Talking Books lending library program (https://www.loc.gov/nls/). Each state has at least one talking book library.
2. Many states offer free radio-reading services in conjunction with a university-sponsored public radio station. Radio-reader services provide a variety of special programming for persons with disabilities, which often includes reading local newspapers.
3. Many telephone carriers will exempt the surcharge for using directory assistance to persons with disabilities; pharmacies will provide large-print medication labels, many restaurants will provide large-print menus, and most businesses will provide statements and bills in large print.

The location of Penny's stroke in the posterior cerebral artery would not typically reduce her visual acuity. However, Penny's diabetes puts her at risk for several eye conditions that can significantly reduce visual acuity. When a review of her medical history indicated that Penny had diabetes, the optometrist in the low vision clinic carefully evaluated the health of Penny's eyes and checked her acuity. The OD completed a very thorough refraction to determine if Penny would benefit from updated lenses. Penny's acuity was 20/30 in her dominant right eye wearing her current bifocal lenses. The ophthalmologist's medical history documented macular edema—an indication of early-stage diabetic retinopathy—which could have contributed to this slight decline in her acuity. The OD updated Penny's eyeglasses prescription to correct her acuity to 20/20. The OD also cautioned Penny that she must maintain her blood glucose levels at the level prescribed by her internist, monitor her diet, and check her blood glucose levels several times a day. The OD asked the OT to evaluate Penny's ability to compensate for her hemianopia when completing diabetes self-management, including drawing insulin and using a glucometer to monitor blood glucose levels and completing meal preparation following her prescribed meal plan.

Oculomotor Function

The purpose of the oculomotor system is to achieve and maintain foveation of an object so that it can be clearly seen.[98] The oculomotor system ensures that the target is located and focused on the fovea of both retinas as long as needed to accomplish the desired goal. Our constant interaction within dynamic moving environments makes this a daunting task because the image is always in danger of slipping off of the fovea as the head or object moves. Eye movements keep the target stabilized on the retina while focusing on stationary and moving targets, when shifting gaze to new targets and during head movement.[98]

Two important functions of the oculomotor system are binocular vision and accommodation. *Binocular vision* ensures that the brain records a single image despite receiving a separate image from each eye. The process of combining two visual images into one is called *sensory fusion*. For sensory fusion to occur, corresponding photoreceptor cells (e.g., cone and rod cells) in the two retinas must be stimulated with the same image. If the photoreceptors are stimulated and if the images match in size and clarity, the brain is able to perceptually fuse the two images into one. The eyes must work together in an integrated binocular system to achieve and maintain sensory fusion. If the eyes do not align with each other or if there is a significant difference in acuity between the eyes, images may appear blurry or doubled (e.g., diplopia).[98]

Accommodation is the ability to zoom in to focus on objects that are close to the face. The natural alignment of the anterior eye structures enables effortless focusing when viewing at a distance, but the structures must change and accommodate to focus at the short distance required for reading or other activities.[98,171] Accommodation occurs through three steps: (1) the eyes *converge* (turn inward) to ensure that the corresponding photoreceptors in the retina are stimulated to capture the image; (2) the lens *thickens* to refract the light rays more strongly and shorten the focal distance, so that the image is focused onto the foveal area of the retina; and (3) the pupil *constricts* to reduce scattering of the light rays and sharpen the image. Multiple areas of the brain are involved in coordinating accommodation, including the cone photoreceptor cells in the retina, optic nerves, lateral geniculate nucleus, occipital lobe, posterior parietal lobe, frontal eye fields, cerebellum, and both nuclei of CN III, the oculomotor nerve.[171]

Oculomotor Impairment

The prevalence of eye movement disorders from acquired brain injury ranges from 50% to 90% in studies.[12] Most oculomotor impairment results from damage to the neural centers that coordinate eye movements.[12] The cortex, thalamus, brainstem, and cerebellum form a complex network to ensure that eye movements are able to attain and maintain foveation.[98,169] The extensiveness and complexity of the pathways controlling

eye movements make them vulnerable to the effects of a brain injury.[98,170] Injury in these areas can cause the person to experience difficulty executing and coordinating eye movements even though the CNs are intact.[12,35,98,169,170] Persons with oculomotor impairment from TBI may also experience other vision-related co-impairments, including light sensitivity, dry eye, visual field deficits, nystagmus, and visuo-vestibular impairment.[f] This section will address two commonly occurring conditions: convergence insufficiency and paralytic strabismus.

Convergence Insufficiency

Studies show that nearly half of all persons with brain injury who are referred for visual assessment have complaints related to focusing.[12,74,171] The most commonly identified focusing disorder is convergence insufficiency,[5,12,35,74,171] which makes it difficult to keep the eyes aligned on the object of interest during accommodation. Persons with convergence insufficiency have difficulty achieving or sustaining adequate focus during near-vision tasks. The client often complains of fatigue, eye pain, or headache after a period of sustained viewing in near tasks, especially reading.[5,30,98,138,169] As the eye muscles fatigue from the exertion of sustaining convergence during reading, the person's ability to fuse images breaks down and the client may experience odd visual phenomena such as print swirling and moving on the page or the page going blank. Because most persons with convergence insufficiency have normal CN function, their reading complaints are often attributed to a perceptual impairment, inattention, or lack of effort, rather than to oculomotor impairment.

Paralytic strabismus. Three pairs of CNs, the oculomotor nerve (CN III), the trochlear nerve (CN IV), and the abducens nerve (CN VI), innervate the seven pairs of striated muscles that move the eye.[98] CN lesions generally occur with moderate to severe brain trauma and account for less than 20% of the oculomotor impairment from TBI or stroke.[141,182] When a CN is damaged, the muscles it innervates are weakened or paralyzed, causing paralytic strabismus.[2,98,146,147] Paralytic strabismus is a misalignment of the eyes (e.g., strabismus) caused by the inability of one eye to move in the direction of the affected (e.g., paralyzed) muscles. Because the eyes must align and move together to maintain sensory fusion, the image breaks apart and the person experiences *diplopia*. Diplopia is a primary characteristic of CN lesions and causes perceptual distortion in which images may appear doubled, distorted, or blurred.[146,147,158] The client's performance limitations depend on whether the diplopia is constant or intermittent and whether it occurs at near or far distances. Milder CN injury may weaken but not paralyze the extraocular muscles (the muscle can still move the eye), enabling the person to maintain sensory fusion when concentrating on a task. However, the weakened muscle often fatigues quickly, causing the client to complain of intermittent diplopia, eye strain, headache, and poor concentration. More severe CN lesions cause significant or complete paralysis of the eye muscles, resulting in constant diplopia and often a noticeable eye turn of the involved eye. Eye doctors use specific medical terms to describe the extent of the strabismus. Phoria describes milder paralysis

---

[f]References 5, 12, 30, 74, 98, 106, 154, 158, 182.

in which the brain's need to maintain sensory fusion keeps the affected eye aligned with the other eye when focusing on an object.[146,147,158] Tropia describes moderate to severe paralysis in which there is a noticeable deviation of the involved eye when focusing.[146,147,158] These terms are combined with four prefixes that describe the direction of the deviation: *eso*, in which the eye turns toward the nose; *exo*, in which the eye turns outward toward the temple; *hypo*, in which the eye turns downward; and *hyper*, in which the eye turns upward. For example, eso*tropia* indicates a constant inward deviation of the eye during focus (e.g., crossed eye), whereas eso*phoria* indicates inward turning of the eye only when the eye muscle becomes fatigued.[147]

CNs 3 and 4 lesions can cause diplopia at close distances, which disrupts reading and activities requiring eye-hand coordination, such as pouring liquids, writing, and grooming. CN 6 and 4 lesions can cause diplopia at a distance beyond arms reach and affect walking, driving, television viewing, and sports such as golf and tennis. Persons with severe paralytic strabismus may be able to eliminate the double image only by assuming a head position that avoids the action of the paretic muscle.[147] For example, a client with a left lateral rectus palsy (CN VI lesion) may turn the head toward the left to avoid the need to abduct the eye; a client with paralysis of the right superior oblique muscle (CN IV lesion) may tilt the head to the right to avoid the downward action of that muscle.[146,147] Without careful assessment of oculomotor function, there is a risk that such alterations in head position will be mistakenly attributed to instability of the neck or trunk rather than a functional adaptation purposely assumed to fuse images.

Neurodegenerative diseases can also cause oculomotor impairment.[98,151] Persons with Parkinson's disease often experience convergence insufficiency early in the course of the disease and develop diplopia—and difficulty moving the eyes as the disease progresses.[98,151,194] Blurred vision and difficulty reading are commonly voiced complaints. Eye movement disorders are common in persons with multiple sclerosis (MS) as a result of the inflammatory demyelinating course of the disease.[40,41] Persons with MS may experience blurred vision, diplopia, nystagmus, and oscillopsia.[40,41,98] Persons with Alzheimer's dementia can experience difficulty executing and controlling saccades.[194]

Evaluation

Much skill and expertise are required to accurately diagnose an oculomotor deficit and determine the appropriate intervention. It is imperative that the client be evaluated by a neuro-ophthalmologist or an optometrist specialized in visual impairment from neurological conditions. The OT is often one of the first members of the rehabilitation team to observe that the client may have an oculomotor impairment affecting occupational performance.[63] This frequently places the OT in the position of requesting further evaluation by an eye care specialist. To make an appropriate referral, the OT must complete a screening to identify patterns of oculomotor impairment that may be contributing to the occupational limitations observed in the client.

The occupational therapist uses a "listen and look" approach to screen the client. The occupational therapist *listens* to the client's complaints about reading and other tasks and *looks* for

changes in oculomotor control that may account for these complaints. The assessment begins with questions about the client's vision before the brain injury. Adults with a childhood history of oculomotor impairment may wear eyeglasses to correct for these deficiencies. The first set of questions to ask is (1) "Do you wear eyeglasses?" (2) "How long have you worn eyeglasses?" (3) "Do you wear them for all activities or only for reading or distance viewing?" Eyeglasses that correct oculomotor deficiencies are generally prescribed to be worn at all times in contrast to eyeglasses that just correct acuity for reading or driving. If a client reports wearing eyeglasses since childhood, follow up with questions that probe whether the eyeglasses were prescribed to correct an oculomotor impairment. These questions include: "Did you have to wear a patch, or have eye surgery or do eye exercises as a child?" "Did anyone ever say that you had a lazy eye?" Affirmative answers suggest that client's eyeglasses may have been prescribed to strengthen oculomotor control and the client must wear them during the rest of the screening to obtain accurate results.

The second set of questions probes whether the client has difficulty focusing or is experiencing diplopia. Persons who have difficulty focusing often complain of blurred vision and visual stress when completing tasks that require a close focusing distance. Ask about the client's comfort when completing occupations that require sustained focus at near distance such as reading, writing a letter, computer work, or quilting; compare these to tasks with longer focal distances such as viewing television, walking the dog, and vacuuming. Look for a pattern that suggests that the client experiences fatigue, eye pain, headache, and reduced concentration during activities that require sustained focusing. If the client reports diplopia, ask about its characteristics. "Do images appear to be doubling, or are they blurry or distorted?" "Does vision clear when one or the other eye is closed?" An affirmative response suggests impairment of the extraocular muscles rather than damage to an eye structure. When images double, do they split side to side or on top of one another? Is the diplopia present only at near distance, far distances, or all of the time? The answers to these questions may suggest CN involvement (Table 24.2), but more importantly

TABLE 24.2 **Summary of Oculomotor Deficits Associated With Cranial Nerve Lesions**		
Oculomotor Nerve III	**Trochlear Nerve IV**	**Abducens Nerve VI**
Impaired vertical eye movements	Impaired downward and lateral eye movements	Impaired lateral eye movements
Lateral diplopia for near-vision tasks	Vertical diplopia for near-vision tasks	Lateral diplopia for far-vision tasks
Dilation of pupil and impaired accommodation		Bilateral lesion: Assumes downward head tilt
Ptosis of the eyelid		

for the OT they suggest the type of performance limitations the client may experience in daily activities. Conclude the initial interview by asking whether the client is experiencing co-impairments such as light sensitivity, headache, or fatigue. Symptom questionnaires can be useful for those who have difficulty clearly describing their symptoms. The 28-item *Brain Injury Vision Symptom Survey*[95] is a comprehensive standardized questionnaire created for persons with traumatic brain injury. The assessment asks the client to rate the frequency of symptoms related to visual clarity, comfort, light sensitivity, dry eyes, depth perception, peripheral vision, and reading.

Observe the client's head position, eyes, and eye movements for signs of impairment. Instruct the client to focus on a distant target and observe the eyes for differences in pupil size, eyelid function, and eye position. Asymmetries such as a dilated pupil in one eye, a droopy eyelid, or an eye turn may indicate CN involvement.[98] Note whether the client has tilted or turned the head to view the target. Next, instruct the client to track the target (a pencil topper works well) as you move it from a central position in front of the nose approximately 8 to 10 inches in each direction vertically, horizontally, and diagonally.[146,147] Observe the client's eyes and note whether both eyes move together the same distance in each direction and stay on target without jerking movement. Assess convergence by instructing the client to track the target as it moves toward the bridge of the nose. The client should be able to easily follow the target in all directions and repeat each movement several times without showing signs of stress such as blinking, tearing, reddening of the eyes, eye rubbing, or sighing. Pay close attention to whether the client has difficulty initiating or maintaining convergence because this may indicate a focusing impairment.[63,147] Comparing the client's distance and reading acuities provides additional information about the client's focusing ability. A reading acuity level 2 to 3 lines lower than the distance acuity level suggests a focusing impairment—for example, reading acuity is 20/50 and distance acuity is 20/20.

If the client complains of diplopia, a cover-uncover and/or alternate cover test helps identify the affected eye and whether the double vision is associated with a phoria or tropia.[146] Cover tests are based on the principle that the brain always uses the fovea to fixate on a target. If a strabismic and drifting eye is suddenly required to fixate on a target, it will achieve foveation by making a saccade toward the target.[146] Requiring the client to fixate with both eyes on a target and then quickly covering one eye can indicate whether both eyes were focused on the target. If the eyes are aligned and fixating on the target, no movement of either eye will be observed when one is covered or uncovered. If the eyes are not aligned, the drifting eye will move to take up fixation when the nonaffected eye is covered. Two cover tests are used: a cover-uncover test identifies a tropia, and an alternate-cover test identifies a phoria.[146,147]

Finally, compare the client's performance on screening assessments with their performance of daily activities to determine if the oculomotor impairment might be contributing to the client's occupational limitations. For example, slowness and effort in converging may help explain why the client has difficulty concentrating when reading. If it appears that an oculomotor impairment may be limiting occupational performance, request a referral to an ophthalmologist or optometrist to evaluate the client's eye movements and provide diagnosis and medical guidance.

Intervention

Oculomotor impairment generally does not prevent the client from independently completing an occupation, but it does affect participation in daily activities and quality of life.[30,32,159,171] The client may experience difficulty coordinating eye movements for reading[134] and other activities; he or she may experience doubling and blurring visual images and may not be able to sustain focus on near objects or quickly switch between near and far focal distances. These difficulties, especially when combined with light sensitivity, can cause the client to experience significant visual stress, which may trigger the onset of headache, eye strain, neck strain, and fatigue.[5,32,63,106] The client may begin to avoid participating in activities that trigger visual stress. The most stressful activities often require reading or take place in community environments that require the person to adjust to bright and changing lighting, such as driving. Computer work and viewing television may also cause significant stress due to sustained focus, light sensitivity, and screen glare.[63]

Ophthalmology/optometry role. Ophthalmologists and optometrists offer interventions to reestablish fusion and binocularity.[75] The intervention selected for a client depends on the prognosis for recovery, the client's ability to participate in therapy, financial resources, and the eye doctor providing the consultation. Both eye doctors use occlusion, prism, and lenses to improve vision but differ in their use of eye exercises or surgery.[g] Most oculomotor dysfunction resolves without intervention within 6 months after the brain injury.[124] Ophthalmologists generally only prescribe prism, lenses, or occlusion during this recovery period. Optometrists hold a different perspective that eye movements and accommodation can be improved through carefully prescribed vision therapy exercises and use them in conjunction with lenses and prism.[36]

Prisms and lenses. Both eye doctors use prism to treat the effects of paralytic strabismus: The prism is applied to the lens of the client's eyeglasses to reestablish single vision in the primary directions of gaze: looking straight ahead and looking down.[36,75,98,126] The prism is placed on the lens of the affected eye to shift the image and fuse the disparate images into a single image.[146,147] A prism is used only as long as it is needed to maintain fusion. If recovery is expected, the eye doctor usually applies temporary plastic Fresnel press-on prisms and gradually weans the client from the need for a prism by reducing the diopter strength of the prism as the muscle weakness resolves. The prism can be permanently ground into the client's eyeglass lens if recovery does not occur. The eye doctors often use lenses to assist clients with accommodative disorders to achieve and maintain focus with less effort.

Occlusion. Diplopia causes images to double and blur; the resulting distortion creates confusion for the client and limits participation in daily activities. Occlusion is used to eliminate

[g] References 36, 63, 98, 127, 140, 141, 143, 146, 147, 170, 171.

the diplopia and visual stress. Eye doctors prescribe occlusion, but in a setting without access to an eye doctor, the OT in collaboration with the rehabilitation team may also apply occlusion to restore single vision to the client. As an OT intervention, occlusion is used to eliminate the stress caused by the diplopia so that the client is willing to participate in daily activities and therapy. It has no therapeutic purpose other than to eliminate the double image. However, it is still considered to be an optometric or ophthalmology intervention; thus, the OT does not prescribe the use of occlusion without physician oversight. The referring physician should be consulted and prescribe using the modification just as is done when applying a splint or a sling.

Either full or partial occlusion is used to eliminate the second image.[63,126,127,146,147] Full occlusion eliminates all of the vision in one eye using a "pirate" patch, a clip-on occluder, or opaque tape. Pirate patches are often used because they are inexpensive and readily available. However, the patch is often poorly tolerated by the client. The first challenge is that the patch also eliminates peripheral vision, disrupting normal mechanisms for control of balance and orientation to space. This may cause the client to feel off balance and disoriented when navigating environments. The second challenge is that most clients cannot tolerate long periods of using one eye alone; the working eye becomes fatigued and the person experiences eye strain and headache. Therefore, for the comfort of the client, the patch is alternated between the eyes. Even though altering occlusion reduces fatigue and eye strain, clients often resist having their dominant eye patched for even short periods because that is the eye used to direct fixation. As a result, the client does not adhere to the occlusion schedule.

Partial occlusion involves covering a portion of the visual field in one eye.[126,127,146,147] Just enough occlusion is applied to eliminate the diplopia and still allow the client to use the eyes together to complete activities.[127] Several types of occluders are used for partial occlusion.[127,147] One technique that can be easily completed by the OT is to apply a strip of translucent material (such as 3 M Transpore surgical tape) to the central portion of the eyeglass lens (Fig. 24.7). The client is instructed to view a target that is doubling while the OT applies the tape from the nasal rim toward the center of the lens until the client reports single vision when viewing the target. The tape is applied to the nondominant eye for the greater comfort of the client. The width of the tape is gradually reduced as the muscle paresis resolves. Partial occlusion provides a kinder, gentler way to achieve single vision without disrupting balance or orientation. Usually the client is more comfortable and therefore more willing to engage in activities. The main disadvantage of partial occlusion is that the tape must be applied to the client prescription lenses or a pair of frames with plano (nonrefractive) lenses. It is important that the OT work with the client and eye doctor to determine the best way to manage diplopia during recovery so that the client will participate in daily occupations. For example, the OT may advocate for partial occlusion instead of total occlusion for a client who must navigate community environments.

Eye exercises. Evidence for the efficacy of using eye exercises to restore binocular function and improve oculomotor

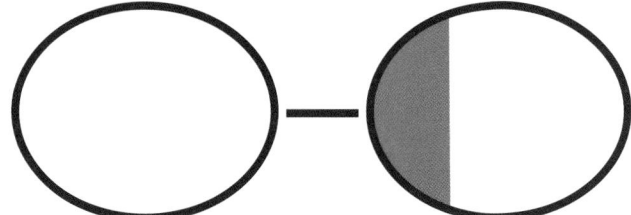

Fig. 24.7 Example of partial occlusion to eliminate diplopia. Translucent tape is applied to the nasal portion of the eyeglass lens on the side of the non dominant eye. (From Warren M: *Brain injury visual assessment battery for adults test manual*, visAbilities Rehab Services, Hoover, AL.)

control after adult acquired brain injury is still limited and inconclusive.[20,140] However, more recent carefully planned studies have shown evidence for the effectiveness of precise exercise protocols to improve vergence and accommodation in persons with mild head trauma.[152,153,170,171] As an optometric intervention, eye exercises are not within the OT scope of practice and should be completed only by the optometrist.

Surgery. Surgery is recommended when the degree of strabismus is too large to be reduced with prism or fusional effort, or when a significant strabismic condition does not resolve in 12 to 18 months.[126] The surgery alters the position of the eye to align with the other eye and create a single image. An ophthalmologist specially trained in strabismus surgery completes this surgery.

Occupational Therapy Role

The occupational therapist focuses on enabling the client to participate in necessary and desired daily occupations despite the challenges and discomfort of oculomotor impairment. Persons with oculomotor impairment can independently complete daily occupations, but they will avoid participating in those activities that cause them to experience considerable visual stress. Co-conditions such as light sensitivity, headache, and blurred vision can persist months to years after the onset of the brain injury even in cases of mild TBI and concussion.[106,159] They can also create significant discomfort that causes the client to alter routines and develop habits that limit or eliminate participation in certain activities. Having to relinquish valued occupations can cause the client to feel depressed and less motivated to engage in daily activities. Ultimately, some clients may experience a debilitating and self-perpetuating cycle in which depression causes activity limitations and activity limitations cause depression.

The occupational therapist can intervene and prevent this cycle from occurring by assisting the client to modify the environment and tasks and devise strategies to complete desired activities with the least amount of visual stress. Intervention begins by observing and interviewing the client to identify stressful occupations and the aspects of the client's performance patterns, context, and environment that aggravate or reduce visual stress in each occupation. Too much lighting, poor quality or glaring light, and fluctuating lighting may all trigger onset of headache in clients who are light sensitive.[159] Clients with blurred vision have difficulty seeing low-contrast features and small visual details. An environment with lots of pattern and clutter forces the client to spend more time searching for items.

The more stress-provoking features there are in an environment, the more likely it is the client will avoid it.

The OT facilitates participation by creating an environment and task that is less stressful and more inviting.[61] Work with the client to add contrast, increase size, reduce pattern, and find sources of comfortable lighting. Remove visually dependent steps in tasks and add structure to the environment to lessen the need to use vision. The OT should also work with the client to establish habits and routines to reduce stress. Teach the client how to pace participation in a stressful activity to avoid onset of a debilitating headache. For example, a client who experiences headache triggered by visual stress when grocery shopping might try shopping for just a few items at a time to reduce the amount of time spent in this stress-provoking environment. Alternatively, the client may prevent headaches by shopping in the early morning when the client is more rested and the grocery store is less crowded. As discussed in the acuity section, fit-over filters and wide-brimmed hats control the light entering the eye and are helpful in community environments for clients with light sensitivity. These practical interventions teach the client how to manage visual stress and build the client's self-efficacy and belief that he or she can control rather than be controlled by their symptoms.

Although Penny's stroke did not cause oculomotor impairment, she is experiencing sensitivity to bright lighting as a result of macular edema caused by her diabetes. She is especially bothered by the lighting in her church sanctuary which has very large windows. She reports that she often has to shut her eyes during the service because the light bothers her so much. She hates that other parishioners might think that she is sleeping but her eyes water if she keeps them open, and she is afraid that people might think she is crying. "I can't win, so we only attend church on cloudy days." The OT took Penny into a room with brightly lit windows and had her try out several pairs of fit-over filters in different tints (manufactured by NoIR Medical Technologies (https://www.noir-medical.com). Penny thought that the filters with a light rose-colored tint provided the greatest comfort in the bright light. The OT loaned the filters to Penny to try out in various settings. Penny reported back that the filters worked well to reduce the glare but she felt self-conscious wearing them because they were so bulky. The OT and Penny explored various styles of fit-over frames, and Penny ordered a more stylish pair. She tried out the new fit-overs in church and excitedly reported that another church member asked her where to get a pair to help him better tolerate the lighting.

Visual Field

The visual field is the external world that we can see when we look straight ahead. It is analogous to the dimensions of a picture imprinted on film in a camera (with the retina representing the film). The normal visual field extends approximately 135 degrees vertically and 160 degrees horizontally. The fields of the two eyes overlap so that most of the visual field is binocular and seen by both eyes (see Fig. 24.1). A small portion of the peripheral field on the temporal (ear) side of the face in each eye is monocular and can be seen only by one eye because the bridge of the nose occludes vision in the other eye (see Fig. 24.1). The central visual field is made up of the macula and fovea (Fig. 24.8). The fovea lies at very center of the macula and provides the highest level of acuity. The central field is packed with cone photoreceptor cells to provide the details and color needed to complete object identification.[109] The remainder of the visual field is the peripheral field. The peripheral visual field comprises rod photoreceptors that detect general shapes and movement in the environment and provide background but not detailed vision.

Visual Field Deficits

Injury to the photoreceptor cells in the retina or to the optic pathway that relays retinal information to the cortex results in a visual field deficit (VFD).[67] Fig. 24.1 illustrates this pathway because it changes from the optic nerve to the optic tract to the GCT. The location and extent of the visual field deficit depends on where damage occurs along the pathway. Although any type of visual field deficit is possible after brain injury, homonymous hemianopia (HH) is the most common deficit occurring in approximately 30% to 50% of persons with stroke.[139] *Hemianopia* (hemi = half; anopia = blindness) means that there has been a loss of vision in half of the visual field in the eye. *Homonymous* means that the deficit is the same in both eyes. A lesion occurring posterior to (e.g., behind) the chiasm within the right hemisphere causes a left HH; the same lesion in the left hemisphere causes a right HH. Hemianopia from stroke typically occurs from occlusion of the posterior or middle cerebral

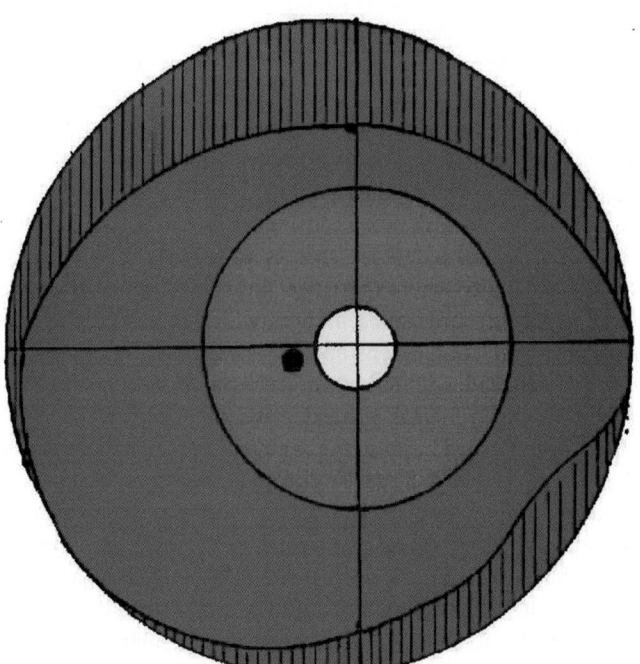

Fig. 24.8 Visual field diagram depicting the acuity divisions of the visual field of the right eye. The *yellow circle* in the center represents the fovea, the area of highest visual acuity containing only cone photoreceptor cells. The *red area* depicts the macula, which contains mostly cone photoreceptor cells. Together the macula and fovea make up the central visual field, which provides the detailed vision and color needed to identify objects. The *blue area* depicts the peripheral visual field, which contains the rod photoreceptor cells and provides the background vision needed to orient to space and maintain balance. The *black dot* is the blind spot located in the temporal portion of the visual field. (Courtesy Josephine C. Moore, PhD, OTR.)

arteries.[139] For example, Penny's hemianopia was caused by occlusion of the posterior cerebral artery. Hemianopia and other types of visual field deficits are also common following TBI.[31,139,182]

Occupational Limitations

Although often considered a mild impairment compared to the dramatic loss of the limbs, hemianopia significantly disrupts search toward the blind side. Changes in visual search include disorganization, multiple fixations, longer search times, and inability to locate relevant objects on the blind side.[200] Instead of spontaneously adopting a wider search strategy, by turning the head farther toward the blind field, the person typically turns the head very little and limits visual search to areas immediately adjacent to the seeing side of the body.[200] The person adopts this ineffective strategy because of the influence of a visual cognitive process called *perceptual completion*.[53,68] The reader will recall that the prefrontal lobes direct voluntary visual search to locate resources and threats in the environment. To increase processing speed, the frontal lobes do not visually catalog every item in the environment but instead visually *sample* the surroundings and use memory of past experiences to fill in (i.e., complete) the rest of the visual scene.[h] By enabling us to rapidly complete a visual scene based on partial visual input, perceptual completion enables us to adapt to fast-paced and dynamic environments. We are unaware that what we are seeing is based on memory and believe our perception is based only on what the retina is recording. Unfortunately, perceptual completion makes it difficult for the client who develops a visual field deficit to realize that their visual field has changed, because he or she perceives a complete visual field without gaps or missing information.[38,79,99,155] In addition, the brain cannot add an unanticipated object to a visual scene if the object was not actually seen during the sampling process. As a result, the client will be unaware of unanticipated objects in the blind side and may, for example, run into a recently placed chair in the blind field. Until the client becomes consciously aware of the field deficit, he or she will experience the odd perception of seeing a complete visual scene wherein objects are always appearing, disappearing, and reappearing without warning on the affected side. Uncertainty regarding the accuracy of visual input from the affected side often causes the client to adopt a protective strategy of attending only to visual input from the intact visual field.[38,200] Focusing on the intact field increases the chance of collisions, especially during dynamic activities such as driving a car or walking through a busy, crowded store.[29,88,110,188] Warren[190] found that 90% of participants with hemianopia experienced collisions with unexpected objects on the affected side during ambulation.

Even when the person becomes aware of a hemianopia, visual search into the blind field often is slow and delayed.[38,122,164,200] Again, the culprit is perceptual completion, which eliminates the presence of a marker to indicate the boundary between the seeing and nonseeing fields. Unable to determine the actual border of the seeing field or where a target might be located within the nonseeing field, the client naturally slows down when searching the blind field. Instead of making a single saccade to locate the target in the blind field, the person may adopt the strategy of making repeated short "stair step" saccades toward the target until it is located.[164,200] Disruption of visual search toward the affected side adds to the difficulties the client has navigating the environment and locating objects for daily occupations.[i]

When the border of the hemianopia extends into the fovea, the client may miss or misidentify visual details when viewing objects because part of the object falls into the blind field. This can create significant challenges in reading.[j] Normally sighted readers view words through a "window" or *perceptual span* that allows them to see approximately 18 characters (letters) with each fixation of the eye.[133] The reader typically moves the eye from the center of one word to the center of the next using a series of alternating fixations and saccadic eye movements. Each fixation lasts approximately 250 milliseconds (ms) and generally only one fixation is needed to decode the word.[133] The brain uses 50 ms to decode the word and 200 ms to plan the saccade to the next word in the sentence.[133] The saccade of a person reading English moves fixation 8 to 9 characters to the right, which is the typical length of English words. The remaining partially decoded letters on the right side of the perceptual span are used to plan the next saccade.[133] The left side of the span is necessary to accurately identify words and navigate through a page of text.

Hemianopia shortens the perceptual span on the side of the deficit causing the client to see only part of a word during fixation and to even miss small words.[96,156,200] For example, a client with a left hemianopia may read the sentence, "She should not shake the juice" as "shake the juice." Right HH can especially hinder reading because the truncated span not only causes the person to miss letters on the right but also disrupts execution of the saccade to the next word causing the eye to land off-center so that only a few letters are seen or to entirely miss the next word.[96,156] Clients who experience these reading errors must stop and reread words and sentences, which reduces their reading speed and comprehension. The same reading challenges occur when reading numbers in series and often with detrimental results. Whereas context alerts the client to an error when reading word because the sentence does not make sense, numbers do not have a precise context, causing mistakes to go unnoticed. For example, price tag of $368 may be misread as $68 and the error missed until purchasing the item; a recipe calling for {1/2} tsp (teaspoon) of salt may be misread as 2 tbsp (tablespoon). Clients making numerical errors quickly lose confidence in the ability to pay bills and manage their checkbook, prepare meals using recipes, or complete medication management and may turn over these important daily occupations to someone else.[79,110,188]

If the hemianopia has occurred on the same side as the dominant hand, the client may have difficulty visually guiding the hand in fine motor activities. The ability to write legibly is a commonly affected performance skill.[110,188] The client

---

[h] References 53, 67, 68, 77, 108, 132.

[i] References 38, 59, 79, 88, 110, 123, 188.
[j] References 25, 38, 79, 81, 110, 123, 129, 141, 156, 188, 200.

experiences difficulty maintaining fixation on the point of the writing instrument as the hand moves into the blind visual field, causing handwriting to drift up and down on the line. Writing over something that was just written and improperly positioning handwriting on a form are also common mistakes. Quilting, hand sewing, pouring liquids, dialing numbers on a smart phone, typing on a keyboard, and other fine motor activities are also frequently impaired.[188]

The client generally experiences only minor limitations completing basic ADLs, which are performed close to the body, but report significant difficulty completing at least one IADL.[k] Reading printed material and functional mobility are the primary performance skills most often disrupted by hemianopia.[79,110,188,200] They are also components of important IADLS, including medication management, financial management, meal preparation, home management, yard work, communication management, shopping, and driving and community mobility. For persons with hemianopia, the more dynamic the environment and the wider the field of view required to complete the occupation, the greater is the limitation. The client's ability to resume driving is always questioned, although research has shown that persons with hemianopia can safely resume driving with specific training.[29] The client's ability to follow the action in sporting events, TV shows, and movies is also impaired.[41,190]

Persons with hemianopia experience ongoing daily challenges that challenge their self-efficacy.[79] They often report feeling anxious when navigating unfamiliar environments.[38,79,188] The anxiety may be so severe that the client experiences shortness of breath, sweating, elevated heart rate in crowded environments. The anxiety can become debilitating, causing the person to withdraw from community activities and limit social participation.[79,123] Clients also report feeling less confident as they continuously make mistakes because they missed seeing something, and many admit they feel frustrated about their inability to complete valued occupations, especially driving and reading.[79] An inability to scan a dynamic scene fast enough to identify landmarks can cause some persons to fear that they will get lost in community environments, and they become reliant on others to guide them.[79,200] The twin effects of anxiety and disorientation can significantly reduce the client's ability to fulfill their varied life roles and reduce their quality of life.

Evaluation

Perimetry testing. The visual field is evaluated using a *perimetry* test. There are many types of perimetry tests ranging from simple bedside assessments, such as a confrontation test, that provide a gross indication of field loss, to the precise imaging of a microperimeter.[144,155,175] Availability, cost, and the client's ability to participate in testing often determine the selection of the test. For example, confrontation testing does not incur any expense and can be performed nearly anywhere, whereas microperimetry must be completed by a specially trained technician in a center that has purchased this expensive instrument. All perimetry testing includes three steps that occur in sequence:

(1) the person fixates on a central target, (2) a second target (or targets) of a specific size and luminosity is presented in a designated area of the visual field, (3) the person acknowledges the second target without breaking fixation on the central target. A static or kinetic test strategy is used to present the target. In a static testing strategy the target appears in a specified area of the visual field without being shown moving to that location; in a kinetic testing strategy, the target moves in from the periphery until it is identified.[200] The number of targets presented during the test can vary from less than 10 for a quick screening test to over 100 for a diagnostic test. Eye doctors use a computerized bowl perimeter such as the Humphrey Visual Field Analyzer to obtain a definitive diagnosis of a hemianopia or other field deficit.[31] For this test, the client places the chin on a chin rest and fixates on a central target inside the bowl-shaped device. As the client fixates on the central target, a second lighted target is displayed inside the bowl at varying locations and intensities. The client responds to each seen target by pushing a small button. When diagnosing a field deficit, lighted targets are often presented in over 100 locations within the field using a step threshold sequence by which the intensity of the light is incrementally increased if it is not identified on the first presentation. The result is an accurate measurement of the areas of absolute loss (no response) and relative loss (decreased retinal sensitivity) within the field.

All perimetry tests require that the person sustain visual attention over an extended period, which means it is impossible to eliminate visual attention from the evaluation process regardless of the type of perimetry test used. Persons with brain injury commonly experience limited visual attention, especially in the acute stages of recovery, and may not be able to reliably complete a diagnostic perimetry test. As a result, a definitive diagnosis often cannot be made until weeks to months into the recovery period, depending on the severity of the brain injury.[31,199]

Screening assessments must be used until the client has sufficient visual attention to complete a diagnostic perimetry test. The occupational therapist can screen for the presence of field deficit using simple standardized assessments in combination with careful observation of client performance in daily occupations. Confrontation testing is often used to provide a rough indication of visual field loss.[175] To complete a static confrontation test, the examiner sits in front of the client at a meter distance and has the client fixate on a centrally placed target (the examiner's nose). The examiner then holds up two targets in each of the four quadrants of the visual field (right upper, right lower, left upper, and left lower). The client indicates whether both targets are visible without breaking fixation on the examiner nose.[189] The examiner must monitor the client's fixation while placing the targets in the correct location. Unfortunately, when the examiner's attention is divided, the client can cheat and look at newly placed targets without the examiner's awareness. Cheating reduces the reliability of the test results. A kinetic version of the confrontation test, the two-person kinetic test, provides a more reliable response by adding a second examiner to monitor the client's fixation on the central target.[189] For this assessment, one examiner stands behind the client and moves a brightly lit penlight in from the periphery while the client fixates

---

[k] References 29, 38, 41, 79, 110, 123, 188.

on a central target held by the second examiner who sits in front of the client and observes for cheating. The first examiner moves the penlight in from the left, right, superior, and inferior field to test these areas of the field. The client indicates as soon as the target appears by saying "now" or making a hand movement. In addition to reducing cheating, the kinetic test strategy assesses the peripheral and central field while the static version only tests the central visual field. Standardized versions of these tests are included in the biVABA. Because a confrontation test can only identify gross defects, the OT must corroborate the test findings by observing client performance. If the confrontation test shows no deficit but client observation suggests that a deficit is present, the observation should carry the greater weight. Client behaviors that suggest a visual field deficit is present include changing head position when asked to view objects placed in a certain location, consistently bumping into objects or missing objects on one side of the field, and making consistent errors in reading such as missing letters and words on the side of the deficit.[189]

The Damato 30-Point Multifixation Campimeter provides a more precise alternative to confrontation testing of the central visual field. The campimeter is included in the biVABA and is also distributed by Good-Lite (https://beta.good-lite.com/search?type=product&q=damato). The test shown in Figs. 24.9 and 24.10 consists of numbered targets that test 30 points in the visual field. The test stimulus is a 6-mm black dot that is shown in a centrally placed window on the chart. The test uses a unique strategy that relies on moving the eye rather than the target. The examiner instructs the client to fixate on one of the numbered targets, then moves the black dot into the central window, and the client indicates if it was seen. If the client does not see the black dot, that point in the visual field is recorded as a loss on the recording form. The client successively moves the eye to view each numbered target until the entire central field is mapped. The campimeter's ability to identify central field deficits was compared against the gold standard Humphrey field Analyzer and found to have a sensitivity of 81% and a specificity of 72%, suggesting good accuracy.[144]

Spontaneous partial recovery of the visual field has been shown to occur in approximately half of persons with hemianopia, but a complete recovery of the visual field is uncommon.[199,200] Most recovery occurs within the first 4 weeks after onset, and the likelihood of improvement significantly decreases beyond 8 weeks.[199] Because of the low rate of complete recovery, hemianopia is generally considered to be a permanent visual impairment.[199,200] Perimetry tests establish only whether a visual field deficit is present and the size and location of the deficit. To develop an intervention plan, the OT must determine the quality and consistency of the client's ability to compensate for the field loss in daily occupations. Hemianopia significantly affects reading and mobility—two important components of many instrumental and community occupations. Therefore, additional assessment should focus on these performance skills.

Reading. The Visual Skills for Reading Test (VSRT; https://www.lowvisionsimulators.com) assesses the influence of central visual field loss on visual word recognition and eye movement control.[25] The test, also known as the Pepper Test, was

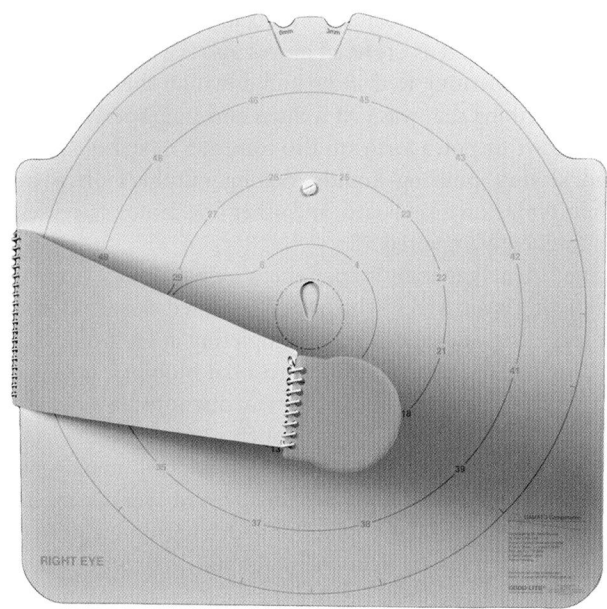

Fig. 24.9 Picture of the Damato 30-point campimeter showing the 30 numbers (arranged in a circular pattern on the board. The arm positions the client at the correct distance from the chart. The black dot appears in the window in the center of the chart. (Courtesy Good-lite; http://good-lite.com.)

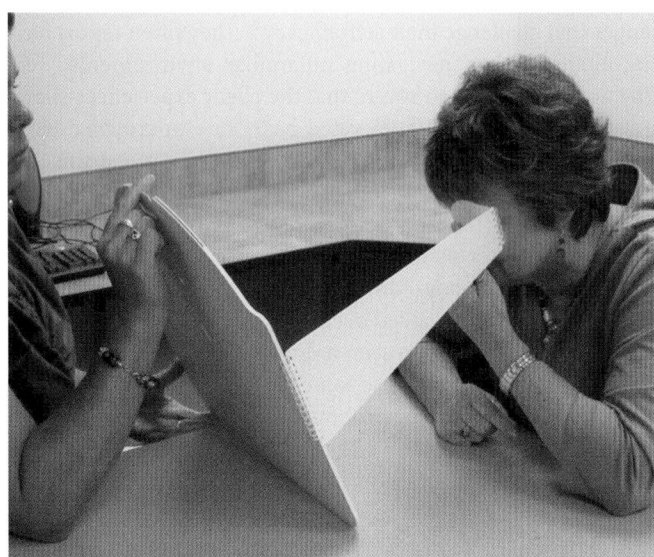

Fig. 24.10 Position of therapist and client for completion of perimetry testing using the Damato 30-point Campimeter. The therapist moves the black dot into the window in the center of the chart while the client fixates the numbered target. Without breaking fixation on the number, the client indicates when the black dot appears in the window.

developed to assess reading performance in persons with central field loss from macular degeneration and was validated as an assessment for persons with hemianopia in 2016.[25] The client is asked to read single letters and words printed on a card. The card contains words that can be transformed into another word if misread. Because the words do not appear within the context of a sentence, the person must rely solely on vision to identify the word. The test includes three versions in varying print sizes to accommodate clients with reduced acuity and to permit retest. The test measures reading accuracy and corrected reading rate and provides information on the prevalent types of reading errors. Clients with hemianopia often make errors on the Pepper test consistent with the side of their field deficit.[25,188] For example, a client with a left hemianopia may read the word "radish" as "dish," and a client with a right hemianopia may read the word "mustard" as "must."

Telephone Number Copy, part of the biVABA, provides information about the client's accuracy in reading numbers. In this test, the client copies down 10 telephone numbers comprising numbers with similar configurations, such as 6, 8, 9, and 3.[189] The OT records the number of errors made in copying down the numbers, provides the client with this feedback, and instructs the client to locate and correct the errors. Persons with hemianopia typically make mistakes accurately reading numbers located on the affected side and often confuse numbers with similar configurations. For example, a client with a left hemianopia may misread the number 9 in 938-2020 and copy down 838-2020 instead. A client should be able to use the feedback from the therapist to locate and correct errors unless their ability to engage visual attention is also impaired.

Mobility. To effectively compensate for the hemianopia, the client must use the intact field to thoroughly search the blind field. For example, a client with a left hemianopia must use the right visual field to search the left half of space. Clients with hemianopia demonstrate difficulty searching both *peripersonal space* (the space immediately around the body) and *extrapersonal space* (the space extending from the body into the environment). Deficiencies in searching peripersonal space may affect performance of ADLS completed close to the body, such as grooming, dressing, reading, and writing. Deficiencies in searching extrapersonal space may have a pronounced impact on mobility and affect activities in outside and community environments, such as driving, shopping, and mowing the yard.[79,110,188]

To safely navigate dynamic and complex community environments, the client must use a wide scanning strategy that quickly and efficiently covers the blind side. The client also must rapidly shift attention back and forth between the central and the peripheral visual fields to keep track of objects moving within the environment. A client who is compensating well for a visual field deficit should be able to symmetrically search both the right and left halves of the visual field with equal speed when standing still or moving. Large interactive light boards, which are primarily used for intervention, are often used in assessment to measure and compare the client's speed in searching the right and left halves of the visual field and ability to divide attention between the central and peripheral field. Clinics use many types of lightboards, including the Dynavision D2,[24] Bioness Integrated Therapy System,[162] and the Neuro VT.[78] The boards use a game format to engage the client while recording the number and speed at which targets are located on the board during the game. Occupational therapists without a light board can create a task analysis using a laser pointer to observe the client's search capability. The OT stands behind the client and randomly projects the laser beam onto various locations on a blank white wall. The client locates and touches the projected laser dot. The OT notes the strategy and the required time to locate the dot and compares performance between the blind and intact fields.

The biVABA ScanCourse is a standardized dual-task assessment with established reliability and validity that determines whether the client equally searches the left and right fields when navigating a hallway.[104,189] The OT constructs the course using 20 targets created by placing a one-inch black stick-on letter or number onto 3- by 5-inch white index cards. Ten targets are placed along each side of the hallway in various locations. The OT instructs the client to identify the targets while walking through the course and observes the client's accuracy in locating the targets on each side. The client is given two trials to complete the scan course. After the first trial, the therapist provides feedback on the client's performance, such as "You missed three targets on the right side; remember to turn your head to make sure you see all of the targets on that side." The client then completes the second trial by reversing and going through the course in the opposite direction. The therapist notes whether the client's performance improves on the second attempt. A client who is unable to use the therapist's feedback to improve performance on the second trial may have an attention deficit.

THREADED CASE STUDY

Penny, Part 2

The ophthalmologist completed a diagnostic perimetry test on Penny that showed a complete left hemianopia in both eyes (homonymous hemianopia) affecting both the central and peripheral fields. Of particular importance was the finding that the border of the hemianopia split the foveal field in half. This finding suggested to the OT that Penny's perceptual span for reading was probably significantly reduced on the left side, which could cause her to miss words and letters to the left of fixation. The OT used the Pepper test to confirm this hypothesis. The results of the Pepper test showed that Penny missed letters and words on the left, reducing her reading accuracy to 83% on the test. Her reading rate was 51 words per minute compared to normal average speed of 90 words per minute for her age group.[102] Because she reported difficulty accurately reading numbers, the OT also administered the biVABA Telephone Number Copy. Penny misread 3 numbers—misidentifying a 3 as an 8, a 4 as a 1, and a 5 as an 8. She was able to find her errors on the test and correct her mistakes.

The OT used a Dynavision lightboard to observe Penny's ability to search for targets in her visual field. Penny demonstrated a reaction time of 2.35 seconds to locate targets on the left half of the board compared to 1.1 seconds in the right half of the board. In observing her locate targets on the board, the OT noted that Penny moved her head very slowly to the left side of the board to locate targets and did not turn her head far enough to see targets on the edge of the board. Penny also completed a ScanCourse. On the first pass through the course, she missed 4 of 10 targets located on the left side (60% accuracy) but easily identified 10/10 targets on the right side (100% accuracy). After receiving feedback on her performance, Penny completed the second trial, walking through the course going the reverse direction. On this trial, she identified 9 of 10 targets (90%) on the left and 10 of 10 targets (100%) on the right. Her performance also indicated that she was able to use feedback to improve her search of the left side of the space and thus demonstrated good rehabilitation potential.

Activities of daily living. Persons with hemianopia typically only experience difficulty completing ADLs that rely on vision to complete. The Self-Report Assessment of Functional Visual Performance (SRAFVP) is a standardized assessment developed specifically to measure a client's ability to complete vision-dependent activities of daily living. Originally developed to assess ADL performance in older adults with age-related eye disease, the assessment was validated on a sample of persons with hemianopia in 2012.[110] The SRAFVP uses an interview format that allows clients to identify the ADLs that they most value. The assessment covers 38 basic and instrumental vision-dependent ADLs. A toolkit containing the assessment and instructions is available as a free download from the Occupational Therapy Department, University of Alabama at Birmingham (https://www.uab.edu/shp/ot/post-professional/low-vision-gc/student-resources).

THREADED CASE STUDY

Penny, Part 3

The OT administered the SRAFVP. Penny reported that she was able to successfully complete basic ADLs but had difficulty completing several IADLs. She reported that she read very slowly and made frequent mistakes, especially when reading numbers. She has difficulty reading bills and financial statements and disclosed that she did not pay a credit card bill correctly and was charged a financing fee. She uses a software program to balance her checkbook and has difficulty reconciling payments because she either incorrectly reads or enters the amount entry and then is unable to find her errors. She estimates that it takes her three times as long to complete financial management as it did before her vision loss; she becomes very anxious and avoids doing it until the last minute. Her difficulty reading numbers also creates other challenges when she renews prescriptions for herself and Pot. She frequently reads the prescription number incorrectly and because of this can no longer use the automated telephone renewal feature and must wait until she can talk to someone in person. This is very embarrassing. She also misread her blood glucometer once and injected insulin when she did not need it, which caused a reaction lasting several hours. She was an avid newspaper reader and read various sections, particularly the sports section, to Pot daily, an activity they both enjoyed, as he would recognize some of the names of local teams and players. She can no longer engage in this daily routine, nor can she read novels to Pot, which was another routine they enjoyed and one that she felt was very therapeutic for Pot. Penny also reported that she is able to complete meal preparation but spends a great deal of time scanning shelves to locate items. She also has difficulty seeing well enough to pour and measure items and occasionally misreads a recipe or enters the wrong time setting on the microwave. She related a time when she was melting chocolate for a cake batter and set the microwave on the wrong time and burned the chocolate. After that experience, she decided to stop baking for the annual church bake sale, even though she was well known for her delicious chocolate brownies.

Penny reported that her greatest limitations revolve around mobility. She is unable to drive and must depend on others for transportation. When a friend takes her shopping, she has difficulty locating the items she needs and reading the labels. Because she does not want to inconvenience her friend and slow her down, she often comes home with the wrong item or without items because she could not find them. She also admits to feeling very uncomfortable in crowded environments, especially with people moving on her left side. She states that her heart pounds and she feels an overwhelming desire to leave. She is afraid that she will collide with someone because she has experienced several instances of this and she sometimes becomes disoriented. She

and Pot attended religious services regularly before her stroke and a neighbor has offered to provide transportation, but she feels too overwhelmed to make the trip.

When asked about her art, Penny became very quiet and finally stated that she felt that this activity was also behind her now. She stated that she had tried drawing again but could not see well enough to complete the intricate line drawings that she used to do. She also could not find the supplies she needed. Instead of a joyful occupation, drawing has become a very frustrating exercise that reminds her of her disability. She stated that she did not want to resume drawing if she could not do it well.

When asked to prioritize her goals for therapy, Penny stated driving was the number one goal and reading was the second goal. She wanted to accurately complete financial management, meal preparation, and diabetes self-management, and she wanted to be able to shop independently, take Pot to appointments, and resume attending church.

Intervention

Persons with hemianopia generally experience performance limitations in mobility and reading. Slowed and inaccurate scanning of the blind side causes clients to experience difficulty navigating independently and safely engaging in daily occupations, especially those completed in dynamic environments, such as driving, shopping, and participating in community events. The client must be able to quickly scan the blind field to safely participate again in these environments. The client's challenges in reading result from an inability to adapt the present saccade strategy to the shortened width of the new perceptual span. The client experiences reduced accuracy and reading speed, which limits participation in occupations such as financial management, meal preparation, and medication management. To overcome reading challenges, the client must develop a new saccade strategy to match the new perceptual span. Because the frontal lobes exercise perceptual completion, the client often initially lacks insight into the extent and boundaries of the field deficit. Successful compensation requires the client to firmly believe that the deficit exists and that the visual input from the blind side cannot be trusted. A client able to develop this level of insight will usually learn to effectively compensate for the deficit. Therefore, every effort must be made through activities and education to make the client aware of the location and extent of the deficit.

Mobility limitations. Mobility limitations occur primarily because the client does not turn the head far enough, fast enough, or often enough toward the blind field to take in the information needed for safe mobility. If the inferior visual field has been affected, as occurs with a hemianopia, the client may also experience difficulty monitoring the support surface on the deficit side. This can result in hesitancy in walking and a tendency to keep the head down and the eyes fixed on the floor directly in front of the client. Although this strategy may keep the client from colliding with objects, it also prevents the client from monitoring the surrounding environment and can add to disorientation during ambulation.

To compensate effectively for these mobility limitations, the client must develop a habit of consciously and regularly

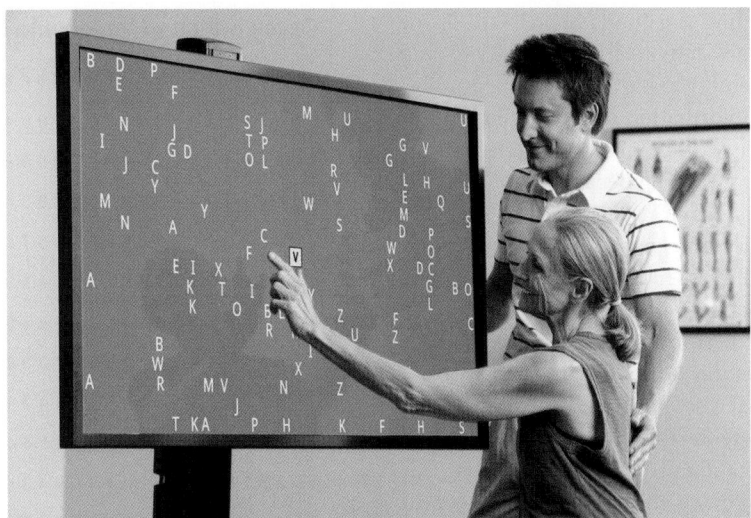

Fig. 24.11 Example of a visual search game on the Bioness Integrated Therapy System (BITS). The client searches for and touches a specified letter target on the board. The client tries to touch as many targets on the board as she can during the time allotted for the game. The game can be used to teach and reinforce efficient search patterns to compensate for visual field deficits and neglect. (Courtesy Bioness Inc., Valencia, CA.)

searching the visual field on the blind side.[l] Specifically, the client must be able to (1) initiate a wide and fast head turn toward the blind field, (2) anticipate visual input from the blind field by increasing head and eye movements toward the blind field, (3) execute an organized and efficient search pattern of the blind side, (4) attend to and detect important visual details on the blind side, and (5) quickly shift attention and search between the central visual field and the peripheral visual field on the blind side.

Combing preparatory methods and tasks with occupation-based intervention can be an effective way to develop these performance skills.[20,178] Preparatory tasks focus on increasing the speed, width, and efficiency of the search pattern toward the blind side.[m] Occupational therapists use light boards to develop the components of efficient search patterns.[24,43,78,162] The large size of the light boards automatically elicits the wide head turn needed to search the blind side. The gaming format challenges clients to give their best effort each time and responsively increases the challenge to facilitate progress. The devices record and analyze performance, identifying where deficiencies exist to enable the client to improve performance on the board. Fig. 24.11 shows a client using the Bioness BITS to improve visual scanning. In a clinic without a light board, the OT can use a laser pointer projected onto the wall and play "tag" games in which the client attempts to locate the red dot as quickly as possible.

As the basic components of the more efficient search strategy are developed, the OT should incorporate them into dual-task activities that require combining search with ambulation. Activities can include completing scan courses using cards with letters taped onto walls in various locations along hallways; activities such as "find red," in which the client points

out every red item in the surrounding environment while navigating toward a destination, and "narrated walks," in which the client points out landmarks, objects, and changes in the environment while navigating toward a destination. These activities reinforce keeping the head up during navigation to improve orientation and avoid collisions. As the client's skill in searching improves, participation in community environments should be added. Create "treasure hunt" activities that require the client to find a specific item in a designated location in the building or campus using landmarks and organized search strategies. As the client becomes more confident navigating areas surrounding the clinic, expand to completing occupations in the community like shopping for groceries, mailing a letter or buying stamps at the post office, or walking through a park. To build the client's self-efficacy, carefully grade the challenge to ensure that the client will successfully complete the task. Begin with simple challenges such as finding a single item in a small shop and expand to more difficult activities such as navigating a large grocery store.

To be successful, the client must develop habits and routines to support performance, especially in high-risk community environments. An essential habit is to stop before entering an unfamiliar environment and slowly scan the environment for potential travel hazards such as temporary and fragile displays or low-contrast features such as curb cuts and other subtle changes in the support surface. This habit helps the client build a mental representation of the space before entering; it should increase the client's confidence and reduce the likelihood of an unexpected collision. Another important habit is to closely observe unique landmarks such as a picture on a wall or a change in wall color to assist in maintaining orientation. Supportive routines include shopping at times of day when the stores are less crowded, choosing well-lighted walkways with minimal obstacles, and arriving at religious services and other events early to settle in before others have arrived.

---

[l]References 46, 75, 82, 128 129, 178, 200.

[m]References 43, 75, 82, 128, 129, 139, 145, 200.

Reading limitations. Reading is a fundamental skill if one wants to participate fully in daily activities. The inability to read not only reduces the person's ability to participate in pleasurable activities but also to acquire information needed to be healthy, safe, and autonomous. Persons with hemianopia often have the language skills to read but stop reading because they must put so much effort into seeing words and navigating text. Research shows that, with daily practice and persistence, persons with HH can improve their reading speed and accuracy.[3,118,156,157] Although not every client can devote the time and energy required to improve reading performance, every client needs to be able to acquire information normally provided in print form. Therefore, a broader goal is set for the OT intervention: to enable the client to compensate for the vision impairment and obtain and understand information provided through text. This goal can be achieved by improving the client's ability to read printed text by using technology to enable the client to obtain needed information via another method.

For clients who are strongly motivated to resume reading print, the occupational therapist can provide a structured home program that provides the practice needed to regain this skill. The client's primary challenges in reading occur because the client is trying to read using a saccade strategy designed for a wider unrestricted perceptual span. To improve reading speed and accuracy the client must learn to adapt the saccade strategy to the new perceptual span—a demanding task that can be extremely frustrating for the client. The OT assists the client to put in the required practice time by breaking the intervention into manageable steps. Preparatory tasks using pre-reading exercises such as those designed by Warren[191] or Wright and Watson[195] and commercially available word and number searches are used in the first stages of the intervention. These are search and find exercises that require the client to locate and mark designated letters, numbers, or words on worksheets (Fig. 24.12). The low cognitive requirements of the exercises enable the client to focus on perfecting the saccade strategy needed to move the new perceptual span across the page. The client completes these worksheets daily, devoting 20 to 30 minutes each day. As the client's ease and accuracy improve, the intervention switches to an occupation-based approach to transition into reading continuous text. The OT assists the client to select a large-print book on a familiar topic and instructs the client to read a chapter a day. The large print format reduces the density of the text, requiring less saccade precision, and the familiar subject matter reduces the cognitive demands on the client. The client should continue reading books on a daily basis until reading becomes less taxing. As the client regains skill in reading, have the client practice reading the materials needed to complete reading-dependent occupations such as financial management, meal preparation, and medication management. Modifications such as drawing a bold red line down the margin of the text can be used as adjuncts to assist the client with a left hemianopia to find the beginning line of text or a client with a right hemianopia find the end of the line of text. Clients who have difficulty staying on line or moving from line to line can use a ruler or card to maintain their place. These aids should be relinquished as reading performance improves because they slow reading speed.

Cross out all of the double numbers 1.5M

```
8 1 2 6 7 2 3 1 2 2 4 5 6 8 8 7 5 6 8 8 4 5 3 2 6 7 8 5 6 7 7 4 5 6 6
5 8 8 3 4 5 2 8 8 3 4 5 8 8 2 1 9 9 4 5 2 3 8 8 5 6 7 6 5 9 9 7 6 5 4
8 9 8 6 3 4 5 8 8 2 3 4 5 2 7 7 9 9 8 7 8 9 5 6 8 8 3 4 5 7 6 8 5 5 4
8 8 6 5 3 4 2 3 7 8 8 6 9 0 3 4 8 8 4 5 2 3 4 5 6 7 8 8 4 6 6 5 4 6 9
3 2 8 8 9 3 4 2 8 8 4 5 7 2 3 5 5 7 8 9 0 0 3 8 3 9 2 3 3 4 3 2 2 1 5
4 8 5 7 3 6 6 7 4 3 2 5 5 3 4 7 8 9 9 2 3 4 2 2 4 5 6 4 3 6 7 8 8 5 4
1 1 2 3 4 5 6 6 5 4 4 4 5 6 7 7 8 8 9 0 0 6 5 6 7 7 4 5 3 4 5 3 3 2 5
4 5 6 6 5 4 4 4 3 3 2 2 5 6 4 7 2 3 4 5 5 9 8 7 6 7 8 8 8 4 5 6 2 2 1
3 4 5 6 5 5 4 6 6 5 4 6 5 6 7 8 4 2 4 5 2 2 4 4 9 9 8 8 7 7 8 6 6 4 3
6 6 4 6 3 7 8 8 5 3 3 3 6 7 7 5 5 4 4 1 1 6 6 9 5 5 3 3 7 1 4 2 3 4 4
5 5 3 3 2 5 7 3 1 1 1 4 4 6 6 8 4 3 5 5 6 6 7 7 3 6 8 5 7 6 5 4 3 2 2
2 3 4 4 5 6 6 7 5 8 7 7 9 8 9 0 0 1 1 1 2 3 4 4 4 3 3 5 6 3 5 4 3 2 2
3 3 4 4 5 4 6 3 7 5 5 7 8 9 0 1 1 8 7 6 5 4 4 1 1 4 5 3 9 6 8 5 4 7 3
4 4 5 3 7 5 5 7 9 9 7 0 9 6 4 5 6 6 8 0 8 0 1 2 2 3 4 4 5 7 8 9 0 1 1
5 5 6 4 5 5 5 4 3 2 2 1 2 4 9 8 9 9 0 0 7 6 5 5 6 7 5 8 4 8 4 4 3 8 3
2 3 4 2 2 1 3 2 5 7 6 8 5 4 4 5 7 3 4 3 2 1 3 5 6 7 7 8 0 0 6 3 2 3 2
3 3 4 4 2 2 5 7 7 8 9 9 0 7 6 5 5 4 4 3 7 7 5 4 3 3 2 2 1 2 3 3 4 5 6
3 3 4 4 4 5 5 6 6 7 4 2 2 5 8 0 7 6 8 6 5 3 3 3 3 7 8 0 6 4 2 4 5 6 6
6 6 4 6 3 7 8 8 5 3 3 3 6 7 7 5 5 4 4 1 1 6 6 9 5 5 3 3 7 1 4 2 3 4 4
5 5 3 3 2 5 7 3 1 1 1 4 4 6 6 8 4 3 5 5 6 6 7 7 3 6 8 5 7 6 5 4 3 2 2
2 3 4 4 5 6 6 7 5 8 7 7 9 8 9 0 0 1 1 1 2 3 4 4 4 3 3 5 6 3 5 4 3 2 2
8 8 6 5 3 4 2 3 7 8 8 6 9 0 3 4 8 8 4 5 2 3 4 5 6 7 8 8 4 6 6 5 4 6 9
3 2 8 8 9 3 4 2 8 8 4 5 7 2 3 5 5 7 8 9 0 0 3 8 3 9 2 3 3 4 3 2 2 8 5
```

© 1996 vis**ABILITIES** Rehab Services Inc.

Fig. 24.12 Example of a pre-reading exercise. The client is instructed to cross out all of the double numbers on the page. (From Warren M: *Pre-Reading and Writing Exercises for Persons with Macular Scotomas.* Courtesy visAbilities Rehab Services Inc., Hoover, AL.)

Assistive devices and technology can enable clients to acquire information without visual reading. The OT assists the client to determine the best device, app, and software to meet his or her needs.[39] Begin by modifying accessibility features on devices the client is already using. Adjust the brightness and background color of the screen; enhance the size, color, and boldness of text, icons, and cursors; and teach the client to use built-in features, such as zoom, voice-over, and speech to text. Locate apps and software that will enable the client to complete a specific task using voice commands. Many types of inexpensive talking devices are readily available. Examples include talking glucose monitors, scales, blood pressure meters, watches, clock, calculators and food scales. Internet-connected virtual assistants such as Apple Siri, Amazon Echo, and Google Home can be programed to perform a variety of functions: setting a timer; telling the time, the outside temperature, and the weather forecast; and ordering items. Be sure to provide instruction on how to use all apps, software, or devices to ensure the client can use it to meet their daily needs. Whenever possible try to eliminate the need for the client to read. *For example, Penny's OT solved the*

THREADED CASE STUDY

Penny, Part 4

Penny received 10 sessions of 1 hour of outpatient OT intervention over a 10-week period. She was motivated to improve her reading performance and was given pre-reading exercises to help her modify her saccade strategy to match her reduced perceptual span. She completed the exercises at home for 30 minutes each day. The Pepper test was repeated at 5 weeks and showed that her reading accuracy had increased to 92% and her corrected reading rate increased to 72 words per minute. The Telephone Number Copy test was also repeated, with 100% accuracy. As Penny's performance improved, the occupational therapist introduced reading large-print books with familiar content to begin the transition to reading continuous text. Penny and Pot loved the Harry Potter books. A friend took Penny to the library to check out a large print version of the first book, and she read the book daily to Pot for an hour. The OT repeated the Pepper test at discharge; Penny demonstrated 100% accuracy with a corrected reading rate of 124 words per minute.

The OT completed a home visit in the third week to evaluate Penny's environment and to meet Pot. A friend from Penny's women's church group and a fellow artist who had been taking her to therapy also attended the session. The assessment showed that Penny's home generally had sufficient lighting, contrast, and organization. However, the kitchen had only a single small round ceiling light that provided insufficient lighting of the countertops and work surfaces., Her cupboards were also packed with food and cookware and her countertops were cluttered with appliances and food items. Penny's studio was also cluttered and had only overhead lighting and a small table lamp. The OT suggested replacing the small overhead lighting fixture in the kitchen with a large 40-inch LED fixture and adding LED under-cabinet lighting to illuminate the countertops. The OT suggested cleaning out the cupboards and removing rarely used items and expired food, and then adding a two-tiered cabinet organizer so that items were stored on rows that were one item deep to make them more visible. The OT also recommended that Penny remove all items from the countertops except those that she used on a daily basis. Although Penny was still resistant to resuming her art, the OT made suggestions to improve the lighting in her studio by adding a 50-watt halogen task lamp on her worktable along with increasing organization and decreasing clutter. The OT also recommended that she purchase a Big Eye lamp—a lamp that combines a low-power magnifier with a high-intensity light (https://www.bigeyelamp.com)—to assist her to see details more clearly. The OT provided detailed information on where to purchase these items, and Penny's friend took notes and shared them with members of their church group; all of the recommendations were implemented within 2 weeks.

Penny's friend contacted the OT and expressed interest in how she might help Penny resume her art. The OT suggested that she could help Penny explore other forms of artistic expression that were not as visually demanding as her detailed line drawings. The next week Penny reported in therapy that she and her friend had attended an art fair on the weekend and she thought she might try watercolor landscapes, something she had done early in her career. Her friend planned to bring her watercolor paints over, and they were going to experiment together.

The OT used environmental and task modification and adaptive devices to address Penny's ability to complete meal preparation, financial management, and diabetes self-management. Penny practiced using the big eye lamp and a talking calculator to verify numbers and reconcile her checkbook. The OT suggested that Penny consider setting up automatic monthly payment withdrawals from her bank account for services that she paid for monthly such as utilities, credit card, and phone. Her son told her that he would set up these accounts when he came to visit in a couple of weeks. The OT also taught Penny how to access and set up the accessibility features on her computer to enlarge the cursor, increase contrast, magnify text and icons on the screen, and use audio descriptions. It was critical that Penny inject the correct insulin amount and accurately monitor her blood glucose levels. To address this, the OT taught Penny how to use the big eye lamp to verify that she had set her insulin pen accurately, The OT also asked Penny's primary care doctor to prescribe a talking glucometer and trained Penny how to use it. The improved lighting and organization implemented after the home assessment greatly improved Penny's ability to complete meal preparation. She was now able to clearly see the touchpad settings for the microwave and more easily locate cooking ingredients and tools. The OT also recommended that she purchase a set of measuring spoons and cups with large high-contrast numbers.

To address mobility, the OT began by having Penny complete a series of exercises on a lightboard for the first 20 minutes of each session. The exercises focused on increasing the speed and efficiency of Penny's search pattern to the left, her ability to shift attention between the center and peripheral areas of the board, and search with cognitive distractions. The OT set up scan courses along the hallways of the center and had Penny engage in "find red," narrated walks, and treasure hunts. As Penny improved on indoor activities, the OT moved outdoors and had Penny navigate sidewalks and areas adjacent to the clinic. Penny practiced consciously turning her head widely and surveying her surroundings to locate potential obstacles and identify landmarks prior to entering an unfamiliar environment. As her comfort and confidence in navigating these environments increased, Penny completed a community outing with the OT to her local grocery store to practice the skills she had learned and receive instruction in how to quickly and efficiently scan shelves to locate needed items. Additional community outings were completed in her local pharmacy and in her church, where she also tried out using the rose-colored filters she had purchased earlier. Two weeks before discharge, Penny excitedly reported that she and Pot had attended church and afterward had lunch with friends with no difficulty.

The OT addressed driving throughout the intervention period. The lightboard exercises Penny completed improved the visual scanning skills she needed for driving: specifically executing frequent, fast, and wide search of the left side. The OT discussed the specific challenges that hemianopic drivers experience, strategies to compensate for these limitations, and vehicle modifications that help compensate for field loss. When Penny had shown sufficient improvement, she was referred to a driving program for an on-the-road evaluation with an occupational therapist credentialed as a certified drivers rehabilitation specialist (CDRS). Penny passed the driving evaluation, and her physician released her to resume driving during daylight hours over familiar routes.

challenge of filling her prescriptions by helping her set up automatic refills at her pharmacy. Penny was also able to alert the pharmacist to her vision loss and need for larger-print labels.

The occupational therapist addresses handwriting by teaching the client to slow down and monitor the pen tip as the hand moves across the page and into the blind side. Preparatory activities that require tracing lines and shapes help the client learn how to position the paper and pen so that the pen tip stays visible on the line. Practice filling out blank checks, addressing envelopes, and filling in a check register helps the client learn to apply handwriting to daily occupations.

The OT also must modify the environment and task to increase visibility and structure as described in the overview on intervention at the beginning of this chapter. Adding color and contrast to the key structures in the environment needed for safe navigation and orientation (e.g., door frames and furniture) will help the client locate these structures more quickly. Using black felt-tip pens and bold-line paper to increase the contrast in writing materials will help the client more accurately monitor the pen tip in handwriting. The simple addition of a high-quality light often increases speed and reduces errors in reading and improves mobility. Reducing pattern in the environment by eliminating clutter and using solid-colored objects enhances the client's ability to locate items more quickly. Creating a structured and predictable environment reduces the need for constant scanning. All of these modifications reduce the amount of effort the client must generate to compensate for the visual field deficit and increases the likelihood that the client will participate in the occupation, which is the ultimate goal.

Visual Attention

Visual attention is the ability to observe objects closely to acquire information about their features and their relationship to self and other objects in the environment. It requires an ability to ignore irrelevant sensory input and random thought processes in order to sustain focus for several seconds to several minutes.[132] Visual attention also entails being able to shift visual focus from object to object in an organized and efficient manner. We engage visual attention through visual scanning or search (these last two terms interchangeable). Although scanning and attention are separated within the visual perceptual hierarchy to help to understand them, they cannot be separated in evaluation and intervention. Any change in visual attention will be observed in the client as a change in the scanning pattern used for visual search.

Visual attention is divided into two broad categories: selective visual attention and global visual attention. Selective attention enables the person to accurately distinguish visual details such as differences between letters, numbers, and faces. It is used to recognize and identify objects.[56,70] Global attention focuses on the location of objects in the environment and their proximity to the person. Its job is to ensure that a person is able to stay oriented and move safely through space, and it depends on seeing the big picture rather than the details.[56,64,70,74] Without global attention, collisions with objects and disorientation when moving would be the norm. To be able to fully engage and learn from the environment, a person must simultaneously employ these two modes of visual attention at all times. The contribution of each is equally important to perceptual processing. Adults without brain injury use an organized, systematic, and efficient pattern to complete visual search.[n] Task demands determine the search pattern we will use; for example, we use a linear strategy to read a book or search for an item on a shelf. [57,94]

Visual Spatial Neglect

Deficits in visual attention commonly occur after brain injury.[70,86,137] Visual spatial neglect is one of the most common attention deficits in persons with acquired brain injury from stroke or head trauma.[179] Kerkhoff and Schenk[90] defined

neglect as the "impaired or lost ability to react to or process sensory stimuli (visual, auditory, tactile olfactory) presented in the hemispace contralateral to a lesion of the human right or left cerebral hemispheres" (p. 1072). There are several key words in this definition that delineate the features of neglect. First, ability can be "impaired" or "lost," implying that there are degrees of severity of the condition ranging from mild to severe. Second, persons can have difficulty "reacting" to stimuli (noticing and responding to it), or difficulty "processing" stimuli (using the sensory information to complete a task). Third, persons can experience inattention to different kinds of sensory input, not just visual. Finally, persons experience impaired attention to incoming sensory input "contralateral" or on the opposite side of the location of the lesion. This means that persons with right hemisphere lesions experience difficulty attending to visual input from the left side of the body midline and vice versa. There is consensus among researchers that neglect represents a heterogeneous disorder characterized by a complex and diverse set of behaviors.[137,164,179] These behaviors can be generally grouped into three broad categories of impairment: (1) a lateralized bias in attending to and searching space, (2) a lateralized inability to map and build internal mental representations of space on the left side of the body, and (3) a nonlateralized impairment in arousal and ability to focus, shift, and sustain attention.[1,18,137,179,180] The diversity of behaviors associated with neglect result from disruptions within the large distributed network that controls visual attention that includes the prefrontal, temporal, parietal, and occipital lobes within the cortex and the brainstem, thalamus, and cerebellum.[179] The diverse areas of the network communicate extensively with each other through the long white matter pathways that connect areas of the brain to each other.[51] Brain injuries damage these pathways, disconnecting areas and disrupting network actions at multiple areas, including those that may not have been directly damaged by the brain injury.[51,198] Visual neglect is predominantly caused by brain injuries affecting the occipital, parietal, temporal, and prefrontal areas of the right hemisphere.[137,179] Visual neglect also may be compounded by neglect of the limbs on the left side of the body or neglect of auditory input from the left side.[27,90,137,179]

Spatial bias. Spatial bias restricts the person's ability to explore the space contralateral (e.g., opposite) to the side of the brain injury. It is the most prominent and consistent behavior associated with neglect caused by right hemisphere lesions and manifests as a difficulty or inability to explore space on the left side of the body.[117,137,179,180] The person may make no attempt to search the left side or make fewer visual fixations and slower eye movements to the left, contributing to slow and incomplete search of the left space.[93,117,186] The person experiences spatial bias toward the right side that alters the normal visual search pattern. Instead of initiating a symmetric left to right search pattern, the client with neglect begins and confines search to the right side of a visual array.[117] This rightward bias creates an asymmetric search pattern depriving the client of needed information on the left side of objects and visual arrays. This can significantly impair the client's ability to complete ADLs that require attention to both sides of the body, such as dressing,

---

[n] References 57, 94, 103, 111, 190, 192.

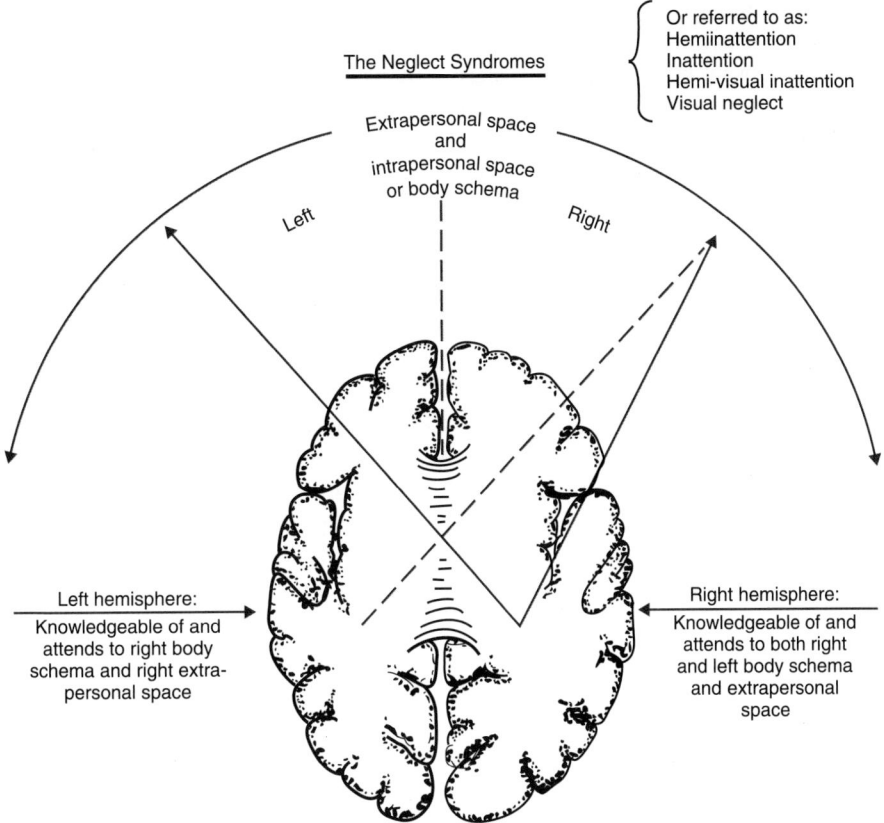

In relation to **movement** and **sensory perceptions** such as vision (visual-spatial and visual-object awareness and recognition), auditory and somesthetic (including body image or schema) cognition and awareness, it appears that the left hemisphere primarily attends to the right extrapersonal space and/or body image parameters, while the right hemisphere attends to both right and left extrapersonal space and body image. Thus **left hemisphere lesions** of the 1°, 2° or 3° areas of the cerebral cortex or associated subcortical fiber tracts concerned with visual, auditory, somesthetic, or motor functions rarely result in a neglect syndrome because the right hemisphere can attend to and compensate for the left hemisphere deficit. However, **right hemisphere lesions** of one or more of these functional areas leave the brain unable to attend to or be aware of the left extrapersonal space and body schema. Visual field deficits (especially left homonymous hemianopia) always compound the neglect syndrome.

Fig. 24.13 Difference in capabilities of the right and left hemispheres to direct visual attention and the relationship of hemisphere lesions to neglect syndrome. (Courtesy Josephine C. Moore, PhD, OTR.)

bathing, eating, grooming, meal preparation, home management, and shopping.[13,92,93]

Left hemisphere cortical lesions can cause right neglect, but the condition occurs with less severe and obvious changes in behavior.[166] The strong association of spatial bias with right hemisphere lesions is thought to occur because of a difference in the way the hemispheres direct visual attention.[51,179,180,198] As illustrated in Fig. 24.13, the left hemisphere directs attention toward the right half of the visual space surrounding the body, while the right hemisphere directs visual attention toward both the right and left halves of space. If a lesion occurs in the left hemisphere, visual attention and search toward the right side are diminished, but the right hemisphere still provides some attentional capability. A similar lesion in the right hemisphere may completely eliminate attentional capability toward the left

because the left hemisphere does not direct attention toward the left side.

Inattention to the left side due to neglect can be confused with the presence of left hemianopia in the client. Although both conditions may cause the client to miss visual information on the left side (and they can occur together), left neglect and left hemianopia are distinctly different conditions that disrupt search performance in different ways.[198] When left hemianopia occurs, the client attempts to compensate for the loss of vision by engaging visual attention.[198] The client directs eye movements toward the left in an attempt to gather visual information from the blind side. Unfortunately, because of perceptual completion, the client may not always move the eyes far enough into the blind visual field to locate objects and features on the left, and this may give the impression of inattention to the left.[198] In contrast, a client with neglect has lost the attentional mechanisms that drive the search for visual information on the left. Even with an intact visual field, the client makes little attempt to search the left side of the visual space.[117] Visual search is most significantly impaired when the two conditions occur together.[179] In this case the client does not receive visual input from the left side because of the hemianopia and does not compensate for the loss of visual input by directing attention toward the left side. Clients who have both conditions show greater inattention toward the left visual space when completing ADLS[14] and experience more difficulty moving the eyes or the head toward the left side.[1,90,137,179]

Impaired mental representation of space. Mental representations of space are internally generated cognitive maps of the space that surrounds the body.[18,26,64,71,83] The maps are continuously updated as the body moves through space. Persons with neglect may experience a disruption of representational space in which objects located on the left side simply disappear from their concept of space. According to Becchio and Bertone,[18] it is as though the mental map of space on the left side did not exist in the past, does not exist in the present, and will never exist in the future. As a result, the client does not attend to landmarks on the left side and does not build a map of environments on the left side. This diminishes the ability to orient to and maintain orientation in space, and clients are often observed at times to be literally "lost in space" as they try to navigate environments.[26]

Difficulty conceptualizing left space may explain the consistency of the client's inattention to the left and also the client's lack of insight regarding the missing space.[18,26] It may also explain another commonly observed behavior associated with spatial neglect called *revisiting*, in which the person repeatedly reexamines objects located on the right side of a visual array while ignoring objects on the left.[137,165] For example, if asked to locate a cup of pudding situated on the left side of the dinner tray, the client will repeatedly search the right side of the tray even though the pudding is not there.

Nonlateralized attention deficit. Persons, especially those with persistent (also called chronic) neglect, often have difficulty generating adequate levels of alertness and sustaining attention.[o] The impairment of attention is nonlateralized, meaning that it does not affect attention to one side differently from the other, but instead affects the brain's overall ability to receive and process visual information. This generalized diminishment of attention impairs the ability to attend to specific tasks, and the client often drifts off and loses focus while completing activities.[135]

Persons with low arousal may have difficulty generating sufficient attention to engage and participate in a task.[180] The energy requirements for the task must be amped up to secure the client's attention. For example, have a client seated on the edge of the mat table rather than seated in a wheelchair to complete a task so that the threat of falling over increases the client's alertness. Inability to sustain attention is particularly detrimental to successful completion of daily occupations because even the simplest ADL requires the sequencing steps over time. The client loses focus and drifts off while completing an activity; this lapse of attention disrupts working

visual memory and sequencing, requiring the occupational therapist to provide continuous redirection to the task. Persons with nonlateralized inattention may also experience difficulty disengaging from one object to shift attention to another object, slowing search performance even when attending to a task.[180] This slowness increases the length and effort required to complete a task, causing fatigue and poor performance.[179]

Occupational Limitations

Visual attention is modulated through an extensive neural network involving the entire brain; therefore, some capacity for visual attention generally is retained even in cases of severe brain trauma.[108] Conversely, because so much of the brain contributes to attention, changes in visual attention occur even with mild brain injuries.[32] Neglect creates asymmetry and gaps in the visual information gathered through visual search. The incomplete search pattern can create challenges completing tasks that require symmetric attention and search. The client misses needed details on the left that can cause confusion when reading and dangerous behavior while navigating through environments.[p] How much the diminishment of visual attention affects occupational performance depends on the circumstances and attentional demands of tasks.[28] For example, reading can require enormous amounts of selective and sustained visual attention when the person is reading a highly technical textbook, and much less when reading comics in the newspaper. Driving requires continuous global attention to monitor the speed and position of other vehicles and objects, and sporadic selective attention to identify landmarks, street signs, and traffic lights.

Evaluation

As a process found at the intermediate level of the visual perceptual hierarchy, visual attention is affected by deficits in the lower-level visual functions of visual acuity, oculomotor function, and visual field. Aphasia and motor impairment can also affect performance on visual attention assessments. Therefore, these client factors must be evaluated first before assessing visual attention. Because visual search is the outward, motor expression of visual attention, it is assessed by observing how the client initiates and carries out visual search when completing a task. The assessment seeks to answer the following questions: (1) "Does the client initiate the normal left-to-right and top-to-bottom search strategy?" (2) "Does the client execute the search strategy in an organized and efficient manner?" (3) "Does the client search symmetrically and obtain complete visual information from both sides of the array?" (4) "Is the client able to sustain visual search, or does the client appear to drift off during search?" (5) "Does the client accurately locate targets?" (6) "Does the client's search ability decrease as the visual complexity of the task increases?"

Cancellation tests are frequently used to evaluate changes in visual search and have been shown to be sensitive to uncovering the spatial bias from neglect.[137,179] Cancellation tests are usually paper and pencil tests consisting of rows of single letters, numbers, or symbols. The examiner instructs the client to search through

---

[o]References 135, 163, 172, 173, 179, 180.

[p]References 26, 131, 138, 177, 179, 193.

NAME: _____B.D._____ DATE:_____

P   F

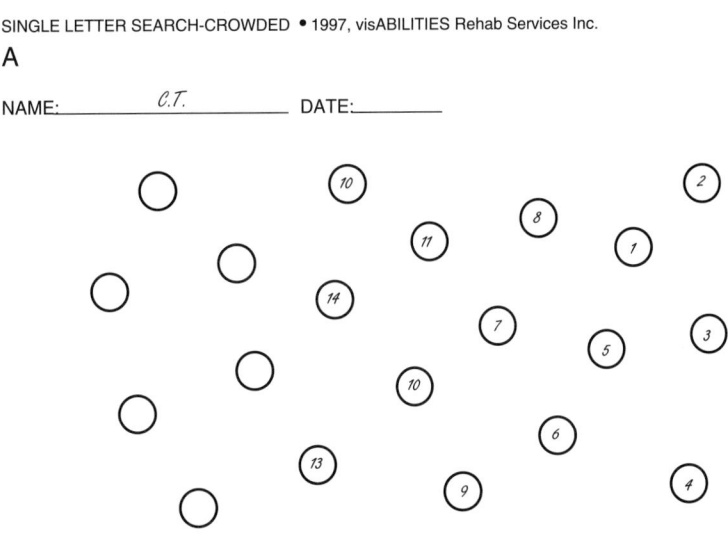

SINGLE LETTER SEARCH-CROWDED • 1997, visABILITIES Rehab Services Inc.

A

NAME: _____C.T._____ DATE:_____

RANDOM PLAIN CIRCLES-SAMPLE   ©1997, visABILITIES Rehab Services Inc.

B

Fig. 24.14 Examples of ineffective search patterns used by clients to complete two visual search subtests of the Brain Injury Visual Assessment Battery for Adults. (A) A client with hemianopia uses an abbreviated search pattern to cross out the letters P and F on the subtest; the client executed an organized left-to-right linear search pattern but failed to locate the beginning of the line on the left side, and as a result failed to cross out targets on that side (the *circled letters*). (B) A client with neglect and left hemianopia who used an asymmetrical abbreviated search pattern was instructed to number open circles consecutively from 1 to 20, choosing any pattern desired. The client began numbering the circles on the right side of the page and proceeded to number only the circles on the right, failing to number the remaining six circles on the left side of the page.

the rows and cross out (e.g., cancel) a specific target (Fig. 24.14) and records completion time and accuracy. Adults without brain injury demonstrate specific characteristics of search strategies on cancellation tests that ensure good accuracy and speed completing the test.[19,166,192] These characteristics include strategies that are linear, organized, symmetric, thorough, and consistent. Warren and colleagues[192] found that the most commonly used strategy on the blVABA cancellation tasks was a left to right and top to bottom linear reading strategy; they also found that most persons consistently employ the same strategy to complete a single cancellation task or a series of cancellation tasks.

When completing a cancellation test, a client with hemianopia may demonstrate an abbreviated search pattern toward the blind side, resulting in an omission of targets and search slowly for targets, especially toward the blind field (see Fig. 24.14A). However, (unless visual attention is diminished), the client's search pattern is organized, consistent, and thorough, resulting in accurate identification of targets in the seen field. The client also responds to a cue such as "be sure to search the left side" to improve performance. A client with neglect will also demonstrate an abbreviated search toward the left side with target omissions but in contrast to the client with hemianopia, the search pattern is often random and unpredictable, reflecting their difficulty selectively focusing and sustaining attention (see Fig. 24.14B).[1,137,166,179] The organization and accuracy of the client's search pattern may also deteriorate when they scan more complex visual arrays. Thus, one way to differentiate between left hemianopia and hemiinattention is to observe the client's search strategies on a cancellation test. Observing the client copy a line drawing of a familiar object like a clock, house, or flower onto a sheet of paper provides additional information about the ability to conceptualize space on the left side.[137,179,189] Clients with neglect often omit details on the left side of their drawings and/or skew the drawing toward the right side, suggesting difficulty accessing a mental representation of the left side of the image.[137,179,198]

Assessments that require the client to scan widely toward the neglected side are needed to determine how the client searches extrapersonal space. The ScanBoard (part of the biVABA) is a simple assessment that can be completed with clients in the early stages of recovery. The test consists of a large (20- by 30-inch) board with 10 numbers displayed in a butterfly type pattern. The OT centers the board at eye level and instructs the client to point out the numbers on the board one at a time as the client sees them. The OT records the pattern the client follows in identifying the numbers. Research comparing adults with brain injury from stroke to a matched cohort of adults without brain injury showed that the control group employed an organized sequential search pattern, beginning on the upper left side of the board and proceeding in either a clockwise or counterclockwise fashion until all of the numbers were identified.[190] In contrast, adults with diminished attention from stroke showed disorganized, random, and often abbreviated search strategies, frequently missing numbers on one side of the board. Light board games also can be used to assess the client's attentional capabilities. Games with multiple, widely scattered targets challenge working visual memory and provide opportunities to observe the client's ability to rapidly shift attention between the left and right fields. Games that extend over several minutes test the person's ability to sustain attention. The biVABA ScanCourse also provides insight into the client's ability to attend. Recall that the client completes the course, is given feedback on the performance, and completes the course a second time. Most clients with left hemianopia can use this feedback to commit fewer errors on the left during the second trial, but clients with neglect often lack the attentional capability to improve their performance.

Information gathered from observing the client complete visual search assessments should reveal a pattern of deficiencies in attention and search that also affect the client's ability to complete ADLs. For example, the client who initiates and confines search to the right side on a cancellation test often demonstrates the same asymmetric pattern while searching for grooming items in the bathroom. The client's level of performance depends on the severity of the attention deficit. Clients with mild inattention generally are able to complete basic and habitual daily activities and experience difficulty only on tasks that are unfamiliar or require search of a complex visual array. In contrast, clients with severe neglect may have difficulty with basic tasks such as locating all the food on their plate.[14] The Catherine Bergego Scale is a widely used validated assessment that measures the impact of neglect on completion of basic ADLS.[14,105,107,198] The occupational therapist observes the client complete 10 ADL and mobility items and assigns each item a point value using a 4-point rating scale (0 = no neglect, 1 = mild, 2 = moderate, 3 = severe neglect). The points are added to provide a cumulative score ranking the client's level of neglect: zero (0 points), mild (1–10), moderate (11–20), and severe (21–30).

THREADED *CASE STUDY*

Penny, Part 5

The ophthalmologist who referred Penny to OT noted that she had neglect in addition to the left hemianopia. Because neglect can interfere significantly with completion of ADLs, especially driving, it was important to determine how much, if any, of Penny's difficulty scanning was due to inattention. To assess this, the OT administered the biVABA visual search subtests, which use a cancellation format. On the first subtest, Penny missed several of the targets located on the left side of the sheet, demonstrating an abbreviated search pattern toward the left. The OT provided a verbal cue "to be sure to look far enough toward the left to see the border of the paper." Penny acknowledged the cue and located the rest of the targets on the left; she also made sure to begin her search on the far-left side on each of the remaining subtests. She consistently used an organized left to right and top to bottom search strategy on all seven subtests. She also carefully looked at each target and rechecked her work for accuracy. These observations suggested normal attention capability, which was verified by her performance on other assessments. For example, although she made mistakes in copying numbers on the Telephone Number Copy test, she was able to search and correct her mistakes without assistance. She also missed targets on the left side during her first pass through the ScanCourse, but after receiving feedback, made no errors on her second trial on the course. On the Dynavision she was able to switch attention easily between the left and right sides of the board, and her ability to search the left side of the board rapidly improved with practice. After analyzing Penny's performance on these assessments, the OT concluded that the severity of Penny's vision loss caused her to appear inattentive toward the left because of perceptual incompletion. But as she gained awareness of the extent of her deficit, she was able to use attention to help compensate for the loss of vision on the left. If Penny's performance had suggested the presence of neglect, the OT would not have set a goal to resume driving and would have explored alternative forms of transportation.

Intervention

The incidence of visual spatial neglect averages between 50% and 70% in the early stages of recovery from a right hemisphere brain injury.[66,87,179] Fortunately, most neglect resolves during the first year of recovery and is significantly diminished by 3 months after injury in most persons.[66,87,116,179] Disruption of the pathways that connect the frontal, temporal, parietal, and occipital lobes together may account for the initially high incidence of neglect immediately after injury and the good potential for recovery.[51] Persons whose neglect persists beyond 3 months may have significant and persistent deficits that reflect structural rather than pathway damage within the brain.[87]

Persons with neglect experience difficulty locating and using resources from the environment to complete daily activities. Performance limitations may include difficulty locating items on the left side in daily tasks,[14] sustaining attention long enough to complete an activity,[180] dividing and shifting attention between tasks,[180] and rapidly and accurately assessing situations in dynamic environments because of limitations in working visual memory.[201] Generally, the more dynamic and ambiguous the environment, the greater the limitations the client will experience due to the demand on visual attention.[28,180] The goal of OT intervention is to enable the client to use his or her attentional capabilities to complete needed daily activities. The OT intervention focuses on creating an environment that supports attention, improving the client's ability to compensate for inattention when searching tasks and environments, improving the client's ability to sustain attention to task completion, and developing habits and routines that reduce visual stress. Before a client can learn to reorganize visual search, he or she must develop insight into how visual search and attention have changed.[92,167,168] Therefore, education is a key component of intervention process that begins during evaluation by using cuing and feedback to alert the client to deficiencies in their search pattern. During intervention the OT can use the client's difficulties or mistakes as teachable moments to improve insight into capabilities and limitations.[89,92,168]

Modify the environment.
The most powerful tool in the occupational therapist's toolkit is creating an environment that supports attention. Intervention focuses on modifying the environment and task to reduce demand on the client's visual attention and helping them use their limited attention capabilities. The key question to ask when planning the intervention is "How can I modify the task/environment to help the client use his or her current attentional capability more effectively to complete occupations?" The first step is to eliminate and minimize features that stress visual processing. These include low-contrast features, insufficient lighting, glare, and too much pattern.[42] Minimizing pattern is a key intervention as dense pattern demands greater selective attention to locate desired objects.[57] The client may not be able to sustain the effort needed to sift through the pattern and subsequently views the environment as filled with "visual noise" rather than meaningful objects. Reducing distractors has been shown to improve effectiveness of the search pattern in persons with neglect.[42,85,161] Another key intervention is to increase the visibility of features that trigger prediction and sequencing. Remember that the neocortex initiates and guides actions by predicting what is going to happen, verifying it through sensory feedback, and modifying as needed.[16] The process begins with detecting and recognizing the environmental feature that will trigger memory and unlock the sequence.

A visible and explicit environment makes it easier for the client to recognize key features and create a meaningful context for action.[57] Research has shown that making targets more explicit elicits an efficient and faster search pattern in persons with neglect by creating a "pop out" effect that grabs the person's attention.[42,57,85,161] An example of using contrast to create a pop out effect would be wrapping a piece of bright orange fluorescent tape around a call button to distinguish it from the bed rail. Strategically adding task lighting to spotlight the components of an ADL task (see Fig. 24.4) helps the client focus attention to complete the task.[73] Adding structure and organization by finding a place for everything and keeping everything in its place is the final critical piece in creating an "attention promoting"

environment.[57] Altogether, making these modifications enables the client to make maximum use of limited attentional capabilities to complete occupations and encourages participation.

Compensation.
Visual scanning training (VST) has a sufficient level of evidence to be considered a practice standard for intervention aimed at reducing the effect of spatial bias on the client's search pattern.[34] VST is a top-down compensatory approach that employs the higher-level functions of language and cognition to help the client learn and employ a structured search pattern that begins on the left side of a visual array and progresses left to right.[q] The use of this structured and proscribed pattern helps the client compensate for the tendency to restrict visual search to the right side and increases the symmetry of the search pattern. The OT can use a variety of preparatory tasks, activities, and occupations to provide practice using this compensatory pattern.[89,178] The following guidelines describe key components to consider when selecting a visual scanning task:

1. *Select activities that require the client to scan as broad a visual space as possible.* To help the client learn to initiate and complete a wide visual search, make the working area of the activity large enough to require the client either to turn the head or to change body positions to accomplish the task. Many activities and games can be enlarged to require head turning to complete visual search. For example, the OT can lay out a deck of playing cards facing up, in rows 3 to 4 feet wide, and ask the client to match the cards with another deck of playing cards, turning the pairs over as the match is made. Ensure that the client initiates a left-to-right, top-to-bottom pattern to locate the matching cards. An occupation-based approach might involve planting, watering or weeding flowers in a garden.

2. *Select activities that require the client to interact physically with the target.* Attention is more focused when the person must act on what is seen. Games such as solitaire and dominoes or video or lightboard games are examples of activities with interactive qualities. Occupations such as cooking, cleaning, and laundry require physical interaction within a wide space.

3. *Select activities that require conscious attention to visual details and careful inspection and comparison of targets.* To facilitate selective attention, require the client to consciously study objects to identify their relevant features. Games such as solitaire, Connect Four, checkers, and dominoes have these qualities. Large piece puzzles, word or number searches, crossword puzzles, adult coloring books, and crafts such as latchet hook, knitting, and paint by number also require selective attention. Encourage the client to recheck his or her work to make sure that critical details are not missed.

4. *Select activities that require the client to sustain attention.* Several influential researchers think that the inability to stay on task underlies neglect and contributes its chronicity, and that rehabilitation focused on sustaining attention can reduce neglect behaviors.[135,163,173,180] Interventions that employ continuously challenging and interactive activities have been shown to increase alertness and the ability to sustain attention.[163,172,180] Fast-paced lightboard and video

---

q References 13, 20, 66, 69, 130, 160.

games that use a go-no-go format are examples of activities that challenge the client to sustain and shift attention.[172,180] All IADLs require sustained attention, and most also require the client to interact with left and right space.

5. *Use visualization to reinforce the correct search pattern.* Niemeier[113] demonstrated that clients with severe chronic neglect could be taught to search left space using a visual imagery technique called the "lighthouse strategy" (p. 40). The intervention placed a simple line drawing of a lighthouse in the client's line of sight to act as a visual cue. The client was instructed to imagine searching like a lighthouse and to scan widely from left to right. All rehabilitation staff cued the client to look at the picture and imagine being a lighthouse before completing an activity. Study participants required various amounts of rehearsal to learn the strategy, but a statistically significant increase in search performance was found after the training. The findings were replicated in a second study that showed statistically significant improvements in route finding, navigation (with or without a wheelchair), and problem-solving tasks.[114]

Occupation.   The goal of OT intervention is to enable the client to complete daily occupations, and this goal is best achieved using occupation. Using occupation as the intervention approach helps the occupational therapist select emotionally relevant and meaningful activities. Emotions tell the brain to "pay attention—this is important," and valued and practiced activities enable the client to tap into expertise and reduce effort and fatigue.[50,79,92,132,148] Evidence for the effectiveness of using occupation to improve attention is still limited but growing, as researchers demonstrate that engaging persons with neglect in emotionally relevant and motivating activities increases attention to the left side.[r] Tham and associates[167] found that participation in everyday activities that were personally relevant and meaningful made it easier for clients with neglect to learn compensatory search strategies because the client was *interested* in using the strategy to complete the task. Klinke and colleagues[92] confirmed the importance of using daily activities in a qualitative study on persons with chronic neglect. Participants reported that it was easier to attend to concrete and meaningful tasks and tasks that held high emotional relevance. For example, one participant reported how much easier it was to hold her baby and make formula to feed her than to make coffee (which she did not drink) and hold a coffee cup. It was also easier to apply compensatory strategies when activities used familiar objects.[167] Activities that place too much demand on attention can exacerbate spatial bias in persons with neglect.[28,180] To avoid overwhelming the client, grade the activity to provide the "just right" attentional challenge; for example, start with preparation of a simple breakfast and progress to a four-course meal. Occupations that incorporate both sides of the body such as playing musical scales on a piano or listening to music played through headphones also have been shown to reduce neglect.[21,27,33,80]

Delivery of the intervention is also important. Tham and Kielhofner[168] and Klinke and associates[92] found that nurturing and positive responses from staff and family increased motivation to learn compensatory strategies to increase awareness of the left side. Persons with neglect respond poorly to ambiguous situations because they put more stress on working memory.[42] Provide explicit instructions and ensure that the activity has a clear outcome. For example, instead of instructing the client to "put the cookies on the baking tray" say "place *12 cookies* on the tray;" instead of "brush your teeth" say "brush your teeth for 10 counts." Repetition is important: the more often the strategy is repeated under varied circumstances, the more the skill is generalized and transferred to new situations.[89,174] Incorporate practice into completing basic ADLs and IADLS. For example, require the client to use a left-to-right search strategy to select clothes from a closet, search for items in a refrigerator, or shop for groceries. Hospital-based rehabilitation programs can use cafeterias, gift shops, and office areas within the facility and surrounding restaurants and shops to expose the client to more demanding visual environments.

Metacognition.   The metacognitive approach has been shown to be an effective intervention for clients capable of using language and cognitive ability to focus attention.[34] The intervention uses a reflective, problem-solving approach that requires the client to plan, execute, and evaluate the successful completion of a task. A simple example of a metacognitive approach would be to require the client to first describe the steps in putting on a shirt, then verbally describe each step out loud while donning the shirt, and conclude by reviewing whether the shirt was donned correctly. Tham and associates[167] used a metacognitive approach to improve ADL performance with clients with chronic neglect. The researchers found that teaching the client to consciously reflect on how to proceed before beginning an activity and then to continue to consciously reflect while completing the activity in order to monitor performance increased the likelihood of a successful outcome. An occupational therapy intervention, the Cognitive Orientation to Occupational Performance (CO-OP), has been used extensively to facilitate occupational performance in persons with neurological conditions[149] and specifically shown to improve performance in persons with mild TBI.[2,34,44,45,84]

Sensory input strategies.   Sensory input strategies use a bottom-up approach that alters sensory input into the brain to reduce rightward spatial bias and increase attention to the left.[13,66,90,160,172] Yoked prism adaptation is the most widely used sensory input intervention.[66] Multiple studies, including several randomized control trials, have been published on the use of this intervention in patients with neglect.[66] The intervention requires the client to wear strong prisms (worn in eyeglasses) that shift images toward the right side while completing a task that requires monitoring of the hand such as placing or painting an object. To successfully complete the task, the client must learn to shift to the left to compensate for the rightward shift of objects. Repetition of tasks using the prism results in increased attention to left space when the prism is removed. Although a majority of studies have shown positive results in increasing attention toward the left, an inconsistency in results suggests the need for further research to establish the best protocols to achieve an optimal outcome.[13,47,66,69,130]

---

[r] References 27, 50, 89, 92, 117, 148, 149, 167.

Small studies have shown that applications of galvanic vestibular or optokinetic stimulation, neck muscle vibration, transcranial magnetic stimulation, and constraint-induced therapy with patching can increase orientation toward the left side in persons with neglect.[s] More research is needed to determine the most appropriate clinical application of these interventions before they will be used widely in rehabilitation.[69,90,184]

Complex Visual Processing

In everyday living, complex visual processing is applied to solve a problem, formulate a plan, or make decisions about specific situations. The OT's understanding of the client's visual processing limitations obtained through standardized assessments and observation is helpful but cannot predict how the client will actually perform within the context of a practiced and valued occupation. Typically, tasks that require complex visual processing also demand complex cognitive processing. The person relies not just on vision, but on a variety of sensory input and memories to determine the right course and complete the task. The more experience a person has had completing a complex task, the better he or she is at recognizing the pertinent, salient features of a visual scene and recalling and formulating a successful plan when returned to the familiar context of the occupation.[108] *For example, an experienced driver such as Penny who has lived in the same area for many years would likely perform*

more competently if asked to drive the familiar roads that she has traveled hundreds of times, than in the artificial context of a driving simulator. Because of the contextual nature of complex visual processing, the best way to evaluate it is to observe the client complete daily tasks that require this level of processing. Thus, for example, if the client is a teacher planning to return to work, the OT should assess the client's ability to develop lesson plans, teach a concept, grade a paper, or other aspects of the job, preferably at the client's place of employment. The OT should also simulate as closely as possible the client's natural context for the task. This will require some creativity and effort, but it is the only way to provide a fair assessment of the client's abilities and determine whether the client is able to resume the desired occupation.

THREADED *CASE STUDY*

Penny, Part 6

This approach was used to determine if Penny was safe to resume driving. The OT/certified driving rehabilitation specialist (CDRS) who evaluated Penny's ability to resume driving conducted a behind-the-wheel evaluation that required Penny to drive for 60 minutes in various types of traffic. During the evaluation the CDRS asked Penny to drive to destinations that she typically traveled to when completing errands, including the grocery store, her church, the doctor's office, the library, and the senior center where her painting guild met.

---

[s]References 66, 69, 90, 130, 196, 198.

SUMMARY

Everything we do as human beings involves sequencing actions over time to accomplish goals. The brain links incoming visual input with past experience to unlock the context for an action and predict what is going to happen next. The process begins with detecting and recognizing the task/environmental feature that will trigger visual memory and unlock the sequence. Brain injury or disease that disrupts visual processing creates gaps in the visual information sent to the brain. The quality of a person's occupational performance decreases because the brain does not have sufficient or accurate visual information to guide actions. Penny's left hemianopia, for example, caused her to misread words and sentences because she did not always see letters and words on the left side. This limited her ability to complete daily occupations that relied on reading, such as medication management, shopping, financial management, and meal preparation. Her inability to quickly and efficiently scan toward her blind field caused her to collide with persons and objects on the left and experience disorientation. This affected her ability to navigate environments safely and to drive. The need for OT intervention depends on whether the visual deficit prevents successful completion of needed and desired daily living activities. As the primary caregiver for an ailing husband, Penny needed to be able to manage the family finances, prepare meals, manage the house, shop, and take care of both of their medical needs. Had Pot been able, he would have assumed most of these responsibilities for Penny. As a caregiver, Penny also needed the

creative outlet and release that her art provided to help her cope with her additional responsibilities.

The framework for assessment and intervention rests on the concept of a hierarchy of visual perceptual processing levels that interact with and subserve one another. Because of the unity of the hierarchy, a process cannot be disrupted at one level without an adverse effect on all visual processing. To understand how the client's vision has changed and, more importantly, how well the client is able to use vision to complete daily activities, OT assessment must measure performance at all levels of the hierarchy and especially the foundation visual functions: acuity, oculomotor control, visual field, and visual attention. For example, Penny's hemianopia caused her to miss objects in the left visual field, creating the impression that she was ignoring the left side, which is a characteristic of neglect. Assessment demonstrated that she had normal attentional capability but had not yet learned to compensate for the hemianopia.

The OT role on the rehabilitation team is to ensure that the client is able to participate in daily occupations. That goal may be achieved through interventions that focus on modification, compensation, adaptation, and, when appropriate, remediation. Penny learned compensatory strategies that improved her ability to use her remaining right visual field to compensate for the left visual field deficit. The most powerful tool in the OT toolkit is to use modification to create a visible and explicit environment that facilitates the client's ability to use vision to complete occupations. Penny learned how to add lighting and contrast, remove pattern, and structure her environment so she could more easily use her remaining vision to complete activities. This improved person-environment fit reduced the stress caused by her vision loss and increased her participation in daily occupations. The client benefits most when a team approach is used to address visual impairment from brain injury. The optimal rehabilitation team includes optometry, ophthalmology, and other vision rehabilitation specialists as needed. Penny's ophthalmologist diagnosed the hemianopia and referred her to a low vision rehabilitation program that treated persons with acquired brain injury; the optometrist in the program completed a comprehensive refraction to ensure that Penny's eyeglasses provided the best possible acuity. A certified driving instructor (CDRS) determined whether Penny was able to resume driving.

There is no guarantee that the client's visual capabilities will recover, and much more research is needed to determine the most efficacious interventions to restore visual processing after acquired brain injury. This means that OT must maximize the client's ability to use their current visual processing to successfully complete valued occupations, keeping in mind that engagement in daily activities promotes neuroplasticity within the brain and improves health-related quality of life.[49,92,150,167,185]

REVIEW QUESTIONS

1. What determines whether intervention is needed for a client with a visual impairment?
2. What aspects of environments/tasks can be modified to create an optimal person-environment fit that promotes the client's ability to use vision in daily activities?
3. When would partial occlusion be used with the client? Describe the technique used to apply partial occlusion.
4. How does convergence insufficiency affect reading performance?
5. What prevents a client from automatically compensating for a hemianopia by turning the head farther to see around the blind field?
6. What is the primary compensatory visual search strategy taught to the client with neglect?
7. What is the most crucial lower-level visual process contributing to the ability to complete visual cognitive processing?
8. What changes occur in the visual search pattern of a client with hemiinattention?

For additional practice questions for this chapter, please visit eBooks.Health.Elsevier.com.

REFERENCES

1. Adair JC, Barrett AM: Spatial neglect: clinical and neuroscience review: a wealth of information on the poverty of spatial attention, *Annals New York Academy of sciences* 1142:21–43, 2008.
2. Ahn S, et al: Comparison of cognitive orientation to daily occupational performance and conventional occupational therapy on occupational performance in individuals with stroke: a randomized controlled trial, *NeuroRehabil* 40:285–292, 2017.
3. Aimola L, et al: Efficacy and feasibility of home-based training for individuals with homonymous visual field defects, *Neurorehabil Neural Repair* 28:207–218, 2014.
4. Albright TD: High-level visual processing: cognitive influences. In Kandel ER, Schwartz JH, Jessell TM, Siegelbaum SA, Hudspeth AJ, editors: *Principles of neural science* ed 5, New York, 2013, McGraw-Hill.
5. Alvarez TL, et al: Concurrent vision dysfunctions in convergence insufficiency with traumatic brain injury, *Optom Vis Sci* 89:1740–1751, 2012.
6. American Academy of Ophthalmology (nd): About ophthalmology & eye. MDS. http://www.aao.org/about/what-is-ophthalmology.
7. American Occupational Therapy Association: Occupational therapy practice framework: domain and process, ed 4, *Am J Occup Ther* 74(Suppl 2):1–87, 2020.
8. American Occupational Therapy Association (nd): Low vision: specialty certified practitioners. https://www.aota.org/Education-Careers/Advance-Career/Board-Specialty-Certifications-Exam/practitioners/specialty-low-vision.aspx.
9. American Optometric Association (nd): Neuro-optometry. https://www.aoa.org/optometrists/tools-and-resources/vision-rehabilitation/neuro.
10. American Optometric Association (nd): What is a doctor of optometry? http://www.aoa.org/about-the-aoa/what-is-a-doctor-of-optometry?sso=y.
11. Arditi A: Improving the design of the letter contrast sensitivity chart, *Invest Ophthalmo Vis Sci* 46:2225–2229, 2005.
12. Armstrong RA: Visual problems associated with traumatic brain injury, *Clin Experi Optom* 101:716–726, 2018.
13. Azouvi P, Jacquin-Courtois S, Luauté J: Rehabilitation of unilateral neglect: evidence-based medicine, *Annals Phys Rehabil Med* 60:191–197, 2017.
14. Azouvi P, et al: Behavorial assessment of unilateral neglect: study of the psychometric properties of the Catherine Bergego Scale, *Arch Phys Med Rehabil* 84:51–57, 2003.
15. Bainbridge D: *Beyond the zonules of Zinn: a fantastic journey through your brain*, Cambridge, MA, 2008, Harvard University Press.
16. Barrett LF: *How emotions are made: the secret life of the brain*, Boston, 2017, Houghton, Mifflin, Harcourt.
17. Beasley IG, Davies LN: Visual stress symptoms secondary to stroke alleviated with spectral filters and precision tinted ophthalmic lenses: a case report, *Clin Exp Optom* 96:117–120, 2013.
18. Becchio C, Bertone C: Time and neglect: abnormal temporal dynamics in unilateral spatial neglect, *Neuropsychologia* 44:2775–2782, 2006.
19. Benjamins JS, et al: Multi-target visual search organisation across the lifespan: cancellation task performance in a large and demographically stratified sample of healthy adults, *Aging Neuropsychol Cogn* 26:731–748, 2019.
20. Berger S, et al: Effectiveness of interventions to address visual and visual-perceptual impairments to improve occupational

performance in adults with traumatic brain injury: systematic review, *Am J Occup Ther* 70, 2016.

21. Bernardi NF, et al: Improving left spatial neglect through music scale playing, *J Neuropsychology* 11:135–158, 2017.

22. Berthold-Lindstedt M, et al: Vision-related symptoms after acquired brain injury and the association with mental fatigue, anxiety and depression, *J Rehabil Med* 51:499–505, 2019.

23. Bertone A, Bettinelli L, Faubert J: The impact of blurred vision on cognitive assessment, *J Clin Exp Neuropsychol* 29:467–476, 2007.

24. Blackwell C, et al: Dynavision normative data for healthy adults: reaction test program, *Am J Occup Ther* 74:1–6, 2020.

25. Blaylock SE, et al: Validation of a reading assessment for persons with homonymous hemianopia or quadrantanopia, *Arch Phys Med Rehabil* 97:1515–1519, 2016.

26. Boccia M, et al: The way to "left" Piazza del Popolo: damage to white matter tracts in representational neglect for places, *Brain Imaging Behav* 12:1720–1729, 2018.

27. Bodak R, et al: Reducing chronic visuo-spatial neglect following right hemisphere stroke through instrument playing. *Front Hum Neurosci.* 8:413, 2014. https://doi.org/10.3389/fnhum.2014.00413.

28. Bonato M, Cutini S: Increased attentional load moves the left to the right, *J Clin Exp Neuropsychol* 38:158–170, 2016.

29. Bowers A: Driving with homonymous visual field loss: a review of the literature, *Clin Exp Optom* 99:402–418, 2016.

30. Brahm KD, et al: Visual impairment and dysfunction in combat-injured servicemembers with traumatic brain injury, *Optom Vis Sci* 86:817–825, 2009.

31. Bruce BB, et al: Traumatic homonymous hemianopia, *J Neuro Neurosurg Psychiatry* 77:986–988, 2006.

32. Cantu R, Hyman M: *Concussions and our kids*, Boston, 2012, Harper Books.

33. Chen M-C, et al: Pleasant music improves visual attention in patients with unilateral neglect after stroke, *Brain Injury* 27:75–82, 2013.

34. Cicerone KD, et al: Evidence-based cognitive rehabilitation: systematic review of the literature from 2009 through 2014, *Arch Phys Med Rehabil* 100:1515–1533, 2019.

35. Ciuffreda KJ, et al: Occurrence of oculomotor dysfunctions in acquired brain injury: a retrospective analysis, *Optometry* 78:155–161, 2007.

36. Ciuffreda KJ, et al: Vision therapy for oculomotor dysfunctions in acquired brain injury: A retrospective analysis, *Optometry* 79:18–22, 2008.

37. Cockerham GC, et al: Eye and visual function in traumatic brain injury, *J Rehabil Res Dev* 46:811–818, 2009.

38. Cole M: When the left brain is not right the right brain may be left: report of personal experience of occipital hemianopia, *J Neuro Neurosurg Psychiatry* 67:169–173, 1999.

39. Copolillo A, Ivanoff SD: Assistive technology and home modification for people with neurovisual deficits, *Neurorehabilitation* 28:211–220, 2011.

40. Costello F: Vision disturbances in multiple sclerosis, *Seminars Neuro* 36:185–195, 2016.

41. Costela FM, et al: People with hemianopia report difficulty with TV, computer, cinema use, and photography, *Optom Vis Sci* 95:428–434, 2018.

42. Cox JA, Davies AM: Keeping an eye on visual search patterns in visuospatial neglect: a systematic review, *Neuropsychologia.* Neuropsychologia. 146:107547, 2020. https://doi.org/10.1016/j.neuropsychologia.2020.107547.

43. Crotty M, et al: Hemianopia after stroke: a randomized controlled trial of the effectiveness of a standardised versus an individualized rehabilitation program, on scanning ability whilst walking, *NeuroRehabilitation* 43:201–209, 2018.

44. Dawson DR, et al: Using the cognitive orientation to occupational performance (CO-OP) with adults with executive dysfunction following traumatic brain injury, *Canadian J Occup Ther* 72:115–127, 2009.

45. Dawson DR, et al: Occupation-based strategy training for adults with traumatic brain injury: a pilot study, *Arch Phys Med Rehabil* 94:1959–1963, 2013.

46. De Haan GA, et al: The effects of compensatory scanning training on mobility in patients with homonymous visual field defects: further support, predictive variables and follow-up, *PLoS ONE* 11:e0166310, 2016.

47. DeWit L, et al: Does prism adaptation affect visual search in spatial neglect patients: a systematic review, *J Neuropsychol* 12:53–77, 2018.

48. Digre KB, Brennan KC: Shedding light on photophobia, *J Neuroophthalmol* 32:68–81, 2012.

49. Doidge N: *The brain that changes itself: stories of personal triumph from the frontiers of brain science*, New York, 2007, Penguin Books.

50. Domínguez-Borràs J, et al: Emotional processing and its impact on unilateral neglect and extinction, *Neuropsychologia* 50:1054–1071, 2012.

51. Doricchi F, et al: White matter (dis)connections and gray matter (dys)functions in visual neglect: gaining insights into the brain networks of spatial awareness, *Cortex* 44:983–995, 2008.

52. Dos Santos N, Andrade SM: Visual contrast sensitivity in patients with impairment of functional independence after stroke, *BMC Neuro* 12(12):90, 2012. https://doi.org/10.1186/1471-2377-12-90.

53. Dowling JE: *Understanding the brain: from cells to behavior to cognition*, New York, 2018, W.W. Norton & Company.

54. Du T, Ciuffreda KJ, Kapoor N: Elevated dark adaptation thresholds in traumatic brain injury, *Brain Inj* 19:1125–1138, 2005.

55. Duffy M: *Making life more livable: simple adaptations for living at home after vision loss*, New York, 2002, American Foundation for the Blind Press.

56. Dutton GN: Cognitive vision, its disorders and differential diagnosis in adults and children: knowing where and what things are, *Eye* 17:289–304, 2003.

57. Eckstein MP: Visual search: a retrospective, *J Vis*, 11:14, 2011. https://doi.org/10.1167/11.5.14.

58. Elliott AF, McGwin G Jr, Owsley C: Vision impairment among older adults residing in assisted living, *J Aging Health* 25:364–378, 2013.

59. Falkenberg HK, et al: "Invisible" visual impairments. A qualitative study of stroke survivors' experience of vision symptoms, health services and impact of visual impairments, *BMC Health Serv Res* 20(1):302, 2020. https://doi.org/10.1186/s12913-020-05176-8.

60. Fimreite V, Willeford KT, Ciuffreda KJ: Effect of chromatic filters in visual performance in individuals with mild traumatic brain injury (mTBI): a pilot study, *J Optom* 9:231–239, 2016.

61. Finn C: An occupation-based approach to management of concussion: Guidelines for practice, *Open J Occup Ther* 7(2), 2019. https://doi.org/10.15453/2168-6408.1550. article 11.

62. Fletcher DC, Colenbrander A: Introducing rehabilitation. In Fletcher DC, editor: *Low vision rehabilitation: caring for the whole person*, San Francisco, 1999, American Academy of Ophthalmology Monograph Series, No 12, pp 1–9.

63. Fox SM, Koons P, Dang SH: Vision rehabilitation after traumatic brain injury, *Phys Med Rehabil Clin North America* 30:171–188, 2019.

64. Freedman DJ, Ibos G: An integrative framework for sensory, motor, and cognitive functions of the posterior parietal cortex, *Neuron* 96:1219–1234, 2018.

65. Frolov A, Feuerstein J, Subramanian PS: Homonymous hemianopia and vision restoration therapy, *Neurol Clin* 35:29–43, 2017.

66. Gammeri R, et al: Unilateral spatial neglect after stroke: current insights, *Neuropsychiatric Dis Treatment* 16:131–152, 2020.

67. Gilbert CD: Intermediate-level visual processing and visual primitives. In Kandel ER, Schwartz JH, Jessell TM, Siegelbaum SA, Hudspeth AJ, editors: *Principles of neural science* ed 5, New York, 2013, McGraw-Hill.

68. Gilbert CD: The constructive nature of visual processing. In Kandel ER, Schwartz JH, Jessell TM, Siegelbaum SA, Hudspeth AJ, editors: *Principles of neural science* ed 5, New York, 2013, McGraw-Hill.

69. Gillen G, et al: Effectiveness of interventions to improve occupational performance of people with cognitive impairments after stroke: an evidence-based review, *Am J Occup Ther* 69:1–9, 2015.

70. Goldberg E: *The new executive brain: frontal lobes in a complex world*, New York, 2009, Oxford University Press.

71. Goldberg ME, Wurtz RH: Visual processing and action. In Kandel ER, Schwartz JH, Jessell TM, Siegelbaum SA, Hudspeth AJ, editors: *Principles of neural science* ed 5, New York, 2013, McGraw-Hill.

72. Greene JDW: Apraxia, agnosias, and higher visual function abnormalities, *J Neuro, Neurosurg, Psychiatry* 76:25–34, 2005.

73. Green M, Barstow B, Vogtle L: Lighting as a compensatory strategy for acquired visual deficits after stroke: two case reports, *Am J Occup Ther* 72:e1–e6, 2018.

74. Greenwald BD, Kapoor N, Singh AD: Vision impairment in the first year after traumatic brain injury, *Brain Injury* 26:1338–1359, 2012.

75. Hanna KL, Hepworth LR, Rowe FJ: The treatment methods for post-stroke visual impairment: a systematic review, *Brain Behavior* 7:e00682, 2017.

76. Hawkins J, Ahmad S: Why neurons have thousands of synapses, a theory of sequence memory in neocortex, *Front Neural Circuits* 10, 2016. https://doi.org/10.3389/fncir.2016.00023.

77. Hawkins J, Ahmad S, Cui Y: A theory of how columns in the neocortex enable learning the structure of the world, *Front Neural Circuits* 1:81, 2017. https://doi.org/10.3389/fncir.2017.00081.

78. Hayes AS, Chen CS, Clarke G, Thompson A: Functional improvements following the use of the NVT vision rehabilitation program for patients with hemianopia following stroke, *NeuroRehabilitation* 31:19–30, 2012.

79. Hazelton C, et al: A qualitative exploration of the effect of visual field loss on daily life in home-dwelling stroke survivors, *Clin Rehabil* 33:1264–1273, 2019.

80. Hegde S: Music-based cognitive remediation therapy for patients with traumatic brain injury, *Front Neurology* 5:e1–7, 2014.

81. Hepworth LR, Rowe FJ: Visual impairment following stroke – the impact on quality of life: a systematic review, *Ophthalmol Res: An Internat J* 5:1–15, 2016.

82. Howard C, Rowe F: Adaptation to poststroke visual field loss: A systematic review, *Brain Behavior* 8:e1–e22, 2018.

83. Huang R-S, Sereno MI: Multisensory and sensorimotor maps. In: Vallar G, Coslett HB, editors: *Handbook of clinical neurology*, 151, 2018, Elsevier. https://doi.org/10.1016/B978-0-444-63622-5.00007-3.

84. Hunt AW, et al: Feasibility and effects of the CO-OP approach in postconcussion rehabilitation, *Am J Occup Ther* 73:1–10, 2019.

85. Hunt LA, Bassi CJ: Near-vision acuity levels and performance on neuropsychological assessments used in occupational therapy, *Am J Occup Ther* 64:105–113, 2010.

86. Husain M, Kennard C: Distractor-dependent frontal neglect, *Neuropsychologia* 35:829–841, 1997.

87. Karnath H-O, et al: The anatomy underlying acute versus chronic spatial neglect: a longitudinal study, *Brain* 134:903–912, 2011.

88. Kasneci E et al: Homonymous visual field loss and its impact on visual exploration: a supermarket study, *Trans Vis Sci Tech* 3:1–10, 2014.

89. Kawabata K, Hoshiyama M: Meaningful occupation: a self-awareness intervention for patients with unilateral spatial neglect, *New Zealand J Occup Ther* 66:4–10, 2019.

90. Kerkhoff G, Schenk T: Rehabilitation of neglect: an update, *Neuropsychologia* 50:1072–1079, 2012.

91. Khan A, et al: Visual complications in diabetes mellitus: beyond retinopathy, *Diabetic Med* 34:478–484, 2017.

92. Klinke ME, et al: "Getting the left right": the experience of hemispatial neglect after stroke, *Qual Health Res*:1–14, 2015.

93. Kortman B, Nicholls K: Assessing for unilateral spatial neglect using eye-tracking glasses: a feasibility study, *Occup Ther Health Care* 30:344–355, 2016.

94. Land MF: Vision, eye movements, and natural behavior, *Vis Neurosci* 26:51–62, 2009.

95. Laukkanen H, Scheiman M, Hayes JR: Brain Injury Vision Symptom Survey (BIVSS) questionnaire, *Optom Vis Sci* 94:43–50, 2017.

96. Leff AP, et al: Impaired reading in patients with right hemianopia, *Ann Neurol* 47:171–178, 2000.

97. Legge GE: *Psychophysics of reading in normal and low vision*, Mahwah, New Jersey, 2007, Lawrence Erlbaum Associates.

98. Leigh RJ, Zee DS: *Neurology of eye movements*, ed. 4, New York, 2006, Oxford University Press.

99. Levine DH: Unawareness of visual and sensorimotor deficits: a hypothesis, *Brain Cogn* 13:233–281, 1990.

100. Lin H, Lema GM, Yoganathan P: Prognostic indicators of visual acuity after open globe injury and retinal detachment repair, *Retina* 36:750–757, 2016.

101. Lotery AJ, et al: Correctable visual impairment in stroke rehabilitation patients, *Age Ageing* 29:221–222, 2000.

102. Lott L, et al: Reading performance in older adults with good acuity, *Optom Vis Sci* 78:316–324, 2001.

103. Lowe MX, et al: Discriminating scene categories from brain activity within 100 miliseconds, *Cortex*:275–287, 2018.

104. Lund P, et al: Evaluating the measurement properties of the ScanCourse, a dual-task assessment of visual scanning, *Am J Occup Ther* 74:7401185040, 2020.

105. Luukkainen-Markkula R, et al: Comparison of the Behavioural Inattention Test and the Catherine Bergego Scale in assessment of hemispatial neglect, *Neuropsychol Rehabil* 21:103–116, 2011.

106. Magone MT, Kwon E, Shin SY: Chronic visual dysfunction after blast-induced mild traumatic brain injury, *J Rehabil Res Dev* 51:71–80, 2014.

107. Marques CLS, et al: Validation of the Catherine Bergego Scale in patients with unilateral spatial neglect after stroke, *Dement Neuropsychol* 13:82–88, 2019.

108. Medina JJ: *Brain rules*, Seattle, WA, 2008, Pear Press.

109. Meister M, Tessier-Lavigne M: Low level visual processing: the retina. In Kandel ER, Schwartz JH, Jessell TM, Siegelbaum SA,

Hudspeth AJ, editors: *Principles of neural science* ed 5, New York, 2013, McGraw-Hill.

110. Mennem TA, Warren M, Yuen HK: Preliminary validation of a vision-dependent activities of daily living instrument on adults with homonymous hemianopia, *Am J Occup Ther* 64:478–482, 2012.

111. Najemnik J, Geisler WS: Eye movement statistics in humans are consistent with an optimal search strategy, *J Vision* 8:1e–14e, 2008.

112. National Eye Institute (nd): *Refractive errors.* https://www.nei.nih.gov/learn-about-eye-health/eye-conditions-and-diseases/refractive-errors.

113. Niemeier JP: The Lighthouse Strategy: use of a visual imagery technique to treat visual inattention in stroke patients, *Brain Injury* 12:399–406, 1998.

114. Niemeier JP, Cifu DX, Kishore R: The Lighthouse Strategy: improving the functional status of patients with unilateral neglect after stroke and brain injury using a visual imagery intervention, *Top Stroke Rehabil* 8:10–18, 2001.

115. Norup A, et al: An interdisciplinary visual team in an acute and sub-acute stroke unit: providing assessment and early rehabilitation, *NeuroRehabilitation* 39:451–461, 2016.

116. Nurmi L, et al: Occurrence and recovery of different neglect-related symptoms in right hemisphere infarct patients during a 1-year follow-up, *J Inter Neuropsychol Soc* 24:617–628, 2018.

117. Ohmatsu S, Takamura Y, Fujii S: Visual search pattern during free viewing of horizontally flipped images in patients with unilateral spatial neglect, *Cortex* 113:83–95, 2019.

118. Ong Y-H, et al: Read-Right: a "web app" that improves reading speeds in patients with hemianopia, *J Neuro* 259:2611–2615, 2012.

119. Osman EA: Glaucoma after open globe injury, *Saudi J Ophthalmol* 29:222–224, 2015.

120. Owsley C: Contrast sensitivity, *Ophthalmol Clin North Am* 16:171–177, 2003.

121. Owsley C, et al: The visual status of older persons residing in nursing homes, *Arch Ophthalmol* 125:925–930, 2007.

122. Pambakian ALM, et al: Scanning the visual world: a study of patients with homonymous hemianopia, *J Neuro, Neurosurg Psychiatry* 69:751–759, 2000.

123. Papageorgiou E, et al: Assessment of vision-related quality of life in patients with homonymous visual field deficits, *Graefe's Arch Clin Exp Ophthalmol* 245:1749–1758, 2007.

124. Park U-C, et al: Clinical features and natural history of acquired third, fourth, and sixth cranial nerve palsy, *Eye* 22:691–696, 2008.

125. Park WL, et al: Rehabilitation of hospital inpatients with visual impairments and disabilities from systemic illness, *Arch Phys Med Rehabil* 86:79–81, 2005.

126. Phillips PP: Treatment of diplopia, *Semin Neuro* 27:288–298, 2007.

127. Politzer TA: Case studies of a new approach using partial and selective occlusion for the clinical treatment of diplopia, *NeuroRehabilitation* 6:213–217, 1996.

128. Pollock A, et al: Interventions for visual field defects in people with stroke, *Cochrane Database Sys Rev*:CD008388, 2019. https://doi.org/10.1002/14651858.CD008388.pub3.

129. Pouget M-C, et al: Acquired visual field defects rehabilitation: critical review and perspectives, *Annals Phys Rehabil Med* 55:53–74, 2012.

130. Priftis K, et al: Visual scanning training, limb activation treatment and prism adaptation for rehabilitating left neglect: who is the winner? *Front Hum Neurosci* 7:1–11, 2013.

131. Qiang W, et al: Reliability and validity of a wheelchair collision test for screening behavioral assessment of unilateral neglect after stroke, *Am J Phys Med Rehabil* 84:161–166, 2005.

132. Ratey JJ: *A user's guide to the brain*, New York, 2001, Vintage Books.

133. Rayner K: Eye movements in reading and information processing: 20 years of research, *Psychol Bull* 124:371–422, 1998.

134. Reddy AVC, et al: Reading eye movements in traumatic brain injury, *J Optom* 13:155–162, 2020.

135. Robertson IH: Do we need the "lateral" in unilateral neglect? Spatially nonselective attention deficits in unilateral neglect and their implications for rehabilitation, *Neuroimage* 14:S85–90, 2001.

136. Roche S, et al: Assessment of the visual status of older adults on an orthopaedic unit, *Am J Occup Ther* 68: 465–471, 2014.

137. Rode G, et al: Semiology of neglect: an update, *Ann Phys Rehabil Med* 60:177–185, 2017.

138. Rodriguez AR, Barton JJS: The 20/20 patient who can't read, *Canadian J Ophthalmol* 50:257–264, 2015.

139. Rowe FJ, et al: A prospective profile of visual field loss following stroke: prevalence, type, rehabilitation, and outcome, *BioMed Res Int*:e1–e12, 2013.

140. Rowe FJ, et al: Interventions for eye movements disorders due to acquired brain injury, *Cochrane Database Sys Rev*:CD011290, 2018.

141. Rowe F: Prevalence of ocular motor cranial nerve palsy and associations following stroke, *Eye* 25:881–887, 2011.

142. Rowe F, et al: Reading difficulty after stroke: ocular and non ocular causes, *International Journal of Stroke* 6:404–411, 2011.

143. Rowe F, et al: Symptoms of stroke-related visual impairment, *Strabismus* 2:150–154, 2013.

144. Rowe FJ, Sueke H, Gawley SD: Comparison of Damato campimetry and Humphrey automated perimetry results in a clinical population, *Brit J Ophthalmol* 94:757–762, 2010.

145. Rowe FJ, et al: A pilot randomized controlled trial comparing effectiveness of prism glasses, visual search training and standard care in hemianopia, *Acta Neurol Scand* 136:310–321, 2017.

146. Rucker JC, Tomsak RL: Binocular diplopia: a practical approach, *The Neurologist* 11:98–110, 2005.

147. Rutstein RP, Daum KM: *Anomalies of binocular vision: Diagnosis and management*, St. Louis, 1998, Mosby.

148. Russell C, Li K, Malhotra PA: Harnessing motivation to alleviate neglect, *Front Hum Neurosci* 7:e1–7, 2013.

149. Saeidi-Borujeni M, et al: Cognitive orientation to daily occupational performance approach in adults with neurological conditions: a scoping review, *Med J Islam Repub Iran* 33(21 Sep):99 e1–8, 2019.

150. Sand KM, et al: Vision problems in ischaemic stroke patients: effects on life quality and disability, *Euro J Neuro* 23(Suppl 1): 1–7, 2016.

151. Savitt J, Mathews M: Treatment of visual disorders in Parkinson disease, *Curr Treat Opt Neuro* 20:30,e1–15, 2018. https://doi.org/10.1007/s11940-018-0519-0.

152. Scheiman MM, et al: Objective assessment of vergence after treatment of concussion-related CI: a pilot study, *Optom Vis Sci* 94:74–88, 2017.

153. Scheiman M, et al: A randomized clinical trial of vision therapy/orthoptics versus pencil pushups for the treatment of convergence insufficiency in young adults, *Optom Vis Sci* 82:e583–e595, 2005.

154. Scherer MR, Schubert MC: Traumatic brain injury and vestibular pathology as a comorbidity after blast exposure, *Phys Ther* 89:980–992, 2009.

155. Schuchard RA: Adaptation to macular scotomas in persons with low vision, *Am J Occup Ther* 49:870–876, 1995.

156. Schuett S: The rehabilitation of hemianopic dyslexia, *Nat Rev Neurol* 5:427–437, 2009.

157. Schuett S, Zihl J: Does age matter? age and rehabilitation of visual field disorders after brain injury, *Cortex* 49:1001–1012, 2013.

158. Sen N: An insight into the vision impairment following traumatic brain injury, *Neurochem Intern* 111:103–107, 2017.

159. Shepherd D, et al: The association between health-related quality of life and noise or light sensitivity in survivors of a mild traumatic brain injury, *Qual Life Res* 29:665–672, 2020.

160. Spaccavento S, et al: Efficacy of visual-scanning training and prism adaptation for neglect rehabilitation, *App Neuropsychol Adult* 23:313–321, 2016.

161. Sprenger A, Kömpf D, Heide W: Visual search in patients with left visual hemineglect, *Prog Brain Res* 140:395–415, 2002.

162. Stephenson S, et al: Pilot study: using the Bioness Integrated Therapy System (BITS) to examine the correlation between skills and success with on-the-road driving evaluations, *Am J Occup Ther* 73(4_Supplement_1):7311515280 2019. https://doi.org/10.5014/ajot.2019.73S1-PO4054.

163. Striemer CL, Ferber S, Danckert J: Spatial working memory deficits represent a core challenge for rehabilitating neglect, *Front Hum Neurosci* 7:1–11, 2013.

164. Tant MLM, et al: Hemianopic visual field defects elicit hemianopic scanning, *Vision Res* 42:1339–1348, 2002.

165. Ten Brink AF, et al: You never know where you are going until you know where you have been: disorganized search after stroke, *J Neuropsychol* 10:256–275, 2016.

166. Ten Brink AF, et al: Differences between left and right-sided neglect revisited: a large cohort study across multiple domains, *J Clin Exp Neuropsychol* 39:707–723, 2017.

167. Tham K, Borell L, Gustavsson A: The discovery of disability: A phenomenological study of unilateral neglect, *Am J Occup Ther* 54:398–406, 2000.

168. Tham K, Kielhofner G: Impact of the social environment on occupational experience and performance among persons with unilateral neglect, *Am J Occup Ther* 57:403–412, 2003.

169. Thiagarajan P, Ciuffreda KJ, Ludlam DP: Vergence dysfunction in mild traumatic brain injury (mTBI): a review, *Ophthalmic Physiol Opt* 31:456–468, 2011.

170. Thiagarajan P, Ciuffreda KJ: Versional eye tracking in mild traumatic brain injury (mTBI): effects of oculomotor training (OMT), *Brain Injury* 28:930–943, 2014.

171. Thiagarajan P, Ciuffreda KJ: Effect of oculomotor rehabilitation on accommodative responsivity in mild traumatic brain injury, *J Rehabil Res Dev* 51:175–192, 2014.

172. Thimm M, et al: Impact of alertness training on spatial neglect: a behavioural and fMRI study, *Neuropsychologia* 44:1230–1246, 2006.

173. Ting DSJ, et al: Visual neglect following stroke: current concepts and future focus, *Surv Ophthalmol* 56:114–134, 2011.

174. Toglia J: Generalization of treatment: a multicontext approach to cognitive perceptual impairment in adults with brain injury, *Am J Occup Ther* 45:505–516, 1991.

175. Trobe JD, et al: Confrontation visual field techniques in the detection of anterior visual pathway lesions, *Ann Neurol* 10:28–34, 1981.

176. Truong JQ, et al: Photosensitivity in mild traumatic brain injury (mTBI): a retrospective analysis, *Brain Injury* 28:1283–1287, 2014.

177. Turton AJ, et al: Walking and wheelchair navigation in patients with left visual neglect, *Neuropsychol Rehabil* 19:274–290, 2009.

178. Turton AJ, et al: Visual search training in occupational therapy – an example of expert practice in community-based stroke rehabilitation, *Brit J Occup Ther* 78:674–687, 2015.

179. Vallar G, Calzolari E: Unilateral spatial neglect after posterior parietal damage, *Handbk Clin Neuro* 151:287–312, 2018. https://doi.org/10.1016/B978-0-444-63622-5.00014-0.

180. Van Vleet TM, DeGutis JM: The nonspatial side of spatial neglect and related approaches to treatment, *Prog Brain Res* 207:327–349, 2013. https://doi.org/10.1016/B978-0-444-63327-9.00012-6.

181. Varma R, et al: Visual impairment and blindness in adults in the United States: demographic and geographic variations from 2015–2050, *JAMA Ophthalmol* 134:802–809, 2016.

182. Ventura RE, Balcer LJ, Galetta SL: The neuro-ophthalmology of head trauma, *Lancet Neuro* 13:1006–1016, 2014.

183. Voleti VB, Hubschman JP: Age-related eye disease, *Maturitas* 75:29–33, 2013.

184. Volkening K, Kerkhoff G, Keller I: Effects of repetitive galvanic vestibular stimulation on spatial neglect and verticality perception – a randomised sham-controlled trial, *Neuropsychol Rehabil* 28:1179–1196, 2018.

185. Wåhlin A, et al: Rehabilitation in chronic spatial neglect strengthens resting-state connectivity, *Acta Neurol Scand* 139:254–259, 2019.

186. Walle KM, et al: Unilateral neglect post stroke: eye movement frequencies indicate directional hypokinesia while fixation distributions suggest compensatory mechanism, *Brain Behav* 9:e01170, 2019. https://doi.org/10.1002/brb3.1170.

187. Warren M: A hierarchical model for evaluation and treatment of visual perceptual dysfunction in adult acquired brain injury, parts I and II, *Am J Occup Ther* 47:42–66, 1993.

188. Warren M: Pilot study on activities of daily living limitations in adults with hemianopsia, *Am J Occup Ther* 63:626–633, 2009.

189. Warren M: *Brain injury visual assessment battery for adults, test manual*, Lawrence, KS, 1998, visAbilities Rehab Services.

190. Warren M: Identification of visual scanning deficits in adults after cerebrovascular accident, *Am J Occup Ther* 44:391–399, 1990.

191. Warren M: *Pre-Reading and writing exercises for persons with macular scotomas*, Lawrence KS, 1996, visAbilities Rehab Services.

192. Warren M, Vogtle L, Moore J: Search performance of healthy adults on cancellation tests, *Am J Occup Ther* 62:580–586, 2008.

193. Webster JS, et al: Effect of attentional bias to right space on wheelchair mobility, *J Clin Exp Neuropsychol* 16:129–137, 1994.

194. Willard A, Lueck CJ: Ocular motor disorders, *Curr Opin Neurol* 27:75–82, 2014.

195. Wright V, Watson G: *Learn to use your vision for reading workbook. LUV reading series*, Trooper, PA, 1995, Homer Printing.

196. Wu C-Y, et al: Effects of constraint-induced therapy combined with eye patching on functional outcomes and movement kinematics in poststroke neglect, *Am J Occup Ther* 67:236–245, 2013.

197. Wu Y, Hallett M: Photophobia in neurologic disorders, *Trans Neurodegen* 6, article 26, 2017. https://doi.org/10.1186/s40035-017-0095-3.

198. Zebhauser PT, et al: Visuospatial neglect: a theory-informed overview of current and emerging strategies and a systematic review on the therapeutic use of non-invasive brain stimulation, *Neuropsychol Rev* 29:397–420, 2019.

199. Zhang X, et al: Natural history of homonymous hemianopia, *Neurology* 66:901–905, 2006.

200. Zihl J: *Rehabilitation of visual disorders after brain injury*, ed 2, United Kingdom, 2011, Psychology Press Ltd.
201. Zimmer HD: Visual and spatial working memory: from boxes to networks, *Neurosci Biobehav Rev* 32:1373–1395, 2008.

SUGGESTED READINGS

Cole M: When the left brain is not right the right brain may be left: report of personal experience with occipital hemianopia, *J Neuro Neurosurg Psychiatry* 67:169–173, 1999.

Duffy M: *Making life more livable: Simple adaptations for living at home after vision loss*, New York, 2002, American Foundation for the Blind Press.

Fox SM, Koons P, Dang SH: Vision rehabilitation after traumatic brain injury, *Phys Med Rehabil Clin North America* 30:171–188, 2019.

Hazelton C, et al: A qualitative exploration of the effect of visual field loss on daily life in home-dwelling stroke survivors, *Clin Rehabil* 33:1264–1273, 2019.

Klinke ME, et al: "Getting the left right": The experience of hemispatial neglect after stroke, *Qual Health Res* 25:1623–1636, 2015.

Turton AJ, et al: Visual search training in occupational therapy – an example of expert practice in community-based stroke rehabilitation, *Brit J Occup Ther* 78:674–687, 2015.

PRODUCT INFORMATION

Brain Injury Visual Assessment Battery for Adults
Warren Pre-Reading and Writing Exercises for Persons With Macular Scotomas
visAbilities Rehab Services
https://www.visabilities.com
Learn to Use Your Vision for Reading Workbook, Wright & Watson
Pepper Visual Skills for Reading Test
http://www.lowvisionsimulators.com
Lea Low Vision Test Charts/Damato Campimeter
https://www.good-lite.com
UV fitover filters
NoIR Medical Technologies

25

Evaluation and Intervention for Perception Dysfunction

Winifred Schultz-Krohn[a]

LEARNING OBJECTIVES

After studying this chapter, the student or practitioner will be able to do the following:

1. Describe how perceptual dysfunction affects participation in occupational performance.
2. Identify standardized and functional evaluation tools for visual perception, visual-spatial perception, tactile perception, body schema perception, and perceptual motor skills.
3. Differentiate between remedial and adaptive approaches to intervention for perceptual dysfunction and how they facilitate engagement in occupation.
4. Describe specific occupational therapy interventions for targeted perceptual motor deficits that facilitate improved performance skills, client factors, and participation in occupation.

CHAPTER OUTLINE

KEY TERMS

Adaptive approaches
Apraxia
Astereognosis
Anosognosia
Asomatognosia
Autotopagnosi
Body scheme/body schema
Color agnosi
Color anomi
Constructional apraxia
Dressing apraxia
Figure-ground discrimination
Finger agnosia
Form constancy
Ideational apraxia

Ideomotor apraxia
Metamorphopsia
Perception
Praxis
Prosopagnosia
Remedial approaches
Right-left discrimination
Simultanagnosia
Spatial relations
Stereognosis
Stereopsis
Visual agnosia
Visual-spatial perception

---

[a]The author wishes to acknowledge the contributions from Shawn Phipps to previous editions of this chapter.

THREADED CASE STUDY

Walt, Part 1

Walt is a 38-year-old man who identifies as male (prefers use of the pronouns he/his/him). Walt sustained a traumatic brain injury from a motor vehicle accident, resulting in right frontal, parietal, temporal, and occipital lobe lesions. His occupational profile included a complex and varied occupational history that consisted of full-time work as a graphic artist in a prestigious architectural firm. Walt is a husband and the father of two young children, as well as an accomplished painter.

After the brain injury, Walt's roles as worker, husband, father, and architect were affected because of impairments with motor and process performance skills and client factors, such as perceptual and cognitive dysfunction. Walt was unable to participate in his most valued areas of occupation, including painting, using a computer, sketching, and playing catch with his children. During the evaluation process, his visual foundation skills, including visual acuity, oculomotor control, and visual field function, were found to be intact. However, he demonstrated difficulty initiating motor actions when playing with his children and interpreting visual information for meaningful visual-spatial relationships when

painting, sketching, or using the computer. In addition, he exhibits clinical signs of unilateral neglect to the left half of his body and is unable to discriminate between different types of materials through touch alone.

During the initial assessment, the occupational therapist (OT) elected to use the Canadian Occupational Performance Measure[56] to obtain client-centered goals that would assist Walt in achieving his occupational performance goals. Walt identified his primary goals in occupational therapy: to submit a painting to a local art gallery, to play with his children, to drive, and to regain computer skills in preparation for resuming part-time work as an architect.

Critical Thinking Questions

1. How would you best evaluate Walt's occupational performance?
2. How would you best evaluate the impact of Walt's perceptual dysfunction on occupational pursuits?
3. How would you assist Walt in achieving his occupational performance goals using remedial and adaptive approaches for his perceptual dysfunction?

Perception is the gateway to cognition.[12]

Perception is the mechanism by which the brain interprets sensory information received from the environment. This perceived information is then processed by the various cognitive centers in the brain (described in Chapter 26). The individual may then choose to respond with a motor act or a verbal expression. For example, when waiting in a checkout line in a grocery store, a person may observe the array of brightly wrapped candy lining the aisle, may remember the sweet taste of the chocolate, may remember a recent resolution to lose weight, and may choose to resist adding any candy bars to the grocery cart. The person may look over to the next aisle, recognize a neighbor, and begin a conversation. In a few minutes, the person may notice that another register has a shorter line and may choose to move over to that line to be able to complete grocery shopping in a shorter amount of time. Perception of the environment provides the information to enable these response options.

In early development, tactile, proprioceptive, vestibular, and visual perception provide an internalized sense of body scheme, which is basic to all motor function.[42,67] Body scheme, also known as body schema, is now viewed as not only the internalized awareness of body and body parts but includes the peripersonal space. This body schema allows the individual to interact within the environment. Highly developed spatial skills are critical to the successful occupational performance in many daily tasks and can be easily seen in the professions of an architect, plumber, designer, or artist.[36] The process of interpreting visual stimuli is a learned skill, as evidenced by blind individuals who, when sight is restored later in life, have difficulty interpreting what they see.[53,76] Acquired perceptual deficits are noted in persons with cerebrovascular accident (CVA), traumatic brain injury (TBI), and other neurological disorders, such as multiple sclerosis and Parkinson's disease.[40,72] Spatial disorders and apraxia of a progressive nature are also seen in Alzheimer's disease.[47]

Severe visual perceptual deficits, frequently combined with cognitive impairments, can affect every area of occupation (e.g.,

activities of daily living [ADLs], instrumental activities of daily living [IADLs], education, work, play, leisure, and social participation) and can present grave safety concerns.[44] For example, an individual who is not able to judge distance and the spatial relationship of the top step of a stairwell may be in danger of a serious fall. Another person who cannot judge the position of the burner on a gas stove when preparing a meal may cause a fire. It is often the occupational therapy practitioner's role to evaluate safe and independent functioning in valued occupations and to assess visual and perceptual skills using standardized instruments along with observations of occupational performance in context.[40]

This chapter describes the client factors of visual perception, visual spatial perception, tactile perception, body schema perception, motor perception, and the potential deficits in occupational performance that result from impairment to these client factors. Suggestions for standardized and functional assessments are provided, and general occupational therapy approaches to intervention are reviewed.

GENERAL PRINCIPLES OF THE OCCUPATIONAL THERAPY EVALUATION

When evaluating visual perception skills, several assessment tools may be required. The optimal battery of standardized assessment tools includes instruments that have a variety of response modes to best fit the client's abilities.[40] Some assessment tools require a verbal response (e.g., naming a picture) or a motor response (e.g., drawing or constructing) or an assessment may allow flexible responses of either mode (multiple choice indicated by verbalizing the number or letter or by pointing to the chosen item). This enables the OT practitioner to assess visual perceptual dysfunction in a client with severe cognitive or communication limitations. With a variety of assessments, the OT practitioner is able to gather information to discriminate between an impairment in the reception of information and an impairment in the motor or verbal output.[25] This information will influence the occupational therapy intervention approach. Observation of the client's occupational performance in context along with analysis of the perceptual-motor demands of functional activities further complement the analysis of perceptual dysfunction obtained from the administration of standardized assessment tools.[88] These data are then integrated to provide a more comprehensive understanding of the deficits in occupational performance. Evaluation methods should be conducted in the specific context of the occupation being performed.

Warren (see Chapter 24) emphasized the importance of using a bottom-up approach to evaluate impairments in visual foundation skills,[91] such as visual acuity, oculomotor function, visual field function, visual attention, and visual scanning, before evaluating the higher-level visual perceptual skills covered in this chapter. For example, a deficit in visual acuity could be the underlying cause of poor performance on a test of perceptual processing. A variety of age-related eye diseases such as macular degeneration, glaucoma, diabetic retinopathy, and cataracts can affect visual acuity or visual field function can interfere with perceptual processing.[52] It is also possible that performance on global perceptual tests may be affected by deficits in cognitive areas such as attention, memory, or executive function (see Chapter 26). For example, an individual with severely limited attention is unlikely to perform well on many standardized assessments, regardless of the modality or nature of the task. Tsurumi and Todd also analyzed the cognitive skills involved in the commonly used assessments of visual perceptual function and warned that an individual's performance using two-dimensional representations of visual stimuli may not predict the person's performance in a dynamic three-dimensional world.[82]

Árnadóttir recommended the observation of ADLs in context to evaluate neurobehavioral dysfunction, including visual perceptual dysfunction and its effect on the performance of tasks essential to functional independence.[7,8] She maintained that it is preferable for occupational therapists to assess neurobehavioral deficits directly from the ADL evaluation. She developed the Árnadóttir OT-ADL Neurobehavioral Evaluation (A-ONE), which evaluates perceptual and perceptual-motor dysfunction in the context of ADLs and functional mobility tasks, including ideational apraxia, ideomotor apraxia, unilateral neglect, body scheme disorders, organization/sequencing dysfunction, agnosia, and spatial dysfunction.[7,8]

Toglia's Dynamic Interactional Model focuses on remediating and compensating for perceptual and cognitive impairments by generalizing functional skills across multiple contexts.[96] Visual processing strategies, task analysis, incorporating the specific learning needs of the client, establishing a criterion for the transfer of learning, metacognitive training, and practicing in multiple environments are key components of Toglia's approach. This approach also assists the client with TBI or stroke to gain self-awareness of perceptual and cognitive strengths and weaknesses to promote the use of strategies for remediation or compensation of skills across multiple contexts.[78,96] Toglia's Dynamic Object Search Test is one assessment that can be used to determine a client's abilities in visual processing, visual scanning, and visual attention.[79]

Another occupation-based assessment tool that can be used to determine the impact of deficient performance skills on functional tasks is the Assessment of Motor and Process Skills (AMPS).[34] This standardized assessment evaluates the performance skills necessary for engagement in areas of occupation by assessing 16 motor skills and 20 process skills (e.g., temporal organization, organizing space and objects). Each performance skill is evaluated in the context of client-identified and culturally relevant IADLs from a list of standardized activities at various levels of difficulty. The AMPS has a high rate of reliability and validity, and the evaluator must be an occupational therapist who has received advanced training and certification to administer this assessment.

The Dynamic Loewenstein Occupational Therapy Cognitive Assessment (DLOTCA)[48–50] and Rivermead Perceptual Assessment Battery[32] provide a comprehensive profile of visual perceptual and motor skills and involve both motor-free and constructional functions. Various other assessment tools require either a verbal or a simple pointing response. The Motor-Free Visual Perception Test, 4th Edition (MVPT-4),[15,24] assesses basic visual perceptual abilities. An alternative version of the test presents the multiple choices in a vertical format (MVPT-V) to reduce the interference of hemianopsia or visual inattention.[23,63] The MVPT-V has been shown to predict on-the-road driving performance and can be used as a screening tool to identify persons who would not be safe drivers.[61] The Test of Visual Perceptual Skills-Upper Level (TVPS-UL)[37] also provides a multiple-choice format and has been normed for adults. Test items require a higher level of visual analysis compared with the MVPT, and the test is untimed.[13,14] The Hooper Visual Organization Test[43,64] requires that the individual mentally assemble fragmented drawings of common objects. The Minnesota Paper Form Board Test[58,65] is a high-level assessment of visual organization, requiring mental rotation of fragmented geometric shapes.

GENERAL APPROACHES TO OCCUPATIONAL THERAPY INTERVENTION

An underlying assumption about perceptual-motor function is that perceptual deficits will adversely affect occupational performance. Further, it is assumed that remediation of or compensation for perceptual deficits will improve occupational performance.[22,23,68,94] In her critical analysis of approaches for treating perceptual deficits, Neistadt described two general classifications: the adaptive and the remedial.[68] Adaptive approaches provide training in occupational performance to facilitate the client's adaptation to unique contextual environments.[3] This compensatory or adaptive approach often includes training in visual scanning for those who have visual field deficits and environmental modifications such as use of high contrast items to enhance functional self-care skills.[94] In contrast, remedial approaches seek to produce some change in central nervous system (CNS) functions.[68] The effectiveness of the various approaches to the remediation of perceptual deficits requires further scientific investigation.[68,75] An example of remedial approaches is seen with the use of virtual reality[23] and prism glasses[33] to improve function for clients who have unilateral spatial neglect. Emerging evidence is seen with the use of prism glasses to improve functional skills and decrease the impact of unilateral neglect following a stroke.[33] Computerized visual perceptual training programs with the use of virtual reality glasses have demonstrated changes in functional skills and in the activation of parietal lobe function identified through fMRI imaging.[90]

The OT practitioner may use one approach or a combination of approaches when designing an intervention plan to address the effects of visual perceptual dysfunction. The remedial and adaptive approaches can be used along a continuum, beginning with remediating basic visual perceptual skills and gradually incorporating compensatory techniques as the deficits persist.[48] The occupational therapy literature suggests specific activities for the intervention of perceptual deficits, but protocols for the use of such activities require further research.[97] For measuring the effectiveness of occupational therapy intervention, criteria are needed for successful performance, task grading, objective methods of evaluating performance, and guidelines for task modification.[52,97] In the absence of objective criteria, the occupational therapist relies on empirical methods to measure and document functional improvement. Several studies have demonstrated the relationship between perceptual deficits and functional performance.[32,75]

Adaptive Approaches for Perceptual Dysfunction

Adaptive approaches are characterized by the repetitive practice of targeted occupational performance tasks that help the person with neurological dysfunction gain independence by using alternative strategies to compensate for perceptual impairments.[22,68,94] The therapist does not retrain specific perceptual skills when using an adaptive approach. Rather, the person is made aware of the problem and is instructed on adaptive strategies to compensate for the perceptual deficit during occupational performance. For example, if the client has difficulty with dressing because of impaired body schema, the therapist may set up a regular dressing routine and provide cues with repetitive practice on how to compensate for the perceptual challenges in context. With these adaptations, the client may learn to dress independently. Adaptation of the physical environment or the specific activity demands (e.g., objects used in the environment and their properties) is another way to compensate for a perceptual deficit. For example, if an individual has difficulty discriminating a white shirt against the white sheets of the bed, the therapist may encourage the person to select a patterned shirt or may lay the white shirt on a colored towel or bedspread to provide a contrasting background.

Remedial Approaches

Remedial, or transfer of learning, approaches assume that multiple practice opportunities with a particular perceptual skill will produce carryover of performance to similar activities or tasks requiring comparable perceptual skills.[23,68] For example, use of VR improved visual perceptual skills on specific assessments during a randomized controlled trial with clients who had sustained a stroke. The capacity for persons to improve their performance on perceptual tests after perceptual training has been documented.[90,96] However, additional research has shown that remedial strategies for optimizing perceptual skills coupled with occupation-based interventions in context are most effective in promoting changes in perceptual awareness and abilities.[22,69,70]

EVALUATION AND INTERVENTION OF SPECIFIC PERCEPTUAL IMPAIRMENTS

Visual Perception Disorders

Visual perception disorder impairs the person's ability to recognize and identify familiar objects and people.[52,97] Although these individuals may have intact visual anatomic structures, objects and people may appear distorted or larger or smaller than they actually are due to neurological damage. These individuals also have difficulty interpreting the meaning of objects in their environment, such as signs and maps. In addition, they can have difficulty recognizing, identifying, or remembering the names of colors in their environment. These visual perception disorders can lead to safety problems in dynamic environments and may affect social skills, because the person has difficulty recognizing family members, friends, and co-workers.

THREADED CASE STUDY

Walt, Part 2

Walt presents with a visual perception disorder. He has difficulty recognizing and differentiating the faces of his two children; he also has difficulties identifying the differences in the brushes he uses for painting. He requires verbal cues to identify the unique features that distinguish the faces of his two children and to identify the appropriate paintbrush to use during an art project. He also has difficulty identifying and recognizing the significance of various traffic signs, which would prevent him from driving safely.

Visual Agnosia

Visual object recognition refers to the ability to verbally identify objects by visual input. An impairment in this area is called visual agnosia, and it is caused by lesions in the right occipital lobe or posterior multimodal association area.[39,40] The individual with agnosia can demonstrate normal visual foundation skills. The inability to name objects is not caused by a language deficit, as noted in aphasic disorders. Rather, the person is unable to recognize and identify an item using only visual means. The person may be able to identify the object using other sensory modalities such as touch.

Visual agnosia is assessed by asking the individual to identify five common objects by sight, such as a pencil, a comb, keys, a watch, and eyeglasses. If the client demonstrates word-finding difficulties, the occupational therapist can offer a choice of three answers and ask the client to indicate the correct choice through a head nod (yes or no). If the client is unable to name four of the five objects, visual agnosia may be indicated.

Occupational therapy intervention for visual agnosia is most often focused on adaptive or compensatory methods of keeping frequently used objects, such as a hairbrush, in consistent locations and teaching the client to rely more heavily on intact sensory modalities, such as stereognosis and tactile discriminatory touch, to seek and find desired items for functional use.[41,77] The use of compensatory intervention approaches requires specific training for specific situations.[41] This approach has the most consistent success in helping clients compensate for visual agnosias and overall visual perceptual deficits. Current research has found that efforts to remediate object recognition have met with limited success.[41,77]

Color Agnosia and Color Anomia

Color agnosia refers to the client's inability to remember and recognize the specific colors for common objects in the environment.[39] For example, Walt was unable to recognize the color of the paints he was using during his landscape painting. He confused the green paint he was using to paint the grass with the blue paint he intended to use for the sky. Alternatively, color anomia refers to the client's inability to name the color of the objects. Although clients understand the differences between the colors of objects, they are unable to name the object accurately. For example, Walt was able to recognize the color red but was not able to name the color.

To assess color agnosia, the occupational therapist can present the client with two common objects that are accurately colored and two objects that are not accurately colored and then ask the client to pick out the objects that are not accurately colored. For example, a stop sign is typically red and presenting a stop sign in blue could assess color agnosia. If the client is unable to choose the objects that are inaccurately colored, color agnosia may be clinically present.

To assess color anomia, the occupational therapist can ask the client to name the color of various objects in the environment. If the patient has aphasia, the therapist will ask him or her to nod yes or no after offering the patient choices of colors. If the client is unable to correctly name the colors of various objects, color anomia may be present.

Occupational therapy intervention for color agnosia and color anomia is focused on functional tasks such as providing the client with opportunities to recognize, identify, and name various colors of objects in the natural environment. Intervention is best provided in a familiar context and can be incorporated functionally during occupational performance. For example, while Walt is painting a landscape, the therapist would provide verbal cues that assist him in recognizing, identifying, and naming the various colors of paint he is using.

Metamorphopsia

Metamorphopsia refers to the visual distortion of objects, such as the physical properties of size and weight.[39,97] For example, when Walt was playing with his two children, he could not distinguish among the basketball, football, baseball, or volleyball. Each of the balls appeared heavier, lighter, larger, or smaller than they actually were, making it difficult to distinguish the differences between them through observation alone.

Assessment for metamorphopsia includes presenting the client with various objects of different weights and sizes (e.g., balls, drinking glasses filled with water, puzzle pieces). The client is asked to place each object in order according to size or weight through visual observation alone. Metamorphopsia may be indicated if the client is unable to visually determine the size and shape of the various objects.

OT intervention for metamorphopsia includes providing the client with opportunities to practice distinguishing objects in the natural environment through intact sensory modalities (e.g., tactile-kinesthetic-proprioception). The functional use of objects during occupational performance will provide the client with feedback about the sizes and shapes of different objects. The occupational therapist should also provide specific verbal descriptors of the object when using this approach. Other treatment modalities include puzzles, board games, and computer games that help the client to gain experience distinguishing the sizes and shapes of different objects.

Prosopagnosia

Prosopagnosia refers to an inability to recognize and identify familiar faces caused by lesions of the right posterior hemisphere.[16,39] The individual with prosopagnosia may have difficulty recognizing their own face, the faces of family members and friends, or the faces of recognizable public figures because the person cannot recognize the unique facial expressions that make each face different. When attempting to identify family members and acquaintances, the person may compensate by relying on auditory cues such as the sound of the family member's voice or a distinctive feature such as long, wavy hair.

Brain lesions can also impair the ability to interpret facial expressions, which can have significant social consequences.[18,95] For example, one client, who identified as male, tended to be very suspicious of others. He had difficulties describing the expressions of various persons depicted in photographs. Because he had immigrated to the United States from another country, his difficulty was originally thought to be a result of cultural differences. He was asked to bring in a newspaper that he regularly received from his native country. The captions of the photographs were occluded, and he was asked to describe the emotional expressions of the persons shown. He was then asked to translate the photo captions and became aware that he was unable to discriminate the emotions apparent on the faces.

A standardized test of facial recognition[11,80] is available, which presents a multiple-choice matching of faces presented in front view and side view and under various lighting conditions. Informal functional assessments could include having the client identify the names of the people in photographs, with family members at a dinner table (e.g., Walt's two children side by side), or by having the client identify his or her own face in a mirror. Photographs of famous public figures also could be used during the assessment. If aphasia is present, the client can communicate through gestures, such as head nodding (e.g., yes or no) in response to a multiple-choice format. If the client is unable to identify self or family members, prosopagnosia may be present. OT interventions for prosopagnosia include remedial approaches such as providing face-matching exercises.[97] Adaptive approaches include providing pictures of family members and famous people with names and assisting the client to associate the family member's face with other unique characteristics and features, such as weight, height, mannerisms, accents, and hairstyle.

Simultanagnosia

Simultanagnosia refers to the inability to recognize and interpret a visual array as a whole, and it is caused by lesions to the right hemisphere of the brain.[39] Clients with simultanagnosia are able to identify the individual components of a visual scene, but they are unable to recognize and interpret the gestalt of the scene. For example, Walt is able to identify the flowers and the trees in one of his paintings, but he is not able to recognize and interpret this painting as the landscape surrounding the family home where he grew up.

Assessment includes presenting the client with a photograph that has a detailed visual array (e.g., Walt's family photograph at the beach), asking the client to describe the scene in detail, and assessing whether the client can describe the scene as a whole. Many clients will be able to identify specific features of the visual array (e.g., the sand castle) but cannot describe the context or meaning of the whole scene (e.g., a family trip to the beach). Simultanagnosia is clinically significant when the client cannot recognize and interpret a visual array as a whole.

OT intervention focuses on helping the client to construct the meaning of a visual array through verbal cues and therapeutic questions to facilitate abstract reasoning. Intervention is best provided in familiar contexts, such as in a client's home, in a work setting, or during a community outing to the shopping mall.

Visual-Spatial Perception Disorders

Visual-spatial perception refers to the capacity to appreciate the spatial arrangement of one's body, objects in relationship to oneself, and relationships between objects in space. Various efforts have been made to subdivide spatial skills into components, but authors acknowledge that spatial skills cannot be isolated easily from one another.[97] It is generally acknowledged that the right hemisphere, which controls spatial abilities, tends to function in the gestalt, whereas the left hemisphere tends to focus on discrete details.[57]

Visual-spatial perception occurs instantaneously to support safe and effective occupational performance. Because of this rapid simultaneous processing of visual and spatial information, it is possible to react quickly to another driver's actions to avoid a collision when operating a motor vehicle. An individual with a mild visual-spatial perception impairment may need additional time to perform a task but processes the information correctly, possibly by compensating with verbal analysis of the perceptual components. Severe impairment may result in an incorrect response despite additional time used in attempting to solve the problem.

Visual-spatial skills are not limited to the visual domain.[91] Sounds can be localized in space, and the mobility and daily occupations of blind individuals are heavily dependent on the tactile appreciation of the spatial arrangements of objects. For example, a blind person's ability to navigate through a familiar room requires awareness of the layout of each piece of furniture

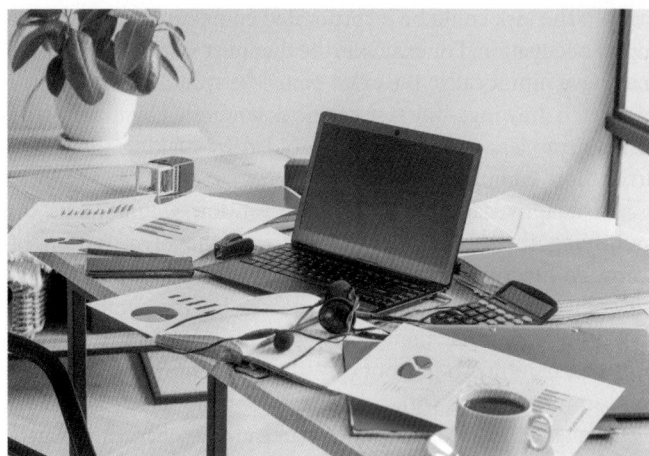

Fig. 25.1 Visual-spatial functions in real life. Note that all components of spatial functions can be found in this scene. (Copyright © iStock/Dina Marozova.)

in the physical environment and continual shifting of the individual's *cognitive map* while changing positions in the room.

As a pencil rolls across a desktop, it is the skill of visual-spatial perception that enables a person to appreciate the relative orientation of the pencil to the table surface as the pencil nears the edge and is about to fall to the floor. Fig. 25.1 illustrates the complexity of visual-spatial perceptual function.

THREADED CASE STUDY

Walt, Part 3

Walt presents with visual-spatial perception dysfunction. He has difficulty distinguishing the right and left sides of his body and often confuses right and left when given directions. He frequently has difficulties navigating novel environments and requires a family member to be with him at all times when he is in unfamiliar community setting. When painting, Walt has been observed to have difficulty distinguishing the foreground and the background in his paintings and is unable to determine the differences between the amounts of paint in each of the cups next to him. In addition, he is often observed missing the canvas in front of him when attempting to apply the paint.

Figure-Ground Discrimination Dysfunction

Figure-ground discrimination allows a person to perceive the foreground from the background in a visual array.[97] For example, Walt is unable to locate a particular painting utensil from the other writing utensils in the pencil holder, thereby demonstrating difficulty distinguishing the targeted object from the background.

Figure-ground discrimination can be assessed functionally in a variety of contexts. During a dressing activity, you may ask the client to identify the white undershirt located on top of his or her white sheets. In the kitchen, you can ask the client to pick out all of the spoons from a disorganized utensil drawer. Figure-ground discrimination dysfunction may be indicated if the client is unable to discriminate the foreground from the background in a complex visual array.

Using a remedial approach, intervention for figure-ground discrimination dysfunction should focus on challenging the client to localize objects of similar color in a disorganized visual array.[97] The task could be incorporated contextually into meaningful occupation. For example, the therapist working with Walt may have him localize the exact pencil he would like to use for his sketch drawings. The task can be downgraded by making the visual array less complex and upgraded by making the visual array more complex.

An adaptive approach[2,66] to intervention would focus on modifying the environment to increase the organization of common functional objects (e.g., placing only the most necessary objects needed for self-care), decreasing the complexity of the visual array that the client has to discriminate (e.g., have only one paintbrush in front of Walt at a given time), or marking common objects with colored tape so that objects are easily distinguished from one another, particularly when the objects are of a similar color.

Toglia's multicontextual approach may be used to help the client gain self-awareness of figure-ground discrimination dysfunction and develop effective organizational and visual scanning strategies for discriminating the foreground and background in the environment.[78,96] This intervention approach also focuses on the generalization of skill to multiple functional contexts by using strategies that the client has identified as effective in locating objects in the environment.

Form-Constancy Dysfunction

Form constancy is the recognition of various forms, shapes, and objects, regardless of their position, location, or size.[97] For example, a person can perceive all of the pencils on a desk, in various sizes or in various positions in the pencil holder.

To assess form constancy, ask the client to identify familiar objects in his or her environment through observation alone when those objects are placed upside down or on their side. For example, in the kitchen, you may ask Walt to identify a cup that is turned upside down or a toaster oven that is placed on its side. Form-constancy dysfunction may be indicated if the client is unable to identify objects in a position that varies from the norm.

Intervention for form-constancy dysfunction includes using tactile cues that will help the client to feel objects in various positions and thereby learn their constancy despite their position, size, or location. Activities can be graded from positioning all objects in an upright position to placing objects in odd positions. Intervention is best provided with common objects that the client uses in everyday occupational performance.

Position in Space

Position in space,[39] or spatial relations,[97] refers to the relative orientation of a shape or object to the self. It is this component of perception that allows a person to recognize that the tip of the pencil is pointed away from him, and so directs the hand to effectively grasp the pencil.

To assess position in space, have the client place common objects in relation to the self or other objects using the following directional terms: top/bottom, up/down, in/out, behind/in front of, and before/after. For example, the occupational therapist can ask Walt to place his paintbrush on top of his computer or his basketball behind his back. Position-in-space dysfunction may

be indicated if the client is unable to discern the relationships of objects to the self or other objects through directional terms.

Intervention for position in space includes providing the client with opportunities to experience the organization of objects in the environment to the self. For example, Walt could practice placing various objects in relation to one another in a graphic design program on the computer so that directional concepts of up/down, in/out, behind/in front of, and before/after can be reinforced.

Right-Left Discrimination Dysfunction

Right-left discrimination is the ability to accurately use the concepts of right and left.[97] An individual with right-left discrimination dysfunction may confuse the right and left side of the body or confuse right and left in directional terms when navigating through the environment.

To assess right-left discrimination, the occupational therapist asks the client to point to various body parts (e.g., left ear) or assess the client's ability to accurately navigate the environment through verbal commands using right and left (e.g., turn right at the end of the hallway). Right-left discrimination dysfunction may be indicated if the client is unable to differentiate between right and left in relation to their own body and the environment.

Intervention for right-left discrimination focuses on assisting the client while engaging in functional tasks such as asking the client to narrate a functional event, for example, the client states: "I am placing my right arm into the shirt sleeve" or "I am now turning left at the stop sign." Remediation of right-left discrimination can significantly improve topographical orientation as the client learns to navigate in a more dynamic home and community environment.

Stereopsis

Stereopsis is the inability to perceive depth in relation to the self or in relation to various objects in the environment.[97] Depth perception is critical to function in a three-dimensional world and to safety in driving and community mobility. Clients with visual dysfunction in one eye or who wear an eye patch to compensate for double vision may demonstrate stereopsis, because binocular visual input from both eyes is required to perceive depth.

To assess depth perception, the occupational therapist places a variety of common objects on a table surface and asks the client to identify which object is closer and which object is farther away. In a community context, depth perception can be assessed by asking the client to identify buildings or landmarks that are closer or farther away. Stereopsis may be indicated if the client is unable to judge the distance between objects in the environment.

Computer-assisted software can help the client develop depth perception by judging the relative distance of objects in relation to one another on a computer screen.[55,90,97] Tactile-kinesthetic approaches also help the client judge distances through the use of tactile input.

Tactile Perception Disorders

Impairment in tactile perception involves tactile discriminative skills of the second somatosensory area of the parietal lobes.[39,93]

These skills require a higher level of synthesis than the basic tactile sensory functions of light touch and pressure described in Chapter 23.

THREADED CASE STUDY

Walt, Part 4

Walt presents with an impairment in tactile perception. He is unable to identify the objects he uses for painting by touch alone. He is unable to discriminate between different types of materials or different forms and shapes by tactile means and must compensate visually to determine the objects he is using during occupational performance.

Stereognosis

Stereognosis,[40] also known as tactile gnosis,[97] is the perceptual skill that enables an individual to identify common objects and geometric shapes through tactile perception without the aid of vision. It results from the integration of the senses of touch, pressure, position, motion, texture, weight, and temperature and is dependent on intact parietal cortical function. Stereognosis is essential to occupational performance because the ability to "see with the hands" is critical to many daily activities. It is the skill that makes it possible to reach into a handbag and find a pen and to find the light switch in a dark room. Along with proprioception, stereognosis enables the use of all fine-motor activities without the need to concentrate visually on the objects being manipulated. Examples of stereognosis are knitting while watching television, reaching into a pocket for house keys, and using a fork to eat while engaged in conversation.

A deficit in stereognosis is called astereognosis.[40] Persons who have astereognosis must visually monitor the use of their hands during activities. This visual monitoring requires additional time and energy during task performance. The purpose of a stereognosis test is to assess a client's ability to identify common objects and perceive their tactile properties.[40] A means to occlude the person's vision is needed, such as a curtain, patch, or folder as described in Chapter 23. Typical objects that could be used for assessment include a pencil, pen, a pair of sunglasses, a key, nail, safety pin, paper clip, metal teaspoon, quarter, nickel, and a button. Any common objects may be used, but it is important to consider the client's social and ethnic background to ensure the client has had previous experience with the objects. Three-dimensional geometric shapes (e.g., a cube, sphere, or pyramid) also can be used to assess shape and form perception.

The evaluation should be conducted in an environment that has minimal distractions. The therapist should sit across from the client being tested. The client's vision is occluded, with the dorsal surface of the hand resting on the table. Objects are presented in random order to the client's palm. Manipulation of objects is allowed and encouraged. The therapist assists with the manipulation of items in the client's hand if the person's hand function is impaired. The client should be asked to name the object, or, if unable to name the object because of aphasia or word finding difficulties, to describe the properties of the object. Clients with aphasia may view a duplicate set of test objects after

each trial and point to a visual choice. The person's response to each of the items presented is scored. The therapist notes if the object is identified quickly and correctly, if there is a long delay before the object is identified, or if the individual can describe only properties (e.g., size, texture, material, and shape) of the object. The therapist also notes if the person cannot identify the object or describe its properties.

Diminished sensory appreciation, particularly tactile discrimination, has a significant negative impact on arm use[83] and participation[20] after a stroke. A systematic approach was used to remediate diminished tactile discrimination, limb position sense, and tactile object recognition.[19] Carey and associates conducted a randomized controlled trial with double blinding to determine if systematic and graded sensory intervention could produce changes in clients after a stroke. The control group received a standard intervention program, and the experimental group received sensory discrimination training addressing textures, limb position, and tactile object recognition. Clients in both groups were at least 6 weeks past a stroke, and most clients were 6 months past a stroke. All 50 enrolled clients received a total of 10 hours of intervention, typically provided for 60 minutes over 3 weeks. The experimental intervention (EI) group received progressively graded sensory input using both vision-occluded training and cross-modal training with vision. Clients in the EI group explored the various sensory experiences of discriminating various textures, recognizing objects through touch, and moving limbs in relation to the body but were also provided with feedback regarding the accuracy of sensory registration and the method of exploration. The graded sensory experiences were an important feature of the EI group. The control group was provided with the same frequency of treatment and the intervention "consisted of nonspecific repeated exposure" to sensory experiences of touch and limb movement. Significant improvements on standardized assessments were noted in the EI group compared to the control group, indicating the importance of systematic sensory training after a stroke. These gains were sustained at 6 weeks and 6 months after the sensory training intervention.

The OT practitioner should provide systematic and graded sensory experiences to support recovery of accurate sensation of touch and position of the limb relative to the body.[19,20,83,84] These skills support occupational performance for clients who sustained a stroke.

Body Schema Perception Disorders

Following a CVA or TBI, a person's sense of body shape, position, and capacity frequently is distorted. This is known as a disorder of body schema, or autotopagnosia.[5,6,39,62] This condition can be noted in attempts to draw a human figure (Fig. 25.2) or in a person's unrealistic expectations of performance abilities.[57] A severe form of body schema distortion is known as asomatognosia and persons may neglect one side of the body or demonstrate generally distorted impressions of the body's configuration.[46] A client may perceive a body part as belonging to another, such as the woman who thought the therapist had stolen her wedding ring, not realizing the hand she was

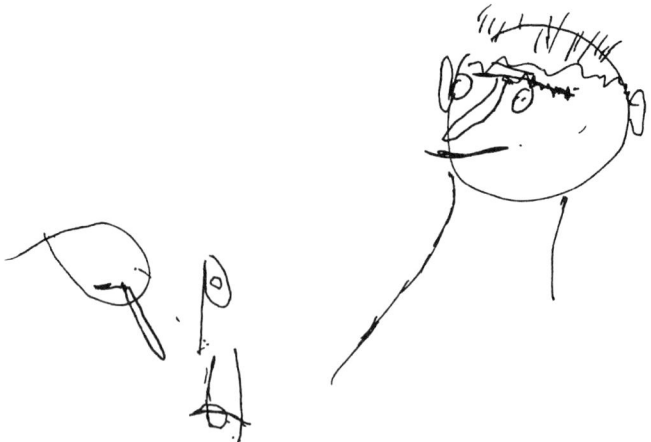

Fig. 25.2 Example of a body schema perception disorder. Drawing on the *left* is the person's first attempt to draw a face. The occupational therapist asked the person to try again. The second effort is the drawing on the *right*.

viewing was her own. **Anosognosia** with hemiplegia can occur in which intellectual function is intact but the client is unable to recognize the inability to move the hemiplegic limb, most often the left arm after a right CVA.[17] Anosognosia occurs in 20% to 30% of individuals after a stroke to the right parietal of right fronto-temporo-parietal areas. Although anosognosia often resolves within a few weeks, the lack of awareness of movement on the hemiplegic side can create unsafe and dangerous situations because the client does not perceive the arm is not moving.[4] **Finger agnosia**, or the inability to discriminate the fingers of the hand, also can be part of the disorder.[11] An impaired body scheme will also affect participation in occupation and performance skills.

Body schema perception disorders can be assessed by asking the individual to draw a human figure (see Fig. 25.2) or point to body parts on command (e.g., "Touch your left hand" and "Touch your right knee"). Finger agnosia is evaluated by occluding the person's vision and asking him or her to name each finger as the therapist touches it. Unilateral body neglect can be observed functionally during occupational performance as the client ignores the affected limb or states that a body part is not his or her own. A body schema perception disorder may be present if the client is unable to correctly identify body parts on self.

A remedial approach to intervention for body schema perception disorders should focus on providing the client with opportunities to reinforce body knowledge through tactile and proprioceptive input.[97] For example, while Walt is dressing or painting, the occupational therapist can incorporate his affected left upper extremity into the activity and verbally acknowledge that his left arm and hand are being used. Tactile-kinesthetic guiding or constraint-induced movement therapy strategies also can be used if the client has difficulty initiating the use of the affected limb. As the client incorporates the use of the affected limb into occupational performance, perceptual awareness of the body and the relationship between various body parts can be enhanced.

THREADED CASE STUDY

Walt, Part 5

Walt demonstrates unilateral inattention to the left side of his body and his environment. He demonstrates asymmetric visual scanning to the left side of his environment, misses details on the left side of his drawings, and routinely neglects the functional use of his left upper extremity during daily tasks. He often states that his left arm is owned by someone else and has difficulty with spatial organization.

Motor Perception Disorders

Praxis is the ability to plan and perform purposeful movement. **Apraxia** has been classically defined as a deficit in "the execution of learned movement that cannot be accounted for by weakness, incoordination, or sensory loss or by incomprehension of or inattention to commands."[38] The disorder can result from damage to either side of the brain or to the corpus callosum, but it is more frequently noted with left hemisphere damage.[54,71] Apraxia has been reported in almost 50% of individuals after a left hemisphere stroke, and clients may have both apraxia and aphasia following a left side lesion. Kusch and associates[54] found that the location of the lesion was associated with remission of apraxia. Those persons with lesions in the left insula area had fewer apraxic deficits 11 days after the stroke when compared to individuals who sustained lesions in the left inferior parietal region. For individuals with lesions in the inferior parietal region, apraxic deficits persisted 11 days after the stroke. Progressive apraxia is also noted with degenerative disorders such as Alzheimer's disease.[71] (See also Chapters 34 and 35).

Apraxia has been strongly correlated with dependence in areas of occupation.[2,27,71] For example, in a severe case of apraxia, Ms. S, who identified as female, initially required total assistance with basic activities of daily living (BADLs). Ms. S was fully cognizant of ongoing events but could not direct her arm and leg movements in a way that would assist the nursing staff during dressing. When asked to pick up a pencil, Ms. S walked around all four sides of the table in an attempt to position her hand correctly to grasp the object. She could describe the desired action in words ("I want to pick up the pencil between my thumb and index finger, with the lead point of the pencil close to the tips of my fingers") but reported after returning to her seat that her hand never "looked like it was in the right position" to take hold of the pencil.

There are different forms of apraxia, but a clear consensus of the different types and operational definitions for each type has not been fully established.[10] The commonality with the various forms of apraxia as the deficit is not singularly the result of a motor, sensory, or cognitive problem.

Ideational Apraxia

Ideational apraxia refers to a conceptual deficit in which the function of objects, or the idea of how objects are used is compromised.[40] The individual may have difficulty sequencing acts in the proper order, such as folding a sheet of paper and inserting it into an envelope. The individual may use the wrong tool for the task or may associate the wrong tool with the object to be acted on, such as by attempting to write with a spoon. This deficit has significant functional implications in a variety of areas of occupation.

Ideomotor Apraxia

Ideomotor apraxia is an inability to carry out a motor act on verbal command or imitation.[73] However, the person with ideomotor apraxia is often able to perform the act spontaneously with the actual object. For example, a person is unable to mime the action of brushing his or her teeth on request but is observed using a toothbrush correctly when performing grooming activities in context. Observation of the person engaged in familiar occupations is critical to the identification of ideomotor apraxia.

Ideomotor apraxia has been related to distorted body schema and representation resulting in impaired functional skills. Romano and colleagues[73] focused on enhancing body schema using a modified mirror box intervention with 13 clients who were several months past a stroke. All clients demonstrated apraxia as measured by the De Renzi test for ideomotor apraxia.[28] A cross-over design was used to stagger the intervention using the mirror box. The mirror box hid the client's apraxic hand from view while the therapist demonstrated motions reflected in the mirror. This use of the mirror box differs from the typical application in which the client watches the less involved hand move in the reflection of the mirror while the more involved hand is hidden by the mirror. This modified mirror box approach had the therapist's hand demonstrate the accurate movements while the client watched the movement in the mirror covering the apraxic hand. Clients were then asked to attempt these motions using the hand shielded by the mirror. This strategy was used to enhance body schema, and all clients demonstrated improved motor performance following use of the modified mirror box therapy.

Dressing Apraxia

Another category of motor perception disorders recognized in the literature is dressing apraxia.[40] Dressing apraxia contributes to the inability to plan effective motor actions required during the complex perceptual task of dressing one's upper and lower body and is often seen as a form of ideomotor apraxia. The classification of dressing impairment as a unique and distinct form

of apraxia has been questioned because the difficulties in ADLs are considered to be caused by perceptual or cognitive dysfunction and an extension of ideomotor apraxia.

General Principles in the Assessment and Treatment of Apraxia

It is important that assessments of sensory function, motor control, and dexterity are completed before the test of praxis because deficits in these areas would complicate any assessment of apraxia. If a person has a hemiplegia, the unaffected hand is used for testing. Input from the speech-language pathologist is important for establishing an individual's capacity for basic comprehension via words or gestures. Because of the frequent association of apraxia with aphasia and left hemisphere brain damage, an apraxia screening is included.

Several apraxia assessments are used in research, such as the De Renzi test of apraxia,[29,31] the Test for Upper Limb Apraxia (TULIA),[85] the Florida Apraxia Screening Test (FAST),[74] the Movement Imitation Test,[29,30] and the Use of Objects Test.[29] The Loewenstein Occupational Therapy Cognitive Assessment, Second Edition (LOTCA-II)[45] includes a praxis subsection. The TULIA contains 48 items and assesses a wide range of tasks, including imitative and pantomime movements, tool use, and gestures.[85] A screen was developed from the TULIA to use at the bedside with clients who have sustained a stroke, known as the Apraxia Screen of TULIA (AST).[86] This screening tool has been translated into Korean[51] and also used with clients diagnosed with Parkinson's disease.[87]

A thorough assessment includes functional items presented, such as those shown in Table 25.1, and involves both transitive movements (actions involving both tool and use, such as writing with an imaginary pen) and intransitive movements (movements for communication, such as waving goodbye). Gestures are often used in standardized assessments and in research protocols.[9,10,85] The type of gestures has been differentiated into transitive and intransitive.[9] Transitive gestures are those arm and hand movements that imply tool use such as asking a client to show how to brush teeth without the actual toothbrush present. Intransitive gestures typically have a communicative intent such as waving goodbye or shrugging shoulders.

Returning to the case of Ms. S, the intervention approach outlined by Aguilar-Ferrándiz and colleagues[2] was used. Occupational therapy services were provided 3 times per week for an 8-week period. The occupational therapy services addressed both restorative functions to recover motor planning skills and compensatory training. The restorative approach included both transitive (using a specific tool or item) and intransitive (communication) gestures of increasing complexity. Compensatory services were also provided to foster functional skills in the home environment. After completing the 8-week intervention program, Ms. S was independent in most areas of occupation, although additional time was needed for each activity.

For another client with apraxia, the occupational therapist used condition and interactive reasoning to guide the intervention. Each task was introduced using verbal instructions and visual demonstration coupled with enhanced sensory input for the object to be used in the functional task. This approach followed the process outlined by Carey and associates[18,19] to promote recovery of function after a stroke using somatosensory discrimination training. This training was provided to enhance texture discrimination, limb position sense, and tactile recognition of objects. The client was also asked to visually monitor the motor performance for functional tasks such as stirring a brownie mix in a bowl or slicing a banana on cereal. As was noted in the randomized control trial investigation completed by Carey and associates,[19] this client demonstrated improved motor performance for functional tasks and the somatosensory approach fostered skill transfer to novel situations.

OT interventions for dressing apraxia involve collaborating with the client[94] on effective dressing strategies, such as distinguishing between right and left or from front to back on specific clothing items. An effective strategy is to have the client position the garment the same way each time (e.g., positioning a shirt with the buttons face up and pants with the zipper face up). Labels, small buttons, or small tags sewn into the inside of the

clothing can be used as cues to differentiate the front from the back of the garment.[97] OT intervention with clients who experience apraxia, or perceptual deficits of any form, is focused on client-driven functional outcomes.[21,66,92]

Constructional Apraxia

The term constructional apraxia refers to the "inability to accurately to reproduce two-dimensional or three-dimensional visual models."[26] Many occupations depend on visual-constructional skills, or the ability to organize visual information into meaningful spatial representations. Constructional deficits refer to the inability to organize or assemble parts into a whole, as in putting together block designs (three dimensional) or drawings (two dimensional). Constructional deficits can result in significant dysfunction in occupations that require constructional ability, such as dressing, organizing food in a refrigerator, following instructions for assembling a toy, and loading a dishwasher.[81] Fig. 25.3, which shows evidence of left inattention, also demonstrates constructional deficits. An individual acts on the contextual environment based on the perceived information. Therefore, deficits in perception become more apparent when a person interacts with the environment in maladaptive ways.

Traditional tests of constructional abilities in a two-dimensional mode are the Test of Visual-Motor Skills, Third Edition[60] the administration of the Benton Visual Retention Test,[1] and the Rey Complex Figure assessment.[57] The latter two tests also are used to evaluate visual memory skills. Use of the Rey Complex Figure has been suggested for a quick screening of visual perceptual function.[59] Nonstandardized tests that may be used are

TABLE 25.1 Elements of a Comprehensive Apraxia Assessment	
Test Condition	**Example**
Gesture to command	"Show me how you would take off your hat." (transitive)
	"Show me how you would throw a kiss." (intransitive)
Gesture to imitation	"Copy what I do." Therapist shrugs shoulders. (intransitive) Therapist flips an imaginary coin. (transitive)
Gesture in response to seeing the tool	"Show me how you would, seeing the tool, use this object." Therapist provides screwdriver for display.
Gesture in response to seeing the object upon which the tool works	"Show me how you would use this object." Therapist provides screwdriver and block of wood with screw partially inserted.
Actual tool use	"Show me how you would use this object." Therapist provides screwdriver for use.
Imitation of the examiner using the tool	"Copy what I do." Therapist makes stirring motion, using a spoon.
Discrimination between correct and incorrect pantomimed movements	"Is this the correct way to blow out a match?" Therapist pantomimes holding a match in an unsafe manner (e.g., match held upside down, with the head of the match near the palm of hand).
Gesture comprehension	"What object am I using?" Therapist pantomimes shaving face with a razor.
Serial acts	"Show me how you would open an imaginary can of soda, pour it into a glass, and take a drink."

From Heilman KM, Rothi LJG: Apraxia. In Heilman KM, Valenstein E, editors: *Clinical Neuropsychology*, New York, 1993, Oxford University Press.

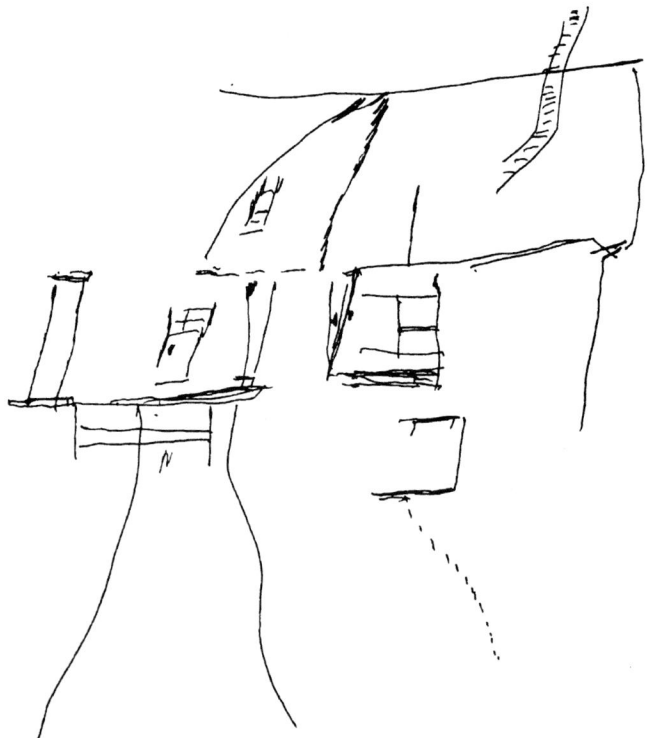

Fig. 25.3 Example of a two-dimensional constructional disorder and left-sided inattention in a drawing of a house by a retired architect who suffered a right cerebrovascular accident.

drawing, constructing matchstick designs, assembling block designs, or building a structure to match a model.[97] In daily living, occupations such as dressing or setting the table require constructional skills. To perform such tasks successfully, an individual must have integrated visual perception, motor planning, and motor execution.

Construction apraxia has been linked to lesions in both the left and right hemispheres.[35] The process involved to construct drawings or block designs is seen as requiring several intact cortical regions to work together effectively.[89] Damage or impairment in the frontal lobe region tends to produce errors in perseveration and planning and poor organization when attempting to replicate the design. Parietal lobe lesions result in errors in the orientation of the design.

The remedial approach to intervention involves the use of perceptual tasks such as paper and pencil activities, puzzles, and three-dimensional craft projects to improve constructional skills. The adaptive approach includes participating in occupational performance and developing compensatory approaches to the functional performance skill impairments. Many areas of occupation are suitable for the treatment of constructional deficits, such as folding towels, hanging up clothing items in a closet, setting the dinner table, and weeding the garden.

BEHAVIORAL ASPECTS OF PERCEPTUAL DYSFUNCTION

Some degree of accurate self-awareness and recognition of the effect of the disability on one's functioning is needed if the person is to invest energy in the therapy process.[17] An individual who is unaware of perceptual deficits may be a serious safety risk and may attempt occupations that are well beyond present physical abilities. Denial of impairment is often noted in early stages of recovery from CVA or TBI in which damage has occurred in the right hemisphere.[17,46] A person's innate trust in the accuracy of perceptions often is a basis for unrealistic self-confidence; demonstrating to the individual that personal perceptions are now distorted and no longer trustworthy can profoundly affect the person's sense of self. An occupational therapist needs to be respectful and sensitive to the individual's sense of self and be prepared to aid the client in understanding the changes in perceptual capacity and in reestablishing an accurate sense of self. Several questionnaires are available to assess an individual's self-awareness.[52] The questionnaires typically are issued to the person with deficits as well as to a family member or close acquaintance. The discrepancies in the two questionnaires are used as a measure of the accuracy of the individual's insight and serve as the basis for intervention. The individual's behavior also may be the result of a disorder in executive function. (See Chapter 26 for additional discussion of this possibility.)

An individual who has some degree of awareness of the disability may be depressed, which seems an appropriate response given the effect of perceptual impairments on participation in occupational roles. The occupational therapist needs to recognize and appreciate this emotional response and assist the individual in achieving an emotional balance to reestablish quality of life through celebrating progress in therapy while acknowledging the impact of the perceptual impairments on participation in occupation. (See also Chapter 6 on the social and psychological aspects.)

THREADED CASE STUDY

Walt, Part 7

1. How would you best assess Walt's occupational performance?

   Walt's performance in his most valued occupations has been affected because of visual perceptual impairment. A combination of skilled observation and formal assessments, such as the A-ONE[7,8] and the AMPS,[34] could be used to assess Walt's occupational performance in a variety of functional contexts. In addition to evaluating occupational performance, these assessments can also appraise Walt's specific perceptual functioning. The Canadian Occupational Performance Measure also can be used to evaluate the client's primary goals in occupational therapy and set the stage for an occupation-based and client-centered approach to intervention.

2. How would you best assess Walt's perceptual function?

   Throughout the chapter, a variety of assessment tools have been presented to evaluate visual perception, visual-spatial perception, tactile perception, body schema perception, and motor perception. In addition, other comprehensive perceptual tests—such as the Motor Free Visual Perceptual Test, Revised,[24] Test of Visual-Motor Skills, Third Edition,[60] the Test for Upper Limb Apraxia

(TULIA),[85] the Florida Apraxia Screening Test (FAST),[74] the Movement Imitation Test,[29,30] the Use of Objects Test,[29] and the Loewenstein Occupational Therapy Cognitive Assessment–Second Edition (LOTCA-II)[45]—could be used to assess global areas of visual processing and perceptual functioning.

3. How would you assist Walt in achieving his occupational performance goals using remedial and adaptive approaches for his perceptual dysfunction?

   To assist Walt in achieving his occupational performance goals of submitting a painting to a local art gallery, playing with his children, driving, and regaining computer skills in preparation for resuming part-time work as a graphic artist at an architectural firm, the therapist would need to use a combination of remedial and adaptive approaches to treat his perceptual impairments. This chapter outlines a variety of intervention possibilities for Walt. The evidence shows that the most successful outcomes for treating visual perceptual impairments are through occupation-based activities that have meaning and offer the client the opportunity to generalize functional skills to multiple contexts through the remediation and adaptation of perceptual dysfunction.[69,70]

REVIEW QUESTIONS

1. Describe the effects of visual perception, visual-spatial perception, tactile perception, body schema perception, and motor perception on occupational performance.

2. Compare the advantages and disadvantages of formal perceptual testing and functional assessment in the context of occupational performance.

3. Describe one assessment used to test perceptual impairments in the following areas: visual perception, visual-spatial perception, tactile perception, body schema perception, and motor perception.

4. Describe the two approaches to treatment of perceptual deficits, and give one example of an occupational therapy intervention for each.

5. Describe an intervention for each of the following types of perceptual dysfunction: visual perception, visual-spatial perception, tactile perception, body schema perception, and motor perception.

REFERENCES

1. Abe M, Kimura N, Sasaki Y, Eguchi A, Matsubara E: Association between Benton Visual Retention Test scores and PET imaging in elderly adults, *Curr Alzheimer Res* 18(11):900–907, 2021. https://doi.org/10.2174/1567205018666211207094121. PMID: 34875990.

2. Aguilar-Ferrándiz ME, Toledano-Moreno S, García-Ríos MC, Tapia-Haro RM, Barrero-Hernández FJ, Casas-Barragán A, Pérez-Mármol JM: Effectiveness of a functional rehabilitation program for upper limb apraxia in poststroke patients: A randomized controlled trial, *Arch Phys Med Rehabil* 102(5):940–950, 2021. https://doi.org/10.1016/j.apmr.2020.12.015. PMID: 33485836.

3. American Occupational Therapy Association: Occupational therapy practice framework: Domain and process (4th ed.), *American Journal of Occupational Therapy*, 74(Suppl. 2), 7412410010 p1–7412410010p87. https://doi.org/10.5014/ajot.2020.74S2001.

4. Antoniello D, Gottesman R: The phenomenology of acute anosognosia for hemiplegia, *J Neuropsychiatry Clin Neurosci* 32(3):259–265, 2020. https://doi.org/10.1176/appi.neuropsych.19010008. PMID: 31662091.

5. Ardila A: Some unusual neuropsychological syndromes: Somatoparaphrenia, akinetopsia, reduplicative paramnesia, autotopagnosia, *Arch Clin Neuropsychol* 31(5):456–464, 2016. https://doi.org/10.1093/arclin/acw021. PMID: 27193360.

6. Ardila A: Gerstmann syndrome, *Curr Neurol Neurosci Rep* 20(11):48, 2020. https://doi.org/10.1007/s11910-020-01069-9. PMID: 32852667.

7. Árnadóttir G: Evaluation and intervention with complex perceptual impairment. In Unsworth C, editor: *Cognitive and Perceptual Dysfunction: A Clinical Reasoning Approach to Evaluation and Intervention*, Philadelphia, 1999, FA Davis.

8. Árnadóttir G: Impact of neurobehavioral deficits on activities of daily living. In Gillen G, editor: *Stroke Rehabilitation: A Function-Based Approach*, ed 4, 2016, Elsevier.

9. Balconi M, Crivelli D, Cortesi L: Transitive versus intransitive complex gesture representation: A comparison between execution, observation and imagination by fNIRS, *Appl Psychophysiol Biofeedback* 42(3):179–191, 2017. https://doi.org/10.1007/s10484-017-9365-1. PMID: 28589287.

10. Baumard J, Le Gall D: The challenge of apraxia: Toward an operational definition? *Cortex.* 141:66–80, 2021. https://doi.org/10.1016/j.cortex.2021.04.001. PMID: 34033988.

11. Benton AL: *Contributions to Neuropsychological Assessment: A Clinical Manual*, Oxford, 1983, Oxford University Press.

12. Blakemore C, Movshon JA: Sensory system: Introduction. In Gazzaniga MS, editor: *The Cognitive Neurosciences*, London, 1996, MIT Press.

13. Brown T, Elliott S: Factor structure of the motor-free visual perception test-3rd edition (MVPT-3), *Can J Occup Ther* 78:26–36, 2011. http://search.proquest.com/docview/859014382?accountid=143111.

14. Brown GT, Rodger S, Davis A: Test of visual perceptual skills—revised: A review and critique, *Scand J Occup Ther* 10:3–19, 2003.

15. Brown T, Peres L: A critical review of the Motor-Free Visual Perception Test–fourth edition (MVPT-4), *Journal of Occupational Therapy, Schools, & Early Intervention* 11(2):229–244, 2018. https://doi.org/10.1080/19411243.2018.1432441.

16. Bruce V, Young A: *In the Eye of the Beholder: The Science of Face Perception*, Oxford, 1998, Oxford University Press.

17. Byrd EM, Jablonski RJ, Vance DE: Understanding anosognosia for hemiplegia after stroke, *Rehabil Nurs.* 45(1):3–15, 2020. https://doi.org/10.1097/rnj.0000000000000185. PMID: 30086101.

18. Calder AJ, Young AW, Rowland D, et al: Facial emotion recognition after bilateral amygdala damage: Differentially severe impairment of fear, *Cogn Neuropsychol* 13:699, 1996.

19. Carey L, Macdonell R, Matyas TA: SENSe: Study of the effectiveness of neurorehabilitation on sensation: A randomized controlled trial, *Neurorehabil Neural Repair* 25(4):304–313, 2011. https://doi.org/10.1177/1545968310397705. PMID: 21350049.

20. Carey LM, Matyas TA, Baum C: Effects of somatosensory impairment on participation after stroke, *Am J Occup Ther* 72(3), 2018. 7203205100p1-7203205100p10. https://doi.org/10.5014/ajot.2018.025114. PMID: 29689179; PMCID: PMC5915232.

21. Cawood J, Visagie S, Mji G: Impact of post-stroke impairments on activities and participation as experienced by stroke survivors in a Western Cape setting, *South African Journal of Occupational Therapy* 46(2):10–15, 2016. https://doi.org/10.17159/2310-3833/2016/v46n2a3.

22. Choi H, Kim D, Yang Y: The effect of a complex intervention program for unilateral neglect in patients with acute-phase stroke: A randomized controlled trial, *Osong Public Health & Research Perspectives* 10(5):265–273, 2019. https://doi.org/10.24171/j.phrp.2019.10.5.02.

23. Choi HS, Shin WS, Bang DH: Application of digital practice to improve head movement, visual perception and activities of daily living for subacute stroke patients with unilateral spatial neglect: Preliminary results of a single-blinded, randomized controlled trial, *Medicine (Baltimore)* 100(6):e24637, 2021. https://doi.org/10.1097/MD.0000000000024637. PMID: 33578583; PMCID: PMC7886475.

24. Colarusso RP, Hammill DD: *Motor-Free Visual Perception Test*, ed 3, Novato, CA, 2003, Academic Therapy Publications.

25. Cooke DM, McKenna K, Fleming J, Darnell R: Criterion validity of the occupational therapy adult perceptual screening test, *Scand J Occup Ther*, 13:38–44, 2006.

26. Cubelli R, Della Sala S: Constructional apraxia, *Cortex*. 104:127, 2018. https://doi.org/10.1016/j.cortex.2018.02.015. PMID: 29587996.

27. De Renzi E: Methods of limb apraxia examination and their bearing on the interpretation of the disorder. In Roy EA, editor: *Neuropsychological Studies of Apraxia and Related Disorders*, Amsterdam, 1985, North-Holland.

28. De Renzi E, Lucchelli F: Ideational apraxia, *Brain* 111(Pt 5):1173–1185, 1988. https://doi.org/10.1093/brain/111.5.1173. PMID: 3179688.

29. De Renzi E, Faglioni P, Sorgato P: Modality-specific and supramodal mechanisms of apraxia, *Brain* 105:301, 1982.

30. De Renzi E, Motti F, Nichelli P, et al: Imitating gestures: A quantitative approach to ideomotor apraxia, *Arch Neurol* 37:6, 1980.

31. Donnelly S: The Rivermead Perceptual Assessment Battery: Can it predict functional performance? *Australian Occupational Therapy Journal* 49:71–81, 2002.

32. Donnelly SM, Hextell D, Matthey S, et al: The Rivermead Perceptual Assessment Battery: Its relationship to selected functional activities, *Br J Occup Ther* 61:27, 1998.

33. Facchin A, Sartori E, Luisetti C, De Galeazzi A, Beschin N: Effect of prism adaptation on neglect hemianesthesia, *Cortex*. 113:298–311, 2019. https://doi.org/10.1016/j.cortex.2018.12.021. PMID: 30716611.

34. Fisher AG: *Assessment of Motor and Process Skills*, Fort Collins, CO, 1995, Three Star Press.

35. Gainotti G, Trojano L: Constructional apraxia, *Handb Clin Neurol* 151:331–348, 2018. https://doi.org/10.1016/B978-0-444-63622-5.00016-4. PMID: 29519467.

36. Gardner H: *Frames of Mind: The Theory of Multiple Intelligences*, New York, 1983, Basic Books.

37. Gardner MF: *The Test of Visual Perceptual Skills—Revised (TVPS-R)*, Hydesville, CA, 1997, Psychological and Educational Publications.

38. Geschwind N: The apraxias: Neural mechanisms of disorders of learned movement, *Am Sci* 63:188, 1975.

39. Gutman SA: *Quick Reference Neuroscience for Rehabilitation Professionals*, ed 3, 2017, Slack, Inc.

40. Gutman SA, Schonfeld AB: *Screening Adult Neurologic Populations*, ed 3, 2019, AOTA Press.

41. Heutink J, Indorf DL, Cordes C: The neuropsychological rehabilitation of visual agnosia and Balint's syndrome, *Neuropsychol Rehabil* 29(10):1489–1508, 2019. https://doi.org/10.1080/09602011.2017.1422272. PMID: 29366371.

42. Holmes NP, Spence C: The body schema and the multisensory representation(s) of peripersonal space, *Cogn Process* 5(2):94–105, 2004. https://doi.org/10.1007/s10339-004-0013-3. PMID: 16467906; PMCID: PMC1350799.

43. Hooper HE: *Hooper Visual Organization Test*, Los Angeles, 1983, Western Psychological Services.

44. Ishihara K, Ishihara S, Nagamachi M, Osaki H: Independence of older adults in performing instrumental activities of daily living (IADLs) and the relation of this performance to visual abilities, *Theoret Iss Ergonomics, Sci* 5:198–213, 2004.

45. Itzkovich M, Elazar B, Averbach S, Katz, N: *Lowenstein Occupational Therapy Cognitive Assessment (LOTCA - II) Battery*. 2nd ed. Pequannock: Maddak; 2000.

46. Jenkinson PM, Moro V, Fotopoulou A: Definition: Asomatognosia, *Cortex*. 101:300–301, 2018. https://doi.org/10.1016/j.cortex.2018.02.001. PMID: 29510834.

47. Jensen L, Padilla R: Effectiveness of environment-based interventions that address behavior, perception, and falls in people with Alzheimer's disease and related major neurocognitive disorders: A systematic review, *American Journal of Occupational Therapy* 71:7105180030 p1–7105180030p10, 2017. https://doi.org/10.5014/ajot.2017.027409.

48. Katz N: *Cognition, Occupation and Participation Across the Lifespan*, ed 3, 2011, AOTA Press.

49. Katz N, Averbuch S, Bar-Haim Erez A: Dynamic Lowenstein Occupational Therapy Cognitive Assessment–Geriatric Version (DLOTCA–G): Assessing change in cognitive performance, *American Journal of Occupational Therapy* 66:311–319, 2012. https://doi.org/10.5014/ajot.2012.002485.

50. Katz N, Livni L, Bar-Haim Erez A, Averbuch S: *Dynamic Lowenstein Occupational Therapy Cognitive Assessment (DLOTCA)*, Pequannock, NJ, 2011, Maddak.

51. Kim SJ, Yang YN, Lee JW, Lee JY, Jeong E, Kim BR, Lee J: Reliability and validity of Korean version of apraxia screen of TULIA (K-AST), *Ann Rehabil Med* 40(5):769–778, 2016. https://doi.org/10.5535/arm.2016.40.5.769. PMID: 27847706; PMCID: PMC5108703.

52. Kline DW, Scialfa CT: Visual and auditory aging. In Birren JE, Schaie KW, editors: *Handbook of the Psychology of Aging*, ed 4, San Diego, CA, 1996, Academic Press.

53. Kremláček J, Šikl R, Kuba M, Szanyi J, Kubová Z, Langrová J, Vít F, Šimecek M, Stodůlka P: Spared cognitive processing of visual oddballs despite delayed visual evoked potentials in patient with partial recovery of vision after 53 years of blindness, *Vision Res* 81:1–5, 2013. https://doi.org/10.1016/j.visres.2012.12.013. PMID: 23395864.

54. Kusch M, Schmidt CC, Göden L, Tscherpel C, Stahl J, Saliger J, Karbe H, Fink GR, Weiss PH: Recovery from apraxic deficits and its neural correlate, *Restor Neurol Neurosci* 36(6):669–678, 2018. https://doi.org/10.3233/RNN-180815. PMID: 30282379.

55. Lannin N, Carr B, Allaous J, Mackenzie B, Falcon A, Tate R: A randomized controlled trial of the effectiveness of handheld computers for improving everyday memory functioning in patients with memory impairments after acquired brain injury, *Clin Rehabil* 28(5):470–481, 2014. https://doi.org/10.1177/0269215513512216. PMID: 24452701.

56. Law M, Baptiste S, McColl M, et al: *The Canadian Occupational Performance Measure*, ed 4, Ottawa, Ontario, 2000, CAOT Publications.

57. Lezak MD: *Neuropsychological Assessment*, ed 5, 2012, Oxford University Press.

58. Likert R, Quasha WH: *The Revised Minnesota Paper Form Board Test*, New York, 1970, Psychological Corporation.

59. Lincoln NB, Drummond AER, Edmans JA, et al: The Rey figure copy as a screening instrument for perceptual deficits after stroke, *Br J Occup Ther* 61:33, 1998.

60. Martin NA: *Test of Visual-Motor Skills. (TVMS-3)*, ed 3, 2010, Western Psychological Services.

61. Mazer BL, Korner-Bitensky NA, Sofer S: Predicting ability to drive after stroke, *Arch Phys Med Rehabil* 79:743, 1998.

62. Mendoza JE: Autotopagnosia. In Kreutzer JS, DeLuca J, Caplan B, editors: *Encyclopedia of Clinical Neuropsychology*, New York, NY, 2011, Springer. https://doi.org/10.1007/978-0-387-79948-3_712.

63. Mercier L, Hebert J, Colarusso RP, et al: *Motor-free Visual Perception Test—Vertical (MVPT-V)*, Novato, CA, 1997, Academic Therapy Publications.

64. Merten T: Factor structure of the Hooper Visual Organization Test: a cross-cultural replication and extension, *Archives of Clinical Neuropsychology* 20(1):123–128, 2005. https://doi.org/10.1016/j.acn.2004.03.001.

65. Mitolo M, Gardini S, Caffarra P, Ronconi L, Venneri A, Pazzaglia F: Relationship between spatial ability, visuospatial working memory and self-assessed spatial orientation ability: A study in older adults, *Cogn Process* 16(2):165–276, 2015. https://doi.org/10.1007/s10339-015-0647-3. PMID: 25739724.

66. Moon J, Park K, Kim H, Na C: The effects of task-oriented circuit training using rehabilitation tools on the upper-extremity functions and daily activities of patients with acute stroke: A randomized controlled pilot trial, *Osong Public Health and Research Perspectives* 9(5):225–230, 2018.

67. Morasso P, Casadio M, Mohan V, Rea F, Zenzeri J: Revisiting the body-schema concept in the context of whole-body postural-focal dynamics, *Front Hum Neurosci* 9:83, 2015. https://doi.org/10.3389/fnhum.2015.00083. PMID: 25741274; PMCID: PMC4330890.

68. Neistadt ME: A critical analysis of occupational therapy approaches for perceptual deficits in adults with brain injury, *Am J Occup Ther* 44:299, 1990.

69. Neistadt ME: Occupational therapy treatments for constructional deficits, *Am J Occup Ther* 46:141, 1992.

70. Neistadt ME: Perceptual retraining for adults with diffuse brain injury, *Am J Occup Ther* 48:225, 1994.

71. Pazzaglia M, Galli G: Action observation for neurorehabilitation in apraxia, *Front Neurol* 10:309, 2019. https://doi.org/10.3389/fneur.2019.00309. PMID: 31001194; PMCID: PMC6456663.

72. Preissner K, Arbesman M, Lieberman D: Occupational therapy interventions for adults with multiple sclerosis, *Am J Occup Ther* 70(3) 7003395010p1–7003395010p4, 2016. https://doi.org/10.5014/ajot.2016.703001. PMID: 27089301.

73. Romano D, Tosi G, Gobbetto V, Pizzagalli P, Avesani R, Moro V, Maravita A: Back in control of intentional action: Improvement of ideomotor apraxia by mirror box treatment, *Neuropsychologia* 160:107964, 2021. https://doi.org/10.1016/j.neuropsychologia.2021.107964. PMID: 34302848.

74. Rothi LJG, Raymer AM, Heilman KM: Limb praxis assessment. In Rothi LJG, Heilman KM, editors: *Apraxia: The Neuropsychology of Action. Brain Damage, Behaviour and Cognition Series*, Hove, UK, 1997, Psychology Press, pp 61–73.

75. Rubio KB, Van Deusen J: Relation of perceptual and body image dysfunction to activities of daily living after stroke, *Am J Occup Ther* 49:551, 1995.

76. Šikl R, Šimeček M, Porubanová-Norquist M, et al. Vision after 53 years of blindness. *i-Perception* 4(8):498–507, 2013. https://www.ncbi.nlm.nih.gov/pmc/articles/PMC4129383/.

77. Schuett S, Heywood CA, Kentridge RW, Dauner R, Zihl J: Rehabilitation of reading and visual exploration in visual field disorders: Transfer or specificity? *Brain* 135(3):912–921, 2012. https://doi.org/10.1093/brain/awr356.

78. Toglia J: Generalization of treatment: A multi-contextual approach to cognitive-perceptual impairment in the brain-injured adult, *Am J Occup Ther* 45:505, 1991.

79. Toglia J: The dynamic interactional model of cognition in cognitive rehabilitation. In Katz N, editor: *Cognition and Occupation Across the Lifespan: Models for Intervention in Occupational Therapy* ed 3, Bethesda, MD, 2011, AOTA Press.

80. Tranel D, Vianna E, Manzel K, Damasio H, Grabowski T: Neuroanatomical correlates of the Benton Facial Recognition Test and Judgment of Line Orientation Test, *J Clin Exp Neuropsychol* 31(2):219–233, 2009. https://doi.org/10.1080/13803390802317542. PMID: 19051129; PMCID: PMC2853018.

81. Trojano L: Constructional apraxia from the roots up: Kleist, Strauss, and their contemporaries, *Neurol Sci* 41(4):981–988, 2020. https://doi.org/10.1007/s10072-019-04186-7. PMID: 31820324.

82. Tsurumi K, Todd V: Theory and guidelines for visual task analysis and synthesis. In Scheiman M, editor: *Understanding and Managing Vision Deficits: A Guide For Occupational Therapists*, Thorofare, NJ, 2011, Slack, Inc.

83. Turville M, Carey LM, Matyas TA, Blennerhassett J: Change in functional arm use is associated with somatosensory skills after sensory retraining poststroke, *Am J Occup Ther* 71(3), 7103190070p1-7103190070p9, 2017. https://doi.org/10.5014/ajot.2017.024950. PMID: 28422633.

84. Turville ML, Cahill LS, Matyas TA, Blennerhassett JM, Carey LM: The effectiveness of somatosensory retraining for improving sensory function in the arm following stroke: A systematic review, *Clin Rehabil* 33(5):834–846, 2019. https://doi.org/10.1177/0269215519829795. PMID: 30798643.

85. Vanbellingen T, Kersten B, Van Hemelrijk B, Van de Winckel A, Bertschi M, Müri R, De Weerdt W, Bohlhalter S: Comprehensive assessment of gesture production: A new test of upper limb apraxia (TULIA), *Eur J Neurol* 17(1):59–66, 2010. https://doi.org/10.1111/j.1468-1331.2009.02741.x. PMID: 19614961.

86. Vanbellingen T, Kersten B, Van de Winckel A, Bellion M, Baronti F, Müri R, Bohlhalter S: A new bedside test of gestures in stroke: The apraxia screen of TULIA (AST), *J Neurol Neurosurg Psychiatry* 82(4):389–392, 2011. https://doi.org/10.1136/jnnp.2010.213371. PMID: 20935324.

87. Vanbellingen T, Lungu C, Lopez G, Baronti F, Müri R, Hallett M, Bohlhalter S: Short and valid assessment of apraxia in Parkinson's disease, *Parkinsonism Relat Disord* 18(4):348–350, 2012. https://doi.org/10.1016/j.parkreldis.2011.11.023. PMID: 22177625; PMCID: PMC4314207.

88. Vancleef K, Colwell MJ, Hewitt O, Demeyere N: Current practice and challenges in screening for visual perception deficits after stroke: a qualitative study, *Disabil Rehabil* 44(10):2063–2072, 2022. https://doi.org/10.1080/09638288.2020.1824245. PMID: 33016779.

89. Van der Stigchel S, de Bresser J, Heinen R, Koek HL, Reijmer YD, Biessels GJ, van den Berg E; on behalf of the Utrecht Vascular Cognitive Impairment (VCI) Study Group. Parietal involvement in constructional apraxia as measured using the pentagon copying task, *Dement Geriatr Cogn Disord* 46(1-2):50–59, 2018. https://doi.org/10.1159/000491634. PMID: 30145597; PMCID: PMC6187841.

90. Wan YT, Chiang CS, Chen SC, Wuang YP: The effectiveness of the computerized visual perceptual training program on individuals with Down syndrome: An fMRI study, *Res Dev Disabil* 66:1–15, 2017. https://doi.org/10.1016/j.ridd.2017.04.015. PMID: 28535411.

91. Warren M, Barstow EA: *Occupational Therapy Interventions for Adults with low Vision*, 2011, AOTA Press.

92. Wheeler S, Acord-Vira A, Arbesman M, Lieberman D: Occupational therapy interventions for adults with traumatic brain injury, *Am J Occup Ther* 71(3), 2017. 7103395010p1-7103395010p3. https://doi.org/10.5014/ajot.2017.713005. PMID: 28422643.

93. Wolf TJ: *Stroke: Interventions to Support Occupational Performance*, 2014, AOTA Press.

94. Yoo PY, Scott K, Myszak F, Mamann S, Labelle A, Holmes M, Guindon A, Bussieres AE: Interventions addressing vision, visual-perceptual impairments following acquired brain injury: A cross-sectional survey, *Can J Occup Ther* 87(2):117–126, 2020. https://doi.org/10.1177/0008417419892393. PMID: 31896281.
95. Young AW, Newcombe F, de Haan EH, et al: Face perception after brain injury: Selective impairments affecting identity and expression, *Brain* 116(Pt 4):941–953, 1993.
96. Zlotnik S, Sachs D, Rosenblum S, Shpasser R, Josman N: Use of the dynamic interactional model in selfcare and motor intervention after traumatic brain injury: Explanatory case studies, *American Journal of Occupational Therapy* 63:549–558, 2009.
97. Zoltan B: *Vision, perception, and cognition*, ed 4, Thorofare, NJ, 2007, Slack.

SUGGESTED READINGS

Gentile M: *Functional Visual Behavior in Adults: An Occupational Therapy Guide to Evaluation and Treatment Options*, ed 2, Bethesda, MD, 2005, AOTA Press.
Scheiman M: *Understanding and Managing Vision Deficits: A Guide for Occupational Therapists*, Thorofare, NJ, 1977, Slack.

26

Evaluation and Treatment of Limited Occupational Performance Secondary to Cognitive Dysfunction

Glen Gillen

LEARNING OBJECTIVES

After studying this chapter, the student or practitioner will be able to do the following:

1. Understand the interplay between cognition and performance in areas of occupation.
2. Choose appropriate standardized, reliable, and ecologically valid tools to measure baseline cognitive status and client progression.
3. Understand the impact of impaired client factors and performance skills on performance in areas of occupation.
4. Develop an evidence-based treatment plan to maximize participation in chosen occupations for individuals with cognitive dysfunction.

CHAPTER OUTLINE

KEY TERMS

Anterograde amnesia
Areas of occupation
Arousal
Attention
Attentional switching or alternating attention
Awareness deficits
Client-centered approach
Cognitive Orientation to Daily Occupational Performance (CO-OP)
Cognitive rehabilitation/retraining model
Cognitive retraining
Declarative memory
Distractibility
Divided attention
Dynamic Interactional Model
Dysexecutive syndrome
Ecological validity
Episodic memory
Explicit memory

Field-dependent behavior
Implicit memory
Long-term memory
Metacognition
Metamemory
Neurofunctional approach
Nondeclarative memory
Procedural memory
Prospective memory
Quadraphonic approach
Retrograde amnesia
Selective attention
Self-awareness
Semantic memory
Short-term memory
Sustained attention (vigilance)
Task-oriented approach
Unilateral neglect
Working memory

THREADED CASE STUDY

Imani, Part 1

Imani, age 28, identifies as female (prefers use of the pronouns she/her/hers). Imani is 6 months from completing her master's degree in social work. She was recently married and lives in a ranch-style house in the suburbs. Approximately 1 week ago, she told her wife, Toni, that she was feeling "off." Later in the day she told Toni that she had the worst headache of her life (i.e., a "thunderclap headache"). She began vomiting and, according to Toni, became confused, so she took her to the hospital. The medical team determined that Imani had sustained a subarachnoid hemorrhage secondary to a ruptured cerebral aneurysm. She had emergency surgery, which involved a craniotomy and clipping of the aneurysm. On postoperative day 8, she was transferred to the brain injury rehabilitation unit at the hospital.

Imani's occupational profile was determined her first day on the rehabilitation unit through interviews with Imani (who was quite drowsy and distracted), Toni, and Imani's sister, Paula. Toni described Imani as "fiercely independent" and reluctant to ask for help. It was determined that, in addition to being a "grade A graduate student," Imani had shared housekeeping responsibilities with Toni, maintained the family garden, was an avid reader of fiction, was responsible for paying the monthly bills online, and loved to cook. Currently Imani could not participate fully in any of these occupations. Her biggest goal has been graduating on time. She has spent a tremendous amount of time and money getting through graduate school. Also, since high school she has been a volunteer working with impoverished children in urban areas. Toni stated that Imani was pursuing a social work degree to build her skills and "give her credibility," so that she could continue to serve these children.

Toni and Paula expressed concern that Imani did not know what day it was, did not remember who had visited earlier in the day, and was slow to respond to questions, to which she sometimes gave inaccurate answers. During the interviews, Imani spent much of the time sleeping. She did not know why she could not "just go home."

Critical Thinking Questions

1. How would you structure Imani's initial evaluation to determine the reasons she cannot currently engage in the occupations meaningful to her? What assessments would you choose, and how would you prioritize them?
2. What are appropriate goals for Imani?
3. What interventions would you use to ensure that Imani meets her initial goals? What is the starting point for intervention?

COGNITION AND OCCUPATIONAL THERAPY

The American Occupational Therapy Association (AOTA) asserts that occupational therapists and occupational therapy assistants, through the use of occupations and activities, facilitate individuals' cognitive functioning to enhance occupational performance, self-efficacy, participation, and perceived quality of life. Cognition is integral to effective performance across the broad range of daily occupations such as work, educational pursuits, home management, and play and leisure. Cognition also plays an integral role in human development and in the ability to learn, retain, and use new information in response to changes in everyday life.

American Occupational Therapy Association[3]

Occupational therapy is one of several professions (e.g., psychology, psychiatry, neuropsychology, speech-language pathology,

and neurology) involved in working with those who are cognitively impaired. However, the approach of occupational therapy to this area of practice is unique and differentiated from other disciplines.[3] The clinical focus of what most professions call cognitive rehabilitation or working on cognition is better described by occupational therapists (OTs) as the process of improving participation and quality of life for individuals with cognitive impairments. In terms of maintaining this unique focus, the reader should consider the following points related to the process and domain of the practice of occupational therapy as they relate to this area of practice.

- Evaluations and assessments should focus on clients' performance of relevant occupations. Simultaneously (as described later), the OT documents what impairment or patterns of impairment in client factors and performance skills are interfering with occupational performance and participation.[11]
- Goals should be related to improving performance in **areas of occupation**, as described by the current version (2020) of the OT Framework, "Occupational Therapy Practice Framework: Domain and Process," fourth edition (OTPF-4).[4]
- Interventions should consist of primarily graded relevant occupations being performed in natural contexts.
- The outcomes of OT intervention for individuals with cognitive impairment should document improved performance in areas of occupation.

Although these points may seem obvious, until recently this area of OT practice focused primarily on impairments in client factors, and the focus of intervention involved the use of contrived "cognitive tasks." Outcomes were measured on the basis of tests of cognition that were not related to daily performance. It was assumed that remediation of an identified impairment or impairments would generalize into the ability to perform meaningful, functional activities. In general, this assumption has not been supported by empirical research.[43] It has become clear that this approach is not consistent with current approaches to occupational therapy.[4] Current practice embraces interventions that focus on strategies for living independently, with a purpose, and with improved quality of life, despite the presence of cognitive impairments. Likewise, outcome measures that focus on documenting improved functioning outside a clinic environment and those that include test items focused on performing functional activities are being embraced.[43] This chapter focuses on areas of occupation, client factors, and performance skills[4] and their relationships (Table 26.1).

OVERVIEW OF MODELS GUIDING THE PRACTICE OF OCCUPATIONAL THERAPY

Various models that guide this OT practice area have been described in the literature. (The reader is referred to Katz for a comprehensive description of these models.[54])

A common theme in OT practice addressing cognitive impairment is maintaining a client-centered approach when providing rehabilitation services. As Law et al.[6] noted, such an approach "embraces a philosophy of respect for, and partnership with, people receiving services. A **client-centered approach** fosters an active partnership where the client joins with the OT

TABLE 26.1	Summary of the OTPF-4 Domains Related to Cognition and Occupation
Domain	**Examples**
Performance in areas of occupation	Activities of daily living (ADLs), instrumental activities of daily living (IADLs), education, work, play, leisure, rest and sleep, and social participation
Client factors (body functions)	**Specific Mental Functions** • Higher level cognitive: Judgment, concept formation, executive functions, metacognition, cognitive flexibility, insight • Attention: Sustained, selective, and divided • Memory: Short-term, long-term, working memory • Perception: Discrimination of sensations • Thought: Control and content of thought, awareness of reality versus delusions, logical and coherent thought • Mental functions to sequence complex movements • Emotional • Experience of self and time **Global Mental Functions** • Consciousness: State of awareness and alertness • Orientation: Orientation to person, place, time, self, and others • Psychosocial: General mental functions, as they develop over the life span, required to understand and constructively integrate the mental functions that lead to the formation of the personal and interpersonal skills needed to establish reciprocal social interactions, in terms of both meaning and purpose • Energy: Energy level, motivation, appetite, craving, impulse • Sleep: Physiological process, quality of sleep • Temperament and personality: Extroversion, introversion, agreeableness, conscientiousness, emotional stability, openness to experience, self-control, self-expression, confidence, motivation, impulse control, appetite
Performance skills	Process skills: Observed as a person (1) selects, interacts with, and uses task tools and materials; (2) carries out individual actions and steps; and (3) modifies performance when problems are encountered. Examples include pace, heeds, attends, chooses, uses, handles, inquirers, initiates, continues, sequences, terminates, search/locates, and gathers.

Adapted from the American Occupational Therapy Association: Occupational therapy practice framework: Domain and process (4th ed.), *Am J Occup Ther* 74(Suppl 2):1–87, 2020.

to design and implement an intervention program to best meet the client's unique needs."

Van den Broek[117] specifically recommended using a client-centered approach as a way to enhance rehabilitation outcomes. He stated that treatment failure may occur secondary to practitioners focusing interventions on what they *believe* the client needs, rather than what the client *actually* wants. Another argument for using a client-centered approach to guide the focus of intervention in cognitive impairment is that the interventions typically used for individuals with cognitive dysfunction are notoriously difficult to generalize to other real-world settings and situations. For example, strategies taught to accomplish a specific task (e.g., using an alarm watch to maintain a medication schedule for those with memory loss) will not necessarily generalize or "carry over" to another task, such as remembering therapy appointments. Finally, in a large number of clients, the level of brain damage precludes generalizing of learned tasks.[74] This issue of task specificity related to treatment interventions must always be considered by practitioners working with clients who have cognitive dysfunction. A client-centered approach helps ensure that the outcomes, goals, and tasks used as the focus of therapy are at least relevant, meaningful, and specific to each *client*, in addition to the *caretaker* or *significant others*, despite their potential lack of generalizability in individuals with cognitive impairment.

Dynamic Interactional Model

The Dynamic Interactional Model views cognition as a product of the interaction among the person, activity, and environment.[114] Therefore, performance of a skill can be promoted by changing either the demands of the activity, the environment in which the activity is carried out, or the person's use of particular strategies to facilitate skill performance.[112,114] Toglia described several constructs associated with this model, including the following:

• Structural capacity, or physical limits in the ability to process and interpret information
• Personal context, or characteristics of the person, such as coping style, beliefs, values, and lifestyle
• Self-awareness, or understanding one's own strengths and limitations, in addition to metacognitive skills, such as the ability to judge the demands of tasks, evaluate performance, and anticipate the likelihood of problems
• Processing strategies, or underlying components that improve the performance of tasks, such as attention, visual processing, memory, organization, and problem solving
• The activity itself with respect to its demands, meaningfulness, and how familiar the activity is
• Environmental factors, such as the social, physical, and cultural aspects

Toglia summarized her conclusions in this way:

To understand cognitive function and occupational performance, one needs to analyze the interaction among person, activity, and environment. If the activity and environmental demands change, the type of cognitive strategies needed for efficient performance changes as well. Optimal performance is observed when there is a match between all three variables. Assessment and treatment reflect this dynamic view of cognition.[114]

This approach may be used with adults, children, and adolescents.

Toglia used the Dynamic Interactional Model to develop the Multicontext Treatment Approach.[112,114] Combining remedial and compensatory strategies, this approach focuses on teaching a particular strategy to perform a task and practicing this strategy across different activities, situations, and environments over time. Toglia summarized the components of this approach:

- Awareness training or structured experiences should be used in conjunction with self-monitoring techniques so that clients may redefine their knowledge of their strengths and weaknesses.
- A personal context strategy should be used. The choice of treatment activities is based on the client's interests and goals. Particular emphasis is placed on the relevance and purpose of the activities. Managing monthly bills may be an appropriate activity for a single person living alone, whereas crossword puzzles may be used as an activity for a retiree who previously enjoyed this activity.
- Processing strategies should be practiced during a variety of functional activities and situations. (Toglia defines processing strategies as strategies that help a client control cognitive and perceptual symptoms such as distractibility, impulsivity, inability to shift attention, disorganization, attention to only one side of the environment, or a tendency to overly focus on one part of an activity.)
- Activity analysis should be used to choose tasks that systematically place increased demands on the ability to generalize strategies that enhance performance.
- Transfer of learning occurs gradually and systematically as the client practices the same strategy during activities that gradually differ in physical appearance and complexity.
- Interventions should occur in multiple environments to promote generalization of learning.

Quadraphonic Approach

The quadraphonic approach was developed by Abreu and Peloquin[1] for use with individuals who were cognitively impaired after brain injury. This approach is described as including both a "micro" perspective (a focus on the remediation of subskills, such as attention and memory) and a "macro" perspective (a focus on functional skills, such as activities of daily living [ADLs] and leisure activities). The approach supports the use of remediation and compensatory strategies.

The micro perspective incorporates four theories:

1. The *teaching-learning theory* describes how clients use cues to increase cognitive awareness and control.

2. The *information processing theory* describes how an individual perceives and reacts to the environment. Three successive processing strategies are described, including detection of a stimulus, discrimination and analysis of the stimulus, and selection and determination of a response.

3. The *biomechanical theory* explains the client's movement, with an emphasis on integration of the central nervous system (CNS), musculoskeletal system, and perceptual-motor skills.

4. The *neurodevelopmental theory* addresses the quality of movement.

The macro perspective involves the use of narrative and functional analysis to explain behavior based on the following four characteristics:

1. Lifestyle status or personal characteristics related to performing everyday activities
2. Life stage status (e.g., childhood, adolescence, adulthood) and marriage
3. Health status (e.g., presence of premorbid conditions)
4. Disadvantage status, or the degree of functional restrictions resulting from impairment

Cognitive Rehabilitation/Retraining Model

The cognitive rehabilitation/retraining model is used for adolescents and adults with neurological and neuropsychological dysfunction.[12] Based on neuropsychological, cognitive, and neurobiological rationales, this model focuses on cognitive training by enhancing clients' remaining skills and teaching cognitive strategies, learning strategies, or procedural strategies.

Neurofunctional Approach

The neurofunctional approach is applied to those with severe cognitive impairments secondary to brain injuries.[38,39] This approach focuses on training clients in highly specific compensatory strategies (not expecting generalization) and specific task training. Contextual and metacognitive factors are specifically considered during intervention planning. The approach does not target the underlying cause of the functional limitation, but rather focuses directly on retraining the skill itself.

Task-Oriented Approach

Although usually discussed in relation to motor control dysfunction, the task-oriented approach has potential application for individuals with cognitive dysfunction.[84] Mathiowetz[69] has discussed this approach in detail. Summary points related to the adoption of a framework for this approach include evaluating the following areas in the order shown[69,70]:

1. Role performance (social participation): Identify past roles and whether they can be maintained or need to be changed; determine how future roles will be balanced
2. Occupational performance tasks (areas of occupation)
3. Task selection and analysis: Determine the client factors, performance skills and patterns, and/or contexts and activity demands that limit or enhance occupational performance
4. Person (client factors, performance skills and patterns): Cognitive (orientation, attention span, memory, problem solving, sequencing, calculations, learning, and generalization); psychosocial; and sensorimotor

5. Environment (context and activity demands): Including physical, socioeconomic, and cultural

In terms of intervention, Mathiowetz and Bass-Haugen[70] and Mathiowetz[69] recommended the following:

- Help clients adjust to their role and to limitations in performing tasks.
- Create an environment that uses the common challenges of everyday life.
- Practice functional tasks or close simulations to find effective and efficient strategies for performance.
- Provide opportunities for practice outside therapy time.
- Remediate a client factor (impairment).
- Adapt the environment, modify the task, or use assistive technology.

Cognitive Orientation to Daily Occupational Performance

The Cognitive Orientation to Daily Occupational Performance (CO-OP) model was developed for children with developmental coordination disorder. More recently, it has been used with neurological and adult clients with various types of dysfunction.[81] CO-OP is a:

- Client-centered problem-solving and
- Performance-based intervention

The goal is performance acquisition through a process of guided discovery of strategies that enable learning of skills. Strategies may be global and provide a general method of approaching any problem (i.e., *goal, plan, do, check*), or they may be domain specific (i.e., relating to one area of dysfunction only, such as attention to doing).

CHOOSING APPROPRIATE ASSESSMENTS

It is important to reiterate that OT outcomes should be focused on areas of occupation. We will use Imani's case to illustrate this point. Potential (noninclusive) outcomes for Imani, based on the OT Framework, may include the following[4]:

- *Outcome 1:* After occupational therapy, Imani has improved her scores on a standardized memory scale (decreased impairment in client factors), but the changes are not detected on measures of instrumental activities of daily living (IADLs) and quality of life (stable performance in areas of occupation).
- *Outcome 2:* After occupational therapy, Imani has no detectable changes on the standardized memory scale (stable impairment in client factors), but changes are detected on measures of IADLs and quality of life (improved performance in areas of occupation).
- *Outcome 3:* After occupational therapy, Imani has detectable changes on the standardized memory scale (decreased impairment in client factors), and changes are detected on measures of IADL and quality of life (improved performance in areas of occupation).

Of the three outcome scenarios, outcome 1 is the least desirable. In the past this type of outcome may have been considered successful (i.e., "Imani's memory has improved"). This outcome may be indicative of an intervention plan that is overly

focused on attempts to remediate memory skills (e.g., memory drills, computerized memory programs) without consideration of generalization to real-life scenarios. If a change at the impairment level of function does not translate or generalize to improved ability to engage in meaningful activities, participate successfully in life roles, or enhance quality of life, the importance of the intervention needs to be reconsidered. Outcomes 2 and 3 are more clinically relevant and arguably more meaningful to Imani and her family, and they represent more optimal results of structured OT services. Outcome 2 may have been achieved by focusing interventions on Imani's chosen tasks. Interventions such as teaching compensatory strategies, including the use of assistive technology, may have been responsible for this outcome. Imani is able to engage in chosen tasks despite stable impairments in memory.

Outcome 3 represents improvement (decreased impairment, improved performance of activities, and improved quality of life) across multiple health domains. Although this outcome may be considered the optimal result, the relationships among the three measures are not clear. Clinicians may assume that the improved status detected by the standardized measure of memory was also responsible for Imani's improved ability to perform household chores and child care. This reasoning is not necessarily accurate, however. The changes in the health domains may in fact occur independently of each other. In other words, Imani's improved ability to manage her household after participating in treatment may be related to the fact that the interventions specifically included teaching Imani strategies to manage her household. Similar to outcome 2, this positive change may have occurred with or without a documented improvement in memory skills.

When choosing assessments, the OT should place particular emphasis on the ecological validity of an instrument. This term refers to the degree to which the cognitive demands of the test theoretically resemble the cognitive demands in the everyday environment (this is sometimes called *functional cognition*). A test with high ecological validity identifies difficulty performing real-world functional and meaningful tasks. Ecological validity also refers to the degree to which existing tests are empirically related to measures of everyday functioning through a statistical analysis.[22]

In terms of a starting point (i.e., which areas of occupation should serve as the basis for assessment), as stated earlier, a client-centered approach is necessary. This can be assessed formally by using the Canadian Occupational Performance Measure[62] (COPM) or informally through an interview with the client and/or significant others. The clinical context also must be considered. OTs working in an acute care setting may be focused on areas such as basic mobility (moving in bed and transfers), bedside self-care, IADLs that can be performed at the bedside (e.g., money management, medication management), and sedentary leisure activities (e.g., reading fiction, doing crossword puzzles). Those working in the home setting may focus on intervention related to community reintegration, more complex IADLs, and returning to work. The OT uses observation skills to determine which underlying cognitive (and other) deficits are interfering with functional performance by using error analysis. In other words, errors in performance (occupational errors[8]) are allowed to occur as long as they are safe and not severe enough to halt performance. Árnadóttir[9] gives the following example of this technique related to observing errors during grooming and hygiene.

Dysfunctions of global and specific mental functions with an effect on grooming and hygiene tasks include ideational apraxia, organization, and sequencing problems related to activity steps, impaired judgment, decreased level of arousal, lack of attention, distraction, field dependency, impaired memory, and impaired intention. Ideational apraxia may appear during grooming and hygiene activities; an individual may not know what to do with the toothbrush, toothpaste, or shaving cream or may use these items inappropriately (e.g., smear toothpaste over the face or spray the shaving cream over the sink). An individual with organization and sequencing difficulties only may have the general idea of how to perform but may have problems timing and sequencing activity steps. Such a client may not complete one activity step before starting another or may perform activities too quickly as a result of problems in timing activity steps, resulting in a poor performance.

Lack of judgment may appear as an inability to make realistic decisions based on environmental information, providing that perception of those impulses is adequate. An individual so affected may leave the sink area without turning off the water taps or may leave the washcloth in the sink, not noticing that the water level is increasing and threatening to overflow.

Field dependency has an attention component and a perseveration component. Individuals with this dysfunction may be distracted from performing a particular task by specific stimuli that they are compelled to act on or incorporate into the previous activity. For example, if an individual with field dependency sees a denture brush while washing the hands, that person may incorporate the brush into the activity and scrub the hands with the denture brush.

An individual with short-term memory problems may not remember the sequence of activity steps or instructions throughout activity performance. The therapist may have to remind an individual several times to comb the hair, even though the individual does not have comprehension problems.

Lack of initiation may occur during performance of grooming and hygiene tasks; the individual may sit by the sink without performing, even after being asked to wash. With repeated instructions to begin, the individual may indicate that the activity is about to start, yet nothing happens. After several such incidents and if the therapist asks for a plan, the individual may state a detailed plan of action in which the water will be turned on, the washcloth will be picked up and put under the running water, soap will be put on the cloth, and washing will begin. The individual has a plan of action but cannot start the plan. This impairment also may be associated with ideational problems.

Traditionally, practitioners and researchers involved in working with those who are cognitively impaired use standardized measures of cognitive impairment (i.e., standardized tests to determine impairments in attention, memory, executive functions, and so on) as the primary outcome measure to document the effectiveness of interventions. These measures tend to be categorized as "pen and paper" or "tabletop" assessments, and they have low ecological validity compared to assessments that use relevant occupations in naturalistic contexts. Although standardized assessments are one important level of measurement, it is critical that clinical programs and research protocols not only include, but also *focus on* measures of activity, participation, and quality of life as key outcomes. As stated, positive changes in these measures are more relevant than an isolated change in an impairment measure; the change in impairment must be associated with a change in other health domains. The individual receiving services, family members, and third-party payers are all likely to be more satisfied with changes in these arguably more meaningful levels of function. Table 26.2 suggests instruments for documenting successful clinical and research outcomes related to improving function in those with functional limitations secondary to the presence of cognitive impairments. (For a thorough review of performance-based measures, see Law et al.[61])

It also is clinically useful to use self-reporting or caregiver reporting measures for clients with cognitive dysfunction. The rationale for this type of assessment is multifold:

- Comparing self-reports with observed performance provides the OT with critical information on the awareness of the severity of impairment and functional status.
- Comparing self-reports and caregiver reports is helpful for getting a "snapshot" of how clients perform in their own environments, which may or may not be congruent with observed performance in an OT clinic.
- It is important that clients and caregivers see benefit from the OT services provided. It is problematic if the OT is documenting improvements that cannot be detected by those to whom services are provided (Table 26.3).

Returning to the case study: the OT had access to Imani's acute care medical record. The OT noted that the day before Imani was transferred to the in-patient rehabilitation unit, the neurology resident administered the Mini-Mental State Examination (a brief, 30-item questionnaire used by multiple disciplines to screen for cognitive impairment). Imani scored 20 of 30, which is indicative of moderate cognitive impairment. She had difficulty on the specific items of orientation, attention and calculation, and recall. An assessment used in many in-patient rehabilitation units is the Inpatient Rehabilitation Facility Functional Outcome Measure (IRF). This tool measures the client's ability to complete specific self-care and also has a measure specifically designed for mobility. The IRF provides information related to *what* tasks Imani can perform and the amount of assistance needed. Imani's OT used this opportunity to also document *why* Imani requires assistance with the various self-care tasks. During the assessment, an error analysis approach, described earlier, was used and objectified the OT findings with the ADL-Focused Occupation-Based Neurobehavioral Evaluation (A-ONE). Imani required minimal physical assistance to *initiate* each self-care task but needed consistent verbal cues to *organize and sequence* the tasks. Additional verbal cues were required to maintain *alertness*, to stay on task secondary to *distractibility*, and to compensate for *short-term memory deficits*, most notably keeping in mind and remembering the tasks the OT had asked her to demonstrate.

TABLE 26.2 **Examples of Instruments for Documenting Improved Participation in Individuals With Functional Limitations Secondary to Cognitive Impairments and Ineffective Performance Skills**

Instrument	Description
Standardized, valid, and reliable measures of quality of life	Measures life satisfaction and well-being. Examples include the Medical Outcomes Study 36-Item Short-Form Health Survey, World Health Organization Quality of Life Scale, and Reintegration to Normal Living.
Standardized, valid, and reliable measures of areas of occupation (e.g., BADLs, IADLs, leisure, work)	Measures performance in areas of occupation. Examples include the Inpatient Rehabilitation Facility Functional Outcome Measure–Self-Care (IRF), the (Modified) Barthel Index, and the Lawton Instrumental Activities of Daily Living Scale.
Standardized, valid, and reliable measures of participation	Measures involvement in life situations. Examples include the Activity Card Sort, Community Integration Questionnaire, and the Canadian Occupational Performance Measure.
Comprehensive Measures to Simultaneously Assess Activity/Participation and Underlying Impairments or Subskills	
Árnadóttir OT-ADL Neurobehavioral Evaluation (more recently referred to as the ADL-Focused Occupation-Based Neurobehavioral Evaluation [A-ONE])[8–11]	A performance-based tool that uses structured observations of upper and lower body dressing, grooming, hygiene, feeding, transfers, mobility, and communication to detect underlying impairments that interfere with function. Examples of impairments include decreased organization and sequencing, short- and long-term memory loss, decreased alertness and arousal, impaired attention, performance latency, confusion, perseveration, distractibility, and impaired initiation, insight, and judgment.
Assessment of Motor and Process Skills (AMPS)[33]	A client-centered performance assessment of both BADLs and IADLs with emphasis on IADL tasks. The AMPS entails the client choosing to perform two or three tasks in collaboration with a therapist from a list of 125 standardized tasks. It evaluates motor and processing skills that affect function. Processing skills are observable actions that a person uses to (1) select, interact with, and use tools and materials; (2) carry out individual actions and steps; and (3) modify performance when problems are encountered. Processing skills should not be confused with cognitive skills.
Brief Measure of Cognitive Functional Performance	
Kettle Test[51]	A brief, performance-based assessment of an IADL task designed to tap into a broad range of cognitive skills. The task consists of making two hot beverages that differ in two ingredients (one for the client and one for the therapist). The electric kettle is emptied and disassembled to challenge problem-solving skills and safety/judgment, and additional kitchen utensils and ingredients are placed as distracters to increase demands on attention.
Assessing Executive Function Impairments	
Executive Function Performance Test (EFPT)[14]	Assesses deficits in executive function during the performance of real-world tasks (cooking oatmeal, making a phone call, managing medications, paying a bill). The test uses a structured cueing and scoring system to assess initiation, organization, safety, and task completion and to develop cueing strategies. More recently tasks were added to create the Alternate EFPT (aEFPT). These include making pasta, calling a doctor's office, sorting medication into a 7-day pill sorter, and ordering a specific item from a catalog.[48]
Weekly Calendar Planning Activity[115]	The calendar planning activity is a higher level simulated IADL task that involves entering 17 appointments and errands into a weekly schedule. It was designed to be sensitive to the effects of executive dysfunction in that it requires planning, organization, and multitasking abilities. In addition to entering appointments, the person must monitor time, keep track of rules, inhibit distractions, and deal with schedule conflicts.
Multiple Errands Test[2,27,59,100]	A multitasking assessment that challenges multiple executive functions. Tasks include purchasing three items, picking up an envelope from reception, using a telephone, mailing the envelope, writing down four items (e.g., price of a candy bar), meeting the assessor, and informing the assessor that the test has been completed.
Executive Function Route-Finding Task[18]	Uses naturalistic observations of route finding to detect dysexecutive symptoms.
Complex Task Performance Assessment[127,128]	An assessment that simulates the task of working in a library. The two primary work tasks are (1) Current Inventory Control and (2) Telephone Messaging. These are administered simultaneously.
Behavioural Assessment of the Dysexecutive Syndrome (BADS)[124]	This battery is designed to assess capabilities typically required in everyday living. It includes six subtests that represent different executive abilities, such as cognitive flexibility, novel problem solving, planning, judgment and estimation, and behavioral regulation. It uses simulated everyday tasks.

TABLE 26.2 Examples of Instruments for Documenting Improved Participation in Individuals With Functional Limitations Secondary to Cognitive Impairments and Ineffective Performance Skills—cont'd

Instrument	Description
Assessing Memory Loss	
Rivermead Behavioral Memory Test—Third Edition[126]	An ecologically valid test of everyday memory. Uses simulations of everyday memory tasks. Modifications are available for those with perceptual, language, and mobility impairments.
Cambridge Behavioural Prospective Memory Test/Cambridge Prospective Memory Test[47]	An objective test of prospective memory
Assessing Impairments in Attention	
Test of Everyday Attention[94]	Considered an ecologically valid test for various types of everyday attention, such as sustained attention, selective attention, attentional switching, and divided attention. Includes several subtests. It is one of the few tests of attention that simulates everyday life tasks. The test is based on the imagined scenario of a vacation trip to the Philadelphia area of the United States.
Moss Attention Rating Scale[50,123]	An observational test of disordered attention that currently includes 22 items. It produces three factor scores and a total score.
Rating Scale of Attentional Behaviour[82]	A short assessment of attention-based impairments that is rated through practitioners' observations of the client's behavior.

BADLs, Basic activities of daily living; *IADLs*, instrumental activities of daily living.

TABLE 26.3 Examples of Self-Reporting and/or Caregiver Reporting Measures

Instrument	Description
Attention Rating and Monitoring Scale[23]	A self-report measure of the frequency of everyday problems related to impairments in attention.
Cognitive Failures Questionnaire[19]	A self-report measure of the frequency of lapses in attention and cognition in daily life. It includes items related to memory, attention, and executive dysfunction.
Prospective Memory Questionnaire[49]	A behaviorally anchored, self-rated evaluation of prospective memory.
Comprehensive Assessment of Prospective Memory[89,95–111,113,119]	An assessment of prospective memory related to BADLs and IADLs.
Everyday Memory Questionnaire[97,109,110]	A subjective report of everyday memory; a metamemory questionnaire. It is self-reported or reported through a proxy.
Prospective and Retrospective Memory Questionnaire[57,102]	A measure of prospective and retrospective failures in everyday life. It is self-rated or proxy rated. Published norms.
Dysexecutive Questionnaire (part of the Behavioral Assessment of the Dysexecutive Syndrome [BADS] test battery)[20,124]	A 20-item questionnaire sampling everyday symptoms associated with impairments in executive functions. Versions for self-rating and rating by significant others are available.
Behavior Rating Inventory of Executive Function—Adult Version[96]	A measure that documents an adult's executive functions or self-regulation in his or her everyday environment. It includes both a self-report and an informant report.

BADLs, Basic activities of daily living; *IADLs*, instrumental activities of daily living.

MANAGING COGNITIVE DYSFUNCTION THAT LIMITS OCCUPATIONAL PERFORMANCE: ASSESSMENT AND INTERVENTIONS

The American Occupational Therapy Association (AOTA) has organized the interventions that OTs may use for clients with performance deficits secondary to cognitive impairment into categories, discussed in the following sections.[3]

Global Strategy Learning and Awareness Approaches

Global strategy learning focuses on improving awareness of cognitive processes and assisting clients to develop higher order compensatory approaches (e.g., internal problem solving and reasoning strategies), rather than attempting to remediate basic cognitive deficits. This approach enables clients to be able to generalize the application of these compensatory strategies to novel circumstances.

Domain-Specific Strategy Training

Domain-specific strategy training focuses on teaching clients particular strategies to manage specific perceptual or cognitive deficits, rather than being taught the task itself.

Cognitive Retraining Embedded in Functional Activity

In cognitive retraining, cognitive processes are addressed in the context of the activity. An example would be working on attention skills while relearning how to use a computer program. The retraining is context specific.

Specific-Task Training

Specific-task training assists clients to perform a specific functional behavior. In specific-task training, the therapist attempts to circumvent the cognitive deficit that hampers performance by teaching an actual functional task. The person can perform the occupation despite having a cognitive impairment.

Environmental Modifications and Use of Assistive Technology

OT intervention involves addressing the complexity of activity demands and altering environmental contexts to enhance the match between the client's abilities and the environmental demands. This includes technology such as cognitive prosthetics (e.g., smart phones, pagers, and alarm watches).

Impact of Awareness Deficits on Daily Function

Management of awareness deficits may be considered a *foundational* intervention for clients with cognitive dysfunction.[43] Findings from standardized assessments of awareness may dictate the overall management of a client's functional limitations (discussed later). Different terminology and definitions related to limited self-awareness are used in the literature, including lack of insight, lack of or impaired self-awareness or unawareness, anosognosia, and denial. Nonimpaired self-awareness has been defined as "the capacity to perceive the self in relatively objective terms, while maintaining a sense of subjectivity."[87-89] The terms *impaired self-awareness* and *anosognosia* are used interchangeably; Prigatano[86] defined this condition as a clinical phenomenon in which a person "does not appear to be aware of impaired neurological or neuropsychological function, which is obvious to the clinician and other reasonably attentive individuals. The lack of awareness appears specific to individual deficits and cannot be accounted for by hyperarousal or widespread cognitive impairment."

Other authors reserve the term *anosognosia* for describing unawareness of physical deficits only (i.e., not including cognitive impairments), such as "anosognosia for hemiplegia" or "anosognosia for hemianopia."

Although impaired self-awareness and anosognosia have clearly been used as overlapping terms in the literature, the term *denial* must be considered separately. Crosson et al.[26] defined psychological denial as "a subconscious process that spares the client the psychological pain of accepting the serious consequences of a brain injury and its unwanted effects on his or her life." Complicating the matter is the fact that impaired self-awareness and denial may occur together. Differentiation between denial (a psychological method of coping) and neurologically based lack of awareness is difficult because some individuals have both types of clinical manifestations.[88]

The pyramid model of self-awareness was developed by Crosson et al.[26] This model includes three interdependent types of awareness:

1. *Intellectual awareness:* The ability to understand at some level that a function is impaired. At the lowest level, one must be aware that one is having difficulty performing

certain activities. A more sophisticated level of awareness is to recognize commonalities between difficult activities and implications of the deficits; it refers to knowing that you have a problem. In the case study, Imani was demonstrating substantial impairment in intellectual awareness on the acute service. Her family reported that she kept repeating, "Why can't I go home? I'm fine." The OT on the rehabilitation service noted that Imani consistently reported that she understood she had had a "stroke." In addition, Imani was reporting that "simple" tasks seemed to take a long time and that she keeps "losing her train of thought." Imani is showing signs of emerging (albeit still severely impaired) intellectual awareness.

2. *Emergent awareness:* The ability to recognize a problem when it is actually happening. Intellectual awareness is considered a prerequisite to emergent awareness in this model because one must first recognize that a problem exists (knowing that you are experiencing a problem when it occurs). Emergent awareness is included in the concept of online awareness or monitoring of performance during the actual task.

3. *Anticipatory awareness:* The ability to anticipate that a problem will occur as the result of a particular impairment in advance of actions. Anticipatory awareness is included in the concept of online awareness.

Individuals with brain injury or cognitive deterioration may be impaired across all three awareness domains[75] or may have better skills in one or more domains of awareness. Crosson et al.[26] further applied this model to the selection of compensatory strategies and categorized compensations appropriate to each type of awareness. They classified compensatory strategies according to the way their implementation is triggered:

- *Anticipatory compensation:* Applied only when needed. This term refers to implementation of a compensatory technique by anticipating that a problem will occur (i.e., requires anticipatory awareness). An example is a person who needs groceries for the week and who is aware that busy environments present a greater challenge to his existing memory and attention deficits; therefore, he decides to defer shopping until 7 pm, when the local store is not as busy.
- *Recognition compensation:* Also applied only when needed. This term refers to strategies that are triggered and implemented because a person recognizes that a problem is occurring (i.e., requires emergent awareness). An example is a client who asks a person to speak more slowly because she realizes she is not processing information quickly enough and is having difficulty following the conversation.
- *Situational compensation:* Applies to compensatory strategies that can be triggered by a specific type of circumstance in which an impairment may affect function. The client is taught to use these strategies consistently, every time a particular event occurs. An example is a student with memory impairments after a traumatic brain injury (TBI) who tape-records all lectures in class.[5] Although recording may not be necessary at times (e.g., for a particularly slow-moving lecture with limited content), the strategy is used anyway because this type of compensation does not rely on the client's judgment. Intellectual awareness is necessary to use this

strategy because one must be aware that a deficit exists to integrate a strategy for overcoming it.

- *External compensation:* Triggered by an external agent or involves an environmental modification. Examples include alarm watches, posted lists of steps related to meal preparation, and so on.

This pyramid model was constructively criticized and expanded on by Toglia and Kirk.[116] Their model, the Dynamic Comprehensive Model of Awareness, suggests a dynamic rather than a hierarchic relationship. The model proposes a dynamic relationship among knowledge, beliefs, task demands, and the context of a situation based on the concept of metacognition. This model differentiates between metacognitive knowledge, or declarative knowledge, and beliefs about one's abilities before performing the task (incorporating aspects of intellectual awareness) and online monitoring and regulation of the performance of a task (i.e., during task performance), which integrates aspects of emergent and anticipatory awareness.

Fleming and Strong[34] discussed a three-level model of self-awareness:

1. Self-awareness of the injury-related deficits themselves, such as cognitive, emotional, and physical impairments (i.e., knowledge of deficits)
2. Awareness of the functional implications of deficits for independent living
3. The ability to set realistic goals; the ability to predict one's future state and prognosis

Most authors recommend that self-awareness be evaluated *before* an intervention program is initiated that focuses on retraining living skills. The findings from standardized evaluations of self-awareness will clearly guide the choices of intervention. For example, a person who exhibits insight into an everyday memory deficit may be a candidate for teaching compensatory strategies, such as using a diary or notebook (discussed later). However, a person who does not realize that he or she has severe unilateral neglect (a lateralized attention deficit) may not be able to learn compensatory strategies and thus may require environmental modifications (e.g., all clothing hung on the right side of the closet) to improve everyday function.

In addition, ascertaining the level of insight into a disability is one factor that may determine how motivated a client is to participate in the rehabilitation process. In the most simplistic interpretation, the client must be aware and concerned about a deficit in everyday function to be motivated to participate in what may be a long and difficult rehabilitation process. Returning to the case study, Imani has goals of returning to school and engaging in complex ADLs on returning home. It is imperative that Imani continue to gain insight so that she can implement strategies to compensate for her persistent deficits. Examples of strategies to return to school may include tape-recording lectures, having a note-taker assigned so Imani can fully attend to the lecture, switching to a part-time school schedule, and using electronic aids to organize her day and assignments.

A variety of assessment measures are typically recommended for ascertaining a person's level of self-awareness, including questionnaires (self or clinician rated); interviews; rating scales; functional observations; comparisons of self-ratings and ratings made by others (e.g., significant others, caretakers, or rehabilitation staff); and comparisons of self-ratings and ratings based on objective measures of function or cognitive constructs. No method is universally accepted for assessing the construct of awareness or lack thereof. In addition, naturalistic observations can provide further information related to how decreased awareness is interfering with the performance of everyday tasks. Table 26.4 presents examples of standardized assessments of awareness.

Although most researchers and scholars agree that interventions focused on improving awareness are critical for maximizing rehabilitation and that greater awareness of deficits is associated with better treatment outcomes,[76] others have documented functional changes through task-specific treatment without concurrent improvement in awareness. Overall, there is a lack of empirical studies that have examined the effectiveness of various interventions aimed at improving awareness. In addition, many of the published studies have not included functional outcomes. As a starting point in managing awareness, the entire team should encourage clients to predict their level of performance before any observed performance in areas of occupation. Those with brain injury or cognitive deterioration most often *underestimate* their level of cognitive impairment and *overestimate* their level of function. Practitioners should leave time at the end of each session to compare actual performance with predicted performance. This comparison of predicted versus actual performance is critical and should be done with all functional tasks. Examples of predictions include questions such as, "How long will the task take?" "How many times will you need to ask for help?" "How many times will the therapist need to physically help you?" and "How many times will the therapist need to verbally help you?" The goal is to reduce the discrepancy between the prediction and the actual performance.

It is important for the OT to remember that the verbal or physical cues used to support participation in meaningful occupations are not provided simply to support the completion of tasks. Cues are used to facilitate insight and to encourage the client to solve problems by developing new strategies to overcome deficit areas (Table 26.5).

Tham et al.[111] developed an intervention to improve awareness related to the effect of neglect (a lateralized attention deficit) on functional performance. Purposeful and meaningful (for the participant) daily occupations were used as therapeutic change agents to improve awareness of disabilities. Specific interventions included encouraging participants to choose motivating tasks as the modality of intervention and discussions about task performance. Examples included the following:

- Encouraging participants to describe their anticipated difficulties
- Linking their earlier experiences of disability to new tasks
- Planning how they would handle new situations
- Asking participants to evaluate and describe their performance
- Asking participants to think about whether they could improve their performance by performing the task in another way
- Providing feedback about the difficulties observed, including verbal feedback, discussion, and the use of

TABLE 26.4   Examples of Standardized Tests of Awareness

Test	Description
Assessment of Awareness of Disability[60]	An assessment based on a semistructured interview that is used in conjunction with the Assessment of Motor and Process Skills (AMPS). It consists of general and specific questions related to the activity of daily tasks, and the interview is conducted after performance of the AMPS.
Awareness Interview[6]	A tool used to evaluate awareness of cognitive and motor defects after cerebral infarction, dementia, or head trauma. Operationally, the authors defined unawareness as a discrepancy between the client's opinion of his or her abilities in the interview and his or her abilities as measured by neuropsychological and neurological examinations.
Awareness Questionnaire[101]	A measure of impaired self-awareness after traumatic brain injury (TBI). The instrument consists of three forms (one form is completed by the client, one by a significant other, and one by a clinician). The self-rated and family/significant others forms contain 17 items, and the clinician form contains 18 items. The client's ability to perform various tasks after the injury, compared with before the injury, is rated on a 5-point scale.
Driving Awareness Questionnaire (DriveAware)[55]	A tool consisting of five questions; the client's responses are compared with the clinician's ratings according to a structured marking guide. The clinician's rating is based on information in the referral and observation of performance on other off-road tests.
Client Competency Rating Scale (PCRS)[85]	A tool that evaluates self-awareness after TBI. It is a 30-item self-report instrument that uses a 5-point Likert scale (1 = can't do and 5 = can do with ease) to self-rate the degree of difficulty in a variety of tasks and functions. More recently, Borgaro and Prigatano[17] developed a modified yet still psychometrically sound version of the PCRS for use in an acute in-client neurorehabilitation unit. This version retains 13 items from the original PCRS.
Self-Awareness of Deficits Interview[34]	An interviewer-rated structured interview is used to obtain quantitative and qualitative data on the status of self-awareness after brain injury. Specifically, it assesses a client's level of intellectual awareness (the ability to understand that a function is decreased from the premorbid level and to recognize the implications of the deficits).
Self-Regulation Skills Interview[78]	A semi-structured, clinician-rated interview based on the model by Crosson and associates[26] discussed earlier. The tool includes six questions that assess metacognitive or self-regulation skills.

TABLE 26.5   Prompts to Promote Awareness of Errors During Functional Activities

Prompt	Rationale
"How do you know this is the right answer/procedure?" or "Tell me why you chose this answer/procedure."	Refocuses the client's attention to task performance and error detection. Can the client self-correct with a general cue?
"That's not correct. Can you see why?"	Provides general feedback about an error but is not specific. Can the client find the error and initiate correction?
"It is not correct because . . . "	Provides specific feedback about an error. Can the client correct the error when it is pointed out?
"Try this [strategy]" (e.g., going slower, saying each step aloud, verbalizing a plan before starting, or using a checklist).	Provides the client with a specific, alternative approach. Can the client use the strategy given?
The task is altered. "Try it another way."	Modifies the task by one parameter. Can the client perform the task? Begin again with grading of prompting described previously.

Data from Brockmann-Rubio K, Gillen G: Treatment of cognitive-perceptual impairments: a function-based approach. In Gillen G, Burkhardt A, editors: *Stroke rehabilitation: a function-based approach*, ed 2, St Louis, 2004, Mosby, pp 427–446; Toglia JP: Attention and memory. In Royeen CB, editor: *AOTA self-study series: cognitive rehabilitation*, Rockville, MD, 1993, American Occupational Therapy Association; and Toglia JP: Generalization of treatment: a multicontext approach to cognitive perceptual impairment in adults with brain injury, *Am J Occup Ther* 45:505, 1991.

compensatory techniques that could improve performance of the task

• Providing opportunities for further practice of the task by using newly learned compensatory techniques
• Using video feedback to improve awareness
• Using interviews to reflect on and heighten awareness

With this approach, awareness of disabilities and ADL ability improved in all four participants; unilateral neglect decreased in three participants; and sustained attention improved in two participants. The authors concluded that training to improve awareness of disabilities might improve the ability to learn the use of compensatory techniques for performing ADLs by clients with unilateral neglect.

Fleming et al.[35] completed a pilot study examining the effect of an occupation-based intervention program on the self-awareness and emotional status of four men after acquired brain injury. Each participant received an individualized program that focused on the performance of three client-chosen occupations (e.g., writing a job application, budgeting, meal preparation, playing lawn bowling, cooking with one hand) for which they had decreased awareness, according to significant others. The intervention was based on Toglia's multicontextual approach, described earlier.[113] Techniques included providing a nonthreatening environment to build positive therapeutic alliances; having the participants analyze their underlying skills, self-predict, and self-evaluate before and after the occupation; setting "just the right challenge"; supported and structured occupational performance; education on brain injury; timely and nonconfrontive verbal feedback in a sandwich format (negative comments are preceded and followed by positive feedback); and video feedback.

Repeated measures of participants' self-awareness and emotional status were performed before and after intervention and analyzed descriptively. The authors found that their results indicated preliminary support for the effectiveness of the program in facilitating participants' self-awareness, although baseline and follow-up data indicated a complex and inconsistent picture. Of note is that slightly increased anxiety was found to accompany improvements in participants' self-awareness in all four cases, and slight increases in depressive symptoms were noted in three participants. These findings are consistent with the literature discussed earlier that focused on the relationships between emotional status and awareness and on the interconnections between denial and self-awareness (Box 26.1).

Imani's OT administered the Self Awareness of Deficits Interview. Toni was present for this session. Imani reported that she was not any different now compared to what she was like before her hospitalization, that her brain injury did not have any effect on everyday life, and that she hoped to be ready to graduate and look for her first job as a social worker in the next 6 months. The findings and ratings were indicative of severely limited self-awareness. The OT chose time as the predictor because Imani had poor initiation, was disorganized, and repeated steps of the tasks. Such behavior increased the amount of time needed to complete tasks. Imani consistently predicted the length of time to complete a task based on her preinjury status. When the OT compared the predicted time with the actual time, Imani reacted with disbelief. As sessions progressed, Imani began to increase her accuracy in predicting the time needed for each task (increased awareness). As her awareness increased, the OT noted that Imani was frequently teary. The OT notified the team that although Imani was developing a better understanding of her current functional status, she required increased emotional support from the team and monitoring for increased levels of depression and anxiety.

Impact of Attention Deficits on Daily Function

Attention in its various forms is one of the most important and basic functions of the human brain, and it constitutes the basis for other cognitive processes. Integrity of the attention system is considered a prerequisite for all other higher cognitive

---

BOX 26.1 Suggestions for Improving Awareness

- Have clients perform tasks of interest and then provide them with feedback about their performance. The goal is to have clients monitor and observe their behavior more accurately so that they can make more realistic predictions about future performance and also gain insight into their strengths and weaknesses.
- Encourage self-questioning during a task and self-evaluation after a task (e.g., "Have I completed all of the steps needed?").
- Provide methods of comparing functioning before and after injury to improve awareness.
- Use prediction methods. Have the client estimate various task parameters (e.g., difficulty, time needed for completion, number of errors, and/or amount of assistance needed before, during, or after a task) and compare those estimates with the actual results.
- Help clients develop and appropriately set their personal goals.
- Allow clients to observe their own performance during specific tasks (i.e., via videotape) and compare the actual performance with what the client had stated he or she could do.
- Use group treatments and peer feedback, which allow one person to receive feedback on performance from multiple individuals.
- Use role reversals: the therapist performs the task and makes errors, and the client must detect the errors.

- Develop a strong therapeutic alliance that is open and based on trust—this is critical in managing both denial and lack of self-awareness. Coach clients to make better choices and understand how defensive strategies affect daily function.
- Use familiar tasks, graded to match the client's cognitive level ("just the right challenge"), to develop self-monitoring skills and error recognition.
- Educate both the client and family members or significant other about the client's deficit areas.
- Integrate experiential feedback experiences. This method (also called "supported risk taking" and "planned failures") is used during daily activities to gently demonstrate impairments. The therapist must provide high levels of support during this intervention.
- Monitor for increased signs of depression and anxiety as awareness increases.
- Increase mastery and control during performance of daily tasks to increase awareness.
- Use emotionally neutral tasks to increase error recognition.
- Use tasks that offer "just the right challenge" to increase error recognition/correction.
- Provide feedback in a sandwich format; that is, negative comments are preceded and followed by positive feedback.

Adapted from Gillen G: Cognitive and perceptual rehabilitation: optimizing function, St Louis, 2009, Mosby.
Data from Fleming JM, Strong J, Ashton R: Cluster analysis of self-awareness levels in adults with traumatic brain injury and relationship to outcome, *J Head Trauma Rehabil* 13:39–51, 1998; Klonoff PS, O'Brien KP, Prigatano GP, et al: Cognitive retraining after traumatic brain injury and its role in facilitating awareness, *J Head Trauma Rehabil* 4:37–45, 1989; Lucas SE, Fleming JM: Interventions for improving self-awareness following acquired brain injury, *Aust Occup Ther J* 52:160–170, 2005; Prigatano GP: Disturbances of self-awareness and rehabilitation of clients with traumatic brain injury: a 20–year perspective, *J Head Trauma Rehabil* 20:19–29, 2005; Sherer M, et al: Assessment and treatment of impaired awareness after brain injury: implications for community re-integration, *NeuroRehabilitation* 10:25–37, 1998; Tham K, Tegner R: Video feedback in the rehabilitation of clients with unilateral neglect, *Arch Phys Med Rehabil* 78:410–413, 1997; Toglia J: A dynamic interactional approach to cognitive rehabilitation. In Katz N, editor: *Cognition, occupation, and participation across the life span*, ed 3, Bethesda, MD, 2011, AOTA Press; Toglia JP: Generalization of treatment: a multicontext approach to cognitive perceptual impairment in adults with brain injury, *Am J Occup Ther* 45:505–516, 1991; and Toglia J, Kirk U: Understanding awareness deficits following brain injury, *NeuroRehabilitation* 15:57–70, 2000.

systems, such as memory, executive functions, and so on.[80] In particular, basic memory functions (e.g., working memory) are dependent on intact attention processes.[23] If a person does not attend to incoming information and cannot hold information in mind, information will not be remembered and cannot be used to guide appropriate behavior or successfully complete daily activities.[72] Attention skills serve as a cognitive foundation and are a prerequisite for engaging in most if not all meaningful activities; also, any impairment in attention processes will result in observable difficulties in everyday life, which may in fact reduce quality of life. Terminology related to attention impairments is shown in Table 26.6.

Compared to controls, impaired attention results in increased rates of off-task behavior during performance of a task (e.g., looking up and away from the task at hand, engaging in unsolicited conversations). Individuals with impairments in attention

---

TABLE 26.6 Terms Related to Attention Impairments

Attention is the voluntary control over more automatic brain systems to be able to select and manipulate sensory and stored information briefly or for sustained periods.[79]

Attention Component	Definition	Functional Examples
Arousal	A state of responsiveness to sensory stimulation or excitability[121]; it is dependent on a widely distributed neural network, including the prefrontal areas and neurotransmitter systems.[116]	• Decreased responsiveness to incoming visual, auditory, or tactile cues during performance of a task • Requires noxious or extreme sensory stimuli (e.g., a cold washcloth applied to the face) to elicit a behavioral response
Selective attention	The type of attention involved in the processing and filtering of relevant information in the presence of irrelevant stimuli[93]; the efficiency with which people can search and focus on specific information while ignoring distracters.[94] Because selective attention is critical for encoding information into memory, retaining and manipulating information in working memory, and successfully executing goal-directed behavior, a deficit in selective attention could contribute to the numerous cognitive deficits observed in individuals with neurological impairments.[93] This skill is linked to the prefrontal and underlying anterior cingulated areas.	• Attending to one conversation during a party • Studying outside with the noise of traffic and children playing • Attending to a therapist's instructions and cues in a crowded therapy clinic • Making dinner while the children watch TV in the background • Playing a board game during recess
Sustained attention (vigilance)	Supports tasks that require vigilance and the capacity to maintain attention over time[7]; often measured by the time spent on a task.[122] In adults this component is linked to prefrontal function in the right hemisphere, and impairment is linked to white matter damage.[94]	• Being able to attend to long conversations, instructions, class lessons, TV shows, or movies • Playing a game of chess • Balancing a checkbook • Watching your child on the playground
Attentional switching or alternating attention	The ability to switch attention flexibility from one concept to another; related to cognitive flexibility. The ability to change attentive focus in a flexible or adaptive manner. The ability to move between tasks with different cognitive requirements. This skill appears to be a function of the prefrontal cortex and the posterior parietal lobe, thalamus, and midbrain.[5,73]	• While typing a paper, a friend comes into your room to discuss a completely different topic; when the conversation is over, you return to typing • Cooking, taking care of a crying child, and then returning to cooking • A unit clerk at the hospital alternating between flagging orders on the medical chart, answering the phone, and writing down phone messages
Divided attention	Dividing attention between two or more tasks simultaneously; dual tasking or multitasking; the capacity to attend to two competing stimuli simultaneously.[7] Deficits occur when limited attentional resources are divided between two tasks.	• Making toast and tea at the same time • Texting while carrying on a conversation • Playing cards while discussing the events of the day
Distractibility	A breakdown in selective attention; an inability to block out environmental or internal stimuli when trying to concentrate on performing a particular task; a symptom of prefrontal damage, particularly the dorsolateral cortex.[68]	• Noise in the hallway takes away your attention while taking notes in class • Inability to attend during a therapy session because of being distracted by watching someone else's session
Field-dependent behavior	Distracted by and acting on an irrelevant impulse that interferes with performance of an activity and takes over goal-directed activity; includes both an attention and a perseveration component.[8]	• While performing oral care, a person becomes distracted by a light switch; the person then stops the oral care activity while turning the light switch on and off (i.e., not relevant to the task at hand)
Unilateral neglect (a lateralized attention deficit)	See Chapter 34	See Chapter 34

Adapted from Gillen G: Cognitive and perceptual rehabilitation: optimizing function, St Louis, 2009, Mosby.

are markedly less attentive than controls both in the presence of distractions (noise, movements) and in their absence.[122] Further compounding this problem is a relationship between attention impairment and awareness of errors. McAvinue et al.[71] investigated the processes of error awareness and sustained attention in individuals with TBI. They found the following:

- In comparison to controls, participants with TBI displayed reduced sustained attention and awareness of error.
- The degree of error awareness strongly correlated with sustained attention capacity, even when the severity of injury was controlled for.
- Error feedback significantly reduces errors.
- TBI leads to impaired sustained attention and error awareness.

The finding of a significant relationship between error awareness and sustained attention deficits in clients with TBI suggests that a link may exist between these two processes.

Posner and Peterson[83] proposed the existence of three main functionally and anatomically distinct attentional control subsystems:

1. An orienting system related to sensory events that relies on the posterior brain areas (superior parietal lobe and temporoparietal junction, in addition to the frontal eye fields). This system is involved in the selection of relevant sensory information. This subsystem brings attention to a specific location in space and generates perceptual awareness. It reflects involuntary orienting or automatic processing. The performance of this system is determined by the reaction time in responding to the detection of stimuli.
2. An executive system focused on selection and involving multiple structures (anterior cingulate, lateral prefrontal cortex, and basal ganglia). This system is responsible for exercising control over lower level cognitive functions and resolving conflicts. The system is prominent in detecting signals for focal or conscious attention. A breakdown in this system results in difficulty managing tasks that require divided attention, screening out interfering stimuli, and responding to novelty.
3. An alerting or sustained attention system involving the frontoparietal regions that are responsible for achieving and maintaining sensitivity to incoming stimuli. Impairments related to this system result in short attention spans.

Dockree et al.[28] summarized the following points:

- Attention deficits are among the most commonly observed deficits after brain injury.
- Damage to the frontal lobes of the brain, particularly the white matter connecting the frontal, parietal, and striatal regions, is partly responsible for these deficits.
- Frontal lobe damage in clients with a brain injury results in a tendency to drift from intended goals and increases the frequency of action slips that were unintended.
- Self-reports from clients with TBI revealed that problems with attention and concentration rate among the highest complaints in this group of clients.

The usual and customary tests of attention include pen and paper measures or laboratory-type tasks, such as the Paced Auditory Serial Addition Test, Trail Making Test Part A, and Wisconsin Card Sorting Task. As discussed earlier, when these measures are used, the question of ecological validity arises regarding the difficulty generalizing the results to everyday living tasks. (Suggested assessments are described in Tables 26.2 and 26.3.) Impairments in attention are manifested as observable errors during performance of tasks and should be documented as such.

In their meta-analysis of attention rehabilitation after an acquired brain injury, Park and Ingles[79] examined two approaches to treating attention deficits:

- *Directly retraining the damaged cognitive function or direct cognitive retraining.* This approach is used under the assumption that practice of carefully selected exercises promotes recovery of damaged neural circuits and restores function in the impaired attentional processes themselves, along with a further assumption that the tasks mediated by those circuits are performed in a way similar to that used by individuals without brain damage. Intervention is then based on a series of repetitive exercises or drills in which clients respond to visual or auditory stimuli. This intervention has received the most attention in the literature with respect to interventions for those with impairments in attention.
- *Having clients learn or relearn how to perform specific skills of functional significance (i.e., specific skill training).* The premise here is that through carefully structured practice of a specific skill that is impaired as a result of brain damage, it is possible for individuals to compensate and develop alternative neuropsychological processes that rely on preserved brain functions (i.e., individuals learn to perform the skill in a way that is different from the way used by individuals without brain damage). In terms of intervention, attention is trained either concurrently with or in the context of the specific skills. In addition, this approach applies behavioral principles and an understanding of how the impairment in attention affects the various skills.

Park and Ingles[79] concluded that specific skills training significantly improved the performance of tasks requiring attention. In comparison, the cognitive retraining methods (i.e., those focused on improving impairments in attention out of context) included in the meta-analysis did not significantly affect outcomes. Further analysis revealed that overall performance improved in 69% of the participants who received specific skills training (e.g., driving, ADLs), whereas performance improved in only 31% of those not so trained. In terms of effect size, the improvements in cognitive functions after direct retraining were small, whereas the improvements in performance after specific skills training were medium or large. These findings demonstrated that acquired deficits in attention are treatable by specific skills training. The authors also proposed clinical implications of their study, including the following:

- The learning that occurs as a function of training is specific and does not tend to generalize or transfer to tasks that differ considerably from those used in training. This specificity of improvement was demonstrated in both the cognitive retraining studies and the specific functional skill-retraining studies.
- Performance of a task after training will improve to the extent that the processing operations required to complete that task overlap with the processes engaged during training

(i.e., performance will improve after training if the training task is similar to the targeted outcome measure).

- Many survivors of brain injury are impaired when performing controlled cognitive processes but not when performing automatic processes. Controlled processing is heavily involved in the early stages of learning a skill and is less involved as a skill becomes more routine with practice. Therefore, training programs that reduce the requirement for controlled processing during learning may be the most effective. Examples of reducing the demands of controlled processing include breaking down a complex functional skill into simpler components, providing practice on these components, and structuring training in such a way that performance feedback can be more easily interpreted. The authors recommended the technique of "shaping" as a way to train people with controlled processing deficits because shaping links the difficulty of a task to the person's performance. As a result of using the technique of shaping, the person may make fewer errors and be able to interpret feedback more easily.
- Rehabilitation procedures should be based on a set of learning principles.

Strategies aimed at modification of task and environments have proved to be beneficial for individuals with cognitive impairment (Box 26.2). Specific strategies include the following:
- *Time pressure management (TPM).* Fasotti et al.[32] noted that after severe closed head injury, deficits in the speed of processing information are common and result in a feeling of

---

BOX 26.2   Strategies for Practitioners and Caretakers in Managing Deficits in Attention

- Avoid overstimulating/distracting environments.
- Face away from visual distracters during tasks.
- Wear earplugs.
- Shop or go to restaurants at off-peak times.
- Use filing systems to enhance organization.
- Label cupboards and drawers.
- Reduce clutter and visual distracters.
- Use self-instruction strategies.
- Use time pressure management strategies.
- Teach self-pacing strategies.
- Control the rate of incoming information.
- Self-manage effort and emotional responses during tasks.
- Teach monitoring or shared attentional resources when multitasking.
- Manage the home environment to reduce auditory and visual stimuli. Keep radios and phones turned off. Close doors and curtains. Keep surfaces, cabinets, closets, and refrigerators organized and uncluttered.
- Use daily checklists for work, self-care, and instrumental activities of daily living.

Data from Cicerone KD: Remediation of "working attention" in mild traumatic brain injury, *Brain Inj* 16:185–195, 2002; Fasotti L, Kovacs F, Eling PATM, et al: Time pressure management as a compensatory strategy training after closed head injury, *Neuropsychol Rehabil* 10:47–65, 2000; Michel JA, Mateer CA: Attention rehabilitation following stroke and traumatic brain injury: a review, *Eura Medicophys* 42:59–67, 2006; and Webster JS, Scott RR: The effects of self-instructional training on attentional deficits following head injury, *Clin Neuropsychol* 5:69–74, 1983.
From Gillen G: Cognitive and perceptual rehabilitation: optimizing function, St Louis, 2009, Mosby.

"information overload" in the performance of daily tasks. The authors tested TPM as an approach for managing slow information processing. TPM uses alternative cognitive strategies to support participation in real-life tasks. The overall focus is to teach people to give themselves enough time to deal with life situations. Specific strategies used to prevent or manage time pressure include enhancing awareness of errors and deficient performance, self-instruction training (e.g., trying to focus, not getting distracted by outside sounds and other information, not getting distracted by irrelevant thoughts, and trying to imagine things that are being said), optimizing planning and organization, rehearsing task requirements, modifying the task environment, and using an overall strategy of "Let me give myself enough time."
- *Self-instruction statements.*[119] Such statements can be suggested to improve listening and to ask for repetition if attention strays:
  - "To really concentrate, I must look at the person speaking to me."
  - "I must also focus on what is being said, not on other thoughts that may want to intrude."
  - "I must concentrate on what I am hearing at any moment by repeating each word in my head as the person speaks."
  - "Although it is not horrible if I lose track of a conversation, I must tell the person to repeat the information if I have not attended to it."

A case study by Webster and Scott[120] demonstrated positive effects of this approach both immediately after treatment and at the 18-month follow-up; the client demonstrated improved attention, which resulted in increased recall, increased sexual function, and improved job performance.
- *Self-management strategies.* Sohlberg and Mateer[105] suggest the use of three self-management strategies:
  1. *Orienting procedures.* Clients are encouraged to consciously monitor activities to prevent or control a lapse in attention. They are taught to ask themselves orienting questions at various intervals (possibly reminded by an alarm watch): "What am I currently doing?" "What was I doing before this?" and "What am I supposed to do next?"
  2. *Pacing.* Pacing is used to decrease task demands. Scheduling uninterrupted work times is one example. Other examples are setting realistic expectations, building in breaks, and self-monitoring fatigue and attention.[105]
  3. *Key ideas log.* Clients are taught to quickly write or tape-record questions or ideas to address later so that the task at hand is not interrupted.

Because there is insufficient evidence to support the use of remediation-based approaches to attention training to improve occupational performance,[44] strategy training is considered a practice standard for the post-acute period of rehabilitation by the American Congress of Rehabilitation Medicine.[25] Intervention should focus on strategy training to compensate for attention deficits in functional situations.

Impact of Memory Deficits on Daily Function

Memory impairment is one of the most common consequences of brain injury and degenerative cognitive disorders. The severity and type of memory loss vary according to the structures affected. Human memory is composed of multiple and distinct systems, which the individual needs to support daily activities and participate in the community (Table 26.7).[107] Examples include remembering your significant other's birthday, remembering to take your medications, remembering to feed the dog, remembering how to type, remembering events that occurred during a vacation, and so on. Even this "simple" list of memory tasks requires intact functioning of multiple memory systems and includes knowledge of facts and events, procedures, and future intentions. Clearly, memory serves as a key cognitive support to facilitate independent living.

TABLE 26.7 Terms Related to Memory Impairments

Term	Definition	Examples of Everyday Behavior
Anterograde amnesia	A deficit in new learning; an inability to recall information learned after acquired brain damage; an inability to form new memories after brain damage occurs	Not able to recall staff names, easily gets lost secondary to topographic disorientation, not able to recall what occurred in therapy this morning, difficulty learning adaptive strategies to compensate for loss of memory
Retrograde amnesia	Difficulty recalling memories formed and stored before the onset of disease; may be worse for recent events than for substantially older memories	Inability to remember autobiographic information (address, social security number, birth order), not able to remember historical events (war, presidential elections, scientific breakthroughs) and/or personally experienced events (weddings, vacations)
Short-term memory	Storage of limited information for a limited time	Difficulty remembering instructions related to the use of adaptive equipment, not able to remember the names of someone just introduced at a dinner party, not able to remember "today's specials" in a restaurant
Working memory	Related to short-term memory; refers to actively manipulating information in short-term storage through rehearsals	While playing a board game, unable to remember and use the rules of the game; not able to perform calculations mentally while balancing the checkbook; difficulty remembering and adapting a recipe
Long-term memory (LTM)	Relatively permanent storage of information with unlimited capacity	May affect declarative memory of knowledge, episodes, and facts or nondeclarative memories such as those related to skills and habits
Nondeclarative memory	Knowing how to perform a skill, retain previously learned skills, and learn new skills; a form of LTM; also called procedural memory	Driving, playing sports, hand crafts, learning to use adaptive equipment or a wheelchair for activities of daily living
Declarative memory	Knowing that something was learned; verbally retrieving a knowledge base (e.g., facts) and remembering everyday events; includes episodic and semantic information; a form of LTM	See episodic and semantic memory
Episodic memory	Autobiographic memory for contextually specific events and personally experienced events; a form of declarative LTM	Remembering the day's events, what one had for breakfast, occurrences on the job, and the content of therapy sessions
Semantic memory	Knowledge of the general world and facts, linguistic skill, and vocabulary; may be spared after injury; a form of declarative LTM	Remembering the dates of holidays, the name of the president, dates of world events
Explicit memory	Memories of events that have occurred in the external world; information about a specific event at a specific time and place	Remembering places and names and various words (see declarative memory)
Implicit memory	Memories necessary to perform events and tasks or to produce a specific type of response; does not require conscious retrieval of the past; knowledge is expressed in performance, without the person being aware of having it	Memory of skills, habits, and subconscious processes (see nondeclarative memory)
Prospective memory	Remembering to carry out future intentions	Remembering to take medications, return phone calls, buy food, pick up the children from school, mail the bills; a critical aspect of memory to support everyday life
Metamemory	Awareness of one's own memory abilities	Knowing when you need to compensate for memory capacity (e.g., making a list of errands or a shopping list, writing down a new phone number or driving directions); recognizing errors in memory, and so on

Data from Baddeley AD: The psychology of memory. In Baddeley AD, Kopelman MD, Wilson BA, editors: *The essential handbook of memory disorders for clinicians*, Hoboken, NJ, 2004, John Wiley; Bauer RM, Grande L, Valenstein E: Amnesic disorders. In Heilman KM, Valenstein E, editors: *Clinical neuropsychology*, ed 4, New York, 2003, Oxford University Press; Markowitsch HJ: Cognitive neuroscience of memory, *Neurocase* 4:429–435, 1998; and Sohlberg MM, Mateer CA: Memory theory applied to intervention. In Sohlberg MM, Mateer CA, editors: *Cognitive rehabilitation: an integrative neuropsychological approach*, New York, 2001, Guilford Press.
From Gillen G: Cognitive and perceptual rehabilitation: optimizing function, St Louis, 2009, Mosby.

TABLE 26.8   Stages of Memory

Stage	Description	Neuroanatomic Areas of Function
Attention	Processes that allow a person to gain access to and use incoming information; includes alertness, arousal, and various attention processes (e.g., selective attention)	• Brainstem • Thalamic structures • Frontal lobes
Encoding	How memories are formed; an initial stage of memory in which the material to be remembered is analyzed (visual versus verbal characteristics); correct analysis of the information is required for proper storage	• Dorsomedial thalamus • Frontal lobes • Language system (e.g., Wernicke's area) • Visual system (e.g., visual association areas)
Storage	How memories are retained; transfer of a transient memory to a form or location in the brain for permanent retention and access	• Hippocampus • Bilateral medial temporal lobes
Retrieval	How memories are recalled; search for or activation of existing memory traces	• Frontal lobe

Data from Sohlberg MM, Mateer CA: Memory theory applied to intervention. In Sohlberg MM, Mateer CA, editors: *Cognitive rehabilitation: an integrative neuropsychological approach*, New York, 2001, Guilford Press.

The steps or stages of memory have been well documented (Table 26.8).[13,105] The flow of these stages is:

$$\text{Attention} \rightarrow \text{Encoding} \rightarrow \text{Storage} \rightarrow \text{Retrieval}$$

Traditional measures of memory have tended to be table-top laboratory-style tools. Contrived tasks commonly used are remembering a string of numbers, a list of words, or the details of a drawn figure and/or paired associate learning (i.e., requiring a person to recognize or recall recently presented material). How the results of these tests relate to everyday memory function is not clear, and associations between scores on this type of test and reports of everyday memory failure are not strong.[109] Similarly, functional gains do not always correlate with improvement in memory processes based on objective testing.[91]

A comprehensive evaluation of how impairments in memory affect everyday function includes the use of standardized assessments, nonstandardized observations, standardized self-reports, and standardized reports of caregivers and significant others. (Tables 26.2 and 26.3 provide descriptions of recommended assessments.) The Contextual Memory Test is a useful screening tool.[113] It allows practitioners to objectify three aspects of memory and screen for possible further evaluation:

1. Awareness of memory: Using general questioning before the assessment, predicting performance before assessment, and estimating memory capacity after performance.
2. Recall of 20 line-drawn aspects: Immediate and delayed (15 to 20 minutes) recall.
3. Strategy use: Probes the use of memory strategies and determines the ability to benefit from strategy recommended by the practitioner.

Interventions focused on individuals with memory deficits can be categorized as (1) restorative approaches to improve underlying memory deficits, (2) strategy training, (3) use of nonelectronic memory aids, and (4) use of electronic memory aids or assistive technology. Techniques aimed at improving the underlying memory impairment (e.g., memory drills) have been unsuccessful in terms of generalization to meaningful activities. In other words, an improvement may be detected on a laboratory-based measure of memory without a corresponding change in daily function or subjective memory reports.

The most promising interventions to improve function in those with memory deficits rely at least partially on compensatory techniques (Box 26.3). When a compensatory approach is used, choosing the correct system of compensation is critical. Kime[58] suggests a comprehensive evaluation that includes:
- Severity of the injury
- Severity of the impairment in memory
- Presence of comorbid conditions, including physical impairments, language deficits, and other cognitive deficits
- Social supports
- Client's needs (e.g., will the system be used for work, home management, or other occupations?)

The following sections discuss specific evidence-based interventions.

Memory Notebooks and Diaries

The use of memory notebooks and diaries has been documented to improve orientation and to support everyday living tasks, such as morning ADLs and simple IADLs.[98] Sohlberg and

BOX 26.3   Suggestions for Working With Individuals With Working Memory Deficits

- Keep directions and instructions short.
- Use real-world functional tasks for training (e.g., adding up monthly bills rather than practicing rote strings of numbers).
- Speak slowly, but not exaggeratedly so.
- Stress target words during training to help the person realize the key part of the instruction. In addition, put key information at the beginning and end of sentences.
- Increase the automaticity of a response through extra practice and rehearsal (e.g., learning to transfer from a wheelchair to a bed).
- Use part-whole learning, or break down a task into components to promote overlearning of the components.
- Teach rehearsal strategies.

Data from Parente R, Kolakowsky-Hayner S, Krug K, Wilk C: Retraining working memory after traumatic brain injury, *NeuroRehabilitation* 13:157–163, 1999.

Mateer[103,104] published a systematic, structured training sequence for teaching individuals with severe memory impairments to independently use a compensatory memory book. The training sequence they proposed incorporates principles of learning theory in addition to procedural memory skills, which may be preserved in many clients with even severe memory impairments. Donaghy and Williams[29] suggested that the diary or notebook include a pair of pages for each day of the week. The notebook is set up to aid scheduling of things to do in the future and to record activities done in the past. For each pair of pages, the left-hand page contains two columns, one with a timetable for the day and the other for to-do items. The right-hand page contains the memory log. A "last week" section at the back stores previous memory log entries. A full year calendar allows appointments to be recorded. Ownsworth and McFarland[77] compared two approaches to memory diary training:

- *Diary-only training.* This approach focuses on functional skill building and compensation-based, task-specific learning. The subjects were taught a behavioral sequence consisting of making a diary entry, checking it, and using the information as needed.
- *Diary and self-instructional training.* This approach emphasizes training of the subjects' capacity for the higher level cognitive skills of self-regulation and self-awareness. The subjects were taught a **WSTC** strategy:
  W: What are you going to do?
  S: Select a strategy for the task.
  T: Try out the strategy.
  C: Check how the strategy is working.

The authors found that during the treatment phase, those in the diary and self-instruction training group consistently made more diary entries, reported fewer memory problems, compensated better through use of strategies, and made more positive ratings associated with the efficacy of treatment. Possible sections for a memory notebook are included in Table 26.9.

Errorless Learning

Errorless learning is a strategy that is in contrast to trial-and-error learning or errorful learning. Interventions using an errorless learning approach are based on differences in learning abilities. It is typical for people with impairments in memory to more successfully remember their own mistakes as results of their own action than they are to remember corrections of their mistakes by explicit means (e.g., a therapist's cue). In other words, people may remember their mistakes, but not the correction. With errorless learning a person learns something by saying or doing it rather than by being told or shown by someone. A meta-analysis of errorless learning for treating memory loss conducted by Kessels and de Haan[56] documented a large and statistically significant effect size for errorless learning treatment. In addition, no significant effect size was demonstrated for the vanishing cues method (i.e., teaching a skill by fading cues over time). It should be noted that the majority of studies analyzed used laboratory-type impairment measures such as word lists, face-name associations, and the like.

TABLE 26.9 Sections of a Memory Notebook

Section	Purpose
Daily log	Used to record, store, and retrieve information about daily activities; forms for charting hourly information and scheduling appointments; forms for prioritizing a list of tasks
Calendar	Used to record appointments and retrieve information about important meetings and upcoming events
Names	Used to record, store, and retrieve identifying information and "name drawings" of new people
Current work	Used to record specific procedures for work assignments that may be needed at a later date
Personal notes	Used to record important personal information (e.g., personal goals, autobiographic information); also used to record addresses, birthdays, and similar information

From Schmitter-Edgecombe M, et al: Memory remediation after severe closed head injury: notebook training versus supportive therapy, *J Consult Clin Psychol* 63:484–489, 1995.

BOX 26.4 Assistive Technology for Individuals With Memory Loss

- Handheld computers
- Smart phones
- Paging systems
- Voice recorders
- Personal digital assistants
- Alarm watches
- Electronic pillboxes
- Microwave with preset times
- Adaptive stove controls that turn off an electric stove after a certain period or when the heat becomes excessive
- A phone with programmable memory buttons (affix pictures to the buttons)
- A phone with buttons programmed to speak the name of the person being called
- A device for locating keys
- A recording to cue a behavioral sequence, such as morning care

From Gillen G: Cognitive and perceptual rehabilitation: optimizing function, St Louis, 2009, Mosby.

Assistive Technology

The literature focused on using technology to improve daily function in those with memory loss is substantial and consistently documents improvement in specifically trained tasks (e.g., managing medication, morning routines, and IADLs). A variety of devices has been used (Box 26.4).

Equipment that formerly was specialized (e.g., paging systems and handheld computers) continues to become commonplace; therefore, there is a larger population who may be amenable to using devices to compensate for memory loss. Typical smart phones have endless possibilities in terms of being used to cue performance of tasks in those with impaired memory. Examples include calendar functions, alarm functions, shopping list applications, dictation systems, map functions, contact lists, and others.

Mnemonics

Mnemonics is a broad term that refers to any strategy used to remember something, including rhymes, poems, acronyms, and imagery techniques. Examples include "Thirty days hath September . . ." (rhymes or poems to remember how many days are in each month), the acronym ROYGBIV to remember the colors of the spectrum, and imagining placing the items you want to remember in specific locations in a room with which you are familiar (method of loci).

Hux et al.[53] assessed the effectiveness of three frequencies of intervention sessions focused on using mnemonics and visual imagery strategies to recall names of people: once per day, 2 times per week, and 5 times per day. The subjects included seven men who had sustained a TBI, ranging in age from 28 to 40 years. The results showed that sessions held daily and twice a week were more effective than sessions held 5 times a day. Mnemonics and visual imagery strategies were effective for 4 of the 7 participants, regardless of the frequency of intervention sessions. More research is required to determine whether mnemonic strategies are generalizable to untrained tasks and also who is an appropriate candidate. At this point it seems that mnemonics are best suited for remembering specific and limited types of information (e.g., staff names).

Task-Specific Training

A series of experiments by Giles and Morgan[40] documented improved daily function in those with severe memory loss using the following interventions:

- An intervention program consisting of chaining nine discrete activities (e.g., shaving, oral care) by using linking phases. The phrases linked the performed activity to the one that immediately followed (e.g., "teeth cleaned, now shave"). The person was then asked to repeat the phrase as a cue to initiate the activity, which was followed by the behavioral techniques of verbal praise and a tangible reward.
- An intervention consisting of a cued ADL sequence determined by the client's preinjury habits and responsiveness to cueing. Washing and dressing were conceptualized as a 16-step program in which the staff would cue the next step if behavior compatible with the next step in the sequence was not evident within approximately 5 seconds of completion of the previous step, or if behavior incompatible with production of the next step in the behavioral chain was demonstrated. Although the client's physical and cognitive status remained unchanged during the program, which lasted for 12 treatment days, he did become independent in washing and dressing. Initially requiring 25 to 30 instructions, in addition to physical assistance, to perform the tasks, the client progressed to independence. Independence was maintained at the 6-month follow-up.[41]

Giles et al.[42] presented further support for these specific retraining protocols. Four clients were treated with the aforementioned washing and dressing protocol. Three had sustained a TBI, and one had brain injury after cerebral bleeding. All

had moderate to severe memory loss. The training program consisted of behavioral observation, task analysis, consistent practice, and cue fading. The Adaptive Behavior Scale was used to measure change in behavior. The authors found that three subjects achieved rapid independence in washing and dressing (requiring 20 days, 37 days, and 11 days of treatment), and one did not show significant clinical improvement. Of note was that all clients admitted to the facility during a 3-year period who required retraining in washing and dressing were treated with the same protocol. The authors further concluded that the consecutive series design prevented researchers from selecting clients they thought were good treatment candidates; therefore, the findings supported the general applicability of the training program. Box 26.5 presents strategies for significant others.

Strategy Training

In addition to the strategies discussed previously, Stringer and Small[108] tested an approach called Ecologically Oriented Neurorehabilitation of Memory, a treatment program that provides a four-step compensatory strategy based on the acronym WOPR: write–organize–picture–rehearse. Performance measures on everyday memory simulations for six declarative

---

BOX 26.5 Strategies for Significant Others of Individuals With Memory Loss

- Understand that in many cases the impairment may not be reversible.
- Become familiar with the specific type of compensatory memory strategies that have been prescribed.
- Keep daily schedules as consistent as possible. Stick with habits and routines.
- Simplify the environment by reducing clutter and keeping the living areas organized.
- Reduce excessive environmental stimuli.
- Help by organizing calendars and having clocks and reminders arranged around the house.
- Be proactive in identifying potential safety issues.
- Use short, direct sentences.
- Make sure the most important information comes at the beginning of the sentence.
- Highlight, cue, and emphasize key aspects of communication (e.g., repeat, point, and so on).
- Avoid conversations that rely on memory (i.e., keep conversations in the present).
- Repetition of sentences may be inevitable.
- Summarize conversations.
- Remember that in many cases intelligence may remain intact.
- Keep "a place for everything, and everything in its place."
- Use photographs, souvenirs, and other appropriate items to help the person access memories.
- Understand that fatigue, stress, sleep disorders, and depression can exacerbate memory loss.
- Keep back-up items (e.g., glasses, spare keys).
- Help create to-do lists. Remind loved ones to check off a task or highlight it when it has been completed.
- Label items, drawers, and shelves.

From Gillen G: Cognitive and perceptual rehabilitation: optimizing function, St Louis, 2009, Mosby.

memory tasks and one prospective memory task were used as outcome measures. Clients in all three diagnostic groups and at all levels of severity showed significant improvement in memory performance.

Impact of Executive Dysfunction on Daily Function

Executive functions is an umbrella term that refers to complex cognitive processing requiring the coordination of several subprocesses to achieve a particular goal.[30] This term has been defined as "a product of the coordinated operation of various processes to accomplish a particular goal in a flexible manner"[37] or "those functions that enable a person to engage successfully in independent, purposive, self-serving behavior."[66] These higher order mental capacities allow a person to adapt to new situations and achieve goals. They include multiple specific functions, such as decision making, problem solving, planning, task switching, modifying behavior in light of new information, self-correction, generating strategies, formulating goals, and sequencing complex actions. Unfortunately, the

published literature is not consistent on whether a particular function is an executive function. Table 26.10 gives an in-depth list of the 20 most commonly reported dysexecutive symptoms and the reported frequencies of these symptoms. Clearly, these executive functions support engagement in daily life activities and participation in the community; they are most important during new, nonroutine, complex, and unstructured situations (Table 26.11).

Recent studies examining meal preparation abilities in those with frontal lobe involvement have supported the importance of executive functions in everyday activities. Godbout et al.[45] examined executive functions and ADLs in 10 clients with excised frontal lobe tumors and 10 normal controls by means of a neuropsychological test battery, a script generation task, and a complex multitask ADL (planning and preparing a meal). The clients manifested numerous basic executive deficits on the pen and paper tests, were unimpaired on the script generation task (despite an aberrant semantic structure), and demonstrated marked difficulties in the meal preparation task. The authors

TABLE 26.10 Frequency of Reporting of Dysexecutive Symptoms[a]

Symptom	Clients Reporting Problem (%)	Caregivers Reporting Problem (%)	Rank of Disagreement[b]	Scaled Disagreement in Rank[c]
Poor abstract thinking	17	21	16.5	−9
Impulsivity	22	22	19.5	−10
Confabulation	5	5	19.5	+3
Planning	16	48	1	+8
Euphoria	14	28	5	+7
Poor temporal sequencing	18	25	15	−8
Lack of insight	17	39	3	+5
Apathy	20	27	13	−5
Disinhibition (social)	15	23	13	−3
Variable motivation	13	15	18	−7
Shallow affect	14	23	10.5	+1
Aggression	12	25	6	+6
Lack of concern	9	26	4	+9
Perseveration	17	26	10.5	−1
Restlessness	25	28	16.5	−6
Can't inhibit responses	11	21	9	+4
Know-do dissociation	13	21	13	−2
Distractibility	32	42	8	+1
Poor decision making	26	38	7	−3
Unconcern for social rules	13	38	2	+10

From Burgess PW, Simons JS: Theories of the frontal lobe executive function: clinical applications. In Halligan PW, Wade DT, editors: *Effectiveness of rehabilitation for cognitive deficits*, Oxford, UK, 2005, Oxford University Press.
[a]Only ratings of 3 or 4 (of a maximum of 4) for each item on the Dysexecutive Questionnaire were considered to indicate a problem. These ratings correspond to classification of the symptom as "often observed" or "very often observed." These results are based on data gathered as part of the study by Wilson et al.[124,125]
[b]This number represents the rank size of the disagreements (in proportions reporting the symptom) between clients and controls, in which 1 represents the greatest disagreement (i.e., 1 means that caregivers reported this symptom much more often than clients did).
[c]This number reflects the relative disagreement in rank frequency of reporting between clients and controls, scaled from −10 to +10, with 0 being absolute agreement in rank position of that symptom. On this scale, −10 means that the symptom was commonly reported by clients but not by caregivers, and +1 means that the symptom was frequently reported by caregivers, but it was relatively uncommon for clients to report it.

TABLE 26.11   **Examples of Executive Functions Related to Daily Life Preparing a Salad**

Executive Function	Associated Tasks
Initiation	Starting the task at the appropriate time without overreliance on prompts
Organization	Organizing the work space and performing the task efficiently (e.g., gathering the necessary vegetables at the same time from the refrigerator)
Sequencing	Sequencing the steps of the task appropriately (e.g., gathering tools and vegetables, washing vegetables, chopping and slicing vegetables, combining vegetables in a bowl, adding dressing)
Problem solving	Solving the problem of using a knife that is too dull to slice

From Gillen G: Cognitive and perceptual rehabilitation: optimizing function, St Louis, 2009, Mosby.

concluded that the difficulties observed in performing a lengthy, complex, multitask ADL can be explained by impairment of several executive functions, generalized slowness in performance, and paucity of behavior.

Similarly, Fortin et al.[36] investigated executive functions in performing ADLs in 10 clients with frontal lobe lesions after a mild to severe closed head injury (CHI), compared with 12 normal controls, by means of a neuropsychological test battery, a script recitation task, and simulation of a complex multitask ADL. These authors found that the groups did not differ on any neuropsychological test by nonparametric testing. However, the clients with CHI manifested marked anomalies in the meal preparation task. Although small sequences of actions were easily produced, large action sets could not be executed correctly. The authors concluded that an outstanding deficit in strategic planning and prospective memory appears to be an important underpinning of the impairment in ADLs observed in clients with CHI with frontal lobe lesions. It also has been found that components of executive functioning (e.g., categorization and deductive reasoning ability) in individuals with brain injury are good predictors of IADL functional performance.[46]

Lezak[65,66] classified the various forms of executive disorders into a four-part schema:

1. *Volition and goal formulation:* Including self-awareness, initiation, and motivation
2. *Planning:* Including the ability to conceptualize change, be objective, conceive alternatives, make choices, develop a plan, and sustain attention
3. *Purposive action:* To implement plans for achieving goals, including productivity, self-regulation, switching, and sequencing of actions
4. *Performance effectiveness:* Including quality control, self-correction, monitoring, and time management

Cicerone et al.[25] also presented a schema for executive functions. It includes four domains based on anatomy and evolutionary development:

1. *Executive cognitive functions* (dorsolateral prefrontal cortex): Involved in the control and direction (planning, monitoring, activating, switching, inhibiting) of lower level functions. Working memory and inhibition mediate executive functions.
2. *Behavioral self-regulatory functions* (ventral/medial prefrontal area): Involved in emotional processing and behavioral self-regulation when cognitive analysis, habit, or environmental cues are not sufficient to determine the best adaptive response.
3. *Activation-regulating functions* (medial frontal areas): Activation through initiative and energizing behavior. Pathology results in a decrease in activation and drive, also known as apathy and abulia.
4. *Metacognitive processes* (frontal poles): Personality, social cognition, and self-awareness as reflected by accurate evaluation of one's own abilities and behavior, rather than objective evaluation or reports by significant others.

People with impairments in executive functions, or **dysexecutive syndrome**, have impaired judgment, impulsiveness, apathy, poor insight, and lack of organization, planning, and decision making, in addition to behavioral disinhibition and impaired intellectual abilities. Specific behavioral characteristics include impulsivity, poor attention, erratic response, lack of flexibility, and poor self-control.[90,106] Of note is that people with impaired executive function may perform normally on pen and paper tests of cognition but unfortunately are found to have catastrophic everyday problems that are particularly evident in situations requiring multitasking and planning.[100]

The usual and customary tests of executive dysfunction include pen and paper measures or laboratory-type tasks, such as the Wisconsin Card Sorting Task, Trail Making Test, and Stroop Test, among others. As discussed earlier, the question of ecological validity arises when these measures are used, in addition to difficulty generalizing the results to everyday living tasks. These measures have only a low to moderate relationship to everyday skills.

Additionally, the standard clinical tests used to assess executive impairments are considered too structured and rater led; therefore, they fail to capture the common problems of initiation, planning, and self-monitoring. (Recommended instruments are summarized in Tables 26.2 and 26.3.)

Interventions for dysexecutive syndrome (Box 26.6) continue to be tested empirically.

Because executive functions act as a manager of other cognitive processes, such as attention, memory, and language,[67] some of the interventions previously described in this chapter are appropriate for those with dysexecutive symptoms, including TPM,[32] self-instruction training,[24] WSTC strategy,[63] external cueing devices (e.g., paging systems, recorded instructions, and checklists),[21,31,99] and manipulation of environmental variables with a focus on level of distraction.[52] Other examples of specific interventions that have been tested and shown to be effective are described in the next three sections.

Problem-Solving Training

The aim of problem-solving training is to substitute a participant's impulsive approach to problem solving with a verbally

BOX 26.6 Categories of Intervention for Clients With Impaired Executive Function

- *Environmental modifications:* Examples include using antecedent control, manipulating the amount of distractions and structure in the environment, organizing work and living spaces, and ensuring balance of work, play, and rest, among others.
- *Compensatory strategies:* Examples include the use of external cueing devices (e.g., checklists, electronic pagers) and the use of reminder systems and organizers.
- *Task-specific training:* Training of specific functional skills and routines, including task modifications.
- Training in metacognitive strategies to promote a functional change by increasing self-awareness and control over regulatory processes. Such strategies include self-instruction strategies, teaching problem solving, and goal management training.

Data from Cicerone KD, Giacino JT: Remediation of executive function deficits after traumatic brain injury, *NeuroRehabilitation* 2:12–22, 1992; Sohlberg MM, Mateer CA: Management of dysexecutive symptoms. In Sohlberg MM, Mateer CA, editors: *Cognitive rehabilitation: an integrative neuropsychological approach*, New York, 2001, Guilford Press; and Worthington A: Rehabilitation of executive deficits: the effect on disability. In Halligan PW, Wade DT, editors: *Effectiveness of rehabilitation for cognitive deficits*, Oxford, UK, 2005, Oxford University Press.

mediated systematic analysis of the goal and the means by which it may be achieved.[118] von Cramon et al.[118] encouraged participants to act in a manner attributed to an intact executive system, with a focus on five aspects of problem solving:

1. *Problem orientation or identifying and analyzing.* The difficulty in general recognition of a task or situation as a problem was the focus. The participant's tendency to oversimplify problems and neglect relevant information was addressed.
2. *Problem definition and formulation.* Participants learned to survey information by reading and rereading directions and formulated questions to augment their understanding of the problem. Main and relevant points were written down. A focus was to teach participants to discriminate between relevant and irrelevant information.
3. *Generating alternatives and solutions.* Participants were asked to generate as many solutions as possible for a given problem. This was done individually, followed by the participants sharing solutions. The goal was to make participants aware that there were more solutions available than they had originally thought.
4. *Decision making.* Solutions were discussed, and the pros and cons of the solutions were weighed. The feasibility of the solutions was also considered.
5. *Solution verification and evaluation.* Participants learned to recognize faulty solutions, self-correct errors, and return to other hypotheses. The focus here was on increased sensitivity to errors and discrepancies.

Others have recommended using problem-solving strategies such as stop and think; asking clear thinking questions; thinking your way through each step; defining the problem; using clear thinking questions to produce, evaluate, and examine the utility of as many alternative solutions as possible; and emotional self-regulation strategies.[92] These problem-solving skills are then reinforced by role playing and the practice of demanding real-life examples.

Goal Management Training

This intervention is aimed at decreasing disorganized behavior and improving the client's ability to maintain intentions in goal-directed behavior (goal management).[64] Such disorganization results in neglect of daily goals, such as never cleaning the house, forgetting to pack a lunch, or never getting around to making a shopping list—all of which compromise functional independence. Goal management training entails five stages that correspond to key aspects of goal-directed behavior:

Stage 1: *Orienting and assessing the current state.* Stop current activity and direct awareness toward the task.
Stage 2: Select the main goal.
Stage 3: Partition the goals and make subgoals.
Stage 4: *Rehearse the steps necessary to complete the task.* Encode, rehearse, and retain goals and subgoals.
Stage 5: *Monitor the outcome.* Compare the outcome of action with the stated goal.

These steps are taught using errorless techniques, and the cues for each stage are gradually faded to make sure the person maintains nearly perfect performance.

Metacognitive Training

Birnboim[15] and Birnboim and Miller[16] tested the effectiveness of a metacognitive therapeutic approach in 10 people with multiple sclerosis and executive dysfunction. This approach focused on the metacognitive aspects of behavior and assumed that metacognitive aspects can and should be learned explicitly through a structured process. Phases of the process included the following:

1. *Understanding:* The participant had to recognize his or her specific metacognitive deficits (e.g., not planning). This was achieved by confronting various tasks in the clinic to increase awareness.
2. *Practice:* Efficient and specific strategies that the participant and therapist identified together (e.g., set priorities) were learned and practiced.
3. *Transfer:* Participants and their therapists considered when and where these strategies could be applied in real-life situations.

Computer strategy games (e.g., Mastermind) and tabletop exercises were used during the first two phases of the training. Individualized daily activities were the focus of the generalization phase (e.g., specific work tasks). Positive results were noted on a strategy application test, tests of attention, memory tests, tests of executive function, and most important, the Occupational Therapy Functional Assessment Compilation Tool, which showed an improved occupational role.

SUMMARY

Imani's case will serve as a summary and a conclusion. Imani's initial evaluation was structured to first and foremost foster a client-centered approach to ensure that her OT sessions were tailored to her goals. Toni, Imani's wife, was also involved in this process because Imani was demonstrating poor self-awareness related to her functional limitations. Toni reported that she worked full-time and that Imani would be alone for part of the day. Toni stated that she would help in any way needed, but was concerned that helping with self-care would change the dynamic in their new marriage, and wanted self-care to be a focus of occupational therapy. Imani reported that she felt "humiliated" when staff members had to help her with personal needs, such as ADLs. Imani was also focused on (sometimes perseverating on) finishing school. It was determined that morning OT sessions would focus on self-care, and afternoon sessions would focus on supporting educational skills.

As described earlier, the IRF self-care outcome measure was administered. The IRF findings were supplemented by the standardized A-ONE, which documented the reasons for Imani's limited performance in areas of occupation. Because it was quickly apparent the Imani was not aware of her limitations (one of Toni's greatest concerns), the standardized Self Awareness of Deficits Interview was also administered as a priority. The OT administered nonstandardized assessments of school tasks with a focus on organizational strategies. To assess performance, the OT requested that Toni bring Imani's current semester requirements and materials to the OT sessions at the end of the second week of therapy. The OT was able to document Imani's reading comprehension, ability to attend to lectures (Imani always recorded lectures, and Toni was able to locate the recordings), ability to structure note taking, and use of her laptop for e-mail functions. Deficits were noted in the areas of sustained attention, short-term memory, and being distracted by environmental stimuli.

The OT, along with Imani and Toni, set the following short-term goals, which focused on documenting improvements in areas of occupation.

Goals to Be Met by Week 1

1. Imani will complete upper body dressing with one tactile cue for initiation and no more than two verbal cues for sequencing.

2. Imani will complete grooming tasks (oral hygiene and hair care) with one tactile cue for initiation and the use of a checklist outlining the steps of the tasks.

3. Imani will persist in feeding herself for 10 minutes after one tactile cue for initiation.

Goals to Be Met by Week 3

1. All self-care tasks except for bathing will be completed with no more than one general verbal cue and external cueing devices as needed.

2. Imani will accurately write down three key points from a 10-minute lecture with one general verbal prompt to stay on task.

3. Imani will retrieve her email from her laptop with no more than one verbal cue for sequencing.

In terms of interventions to meet the aforementioned goals and others, the general treatment approach chosen by Imani's OT was the multicontext approach described earlier. This model was chosen primarily because of its emphasis on awareness training so that Imani could redefine her knowledge of her strengths and weaknesses. The OT hypothesized that improving awareness would be the starting point for intervention because he felt confident that if Imani were aware of her errors, he could teach her strategies that would allow her to meet her goals. In addition, the choice of intervention activities was based on Imani's interests and goals (school tasks, reading fiction, cooking). Various processing strategies were practiced during a variety of functional activities and situations. Processing strategies were chosen to allow Imani to control the cognitive symptoms detected on her assessment. As Imani's awareness improved, the OT was vigilant in monitoring her for signs of depression and anxiety. Imani's OT began to place emphasis on teaching specific strategies to keep Imani "on task" (sustained attention), in addition to determining which external cueing devices would allow Imani to stay organized and perform the steps of various tasks in the proper sequence. The OT planned interventions to occur in multiple environments (bedside, OT clinic, hospital gift store, staff office, hospital library) to promote generalization of learning.

REVIEW QUESTIONS

1. Name the three levels of the pyramid model of self-awareness.
2. How does the concept of ecological validity relate to cognitive assessment?
3. List some of the rationales for using self-report/caregiver report measures for individuals with cognitive impairment.
4. How does the OT approach for individuals with cognitive impairments differ from that used by other disciplines?

REFERENCES

1. Abreu BC, Peloquin SM: The quadraphonic approach: a holistic rehabilitation model for brain injury. In Katz N, editor: *Cognition and occupation across the life span*, Bethesda, MD, 2005, AOTA Press.

2. Alderman N, Burgess PW, Knight C, Henman C: Ecological validity of a simplified version of the Multiple Errands Shopping Test, *J Int Neuropsychol Soc*, 9:31–44, 2003.

3. American Occupational Therapy Association: Cognition, cognitive rehabilitation, and occupational performance, *Am J Occup Ther* 67:S9–S31, 2013.

4. American Occupational Therapy Association: Occupational therapy practice framework: Domain and process (4th ed.), *American Journal of Occupational Therapy* 74(Suppl. 2):1–87, 2020.

5. Amos A: Remediating deficits of switching attention in clients with acquired brain injury, *Brain Inj* 16:407–413, 2002.

6. Anderson SW, Tranel D: Awareness of disease states following cerebral infarction, dementia, and head trauma: standardized assessment, *Clin Neuropsychol* 3:327–339, 1989.

7. Anderson V, Fenwick T, Manly T, Robertson I: Attentional skills following traumatic brain injury in childhood: a componential analysis, *Brain Inj* 12:937–949, 1998.

8. Árnadóttir G: *The brain and behavior: assessing cortical dysfunction through activities of daily living*, St Louis, 1990, Mosby.

9. Árnadóttir G: Impact of neurobehavioral deficits of activities of daily living. In Gillen G, editor: *Stroke rehabilitation: a function-based approach* ed 4, St Louis, 2016, Elsevier.

10. Árnadóttir G, Fisher AG: Rasch analysis of the ADL scale of the A-ONE, *Am J Occup Ther* 62:51–60, 2008.

11. Árnadóttir G, Fisher AG, Löfgren B: Dimensionality of nonmotor neurobehavioral impairments when observed in the natural contexts of ADL task performance, *Neurorehabil Neural Repair* 23:579–586, 2009.

12. Averbuch MA, Katz N: Cognitive rehabilitation: a retraining model for clients with neurological disabilities. In Katz N, editor: *Cognition, occupation, and participation across the life span* ed 3, Bethesda, MD, 2011, AOTA Press.

13. Baddeley AD: The psychology of memory. In Baddeley AD, Kopelman MD, Wilson BA, editors: *The essential handbook of memory disorders for clinicians*, Hoboken, NJ, 2004, John Wiley.

14. Baum CM, Tabor Connor L, Morrison T, et al: The reliability, validity, and clinical utility of the Executive Function Performance Test: a measure of executive function in a sample of persons with stroke, *Am J Occup Ther* 62:446–455, 2008.

15. Birnboim SA: Metacognitive approach to cognitive rehabilitation, *Br J Occup Ther* 58:61–64, 1995.

16. Birnboim S, Miller A: Cognitive rehabilitation for multiple sclerosis clients with executive dysfunction, *J Cogn Rehabil* 22:11–18, 2004.

17. Borgaro SR, Prigatano GP: Modification of the Client Competency Rating Scale for use on an acute neurorehabilitation unit: the PCRS-NR, *Brain Inj* 17:847–853, 2003.

18. Boyd TM, Sautter SW: Route-finding: a measure of everyday executive functioning in the head-injured adult, *Appl Cogn Psychol* 7:171–181, 1993.

19. Broadbent DE, Cooper PF, FitzGerald P, Parkes KR: The Cognitive Failures Questionnaire (CFQ) and its correlates, *Br J Clin Psychol* 21:1–16, 1982.

20. Burgess PW, Wilson BA, Evans JJ, Emslie H: The Dysexecutive Questionnaire. In Wilson BA, Alderman N, editors: *Behavioural assessment of the dysexecutive syndrome*, Bury St Edmunds, UK, 1996, Thames Valley Test Co.

21. Burke WH, Zencius AH, Wesolowski MD, Doubleday F: Improving executive function disorders in brain-injured clients, *Brain Inj* 5:241–252, 1991.

22. Chaytor N, Schmitter-Edgecombe M: The ecological validity of neuropsychological tests: a review of the literature on everyday cognitive skills, *Neuropsychol Rev* 13:181–197, 2003.

23. Cicerone KD: Remediation of "working attention" in mild traumatic brain injury, *Brain Inj* 16:185–195, 2002.

24. Cicerone KD, Giacino JT: Remediation of executive function deficits after traumatic brain injury, *NeuroRehabilitation* 2:12–22, 1992.

25. Cicerone KD, Dahlberg C, Malec JF, et al: Evidence-based cognitive rehabilitation: updated review of the literature from 1998 through 2002, *Arch Phys Med Rehabil* 86:1681–1692, 2005.

26. Crosson B, Barco PP, Velozo CA, et al: Awareness and compensation in postacute head injury rehabilitation, *J Head Trauma Rehabil* 4:46–54, 1989.

27. Dawson DR, Anderson ND, Burgess P, et al: Further development of the Multiple Errands Test: standardized scoring, reliability, and ecological validity for the Baycrest version, *Arch Phys Med Rehabil* 90(Suppl 11):S41–S51, 2009.

28. Dockree PM, Kelly SP, Roche RA, et al: Behavioural and physiological impairments of sustained attention after traumatic brain injury, *Cogn Brain Res* 20:403–414, 2004.

29. Donaghy S, Williams W: A new protocol for training severely impaired clients in the usage of memory journals, *Brain Inj* 12:1061–1076, 1998.

30. Elliott R: Executive functions and their disorders, *Br Med Bull* 65:49–59, 2003.

31. Evans JJ, Emslie H, Wilson BA: External cueing systems in the rehabilitation of executive impairments of action, *J Int Neuropsychol Soc* 4:399–408, 1998.

32. Fasotti L, Kovacs F, Eling PATM, et al: Time pressure management as a compensatory strategy training after closed head injury, *Neuropsychol Rehabil* 10:47–65, 2000.

33. Fisher AG, Jones KB: Assessment of motor and process skills, ed 8, *Development, standardization, and administration manual*, vol 1, Fort Collins, CO, 2014, Three Star Press.

34. Fleming J, Strong J: Self-awareness of deficits following acquired brain injury: considerations for rehabilitation, *Br J Occup Ther* 58:55–60, 1995.

35. Fleming JM, Lucas SE, Lightbody S: Using occupation to facilitate self-awareness in people who have acquired brain injury: a pilot study, *Can J Occup Ther* 73:44–55, 2006.

36. Fortin S, Godbout L, Braun CM: Cognitive structure of executive deficits in frontally lesioned head trauma clients performing activities of daily living, *Cortex* 39:273–291, 2003.

37. Funahashi S: Neuronal mechanisms of executive control by the prefrontal cortex, *Neurosci Res* 39:147–165, 2001.

38. Giles GM: A neurofunctional approach to rehabilitation following severe brain injury. In Katz N, editor: *Cognition and occupation across the life span*, Bethesda, Md, 2005, AOTA Press.

39. Giles GM: Cognitive versus functional approaches to rehabilitation after traumatic brain injury: commentary on a randomized controlled trial *Am J Occup Ther* 64, 2010. pp 182–185.

40. Giles GM, Morgan JH: Training functional skills following herpes simplex encephalitis: a single case study, *J Clin Exp Neuropsychol* 11:311–318, 1989.

41. Giles GM, Shore M: The effectiveness of an electronic memory aid for a memory-impaired adult of normal intelligence, *Am J Occup Ther* 43:409–411, 1989.

42. Giles GM, Ridley JE, Dill A, Frye S: A consecutive series of adults with brain injury treated with a washing and dressing retraining program, *Am J Occup Ther* 51:256–266, 1997.

43. Gillen G: *Cognitive and perceptual rehabilitation: optimizing function*, St Louis, 2009, Mosby.

44. Gillen G, Nilsen DM, Attridge J, et al: Effectiveness of interventions to improve occupational performance of people with cognitive impairments after stroke: an evidence-based review, *Am J Occup Ther* 69:1–9, 2015.

45. Godbout L, Grenier MC, Braun CMJ, Gagnon S: Cognitive structure of executive deficits in patients with frontal lesions performing activities of daily living, *Brain Inj* 19:337–348, 2005.

46. Goverover Y, Hinojosa J: Categorization and deductive reasoning: can they serve as predictors of instrumental activities of daily living performance in adults with brain injury? *Am J Occup Ther* 56:509–516, 2002.

47. Groot YC, Wilson BA, Evans J, Watson P: Prospective memory functioning in people with and without brain injury, *J Clin Exp Neuropsychol* 8:645–654, 2002.

48. Hahn B, Baum C, Moore J, et al: Brief report: development of additional tasks for the Executive Function Performance Test, *Am J Occup Ther* 68:e241–e246, 2014.

49. Hannon R, Adams P, Harrington P, et al: Effects of brain injury and age on prospective memory self-rating and performance, *Rehabil Psychol* 40:289–298, 1995.

50. Hart T, Whyte J, Millis S, et al: Dimensions of disordered attention in traumatic brain injury: further validation of the Moss Attention Rating Scale, *Arch Phys Med Rehabil* 87: 647–655, 2006.

51. Hartman-Maeir A, Harel H, Katz N: Kettle Test: a brief measure of cognitive functional performance—reliability and validity in stroke rehabilitation, *Am J Occup Ther* 63:592–599, 2009.

52. Hayden ME, Moreault AM, LeBlanc J, Plenger PM: Reducing level of handicap in traumatic brain injury: an environmentally based model of treatment, *J Head Trauma Rehabil* 15: 1000–1021, 2000.

53. Hux K, Manasse N, Wright S, Snell J: Effect of training frequency on face-name recall by adults with traumatic brain injury, *Brain Inj* 14:907–920, 2000.

54. Katz N: *Cognition, occupation, and participation across the life span*, Bethesda, MD, 2011, AOTA Press.

55. Kay LG, Bundy AC, Clemson L: Validity, reliability and predictive accuracy of the Driving Awareness Questionnaire, *Disabil Rehabil* 31:1074–1082, 2009.

56. Kessels RP, de Haan EH: Implicit learning in memory rehabilitation: a meta-analysis on errorless learning and vanishing cues methods, *J Clin Exp Neuropsychol* 25:805–814, 2003.

57. Kim HJ, Craik FI, Luo L, Ween JE: Impairments in prospective and retrospective memory following stroke, *Neurocase* 15:145–156, 2009.

58. Kime SK: *Compensating for memory deficits using a systematic approach*, Bethesda, MD, 2006, AOTA Press.

59. Knight C, Alderman N, Burgess PW: Development of a simplified version of the Multiple Errands Test for use in hospital settings, *Neuropsychol Rehabil* 12:231–256, 2002.

60. Kottorp A, Tham K: *Assessment of Awareness of Disability (AAD): manual for administration, scoring, and interpretation*, Stockholm, 2005, Karolinska Institute, NEUROTEC Department, Division of Occupational Therapy.

61. Law M, Baum C, Dunn W: *Measuring occupational performance: supporting best practice in occupational therapy*, Thorofare, NJ, 2005, Slack.

62. Law M, Baptiste S, Carswell A, et al: *The Canadian Occupational Performance Measure*, ed 4, Ottawa, ON, 2005, CAOT Publications ACE.

63. Lawson MJ, Rice DN: Effects of training in use of executive strategies on a verbal memory problem resulting from closed head injury, *J Clin Exp Neuropsychol* 11:842–854, 1989.

64. Levine B, Robertson IH, Clare L, et al: Rehabilitation of executive functioning: an experimental-clinical validation of goal management training, *J Clin Exp Neuropsychol* 6: 299–312, 2000.

65. Lezak MD: Newer contributions to the neuropsychological assessment of executive functions, *J Head Trauma Rehabil* 8:24–31, 1993.

66. Lezak MD: Executive function and motor performance. In Lezak MD, Howieson DB, Loring DW, editors: *Neurological assessment*, New York, 2004, Oxford University Press.

67. Manchester D, Priestley N, Jackson H: The assessment of executive functions: coming out of the office, *Brain Inj* 18:1067–1081, 2004.

68. Manly T, Ward S, Robertson IH: The rehabilitation of attention. In Eslinger PJ, editor: *Neuropsychological interventions: emerging treatment and management models for neuropsychological impairments*, New York, 2000, Guilford Press.

69. Mathiowetz V: Task oriented approach to stroke rehabilitation. In Gillen G, editor: *Stroke rehabilitation: a function-based approach* ed 4, St Louis, 2016, Elsevier.

70. Mathiowetz V, Bass-Haugen J: Assessing abilities and capacities: motor planning and performance. In Radomski MV, Latham CAT, editors: *Occupational therapy for physical dysfunction* ed 7, Baltimore, MD, 2014, Lippincott Williams & Wilkins.

71. McAvinue L, O'Keeffe F, McMackin D, Robertson IH: Impaired sustained attention and error awareness in traumatic brain injury: implications for insight, *Neuropsychol Rehabil* 15:569–587, 2005.

72. Michel JA, Mateer CA: Attention rehabilitation following stroke and traumatic brain injury, a review, *Eura Medicophys* 42: 59–67, 2006.

73. Mirsky AF, Anthony BJ, Duncan CC, et al: Analysis of the elements of attention: a neuropsychological approach, *Neuropsychol Rev* 2:109–145, 1991.

74. Neistadt ME: Perceptual retraining for adults with diffuse brain injury, *Am J Occup Ther* 48:225–233, 1994.

75. O'Keeffe F, Dockree P, Moloney P, et al: Awareness of deficits in traumatic brain injury: a multidimensional approach to assessing metacognitive knowledge and online awareness, *J Int Neuropsychol Soc* 13:38–49, 2007.

76. Ownsworth T, Clare L: The association between awareness deficits and rehabilitation outcome following acquired brain injury, *Clin Psychol Rev* 26:783–795, 2006.

77. Ownsworth TL, McFarland KM, Young RM: Memory remediation in long-term acquired brain injury: two approaches in diary training, *Brain Inj* 13:605–626, 1999.

78. Ownsworth TL, McFarland KM, Young RM: Development and standardization of the Self-regulation Skills Interview (SRSI): a new clinical assessment tool for acquired brain injury, *Clin Neuropsychol* 14:76–92, 2000.

79. Park NW, Ingles JL: Effectiveness of attention rehabilitation after an acquired brain injury: a meta-analysis, *Neuropsychology* 15:199–210, 2001.

80. Penner IK, Kappos L: Retraining attention in MS, *J Neurol Sci* 245:147–151, 2006.

81. Polatajko HJ, Mandich A, McEwen SE: Cognitive orientation to occupational performance (CO-OP): a cognitive-based intervention for children and adults. In Katz N, editor: *Cognition, occupation, and participation across the life span* ed 3, Bethesda, MD, 2011, AOTA Press.

82. Ponsford J, Kinsella G: The use of a rating scale of attentional behaviour *Neuropsychol Rehabil* 1:241–257, 1991.

83. Posner MI, Peterson SE: The attention system of the human brain, *Annu Rev Neurosci* 13:25–42, 1990.

84. Preissner K: Use of the occupational therapy task-oriented approach to optimize the motor performance of a client with cognitive limitations, *Am J Occup Ther* 64:727–734, 2010.

85. Prigatano GP: *Neuropsychological rehabilitation after brain injury*, Baltimore, MD, 1986, Johns Hopkins University Press.

86. Prigatano GP: Anosognosia. In Beaumont JG, Kenealy PM, Rogers MJC, editors: *The Blackwell dictionary of neuropsychology*, Cambridge, MA, 1996, Blackwell.

87. Prigatano GP: Disturbances of self-awareness and rehabilitation of clients with traumatic brain injury: a 20–year perspective, *J Head Trauma Rehabil* 20:19–29, 2005.

88. Prigatano GP, Klonoff PS: A clinician's rating scale for evaluating impaired self-awareness and denial of disability after brain injury, *Clin Neuropsychol* 12:56–67, 1998.

89. Prigatano GP, Schacter DL: *Awareness of deficit after brain injury: clinical and theoretical implications*, New York, 1991, Oxford University Press.

90. Proctor A, Wilson B, Sanchez C, Wesley E: Executive function and verbal working memory in adolescents with closed head injury (CHI), *Brain Inj* 14:633–647, 2000.

91. Quemada JI, Muñoz Céspedes JM, Ezkerra J, et al: Outcome of memory rehabilitation in traumatic brain injury assessed by neuropsychological tests and questionnaires, *J Head Trauma Rehabil* 18:532–540, 2003.

92. Rath JF, Simon D, Langenbahn DM, et al: Group treatment of problem-solving deficits in outclients with traumatic brain injury: a randomised outcome study, *Neuropsychol Rehabil* 13:461–488, 2003.

93. Ries M, Marks W: Selective attention deficits following severe closed head injury: the role of inhibitory processes, *Neuropsychology* 19:476–483, 2005.

94. Robertson IH, Ward T, Ridgeway V, Nimmo-Smith I: The structure of normal human attention: the Test of Everyday Attention, *J Clin Exp Neuropsychol* 2:525–534, 1996.

95. Roche NL, Fleming JM, Shum DH: Self-awareness of prospective memory failure in adults with traumatic brain injury, *Brain Inj* 16:931–945, 2002.

96. Roth RS, Geisser ME, Theisen-Goodvich M, Dixon PJ: Cognitive complaints are associated with depression, fatigue, female sex, and pain catastrophizing in clients with chronic pain, *Arch Phys Med Rehabil* 86:1147–1154, 2005.

97. Royle J, Lincoln NB: The Everyday Memory Questionnaire—revised: development of a 13-item scale, *Disabil Rehabil* 30:114–121, 2008.

98. Sandler AB, Harris JL: Use of external memory aids with a head-injured client, *Am J Occup Ther* 46:163–166, 1992.

99. Schwartz SM: Adults with traumatic brain injury: three case studies of cognitive rehabilitation in the home setting, *Am J Occup Ther* 49:655–667, 1995.

100. Shallice T, Burgess PW: Deficits in strategy application following frontal lobe damage in man, *Brain* 114(Pt 2):727–741, 1991.

101. Sherer M, Bergloff P, Boake C, et al: The Awareness Questionnaire: factor structure and internal consistency, *Brain Inj* 12:63–68, 1998.

102. Smith G, Della Sala S, Logie RH, Maylor EA: Prospective and retrospective memory in normal ageing and dementia: a questionnaire study, *Memory* 8:311–321, 2000.

103. Sohlberg MM, Mateer CA: Training use of compensatory memory books: a three stage behavioral approach, *J Clin Exp Neuropsychol* 11:871–891, 1989.

104. Sohlberg MM, Mateer CA: Management of attention disorders. In Sohlberg MM, Mateer CA, editors: *Cognitive rehabilitation: an integrative neuropsychological approach*, New York, 2001, Guilford Press.

105. Sohlberg MM, Mateer CA: Memory theory applied to intervention. In Sohlberg MM, Mateer CA, editors: *Cognitive rehabilitation: an integrative neuropsychological approach*, New York, 2001, Guilford Press.

106. Sohlberg MM, Mateer CA: Management of dysexecutive symptoms. In Sohlberg MM, Mateer CA, editors: *Cognitive rehabilitation: an integrative neuropsychological approach*, New York, 2001, Guilford Press.

107. Squire LR: Memory systems of the brain: a brief history and current perspective, *Neurobiol Learn Mem* 82:171–177, 2004.

108. Stringer AY, Small SK: Ecologically-oriented neurorehabilitation of memory: robustness of outcome across diagnosis and severity, *Brain Inj* 25:169–178, 2011.

109. Sunderland A, Harris JE, Baddeley AD: Do laboratory tests predict everyday memory? a neuropsychological study, *J Verbal Learning Verbal Behav* 22:341–357, 1983.

110. Sunderland A, Harris JE, Baddeley AD: Assessing everyday memory after severe head injury. In Harris JE, Morris PE, editors: *Everyday memory, actions, and absent-mindedness*, London, 1984, Academic Press.

111. Tham K, Ginsburg E, Fisher AG, Tegnér R: Training to improve awareness of disabilities in clients with unilateral neglect, *Am J Occup Ther* 55:46–54, 2001.

112. Toglia J: Generalization of treatment: a multicontext approach to cognitive perceptual impairment in adults with brain injury, *Am J Occup Ther* 45:505–516, 1991.

113. Toglia J: *Contextual Memory Test*, San Antonio, 1993, Harcourt Assessments.

114. Toglia J: The Dynamic Interactional Model of cognition in cognitive rehabilitation. In Katz N, editor: *Cognition, occupation, and participation across the life span* ed 3, Bethesda, MD, 2011, AOTA Press.

115. Toglia J: *Weekly calendar planning activity*, Bethesda, MD, 2015, AOTA Press.

116. Toglia J, Kirk U: Understanding awareness deficits following brain injury, *NeuroRehabilitation* 15:57–70, 2000.

117. van den Broek MD: Why does neurorehabilitation fail? *J Head Trauma Rehabil* 20:464–473, 2005.

118. von Cramon DY, Matthes-von Cramon G, Mai N: Problem-solving deficits in brain-injured clients: a therapeutic approach, *Neuropsychol Rehabil* 1:45–64, 1991.

119. Waugh N: *Self report of the young, middle-aged, young-old, and old-old individuals on prospective memory self-rating performance*, honours thesis, Brisbane, Australia, 1999, School of Applied Psychology, Griffith University.

120. Webster JS, Scott RR: The effects of self-instructional training on attentional deficits following head injury, *Clin Neuropsychol* 5:69–74, 1983.

121. Whyte J: Attention and arousal: basic science aspects, *Arch Phys Med Rehabil* 73:940–949, 1992.

122. Whyte J, Polansky M, Flemin M, et al: Sustained arousal and attention after traumatic brain injury, *Neuropsychologia* 33:797–813, 1995.

123. Whyte J, Hart T, Bode RK, Malec JF: The Moss Attention Rating Scale for traumatic brain injury: initial psychometric assessment, *Arch Phys Med Rehabil* 84:268–276, 2003.

124. Wilson BA, Evans JJ, Alderman N, Burgess P: The development of an ecologically valid test for assessing clients with dysexecutive syndrome, *Neuropsychol Rehabil* 8:213–228, 1998.

125. Wilson BA, Alderman N, Burgess P, et al: *Behavioural assessment of the dysexecutive syndrome*, Flempton, UK, 1996, Thames Valley Test Co.

126. Wilson BA, Greenfield E, Clare L, et al: *The Rivermead Behavioural Memory Test*, ed 3, London, 2008, Pearson Assessment.

127. Wolf T, Morrison T, Matheson L: Initial development of a work-related assessment of dysexecutive syndrome: the Complex Task Performance Assessment, *Work* 31:221–228, 2008.

128. Wolf TJ, Dahl A, Auen C, Doherty M: The reliability and validity of the Complex Task Performance Assessment: a performance-based assessment of executive function, *Neuropsychol Rehabil* 27:707–721, 2017.

27

Eating and Swallowing

Jerilyn (Gigi) Smith

LEARNING OBJECTIVES

After studying this chapter, the student or practitioner will be able to do the following:

1. Name and locate oral structures concerned with eating and swallowing.
2. Name and describe the stages of normal eating and swallowing.
3. List the components of the swallowing assessment.
4. Name and describe normal and abnormal oral reflexes.
5. Describe the role of the occupational therapist in the clinical assessment of eating and swallowing.
6. Describe four steps in the swallowing assessment.
7. Describe the appropriate progression of foods and liquids in the assessment and intervention of deglutition and dysphagia.
8. Name two types of tracheostomy tubes, and list the advantages and disadvantages of each.
9. List symptoms of swallowing dysfunction.
10. Identify basic intervention goals for clients with eating and swallowing dysfunction.
11. Describe the roles of the dysphagia team members.
12. Describe proper positioning for safe feeding and swallowing.
13. Describe two methods of nonoral feeding.
14. List principles of oral feeding.
15. List and describe intervention techniques for the management of eating and swallowing dysfunction.

CHAPTER OUTLINE

KEY TERMS

Anticipatory phase
Aspiration
Bolus
Compensatory strategies
Deglutition
Dysphagia
Dysphagia diet

Dysphagia team
Eating
Esophageal phase
Feeding
Fiberoptic endoscopy
Gastrostomy tube
Hyoid bone

Instrumental assessment

Larynx

Nasogastric tube

Oral phase

Oral preparatory phase

Pharyngeal phase

Pyriform sinuses

Sulcus

Swallow response

Tracheostomy

Valleculae

Velopharyngeal port

Velum

Videofluoroscopy

THREADED CASE STUDY

Mattias, Part 1

Mattias, a 65-year-old man (prefers use of the pronouns he/him/his), experienced a right cerebrovascular accident (CVA) 3 days ago, which resulted in left hemiplegia. During his occupational therapy evaluation of activities of daily living (ADLs), it was determined that Mattias had difficulties with self-feeding, chewing, and swallowing at meals. He had frequent episodes of coughing and pocketing of food in the left cheek, and he often had food on the left side of his face. His oral intake is below the normal calorie range at this time. He complains that he chokes on many foods, including water.

An occupational profile provided the following background information. Mattias is married and has two daughters. Until onset, he was working full time as a vice president for marketing in the computer industry. He and his wife are active socially in their golf and tennis club. They also entertain with frequent dinner parties, and both are exceptional cooks. Their oldest daughter is engaged and planning to be married in 4 months.

During the occupational therapy assessment, Mattias was asked to prioritize his concerns regarding his occupational performance. Mattias wants to be able to attend and participate in his daughter's wedding in 4 months. His goal is to be able

to escort her down the aisle. He wants to be able to eat and drink without concerns about choking or coughing, particularly because he and his wife were going to prepare the dinner for the wedding rehearsal party. He also wants to be able to make and drink a toast to his daughter and her new husband without risk of choking. He had planned to work to the end of the year and then retire. Upon retirement he and his wife planned to travel to Italy to attend a 1-week cooking class.

Critical Thinking Questions

1. What evaluations would you perform to develop an intervention plan for Mattias' eating and swallowing needs based on the information described?
2. What interventions would you consider to address his goal to participate in his daughter's wedding?
3. How does context influence Mattias' need to eat safely and eat a variety of foods? How would you incorporate this knowledge into your intervention plan?
4. How would you systematically grade the challenges in the intervention program for Mattias?

ETHICAL CONSIDERATIONS

Continuing education and special training are required for competence in assessing and intervening with clients who have dysphagia.

Eating is the most basic activity of daily living (ADL), necessary for survival from birth until death. Eating occurs throughout life in a variety of contexts and in every culture and is an essential activity of daily living that facilitates an individual's basic survival and well-being.[1] Although eating and feeding are closely related, these terms are not synonymous. The *Occupational Therapy Practice Framework: Domain and Process*, Fourth Edition (OTPF-4) defines feeding as "setting up, arranging, and bringing food (fluids) from vessel to the mouth (includes self-feeding and feeding others)" and swallowing/eating is defined as "keeping and manipulating food or fluid in the mouth, swallowing it (i.e., moving it from the mouth to the stomach" (p. 30).[1] Swallowing is a complicated act that involves moving food, fluid, medication, or saliva through the mouth, pharynx, and esophagus into the stomach. Feeding, eating, and swallowing are influenced by contextual issues, including psychosocial, cultural, and environmental factors. Dysphagia is a medical term that means difficulty with swallowing. This difficulty can occur at any stage (oral, pharyngeal, or esophageal) of the swallow. Dysphagia is not a primary medical diagnosis; rather, it is

a symptom of underlying disease and is often identified by its clinical characteristics.[15]

Feeding, eating, and swallowing are within the domain and scope of practice of occupational therapy, and occupational therapists are trained to assess and provide intervention for the performance issues involved in these activities.[2,3] Areas addressed in occupational therapy include *performance skills* such as motor and process skills; social interaction skills; *client factors* such as values and beliefs; mental functions (cognitive, attention, memory, perception); global mental functions (consciousness, energy), sensory functions, muscle strength, endurance and motor control, muscle tone, normal and abnormal motor reflexes, respiratory system function, and digestive system function; *activity demands* such as social demands relating to the social environment and cultural contexts, sequence and timing, and required body functions and structures; and *performance patterns*, including the habits, routines, and rituals that support or influence the eating process. The *contexts* and *environments*, including those that are cultural, personal, and social, that may influence the client's successful engagement in eating also must be considered when assessing and designing interventions for individuals with feeding, eating, and swallowing problems.

This chapter provides the occupational therapist with a foundation for the assessment and intervention process of the adult client with eating and swallowing dysfunction. Conditions that can result in eating and swallowing problems include cerebrovascular accident (CVA), traumatic brain injury, brain tumor, anoxia, Guillain-Barré syndrome, Huntington's disease, Alzheimer's disease, multiple sclerosis, amyotrophic lateral sclerosis, Parkinson's disease, myasthenia gravis, poliomyelitis, postpolio syndrome/muscular atrophy, and quadriplegia. Structural, iatrogenic, and developmental causes of dysphagia are not discussed in this chapter.

ANATOMY AND PHYSIOLOGY OF NORMAL EATING SWALLOW

Deglutition, the normal consumption of solids or liquids, is a complex sensorimotor process involving the brainstem, the cerebral cortex, six cranial nerves, the first three cervical nerve segments, and 48 pairs of muscles.[23] A normal swallow requires all of these structures to be intact (Fig. 27.1). Therefore, occupational therapists who work with clients with eating and swallowing problems must have a thorough understanding of the anatomy and physiology of all phases of the swallow (Table 27.1). The eating and swallowing process can be divided into four stages: oral preparatory phase, oral phase, pharyngeal phase, and esophageal phase (Fig. 27.2). An additional phase, the anticipatory phase, also will be discussed.

Anticipatory Phase

Psychological factors, social interactions, dining environment, personal preferences around eating and dining, and cultural influences contribute to the eating experience. The psychological, emotional, and social aspects surrounding mealtime can have a huge impact on an older individual's participation in the feeding process as well as on oral intake. The anticipatory phase takes place before feeding or eating takes place. Factors to be considered that may have an effect on the anticipatory phase include the variety of foods offered, presentation of food, seating during meals, mealtime atmosphere, attention to food preferences, cultural aspects around eating and food choices, and mealtime habits and routines.

The anticipatory phase begins even before the client enters the dining area. The client's expectations of the eating experience will influence their reaction to the dining environment (sounds, smells, seating arrangement, lighting) and to the foods presented. Appetite/hunger; the sensory qualities of the food; the sensory qualities of the utensils, cups, and plates; the client's motivation to eat; and cognitive awareness of the eating activity will all have an impact on the degree to which the client engages

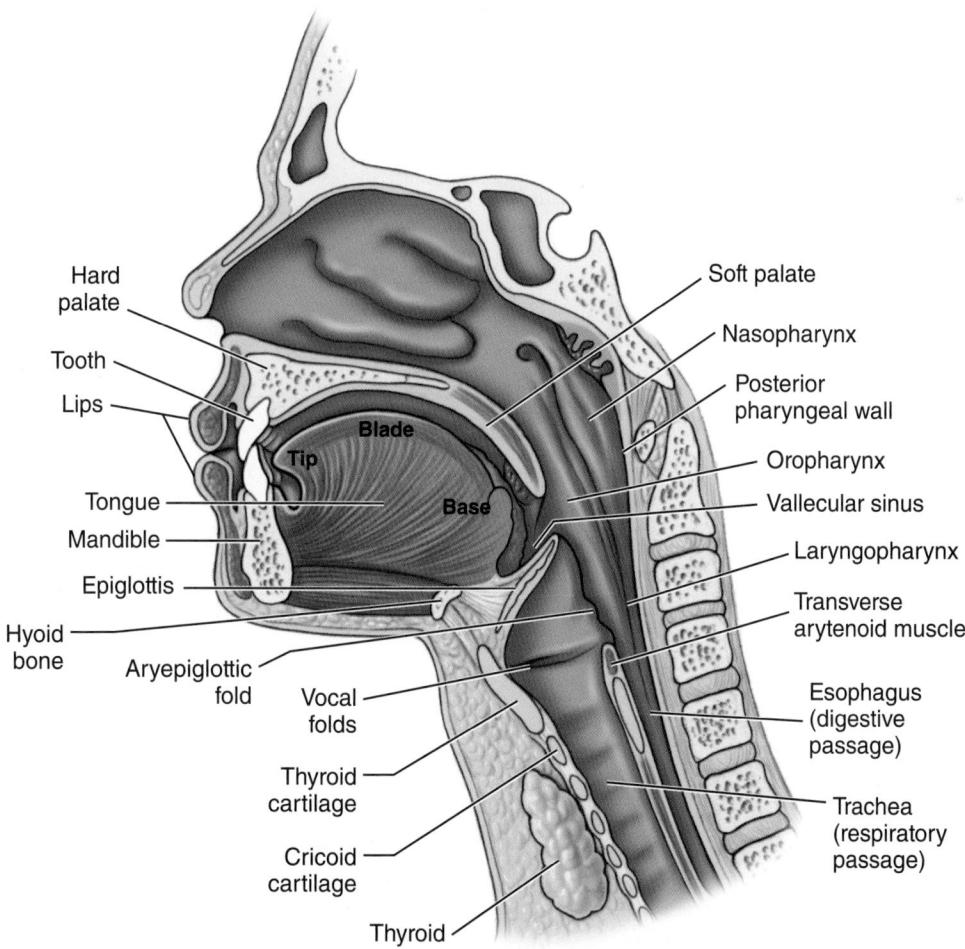

Fig. 27.1 Oral structures, swallowing mechanism at rest. (From Herlihy B: *The human body in health and illness*, ed 7, St. Louis, 2022, Elsevier.)

TABLE 27.1 Swallowing Process

		ORAL PREPARATORY STAGE		
Structure	**Muscle**	**Movement**	**Cranial Nerve**	**Sensation**
Jaw	Pterygoideus medialis	Opens jaw	Trigeminal (V)	Face, temple, mouth, teeth, mucus
	Pterygoideus medialis and lateralis	Protrudes lower jaw; moves jaw laterally		
	Masseter	Closes jaw		
	Digastricus, mylohyoideus, geniohyoideus	Depresses lower jaw		
Mouth	Orbicularis oris	Compresses and protrudes lips	Facial (VII)	
	Zygomaticus minor	Protrudes upper lip		
	Zygomaticus major	Raises lateral angle of mouth upward and outward (smile)		
	Levator anguli oris	Moves angle of mouth straight upward		
	Risorius	Draws angle of mouth backward (grimace)		
	Depressor labii inferioris	Draws lower lip downward and outward		
	Mentalis	Protrudes lower lip (pouting)		
	Depressor anguli oris	Draws down angles of mouth		
Tongue	Superior longitudinal	Shortens tongue; raises sides and tip of tongue	Facial (VII)	Taste, anterior two thirds of tongue
	Transverse	Lengthens and narrows tongue	Glossopharyngeal (IX)	Taste, posterior third of tongue
	Vertical	Flattens and broadens tongue	Hypoglossal (XII)	
	Inferior longitudinal	Shortens tongue; turns tip of tongue downward		
Oral Stage				
Tongue	Styloglossus	Elevates and pulls tongue posteriorly	Accessory (XI)	
	Palatoglossus	Elevates and pulls tongue posteriorly; narrows fauces (faucial arches)		
	Genioglossus	Depresses, protrudes, and retracts tongue; elevates hyoid	Hypoglossal (XII)	
	Hyoglossus	Depresses and pulls tongue posteriorly		
Soft palate	Tensor veli palatini	Tenses soft palate	Trigeminal (V)	Mouth
	Levator veli palatini	Elevates soft palate	Accessory (XI)	
	Uvulae	Shortens soft palate		
Pharyngeal Stage				
Fauces (Faucial Arches)	Palatoglossus Membranes of pharynx	Narrows fauces	Vagus (X)	Fauces
	Palatopharyngeus	Elevates larynx and pharynx		
Hyoid	Suprahyoideus Stylohyoideus	Elevates hyoid anteriorly, posteriorly	Trigeminal (V)	
	Sternothyroideus	Depresses thyroid cartilage	Cervical 1, 2, 3	
	Omohyoideus	Depresses hyoid		
Pharynx	Salpingopharyngeus	Pharynx elevation	Glossopharyngeal (IX)	
	Palatopharyngeus	Pharynx elevation		
	Stylopharyngeus	Pharynx and larynx elevation		
	Constrictor pharyngeus Membranes of pharynx Constrictor pharyngeus medius Constrictor pharyngeus inferior	Sequentially constricts the superior nasopharynx, oropharynx, laryngopharynx	Vagus (X)	Laryngeal and nasal pharynx
	Cricopharyngeus	Relaxes during swallow; prevents air from entering esophagus		

TABLE 27.1   Swallowing Process—cont'd

ORAL PREPARATORY STAGE

Structure	Muscle	Movement	Cranial Nerve	Sensation
Larynx	Aryepiglotticus Membranes of larynx Thyroepiglotticus	Closes inlet of larynx	← Vagus (X) →	
	Thyroarytenoideus	Closes glottis; shortens vocal cords		
	Arytenoid-oblique, transverse	Adducts arytenoid cartilages		
	Lateral cricoarytenoid	Adducts and rotates arytenoid cartilage		
	Vocalis	Controls tension of vocal cords		
	Postcricoarytenoideus	Widens glottis		
	Cricothyroideus-straight, oblique	Elevates cricoid arch		
Esophageal Stage				
Esophagus	Smooth	Peristaltic wave	← Vagus (X)	

Data from Finsterer J, Griswold W: Disorders of the lower cranial nerves, *J Neurosci Rural Pract* 6:377–391, 2015; Groher M: Normal swallowing in adults. In Groher M, Crary M, editors: *Dysphagia: clinical management in adults and children*, ed 2, St. Louis, 2016, Elsevier; and Gutman SA, Schonfeld AB: *Screening adult neurologic populations*, ed 2, Bethesda, MD, 2009, American Occupational Therapy Association.

in the feeding process. The anticipatory phase is an important precursor to successful eating. The occupational therapist can be instrumental in identifying environmental and contextual modifications that can positively influence the client's response to the eating experience.

Oral Preparatory Phase

In the oral preparatory phase of the swallow, food is masticated by the teeth and gums (if necessary) and manipulated by the lips, cheek, and tongue to form a bolus of appropriate texture for swallowing.[14] Visual and olfactory information stimulates salivary secretions from three pairs of salivary glands. Saliva is mixed with the food to prepare the bolus for the swallow. As tactile contact is made with the food, the jaw comes forward to open. The lips close around the glass or utensil to remove the food or liquid. The labial musculature forms a seal to prevent any material from leaking out of the oral cavity. This phase reflects the close relationship between feeding and eating. As Mattias brought food to his mouth, he did not have symmetrical lip closure on utensils or a glass, and often food or fluid would dribble from the left side of his mouth.

As chewing begins, the mandible and tongue move in a strong, combined rotary and lateral direction. The upper and lower teeth shear and crush the food. The tongue moves laterally to push the food between the teeth. The buccinator muscles of the cheeks contract to act as lateral retainers, to prevent food particles from falling into the sulcus between the jaw and cheek. The tongue sweeps through the mouth, gathering food particles and mixing them with saliva. Recall that Mattias frequently had food remaining in his cheek after swallowing. Retention of food in the cheek may occur from diminished motor control of the tongue to manipulate the bolus or may indicate diminished sensory appreciation for food remaining in the sulcus. Sensory receptors throughout the oral cavity carry information of taste, texture, and temperature of the food or liquid through the seventh and ninth cranial nerves to the brainstem. The

chewing action of the mandible and tongue is repeated rhythmically, repositioning the food until a cohesive bolus is formed. The length of time needed to form a bolus one can safely swallow varies with the viscosity of the food. Less time is required to orally manage soft foods, and a longer time is needed for more textured or dense foods. Large amounts of thick liquids or thick and dense foods require the tongue to divide the food into smaller parts to be swallowed one at a time. The posterior portion of the tongue forms a tight seal with the velum, preventing slippage of the bolus or liquid into the pharynx.[14] Foods that are a mixture of liquid and solids (e.g., soup with chunks of vegetables) require greater oral motor control and often present more difficulty for clients with oral preparatory phase swallowing problems.

In preparation for the next stage, the solid or liquid bolus, having been formed into a cohesive and easily swallowed mass, may be held between the anterior tongue and palate, with the tongue tip either elevated or dipped toward the floor of the mouth.[23] The tongue cups around the bolus to seal it against the hard palate. The larynx and the pharynx are at rest during this phase of the swallowing process, and the airway is open.

THREADED CASE STUDY

Mattias, Part 2

As Mattias brought food to his mouth, he did not have symmetric lip closure on utensils or a glass, and often food or fluid would dribble from the left side of his mouth. Mattias frequently has food remaining in his cheek after swallowing.

Problems at the oral preparatory phase can disrupt the normal swallow sequence. Mattias has problems with this phase of the eating process. Of additional concern to Mattias is the embarrassment of having food or fluid dribble from the left side of his mouth. His decreased sensory awareness compromises his ability to notice foods/fluids and use a napkin to wipe the remaining food from his face.

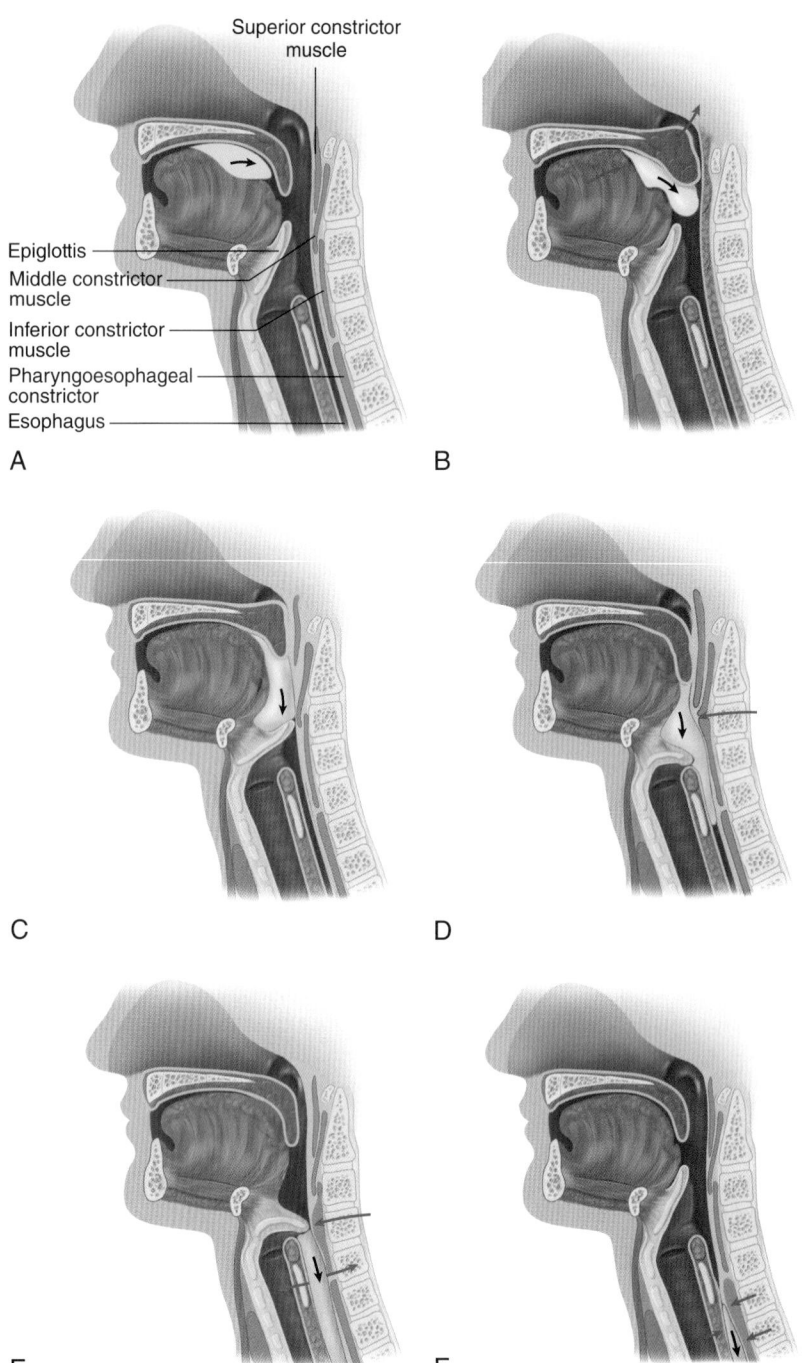

Fig. 27.2 (A) A bolus of food *(yellow)* is pushed against the hard palate and posteriorly toward the oropharynx by a stripping action of the tongue against the palate. (*Black arrows* indicate movement of the bolus.) (B) to (E) The soft palate is elevated, closing off the nasopharynx, and the pharynx is elevated by the palatopharyngeal and salpingopharyngeal muscles. Successive contractions of the pharyngeal constrictors (C) and (D) force the bolus through the pharynx and into the esophagus. As this occurs, the epiglottis is bent down over the opening of the larynx, largely by the force of the bolus pressing against it. (*Red arrows* indicate muscle movement.) E, The tonically active pharyngoesophageal constrictor relaxes *(outward direction red arrows)*, allowing the bolus to enter the esophagus. (F) During the esophageal phase, the bolus is moved by successive contractions of the esophagus toward the stomach. (From Schapira AHV: Neurology and clinical neuroscience, Philadelphia, 2007, Mosby.)

Oral Phase

The oral phase of swallowing begins when the tongue initiates posterior movement of the bolus toward the pharynx.[23] The tongue elevates to squeeze the bolus up against the hard palate and forms a central groove to funnel the bolus posteriorly. As the viscosity of the food increases, the amount of pressure created by the tongue against the palate increases. Thicker foods require more pressure to propel them efficiently through the oral cavity.

The oral phase of the swallow is voluntary, requiring the person to be alert and involved in the process. A normal voluntary oral phase is necessary to elicit a strong swallow response during the pharyngeal stage that follows. This stage of the swallow requires intact labial musculature to maintain food or liquid inside of the oral cavity, intact lingual movement to propel the bolus toward the pharynx, intact buccal musculature to prevent material from falling into the lateral sulci, and the ability to comfortably breathe through the nose. The oral phase takes approximately 1 second to complete with thin liquids and slightly longer with thick liquids and textured foods.

THREADED CASE STUDY

Mattias, Part 3

Mattias is alert but has difficulties maneuvering food within his mouth during the oral phase. His ability to chew textured foods is compromised, and he requires additional time to chew foods. This contributes to the decreased oral intake.

Pharyngeal Phase

Both voluntary and reflexive components are necessary for a normal swallow. Both must be functioning efficiently to produce an immediate, consistent and safe swallow necessary for normal eating.[23] The pharyngeal phase marks the beginning of the reflexive portion of the swallowing process.

This phase of swallowing typically begins when the bolus passes any point between the anterior faucial arches and where the tongue base crosses the lower rim of the mandible into the pharynx, marking the start of the reflexive component of the swallow.[25] After the swallow response has been triggered, it continues with no pause in bolus movement until the total act has been completed. The pharyngeal swallow is controlled by central pattern-generating (CPG) circuitry of the brainstem and peripheral reflexes.[38] Within the medulla oblongata the medullary reticular formation is responsible for screening out all extraneous sensory patterns and for responding only to those patterns that indicate the need to swallow. The reticular formation also assumes control of all motor neurons and related muscles needed to complete the swallow. Higher brain functions such as speech and respiration are preempted.

When the swallow response is triggered, several physiological functions occur simultaneously. The velum elevates and retracts, closing the velopharyngeal port to prevent regurgitation of material into the nasal cavity. The tongue base elevates to direct the bolus into the pharynx. The hyoid and the larynx elevate and move anteriorly. There is closure of the larynx at the vocal folds, the laryngeal entrance, and the epiglottis to prevent material from entering the airway. The pharyngeal tube elevates and contracts from the top to the bottom in the pharyngeal constrictors, using a squeezing motion to move the bolus through the pharynx toward the esophagus. The bolus passes through the pharynx, dividing in half at the valleculae and moving down each side through the pyriform sinuses toward the esophagus. The upper esophageal sphincter (UES) relaxes and opens, allowing the material to enter the esophagus.[14] This movement must be rapid and efficient so that respiration is interrupted only briefly. The pharyngeal phase of the swallow takes approximately 1 second to complete for thin liquids.

THREADED CASE STUDY

Mattias, Part 4

Mattias frequently coughs, indicating difficulties with the timing and coordination of the pharyngeal phase. His problems swallowing water may indicate diminished laryngeal elevation and decreased airway protection during the swallow.

Esophageal Phase

The esophageal phase of the swallow starts when the bolus enters the esophagus through the cricopharyngeal juncture or UES. The esophagus is a straight tube, approximately 10 inches long, that connects the pharynx to the stomach. The pharynx is separated from the esophagus by the UES. The lower esophageal sphincter (LES) separates the esophagus from the stomach. During the swallow, the strong muscles of the esophagus contract and the bolus is transported through the esophagus by peristaltic wave contractions. The overall transit time needed for the bolus to reach the stomach varies from 8 to 20 seconds. As the food enters the esophagus, the epiglottis returns to the relaxed position, and the airway opens.[14]

THREADED CASE STUDY

Mattias, Part 5

Mattias complains of frequently coughing and choking on food and fluid. This may be due to problems with the preoral, oral, pharyngeal, or esophageal phase of eating. As you read the section on eating and swallowing assessment, use the case presentation of Mattias and consider what assessment results you would look for to identify which phase is producing the episodes of coughing and choking.

EATING AND SWALLOWING ASSESSMENT

When a physician refers a client to occupational therapy for a suspected swallowing or feeding problem, a thorough eating and swallowing assessment must be completed. The occupational therapist reviews the client's medical history and assesses the client's perceptual and cognitive skills; physical control of head, trunk, and extremities; oral structures; oral motor control; sensation; swallowing ability; and risk for aspiration.

Medical Chart Review

A careful review of the client's medical chart before initiating the bedside assessment reveals important information. The therapist should take note of the client's diagnosis, pertinent medical history (including prior incidents of aspiration), prescribed medications, and current hydration and nutritional status.

The medical diagnosis may indicate the cause of the client's eating or swallowing problems. For example, a diagnosis of a neurologic disorder such as a CVA or a degenerative disease/disorder, such as Parkinson's, Huntington's or Alzheimer's disease, should alert the therapist that eating or swallowing problems may exist.[34] It is important to know whether problems developed suddenly or gradually. The therapist should seek information regarding the duration of the client's swallowing difficulties and note any secondary diagnoses that could contribute to dysphagia, such as gastrointestinal or respiratory problems or changes in medication. A diagnosis of dehydration, weight loss, or malnutrition may indicate a chronic problem with eating or swallowing.

Particular attention should be paid to reported episodes of pneumonia or aspiration (entry of food or material into the airway below the level of the true vocal folds). Aspiration pneumonia occurs when food or material enters into the lung and can be a serious medical complication that is identified by x-ray examination and treated with antibiotics.[13] Predictors of aspiration pneumonia include the need for frequent suctioning, chronic obstructive pulmonary disease, congestive heart failure, use of a feeding tube, swallowing problems, multiple medications, and eating dependence. A smoking history, underweight status, abnormal pharyngeal delay time, and laryngeal penetration during the swallow are also associated with aspiration pneumonia.[20] An elevated temperature may also indicate that a client is aspirating.

An examination of the client's current hydration and nutritional status provides valuable information about the client's ability to manage oral intake. This information can be found in the dietary section of the chart or in the nursing progress notes in the intake and output (I&O) record. An altered diet texture (puréed food or thickened liquids) alerts the therapist to a potential problem with the client's ability to safely eat a regular diet. The presence of an intravenous (IV) fluid may indicate dehydration. Weight loss is frequently a result of a swallowing or feeding problem. Consideration should be given to prescribed medications that may alter the client's alertness, orientation, saliva production, appetite, and muscle control. The nursing notes may also indicate whether the client coughs or chokes when taking medications. How the client receives nutrition is also important—for example, the presence of a nonoral feeding device such as a nasogastric tube (NG tube) or gastrostomy tube (G tube) is an indication of a serious dysphagia problem.

Occupational Profile

In the beginning of the evaluation process, the therapist obtains information from the client to develop the occupational profile. Information gathered for the profile is designed to help the therapist understand what is meaningful and important to the client.[2] Prior eating habits and routines and the importance of eating to the client (and the client's family or significant other) are essential to know so that interventions can be established to meet the client's needs. The occupational therapist must take into consideration the cultural values, beliefs, habits, and routines of the client revolving around food and eating. The client may have strong feelings about particular foods, food temperatures, or food textures. Food and food preparation methods may be symbolically meaningful to clients and may have a strong impact on the client's oral intake. The presentation of food may have a significant influence on the individual's desire to eat. Most adults have firmly rooted routines surrounding the activity of eating. For example, an elderly person may eat a late breakfast, a larger meal at midday, and only a light meal in the evening. He or she may watch TV while eating. This routine can be severely disrupted in an institutionalized setting.

THREADED CASE STUDY

Mattias, Part 6

The intervention program is developed based on information provided to the therapist in the occupational profile. Mattias clearly identified his intervention priorities and discussed his concerns about participating in his daughter's wedding. The issues related to eating and drinking are closely tied to the cultural and social expectations for the father of the bride.

Cognitive-Perceptual Status

The client's cognitive and perceptual abilities are assessed to determine the degree to which the client can actively participate in an eating and swallowing assessment and intervention program. The therapist should establish whether the client is alert, oriented, and able to follow simple directions, either verbal, with demonstration, or with manual guidance. It is important to assess the client's memory to determine if he or she will be able to recall strategies for safe eating. The therapist should also evaluate the client's visual function, visual-perceptual skills, and motor planning skills, because they are important for independent feeding. An individual who exhibits confusion, dementia, poor awareness of the eating task, poor attention span, or impaired perception or memory will require close supervision and assistance during eating for safe consumption and adherence to any eating strategies that will facilitate intake and reduce aspiration risk.

Physical Status

Head and neck control is an important component of a safe swallow. To assess head control, the therapist asks the client to turn the head from side to side and up and down. The therapist assesses the client's range of motion (ROM) and motor control. Assessment should include the quality of head movement without physical assistance or with assistance, if needed. The therapist should also gently move the client's head passively from side to side and up and down to look for stiffness or abnormal muscle tone. Poor head control may indicate decreased strength, decreased or increased muscle tone, or decreased awareness of posture. Appropriate head control is necessary to provide a stable base for adequate jaw and tongue movement, allowing an optimal swallow response. Head control is also necessary to anatomically position the client in the safest posture to reduce the risk of aspiration.

In assessing the client's trunk control, the therapist observes whether the client is able to sit in the upright position in midline with equal weight bearing on both hips. The therapist assesses the client's ability to maintain the midline position independently when involved in eating and whether he or she requires the use of postural supports (e.g., wheelchair trunk supports or a lap board) or physical assistance. It is also important to determine if the client can return to midline if a loss of balance occurs. To participate in an eating and swallowing intervention program, the client must maintain an upright position with the head and trunk in midline to provide correct alignment of the swallowing structures and reduce the risk of aspiration caused by poor positioning. The client's endurance for sitting upright and participating in an eating activity is assessed, and the impact of fatigue on the swallow is determined.

THREADED CASE STUDY

Mattias, Part 7

Mattias is able to independently sit in a chair and at the side of the bed. His head control appears adequate, but he tends to sit shifted to his right side, and his head is most often facing to the right side instead of positioned in midline. This indicates poor trunk and head alignment and can affect eating.

Oral Assessment

Outer Oral Status

The face and mouth are sensitive areas to assess. Most adults are cautious about or even threatened by having another person touch their face. Therefore, each step of the assessment process should be carefully explained before touching the client, using terms that the individual understands. The therapist also should tell the client how long they will be touching the face—for example, "For a count of three." The therapist assesses the outer oral structures, including the facial musculature and mobility of the cheeks, jaw, and lips. Working within the client's visual field, the therapist moves their hand(s) slowly toward the client's face. This allows the individual time to process and acknowledge the approach.

Sensation. Indications of poor oral sensation include drooling, food remaining on the lips, and food falling out of the mouth without the client being aware that this is happening. To assess the client's awareness of touch, the therapist occludes the client's vision and uses a cotton-tipped swab to gently touch different areas of the face. The individual is asked to point to where they were touched. If pointing is difficult, the client is asked to nod or say yes or no when touched. The client with intact sensation responds accurately and quickly, unless there are compromises in communication or cognition.

The client's ability to sense hot and cold should be assessed. The therapist may use two test tubes, one filled with hot water and one with cold water. A laryngeal mirror that is first heated and then cooled using hot and cold water may also be used. The client's face or lips are touched in several places, and the client is asked to indicate whether the touch was hot or cold. A client with aphasia or cognitive impairment may have difficulty responding accurately. In this instance, the therapist must make an assessment from clinical observations.

Poor sensory awareness can affect the client's ability to move facial musculature appropriately. The client's self-esteem may be affected, especially in social situations, if decreased awareness causes the client to ignore saliva, food, or liquids remaining on the face or lips.

THREADED CASE STUDY

Mattias, Part 8

Consider Mattias and his personal goal of eating at his daughter's wedding rehearsal dinner. The diminished sensation around Mattias' face will need to be addressed to avoid his embarrassment during this important event. Strategies that promote compensatory habit formation should be used, such as having Mattias wipe his face after every second or third bite of food to remove any food on his face. This strategy provides further sensory input to the face in addition to decreasing the potential embarrassment of having food remain on his face.

Musculature. An assessment of the facial musculature provides the therapist with information about the movement, strength, and tone available to the client for chewing and swallowing. The therapist first observes the client's face at rest and notes any visible asymmetry. If a facial droop is obvious, the therapist should observe whether the muscles feel slack or taut. A masked appearance, with little change in facial expression, also may be observed. The therapist should observe whether the client appears to be frowning or grimacing with the jaw clenched and the mouth pulled back.

The therapist tests the facial musculature by asking the client to perform the movements listed in Table 27.2. The therapist should note how much assistance the client needs to perform these movements. As the client moves through each task, symmetry of movement is assessed. Asymmetry could indicate weakness or increased tone. Musculature is palpated for abnormal resistance to the movement.

If the client is able to hold the position at the end of the movement, the therapist applies gentle pressure against the muscle to determine strength. An individual with normal strength is able to hold the position throughout the applied resistance. The person who is only able to hold the position briefly against pressure may have adequate strength for chewing and swallowing but may require an altered diet.

Oral reflexes. A client who has sustained damage to brainstem or cortical structures may demonstrate primitive oral reflexes that will interfere with a dysphagia-retraining program. The presence of the rooting, bite, or suck-swallow reflex, normal from 0 to 5 months of age, will interfere with oral motor control in adults. Persistence of these primitive oral reflexes interferes with the client's isolated oral motor control, which is needed for chewing and swallowing. The gag, palatal, and cough reflexes should be present in adults and contribute to airway protection. The absence or impairment of these important reflexes may interfere with a safe swallow. Specific assessment techniques are presented in Table 27.3.

TABLE 27.2 Outer Oral Motor Assessment

Function	Instruction to Client	Testing Procedure*
Facial expression	"Lift your eyebrows as high as you can."	Place one finger above each eyebrow. Apply downward pressure.
	"Bring your eyebrows toward your nose in a frown."	Place one finger above each eyebrow. Apply pressure outward.
	"Wrinkle your nose upward."	Place one finger on tip of nose and apply downward pressure.
	"Suck in your cheeks."	Apply pressure outward against each inside cheek.
Lip control	"Smile."	Observe for symmetric movement. Palpate over each cheek.
	"Press your lips together tightly and puff out your cheeks."	Place one finger above and one finger below lips. Apply pressure, moving fingers away from each other; check for ability to hold air.
	"Pucker your lips as in a kiss."	Apply pressure inwardly against lips (toward teeth).
Jaw control	"Open your mouth as far as you can."	Help patient maintain head control. Apply pressure from under chin upward and forward.
	"Close your mouth tightly. Don't let me open it."	Help client maintain head control. Apply pressure on chin downward.
	"Push your bottom teeth forward."	Place two fingers against chin and apply pressure backward.
	"Move your jaw from side to side."	Place one finger on left cheek and apply pressure to right.

*Apply resistance only in the absence of abnormal muscle tone.
Data from Avery W: *Dysphagia care and related feeding concerns for adults*, ed 2, Bethesda, MD, 2010, American Occupational Therapy Association; and Gutman SA, Schonfeld AB: *Screening adult neurologic populations*, ed 2, Bethesda, MD, 2009, American Occupational Therapy Association.

TABLE 27.3 Oral Reflexes

Reflex	Assessment	Functional Implications
Rooting (0–4 mo)	*Stimulus:* touch client on right or left corner of mouth	Limits isolated motor control of lip muscles
	Response: client moves lips and head in direction of stimulus	Moves head out of midline, which alters alignment of swallowing mechanism
Bite (4–7 mo)	*Stimulus:* touch crowns of teeth with unbreakable object *Response:* client involuntarily clamps teeth shut	Prevents normal forward, lateral, and rotary movements of jaw necessary for chewing
Suck-swallow (0–4 mo)	*Stimulus:* introduction of food and liquid *Response:* sucking	Prevents development of normal voluntary swallow
Tongue thrust (abnormal)	*Stimulus:* introduction of food and liquid	Interferes with ability to keep lips and mouth closed
	Response: tongue comes forward to front of teeth	Prevents tongue from propelling food to back of mouth in preparation for swallow; prevents formation of bolus, loss of tongue lateralization
Gag (0–adult)	*Stimulus:* pressure on back of tongue *Response:* tongue humping, pharyngeal constriction	Protects airway (not always present in normal adult); hypersensitive gag reflex can interfere with chewing, swallowing
Palatal (0–adult)	*Stimulus:* stroke along faucial arches *Response:* constriction of faucial arches; elevation of uvula	Protects airway, closes off nasal passages, triggers swallow response

Data from Avery W: *Dysphagia care and related feeding concerns for adults*, ed 2, Bethesda, MD, 2010, American Occupational Therapy Association; and Logemann J: *Evaluation and treatment of swallowing disorders*, Austin, TX, 1998, Pro-Ed.

Intraoral Status

An assessment of the client's intraoral status includes an examination of oral structures, including the tongue and palatal function. The therapist first explains each procedure to the client, then works within the client's visual field and gives sufficient time to process the instructions found in Table 27.4.

Standard precaution techniques are used throughout the assessment and include the use of examination gloves and careful hand-washing. The therapist should check for allergies to latex before examining the person's mouth and use an examination glove made of appropriate material for an intraoral examination. The therapist must place only a wet, gloved finger or dampened tongue blade into the client's mouth. The mouth is normally a wet environment, and a dry finger or tongue blade can be uncomfortable. After a count of three, the therapist removes the finger and allows the client to swallow the secretions that may have accumulated.

Dentition. Because the adult uses teeth to shear and grind food during bolus formation, it is important for the therapist to assess the condition and quality of the client's teeth and gums. Poor dental status or inadequate denture fit can contribute to dysphagia, discomfort or pain with swallowing, dehydration, malnutrition, low dietary intake, poor nutritional status, and weight loss.[11]

For assessment purposes, the mouth is divided into four quadrants: right upper, right lower, left upper, and left lower. The therapist visually notes whether the client's gums are bleeding, tender, or inflamed and by sliding a gloved finger between the cheek and gums, assesses whether the gums feel spongy or firm. Loose teeth and sensitive or missing teeth are also noted.

TABLE 27.4   Intraoral Motor Assessment

Function	Instruction to Client	Testing Procedure*
Tongue		
Protrusion	"Stick out your tongue."	Apply slight resistance toward the back of the throat with tongue blade after client exhibits full range of motion.
Lateralization	"Move your tongue from side to side."	Apply slight resistance in opposite direction of motion with tongue blade.
	"Touch your tongue to your inside cheek—right, then left; move your tongue up and down."	Using finger on outside of cheek, push against tongue inwardly.
Tipping	"Touch your tongue to your upper lip."	With tongue blade between tongue tip and lip, apply downward pressure.
	"Open your mouth. Touch your tongue behind your front teeth."	With tongue blade between tongue and teeth, apply downward pressure on tongue.
Dipping	"Touch your tongue behind your bottom teeth."	With tongue blade between tongue and bottom teeth, apply upward pressure.
Humping	"Say, 'ng'; say, 'ga.'"	Observe for humping of tongue against hard palate. Tongue should flow from front to back.
	"Run your tongue along the roof of your mouth, front or back."	Observe for symmetry and ease of movement.
Swallow		
Hard palate	"Open your mouth and hold it open."	Using flashlight, gently examine for sensitivity by walking finger from front to back.
Soft palate	"Say, 'ah' for as long as you can (5 seconds). Change pitch up an octave."	Observe for tightening of faucial arches, elevation of uvula. Using laryngeal mirror, stroke juncture of hard and soft palate to elicit palatal reflex. Observe for upward and backward movement of soft palate.
Hyoid elevation (base of tongue)	"Can you swallow for me?"	Place finger at base of client's tongue underneath the chin, and feel for elevation just before movement of the larynx.
Laryngeal		
Range of motion	"I am going to move your Adam's apple side to side."	Grasp larynx by placing fingers and thumb along sides. Move larynx gently side to side; evaluate for ease and symmetry of movement.
Elevation	"Can you swallow for me?"	Place fingers along the larynx: first finger at hyoid, second finger at top of larynx, and so on. Feel for quick and smooth elevation of larynx as the client swallows.
Cough		
Voluntary	"Can you cough?"	Observe for ease and strength of movement, loudness of cough, swallow after cough.
Reflexive	"Take a deep breath."	As client holds breath, using palm of hand, push downward (toward stomach) on the sternum. Evaluate strength of reaction.

*Apply resistance in absence of abnormal muscle tone.
Data from Avery W: *Dysphagia care and related feeding concerns for adults*, ed 2, Bethesda, MD, 2010, American Occupational Therapy Association; and Gutman SA, Schonfeld AB: *Screening adult neurologic populations*, ed 2, Bethesda, MD, 2009, American Occupational Therapy Association.

OT PRACTICE NOTES

The therapist should avoid placing a finger between the client's teeth until it has been determined that the client does not have a bite reflex.

After assessing the gums, the therapist turns over the gloved finger, slides the pad of the finger against the inside of the client's cheek, and gently pushes the cheek outward to feel the tone of the buccal musculature. The therapist notes whether the cheek is firm with an elastic quality, too easy to stretch, or tight without any stretch. The therapist observes the condition of the inside of the client's mouth, checking for bite marks on the tongue, cheeks, and lips. Next, the therapist should remove the finger from the client's mouth, allow or assist the client to swallow saliva, and assist the client to move the lip and cheek musculature into the normal resting position. This procedure is repeated for each quadrant.

If the client has dentures, the therapist must determine whether the fit is adequate for chewing. Because dentures are held in place and controlled by normal musculature and sensation, changes in these areas, or marked weight loss, affect the client's ability to use dentures effectively for eating. Dentures should fit over the gums without slipping or sliding during eating or talking. Clients should always wear well-fitting dentures during oral intake. A dental consultation may be needed to ensure appropriate fit if dentures cannot be held firmly with commercial adhesive creams or powders. Loose dentures or teeth may necessitate changes in food consistencies that the client may have otherwise managed. Clients who have gum or dental problems require appropriate follow-up and excellent oral hygiene to participate in a feeding and eating program. Poor oral hygiene can lead to the development of bacteria, which, if aspirated, contributes to the increased risk of bacterial pneumonia.[30] It is particularly important to ensure that the oral cavity is clear of any residual food after a swallowing, feeding, or eating assessment or session. It is also important to educate caregivers about the importance of good oral hygiene after eating, particularly for an individual with dysphagia.

Tongue movement. The tongue has a critical role in the normal chewing and swallowing process. Controlled lingual movement is necessary to assist in the preparation and movement of food in the mouth. The extrinsic muscles of the tongue control the position of the tongue in the oral cavity, and the intrinsic muscles are responsible for changing the shape of the tongue, which is necessary in propelling the bolus posteriorly.[33] Lingual discoordination is one of the most commonly reported problems affecting the oral stage of swallowing.[34] A thorough assessment of the tongue's strength, range of motion, control, and tone is an important component of the swallowing assessment.

The client is asked to open the mouth, and the therapist assesses the appearance of the tongue using a flashlight and notes whether the tongue is pink and moist, red, or heavily coated and white. A heavily coated tongue decreases the client's sensations of taste, temperature, and texture and may indicate poor tongue movement or be a sign of infection.

When examining the shape of the tongue, the therapist notes whether it is flattened, bunched, or rounded. Normally, the tongue is slightly concave with a groove running down the middle. The therapist observes the tongue at rest in the mouth and determines whether it is in the normal position of midline, resting just behind the front teeth, retracted or pulled back away from the front teeth, or deviated to the right or left side. A retracted tongue may indicate an increase of abnormal muscle tone or a loss of range of motion as a result of soft-tissue shortening. The client exhibiting tongue deviation with protrusion may have muscle weakness on the affected side, causing the tongue to deviate toward the unaffected side because the stronger muscles dominate. The client also may have abnormal tone, causing the tongue to deviate toward the affected side.

Using a wet gauze pad to grasp the tongue gently between the gloved forefinger and thumb, the therapist pulls the tongue slowly forward. Next, the therapist walks a wet finger along the tongue from front to back to determine whether the tongue feels hard, firm, or mushy. The tongue should feel firm. An abnormally hard tongue may be the result of increased muscle tone, and a mushy tongue is associated with low muscle tone. The right side of the tongue is compared with the left side for symmetry.

While continuing to grip the tongue between forefinger and thumb, the therapist assesses the client's range of motion by moving the tongue forward, side to side, and up and down. The tongue with normal range will move freely in all directions without resistance. Moving the tongue through its range, the therapist can simultaneously evaluate tone. The therapist gently pulls the tongue forward, assessing whether it is easily moved or whether resistance is noted. If the tongue pulls back against the movement, this indicates increased tone. If the tongue seems to stretch far beyond the front teeth, this indicates decreased tone. When moving the tongue side to side, the therapist notes whether it is easier to move in one direction or the other. Increased tone makes it difficult for the therapist to move the tongue in any direction without feeling resistance against the movement. Be aware that clients who are confused or apraxic may resist this passive motion yet not have abnormal tone.

To assess the tongue's motor control (strength and coordination), the therapist asks the client to elevate, stick out, and move the tongue laterally (see Table 27.4). If the client has difficulty understanding verbal directions, the therapist can use a wet tongue blade to guide the client through the desired movements.

Poor muscle strength or abnormal tone decreases the tongue's ability to sweep the mouth and gather food particles to form a cohesive bolus. If the tongue loses even partial control of the bolus, food may fall into the valleculae, the pyriform sinuses, or the airway, possibly leading to aspiration before the actual swallow.[23] The back of the tongue must also elevate quickly and strongly to propel the bolus past the faucial arch into the pharynx to trigger the swallow response.[14] The client with poor tongue control may not be a candidate for eating or may need altered food or liquid textures. Close supervision by an experienced therapist is required for a client with impaired tongue control to participate in eating.

THREADED CASE STUDY

Mattias, Part 9

Mattias had decreased tongue mobility and control. When he protruded his tongue, it was deviated toward the left, which indicates diminished motor control on the left side of his tongue. An additional indication of diminished tongue control is the pocketing of food in his mouth following a swallow.

Clinical Assessment of Swallowing

Because aspiration is a primary concern in swallowing, the occupational therapist must carefully assess the client's ability to swallow safely. A swallow screening should be conducted as soon as medically appropriate followed by a more comprehensive assessment. Before the therapist presents the client with material to swallow, he or she should assess the client's ability to protect the airway. The client must have an intact palatal reflex, elevation of the larynx, and a productive cough. The purpose of a productive cough is to remove any food or liquid from the airway. Individuals with a weak or nonproductive cough are at a higher risk for aspiration.[6] Directions for assessing all the components of the swallow are described in Table 27.4. The therapist should note the speed and strength of each component. The client with intact cognitive skills may accurately report to the therapist where and when difficulty occurs with the swallow.

The occupational therapist integrates all the information from the assessment process. Clinical judgment plays an important role in the accurate assessment of dysphagia.[2] The following questions should be asked:

1. Is the client alert and able to participate in a swallowing assessment?
2. Does the client maintain adequate trunk and head control, with or without assistance?

3. Does the client display adequate tongue control to form a cohesive bolus and move the bolus through the oral cavity?
4. Is the larynx mobile enough to elevate quickly and with sufficient force during the swallow?
5. Can the client handle saliva with minimal drooling?
6. Does the client have a productive cough, strong enough to expel any material that may enter the airway?

If the answer is yes to all of these questions, the therapist then assesses the client's oral-motor skills and ability to swallow a variety of food and liquid consistencies.

An assessment tray with a variety of textures can be ordered from dietary services. The following foods are merely suggestions, and the therapist must consider cultural factors and dietary restrictions that might influence the selection of foods. For example, a vegan or an individual who is lactose intolerant will require an appropriate selection of foods. The tray should contain a sample of foods of various textures, including puréed food such as pudding or applesauce, soft foods such as a banana or macaroni and cheese, and a mechanical soft-textured food such as ground tuna with mayonnaise or chopped meat with gravy. The tray should also include a thick drink such as nectar blended with half of a banana for a 7-oz drink; a semi-thick drink such as fruit nectar or a yogurt drink; and a thin, flavored liquid such as juice and water.

To minimize the risk of aspiration, puréed foods are chosen for clients with decreased oral motor control, chewing difficulties or apraxia. Clients who have poor endurance, breathing difficulties, or difficulty attending to the task of eating may also require puréed foods. Soft foods are more easily formed into a bolus and require less chewing than ground or regular textures for clients who have impaired oral motor strength or control. Soft foods are also easier to keep in a cohesive bolus as they are moved through the oral cavity. Ground foods allow the therapist to assess a client's ability to chew, form a cohesive bolus, and move it in the mouth. Thick liquids move more slowly from the front of the mouth to back, giving the client with a delayed swallow or impaired oral motor skills more time to control the liquid until the swallow response is triggered. Thin liquids are the most difficult to control because they move quickly through the oral cavity and pharynx and require intact oral motor strength and coordination, and an intact swallow to prevent aspiration.

For the client who appears to have some ability to chew, the therapist should start with puréed and soft textures. Solid textures may be introduced next if the client is able to safely and efficiently swallow the puréed and soft food textures. The following procedures should be followed for each swallow of food or liquid during the initial assessment:

1. The therapist places a small amount (⅓ teaspoon) of food or liquid on the middle of the client's tongue. The client is asked to swallow. Two to three bites are presented of each texture to check for fatigue in controlling that texture.
2. The therapist evaluates oral transit time by noting when food entered the mouth, when tongue movement was initiated, and when the elevation of the hyoid notch was felt, which indicates the beginning of the swallow process. The therapist palpates for the swallow by placing the index finger at the hyoid notch, the second finger at the top of the larynx,

and the third finger along the midlarynx.[8] The strength and smoothness of the swallow is assessed, and the therapist can feel if the client requires subsequent or additional swallows to clear the bolus. The therapist can time the swallow from the time that hyoid movement begins to when laryngeal elevation occurs, indicating triggering of the swallow response. A normal pharyngeal swallow takes only 1 second to complete for thin liquids and slightly longer for textured foods.[23]

3. The therapist asks the client to open the mouth to check for remaining food. Food is commonly seen in the lateral sulci, under the tongue, on the base of the tongue, and against the hard palate. Food remaining in the mouth indicates decreased sensation or impaired oral transit skills. The client who exhibits oral motor deficits has increasing difficulty with chewing, shaping a bolus, and moving the bolus in and through the oral cavity as textured foods requiring chewing are introduced. They usually also have difficulty with safely and efficiently moving thin liquids through the mouth, resulting in spillage from the mouth or coughing as the uncontrolled liquid bolus splashes into the throat.
4. The therapist asks the client to say "ah." By listening carefully, the therapist can assess the client's voice quality and classify the sound production as strong, clear, gurgly, or gargling.[23]

A wet-sounding voice may result from a delayed swallow response, which allows material to collect in the larynx before the initiation of the swallow. The therapist asks the client to take a second "dry" swallow to clear any pooling of material. Asking the client to say "ah" again enables the therapist to assess whether the voice quality remains wet-sounding for any length of time after the dry swallow. In addition, the therapist asks the client to pant for a few seconds. This may shake loose any material that may remain in the pyriform sinuses or valleculae. If the voice quality is still affected, the therapist should be concerned that material has come into contact with or is resting on the vocal cords, putting the client at risk for aspiration after the swallow.[23]

A client with central nervous system damage, motor impairment or impaired sensation may have difficulty with puréed food because this texture does not stay together as a bolus as it is manipulated in the mouth. The consistency and weight of soft foods, which are denser than puréed foods, may provide increased sensation to help to trigger the swallow response.

A client with an impaired swallow may aspirate immediately or may pool residuals in the pyriform sinuses and valleculae, which, when full, may overflow into the laryngeal vestibule and down into the trachea. It is appropriate to introduce swallowing strategies and techniques to facilitate a safe swallow at this point. If a client continues to have a wet-sounding voice after a second dry swallow or has substantial coughing with any of the consistencies offered, the assessment with food should be discontinued and further assessment without food or via and instrumental swallowing assessment such as videoflouroscopy or fiberoptic endoscopic evaluation of swallowing (FEES) should be considered. If the client is unable to demonstrate the ability to safely swallow during the assessment, alternative methods for nutrition and hydration would be recommended by the swallowing therapist to the physician. An appropriate intervention at this point would be a pre-feeding program to address areas of impairment that are contributing to dysphagia. Frequent reevaluation is important to assess the feasibility of safely introducing oral intake.

It is important to assess the client on all appropriate textures during the swallowing evaluation. A client who has difficulty managing solid consistencies may or may not have difficulty with liquids. To assess the client's swallow with liquids, the therapist starts with a thickened (thick) nectar, then a pure nectar (semithick), and finally a thin liquid such as water or juice, presented later in the chapter). Small amounts of the liquid are placed on the middle of the client's tongue with a spoon. The therapist proceeds by following the four-step sequence described earlier for solid foods. The therapist assesses the client's skill at moving material from front to back, the time of oral transit, the timing and effectiveness of the swallow, and the voice quality after each swallow. Each liquid consistency is assessed for two or three swallows to check for fatigability. If the client tolerates and swallows liquids by spoon without difficulty, the therapist assesses the client's ability to tolerate liquids from a cup or with a straw. The client's voice quality is checked after each swallow. The taste and temperature of the liquid can affect the client's ability to safely swallow and must be considered during the assessment.

The therapist must also assess the client's ability to alternate between liquids and solids, which occurs naturally during meals. The therapist presents the client with an easily managed food bolus, followed by the safest type of liquid tolerated, and then assesses the client's ability to safely swallow when the consistency of the food is changed.

A client with a tracheostomy tube in place can be assessed as previously described. The same criteria must be met before the therapist assesses the client's eating and swallowing of food or liquids. The therapist must have a thorough understanding of the types of tracheostomy tubes and varied functions. The therapist also must be aware that clients who have had a tracheostomy tube, especially those on ventilation for any length of time, may experience changes in the swallowing mechanism such as muscle atrophy, decreased sensation, and laryngeal damage.[40]

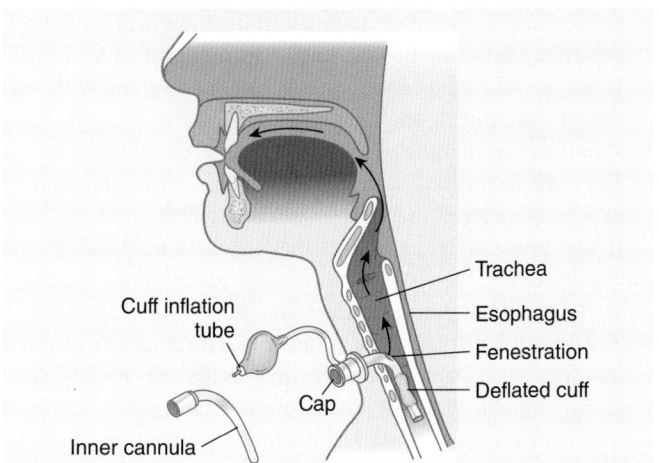

Fig. 27.3 Fenestrated tracheostomy. (From Lewis SL, Bucher L, Heitkemper MM, et al: *Medical-surgical nursing: assessment and management of clinical problems*, ed 9, St. Louis, 2014, Mosby.)

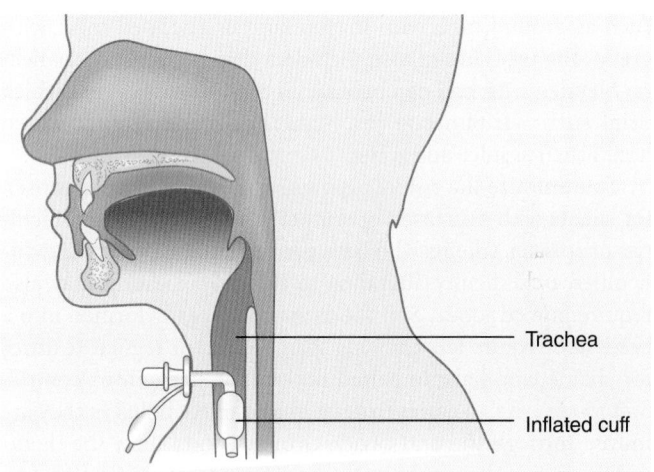

Fig. 27.4 Cuffed tracheostomy. (Modified from Harding, MM, et al: *Lewis's medical-surgical nursing: assessment and management of clinical problems*, ed 12, St. Louis, 2023, Elsevier.)

THREADED CASE STUDY

Mattias, Part 10

Although Mattias had frequent episodes of coughing during the bedside evaluation, no gurgly or raspy vocal quality was noted during speech. He is able to clear material from his vocal folds with a strong protective cough. He is able to swallow his secretions, but drooling was noted from the left corner of his mouth, which indicates diminished sensation.

Because Mattias is able to safely manage a modified diet texture using positioning strategies and does not have signs and symptoms of aspiration, a videofluoroscopy was not deemed necessary.

Two main types of tracheostomy tubes exist: fenestrated and nonfenestrated.[13] A fenestrated tube (Fig. 27.3) is designed with an opening in the middle to allow increased air flow. This type of tube is frequently used for clients being weaned from a tube because it allows a client to breathe nasally as he or she relearns a normal breathing pattern. Placement of an inner cannula piece into the tracheostomy tube allows the fenestrated opening

to be closed off. With the inner cannula removed, a trachea button may be used to allow the client to talk. A nonfenestrated tube has no opening. A fenestrated tube is preferred for treating a client with dysphagia.

A tracheostomy tube may be cuffed or uncuffed. A cuffed tube has a balloon-like cuff surrounding the bottom of the tube (Fig. 27.4). When inflated, the cuff comes into contact with the trachea wall, preventing the aspiration of secretions into the airway.[13] A cuffed tube is used in cases in which aspiration has occurred. The therapist should consult with the client's physician to see whether the client is still at risk of aspiration or if it is safe to deflate the cuff for an eating and swallowing assessment.

The presence of a tracheostomy tube may affect a client's ability to swallow because laryngeal elevation is impeded due to the presence of the tube, loss of upper airway sensitivity, inability of the larynx to effectively close during the swallow, and reduced subglottal air pressure atrophy of the laryngeal muscles due to disuse.[13]

Before assessing swallowing with a client who has a tracheostomy, it is important to consult with the medical team regarding guidelines and precautions for this specific individual. The physician will write orders for how the tracheostomy tube is to be managed during the presentation of food or liquid. It is very important to follow the physician's orders for tracheostomy management during all oral feeding trials. The respiratory therapist is often present during the assessment to assist with suctioning.

When presenting food or liquids, the therapist should assess oral transit skills and the pharyngeal swallow. If approved by the physician, blue food coloring may be added to food or liquids presented orally if the client is not allergic to dyes. This can help the therapist identify aspirated material in the trachea. During the swallow, the client or the therapist can use a gloved finger to cover the trachea opening and thereby achieve a more normal tracheal pressure, which has been shown to improve the pharyngeal swallow.[40]

If the tracheostomy tube is cuffed and inflated during the assessment, the cuff is slowly deflated after the client has swallowed. The airway is suctioned through the tracheostomy tube to determine whether any material entered the airway. The swallow assessment should not be continued if material is found in the trachea. When the assessment is complete, the airway is thoroughly suctioned. The inner cannula is removed from the fenestrated tube, or the cuff is inflated to the level prescribed by the physician.

The client's performance on the swallowing assessment determines whether he or she is able to participate in a feeding program and which diet texture is the most appropriate to ensure a safe, efficient swallow. The safest consistency is that which the client is able to chew, move through the oral cavity, and swallow with the least risk of aspiration.

Indicators of Eating and Swallowing Dysfunction

Symptoms of oropharyngeal dysphagia include (but are not limited to) the following:
1. Difficulty with bringing food to the mouth
2. Difficulty or inability to shape food into a cohesive bolus-prolonged chewing
   Loss of food or liquids from the mouth; drooling
   Loss of food or liquids from the nose (nasal regurgitation)
3. Coughing or frequent throat clearing before, during, or after the swallow
4. Wet or gurgling voice quality after eating or drinking
5. Changes in mealtime behaviors
   Food residue remaining in the mouth (cheeks, gums, teeth, tongue)
   Loss of appetite; dehydration or weight loss
   Discomfort or pain when swallowing
   Difficulty breathing while eating
   Unusual head or neck movements when swallowing
6. Delayed or absent swallow response
7. Weak cough
8. Reflux of food after meals
   Heartburn
   Changes in eating—for example, eating slowly or avoiding social occasions
   Food avoidance
   Prolonged mealtimes
   Recurrent episodes of pneumonia

Aspiration

Swallowing dysfunction can lead to aspiration of food or liquid into the airway, below the level of the vocal cords. Material that falls into the larynx, but does not continue past the level of the vocal cords is called *penetration*. Aspiration can occur at any point during the swallowing process (Fig. 27.5). Aspiration can occur before the swallow because of poor tongue control, pooled material in the valleculae, or a delayed or absent swallow response. Poor laryngeal closure can result in aspiration during the swallow. Aspiration after the swallow is the result of pooled material in the pyriform sinuses or in the valleculae overflowing into the trachea. Repeated aspiration, even in small amounts, can lead to aspiration pneumonia, a serious lung infection that requires immediate medical intervention. The following are acute clinical signs of aspiration that may occur before, during, or after the swallow[40]:
1. Any change in the client's color, particularly if the airway is obstructed
2. Coughing while drinking liquids or eating solids
3. Coughing or wheezing during after eating
4. Gurgling voice and extreme breathiness, dysphonia, changes in voice quality, loss of voice
5. Excessive secretions
6. Chest discomfort or heartburn

Many individuals with dysphagia silently aspirate, which means they show no clinical symptoms of aspiration during swallowing. For these individuals, aspiration and the cause of aspiration can be determined only through an instrumental assessment, such as videoflouroscopy. Predictors of silent aspiration include dysarthria, abnormally depressed gag reflex, weak or ineffective volitional cough, and dysphonia.[28,36]

During the 24 hours immediately after the consumption of oral intake by an individual with swallowing difficulties, the therapist, caregiver, and medical staff must observe the client for signs of aspiration. Clinical signs of aspiration pneumonia include fever, chest pain, shortness of breath with a rapid heart rate, mental confusion, and incontinence, although not all of these symptoms are always present, especially in older clients.[13] If aspiration pneumonia develops, the client must be reevaluated for a change in diet levels and swallowing strategies, or taken off the feeding program, if necessary. An alternative feeding method may be necessary to ensure adequate hydration and nutrition.

The occupational therapist is an important member of the dysphagia team who provides input and recommendations to reduce aspiration risk through interventions such as positioning, diet texture modification, feeding techniques and swallowing strategies.

INSTRUMENTAL ASSESSMENT

Instrumental assessments are important techniques for evaluating biomechanical and physiological function and for determining swallow safety and assessing the effects of compensatory strategies (i.e., posture and bolus texture) on swallowing. They are performed in conjunction with the clinical bedside assessment to assess the swallow at the oral and pharyngeal phases

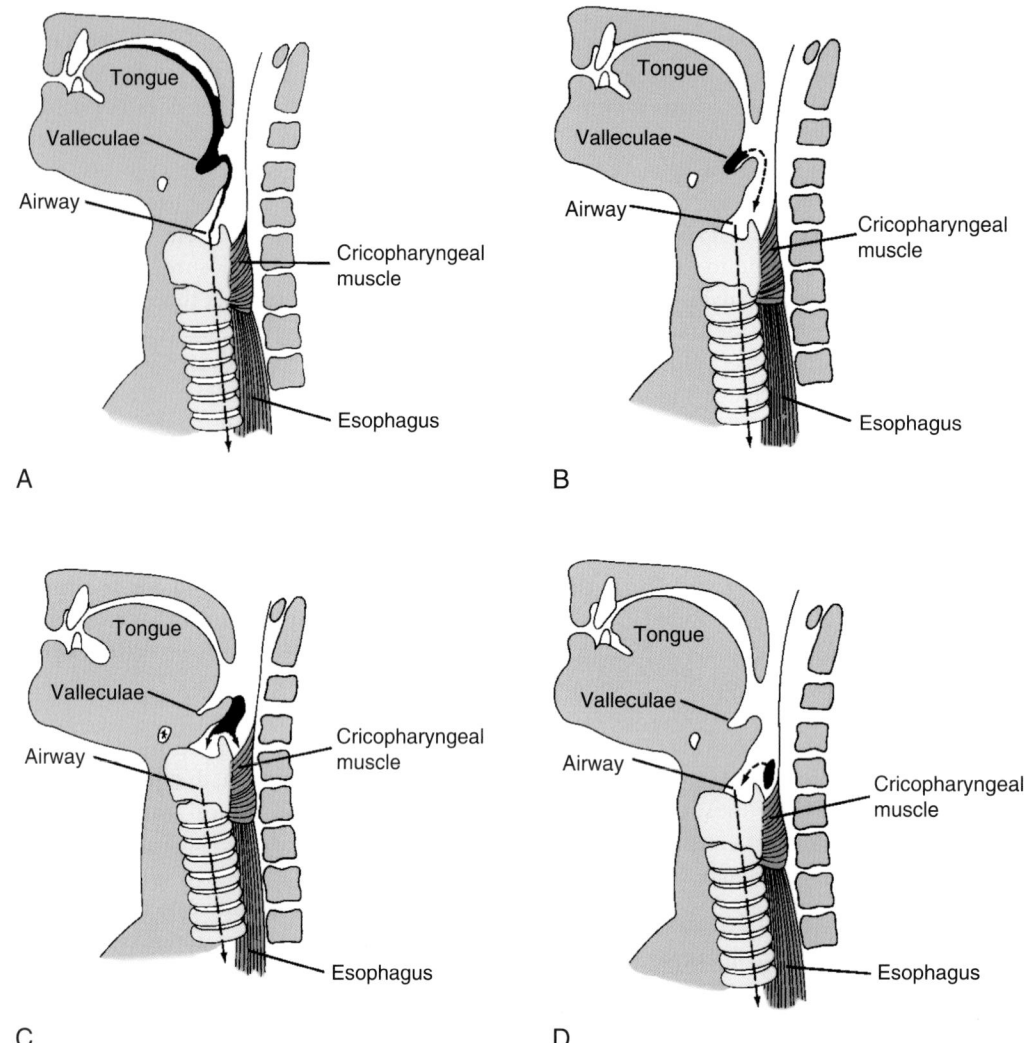

Fig. 27.5 Types of aspiration. (A) Aspiration before swallow caused by reduced tongue control. (B) Aspiration before swallow caused by absent swallow response. (C) Aspiration during swallow caused by reduced laryngeal closure. (D) Aspiration after swallow caused by pooled material in pyriform sinuses overflowing into airway. (From Logemann J: *Evaluation and treatment of swallowing disorders*, San Diego, 1998, College-Hill Press.)

and to rule out or identify silent aspiration. Silent aspiration may not always be accurately identified solely through a clinical bedside assessment. Studies have shown that up to 33% of individuals with neurological impairment were found to be silent aspirators during the instrumental assessment, which was difficult to detect by bedside screening tests.[27,36]

Understanding why a client is aspirating helps the occupational therapist plan appropriate intervention. Instrumental evaluations provide valuable information about a client's swallow during a specific period and under specific conditions. They allow the therapist to try different intervention strategies and to assess the results of these strategies on the swallow. This information is considered part of the complete evaluation process, which includes the bedside assessment and client performance during intervention sessions and meal activities.

The two most common instrumental evaluations used, videofluoroscopy swallow study (VFSS) and fiberoptic endoscopy (FEES), are described next.

ETHICAL CONSIDERATIONS

Instrumental assessment procedures require advanced knowledge and training in techniques, purpose, and indications for use. Only occupational therapists who have these advanced skills may use instrumental evaluation procedures.[1]

Assessment With Videofluoroscopy

The videofluoroscopic swallow study (VFSS) is the most commonly used instrumental assessment tool to examine oropharyngeal swallowing disorders.[12] This assessment uses fluoroscopy to examine the client's ability to safely and effectively swallow a variety of foods and textures. The VFSS allows the therapist to see the client's jaw and tongue movement, measure the transit times of the oral and pharyngeal stages, observe the stages of the swallow, note any residue in the valleculae and the pyriform sinuses after the swallow, and identify aspiration. With **videofluoroscopy**, the therapist can determine the anatomic or physiological cause of aspiration. Various compensatory techniques and swallowing strategies also may be used during the videofluoroscopy study to determine if the airway can be protected and if swallow function can be improved, which may allow the therapist to initiate a feeding program.[28] Videofluoroscopy, in conjunction with the clinical assessment, may be used to select appropriate intervention techniques and assist the therapist in determining the safest diet level to help the client achieve a safe swallow.

The VFSS is conducted in the hospital radiology department. The radiologist, the radiology technician, and the swallowing therapist are present during the evaluation. Equipment necessary for the VFSS includes the fluoroscopy x-ray machine, a monitor for viewing the movement of the bolus in real time. The images are usually videotaped or digitally recorded to allow the radiologist and the therapist to review the recording in slow motion or frame by frame for more in-depth analysis. Other pieces of equipment normally available in a radiology department are lead-lined aprons, lead-lined gloves, and foam positioning wedges. Although VFSS subjects the client to radiation, the doses are relatively small and are considered to be safe for both the client and the others involved with the procedure.[16]

The client is positioned in a seated, upright position to allow a lateral view, with the fluoroscopy tube focused on the lips, hard palate, and posterior pharyngeal wall. The lateral view is most frequently used because it allows the therapist to evaluate all four stages of the swallow. This view clearly shows the presence and cause of aspiration. A posteroanterior view also may be needed to evaluate asymmetry in the vocal cords and pooling in the valleculae or pyriform sinuses.

During the VFSS, the therapist presents the client with food or liquid to which barium paste or powder has been added. The barium contrast allows the bolus to be visible on videofluoroscopy. The therapist mixes or spreads small amounts of paste or powder onto or into each food or liquid consistency. Premixing the consistencies with the barium paste or powder prevents time-consuming interruptions during the actual assessment procedure.

Food and liquids are presented in the same sequence used for the clinical assessment. Starting with puréed foods, the client is given ½ to ⅓ teaspoon at a time of each consistency and asked to swallow when instructed. Liquids are tested separately, beginning with the thickened substance. Material is given in small amounts to reduce the risks of aspiration. An experienced dysphagia therapist may choose to use only foods or liquids that the client had difficulty with during the clinical examination, rather than to proceed through the entire sequence. The therapist continues to present each consistency to determine if the client can swallow safely and efficiently without aspirating. If aspiration occurs, the therapist should try compensatory strategies and reassess with the same texture. If greater than 10% aspiration occurs while using the strategies, the assessment with this texture is discontinued.

The videofluoroscopy procedure also can be used to observe for fatigue of the oral or pharyngeal musculature or the swallow response. The client is asked to take repeated or serial swallows of solids and liquids. The therapist also assesses the client's ability to control mixed consistencies of solids and liquids such as soups with broth and bits of vegetables, as well as the ability to alternate between solids and liquids. The solid and liquid consistency that the client manages without aspiration is selected as the starting point for eating and swallowing intervention. A client who aspirates on puréed or soft foods and aspiration risk cannot be reduced or eliminated through various strategies may not be suited for an oral feeding program. The client who aspirates on even the thickest liquid texture is not a candidate for safe liquid intake. During the VFSS, the therapist must try different strategies, including postural adjustments, food and liquid texture adjustments, and swallowing strategies before determining that a client may not safely consume oral intake. The ability to safely orally manage medications also may be assessed during VFSS.

VFSS is a valuable tool to be used in conjunction with the clinical examination. It can provide the therapist with additional information regarding the client's difficulties. By identifying silent aspiration, the therapist can feel comfortable with the decisions made in determining a course of treatment. The therapist must keep in mind that VFSS records the client's performance in an isolated instance, in an abnormal eating environment, and is not a conclusive indicator of the client's potential ability in a feeding program, or how other variables involved in eating a meal might influence safe oral intake. Many factors may interfere with an individual's ability to participate in a VFSS, including a poor level of awareness, poor endurance, impaired cognitive status, or inability to physically be positioned for the assessment. Additionally, there may not be access to a hospital where the assessment can take place. A second VFSS may be indicated in some situations to reevaluate a client who previously was initially unable to safely swallow on video but now shows signs of readiness to participate in a feeding program.

When the results of a VFSS test are documented, foods that were presented, problems that occurred at each stage, and the number of swallows taken to clear the food or liquid are recorded. The presentation of any aspiration is also noted, as is the client's response to the aspiration. The therapist also should document compensatory strategies or facilitation techniques that worked effectively to elicit a safe swallow or reduce aspiration risk. Occupational therapists and speech pathologists can receive special training in administering VFSS.

Assessment With Fiberoptic Endoscopy

Fiberoptic endoscopy (FEES) is a nonradioactive alternative to the VFSS. FEES allows for direct assessment of the motor and sensory aspects of the swallow. It can be repeated as often as necessary without exposure to radiation. FEES has been shown to be highly effective in detecting aspiration and critical features of pharyngeal dysphagia.[26,41] The equipment needed for FEES includes a flexible fiberoptic nasopharyngolaryngoscope, a portable light source, a video camera, a video recorder, and a monitor. Placed on a rolling cart, this system can be brought directly to the client's bedside. The therapist passes a flexible fiberoptic tube through the nasal fossa, along the floor of the nose through the velopharyngeal port, ending in the hypopharynx. The scope allows the therapist to observe the oral cavity, the base of the tongue, and the swallowing structures. The client is given foods and liquids. As the client the swallows, the therapist is able to observe on the monitor tongue movement, pharyngeal and laryngeal function both before and after the swallow, and assess for penetration and aspiration.[10]

The results of a thorough assessment determine the course of intervention to increase a client's ability to safely eat. Upon completion of the dysphagia assessment, the therapist should clearly document the client's strengths, major problems, goals and objectives, and intervention plan. The objectives should be concise and measurable. The intervention plan should include the type of diet needed, the training and facilitation that the client requires, positioning techniques to be used during feeding, and the type of supervision that must be provided. Recommendations should be communicated to the appropriate nursing and medical staff.

INTERVENTION

Because a client may display more than one problem at each stage of deglutition, the intervention program for eating and swallowing problems is multifaceted. Intervention for the client with dysphagia involves trunk and head positioning techniques to facilitate oral performance, improve pharyngeal swallow, and reduce the risk of aspiration. The occupational therapist uses clinical reasoning skills to evaluate the interplay of physical, cognitive, environmental, and sociocultural factors that have an impact on feeding, eating, and swallowing.[1] Clients with severe problems can require a prolonged course of intervention before they reach optimal recovery.

Intervention falls into two broad categories: rehabilitation techniques and compensatory strategies. Rehabilitation techniques include the use of exercise to improve strength and function.[5] Oral motor exercises are specifically designed to improve the strength and coordination of facial musculature, the tongue, and jaw. An effortful swallow in which the client is instructed to swallow with maximal effort either with or without food has been shown to increase tongue base retraction and oral and pharyngeal pressure to improve the swallow.[4] Other swallowing maneuvers such as the Mendelsohn maneuver, the Masako maneuver, and the Shaker head lift are rehabilitative techniques used to physically change swallow function. Compensatory swallowing strategies increase swallow safety and decrease the client's symptoms, such as aspiration, but do not change the physiology of the swallow. Postural techniques such as those listed in Table 27.5 have been found to redirect bolus flow and reduce aspiration risk.[19,24] Rehabilitative techniques and compensatory strategies are often both used during the client's therapy program.

Goals

The overall goals of occupational therapy in the remediation of eating and swallowing dysfunction are as follows:
1. Facilitation of appropriate positioning during eating
2. Improvement of motor control at each stage of the swallow, through normalization of tone, facilitation of quality movement, and strengthening of oral musculature

TABLE 27.5 Postural Techniques Used in Dysphagia Management

Problem	Posture	Rationale
Impaired oral transit	Head back	Utilizes gravity to clear oral cavity
Delay in triggering of pharyngeal swallow	Chin down	Widens valleculae to prevent bolus from entering airway; narrows airway entrance; pushes epiglottis posteriorly
Residue in valleculae after the swallow	Chin down	Pushes tongue base backward
Reduced laryngeal closure	Chin down, head rotated to weak side	Narrows laryngeal entrance, increases vocal fold closure
Reduced pharyngeal contraction (residue in pharynx)	Lying down on side	Eliminates gravitational effect in pharynx
Unilateral oral and pharyngeal weakness	Head tilt to stronger side	Directs bolus down stronger side
Cricopharyngeal dysfunction (residue in pyriform sinuses)	Head rotated	Pulls cricoid cartilage away from posterior pharyngeal wall, reducing resting pressure in cricopharyngeal sphincter

Adapted from Logemann J: *Evaluation and treatment of swallowing disorders*, Austin, TX, 1998, Pro-Ed.

3. Maintenance of an adequate hydration and nutritional intake
4. Prevention or reduction of aspiration risk
5. Reestablishment of oral eating to the safest, optimum level on the least restrictive diet texture
6. Increase independence for safe, efficient eating

Team Management

Because of the complex nature of dysphagia treatment, the client's optimal progress is facilitated by the use of a team approach.[35,39] The dysphagia team should include the client's physician, the occupational therapist, the dietitian, the nurse, the physical therapist, the speech-language pathologist, the radiologist, and the client's family. Each professional contributes expertise to facilitate client improvement. All members of the dysphagia team should have the training and knowledge necessary to work with clients with dysphagia. Interdepartmental in-service education is frequently required so that team members have a similar frame of reference.

The occupational therapist's role is to select, administer, and interpret assessment measures; develop specific intervention plans; and provide therapeutic interventions.[1] The American Occupational Therapy Association (AOTA) has prepared a document, *The Practice of Occupational Therapy in Feeding, Eating and Swallowing*, that clarifies the role and describes the unique perspective of occupational therapy practitioners in the delivery of services for individuals with feeding, eating, and swallowing problems. This includes selecting, administering, and interpreting assessment measures; developing an intervention plan; and providing therapeutic interventions.[1] The occupational therapist also may be responsible for coordinating the team effort, which includes obtaining physician's orders as needed, communicating with other team members and staff, providing family education to ensure proper follow-through, and selecting the appropriate diet.

The physician's role involves the medical management of the client's health and safety. The physician gives the orders for clinical and instrumental assessments and approves intervention and program recommendations. The physician oversees all decisions regarding treatment for diet level selection, oral and nonoral feeding procedures, and the progression of treatment as recommended by the team. The physician also reinforces the course of treatment with the client and the family.[15]

The dietitian is responsible for monitoring the client's caloric intake. This member of the dysphagia team makes recommendations to ensure that the client receives a balanced, nutritional diet in accordance with the medical condition. The dietitian is involved in suggesting types of feeding formulas for the nonoral client. Diet supplements to augment oral intake may be recommended. In conjunction with the dysphagia team, the dietitian ensures that the client receives the proper food and liquid consistencies. Additional training may be necessary for the dietary staff, because dysphagia diets vary from traditional medical diets.

The client's physical therapist is involved in muscle reeducation and tone normalization techniques. The client receives treatment in balance, strength, and control. The physical therapist and the occupational therapist collaborate on positioning options. The physical therapist is involved in increasing the client's pulmonary status for breath support, chest expansion, and cough.

The role of the speech-language pathologist (SLP) involves reeducating the oral and laryngeal musculature used in speaking, voice production, and swallowing. The SLP is a key member of the dysphagia team.

The nurse is another important member of the dysphagia team. The nursing staff is responsible for monitoring the client's medical and nutritional status. Nurses who are available on a 24-hour basis in the hospital setting and who are trained in dysphagia screening are in a key position to administer initial swallowing screenings.[7,42] The nurse usually is the first to notice changes in the client's condition, such as an elevated temperature; an increase in pulmonary congestion; and an increase in secretions, which indicates swallowing dysfunction. The nurse informs the physician and the dysphagia team of these changes. The nurse records the client's oral and fluid intake and notifies the dysphagia team when the client's nutritional status is adequate or inadequate. The nursing staff members administer supplemental tube feedings that have been ordered by the physician; the staff also provides oral hygiene, tracheostomy care, and supervision for appropriate clients during meals.

The client's family is included on the team to act as program supporters. Families frequently underestimate the danger of aspiration. Therefore, both the family and the client must be educated, beginning with the first day of assessment. The family and client should understand which food consistencies are safe to eat and which foods must be avoided, including the reasons behind the food and liquid texture recommendations.

The roles of the team members may vary from one treatment facility to another. Designated roles must be clearly defined to ensure a coordinated team approach. Therapists who are responsible for direct treatment should have advanced knowledge and training in dysphagia treatment procedures.

Positioning

Proper positioning is essential when working with the client who has dysphagia. This is an important role for the occupational therapy practitioner as a member of the dysphagia team. The client should be positioned symmetrically with normal alignment between the head, neck, trunk, and pelvis. The ideal position is as follows:

1. The client is seated on a firm surface, such as a chair.
2. The client's feet are flat on the floor.
3. The client's knees are at 90-degree flexion.
4. There is equal weight bearing on both ischial tuberosities of the hips.
5. The client's trunk is flexed slightly forward (100-degree hip flexion) with the back straight.
6. Both of the client's arms are placed forward on the table.
7. The head is erect, in midline, and the chin is slightly tucked (Fig. 27.6).

For the client who may be restricted to bed but is able to sit in a semi-reclined position, the same positioning principles apply: equal weight bearing on both ischial tuberosities for the hips, the trunk flexed slightly forward (100-degree hip flexion) with the back straight, knees slightly flexed, and both arms placed forward on a bedside table. The head and neck should be aligned appropriately to reduce the risk of aspiration.

For the client who must remain completely supine in bed, oral feeding is usually contraindicated. If the client can be positioned side-lying in bed, appropriate head and neck alignment

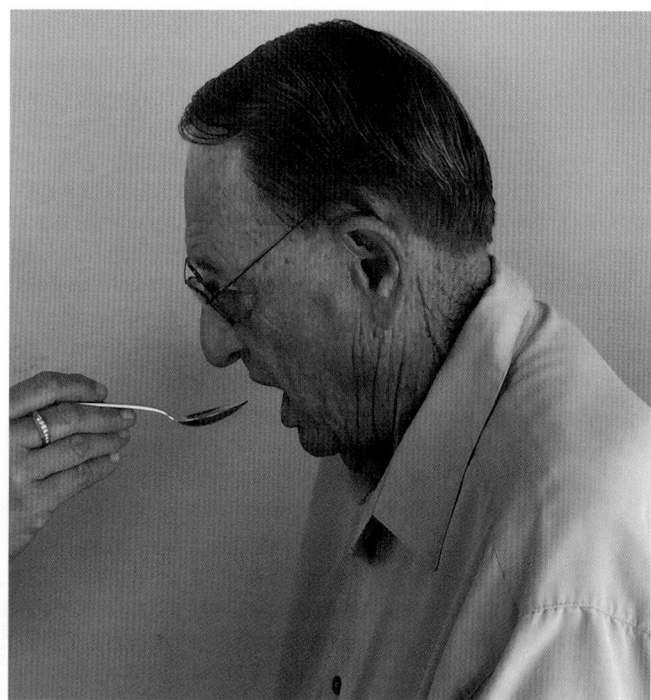

Fig. 27.6 Proper head position for a client with dysphagia.

must be achieved before the assessment of feeding skills. The client's knees and hips should be slightly flexed and trunk aligned while supported in the side-lying position. The use of additional pillows, rolls, and supports may be required to maintain the appropriate alignment.

A client who has difficulty moving into the correct position or maintaining the position presents a challenge to the occupational therapist. A careful analysis of the client is needed to determine the major problem preventing proper positioning. Poor positioning may be a result of decreased control, strength or balance secondary to hypertonicity, hypotonicity, or weakness or poor body awareness in space secondary to perceptual dysfunction (Fig. 27.7). Poor endurance is often a complicating factor in maintaining an optimal position for safe swallowing. The therapist develops an intervention plan to address the specific positioning problems identified. Treatment suggestions are described later in this chapter.

Fig. 27.8 shows different supportive positions that allow the therapist to help the client maintain head control. Correct positioning allows more appropriate muscular action, which thereby facilitates quality motor control and function of the facial musculature, jaw and tongue movement, and the swallowing process, all of which minimize the potential for aspiration.

THREADED CASE STUDY

Mattias, Part 11

Mattias was able to sit in a chair and responded well to physical prompts to sit aligned with both arms supported on the tabletop. Although he was concerned that resting his arms on the table was impolite, his therapist suggested using a chair with armrests. He typically would slightly extend his neck when attempting to swallow foods, and using the technique of a slight chin tuck diminished the coughing and choking episodes when he ate textured foods.

Oral Hygiene

Oral care by nursing and therapy team members prevents gum disease, the accumulation of secretions, the development of plaque, and the aspiration of food particles that remain after eating. Poor or inadequate oral hygiene has been linked with oral infections, bacterial pneumonia, respiratory tract infections, heart disease, and influenza in elderly people.[9,30] The client who is hypersensitive or resistant to having anything in the mouth may require intervention from the occupational therapist. Preparation steps may include firmly stroking outside the client's mouth or lips with the client's or therapist's finger. Sensitive gums also can be firmly rubbed, preparing the client for the toothbrush.

For cleaning purposes, the mouth can be divided into four quadrants. A toothbrush with a small head and soft bristles is used to clean each quadrant, starting with the top teeth and moving from front to back. When brushing the bottom teeth, the therapist brushes from back to front. Next, holding the toothbrush at a vertical angle, the therapist brushes the inside teeth downward from gums to teeth. Finally, the cutting surfaces of the teeth are brushed. An electric toothbrush can be more effective, if the client can tolerate it.

After each procedure the client is allowed to dispose of secretions. After brushing, the client is carefully assisted in rinsing the mouth. If the client can tolerate thin liquids, small amounts of water can be given. Having the client flex the chin slightly toward the chest helps prevent the water from being swallowed. The therapist can help the client expel the water by placing one hand on each cheek and simultaneously pushing inward on the cheeks while the chin remains slightly tucked. If the client has no ability to manipulate liquids, a dampened sponge oral swab can be used.

Oral hygiene for the nonoral or oral client can be used as effective sensory stimulation of touch, texture, temperature, and taste. It can be used to facilitate beginning tongue movements and to encourage an automatic swallow. Lack of oral stimulation

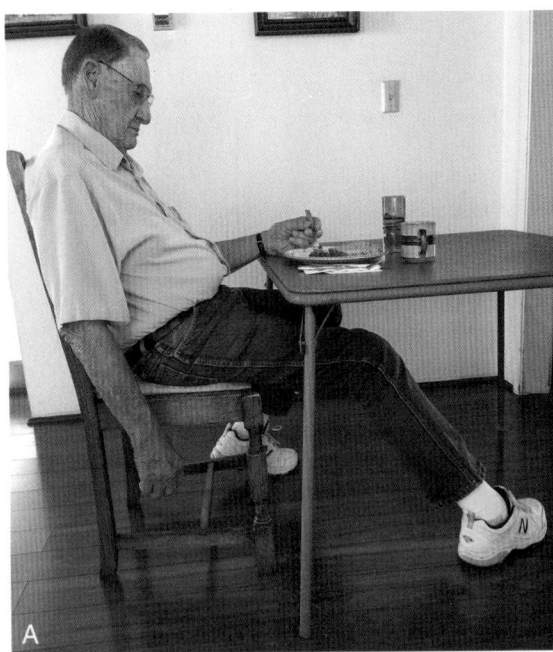
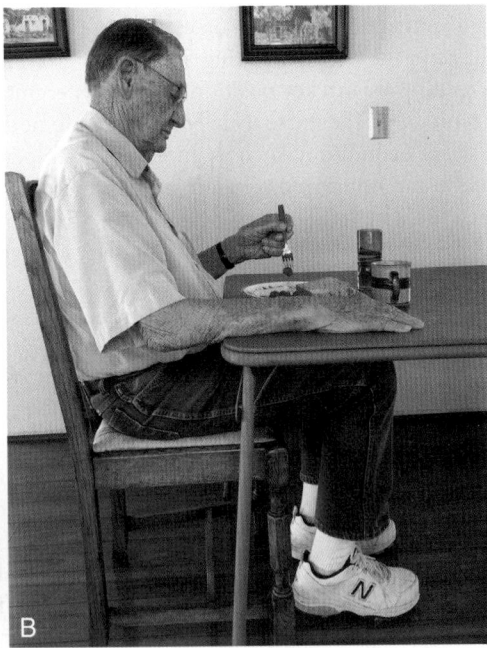

Fig. 27.7 Positioning of the client with dysphagia. (A) Incorrect positioning. (B) Correct positioning.

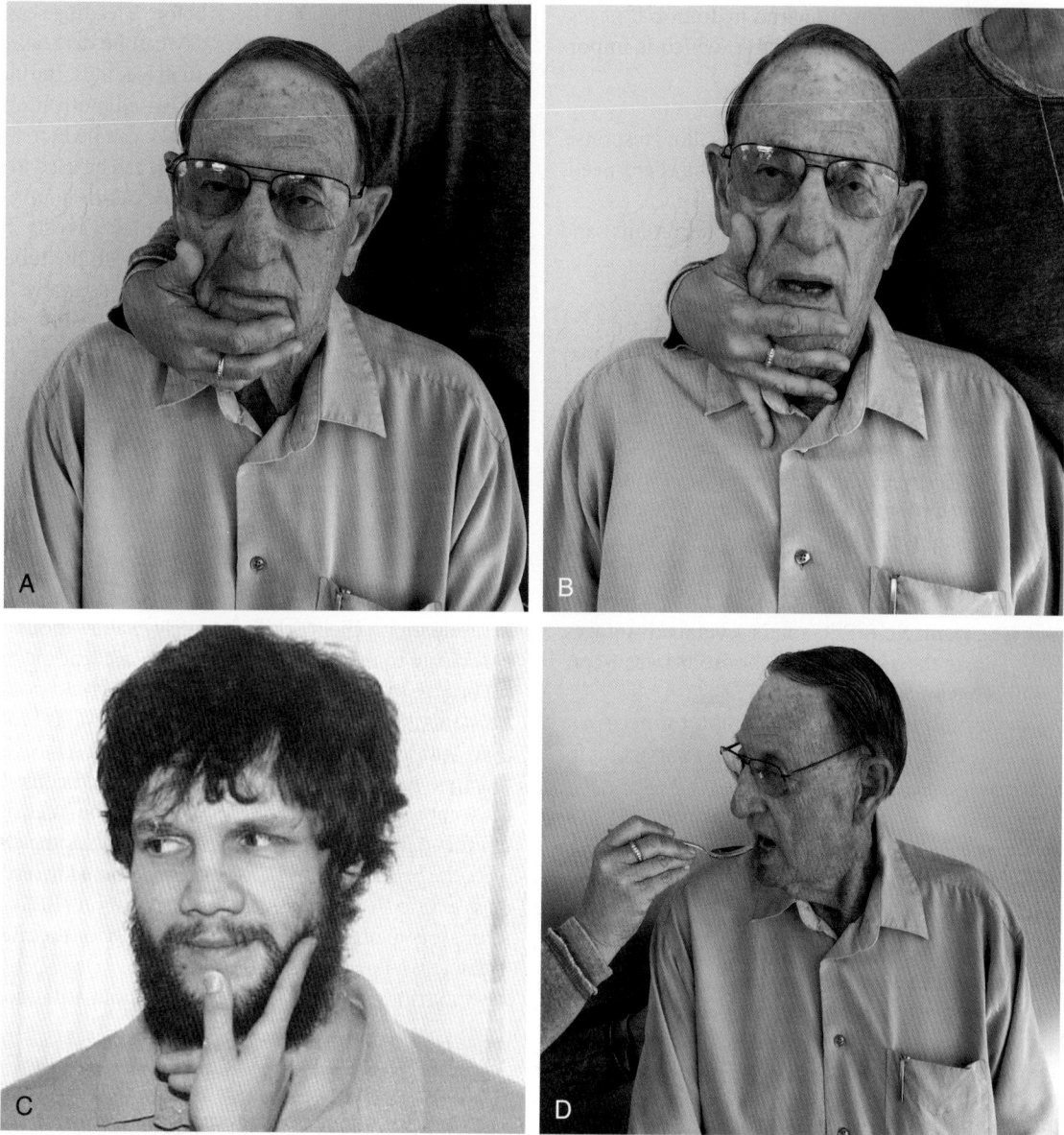

Fig. 27.8 Different supportive positions allow the therapist to help the client maintain head control. (A) and (B) Side hold position for clients requiring maximum to moderate assistance. (C) Front hold position for clients requiring minimal assistance. (D) Turning the head toward the more involved side for an individual who sustained a cerebrovascular accident.

over a prolonged time leads to hypersensitivity within the oral cavity. Clients who display poor tongue movement or decreased oral sensation and who are able to eat frequently have food remaining on their teeth or dentures or between the cheek and gum. A client with decreased sensation is not aware of the remaining food. A thorough cleaning of the oral cavity should follow each time the client eats.

Nonoral Feedings

A client who aspirates more than 10% of food or liquid consistencies or whose combined oral and pharyngeal transit time is more than 10 seconds, regardless of positioning or facilitation techniques, is an inappropriate candidate for oral eating.[23] This client needs a nonoral nutritional method until safe eating and drinking ability is regained. Clients who lack the endurance to

take in sufficient calories also may require nonoral feedings or supplements.

The two most common procedures for nonoral feedings involve the nasogastric (NG) tube and the percutaneous endoscopic gastrostomy (PEG) tube. The NG tube is passed through the nostril, through the nasopharynx, and down through the pharynx and esophagus to rest in the stomach. The NG tube is a temporary measure that should not be used for longer than 1 month.[13] The NG tube has several advantages:

1. The NG tube can be inserted and removed nonsurgically.
2. The NG tube allows the physician to choose between continuous or bolus feedings (a feeding that runs no more than 40 minutes).
3. The NG tube allows the therapist to begin pre-feeding and feeding training while the tube is in place.

4. The NG tube provides full nutrition and hydration if necessary and keeps the digestive system active, which is important for moving to oral feedings.

The NG tube also has some disadvantages[21]:

1. It can desensitize the cough reflex and the swallow response.
2. It can interfere with a positioning program (the client needs to be elevated to 30 degrees during feeding).
3. It can increase aspiration risk, pharyngeal secretions, and nasal reflux.
4. It can decrease the client's self-esteem.
5. It can be uncomfortable.
6. It distends pharyngeal esophageal segment and UES; it may promote reflux.
7. It can cause nasal ulceration.

If nonoral feeding is required for longer than 3 to 4 weeks, the physician may choose to insert a PEG that offers a more permanent option for long term nutritional support.[13] Placement of a PEG is a minor surgical procedure. The client receives a local anesthetic, and a small skin incision is made to create an external opening in the abdominal wall. A tube is passed through the opening into the stomach. A PEG offers several advantages:

1. Using a PEG allows the physician to choose between continuous or bolus feedings.
2. The PEG provides full nutrition and hydration if necessary and keeps the digestive system active, which is important for moving to oral feedings.
3. It allows the therapist to begin a pre-feeding or feeding program while the tube is in place.
4. It carries less risk of reflux and aspiration.
5. It does not irritate or desensitize the swallowing mechanisms.
6. It does not interfere with a positioning program.
7. It can be removed when the client no longer requires supplemental feedings or liquids.

However, use of a PEG also has some disadvantages[13]:

1. It requires surgical placement.
2. The stoma site can become irritated or infected.
3. Reflux can occur if the stomach fills too fast.
4. The family can perceive the tube as being permanent.

A commercially prepared liquid formula that provides complete nutrition typically is used for tube feedings. Many types and brands are available. The physician and dietitian determine which formula is best suited to the client. The feedings are administered by either a bolus or a continuous method. A bolus feeding takes 20 to 40 minutes to run through either the NG tube or the PEG tube. It can be gravity assisted or run through a feeding pump. Bolus feedings can be scheduled at numerous times throughout a 24-hour period.

Continuous feedings, which the client may better tolerate, provide smaller amounts that are administered continuously by a feeding pump. The feeding pump can be set to regulate the rate at which the formula is dripped into the tube. A disadvantage of continuous feedings is that the client must be attached to the feeding pump during tube feedings, which limits mobility.

As a client begins to eat enough to require an adjustment in the intake amount of formula, bolus feedings become the preferred method. A bolus feeding allows the therapist to work with the physician to wean the client from formula feeding. A bolus feeding can be held back before a feeding session, and the number of bolus feedings per day can be decreased as the client improves. If satisfied by the tube feedings, the client will not have an appetite and will have decreased motivation to eat.

As the client improves, oral intake can be increased, and the formula feeding can be decreased and can be used to supplement the client's caloric intake. An accurate calorie count, determined by recording the percentage of oral intake, assists the physician in decreasing the calories received through the tube feedings as the client begins to meet nutritional needs orally. The occupational therapist works closely with the dietitian to ensure that all hydration and caloric needs are being met. If the client has progressed only enough to handle solids, the NG or PEG tube can be used to meet the client's total or partial fluid requirements. When the client is able to meet nutrition and hydration needs through oral feedings, the NG or PEG tube can be removed.

Oral Feedings

For a client to be an appropriate candidate for oral feeding, several criteria must be met. The therapist can use the following criteria for evaluating a client's ability to safely swallow foods or liquids. To participate in an oral feeding program, a client must (1) be alert, (2) be able to maintain adequate trunk and head positioning with assistance, (3) have beginning tongue control, (4) manage secretions with minimal drooling, and (5) have a reflexive cough. The therapist needs to identify the food or liquid consistency that is most appropriate for the client. The safest consistency with which to initiate the oral program is one that enables the client to complete the oral and pharyngeal stages combined in less than 10 seconds and to swallow with minimal aspiration (10% or less).[23] The ultimate goal of an oral feeding program is for the client to be able to safely swallow the least restrictive diet in sufficient amounts to meet nutrition and hydration needs without aspiration.

Diet Selection

For those diagnosed with dysphagia, the texture of their food may need to be modified to help make swallowing safer and more efficient and to help prevent aspiration. A dysphagia diet must be carefully selected to reflect the needs of the client, which are obtained from the comprehensive clinical swallowing assessment. In general, foods chosen for dysphagia diets should (1) be uniform in consistency and texture, (2) provide sufficient density and volume, (3) remain cohesive, (4) provide pleasant taste and temperature, and (5) be easily removed or suctioned when necessary.

The following foods are contraindicated for dysphagia diets: foods with multiple textures, such as vegetable soup and salads; fibrous and stringy vegetables, meats, and fruits; crumbly and flaky foods; foods that liquefy, such as gelatin and ice cream; and foods with skins and seeds.

The therapist should work closely with the dietitian to identify the appropriate dysphagia diet for the client. Because many disciplines are involved in the care of an individual with dysphagia, standardized language is needed when describing food and liquid textures to facilitate the diagnostic and nutritional management of the client. The International Dysphagia Diet Standardization Initiative[17] has developed an evidence-based, multilevel framework to describe texture-modified foods and thickened liquids for individuals with dysphagia of all ages, in all settings and all cultures.[17] This framework offers standardized, globally accepted terminology and definitions to describe the qualities of food and liquids to provide consistent language and definitions for food textures used in a dysphagia diet to improve the safety and care for individuals with dysphagia. This framework describes an eight-level continuum of liquid and solid consistencies. Textures are described on a continuum of eight levels; from 0 (thin liquids) to 7 (regular foods) with descriptors provided for each level. For each level, the characteristics of the food or liquid is described. The physiological rationale and oral motor skills required to manage the texture is provided and examples of appropriate foods for each level are listed. Although the International Dysphagia Diet Standardisation Initiative (IDDSI) provides the standardized language to describe liquid and food textures for use in dysphagia diets, it does not suggest a particular diet, nor does it make recommendations for diet progression. The swallowing therapist has the responsibility to determine the appropriate diet level and foods or liquids for a particular client based on a comprehensive clinical assessment. Once the therapist has determined the appropriate level for the client, all members of the team, including the family and the client, should be educated about which foods are acceptable and which foods should be avoided to ensure the client's safety. Liquid diet levels also should be established. When requesting a dysphagia diet, the therapist should specify which level is required for both liquids and solids, including any unique recommendations for the specific client (e.g., spices, temperatures, food preferences).

Diet Progression

Diet texture progression is determined based on clinical assessment of the client. Many different things must be taken into consideration when evaluating changing or upgrading diet textures. The client's endurance, oral motor skills, cognitive status, oral sensory status, postural control, oral and pharyngeal swallow status, and ability to protect the airway must be continually reassessed before advancing the diet texture. Additionally, the context in which the client eats must be evaluated to determine if it supports the safe transition to a more challenging diet. Although the IDDSI Framework is not intended to be used as a model for diet progression, the various levels that provide the description of the food texture are included in this section.

Individuals with moderate to severe dysphagia who may need special positioning and feeding strategies to safely swallow typically begin the swallowing program on a puréed diet (Level 4 foods in the IDDSI Framework). This food group is best for individuals with little to no jaw or tongue control, a moderately delayed swallow, and a decreased pharyngeal transit, resulting in pooling in the valleculae and/or pyriform sinuses. Puréed foods move more slowly past the faucial arches and into the pharynx, which allows time for the swallow response to trigger. Puréed foods should be homogenous, pudding-like in consistency. No coarse textures, raw fruits or vegetables, nuts, or foods requiring any mastication should be included at this stage. Food that is puréed should hold its shape on a spoon, flow very slowly off the spoon when tilted in a single spoonful, not separate into a liquid and a solid, not have any textured pieces,

and is unable to be sucked through a straw. Puréed foods may be commercially purchased or prepared by preparing regular foods in the blender. Puréed foods may be unappetizing and unfamiliar to the client, so care must be taken when choosing and preparing foods to include in the client's diet. A more visually appealing way to present puréed foods includes using a piping bag and piping foods such as mashed potato, puréed carrots, or pumpkin on a plate in bite-sized portions. Adding a sauce or gravy to puréed meat will not only make it look more appetizing but will also add extra flavor and moisture. Some foods are naturally puréed in texture, such as puréed fruits, whipped or smooth mashed potatoes, cream of wheat, yogurt, and puddings, and these are often better accepted by individuals who must be on an altered diet. The occupational therapist can work with the client, dietary staff, caregivers and others involved with preparing food for the client to ensure that the food is tasteful, aesthetically presented and nutritional. There are many resources (e.g., cookbooks, web-based recipes) that provide ideas or recipes for preparing puréed foods. There are also commercially prepared puréed food for adults that are available as frozen meals. Formed or shaped puréed foods are puréed foods that are prepared in such a way to look like the actual food item (e.g., pancakes, waffles, chicken). However, when placed in the mouth, these foods convert to a puréed texture.

When the client is able to chew and efficiently manipulate and move food in the mouth, minced and moist foods (Level 5 IDDSI Framework) may be introduced. Minced foods are those that require little chewing and stay together as a cohesive bolus, thus decreasing the possibility of particles spilling into the airway. This texture is best for clients with a beginning rotary chew, enough tongue control to propel food back toward the pharynx, and a minimally delayed swallow. Bite-sized soft foods (Level 6 IDDSI Framework) reduce the risk of aspiration in individuals who have both a motor and a sensory loss. Bite-sized or mechanical soft foods have increased density, which provides increased proprioceptive input throughout the mouth, which often enhances oral motor awareness. Meats should be ground or minced and kept moist with gravies and sauces. Mashed soft and mechanical soft foods are indicated for individuals with mild to moderate swallowing difficulties.

As oral motor skills improve and the client is able to chew using a rotary chew pattern with increased strength and efficiency, and has the ability to form a cohesive bolus of textured food and move the bolus posteriorly in the oral cavity, a greater variety of textured foods can be introduced. Chopped meats, vegetables, and fruit can be added to the diet. Bread and rice are often introduced at this stage. This food group offers a wider variety of consistencies and food choice and works well for the client who has minimal problems with jaw or tongue control and may have a mildly delaying but otherwise intact swallow response.

The next progression in diet texture advancement for foods is a regular diet (Level 7 IDDSI Framework) that consists of all food, unless there are specific food items that the individual continues to have difficulty with. A client should progress to a regular diet when oral motor control is within functional limits, allowing the client to chew and form any consistency of food into a bolus and propel it back toward the faucial arches. The client at this level should be able to swallow all food and liquid consistencies with only occasional coughing.

Strategies for positioning and swallowing techniques may be used with any type of food texture. The swallowing therapist should work collaboratively with the other members of the team to ensure that the client is meeting nutritional needs when moving through the progression of diet textures. Not all individuals with swallowing problems will progress through all of the textures, and not all will resume eating a normal diet. The client's unique swallowing profile compiled from thorough assessment and reassessment will guide the therapist in determining the appropriate diet texture. The overarching goal of swallowing therapy is that the client is able to eat the least restrictive diet with the least risk for aspiration.

THREADED CASE STUDY

Mattias, Part 12

Mattias agreed to eat puréed foods to increase his caloric intake and joked with his wife that his occupational therapist gave him permission to eat ice cream. He was progressed to textured foods (minced meats and soft finely chopped vegetables) but continued to use the puréed foods as a supplement because of the effort required to eat a sufficient quantity of textured foods.

After 3 weeks of intervention, Mattias progressed to a soft foods that greatly increased the variety of foods he could eat and increased his overall satisfaction with meal selections. He continued to support caloric intake using puréed and soft foods because of motor coordination and fatigue issues. His daughter selected foods for the wedding meal that required minimal chewing, including baked sole and crème brûlée in addition to the wedding cake.

The IDDSI Framework[17] also provides universal terminology for describing the characteristics of the various viscosities of liquids. The properties of liquids are categorized from 0 to 4. Thin liquids such as water, coffee, tea and milk that have a fast flow (like water) and can be consumed by cup or straw are identified as Level 0. Individuals with an intact swallow are usually able to safely drink thin liquids at this level, although there may be a preferred drinking method to increase safe intake. Level 1, "slightly thick" liquids are thicker than water, but they can still flow through a straw. Thin liquids can be thickened to the slightly thick levels. Thinner nectars fall into this category.

Level 2, "mildly thick" liquids pour quickly from a spoon but slower than slightly thick drinks. They are "sippable," and it requires some effort to drink them using a wide-diameter straw. Some thick milkshakes may fall into this level, others will require further thickening. Level 3, "moderately thick" liquids can be taken with a spoon or drunk from a cup. Individuals who have difficulty with tongue movement or oral motor coordination often require this level of liquid texture. Level 4 "extremely thick" liquids must be taken with a spoon. They cannot be sucked up through even a wide-diameter straw. These liquids have a smooth texture with no lumps. Level 4 liquids are usually prepared using a commercial thickener.

The liquid consistency chosen depends on the client's swallowing problems. Many individuals with dysphagia have

difficulty with thin liquids, because this texture requires greater oral motor and pharyngeal control, as well as an intact sensation and an intact swallow response. Increasing the viscosity of the liquid is often used as a strategy to decrease aspiration risk.

Thicker liquids are the appropriate choice for clients with cognitive problems that interfere with bolus preparation or who have moderate to severely impaired oral motor skills, markedly delayed swallow response, or diminished ability to protect the airway.[29] Thick liquids moves more slowly through the oral cavity, which allows the client with impaired motor skills to have greater control of the bolus, preventing it from entering the pharynx and open airway before the swallow has been triggered. Videofluoroscopic studies show higher aspiration rates for thin liquids compared to thicker liquid consistencies for individuals with dysphagia.[22] Care must be taken when a client is on modified liquids to ensure that adequate hydration is maintained. Many clients dislike thickened liquids and do not take them in sufficient amounts, putting them at risk for dehydration.

Thickened liquids are made by adding thickening agents such as banana, puréed fruit, yogurt, dissolved gelatin, baby cereal, cornstarch, or a commercial thickener to achieve the appropriate viscosity. The thickened drink or soup should stay blended and not separate or liquefy. It is important that everyone involved in the client's care understands what constitutes the various liquid levels so that the correct amount of thickening agent is added. Commercially prepared thickened liquids (all levels) are available for use in the hospital setting and at home. Using a commercially prepared product guarantees the proper viscosity.

Principles of Oral Feeding

The therapist should incorporate certain principles into the oral feeding program. An important aspect of the oral preparation stage is looking at, recognizing, and reaching for food. The client must actively participate in the eating process. Food should be presented within the client's visual field. If the client has a severe visual field deficit or unilateral neglect, the therapist must help the client to scan the plate or tray visually.

When physically possible, the client should self-feed, even if assistance is necessary. If the client does not have a normal hand-to-mouth movement pattern, the therapist must help the client achieve these skills by guiding the extremity in the correct pattern. Abnormal movement of the upper extremity influences abnormal movement in the trunk, head, face, tongue, and pharynx and decreases the client's ability to safely swallow.

If the client is not capable of self-feeding, the therapist can keep the client actively involved by allowing the choice of which food or liquid is preferred for each bite. Food is presented by moving the utensil slowly from the front, toward the mouth, so that the food can be seen the entire time. The client should be allowed as much control of the eating situation as possible.

For adults, eating is often a social activity shared with friends and family. A normal, familiar dining environment facilitates normal eating. If the client has difficulty in this environment, intervention can be directed toward reducing distractions and identifying environmental modifications that will allow them to be successful. Cultural preferences must be taken into account when selecting foods and dining settings. The client's normal eating habits and routines should be considered in the development of the eating program. Special care must be taken to obtain this information during the initial assessment.

The occupational therapist must continually assess the client's positioning, muscle tone, oral control, and swallow. If the client displays poor oral motor skills, the therapist assesses for food pocketing after every few bites. The ability to cough should also be assessed. A strong cough reflex is essential in preventing aspiration.[6] The rate of the client's intake is monitored. The therapist should determine when too much food is in the mouth and when the client puts food into the mouth before the previous bite has been cleared. The therapist feels for the swallow with a finger at the hyoid notch if the client displays abnormal laryngeal movement or a delayed swallow. The therapist also assesses the client's vocal quality by having them say "ahh" upon completion of the swallow to assess for possible penetration into the laryngeal vestibule.

The frequency with which the therapist must check each component depends on the skill level and performance of the client. The more difficulty the client exhibits, the more frequent the assessment. The therapist may find it necessary to assess after each bite or sip, after a few bites or sips, or after each food item. Use of skilled observational skills allows the therapist to make the appropriate clinical decision. Specific techniques for assessment during feeding trials can be found in the swallowing assessment section of this chapter. After completing the feeding process, the client should remain in an upright position for 15 to 30 minutes to reduce the risk of refluxing food and of aspirating small food particles that may remain in the throat.

The therapist must observe the client for signs of aspiration while eating and monitor for the development of aspiration pneumonia over time. Clients vary in the amount of aspiration they can tolerate before developing aspiration pneumonia, according to age, health, and pulmonary status. The signs of acute and chronic aspiration were outlined previously.

When a client with compromised swallow function is participating in oral feedings, careful monitoring of the nutritional status is necessary. Nutrient requirements and fluid intake needs are determined by a nutrition assessment.[31,32] Nutritional deficiency is a concern, especially for older individuals, and places the client at risk for adverse health outcomes such as malnutrition, dehydration, decreased functional ability, increased use of health wcare services, and increased morbidity.[37] The client's caloric needs are determined by the dietitian and the physician and depend on the client's height, weight, activity level, and medical condition. Caloric and fluid intake is monitored by having the physician order a calorie count and a liquid intake and output (I & O) hydration count. Each person who works with the client with oral intake should record the percentage of each item the client eats or drinks. The dietitian converts the percentages into a daily calorie total. The client also should be monitored for physical signs of nutritional deficiency and dehydration. These symptoms include weakness, irritability, depression, decreased alertness, changes in eating habits, hunger, thirst, decreased turgor, and changes in amounts or color of urine. If a client is not able to take in the necessary calories, supplemental feedings are necessary to make up the difference. The physician and dietitian decide on the number of supplemental feedings.

Techniques for the Management of Dysphagia

Tables 27.6 through 27.9 provide intervention techniques for the management of dysphagia. These techniques are not intended to be used in all situations. Each client presents a different clinical picture and may display one deficit or a combination of deficits. After careful assessment, the therapist must determine the primary cause of the client's deficits and intervene accordingly. The occupational profile determines the focus of occupational therapy services and identifies the importance of dysphagia intervention taking into account the client's priorities, values, and goals as they relate to feeding and eating.

Intervention for clients with dysphagia is multifaceted and may involve rehabilitative techniques and compensatory strategies.[5] It is essential to have an excellent understanding of the underlying problems causing the swallowing disorder so that an intervention program can be designed that directly addresses these problems. The overarching goal of dysphagia intervention is the resumption of safe oral intake with the least restrictive diet. The therapist should strive toward facilitating the return of normal eating habits and routines for each client. Establishing proper positioning for safe swallowing is often the first therapeutic intervention in dysphagia management. This may involve the use of positioning equipment, therapeutic exercises to improve trunk and head control, and physical positioning by feeding staff.

When a client is unable to orally manage food, an *indirect swallowing intervention* program is initiated. Indirect intervention does not involve the ingestion of food or liquid. Indirect intervention techniques include facilitation of tone and movement for hypotonic muscles, desensitization for hypersensitive areas of the face and oral cavity, sensory stimulation to heighten sensation and proprioception, range-of-motion and gentle resistive exercises to strengthen weak oral and pharyngeal musculature, swallowing stimulation (without food), and oral motor exercises and tasks.[10]

Intervention for swallowing performance is called *direct intervention* because it involves the ingestion of food or liquid. These interventions are aimed at facilitating oral performance, improving the pharyngeal swallow, and reducing the risk of aspiration. Examples include compensatory swallowing techniques and strategies, thermal or tactile stimulation, gradation or alteration of the bolus size/texture/consistency, or method of food presentation and specialized positioning.

Compensatory techniques are introduced to improve swallow safety by helping to control the flow of food and liquid and reduce the risk of aspiration. They do not change the physiology

TABLE 27.6 Dysphagic Treatment: Oral Preparatory Stage

Structure	Symptoms	Problem	Pre-feeding Technique	Feeding Technique
Trunk	Leaning to one side	Decreased trunk tone Ataxia Increased trunk tone Poor body awareness in space	Facilitate trunk strength Exercises at midline Have client clasp hands, lean down, and touch foot, middle, other foot; rotate trunk with hands clasped and shoulders flexed to decrease or normalize tone	Assist client to hold correct position; assist with head control Assist client to hold correct feeding position; provide with perceptual boundary; consider lateral trunk support
	Hips sliding forward out of chair	Increased tone in hip extensors Poor body awareness in space	See previous entry Provide firm seating service	Adjust positioning so that client leans slightly forward at hips, arms forward on table
Head	Inability to hold head in midline	Decreased tone Weakness	Facilitate strength through neck and head exercises in flexion, extension, and lateral flexion	Assist with head control
	Inability to move head	Increased tone Poor range of motion	Tone reduction of head, shoulders, and trunk Facilitate normal movement Myofascial release techniques Soft tissue mobilization	Assist with head control
Upper extremity	Spillage of food from utensils	Decreased tone Apraxia Decreased coordination	Facilitate increased tone through weight bearing, sweeping, or tapping muscle belly of desired muscle	Guide client through correct movement pattern Provide adaptive equipment or utensils as needed
	Inability to self-feed	Increased tone Abnormal movement patterns Weakness or decreased motor control	Reduce proximal tone with scapula mobilization, weight bearing through arm strengthening exercises Facilitation of normal movement	Guide client through correct movement pattern Provide adaptive equipment or utensils as needed
Face	Drooling, food spillage from mouth	Decreased lip control Poor lip closure secondary to decreased tone, poor sensation Apraxia	Place a wet tongue blade between client's lips; ask client to hold tongue blade while therapist tries to pull it out Vibrate lips with back of electric toothbrush down cheek and across lips Lip exercises: movements described in outer oral motor evaluation; client performs repetitions two to three times daily Blow bubbles into glass of liquid with straw	Using side handgrip for head control, the therapist approximates lip closure by guiding and assisting with jaw closure Have client use a straw when drinking liquids until control improves Place food to unimpaired side Use cold food or liquids
		Decreased sensation	Fan lips so that client feels drool or wetness on lips or chin to increase awareness	Teach client to pat mouth (versus wiping mouth) and chin every few bites or sips
Tongue	Pocketing of food in cheeks or sulci Poor bolus formation	Poor tongue control for lateralization or tipping Decreased tone Poor sensation	Tongue exercises: use movements described in inner oral motor evaluation	Avoid crumbly foods Stroke client's outside cheek where pocketing occurs with index finger back and up toward client's ear; instruct client to check cheek for pocketing
	Retracted tongue	Increased tone Retracted jaw	Tongue range of motion: wrap tip of tongue in wet gauze; gently pull tongue forward, side to side and up and down; move slowly Pull tongue wrapped in wet gauze forward past front teeth, using index and middle fingers to vibrate tongue back and forth sideways to decrease tone and facilitate protrusion	Avoid crumbly foods Reduce tone as needed during meal Double swallow Resist head flexion to facilitate jaw closure Resist head extension to facilitate jaw opening

Data from Daniels S, Huckabee ML: *Dysphagia following stroke (clinical dysphagia)*, ed 2, San Diego, CA, 2013, Plural Publishing; and Logemann J: *Evaluation and treatment of swallowing disorders*, ed 2, Austin, TX, 1998, Pro-Ed.

TABLE 27.7   Dysphagic Treatment: Oral Stage

Structure	Symptoms	Problem	Pre-feeding Technique	Feeding Technique
Tongue	Slow oral transit	Poor anterior to posterior movement; decreased tone, poor sensation	Practice "ng-ga" sounds	Tuck chin toward chest
	Tongue retraction	Increased tone	Grasping tongue wrapped in gauze, pull it forward past front teeth; use finger or tongue blade to vibrate base of tongue back and forth sideways Improve tongue range of motion	Position food in center, mid-tongue Avoid crumbly foods Use cold or hot foods instead of warm Correct positioning Place index finger at base of tongue under chin; stroke up and forward
	Slow oral transit time Inability to channel food back toward pharynx	Inability to form central groove in tongue Apraxia	Grasping tongue wrapped in gauze, pull forward to front teeth; stroke firmly down middle of tongue with edge of tongue blade	Tuck chin toward chest Position food in center, mid-tongue Avoid crumbly foods Use cold or hot foods instead of warm Correct positioning Place index finger at base of tongue under chin; stroke up and forward
	Repetitive movement of tongue; food is pushed out front of mouth	Tongue thrust	Facilitate tongue retraction to bring tongue back into normal resting position; vibrate on either side of the frenulum found inside the mouth, under the tongue with finger Increase jaw control; teach isolated tongue movements	Correct positioning Place food away from midline of tongue toward back of mouth Provide downward and forward pressure to back of tongue with spoon after food placement
	Food falls off tongue into sulci or food remains on tongue without the client's awareness	Poor sensation	Ice tongue with ice chips placed in gauze to prevent ice chips from slipping into pharynx Brush tongue with toothbrush to stimulate receptors	Use foods with high viscosity or density Alternate presentation of cold and hot foods during meal
	Slow oral transit time; food remains on hard palate; coughing before swallow	Poor tongue elevation; decreased tone	Ask client to practice "k," "g," "n," "d," and "t" sounds Lightly touch tongue blade or soft toothbrush to roof of mouth at back of tongue; instruct client to press spot with tongue; resist movement with blade or brush to increase strength Vibrate tongue at base below chin; provide quick stretch by pushing down on base of tongue	Correct positioning With finger under chin at base of tongue, move finger upward and forward to facilitate elevation Avoid crumbly foods Double swallow
	Slow oral transit time Food remains on back of tongue because client is unable to elevate tongue to push food to hard palate Coughing before the swallow Retracted tongue	Decreased sensation Increased tone Decreased range of motion Soft tissue shortening	Tone tongue with gauze reduction; grasping wrapped tongue forward with around tip, pull finger or tongue blade Apply pressure to base of tongue right to left Grasping base of tongue under chin between two fingers, move it back and forth to decrease tone Tone reduction Range of motion exercises Place a variety of tastes on lips to facilitate tongue licking lips	Adjust correct positioning by increasing forward flexion at hips, arms forward to decrease tone Reduce tone as needed; give client breaks because tone increases with effort With finger under chin at base of tongue, move finger upward and forward to facilitate tongue elevation

Data from Logemann J: *Evaluation and treatment of swallowing disorders*, ed 2, Austin, TX, 1998, Pro-Ed; Wheeler-Hegland K, Ashford J, Frymark T, et al: Evidence-based systematic review: oropharyngeal dysphagia behavioral treatments. Part II: Impact of dysphagia treatment on normal swallow function, *J Rehabil Res Dev* 46:185–194, 2009.

TABLE 27.8 Dysphagia Treatment: Pharyngeal Stage

Structure	Symptoms	Problem	Pre-feeding Technique	Feeding Technique
Soft palate	Tight voice; nasal regurgitation; Air felt through nose or mist seen on mirror when client says "ah"; Decreased tone; Nasal speech	Increased tone; Decreased tone; Rigidity	Facilitate normal head/neck positioning; Have client tuck chin into therapist's cupped hand, then push into hand as therapist applies resistance; client says, "ah" afterward; speed and height of uvula elevation should increase; follow by thermal application	Facilitate normal head and neck positioning; With head and neck in midline, have client tuck chin slightly to decrease rate of food entering into pharynx
	Delayed swallow	Decreased triggering of swallow response	Thermal application: using a laryngeal mirror size 00 after being placed in ice water or chips for 10 seconds, touch base of faucial arch; repeat up to 10 times; process can be repeated several times a day	Alternate presentation of food; start with a very cold substance, then warm; cold substance can increase sensitivity of faucial arches; tuck chin slightly forward to prevent bolus entering airway
Hyoid	Delayed elevation of **hyoid bone**; Poor tongue elevation	Delayed swallow; Incomplete swallow	Increase tongue humping because elevation of tongue and hyoid stimulates triggering of response	Place index finger under chin at base of tongue and push up and forward to facilitate tongue elevation
	Tongue retraction	Abnormal tongue tone; poor range of motion	Tone reduction and range-of-motion exercises	
Pharynx	Coughing after swallow	Decreased pharyngeal movement; Penetration into laryngeal vestibule	None	If appropriate, alternate presentation of liquid with stage II or stage III solids; liquid material moves solids through pharynx
	Coating of pharynx seen on videofluoroscopy; Gurgling voice	Pharyngeal weakness	Isometric or resistive head and neck exercises	Have client take second dry swallow to clear valleculae and pyriform sinuses; Tilt head to stronger side; Supraglottic swallow
	Seen on videofluoroscopy, anteroposterior view; material residue seen on one side; weak or hoarse voice	Unilateral pharyngeal movement	None	Compensatory technique for clients with low tone: have client turn head toward affected side during swallow to prevent pooling in affected pyriform sinuses; evaluate technique against its effect on client positioning and tone in trunk, upper extremities
Larynx	Coughing, choking after swallow	Decreased laryngeal elevation; Decreased tone; Weakness	Quickly ice up sides of larynx; ask client to swallow; assist movement by guiding larynx upward; Vibrate laryngeal musculature from under chin, downward on each side to sternal notch	Teach client to clear throat immediately after swallow to move residual; Use supraglottic swallow, Mendelsohn maneuver, effortful swallow
	Noisy or audible swallow	Increased tone; Rigidity; Uncoordinated swallow	Range of motion—place fingers and thumb along both sides of larynx and gently move it back and forth until movement is smooth and easy tone decreased; Using chipped ice, form pack in washcloth and place around larynx for 5 min	Placing fingers and thumb along both sides of larynx, assist client with upward elevation before swallow; Double swallow
Trachea	Continuous coughing before, during, after swallow	Aspiration—before: poor tongue control; during: delayed swallow response; after: decreased pharyngeal movement	Teach client how to produce a voluntary cough; ask client to take a deep breath and cough while breathing out; therapist uses palm of hand to push downward (toward stomach) on the sternum	Encourage client to keep coughing; facilitate reflexive cough; push downward on sternum as client breathes out; suction client if problem increases; Push into client's sternal notch to assist with cough
	Client grabs or reaches for throat; Reddening in the face; No voice or cough	Blocked airway	None	Perform Heimlich maneuver (abdominal thrusts) Seek medical assistance

Data from Crary M: Imaging swallowing examinations: videofluoroscopy and endoscopy. In Groher ME, Crary MA: *Dysphagia: clinical management in adults and children*, ed 2, St. Louis, 2016, Elsevier; Logemann J: *Evaluation and treatment of swallowing disorders*, Austin, TX, 1998, Pro-Ed; and Wheeler-Hegland K, Ashford J, Frymark T, et al: Evidence-based systematic review: oropharyngeal dysphagia behavioral treatments. Part II: Impact of dysphagia treatment on normal swallow function, *J Rehabil Res Dev* 46:185–194, 2009.

TABLE 27.9 Dysphagia Treatment—Esophageal Stage

Structure	Symptoms	Problem	Pre-feeding Technique	Feeding Technique
Esophagus	Frequent regurgitation of food or liquid and coughing or choking after the swallow; material collecting in a side pocket in esophagus	Esophageal diverticulum	Requires a medical diagnosis; problem can be seen through traditional barium x-ray examination Surgical correction is needed	Report symptoms to medical staff (therapist cannot treat)
	Regurgitation of food, coughing, or choking on food after the swallow: inability of food to pass through the pharynx, esophagus, or stomach	Partial or total obstruction of the pharynx or esophagus Impaired esophageal peristalsis	Requires a medical diagnosis; problem can be seen through traditional barium x-ray examination Surgical correction is needed	Report symptoms to medical staff (therapist cannot treat)

Data from Crary M: Imaging swallowing examinations: videofluoroscopy and endoscopy. In Groher M, Crary M, editors: *Dysphagia: clinical management in adults and children*, ed 2, St. Louis, 2016, Elsevier; and Logemann, J: *Evaluation and treatment of swallowing disorders*, Austin, TX, 1998, Pro-Ed.

BOX 27.1 Bolus Textures and Swallow Problems

Texture	Disorders for Which This Texture Is Most Appropriate
Thin liquid	Tongue dysfunction (ROM, strength, coordination) Reduced tongue base retraction Reduced pharyngeal wall contraction Reduced laryngeal elevation Reduced cricopharyngeal opening
Thickened liquid	Tongue dysfunction (ROM, strength, coordination) Delayed pharyngeal swallow
Puréed	Oral motor impairment Delayed pharyngeal swallow Impaired cognition Decreased endurance
Mechanical soft	Oral motor impairment (decreased chew) Decreased endurance

Adapted from Logemann J: *Evaluation and treatment of swallowing disorders*, ed 2, Austin, TX, 1998, Pro-Ed; and Crary MA: Imaging swallowing examinations: videofluoroscopy and endoscopy. In Groher M, Crary M, editors: *Dysphagia: clinical management in adults and children*, ed 2, St. Louis, 2016, Elsevier.
ROM, Range of motion.

BOX 27.2 Techniques to Improve Oral Sensory Awareness

- Downward pressure of metal spoon on tongue during presentation of food
- Cold bolus
- Sour bolus
- Larger bolus
- Bolus that requires chewing
- Thermal-tactile stimulation*

*Tactile stimulation provided directly to the anterior faucial arch using a cold, size 00 laryngeal mirror before the presentation of the bolus. This technique heightens oral awareness and provides an alerting sensory stimulus to the cortex and brainstem to facilitate the triggering of the swallow response.
Adapted from Logemann J: *Evaluation and treatment of swallowing disorders*, ed 2, Austin, TX, 1998, Pro-Ed.

of the individual's swallow. Compensatory strategies used in dysphagia intervention include (1) postural techniques (e.g., turning the head toward the more involved side for an individual who sustained a CVA closes off the weaker pharyngeal wall and allows safer swallowing (see Figs. 27.8, D), (2) techniques to improve oral sensory awareness, (3) modification of bolus volume and speed of presentation, and (4) texture modifications (Box 27.1). Compensatory strategies often allow a client to safely engage in oral eating while continuing to work on

remediation of the underlying problems. The client and those involved with assisting the client to eat are trained in the use of these strategies.

Rehabilitative or remediation techniques include oral motor and range-of-motion exercises, oral motor strengthening exercises, bolus control exercises, vocal fold adduction and laryngeal elevation exercises, neuromuscular electric stimulation, and exercises to improve pharyngeal pressure.[4,18,19,24] Swallow maneuvers also may be introduced to improve laryngeal closure and bolus movement through the pharynx. Box 27.2 presents examples of swallow maneuvers.

The therapist continually assesses the client's response to intervention and makes necessary modifications to the eating and swallowing program. The therapist must develop excellent clinical observation skills. For complex clients, the clinician should seek a consultation with an experienced dysphagia therapist. To develop expertise in dysphagia management, it is recommended that the therapist seek continued education in this area.

CASE STUDY

Nick

Nick is a 65-year-old man (prefers the pronouns he/him/his) who suffered a right cerebrovascular accident (CVA) with left hemiplegia 2 weeks ago. He has a percutaneous endoscopic gastrostomy (PEG) tube in place for nutrition. He recently retired from his position as vice president of a local marketing company. Nick lives with his wife. He and his wife have two grown children living in the area. Before the onset of the CVA, Nick was independent in all ADLs and instrumental activities of daily living (IADLs). He was an active member of the community.

Results of the occupational therapy evaluation indicate that Nick needs moderate to maximum assistance in dressing, toileting, bathing, eating and swallowing, and transfers. The clinical assessment of eating indicates that the client has a mild to moderate increase in jaw and facial tone with poor rotary chew, poor isolated tongue control, and a mild increase in laryngeal tone with delayed swallow.

The videofluoroscopy confirmed that the client had a mildly delayed swallow with minimal pooling in the valleculae and pyriform sinuses. Aspiration was less than 10% on puréed foods. The occupational therapist saw the client three times a week for 6 weeks. A summary of evaluation results and a treatment plan are shown in Fig. 27.9.

The client responded well to treatment. The PEG was removed after 5 weeks. The client achieved all treatment goals by the time of discharge. He went home with family supervision for correct diet, positioning, and swallowing techniques during meals. The client was referred to home health occupational therapy for 2 to 3 weeks for ADLs and home modification so that he could achieve independence at home. The client returned for follow-up outpatient visits.

DYSPHAGIA EVALUATION AND INTERVENTION PLAN

Name: N.X.
Dx: R CVA
Age/Onset: 65 y/o male, 1 week ago

Medical hx:
Elevated BP x 5 years. Elevated blood lipids. Otherwise unremarkable. Independent in ADL & IADL prior to onset. No previous swallowing problems. Previously ate a regular diet.

Current nutritional status:	NG tube, NPO until swallowing evaluation

---

Mental status:

Alert/oriented	Oriented to self only
Direction following	Follows 1-2 step directions well

Physical status (symmetry, control, tone)

Head control	Slight increase in tone with head turning.
Trunk control	Poor trunk control. Leans to the right, unable to bring self to midline
Endurance	Fatigues after 20 minutes of activity
Respiratory	No SOB noted

Outer oral status:

Facial expressions	Flat affect. Unable to mimic facial expressions. Drooping right side
Jaw movement	Poor rotary chew pattern, poor jaw glide, uses up and down movement
Lip movement	Asymmetrical purse and retract, poor lip compression with closure
Sensation	Decreased-absent touch on right side
Abnormal reflexes	Absent

Inner oral status (symmetry, control, tone)

Dentition		Dentures, fit well
Tongue		
	Appearance	White coating, deviated to right
	Tone	Hypotonic
	Movement: Protrusion	To just past lips, poor anterior to posterior sweep on palate
	Lateralization	Reduced ROM both sides, deviated to right at rest
	Elevation	With effort, fatigues with repetition

Fig. 27.9 Dysphagia evaluation and intervention plan.

DYSPHAGIA EVALUATION AND INTERVENTION PLAN	

Soft palate/gag reflex:	Uvula rises symmetrically but with slight delay "ah". Gag present
Cough (reflexive/voluntary):	Weak voluntary cough to command

Swallow:

Spontaneous	Intact
Voluntary	Slight delay with effort
Laryngeal movement	Mild reduction in laryngeal excursion

Food management:

Puree	Requires verbal cues to attend to food in mouth. Increased oral transit
Mechanical soft	Requires increased effort, verbal cues, transit time, residuals after sw.
Regular	Not tested
Liquids: Thick	With straw, 5 second delay, no cough
Semi-thick	With straw, 5 second delay, cough; by spoon, 5 second delay, no cough
Thin	Not tested

Required assistance with feeding to utilize strategies (chin tuck, clearing swallow). Decreased sensory awareness of food and liquid in mouth. Weak cough reduces airway protection. Limited amounts of PO provided during testing.

Major problems:
1. Poor sitting balance
2. Poor endurance for eating
3. Weak cough
4. Impaired cognition for attention and awareness of food in mouth
5. Decreased intra-oral and extra-oral sensation
6. Poor isolated tongue movements for lateralization, elevation and protrusion
7. 3-second delay in pharyngeal swallow as per videofluoroscopy evaluation
8. 5-10% residuals in valleculae and pyriform sinus after the swallow as per videofluoroscopy

Recommendations/methods:
(positioning, diet texture modifications, environmental modifications, sensory stimulation, compensatory strategies to improve pharyngeal swallow, client/caregiver training)

1. Positioning – Upright on a solid seating surface, feet flat on the floor, trunk and head in midline, arms supported with slight forward flexion at hips
2. Diet texture – Pureed and mechanical soft (finely chopped) foods, nectar thick liquids. P.O. intake with nursing or therapist only
3. Environmental modifications – quiet eating environment without distractions
4. Alternate cold, frozen textured liquid with food to increase sensory awareness in the mouth.
5. Small frequent meals
6. Oral motor exercises to increase tongue ROM and strength
7. Chin tuck during swallow to reduce risk of aspiration due to delayed swallow
8. Clearing (double) swallow to clear pharyngeal residuals
9. Monitor for signs of aspiration
10. Check mouth for pocketing or residuals after oral intake
11. Advance diet texture as client status improves

Long term goals:
1. Good trunk and head control for safe eating
2. Good awareness of food and liquid in mouth – no food/liquid loss from mouth during eating
3. Good attention to task of eating in a variety of eating environments without verbal cues
4. Improved endurance for eating so that client can eat a full meal without signs of fatigue
5. Adequate strength and coordination of oral musculature to safely manage a soft diet
6. Able to safely drink thin liquids via straw and cup
7. Able to meet nutrition and hydration needs P.O.
8. No signs or symptoms of aspiration
9. Safe eating with caregivers

Fig. 27.9 cont'd

SUMMARY

Eating is the most basic activity of daily living. Several performance components are required for the client to eat and swallow effectively. Dysphagia refers to difficulty with swallowing or an inability to swallow. The occupational therapist is trained to assess and provide intervention for many of the problems that interfere with normal eating. An understanding of the normal anatomy and physiology of swallowing and advanced training in eating and swallowing disorders are required to effectively treat dysphagia.

Assessment of the client with dysphagia includes testing of head and trunk control, sensation, perception, cognition, intraoral and extraoral structures, oral reflexes, and swallowing. Instrumental assessment may also include videofluoroscopy or fiberoptic endoscopy.

Several members of the rehabilitation team are involved in the treatment of the client with dysphagia. Positioning, selection of appropriate feeding procedures, diet texture selection, diet progression, and special techniques to facilitate normal patterns of swallowing are part of the intervention plan. The social, cultural, contextual, and psychological aspects of eating are also important considerations in the intervention program.

REVIEW QUESTIONS

1. List the components of dysphagia.
2. List the four stages of swallowing and the characteristics of each.
3. List the physiologic functions that occur when the swallow response triggers, and explain why these functions are necessary.
4. Why is it necessary to assess a client's mental status during a dysphagia evaluation?
5. Describe what the therapist should look for when evaluating the trunk and head during the dysphagia evaluation.
6. What information can the therapist gain when assessing the client's facial motor control?
7. How does poor tongue control contribute to aspiration?
8. Name the components required to protect the airway.
9. What is the safest food sequence to follow for a swallowing evaluation?
10. Describe the finger placement that a therapist can use to feel the strength and smoothness of the swallow.
11. Why should the therapist assess voice quality after a swallow?
12. Will a client who has difficulty handling solids also have difficulty with liquids?
13. List the indicators of swallowing dysfunction.
14. List the acute symptoms of aspiration.
15. When is videofluoroscopy necessary?
16. List the types of intervention used with clients with dysphagia.
17. Describe how the client should be optimally positioned for eating and give the rationale.
18. What are the indications for placing a client on a nonoral treatment program?
19. Name five important criteria a client must meet to participate in an oral feeding program.
20. List the properties of food preferred for diets for clients with dysphagia.
21. Why is it important to involve the client in the eating process?
22. What are the symptoms of nutritional deficiency?
23. Name three treatment techniques the occupational therapist can use for poor rotary jaw movement and increased tone.
24. Describe two ways a therapist can decrease abnormally high tone in the tongue.
25. Describe thermal application as a treatment technique. For which problem is it used?
26. When is use of the dry swallow technique appropriate?

REFERENCES

1. American Occupational Therapy Association: The practice of occupational therapy in feeding, eating, and swallowing, *Am J Occup Ther* 71(suppl 2), 2017.
2. American Occupational Therapy Association: Occupational therapy practice framework: domain and process, ed 4, *Am J Occup Ther* 74(suppl 2), 2020.
3. American Occupational Therapy Association: Scope of practice, *Am J Occup Ther* 75(Suppl 3), 2021, 7513410030. https://doi.org/10.5014/ajot.2021.75S3005.
4. Bahia M, Lowell S: A systematic review of the physiological effects of the effortful swallow maneuver in adults with normal and disordered swallowing, *Am J Speech-Language Pathol* 29(3), 2020. https://doi.org/10.1044/2020_AJSLP-19-00132.
5. Banik A: Outcomes of swallowing rehabilitation in patients with dysphagia: A retrospective study, *Bengal J Otolaryngol Head Neck Surg* 28(2):151–156, 2020.
6. Belal E, Selim S, Aboul Fotouh A: Detection of airway protective level of the cough reflex in acute stroke patients, *The Egypt J Neurol, Psychiatry Neurosurg* 56:21, 2020. https://doi.org/10.1186/s41983-020-0157-9.
7. Benfield J, Everton L, Bath P, England T: Accuracy and clinical utility of comprehensive dysphagia screening assessments in acute stroke: A systematic review and meta-analysis, *J Clinic Nurs* 29(9-10):1527–1538, 2020. https://doi.org/10.1111/jocn.15192.
8. Brates D, Molfenter S, Thibeault S: Assessing hyolaryngeal excursion: Comparing quantitative methods to palpation at the bedside and visualization during videofluoroscopy, *Dysphagia* 34:298–307, 2019. https://doi.org/10.1007/s00455-018-9927-2.
9. Coll P, Lindsay A, Meng J, Gopalakrishna A, Raghavendra S, Bysani P, O'Brien D: The prevention of infections in older adults: oral health. *J Am Geriatrics Soc*, 68(2), 411–416. https://doi.org/10.1111/jgs.16154.
10. Crary M: Imaging swallowing examinations: videofluoroscopy and endoscopy. In Groher M, Crary M, editors: *Dysphagia:*

clinical management in adults and children, ed 3, St. Louis, 2021, Elsevier.

11. Darjanki C, Perdana S, Purwaningsih Y, Palupi R: Relationship between age in patients with dental and oral health problems with quality of life, *Eur J Mol Clin Med* 7(05):699–708, 2020.

12. Fairfield C, Smithard D: Assessment and management of dysphagia in acute stroke: An initial service review of international practice, *Geriatrics* 5(1):4, 2020. https://doi.org/10.3390/geriatrics5010004.

13. Groher M: Ethical considerations. In Groher M, Crary M, editors: *Dysphagia: clinical management in adults and children*, ed 3, St. Louis, 2021, Elsevier.

14. Groher M: Normal swallowing in adults. In Groher M, Crary M, editors: *Dysphagia: clinical management in adults and children*, ed 3, St. Louis, 2021, Elsevier.

15. Groher M, Puntil-Sheltman J: Dysphagia unplugged. In Groher M, Crary M, editors: *Dysphagia: clinical management in adults and children*, ed 3, St. Louis, 2021, Elsevier.

16. Hong JH, Hwang NK, Lee G, Park JS, Jung Y-J: Radiation safety in videofluoroscopic swallowing study: Systemic review, *Dysphagia*, 2020. https://doi.org/10.1007/s00455-020-10112.

17. International Dysphagia Diet Standardisation Initiative (IDDSI) Framework. (2019). Retrieved from: https://iddsi.org/framework/.

18. Jeon Y, Cho K, Park S: Effects of neuromuscular electrical stimulation (NMES) plus upper cervical spine mobilization on forward head posture and swallowing function in stroke patients with dysphagia, *Brain Sci* 10:478, 2020. https://doi.org/10.3390/brainsci10080478.

19. Jongprasitkul H, Kitisomprayoonkul W: Effectiveness of conventional swallowing therapy in acute stroke patients with dysphagia, *Rehabil Res Pract,* 2020, Article ID 2907293, 2020. https://doi.org/10.1155/2020/2907293.

20. Kim J, Choi H, Jung J, Kim H: Risk factors for aspiration pneumonia in patients with dysphagia undergoing videofluoroscopic swallowing studies: A retrospective cohort study, *Medicine* 99(46), e23177, 2020.

21. Kohli M, Andrade A, Dharmarajan T: Enteral nutrition. In Pitchumoni C, Dharmarajan T, editors: *Geriatric Gastroenterology*, Switzerland, 2020, Springer.

22. Langmore S, Krisciunas G, Warner H, White SD, Dvorkin D, Fink D, McNally E, Scheel R, Higgins C, Levitt J, McKeehan J, Deane S, Siner J, Vojnik R, Moss M: Abnormalities of aspiration and swallowing function in survivors of acute respiratory failure, Dysphagia, 2020. https://doi.org/10.1007/s00455-020-10199-8.

23. Logemann J: Evaluation and treatment of swallowing disorders, *Austin, TX*, 1998, Pro-Ed.

24. Lopez-Liria R, Parra-Egeda J, Vega-Ramirez F, Aguilar-Parra J, Trigueros-Ramos R, Morales-Gazquez M, Rocamora-Perez P: Treatment of dysphagia in Parkinson's disease: A systematic review, *Int J Environ Res Public Health* 17(11):4104, 2020. https://doi.org/10.3390/ijerph17114104.

25. Matsuo K, Palmer J: Anatomy and physiology of feeding and swallowing-normal and abnormal, *Phys Med Rehabi ClinNorth Am* 19(4):691–707, 2008.

26. Miller C, Schroeder J, Langmore S: Fiberotpic evaluation of swallowing across the age spectrum, *Am J Speech Lang Patho* 29(2S), 2020. https://doi.org/10.1044/2019_AJSLP-19-00072.

27. Moon M, Min J, Shin Y, Ko S: Frequency and characteristics of videofluoroscopic swallow study in patients with aspiration pneumonia, *J Korean Dysphagia Soc* 8(1):48–55, 2018.

28. Mulheren R, Azola A, Gonzalez-Fernandez M: Avoiding the downward spiral after stroke: Early identification and treatment of dysphagia, *Curr Phys Med Rehabil Rep* 8:469–477, 2020. https://doi.org/10.1007/s40141-020-00290-4.

29. Nagy A, Molfenter SM: Péladeau-Pigeon, et al: The effect of bolus consistency on hyoid velocity in healthy swallowing, *Dysphagia* 30:445–451, 2015.

30. Nakajima M, Umezaki Y, Takeda S, Yamaguchi M, Suzuki N, Yoneda M, Hirofuji T, Sekitani H, Yamashita Y, Morita H: Association between oral candidiasis and bacterial pneumonia: A retrospective study, *Oral Diseases* 26(1):234–237, 2020.

31. Nazarko L: Maintaining or improving nutrition and hydration in dysphagia, *Independent Nurse* 9, 2018. https://doi.org/10.12968/indn.2018.9.17.

32. Nazarko L: Dysphagia: addressing nutritional, hydration and medication difficulties, *J Prescrib Pract* 2(supp 10), 2020. https://doi.org/10.12968/jprp.2020.2.Sup10.S2.

33. Orsbon C, Gidmark N, Gao T, Ross C: XROMM and diceCT reveal a hydraulic mechanism of tongue base retraction in swallowing, *Scientific Reports* 10:8215, 2020. https://doi.org/10.1038/s41598-020-64935-z.

34. Panebianco M, Marchese-Ragona R, Masiero S, Restivo D: Dysphagia in neurological diseases: a literature review, *Neurol Sci* 41:3067–3073, 2020. https://doi.org/10.1007/s10072-020-04495-2.

35. Patel B, Legacy J, Hegland K, Okun M, Herndon N: A comprehensive review of the diagnosis and treatment of Parkinson's disease dysphagia and aspiration, *Exp Rev Gastroenterol Hepatol* 14(6), 2020. https://doi.org/10.1080/17474124.2020.1769475.

36. Ramsey D, Smithard D, Kalra L: Silent aspiration. What do we know? *Dysphagia* 20:218–225, 2005. https://doi.org/10.1007/s00455-005-0018-9.

37. Salinas Jimenez M: General nutritional recommendations in care of neurological elderly patients with dysphagia. Jamk.fi (Masters thesis), 2020. Retrieved from: http://urn.fi/URN:NBN:fi:amk-2020062319252.

38. Sasegbon A, Hamdy S: The role of the cerebellum in swallowing, *Dysphagia,* 2021. https://doi.org/10.1007/s00455-021-10271-x.

39. Schwarz M, Coccetti A, Cardeil E, Hirst T, Lyons L: A retrospective cohort study of complex feeding decisions: Informing dysphagia decision-making through patient experiences, *J Clin Pract Speech-Lang Pathol* 21(3):154–158, 2019.

40. Skoretz S, Riopelle S, Wellman L, Dawson C: Investigating swallowing and tracheostomy following critical illness: A scoping review, *Critical Care Med* 48(2):141–151, 2020. https://doi.org/10.1097/CCM.0000000000004098.

41. Tye C, Gardner P, Dion G, Simpson CB, Dominguez L: Impact of fiberoptic endoscopic evaluation of swallowing outcomes and dysphagia management in neurodegenerative diseases, *The Laryngoscope*, 2020. https://doi.org/10.1002/lary.28791.

42. Zuercher P, Dziewas R, Schefold J: Dysphagia in the intensive care unit: a (multidisciplinary call to action, *Intens Care Med* 46:554–556, 2020. https://doi.org/10.1007/s00134-020-05937-3.

28

Pain Management

Joyce M. Engel

LEARNING OBJECTIVES

After studying this chapter, the student or practitioner will be able to do the following:

1. Discriminate acute from chronic pain.
2. Explain Loeser and Fordyce's model of pain.
3. Describe two chronic pain interventions.
4. Summarize two domains for pain assessment.
5. Describe occupationally based approaches to pain intervention.

CHAPTER OUTLINE

KEY TERMS

Acute pain
Biopsychosocial model of pain
Chronic pain
Nociception

Pain
Pain Assessment
Pain Behavior
Pain Intervention

Quota Programs
Suffering

THREADED CASE STUDY

Susan, Part 1

Susan is a 34-year-old who identifies as female (prefers use of the pronouns she/her/hers). Susan is single, works in an office, and presented with fibromyalgia, including severe constant pain of the shoulder and neck regions. She also reported generalized joint stiffness, body aches, and fatigue. Susan has tried analgesics and cryotherapy without relief. She was referred by her physician to occupational therapy (OT) so she could "learn to live with the pain." Susan reported being mildly depressed. Use of the Brief Pain Inventory was found to reveal moderate pain interference with Susan's activities of daily living (ADLs) with general activity, work, self-care, and enjoyment of life. Her current overall numerical pain intensity score was 5 (moderate) on a scale of 0 to 10. She reported pain exacerbating factors as shoulder flexion greater than 90 degrees when washing her hair and being active more than 30 minutes. She was capable of only 5 minutes swimming, a previously enjoyed activity because she felt invigorated afterward. Susan's goals are to wash her hair with less pain and be more active, especially in swimming. She demonstrated poor posture, body mechanics, and energy conservation skills.

Critical Thinking Questions

1. How would you best evaluate Susan's pain?
2. How would you apply Loeser and Fordyce's model of pain[25] to the case?
3. Describe a hierarchy of three interventions for Susan.

Pain is a primary reason for seeking healthcare and a reason for avoiding it. The treatment of chronic pain resulting from trauma, disease, or unknown etiology is a significant healthcare problem in the United States. Population-based estimates of chronic pain among American adults range from 11% to 40%.[21] No doubt this is a conservative estimate of pain because it does not include data on youths or individuals experiencing acute pain. The obligation to manage pain and relieve a client's suffering is fundamental to healthcare.[12] Pain may coexist with a medical condition (e.g., arthritis) or a rehabilitative procedure (splinting), and it may be the primary problem (e.g., low back pain) or a secondary disability (e.g., chronic pain associated with cerebral palsy). Occupational therapy practitioners may suspect that pain is impeding the client's occupational performance but are unsure about how best to evaluate the condition and intervene. This chapter defines pain, discusses the biopsychosocial model of pain, describes common pain syndromes, outlines assessment procedures, and suggests interventions.

DEFINITION OF PAIN

The word *pain* refers to an endless variety of qualities that are categorized under a single linguistic label. The International Association for the Study of Pain defines pain as an unpleasant sensory and emotional experience associated with, or resembling that associated with, actual or potential tissue damage.[20] This definition conveys the multidimensional and subjective nature of pain. Pain is recognized as a private experience that is influenced to varying degrees in biological, psychological, and social factors. Through life experiences, individuals learn the concept of pain. Individual variables such as mood, attention, prior pain experiences, and familial and cultural factors are known to affect one's experience of pain.[1]

There are many types of pain. Most researchers differentiate *acute* from *chronic pain*, which is critical for selecting appropriate evaluation and intervention strategies. Acute pain and its associated physiological, psychological, and behavioral responses are typically caused by tissue irritation or damage related to injury, disease, rehabilitative, or medical procedures. Acute pain has a well-defined onset and serves a biologic purpose alerting the individual for the need for immobilization and protection of the body part. It follows a predictable course of recovery. Acute pain has a duration of less than 12 weeks.[9]

In contrast, chronic pain does not appear to serve a biological purpose. It is unpredictable and not amenable to routine interventions. It lasts more than 12 weeks. Chronic pain often results in changes in quality of life (e.g., emotions, thoughts, attitudes, environment, lifestyle), including a negative effect on occupational performance.[8]

BIOPSYCHOSOCIAL MODEL OF PAIN

Occupational therapy has long embraced the biopsychosocial model for its emphasis on the interaction of the individual's mind, body, and environment.[28] Conceptualizing pain using a biopsychosocial model can clarify the complex, multifaceted nature of pain that is critical to accurate evaluation and effective intervention.

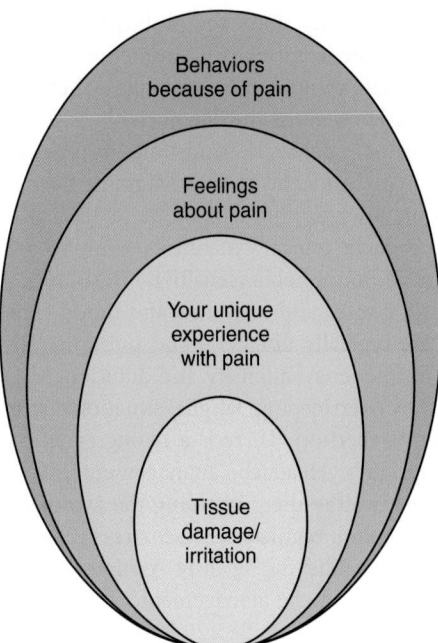

Fig. 28.1 Loeser's model of pain. (Adapted from Loeser JD: Concepts of pain. In Stanton-Hicks M, Boas R, editors: *Chronic low back pain*, New York, 1982, Raven Press.)

Loeser and Fordyce (in 1983) proposed that the phenomenon of pain could be divided into four distinct domains: nociception, pain, suffering, and pain behavior[25] (Fig. 28.1). Nociception is the perception of pain. Specialized sensory receptors in the skin and deeper structures detect current or impending tissue damage or irritation and transmit this information by A-delta and C fibers in the peripheral nerves. Nociception alerts the body to do something or to cease doing something. Pain is the perceived noxious input to the nervous system. Specifically, it is the individual's unique unpleasant sensory and emotional experience. Suffering is the negative affective response to pain. Pain is always a personal experience. Pain may cause depression, anxiety, fear, or substance use or dependence. Pain behavior is what a person says or does (e.g., taking medication) or does not do (e.g., job absenteeism) that communicates the occurrence of pain. These behaviors are observable and readily influenced by cultural, spiritual, familial, and environmental factors.[9,10] Loeser and Fordyce's biopsychosocial model purports that an individual can experience some but not all domains at any given time.[25] As illustrated, Susan may experience tissue irritation and decreased occupational performance, but have no emotional response to the pain.

PAIN SYNDROMES

Numerous pain syndromes result from disease, trauma, or an unknown cause. Several common pain syndromes are described in the next section.

Headache Pain

Recurrent headaches are one of the most common reports of pain. More than half of persons with headache do not seek treatment because they think the problem is too trivial, have concerns about medications (e.g., addiction, side effects), or think no adequate treatment is available. A headache diary is commonly used in making the diagnosis.[9,16]

The two primary headache syndromes or types are migraine and tension-type headache (TTH). Migraine headaches are an episodic brain disorder that affect 12% to 15% of the population.[16] The headache typically manifests with photophobia (sensitivity to light), sonophobia (sensitivity to sound), intolerance to movement, nausea and vomiting, and mood changes. These headaches are typically unilateral and pulsatile. The pain episodes vary in frequency, intensity, and duration. Migraines may be triggered by oversleeping, fatigue, situational stress, skipped meals, and overexertion. There is a strong genetic predisposition for migraines. Headache management involves regular sleep patterns; healthy diet, including the avoidance of excess caffeine and alcohol; regular exercise; stress management; and medication.[9,16] Establishing healthy routines is an important part of migraine headache management.

Tension-type headaches affect 20.8% of the population. These headaches are usually mild to moderate in intensity. The pain is perceived as bilateral and of a pressing nature. Precipitating headache factors include sleep deprivation, situational stress, missed meals, and noxious stimuli (e.g., heat exposure). TTH has been attributed to a disorder of central nervous system modulation. Medication management (e.g., acetaminophen) and stress management are the typical course of treatment.[9,16] As with management of migraines, establishing healthy routines is an important part of the intervention process.

Low Back Pain

Low back pain (LBP) is a very common disabling condition, and individuals may live years with this disability. The lifetime prevalence of LBP is estimated to be 60% to 70% in industrialized countries.[7] Mechanical issues and soft-tissue injuries are the most common cause of LBP. These injuries may result in damage to the intervertebral discs, compression of nerve roots, and improper movement of the spinal joints. Common causes of strain and sprain can develop over time from repetitive movements or suddenly. Common causes of sprain or strain include heavy lifting, sudden movements, poor posture, and sports injuries. The resultant acute pain can be significant. Job absenteeism, loss of productive activity, and decreased participation are common pain consequences. Clients may restrict occupational engagement because of a fear that the cause of pain, the interventions, and the restricted social consequences may be harmful. Fortunately, LBP tends to improve spontaneously. Functional restoration is vital for the client with chronic back pain. Medication management, physical therapy (e.g., exercise, traction), and self-care education are common treatment approaches.[7,24]

Arthritis

An estimated 22.7% of adults have arthritis.[3] Primary osteoarthritis (OA) has no known cause. It may affect one or two joints or be generalized (three or more joints). Secondary OA can result from trauma, anatomic abnormalities, septic necrosis,

and infection. It is characterized by a dull ache and swelling, typically affecting the fingers, elbows, hips, knees, and ankles. Excessive movement may exacerbate OA. Degeneration of the articular cartilage leading to joint pain, reduced mobility, and swelling occur, typically affecting weight-bearing joints in persons after age 45.[15,35] Rheumatoid arthritis (RA) is a chronic, systemic inflammatory disease.[5] The etiology of RA is not well known. RA typically has a slow insidious onset, characterized by aches and pains, stiffness, and swelling. The disease involves exacerbations and remissions. The Centers for Disease Control Prevention supports self-management programs (e.g., activity, exercise, cognitive-behavioral therapy), weight loss, and over-the-counter medication (e.g., acetaminophen) for pain control for both OA and RA.[3]

Cancer Pain

Cancer is the second leading cause of death in the United States. From a large meta-analysis on pain, cancer pain prevalence rates were 39.3% after curative treatment, 55% during anticancer treatment, and 66.4% in advanced, metastatic terminal disease. Moderate-to-severe pain was reported by 38% of all patients.[39] Clients with cancer typically have multiple pain locations. Cancer pain varies in frequency, duration, and intensity. Pain from the cancer can be caused by a tumor pressing on nerves, bones, or organs.[29] The impact of pain includes decreased occupational performance (e.g., job absenteeism), sleep disturbance, poor appetite, and mood changes (e.g., anger, irritability, sadness, frustration). There are many types of cancer treatments. The type of treatment (surgery, radiation therapy, chemotherapy) pursued depends on the type of cancer the client has, the progression of the disease, and the stage of the disease.

Fibromyalgia

Fibromyalgia affects about 10 million Americans. Fibromyalgia is the current term for individuals with chronic widespread musculoskeletal pain, for which no clear cause is known.[4] It has been hypothesized that skeletal muscles are the cause of fibromyalgia. Abnormalities of the neuroendocrine, autoimmune dysfunction, immune regulation, central blood flow difficulties,

THREADED CASE STUDY

Susan, Part 2

Susan and the occupational therapy (OT) practitioner developed an intervention plan. A systematic graded tolerance (quota) program was designed for mobility, swimming, and ambulation. Susan would listen to music to distract herself from the pain when walking. She would go for a daily walk beginning with a 30-minute duration and gradually increasing in 5-minute increments every few days until she reached a 1-hour goal. She would often do this in the swimming pool. She was able to wash her hair but experienced moderate-to-severe pain while doing so. To address the pain during this self-care task, Susan would allow warm water to run down the back of her neck and shoulders for 5 minutes before shampooing her hair. Susan was also instructed in abdominal breathing for relaxation purposes and autogenic relaxation. When her pain would start to escalate, Susan was to practice these relaxation techniques. Treatment also included instruction in proper posture, body mechanics, and energy conservation techniques.

and sleep disturbances have been suggested.[17] Genetic factors, physical trauma, peripheral pain syndromes, hormonal changes, infections, and emotional distress are capable of triggering fibromyalgia. Pharmacological therapies, exercise, and cognitive-behavioral therapy have all proved beneficial.[9]

EVALUATION

Whatever intervention methods (e.g., biomechanical, cognitive behavioral) are used, effective management of pain depends on accurate evaluation. Effective pain control is more likely to occur if pain were assessed on a regular basis like vital signs. Pain behaviors are often targeted in evaluation and intervention.[13] Pain behaviors include guarded movement, bracing, posturing, limping, rubbing, and facial grimacing[13] and are in response to pain and distress.

Numerous standardized pain evaluations exist. An evaluation tool must be valid, reliable, and sensitive. The tool should

be easy to understand, simple to use, and not too time consuming. The evaluation serves as a baseline for determining whether progress has been made. Evaluation is facilitated by qualitative input (e.g., clinical interviews) that can be used in conjunction with evaluations. Popular adult evaluations include the numerical rating scale (NRS), visual analogue scale (VAS), verbal rating scale (VRS), the Brief Pain Inventory (BPI), and pain diaries. See Boxes 28.1 and 28.2 for examples. Information on activity patterns, time use, occupational performance, and changes in habits, roles, and routines can be used in collaborative goal setting. Pain intensity is the primary focus of these evaluations.[10]

Numerical Rating Scale

Self-report is the primary approach to pain assessment. The numerical rating scale (NRS) was developed for individuals ages 6 years and older. The NRS consists of a series of whole numbers ranging from 0 (no pain) to 10 (worst pain possible). The client indicates which number best describes the pain

---

BOX 28.1 Examples of Pain Intensity Scales

Simple Descriptive Pain Intensity Scale*

| No pain | Mild pain | Moderate pain | Severe pain | Very severe pain | Worst pain possible |

0–10 Numeric Pain Intensity Scale*

| 0 | 1 | 2 | 3 | 4 | 5 | 6 | 7 | 8 | 9 | 10 |

No pain — Moderate pain — Worst pain possible

Visual Analogue Scale (VAS)†

No pain — Pain as bad as it could possibly be

*If used as a graphic rating scale, a 10-cm baseline is recommended.
†A 10-cm baseline is recommended for VAS scales.
From U.S. Department of Health and Human Services, Acute Pain Management Guideline Panel: *Acute pain management in adults: operative procedures. Quick reference guide for clinicians*, AHCPR Pub No. 92-0019, Rockville, MD, 1995, U.S. Government Printing Office.

BOX 28.2 Pain Interference Scales

A. *In the past week*, how much has pain interfered with your daily activities?

0–10 Numeric Pain Intensity Scale

| 0 | 1 | 2 | 3 | 4 | 5 | 6 | 7 | 8 | 9 | 10 |

No interference — Unable to carry out any activities

B. *In the past week*, how much has pain interfered with your ability to take part in recreational, social, and family activities?

0–10 Numeric Pain Intensity Scale

| 0 | 1 | 2 | 3 | 4 | 5 | 6 | 7 | 8 | 9 | 10 |

No interference — Unable to carry out any activities

C. *In the past week*, how much has pain interfered with your ability to work (including housework)?

0–10 Numeric Pain Intensity Scale

| 0 | 1 | 2 | 3 | 4 | 5 | 6 | 7 | 8 | 9 | 10 |

No interference — Unable to carry out any activities

From National Institutes of Health, National Institute of Child Health and Human Development, National Institute of Neurological Disorders and Stroke: Ongoing research (Grant No. 1 PO1 HD/NS33988), Pain Management.

intensity for a given time interval (e.g., current, past week). In most client samples, ratings in the range of 1 to 4 have a minimal impact on function and can be termed "mild" pain. At 5 or 6, the client reports the pain has a greater impact; this would be termed "moderate" pain. Ratings ranging from 7 to 10 have the greatest impact on function and are labeled "severe" pain. The NRS has high reliability and validity.[22]

Visual Analogue Scale

The visual analogue scale (VAS) was developed for persons ages 10 and older. This scale consists of a horizontal or vertical line, typically 100 mm long, with each end of the line labeled with descriptors representing the extremes of pain intensity (e.g., "no pain" on one end and "worst pain imaginable" on the other end of the line). The client places a mark on the line that best describes the pain. The distance measured from the "no pain" mark to the mark placed by the client along the line becomes the individual's VAS pain score. The VAS has a high number of response categories, demonstrated score changes reflecting response to intervention, and high test-retest reliability. However, for some individuals, understanding and completing the measure is difficult. Scoring is more time consuming than other pain intensity measures.[22]

Verbal Rating Scale

The verbal rating scale (VRS) of pain intensity consists of a list of verbal descriptors. The scale was developed for individuals as young as age 6 years. The client selects the one word that best describes the pain intensity. Clients should be cautioned that the list could be lengthy and that the individually preferred descriptor may not be on the list. VRSs are adequately valid and reliable.[10] For both the VAS and VRS, decreases between 30% and 35% appear to indicate meaningful change in pain.[22]

Brief Pain Inventory (BPI) Pain Interference Scale

Pain interference refers to the extent pain interferes with one's day-to-day occupational performance. The BPI Pain Interference scale is used to measure pain interference. The BPI scale consists of seven items that assess the extent to which pain has interfered with general activity, mood, walking ability, normal work (both work outside the home and housework), relations with other people, sleep, and enjoyment of life. Clients rate the degree of interference for each item on a numerical scale of 0 (does not interfere) to 10 (completely interferes). The responses to the seven items are then averaged to form the Pain Interference score. The BPI scale's mobility category was modified to "ability to get around," making it possible for individuals with mobility restrictions unrelated to pain to rate the impact of pain on their mobility. The scale also has been modified to include self-care, recreational activities, social activities, communication, and learning new skills. This information may be helpful in establishing baseline levels for specific occupations and participation that might be targeted in treatment as well as an outcome measure. There are both short (for clinical use) and long forms. The BPI is available in numerous languages.[22]

Pain Diaries

Paper and electronic pain diaries provide another way for clients to communicate their private pain experiences to the healthcare team. The client is requested to make routine entries that can be used to track precipitating and exacerbating pain factors; activity levels; the frequency, duration, intensity of pain episode; pain medication use; and rest time. For some individuals, keeping a diary might exacerbate pain because of their increased attention to it.[11] Pain diaries can be used with people as young as age 12 years.[10]

Measuring Outcomes

The evaluations described previously can be used to measure the effectiveness of pain interventions. Clinical improvement in pain intensity can be measured as described in the NRS paragraph. Changes in occupational performance and pain interference can be assessed with the BPI. Pain diaries can be used to determine activity levels, social participation, and time use. The outcome measures should be statistically and clinically significant.[40]

Regardless of the pain assessment instrument used, any pain evaluation must acknowledge that cultural and ethnic disparities in pain experiences and treatment exists.[26] Persons with a lower socioeconomic status (SES) tend to be sicker and overall have more chronic health problems compared to those at a higher SES level. Additionally, pain frequently has been overlooked and therefore undertreated in children and the elderly.[37] These differences have been attributed to numerous causes such as limited access to healthcare and poor coping skills.

THREADED CASE STUDY

Susan, Part 3

Susan's initial daily treatment program consisted of 10 shoulder flexion exercises of 95 degrees and washing her hair in a forward bent position. Susan would allow warm water as tolerated to the back of her neck and shoulders for 5 minutes. She performed abdominal breathing throughout the activities as a means to decreasing pain. Each day she would go for a walk or swim, which eventually gave her pleasure. Susan would assume correct posture and body mechanics during sitting, standing, and walking.

INTERVENTION

The obligation to manage pain and relieve a client's suffering is fundamental in providing client-centered services.[18] Pain is a complex problem that warrants biopsychosocial interventions. The biopsychosocial model states pain is an interaction of physical (e.g., tissue damage), psychological (e.g., anxiety), and socioenvironmental (e.g., role obligations) factors. The choice of intervention depends on objective findings, pain characteristics (frequency, duration, intensity of pain), the client's overt management (e.g., taking medication), covert responses (e.g., depression), and physiological (e.g., muscle tension) behaviors in addition to the practitioner's training.[10] The ultimate goal of treatment is to reestablish the client's occupational roles, occupational performance, and participation despite the pain.[10,30]

Multidisciplinary Treatment

A multidisciplinary pain clinic is a healthcare delivery facility staffed by physicians of different specialties and other healthcare professionals (e.g., nurses, occupational therapists [OTs], physical therapists, psychologists) who specialize in the evaluation and treatment of chronic pain. Treatment may occur on an inpatient or outpatient basis.[19]

Medication

Medications are typically the treatment of choice for acute pain and often prescribed by the physician. Occupational therapists need to observe clients for possible drug reactions. To ease pain from rehabilitative procedures, practitioners should check if the client is adequately medicated before treatment. Acetaminophen and aspirin are used in the treatment of mild pain (e.g., headache) because of their high level of effectiveness, low level of toxicity, and low abuse potential. Nonsteroidal antiinflammatory drugs (NSAIDs) are used to treat inflammation of a musculoskeletal nature and arthritis. Codeine may be used for moderate intensity pain that has not responded to acetaminophen and aspirin. Morphine is the standard medication for severe pain. Finally, the use of opioids (narcotics) for severe short-lived pain is controversial because of concerns about addiction. Behavioral and physical interventions should be pursued over opioids.[9]

Activity Tolerance

In the past, clients with chronic pain were instructed to rest. Current advice now is to keep active, whether to relieve the pain or to combat related problems (e.g., decreased strength). Activity levels are gradually increased with the client working to "tolerance" (i.e., gradual increase in task demands such as mobility) as opposed to "pain" before a scheduled rest break.[13] Rest at the onset of pain is avoided because it may reinforce pain behaviors. A gradual increase in activity decreases the likelihood of a pain flare-up. Fordyce provided guidelines for *quota programs*. Quota programs typically provide a target of the number of repetitions and gradually increase the target. Regular gentle exercise (e.g., walking, swimming) is prescribed. Detailed baselines are recorded. The practitioner then establishes a quota for each exercise. Initial quotas are slightly lower than baseline trials (e.g., about 75% of baseline mean) and are gradually increased by predetermined small amounts (e.g., about 10% every few days). Modalities such as heat and cold may be used before activity as a means of enhancing functional performance. When an individual is distracted in purposeful activity, that person may become more relaxed, less preoccupied with the pain, and more fluid in movement. Task selection based on occupational roles, interests, and abilities is a unique contribution of occupational therapy in pain control.[9,10,36]

Therapeutic Modalities

Occupational therapists may use physical agent modalities (PAMs) in preparation for therapeutic activities. Appropriate postprofessional education is required to ensure the practitioner is competent (see Chapter 29). Heat and ice are known to relieve pain and muscle spasm. Hot packs, heating pads, paraffin wax, fluidotherapy, hydrotherapy, whirlpool, and heat lamps can conduct superficial heat. The application of heat increases local metabolism and circulation. Vasoconstriction is followed by vasodilatation, resulting in muscle relaxation. Heat is used in the treatment of subacute and chronic traumatic and inflammatory conditions (e.g., muscle spasms). Heat has been found helpful in the relief of muscle spasms, arthritis of the small and large joints of the hands and feet, tendinitis, and bursitis.[2]

Heat is contraindicated in acute inflammatory diseases, malignancies, cardiac insufficiency, or peripheral vascular disease. Heat may aggravate preexisting edema and cause malignancies to spread. Heat should not be used with clients who are insensate.

Cold affords pain relief through increasing the pain threshold (i.e., minimal level of noxious stimulation at which the client initially reports pain). Local vasoconstriction occurs in response to cryotherapy. In addition, cold applications decrease local metabolism, slow nerve conduction velocity, decrease muscle spasm, decrease edema, and diminish tissue damage. Cold can be applied via ice cups, massage sticks, sprays, or commercial packs.[2]

There are numerous contraindications in the use of cryotherapy. Clients who are extremely sensitive may not be able to tolerate the cold. Cryotherapy cannot be used in an area with a history of frostbite. If a client has Raynaud disease, severe pain might result in the affected area. Cryotherapy is contraindicated in the very young and old because their thermoregulatory responses may not function sufficiently.[33,34]

Transcutaneous Electrical Nerve Stimulation

Transcutaneous electrical nerve stimulation (TENS) is a nonpharmacological intervention for acute and chronic pain. This battery-powered device delivers alternating currents via cutaneous electrodes positioned near the painful area. Some success has been demonstrated with using TENS to relieve specific chronic painful conditions caused by disease or injury of nervous system structures or the skeleton, muscle pain of ischemic origin in the extremities. The evidence for TENS efficacy is incomplete, and continued research is advocated to determine correct dosing and use for specific conditions.[38] Emerging evidence exists to support the use of TENS with individuals who have diabetic peripheral neuropathy, fibromyalgia, and complex regional pain syndrome. Use of TENS to relieve pain in individuals with neuropathic pain and osteoarthritis is inconclusive.[27]

Posture and Body Mechanics

Posture refers to keeping bones in the back in their natural curves. Proper posture reduces the risk of back pain, resulting in better respiration and increased energy. Guidelines for standing posture (e.g., avoid learning to one side), sitting posture (e.g., keep feet supported), and sleeping posture (e.g., use pillows to support curves) exist. Body mechanics refers to maintaining good posture when moving. Basic body mechanics emphasize keeping the backbones in line, keeping a wide base of support, and avoiding bending and twisting the back. The intervention plan should include practicing using proper posture and body mechanics safely and to maximize performance during routine tasks in natural environments such as home and work.[9,31]

Energy Conservation, Pacing, and Joint Protection

Instruction in energy conservation, pacing, and joint protection may be beneficial for achieving recommended amounts of rest during task completion, recommended time spent physically active, and balance between rest and physical activity. Clients, especially those with rheumatoid arthritis, are taught to use these strategies before they experience pain and fatigue so that occupational performance can continue as long as possible without pain and fatigue.[14]

Splints

Splints are low-cost aides that may provide relief of chronic pain. Splints reduce swelling and provide joint support. The splint immobilizes the affected joint in the proper position so as to promote healing. Splints have been used in the treatment of osteoarthritis and rheumatoid arthritis.

Relaxation

Relaxation training can decrease muscle tension, a known precipitating and exacerbating pain factor. There are a variety of relaxation techniques. Deep breathing can induce relaxation. The process is as follows: the client assumes a comfortable position; the client is instructed to notice the breathing pattern without trying to change it; the client is then asked to breathe through the nose, place hands on the abdomen while relaxing the stomach muscles. The client is instructed to continue deep breathing and while breathing, imagines tension being breathed away.

Progressive muscle relaxation involves the systematic tensing of major skeletal muscles for a few seconds, passive focusing of attention on how the tension feels, and then release of the muscles and passive focusing on the sensation of relaxation.[9]

Autogenic relaxation is another relaxation option. It involves the silent repetition of self-directed positive phrases that describe the psychophysiological aspects of relaxation (e.g., "My arms and legs are warm with relaxation.") The client passively concentrates on these phrases while assuming a comfortable body position with eyes closed, arms and legs uncrossed, and while doing abdominal breathing.[9] Susan was instructed in how to use autogenic relaxation techniques in her daily activities as a means of diminishing the pain.

Another relaxation option is imagery. This technique involves assuming a comfortable position, gently closing the eyes, uncrossing the arms and legs, and gently breathing. The client imagines a beautiful place that can be gone to anytime. The client is aware of his or her senses. When ready to return to one's normal level of awareness, one takes in a deep breath, gently exhales, gradually opens eyes, and stretches.[6]

Finally, mindfulness involves focusing one's awareness on the present moment while calmly accepting one's feelings, thoughts, and bodily sensations. With all of these techniques the client learns to recognize tension and with one's first awareness, he or she can focus on relieving it. A variety of chronic pain complaints, including low back pain, headaches, myofascial pain, arthritis, and cancer pain have responded to relaxation training.[9,32]

Biofeedback

Biofeedback refers to instrumentation used to measure physiological changes (e.g., hand temperature) as they occur. The signals increase the client's awareness of these changes so the changes come under voluntary control. Biofeedback is based on the assumption that a maladaptive psychophysiological results in pain. Biofeedback has been found effective in the treatment of headache disorders, low back pain, arthritis, and myofascial pain.[9]

Distraction

Distraction is used to divert an individual's attention away from mild-to-moderate pain, especially during medical and rehabilitative procedures. Listening to music, visualization, blowing bubbles, and counting numbers are simple diversion techniques.

Relapse

Chronic pain can be very uncontrollable, with flare-ups occurring. A flare-up is a period of severe pain that is more intense than daily chronic pain. Typically, the pain has a sudden onset with a gradual regression. Flare-ups accompany many conditions such as arthritis, LBP, and fibromyalgia. Flare-ups affect activity participation. There are numerous steps when implementing a plan to address a flare-up: (1) pay attention to what may cause the flare-up, (2) find patterns in pain onset and relief, (3) develop an action plan (e.g., temporarily decreasing aerobic activity, (4) practice relaxation techniques, and (5) use distraction strategies.

Prevention

Approximately 19.6 million persons have high-impact chronic pain (e.g., peripheral neuropathy, cancer pain). The entire person and the environment are affected by chronic pain. The impact of pain on an individual's life depends on the severity and duration of pain and the individual's ability to cope with pain. Chronic pain can result in reduced activity performance and social isolation. Numerous physical, genetic, environmental, psychological, and social factors interact with pathophysiology to contribute from acute to chronic pain. Physical factors include inflammation and muscle tension. Psychological factors include depression and anxiety. Environmental factors are abuse and exposure to disease. Any of these factors initiate acute pain and allow for the transition to chronic pain. As these conditions persist, the pain may change and it is thought that around 3 months of persistent pain in a local body region changes in the central nervous system begin to occur. The changes involve the rewiring of the neural pathways to compensate for ongoing pain. General health guidelines on how to reduce the chance of developing chronic pain are as follows: maintain healthy diet and weight, exercise regularly, eliminate alcohol and smoking, work and rest in healthy postures, manage stress, and seek psychological counseling.[20]

SUMMARY

Pain is a significant healthcare problem. Occupational therapists bring their understanding of a biopsychosocial model and of function to the comprehensive evaluation and intervention of pain. Treatment emphasizes pain relief, improving occupational performance, and enhancing coping. Data are needed to support the use of occupational therapy interventions.

REVIEW QUESTIONS

1. How does acute pain evolve into chronic pain?
2. Describe a pain syndrome according to Loeser and Fordyce's model of pain.
3. List three components of a comprehensive pain evaluation.

For additional practice questions for this chapter, please visit eBooks.Health.Elsevier.com.

REFERENCES

1. Baptiste S: Chronic pain, activity and culture, *Can J Occup Ther* 55:179–184, 1988.
2. Breines EB: Therapeutic occupations and modalities. In Pendleton HM, Schultz-Krohn W, editors: *Pedretti's occupational therapy; practice skills for physical dysfunction* ed 6, St. Louis, 2006, Mosby.
3. Centers for Disease Control and Prevention. Arthritis-related statistics, 2021. https://www.cdc.gov/arthritis/data_statistics/arthritis-related-stats.htm.
4. Clauw D, Brummett C: Fibromyalgia: a discrete disease at the end of the continuum. In Ballantyne JC, Fishman SM, Rathmell JP, editors: *Bonica's management of pain* ed 5, Philadelphia, 2019, Wolters Kluwer, pp 525–542.
5. Deshaies L: Arthritis. In Pendleton HM, Schultz-Krohn W, editors: *Pedretti's occupational therapy: practice skills for physical dysfunction* ed 8, St. Louis, 2018, Elsevier, pp 945–971.
6. Dunford E, Thompson M: Relaxation and mindfulness in pain: a review, *Rev Pain* 4(1):18–22, 2010.
7. Duthey B, Scholten W: Adequacy of opioid analgesic consumption at country, global, and regional levels in 2010, its relationship with development level, and changes compared with 2006. *Journal of Pain and Symptom Management* 47(2):283–297, 2014. http://dx.doi.org/10.1016/j.jpainsymman.2013.03.015.
8. Engel, JM: Pain management. In Pedretti LW, Early MB, editors: *Occupational therapy: practice skills for physical dysfunction*, ed 5. St. Louis, 2001, Elsevier, pp 493–500.
9. Engel, JM: Pain management. In Pendleton HM, Schultz-Krohn W, editors: *Pedretti's occupational therapy: practice skills for physical dysfunction*, ed 8, St Louis, 2018, Elsevier, pp 701–709.
10. Engel, JM: Pain. In Brown C, Stoffel VC, Munoz JP, editors: *Occupational therapy in mental health: a vision for participation*, ed 2, Philadelphia, 2019, FA Davis, pp 421–434.
11. Ferrari R: Effect of a pain diary use on recovery from acute low back (lumbar) sprain, *Rheumatology International* 35(1):55–59, 2015.
12. Fishman S: Forensic pain medicine, *Pain Med* 5:212–213, 2004.
13. Fordyce WE: *Behavioral methods for chronic pain and illness*, St. Louis, 1976, Mosby.
14. Furst GP, et al: A program for improving energy conservation behaviors in adults with rheumatoid arthritis, *Am J Occup Ther* 41(2):102–111, 1987.
15. Gardner GC: Joint pain. In Fishman SM, Ballantyne JC, Rathmell JP, editors: *Bonica's management of pain*, ed 4, Philadelphia, 2010, Lippincott Williams & Wilkins, pp 431–450.
16. Goadsby PJ: Headache. In Ballantyne JC, Fishman SM, Rathnell JP, editors: *Bonica's management of pain*, ed 5, Philadelphia, 2019, Wolters Kluwer.
17. Hernandez-Garcia JM: Fibromyalgia. In Warfield CA, Fausett HJ, editors: *Manual of pain management* ed 2, Philadelphia, 2002, Lippincott Williams & Wilkins.
18. International Association for the Study of Pain. Declaration of Montreal. http://www.iasp-pain.org/DeclarationofMontreal,2018.
19. International Association for the Study of Pain. Pain clinic guidelines, 2021. http://www.iasp-pain.org/Education/Content.aspx?ItemNumber=1471.
20. International Association for the Study of Pain. 2020 Global Year for the Prevention of Pain Factsheet. https://www.sip-platform.eu/resources/details/iasp-2020-global-year-for-the-prevention-of-pain.
21. Intragency Pain Research Coordinating Committee: *National pain strategy: A comprehensive population health-level strategy for pain*, Washington, D.C., 2016, U.S. Department of Health and Human Services, National Institutes of Health.
22. Jensen MP: Measurement of pain. In Ballantyne JC, Fishman SM, Rathmell JP, editors: *Bonica's management of pain* ed 5, Philadelphia, 2019, Wolters Kluwer, pp 272–294.
23. Keefe FJ, Block AR: Development of an observation method for assessing pain behavior in chronic low back pain patients, *Behav Ther* 13:363, 1982.
24. King W, Bogduk N: Chronic low back pain. In Ballantyne JC, Fishman SM, Rathnell JP, editors: *Bonica's management of pain* ed 5, Philadelphia, 2019, Wolters Kluwer, pp 1259–1282.
25. Loeser JD, Fordyce WE: Chronic pain. In Carr JE, Dengerink HA, editors: *Behavioral science in the practice of medicine*, New York, 1983, Elsevier.
26. Meints SM, Cortes A, Morais CA, Edwards RR: Racial and ethnic differences in the experience and treatment of noncancer pain, *Pain Management* 9:317–334, 2019. https://doi.org/10.2217/pmt-2018-0030.
27. Mokhtari T, Ren Q, Li N, Wang F, Bi Y, Hu L: Transcutaneous electrical nerve stimulation in relieving neuropathic pain: basic mechanisms and clinical applications, *Current Pain and Headache Reports* 24(4):14, 2020. https://doi.org/10.1007/s11916-020-0846-1.
28. Mosey AC: An alternative: the biopsychosocial model, *American Journal of Occupational Therapy* 28:137–140, 1974.
29. National Cancer Institute. Cancer treatment. http://www.cancer.gov/about-cancer/treatment,2020.
30. National Institute of Neurological Disorders and Stroke. Pain: hope through research, 2020, https://www.ninds.nih.gov/current-research/focus-disorders/focus-pain-research.

31. Occupational and Physiotherapy Departments and Educational Services for the Respiratory Rehabilitation Program. Back pain, posture and body mechanics, 2020, https://www.stjoes.ca/patients-visitors/patient-education/a-e/PD%205844%20Resp%20Rehab%20-%20Back%20Pain%20and%20Posture.pdf.

32. Payne RA: *Relaxation techniques: a practical handbook for the health care professional*, New York, 2000, Churchill Livingstone.

33. Prentice WE: *Therapeutic modalities in rehabilitation*, New York, 2018, McGraw-Hill Education.

34. Rakel B, Barr JO: Physical modalities in chronic pain management, *Nurs Clin North Am* 38(3):477–494, 2003.

35. Spencer EA: Upper extremity musculoskeletal impairments. In Crepeau EB, Cohn ES, Schell BAB, editors: *Willard & Spackman's occupational therapy* ed 10, Philadelphia, 2003, Lippincott.

36. Strong J: *Chronic pain: the occupational therapist's perspective*, New York, 1996, Churchill Livingstone.

37. Szafran SH: Physical, mental, and spiritual approaches to managing pain in older clients, *OT Practice* 16:CE-1–CE-8, 2011.

38. Vance CGT, Dailey DL, Rakel BA, Sluka KA: Using TENS for pain control; the state of the evidence, *Pain Manag* 4(3):197–209, 2014.

39. Van den Beuken-van Everdingen MH, Hochstenbach LM, Joosten EA, Tjan-Heijnen VC, Janssen DJ: Update on prevalence of pain in patients with cancer: a systematic review and meta analysis, *J Pain Symptom Manage* 51(6):1070–1090, 2016.

40. Younger J, McCue R, Mackey S: Pain outcomes: a brief review of instruments and techniques, *Curr Pain Headache Rep* 13(1):39–43, 2009.

Therapeutic Occupations and Modalities

Jacqueline Reese Walter and Kristin Winston

LEARNING OBJECTIVES

After studying this chapter, the student or practitioner will be able to do the following:

1. Recognize and differentiate occupation, activity, and interventions to support occupation as they relate to intervention choices.
2. Discuss the role of occupational analysis and activity analysis in the selection of intervention strategies.
3. Understand the similarities and distinctions between therapeutic activity and therapeutic exercise as intervention strategies.
4. Describe how grading and adapting intervention choices heighten occupational performance.
5. Describe how occupation, activity, and interventions to support occupation are used in practice in different contexts through case study exploration.
6. Differentiate between the various types of therapeutic exercise as intervention strategies.
7. Describe how and why intervention to support occupation, such as physical agent modalities (PAMs), are used in occupational therapy practice.
8. Identify the role of physical agent modalities in OT practice.
9. Identify the requirements established by the American Occupational Therapy Association for the use of physical agent modalities in occupational therapy practice.

KEY TERMS

Adapting	Occupation	Therapeutic activity
Grading	Physical agent modalities	Therapeutic exercise

THREADED CASE STUDY

Fareed

Fareed is a 66-year-old who identifies as male (prefers use of the pronouns he/him/his). Fareed is a semi-retired (working part time) bookkeeper whose primary diagnosis is status post (s/p) right cerebrovascular accident (CVA). The stroke resulted in his hospitalization and subsequent admission to a subacute facility. He has a medical history of hypertension and prostate cancer, and he has exhibited reactive depression since his recent hospitalization.

Before this recent hospitalization, Fareed lived with his wife in a private two-story home in a suburban neighborhood and was fully independent for activities of daily living (ADLs) and instrumental ADLs (IADLs). He has a master's degree in finance and a strong value for education. Fareed's Islamic faith is an important part of his spirituality, including personal and environmental contextual factors related to his spiritual practices. One of his children lives in a nearby town and visits weekly. His other two children and their families live in cities within a day's drive and visit several times a year. Since his change to semi-retirement and working part time as a bookkeeper, Fareed has developed or expanded several interests, including woodworking, gardening, cooking, and traveling. In all, before the CVA, Fareed had an active schedule and was engaged in varied occupations before his recent hospitalization.

The initial evaluation in the subacute facility revealed that Fareed requires moderate assistance for dressing and bathing. He requires set-up for grooming and mealtimes (e.g., opening containers, positioning the tray, and cutting foods as needed). Once items are set up, Fareed is able to independently feed himself using a spoon and a fork; he requires assistance with cutting. He is also independent with drinking from a cup. He exhibits a mild left visual field cut.

He requires minimum (min) assistance for bed mobility. Results of the Berg Balance Scale indicate that Fareed is able to move from sit to stand with min assistance to stand or stabilize, and one-person min assist to complete a stand and pivot transfer. He is able to sit unsupported at the edge of the bed (EoB) with arms folded for up to 30 seconds. When interacting within his environment, he requires min assist to maintain his dynamic sitting balance. Fareed requires several attempts to maintain a standing position for 30 seconds unsupported. When engaging in occupations, he requires min assist from another person to maintain dynamic standing balance.

Evaluation of upper extremity function revealed residual shoulder and hand pain of his left upper extremity (LUE). Fareed's range of motion (ROM) and strength are within normal limits in his right upper extremity (RUE). In the LUE he has full passive range of motion (PROM) but limited active ROM (AROM) to 100 degrees because of weakness and pain near the end of the range. His L shoulder strength is 3/5. Although active ROM is limited in the LUE, Fareed is able to maintain a gross grasp; however, he requires assistance to initiate opening his fingers secondary to increased tone. He is able to pronate his forearm, flex the elbow, and internally rotate the shoulder with a gross manual muscle grade of 3/5. Although his prospects for recovery are positive, Fareed expresses feelings of grief over his loss of function and discouragement about regaining his ability to resume his independence, roles, and occupations.

The focus of occupational therapy (OT) intervention included the following:
- Prepare Fareed and family with skills needed for him to return home through client and family education
- Engage in meaningful occupations to reduce feelings of grief over his loss of function and discouragement
- Adapt and grade occupations and activities
- Reduce pain associated with movement to enable use of LUE in occupations through the use of preparatory methods and modalities
- Increase ROM and strength of LUE to facilitate occupational performance in ADLs, leisure, and work
- Improve balance and mobility through participation in occupations and activities to facilitate occupational performance in ADLs, leisure, and work
- Prepare Fareed to resume occupations and social participation with family, friends, and co-workers

Critical Thinking Questions

1. Using the OTPF-4, explore the contextual factors that influence Fareed in resuming the occupation of gardening.
2. Describe how the occupation and activities of gardening (a favored occupation) could be graded to address concerns in performance skills.
3. Identify and describe the hierarchy of interventions the occupational therapist might use to address the limitations Fareed is experiencing in his LUE. Specifically, the limitations Fareed is experiencing include L shoulder pain, decreased L shoulder AROM (especially at end range), decreased strength in LUE, and decreased functional use of the LUE.

OCCUPATIONAL THERAPY INTERVENTION

OTPF-4 as the Foundation for Intervention Planning and Implementation

In 2020 the American Occupational Therapy Association (AOTA) developed the fourth edition of the "Occupational Therapy Practice Framework: Domain and Process"[1] (OTPF-4), a document that describes occupational therapy practice. The Framework describes the domain of occupational therapy practice as the "profession's purview and the areas in which its members have an established body of knowledge and expertise" (OTPF-4, p. 4). In addition, the Framework explores the occupational therapy process, which describes "the actions practitioners take when providing services that are client centered and focused on engagement in occupations"[1] (OTPF-4, p. 4). This chapter will focus primarily on aspects of intervention related to the process of occupational therapy.

Occupation

Occupation is the foundation of OT practice.[28] Occupations may include personal care, caregiving, leisure occupations (e.g.,

reading, bowling, games, crafting), schoolwork (including the use of technology such as computers and iPads), work, and vocational pursuits. In support of engagement in a variety of occupations, Wilcock[34] states that "a varied and full occupational lifestyle will coincidentally maintain and improve health and well-being if it allows people to be creative and adventurous physically, mentally, and socially."

When clients face a physical disability and occupational performance becomes impaired, the OT practitioner works with clients to regain skills, using occupation as both means and ends. Trombly[31] describes occupation as end as "not only purposeful but also meaningful because it is the performance of activities or tasks that a person sees as important" (p. 963). Gillen[10] refers to this as the use of occupations that are the end product of the intervention. For example, an intervention focused on improving a client's ability to complete a meal for the family would be considered an end product. Occupation as means "refers to occupation acting as the therapeutic change agent to remediate impaired abilities or capacities"[31] (p. 964). For example, cooking (mixing and stirring) may be used to improve shoulder range of motion (ROM) and strength for a client who enjoys cooking.

Ultimately the focus of OT intervention is to design an intervention that enables clients to assume or resume their ability to engage in their desired life occupations.[28] The needs and interests of clients guide the selection of occupations used as intervention in therapy. These needs are often governed by the roles clients play in their worlds. The clients' needs and interests are tied to the societies in which they live. In a society in which independence, leisure, and work are all valued, the interests of clients are variable and include self-care, hobbies, and work-related tasks. Thus, OT practitioners must remember that clients have an inner drive to engage in occupations beyond self-care or self-maintenance, which Tubbs and Drake[32] point out is "too often the starting and stopping point of most traditional rehabilitation programs" (p. 12). As OT practitioners working with clients with physical dysfunction, it is important to have a broad focus with regard to the scope of intervention.

RELATIONSHIPS AMONG PERSON, ENVIRONMENT, AND OCCUPATION AS THEY RELATE TO INTERVENTION CHOICES

There are many factors that OT practitioners address as a part of the intervention planning process. Occupational therapy practitioners complete a thorough analysis of each client's interests and abilities and the contexts within which the client engages in occupations. Intervention choices are based on this analysis and may address aspects of the person, the environment or context, and/or occupations themselves. Intervention decisions should be made in collaboration with the client, family, and other important people in the client's life as appropriate and as feasible.

Aspects of the person that may influence the OT process include the client's values, beliefs, and spirituality[1] (OTPF-4). What a client values or believes about his or her health, sense of purpose or meaning, and roles in life, for example, will be important factors for the OT practitioner to understand in terms of how these factors will influence intervention choices. In addition, understanding how a diagnosis or disease process may influence the client's body functions and body structures will affect intervention decisions. For example, in the case study, given Fareed's limitations in ROM of his left upper extremity, it will be important to assess the structure of the shoulder girdle as it relates to joint ROM at the shoulder for engagement in occupations.

OT practitioners will also assess the client's performance skills within a variety of occupations, depending on the setting in which they practice. Occupations within an acute care setting may differ from those within a home health setting, based on the client's goals and health status. The Framework describes performance skills as "goal directed actions that result in a client's quality of performing desired occupations"[1] (OTPF-4, p. 89). In the case study, Fareed demonstrates concerns in the area of motor performance skills, such as stabilizing and positioning, reaching and grasping, and moving about his environment. Performance skill deficits may exist in many different areas,

including motor and process skills. It is also important, when planning intervention, to consider what performance skills may be assets for the client in regard to recovery and participation in OT intervention. Performance skills that assist Fareed in his recovery include intact motor skills in his right upper extremity and social interaction skills.

Aspects of context that may influence intervention include environmental factors and personal factors.[1] The environment encompasses natural and human-made aspects of the environment. The OTPF-4 outlines the many facets of context related to the environment. An example of environmental aspects of context to consider for Fareed includes the accessibility of his home, given the two stories, his workplace environment, technology that he needs to access, and the many facets of his social support and relationships. Personal factors are also considered in the provision of occupational services. These factors are "unique aspects of the person that are not part of a health condition or health state" (AOTA, 2020 p. 52). Examples that illustrate Fareed's personal context include his age (66), his gender (he identifies as male), cultural identification or attitudes (his Islamic faith), education (he has a master's degree), and upbringing and life experiences.

How various factors come together to support or inhibit a client's participation in desired and meaningful occupations is at the center of OT practice. Thus, OT practitioners need to develop a wide range of skills related to understanding and facilitating participation and engagement in a variety of occupations across the lifespan and across multiple contexts. For persons with disabilities, participation may require relearning skills, learning new skills, or learning to perform activities in new ways. Therefore, the OT practitioner must be prepared with a broad knowledge of occupations, activities, and techniques that may be used as intervention strategies in a client-centered approach.

TYPES OF OCCUPATIONAL THERAPY INTERVENTION

1. Occupations are described as "the everyday personalized activities that people do as individuals, in families, and with communities to occupy time and bring meaning and purpose to life"[1] (OTPF-4, p. 88). An occupation focus for Fareed might include a focus on his prior independence with self-care, his bookkeeping work, and his leisure interests, including gardening, cooking, traveling, and woodworking.
2. Activities are described as "actions designed and selected to support the development of performance skills and performance patterns to enhance occupational engagement"[1] (OTPF-4, p. 83).
3. Interventions to support occupations are described as "methods and tasks that prepare the client for occupational performance"[1] (OTPF-4, p. 73). The OTPF indicates that these interventions may include the use of physical agent modalities (PAMs) (discussed in detail in this chapter), construction of orthotics or use of prosthetics, assistive technology, wheeled mobility, and self-regulation. Application of PAMs such as hot or cold packs at the beginning of an intervention

session aimed at decreasing pain, improving range of motion, or decreasing edema is an example of an intervention that will prepare a client for participation in occupation. As an example with Fareed, before beginning the activity, to reduce pain in his LUE and improve his tolerance for movement, the OT practitioner applied heat to his shoulder using hot packs as a preparatory aspect of intervention.

4. Education is described as "imparting of knowledge and information about occupation, health, well-being, and participation to enable the client to acquire helpful behaviors, habits, and routines"[1] (OTPF-4, p. 74).

5. Training is described as "facilitation of the acquisition of concrete skills for meeting specific goals in a real-life, applied situation"[1] (OTPF-4, p. 75).

6. Advocacy is described as "efforts directed toward promoting occupational justice and empowering clients to seek and obtain resources to support health, well-being, and occupational participation"[1] (OTPF-4, p. 75).

OCCUPATIONAL ANALYSIS AND ACTIVITY ANALYSIS

Participation in everyday occupation is quite complex when one stops to consider all the aspects that must work smoothly together to be successful. Careful analysis is essential to the selection of appropriate intervention strategies. Analysis should yield information about various occupations and activities as potential intervention strategies for addressing physical dysfunction and facilitating health and wellness. As discussed previously, analysis as a part of intervention planning should be done at the person level, the environment level, and finally the occupation level.

Activity analysis and occupational analysis are important for many reasons. Baum and Christiansen[3] state that "people are naturally motivated to explore their world and demonstrate mastery within it." They go on to state that "situations in which people experience success help them feel good about themselves." Analysis of clients' desired occupations will allow practitioners to create intervention sessions that motivate their clients and help clients experience success. Having done the analysis, practitioners can anticipate and address potential barriers at the person level and the environment level to facilitate self-efficacy in their clients. When people perceive themselves as competent and capable, they are more likely to want to continue to participate in the therapy process.[3] A thorough analysis facilitates OT practitioners' abilities to design and implement intervention strategies that help clients engage or reengage in occupations, roles, and routines that are meaningful and valuable to everyday life.

Occupational and activity analyses facilitate the ability to understand the complex nature of the things we do on a daily basis. For example, understanding the interaction of multiple factors is needed for Fareed to return to his prior level of function in self-care or his computer skills to stay in touch with his family. In addition, this type of analysis allows practitioners to consider the potential meaning that occupations have for clients. As such, intervention strategies cannot be chosen or designed without careful and thorough analysis, the process of looking at all the components and requirements of an activity/occupation, and synthesis, the process of combining all of those factors to facilitate performance.[13]

Activity Analysis

Activity analysis considers activities and tasks in the abstract, or how these things might be done within a certain culture or a given situation.[1,3] Through activity analysis, OT practitioners can begin to anticipate what may facilitate a client's performance and participation. OT practitioners can anticipate where barriers to performance and participation may exist and, through careful selection of intervention strategies, can increase the likelihood of a "just right challenge" for the client in intervention.[30] The just right challenge occurs when OT practitioners design interventions that challenge clients just enough so that they do not become bored or do not see the need for therapy, but the challenge does not result in the client feeling defeated or having a loss of self-efficacy. Completing a general analysis of a variety of activities and tasks allows OT practitioners to prepare options and generate ideas/strategies that may or may not work for clients. Additionally, it provides practitioners with a starting point from which they can then individualize assessment, intervention, and discharge plans. Thomas[30] states that activity analysis can help us to:

- Determine what equipment, materials, space, and time are needed for the activity
- Consider how we might prepare for instructing another by having knowledge of the steps involved in the activity
- Think about how the activity might be therapeutic and for what type of client
- Consider grading and or adapting the activity for greater success
- Identify options for clear documentation
- Think about how context might influence performance
- Consider the just right challenge
- Consider where the client may need help or where he or she will most likely do well (p. 8)

Occupational analysis, in contrast to activity analysis, helps OT practitioners understand the circumstances of the client with whom they are working.[3] In occupational analysis the practitioner considers several questions: What the client wants or needs to do, how the client did things before coming to occupational therapy, what they feel has changed, what environments are typical for the occupations, and where the client envisions occupations taking place in the future. Occupational analysis is about how the individual engages in daily life. Once OT practitioners have completed the analysis, the next step in designing an appropriate intervention is to determine how to structure the intervention strategies to facilitate improvement and participation. One way to do this is through grading and adapting of intervention strategies.

GRADING AND ADAPTING OCCUPATIONS AND ACTIVITIES AS AN INTERVENTION APPROACH

Grading and adapting of occupations and activities is the crossroad where client-centered practice and clinical reasoning meet.

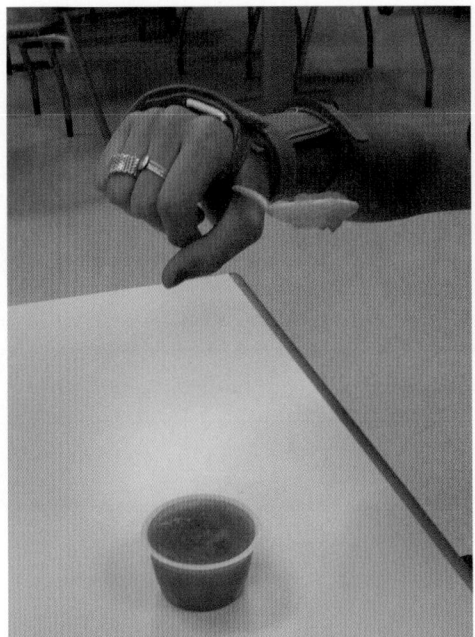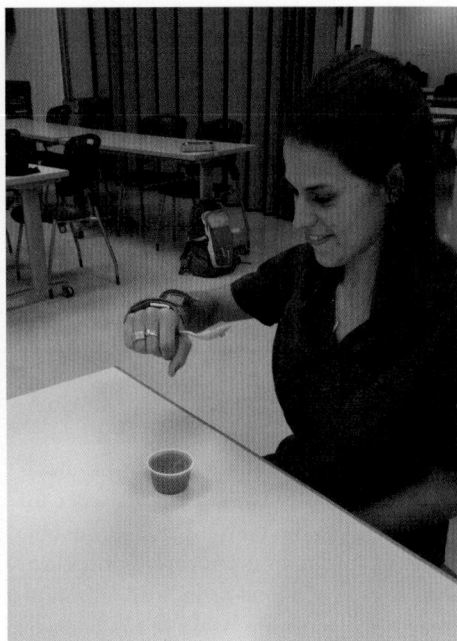

Fig. 29.1 Eating with a special orthosis using a utensil holder fitted to the hand.

The overall goal of grading is to find the just right challenge for the client; that is, one that encourages progress without causing the person to become frustrated or lose self-efficacy, but at the same time creates enough challenge so that the client does not become bored, lose interest, or fail to see the value in participating in the OT session. The overall goal of adapting a client's participation in an occupation or activity is to increase the individual's performance within that occupation or activity.

Adapting (Compensating)

As stated previously, the overall goal of adapting an intervention strategy is to change the occupation or activity to enable a client to continue to participate in that valued occupation and/or activity or find new occupations to participate in. When practitioners adapt an activity or occupation, the intent is to allow for greater participation and independence within the chosen occupation.

The use of adaptation as an intervention strategy requires flexibility on the part of the clinician and the client. Some clients will not want to participate in an occupation if they cannot do so the way they have always participated, "their typical way." For some this means that they may continue to participate in a way that increases their symptoms; for others it may mean that they will give up valued occupations. One concern OT practitioners have is being aware of clients' safety if they choose to continue with previous patterns.

Adaptations to occupations must maintain the intrinsic value and meaning for the client. Many clients will find meaning in new occupations once they see what is possible. In the OTPF-4 section describing Approaches to Intervention,[1] adapting is also seen as modifying or compensating.

It may be necessary to adapt activities to suit the special needs of the client or the environment. An occupation may have to be performed in a special way to accommodate the client's abilities; for example, eating using a special orthosis with a utensil holder fitted to the hand (Fig. 29.1). An occupation may have to be adapted to the positioning of the client or to the environment; for instance, by setting up a special reading stand and providing prism glasses to enable a client to read while supine in bed. The problem-solving ability, creativity, and ingenuity of OT practitioners in making adaptations are some of their unique skills.

As practitioners it is important to remember that for adaptations to be effective, the OT practitioner should collaborate with the client to develop adaptations that will be most applicable to their situation. The client must understand the need and purpose of the activity and the adaptations and must be willing to perform the activity with the modifications. In most cases simpler adaptations are more useful for the client compared to complicated adaptations. The complexity of the adaptation must be decided with the client, not for the client.

GRADING (REMEDIATING)

The overall goal of grading is to "increase or decrease the activity demands on the person while he or she is performing an activity."[30] Grading participation or engagement in an occupation or activity within interventions allows for the just right challenge.[30] Grading allows for the development of skills while at the same time ensuring the client's success within individual sessions. In other words, grading refers to structuring an activity such that the challenge or demand will gradually facilitate improvement in the client's function and participation. There is no one correct way to grade an occupation or activity because multiple factors can be considered in terms of how participation is graded. The clients' goals, current level of function, and the occupational model or frame of reference a practitioner uses will help determine how and what aspects of the occupation or activity are graded within intervention choices.

How does a practitioner begin to grade an intervention strategy? First, the practitioner needs to understand the strengths and needs of the client. Second, the practitioner needs to thoroughly understand the multiple demands of the chosen intervention. Finally, there is the need to determine what factors support the client's participation and what factors hinder their participation. In the OTPF-4, grading is also seen as establishing, restoring, or remediating a skill.[1]

Grading Down

When choosing to "grade down," the OT practitioner seeks to make components or aspects of an intervention strategy easier for the client. For an adult experiencing difficulty with clothing fasteners secondary to muscle weakness or incoordination, the strategy may be to use pull-on clothing or clothing items with large fasteners (e.g., large buttons), making it easier for the client to hold and manipulate the button through the buttonhole until strength and coordination improve. For a client with muscle weakness as a result of a long-term hospitalization, the OT practitioner may begin morning ADLs at the bedside, as opposed to the bathroom, to conserve strength and energy. These are both examples of grading to make participation easier for a client the therapy practitioner believes has the potential to work up to a higher level of skill within these occupations.

Grading Up

When choosing to "grade up," the OT practitioner seeks to make components or aspects of an intervention more challenging for the client. A client recovering from a post-traumatic brain injury who demonstrates the ability to make decisions about meal choices in a quiet clinic environment from a set menu with limited choice needs to be able to do so in the community. To grade up, the intervention session moves from the clinic to working on making meal choices in the hospital cafeteria or a local restaurant, where choices are greater and

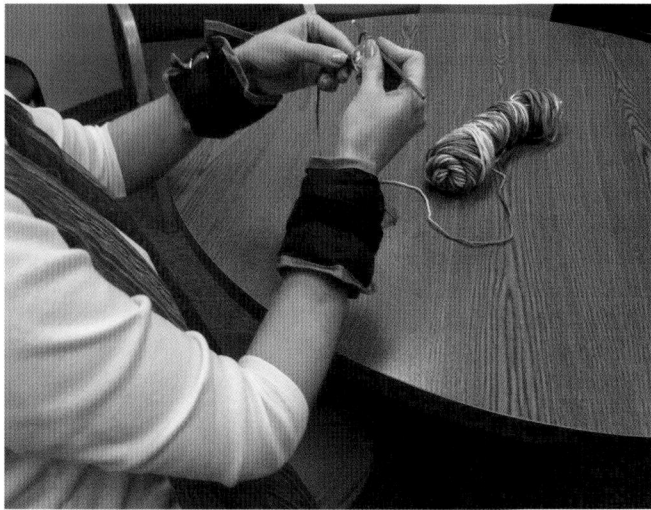

Fig. 29.2 Weight attached to the wrist increases resistance during needlework or crocheting.

the client must deal with multiple factors. This is a busier and more complex environment, thereby increasing the demands on the client. An additional example might be the case of a client with decreased activity tolerance who heretofore has been dressing at the bedside, with all items arranged. The OT practitioner now changes the intervention's focus to work on accessing clothing from the closet and carrying clothing items to a chair beside the bed to increase the demands on the client, with the expectation that they will be able to improve their level of function.

Examples of Grading

Strength

Strength may be graded by an increase or decrease in resistance. Methods to modify the resistance for strengthening can include changing the plane of movement from gravity eliminated, to gravity minimized, to against gravity by adding weights to the equipment or to the client, or by using tools of increasing weights. For example, a weight attached to the wrist by a strap increases resistance to arm movements during needlework or leatherwork (Fig. 29.2) to improve muscle strength while engaged in occupation. When grasp strength is inadequate, grasp mitts may be used to fasten the hand to a tool or equipment handle to assist grip strength and allow arm motion.

Range of Motion

Activities for increasing or maintaining joint ROM may be graded by positioning materials and equipment to demand greater reach or excursion of joints. As the work progresses, the activity itself establishes increased demands on active range. Positioning objects, such as dominos used in a game, at increasing or decreasing distances from the client, changes the range needed to reach the materials (Fig. 29.3). Tool handles, such as those used in eating or painting, may be increased in size by padding the handle with foam tubing to accommodate limited ROM or to facilitate grasp for clients the practitioner thinks will gain ROM as they progress in therapy (Fig. 29.4). Reducing the

---

CAUTION!

When grading an intervention, be sure not to grade down to the extent that the client is not engaged, challenged, or motivated. Conversely, be sure not to grade up such that the client experiences unnecessary struggles, resulting in frustration, a loss of self-efficacy, or loss of motivation. In addition, select only one or two aspects to grade within the occupation/activity at any one time. Grading or changing too many aspects of any intervention/occupation will make it difficult to know what is working or not working as the practitioner documents the client's progress. The example of the client working on meal choices first in the therapy setting and then in the hospital cafeteria or community may change too many parts of the task at one time. If the client is asked to work on making choices in a quiet therapy setting while seated, the task demands are limited compared to maneuvering through a hospital cafeteria or restaurant and making choices for a meal. This client might be experiencing difficulties not only with meal choice, but also with mobility, following directions, balance, or sensory integration concerns. It then becomes difficult to determine which factor to grade for improved performance. The practitioner needs to be confident the client can handle the other factors that have changed in the context. This is where the connection between activity/occupational analysis, clinical reasoning, and grading and adapting becomes most apparent.

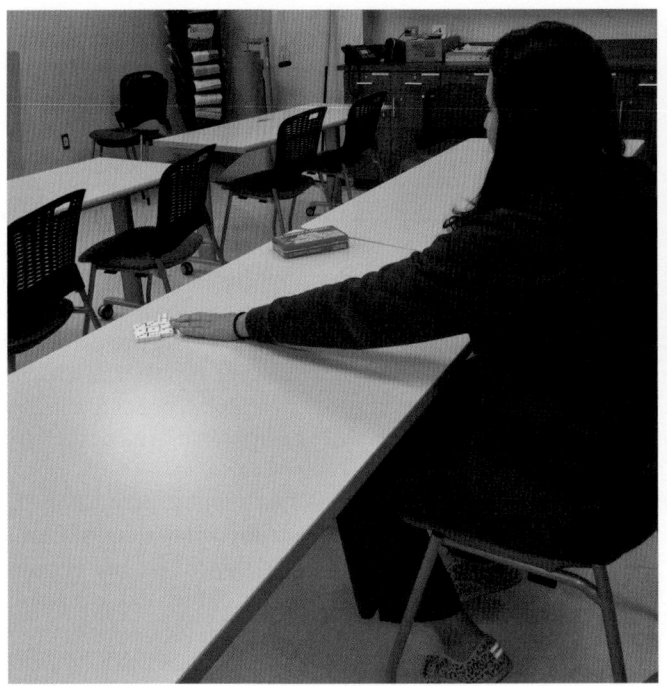
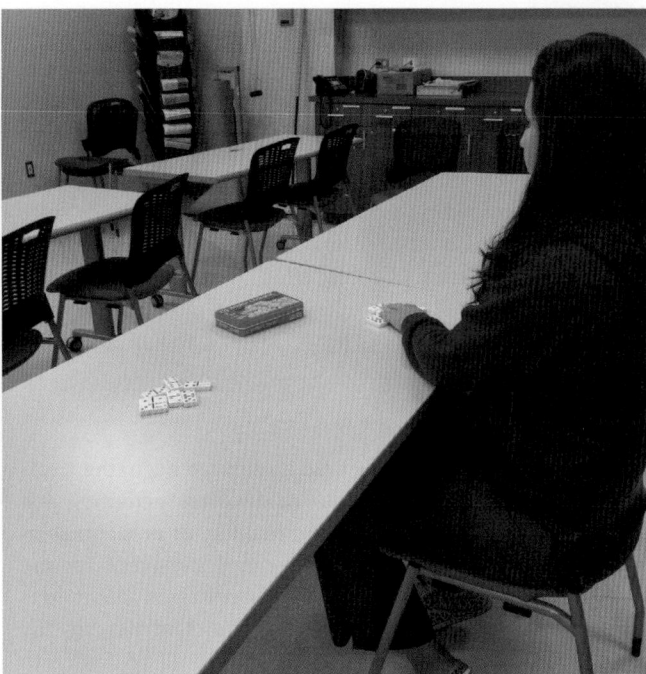

Fig. 29.3 Placing objects at alternate distances changes the range needed to reach materials.

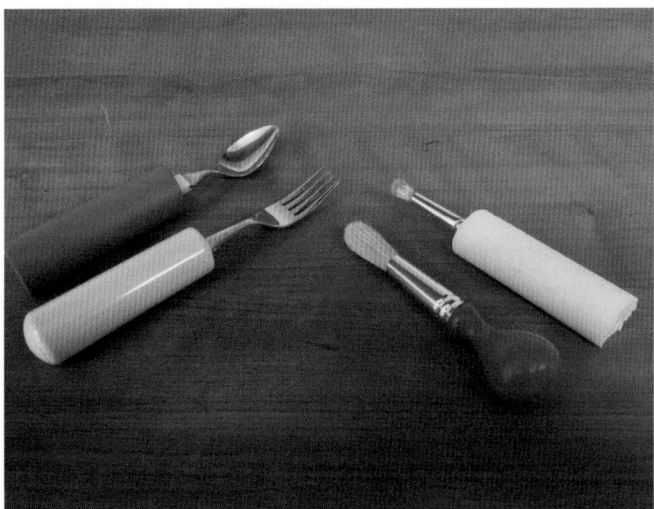

Fig. 29.4 The size of tool handles may be increased by padding the handle with foam tubing.

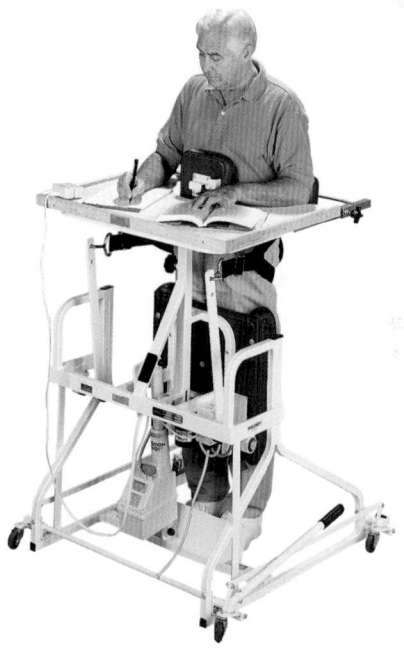

Fig. 29.5 Midland Electric Stand-In Table. Four-point support system stabilizes clients at the feet, knees, buttocks, and chest. (Courtesy Performance Health, Warrenville, IL.)

amount of padding as range or grasp improves is an example of grading up, changing the participation to require increased ROM as ROM becomes available to the client. Reaching for clothing items hung in a closet as opposed to items in a bureau drawer can be used to require an increase in a client's shoulder ROM.

Endurance and Tolerance

Endurance may be graded by moving from light to heavy work and increasing the duration of the work period. Standing and walking tolerance may be graded by an increase in the time spent standing to work, perhaps at first at a standing table (Fig. 29.5), and an increase in the time and distance spent in activities requiring walking, such as home management and gardening activities. Medical conditions that are progressively degenerative, such as muscular dystrophy, multiple sclerosis, or Parkinson's disease, require grading endurance task demands down to make aspects of participation easier for the client. The practitioner and client may decide to begin by discussing how to adapt participation or changing participation to an occupation or activity that requires less effort instead of grading participation.

Coordination

Coordination and muscle control may be graded by decreasing the gross resistive movements and increasing the fine controlled movements required. An example for a client with an interest in craftsmanship is progressing from sawing wood with a cross-cut saw to using a jeweler's saw. Dexterity and speed of movement may be graded by practicing at increasing speeds once movement patterns have been mastered through coordination training and neuromuscular education. Occupational therapy practitioners may wish to consider aspects of motor control and motor learning theory (see Chapter 33) as a way to grade the demands on motor coordination within participation.

Perceptual, Cognitive, and Social Skills

In grading cognitive skills, the practitioner can begin the treatment program with simple one- or two-step activities that require minimal judgment, decision making, or problem solving and progress to activities with several steps that require some judgment or problem-solving processes. A client in a lunch preparation group may butter bread that has already been placed on the work surface. This task could be graded to increase task demands by asking the client to position the bread, butter it, and place a slice of lunch meat on it, and, ultimately, to make several sandwiches.

For grading social interaction, the intervention plan may begin with an activity that demands interaction only with the OT practitioner. The client can progress to activities that require dyadic interaction with another client and, ultimately, to small group activities. The practitioner can facilitate the client's progression from the role of observer to that of participant and then to leader. At the same time, the practitioner decreases the supervision, guidance, and assistance to facilitate more independent functioning in the client.

Multiple factors influence the decision to adapt or grade intervention strategies to support a client's occupational performance. Knowing the client's desired outcomes and understanding the client's ability to change may determine whether the OT practitioner grades or adapts. If there is a belief that the client's condition can change for the better or the diagnosis is static in nature, the choice may be to grade participation with increasing demands. If it is determined that the client's condition will likely not improve, the decision may be to adapt participation. The OT practitioner, in collaboration with the client, will determine the client's interest in new ways of participating in previous occupations through adaptation. The OT practitioner may choose to adapt if the client's skill level is not likely to change or change in the near future or if the diagnosis is degenerative in nature. The choice to grade or adapt may also depend on the length of time established for the client's OT services. If there are multiple visits, the goal may be to grade participation as improvements occur. If there are limited visits, the decision may be made to adapt for safety or independence within an occupation.

The second half of this chapter will focus on the intervention strategies that prepare a client for participation and engagement in occupation, including therapeutic exercise, therapeutic activity, and physical agent modalities. The concepts of analysis, grading, and adapting can be applied to all of these intervention strategies.

INTERVENTIONS TO SUPPORT OCCUPATIONS

Interventions to support occupations are used by the OT practitioner to prepare the client for occupational performance and are carefully selected to address client factors or performance skills that the OT practitioner and the client have identified as barriers to the client's desired occupational performance (OTPF-4). Examples in which the client is an active participant may include using resistive Thera-Bands to increase strength, performing active stretching to restore ROM, opening and closing various-sized jars to improve hand strength and dexterity, or folding and sorting towels on a linen cart.

An example of interventions that support occupation that are more therapist directed include the application of heat to prepare soft tissue for movement or stretch; the use of physical agent modalities such as paraffin or ultrasound to influence soft tissue extensibility and prepare muscles for stretch or movement; the application of a mechanical device, such as a continuous passive motion machine to restore ROM and improve flexibility; and the use of various manual techniques to prepare the client for occupational performance, such as manual edema mobilization or manual lymphatic drainage.

The following sections will further discuss the use of interventions such as therapeutic exercise and therapeutic activity. Additionally, interventions, including physical agent modalities, manual interventions, and the application of mechanical devices and orthoses, will be discussed.

THERAPEUTIC EXERCISE AND THERAPEUTIC ACTIVITY

Therapeutic exercise and therapeutic activity often complement one another in a single intervention plan. Therapeutic exercises and therapeutic activities are used to remediate sensory and motor dysfunction and augment purposeful activity. It is important to remember that interventions, such as exercise and simulated activities, are used to prepare the client for occupational engagement and should always be performed in connection with the restoration of the client's desired occupations.

In practice, therapeutic exercise and therapeutic activities are considered to be different therapeutic approaches and are coded and billed differently. Although both are considered interventions that support occupation, they take on slightly different meanings clinically. The term *therapeutic exercise* usually describes interventions that are used to develop strength and endurance, ROM, and flexibility. Therapeutic activity usually describes dynamic activities to improve functional performance. Therapeutic exercises tend to include rote exercises, such as resistive Thera-Band exercises or pinching Theraputty. Therapeutic activities tend to include simulated occupations or components of occupations. For example, pinching clothespins to improve finger strength or manipulating coins to improve dexterity. In both of these examples, the activities performed are possible components of large occupations, such as the instrumental daily activities (IADLs) of laundry and manipulating money while paying for items at a store.

The occupational therapy practitioner must have a comprehensive understanding of the principles of kinesiology and exercise physiology to develop and apply therapeutic exercise and therapeutic activity. Therapeutic exercise and therapeutic activities are carefully selected to target body movements and/or muscle actions to prevent or correct a physical impairment, improve musculoskeletal function, and maintain a state of well-being.[18] A wide variety of exercise options are available, and each should be tailored to meet the goals of the intervention plan and the specific capacities and precautions relative to the client's physical condition.

Purposes

The general purposes of therapeutic exercise and therapeutic activity are:

- To develop or restore normal movement patterns and improve voluntary, automatic movement responses
- To develop or restore strength and endurance in patterns of movement that are acceptable and necessary and do not produce deformity
- To improve, develop, or restore coordination
- To increase muscle power
- To increase muscle endurance
- To remediate ROM deficits
- To increase work tolerance and physical endurance through increased strength
- To prevent or eliminate contractures

Indications for Use

Therapeutic exercises and therapeutic activities can be implemented when the client is experiencing limitations in ROM, decreased strength, decreased coordination, and/or decreased endurance. These deficits may be observed in orthopedic disorders resulting in contractures and arthritis and in lower motor neuron disorders that produce weakness and flaccidity. Examples of the latter are peripheral nerve injuries and diseases, Guillain-Barré syndrome, infectious neuritis, and spinal cord injuries and diseases.

The candidate for therapeutic exercise must be medically able to participate in the exercise regimen, able to understand the directions and purposes, and interested and motivated to perform the exercise. The client must have available motor pathways and the potential for recovery or improvement of strength, ROM, coordination, or movement patterns, as applicable. Some sensory feedback must be available to the client; that is, sensation must be at least partially intact so that the client can perceive motion and the position of the exercised part and sense superficial and deep pain. Muscles and tendons must be intact, stable, and free to move. Joints must be able to move through an effective ROM for those types of exercise that use joint motion. The client should be relatively free of pain during motion and should be able to perform isolated, coordinated movement. The type of exercise selected depends on the client's muscle grade, muscle endurance, joint mobility, diagnosis and physical condition, treatment goals, position of the client, and desirable plane of movement.

Contraindications

Therapeutic exercise and therapeutic activity are contraindicated for clients who are in a fragile medical state. Other contraindications include, but are not limited to, recent joint surgery, recent tendon or nerve repair, inflamed joints, and certain cardiopulmonary diagnoses and surgical interventions. Therapeutic exercise and therapeutic activities may not be useful where joint ROM is severely limited, as in the case of a long-standing, permanent contracture. Careful consideration is required to determine the appropriateness of the use of therapeutic exercise and therapeutic activities with those who have severe spasticity and severe lack of controlled movement. If the motor control in such cases is severely impaired, the therapeutic exercise or therapeutic activity cannot be executed in a controlled fashion, and therefore benefit from engagement in this intervention will not be gained.

Exercise Programs
Progression of Exercise Programs

If a client lacks both ROM and strength, it is important that the therapeutic exercise program focus on restoration of the available joint ROM before emphasis on progressive strengthening. When therapeutic exercises and therapeutic activities are performed, the most effective strength benefit will be gained if the individual is able to exercise the muscle or muscles through the full range of motion. Therefore, the progression of therapeutic exercises and therapeutic activities begins with resolution of ROM deficits and then progresses to muscle strength and endurance. The emphasis on improving coordinated movement occurs last in this progression because the individual would have to be able to move freely (resolution of ROM deficits) and be able to tolerate movement (muscle strength and endurance) before achieving the ability to develop or improve coordinated movement.

Range of Motion and Joint Flexibility

There are three main types of movement the OT practitioner may use to improve or maintain joint ROM and flexibility. The three main types of movement include passive ROM, active-assistive ROM, and active ROM.

Passive range of motion (PROM) occurs when the client does not exert any effort to move independently, but rather an outside force, typically the OT practitioner, moves the client's body segment for them. The purpose of PROM is to improve or maintain joint ROM and to prevent joint contracture or capsular adhesion. During PROM no muscle contraction occurs within the body segment being moved, either because the client is unable to generate a muscle contraction independently (muscle grade 0 or 1) or because it is contraindicated for the client to produce muscle force and/or active movement because generation of muscle force could cause damage to intracapsular or extracapsular joint structures (as in the case of tendon repair or rotator cuff repair). PROM may be performed in several different ways. First, PROM may be

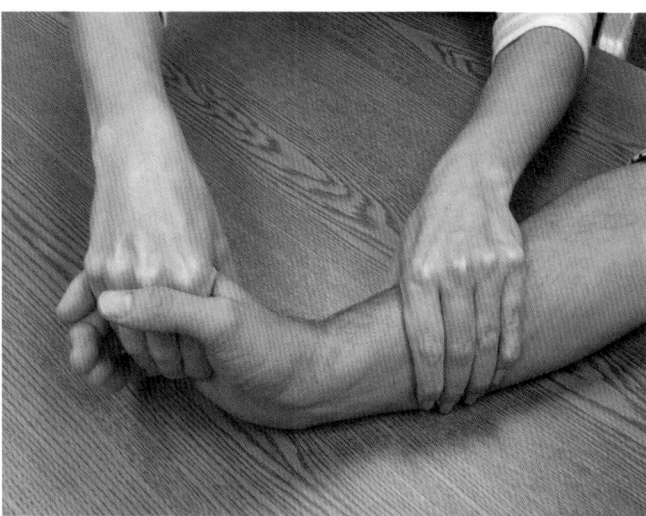

Fig. 29.6 Passive exercise of the wrist with stabilization of the joint proximal to the one being exercised.

performed when the therapist moves the client's body part through the ROM. The joint proximal to the joint being exercised should be stabilized during the procedure (Fig. 29.6). Next, the client may perform self-initiated PROM. During self-initiated PROM, the client uses the unaffected extremity to move the affected extremity when no active movement of the affected extremity is available or permitted. Our case study client, Fareed, would be able to support his left upper extremity with his right upper extremity and gently perform PROM to his left shoulder. Last, PROM may be performed by an external mechanical force, such as a continuous passive motion (CPM) machine. A CPM machine is an electrically powered mechanical device that is attached to the client's affected extremity and moves the extremity through a preset ROM. A CPM machine is considered to be a preparatory method that is used when a client is unable to generate active muscle force independently or when it is contraindicated for the client to generate internal active muscle force. It is important to note that the use of such a mechanical device requires skillful application and careful monitoring, which are achieved through specialized training.

Active-assistive range of motion (AAROM) occurs when the client is able and permitted to move the affected extremity under their own muscle power but requires the assistance of an outside force to complete the range of motion. The outside force needed to complete the ROM may be provided by the practitioner or by the client's unaffected extremity. As Fareed gains control over his left upper extremity, the support provided by his right upper extremity can be reduced. The outside force needed to complete the ROM also may be provided by a mechanical device or external force, such as pulleys.

Active range of motion (AROM) is performed when the client is able to generate enough muscle force to independently move the extremity through the range of motion without the assistance of an outside force. AROM is performed when the client is able to generate muscle force independently and when generating internal muscle force is not contraindicated. AROM can be used to maintain full joint ROM.

Active and Passive Stretch

If the OT practitioner determines that the client has limited joint ROM during the initial evaluation, the practitioner may opt to perform passive stretch or active stretch to restore the joint movement. Passive stretch, like PROM, may be performed in several different ways, including passive stretch performed by the practitioner, passive stretch performed by the client, or passive stretch performed by an external mechanical device. Passive stretch is performed by the practitioner when moving the client's body segment through the available joint ROM and holding the segment at the end of the ROM while applying gentle but firm force or stretch. Passive stretch also may be performed by the client. This is performed when the client uses the unaffected extremity to move the affected extremity through the available range of motion and holds the stretch at the end of the ROM. Last, passive stretch may be performed through the use of an outside mechanical device, which may include CPM machines, pulleys, or static or dynamic orthotic devices.

It is important to note that passive stretch is meant to increase ROM and is not needed when full range of motion is available within the joint. It is used only when a loss of joint ROM is evidenced through comparison to the contralateral side and stretching is not contraindicated. Passive stretching requires a good understanding of joint anatomy and muscle function because incorrect stretching may cause damage to the joint and/or surrounding structures. Passive stretching should be carried out cautiously and is often specifically prescribed by the referring medical professional. The OT practitioner should never force movement when pain is present unless ordered by the physician to work through pain. Slow, gentle, and firm stretching held at the end of the range of motion is required to elongate the soft tissue responsible for limiting the joint ROM and to increase the joint angle. The amount of time a stretch should be held at the end of the range of motion is somewhat controversial and largely depends on the velocity, force, and frequency of the stretch. Current evidence suggests that effective stretching can occur when the limb is held in the maximal end range position for as little as 15 seconds or for as long as 2 minutes.[17] It is important to stabilize the body parts around the joint being stretched, to prevent extraneous or compensatory movements.

As with passive stretching, the OT practitioner may choose to initiate active stretching. The purpose of active stretching is also to increase joint ROM. In active stretching the client uses the force of the agonist muscle to increase the length of the antagonist muscle. This requires good to normal strength of the agonist muscle, relatively good coordination, and motivation of the client. For example, forceful contraction of the triceps could be used to stretch the bicep muscles. Another stretching technique is the proprioceptive neuromuscular facilitation technique referred to as contract relax (CR) stretching or contract relax-agonist stretching. To perform this technique, the practitioner passively brings the muscle to the point of stretch, and the client is asked to contract and hold the muscle in an isometric contraction. This procedure is followed by relaxation of the isometric contraction and manual stretch toward the end of the range of motion.[14,15] Research has shown that the CR method is an effective technique that can be used to increase joint ROM;

however, there is controversial evidence regarding the length of time the stretch and/or the isometric contraction should be held and the intensity of the isometric contraction and stretch performed.[7]

When performing passive or active stretching, the OT practitioner must take care not to overstretch joints. Thorough assessment of the joint mobility and end feel must be performed, with careful comparison to the contralateral side, before initiating stretching. A thorough evaluation will inform the OT practitioner of preexisting joint hypermobility or instability. Such conditions easily allow for overstretching with little force, resulting in injury and damage to the surrounding soft tissue.

It is important that the OT practitioner begin to include functional activities and meaningful occupations that use the target movement or movements to maintain joint ROM gains achieved through passive and active stretching. Such gains will not last unless the client continues to move through the full available range of motion, which is most effectively accomplished through engagement in meaningful occupations.

Muscle Strengthening

The OT practitioner may opt to use muscle strengthening exercises when the client's muscle strength has decreased because of inactivity or disuse secondary to injury or disease. The OT practitioner may also choose to perform strengthening exercises when joint instability is present. Strengthening the muscles on either side of an unstable joint can improve the stability of that joint. The OT practitioner is particularly concerned with muscle weakness when it prevents or inhibits the client's ability to engage in meaningful occupations. Three primary types of muscle actions may be used to improve muscle strength: isometric contractions, concentric contractions, and eccentric contractions.

During an isometric contraction the muscle fibers generate tension; however, no joint motion occurs, and the muscle length remains the same. The limb is set or held taut as agonist and antagonist muscles are contracted simultaneously such that the joint ROM remains constant. This action may be performed without resistance or against some outside resistance, such as the therapist's hand or a fixed object. Isometric exercises are appropriate to use under a variety of circumstances. First, isometric exercises are useful when AROM, which produces joint movement, is contraindicated, as in the case of tendon rehabilitation or an unhealed fracture. Performing isometric exercise under these circumstances, when prescribed by the referring medical professional, will improve muscle strength while producing controlled stress, which has the potential to facilitate tendon and bone growth and improved function in the early stages of recovery.[8,29] Isometric exercises are also useful when first initiating active movement and strengthening in the early stages of the rehabilitation process, particularly in clients in whom the bone may be fragile as a result of prolonged immobilization or when extremely gentle exercises are indicated to prevent reinjury. Isometric exercises also may be used when it is not possible to apply resistance to the targeted muscle or muscle groups, as in the case of Kegel exercises to strengthen the pelvic floor.

There are many ways to incorporate functional tasks while performing isometric exercises. For example, isometric strengthening of the bicep occurs when an individual is holding a grocery bag draped from the forearm while maintaining elbow flexion. Isometric strengthening of the shoulder can be achieved while an individual maintains shoulder flexion, external rotation, and abduction to perform hair care tasks. Isometric grip strengthening can be achieved while an individual maintains a static grasp on an object during a functional activity such as holding onto a spoon while stirring.

Isometric exercises may be graded as the individual's strength increases. This is done by altering the amount of external resistance needed to maintain the targeted static contraction and/or the amount of time the client is able to maintain the contraction. For example, to facilitate grip strength during cooking tasks, the practitioner may opt to begin with using an isometric contraction on a spoon to stir soup and progress to an isometric contraction to maintain grasp on a mixing spoon to stir cookie batter. The amount of force needed to maintain the grasp on the spoon is greater when stirring cookie batter than it is to stir soup. It is important to note that isometric exercises may affect the cardiovascular system, which may be a contraindication for some clients.

Muscle strengthening also may be accomplished through the use of concentric contractions. Exercising muscles using concentric contractions is a very common method of strengthening and can be performed with or without resistance, depending on the client's muscle grade. During concentric contractions the muscle fibers generate force, which shortens the muscle and creates joint movement, provided the force generated by the muscle is strong enough to overcome the resistance provided by the outside force. If the client's strength allows movement through the full ROM against gravity (muscle grade 3/5), the practitioner may use AROM to strengthen a particular muscle or muscle group. Depending on the muscle or muscles targeted for strengthening, the OT practitioner may need to position the client correctly to challenge the muscle or muscles to move the body segment against the force of gravity. For example, when aiming to strengthen the wrist flexors, the practitioner must position the forearm in supination so that the wrist flexors have to overcome the force of gravity in order to pull the wrist up into flexion. If the client can tolerate resistance during manual muscle testing (muscle grades 3+/5 or 4/5), resistance may be added to the movement against gravity. Outside resistance may be added by using dumbbells or resistive elastic bands. In a more occupation-based approach, resistance may be added by applying wrist weights while the client performs a functional task or meaningful occupation. To strengthen the targeted muscle or muscles, the contraction must be forceful enough to overcome the pull of gravity with the additional weight. It is important that the weight be heavy enough to challenge the muscle but not too heavy, such that the individual cannot complete the full movement. Optimal strengthening occurs when resistance is overcome throughout the entire range of motion.

If the client cannot move through the full ROM against gravity (muscle grade below 3/5), the OT practitioner may still opt to use concentric strengthening; however, rather than have the client move against gravity, the practitioner places the targeted muscle or muscles in a gravity-modified position. For example, if the aim is to strengthen the elbow flexors (the bicep muscles), the client could be given a task that would require AROM with the arm supported on the table in front of the client. In this example, as the client performs elbow flexion and extension, the arm is supported by the table, and therefore the client does not need to overcome the force of gravity to complete elbow flexion. When the client is performing exercises in a gravity-modified position, the OT practitioner must monitor for and eliminate friction that may occur between the client's extremity and the table or mat surface on which he or she is working. If the friction is significant, it will generate resistance and prohibit movement. Friction may be reduced by using a powder board, placing a cloth under the extremity, or resting the extremity on a skateboard configured to support the hand and arm.

In some instances, the OT practitioner may opt to have the client perform exercises through the use of eccentric muscle contractions. During an eccentric muscle contraction, the muscle generates force that creates a change in the joint angle; however, during an eccentric contraction the muscle belly is actually elongating, rather than shortening (as happens in a concentric contraction). For example, if a client is lowering a can of soup from a shelf to the countertop and the elbow is extending, the bicep muscle is elongating as it controls the descent of the soup can toward the counter.

Although eccentric contractions are a typical component of normal movement patterns, the use of resistive eccentric exercises is somewhat controversial. There is some evidence that eccentric exercise programs generate superior results in muscle strength compared to concentric strengthening.[27] Additional evidence indicates that eccentric exercise may also be useful in the rehabilitation of tendon pathology and for strength training around arthritic joints.[7,12] Conversely, there are also studies that indicate that more research is needed to conclude that eccentric exercises are superior to concentric exercises in regard to strength training, the management of tendinopathies, and the prevention of injuries.[11,14] It is recommended that the OT practitioner stay abreast of the current evidence in regard to the use of concentric and eccentric resistive strength training to understand the proper application of each technique to prevent soft tissue damage and injury to the client.

When a client performs ROM or strengthening exercises, it is important that the OT practitioner watch for compensatory movements or substitution patterns of movement made by the client. For example, if the exercises are targeted to strengthen shoulder flexion, the practitioner should watch that the client does not use shoulder elevation and/or protraction to complete the movement. Another example is using shoulder abduction to achieve a hand-to-mouth movement if elbow flexors cannot move through the ROM against gravity (Fig. 29.7). Such substitutions do not strengthen the targeted muscles and can perpetuate muscle imbalance or weakness, which may further inhibit functional performance. Typically, it is the practitioner's aim to prevent or correct compensatory movements; however, when muscle loss is permanent, some substitution patterns may be desirable. For example, the practitioner may work on tenodesis as a compensatory measure to develop a functional grasp,

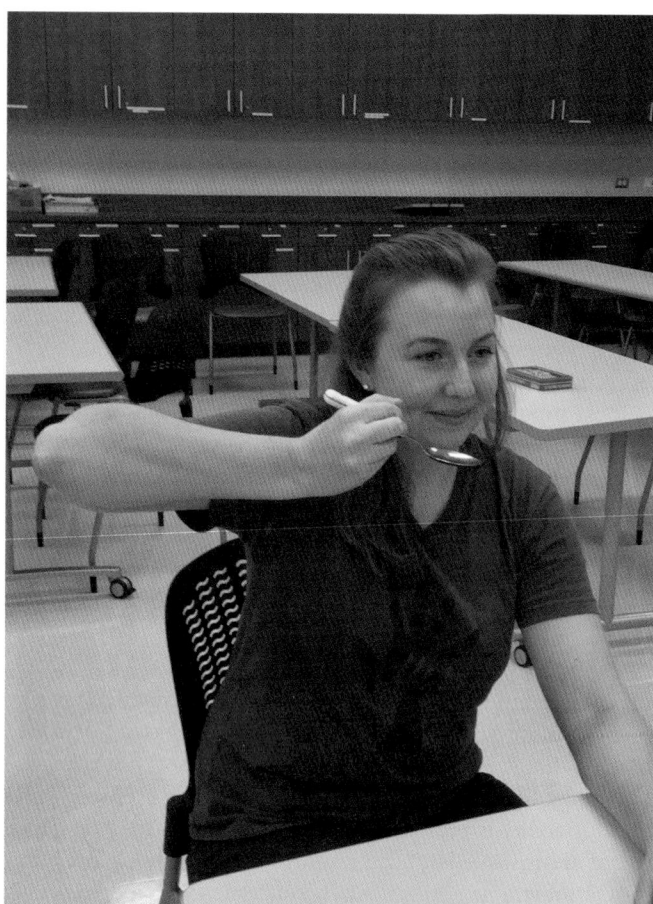

Fig. 29.7 Using shoulder abduction as compensation to achieve hand-to-mouth movement.

which in turn will enable engagement in occupations such as self-feeding.

It is important for the OT practitioner to remember that performing ROM and strengthening exercises is a preparatory task. Preparatory tasks are intended to prepare the client for occupational performance and should always be performed in connection to the restoration of the client's ability to perform functional tasks and meaningful occupations. Whenever possible, the OT practitioner should incorporate functional tasks and/or meaningful occupations into the treatment plan to improve client motivation, facilitate carryover of the exercises and, ultimately, enhance long-term functional gains.

Implementing Therapeutic Exercises and Therapeutic Activities

The OT practitioner may choose to use therapeutic exercises or therapeutic activities for several reasons. Therapeutic exercise and therapeutic activities may be used to increase muscle strength, increase muscle endurance, provide overall physical conditioning, and improve cardiovascular endurance, or to improve coordination and neuromuscular control. Before initiating therapeutic exercises or therapeutic activities, the occupational therapy practitioner must thoroughly evaluate the client's muscle strength and occupational desires to determine the most appropriate therapeutic exercises or therapeutic activities to use.

Improving Muscle Strength

If the aim of the exercise is to increase muscle strength, the client is asked to perform exercises with a relatively high load over few repetitions. To correctly strengthen a muscle, the amount of resistance must allow the client to overcome the resistance force and perform exercise through the entire range of motion. The type of exercise must suit the muscle grade and the client's fatigue tolerance level. It is important to note that there are specific techniques used in strength training known as progressive resistive exercises.[25] Progressive resistive exercises are specific protocols that are performed by incrementally increasing or decreasing the amount of resistance applied during the exercise. Progressive resistive exercises have been found to improve muscle strength in individuals with a wide variety of musculoskeletal injuries and disorders.[16,25]

Muscle strengthening exercises are graded by gradually increasing the amount of resistance as the client's strength improves. For example, if the client enjoys painting, the OT practitioner may opt to apply 3-lb wrist weights while the client participates in painting on a vertical surface using several large brush strokes. As the client's strength progresses and improves, the wrist weight may be increased to 5 lb with the same number of repetitions. When grading muscle strengthening exercises and activities, the OT practitioner gradually increases the amount of weight used but the number of repetitions remains the same.

Improving Muscle Endurance

Muscle endurance is the ability of the muscle to tolerate activity over time, work for prolonged periods, and resist fatigue. If the aim of the exercise is to increase muscle endurance, the exercises are performed in a relatively low-load, high-repetition regimen that is generally performed over an extended period.[16] It is important to differentiate muscle strength from muscle endurance because the two are not always correlated with one another.[16] For example, an individual who is able to lift a 25-lb bag of dog food one time to fill their dog's dish may not necessarily be able to carry several 5-lb grocery bags into the house, over two or three trips to and from the car, without experiencing extreme fatigue in the muscles of the upper extremities. To grade muscle endurance exercises and activities, the OT practitioner will increase the length of time the client performs an exercise or activity and/or the number of repetitions.

Physical Conditioning and Cardiovascular Fitness

Improving general physical endurance and cardiovascular fitness requires the use of large muscle groups in sustained, rhythmic aerobic exercise or activity. Examples are swimming, walking, bicycling, jogging, and some games and sports. This type of activity is often used in cardiac rehabilitation programs in which the parameters of the client's physical capacities and tolerance for exercise should be well defined and medically supervised. To improve cardiovascular fitness, exercise should be done 3 to 5 days per week at 60% to 90% of maximum heart rate or 50% to 85% of maximum oxygen uptake. Between 15 and 60 minutes of exercise or rhythmic activities using large muscle groups is desirable.[6] Grading of exercises and activities used to target overall physical conditioning and cardiovascular fitness involves gradually increasing the aerobic demands of the activity with careful monitoring of the client's response to activity, especially in the acute rehabilitation phases.

General Exercise and Activity Precautions

During therapeutic exercises and activities the OT practitioner must carefully monitor the client's response to the intervention. Excessive repetitions of strengthening exercises may result in muscle fatigue, pain, and temporary reduction of strength. If a muscle is overworked, it becomes fatigued and is unable to contract. Other signs of fatigue include slowed performance, distraction, perspiration, an increase in the rate of respiration, performance of an exercise pattern through a decreased ROM, and inability to complete the prescribed number of repetitions. It is important to realize that various disease states may significantly alter a person's endurance capacity and tolerance for activity. Many clients may not be sensitive to fatigue or may push themselves beyond tolerance in the belief that this approach hastens recovery. Therefore, the occupational therapist must carefully assess the client's muscle power, capacity for performance, and response to the therapeutic exercise or activity.

Neuromuscular Control and Coordination

Coordination is the combined activity of many muscles into smooth patterns and sequences of motion. Coordination is an automatic response monitored primarily through proprioceptive sensory feedback. Kottke[20] defined control as "the conscious activation of an individual muscle or the conscious initiation of a pre-programmed engram." Control involves conscious attention to and guidance of an activity.

A pre-programmed pattern of muscular activity represented in the central nervous system (CNS) has been described as an engram. An engram is formed only if many repetitions of a specific motion or activity occur. With repetition, conscious effort by the client is decreased and the motion becomes increasingly more automatic. Ultimately the motion can be carried out with little conscious attention. It has been hypothesized that when an engram is excited, the same pattern of movement is produced automatically.

Procedures for the development of neuromuscular control and neuromuscular coordination are briefly outlined in the following paragraphs. The reader is referred to original sources for a full discussion of the neurophysiologic mechanisms underlying these exercises. Neuromuscular education or control training involves teaching the client to control individual muscles or motions through conscious attention. Coordination training is used to develop pre-programmed multimuscular patterns or engrams, thereby creating a motor memory.[19]

Neuromuscular Control

It may be desirable to teach control of individual muscles when the muscle is so weak that it cannot be used normally. The purpose is to improve muscle strength and muscle coordination to new patterns. To achieve these ends, the person must learn precise control of the muscle, an essential step in the development of optimal coordination for persons with neuromuscular disease.

To participate successfully the client must be able to learn and follow instructions, cooperate, and concentrate on the muscular retraining. Before beginning, the client should be comfortable and securely supported. The exercises should be carried out in a nondistracting environment. The client must be alert, calm, and rested and should have an adequate, pain-free arc of motion of the joint on which the muscle acts, in addition to good proprioception. Visual and tactile sensory feedback may be used to compensate or substitute for limited proprioception, but the coordination achieved will never be as great as when proprioception is intact.[19]

Awareness of the desired motion and the muscles that produce it is first taught to the client using passive motion to stimulate the proprioceptive stretch reflex. This passive movement may be repeated several times. The client's awareness may be enhanced if the practitioner also demonstrates the desired movement and if the movement is performed by the analogous unaffected part. The skin over the muscle belly and tendon insertion may be stimulated to enhance the effect of the stretch reflex. Stroking and tapping over the muscle belly may be used to facilitate muscle action.[19]

The occupational therapy practitioner should explain the location and function of the muscle, its origin and insertion, line of pull, and action on the joint. The practitioner should then demonstrate the motion and instruct the client to think of the pull of the muscle from insertion to origin. The skin over muscle insertion can be stroked in the direction of pull while the client concentrates on the sensation of the motion during the passive movement performed by the practitioner.

The exercise sequence begins with instructions to the client to think about the motion while the OT practitioner carries it out passively and strokes the skin over the insertion in the direction of the motion. The client is then instructed to assist by contracting the muscle while the practitioner performs passive motion and stimulates the skin as before. Next the client moves the part through ROM with assistance and cutaneous stimulation while the practitioner emphasizes contraction of the prime mover only. Finally the client carries out the movement independently, using the prime mover.

The exercise must be initiated against minimal resistance if activity is to be isolated to prime movers. If the muscle is very weak (trace to poor muscle grade), the procedure may be carried out entirely in an active-assisted manner so that the muscle contracts against no resistance and can function without activating synergists. Progression from one step to the next depends on successful performance of the steps without substitutions. Each step is carried out 3 to 5 times per session for each muscle, depending on the client's tolerance.

Coordination Training

The goal of coordination training is to develop the ability to perform multimuscular motor patterns that are faster, more precise, and stronger than those performed when control of individual

muscles is used. The development of coordination depends on repetition. Initially in training, the movement must be simple and slow so that the client can be conscious of the activity and its components. Good coordination does not develop until repeated practice results in a well-developed activity pattern that no longer requires conscious effort and attention.

Training should take place in an environment in which the client can concentrate. The exercise is divided into components that the client can perform correctly. Kottke[20] calls this approach desynthesis. The level of effort required should be kept low, by reducing speed and resistance, to prevent the spread of excitation to muscles that are not part of the desired movement pattern. Other theorists offer contrary advice, which emphasizes the integration of movements that customarily occur during activity. The practitioner's experience and judgment are important in determining which method to use.

When the motor pattern is divided into units that the client can perform successfully, each unit is trained by practice under voluntary control, as described previously for training of control. The practitioner instructs the client in the desired movement and uses sensory stimulation and passive movement. The client must observe and voluntarily modify the motion. Slow practice is imperative to make this monitoring possible. The practitioner offers enough assistance to ensure precise movement while allowing the client to concentrate on the sensations produced by the movements. When the client concentrates on movement, fatigue occurs rapidly and the client should be given frequent, short rests. As the client masters the components of the pattern and performs them precisely and independently, the sequence is graded to subtasks or several components that are practiced repetitively. As the subtasks are perfected, they are linked progressively until the movement pattern can be performed.

The protocol can be graded for speed, force, or complexity, but the practitioner must be aware that the increased effort put forth by the client may result in incoordinated movement. Therefore, the grading must remain within the client's capacity to perform the precise movement pattern. The motor pattern must be performed correctly to prevent the development of faulty patterns.

If CNS impulses are generated to muscles that should not be involved in the movement pattern, incoordinated motion results. Constant repetition of an incoordinated pattern reinforces the pattern, resulting in a persistent incoordination. Factors that increase incoordination are fear, poor balance, too much resistance, pain, fatigue, strong emotions, prolonged inactivity,[19] and excessively prolonged activity.

PHYSICAL AGENT MODALITIES

According to the OTPF-4, **physical agent modalities (PAMs)** are interventions that the OT practitioner may use to prepare the client for occupational engagement.[1] The AOTA recognizes and supports the use of PAMs by OT practitioners as outlined in its position paper on physical agent modalities.[2] If an OT practitioner chooses to implement a PAM in treatment, it must be connected to a preparatory task or occupation. The AOTA's position paper clearly states that "[the] exclusive or stand-alone use of PAMs without linking it to a client-centered, occupation-based intervention plan and outcomes is not occupational therapy."[2] Furthermore, although the foundational knowledge leading to the safe application of PAMs by an OT practitioner is provided in entry-level educational programs, application and use of PAMs by an OT practitioner is permitted only after the practitioner has obtained additional education and training through continuing education and has demonstrated competence in the use of PAMs.[2] Before an OT practitioner may use PAMs, it is mandatory that he or she comply with the guidelines outlined by the AOTA.

PAMs may be used before or during functional activities to enhance the effects of the OT intervention program to facilitate occupational engagement. PAMs are often used by OT practitioners working in orthopedic settings (e.g., hand therapy) but also may be used in other settings, such as neurological rehabilitation and wound management. This section introduces the reader to basic techniques and when and why they may be applied. The following sections are divided into the four main areas outlined in the AOTA position paper on PAMs: superficial thermal agents, deep thermal agents, electrotherapeutic agents, and mechanical devices. Because modalities are commonly used by OT practitioners for treatment of hand injuries and diseases, the examples provided are focused on intervention to improve upper extremity function. The use of PAMs is not limited to the treatment of hands, however.

Therapeutic Modalities and Thermal Agents

The AOTA position paper defines therapeutic modalities as follows:

> *Therapeutic modalities refer to the systematic application of various forms of energy or force to effect therapeutic change in the physiology of tissues. Physical agents such as heat, cold, water, light, sound, and electricity may be applied to the body to impact client factors, including the neurophysiologic, musculoskeletal, integumentary, circulatory, or metabolic functions of the body."[2]*

Thermal agents may be divided into two overarching categories: superficial thermal agents and deep thermal agents. The following sections will further discuss the various thermal agents, their properties, and their applications within the practice of occupational therapy.

Superficial Thermal Agents

There are two primary ways by which superficial thermal agents may alter the temperature of soft tissue. Superficial thermal agents may change soft tissue temperature through a process known as convection or through a process known as conduction. The process of convection and the process of conduction each have the ability to cool soft tissue, known as cryotherapy, or to heat soft tissue.

Convection

Convection includes superficial thermal modalities such as hydrotherapy and Fluidotherapy. Convection transfers heat or cold to the tissues by fluid motion around a body segment. The practitioner may choose to use convection techniques to cool the soft tissue (heat abstraction) or to heat the soft tissue (heat transmission), depending on the aim of the modality. The most common example of convection for cryotherapy (cold therapy) is cold whirlpool.[9] When a cold whirlpool is used, the client's extremity is submerged in a tub of cold water and turbine jets are used to circulate the cold water around the extremity. The OT practitioner may choose to use a cold whirlpool to decrease inflammation, decrease pain, and/or decrease edema. Cold whirlpools are typically used for cooling distal extremities, such as the wrist or elbow, particularly when the aim is to cool large portions of the extremity evenly.[9] The client's comfort with and tolerance to the cold temperatures will serve to guide the therapeutic use of this modality. Additional uses of cryotherapy will be discussed in the following section.

As previously stated, convection also may be used to heat soft tissue. The most common example of convection for heating soft tissue is Fluidotherapy. Fluidotherapy involves a machine that agitates finely ground corn husk particles by blowing warm air through them. This modality feels similar to a water whirlpool, but corn particles are used instead of water. The temperature is thermostatically maintained, with the therapeutic range between 102° and 118° F.[27] Fluidotherapy units are available in various sizes to accommodate various body parts,[27] but heating the elbow or hand is the most common use of this heat modality. An additional benefit of Fluidotherapy is its effect on desensitization. The agitator can be adjusted to decrease or increase the flow of the corn particles, thus controlling the amount of stimulation to the skin. Because an extremity can be heated gradually, this technique is effective as a warm-up before exercises, dexterity tasks, functional activities, and work simulation tasks.

Conduction

Conduction includes superficial thermal modalities such as cold packs (cryotherapy), hot packs, and paraffin. Conduction transfers heat or cold from one object to another through direct contact.

Cryotherapy, the use of cold therapy, is often used in the treatment of edema, pain, and inflammation. The cold produces a vasoconstriction, which decreases the amount of blood flow into the injured tissue. Cold decreases muscle spasms by decreasing the amount of firing from the afferent muscle spindles. Cryotherapy is contraindicated for clients with cold intolerance or vascular repairs. The use of cryotherapy may be incorporated into intervention programs provided in the clinical setting; however, it is particularly useful in a home program.

Cold packs can be applied in a number of ways. Many commercial packs exist, which range in size and cost. An alternative to purchasing a cold pack is to use a bag of frozen vegetables or to combine crushed ice and alcohol in a plastic bag to make a reusable slush bag. Ice packs should be covered with a towel to prevent tissue injury. The benefit of commercial packs is that they are easy to use, especially if the client must use them frequently during the day. When clients are working, it is recommended that they keep cold packs at home and at work to increase the ease of use.

Other forms of cryotherapy include ice massage and cooling machines. Ice massage is used when the area to be cooled is small and very specific; for example, inflammation of a tendon specifically at its insertion or origin. The procedure entails using a large piece of ice (e.g., water frozen in a paper cup) to massage the area with circular motions until the skin is numb, usually for 4 to 5 minutes. Care must be taken to keep the ice moving to prevent damage to tissues that are most superficial. Cooling devices, which circulate cold water through tubes in a pack, are available through vendors. These devices maintain their cold temperatures for a long time, but they are expensive to rent or purchase. They are effective in reducing edema immediately after surgery or injury, during the inflammatory phase of wound healing.

Contrast baths combine the use of heat and cold. The physical response is alternating vasoconstriction and vasodilation of the blood vessels. For example, the client is asked to submerge the arm, alternating between two tubs of water. One contains cold water (55° to 65° F), and the other contains warm water (100° to 110° F).[5] The purpose is to increase collateral circulation, which effectively reduces pain and edema. As with the use of cold packs, contrast baths are a beneficial addition to a home therapy program. This technique is contraindicated for clients with vascular disorders or injuries.

Alternatively, the OT practitioner may choose to use heat as a therapeutic modality. Hot packs and paraffin provide heat through conduction. Heat may be used to increase circulation and promote healing. The increase in blood flow will also increase elasticity of soft tissue and improve soft tissue extensibility before stretch. This will more easily allow for permanent soft tissue elongation, resulting in improved joint movement and decreased joint stiffness. Heat also may be used to relieve muscle spasms and decrease pain.[27] To obtain maximum benefits from heat, the tissue temperature must be raised to 104° to 113° F.[27] Precautions must be taken with temperatures above this range to prevent tissue destruction.

Contraindications to the use of heat include acute inflammatory conditions of the joints or skin, sensory losses, impaired vascular structures, malignancies, and application to the very young or very old. The use of heat may substantially enhance the effects of orthotic interventions and therapeutic activities that attempt to increase ROM and functional abilities.

Paraffin is another form of heat modality. Paraffin is stored in a tub that maintains a temperature between 113° and 129° F.[27] The client repeatedly dips his or her hand into the tub until a thick, insulating layer of paraffin has been applied to the extremity. The hand is then wrapped in a plastic bag and towel for 15 to 30 minutes.[26] This technique provides an excellent conforming characteristic, so it is ideal for use in hands and digits. Partial hand coverage is possible. The paraffin transfers its heat to the hand, and the bag and towel act as an insulator against dissipation of heat to the air. An additional benefit to the use of paraffin is that it provides moisturization to the skin, which is especially beneficial in scar management or for improving skin elasticity, as in the case of scleroderma.

Care must be taken to protect insensate parts from burns. To prevent excessive vasodilation, paraffin should not be applied when moderate to severe edema is present. It cannot be used if open wounds are present. Paraffin can be used in the clinic or incorporated into a home program. The tubs are small, and the technique is safe and easy to use in the home. It is an excellent adjunct to home programs that include dynamic splinting, exercises, or general ADLs. It may be used in the clinic before therapeutic exercises and functional activities.

Hot packs contain either a silicate gel or a bentonite clay wrapped in a cotton bag and submerged in a Hydrocollator, a water tank that maintains the temperature of the packs at 158° to 167° F.[27] Because tissue damage may occur at these temperatures, the packs are separated from the skin by layers of towels. As with paraffin, precautions should be taken in application of hot packs to insensate tissue that has sustained vascular damage. Hot packs are commonly used for myofascial pain, before soft tissue mobilization, and before any activities aimed at elongating contracted tissue. For a client with a hand injury the packs may be applied to the extrinsic musculature to decrease muscle tone caused by guarding, without also heating the hand. Unless contraindicated, hot packs can be used (with precautions) when open wounds are present.

Deep Thermal Agents

Deep thermal agents use conversion to apply heat deep into the tissues. Conversion occurs when energy is converted from one form to another. For example, in ultrasound therapy, acoustic energy (sound waves) is converted internally to heat. As the sound waves penetrate the tissue, they vibrate the tissue molecules, causing them to rub against one another and create friction, which in turn generates heat.[22] The energy of sound waves is thus converted to heat energy. The sound waves are applied with a transducer, which glides across the skin in slow, continuous motions. Gel is used to improve the transmission of the sound waves to the tissues. Ultrasound is considered a deep heating agent. Most ultrasound machines are dual-frequency units, allowing the therapist to choose between a 1-MHz or a 3-MHz sound head or transducer. The OT practitioner selects the frequency of the sound head based on the depth of the structures targeted for treatment. The 3-MHz transducer is selected when the target tissue is relatively superficial (1 to 3 cm below the skin), and the 1-MHz transducer is selected to heat tissues more than 2 cm below the skin.[29] Because of its ability to heat deeper tissues, ultrasound is excellent for treating problems associated with joint contractures, scarring and its associated adhesions, and muscle spasms. When ultrasound is used, the OT practitioner should apply a stretch to the tissues while they are being heated. The gains made through this type of stretching are best maintained when they are followed by activities, exercises, or the application of an orthosis to maintain the stretch.

Ultrasound also may be used in a nonthermal application. For example, ultrasound has been shown to increase circulation, promote healing, and reduce inflammation.[22] Evidence suggests that nonthermal ultrasound is effective to facilitate wound healing, peripheral nerve healing, and soft tissue repair after injury. Nonthermal ultrasound also has been shown to facilitate tendon and bone healing.[22] One additional use of ultrasound involves using the sound waves to drive antiinflammatory medications into the tissue. This process is called phonophoresis.

There are many useful and effective applications for ultrasound; however, the OT practitioner must have a good understanding of this modality and be well aware of the precautions and contraindications for its use. Ultrasound at frequencies higher than recommended standards or failure to continually move the applicator during treatment can generate too much heat and can destroy tissue. Ultrasound can be used to facilitate bone healing, but if it is used with the wrong parameters, it can vibrate the bone, cause pain, and delay the healing process. When ultrasound is used over bone in children, precautions must be taken to avoid the growth plates in the client's bones. Ultrasound should never be used over an unprotected spinal cord or freshly repaired structures such as tendons and nerves. If ultrasound is being used to facilitate wound healing, the wound should be free from infection because increasing circulation has the potential to spread the infection. Finally, because ultrasound can facilitate cell proliferation, it should never be used over a malignancy.

Electrotherapeutic Agents

The AOTA has defined electrotherapeutic agents in this way:

Electrotherapeutic agents use electricity and the electromagnetic spectrum to facilitate tissue healing, improve muscle strength and endurance, decrease edema, modulate pain, decrease the inflammatory process, and modify the healing process. Electrotherapeutic agents include but are not limited to neuro-muscular electrical stimulation (NMES), functional electrical stimulation (FES), transcutaneous electrical nerve stimulation (TENS), high-voltage galvanic stimulation for tissue and wound repair (HVGS), high-voltage pulsed current (HVPC), direct current (DC), [and] iontophoresis . . .[2]

As with all PAMs, the OT practitioner must use these interventions to improve the client's functional performance and facilitate engagement in occupation. Many techniques are available; those most commonly used are presented here. It is important to note that electrical modalities should never be used with clients with pacemakers or cardiac conditions.

Transcutaneous Electrical Nerve Stimulation

Transcutaneous electrical nerve stimulation (TENS) uses electrical current to decrease pain. Pain is a very complex phenomenon and can cause severe functional impairment. Pain is considered to be acute when it immediately follows trauma. Individuals may also experience chronic pain, which is longstanding. When trauma occurs, an individual responds to the initial pain by guarding the painful body part, often by restricting motion of the body part or assuming a posture that limits use of the painful body part. This guarding may result in muscle spasms and fatigue of the muscle fibers, especially after prolonged guarding. The supply of blood and oxygen to the affected area decreases, and resultant soft tissue and joint dysfunction may occur. These reactions magnify and compound the problems associated with the initial pain response. The therapist's goal after an acute injury is to prevent this cycle. In the case of chronic pain, the goal is to stop the cycle that has been established.

TENS is commonly used to decrease acute pain and control chronic pain. It should be noted that there is inconclusive evidence regarding the use of TENS for pain control. The lack of such evidence is likely due to the fact that pain is a difficult construct to study because it is a subjective measure and manifests very differently, depending on a wide variety of individual factors.[24] Many individuals respond favorably to TENS and report effective pain relief without the side effects of medications. TENS units are portable, safe to use, and clients can be educated in independent home use.

TENS units provide constant electrical stimulation with a modulated current that is directed to the peripheral nerves through electrode placement. The practitioner can control several attributes of the modulation waveform, such as the frequency, amplitude, and pulse width. When TENS is applied at a low-fire setting, it creates an "electroanalgesia" effect.[24] When this occurs, the brain releases endorphins, which in turn reduce the sensation of pain. The effects of high-frequency TENS are based on the gate control theory. This theory describes how the electrical current from the TENS unit, applied to the peripheral nerves, blocks the perception of pain in the brain. Nociceptors (pain receptors) transmit information to the CNS through the A-delta and C fibers. A-delta fibers transmit information about pressure and touch. It is thought that TENS stimulates the A fibers, effectively saturating the gate to pain perception, and the transmission of pain signals via the A-delta and C fibers is blocked at the level of the spinal cord.[33] TENS can be applied for acute or chronic pain. TENS is frequently used postsurgically for orthopedic conditions when it is mandatory that ROM be initiated within 72 hours following surgery, such as in tenolysis and capsulotomy surgeries, or when it is important to maintain tendon gliding through the injured area after fractures. In these cases TENS may be useful in controlling pain so that the client can tolerate immediate postsurgical movement. TENS can be especially helpful for clients with a low threshold to pain by making exercising easier. TENS also may be useful when working with clients with complex regional pain syndrome.

TENS can be used to decrease pain from an inflammatory condition such as tendinitis or a nerve impingement; however, the client must be educated in tendon and nerve protection and rest, with a proper home program of symptom management, positioning, and ADL and work modification. Without the sensation of pain the client may overdo and stress the tissues; therefore, education regarding activity level is important.

Neuromuscular Electrical Stimulation

Neuromuscular electrical stimulation (NMES) is the use of electrical current to activate muscles. It is applied through an electrode to the motor point of innervated muscles to provide a muscle contraction. The current is interrupted to enable the muscle to relax between contractions, and the durations of the on and off times can be adjusted by the therapist. Adjustments also can be made to control the rate of the increase in current (ramp) and intensity of the contraction.

NMES is used to increase ROM, facilitate muscle contractions, and strengthen muscles.[15] It may be used postsurgically to provide a stronger contraction for improved tendon gliding, for example, after a tenolysis. It also may be used later in the tendon repair protocol once the tendon has healed sufficiently to tolerate stress. NMES may be used to lengthen a muscle that has become weakened because of disuse. During the reinnervation phase after a nerve injury this technique may be used to help stimulate and strengthen a newly innervated muscle. Care must be taken not to overfatigue the muscle. NMES can be applied during a dexterity or functional activity, which allows the muscle to be retrained in the purpose of its contraction. NMES is particularly beneficial when it is used to facilitate movement during functional activities or meaningful occupations. As with TENS, there are portable NMES units that can be prescribed for home use.

Other techniques that use an electrical current include high-voltage galvanic stimulation (HVGS) and inferential electrical stimulation. These techniques are applied to treat pain and edema.[23] Iontophoresis is yet another electrotherapeutic agent. Iontophoresis uses electrical current to drive ionized medication into the tissue. The medications most often used are antiinflammatory drugs and agents to decrease scar tissue. The technique uses an electrode filled with the medication of choice. The medicine is transferred by applying an electric field that propels the ions into the tissues.

MECHANICAL DEVICES

The OT practitioner also may choose to use a mechanical device to increase ROM to facilitate functional movement and engagement in occupational performance. The most common device used by OT practitioners is the CPM machine. A CPM machine is a mechanical device that is electrically powered and provides passive movement to the client's extremity. The machine can be programmed to move the extremity through a specific ROM according to the parameters the therapist sets. CPM machines are particularly useful when a joint must be moved immediately after surgery to prevent stiffness and soft tissue scarring or when the client has difficulty performing full ROM independently.

▮ SUMMARY

Engagement in occupation is the primary tool and objective of occupational therapy practice. OT practitioners use occupational analysis, activity analysis, adaptation, grading of activities, therapeutic exercise, and adjunctive modalities in the continuum of intervention, and they may use these methods simultaneously toward these ends. For example, one possible hierarchy of interventions for our case study client, Fareed, may proceed as follows. The OT may first opt to use TENS in an effort to control Fareed's left shoulder pain and to prepare Fareed for engagement in therapeutic exercise, therapeutic activities, or engagement in occupations. Once Fareed's pain is better controlled, the therapist may then decide to use work strengthening. It is important for the therapist to note that Fareed's lack of ROM in the left shoulder is caused by pain and weakness and not limitations in the available ROM in the left shoulder joint itself. There are several ways in which the therapist may decide to work on strength. In view of the fact that Fareed enjoys gardening, the therapist could use a gardening activity such as transferring soil into a container for potting. In this activity, Fareed could participate in grasping the container and spade with his left hand and use the LUE to shovel the soil into the container, thus working on strength of the LUE. We also know that Fareed requires assistance for dressing. The therapist also may use the activity of donning an overhead shirt or washing his hair to work on LUE strength and promote independence in self-care. Through this breadth of practice skills, based on the client's personal and social needs, the OT practitioner helps the client apply newly gained strength, ROM, and coordination during the performance of occupation and activity to assume or reassume life roles.

Appropriate intervention strategies are individualized and designed to be meaningful to the client while meeting therapeutic goals and objectives designed collaboratively by the client and the practitioner. One way to ensure choices are meaningful to the client is to explore contextual factors that influence participation and engagement in occupation. Personal and environmental contextual factors are important to consider in terms of how they might facilitate or inhibit a client's participation in preferred occupations. Contextual considerations that influence Fareed's participation in gardening might include the following:

Environmental factors:

- *Natural and built environment:* The fact that Fareed is a long-time gardener would indicate that he has access to gardening spaces that likely include natural and built elements. The OT practitioner would gather information about his garden to include or replicate contextual features of his gardening in his intervention.
- *Support and relationships:* Fareed has a supportive immediate and extended family that will likely support his return to gardening. His family can be helpful in gathering information about his current garden and ideas for how to encourage participation moving forward.

Personal factors:

- Fareed's participation in gardening may be influenced by his identity as a gardener, habits he may have about gardening, and his upbringing and life experiences related to gardening. The OT should consider these factors as a part of planning client-centered intervention strategies.

Intervention strategies may be adapted to meet the individual needs of the client or the environment. Strategies may be graded for a number of factors, including physical, perceptual, cognitive, and social factors, to keep the client functioning at maximal potential at any point in the intervention program. To assist Fareed in engaging in gardening, one of his favored occupations, the OT practitioner can consider grading any number of factors that the OT believes has the potential to improve. For example we can look at grading participation in gardening to address concerns with the motor performance skills such as stabilizing, aligning, and balancing. Given the need for minimal assistance with dynamic sitting and standing balance, the OT may choose to start by grading down to have gardening activities take place in a supported seated position while working on reaching and weight shifts. This might be using a raised bed garden or gardening containers on a low table or other surface. As Fareed gains skill, he can transition to working in a seating position with less support either from the OT or changing surfaces, increasing the skills needed for dynamic sitting balance while reaching and weight shifting. As performance skills continue to improve, the OT can continue to grade up by beginning to work on gardening activities such as watering a hanging plant or repotting plants at a gardening bench where Fareed needs to stand for short periods of time to reach and actively weight shift. The amount of assistance given to Fareed can be decreased as skills increase. The ability to work in a standing position or shift from sitting to standing can gradually be increased from the current level of 30 seconds with min assist to longer periods of time with contact guard support, close supervision, distant supervision, to independent or modified independence as appropriate.

The uniqueness of occupational therapy lies in its extensive and intentional use of occupation and goal-directed strategies as treatment modalities. In practice, OT practitioners' roles may not be clearly defined because they are subject to variations in expectations that stem from regional differences, healthcare developments, legislation, institutional philosophy, and the roles and responsibilities assigned by the treatment facility. In all instances, OT practitioners must be well trained and well qualified to deliver all aspects of practice. They should not hesitate to refer clients to experts for treatment whenever appropriate.

REVIEW QUESTIONS

1. Define modality.
2. Define occupation, activity, and interventions to support occupations.
3. Name two reasons occupation is valuable.
4. Compare and contrast activity analysis and occupational analysis.
5. What term best describes how activities and environments are modified to meet the individualized needs of clients?
6. What is used to create the "just right" challenge in performance?
7. When are adjunctive modalities appropriately used by occupational therapy practitioners?
8. For which types of disabilities would therapeutic exercise (as defined in this chapter) be inappropriate?
9. List and define three types of muscle contraction.
10. Identify an activity that can be used to provide resistive exercise and describe how it could be done.
11. List four general categories of physical agent modalities.
12. What kinds of symptoms are treated with cryotherapy?

REFERENCES

1. American Occupational Therapy Association. Occupational therapy practice framework: Domain and process (4th ed.). *American Journal of Occupational Therapy*, 74(Supplement 2), 2020. Advance online publication.
2. American Occupational Therapy Association: Physical agent modalities. 2018. https://www.aota.org/~/media/Corporate/Files/Secure/Practice/OfficialDocs/Position/PAM-Interim-20181112.pdf.
3. Baum CM, Christiansen CH: Person-environment-occupation-performance. In Christiansen CH, Baum CM, editors: *Occupational therapy: performance, participation, and well-being*, Thorofare, NJ, 2005, Slack, pp 243–268.
4. Boyt-Schell BA, Gillen G, Crepeau EB, Scaffa ME: Analyzing occupations and activity. In Boyt-Schell BA, Gillen G, editors: *Willard and Spackman's occupational therapy* ed 13, Philadelphia, 2019, Lippincott Williams & Wilkins, pp 320–334.
5. Bukowski E, Nolan T Jr: Hydrotherapy: the use of water as a therapeutic agent. In Michlovitz S, Bellew J, Nolan T, editors: *Modalities for therapeutic intervention* ed 5, Philadelphia, 2012, FA Davis.
6. Ciccone CD, Alexander J: Physiology and therapeutics of exercise. In Goodgold J, editor: *Rehabilitation medicine*, St Louis, 1988, Mosby.
7. Cullinane FL, Boocock MG, Trevelyan FC: Is eccentric exercise an effective treatment for lateral epicondylitis? A systematic review, *Clin Rehabil* 28:3–19, 2014.
8. Feehan LM, Bassett K: Is there evidence for early mobilization following an extraarticular hand fracture? *J Hand Ther* 17:300–308, 2004.
9. Fruth S, Michlovitz S: Cold therapy. In Michlovitz S, Bellew J, Nolan T Jr, editors: *Modalities for therapeutic intervention* ed 5, Philadelphia, 2012, FA Davis.
10. Gillen G: Occupational therapy interventions for individuals. In Boyt-Schell BA, Gillen G, editors: *Willard and Spackman's occupational therapy* ed 13, Philadelphia, PA, 2019, Wolters Kluwer, pp 413–435.
11. Habets B, van Cingel REH: Eccentric exercise training in chronic mid-portion Achilles tendinopathy: a systematic review on different protocols, *Scand J Med Sci Sports* 25:3–15, 2015.
12. Hernandez HJ, McIntosh V, Leland A, Harris-Love MO: Progressive resistance exercise with eccentric loading for the management of knee osteoarthritis, *Front Med (Lausanne)* 2:45, 2015.
13. Hersch GI, Lamport NK, Coffey MS: *Activity analysis: application to occupation*, ed 5, Thorofare, NJ, 2005, Slack.
14. Hibbert O, Cheong K, Grant A, et al: A systematic review of the effectiveness of eccentric strength training in the prevention of hamstring muscle strains in otherwise healthy individuals, *N Am J Sports Phys Ther* 3:67–81, 2008.

15. Johnston T: NMES and FES in patients with neurological diagnoses. In Michlovitz S, Bellew J, Nolan T Jr, editors: *Modalities for therapeutic intervention* ed 5, Philadelphia, 2012, FA Davis.

16. Kisner C, Colby LA: Resistance exercise for impaired muscle performance. In Kisner C, Colby LA, editors: *Therapeutic exercise: foundations and techniques* ed 6, Philadelphia, 2012, FA Davis.

17. Kisner C, Colby LA: Stretching for improved mobility. In Kisner C, Colby LA, editors: *Therapeutic exercise: foundations and techniques* ed 6, Philadelphia, 2012, FA Davis.

18. Kisner C, Colby LA, editors: *Therapeutic exercise: foundations and techniques* ed 6, Philadelphia, 2012, FA Davis.

19. Konrad A, Gad M, Tilp M: Effect of PNF stretching training on the properties of human muscle and tendon structures, *Scand J Med Sci Sports* 25:346–355, 2015.

20. Kottke FJ: Therapeutic exercises to develop neuromuscular coordination. In Kottke FJ, Lehmann JF, editors: *Krusen's handbook of physical medicine and rehabilitation* ed 4, Philadelphia, 1990, Saunders.

21. Reference deleted in proofs.

22. Michlovitz S, Sparrow K: Therapeutic ultrasound. In Michlovitz S, Bellew J, Nolan T, editors: *Modalities for therapeutic intervention* ed 5, Philadelphia, 2012, FA Davis.

23. Mullins PT: Use of therapeutic modalities in upper extremity rehabilitation. In Hunter JM, editor: *Rehabilitation of the hand* ed 3, St Louis, 1990, Mosby.

24. Petterson S, Michlovitz S: Pain and limited motion. In Michlovitz S, Bellew J, Nolan T Jr, editors: *Modalities for therapeutic intervention* ed 5, Philadelphia, 2012, FA Davis.

25. Rancho Los Amigos Hospital: Progressive resistive and static exercise: principles and techniques (unpublished), Downey, CA, The Hospital.

26. Rennie S, Michlovitz S: Therapeutic heat. In Michlovitz S, Bellew J, Nolan T Jr, editors: *Modalities for therapeutic intervention* ed 5, Philadelphia, 2012, FA Davis.

27. Roig M, O'Brien K, Kirk G, et al: The effects of eccentric versus concentric resistance training on muscle strength and mass in healthy adults: a systematic review with meta-analysis, *Br J Sports Med* 43:556–568, 2009.

28. Spackman CS: Occupational therapy for the restoration of physical function. In Willard HS, Spackman CS, editors: *Occupational therapy* ed 4, Philadelphia, 1974, JB Lippincott.

29. Sultana SS, MacDermid JC, Grewal R, Rath S: The effectiveness of early mobilization after tendon transfers in the hand: a systematic review, *J Hand Ther* 26:1–21, 2013.

30. Thomas H: *Occupation-based activity analysis*, ed 2, Thorofare, NJ, 2015, Slack.

31. Trombly CA: Occupation: purposefulness and meaningfulness as therapeutic mechanisms: 1995 Eleanor Clarke Slagle Lecture, *Am J Occup Ther* 49:960–972, 1995.

32. Tubbs CC, Drake M: *Crafts and creative media in therapy*, ed 5, Thorofare, NJ, 2017, Slack.

33. Wietlisbach CM: *Cooper's fundamentals of hand therapy*, ed 3, St Louis, 2020, Elsevier.

34. Wilcock AA: *An occupational perspective of health*, ed 2, Thorofare, NJ, 2006, Slack.

SUGGESTED READINGS

Kwak DH, Ryu YU: Applying proprioceptive neuromuscular facilitation stretching: optimal contraction intensity to attain the maximum increase in range of motion in young males, *J Phys Ther Sci* 27:2129–2132, 2015.

Magnusson SP, et al: Mechanical and physiological responses to stretching with and without preisometric contraction in human skeletal muscle, *Arch Phys Med Rehabil* 77:373–378, 1996.

30

Orthotic Fabrication for the Upper Extremity

Deborah A. Schwartz and Donna Lashgari

LEARNING OBJECTIVES

After studying this chapter, the student or practitioner will be able to do the following:

1. Describe the basic knowledge base required by an occupational therapy practitioner before orthotic fabrication.
2. Describe three major goals of immobilization orthoses.
3. Describe three major goals of mobilization orthoses.
4. Describe the steps of orthotic fabrication in order from pattern making to critique of the completed orthosis.
5. Identify three characteristics of low-temperature thermoplastic material.
6. Describe 3 to 5 clinical conditions of the hand and/ or wrist that benefit from orthotic fabrication.
7. Demonstrate how to determine the proper length of a forearm-based orthosis.

CHAPTER OUTLINE

KEY TERMS

Axis of motion
Boutonnière deformity
Carpal tunnel syndrome
Carpal-metacarpal (CMC) joint
De Quervain's tenosynovitis
Distal interphalangeal (DIP) joint
Dupuytren's contracture
Dynamic orthoses
Force
Friction

Immobilization orthoses
Mallet finger
Metacarpophalangeal (MCP) joint
Mobilization orthoses
Orthosis
Osteoarthritis (OA)
Proximal inter-phalangeal (PIP) joint
Radial nerve palsy
Rheumatoid arthritis (RA)
Serial static orthosis

Static orthosis
Static progressive orthosis
Tenodesis
Torque
Swan neck deformity
Trigger finger
Ulnar drift deformity
Ulnar nerve palsy

THREADED CASE STUDY

Johanna, Part 1

Johanna (prefers use of the pronouns she/her/hers) is a pleasant, woman of 56 years who lives with her husband in a ranch style family home. Johanna is an elementary school teacher and currently teaches third grade at the local neighborhood school. Johanna's husband is an engineer with the county. Their three young adult children are all living on their own. The eldest son is married with small children and lives in a nearby community, and Johanna's younger son and daughter each live about an hour away. Johanna's hobbies include sewing and quilting, reading and participating in a local book club, swimming and walking for exercise, and baking. She often babysits her young grandchildren. She has recently taken up knitting and her goal is to knit sweaters for everyone in the family as gifts.

Johanna noticed increasing pain and discomfort in her thumb while doing her activities. The pain would last even when she stopped sewing or knitting. She was also having trouble lifting her grandchildren. Both of her thumbs would hurt, and often she would awaken at night with a dull ache that did not go away quickly. The left thumb often felt worse than the right even though she was right handed. Reluctantly, she made an appointment with her general practitioner who in turn recommended that Johanna see an orthopedic surgeon for evaluation.

The orthopedic surgeon did a thorough evaluation of both of Johanna's upper extremities and obtained x-ray films. The results of the examination were shared with Johanna and explained that her diagnosis was osteoarthritis of the base of the thumb, the carpometacarpal (CMC) joint. Johanna was informed that CMC joint osteoarthritis and thumb pain is a common diagnosis among women

in the fourth through sixth decades of life. It was recommended that Johanna see an occupational therapist for evaluation and prescribed hand-based short thumb opponens orthoses for the right and left thumbs to support and immobilize the problematic CMC joints.

Critical Thinking Questions

1. As you learn more about treatment strategies for clients with osteoarthritis of the thumb CMC joints, you will be introduced to a variety of possible procedures for this condition, including medications, injections, and surgeries, as well as occupational therapy interventions for patient education, activity modifications as needed, joint protection techniques and fabrication of supportive orthoses. Why do you think the orthopedic surgeon would select occupational therapy for the first intervention?

2. Johanna performs many occupations throughout her day that include heavy use of the thumbs, including knitting, baking, caring for grandchildren, holding books, and her normal self-care activities. According to the current available evidence, in addition to wearing supportive CMC orthoses, what other adaptations might Johanna consider to continue engaging in her chosen occupations with less pain?

3. Johanna is an elementary school teacher. What occupations does she engage in while on her job, and what modifications or adaptations would you suggest to decrease CMC joint stress in these tasks?

A client-centered focus is at the core of occupational therapy practice. The case of Johanna illustrates how the use of immobilization orthoses helped a client achieve her goals and resume her independent occupations and activities.

The human hand is the brain's most important instrument for exploring and mastering the world. Hands are critical for communication and function, for expression and exploration. When there is dysfunction of the upper extremity, it can affect every aspect of an individual's performance in occupations and activities of importance. Fine motor functions and dexterity of the fingers and thumbs depend on stability and control of the shoulder, elbow, and wrist, which are needed to position the hand in space. Dysfunction anywhere from the brain to the fingertips may impair function of the hand.

An orthosis is a support or brace placed upon a body part to immobilize, protect, position, and/or maintain joint alignment to assist in the rehabilitation process, and/or to assist in aiding an individual to participle and engage in activities of importance.[16]

Occupational therapy practitioners often design and fabricate orthoses (plural form of orthosis). The *Occupational Therapy Practice Framework: Domain & Process*, fourth edition, (OTPF-4) supports occupational therapy's role in this intervention, stating that "occupational therapy practitioners . . . design occupation based intervention plans that facilitate change or growth in the client factors (body functions, body structures) and skills (motor, process, and social interaction) needed for successful participation."[2]

According to the OTPF, orthotic fabrication falls into the category of interventions to support occupations and are used to facilitate "*participation in life through engagement in occupation.*"

Orthoses can offer support to a weakened upper extremity or protection of injured structures to allow the client to participate more fully in occupations that are meaningful to him or her. Occupational therapy practitioners fabricate orthoses for clients in hand therapy clinics, outpatient rehabilitation centers, inpatient and outpatient hospital departments, pediatric settings, and skilled nursing facilities. Clients across the lifespan in all types of settings often require and benefit from having an orthosis as an intervention to help facilitate more independent living.[2]

Orthotic fabrication is an important treatment intervention that occupational therapy practitioners use to minimize and/or correct impairment, to restore and/or augment function, to protect after injury, and/or position against deformity. The clinical reasoning and critical thinking behind every decision to provide or fabricate an orthosis requires an in-depth understanding of normal anatomy of the upper extremity, a variety of different pathological conditions that can affect the upper extremity, and a core understanding of orthotic fabrication principles along with knowledge of the many orthotic designs available. Consider that instruction in orthotic fabrication begins in the classroom, but continued practice and experience gained in the clinic will lead to increased competence and improved skills[16] (Table 30.1).

This chapter introduces the key background information necessary for orthotic fabrication, including a brief review of anatomic structures of the upper extremity, types of orthoses for different goals, the biomechanical principles involved in orthotic fabrication, pattern making, material choices, and steps of fabrication and molding.

TABLE 30.1 Common Orthoses for the Upper Extremity[15]

Name of Orthosis	Body Parts Included	Positioning
Resting hand orthosis	Forearm, wrist, hand, and fingers	Wrist in extension: 10–15 degrees MCP joints in flexion 40–60 degrees PIP and DIP joints in slight flexion Thumb in abduction and opposition
Long thumb opponens orthosis	Wrist and thumb CMC and MCP joints (IP usually free)	Wrist in extension and thumb in abduction and opposition
Short thumb opponens orthosis	Thumb CMC and MCP joints (IP usually free)	Thumb in abduction and opposition
Volar wrist cock-up orthosis	Wrist joint	Wrist in functional extension: 10–30 degrees
Boutonnière orthosis	PIP joint	PIP joint in maximum extension
Mallet orthosis	DIP joint	DIP joint in maximum extension or slight hyperextension
Radial gutter orthosis	Forearm (wrist and hand) on radial side	Wrist in functional extension MCP joints in flexion, PIP, DIPs can be free
Ulnar gutter orthosis	Forearm (wrist and hand) on ulnar side	Wrist in functional extension MCP joints in flexion, PIP, DIPs can be free
Anti–swan neck orthosis	PIP joint	PIP joint in slight flexion
Anti–ulnar claw orthosis	MCP joints (usually of ring and little)	MCP joints in flexion: 45–60 degrees

UPPER EXTREMITY ANATOMY

The following is a brief review of the anatomy and movement patterns in the hand and wrist that are pertinent to orthotic fabrication. (For more in-depth understanding of this, refer to Chapters 20, 21, 22, and 40.)

Bones

The wrist and hand are a complex of 27 bones that contribute to the mobility and adaptability of the upper extremity; the 54 bones that make up both hands and wrists account for approximately one-fourth of the total bones of the human body. The wrist is a complex that consists of the distal ulna and radius and the eight carpal bones arranged in two rows. The carpal bones form the concave transverse arch and, with the configuration of the distal radius, contribute substantially to the conformability of the hand. The distal ulna does not articulate with any carpal bone, and its contribution to wrist stability is made through the attachments of the ulnar collateral ligaments, which places a check on radial deviation.[3]

Joints

The Wrist Joint

The wrist complex (Fig. 30.1) allows a greater arc of motion than any other joint complex except the ankle. This mobility is the result of a unique skeletal configuration and an involved ligamentous system. All motion at the wrist is component motion that occurs in more than one anatomic plane; no pure or isolated motions occur. This concept is key in any treatment directed at the wrist. Extension occurs with a degree of radial deviation and supination. Wrist flexion includes ulnar deviation and pronation. The wrist is contiguous and continuous with the hand. The distal carpal row (the trapezium, trapezoid, capitate, and hamate) articulates firmly with the metacarpals. Motion is produced across these articulations by muscles that cross the

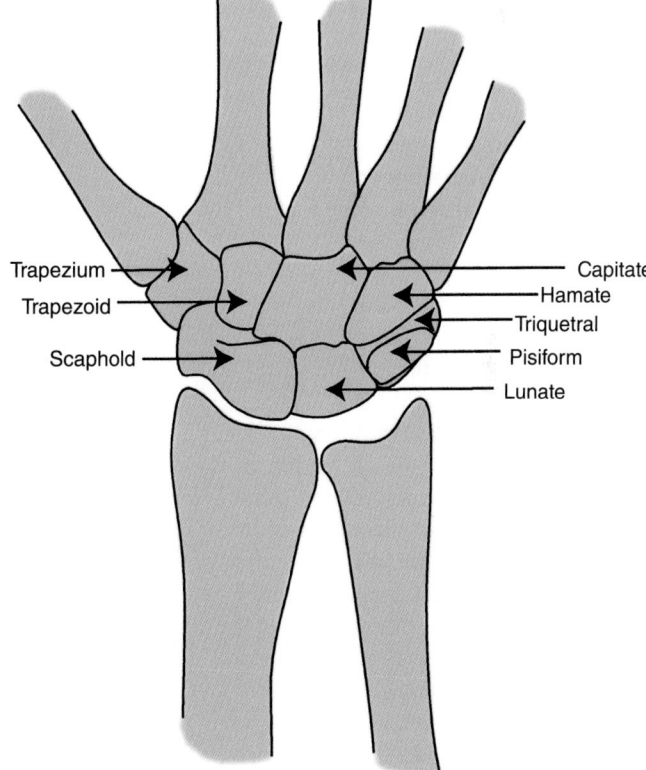

Fig. 30.1 Skeletal structures of the wrist, dorsal view.

carpals and attach to the metacarpals. The proximal carpal row (the scaphoid, lunate, and triquetrum) articulates distally with the distal carpal row and proximally with the radius and the triangular cartilage. Gliding motions occur between the carpal rows during flexion, extension, and deviation, and the carpal ligaments check excessive motion.

Placement of the hand for functional tasks is reliant on the stability, mobility, and precision of placement permitted by the

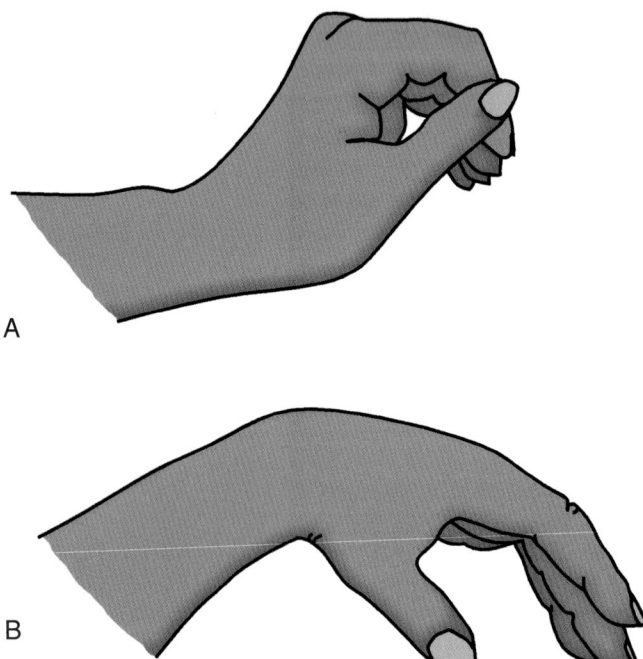

Fig. 30.2 Tenodesis. (A) Active wrist extension results in passive finger flexion. (B) Active wrist flexion results in passive finger extension.

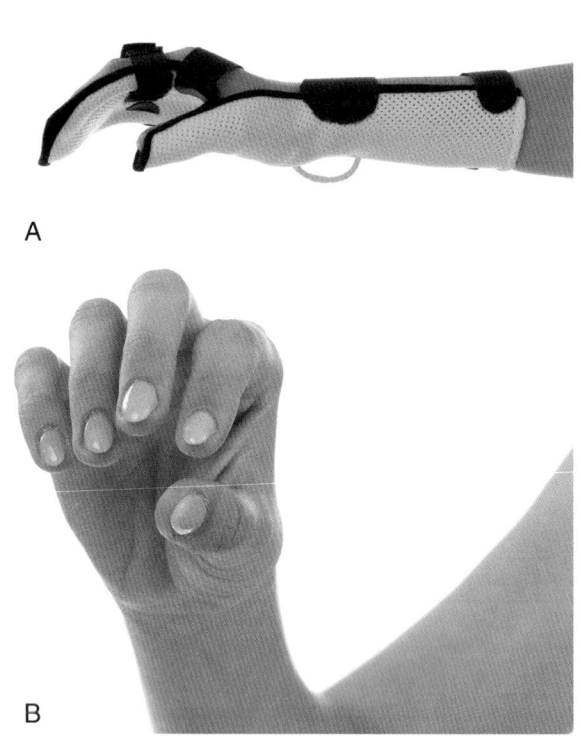

Fig. 30.3 (A) Resting hand orthosis. (B) Functional position of the hand. (With permission from Orfit Industries.)

wrist complex. Any mechanism of injury or disease that alters this complex system, such as rheumatoid arthritis, translates into some level of dysfunction. Even the simplest orthosis that crosses the wrist alters in some way the functional abilities of the hand.[3]

Wrist tenodesis. Tenodesis is the reciprocal motion of the wrist and fingers that occurs during active or passive wrist flexion and extension. Tenodesis is the action of wrist extension producing finger flexion and wrist flexion producing finger extension. It is caused by a lack of change in length of the long finger muscles during wrist flexion or extension (Fig. 30.2).[12]

The extrinsic finger muscle tendon units have a fixed resting length; because they cross multiple joints before inserting onto the phalanges, they can affect the position of several joints with no contraction or length change required of the muscles. This concept is crucial for understanding how passive positioning of the wrist affects the resting position of the digits. In the nerve-injured hand, tenodesis is often harnessed by orthoses to provide function. The client with spinal cord injury with sparing of a wrist extensor (C6 or C7 functional level) gains considerable function from a tenodesis, or wrist-driven flexor hinge hand orthosis. In a dynamic orthosis, such as a tenodesis orthosis, the effect that tenodesis has on tendon length will dictate in part the wrist position that will optimize forces directed at the digits (flexion/extension).

Metacarpal and Metacarpophalangeal Joints

The distal heads of the metacarpals articulate with the proximal phalanges to form the metacarpophalangeal (MCP) joints. Active motion is possible along an axis of flexion and extension and along an axis of abduction and adduction. The distal transverse arch of the hand lies obliquely across the metacarpal

heads. This obliquity is crucial to the ability of the hand to adapt its shape to objects. This concept is most important when determining the distal trim lines for a wrist support when full MP flexion is desired. In addition, a small degree of rotation is present in the MP joints. These axes of motion allow for the hand to conform to different shapes and sizes of objects. When MCP joints are immobilized in extension, a strong tendency exists for secondary shortening of the lax collateral ligaments, in addition to contraction and adherence of the volar plate, which results in limited MP flexion and loss of functional grasp patterns. The resting hand orthosis positions the wrist in 10 degrees to 15 degrees of extension, the MP joints at 40 to 60 degrees of flexion, and the PIP and DIP at 10 degrees to 25 degrees of flexion (Fig. 30.3). This position is designed to prevent shortening and to maintain the joints in midrange for optimal function. An important consideration is to ensure that the mobile fourth and fifth digits are positioned in the orthosis to accommodate their additional degree of mobility by allowing somewhat greater flexion at their MP joints.[3]

Proximal Interphalangeal Joints

The proximal interphalangeal (PIP) joint capsule and ligaments provide stability and allow mobility in one plane only. Collateral ligaments on each side of the joint run in a dorsal-to-palmar direction, inserting into the fibrocartilage plate of the PIP. These ligaments and the plate are lax with the PIP joint in flexion and taut with it in extension. The seemingly simple joint is made more complex by inclusion of the extensor mechanism passing through the capsule dorsally and contributing slips to the system of ligaments affecting this joint. The potential for disruption of the extensor mechanism is high. Many finger injuries to this area of the dorsal extensor mechanism (zones III) can be treated with orthotic interventions, including injuries such as Boutonnière deformity and swan neck deformity (Figs. 30.4 to 30.6).[11,15]

Distal Interphalangeal Joints

The distal interphalangeal (DIP) joint capsule and ligaments are similar to the PIP joint but have less structural strength to

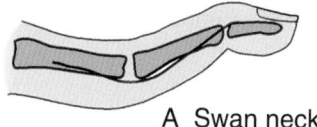

A Swan neck

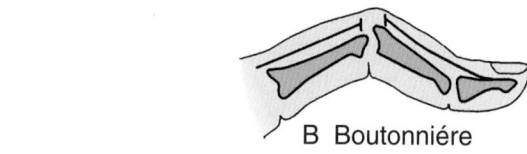

B Boutonnière

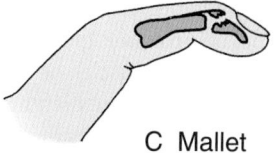

C Mallet

Fig. 30.4 (A) Swan-neck deformity, or joint change, with proximal interphalangeal joint hyperextension and distal interphalangeal joint flexion. (B) Boutonnière deformity, or joint change, characterized by proximal interphalangeal joint flexion and distal interphalangeal joint hyperextension. (C) Mallet finger with distal interphalangeal joint flexion and loss of active extension.

the terminal insertions of the palmar plate and collateral ligaments. As the structures become smaller, they lose integrity and strength. One of the most frequent injuries to the digits is disruption of the terminal end of the extensor tendon, which results in a mallet or "baseball" finger (Fig. 30.7).[5]

Thumb Joints

The thumb includes the CMC, the MCP joint and the interphalangeal (IP) joint. The base of the first metacarpal articulates with the trapezium to form a highly mobile joint that often is compared with the shape of a saddle. The base of the first metacarpal is concave in the anteroposterior plane and convex in the lateral plane. This surface is met by reciprocal surfaces on the trapezium. This configuration allows for a wide arc of motion, with the thumb able to rotate not only for pad-to-pad opposition but also for full extension and abduction to move away from the palm. Both motions are important for function.[12]

Ligaments

The ligamentous structures of the hand act as checkreins for the hand and wrist; this limits extremes of motion and provides stability. The complex motions of the wrist depend in large part on the ligaments that restrain them, rather than on the contact surfaces between the carpals and metacarpals. Three groups of

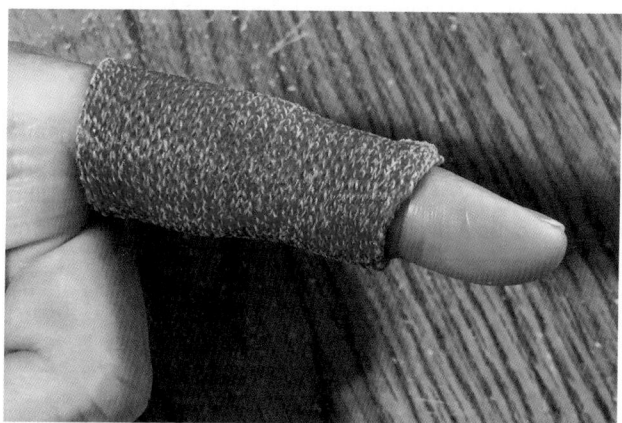

Fig. 30.6 Boutonniere orthosis. (With permission from Orfit Industries.)

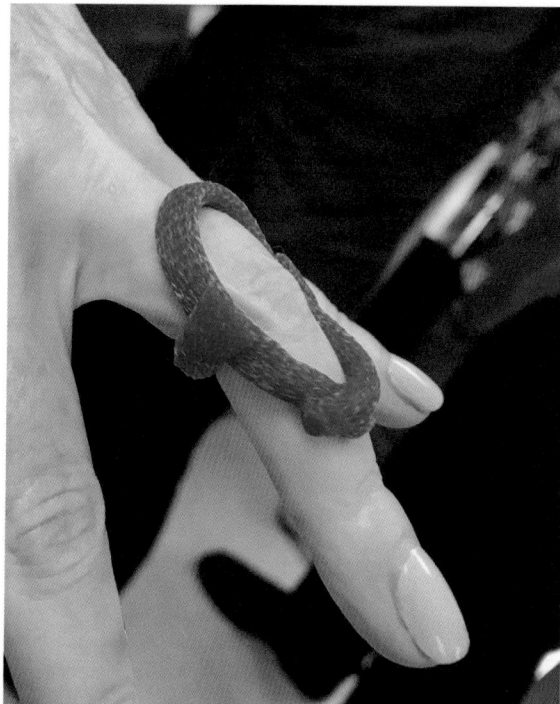

Fig. 30.5 Anti–swan neck orthosis, which blocks hyperextension but allows full flexion. (Even the simplest orthoses addressing the muscles/tendons that cross the wrist will alter functional abilities.)

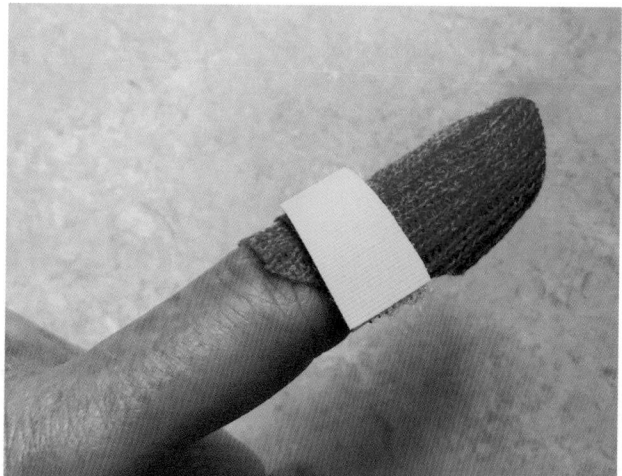

Fig. 30.7 Mallet orthosis. (With permission from Orfit Industries.)

ligaments are discussed briefly to highlight their contribution to wrist stability and mobility[3]:

1. The palmar ligaments include the radio-scapho-capitate ligament, which contributes support to the scaphoid; the radio-lunate ligament, which supports the lunate; and the radio-scapho-lunate ligament, which connects the scapholunate articulation with the palmar surface of the distal radius. The stability and mobility of the thumb and radial carpus depend on the integrity of these ligaments. Disruption of the ligaments results in instability and pain at the wrist and in significant dysfunction of the thumb. Use of orthotics is frequently the treatment of choice to supply stability for pain reduction.

2. The radial and ulnar collateral ligaments provide dorsal stability. These capsular ligaments, along with the radiocarpal and dorsal carpal ligaments, provide carpal stability and permit range of motion (ROM). Disruption of any of these ligaments may result in pain, loss of strength, and functional impairment.

3. The triangular fibrocartilage complex (TFCC) includes the ligaments and the cartilaginous structures that suspend the distal radius from the distal ulna and the proximal carpus. Tears or strains in this complex are evidenced by pain and weakness with resultant loss of function in resistive tasks. The advent of new imaging techniques has made the diagnosis of TFCC tears more common; orthoses are often provided for support and pain relief.

Muscles

Balance in the hand must be considered when the hand is assessed for an orthosis. Two groups of muscles act on the wrist and hand: (1) the extrinsic muscles that arise from the elbow and the proximal half of the mid-forearm and (2) the intrinsic

muscles with origins and insertions entirely in the hand. The extrinsic muscles include both a flexor and an extensor group acting on the wrist and on the digits. The intrinsic muscles include the lumbricals, the dorsal and palmar interossei, and the thenar and hypothenar groups. Smooth, coordinated motions of the hand in functional activities depend on a well-integrated balance between and within these two muscle groups.[12] Many of the contractures that occupational therapists work to correct with orthoses are caused by neurological dysfunction (central or peripheral), which results in an imbalance of muscle tone or innervation. (See Table 30.2.)

Nerves

A discussion of the nerve supply to the hand should include mention of the continuity of the brachial plexus from its origins in the spinal cord to its terminal innervations in the hand. There are three main peripheral nerves that supply motor and sensory function to the upper extremity; the radial nerve, the median nerve and the ulnar nerve (Fig. 30.8). The radial nerve is the primary motor supplier to the extensor and supinator muscles. The sensory fibers of the radial nerve supply the dorsum and the radial border of the hand. The median nerve provides motor supply to the flexor-pronator group, which includes most of the long flexors and the muscles of the thenar eminence. The sensory distribution of the median nerve is functionally the most important because it includes the palmar surface of the thumb, index, and long fingers and the radial half of the ring finger. The ulnar nerve supplies most of the intrinsic muscles, the hypothenar muscles, the ulnar most profundi, and the adductor pollicis brevis. The sensory supply of the ulnar nerve includes the palmar surface of the ulnar half of the ring finger, the little finger, and the ulnar half of the palm. Injuries or compressions that occur anywhere along pathways of these

TABLE 30.2	Forearm and Hand Extrinsic and Intrinsic Muscles and Nerve Innervations[12]		
	Radial Nerve	**Median Nerve**	**Ulnar Nerve**
Extrinsic muscles	Extensor carpi radialis longus	Flexor carpi radialis	Flexor carpi ulnaris
	Extensor carpi radialis brevis	Palmaris longus	Flexor digitorum profundus (ring and little)
	Extensor carpi ulnaris (pin)	Flexor digitorum superficialis	
	Extensor digitorum (pin)	Flexor digitorum profundus (AIN) (index and middle)	
	Extensor indicis (ping)	Flexor pollicis longus (AIN)	
	Extensor pollicis brevis (pin)		
	Extensor pollicis longus (pin)		
	Abductor pollicis longus (pin)		
	Extensor digiti minimi (pin)		
Intrinsic muscles		Lumbricals (index and middle)	Lumbricals (ring and little)
		Thenar muscles: abductor pollicis brevis, flexor pollicis brevis, opponens pollicis	Palmar interossei
			Dorsal interossei
			Hypothenar muscles: abductor digiti minimi, flexor digiti minimi, opponens digiti minimi

PIN, Posterior interosseous nerve; *AIN*, anterior interosseous nerve.

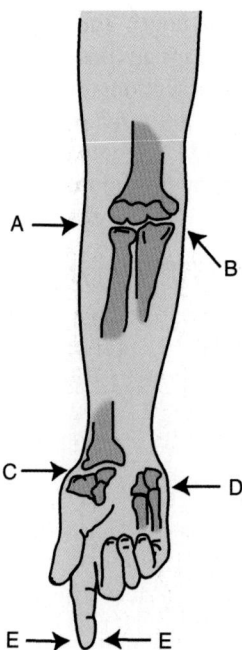

Fig. 30.8 Potential sites for nerve compression from improperly fitted orthoses. *A*, Radial nerve. *B*, Ulnar nerve. *C*, Radial digital nerve in anatomic snuffbox. *D*, Ulnar nerve in Guyon's canal. *E*, Digital nerves.

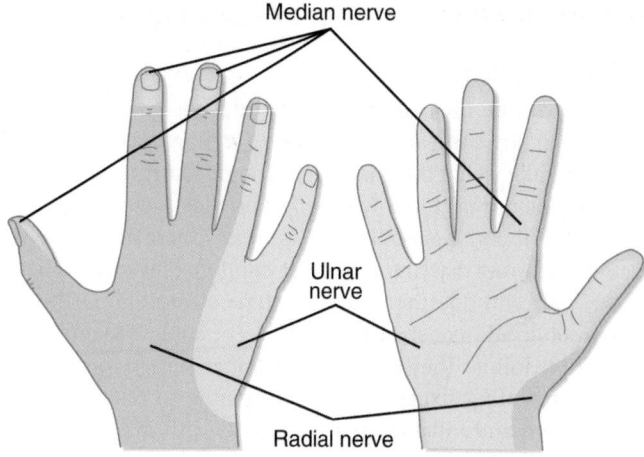

Fig. 30.9 Sensory distribution in hand. Median nerve distribution includes most of the prehensile surface of the palm. (From Adams JG: *Emergency Medicine: Clinical Essentials*, ed 2, Philadelphia, 2013, Saunders.)

nerves may result in motor or sensory dysfunction. When providing an orthosis for the upper extremity, the occupational therapist must give attention to the pathways of the nerves and to potential sites for nerve entrapment. In the fabrication of any orthotic device, care must be taken to avoid applying pressure over sites where the nerves are superficial and prone to compression. These sites include the ulnar nerve at the elbow in the cubital tunnel and in Guyon's canal at the ulnar border of the wrist, the radial nerve at the elbow and in the thenar snuffbox, and the digital nerves along the medial and lateral borders of the digits (Fig. 30.9).[10]

Circulation

Blood supply to the hand is contributed by the radial and ulnar arteries. The ulnar artery lies just lateral to the flexor carpi ulnaris tendon, where it divides into a large branch that forms the superficial arterial arch and a small branch that forms the lesser part of the deep palmar arch. The ulnar artery is vulnerable to trauma where it passes between the pisiform and the hamate (Guyon's canal). The radial artery divides at the proximal wrist crease into a small, superficial branch and a larger, deep radial branch. The superficial arterial arch further divides into common digital branches and then into proper digital branches.

Venous drainage of the hand is accomplished by two sets of veins: a superficial and a deep group. Occupational therapists are more likely to be concerned with the superficial venous system because it lies superficially in the dorsum of the hand. Disruption of this superficial system may result in extensive fluid edema in the dorsum of the hand, which requires the occupational therapist's intervention. Care must be taken not to strap orthotics too tightly over the dorsum of the hand; this traps fluids from draining.[3]

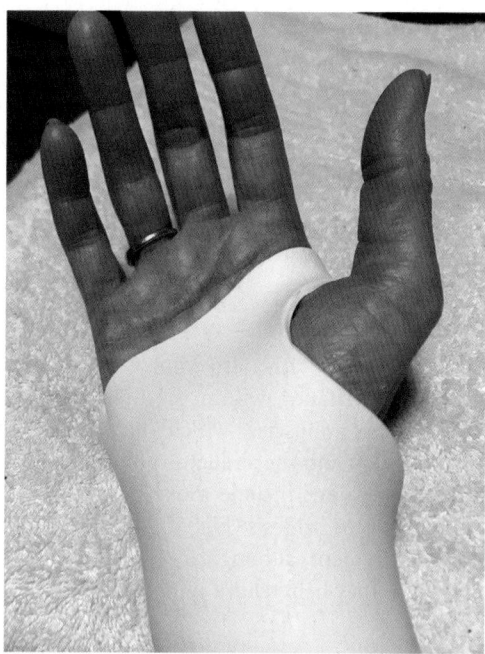

Fig. 30.10 Distal palmar crease line visible and distal edge of orthosis angled to allow full flexion of all MCP joints. (With permission from Orfit Industries.)

Superficial Anatomy and Landmarks

Creases on the volar surface of the wrist and hand serve as important landmarks for where orthoses are placed and their proximal and distal borders. The cascade of the fingers is a direct result of the oblique angle formed at the metacarpal heads (sloping angle, not parallel to the wrist). This concept is most important when determining the distal trim lines for a wrist support when full MP flexion is desired. Distal borders of a wrist orthosis should allow for the distal palmar crease to be visible (Fig. 30.10).[3]

ORTHOTIC FABRICATION: TYPES AND GOALS

Types of Orthoses

Orthoses can be divided into two distinct categories depending on their structure and goals of use. Occupational therapists must carefully weigh the goals of the intended orthosis and the diagnosis before deciding whether to provide a client with an immobilization or a mobilization orthosis. There are immobilization orthoses that are a brace or support that immobilizes a body part and does not allow any type of motion. Orthoses for immobilization or static orthoses can be applied to one joint or multiple joints. They are often used after surgery or trauma to protect healing structures, for positioning to relieve symptoms of pain and inflammation for clients with different types of arthritis, for functional positioning and tone management for clients with neurological diagnoses and for a variety of other diagnoses and goals.[12]

IMMOBILIZATION ORTHOSES

Common Goals and Clinical Conditions for Immobilization Orthoses

A common goal of orthotic fabrication is to limit or reduce pain by providing rest and support in a position of healing. The goals for immobilization orthoses can be found in Box 30.1.

There are several examples of different clinical conditions that may benefit from an orthosis based on this specific goal of treatment.

De Quervain's Tenosynovitis

De Quervain's tenosynovitis, also known as stenosing tenosynovitis, involves irritation within the first dorsal compartment of the extensor muscles, which includes the extensor pollicis brevis tendon and the abductor pollicis longus tendon. Therapeutic interventions include moist heat, modalities, and a *long thumb opponens orthosis* (Fig. 30.11) to rest the specific tendons from movement, although in some case a corticosteroid injection also may help relieve symptoms.[9]

Trigger Finger

Digital flexor tendinitis and tenosynovitis refer to inflammation, sometimes with subsequent fibrosis, of tendons and tendon sheaths of the digits. Pathologic changes begin with a thickening or nodule within the tendon. When located at the site of the tight first annular (A1) pulley, the nodule blocks

smooth extension of the finger. The finger may lock in flexion, or suddenly extend with a snap (hence the term trigger finger). Typical therapeutic interventions include moist heat, modalities, and an *orthosis that limits full composite flexion* in order to block triggering (Fig. 30.12). Some clients may need a steroid injection and or a surgical procedure typically followed with an orthosis.[9]

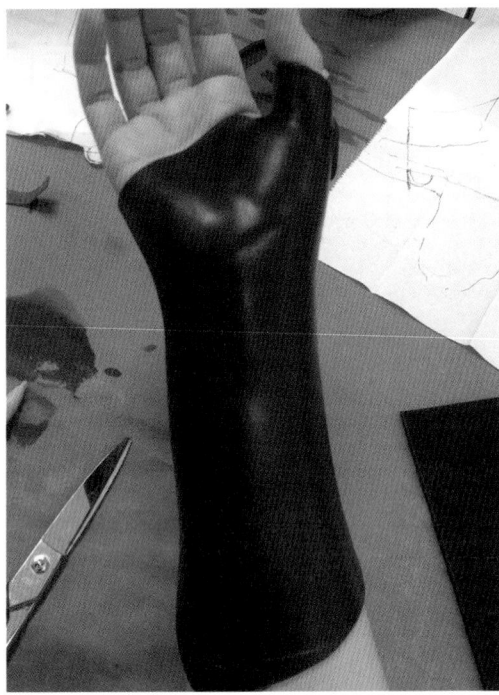

Fig. 30.11 Long thumb opponens orthosis. (With permission from Orfit Industries.)

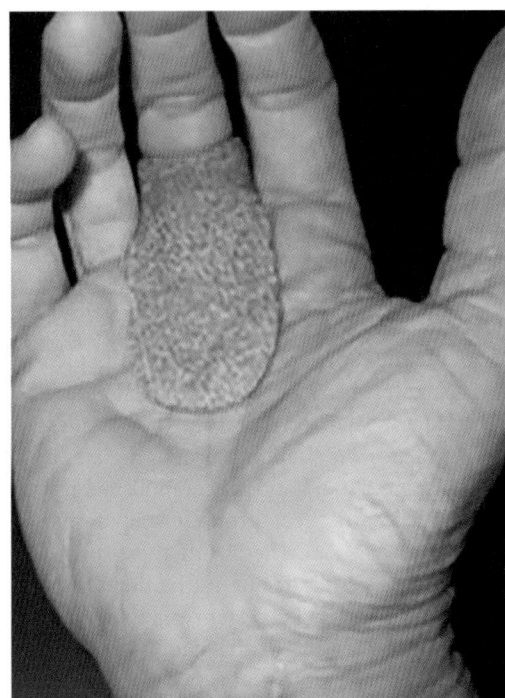

Fig. 30.12 Trigger finger orthosis. (With permission from Orfit Industries.)

BOX 30.1   **Goals of Immobilization Orthoses**
• Symptom relief
• Protection and positioning
• Maximize function
• Improve and/or preserve joint alignment
• Contracture management
• Block and/or transfer muscle force for improved function

Osteoarthritis of the Thumb Carpometacarpal Joint

Pain is the earliest symptom of osteoarthritis (OA) at the base of the thumb, sometimes described as a deep ache. Additional characteristics of osteoarthritis are loss of joint cartilage and bone hypertrophy. Therapeutic interventions address the symptoms and provide pain relief with moist heat, modalities, activity analysis and modifications, and patient education in joint protection techniques. *A thumb orthosis, known as a short thumb opponens orthosis that stabilizes the CMC joint and often the MCP joint*, as well, helps with positioning and immobilizing and/or supporting the joint (Fig. 30.13).[9]

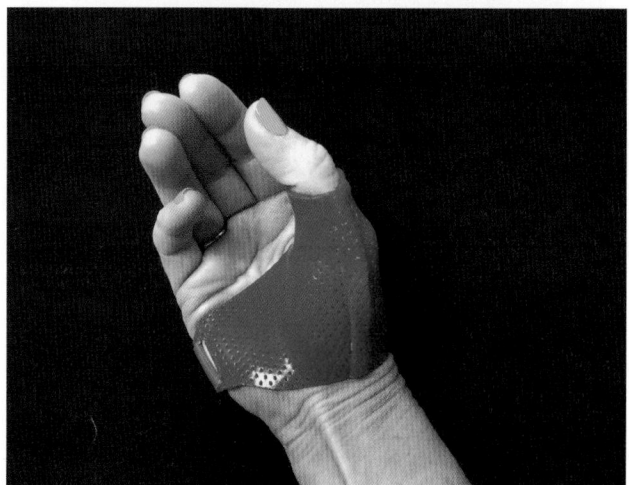

Fig. 30.13 Short thumb opponens orthosis. (With permission from Orfit Industries.)

Immobilizing Orthoses for Positioning

Another common goal of orthotic fabrication is to provide positioning for improved function or healing. Common clinical conditions include the following.

Carpal Tunnel Syndrome

Carpal tunnel syndrome refers to compression of the median nerve as it passes through the carpal tunnel in the wrist. Symptoms include pain and paresthesias in the median nerve distribution. Therapeutic interventions include ergonomic improvements, avoidance of wrist flexion and repetitive motion activities, and use of a *wrist cock-up orthosis* to prevent posturing in wrist flexion (worn at night or during the day as needed) (Fig. 30.14).[8,9]

Mallet Finger

A mallet finger is an extensor tendon injury in zone 1 on the dorsum of the hand that causes a flexion deformity at the DIP joint. It is caused by avulsion of the extensor tendon, with or without a small bony fragment. The usual mechanism of injury is forced flexion of the distal phalanx, typically when hit with a ball. Therapeutic intervention includes an *orthosis that positions the DIP joint in full extension or slight hyperextension* for a period of 6 to 8 weeks (see Fig. 30.7). The DIP joint cannot be allowed to flex during this time.[5]

Boutonnière Deformity

A boutonnière deformity consists of flexion of the proximal interphalangeal (PIP) joint accompanied by hyperextension of the distal interphalangeal (DIP) joint. It is caused by disruption of the central slip attachment of the

THREADED CASE STUDY

Johanna, Part 2

Johanna made an appointment to see an occupational therapist the following week. Using the Occupational Therapy Practice Framework, the occupational therapist prepared an occupational profile of the client to establish her needs, priorities, and goals, which included the ability to have less pain and resume fine motor activities, pick up her grandchildren and be able to perform her normal activities of daily living without discomfort. The occupational therapist evaluated Johanna's range of motion, muscle strength, grip, and pinch strength and discussed her daily routine. Johanna was asked to complete a client-rated functional outcome measure to describe her performance on certain regular tasks that she performed at home. The occupational therapist then shared the analysis of Johanna's occupational performance and discussed an intervention plan with Johanna.

The occupational therapist commented that although grip strength was within normal limits on both the right and left hands, Johanna's pinch strength was markedly weak in both right and left sides, and Johanna had reported pain while performing the testing. The occupational therapist also pointed out that her active and passive joint range of motion for fingers and thumbs was within normal limits, but her left thumb did not oppose or flex quite as much as the thumb on the right. Physical evaluation revealed some swelling around the base of each thumb, more on the right than the left. There was also decreased ability on both right and left to actively abduct the thumb in palmar and radial abduction, and the left thumb CMC joint was showing signs of beginning subluxation.

The client-rated functional outcome measure that Johanna filled out is called the Patient Rated Wrist and Hand Evaluation (PRWHE).[7] This is a 15-question survey asking about pain and function doing normal everyday activities and asks clients to fill out their answers using a Likert scale of 1 to 10. They self-rate their performance on tasks such as lifting a heavy object, buttoning buttons, and turning a door knob. The lower scores indicate a better overall performance of activities of daily living. Johanna had rated her performance overall as 120 of a possible 150, indicating that she was having difficulty and pain performing many of her regular activities and doing her normal occupations. She recently had to stop knitting and was having trouble holding books to read. She could not pick up her grandchildren when they visited. Johanna's goals were to have less pain in her thumbs so that she could resume her normal activities, and finish knitting sweaters for her family.

The occupational therapist recommended that Johanna attend therapy for a few visits to review joint protection techniques and learn some pain management strategies. Also recommended was the use of hand-based short opponens orthoses, which would help to immobilize the CMC joint while still allowing a great deal of function. The orthoses should initially be worn all of the time to help calm the irritated tissues around each CMC joint. In the future, Johanna might be able to wean off the orthoses and wear them on an as-needed schedule.

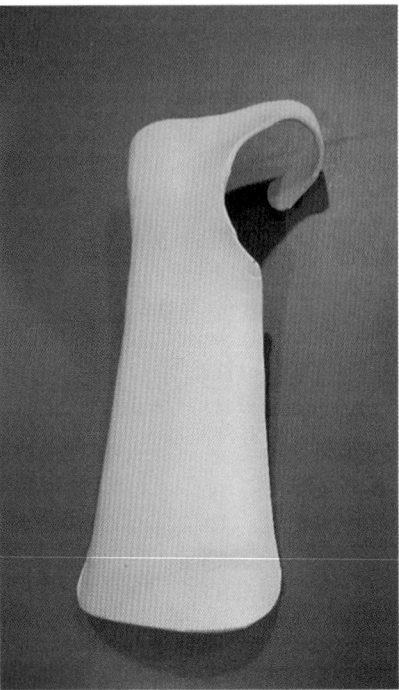

Fig. 30.14 Wrist cock-up orthosis. (With permission from Orfit Industries.)

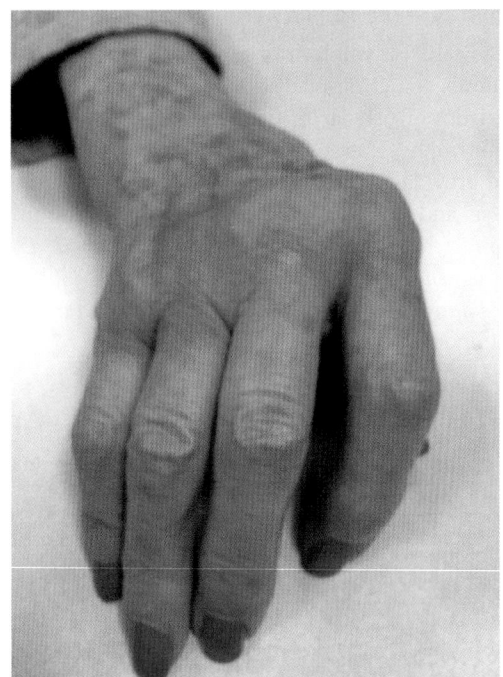

Fig. 30.15 Patient with ulnar drift of digits. (With permission from Orfit Industries.)

extensor tendon to the base of the middle phalanx, allowing the proximal phalanx to protrude (buttonhole) between the lateral bands of the extensor tendon. Therapeutic intervention includes an *orthosis that immobilizes the PIP joint in extension* (see Fig. 30.6).[5]

Swan-Neck Deformity

A swan neck deformity consists of hyperextension of the proximal interphalangeal (PIP) joint, flexion of the distal interphalangeal (DIP) joint, and sometimes flexion of the metacarpophalangeal (MCP) joint. It can be caused by rheumatoid arthritis, untreated mallet finger, laxity of the ligaments of the volar aspect of the PIP, or rupture of the flexor tendon of the PIP. A therapeutic intervention includes fabrication of an *orthosis called a figure-of-8 orthosis, which blocks hyperextension but allows full flexion* (see Fig. 30.5).[5]

Ulnar Drift of the Digits

Patients with rheumatoid arthritis often develop ulnar drift at their MCP joints (Fig. 30.15). Ulnar drift (also called ulnar drift deformity) may occur as a result of the following progression: joint synovitis and stretching of the joint capsule and radial collateral ligaments with subsequent subluxation of the extensor tendons in an ulnar direction, destruction of the metacarpal heads, and volar dislocation of the proximal phalanxes. Additionally, many activities of daily living place excessive ulnar and volar deviating forces across the MCP joints when the thumb pinches against the side of the index finger, thereby increasing the deforming forces. An *anti-ulnar drift orthosis* can position the MCP joints into a neutral position provided the joints can be passively aligned (Fig. 30.16). An orthosis cannot correct a fixed deformity.[1]

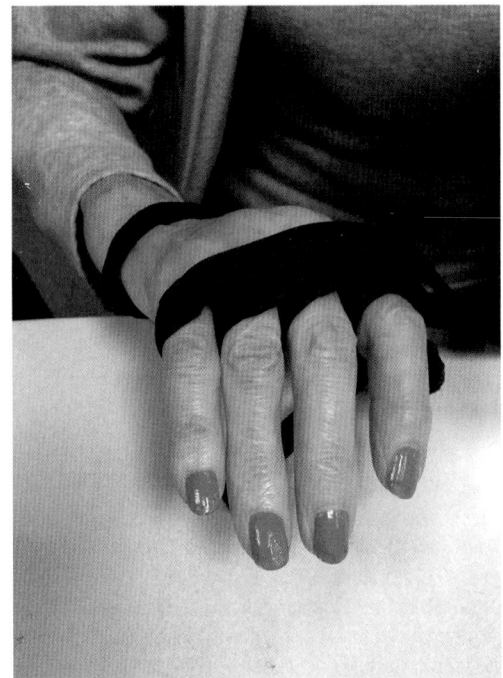

Fig. 30.16 Anti–ulnar drift orthosis. (With permission from Orfit Industries.)

Ulnar Nerve Palsy

Ulnar nerve palsy is caused by compression or disruption of the ulnar nerve usually at the cubital tunnel in the elbow or Guyon's canal in the wrist or by injury along this pathway. Ulnar clawing, or hyperextension of the MCP joints with flexion of the PIP and DIP joints, is caused by the lack of innervation to the interosseus muscles in the presence of functioning extrinsic finger

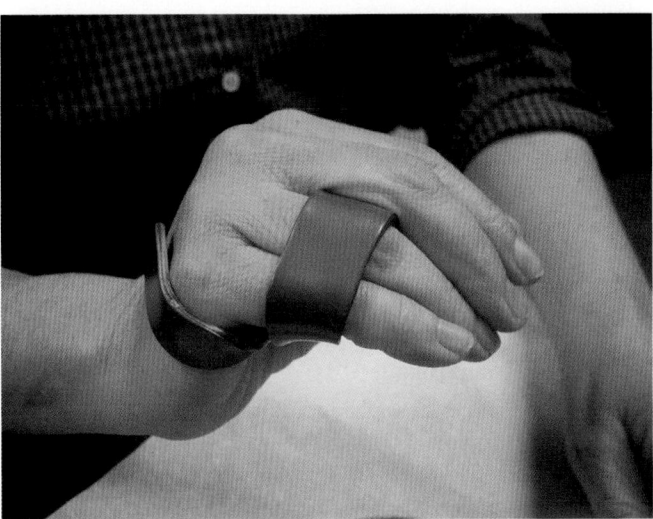

Fig. 30.17 Anti-claw orthosis for ulnar nerve palsy. (With permission from Orfit Industries.)

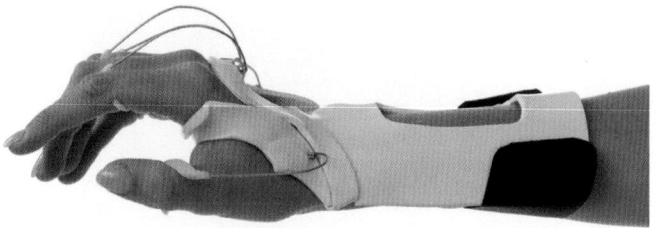

Fig. 30.18 Outrigger orthosis for radial nerve palsy. (With permission from Orfit Industries.)

BOX 30.2 Goals for Mobilization Orthoses

- Substitute for weak or absent muscle
- Remodel long-standing dense mature scar tissue
- Elongate soft-tissue contractures
- Increase passive joint range of motion

---

flexors. This results in a loss of active IP joint extension and MCP joint flexion, which prevents the patient from cupping the hand and holding any objects. Because the MP joints of (usually) the ring and small fingers are pulled back into extension or hyperextension, the force translates into forced finger flexion (claw), and the client cannot flex the MP joints to grasp objects. The *anti-claw orthosis* positions the MCP joints in flexion and helps to transmit the extensor force distally to the IP joints (Fig. 30.17).[10]

MOBILIZATION ORTHOSES

Mobilization orthoses are constructed with a base similar to that of orthoses for immobilization but have added components often called outriggers to apply force or traction to various parts of the body to gain passive joint motion or assist in active function. The goals of these orthoses are very different from goals for immobilization orthoses. Often, these orthoses are more complex to fabricate and fit to clients. They require additional skill in understanding the application of force through pulleys and finger cuffs. But more importantly, they require that occupational therapy practitioners recognize the need for these mobilization orthoses and know how to select the appropriate one to best serve the client's needs.[12] Goals for mobilization orthoses can be found in Box 30.2.

Dynamic, Static Progressive, and Serial Static Designs

Dynamic orthoses include one or more resilient components (elastics, rubber bands, or springs) that produce motion (Fig. 30.18). The force applied from the resilient component is constant even when tissues have reached end range. Dynamic orthoses are designed to increase passive motion, to augment active motion by assisting a joint through its range, or to substitute for lost motion. Dynamic orthoses generally include a static base on which movable, resilient components can be attached. A common use of dynamic orthotics is to gain greater finger

range of motion by adding dynamic MP extension or MP flexion components.[12]

A serial static orthosis achieves a slow, progressive increase in ROM by repeated remolding of the orthosis or cast. The serial static orthosis has no movable or resilient components but rather is a static orthosis whose design and material allow repeated remolding. Each adjustment repositions the part at the end of the available range to progressively gain passive motion. A cylindrical cast designed to reduce a PIP joint flexion contracture through frequent removal and recasting is a classic example of a serial static orthosis (Fig. 30.19).[12]

Static progressive orthoses include a static mechanism that adjusts the amount or angle of traction acting on a part (Fig. 30.20). This mechanism may be a turnbuckle, a cloth strap, nylon line, or a buckle. The static progressive orthosis is distinguished from the dynamic orthosis by its lack of a resilient force. It is distinguished from a serial static orthosis in having a built-in adjustment mechanism, so that the part can be repositioned at end range without the need to remold it. Generally, the client can adjust the static progressive mechanism as prescribed or as tolerated.[13]

Common Clinical Conditions for Mobilization Orthoses
Radial Nerve Palsy

An injury to the radial nerve (sometimes referred to as radial nerve palsy depending on severity of the injury) is a relatively common occurrence and can be caused by humeral fracture, laceration, injections, traction, shoulder or elbow joint dislocations, and compression.

Because of the lack of innervation to the extensor muscles, the wrist assumes a flexed posture. This "wrist drop" position causes elongation of the extensor muscles and a flexion posture of the flexor muscles, causing them to shorten. Orthoses are provided to assist in lost motor power and to provide support for the wrist.[8] The fingers and thumb can be fitted with dynamic extension cuffs to allow assisted extension of the MCP joints.[6,8]

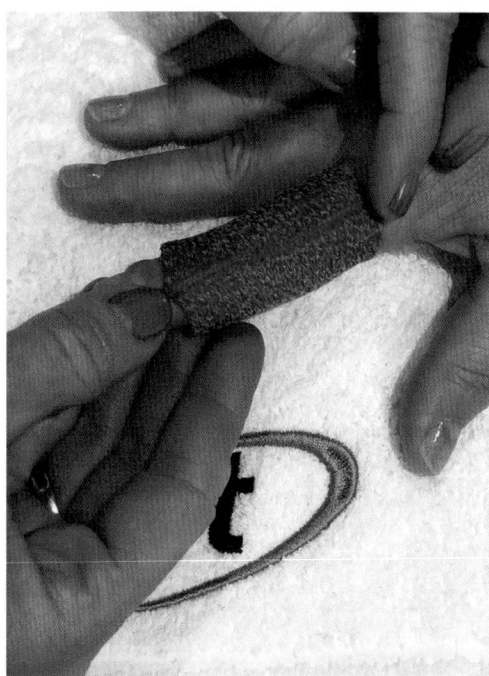

Fig. 30.19 Serial orthosis for PIP extension. (With permission from Orfit Industries.)

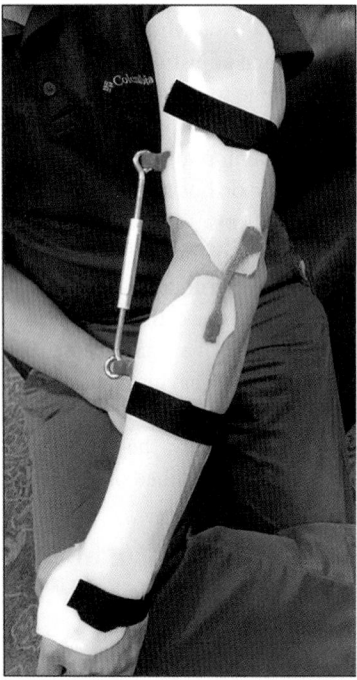

Fig. 30.20 Static progressive orthosis for elbow extension. (With permission from Orfit Industries.)

Limitations in Joint Range of Motion

Limitations in joint range of motion, although they can be congenital, are usually the result of either an ongoing disease process such as rheumatoid arthritis slowly affecting the joints or injuries such as fractures, especially in the elbow, wrist, and fingers, because of the length of time the body part must be immobilized for healing, resulting in tightened and contracted ligaments or in changes to the joint integrity or structure. Neurological

diagnoses resulting in abnormal muscle tone or hemiplegia can result in range of motion changes as a result of lack of normal movement and/or poor positioning. An example of limited wrist range of motion might be a client who fractures the wrist and has difficulty regaining functional wrist extension after immobilization in a cast, or clients who have had a CVA and have spasticity in their affected upper extremity. A serial static, dynamic, or static progressive orthosis might be incorporated into the treatment to provide a low load of prolonged stretch to help regain passive joint motion.[14]

Decreased Tissue Length

In the same manner of applying low load and prolonged stress to a stiff joint, mobilization orthoses also can be used to help with regaining tissue length. Decreased tissue length can be caused by a number of conditions, including lengthy immobilization that allows the tissue to contract, scar formation after wound contraction, dense scar tissue formation from burns or large wounds that contract as they remodel, and from disease processes such as Dupuytren's contracture, which is a connective tissue disorder of the palmar fascia. Dupuytren's contracture can affect the ability to fully open the palm and extend the digits. Although an orthosis will not prevent the original contracture of a progressive Dupuytren's contracture, a client might be seen after collagenase injection or surgery for therapy to help regain finger motion. An occupational therapist can provide a mobilization orthosis for this purpose: a serial static orthosis to help regain length of the palmar tissue, and/or a static progressive or dynamic finger orthosis to help with increasing tendon length of the involved digits.[12]

PRINCIPLES OF ORTHOTIC FABRICATION

Biomechanics

Mechanics deals with the application of force, and biomechanics may be viewed as the body's response to those forces. In the hand, muscles supply the force required to produce motion. The force then is transmitted by the tendons to the bones and joints, with control supplied by the skin and pulp of the fingers and palm. How the application of an orthotic affects the transmission of force to produce motion depends on the relationship between the axis of rotation of joints and anatomic planes and the forces imposed on the hand.[4]

Axis of Motion

Each joint in the body rotates around what is called the axis of motion, or a single line that does not move while the bones of a joint move around it, in relation to each other. Consider a car tire that is perfectly balanced around its axis of motion. When a tire is perfectly balanced, it does not wobble; it has pure motion around a single point.

In a single-axis joint, motion occurs in only one plane. The PIP joint is an example of a single-axis joint in alignment with an anatomic plane. It moves only in the plane of flexion and extension.

Joints that have more than one axis of motion may move in more than one plane at a time. For example, the wrist complex has two axes of motion: flexion-extension and radial-ulnar deviation. A joint with multiple axes has conjoint motions that occur in addition to the primary motions described by the joint. Wrist flexion occurs with a moment of ulnar deviation and with a small degree of pronation. Wrist extension occurs with radial deviation and slight supination.[4]

Application of Force

It is crucial to understand basic principles of force and apply them correctly in the fabrication of orthoses. An understanding of the forces applied by levers and the stresses that occur between opposing surfaces can help to explain what happens as forces are applied within the body by muscles and externally by orthoses.[4]

Definitions. The term *force*, as it relates to orthotic fabrication, describes the effects that materials and dynamic components have on bone and tissue. *Force* is a measure of stress, friction, or torque. *Stress* is resistance to any force that strains or deforms tissue. Shear stress occurs when force is applied to tissues at an angle or in opposing directions. Pinching skin between the surface of an orthosis and the underlying bony structures causes shear stress.

Area. When the area over which a force is distributed is made larger, the pressure is reduced. Occupational therapists take this into account by creating orthotic designs that allow for the best possible pressure distribution over larger surface areas.

Lever Arms

Most orthoses follow the concept of a first class lever system with the joint positioned between two lever arms. The length of the bones serves as the lever arms and the joint serves as the fulcrum or center of rotation. The proximal and distal components of the orthoses are known as the lever arms representing the force and the resistance.[4]

Friction occurs when one surface impedes or prevents gliding of a surface on another. Friction is produced in the stiff or contracted joint when soft tissue restriction prevents gliding of the bones. Orthotics may contribute to friction if they are misaligned in relation to a joint axis. For example, a hinged orthosis that is not properly aligned with the axis of rotation will limit motion by producing friction as the joint attempts to move.[4]

Torque is a measure of the force that results in rotation of a lever around its axis of motion. The torque created when a lever rotates depends on the force used and the length of the lever employed. In the body, muscles are the levers that create torque when they act to move a joint. Externally, orthoses may act as levers to apply the force necessary to move a bone around its joint axis. The measure of torque is given by the following formula[12]:

$$\text{Torque} = (\text{amount of}) \text{ Force} \times (\text{length of}) \text{ Lever arm}$$

Internally, the length of the lever arm is measured as the perpendicular distance from the axis of the joint to the tendon. Externally, the length of the lever arm is measured as the estimated distance from the joint axis to point of application of force. In orthotic fabrication, force to a finger joint is usually applied with a molded finger cuff. For example, a mobilization orthosis with an outrigger system will apply force with a finger cuff, to help gain passive motion after an injury that resulted in joint stiffness. This application of force to the stiff joint must be applied at a **right angle (a 90-degree angle) to the long axis of the bone distal to the joint** (Fig. 30.21A–B).[4]

This ensures that the joint surface and ligaments will not be damaged. One additional key concept regarding mobilization orthoses is that longer lever arms lessen the amount of force or torque required to move the bones through the joint axis of motion. The greater the length of the lever arm between the finger cuff or strap and the joint axis, the less force is required to

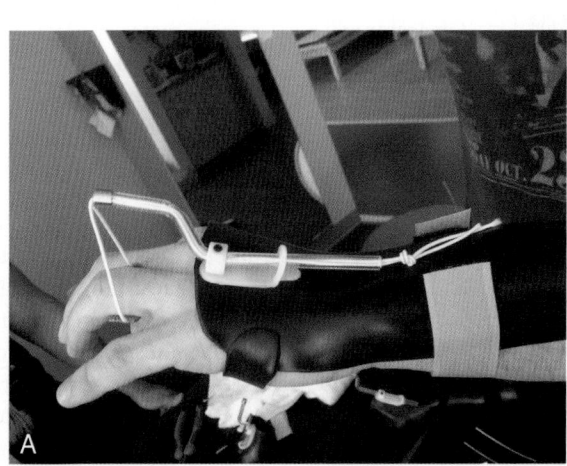
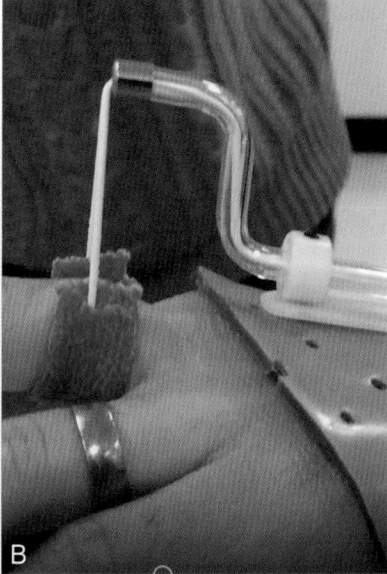

Fig. 30.21 (A) Dynamic orthosis with finger cuff. (B) Finger cuff highlighting 90-degree angle. (With permission from Orfit Industries.)

achieve motion. This makes an orthosis more comfortable on the client.[12]

THE ORTHOSIS FABRICATION PROCESS

The orthotic fabrication process typically begins with a written referral or script from a physician requesting an orthosis for a client. Following the guidelines of the OTPF, the occupational therapist conducts an evaluation and assessment of the client and determines the appropriate orthosis and the best design to match the needs of the client.[2]

Step One: Creating a Pattern

Once the decision has been reached to fabricate a specific orthosis, a critical step in the fabrication process is deciding on and creating a pattern. The pattern, if well drawn, can determine the success of the orthosis in terms of fit and function. Allowing the time to make a well-thought-out and properly fitted pattern gives the occupational therapist time to establish the goals of the orthosis and determine how it will be fit to the client to accomplish the goals. Ultimately a properly fitted pattern makes the entire fabrication process easier and faster and increases the chance of success (Box 30.3).

OT PRACTICE NOTES

Creation of a pattern involves an understanding of the anatomy and biomechanics of the hand, the materials to be used, and a bit of creativity.

Steps for making a pattern for a wrist cock up orthosis (Fig. 30.22) are as follows:

1. Drawing the pattern (see Fig. 30.22A)
2. Pattern drawn on thermoplastic material (see Fig. 30.22B)
3. Molding the orthosis (see Fig. 30.22C)
4. Molding the orthosis (see Fig. 30.22D)

BOX 30.3   Steps of Making a Pattern

1. Have patient place the involved hand (if they are unable to do so use their opposite hand or even your own hand) palm down on a paper towel.
2. Draw an outline of the hand.
3. Add extra width on the sides of the forearm (typically half the height of the forearm) and around the fingers as needed to encompass the extremity.
4. Mark relevant anatomic landmarks (first web, thenar crease, MCP joints of the index and little finger). Marking the MCP joints of the index and little fingers will help to locate the distal palmar crease, which is about a finger's width proximal to these joints. Remember that this line is angled.
5. Draw the specific pattern marks of the chosen orthosis.
6. Cut out the pattern and assess the fit on the patient. Make sure to place the patient's extremity in the desired position of the finished orthosis to assess correct length and width. Make corrections as needed.
7. Trace the pattern on thermoplastic material, drawing or etching lightly with an awl or a marker. Leave a slight amount of room so that cutting can be done within the lines to make sure that no drawn lines remain on the material.
8. Briefly heat the thermoplastic material in hot water to soften for cutting.
9. Cut out the orthosis using long and even scissor strokes. Keep the edges smooth and round all corners.

MCP, Metacarpophalangeal.

The radial and ulnar borders of a forearm-based orthosis should reach midway around the circumference, and the length should equal about two-thirds of the forearm, as measured from the wrist proximally.

For trim lines, adequate material must be allowed around the musculature of the forearm to reach the midline on both sides (Fig. 30.23). The pattern should reflect widening of the material along the sides of the forearm (Fig. 30.24). **A good rule to remember is to bend the client's elbow fully and mark where the forearm and the biceps muscle meet**. The orthosis should be trimmed one-quarter inch below this point to avoid limiting elbow flexion and to prevent the orthosis from being pushed distally when the elbow is flexed (Fig. 30.25).

Most low-temperature thermoplastic materials used to make orthotics will stretch to conform around angles and contours. Creating a well-fitting pattern and choosing the most appropriate thermoplastic material for the design will result in a quicker and easier fabrication process.

Step Two: Choosing Appropriate Material

The materials commonly used for custom-fabricated orthoses are low-temperature thermoplastic materials (LTTPs) that can be molded directly onto the skin. These materials have certain characteristics that can be defined according to how a material reacts or handles when warm and how it reacts once molded. Choosing the optimal material for a given orthotic application can make the difference between a quick and easy fabrication process and one that requires extensive adjustments and reheating. Occupational therapists are encouraged to sample a variety of materials and test the handling characteristics so that they are familiar with the most appropriate material to select for a specific client and goal.

Characteristics of Low-Temperature Thermoplastic Materials

Each low-temperature thermoplastic material (LTTP) has specific handling characteristics, which are described in the following.

Resistance to stretch.   Resistance to stretch describes the extent to which a material resists pulling or stretching. The greater the resistance, the greater is the degree of control that the fabricator will have over the material. Materials that resist stretch tend to hold their shape and thickness while warm and can be handled more aggressively without the material thinning. More resistant materials are recommended for large orthotics and for orthotics made for persons who are unable to cooperate in the fabrication process. In contrast, the less resistance to stretch a material has, the more the material is likely to thin during the fabrication process, and the more delicately it must be handled. The advantage of stretch is seen in the greater degree of conformability attained with less effort on the part of the fabricator.

Conformability or drape.   Resistance to stretch and conformability or drape describe nearly the same characteristic—that is, if a material stretches easily, it will have better drape and conformability. The great advantage of materials with a high degree of drape or conformability is that with a light, controlled touch or simply the pull of gravity, they readily conform around a

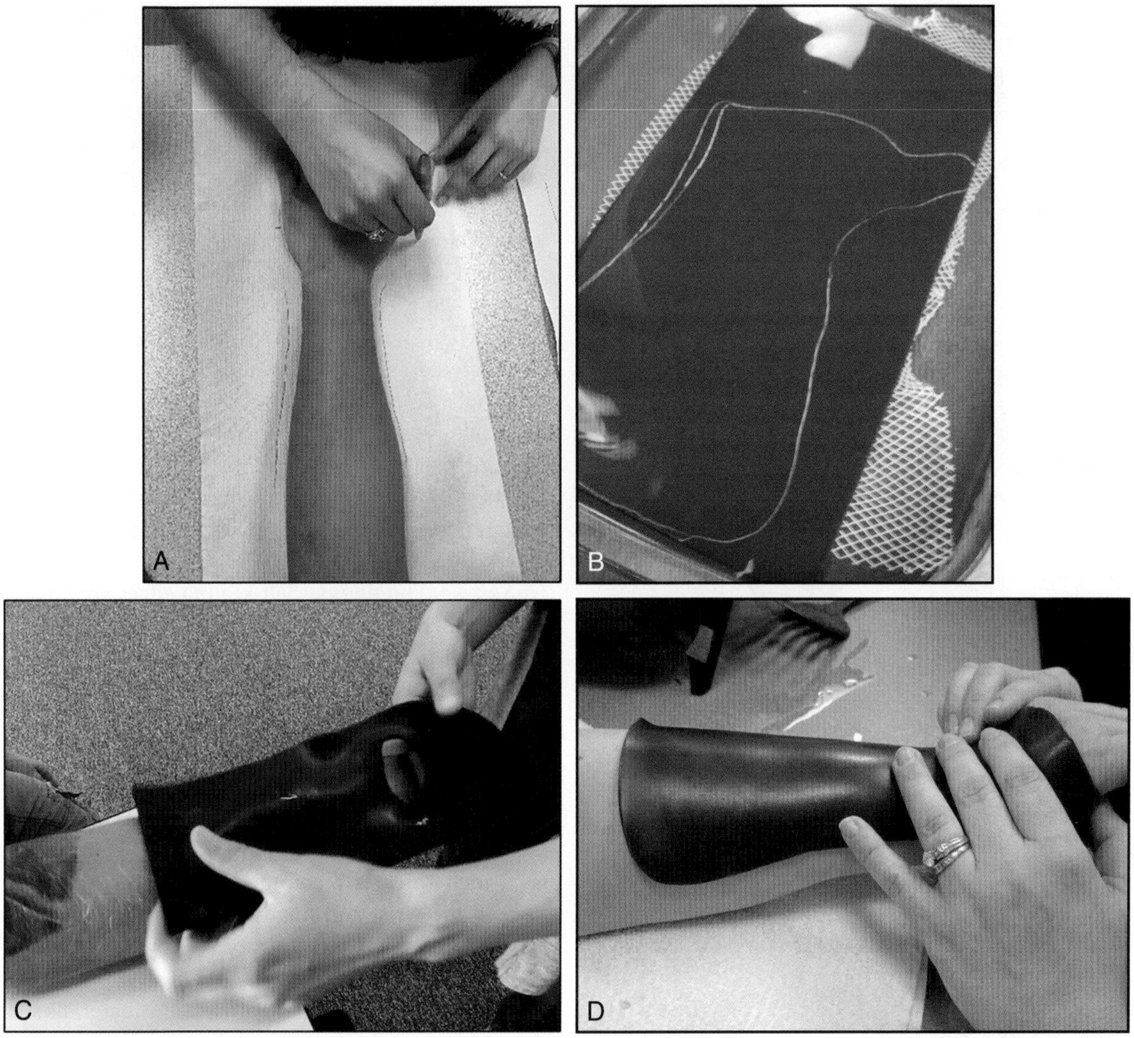

Fig. 30.22 Pattern making. (A) Drawing a pattern. (B) Pattern drawn on material. (C) Molding the orthosis. (D) Molding the orthosis. (With permission from Orfit Industries.)

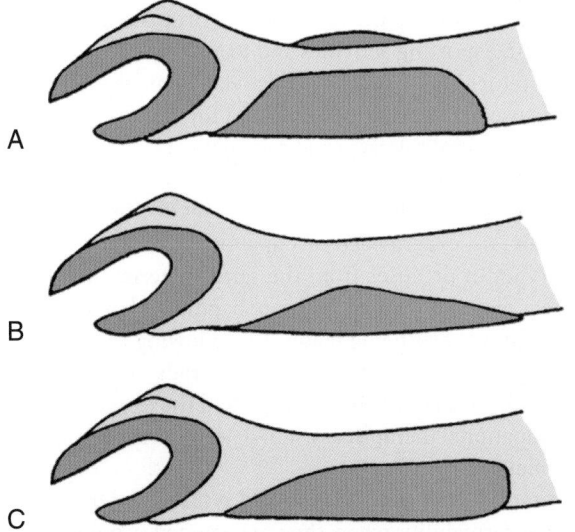

Fig. 30.23 Forearm trim lines. (A) Trim lines are too high, extending above forearm. Straps will bridge arm and will be ineffective. (B) Trim lines are too low. Straps cannot substitute for trim lines that are too low without applying excessive pressure. (C) Midline trim lines ensure that straps properly secure splint on arm and hand.

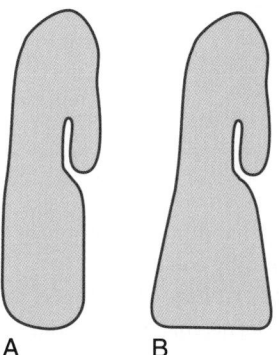

Fig. 30.24 (A) Narrowing the proximal pattern will cause trim lines to drop below midline. (B) Flaring the proximal border of the splint maintains trim lines at midline.

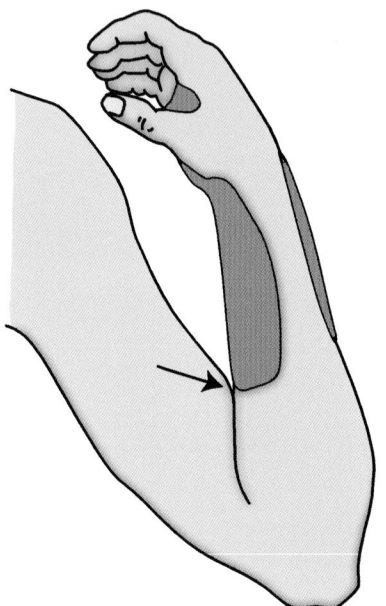

Fig. 30.25 Length of forearm-based orthosis is checked by flexing elbow and noting where biceps meet forearm.

part for a precise fit. The disadvantage of materials with a high degree of drape (and generally also low resistance to stretch) is that they tolerate only minimal handling, and care must be taken to prevent overstretching and fingerprints in the material. Materials with a high degree of drape are not recommended for large orthotics or for clients who are unable to participate in the fitting process. They are ideal, however, for use with postoperative clients when minimal pressure is desired, and for dynamic orthosis bases, in which conformability secures the orthosis against migration (movement distally) when components are attached. Materials with a low degree of drape must be handled continuously until the materials are fully cooled to achieve a contoured fit; often they will not conform intimately around small parts such as the fingers.

Memory. Memory is the ability of a material, when reheated, to return to its original, flat shape after it has been stretched and molded. The advantage of high memory in a material is that the orthosis can be remolded repeatedly without thinning and weakening of the material. Materials with memory require handling throughout the fabrication process because until they are fully cooled and molded, they tend to return to a flat shape. This and the slightly longer cooling time of materials with high memory can be used to advantage with clients who require more aggressive handling to achieve the desired position. Disadvantages of materials with excellent memory are their tendency to return to a flat sheet state when an area is spot heated for adjustment and their need for longer handling to ensure that they maintain their molded shape until fully cooled.

Rigidity versus flexibility. *Rigidity* and *flexibility* in thermoplastic material are terms that describe the amount of resistance a material gives when force is applied to it. A highly rigid material is very resistive to applied force and may, with enough force, break. A highly flexible material bends easily when even small force is applied to it, and it is not apt to break under high stress. Materials are available that fall all along this continuum.

Generally, the thicker a thermoplastic and the more plastic its formula contains, the more rigid the material will be. Flexibility in a material allows for easier donning and doffing of orthoses and may be desirable for clients unable to tolerate the more unforgiving rigid materials. Rigidity is also a factor of the number and depth of contours included in the design. The same material may yield a semiflexible orthosis when used to make a volar or dorsal orthosis with shallow contours or a rigid orthosis when used to make a tightly filled circumferential orthosis.

Bonding. Bonding is the ability of a material to adhere to itself when warmed and pressed together. Many materials are coated to resist accidental bonding and require solvents or surface scraping to remove the coating to bond. Uncoated materials, which require no solvents or scraping, have strong bonding properties when two warm pieces are pressed together. Self-bonding is helpful when outriggers or overlapping corners are applied to form acute angles, but it can be a problem if two pieces adhere accidentally.

Self-sealing edges. Self-sealing edges are edges that round and seal themselves when heated material is cut. This time-saving characteristic produces smooth edges that require no additional finishing. Materials with little or no memory and high conformability generally produce smooth, sealed edges when cut while warm. Materials with memory and those with high resistance to stretch resist sealing, requiring additional finishing.

Thicknesses. Thermoplastic materials are available in various thicknesses and different perforation patterns. Material that is $\frac{1}{8}$-inch thick is recommended to obtain sufficient rigidity to hold the wrist and finger joints firmly in position; $\frac{1}{12}$- and $\frac{1}{16}$-inch materials are appropriate for the thumb and fingers and pediatric clients.

Soft orthotic materials. Soft, flexible materials such as cotton duck, neoprene, knit elastics, and plastic-impregnated materials may be used alone or in combination with metal or plastic stays to fabricate semiflexible orthotics. These materials allow fabrication of orthotics that permit partial motion around a joint yet limit or protect the part. Semi-flexible orthoses are sometimes used during sporting activities and to assist clients with chronic pain in returning to functional activity. Semi-flexible orthoses are also used for geriatric clients and for clients with arthritis, who often cannot tolerate rigid material.

Choosing the Best Category of Material for the Orthosis

Although an experienced occupational therapist can make many types of orthoses from the same material, it is better to choose a material with appropriate handling characteristics for the type of orthosis being made. The following can be used as a guide from which to start choosing materials for different applications. The availability of materials and the experience level of the occupational therapist assist in determining the most appropriate material.

Forearm-based and hand-based orthoses. Orthoses need close conformability when they are molded around the intricate anatomy of the thumb musculature, or when they are to serve as a base for a dynamic orthosis, stabilize a part of the body, reduce contractures, remodel scar tissue, or immobilize to facilitate healing of an acute condition. Such orthoses should be made from a material with a high degree of conformability to achieve an accurate fit. When conformability is not crucial, the orthosis can be made from a material with high resistance to stretch and low to moderate drape. Orthoses fabricated for burns and other acute trauma do not require as conforming a fit and can be made from low-drape materials. Materials that resist stretch and tolerate aggressive handling are recommended for positioning of a spastic body part, because such materials will not stretch and thin during the fabrication process.

Large upper and lower extremity orthoses. Long orthoses fabricated for the elbow, shoulder, knee, or ankle generally should be made of materials that have high resistance to stretch, to provide the control necessary for dealing with large pieces of material. Such orthoses generally do not need to be highly conforming because they are molded over broad expanses of soft tissue. Care must be taken to provide relief for bony prominences or to provide padding to distribute pressure.

Circumferential orthoses. Circumferential orthoses encompass both volar and dorsal surfaces of the extremity and can be fabricated from thinner materials. Materials with high elasticity and memory will tolerate stretching without forming thin spots. The materials should be highly perforated, to allow ventilation. After being stretched, these materials will cinch in around the body part while still allowing sufficient flexibility for easy donning and doffing. Circumferential orthoses work well for protection of healing fractures, and for stabilizing or immobilizing joints. They also work well for contracture reduction and as a base for outrigger attachments. Another choice for making less restrictive circumferential orthoses is the use of semi-flexible materials, which facilitate easy donning and doffing and allow limited motion within the available arc of motion.

Serial orthoses. Serial orthoses that require frequent remolding to accommodate increases in joint ROM should be made from a material that has considerable memory or is highly resistant to stretch to avoid thinning with repeated remolding. The chosen material should have moderate to high rigidity when molded to resist forces from contracted joints or from spastic muscle tone.

Pressure from the orthosis over a bony prominence may cause ischemia (localized anemia caused by obstruction of blood supply to tissues). Pressure may also increase when the material does not conform uniformly, or when it does not cover a broad enough area of soft tissue. Orthoses that migrate or move on the hand because of insufficient strapping or contouring may actually apply pressure in areas that the orthosis was designed to relieve. Tight strapping can affect the circulation and the nerve supply. Table 30.3 presents areas of concern and corrections.

Step Three: Molding the Orthosis
Cutting and Molding the Wrist Cock-Up Orthosis
An orthosis can be placed on the volar or dorsal surface, ulnar or the radial side of the arm and hand or even circumferentially around the body part. Orthoses should have gentle contours matching the underlying anatomy, and cover as broad an area as possible to distribute pressure.

1. Reheat the material to activate it for molding on the client. Dry briefly on a towel to remove excess hot water and heat. Place the material on the forearm and hand with the forearm

TABLE 30.3	Areas of Concern and Corrections	
Area of Concern	**Correction**
Lack of conformity of the material	Reheat and remold Select a more conforming material
Tingling and numbness/ color changes in fingers	Check and loosen straps
Migration of orthosis	Readjust strapping
Pressure over bony prominences	Reheat material and bump out with fingers to create more space
Red marks on skin	Reheat all edges and smooth them with fingers; round all corners. Consider adding slight padding to each side of the orthosis leaving the marks to raise it.
Skin maceration	Increase perforations/use perforated materials to add ventilation, have client wear a cotton sleeve or sock under orthosis

in supination so that gravity can assist the initial molding. Some occupational therapists prefer the elbow propped on a table with the hand in the air. Take care not to squeeze the material around the wrist or forearm.

2. Let the material harden in the desired position. Check that the trim lines fall at the midline. Mark where excess material needs to be removed. Trim the material before it cools. Note areas that will need to be trimmed for clearance and for creation of smooth edges. Mark the placement of the straps.

3. Reposition the hardened orthosis on the forearm. Maintaining control on the wrist and forearm sections, carefully pronate the forearm. If necessary, rotate the forearm section to ensure that the trim lines are at midline (Fig. 30.26). Also see Fig. 30.23 and Fig. 30.24 to reconfirm appropriate trim lines on the forearm.

See Fig. 30.25 to review the importance of the changing shape of the forearm from a supinated to a pronated position.

4. Apply the straps, using a heat gun to heat both the adhesive-backed hook and the spot on the orthosis to assist with bonding. Smooth all edges and round all corners.

Step 4: Finishing Steps and Critique
Strapping
Adhesive-backed hook and loop strapping are applied to the base orthosis for easy donning and doffing as needed. Most commonly, straps are be placed proximally, distally, and in the middle of the orthosis to firmly support the body part (Fig. 30.27).

The width of the loop strapping should match the size of the body part. Loop strapping should be narrow for the fingers and wider for larger body parts. The proximal forearm strap is typically angled to accommodate the wider forearm musculature (Fig. 30.28). Critique the completed orthosis for comfort and fit.

Skin Tolerance and Hypersensitivity
The occupational therapist should assess the client's skin condition and sensitivity to the completed orthosis. Clients who experience a high degree of perspiration that may lead to skin

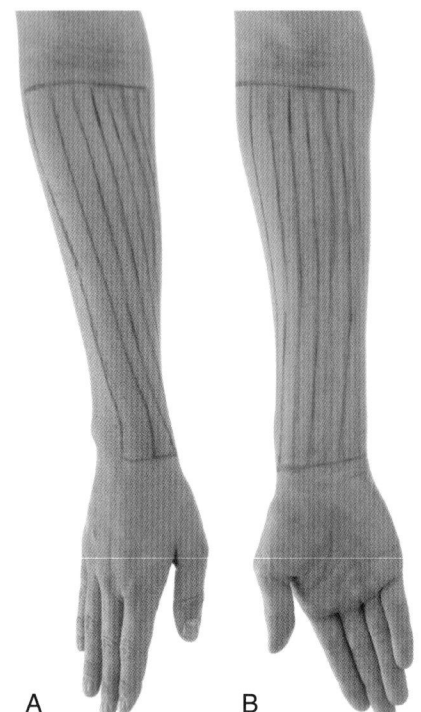

Fig. 30.26 The shape of the forearm is altered as it moves from (A) pronation to (B) supination. Forearm-based orthoses must accommodate this movement pattern by adequate strapping and fitting. (With permission from Orfit Industries.)

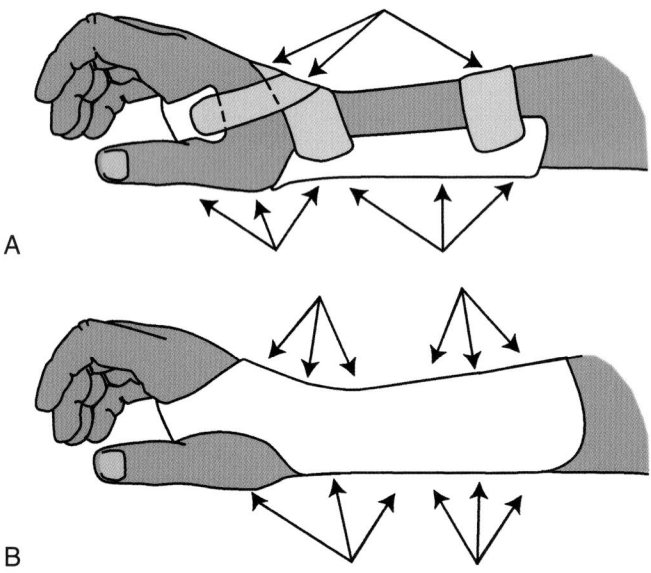

Fig 30.27 (A) A volar-based orthosis requires properly placed straps to create three-point pressure systems to secure orthosis and ensure distribution of pressure. (B) Circumferential orthoses create multiple three-point pressure systems to secure orthosis for immobilization.

maceration need to be evaluated more carefully for orthotic consideration and type, such as ventilated plastics and absorbent padding. Some clients are intolerant of any pressure because of extremely fragile skin or sensory dysfunction. Many clients do well with stockinette sleeves or cotton socks worn underneath the orthosis.

Step Five: What to Tell Your Client
Instructions and Precautions

Instruct the client regarding the wearing schedule, duration of expected use, and the proper care of the orthosis. Explain in terms that the client can understand. Make sure to explain the benefits of wearing the orthosis and potential outcomes for not wearing the orthosis as directed. Many occupational therapists now require that clients sign a document for their records that they were informed of the purpose of the orthosis and the wearing schedule to avoid possible misinterpretations. The client should be cautioned to check the fit of the orthosis regularly, looking for red marks and signs of irritation. Clients with nerve injuries and/or areas of lack of sensation should visually check several times a day for signs of skin breakdown.

Occupational therapists should inform clients not to leave the orthosis near any sources of heat as the material can easily soften and lose its shape. Orthoses left in a car on a sunny day are often ruined in this manner.

Your client should also be instructed to clean the orthosis with warm water and soap regularly or to use disinfectant wipes to remove surface dirt and bacteria.

Wearing Schedules

The occupational therapist should decide on the optimum wearing schedule for the orthosis based on the client's condition, the diagnosis, and the goals of the orthosis. Some orthoses should be worn full time and not removed at all until adequate healing has occurred. Other conditions may warrant nighttime use only or during functional activities as an assist. Nighttime may be the best time for a client to wear a static orthosis designed to change ROM. It is also the time when some clients may benefit from using resting orthoses for better positioning. During the daytime, the client may wear a dynamic orthosis or an orthosis designed to assist function. If allowed per the diagnosis, the client should be instructed to remove the orthosis and perform exercises and light activities to use the hand as normally as possible. Clients who require orthotic use in both hands should be instructed to alternate wearing orthoses on one hand at a time so that the individual is not left without the sensory input and function of an orthosis-free hand. Although this might not be the ideal orthosis-wearing schedule, for meeting therapeutic goals, it may at least offer a compromise for better compliance.

Precautions and Contraindications

The occupational therapist is responsible for deciding which orthosis style and design is appropriate for the client but also should use clinical reasoning and critical thinking to determine whether the client is a good candidate for wearing an orthosis. Several issues should be examined in this regard.

Compliance Issues

First, the occupational therapist must consider whether the client is likely to comply with the orthosis wearing program. The orthosis may have a negative effect on the client's ability to be independent in self-care or to function at work. Some clients are sensitive about their appearance and may refuse to wear an orthosis if it offends their aesthetic sense or negatively affects their body image.

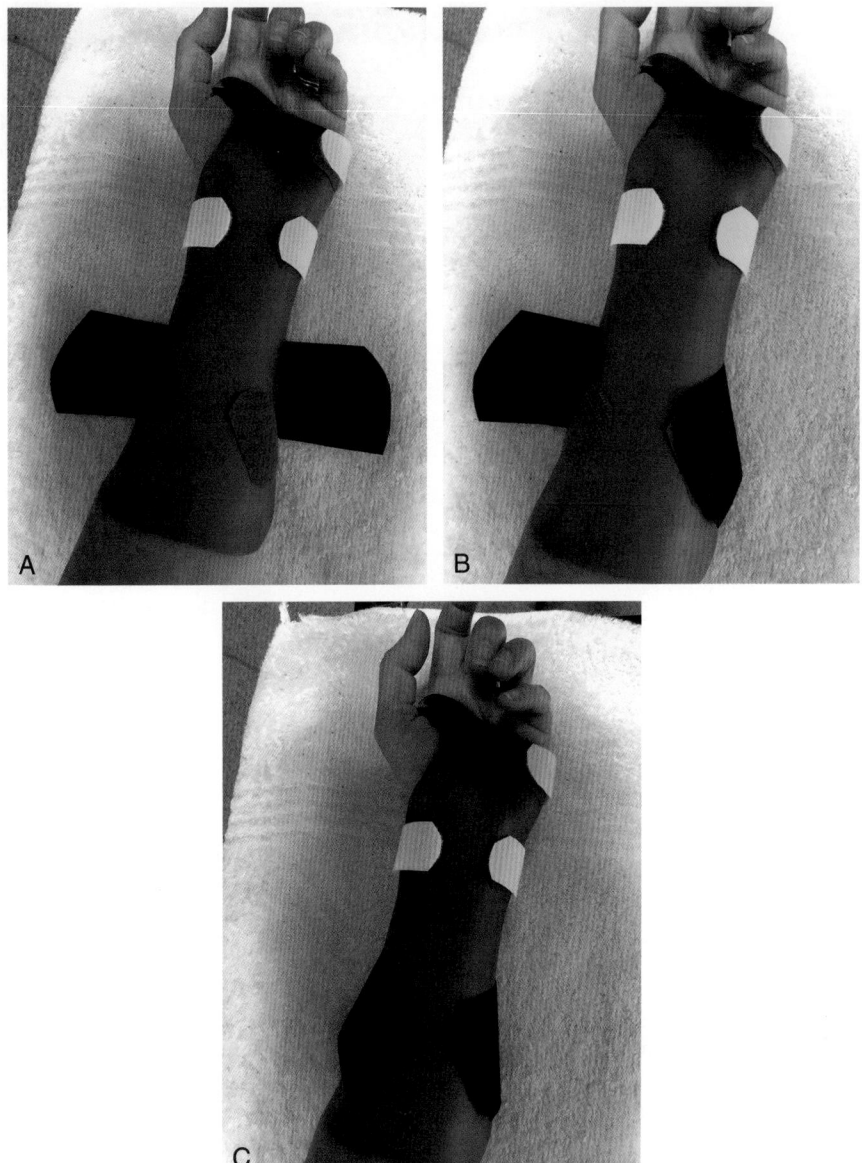

Fig. 30.28 (A) to (C) Forearm strapping at an angle to accommodate wider musculature in proximal forearm. (With permission from Orfit Industries.)

Motivation Level

Compliance with an orthosis wearing program may be poor if the client's general level of motivation to get better is low. On the other hand, some clients are so highly motivated that they will overdo the wearing program and cause themselves damage.

Cognitive Level

Finally, the client's cognitive and perceptual ability to follow an orthosis wearing program should be considered, especially if no responsible care provider is available to supervise the orthosis-wearing precautions. The occupational therapist should make every effort to explain the purpose of the orthosis and the benefits of wearing it to help with client compliance. Care in fabrication of the orthosis and making an effort to allow the client some choices in color or design may improve compliance and acceptance.

COMMERCIALLY AVAILABLE ORTHOSES

Many distributors that sell rehabilitation products for therapy also offer commercially available orthoses made with a variety of different materials. Refer to the company catalogs or websites to see the numerous choices of resting hand, wrist, and thumb supports. These are options when it might not be feasible to fabricate a custom-fitting orthosis on a client. Although available in different sizes, orthoses that come in large, medium, and small rarely have as good a fit as a custom-made orthosis. It is highly recommended that an occupational therapist check the fit of a prefabricated orthosis on each individual client and recommend an appropriate wearing schedule.

THREADED CASE STUDY

Johanna, Part 3

Johanna was in agreement with the intervention plan and attended several visits of occupational therapy. She received heat treatments through paraffin and heat packs and performed gentle range-of-motion exercises to stretch her fingers and thumbs. The occupational therapist instructed Johanna in joint protection techniques and helpful strategies for activities of daily living. The therapist reviewed guidelines for activities by which Johanna could eliminate some pain by holding objects (baking tools or knitting needles) in a different manner to lessen the forces across the CMC joint. The client was instructed to hold bowls from underneath or use larger handled spoons instead of smaller ones, which require pinching to stabilize. It was also recommended that Johanna read from hardcover books while sitting as opposed to reading paperback books while lying down to eliminate forceful pinching to hold the pages. Knitting with larger needles was also another well-advised strategy to lessen forces across the CMC joints.

Johanna was fitted with custom fabricated hand-based short opponens orthoses fabricated from a lightweight and conforming material. She chose pink straps to help remind herself to wear them.

After a few weeks of therapy sessions, Johanna reported a reduction of pain and aching especially at night. She was instructed to continue to wear the orthoses full time until she felt she could wean out of them and resume limited activities without discomfort. She scheduled a follow-up appointment with the occupational therapist for the following month for a reevaluation.

Critical Thinking Questions

1. What is the value of a client-rated performance outcome measure?
2. How important is reviewing strategies for clients to perform their regular activities in different manners?
3. How did the occupational therapist utilize the OTPF to evaluate this client?
4. What will be the main goal of the orthoses in this case study?

SUMMARY

Engagement in meaningful occupations is beneficial to the physical, mental, and emotional health of an individual, and every effort should be taken to promote continued engagement in one's chosen activities. If physical conditions such as slowly deteriorating and painful thumb CMC joints begin to interfere with these activities, the occupational therapist and the client should work together to modify and adapt specific and stressful activities so that enjoyment and participation can continue. Early intervention by an occupational therapist is usually the first avenue chosen by the orthopedic or hand surgeon, because this referral for supportive orthoses and activity analysis and modification may potentially delay more invasive interventions for years. There are now a wide variety of specially designed ergonomic utensils available with larger and softer handles for cooking and gardening to lessen grip force, electric can openers to reduce thumb stress, and door knobs or key holders with levers all designed to reduce stress on painful joints. Education in activity modification strategies can include simple techniques such as using scissors to open boxes instead of pinching tabs, using book holders for reading, employing larger knitting needles and yarns, and applying easy computer dictation software to reduce some computer workload with the hands. A few visits with an occupational therapist for instruction in joint protection techniques, activity modification ideas, and the fabrication of CMC joint supporting orthoses can benefit a client for years.

REVIEW QUESTIONS

1. Describe the role of the occupational therapist in the orthoses-making process.
2. What is wrist tenodesis, and how do we use this motion functionally?
3. Name the three major nerves that supply the hand, and describe their sensory innervation patterns.
4. Name three intrinsic muscles and three extrinsic muscles of the upper extremity.
5. Name three common orthoses for the upper extremity and include the parts of the body that are included.
6. Define the terms *friction, torque,* and *stress.*
7. How is force applied to a body part in a mobilization orthosis?
8. Describe the difference between a dynamic and a static progressive orthosis.
9. How does the amount of drape in a low-temperature thermoplastic material affect the making of an orthosis?
10. What is the recommended thickness of material for small finger orthoses? Why?
11. What is the recommended thickness of material for large elbow orthoses? Why?

For additional practice questions for this chapter, please visit eBooks.Health.Elsevier.com.

REFERENCES

1. Adams J, Hammond A, Burridge J, Cooper C: Static orthoses in the prevention of hand dysfunction in rheumatoid arthritis: A review of the literature, *Musculoskeletal Care* 3(2):85–101, 2005.

2. American Occupational Therapy Association: Occupational therapy practice framework: Domain and process (4th ed.), *Am J Occup Ther* 74(Supplement 2): 7412410010p1–7412410010p87, 2020.

3. Austin NM: Anatomical principles. In Jacobs MA, Austin NM, editors: *Orthotic Intervention for the Hand and Upper Extremity: Splinting Principles and Process,* 2nd ed, 2014, Lippincott Williams & Wilkins.

4. Coppard BM, Lohman H: *Introduction to orthotics: a clinical reasoning and problem-solving approach.* St. Louis, 2019, Elsevier.

5. Jacobs MA, Austin NM: *Orthotic intervention for the hand and upper extremity: splinting principles and process*, 2014, Lippincott Williams & Wilkins.

6. Klein L: Extensor tendon injury. In Wietlisbach CM, editor: *Cooper's fundamentals of hand therapy: clinical reasoning and treatment guidelines for common diagnoses of the upper extremity,* St. Louis, 2019, Elsevier.

7. MacDermid, J. (2007) *The patient-rated wrist evaluation (PRWE)© user manual.* McMaster University, Hamilton, Ontario, Canada Clinical Research Lab, Hand and Upper Limb Centre, St Joseph's Centre, London, Ontario, Canada. http://www.handweb.nl/wp-content/uploads/2015/10/PRWE_PRWHEUserManual_Dec2007.pdf.

8. McKee P, Nguyen C: Customized dynamic splinting: Orthoses that promote optimal function and recovery after radial nerve injury: A case report, *J Hand Ther* 20(1):73–88, 2007.

9. Mee S: Wrist instabilities. In Wietlisbach CM, editor: *Cooper's fundamentals of hand therapy: clinical reasoning and treatment guidelines for common diagnoses of the upper extremity*, St. Louis, 2019, Elsevier.

10. Merck Manual Professional Version, revised May 2020. Steinberg, David. Merckmanuals.com/professional/musculoskeletal-and-connective-tissue-disorders/handdisorders/.

11. Moscony AM: Peripheral nerve problems. In Wietlisbach CM, editor: *cooper's fundamentals of hand therapy: clinical reasoning and treatment guidelines for common diagnoses of the upper extremity*, St. Louis, 2019, Elsevier.

12. Schofield KA, Schwartz DA: Teaching orthotic design and fabrication content in occupational therapy curricula: Faculty perspectives, *J Hand Ther* 33(1):119–126, 2018.

13. Schofield KA, Schwartz DA: *Orthotic design and fabrication for the upper extremity: a practical guide*, Thorofare, NJ, 2019, Slack Incorporated.

14. Schwartz DA: Static progressive orthoses for the upper extremity: A comprehensive literature review, *Hand* 7(1):10–17, 2012.

15. Solomon G: Finger sprains and deformities. In: Wietlisbach CM, editor: *Cooper's fundamentals of hand therapy: clinical reasoning and treatment guidelines for common diagnoses of the upper extremity*, St. Louis, 2019, Elsevier.

16. Solomon JW, O'Brien JC: *Pediatric skills for occupational therapy assistants–e-book* St. Louis, 2015, Elsevier.

31

Therapeutic Arm Supports and Robotic-Assisted Therapy

Michal S. Atkins and Jane Baumgarten

LEARNING OBJECTIVES

After reading this chapter, the learner will be able to:

1. Identify clients who may benefit from static or dynamic arm supports.
2. Describe the general physical principles of dynamic arm supports.
3. Describe three types of dynamic arm supports and how they differ.
4. List the challenges of using dynamic arm supports for individuals who are ambulatory and for those who use a wheelchair.
5. Describe the occupations in which a client with very weak upper extremities can engage.
6. List the client factors that must be considered before recommending a mobile arm support for home use.
7. Identify the benefits and limitations of robot-assisted therapy.
8. Identify clients who may benefit from robot-assisted therapy.
9. List robot-assisted therapy training modalities.
10. Identify the concepts in the OTPF-4 that are most relevant to this therapeutic intervention.

CHAPTER OUTLINE

KEY TERMS

Dynamic arm supports
Freestanding dynamic arm supports
Mobile arm supports

Robot-assisted therapy
Static arm supports
Suspension arm devices

THREADED CASE STUDY

Matt, Part 1

Matt is a 38-year-old man (prefers use of the pronouns he/him/his) has been married for 10 years and has a 9-year-old daughter and a 7-year-old son. He has been working for 15 years as a high school math teacher and was recently promoted to the position of assistant principal. Matt's wife is a speech and language pathologist (SLP) and works at a local hospital. His daughter is in third grade, and his son is a first grader. Matt and his family love to take bicycle rides or go hiking on the weekends and play computer and board games. Both children play soccer, and Matt is an assistant coach for his daughter's team.

One month ago, Matt sustained a spinal cord injury (SCI) in a motor vehicle accident. His injury was identified as C4 AIS A using the American Spinal Injury Association (ASIA) Impairment Scale. Matt has complete C4 quadriplegia/tetraplegia and is unable to lift his arms to a tabletop level or to his face and head.[3] (Please see Chapter 37 for more on SCI).

He was admitted to an acute hospital for 2 weeks and was just transferred to an inpatient rehabilitation facility near his family and friends. During his initial occupational therapy (OT) evaluation, Matt was asked to identify his most important roles and the occupations in which he would like to participate on his

Matt, Part 1

return home. Matt wanted to resume the roles of husband, father, and worker. The occupation of greatest importance to Matt was to return to teaching, so that he could support his family financially and be active in the community.

During his first evaluation, Matt was overwhelmed. Overnight, his life had turned upside down. The therapist listened empathetically to Matt's bleak assessment of his future life and encouraged him to take 1 day at a time as he gains strength and sees some improvements. In addition to returning to teaching, he expressed concern about being able to do things for himself.

To improve Matt's immediate state of mind, the therapist redirected the initial interview, focusing on more pressing goals. Matt had to feel that he was more in control of his body and his immediate environment. Using the Canadian Occupational Performance Measure (COPM), the initial goals identified by Matt were to be able to use his call light, phone, and iPad and to feed himself. Matt also placed high importance on seeing his wife and children. He said that he did not want his friends to visit him in the hospital. On admission to the acute rehabilitation unit, Matt was unable to participate in any of these activities.

Occupational assessment determined that Matt was unable to complete any activities of daily living (ADLs) or instrumental activities of daily living (IADLs). Evaluation of client factors revealed that Matt's passive range of motion (ROM) was within normal limits (WNL) throughout his upper extremities (UEs) except for 15- to 25-degree limitations in shoulder flexion, abduction, and external rotation bilaterally. Bilateral UE strength was 2/5 (poor) in the anterior, middle, and

posterior deltoids; 2/5 (poor) in the biceps and brachioradialis; 2−/5 (poor minus) in the supinators; 0/5 in the triceps; and 0/5 in all wrist and hand musculature. Assessment of muscle tone revealed the presence of mild spasticity in multiple muscle groups in his UEs. Matt's sensation regarding light touch and superficial pain was intact through C4 bilaterally, impaired bilaterally at C5, and absent bilaterally at C6 and below. Proprioception was intact at the shoulders, impaired in the elbows, and absent in the wrists, fingers, and thumbs.[3] (See Chapter 23 for Sensory Evaluation.)

Critical Thinking Questions
As you read through the chapter, keep the following questions regarding Matt's situation in mind.
1. Given Matt's status on initial evaluation, what equipment can support the weight of his arm and allow him to begin engaging in basic activities?
2. Are there any devices that would enable him to resume use of his personal electronic devices?
3. What equipment and setup would allow Matt to play with his children and be involved with their school and extracurricular activities, while continuing to strengthen his arms?
4. What series of interventions would you provide to enable Matt to return to role of assistant principal, where the teachers and district administrators are concerned about his ability to manage the many aspects of the job?

THERAPEUTIC ARM SUPPORTS

Introduction and Clinical Reasoning

Therapeutic arm supports are static or dynamic devices that support, protect, and/or enhance arm function for individuals with weak upper extremities. In the Occupational Therapy Practice Framework-4 (OTPF-4), arm supports would be most closely associated with the intervention types Orthotics and Prosthetics and Assistive Technology and Environmental Modification to restore the client's participation in chosen occupations.[1] Static devices are used to support, align, or prevent/decrease deformity of the arm. Dynamic devices provide support as well; however, their primary function is to allow clients with significant upper extremity (UE) weakness to move their arms and engage in meaningful occupations. The main challenge for people who need these orthoses is achieving the shoulder and/or elbow motion necessary for functional arm use, which typically requires the hands to be placed at a tabletop level or in close proximity to the face and head.

Many functions that once had to be accomplished with arm movement are now possible with the advent of sophisticated switches that do not depend on touch. Voice and gaze activation, WiFi, and Bluetooth technology can eliminate the need for wires and the limitations of connectivity in one location only. This enables the person with severe upper extremity (UE) weakness to perform a myriad of tasks without the use of their UEs. However, this is not the case with many basic activities of daily living (ADLs). To eat, brush teeth, comb or brush hair, and touch the face of others, clients must be able to reach their head. In addition, when given the option, many clients would

rather use their hands than depend on high-tech equipment to accomplish tasks such as using a keyboard or propelling a power wheelchair (WC).

Commercially available products range from simple to complex and can be prescribed for temporary or permanent use. They can be home-based or clinic-based in their application, and the indications for their use may be positional, therapeutic, occupation based, or any combination of these uses. Static positional devices provide support for weak UEs, prevent or reduce pain, and help to maintain range of motion (ROM). Goals for the use of dynamic arm supports may include decreasing pain, increasing strength and/or ROM, engagement in meaningful occupations, or any combination of these potential benefits. These goals are accomplished through a combination of supporting the weight of the arm and minimizing the effect of gravity.

The challenge to the occupational therapist is to combine a thorough occupational history, called the occupational profile, with in-depth assessment and collaborative goal setting to establish the best choice of arm support for each client.[1] A trial-and-error approach to finding the optimal arm support for each patient is often required, weighing the variables involved, to optimize function and prevent injury or pain.

Unfortunately, there is a paucity of evidence-based data comparing different arm supports to assist the therapist in choosing the optimal device.[4] Garber and Gregorio[14] studied the prescription and use of upper limb devices in persons with quadriplegia. Although these authors did not provide specific information on mobile arm supports (MASs), they stated "The devices retained in use most often were the more costly orthoses such as reciprocal orthoses and ball-bearing feeders" (pg. 126).[14]

The following process is critical to the optimal selection of arm supports. For each patient, the therapist must carefully consider the nature of the trauma or the condition and its likely course. Will the client get stronger? Is the condition static, or is it a degenerative condition with an expected decrease in function? Are arm supports a short-term or long-term/permanent solution to decreased UE function and occupational engagement?

The next step is to identify the goal of the intervention with respect to the use of an arm support. Is the goal of the treatment to provide comfortable positioning and pain reduction? Is it to provide a strengthening program in preparation for occupational engagement? Is it to achieve mastery of a specific task or tasks? Is it to combine both meaningful occupation and exercise? Are the goals subject to repeated revision as the client's physical status changes?

Once the primary goal for the use of arm supports is established, the acuity of the trauma or medical condition is considered. Immediately after a traumatic injury, the priority must be to manage pain and to prevent further complications. Static positioning devices provide support and stability but will limit mobility when the arms are very weak. Dynamic arm supports are necessary to increase function in the UEs and to increase strength and active movement of the arms, but their effect on pain must be carefully evaluated.

Expense and available funding source(s) can be a significant factor in the prescription and use of arm supports, as is the setting in which the client is receiving treatment. Sample clinic equipment may be available for use in the inpatient rehabilitation setting, but not funded for long-term use. If the optimal arm supports will not be available to a client, less expensive or homemade options must be considered.

It is crucial to evaluate where the arm device will be used and, if necessary, where it will be mounted. Will the client always be in a WC when out of bed, or will the client be independent in household and/or community ambulation and require an alternative mounting location?

Thorough assessment of client factors, including motor control, muscle strength, ROM, muscle tone, and sensation will round out the evaluation process for determining the appropriate arm support. The therapist must ascertain if the client has adequate motor control and muscle strength to benefit from a particular dynamic arm support, as well as the space to use it, an adequate mounting surface, and the motivation to engage in the training necessary to maximize the benefits of an arm support.

Careful consideration of each of these factors will result in optimal prescription of static or dynamic arm supports, maximizing both therapeutic and functional benefits for the client.

Static Arm Supports

Optimal early static positioning is critical to maximizing later functional use of weak UEs. **Static arm supports** provide support for the UEs in a comfortable, protected position to minimize pain and subluxation.[7] They also can be used to stretch the shoulder(s) and/or elbow(s) to maintain or increase ROM.

Pillows are often the first and most readily available solution for providing static support to the upper limbs. While in bed,

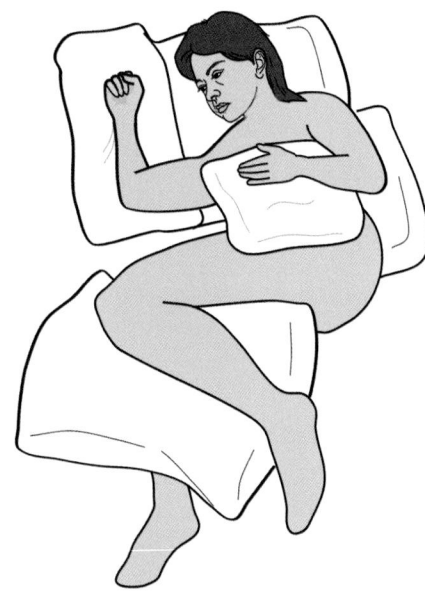

Fig. 31.1 Static arm support with carefully placed pillows. (Courtesy Department of Occupational and Recreational Therapy; Rancho Los Amigos National Rehabilitation Center, Downey, CA.)

clients tend to rest their arms close to their body with the shoulder positioned in adduction and internal rotation. To prevent a functionally significant loss of ROM, the UEs must be positioned in abduction and external rotation for part of the day (Fig. 31.1).

Static arm supports also must be considered when the client is first seated, because the weight of the arm in an upright position may cause increased pain, swelling, and/or shoulder subluxation (Fig. 31.2).[7] The priority is to reduce pain and prevent further complications, because this may lead to decreased functional capabilities in the future. At times simple solutions such as using an over-the-bed table is cheaper and more practical for some individuals (Fig. 31.3). If the shoulders are weak but clients have functional elbow flexion and some wrist and/or hand function, the elbows can be propped on the table, allowing the person to eat and engage in hygiene and grooming activities. With the elbows supported, the person can also perform activities such as writing, drawing, and playing board games. Static positioning while in a WC can be achieved with lap trays or arm rests. Half lap trays are available for clients who need unilateral support, such as survivors of stroke. Full lap trays are used when support for both arms is required, as with individuals with spinal cord injury (SCI) resulting in tetraplegia (also known as quadriplegia) or Guillain Barré syndrome (GBS). Static positioning devices provide support and stability, but do not enhance mobility when the arms are very weak. Dynamic arm supports are necessary to allow clients with significant UE weakness to engage in functional and therapeutic activities.

Dynamic Arm Supports

Dynamic arm supports are devices that support the weight of the arm and minimize the negative effect of gravity on the functional use of weak UEs. They enable clients to move their arms despite significant weakness, to exercise, and to engage in ADL

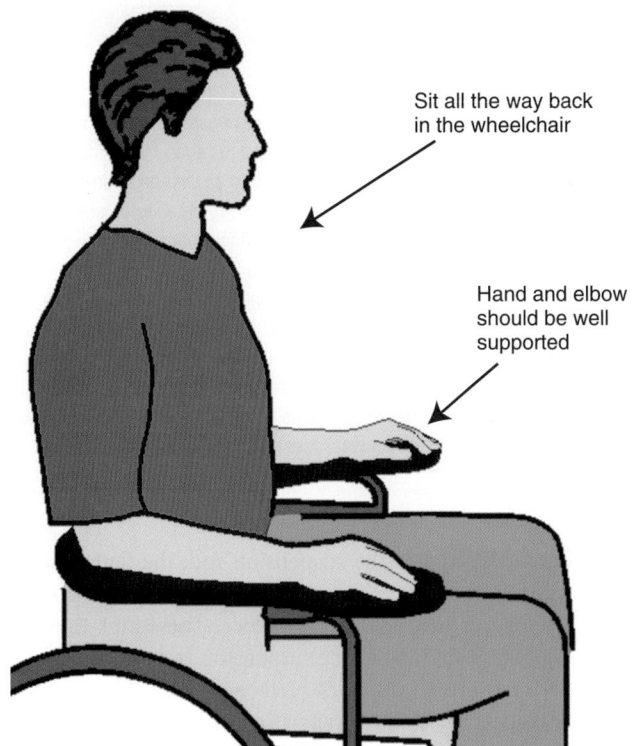

Sit all the way back in the wheelchair

Hand and elbow should be well supported

Fig. 31.2 Correct static arm support positioning in the wheelchair. (Courtesy Department of Occupational and Recreational Therapy; Rancho Los Amigos National Rehabilitation Center, Downey, CA.)

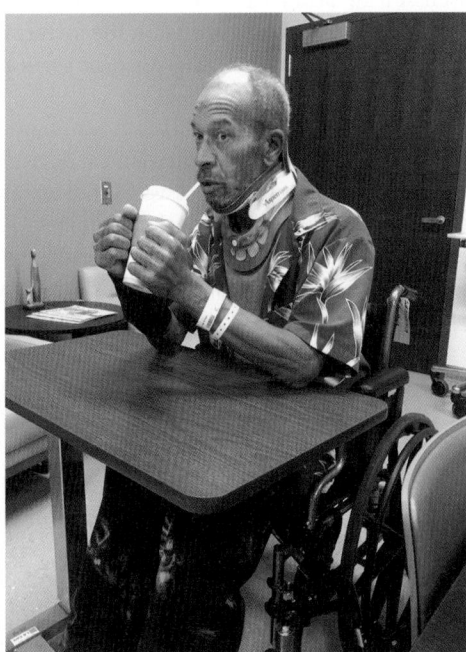

Fig. 31.3 A client supports his weak shoulders with an over-bed table. Strong elbow flexors allow him to bring his drink to his mouth.

and tabletop activities. Although these devices vary in design, complexity, and cost, all assist the upper limb in moving as freely as possible. In the past decade, the use of robotic devices (computerized dynamic arm supports) has been introduced in an increasing number of therapy clinics to further enhance the

benefits of therapy. Terminology associated with dynamic arm supports is inconsistent and confusing as the field continues to develop.[32] This is due in part to the different "languages" spoken by the engineers who develop the devices, and the therapists and their clients who use them. It is the responsibility of the purchasing institution and the therapists to educate themselves regarding the capabilities of any device they are considering for use in treatment. Video demonstrations of various devices can be helpful in this process. In a recent attempt to identify and categorize the currently existing dynamic arm supports, Van der Heide et al. identified 97 commercially available devices to support weak UEs.[32] The article classifies dynamic arm supports in three categories: (1) nonactuated devices, which provide no external power; (2) passively actuated devices, which assist the UE with rubber bands, springs, or weights; and (3) actively actuated devices that use electrical power, such as robotic arms.[32]

In this chapter we will discuss only the most commonly used devices and those that are available for purchase in the United States.

Suspension Arm Devices

Suspension arm devices are orthoses that hang from a bed frame or an overhead suspension rod attached to a WC or table and support the arm. They are reasonably priced and easily adjustable, offering a myriad of potential therapeutic and functional benefits for clients with significant UE weakness and/or motor control impairment. These devices support the shoulder, elbow, and forearm and wrist, allowing increased motion in weak proximal muscles. In addition, they prevent disuse atrophy, maintain ROM, and provide pain relief. Suspension arm devices provide proximal support, allowing for distal function with or without additional equipment. They enable occupational engagement for individuals who would otherwise be unable to move their arms against gravity. With minimal training, suspension arm devices allow clients with very weak UEs to recognize early in their rehabilitation program that they can successfully engage in an occupation of choice, decreasing feelings of helplessness and hopelessness. Because of the mechanical principles on which they operate, suspension arm devices are generally more effective for positioning and exercise than for occupational performance. Because the upper limb swings as a pendulum from straps or springs attached to the suspension rod, it is difficult to make fine adjustments in movement.[23]

Suspension arm slings. The JAECO suspension arm sling (Fig. 31.4) has a single strap or spring suspended from an over-bed frame for use in bed, or a WC-mounted suspension rod for use while the person is seated out of bed.[20] Attached to the strap is an adjustable balance bar with two leather cuffs, which are placed around the elbow and wrist or hand. These cuffs provide separate support for the wrist and elbow, allowing gravity eliminated movement of weak proximal muscles.[20]

Suspension arm supports. The JAECO suspension arm support (Fig. 31.5) has a single forearm support with an adjustable fulcrum instead of the two slings, which allows for greater customized adjustment in elbow flexion and extension. It is suspended from a single point on the suspension rod or over-bed

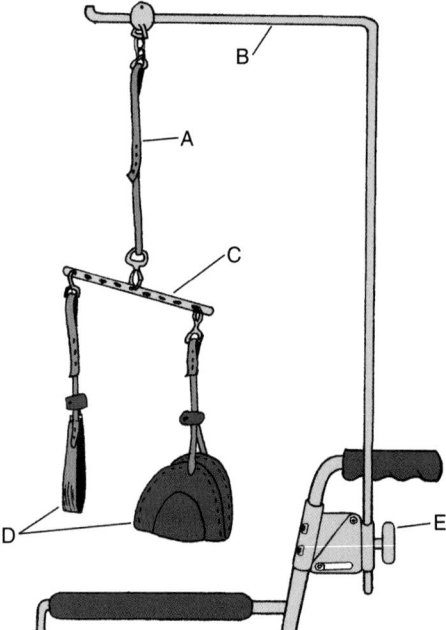

Fig. 31.4 Suspension sling. *A*, Strap. *B*, Suspension rod. *C*, Horizontal bar (adjustable balance bar). *D*, Wrist and elbow suspension slings. *E*, Adjustable suspension mount. (Adapted with permission from Department of Occupational and Recreational Therapy; Rancho Los Amigos National Rehabilitation Center, Downey, CA.)

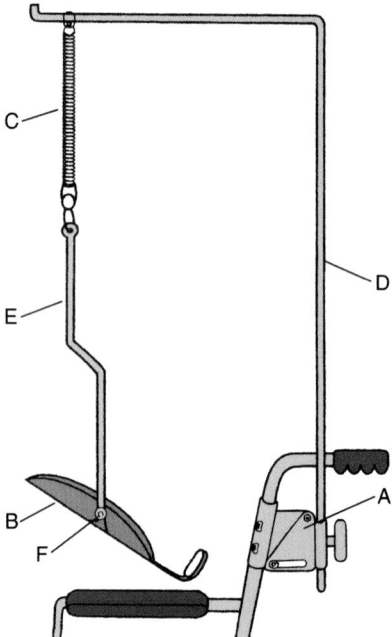

Fig. 31.5 Suspension arm support. *A*, Adjustable suspension mount. *B*, Forearm support. *C*, Springs. *D*, Suspension rod. *E*, Suspension bar. *F*, Rocker arm (offset swivel). (Adapted with permission from Department of Occupational and Recreational Therapy; Rancho Los Amigos National Rehabilitation Center, Downey, CA.)

frame and allows the client to perform simple tabletop activities and occupations such as feeding or grooming.[20]

Adjustment of suspension arm devices. Suspension arm devices are simple to adjust. The overall height of the device is adjusted at the interface between the suspension rod and the

THREADED CASE STUDY

Matt, Part 2

When Matt was first cleared to sit in bed, he was frustrated that he could feel his muscles contracting but was unable to move his arms. When Matt's arms were placed in the suspension slings mounted to an over-bed frame, he was immediately able to move them. He was excited to be able to "exercise my arms." When asked what he would like to do with his arms in the slings, Matt decided that he would like to try and use his iPad. The iPad was positioned on an over-bed table, and with his arms in the suspension slings and a short training session, Matt was able to FaceTime with his wife and children. With practice he was able to listen to music and connect with friends on Facebook, by moving his shoulders and activating the screen with the dorsum of his fingers or his thumb. This successful experience helped Matt realize that he could use his arms, despite the significant weakness and remaining paralysis.

WC mount. The higher the suspension rod, the flatter the arc of pendulum swing when the arm is in motion, enhancing the capability for occupational performance. The straps that connect the forearm support to the suspension rod can be adjusted to allow for use at various work surfaces and for specific activities. The placement of the straps along the horizontal balance bar will position the elbow in greater or lesser degrees of flexion, and if edema is present, the hand is held higher than the elbow. The forearm support used with the suspension arm support is the same as that used with a mobile arm support (MAS), which will be discussed in detail later in this chapter. The attached rocker arm can be adjusted lengthwise on the forearm support, which permits greater directional assistance for vertical motion.

Mobile Arm Supports

A mobile arm support (MAS) is a mechanical device that supports the weight of the arm and assists shoulder and elbow motions through a linkage of low-friction joints (Fig. 31.6). Mobile arm supports (MASs) are used for persons with weakness of the shoulder and elbow that limits their ability to

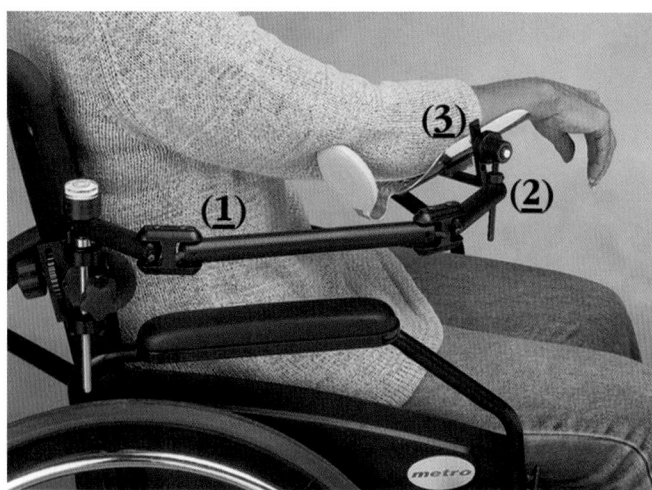

Fig. 31.6 The JAECO/Rancho MultiLink MAS mounted on a wheelchair. *(1)* MultiLink arm, *(2)* offset swivel with forearm support slide, *(3)* forearm support. (Courtesy North Coast Medical, Inc., Gilroy, CA.)

position the hand in space. They were developed early in the 1950s and have been known by other names, including ball-bearing feeder, ball-bearing arm support, and balanced forearm orthosis (BFO).

A MAS can increase UE function for persons with severe arm weakness caused by conditions such as cervical spinal cord injury, muscular dystrophy, Guillain-Barré Syndrome, amyotrophic lateral sclerosis, poliomyelitis, and polymyositis.[16,33,34] The MAS also has been used for pain relief in the shoulder and elbow during occupational performance for clients with arthritis and other painful conditions. Motor control problems such as ataxia, the inability to generate coordinated motor activity during voluntary movement, can significantly interfere with successful occupational performance. There are also commercially available arm supports that provide dampening of extraneous motion, although results with these devices have been mixed.

How the MAS works. MASs compensate for proximal weakness in the UEs in three ways: (1) they allow for a significant increase in active movement in the shoulder and elbow, (2) they enable hand placement in a variety of positions, and (3) they allow persons with significant weakness to engage in functional tasks. MASs can be used for occupational performance (allowing engagement in desktop tasks and ADLs such as feeding, hygiene, and grooming) and/or for therapeutic exercises (improving ROM, strength, endurance). Their use may be temporary or permanent.[4,6,33] The mechanical principles on which the MAS functions are threefold. The devices (1) use gravity to assist weak muscles, (2) support the weight of the arm to reduce the load on weak muscles, and (3) use friction reduced bushings in the arm support joints to increase the ease of movement.[23]

Some devices also use springs and/or rubber bands to assist weak muscles.

Criteria for use. Several criteria must be met for a person to be considered for MAS use. Many of these criteria apply to use of other devices to assist weak arms, but they were initially developed for MAS use.[33,34] These include:

Client goals, occupational performance, and motivation. The person must have a goal and/or need to perform specific occupations and motions of the arm that cannot otherwise be accomplished because of weak shoulder and elbow musculature. To optimize chances for successful use of a MAS, the client must *want* to use the device and must have sufficient motivation for training to use it proficiency.[4] Atkins et al. surveyed therapists who specialize in treating clients with spinal cord injury, and the most frequently identified activities in which MAS users engaged were (in descending frequency) exercise, eating, page turning, power WC propulsion, brushing teeth, and keyboarding.[4]

Adequate motor control. To use a MAS, the person must possess selective volitional control of the existing muscles, which will power the MAS. People with conditions such as cerebral palsy, stroke, or traumatic brain injury who do not possess isolated selective motor control are typically not good candidates for use of a MAS.

Adequate source of power. The potential MAS user must have adequate strength to move the MAS with the arm secured

in it. Movement is typically generated by the shoulder and elbow muscles, although the source of power can also come from a combination of functioning muscles in the neck, trunk, and shoulder girdle. Neck and/or trunk musculature alone is seldom adequate for performance of ADLs using a MAS but can enhance function in combination with other muscles. Muscle strength of 2–/5 (poor minus) in the available scapular, shoulder, and elbow muscles is typically the minimum for successful use of the MAS.

Sufficient passive range of motion. To operate a MAS, the potential user must have sufficient passive range of motion (PROM) in shoulder flexion, abduction, and external rotation, elbow flexion and extension, and forearm pronation. Adequate available PROM for functional use of the MAS includes at least 0 to 90 degrees of shoulder flexion and abduction, external rotation of 0 to 30 degrees or more, normal shoulder internal rotation and elbow flexion, and 0 to 80 degrees of forearm pronation. PROM of 0 to 90 degrees in hip flexion allows for an upright sitting position and provides an optimal base of support for UE function.

Stable trunk positioning. An upright sitting posture is ideal, but initially clients may have difficulty tolerating this position. Using the MAS in a semi-reclined (5–20 degrees) sitting position is possible, but more challenging. In addition to presenting with weakness in the UEs, clients may present with absent or weak trunk musculature, as in the case of those with complete quadriplegia/tetraplegia. Clients with significant trunk weakness will require lateral trunk supports to be mounted on their WC for optimal use of the MAS.

Freedom from interfering pain. Thorough evaluation of pain level, pain triggers, and pain buffers assists the therapist in deciding whether a client is a candidate for MAS use. Using MASs may decrease chronic pain, because the device supports the weight of the arm and allows the person to move more freely. However, freer movement also may have the opposite effect, increasing pain from overuse of weak muscles, because the MAS allows the person to engage in repetitive motion despite severe weakness. When introducing the MAS, pain level must be carefully considered and monitored.

Adequate cognition. A basic understanding of the device, how it works, and its basic adjustments is crucial for clients who use the device at home. With young children, or adults with cognitive impairment, a family member or a caregiver may receive training to assist with setting up and adjusting the MAS.

Potential client populations. Any person who presents with significant upper extremity weakness who meets the previously described criteria for use is a candidate for use of a MAS. Use can be unilateral or bilateral, depending on the goals of the client and the environment in which it will be used.

One of the most common uses of MASs is with people who have sustained a spinal cord injury at the C4 level with emerging strength in the C5 musculature, particularly the deltoids and biceps. With proper training, these clients can engage in multiple hand to face or head activities, as well as tabletop/desk activities. Strengthening exercises also can be done while in the MAS. (In addition see Chapter 37.)

Individuals with Guillain Barre Syndrome (GBS) are often ideal candidates for use because as their return of muscle function is typically proximal to distal, starting with the trunk. Functional strength in the trunk makes use of a mobile arm support much easier because clients can reposition their trunk independently, expanding their reach when using the MAS.

People with Amyotrophic Lateral Sclerosis (ALS) experience a loss of ability to participate in activities as a result of decreasing upper extremity strength, which is frequently accompanied by feelings of hopelessness.[19] Although ALS is a progressive, terminal disease, use of a MAS may prolong a client's ability to engage in meaningful occupations. Ivy et al. reported on the orthotic needs and use in three individuals with ALS, concluding that orthotic devices such as the MAS may be beneficial for this population, providing the client receives early intervention, as well as reassessment and revision throughout the course of the disease.[19]

Cruz et al. interviewed four individuals with Duchenne's muscular dystrophy (DMD) who were current or past users of a MAS.[12] Three of the participants benefitted from using the MAS, citing increased upper extremity function and independence with ADLs, most notably eating and drinking. Access to experienced professionals for setup and ongoing consultation were important to successful use. Barriers to success included inadequate strength, the device interfering with WC controls, and funding challenges.[12] (See Chapter 38 for further information on disorders of the motor unit mentioned in the above three paragraphs.)

Van der Heide et al. studied the use of various dynamic arm supports available in the Netherlands with 19 individuals.[32] Diagnoses of the participants included spinal muscular atrophy (SMA), spinal cord injury (SCI), postpolio syndrome, multiple sclerosis (MS), limb-girdle muscular dystrophy (LGMD), and Ehlers-Danlos syndrome (EDS). Five study participants reported a large perceived functional benefit from the device, 5 participants did not perceive a functional benefit, and the remaining 9 participants reported a minor functional benefit from using the device. Conclusions from this study were that people with the greatest functional limitations benefitted the most from dynamic arm supports, and those who did not perceive functional benefit indicated that they were able to perform ADLs without the device. Results suggested that incorrectly chosen devices (poor user-device match) was a factor for several participants, reinforcing the need to carefully assess functional abilities, need for the device, and the environment in which the device will be used.[32]

The client populations described in this section represent several diagnoses for which MASs have been found to be valuable. MASs can be used by any client with demonstrated functional limitations as a result of proximal upper extremity weakness who meets the criteria for use described earlier in this chapter.

Barriers to successful use. Several barriers to successful use have been identified by clients who use or have used MASs. An optimal match between the client and the device is essential for maximizing or maintaining function, and to achieve this, clients must have access to knowledgeable clinicians.[32]

The need for repeated readjustment of the device, particularly among users with progressive conditions was also identified as a barrier. Routine follow-up with an experienced clinician can enable continued occupational engagement for this population of clients.[19] Cosmetic appearance and the resultant negatively affected body image as well as a perceived appearance of greater disability with the device has been reported as a barrier by some clients.[4] Another significant barrier is the increased WC width because of the device, and the resultant inability to move freely from room to room because of doorway width. If strength permits, individuals can cross their arms while navigating doorways, propelling the WC with the opposite hand if a hand control is being used. For adult clients who need a MAS but are ambulatory, the weight and discomfort of the device and back brace to which it attaches presents a barrier to successful use.[29] Finally, access to an adequate funding source presents a barrier for numerous clients. The most common design limitations that can interfere with successful use of the MAS included the MAS hitting the work surface, blocking of the WC armrest or joystick, difficulty managing the MAS when reclining for pressure relief, difficulty mounting the MAS, and adjustments needing to be made to the MAS when transitioning between activities.[4]

THREADED CASE STUDY

Matt, Part 3

> Matt meets all the criteria listed for using a mobile arm support (MAS). He has identified goals such as using a computer, writing, feeding himself, and brushing his teeth, that can be accomplished using a MAS and additional equipment to compensate for loss of hand function. Client factors, including motor control, strength, ROM, and stable trunk positioning, are sufficient to allow him to use a MAS. He has minimal pain in his arms, and his cognition is intact. He is highly motivated to return to work and to be able to engage with family and friends. His family is incredibly supportive of these goals.

The JAECO/Rancho MultiLink MAS. The most used MASs in the United States during the past 60 years have been manufactured by JAECO Orthopedics (Fig. 31.6 and Fig. 31.8). The newer JAECO/Rancho MultiLink MAS, developed in the early 2000s, is easy to adjust and comes with a clearly written manual detailing its setup and basic adjustments. In addition, the manufacture's website, https://jaecoorthopedic.com/, has videos addressing the evaluation process and device assembly. All parts of the MultiLink MAS are interchangeable for application between the right and left side of the mounting surface (i.e., WC or table). The MultiLink Mount (Fig. 31.7B) is attached to the WC or a standard chair, and is the interface between the chair and the MAS arm. The MultiLink arm (see Fig. 31.7A-3) is then connected to the mount (see Fig. 31.7A-1) using the proximal shaft (see Fig. 31.7A-2), and allows for friction-reduced movement. The MultiLink arm is available in a standard or elevating model, and differences in functionality between the two models will be described. The adjustable forearm support is connected to an adjustable offset swivel (see Fig. 31.7C), which is inserted into the distal end of the MultiLink arm. The MAS user's arm is placed in the forearm support.

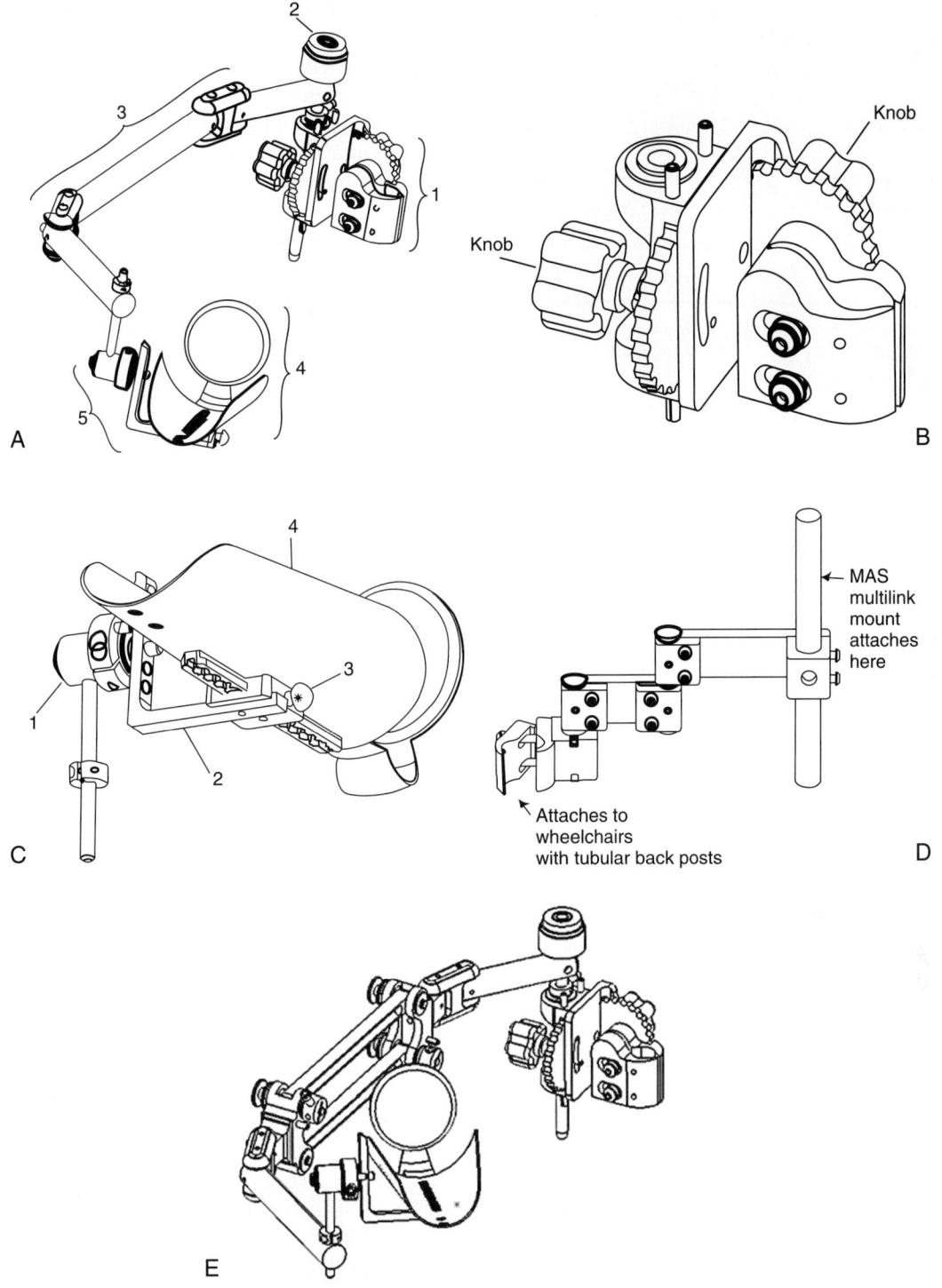

Fig. 31.7 (A) JAECO/Rancho Multilink Mobile Arm Support. *1,* MAS mount. *2,* Proximal shaft with bubble level. *3,* MultiLink. *4,* Forearm support with elbow dial. *5,* Offset swivel with adjustable slide. (B) JAECO/ Rancho MultiLink Mobile Arm Support mount. Two knobs control adjustment without use of tools. (C) JAECO/ Rancho MultiLink Mobile Arm Support offset swivel with adjustable slide. *1,* Offset swivel with *(2)* adjustable slide. *3,* Spring-loaded pullout knob to adjust position on the forearm support *(4).* (D) JAECO Mount Adapter MR-10 enables the JAECO/Rancho mount to attach to wheelchairs with tubular back posts. (E) The JAECO/ Rancho MultiLink Arm with Elevation Assist. (Courtesy JAECO Orthopedic, Inc., Hot Springs, AR.)

It is of greatest importance that the therapist understands the adjustment capabilities of each component of the MAS, because it is these adjustments that customize the MAS to meet the needs and goals of each individual MAS user and augment the user's available internal source of power (muscle strength).

Adjustment capabilities of individual parts (JAECO Orthopedic, 2008)

MultiLink mount. The mount comes with two adjustable scroll wheels that tilt the MAS, using gravity to assist the user to move in the direction in which they are weaker (see Fig. 31.7B).

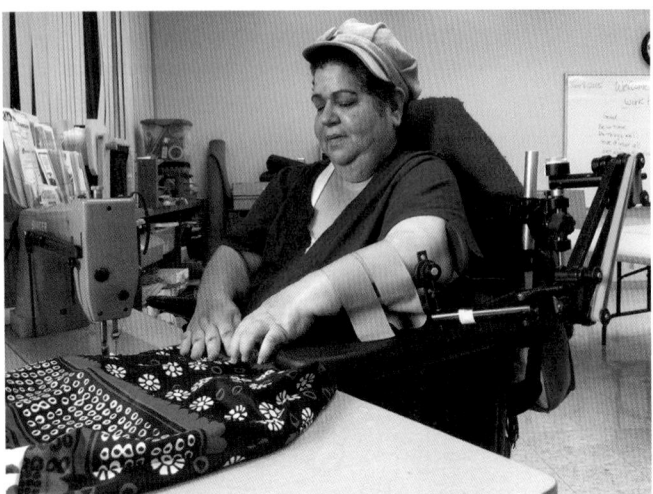

Fig. 31.8 Sewing using the JAECO/Rancho MultiLink Arm with Elevation Assist.

It is important to note that the user must have adequate strength to move against the assisted motion. These adjustments allow for optimal forward reach and return movements and side to side movements. Once overall functional range of the MAS is maximized, the scroll wheels are tightened (locked) in place.

MultiLink arms. Based on client factors and the client's individual goals, the therapist will choose between two types of MultiLink Arms.[1] The Standard MultiLink Arm (see Fig. 31.6 and 31.7A) provides horizontal movement, however vertical motion is limited to that which is generated by shoulder external rotation and elbow flexion and extension. The MultiLink Arm with Elevation Assist (see Fig. 31.7E and 31.8) attaches to the mount in the same manner as the standard MultiLink arm but allows for assisted elevation of the arm at the shoulder in both flexion and abduction. According to 2020 data, this is the most frequently ordered type of multilink arm, accounting for approximately 50% of all MAS orders. (M. Conry, personal communication, May 2015 and July 2020). The MultiLink Arm with Elevation Assist is useful for the person who has deltoid strength between 2–/5 (poor–) and 3/5 (fair). This multilink arm allows for significantly greater freedom of movement and thus expanded functional use (see Fig. 31.8). The client initiates the elevating motion (shoulder flexion or abduction), and the rubber bands attached to the middle section of the MultiLink arm assist the client to flex or abduct the shoulder through greater active ROM. The MultiLink Arm with Elevation Assist has stops that can be adjusted to limit the amount of upward and downward motion. It is important to note that the client must have sufficient muscle power combined with the weight of the arm to return to the resting position. For this reason, not all persons with 2–/5 to 3/5 deltoid strength are good candidates for this MAS component. Individuals who have strong shoulder extensors/depressors to oppose the force of the rubber bands and return the arm to the side (e.g., persons with GBS) are exceptionally well suited to successfully use the MultiLink Arm with Elevation Assist.[20]

Forearm support and offset swivel. Optimal vertical (hand to mouth) movements are achieved by adjusting the offset

swivel along the slide that is affixed to the bottom of the forearm support (see Fig. 31.7C-2). Moving the rocker arm along the slide toward the wrist aids in upward motion, and moving it toward the elbow aids the downward motion. As with the previously mentioned adjustments, the MAS user must have sufficient strength to move against the assisted motion. Each of these basic adjustments is made with the person's arm secured in the MAS.[20]

MAS mount relocator. Mounting the MAS to a WC is frequently a challenge because WC backs and back posts vary in design and because other equipment such as lateral trunk supports also must be attached to the WC in the same area (see Fig. 31.7D). The MAS can be attached to most common WCs and mobility seating systems using one of the three mount bases provided with the arm. Before ordering the MAS, the therapist must be familiar with the backrest design of the client's WC.[20]

Other MASs

The WREX. More recently, a newer design of MAS, the Wilmington Robotic Exoskeleton (WREX) (Fig. 31.9), has been shown to allow freer shoulder movement[29] (M. Conry, personal communication). The WREX WC mount is attached higher than the shoulder and has 2 links and four degrees of motion, similar to typical human anatomy, which allows the arm to "float." This is an excellent MAS alternative for individuals who are somewhat stronger, but still in need of assistance for vertical movement. Like the JAECO/Rancho MultiLink MAS, the WREX is effective for people with upper limb neuromuscular weakness such as muscle disease, spinal cord injury, multiple sclerosis and amyotrophic lateral sclerosis. The WREX can be attached to most WCs and mobility seating systems using one of the three mount bases provided with the arm.

The mobility arm. The Mobility Arm (Fig. 31.10A) is a simpler WC-mounted arm support. Like the freestanding Swedish HelpArm (see Fig. 31.10B) described later in this chapter, it uses a weight to counterbalance the weight of the arm, allowing greater vertical movement from weak shoulder musculature. However, it lacks the fine adjustment of the JAECO/Rancho Multilink MAS. Achieving the optimal match between equipment and client has a significant impact on functional benefit continued use.

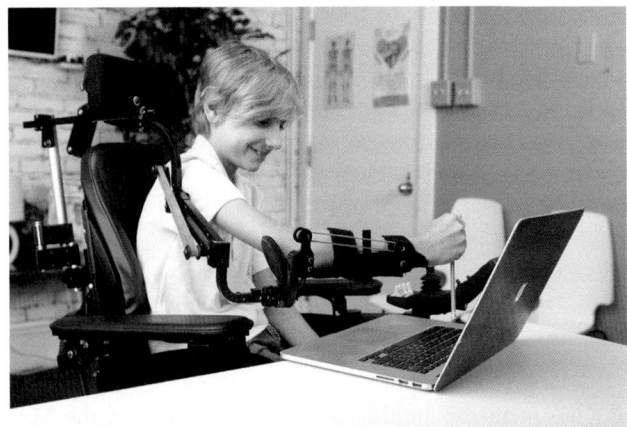

Fig. 31.9 WREX Wilmington Robotic Exoskeleton Arm. (Used with permission of Jaeco Orthopedic. All rights reserved.)

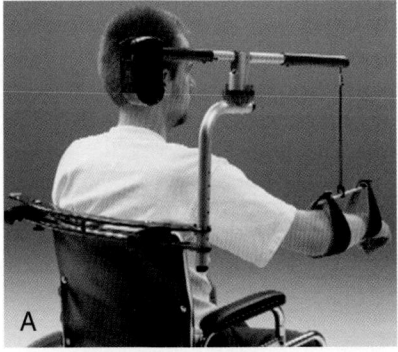

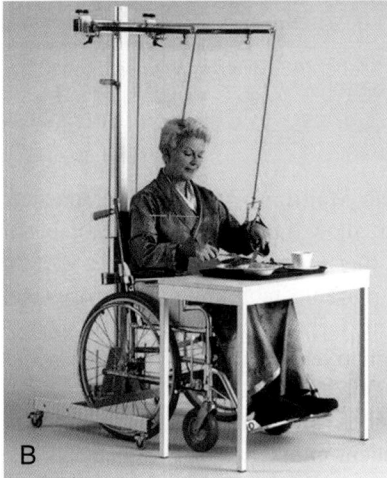

Fig. 31.10 (A) Mobility arm sling mounted on a wheelchair. (B) The Swedish HelpArm is similar in design to a traditional deltoid aid. (A and B Courtesy Performance Health, Warrenville, IL.)

THREADED CASE STUDY

Matt, Part 4

After 2 weeks in rehabilitation, Matt was able to sit upright in a WC for 5 hours a day. He was given a power WC, which he operated independently with a head control, for both mobility and reclining the WC for pressure relief. He was still unable to participate in any of the most important occupations he identified on admission.

A JAECO/Rancho MultiLink MAS was mounted on Matt's WC, and he was given a lapboard for his WC as well. With the MAS and his wrist-hand orthosis, Matt was able to use his iPad more easily and for an increasing variety of applications. His wife brought his laptop computer to the hospital, and with training and further MAS adjustment Matt was able to send emails to his wife, co-workers, and friends. Activities requiring hand-to-mouth skills are more challenging and complex than tabletop activities, so these occupations were introduced more gradually as Matt worked on reaching higher and higher. Once Matt could reach his mouth using the MAS, eating activities were introduced. After training, Matt was able to feed himself following set-up, using a wrist-hand orthosis and a universal cuff to hold a fork or spoon. When Matt's children came to visit, the OT planned some treatment sessions to encourage Matt to use his MAS to play games on the computer with them. Matt was encouraged by being able to play with his children, affirming the resumption of his role as a father.

Another of Matt's goals was to drive his power WC using a hand control instead of the head control. This entailed in-depth discussion with his OT regarding the energy required to drive the WC all day using a hand control, as well as returning to full time employment. Careful consideration had to be given to community WC use, regarding uneven terrain (hills and ramps) and endurance. Matt practiced using the MAS to drive his WC until he accomplished this task, but ultimately decided to stay with the head control, recognizing how fatiguing full time WC propulsion with the hand control was for him. With practice, Matt was able to use his iPad and his laptop computer, turn pages, manage a speakerphone, feed himself simple meals, and drive his power WC.

Training. Selecting the appropriate equipment and providing the user with an optimally adjusted device is key to continued use and maximizing the functional benefit of a MAS.[32] Training includes therapist-supervised practice in all occupations that interest the client and that need to be performed.[6,32,33] Any of these occupations may require fine adjustments to the MAS until the optimal settings are achieved, maximizing quality of performance and engagement in a variety of activities. If strength or ROM increases during the training period, further adjustments will be needed. A wrist-hand orthosis and/or occupation-specific adaptive equipment may be necessary for use with the MAS.[6,33] When using a MAS to propel a power WC, training must include a variety of environments to ensure that the client can successfully negotiate hills and rough terrain. Because MASs rely on gravity to assist weak muscles, inclined terrain may pose significant challenges to the very weak client. Follow-up assessment and training is indicated, especially for a growing child or for any client whose physical status may change.

Freestanding Dynamic Arm Supports

Freestanding dynamic arm supports that do not attach to the WC allow the therapist to assess the potential benefit of a MAS and initiate treatment earlier in the rehabilitation process. These devices allow for quicker set-up than a WC mounted MAS, maximizing inpatient therapy time. The rapid set-up allows the client to begin engaging in self-care and tabletop activities and exercise as soon as minimal WC sitting tolerance is established.

Freestanding devices vary in their complexity and ease of adjustment. All provide support to the arm, allowing the client to engage in activities. These devices use rubber bands, springs, ball bearings and other mechanical elements to negate the effects of gravity on weak proximal UE musculature.

The SaeboMAS has an adjustable parallelogram design offering various levels of assistance (Fig. 31.11). The mechanism is spring based, allowing for multidirectional activities. It features a mechanical tension scale, which allows the therapist to grade the activity and track and document progress. Height adjustment allows the client to practice skills in either a sitting or standing position.

The JAECO/Rancho MultiLink MAS can be mounted to a lightweight, portable, and height-adjustable floor stand that is placed next to the WC (Fig. 31.12). This allows the seated client to engage in activities immediately, and to evaluate whether a WC or table-mounted MAS would be most beneficial.

The Swedish HelpArm (similar to what was once called a Deltoid Aid) uses weights to assist with upward motion of the arm (see Fig. 31.10B). Increasing or decreasing the weights provides the optimal amount of assistance to the arm. This device

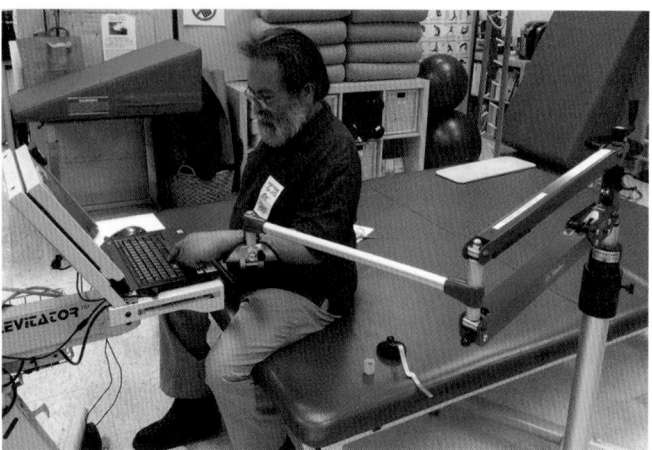

Fig. 31.11 The SaeboMAS floor model allows for a quick setup supporting the arm.

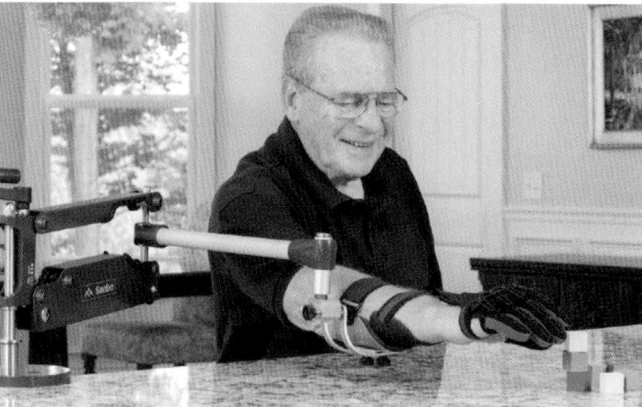

Fig. 31.13 The SaeboMAS Mini mounted on a table. (Courtesy Saebo, Inc., Charlotte, NC.)

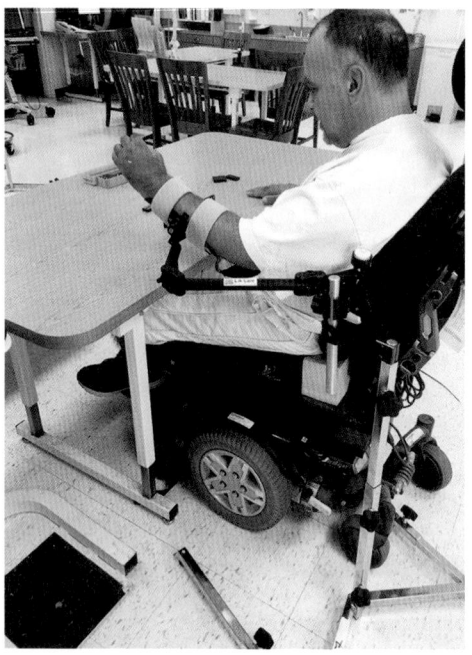

Fig. 31.12 The JAECO/Rancho MultiLink mounted to a stand allowing for a quick setup in the clinic.

can be used while the person is sitting in bed or in a chair. The therapist can limit the available motion, allowing clients with very weak muscles to exercise and engage in self-care and table-top activities.

Dynamic Arm Supports for the Ambulatory Client

Ambulatory clients with weak proximal UE musculature are unable to reach their upper torso and head, engage in tabletop activities, and reach for objects that are above waist height. If only one arm is significantly affected, the person can easily use the less affected side. However, when both shoulders are weak, the hands may have functional strength, but the arms rest by the side of the body in a dependent position, making reaching for objects and lifting them impossible. Clients with bilateral proximal weakness may use table-mounted arm supports to allow them to position the hand in space for function. The

JAECO/Rancho MultiLink MAS can be attached to a special table mount to allow the person to sit at a table and engage in activities. Another such device is the SaeboMAS Mini, which is a lightweight, portable, table-mounted device (Fig. 31.13). Like the freestanding Saebo, it has an adjustable spring-based parallelogram design, offering graded levels of assistance in multiple planes of movement.

When using a table-mounted dynamic arm device, the ambulatory client must dedicate one location in which to engage in all desired activities. An activity center or desk with the dynamic arm support attached is a good solution for a person who spends hours in one area, such as at work. However, what is the solution for a person to brush his or her teeth at the sink, use an ATM machine, and reach for a box of cereal at the supermarket? This is an as-yet unsolved dilemma.

Dynamic arm supports can be attached to the trunk by a custom-made body orthosis, but they are heavy and cumbersome. These devices have primarily been studied and developed for children. A commercially available example is the Wilmington Robotic Exoskeleton (WREX). It is typically attached to a WC but can be attached to a custom back brace for ambulatory clients. The ambulatory WREX has been fitted on children as young as 6 years old, allowing them to engage in activities while sitting, standing, or walking.[15,29] For the past two decades, Tariq Rahman, PhD, and his team at the Alfred I. DuPont Hospital for Children have been improving the WREX to allow children with arthrogryposis, myopathy, and spinal muscular atrophy (SMA) to eat, play, and study using the device. The mobile arm supports are custom made for each child with three-dimensional printing.[29] This device is large and visible however, and potential users, parents and therapists must weigh the benefits against the negative social impact in deciding whether to use it.[15,29]

With the ongoing development of new materials and technologies, it is the hope of these authors that better equipment solutions for ambulatory, actively engaged adults with weak proximal UE musculature will be developed and marketed soon.

Cost of Equipment

Recommending the optimal equipment for home use is critical for maximizing both UE strength and occupational performance. Cost and funding sources must always be considered. The therapist must establish whether equipment will be covered by insurance; if the first attempt to procure equipment through insurance fails, the therapist may resubmit the request with a stronger justification. When arm supports and additional adaptive equipment are not covered by insurance, and the client has no means to pay for the orthosis, alternative funding sources such as community fundraising and nonprofit grant assistance should be explored.

Alternatives to purchasing expensive devices are cheaper or homemade equipment. At times simple solutions such as using an over-bed table is cheaper and more practical for some individuals. If the shoulders are weak but clients have functional elbow flexion and some wrist and/or hand function, the elbows can be propped on the table allowing the person to eat and engage in hygiene and grooming. With the elbows supported, the person can perform activities such as writing, drawing, and playing board games. Despite not meeting all the capabilities of a well-designed orthosis, homemade solutions may provide an adequate substitute for an expensive device.

All types of equipment are not available at every facility; therefore, therapists must familiarize themselves with the devices that are available in their clinic and have their department purchase or arrange a loan of trial equipment as necessary for patient evaluation. To achieve the optimal desired therapeutic outcome, the therapist must combine a clear understanding of the equipment at hand with the desired therapeutic goals.

ROBOT-ASSISTED THERAPY

Robot-assisted therapy (RT), also called robot-mediated therapy, primarily includes a variety of complex and expensive devices for the upper limb (Figs. 31.14 to 31.18). They provide automated, goal-directed, repetitive movements with highly adjustable levels of assistance or resistance.[27] In the past few years, smaller, portable, and less expensive robots have been developed with the introduction of lighter materials and more affordable computer systems.[11] RT allows for systematic adjustment of treatment parameters and provides the client with feedback and thus motivation to reach a goal.[24,27] In addition, it provides kinetic measurements that can assist the therapist in grading the therapy program and monitoring and documenting progress.

RT produces high-intensity and goal-directed repetition without boredom, because of the interactive component of the treatment. The feedback can promote patient engagement, motivating the client to reach targets beyond their comfortable reach, while providing assist-as-needed help. Assist-as-needed parameters estimate patient effort and impairment in real time based on data collected by the robot, thus adjusting the level of assistance provided.[8]

The interest in RT began two decades ago, with the emergence of evidence indicating that brain neuroplasticity can occur in adults, and not only in children, as was previously thought. Unlike the mechanical arm supports discussed earlier in this chapter, RT development, research, and intervention has been focused primarily on survivors of cerebral vascular accident (CVA).[26] Research showed that rote, repetitive exercise of an

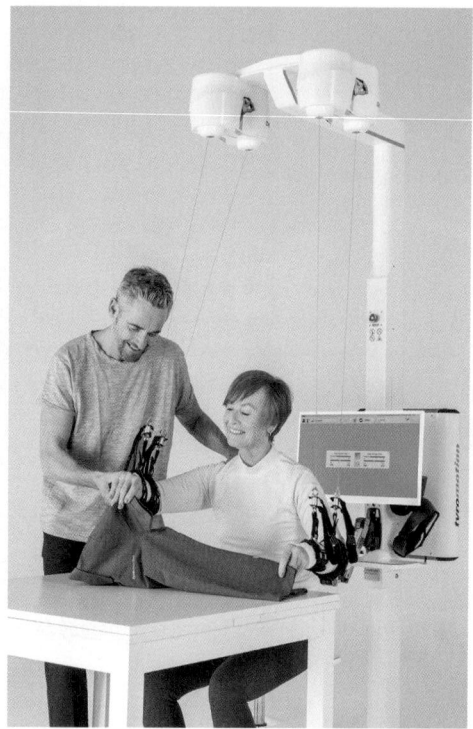

Fig. 31.14 The Tyromotion "DIEGO" allows the client to interact with the computer screen or to engage in functional activities away from the screen. (Used with permission of Tyromotion. All rights reserved.)

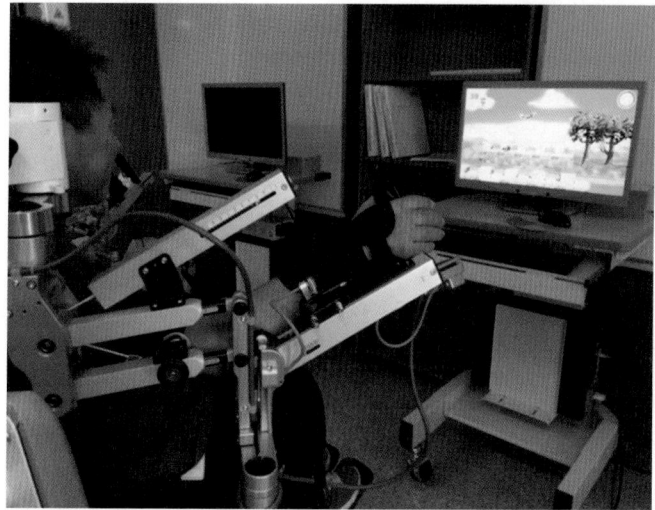

Fig. 31.15 The ArmeoSpring mobile arm support by Hocoma.

affected limb, shortly after trauma, leads to increased brain activity and improved function. Initial studies focused on gait training after neurologic injuries such as CVA and incomplete SCI. The use of RT for the upper limbs began with stroke survivors, after initial evidence showed that (as with the lower extremities) it reduced motor impairments in the upper limbs when administered shortly after onset of the CVA. Recent small, yet promising studies show neural and some functional improvement following RT after stroke.[2,18,21,28] However, most authors caution against overreliance on robotics because they acknowledge that transfer of repetitive, predictable range of motion is vastly different from

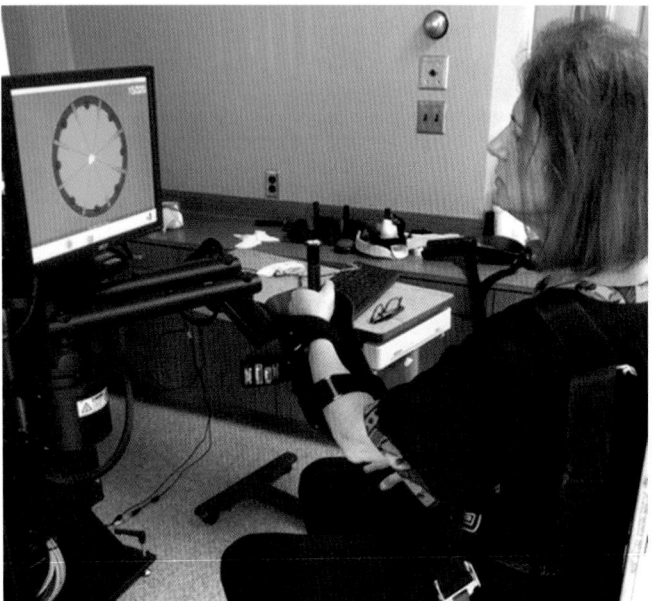

Fig. 31.16 The InMotion Arm Interactive Therapy System.

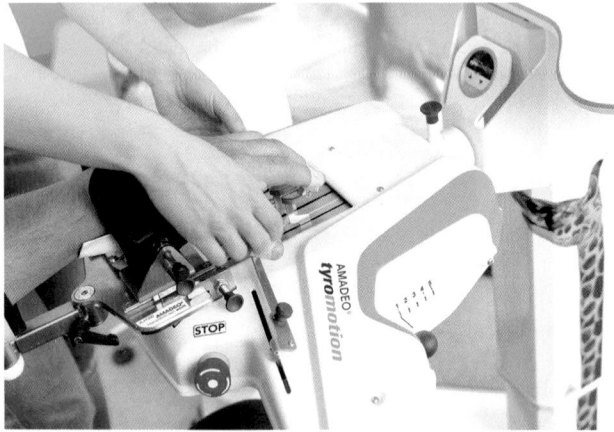

Fig. 31.17 The Tyromotion "AMADEO" is an an end-effector hand rehabilitation device that allows for active, assistive, and passive therapies for individual finger and thumb movements. (Used with permission of Tyromotion. All rights reserved.)

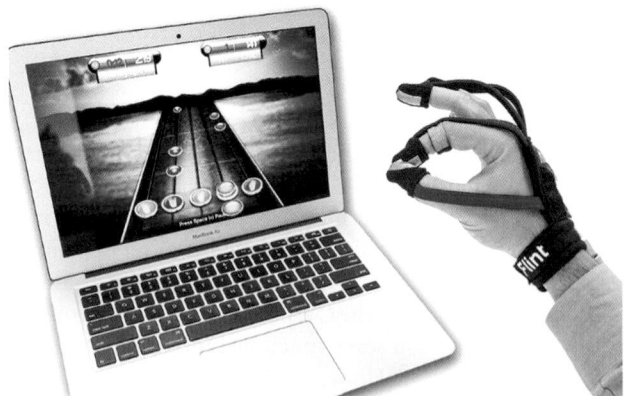

Fig. 31.18 The Flint Rehab MusicGlove device opens up the possibility for a sensorized home exercise program. (Used with permission of Flint Rehab. All rights reserved.)

performing ADLs and other activities.[28,36] The engineers who study, create, and improve robotic products also grapple with mechanical and material problems. The complexity of the arm (most notably the shoulder and hand) poses many challenges in developing portable, lightweight robots.[26,36]

It is important to note that RTs are not meant to replace the therapist but rather to augment traditional therapies and enable the therapist to provide more intensive therapy than was previously possible.[28] RT is frequently combined with neuromuscular electrical stimulation to facilitate and strengthen movement and to provide greater feedback to the client.

Most of the robots allow the client to interact with a computer monitor, offering games, target practices, and other goal-oriented tasks. Some robots offer virtual reality goggles to enhance clients' motivation and to facilitate movements outside of a narrow screen. The Tyromotion DIEGO (see Fig. 31.14) is unique in its ability to allow patients to practice skills a little farther away from the monitor, enabling the client to engage in other tabletop activities such as eating or folding clothes. The arms are suspended in air much like mechanical slings, allowing the therapist to fine tune training modalities and parameters. An RT session may include the therapist and client collaborating on a specific goal such as reaching a target by moving the arm in a prescribed direction. When the arm is weak, the robot can provide adequate assistance to allow the motion to be completed repeatedly.

Some devices, such as the ArmeoSpring, use hybrid technology, combining traditional MAS type components with interactive computerized elements to provide valuable feedback and monitoring of client performance (see Fig. 31.15). Electrical sensors in the mechanical arm which are connected to a computer allow the client to focus on a clear goal, and the therapist to monitor and record progress, optimizing the therapeutic session.

In the past two decades more companies have been developing and marketing RT devices. These robots are expensive (approximately 80,000–200,000 dollars) and are usually purchased by large rehabilitation hospitals and research institutions. More affordable alternatives have been developed and are available in Europe such as the ArmAssist (TECNALIA R&I, Spain), an arm "skateboard" allowing the client to move the limb on a flat surface much like a traditional therapy skateboard. A computer monitor enhances client engagement and feedback.[31]

Considerations for Use

Patient safety is of outmost concern, and therefore the therapist must carefully evaluate the patient-machine fit and interaction.[36] The therapist must set the correct parameters for optimal arm-robot movement and force and monitor the session carefully. An emergency stop button (kill switch) is important to enable either the client or the therapist to stop the machine at any time. This is essential for unexpected situations such as UE muscle spasm or sudden severe pain.

As stated previously, motor control problems such as ataxia pose a continual challenge to both therapist and client. Some robotic devices can be adjusted to damp extraneous movements, allowing for greater function in certain clients.

Suggested protocols for frequency and duration of treatment have been developed for individuals recovering from CVAs[10,25]; however, at this time, there is no conclusive evidence to guide the therapist in determining what specific regimen is optimal for each client.[10,24] With the successful outcomes of RT for stroke survivors, some studies analyze the its efficacy with individuals with traumatic brain injury, spinal cord injury,[13] and cerebral palsy.[22] Despite their small sample size limitations, these studies show promise for more versatile use of RT with various patient diagnoses.

Clinical Reasoning and Training Modalities

The decision to augment treatment using RT must be carefully evaluated, answering the following questions:

- How does RT use meet the patient-therapist overall goals?
- What is achieved by RT use that cannot be achieved with engagement in meaningful occupations?
- Will repetitive motion enhance the return of voluntary motor strength and control and enhance function?
- When should RT be introduced and how much therapy time should be devoted to RT?
- What kind of RT-like home program can be replicated after discharge and embedded in a person's daily routine?
  RT training modalities are shown in Table 31.1.

THREADED CASE STUDY

Matt, Part 5

Matt, who's goal was to reach for objects away from his body, to touch his face, eat, brush his teeth, and be able drive his power WC with his hand, enjoyed using the robot. Matt's OT used a shoulder-elbow robot several times a week for part of his treatment session. The goal of the sessions was to help Matt improve forward reach at the shoulder, and elbow flexion. The settings of the robot were frequently adjusted in response to Matt's changing status, providing continual challenge as his strength and endurance increased. He initially required active-assistive exercise, moving his arm through part of a predetermined pathway for reaching and returning his arm to his side, with assistance provided by the robot at the end of his available active ROM. Eventually Matt was able to complete the entire motion independently, and finally the therapist adjusted the parameters by introducing light resistance to his movement. Matt was highly motivated to train on the robot, and he liked the visual and auditory feedback he received when he reached his daily goals. Interacting with the robot provided Matt with the just-right challenge.

TABLE 31.1 Robotic-Assisted Therapy Training Modalities

Modality	Client's Effort	Robot Effort
Passive[a]	No voluntary effort required. May be valuable if sensation is intact and muscle strength is emerging, to facilitate muscle reeducation. Can also provide passive range of motion (PROM)	Robot executes the full movement An option for continuous passive motion (CPM)
Assisted[a]	Voluntary effort needed throughout the movement	Robot provides limb weight support and/or some force assistance for task completion
Active-assistive[a]	Clients perform the task as much as they are able	Robot completes the task
Active[a]	Full effort by the client	Robot is used for tracking and measuring performance
Corrective[a]	The client is stopped by the robot and is required to actively correct the movement	Robot stops and/or corrects the course of the movement
Path guidance[a]	Client has a predetermined route to perform the movement	Robot dictates the path parameters of the movement
Resistive[a]	Client must push through resistance to achieve the target	Robot resists the movement, and therapist sets a predetermined resistance force
Mirror guidance[b] Only available with bimanual robots	With bilateral robotic arms the affected arm moves symmetrically with the unaffected arm. The client leads the impaired UE with the unimpaired UE	Robot assists in mirroring the motion of the unaffected arm, providing support to the limb and/or assistance with task completion
Vibration[c]	None	Robot provides focal vibration (mechanical oscillation) over a target muscle after stroke.
Electromyography (EMG) driven[d] EMG electrodes guide desired movement.	Clients perform the task as much as they are able	The robot provides some assistance to complete the task along with neuromuscular focal stimulation on specific muscles to enhance power

Modalities of each robot vary; some can be set to provide a combination of above modalities.

[a]Basteris A, Nijenhuis SM, Stienen AH, et al: Training modalities in robot-mediated upper limb rehabilitation in stroke: a framework for classification based on a systematic review. *J Neuroeng Rehab* 11(1):111, 2014.[5]
[b]Simkins M, Kim H, Abrams G, Byl N, Rosen J: (2013, June). Robotic unilateral and bilateral upper-limb movement training for stroke survivors afflicted by chronic hemiparesis. *IEEE Int Conf Rehab Robot* 2013:6650506, 2013.[30]
[c]Celletti C, Suppa A, Bianchini E, et al: Promoting post-stroke recovery through focal or whole-body vibration: criticisms and prospects from a narrative review. *Neurol Sci* 41(1), 11–24, 2020.[9]
[d]Huang Y, Lai WP, Qian Q, Hu X, et al: Translation of robot-assisted rehabilitation to clinical service in upper limb rehabilitation. In *Intelligent Biomechatronics in Neurorehabilitation*, San Diego, 2020, Academic Press, pp 225–238;[17] and Huang Y, Lai WP, Qian Q, et al: Translation of robot-assisted rehabilitation to clinical service: a comparison of the rehabilitation effectiveness of EMG-driven robot hand assisted upper limb training in practical clinical service and in clinical trial with laboratory configuration for chronic stroke. *Biomed Eng Online*, 17(1):91, 2018.[18]

Robotic-Assisted Therapy for the Hand

The development of hand robotics has trailed behind shoulder and elbow technology. This is in part because of the complexity of hand movements and the nature of hand tasks, demanding small, dexterous motions. The overall goal of hand RT is to facilitate grasp and release and to achieve the independent finger movements needed for functional performance of ADLs, IADLs, and other specific tasks.

The AMADEO by Tyromotion (see Fig. 31.17) allows isolation of finger movements, changes in modalities (EMG-integration, CPM, assistive, active), various measurements, and feedback. Smaller robots have less capacity for variations in modes and parameters, limiting the range of patients who can work with it. Soft, lighter hand robotic devices in the form of a glove have recently been introduced, increasing portability and allowing freedom of motion that is impossible with rigid devices. The thumb for example, with its complex circumduction, is freer to move in all directions in a soft glove, compared to a rigid metal structure that allows only flexion and extension. In contrast to that, patients who are barely able or unable to grasp can perform hundreds of robot-assisted grasping movements with devices like the AMADEO.

The advent of portable robotic and sensorized devices for the hand has the potential for seamless implementation in a home setting. Zondervan et al. conducted a randomized controlled study to determine the feasibility and efficacy of a 1-month home therapy intervention using the MusicGlove (see Fig. 31.18) compared to a conventional home exercise program.[37] Although there was no significant difference between the groups in the post-treatment Box and Blocks test, the MusicGlove group demonstrated significantly greater improvement in the postintervention Motor Activity Log Quality of Movement and Amount of Use scores. In addition, the MusicGlove treatment resulted in a significantly greater increase in self-driven repetitions, self-reported quality of movement, and functional use. After specific training and instructions, clients may develop a daily routine of RT at home, with or without the supervision of a therapist. Telehealth sessions allow the therapist to visually monitor program implementation and progress. One of the most significant of Zondervan's findings was the increase in frequency of repetitions, suggestive of clients' greater motivation for self-management.[37]

In an extensive literature review, Chu and Patterson analyzed features of 44 soft robotic hand devices, concluding that their primary use is facilitating beginning functional hand use through task-specific training (TST).[11] Increasing passive range of motion (PROM) was the second most frequent purpose for using a hand robot because of the ease of implementing and executing a repetitive PROM program. Because this technology is relatively new and in continuous development, special precautions must be taken to ensure client safety. Chu and Patterson expressed concern that only 12 of the 44 robots mentioned the presence of emergency stop mechanisms in their devices. The ability to stop the robot is especially important when robots are used at home without supervision.[11]

As with shoulder and elbow RT, evidence-based data on the development and efficacy of hand robots focuses on stroke survivors and is carried out mostly by engineers. The authors acknowledge that hand RT is still early in its development and that further study and device improvements are necessary to enable these devices to be fully integrated in therapy.[11,35]

In summary, RTs, if available, can augment traditional therapies. They can provide the client with a motivating platform to engage in goal-directed, repetitive movements. Additionally, they allow the therapist to assess, monitor, and obtain objective measurements of client progress, assisting with documentation. Although evidence shows that clinic-based robotic arms can facilitate positive neural changes and functional improvement after stroke, it is important to note that most published studies are conducted by engineers under strict protocols. These studies provide subjects with optimal conditions that are challenging to duplicate in a busy OT clinic. Recent evidence suggests that a combination of conventional therapy interventions and RT will most likely yield the best overall result for the patient.[28]

THREADED CASE STUDY

Matt, Part 6

Matt was first able to benefit from using suspension arm supports in bed and using adapted equipment to access his iPad. Once he established adequate sitting tolerance in a power WC, he was fitted for a MAS. Additional adaptive equipment and adequate training and practice allowed him to engage in many of his desired occupations, including feeding, hygiene/grooming activities, computer use, and controlling aspects of his home and office environments, including operating light switches and using electronic devices. His children's visits always included special playtime using the MAS for computer and board games. Robot-assisted therapy sessions were used to strengthen weak muscles and to provide precise feedback that quantified gains in both strength and endurance. After discharge, Matt was referred to the assistive technology service, where a plan was formulated for Matt and the occupational therapist to visit his home office and school, to determine how he could manage his required work functions. In addition to the equipment he obtained as an inpatient, it was recommended that Matt would benefit from an adjustable desk, which would allow him to independently access his phone, computer, and files. He was also instructed in the procedure to obtain free specialized adaptive equipment from his telephone company, for both work and home and was trained in the use of voice recognition software installed on his computer and available for him to compose materials for his classroom, attend meetings by Zoom, and keep up with reading and answering his email. Even with this software, being able to access controls with his arm by the MAS was very valuable to Matt and maximized his feeling of control in his job. This visit and the implementation of equipment recommendations resulted in Matt's return to his job as a high school assistant principal 8 months after discharge.

SUMMARY

Clients with weak UEs benefit greatly from the use of carefully prescribed therapeutic arm supports. Static arm positioning provides support for weak musculature, helps to prevent shoulder subluxation, and assists with the management of pain in the UEs. Dynamic arm supports allow the client with weak upper limbs to engage in meaningful occupations and may also be used for strengthening. Suspension Arm Supports are inexpensive and easy to adjust, but do not allow for the discrete adjustments required for clients with severe weakness. MASs are highly adjustable devices that support the weight of the arm and minimize the effects of gravity on weak proximal UE muscles. Depending on the diagnosis and prognosis of the client, the use of MASs may be temporary or permanent. Clients must have an occupational goal and strong motivation to successfully use MASs. Freestanding dynamic arm supports are used in therapy clinics and allow quick setup and early therapeutic intervention. It is the role of the occupational therapist to select the arm support that best meets the needs of each client, through careful evaluation and the assurance that they meet the minimum criteria for optimal use.

Client concerns about MASs include increased overall WC dimensions and a heightened appearance of disability. With adequate training, however, clients who experience occupational benefits accept and use the device.

RT is a rapidly growing field with mounting evidence supporting its efficacy as an adjunct to traditional therapy. Intervention can provide the client with a motivating platform to engage in goal-directed repetitive movements. Additionally, robots allow the therapist to assess, monitor, and obtain objective measurements of client progress, assisting with documentation. Currently, most robots are expensive and available only in well-funded clinical settings. The therapist must have a clear understanding of client-therapist goals when deciding if and how to use RT. This is especially true because the carryover to functional tasks has not been fully studied. As technology continues to evolve, robots are becoming lighter and less expensive. Future research should continue to examine the effectiveness of RTs and lay the foundation for evidence-based patient-specific protocols.

REVIEW QUESTIONS

1. Why is optimal early static positioning important?
2. What are the main purposes of dynamic arm supports?
3. Where can suspension arm devices be attached?
4. What are the benefits of a MAS?
5. How does a mobile arm support work?
6. What are the criteria for successful MAS use?
7. What occupations can be achieved with the use of a MAS?
8. What are the parts of the JAECO/Rancho MultiLink MAS?
9. What are the benefits and limitations of freestanding dynamic arm supports?
10. What dynamic arm supports are available for the ambulatory client? What are their benefits and limitations?
11. What strategies can the therapist employ to encourage a reluctant client to try using a MAS?
12. What are the benefits and limitations of robot-assisted therapy?
13. How can robot-assisted therapy improve clients' engagement in therapy?
14. What training modalities can be used with robot-assisted therapies?

For additional practice questions for this chapter, please visit eBooks.Health.Elsevier.com.

ACKNOWLEDGMENTS

We would like to thank Y. Lynn Yasuda, MA, OTR/L, FAOTA, and the staff and clients at Rancho Los Amigos National Rehabilitation Center, who have taught us so much.

We would also like to thank Mark Conry and his family for their commitment to improving the JAECO MAS throughout the years, and by so doing, improving the lives of many individuals.

REFERENCES

1. American Occupational Therapy Association: Occupational therapy practice framework: domain and process, ed 4, *Am J Occup Ther.* 74(Supplement_2):7412410010, 2020. https://doi.org/10.5014/ajot.2020.74S2001.
2. Amirabdollahian F, Loureiro R, Gradwell E, Collin C, Harwin W, Johnson G: Multivariate analysis of the Fugl-Meyer outcome measures assessing the effectiveness of GENTLE/S robot-mediated stroke therapy, *Journal of NeuroEngineering and Rehabilitation* 4(1):4, 2007.
3. Atkins M: Spinal cord injury. In Trombly C, Vining Radomsky M, editors: *Occupational Therapy for Physical Dysfunction* ed 7, Philadelphia, 2014, Lippincott Williams & Wilkins.
4. Atkins MS, Baumgarten JM, Yasuda YL, et al: Mobile arm supports: evidence-based benefits and criteria for use, *J Spinal Cord Med* 31:388–393, 2008.
5. Basteris A, Nijenhuis SM, Stienen AH, et al: Training modalities in robot-mediated upper limb rehabilitation in stroke: a framework for classification based on a systematic review, *Journal of Neuroengineering and Rehabilitation* 11(1):111, 2014.

6. Baumgarten JM: Upper extremity adaptations for the person with quadriplegia. In Adkins H, editor: *Spinal Cord Injury Clinics in Physical Therapy*, New York, 1985, Churchill Livingston.

7. Bender L, McKenna K: Hemiplegic shoulder pain: defining the problem and its management, *Disability and Rehabilitation* 23(16):698–705, 2001. https://doi.org/10.1080/09638280110062149.

8. Blank AA, French JA, Pehlivan AU, O'Malley MK: Current trends in robot-assisted upper-limb stroke rehabilitation: promoting patient engagement in therapy, *Current Physical Medicine and Rehabilitation Reports* 2(3):184–195, 2014.

9. Celletti C, Suppa A, Bianchini E, Lakin S, Toscano M, La Torre G, Camerota F: Promoting post-stroke recovery through focal or whole-body vibration: criticisms and prospects from a narrative review, *Neurological Sciences* 41(1):11–24, 2020.

10. Cheng HJ, Lin TA, Lee MT, et al: Effects of robot-assisted bilateral arm training on UE motor functions in clients with stroke: A literature review, *Journal of Taiwan Occupational Therapy Research and Practice* 10(2):115–126, 2014.

11. Chu CY, Patterson RM: Soft robotic devices for hand rehabilitation and assistance: a narrative review, *Journal of Neuroengineering and Rehabilitation* 15(1):9, 2018.

12. Cruz A, Callaway L, Randall M, Ryan M: Mobile arm supports in Duchenne muscular dystrophy: a pilot study of user experience and outcomes, *Disability and Rehabilitation: Assistive Technology* 16(8):880–889, 2021.

13. Dobkin BH: Motor rehabilitation after stroke, traumatic brain, and spinal cord injury: common denominators within recent clinical trials, *Curr Opin Neurol* 22(6):563–569, 2009. https://doi.org/10.1097/WCO.0b013e3283314b11.

14. Garber S, Gregorio T: Upper extremity assistive devices: Assessment of use by spinal cord-injured patients with quadriplegia, *Am J Occup Ther* 44:126–131, 1990.

15. Haumont T, Rahman T, Sample W, King MM, Church C, Henley J, Jayakumar S: Wilmington robotic exoskeleton: a novel device to maintain arm improvement in muscular disease, *Journal of Pediatric Orthopaedics* 31(5):e44–e49, 2011.

16. Haworth R, Dunscombe S, Nichols PJR: Mobile arm supports: an evaluation, *Rheumatol Rehabil* 17:240, 1978.

17. Huang Y, Lai WP, Qian Q, Hu X, Tam EW, Zheng Y: Translation of robot-assisted rehabilitation to clinical service in upper limb rehabilitation. In *Intelligent Biomechatronics in Neurorehabilitation*, 2020, Academic Press, pp 225–238.

18. Huang Y, Lai WP, Qian Q, Hu X, Tam EW, Zheng Y: Translation of robot-assisted rehabilitation to clinical service: a comparison of the rehabilitation effectiveness of EMG-driven robot hand assisted upper limb training in practical clinical service and in clinical trial with laboratory configuration for chronic stroke, *Biomedical Engineering Online* 17(1):91, 2018.

19. Ivy CC, Smith SM, Materi MM: Upper extremity orthoses use in amyotrophic lateral sclerosis/motor neuron disease: three case reports, *Hand* 9(4):543–550, 2014.

20. JAECO Orthopedic, Inc. *Set-up instructions for MultiLink Mobile Arm Support*, Hot Springs, Ark, 2008, JAECO.

21. Kahn LE, Zygman ML, Rymer WZ, Reinkensmeyer DJ: Robot-assisted reaching exercise promotes arm movement recovery in chronic hemiparetic stroke: a randomized controlled pilot study, *Journal of Neuroengineering and Rehabilitation* 3(1):12, 2006.

22. Krebs H, Ladenheim B, Hippolyte C, et al: Robot-assisted task-specific training in cerebral palsy, *Developmental Medicine & Child Neurology* 51(suppl. 4):140–145, 2009. https://doi.org/10.1111/j.1469-8749.2009.03416.x.

23. Long C: Upper limb bracing. In Licht S, editor: Orthotics etcetera, Baltimore, MD, 1966, Waverly Press.

24. Marchal-Crespo L, Reinkensmeyer D: Review of control strategies for robotic movement training after neurologic injury, *Journal of NeuroEngineering and Rehabilitation* 6:20, 2009. https://doi.org/10.1186/1743-0003-6-20.

25. Masiero S, Armani M, Rosati G: Upper-limb robot-assisted therapy in rehabilitation of acute stroke clients: Focused review and results of new randomized controlled trial, *Journal of Rehabilitation Research & Development* 48:355–366, 2011. https://www.rehab.research.va.gov/jour/11/484/masiero484.html.

26. McConnell AC, Moioli RC, Brasil FL, et al: Robotic devices and brain–machine interfaces for hand rehabilitation post-stroke, *J Rehabil Med* 49:449–460, 2017.

27. Munih M, Bajd T: Rehabilitation robotics, *Technology & Health Care* 19(6):483–495, 2011.

28. Norouzi-Gheidari N, Archambault PS, Fung J: Effects of robot-assisted therapy on stroke rehabilitation in upper limbs: Systematic review and meta-analysis of the literature, *Journal of Rehabilitation Research and Development* 49:479–496, 2012.

29. Rahman T, Sample W, Jayakumar S, et al: Passive exoskeletons for assisting limb movement, *Journal of Rehabilitation Research and Development* 43:583–590, 2006.

30. Simkins M, Kim H, Abrams G, Byl N, Rosen J: Robotic unilateral and bilateral upper-limb movement training for stroke survivors afflicted by chronic hemiparesis. In *2013 IEEE 13th International Conference on Rehabilitation Robotics (ICORR)*, 2013, June, IEEE, pp 1–6.

31. Tomić TJD, Savić AM, Vidaković AS, Rodić SZ, Isaković MS, Rodríguez-de-Pablo C, Konstantinović LM: ArmAssist robotic system versus matched conventional therapy for poststroke upper limb rehabilitation: a randomized clinical trial, *BioMed Research Int* 2017:7659893, 2017.

32. van der Heide LA, Gelderblom GJ, de Witte LP: An overview and categorization of dynamic arm supports for people with decreased arm function, *Prosthetics and Orthotics Int* 38:287–302, 2014.

33. Wilson DJ, McKenzie MW, Barber LM: *Spinal Cord Injury: a Treatment Guide for Occupational Therapists, rev ed*, Thorofare, NJ, 1984, Slack.

34. Yasuda YL, Bowman K, Hsu JD: Mobile arm supports: criteria for successful use in muscle disease clients, *Arch Phys Med Rehabil* 67:253, 1986.

35. Yue Z, Zhang X, Wang J: Hand rehabilitation robotics on poststroke motor recovery, *Behavioural Neurology* 2017:3908135, 2017. https://doi.org/10.1155/2017/3908135.

36. Zhang K, Chen X, Liu F, Tang H, Wang J, Wen W: System framework of robotics in upper limb rehabilitation on poststroke motor recovery, *Behavioural Neurology*, 6737056, 2018.

37. Zondervan DK, Friedman N, Chang E, Zhao X, Augsburger R, Reinkensmeyer DJ, Cramer SC: Home-based hand rehabilitation after chronic stroke: Randomized, controlled single-blind trial comparing the MusicGlove with a conventional exercise program, *Journal of Rehabilitation Research and Development* 53(4):457–472, 2016.

Traditional Sensorimotor Approaches to Intervention[a]

Winifred Schultz-Krohn and Luis de Leon Arabit

LEARNING OBJECTIVES

After studying this chapter, the student or practitioner will be able to do the following:

1. Describe the four general processes of information flow related to control of movement.
2. Define motivational urge, and name the locus of this function in the brain.
3. Trace the flow of information in the central and peripheral nervous systems that leads to purposeful movement.
4. Define the sensorimotor system, its locus in the brain, and its function during motor performance.
5. List the structures that constitute the higher, middle, and lower levels of the central nervous system components for movement.
6. Name the four traditional sensorimotor approaches to intervention and the theorist(s) responsible for each.
7. Name the two models of motor control that form the basis for the sensorimotor approaches to treatment.
8. Briefly describe each of the four traditional sensorimotor approaches to intervention; compare and contrast their similarities and their differences.
9. Understand and apply proprioceptive neuromuscular facilitation (PNF) as a preparatory method to facilitate client participation in desired occupations.
10. Define PNF and how this approach facilitates adaptive responses that are performed in daily occupations.
11. Understand the principles of PNF and how to apply them to enhance client performance.
12. Describe the influence of sensory input on motor learning.
13. Use the PNF evaluation to determine factors limiting clients' participation in their occupation.
14. Recognize upper and lower extremity diagonal patterns in daily performance skills.
15. Name the theorists who developed the PNF approach.
16. Discuss the historical background and current use of Neuro-Developmental Treatment (NDT) within occupational therapy.
17. Identify theoretical foundations of NDT and current principles of evaluation and intervention.
18. Identify management strategies associated with NDT intervention and treatment techniques.
19. Integrate NDT within an occupation-centered and client-centered approach to evaluation and intervention.
20. Discuss the relationship between evidence-based practice and NDT, and discuss the types of evidence available to support the use of NDT in occupational therapy.

CHAPTER OUTLINE

[a] The authors wish to gratefully acknowledge the contributions from Julie McLaughlin Gray, Judy M. Jourdan, and Sara A. Pope-Davis.

KEY TERMS

Approximation	Maximal resistance	Sensory stimulation
Asymmetric patterns	Motivational urge	Slow reversal
Bilateral patterns	Motor program	Slow reversal-hold-relax
Co-contraction	Movement strategy	Stabilizing reversals
Combined movements	Part-task practice	Stepwise procedures
Conation	Proprioceptive neuromuscular	Stretch
Contract-relax	facilitation	Symmetric patterns
Diagonal patterns	Reciprocal inhibition	Therapeutic handling
Generalizability	Reciprocal patterns	Traction
Handling techniques	Reflex and hierarchical models	Unilateral patterns
Hold-relax	Repeated contractions	Upper motor neuron
Inhibitory techniques	Rhythmic initiation	Verbal commands
Lower motor neurons	Rhythmic rotation	Verbal mediation
Manual contacts	Rhythmic stabilization	Whole-task practice
Mass movement patterns	Sensorimotor system	

OVERVIEW

Winifred Schultz-Krohn

CASE STUDY

Carlos

Carlos, a 59-year-old construction supervisor, who identifies as male (prefers use of the pronouns of he/him/his), sustained a right cerebrovascular accident 3 days earlier and currently requires maximum assistance for most self-care tasks. He is able to speak and recognizes his wife and two adult children, but he appears easily confused when expected to participate in self-care activities. He has no functional motor control of his left arm or hand, and sensation is markedly impaired on his left extremities. He exhibits a decorticate posture in both left extremities, with flexion tone dominating his arm and extensor tone dominating his leg. He is able to partially roll to the right side of the hospital bed and push up on his right arm to a sitting position, but at home he sleeps on the opposite side of the bed. He is able to stand by using a quad cane in his right hand but is unable to safely walk from the bed to the bathroom in his hospital room.

As Carlos' occupational therapist (OT), you are expected to design and implement an intervention plan based on the best evidence available. Occupational therapists working with clients who have sustained damage to the central nervous system are often concerned with enhancing functional movement as a means of promoting independence in occupational performance.[23] To achieve this objective, a variety of intervention approaches are available from which the therapist may choose. This chapter reviews the traditional sensorimotor approaches and presents a brief description of each.

Critical Thinking Questions

1. How can a traditional intervention approach improve Carlos' occupational performance?
2. What potential difficulties should be anticipated when using a traditional intervention approach?
3. What current knowledge of central nervous system function could be used to support the selection and implementation of traditional sensorimotor intervention methods?

Occupation performance frequently requires precise voluntary movement that is controlled and monitored by both the central and peripheral nervous systems. Various structures within the nervous system are coordinated to activate specific muscles to initiate, perform, and complete a desired task or activity. If a movement is poorly performed and thereby compromises task performance, feedback occurs through knowledge of the results of the action, and the neurologic commands to the muscles are modified so that accuracy of movement is achieved. Knowledge of the intricate working of the nervous system is of special importance to the occupational therapist (OT) concerned with refinement and improvement of the motor performance of clients with neurologic conditions.[3] A brief overview of the flow of information associated with the control of movement is described in the following sections.

CENTRAL NERVOUS SYSTEM CONTROL OF MOVEMENT

The firing of motor neurons located in the anterior horn of the spinal cord innervates muscular tissue to produce movements.[89] The activity of the spinal or lower motor neurons can be modulated by segmental spinal circuitry and by the descending influence of the upper motor neurons (UMNs) located in the motor cortex and brainstem.[60,61] Two other structures, the basal ganglia and the cerebellum, and their associated pathways, are also intimately involved with motor control. Lesions in these structures are associated with characteristic movement disorders.

Movement production does not begin and end with the upper motor neurons or lower motor neurons. Many central nervous system (CNS) structures contribute to the development of the signals that activate muscles. Although much about the control of movement is still unknown, animal and human research suggests that four general processes are related to the flow of information needed to control movement. The four general processes of information flow are motivation, ideation, programming, and execution.[19,25] A schematic diagram that indicates the main direction of information flow to produce goal-directed movement and the connection among various motor centers appears in Fig. 32.1.

The motivation or emotive component of the movement is a function of the limbic system.[19,83] The motivational urge or impulse to act associated with the limbic system is transformed to ideas by the cortical association areas. This connection of knowledge and affective behavior is also referred to as conation.[46] Conation represents the intentional, deliberate, and goal-directed aspect of behavior and is related to the individual's reason for the motor performance. The association areas of the frontal, parietal, temporal, and occipital lobes are concerned with ideation, or the goal of the movement, and the programming or movement strategy (plan) that best achieves the goal. Programming of a movement strategy also involves the premotor areas, the basal ganglia, and the cerebellum. The motor program is the procedure or the spatiotemporal order of muscle activation that is needed for smooth and accurate motor performance. The execution level, represented by the motor cortex, the cerebellum, and the spinal cord, is concerned with the activation of the spinal motor neurons and interneurons that generate the goal-directed movement and the necessary postural adjustments.

To appreciate the flow of information leading to purposeful movement, consider the actions of your client Carlos, who sustained a right cerebrovascular accident (CVA) with resultant left hemiplegia, is thirsty, and is reaching out for a glass of water

while seated at a table for support (Fig. 32.2). The limbic system, which connects with the areas of the midbrain and brainstem that control vital functions such as hunger and thirst, has registered the need for water.[44] This need for drinking water has been conveyed to the cortical association areas, which also received visual, auditory, somatosensory, and proprioceptive information about precisely where the body is in space and where the glass of water is relative to the body.[48] This sensory information is needed before the movement is initiated. Strategies or motor plans are formulated to move the arm and hand from their immediate location in space to one in which the glass of water is picked up and moved to the mouth. Motor programs are generated by the association cortex in conjunction with the basal ganglia, lateral cerebellum, and premotor cortex. Once a strategy is selected, the motor cortex is activated. The motor cortex, in turn, conveys the action plan to the brainstem and spinal cord. Activation of the cervical spinal neurons generates a coordinated and precise movement of the shoulder, elbow, wrist, and fingers. Input from the brainstem and cerebellum ensures that the axial musculature makes the necessary postural adjustments. Sensory information during the movement is necessary to ensure smooth performance throughout reaching for the glass and bringing the glass to the mouth, including the acceleration and deceleration of movement, direction, and force. This sensory information is used to improve subsequent similar movements. Because the motor areas rely heavily on sensory feedback provided by exteroceptors and proprioceptors regarding the accuracy of movement, the structures of the brain that control movement are often referred to as the sensorimotor system. Carlos is able to use his right hand to pick up the glass of water but has compromised postural control. When he is supported, sitting at the table, he is able to complete this task, but when standing and holding his cane in his right hand he is unable to use his left arm and hand to reach and pick up the glass of water. The resultant motor problems from the right CVA further compromise his ability to perform a bimanual task such as pouring liquid into a glass even when he has the necessary motivational urge or intention for movement.

Given the motivation-ideation-programming-execution scheme of how information is organized through the nervous system, it is obvious that control of voluntary movement involves almost all of the neocortex. Voluntary movement depends on knowledge of where the body is in space, where the body intends to go with respect to this external space, the internal and external loads that must be overcome, and formulation of a strategy or plan to perform the movement. Once a strategy or plan has been formulated, it must be held in memory until execution, at which point appropriate instructions are sent to the spinal motor neurons. The primary functional aspects of the sensorimotor areas involved in motor control are examined next.[19,53,83]

Sensorimotor Cortex

The sensorimotor cortex is the major integrating center of sensory input and motor output. It is composed of cortical areas located immediately anterior and posterior to the central sulcus (Fig. 32.3). The three principal motor regions located in the frontal lobe are the primary motor area, the supplementary motor area, and the premotor area. The two principal sensory regions located in the parietal lobe are the primary somatosensory cortex and the posterior parietal cortex. Each area of the sensorimotor cortex (primary motor cortex, primary somatosensory cortex, posterior parietal cortex, supplementary motor area, and premotor cortex) is arranged in a manner that provides a topographical representation of the contralateral body segments.[53,76] Each of these areas is responsible for certain aspects of movement generation. In the previous example of reaching out for the glass of water, Carlos had a mental image of his body and its relation to the surrounding

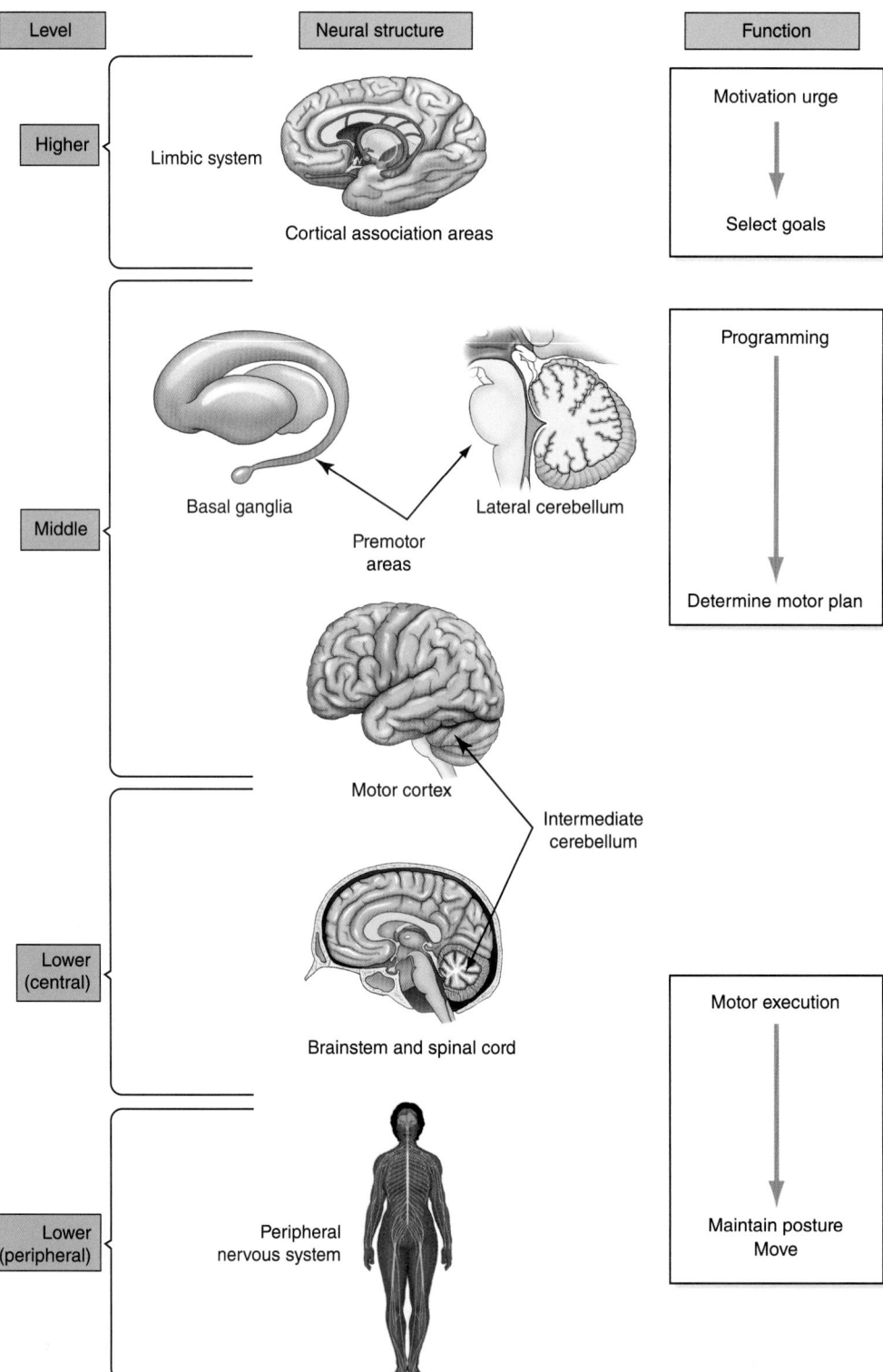

Fig. 32.1 Schematic representation of the hierarchy of the neural structures involved in motor control. The *left column* indicates the hierarchical level and the *right column* the major function of the neural structures shown in the center column during motor performance. (Based on work from Cheney PD: Role of cerebral cortex in voluntary movements: A review, *Phys Ther* 65:624, 1985.)

space by integrating the information supplied through somatosensory, proprioceptive, and visual inputs to the posterior parietal cortex. Clients with a lesion in this area demonstrate impairment of body image and its relation to extrapersonal space, and, in the extreme situation, neglect of the contralateral body segments.

The posterior parietal cortex integrates and translates sensory information so that the ensuing movements are directed appropriately in extrapersonal space. It is extensively interconnected with the association areas of the frontal lobe that are considered to be involved in determining the consequences of movement strategies such as moving the arm forward, curling the fingers around the glass, and lifting the glass to the mouth. The fingers begin to curl appropriately before any contact occurs with the glass; therefore, the size and shape of the glass must

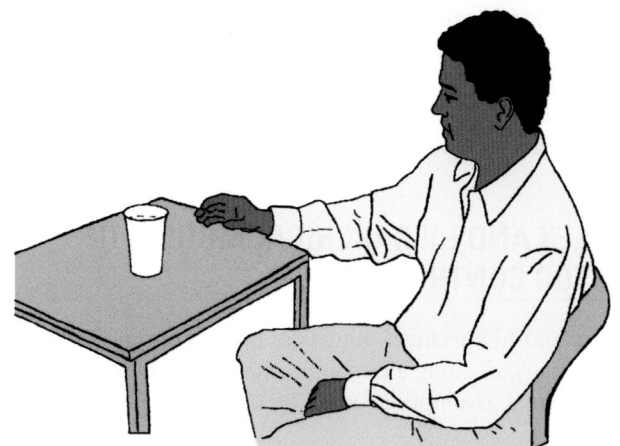

Fig. 32.2 A person reaching for a glass of water.

be recognized before grasping. The prefrontal association areas and the posterior parietal cortex project to the premotor area, which is thought to be concerned with the orientation of body segments before the initiation of movement. The input of the posterior parietal cortex to the premotor area may be important in the somatosensory guidance of movement.[25] Lesions of the premotor area or posterior parietal cortex have been demonstrated to generate an inappropriate movement strategy.[50]

Planning of movement is considered to be the function of the supplementary motor area. In animal studies, the electrophysiological recordings of cells in this area indicate that the cells typically increase discharge rates about a second before the observable execution of movement of either hand.[94] The same findings have been corroborated in humans with the use of imaging techniques to study patterns of cortical activation. Imaging studies using positron emission tomography (PET) monitor changes in local blood flow, because an increase in the local cerebral blood flow is associated with increased neuronal activity. Under these conditions, when subjects were asked to imagine a movement without actually moving the finger, the blood flow to the supplementary motor cortex increased and no comparable increase in blood flow was seen in the primary motor area.[79] When subjects were asked to perform a series of finger movements from memory, blood flow to the supplementary motor cortex increased in advance of the movement but not during the performance of the movement. Unilateral lesions of the supplementary motor area result in apraxia (the loss of the ability to perform movement in the absence of motor or sensory impairments). Another effect of such lesions is the inability to produce the correct sequence of muscle activation for complex

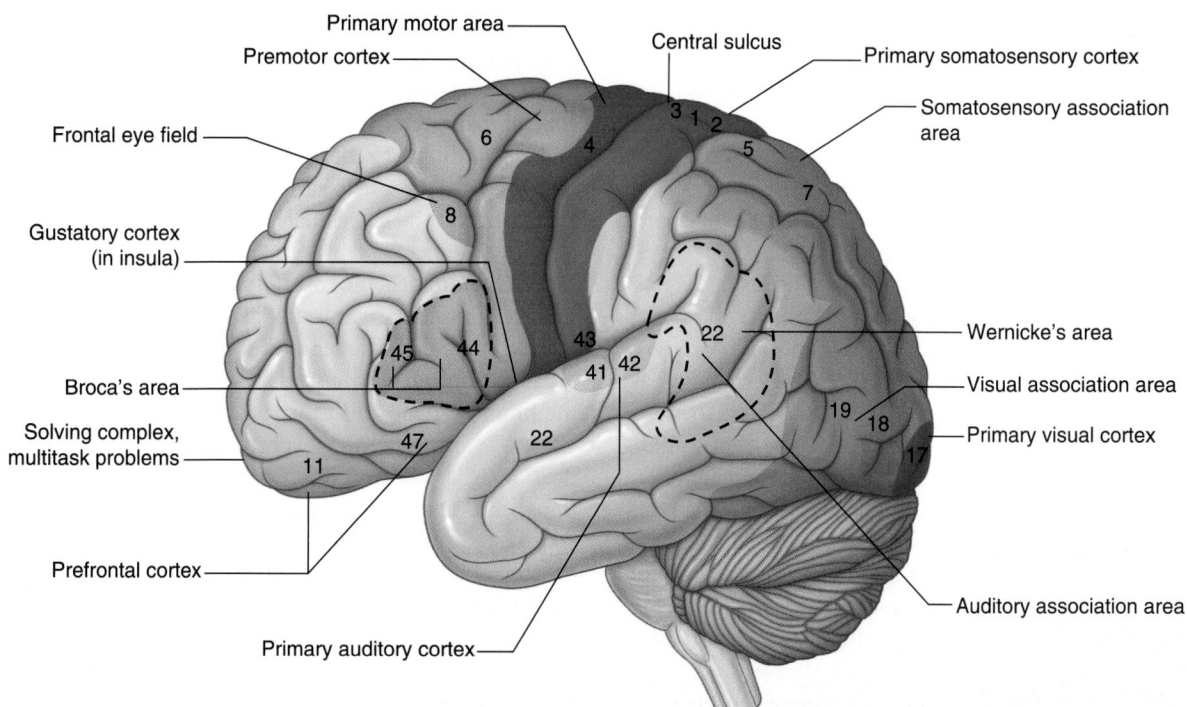

Fig. 32.3 Areas of the neocortex intimately involved in planning of and instruction for voluntary movement. Areas 4 and 6 constitute the motor cortex. (*Red:* motor cortex; *blue:* sensory cortex; *pale blue and pale red:* association cortex.) (From Naish J, Syndercombe D, editors: *Medical Sciences*, ed 2, Edinburgh, 2015, Saunders.)

motor activities such as speaking, writing, buttoning, typing, sewing, and playing the piano.

The primary somatosensory cortex projection to the primary motor cortex and association areas provides the sensory input needed for motor planning, movement initiation, and regulation of ongoing movement.[38] The primary motor cortex integrates the information it receives from other areas of the brain and generates the descending command for the execution of movement. Not only is this descending command sent to the brainstem and spinal cord, but a copy of it is also sent to the basal ganglia and cerebellum. The descending command specifies the muscles to be activated and the direction, speed, and required force.[25] Lesions of the primary somatosensory cortex typically result in contralateral sensory loss. Movements are uncoordinated because the ability to register sensory feedback during and after the movement is compromised. Damage to the primary motor area results in motor execution deficits. The client presents the classic picture of contralateral muscle weakness, spasticity, and poor isolation of movement with corresponding loss of function.

RELATION TO SENSORIMOTOR INTERVENTION APPROACHES

The CNS structures involved with movement can be grouped functionally into higher, middle, and lower levels. The higher level consists of the limbic system and association areas, where the motivation for action is generated. The sensorimotor areas, along with the basal ganglia and cerebellum, form the middle level, and the lower level consists of the nuclei in the brainstem and spinal cord. Under normal circumstances, an individual's repertoire of motor activity is varied and complex, meeting the unique task and environmental demands. After damage to the CNS regions involved with movement, the coordinated efforts between the various levels of motor control are disrupted, and the motor response may be limited or stereotyped. Traditional sensorimotor approaches, specifically Rood, Brunnstrom, Proprioceptive Neuromuscular Facilitation, and Bobath, can be viewed as targeting the middle sensorimotor level, the motor planning–strategy formulation process, and the lower level–execution process, with the aim of reintegrating, as far as possible, a complete motor control hierarchy. A motor relearning program (discussed in Chapter 33) also should be cognitively oriented and targeted toward achieving a goal or "occupational" task and include all three levels of CNS function related to motor control. This represents the inherent limitation of the traditional sensorimotor approaches that do not actively engage the client's volitional intent or motivation to perform a motor act. The limitations of traditional sensorimotor approaches must be carefully considered before selecting this form of intervention for the client. The OT practitioner must include activities to foster the generalizability of movement patterns to functional and meaningful tasks for clients.

The foundational premise of these traditional sensorimotor approaches posits that clients need to be taught motor strategies or compensatory mechanisms to adapt to the deficits produced by a lesion. Compensatory mechanisms and the shaping of

motor programs are brought about by the use of sensory inputs. The sensorimotor approaches use sensory stimulation to elicit specific movement patterns. Early in the intervention phase, the emphasis is on the use of external sensory stimuli. Once a movement response is obtained, to reinforce and strengthen the response, the focus shifts to the use of intrinsic sensory information, which thereby encourages voluntary motor control.

Two traditional sensorimotor intervention approaches, proprioceptive neuromuscular facilitation (PNF) and the Bobath or Neuro-Developmental Treatment approach, were historically used by occupational therapists (OTs). These approaches, developed in the 1950s and 1960s, have their theoretical basis in the reflex and hierarchical models of motor control. The Rood and Brunnstrom approaches are briefly presented with a discussion of current views of these approaches. Although more contemporary models are typically used to guide intervention with clients who demonstrate CNS dysfunction, an understanding of these traditional approaches is warranted to appreciate their contributions to clinical practice and to recognize the appropriate application of these approaches in selected populations.

REFLEX AND HIERARCHICAL MODELS OF MOTOR CONTROL

Reflex and hierarchical models of motor control view movement strategies along a developmental continuum. Two major fundamental assumptions underlie the reflex and hierarchical models.

The basic units of motor control are reflexes. Reflexes are motor responses that occur in response to specific sensory stimuli. Reflexes are automatic, predictable, and stereotypical; they are normal responses seen from early infancy. As the CNS matures, a greater variety of movement patterns emerge but many view reflexes as the foundation for volitional motor control. Volitional (purposeful) movement is the summation and integration of reflexive movement. When damage to the CNS occurs, the great variety of possible movement options decreases and the individual is often limited to the use of reflexive movements.

In a hierarchical model of motor control, the CNS is thought to have a specific organizational structure and motor development and function depend on that structure. This hierarchical organization refers to a system in which the higher centers of the brain regulate and exert control over lower centers of the CNS. The higher centers, specifically the cortical and subcortical areas, are responsible for regulation and control of volitional, conscious movement. The lower levels regulate and control reflexive, automatic, and responsive movement. Based on this conceptualization, when damage occurs to the CNS, the damaged area can no longer regulate and exert control over the underlying areas. Motor control, according to this belief, becomes a function of the next lower functioning level of the CNS. Typically this means a return to more reflexive and primitive movement patterns.

These traditional sensorimotor intervention strategies rely heavily on these basic assumptions about motor development

TABLE 32.1 **Comparison of Key Treatment Strategies Used in the Traditional Sensorimotor Approaches**

Key Treatment Strategies	Rood Approach	Brunnstrom Approach (Movement Therapy)	Proprioceptive Neuromuscular Approach	Neuro-Developmental Treatment
Sensory stimulation used to evoke a motor response	YES (uses direct application of sensory stimuli to muscles and joints)	YES (movement occurs in response to sensory stimuli)	YES (tactile, auditory, and visual sensory stimuli promote motor responses)	YES (abnormal muscle tone occurs, in part because of abnormal sensory experiences)
Reflexive movement used as a precursor for volitional movement	YES (reflexive movement achieved initially through the application of sensory stimuli)	YES (move the patient along a continuum of reflexive to volitional movement patterns)	YES (volitional movements can be assisted by reflexive supported postures)	NO
Treatment directed toward influencing muscle tone	YES (sensory stimuli used to inhibit or facilitate tone)	YES (postures, sensory stimuli used to inhibit or facilitate tone)	YES (movement patterns used to normalize tone)	YES (handling techniques and postures can inhibit or facilitate muscle tone)
Developmental patterns/ sequences used for the development of motor skills	YES (ontogenic motor patterns used to develop motor skills)	YES (flexion and extension synergies; proximal to distal return)	YES (patterns used to facilitate proximal to distal motor control)	YES
Conscious attention is directed toward movement	NO	YES	YES	YES
Treatment directly emphasizes the development of skilled movements for task performance	NO	NO	NO	YES

and motor control. Consequently, intervention strategies used in these approaches frequently involve the application of sensory stimulation to muscles and joints to evoke specific motor responses, handling and positioning techniques to effect changes in muscle tone, and the use of developmental postures to enhance the ability to initiate and carry out movements. Table 32.1 presents a comparison and summary of key treatment strategies used in each of the four traditional sensorimotor approaches.

SECTION 1: TRADITIONAL SENSORIMOTOR INTERVENTION APPROACHES

Winifred Schultz-Krohn

ROOD APPROACH

Margaret Rood drew heavily from both the reflex and the hierarchical models in designing her intervention approach.[80-82] Key components of the Rood approach are the use of sensory input to evoke a motor response and the use of developmental postures to promote changes in muscle tone. Sensory stimulation is applied to muscles and joints to elicit a specific motor response. This sensory input has the potential to have either an inhibitory or a facilitatory effect on muscle tone. Rood described various types of sensory input, including the use of slow rolling,

neutral warmth, deep pressure, tapping, and prolonged stretch. Examples of how this sensory input may be applied include tapping over a muscle belly to facilitate (increase) muscle tone and applying deep pressure to a muscle's tendinous insertion to elicit an inhibitory (decreased) effect. Rood also advocated the use of specific developmental sequences to promote motor responses.[80] Although the use of developmental postures does not promote increased function, several interventions methods developed by Rood have continued to be used to improve motor function.[18] Specific Rood techniques, such as cryotherapy and slow stretch to decrease spasticity, have been successfully used but the explanatory mechanism is focused on the muscular tissue, not a reflexive model. Slow stretch was provided for 27 individuals, several months after a stroke (3–18 months), using an externally actuated glove to provide the slow passive stretch.[95] The slow stretch resulted in immediate changes in spasticity and improved function as measured by the Graded Wolf Motor Function Test and the Box and Block Test. Sustained benefit was noted for individuals whose status was considered subacute (3–6 months after stroke) compared to chronic (over 7 months after stroke). Essentially, many of the sensory techniques described by Rood continue to be used with a more contemporary explanation of how the technique supports motor function. Rood contended that reduction of spasticity was an important part of intervention and could be promoted through the use of sensory input. A randomized controlled trial with 36 individuals, a minimum of 4 months after stroke, found that the use of vibration applied to spastic hand and arm flexor muscles produced greater reduction in spasticity compared to rest and sustained stretch.[72] Spasticity was measured by electromyography F-waves amplitude and the Modified Ashford Scale.

In current clinical practice, practitioners may use selected principles from Rood's work as adjunctive or preliminary interventions to prepare an individual to engage in a purposeful activity—for example, the application of quick stretch over the triceps before instructing a client to reach for a cup or glass to improve elbow extension.[92] A client may be instructed in ways to apply his or her own sensory stimulation to enhance activities of daily living (ADLs) performance. For example, during upper extremity dressing, the occupational therapist may ask Carlos to perform a prolonged stretch to the left biceps, which reduces muscle tone, which may in turn increase the ease with which the arm is moved through the sleeve of his shirt.

Limitations in the use of Rood's approach are numerous and include the passive nature of the sensory stimulation (it is applied *to* an individual) and the short-lasting and unpredictable effect of some of the sensory stimulation.

BRUNNSTROM (MOVEMENT THERAPY) APPROACH

Signe Brunnstrom, a physical therapist (PT), developed an intervention approach specifically for individuals who had sustained a cerebrovascular accident (CVA).[20,21] The approach she designed draws strongly from both the reflex and hierarchical models of motor control. Brunnstrom conceptualized clients who had sustained a CVA as going through an "evolution in reverse." Spastic or flaccid muscle tone and the presence of reflexive movements that may be evident after a client sustains a CVA are considered part of the normal process of recovery and are viewed as necessary intermediate steps in regaining volitional movement.[86] Brunnstrom clearly detailed stages of motor recovery after a CVA (Table 32.2). These stages include the description of flexor synergy patterns and extensor synergy patterns for the upper and lower limbs and are used as descriptors of change following a CVA.[41] Carlos currently displays flexor tone dominating his left arm and extensor tone dominating his left leg. This dominating tone interferes with isolated control of his left extremities.

In the Brunnstrom approach, emphasis is placed on facilitating the progress of the individual by promotion of movement, from reflexive to volitional. In the early stages of recovery, this may include the incorporation of reflexes and associated reactions to change tone and achieve movement. For example, to generate reflexive movement in the arm, resistance may be applied to one side of the body to increase muscle tone on the opposite side. This technique is applied until the client demonstrates volitional control over the movement pattern. A randomized control trial compared the outcomes of Brunnstrom's Hand Manipulation (BHM) intervention to the motor relearning program (MRP) developed by Carr & Shepherd.[75] All 30 clients

TABLE 32.2 Brunnstrom Recovery Stage of Hand Function

Stage	Arm Function[71]	Hand Function[75]
1	Flaccidity is present and no movements of the limbs can be initiated.	Flaccidity.
2	The basic limb synergies or some of their components may appear as associated reactions or minimal voluntary movement responses may be present. Spasticity begins to develop.	Little or no active finger flexion.
3	The patient gains voluntary control of the movement synergies, although full range of all synergy components does not necessarily develop. Spasticity is severe.	Mass grasp; use of hook grasp but no release; no voluntary finger extension; possible reflex extension of digits.
4	Some movement combinations that do not follow the synergies are mastered, and spasticity begins to decline.	Lateral prehension, release by thumb movement; semi-voluntary finger extension of digits, variable range.
5	More difficult movement combinations are possible as the basic limb synergies lose their dominance over motor acts."	Palmar prehension; possibly cylindrical and spherical grasp, awkwardly performed and with a limited functional use; voluntary mass extension of the digits, variable range.
6	"Spasticity disappears and individual joint movements become possible."	All prehensile types under control; skills improving; full range voluntary extension of the digits; individual finger movements present, less accurate than on the opposite side.

Naghdi S, Ansari NN, Mansouri K, et al: A neurophysiological and clinical study of Brunnstrom recovery stages in the upper limb following stroke, *Brain Inj* 24:1372–1378, 2010; and Pandian S, Arya KN, Davidson EW: Comparison of Brunnstrom movement therapy and motor relearning program in rehabilitation of post-stroke hemiparetic hand: a randomized trial, *J Bodywork Movement Ther* 16:330–337, 2012.

had sustained a stroke, and hand function was at Brunnstrom Stage 3 with mass grasp but no voluntary release or finger extension. Both groups were evaluated by an independent examiner using the Fugl-Meyer Assessment (FMA), range-of-motion (ROM) measurements, and the Brunnstrom Hand Function grading mechanism. Each group received 12 intervention sessions, 1 hour each in length. Clients in both treatment groups improved but those who received the BHM intervention had significantly better performance on the FMA compared to the group who received MRP. Authors concluded that the BHM intervention was a more effective intervention to recover hand function compared to MRP.

PROPRIOCEPTIVE NEUROMUSCULAR FACILITATION APPROACH

The proprioceptive neuromuscular facilitation (PNF) approach is grounded in the reflex and hierarchical models of motor control. Developed through the collaborative efforts of a physician, Dr. Herman Kabat, and two PTs, Margaret Knott and Dorothy Voss, in the 1950s, this intervention approach continues to be used but has not been revised since its origins. Major emphasis in this approach is on the developmental sequencing of movement and the balanced interplay between agonist and antagonist in producing volitional movement.[101] PNF describes mass movement patterns, which are diagonal, for the limbs and trunk. Intervention strategies use these patterns to promote movement. The use of sensory stimulation, including tactile, auditory, and visual inputs, is also actively incorporated into treatment to promote a motor response.

In OT clinical practice the inclusion of PNF patterns often can be seen in the way functional activities are designed, especially in the placement of objects during purposeful activities. For example, a client is asked to reach into a shopping bag placed on his left side to retrieve objects that will then be placed into a cabinet on the right side. Specific information regarding the application of PNF is discussed later in Section 2. This approach has been successfully used to increase range of motion and to stretch tightened muscles.[88] The application of PNF also has been demonstrated to reduce falls in older adults.[90]

NEURO-DEVELOPMENTAL TREATMENT APPROACH

Neuro-Developmental Treatment (NDT), also known as the Bobath treatment approach, is based on normal development and movement. The treatment approach was developed by the Bobaths to guide therapists in managing and treating persons diagnosed with stroke and cerebral palsy. Berta Bobath, a gymnast who later became a PT, and her husband, Karel Bobath, a physician, provided the initial theoretical foundations of NDT in the 1950s.[45] At that time they drew from the hierarchical model of motor control. The primary objectives of Neuro-Developmental Treatment are to normalize muscle tone, inhibit primitive reflexes, and facilitate normal postural reactions.[14] Improving the quality of movement and helping clients relearn normal movement patterns are key objectives of this approach. To achieve these objectives, therapists employ numerous techniques, including handling techniques, use of inhibitory techniques to diminish the negative impact of spasticity on normal movement, weight bearing over the more affected limb, the use of positions that encourage the use of both sides of the body, and the avoidance of any sensory input that may adversely affect muscle tone.[30] In clinical practice today, many of these techniques and strategies are used within the context of purposeful activities and occupations that are meaningful to the client.

NDT continues to revise its theoretical framework in response to new evidence on the function of the CNS.[45] Discussions on the rationale for NDT include the current understanding of motor systems and motor learning, as well as the introduction of the NDT Practice Model and its application to occupational therapy practice. See Section 3 for further descriptions.

■ SECTION 1 SUMMARY

Movement takes place within an occupational context. Emotional needs influence motor strategies. The spinal cord or brainstem can mediate reflexive responses, but interpretation and transformation of sensory signals by all areas of the sensorimotor system are essential for voluntary movement to occur with precision. The primary somatosensory cortex and posterior parietal cortex are primarily responsible for processing sensory information. The premotor area uses sensory information for the planning of movements, the supplementary motor area is important for bimanual coordination, and the motor cortex is important for execution.

The traditional sensorimotor intervention approaches have their theoretical basis in reflex and hierarchical models of motor control. These approaches offer a valuable link between neurophysiological principles and the rehabilitation treatment of clients with CNS dysfunction. In contemporary practice, many of the techniques described in these approaches are used as adjunctive or preliminary techniques or are incorporated into more task-directed treatment activities.

SECTION 2: PROPRIOCEPTIVE NEUROMUSCULAR FACILITATION APPROACH

Winifred Schultz-Krohn

THREADED CASE STUDY

Leticia, Part 1

Leticia identifies as a woman (prefers use of the pronouns she/her/hers). Leticia, a 34-year-old married mother of two, was involved in an automobile accident in which she sustained a brain injury and fractures of her left wrist and several ribs. Leticia's injuries resulted in diplopia, poor trunk control, and severely limited motor control in all extremities as a result of ataxia. As a mother, Leticia had always been involved with her children and was employed as a teacher's aide at their grade school. It is important to Leticia that she resume her parenting role, including caring for their home, driving a car, and resuming her work in the classroom. Unfortunately, she experiences fatigue quickly and struggles to engage in the routine daily activities she used to enjoy with her family. She specifically expressed her desire to be able to play games with her children, prepare family meals, and tutor children in the third grade class in which she assisted before her accident.

Critical Thinking Questions
1. Which movement patterns would you select to help Leticia regain the ability to perform these family- and work-related occupations or tasks?
2. Which PNF techniques will most effectively address Leticia's impairments, and how do you select a PNF technique to facilitate the desired performance of a task?
3. How do you determine the progression of intervention from a PNF perspective?

Based on normal movement and motor development, PNF is more than a technique; it is a philosophy of intervention. Through the case study of Leticia we will discuss the application of PNF to the evaluation and intervention of occupational therapy. Basic principles, diagonal patterns, and more commonly used techniques will be introduced, and their application and presence in routine daily life skills will be demonstrated. PNF addresses the client factors of posture, mobility, strength, effort, and coordination. To use PNF effectively, it is necessary to understand normal development, learn the motor skills to use the techniques, and apply the concepts and techniques to OT activities.[5] This section should form the basis for further reading and training under the supervision of a therapist experienced in PNF.

PNF is based on normal movement and motor development. In normal motor activity the brain registers total movement and not individual muscle action.[49] Encompassed in the PNF approach are mass movement patterns that are spiral and diagonal and resemble movement seen in functional activities. In this multisensory approach, facilitation techniques are superimposed on movement patterns and postures through the therapist's manual contacts, verbal commands, and visual cues. These facilitation techniques and movement patterns can be preparatory methods that prepare clients to participate more effectively in their daily occupations, or they can be applied within the performance of a task.

PNF is used as an intervention technique for numerous conditions, including Parkinson's disease, spinal cord injuries, arthritis, stroke, head injuries, and hand injuries. It has been effectively combined with neuromobilization techniques to reduce sensory deficits in individuals who sustained a CVA.[104]

HISTORY

PNF originated in the 1940s with Dr. Herman Kabat, a physician and neurophysiologist. He applied neurophysiological principles, based on the work of Sherrington, to the intervention of paralysis secondary to poliomyelitis and multiple sclerosis. In 1948, Kabat and Henry Kaiser founded the Kabat-Kaiser Institute in Vallejo, California. Here Kabat worked with Margaret Knott, a physical therapist (PT) to develop the PNF method of intervention. By 1951, the diagonal patterns and core techniques were established. PNF is now used to treat numerous neurological, musculoskeletal, and general medical conditions.

In 1952, Dorothy Voss, a PT, joined the staff at the Kaiser-Kabat Institute. She and Knott undertook the teaching and supervision of staff therapists. In 1954, Knott and Voss presented the first 2-week course in Vallejo. Two years later, the first edition of *Proprioceptive Neuromuscular Facilitation* by Margaret Knott and Dorothy Voss was published.

During this same period, several reports in the *American Journal of Occupational Therapy* described PNF and its application to OT intervention.[5,24,26,52,98,103] In 1984, PNF was first taught concurrently to both PTs and OT practitioners at the Rehabilitation Institute in Chicago.[70,101] Today courses are offered throughout the United States, as well as Europe, Asia, and South America. Currently, four main theoretical models are used to explain the beneficial effects of PNF to improve motor performance: autogenic inhibition, reciprocal inhibition, stress relaxation, and the gate control theory.[43]

PRINCIPLES OF INTERVENTION

Voss presented 11 principles of PNF developed from concepts in the fields of neurophysiology, motor learning, and motor behavior.[99]

1. All humans have potentials that have not been fully developed. This philosophy is the underlying basis of PNF. Therefore, in evaluation and intervention planning, the client's abilities and potentials are emphasized. For example, the client who has weakness on one side of the body can use the intact side to assist the weaker part. Likewise, the client who has hemiplegia with a flaccid arm can use the intact head, neck, and trunk musculature to begin reinforcement of the weak arm in weight-bearing activities.

2. Normal motor development proceeds in a cervicocaudal and proximodistal direction. This motor developmental progression is followed in evaluation and intervention. When severe disability is present, attention is first given to the head and neck region, with its visual, auditory, and vestibular receptors, and then to the upper trunk and extremities following a cervicocaudal progression.[101] The proximodistal direction is followed by developing adequate function in the head, neck, and trunk before developing function in the extremities. This approach is of particular importance in intervention that facilitates fine motor coordination in the upper extremities. Unless adequate control exists in the head, neck, trunk, and shoulder complex, fine motor skills cannot be developed effectively. For example, Leticia needs to strengthen her head, neck, and trunk muscles to regain adequate postural control before she can adequately perform fine motor tasks required in her job such as cutting with scissors. This illustrates how addressing a specific client factor of postural control can influence occupational performance.

3. Early motor behavior is dominated by reflex activity. Mature motor behavior is supported or reinforced by postural reflexes. As the human being matures, primitive reflexes are integrated and available for reinforcement to allow for progressive development such as that of rolling, crawling, and sitting. For example, Leticia is seated in a car and extends her right arm to reach for the handle to close the car door while turning her head to the right using the motor pattern of the asymmetrical tonic neck reflex for this functional movement.

4. Early motor behavior is characterized by spontaneous movement, which oscillates between extremes of flexion and extension. These movements are rhythmic and reversing in character. In intervention it is important to attend to both directions of movement. When the OT practitioner is working with the client to safely stand up from a chair, attention also must be given to sitting back down. Often with an injury, the eccentric contraction (e.g., sitting down) is lost and becomes very difficult for the client to regain. If the eccentric contraction is not addressed, the

client may be left with inadequate motor control to sit down smoothly and, thus, may "drop" into a chair. This eccentric control would be particularly important for Leticia because she is required to sit in low chairs at her children's school. Similarly, in training for ADLs the client must learn how to get undressed and dressed.

5. Goal-directed behavior is constructed with reversing movements such as Leticia reaching for a glass by extending her elbow and then bringing the glass to her mouth to take a drink by flexing her elbow. In this process of reach, grasp, and moving the object, there is a need to control forearm supination and pronation to avoid spilling the contents of the glass.

6. Developing motor behavior is expressed in an orderly sequence of total patterns of movement and posture. In the normal infant the sequence of total patterns is demonstrated through the progression of locomotion. The infant learns to roll, to crawl, to creep, and finally to stand and walk. Initially the hands are used for reaching and grasping within the most supported postures, such as supine and prone. As postural control develops, the infant begins to use the hands in side-lying, sitting, and standing positions to manipulate objects. In intervention, to maximize motor performance, clients should be given opportunities to work in a variety of developmental postures. The use of extremities in various body positions requires interaction with component patterns of the head, neck, and trunk.

7. The growth of motor behavior has cyclic trends, as evidenced by shifts between flexor and extensor dominance. The shifts between antagonists help to develop muscle balance and control. One of the main goals of the PNF intervention approach is to establish a balance between antagonists. Developmentally the infant establishes this balance before creeping (i.e., when rocking forward [extensor dominant] and backward [flexor dominant] on hands and knees).[73] Postural control and balance must be achieved before movement can begin in this position. In intervention it is important to establish a balance between antagonistic muscles by first observing where imbalance exists and then facilitating the weaker component. For example, if the client who has a stroke demonstrates a flexor synergy (flexor dominant), extension should be facilitated. Leticia has ataxia, which compromises the smooth contraction of the antagonists muscle group during movement.

8. Normal motor development has an orderly sequence but lacks a step-by-step quality. Overlapping of skills occurs. The child does not thoroughly master one activity before beginning another, more advanced activity. In trying to ascertain the position of the client for any task, normal motor development should be heeded. If one developmental posture is not effective in obtaining the desired result, it may be necessary to try the activity in another developmental posture. For example, if a client who has ataxia, such as Leticia, is unable to perform a fine motor task while sitting on a bench, it may be necessary to practice skills in a more supported posture, such as sitting in a chair with armrests, prone on the elbows, or with her elbows supported on a surface such as a table. Just as the infant reverts to a more

secure posture when attempting a complex fine motor task, the client also needs a secure posture when attempting more challenging tasks. It is natural for the client to move up and down the developmental sequence, and this allows multiple and varied opportunities for practicing motor activities. The cognitive demands of the task in relation to the developmental posture also must be considered. When the client's position is varied, either by changing the base of support or by shifting weight on different extremities, the quality of visual and cognitive processing is influenced.[1]

9. Improvement in motor ability is dependent on motor learning. Multisensory input from the therapist facilitates the client's motor learning and is an integral part of the PNF approach. For example, the therapist may work with a client on a shoulder flexion activity such as reaching into the cabinet for a cup. The therapist may say, "Reach for the cup," to add verbal input. This approach also encourages the client to look in the direction of the movement to allow vision to enhance the motor response. Thus, tactile, auditory, and visual inputs are used. Motor learning has occurred when these external cues are no longer needed for adequate performance.

10. Frequency of stimulation and repetitive activity are used to promote and retain motor learning and to develop strength and endurance. Just as the therapist who is learning PNF needs the opportunity to practice the techniques, the client needs the opportunity to practice new motor skills. With practice, habits will be formed that support motor performance in occupation. In the process of development, the infant constantly repeats a motor skill in many settings and developmental postures until it is mastered, as becomes apparent to anyone who watches a child learning to walk. Numerous attempts fail, but the child repeats the efforts until the skill is mastered. After the activity is learned, it becomes part of the child's motor repertoire and requires less energy to execute.[101] The same is true for the person learning to play the piano or to play tennis. Without the opportunity to practice, motor learning cannot successfully occur. Just as Leticia's students may be given homework to help them practice the material they learn in school, Leticia will also need to be given a home program that encourages her to practice the postures and movements facilitated in therapy.

11. Goal-directed activities coupled with techniques of facilitation are used to hasten learning of total patterns of walking and self-care activities. When facilitation techniques are applied to self-care, the objective is improved functional ability, but improvement is obtained by more than instruction and practice. Deficiencies are corrected by the direct application of manual contacts and techniques to facilitate a desired response.[47] During an intervention session, this approach may mean applying stretch to finger extensors to facilitate the release of an object or providing joint approximation through the shoulders and pelvis of a client who has ataxia to provide stability while the client is standing to wash dishes. With repetition of appropriate facilitation techniques, Leticia will have the opportunity to feel more normal movement and need to rely less on the therapist's external input.

MOTOR LEARNING

Motor learning requires a multisensory approach. Auditory, visual, and tactile systems are all used to achieve the desired response. The correct combination of sensory input with each client should be ascertained, implemented, and altered as the client progresses. The developmental level of the client and the ability to cooperate also should be taken into consideration.[101] The approach used with a client who has aphasia differs from the approach used with a client who has a hand injury. For example, the client with a hand injury would better understand verbal instructions than would the client with receptive aphasia. Fewer verbal and more tactile and gestural cues would be appropriate with the client who has aphasia. Similarly, the approach used with a child varies greatly from that used with an adult. Interventions with Leticia must take into consideration her visual deficits in addition to any cognitive impairment as a result of her head injury.

Auditory System

Verbal commands should be brief and clear. It is important to time the command so that it does not come too early or too late in relation to the motor act. Tone of voice may influence the quality of the client's response. Buchwald[22] stated that tones of moderate intensity evoke gamma motor neuron activity and that louder tones can alter alpha motor neuron activity. Strong, sharp commands simulate a stress situation and are used when maximal stimulation of motor response is desired. A soft tone of voice is used to offer reassurance and to encourage a smooth movement, as in the presence of pain (e.g., when techniques are used to increase the mobility in Leticia's left wrist). When a client is giving the best effort, a moderate tone can be used.[101]

Another effect of auditory feedback on motor performance was studied by Loomis and Boersma.[61] They used a **verbal mediation** strategy to teach wheelchair safety before transferring out of the chair to clients with right CVA. Loomis and Boersma taught clients to say aloud the steps required to leave the wheelchair safely and independently. They found that only clients who used verbal mediation learned the wheelchair drill sufficiently to perform safe and independent transfers. These clients also had better retention of the sequence of steps, which suggests that verbal mediation is beneficial in reaching independence with better sequencing and fewer errors.

When Leticia first arrived in therapy, she suffered considerable pain at the site of her wrist fracture. Early PNF intervention should use soft verbal commands when activities that involve wrist mobility are performed. In contrast, when facilitating Leticia's ability to assume postures (i.e., moving from side-lying to tall kneeling), more forceful, sharp commands may be needed.

Visual System

Visual stimuli assist in initiation and coordination of movement. Visual input should be monitored to ensure that the client is tracking in the direction of movement. For example, the therapist's position is important because the client often uses the therapist's movement or position as a visual cue. If the therapist desires Leticia to move in a forward direction, he or she should be positioned diagonally in front of the client. In addition to the therapist's position, placement of the OT activity also should be considered. Using one of her children's favorite board games, the therapist could place it in front and to the left of Leticia to increase head, neck, and trunk rotation while Leticia plays the game with her children. Because occupational therapy is activity oriented, an abundance of visual stimuli is offered to the client.

Special consideration will need to be given to the use of vision when working with Leticia. Her stronger head and neck musculature can be used to reinforce oculomotor control. Total body and extremity diagonal patterns can be used to reinforce eye teaming.

Tactile System

Developmentally the tactile system matures before the auditory and visual systems.[32] Furthermore, the tactile system is more efficient. This is because it has temporal and spatial discrimination abilities, as opposed to the visual system, which can make only spatial discriminations, and the auditory system, which can make only temporal discriminations.[40] Affolter[2] stated that during development, processing of tactile-kinesthetic information can be considered fundamental for building cognitive and emotional experience. Looking at and listening to the world do not result in change; however, the world cannot be touched without some change taking place. A Chinese proverb often cited at PNF courses reinforces this viewpoint: "I listen and I forget, I see and I remember, I do and I understand."

It is important for the client to feel movement patterns that are coordinated and balanced. This is particularly important for clients with ataxia, such as Leticia. With the PNF approach, tactile input is supplied through the therapist's manual contacts to guide and reinforce the desired response. This approach may involve gently touching the client to guide movement, using stretch to initiate movement, and providing resistance to strengthen movement. The type and extent of manual contacts depend on the client's clinical status, which is determined through evaluation and reevaluation. For example, the use of stretch or resistance in the presence of musculoskeletal instability may be contraindicated, as in the early healing phases of Leticia's fractures. Likewise, stretch or resistance should not be used if they cause increased pain or tone imbalance.

To increase speed and accuracy in motor performance, the client needs the opportunity to practice. Through repetition, habit patterns that occur automatically without voluntary effort are established. The PNF approach uses the concepts of **part-task practice** and **whole-task practice**. In other words, to learn the whole task, emphasis is placed on the parts of the task that the client is unable to perform independently. The term **stepwise procedures** describes the emphasis on a part of the task during performance of the whole.[101] Performance of each part of the task is improved by combining practice with appropriate sensory cues and techniques of facilitation. For example, the client learning to transfer from a wheelchair to a tub bench may have difficulty lifting the leg over the tub rim. This part of the task should be practiced, with repetition and facilitation techniques to the hip flexors, during performance of the transfer.

When the transfer becomes smooth and coordinated, it is no longer necessary to practice each part individually. It is also unnecessary for the therapist to facilitate.

Leticia has difficulty getting down on the floor to play games with her children. In intervention, she should be provided with facilitation and practice of moving from sitting on a chair to tall kneeling to side-sitting on the floor. She will initially require considerable manual facilitation by the therapist to move through and achieve these various movement patterns. As she develops more skill, the therapist will reduce and adjust the intensity of the tactile input.

In summation, several components are necessary for motor learning to occur. In the PNF intervention approach, these components include multisensory input from the therapist's verbal commands, visual cues, and manual contacts. Touch is the most efficient form of stimulation and provides the opportunity for the client to feel normal movement. Current motor-learning theory argues that for motor learning to occur, the client cannot be a passive recipient of intervention. Therefore, the client needs opportunities to practice motor skills in the context of functional life situations. Initially the therapist's manual contacts and sensory input are needed. These should be decreased, however, as the client demonstrates and learns skilled movement. The amount of feedback from the therapist should also be decreased as the client learns to rely on his or her own internal feedback system for error detection and correction.

ASSESSMENT

Assessment requires astute observational skills and knowledge of normal movement. An initial assessment is completed to determine the client's abilities, deficiencies, and potential. After the intervention plan is established, ongoing assessment is necessary to ascertain the effectiveness of intervention and to make modifications as the client changes.

The PNF assessment follows a sequence from proximal to distal. First, vital and related functions are considered, such as breathing, swallowing, voice production, facial and oral musculature, and visual-ocular control. Any impairment or weakness in these functions is noted. Because Leticia fatigues quickly, breathing patterns and efficiency need to be closely evaluated as she engages in her daily activities.

The head and neck region is observed after vital functions. Deficiencies in this area directly affect the upper trunk and extremities. Head and neck positions are observed in varying postures and total patterns during functional activities. It is important to note (1) dominance of tone (flexor or extensor), (2) alignment (midline or shift to one side), and (3) stability and mobility (more or less needed).[68]

After observation of the head and neck region, the assessment proceeds to the following parts of the body: upper trunk, upper extremities, lower trunk, and lower extremities. Each segment is assessed individually in specific movement patterns, in addition to in developmental activities in which the body segments interact. For example, shoulder flexion can be observed in an individual upper-extremity movement pattern, in addition to during a total developmental pattern such as rolling.

During assessment of developmental activities and postures, the following issues should be addressed:

- Is there a need for more stability or mobility?
- Is there a balance between flexors and extensors, or is one more dominant?
- Is the client able to move in all directions?
- What are the major limitations (e.g., weakness, incoordination, spasticity, and contractures)?
- Is the client able to assume a posture and to maintain it? If not, which total pattern or postures are inadequate?
- Are the inadequacies more proximal or distal?
- Which sensory input does the client respond to most effectively: auditory, visual, or tactile?
- Which techniques of facilitation does the client respond to best?

When applying these questions to Leticia's evaluation, the following observations can be made. First, Leticia will need to develop stability to diminish the effects of her ataxia. She is not dominated by either flexor or extensor tone, but when fatigued she has more difficulty maintaining upright posture. She will therefore need to have facilitation of head, neck, and trunk extensors when fatigued. She can move in all directions but has less stability when walking backward. Her major limitations are poor motor control and rigidity, but prevention of a wrist contracture is also a concern. Leticia is having difficulty assuming kneeling, sitting, and standing postures because of her instability. Once in an upright posture, she can maintain it for a few minutes, but then fatigue sets in. She will therefore need to build endurance in more supported lower developmental postures. When moving into more upright postures, she will need PNF techniques to build strength and endurance. Her inadequate proximal control and trunk rigidity affect her ability to effectively use her extremities, especially in higher developmental positions. Visual sensory input may not be the best to start with because of her diplopia; however, facilitation of oculomotor control using PNF techniques will be of benefit as she progresses. Facilitation techniques that Leticia responds to best are rhythmic stabilization, stabilizing reversals, and approximation.

Finally the client is observed during self-care and other ADLs to determine whether performance of individual and total patterns is adequate within the context of a functional activity. The client's performance may vary from one setting to another. After the client leaves the structured setting of the OT or PT clinic for the less structured home or community environment, deterioration of motor performance is not unusual. Thus the intervention plan must accommodate the practice of motor performance in a variety of settings in locations appropriate to the specific activity.

INTERVENTION IMPLEMENTATION

After assessment, an intervention plan is developed that includes goals the client hopes to accomplish. The techniques and procedures that have the most favorable influence on movement and posture are used. Similarly, appropriate total patterns (developmental postures) and patterns of facilitation are selected to enhance performance.

Diagonal Patterns

The diagonal patterns used in the PNF approach are mass movement patterns observed in most functional activities. Part of the challenge in OT assessment and intervention is recognizing the diagonal patterns in ADLs. Knowledge of the diagonals is necessary for identifying areas of deficiency. Two diagonal motions are present for each major part of the body: head and neck, upper and lower trunk, and extremities. Each diagonal pattern has a flexion and extension component, together with rotation and movement away from or toward the midline.

The head, neck, and trunk patterns are referred to as (1) flexion with rotation to the right or left and (2) extension with rotation to the right or left. These proximal patterns combine with the extremity diagonals. The upper and lower extremity diagonals are described according to the three movement components at the shoulder and hip: (1) flexion and extension, (2) abduction and adduction, and (3) external and internal rotation. Voss[99] introduced shorter descriptions for the extremity patterns in 1967 and referred to them as diagonal 1 (D_1) flexion/extension and diagonal 2 (D_2) flexion/extension. The reference points for flexion and extension are the shoulder and hip joints of the upper and lower extremities, respectively.

The movements associated with each diagonal and examples of these patterns seen in self-care and other ADLs are presented in the following sections. Note that in functional activities, not all components of the pattern or full range of motion (ROM) are necessarily seen. Furthermore, the diagonals interact during functional movement, changing from one pattern or combination to another, when they cross the transverse and sagittal planes of the body.[70]

Unilateral Patterns

Various unilateral patterns can be applied:

1. *Upper extremity (UE) D_1 flexion (shoulder flexion-adduction-external rotation)*: scapula elevation, abduction, and rotation; shoulder flexion, adduction, and external rotation; elbow in flexion or extension; forearm supination; wrist flexion to the radial side; finger flexion and adduction; thumb adduction (Fig. 32.4A). Examples in functional activity: hand-to-mouth motion in feeding, tennis forehand, combing hair on the left side of the head with right hand (Fig. 32.5A), rolling from supine to prone.

2. *UE D_1 extension (shoulder extension-abduction-internal rotation)*: scapula depression, adduction, and rotation; shoulder extension, abduction, and internal rotation; elbow in flexion or extension; forearm pronation; wrist extension to the ulnar side; finger extension and abduction; thumb in palmar abduction (see Fig. 32.4B). Examples in functional activity: pushing a car door open from the inside (see Fig. 32.5B), tennis backhand stroke, rolling from prone to supine.

3. *UE D_2 flexion (shoulder flexion-abduction-external rotation)*: scapula elevation, adduction, and rotation; shoulder flexion, abduction, and external rotation; elbow in flexion or extension; forearm supination; wrist extension to the radial side; finger extension and abduction; thumb extension (Fig. 32.6A). Examples in functional activity: combing hair on the right side of the head with the right hand (Fig. 32.7A), lifting a racquet in tennis serve, backstroke in swimming. The D_2 flexion pattern would be emphasized with Leticia in her left

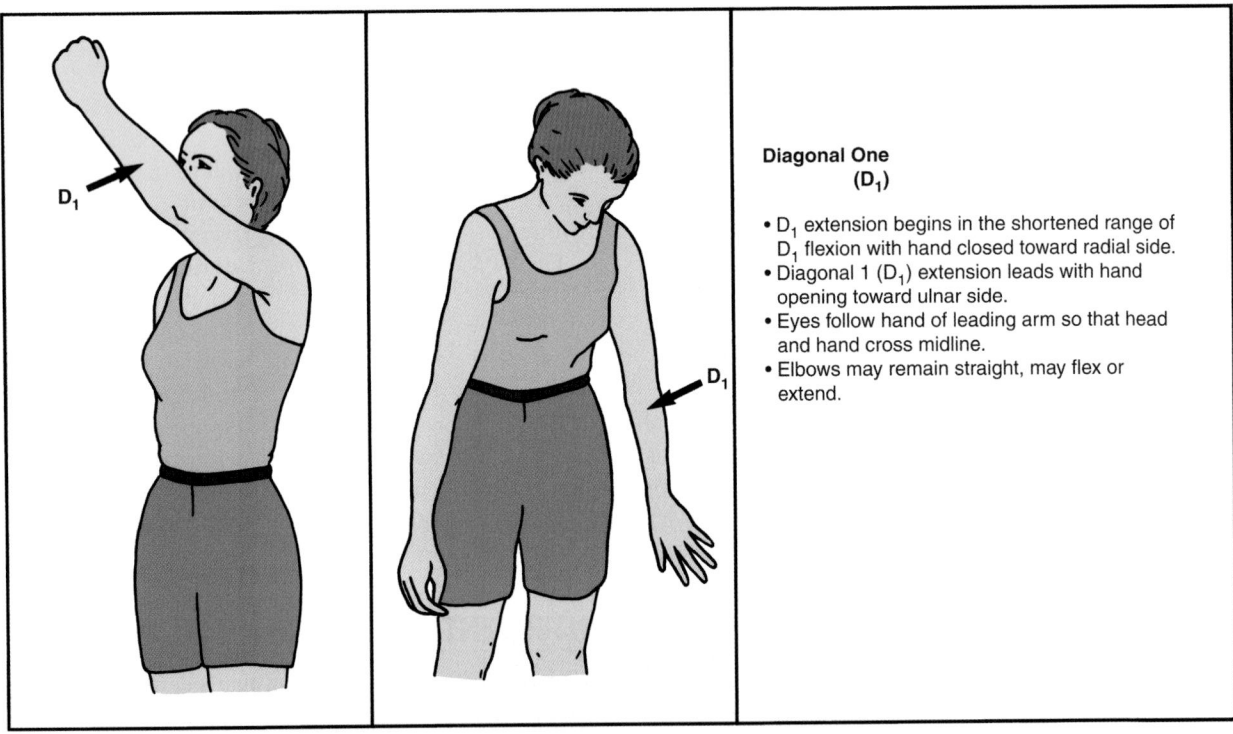

Diagonal One (D_1)

- D_1 extension begins in the shortened range of D_1 flexion with hand closed toward radial side.
- Diagonal 1 (D_1) extension leads with hand opening toward ulnar side.
- Eyes follow hand of leading arm so that head and hand cross midline.
- Elbows may remain straight, may flex or extend.

A   B

Fig. 32.4 (A) Upper extremity D_1 flexion pattern. (B) Upper extremity D_1 extension pattern. (From Myers BJ: Unit I: *PNF Diagonal Patterns and their Application to Functional Activities, Videotape Study Guide,* Chicago, 1982, Rehabilitation Institute of Chicago.)

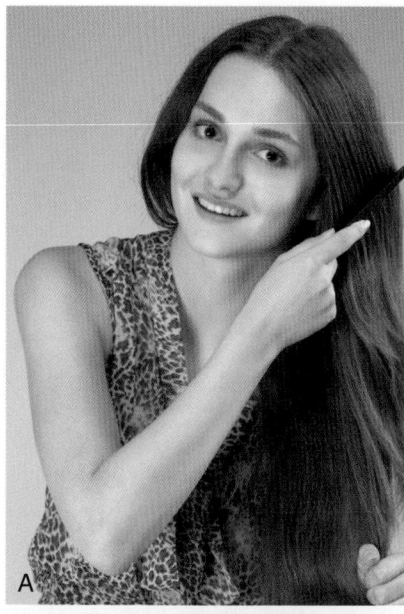

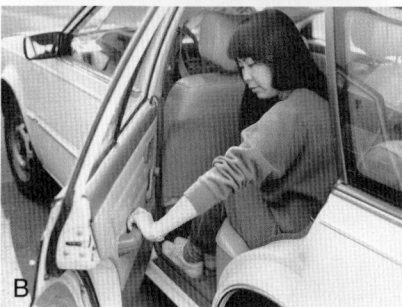

Fig. 32.5 (A) Upper extremity D_1 flexion pattern used to comb the hair, opposite side. (B) Upper extremity D_1 extension pattern used to push a car door open. (*A*, From iStock.com.)

upper extremity to facilitate supination and wrist extension, which are weak secondary to her wrist fracture.

4. *UE D_2 extension (shoulder extension-adduction-internal rotation)*: scapula depression, abduction, and rotation; shoulder extension, adduction, and internal rotation; elbow in flexion or extension; forearm pronation; wrist flexion to the ulnar side; finger flexion and adduction; thumb opposition (see Fig. 32.6B). Examples in functional activity: pitching a baseball, hitting a ball in tennis serve, buttoning pants on the left side with the right hand (see Fig. 32.7C). The rotational component in lower extremity (LE) D_1 flexion and extension parallels the UE patterns.

5. *LE D_1 flexion (hip flexion-adduction-external rotation)*: hip flexion, adduction, and external rotation; knee in flexion or extension; ankle and foot dorsiflexion with inversion and toe extension. Examples in functional activity: kicking a soccer ball, rolling from supine to prone, putting on a sock with legs crossed (Fig. 32.8A).

6. *LE D_1 extension (hip extension-abduction-internal rotation)*: hip extension, abduction, and internal rotation; knee in flexion or extension; ankle and foot plantar flexion with eversion and toe flexion. Examples in functional activity: putting leg into pants (see Fig. 32.8B), rolling from prone to supine. The rotational component of LE D_2 flexion and extension is opposite to the UE patterns.

7. *LE D_2 flexion (hip flexion-abduction-internal rotation)*: hip flexion, abduction, and internal rotation; knee in flexion or extension; ankle and foot dorsiflexion with eversion and toe extension. Examples in functional activity: karate kick (Fig. 32.9A), drawing the heels up during the breaststroke in swimming.

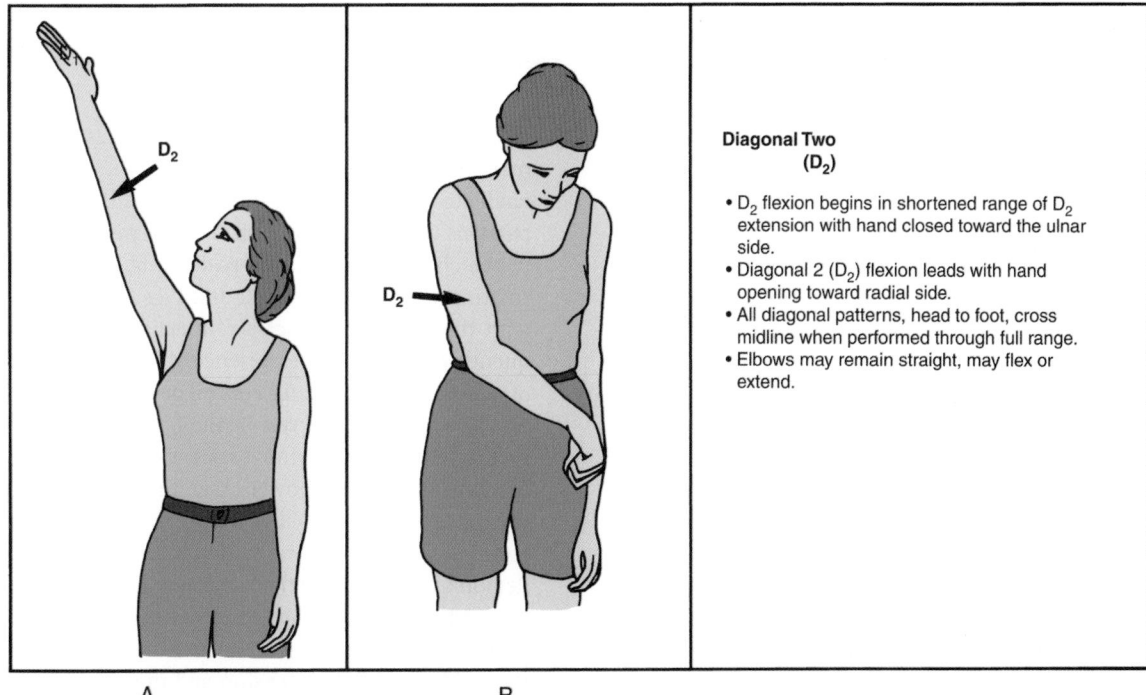

Diagonal Two
(D_2)

• D_2 flexion begins in shortened range of D_2 extension with hand closed toward the ulnar side.
• Diagonal 2 (D_2) flexion leads with hand opening toward radial side.
• All diagonal patterns, head to foot, cross midline when performed through full range.
• Elbows may remain straight, may flex or extend.

A   B

Fig. 32.6 (A) Upper extremity D_2 flexion pattern. (B) Upper extremity D_2 extension pattern. (From Myers BJ: Unit I: *PNF Diagonal Patterns and their Application to Functional Activities, Videotape Study Guide,* Chicago, 1982, Rehabilitation Institute of Chicago.)

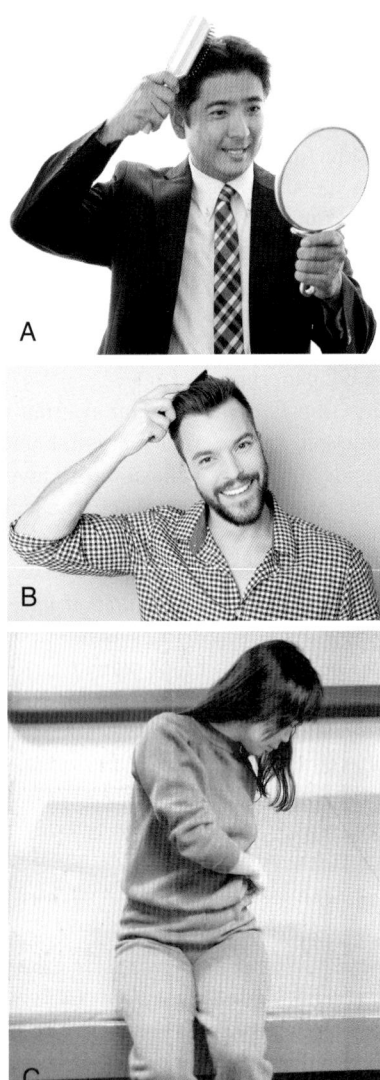

Fig. 32.7 (A–B) Upper extremity D_2 flexion pattern used to comb the hair, same side. (C) Upper extremity D_2 extension pattern used to button trousers, opposite side. (A from iStock.com. B from Shutterstock.com.)

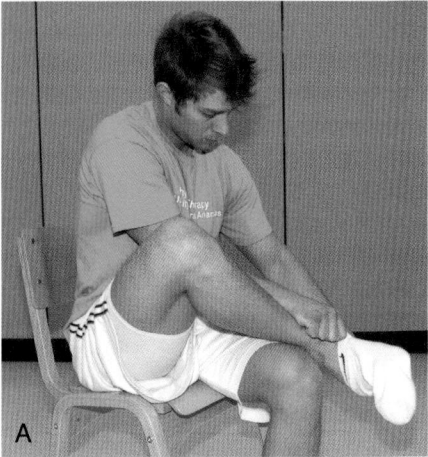

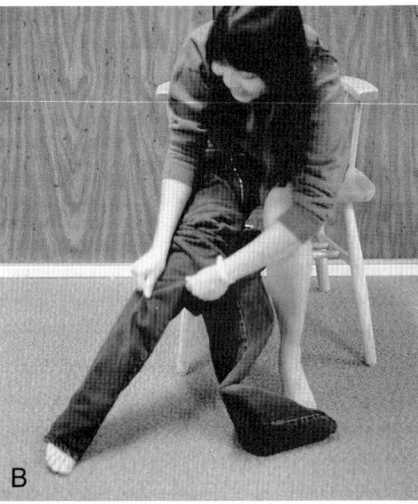

Fig. 32.8 (A) Lower extremity D_1 flexion pattern demonstrated when crossing the leg to put on a sock. (B) Lower extremity D_1 extension pattern used when pulling on trousers. (A from Reese NB, Bandy WD: *Joint Range of Motion and Muscle Length Testing*, ed 3, St. Louis, 2017, Elsevier.)

8. *LE D_2 extension (hip extension-adduction-external rotation):* hip extension, adduction and external rotation: knee in flexion or extension; ankle and foot in plantar flexion with inversion and toe flexion. Examples of functional activity: push-off in gait, the kick during the breaststroke in swimming, long sitting with legs crossed (see Fig. 32.9B).

Bilateral Patterns

Movements in the extremities may be reinforced by combining diagonals in bilateral patterns as follows:

1. **Symmetric patterns:** Paired extremities perform similar movements at the same time (Fig. 32.10A). Examples: bilateral symmetric D_1 extension, such as pushing off a chair to stand (Fig. 32.11A); bilateral symmetric D_2 extension, such as starting to take off a pullover sweater (see Fig. 32.11B); bilateral symmetric D_2 flexion, such as reaching to lift a large item off a high shelf (see Fig. 32.11C). Bilateral symmetric UE patterns facilitate trunk flexion and extension.

2. **Asymmetric patterns:** Paired extremities perform movements toward one side of the body at the same time, which facilitates trunk rotation (see Fig. 32.10B). The asymmetric patterns can be performed with the arms in contact, such as in the chopping and lifting patterns in which greater trunk rotation is seen (Figs. 32.12 and Figs. 32.13). Furthermore, with the arms in contact, self-touching occurs. This is frequently observed in the presence of pain or in reinforcement of a motion when greater control or power is needed.[101] This phenomenon is observed in the baseball player at bat and in the tennis player who uses a two-handed backhand to increase control and power. Asymmetric patterns with arms in contact would be beneficial for Leticia to control ataxia. Examples of asymmetric patterns are bilateral asymmetric flexion to the left, with the left arm in D_2 flexion and the right arm in D_1 flexion, such as when putting on a left earring (Fig. 32.14), and bilateral asymmetric extension to the left, with the right arm in D_2 extension and the left arm in D_1 extension, such as when zipping a left-side zipper.

3. **Reciprocal patterns:** Paired extremities move in opposite directions simultaneously, either in the same diagonal or in

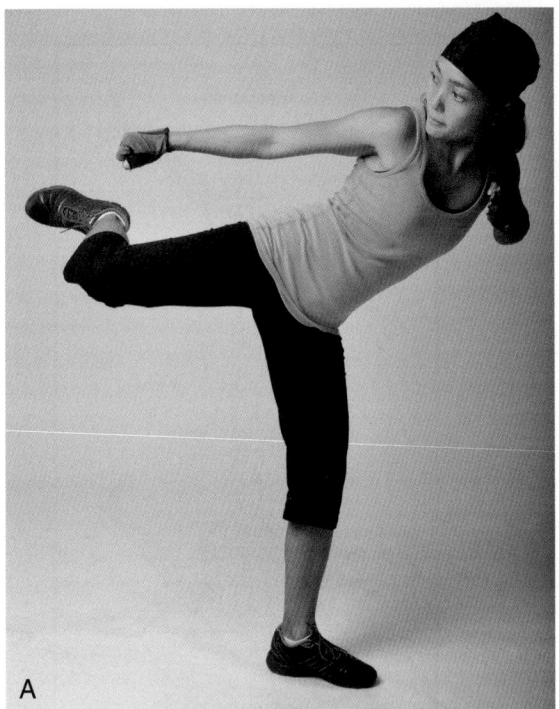

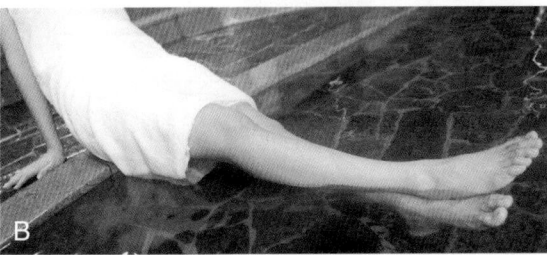

Fig. 32.9 (A) Lower extremity D_2 flexion pattern shown in a karate kick. (B) Lower extremity D_2 extension pattern used in long sitting with the legs crossed. (A from Shutterstock.com. B from DAJ [via Thinkstock. com].)

combined diagonals. If paired extremities perform movements in combined diagonals (see Fig. 32.10C), a stabilizing effect occurs on the head, neck, and trunk because movement of the extremities is in the opposite direction while head and neck remain in midline. During activities requiring high-level balance, the reciprocal patterns with combined diagonals come into play with one extremity in D_1 extension and the other extremity in D_2 flexion. Examples of this are pitching in baseball, sidestroke in swimming, and walking on a narrow walkway with one extremity in a diagonal flexion pattern with the other in a diagonal extension pattern (Fig. 32.15). In contrast, reciprocal patterns in the same diagonal, such as D_1 in arm swing during walking, facilitate trunk rotation. Leticia needs to work with reciprocals of D_1 to improve rhythm of arm swing and trunk rotation during walking.

Combined Movements of Upper and Lower Extremities

Interaction of the upper and lower extremities results in (1) ipsilateral patterns, with extremities of the same side moving in the same direction at the same time; (2) contralateral patterns, with

extremities of opposite sides moving in the same direction at the same time; and (3) diagonal reciprocal patterns, with contralateral extremities moving in the same direction at the same time while opposite contralateral extremities move in the opposite direction (see Fig. 32.10D–E, and F).

The combined movements of the upper and lower extremities are observed in activities such as crawling and walking. Awareness of these patterns is important in the assessment of the client's motor skills. The ipsilateral patterns are more primitive developmentally and indicate a lack of bilateral integration. Less rotation also is observed in ipsilateral patterns. Therefore, the goal in intervention is to progress from ipsilateral to contralateral to diagonal reciprocal patterns.

Several advantages exist to the use of the diagonal patterns in intervention. First, crossing of midline occurs. This movement is of particular importance in the remediation of perceptual motor deficits such as unilateral neglect, in which integration of both sides of the body and awareness of the neglected side are intervention goals. Second, each muscle has an optimal pattern in which it functions. For example, the client who has weak thumb opposition benefits from active movement in D_2 extension. Similarly, D_1 extension is the optimal pattern for ulnar wrist extension. Leticia should work in D_2 flexion after her Colles wrist fracture is stable. This pattern will increase range of motion and strengthen supination and radial wrist extension. Third, the diagonal patterns use groups of muscles, which is typical of movement seen in functional activities. For example, in eating, the hand-to-mouth action is accomplished in one mass movement pattern (D_1 flexion) that uses several muscles simultaneously. Therefore, movement in the diagonals is more efficient than movement performed at each joint separately. Finally, rotation is always a component in the diagonals (e.g., trunk rotation to the left or right and forearm pronation and supination). With an injury or with the aging process, rotation frequently is impaired and can be facilitated with movement in the diagonals. In intervention, attention should be given to the placement of activities so that movement occurs in the diagonal. For example, if the client is working on a wood-sanding project, trunk rotation with extension can be facilitated by placing the project on an inclined plane in a diagonal. Leticia can incorporate rotational movements into homemaking activities such as unloading the dishwasher.

Total Patterns

In PNF, developmental postures also are called total patterns of movement and posture.[69] Total patterns require interaction between proximal (head, neck, and trunk) and distal (extremity) components. The assumption of postures is important, as is the maintenance of postures. When posture cannot be sustained, emphasis should be placed on the assumption of posture.[100] For example, before the client can be expected to sustain a sitting posture, he or she must be able to perform lower developmental total patterns of movement, such as rolling and moving from side-lying to side-sitting.

The active assumption of postures can be included in OT activities. For example, a reaching and placing activity could be set up so that the client must reach for the object in the supine

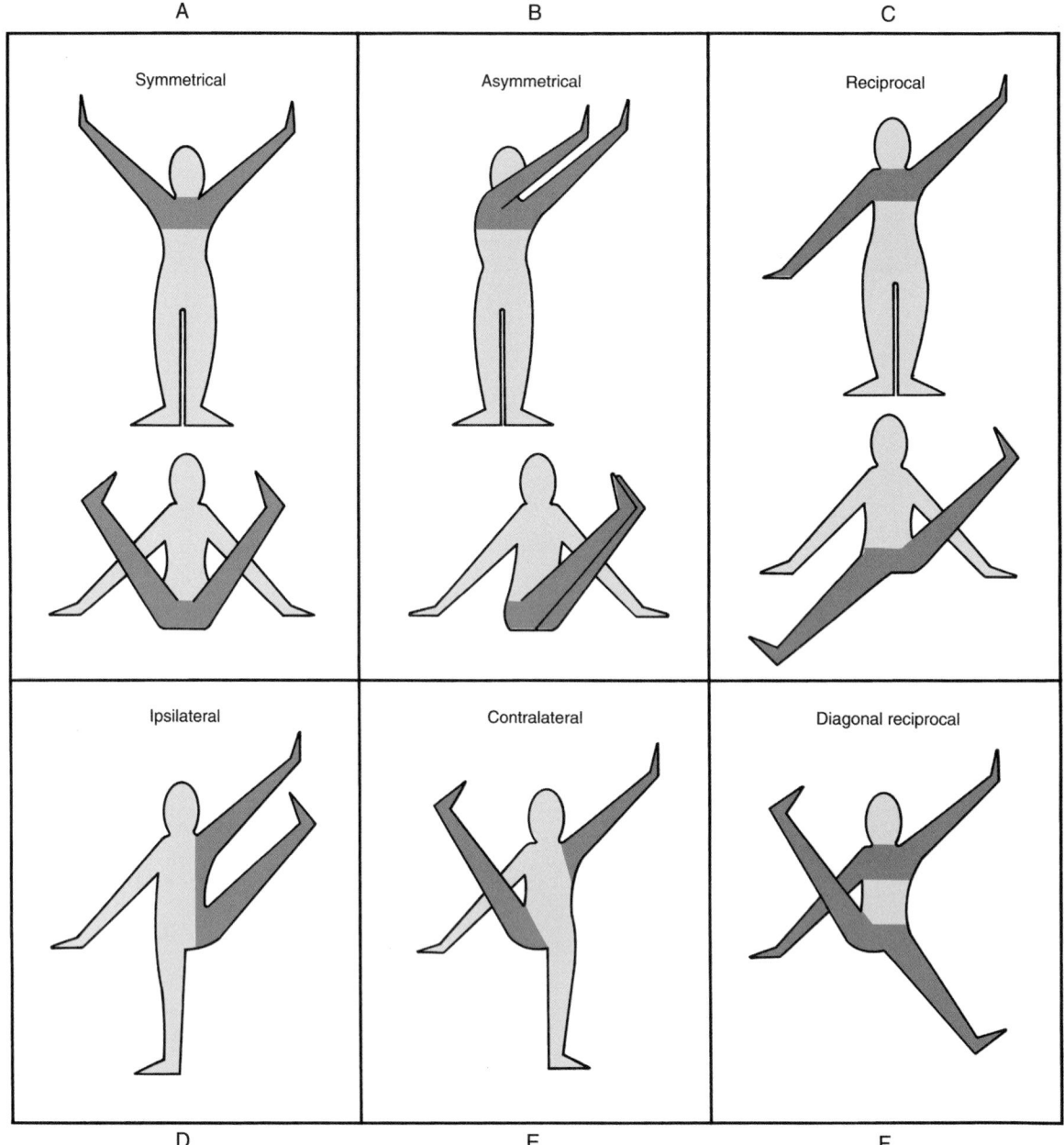

Fig. 32.10 (A) Symmetrical patterns. (B) Asymmetrical patterns. (C) Reciprocal patterns. (D) Ipsilateral pattern. (E) Contralateral pattern. (F) Diagonal reciprocal pattern. (From Myers BJ: Unit I: *PNF Diagonal Patterns and their Application to Functional Activities, Videotape Study Guide*, Chicago, 1982, Rehabilitation Institute of Chicago.)

posture and place it in the side-lying posture. The use of total patterns also can reinforce individual extremity movements. For example, in an activity such as wiping a tabletop, wrist extension is reinforced when the client leans forward over the supporting arm. This would be a way to make homemaking activities part of Leticia's home exercise program for her wrist in the later stages of recovery.

Several facts support the use of total patterns in the PNF intervention approach.[69] First, total patterns of movement and posture are experienced as part of the normal developmental process in all humans. Therefore, recapitulation of these postures is meaningful to the client and acquired with less difficulty.

Second, movement in and out of total patterns and the ability to sustain postures enhance components of normal development, such as reflex integration and support, balance between antagonists, and development of motor control in a cephalo-caudal, proximodistal direction. Third, the use of total patterns improves the ability to assume and maintain postures, which is important in all areas of occupation.

Voss developed the sequence and procedures for assisting clients with developmental postures. In 1981, Myers developed a videotape that shows the use of the sequence and procedures in OT.[69] This video demonstrates more information on the application of the total patterns and postures to OT.

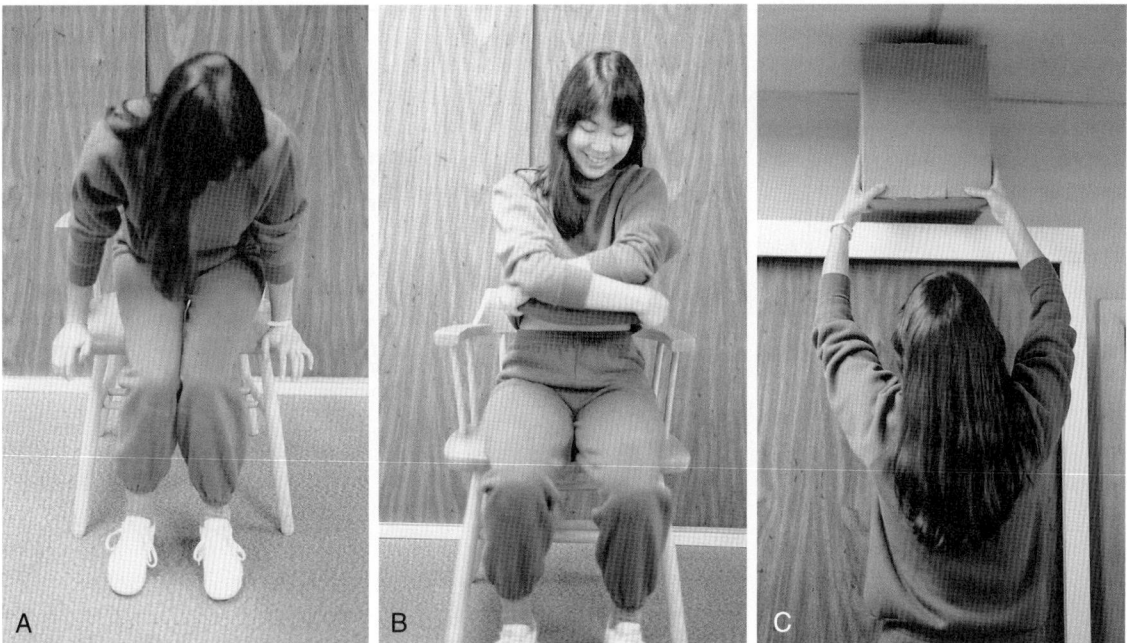

Fig. 32.11 (A) Upper extremity bilateral symmetric D_1 extension pattern shown when pushing off from a chair. (B) Upper extremity bilateral symmetric D_2 extension pattern used when starting to take off a pullover shirt. (C) Upper extremity bilateral symmetric D_2 flexion pattern used when reaching to lift a box off a high shelf.

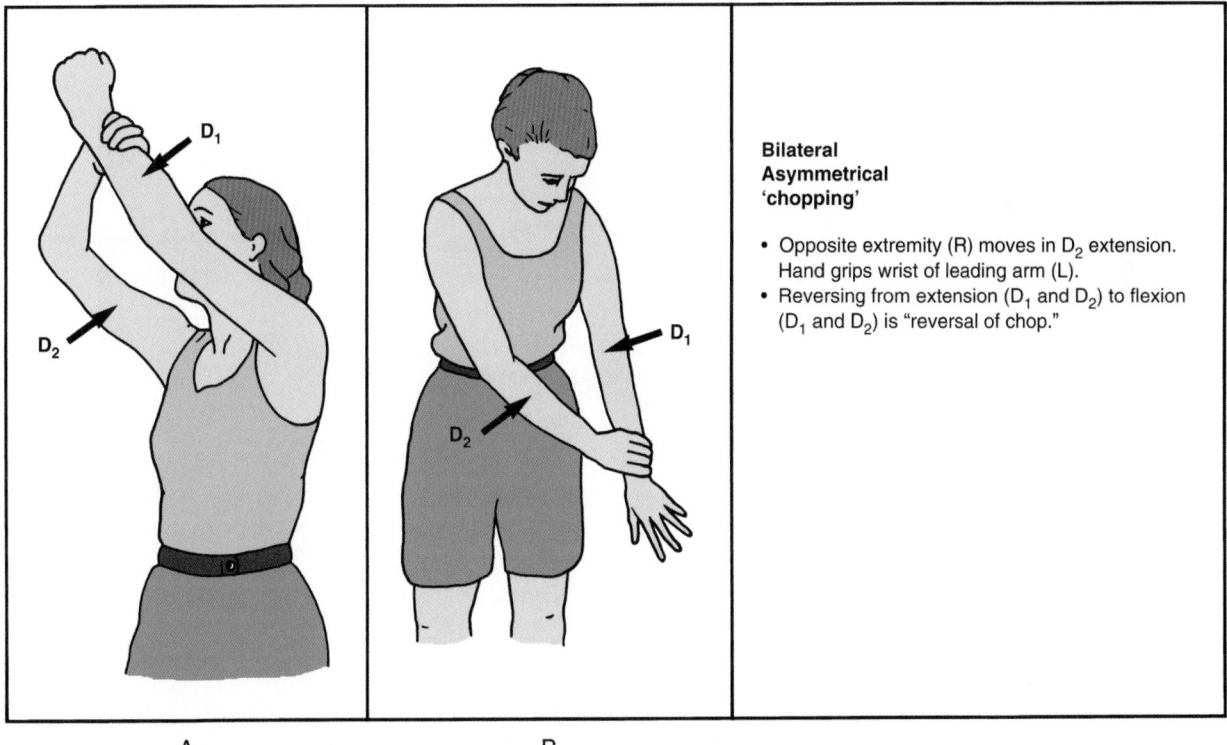

Bilateral Asymmetrical 'chopping'

- Opposite extremity (R) moves in D_2 extension. Hand grips wrist of leading arm (L).
- Reversing from extension (D_1 and D_2) to flexion (D_1 and D_2) is "reversal of chop."

Fig. 32.12 Bilateral asymmetric chopping. (From Myers BJ: Unit I: *PNF Diagonal Patterns and their Application to Functional Activities, Videotape Study Guide*, Chicago, 1982, Rehabilitation Institute of Chicago.)

Procedures

PNF techniques are superimposed on movement and posture. Among these techniques are basic procedures considered essential to the PNF approach. Two procedures, verbal commands and visual cues, were discussed previously. Other procedures are described in the following sections.

Manual contacts refer to the placement of the therapist's hands on the client. These contacts are most effective when

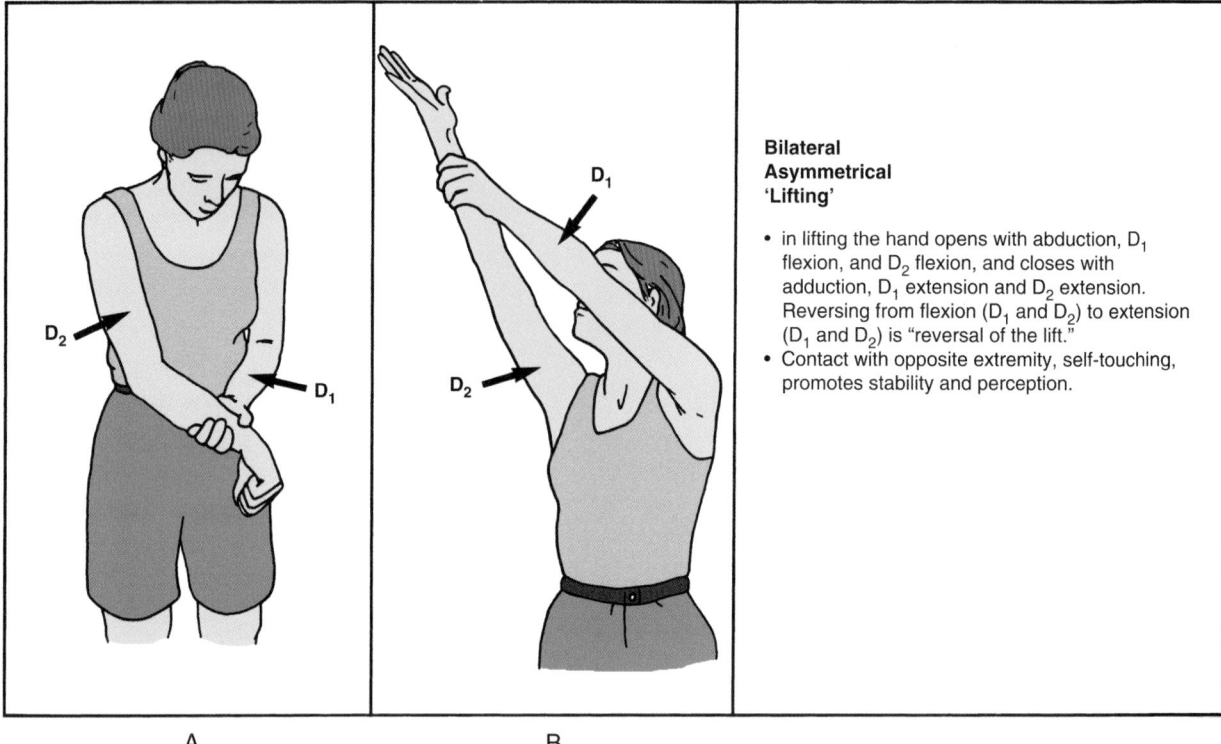

Bilateral Asymmetrical 'Lifting'

• in lifting the hand opens with abduction, D_1 flexion, and D_2 flexion, and closes with adduction, D_1 extension and D_2 extension. Reversing from flexion (D_1 and D_2) to extension (D_1 and D_2) is "reversal of the lift."
• Contact with opposite extremity, self-touching, promotes stability and perception.

Fig. 32.13 Bilateral asymmetric lifting. (From Myers BJ: Unit I: *PNF Diagonal Patterns and their Application to Functional Activities, Videotape Study Guide,* Chicago, 1982, Rehabilitation Institute of Chicago.)

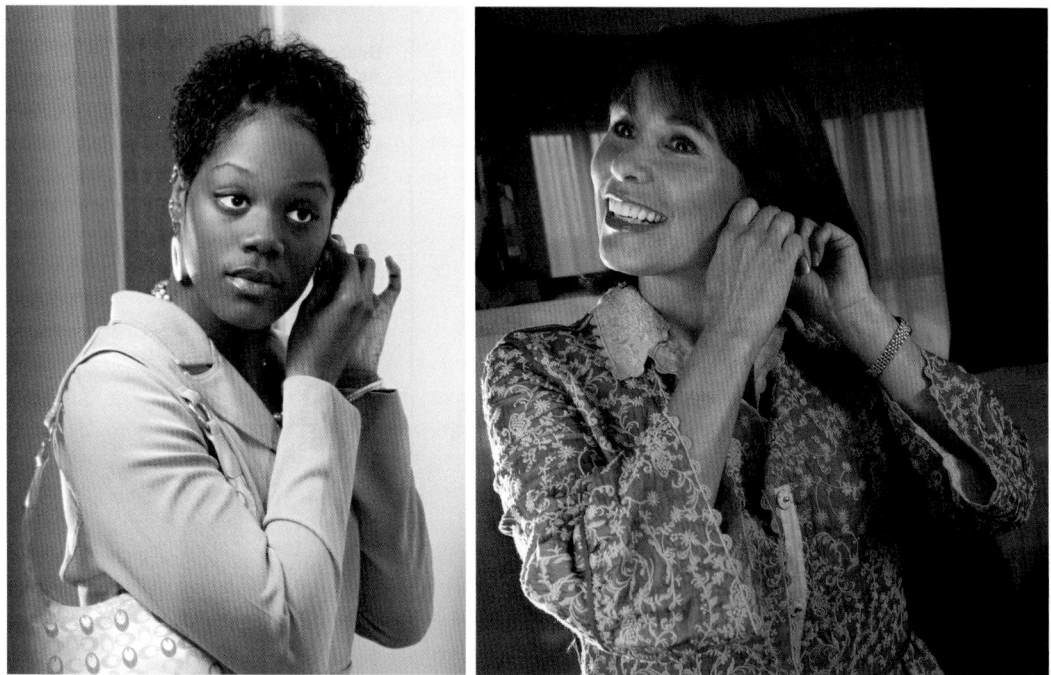

Fig. 32.14 Putting on an earring requires use of the upper extremity bilateral asymmetric flexion pattern. (*Left,* From iStock.com. *Right,* From Jupiterimages [via Thinkstock.com].)

applied directly to the skin. Pressure from the therapist's touch is used as a facilitating mechanism and serves as a sensory cue to help the client understand the direction of the anticipated movement.[101] The amount of pressure applied depends on the specific technique being used and on the desired response. The location of manual contacts is chosen according to the groups of muscles, tendons, and joints responsible for the desired movement patterns. If the client is having difficulty reaching to comb the back of the hair because of scapular weakness, the desired movement pattern is D_2 flexion. Manual contacts should be on

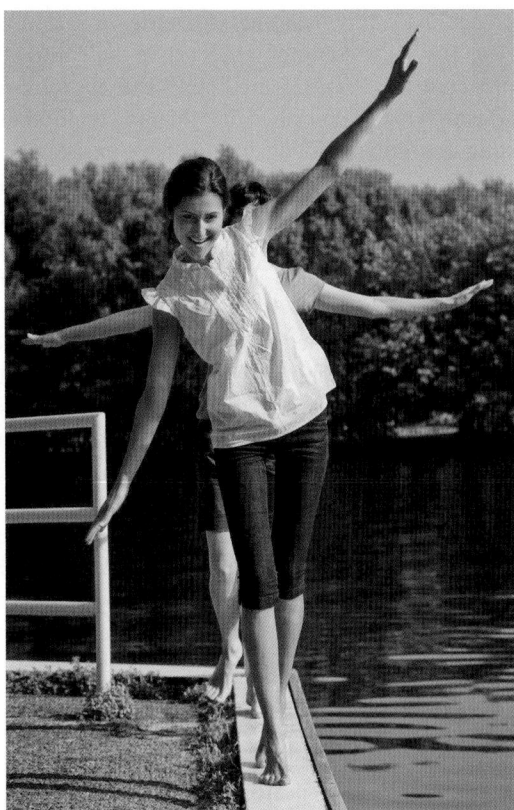

Fig. 32.15 A bilateral reciprocal pattern of the upper extremities is used to maintain balance when walking on a narrow walkway. (From Jupiterimages [via Thinkstock.com].)

the posterior surface of the scapula to reinforce the muscles that elevate, adduct, and rotate the scapula.

Stretch is used to initiate voluntary movement and enhance speed of response and strength in weak muscles. This procedure is based on Sherrington's neurophysiological principle of reciprocal innervation.[89] When a muscle is stretched, the Ia and II fibers in the muscle spindle send excitatory messages to the alpha motor neurons, which innervate the stretched muscle. Inhibitory messages are sent to the antagonistic muscle simultaneously.[32]

When stretch is used in the PNF approach, the part to be facilitated is placed in the extreme lengthened range of the desired pattern (or where tension is felt on all muscle components of a given pattern). This range is the completely shortened range of the antagonistic pattern. Special attention is given to the rotatory component of the pattern because it is responsible for elongation of the fibers of the muscles in a given pattern. After the correct position for the stretch stimulus has been achieved, stretch is superimposed on the pattern. The client should attempt the movement at the exact time that the stretch reflex is elicited. The use of verbal commands also should coincide with the application of stretch, to reinforce the movement. Discrimination should be exercised with the use of stretch to prevent an increase in pain or muscle imbalances.

Traction facilitates the joint receptors by creating a separation of the joint surfaces. It is thought that traction promotes movement and is used for pulling motion.[101] In activities such

as carrying a heavy suitcase or pulling open a jammed door, traction can be felt on joint surfaces. Although traction may be contraindicated for clients with acute symptoms, such as after surgery or a fracture, it can sometimes relieve pain and promote greater ROM in painful joints.

Approximation facilitates joint receptors by compressing joint surfaces. It promotes stability and postural control and is used for pushing motion.[101] Approximation is usually superimposed on a weight-bearing posture. For example, to enhance postural control in the prone-on-elbows posture, approximation may be given through the shoulders in a downward direction. As part of a home program to enhance proximal stability, Leticia could play board games on the floor with her children in weight-bearing positions such as prone on elbows or side-sitting. A weighted vest could be used in place of the therapist's manual contacts to provide approximation.

Maximal resistance involves Sherrington's principle of irradiation—namely, that stronger muscles and patterns reinforce weaker components.[89] This procedure is frequently misunderstood and applied incorrectly. It is defined as the greatest amount of resistance that can be applied to an active contraction while allowing full ROM to occur or to an isometric contraction without defeating or breaking the client's hold.[101] Maximal resistance is not the greatest amount of resistance that the therapist can apply. The objective is to obtain maximal effort on the part of the client because strength is increased by movement against resistance that requires maximal effort.[42]

If the resistance applied by the therapist results in uncoordinated or jerky movement or if it breaks the client's hold, too much resistance has been given. Movement against maximal resistance should be slow and smooth. To use this technique effectively, the therapist must sense the appropriate amount of resistance. For clients with neurologic impairment or pain, the resistance may be very light, and light resistance is probably maximal for the client's needs. The therapist's manual contacts may offer light resistance that actually assists by providing the client with a way to track the desired movement. In the presence of spasticity, resistance may increase existing muscle imbalance and thus needs to be monitored. For example, if an increase in finger flexor spasticity is noted with resisted rocking in the hands-knees position, resistance should be decreased or eliminated or an alternative position should be used.

Techniques

Specific techniques are used in conjunction with these basic procedures. A few have been selected for discussion. These techniques are divided into three categories: those directed to the agonists, those that are a reversal of the antagonists, and those that promote relaxation.[101]

Techniques Directed to the Agonist

Repeated contractions is a technique based on the assumption that repetition of an activity is necessary for motor learning and helps develop strength, ROM, and endurance. The client's voluntary movement is facilitated with stretch and resistance, using isometric and isotonic contractions. This is also referred to as the contract-relax (CR) method in which the targeted muscles for lengthening are contracted by the client against resistance for a short period of time.[43] Following the contraction against a stable resistance (isometric contractions), stretch is gently applied to lengthen the targeted muscle. The process of repeatedly contracting against a force and then relaxing and stretching has been effective in increasing muscle length. Repeated contractions could be used to increase trunk flexion with rotation in the client who has difficulty reaching to put on a pair of shoes from the sitting position. The client bends forward as far as possible. At the point at which active motion weakens, the client is asked to hold with an isometric contraction. This action is followed by isotonic contractions, facilitated by stretch, as the client is asked to "reach toward your feet." This sequence is repeated either until fatigue is evident or until the client is able to reach the feet. The pattern can be reinforced further by asking the client to hold with another isometric contraction at the end of the sequence.

The use of PNF with older adults residing in assisted-living settings has been investigated.[56] Residents were provided with a 10-week training period using PNF to improve sit-to-stand, shoulder, and ankle range of motion and strength. Using repeated measures analysis of variance (ANOVA), statistically significant improvements were noted in all mentioned areas. The skills allowed individuals to engage in instrumental activities of daily living (IADLs) with improved postural control.

Elderly clients who had sustained falls were provided with training using PNF.[90] When compared to older adults who were provided only with general exercise, the older adults who had PNF training had statistically significant improvements in various measures related to fall prevention. Authors concluded that PNF training was beneficial in enhancing physical conditioning of older adults who had experienced falls.

Rhythmic initiation is used to improve the ability to initiate movement, which may be a problem with clients who have Parkinson's disease or apraxia. This technique involves voluntary relaxation, passive movement of the extremity by the therapist, and repeated isotonic contractions of the agonistic pattern. The verbal command is, "Relax and let me move you." As relaxation is felt, the command is, "Now you do it with me." After several repetitions of active movement, resistance may be given to reinforce the movement. Rhythmic initiation allows the client to feel the pattern before beginning active movement. Thus, the proprioceptive and kinesthetic senses are enhanced. This rhythmic initiation was used with clients who had chronic strokes to enhance controlled movements.[102] When compared to healthy adults, the use of PNF effectively reduced the muscle stiffness noted in individuals who have chronic stroke. The muscle stiffness contributes to increased effort when attempting to move and compromises functional skills.

Reversal of Antagonist Techniques

Reversal of antagonist techniques employ a characteristic of normal development—namely, that movement is reversing and changes direction. These techniques are based on Sherrington's principle of successive induction, according to which the stronger antagonist facilitates the weaker agonist.[89] The agonist is facilitated through resistance to the antagonist. The contraction

of the antagonist can be isotonic, isometric, or a combination of the two. The most common approach is the contract-relax-antagonist-contract (CRAC) method.[43] The contract-relax is the same as previously described, but then the method includes contracting the antagonist against a stable resistance. These techniques may be contraindicated for clients in whom resistance of antagonists increases symptoms such as pain and spasticity. For example, the facilitation of finger extension (agonist) would not be achieved effectively through resistance applied to spastic finger flexors (antagonist). In this situation, finger extension may be better facilitated through the use of repeated contractions, in which the emphasis is only on the extensor surface.

Slow reversal is an isotonic contraction (against resistance) of the antagonist followed by an isotonic contraction (against resistance) of the agonist. Slow reversal–hold is the same sequence, with an isometric contraction at the end of the range. For the client who has difficulty reaching his or her mouth for oral hygiene because of weakness in the D_1 flexion pattern, the slow reversal procedure is as follows: an isotonic contraction against resistance in D_1 extension with the verbal command "Push down and out," followed by an isotonic contraction of D_1 flexion against resistance with the verbal command "Pull up and across." An increase or buildup of power in the agonist should be felt with each successive isotonic contraction. Slow reversal used in conjunction with repeated contractions could be applied to trunk movement patterns to help Leticia overcome her rigidity and improve the balance of antagonists. This sequence of techniques could also be used to increase Leticia's wrist range of motion and strength once her fracture is stable.

Stabilizing reversals are characterized by alternating isotonic contractions opposed by enough resistance to prevent motion. In practice, the therapist gives resistance to the client in one direction while asking the client to oppose the force, allowing no motion. Once the client is fully resisting the force, the therapist gradually moves the resistance in another direction. Each time the client is able to respond to the new resistance, the therapist moves the hand to resist a new direction, reversing directions as often as needed to achieve the client's stability. This technique is used to increase stability, balance, and muscle strength.

Rhythmic stabilization is used to increase stability by eliciting simultaneous isometric contractions of antagonistic muscle groups. Co-contraction results if the client is not allowed to relax. This technique requires repeated isometric contractions, leading to increased circulation or the tendency for the client to hold his or her breath, or both. Therefore rhythmic stabilization may be contraindicated for clients with cardiac involvement, and no more than three or four repetitions should be done at a time on any clients.

In rhythmic stabilization, manual contacts are applied on both agonist and antagonist muscles, with resistance given simultaneously. The client is asked to hold the contraction against graded resistance. Without allowing the client to relax, manual contacts are switched to opposite surfaces. Rhythmic stabilization is useful with clients lacking postural control because of ataxia or proximal weakness. Used intermittently during an activity requiring postural stability, such as meal preparation in standing posture, this technique enhances muscle balance, endurance, and control of movement. Rhythmic stabilization techniques were found to be effective in improving postural control and reducing pain for individuals who had chronic low back pain.[57]

Because these two stabilizing techniques can be superimposed on activity-based movements, they could be used to facilitate Leticia's ability to perform numerous daily activities. For example, rhythmic stabilization could be used to improve trunk endurance and stability when Leticia experiences fatigue while standing at the sink to do the dishes.

Relaxation Techniques

Relaxation techniques are an effective means of increasing ROM, particularly in the presence of pain or spasticity, which may be increased by passive stretch.

Contract-relax involves passive motion to the point of limitation in movement patterns. This is followed by an isotonic contraction of the antagonist pattern against maximal resistance, with only the rotational component of the diagonal movement allowed. This action is followed by relaxation, then by further passive movement into the agonistic pattern (e.g., contract-relax could involve passive motion to the point of limitation in D_2 flexion, which would be followed by an isotonic contraction of D_2 extension, then by further passive movement into D_2 flexion). This procedure is repeated at each point in the ROM in which limitation is thought to occur.[101] Contract-relax is used when no active range in the agonistic pattern is present. However, the ultimate goal is active movement through the full range. Therefore, once relaxation and increased ROM occur, active movement should be facilitated. The contract-relax (CR) technique has been demonstrated as an effective means to gain ROM when compared to passive stretch, but the mechanism underlying this technique is not clear.[67]

Hold-relax is performed in the same sequence as contract-relax but involves an isometric contraction (no movement allowed) of the antagonist, followed by relaxation and then active movement into the agonistic pattern. It has been recommended that the static contraction be held for 3 seconds to achieve the greatest improvement in ROM.[88] Because this technique involves an isometric contraction against resistance, it is particularly beneficial in the presence of pain or acute orthopedic conditions. For the client with reflex sympathetic dystrophy (RSD) who has pain with shoulder flexion, abduction, and external rotation, the therapist asks the client to hold against resistance in the D_2 extension pattern, then to initiate active movement into the D_2 flexion pattern. This technique is beneficial for the client with RSD during self-care activities such as shampooing hair and zipping a shirt in back.

Slow reversal-hold-relax begins with an isotonic contraction, followed by an isometric contraction, relaxation of the antagonistic pattern, and then active movement of the agonistic pattern. When the client has the ability to move the agonist actively, this technique is preferred. For example, to increase active elbow extension in the presence of tight elbow flexors, the therapist asks the client to perform D_1 flexion with elbow flexion as resistance is applied. When the ROM is complete, the client is asked to hold with an isometric contraction, followed immediately by relaxation. When the client relaxes, he or she moves actively into D_1 extension with elbow extension. This technique

THREADED CASE STUDY

Leticia, Part 2

To respond to the initial three questions at the beginning of this section, we need to review our assessment of Leticia. To determine the most effective movement patterns, we need to observe Leticia in her daily tasks, in addition to her performance of specific diagonal patterns and total patterns of movement. Techniques and procedures that best address Leticia's key deficits in motor control and rigidity should be selected. In addition to a focus on these key areas, special attention should be given to whether more mobility or stability is needed. Trunk ataxia would respond best to stabilizing techniques such as rhythmic stabilization, stabilizing reversals, and approximation. Rigidity would need mobilizing techniques such as slow reversal, slow reversal–hold, and repeated contractions. These techniques can be applied to clients during occupation-based activity.

The progression of intervention begins at the time of evaluation and considers the client's abilities as well as deficiencies. In Leticia's case, intervention will need to follow PNF principles. Intervention should initially address proximal control and start in lower developmental positions where she has the ability to perform coordinated movement. Once she has achieved more proximal stability, intervention can progress to work in higher developmental postures such as standing. Integrated into this progression of movement patterns and techniques are selected procedures that facilitate the desired motor response or activity performance.

helps increase elbow extension for such activities as reaching to lock the wheelchair brakes or picking up an object off the floor.

Rhythmic rotation is effective in decreasing spasticity and increasing ROM. The therapist passively moves the body part in the desired pattern. When the client feels tightness or restriction of movement, the therapist rotates the body part slowly and rhythmically in both directions. After the client relaxes, the therapist continues to move the body part into the newly available range. This technique prepares the paraplegic client with LE spasticity or clonus to put on a pair of pants. The technique is also effective in preparing for splint fabrication on a spastic extremity.

SECTION 2 SUMMARY

The PNF approach emphasizes the client's abilities and potential so that strengths assist weaker components. Strengths and deficiencies are assessed and addressed in intervention within total patterns of movement and posture. Carefully selected techniques are superimposed on these total patterns to enhance motor response and facilitate motor learning.

PNF uses multisensory input. The coordination and timing of sensory input are important in eliciting the desired response from the client. The client's performance should be monitored, and sensory input should be adjusted accordingly.

To use PNF effectively, the therapist must understand the developmental sequence and the components of normal movement. The therapist must learn the diagonal patterns and how they are used in ADL, must know when and how to use the techniques of facilitation and relaxation, and must be able to apply patterns and techniques of facilitation to OT evaluation and intervention. Attaining these skills requires observation and practice under the supervision of a therapist experienced in the PNF approach.

CASE STUDY

Sophia

Sophia, a 50-year-old who identifies as female (prefers use of the pronouns she/her/hers), was referred for occupational therapy (OT) services after a right cerebrovascular accident (CVA) resulting in left hemiplegia. Before the CVA she had a history of hypertension but otherwise good health. Referral to occupational therapy was made 3 days after onset of the CVA for evaluation and intervention in ADLs, visual perceptual skills, and left upper extremity function.

Assessment

Initial assessment revealed intact vital and related functions, such as the oral and facial musculature and swallowing. Voice production was good. Sophia had a tendency to hold her breath during activities, and subsequent decreased endurance was noted. Visual tracking was impaired, with an inability to scan past midline and apparent left-sided neglect.

Her head and neck were observed to be frequently rotated to the right and slightly flexed because of weak extensors. Her trunk was noted to be asymmetric in a sitting posture, with most of the weight supported on her right side. Sophia's posture was flexed because of weak extensors. Static sitting balance was fair and dynamic sitting balance was poor, with Sophia leaning forward and to the left.

Upon assessment, Sophia's right arm had normal sensation and strength, although motor planning was impaired with her right hand. Her left arm was essentially flaccid, with impaired light touch, pain, and proprioceptive sensation. Sophia complained of mild left glenohumeral pain during passive movement at the end ranges of shoulder abduction and flexion. Scapular instability was noted. No active movement could be elicited in her left arm.

Perceptual testing showed apraxia (especially during activities requiring crossing of the midline) and left-sided neglect. Sophia was alert and oriented, with a good attention span and memory. She was able to follow directions and carryover in tasks was adequate.

Sophia needed moderate assistance in ADLs and moderate to maximum assistance in transfers. Impaired balance and apraxia were the most limiting factors in performance of ADLs. She stated her immediate goal as being able to get herself ready in the morning with less time and effort.

Intervention Implementation

Following the cervicocaudal direction of development, alignment of her head and neck was the appropriate starting point for intervention. Left-sided awareness, sitting posture, and trunk balance were directly influenced by the position of her head and neck. Before the start of self-care activities, Sophia completed gentle ROM exercises of head and neck patterns of flexion and extension with rotation. To reinforce neck and trunk rotation to the left, the therapist was positioned to the left of Sophia. Clothing and hygiene articles were also placed to Sophia's left.

Lack of trunk control was another problem. During bending activities while seated, Sophia reported a fear of falling and was unsure of her ability to return to the upright seated position. Consequently, she had difficulty leaning forward to transfer from the wheelchair. The slow reversal–hold technique was used to reinforce trunk patterns during ADLs. For example, as a preparatory method to facilitate the trunk control needed for donning pants over legs, the therapist was positioned in front and to the left of Sophia. Manual contact was on the anterior aspect of either scapula at the glenohumeral joint. The therapist moved with Sophia and applied slight resistance as she leaned forward. At the end of the range, Sophia was instructed to hold with isometric contraction. Manual contact was then switched to the posterior surface of either scapula. Resistance was applied as Sophia returned to the upright position. The verbal command

was, "Look up and over your left shoulder." When she was upright, she was again instructed to hold with isometric contraction. In addition to reinforcing trunk control, this technique alleviated Sophia's fear of leaning forward because the therapist was in continual contact with her.

An indirect benefit of the flexion and extension patterns of the head, neck, and trunk was the reinforcement of respiration. Sophia was encouraged to inhale during extension and exhale during flexion. This approach eliminated Sophia's tendency to hold her breath when engaged in functional activities.

Intervention consisted of total patterns and techniques to facilitate proximal stability in the left UE and to provide proprioceptive input. Weight-bearing activities were selected because no active movement was available in her left arm. Sophia used her right UE in diagonal patterns to perform repetitive perceptual tasks, such as a mosaic tile design, paper-and-pencil activities, and board games. These activities were performed to include the side-lying posture on the left elbow, the prone posture on elbows, the side-sitting posture with weight on the left arm, and posture on all fours. To reinforce stability at the shoulder girdle, approximation and rhythmic stabilization were used with manual contact at both shoulders and then at the shoulder and pelvis. The performance of perceptual tasks in diagonals improved Sophia's motor planning, left-sided awareness, and trunk rotation.

Sophia was instructed in bilateral asymmetric chopping and lifting patterns to support her scapula and left UE in rolling and other activities. These patterns also enhanced left-sided awareness and trunk rotation. To facilitate scapular movement during chop and lift patterns, the therapist applied stretch to initiate movement, followed by the slow-reversal technique. In preparation for the lift pattern, manual contact was placed on the posterior surface of the scapula. Stretch was applied in a lengthened range. As Sophia initiated the lifting pattern, resistance was provided and maintained throughout the ROM. This procedure was repeated for the antagonistic or reverse-of-lift pattern, with manual contact switching to the anterior surface of the scapula.

About 3 to 4 weeks after the injury, Sophia was able to initiate left UE movement in synergy with a predominance of flexor tone. Weight-bearing activities and rhythmic rotation were helpful in normalizing tone, and both techniques were used with ADLs such as dressing and bathing. Wrist and finger extensions were facilitated in the D_1 extension and D_2 flexion patterns by using repeated contractions.

Outcomes

Reevaluation after 5 weeks of occupational therapy revealed increased endurance and ability to coordinate breathing with activity and consistency in crossing the midline during visual scanning activities. Sophia was able to turn her head and neck to the left without cues from the therapist. The fear of falling forward with bending had diminished, and she automatically turned her head to look up and over her left shoulder to reinforce assumption of the upright position. As trunk strength continued to improve, reinforcement with head and neck rotation was no longer necessary. Visual tracking alone, in the direction of movement, was sufficient to reinforce assumption of the upright position. Eventually, Sophia was able to achieve an upright position without apparent visual or head and neck reinforcement. Sitting balance improved with bilateral weight bearing through both hips. Shoulder pain decreased and scapular stability improved during weight-bearing activities. Sophia initiated left UE movement out of a flexor synergy pattern. Right UE motor planning was within functional limits for ADLs. Transfers and self-care required only minimal assistance, and cues were no longer needed for left UE awareness.

SECTION 3: NEURO-DEVELOPMENTAL TREATMENT APPROACH

Luis de Leon Arabit, with contributions from Julie McLaughlin Gray

CASE STUDY

Charlotte

Charlotte, a 69-year-old who identifies as female (prefers use of the pronouns of she/her/hers), sustained a left CVA with resultant right hemiplegia 4 months ago. She is able to move her right arm in a synergistic manner but does not have smooth coordinated movements. When she attempts to use her right arm as an assist for functional tasks, the movement of her arm is dominated by hypertonicity in flexor muscles and it is difficult for her to extend her elbow or open her hand to grasp objects. Charlotte is able to stand and walk but tends to maintain more weight on her left lower extremity and take small steps with her right. She is right hand dominant and is having difficulties completing both ADL and IADL tasks that require the use of both hands. In particular, Charlotte reports that it is difficult for her to cook meals and dress herself. Although she was instructed in one-hand dressing techniques, she reports that it is very time consuming and tiring to use these strategies. Charlotte reports that she misses not being able to paint, play the piano, or engage in gardening. She would like to improve the control of her right arm and hand.

Critical Thinking Questions

1. What additional information would be useful in designing an intervention plan to foster improved right hand function?
2. Which assessments would be useful to evaluate Charlotte's upper extremity function in relation to her occupational goals? How would the occupational therapist best evaluate Charlotte's upper extremity function in relation to her occupational goals?
3. What intervention would support the best outcomes to meet the client's goals?
4. Through skilled analysis of client factors and performance skills, what client abilities can be fostered during intervention and used to support the client's engagement in occupations?

DEFINITION OF NEURO-DEVELOPMENTAL TREATMENT

Neuro-Developmental Treatment (NDT) is a clinical practice model used by occupational, physical, and speech and language therapists who work with people with motor control problems due to a stroke, traumatic brain injury, cerebral palsy, and other related neurological disorders.[8] NDT is defined as a holistic and interdisciplinary clinical practice model informed by current and evolving research that emphasizes individualized therapeutic handling based on movement analysis for habilitation and rehabilitation of individuals with neurological pathophysiology. The International Classification of Functioning, Disability and Health (ICF) model is incorporated by the therapist in a problem-solving approach to assess activity and participation to identify and prioritize relevant integrities and impairments as a basis for establishing achievable outcomes with clients and caregivers. An in-depth knowledge of the human movement system, including the understanding of typical and atypical development, and expertise in analyzing postural control, movement, activity, and

participation throughout the lifespan, form the basis for examination, evaluation, and intervention using an NDT approach. Therapeutic handling, used during evaluation and intervention, consists of tactile cues and touch and touch in a dynamic and reciprocal interaction between the client and therapist for activating optimal sensorimotor processing, task performance, and skill acquisition to enable participation in meaningful activities.[8]

Neuro-Developmental Treatment Practice Model

The NDT Practice Model (Fig. 32.16) illustrates the interconnectedness of communication, observation, thinking, analysis, and actions that can move in any direction as the clinician and client interact.[91] It depicts how therapists who use the NDT philosophy gather, synthesize, and analyze information relevant to support their clients. Information gathering, examination, evaluation and intervention are components of practice that are interwoven and connected processes rather than discrete and separate ones. The partnership and communication between the client, family/caregiver and the therapist is an essential ongoing process with each entity responsible toward effective and meaningful results. The NDT Practice Model is divided into four sections: *Information Gathering, Examination, Evaluation, and Intervention.*

Information gathering, in the NDT Practice Model, often begins before meeting with the client through a review of information provided by other members of the team or significant others in the client's life. If this is not possible, this process begins during the initial meeting among the therapist, the client, and family/caregiver. Listening carefully and intently to the client and family's verbal and nonverbal communication helps develop rapport and provides the therapist information that meets the NDT philosophy of individualized care. Therapists deepen their understanding of the client's daily life routines that takes into consideration the environmental conditions where occupations are performed, how they are performed, and the degree of assistance or support that is needed.

The process of *examination* in the NDT Practice Model emphasizes learning the specific details regarding how the client participates in daily occupations, taking into consideration current abilities as well as limitations. The therapist observes the client's occupational participation capacities and restrictions/limitations and records and assesses body structures and functions, noting integrity and impairments. Based on the results from skilled observation, the therapist hypothesizes about the origins of the impairments caused by body system interactions such as movement and posture. Therapists who practice NDT acknowledge that functional abilities are shaped by the client's past and that the future functioning depends on several variables. The client's progress is influenced by how successfully the client, family, and the team can build on the client's abilities while intervening to improve current skills.[91]

The process of *evaluation* in the NDT Practice Model focuses on analysis and problem solving. The evaluation process is where the therapist categorizes and prioritizes the information gathered, analyzes the relationships of human functioning and contextual factors using the ICF model with the addition of analysis of the client's movement and posture.

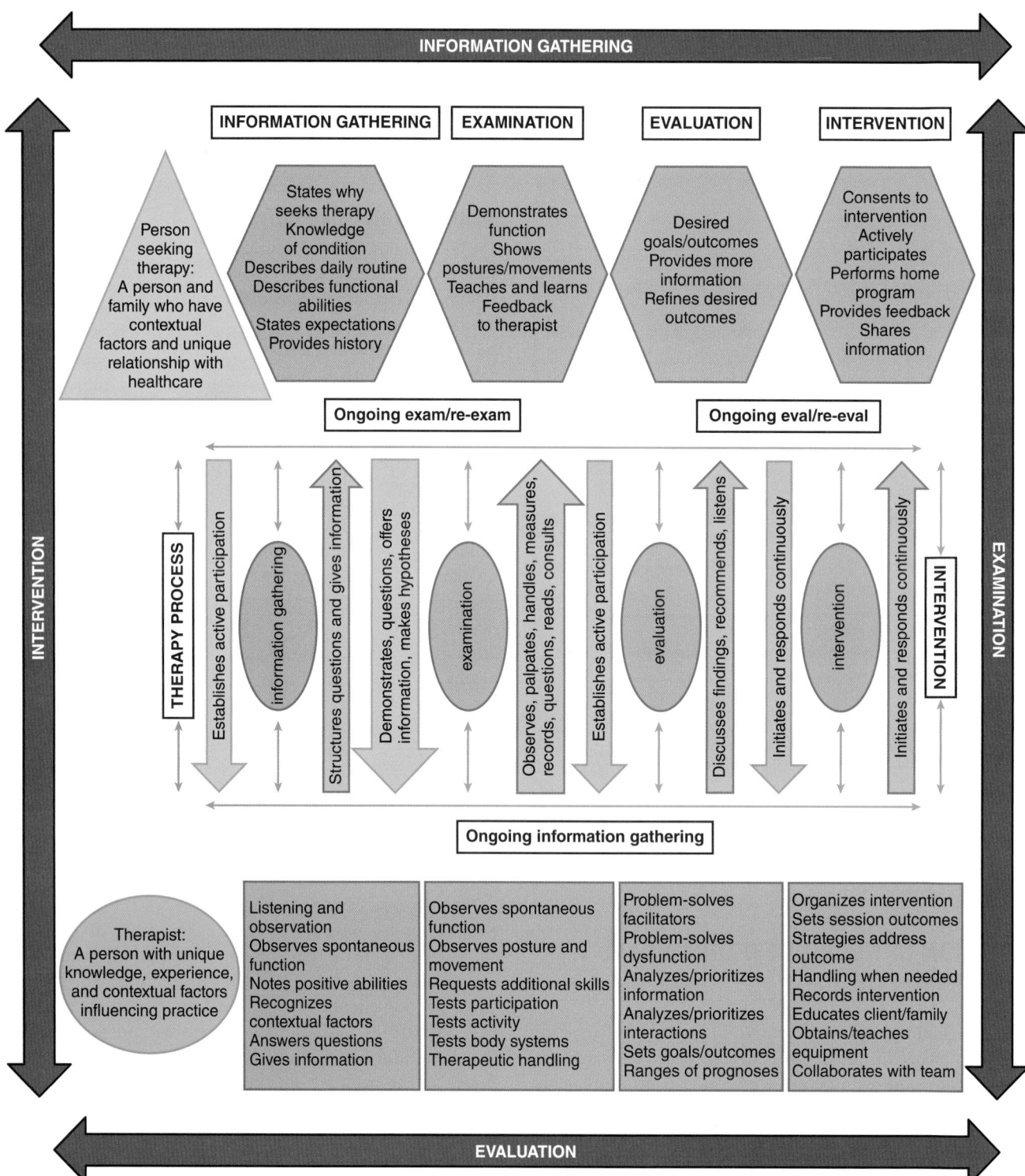

Fig. 32.16 The NDT Practice Model. (Reprinted with Permission granted by Thieme Group, Stuttgart, Germany.)

The *intervention* process of the NDT Practice Model is organized around a functional outcome, and all sessions aim to move toward multiple functional outcomes identified by the client. The intervention process is built using a collaborative approach with the client, the family/significant others, and the therapist. All parties are involved in the initiation of services, developing goals with intended outcomes, and assessing the response to the intervention. The therapist plans the intervention in collaboration with the client

and the family. There is a need for ongoing communication among all parties about the client's health conditions, changes in participation and engagement in activities, the results of the individually designed home programs, any team members' communication reports, and what the client and family desires to focus on in the next few sessions. The therapist addresses the impairments that interfere with the client's meaningful engagement in occupations using intervention strategies that include therapeutic handling skills. The term *handling techniques* refers to the therapist's ability to detect changes in the client's movement while simultaneously providing support for efficient movement. These techniques require the therapist to provide physical contact with hands, either intermittent or sustained, typically placed on the client's arm/hand, leg/foot, or the client's trunk. This physical contact is used as a support to help the client move more efficiently. Handling techniques are used to assess the responses to intervention and to provide guidance and assistance to participation and engagement in occupations, movements and postures, body structures, and functions across various contexts. Through handling techniques, therapists continuously update and monitor the intervention by observing client responses, changes in behavior and any alterations in function.

Handling is a highly developed assessment and intervention skill taught in NDT educational courses.[91] Handling involves the therapist's ability to perceive discrete sensorimotor responses; assist the client to initiate, sustain, and terminate muscle activity; assist the client to use more effective postures and movement synergies; assist the client to grade movement appropriately from powerful and ballistic to smooth and sustained as needed; and the ability to practice repetitive movements for strengthening, perceptual accuracy, and motor learning.[91] The *key points of control* is the term used in referring to the therapist's hand placement to offer the client the needed support and guidance. The key points of control in handling are modified as the therapist senses or perceives any changes in the client's movements and posture. The therapist makes the determination whether handling is to be provided in a continuous manner or intermittently during an intervention.

HISTORICAL CONTEXT OF THE NEURO-DEVELOPMENTAL TREATMENT APPROACH

Neuro-Developmental Treatment (NDT), as it is currently referred to in the United States, originally began as the "Bobath concept," a treatment approach developed by Berta and Karel Bobath in the 1940s for individuals with neurological disorders of movement and posture. Berta Bobath received her early training as a remedial gymnast at the Anna Herrmann School of gymnastics in Germany, where she stayed on as an instructor of gymnastics upon graduation.[87] She described the focus of her educational program at Anna Herrmann:

> We were taught about the analysis of normal movements and various ways of relaxation. We learned to feel and evaluate degrees of relaxation not only on tight muscles but its effect on the strength and activity of their antagonists. This was done by a special way of handling a person, inducing movements in response to being moved.

In the 1930s, when the Nazis came to power in Germany, Berta Bobath lost her job as a gymnastics instructor; the school would not retain a Jewish teacher. She subsequently moved to London, eventually working at the Princess Louise Hospital.

Based on her background and skills in analyzing normal movement, Berta Bobath was repeatedly asked to see special cases of both children with cerebral palsy (CP) and adults with hemiplegia. At the time, it was assumed that individuals with upper motor neuron (UMN) lesions could not recover from their motor deficits. Because of her background in dance, her training in posture and the analysis of movement, and likely also her "heretical or eccentric"[93] views, Berta Bobath did not ascribe to this belief. She began by using her hands and body to reposition these clients into neutral and symmetric alignment. She examined the impact of her positioning and handling on their muscle tone and ability to move. Berta found that it was possible to change the abnormal muscle tone in individuals who had a stroke or CP.[8–10,12,15,16,28] This was contrary to the medical understanding of the time that CNS damage produced irreversible changes in posture and motor control.[17] She described the basis of her approach as "the inhibition of released and exaggerated abnormal reflex action, the counteraction of abnormal patterns, and the facilitation of more normal automatic voluntary movements."[87]

After success with her techniques, Berta ultimately studied to become a physiotherapist and passed the examination in 1950. Dr. Karel Bobath, Berta's husband and a psychiatrist, wrote the theoretical explanations for his wife's clinical findings and made recommendations based on his readings and understanding of how she could improve her clinical practice. The revised clinical practice led to more questions and additional exploration of the literature that again modified the treatment approach.[8] Together, Berta and Karel Bobath are credited with the development of the Bobath concept and the NDT approach. They established the first Bobath Centre in London in 1951 and soon began training other physiotherapists on her approach to the treatment of children with cerebral palsy and adults with hemiplegia. Today, courses on this approach are taught internationally to occupational and physical therapists, speech and language pathologists (SLPs), and, in some countries, nurses, physicians, and teachers.[45] Information regarding specialized certification and continuing education courses in the United States can be found at the Neuro-Developmental Treatment Association (NDTA) website: http://www.ndta.org.

Given the period when NDT was developed, several contemporary authors described NDT as a treatment approach based on a hierarchical view of the nervous system. Although the accepted view of the nervous system when the NDT approach began reflected a hierarchical model, it does not appear true, or consistent with the writings of the Bobaths and other historians. The NDT approach was *not originally based on* a hierarchical perspective. The approach was based on Berta Bobath's experiences—her skilled observations of alignment, posture, and movement—and she achieved remarkable results in helping clients improve functional movement is spite of having damage to upper motor neurons. The gains noted would not be considered possible using a hierarchical model. The results were then interpreted using the reflex-hierarchical model, which, at that time, was the proposed explanation of how the CNS was organized.[78,87] This inductive sequence, from observations to theory development, is discussed in many historical accounts of the approach. Although dynamic models of central nervous system function and specifically motor control did not exist at the time, contemporary dynamic perspectives support Berta Bobath's original observations and experiences more accurately than reflex-hierarchical models. Her handling resulted in changes in tone and movement capacity that were unlikely (or could not have resulted) if the client's tone and movement patterns were exclusively reflexive in nature. Her handling tapped into the dynamic system influencing motor output that is reflected in contemporary models of motor control.[89]

Whether the original NDT approach was founded upon a reflex-hierarchical perspective or simply explained in terms of that model accepted at that time, it was clearly suggested as a "living concept" from its inception[45]; theoretical and intervention concepts were intended as "working hypotheses." Dr. Bobath used this terminology to stress the need for the approach to change across time based on changes in the populations served, the healthcare system, new clinical experiences, and evidence from scientific research.[8] Because the approach was grounded in an understanding of and appreciation for normal movement rather than pathological condition, Dr. Bobath emphasized that NDT would continue to evolve as the understanding of normal movement advances through new discoveries and theory development. The Bobath's discoveries were formalized in their writings, and the underpinnings of the approach were outlined in descriptions of an overall philosophy, theoretical assumptions, and specific recommendations for the practice of NDT.[8]

BERTA BOBATH'S DEVELOPING THEORY: ORIGINAL CONCEPTS AND CHANGES OVER TIME

When Berta Bobath began working with people with UMN lesions, in the 1950s, most people believed that these individuals would not recover and practices reflected this perspective. Individuals were either not provided rehabilitation services or were provided a compensatory approach exclusively. Any remedial intervention was from an orthopedic frame of reference—primarily stretching and strengthening—and, therefore, did not address the neurological basis underlying the movement problems.[45,78] Contrary to these views and practices and related to her clinical observations and experiences, Berta Bobath thought these individuals could regain control of movement, given the right opportunities.

Part of the NDT philosophy is *a belief in recovery*, in the client's potential. This belief was coupled with a belief in the influence that normal movement could have on a person's quality of life. In the foreword to Bobath's first book,[11] Dr. P.W. Nathan eloquently discussed some of the philosophical underpinnings of the approach, the essence of which remain today:

Whether the doctor knows he is doing so or not, he chooses either a policy of persuading the client to use the hemiplegic limbs and re-train his affected side, or else a policy of encouraging the client to neglect the hemiplegic side and to use the unaffected side for all tasks previously done by the limbs of both sides. The choice affects only the upper limb and the general posture of the client. There is no choice about the lower limb; the client has to learn to use it. That being so, it is best for him to learn to use it properly. . . . If he learns to retrain his hemiplegic side, he returns to life.

Philosophical Tenets of Neuro-Developmental Treatment

The NDT approach is now widely described as a problem-solving method for restoring movement and participation for individuals with UMN lesions, specifically cerebral palsy and hemiplegia.[45] The approach is aimed at restoration of function through identifying and correcting underlying impairments that interfere with movement and participation in everyday activities. The emphasis is on regaining normal movement and postural control, and quality of movement in general. Compensations are discouraged.[39] Clinicians studying the approach are instructed in Berta Bobath's belief in the potential of the hemiplegic side to recover movement and her emphasis on addressing the whole body and the whole person.[9] According to Tallis,[93] the "fundamental ethos of Bobath [remains today as] . . . the client as partner, rehabilitation tailored to the client's current situation, and rehabilitation as a 24/7 activity." In 2002, the NDTA published *Neuro-Developmental Treatment Approach: Theoretical Foundations and Principles of Clinical Practice*, which updated the theoretical basis of NDT practice. In addition, the first textbook on NDT, *Neuro-Developmental Treatment: A Guide to Clinical Practice*, was published in 2016.

Although the basic principles of collaborative intervention remain the same, ideas regarding the nature of the client's movement deficits and how movement is controlled and learned have evolved over time in response to scientific advances. Primary changes to the approach can be tied to discoveries in neuroscience and motor learning research, specifically a dynamic and interactive understanding of the way in which movement is controlled and executed, and feedback is used. Intervention is no longer directed at reducing spasticity; merely reducing spasticity will not foster improvements in the client's motor control.[14,39] However, there appear to be other aspects of hypertonicity that are nonneural, such as changes in muscle length (shortening or contractures), joint alignment, and recruitment patterns, that tend to be amenable to handling strategies. Motor output is organized around task goals, and therefore motor skills are practiced in function as much as possible. Errors are required for motor learning, as is active participation on the part of the client; therefore, passive movement of the client is minimized and handling is graded to ensure increasing autonomy on the part of the client (Fig. 32.17).

NDT continues to accumulate evidence that supports its effectiveness regardless of age or diagnosis.[8] In 2012, Franki and colleagues[36,37] found evidence that NDT was effective in making positive changes in all domains described in the International Classification of Functioning, Disability and Health (ICF) developed by the World Health Organization (WHO). NDT uses a holistic and client-centered approach by viewing clients as unique individuals with various needs and distinct occupational histories. A key philosophical tenet of NDT is to focus on the whole person in intervention planning and implementation as a key element at every stage of the evaluation and intervention process. There is also increasing emphasis on addressing and improving the client's participation in functional activities by addressing specific impairments in the client's posture and

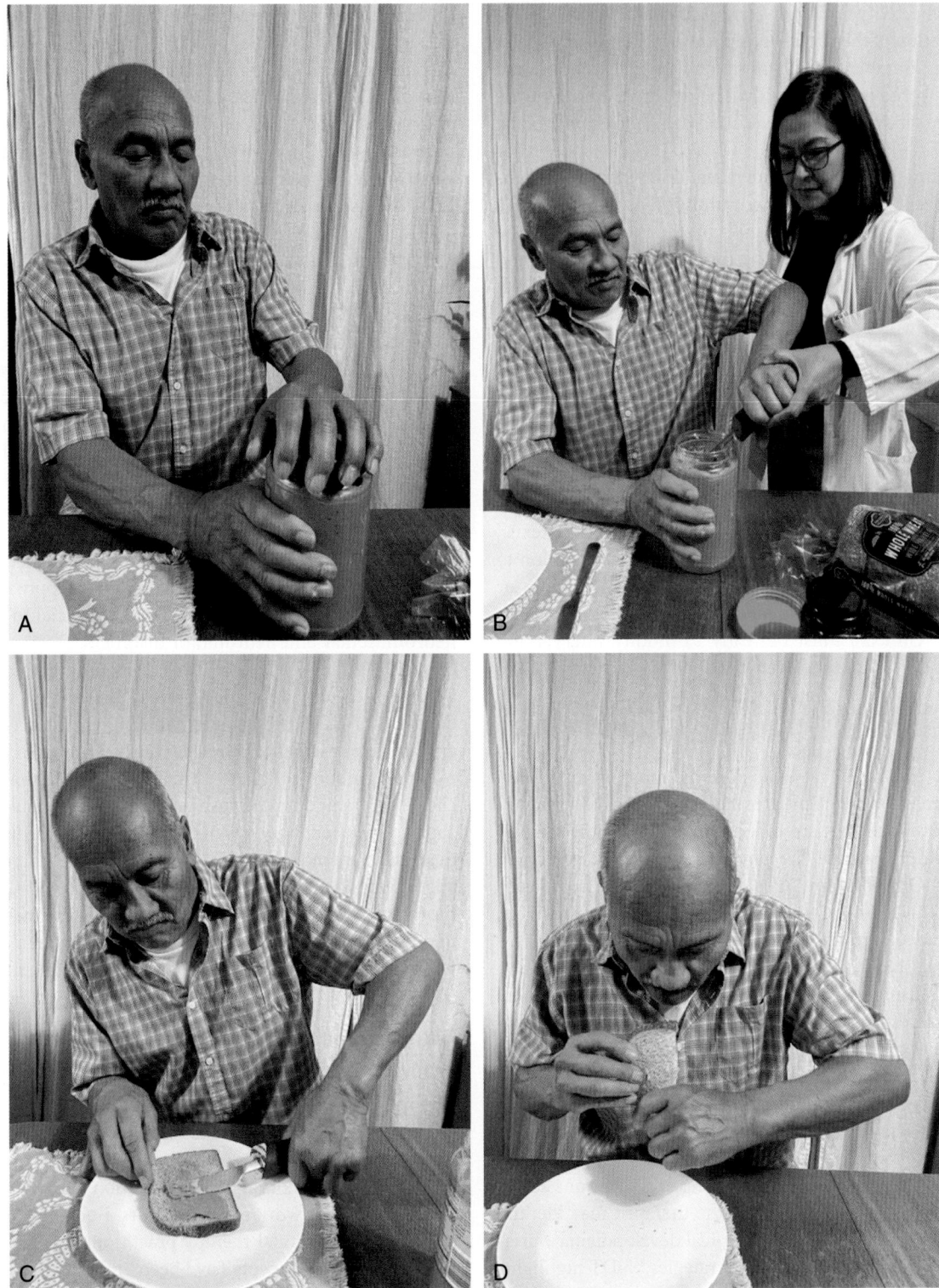

Fig. 32.17 Meal preparation—making a sandwich. (A) Opening a jar of peanut butter. (B) Occupational therapist facilitating (handling) client's left arm/hand to scoop peanut butter from the jar using an adapted knife. (C) Spreading peanut butter on the bread. (D) Eating the peanut butter sandwich using both hands. (Photographs courtesy Marie Arabit-Ball, OTR/L.)

movement, as well as individual body system impairments. NDT addresses the impairments and builds on the client's strengths. Capitalizing on this perspective, the NDT-educated therapist anticipates and takes advantage of those strengths in every client

and develops and fosters an intervention plan of care based on those strengths. NDT also believes in individualizing interventions and therefore requires a problem-solving process with ongoing evaluation and modification of the intervention based on the client's activity limitations and participation restrictions. Individualization of the client's treatment is built into all aspects of evaluation; intervention planning and implementation and are modified based on the individual being served, the clinician providing the services, and all the contextual factors influencing the case.[8]

While taking into account individual differences in designing the intervention plan, another philosophical tenet of NDT simultaneously considers the client's past, present, and future state. The importance of considering the past, present, and future state of the client in NDT is mainly based on the belief that the client is a dynamic, evolving, and ever-changing entity. This means the client's personal history, their immediate concerns and their future plans can have a significant influence and bearing in the manner of how the therapist will appropriately choose to implement NDT intervention strategies. It is therefore important for occupational therapists to understand the client's occupational profile. The occupational profile is a summary of the client's occupational history and experiences, patterns of daily living, interests, values, needs, and relevant contexts.[3] The occupational profile provides the therapist a foundation to understand the client's needs and serves as a guide to alter or adapt the NDT intervention to meet the client's evolving needs. In NDT, the clinician must be ready to modify intervention based on the day-to-day and even moment-to-moment changes in the client's abilities.[8] Similarly, the person's hopes, dreams, and aspirations for the future will change the overall plan and the specific interventions used.[8]

NDT also promotes that to achieve the most optimal functional outcomes for the client, it is necessary to have a team of service professionals that are called into action. These team of service providers include the physician, nurses, psychiatrist, psychologist, OTs, PTs, and SLPs, to name a few. Also considered part of this team are the client, the family, and caregivers, who are included as much as possible in every practicable manner in the assessment, planning, and intervention process.

Therapists using the NDT Practice Model recognize there are general patterns of skill acquisition during typical development and maturation.[8] The Bobaths originally applied a rigid approach in the development of intervention plans based on sequential acquisition of motor skills. This premise has since shifted with therapists examining the emergence or loss of functional activities based on the relationships of posture and movement and the body system structures and functions across the lifespan.[8] Through examination, the therapist may identify the differences in individuals with typical developmental variations and those with atypical motor strategies.[8] NDT highlights the analysis of typical movement and its progression across the life span to support the analysis of why individuals with various neurological conditions move the way they do while engaged in an occupation or activity.[7]

Another philosophical tenet of NDT is the importance of active carryover and transition of therapeutic functional activities into real daily life conditions and situations. This can be achieved by engaging the client in a variety of personal and environmental contexts, such as in the home, work, community, and recreational spaces. Achieving performance standards

during therapy is worthwhile but does not have the same value as promoting functional activities in real-life situations or in increasing participation in various environments.[8] Based on this principle, NDT sessions should incorporate therapeutic activities and occupations that are relevant to the client. The purpose is not to perform a series of exercises, but to support clients in real-life occupations or activities, such as how clients dress themselves or sit at the table or how parents carry a child. The focus of NDT is to help the person achieve more efficient and effective movement to enhance function and minimize impairment.[8]

The NDT approach uses therapeutic handling techniques to support a person in achieving effective and efficient movement, which is a significant element of the intervention process. A central NDT philosophical tenet is that handling is a natural method to help others learn the optimal or necessary postures and movements for specific functional activities.[8] This tenet assumes that physical guidance, with active participation between the person and therapist, is a part of human relationships in teaching and learning situations that can support individuals who have disorders of posture and movement.[8] What separates NDT from other rehabilitative approaches is the principle that therapeutic handling is beneficial to clients with neuromuscular and neuromotor disorders. During therapeutic handling, the client is at all times encouraged to actively participate in the activity or occupation. The client is not a passive recipient of NDT therapeutic handling but rather an engaged and active participant in the intervention process. The therapist may provide subtle therapeutic handling cues in the trunk of the client while standing to brush teeth in front of a sink to facilitate shifting the client's body weight from one side to the other or to make adjustments anteriorly or posteriorly to improve postural alignment. The clinician practicing within the NDT framework monitors the response to the handling and systematically works to reduce the amount of handling provided to the person to foster greater independence and therefore a better quality of life.[8]

The Practice of Neuro-Developmental Treatment From An Occupational Therapy Lens

The profession of occupational therapy and the practice of NDT are a perfect match in the rehabilitation of neurological impairments because they focus on improving ability to function while promoting and encouraging participation in the client's desired occupations. The work of Dr. and Mrs. Bobath were first introduced to occupational therapy practitioners in the 1960s, and since then their concepts have been embraced by the OT profession worldwide.[7] The Bobaths believed in the importance of an interdisciplinary approach to intervention to provide best practice and care to the client. The foreword of Egger's book, *Occupational Therapy in the Treatment of Adult Hemiplegia*, written by Karel and Berta Bobath states, "It requires teamwork and the close collaboration of physiotherapists, speech therapists and occupational therapists. We have long awaited this book, which meets a need in the area of total management by relating physiotherapy and occupational therapy. It will be of special value to occupational therapists who are working in hospitals where each member of the team follows the same concept and principles."[7]

An American OT, Judy Murray, who resided in London and had conversations with the Bobaths, merged the concepts of activities of daily living (ADLs), play, vision, sensory, perceptual, and adaptive equipment in the NDT treatment approach.[7] Mecthild Rast, an NDTA-certified OT instructor, also helped shape the original theory by incorporating the importance of upper extremity performance.[7] The profession of occupational therapy has influenced, and continues to influence, the NDT curriculum, accentuating the need for an interdisciplinary team approach to effectively serve the needs of the client.[7]

Because NDT uses a dynamic therapeutic handling approach, this process guides the occupational therapist in the evaluation and intervention of persons with neurological deficits. Guided by the WHO's International Classification of Functioning, Disability and Health (ICF), an occupational therapist using the NDT Practice Model will examine body functions and structure, and the domains of activity and participation, identifying which tasks the individual has not yet learned to do or is no longer able to accomplish.[7] Through examination, the occupational therapist is able to identify deficits within the domains of motor and body structure such as cognitive, perceptual, neuromotor, and sensory systems that may interfere with the client's engagement in desired occupations.

Activity or Task Analysis

Occupational therapists are professional experts in analyzing components of occupational tasks or activities using task analysis, which also includes the environment. Through analysis of inherent specific subtasks, the NDT-trained/educated occupational therapist will be able to judiciously select therapeutic activities and occupations to avoid the likelihood of excessive effort on the part of the client, resulting in atypical muscle substitution with inefficient strategies for posture and movement. For example, during the intervention process with persons with neurological impairments, the subtask of cutting vegetables within the occupation of meal preparation may provide insight on how an occupational therapist may be able to alter, adjust, or adapt the environment (height of counter surfaces, position of the client, the textures of the vegetables being cut). During the intervention process, the occupational therapist is providing therapeutic handling to the client's postural system while also continuing to evaluate and modify the environment and the task itself, which can either facilitate or inhibit movement patterns to develop independent motor control for occupational performance. It is important for the therapist to provide the "just right" challenge within the selected or chosen activity with opportunities for repetition as well as carryover in various environmental contexts capitalizing on the client's newly learned movements. The just right challenge means an optimal fit between the demands of the occupation and the skills of the person necessary for initial and sustained engagement in occupation.[105]

Sensory Processing for Occupational Performance

Occupational therapists are also experts in understanding the importance and influences of sensory processing on posture and movement during occupational performance. For persons with neurological challenges, any disturbance in sensory information processing can contribute to substantial motor control deficits, which gives rise to maladaptive posture and movement. Disorders of the sensory processing systems may result in challenges with anticipatory posture and movements as well as sensory feedback from movements necessary for functional performance.[7]

The processing of tactile, proprioceptive and vestibular sensations at various levels sends signals throughout the body's nervous system and contributes to the client's perception, movement, cognition, and emotion. Reactions of clients may range from either no response to slight response or hypersensitivity to sensory input. For example, a client with stroke may exhibit diminished proprioceptive awareness, which may delay participation in desired occupations and impede motor learning. When there is limited appreciation of a body part related to the body position, the client's capacity and willingness to engage in their environment may be compromised.

During NDT handling techniques, the occupational therapist must be sensitive to the individual responses of clients and have knowledge to help modulate sensory processing issues to prepare for function. Therapists must pay close attention to the amount of pressure provided during handling, minimizing the speed and frequency with which they change key points of control while monitoring the individual's stress response to handling.[7] Deliberate and mindful provision of deep-pressure touch to an individual's body is typically perceived as a calming and organizing stimulus.[7] Interchangeably, clients also may have minimal to no response to the tactile stimulation provided by the therapist. Clients who are unable to perceive or respond to tactile and vestibular stimuli may seek touch and movement opportunities to engage with the environment. For example, clients with TBI may experience sensory deficits on one part of their body and may not use that body part in functional activities, which affects muscle activation and initiation of the movement.

Therefore, activities that provide tactile sensory experiences to the client, which are either bilateral or bimanual, are highly encouraged to enhance the tactile sensory system, increase body awareness, and provide feedback for motor control. Tasks such as kneading dough to make pizza (Fig. 32.18), rolling a pie crust, making tortillas, braiding hair, playing mahjong, sewing, knitting, or playing a card game are all excellent activities that can be introduced.

Proprioceptive and vestibular processing are also frequently altered by neuropathology, affecting motor control.[7] Information about direction, force and speed of movement sends signals to muscles responsible for postural control to respond appropriately to shifting posture to retain balance. Clients who are hypersensitive to vestibular stimulation can feel dizzy, which may effectively process the sensation of position in space, which challenges their vestibular system against gravitational forces. If not addressed during NDT intervention, this hypersensitivity can lead to disruptions to the client's ability to learn and experience more efficient and effective movement strategies. Occupational therapists typically label this type

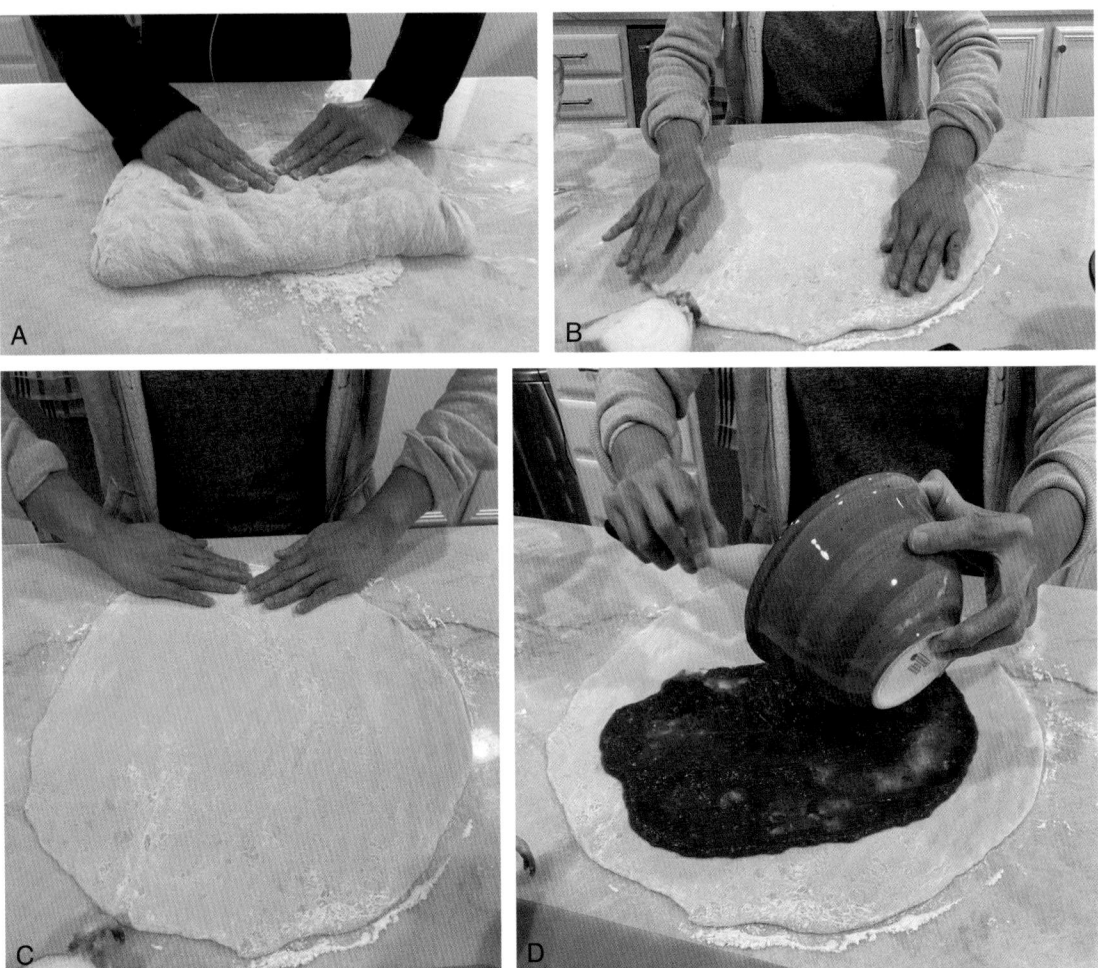

Fig. 32.18 Kneading dough to make pizza requires bimanual and bilateral coordination while providing tactile sensory experiences to increase body awareness and feedback for motor control.

of sensory processing challenge gravitational insecurity.[6,7] An individual experiencing gravitational insecurity will feel uneasy and frightened when they move off a supporting surface, resulting in a tense body, trying to guard their position to offset their feelings or sensation of falling. In individuals with neuropathology who are experiencing impairments in the sensory vestibular system, atypical movement patterns can develop because of the fear of falling or the lack of midline orientation.

The occupational therapist must evaluate sensory sensitivity by identifying specific movements that produce reports of dizziness by the client. Vestibular and balance problems do not need to disappear before initiating NDT intervention. The client with a neurological impairment such as a stroke can experience fear of falling either forward or backward most especially during the initial stages of acute recovery. This often is exhibited in a compensatory manner of an atypical movement pattern of leaning to one side of the body or pushing backward to find their center of gravity. Such occurrence can result in a postural bias, in which the client favors either the affected or unaffected limb depending on the area of the lesion caused by the stroke. Therefore, the NDT-educated occupational therapist may provide support, using their own body, to facilitate the client's weight shifting/bearing. An example of this is when the client

is sitting on a couch and attempts to stand up from the couch using only one side of the body. To improve the safety and efficiency of moving from sit to stand, the occupational therapist sits next to the client on the more involved side. The occupational therapist provides support to the client to assume and remain in appropriate alignment while sitting on the couch and then supports this alignment while both the client and occupational therapist move from sitting to standing.

Sensory input from the somatosensory systems converges with visual and auditory information at varying levels throughout the central nervous system, increasing integration and perception in preparation for action.[7] The visual and vestibular system provides an excellent partnership and works collaboratively to stabilize visual gaze, maintain a stable visual horizon, and orient the eyes toward a target. Because of the integrated nature of interaction of these two systems, deficits in either system can change the function of their partnership.

The vestibular system has the job of interpreting the orientation of the head and body in relation to gravitational forces so that the individual can orient the body to what is observed through the visual system.[7,27] Occupational performance is influenced by the interaction of the visual system with posture and movement.

USING NEURO-DEVELOPMENTAL TREATMENT PRACTICE MODEL TO RESTORE PARTICIPATION IN OCCUPATION

There has been a fair amount of controversy in the literature not only about the efficacy of NDT, which is addressed in the next section, but also about the approach.[29,63,64] Given the dynamic and evolving changes in the NDT approach over time, questions arise as to which aspects of the approach have remained constant. What are the current NDT strategies used to promote recovery of functional movement and therefore participation in occupation? What makes something NDT versus an entirely new approach to intervention? Because NDT has changed over time, other approaches have evolved from NDT. Additionally, NDT is often used in combination with other approaches, making it challenging to specify exactly which specific strategies are NDT. Physiotherapists who use the Bobath concept were surveyed and agreed that the following interventions are definitely or probably part of the NDT approach: facilitation, mobilization, practicing motor skills of certain activities, practicing activities themselves, and teaching caregivers how to position the client.[97] Based on a review of the literature, the content of NDTA-approved courses (http://www.ndta.org), and information from the most recent NDT textbook, *Neuro-Developmental Treatment: A Guide to Clinical Practice* (2016), the next section discusses the contemporary approach using NDT and the components of the NDT Practice Model.

The NDT Practice Model can readily be incorporated into the practice of occupational therapy and reflects the ongoing interrelationships of communicating, observing, thinking, analyzing, and actions that can possibly change or shift in various directions as the therapist, client, and family interact. The processes of information gathering, examination, evaluation, and intervention are components of the NDT Practice Model that are interconnected with each other rather than in isolation. When providing service using the NDT practice model, these processes occur in every session at any given time. Occupational therapists gather information, examine and evaluate the client's occupational performance, and design and implement an intervention plan to address problems of motor control and functional movement related to occupational performance. The NDT Practice Model can be used in concert with other theoretical models to provide a comprehensive occupational therapy program. It also should be combined, as appropriate, with other interventions supported by the best available contemporary research, to effectively manage the client's needs and responses.

The following are important considerations in each process of information gathering, examination, evaluation, and intervention as part of the NDT Practice Model.

Information Gathering

An occupational therapist, using the NDT Practice Model, begins with a client's occupational profile and history interview as part of information gathering. During information gathering, therapists express the belief that people with disabilities and those with impaired functions have value and worth. This also includes the knowledge of the positive influence of therapeutic interventions to support a client's engagement in meaningful occupations. Therapists must be able to build trust so the client/family can feel comfortable expressing their concerns, needs, and goals. Additionally, therapists must be able to establish good communication with the client/family in all aspects of care, especially encouraging the client/family to take the lead during the intervention planning and implementation. In Charlotte's case, we were able to gather information in her occupational profile about her desire to paint, play the piano, and engage in gardening activities. Charlotte's goals provide the therapist with valuable information that can be used as part of the NDT process.

Examination

Grounded in the occupational profile and the client's goals, the therapist would then observe and analyze the client's performance in a variety of client-selected occupations. This examination also considers the client's ability to function and perform desired occupations in the future. During the examination process, the therapist is able to streamline and tailor the examination based on the initial interview, occupational profile, and observations made during the information gathering process. Therapists must possess knowledge of effective and ineffective postural control and movement strategies, body system integrities, and impairments. Therapists must know how and why multiple systems develop compensatory responses and the impact of handling skills and key points of control on function, posture, and movement. In Charlotte's case, the therapist is able to examine and use handling skills to determine Charlotte's abilities for postural control, alignment, and movement integrities during performance of her chosen occupations as gleaned from the occupational profile.

Evaluation

The evaluation process of the NDT Practice Model emphasizes analysis and problem solving, in which the therapist works to categorize and prioritize all of the information gathered. The therapist analyzes the relationships among the domains of human functioning and contextual factors using the ICF with the added analysis of postures and movements. The therapist records hypotheses regarding these relationships, leading to a prognosis of a range of outcomes. Based on the NDT Practice Model, the evaluation includes not only the client's level of assistance and the amount of movement present, but also of the *quality* of their movement and postural control. As the therapist, client, and the entire team work and interact collaboratively, these predictions can be either revised or refined further to suit the client's needs. The therapist should summarize and prioritize the client/family's needs and views of participation and activity limitations according to its importance in the lives of the client/family. During evaluation, the therapist analyzes the relationship among participation, activity, and body system integrities, and impairments, which includes effective and ineffective postures and movements. A plan of care must be developed and included in the evaluation that identifies specific intervention strategies, postures and movements that need to be addressed, occupations or activities to be practiced, and any equipment that may be needed. The plan of care organizes the hypotheses generated during the information gathering and examination process to address specific causes of participation restrictions and activity limitations. Specifically, the clinician would evaluate the following:

1. The client's ability to maintain postural alignment required for the occupation. Consider Charlotte and her alignment when standing; the majority of her weight is shifted to her left leg, and her right arm predominantly exhibits flexion hypertonicity.
2. The "normal" or typical motor performance skills required for the tasks or activities that will be addressed. NDT-educated therapists analyze movement in terms of the whole body and the stability-mobility relationships between body segments in a task.
3. The client's alignment and movement while performing basic motor skills necessary in everyday activity such as reaching, sit-to-stand, and transferring, as well as during occupational performance tasks.
4. Underlying impairments that are contributing to movement dysfunction. Ryerson and Levit[84] outlined the four primary impairments resulting from CNS lesions as "changes in muscle strength, muscle tone, and muscle activation, and changes in sensory processing." It is these impairments that result in compensatory movements observed after CNS lesion and, without intervention, often result in secondary impairments such as "changes in orthopedic alignment and mobility, changes in muscle and tissue length, edema, and pain." Impairments are typically assessed during functional activity, through observation, handling, and the client/family's subjective report. A common method for assessing tone is *placing*, in which the therapist guides the limb in space and asks the client to hold against gravity. If tone is too low, the client cannot hold the limb against gravity; if it is too high, the therapist will feel resistance during placing.[13]
5. The NDT-educated therapist must also assess environmental factors and the task demands that may influence the selection of posture and movement sequences. For instance, having a client reach with the more involved hand to a lower countertop may increase the possibility of success when compared to the increased demands of reaching for an object in a cupboard overhead. Another example of environmental factors can be seen with the orientation of the shower head and the person's ability to transfer in and out of the tub/shower to face the shower head.

Intervention

Intervention integrates decision-making and the previous parts of the NDT Practice Model. In the intervention process the client and the therapist work collaboratively to make logical choices toward meeting favorable outcomes. It is important to note that other components of the NDT Practice Model continue to be present during the intervention process, allowing the therapist to continually gather information, examine, and evaluate and therefore alter the plan of care as appropriate and needed, throughout the intervention session.

Berta Bobath[13] believed that you cannot "superimpose normal patterns on abnormal ones" and that there is a desire to minimize abnormal movement patterns of movement from the beginning. The NDT Practice Model promotes the constant integration of communicating, observing, thinking, and analyzing to support the functional use of normal movement patterns.[51] Although "normal" movement has been emphasized since the inception of the approach, more recent descriptions emphasize efficient and functional movement, minimizing compensatory movement patterns.[66] Intervention typically includes facilitation of normal motor performance skills involved in a task and practice of tasks themselves—or occupations—with manual guidance or handling.[59] An occupational therapist also uses the NDT Practice Model when providing strategies to promote modified independence in necessary and valued occupations while remediating motor skills. Motor interventions based on an NDT approach stress incorporating the hemiplegic side as much as possible; avoiding repetition of abnormal movement patterns, many of which lead to orthopedic impairments over time; and neutral/symmetric alignment during activities.[84] After discussions and consultations with the client/family and analyzing the client's posture, movement, body system integrities, activity abilities, problems, and tendencies, as well as contextual preferences, both outside of and within the occupational goal, the intervention session is structured according to the following concepts: environmental setup, preparation, practice as well as achieving carry over.[8] These concepts may overlap or repeat and do not follow a linear sequence, nor do they reflect completely separate concepts within the intervention process.

Careful thought and planning must be given to the environmental setup to achieve successful outcomes. Would the intervention session occur at a hospital or clinic setting or would it occur at home in the client's bedroom with other people present? Would it be a quiet environment or a location with numerous distractions? The therapist must also consider tools and equipment that might be needed to complete the chosen task for the intervention. If the client is a chef, careful selection of real-life objects, tools, furniture, and other items needed for a meal preparation task, while considering movement, posture, and subtasks will optimize outcomes for the client. In Charlotte's case, she loves to engage in gardening activities, therefore gardening tools must be at hand to complete the gardening task during intervention.

Preparation is the process of addressing the impairments in body system structures and functions.[8] Preparation encompasses all of the activities that are necessary for the client to actively work on motor skills required for the task and the task itself. Preparation might include the following:

1. The therapist's careful analysis of the movement components required for the task or occupational goal. A helpful way to organize this analysis is using segments of the body and analyzing the flow of movement that occurs within body segments and between body segments.

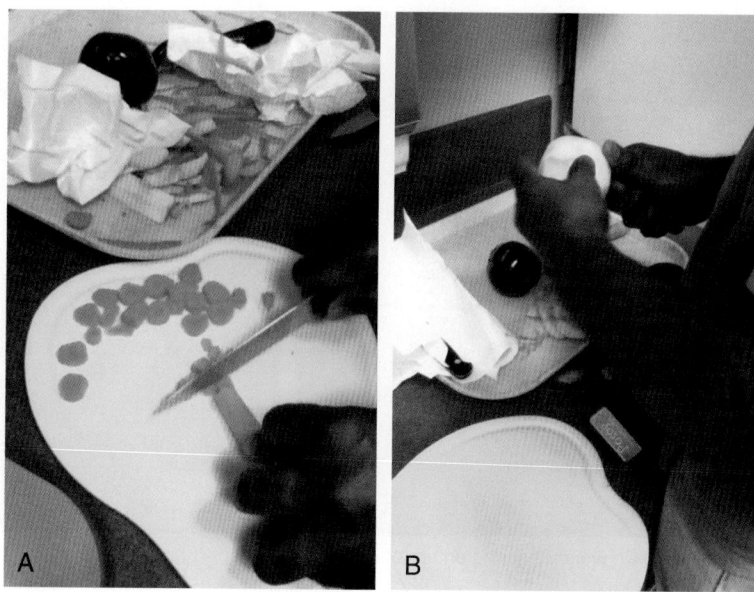

Fig. 32.19 Preparing for a meal using both hands to chop (A) and peel (B) vegetables.

2. Promote active participation on the part of the client as well as attention to the client's starting alignment for activity. Consider the task of preparing vegetables for a meal. Although compensatory strategies may be used, incorporating the use of both hands while preparing vegetables provides a more functional approach (Fig. 32.19).
3. Mobilization to give the client access to the range of motion required for the task.

Following preparation, the therapist will structure the session to work on specific motor skills required for the task. Often these are partially addressed outside of the occupation itself, in preparation for practice of the whole task, which is congruent with motor learning guidelines regarding part and whole-task practice.[34] Along with verbal cues, demonstration, and structure of the environment, facilitation of motor skills is done with *handling*. Therapists who use the NDT Practice Model constantly update and modify intervention through handling, observing responses, monitoring changes in any aspect of the client's behavior and function.[91] In handling, the therapist uses his or her body in contact with the client's to promote more efficient movement and avoid unwanted motor responses or alignments. Specifically, therapists use handling to add to the sensorimotor information that the client experiences during the performance of task, to make the client more aware of his or her body and incorporate the hemiplegic side, and to assist with the coordination and timing of movement patterns.[66] Continuing education courses and textbooks based on the NDT approach instruct clinicians on precise choices for hand placement that result in desired movement outcomes. These choices are referred to as *key points of control* (Fig. 32.20). Key points can include the therapist's hands, which are viewed as clinical tools but can also include any avenue of contact using the therapist's body on the client. Although the therapist uses manual handling and guiding, the client should be active in the process. Handling and guiding should be graded to provide just enough assistance and input to give the client a feel for a more efficient movement pattern and

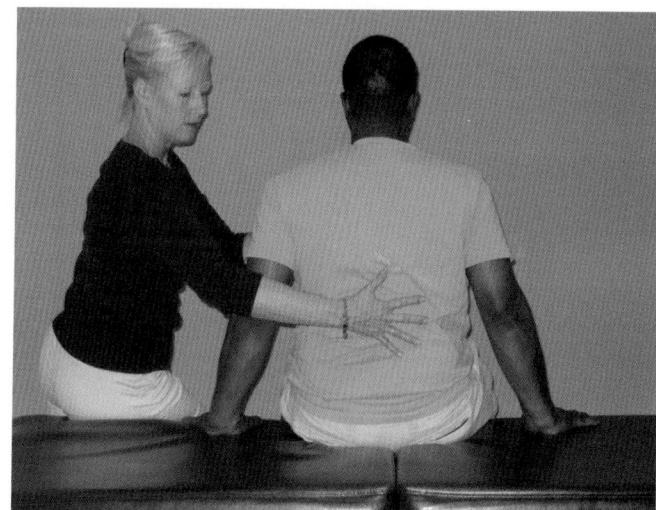

Fig. 32.20 Key points of control. Trunk extension.

gradually withdrawn as the client progresses and is able to do more of the movement pattern and task independently.[39] The unique handling and clinical reasoning skill set rooted in NDT is a powerful adjunct to the practice of occupational therapy for individuals experiencing neurological impairment.[7]

Intervention for limb movements is also graded from closed-chain patterns of movement to open-chain patterns. A closed-chain movement is one in which the distal part of a joint, or "chain" of joints, is fixed, and the proximal part is moving.[77] An example of a closed-chain pattern for the upper extremity (UE) would be incorporating the arm in a weight-bearing alignment for postural support and to assist with balance during an activity such as standing at a counter, weight bearing on one hand for support while reaching with the other hand overhead into a cupboard for an item (Fig. 32.21). Muscles in the weight-bearing arm must be active. Clinicians using an NDT approach include the UE in weight bearing as part of the base of support to assist

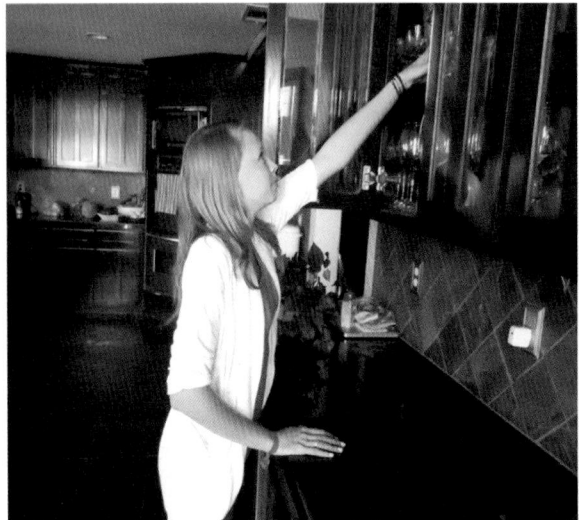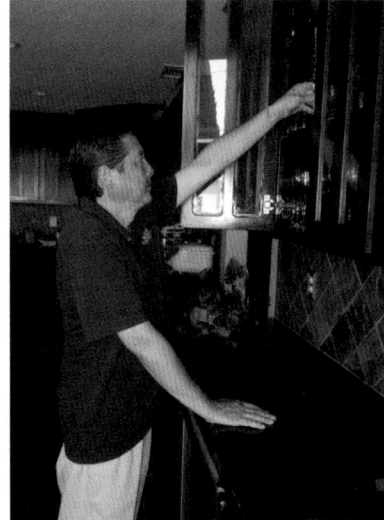

Fig. 32.21 Closed chain with weight bearing on upper extremity to support postural control.

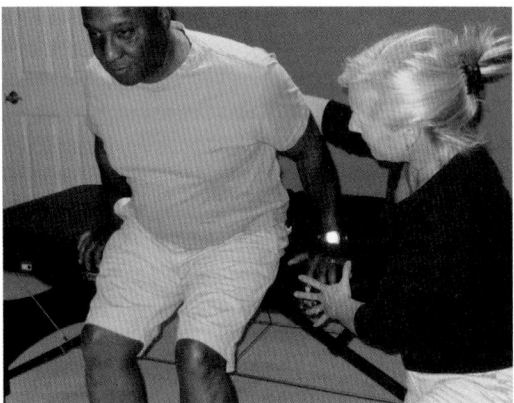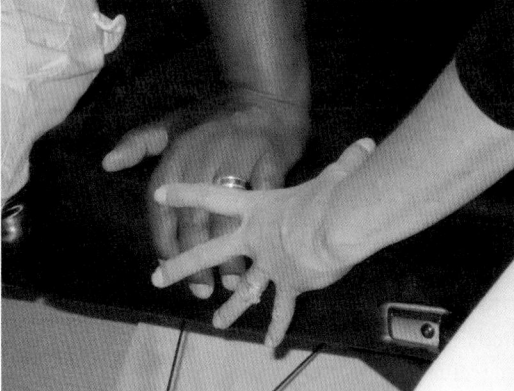

Fig. 32.22 Weight bearing on the hand to mobilize and stretch wrist and finger flexors while supporting postural control.

with postural control and to promote sensory input and isometric and eccentric control in the limb. Use of the weight-bearing or closed-chain strategy requires muscle activity in the arm; it is not passive positioning. Closed-chain weight-bearing positions are often combined with movement over the base of support to encourage activation of the UE musculature to maintain balance.

Positioning the UE with the hand in contact with a stable surface also can be a useful position for mobilization and stretching the distal UE and to grade facilitation of isolated movement patterns in the arm. During mobilization and stretching, particularly of the wrist and hand, moving the arm on a fixed hand (hand, placed on a surface and actively supporting the body) allows the therapist to stretch the extrinsic finger, thumb, and wrist flexors (Fig. 32.22). Muscle lengthening and active stretching may lead to decreased hypertonicity. Like handling and other forms of sensory input and feedback, this support provided while the client is in a weight-bearing position must be gradually withdrawn for muscle strengthening and motor learning to occur. The intervention should incorporate the learned movement patterns into an occupation or functional task.

In addition, simulation is the use of an activity or series of activities that are similar to the functional outcomes yet different in some aspect to make performance easier or more motivating

initially for the client.[8] For example, a client might have difficulty donning sleeves on a pullover shirt and have repeatedly struggled in past sessions, showing signs of increasing frustration. A simulation activity that requires the same postural movement components with reduced motor planning might be a simple activity such as applying lotion on the forearms or sliding a bracelet or a wristwatch over the hand to the wrist. In this manner the client is simulating the movements patterns and postures related to the original activity of donning sleeves on a pullover shirt with success, but the full motor plan is not accomplished. It is important to remember when planning on a simulation activity, the client needs to be engaged and invested in the task to be beneficial. Not all clients respond well to simulation despite its opportunities to address the impairments. The client must be able to generalize motor learning of the activity, otherwise simulation will not be as effective and may not be the correct choice for intervention.

Practice and achieving carryover in the NDT Practice Model of intervention is the ability of the client to reach and perform their desired and chosen functional task(s) during each session. When the therapist plans the intervention session, environmental setup, and preparation tasks are performed with the client actively engaged while taking into consideration the client's values that are related to the outcome of the task. It is not the intention of NDT interventions to divide and separate preparation tasks or activities in one session and practice the performance of functional tasks and outcomes at the next session. The performance of the functional outcome task should be done before the end of the session to enable clients to perform or practice their chosen functional skill, provided under varying conditions. It is important to remember that motor learning and carryover of occupational task performance requires practice and numerous repetitions to be successful and for permanent learning to occur.[54]

NEURO-DEVELOPMENTAL TREATMENT AND EVIDENCE-BASED PRACTICE

Evidence-based practice is a clinical reasoning process that combines the best available research, a clinician's expertise, and the client's preferences and values to make decisions about intervention with individual cases to provide the most effective and efficient care.[85] The best available research for clinical decision-making regarding the effectiveness of specific interventions is a systematic review of randomized clinical trials or a randomized clinical trial.[33,88] Few studies have addressed the effect of NDT on client outcomes. At the present time, a great majority of the evidence for the effectiveness of NDT is at a lower level on the evidence scale—expert opinion. The experts include many practitioners, as well as clients and caregivers—who could be considered experts on their own lived experiences with the condition—who report positive outcomes as a result of incorporating NDT principles and management strategies into intervention. More recently, there are published adult and pediatric NDT case reports, which are written by clinicians and provide real examples of how the NDT Practice Model can serve as a decision-making framework for daily practice.[35]

The limited number of systematic reviews and clinical trials addressing the effectiveness of the NDT approach has yielded mixed results. One systematic review of the literature by Kollen et al.[58] examined 16 studies encompassing 813 clients and concluded that "there was no evidence of superiority of Bobath on sensorimotor control of upper and lower limb, dexterity, mobility, activities of daily living, health-related quality of life, and cost-effectiveness." Intervention studies have reported positive effects of NDT on gross motor skills in children and gait patterns in adults with CP.[55,96] Luke et al.[62] indicated that although the Bobath concept was found to have slightly better results than other approaches or no intervention at all in reducing shoulder pain and tone, the Bobath concept was one approach among several and did not demonstrate "superiority of one approach over the other at improving upper limb impairment, activity or participation." Similarly, Paci,[74] in his review of 15 trials, found no evidence to support NDT as an optimal type of treatment but also no conclusive support for the idea that the approach is not effective. In a study using a large randomized controlled trial by Arya et al.[4] in 2012 found that NDT was inferior when compared with meaningful task-related training, an approach clearly aligned with the tenets of occupational

therapy. Researchers agree that additional higher-level research, with more rigorous methodologies that define and detail NDT methods, is needed to provide evidence-based guidelines for practice. To systematize such research, Tyson et al.[97] outlined a "typical treatment package" for future clinical trials based on their study of physiotherapists using the Bobath concept. The focus of the intervention package would be "facilitation, mobilization, practicing the components of movement, practicing a few whole activities, and teaching clients and caregivers on how to position the client." It has also been suggested that researchers study specific intervention techniques, rather than the NDT concept or approach as a whole.[97]

Neuro-Developmental Treatment is not alone in lacking evidence. As Mayston stated,[65] "the reality is that there is only partial evidence to support current modalities such as task-specific training, constraint-induced movement therapy, treadmill training and muscle strengthening." The present evidence for use of the NDT approach consists of widespread clinical observations and expertise along with limited clinical trials and systematic reviews. In spite of a lack of high-level evidence supporting its efficacy, according to authors of one systematic literature review, "in the Western world, the Bobath Concept or Neuro-Developmental Treatment is the most popular treatment approach used in stroke rehabilitation."[58] This evidence, although useful and substantial, is not enough to warrant continued and isolated use of this approach as research demonstrating more effective or efficient methods at higher levels of evidence becomes available. Based on dynamic models integrating multiple systems within and outside the person that contribute to the control of movement, as well as occupational performance, contemporary clinical reasoning and intervention planning for individuals with UMN lesions must consider the complex web of factors contributing to function and integrate all available resources and intervention methods, supported by evidence, that contribute to effectively restoring participation in desired occupations (Fig. 32.23).

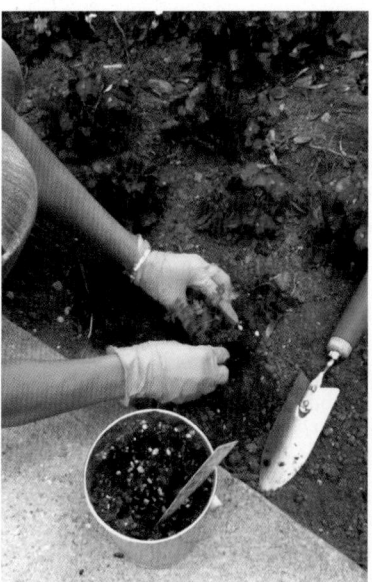

Fig. 32.23 Client participating in an enjoyed occupation, gardening.

REVIEW QUESTIONS

1. What are the four general processes of information flow related to control of movement?
2. Define motivational urge and name the locus of this function in the brain.
3. Trace the flow of information in the central and peripheral nervous systems that leads to purposeful movement.
4. What is the sensorimotor system?
5. List the areas of the sensorimotor cortex.
6. List the structures that constitute the higher, middle, and lower levels of the CNS components for movement.
7. Name the four traditional sensorimotor approaches to treatment and the theorist responsible for each.
8. Which two models of motor control form the basis for the sensorimotor approaches to treatment?
9. Briefly describe each of the four traditional sensorimotor approaches to treatment. Compare and contrast their similarities and differences.
10. List some techniques used by therapists to influence or modify motor responses in each of the traditional sensorimotor approaches.
11. How are the sensorimotor approaches used in current clinical practice?
12. In clients with pain, what tone of voice should be used when giving verbal commands?
13. Discuss the significance of auditory, visual, and tactile input in motor learning.
14. Which UE diagonal pattern is used for the hand-to-mouth phase of eating? For zipping front-opening pants?
15. Discuss the advantages of using the chop and lift patterns.
16. Which trunk pattern is used when donning a left sock?
17. List three advantages of using the diagonal patterns.
18. What is the developmental sequence of total patterns?
19. If a client needs more stability, which of the following total patterns should be chosen: side lying or prone posture on elbows?
20. Which PNF technique facilitates postural control and co-contraction?
21. Discuss the neurophysiological principles of Sherrington on which the PNF techniques of facilitation are based.
22. What is an effective technique to prepare a client with UE flexor spasticity to don a shirt?
23. Define maximal resistance.
24. Name two PNF techniques that facilitate initiation of movement.
25. What are the key principles of the NDT approach?
26. What are the four processes/components of the NDT Practice Model?
27. What is the difference between a closed and open kinetic chain?
28. Identify a task in which you would use a closed kinetic chain and a task in which you would use an open kinetic chain.

For additional practice questions for this chapter, please visit eBooks.Health.Elsevier.com.

REFERENCES

1. Abreu BF, Toglia JP: Cognitive rehabilitation: A model for occupational therapy, *Am J Occup Ther* 41:439, 1987.
2. Affolter F: Perceptual processes as prerequisites for complex human behavior, *Int Rehabil Med* 3:3, 1981.
3. American Occupational Therapy Association: Occupational therapy practice framework: Domain and process (4th ed.), *American Journal of Occupational Therapy* 74(Suppl. 2): 7412410010, 2020. https://doi.org/10.5014/ajot.2020.74S2001.
4. Arya KN, Verma R, Garg RK, Sharma VP, Agarwal M, Aggarwal GG: Meaningful task-specific training (MTST) for stroke rehabilitation: A randomized controlled trial, *Topics in Stroke Rehabilitation* 19:193–211, 2012. https://doi.org/10.1310/tsr1903-193.
5. Ayres AJ: Proprioceptive neuromuscular facilitation elicited through the upper extremities. I. Background, II. Application, III. Specific application to occupational therapy, *Am J Occup Ther* 9:1, 1955.
6. Ayres AJ, Robbins J: *Sensory Integration and the Child: Understanding Hidden Sensory Challenges*, Torrance, CA, 2005, Western Psychological Services.
7. Barthel K, Cayo C, Gellert K, Tarduno B: The practice of occupational therapy from a neuro-developmental treatment perspective. In Bierman JC, Franjoine MR, Hazzard CM, Howle JM, Stamer M, editors: *Neuro-developmental Treatment: A Guide to NDT Clinical Practice*, Stuttgart, 2016, Thieme Publishers, pp 4–16.
8. Bierman JC: Neuro-developmental treatment: Definitions and philosophical foundations. In Bierman JC, Franjoine MR, Hazzard CM, Howle JM, Stamer M, editors: *Neuro-developmental Treatment: A Guide to NDT Clinical Practice*, Stuttgart, 2016, Thieme Publishers, pp 4–16.
9. Bobath B: Observations on adult hemiplegia and suggestions for treatment, *Physiotherapy* 45:279–289, 1959.
10. Bobath B: Treatment principles and planning in cerebral palsy, *Physiotherapy* 49:122–124, 1963.
11. Bobath B: *Adult Hemiplegia: Evaluation and Treatment*, London, 1970, Heinemann Medical Books.
12. Bobath B: Treatment of adult hemiplegia, *Physiotherapy* 63(10):310–313, 1977.
13. Bobath B: *Adult Hemiplegia: Evaluation and Treatment*, ed 2, London, 1978, Heinemann Medical Books.
14. Bobath B: *Adult Hemiplegia: Evaluation and Treatment*, ed 3, Boston, 1990, Heinemann Medical Books.
15. Bobath K, Bobath B: An analysis of the development of standing and walking patterns in patients with cerebral palsy, *Physiotherapy* 48:144–153, 1962.
16. Bobath B, Finnie N: Re-education of movement patterns for everyday life in treatment of cerebral palsy, *British Journal of Occupational Therapy* 21(6):23–30, 1958.
17. Bobath K, Bobath B, Davis J: *Part 1: Karl and Berta Bobath, Part 2: Adult Hemiplegia: Principles of Treatment* (VHS Video). 1988, CA: International Clinical Educators.
18. Bordoloi K, Deka RS: Scientific reconciliation of the concepts and principles of Rood approach, *Int J Health Sci Res* 8(9):225–234, 2018.

19. Brooks VB: *The Neural Basis of Motor Control*, New York, 1986, Oxford University Press.

20. Brunnstrom S: Motor behavior in adult hemiplegic patients, *Am J Occup Ther* 15:6, 1961.

21. Brunnstrom S: *Movement Therapy in Hemiplegia*, New York, 1970, Harper & Row.

22. Buchwald J: Exteroceptive reflexes and movement, *Am J Phys Med* 46:141, 1967.

23. Carmena JM, Lebedev MA, Crist RE, et al: Learning to control a brain-machine interface for reaching and grasping in primates, *Public Library Sci Bio* 1(2):E42, 2003.

24. Carroll J: The utilization of reinforcement techniques in the program for the hemiplegic, *Am J Occup Ther* 4:211, 1950.

25. Cheney PD: Role of cerebral cortex in voluntary movements: A review, *Phys Ther* 65:624, 1985.

26. Cooke DM: The effects of resistance on multiple sclerosis patients with intention tremor, *Am J Occup Ther* 12:89, 1958.

27. Crivelli F, Omlin X, Rauter G, et al: Somnomat: A novel actuated bed to investigate the effect of vestibular stimulation, *Med Biol Eng Comput* 54:877–889, 2016. https://doi.org/10.1007/s11517-015-1423-3.

28. Curtis DJ, Butler P, Saavedra S, et al: The central role of trunk control in the gross motor function of children with cerebral palsy: A retrospective cross-sectional study, *Developmental Medicine and Child Neurology* 57(4):351–357, 2015.

29. Damiano D: Pass the torch, please! *Dev Med Child Neurol* 49:723, 2007.

30. Eggers O: *Occupational Therapy in the Treatment of Adult Hemiplegia*, Rockville, MD, 1987, Aspen.

31. Reference deleted in proofs.

32. Farber SD: *Neurorehabilitation: A Multisensory Approach*, Philadelphia, 1982, WB Saunders.

33. Fineout-Overholt E, Melnyk B, Schultz A: Transforming health care from the inside out: Advancing evidence-based practice in the 21st century, *J Prof Nurs* 21:335–344, 2005.

34. Fletcher L, Cornall C, Armstrong S: Moving between sitting and standing. In Raine S, Meadows L, Lynch-Ellerington M, editors: *Bobath Concept: Theory and Clinical Practice in Neurological Rehabilitation*, Oxford, 2009, Blackwell, pp 83–116.

35. Franjoine MR: Case reports. In Bierman JC, Franjoine MR, Hazzard CM, Howle JM, Stamer M, editors: *Neuro-developmental Treatment: A Guide to NDT Clinical Practice*, Stuttgart, 2016, Thieme Publishers, pp 4–16.

36. Franki I, Desloovere K, De Cat J, et al: The evidence-base for basic physical therapy techniques targeting lower limb function in children with cerebral palsy: A systematic review using the International Classification of Functioning, Disability and Health as a conceptual framework, *Journal of Rehabilitation Medicine* 44(5):385–395, 2012.

37. Franki I, Desloovere K, De Cat J, et al: The evidence-base for conceptual approaches and additional therapies targeting lower limb function in children with cerebral palsy: A systematic review using the ICF as a framework, in children with cerebral palsy, *Journal of Rehabilitation Medicine* 44(5):396–403, 2012.

38. Fromm C, Wise SP, Evarts EV: Sensory response properties of pyramidal tract neurons in the precentral motor cortex and postcentral gyrus of the rhesus monkey, *Exp Brain Res* 54:177, 1984.

39. Graham J, Eustace C, Brock K, et al: The Bobath concept in contemporary clinical practice, *Top Stroke Rehabil* 16:57–68, 2009.

40. Hagbarth KE: Excitatory and inhibitory skin areas for flexor and extensor mononeurons, *Acta Physiol Scand* 26(Suppl 94):1, 1952.

41. Hashimoto K, Higuchi K, Nakayama Y, Abo M: Ability for basic movement as an early predictor of functioning related to activities of daily living in stroke patients, *Neurorehabil Neural Repair* 21:353–357, 2007.

42. Hellebrandt FA: Physiology. In Delorme TL, Watkins AL, editors: *Progressive Resistance Exercise*, New York, 1951, Appleton, Century, & Crofts.

43. Hindle KB, Whitcomb TJ, Briggs WO, Hong J: Proprioceptive neuromuscular facilitation (PNF): Its mechanisms and effects on range of motion and muscular function, *J Hum Kinet* 31:105–113, 2012.

44. Holstege G: The emotional motor system, *Eur J Morphol* 30:67, 1992.

45. Howle JM: *Neuro-developmental Treatment Approach: Theoretical Foundations and Principles of Clinical Practice*, Laguna Beach, CA, 2002, NDTA Association.

46. Huitt W: Conation as an important factor of mind. *Educational Psychology Interactive*, Valdosta, GA, 1999, Valdosta State University. http://www.edpsycinteractive.org/topics/conation/conation.html.

47. Humphrey TL, Huddleston OL: Applying facilitation techniques to self care training, *Phys Ther Rev* 38:605, 1958.

48. Huss AJ: Sensorimotor approaches. In Hopkins H, Smith H, editors: *Willard and Spackman's Occupational Therapy*, Philadelphia, 1978, JB Lippincott.

49. Jackson JH:. In Taylor J, editor: *Selected Writings (vol 1)*, London, 1931, Hodder & Stoughton.

50. Jeannerod M: *The Neural and Behavioral Organization of Goal-Directed Movements*, Oxford, 1988, Clarendon Press.

51. Johnson P: Assessment and clinical reasoning in the Bobath concept. In Raine S, Meadows L, Lynch-Ellerington M, editors: *Bobath Concept: Theory and Clinical Practice in Neurological Rehabilitation*, Oxford, 2009, Blackwell, pp 43–63.

52. Kabat H, Rosenberg D: Concepts and techniques of occupational therapy for neuromuscular disorders, *Am J Occup Ther* 4:6, 1950.

53. Kandel ER, Schwartz JH, Jesell TM, editors: *Principles of Neural Science,* ed 4, New York, 2000, Elsevier.

54. Kawahira K, Shimodozono M, Etoh S, Kamada K, Noma T, Tanaka N: Effects of intensive repetition of a new facilitation technique on motor functional recovery of the hemiplegic upper limb and hand, *Brain Inj* 24(10):1202–1213, 2010. https://doi.org/10.3109/02699052.2010.506855. PMID: 20715890; PMCID: PMC2942772

55. Kim SJ, Kwak EE, Park EC, Cho S-R: Differential effects of rhythmic auditory stimulation and neurodevelopmental treatment/Bobath on gait patterns in adults with cerebral palsy: A randomized controlled trial, *Clin Rehabil* 26:904–914, 2012.

56. Klein DA, Stone WJ, Phillips WY, Gangi J, Hartman S: PNF Training and physical function in assisted-living older adults, *J Aging Phys Act* 10:476–488, 2002.

57. Kofotolis N, Kellis E: Effects of two 4-week proprioceptive neuromuscular facilitation programs on muscle endurance, flexibility, and functional performance in women with chronic low back pain, *Phys Ther* 86:1001–1012, 2006.

58. Kollen BJ, Lennon S, Lyons B, et al: The effectiveness of the Bobath concept in stroke rehabilitation: What is the evidence? *Stroke* 40(4):e89–e97, 2009.

59. Lennon S, Ashburn A: The Bobath concept in stroke rehabilitation: A focus group study of the experienced physiotherapists' perspective, *Disabil Rehabil* 22:665–674, 2000.

60. Levy CE, Nichols DS, Schmalbrock PM: Functional MRI evidence of cortical reorganization in upper-limb stroke

hemiplegia treated with constraint-induced movement therapy, *Am J Phys Med Rehabil* 80:4, 2000.

61. Loomis JE, Boersma FJ: Training right brain damaged patients in a wheelchair task: Case studies using verbal mediation, *Physiother Can* 34:204, 1982.

62. Luke C, Dodd K, Brock K: Outcomes of the Bobath concept on upper limb recovery following stroke, *Clin Rehabil* 18:888–898, 2004.

63. Mayston MJ: Letter: Motor learning now needs meaningful goals, *Physiotherapy* 86:492–493, 2000.

64. Mayston MJ: Letter: Fusion not feuding, *Physiother Res Int* 6:265–266, 2001.

65. Mayston MJ: Raine: A response, *Physiother Res Int* 11:183–186, 2006.

66. McCloskey DI: Kinesthetic sensibility, *Physiol Rev* 58:763, 1978.

67. Mitchell UH, Myrer JW, Hopkins JT, et al: Neurophysiological reflex mechanisms' lack of contribution to the success of PNF stretches, *J Sport Rehabil* 18:343–357, 2009.

68. Myers B.J.: Proprioceptive neuromuscular facilitation: Concepts and application in occupational therapy as taught by Voss. Notes from course at Rehabilitation Institute of Chicago, September 8–12, 1980.

69. Myers BJ: *Assisting to Postures and Application in Occupational Therapy Activities*, Chicago, 1981, Rehabilitation Institute of Chicago (videotape).

70. Myers BJ: *PNF: Patterns and Application in Occupational Therapy*, Chicago, 1981, Rehabilitation Institute of Chicago (videotape).

71. Naghdi S, Ansari NN, Mansouri K, Hasson S: A neurophysiological and clinical study of Brunnstrom recovery stages in the upper limb following stroke, *Brain Injury* 24:1372–1378, 2010.

72. Noma T, Matsumoto S, Shimodozono M, Etoh S, Kawahira K: Anti-spastic effects of the direct application of vibratory stimuli to the spastic muscles of hemiplegic limbs in post-stroke patients: A proof-of-principle study, *J Rehabil Med* 44(4):325–330, 2012. https://doi.org/10.2340/16501977-0946. PMID: 22402727

73. Omlin X, Crivelli F, Heinicke L, Zaunseder S, Achermann P, Riener R: Effect of rocking movements on respiration, *PLoS ONE* 11(3):e0150581, 2016. https://doi.org/10.1371/journal.pone.0150581.

74. Paci M: Physiotherapy based on the Bobath concept for adults with post-stroke hemiplegia: A review of effectiveness studies, *J Rehabil Med* 35:2–7, 2003.

75. Pandian S, Arya KN, Davidson EW: Comparison of Brunnstrom movement therapy and motor relearning program in rehabilitation of post-stroke hemiparetic hand: A randomized trial, *J Bodywork Movement Ther* 16:330–337, 2012.

76. Penfield W: *The Excitable Cortex in Conscious Man*, Liverpool, 1958, Liverpool University Press.

77. Prentice WE: Open- versus closed-kinetic-chain exercise in rehabilitation. In Prentice WE, editor: *Rehabilitation Techniques for Sports Medicine and Athletic Training* ed 4, New York, 2004, McGraw-Hill.

78. Raine S: The Bobath concept: Developments and current theoretical underpinning. In Raine S, Meadows L, Lynch-Ellerington M, editors: *Bobath Concept*, Oxford, 2009, Blackwell, pp 1–22.

79. Roland P, Ansari NN, Mansouri K, Hasson S: Supplementary motor area and other cortical areas in organization of voluntary movements in man, *J Neurophysiol* 43:118, 1980.

80. Rood M: Occupational therapy in the treatment of the cerebral palsied, *Phys Ther Rev* 32:220, 1952.

81. Rood M: Neurophysiological mechanisms utilized in the treatment of neuromuscular dysfunction, *Am J Occup Ther* 10:4, 1956.

82. Rood M: The use of sensory receptors to activate, facilitate and inhibit motor responses, automatic and somatic, in developmental sequence. In Sattely C, editor: *Approaches to the Treatment of Patients with Neuromuscular Dysfunction*, Dubuque, IA, 1962, William C Brown.

83. Rothwell JC: *Control of Human Voluntary Movement*, ed 2, London, 1994, Chapman & Hall.

84. Ryerson S, Levit K: *Functional Movement Reeducation*, Philadelphia, 1997, Churchill Livingstone.

85. Sackett D, Straus SE, Richardson WS, et al: *Evidence-based Medicine: How to Practice and Teach EBM*, ed 2, New York, 2000, Churchill Livingstone.

86. Sawner K, LaVigne J: *Brunnstrom's Movement Therapy in Hemiplegia: a Neurophysiological Approach*, ed 2, Philadelphia, 1992, JB Lippincott.

87. Schleichkorn J: *The Bobaths: a Biography of Berta and Karel Bobath*, Tucson, AZ, 1992, Therapy Skill Builders.

88. Sharman MJ, Cresswell AG, Riek S: Proprioceptive neuromuscular facilitation stretching: Mechanisms and clinical implications, *Sports Med* 36:929–939, 2006.

89. Shumway-Cook A, Woolacott MH: *Motor Control: Translating Research into Clinical Practice*, ed 3, Philadelphia, 2007, Lippincott Williams & Wilkins.

90. Song H, Park S, Kim J: The effects of proprioceptive neuromuscular facilitation integration pattern exercise program on the fall prevention and gait ability of the elders with experienced fall, *J Exerc Rehabil* 10:236–240, 2014.

91. Stamer M: Neuro-developmental treatment practice model. In Bierman JC, Franjoine MR, Hazzard CM, Howle JM, Stamer M, editors: *Neuro-developmental Treatment: A Guide to NDT Clinical Practice*, Stuttgart, 2016, Thieme Publishers, pp 4–16.

92. Stockmeyer S: An interpretation of the approach of Rood to the treatment of neuromuscular dysfunction, NUSTEP proceedings, *Am J Phys Med* 46:900, 1967.

93. Tallis R: Forward. In Raine S, Meadows L, Lynch-Ellerington M, editors: *Bobath Concept*, Oxford, 2009, Blackwell, pp viii–ix.

94. Tanji J, Taniguchi K, Saga T: Supplementary motor area: Neuronal response to motor instructions, *J Neurophysiol* 43:60, 1980.

95. Triandafilou KM, Kamper DG: Carryover effects of cyclical stretching of the digits on hand function in stroke survivors, *Archive of Physical Medicine and Rehabilitation* 95:1571–1576, 2014. https://doi.org/10.1016/j.apmr.2014.04.008.

96. Tsorlakis N, Evaggelinou C, Grouios G, Tsorbatzoudis C: Effect of intensive neurodevelopmental treatment in gross motor function of children with cerebral palsy, *Dev Med Child Neurol* 46:740–745, 2004.

97. Tyson S, Connell L, Busse M, Lennon S: What is Bobath? A survey of UK stroke physiotherapists' perceptions of the content of the Bobath concept to treat postural control and mobility problems after stroke, *Disabil Rehabil* 31:448–457, 2009.

98. Voss DE: Application of patterns and techniques in occupational therapy, *Am J Occup Ther* 8:191, 1959.

99. Voss DE: Proprioceptive neuromuscular facilitation, *Am J Phys Med* 46:838, 1967.

100. Voss DE: Proprioceptive neuromuscular facilitation: The PNF method. In Pearson PH, Williams CE, editors: *Physical Therapy Services in the Developmental Disabilities*, Springfield, IL, 1972, Charles C Thomas.

101. Voss DE, Ionta MK, Myers BJ: *Proprioceptive Neuromuscular Facilitation*, ed 3, Philadelphia, 1985, Harper & Row.
102. Wang J, Lee S, Moon S: The immediate effect of PNF pattern on muscle tone and muscle stiffness in chronic stroke patient, *J Phys Ther Sci* 28:967–970, 2016.
103. Wilson-Panwells A, Akesson EJ, Stewart PA: *Cranial Nerves: Anatomy and Clinical Comments*, Toronto, 1988, BC Decker, p 42.
104. Wolny T, Saulicz E, Gnat R, Koksz M: Butler's neuromobilizations combined with proprioceptive neuromuscular facilitation are effective in reducing of upper limb sensory in late-stage stroke subjects: A three-group randomized trial, *Clin Rehabil* 24:810–821, 2010.
105. Yerxa EJ, Clark F, Frank G, et al: An introduction to occupational science: A foundation for occupational therapy in the 21st century. In Johnson J, editor, & Yerxa EJ, co-editor: *Occupational Science: The Foundation for New Models of Practice*, Binghamton, NY, 1990, Haworth Press, pp 1–17.

SUGGESTED READINGS

Adler SS, Beckers D, Buck M: *PNF in Practice: An Illustrated Guide*, Berlin, Germany, 1993, Springer-Verlag.
Byl N, Roderick J, Mohamed O, et al: Effectiveness of sensory and motor rehabilitation of the upper limb following the principles of neuroplasticity: Patients stable poststroke, *Neurorehabil Neural Repair* 17:196, 2003.
Clautti C, Baron JC: Functional neuroimaging studies of motor recovery after stroke in adults: A review, *Stroke* 34:1553, 2003.
Cramer SC, Bastings EP: Mapping clinically relevant plasticity after stroke, *Neuropharmacology* 39:842, 2000.
Gjelsvik B: *The Bobath Concept in Adult Neurology*, New York, 2008, Thieme.
Goloszewwski S, Kremser C, Wagner M, et al: Functional magnetic resonance imaging of the human motor cortex before and after whole-hand electrical stimulation, *Scand J Rehabil Med* 31:165, 1999.
Greenwood RJ, McMillan TM, Barnes MP, Ward CD: *Handbook of Neurological Rehabilitation*, ed 2, New York, 2003, Psychology Press, p 577.
Hwangbo PN, Kim KD: Effects of proprioceptive neuromuscular facilitation neck pattern exercise on the ability to control the trunk and maintain balance in chronic stroke patients, *J Phys Ther Sci* 28:850–853, 2016.
Luft AR, McCombe-Waller S, Whitall J, et al: Repetitive bilateral arm training and motor cortex activation in chronic stroke: a randomized controlled trial, *J Am Med Assoc* 292:1853, 2004.
Mathews PB: Proprioceptors and their contribution to somatosensory mapping: Complex messages require complex processing, *Can J Physiol Pharmacol* 66:430, 1988.
Meadows L, Williams J: An understanding of functional movement as a basis for clinical reasoning. In Raine S, Meadows L, Lynch-Ellerington M, editors: *Bobath Concept: Theory and Clinical Practice in Neurological Rehabilitation*, Oxford, 2009, Blackwell, pp 23–42.
Oken B: *Complementary Therapies in Neurology: An Evidence Based Approach*, Boca Raton, FL, 2004, Parthenon, p 95.
Sherrington C: *The Integrative Action of the Nervous System*, ed 2, New Haven, CT, 1961, Yale University Press.
Weiss PL, Naveh Y, Katz N: Design and testing of a virtual environment for patients with unilateral spatial neglect to cross a street safely, *Occup Ther Int* 10:39, 2003.

33

Motor Learning

Pamela Roberts and Debra S. Ouellette

LEARNING OBJECTIVES

After reviewing this chapter, the student or practitioner will be able to do the following:

1. Describe how motor control affects occupational performance.
2. Describe dynamic systems theory and how it explains motor control.
3. Describe the task-oriented approach to motor learning.
4. Describe constraint-induced movement therapy as an intervention targeting functional use of a hemiparetic upper extremity after a neurological insult to the brain.
5. Describe the role of robotics in the use of upper extremity motor control.
6. Describe the role of virtual reality technology in the use of upper extremity motor control.
7. Describe the use of bilateral training techniques for improving upper extremity motor control.
8. Describe the use of action observation, mirror therapy, and mental practice in the management of motor control.
9. Develop client-centered and occupation-based treatment programs to facilitate motor learning.

CHAPTER OUTLINE

KEY TERMS

Action observation
Bilateral training techniques
Brain plasticity
Constraint-induced movement therapy (CIMT)
Dynamic systems theory
Feedback

Heterarchical model
Hierarchical model
Knowledge of results
Learned nonuse
Mental practice
Mirror therapy
Motor control

Motor learning
Robotics in rehabilitation
Shaping
Task-oriented approach
Virtual reality technology

THEORETICAL FOUNDATIONS OF MOTOR LEARNING

Motor learning is the acquisition and modification of learned movement patterns over time.[64] It involves cognitive and perceptual processes to code various motor programs. Motor learning requires practice and experience, which leads to permanent changes in the person's ability to produce movement sufficient to meet the demands of occupational performance. Motor control is the outcome of motor learning and involves the ability to produce purposeful movements of the extremities and postural adjustments in response to activity and environmental demands.[7] Despite the vast advances in the acute management of stroke, neurological functions impaired by stroke still has motor disability as the most common. Stroke survivors may experience deficits for months following a stroke that may have an impact on the long-term needs of return to the community.[8] Much of stroke rehabilitation protocols and guidelines are based on motor learning that induces neural plasticity. This signifies the ability of the brain to develop new

THREADED CASE STUDY

Richard, Part 1

Client Factors

Richard, a 76-year-old African American who identifies as male (prefers use of the pronouns he/his/him), was admitted to a rehabilitation hospital on July 21, 2020, because of the onset of a left cerebrovascular accident with resulting right-sided hemiparesis.

Before admission, the client lived with his wife in an apartment with four steps at the entrance. They have four grown children who do not live in the area. They also have three grandchildren. Richard's occupational and client's factors include being a retired electrician, and he was independent in all activities of daily living (ADLs) before admission. He was responsible for meal preparation, household maintenance, and finances. He enjoys gardening, playing cards, and cooking. His personal interest, values, and social participation consisted of doing the weekly grocery shopping and attending church every Sunday. Richard valued staying connected to his family through use of weekly posts on social media platforms and using email and weekly video/face time with his children and grandchildren and going to the theater with his wife. His extended family frequently gets together to celebrate special events during the year.

Richard's symptoms include right-sided hemiparesis. He has selective motion at the shoulder, elbow, wrist, and hand. He can lift his right arm above his head and grasp and release objects of all sizes; however, he has difficulty manipulating smaller objects. He is right hand dominant.

Richard's pattern of engagement for his daily routine consisted of getting up each morning at 6:00 am and walking the dog for about a mile. He then cooked breakfast for himself and his wife. After breakfast, he was responsible for cleaning the kitchen. He often spent time during the day writing content for the church's blog and weekly newsletter, following the stock market, and managing their finances. He maintained a list of what was needed at the grocery store and would compile the grocery list and drive a short distance to the local grocery store. He spends time daily ensuring that both he and his wife adhere to their medication routine, and in the evening both he and his wife completed their showering activities and then played cards, games, or puzzles. Additionally, he is an avid reader and reads at least three books a week and often was found "tinkering" with household maintenance projects and working in his garden.

Using the Canadian Occupational Performance Measure (COPM),[30] Richard identified the following occupational performance problems:

- Inability to perform cooking tasks with both upper extremities
- Difficulty with fasteners and with the manipulation of objects of different textures and sizes greater than 1 inch
- Difficulties with computer/keyboard use for church blog and with handwritten notes
- Inability to turn the pages of a prayer book while in church
- Difficulty performing the transition movements of sitting to standing to kneeling and kneeling to standing to sitting while in church
- Inability to perform transition movements during gardening activities
- Inability to perform fine motor movements to manipulate game and puzzle pieces
- Inability to manipulate cards with the more involved right upper extremity

Critical Thinking Questions

1. How would you use the occupational therapy process, and having completed your evaluation, what evidence-based interventions would you use to achieve your targeted outcomes (e.g., motor control, muscle strength, activities of daily living, etc.)?
2. How has Richard's motor control affected his ability to engage in meaningful occupation?
3. What motor control intervention strategies would enable Richard to engage in his daily occupations more effectively?

neuronal connections, ability to acquire new functions, and address motor impairments. An aspect that is important is the practice or intervention method that is meaningful, repetitive, and intensive.[67]

The process of motor learning after a cerebrovascular accident (CVA), traumatic brain injury, cerebral palsy, and other neurological insults to the brain has received a great deal of attention in research and occupational therapy (OT) practice. Researchers have found that 5 years after the onset of a stroke, approximately 56% of clients continue to have severe hemiparesis.[14] The initial degree of motor impairment is a predictor of motor recovery. Dominkus and colleagues[12] assessed motor recovery in the upper extremity with the Motricity Index[11] and found that a client with initial paresis was 4.58 times more likely to achieve motor recovery than a client with initial paralysis. Furthermore, nearly 400,000 people survive with some level of neurological impairment and disability.[23] The explosion of new research on brain plasticity, or the ability of the brain to reorganize and develop new pathways, has paved the way for evolving approaches that target the ability of the individual to regain movement that enhances occupational performance, participation, and quality of life.[64] Recent studies support the theory that a form of brain plasticity known as cortical map reorganization plays a major role in regaining functional use of a hemiparetic upper extremity after a stroke.[9,34]

Overall, rehabilitation after a stroke increases motor reorganization. Most studies have found clinically that therapy intensity improves outcomes. There have not been any studies that have systematically determined a critical threshold[39] of rehabilitation intensity to obtain benefit.[62] There have been studies that have noted that if the threshold is not reached, there is less recovery of the affected arm.[62] Lang et al.[29] found practice of task-specific, functional upper extremity movements occurred in only 51% of rehabilitation sessions and that the average number of repetitions per session was 32. Other forms of therapy using technology (e.g., robotics, virtual reality) may be needed to increase the repetitions.[61]

Dynamic Systems Theory

Modern motor control approaches are based on dynamic systems theory, which views motor behavior as a dynamic interaction between client factors (e.g., sensorimotor, cognitive, perceptual, and psychosocial), the context (e.g., physical, cultural, spiritual, social, temporal, personal, and virtual), and the occupations that must be performed to enact the client's roles.[40,41] Dynamic systems theory is based on a heterarchical model in which each component (e.g., client, environment, and occupational performance) is viewed as being critical in a dynamic interaction to support the client's ability to engage in occupation.[7,64] Thus, movement and motor control are the result of a dynamic interaction between each of the subsystems. In addition, any change in the system influences all the subsystems. For example, a stroke can lead to changes in the client's sensorimotor, cognitive, and perceptual skills, which affects motor control, engagement in occupation, and the person's ability to master the environment.

The heterarchical model is contrasted to the hierarchical model, which views higher centers in the central nervous system as having control over the subordinate lower centers.[41] The traditional sensorimotor approaches, such as neurodevelopmental treatment, proprioceptive neuromuscular facilitation, and the theories developed by Rood and Brunnstom, are based on a hierarchical model. Recent research supports a dynamic systems theory approach in which motor learning plus the development of motor control is a dynamic process that involves interaction of the person, environment, and occupations that the client needs to perform or wants to perform.

Task-Oriented Approach

The task-oriented approach to motor recovery is based on dynamic systems principles in which occupational performance and motor recovery are achieved by a dynamic interaction of the person, the environment, and the occupations that the person is performing.[40,41] In occupational therapy, this approach is occupation based and client centered and focuses on enabling the client to achieve motor recovery through occupational performance using real objects, environments, and meaningful occupations.[58,60] Research shows that the use of real objects from the environment versus simulated objects produces better functional movement.[88] The client must also have the opportunity to attempt to solve motor problems in the context of multiple environments by using a variety of strategies. For example, Richard (see the case study) would need to be able to turn the pages in the prayer book in the environmental context of his place of worship to engage in his spiritual practices, in addition to using motor strategies that allow him to move from sitting to standing to kneeling. Research has shown that the environmental context plays a key role in the transfer of motor skill acquisition.[17,38]

Occupations that the client has identified as being important through the COPM[30] can be used to motivate the client to problem-solve various motor strategies. An intervention plan that is developed collaboratively between the client and the therapist can aid the client in taking a more proactive role in making progress toward his or her outcomes and can facilitate more effective follow-through. Research has shown that a client-centered and occupation-based approach can assist clients in attaining their personal goals.[76,77] Emerging research is also demonstrating that an occupation-based approach is more effective than rote exercise in remediating motor control impairments.[10,18,51,52,63,74,75,89] In addition, engaging in an occupation or activity from start to finish has been shown to elicit a more efficient, forceful, and coordinated motor response than has performing only small portions of an activity.[37]

Activity analysis must be used to analyze the necessary movements that the client must perform to complete the task successfully. Effective upgrading and downgrading of the activity must be incorporated for clients to feel that they are successfully

moving toward their goals. In addition, motor learning can take place only if the client has multiple practice opportunities across several real environmental contexts.[17,32]

Qualitative (e.g., verbal encouragement) and quantitative (e.g., concrete measures of success or failure during a motor task) analyses have been shown to produce knowledge of results, which enables the client to cognitively reflect on the strengths and weaknesses of a particular motor strategy and implement a more effective strategy for completing an activity.[24,81,82] Through this dialogue, the client can learn to transfer various motor skills across multiple contexts. In a more recent study involving patients with moderate upper extremity motor control limitations, it was found that use of a structured task-oriented approach did not significantly improve motor function beyond the equivalent or lower dose of usual and customary upper extremity interventions.[84] Feedback and analysis of factors that promote success or failure in a particular motor strategy must be a central problem-solving dialogue between the OT practitioner and the client.[20-22,43]

CONSTRAINT-INDUCED MOVEMENT THERAPY

Constraint-induced movement therapy (CIMT), or forced use, is a therapeutic strategy designed to promote functional use of a hemiparetic upper extremity and has been credited with speeding up the cortical map reorganization process in nonhuman primates[72] and in humans.[28] CIMT is based on the principles of dynamic systems theory and a task-oriented approach to the acquisition of motor control. In other methods of stroke rehabilitation, clients learn to use the more functional or less involved upper extremity for daily activities, thus employing a compensatory approach. This compensatory treatment approach may foster learned nonuse of the more involved (more affected) upper extremity. Learned nonuse is a phenomenon in which the individual neglects to use the affected or more involved extremity because of the extreme difficulty coordinating movement after the onset of a stroke, brain injury, or other neurological condition.[28]

As a person or animal moves through its environment and manipulates objects, sensory feedback is received from various sources simultaneously. Vision, audition, proprioception, and kinesthesia provide important sensory information for skilled movement. The importance of sensory information on motor action was demonstrated in the classic experiment carried out by Mott and Sherrington.[50] The afferent (sensory) input enters the spinal cord through the dorsal roots of the spinal nerves. By selectively severing the dorsal roots, sensory input was effectively eliminated while leaving motor innervation basically intact. Experiments conducted before 1955 demonstrated that deafferentation of a single forelimb in rhesus monkeys resulted in an unused extremity when the animal is unrestricted.

Animal research has led to the discovery that cortical reorganization occurs after injury to the nervous system.[34] Research on somatosensory deafferentation in monkeys has shown that if a single monkey forelimb is deafferented, the monkey will not use that extremity.[25,26] In other words, the procedure left the monkeys with intact motor nerves but no sensation in the affected upper extremity. The initial shock to the nervous system prevented movement. Even after the nervous system recovered, the monkeys failed to use their affected limb. Taub[68] theorized that use of the deafferented extremity could be retrained if the intact extremity is restrained and the monkey is forced to use the affected extremity. If the restraint were used for a specific time, between 1 and 2 weeks, the functional improvement could be permanent. These studies have shown that certain training procedures can be used to enable monkeys to regain use of their deafferented extremity.[25,26,69,70] Experimental evidence indicates that the persistent loss of motor function caused by deafferentation was due to learned behavioral suppression, a phenomenon called learned nonuse.[68] Conditioned response techniques did not show promise in restoring use of the extremity for daily activities.

Another therapeutic strategy, shaping, did result in significant improvements in motor function during ADL. **Shaping** procedures are behavioral techniques that approach a desired motor outcome in small, successive increments.[47,55,71] Shaping strategies allow subjects to experience successful gains in performance with relatively small amounts of motor improvement. Explanations from several studies have led to the development of a hypothesis that explains why the constraint and training procedures improve motor recovery after deafferentation.

The theory of learned nonuse was first described by Taub and is thought to extend to humans after central nervous system damage (Fig. 33.1).[68–70,85] Animal research has demonstrated that when the forelimb is not functional, the animal no longer uses the affected upper extremity for everyday tasks. This tendency has led to reinforcement and persistence of nonuse of the affected limb. Constraining the unaffected limb of the monkeys provided the early evidence for reversing learned nonuse.

To date, rehabilitation methods for those who have sustained a cerebrovascular accident (CVA) or other neurological insult to the brain have included but are not limited to biofeedback, neuromuscular facilitation, and operant conditioning. These various forms of rehabilitation are often used in conjunction with methods that teach clients to compensate by using their intact upper extremity to perform their day-to-day functional activities. Compensatory rehabilitation strategies may improve the efficiency of the intact upper extremity, but at the same time they encourage learned nonuse of the affected upper extremity. At present, there is minimal experimental evidence demonstrating the positive benefits of these forms of therapy.

An alternative therapeutic approach, CIMT, has been used extensively for rehabilitation. Unlike more traditional rehabilitation therapies, CIMT forces the client to use the more involved upper extremity by immobilizing the less involved or unaffected upper extremity in a sling, mitt, or a combination of both (Fig. 33.2). Clients then practice using their affected upper extremity on an intensive basis for several consecutive weeks by using shaping movements with the affected upper extremity. The improvements noted in the more involved extremity after this program were attributed to the learned nonuse phenomenon described by Taub[68]; thus, part of the theoretical framework of CIMT is taken from the neurophysiological and

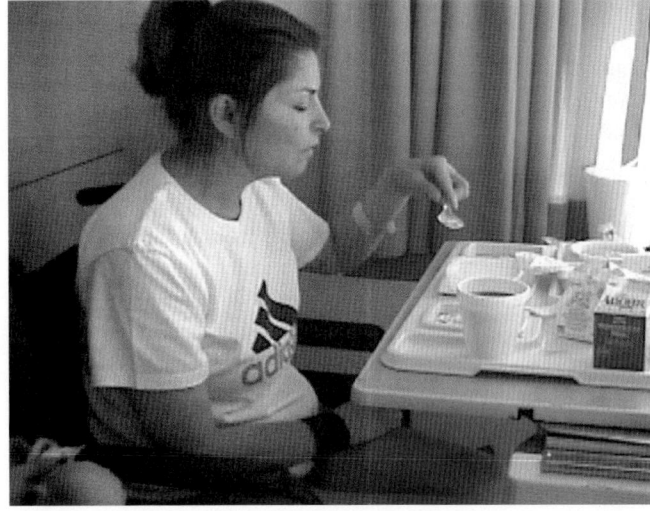

Fig. 33.1 Client with a left cerebrovascular accident and right hemiparesis before initiation of the constraint-induced movement therapy (CIMT) program. The client demonstrates learned nonuse by using her stronger, uninvolved left upper extremity during self-feeding. (Courtesy Remy Chu, OTR/L.)

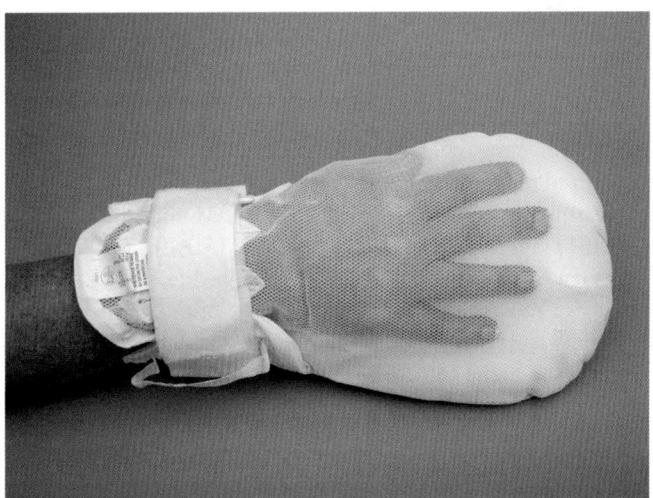

Fig. 33.2 Constraint-induced movement therapy forces the individual to use the affected upper extremity by immobilizing the unaffected upper extremity in a mitt. (From Sorrentino SA, Remmert LN: *Mosby's workbook for nursing assistants*, ed 10, St Louis, 2021, Elsevier.)

behavioral studies of the learned nonuse of the more affected limb seen in animal experiments. Constraining the intact forelimb of these monkeys provided the first evidence of the ability to overcome the learned nonuse phenomenon. This success led to further studies involving humans with hemiparesis that developed after a stroke, brain injury, and other neurological conditions.

Wolf[85,87] and Miltner and associates[46] demonstrated the positive effects of using CIMT in individuals with stroke. Liepert and co-workers[34] demonstrated cortical reorganization in humans undergoing CIMT. In 1993, Taub and colleagues[73] found significant results when using CIMT in a randomized clinical trial of nine individuals after stroke. These subjects had experienced strokes from 1 to 18 years before participation in

CIMT and were required to meet inclusion criteria similar to those used by Wolf and et al. (e.g., possessing some wrist and finger extension while still demonstrating significant disability).[11] Additionally, the subjects had to demonstrate good balance because they would be wearing a sling and would therefore be unable to use their less affected or unaffected upper extremity to protect themselves in the event of a fall. The subjects were randomly assigned to either an experimental group or a control group. The subjects assigned to the experimental group wore a sling on the less involved upper extremity for a period of 12 days. During the 12 days the sling was worn throughout all waking hours except when specific activities were being carried out, such as when it was unsafe or extremely difficult to use the more affected arm exclusively. The study also used a behavioral contract that included an agreement from the subjects to wear the restraint device for at least 90% of their waking hours during the 12-day intervention period. The behavioral contract specifically identified activities during which the subject was to use the more involved arm exclusively, to use both arms, and/or to use the less involved arm (for safety reasons). Participants in the control group were instructed to focus attention on the more involved upper extremity and were encouraged to attempt to use the more involved upper extremity for as many new functional activities as possible at home. Activities were recorded throughout the 2-week period. Those in the control group also received two sessions involving activities requiring active movement of the more involved extremity and were provided an individualized range-of-motion exercise program. The effectiveness of treatment was measured with the Wolf Motor Function Test (WMFT) and the Motor Activity Log (MAL), a structured interview exploring functional use in the life setting. Speed, quality of movement, and functional use of the affected upper extremity were significantly improved in the research group in comparison to the control group, and functional movement was maintained over a 2-year period. In 1999, Kunkel and associates[28] also demonstrated a greater than 100% increase in the amount of use of the affected upper extremity in real-world environments. The effective factor in all forms of CIMT appears to be intensive practice and functional use of the affected upper extremity repeatedly across multiple contexts for many hours a day for a period of consecutive days.[88]

Over the past 30 years, numerous studies have further confirmed the effectiveness of CIMT versus traditional rehabilitation therapy in improving the client's functional motor control after stroke.[63] More recently, however, research involving CIMT has used various populations, altered the inclusion criteria, and modified the intensity of treatment and the length of the therapy program from the original research protocol. For example, Pierce and colleagues[57] found that the forced-use component of CIMT in conjunction with a home program may be effectively incorporated into the traditional outpatient setting. Furthermore, Page and associates[54] found that repeated task-specific practice is more critical than intensity in improving upper extremity function.

In the Very Early Constraint-Induced Movement during Stroke Rehabilitation (VECTORS) study,[13] 52 subjects were randomized to one of three groups an average of 9.7 days after stroke. The three groups included (1) standard CIMT in which subjects received 2 hours of shaping therapy and wore a mitt for 6 hours per day, (2) high-intensity CIMT in which clients underwent 3 hours of shaping exercise per day and wore a mitt for 90% of waking hours, and (3) the control treatment consisting of 1 hour of ADL training and 1 hour of upper extremity bilateral training exercises. All treatment was provided for 2 weeks. The primary end point measure was the total Action Research Arm Test (ARAT) score on the more affected side at 90 days after stroke onset. In all groups the total ARAT score improved with time. Subjects in the standard CIMT and control treatment groups achieved similar gains in total ARAT score (24.2 and 25.7, respectively), whereas subjects in the high-intensity CIMT group exhibited an average gain of just 12.6 points.[13] Overall, there is conflicting evidence of the benefit of CMIT over traditional therapies in the acute stage of stroke; however, there is strong evidence of the benefit of CIMT and modified CIMT over traditional therapies in the chronic stage of stroke. The benefits appear to be confined to stroke patients with some active wrist and hand movements, particularly those with sensory loss and neglect. These findings have broadened the scope and applicability of CIMT to various populations.

Although recent CIMT research has expanded the scope to include different diagnostic criteria, different treatment regimens, and different inclusion criteria, little of the current CIMT research has addressed the participant's self-reported satisfaction in life roles after completing a CIMT program. After individuals have a stroke or other neurological condition, they experience a disruption in their life roles. This disruption can lead to feelings of ineffectiveness, incompetence, and helplessness. To restore health and quality of life, one must identify and alter one's lifestyle to improve the fit between oneself and the environment. CIMT has been proved to be effective in improving motor control in individuals who have experienced a stroke or other neurological condition. Functional carryover of CIMT from the clinic to the natural environment has been demonstrated. Research has shown significant improvement in daily use of the affected upper extremity and an increase in the speed at which the individual carries out activities after participating in a CIMT program. Increased life satisfaction resulting from an increased ability to use the affected upper extremity has been noted in individuals who reported satisfaction in performance of meaningful daily activities and life roles.[53,59]

To determine whether a subject meets the inclusion criteria for CIMT, a telephone screening protocol is often administered.[58] Many research studies use a CIMT protocol that contains typical inclusion criteria for use of this therapeutic strategy. These criteria can include (1) a first-time stroke that occurred more than 1 year earlier; (2) not currently receiving any therapeutic intervention; (3) a score of higher than 44 on the Berg Balance Test[3] or limited balance problems requiring an assistive device for mobility in clients who had a full-time caregiver to assist in any balance issues; (4) ability to move the affected arm in 45 degrees of shoulder flexion and abduction, 90 degrees of elbow flexion and extension, 20 degrees of wrist extension, and 10 degrees of extension at the metacarpal phalanges and interphalanges as determined by the client's available active range of motion (Fig. 33.3); (5) no significant cognitive impairments as demonstrated by a Mini-Mental State Examination score of at least 19 points or other type of cognitive test; (6) no preexisting comorbid conditions that might interfere with mobility or function; (7) limited spasticity (score of 0 or 1) as measured by the Modified Ashworth Scale[4]; and (8) the ability to identify an individual or caregiver who could assist in the home program.[48,59] In summary, potential reasons for a person to be excluded may include motor ability that is too high or too low, cognitive deficits that prevent adequate participation, and an existing high degree of functional use of the affected upper extremity.

A battery of assessments are typically administered to all clients included in a CIMT treatment program.[49] Results from these assessments are used to test certain research hypotheses, whereas other assessments are used for diagnostic purposes or to generate new hypotheses. Some typical assessments include the WMFT and MAL.

The WMFT consists of 15 motor items that examine contributions from the distal and proximal muscles of the arm. The tasks in this assessment are sequenced from proximal to distal and gross to fine motor. The majority of tasks are completed with the subject seated in a chair. Standard tasks such as lifting the forearm to the table, reaching for an object, or lifting a pencil are rated on a scale from 0 (does not attempt with the weaker arm) to 5 (movement appears normal), and the time to complete the task is measured (Fig. 33.4). The WMFT uses a grid or template that is taped to the desk to specify standardized measurements. The WMFT is administered before the intervention, immediately after the intervention, and at a designated follow-up time.

The MAL was developed for the purpose of assessing activities attempted outside the clinical setting. The MAL is a self-reported, 30-item instrument administered in an interview format. Subjects are asked to rate their performance on each activity reported, and emphasis is placed on clients' functional use of the hemiparetic upper extremity in their home environment. The assessment is administered approximately 10 times throughout the course of CIMT intervention. The instrument consists of specific functional activities, such as turning on a light switch or opening a drawer. The amount of functional use of the more involved upper extremity is rated by the participant from 0 (never used) to 5 (involved arm used the same as it was before the stroke). Quality of movement (how well) is also self-rated from 0 (not used) to 5 (normal movement).

Therapeutic procedures using CIMT in the clinic are performed under the supervision of an OT practitioner (Fig. 33.5). The procedures are effective only if use of the affected upper extremity is carried over to the client's home and community environment. Clients are asked about their compliance in incorporating their affected upper extremity into functional activities as noted in a log or personal diary. The home diary is used to outline the clients' activities from the time at which they are discharged from the clinic until they return for their CIMT sessions. A typical daily schedule is often used. The schedule includes the time and length of rest periods. Furthermore, specific shaping task practice is also listed on the daily schedule. A desired motor or behavioral objective is approached in small steps with an individualized shaping plan. During shaping, explicit feedback is provided to identify small improvements in motor or functional performance. The shaping task selected depends on the specific joint movements exhibiting impairment that have the greatest chance of improving and the client's preference among tasks that have a similar potential for producing specific improvements. Applying CIMT and shaping requires repetitive, supervised, constant practice. CIMT study protocols call for 6 hours of continuous task practice per day (Figs. 33.6 and 33.7).

An important component of interventions designed to enhance motor learning is the feedback received by the client while attempting a movement strategy and the results of the movement action.[64] Feedback refers to the sensory experiences intrinsic to the client and the external information provided by the environment, which includes verbal comments from the OT practitioner. This combined type of feedback can be seen when a client attempts to place a hemiparetic arm into the wrong sleeve of a button-front shirt and receives the visual information that something does not "look correct," along with verbal directions by the OT practitioner that placing the arm in the other sleeve will make the task easier. Knowledge of the results is a form of external feedback in which the client assesses whether the correct results were achieved after completion of the motor action. The OT practitioner assists the client by providing feedback during performance of the motor task and on completion of the motor task to assess the results. These strategies are combined with shaping to foster a higher frequency of successful motor practice for functional tasks.

A more recent study that evaluated the immediate and long-term effects of upper extremity rehabilitation approaches for

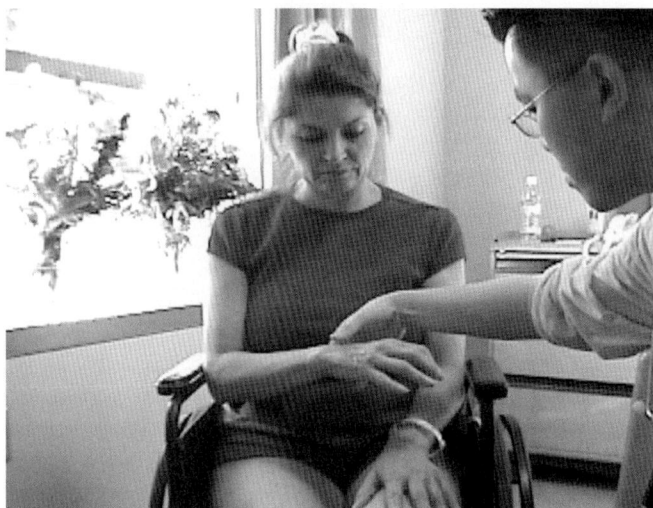

Fig. 33.3 The client is asked to demonstrate active wrist and finger extension in her dominant right hand. The client is able to achieve 20 degrees of wrist extension and 10 degrees of finger extension (at the metacarpal phalanges) from a flexed position. (Courtesy Remy Chu, OTR/L.)

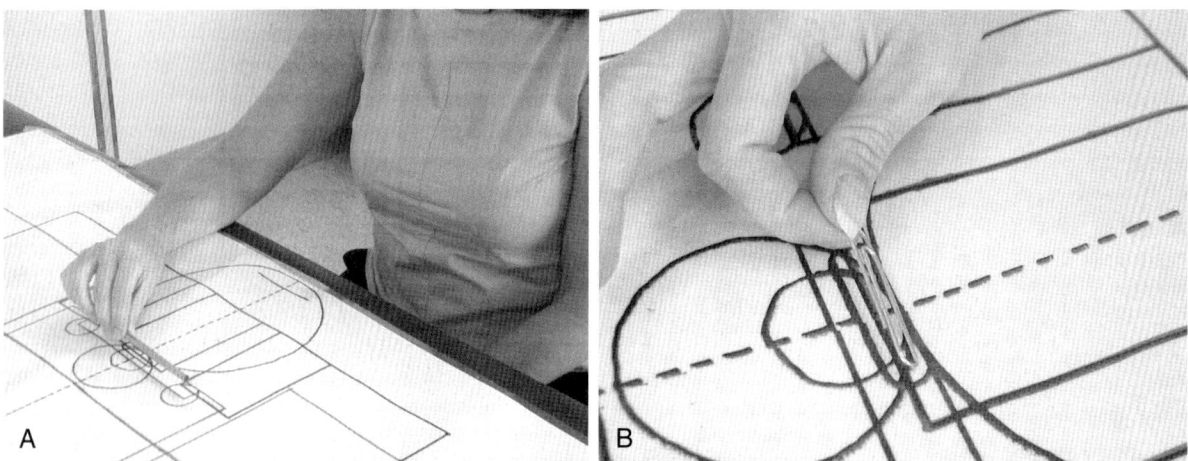

Fig. 33.4 The Wolf Motor Function Test includes standard tasks such as lifting the forearm to the table and reaching for an object.

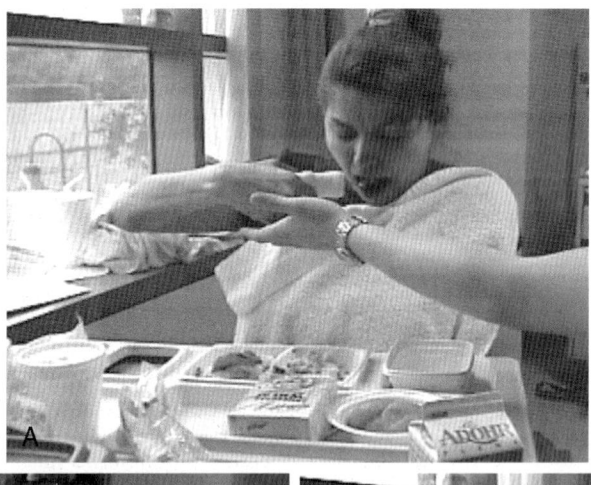

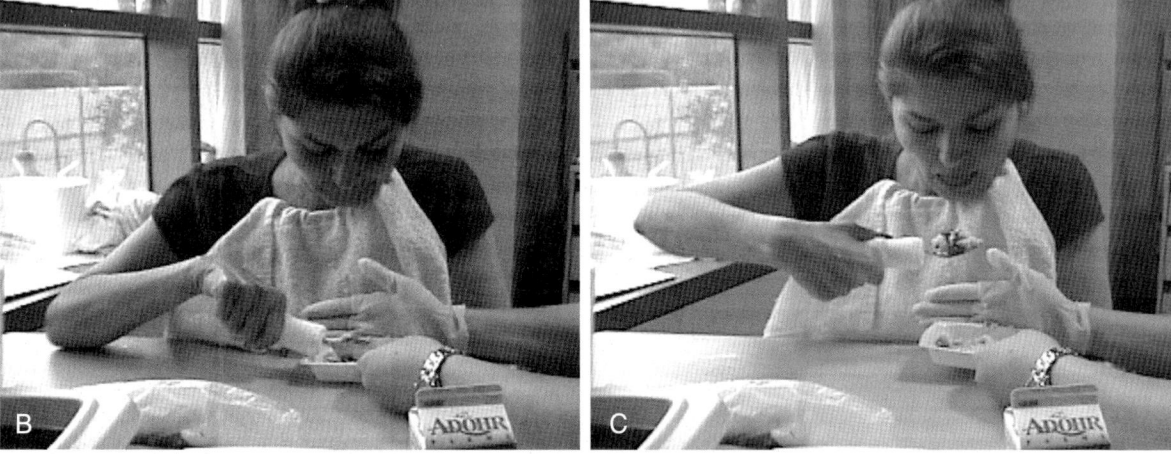

Fig. 33.5 (A) Initiation of the constraint-induced movement therapy (CIMT) program during a self-feeding activity. The client requires minimal hand-over-hand physical assistance to take her first bite with her weaker right hand. Hand-over-hand physical assistance focuses on eliminating gravity as the client brings the spoon to her mouth. (B–C) After 10 CIMT trials, the client is attempting to feed herself without physical assistance from the occupational therapist. (Courtesy Remy Chu, OTR/L.)

stroke compared functional task practice and strength training with standard care and found that task specificity and stroke severity are important factors in rehabilitation of arm use after an acute stroke.[83] Another recent approach that involves repetitive training of the paretic upper extremity on task-oriented activities has provided evidence of efficacy in stroke survivors. The Effect of Constraint-Induced Movement Therapy on Upper Extremity Function (EXCITE) trial of individuals 3 to 9 months after stroke found that CIMT produced statistically and clinically relevant improvements in arm motor function

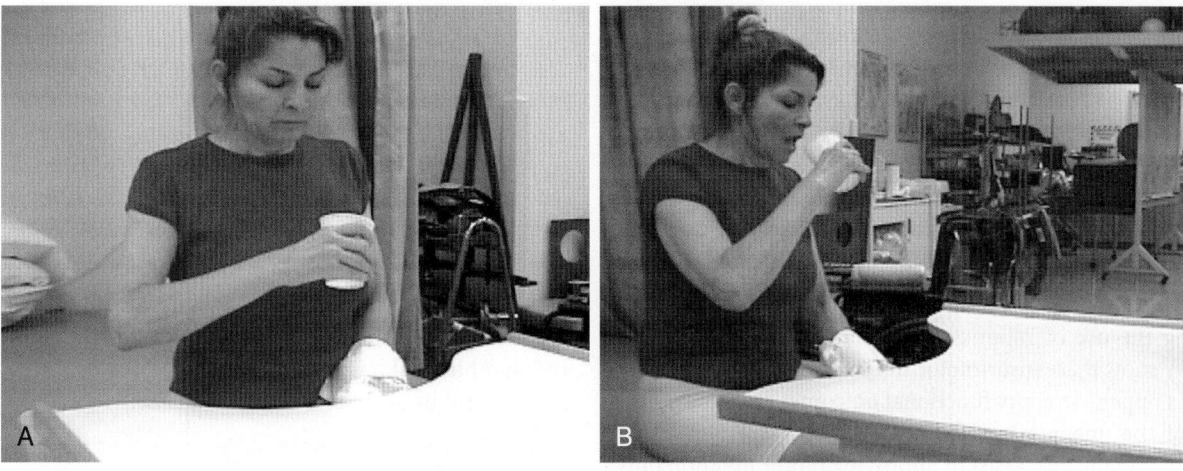

Fig. 33.6 The client is performing a block trial (cup-to-mouth trial). The client demonstrates less strain in her neck and shoulder while bringing the cup to her mouth. (Courtesy Remy Chu, OTR/L.)

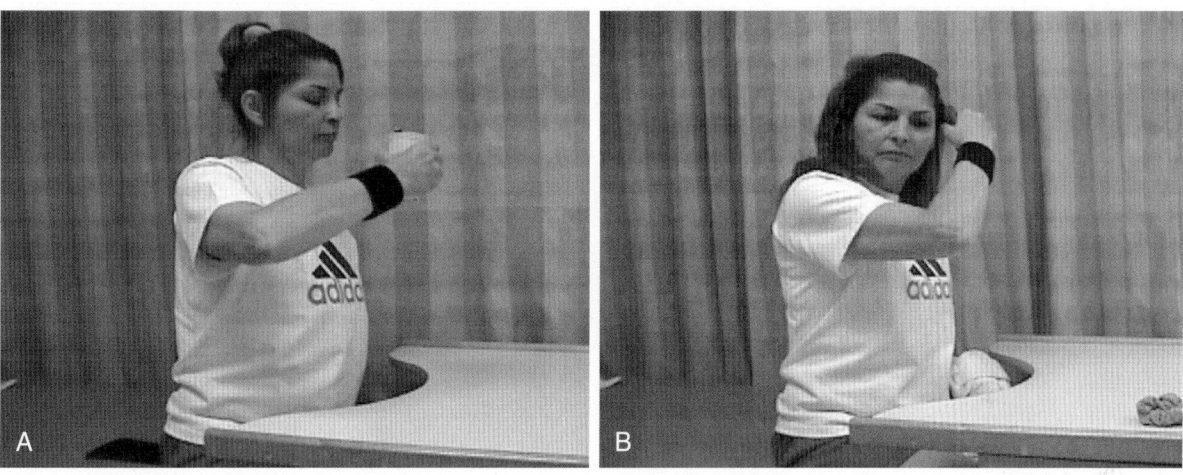

Fig. 33.7 (A) After 1.5 weeks of constraint-induced movement therapy (CIMT), the client is able to bring a cup to her mouth independently with the weaker right upper extremity. (B) She is also able to bring her right hand to her head to brush her hair. (Courtesy Remy Chu, OTR/L.)

that persisted for at least 1 year.[87] More recently, Wolf and colleagues[86] compared functional improvements between stroke participants that are randomized to receive CIMT within 3 to 9 months poststroke compared to participants randomized to receive the identical intervention 15 to 21 months after their stroke. The results of this study showed that both groups had approximately the same level of arm motor function 24 months after enrollment.

ROBOTICS IN REHABILITATION

Robotics in rehabilitation therapies involve the use of a robot to assist in initiation of movement, guidance, and resistance to movement, as well as to provide feedback. Mirror-image motion enabler (MIME) robotic devices were developed to enable unrestricted unilateral or bilateral shoulder or elbow movement. The robotic unit applies force to the more affected forearm during goal-directed movements. A randomized study involving the use of a robotic device and a control group found that there were no significant differences between the groups on either of the ADL assessments but that the clients

in the robotic group exhibited a trend toward greater improvement in Fugl-Meyer scores. These differences achieved statistical significance only if the shoulder and elbow portions of the Fugl-Meyer test were considered.[6] Another study examined robot-assisted movement therapy versus conventional therapy in individuals with chronic hemiparesis. This study found that after the first and second months of treatment, the group using robot-assisted therapy had significantly greater improvements in the proximal movement portion of the Fugl-Meyer test. The clients using the robots also had larger gains in strength and larger increases in reach extent after 2 months of treatment. At 6 months, no significant differences were seen between the two groups on the Fugl-Meyer test, although the robot group did have significantly greater improvements on the Functional Independence Measure.[36] In two other studies using robotic therapy, one found that significantly greater gains were attained after treatment in the robot-combined group than in the control group; however, the gains were not maintained at 6 months' follow-up.[35] The other study examined 19 clients following stroke with resultant hemiplegia who underwent a standardized passive exercise program using a robotic arm targeting the upper extremity. This study found no significant changes in preexercise and postexercise responses.[56] In a more recent systematic review, 34 randomized control trials of low to very low quality evaluated 19 different electromechanical assistive devices for their efficacy and ability to improve upper extremity control. The results showed that robotic devices that target arm and hand movement produced improvements in activities of daily living (ADLs) and recovery of function and muscle strength.[42] Another study found summary effects sizes for proximal but not distal motor function.[78] The conclusions regarding the use of robotics for rehabilitation of the upper extremity show that sensorimotor training with robotic devices improves upper extremity functional outcomes and motor outcomes of the upper extremity. Overall, robot-assisted upper extremity therapy may assist in improving motor function during the inpatient period after a stroke.[1,16,79]

VIRTUAL REALITY TECHNOLOGY

Virtual reality technology allows individuals to experience and interact with three-dimensional environments. Merians et al.[44,45] found that computerized virtual environments have opened the doors to an "exercise environment where the intensity of practice and positive feedback can be consistently and systematically manipulated and enhanced to create the most appropriate, individualized motor learning approach. Adding computerized virtual reality to computerized motor learning activities provides a three-dimensional spatial correspondence between the amount of movement in the real world and the amount of movement seen on the computer screen. This exact representation allows for visual feedback and guidance for the patient." There have been studies in which virtual reality training as compared to conventional training on measures of upper extremity motor function have shown no effect.[27,61] Virtual reality is an innovative treatment approach that is in its early stages, but it has shown varying results in improving motor function in clients after a stroke and experiencing chronic hemiparesis. Virtual reality may be useful as an adjunct to other interventions enabling opportunities for increasing repetition, intensity, and use of task-oriented training.

BILATERAL TRAINING TECHNIQUES

As new theories of neural plasticity have developed, the use of bilateral training techniques for the upper limb following stroke has been discussed. Bilateral upper limb training is a technique in which clients practice the same activities with both upper limbs simultaneously. Theoretically, use of the intact limb assists in promoting functional recovery of the impaired limb through facilitative coupling effects between the upper limbs. Practicing bilateral movements allows activation of the intact hemisphere to facilitate activation of the damaged hemisphere through neural networks linked via the corpus callosum.[49,66] In a systematic review that examined 11 clinical trials, Stewart and colleagues[65] found that bilateral movement training alone or in combination with sensory feedback is an effective stroke rehabilitation protocol during the subacute and chronic phases of motor recovery. Lastly, bilateral arm training along with usual and customary occupational therapy may be more effective than occupational therapy alone for improving upper limb function and ADLs performance in hemiplegic stroke patients.[31] Overall, bilateral activities in daily life has an important contribution in the neural recovery to improve outcomes.[80] Sequencing and combining unilateral and bilateral approaches are needed for participation and engagement in ADLs and instrumental activities of daily living (IADLs).

ACTION OBSERVATION, MIRROR THERAPY, AND MENTAL PRACTICE

Action observation has been shown to facilitate motor learning. That is, observations of actions performed by others activate the same internal representations of actions. The neural network involves motor regions, and the main function is that it activates during the execution of the action and during the observation of the same action. This mechanism was first described in the premotor cortex and over the last decades has continued to evolve. Currently, there is agreement about the existence of a neural network formed by regions that present the mirror mechanism.[5] Action observation is designed to increase the excitability in the primary motor cortex by activating representations of actions through the mirror neuron system.[5] Franceschini et al.[20] found that action observation may be favorable for improving dexterity and spasticity; however, the evidence for improving motor function and ADLs is mixed. Mirror therapy involves using mirror visual feedback or visual imagery of normal movement patterns in the nonaffected limb to trick the brain into perceiving normal movement patterns in the affected limb. It uses the mirror neurons that fire during action observation. Mirror therapy has been shown to improve motor recovery, sensory function, and visuospatial attention and has been shown with mixed results for ADLs performance, spasticity, and muscle strength.[90] Mental practice is the ability to create mental representations of people, objects, and places that are absent from the individual's visual field. Mental practice encompasses rehearsing a specific task or series of tasks mentally, that is, imaging your body or limb moving or performing an activity while at rest. It has been found that imagery and perception share many of the same areas of the brain that function similarly during imagery and perception. Barclay-Goddard et al.[2] showed that based on the results of six randomized, controlled trials that mental practice in combination with other treatments appeared to be more effective in improving upper extremity function. Further, a study using mental practice with imagery in stroke recovery may improve motor function and muscle strength.[33]

THREADED CASE STUDY

Richard, Part 2

At screening, Richard was eligible to participate in a CIMT program because his stroke occurred more than 1 year earlier. He had residual right hemiparesis with selective motion in all joints. He was able to touch the top of his head with his weaker arm, bend his wrist, and grasp or release with slow movements. He had completed an inpatient and outpatient rehabilitation program. Richard has not had any major medical complications, has not suffered any falls within the past 6 months, and is able to walk without an assistive device. After screening, an upper extremity range-of-motion assessment, tone assessment using the Modified Ashworth Scale,[4] Berg Balance Test, and a functional cognition test using the Menu Task[15] were completed. Richard met all the criteria and was therefore a good candidate for CIMT.

Richard participated in the MAL interview throughout the intervention. Each task was modeled twice before the participant's performance, and the task was videotaped for scoring purposes. Specific tasks to determine grip strength and the amount of weight added to the task of lifting a box with shoulder flexion were also scored separately. He also completed the WMFT. After completion of the pretraining assessment, Richard and his wife were taught how to don and doff the mitt and use the home diary, and they both signed a behavioral contract. Richard was then scheduled for 14 days of consecutive intervention in which his less involved left arm was constrained by a mitt so that he was required to complete his daily activities with his more involved right arm. The behavioral contract stipulated that Richard would wear the mitt for 90% of waking hours. There was also a home program contract that included exceptions to wearing the mitt, such as while bathing and sleeping. Richard also kept a diary to record which upper extremity was used and the amount of time used during various daily activities, as well as the amount of time that the mitt was worn. Richard recorded all activities completed from the time that he left the clinic until his return the following day.

In addition to the activity-based home program, Richard's intervention involved both a group setting and individual sessions. Each of the sessions lasted 6 hours. Tasks during the 6-hour sessions included shaping activities to ensure success in performance. Each small improvement in motor performance was reinforced with positive feedback. Tasks were progressively increased in difficulty as Richard's motor performance improved. To ensure that the activities were occupation based and client centered, they were developed according to the information provided and identified by the COPM.

After Richard arrived at the clinic, the therapist reviewed his diary and performed the MAL. The CIMT activities were identified through information obtained from the COPM. For example, Richard participated in group activities such as playing cards and board games, which required him to use his more

affected hand to manipulate the cards while his less affected hand was constrained in the mitt. He further participated in activities such as cooking. He was responsible for set-up, preparation, and clean-up of the meal with his right upper extremity. His left upper extremity was constrained in the mitt, which necessitated use of his more affected right hand to chop vegetables. Richard would often attempt to use his less affected hand in the mitt and would require prompting from the therapist. To focus on activities that were meaningful for Richard, all activities during the 6-hour intervention session were based on his goals from the COPM. His CIMT activities became progressively more challenging, with repetitions of task practice requiring range of motion, strength, activity tolerance, and coordination. Verbal acknowledgment of daily achievements was provided.

After the 2-week intervention program, Richard learned to incorporate his more affected right upper extremity into meaningful daily occupations. It became routine for Richard to initiate activities with his right upper extremity, although he primarily used his left upper extremity before the intervention. Richard's level of participation grew to include gardening, attending church, participation in social media activities in order to have continued connections with his children and grandchildren, and turning the pages of the prayer book with his right hand. He also resumed his roles in cooking and performing household maintenance.

How Has Richard's Motor Control Affected His Ability to Engage in Meaningful Occupation?

Because of impairments in motor control in his right upper extremity, Richard was unable to perform cooking tasks with both upper extremities. He also had difficulty with fasteners and manipulation of objects of different textures and sizes greater than 1 inch and with typing on the computer. Richard was unable to turn the pages of his prayer book while in church or when reading his books and had difficulty with the transitional movements of sitting to standing and standing to sitting while in church. He was also unable to perform transition movements during gardening activities and was not able to manipulate cards and game or puzzle pieces with the affected upper extremity.

What Motor Control Treatment Strategies Would Enable Richard to Engage More Effectively in His Daily Occupations?

Richard's CIMT program consisted of restricting movement of the unaffected upper extremity by placing it in a splint, sling, or mitt for more than 90% of his waking hours. He complied with this protocol for a period of 14 days and participated in training of the affected upper extremity through shaping for approximately 7 hours per day during the 10 weekdays of that period. This approach enabled Richard to regain functional use of his right dominant upper extremity for occupations such as preparing meals, dressing, and opening the pages of a prayer book.

SUMMARY

Dynamic systems theory supports a heterarchical model of motor control in which motor acquisition is influenced by the client, the environment, and the occupations that the client needs to perform or wants to perform. A task-oriented approach supports the use of occupation-based and client-centered interventions to assist clients in problem solving (e.g., learning how they will perform their desired occupations in a variety of contexts to support transfer of motor learning). CIMT is a task-oriented approach that focuses on constraining use of the unaffected upper extremity to facilitate motor recovery in the affected upper extremity during occupational performance.

More research is needed in occupational therapy to support the use of a task-oriented CIMT approach to motor recovery to improve participation in occupation. Sensorimotor training with the use of robotic devices improves functional and motor outcomes of the shoulder and elbow; however, it does not improve functional and motor outcomes of the wrist and hand. In virtual reality technology, evidence has shown that this form of intervention may improve motor outcomes. Bilateral arm training uses the intact extremity to assist the impaired extremity through facilitative coupling effects between both upper extremities. Action observation, mirror therapy, and mental practice are useful for improving motor control but do have limitations. Action observation has been shown to improve dexterity and spasticity. Similarly, mirror therapy may improve motor function, dexterity, proprioception, and stroke severity. Finally, mental practice has evidence for improvement in motor function and muscle strength. Action observation, mirror therapy, and mental practice have varied results for improving activities of daily living.

REVIEW QUESTIONS

1. How does motor control affect occupational performance?
2. What is the task-oriented approach to motor learning?
3. What is dynamic systems theory and how does it explain motor control?
4. What is constraint-induced movement therapy and how does this approach increase functional use of a hemiparetic upper extremity after a neurologic insult to the brain?
5. What is robot-assisted therapy and how does this approach improve motor control of the upper extremity?
6. What is virtual reality technology and how is this used to improve upper extremity motor control?
7. How are bilateral training techniques used to improve upper extremity motor control?
8. How are action observation, mirror therapy, and mental practice used to improve upper extremity motor control?
9. How would you develop a client-centered and occupation-based treatment program to facilitate motor learning?

For additional practice questions for this chapter, please visit eBooks.Health.Elsevier.com.

REFERENCES

1. Aisen ML, Krebs HI, Hogan N, et al: The effect of robot-assisted therapy and rehabilitative training on motor recovery following stroke, *Arch Neurol* 54:443–446, 1997.
2. Barclay-Goddard RE, Stevenson TJ, Poluha W, Thalman L: Mental practice for treating upper extremity deficits in individuals with hemiparesis after stroke, *Cochrane Database of Systematic Reviews* (Issue 5), 2011. Art. No.: CD005950. https://www.ahajournals.org/doi/10.1161/STROKEAHA.111.627414.
3. Berg KO, Wood-Dauphinee SL, Williams JI, Maki B: Measuring balance in the elderly: validation of an instrument, *Can J Public Health* 83(Suppl 2):S7, 1992.
4. Bohannon RW, Smith MB: Interrater of a Modified Ashworth Scale of muscle spasticity, *Phys Ther* 67:206, 1986.
5. Buccino G: Action observation treatment: a novel tool in neurorehabilitation. Phil. Trans. R. Soc. B 369: 20130185. https://doi.org/10.1098/rstb.2013.0185.
6. Burgar CG, Lum PS, Shor PC, et al: Development of robots for rehabilitation therapy: the Palo Alto VA/Stanford experience, *J Rehabil Res Dev* 37:663–673, 2000.
7. Carr JH, Shepherd RB: *Neurological rehabilitation: optimizing motor performance.* In Oxford, 1998, Butterworth-Heinemann.
8. Chen T, Zhang B, Deng Y, Fan JC, Zhang L, Song F: Long-term unmet needs after stroke: systematic review of evidence from survey studies, *BMJ Open* 9:028137, 2019.
9. Cramer SC, Moore CI, Finklestein SP, Rosen BR: A pilot study of somatotopic mapping after cortical infarct, *Stroke* 31:668, 2000.
10. Dearn CM, Shepherd RB: Task-related training improves performance of seated reaching tasks after stroke: a randomized controlled trial, *Stroke* 28:722, 1997.
11. Demeurisse G, Gemol O, Robaye E: Motor evaluation in vascular hemiplegia, *Eur Neurol* 19:382–389, 1980.
12. Dominkus M, Grisold W, Jelinek V: Transcranial electrical motor evoked potentials as a prognostic indicator for motor recovery in stroke patients, *J Neurol Neurosurg Psychiatry* 53:745–748, 1990.
13. Dromerick AW, Lang CE, Birkenmeier RL, et al: Very Early Constraint-Induced Movement during Stroke Rehabilitation (VECTORS): a single-center RCT, *Neurology* 73:195–201, 2009.
14. Duncan PW, Goldstein LB, Matchar D, et al: Measurement of motor recovery after stroke. Outcome assessment and sample size requirements, *Stroke* 23:1084, 1992.
15. Edwards DF, Wolf TJ, Marks T, Alter S, Larkin V, Padesky BL, Spiers M, Al-Heizan MO, Giles GM: Reliability and validity of a functional cognition screening tool to identify the need for occupational therapy, *American Journal of Occupational Therapy* 73:1–10, 03 2019. https://doi.org/10.5014/ajot.2019.028753.
16. Fasoli SE, Krebs HI, Ferraro M, et al: Does shorter rehabilitation limit potential recovery poststroke? *Neurorehabil Neural Repair* 18:88–94, 2004.
17. Ferguson MC, Rice MS: The effect of contextual relevance on motor skills transfer, *Am J Occup Ther* 55:558, 2001.
18. Flinn NA: Clinical interpretation of effect of rehabilitation tasks on organization of movement after stroke, *Am J Occup Ther* 53:345, 1999.
19. Folstein MF, Folstein SE, McHugh PR: "Mini mental state." A practical method for grading the cognitive state of patients for the clinician, *J Psychiatr Res* 12:189, 1975.
20. Franceschini M, Ceravolo MG, Agosti M, Cavallini P, Bonassi S, Dall'Armi V, Massucci M, Schifini F, Sale P: Clinical relevance of action observation in upper-limb stroke rehabilitation: a possible role in recovery of functional dexterity, *A randomized clinical trial. Neurorehabil Neuro Repair* 26(5):456–462, 2012.
21. Jarus T: Motor learning and occupational therapy: the organization of practice, *Am J Occup Ther* 48:810, 1994.
22. Jarus T: Is more always better? Optimal amounts of feedback in learning to calibrate sensory awareness, *Occup Ther J Res* 15:181, 1995.
23. Kelly-Hayes M, Robertson JT, Broderick JP, et al: The American Heart Association Stroke Outcome Classification, *Stroke* 29:1274–1280, 1998.
24. Kilduski NC, Rice MS: Qualitative and quantitative knowledge of results: effects on motor learning, *Am J Occup Ther* 57:329, 2003.
25. Knapp HD, Taub E, Berman AJ: Effect of deafferentation on a conditioned avoidance response, *Science* 128:842, 1958.
26. Knapp HD, Taub E, Berman AJ: Movement in monkeys with deafferented forelimbs, *Exp Neurol* 7:305, 1963.

27. Kong KH, Loh YJ, Thia E, Chai A, Ng CY, Soh YM, Toh S, Tjan SY: Efficacy of a virtual reality commercial gaming device in upper limb recovery after stroke: A randomized controlled study, *Topics in Stroke Rehabilitation* 23(5):333–340, 2016.

28. Kunkel A, Kopp B, Müller G, et al: Constraint-induced movement therapy for motor recovery in chronic stroke patients, *Arch Phys Med Rehabil* 80:624, 1999.

29. Lang CE, MacDonald JR, Reisman DS, et al: Observation of amounts of movement practice provided during stroke rehabilitation, *Arch Phys Med Rehabil* 90:1692–1698, 2009.

30. Law M, Baptiste S, Carswell A, et al: *The Canadian occupational performance measure*, ed 4, Ottawa, Canada, 2005, CAOT Publications.

31. Lee MJ, Lee JH, Koo HM, Lee SM: Effectiveness of bilateral arm training for improving extremity function and activities of daily living performance in hemiplegic patients. *Journal of Stroke and Cerebrovascular Diseases*, 26(5):1020-1025. https://doi.org/10.1016/j.jstrokecerebrovasdis.2016.12.008.

32. Lee TD, Swanson LR, Hall AL: What is repeated in a repetition? Effects of practice conditions on motor skills acquisition, *Phys Ther* 71:150, 1991.

33. Ietswaart M, Johnston M, Dijkerman HC, et al: Mental practice with motor imagery in stroke recovery: randomized controlled trial of efficacy, *Brain* 134(5):1373–1386, 2011.

34. Liepert J, Bauder H, Wolfgang HR, et al: Treatment-induced cortical reorganization after stroke in humans, *Stroke* 31:1210, 2000.

35. Lum PS, Burgar CG, Van der Loos MV, et al: MIME robotic device for upper limb neurorehabilitation in subacute stroke subjects: a follow-up study, *J Rehabil Res Dev* 43:631–642, 2006.

36. Lum PS, Burgar CG, Shor PC, et al: Robot-assisted movement training compared with conventional therapy techniques for the rehabilitation of upper-limb motor function after stroke, *Arch Phys Med Rehabil* 83:952–959, 2002.

37. Ma HI, Trombly CA: The comparison of motor performance between part and whole tasks in elderly persons, *Am J Occup Ther* 55:62, 2001.

38. Ma HI, Trombly CA, Robinson-Podolski C: The effect of context on skill acquisition and transfer, *Am J Occup Ther* 53:138, 1999.

39. MacLellan CL, Keough MB, Granter-Button S, Chernenko GA, Butt S, Corbett D: A critical threshold of rehabilitation involving brain-derived neurotropic factor is required for post-stroke recovery, *Neurorehabil Neural Repair* 25(8):740–748, 2011.

40. Mathiowetz V: OT task-oriented approach to person post-stroke. In Gillen G, Burkhardt A, editors: *Stroke rehabilitation: a function-based approach* ed 2, St Louis, Mo, 2004, Mosby.

41. Mathiowetz V, Bass Haugen J: Motor behavior research: implications for therapeutic approaches to CNS dysfunction, *Am J Occup Ther* 47:733, 1994.

42. Mehrholz J, Pohl M, Platz T, Kugler J, Elsner B: Electromechanical and robot-assisted arm training for improving activities of daily living, arm function, and arm muscle strength after stroke, *Cochrane Database Syst Review* (9):CD006876, 2015.

43. Merians A, Winstein CJ, Sullivan K, Pohl PS: Effects of feedback for motor skills learning in older healthy subjects and individuals post-stroke, *Neurol Rep* 19:23, 1995.

44. Merians AS, Jack D, Boian R, et al: Virtual reality-augmented rehabilitation for patients following stroke, *Phys Ther* 82:898–915, 2002.

45. Merians AS, Poizner H, Boian R, et al: Sensorimotor training in a virtual reality environment: does it improve functional recovery poststroke? *Neurorehabil Neural Repair* 20:252–267, 2006.

46. Miltner WH, Bauder H, Sommer M, et al: Effects of constraint-induced movement therapy on patients with chronic motor deficits after stroke: a replication, *Stroke* 30:586, 1999.

47. Morgan GW: The shaping game: a technique, *Behav Ther* 5:481, 1974.

48. Morris DM, Crago JE, DeLuca SC, et al: Constraint-induced movement therapy for motor recovery after stroke, *NeuroRehabilitation* 9:29, 1997.

49. Morris JH, van Wijck F, Joice S, Ogston SA, et al: A comparison of bilateral and unilateral upper-limb task training in early poststroke rehabilitation: a randomized controlled trial, *Arch Phys Med Rehabil* 89:1237–1245, 2008.

50. Mott FW, Sherrington CS: Experiments upon the influence of sensory nerves upon movement and nutrition of the limbs, *Proc R Soc Lond* 57:481, 1895.

51. Nagel MJ, Rice MS: Cross-transfer effects in the upper extremity during an occupationally embedded exercise, *Am J Occup Ther* 55:317, 2001.

52. Neistadt M: The effects of different treatment activities on functional fine motor coordination in adults with brain injury, *Am J Occup Ther* 48:877, 1994.

53. Ostendorf CG, Wolf SL: Effect of forced use of the upper extremity of a hemiplegic patient on changes in function: a single-case design, *Phys Ther* 61:1022, 1981.

54. Page SJ, Sisto S, Levine P, McGrath RE: Efficacy of modified constraint-induced movement therapy in chronic stroke: a single-blinded randomized controlled trial, *Arch Phys Med Rehabil* 85:14, 2004.

55. Panyan MV: *How to use shaping*, Lawrence, Kan, 1980, H & H Enterprises.

56. Patel S, Ho JT, Kumar R, et al: Changes in motor neuron excitability in hemiplegic subjects after passive exercise when using a robotic arm, *Arch Phys Med Rehabil* 87:1257–1261, 2006.

57. Pierce SR, Gallagher KG, Schaumburg SW, et al: Home forced use in an outpatient rehabilitation program for adults with hemiplegia: a pilot study, *Neurorehabil Neural Repair* 17:214, 2003.

58. Poole JL: Application of motor learning principles in occupational therapy, *Am J Occup Ther* 45:531, 1991.

59. Roberts PS, Vegher JA, Gilewski M, et al: Client-centered occupational therapy using constraint-induced therapy, *J Stroke Cerebrovasc Dis* 14:115, 2005.

60. Sabari JS: Motor learning concepts applied to activity-based intervention with adults with hemiplegia, *Am J Occup Ther* 45:523, 1991.

61. Saposnik G, et al: Efficacy and safety of non-immersive virtual reality exercising in stroke rehabilitation (EVREST): A randomized multicentre, single-blind, controlled trial, *Lancet Neurology* 15(10):1019–1027, 2016.

62. Schweighofer N, Han CE, Wolf SL, Arbib MA, Winstein CJ: A functional threshold for long-term use of hand and arm function can be determined: predictions from a computational model and supporting data from the Extremity Constraint-Induced Therapy Evaluation (EXCITE) Trial, *Phys Ther* 89(12):1327–1336, 2009.

63. Shepherd RB: Exercise and training to optimize functional motor performance in stroke: driving neural reorganization?, *Neural Plast* 8:121, 2001.

64. Shumway-Cook A, Woollacott M: *Motor control: theory and practical applications*, ed 3, Philadelphia, 2007, Lippincott Williams & Wilkins.

65. Stewart KC, Cauraugh JH, Summers JJ: Bilateral movement training and stroke rehabilitation: a systematic review and meta-analysis, *J Neurol* 244:89–95, 2006.

66. Summers JJ, Kagerer FA, Garry MI, et al: Bilateral and unilateral movement training on upper limb function in chronic stroke patients. A TMS study, *J Neurol Sci* 252:76–82, 2007.

67. Takeuchi N and Izumi SI: Rehabilitation with poststroke motor recovery: A review with a focus on neural plasticity. *Stroke Research and Treatment*, Vol 2013, Article ID 128641, https://doi.org/10.1155/2013/128641.

68. Taub E: Movement in nonhuman primates deprived of somatosensory feedback, *Exerc Sport Sci Rev* 4:335, 1977.

69. Taub E, Berman AJ: Avoidance conditioning in the absence of relevant proprioceptive and exteroceptive feedback, *J Comp Physiol Psychol* 56:1012, 1963.

70. Taub E, Bacon R, Berman AJ: The acquisition of a trace-conditioned avoidance response after deafferentation of the responding limb, *J Comp Physiol Psychol* 58:275, 1965.

71. Taub E, Goldberg IA, Taub PB: Deafferentation in monkeys: pointing at a target without visual feedback, *Exp Neurol* 46:178, 1975.

72. Taub E, Crago JE, Burgio LD, et al: An operant approach to rehabilitation medicine: overcoming learned nonuse by shaping, *J Exp Anal Behav* 61:281, 1994.

73. Taub E, Miller NE, Novack TA, et al: Technique to improve chronic motor deficit after stroke, *Arch Phys Med Rehabil* 74:347, 1993.

74. Thielman GT, Dean CM, Gentile AM: Rehabilitation of reaching after stroke: task-related training versus progressive resistive exercise, *Arch Phys Med Rehabil* 85:1613, 2004.

75. Trombly C, Wu CY: Effect of rehabilitation tasks on organization of movement after stroke, *Am J Occup Ther* 53:333, 1999.

76. Trombly CA, Radomski MV, Davis ES: Achievement of self-identified goals by adults with traumatic brain injury: phase I, *Am J Occup Ther* 52:810, 1998.

77. Trombly CA, Radomski MV, Trexel C, et al: Occupational therapy and achievement of self-identified goals by adults with acquired brain injury: phase II, *Am J Occup Ther* 56:489, 2002.

78. Veerbeek JM, van Wegen E, van Peppen R, van der Wees PJ, Hendriks E, Rietberg M, Kwakkel G: What is the evidence for physical therapy poststroke? A systematic review and meta-analysis, *PloS One* 9(2):e87987, 2014.

79. Volpe BT, Krebs HI, Hogan N, et al: Robot training enhanced motor outcome in patients with stroke maintained over three years, *Neurology* 53:1874–1876, 1999.

80. Waller SM and Whitall J: Bilateral arm training: why and who benefits? *NeuroRehabilitation.* 23(1):29–41, 2008.

81. Winstein CJ: Knowledge of results and motor learning: implications for physical therapy, *Phys Ther* 71:140, 1991.

82. Winstein CJ, Schmidt RA: Reduced frequency of knowledge of results enhances motor skills learning, *J Exp Psychol Learn Mem Cogn* 16:677, 1990.

83. Winstein CJ, Rose DK, Tan SM, et al: A randomized controlled comparison of upper extremity rehabilitation strategies in acute stroke: a pilot study of immediate and long term outcomes, *Arch Phys Med Rehabil* 85:620–628, 2004.

84. Winstein CJ, Wolf SL, Dromerick AW, Lane CJ, Nelsen MA, Lewthwaite R, Yongcen S, Azen SP: Interdisciplinary comprehensive arm rehabilitation evaluation ICARE investigative team: Effect of a task-oriented rehabilitation program on upper extremity recovery following motor stroke: the ICARE randomized clinical trial, *JAMA* 315(6):571–581, 2016.

85. Wolf SL, Lecraw DE, Barton LA, Jann BB: Forced use in hemiplegic upper extremities to reverse the effect of learned non-use among chronic stroke and head injured patients, *Exp Neurol* 104:125, 1989.

86. Wolf SL, Thompson PA, Winstein CJ, Miller JP, Blanton SR, Nichols-Larsen DS, Morris DM, Uswatte G, Taub E, Light KE, Sawaki L: The EXCITE stroke trial: Comparing early and delayed constraint induced movement therapy. *Stroke* 41(10): 2309–2315, 2010.

87. Wolf SL, Winstein CJ, Miller JP, et al: Effect of constraint-induced movement therapy on upper extremity function 3 to 9 months after stroke. The EXCITE randomized clinical trial, *JAMA* 296:2095–2104, 2006.

88. Wu C-Y, Trombly CA, Lin K-C, Tickle-Degnen L: A kinematic study of contextual effects on reaching performance in persons with and without stroke: influences of object availability, *Arch Phys Med Rehabil* 81:95, 2000.

89. Wu CY, Wong MK, Lin KC, Chen HC: Effects of task goal and personal preference on seated reaching kinematics after stroke, *Stroke* 32:70, 2001.

90. Yavuzer G, Selles R, Sezer N, Sütbeyaz S, Bussmann JB, Köseoglu F, Atay MB, Stam HJ: Mirror therapy improves hand function in subacute stroke: a randomized controlled trial, *Arch Phys Med Rehabil* 89(3):393–398, 2008.

34

Cerebrovascular Accident (Stroke)

Daniel Geller and Glen Gillen

LEARNING OBJECTIVES

After studying this chapter, the student or practitioner will be able to do the following:

1. List and describe evaluation procedures for survivors of a stroke.
2. Discuss the neuropathology of a stroke.
3. Identify risk factors associated with a stroke.
4. Identify multiple factors (e.g., impaired client factors, performance skills) that impede performance in areas of occupation after a stroke.
5. Describe evaluation procedures for impaired body functions related to neurobehavioral deficits.

6. Identify balance strategies (a body function) that support performance of areas of occupation.
7. Describe the motor control dysfunction (impaired body function) associated with stroke.
8. Identify standardized stroke assessments for multiple areas of dysfunction.
9. Apply a client-centered approach to stroke rehabilitation.
10. Develop comprehensive, occupation-based treatment plans to remediate or compensate for underlying deficits.

CHAPTER OUTLINE

KEY TERMS

Aphasia
Client-centered practice
Dysarthria
Impingement syndrome
Ischemia
Motor control
Neurobehavioral deficit

Postural strategies
Subluxation
Task-oriented approach
Top-down approach to assessment
Transient ischemic attack
Weight bearing

This chapter focuses on occupational therapy (OT) assessment and intervention for individuals who have sustained a stroke. Specifically, it focuses on improving participation in chosen areas of occupation. After a person has a stroke, multiple client factors and performance skills are affected and potentially limit participation and engagement in occupation.[4] These multiple problems are addressed throughout this chapter.

THREADED CASE STUDY

Jasmine, Part 1

Jasmine is a 39-year-old single mother of a 2-year-old boy. Jasmine identifies as female (prefers use of the pronouns she/her/hers). They live in a two-bedroom rented apartment. She converted the dining area into a home office, where she works at her home-based business in desktop publishing. Jasmine drives her son to preschool each morning and shops on the way home before working for the rest of the day from home. While working on her computer, Jasmine experienced tingling and "clumsiness" in her left hand. She attributed this to long work hours. Still feeling "not quite right," she attempted to stand to go to the bathroom and collapsed on the floor. She was able to crawl to the phone to call 911.

Jasmine next remembers waking up in the emergency department, where she was told that she had just experienced a stroke. Her neuroimaging studies eventually documented the presence of a right frontal-parietal infarct. Jasmine is unable to move or feel the left side of her body, has a left visual field cut, and tends to not respond to sensory stimuli on the left side of her body. The nursing staff are lifting Jasmine out of bed and providing full assistance for self-care and mobility. Jasmine was told that by the end of the week she will be transferred to the local rehabilitation hospital and will require "aggressive" occupational and physical therapy. Her son is under the care of his aunt and uncle. Jasmine has been crying often and is concerned that she will not be able to work or take care of her son. She is also concerned about losing her apartment; she explains that she has been "just getting by" recently. Jasmine is most concerned about returning home, being able to care for herself and her son, and returning to work.

Critical Thinking Questions

1. How will Jasmine's impaired body functions and body structures (e.g., loss of motor control, sensory loss, visual dysfunction, and neglect) affect her ability to return to her previous lifestyle and engage in chosen areas of occupation?
2. What three assessments are most critical to administer? Why?
3. Which interventions should be considered to address Jasmine's inability to participate in activities of daily living such as self-care (e.g., toileting, dressing), mobility (e.g., bed mobility, transfers), instrumental activities of daily living (e.g., meal preparation, childcare), and work throughout her rehabilitation stay?

Cerebrovascular accidents (CVAs), or strokes, continue to be a national health problem despite recent advances in medical technology. The American Heart Association[103] publishes stroke statistics that demonstrate the severity of this problem. Selected statistics include the following[103]:

- Stroke is a leading cause of long-term disability.
- On average, a U.S. citizen experiences a stroke every 40 seconds.
- Each year 795,000 people experience a new or recurrent stroke. Approximately 610,000 strokes are first attacks, and 185,000 are recurrent.
- The vast majority (87%) of strokes are due to a blockage (ischemic stroke) restricting blood flow to the brain
- An estimated 7 million Americans over age 20 have had a stroke.
- Women have a higher lifetime risk of stroke than men. After stroke, women have greater disability than men.
- Incidence of first ischemic stroke per 1000 was 0.88 in Whites, 1.91 in Blacks and 1.49 in Hispanics.
- Of people who experience a stroke, 28% are younger than 65 years and 17% are older than 85 years. For people older than 55 years, the incidence of stroke more than doubles with each successive decade.
- The estimated overall annual incidence of stroke in U.S. children is 6.4 per 100,000 children (0–15 years).
- The incidence of stroke is about 1.25 times higher in men than in women.
- The aftermath of a stroke is a substantial public health and economic problem; stroke is a leading cause of serious, long-term disability in the United States.
- Stroke accounts for more than half of all clients hospitalized for acute neurological disease.
- Among long-term clients who sustained a stroke, 50% have hemiparesis, 30% cannot walk, 26% are found to be dependent in activity of daily living (ADL) scales, 19% are aphasic, 35% are clinically depressed, and 26% require home nursing care.

Stroke rehabilitation as a practice area for occupational therapists is a specialization that crosses multiple settings, from the intensive care unit to community-based programs.

DEFINITION OF STROKE

A CVA, or stroke, is a complex dysfunction caused by a lesion in the brain. The World Health Organization (WHO) defines stroke as an "acute neurological dysfunction of vascular origin with symptoms and signs corresponding to the involvement of focal areas of the brain."[107] Stroke results in upper motor neuron dysfunction that produces hemiplegia, or paralysis of one side of the body, including the limbs and trunk and sometimes the face and oral structures that are contralateral to the hemisphere of the brain with the lesion. Thus, a lesion in the left cerebral hemisphere (left CVA) produces right hemiplegia. Conversely, a lesion in the right cerebral hemisphere (right CVA) produces left hemiplegia. When reference is made to the client's disability as right or left hemiplegia, the reference is to the paralyzed side of the body and not to the locus of the lesion.

Accompanying the motor paralysis may be a variety of dysfunctions other than the motor paralysis. Some of these dysfunctions include sensory disturbances, cognitive and perceptual dysfunction, visual disturbances, personality and intellectual changes, and a complex range of speech and associated language disorders. The neurological deficits must persist longer than 24 hours to be labeled a CVA.

CAUSES OF STROKE

Rief et al.[83] describe a stroke as "essentially a disease of the cerebral vasculature in which failure to supply oxygen to the brain cells, which are the most susceptible to ischemic damage, leads to their death. The syndromes that lead to stroke comprise two broad categories: ischemic and hemorrhagic stroke." Ischemic strokes account for the vast majority of strokes.

Ischemia

Ischemia refers to insufficient blood flow to meet metabolic demand. Ischemic strokes may be the result of embolism to the brain from cardiac or arterial sources. Cardiac sources include atrial fibrillation (pooling of blood in the dysfunctional atrium leads to the production of emboli), sinoatrial disorders, acute myocardial infarction, endocarditis, cardiac tumors, and valvular (both native and artificial) disorders. Cerebral ischemia caused by perfusion failure occurs with severe stenosis of the carotid and basilar arteries, and with microstenosis of the small deep arteries.[83,103]

Age, race, ethnicity, and heredity are considered nonmodifiable risk factors for ischemic strokes. In contrast, a major focus of stroke prevention and education programs are the potentially modifiable risk factors discussed in the following list.[53,103]

1. Hypertension is considered the single most important modifiable risk factor for ischemic stroke. Those with a blood pressure lower than 120/80 mm Hg have about half the lifetime risk for stroke as those with high blood pressure.[103]
2. Management of cardiac diseases, particularly atrial fibrillation, mitral stenosis, and structural abnormalities (patent foramen ovale and atrial septal aneurysm), can reduce the risk for stroke.
3. Management of diabetes and glucose metabolism can also reduce the risk for stroke.
4. Cigarette smoking increases the relative risk for ischemic stroke nearly 2 times.

5. Although excessive use of alcohol is a risk factor for many other diseases, moderate consumption of alcohol may reduce the incidence of cardiovascular disease, including stroke.
6. Use of illegal drugs, particularly cocaine, is commonly associated with stroke. Other drugs linked to stroke include heroin, amphetamines, lysergic acid diethylamide (LSD), phencyclidine (PCP), and marijuana.
7. Lifestyle factors (e.g., obesity, physical inactivity, diet, and emotional stress) are associated with a risk for stroke.

The responsibility for stroke prevention education (including prevention of recurrence) falls on each member of the stroke rehabilitation team.

Hemorrhage

Hemorrhagic strokes include subarachnoid and intracerebral hemorrhages, which account for only 13% of the total number of strokes.[103] This type of stroke has numerous causes. The four most common are deep hypertensive intracerebral hemorrhages, ruptured saccular aneurysms, bleeding from arteriovenous malformations, and spontaneous lobar hemorrhages.[89]

Related Syndromes

Cerebral anoxia and aneurysm can also result in hemiplegia. Some of the treatment approaches outlined in this chapter may be applicable to hemiplegia resulting from causes other than CVA or stroke, such as head injuries, neoplasms, and infectious diseases of the brain.

Transient Ischemic Attacks

Vascular disease of the brain can result in a completed stroke or in transient ischemic attacks (TIAs). A TIA is characterized by mild, isolated, or repetitive neurological symptoms that develop suddenly, last from a few minutes to several hours but not longer than 24 hours and clear completely. A TIA is seen as a sign of an impending stroke.[103] Most TIAs occur in people with atherosclerotic disease. Of those who experience TIAs and do not seek treatment, an estimated one-third will sustain a completed stroke; another one-third will continue to have TIAs without a stroke; and one third will experience no further attacks.[84] If the TIA is caused by extracranial vascular disease, surgical intervention to restore vascular flow (carotid endarterectomy) may be effective in preventing the stroke and resultant disability.

EFFECTS OF STROKE

The outcome of a stroke depends on which artery supplying the brain was involved (Fig. 34.1). Stroke diagnostic workups help localize the lesion and find a cause of the stroke. Techniques include cerebrovascular imaging such as computed tomography (CT), CT angiography, and magnetic resonance imaging (MRI).[83] The information collected with these techniques (e.g., the extent of damage and location of the lesion) may help the occupational therapist identify neurological deficits that affect function. The information may also help the therapist develop hypotheses regarding recovery and plan appropriate treatment. Initial information may be collected during a medical record review that focuses on the chief complaint of the client on

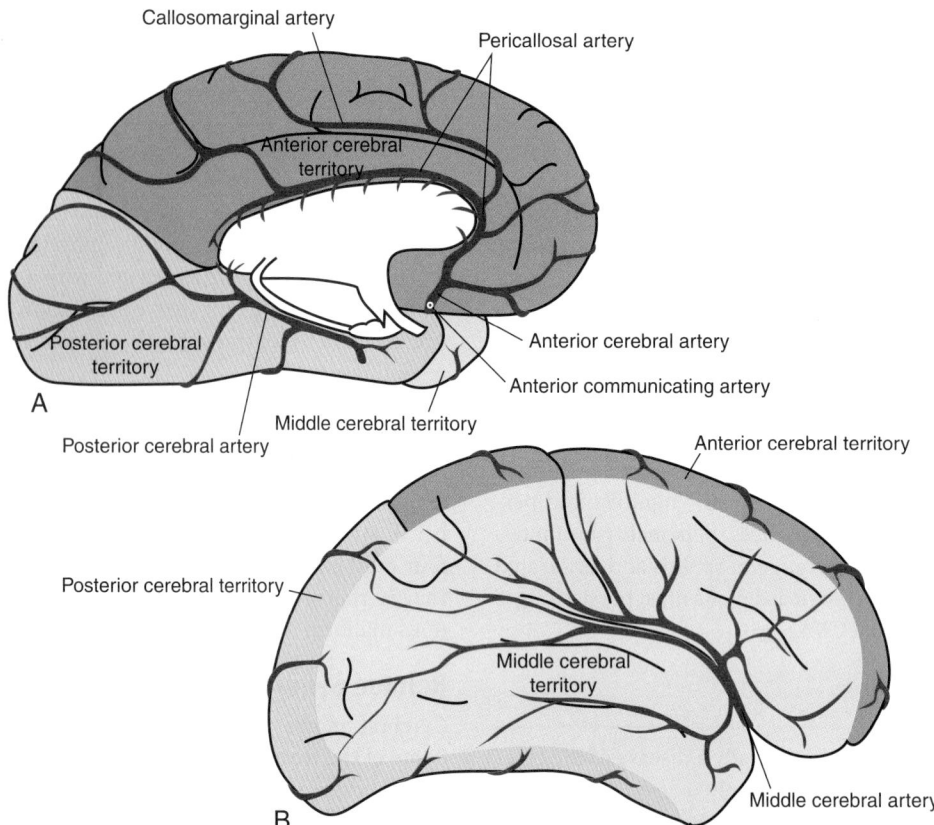

Fig. 34.1 Blood supply to the brain. The middle cerebral, anterior cerebral, and posterior cerebral arteries supply blood to the cerebral hemispheres. (A) Medial surface. (B) Lateral surface. (Modified from Mettler FA: *Neuroanatomy*, ed 2, St Louis, 1948, Mosby. In Vanderah T, Gould D, editors: *Nolte's the human brain: an introduction to its functional anatomy*, ed 7, Philadelphia, 2016, Elsevier.)

admission, medical and surgical history, results of diagnostic tests, and current pharmacological management. The following section and Tables 34.1 and 34.2 explain patterns of impairment resulting from stroke in both the cortical and subcortical areas.

Internal Carotid Artery

In the absence of adequate collateral circulation, occlusion of the internal carotid artery results in contralateral hemiplegia, hemianesthesia, and homonymous hemianopia.[6,83] Additionally, involvement of the dominant hemisphere (i.e., the cerebral hemisphere containing the representation of speech/language and controlling the arm and leg used preferentially in skilled movements, usually the left hemisphere) is associated with aphasia, agraphia or dysgraphia, acalculia or dyscalculia, right-left confusion, and finger agnosia. Involvement of the nondominant hemisphere is associated with visual perceptual dysfunction, unilateral neglect, anosognosia, constructional or dressing apraxia, attention deficits, and loss of topographic memory.

Middle Cerebral Artery

Involvement of the middle cerebral artery (MCA) is the most common cause of stroke.[5,19,83] Ischemia in the area supplied by the MCA results in contralateral hemiplegia with greater involvement of the arm, face, and tongue; sensory deficits; contralateral homonymous hemianopia; and aphasia if the lesion is in the

language-dominant hemisphere. There is pronounced deviation of the head and neck toward the side on which the lesion is located during the initial phase of the stroke.[20,27] Perceptual deficits, such as anosognosia, unilateral neglect, impaired vertical perception, visual spatial deficits, and perseveration, are seen if the lesion is in the nondominant hemisphere.[6]

Anterior Cerebral Artery

Occlusion of the anterior cerebral artery (ACA) produces contralateral lower extremity weakness that is more severe than that of the arm. Apraxia, mental changes, primitive reflexes, and bowel and bladder incontinence may be present. Total occlusion of the ACA results in contralateral hemiplegia with severe weakness of the face, tongue, and proximal arm muscles and marked spastic paralysis of the distal end of the lower extremity. Cortical sensory loss is present in the lower extremity. Intellectual changes, such as confusion, disorientation, abulia, whispering, slowness, distractibility, limited verbal output, perseveration, and amnesia, may be seen.[6,83]

Posterior Cerebral Artery

The scope of posterior cerebral artery (PCA) symptoms is potentially broad and varied because this artery supplies the upper brainstem region and the temporal and occipital lobes. Possible results of PCA involvement depend on the arterial branches affected and the extent and area of cerebral compromise. Some

TABLE 34.1   Cerebral Artery Dysfunction: Cortical Involvement and Patterns of Impairment

Artery	Location	Possible Impairments

Middle cerebral artery: upper trunk	Lateral aspect of the frontal and parietal lobe	• Dysfunction of either hemisphere:
		  • Contralateral hemiplegia, especially of the face and upper extremity
		  • Contralateral hemisensory loss
		  • Visual field impairment
		  • Poor contralateral conjugate gaze
		  • Ideational apraxia
		  • Lack of judgment
		  • Perseveration
		  • Field dependency
		  • Impaired organization of behavior
		  • Depression
		  • Lability
		  • Apathy
		• Right hemisphere dysfunction:
		  • Left unilateral body neglect
		  • Left unilateral visual neglect
		  • Anosognosia
		  • Visuospatial impairment
		  • Left unilateral motor apraxia
		• Left hemisphere dysfunction:
		  • Bilateral motor apraxia
		  • Broca's aphasia
		  • Frustration

Middle cerebral artery: lower trunk	Lateral aspect of the right temporal and occipital lobes	• Dysfunction of either hemisphere:
		  • Contralateral visual field defect
		  • Behavioral abnormalities
		• Right hemisphere dysfunction:
		  • Visuospatial dysfunction
		• Left hemisphere dysfunction:
		  • Wernicke's aphasia

Middle cerebral artery: both upper and lower trunks	Lateral aspect of the involved hemisphere	• Impairments related to both upper and lower trunk dysfunction, as listed in previous two sections
Anterior cerebral artery	Medial and superior aspect of the frontal and parietal lobes	• Contralateral hemiparesis, greatest in the foot • Contralateral hemisensory loss, greatest in the foot • Left unilateral apraxia • Inertia of speech or mutism • Behavioral disturbances
Internal carotid artery	Combination of the middle cerebral artery distribution and anterior cerebral artery	• Impairments related to dysfunction of the middle and anterior cerebral arteries, as listed in previous sections
Anterior choroidal artery (a branch of the internal carotid artery)	Globus pallidus, lateral geniculate body, posterior limb of the internal capsule, medial temporal lobe	• Hemiparesis of the face, arm, and leg • Hemisensory loss • Hemianopia

(Continued)

TABLE 34.1   Cerebral Artery Dysfunction: Cortical Involvement and Patterns of Impairment—cont'd

Artery	Location	Possible Impairments

Posterior cerebral artery	Medial and inferior aspects of the right temporal and occipital lobes, posterior corpus callosum, and penetrating arteries to the midbrain and thalamus	• Dysfunction of either side:
		  • Homonymous hemianopia
		  • Visual agnosia (visual object agnosia, prosopagnosia, color agnosia)
		  • Memory impairment
		  • Occasional contralateral numbness
		• Right-sided dysfunction:
		  • Cortical blindness
		  • Visuospatial impairment
		  • Impaired left-right discrimination
		• Left-sided dysfunction:
		  • Finger agnosia
		  • Anomia
		  • Agraphia
		  • Acalculia
		  • Alexia

Basilar artery, proximal	Pons	• Quadriparesis • Bilateral asymmetric weakness • Bulbar or pseudobulbar paralysis (bilateral paralysis of the face, palate, pharynx, neck, or tongue) • Paralysis of the eye abductors • Nystagmus • Ptosis • Cranial nerve abnormalities • Diplopia • Dizziness • Occipital headache • Coma
Basilar artery, distal	Midbrain, thalamus, and caudate nucleus	• Papillary abnormalities • Abnormal eye movements • Altered level of alertness • Coma • Memory loss • Agitation • Hallucination
Vertebral artery	Lateral medulla and cerebellum	• Dizziness • Vomiting • Nystagmus • Pain in ipsilateral eye and face • Numbness in face • Clumsiness of ipsilateral limbs • Hypotonia of ipsilateral limbs • Tachycardia • Gait ataxia
Systemic hypoperfusion	Watershed region on the lateral side of the hemisphere, hippocampus, and surrounding structures in the medial temporal lobe	• Coma • Dizziness • Confusion • Decreased concentration • Agitation • Memory impairment • Visual abnormalities caused by disconnection from the frontal eye fields • Simultanagnosia • Impaired eye movements • Weakness of shoulder and arm • Gait ataxia

From Gillen G, Nilsen DM, editors: *Stroke rehabilitation: a function-based approach*, ed 5, Philadelphia, 2021, Elsevier.

TABLE 34.2 Cerebrovascular Dysfunction in Noncortical Areas: Patterns of Impairment

Location	Possible Impairments
Anterolateral thalamus	• Either side: 　• Minor contralateral motor abnormalities 　• Long latency period 　• Slowness • Right side: 　• Visual neglect • Left side: 　• Aphasia
Lateral thalamus	• Contralateral hemisensory symptoms • Contralateral limb ataxia
Bilateral thalamus	• Memory impairment • Behavioral abnormalities • Hypersomnolence
Internal capsule or basis pontis	• Pure motor stroke
Posterior thalamus	• Numbness or decreased sensibility of the face and arm • Choreic movements • Impaired eye movements • Hypersomnolence • Decreased consciousness • Decreased alertness • Right side: 　• Visual neglect 　• Anosognosia 　• Visuospatial abnormalities • Left side: 　• Aphasia 　• Jargon aphasia 　• Good comprehension of speech 　• Paraphasia 　• Anomia
Caudate	• Dysarthria • Apathy • Restlessness • Agitation • Confusion • Delirium • Lack of initiative • Poor memory • Contralateral hemiparesis • Ipsilateral conjugate deviation of the eyes
Putamen	• Contralateral hemiparesis • Contralateral hemisensory loss • Decreased consciousness • Ipsilateral conjugate gaze • Motor impersistence • Right side: 　• Visuospatial impairment • Left side: 　• Aphasia
Pons	• Quadriplegia • Coma • Impaired eye movement
Cerebellum	• Ipsilateral limb ataxia • Gait ataxia • Vomiting • Impaired eye movements

From Gillen G, Nilsen DM, editors: *Stroke rehabilitation: a function-based approach*, ed 5, Philadelphia, 2021, Elsevier.

possible outcomes are sensory and motor deficits, involuntary movement disorders (e.g., hemiballism, postural tremor, hemichorea, hemiataxia, and intention tremor), memory loss, alexia, astereognosis, dysesthesia, akinesthesia, contralateral homonymous hemianopia or quadrantanopia, anomia, topographic disorientation, and visual agnosia.[6,27,83]

Cerebellar Artery System

Occlusion of the cerebellar artery results in ipsilateral ataxia, contralateral loss of pain and temperature sensitivity, ipsilateral facial analgesia, dysphagia and dysarthria caused by weakness of the ipsilateral muscles of the palate, nystagmus, and contralateral hemiparesis.[6,20,27,83]

Vertebrobasilar Artery System

A stroke in the vertebrobasilar artery system affects brainstem functions. The outcome of the stroke is some combination of bilateral or crossed sensory and motor abnormalities, such as cerebellar dysfunction, loss of proprioception, hemiplegia, quadriplegia, and sensory disturbances, along with unilateral or bilateral involvement of cranial nerves III to XII.

MEDICAL MANAGEMENT

Specific treatment of stroke depends on the type and location of the vascular lesion, the severity of the clinical deficit, concomitant medical and neurological problems, the availability of technology and personnel to administer special types of treatment, and the cooperation and reliability of the client.

Early medical treatment involves maintenance of an open airway, hydration with intravenous fluids, and treatment of hypertension. Appropriate steps should be taken to evaluate and treat coexisting cardiac or other systemic diseases. Measures should be taken to prevent the development of deep venous thrombosis (DVT). DVT is the formation of a blood clot (thrombus) in a deep vein, usually in the lower extremity, a common risk in clients who have prolonged periods of bed rest and immobility. The incidence of DVT in individuals with stroke ranges from 22% to 73%. Emboli that are released from deep veins and subsequently lodge in the lungs are referred to as pulmonary emboli. Pulmonary embolism is the most common cause of death in the first 30 days after a stroke.[18,83]

The physician oversees routine surveillance for thrombosis, which includes daily evaluation of leg temperature, color, circumference, tenderness, and appearance. Preventive treatments for DVT may involve medication, the use of elastic stockings, the use of reciprocal compression devices, and early mobilization of the client.

Respiratory problems and pneumonia may complicate the early poststroke course. The National Survey of Stroke reported that one third of clients who had sustained strokes also had respiratory infections.[82] More recently, there has been an association between COVID-19 and stroke; thus, clients with the dual diagnosis have more complicated respiratory conditions.[36]

Symptoms are a low-grade fever and increased lethargy. Medical management involves the administration of fluids and antibiotics, aggressive pulmonary hygiene, and mobilization of the client. Ventilatory insufficiency is a major factor contributing to the high frequency of pneumonia. The hemiparesis associated with stroke involves the muscles of respiration. Exercise programs that involve strengthening and endurance training of both the inspiratory and expiratory muscles help improve breathing and cough effectiveness and reduce the frequency of pneumonia.[18]

Cardiac disease is another frequently occurring condition that complicates the post-stroke course. The stroke itself may cause the cardiac abnormality, or the client may have had a preexisting cardiac condition. The former is treated in the same manner as any new cardiac diagnosis. A preexisting cardiac condition is reevaluated and the treatment regimen modified as appropriate. Monitoring of the heart rate and blood pressure, in addition to an electrocardiogram (ECG) during self-care evaluations, is frequently indicated to determine the cardiac response to activity.

During the acute phase, bowel and bladder dysfunction is common. The physician is responsible for ordering a specific bowel program that includes a time schedule, adequate fluid intake, stool softeners, suppositories, oral laxatives, and medications or procedures to treat fecal impaction. A timed or scheduled toilet program is essential in treating urinary incontinence. Catheterization may be necessary during stroke rehabilitation.

EVALUATION AND INTERVENTION PROCEDURES FOR CLIENTS WHO SUSTAINED A STROKE

Tables 34.1 and 34.2 provide information related to patterns of impairments that are typically observed and that vary depending on the area of the brain that has been damaged. The location of the stroke is determined by CT or MRI and is generally documented in the medical record. Understanding this information is the first step of the evaluation process; it should take place before the OT practitioner meets the client because it helps the therapist focus the evaluation procedures and begin to understand which client factors are impaired and affecting performance in areas of occupation.

For example, Jasmine has documented damage in her right frontal and parietal lobes (most likely secondary to MCA occlusion). Patterns of impairment that are typically observed with this type of stroke include contralateral motor loss, contralateral sensory loss, difficulty interpreting spatial relationships (e.g., depth/distance, foreground from background), decreased attention or neglect of left-sided information (personal and extrapersonal), and left limb motor-planning deficits. These impairments may in turn affect Jasmine's ability to engage in meaningful areas of occupation. Her sensory-motor loss may prevent her fulfilling her role as a mother (e.g., assisting her child in the bath, lifting her son into the crib, preparing meals) and as a worker (e.g., typing, filing). Simultaneously, her attention deficits (left-sided neglect) will make driving unsafe, interfere with self-care and care of her child, affect her computer use (e.g., finding information on the left side of the screen), and impede her ability to manage her household (e.g., read and write bills and checks, prepare meals.)

Typically, a client's clinical findings immediately after a stroke (the acute stage) represent the worst-case scenario. In other words, once the stroke is complete and the client who sustained the stroke has been medically stabilized, the lesion is considered static or not progressive. At this point, a client who sustained a stroke in one of the cerebral hemispheres may exhibit little or no contralateral motor function (hemiparesis or hemiplegia) because of severe weakness, no response to contralateral sensory stimuli, and a severe attention deficit; the client may also require assistance performing any work-related tasks. Fortunately, barring another neurological insult, the client is usually expected to improve from both a neurological and functional perspective. Unfortunately, predicting the amount of improvement and the length of time necessary for improvement to take place is difficult. Clinicians generally agree that the first 3 to 6 months after a stroke is the most crucial time and that the greatest improvement takes place during this period. This time frame remains controversial and should be used only as a general guideline. For example, studies[72] have documented improvements in upper extremity (UE) function in clients who sustained a stroke many years earlier. It is important to note that some clients may recover only slightly and slowly, whereas others may recover fully.

Given this information, it is important to understand that neurological recovery and functional recovery are different aspects to consider. An example of motor control (i.e., the process that must be performed to achieve movement) will be used to illustrate this point. Clients A and B may share similar findings (no motor function on the left side of the body) immediately after experiencing a stroke. Client A may recover substantial motor function and resume engagement in previous occupations, such as shopping and dressing, with few residual impairments (perhaps mild gait problems or clumsiness) resulting from the stroke. Client B may not experience the same level of neurological motor recovery and yet still be able to resume engagement in previous occupations by using adaptive methods. Dressing may require learning new one-handed techniques, wearing clothing with a looser fit, and using adaptive equipment such as a reacher. Shopping may be accomplished with the use of powered mobility (e.g., scooter or wheelchair), an ankle-foot orthotic and a cane, or the internet. Despite these differences, both client A and client B are able to participate in meaningful occupations.

Client-Centered Assessments

Law et al.[65] involved with the development of the Canadian Occupational Performance Measure (COPM), stated:

Client-centered practice is an approach to providing occupational therapy which embraces a philosophy of respect for, and partnership with, people receiving services. Client-centered practice recognizes the autonomy of individuals, the need for client choice in making decisions about occupational needs, the strengths clients bring to a therapy encounter, the benefits of client-therapist partnership, and the need to ensure that services are accessible and fit the context in which a client lives.

Both Law et al.[64] and Pollack[79] suggest that therapists implementing this approach to evaluation include the following concepts:

1. Recognize that recipients of OT are uniquely qualified to make decisions about their occupational functioning.
2. Offer the client a more active role in defining goals and desired outcomes.
3. Make the client-therapist relationship an interdependent one to enable the solution of performance dysfunction.
4. Shift to a model in which occupational therapists work with clients to enable them to meet their own goals.
5. Focus the evaluation (and intervention) on the contexts in which clients live, their roles and interests, and their culture
6. Allow the client to be the "problem definer" so that he or she will in turn become the "problem solver".
7. Allow the client to evaluate his or her own performance and set personal goals.

Through the use of these strategies, the evaluation process becomes more focused and defined, clients become immediately empowered, the goals of therapy are understood and agreed on, and a client-tailored treatment plan may be established. The COPM[65] is a standardized tool that uses a client-centered approach to allow the recipient of treatment to identify areas of difficulty, rate the importance of each area, and rate his or her satisfaction with current performance. It is a particularly useful tool to use with clients who sustained a stroke because of the multiple and extensive problems that this population experiences in performance of areas of occupation.

The COPM would be a good assessment to use with Jasmine. It would give the occupational therapist insight into the occupations that should be prioritized, assist in goal writing, and facilitate treatment planning. In addition, use of the COPM would empower Jasmine as an active participant in the rehabilitation process. Jasmine completed the COPM, and the results identified toilet transfers, computer use, grooming, feeding, and child care as the occupations that she wanted to pursue first; in other words, these occupations would be the focus of her initial OT services. Jasmine indicated that gaining mastery in the occupations would make her feel better about herself ("boost my self-esteem") and give her hope that she could return to work ("and provide for my child").

Top-Down Approach to Assessment

A **top-down approach to assessment** has been described in the literature[97] and is applicable to the evaluation of clients who sustained a stroke. Principles of this approach include the following:

1. Inquiry into role competency and meaningfulness is the starting point for evaluation.
2. Inquiry is focused on the roles that are important to the client who sustained a stroke, particularly those in which the client was engaged before the stroke.
3. Any discrepancy of roles in the past, present, or future is identified to help determine a treatment plan.
4. The tasks that define the person are identified, in addition to whether those tasks can be performed and the reasons that the tasks are problematic.
5. A connection is determined between the components of function and occupational performance.

A top-down approach to evaluation is in contrast to a bottom-up approach, which first focuses on dysfunction of client factors.[97]

Effects of Neurological Deficits on Performance in Areas of Occupation

Using activity analysis and keen observation allows therapists to identify errors during task performance and to analyze the errors and determine the underlying deficits blocking independent functioning. Árnadóttir states that:

> Therapists can benefit from detecting errors in occupational performance while observing ADL and thereby gain an understanding of the impairments affecting the patient's activity limitation. Therapists can use the information based on observed task performance in a systematic way as a structure for clinical reasoning to help them assess functional independence related to the performance and to subsequently detect impaired neurological body functions. Such information can be important when intervention methods are aimed at addressing occupational errors[6] (Fig. 34.2).

Because performance of a single functional task (e.g., donning a shirt) requires the use of multiple underlying client factors and performance skills that may have been affected by a stroke, multiple variables may be evaluated in the context of one client-chosen activity (Fig. 34.3).[5,6]

Standardized Tools

Occupational therapists use assessment tools that are reliable, valid, and sensitive to change. In addition, assessment tools focused on task performance should be used. Tools that are focused on evaluation of client factors in isolation from performance of occupations, that use novel nonfunctional tasks, and that do not consider the effect of environmental context should be interpreted with caution. Tools are available to the occupational therapist that directly relate performance dysfunction observed during ADLs to the effect of underlying skills necessary for independent performance of activities.

The Arnadottir Occupational Therapy Neurobehavioral Evaluation[5,6] (A-ONE) objectively documents the way that dysfunction of client factors (e.g., left-sided neglect, apraxia, and spatial dysfunction) affects self-care and mobility tasks. The A-ONE also has been referred to as the ADL-focused Occupation-Based Neurobehavioral Evaluation.[7,8] The Assessment of Motor and Process Skills[39] (AMPS) uses predominantly instrumental activities of daily living (IADLs) to evaluate underlying performance skills related to the completion of various IADLs (e.g., reaching, grasping, and posture) and process skill dysfunction (e.g., using items and searching and locating). Table 34.3 provides a summary of standardized assessments used with clients who have sustained a stroke.

The A-ONE was used to objectively document the ways that Jasmine's various impairments (e.g., neglect, spatial relationship dysfunction, loss of motor control, and topographical disorientation) affected her ability to perform basic activities

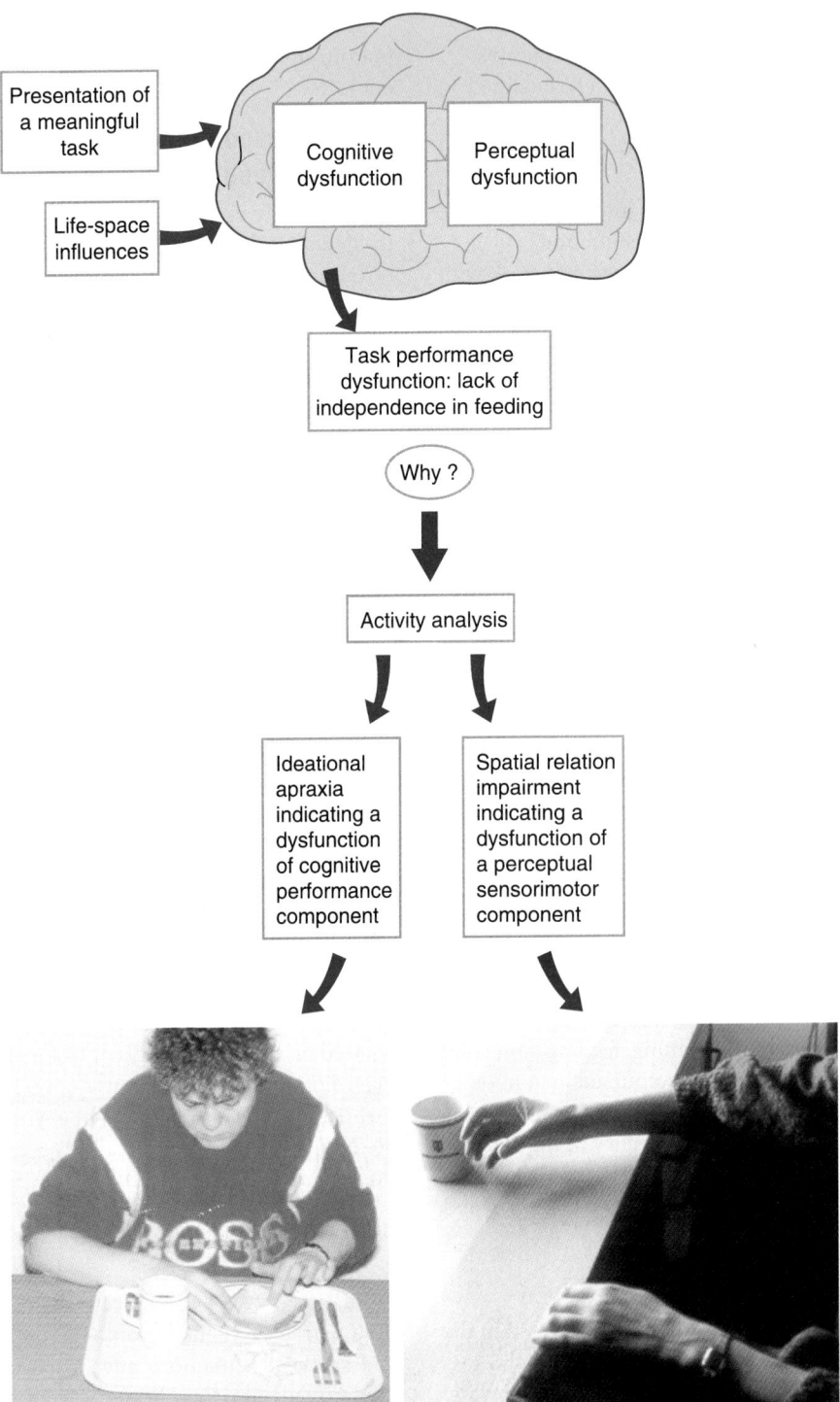

Fig. 34.2 Dysfunction of multiple client factors, such as ideational apraxia and spatial relationships, can be revealed by activity and error analysis during functional tasks such as feeding. (Modified from Árnadóttir G: *The brain and behavior: assessing cortical dysfunction through activities of daily living*, St Louis, 1990, Mosby.)

of daily living (BADLs) and mobility (e.g., bed mobility, transfers, wheelchair mobility, and walking when applicable). Errors observed and documented included not dressing the left side of her body, inability to locate grooming items on the left side of the sink, and difficulty dressing the lower part of her body and getting out of bed secondary to loss of motor control in her left limbs and trunk.

ADOPTING A FRAMEWORK FOR INTERVENTION

Therapists should consider overarching themes when deciding which interventions to use to address a client's inability to resume meaningful roles and successfully participate in chosen occupations. Evidence-based practice should serve as the foundation for all OT interventions.[57] To be successful in this endeavor, practitioners must remain abreast of new and emerging research

Possible behavioral deficits interfering with function

Premotor perseveration: pulling up sleeve

Spatial-relation difficulties: differentiating front from back on shirt

Spatial-relation difficulties: getting an arm into the right armhole

Unilateral spatial neglect: not seeing shirt located on neglected side (or a part of the shirt)

Unilateral body neglect: not dressing the neglected side or not completing the dressing on that side

Comprehension problem: not understanding verbal information related to performance

Ideational apraxia: not knowing what to do to get shirt on or not knowing what the shirt is for

Ideomotor apraxia: having problems with the planning of finger movements in order to perform

Tactile agnosia (astereognosis): having trouble buttoning shirt without watching the performance

Organization and sequencing: dressing the unaffected arm first; getting into trouble with dressing the affected arm; inability to continue the activity without being reminded

Lack of motivation to perform

Distraction: becomes interrupted by other things

Attention deficit: difficulty attending to task and quality of performance

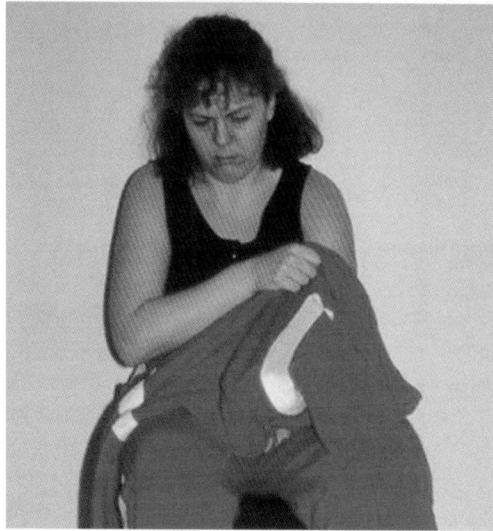

Irritated or frustrated when having trouble performing or when not getting the desired assistance

Aggressive when therapist touches patient in order to assist her (tactile defensiveness)

Difficulties recognizing foreground from background or a sleeve of a unicolor shirt from the rest of the shirt

Fig. 34.3 Possible behavioral deficits interfering with function while donning a shirt. (From Árnadóttir G: *The brain and behavior: assessing cortical dysfunction through activities of daily living*, St Louis, 1990, Mosby.)

TABLE 34.3   Sample Assessments Used With Clients Who Sustained a Stroke

Instrument	Description and Use
Activity Card Sort (ACS)[11]	Uses a Q-sort methodology to assess participation in 80 instrumental, social, and high and low physical demand leisure activities. The cards have pictures of tasks people do every day, and clients sort the cards into different piles to identify activities they did before the stroke, activities they now do less often, and those they have given up since the stroke.
Arm Motor Ability Test (AMAT)[62]	Arm function evaluated by functional ability and quality of movement; test involves performance of 28 tasks (e.g., eating with a spoon, opening a jar, tying a shoelace, using the telephone)
Árnadóttir Occupational Therapy Neurobehavioral Evaluation (A-ONE)[5]	Evaluates apraxias, neglect syndromes, body scheme disorders, organization/sequencing dysfunction, agnosias, and spatial dysfunction via basic activities of daily living (BADLs) and mobility tasks; directly correlates impairment and disability levels of dysfunction
Assessment of Motor and Process Skills[39]	Assessment tool covering 16 motor skills (e.g., reach, manipulation, calibration, coordination, posture, mobility) and 20 process skills (e.g., attends, organizes, searches and locates, initiates, sequences) that are evaluated within the context of client-chosen instrumental activities of daily living (IADLs) skills; clients choose familiar and culturally relevant tasks from a list of 50 standardized activities of various difficulties
Barthel Index[69]	Measure of disability in performing BADLs that ranges from 0 to 20 or 0 to 100 (by multiplying each item by 5); includes 10 items: bowels, bladder, feeding, grooming, dressing, transfer, toileting, mobility, stairs, and bathing
Beck Depression Inventory[12]	Self-rating scale of 21 items that has attitudinal, somatic, and behavioral components
Berg Balance Scale[13]	Balance assessment of 14 items scored on a 0- to 4-point ordinal scale
Boston Diagnostic Aphasia Examination[50]	Assesses sample speech and language behavior, including fluency, naming, word finding, repetition, serial speech, auditory comprehension, reading, and writing
Canadian Neurological Scale[30]	Stroke deficit scale that scores 8 items (e.g., consciousness, orientation, speech, motor function, facial weakness)
Canadian Occupational Performance Measure (COPM)[64]	Client-centered assessment tool based on clients' identification of problems in performance in areas of occupation (clients rate importance of self-care, productivity, and leisure skills and also their perception of performance and satisfaction with performance) Used as an outcome measure and a client satisfaction survey

(Continued)

TABLE 34.3 Sample Assessments Used With Clients Who Sustained a Stroke—cont'd

Instrument	Description and Use
Family Assessment Device[37]	Family assessment of problem solving, communication, roles, affective responsiveness, affective involvement, behavioral control, and general functioning
Frenchay Activities Index[55]	A 15-item scale for IADLs that evaluates domestic, leisure, work, and outdoor activities
Fugl-Meyer Test[42]	Motor function assessment that uses a 3-point scale to score the domains of pain, range of motion, sensation, volitional movement, and balance
Functional Independence Measure (FIM)[58]	Measure of disability in performing BADLs that includes 18 items scored on a 7-point scale; includes subscores for motor and cognitive function; performance areas include self-care, sphincter control, mobility, locomotion, cognition, and socialization
Functional Reach Test[35]	Balance evaluation; objectively measures length of forward reach in the standing posture
Functional Test for the Hemiparetic Upper Extremity[105]	Assessment of arm and hand function via 17 hierarchic functional tasks based on Brunnstrom's view of motor recovery; sample tasks are folding a sheet, screwing in a light bulb, stabilizing a jar, and zipping a zipper
Functional Upper Extremity Levels (FUEL)[102]	A classification tool to assess the client's ability to use their upper extremity during functional tasks. The FUEL includes 7 levels of upper extremity use: nonfunctional, dependent stabilizer, independent stabilizer, gross assist, semifunctional assist, functional assist, and fully functional
Geriatric Depression Scale[109]	Self-rating depression scale of 30 items in a yes/no format
Glasgow Coma Scale[92]	Level of consciousness scale that includes 3 sections scoring eye opening, motor, and verbal responses to voice commands or pain
Inpatient Rehabilitation Facility-Patient Assessment Instrument (IRF-PAI)[99]	This assessment, required by the U.S. Centers for Medicare and Medicaid Services, is used to collect patient data from inpatient rehabilitation facilities to determine reimbursement for Medicare services. Included is a self-care and mobility section which is scored on a 6-point scale (e.g., upper dressing, eating, toilet transfer, and sit to lying)
Jebsen Test of Hand Function[56]	Hand function evaluation; includes 7 test activities: writing a short sentence, turning over index cards, simulated eating, picking up small objects, moving empty and weighted cans, and stacking checkers during timed trials
Kohlman Evaluation of Living Skills (KELS)[93]	Living skills evaluation that includes ratings of 17 tasks (e.g., safety awareness, money management, phone book use, money and bill management)
Medical Outcomes Study/Short-Form Health Survey (SF-36)[104]	Quality of life measure that includes the domains of physical functioning, physical and emotional problems, social function, pain, mental health, vitality, and health perception
Mini-Mental State Examination[40]	Mental status screening test for orientation to time and place, registration of words, attention, calculation, recall, language, and visual construction
Motor Assessment Scale[23]	Motor function evaluation; includes disability and impairment measures, arm and hand movements, tone, and mobility (bed, upright, and ambulation)
Motricity Index[32]	Measures impairments in limb strength with a weighted ordinal scale
Neurobehavioral Cognitive Status Examination (NCSE)[60]	Mental status screening test that includes the domains of orientation, attention, comprehension, naming, construction, memory, calculation, similarities, judgment, and repetition
NIH Stroke Scale[21]	Stroke deficit scale that scores 15 items (e.g., consciousness, vision, extraocular movement, facial control, limb strength, ataxia, sensation, speech, and language)
The Lawton Instrumental Activities of Daily Living[66]	IADL evaluation of telephone use, walking, shopping, food preparation, housekeeping, laundry, public transportation, and medication management
Modified Rankin Scale[17]	Global disability scale with 6 grades indicating degrees of disability
Rivermead Mobility Index[28]	Uses a "pass" or "fail" scale to measure bed mobility, sitting, standing, transfers, and walking
Sickness Impact Profile[14]	Quality of life measure in the format of a 136-item scale with 12 subscales that measure ambulation, mobility, body care, emotion, communication, alertness, sleep, eating, home management, recreation, social interactions, and employment
Stroke Impact Scale[63]	A stroke-specific measure that incorporates function and quality of life into one measure. It is a self-report measure with 59 items and 8 subgroups, including strength, hand function, BADLs and IADLs, mobility, communication, emotion, memory and thinking, and participation
TEMPA[33,34]	Upper extremity performance test composed of 9 standardized tasks (bilateral and unilateral) measured by 3 criteria: length of execution, functional rating, and task analysis; sample tasks are handling coins, picking up a pitcher and pouring water, writing and stamping an envelope, and unlocking a lock
Tinetti Test[94]	Evaluates balance and gait in the older adult population
Trunk Control Test[41]	Trunk control evaluated on a 0- to 100-point scale; tasks used include rolling, supine to sitting, and balanced sitting
Western Aphasia Battery[59]	Includes an "Aphasia Quotient" and a "Cortical Quotient," scored on a 100-point scale; assesses spontaneous speech, repetition, comprehension, naming, reading, and writing

in the OT literature and in related fields. Review papers[a] and evidence-based libraries and search engines (e.g., the Cochrane Library) are sources of up-to-date information.

Over the past several years there has been a paradigm shift related to the intervention philosophies typically used with clients who sustained a stroke. In the past, sensorimotor approaches were used to treat individuals who sustained a stroke (see Chapter 32). These sensorimotor approaches were developed based on the understanding of the central nervous system (CNS) dysfunction at the time these clinicians were doing their research (mid-1900s). Although these interventions are commonly used, their effectiveness has been challenged as occupational therapists move toward models of evidence-based practice.[80] At present there is limited to no research to support these neurofacilitation approaches. Indeed, the Bobath approach (neurodevelopmental treatment [NDT]), although commonly used in the clinic, has not been shown to be superior to other treatment approaches and in fact is inferior to more current models of practice. For example, a large, nonrandomized, parallel-group study[51] ($N = 324$) compared the NDT approach with conventional treatment. Subjects were monitored for 12 months. The authors concluded that "the NDT approach was not found effective in the care of stroke patients in the hospital setting. Healthcare professionals need to reconsider the use of this approach."[51] Similarly, a systematic review of 16 studies involving 813 patients with stroke concluded that "there was no evidence of superiority of Bobath on sensorimotor control of upper and lower limb, dexterity, mobility, ADLs, health-related quality of life, and cost-effectiveness. Only limited evidence was found for balance control in favor of Bobath. This systematic review confirms that overall the Bobath concept is not superior to other approaches."[61]

In contrast, approaches that focus on the use of functional activities as the therapeutic change agent (e.g., task-oriented approaches) show promise from both a research and a clinical perspective.[70,71] A systematic review of task-oriented approaches concluded that "studies of task-related training showed benefits for functional outcome compared with traditional therapies. Active use of task-oriented training with stroke survivors will lead to improvements in functional outcomes and overall health-related quality of life."[81] The authors recommended "creating opportunities to practice meaningful functional tasks outside of regular therapy sessions."[81] A more recent evidence review concluded that "task-oriented training may be considered the foundation of interventions focused on improving occupational performance for those with motor impairment after stroke."[78] The authors further summarized that "commonalities among several of the effective interventions include the use of goal-directed, individualized tasks that promote frequent repetitions of task-related or task-specific movements."[78] One final note on the subject is that approaches focused on the use of functional tasks are more consistent with traditional and current principles of OT.[4]

Mathiowetz[70,71] outlined a series of intervention principles based on use of the OT task-oriented approach. These principles include the following:

- Help clients adjust to role and task performance limitations by exploring new roles and tasks.
- Create an environment that includes the common challenges of everyday life.
- Practice functional tasks or close simulations that have been identified as important by participants to find effective and efficient strategies for performance.
- Provide opportunities for practice outside therapy time (e.g., homework assignments).
- Minimize ineffective and inefficient movement patterns.

FUNCTIONAL LIMITATIONS COMMONLY OBSERVED AFTER STROKE

Multiple factors can impede effective and efficient performance of various tasks on which the client desires to focus during OT. The following sections review problem areas that are typically observed during work with clients who have sustained a stroke.

Inability to Perform Chosen Occupations While Seated

A commonly observed deficit after stroke is loss of trunk and postural control. Trunk and postural control may be considered a foundation for occupational performance. We require postural control to roll and get out of bed the first thing in the morning, feed a baby, sit at a desk to type, propel a wheelchair, eat, and so on. Impairment of trunk control may lead to the following problems[46]:

1. Dysfunction of limb control
2. Increased risk for falls
3. Impaired ability to interact with the environment
4. Visual dysfunction secondary to resultant head and neck malalignment
5. Symptoms of dysphagia secondary to proximal malalignment
6. Decreased independence in ADLs

Loss of trunk and postural control (i.e., "controlling the body's position in space for the dual purposes of stability and orientation"[47]) after a stroke may be manifested as an inability to sit in proper alignment, loss of righting and equilibrium reactions, inability to reach beyond the arm span because of lack of postural adjustments, and falling during attempts to function.

Clients who sustained a stroke and lose trunk control need to use the more functional UE for postural support to remain upright and prevent falls. In these cases, the client effectively eliminates the ability to engage in ADLs and mobility tasks because lifting the more functional arm from the supporting surface can result in a fall. As Franchignoni et al.[41] noted, "Trunk control appears to be an obvious prerequisite for the control of more complex limb activities that in turn constitute a prerequisite to complex behavioral skills." Studies have found trunk control to be a predictor of gait recovery, sitting balance,[67] Functional Independence Measure (FIM) scores,[41] and scores on the Barthel Index[85] after a stroke.

Specific effects of a stroke on the trunk include the following:

1. Inability to perceive the midline as a result of spatial relationship dysfunction, leading to sitting postures that are misaligned from the vertical
2. Assumption of static postures that do not support engagement in functional activities (e.g., posterior pelvic tilt, kyphosis, lateral flexion)
3. Multidirectional trunk weakness[16]
4. Spinal contracture secondary to soft tissue shortening
5. Inability to move the trunk segmentally (i.e., the trunk moves as unit; examples of this phenomenon are clients using "logrolling" patterns during bed mobility and an inability to rotate the trunk while reaching for an item across the midline)
6. Inability to shift weight through the pelvis anteriorly, posteriorly, and laterally

Specific deficits in trunk control are evaluated during observation of task performance (Box 34.1). Observing tasks allows the therapist to evaluate trunk control in many directions (i.e., isometric, eccentric, and concentric control of the trunk muscle groups [extensors, abdominal muscles, and lateral flexors]) and the client's limits of stability. The phrase "limits of stability" refers to an area about which the center of mass may be moved over any given base of support without disrupting equilibrium.[77] The therapist must differentiate between the client's perceived limits of stability and the actual limits of stability. After a stroke, it is common to experience a disparity between the two because of body scheme disorder, fear of falling, or lack of insight into or awareness of disability. If the client's perceived limits are greater than his or her actual limits, there is a risk for falls. In other cases, the client's perceived limits are less than the actual limits. In such instances the client will not attempt more dynamic activities or will rely too greatly on adaptive equipment.

BOX 34.1 Trunk Control Evaluation During Task Performance

Examples of Postural Adjustments That Support Participation in Chosen Activities

Feeding
Anterior weight shift occurs to bring the upper part of the body toward the table, to prevent spillage of food from utensils, and to support a hand-to-mouth pattern.

Dressing
Lateral weight shift to one side of the pelvis occurs so that pants and underwear can be donned over the hips.

Oral Care
Anterior weight shift occurs so that saliva and toothpaste may be expectorated.

Transfer
The trunk extends with concurrent hip flexion to initiate a sit-to-stand transition.

Meal Preparation
The trunk flexes into gravity in a controlled fashion to support a reach pattern to the lower shelf of the refrigerator.

Treatment interventions aimed at increasing the client's ability to perform chosen tasks in seated postures include the following[46]:

1. Establishing a neutral yet active starting alignment (i.e., a position of readiness to function). This starting alignment (similar to a typist's posture) is a prerequisite to engaging the limbs in an activity. The desirable posture is as follows:

   Feet flat on the floor shoulder distance apart and bearing weight

   Equal weight bearing through both ischial tuberosities

   Neutral to slight anterior pelvic tilt

   Erect spine

   Head over the shoulders and shoulders over the hips

   The client should attempt reaching activities from the previously described posture (Fig. 34.4).

2. Establishing the ability to maintain the trunk in the midline by using external cues. Many clients have difficulty assuming and maintaining the correct posture. The therapist can provide verbal feedback (e.g., "Sit up nice and tall"). Visual feedback (e.g., using a mirror or the therapist assuming the same postural misalignment as the client) may be helpful. Environmental cues may be used to correct the posture. For example, the client may be instructed to maintain contact between the shoulder and an external target such as a bolster or wall, positioned so that the trunk is in the correct posture.

3. Maintaining trunk range of motion (ROM) by wheelchair and armchair positioning that maintains the trunk in proper alignment. The therapist can provide an exercise program focused on trunk ROM and flexibility. Activities that elicit the desired movement patterns can be chosen, and hands-on mobilization of the trunk can be used if needed. Types of trunk ROM that should be addressed include flexion, extension, lateral flexion, and rotation.

4. Prescribing dynamic weight-shifting activities to allow practice of weight shifts through the pelvis. The most effective way to train the client in weight shifts is to coordinate the trunk and limbs. Randomized controlled trials have confirmed that sitting training protocols that involve practice in reaching tasks beyond arm's length significantly improve function.[31] Successfully engaging in meaningful occupations that require reach beyond the span of either arm requires clients to adjust their posture. The client is encouraged to reach beyond arm span in all directions while seated (preferably while reaching for an object) and to analyze the corresponding postural adjustment of the pelvis and trunk. The position and goal of the task will dictate the required weight shift (Table 34.4).

5. Strengthening the trunk, best achieved by tasks that require the client to control the trunk against gravity. Some examples are bridging the hips in the supine position to strengthen the back extensors and initiating a roll with the arm and upper part of the trunk to strengthen the abdominal muscles. Strengthening occurs within the context of an activity.

6. Using compensatory strategies and environmental adaptations when trunk control does not improve to a sufficient level and the client is at risk for injury. Examples of interventions include wheelchair seating systems (e.g., lateral

supports, lumbar rolls, chest straps, tilt-in-space frames with head supports) and adaptive ADL equipment (e.g., reachers, long-handled equipment) to decrease the amount of required trunk displacement (see Chapter 10).

For Jasmine, occupational therapy first focused on her ability to keep her trunk stable (i.e., not moving) while using her limbs to engage in occupations. Occupations that do not require substantial weight shifting while sitting (e.g., hair care, upper

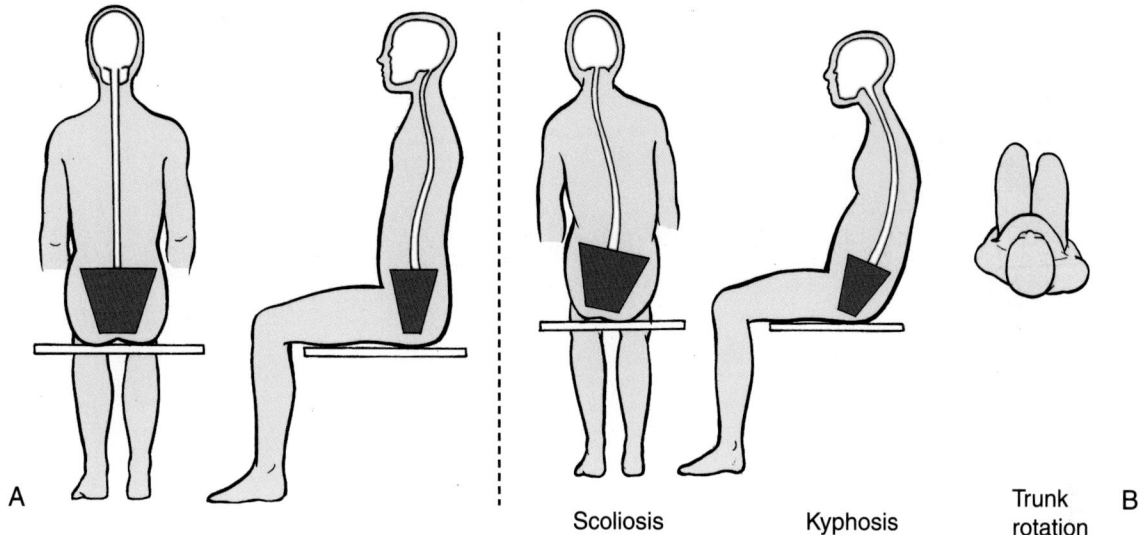

A   Scoliosis   Kyphosis   Trunk   B
                                                                                                                 rotation

Fig. 34.4 Normal (A) and poststroke (B) sitting alignment. (From Nilsen DM, Donato SM, Pulaski KH, Gillen G: Standing postural control: supporting functional independence. In Gillen G, Nilsen DM, editors: *Stroke rehabilitation: a function-based approach*, ed 5, Philadelphia, 2021, Elsevier.)

TABLE 34.4	**Effects of Object Positioning on Trunk Movements and Weight Shifts During Reaching Activities**[a]
Position of Object	**Trunk Response/Weight Shift**
Straight ahead at the forehead level, past arm's length 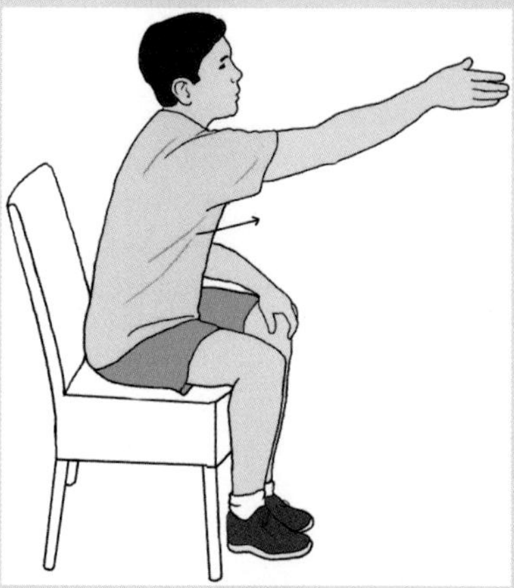	• Trunk extension, anterior pelvic tilt • Anterior weight shift
On the floor, between the feet 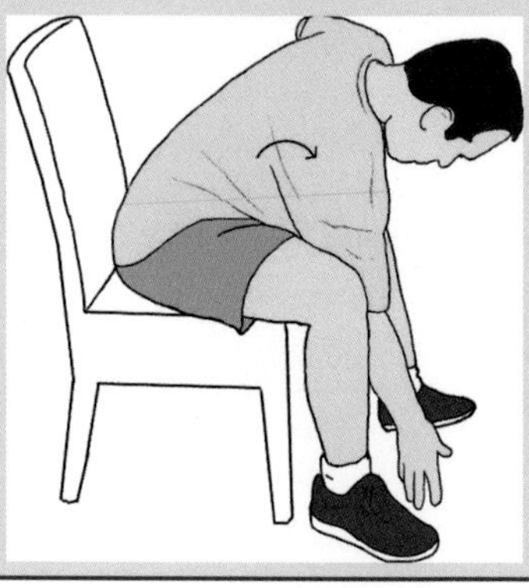	• Trunk flexion • Anterior weight shift

(Continued)

Position of Object	Trunk Response/Weight Shift
To the side at the shoulder level, past arm's length 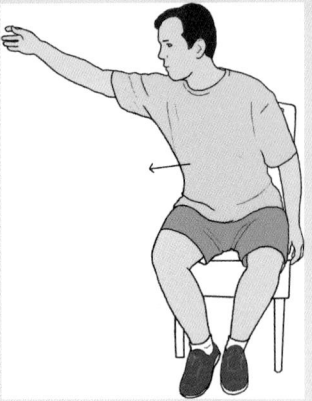	• Left trunk shortening, right trunk elongation, left hip hiking • Weight shift to the right
On the floor, below the right hip 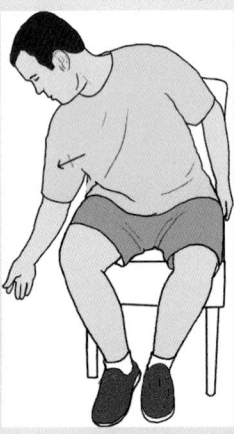	• Right trunk shortening, left trunk elongation
Behind the right shoulder, at arm's length 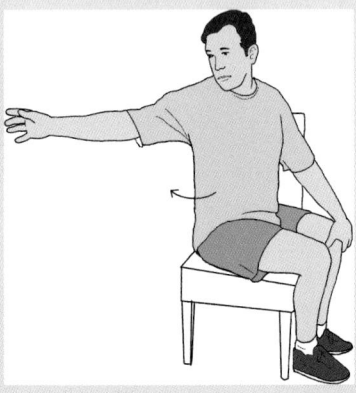	• Trunk extension and rotation (right side posteriorly) • Weight shift to the right
At shoulder level, to the left of the left shoulder 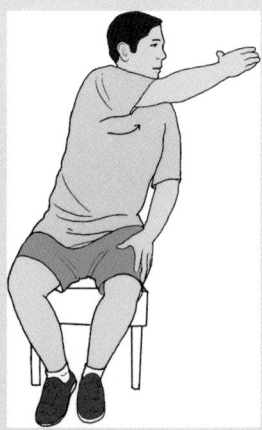	• Trunk extension and rotation (left side posteriorly) • Weight shift to the left

TABLE 34.4   Effects of Object Positioning on Trunk Movements and Weight Shifts During Reaching Activities[a]—cont'd

Position of Object	Trunk Response/Weight Shift
On floor, to left of left foot 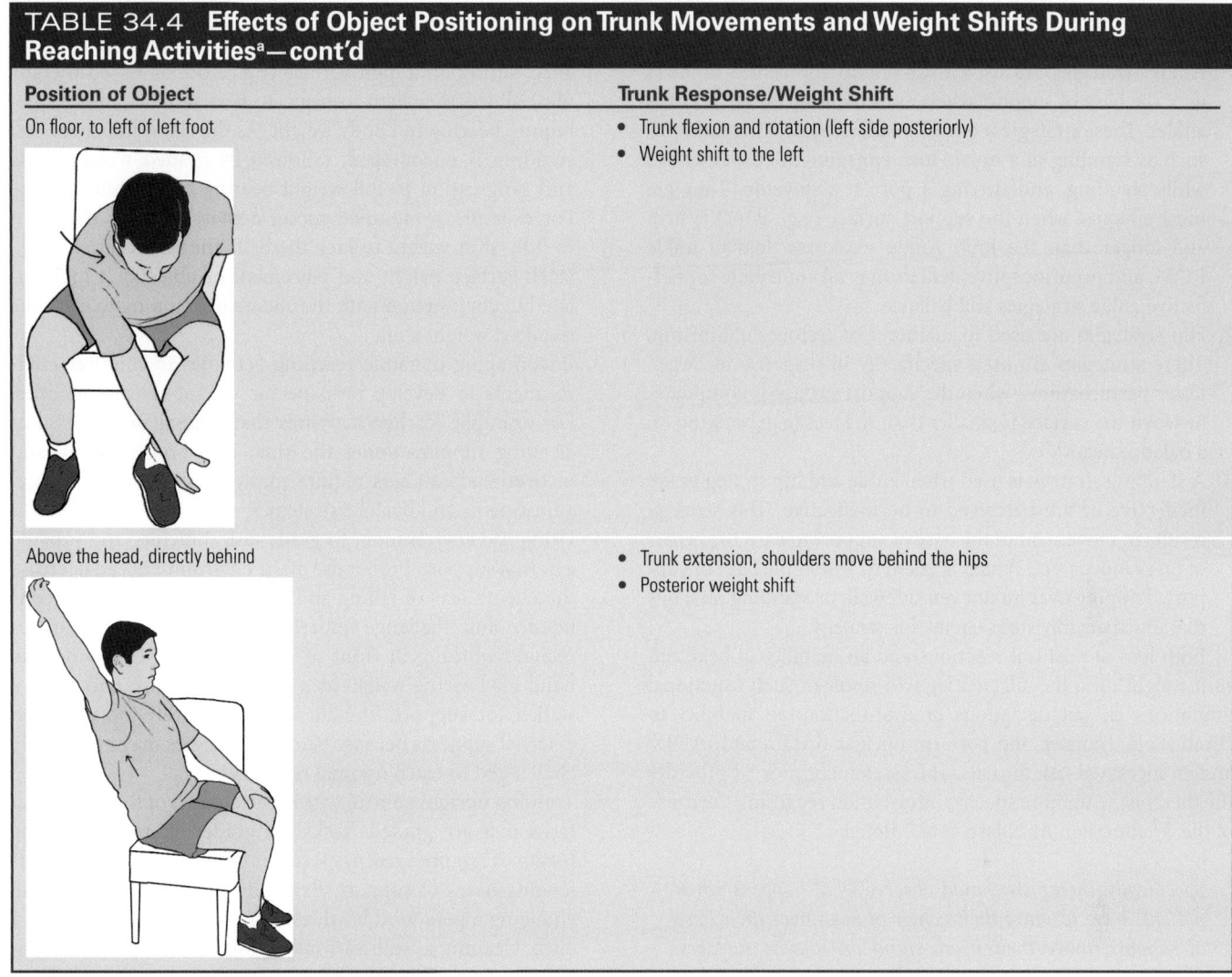	• Trunk flexion and rotation (left side posteriorly) • Weight shift to the left
Above the head, directly behind	• Trunk extension, shoulders move behind the hips • Posterior weight shift

From Gillen G, Nilsen DM, editors: *Stroke rehabilitation: a function-based approach*, ed 5, Philadelphia, 2021, Elsevier.
[a]These examples are for a patient with left hemiplegia. The left-hand column indicates where to position objects during a reaching task (with the right upper extremity). The right-hand column indicates the resultant trunk position and weight shift.

body washing, feeding, card playing) were chosen first, followed by those that required progressively more weight shifting in all directions (e.g., wiping after use of the toilet, lower body dressing, scooting, reaching to the floor to pick up shoes, washing her feet). As needed, the occupational therapist provided external support at Jasmine's shoulders during these activities to increase her confidence, prevent falls, and provide necessary support to compensate for Jasmine's weakness. As Jasmine improved, more challenging seated activities were chosen and external support was diminished.

Inability to Engage in Chosen Occupations While Standing

An inability to assume and maintain a standing posture has a significant effect on the type of activities in which a person may engage; it may also play a significant role in the eventual discharge destination for a hospitalized client recovering from a stroke. Impaired upright control has been correlated with an increased risk for falls[108] and with less than optimal functional outcomes[71]

on the Barthel Index. Because many BADLs and IADLs, work, and leisure skills require control of standing postures, early training in upright control is a necessary component of stroke rehabilitation programs. Postural strategies (e.g., ankle, hip, and stepping strategies) are typically impaired after a stroke.

Similar to the deficits seen while sitting, upright standing postures are characterized by asymmetric weight distribution; unlike deficits occurring while sitting, the weight distribution while standing is seen through the lower extremities,[108] in addition to the trunk. Clients who sustained a stroke often experience an inability to bear weight through the affected leg. Reasons for this disability include fear of falling or buckling of the knee, patterns of weakness that will not support the weight of the body, spasticity impeding proper alignment (i.e., plantar flexion spasticity that effectively blocks weight bearing through the sole of the foot),[43] and perceptual dysfunction.

In addition to asymmetry and an inability to bear weight or shift weight through the affected leg, many clients who have sustained a stroke lose upright postural control and balance strategies. Effective upright control depends on the following automatic postural reactions.[77,88]

1. Ankle strategies are used to maintain the center of mass over the base of support when movement is centered on the ankles. These strategies control small, slow, swaying motions, such as standing in a movie line, engaging in conversations while standing, and stirring a pot on a stovetop. They are most effective when the support surface (e.g., floor) is firm and longer than the foot. Ankle weakness, loss of ankle ROM, and proprioceptive deficits may all contribute to ineffective ankle strategies and balance.

2. Hip strategies are used to maintain or restore equilibrium. These strategies are used specifically in response to larger, faster perturbations, when the support surface is compliant, or when the surface is smaller than the feet (e.g., walking on a balance beam).[9]

3. A stepping strategy is used when ankle and hip strategies are ineffective or are perceived to be ineffective. This strategy results in movement of the base of support toward the center of mass movement. A step is taken to widen the base of support. Tripping over an uneven sidewalk or standing on a bus that unexpectedly stops elicits this strategy.

Both loss of postural reactions and an inability to bear and shift weight onto the affected leg will result in such functional limitations as gait deviations or dysfunction; an inability to climb stairs, transfer, and perform upright BADLs and IADLs; and an increased risk for falls. The assessment process provides the therapist with more specific information regarding the cause of the dysfunction. As Nilsen et al.[77] noted:

Specifically, therapists should observe what happens when patients have to move their center of mass over their base of support, move their head, stand on uneven surfaces, function in lower lighting, move from one type of surface to another, or function on a narrower base of support. Therapists should also observe patients' postural alignment, whether a bias in posture exists and in which direction that bias occurs, patients' limits of stability, the width between their feet during functional tasks, and what patients do after losing their balance.

Treatment strategies aimed at improving the patient's ability to perform chosen tasks in standing postures include the following[77]:

1. Establishing a symmetric base of support and proper alignment to prepare to engage in occupations. This starting alignment is assumed to provide ample proximal stability and to support engagement in functional tasks. The therapist may use hands-on support or visual or verbal feedback to establish proper alignment as follows:
   Feet approximately hip width apart
   Equal weight bearing through the feet
   Neutral pelvis
   Both knees slightly flexed
   Aligned and symmetric trunk

2. Establishing the ability to bear and shift weight through the more affected lower extremity. The ability to bear weight may

be graded at first. For example, if a client cannot assume a standing position because of postural insecurity or imbalance, sitting on a high surface (e.g., stool or raised therapy mat) allows the client to begin to bear weight but does not require bearing full body weight. As the client improves, full standing is encouraged, followed by graded weight shifts and progression to full weight bearing on the affected leg. For example, a modified soccer activity requires the client to fully shift weight to kick the ball. The environment (e.g., work surface height and placement of objects) is manipulated in conjunction with the client's positioning to elicit the required weight shift.

3. Encouraging dynamic reaching activities in multiple environments to develop task-specific weight-shifting abilities. For example, kitchen activities that necessitate retrieval of cleaning supplies under the sink, in a broom closet, and in overhead cabinets require mastery of multiple postural adjustments and balance strategies.

4. Using the environment to grade task difficulty and provide external support. Proper use of the environment can decrease the client's fear of falling and simultaneously improve confidence and challenge underlying balance skills. Examples include working in front of a high countertop, using one hand for bearing weight as a postural support, and using a walker for support. The client must not rely too much on external supports because balance strategies may not be fully challenged to reach optimal recovery.

5. Training upright control within the context of the functional tasks that are graded. Tasks are graded in relation to the length of required reach, speed, and progressively more challenging bases of support. Examples include making a bed, changing a pet's food bowl, setting a table, stepping up on a curb, cleaning a wall mirror, playing horseshoes or shuffleboard, and doffing slippers in a standing posture. All these activities require shifting of body weight, balance strategies, and the ability to bear weight through both lower extremities. The choice of activity is driven by the client's desires, and the therapist designs positioning and setup of the activity to elicit the desired postural strategies (Fig. 34.5).

Jasmine was quickly engaged in activities that required standing despite persistent issues related to sitting balance. Standing was first attempted in front of stable work surfaces (e.g., kitchen counter, sink) to provide a balance point, increase Jasmine's feeling of security and safety, and highlight the functional relevance of standing. As needed, the therapist stabilized the weak joints (e.g., hip and knee) with manual support, and Jasmine wore an ankle-foot orthotic to protect the integrity of her ankle. As Jasmine improved, she was asked to begin to use the upper part of her body for function while controlling her standing. Examples include wiping the counter, organizing a shelf, and grooming while standing. Progressively more demanding occupations from a standing balance perspective were chosen (e.g., modified games, such as volleyball and Wii tennis; vacuuming; emptying a dishwasher; and stand-pivot transfers), and external manual and environmental support was decreased as Jasmine improved. All occupations were chosen to improve Jasmine's ability to accept and shift weight through her left lower extremity.

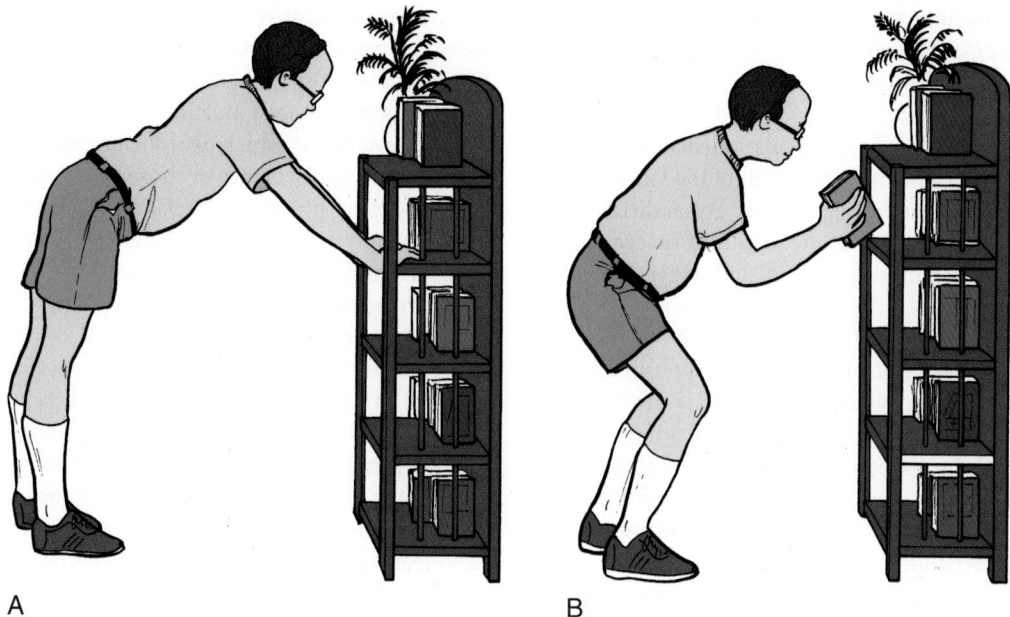

Fig. 34.5 Activity is positioned to elicit the desired postural strategies. (From Nilsen DM, Donato SM, Pulaski KH, Gillen G: Standing postural control: supporting functional independence. In Gillen G, Nilsen DM, editors: *Stroke rehabilitation: a function-based approach*, ed 5, Philadelphia, 2021, Elsevier.)

Inability to Communicate Secondary to Language Dysfunction

Stroke may result in a wide variety of speech or language disorders, ranging from mild to severe. These deficits occur most frequently with stroke resulting from damage to the left hemisphere of the brain. They occur far less frequently after damage to the right hemisphere. All persons with stroke should be evaluated by a speech-language pathologist for the presence of speech and language disorders. The speech-language pathologist can provide valuable information to other members of the rehabilitation team and to the family regarding the best techniques for communicating with a particular client. The occupational therapist should continue the work of the speech therapist in the treatment sessions, as appropriate. Carryover may occur in reinforcing communication techniques that the client is learning and in presenting instruction in ways that the client is able to understand and integrate.[90]

The specific speech and language dysfunctions described in the following sections can exist in mild to severe forms and in combination with one another.

Aphasia

Aphasia is an acquired communication disorder caused by brain damage that is characterized by impairment of language modalities (i.e., speaking, listening, reading, and writing); it is not the result of a sensory or motor deficit, a general intellectual deficit, confusion, or a psychiatric disorder.[52]

Global aphasia. Global aphasia is characterized by loss of all language skills. Oral expression is lost, except for some persistent or recurrent utterance. Global aphasia is usually the result of involvement of the MCA of the dominant cerebral hemisphere. A client with global aphasia may be sensitive to gestures,

vocal inflections, and facial expression. Consequently, the client may appear to understand more than he or she actually does.

Broca's aphasia. Poor speech production and agrammatism characterize Broca's aphasia. This aphasia manifests as slow, labored speech with frequent misarticulations. Syntactic structure is simplified because of the agrammatism, sometimes referred to as telegraphic speech. A client with this form of aphasia demonstrates good auditory comprehension except when speech is rapid, grammatically complex, or lengthy. Reading comprehension and writing may be severely affected, and a client with Broca's aphasia usually has deficits in monetary concepts and the ability to perform calculations.[90]

Wernicke's aphasia. Wernicke's aphasia is characterized by impaired auditory comprehension and feedback, along with fluent, well-articulated paraphasic speech. Paraphasic speech consists of word substitution errors. Speech may occur at an excessive rate and may be hyperfluent. The client uses few substantive words and many function words. The client produces running speech composed of English words in a meaningless sequence. English-speaking clients produce neologisms (non-English nonsense words) interspersed with real words. Reading and writing comprehension is often limited, and mathematical skills may be impaired.[90]

Anomic aphasia. Persons with anomic aphasia have difficulty in word retrieval. Anomia, or word-finding difficulty, occurs in all types of aphasia. However, clients in whom word-finding difficulty is the primary or only symptom may be said to have anomic aphasia. Clients with this form of aphasia have fluent, grammatically correct, and well-articulated speech patterns but display significant difficulty in word finding. This problem can result in hesitant or slow speech and the substitution of descriptive phrases for the actual names of things. Mild to severe deficits in reading comprehension and written expression occur, and mild deficits in mathematical skills may be present.[90]

Dysarthria

Clients with dysarthria have an articulation disorder, in the absence of aphasia, because of dysfunction of the CNS mechanisms that control the speech musculature. Dysarthria results in paralysis and incoordination of the organs of speech, which causes the speech to sound thick, slurred, and sluggish.

Communication With Clients Who Have Aphasia

Although the speech-language pathologist is responsible for the treatment of speech and language disorders, the occupational therapist can facilitate communication and meaningful interaction with clients who have aphasia. The use of gestures for communication should be encouraged. Having the client demonstrate through performance is the best way to ensure that the instructions are understood.

The occupational therapist can use routine ADLs as opportunities to encourage speech. The client should be reassured that the language disorder is part of the disability, not a manifestation of mental illness. Additional strategies for the occupational therapist to use with clients and their caregivers include the following[90]:

- Understanding is facilitated when one person talks at a time. Extra noise creates confusion.
- Give the client time to respond.
- Carefully phrase questions to make it easier for the client to respond; for example, use "yes/no" and "either/or" questions.
- Use visual cues or gestures with speech to help the client understand.
- Never force a response.
- Use concise sentences.
- Do not rush communication because this may increase frustration and decrease the effectiveness of communication.

Given that Jasmine sustained a right hemispheric stroke, aphasia would not typically be expected. Jasmine did exhibit severe sensory motor loss related to her left oral structures. She had moderate dysarthria, occasional drooling, and difficulty managing food (chewing) on the left side of her mouth. Jasmine was encouraged to speak slowly and overenunciate. In addition, her occupational therapist taught her safe feeding strategies, including eating slowly, alternating between solids and liquids, shifting food to the right side of her mouth, tilting her head to the right at a 45-degree angle, using her finger to sweep her mouth and clear out food pocketing on the left, and performing supervised oral care after each meal.

INABILITY TO PERFORM CHOSEN OCCUPATIONS SECONDARY TO NEUROBEHAVIORAL/COGNITIVE-PERCEPTUAL IMPAIRMENTS

A neurobehavioral deficit is defined as "a functional impairment of an individual manifested as defective skill performance resulting from a neurological processing dysfunction that affects performance components such as affect, body scheme,

cognition, emotion, gnosis, language, memory, motor movement, perception, personality, sensory awareness, spatial relations, and visuospatial skills."[6] A major responsibility of the occupational therapist treating a client who has sustained a stroke is evaluating which neurobehavioral deficits are blocking independent performance of chosen occupations.

Árnadóttir[6] proposed a relationship among the ability to perform daily activities, neurobehavioral impairments, and the CNS origin of the neurobehavioral dysfunction (a stroke, for the purposes of this chapter). She supported this theory with the following relational statements:

1. Behaviors required for task performance are related to neuronal processing at the CNS level. Therefore, a relationship also exists between the defective behavioral responses of an individual with CNS damage during performance of ADLs and the dysfunction of neuronal processing and performance components resulting from the CNS damage.
2. Performance of daily activities requires adequate function of specific parts of the nervous system. Consequently, CNS impairment may result in dysfunction of specific aspects of ADLs. For example, a stroke caused by a lesion of the posteroinferior parietal lobe of the left hemisphere commonly results in bilateral motor apraxia. "This neurobehavioral impairment may make manipulation of objects difficult during functional activities such as combing hair, brushing teeth, or holding a spoon while eating."[6]
3. Neurological impairment can be observed through the client's engagement in daily activities. Thus, by analysis of ADLs, the integrity of the CNS can be evaluated (Box 34.2 and Table 34.5).

To properly evaluate the effect of neurobehavioral deficits on task performance, the therapist must develop activity analysis skills with the goal of analyzing which components of performance are necessary to achieve an outcome that is satisfactory to the client. Even the simplest of BADL tasks challenges multiple underlying skills (Boxes 34.3 and 34.4; also see Fig. 34.3).[6,47]

Árnadóttir[5,6] proposed a system of observing clients engaged in functional activities in which errors are allowed to occur (safe errors), the errors are analyzed, and, finally, impairments that are interfering with performance of tasks are detected so that an appropriate treatment plan can be developed. She cautioned that when the therapist analyzes errors and observed behavior, knowledge of neurobehavior, cortical function, activity analysis, and clinical reasoning must be considered in the results of the evaluation (see Table 34.5).

Treatment aimed at counteracting the effects of neurobehavioral dysfunction may be based on an adaptive and compensatory approach or on a restorative and remedial approach.[44,47,74,76] A combination of approaches also has been suggested (Table 34.6).[1]

Decisions regarding the selection of a particular treatment approach may be difficult. Neistadt[75,76] suggested evaluating a client's learning potential in the context of ADL evaluation and training, with a focus on such issues as the number of repetitions needed to learn new approaches to tasks and the type of transfer of learning that is demonstrated.

BOX 34.2 Toothbrushing Task

Treatment of Neurobehavioral Impairments

Spatial Relationships and Spatial Positioning
- Positioning of the toothbrush and toothpaste while applying paste to the brush
- Placement of the toothbrush in the mouth
- Positioning of bristles in the mouth
- Placement of the brush under the faucet

Spatial Neglect
- Visual search for and use of the brush, paste, and cup in the affected hemisphere
- Visual search for and use of the faucet handle in the affected hemisphere

Body Neglect
- Brushing of the affected side of the mouth

Motor Apraxia
- Manipulation of the toothbrush during task performance
- Manipulation of the cap from the toothpaste
- Squeezing of toothpaste onto the brush

Ideational Apraxia
- Appropriate use of objects (e.g., brush, paste, cup) during a task

Organization and Sequencing
- Sequencing of the task (e.g., removal of the cap, application of paste to the brush, turning on the water, putting the brush in the mouth)
- Continuation of task to completion

Attention
- Attention to the task (to increase difficulty, distractions such as conversation, flushing the toilet, or running water may be added)
- Refocusing on the task after the distraction

Figure-Ground
- Distinguishing a white toothbrush and toothpaste from the sink

Initiation and Perseverance
- Initiation of the task on command
- Cleaning parts of the mouth for an appropriate period, then moving the bristles to another part of the mouth
- Discontinuation of the task when complete

Visual Agnosia
- Use of touch to identify objects

Problem Solving
- Search for alternatives if the toothpaste or toothbrush is missing

From Gillen G, Nilsen DM, editors: *Stroke rehabilitation: a function-based approach*, ed 5, Philadelphia, 2021, Elsevier.

TABLE 34.5 Evaluating the Effect of Neurobehavioral Dysfunction on Task Performance

Performance Area	Observed Behavior	Possible Impairment
Grooming	Difficulty adjusting grasp on razor or toothbrush	Motor apraxia
	Using a comb to brush teeth	Ideational apraxia
	Repetitive brushing of one side of mouth	Premotor perseveration
Feeding	Not eating food on left side of plate	Spatial neglect
	Overestimating or underestimating distance to glass, resulting in knocking over glass	Spatial relationship dysfunction
	"Forgetting" that a glass of orange juice is in hand, resulting in spillage as client attends to another aspect of meal	Body neglect
	Placing hand in cereal bowl	
Dressing	Client attempting to put socks on after sneakers	Organization and sequencing dysfunction
	Client unable to locate armholes in undershirt	Spatial relationship dysfunction
	Dressing only right side of body	Body neglect
	Client attempting to dress therapist's arms instead of his or her own	Somatoagnosia
Mobility	Client unable to locate bathroom in his or her hospital room	Topographic disorientation
	Client neglecting to lock brakes or remove wheelchair footrests before attempting to transfer	Organization and sequencing dysfunction
	After a transfer, only intact buttock is in contact with seat of chair	Body neglect

From Árnadóttir G: The brain and behavior: assessing cortical dysfunction through activities of daily living, St Louis, 1990, Mosby; and Gillen G, Nilsen DM, editors: *Stroke rehabilitation: a function-based approach*, ed 5, Philadelphia, 2021, Elsevier.

Toglia[95] has suggested that transfer of learning from one context to another (e.g., transferring skills learned from making a cup of tea in the OT clinic to meal preparation at home) may be facilitated by the therapist through the following methods:

1. Varying treatment environments
2. Varying the nature of the task
3. Helping clients become aware of how they process information
4. Teaching processing strategies
5. Relating new learning to previously learned skills

Toglia[95] has identified degrees of transfer of learning. The degree of transfer is defined by the number of task characteristics that differ from those of the original task. Examples of these characteristics are spatial orientation, mode of presentation (e.g., auditory or visual), movement requirements, and environmental context.

BOX 34.3　Examples of Environmental and Task Manipulation to Challenge Component Skills During Meal Preparation

Spatial Neglect
- Place ingredients in both visual fields.
- Choose a task that requires use of the right and left burners.

Figure-Ground
- Place necessary utensils in a cluttered drawer.
- Use utensils that match the color of the counter.

Spatial Dysfunction
- Prepare items that require the client to pour ingredients from one container to another (e.g., pour pasta into a bowl or fill a pot with water).

Motor Apraxia
- Choose recipes that require manipulation of food items.
- Choose recipes that require control of distal extremity adjustments (e.g., using a ladle, whisking, and stirring).

BOX 34.4　Sample Compensatory Strategies for Neurobehavioral Deficits Affecting Dressing Skills

Spatial Neglect
- Place necessary clothing on the right side of the closet and drawers.
- Move the dresser to the right side of the room.

Motor Apraxia
- Use loose-fitting clothing without fasteners.
- Use Velcro closures.

Spatial Dysfunction
- Use shirts with a front emblem to identify proper orientation.
- Lay out clothing in the proper orientation.

TABLE 34.6　Treatment Approaches for Neurobehavioral Deficits After Stroke

Compensatory and Adaptive Approach	Restorative and Remedial Approach	Combination Approach
• Repetitive practice of tasks • Top-down approach • Emphasizes intact skill training • Emphasizes modification • Uses environmental or task modifications to support optimal performance • Choice of activity driven by performance challenges, not by component deficits • Treats symptoms, not the cause • Client-driven compensatory strategies • Caregiver-therapist environmental adaptations • Task specific and not generalizable	• Restoration of component skills • Bottom-up approach • Deficit specific • Targets cause of symptoms and emphasizes components • Assumes that transfer of training will occur • Assumes that improved component performance will result in increased skill • Choice of activity driven by component deficits • Research demonstrates short-term results with skills generalizable to very similar tasks	• Rejects dichotomy between compensatory and restorative approaches • Uses optimally relevant occupations and environments as the treatment modality to challenge components • Choice of treatment driven by tasks relevant to client needs; tasks presented so that the underlying deficits are challenged via the task • Rejects use of contrived activities

A near transfer of learning involves transfer between two tasks that have one or two differing characteristics. Intermediate transfer involves transfer of learning to a task that varies by three to six characteristics. A far transfer involves a task that is conceptually similar but has one or no characteristics in common. Finally, a very far transfer involves the "spontaneous application of what has been learned in treatment to everyday living."[95]

From her review of the literature, Neistadt[74] reached the following conclusions:

1. Near transfer from remedial tasks to similar tasks is possible for all clients with brain injury.
2. Intermediate, far, and very far transfer from remedial to functional tasks will occur only in clients with localized brain lesions and good cognitive skills and after training with a variety of treatment tasks.
3. Far and very far transfer from remedial to functional tasks will not occur in clients with diffuse injury and severe cognitive deficits.

Using a functional and meaningful task as a treatment modality promotes the acquisition of a desired skill, and the therapist may use this task to challenge multiple underlying impairments.[1,44,47] It is up to the therapist to present the task by manipulating the environment in a way that challenges the underlying skills (see Box 34.3). If a compensatory approach is chosen, adaptive techniques are used to counteract the effects of the underlying neurobehavioral deficits (see Box 34.4).

Jasmine's left-sided neglect had a substantial impact on her ability to perform relevant occupations independently and safely. A variety of strategies was used to improve her ability to attend to the left side. Organized visual scanning was taught during daily activities such as feeding and grooming.[49] Occupations were chosen that required scanning to both the left and the right to be successful (e.g., finding ingredients in the refrigerator, locating the toothbrush on the left side of the sink and toothpaste on the right, reading, and describing a room). Vanishing physical and verbal cues were used as Jasmine progressed. Another strategy that was helpful for Jasmine was the use of a left-sided anchor. A red strip of tape was placed on the left side (e.g., the left side of the computer monitor, placemat, sink, book), and Jasmine focused on scanning to the anchor to ensure that she was attending to all of the information required to be successful at performing each occupation. Because Jasmine's neglect persisted, driving was not an option. Other modes of transportation were considered, including supervised use of public transportation, assistance with transport by friends and neighbors, and local Access-A-Ride companies. (See Chapter 11.)

INABILITY TO PERFORM CHOSEN TASKS SECONDARY TO UPPER EXTREMITY DYSFUNCTION

Loss of UE control is the most common and challenging consequence of stroke. In the Copenhagen Stroke study (515 stroke patients), 32% had severe and 37% had mild UE dysfunction.[73] The client's ability to integrate the affected arm into chosen tasks may be limited by multiple factors, including the following[48]:

1. Pain
2. Contracture and deformity
3. Loss of selective motor control
4. Weakness[19]
5. Superimposed orthopedic limitations
6. Loss of postural control to support UE control
7. Learned nonuse[91]
8. Loss of biomechanical alignment[22]
9. Inefficient and ineffective movement patterns

Integration Into Function

UE evaluation procedures should focus primarily on assessing the client's ability to integrate the UE into the performance of functional tasks—in other words, to use the affected UE to support performance in areas of occupation. The Functional Upper Extremity Levels (FUEL)[102] is a valid and reliable classification tool to assess a client's ability to use the UE during functional tasks after stroke. The FUEL includes 7 levels of use, ranging from nonfunctional to fully functional, and provides a description of each level about how to classify the UE during a task. This tool can be used for any functional task that requires arm use as long as the levels and definitions are adhered to.[102] Other standardized evaluations, such as the Test d'Evaluation des Membres Supérieurs de Personnes Agées (TEMPA),[33,34] Arm Motor Ability Test (AMAT),[62] and Jebsen Test of Hand Function[56] (see Table 34.3), are available to objectively measure the client's ability to use the affected extremity during performance of tasks. In addition, self-reported measures of UE function are recommended. Examples include the following:

1. The Motor Activity Log is a self-reported questionnaire (reported by the patient or family) related to actual use of the involved UE outside structured therapy time. It uses a semi-structured interview format. Quality of movement ("how well" scale) and the amount of use ("how much" scale) are graded on a 6-point scale. At present there are 30-, 28-, and 14-item versions of the tool. Sample items include holding a book, using a towel, picking up a glass, writing/typing, and steadying oneself.[100,101]
2. The 36-item Manual Ability Measure (MAM-36) is a new Rasch-developed, self-reported disability outcome measure.[25,26] It contains 36 gender-neutral, commonly performed everyday hand tasks. The patient is asked to report the ease or difficulty of performing such tasks. It uses a 4-point rating scale, with 1 indicating "unable" (I am unable to do the task all by myself); 2 indicating "very hard" (It is very hard for me to do the task, and I usually ask others to do it for me unless no one is around); 3 indicating "a little hard" (I usually do the task myself, although it takes longer or more effort now than before); and 4 indicating "easy" (I can do the task without

any problem). The MAM-36 has been validated and is psychometrically sound, reflecting the use of occupation-based tasks to determine hand function.[25]

The UE may be used during functional performance in different ways (Table 34.7), including, but not limited to, the following[48]:

1. *Weight bearing or accepting partial body weight through a limb.* Weight bearing through the hand and forearm with an extended elbow is a pattern used during ADLs and mobility tasks. Establishment of weight bearing is a goal of UE rehabilitation.[15] Effective control of weight bearing depends on the presence of sufficient trunk and scapula stability to accept partial body weight, control of active elbow extension, and ability of the hand to bear weight without losing the palmar arches. Once weight bearing has been established, the client can effectively use the arm as a postural support (e.g., by supporting upper body weight with the affected arm while wiping crumbs from the table with the more functional arm), as an aid during transitional movements (e.g., while pushing up from lying on the side to sitting), and for preventing falls (increased postural support is provided).[48]

2. *Moving objects across a work surface with a static grasp (supported reach).* Activities such as ironing clothes, opening or closing a drawer, polishing furniture, and sliding a paper across the table are examples of UE control of movement that do not occur with the arm in space. The hand is in contact with the objects involved in the task or is supported on the work surface; therefore, these types of tasks do not require the same control as (and may require less effort than)

TABLE 34.7 Suggestions for Categorizing Upper Extremity Tasks

Category	Tasks
No functional use of the arm	• Teach shoulder protection • Self range of motion • Positioning
• Postural support/weight bearing (forearm or extended arm)	• Bed mobility assistance • Support upright function (e.g., work, leisure, activities of daily living [ADLs]) • Support during reach with the opposite hand • Stabilize objects
• Support reach (hand on a work surface)	• Wiping a table • Ironing • Polishing • Sanding • Smoothing out laundry • Applying body lotion • Washing body parts • Vacuuming • Locking wheelchair brakes
• Reach	• Multiple possibilities to engage the upper extremity in ADLs, leisure, and mobility; grade tasks by height/distance reached, weight of object, speed, and accuracy

From Gillen G, Nilsen DM, editors: *Stroke rehabilitation: a function-based approach*, ed 5, Philadelphia, 2021, Elsevier.

activities performed while the client is reaching in space, such as removing dishes from a cabinet or reaching for food in the refrigerator. This movement pattern can be used for multiple tasks and at the same time strengthens the various muscle groups used to eventually support reach in space.[48]

3. *Reach and manipulation.* Reviews of research on UE motor control[2,48] have identified two components of function during reaching activities. The first is the transportation component, which is defined as the trajectory of the arm between the starting position and the object. The second is the manipulation component, which is the formation of grip by combined movements of the thumb and index finger during arm movement. Finger posturing anticipates the real grasp and occurs during transportation of the hand toward the object.[2] Shaping of the hand is independent of the manipulation itself. A systematic review and meta-analysis study of kinematic components of reach to target movement showed that clients with hemiparesis had significantly less ability to reach smoothly and with coordination as compared to healthy adults.[29] The continuous movement strategy was lost, movement time was longer, peak velocity occurred earlier, and there was greater trunk displacement.

Trombly[96] demonstrated that although muscular activity did not improve in the clients in her study, the discontinuity improved over time. She stated that the "level and pattern of muscle activity of these subjects depended on the biomechanical demands of the task rather than any stereotypical neurological linkages between the muscles."

Clients are commonly observed demonstrating the use of stereotypical movement patterns of the UE. These patterns are characterized by scapula elevation and fixation, humeral abduction, elbow flexion, and wrist flexion. Mathiowetz and Bass Haugen[70] suggested that the use of these movement patterns is evidence of attempts to use the remaining systems to complete tasks. They gave an example of a client with weak shoulder flexors trying to lift an arm. The client flexes the elbow when trying to raise the arm because this movement strategy shortens the lever arm and eases shoulder flexion.

An evidence-based review[78] documented that the following interventions resulted in improved occupational performance for those with motor control limitations:

- *Repetitive task practice:* This term was used to describe training approaches that included performance of goal-directed, individualized tasks with frequent repetitions of task-related or task-specific movements.
- *Constraint-induced movement therapy (CIMT) or modified constraint-induced movement therapy (mCIMT):* A method of training that involves restraint of the unaffected limb for approximately 90% of waking hours, forcing use of the affected limb during daily activities. The other components of CIMT include shaping and intensive and repetitive task training using the affected limb for 6 hours per day for 2 weeks. Modified CIMT is a shortened version of the original CIMT. During mCIMT, the amount of time for intensive training of the affected limb, the restraint time of the nonaffected limb, or both are decreased and/or distributed over a longer period of time (Box 34.5).

BOX 34.5   Main Points of Constraint-Induced Movement Therapy

1. **Counteracts learned nonuse.** Hypothesized causes of learned nonuse include therapeutic interventions implemented during the acute period of neurological suppression after a stroke, an early focus on adaptations to meet functional goals, negative reinforcement experienced by patients as they unsuccessfully attempt to use the affected limb, and positive reinforcement experienced by using the less involved hand and/or successful adaptations.
2. **Motor inclusion criteria.** Control of the wrist and digits is necessary to engage in this type of intervention. Current and past protocols have used the following inclusion criteria: 20 degrees of extension of the wrist and 10 degrees of extension of each finger; 10 degrees of extension of the wrist, 10 degrees of abduction of the thumb, and 10 degrees of extension of any two other digits; or the ability to lift a washrag from a table using any type of prehension and then release it.
3. **Main therapeutic factor.** Massed practice and shaping of the affected limb during repetitive functional activities appear to be the therapeutic change agents. "There is thus nothing talismanic about use of a sling or other constraining device on the less-affected limb."[48]
4. **Choices of activity and the therapist's interventions.** Select tasks that address the motor deficits of the individual client, assist clients in carrying out parts of a movement sequence if they are incapable of completing the movement on their own at first, provide explicit verbal feedback and verbal reward for small improvements in task performance, use modeling and prompting of task performance, use tasks that are of interest and motivational to the patient, ignore regression of function, and use tasks that can be quantified related to improvements.
5. **Outcome measures.** The Motor Activity Log (actual use outside of structured therapy, or "real-world" use), Arm Motor Ability Test, Wolf Motor Function Test, and Action Research Arm Test have been used to document outcomes.
6. **Cortical reorganization.** Constraint-induced movement therapy is the first rehabilitation intervention that has been demonstrated to induce changes in the cortical representation of the affected upper limb.
7. **Research validity.** The rigorous research that has been and continues to be carried out to demonstrate the effectiveness or efficacy of constraint-induced movement therapy should be used as a gold standard for other rehabilitation interventions that are used traditionally (e.g., neurodevelopmental therapy) but have little or no research support.
8. **Evidence-based support.** On the basis of available evidence, constraint-induced movement therapy appears to be an effective intervention for those living with stroke who have learned nonuse and fit the motor inclusion criteria.

From Gillen G, Nilsen DM: Upper extremity function and management. In Gillen G, Nilsen DM, editors: *Stroke rehabilitation: a function-based approach*, ed 5, Philadelphia, 2021, Elsevier.

- *Strengthening and exercise:* All forms of strengthening and exercise, including yoga and tai chi, were combined into the intervention category of strengthening and exercise in this review.
- *Mental practice:* A training method during which a person cognitively rehearses a physical skill in the absence of actual movements. Most often this type of training is coupled with traditional task-oriented practice.
- *Virtual reality:* Participants take part in various goal-directed activities in a computer-based, interactive, multisensory-simulated environment designed to replicate real-world experiences.

- *Mirror therapy:* During mirror therapy, a mirror or mirror box is placed in the midsagittal position between the extremities of interest. The individual is then encouraged to concentrate on the mirror reflection of the uninvolved extremity performing movements or receiving sensory stimulation while the involved extremity remains hidden out of sight behind the mirror. This procedure creates a visual illusion whereby the activities of the uninvolved extremity are attributed to the involved extremity.

- *Action observation:* Participants watch another person performing common functional actions (most often by watching a prerecorded video) with the intention of imitating the observed actions. Accordingly, action observation is followed by actual task performance.

The following are examples of using treatment activities to improve the client's ability to integrate the UE into tasks.[2,24,44,46,88]

1. Using objects of different sizes and shapes to encourage control of the hand during reach and manipulation.

2. Choosing activities that are appropriate to the client's level of available motor control.

3. Using CIMT techniques (see Box 34.5): techniques in which the less affected UE is constrained (e.g., with a sling and splint or similar device) to compel use of the affected extremity, thereby providing massed practice of graded activities for the affected side to increase functional use.[72]

4. Specifically training the arm to be used in weight bearing, reach, and manipulation situations within the context of ADLs and mobility.

5. Presenting the client with graded tasks related to the number of degrees of freedom, the level of antigravity control required, and the resistance involved in the task (Fig. 34.6).

Jasmine had very little motor activity throughout her left UE. Therapy focused on having Jasmine position her arm correctly (on the work surface and within her sight lines) during activities to prevent it from dangling all day and to use her arm as a stabilizer (e.g., using the weight of her arm to stabilize a paper while writing or holding a book open). As Jasmine improved, she was encouraged to use her arm in weight bearing as a postural support (e.g., pushing up when transitioning from the supine position to a seated position, pushing up to stand, reaching back to sit, and using the arm as support when standing at a sink or counter). Occupations were chosen that matched her available motor control and challenged her current level.

Upper Extremity Complications After Stroke

Subluxation. Subluxation, or malalignment caused by instability of the glenohumeral joint, is a common occurrence after stroke. The subluxation may be inferior (head of the humerus below the glenoid fossa), anterior (head of the humerus anterior to the fossa), or superior (head of the humerus lodged under the acromion-coracoid).[48] Cailliet[22] and Basmajian[10] described the mechanism of inferior subluxation, in which the humeral head drifts inferior to the glenoid fossa. This common subluxation occurs as a result of malalignment of the scapula and the trunk. The normal position of the scapula is one of upward rotation, an orientation that cradles the head of the humerus and stabilizes it in alignment. The weight of the arm combined with instability and malalignment contributes to subluxation.

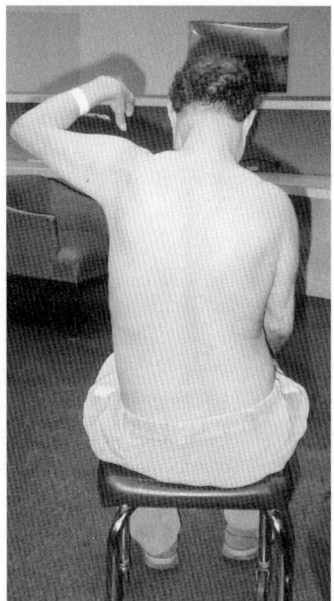
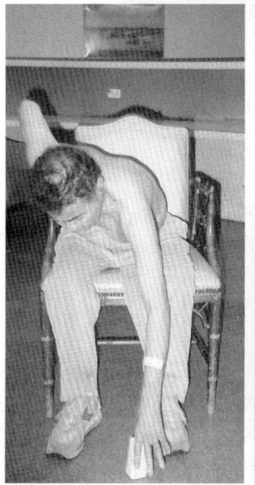
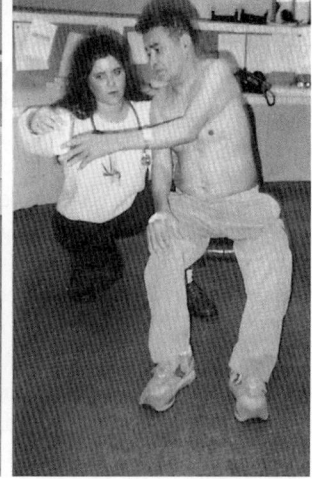

Fig. 34.6 The task is designed to elicit the desired motor pattern; the purpose of the task drives the motor output. (From Gillen G, Nilsen DM: Upper extremity function and management. In Gillen G, Nilsen DM, editors: *Stroke rehabilitation: a function-based approach*, ed 5, Philadelphia, 2021, Elsevier.)

A common misunderstanding about subluxation is that it is associated with pain. The literature does not support this relationship.[110] Because the shoulder is unstable after a stroke, care must be taken to support the flail shoulder in bed (e.g., using pillows to maintain alignment), in a wheelchair (e.g., with lap boards or pillows), and in the upright position (e.g., putting the hands in a pocket, taping the shoulder, GivMohr Sling). Treatment to reduce subluxation should focus on achieving trunk alignment and scapula stability in a position of upward rotation.[48]

Abnormal skeletal muscle activity. A change in the resting state of the limb and postural muscles is common after stroke.[15] Immediately after a stroke, a change in available, or resting, skeletal muscle activity occurs. Most commonly, the acute state is characterized by low tone (low-tone stage). During this low-tone stage, the limbs and trunk become increasingly influenced by the pull of gravity. Little or no muscle activity is available at this stage, which results in deviations from the normal resting alignment of the musculoskeletal system.

An inability to recruit and maintain muscle activity is generally the greatest limiting factor at this stage. Because of the generalized lack of muscle activity and the dependent nature of the trunk and limbs, secondary problems can occur,[43] including the following:

1. Edema affecting the dorsal surface of the hand and pooling of fluids under the extensor tendons, thereby effectively blocking active or passive digit flexion

2. Overstretching of the joint capsule of the glenohumeral joint

3. Eventual shortening of muscles that are passively positioned in an effort to support a weak limb (Commonly, flaccid UEs are positioned in the client's lap, on a pillow, on a lap tray, or in a sling. Although these support the arm, the static positions result in prolonged positioning of certain muscle groups [internal rotators, elbow flexors, and wrist flexors] in a shortened position, which places them at risk for mechanical shortening. Interestingly, these are the muscle groups that tend to become spastic as time progresses.)

4. Overstretching of the antagonists to the previously mentioned muscles

5. Risk of joint and soft tissue injury during ADLs and mobility tasks (Because of the lack of control associated with a low-tone stage, the arm dangles and is not positioned appropriately during dynamic activities. Common examples include an arm being caught in the wheel during wheelchair mobility, pinning of the arm during bed mobility or rest, sitting on the arm after a transfer, or weight bearing through a flexed wrist during engagement in self-care activities.)

Progression to a state of increased or excessive skeletal muscle activity (increased tone), such as clonus, stereotypic posturing of the trunk and limbs, hyperactive stretch reflexes, and increased resistance to passive limb movements that are dependent on velocity, may occur within several days or months of the stroke.[43]

As spasticity increases, the risk for soft tissue shortening is heightened. This factor may lead to a vicious circle of spasticity to soft tissue shortening to over-recruitment of shortened muscles to increased stretch reflexes. Secondary problems that may occur if the spasticity is not managed in a therapy program include the following[43]:

1. Deformity of the limbs, specifically the distal end of the upper limb (elbow to digits)

2. Maceration of palm tissue

3. Possible masking of underlying selective motor control

4. Pain syndromes resulting from loss of normal joint kinematics (These syndromes are usually related to soft tissue contracture that blocks full joint excursion. A typical example is loss of full passive external rotation of the glenohumeral joint. Attempts at forced abduction in these cases will result in a painful impingement syndrome of the tissues in the subacromial space.)

5. Impaired ability to manage BADL tasks, specifically UE dressing and bathing of the affected hand and axilla when flexor posturing is present

6. Loss of reciprocal arm swing during gait activities

Prevention of pain syndromes and contracture. Protection of unstable joints. During the low-tone stage, joints tend to become malaligned secondary to loss of muscular stabilization. In these cases, clients are at risk for injury to unstable joints

(e.g., traction injuries and joint trauma) because of the joint instability. The glenohumeral and wrist joints are particularly at risk. The glenohumeral joint (usually already inferiorly subluxated at this stage) is at risk for a superimposed orthopedic injury if another individual unknowingly pulls on the affected arm during self-care and mobility or during unskilled passive range of motion (PROM) of the joint. The unstable glenohumeral joint is in a malaligned state, which puts the client at risk for an impingement syndrome during PROM if normal joint mechanics is not addressed. Key joint motions of concern are upward rotation of the scapula and external (lateral) rotation of the shoulder. If these motions are not present and ROM is forced, the client is at risk for the development of an impingement and pain syndrome.[43]

Clients with low tone also have an unstable wrist. Care should be taken to protect the wrist if the client is not controlling the joint during ADL and mobility tasks. Clients commonly practice a bed mobility or lower extremity dressing sequence and then complete the task while bearing weight through a misaligned flexed wrist. These clients are at risk for orthopedic injury (traumatic synovitis) and may be considered candidates for splinting to protect the wrist.[48]

Maintaining soft tissue length. Clients who have both increased and decreased skeletal muscle activity are at risk for soft tissue contracture secondary to the immobilization that occurs during both low-tone and increased-tone stages. Maintenance of tissue length is a 24-hour regimen. It involves frequent variations in resting postures during waking hours, teaching the client and significant others appropriate ROM procedures, daytime and nighttime positioning programs, and staff and family education so that positioning and exercise programs may be carried out in the home environment.[43]

Prolonged static positioning (e.g., prolonged use of a sling) must be avoided. Teaching clients to adjust their resting postures during the day will help prevent soft tissue tightness.

Positioning programs. The same wheelchair and bed positioning programs should not be applied to every client. Instead, positioning should be individualized and should focus on (1) promoting normal resting alignment of the trunk and limbs in an effort to maintain tissue length on both sides of the joints; (2) providing stretch to muscle groups that have been identified as being prone to contracture or already shortened; and (3) placing particular focus on maintaining passive external rotation of the shoulder.[3]

Soft tissue elongation. If soft tissue shortening and length-associated changes have already developed, the treatment of choice is low-load/prolonged stretch (LLPS). LLPS involves placing the soft tissues in question on submaximal stretch for prolonged periods. This technique is quite different from the common PROM with terminal stretch (high-load/brief stretch) programs commonly used to treat this population.[45]

LLPS can be implemented in various ways, including splinting, casting, and positioning programs. For example, during a UE assessment a client is noted to have tightness in the internal rotators, overactive internal rotation during attempts to move, and weakened external rotators. An effective LLPS program would involve having the client rest in a supine position with the arm abducted to 45 degrees and in external rotation. This position has been shown to decrease the potential for contracture.[3]

LLPS also can be achieved through splinting programs. A common example is the use of a splint designed to elongate the long flexors of the hand during sleeping hours.

Orthotics. Commonly a controversial subject in the management of stroke, orthotics should be considered on a case-by-case basis and may be quite effective for many clients.[45] The most common uses for orthotics during the low-tone stage are for maintaining joint alignment, protecting the tissues from shortening or overstretching, preventing injury to the extremity, and serving as an adjunctive treatment to control edema.[45] Specifically, orthotic support may be needed to provide palmar arch support and maintain neutral wrist deviation and a neutral position of the wrist between flexion and extension. In most cases the fingers do not require splinting in this stage of recovery.[45]

Orthotics also may be effective for clients in whom spasticity is developing. In these cases, the splints may be used to maintain soft tissue length, provide LLPS, place muscles at their resting lengths on both sides of the joints, and attempt distal relaxation by promoting proximal alignment.[45]

Client management. In addition to the interventions already described, it is helpful to train the client to manage the UE. For a client with low tone, the most important information to share with the client and significant others is the method for protecting the unstable joints and maintaining full ROM. In the spastic stage, the treatment of choice is to teach positioning that will provide prolonged elongation of the overactive muscles and prevent contracture. Examples of positions that may be prescribed during leisure or self-care activities include the following[43]:

1. Weight bearing on the extended arm (elongates the commonly shortened UE musculature)
2. In the supine position, hands behind the head while allowing the elbows to drop toward the bed (provides stretch of the internal rotators)
3. In the supine position, a pillow protracting the scapula and under the elbow to promote glenohumeral joint alignment
4. Lying on a protracted scapula to maintain stretch of the retractors and scapulothoracic mobility
5. Supporting the involved wrist with the more functional hand and reaching down toward the floor with both hands (This pattern will elongate muscles that tend to contract during difficult activities, which is particularly helpful after gait activities or difficult self-care activities.)
6. Cradling the affected arm with the stronger arm, lifting it to chest level, and gently raising and lowering (staying below 90 degrees) and gently abducting or adducting the arm (Fig. 34.7). *Cautionary note:* Clasping the hands and lifting the affected arm overhead should be discouraged because of the risk for increasing pain, causing an impingement syndrome, and stressing the carpal ligaments (Fig. 34.8). Similarly, overhead pulleys should be avoided.

The keys to prescribing a proper resting posture are (1) to identify muscle groups in the trunk and upper limb that are shortening, overactive, or at risk for the development of shortening and (2) to select a comfortable posture that elongates the muscle group for a prolonged period.

Jasmine and her family were taught appropriate positioning when Jasmine is in bed and when seated on chairs and during upright activities. In addition, Jasmine learned how to safely perform self-ROM exercises and was provided with a resting hand orthotic for nighttime use.

Nonfunctional Upper Extremity

Although restoration of UE control is a realistic goal for some clients, many clients will not regain enough control to integrate the affected UE into ADL and mobility tasks. Clients who will not regain sufficient control require extensive retraining in BADLs and IADLs (see Chapter 10) with one-handed techniques and prescription of appropriate assistive devices (Box 34.6). Persons in this population are also candidates for dominance retraining. Control of deformity to prevent body image issues is paramount for these clients.

INABILITY TO PERFORM CHOSEN TASKS SECONDARY TO VISUAL IMPAIRMENT

Processing of visual information is a complex act that requires intact functioning of multiple peripheral nervous system and CNS structures to support functional independence. The site of the lesion determines the visual dysfunction and the effect on performance of tasks (Fig. 34.9).[5]

Visual dysfunction and its treatment are detailed in Chapter 24. In general, treatment approaches may focus on remediation, such as eye calisthenics, fixations, scanning, visual motor techniques, and bilateral integration. Adaptive techniques are also used, including a change in working distance, the use of prisms, adaptations for driving and reading, changes in lighting, and enlarged print.[87]

PSYCHOSOCIAL ADJUSTMENT

The psychological consequences of a stroke are substantial. The incidence of depression in this population is 33%, according to statistics collected by the American Heart Association.[103] The highest reported incidence is found in clients in acute and rehabilitation hospitals, and the lowest is in samples of those living in the community after stroke. Other psychological manifestations that have been documented in survivors of stroke include anxiety, agoraphobia, substance abuse, sleep disorders, mania, aprosodia (difficulty expressing or recognizing emotion), behavioral problems (e.g., sexual inappropriateness, verbal outbursts, aggressiveness), lability (alteration between pathological laughing and crying), and personality changes (e.g., apathy, irritability, social withdrawal).[38]

A critical role of the occupational therapist is to help the client adjust to hospitalization and, more important, to disability. Much patience and a supportive approach by the therapist are essential. The therapist must be sensitive to the fact that the client has experienced a devastating and life-threatening illness that has caused sudden and dramatic changes in his or her life roles and performance. The therapist must be cognizant of the

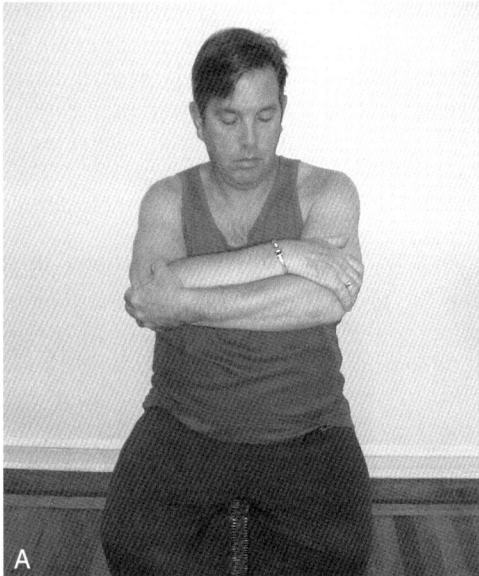

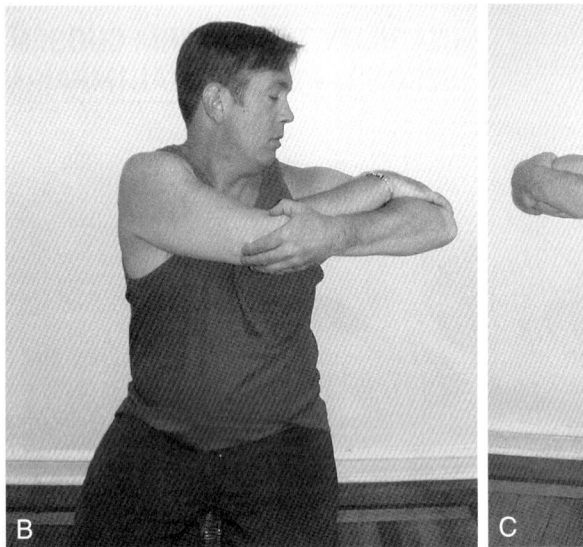
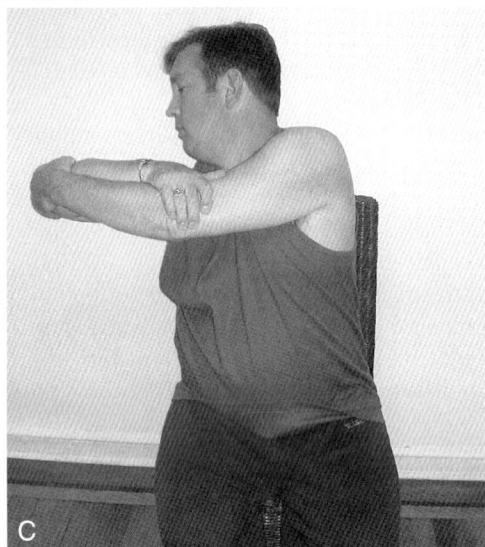

Fig. 34.7 "Rock the baby." The client lifts the right upper extremity to chest level (A), adducts (B), and abducts (C) horizontally to allow trunk rotation.

normal adjustment process and must gear the approach and expectations of performance to the client's level of adjustment. Frequently, the client is not ready to engage in rehabilitation measures with wholehearted effort until several months after the onset of the disability.

Family education is extremely important throughout the treatment program. Family members are better equipped to assist their loved one in adjusting to disability when they are knowledgeable about the disability and its implications.

Many clients dwell on the possibility of full recovery of function; they should gradually be made aware that some residual dysfunction is likely. The therapist may approach this probability by discussing in objective terms what is known about the prognosis for functional recovery after stroke. It may be necessary to review this information many times before the client begins to apply it to his or her recovery. This education should be done in a way that is honest and yet does not destroy all hope.

Falk-Kessler[38] has provided occupational therapists with guidelines related to interventions for the psychological manifestations of stroke, including the following:
- Fostering an internal locus of control related to recovery
- Using therapeutic activities to improve self-efficacy or confidence in the performance of specific activities
- Promoting the use of adaptive coping strategies, such as seeking social support, information seeking, positive reframing, and acceptance
- Promoting success in chosen occupations to improve self-esteem
- Encouraging social support networks, such as families, friends, or support groups
- Using occupations to promote social participation

In addition to the aforementioned interventions, it is important to remember that pharmacological interventions have been shown to be effective in this population and should not be overlooked[38] as part of a team approach. Such interventions include,

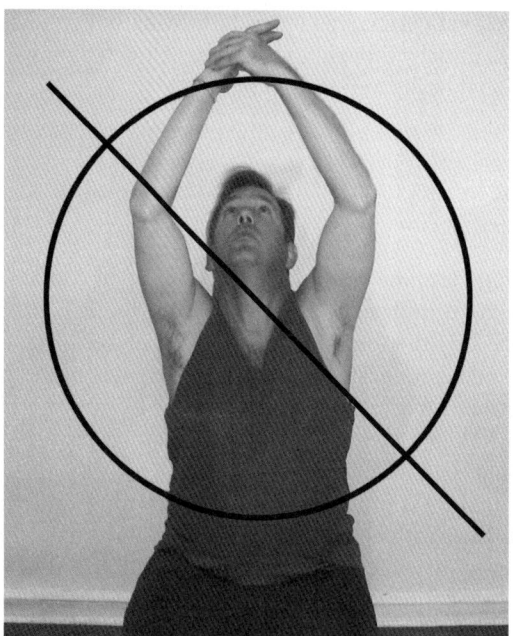

Fig. 34.8 Because of multiple biomechanical concerns (e.g., impingement), self–overhead range of motion is discouraged.

but are not limited to, antidepressants for depression or for individuals with a pathological affect, benzodiazepines for generalized anxiety disorder, and neuroleptic medications for those with poststroke psychosis.[24]

The OT program should focus on supporting and fostering the client's participation in preferred occupations. The client's attention should be focused, through the performance of activity, using remaining and newly learned skills. The OT program

---

BOX 34.6 Examples of Assistive Devices Used After Stroke to Improve Occupational Performance

- Rocker knife
- Elastic laces and lace locks
- Adapted cutting board
- Dycem
- Plate guards
- Pot stabilizer
- Playing card holder
- Suction devices to stabilize mixing bowls and cleaning brushes

---

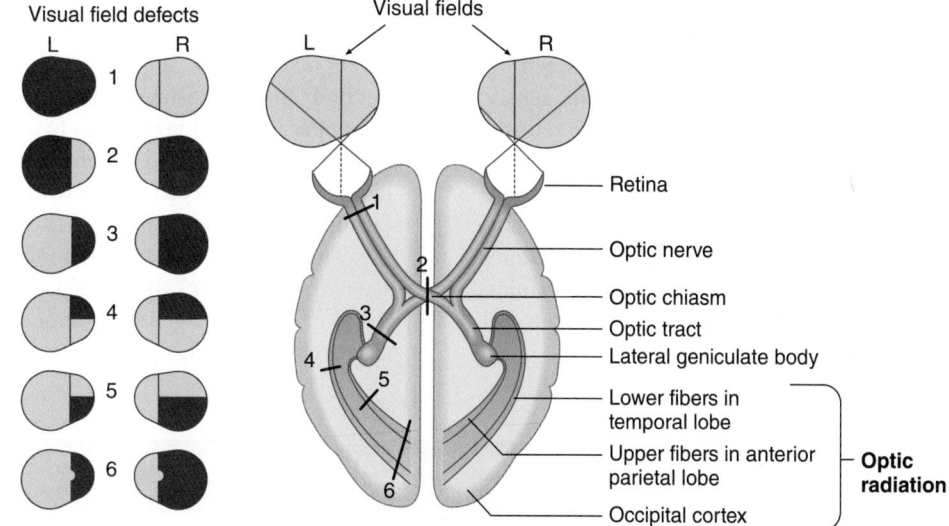

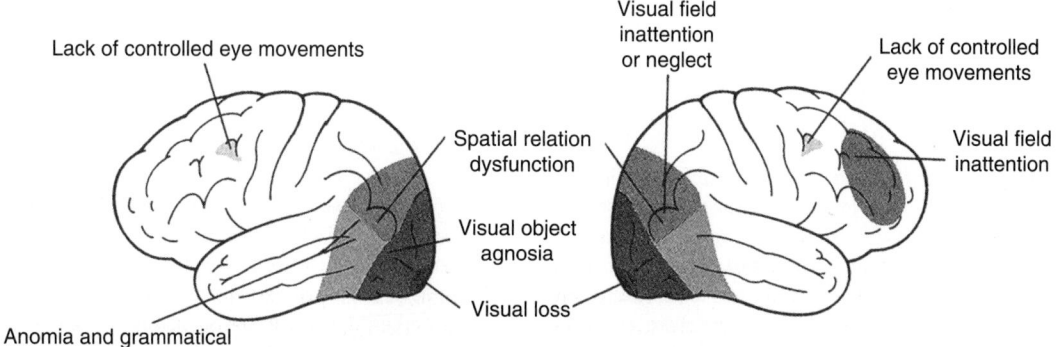

Fig. 34.9 Visual processing deficits. (Top from Walker BR, et al: *Davidson's principles and practice of medicine*, ed 22, Edinburgh, 2014, Churchill Livingstone; Bottom from Árnadóttir G: *The brain and behavior: assessing cortical dysfunction through activities of daily living*. St Louis, 1990, Mosby.)

also can include therapeutic group activities for socialization and sharing of common problems and their solutions. The discovery that there are residual abilities and perhaps new abilities and success at performing many daily living skills and activities that were initially thought to be impossible can improve the client's mental health and outlook.

SUMMARY

Stroke is a complex disability that challenges the skills of professional healthcare workers. Although the number and effectiveness of approaches for the remediation of affected motor, sensory, perceptual, cognitive, and performance dysfunctions have increased considerably (Box 34.7), many limitations in treatment remain. The occupational therapist must bear in mind that the degree to which the patient achieves treatment goals depends on the CNS damage and recovery, neurological impairment residuals, psychosocial adjustment, and the skilled application of appropriate treatment by all concerned health professionals.

Some patients remain severely disabled despite the noblest efforts of rehabilitation workers, whereas others recover quite spontaneously with minimal help in a short period. Most patients benefit from the professional skills of occupational therapists and other rehabilitation specialists and achieve improvement of performance skills and resumption of meaningful occupational roles.

Jasmine demonstrated a clear relationship between her impaired body functions (e.g., loss of motor control, sensory loss, visual dysfunction, and neglect) and her ability to return to her previous lifestyle and engage in chosen areas of occupation. Through the development of an occupational profile, standardized assessments, and skilled observation made while Jasmine was performing her chosen occupations of feeding, grooming, toilet transfers, computer use, and child care, it was determined that several impairments were affecting Jasmine's ability to perform independently:

- *Feeding:* Jasmine was unable to cut or open containers secondary to unilateral UE weakness on the left; she tended to eat only the food on the right side of her plate; and she was unable to locate utensils on the left side of the plate. In addition, food remained between her left gums and cheek ("pocketing") after meals, resulting in oral hygiene issues and putting Jasmine at risk for aspiration.
- *Grooming:* Jasmine had difficulty opening and applying toothpaste with one hand. She attended only to the right side of her body while grooming, with the left side of her mouth and hair not being cared for during oral and hair care.
- *Toilet transfers:* Jasmine required moderate physical assistance to transfer to the toilet secondary to an inability to bear weight on her left leg and an inability to control her trunk (she falls laterally when sitting on the toilet). The occupational therapist also noted that when Jasmine "completed" the transfer to the toilet, only the right side of her body was sitting on the toilet. She neglected to include the left side of her body in the transfer and left it in the wheelchair.
- *Computer use:* During attempts to use the computer, Jasmine became easily frustrated and made comments such as, "I feel like a failure" and "I can't even provide for my child anymore." Jasmine agreed to attempt to write a letter to her friend on the computer. Multiple mistakes were noted because Jasmine seemed to "not see" the left-sided keys, could not control the shift keys, and generally appeared disorganized in her approach to the task.

BOX 34.7   Summary of Reviews of Evidence-Based Interventions to Improve Occupational Performance After Stroke

- *Motor impairments limiting occupational performance:* Evidence suggests that repetitive task practice, constraint-induced or modified constraint-induced movement therapy, strengthening and exercise, mental practice, virtual reality, mirror therapy, and action observation can improve upper extremity function, balance and mobility, and/or activity and participation. Commonalities among several of the effective interventions include the use of goal-directed, individualized tasks that promote frequent repetitions of task-related or task-specific movements.[78]
- *Cognitive impairments affecting occupational performance:* Evidence is available from a variety of clinical trials to guide interventions regarding general cognition, apraxia, and neglect. The evidence regarding interventions for executive dysfunction and memory loss is limited. There is insufficient evidence regarding impairments of attention and mixed evidence regarding interventions for visual field deficits. The effective interventions have some commonalities, including being performance focused, involving strategy training, and using a compensatory as opposed to a remediation approach.[78]
- *Psychological/emotional impairments affecting occupational performance:* Evidence from well-conducted research supports the use of problem-solving or motivational interviewing behavioral techniques to address depression. The evidence is inconclusive for using multicomponent exercise programs to combat depression after stroke and for the use of stroke education and care support and coordination interventions to address poststroke anxiety. One study provided support for an intensive multidisciplinary home program in improving depression, anxiety, and health-related quality of life.[54]
- *Improving performance in areas of occupation and participation:* Most of the literature targeted interventions based on activities of daily living (ADLs) and collectively provided strong evidence for the use of occupation-based interventions to improve ADL performance. The evidence related to instrumental activities of daily living (IADLs) was much more disparate, with limited evidence to support the use of virtual reality interventions and emerging evidence to support driver education programs to improve occupational performance after a stroke. Only six studies addressed leisure, social participation, or rest and sleep, and evidence was sufficient to support only leisure-based interventions.[106]

- *Simulated child care:* A weighted doll was used to observe Jasmine's ability to care for her child. It was quickly decided that this area of occupation would be deferred until Jasmine's status improved. Jasmine and her occupational therapist made this decision collaboratively on the basis of safety concerns and Jasmine's emotional status. Jasmine was gravely concerned about her ability to care for her child. The occupational therapist wanted to focus on occupations that Jasmine could master, build her confidence, and upgrade her occupations systematically according to Jasmine's abilities.

These findings were determined based on the initial assessment choices. The first assessment administered was the COPM.[64,65] Because multiple areas of occupation are limited after a stroke, it is imperative to use a tool such as this to determine the client's priorities for intervention. These priorities, in turn, become the client's initial goals. In addition, the Inpatient Rehabilitation Facility Patient Assessment Instrument (IRF-PAI)[99] and the A-ONE[6,8] were used to objectify limitations in daily function and to determine limiting factors. The IRF-PAI is typically used in inpatient rehabilitation settings and documents the level of caregiver burden related to BADLs and mobility. The A-ONE is complementary to the IRF-PAI and determines the reasons for lack of independence by evaluating client factors that result in errors in occupational performance by skilled observations of tasks performed in natural contexts.

Several interventions were considered to address Jasmine's inability to participate in chosen occupations (toilet transfers, computer use, grooming, feeding, and child care). Task-specific training of grooming, feeding, and toileting served as the basis for her initial OT. A system of vanishing physical and verbal cues was used as Jasmine relearned the tasks at hand. Jasmine had substantial motor loss in her left limbs, thus making training with adaptive equipment imperative. Examples included a rocker knife and Dycem for feeding and a grab bar and raised toilet seat. To ensure continued integration of her affected upper limb, Jasmine was taught to use her left limb as a stabilizer during tasks. She was also taught to keep her arm positioned on a surface and in her line of sight. A strategy that was used to help Jasmine overcome her neglect was use of a perceptual anchor. In addition to her left arm being positioned on the left side of a surface, a strip of red tape was placed on the left edge of work surfaces (e.g., on the table to the left of her place setting and on the left side of the sink). As Jasmine gained mastery of these tasks, task-specific training of work tasks via similar strategies was introduced.

REVIEW QUESTIONS

1. Define stroke and list two of its causes.
2. Name three modifiable risk factors associated with stroke.
3. Define TIA.
4. Name three functional deficits that occur as a result of loss of trunk control.
5. Name two components of a client-centered approach to evaluation.
6. What are two frames of reference used to treat neurobehavioral impairments after stroke?
7. Name three postural reactions that support standing activities.
8. How does aphasia differ from dysarthria?

REFERENCES

1. Abreu B, et al: Occupational performance and the functional approach. In Royeen C, editor: *AOTA self-study: cognitive rehabilitation*, Bethesda, MD, 1994, American Occupational Therapy Association.
2. Ada L, Carr J, Kilbreath S, Shepherd R: Task-specific training of reaching and manipulation. In Bennett KMB, Castiello U, editors: *Insights into the reach to grasp movements*, New York, 1994, Elsevier Science.
3. Ada L, Goddard E, McCully J, et al: Thirty minutes of positioning reduces the development of shoulder external rotation contracture after stroke: a randomized controlled trial, *Arch Phys Med Rehabil* 86:230–234, 2005.
4. American Occupational Therapy Association. Occupational therapy practice framework: domain and process, ed 4, *Am J Occup Ther* 74:1–87, 2020.
5. Árnadóttir G: The Brain and Behavior: Assessing Cortical Dysfunction through Activities of Daily Living, St Louis, 1990, Mosby.
6. Árnadóttir G: Impact of neurobehavioral deficits of activities of daily living. In Gillen G, Nilsen DM, editors: *Stroke rehabilitation: a function-based approach* 5th ed., Philadelphia, 2021, Elsevier.
7. Árnadóttir G, Fisher AG: Rasch analysis of the ADL scale of the A-ONE, *Am J Occup Ther* 62:51–56., 2008.
8. Árnadóttir G, Fisher AG, Löfgren B: Dimensionality of nonmotor neurobehavioral impairments when observed in the natural contexts of ADL task performance, *Neurorehabil Neural Repair* 23:579–586, 2009.
9. Barros de Oliveira C, Torres de Medeiros IR, Frota NAF, et al: Balance control in hemiparetic stroke patients: main tools for evaluation, *J Rehabil Res Dev* 45(8):1215–1226, 2008.
10. Basmajian JV: The surgical anatomy and function of the arm-trunk mechanism, *Surg Clin North Am* 43:1471, 1963.
11. Baum CM, Edwards DF: *Activity card sort*, ed 2., Bethesda, MD, 2008, AOTA Press.
12. Beck AT, Steer RA: *Beck depression inventory manual*, rev ed., New York, 1987, Psychological Corp.
13. Berg K, Wood-Dauphinee S, Williams JI, Gayton D: Measuring balance in the elderly: preliminary development of an instrument, *Physiother Can* 41:304–311, 1989.
14. Bergner M, Bobbitt RA, Carter WB, Gilson BS: The sickness impact profile: development and final revision of a health status measure, *Med Care* 19:787–805, 1981.
15. Bobath B: *Adult hemiplegia: evaluation and treatment*, ed 3, Oxford, England, 1990, Butterworth-Heinemann.

16. Bohannon RW, Cassidy D, Walsh S: Trunk muscle strength is impaired multidirectionally after stroke, *Clin Rehabil* 9:47–51, 1995.

17. Bonita R, Beaglehole R: Modification of Rankin Scale: recovery of motor function after stroke, *Stroke* 19:1497–1500, 1988.

18. Bounds JV, Wiebers DO, Whisnant JP: Mechanisms and timing of deaths from cerebral infarction, *Stroke* 12:474–477, 1981.

19. Bourbonnais D, Vanden Noven S: Weakness in patients with hemiparesis, *Am J Occup Ther* 43:313–319, 1989.

20. Branch EF: The neuropathology of stroke. In Duncan PW, Badke MB, editors: *Stroke rehabilitation: the recovery of motor control*, Chicago, 1987, Year Book.

21. Brott T, Adams HP, Olinger CP, et al: Measurements of acute cerebral infarction: a clinical examination scale, *Stroke* 20:864–870, 1989.

22. Cailliet R: *The shoulder in hemiplegia*, Philadelphia, 1980, FA Davis.

23. Carr JH, Shepherd RB, Nordholm L, Lynne D: Investigation of a new motor assessment scale for stroke patients, *Phys Ther* 65:175–180, 1985.

24. Chemerinski E, Robinson RG: The neuropsychiatry of stroke, *Psychosomatics* 41:5–14, 2000.

25. Chen CC, Bode RK: Psychometric validation of the Manual Ability Measure-36 (MAM-36) in patients with neurologic and musculoskeletal disorders, *Arch Phys Med Rehabil* 91:414–420, 2010.

26. Chen CC, Palmon O, Amini D: Responsiveness of the Manual Ability Measure-36 (MAM-36): changes in hand function using a self-reported and clinician-rated assessment, *Am J Occup Ther* 68(2):187–193, 2014.

27. Chusid J: *Correlative neuroanatomy and functional neurology*, ed 19, Los Altos, CA, 1985, Lage.

28. Collen FM, Wade DT, Robb GF, Bradshaw CM: The Rivermead Mobility Index: a further development of the Rivermead Motor Assessment, *Int Disabil Stud* 13:50–54, 1991.

29. Collins KC, Kennedy NC, Clark A, et al: Kinematic components of the reach-to-target movement after stroke for focused rehabilitation interventions: systematic review and meta-analysis, *Front Neurol* 9:472, 2018.

30. Côté R, Hachinski VC, Shurvell BL, et al: The Canadian Neurological Scale: a preliminary study in acute stroke, *Stroke* 17:731–737, 1986.

31. Criekinge TV, Truijen S, Schröder J, et al: The effectiveness of trunk training on trunk control, sitting and standing balance and mobility post-stroke: a systematic review and meta-analysis, *Clinic Rehabil* 33(6):992–1002, 2019.

32. Demeurisse G, Demol O, Robaye E: Motor evaluation in vascular hemiplegia, *Eur Neurol* 19:382–389, 1980.

33. Desrosiers J, Hébert R, Bravo G, Dutil E: Upper extremity performance test for the elderly (TEMPA): normative data and correlates with sensorimotor parameters, *Arch Phys Med Rehabil* 76:1125–1129, 1995.

34. Desrosiers J, Hébert R, Dutil E, Bravo G: Development and reliability of an upper extremity function test for the elderly: the TEMPA, *Can J Occup Ther* 60:9–16, 1993.

35. Duncan PW, Weiner DK, Chandler J, Studenski S: Functional reach: a new clinical measure of balance, *J Gerontol* 45:M192–M197, 1990.

36. Ellul MA, Benjamin L, Singh B, et al: Neurological associations of COVID-19, *Lancet Neurology* 19:767–783, 2020.

37. Epstein NB, Baldwin LM, Bishop DS: The McMaster Family Assessment Device, *J Marital Fam Ther* 9:171–180, 1983.

38. Falk-Kessler J: Psychological aspects of stroke rehabilitation. In Gillen G, Nilsen DM, editors: *Stroke rehabilitation: a function-based approach* ed 5, Philadelphia, 2021, Elsevier.

39. Fisher AG, Jones KB: Assessment of motor and process skills, 7th ed. *Development, standardization, and administration manual*, Vol. 1, Fort Collins, CO, 2012, Three Star Press.

40. Folstein MF, Folstein SE, McHugh PR: Mini-mental state: a practical method for grading the cognitive state of patients for the clinician, *J Psychiatr Res* 12:189–198, 1975.

41. Franchignoni FP, Tesio L, Ricupero C, Martino MT: Trunk control test as an early predictor of stroke rehabilitation outcome, *Stroke* 28:1382–1385, 1997.

42. Fugl-Meyer AR, Jääskö L, Leyman I, et al: The post-stroke hemiplegic patient: a method for evaluation of physical performance. *Scand J Rehabil Med* 7:13–31, 1975.

43. Gillen G: Managing abnormal tone after brain injury, *OT Pract* 3:8, 1998.

44. Gillen G: *Cognitive and perceptual rehabilitation: optimizing function*, St Louis, 2009, Mosby.

45. Gillen G: Orthotic devices after stroke. In Gillen G, Nilsen DM, editors: *Stroke rehabilitation: a function-based approach* ed 5, Philadelphia, 2021, Elsevier.

46. Gillen G: Seated postural control: supporting functional independence. In Gillen G, Nilsen DM, editors: *Stroke Rehabilitation: a function-based approach* ed 5, Philadelphia, 2021, Elsevier.

47. Gillen G: Treatment of cognitive-perceptual deficits: a function-based approach. In Gillen G, Nilsen DM, editors: *Stroke rehabilitation: a function-based approach* ed 5, Philadelphia, 2021, Elsevier.

48. Gillen G, Nilsen DM: Upper extremity function and management. In Gillen G, Nilsen DM, editors: *Stroke rehabilitation: a function-based approach* ed 5, Philadelphia, 2021, Elsevier.

49. Gillen G, Nilsen DM, Attridge J, et al: Effectiveness of interventions to improve occupational performance of people with cognitive impairments after stroke: an evidence-based review, *Am J Occup Ther* 69(1):1–9, 2015. https://doi.org/10.5014/ajot.2015.012138.

50. Goodglass H, Kaplan E: *Boston Diagnostic Aphasia Examination*, Philadelphia, 1983, Lea & Febiger.

51. Hafsteinsdóttir TB, Algra A, Kappelle LJ, Grypdonck MHF: Neurodevelopmental treatment after stroke: a comparative study, *J Neurol Neurosurg Psychiatry* 76:788–792, 2005.

52. Hallowell B, Chapey R: Delivering language intervention services to adults with neurogenic communication disorders. In Chapey R, editor: *Language intervention strategies in aphasia and related neurogenic communication disorders* ed 5, Philadelphia, 2008, Wolters Kluwer/Lippincott Williams & Wilkins.

53. Helgason CM, Wolf PA: *American Heart Association Prevention Conference IV: prevention and rehabilitation of stroke*, Dallas, 1997, American Heart Association.

54. Hildebrand MW: Effectiveness of interventions for adults with psychological or emotional impairment after stroke: an evidence-based review, *Am J Occup Ther* 69(1):1–9, 2015. https://doi.org/10.5014/ajot.2015.012054.

55. Holbrook M, Skilbeck CE: An activities index for use with stroke patients, *Age Ageing* 12:166–170, 1983.

56. Jebsen RH, Taylor N, Trieschmann RB, et al: An objective and standardized test of hand function, *Arch Phys Med Rehabil* 50:311–319, 1969.

57. Juckett LA, Wengerd LR, Faieta: Evidence-based practice implementation in stroke rehabilitation: a scoping review of barrier and facilitators, *Am J Occup Ther* 74(1):1–14, 2020.

58. Keith RA, Granger CV, Hamilton BB, Sherwin FS: The Functional Independence Measure: a new tool for rehabilitation, *Adv Clin Rehabil* 1:16–18, 1987.

59. Kertesz A: *Western aphasia battery*, New York, 1982, Grune & Stratton.

60. Kiernan RJ, Mueller J, Langston JW, et al: The Neurobehavioral Cognitive Status Examination: a brief but quantitative approach to cognitive assessment, *Ann Intern Med* 107(4):481–485, 1987.

61. Kollen BJ, Lennon S, Lyons B, et al: The effectiveness of the Bobath concept in stroke rehabilitation: what is the evidence? *Stroke* 40:e89–e97, 2009.

62. Kopp B, Kunel A, Platz T, et al: The Arm Motor Ability Test: reliability, validity, and sensitivity to change of an instrument for assessing disabilities in activities of daily living, *Arch Phys Med Rehabil* 78:615–620, 1997.

63. Lai SM, Studenski S, Duncan PW, Perera S: Persisting consequences of stroke measured by the stroke impact scale, *Stroke* 33:1840–1844, 2002.

64. Law M, Baptiste S, Mills J: Client-centered practice: what does it mean and does it make a difference? *Can J Occup Ther* 62:250–257, 1995.

65. Law M, Baptiste S, McColl M, et al: The Canadian Occupational Performance Measure: an outcome measure for occupational therapy, *Can J Occup Ther* 57(2):82–87, 1990.

66. Lawton MP, Brody EM: Assessment of older people: self-maintenance and instrumental activities of daily living, *The Gerontologist* 9(3):179–186, 1969.

67. Lee HH, Lee JW, Kim BR, et al: Predicting independence of gait by assessing sitting balance through sitting posturography in patients with subacute hemiplegic stroke, *Topics Stroke Rehabil* 28(4):258–267, 2021. https://doi.org/10.1080/10749357.2020.1806437.

68. Ma HI, Trombly CA: A synthesis of the effects of occupational therapy for persons with stroke, part II: Remediation of impairments, *Am J Occup Ther* 56:260, 2002.

69. Mahoney FI, Barthel DW: Functional evaluation: the Barthel Index, *Md State Med J* 14:61–65, 1965.

70. Mathiowetz V, Haugen JB: Motor behavior research: implications for therapeutic approaches to central nervous system dysfunction, *Am J Occup Ther* 48:733–745, 1994.

71. Mathiowetz V, Nilsen DM, Gillen G: Task-oriented approach to stroke rehabilitation. In Gillen G, Nilsen DM, editors: *Stroke rehabilitation: a function-based approach* ed 5, Philadelphia, 2021, Elsevier.

72. McIntyre A, Viana R, Janzen S, et al: Systematic review and meta-analysis of constraint-induced movement therapy in the hemiparetic upper extremity more than six months post stroke, *Top Stroke Rehabil* 19(6):499–513, 2012.

73. Nakayama H, Jørgensen HS, Raaschou HO, et al: Recovery of upper extremity function in stroke patients: the Copenhagen stroke study, *Arch Phys Med Rehabil* 75(4):394–398, 1994.

74. Neistadt ME: A critical analysis of occupational therapy approaches for perceptual deficits in adults with brain injury, *Am J Occup Ther* 44:299–304, 1990.

75. Neistadt ME: Occupational therapy treatments for constructional deficits, *Am J Occup Ther* 46:141–148, 1992.

76. Neistadt ME: Perceptual retraining for adults with diffuse brain injury, *Am J Occup Ther* 48:225–233, 1994.

77. Nilsen DM, Donato SM, Pulaski KH, Gillen G: Standing postural control: supporting functional independence. In Gillen G, Nilsen DM, editors: *Stroke rehabilitation: a function-based approach* ed 5, Philadelphia, 2021, Elsevier.

78. Nilsen DM, Gillen G, Geller D, et al: Effectiveness of interventions to improve occupational performance of people with motor impairments after stroke: an evidence-based review, *Am J Occup Ther* 69(1):1–9, 2015. https://doi.org/10.5014/ajot.2015.011965.

79. Pollock N: Client-centered assessment, *Am J Occup Ther* 47:298–301, 1993.

80. Rao A: Approaches to motor control dysfunction: an evidence-based review. In Gillen G, Nilsen DM, editors: *Stroke rehabilitation: a function-based approach* ed 5, Philadelphia, 2021, Elsevier.

81. Rensink M, Schuurmans M, Lindeman E, Hafsteinsdóttir T: Task-oriented training in rehabilitation after stroke: systematic review, *J Adv Nurs* 65:737–754, 2009.

82. Roth EJ: Medical complications encountered in stroke rehabilitation, *Phys Med Rehabil Clin North Am* 2:563–578, 1991.

83. Rief K, Bartels MN, Duffy CA, Beland HE, Stein J: Pathophysiology, medical management and acute rehabilitation of stroke survivors. In Gillen G, Nilsen DM, editors: *Stroke rehabilitation: a function-based approach* ed 5, Philadelphia, 2021, Elsevier.

84. Rubenstein E, Federman D, editors: *Neurocerebrovascular diseases*, New York, 1994, Scientific American.

85. Sandin KJ, Smith BS: The measure of balance in sitting in stroke rehabilitation prognosis, *Stroke* 21:82–86, 1990.

86. Sarfo F, Ulasavets U, Opare-Sem OK, et al: Tele-Rehabilitation after stroke: an updated Systematic review of the literature, *J Stroke Cerebrovasc Dis* 27(9):2306–2318, 2018.

87. Scheiman M: *Understanding and managing vision deficits: a guide for occupational therapists*, ed 3, Thorofare, NJ, 2011, Slack.

88. Shumway-Cook A, Woollacott M, editors: *Motor control: translating research into clinical practice*, 5, Philadelphia, 2017, Wolters Kluwer.

89. Smith WS, Johnston SC, Hemphill JC: Cerebrovascular disease. In Jameson LJ, Fauci AS, Kasper DL, editors: *Harrison's principles of internal medicine* ed 20, New York, 2018, McGraw-Hill Education.

90. Stewart C, Riedel K: Managing speech and language deficits after stroke. In Gillen G, Nilsen DM, editors: *Stroke rehabilitation: a function-based approach* ed 5, Philadelphia, 2021, Elsevier.

91. Taub E, Uswatte G, Mark VW, et al: The learned nonuse phenomenon implications for rehabilitation, *Eura Medicophy* 42(3):241–256, 2006.

92. Teasdale G, Jennett B: Assessment of coma and impaired consciousness: a practical scale, *Lancet* 2:81–84, 1974.

93. Thomson-Kohlman L: *The Kohlman evaluation of living skills*, ed 4, Bethesda, MD, 2016, American Occupational Therapy Association.

94. Tinetti ME: Performance-oriented assessment of mobility problems in elderly patients, *J Am Geriatr Soc* 34:119–126, 1986.

95. Toglia J: Generalization of treatment: a multicontext approach to cognitive perceptual impairment in adults with brain injury, *Am J Occup Ther* 45:505–516, 1991.

96. Trombly CA: Deficits in reaching in subjects with left hemiparesis: a pilot study, *Am J Occup Ther* 46:887–897, 1992.

97. Trombly CA: Anticipating the future: assessment of occupational function, *Am J Occup Ther* 47:253–257, 1993.

98. Trombly CA, Ma HI: A synthesis of the effects of occupational therapy for persons with stroke, Part I: restoration of roles, tasks, and activities, *Am J Occup Ther* 56:250–259, 2002.

99. U.S. Centers for Medicare and Medicaid Services: IRF-PAI and IRF QRP Manual. CMS.gov Centers for Medicare & Medicaid

Services. https://www.cms.gov/Medicare/Medicare-Fee-for-Service-Payment/InpatientRehabFacPPS/IRFPAI.

100. Uswatte G, Taub E, Morris D, et al: Reliability and validity of the upper-extremity Motor Activity Log-14 for measuring real-world arm use, *Stroke* 36:2493–2496, 2005.

101. Uswatte G, Taub E, Morris D, et al: The Motor Activity Log-28: assessing daily use of the hemiparetic arm after stroke, *Neurology* 67:1189–1194, 2006.

102. Van Lew S, Geller D, Feld-Glazman R, et al: Development and preliminary reliability of the Functional Upper Extremity Levels (FUEL), *Am J Occup Ther* 69(6):1–5, 2015.

103. Virani S, Alonso A, Benjamin EJ, et al: Heart disease and stroke statistics: 2020 update, *Circ* 141:e139–e596, 2020.

104. Ware JE, Sherbourne CD: The MOS 36-Item Short Form Health Survey: conceptual framework and item selection, *Med Care* 30:473–483, 1992.

105. Wilson DJ, Baker LL, Craddock JA: Functional test for the hemiparetic upper extremity, *Am J Occup Ther* 38:159–164, 1984.

106. Wolf TJ, Chuh AC, Floyd T, et al: Effectiveness of occupation-based interventions to improve areas of occupation and social participation after stroke: an evidence-based review, *Am J Occup Ther* 69(1):1–11, 2015. https://doi.org/10.5014/ajot.2015.012195.

107. World Health Organization: *International classification of diseases (ICD-10)*, Geneva, 2007, WHO.

108. Xu T, Clemson L, O'Loughlin K, et al: Risk factors for falls in community stroke survivors: a systematic review and meta-analysis, *Arch Phys Med Rehabil* 99:563–573, 2018.

109. Yesavage JA, Brink TL, Rose TL, et al: Development and validation of a geriatric depression screening scale: a preliminary report, *J Psychiatr Res* 17:37–49, 1982-1983.

110. Zorowitz RD, Hughes MB, Idank D, et al: Shoulder pain and subluxation after stroke: correlation or coincidence? *Am J Occup Ther* 50:194–201, 1996.

35

Traumatic Brain Injury

Michelle Tipton-Burton and Brenna Craig[a]

LEARNING OBJECTIVES

After studying this chapter, the student or practitioner will be able to do the following:

1. Describe the pathological processes underlying traumatic brain injury (TBI).
2. State current medical, surgical, and pharmaceutical interventions for acute TBI.
3. Identify levels of consciousness in individuals with TBI by using standard scales.
4. Describe the clinical picture of individuals with TBI, including common physical, cognitive, and psychosocial sequelae.
5. Identify occupational therapy (OT) evaluation methods for lower, intermediate, and higher functioning individuals with TBI.
6. Identify several standard OT assessments for physical, cognitive, and psychosocial impairment after TBI.
7. Describe OT intervention methods for lower, intermediate, and higher functioning individuals with TBI.
8. Describe the continuum of care services available for an individual with TBI in the acute, subacute, and postacute stages of rehabilitation.

CHAPTER OUTLINE

[a] The author wishes to gratefully acknowledge the contributions by Rochelle McLaughlin and Jeffrey Englander.
[b] The Rancho Los Amigos Scale of Cognitive Functioning is a means of describing the level of activity of a person with a brain injury. The RLA scale measures the levels of awareness, cognition, behavior, and interaction with the environment.

KEY TERMS

Compensatory model
Decerebrate rigidity
Decorticate rigidity
Diffuse axonal injuries (DAIs)
Environmental interventions
Ideational apraxia
Ideomotor apraxia
Impaired initiation
Interactive interventions
Modified Ashworth Scale

Neuromuscular reeducation
Neuroplasticity
Pelvic alignment
Post-Traumatic amnesia (PTA)
Postural deficits
Rehabilitative model
Sensory regulation
Tone normalization
Traumatic brain injury (TBI)
Unilateral neglect syndrome

CASE STUDY

Maria

Maria, an 18-year-old Hispanic who identifies as female (prefers use of the pronouns she/her/hers). Maria was an unrestrained passenger in a sport utility vehicle involved in an accident. Maria sustained a severe brain injury in the crash. She is a high school graduate who lives with her boyfriend and works as a waitress. A computed tomography (CT) scan showed a basilar skull fracture and diffuse subdural hematoma. Approximately 2 weeks after she had been injured, she was transferred to an acute rehabilitation unit to participate in a journey to recovery program, which is designed for clients whose progress is expected to be slower than that of typical acute care clients. This is determined by the extent of the injury; typically these clients are at level II or III on the Rancho Los Amigos (RLA) Scale.

The results of the occupational therapy (OT) evaluation indicated that Maria was dependent for all mobility and activities of daily living (ADLs) as a result of deficits in motor and process skills. She also displayed significant deficits in various client factors. Her right upper extremity had full active and passive range of motion (ROM), with minimal ataxia in all joints. Her left upper extremity had decreased range of motion at her shoulder, elbow, and wrist. Severe spasticity was noted throughout her left upper extremity. Maria was alert and able to visually attend and track. She was nonverbal and being fed through a gastrointestinal (GI) tube. When positioned at the edge of the bed, she required total assistance to maintain a sitting position, including support of her head and trunk. She did not display sitting balance.

Occupational therapy was begun to foster Maria's ability to engage in self-care and some instrumental activities of daily living (IADLs) by accomplishing the following: (1) improving her left upper extremity range of motion, (2) reducing spasticity in her left upper extremity, (3) improving functional use of her right upper extremity to facilitate participation in self-care tasks, (4) improving head and trunk control so that she could sit upright in a wheelchair, (5) participating in bed mobility and transfers, and (6) improving cognition such that she could participate in a self-care and self-feeding program and communicate with others.

Critical Thinking Questions
1. How should Maria's injury be characterized?
2. What is her cognitive state?
3. How might Maria's progress be measured?
4. How will her various problems be treated?

EPIDEMIOLOGY

Traumatic brain injury (TBI) is defined as an alteration in brain function or other evidence of brain pathological condition caused by an external force. There may be a resultant loss of consciousness, post-traumatic amnesia (PTA), skull fracture, or objective neurological findings that can be attributed to the traumatic event on the basis of radiologic findings or a physical or mental status examination.[28,73,78]

TBI is the most common cause of death and disability in young people.[28] TBI is a contributing factor to a third (30%) of all injury-related deaths in the United States. Typically, more than 60,000 Americans die each year from a TBI according to the Centers for Disease Control and Prevention,[16] 288,000 are hospitalized, and 2.5 million are treated and released from an emergency department (ED). Among children up to age 14, TBI results in an estimated 2685 deaths, 37,000 hospitalizations, and 435,000 ED visits. The number of people with TBI who are not seen in an ED or who receive no care is unknown. The direct and indirect costs of TBI in the United States have been estimated to be in excess of $76 billion annually.[4] Survivor costs account for more than $31 billion, and fatal brain injuries cost another $16.6 billion (Dawn Newmann, Assistant Research Professor, Indiana University School of Medicine, personal communication, 2015).[80] The Centers for Disease Control and Prevention (CDC) estimates that at least 5.3 million Americans currently have a long-term or lifelong need for help to perform activities of daily living (ADLs) as a result of TBI.[12]

According to the CDC, the leading causes of TBI are falls (48%), struck by or against an object (17%), motor vehicle accidents (14.3%), assaults (10.7%), and other (19%).[12] Men are three times more likely to die as a result of TBI than are women. The highest rate of TBI is among those age 65 or older, and the leading cause of TBI varies by age group: age 65 or older—falls; ages 5 to 24—motor vehicle accidents; and newborn to 4 years—assault.[12]

The cause of TBI is closely associated with age and gender. Children younger than age 5 tend to be injured in falls and motor vehicle crashes and by adults inflicting violence. Those ages 5 to 15 are also injured on bicycles, skateboards, and horses; as pedestrians; and during sports activities. From age 15 to 40, high-speed motor vehicle and motorcycle crashes are the most common causes of TBI. After age 40, the incidence of violence-related injury approaches that of motor vehicles, particularly in metropolitan areas. Young and middle-aged males are 1.5 times more likely to be injured than their female counterparts. The two age groups at highest risk for TBI are newborns to age 4 and teens from age 15 to 19.[12] Elderly individuals are injured just as often (80%) by a fall or during a pedestrian mishap as they are in motor vehicle accidents.[23,50] Blasts are a leading cause of TBI in active duty military personnel in war zones.[12]

Nontraumatic or acquired brain injuries include toxicity from drug overdose, chronic substance abuse, carbon monoxide poisoning, and environmental exposure; anoxia from cardiopulmonary arrest or near-drowning; brain abscess or tumors, meningitis, and encephalitis from bacteria, viruses, acquired immunodeficiency syndrome (AIDS), fungi, or parasites; nutritional deficiencies; genetic and congenital disorders; chronic epilepsy; and degenerative neurological diseases.[53]

Concussions

A concussion is an injury to the brain that occurs because of a blow to the head or because a fall or blow to another part of the body causes rapid back-and-forth movement of the head. When a concussion occurs, the individual may experience symptoms such as headache, dizziness, blurred vision, memory lapses or loss, alterations in judgment or decision making, or changes in coordination. It is important to know that loss of consciousness frequently does not accompany a concussion. Concussions can be difficult to identify because the symptoms can be vague, and often individuals minimize or fail to report symptoms. Concussions are difficult to treat. Rest is usually the best intervention, although a physician may recommend that the individual refrain from contact sports and avoid strenuous or challenging cognitive activities, such as exercise and driving. The symptoms of a concussion can last several days or even weeks or months. Repeated concussions can have greater effects on the trauma to the brain and require even longer recovery times. Long-term effects of concussions can include attention deficits and symptoms of other types of nerve and brain damage.

Chronic Traumatic Encephalopathy

Chronic traumatic encephalopathy (CTE) is a progressive degenerative disease seen in people with a history of repetitive brain trauma, including symptomatic concussions and subconcussive hits to the head that do not cause symptoms.[57]

Individuals with CTE may show symptoms of dementia (e.g., memory loss, aggression, confusion, and depression), which generally appear years or many decades after the trauma. Baseline tests, such as the imPACT test (Immediate Post-Concussion Assessment and Cognitive Testing[42]), have been created to assess potential cognitive impairment in athletes in contact sports. However, as of yet no test is available to detect CTE in a living person; the condition can be determined only by autopsy.

Although the aforementioned conditions often have characteristics similar to those resulting from TBI (particularly with regard to rehabilitation approaches), this chapter's primary focus is assessment of and intervention for individuals with TBI.

Substance abuse is strongly linked to TBI. At least 45% of individuals with a TBI requiring rehabilitation were intoxicated at the time of their injury.[12,47] An even greater number of individuals have a history of alcohol or other substance abuse in the year preceding the injury. The American Psychiatric Association's *Diagnostic and Statistical Manual of Mental Disorders*, fifth edition (DSM-5) defines substance abuse as (1) failure to fulfill major role obligations at work, school, or home; (2) use of a substance in situations in which it is physically hazardous; (3) substance-related legal problems; or (4) continued use despite persistent or recurrent social or interpersonal problems related to use.[5,20,47,51] Therefore, knowledge of the acute and chronic sequelae of substance abuse disorders is crucial when assessing and treating individuals with brain injuries. Unsurprisingly, individuals who use alcohol or other drugs after sustaining a brain injury do not recover as well as those who do not use alcohol or other drugs.

Recovery from any type of brain injury depends on the client's age and preinjury capabilities, the severity of the injuries incurred, and the quality of intervention and support available during recovery. Unfortunately, recurrent brain injury is all too common and occurs in those who have previously sustained trauma, have developmental disabilities, or have acquired disabilities associated with other causes.

Prevention of secondary complications is critical throughout all stages of the recovery process—at the time the person is resuscitated (i.e., at the site of injury), in acute medical care settings, during acute and postacute rehabilitation programs, and when the individual is trying to reintegrate into their family and community. Many of the available medical and therapeutic interventions target these secondary complications. A well-coordinated team of knowledgeable professionals, family members, and supportive community caregivers can optimize the outcome for a given individual.[14]

PATHOPHYSIOLOGY

Neuropathologists and neurosurgeons currently categorize the early stages of TBI as primary (occurring at the moment of impact) and secondary (occurring in days to several weeks after the injury). Prevention of primary injury includes never driving under the influence; reducing distractions while driving (e.g., texting, phone calls); using safety belts in vehicles with intact air bags; and wearing protective helmets during sports such as bicycling, snowboarding, skateboarding, roller blading, and skiing; all these measures can minimize the impact of the initial cause of injury. Prevention also includes making living areas safer for older adults, such as removing fall hazards and installing grab bars.

Prevention of secondary injury typically begins at the point of contact, with those providing first aid at the scene of the trauma. It continues with emergency medical services (EMS), resuscitation and transport, and acute medical and surgical management; it then carries over to rehabilitation settings. The section on medical interventions, presented later in the chapter, particularly discusses secondary interventions to prevent further disability.

An individual with TBI will typically have some combination of primary focal and diffuse brain injury, depending on the cause and mechanism of the initial injury. In the best case scenario, a minimal amount of secondary brain damage and functional disability occurs as a result of brain swelling, hypotension, hypoxia, and systemic injury; prompt recognition of these complications and appropriate intervention improve survival and the functional outcome.[28]

Focal Brain Injury

Focal brain injury is caused by a direct blow to the head after collision with an external object or a fall, a penetrating injury resulting from a weapon, or collision of the brain with the inner surface of the skull. The bones of the face or skull may or may not be fractured. Common findings in individuals with a focal injury resulting from falls include intracerebral and brain surface contusions, particularly in the inferior and dorsolateral frontal lobes, the anterior and medial temporal lobes, and less commonly, the inferior cerebellum. Assault and missile wounds can occur anywhere in the brain, depending on the direction of force. Other surface areas of the brain, including those not directly affected by the blow to the head, can also suffer contusions as a result of collision of the brain with the interior surface of the skull. The directly injured area is referred to as the *coup*, and the site of the indirect injury is known as the *contrecoup*.[33,34]

If there are injuries to the coverings of the brain, especially the dura, pia, and arachnoid, other focal hemorrhages often occur. Epidural hematomas (EDHs) are associated with skull fractures in adults with disruption of the integrity of the meningeal arteries; children may have arterial disruption with or without a skull fracture. Individuals with an EDH may initially be alert after the blow to the skull; as the hematoma develops between the skull and the dura, it can cause pressure on underlying brain tissue (secondary injury) with rapid deterioration in mental and physical status. Prompt recognition and neurosurgical treatment can save lives and limit morbidity.[39]

Subdural hematomas (SDHs) occur between the dura and the brain surface through tearing of bridging veins. The rate of hemorrhage is often slower than that of an EDH because venous bleeding is more gradual than arterial. An SDH may occur just as frequently on the side of the head opposite the direct blow (contre coup); therefore, an EDH can occur on one side of the brain adjacent to the trauma and an SDH on the other. SDHs tend to spread around the entire surface of one hemisphere or, less commonly, in the posterior fossa. Acute SDH is diagnosed within 48 hours of injury, subacute SDH within 2 to 14 days after injury, and chronic SDH after 2 weeks. The fall or blow to the head in individuals with subacute or chronic SDH may have occurred days before the person arrives at the hospital with symptoms typical of changes in mental status. The urgency of treatment for SDH depends on the clinical condition of the

individual and the extent of adjacent brain tissue affected, as observed radiologically.[72]

Multifocal and Diffuse Brain Injury

In multifocal and diffuse brain injuries, there may be sudden deceleration of the body and head, with variable forces transmitted to the surface and deeper portions of the brain. Motor vehicle, bicycle, and skateboard crashes are typical causative factors, but falls off a horse or from a high surface, such as a roof or ladder, can produce multifocal and diffuse injuries.

Intracerebral hemorrhage (ICH) is nearly always a focal injury with missile wounds and is common after falls and assaults. Within the first week after TBI, particularly in clients with blood-clotting abnormalities, ICH may appear on followup CT scans. With a high-speed deceleration injury, multiple small, deep ICHs occur throughout the neuraxis; on high-resolution CT or magnetic resonance imaging (MRI), they are typically visible at the junction between gray and white matter and in the basal ganglia, corpus callosum, midbrain, and/or cerebellum.

Subarachnoid hemorrhage (SAH) and intraventricular hemorrhage (IVH) occur when the pia or arachnoid is torn. SAH caused by trauma is less frequently associated with vasospasms than is SAH caused by rupture of an aneurysm. A large IVH can block the flow of cerebrospinal fluid (CSF) and result in acute hydrocephalus. Thus, clinical evaluation for a possible ruptured aneurysm causing brain dysfunction, which may result from a fall or motor vehicle crash, is important with either of these entities.

Diffuse axonal injuries (DAIs) are prototypical lesions caused by rapid deceleration. The degree of injury may vary from primary axonotomy, with complete disruption of the nerve, to axonal dysfunction, in which the structural integrity of the nerve remains intact but there is loss of ability to transmit normally along neuronal pathways. The clinical severity of DAI is measured by the depth and length of coma (i.e., the time from the onset of injury until the individual performs purposeful activity) and associated signs, such as pupillary abnormalities.[51]

Prevention of Secondary Brain Injuries

The brain, like any body tissue, reacts to injury with swelling or edema, neurochemical injury cascades, changes in blood flow, and inflammation. Unlike other tissues, however, the brain is confined in a closed container, the skull; this protects it from outside injury but also restricts the amount of swelling or blood accumulation that can occur. The brain is also the organ least able to tolerate loss of blood flow or oxygen. Secondary injury occurs as a result of the effects of brain swelling in a closed space, loss of perfusion, and decreased delivery of oxygen to healthy and damaged tissue. Recovery is related to the extent of the initial pathology and secondary injury.[27] Improved outcomes result when secondary, delayed insults are prevented or respond to treatment.

Guidelines for the management of severe TBI to minimize the impact of secondary injury have been developed over the past 10 years by the American Association of Neurological Surgeons (AANS) and the Brain Trauma Foundation. Some of the areas addressed include resuscitation of blood pressure and oxygenation, management of elevated intracranial pressure (ICP) or hypertension, nutrition after acute trauma, and seizure prophylaxis. These care recommendations are based on a critical review of the available literature on the management of individuals with TBI, and they are categorized into three groups: *standards*, which represent a high degree of clinical certainty; *guidelines*, which represent a moderate degree of clinical certainty; and *options*, which represent a low degree of clinical certainty.[13] Each of these terms (standards, guidelines, and options) is used as a label for forms of intervention for individuals who have sustained a TBI.

Areas of intervention that are considered standards are relatively few and relate to interventions that may be more harmful than helpful. They include the following:

- In the absence of increased ICP, chronic prolonged ventilation should be avoided.
- Steroids are not recommended to reduce ICP.
- Prophylactic anticonvulsants are not recommended for preventing late (i.e., after the first week) post-traumatic seizures (PTSs).[44]

Guidelines that have a moderate degree of certainty regarding efficacy include the following for individuals with severe TBI: (1) all geographic regions should have an organized trauma care system to provide emergency care; (2) hypotension (systolic blood pressure [SBP] below 90 mm Hg) or hypoxia (apnea, cyanosis, oxygen saturation below 90% in the field, or a partial arterial oxygen pressure [Pao$_2$] of 60 mm Hg) must be corrected immediately and the condition monitored; (3) ICP monitoring is appropriate for injuries in individuals younger than age 40 with a systolic blood pressure (SBP) below 90 mm Hg, with a Glasgow Coma Scale (GCS) score between three and eight, or when CT scans show hematomas, contusions, edema, herniation, or compressed basal cisterns; (4) intervention should be initiated to lower the ICP if it exceeds 20 to 22 mm Hg; (5) effective ICP treatments include mannitol, high-dose barbiturate therapy, ventriculostomy for drainage of CSF, and craniectomy (i.e., removal of portions of the skull to allow external brain swelling [bone flap]); and (6) enteral or parenteral nutritional support at 140% of the basal rate in nonparalyzed and 100% in paralyzed individuals, with 15% of calories provided as protein before maximum 7 days of TBI.

PTSs are classified as *immediate* when they occur during the first 24 hours after injury, *early* when they occur during the first 7 days, and *late* after the first 7 days. Prophylactic treatment with phenytoin or carbamazepine during the first week after TBI is an intervention option recognized by both the AANS and the American Academy of Physical Medicine and Rehabilitation (AAPM&R). Both organizations recognize that the efficacy of prophylactic treatment diminishes greatly after the first week and therefore recommend discontinuation of anticonvulsant medication as standard treatment after the first week.[4,13] If late PTSs develop, treatment is warranted because the recurrence rate is greater than 80%.[36] All clients and caregivers should learn recognition of and first aid for seizures, in addition to risk modification. Avoidance of alcohol, street drugs, and prescribed medications that lower the seizure threshold is important for

CASE STUDY

Victor

Victor, an 18-year-old who identifies as male (prefers use of the pronouns he/him/his) sustained multiple cerebral contusions, has right arm and leg tremors with intentional movement and severe rigidity. He also has increased tone in his left arm and leg. He is dependent for all self-care and mobility.

After a baseline evaluation conducted over 2 days, both occupational and physical therapists note that the tremors increase with any voluntary movement. Medication is introduced to reduce the tremors, and feedback is provided to the prescribing physician about Victor's performance of self-care activities and bed mobility. Over the next 2 weeks, Victor developed the ability to use his right hand to wipe his face with minimal assistance, which takes 10 seconds, and his medication dose is tapered, with no worsening of the tremor.

Meanwhile, the flexor tone on his left side is increasing, especially at the elbow; this prevents progress in upper body dressing. A temporary musculocutaneous nerve block with bupivacaine results in increased ability to extend his left arm so that dressing now requires only moderate assistance; the next day, a phenol nerve block is performed, at the therapist's suggestion, for longer-term relief of the elbow flexion tone. This intervention is directed toward a focal area of difficulty for the client, which is his ability to use his left arm for upper body self-care.

Alternative interventions include systemic tone-reducing medications, which may have adverse side effects, and inhibitive casting of the elbow, which may help but makes the limb less useful while casted.

clients recovering from TBI. The groups at highest risk of developing PTS are those with a history of chronic substance abuse, penetration of metal and bone into the brain tissue, biparietal contusions, multiple intracranial operations, epidural hematoma, severe TBI, and any injury that causes more than a 5-mm lateral shift on CT scans.[25]

Implementation of the aforementioned standards and guidelines more typically takes place in designated trauma centers, where physicians, nurses, and allied health providers are accustomed to treating large numbers of individuals with TBI. Studies in both academic and community hospital settings have shown that morbidity and mortality can be reduced appreciably by following the AANS guidelines.[64]

Ongoing optimal medical and health management can facilitate individuals' recovery and ability to participate in their own rehabilitation. Early detection and prompt management of sleep and mood disorders, pain, hydrocephalus, heterotopic ossification, and endocrinopathies, all common sequelae of TBI, must be addressed. Medical therapeutic interventions should be based on behavioral, cognitive, and functional performance factors that are observable and measurable by members of a rehabilitation team.

COMA AND LEVELS OF CONSCIOUSNESS

A TBI typically results in an altered level of consciousness. The continuum of consciousness ranges from coma to conscious awareness. After a brain injury, an individual's progression along this continuum of consciousness depends on the client's age and previous health status, the severity of the injury, and the methods of medical, therapeutic, and environmental management.

TABLE 35.1   Glasgow Coma Scale

Examiner's Test		Individual's Response	Assigned Score
Eye opening	Spontaneous	Opens eyes on own	4
	Speech	Opens eyes when asked to in a loud voice	3
	Pain	Opens eyes when pinched	2
	Pain	Does not open eyes	1
Best motor response	Commands	Follows simple commands	6
	Pain	Pulls examiner's hand away when pinched	5
	Pain	Pulls a part of the body away when pinched by examiner	4
	Pain	Flexes body inappropriately to pain (decorticate posturing)	3
	Pain	Body becomes rigid in an extended position when examiner pinches (decerebrate posturing)	2
	Pain	Has no motor response to pinch	1
Verbal response (talking)	Speech	Carries on a conversation correctly and tells examiner where and who he or she is and the month and year	5
	Speech	Seems confused or disoriented	4
	Speech	Talks so examiner can understand but makes no sense	3
	Speech	Makes sounds that examiner cannot understand	2
	Speech	Makes no noise	1

Adapted from Rosenthal M: *Rehabilitation of the head-injured adult*, Philadelphia, 1984, FA Davis.

Consciousness is a state of environmental awareness and self-awareness. Coma is the absence of awareness of self and the environment despite maximal external stimuli. No periods of wakefulness occur in the coma state.[65,66] When sedating and hypnotic medications are discontinued, the coma rarely lasts longer than 4 weeks. When the coma resolves, the person becomes either partially aware of self and the environment (minimally conscious) or, if no awareness is present, "vegetative."

The Glasgow Coma Scale (GCS) has been the traditional method used by healthcare professionals to assess levels of consciousness after TBI (Table 35.1). The GCS has been used to quantify the severity of brain injury and predict outcome. The three behavioral areas assessed in the GCS are best motor response, verbal response (talking), and eye opening. The most reliable is the motor score of 5 or 6; a score of 5 signifies a purposeful response to stimuli such as pain or pressure (e.g., pushing away noxious stimuli), and 6 represents an ability to follow simple commands. When these scores are reached by injured individuals, they are considered to no longer be in a coma or vegetative state. This is an important landmark in recovery from TBI.[80]

The vegetative state is most succinctly described as wakefulness without awareness. A person in a vegetative state has the following characteristics: (1) no awareness of self or the environment and inability to interact with others; (2) no sustained, reproducible, or voluntary behavioral responses to sensory stimuli; (3) no language comprehension or expression; (4) sleep/wake cycles of variable length; (5) ability to regulate temperature, breathing, and circulation to permit survival with routine medical and nursing care; (6) incontinence of bowel and bladder; and (7) variably preserved cranial nerve and spinal reflexes. A persistent vegetative state refers to a condition of past and continuing disability with an uncertain future; the typical onset is within 1 month of a TBI or non-TBI or after a month-long metabolic or degenerative condition. The condition may improve, and the client may achieve a minimally conscious state (MCS) over time. If the client does not improve, the term permanent vegetative state is appropriate and signifies that the chance of regaining consciousness before death is exceedingly small.[71] Recovery of consciousness is rare for individuals in a persistent vegetative state 12 months after a TBI or 3 to 6 months after a non-TBI.[77]

Practice parameters for the care of individuals in a persistent vegetative state indicate that appropriate diagnosis of the condition is crucial; a physician with experience in this area should participate in the determination. Once the diagnosis has been established, the prognosis should be explained in detail to the family, surrogates, and caregivers. Appropriate care respects the individual's comfort, hygiene, and dignity. Careful observation of any signs of emergence to MCS is important in determining the intensity of therapeutic interventions. Positioning and other interventions to manage tone and prevent contractures should be included. The amount of extraordinary care is guided by the advance directives or presumed directives supplied by the client's surrogate.[3]

Many individuals emerge from a persistent vegetative state to MCS in which there is definite behavioral evidence of awareness of self, environment, or both. Clearly discernible, reproducible behavior in one or more of the following areas must be demonstrated: (1) ability to follow commands, (2) gestural or verbal yes/no responses (regardless of accuracy), (3) intelligible verbalizations, and (4) purposeful movements or affective responses that are appropriate reactions to environmental stimuli. Examples include reaching for objects; touching or holding objects and accommodating for their size and shape; engaging in eye pursuit movements or sustained fixation in direct response to stimuli; and smiling, crying, vocalizing, or gesturing in response to relevant stimuli. Convenient ways to assess for MCS are testing an individual with situational orientation questions ("Are you standing?" "Are you in a chair?") and giving the individual an object of common use (e.g., washcloth or comb) to see whether he or she tries to use it appropriately. Testing for MCS should be done in a quiet environment when the client is alert (i.e., not under sedating medication or in a physical position that encourages inattention). Requested commands should not exceed the client's physical capabilities and should not involve reflexive movements.[30] Serial assessment tools that can be useful for measuring the cognitive progress of individuals in MCS include the JFK Coma Recovery Scale–Revised (JFK-Revised), Wessex Head Injury Matrix (WHIM), Coma–Near Coma Scale, Sensory Stimulation Assessment Measure, and the Western Neuro Sensory Stimulation Profile.[17,29,62]

Another important landmark in recovery is posttraumatic amnesia (PTA), which is probably the single best measurable predictor of functional outcome in the research literature (Table 35.2). PTA is the length of time from the injury to the moment when the individual regains ongoing memory of daily events. Some evidence suggests that the duration of PTA is highly correlated with individual outcomes. A longer PTA is associated with poorer long-term cognitive and motor abilities and a decreased ability to return to work and school. PTA that lasts 4 weeks or longer is correlated with significant long-term disability.[59] PTA is measured with the Galveston Orientation and Amnesia Test (GOAT) or the Orientation Log.[52] The latter test is easier to administer to individuals with moderate to severe TBI in which the examiner may not know the details of circumstances immediately before the injury and in which the injured individual has begun to remember events.[43,52]

The Rancho Los Amigos (RLA) Scale of Cognitive Functioning is a descriptive measurement of eight (and sometimes 10) levels of awareness and cognitive function.[68] Progression through the levels occurs most typically with traumatic injuries.

TABLE 35.2 Relationship of Severity of Injury to Duration of Post-Traumatic Amnesia

Severity of Injury	Duration of PTA
Very mild	<5 min
Mild	5–60 min
Moderate	1–24 hr
Severe	1–7 days
Very severe	1–4 wk
Extremely severe	>4 wk

PTA, Post-traumatic amnesia.
From Rosenthal M: *Rehabilitation of the head-injured adult*, Philadelphia, 1984, FA Davis.

However, in some very severely injured individuals, the recovery curve may actually skip a level (typically level IV, an agitated confused state). Other clients may never be as low as level I or II, but they may be agitated and confused for several weeks (level IV). These individuals may experience periods during which they also function at level V or VI. Thus, this scale can be helpful to staff and family members in designing specific behavioral interventions for a given client. Table 35.3 presents a complete description of the RLA scale.

Many studies have analyzed factors such as the client's age, the severity and cause of the injury, substance abuse, and the client's psychosocial status in predicting outcomes after TBI; however, these factors have definite limitations in predicting the recovery of an individual.[c]

Individuals with TBI improve over a period of months to years, especially once individuals become aware of their altered capabilities.[67] Monitoring an individual's personal rate of recovery is probably more predictive of future recovery than any other factor.

CLINICAL PICTURE

Physical Status

An individual with TBI may exhibit a variety of symptoms, depending on the type, severity, and location of the injury. Individuals may have limitations in most of the areas discussed in the following sections, or they may have subtle deficits evident only during more complex activities.

Table 35.4 shows some of the most common clinically diagnosed physical signs and symptoms of a client who has sustained a TBI.

Decorticate, Decerebrate, and Motor Rigidity

Rigidity is the presence of increased resistance to passive movement throughout most of the range that is independent of stretch velocity.[51] Comatose individuals often display one of two common positions, decorticate rigidity or decerebrate rigidity. In decorticate rigidity, the upper extremities (UEs) are in a spastic flexed position with internal rotation and adduction. The lower extremities (LEs) are in a spastic extended position but also internally rotated and adducted.

Decorticate rigidity results from damage to the cerebral hemispheres, particularly the internal capsules, which causes an interruption in the corticospinal tracts (which emerge from the cortex and send voluntary motor messages to all extremities).

In decerebrate rigidity, both the UEs and LEs are in a position of spastic extension, adduction, and internal rotation. The wrists and fingers flex, the ankles are in plantar flexion with the feet inverted, the trunk and neck extend, and the head retracts. Decerebrate rigidity occurs as a result of damage to the brainstem and extrapyramidal tracts (which send involuntary motor messages from the brainstem to the extremities). Individuals with decerebrate rigidity have a poorer prognosis than do those exhibiting decorticate rigidity.[18,33]

[c]References 11, 14, 20, 24, 38, 84.

TABLE 35.3   Rancho Los Amigos Levels of Cognitive Functioning

Level I No response	These individuals appear to be in a deep sleep and are completely unresponsive to any stimuli presented.
Level II Generalized response	These individuals react inconsistently and nonpurposefully to stimuli in a nonspecific manner. Responses are limited and are often the same, regardless of the stimulus presented. Responses may be physiological changes, gross body movements, or vocalization. Often the earliest response is to deep pain. Responses are likely to be delayed.
Level III Localized response	These individuals react specifically but inconsistently to stimuli. Responses are directly related to the type of stimulus presented, as in turning the head toward a sound or focusing on an object presented. These individuals may withdraw an extremity or vocalize when presented with a painful stimulus. They may follow simple commands in an inconsistent, delayed manner, such as closing the eyes, squeezing, or extending an extremity. After the external stimulus has been removed, these individuals may lie quietly. They may also show a vague awareness of self and body by responding to discomfort by pulling at a nasogastric tube or catheter or resisting restraints. They may show bias by responding to some people (especially family and friends) but not to others.
Level IV Confused, agitated	These individuals are in a heightened state of activity with a severely decreased ability to process information. They are detached from the present and respond primarily to their own internal confusion. Behavior is frequently bizarre and nonpurposeful relative to the immediate environment. The individual may cry out or scream out of proportion to the stimuli even after removal and may exhibit aggressive behavior, attempt to remove restraints or tubes, or crawl out of bed in a purposeful manner. However, the individual does not discriminate among people or objects and is unable to cooperate directly with treatment effort. Verbalization is frequently incoherent and inappropriate to the environment. Confabulation may be present; these individuals may be euphoric or hostile. Thus, gross attention is very short and selective attention is often nonexistent. Being unaware of present events, these individuals lack short-term recall and may be reacting to past events. They are unable to perform self-care (e.g., feeding and dressing) without maximal assistance. If not disabled physically, these individuals may perform motor activities (e.g., sitting, reaching, and ambulating), but as part of the agitated state and not as a purposeful act or on request.
Level V Confused, inappropriate, nonagitated	These individuals appear alert and are able to respond to simple commands fairly consistently. However, with increased complexity of commands or lack of any external structure, responses are nonpurposeful, random, or at best fragmented toward any desired goal. These individuals may exhibit agitated behavior, not on an internal basis (as in level IV) but rather as a result of external stimuli and usually out of proportion to the stimuli. These individuals have gross attention to the environment but are highly distractible and lack the ability to focus attention on a specific task without frequent redirection back to it. With structure, these individuals may be able to converse on a social, automatic level for short periods. Verbalization is often inappropriate; confabulation may be triggered by present events. Memory is severely impaired, with confusion of past and present in the reaction to ongoing activity. These individuals lack initiation with regard to functional tasks and often show inappropriate use of objects without external direction. They may be able to perform previously learned tasks when they are structured for them, but the individual is unable to learn new information. They respond best to self, body, comfort, and often family members. They can usually perform self-care activities with assistance and may accomplish feeding with maximal supervision. Management on the unit is often a problem if these individuals are physically mobile because they may wander off either randomly or with the vague intention of going home.
Level VI Confused, appropriate	These individuals show goal-directed behavior but are dependent on external input for direction. The response to discomfort is appropriate, and they are able to tolerate unpleasant stimuli (e.g., nasogastric tube) when the need is explained. These individuals follow simple directions consistently and show carryover for tasks that have been relearned (e.g., self-care). They are at least supervised with old learning but are unable to maximally assist in new learning with little or no carryover. Responses may be incorrect because of memory problems, but they are appropriate to the situation. Responses may be delayed, and these individuals show a decreased ability to process information with little or no anticipation or prediction of events. Older memories have more depth and detail than recent memory. These individuals may show beginning awareness of their situation by realizing that they do not know an answer. These individuals no longer wander and are inconsistently oriented to time and place. Selective attention to tasks may be impaired, especially with difficult tasks and in unstructured settings, but they are now functional for common daily activities (30 minutes with structure). They show at least vague recognition of some staff members and have increased awareness of self, family, and basic needs (e.g., food), again in an appropriate manner, in contrast to level V.

TABLE 35.3   Rancho Los Amigos Levels of Cognitive Functioning — cont'd

Level VII Automatic, appropriate	These individuals appear appropriate and oriented in the hospital and home settings and go through the daily routine automatically but are frequently robot-like. They exhibit minimal to absent confusion, but have shallow recall of what they have been doing. They show increased awareness of self, body, family, foods, people, and interaction in the environment. These individuals have superficial awareness of, but lack insight into, their condition, demonstrate decreased judgment and problem solving, and lack realistic planning for the future. They show carryover for new learning, but at a decreased rate. They require at least minimal supervision for learning and for safety purposes and are independent in self-care activities and supervised in home and community skills for safety. With structure these individuals are able to initiate tasks in social and recreational activities in which they now have an interest. Judgment remains impaired, such that these individuals are unable to drive a car. Prevocational or avocational evaluation and counseling may be indicated.
Level VIII Purposeful and appropriate	These individuals are alert and oriented, are able to recall and integrate past and recent events, and are aware of and responsive to their culture. They show carryover for new learning if it is acceptable to their life role. These individuals need no supervision after activities are learned within their physical capabilities. They are independent in home and community skills, including driving. Vocational rehabilitation is indicated, to determine ability to return as a contributor to society (perhaps in a new capacity). These individuals may continue to show decreased ability, relative to premorbid abilities, in reasoning, tolerance for stress, judgment in emergencies, or unusual circumstances. Their social, emotional, and intellectual capacities may continue to be at a decreased level but are functional for society.
	**Levels IX and X are used at some out-client facilities to identify higher functioning individuals.**
Level IX Purposeful, appropriate stand-by assistance on request	Independently shifts back and forth between tasks and completes them accurately for at least 2 consecutive hours. • Use assistive memory devices to recall daily schedule and to-do lists and to record critical information for later use with assistance when requested. • Initiate and carry out steps to complete familiar personal, household, work, and leisure tasks independently and unfamiliar personal, household, work, and leisure tasks with assistance when requested. • Aware of and acknowledge impairments and disabilities when they interfere with task completion and take appropriate corrective action, but require stand-by assistance to anticipate a problem before it occurs and take action to prevent it. • Able to think about the consequences of decisions or actions with assistance when requested. • Accurately estimate abilities but require stand-by assistance to adjust to task demands. • Acknowledge others' needs and feelings and respond appropriately with stand-by assistance. • Depression may continue. • May be easily irritable. • May have low tolerance for frustration. • Able to self-monitor appropriateness of social interaction with stand-by assistance.
Level X Purposeful, appropriate: modified independent	• Able to handle multiple tasks simultaneously in all environments, but may require periodic breaks. • Able to independently procure, create, and maintain own assistive memory devices. • Independently initiate and carry out steps to complete familiar and unfamiliar personal, household, community, work, and leisure tasks, but may require more than the usual amount of time and/or compensatory strategies to complete them. • Anticipate impact of impairments and disabilities on ability to complete daily living tasks and take action to prevent problems before they occur, but may require more than the usual amount of time and/or compensatory strategies. • Able to independently think about the consequences of decisions or actions, but may require more than the usual amount of time and/or compensatory strategies to select the appropriate decision or action. • Accurately estimate abilities and independently adjust to task demands. • Able to recognize the needs and feelings of others and automatically respond in appropriate manner. • Periods of depression may occur. • May show irritability and low tolerance for frustration when sick, fatigued, and/or under emotional stress. • Social interaction behavior is consistently appropriate.

Adapted from the Adult Brain Injury Service: *Original scale, levels of cognitive functioning*, Downey, CA, 1980, Rancho Los Amigos Medical Center.

TABLE 35.4   Clinical Signs and Symptoms Commonly Seen in a Client With a Traumatic Brain Injury

Sign	Lesion Location	Clinical Characteristics	Interventions
Decerebrate rigidity	Midbrain, pons, diencephalon	Extended internally rotated shoulders; extended elbows; flexed wrists, fingers; extended internally rotated hips, extended knees, ankle plantar flexion, inversion; increased rigidity when awake	Positioning, range of motion (ROM), neuromuscular blocks, early casting
Decorticate rigidity	Cortical white matter, internal capsule, thalamus, cerebral peduncle, basal ganglia	Internally rotated shoulder; flexed elbow, wrists, fingers; extended, internally rotated hips; knee flexion; ankle plantar flexion, inversion; increased rigidity when awake	Positioning, ROM, neuromuscular blocks, early casting
Bruxism	—	Persistent jaw clenching, grinding of teeth with or without temporomandibular dislocation or subluxation	Neuromuscular blocks, oral orthotics
Spasticity	Upper motor neuron syndrome; corticospinal pathways	Velocity-dependent resistance, hyperreflexia/clonus, muscle shortening; present in face, neck, trunk, limbs; worse when awake and with effort	Bed/chair positioning, ROM, weight bearing, neuromuscular blocks, inhibitive casting, enteral and intrathecal medications, tendon releases, relaxation techniques
Rigidity and bradykinesia; parkinsonism	Substantia nigra, extrapyramidal pathways; also with medications that block dopamine	Velocity-independent resistance; lead pipe, cogwheel types of rigidity; worse when awake	Positioning, ROM, functional activities, medications
Torticollis		Dystonic posture of the neck; spasticity and/or contracture of the sternocleidomastoid, splenius muscles	Positioning, modalities and ROM, medications, neuromuscular blocks
Myoclonus	Variable	Abrupt, shocklike involuntary jerks in large (limb) or small muscles when sleep or awake	Medications, neuromuscular blocks
Tremor	Variable	Involuntary rhythmic oscillations while awake	Weighted devices, weight bearing, medications, neuromuscular blocks, appropriate assistive devices
Dystonia	Variable	Dynamic contraction/relaxation of muscles with slow, writhing or repetitive twisting movements or sustained contortions; usually distal limb(s)	Positioning, ROM, neuromuscular blocks, medications, appropriate assistive devices
Athetosis	Basal ganglia, medications with effect on dopamine	Slow, sinuous movements of the face, tongue, or limbs	Relaxation techniques, taper offending medications
Chorea	Contralateral neostriatum, thalamus	Involuntary dancelike or jerky movements without rhythmic pattern; distal	Medications
Hemiballismus/ballismus	Contralateral subthalamic nucleus, thalamus, cerebellum	Sudden irregular flinging movements starting in the hip or shoulder, occasionally facial or oral with or without rotator component; worse with arousal/excitement, absent in sleep	Medications

TABLE 35.4   Clinical Signs and Symptoms Commonly Seen in a Client With a Traumatic Brain Injury—cont'd

Sign	Lesion Location	Clinical Characteristics	Interventions
Tics	Variable	Sudden stereotypic coordinated automatic movements or vocalizations while awake	Medications, behavioral management, Relaxation techniques
Pseudobulbar athetoid syndrome	Bilateral pyramidal tract	Postural dystonia with fragmentary athetosis, with or without bradykinesia; often preserved intellect/personality	Positioning, appropriate assistive devices

Data from Mayer NH, Keenan MAE, Esquenzi A: Limbs with restricted or excessive motion after traumatic brain injury. In Rosenthal M, Griffith ER, Kreutzer JS, Pentland B, editors: *Rehabilitation of the adult and child with traumatic brain injury*, ed 3, Philadelphia, 1999, FA Davis; Mayer NH: Choosing upper limb muscles for focal intervention after traumatic brain injury, *J Head Trauma Rehabil* 19:119, 2004; and Zafonte R, Elovic E, Lombard L: Acute care management of post-TBI spasticity, *J Head Trauma Rehabil* 19:89, 2004.

Cogwheel or lead pipe rigidity resembling Parkinson's disease can occur, typically in individuals with severe TBI. It may respond to dopamine agonists, such as levodopa/carbidopa or amantadine. Dystonia of the neck (torticollis), jaw, or distal ends of the limbs can also occur and may require treatment with motor point blocks.[56]

Abnormal Muscle Tone and Spasticity

Although decorticate rigidity and decerebrate rigidity are associated with the most severe types of abnormal muscle tone and tend to occur in comatose individuals, hypertonicity may range from minimal to severe in any muscle group. Individuals functioning at a higher cognitive level than coma generally display a combination of hypotonicity (i.e., decreased tone, or flaccidity) and hypertonicity (i.e., increased tone, or spasticity). Flaccidity (hypotonicity) is a decrease in normal muscle tone. It is usually attributed to peripheral nerve injury resulting in soft muscle feel, in which the muscles offer no resistance to passive movement. Spasticity (hypertonicity or hypertonia) is an involuntary increase in muscle resistance that is dependent on velocity.[51] The Modified Ashworth Scale, a widely used assessment of muscle tone, scores muscle tone on a scale of 0 to 4[10]:

0	No increase in muscle tone
1	Slight increase in muscle tone, manifested by a catch and release or by minimal resistance at the end of the range of motion (ROM) when the affected part or parts are moved in flexion or extension
1+	Slight increase in muscle tone, manifested by a catch, followed by minimal resistance throughout the remainder (less than half) of the ROM
2	More marked increase in muscle tone through most of the ROM, but the affected part or parts are easily moved
3	Considerable increase in muscle tone, passive movement difficult
4	Affected part or parts rigid in flexion or extension

Because individuals with spasticity cannot voluntarily relax their limbs, voluntary movement of an affected limb may be impossible. Spasticity can be seen as early as a few days after brain injury, or it may take 3 to 6 months to develop. In as little as 2 weeks, spasticity may cause muscles to shorten permanently, which in turn can cause joints to lose motion. The condition of permanent shortening is called a *muscle contracture*.

OT PRACTICE NOTES

It is important to instruct all staff members involved in the client's care that tone can fluctuate as a result of changes in position, volitional movement, medication, infection, menstruation, illness, pain, environmental factors (i.e., ambient temperature), and emotional state.[9]

Primitive Reflexes

If damage to the midbrain has occurred, impaired righting reactions are commonly observed. Damage to the brainstem can result in the absence of equilibrium reactions and protective extension. The absence of righting reactions, equilibrium reactions, and protective extension places the individual at significant risk for further injury from falls during such activities as transfers, getting out of bed, toileting, bathing, and dressing.

Muscle Weakness

A decrease in muscle strength without the presence of spasticity can occur as a result of peripheral nerve or plexus injuries and lack of physical activity caused by secondary factors associated with TBI (e.g., compromised respiration, fractures, and infection). A functional muscle and sensory test may be indicated when an individual exhibits decreased strength in the limbs. Additionally, impaired gross and fine motor coordination will be evident and should be assessed.

Decreased Functional Endurance

Decreased endurance and vital capacity usually accompany reduced muscle strength as a result of medical complications such as infections, poor nutrition, or prolonged bed rest. Increasing the individual's muscle strength and endurance is a primary goal in the acute stage and in the initial stages of rehabilitation.

Ataxia

Ataxia results from impairment of the cerebellum itself or the motor pathways leading to and from the cerebellum; it can also occur with impaired proprioception. Ataxia is a movement abnormality characterized by incoordination, impaired sitting and standing balance, or both.[9] Ataxia can occur in the entire body, in the trunk, or in the UEs and LEs; it presents as jerkiness during movement. An individual with ataxia has lost the ability to perform the small adjustments between agonist and antagonist muscles of extremities that are necessary for smooth, coordinated movement.

The degree of ataxia ranges from mild to severe. An individual with ataxia in the trunk displays impaired postural stability when sitting and standing. They have difficulty maintaining the trunk in a stable position to free the UEs or LEs for activities. The individual may compensate for this deficit by grasping a stable surface, such as a tabletop. Ataxia in the UEs causes dysfunction in activities in which the person attempts to perform a combination of gross and fine motor movements, such as bringing a glass of water to the mouth. The UE oscillates back and forth, causing the water to spill. Ataxia in the LEs results in an impaired ability to ambulate while maintaining balance; falls can easily occur with this condition.

Postural Deficits

Postural deficits develop as a result of an imbalance in muscle tone throughout the body. An individual may inadvertently accentuate the postural deficits by using ineffective strategies to compensate for impaired motor control; delayed or absent righting reactions; or impaired vision, cognition, or perception. Therapists must have a thorough knowledge of the postural deficits of their clients to position them properly in a wheelchair with the appropriate seating system; this is a necessary step to obtain an upright posture, maintain good postural alignment, and prevent further postural deformities. Frequently exhibited abnormal postures include the following:

1. *Pelvis.* Posterior pelvic tilt is often due to prolonged bed rest in the supine position, which causes loss of ROM in the lower part of the back. Posterior pelvic tilt reduces or eliminates the typical sacral curvature that results in sacral sitting and potentially kyphosis. Pelvic obliquity is observed when one side of the pelvis sits lower than the other side as a result of hypertonicity of the quadratus lumborum on the involved side.
2. *Trunk.* Kyphosis, scoliosis, and lordosis all may be present as a result of weak or spastic trunk muscles (e.g., pectoralis, abdominal, spinal, and paraspinal). It is also common to observe lateral flexion toward the involved side (trunk shortening) with elongation of muscle on the opposite side.

3. *Head and neck.* Forward flexion or hyperextension of the neck and lateral flexion of the head often accompany lateral flexion of the trunk.
4. *Scapula.* The scapula may be depressed, protracted or retracted, downwardly rotated, or all of these at once. This results from an imbalance in scapular muscle tone; some muscles are hypertonic, whereas others are hypotonic.
5. *Upper extremities.* UEs may be bilaterally or unilaterally involved. In unilateral involvement, it is common to see variations in ROM, tone, and strength in each muscle group and joint of the arm, forearm, wrist, and hand.
6. *Lower extremities.* Severe extension patterns are often observed in both LEs, which can pose a problem with wheelchair positioning; this is evident when the individual thrusts forward and slides out of the seating system. Hip adduction, internal rotation, knee flexion, plantar flexion, and inversion of the feet can all be observed.

Limitations of Joint Motion

Loss of ROM in the joints is a common problem. It is often difficult to distinguish between several possible causes of decreased ROM, such as increased muscle tone, volitional resistance, contractures, heterotopic ossification, fractures or dislocations, and pain. Because the intervention addressing decreased ROM depends on the cause, the therapist should consult a physician to determine the cause of the decreased ROM before initiating intervention. Distal limb fractures are often overlooked in acute trauma settings when clients are unable to communicate because of cognitive deficits. Therapists are typically the first to detect the hard end feeling of joints with limited ROM typical of heterotopic ossification, the formation of lamellar bone in soft tissue.[37]

Sensation

Clients with TBI may exhibit signs of absent or diminished sensation, including problems with light touch, differentiation between sharp and dull sensations, proprioception, temperature, pain, and kinesthesia. Additionally, impaired senses of taste and smell, caused by cranial nerve injury, may be observed.[9] Lost or diminished stereognosis, two-point discrimination, and graphesthesia (i.e., the ability to interpret letters written on the hand without visual input) may be present. Hypersensitivity, which can often interfere with postural alignment, may also occur.

Integration of Total Body Movements

Total body movements involve the integration of head, neck, and trunk control with dynamic sitting and standing balance while reaching, bending, stooping, and ambulating. To perform total body movements, the individual must coordinate and modulate gross and fine motor movements of the trunk, head, neck, and limbs while performing ADLs. An individual with severe physical involvement often displays poor sitting and standing balance and is unable to maintain an upright position to free the UEs for activities. Individuals functioning at a more advanced level may exhibit subtle deficits in total body movements that make it difficult to bend down, reach overhead to retrieve items in a cabinet, or stoop to retrieve an item that has fallen to the floor. Integrated total body movements are necessary for the performance of all ADLs.

Dysphagia

Dysphagia, or difficulty completing the four stages of chewing and swallowing, is caused by damage to the cranial nerve or brainstem (see Chapter 27). There is a higher incidence of oral preparatory–stage, oral-stage, and pharyngeal-stage dysphagia than esophageal-stage dysphagia for individuals with TBI. Typically, more than one stage of chewing and swallowing is impaired.[7,8] An individual may display oral motor impairments that prevent or impair the activity of speaking or eating; such impairments include muscular hypotonicity or hypertonicity, instability of the jaw, and abnormal oral reflexes, including rooting, biting, sucking, gagging, and coughing. As a result of cognitive deficits, the individual may experience difficulty sequencing chewing, swallowing, and breathing.

Self-Feeding

Clients with TBI may be unable to sustain attention long enough to feed themselves. If impulsivity is apparent, these clients will have difficulty monitoring the amount and rate of food brought to the mouth, thus causing coughing and possibly aspiration. Oral apraxia, an inability to perform an intended action or execute an act on command with the mouth or lips, may occur. If clients have ideational apraxia, they will have difficulty understanding the demands required of the self-feeding activity and will be unable to recognize utensils as tools for eating. Because they may also have lost the motor plan for self-feeding (ideomotor apraxia), they may be unable to gain access to the neurological motor pattern for bringing food to the mouth. Hemianopia (visual field cut) or visual neglect may prevent them from seeing half of the plate of food.

Cognitive Status

Cognitive deficits are always evident to varying degrees after a TBI and can affect many aspects of the individual's quality of life, as mentioned in previous sections. The most common cognitive deficits include decreased attention and concentration, impaired memory, impaired initiation and termination of activities, decreased safety awareness and poor judgment, impulsivity, and difficulty with executive functions and abstract thinking (e.g., problem solving, planning, integration of new learning, and generalization).

Attention and Concentration

Reduced attention and concentration impair the ability to maintain focus on an activity without becoming distracted and the ability to resume an activity when interrupted. Clients with TBI often lose the ability to concentrate for a length of time and the ability to filter out distractions from the surrounding environment. The inability to attend to and concentrate on activities severely impedes the ability to function at work and school and complete ADLs. Although deficits in attention and concentration can diminish as neurological recovery progresses, such deficits can remain to varying degrees throughout an individual's life. Even clients who experience mild TBI can demonstrate subtle deficits in attention and concentration that often linger for years after the injury and can affect daily functioning.

Memory

Impaired memory, the most frequently observed cognitive deficit in clients with TBI, can remain a lifelong problem. Memory impairment ranges from forgetting several words just heard (immediate memory), to forgetting which family members visited the night before (short-term memory), to forgetting events that occurred years before the injury (long-term memory). Despite neurological recovery, most of these clients continue to demonstrate difficulty learning new information. Safety concerns include getting lost, leaving doors unlocked, and leaving a stove on; clients with impaired memory typically require supervision if compensatory methods cannot be used. This loss of independence can be emotionally devastating because clients with TBI often have insight into both who they were before the injury and their accomplishments, goals, and plans for the future, many of which are severely disrupted and perhaps lost as a result of TBI.

Memory losses are also labeled in relation to the time of the injury or brain damage. Loss of memories for events before the time of the specific injury is referred to as retrograde amnesia. The client may forget events that occurred just before the accident or forget events that happened several days, weeks, and even months before the accident. After TBI the client is often unable to form new memories, and this is referred to as anterograde amnesia; this period can last for days, weeks, or even months after the injury.

Initiation and Termination of Activities

Impaired initiation and termination of activities affect the ability to start and end activities. An inability to initiate activities without assistance affects the individual's ability to live independently. In general, clients who exhibit deficits in initiation demonstrate the greatest progress in a rehabilitation setting that provides assistance and structure. After returning home, these individuals may regress and have difficulty completing basic daily activities if the necessary structure has not been set up. Similarly, clients may exhibit difficulty terminating an activity once it has been started, which is a type of perseveration. For example, a client may begin brushing the teeth but may be unable to end the task because of feeling compelled to continue. Perseveration sometimes involves a thought process. Clients may be unable to concentrate on one activity because they are perseverating on the idea that another activity (e.g., the laundry) must be completed.

Safety Awareness and Judgment

Frontal lobe damage often results in an impairment in insight about a person's limitations and in impulsivity, or the inability to consider consequences before acting. Such individuals demonstrate poor safety awareness and judgment. For example, the client may attempt to rise out of a wheelchair without locking the brakes or moving the footrests. A more mobile client who has been reintegrated into the community may attempt to cross streets without observing traffic signals or remove pots from the stove or oven without using protective oven mitts or pot holders. It is important for the OT to structure the client's environment to reduce accidents and increase the client's awareness of their limitations through repeated opportunities to practice and relearn safe and appropriate behavior.

Processing of Information

Most people with TBI experience some degree of difficulty processing external information from the environment. A delay in response time is often noted and can range from a few seconds to several minutes. It is important for the therapist to recognize the presence of delayed processing and distinguish the delay from the absence of function. For example, during sensory evaluation a client may exhibit a delay in response to a dull stimulus. The therapist may mistakenly interpret the individual's delayed processing time as an absence seizure or impairment of sensory awareness. A delay in the processing of external information from the environment can involve visual, auditory, sensory, and perceptual processing.

Executive Functions and Abstract Thought

Executive function skills include the ability to plan, organize, set goals, understand the consequences of one's actions, and modify behavior in accordance with environmental responses. Abstract thinking is the ability to hold and manipulate a concept in one's mind by using critical reasoning and analytic skills, which can be challenging for many TBI clients. As a result, many clients with TBI exhibit concrete thinking, in which they are able to interpret information only at the most literal level. For example, individuals with impaired executive and abstract functions may be able to complete a meal preparation activity accurately and safely only if step-by-step directions are provided. If the directions do not specifically direct the reader to modify the cooking temperature, these individuals may burn the food because they are unable to foresee the consequences of maintaining the stove on a high setting.

Generalization

Generalization of new learning is the ability to learn to transfer the skills needed for a specific task to another similar activity. Deficits in executive function skills, abstract thinking, and short-term memory significantly impair the generalization of new learning. For example, an individual who has learned in a day treatment setting the skills for completing a laundry task may be unable to transfer the skills at home or at a different laundromat. Such deficits often occur as a result of concrete thinking and the inability to form abstractions. Although the cognitive pattern for completing laundry tasks with the laundry machine in the clinical setting is established, the individual cannot transfer that cognitive pattern to a similar but unfamiliar laundry machine in a different environment. Impaired generalization of new learning is one of the most significant problems impeding the individual's ability to resume independent functioning in a community setting.

Visual Status

Visual skills involve the ability to accurately see stimuli from the external environment (see Chapter 24). Visual skills do not involve the identification of objects, which is a function of perception. Among the many deficits in visual skills that may result from TBI are accommodative dysfunction (causing blurred vision), convergence insufficiency (the inability to maintain a single vision while fixating on an object), lateral or medial strabismus, nystagmus, hemianopia, impaired vestibulo-ocular reflex (maintaining gaze on an object during opposite head movement), and impairment of scanning and pursuits. Saccades (fast, jerky movements of the eyes as they change from one position of gaze to another, as is needed to read a book) as well as antisaccades (the ability to look away from a stimuli) also may be compromised by TBI. Reduced blink rate, ptosis (drooping of the eyelid), and lagophthalmos (incomplete eyelid closure) are also common visual deficits resulting from damage to the oculomotor nerve.[9] Dysfunction in any of these visual elements can profoundly affect daily life function.

Individuals rely on vision indirectly in social and interpersonal interactions. Vision is used as a cueing and feedback system for motor skills such as ambulation and for eye-hand coordination activities. Deficits in vision can affect all daily life activities, including the areas of hygiene and grooming, meal preparation and eating, wheelchair mobility, reading and writing, and driving.

Perceptual Skills

Perception is the ability to interpret stimuli from the external environment (see Chapter 25). Perception is a function of the secondary cortical areas of the right hemisphere, including the secondary visual area, the secondary somatosensory area, the secondary auditory area, and the multimodal parietal-occipital-temporal area. Perceptual deficits are more often a result of right hemisphere damage but may also occur with lesions in the left hemisphere. Perception can be grouped into the following categories: visual perception, body schema perception, motor perception, and speech and language perception. An individual with impairments in visual perceptual may exhibit difficulty in right-left discrimination, figure-ground discrimination, form constancy, position in space, and topographic orientation. Visual perceptual deficits also include visual agnosia, in which the individual displays difficulty recognizing familiar objects and people. For example, prosopagnosia is the inability to connect faces with names. Prosopagnosia results from damage to the multimodal association area.[9] Visual perceptions in recognizing and interpreting the facial expressions of others also may be affected.

Body schema perception is awareness of the spatial characteristics of a person's own body. This awareness is derived from the neural synthesis of tactile, proprioceptive, and pressure sensory associations about the body and its individual parts. A common problem in people with TBI is anosognosia, a failure to recognize deficits or limitations. This may lead to the body schema perceptual dysfunction of **unilateral neglect syndrome**, in which the individual has lost the ability to integrate perceptions from one side of the body or environment (usually the left).

Unilateral neglect is commonly caused by a lesion in the right parietal lobe but also can occur as a result of frontal and occipital lobe damage. Clients with left unilateral neglect may disown their left extremities and treat them as though they belong to someone else. For example, these individuals may shave only the right side of their face or dress only the right side of their body.[8] Aphasia is a disturbance in the comprehension (receptive) or formulation (expressive) of language (or both) caused by dysfunction in specific brain regions, typically the left hemisphere.[22] A few left-handed individuals have language dominance in the right hemisphere. Establishing reliable communication is crucial in treating a person with aphasia. If auditory comprehension is compromised, gestural demonstration of instructions or activities is more reliable. Common types of aphasia involving disorders of comprehension include the Wernicke and transcortical sensory types. Individuals affected with these types of aphasia have longer periods of PTA because they do not understand orientation questions. Although their spoken language may be fluent, such individuals could struggle with verbal paraphasias or word substitutions. Clients with aphasia may also misinterpret speech and become suspicious and agitated. Insight into their communication deficit may be limited.

The nonfluent aphasias (Broca's aphasia and transcortical motor aphasia) are characterized by relatively preserved comprehension but effortful or explosive speech with phonemic paraphasias (e.g., "bork" for "fork"). Broca's aphasia specifically is characterized by coordination deficits in oral motor skills resulting in impaired speech. Conduction aphasia (i.e., intact comprehension, fluent speech, impaired repetition) and anomic aphasia are characterized by circumlocution and frequent paraphasias. Individuals with these types of aphasia are typically aware of their problems and are often frustrated by their limitations. They should be encouraged to use gestures to express their immediate desires and needs.

Dyslexia (disturbance in reading), agraphia (disorder of writing), and dyscalculia (disturbance in calculation) frequently accompany the aphasias. However, with traumatic aphasias, these capabilities may be better preserved than with stroke; treating therapists should always attempt alternative modes of communication.

Dysprosody, or aprosody, is impaired production or comprehension of the tonal inflections or emotional tone of speech. Executive dysprosody is an inability to inflect one's voice to convey emotion. It can occur with cerebellar, basal ganglia, or right frontal lobe injury. Receptive dysprosody is an inability to perceive the emotional content of other people's spoken language. It occurs with right temporal or parietal injury and less often with left hemisphere injury. Individuals with this disorder may miss the point of a joke or story because they cannot comprehend the subtle innuendos and implicit meanings conveyed through tonal qualities and inflections.[81] Even more disabling is the inability to interpret anger, humor, or sarcasm during communication with others.[21] Perceptual motor dysfunction is impairment in motor planning, or an apraxia. It is a disorder of learned movement that cannot be explained by weakness, lack of sensation, inattention, or comprehension of the requested task.[21]

The apraxias are usually a result of impairment of the premotor cortex, corpus callosum, or connections between the temporal and parietal lobes and frontal motor cortex.[40] It is in these cortical areas that established motor patterns for specific activities are stored and accessed for the execution of common movement patterns. Ideational apraxia is an inability to understand the demands of a task or use of the wrong motor plan for a specific task. For example, individuals suffering from ideational apraxia may not understand that a shirt is an item of clothing to be placed on the torso and UEs. Not understanding the demands of the task, they may be unable to activate the motor plan for UE dressing or may activate the wrong plan and attempt to place their legs through the sleeve holes. This deficit is sometimes referred to as a dressing apraxia.

Ideomotor apraxia is loss of the kinetic memory of a movement pattern for a specific activity. Individuals with this disorder may understand that a shirt is an item of clothing to be placed on the torso and UEs, but they may be unable to execute the appropriate movement plan because it is no longer accessible. Constructional apraxia is an inability to accurately assemble pieces of an object to form a three-dimensional whole. For example, a former carpenter who suffers from constructional apraxia may be unable to put together the wooden pieces of a basic birdhouse kit.

Psychosocial Factors

Researchers have found that the greatest concerns of clients 1 year or more after TBI are the psychosocial deficits that prevent them from rebuilding a satisfactory quality of life. As the time after injury increases, clients and family members view such psychosocial factors as more detrimental than both the physical and cognitive sequelae of TBI.

In Maria's case, it was initially difficult to assess her psychosocial status because she was nonverbal. The team was able to assess her mood on the basis of her level of participation and affect during therapy. Maria would laugh appropriately and become visibly more interactive, with brighter affect, when her boyfriend arrived to visit.

Maria continued to engage in positive interactions throughout her 4-month in-patient and day treatment stay. Her discharge plan involved moving to another state to live with her mother. When the move was discussed with Maria, it was evident that she was quite saddened by the knowledge that she would no longer be able to see her boyfriend. The team observed her closely to assess whether her sadness would eventually culminate in depressive symptoms.

Self-Concept

One of the most difficult psychosocial sequelae of TBI is alteration of the individual's self-concept. Self-concept is the internal image people hold about their human identity, sexual and gender identity, body image, personal strengths and limitations, and position in the family, peer group, and community systems. An individual's self-concept changes drastically after TBI. One of the most difficult characteristics of TBI is that although short-term memory is often impaired, long-term memory commonly remains intact. Individuals with TBI often have a clear memory of who they were before their injury and must now resolve the emotional conflict of having to replace their preinjury self-concept with a postinjury self-concept that is both meaningful and satisfying. Affected individuals sometimes describe this process as an unwanted death and rebirth. They say that the person who lived before the injury is now gone, replaced by someone who is very different from the person they remember themselves to have been.[63]

Social Roles

Self-concept is derived largely from the social roles the person attains in the family, peer group, and larger community systems. Frequently, an individual with TBI loses most preinjury roles and the activities that supported those roles. Family and peer group roles change. Family members and friends are often readily visible during the acute and subacute stages of TBI rehabilitation. However, as the time after injury increases, family and friends become progressively less involved with the individual, which frequently leads to feelings of isolation and abandonment. Many individuals with TBI report that the feeling of isolation and the inability to form and maintain social relationships are their most troubling postinjury concerns. Loss of the role of dating partner or spouse commonly leaves clients with TBI with a deep sense of loss and failure if they cannot rebuild a postinjury life that includes intimacy with another human being, partnership in a committed relationship, and parenting of children. Loss of the work role and inability to support oneself are intimately tied to feelings of dependence and lack of personal control.[48]

Independent Living Status

As a result of the physical, cognitive, and psychosocial sequelae of TBI, many affected individuals find they require supportive living arrangements or must live with their parents. Loss of the ability to live independently in the community further reinforces feelings of dependence and decreased personal control. As a result of these role losses, adults who sustain TBI commonly experience role strain and feel that they cannot reenter their communities. The TBI, particularly if it occurred between the ages of 18 and 30, disrupts the developmental transition from adolescence to adulthood and leaves individuals feeling inadequate and unable to attain a postinjury adult status. Depression, withdrawal, and apathy are common psychosocial sequelae of the alterations in self-concept discussed earlier and of the loss of desired social roles.[58]

Dealing With Loss

People with TBI and their family members often go through a process that resembles the stages of death and dying experienced by the terminally ill.[49] These stages begin with denial, in which affected individuals deny that they are experiencing physical, cognitive, or psychosocial deficits. Denial can impede therapy because these clients may refuse to participate, in the belief that it is unnecessary. Denial gradually subsides as they continually confront their limitations in ADLs. Anger follows denial. Clients grow increasingly aware of their deficits and become frustrated and angry because recovery is slower than desired. Bargaining is the next stage. Clients strike a deal with the Creator or fate and offer to work as diligently as possible in

therapy if only their preinjury lifestyle could be restored. The bargaining stage is often marked by increased motivation and optimism. Depression tends to emerge next. Eventually, clients begin to realize the severity of the injury and its effect on the rest of their lives. Acceptance of the injury and its resultant limitations, the next stage in the process, is necessary for clients to become sufficiently motivated to attempt to build a postinjury life that, although drastically different from their preinjury goals and expectations, is nevertheless meaningful and personally valuable. These stages may require years of transition. Frequently, denial, anger, and bargaining occur in the first few months to a year after the injury. Depression sets in as the individual is able to let go of some of the denial and becomes aware of the effect that the injury will have on the future. It may take years before they can truly accept the injury and alterations in personality, skill, and lifestyle and move on to rebuild a new life.

The process of denial, anger, depression, and acceptance does not generally proceed in a linear fashion. Clients with TBI commonly experience repeated periods of denial, anger, and depression throughout their years of rehabilitation. Renewed denial, anger, and depression may occur in response to a new environmental demand, such as a change in life condition (e.g., a need to move from the parental home to a community group home) or the development of further physical, cognitive, or psychosocial deterioration over time (e.g., the need for increased ambulatory assistance because of deterioration in visual skills).

Affective Changes

Depression, increased emotional lability, involuntary emotional displays of mood that are overly frequent and excessive, and decreased effect can result from the neurological damage. Individuals with left hemisphere damage tend to exhibit increased depression and emotional lability. Lesions of the left orbitofrontal lobe often cause severe depression and heightened affect (including excitement, agitation, and tearfulness). Lesions of the left dorsolateral frontal lobe commonly result in a decreased or flat affect. Individuals with these lesions may appear depressed even though they feel fine. Neurological damage to the right hemisphere frequently causes a strange sense of euphoria or lack of emotional response to the severity of injury.[63] People with brain injury often have difficulty recognizing others' emotions. Because this ability is essential for guiding appropriate emotional and behavioral responses toward others, this type of impairment poses various psychosocial and emotional problems (Dawn Newmann, Assistant Research Professor, Indiana University School of Medicine, personal communication).

Behavioral Status

Behavioral impairments are a natural part of the recovery process. The Rancho Los Amigos (RLA) cognitive level IV is typically described by the rehabilitation team as the "agitated, confused" level.[68] During this stage of recovery, affected individuals can be described as restless and combative. They may be responding to internal body experiences, or some external environmental stimuli may be provoking the agitation. Commonly observed behavior includes yelling, swearing, grabbing, and biting. Behavioral problems can be disturbing to

ETHICAL CONSIDERATIONS

Working with clients who have behavior problems can be frustrating and sometimes frightening. Untrained staff members can be injured, and they often reinforce the client's negative behavior through their own actions and responses.

both the individual's family and the intervention team; therefore, behavioral management is an essential component of TBI rehabilitation.

A comprehensive behavior management program should be established for anyone who exhibits behavior that interferes with active participation in therapy and achievement of goals. The goals and objectives of a comprehensive program include maintaining a safe environment for individuals and staff members at all times, developing and consistently implementing behavior management techniques, minimizing the use of all restrictive modalities, and providing an environment that facilitates participation and appropriate behavior in the hospital setting and after discharge.[70]

Interventions used in an effective behavior management program include one-on-one coaching, intervention with psychotropic medications, and individually designed behavior management guidelines and interventions. One-on-one coaching, usually performed by a trained nursing assistant or rehabilitation technician, is especially necessary for clients who are at risk of harming themselves or others. In many cases, implementation of a behavior management program is necessary 24 hours a day, 7 days a week. A coach helps reinforce the client's behavior plan and redirects inappropriate or maladaptive behavior. Medications are required to regulate sleep and minimize agitation and combative behavior until clients can control the behavior on their own. Because pain may often provoke agitation, assessing a client's level of pain and providing appropriate medication may resolve the restlessness, agitation, and/or inability to sleep. Medications must be chosen carefully to prevent side effects such as clouding of awareness and psychomotor slowing. Clients should have specific behavioral endpoints, such as establishing adequate sleep at night, facilitating attention during functional activities, and reducing the frequency of verbal or physical outbursts.

Environmental modifications are a proactive approach to prevent and minimize undesirable behavior. Such modifications may include use of a cubicle or net bed, an alarm system, a helmet, and walkie-talkies. A drug and alcohol policy is frequently necessary; it is well documented that many individuals with TBI have preexisting alcohol or drug problems (or both).[71]

The first step in becoming more comfortable when working with clients who have behavior problems is to understand why the problems occur and how they manifest themselves.

Clients exhibiting agitation, combativeness, disinhibition, and refusal to cooperate and participate in activities typically have difficulty filtering distractions and can become agitated in noisy environments. Providing a quiet room during interventions and use of a cubicle bed may help minimize noise and reduce outbursts.

A disinhibited individual may lack awareness of the external environment and may make indiscriminate sexual remarks

or gestures to others. Ignoring comments, redirecting inappropriate behavior, and modeling acceptable behavior are typical therapeutic interventions.

Clients who refuse to cooperate and participate in interventions can be the most challenging because this behavior may affect their ability to remain in an acute rehabilitation program. The lack of participation is typically organically based and due to cognitive deficits such as impaired initiation and lack of insight into the disability. It is important to document such behavior throughout the course of care; however, when clients refuse to participate, documenting progress can be challenging. Interventions include providing consistent structure through daily schedules and goal sheets that provide visual cues for expectations and also visual and physical guidance through activities until clients are capable of completing tasks without assistance.

OT PRACTICE NOTES

Behavior management is essential in all TBI rehabilitation programs. It is important to develop and implement a behavioral program, whether the behavior is passive (decreased initiation), active (agitation), or somewhere along the continuum. An effective program includes comprehensive staff training, tools that track and monitor behavior and techniques, and consistent multidisciplinary communication (behavior management meetings) to ensure that the individualized behavior plan is effective and goal oriented.[71]

EVALUATION OF THE INDIVIDUAL AT A LOWER RLA LEVEL

Clients emerging from coma and at the beginning stages of the injury (RLA levels I through III) may exhibit minimal arousal and limited purposeful movements. It may be necessary to evaluate such individuals in short sessions and at different times of the day. A quiet environment with minimal distractions will enhance the client's ability to attend to and follow commands.

Evaluation includes assessment of the following:

1. *Level of arousal and cognition:* Can the client visually attend to the speaker and follow commands such as "Open your mouth" and "Squeeze your eyes closed"? Can the client communicate through verbalizations, gestures, or eye movements? Do they demonstrate purposeful movements, such as pulling at vital tubes? How easy or difficult is it to wake the client, and how long can the client stay awake?
2. *Vision:* Is the client able to visually scan or attend to a person, object, or activity? Can the client maintain eye contact?
3. *Sensation:* Does the client respond to external stimulation, such as pain, temperature, and movement of the joints?
4. *Joint ROM:* Has the client lost ROM in certain joints as a result of decorticate or decerebrate posturing, increased tone or spasticity, contractures, or heterotopic ossification?
5. *Motor control:* Does the client exhibit decorticate or decerebrate posturing? Is there an increase in tone and spasticity? Is there decreased tone and hypotonicity? Are deep tendon responses present, diminished, or absent? Does the client exhibit the presence of primitive reflexes? Does the client engage in spontaneous motor movements, such as scratching the face?

6. *Dysphagia:* Does the client handle secretions, drool, or swallow spontaneously? Does the client demonstrate poor oral motor control? Answers to these questions provide valuable information on whether a swallowing evaluation is indicated.

7. *Emotional and behavioral factors:* Is the client's affect flat or expressive? Are responses such as crying or laughing observed in response to interactions with the rehabilitation team or family members?

Evaluation of lower level individuals with TBI is generally accomplished with tools such as a goniometer, clinical muscle and tone testing, traditional neurological screening, and clinical observations. Many acute TBI rehabilitation facilities have developed their own initial evaluation forms. A variety of scales can be used to establish a baseline and predict recovery. The GCS and RLA scale are commonly used; however, newer cognitive scales are also being used (e.g., the JFK-Revised and WHIM).[3] Some clients tend to emerge quickly and move expeditiously through the RLA levels, whereas others (e.g., those with anoxia) may demonstrate limited or slow recovery. A subacute program or a rehabilitation center that specializes in working with clients who are slow to recover may be necessary. In either case, a rehabilitation program with active therapeutic intervention is necessary to prevent contractures, encourage activity, and facilitate the client's progress through the rehabilitative process.

In the case of Maria, the team decided to address her spasticity and joint contractures first by providing appropriate medical interventions, including blockade of her musculocutaneous nerve to decrease her left UE spasticity. This was followed by casting to reduce her elbow contracture. The team also gave Maria a comprehensive activity schedule in a multi-stimulus environment. This schedule involved transferring her out of bed and into a customized wheelchair, in which she would remain 6 to 8 hours a day, getting up into a standing frame daily, and requiring active participation in all therapies 4 hours per day. Her cognitive level was assessed weekly with the JFK-Revised scale, and her ability to follow through with basic mobility and self-care tasks also was assessed.

INTERVENTION FOR THE INDIVIDUAL AT A LOWER RLA LEVEL

The general aim of intervention for those at RLA levels I through III is to increase the individual's level of response and overall awareness of self and environment. All stimulation should be well structured and broken down into simple steps and commands. Allotting sufficient time for an individual's response is necessary because cognitive processing is often significantly delayed during this phase of recovery. Intervention at this stage can be grouped into six areas: sensory stimulation, bed positioning, casting or splinting, wheelchair positioning, management of dysphasia, and emotional and behavioral management; family and caregiver education also begins. Interventions may occur simultaneously to optimize progress. Each intervention affects and enhances the next. Because clients often respond more to the familiar and routine, it is important to involve close family members and friends in the sessions.

Sensory Stimulation

Intervention for clients emerging from coma should start as soon as they are medically stable. Intervention generally begins in the intensive care unit. At this stage, clients frequently lack responsiveness to pain, touch, sound, or sight. They may exhibit a generalized response to pain that appears reflexive (e.g., attempting to pull away from painful stimuli). The goal of intervention is to increase the client's level of awareness by trying to increase arousal with controlled sensory input. **Sensory regulation** increases neurological signals to the reticular activation system, the structure of the brainstem that alerts the brain to important sensory input from the external environment.

Sensory stimulation can be introduced in a variety of ways and methods. Introducing isolated visual, auditory, tactile, olfactory, and gustatory stimulants to the individual may heighten arousal. For example, a flashlight may be used to elicit eye opening and visual tracking. Playing familiar music may facilitate autonomic responses, such as a change in the respiratory rate or changes in blood pressure. Introducing olfactory stimulation through a variety of scents may elicit eye opening or head turning. Gustatory stimulation involves the controlled presentation of taste to the client's lips and tongue using a cotton swab. Such stimulants may include salty, sweet, bitter, and sour tastes. Any response from the client is noted.

OT PRACTICE NOTES

The most effective types of sensory stimulants are those that have personal meaning to the client, such as favorite songs or stories. Family members often bring in familiar objects and pictures that can facilitate responses from the client. It is helpful to learn about the client's preinjury history to incorporate familiar items and routines into the intervention plan.

Kinesthetic input is incorporated early in the intervention. One of the most effective ways to facilitate volitional movement is by actively guiding movements in a normalized fashion while performing functional activities. The therapist actively helps the client perform simple movements (e.g., rolling from side to side) and simple functional activities (e.g., wiping the mouth with a washcloth, combing the hair, and applying lotion to the skin). The theoretical aim of functional sensory stimulation is to reactivate highly processed neural pathways that had been established before the injury. Other activities related to functional sensory stimulation include sitting the individual up at the edge of the bed and having the client stand by using a tilt table or a hydraulic standing frame. During all these activities, the therapist observes the client for any changes, such as visual tracking, turning of the head, physical responses, vocalizations, and ability to follow verbal commands.

Wheelchair Positioning

Seating and positioning are important components of treatment in clients at lower RLA levels. Proper positioning in a wheelchair allows these clients to interact with their immediate environment in an upright, midline posture. Proper positioning facilitates head and trunk control so that clients can see and interact with people and objects in the environment. A proper

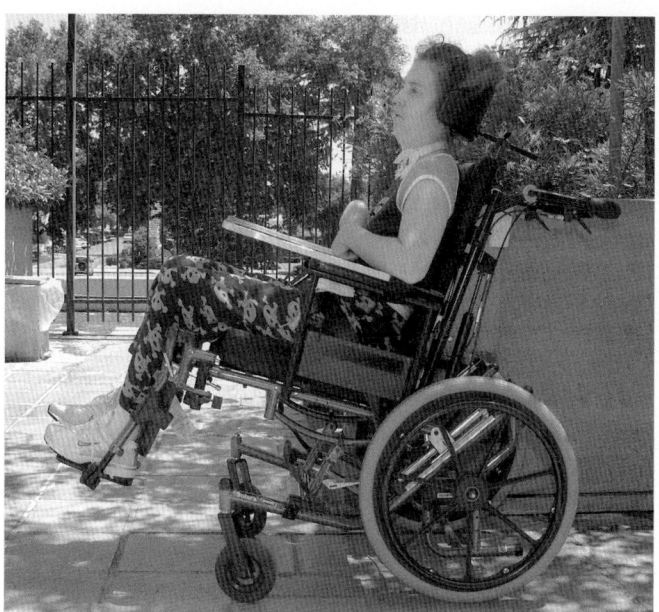

Fig. 35.1 Proper wheelchair seating position.

wheelchair seating position helps prevent skin breakdown and joint contractures, facilitate normal muscle tone, inhibit primitive reflexes, increase sitting tolerance, enhance respiration and swallowing function, and promote function (Fig. 35.1).

Effective seating and positioning require a stable base of support at the pelvis, maintenance of the trunk in the midline, and facilitation of the head in an upright, midline position. This position frees the UEs for use and allows the client to visually scan the environment. Once the client has a seating system that encourages and promotes function, therapy sessions can be more effective and beneficial. For example, clients generally find it easier to handle their secretions in this position, so swallowing trials may be safer and more effective.

Maria required a wheelchair and specific positioning devices when she entered the acute rehabilitation program. Given her motor abilities and deficits, what type of wheelchair setup would you prescribe?

Pelvis

Wheelchair positioning should begin at the pelvis. Poor hip placement adversely alters trunk and head alignment and influences tone in the extremities. Because sling-seat wheelchairs contribute to internal rotation and adduction of the hips, it is important to insert a firm, solid seat (padded with foam and covered by vinyl) to facilitate a neutral to slightly anterior pelvic tilt. A lumbar support may also help maintain the natural curve in the lumbar spine. A wedged seat insert (with the downward slope pointing toward the back of the chair) can be used to facilitate hip flexion and inhibit extensor tone in the hips and lower extremities (LEs). The individual's buttocks should bear weight evenly, with both ischial tuberosities firmly resting on the wheelchair seat. A seat belt angled across the pelvis helps maintain this desired position. Because these clients have spent a significant amount of time in bed, loss of anterior pelvic tilt is present. Before clients are positioned in a wheelchair, significant

stretching of the pelvis and trunk often is necessary to achieve neutral pelvic alignment and upper trunk extension. These stretches often facilitate upright, symmetric trunk alignment, which may have occurred secondarily to prolonged bed rest and abnormal tone, reflexes, and patterns.

Trunk

The trunk should be positioned after the pelvis because it is the next most proximal body structure. A solid back insert or firm contoured back should be placed behind the client's back to maintain the spine in an erect posture. A back insert contoured to the curves in the spine will maintain the lumbar and thoracic curves. Lateral trunk supports can be used to reduce scoliosis and lateral trunk flexion caused by imbalanced tone of the intrinsic muscles of the back. A chest strap (with easily opened Velcro fasteners) can be used to reduce kyphosis, facilitate shoulder retraction and abduction, and expand the upper part of the chest for proper diaphragmatic breathing and UE use.

Lower Extremities

An abductor wedge placed between the LEs just proximal to the knees may be used to reduce hip adduction and internal rotation. If hip abduction is present, a padded abductor wedge can be placed along the lateral aspect of the thigh to reduce LE abduction. Ideally, the knees should be positioned at 90 degrees, with the heels slightly behind the knees while sitting. Both feet should be maintained securely on the foot plates to provide proprioceptive input and facilitate weight bearing in both heels to normalize tone.

Upper Extremities

The upper extremities (UEs) should be positioned with the scapulae in a neutral position (neither elevated nor depressed), the shoulders slightly externally rotated and abducted, the elbows in a neutral position of slight flexion with forearm pronation, and the wrists and digits in a functional position. This position is often difficult to achieve because of severe spasticity and soft tissue contractures of the UEs. A splint or cast may be applied to reduce spasticity and facilitate a functional position of the UEs. Frequently, a lap tray is used to provide support for the UEs and encourage bilateral UE weight bearing and use.

Head

Lower functioning clients with TBI often have little or no active head control. Attaining a neutral-midline head position, which allows optimal visual contact with the environment, is difficult. A dynamic head-positioning device (Fig. 35.2) can be used to maintain neutral head alignment and facilitate head control. A contoured headrest that cradles the head posteriorly and laterally may be used to support the head in a midline position. A forehead strap (fabricated from soft, padded material) may be used to prevent the head from falling forward. Slightly reclining the wheelchair also prevents the client's head from falling forward and facilitates visual interaction with the environment. The client should be reclined 10 to 15 degrees; reclining the client beyond this point reduces weight bearing through the trunk

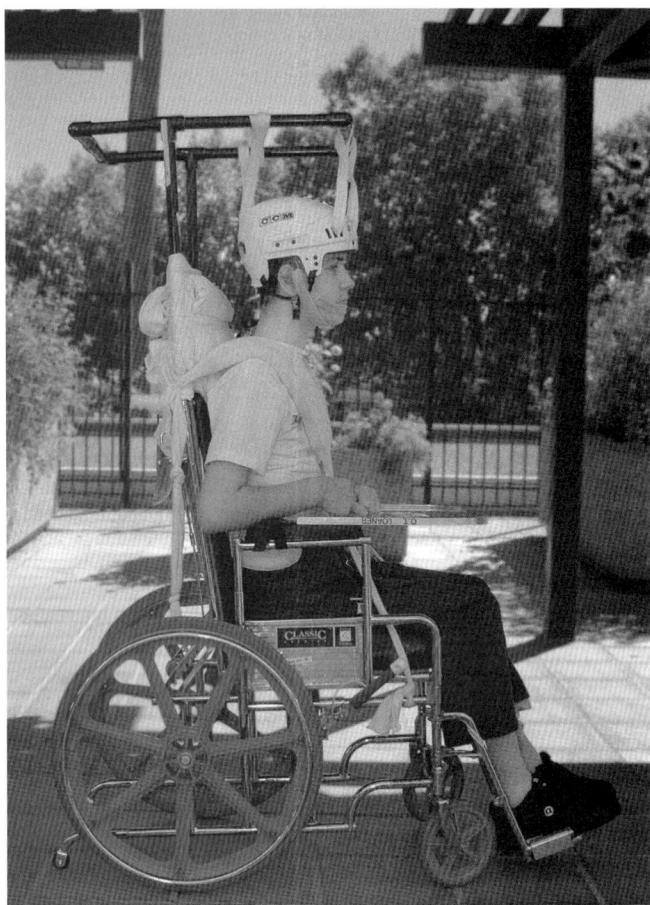

Fig. 35.2 A dynamic head-positioning device maintains neutral head alignment and facilitates head control.

any medical precautions that must be followed while the client is in bed.

If the client exhibits abnormal tone or posturing, a side-lying or semiprone position is preferable. This position assists in normalizing tone and providing sensory input. A supine position may elicit a tonic labyrinthine reflex and extensor tone. A supine position with the head in a lateral position could elicit an asymmetric tonic neck reflex. Clients with TBI generally have bilateral involvement, requiring a program for side-lying on both sides. The traditional bed-positioning techniques used for clients who sustained a cerebrovascular accident may require modification, depending on the extent of bilateral involvement. Pillows, foam wedges, and splints may be incorporated into the bed-positioning program to facilitate normal positions and prevent abnormal postures, such as extreme elbow flexion, head and neck extension, and footdrop deformity.

OT PRACTICE NOTES

Because all clients have unique needs, each should be assessed and set up with an ideal positioning program. It often helps to take a photo of the client once positioned and post it to ensure that it can be easily duplicated and carried out by staff and family members.

Splinting and Casting

Splinting or casting may be indicated when (1) spasticity interferes with functional movement and independence in ADLs, (2) joint ROM limitations are present, and (3) soft tissue contractures are possible. Splints have been thought to provide elongation and inhibition by positioning the joint in a static position with the muscles and soft tissues on stretch. Splinting of the elbows, wrists, and hands is often implemented to maintain a functional position at rest and to reduce tone. Serial casting is a more aggressive intervention to increase ROM in the joints when contractures have formed or spasticity is present (or both). Splinting and casting not only reduce contractures and increase ROM but also prevent skin breakdown. Because clients with TBI often have limited active ROM, the UE joints often assume a position of flexion (particularly when severe finger flexor spasticity has caused the fingers and nails to embed in the palmar surface of the hand), and this may cause moisture, redness, and breakdown of the skin.

A resting wrist-hand orthosis (Fig. 35.3) or antispasticity splint (Fig. 35.4) is worn when the client is not involved in active movements or functional tasks. The rest hand orthosis can be adjusted and readjusted to different degrees of extension or flexion of the wrist and fingers joints as desired; this is especially helpful when a client's spasticity level tends to fluctuate. In comparison, the antispasticity splint maintains the hand and fingers in reflex-inhibiting position and wrist in neutral position to reduce spasticity. Once the splint has been fitted, a wearing schedule must be established for the rehabilitation team and caregivers to follow. A typical splint schedule during the day requires the client to wear the splint for repeated, alternating 2-hour periods (2 hours on, followed by 2 hours off). The client must be monitored frequently for any skin breakdown or tonal

and pelvis and tends to encourage extensor tone, a posterior pelvic tilt, and sacral sitting. If the client has had a portion of the skull removed, a helmet is necessary to protect the brain during all mobility and when getting the client out of bed into a wheelchair.

As the client progresses in rehabilitation, wheelchair seating and positioning should be continually reevaluated to better meet the client's specific needs. Devices should be modified gradually or removed as the client begins to control the body actively and manipulate more items in the environment. A schedule is necessary to indicate the length of time the client can tolerate being seated in the wheelchair. Keeping the client in a wheelchair longer than can be tolerated may result in fatigue, which can subsequently interfere with active participation in therapy.

Bed Positioning

Proper bed positioning is critical in the early stages of TBI. Because the client tends to spend a lot of time in bed, proper bed positioning is crucial to prevent pressure sores, facilitate normal muscle tone, and prevent loss of pelvis and trunk ROM and mobility. It is often difficult to maintain optimal positioning because of spasticity and abnormal posturing. Other complications that may interfere with proper positioning are casts or splints, intravenous tubes, nasogastric tubes, fractures, and

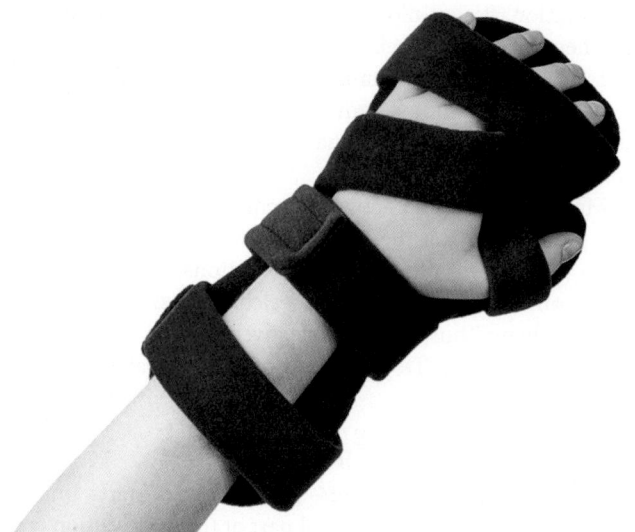

Fig. 35.3 Resting splint. (Courtesy Comfy Splints. All rights reserved. https://www.comfysplints.com/product/rest-hand/.)

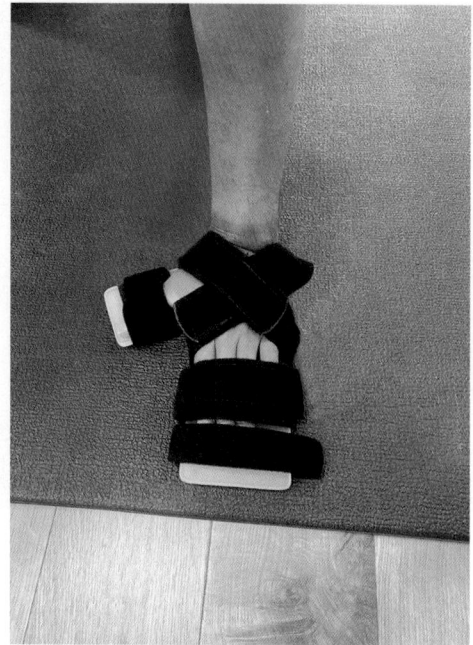

Fig. 35.5 Hand paddle splint. (Courtesy Lisa Bullard.)

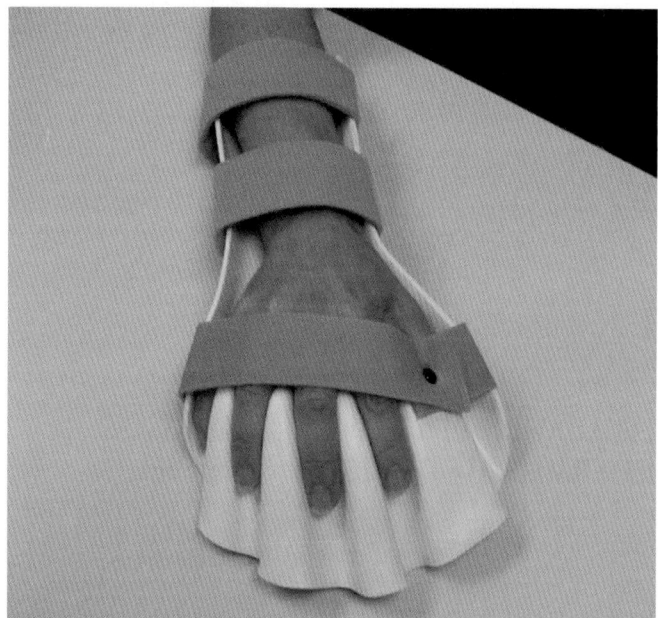

Fig. 35.4 Antispasticity splint. (From Skirven TM, Osterman AL, Fedorczyk JF, et al: *Rehabilitation of the hand and upper extremity,* ed 6, Philadelphia, 2011, Mosby.)

changes that may change the initial fit of the splint. Another option is a hand paddle splint. This orthotic is specifically designed to decrease the effects of hypertonicity in the finger wrist flexors and can be used during therapy sessions to incorporate weight bearing through the affected limb while performing functional activities with the unaffected limb (Fig. 35.5).

Other common splints worn at this stage of recovery are cone splints, which are used in the palm of the hand to keep the fingers from digging into the palmar surface. Frequently, rolled cloth is put into the clenched hand; however, because this may facilitate increased spasticity, a hard cone splint is more appropriate. An antispasticity splint (see Fig. 35.4) not only positions

the hand and wrist in a functional position, but also abducts the fingers to further reduce spasticity. Splints are modified as needed and may eventually be discontinued if the individual's motor control and tone improve.

A serial casting program is indicated when moderate to severe spasticity cannot be managed by splints. The goal of casting is to increase ROM and decrease tone gradually by using a progressive succession of separately fabricated casts, each worn continuously for a period of weeks. Casts are often left on for 5 to 7 days, which places the muscle and tendons on prolonged stretch and reduces tone. Successive casts are designed to increase ROM further until a functional joint range is achieved and maintained. A common difficulty that prevents success with serial casting is skin breakdown. If skin breakdown occurs because of a cast that is worn for several days, the cast must be removed until the skin has healed. While wound healing is occurring, spasticity again increases, and any gain in joint ROM is often lost.

The most common UE casts are the elbow cast, which is used for loss of passive range of motion (PROM) in the elbow flexors, and the wrist-hand cast, which is used for loss of PROM in the wrist and finger flexors. Variations of these casts include elbow dropout wrist, thumb, hand, and individual finger casts. However, casting of more than one joint at a time often leads to skin breakdown as a result of multiple pressure points. Therefore, casting should be applied to one joint at a time.[32]

Casting is frequently used in conjunction with motor point blocks, nerve blocks, or botulinum toxin injections. Blocks involve the injection of a chemical substance (e.g., lidocaine, bupivacaine, phenol) into the nerve or motor point to temporarily inhibit the innervation of spastic muscles. Botulinum toxin is injected directly into the target muscle and works by causing presynaptic blockade of acetylcholine release.

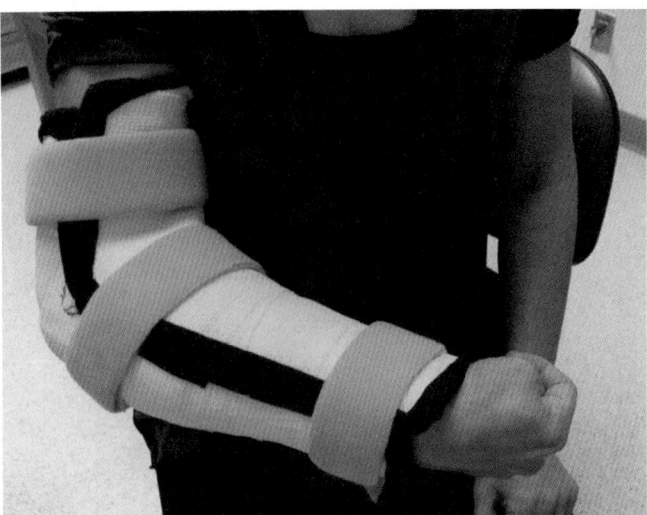

Fig. 35.6 Bivalved split to reduce spasticity. (From Skirven TM, Osterman AL, Fedorczyk JF, et al: *Rehabilitation of the hand and upper extremity,* ed 6, Philadelphia, 2011, Mosby.)

Indications for termination of a casting program include achieving functional ROM or plateauing (e.g., the individual has not gained significant improvement in ROM after two consecutive casts). When improvement in ROM has been made and the goal has been achieved, the final cast is cut in half lengthwise, the edges are finished, and the cast is used as a bivalve splint to maintain the functional position. Velcro straps or elastic wrap bandages are used to secure them in place (Fig. 35.6). A wearing schedule is then established for the bivalve splint (cast).

Casting is an advanced intervention technique that carries some risk. Competent application of the technique requires knowledge and advanced clinical training.

Maria had increased spasticity and reduced function in her UEs. What splint or cast (or both) would best suit her needs initially?

Dysphagia

Clients emerging from coma are fed through a nasogastric or gastrointestinal (GI) tube. Once the client is alert and more oriented, the physician decides when evaluation for dysphagia is indicated. Dysphagia programs usually begin when the client has moved into the intermediate or advanced levels of rehabilitation (see Chapter 27).

Behavior and Cognition

As clients emerge from coma and become more alert and aware of their surroundings, it is important to track their improvement and attempt to establish a form of communication. In acute rehabilitation, tracking the level of arousal and awareness is important because it demonstrates progress. Several scales and assessments are available, including the WHIM, JFK-Revised, and Orientation Log. These measurement tools document improvements in visual attention, visual tracking, and ability to follow commands.

Establishing a way for the client to communicate wants and needs is of the utmost importance because it helps guide

intervention. It also allows the team to more accurately assess the client's cognitive level. A reliable yes/no system should typically be implemented. Examples include eye blinks, eye gaze, head nods, and motor movements, such as thumb up and thumb down. Once a system has been established, communication is possible.

Maria gained some active movement of her right UE and with guiding was able to use large colored buttons to answer yes or no to questions. The yes and no buttons, which were positioned on the lap tray of her wheelchair, buzzed when Maria touched them. Thus, she was effectively able to answer simple questions, such as, "Do you need to use the bathroom?" and "Are you in pain?"

Family and Caregiver Education

Education of family members and caregivers starts immediately because they are an integral part of the intervention team. Family members often play an essential role in eliciting the client's responses and implementing the sensory regulation program, positioning the client in bed, and contributing to the ROM program. At the earliest stage after injury, therapy may be limited; therefore, setting up a simple intervention plan for the family to implement is important in fostering the client's recovery and maintaining passive joint motion. Family members often feel helpless, and allowing them to be actively involved helps alleviate their feelings of helplessness and focuses their array of emotions. Later, when the individual is more alert and mobile, family members can be involved in transfers, wheelchair positioning, feeding programs, and ADL retraining. Providing several education materials is helpful for family members. Brain injury education booklets and Internet websites are effective tools in educating clients and family members.

EVALUATION OF THE INDIVIDUAL AT AN INTERMEDIATE OR HIGHER RLA LEVEL

During the intermediate and advanced levels of recovery (RLA levels IV to VIII), the client is alert but often displays confused, agitated, and inappropriate responses. The client may be able to follow simple two- or three-step verbal commands but is easily distracted. Minimal or moderate cues are often necessary to assist clients at an intermediate or a higher level in the performance of ADLs. In general, they can complete most components of the OT evaluation; however, they may require several breaks during the evaluation process because of distractibility or agitation. The evaluation is similar to that for clients in the earlier recovery levels in that physical status, dysphagia, psychosocial and behavioral factors, vision, sensation, and perception are all assessed. However, clients at intermediate or higher levels require more extensive evaluation of ADLs (including driving), work readiness, and ability to reintegrate into the community.

Physical Status

The physical status evaluation includes an assessment of joint ROM, muscular strength, sensation, proprioception, kinesthesia, fine and gross motor control, and total body control (i.e., dynamic sitting or standing balance). Limitations in physical status are usually the result of abnormal tone, spasticity, and muscle weakness without abnormal tone, heterotopic ossification, fractures, soft tissue contractures, and peripheral nerve compression. Tools to assess physical status include goniometers, dynamometers, manual muscle testing, and clinical observation.

Dysphagia

The dysphagia assessment may include both clinical (bedside) evaluation and videofluoroscopy. The bedside examination provides the therapist with a variety of information. For example, aspiration can be caused by impulsivity because the client may gulp large portions of food quickly. Pocketing food and drooling may be apparent and are a result of impaired oral motor control. The dysphagia examination can also provide the therapist with information about cognitive status. Does the client appear to understand what to do with the utensils and food items? Is neglect present and causing the client to leave one side of the plate untouched? Does the client know the names of the utensils and food items or is aphasia suspected?

Performed by a speech pathologist or a trained occupational therapist, videofluoroscopy provides information about the anatomy and physiology of the oral, pharyngeal, and esophageal stages of swallowing. Videofluoroscopy is the primary dysphagia assessment tool that can provide information on the individual's ability to manage liquids and solid foods, particularly during the oral, pharyngeal, and esophageal phases of the swallow. This information is used to design a feeding program, which may require a diet of thick liquids and pureed foods. Swallowing status should be reevaluated as the individual improves in rehabilitation and can progress to thin liquids and solid foods. (See Chapter 27 for more information on dysphagia.)

Improper positioning, behavioral disorders, and cognitive-perceptual impairment have all been implicated as factors contributing to swallowing disorders. Dysphagia intervention must address seating and positioning and cognitive-perceptual distortions. Formal assessments to evaluate dysphagia include the Dysphagia Evaluation Protocol[8] and the Evaluation of Oral Function in Feeding.[74]

Cognition

Cognitive skills are assessed within functional tasks (e.g., ADLs, meal preparation, money management, and community skills). Tasks that involve paper and pencil can also provide valuable information, although they are only part of the equation. Assessment of a client's cognition during preparation of a cold meal may include the following skills: (1) following two- or three-step written or spoken directions, (2) correctly sequencing the order of steps, (3) attending to the task with minimal distraction, and (4) displaying good safety and judgment. The therapist may evaluate the client's cognitive status by using any of the following: (1) counting the number of errors and correct responses, (2) assessing the amount of assistance or cueing required (minimal, moderate, or maximal), and (3) determining the percentage of the task that was completed correctly. Assessment of the complexity of the activity (simple versus multistep or basic to complex) and the conditions of the environment (isolated versus multistimulus or quiet to distracting) is also important.

When assessing an individual's cognitive skills, the therapist must consider and document other factors that may affect performance, such as language barriers (e.g., the presence of aphasia, a primary language other than English), visual-perceptual deficits, the effects of medication on cognitive level, educational and cultural background, and previous experience with the task. Formal cognitive assessments that may be used with clients with a TBI include the Allen Cognitive Level Test,[2] Loewenstein Occupational Therapy Cognitive Assessment,[55] Rivermead Behavioral Memory Test,[82,83] Kohlman Evaluation of Living Skills,[46] and Cognitive Assessment of Minnesota.[69]

Vision

Clients with TBI should undergo vision screening. This screening should be completed as early as possible in the rehabilitation process because early detection of visual deficits allows the intervention team to obtain more reliable information about the client's overall health status. For example, diplopia (double vision) or accommodative dysfunction (inability to adjust focus for changes in distance) will probably influence the results of the neuropsychology or speech-language pathology assessments.

Vision screening is a tool that allows therapists to identify potential deficits in vision. Although therapists cannot diagnose conditions of vision dysfunction, they can determine whether an individual passes or fails a visual screening based on standard criteria. The screening is a means of determining which clients require referral to an optometrist or ophthalmologist for a complete evaluation and intervention. A comprehensive vision intervention program is designed by an optometrist and implemented by an occupational therapist or vision therapist. A visual history questionnaire also should be completed. The questionnaire should contain an ophthalmologic history, questions about the use of glasses and contact lenses, and questions about the presence of blurred vision, dizziness, headaches, eyestrain, diplopia, and visual field loss.

Common areas evaluated in a vision screening include visual attention, near and distant acuity, ocular movement (e.g., pursuits and saccades), convergence, accommodation, ocular alignment, depth perception (stereopsis), and visual field function. Visual dysfunction also can be identified during clinical observation of the individual's performance in functional activities. Tilting the head as a result of a field deficit, closing or covering one eye to reduce blurred vision, and bumping into walls or objects in the environment because of a field deficit or unilateral neglect are all easily observed behaviors indicative of visual dysfunction.

Perceptual Function

Perceptual evaluation should be performed when the therapist has obtained a clear understanding of the individual's cognitive, sensory, motor, and language status because deficits in these areas may skew the client's performance on a perceptual evaluation. Evaluation of visual perception should include right-left discrimination, form constancy, position in space, topographical orientation, and naming of objects. Evaluation of perceptual speech and language function should assess for aphasia and anomia. Evaluation of perceptual motor function should include the functions of ideational praxis, ideomotor praxis, three-dimensional constructional praxis, and body schema perception (including identification of unilateral neglect). Formal perceptual assessments that can be used for adults with TBI include the Hooper Visual Organization Test,[41] Motor-Free Visual Perception Test–Revised,[19] Rivermead Perceptual Assessment Battery,[76] and Loewenstein Occupational Therapy Cognitive Assessment.[55]

Activities of Daily Living

Clients at an intermediate RLA level should be assessed in all basic ADLs (e.g., grooming, oral hygiene, bathing, toileting, dressing, functional mobility, and emergency response). Clients at an advanced RLA level also should be assessed in IADLs, such as hot and cold meal preparation, money management, community shopping (Fig. 35.7), household maintenance, cleaning and clothing care, safety procedures, medication routine, and work readiness. The therapist will have ample opportunity during assessment to observe cognitive skills, perceptual skills, and behavioral appropriateness.[35] Formal assessments that can be used for clients with TBI to assess ADL skills include the Árnadóttir OT-ADL Neurobehavioral Evaluation (A-ONE),[6] Assessment of Motor and Process Skills (AMPS),[26,28] Functional Independence Measure (FIM),[38] and the Klein-Bell Activities of Daily Living Scale.[45] Clients with a history of alcohol abuse require assessment of leisure patterns. An interest history and interest checklist may reveal healthful leisure interests that can replace alcohol use. The combination of leisure skills development and substance abuse rehabilitation will help clients manage time more effectively and thereby refrain from using alcohol after discharge.

Driving

Many states require physicians to report anyone to the Department of Motor Vehicles who has lapses of consciousness,

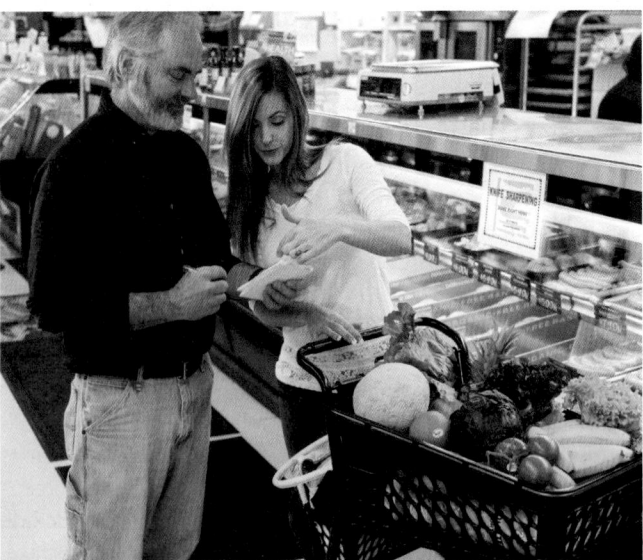

Fig. 35.7 Community shopping. (Courtesy iStock.com.)

seizure disorders, and cognitive, visual, and perceptual dysfunction caused by TBI. Regulations that apply to clients with such disorders often mandate that the driver's license be revoked until further assessment confirms that the person can drive without posing a safety risk to himself or herself or others. These laws vary from state to state.

Clients with TBI who are at an advanced RLA level and who do not have seizure disorders or severe cognitive deficits must undergo a comprehensive driving evaluation to assess their ability to resume driving. Two types of driving evaluation can be performed: a clinical assessment (evaluation of the individual's visual, cognitive, perceptual, and physical status as these relate to driving) and an on-road assessment. Both types of evaluation are necessary because the client may fail the clinical assessment but pass the on-road assessment by using compensatory strategies. Conversely, the client may perform successfully on the clinical assessment but fail the on-road assessment (see Chapter 11).

Clients with TBI frequently exhibit deficits (e.g., visual processing disorders, figure-ground discrimination dysfunction, and impulsivity) that significantly affect their ability to drive safely. Individuals with delayed visual processing hesitate during driving maneuvers and stop in an unsafe manner (e.g., in the middle of the road or at a corner) to allow themselves adequate time to process visual information. Those with figure-ground impairments may be unable to identify stop signs and traffic signals at intersections or locate the gearshift near the dashboard. Impulsive individuals may respond aggressively rather than defensively when driving, increasing the risk of accidents. They may use poor judgment when making driving decisions and may be unable to inhibit inappropriate responses. The Elemental Driving Simulator[31] and Driving Assessment System[31] are off-the-road clinical driving assessments that can be used with an on-road assessment to determine a client's ability to resume driving after brain injury.

Occasionally clients have a strong desire to drive but poor insight into whether they have the safety skills to resume driving. Because most rehabilitation centers and out-settings do not have an adaptive driving program and expensive driving simulators, occupational therapists need to use low-tech options to determine driving readiness and educate clients on whether they are safe to drive. There are many commercially available computerized driving assessments and training tools that are easy to download and inexpensive. One option is the Roadwise Review, distributed by the American Automotive Association (AAA).[1] This computer-based tool measures the functional abilities scientifically linked to the risk of crashing in older drivers. Because it assesses useful field of view, visual-perceptual skills, and reaction times, it is an excellent tool that can be used for adults with TBI.

Vocational Rehabilitation

Clients at an advanced RLA level may be evaluated to determine whether they are ready to return to work. It has been well documented that return to work after moderate to severe TBI is generally unsuccessful. The high unemployment rate among individuals with TBI has been attributed to the adverse emotional, behavioral, and neuropsychological changes arising from brain injury. Substance abuse in clients with TBI is another major factor inhibiting the person's ability to return to and maintain employment.[30]

Vocational assessment for clients at an advanced RLA level must involve assessment in the actual work setting because psychometric tests and job simulations in themselves do not accurately determine work potential. The client is often able to compensate in a familiar work setting for deficits that may appear to be significant impairments on a psychometric test. The therapist's vocational evaluation should summarize the individual's interests, strengths, and areas of deficit. The report should conclude with recommendations stating the modifications required, realistic job goals, and a plan for achieving these goals with professional assistance as needed.

Psychosocial Skills

Clients at an advanced RLA level who will be discharged to the home or to a community supportive living residence should also undergo a psychosocial skill evaluation. Such an evaluation should assess role loss, social conduct, interpersonal skills, self-expression, time management, and self-control. In addition, the therapist should assess the client's social support system, ability to form and maintain friendships, and resources for reducing feelings of isolation (e.g., TBI support groups). The ability to form and maintain intimate and sexual relationships after TBI will be of paramount concern to single clients who sustained a TBI between the ages of 18 and 30. Childrearing and care of family members will be of concern for clients who are responsible for children and other family members.

Assessment of psychosocial skills in clients with TBI is critical. For 1 or more years after injury, clients with TBI report that their psychosocial deficits significantly diminish life satisfaction and are a greater problem than the physical and cognitive deficits combined.

Psychosocial impairment is often neglected in the rehabilitation setting, which prioritizes intervention for acute physical, cognitive, and perceptual deficits. Psychosocial difficulties are more apparent after discharge, when the individual has left the structured and safe setting of the rehabilitation hospital to reenter the community. It is important to address psychosocial difficulties before the individual is discharged. Psychosocial assessment tools that can be used for these clients include the Assessment of Communication and Interaction Skills,[70] Occupational Role History,[27] and Role Checklist.[61,75]

Maria received skilled OT intervention throughout a 3-month in-patient rehabilitation stay, followed by 6 weeks in a day treatment program. Maria participated in a multifaceted spasticity reduction program and neuromuscular reeducation, which improved ROM and functional use of her right UE. As her ROM and selective movement improved, Maria learned how to feed, dress, and bathe herself with minimal assistance. As Maria's head and trunk control improved, she was able to participate in all aspects of bed mobility and transfers. Daily guided self-care tasks were a critical part of her morning schedule. Performing meaningful, routine tasks allowed Maria to work on her basic cognitive abilities. Spontaneous neurological recovery,

cognitive reeducation, and memory strategies improved Maria's ability to plan, organize, and sequence her ADLs and recall her daily therapy schedule, with occasional verbal cues. Maria was referred to an out-client OT program after discharge from the day treatment program.

INTERVENTION FOR THE INDIVIDUAL AT AN INTERMEDIATE OR HIGHER RLA LEVEL

Intervention for individuals at an intermediate or higher RLA level (IV through VIII) involves two primary approaches: the rehabilitative model and the compensatory model. The rehabilitative model is supported by the theory of neuroplasticity, which holds that the brain can repair itself or reorganize its neural pathways to allow relearning of functions lost as a result of neural damage sustained in the accident. The compensatory model holds that repair of damaged brain tissue either has occurred to its fullest extent or cannot occur, with the individual being left unable to perform lost functions without external assistance. Tools used in the compensatory model are adaptive equipment, environmental modification, and compensatory strategies that allow the client to perform ADLs. It is valuable to approach intervention using both the rehabilitative and compensatory approaches by addressing neuromuscular impairment, cognitive deficits, perceptual deficits, vision dysfunction, and behavioral disorders. In general, a rehabilitative approach is used in the acute stage of TBI recovery until the client has plateaued or progress has slowed, at which time a compensatory approach is attempted.

Neuromuscular Impairments

As with clients at lower RLA levels, clients at intermediate or advanced levels can have numerous types of neuromuscular impairment. Spasticity, rigidity, soft tissue contractures, primitive reflexes, diminished or lost postural reactions, muscular weakness, and impaired sensation affect the ability to perform activities independently and with normal control (see Table 35.4). The prerequisites for normal movement include normal postural tone, balanced integration of flexor control (reciprocal innervation), normal proximal stability, and the ability to implement selective movement patterns.

The common principles of intervention for neuromuscular impairment are to facilitate control of muscle groups, progressing proximally to distally; encourage symmetric posture; facilitate integration of both sides of the body into activities; encourage bilateral weight bearing; and introduce a normal sensory experience. Effective rehabilitation techniques for such individuals include neurodevelopmental treatment (NDT), proprioceptive neuromuscular facilitation (PNF), myofascial release, and some physical agent modalities (see Chapters 29 and 32). These clinical interventions require education beyond the entry level and must be either incorporated into or followed by a meaningful functional activity that requires the same movement. The following brief overview of principles is merely an introduction and cannot substitute for training in the specific techniques.

Intervention for impaired neuromuscular control should begin at the pelvis because positioning of the pelvis affects the motor control of all other body parts. A variety of approaches may be used to normalize pelvic positioning. For example, clients with TBI commonly have a posterior pelvic tilt. To move the client to a more functional erect pelvic position, a therapist trained in NDT might use anterior pelvic tilt mobilization. A therapist with a different approach might use a bed sheet behind the pelvis to lift and rotate the pelvis forward over the heads of the femurs. In either case, the client would be directed to raise the head and sit up tall.

The trunk is positioned after the pelvis. Proper positioning of the trunk frees the UEs for functional activities. Major principles include (1) facilitating trunk alignment, (2) stimulating reciprocal trunk muscle activity, (3) encouraging the individual to shift weight out of a stable posture into all directions (bending forward, bending backward, reaching to each side while laterally flexing the trunk), and (4) helping the individual move the lower part of the trunk on a stable upper trunk or move the upper trunk on a stable lower trunk. Once trunk control improves, intervention should progress to the UEs.

Competent practitioners may apply rehabilitative techniques in a variety of ways. A client with soft tissue contractures or spasticity in a particular muscle group may benefit from NDT mobilization and inhibitory techniques for the agonistic muscle group. A client with low tone or weak muscles (without spasticity) may benefit from NDT, PNF, and physical agent modalities.

Kinesiotaping can assist in providing stability to weak muscle groups. Neuromuscular electrical stimulation can effectively stimulate UE muscle groups (i.e., the triceps, pronators, supinators, and wrist and finger extensors) to enhance muscle strength, increase sensory awareness, and assist in motor learning and coordination.[15] Many clients at an advanced RLA level have fairly intact motor control and are able to ambulate independently and use both UEs in functional activities. However, close observation reveals subtle trunk and extremity deficits related to coordination and speed of movement. The intervention for trunk control focuses on developing full isolated movements of the trunk and extremities, good dynamic standing balance for all activities (including reaching and bending to high and low surfaces), and the ability to shift weight naturally from one LE to the other during activities. UE intervention programs are designed to increase scapular stability and improve fine motor control. A goal of intervention is to improve the client's speed while maintaining good coordination and minimizing compensatory strategies (Fig. 35.8).

Ataxia

Ataxia is a common motor dysfunction that occurs primarily as a result of damage to the cerebellum or to the neural pathways leading to and from the cerebellum. Ataxia develops early in the acute stage of recovery and may remain permanently. It is a clinical problem for which rehabilitation methods are generally ineffective. More often, therapists train the client to use compensatory strategies to control the effects of ataxia. For example, weighting body parts and using resistive activities often improve

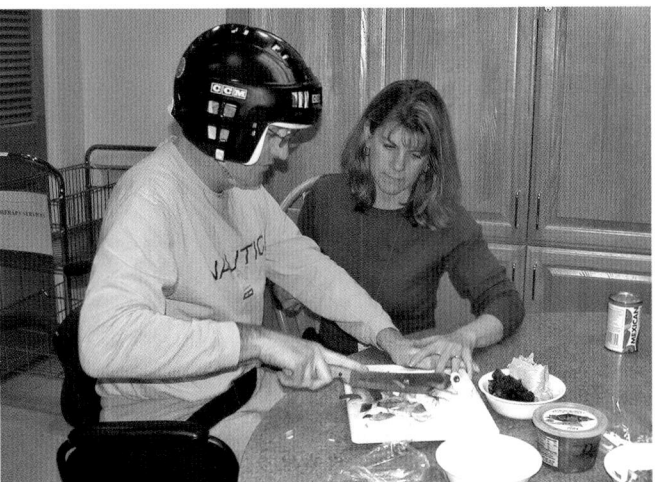

Fig. 35.8 Use of both hands during meal preparation.

control during the performance of tasks but show inconsistent carryover of muscular control when the resistance is removed.

When applying weights to clients, the therapist must identify at which joint (or joints) the tremor originates. Applying weights to clients' wrists when the tremor emerges from the trunk and shoulders is ineffective. Weighted eating utensils and cups are also used as compensatory aids to reduce the effects of ataxia on the UEs; however, these assistive devices are limited in their effectiveness.

Cognition

Intervention designed to enhance cognitive skills should be implemented through functional ADLs and IADLs. A common impairment in cognition is concrete thinking, in which the individual is likely to have difficulty with abstract concepts. Activities that require generalization of skills from one task to another are difficult for clients with TBI. It is best to engage these clients in activities of everyday life in which they need to participate. For example, if the client will return to a community environment in which it is necessary to use public transportation, interpreting bus schedules is a meaningful and relevant activity that addresses many critical cognitive skills, including problem solving, planning, organization, concentration, tolerance of frustration, sequencing, money management, and categorization. Another way to address the aforementioned cognitive skills is by planning a trip to the hardware store to purchase supplies necessary to install a handheld showerhead.

Clients at an advanced level of recovery who demonstrate high-level cognitive skills often display subtle cognitive deficits in the areas of organization, planning, sequencing, and short-term memory. Their executive functioning skills also could be affected.

Executive function encompasses a set of interrelated cognitive abilities that are critical to the control, coordination, and regulation of thoughts, emotions, and goal-directed actions.[85] This can include working memory, initiation, inhibition, cognitive flexibility, insight into deficits, and self-monitoring. These components contribute to self-regulation and cognitive control that is required for problem solving, planning, sequencing, and organization. There are a limited number of specific evaluation tools that are available to assess executive functioning in the context of instrumental activities of daily living (IADLs). One such assessment is The Weekly Calendar Planning Activity (WCPA), which is a performance-based assessment of executive function. Observations made during the WCPA provide in-depth information about performance on a complex, cognitive IADL.[79]

OT PRACTICE NOTES

Activities such as establishing a monthly budget to live independently to pay a utility bill and negotiating the community public transportation system provide a context for cognitive retraining to address subtle cognitive deficits. Activities should be challenging, age appropriate, and relevant to the individual's real-life needs. Compensatory strategies for cognitive deficits such as poor initiation and memory may include the use of applications on mobile devices for items such as managing schedules, setting alarms as reminders for important dates, using activated assistance, and obtaining simplified maps or GPS navigation of the client's community. For optimal results, the system chosen must take into account the client's familiarity with and motivation to use the given strategy. For example, a client may have used a high-tech cell phone as a day planner before the injury and may also prefer to use this system after the injury.

Generally, neuropsychologists and cognitive educators have implemented the use of computers in cognitive retraining. However, use of computer programs has not been shown to generalize to the cognitive skills needed to improve performance in IADLs.[60] Computers can be used in therapy if they are meaningful in the client's daily life; the therapist should address the client's specific computer needs. For example, by simplifying toolbars and menus and programming step-by-step written directions that appear on the screen, therapists may reprogram a client's home computer to make it less complicated to use. Software programs that do not represent functional activities should be avoided. With that said, computer programs can be used as a preparation tool to target specific cognitive deficits, such as vision, attention, and coordination of movements.

Computers in the home are now commonplace, and Americans with disabilities are likely to benefit from the use of accessible technology; it is important to introduce computer use into intervention sessions as a therapeutic modality.[54] Not only can occupational therapists set up a computer using the built-in accessibility options and utilities but they also can provide specialty assistive technology products (e.g., voice recognition, alternative keyboards, and trackballs) to allow clients to access and use a computer successfully.[34] Computer access not only facilitates cognitive retraining opportunities but also can serve as a source of communication and can address visual, perceptual, and motor deficits.

Vision

Intervention alternatives for clients with TBI and visual dysfunction include the use of corrective lenses, occlusion (e.g., patching one eye), prism lenses, vision exercises, environmental adaptations, and corrective surgery. An optometrist or ophthalmologist can evaluate the client's vision and prescribe glasses to address any accommodative dysfunction caused by brain injury. However, the glasses should not be prescribed until the client has passed the subacute phase of rehabilitation because an accommodative dysfunction that appears in the acute stage of brain injury may improve during the recovery process.

A common technique for eliminating double vision (diplopia) is patching, or occlusion. The client wears a patch over one eye to block the image seen by that eye and eliminate diplopia. Patching is a temporary compensatory strategy. An optometrist may prescribe prism glasses or binasal occluders for clients with consistent diplopia resulting from permanent oculomotor nerve damage. The prisms assist the eyes in fusing images. Prism glasses are not effective for those with significant lateral strabismus or exotropia (outward eye turn). Binasal occluders encourage the malaligned eye to fixate centrally. Prism glasses and binasal occluders are used with vision exercises. The goal of this intervention is to reduce the diplopia and eventually eliminate the need for prisms or occluders.

Vision exercises consist of a series of activities that (1) maximize residual vision, (2) enhance impaired vision skills (the rehabilitative approach), (3) increase the client's awareness of their visual deficits, and (4) help the client learn compensatory strategies. Intervention progresses from monocular to binocular vision and follows a developmental progression (supine to sitting to standing). Exercises initially address basic skills, such as visual attention, pursuits, and saccades, and may progress to more difficult skills, such as fusion and stereopsis. These vision exercises are based on the rehabilitative model, which holds that impaired visual skills can improve with training.

Environmental adaptations for visual deficits are based on the compensatory model. Compensatory strategies for visual deficits include using a colored border along one side of a page to facilitate reading. A colored strip of tape along one side of a plate or meal tray to promote self-feeding is one option. Use of large objects, such as a clock with bold numbers or a telephone with enlarged buttons, is another compensatory technique. Using contrasting colors to highlight controls and knobs (e.g., marking TV/DVD remote control buttons with fluorescent paint) may be helpful. Increasing lighting in an environment and using textures as cues (e.g., placing textured tape on a banister by the bottom step to alert the individual that the bottom step is coming and thereby reduce falls) may be used for clients with low vision. The latter compensatory strategy is also valuable for clients with vertical gaze paralysis who can look neither up nor down. Those who have lost pupil constriction should wear sunglasses whenever they are in bright light.

Corrective surgery performed by an ophthalmologist may be indicated to align the eyes and eliminate double vision; however, the individual must wait at least a year after the injury to allow any improvement that may occur naturally in the course of recovery.

Perception

Treatment of perceptual deficits involves both rehabilitative and compensatory intervention. For example, impairment of figure-ground perception might be treated using a rehabilitative approach through the repeated practice of locating objects against a similar background (e.g., finding a white shirt on a bed with white sheets or finding a spoon in a drawer of similar stainless steel utensils). Using a compensatory approach, the therapist would help the client arrange the kitchen drawers so that utensils are categorized (perhaps color coded) and distinctly divided to facilitate identification.

Aphasia (a perceptual speech disorder) also can be treated by both rehabilitative and compensatory approaches. Expressive aphasia may be treated through a rehabilitation approach by using repeated conversation exercises in which clients are given feedback about their incorrect spoken words and challenged to express the words they meant to verbalize. If the client has not made significant gains in expressive speech through use of the rehabilitative approach, the compensatory approach should be used to help the client articulate needs to caregivers. For example, a chart with letters, words, or pictures (or a combination of the three) of important items in the client's environment can be used to help the client identify needs such as eating, toileting, and medications. Such a chart may be used along with rehabilitative approaches.

Through a rehabilitative approach, apraxia can be treated by helping the client perform specific tasks (e.g., brushing the hair) hand over hand (i.e., the therapist's hands guide the client's hands during brushing). The rehabilitative approach holds that through repeated hand-over-hand exercise, the client's brain can repair the neural pathways that mediate specific motor patterns, such as those needed for brushing the hair, or can reorganize pathways so that different, undamaged areas of the brain can establish new pathways for specific motor patterns. In a compensatory approach, the client may brush the hair by following steps through the visual interpretation of sequentially depicted (pictures) or listed (words) on a poster or note card.

Neglect syndrome (a disorder of body schema) also can be addressed by using rehabilitative and compensatory strategies. Severe neglect syndromes tend to decline as a natural part of the recovery process. However, some neglect syndromes may continue into the postacute rehabilitation stage. With a rehabilitative approach, the client is encouraged to use the neglected extremity for all ADLs. The client's room may be rearranged to encourage interaction with the neglected part of the environment (e.g., placing the television or standing bed tray on the left side of the room if the client has left-sided neglect). A compensatory model is used when the client has not demonstrated significant improvement in attending to the neglected side of the body or environment. The meal tray may be placed within the client's field of vision to maximize success. A colored border may be placed on the left side of book pages to cue the individual to scan the entire line while reading.

Behavioral Management

The types of intervention strategies used to reduce or eliminate problem behavior may be divided into two categories: environmental and interactive. Environmental interventions alter objects or other environmental features to facilitate appropriate behavior, inhibit unwanted behavior, and maintain individual safety. Agitated clients should be placed in a quiet, isolated room without a roommate. All extraneous stimuli (e.g., radios and televisions) should be removed. Similarly, therapy is provided

in a private, quiet room away from other people and extraneous stimuli.

An agitated client who demonstrates severe behavioral problems may require one-to-one care. The client is assigned a rehabilitation aide who remains with the client throughout the day (including during therapy) to monitor and regulate the client's behavior. The rehabilitation aide may wear an alarm bracelet that signals staff when the client attempts to wander away from the appropriate floor or out of the building. Walkie-talkies, pagers, and wander guards may be used with those who are at risk of eloping. One walkie-talkie or pager remains in the nursing station; the other is held by the therapist or staff member who is providing one-to-one care to the client. If the client begins to act aggressively or attempts to elope, the rehabilitation aide can alert the staff that assistance is needed.

Interactive interventions are the approaches staff members and caregivers use to interact with the client. The entire team should implement these interventions in a consistent way. Consistent implementation includes speaking in a calm and concise manner and deliberately refraining from detailed explanations that will only increase the client's confusion and frustration. For safety's sake, therapists should also keep the door open when working with the client at the bedside and should always maintain awareness of the individual in relation to self.

A client in the postacute stages of rehabilitation who continues to exhibit behavioral problems should be placed in a behavioral management program. Such a program should allow the client to experience the natural consequences of inappropriate behavior (e.g., losing community recreational privileges) in an effort to encourage more appropriate responses. Drug therapy may be used for those who do not make significant improvements in their behavior and who present a safety risk to themselves and others.

Dysphagia and Self-Feeding

Intervention strategies for dysphagia follow the same guidelines as for other neurological impairments; however, intervention may be more complex for these clients because of bilateral neurological involvement, cognitive and behavioral issues, and severe neuromuscular impairments.[7,8] A self-feeding program may begin in a quiet area, such as the client's room. Eating is then advanced to more social situations, such as the hospital dining room. Common pieces of adaptive equipment, such as a rocker knife, plate guard, and nonspill mug, may be used if the client demonstrates diminished strength, coordination, or perceptual deficits. If the client displays decreased attention, introducing one piece of adaptive equipment at a time may help. Clients with heightened impulsivity may benefit from the strategy of placing the fork down after each bite to ensure that they completely chew and swallow before initiating the next bite. Depending on the client's level of dysphagia (i.e., preoral, oral, pharyngeal, or esophageal), a diet of thick liquids or pureed foods may be indicated until the client makes progress toward recovery.

Functional Mobility

Mobility training can be subdivided into bed mobility, transfer training, wheelchair mobility, functional ambulation during performance of ADLs, and community mobility. The NDT principles of bilateral extremity use, equal weight bearing, and **tone normalization** are used in intervention strategies that address functional mobility. The rehabilitation model based on the principles of NDT and PNF should be used for intermediate-level clients with TBI in the acute and subacute stages of rehabilitation. Allowing a client with loss of function to use compensatory strategies, such as grabbing a bed rail with one hand and rolling or standing on one leg to transfer, may appear to enable the client to function more independently earlier. However, use of such strategies diminishes the client's ability to perform activities with a bilateral UE pattern at a later point. In time, unilateral performance of activities results in hemiplegic postures, contractures, and abnormal gait deviations. Compensatory strategies should be used only in the later stages of recovery and when the client has not been able to demonstrate significant improvement in functional mobility skills and thus must learn compensatory strategies to enhance the ability to live independently in the community.

Bed Mobility

An intermediate-level client with TBI may require training in bed mobility skills, including (1) scooting up and down in bed, (2) rolling, (3) bridging, and (4) moving from a supine position to and from sitting and standing positions.

Wheelchair Management

Wheelchair management includes the ability to manage wheelchair parts (e.g., removing footrests and locking brakes) and propelling the wheelchair both indoors and outdoors on a variety of surfaces (e.g., low-pile carpeting, sidewalks, and ramps). Customized wheelchairs may be ordered for a client who is in the postacute stage of rehabilitation and continues to exhibit neuromuscular impairment that requires the use of a wheelchair for long-term mobility needs. A custom wheelchair provides a seating and positioning system that contours the client's body for comfort and skin protection, includes adaptive supports for proper pelvic and trunk alignment, and offers a seating position that enhances the client's ability to interact with the environment.

Clients who cannot propel or control a manual wheelchair may require a power wheelchair for independent home or community mobility.

Functional Ambulation

Functional ambulation refers to the ability to walk during functional activities. Physical therapists address gait training, whereas occupational therapists facilitate the carryover of ambulation skills into ADLs. Ambulation during performance of ADLs often requires the integrated use of UEs and LEs to carry and manipulate objects (e.g., carrying a plate to a table, holding a book bag or purse, sweeping with a broom or vacuum cleaner, and carrying an infant). Functional ambulation also requires the ability to negotiate an ambulatory device (e.g., straight or quad cane and walker) with one or both UEs during performance of ADLs. This is a high-level activity that requires eye-hand coordination and the integration of total body movements. Compensatory aids to improve the client's ability to

negotiate an ambulatory device while performing ADLs include walker bags and baskets, wheeled carts (to provide balance and support during transport of items such as plates to a table), canes with built-in reachers, pouch belts (to hold keys, wallet, and memory books), and an apron during meal preparation (see Chapter 10).

Community Travel

For clients who will be discharged to home or a community supportive living arrangement, the ability to negotiate their environment must be considered. Negotiating uneven sidewalks and curb cutouts and correctly interpreting traffic light signals and the direction and speed of oncoming traffic are important skills to practice for safe and independent community mobility. Functional ambulation in the community requires the client to respond and initiate actions quickly; for example, to cross the street after the light turns green and before it turns red. Clients must perceive depth and spatial relationships (to correctly judge the distance and speed of oncoming and turning traffic) and visually identify and avoid environmental hazards that could cause falls (e.g., potholes and cracks in the sidewalk). Power mobile scooters or power wheelchairs are often recommended for clients who need long-distance mobility in the community but who fatigue easily or are unable to walk independently. Use of a power mobile scooter or power wheelchair requires good static sitting balance and the ability to quickly integrate UE hand control and cognitive decisions about the environment. Practicing with clients during the wheelchair evaluation is crucial to determining whether they are able to safely propel a power system in the community.

Transfers

All transfers, whether from bed to chair, from wheelchair to toilet, or from lying in bed to sitting on the edge of the bed, need to be performed in a safe manner. Individuals with TBI commonly have memory deficits and limited carryover of information; therefore, transfer training should be consistent (in technique and sequence) among all staff members treating the client. It is preferable that transfers for intermediate- and advanced-level clients be practiced while moving to both the right and the left sides of the body. Without such practice, clients who become proficient in a transfer toward the uninvolved side (in the hospital) may be dismayed to find that the home setting or public restroom requires transfers toward the opposite side. Additionally, teaching clients to transfer to both sides provides weight bearing on both LEs, the use of bilateral trunk muscles, and bilateral sensory input.

Family members and caregivers should be trained in proper transferring techniques (including proper body mechanics) by a therapist before transferring the individual alone. The decision on when to begin caregiver training depends on the client's functional level and ability to cooperate, the discharge date, and the caregiver's physical and cognitive abilities.

Home Management

As the client's skills and independence in self-care, dressing, self-feeding, and functional mobility increase, intervention is expanded to include home management skills in preparation for discharge to the community. Home management skills include meal preparation, laundry, cleaning, money management (e.g., balancing a checkbook, paying bills, and budgeting), home repairs (e.g., changing a washer in a leaking faucet), and community shopping (making a shopping list, locating the correct items in the store, and paying the correct amount of money at the cash register). Examples of high-level activities include planning a monthly budget, organizing a file cabinet, ordering from a catalog or the internet, and filing income taxes. These are skills that adults need to live independently in the community and are thus relevant for most clients with TBI.

The degree to which clients participate in home management activities varies. For example, some prepare only simple meals using a microwave oven. For those who must prepare meals to live independently in the community but who are not interested in cooking, the goal is to help them safely prepare simple hot and cold meals at home. Some clients perform no household cleaning activities other than making their bed and doing the laundry. Common sense dictates that therapeutic interventions first address the activities that the client performed before the injury.

As in all other areas of intervention, home management skills are graded to accommodate the client's functional level. Beginning meal preparation tasks may involve making a cold sandwich, whereas beginning money management skills may involve learning to perform basic cash transactions. As clients progress in home management skills, the meal preparation task may be upgraded to preparing a two-item hot meal using a stovetop, oven, or microwave oven. Money management skills may be upgraded to writing checks and balancing a checkbook. As the client continues to gain skills, activities requiring higher level demands are performed until the client reaches the desired goals.

Child care, if appropriate, must not be overlooked as an area of intervention. Family involvement is critical if a father or mother is to return effectively to his or her role as a spouse and parent. Sensory overload and its resultant agitation in a parent with TBI are a commonly reported problem for families. OT sessions should gradually reintroduce parents to their role of caring for their children. Some hospitals have a family suite in which family members can practice ADLs and interpersonal skills with the client on weekends in preparation for discharge. This allows family members to gain a greater awareness of their loved one's impairments and need for assistance. It also makes the transition from hospital to home less stressful for both clients and family members.

The occupational therapist can also assist parents with TBI in the adaptation of strollers, cribs, and child care equipment to make handling of such items easier. Safely bathing or carrying a baby, preparing a meal while simultaneously caring for children, and one-handed diapering and dressing techniques are all examples of areas that could be addressed by OT services.

Community Reintegration

Clients who will be discharged from the acute rehabilitation hospital to home or to a postacute residential supportive living arrangement should receive training to facilitate the transition from the hospital to the community. Clients who achieve a maximal level of independence in the protected and structured environment of the rehabilitation hospital may find that community reintegration holds even greater challenges. Community trips, in which an advanced-level client with TBI is accompanied by the occupational therapist (and perhaps a family member) to practice IADLs in the natural environment, should be implemented to provide the client with the opportunity to rebuild daily life skills. Depositing or withdrawing money from the bank or ATM, using the public transportation system, planning a shopping list, and purchasing items at the grocery or hardware store are activities that can facilitate initiation of the client's reentry into the community. Having the client perform ADLs in the community setting also allows the therapist to observe the client's ability to interact successfully or otherwise with the environment. The client is provided a chance to receive valuable feedback from others in the community about his or her behavior.

Some clients are discharged from the acute rehabilitation center to a transitional living center. Transitional living centers are designed to develop daily life skills by providing the client an opportunity to temporarily live in a community group setting with 24-hour staff supervision and assistance. The goal of transitional living centers is to facilitate progression from supervised living to greater independence in community living. The client is usually discharged from the transitional living center to a relative's home or to a residential supportive living facility that provides various levels of living arrangements (e.g., community apartments and shared community group homes). Because long-term residential community facilities for people with TBI are expensive and not covered by most insurance companies, many are discharged home, where they receive continued intervention in out-rehabilitation or in day treatment programs that provide community, work, and school reentry training.

Psychosocial Skills

One year or more after their injury, individuals with TBI commonly report that psychosocial impairment is the greatest obstacle to rebuilding a meaningful lifestyle. Many report feeling a deep sense of isolation and loneliness. Loss of roles such as partner or spouse, worker or student, independent home maintainer, friend, and community member often leaves individuals feeling as though they have lost their identity. The goal of the occupational therapist, particularly in postacute TBI centers (e.g., day treatment programs, out-rehabilitation, transitional living sites, and long-term community supportive living arrangements), is to help rebuild desired occupational and social roles. This involves a three-step process: (1) identifying the desired roles that were lost as a result of TBI, (2) identifying activities that would support the desired roles, and (3) identifying rites of passage that were either lost or never transitioned through as a result of the TBI. Rites of passage are socially recognized events that mark the transition from one life stage to another. Common rites of passage in Western society include obtaining a driver's license, graduating from secondary school or obtaining a higher education degree, securing full-time employment, living independently in the community, dating, marrying, and parenting.

Once the desired occupational and social roles, activities, and rites of passage have been identified, the therapist facilitates the client's use of adaptation, compensatory strategies, and integration of new learning. The therapist will also help the client enhance or regain interpersonal skills, self-expression, social appropriateness, time management, and self-control. Such psychosocial skills are critical if the client is to reenter the community; that is, to live in a neighborhood setting, hold a job, perform volunteer work in the community, and participate in desired recreational opportunities along with other adult community members.

Group intervention is beneficial because it enables the client to meet others experiencing the same life concerns (thereby reducing feelings of isolation). Groups can offer exposure to peer reactions, which is particularly helpful if the client exhibits socially inappropriate behavior. Groups may also facilitate problem solving by providing the opportunity to speak with others who have successfully dealt with the same or similar problems. Participants who have been in the group longer can become peer mentors to new group members. The opportunity to help others—that is, to share one's experience of having a brain injury with others who can benefit from that knowledge—has been shown to enhance an individual's life satisfaction, feelings of competence, and sense of usefulness. Many states have state associations for brain injury that provide support groups for individuals with TBI and their families.

Substance Use

If clients' preinjury history includes substance use, they should receive drug and rehabilitation services specifically designed for individuals with TBI. Clients with a history of substance use may not display any signs of a desire to return to substance use while in the structured and protective environment of the subacute rehabilitation facility. Substance use may become a problem only after the client is discharged to the home, a community-supported living arrangement, or any residential situation in which long periods may be spent alone and unsupervised. Drug rehabilitation services are critical for clients with a substance abuse history because return to substance use after brain injury has been closely implicated in the occurrence of a second TBI.

Discharge Planning

Planning for discharge from OT services begins at the initial evaluation and continues until the last day of intervention. Components of discharge planning include a home safety evaluation (if the client will be discharged home), equipment evaluation and ordering, family and caregiver education, recommendations for a driver's training program (if indicated), and recommendations for a successful return to school or vocational retraining and work skills.

Home Safety

If the client is to be discharged home, the therapist should visit the home (or transitional living setting) to recommend modifications for increased safety. For example, clients with

balance difficulties should have grab bars in the shower stall. Increased lighting should be provided as necessary for clients with visual deficits because low lighting has been linked to falls. Recommendations also should be made regarding the client's ability to handle sharp items (e.g., knives or glass items that could shatter easily), use the stove, and remember to turn off the faucet and other appliances. The temperature for the hot water system should be set at 120° F or lower to prevent scalding.

Anything the client could trip over (e.g., throw rugs, appliance cords, furniture legs, objects placed on steps) should be removed. If feasible, nonslip flooring should be added to slippery surfaces (e.g., bathroom and kitchen tiles). If a wheelchair is indicated, the therapist should recommend modifications to doorways and bathroom spaces and should suggest replacement of high-pile carpeting with tile, wood, or other surfaces that can be easily traversed by a wheelchair.

Additionally, family members and caregivers should be educated in the appropriate steps to follow during a seizure, should understand how to evacuate the individual in case of emergency, and should practice methods by which to transfer the individual safely. Caregivers should be able to identify unsafe activities in which their loved one should not participate, and they should know the length of time the person can be safely left alone if that is possible at all.

Equipment Evaluation and Ordering

If a client will be discharged from the acute rehabilitation facility, an evaluation of the equipment needed in the next setting is required. This may necessitate reevaluation of the client's equipment needs because many of the adaptive devices that were valuable in the beginning and intermediate stages of rehabilitation may be discarded as the client improves. For example, a tub bench or shower chair may have been needed initially because of dynamic standing balance difficulties. The client may have progressed sufficiently during the course of rehabilitation to stand in the shower while using only a grab bar. Because clients with TBI may demonstrate improvements over the course of many months, a rental wheelchair may be considered.

Family and Caregiver Education

Family members and caregivers should be involved in the client's rehabilitation from the beginning of treatment and should be considered members of the intervention team. Education of caregivers in such activities as transfers, wheelchair mobility, ADLs, bed positioning, splint schedules, use of equipment, ROM exercises, and self-feeding techniques facilitates follow-through with the skills the client has learned in the rehabilitation hospital. Individual safety is of primary importance for caregiver education. The caregiver should be trained in implementation of the home program (in either written or videotape form). Home programs may include the areas listed previously, in addition to specific activities for the improvement of cognition, vision, perception, and motor control.

Recommendations for Driver's Training

If the client passes the clinical driver's evaluation, the occupational therapist may recommend a specific number of hours of driver's training. An occupational therapist or a driving instructor who has experience working with individuals with TBI (see Chapter 11) should implement the driver's training.

Recommendations for Vocational Training and Work Skills

If indicated, an OT may make recommendations for vocational training if the client is discharged to a day treatment program, an out-rehabilitation center, or a transitional living site. Vocational training is an extended process that requires the involvement of an OT and possibly a vocational counselor. The client's eventual return to work may require the assistance of a job coach. The success of a client's return to work depends highly on the environment to which they are returning and the supportiveness of the environment. These are all aspects that must be considered when a client's potential is evaluated.

SUMMARY

Treatment of adults with TBI is challenging and requires flexibility, stamina, and creativity. Behavioral and psychosocial deficits greatly influence recovery. Substance abuse, a possible contributing factor, must be assessed and addressed. Most clients have a multitude of problems requiring intervention. Coordination of evaluation and goal setting with the interdisciplinary team (including the client and family) is assumed. Intervention should be individualized and oriented toward functional outcomes that are meaningful to the client. An effective transition from acute care to intermediate care and then to the community requires the therapist to plan thoughtfully and communicate clearly. For some people with TBI, recovery and adjustment are lifelong challenges; for this reason, and because the needs of these individuals continue to evolve, providing resources throughout the continuum is essential for an ongoing productive outcome.

REVIEW QUESTIONS

1. What are two important measurable landmarks of recovery from TBI?
2. Name five types of neuromuscular impairment that may be present in a client with TBI.
3. Describe the types of care settings available for clients with TBI in the acute, subacute, and postacute stages of rehabilitation.
4. Describe the psychosocial deficits that may be present in a client with TBI.
5. List two components of a behavioral management program.
6. Name three standard assessments for individuals with TBI and describe the performance components and areas they assess.
7. List four visual skills that are evaluated in a vision screening.
8. Why is it important for a client with TBI to complete an on-road driving assessment?
9. What are the goals of a proper wheelchair positioning program?
10. What are the indications for splinting? For casting?
11. Describe three areas that should be addressed during discharge planning.
12. Why is it important to address substance use in individuals with TBI?

REFERENCES

1. AAA Foundation for Traffic Safety: https://aaafoundation. org/?s=road+wise.
2. Allen C: *Occupational therapy for psychiatric diseases: measurement and management of cognition disabilities*, Boston, MA, 1985, Little, Brown and Co.
3. American Academy of Neurology: Quality Standards Subcommittee: Practice parameters: assessment and management of patients in the persistent vegetative state (summary statement), *Neurology* 45:1015–1018, 1995.
4. American Academy of Physical Medicine and Rehabilitation: Brain Injury Special Interest Group: Practice parameter: antiepileptic drug treatment of posttraumatic seizures, *Arch Phys Med Rehabil* 79:594, 1998.
5. American Psychiatric Association: *Diagnostic and statistical manual of mental disorders, fifth edition: DMS-5*, Washington, D.C., 2013, American Psychiatric Association.
6. Árnadóttir G: *The brain and behavior: Assessing cortical dysfunction through activities of daily living (ADL)*. St. Louis, 1990, Mosby.
7. Avery-Smith, W, Dellarosa, D: Approaches to treating dysphagia in patients with brain injury. *American Journal of Occupational Therapy*, 48(3):235–239, 1994. https://doi.org/10.5014/ ajot.48.3.235.
8. Avery-Smith W, Dellarosa DM, Brod Rosen A: *Dysphagia evaluation protocol*, San Antonio, TX, 1996, Therapy Skill Builders.
9. Bennett SE, Karnes JL: *Neurological disabilities*, Philadelphia, 1998, Lippincott.
10. Bohannon R, Smith M: Interrater reliability of a modified Ashworth Scale of muscle spasticity, *Phys Ther* 67:206, 1987.
11. Bombardier CH, Temkin NR, Machamer J, Dikmen SS: The natural history of drinking and alcohol-related problems after traumatic brain injury, *Arch Phys Med Rehabil* 84:185, 2003.
12. Brain Injury Association: *Fact sheets*, Washington, D.C., 2006, The Association.
13. Brain Trauma Foundation and American Association of Neurological Surgeons: *Management and prognosis of severe traumatic brain injury*, 2010, Brain Trauma Foundation. http:// www.braintrauma.org.

14. Brain Trauma Foundation and American Association of Neurological Surgeons: *Management and prognosis of severe traumatic brain injury. II. Early indicators of prognosis in severe brain injury*, 2000, Brain Trauma Foundation. http://www.braintrauma.org.

15. Carmick J: Clinical use of neuromuscular electrical stimulation for children with cerebral palsy. Part 2, Upper extremity, *Phys Ther* 73:514, 1993.

16. Centers for Disease Control and Prevention [CDC] (2021). National Center for Health Statistics: Mortality Data on CDC WONDER. https://wonder.cdc.gov/mcd.html.

17. Center for Outcome Measures in Brain Injury, Santa Clara Valley Medical Center: http://www.tbims.org/combi/.

18. Chestnut RM: The management of severe traumatic brain injury, *Emerg Med Clin North Am* 15:581, 1997.

19. Colarusso RP, Hammill DD, Mercier L: *Motor-Free Visual Perception Test–Revised*, Novato, CA, 1995, Academic Therapy Publications.

20. Corrigan JD, Bogner JA, Mysiw WJ, et al: Systemic bias in outcome studies of persons with traumatic brain injury, *Arch Phys Med Rehabil* 78:132, 1997.

21. Cummings JL, Mega MS: *Neuropsychiatry and behavioral neuroscience*, Oxford, 2003, Oxford University Press.

22. Damasio AR: Aphasia, *N Engl J Med* 326:531, 1992.

23. Englander J, Cifu DX: The older adult with traumatic brain injury. In Rosenthal M, Griffith ER, Kreutzer JS, Pentland B, editors: *Rehabilitation of the adult and child with traumatic brain injury* ed 3, Philadelphia, 1999, FA Davis.

24. Englander J, Cifu DX, Wright JM, Black K: The association of early computed tomography scan findings and ambulation, self-care and supervision needs at rehabilitation discharge and at 1 year after traumatic brain injury, *Arch Phys Med Rehabil* 84:214, 2003.

25. Englander J, Bushnik T, Duong TT, et al: Analyzing risk factors for late posttraumatic seizures: a prospective, multicenter investigation, *Arch Phys Med Rehabil* 84:365, 2003.

26. Fisher AG: *Assessment of motor and process skills*, Fort Collins, CO, 1994, Colorado State University.

27. Florey LL, Michelman SM: Occupational role history: a screening tool for psychiatric occupational therapy, *Am J Occup Ther* 36:301, 1982.

28. Ghajar J: Traumatic brain injury, *Lancet* 356:923, 2000.

29. Giacino JT, Kalmar K, Coma JFK: *Recovery Scale–Revised*, Edison, NJ, 2004, Johnson Rehabilitation Institution.

30. Giacino JT, Ashwal S, Childs N, et al: The minimally conscious state: definition and diagnostic criteria, *Neurology* 58:349, 2002.

31. Giatnutsos R: *Elemental Driving Simulator and Driving Assessment System*, Bayport, NY, 1994, Life Sciences Associates.

32. Goga-Eppenstein P: *Casting protocols for the upper and lower extremities*, Gaithersburg, MD, 1999, Aspen.

33. Graham DI: Pathophysiological aspects of injury and mechanisms of recovery. In Rosenthal M, Griffith ER, Kreutzer JS, Pentland B, editors: *Rehabilitation of the adult and child with traumatic brain injury* ed 3, Philadelphia, 1999, FA Davis.

34. Graham DI, Adams JH, Nicoll JA, et al: The nature, distribution and causes of traumatic brain injury, *Brain Pathol* 5:397, 1995.

35. Granger CV, Cotter AC, Hamilton BB, Fiedler RC: Functional assessment scales: a study of persons after stroke, *Arch Phys Med Rehabil* 74:133, 1993.

36. Haltiner AM, Temkin NR, Dikmen SS: Risk of seizure recurrence after the first late posttraumatic seizure, *Arch Phys Med Rehabil* 78:835, 1997.

37. Hammond FM, McDeavitt JT: Medical and orthopedic complications. In Rosenthal M, Griffith ER, Kreutzer JS, Pentland B, editors: *Rehabilitation of the adult and child with traumatic brain injury* ed 3, Philadelphia, 1999, FA Davis.

38. Hart T, Millis S, Novack T, et al: The relationship between neuropsychologic function and level of caregiver supervision at 1 year after traumatic brain injury, *Arch Phys Med Rehabil* 84:221, 2003.

39. Haselsberger K, Pucher R, Auer LM: Prognosis after acute subdural or epidural haemorrhage, *Acta Neurochir (Wien)* 90:111, 1988.

40. Heilman KM, Gonzales Rothi LJ: Apraxia. In Heilman KM, Valenstein E, editors: *Clinical neuropsychology* ed 4, New York, 2003, Oxford University Press.

41. Hooper HE: *Hooper Visual Organization Test*, Los Angeles, 1983, Western Psychological Services.

42. ImPACT: FDA Approved Concussion Assessment. https://www.impacttest.com/.

43. Jackson WT, Novack TA, Dowler RN: Effective serial management of cognitive orientation in rehabilitation: the Orientation Log, *Arch Phys Med Rehabil* 79:718, 1998.

44. Khan A, Banerjee A: The role of prophylactic anticonvulsants in moderate to severe head injury, *International Journal of Emergency Medicine* 3(3):187–191, 2010. https://doi.org/10.1007/s12245-010-0180-1.

45. Klein RM, Bell BJ: *Klein-Bell Activities of Daily Living Scale*, Seattle, 1982, Health Science Center for Educational Resources.

46. Kohlman Thomson L: *The Kohlman Evaluation of Living Skills*, ed 3, Bethesda, MD, 1992, American Occupational Therapy Association.

47. Kraus JF, Morgenstern H, Fife D, et al: Blood alcohol tests, prevalence of involvement, and outcomes following brain injury, *Am J Public Health* 79:294, 1989.

48. Kreuter M, Sullivan M, Dahllöf AG, Siösteen A: Partner relationships, functioning, mood and global quality of life in persons with spinal cord injury and traumatic brain injury, *Spinal Cord* 36:252, 1998.

49. Kübler-Ross E: *On death and dying*, New York, 1969, Macmillan.

50. Langlois JA, Kegler SR, Butler JA, et al: Traumatic brain injury–related hospital discharges: Results from a 14-state surveillance system, 1997, *MMWR Surveill Summ* 52:1, 2003.

51. Levi L, Guilburd JN, Lemberger A, et al: Diffuse axonal injury: analysis of 100 patients with radiological signs, *Neurosurgery* 27:429, 1990.

52. Levin HS, O'Donnell VM, Grossman RG: The Galveston Orientation and Amnesia Test: a practical scale to assess cognition after head injury, *J Nerv Ment Dis* 167:675, 1979.

53. Levy DE, Bates D, Caronna JJ, et al: Prognosis in nontraumatic coma, *Ann Intern Med* 94:293, 1981.

54. Li K, Alonso J, Chadha N, Pulido J: Does generalization occur following computer-based cognitive retraining?—An exploratory study, *Occup Ther Health Care* 29(3):283–296, 2015.

55. Loewenstein Rehabilitation Hospital, Israel: *Loewenstein Occupational Therapy Cognitive Assessment*, Second Edition, Pequannock, NJ, 2000, Maddak.

56. Mayer NH, Keenan ME, Esquenazi A: Limbs with restricted or excessive motion after traumatic brain injury. In Rosenthal M, Griffith ER, Kreutzer JS, Pentland B, editors: *Rehabilitation of the adult and child with traumatic brain injury* ed 3, Philadelphia, 1999, FA Davis.

57. Mayo Clinic. Chronic traumatic encephalopathy. (n.d.). https://www.mayoclinic.org/diseases-conditions/chronic-traumatic-encephalopathy/symptoms-causes/syc-20370921?p=1

58. Mazaux JM, Masson F, Levin HS, et al: Long-term neuropsychological outcome and loss of social autonomy after traumatic brain injury, *Arch Phys Med Rehabil* 78:1316, 1997.

59. McKinlay WM, Watkiss AJ: Cognitive and behavioral effects of brain injury. In Rosenthal M, Griffith ER, Kreutzer JS, Pentland B, editors: *Rehabilitation of the adult and child with traumatic brain injury* ed 3, Philadelphia, 1999, FA Davis.

60. Novack TA, Caldwell SG, Duke LW, et al: Focused versus unstructured intervention for attentional deficits after traumatic brain injury, *J Head Trauma Rehabil* 11:52, 1996.

61. Oakley F, Kielhofner G, Barris R, Reichler RK: The Role Checklist: development and empirical assessment of reliability, *Occup Ther J Res* 6:157, 1986.

62. O'Dell MW, Jasin P, Lyons N, et al: Standardized assessment instruments for minimally-responsive, brain-injured patients, *NeuroRehabilitation* 6:45, 1996.

63. Ownsworth TL, Oei TP: Depression after traumatic brain injury: conceptualization and treatment considerations, *Brain Inj* 12:735, 1998.

64. Palmer S, Bader MK, Qureshi A, et al: The impact on outcomes in a community hospital setting of using the AANS traumatic brain injury guidelines, *J Trauma* 50:657, 2001.

65. Parmontree P, Tunthanathip T, Doungngern T, Rojpitbulstit M, Kulviwat W, Ratanalert S: Predictive risk factors for early seizures in traumatic brain injury, *Journal of Neurosciences in Rural Practice* 10(4):582–587, 2019. https://doi.org/10.1055/s-0039-1700791.

66. Plum F, Posner JB, editors: *The diagnosis of stupor and coma* ed 3, Philadelphia, 1980, FA Davis.

67. Prigatano GP, Schacter DL: *Awareness of deficit after brain injury: clinical and theoretical issues.* In *New York*, 1991, Oxford University Press.

68. Ranchos Los Amigos Medical Center: *Levels of cognitive functioning*, Downey, CA, 1997, The Medical Center.

69. Rustad RA, DeGroot TL, Jungkunz ML, et al: *Cognitive Assessment of Minnesota*, San Antonio, TX, 1999, Therapy Skill Builders.

70. Salamy M, et al: *Assessment of communication and interaction skills*, Chicago, IL, 1993, Department of Occupational Therapy, University of Illinois at Chicago.

71. Santa Clara Valley Medical Center: *Behavior management program policy and procedure manual*, San Jose, CA, 2006, The Medical Center.

72. Seelig JM, Becker DP, Miller JD, et al: Traumatic acute subdural hematoma: major mortality reduction in comatose patients treated within four hours, *N Engl J Med* 304:1511, 1981.

73. Sosin DM, Sniezek JE, Thurman DJ: Incidence of mild and moderate brain injury in the United States, 1991, *Brain Inj* 10:47, 1996.

74. Stratton M: Behavioral assessment scale of oral functions in feeding, *Am J Occup Ther* 35:719, 1981.

75. Teasdale G, Allen D, Brennan P, et al: Nursing Practice Review Neurology. (2015, Oct. 14). Forty years on: updating the Glasgow Coma Scale, *Nursing Times* 110(42):12, 2015. https://cdn.ps.emap.com/wp-content/uploads/sites/3/2014/10/141015Forty-years-on-updating-the-Glasgow-coma-scale.pdf.

76. The Multi-Society Task Force Report on PVS: Medical aspects of the persistent vegetative state (first of two parts), *N Engl J Med* 330:1499, 1994.

77. The Multi-Society Task Force Report on PVS: Medical aspects of the persistent vegetative state (second of two parts), *N Engl J Med* 330:1499–1508, 1994.

78. Thurman DJ, Sniezek JE, Johnson D, et al: Guidelines for surveillance of central nervous system injury, Atlanta, 1995, Centers for Disease Control and Prevention (CDC).

79. Toglia J: *Weekly calendar planning activity.* Bethesda, MD, 2015, AOTA Press.

80. Traumatic Brain Injury Model Systems National Data and Statistical Center, 2008. https://www.tbindsc.org/.

81. Tucker FM, Hanlon RE: Effects of mild traumatic brain injury on narrative discourse production, *Brain Inj* 12:783, 1998.

82. Ventura RE, Balcer LJ, Galetta SL: The neuro-ophthalmology of head trauma, *Lancet Neurol* 13(10):1006–1016, 2014. https://doi.org/10.1016/S1474-4422(14)70111-5.

83. Wilson B, Cockburn J, Baddeley A: *The Rivermead Behavioural Memory Test–Third Edition*, Gaylord, MN, 2008, National Rehabilitation Services.

84. Zasler ND: Prognostic indicators in medical rehabilitation of traumatic brain injury: a commentary and review, *Arch Phys Med Rehabil* 78(8 Suppl 4):S12–S16, 1997.

85. Zelazo PD, Carlson, SM: Hot and cool executive function in childhood and adolescence: Development and plasticity. *Child Development Perspectives*, 6(4), 2012. https://doi.org/10.1111/j.1750-8606.2012.00246.x.

SUGGESTED READINGS

Green JL: *Technology for communication and cognitive treatment: the clinician's guide*, Potomac, MD, 2007, Innovative Speech Therapy.

Jebsen RH, Taylor N, Trieschmann RB, et al: An objective and standardized test of hand function, *Arch Phys Med Rehabil* 50:311, 1969.

Minnesota rate of manipulation tests, Circle Pines, MN, 1969, American Guidance Service.

Tiffan J: *Purdue pegboard*, Lafayette, IN, 1960, Lafayette Instruments.

Whiting S, Lincoln NB, Bhavnani G, Cockburn J: *Rivermead Perceptual Assessment Battery*, Los Angeles, 1985, NFER-Nelson.

36

Degenerative Diseases of the Central Nervous System

Winifred Schultz-Krohn and Katrina M. Long

LEARNING OBJECTIVES

After studying this chapter, the student or practitioner will be able to do the following:

1. Describe the course of amyotrophic lateral sclerosis (ALS).
2. Describe the differences between familial ALS (FALS) and sporadic ALS (SALS).
3. Describe the role of the occupational therapist (OT) for a client with ALS.
4. Describe the three subtypes of ALS.
5. Identify the symptoms and incidence of Alzheimer's disease.
6. Describe the pathophysiology of Alzheimer's disease.
7. Describe the overall model of medical management used by primary care providers and other healthcare professionals.
8. Describe an approach to evaluation used by OTs.
9. Identify stages of disease progression and general treatment interventions associated with stages of dementia.
10. Describe the course and stages of Huntington's disease (HD).
11. Identify current research regarding the cause of HD.
12. Describe the medical management of HD.
13. Describe the purpose of occupational therapy for a client with HD.
14. Describe the three typical forms of multiple sclerosis (MS).
15. Describe current research regarding the cause of MS.
16. Describe the symptoms of MS.
17. Describe complications that may occur as a result of MS.
18. Describe the role of the OT for the person with MS.
19. Describe the course and stages of Parkinson's disease (PD).
20. Identify current research regarding the cause of PD.
21. Describe the medical management of PD.
22. Describe the role of the OT for a client with PD.

CHAPTER OUTLINE

KEY TERMS

Akinesia

Alzheimer's disease

Amyotrophic lateral sclerosis

Bradykinesia

Chorea

Emotional lability

Exacerbation

Fasciculations

Festinating gait

Hypomimia

Huntington's disease

Motor neuron disease

Multiple sclerosis

Parkinson's disease

Relapse

Remission

Resting tremor

Rigidity

Stereotactic surgery

CASE STUDY

Marguerite

Marguerite is a 35-year-old who identifies as female (prefers use of the pronouns she/her/hers). She was diagnosed with multiple sclerosis (MS) at age 26. Although Marguerite was initially identified as having the relapsing and remitting form of MS, her neurologist recently diagnosed her with the secondary progressive form of MS and referred Marguerite to occupational therapy (OT). Marguerite now uses an ankle-foot orthosis on her right lower extremity when walking and has diminished sensation and dexterity in her nondominant left hand.

An occupational profile revealed the following background information about Marguerite. She is married and has two boys, ages 8 and 6. Both children participate in soccer and swimming on a weekly basis. Her husband travels every month for his job as a sales manager at an insurance company. Marguerite is a special education teacher in an elementary school and works full time, although she was unable to work during relapses. She cares for her 69-year-old mother, who has been diagnosed with Alzheimer's disease (AD). Her mother lives alone in her own apartment in the same city. Although Marguerite has two sisters, neither lives within driving distance; Marguerite has the primary responsibility of caring for her mother.

Marguerite was asked to identify what areas of occupational performance were problematic or successful. She quickly replied that being a chauffeur for her children, a manager of her mother's medical care, and a housekeeper for her family were problematic. She felt as though she was constantly juggling schedules; recently, her children's swimming class changed to a different day, causing a big change in the schedule. Although she wants her children to have

the opportunity to pursue sports, Marguerite finds it difficult to supply snacks every month for these extracurricular activities, an obligation that each participant's mother is expected to fulfill. Her husband does try to help with household chores when he is home, but he works long hours and does not have time to shop for the family's groceries. Marguerite is also responsible for arranging all of her mother's medical appointments; shopping for her mother, who no longer drives; and visiting her mother daily. Marguerite reports that she often feels so tired after teaching all day and running all of her errands that she has trouble making dinner when she returns home.

Marguerite was most comfortable with her work situation and reported that many of her colleagues had offered to help with various tasks such as playground duty or monitoring the students during lunchtime. This allowed Marguerite to have a brief break during the day to rest.

Critical Thinking Questions

1. What evaluations would you perform to collect additional data to develop an intervention plan?
2. Where would you start your intervention plan, considering Marguerite's report of her occupational profile?
3. How would the change in Marguerite's diagnosis from the relapsing and remitting form to the secondary progressive form of MS affect her current occupational roles?
4. How would the strategies you select for Marguerite be applied to other clients who have degenerative neurological disorders?

INTRODUCTION

This chapter addresses the impact of degenerative neurological disorders on a person's occupational performance and outlines the role of occupational therapy (OT) in providing services to clients with these disorders. The specific disorders discussed in this chapter are amyotrophic lateral sclerosis (ALS), Alzheimer's disease (AD), Huntington's disease (HD), multiple sclerosis (MS), and Parkinson's disease (PD).

In degenerative neurological disorders, the disease progresses and an individual's occupational performance is often increasingly compromised. OT aims to help the client compensate and adapt as function declines secondary to the disease process. Environmental adaptations and modifications are often necessary to maintain functional skills for as long as possible.

Degenerative neurological diseases may occur because of structural or neurochemical changes within the central nervous system (CNS).[74] In the disorders discussed in this section, the client's CNS usually functions normally during childhood and

early adolescence. After these years, the client experiences signs and symptoms indicating that CNS functions are deteriorating. The progressive nature of the disorder varies from person to person. Some clients have a rapid decline in function, whereas others maintain functional skills for many years.

The decline in function may compromise the individual's sense of self-efficacy in performing various tasks.[179] No longer is the individual able to perform personal or instrumental activities of daily life at the same level of independence. Dependence on others can alter the client's concept of self-worth and self-control. The OT practitioner serves an important role in reframing the client's sense of self with the potential of declining functional independence. A man with PD who is unable to dress independently may now direct a personal care attendant or home health aide to perform these tasks. A woman with MS, who was previously responsible for household finances, may need to instruct a member of the family to complete these activities.

The disorders discussed in this chapter are most often diagnosed during adult or later adult life, after habits, routines, and patterns of independent behavior are well established. Although MS and HD have been identified in children and adolescents, the majority of clients diagnosed with MS or HD are adults, as is seen with ALS, AD, and PD. An adult client may encounter a significant change in social relationships and interactions secondary to a decline in functional abilities. The OT practitioner must consider the ways in which progressive loss of function affects the client's social and occupational roles, whether those roles are as a partner, parent, adult child, worker, sibling, or friend. OT must address the needs of the client within the context of the social, physical, and cultural environment.

OT intervention aims to support the client's ability to function within the environment. The rate at which the client's symptoms progress influences the intervention plan. A client who displays a progressive loss of fine motor skills over 20 years has a much different profile than a client who loses all upper extremity function within 2 years. Use of adaptive equipment must be carefully evaluated against the rate of deteriorating skills.

The OT practitioner must be knowledgeable about support services and respite care available to clients with a degenerative neurological disorder. A PD support group may provide the necessary social support for both the person with this disorder and the individual's family. MS support groups may offer clients information regarding new intervention methods available, along with the opportunity to share life experiences.

An OT intervention plan should address not only the physical limitations associated with various disorders but also their cognitive, social, and emotional implications. Many individuals with neurodegenerative disorders have concomitant depression. Depression can be a reaction to the loss of function associated with some disorders or the primary symptom of other disorders. OTs should regularly screen for depressive features. An instrument such as the Beck Depression Inventory can effectively evaluate this factor.[25] In addition to the evaluation of depression in clients with neurodegenerative disorders, cognitive abilities should be evaluated. Clients may have concomitant cognitive problems because of the destruction of neurological structures, and these deficits can have a dramatic effect on intervention. Brief assessments such as the Mini-Mental State Examination (MMSE)[68] or the Cognistat[154] can be used to determine cognitive abilities and establish a baseline of performance.

In most cases, the occupational therapist (OT) is a member of a team providing services to the individual with a degenerative neurological disorder.[179] As a team member, the OT must consider the roles other professionals and family members play in the client's life and incorporate this knowledge into the intervention plan. OT practitioners provide a unique and needed service to individuals with degenerative neurological disorders. A client who is able to engage in meaningful occupations despite deteriorating skills reflects the significant contribution of OT.

Three case studies are presented to illustrate the similarities and differences among clients faced with degenerative neurological disorders. The first case discussion describes Marguerite, who has MS. That case is presented at the beginning of the chapter to consider how progressive neurodegenerative disorders affect occupational engagement. The second case presentation is Marcus, who has ALS and is presented at the beginning of Section 1 on ALS to provide context for the chapter content. The third case illustration is Carl, diagnosed with PD, and is presented at the end of the chapter to serve as a review. The cases are designed to prompt clinical reasoning and decision-making as you read this chapter.

SECTION 1: AMYOTROPHIC LATERAL SCLEROSIS

Winifred Schultz-Krohn

The role of the OT when working with an individual diagnosed with ALS (such as Marcus in the case study) is to focus on the occupations most important to the individual and on the adaptation methods he will need to apply as his performance skills decline.[11] Occupations that are addressed by the OT practitioner are as diverse as the individuals' personal interests, goals, and priorities. The novice OT should not assume that basic ADLs are a priority but should listen to what motivates, drives, and frustrates the client and family. The therapist will have the opportunity to use the expanse of OT skills through the evaluation and intervention process, which may include ADLs/IADLs adaptation; hand splinting; adaptive equipment; cognitive assessment and strategies; psychosocial assessment; environmental modifications for work, home, and leisure; and wheelchair seating and positioning. Most critical is to listen to the client and family about their needs and make those a priority. The personal context of the individual will significantly influence the choices an individual makes regarding home modification and choice of power versus manual wheelchair mobility. For example, a person with limited financial means may choose to not make significant home modifications. Diagnosis and progression of disease are described in terms of the loss of performance skills, whereas Box 36.1 describes the OT interventions in relation to both occupation and performance skills as identified in the Occupational Therapy Practice Framework.[11]

The term amyotrophic lateral sclerosis (ALS) is used to identify a group of progressive, degenerative neuromuscular diseases. The underlying neurological process involves destruction of the upper and lower motor neurons within the spinal cord, brainstem, and motor cortex.[127] Affected individuals exhibit a combination of both upper motor neuron (UMN) and lower motor neuron (LMN) deficits at some point in the progression of the disease. As the disease progresses, approximately 50% of those diagnosed with ALS experience changes in behavior, executive functioning, and language problems.[127]

In the United States, ALS is also known as Lou Gehrig's disease.[163] The term motor neuron disease refers to a group of diseases that includes the three subtypes of ALS (progressive bulbar palsy, progressive spinal muscular atrophy, primary lateral sclerosis).[149] These three subtypes often do not remain distinct over the course of the disease and as the disease progresses, the person may exhibit symptoms of all three subtypes.[127] Table 36.1 describes each of these distinct subtypes of ALS. The classic forms

CASE STUDY

Marcus

Marcus is a 61-year-old who identifies as male (prefers use of the pronouns of he/him/his). Marcus is diagnosed with ALS and is married and has two adult children. He works as the supervisor at an automotive parts outlet store that is a small local family business. He was planning to retire in 6 months when he turns 62. He shares all of the household chores with his wife, Sandy, who also works full time. He loves to garden, goes to church, reads, and plays harmonica.

About 6 months before his diagnosis he noticed that he was having difficulties sustaining his grasp on tools and was often dropping things at work. He also reported he was having a harder time lifting boxes off of shelves taller than shoulder height. He fell two times, once at work tripping on a step and once in the garden. His primary doctor noticed the fasciculations in his forearms and calves along with slight atrophy of the intrinsics of his hands. He was referred to a neurologist who made the definitive diagnosis of ALS. The neurologist referred Marcus to OT and physical therapy (PT) in the outpatient department. The OT referral was for evaluation and treatment of activities of daily living (ADLs) with a specific focus on Marcus' desire to keep working for at least 6 additional months. The PT referral was for an ankle-foot orthosis and gait evaluation.

The OT evaluation included learning which occupations were the most important and most problematic for Marcus. This allowed the OT to collaborate and prioritize goals with him. The OT asked Marcus to describe his understanding of his condition. Marcus said he was not sure if the neurologist's diagnosis was correct so he was seeking a second opinion. Either way, he decided it would not hurt to come to his OT and PT appointments. He stated the doctor told him he would get weaker, but Marcus thought if he just exercised enough he could improve his hand, shoulder, and leg weakness and prevent it from getting worse.

Along with a discussion of Marcus' work, family, and home environments, the OT assessed his motor and sensory skills and completed a cognitive screening. The OT presented the cognitive screening as a tool to help determine how Marcus best learns. The cognitive screening was within normal limits, without evidence of impaired short-term memory, spatial deficits, attention deficits, or problem-solving issues.

The OT practitioner found Marcus had intrinsic weakness bilaterally; Marcus reported he was right-handed. He had a weak key pinch (lateral pinch). His gross grasp strength was 3+/5. He was able to pick up small coins but could not manipulate them in his hands. He also had 4/5 shoulder flexion strength. The OT also noted hip and ankle dorsiflexion weakness. When he got up from a chair, he used his hands to push off and tended to shuffle his feet.

Marcus reported that most of his socialization beyond his family occurred at work with his buddies. He had known some of them for 20 years. He went to church regularly but did not socialize there. He stated church was a personal quiet introspective time, not a time to socialize.

Marcus and his wife live in a two-story house with a half-bath downstairs and his bedroom upstairs. The full bathroom with tub and shower was upstairs. There are two steps to enter and exit the house. He has lived in this house for 15 years. One of his sons and a daughter-in-law live down the street with their two children.

Marcus' daily routine includes having coffee in the garden or in the sunroom and dropping off his two grandchildren at school on his way to work. Typically, when he returns home from work, he would either take a walk with his wife and dog or work in the garden. On the weekends Marcus goes for long walks with his wife and spends time playing harmonica.

Functional deficits noted during the initial evaluation are as follows:
- Home: ADLs/instrumental activities of daily living (IADLs)
  - Difficulty fastening buttons and zippers
  - Difficulty with handwriting
  - Increased effort to get off of the toilet, chair, couch
  - Difficulty handling tools for repairs at home
- Leisure
  - Difficulty shoveling dirt
  - Difficulty getting off the ground when weeding
  - Fatigues rapidly when playing harmonica
- Work
  - Dropping small auto parts that need to be stored at the shop
  - Difficulty carrying boxes greater than 15 lb and walking
  - Extreme fatigue at the end of the day and needs to take a nap when he gets home

OT interventions during the initial evaluation included the following:
- Prioritizing goals with Marcus
- Instruction in energy-conservation principles in all occupations
- Hand splint option of using a custom-made short opponens splint to improve key pinch
- General hand strengthening with soft Theraputty with instruction not to overdue the repetitions
- Instruction in compensatory strategies for sit to stand
- Resources for bathroom equipment, including a shower seat, low/small-diameter grab bars (to function as long as possible with progression of the disease), shower hose, rubber mat, and rationale for implementing equipment as energy-conservation technique and fall prevention
- Recommendations for easy-to-don clothing and instruction in use of a button hook
- Education on Americans with Disabilities Act (ADA) and work accommodations
- The future need for a home evaluation or lengthy discussion about potential access issues in his home
- Discussing frequency of follow-up appointments and alternative methods of communicating via the secure healthcare message system
- Education on the scope of OT and how the OT practitioner will work with Marcus throughout the course of the ALS to make ongoing adaptations to the activities he thinks are important

The therapist continued to work with Marcus and his family throughout the course of his disease. The frequency of services depended on his current needs. Marcus and his wife frequently communicated with the OT via e-mails asking about different adaptive equipment and ideas to remain functional. He eventually was followed by an OT who worked for home health and hospice. At that time Marcus used a power wheelchair full time with a chin switch and a Hoyer lift for transfers; he was dependent with all ADLs and IADLs except using an adapted phone and tablet. He had a percutaneous endoscopic gastrostomy (PEG) feeding tube. Marcus entered the hospice program approximately 2 years after initial diagnosis. His goals at that time were to be more comfortable, continue to use his tablet to connect with friends at work, connect with his grandchildren on Facebook, and do online grocery shopping for the family.

Critical Thinking Questions

1. What evaluations would you perform to collect additional data for developing an intervention plan? What events would indicate a need for reevaluations?
2. Where would you start your intervention plan in light of Marcus' report of his occupational concerns?
3. The early and late stages of ALS are briefly described in the case study. What types of participation and performance skill deficits will likely arise during the middle stage of ALS?
4. When would you begin to include Marcus' family in treatment?

BOX 36.1 Persons With Cognitive Dysfunction Benefit From the Following Approaches

- Use simpler tools for communication than you would use for patients who do not have cognitive deficits.
- Use simpler and more straightforward language and communicate clearly and directly.
- Supervise eating more closely. Patients with frontal lobe abnormalities and poor swallowing ability may have difficulty following medical advice to limit solid foods, or they may place too much food in their mouth.
- Assess patients' ability to make decisions by talking with them and the caretaker because patients with neurological disorders are faced with complicated medical, financial, and sometimes legal issues.
- Even patients with subthreshold cognitive deficits who do not meet the criteria for dementia may lack the ability to make sound judgments about their care. Poor insight is common, so caregiver involvement may be appropriate.
- Supervise walking. Patients with cognitive deficits often have a loss of impulse control and may make poor decisions about where to walk, how far to walk, or when to use equipment such as a walker.
- Remind caregivers and family to avoid taking the person's behavior personally.
- Help them understand that there is a physiological cause for the behavior.
- Encourage the caregiver and the family to build an atmosphere of comfort and love with a calm and orderly environment.

Modified from ALS Association: *ALS, cognitive impairment (CI) and frontotemporal lobar dementia (FTLD): a professional's guide*, 2005, 27001 Agoura Road, Suite 250, Calabasas Hills, CA 91301-5104. Phone: (800) 782-4747. Website: https://www.als.org/navigating-als/resources/fyi-als-cognitive-impairment-dementia.

TABLE 36.1 Clinical Subtypes of Amyotrophic Lateral Sclerosis

Name	Area of Destruction	Symptoms
Progressive bulbar palsy (PBP; bulbar form)	Corticobulbar tracts and brainstem motor	Dysarthria, dysphagia, facial and tongue weakness, bulbar (brainstem) nuclei involved with muscular wasting
Progressive spinal muscular atrophy	Lower motor neurons in the spinal cord	Marked muscle wasting of the limbs, trunk (PMA or PSMA) (LMN form), and sometimes the brainstem and/or the bulbar muscles
Primary lateral sclerosis (PLS; UMN form)*	Destruction of the cortical motor neurons; progressive spastic paraparesis may involve both corticospinal and corticobulbar regions	Progressive spastic paraparesis

*The World Federation of Neurology Classification of spinal muscular atrophy and other disorders of the motor neurons does not identify primary lateral sclerosis (PLS) as a subtype of amyotrophic lateral sclerosis (ALS). This author is including PLS in the list in recognition of the many other articles and books that recognize it as a subtype of ALS.
LMN, Lower motor neuron; *PMA*, progressive muscular atrophy; *PSMA*, progressive spinal muscular atrophy; *UMN*, upper motor neuron.
From Belsh JM, Schiffman PL, editors: *ALS diagnosis and management for the clinician*, Armonk, NY, 1996, Futura Publishing; Guberman A: *An introduction to clinical neurology, pathophysiology, diagnosis, and treatment*, Boston, 1994, Little, Brown.

of ALS are presented in this section. The prevalence or number of people living with ALS in the United States is about 5 in every 100,000.[163] ALS incidence increases after age 40, with cases peaking among those in their 60s and 70s. ALS is more common in males than females by a 1.5 factor. Veterans have both a higher incidence and prevalence of ALS compared to the general population.[24,133,194] One investigation found that both the incidence and prevalence of ALS were significantly higher in Air Force personnel compared to other branches of armed forces.[194]

Two primary forms of ALS are recognized: sporadic and familial.[42,127] Sporadic ALS makes up about 90% to 95% of ALS cases. Between 5% and 10% of individuals with ALS are found to have a family history of the disease. There is no difference in the symptoms or course of the disease for clients with the familial and sporadic types.

There is no specific diagnostic test to confirm ALS, and the diagnosis is primarily determined by clinical symptoms, electrophysiological examination, and ruling out other neurological disorders.[42] Criteria established by the World Federation of Neurology and revised by Costa and colleagues state that it is critical for the diagnosis to document both UMN and LMN involvement with progressive weakness and to exclude all alternative diagnoses.[48] Definite ALS occurs when motor neurons from three or four of the following regions are involved and display signs of neurodegeneration: bulbar (jaw, face, palate, larynx, and tongue); cervical (neck, arm, hand, and diaphragm); thoracic (back and abdomen); and lumbosacral (back, abdomen, leg, and foot). The presence of upper and lower motor

neuron involvement but intact bowel and bladder, the absence of sensory changes, and a normal spinal x-ray film all support a positive diagnosis for ALS.[207]

PATHOPHYSIOLOGY

The familial presentation of ALS has been linked to genetic markers but the cause for sporadic ALS has not been established. Over 20 genes have been associated with ALS.[127] Multiple theories have been proposed as the cause of the motor neuron destruction, including gene mutation, environmental factors, and the interaction of several factors.[163]

CLINICAL PICTURE

The symptoms of ALS vary, depending on the initial area of motor neuron destruction. An individual with ALS typically has a focal weakness beginning in the arm, leg, or bulbar muscles. The individual may trip or drop things as in the case of Marcus and may have slurred speech, abnormal fatigue, shortness of breath, and emotional lability, which is uncontrollable periods of laughing or crying. As the disease progresses, marked muscle atrophy, weight loss, spasticity, muscle cramping, and fasciculations (i.e., twitching of the muscle fascicles at rest) ensue

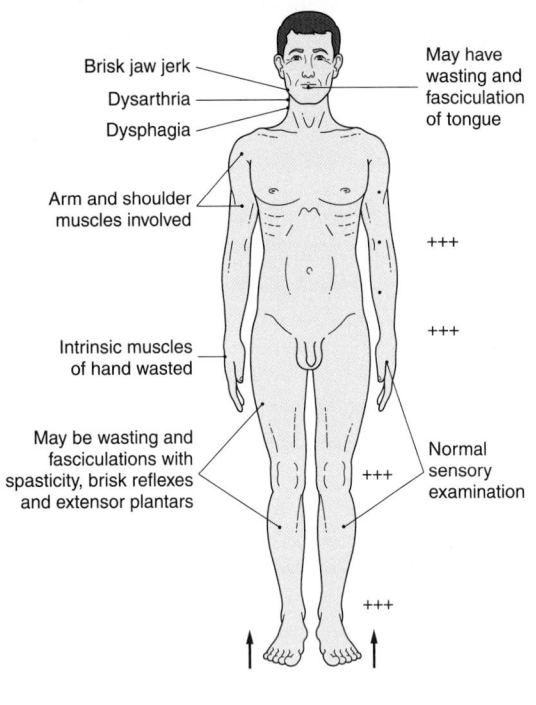

Brisk jaw jerk

Dysarthria

Dysphagia

May have wasting and fasciculation of tongue

Arm and shoulder muscles involved

+++

+++

Intrinsic muscles of hand wasted

May be wasting and fasciculations with spasticity, brisk reflexes and extensor plantars

+++

Normal sensory examination

+++

++, Normal; +++, pathologically brisk reflex; ⥮, extensor plantar

Fig. 36.1 Clinical findings in a patient with classic amyotrophic lateral sclerosis with a mixture of upper and lower motor neuron signs. (From Vivekananda U: *Crash course: neurology*, ed 5, Edinburgh, 2019, Elsevier Ltd.)

(Fig. 36.1). To better understand the condition, the OT practitioner may want to research videos that show fasciculation. This will improve the OT practitioner skills when assessing function and reporting symptoms and deficits to the physician. Performance areas may be affected as the individual has greater difficulty with walking, dressing, fine motor activities, and swallowing. In the end stages the individual may elect to use complex, life-prolonging interventions such as tube feedings and a ventilator for respiration. ALS is a rapidly progressive disease, with the majority of clients dying of respiratory failure in 2 to 5 years after the onset of symptoms if additional support such as a tracheostomy and ventilation are not used. Approximately 10% of the population will live 10 to 20 years or longer.[145] As ALS progresses, the disorder does not affect a person's eye or sensory function; bowel and bladder remain intact but constipation and urinary urgency are often reported.

Research has found that mild to moderate cognitive changes occur in 35% to 40% of the population with ALS and as much as 20% of the population has dementia.[127] Specific cognitive deficits have been identified, such as frontotemporal lobe dysfunction and disorders of executive function. Executive function impairment includes reasoning, judgment, sequencing, ordering, inferring, regulating emotions, planning, retrieval inefficiency, and a person's ability to have insight regarding personal behaviors. A clinician or family member may observe repetition of questions, actions, or phrases; getting stuck on an idea; and an overly emotional response to a situation. Risk factors for developing

cognitive problems, behavior changes, or a full-fledged dementia syndrome may include older age, bulbar onset ALS, a reduction in functional vital capacity, and a family history of dementia.[127]

The prognosis is difficult to predict. Generally, individuals with early bulbar involvement have a poorer prognosis.[127] A more positive prognosis is usually associated with the following factors: younger age at onset; onset involving LMNs located in the spinal cord; deficits in either UMNs or LMNs, not a combination of both areas; absent or slow changes in respiratory function; fewer fasciculations; and a longer time from the onset of symptoms to diagnosis.

The loss of function with ALS is more rapid, without episodes of remission or plateauing as may be seen with individuals diagnosed with MS. A person with ALS must cope with a fatal disease, whereas a person with MS or PD must cope with a chronically disabling condition.

MEDICAL MANAGEMENT

The American Academy of Neurology has established practice parameters and standards to address major management issues for persons with ALS. An OT practitioner working with this population should be familiar with the standards to better understand the approaches and rationale for intervention. The parameters cover the following topics: how to inform the client of the diagnosis, when to consider noninvasive and invasive ventilator support, evaluation of dysphagia and intervention with a feeding tube, management of saliva and pain, and use of hospice services.[135] Symptoms such as muscle cramping, excessive saliva, depression, lability, and pain are managed with medication. The client's respiratory status should be reevaluated frequently to determine when noninvasive and invasive ventilator support is necessary. Swallowing function should also be evaluated frequently to prevent aspiration and to determine when and whether a feeding tube should be placed.

The U.S. Food and Drug Administration (FDA) approved the drug riluzole (Rilutek) in 1995. Riluzole, an antiglutamate, was the first drug used specifically to alter the course of the disease by prolonging survival. Researchers thought that the success of riluzole indicates that an excess of glutamate leads to the death of motor neurons.[100] Riluzole comes in several forms, including a tablet, an oral suspension that can be more easily swallowed or delivered via a syringe, and an oral film placed on the tongue to dissolve. Research has shown that riluzole prolongs the life of clients with ALS by at least a few months.[6] Most recently, as of 2017, the FDA approved an intravenous drug, edaravone (Radicava) that acts as a free radical scavenger and antioxidant. Edaravone slowed the progression of ALS motor deterioration symptoms.[163,240] Although additional medications may be used to manage symptoms, there is no cure for ALS and no medication to reverse the course of the disease.

Many clinical trials have been funded for research on extending survival, slowing the decline associated with the disease, and assessing and treating the resulting deficits. A comprehensive list of current studies can be found on the National Institutes of Health, https://www.clinicaltrials.gov, and the alsconsortium.org websites.

OCCUPATIONAL THERAPY EVALUATION AND INTERVENTION

It is essential to work with the client and family throughout progression of the disease as client factors and performance skills become impaired. The case study of Marcus illustrates OT intervention for a newly diagnosed individual and the changing needs for OT services through the progression of ALS; there are opportunities for the client to benefit from OT at all stages of ALS (Table 36.2). The client factors, including cultural, social, and spiritual values, must be understood because these factors will influence ongoing decisions about personal care and life support. When working with Marcus, the OT practitioner should recognize that the worksite is Marcus's primary social networking opportunity and that he has a consistent role as a grandfather driving his grandchildren to school.

The client and family members must regularly update decisions about care. Decisions range from when or whether a wheelchair or adaptive eating device should be used to whether the client should undergo a tracheostomy, choose tube feeding, or use a ventilator. The entire healthcare team should provide psychosocial support regarding decisions about the extent of life support and medical intervention, with the client having the primary responsibility for decisions about life support. As the OT practitioner works with Marcus to consider ADL adaptations and home modifications, opportunities will arise to discuss how much intervention the client wants and what type. Several studies have shown that caregivers and clients have different needs

TABLE 36.2 Amyotrophic Lateral Sclerosis Interventions

Patient Characteristics	Interventions With Focus on Performance Areas of Occupation	Interventions With Focus on Client Factors
Phase I (Independent) Stage I Mild weakness Clumsiness Ambulatory Independent with ADLs	Continue normal activities or increase activities if client is sedentary to prevent disuse atrophy and prevent depression. Integrate energy conservation into daily activities, work, and leisure. Provide opportunity for individual to voice concerns (provide psychological support as needed).	Begin range-of-motion program (e.g., stretching, yoga, tai chi). Add strengthening program of gentle resistance exercise to all musculature, using caution to prevent overwork fatigue.
Stage II Moderate, selective weakness Slightly decreased independence in ADLs; for example, difficulty climbing stairs, difficulty raising arms, difficulty buttoning clothing	Assess self-care, work, and leisure skills impaired by loss of function; if patient continues to work, focus on how to adapt tasks with current deficits; assist with balance between work, home, and leisure activities; include significant others in treatment. Use adaptive equipment to facilitate ADLs (e.g., button hook, reacher, built-up utensils, shower seat, grab bar). Integrate hand orthotic use into daily activities. Perform baseline dysphagia evaluation; reevaluate throughout each stage of the disease.	Continue stretching to avoid contractures. Continue cautious strengthening of muscles with MMT grades above F+ (3+). Monitor for overwork fatigue. Consider orthotic support (e.g., AFOs, wrist or thumb splints—short opponens splint).
Stage III Severe, selective weakness in ankles, wrists, and hands Moderately decreased independence in ADLs Tendency to become easily fatigued with long-distance ambulation Slightly increased respiratory effort	Prescribe manual or power wheelchair with modifications to eventually allow recline or tilt posture with headrest, elevating leg rests, adequate trunk and arm support. Help patient prioritize activities and provide work simplification. Reassess for adaptive equipment needs (universal cuff to eat). Assess and adapt use of communication devices (e.g., regular phone to cordless or speaker phone; pen and paper to computer with adapted typing aid). Provide support if there is loss of employment or other activities; explore alternative activities. Begin discussing need for home modification, such as installing ramps or moving the bedroom to the lowest floor. Provide education regarding the types of bathroom equipment available for energy conservation and safety.	Keep patient physically independent as long as possible through pleasurable activities and walking. Encourage deep breathing exercises, chest stretching, and postural draining if needed.

(Continued)

TABLE 36.2   Amyotrophic Lateral Sclerosis Interventions—cont'd

Patient Characteristics	Interventions With Focus on Performance Areas of Occupation	Interventions With Focus on Client Factors
Phase II (Partially Independent) Stage IV Hanging-arm syndrome with shoulder pain and sometimes edema in the hand Wheelchair dependent Severe lower extremity weakness (with or without spasticity) Able to perform some ADLs, but fatigues easily	Evaluate need for arm slings, overhead slings, mobile arm supports for eating, typing, page turning. Prescribe power wheelchair if the patient wants to be independent with mobility; controls must be adaptable from hand to other mode of control. Evaluate need for assistive technology such as environmental control systems, voice-activated computer; augmentative communication device. Help the patient prioritize activities, and consider negotiating roles with significant others. Reinforce the need for home modifications. Reinforce the need for shower seat or transfer tub bench and shower hose. Assist with patient's ability to participate in closure activities, such as writing letters or making tapes for children, completing a life history, and writing a log on household management for family.	If arm supports are not used, provide arm troughs or wheelchair lap tray for wheelchair positioning; wrist cock-up splints for full resting; hand splints may be needed for positioning. Provide pain and spasm management through the following: • Heat, massage as indicated to control spasm and pain • Anti-edema measures • Active assisted or passive range-of-motion exercises to the weak joints; caution to support and rotate shoulder during abduction and joint accessory motions • Isometric contractions of all musculature to tolerance
Stage V Severe lower extremity weakness Moderate to severe upper extremity weakness Wheelchair dependent Increasingly dependent in ADLs At risk for skin breakdown caused by poor mobility	Instruct family in methods to assist patient with self-care, especially bathing, dressing, and toileting; aim to minimize caregiver's burden and stress. Family training to learn proper transfer, positioning principles, and turning techniques. Instruct in use of mechanical lift if needed for transfers out of bed (patients in slings require head support). Adapt and select essential control devices for telephone, stereo, television, electric hospital bed controls for independent use. Adapt wheelchair for respiratory unit if needed to allow for continued community access.	Instruct family and patient in skin inspection techniques. Instruct in use of electric hospital bed and antipressure device. Adapt wheelchair for respiratory unit if needed; reassess adequacy of wheelchair cushion for pressure relief.
Phase III (Dependent) Stage VI Dependent, with all positioning in bed or wheelchair Completely dependent in ADLs Extreme fatigue	Eating: Evaluate dysphagia and recommend appropriate diet; therapist may recommend tube feedings if patient is at high risk for aspiration; recommend suction machine for handling secretions and preventing aspiration. Augmentative speech devices may be recommended, in addition to speech therapy.	Continue with passive range-of-motion exercises for all joints. Provide sensory stimulation with massage and skin care.

ADLs, Activities of daily living; *AFO*, ankle-foot orthosis; *MMT*, Manual Muscle Testing.
Modified from Yase Y, Tsubaki T, editors: *Amyotrophic lateral sclerosis: recent advances in research and treatment*, Amsterdam, 1988, Elsevier Science. In Umphred DA, editor: *Neurological rehabilitation*, ed 3, St. Louis, 1995, Mosby.

and perceptions of quality of life. It may be beneficial for clients and caregivers to have time for education and support separately to meet their individual needs.[29,160] Additionally, given the costs of equipment and variety of options, the OT practitioner needs to carefully match the equipment to the client's interest and acceptance. Pousada and colleagues[178] found carefully matching the equipment to the client resulted in a positive impact in acceptance and use of the equipment.

Initial and ongoing OT assessment is essential to educate the client about ways to adapt functional activities as the disease progresses. As Marcus declines in physical function and relies more on caregivers, the emphasis is on caregiver training.

Education is needed for nursing staff and physicians to understand the role of OT in the treatment of clients with ALS.

Steady deterioration in the ability to speak, swallow, move, and perform ADLs makes it easy to overlook the presence of some common signs of cognitive or behavioral dysfunction, such as poor insight and deficits in planning.[5] Multiple cognitive domains may be affected in persons with ALS, including psychomotor speed, fluency, language, visual memory, immediate verbal memory, and executive function.[185]

With impaired executive function, a person with ALS may have difficulty handling the visual, auditory, and other sensory data required for complex decision making.[161] These cognitive and behavioral issues are pertinent when considering teaching strategies and the need for caregiver counseling and support.

ROLE OF THE OCCUPATIONAL THERAPIST

ALS progresses rapidly, within 2 to 5 years after diagnosis, with ongoing deterioration in physical status and possibly cognitive deficits. The intervention plan should focus on the client's participation in occupational performance because the client's functional status changes frequently and intervention focused on physical performance is limited. Addressing the energy expenditure for preferred occupations is an important foundation for OT services, and equipment may allow the client to continue in preferred occupations for a longer period.[208] As the client's function declines, there is a greater need for environmental support through providing durable medical equipment, modifying the home, and providing adaptive equipment. Investigations have demonstrated the importance of the client having a sense of control in the decision-making process as an important element in the quality of life.[206] Some studies have shown that exercise, including passive range of motion and light resistive exercise, improves an individual's function and reduces spasticity. Daily range of motion to reduce spasticity and prevent contractures is important during the middle to late stages of the disease.[14] Depending on the client's level of understanding, life support choices, and acceptance of the disease, the OT intervention may initially focus on structuring the client's environment to support independence, and in middle to later stages attention may shift to caregiver training and adaptation to ADLs with assistance. Some clients with ALS may choose to have the maximum environmental and life support available to extend life. In this case, the OT may provide periodic reevaluations to determine the client's need for adapting self-care, work, and leisure activities. Other clients may request that no extraordinary life support be used, in which case the OT would assume a supportive role, perhaps helping these clients create a memory book to give to their loved ones. Table 36.2 provides a list of the functional deficits at various stages of the disease and interventions that may be required. When referring to this table, the OT practitioner must remember that each client's clinical picture is unique and that symptoms may appear in a different sequence than the table indicates. For example, a client with early-onset bulbar signs will require earlier intervention regarding swallowing assessment and communication devices; another client may not need a wheelchair until the very late stages. The ALS Association website (https://www.als.org/support) provides practical solutions for ADLs and a variety of resources that address many of the problems that this population faces, and it is an invaluable resource for practitioners, patients, and families.

Individuals and their families require an interdisciplinary approach to the rapid changes in function, complex psychosocial factors, and quality-of-life issues associated with ALS. The impact of the disease on the client's quality of life has been examined frequently. One study indicated that those who were less distressed and less depressed[41] and had a more positive attitude lived longer.[90] Fatigue and depression have been associated with a poor quality of life for an individual with ALS.[122] Research

has found that level of disability was not directly correlated with degree of anxiety and depression.[41] Hecht and colleagues found that social withdrawal correlated with levels of disability; based on the results of this investigation, the authors recommended that mobility be improved with power wheelchairs and public transportation to prevent social withdrawal.[90] Studies have also examined the impact of hope, spirituality, and religion as a means of coping with the disease.

OT PRACTICE NOTES

Formulation of an occupational profile during the OT evaluation can promote better understanding of the client's outlook and help determine the most appropriate interventions to improve quality of life with this rapidly progressing disease.

SECTION 1 SUMMARY

The Marcus case study demonstrates how ALS symptoms manifest and the impact on occupations and client factors. As ALS progresses rapidly, OT reassessment and interventions are needed throughout the process. OT aims to maximize the client's function by providing interventions and periodic reassessment to compensate for declining motor function through modification of the environment, occupations, and tasks and by helping the client and family achieve their client-centered goals.

SECTION 2: ALZHEIMER'S DISEASE

Winifred Schultz-Krohn

Dementia is the general word used for a group of symptoms caused by serious disorders of the brain. Memory loss and other related problems in language, perception, thinking, executive functioning and judgment interfere with learning, communicating, relating, and even caring for self. Dementia is not just one disease but includes a number of diseases (e.g., vascular dementia, Lewy body dementia, frontotemporal dementia). The most common cause of dementia is Alzheimer's disease (AD), especially in persons over 65 years of age.

AD is considered a primary dementia because it does not result from other diseases. Secondary dementia is a word that may be used to refer to symptoms of dementia that are associated with other physical diseases (PD, HD, ALS, MS) and are discussed elsewhere in this chapter. AD, unlike the other neurological disorders discussed in this chapter, is formally classified as a mental disorder by the American Psychiatric Association.[12] The exact cause of AD is still unknown, although various pathological changes have been identified, including the accumulation of amyloid beta plaques in the CNS.[7] In addition to the increased protein deposits (amyloid beta plaques) outside the neuron, there is an increase in tangled protein elements within the neuron, tau tangles, that compromise neuronal synaptic transmission and block the transport of nutrients required for neuronal survival.[7] The progressive neuronal death results in atrophy of the cerebral hemispheres along with a decrease in the brain's ability to metabolize glucose. Because of the damage to brain cells and irreversible cognitive decline, the disease results in impaired cognitive processes, altered behavior, and disturbances in mood. The disorder progresses gradually, producing multiple cognitive deficits, a significant decline from previous levels of functioning, and noticeable impairment in social and occupational functioning is seen over the course of time.[7] Effects on the motor and sensory systems are not apparent until later in the disease process.

Dementia is a significant healthcare problem because of the increasing number of individuals who are living longer, the higher incidence of dementia among older persons, the very high cost of supervised care, and the extensive use of medical resources.[7,196,197,217] Medicare spends almost three times as much on persons with AD and other dementias than on beneficiaries without AD.[7] Early recognition of cognitive decline by physicians, OTs, and all other healthcare professionals is critical.[58,243] Potential slowing the progression of the disease, greater understanding of functional decline, improved quality of life, and time to prepare for the future for older adults and their families could be an outcome of early recognition. The AD diagnosis is often overlooked or mistaken for other disorders, especially in the early stages.

OT PRACTICE NOTE

OTs have an essential role in helping the client with AD enjoy life and remain as self-sufficient as possible and in supporting families and caregivers over the course of this difficult disease.

INCIDENCE AND PREVALENCE

AD accounts for more than two-thirds of the cases of dementia, and the incidence increases dramatically as people age.[7,213] It is projected that 12.7 million adults 65 years of age and older will have AD by 2050.[7] The disease is estimated to impact more than 6.2 million people in the United States in 2021 for persons over 65 years of age. Of this group, 3.8 identify as women and 2.4 million identify as men, and it has been hypothesized that the difference is primarily due to women living longer than men. Age is the strongest primary risk factor. The incidence of AD increases with age, and 76 of every 1000 persons over 85 years have AD. As the population of older adults continues to grow, the number of persons with AD is also expected to grow. Family history and genetics are other risk factors for AD.[7,79] Two general forms of AD are reported and are primarily determined by the age of onset of the disease. Early-onset AD is diagnosed before the age of 65 and can be seen in persons as young as 35 to 40 years. Individuals with trisomy 21, a genetic alteration, exhibit signs of AD at an earlier age with estimates that 50% of those with trisomy 21 have AD by age 50.[7] The early-onset form is seen in less than 10% of all AD cases. Late-onset AD is diagnosed after the age of 65 and is the most common form of AD.[37] Approximately 35% of persons over the age of 85 have AD dementia.[7] A variant of early-onset AD presents with a familial transmission, familial AD (FAD). FAD accounts for less than 1% of all AD cases, is linked to genetic mutations of the amyloid precursor protein (APP), and presenilin-1 and 2 (PS-1, PS-2) genes.[153] Late-onset AD has been linked to the apolipoprotein E-4 (APOE-4) allele. Currently over 20 genetic markers have been associated as a risk factor for late-onset AD, and this form is considered multifactorial in cause. Previous head trauma is a well-established risk factor for AD; other factors that increase risk include diabetes mellitus, APOE gene variation, current smoking, and depression.

Although the incidence of dementia is growing rapidly, it does not occur in all older adults. Many older adults experience a normal slowing of information processing, called age-related cognitive decline. They do not develop clinically significant cognitive deficits.[12,117]

A portion of the older adult population will develop mild cognitive impairment (MCI), a condition that involves problems with memory, language, or other essential cognitive functions that is serious enough to be noticeable to others and to show up on tests, but this impairment is not severe enough to interfere with daily life.[7] Some, but not all, persons with MCI go on to develop AD. Driscoll and colleagues found that persons with MCI showed brain atrophy, but the group who went on to develop AD showed a distinct pattern of atrophy in the region of the temporal lobes.[57] A term sometimes used by laypersons to talk about older adults with memory loss or cognitive impairments is *senility*. Senility is not a medical term. The use of the word *senility* perpetuates stereotypical impressions that progressive cognitive decline occurs in normal aging. Such ideas prevent early recognition and accurate diagnosis of dementia.

PATHOPHYSIOLOGY

AD is the result of degenerative changes in the CNS. Neuroanatomic and neurochemical changes occur with neuronal disruptions in synaptic connections and cellular death. The result of these changes is progressive and diffuse neuronal loss in the cerebral cortex and the hippocampus.[147,198] Three noticeable pathological changes have been found through microscopic examination of brain tissue after death. These changes include accumulation of amyloid in the space between neurons, increased neuritic plaques, and neurofibrillary tangles, with loss of neurons and synapses. Early stages of AD are associated with decreased cholinergic markers in areas of the brain where there is also increased distribution of plaques and tangles. Many of the changes in the brains of persons with AD, such as enlarged ventricles, can be seen through neuroimaging techniques (e.g., computed tomography [CT], magnetic resonance imaging [MRI], and positron emission tomography [PET]) (Fig. 36.2). Degenerative changes in the brain involve several processes that affect neurotransmission and result in neuronal death.[198]

The amyloid deposits can occur in the preclinical stage of AD before signs of mild cognitive impairment.[7] Later there is an accumulation of abnormal tau, causing loss of synaptic connections, neurons, and brain volume. An inflammatory process causes the tau proteins in the cortical and limbic neurons to undergo microtubular dysfunction, preventing the neurons from sending nutrients along the axons. The paired filaments of these intracellular proteins actually become cross-linked in an abnormal metabolic process. These filaments form neurofibrillary tangles that eventually lead to neuron death as the

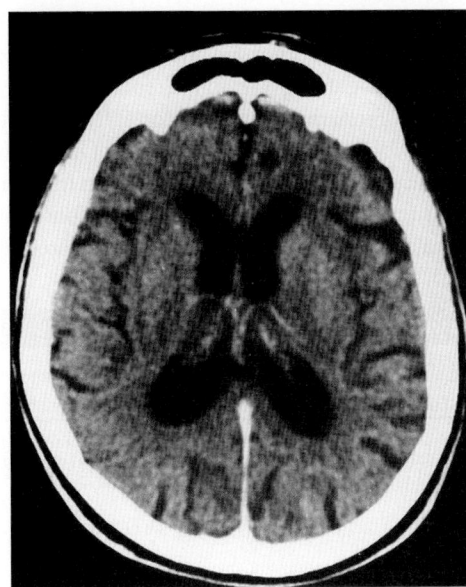

Fig. 36.2 Alzheimer's disease. Noncontrast CT scan of a 56-year-old woman with progressive dementia shows generalized enlargement of ventricular system and sulci. (From Eisenberg RL, Johnson N: *Comprehensive radiographic pathology*, ed 7, St. Louis, 2021, Elsevier.)

neuron-transport system collapses. Neurofibrillary tangles are also seen in the temporal areas and to a lesser degree in the parietal association areas. Neuritic plaques are large, extraneuronal bodies consisting of accumulated amyloid beta proteins and neuronal debris—small axons and dendrites. Distribution of neuronal plaques predominates in the temporal and parietal areas in early AD. When neurons lose their connections, they cannot function and eventually die. The neuron degeneration and death spreads through the brain, connections between other neurons break down, and affected regions begin to shrink in a process called brain atrophy. By the final stage of AD, damage is widespread and brain tissue has shrunk significantly.

CLINICAL PICTURE

Initially, the presentation of AD may seem puzzling, because it can affect different people in different ways.[7] The most prominent symptom is the progressive inability to remember new information. The Alzheimer's Association has compiled a checklist "Know the 10 Signs," an Early Detection Matters education campaign that assists older adults and their families with early recognition and contact with their primary care physician.[8] Symptoms and patterns of behavior in AD are often described in terms of stages, but it is important to recognize that it can be difficult to place a person with Alzheimer's in a specific stage, as stages may overlap. The Alzheimer's Association provides a description of the disease progression as five stages from preclinical AD to severe dementia as a result of AD.[7] This continuum recognizes that AD begins several years before clinical signs are noticeable. During the preclinical stage (stage 1) changes in the brain can be noted through detection of abnormal levels of amyloid beta plaques and with PET scans. Stage 2 is marked by subtle cognitive changes noticed by family members

and significant others, but the person with AD is still able to complete the majority of ADLs and IADLs. The second stage, in which MCI is noted, is of particular interest in pharmacological research because the individual is still functionally independent. Delaying the progression from stage two (MCI) to stage 3, in which mild dementia is seen, would improve the quality of life for the person and caregivers. Approximately a third of individuals with MCI develop AD dementia within 5 years. In stage 3, mild signs of dementia are noted from AD. The person is often able to perform basic ADLs and some IADLs but requires assistance for safety. As the disease progresses, the severity of dementia also progresses. In stage 4 the person displays moderate signs of dementia and requires assistance with routine ADLs such as bathing and dressing. Behavioral changes and increased levels of agitation may be seen during this stage. The final stage (stage 5) is marked by severe dementia and significant difficulties with motor function. The person with AD may be unable to ambulate independently and have significant difficulties with safe swallowing. Aspiration becomes a risk at this stage.

The primary symptom of AD is impairment in recent memory that worsens as the disease progresses and includes at least one other cognitive deficit such as apraxia, aphasia, agnosia, or impaired executive function, according to the American Psychiatric Association.[12] Memory impairment involves increased difficulty learning new information and recalling information after more than a few minutes.[147] Over time, the ability to learn deteriorates further and the ability to recall old memories also declines. Symptoms such as speech and language problems, impaired recognition of previously familiar objects, and impaired ability to perform planned motor movement are more variable and may not be seen in all persons with AD. The expression of symptoms depends on the areas of the brain most affected by the disease. Executive function (the ability to initiate, plan, organize, safely implement, and judge and monitor performance) inevitably deteriorates as AD progresses. Visuospatial dysfunction is common. Mood and behavioral changes are often observed in the early stages of AD, with personality shifts and the development of depression, anxiety, and increased irritability. Later in the course of the disease, troubling behavioral problems such as agitation, psychosis (i.e., delusions and hallucinations), aggression, and wandering can emerge.[7,147] Motor performance areas such as gait and balance may become impaired, and sensory changes usually arise in the middle to later stages in the course of AD (Table 36.3). Frequently, delirium and depression complicate the clinical picture. The life expectancy after the diagnosis of AD is typically from 8 to 10 years but can range from 3 to 20 years, with a variable rate of progression.

Deterioration in the individual's functional performance usually occurs in a hierarchical pattern. This pattern of decline consists of initially a gradual progression from mild impairments in work and leisure performance to more moderate difficulties in performing IADLs, especially with finances and driving. Eventually, there is a progressive loss of the ability to perform even basic self-care tasks in ADLs. The disability pattern is usually characterized by lower extremity ADL problems (walking) before decline in upper extremity ADL functions.[86] The trend in AD is for cognitive deficits to increase and executive function to become more impaired (see Table 36.3). Motivation and perception can influence functional performance but may not be routinely considered in individuals with AD.[117]

MEDICAL MANAGEMENT

According to Larson,[113] medical management of the individual with AD in primary care settings generally includes several areas.

Many aspects of what is termed medical management also may be performed by certain other members of an interdisciplinary healthcare team, including the nurse, social worker, physical therapist, or OT. First, there is a need for early recognition and diagnosis of AD.[113] Second, there is the issue of how to intervene on behalf of the person with AD who is living in the community, before more supportive and restrictive care becomes necessary. The third area concerns timely modifications of interventions as

TABLE 36.3 Progression of Alzheimer's Disease and Intervention Considerations

Client Characteristics	Intervention Using Occupational Performance Patterns and Client Factors	Intervention Using Performance Patterns and Client Factors
Stage 1: Preclinical Stage of AD: Changes in brain function are detected by imaging, etc., but clinical signs are not seen in the individual		
Stage 2: MCI Due to AD		
Feels loss of control, less spontaneous; may become more anxious and hostile if confronted with losses	Listen to client concerns; collaborate with client in identifying areas that are challenging and identify associated feelings (depression or anxiety).	Encourage physical exercise and wellness behavior.
Mild problems with memory and less initiative; difficulty with word choice, attention, and comprehension; repetition sometimes necessary; conversation more superficial; mild problems with gnosis or praxis	Begin training the caregiver to serve as a case manager.	Help client and caregiver establish a daily routine and post it in a central place.
Seems socially and physically intact except to intimates; decline in job performance	Provide educational and other resources for disease information, support and relaxation, support groups, or activities for both client and caregiver.	Use environmental aids such as calendars, appointment books, adhesive notes, and notebooks to enhance memory and reinforce engagement in occupation.
	Identify roles, activity frequency, and configuration; encourage continuation of or increase in enjoyable activities by keeping a log and planning enjoyable activity daily or weekly; use activity or task as a focus in socialization.	Identify appropriate environments or adapt for activities that are currently challenging.
	Explore meaning of occupations and occupational role changes with client and caregiver.	In teaching new tasks, use auditory, visual, and kinesthetic input, and provide supportive or positive feedback; grade activity for success to decrease anxiety.
	Identify needs, preferences, and goals of the caregiver. Discuss driving skills, and plan for future evaluation and restrictions.	During communication training, rehearse with client how to use "I" statements and assertively express self and needs in response to changed ability and the feelings aroused.
		Educate and train caregiver in how to empower client to keep active and facilitate initiation of tasks.
Stage 3: Mild Dementia Due to AD		
Use of denial, labile moods, anxious or hostile at times; excessive passivity and withdrawal in challenging situations; possible development of paranoia	Emphasize to caregiver the importance of environment in managing dementia at home.	Maintain routines and design environmental support (e.g., lists, posters, and pictures) and level of assistance for cues to remember daily routine and important events.
Moderate memory loss, with some gaps in personal history and recent or current events; decreased concentration; possible tendency to lose valued objects; difficulty with complex information and problem solving; difficulty learning new tasks; visuospatial deficits more apparent	Analyze and adapt meaningful leisure, home management, and other productive activities so as to allow the client to safely participate and exert initiation, independence, and control.	Avoid tasks involving new learning; help to simplify surroundings and tasks; make objects accessible, establish expectations for object use, simplify instructions, and clarify the meaning of "success."

TABLE 36.3 Progression of Alzheimer's Disease and Intervention Considerations—cont'd

Client Characteristics	Intervention Using Occupational Performance Patterns and Client Factors	Intervention Using Performance Patterns and Client Factors
Need for supervision slowly increases; decreased sociability; moderate impairment in IADLs that are complicated and mild impairment in some ADLs (e.g., finances, shopping, medications, community mobility, cooking complex meals); no longer employed; complicated hobbies dropped	Identify needs, and design ways to adapt and grade activity by simplifying complex tasks; train the caregiver to provide cognitive support (verbally) with the client on IADLs and some ADLs.	Help caregiver interpret behavioral problems by understanding source of frustration and the effects of memory loss on behavior.
	Encourage scrutiny of family structure and resources to respond to increasing need for supervision; consider outside resource (e.g., daycare, legal planning, friendly visitor volunteer, public transportation for the disabled).	Maintain socialization, and structure opportunities in which others initiate socialization to ensure satisfying relationships in group activity and other social activities.
		Use reality orientation activities, photo albums, and pictures around the home as a reminder of the past, past competence, and opportunities for socializing.
		Encourage stretching, walking, and other balance activities.

Stage 4: Moderate Dementia Due to AD

Reduced affect, increased apathy; sleep disturbances; repetitive behaviors; hostile behavior, paranoia, delusions, agitation and violence possible if client becomes overwhelmed	Maintain involvement in meaningful activity and reactivate alternative roles; identify and design tasks in home management activity; client can assist caregiver with design of productive activity related to former work role.[118]	In managing problem behaviors (e.g., assaultive behavior), teach caregivers to identify problem, understand and consider possible precipitants for the behavior (e.g., feelings; antecedent events; who, where, when; medical problem or task; environment; or communication problem), and adapt own behavior or change the environment.
Progressive memory loss of well-known material; some history retained; client unaware of most recent events; disorientation to time and place and sometimes extended family; progressively impaired concentration; deficits in communication severe; apraxia and agnosia more evident	Help caregiver problem-solve and recognize degree of need for initiation, verbal cues, physical assistance, and ADLs; provide time orientation; simplify environment.	It is essential to maintain consistent daily routines as means of facilitating participation in overlearned tasks, maintain function, and continue to define the self.
Slowed response, impaired visual and functional spatial orientation	Support socialization at home and with family or in structured settings outside of the home.	Teach family that overlearned tasks are possible but require safe environment; overall, tasks take longer, need to be simplified, and require setup and grading to comprise two steps or less.
Unable to perform most IADLs; in ADLs, assistance eventually needed with toileting, hygiene, eating, and dressing; beginning signs of urinary and fecal incontinence; wandering behavior	Ensure safety in the home and other environments by making adaptations suited to level of client functioning (e.g., alarms, restricted use of heating devices and sharps, cabinet latches, ID bracelet, visual cues for item location, and visual camouflaging).[97]	Make further environmental adaptations to compensate for perceptual deficits and ensure safe mobility.
		Rehearse and review names of family and others, using pictures.
		Encourage standby or assisted ambulation, stretching, and exercise on a regular basis.
		In new environments, cue and assist client in navigation, and provide more light and pictorial representations to cue.

Stage 5: Severe Decline and Moderate to Severe Physical Decline Due to AD

Memory impairment severe; may forget family member's name but still recognize familiar people; can become confused even in familiar surroundings	For ADLs (hygiene, feeding), instruct caregivers (family or nursing assistants) regarding need for simple communication, one-step commands, step-by-step verbal cues, and physical guidance.	Encourage caregiver to use respite programs and maintain recreation and leisure activity for himself or herself.

(Continued)

	Intervention Using Occupational Performance Patterns and Client Factors	Intervention Using Performance Patterns and Client Factors
TABLE 36.3 **Progression of Alzheimer's Disease and Intervention Considerations—cont'd**		
Client Characteristics	**Intervention Using Occupational Performance Patterns and Client Factors**	**Intervention Using Performance Patterns and Client Factors**
Gait and balance disturbances; difficulty negotiating environmental barriers; generalized motoric slowing	Encourage continued socialization by family; socialization depends on initiation of conversation by others and may not consistently include a response from the client.	Encourage assisted ambulation methods until client is no longer able to use them.
Often unable to communicate except by grunting or saying single word; psychomotor skills deteriorate until unable to walk; incontinent of both urine and feces; unable to eat; often becomes necessary to place client in nursing home at this time	Use dysphagia techniques to promote swallowing, prevent choking, and encourage eating.	Maintain proper positioning in bed and wheelchair; instruct family in skin inspection.
	Instruct family in transfer techniques.	Provide controlled sensory stimulation involving sound, touch, vision, and olfaction to maintain contact with reality.
		Begin program of active and assisted and passive ROM exercises.

ADLs, Activities of daily living; *IADLs*, instrumental ADLs; *ROM*, range of motion.
Adapted from Alzheimer's Association, 2021; Baum C: Addressing the needs of the cognitively impaired elderly from a family policy perspective, *Am J Occup Ther* 45:594, 1991; Corocoran M, Giles G: *Neurocognitive disorder (NCD): interventions to support occupational performance*, Washington, D.C., 2014, AOTA Press; Glickstein J: *Therapeutic interventions in Alzheimer's disease*, Gaithersburg, MD, 1997, Aspen.

the disease progresses. Last is the role of healthcare providers in recognizing and addressing other conditions that contribute to excess disability for the person with AD.

A comprehensive physical examination, laboratory evaluation, mental status examination, brief neurological examination, and informant interview are essential in diagnosing AD.[8] It is important to identify and treat medical conditions (e.g., metabolic disturbances, infections, alcohol use, vitamin deficiencies, chronic obstructive pulmonary disease [COPD], heart disease, and drug toxicity) that can contribute to comorbidity. MRI, PET, and CT scan results can be useful, but overreliance on these techniques should be avoided because their value is in identifying relatively uncommon, treatable causes of cognitive impairment. A comprehensive and skillful interview with a reliable informant is essential to the evaluation and diagnostic process in order to recognize decline by comparing current changes with past performance. Informant questionnaires, interviews, and screening measures may be performed by many healthcare professionals other than physicians and are important to the diagnostic process.

The goal of OT practitioners in the successful management of an individual with cognitive problems, whether in the community or in a semi-institutional or institutional setting, is to minimize behavior disturbances, maximize function and independence, and foster a safe and secure environment.[117] Increased mortality is associated with dementia.[7] Regular health maintenance visits in primary care settings to identify treatable illnesses such as depression, PD, low folate levels, arthritic conditions, urinary tract infections, and other conditions that may exacerbate dementia are important for all older adults, but especially those with AD.[116,198]

Depression and dementia easily may be mistaken for each other or they may coexist. Careful attention to whether the onset of symptoms has been gradual (dementia) or more recent (depression) is an important diagnostic issue because affective and cognitive symptoms frequently occur together.[188] Cognitive impairments and especially functional performance may improve in individuals with both dementia and depression after they are treated for depression. Delirium (i.e., impairment in attention, alertness, and perception) and dementia frequently coexist as well, especially in hospital settings.[7] Both conditions involve global cognitive impairment, but delirium is usually acute in onset, shows fluctuating symptoms, disrupts consciousness and attention, and interferes with sleep. Adverse drug reactions are more common in AD because of the impaired brain function.[96] Often, a cause of delirium, such as drug toxicity, is treatable.

Hearing, vision, and other sensory impairments are known to make dementia worse and cause greater strain on the caregiver.[114] Falls with hip fractures are 5 to 10 times more common in persons with AD than in normal persons of the same age and often result in earlier institutionalization for the individual and the need for higher levels of care.[3,102] Unsafe mobility quickly becomes an overwhelming burden for caregivers, especially those who are aged.

Although there have been decades of research addressing pharmacological interventions for the individuals with AD, there is limited effectiveness in pharmacotherapy.[96] Any pharmacotherapy provided should be assessed carefully and justified at regular intervals. Although OT practitioners do not prescribe medications, knowledge of pharmacotherapy for individuals with AD is useful when providing OT intervention.[39]

Sundowning, or sundown syndrome, is a fairly common problem during the middle stages of AD when the person becomes restless, agitated, irritable, or confused in the late afternoon or early evening.[147,222] The person with AD may have increased levels of anxiety or confusion and may wander. Various interventions can reduce the anxiety associated with sundowning symptoms such as cognitive and exercise-based services.[228] An investigation completed by Menegardo and colleagues[134] found irritability was the most common behavior observed in persons with AD who had sundown syndrome. These episodes of irritability and aggressiveness occurred daily for the majority of the sample or several times per week. The management of sundown syndrome places an extraordinary burden on caregivers.[148] Although the cause for sundown syndrome is not understood, the level of melatonin decreases with the aging process and is far more reduced in persons with AD compared to peers. Shih and associates[202] found that walking 30 minutes, four times a week, significantly decreased sundowning symptoms for clients with AD compared to clients with AD who did not walk. The 30 minutes of walking occurred either in the morning or afternoon, depending on the caregiver's preference. This simple routine may serve as a means to decrease sundown syndrome for clients with AD.

ROLE OF THE OCCUPATIONAL THERAPIST

Most individuals with AD live in the community, alone, or with family and friends, rather than in institutions. A predominant feature of AD is significant and progressive deterioration of function from previous levels of performance because of advancing brain atrophy and pathological tissue changes. Families and significant others connected with persons who have AD become progressively involved as the disease progresses. Family and significant others provide increasing oversight and personal assistance.[7,39,80] Changes in the brain caused by AD result in deficits in client factors, which in turn lead to deterioration in occupational performance skills, engagement in occupations, and major changes in occupational roles. Over time, more structured, supervised living environments are needed. Increased difficulties in performing everyday functions create challenges for the individual with AD and impact the quality of life for the client, family, and caregivers as the disease progresses. Effective OT interventions must be directed at supporting occupational performance for the individual and creating as much quality of life as possible. Intervention should focus on supporting and maintaining capabilities, adapting tasks and environments, and otherwise compensating for declining function in individuals with AD while trying to help them retain as much control as possible over their lives in the least restrictive environment.[172,173]

ETHICAL CONSIDERATIONS

Support for the caregiver is a must. Collaboration with and training of the caregiver is essential in the management of clients with dementia. Family members should encounter an open and encouraging environment in which to discuss safety, security, and dependence issues. Legal, financial, and health concerns that require advance directives (e.g., medical and legal), trusts, activity restrictions (e.g., driving, financial matters, and medication management), and contingency and transitional care plans (e.g., daycare, residential care, and long-term care) are important in preparation for the inevitable progression of the disease.[113,172,173]

Behavioral problems can be expected in the client with AD until the terminal or bed-bound stage. Encouragement to use respite care, in-home support services, and support groups is important. Caregivers also need effective strategies for dealing with behavioral disturbances and disruptions in mood.[114] The use of environmental adaptations, therapeutic interpersonal approaches, referral to other disciplines, and resource sharing helps in collaborating with the client's family and handling these problems. Health professionals use education, training, counseling, and support to help caregivers deal with their feelings, manage behaviors, and maintain quality of life for themselves and for the client with AD. Awareness of the multidimensional effects of this illness on the individual, the family, and the society at large is important to promote more effective and efficient care.[40,47]

EVALUATION

OT services are indicated for individuals who have demonstrated a recent decline in function; whose behaviors pose a safety hazard to family, staff, other residents, or self; or who may experience improved quality of life.[205]

The type of assessment and the depth of the evaluation process used are influenced by the setting, the stage of progression of AD, the reimbursement process, the presence of other medical and mental health disorders, and the cooperation and interest of the caregiver or care staff. An instrument used to detect changes in progression of the disease process is the Alzheimer's Disease Assessment Scale–Cognitive subscale (ADAS-Cog).[175] This 11-item instrument has been successfully used to detect decline in cognitive function over the course of time and has good sensitivity. This tool is often part of an interdisciplinary assessment, and the psychologist or the OT practitioner may be involved in administering this instrument. The Integrated Alzheimer's Disease Rating Scale (iADRS) is another tool used in clinical trials in which the ADAS-Cog is combined with the Alzheimer's Disease Cooperative Study–Instrumental Activities of Daily Living (ADCS-iADL).[235] Additional assessment tools that may be useful include the Loewenstein Occupational Therapy Cognitive Assessment-Geriatric (LOTCA-G),[18] the Mini-Mental Status Exam (MMSE), the Short Geriatric Depression Scale (SGDS), and various instruments to assess ADL and IADL status along with quality of life assessment tools.

Providing OT services in community settings and in long-term care facilities requires the OT practitioner to consider the "client" as the person with AD along with caregivers, family members, and significant others supporting the person with AD. The OT intervention is often focused on helping families and caregivers develop strategies and environmental adaptations to cope with the overwhelming stresses of safely managing a cognitively impaired individual.[111,205] The consequences of caregiving and the needs of the caregiver can vary greatly, depending on gender, family relationships, culture, and ethnicity.[7] The caregiver's understanding of dementia, reaction to dementia-related behaviors, use of problem-solving skills, use of the environment, use of formal and informal support systems, and decision-making style greatly affect the caregiver's ability to participate in the care plan and treatment of persons with dementia.[46] The Activities of Daily Living Inventory is a 23-item inventory that assesses both ADLs and IADLs using the caregiver interview.[39] This instrument does not focus on what the individual might be able to do but rather asks for specific information on what the individual with AD actually does in day-to-day life. It has been used as a primary outcome measure in research regarding the efficacy of OT services provided to individuals with AD and their respective caregivers.

Evaluations for individuals who have AD should be comprehensive despite changing reimbursement requirements. Substantial information can be gathered before an interview and intervention session by asking caregivers, family members, and staff informants to complete questionnaires and rating scales. These scales assess occupational performance, functional abilities, and skills using measures such as the Functional Behavior Profile,[23] the Modified Caregiver's Strain Questionnaire,[220] the Katz Activities of Daily Living Scale (KADL),[108] and the Instrumental Activities of Daily Living (IADL) Scale.[115] Informant rating measures should routinely be followed by an interview either before or during the first visit. The use of a few brief screening instruments for mental status (e.g., the MMSE),[68] depression,[25,239] and anxiety[116] provides baseline data and a wealth of information about factors that are likely to influence performance.

The functional evaluation of an individual with AD depends on the stage of cognitive decline. OT services for persons with AD during the early stages of the disease should be focused on tasks involving work, home management, driving skills, and safety. Driving has been specifically identified as an area in which OT practitioners should provide not only ongoing assessment but also intervention.[93] Although the on-road driving assessment is considered the gold standard, standardized off-road assessments are available to determine the safety of drivers who have cognitive impairments. In the later stages, the focus shifts to self-care, mobility, communication, and leisure skills.

The concerns and observations of the caregiver are important, but the therapist's observation of task performance is also necessary. Many of the functional ADL scales developed for use with older adults have targeted physical performance in the assessment process and are not appropriate for persons experiencing cognitive decline.[75] Fortunately, several excellent, standardized measures that determine whether individuals are able to use their cognitive skills to perform tasks in ADLs and IADLs have been developed. The Kitchen Task Assessment (KTA) determines the level of cognitive support a person with AD needs to complete a cooking task successfully. Baum and colleagues created the Executive Function Performance Test (EFPT) with standardized administration and scoring.[23] The Allen Cognitive Level (ACL)[4] test determines the quality of problem solving a person uses while engaged in perceptual motor tasks. Levy[117,118] has extensively discussed the use of the ACL for clients with cognitive impairments. Consistent with the Allen theoretical approach, the Cognitive Performance Test (CPT)[5,36] was developed to identify cognitive deficits that are predictive of functional capacity using several ADLs and IADLs tasks. Another measure, the Assessment of Motor and Process Skills (AMPS),[66] has been used with individuals who have dementia.[66,157] The AMPS measures motor (e.g., posture, mobility, and strength) and process (e.g., attentional, organizational, and adaptive) skills by using task performance in IADLs. The Disability Assessment for Dementia (DAD)[75] uses informant ratings to determine the ability of the individual with AD

to complete tasks in both ADLs and IADLs. The DAD also provides information relevant to executive functioning, such as the person's ability to initiate, plan, and execute the activity. Further information regarding the evaluation of cognitive function and ADL performance is given in Chapters 10 and 26. After obtaining a good understanding of the functional level of the person with AD, the therapist can begin to look at what aspects of the occupational performance context, especially the environment and care provider interactions, must be modified to optimize function of the person with AD.[157]

INTERVENTION METHODS

The goals of OT are to provide services to persons with dementia and their families and caregivers to emphasize remaining strengths, maintain physical and mental activity for as long as possible, decrease caregiver stress, and keep the person in the least restrictive setting possible.[87,104] Although AD is the primary presenting problem, the OT practitioner has to consider the complexities of developing interventions with an older adult who may be experiencing additional sensory losses and numerous medical problems such as arthritis, orthopedic issues, COPD, diabetes, and heart disease in addition to AD.[56,102,103] Intervention planning takes into account the physical issues associated with aging, co-occurring disorders such as depression and anxiety, the progressive nature of the disorder, the expected decline in function, and the care setting itself. OT interventions for clients with dementia are directed toward maintaining, restoring, or improving functional capacity; promoting participation in occupations that are satisfying and that optimize health and well-being; and easing the burdens of caregiving.[114,120] The caregivers need to be included as an important member in developing the intervention plan, and OT services may be focused on reducing the caregiver distress and enhancing caregiver coping strategies.[120] A program developed specifically for caregivers focused on the level of stress and dysfunctional coping strategies. When caregivers were supported, the burden of caring for the person with AD was reduced.[120] Gitlin and colleagues instituted a program to improve the overall pleasure of persons living at home with dementia in an effort to decrease the distress of the caregivers who are affected by the behaviors of the persons with AD for whom they were caring.[80] A program called the Tailored Activity Program (TAP), an OT service that evaluates the interests and capabilities of persons with dementia, provides customized activities for each individual. TAP then trains their families to use those activities as part of their daily care routines. The methods therapists use in the intervention process include activity analysis, caregiver training, behavior management techniques, environmental modification, use of purposeful activity, and the provision of resources and referrals. Services are provided in many settings, such as home care, adult daycare, and semi-institutional or institutional long-term care. The intervention setting and the stage of the illness help frame the focus of intervention, determine the recipients of service, and prescribe the methods used (see Table 36.3). Ávila and colleagues[18] demonstrated significant gains in functional independence and cognitive function for persons with AD when provided with short-term, intensive (2 times per week for 12 weeks) OT services focused on functional task performance, cognitive stimulation, and caregiver training. In France, a multicenter randomized controlled trial is investigating the effect of providing home-based OT services for persons with mild to moderate AD.[173] The OT services address caregiver training along with individualized tailored environmental modifications, behavior management, and emotional support. In Korea, a randomized controlled trail examined the use of a systematic recollection-based OT program provided daily for persons with mild AD who attended an adult daycare program.[111] The group receiving OT services demonstrated significantly better outcomes on standardized assessments when compared to a control group who received usual services at the daycare program. Shih and associates[202] used a quasi-experimental design to diminish sundown syndrome by having persons with AD engage in walking for a 30-minute duration four times a week. The walking significantly reduced the sundown syndrome symptoms. Jensen and Padilla[102] completed a systematic review of the existing literature, and strong to moderate evidence was found to support various OT strategies based on person-centered, individually tailored interventions. These strategies included use of environmental modifications such as covering doors and door knobs to reduce wandering and exiting, moderation of noise levels within the environment, use of ambient music particularly at mealtime, and use of visual displays as cues for room use such as dining room for meal or bathroom for toileting.

SECTION 2 SUMMARY

AD is a neurological condition characterized by the development of multiple cognitive impairments with a gradual onset. The effect of these impairments is a significant and progressive decline from previous levels of functioning. The course of the disorder is variable, but loss of function generally occurs in a hierarchical pattern, beginning with work and progressing to difficulties with home management, driving, and safety until even basic self-care skills such as dressing, functional mobility, toileting, communication, and feeding are affected.

OT interventions should be directed at enhancing the abilities of the client with AD by continually adapting tasks of daily living and modifying the physical and social environment as the client experiences progressive loss of function. Given many of the current limitations in treatment time imposed by third-party payment, therapists may find it useful to employ some of the self-report and informant report measures identified in this chapter as a means of gathering information more efficiently during the evaluation process. Several standardized measures also have been identified to assist with the assessment of functional performance and the establishment of a baseline of performance. Recommendations for OT intervention with those who have AD have been identified. The focus of intervention must be flexible and depends on an understanding of the disease process in the client, the specific treatment setting, and the needs of the caregiver. Generally, the goals of OT services for persons with dementia are to maintain or enhance function,

promote continued participation in meaningful occupation, optimize health and quality of life, and work collaboratively with the caregiver to ease the burden of caregiving.

SECTION 3: HUNTINGTON'S DISEASE

Winifred Schultz-Krohn

INCIDENCE

Huntington's disease (HD) is a fatal, degenerative neurological disorder that affects 5 to 10 of every 100,000 individuals.[62,191] The disorder is transmitted in an autosomal dominant pattern. Each offspring of an affected parent has a 50% chance of having HD. Genetic studies have identified a mutation (cytosine-adenine-guanine [CAG]) on the Huntington gene *(HTT)* of chromosome 4 as the cause of this disease.[144,171,191,227] Presymptomatic diagnosis of HD is possible with genetic testing when the family history shows this disease.[169,171] Diagnosis is also made through clinical examination when the family history is unavailable or unknown.

PATHOPHYSIOLOGY

The neurological structure associated with HD is the corpus striatum (Fig. 36.3). Deterioration of the caudate nucleus is more severe and occurs earlier than atrophy of the putamen.[43,165] The corpus striatum plays an important role in motor control, and deterioration in this area contributes to the chorea associated with HD. The caudate nucleus is also linked to cognitive and emotional function through connections with the cerebral cortex. Thinning of the gray matter in the caudate and dorsolateral prefrontal cortex has been identified with the progression of HD.[49] A progressive loss of tissue occurs in the frontal cortex, globus pallidus, and thalamus as the disease advances.[171] The degeneration of the corpus striatum results in a decrease in the neurotransmitter gamma-aminobutyric acid (GABA). Additional deficiencies in acetylcholine and substance P, both

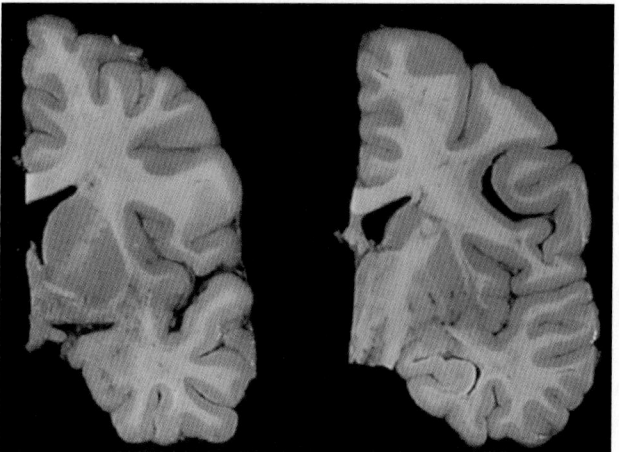

Fig. 36.3 Huntington's disease. *Left,* The coronal section from person with Huntington's disease shows atrophy of the caudate, putamen, and globus pallidus. *Right,* Normal coronal section for comparison. (From Perkin GD: *Mosby's color atlas and text of neurology,* St. Louis, 2002, Mosby.)

neurotransmitters, are noted in clients with HD. The triggering mechanism for the neuronal degeneration has not been clearly identified, but it is linked to genetic coding on the HTT chromosome.

CLINICAL PICTURE

HD is characterized as a progressive disorder involving both voluntary and involuntary movement, in addition to a significant deterioration of cognitive and behavioral abilities.[171] A client usually experiences an insidious onset of symptoms in the third to fourth decade of life, but cases have been reported in teenage and younger clients.[237] Clients who are positively identified by genetic testing should be carefully monitored for the first indications of HD symptoms. Not all individuals who have the potential to develop HD, because of family history, elect to undergo genetic testing, and this may negatively affect the time at which first symptoms are identified. The course of progression of HD is often divided into three stages, early, middle, and late, but with the advent of genetic testing, a presymptomatic stage has been added.[230] During the presymptomatic stage, monitoring symptoms is critical, and a decrease in the speed of finger tapping (an item on the Unified Huntington's Disease Rating Scale [UHDRS]) may mark the beginning of the early stage of HD. The UHDRS has been used to divide the course of the disease into five stages.[227] The presymptomatic stage is considered stage I. The early stage of the disease process is sometimes referred to as stage II. The middle stage of the disease is stage III, and the late stages, marked by little to no functional capacity, are stages IV and V. The stages refer to specific scores obtained on the UHDRS Functional Assessment. Regardless of the method used to indicate the stage of the disease, symptoms progress over a 15- to 20-year period, ultimately necessitating long-term care or hospitalization for the client.[171] Death is often the result of secondary causes, such as pneumonia.[169]

The initial symptoms vary but are most often reported as alterations in behavior, changes in cognitive function, and choreiform movements of the hands.[139,230,237] The early symptoms of cognitive disturbances are most likely related to the degeneration of the caudate nucleus. The client may appear forgetful or display difficulty concentrating. During the early stages of HD, a client may have difficulty maintaining adequate work performance. Family members often identify the initial behavioral changes in the person with HD as increased irritability or depression.[139] Irritability and depression may be attributed inappropriately to the decline in work performance rather than to the disease process.[49] Emotional and behavioral changes are often the earliest symptoms of HD.[20] Chorea, seen in clients with HD, consists of rapid, involuntary, irregular movements.[170] During the early stages of HD, chorea is often limited to the hands. A client may mask the initial chorea by engaging in behaviors such as manipulating small objects within the hands. These irregular movements are exacerbated during stressful conditions and decrease during voluntary motor activities in the early stages of HD. Chorea is absent when the client is sleeping. Onset of HD in teenage years is associated more often with early symptoms of rigidity than with chorea.[230,237]

Cognitive and emotional abilities progressively deteriorate over the course of the disease.[237] Disturbances in memory and in decision-making skills become more apparent during the middle stages of HD. Establishing and maintaining meaningful habits and routines for the individual who has HD are important ways to support continued participation in occupational pursuits. A client may be able to complete familiar tasks at work or in the home, but if the environment is changed or if additional demands are placed on the individual, task performance is significantly compromised. Further deterioration of cognitive abilities in the person with HD may result in dismissal from employment. The cognitive deficits most frequently associated with HD are problems with mental calculations, the performance of sequential tasks, and memory. Verbal comprehension is often spared until the middle or later stages of the disease, and even then, dysarthria manifests as a more significant issue than difficulty in comprehension until the late stages of HD.

Over the course of HD, depression often worsens and suicide is not uncommon.[230,237] Clients with HD are often hospitalized because of various psychiatric problems, including depression, emotional lability, and behavioral outbursts. Although the loss of function may contribute to the client's level of depression, depression is clearly identified as a specific characteristic of HD.[139,143] This affective disorder frequently is treated with various antidepressants. Periods of mania also have been reported in approximately 10% of individuals diagnosed with HD.

As the disease progresses, the chorea becomes more severe and may be observed throughout the entire body, including the face (Fig. 36.4).[171] Disturbances in gait are often observed during the middle stages of the disease, and balance is frequently compromised.[139] The individual with HD may display a wide-based gait pattern and have difficulties walking on uneven

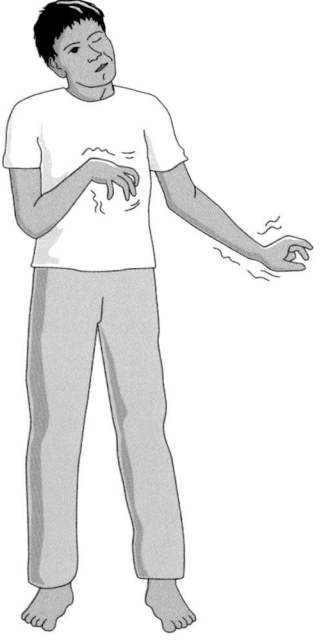

Fig. 36.4 Typical chorea movements in a patient with Huntington's disease. (From Schindelmeiser J: *Neurologie für sprachtherapeuten*, ed 2, München, 2012, Elsevier GmbH, Urban & Fischer.)

terrain. This staggering gait is at times misinterpreted by others in the client's life as evidence of alcoholism.[170] The client also has progressive difficulty with voluntary movements.[171] The performance of voluntary motor tasks is slowed (bradykinesia), and the initiation of movement is compromised (akinesia). Although handwriting ability may be spared initially, the client displays increasing difficulties with this task as the disease progresses. Letter size is enlarged, and letter formation, such as slant and shape, is distorted. Saccadic eye movements and ocular pursuits may be slowed at this stage of HD.[169] Slight dysarthria may be noted, which compromises communication. Dysphagia is seen, and the client may choke on various foods. Difficulties may be noted with the coordination of both chewing and breathing while eating.

In the later stages of HD, choreiform movements may be reduced because of the further deterioration of the corpus striatum and globus pallidus.[171] Hypertonicity and rigidity often replaces the chorea as the disease progresses, and the client experiences a severe reduction in voluntary movements. Severe difficulties in eye movement are common during the final stage of the disease.[169] At this stage, the client often needs significant support from others or resides in a long-term care facility. The client is usually unable to talk, walk, or perform basic ADLs without significant assistance.[144]

MEDICAL MANAGEMENT

Medical management of clients with HD can address symptoms, but no effective course of treatment has been identified to arrest the progression of this disease.[49,191,229] Intervention based on replacing the deficient neurotransmitters has not been effective in changing the course or rate of progression of HD. Tricyclic antidepressants are often used to treat the depression seen in clients with HD, but monoamine oxidase inhibitors are contraindicated because of possible exacerbation of chorea.[237] Haloperidol may be used to decrease the negative effects of chorea on the performance of functional activities.[171] Tetrabenazine also has been approved as a treatment for chorea.[191,229] Medical management focuses on three areas: managing symptoms and reducing the burden of the symptoms, maximizing function, and providing education to the client and significant others regarding the course of the disease progression.[143] A team of professionals, including OTs, is advocated when working with a client who has HD.

Investigations have noted how active engagement in activities, through the use of a multidisciplinary team approach, improved function for the client with HD.[49] OT services were provided once every 2 weeks to clients diagnosed with HD to improve cognitive skills and executive functioning. Clients also participated in home exercises designed to improve overall muscle strength and fine motor skills. After 9 months of intervention, clients had a significant increase in gray matter of the caudate and prefrontal cortex. Significant gains were also noted in learning and memory skills after the 9 months of multidisciplinary intervention services.

A team of various medical professionals is needed to support the individual who has HD and support the family members and significant others in the client's life.[91,106] The perception of the illness experience and coping strategies used by the client who has HD is an important part of the overall medical services provided.[91] Likewise, the significant others in the client's life need support and guidance in developing coping strategies as their loved one experiences progressive deterioration.[106]

Systematic evaluation of a client with HD must be performed at regular intervals to identify the rate of symptom progression and modify intervention strategies. Standardized instruments are available for determining the presence and severity of various symptoms.[88,95,99] The UHDRS is an evaluation tool that combines aspects from several instruments into a scale that can be administered within 30 minutes. The UHDRS is often administered by a team. This tool provides an accurate means of determining a change in the areas of "motor function, cognitive function, behavioral abnormalities, and functional capacity."[95] The UHDRS has been used to assess the rate of decline, and it demonstrates good reliability.[112] The OT should complete additional assessments before an intervention plan is developed. An evaluation would address functional daily living skills; cognitive abilities such as problem solving, motor performance, and strength; and personal interests and values. The OT must consider the client's role within the family and community and incorporate these data into the intervention plan. An evaluation at both the home and worksite would provide needed information that could be modified if necessary.

ROLE OF THE OCCUPATIONAL THERAPIST

The role of the OT practitioner varies depending on the stage of the disease.[99] During the early stages of HD, an OT should address the cognitive components of memory and concentration. A client may still be employed at this stage. Strategies such as establishment of a daily routine, the use of checklists, and task analysis to break down tasks into manageable steps can be very helpful. These strategies provide the external structure and support to help the person with HD maintain functional abilities at both the workplace and home. Specific OT intervention to help clients develop verbal strategies and problem-solving skills have significantly improved functional abilities for individuals who have HD.[49] A worksite evaluation can identify changes that would allow the person with HD to continue working. Modifications may include the use of tools such as organizers, electronic planners, and reminders to prompt an individual to complete regularly occurring tasks in the workplace. Family members also should be instructed in the use of these techniques. Environmental modifications such as providing a quiet workplace and reducing extraneous stimuli will decrease the impact of compromised memory and concentration on performing functional tasks in the workplace. Even during the early stages, work performance may deteriorate and the client may be dismissed because of an inability to meet the job essentials. This increases the stress experienced by the client from a financial perspective and from the loss of a role as a worker.

Psychological issues during this stage of the disease often include anxiety, depression, and irritability.[88,91,106] A client may express guilt that any of his or her children have a 50% chance of having HD.[170] The diagnosis of HD often is not confirmed until a person is 30 to 40 years old unless genetic testing is completed and confirms HD. The client may already be married and have children by that time. Decisions as to whether to complete predictive genetic testing on children may be a significant stressor for the client with HD and for his or her family members. As mentioned previously, not all individuals elect to be genetically tested, and sporadic presentations of HD do exist in which no family member has HD. During this early stage of HD, clients may use denial as a coping strategy even though choreiform movements are present in the hands.[91]

Maintaining social contacts and engaging in purposeful activities are important in designing interventions for clients with HD.[170] Changes in cognitive abilities and unpredictable or exaggerated emotional responses may result in the loss of a job and decreased income for the family, even during this early stage of the disease.[139] This additional stress also should be considered when developing an intervention plan. The OT intervention plan must include community support services for the client with HD. OT services should include providing clients with information regarding support groups, opportunities to engage in community activities, and virtual resources accessible through the internet. During the early and middle stages of the disease, rehabilitation services focused on cognitive skills, quality of life, physical strength, and endurance have shown positive results for individuals with HD.[49,183,219] OT services were able to support cognitive as well as physical function.[49,132]

The motor disturbances during the early stages of HD are usually limited to fine motor coordination problems.[146] The characteristic chorea may be noticed only as a twitching of hands when the client is anxious. OT should provide modifications to diminish the effect of chorea and fine motor incoordination on performance of functional activities.[99] This would include modifications to clothing and selection of clothing that does not require small fasteners such as small buttons, snaps, or hooks. Shoes with Velcro closures or elastic closures are recommended to compensate for diminished fine motor skills. Home modifications should be instituted at this stage to allow the client with HD to become familiar with the changes. Developing the skills of using adaptive equipment or modifications and then converting these skills into habits are critical during the early stage of HD. Typical modifications are the use of cooking and eating utensils with built-up handles, unbreakable dishes, a shower bench or seat with tub safety bars, and sturdy chairs with high backs and armrests. Throw or scatter rugs should be eliminated wherever possible in the home, and walkways should be kept free of clutter.

In the area of health management, the OT plays a key role in supporting physical activity participation and should work with the client to establish an individualized home exercise program to address the flexibility and endurance of the entire body.[110] The therapist can additionally support the client's self-management of their newly established exercise routine. In a randomized controlled pilot investigation, individuals who were in the middle stage of HD engaged in a regular home exercise program to improve balance, gait, and level of physical activity. After completing 8 weeks of home exercises, substantial

improvements were noted in physical abilities, but no significant change in quality of life was seen on the Short Form-36 (SF-36) instrument. The OT should develop home exercises that can be incorporated into the client's daily routine. As the movement disorder progresses with increased chorea and difficulties with oculomotor control, the client will no longer be safe driving a car and may experience further losses of community mobility. These further losses of independent function and control must be considered within the OT intervention plan. Alternative methods of community mobility must be explored.

As HD progresses, the role of OT changes to meet the client's needs.[99] During the middle stages of HD, further deterioration of cognitive abilities often requires the person to resign from a job. Engagement in purposeful activities is greatly needed at this stage and should be a focus of the OT intervention plan.[49,88,170] Decision-making and arithmetic skills show further deterioration, and family members may need to arrange for others to handle the client's financial matters.[91,146] Generally, comprehension of verbal information is better preserved than ability to complete sequential tasks during this stage. The OT should encourage the family to use simple written cues or words to help the family member with HD complete self-care and simple household activities. For example, selecting clothing items for the person with HD and placing the clothes in a highly visible area can prompt the individual to change from pajamas to daytime clothes in the morning. Arranging the bathroom with visual cues, such as putting the toothpaste and toothbrush by the sink, can remind the client to brush his or her teeth in the morning and evening.

During the middle stage of HD, the client may display increasing levels of irritability and depression.[237] Clients with HD may attempt suicide. The OT intervention plan should focus on the client's engagement in purposeful activities, particularly leisure activities.

When selecting craft activities, the therapist should always consider the client's interests but should also strive to ensure that no sharp instruments are required.[88,146] Modification of craft activities allows the client with HD to successfully complete a task with minimal support.[27] Materials often require additional stabilization to compensate for the client's movement disorders, and any tools used in the leisure activity, such as a wood sander and paintbrushes, should have enlarged or built-up handles. New leisure activities can be explored during the middle stage of HD.[210] In one study, clients in the middle stage of HD were provided with the opportunity to engage in gardening activities. A multidisciplinary team designed these activities, and OT figured prominently in the assessment and design of the program. Positive results were noted after the use of this program.[210]

Motor problems become more apparent during the middle stage of HD, necessitating further modifications in daily living tasks.[49,99] The client's compromised balance may require that tasks such as dressing, brushing teeth, shaving, and combing hair be performed while the client is seated. The client may require the use of a walker or wheelchair at this stage. A rollator walker is preferred to a standard walker without wheels. The walker may need to be fitted with forearm supports to provide additional stability when the client is ambulating. When a wheelchair becomes necessary, it should have a firm back and seat; however, additional padding is often required on the armrests because of the client's chorea. Many clients with HD are better able to move the wheelchair with their feet than with their hands. The seat height of the wheelchair should be fitted to allow the client to use his or her feet to move the chair, if possible.

Fatigue is a common issue during the middle stage of HD and can be addressed by taking frequent breaks during the day. Breaks must be scheduled because the person with HD may not readily recognize fatigue. Clothing should have few or no fasteners, and shoes should be sturdy with low heels.[146] Additional adapted equipment that may prove helpful for the client with HD includes shower mitts, an electric razor or chemical hair removal method, covered mugs, and nonslip placemats.[99] The choreic movements may become so severe as to necessitate the use of a bed with railings. Padding should be used on the railings, and additional cushions should be used in the bed.

Because of excessive movements associated with chorea, the client with HD often needs to consume 3000 to 5000 calories per day to maintain weight.[146] Clients with HD display a higher energy expenditure than individuals without HD and consequently have issues with weight loss and difficulties maintaining appropriate weight.[224] Smaller, high-calorie meals should be provided five times a day. This schedule may require additional support from family members or a personal care attendant. Dysphagia, poor postural control, and deficient fine motor coordination compromise the client's ability to eat.[99] Positioning during feeding is crucial, and the trunk should be well supported during mealtime. The client with HD should be able to support his or her arms on the table while the feet are stabilized. Feet may be supported on the floor, or the client may wrap the feet around the legs of the chair for additional support. Problems with dysphagia can be addressed with positioning, oral motor exercises, and changes in diet consistency. Soft foods and thickened fluids are preferable to chewy foods, foods with mixed textures, and thin liquids. Nutritional support has been successfully used for clients with HD to maintain appropriate weight.[224] Appropriate body weight is important to maintain overall health for the client with HD.

During the final stages of HD, the client often depends on others for all self-care tasks because of the lack of voluntary motor control.[99,106,144] In some clients, the chorea may diminish, leading to rigidity. The OT provides important input on positioning and the use of splints to prevent contractures at this stage. Because of the risk of aspiration, oral feedings are provided by trained personnel; alternatively, the client may receive nutrition through a feeding tube.[146] A combination of oral feedings and tube feedings may be used during this stage.

Although cognitive abilities continue to deteriorate, the level of functional decline is difficult to assess because of dysarthria and the loss of motor control.[91,95,112,146] Dementia is part of the HD profile and must be considered in the development of the intervention plan. For example, a person in the late stage of HD may still recognize family members and enjoy watching television. The OT should explore the use of various environmental controls to allow the client control of and access to the immediate environment. Providing adaptive access through the use of a touch pad, switch, eye gaze, or retinal scanning to select entertainment options may prove beneficial for the client.

Behavioral outbursts have been reported in approximately one-third of clients with HD living in long-term care facilities.[144] OT can decrease the frequency of these outbursts by organizing consistent daily schedules and routines for the client with HD.

SECTION 3 SUMMARY

Although HD is a progressive, degenerative process, OT has much to offer clients with this disease.[88,99,146,170] The diminishing ability to control the environment has been identified as one of the variables contributing to the deterioration of function in clients with HD. Throughout the course of the disease, OT addresses the client's ability to exercise a degree of control over the environment and engage in purposeful activity.

SECTION 4: MULTIPLE SCLEROSIS

Winifred Schultz-Krohn with contributions from Diane Foti

INCIDENCE

Multiple sclerosis (MS) is a progressive, autoimmune, inflammatory neurological disease most often first diagnosed in young adults.[151] Almost 70% of cases show signs and symptoms between the ages of 20 and 40 years of age; however, the disease has been identified in children as young as 3 years[59] and adults as old as 67.[187] The prevalence in the United States is approximately 750,000,[231] and over 2.8 million people are living with MS worldwide.[232] It is more prevalent in women than in men by an approximately 2:1 ratio overall but differences are noted with the initial presentation of MS. Men and women are equally identified with the primary-progressive form of MS, whereas women have a much higher prevalence of the relapsing form of MS, with a ratio of 3:1. There is a geographic distribution of MS in which those residing farther from the equator have a higher risk of developing MS.

Typically, MS has been considered a disease of the white matter, but research now shows there are also lesions in the gray matter structures.[151] Large lesions, known as plaques, are often seen in the spinal cord (50%), optic nerves (25%), brainstem/cerebellum (20%), and periventricular white matter (Fig. 36.5). The myelin is typically damaged in discrete regions of the white matter, with relative preservation of the axons and astrocytic gliosis.[187] Disruption of the myelin sheath has differing effects on axonal conduction, depending on the amount of myelin deterioration or inflammation and the length of the damaged segment.[35,38] When axons are conducting impulses in a slower manner because of inflammation of the myelin sheath, a person with MS may have intermittent symptoms of sensory distortion, incoordination, visual loss, or weakness. This inflammatory process accounts for the unpredictability of the disease.

In advanced cases of MS, acute and chronic plaques develop throughout the white matter, including the corpus callosum. Axons may be damaged and severed in advanced cases of MS

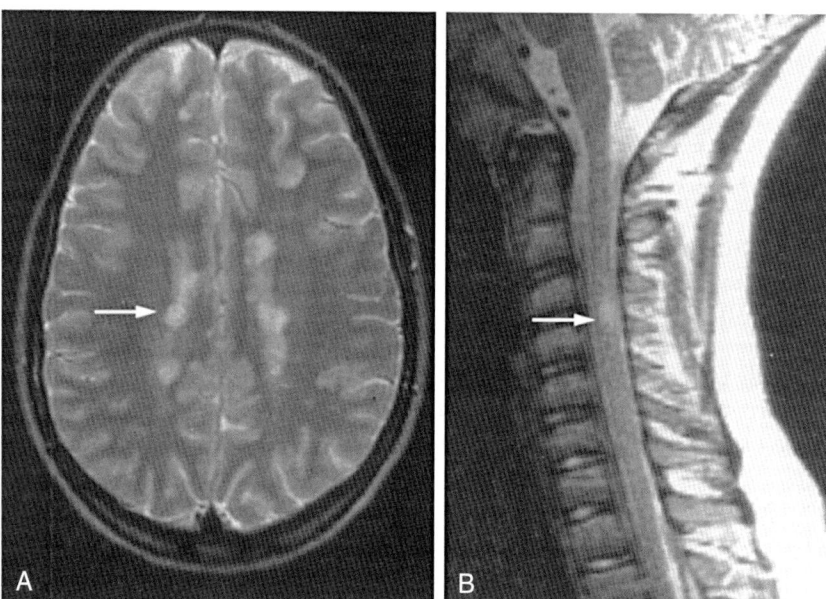

Fig. 36.5 Multiple sclerosis. (A) MRI scan of brain demonstrates multiple lesions located in the white matter characteristic of multiple sclerosis *(arrow)*. (B) MRI scan of spine indicates a demyelinating plaque of multiple sclerosis in the midcervical region *(arrow)*. (From Kliegman RM, Behrman RE, Jenson HB, Stanton BF, eds: *Nelson textbook of pediatrics*, ed 18, Philadelphia, 2007, Saunders.)

and result in extensive loss of function. MRI may show lesions and changes in brain volume.[26]

ETIOLOGY

The specific cause of MS is unknown. Current theories include environmental, immunological, infectious, and genetic factors. Environment is considered a factor because there is a higher incidence of MS among individuals living farther north of the equator. Studies have shown that 30% to 60% of new clinical attacks of the disease occur after a cold, flu, or common viral illness. Genetics plays an important factor, because identical twins have over a 30% chance of developing the disease, whereas an average person in the United States has a 0.1% chance of developing MS.[142]

CLINICAL PICTURE

The symptoms that occur in individuals with MS are related to the area of the CNS affected. These symptoms may include the following[130]:

- Fatigue
- Numbness or weakness in one or more limbs that typically occurs on one side of the body at a time, or the legs and trunk
- Partial or complete loss of vision, usually in one eye at a time, often with pain during eye movement
- Double vision or blurring of vision
- Tingling or pain in parts of the body
- Electric-shock sensations that occur with certain neck movements, especially bending the neck forward
- Tremor, lack of coordination, or unsteady gait
- Slurred speech
- Dizziness
- Problems with bowel and bladder function

Symptoms may temporally worsen when body temperature is elevated but resolve with time. Cognitive deficits are reported to occur in 30% to 70% of persons with MS but do not necessarily correlate with a physical decline.[9,98,128,156] Cognitive deficits have been documented in individuals during early stages of the disease.[200] In advanced stages of the disease process, the individual may have varying degrees of paralysis, from total lower extremity paralysis to involvement of the upper extremities, dysarthria, dysphagia, severe visual impairment, ataxia, spasticity, nystagmus, neurogenic bladder, and impaired cognition.

The course of MS is unpredictable. It is marked by episodes of exacerbation and remission.[156] An **exacerbation** is when symptoms intensify or when new symptoms emerge and may be an episode as minor as fatigue and slight sensory loss or as extensive as total paralysis of all extremities and loss of bladder control.[17] **Remission**, when symptoms diminish or resolve, may involve total resolution of the symptoms, slight return of some function with the symptoms remaining, or a short plateau in which no new symptoms occur but the current symptoms remain.

Four patterns seen in MS are (1) relapsing and remitting, (2) secondary progressive, (3) primary progressive, and (4) progressive relapsing.[151] The relapsing and remitting form of MS involves 85% of the MS population and leads to episodes of exacerbation and remission of symptoms that result in a slow, stepwise progression as the deficits accumulate. The secondary progressive course of the disease begins with a pattern of **relapses** and remissions but evolves into the progressive form of the disease given time. Before the introduction of disease-modifying drugs, approximately 50% of clients with relapsing and remitting MS progressed to the secondary progressive form of the disease. Marguerite, introduced in the beginning of this chapter, was first diagnosed with the relapsing and remitting form of MS and was later diagnosed with the secondary progressive course of the disease. She is now experiencing sustained diminished fine motor abilities and sensation in her left hand. She also has weakness in one lower extremity, requiring the use of an ankle-foot orthosis and a quad cane.

Although not as common as adult-onset MS, childhood MS does occur, and children account for 3% to 10% of the MS population.[76,174] Of children with MS, 95% initially experience a relapsing and remitting course of the disease. Over time, secondary progressive MS will develop in approximately 60% of children.[218]

The primary progressive form of MS (10% of the MS population) is distinguished by a downward course with episodes of exacerbations or remissions. Individuals with this form eventually become nonambulatory and incontinent of urine and may have dysphagia and dysarthria, severely compromised lower extremity function, and varying limitations in upper extremity function. These individuals have difficulty remaining in the workforce and require more assistance with ADLs.

The progressive relapsing form of MS is the least common of the four types of MS. This type of MS accounts for approximately 5% of the MS population. These individuals experience a steady worsening of symptoms but with episodes of exacerbations.[225]

Kaufman and colleagues found that individuals with MS typically live 6 years less than those without MS.[109] Approximately 50% of individuals with MS live for at least 30 years after onset of the disease, and 50% die of complications of MS. Most people with MS will live to experience other changes related to normal aging, which can complicate the clinical picture. Typically, the course of the disease can generally be determined after 5 years of the initial symptoms (Box 36.2).

MEDICAL MANAGEMENT

Medical management depends on the type of MS. Disease-modifying drugs are used in those with relapsing and remitting MS, and for all forms of the disease antiinflammatories are used to treat exacerbations.[156] The antiinflammatory medications, such as prednisone and methylprednisolone, help reduce

symptoms and shorten the duration of the exacerbation.[38,130] For the relapsing and remitting form of MS, disease-modifying medications are thought to have an effect in slowing progression of the disease. These medications are available in injectable, oral, and infusible forms. Clients treated with these medications, administered by self-injection, showed a one-third reduction in frequency of exacerbations. Studies regarding the effectiveness of these medications in individuals with the progressive form of the disease are ongoing. The physician and patient determine which is the most appropriate form of treatment. It is important for the OT practitioner to understand that some individuals experience side effects from the medications, which affect function for a day or so following application.

Medical management primarily focuses on treating the symptoms of the disease. Symptom management includes treatment of spasticity, bladder management, prevention of bladder infection, and management of pain and fatigue. Symptom-specific medications may be prescribed. The OT practitioner can learn more specifically about all of the medications from the MS Society medication site.[150] Spasticity is often managed with medications; unfortunately, this may also worsen the muscle weakness. Bladder management may involve the use of incontinence pads or catheters, along with prevention of bladder infections. Fatigue should be managed with good nutrition, prevention of over-fatigue with energy-conservation methods, regular exercise, establishment of routines for rest and sleep, and control of stress; in addition, several medications are available that may help with fatigue.[151] The ADL evaluation for Marguerite should include questions about bowel and bladder management and how it affects her function at work, at home, and during sleep.

Changes in cognition and mood often occur in persons with MS.[53,60,98] The volume of lesions seen on MRI correlates with cognitive decline in the areas of complex attention, processing speed, and verbal memory.[209] One investigation evaluated overall brain atrophy and size of the ventricles in relation to cognitive abilities. The results suggested a relationship between an increase in the size of the third ventricle and a decrease in cognition.[26]

BOX 36.2 Predictors of Poor or Favorable Prognosis at the Onset of Multiple Sclerosis

Predictors of a Poor Prognosis
- Progressive course
- Age at onset older than 40 years
- Cerebellar involvement
- Polysymptomatic onset
- Male sex

Predictors of a Favorable Prognosis
- Minimal disability 5 years after onset of the disease
- Complete, rapid remission of the initial symptoms
- Age at onset younger than 40 years
- Only one symptom during the first year
- Onset with sensory symptom or mild optic neuritis

From Multiple sclerosis and the aging process, *Formulary* 40(11):S17, 2005. Formulary is a copyright publication of Advanstar Communications, Inc. dba UBM, LLC.

ETHICAL CONSIDERATIONS

Consider the following situation: a client with MS is able to drive the car but has cognitive deficits that are exacerbated by fatigue in the afternoon. Because the client has discontinued work, the family members do not want to take away driving privileges as well. However, by continuing to drive, the client places self and others at risk for injury. The OT may need to educate the family about the deficits by providing examples of the ways in which cognition is evaluated and by discussing the ways in which cognitive deficits affect driving and other daily activities. The OT is responsible for reporting the driving risk to the client's physician.

Emotional changes such as depression also may be present. Persons with MS and other chronic conditions experience a higher rate of depression than the general population.[105,151] Depression may have different causes and should be assessed by the team. Depression may be caused by a physiological response to the disease process, may be a psychological response to the diagnosis, or might be a side effect of one of the disease-modifying medications.[105] Depression may occur at any stage of the disease process. It should be addressed promptly because it may contribute to fatigue and an inability to cope with challenges and make adaptations as needed.[151]

The most widely accepted tool to measure clinical impairment in a person with MS is the Expanded Disability Status Scale (EDSS).[168] The EDSS combines an assessment of neurological function and a scale to measure a client's ambulatory and functional mobility status. There are limitations with this tool; it does not allow specific assessment of all ADLs and is not sensitive to potential cognitive and sexual deficits in MS.[168] The OT practitioner should be familiar with the EDSS because it is often mentioned in the literature as a baseline for evaluating disability.[233] The MS Functional Composite was developed to measure leg function and ambulation, arm and hand function, and cognition.[45,152,221] It can be used for periodic baseline function and may be more sensitive for use as baseline cognitive evaluation than the EDSS.

ROLE OF THE OCCUPATIONAL THERAPIST

OT practitioners provide services for persons with MS in a number of settings. The type and degree of intervention provided will be determined by the setting, the type of reimbursement, and the client's and caregiver's responses to intervention. Preissner provides an overview of the OT role for persons with MS. This reference is a starting point for the beginning practitioner.[179]

Evaluation includes an occupational profile to guide the evaluation process. The OT then selects the necessary instruments to assess occupational performance of ADLs, IADL education, work, play, leisure, and social participation. During the performance of various occupations, the following skills should be evaluated: motor and praxis, sensory-perceptual, emotional regulation, cognitive, and communication skills. This is generally accomplished with a combination of standardized and nonstandardized assessments, through the use of interviews with the family and client, and by observation. The MS Society recommends a number of standardized evaluations appropriate for the OT evaluation.[152] Optimally, a home evaluation should be completed. Because not all settings allow a home evaluation, the OT should interview the client and caregiver regarding the home environment and potential barriers. MS has an unpredictable course and the client may need referral for other resources and will benefit from periodic reevaluation by an OT.[15] If the client has a cognitive deficit, a family member or significant other should be included in the evaluation process to provide accurate information, if the client allows. It is essential that actual performance evaluations be used for persons with MS because studies have shown that self-report is frequently inaccurate.[83] Understanding the client's cultural, social, and spiritual perspective will provide insight into available support systems and their impact on the client's adaptation to the disability.

Assessment of sensorimotor skills is discussed thoroughly in previous chapters. Because endurance and fatigue are such significant factors, it is important to not rely solely on the results of assessment of a specific client factor. For example, a manual muscle test is not likely to accurately reflect the degree of weakness experienced throughout the day. Observing a client performing a functional activity over a certain period or gathering information about the client's daily activity patterns will provide the clinician with a more accurate evaluation of fatigue.[92] The National Multiple Sclerosis Society recommends use of the Modified Fatigue Scale (MFS) or the Fatigue Questionnaire to understand specific problems resulting from fatigue.[151] In Marguerite's case, the MFS assessment may help determine the impact of fatigue on her daily activities.

When evaluating a client's activity patterns, the OT practitioner should also ask about sleep patterns because sleep difficulties are often seen in persons with MS.[2] Disrupted sleep patterns sometimes contribute to fatigue in the MS population. The information can be shared with the client's physician so that appropriate intervention can be undertaken to address the habits and routines that may contribute to the client's disrupted sleep.[2] Marguerite's OT practitioner may ask whether toileting issues also disrupt sleep.

MS may also affect visual abilities, and compromises may be noted in visual tracking, scanning, and acuity. An objective evaluation will help determine the type of deficits, when the deficits occur, and more specifically how they affect ADLs and IADLs.

Perceptual processing and cognitive status should be reassessed periodically. The data gathered will help identify specific deficits and their potential impact on functional activities so that the OT practitioner can incorporate this information into family training.[155] Cognitive deficits vary from a slight decrease in short-term memory and attention span to poor orientation and severely impaired short-term memory. The literature is mixed on the relationship between cognitive deficits and the degree of physical deficits.[51] Assumptions should not be made regarding the presence or absence of cognitive deficits based on physical deficits or abilities or on an individual's basic social skills. A person with significant physical deficits may have fewer cognitive deficits than an ambulatory person with MS. The client's perceptual and cognitive deficits are factors that must be considered when deciding whether the client needs close, constant supervision or can stay home alone. Various standardized cognitive and perceptual assessments are included in previous chapters of this text. Basso developed a screening tool for cognitive dysfunction in individuals with MS. Basso's tool was found to be both sensitive to functional impairment and cost-effective.[22] OTs or practitioners in other disciplines can use this tool when evaluating a person with MS for cognitive deficits. ADLs may be evaluated using AMPS[54] or other standardized assessments for ADLs.[16]

Marguerite's OT should consider completing a cognitive screening or, as appropriate, a full cognitive evaluation. Compensation for mild cognitive deficits may contribute to fatigue. If the results of the cognitive screen indicate deficits, Marguerite may also benefit from a full cognitive assessment administered by a psychologist or neuropsychologist to help her better understand deficits and obtain a baseline of her current cognitive abilities. These assessments could help Marguerite receive disability benefits if her MS deficits progress to the point at which she is unable to work. The OT practitioner should also teach compensatory strategies for cognitive deficits along with how fatigue may contribute to cognitive difficulties. Bonzano and associates[31] found that adaptive memory training produced changes in brain activity for clients with MS.

Evaluation of the cultural, social, and physical environment is important to consider with each client. MS is usually identified during the phase of life in which a person is raising a family and developing a career, as was seen with Marguerite. Because the disease is unpredictable and fluctuating, it leads to disruptions in normal daily activities and in family life. These disruptions create stress for the spouse or partner, children, and other family members. The OT must determine the type of support the client can expect from family members. The therapist may recommend that Marguerite begin to teach her teenage children to help prepare dinner as an energy-conservation technique.

The occupational performance assessment should include listening to the client and family members describe performance patterns to identify the activity demands, typical daily habits, routines, and roles. Assessment and treatment should also focus on the client's engagement in the occupations and the impact on life, sense of self-identity, and sense of competency.[119]

Evaluating and treating the client at different times during the day will often reflect different levels of fatigue. Understanding the performance patterns of rest periods; quality and amount of sleep; exercise patterns; intensity of activity (activity demands) during various times of the day, week, or month; and the time of the day when activities are most challenging is critical in developing treatment planning strategies. Understanding the performance patterns may help the OT practitioner understand how the side effects of the disease-modifying medications affect activity and also how to encourage integrating use of the medication into daily routines while managing side effects.

Emotional and behavioral issues vary depending on the premorbid personality, progression of the disease, coping skills, and social environment of the person with MS. Cognitive deficits and denial of the progressive nature of the disease may create safety issues for the client, given the unpredictable nature of MS. If family members do not understand or recognize the client's behavioral problems, further complications may arise when the behavior is not restricted or modified by the family. Other emotional and cognitive issues include a client who is depressed or labile, has poor memory, refuses assistance from outside caregivers, or uses poor judgment regarding safety with medications and transfers. Each client demonstrates a unique set of behavioral issues and requires individual evaluation and an intervention approach that encompasses the client and caregivers.

GOAL SETTING AND INTERVENTION

For a client with a progressive disease such as MS, goal setting focuses on the client's need to adapt as the disability progresses and during the relapse phases. Goal setting should be client centered and client driven, and it should be short term

with follow-up provided and focused on self-directed participation.[1,15,107] Families often need to negotiate role changes to accommodate the person with MS who may not be able to participate consistently in a previously established family role. For example, with Marguerite's family, her husband may consider taking over the job of grocery shopping. Marguerite and her children can add items to a phone application that allows her husband to have a comprehensive grocery list. Hwang and colleagues found that support from family and friends helped clients adjust to the diagnosis, maintain their health, and participate in productive and social activities.[97] The client's ability to adapt depends on the family's and client's acknowledgment of deficits and willingness to consider alternatives. OT intervention may include (1) problem-solving compensatory strategies,[98] (2) fatigue management group treatment intervention,[65,92,241,242] including habits to support sleep,[2] (3) role delegation,[1] and (4) the use of adaptive equipment to compensate for motor, sensory, endurance, cognitive, and visual deficits.[10,19,137,167] The National Multiple Sclerosis Society has developed guidelines and recommendations for care at home that address many ADLs issues requiring OT treatment. These guidelines are by no means all-encompassing regarding interventions for ADLs and IADLs but provide a solid starting point to problem-solve with the patient and family.[155] For specific techniques related to the individual's deficits, see Chapter 10.

Marguerite may be referred to an OT group designed for persons who have MS to learn fatigue management techniques and sleep strategies.[2,129] The fatigue management group intervention may involve analyzing daily and weekly routines to identify activities that can be eliminated, modified, or delegated. Marguerite may be asked to set short-term realistic goals. She may consider grocery shopping online or delegating this task to her husband. Marguerite will need to evaluate the number of activities in which her teenagers participate and the possibility of carpooling so her teenage children can participate in various activities. She may need adaptive equipment for activities that require bilateral strength and dexterity because of the loss of sensation and dexterity in her left hand. Because Marguerite is receptive to potential home modifications, she and her husband can work with the OT practitioner to determine the most important immediate changes and future changes that may be needed. Long-term changes and home modifications should be discussed in light of her MS diagnosis being changed from relapsing and remitting to secondary progressive.

The benefits of an exercise program should be discussed with clients who have MS. The OT role may develop an exercise program and involve the clients with fatigue management issues to fit the exercise program into their usual routine.[92,195] Fatigue management recommendations should include assessment of the client's typical exercise routine. It has long been thought that exercise will exacerbate and worsen symptoms, but recent studies report benefits such as improved quality of life, reduced fatigue, and improved ambulation from a regular exercise program.[84,140,158] Bonzano and associates[32] found active exercise routines of three times per week for 8 weeks actually enhanced functional brain reorganization.

As a method of learning coping strategies, Marguerite may benefit from attending a cognitive-behavioral therapy (CBT) support group. Evidence shows that participation in CBT may help with depression, which is common among individuals with MS.[241,242]

SECTION 4 SUMMARY

Because MS affects each person in a unique way, an individualized evaluation is essential to determine the client's deficits and strengths. Individuals with MS may range from being ambulatory with limited symptoms, primarily fatigue and energy management issues, to partially limited in mobility and hand function, to using a wheelchair and needing assistance with ADLs. Working with clients who have MS requires the OT practitioner to use expertise in evaluation and intervention from all areas of occupational performance. A comprehensive evaluation will include the occupational status of ADLs/IADLs, rest and sleep, health management, work, leisure, social participation, along with the performance patterns and skills and client factors of sensorimotor, visual-perceptual, and cognitive and depression screens. The social, cultural, and physical environment also must be considered. Because Marguerite's occupational profile indicates many areas are affected by her MS symptoms, the therapist may ask her to prioritize them. If her husband is present, he may also prioritize the issues he sees as most problematic.

With a pattern of relapses and remissions over the course of the disease process, development of an OT intervention plan is particularly challenging. The OT practitioner should know the client's specific type of MS diagnosis, because this will drive the clinical interventions. If the client has the relapsing/remitting form of MS and is currently experiencing a relapse, minimal changes to the home environment may be made, as the client is expected to improve. If an individual has progressive MS or secondary progressive MS, the OT practitioner may strongly recommend more extensive home modifications such as a roll-in shower. Because the client may expect return of function, he or she may deny deficits and refuse to adapt to a change in status; this attitude can create safety problems. The OT practitioner focuses on assessing the current level of functioning and the best methods for the client to adapt to current changes in status.[180,182] The OT may also assist the family in making long-range, realistic plans. For example, if the family is planning to remodel the bathroom, the therapist may encourage consideration of a roll-in shower and not just a standard shower stall with a shower seat.

As with the other progressive neurological conditions, working with clients who have MS requires a multidisciplinary approach. In addition to the OT, a physician, physical therapist, registered nurse, social worker, and psychologist may be involved as team members. Because the social environment may create complex and difficult problems, good communication among all team members is needed to ensure that the team goals are congruous. The OT has a unique perspective to offer the team regarding the client's strengths and weaknesses when cognitive, perceptual, psychosocial, and motor abilities are assessed and treated in a functional context.

SECTION 5: PARKINSON'S DISEASE

Winifred Schultz-Krohn and Katrina Long

PREVALENCE

Parkinson's disease (PD) is one of the most common adult-onset, degenerative neurological disorders, second only to AD.[73,166] PD affects multiple systems, including physical, mental, and behavioral, and as a result produces both motor and non-motor symptoms.[124] Three classic motor symptoms associated with PD include tremor, rigidity, and bradykinesia. There are over 10 million people living with PD worldwide.[166] Prevalence increases with age, but approximately 3% of all PD cases are initially recognized in individuals younger than 50 years of age.[203] Diagnosis is most often made after the age of 60. Approximately 10% to 30% of clients with PD report first-degree relatives who also have PD. Sex differences have been noted; the prevalence of PD is 1.5 times higher in men than in women of the same age.

The cause for PD has not been definitively established.[21,82] Previous literature referred to familial and sporadic forms of PD, but those distinctions are being revised in light of current genetic research. Although a positive family history has been established as a risk factor for PD, a single predictive genetic marker has not been absolutely identified. To date, mutations have been found in several genes that are associated with PD and include alpha-synuclein, parkin, ubiquitin carboxyl terminal hydrolase, SCA2, and DJ-1.[203] These mutations have been found to have a role in abnormal protein processing in cells.[21] Current genetic work has identified a gene mutation in familial PD, and this genetic mutation also has been identified in clients with sporadic PD, providing further evidence of a genetic determination for this disease process.[203] Genetic causes explain 3% to 5% of PD in most populations, and 90 genetic risk variants together explain 16% to 36% of the heritable risk.[28]

Previously, environmental factors were considered as a possible cause of PD.[82] The possibility of an exogenous agent's producing PD gained considerable recognition when narcotic addicts began using 1-methyl-4-phenyl-1,2,3,6-tetrahydropyridine (MPTP). After using MPTP, many addicts quickly exhibited parkinsonism that "strictly mimics the clinical and anatomic features of PD."[82] Other factors, such as environmental pesticides and metal elements factors, have not been completely eliminated as contributing factors in the cause of PD; these appear to play less of a role when compared to various genetic mutations.[226]

PATHOPHYSIOLOGY

The neurological structure associated with PD is the substantia nigra, specifically the pars compacta portion, located within the basal ganglia.[159] The basal ganglia mainly helps with the planning, preparation, initiation, and sequencing of movements. The pars compacta receives input from other basal ganglia nuclei and appears to serve as a modulator of striatal activity.[171] This system is responsible for the coordination of smooth balanced movements and is also involved in learning, memory, and motivation.[124,131] Nerve cells in the substantia nigra generate the neurotransmitter dopamine and are responsible for sending messages that plan and control body movement. The substantia nigra nuclei undergo significant deterioration as the disease progresses. Hence, progressive malfunctioning of this system results in the motor impairments seen in PD, including bradykinesia, rest tremor, and rigidity. The significant reduction in the dopaminergic neurons in the substantia nigra pars compacta produces a decrease in activity within the basal ganglia and an overall "reduction in spontaneous movement."[171] The substantia nigra serves as one of the major output nuclei for the basal ganglia to other structures.[165] Dopamine also has a role in other cognitive processes, including drive and motivation, mood, maintaining and switching attention, visual perception, problem-solving, and decision-making.[33,162,236]

In addition to the loss of dopaminergic neurons, intracytoplasmic inclusions are found on postmortem examination within the substantia nigra.[159] These intracytoplasmic inclusions are also known as Lewy bodies.[89] Although the greatest amount of neurodegeneration is found in the pars compacta substantia nigra, destruction of other neurological structures has been reported.[159] Deterioration is also seen in the remainder of the substantia nigra, locus ceruleus, nucleus basalis, and hypothalamus. It is suspected that there are additional changes in associated brain regions and in other neurotransmitters, such as glutamate, GABA, noradrenaline, and serotonin.[70]

CLINICAL PICTURE

PD is characterized as a slowly progressive, degenerative movement disorder.[89,171] The diagnosis of PD is usually made after the age of 55. Although PD is not considered fatal, the degeneration of various neurological structures may severely compromise performance of functional tasks over time. An extensive longitudinal study over 12 years investigated potential changes in life expectancy for those diagnosed with PD.[55] Those diagnosed with PD at 65 years old had a reduced life expectancy of approximately 6 years compared to peers, but those diagnosed with PD at 85 years old had a reduced life expectancy of approximately 1 year compared to peers. A person diagnosed with PD may live an additional 20 to 30 years, with a progressive loss of motor function that eventually requires specialized care.[89] In addition to motor symptoms, there is a substantial number of nonmotor symptoms associated with PD, some of which manifest before motor symptoms. Most individuals experience just a few of the nonmotor symptoms. The most commonly reported and troublesome nonmotor symptoms include autonomic failure, continence problems, sexual health issues, fatigue, pain, sleep and nighttime problems, cognitive changes, emotional and neuropsychiatric problems, and dementia.[13,89] Motor symptoms will be discussed in detail, followed by a description of the nonmotor symptoms, and then the stages of progression.

PD is characterized by dysfunction in both voluntary and involuntary movements.[171] A classic triad of motor symptoms includes tremor, rigidity, and disorder of voluntary movements (Fig. 36.6). Motor symptoms are typically seen clinically after 60% of dopaminergic cells have deteriorated in the substantia nigra.[203] Disturbances in voluntary movement are identified as

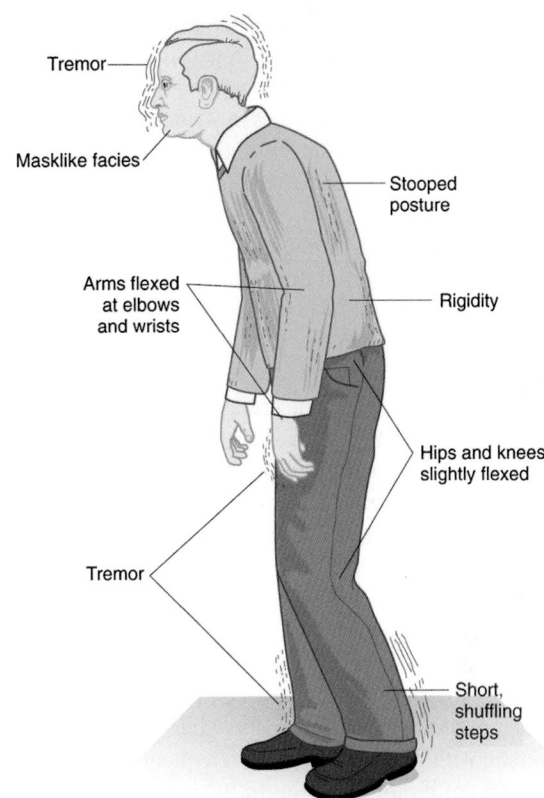

Fig. 36.6 Symptoms and signs of Parkinson's disease. (From Davis K, Guerra A: *Mosby's pharmacy technician: principles and practice*, ed 6, St. Louis, 2022, Elsevier.)

difficulty initiating movement (**akinesia**) and slowness in maintaining movement (bradykinesia). Bradykinesia and akinesia are often the most disabling motor symptoms for the client with PD.[52] The delay in initiating movement patterns and the slowness in executing the motion compromise functional tasks such as driving, dressing, and eating. In addition, akinesia causes people with PD to often develop **hypomimia**, also known as masked facies, which is the loss of facial expressions.[85] Because of decreased speed and coordination of the facial musculature, hypomimia restricts the accurate expression of emotion, which can have an impact on communication for people with PD. Initially decreased facial expressions are seen unilaterally, but as the disease progresses, diminished spontaneous facial expressions are seen bilaterally. Respiratory support is diminished and speech volume is decreased and persons with PD seem to whisper. Articulation is imprecise and speech prosody and intonations are substantially reduced often resulting in monotone speech. Dysphagia tends to occur in the later stages of PD, and clients may be at risk for choking and aspiration pneumonia from dysphagia.

Rigidity is the stiffness within a muscle that impedes smooth movement. This stiffness occurs in both directions for each plane of motion at a specific joint.[181] The characteristic **resting tremor** with a rate between 4 and 5 Hz is a disturbance of involuntary movement.[136] This tremor often diminishes with activity, but in some clients the tremor persists during performance of functional activities.

Additional symptoms of PD are disturbances in gait and postural reactions.[81,171] Deterioration in gait is seen throughout the course of the disease.[192] Initially, gait may be fairly normal, but as the disease progresses, changes in stride length and speed of gait are apparent. The characteristic festinating gait is often seen; as the client walks, the stride length decreases in length and the speed slightly increases, creating a shuffling effect. A reduced arm swing during ambulation is evident, and trunk rotation is markedly decreased during walking. Another motor disturbance associated with gait is the phenomenon of "freezing."[77] Freezing occurs when the person ceases to move, often after attempting to initiate, maintain, or alter a movement pattern. During gait, freezing may be seen as the client attempts to change directions or approach a narrow hallway or stairs. As the client attempts to alter the trajectory of walking to turn to enter another room, he or she may cease moving. Freezing also can be seen during other motor tasks, such as writing, brushing teeth, and speaking.

Postural abnormalities associated with PD include a flexed, stooped posture with the head positioned forward.[141] The client tends to stand with flexion at the knees and hips. In addition to the stooped posture, balance reactions are compromised.[177] Righting and equilibrium reactions are markedly reduced in effectiveness, and the person with PD may experience frequent falls.

A common nonmotor symptom in PD is pain, with moderate to severe pain being reported in half the patients during the disease course. Intense and persistent pain is sometimes attributed to muscle rigidity or dystonic muscle cramp (dystonia). Areas commonly affected include the foot, lower back, or one side of the neck (cervical dystonia).

Emotional and neuropsychiatric problems are other important nonmotor symptoms to consider, and include anxiety, depression, apathy, irritability, and psychosis.[81,171] Approximately 50% of individuals with diagnosed PD exhibit depression,[177] which is not merely reactive to the severity of symptoms or the chronic nature of the disease. The depression seen in individuals with PD appears to be related to a serotonergic deficit, which is similar to that in clients without PD who have depression. Complicating the feature of depression is the decrease in facial expressiveness caused by akinesia and hypomimia, mentioned earlier.[177] Individuals with PD may also self-limit social interaction because they are embarrassed by their decreased facial expressions and movement disorders. Psychosis is also a common complication for clients with PD, and they may experience hallucinations and delusions.[81,89] These disturbances compromise cognitive abilities and often limit functional skills.

Mental status is fairly normal throughout the early stages of PD, but visuospatial perception is often compromised.[177] Higher-order cognitive disorders are common in clients with PD. Clients with PD often have difficulty shifting attention among various stimuli. Processing simultaneous information is often difficult for the individual with PD, and tasks that require a sequential process are somewhat easier to perform. Driving a car presents a particular challenge because it necessitates the processing of multiple forms of information in a simultaneous manner. Some self-care tasks, such as brushing teeth, have a clear sequence that can be followed; these activities can be performed

with less demand on cognitive functioning. Although dementia is seldom seen in clients with an earlier-onset form of PD, approximately one-third of people over 70 years old who have PD display dementia.

Another common nonmotor symptom is autonomic dysfunction (also called dysautonomia), which is dysfunction of the autonomic nervous system (ANS).[177] For example, a person with PD may experience a drop in blood pressure when rising from lying or sitting (known as orthostatic hypotension or postural hypotension).[212] Orthostatic hypotension increases risk of falling, though syncope is rare. In addition, people with PD may experience periods of sweating and abnormal tolerance of heat and cold.[177] People with PD may also have issues with their ability to control bowel and bladder movements (continence), with reduced intestinal motility producing constipation and an increase in the frequency and urgency of urination. There can be an increase in frequency of urine at night (nocturia) and the majority of urine can be passed at night instead of during the day (diurnal bladder rhythm). In addition, when using the toilet, there may be a delay in sphincter response.

Nocturia adds to the list of sleep and nighttime problems that are commonly experienced by people with PD, including insomnia; sleep fragmentation, vivid or disturbing dreams, and restless legs.[13] In addition, they may experience rapid eye movement (REM) sleep behavior disorder (RBD) secondary to brainstem changes that disrupt normal sleep paralysis that occurs when dreaming. This causes dreams to be acted out physically and may result in injuries to the person with PD or the bedpartner.[215] Fatigue is another independent nonmotor symptom that has been associated with sleep disturbances and daytime sleepiness, in addition to apathy, anxiety, and poorer quality of life.[204] Fatigue appears early in the disease and is persistent. Sexual health issues, including reduced libido or erectile dysfunction, are other impactful nonmotor symptoms in PD.[34] Hypersexuality may develop as a side effect of some anti-Parkinson's medications and is estimated to occur in about 3.5% of people with PD.[44]

The course of the disease varies from person to person, but the first clinical symptom identified is typically a motor symptom, such as unilateral resting tremor in the hand.[136] Hoehn and Yahr[94] established a scale identifying the progression of motor symptoms in PD. The Hoehn and Yahr (H&Y) scale[94] is a commonly used system for describing the stages of PD and consists of five stages (Table 36.4). Although symptoms typically get worse over time, not everyone with PD progresses to H&Y stage 5.

A client at H&Y stage 1 exhibits unilateral involvement, typically a hand tremor, but no impairment of functional abilities is reported. A client is able to complete personal ADLs and IADLs, but performance often requires additional effort and energy. Depending on job demands, a client with PD at stage 1 is often employed but may require modifications to the worksite. During this stage the client's handwriting may become very small, with letters that are cramped together. This change in handwriting is referred to as micrographia.[89] The client may also complain of muscle cramping when required to write for extended periods. Slight rigidity may be seen when the client is asked to rapidly open and close the involved hand.

TABLE 36.4 **Progression of Symptoms in Parkinson's Disease**		
Stage	Symptoms	OT Management
1	Unilateral tremor, micrographia, poor endurance for previous occupations, fatigue	Work evaluation if client is employed; work simplification for work and home settings; develop the habit of taking frequent rest breaks; use of utensils with enlarged handles
2	Bilateral motor disturbances, mild rigidity reported, difficulties with simultaneous tasks, difficulties with executive function	Energy conservation techniques related to ADLs; develop daily flexibility exercises focused on trunk rotation; driving assessment and alternatives for community mobility, use of task analysis to structure sequential tasks
3	Balance problems with delayed reactions, difficulties with skilled sequential tasks	Environmental modifications in the home, including raised toilet seats, chairs with armrests, removal of throw rugs; use of visual cues and supports for sequential tasks
4	Fine motor control severely compromised, oral motor deficits	Modifications to support participation in self-care tasks, changes in food textures
5	Client severely compromised in regard to motor skills, dependent with ADLs	Use of environmental controls to allow access to environment

ADLs, Activities of daily living.

Stage 2 denotes a progression of symptoms and the development of bilateral motor disturbances.[94] Although the course of PD is variable, this stage is usually seen 1 to 2 years after initial diagnosis. Even though tremors or rigidity may be noted bilaterally, the client can still perform ADL skills. Performance of IADL skills may require modification because of motor difficulties. Work, depending on the job requirements, often requires additional modifications, and the client may require several rest breaks during the day. The client should make decisions at this point regarding the benefits of remaining employed relative to the energy expenditures. Posture becomes slightly stooped, with flexion at the knees and hips. The person with stage 2 PD is still able to ambulate independently.

As PD progresses to stage 3, the client experiences delayed righting and equilibrium reactions. Balance is impaired; the client has difficulty performing daily tasks that require standing, such as showering and meal preparation. Employment may be difficult because of its energy demands. Safety in walking is a concern because of the client's reduced balance, and home modifications are necessary at this stage. A person with stage 4 PD has significant deficits in completing daily living tasks. The client is still able to ambulate at this stage, but motor control is severely compromised and negatively affects dressing, feeding, and hygiene skills. Stage 5 is the final stage of PD. The client is typically confined to a wheelchair or bed and depends on others for most self-care activities. The rate of progression through these stages varies from person to person, but PD is a slowly progressive disorder.

The extent of PD symptoms in individual clients has been measured using the UPDRS.[63] This scale evaluates a client's motor skills, functional status, and extent of disability. Motor skills are evaluated by a trained observer.[189] The functional status and extent of disability are measured through a client interview that includes items addressing ADL skills and cognitive and emotional factors.[123] This instrument has been used for research and clinical practice to measure the effectiveness of various interventions in reducing PD symptoms (see Table 36.4).

MEDICAL MANAGEMENT

The most frequently used medical management strategy for PD is the provision of a dopamine agonist to make up for the depletion of dopamine caused by the destruction of the substantia nigra.[193] Levodopa is the medication most commonly used in the treatment of PD.[176] This oral medication is actually a precursor to dopamine because dopamine is too large to cross the blood-brain barrier. Levodopa provides substantial relief from tremors and rigidity during the initial stages of PD. After approximately 5 to 10 years of chronic use of levodopa, motor side effects are reported.[177] Those most often reported are dyskinesias and motor fluctuations. This "on-off" phenomenon is related to the levodopa dosage. A decrease in tremors and rigidity occurs during the "on" period after administration of levodopa, but the client may also experience various dyskinesias, such as abnormal movements of the limbs. As the dosage of levodopa wears off, the motor symptoms, specifically tremors and rigidity associated with PD, return.

Timing of the medication and the periods of "on-off" are important considerations in planning the client's daily activities. Even though abnormal movements are observed during the "on" period, the client has greater freedom of movement to complete functional activities.

As PD progresses, control of various motor symptoms through the use of levodopa becomes less effective.[177] Deep brain stimulation has been used for decades to reduce the tremors and motor fluctuations associated with PD.[64,78,126] This process involves surgically inserting electrodes into a specific portion of the brain, typically the thalamus, subthalamic nucleus, or the internal globus palliudus. Using a remote device, specific stimulation is provided to the brain to reduce tremors, rigidity, slow movements and festinating gait. It does not reverse or slow the progression of the disease but minimizes the motor problems that can no longer be managed using medications.[64,78,89,126] Surgical intervention, known as **stereotactic surgery**, has been used in the past to lesion portions of the globus pallidus and subthalamic nucleus to decrease the severity of PD symptoms. Stereotactic surgery decreased the severity of motor symptoms associated with PD and thus reduced the needed dosage of levodopa.[159] A noninvasive procedure uses magnetic resonance (MR) guided focused ultrasound to create specific lesions in portions of the ventral intermediate nucleus of the thalamus, the subthalamic nucleus, and the internal globus pallidus.[138] These lesions reduce the tremors and rigidity associated with PD.

ROLE OF THE OCCUPATIONAL THERAPIST

OT services vary depending on the client's stage of PD. Typically an OT program would provide compensatory strategies, client and family education, environmental and task modifications, and community involvement. It is at the earlier, less severe stages of PD (H&Y stage 1 and 2) that the importance of exercise is emphasized for its potential neuroprotective, neurorestorative, and disease-modifying effects.[71,199] Although OT services have been shown to be beneficial, there are still inconsistent referrals to provide OT services to those who have PD,[186] and most referrals for OT treatment are made later in the disease stage when occupational performance dysfunction is most apparent and problematic. More recently, OT has a clear role addressing health-related quality of life for clients with PD and their caregivers.[101] In a multisite randomized control trial, Sturkenboom and colleagues provided 10 weeks of OT for 124 clients diagnosed with PD.[211] A control group of 67 clients with PD served as the comparison for the investigation. The Canadian Occupational Performance Measure (COPM) was used as both the assessment and outcome measure for this investigation. Following the 10 weeks of intervention, those who received OT services had significant improvements when compared to the control group for "self-perceived performance on prioritised activities." This multisite investigation provided strong evidence of the effectiveness of OT services in fostering functional, self-identified activities.

During the initial stages of the disease, the OT should develop an occupational profile with the client and significant others to establish intervention priorities.[190] Clients have expressed the desire to retain a sense of self and normalcy within their family, even in the face of deteriorating abilities. The focus of intervention is developing the habits and routines to foster participation in desired occupations as the disease process progresses. Educating the client and significant others regarding the course of the disease is an important step in this process, one that aids in the selection of occupations. For example, the case study at the end of this section introduces Carl, who identifies as male (prefers use of the pronouns he/his/him). He identified traveling and painting as important occupations, and interventions were designed to help him continue participating in these occupations as the disease progressed.

During the early stages of the disease, the client and family should be informed of community resources and support groups. In one study, clients with PD were found to be far more dependent on others for personal care and household activities than were same-age peers without PD.[166] This dependence can place additional stress on the family. Involvement in a community-based group may provide the support needed to accommodate the changes in family roles and interaction.[190]

Even during the early stages of the disease process, clients with PD have difficulties with executive functioning.[69] An investigation by Foster and Hershey compared clients who had PD, but no dementia, with age-matched controls on several assessments of executive functioning. Clients with PD included in this investigation were in stage 1 or 2. Clients with PD performed significantly worse on working memory and executive functioning compared to age-matched controls. Furthermore, lower executive functioning "was associated with reduced activity after controlling for motor dysfunction and depressive symptoms." The authors urge OT to assess executive functioning even during the early stages of PD and develop strategies to support client participation in desired occupations.

Modification of household items may decrease the impact of tremors during the initial stage of the disease process. Built-up handles for eating and writing utensils should be introduced during the initial stages of PD. Handwriting often becomes small and difficult to read during the initial stage of PD. Time management techniques should be introduced at this stage. Paying bills, signing forms, or doing other written work should be completed soon after taking levodopa, using utensils with built-up handles. Even though tremors are not severe during the early stages of PD, clothing fasteners should be modified. The use of slip-on shoes or Velcro closures for clothing should be considered at this time. Although a client may be able to fasten clothing during this stage of PD, the OT must consider the amount of energy and time needed to perform such a task.

Hand function for the client with PD is often difficult, and OT services can substantially improve dexterity.[72] Franciotta and associates completed a pretest/posttest investigation of 482 clients with PD and revealed the gains that could be achieved with daily OT services over a 4-week period. Clients were divided by H&Y scale, and all pretest scores on standardized assessments of dexterity and hand function were significantly lower compared to posttest scores. The OT services provided specifically focused on functional hand use.

In addition to the modification of specific tasks, household changes should be made at this time. Loose rugs should be removed from floors and furniture placed close to the wall to decrease obstacles. Chairs should have armrests to allow the client to push up from the chair to stand. Although balance is not significantly compromised during the early stages of PD, the family and client should become familiar with the new arrangement of furniture before this becomes a necessity. Bath and toilet railings and a raised toilet seat should be provided within the home. Because fatigue is a common complaint, clients should develop the habit of taking frequent breaks during the day. Modifying the household setting early in the course of PD allows the client and family members to adjust to changes and incorporate these changes into daily routines before they become a necessity.

A work evaluation should be performed during the early stage of the disease process to assess safety risks, potential hazards, and work simplification techniques that could be used. An ergonomic assessment of the worksite and modifications to the tools would be appropriate. In the case of Carl, computer modifications were considered. A client may have the option of reducing the number of work hours, but that decision may reduce medical benefits. These decisions and available options are part of the OT intervention process during the early stage of the disease.

An important area to address within health management is participation in physical activity. In particular, exercise can be an effective adjunctive treatment to lessen both cognitive and motor symptoms in PD.[30] Isolated benefits from aerobic exercise, stretching, and resistance training have shown functional improvements in mobility, ADLs, depression, and reduced rates of falls for persons with PD.[30,61,201,238] Physical activity can produce an array of positive effects in persons with PD, including improvements in motor and mental functions and reduced symptoms of PD.

During the initial stage of PD (H&Y stages 1 and 2), the OT should work with the client to establish a daily exercise routine that includes stretching for full range of motion, resistance exercise, neuromotor balance training, and aerobic exercise.[61,199] The OT must recognize that physical and psychological symptoms of PD create challenges to participation in physical activity. However, the OT practitioner can assist their clients to identify supports and overcome barriers to attain meaningful engagement in physical activity.[121,184]

It is preferable to have a client with PD perform a short exercise program for 5 to 10 minutes daily rather than a longer program three times a week. Exercises should include alternating movements from various planes, because many clients with PD display difficulties with smooth shifting of movements.[125] Postural flexibility exercises should be included in the program, with specific attention given to trunk extension. The most common postural change noted with the progression of PD is a stooped posture. In addition to the flexibility exercises, OTs should instruct clients in the use of relaxation techniques and controlled breathing. Inhaling slowly through the nose and exhaling through pursed lips two or three times in succession, combined with improved postural alignment, can promote relaxation. Swink and associates[214] used a combination of an OT fall prevention programming and yoga with clients for 8 weeks. Each client served as their own control before the initiation of the program and a substantial reduction in falls was noted.

As the disease progresses, additional exercises can improve gait.[216] Rhythmic auditory stimulation in the form of music with an accentuated initial beat has been found to significantly improve stride length and speed in clients with PD. Dancing can also enhance gait patterns, in addition to providing a social environment for the client with PD. As akinesia becomes more apparent, the client with PD should be instructed to use a rocking motion to begin movement activities. Rocking forward and backward a few times while seated can produce the momentum needed to rise from a chair.

As a person with PD progresses to the middle stages of the disease, the client experiences further deterioration of motor skills, particularly the execution of skilled sequential movements.[50] These types of movements are needed to complete personal care and household tasks. Curra and associates[50] found that external cues improved the speed and sequential performance of novel motor tasks. The OT should suggest modifying activities to include visual cues, verbal prompts, and rehearsal of movements. These strategies increase a client's ability to perform personal care and household activities.

During the middle stages of PD, clients may have decreased oral motor control.[177] Dysphagia and drooling may embarrass them and further restrict social engagements. The OT should encourage oral motor exercises and provide education regarding food selection. Food consistencies can be altered to improve the client's ability to eat.

The ability to complete personal care tasks has been identified as a critical variable in a client's perception of quality of life.[67] Although progressive movement problems are characteristic of PD, the OT can minimize the impact the movement disorder has on functional activities. Tremors have less effect on the completion of personal care tasks than compensations for postural instability. The use of group OT sessions has been demonstrated to be effective in reducing the impact of postural instability in clients with PD.[214] An additional benefit of these group sessions is the reported improvement in the perception of quality of life in clients attending the sessions.

Access to community mobility and support programs should be included in the OT intervention plan during the middle stages of PD. A client with PD is often dependent on others for transportation. The use of community mobility services can decrease the client's dependence on family members for shopping and errands.

During the last stages of PD, movement disorders and rigidity may eliminate the client's ability to perform personal care tasks such as dressing and grooming.[94] Depression caused by the decreased ability to perform these tasks can significantly compromise a person's quality of life.[67] OT services should be provided to further modify the home environment for access and control. The use of environmental control units, such as a switch-operated television or radio, can be helpful. The switch plate should be activated with only light touch. Voice- or sound-activated environmental control units may not be as useful because of decreased vocal volume and poor articulation control during speech production. The client's ability to control the immediate environment can compensate for the losses experienced during the final stages of PD. The client may no longer be able to dress himself or herself, but through the use of various switches the client can select preferred television or radio programs, control room lighting, and operate a computer by using minimal motor action.

SECTION 5 SUMMARY

Although PD is a progressive, neurodegenerative disorder, OT has much to offer the client with this disease.[67,72,101,164,214,223,234] The diminishing ability to perform personal care activities and engage in self-selected tasks has been identified as one of the variables contributing to depression and the decreased quality of life in clients with PD. Throughout the progressive course of PD, OT addresses the ability of the client to engage in meaningful activities. The client's wishes and family circumstances are incorporated into the OT intervention plan at every stage of the disease process.

CASE STUDY

Carl

Carl is a 62-year-old college professor diagnosed with PD at the age of 57. Carl identifies as male (prefers use of the pronouns he/his/him). He is married and lives in a small one-story home with his wife. He has two adult children, who live in another state. Carl enjoys traveling, reading, painting, and attending concerts.

Carl recently considered taking early retirement because of the increase in tremors in both of his hands, which made correcting papers difficult. He also reports some problems with endurance as a result of stiffness. Carl indicates that he is no longer able to paint because of the tremors in his hands. He also reports that he is unsure whether he should continue driving because of the tremors.

Results of the OT evaluation indicate that Carl is cooperative and motivated for therapy. Although he does not indicate that he is depressed, his wife notes features of depression, such as a decreased interest in going to concerts and planning summer vacations to see their adult children and grandchildren. His wife also reports that Carl seems depressed about his possible early retirement and loss of status as a college professor.

Carl is able to complete most personal ADLs independently but has difficulties stepping into and out of the tub to shower. His wife reports that she is afraid he will fall and that she often assists him in getting into and out of the shower. Carl also has difficulty tying his shoes and buttoning his shirt. Tremors are noted bilaterally in his hands, and slight rigidity is present during passive range of motion. Dynamic balance is slightly compromised on uneven surfaces and stairs.

Carl has been taking Sinemet (levodopa and carbidopa medication) for the past 3 years to decrease the rigidity and tremors. He does not report any dyskinesias.

When asked about his personal goals, Carl replies, "I guess I'll have more time to read now."

OT was initiated to accomplish the following:

1. Improve ADL performance
   a. Instruct in use of a buttonhook
   b. Make suggestions regarding clothing modifications such as slip-on shoes
   c. Instruct in use of momentum to initiate movement, such as rocking back and forth to rise from a chair
2. Modify home environment
   a. Remove throw rugs and obstacles in walkways
   b. Provide a tub seat and shower extension hose
   c. Provide a raised toilet seat
   d. Provide a cushion on dining room chairs
3. Assess work setting for modifications
   a. Assess for computer access
   b. Instruct in energy conservation, urging him to take frequent breaks and schedule activities during "on" phase of medications
4. Investigate leisure pursuits
   a. Provide modifications to his easel, using forearm supports to allow him to continue to paint
   b. Provide information regarding community-based PD support groups
5. Instruct in a daily active range-of-motion exercise program
   a. Trunk extension and rotation exercises
   b. Bilateral upper extremity exercise
   c. Use of music during exercise program

Carl responded well to OT intervention. Although he was able to complete the academic school year, he decided to retire afterward. He stopped driving, but his wife began to drive them to concerts and art exhibits. He was able to complete personal ADLs safely with the use of adapted equipment and home modifications. He resumed painting during the "on" periods of his medications schedule, using the forearm supports attached to an angled table. He attended a Parkinson's support group two times a week and began to socialize with members from that group. Carl reported that the daily exercises seemed to decrease his stiffness, and he and his wife took frequent strolls in the park when weather permitted. He and his wife also joined a book club.

■ REVIEW QUESTIONS

1. What are the symptoms of ALS at onset?
2. What is the underlying neurological process in ALS?
3. What bodily functions remain intact throughout the disease process?
4. What is the prognosis for ALS? Given this prognosis, what is the goal of the occupational therapist?
5. What are the symptoms of ALS at each stage of the disease?
6. What interventions are appropriate at each stage of ALS?
7. What are the initial symptoms of AD?
8. What underlying degenerative neurological process is associated with AD?
9. What changes in symptoms occur over the course of AD?
10. How do the changes in symptoms affect occupational performance in clients with AD?
11. What is the prognosis for a client with AD?
12. What OT interventions are appropriate for the client at each stage of AD?
13. What environmental modifications should be made to accommodate the client with AD?
14. What are the symptoms of MS at onset?
15. What is the underlying neurological process in MS?
16. What are the three typical patterns of MS? How do they differ?
17. What symptoms of MS are managed with medication? What are the side effects of medication management?
18. How is medication management in the relapsing and remitting form of MS different than in the other forms of MS?
19. What does the OT evaluation include for the person with MS?
20. Why is it important to include the family in the evaluation and treatment process for the client with MS?
21. What are the initial symptoms of HD?
22. What underlying degenerative neurological process is associated with HD?
23. What changes in symptoms occur over the course of the disease?
24. How do the changes in symptoms affect occupational performance?
25. What is the prognosis for a client with HD?
26. What OT interventions are appropriate for the client with HD at the various stages of the disease?

27. What environmental modifications should be made to accommodate the client with HD?
28. What are the initial symptoms of PD?
29. What underlying degenerative neurological process is associated with PD?
30. What changes in symptoms occur over the course of PD?
31. How do the changes in symptoms affect occupational performance?

32. What is the prognosis for a client with PD?
33. What OT interventions are appropriate for the client with PD?
34. How does the medication schedule of levodopa affect a client's daily routine?
35. What environmental modifications should be made to accommodate the client with PD?

For additional practice questions for this chapter, please visit eBooks.Health.Elsevier.com.

REFERENCES

1. Abdullah EJ, Badr HE, Manee F: MS People's Performance and Satisfaction With Daily Occupations: Implications for Occupational Therapy, *OTJR (Thorofare N J)* 38(1):28–37, 2018. https://doi.org/10.1177/1539449217719867. PMID: 28770646.hh.
2. Akbarfahimi M, Nabavi SM, Kor B, Rezaie L, Paschall E: The effectiveness of occupational therapy-based sleep interventions on quality of life and fatigue in patients with multiple sclerosis: a pilot randomized clinical trial study, *Neuropsychiatric Disease and Treatment* 2020(16):1369–1379, 2020. https://doi.org/10.2147/NDT.S249277.
3. Allan LM, Wheatley A, Flynn E, Smith A, Fox C, Howel D, Barber R, Homer TM, Robinson L, Parry SW, Corner L, Connolly JA, Rochester L, Bamford C: Is it feasible to deliver a complex intervention to improve the outcome of falls in people with dementia? A protocol for the DIFRID feasibility study, *Pilot Feasibility Stud.* 4:170, 2018. https://doi.org/10.1186/s40814-018-0364-7. PMID: 30455976; PMCID: PMC6230281.
4. Allen C: *Allen Cognitive Level (ACL) test*, Rockville, MD, 1991, American Occupational Therapy Foundation.
5. Allen CK, Earhart CA, Blue T: *Occupational therapy treatment goals for the physically and cognitively disabled*, Rockville, MD, 1992, American Occupational Therapy Association.
6. ALS Today Newsletter, May 6, 2020. https://alsnewstoday.com/approved-treatments/.
7. Alzheimer's Association. *2021 Alzheimer's & Dementia.* https://www.alz.org/alzheimers-dementia/10_signs.
8. Alzheimer's Association: *2021 Know the 10 signs.* https://www.alz.org/alzheimers-dementia/10_signs.
9. Amato MP, Ponziani G, Siracusa G, Sorbi S: Cognitive impairment in early-onset multiple sclerosis: a reappraisal after 10 years, *Arch Neurol* 58:1602–1606, 2001.
10. Amatya B, Khan F, Galea M: Rehabilitation for people with multiple sclerosis: an overview of Cochrane Reviews, *Cochrane Database of Systematic Reviews*(Issue 1), 2019. https://doi.org/10.1002/14651858.CD012732.pub2. Art. No.: CD012732
11. American Occupational Therapy Association: Occupational therapy practice framework: Domain and process – fourth edition, *American Journal of Occupational Therapy* 74(Suppl. 2):1–87, 2020. https://doi.org/10.5014/ajot.2020.74S2001.
12. American Psychological Association: *Diagnostic and statistical manual of mental disorders*, ed 5, Arlington, VA, 2013, American Psychological Association.
13. Aragon A, & Kings J: *Occupational therapy for people with Parkinson's*, ed 2, In The Royal College of Occupational Therapists, 2018. https://www.rcot.co.uk/publications.
14. Arbesman M, Sheard K: Systematic review of the effectiveness of occupational therapy-related interventions for people with amyotrophic lateral sclerosis, *Am J Occup Ther* 68:20–26, 2014.

15. Asano M, Preissner K, Duffy R, Meixell M, Finlyason M: Goals set after completing a teleconference-delivered program for managing multiple sclerosis fatigue, *Am J Occup Ther* 69:1–8, 2015.
16. Asher IE: *Occupational therapy assessment tools: an annotated index*, ed 4, Bethesda, MD, 2014, American Occupational Therapy Association.
17. Attarian HP, Brown KM, Duntley SP, Carter JD, Cross AH: The relationship of sleep disturbances and fatigue in multiple sclerosis, *Arch Neurol* 61:525–528, 2004.
18. Ávila A, De-Rosende-Celeiro I, Torres G, et al: Promoting functional independence in people with Alzheimer's disease: outcomes of a home-based occupational therapy intervention in Spain, *Health Soc Care Community* 26(5):734–743, 2018. https://doi.org/10.1111/hsc.12594. PMID: 29998539.
19. Azimian M, Yaghoubi Z, Ahmadi Kahjoogh M, Akbarfahimi N, Haghgoo HA, Vahedi M: The effect of cognitive rehabilitation on balance skills of individuals with multiple sclerosis, *Occup Ther Health Care* 35(1):93–104, 2021. https://doi.org/10.1080/07380577.2021.1871698. PMID: 33433260.
20. Baker M, Blumlein D: Huntington's disease part 1: what is it? *Br J Healthcare Assistants* 35:223–227, 2009.
21. Bandmann O, Marsden CD, Wood NW: Genetic aspects of Parkinson's disease, *Mov Disord* 13:203, 1998.
22. Basso MR, Beason-Hazen S, Lynn J, Rammohan K, Bornstein RA: Screening for cognitive dysfunction in multiple sclerosis, *Arch Neurol* 53:980–984, 1996.
23. Baum MC, Edwards DF: Documenting productive behaviors. Using the functional behavior profile to plan discharge following stroke, *J Gerontol Nurs* 26(4):34–40, 2000. quiz 41-3. https://pubmed.ncbi.nlm.nih.gov/11272964/. Erratum in: *J Gerontol Nurs* 2000;26(8):54. PMID: 11272964.
24. Beard JD, Engel LS, Richardson DB, Gammon MD, Baird C, Umbach DM, Allen KD, Stanwyck CL, Keller J, Sandler DP, Schmidt S, Kamel F: Military service, deployments, and exposures in relation to amyotrophic lateral sclerosis survival, *PLoS One* 12(10):e0185751, 2017. https://doi.org/10.1371/journal.pone.0185751. PMID: 29016608; PMCID: PMC5634564.
25. Beck AT, Steer RA: *Beck Depression Inventory*, rev ed, San Antonio, TX, 1987, Psychological Corporation.
26. Berg D, Mäurer M, Warmuth-Metz M, Rieckmann P, Becker G: The correlation between ventricular diameter measured by transcranial sonography and clinical disability and cognitive dysfunction in patients with multiple sclerosis, *Arch Neurol* 57:1289–1292, 2000.
27. Blacker D, Broadhurst L, Teixeira L: The role of occupational therapy in leisure adaptation with complex neurological disability: a discussion using two case study examples, *NeuroRehabilitation* 23:313–319, 2008.

28. Bloem BR, Okun MS, Klein C: Parkinson's disease, *The Lancet* 397(10291):2284–2303, 2021. https://doi.org/10.1016/S0140-6736(21)00218-X.

29. Bolmsjö I, Hermerén G: Interviews with patients, family, and caregivers in amyotrophic lateral sclerosis: comparing needs, *J Palliat Care* 17:236–240, 2001.

30. Bonavita S: Exercise and Parkinson's disease, *Adv Exp Med Biol* 1228:289–301, 2020. https://doi.org/10.1007/978-981-15-1792-1_19. PMID: 32342465.

31. Bonzano L, Pedullà L, Pardini M, Tacchino A, Zaratin P, Battaglia MA, Brichetto G, Bove M: Brain activity pattern changes after adaptive working memory training in multiple sclerosis, *Brain Imaging Behav* 14(1):142–154, 2020. https://doi.org/10.1007/s11682-018-9984-z. PMID: 30377931; PMCID: PMC7007888.

32. Bonzano L, Pedullà L, Tacchino A, Brichetto G, Battaglia MA, Mancardi GL, Bove M: Upper limb motor training based on task-oriented exercises induces functional brain reorganization in patients with multiple sclerosis, *Neuroscience* 410:150–159, 2019. https://doi.org/10.1016/j.neuroscience.2019.05.004. PMID: 31085282.

33. Bradshaw JL, Georgiou N, Phillips JG, Iansek R, Chiu E, Cunnington R, Sheppard D: Motor sequencing problems in Parkinson's disease, Huntington's disease, and Tourette's syndrome 1: a review of the basal ganglia. In Piek JP, editor: *Motor behavior and human skill: a multidisciplinary approach*, Champaign, IL, 1998, Human Kinetics, pp 305–317.

34. Bronner G, Vodušek DB: Management of sexual dysfunction in Parkinson's disease, *Therapeutic Advances in Neurological Disorders* 4(6):375–383, 2011.

35. Burks J, Bigley GK, Hill H: Multiple sclerosis. In Lin V, editor: *Spinal cord medicine principles and practice*, New York, 2003, Demos Medical.

36. Burns T, Mortimer JA, Merchak P: Cognitive performance test: a new approach to functional assessment in Alzheimer's disease, *J Geriatr Psychiatry Neurol* 7(1):46–54, 1994.

37. Cacace R, Sleegers K, van Broeckhoven C: Molecular genetics of early-onset Alzheimer's disease revisited, *Alzheimer's Dement* 12:733–748, 2016.

38. Calabresi P: Diagnosis and management of multiple sclerosis, *Am Fam Physician* 15:1935, 2004.

39. Callahan CM, Boustani MA, Schmid AA, et al: Alzheimer's disease multiple intervention trial (ADMIT): study protocol for a randomized controlled clinical trial, *Trials* 13:92, 2012.

40. Callahan CM, Boustani MA, Schmid AA, LaMantia MA, Austrom MG, Miller DK, Gao S, Ferguson DY, Lane KA, Hendrie HC: Targeting Functional Decline in Alzheimer Disease: A Randomized Trial, *Ann Intern Med* 166(3):164–171, 2017 Feb 7. https://doi.org/10.7326/M16-0830. Epub 2016 Nov 22. PMID: 27893087; PMCID: PMC5554402.

41. Chen D, Guo X, Zheng Z: Depression and anxiety in amyotrophic lateral sclerosis: Correlations between the distress of patients and caregivers, *Muscle Nerve* 51:353–357, 2015.

42. Cho H, Shukla S: Role of edaravone as a treatment option for patients with amyotrophic lateral sclerosis, *Pharmaceuticals* 14:29, 2021. https://doi.org/10.3390/ph14010029.

43. Cicchetti F, Parent A: Striatal interneurons in Huntington's disease: selective increase in the density of calretinin-immunoreactive medium-sized neurons, *Mov Disord* 11:619, 1996.

44. Codling D, Shaw P, David AS: Hypersexuality in Parkinson's disease: systematic review and report of 7 new cases, *Mov Disord Clin Pract* 2(2):116–126, 2015. https://doi.org/10.1002/mdc3.12155. PMID: 30363884; PMCID: PMC6183311.

45. Cohen JA, et al: Intrarater and interrater reliability of the MS functional composite outcome measure, *Neurology* 54:802–806, 2000.

46. Connors MH, Seeher K, Teixeira-Pinto A, Woodward M, Ames D, Brodaty H: Dementia and caregiver burden: A three-year longitudinal study, *Int J Geriatr Psychiatry* 35(2):250–258, 2020. https://doi.org/10.1002/gps.5244. PMID: 31821606.

47. Corvol A, Netter A, Campeon A, Somme D: Implementation of an occupational therapy program for Alzheimer's disease patients in France: patients' and caregivers' perspectives, *J Alzheimers Dis* 62(1):157–164, 2018. https://doi.org/10.3233/JAD-170765. PMID: 29439340.

48. Costa J, Swash M, de Carvalho M: Awaji criteria for the diagnosis of amyotrophic lateral sclerosis: a systematic review, *Arch Neurol* 69:1410–1416, 2012.

49. Cruickshank TM, Thompson JA, Domínguez DJF, Reyes AP, Bynevelt M, Georgiou-Karistianis N, Barker RA, Ziman MR: The effect of multidisciplinary rehabilitation on brain structure and cognition in Huntington's disease: an exploratory study, *Brain Behav* 5(2):e00312, 2015. https://doi.org/10.1002/brb3.312. PMID: 25642394; PMCID: PMC4309878.

50. Curra A, Berardelli A, Agostino R: Performance of sequential arm movements with and without advanced knowledge of motor pathways in Parkinson's disease, *Mov Disord* 12:646, 1997.

51. Deloire M, et al: Early cognitive impairment in multiple sclerosis predicts disability outcome several years later, *Mult Scler* 16:581–587, 2010.

52. Delwaide PJ, Gonce M: Pathophysiology of Parkinson's signs. In Jankovic J, Tolosa E, editors: *Parkinson's disease and movement disorders* ed 3, Baltimore, 1998, Williams & Wilkins.

53. DiGiuseppe G, Blair M, Morrow SA: *Short report:* prevalence of cognitive impairment in newly diagnosed relapsing-remitting multiple sclerosis, *Int J MS Care* 20(4):153–157, 2018. https://doi.org/10.7224/1537-2073.2017-029. PMID: 30150898; PMCID: PMC6107340.

54. Doble SE, Fisk JD, Fisher AG, Ritvo PG, Murray TJ: Functional competence of community-dwelling persons with multiple sclerosis using the Assessment of Motor and Process Skills, *Arch Phys Med Rehabil* 75:843–851, 1994.

55. Dommershuijsen LJ, Heshmatollah A, Darweesh SKL, Koudstaal PJ, Ikram MA, Ikram MK: Life expectancy of parkinsonism patients in the general population, *Parkinsonism Relat Disord* 77:94–99, 2020. https://doi.org/10.1016/j.parkreldis.2020.06.018. PMID: 32712564.

56. Döpp CME, Graff MJL, Olde Rikkert MGM, et al: Determinants for the effectiveness of implementing an occupational therapy intervention in routine dementia care, *Implement Sci* 8:131, 2013.

57. Driscoll I, Davatzikos C, An Y, et al: Longitudinal pattern of regional brain volume change differentiates normal aging from MCI, *Neurology* 72:1906–1913, 2009.

58. Dubois B, Hampel H, Feldman HH, et al: Preclinical Alzheimer's disease: definition, natural history, and diagnostic criteria, *Alzheimers Dement* 12:292–323, 2016.

59. Duignan S, Brownlee W, Wassmer E, Hemingway C, Lim M, Ciccarelli O, Hacohen Y: Paediatric multiple sclerosis: a new era in diagnosis and treatment, *Dev Med Child Neurol* 61(9):1039–1049, 2019. https://doi.org/10.1111/dmcn.14212. PMID: 30932181.

60. Dwyer CP, Alvarez-Iglesias A, Joyce R, Counihan TJ, Casey D, Hynes SM: Evaluating the feasibility and preliminary efficacy

of a Cognitive Occupation-Based programme for people with Multiple Sclerosis (COB-MS): protocol for a feasibility cluster-randomised controlled trial, *Trials* 21(1):269, 2020. https://doi.org/10.1186/s13063-020-4179-5. PMID: 32183874; PMCID: PMC7077165.

61. Ellis T, Rochester L: Mobilizing Parkinson's disease: the future of exercise, *J Parkinsons Dis* 8(s1):S95–S100, 2018. https://doi.org/10.3233/JPD-181489. PMID: 30584167; PMCID: PMC6311359

62. Exuzides A, Reddy SR, Chang E, Ta JT, Patel AM, Paydar C, Yohrling GJ: Healthcare utilization and cost burden of Huntington's disease among Medicare beneficiaries in the United States, *J Med Econ* 24(1):1327–1336, 2021. https://doi.org/10.1080/13696998.2021.2002579. PMID: 34730477.

63. Fahn S, Elton RL: The Unified Parkinson's Disease Rating Scale. In: Fahn S, editor: *Recent developments in Parkinson's disease*, vol 2, Florham Park, NJ, 1987, Macmillian Healthcare Information.

64. Fasano A, Lozano AM, Cubo E: New neurosurgical approaches for tremor and Parkinson's disease, *Curr Opin Neurol* 30(4):435–446, 2017. https://doi.org/10.1097/WCO.0000000000000465. PMID: 28509682.

65. Finlayson M, Preissner K, Cho C: Outcome moderators of a fatigue management program for people with multiple sclerosis, *Am J Occup Ther* 66:187–197, 2012.

66. Fisher A: *The Assessment of Motor and Process Skills (AMPS) in assessing adults: functional measures and successful outcomes*, Rockville, MD, 1991, American Occupational Therapy Foundation.

67. Fitzpatrick R, Peto V, Jenkinson C: Health-related quality of life in Parkinson's disease: a study of outpatient clinic attenders, *Mov Disord* 12:916, 1997.

68. Folstein MF, Folstein SE, McHugh PR: Mini-mental state: a practical method for grading the cognitive state of patients for the clinician, *J Psychiatr Res* 12:189, 1975.

69. Foster ER, Hershey T: Everyday executive function is associated with activity participation in Parkinson disease without dementia, *OTJR (Thorofare N J)* 31:S16–S22, 2011.

70. Fox SH, Chuang R, Brotchie JM: Serotonin and Parkinson's disease: on movement, mood, and madness, *Movement Disorders* 24(9):1255–1266, 2009.

71. Francardo V, Schmitz Y, Sulzer D, Cenci MA: Neuroprotection and neurorestoration as experimental therapeutics for Parkinson's disease, *Exp Neurol* 298(Pt B):137–147, 2017. https://doi.org/10.1016/j.expneurol.2017.10.001. PMID: 28988910.

72. Franciotta M, Maestri R, Ortelli P, Ferrazzoli D, Mastalli F, Frazzitta G: Occupational therapy for Parkinsonian patients: a retrospective study, *Parkinsons Dis* 2019:4561830, 2019. https://doi.org/10.1155/2019/4561830. PMID: 31781364; PMCID: PMC6875269.

73. Fu P, Gao M, Yung KKL: Association of intestinal disorders with Parkinson's disease and Alzheimer's disease: a systematic review and meta-analysis, *ACS Chem. Neurosci.* 11(3):395–405, 2020. https://doi.org/10.1021/acschemneuro.9b00607.

74. Gelb DJ: *Introduction to clinical neurology*, ed 5, Oxford, UK, 2016, Oxford University Press.

75. Gélinas I, et al: Development of a functional measure for persons with Alzheimer's disease: the disability assessment for dementia, *Am J Occup Ther* 53:471, 1999.

76. Ghezzi A: Therapeutic strategies in childhood multiple sclerosis, *Ther Adv Neurol Disord* 3(4):217–228, 2010. https://doi.org/10.1177/1756285610371251. PMID: 21179613; PMCID: PMC3002659.

77. Giladi N, Kao R, Fahn S: Freezing phenomenon in patients with Parkinsonian syndromes, *Mov Disord* 12:302, 1997.

78. Giordano M, Caccavella VM, Zaed I, Foglia Manzillo L, Montano N, Olivi A, Polli FM: Comparison between deep brain stimulation and magnetic resonance-guided focused ultrasound in the treatment of essential tremor: a systematic review and pooled analysis of functional outcomes, *J Neurol Neurosurg Psychiatry* 91(12):1270–1278, 2020. https://doi.org/10.1136/jnnp-2020-323216. PMID: 33055140.

79. Giri M, Zhang M, Lü Y: Genes associated with Alzheimer's disease: an overview and current status, *Clin Interv Aging* 11:665–681, 2016. https://doi.org/10.2147/CIA.S105769. PMID: 27274215; PMCID: PMC4876682.

80. Gitlin LN, Winter L, Earland TV, et al: The Tailored Activity Program to reduce behavioral symptoms in individuals with dementia: feasibility, acceptability, and replication potential, *Gerontologist* 49:428–439, 2009.

81. Goldman JG: New thoughts on thought disorders in Parkinson's disease: review of current research strategies and challenges, *Parkinsons Dis* 2011:675630, 2011.

82. Goldman SM, Tanner C: Etiology of Parkinson's disease. In Jankovic J, Tolosa E, editors: *Parkinson's disease and movement disorders* ed 3, Baltimore, 1998, Williams & Wilkins.

83. Goverover Y, O'Brien AR, Moore NB, DeLuca J: Actual reality: a new approach to functional assessment in persons with multiple sclerosis, *Arch Phys Med Rehabil* 91:252–260, 2010.

84. Green E, Huynh A, Broussard L, Zunker B, Matthews J, Hilton CL, Aranha K: Systematic review of yoga and balance: effect on adults with neuromuscular impairment, *Am J Occup Ther* 73(1):1–11, 2019. https://doi.org/10.5014/ajot.2019.028944. PMID: 30839270.

85. Gunnery SD, Habermann B, Saint-Hilaire M, Thomas CA, Tickle-Degnen L: The relationship between the experience of hypomimia and social wellbeing in people with Parkinson's disease and their care partners, *Journal of Parkinson's Disease* 6(3):625–630, 2016. https://doi.org/10.3233/JPD-160782.

86. Gure T, Kabeto MU, Plassman BL, et al: Differences in functional impairments in subtypes of dementia, *J Gerontol A Biol Sci Med Sci* 65A:431–441, 2010.

87. Hasselkus B: Occupation and well-being in dementia: the experience of day-care staff, *Am J Occup Ther* 52:423, 1998.

88. Hayden MR: *Huntington's chorea*, New York, 1996, Springer-Verlag.

89. Hayes MT: Parkinson's disease and Parkinsonism, *Am J Med* 132(7):802–807, 2019. https://doi.org/10.1016/j.amjmed.2019.03.001. PMID: 30890425.

90. Hecht M, Hillemacher T, Gräsel E, et al: Subjective experience and coping in ALS, *Amyotroph Lateral Scler Other Motor Neuron Disord* 3:225–231, 2002.

91. Helder DI, Kaptein Ad A, Van Kempen GMJ, et al: Living with Huntington's disease: illness perceptions, coping mechanisms, and patients' well-being, *Br J Health Psychol* 7:449–462, 2002.

92. Hersche R, Weise A, Michel G, Kesselring J, Barbero M, Kool J: Development and preliminary evaluation of a 3-week inpatient energy management education program for people with multiple sclerosis-related fatigue, *Int J MS Care* 21(6):265–274, 2019. https://doi.org/10.7224/1537-2073.2018-058. PMID: 31889931; PMCID: PMC6928585.

93. Hines A, Bundy A: Predicting driving ability using DriveSafe and DriveAware in people with cognitive impairments: a replication study, *Aust Occup Ther J* 61:224–229, 2014.

94. Hoehn MM, Yahr MD: Parkinsonism: onset, progression and mortality, *Neurology* 17:427, 1967.

95. Huntington Study Group: Unified Huntington's Disease Rating Scale: reliability and consistency, *Mov Disord* 11:136, 1996.

96. Husna Ibrahim N, Yahaya MF, Mohamed W, Teoh SL, Hui CK, Kumar J: Pharmacotherapy of Alzheimer's disease: seeking clarity in a time of uncertainty, *Front Pharmacol* 11:261, 2020. https://doi.org/10.3389/fphar.2020.00261. PMID: 32265696; PMCID: PMC7105678.

97. Hwang JE, Cvitanovich DC, Doroski EK, Vajarakitipongse JG: Correlations between quality of life and adaptation factors among people with multiple sclerosis, *Am J Occup Ther* 65:661–669, 2011.

98. Hynes SM, Forwell S: A cognitive occupation-based programme for people with multiple sclerosis: a new occupational therapy cognitive rehabilitation intervention, *Hong Kong J Occup Ther* 32(1):41–52, 2019. https://doi.org/10.1177/1569186119841263. PMID: 31217761; PMCID: PMC6560833.

99. Imbriglio S: *Physical and occupational therapy for Huntington's disease*, New York, 1997, Huntington's Disease Society of America.

100. Jaiswal MK: Riluzole and edaravone: A tale of two amyotrophic lateral sclerosis drugs, *Med Res Rev* 39(2):733–748, 2019. https://doi.org/10.1002/med.21528. PMID: 30101496.

101. Jansa J, Aragon A: Living with Parkinson's and the emerging role of occupational therapy, *Parkinsons Dis* 2015:196303, 2015. https://doi.org/10.1155/2015/196303. PMID: 26495151; PMCID: PMC4606403.

102. Jensen L, Padilla R: Effectiveness of environment-based interventions that address behavior, perception, and falls in people with Alzheimer's disease and related major neurocognitive disorders: a systematic review, *American Journal of Occupational Therapy* 71:1–10, 2017. https://doi.org/10.5014/ajot.2017.027409. 7105180030.

103. Jensen LE, Padilla R: Effectiveness of interventions to prevent falls in people with Alzheimer's disease and related dementias, *Am J Occup Ther* 65:532–540, 2011.

104. Joiner C, Hansel M: Empowering the geriatric client, *OT Practice* 1:34–39, 1996.

105. Kalb R, Feinstein A, Rohrig A, Sankary L, Willis A: Depression and suicidality in multiple sclerosis: red flags, management strategies, and ethical considerations, *Current Neurology and Neuroscience Reports* 19:77, 2019. https://doi.org/10.1007/s11910-019-0992-1.

106. Kaptein AA, Scharloo M, Helder DI, et al: Quality of life in couples living with Huntington's disease: the role of patients' and partners' illness perceptions, *Qual Life Res* 16:793–801, 2007.

107. Karhula ME, Tolvanen A, Hämäläinen PI, Ruutiainen J, Salminen AL, Era P: Predictors of participation and autonomy in people with multiple sclerosis, *Am J Occup Ther* 73(4), 2019. 7304205070p1-7304205070p8. https://doi.org/10.5014/ajot.2019.030221. PMID: 31318671.

108. Katz S, Ford AB, Moskowitz RW, Jackson BA, Jaffe MW: Studies of illness in the aged. The index of ADL: a standardized measure of biological and psychological function, *JAMA* 135:75, 1963.

109. Kaufman DW, Reshef S, Golub HL, et al: Survival in commercially insured multiple sclerosis patients and comparator subjects in the US, *Mult Scler Relat Disord* 3:364–371, 2014.

110. Khalil H, Quinn L, van Deursen R, et al: What effect does a structured home-based exercise programme have on people with Huntington's disease? A randomized, controlled pilot study, *Clin Rehabil* 27:646–658, 2013.

111. Kim D: The effects of a recollection-based occupational therapy program of Alzheimer's disease: a randomized controlled trial, *Occup Ther Int* 2020:6305727, 2020. https://doi.org/10.1155/2020/6305727. PMID: 32821251; PMCID: PMC7416254.

112. Klempír J, Klempírova O, Spaková N, Zidovská J, Roth J: Unified Huntington's Disease Rating Scale: clinical practice and critical approach, *Funct Neurol* 21:217–221, 2006.

113. Larson E: Management of Alzheimer's disease in primary care settings, *Am J Geriatr Psychiatry* 6:S34, 1998.

114. Laver K, Cumming R, Dyer S, Agar M, Anstey KJ, Beattie E, Brodaty H, Broe T, Clemson L, Crotty M, Dietz M, Draper B, Flicker L, Friel M, Heuzenroeder L, Koch S, Kurrle S, Nay R, Pond D, Thompson J, Santalucia Y, Whitehead C, Yates M: Evidence-based occupational therapy for people with dementia and their families: what clinical practice guidelines tell us and implications for practice, *Aust Occup Ther J* 64(1):3–10, 2017. https://doi.org/10.1111/1440-1630.12309. PMID: 27699792.

115. Lawton M, Brody E: Assessment of older people: self-maintaining and IADL, *Gerontologist* 9:179, 1969.

116. LeBarge E: A preliminary scale to measure degree of worry among mildly demented Alzheimer disease patients, *Phys Occup Ther Geriatr* 11:43, 1993.

117. Levy LL: Cognitive aging. In Katz N, editor: *Cognition, occupation, and participation across the life span* ed 3, 2011, American Occupational Therapy Association, pp 117–142.

118. Levy LL, Burns T: The cognitive disabilities reconsidered model: rehabilitation of adults with dementia. In Katz N, editor: *Cognition, occupation, and participation across the life span* ed 3, 2011, American Occupational Therapy Association, pp 407–441.

119. Lexell EM, Lund ML, Iwarsson S: Constantly changing lives: experiences of people with multiple sclerosis, *Am J Occup Ther* 63:772–781, 2009.

120. Li R, Cooper C, Barber J, et al: Coping strategies as mediators of the effect of the START (strategies for RelaTives) intervention on psychological morbidity for family carers of people with dementia in a randomised controlled trial, *J Affect Disord* 168:298–305, 2014.

121. Long K. (2020). Pre-active PD: A therapist delivered physical activity behavior change program for people with early stage Parkinson's disease. Available from ProQuest Dissertations & Theses Global. (2359437963). https://tc.idm.oclc.org/login?url=https://search-proquest-com.tc.idm.oclc.org/docview/2359437963?accountid=14258.

122. Lou JS, Reeves A, Benice T, Sexton G: Fatigue and depression are associated with poor quality of life in ALS, *Neurology* 60:122–123, 2003.

123. Louis ED, et al: Reliability of patient completion of the historical section of the Unified Parkinson's Disease Rating Scale, *Mov Disord* 11:185, 1996.

124. Magrinelli F, Picelli A, Tocco P, Federico A, Roncari L, Smania N, Zanette G, Tamburin S: Pathophysiology of motor dysfunction in Parkinson's disease as the rationale for drug treatment and rehabilitation, *Parkinson's Disease*:1–18, 2016. https://doi.org/10.1155/2016/9832839.

125. Maitra KK, Dasgupta AK: Incoordination of a sequential motor task in, Parkinson's disease, *Occup Ther Int* 12:218–233, 2005.

126. Malek N: Deep brain stimulation in Parkinson's disease, *Neurol India* 67(4):968–978, 2019. https://doi.org/10.4103/0028-3886.266268. PMID: 31512617.

127. Masrori P, Van Damme P: Amyotrophic lateral sclerosis: a clinical review, *European Journal of Neurology* 27:1918–1929, 2020. https://doi.org/10.1111/ene.14393.

128. Matias-Guiu JA, Cortés-Martínez A, Valles-Salgado M, Oreja-Guevara C, Pytel V, Montero P, Moreno-Ramos T, Matias-Guiu J: Functional components of cognitive impairment in multiple sclerosis: a cross-sectional investigation, *Front Neurol* 8:643, 2017. https://doi.org/10.3389/fneur.2017.00643. PMID: 29234305; PMCID: PMC5712315.

129. Matuska K, Mathiowetz V, Finlayson M: Use and perceived effectiveness of energy conservation strategies for managing multiple sclerosis fatigue, *Am J Occup Ther* 61:62–69, 2007.

130. Mayo Clinic: Multiple sclerosis. https://www.mayoclinic.org/diseases-conditions/multiple-sclerosis/symptoms-causes/syc-20350269.

131. Mazzoni P, Shabbott B, Corte JC: Motor control abnormalities in Parkinson's disease, *Cold Spring Harb Perspect Med* 2:1–17, 2012.

132. McCraith DB, Austin SL, Earhart CA: The cognitive disabilities model in 2011. In Katz N, editor: *Cognition, occupation, and participation across the life span* ed 3, 2011, American Occupational Therapy Association, pp 382–406.

133. McKay KA, Smith KA, Smertinaite L, Fang F, Ingre C, Taube F: Military service and related risk factors for amyotrophic lateral sclerosis, *Acta Neurol Scand* 143(1):39–50, 2021. https://doi.org/10.1111/ane.13345. PMID: 32905613; PMCID: PMC7756624.

134. Menegardo CS, Friggi FA, Scardini JB, Rossi TS, Vieira TDS, Tieppo A, Morelato RL: Sundown syndrome in patients with Alzheimer's disease dementia, *Dement Neuropsychol* 13(4):469–474, 2019. https://doi.org/10.1590/1980-57642018dn13-040015. PMID: 31844502; PMCID: PMC6907707.

135. Miller RG, Jackson CS, Kasarskis EJ, et al: Practice Parameter update: the care of the patient with amyotrophic lateral sclerosis: multidisciplinary care, symptom management, and cognitive/behavioral impairment (an evidence-based review): report of the Quality Standards Subcommittee of the American Academy of Neurology, *Neurology* 73:1227–1233, 2009.

136. Misulis KE: *Neurologic localization and diagnosis*, Boston, 1996, Butterworth-Heinemann.

137. Momsen AH, Ørtenblad L, Maribo T: Effective rehabilitation interventions and participation among people with multiple sclerosis: an overview of reviews, *Ann Phys Rehabil Med* 65:101529, 2022. https://doi.org/10.1016/j.rehab.2021.101529. PMID: 33940247.

138. Moosa S, Martínez-Fernández R, Elias WJ, Del Alamo M, Eisenberg HM, Fishman PS: The role of high-intensity focused ultrasound as a symptomatic treatment for Parkinson's disease, *Mov Disord* 34(9):1243–1251, 2019. https://doi.org/10.1002/mds.27779. PMID: 31291491.

139. Moskowitz CB, Rao AK: Making a measurable difference in advanced Huntington disease care. In AS Feigin & KE Anderson (eds) *Handbook of clinical neurology*, Vol 144 Huntington Disease 183–196. https://doi.org/10.1016/B978-0-12-801893-4.00016-X. PMID: 28947117.

140. Motl RW, Gosney JL: Effect of exercise training on quality of life in multiple sclerosis: a meta-analysis, *Mult Scler* 14:129–135, 2008.

141. Müller V, Mohr B, Rosin R, et al: Short-term effects of behavioral treatment on movement initiation and postural control in Parkinson's disease: a controlled clinical study, *Mov Disord* 12:306, 1997.

142. Multiple Sclerosis Association of America (2021) Who gets multiple sclerosis? https://mymsaa.org/ms-information/overview/who-gets-ms/.

143. Nance MA: Comprehensive care in Huntington's disease: a physician's perspective, *Brain Res Bull* 72:175–178, 2007.

144. Nance MA, Sander G: Characteristics of individuals with Huntington's disease in long-term care, *Mov Disord* 11:542, 1996.

145. National Institutes of Health: Amyotrophic lateral sclerosis, https://www.ninds.nih.gov/Disorders/All-Disorders/Amyotrophic-Lateral-Sclerosis-ALS-Information-Page.

146. National Institutes of Health: Huntington's disease: hope through research, https://www.ninds.nih.gov/Disorders/Patient-Caregiver-Education/Hope-Through-Research/Huntingtons-Disease-Hope-Through.

147. National Institutes of Health: *2009 progress report on Alzheimer's disease: translating new knowledge*, Bethesda, MD, 2010, National Institute of Aging.

148. National Institutes of Health (NIH) 2021. National Institute on Aging. https://www.nia.nih.gov/health/tips-coping-sundowning.

149. National Institute of Neurological Disorders and Stroke. https://www.ninds.nih.gov/health-information/disorders/motor-neuron-diseases?search-term=motor%20neuron%20disease.

150. National Multiple Sclerosis Society: Medications. http://www.nationalmssociety.org/Treating-MS/Medications.

151. National Multiple Sclerosis Society: What is MS? https://www.nationalmssociety.org/What-is-MS.

152. National Multiple Sclerosis Society: Clinical study measures (2021). https://www.nationalmssociety.org/For-Professionals/Researchers/Resources-for-MS-Researchers/Research-Tools/Clinical-Study-Measures.

153. Nikolac Perkovic M, Pivac N: Genetic Markers of Alzheimer's Disease, *Frontiers in Psychiatry: Adv Exp Med Biol* 1192:27–52, 2019. https://doi.org/10.1007/978-981-32-9721-0_3. PMID: 31705489.

154. Novatek Medical Data Systems: Cognistat: the neurobehavioral cognitive status examination, https://www.cognistat.com/.

155. Northrup D., Frankel D.: Guidelines & recommendations for home care providers and personal care assistants, 2008, National Multiple Sclerosis Society Clinical Programs Department. https://pdfroom.com/books/home-care-providers-and-personal-care-assistants/JZOgZpLN5kb.

156. Noseworthy JH, Lucchinetti C, Rodriguez M, Weinshenker BG: Multiple sclerosis, *N Engl J Med* 343:938–952, 2000.

157. Nygard L, Bernspång B, Fisher AG, Winblad B: Comparing motor and process ability of persons with suspected dementia in home and clinic settings, *Am J Occup Ther* 48:689, 1994.

158. Oken BS, Kishiyama S, Zajdel D, et al: Randomized controlled trial of yoga and exercise in multiple sclerosis, *Neurology* 62:2058–2064, 2004.

159. Olanow CW, et al: Neurodegeneration and Parkinson's disease. In Jankovic J, Tolosa E, editors: *Parkinson's disease and movement disorders* ed 3, Baltimore, 1998, Williams & Wilkins.

160. Olsson AG, Markhede I, Strang S, Persson LI: Differences in quality of life modalities give rise to needs of individual support in patients with ALS and their next of kin, *Palliat Support Care* 8:75–82, 2010.

161. Orsini M, Oliveira AB, Nascimento OJM, et al: Amyotrophic lateral sclerosis: new perspectives and update, *Neurol Int* 7:5885, 2015.

162. O'Shea S, Morris M, Iansek R: Dual task interference during gait in people with Parkinson's disease: effects of motor versus cognitive secondary tasks, *Physical Therapy* 72(9):888–897, 2002.

163. Oskarsson B, Gendron TF, Staff NP: Amyotrophic Lateral Sclerosis: An Update for 2018, *Mayo Clin Proc* 93(11):1617–1628, 2018. https://doi.org/10.1016/j.mayocp.2018.04.007. PMID: 30401437.

164. Ott KR, Kolodziejczak S: Occupational therapy interventions for people with Parkinson's disease, *Am J Occup Ther* 76(1), 2022. 7601390010. https://doi.org/10.5014/ajot.2022.049390. PMID: 34964837.

165. Parent A, Cicchetti F: The current model of basal ganglia organization under scrutiny, *Mov Disord* 13:199, 1998.

166. Parkinson's Foundation. Parkinson's Foundation: Understanding Parkinson's 2021. https://www.parkinson.org/understanding-parkinsons.

167. Patt N, Kool J, Hersche R, Oberste M, Walzik D, Joisten N, Caminada D, Ferrara F, Gonzenbach R, Nigg CR, Kamm CP, Zimmer P, Bansi J: High-intensity interval training and energy management education, compared with moderate continuous training and progressive muscle relaxation, for improving health-related quality of life in persons with multiple sclerosis: study protocol of a randomized controlled superiority trial with six months' follow-up, *BMC Neurol* 21(1):65, 2021. https://doi.org/10.1186/s12883-021-02084-0. PMID: 33573608; PMCID: PMC7877079.

168. Paty D, Willoughby E, Whitaker J: Assessing the outcome of experimental therapies in multiple sclerosis patients. In Rudick RA, Goodkin DE, editors: *Treatment of multiple sclerosis: trial design, results, and future perspectives*, London, UK, 1992, Springer-Verlag.

169. Penney JB, Young AB: Huntington's disease. In Jankovic J, Tolosa E, editors: *Parkinson's disease and movement disorders* ed 3, Baltimore, 1998, Williams & Wilkins.

170. Phillips DH: *Living with Huntington's disease*, Madison, WI, 1982, University of Wisconsin Press.

171. Phillips JG, Stelmach GE: Parkinson's disease and other involuntary movement disorders of the basal ganglia. In Fredericks CM, Saladin LK, editors: *Pathophysiology of the motor systems*, Philadelphia, 1996, FA Davis.

172. Piersol CV, Jensen L, Lieberman D, Arbesman M: Occupational therapy interventions for people with Alzheimer's disease, *Am J Occup Ther* 72(1), 2018. 7201390010p1–7201390010p6. https://pubmed.ncbi.nlm.nih.gov/29280729/. PMID: 29280729.

173. Pimouguet C, Sitta R, Wittwer J, Hayes N, Petit-Monéger A, Dartigues JF, Helmer C: Maintenance of occupational therapy (OT) for dementia: protocol of a multi-center, randomized controlled and pragmatic trial, *BMC Geriatr* 19(1):35, 2019. https://doi.org/10.1186/s12877-019-1046-x. PMID: 30727947; PMCID: PMC6366025.

174. Pinhas-Hamiel O, Sarova-Pinhas I, Achiron A: Multiple sclerosis in childhood and adolescence: clinical features and management, *Paediatr Drugs* 3:329, 2001.

175. Podhorna J, Krahnke T, Shear M, et al: Alzheimer's Disease Assessment Scale—cognitive subscale variants in mild cognitive impairment and mild Alzheimer's disease: change over time and the effect of enrichment strategies, *Alzheimers Res Ther* 8:8, 2016.

176. Poewe W, Wenning G: Levodopa in Parkinson's disease: mechanisms of action and pathophysiology of late failure. In Jankovic J, Tolosa E, editors: *Parkinson's disease and movement disorders* ed 3, Baltimore, 1998, Williams & Wilkins.

177. Pollak P: Parkinson's disease and related movement disorders. In Bogousslasky J, Fisher M, editors: *Textbook of neurology*, Boston, 1998, Butterworth-Heinemann.

178. Pousada T, Garabal-Barbeira J, Martínez C, Groba B, Nieto-Riveiro L, Pereira J: How loan bank of assistive technology impacts on life of persons with amyotrophic lateral sclerosis and neuromuscular diseases: a collaborative initiative, *Int. J.* *Environ. Res. Public Health* 18:763, 2021. https://doi.org/10.3390/ijerph18020763.

179. Preissner K: *Occupational therapy practice guidelines for adults with neurodegenerative diseases*, Bethesda, MD, 2014, American Occupational Therapy Association.

180. Preissner K, Arbesman M, Lieberman D: Occupational therapy interventions for adults with multiple sclerosis, *Am J Occup Ther* 70(3), 2016. 7003395010p1–4. https://doi.org/10.5014/ajot.2016.703001. PMID: 27089301.

181. Prochazka A, Bennett DJ, Stephens MJ, et al: Measurement of rigidity in Parkinson's disease, *Mov Disord* 12:24, 1997.

182. Quinn É, Hynes SM: Occupational therapy interventions for multiple sclerosis: A scoping review, *Scand J Occup Ther* 28(5):399–414, 2021. https://doi.org/10.1080/11038128.2020.1786160. PMID: 32643486.

183. Quinn L. & Busse, M. (2017) The role of rehabilitation in Huntington disease. In AS Feigin & KE Anderson (eds) *Handbook of Clinical Neurology*, Vol 144 Huntington Disease, pp 151–165. https://doi.org/10.1016/B978-0-12-801893-4.00013-4.

184. Quinn L, Macpherson C, Long K, Shah H: Promoting physical activity via telehealth in people with parkinson disease: the path forward after the COVID-19 pandemic? *Physical Therapy* 100:1730–1736, 2020. https://doi.org/10.1093/ptj/pzaa128.

185. Raaphorst J, de Visser M, Linssen WHJP, de Haan RJ, Schmand B: The cognitive profile of amyotrophic lateral sclerosis: a meta-analysis, *Amyotroph Lateral Scler* 11:27–37, 2010.

186. Rao AK: Enabling functional independence in Parkinson's disease: update on occupational therapy intervention, *Mov Disord* 25(Suppl 1):S146–S151, 2010.

187. Reidak K, Jackson S, Giovannoni G: Multiple sclerosis: a practical overview for clinicians, *Br Med Bull* 95:79–104, 2010.

188. Reifler B: Detection and treatment of mixed cognitive and affective symptoms in the elderly: is it dementia, depression or both? *Clin Geriatr* 6:17, 1998.

189. Richards M, Marder K, Cote L, Mayeux R: Interrater reliability of the Unified Parkinson's Disease Rating Scale motor examination, *Mov Disord* 9:89, 1994.

190. Roger KS, Medved MI: Living with Parkinson's disease: managing identity together, *Int J Qual Stud Health Well-being* Mar 30:5, 2010.

191. Rosenblatt A, Frank S: Huntington's disease: Emerging concepts in diagnosis and treatment, *Supplement to Neurology Review*:S1–S8, 2015.

192. Rosin R, Topka H, Dichgans J: Gait initiation in Parkinson's disease, *Mov Disord* 12:682, 1997.

193. Sage JI, Duvoisin RC: The modern management of Parkinson's disease. In Chokroverty S, editor: *Movement disorders*, New Brunswick, NJ, 1990, PMA.

194. Sagiraju HKR, Živković S, VanCott AC, Patwa H, Gimeno Ruiz de Porras D, Amuan ME, Pugh MJV: Amyotrophic lateral sclerosis among veterans deployed in support of post-9/11 U.S. conflicts, *Mil Med* 185(3-4):e501–e509, 2020. https://doi.org/10.1093/milmed/usz350. PMID: 31642489.

195. Salomè A, Sasso D'Elia T, Franchini G, Santilli V, Paolucci T: Occupational therapy in fatigue management in multiple sclerosis: an umbrella review, *Mult Scler Int* 2019:2027947, 2019. https://doi.org/10.1155/2019/2027947. PMID: 31016045; PMCID: PMC6448334.

196. Sarkar A, Irwin M, Singh A, Riccetti M, Singh A: Alzheimer's disease: the silver tsunami of the 21st century, *Neural Regen Res* 11:693–697, 2016.

197. Scheltens P, De Strooper B, Kivipelto M, et al: Alzheimer's disease, *Lancet* 388:505–517, 2016.

198. Schneider L: Cholinergic deficiency in Alzheimer's disease: pathogenic model, *Am J Geriatr Psychiatry* 6(2 Suppl 1):S49–S55, 1998.

199. Schootemeijer S, van der Kolk NM, Bloem BR, de Vries NM: Current perspectives on aerobic exercise in people with Parkinson's disease, *Neurotherapeutics* 17(4):1418–1433, 2020. https://doi.org/10.1007/s13311-020-00904-8. PMID: 32808252; PMCID: PMC7851311.

200. Schulz D, Kopp B, Kunkel A, Faiss JH: Cognition in the early stage of multiple sclerosis, *J Neurol* 3:1002–1010, 2006.

201. Sherrington C, Michaleff ZA, Fairhall N, Paul SS, Tiedemann A, Whitney J, Cumming RG, Herbert RD, Close JCT, Lord SR: Exercise to prevent falls in older adults: an updated systematic review and meta-analysis, *Br J Sports Med* 51(24):1750–1758, 2017. https://doi.org/10.1136/bjsports-2016-096547. PMID: 27707740.

202. Shih YH, Pai MC, Lin HS, Sung PS, Wang JJ: Effects of walking on sundown syndrome in community-dwelling people with Alzheimer's disease, *Int J Older People Nurs* 15(2):e12292, 2020. https://doi.org/10.1111/opn.12292. PMID: 31814316.

203. Shulman JM, DeJager PL, Feany MB: Parkinson's disease: genetics and pathogenesis, *Annu Rev Pathol* 6:193–222, 2010.

204. Siciliano M, Trojano L, Santangelo G, De Micco R, Tedeschi G, Tessitore A: Fatigue in Parkinson's disease: A systematic review and meta-analysis, *Movement Disorders* 33(11):1712–1723, 2018. https://doi.org/10.1002/mds.27461.

205. Smallfield S, Heckenlaible C: Effectiveness of occupational therapy interventions to enhance occupational performance for adults with Alzheimer's disease and related major neurocognitive disorders: a systematic review, *Am J Occup Ther* 71(5), 2017. 7105180010p1-7105180010p9. https://doi.org/10.5014/ajot.2017.024752. PMID: 28809651.

206. Soofi AY, Bello-Haas VD, Kho ME, Letts L: The impact of rehabilitative interventions on quality of life: a qualitative evidence synthesis of personal experiences of individuals with amyotrophic lateral sclerosis, *Qual Life Res* 27(4):845–856, 2018. https://doi.org/10.1007/s11136-017-1754-7. PMID: 29204783.

207. Sorenson E, Thurman DJ: Amyotrophic Lateral Sclerosis (ALS) Continuing Education Module. http://www.atsdr.cdc.gov/emes/ALS.

208. Soriani MH, Desnuelle C: Care management in amyotrophic lateral sclerosis, *Revue Neurologique* 173:288–299, 2017. https://doi.org/10.1016/j.neurol.2017.03.031.

209. Sperling RA, Guttmann CR, Hohol MJ, et al: Regional magnetic resonance imaging lesion burden and cognitive function in multiple sclerosis: a longitudinal study, *Arch Neurol* 58:115–121, 2001.

210. Spring JA, Baker M, Dauya L, et al: Gardening with Huntington's disease clients: creating a programme of winter activities, *Disabil Rehabil* 33:159–164, 2011.

211. Sturkenboom IH, Graff MJL, Hendriks JCM, et al: Efficacy of occupational therapy for patients with Parkinson's disease: a randomised controlled trial, *Lancet Neurol* 13:557–566, 2014.

212. Sturkenboom IHWM, Thijssen MCE, Gons-van Elsacker, JJ, Jansen IJH, Maasdam A, Schulten M, Vijver-Visser D, Steultjens EJM, Bloem BR, & Munneke M. (2011). Guidelines for Occupational Therapy in Parkinson's Disease Rehabilitation. In ParkinsonNet/National Parkinson Foundation (NPF). https://www.movementdisorders.ch/index/wp-content/uploads/2019/09/Guidelines_OT_Parkinsons-disease_2012.pdf.

213. Sun HQ, Zhang X, Huang WJ, Chen WW: The news advances on Alzheimer's disease's therapeutics, *Eur Rev Med Pharmacol Sci* 20:1903–1910, 2016.

214. Swink LA, Fling BW, Sharp JL, Fruhauf CA, Atler KE, Schmid AA: Merging yoga and occupational therapy for Parkinson's disease: a feasibility and pilot program, *Occup Ther Health Care* 34(4):351–372, 2020. https://doi.org/10.1080/07380577.2020.1824302. PMID: 32965143.

215. Tekriwal A, Kern DS, Tsai J, Ince NF, Wu J, Thompson JA, Abosch A: REM sleep behaviour disorder: prodromal and mechanistic insights for Parkinson's disease, *Journal of Neurology, Neurosurgery and Psychiatry* Vol. 88(Issue 5):445–451, 2017. https://doi.org/10.1136/jnnp-2016-314471.

216. Thaut MH, McIntosh GC, Rice RR, et al.: Rhythmic auditory stimulation in gait training for Parkinson's disease patients, *Mov Disord* 11:193, 1996.

217. Thinnes A, Padilla R: Effect of educational and supportive strategies on the ability of caregivers of people with dementia to maintain participation in that role, *Am J Occup Ther* 65:541–549, 2011.

218. Thomas T, Banwell B: Multiple sclerosis in children, *Semin Neurol* 28:70, 2008.

219. Thompson JA, Cruickshank TM, Penailillo LE, et al: The effects of multidisciplinary rehabilitation in patients with early-to-middle-stage Huntington's disease: a pilot study, *Eur J Neurol* 20:1325–1329, 2013.

220. Thornton M, Travis SS: Analysis of the reliability of the modified caregiver strain index, *J Gerontol B Psychol Sci Soc Sci* 58(2):S127–S132, 2003. https://doi.org/10.1093/geronb/58.2.s127. PMID: 12646602.

221. Tiftikçioğlu Bİ: Multiple Sclerosis Functional Composite (MSFC): Scoring Instructions, *Arch Neuropsychiatry* 55(Supplement 1):S46–S48, 2018. https://doi.org/10.29399/npa.23330.

222. Todd WD: Potential pathways for circadian dysfunction and sundowning-related behavioral aggression in Alzheimer's disease and related dementias, *Front Neurosci* 14:910, 2020. https://doi.org/10.3389/fnins.2020.00910. PMID: 33013301; PMCID: PMC7494756.

223. Tofani M, Ranieri A, Fabbrini G, Berardi A, Pelosin E, Valente D, Fabbrini A, Costanzo M, Galeoto G: Efficacy of occupational therapy interventions on quality of life in patients with Parkinson's disease: A Systematic Review and Meta-Analysis, *Mov Disord Clin Pract* 7(8):891–901, 2020. https://doi.org/10.1002/mdc3.13089. PMID: 33163559; PMCID: PMC7604677.

224. Trejo A, Boll M-C, Alonzo ME, Ochoa A, Velásquez L: Use of oral nutritional supplements in patients with Huntington's disease, *Nutrition* 21:889–894, 2005.

225. Tullman MJ, Oshinsky RJ, Lublin FD, Cutter GR: Clinical characteristics of progressive relapsing multiple sclerosis, *Mult Scler* 10:451–454, 2004.

226. Ullah I, Zhao L, Hai Y, Fahim M, Alwayli D, Wang X, Li H: Metal elements and pesticides as risk factors for Parkinson's disease – a review. *Toxicology Reports*, Vol. 8, 2021, Elsevier, pp 607–616. https://doi.org/10.1016/j.toxrep.2021.03.009.

227. Van Walsem MR, Howe EI, Iversen K, Frich JC, Andelic N: Unmet needs for healthcare and social support services in patients with Huntington's disease: a cross-sectional population-based study, *Orphanet J Rare Dis* 10:124, 2015.

228. Venturelli M, Sollima A, Cè E, Limonta E, Bisconti AV, Brasioli A, Muti E, Esposito F: Effectiveness of exercise- and cognitive-based treatments on salivary cortisol levels and sundowning

syndrome symptoms in patients with Alzheimer's disease, *J Alzheimers Dis* 53(4):1631–1640, 2016. https://doi.org/10.3233/JAD-160392. PMID: 27540967.

229. Videnovic A: Treatment of Huntington disease, *Curr Treat Options Neurol* 15(4):424–438, 2013. https://doi.org/10.1007/s11940-013-0219-8. 2013.

230. Walker FO: Huntington's disease, *Lancet* 369:218–228, 2007.

231. Wallin MT, Culpepper WJ, Campbell JD, Nelson LM, Langer-Gould A, Marrie RA, Cutter GR, Kaye WE, Wagner L, Tremlett H, Buka SL, Dilokthornsakul P, Topol B, Chen LH, LaRocca NG: US Multiple Sclerosis Prevalence Workgroup. The prevalence of MS in the United States: A population-based estimate using health claims data, *Neurology* 92(10):e1029–e1040, 2019. https://doi.org/10.1212/WNL.0000000000007035. Erratum in: Neurology. 2019;93(15):688. PMID: 30770430; PMCID: PMC6442006.

232. Walton C, King R, Rechtman L, Kaye W, Leray E, Marrie RA, Robertson N, La Rocca N, Uitdehaag B, van der Mei I, Wallin M, Helme A, Angood Napier C, Rijke N, Baneke P: Rising prevalence of multiple sclerosis worldwide: Insights from the Atlas of MS, third edition, *Mult Scler* 26(14):1816–1821, 2020. https://doi.org/10.1177/1352458520970841. PMID: 33174475; PMCID: PMC7720355.

233. Weinshenker BG, Issa M, Baskerville J: Long-term and short-term outcome of multiple sclerosis, *Arch Neurol* 53:353, 1996.

234. Welsby E, Berrigan S, Laver K: Effectiveness of occupational therapy intervention for people with Parkinson's disease: systematic review, *Aust Occup Ther J* 66(6):731–738, 2019. https://doi.org/10.1111/1440-1630.12615. PMID: 31599467.

235. Wessels AM, Andersen SW, Dowsett SA, Siemers ER: The Integrated Alzheimer's Disease Rating Scale (iADRS) findings from the EXPEDITION3 trial, *J Prev Alzheimers Dis* 5(2):134–136, 2018. https://doi.org/10.14283/jpad.2018.10. PMID: 29616706.

236. Wichmann T, DeLong MR: Functional and pathophysiological models of the basal ganglia, *Current Opinion in Neurobiology* 6(6):751–758, 1996.

237. Wiederholt W: Parkinson's disease and other movement disorders. In *Neurology for non-neurologists*, ed 4, Philadelphia, 2000, WB Saunders.

238. Wu P-L, Lee M, Huang T-T: Effectiveness of physical activity on patients with depression and Parkinson's disease: A systematic review, *PLoS One* 12(7):e0181515, 2017. https://doi.org/10.1371/journal.pone.0181515.

239. Yesavage JA, Brink TL, Rose TL, et al: Development and validation of a geriatric depression scale: a preliminary report, *J Psychiatr Res* 17:37, 1982–1983.

240. Yoshino H: Edaravone for the treatment of amyotrophic lateral sclerosis, *Expert Rev Neurother* 19(3):185–193, 2019. https://doi.org/10.1080/14737175.2019.1581610. PMID: 30810406.

241. Yu C-H, Mathiowetz V: Systematic review of occupational therapy–related interventions for people with multiple sclerosis: part 1. Activity and participation, *Am J Occup Ther* 68:27–32, 2014.

242. Yu C-H, Mathiowetz V: Systematic review of occupational therapy–related interventions for people with multiple sclerosis: part 2. Impairment, *Am J Occup Ther* 68:33–38, 2014.

243. Zucchella C, Sinforiani E, Tamburin S, Federico A, Mantovani E, Bernini S, Casale R, Bartolo M: The multidisciplinary approach to Alzheimer's disease and dementia. a narrative review of non-pharmacological treatment, *Front Neurol* 9:1058, 2018. https://doi.org/10.3389/fneur.2018.01058. PMID: 30619031; PMCID: PMC6300511.

SUGGESTED READINGS

Beghi E, Chiò A, Couratier P, et al: The epidemiology and treatment of ALS: Focus on the heterogeneity of the disease and critical appraisal of therapeutic trials, *Amyotroph Lateral Scler* 12:1–10, 2011.

Bello-Haas VD, Kloos AD, Mitsumoto H: Physical therapy for a patient through six stages of amyotrophic lateral sclerosis, *Phys Ther* 78:1312, 1998.

Borasio GD, Votz R, Miller RG: Palliative care in amyotrophic lateral sclerosis, *Neurol Clin* 19:829, 2001.

Brown RH Jr: Amyotrophic lateral sclerosis and other motor neuron diseases. In Fauci A, Braunwald E, editors: *Harrison's principles of internal medicine* ed 17, New York, 2008, McGraw-Hill.

Corcoran, MA (ed.) *Neurocognitive Disorder (NCD): Interventions to Support Occupational Performance.* AOTA Press.

LaBan MM, Martin T, Pechur J, et al: Physical and occupational therapy in the treatment of patients with multiple sclerosis, *Phys Med Rehabil Clin N Am* 9:603, 1998.

Lechtzin N, Rothstein J, Clawson L, et al: Amyotrophic lateral sclerosis: evaluation and treatment of respiratory impairment, *Amyotroph Lateral Scler Other Motor Neuron Disord* 3:5, 2002.

Mitsumoto H: *Amyotrophic lateral sclerosis: a guide for patients and families*, ed 3, New York, 2001, Demos Medical Publishing.

RESOURCES

Amyotrophic Lateral Sclerosis Association: http://www.alsa.org.

National Multiple Sclerosis Society: https://secure.nationalms-society.org/site/Donation2?df_id=65831&65831.donation=form1&s_src=dmp-fy23-HOM-don-cpc&s_subsrc=SEM-General-Headline&utm_source=SEM&utm_medium=cpc&utm_campaign=dmp-fy23-HOM-don&utm_content=General-Headline&gclid=COnPtMXhwoIDFeA_rQYd5e4Eeg&gclsrc=ds.

37

Spinal Cord Injury

Jennifer Bashar and Heidi A. Dombish

LEARNING OBJECTIVES

After studying this chapter, the student or practitioner will be able to do the following:

1. Understand the difference between a complete and an incomplete spinal cord injury and the classification system used to describe such levels of injury.
2. Recognize and identify the various spinal cord injury syndromes.
3. Briefly describe the medical and surgical management of the individual who has experienced a traumatic spinal cord injury.
4. Identify some of the complications that can limit optimal functional potential.
5. Describe the changes in sexual functioning in males and females after a spinal cord injury.
6. Identify the specific assessment areas that must be considered before developing intervention objectives.
7. Analyze the critical issues to consider when developing intervention objectives during the acute, post-acute, and outpatient phases of the rehabilitation process.
8. Identify the functional outcomes, including equipment considerations and personal and home care needs that can be reached at each level of complete injury under optimal circumstances.
9. Describe some of the special considerations that arise for a spinal cord injury in the pediatric population.
10. Analyze how the effects of a spinal cord injury accelerate the normal aging process and explain how functional status may change.

CHAPTER OUTLINE

KEY TERMS

Autonomic dysreflexia (AD)

Durable medical equipment provider

Heterotopic ossification (HO)

Paraplegia

Pressure injury

Quadriplegia

Spasticity

Tetraplegia

THREADED CASE STUDY

Jack, Part 1

Jack (prefers the pronouns he/him/his) is a 23-year-old White male who sustained a C6 complete (AIS A) spinal cord injury (SCI) as a result of a motor vehicle accident. He works full-time in a bank and is studying to get a degree in business administration. He lives alone in a two-story house that he recently purchased and plans to renovate. His mother and stepfather live in the same city, and both work full-time.

Jack was initially airlifted from the accident site to a trauma hospital, where he underwent a posterior spinal fusion from C5–T1. While in the intensive care unit he was referred to and evaluated by occupational therapy providers (OT). OT services provided during the acute stage focused on addressing Jack's physical needs (providing range of motion and positioning devices to protect joint integrity and prevent skin breakdown) and environmental needs (nurse call light, television control, phone access). Spinal injury education with Jack and his family was initiated.

Upon his transfer to the inpatient rehabilitation unit, a comprehensive OT evaluation was conducted. Jack's occupational profile and history were obtained, in addition to a comprehensive evaluation of his strength, sensation, cognition, and vision. His specific manual muscle test revealed 3+ (Fair+) to 4 (Good) strength in deltoids, biceps, and radial wrist extensors and 2– (Poor–) strength in triceps. Sensory examination was intact to the C6 dermatome. He initially required assistance for all aspects of his activities of daily living (ADLs), including bed

and wheelchair mobility. Jack's goals included being able to feed himself, get dressed by himself, be strong enough to push a manual wheelchair, live in his house again, and return to school to complete his degree.

Throughout this chapter, consider the short- and long-term consequences of Jack's injury to his ability to successfully engage and participate in his occupations and life contexts. Keep in mind the effects of his SCI on client factors, performance skills and patterns, and the relationship of activity demands to the selection of optimal equipment to enhance mobility and other areas of occupation.

Critical Thinking Questions

1. Considering Jack's level of SCI, what expectations would there be for functional recovery, and what interventions could the therapist provide to maximize his independence in performance of ADLs and instrumental activities of daily living (IADLs)?
2. What durable medical equipment and adaptive equipment will maximize efficiency in his mobility and ADLs?
3. How will the therapist approach OT interventions and realistic expectations regarding his specific goals of achieving independence in self-care, returning to school, living independently, and other important lifestyle options?

DEFINITION OF SPINAL CORD INJURY

A spinal cord injury (SCI) is a catastrophic and life-changing event that is defined as an injury to the spinal cord or spinal nerve roots that results in temporary or permanent change in an individual's motor, sensory, and/or autonomic function. According to the National Spinal Cord Injury Statistical Center (2020), there are approximately 294,000 people in the United States living with SCI, and an estimated 17,810 new cases occur each year.[41] SCI can be the result of a traumatic or nontraumatic event. Motor vehicle accidents are the most common cause of traumatic SCI, followed by accidental falls, acts of violence (e.g., gunshot and stab wounds), and sports accidents. The average age at onset has risen from 29 years old in the 1970s to 43 years old since 2015; approximately 78% of SCIs occur among males.[41] Nontraumatic spinal cord dysfunction may be a result of multiple sclerosis, degenerative central nervous system diseases, tumors, vascular disease, inflammatory disease, spinal stenosis, myelomeningocele, or hydrosyringomyelia.[23] Although some of the intervention principles discussed may apply to the nontraumatic spinal cord conditions, this chapter will focus primarily on rehabilitation of the individual with a traumatic SCI.

SCI can result in neurological impairment below the level of injury to the spinal cord. Tetraplegia (also known as quadriplegia) is paralysis caused by a cervical injury and involves any degree of paralysis of the four limbs and trunk musculature. There may be partial upper extremity function, depending on the level of the cervical lesion. Paraplegia is paralysis caused by a thoracic, lumbar, or sacral injury and involves any degree of paralysis of the lower extremities with involvement of the trunk, legs, feet, and toes, depending on the level of the lesion.[37,38]

The extent of neurological damage depends on the location and severity of the injury (Fig. 37.1). The neurological level of injury is determined by the International Standards for Neurological Classification of Spinal Cord Injury (ISNCSCI).

A neurological examination is completed by a trained medical professional that involves testing of key muscles and sensory points (Fig. 37.2).[7] SCIs are referred to in terms of the regions (*C*, cervical; *T*, thoracic; *L*, lumbar; and *S*, sacral) of the spinal cord in which they occur and the numerical order of the neurological segments. The neurological level given is the most caudal segment of the cord where sensation is intact and muscle strength is at least 3/5 (Fair). The results of the ISNCSCI examination also determine whether the injury is complete or incomplete and its classification on the ASIA Impairment Scale (AIS), which was established by the American Spinal Injury Association (ASIA).

Complete Versus Incomplete Neurological Classification

The difference between a complete and an incomplete injury is whether the individual has voluntary motor control or sensation in the anal area (S4–S5 segments of the spinal cord). A complete injury, classified as an AIS A, indicates that there is no motor or sensory function preserved at S4–S5. An individual with an AIS A SCI may have preservation of strength or sensation below the neurological level of injury; this is referred to as the zone of partial preservation (ZPP).[7]

In an incomplete injury, the individual has some degree of voluntary motor control or sensation preserved at S4–S5. An AIS B SCI (sensory incomplete) indicates that there is sensation, but not motor control, below the neurological level of injury, including at S4–S5. An AIS C SCI (motor incomplete) indicates that there is motor function preserved below the neurological level of injury, and more than half of the key muscles below the neurological level have a muscle grade of less than 3 (Fair). An AIS D SCI (motor incomplete) indicates that there is motor function preserved below the neurological level of injury, and more than half of the key muscles have a muscle grade of 3 (Fair) or more. An AIS E SCI indicates that the individual tests

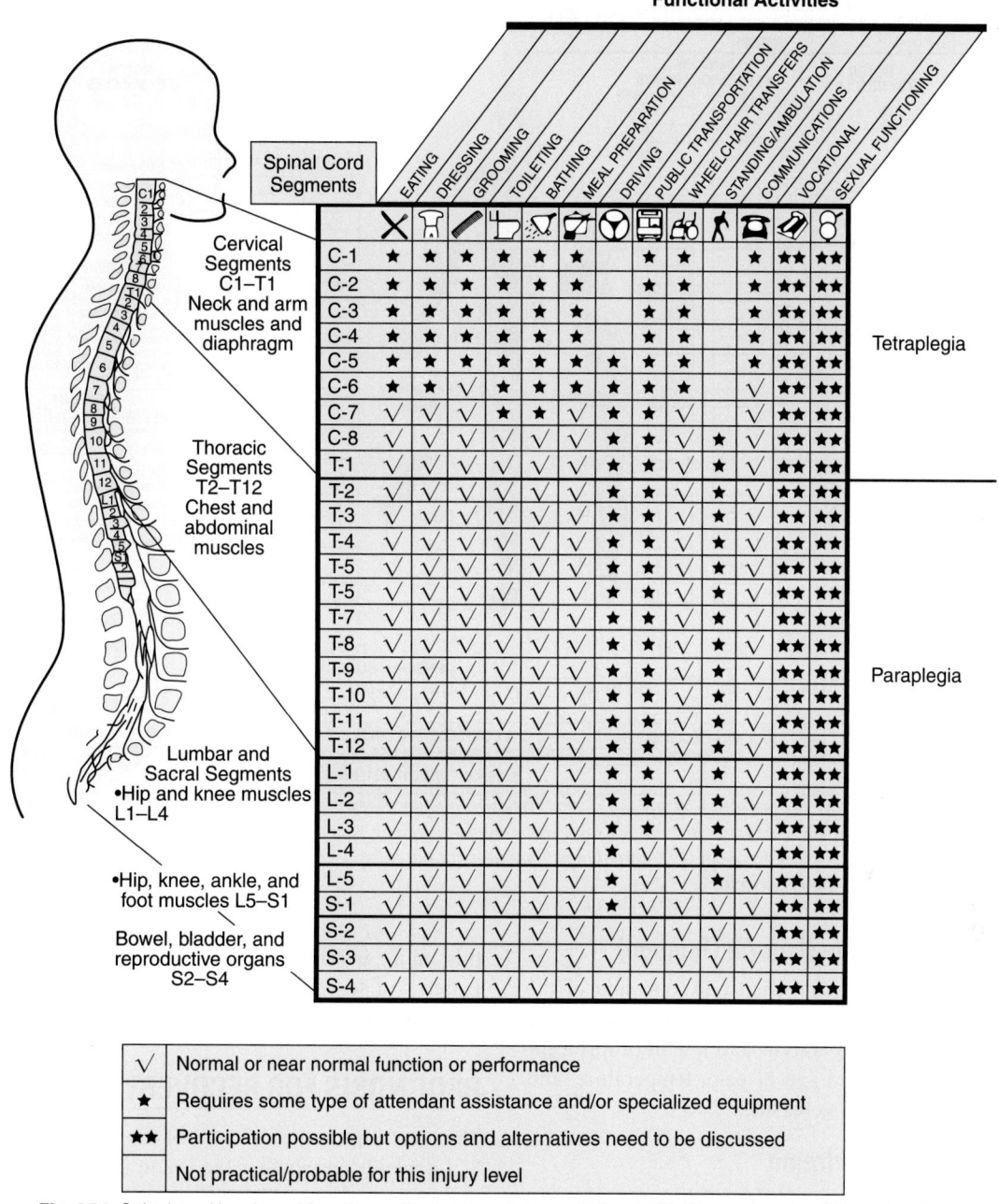

Fig. 37.1 Spinal cord levels and functions affected by spinal cord injury (SCI). (From Monahan FD, et al, editors: *Phipps' medical-surgical nursing health and illness perspectives*, ed 8, St Louis, 2007, Mosby.)

as having normal sensation and motor control.[7] Incomplete tetraplegia is the most frequently occurring neurological category, accounting for 47.2% of SCI since 2015.[41] Incomplete paraplegia and complete paraplegia each account for approximately 20% of SCIs since 2015.[41]

An ISNCSCI examination was completed with Jack upon arrival at the trauma center and at 72 hours post onset. For both examinations his sensory examination was intact to the C6 dermatome and absent below. The key muscles innervated at C6, radial wrist extensors, were graded at 3+/5 (Fair+). Because he had 2−/5 (Poor−) strength in his triceps (C7 key muscle) at the 72-hour examination, he was given a neurological level of C6 AIS A with a ZPP at C7.

CLINICAL SYNDROMES

Central Cord Syndrome

Central cord syndrome (CCS) is the most common incomplete SCI and occurs when there is more damage in the center of the cord than in the periphery. This damage is most frequently a result of a cervical hyperextension injury, such as a fall, and is commonly seen in older adults with arthritic changes that have caused a narrowing of the spinal canal. Symptoms include paralysis that is greater in the hands and arms than in the trunk and legs, bladder dysfunction, sensory loss below the level of injury, and painful sensations, including tingling, burning, or dull aching.[32,40]

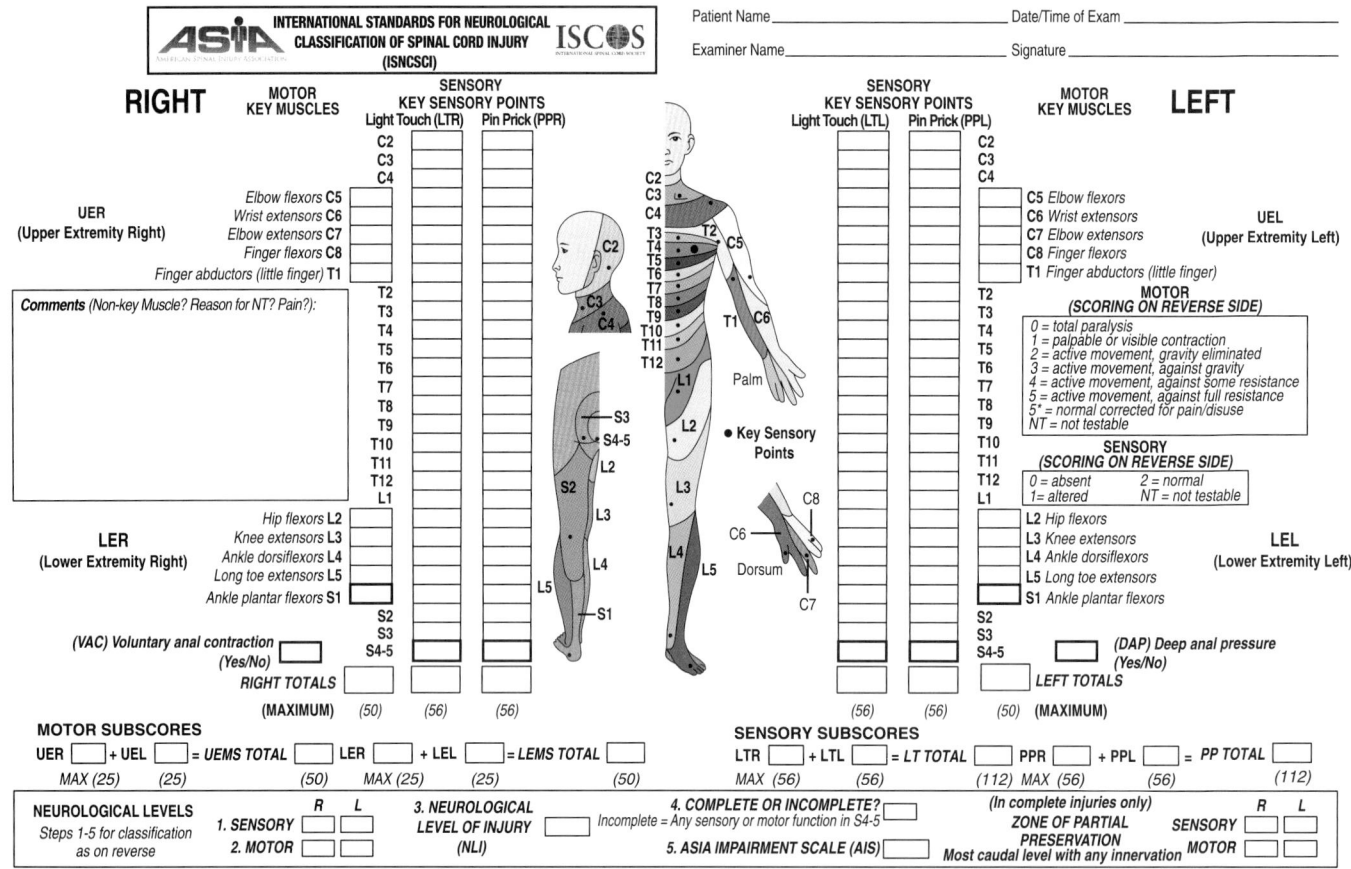

Fig. 37.2 International Standards for Neurological Classification of Spinal Cord Injury (ISNCSCI). (From American Spinal Injury Association: *International standards for neurological classification of spinal cord injury*, Atlanta, 2008, The Association.)

Brown-Séquard Syndrome (Lateral Damage)

Brown-Séquard syndrome results when only one side of the cord is damaged, as in a stabbing or gunshot injury. Below the level of injury there is motor paralysis and loss of proprioception on the ipsilateral side and loss of pain, temperature, and touch sensation on the contralateral side.

Anterior Spinal Cord Syndrome

Anterior spinal cord syndrome results from injury that damages the anterior spinal artery or the anterior aspect of the cord. This syndrome involves paralysis and loss of pain, temperature, and touch sensation. Proprioception is preserved.

Conus Medullaris Syndrome

Conus medullaris syndrome involves injury of the sacral cord (conus) and lumbar nerve roots within the neural canal, which usually results in an areflexic bladder, bowel, and lower extremities.

Cauda Equina Syndrome

Cauda equina injuries involve peripheral nerves rather than directly involving the spinal cord. This type of injury usually occurs with fractures below the L2 level and results in a flaccid-type paralysis. Because peripheral nerves possess a regenerating capacity that the cord does not (at a rate of 1–2 mm/day),[34]

this injury is associated with a better prognosis for recovery. Patterns of sensory and motor deficits are highly variable and asymmetric in cauda equina injuries.

PROGNOSIS FOR RECOVERY

The most important indicator of the long-term prognosis after SCI depends on whether the lesion is complete or incomplete, as determined by an ISNCSCI examination completed 72 hours to 1 week post injury.[21,28] If there is no sensation or return of motor function below the level of lesion during this period in carefully assessed complete lesions, motor function is less likely to return. However, partial to full return of neurological function one spinal nerve root level below the vertebral fracture can be gained and may occur in the first 6 to 9 months after injury. The majority of improvements will occur within the first year post injury but may continue up to 3 to 4 years after the injury.[21] Among individuals with complete tetraplegia, 70% to 85% will gain at least one level by 1 year post injury. The rates of conversion from complete (AIS A) to incomplete (AIS B, C, or D) status at 1 year post injury range from 4% to 22%; the rates of conversion from incomplete (AIS B) to motor incomplete (AIS C or D) status range from 33.3% to 71.3%.[27,30] For Jack, it is reasonable to anticipate that he will regain one neurological level, from C6 AIS A to C7 AIS A, within the next year.[38]

With incomplete lesions, progressive return of motor function is possible but varies, depending on the type of lesion. Brown-Séquard syndrome has the best prognosis; 75% to 90% of individuals ambulate independently at discharge from inpatient rehabilitation.[32] CCS also has a good prognosis for recovery but is age dependent; 97% who are younger than 50 years will ambulate, compared with 41% of individuals older than age 50.[32] Anterior cord syndrome has a poor prognosis for functional improvement, with only a 10% to 20% chance of motor recovery.[32] Frequently, chances for a better recovery are greater the earlier recovery begins.

Questions regarding the prognosis can be expressed at any point in time along the rehabilitation continuum by the individual with SCI, the client's family, or friends. The therapist's response will depend on many factors, including the age, educational level, level of adjustment, and stage of recovery of the individual. It is important to acknowledge and respect any expressions of hope, uncertainty, loss, and helplessness while simultaneously fostering effective coping strategies and feelings of independence.[15] As you build a partnership with the individual, actively promote the client's understanding of the rehabilitation process. Take opportunities to educate the client in self-management and directing care strategies. Emphasize that the purpose of rehabilitation is to prevent further medical complications through education, to maintain and improve the strength and skills that are present, to maximize function and facilitate mobility, and to optimize lifestyle options for the individual and the family.

MEDICAL AND SURGICAL MANAGEMENT OF THE PERSON WITH A SPINAL CORD INJURY

After a traumatic event in which SCI is likely, careful examination, stabilization, and transportation of the patient may keep a temporary or minimal SCI from becoming more severe or permanent. Emergency medical technicians, paramedics, and air transport personnel are trained in SCI precautions and extrication techniques for moving a person who has sustained a possible SCI from an accident site. Axial traction on the neck should be maintained, and any movement of the spine and neck prevented during this process. Initial care is directed toward preventing further damage to the spinal cord and reversing neurological damage, if possible, by stabilization or decompression of the injured neurological structures.[15,25] The effects of steroids administered within the first 24 to 48 hours post injury continue to be actively researched and, while still used, are not definitively recommended.[15,21,25] Emerging acute medical therapies include the use of cooling measures (hypothermia) and pharmacological neuroprotective agents; both are still in experimental phases.[21,24]

Anteroposterior and lateral x-ray films are commonly taken with the individual's head, neck, or spine immobilized to help determine the type of injury. A computed tomography (CT) scan or magnetic resonance imaging (MRI) may be needed to further determine the extent of injury. Open surgical reduction with internal fixation and spinal fusion are sometimes indicated to decompress the spinal cord and achieve spinal stability and normal bony alignment. Surgery is not always necessary,

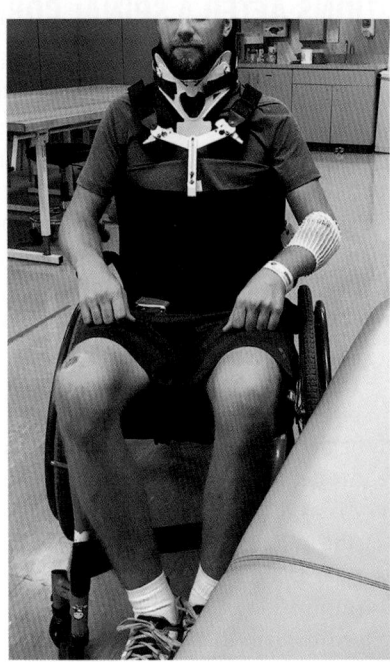

Fig. 37.3 Cervical collar and thoracolumbosacral orthosis (TLSO). (Courtesy Rancho Los Amigos National Rehabilitation Center, Downey, CA.)

and adequate immobilization may allow the individual to heal. Specialized beds are recommended for patients with an unstable spine if they are going to be immobilized for an extended length of time.[15] As soon as possible a means of portable immobilization is provided, usually a cervical collar or halo vest for cervical injuries and a thoracic brace or body jacket for thoracic injuries (Fig. 37.3). This approach enables the client to be transferred to a standard hospital bed and, subsequently, to be upright in a wheelchair and involved in an active therapy program as soon as there is medical and spinal stability.[15] Initiating an upright sitting tolerance program shortly after injury can substantially reduce the incidence and severity of further medical complications, such as deep vein thrombosis, joint contractures, and the general deconditioning that can result from prolonged bed rest.

The benefits of early transport to a specialized SCI center have been documented and include improved outcomes and fewer complications.[15,49] Spinal cord centers are equipped to offer a complete, multidisciplinary program executed by an experienced team of professionals who specialize in this unique and demanding disability. Clients treated in specialized SCI centers demonstrate reduced total lengths of stay, reduced incidence of pressure injuries, lower rates of joint contractures, and increased neurological recovery. It also has been found that individuals sent to rehabilitation centers specializing in the treatment of SCI make functional gains with greater efficiency.[15,24]

Jack was airlifted from the accident site to a trauma hospital, where a CT scan revealed significant fractures at C5–C6. He was intubated due to signs of respiratory failure, and a catheter was placed in his bladder to drain urine. He underwent posterior spinal stabilization and fusion from C5–T1. After his surgery he was placed on a specialty bed to prevent pressure injuries.

COMPLICATIONS AFTER A SPINAL CORD INJURY

After an SCI there is potential for the individual to experience secondary complications as the body adjusts to disturbances in both body functions and body structures. It is imperative that the therapist understand the signs, symptoms, and potential effects these secondary complications could have on occupational performance. During each interaction the therapist must be vigilant in detecting the signs and symptoms of these complications, proactive in preventing their occurrence, and diligent about educating the client and identified caregivers.

Autonomic Dysreflexia

Autonomic dysreflexia (AD), an abnormal response to a problem in the body below the level of the SCI, is a medical emergency and can be life-threatening. It is a phenomenon seen in individuals whose injury is at the T6 level and above. AD is caused by reflex action of the autonomic nervous system in response to some stimulus, such as a distended bladder or bowel, kidney or bladder stone, constipation or bowel impaction, infection, pressure sore, ingrown toenail, thermal or pain stimuli, deep vein thrombosis, or broken bone. The most dangerous sign of AD is a rapid rise in systolic blood pressure that is 20 to 40 mm Hg or higher than the individual's normal blood pressure; most individuals with SCI have a baseline systolic blood pressure in the range of 90 to 110 mm Hg. Other symptoms are an immediate pounding headache, anxiety, perspiration, flushing, goose bumps above the level of injury, nasal congestion, and bradycardia.[11,28]

If AD is suspected, the client should be placed in an upright position with removal of anything restrictive or noxious, such as abdominal binders or antiembolism stockings, to reduce blood pressure. The bladder should be drained or leg bag tubing checked for obstruction. Blood pressure and other symptoms should be monitored until they return to normal. The occupational therapist must be aware of symptoms and treatment because AD can occur at any time after the injury. Individuals who are susceptible to this condition are encouraged to carry an emergency card describing the condition and treatment because many emergency departments and medical personnel may be unfamiliar with it.

Orthostatic Hypotension

Orthostatic hypotension is defined as a decrease of 20 mm Hg or more of systolic blood pressure and is common during the acute phase of rehabilitation when the patient moves from a supine to an upright position or changes body position too quickly.[19] A lack of muscle tone in the abdomen and lower extremities leads to pooling of blood in these areas, with a resultant decrease in blood pressure (hypotension). Risk factors are prolonged bed rest, rapid changes in position, dehydration, and eating heavy meals.[19] Symptoms are dizziness, nausea, and loss of consciousness. With time this problem can diminish as sitting tolerance and level of activity increase; however, some people continue to have hypotensive episodes.

Therapists frequently encounter orthostatic hypotensive episodes when assisting the patient to sit upright for the first time. If this occurs, the patient must be reclined quickly and, if sitting in a wheelchair, should be tipped back with the legs elevated until symptoms subside. Abdominal binders, compression garments, antiembolism stockings, and medications can help reduce symptoms. Allowing the patient's body to adjust to upright sitting more gradually by elevating the head of the bed before therapy interventions can also help reduce symptoms.

Neurogenic Bladder and Bowel

SCI interrupts the communication between the nerves in the spinal cord that control bladder and bowel function. Signs of a neurogenic bladder include the inability to empty the bladder, incontinence, urinary frequency, and urinary tract infections. Signs of a neurogenic bowel include bowel incontinence, constipation, and impaction. After the onset of SCI the manner by which the bladder and bowel works depends on the level of injury.

A spastic (reflex) bladder usually occurs in clients with SCI at T12 and above; these individuals will have no control over when the bladder empties. A flaccid bladder usually occurs in clients with SCI T12 to L1, and they lose the ability to detect when the bladder is full. These individuals are at risk for the bladder wall to be overstretched and, in extreme cases, ruptured. The most common approach to managing both types of SCI bladder is intermittent catheterization.

The reflex or upper motor neuron bowel occurs in lesions above T12. The anal sphincter remains closed but opens on a reflex basis when the rectum is full. Management of the reflex bowel typically involves using digital rectal stimulation and stimulant medications. The areflexic bowel occurs in lesions in the lumbar or sacral level. There is reduced reflex control of the anal sphincter, and the individual is prone to accidental defecation. The areflexic bowel is typically managed by digital stimulation.

Occupational therapists are frequently involved in assisting clients with lesions below C5 to achieve independence with bladder and bowel management. The clinical practice guidelines of the Consortium for Spinal Cord Medicine—"Bladder Management for Adults with Spinal Cord Injury: A Clinical Practice Guideline for Health-Care Providers" and "Neurogenic Bowel Management in Adults with Spinal Cord Injury"—are comprehensive and valuable resources in SCI bladder and bowel management.[12,14]

Pressure Injuries

A pressure injury (also referred to as pressure ulcer, pressure sore, decubitus ulcer, bedsore, or skin breakdown) is a lesion or an injury to the skin or underlying tissue that is caused by a loss of blood flow to the area. Sensory loss after SCI prevents messages of pain or discomfort from reaching the brain and increases the risk of a pressure injury. Too much pressure on the skin, shearing forces, and trauma (cuts, burns, bumps) are all causes of pressure injuries. The areas most likely to develop skin breakdown are bony prominences over the sacrum, ischium, trochanters, elbows, and heels; however, other bony prominences, such as the iliac crest, scapula, knees, toes, occiput, and rib cage, are also at risk.

Pressure injuries are life-threatening, but most are preventable. All rehabilitation personnel must be aware of the signs of developing skin problems. Box 37.1 presents a description of the stages of pressure injuries. Pressure injuries can be prevented by having the client perform the following measures: regular pressure reliefs when seated (also referred to as weight shifts, pressure reduction, or pressure redistribution); complete skin inspections; routine turning and repositioning in bed; keeping the skin clean and dry; maintaining adequate nutrition and hydration; and wearing properly fitting clothing and shoes. Specialized mattresses and wheelchair seat cushions, proper transfer techniques, and protection of bony prominences with various types of padding are also essential to pressure injury prevention.

Occupational therapists play a key role in pressure injury prevention. During activities of daily living (ADLs) training sessions the therapist will teach clients how to examine their skin using adaptive equipment, such as a mirror, and how to integrate skin inspection into their daily routine. Other strategies, such as directing others to watch for signs of developing problems or using technology such as smart phone apps for pressure relief reminders, may be introduced. Additional skin inspection is necessary when orthoses such as hand splints and body jackets are used because they can cause skin breakdown, particularly when protective sensation in those areas is impaired.

Decreased Vital Capacity

Acute respiratory compromise and subsequent decreased vital capacity is a problem among individuals who have sustained cervical and high thoracic lesions. Individuals with injuries at C4 and above require mechanical ventilation to breathe secondary to paralysis of the diaphragm, intercostal muscles, and abdominal muscles. They will require caregiver assistance to maintain a patent airway (free of secretions). Individuals with injuries between C4 and T6 may have a tracheostomy. They will be able to breathe on their own but will have limited chest expansion and a decreased ability to cough because of weakness of the intercostal and abdominal muscles. Individuals with tetraplegia who breathe on their own may still require the assistance of a caregiver to cough (assisted cough). Individuals with injuries between T6 and T12 will have an impaired cough due to weakness of intercostal and abdominal muscles. Sequelae of respiratory compromise include an increased risk for respiratory tract infections and a decreased endurance level for activity. Strengthening of the sternocleidomastoids and the diaphragm, manually assisted cough, and deep breathing exercises are essential to maintain optimal vital capacity.[21]

Jack's vital capacity was 50% of normal capacity for a person of his size. He required assistance to cough because he did not have the force to clear his secretions upon exhaling. His endurance was low, and he initially required frequent rest breaks during treatment sessions.

Spasticity

Spasticity is an involuntary muscle contraction below the level of injury that results from a disruption in the flow of signals between the spinal cord and the brain. Patterns of spasticity change over the first year, gradually increasing in the first 6

months and reaching a plateau approximately 1 year after the injury. Moderate spasticity can be helpful in the overall rehabilitation of the individual with SCI. It helps to maintain muscle mass, assists in the prevention of pressure injuries by facilitating blood circulation, and can be used to assist in range of motion (ROM) and bed mobility. A sudden increase in spasticity can alert the individual to other medical problems, such as urinary tract infections, constipation, skin breakdown, and fractures or other injuries below the level of injury.[36]

Severe spasticity can be frustrating to the client because it can be painful, cause a loss of joint ROM, interrupt sleep, and interfere with activities such as self-feeding and transferring to a wheelchair. Therapeutic interventions include consistent ROM exercises and stretching to help maintain flexibility; splints, braces, or serial casting can be used to provide continuous stretch to the muscle. Severe spasticity may need to be treated more aggressively with a variety of medications (e.g., baclofen, dantrolene, benzodiazepines) or with nerve or motor point blocks using chemodenervative agents such as strains of botulinum toxin. In severe cases intrathecal medication therapy (e.g., baclofen pump) or neurosurgical procedures (e.g., myelotomy, rhizotomy, tendon lengthening) may be indicated.[28,36]

Heterotopic Ossification

Heterotopic ossification (HO) is bone that develops in abnormal anatomic locations. HO occurs in 16% to 53% of individuals with SCI. It is most commonly seen in the muscles around the hip and knee, but it can also develop at the elbow and shoulder.[28] The onset of HO is usually 1 to 6 months after injury, and the first symptoms are pain, swelling, warmth, and decreased joint ROM. Symptoms are often discovered during physical therapy (PT) or OT sessions, even when radiologic findings are negative. Early diagnosis and initiation of treatment can minimize complications. Treatment consists of medication and the maintenance of joint ROM during the early stage of active bone formation to preserve the functional ROM necessary for good wheelchair positioning, symmetric position of the pelvis, and maximal functional mobility.[26]

Pain

Pain is a serious obstacle for many individuals with SCI and has the potential to negatively affect engagement in meaningful occupations. Acute pain begins suddenly and is usually described as a sharp pain; it may be mild or severe and usually disappears after the underlying cause of the pain is treated or healed. For individuals with SCI, acute pain could be a result of broken bones, surgery, pressure areas or sores, burns, or a muscle tear. Chronic pain is persistent pain that does not go away and lasts months to years.[10] It is usually the result of nerve damage related to the SCI, but the cause may be unknown.

Types of pain an individual with SCI may experience can be further differentiated between musculoskeletal pain, neuropathic (or neurogenic) pain, and visceral pain. Musculoskeletal pain is a result of muscular, joint, or bone damage and will usually get worse with movement and get better with rest.[35] Neuropathic pain is a result of damage to the nerve fibers; this damage creates abnormal communication between the spinal cord and the brain, causing the brain to misinterpret the intensity of signals it receives from the area of injury. Neuropathic pain is usually described as burning, stabbing, or tingling pain.[1] Visceral pain is usually described as cramping or aching in the abdomen and can be a result of a medical problem such as constipation, a kidney stone, ulcer, gallstone, or appendicitis.[35]

Neck and/or back pain is often reported by individuals with SCI. Causes of neck and back pain include recent surgery to fuse the spine, soft tissue involvement (e.g., muscle strain, bruising), increased motion above and below the spinal fusion, and overuse by individuals who use mouth- or chin-operated joysticks to control their power wheelchairs.

The shoulder is the most common location of pain after onset of SCI, with the incidence and severity increasing over time after injury.[39] During the acute and post-acute phases of rehabilitation, shoulder pain is extremely common in individuals with C4 through C7 tetraplegia, causing decreased shoulder and scapular ROM and impacting participation in functional activities. Possible causes include scapular immobilization resulting from prolonged bed rest, nerve root compression subsequent to the injury, and subluxation at the glenohumeral joint. During the outpatient phase of rehabilitation, shoulder pain is common in individuals with C5 through C8 tetraplegia and all levels of paraplegia. Repetitive movements, such as pushing a manual wheelchair, doing pressure reliefs, and transfers, can cause muscle overuse and strain, chronic impingement syndrome, rotator cuff tears, and arthritic changes.[35] Shoulder pain should be thoroughly assessed and diagnosed so that proper intervention and activity or equipment modifications can be provided before the onset of chronic discomfort and functional loss.

SPINAL CORD INJURY REHABILITATION

Rehabilitation Team

SCI rehabilitation is best delivered under the auspices of a highly cohesive interdisciplinary team. The team, with the client at its center, is ideally composed of a rehabilitation physician (physiatrist) experienced in SCI, a rehabilitation nurse, occupational therapist (OT), physical therapist (PT), speech therapist, recreation therapist, psychologist, social worker, and case manager. Team members should understand the ISNCSCI classification system and how it applies to recovery; of common medical complications of SCI and how to prevent them; and of the psychological and social ramifications of SCI and how to assist clients and their families during the adjustment process. Team members also should be actively involved in the education of the client throughout the rehabilitation process.[5]

Goal of Rehabilitation

The goal of all phases of rehabilitation is to help the individual with SCI reach his or her full potential after the injury. Because every individual is unique and each injury is different, the rehabilitation program can differ markedly from one individual to the next. The severity of injury, functional goals, adjustment to injury, and discharge options will all have an impact on the length of time an individual spends in any one phase of rehabilitation.

- Occupational profile: Client factors, context, goals
- Sensation: Light touch, pinprick (per the guidelines established by the International Standards for Neurological Classification of Spinal Cord Injury [ISNCSCI])
- Pain: Type, location, rating scale
- Range of motion: Active, passive
- Manual muscle test
- Grip and pinch strength
- Modified Ashworth Scale (MAS)
- Self-care function
- Vision
- Cognition

Occupational Therapy Evaluation

The OT evaluation of the SCI client begins during the initial contact, continues during each subsequent interaction with the client, and lasts long after discharge on an outpatient follow-up basis. It is an ongoing, fluid process that requires the OT to continually evaluate the client's functional progress, the appropriateness of any OT intervention, and the utility of recommended adaptive equipment. The top-down and client-centered approaches outlined in the current Occupational Therapy Practice Framework (OTPF-4)[4] recommend that the OT evaluation contain a thorough occupational profile and analysis of occupational performance. Box 37.2 presents key OT assessments for SCI.

Before treating the client, the therapist must gather pertinent data from the medical chart, including personal information, a medical diagnosis, and a history of other relevant medical information. Specific medical precautions will be obtained from the primary and consulting physicians. Skeletal instability and related injuries or medical complications will affect the way in which the client is moved and the active or resistive movements allowed.

Occupational Profile

The occupational profile is the key to the evaluation process and will help shape and guide all therapeutic interventions. It is developed in close collaboration between the therapist and the client and should include the following information about the client: (1) occupational history and life experiences; (2) patterns of daily living (i.e., daily life roles, typical day); (3) values, interests, and needs; and (4) current understanding of his or her issues and problems.[4] This information can be gathered formally through a structured interview or informally during casual conversation. Often it is helpful to involve the client's family and friends if the client is unable to participate; however, once the client is able to participate in the process, his or her input is prioritized.

Keeping the client's priorities, occupational goals, and desired outcomes central to the intervention plan will maximize the individual's engagement in the rehabilitation program, and the more physical aspects (body structure and body functions) will be put into perspective as underlying and supportive to these occupational goals.

Psychosocial Status

By gathering the information required to build the client's occupational profile and beginning OT interventions, the occupational therapist has the opportunity to learn about and observe the client's psychosocial adjustment to the disability and life in general through the nature of the activities and occupations in which the client participates.[42] The evaluation phase is important for establishing rapport and mutual trust, which will facilitate participation and progress in later and more difficult phases of rehabilitation. The client's motivation, determination, and contexts—including socioeconomic background, education, family support, personal attitudes toward disability, problem-solving abilities, and financial resources—can prove to be invaluable assets or limiting factors in determining the outcome of rehabilitation. A therapist must carefully observe the client's status in each of these areas before recommending the course of intervention. In preparation for understanding the gamut of issues affecting a client's short- and long-term psychosocial health after SCI, it is recommended to the reader to study Chapter 6, in which the "Lived Experience of Disability" is presented by examining the "Intersection of Disability Perspectives and Occupational Justice."

Clinical Picture

Body Functions and Structures

A thorough physical assessment of a client with SCI will address (1) sensory functions, (2) neuromusculoskeletal and movement-related functions (joint mobility and joint stability), (3) muscle functions (power, endurance, tone), (4) movement functions (control of voluntary movement motor skills, involuntary movement reactions, gait patterns), and (5) mental functions (cognition, affect). It is also important to understand how the SCI is affecting the individual's cardiovascular, respiratory, voice and speech, digestive, genitourinary, reproductive, and skin functions (refer to previous section on medical complications of SCI).

Key sensory functions to be assessed include pain, touch (light touch, superficial pain), and proprioception (see Chapter 23). Vision should be screened for impairment, particularly in clients with a dual diagnosis (SCI and traumatic brain injury [TBI]) and in clients with C1–C4 tetraplegia in which there may have been trauma to the brainstem (see Chapter 24).

The presence or absence of pain must be established before and during each intervention. If pain is present, a quantifiable client self-report measure, such as the Numeric Rating Scale or Visual Analog Scale, should be used to establish severity and track changes in pain in response to therapeutic intervention (see Chapter 28). The OT must take careful note of how the client describes his or her pain to differentiate neuropathic pain (described as burning, stabbing, or tingling), musculoskeletal pain (usually gets worse with movement and improves with rest), and visceral pain (located in the abdomen).

Sensation is evaluated for light touch and superficial pain (pin prick) according to ISNCSCI guidelines and determines areas of absent, impaired, and intact sensation. These findings are useful in establishing the level of injury and determining functional limitations (see Fig. 37.1).[7] Proprioception and kinesthesia testing (particularly with incomplete lesions), stereognosis testing, and monofilament testing (particularly with peripheral nerve

injuries) also may be indicated to obtain an accurate picture of upper extremity functional use.

Passive range of motion (PROM) and active range of motion (AROM) should be measured before specific manual muscle testing to determine available pain-free movement. This evaluation also identifies the presence of or potential for joint contractures, which could suggest the need for preventive or corrective splinting and positioning (see Chapter 21).

Accurate assessment of muscle power, or strength, is critical in determining a precise diagnosis of neurological and functional level and for establishing a baseline for physical recovery and functional progress. Because the occupational therapist's skills in activity analysis greatly enhance the therapist's effectiveness in treating the client with SCI, a precise working knowledge of musculoskeletal anatomy and specific manual muscle testing techniques is essential. Use of accepted muscle testing protocols ensures accurate technique during performance of this complex evaluation. The muscle test should be repeated as often as is necessary to provide an ongoing picture of the client's strength and progress (see Chapter 22).

Muscular endurance, the muscle's ability to perform contractions repeatedly over time before fatigue sets in, is important to consider before planning interventions. Endurance is assessed by engaging the client in various activities or exercises and tracking the length of time that the specific muscle group can be used to continue the activity. For example, Jack was only able to feed himself three bites of his meal during his first self-feeding session. Over time his endurance increased, and after 1 week he was able to feed himself an entire meal (see Chapter 20 for occupation-based functional assessments).

Spasticity is rarely noted in the acute phase because the client is still in spinal shock. When spinal shock subsides, increased muscle tone may be present in response to stimuli. The therapist should then determine whether the spasticity interferes with or enhances function. Use of a quantifiable measure, such as the Modified Ashworth Scale (see Chapter 19), will help track changes in spasticity and help justify specific interventions.

An evaluation of upper extremity function determines the degree to which a client can perform functional movement and manipulate objects. Formal assessment of tetraplegic hand function is strongly recommended and can be used to track a client's progress over time and as an outcome measure in clinical research. Factors such as the client's upright sitting tolerance and adjustment to disability will influence the selection of the appropriate outcome measure. Information on websites such as http://www.rehabmeasures.org and http://www.scireproject.com can be used to guide selection of the most appropriate measure. Gross grasp and pinch measurements indicate functional abilities and may be used as an adjunct to manual muscle testing to provide objective measurements of baseline status and progress for clients who have active hand musculature. Additional assessment of wrist and hand function is completed through observation of the client interacting with and moving objects around the immediate environment. Note whether any compensatory strategies are being used to manipulate and grip objects, such as using a two-hand hold, using extreme ranges, weaving objects, dragging objects, using the teeth or a table to stabilize an object, and/or tenodesis.[18] This information is used to suggest the need for equipment such as positioning splints or adaptive devices. (See Chapters 30, 10, and 17 for splinting and assistive device and technology information.)

Clinical observation is used to assess oral motor control, head control, trunk control (righting reactions and static/dynamic sitting balance), lower extremity functional muscle strength, and total body function. Additional variables such as age, body morphology, limb length, and general flexibility could have an impact on the client's ability to achieve independence and should be recorded. More specific assessment in any of these areas may be required depending on the client's specific needs.

Mental (cognitive, affective, and perceptual) function should be screened in all individuals with SCI. From 25% to 64% of individuals with SCI have some degree of TBI and are referred to as having a dual diagnosis.[28] Variables that may indicate the presence of a TBI include loss of consciousness at the time of injury, tetraplegia from a high-energy deceleration crash, evidence of brainstem or cortical damage, and/or the need for initial respiratory support.[28] Others may have a history of mental illness, such as schizophrenia, bipolar affective disorder, or depression, and still others may be showing early signs of age-related dementia. It is important to assess the client's ability to initiate tasks, follow directions, carry over learning day to day, and handle problem-solving tasks. Understanding the client's learning style, coping skills, and communication style is also essential and contributes to the information base necessary for appropriate and realistic goal setting (see Chapters 25 and 26).

Because of the nature of Jack's injury (motor vehicle accident), a screening of mental function was completed both in the intensive care unit and in the inpatient rehabilitation unit. The occupational therapist in the intensive care unit noted that Jack required additional time to process new information and also verbal cues to carry over tasks between sessions, such as remembering to use his universal cuff to hold his fork. By the time Jack was transferred to inpatient rehabilitation, his affect had improved and he was able to consistently demonstrate carryover of new learning between treatment sessions.

Functional Status

Observing as the client performs ADLs is an important part of the OT evaluation. The purpose of this observation is to determine present and potential levels of functional ability. If the client is cleared of bed rest precautions, evaluation and simultaneous intervention should begin as soon as possible after injury. Light activities such as feeding, light hygiene at the sink, and object manipulation may be appropriate, depending on the level of injury (see Chapter 10). Performance is scored using outcome measures such as the Inpatient Rehabilitation Facility-Patient Assessment Instrument (IRF-PAI) Quality Indicators, or the Spinal Cord Independence Measure (SCIM). Table 37.1 presents the IRF-PAI QI scoring guidelines.

ESTABLISHING INTERVENTION OBJECTIVES

Establishing intervention objectives in concert with the client and the rehabilitation team is vital. The primary objectives of the rehabilitation team may not be those of the client. Psychosocial

TABLE 37.1   Scoring of the Inpatient Rehabilitation Facility Patient Assessment Instrument (IRF-PAI): Self-Care Quality Indicators

Score	Assistance Level Required
6	Independent
5	Set-up or clean up assistance
4	Supervision or touching assistance
3	Partial/moderate assistance (helper does less than half the effort)
2	Substantial/maximal assistance (helper does more than half the effort)
1	Dependent (helper does all of the effort)

factors, cultural factors, cognitive deficits, environmental limitations, and individual financial considerations must be identified and integrated into a comprehensive intervention program that will meet the unique needs of each individual. Every client is different; therefore, a variety of intervention approaches and alternatives may be necessary to address each factor that may affect goal achievement.[15] Tools for client-driven goal setting, such as the Canadian Occupational Performance Measure (COPM),[29] should be used to aid the client in identifying and prioritizing occupations that are meaningful at this point in his or her rehabilitation. Increased participation can be expected if the client's priorities are respected to the extent that they are achievable and realistic.

General objectives for OT intervention with the individual with SCI are as follows:

1. Maintain or increase joint ROM and prevent problems associated with body functions and other body structures (skin) via preparatory activities, such as active and passive ROM, splinting, positioning, and client education.
2. Increase the strength of all innervated and partially innervated muscles and address problems associated with other body functions (e.g., sensation, higher-level cognitive functions, psychosocial functions) through preparatory activities and engagement in purposeful activities and occupations.
3. Increase physical endurance and other performance skills and performance patterns through engagement in purposeful activities and occupations.
4. Maximize independence in performance in all areas of occupation, including ADLs, instrumental activities of daily living (IADLs), rest and sleep, education, work, play, leisure, and social participation.
5. Aid in the psychosocial adjustment to disability.
6. Evaluate, recommend, and educate the client in the use and care of necessary durable medical and adaptive equipment.
7. Ensure safe and independent home and environmental accessibility through consultation and safety and accessibility recommendations.
8. Assist the client in developing the communication skills necessary for training caregivers to provide safe assistance.
9. Educate the client and family regarding the benefits and consequences of maintaining healthy and responsible lifestyle habits in relation to long-term function and the aging process.

OCCUPATIONAL THERAPY INTERVENTION

Phases of Recovery

Occupational therapists provide services across the continuum of care for individuals with SCI. The acute care phase begins in the intensive care unit and is the time when the individual is most medically fragile. Once the client is medically stable, the post-acute/rehabilitation recovery phase begins; it is during this phase that the individual receives intense inpatient therapy (at least 3 hours a day, 5 to 6 days a week). The length of time spent in the post-acute/rehabilitation recovery phase depends on many factors and varies from individual to individual. The outpatient rehabilitation phase begins after discharge from acute/post-acute hospitalization and can take place in a variety of settings, including clinics, private or group homes, and specialty gyms. Beyond the outpatient phase, lifetime follow-up emphasizes keeping clients healthy and active.

Acute Phase

The role of the Occupational therapist in the acute care setting with individuals with SCI includes preserving joint integrity and mobility with positioning and early mobilization, restoring function through self-care training, initiating education and training of families and caregivers, and coordinating care, including preparation for transition to the next level of care.[3] The OT evaluation during this phase will give priority to determining the baseline neurological, clinical, and functional status from which to formulate an early intervention program. Although initially addressing these critical physical client factors, the OT can be simultaneously engaging the client in an occupational profile, learning the client factors related to values, beliefs, and spirituality, along with the areas of occupation that comprise and give meaning to the client's life. Medical precautions must be followed at all times. The individual may be in traction, wearing a stabilization device (e.g., halo brace or body jacket), or have limitations in joint mobility and body movement.

Preservation of joint integrity and mobility includes an evaluation of total body positioning and hand splinting needs. For individuals with tetraplegia, the arms should be intermittently positioned in 80 degrees of shoulder abduction, external rotation with scapular depression, and full elbow extension to prevent the development of ROM limitations and shoulder pain (Fig. 37.4). Hand splints are introduced when muscle strength is not adequate to support the wrist and hands properly. If wrist extension strength is less than 3+/5 (Fair+/Normal), a splint that supports the wrist at neutral, keeps the thumb in opposition to maintain the thumb web space, and allows the fingers to flex slightly at the metacarpophalangeal (MP) and proximal interphalangeal (PIP) joints should be used (Figs. 37.5 and 37.6). If wrist extension strength is 3+/5 (Fair+/Normal) or greater, a short opponens splint should be considered to maintain the web space and support the thumb in opposition during functional tenodesis training. Passive, active-assisted, and active ROM of all joints should be performed within strength, ability, and tolerance levels. Muscle reeducation techniques for the wrists and elbows should be used when indicated. Light progressive resistive exercises may be introduced as permitted by the medical team. During this time families and caregivers can be trained to assist with ROM exercises, splint use, and skin inspection.

The client should be encouraged to engage in self-care activities (e.g., self-feeding, hygiene) using simple devices such as a universal cuff or built-up handle (Fig. 37.7). When indicated, access to bedside activities that might be of interest to the client, such as modified call systems, laptop computer setup on bedside

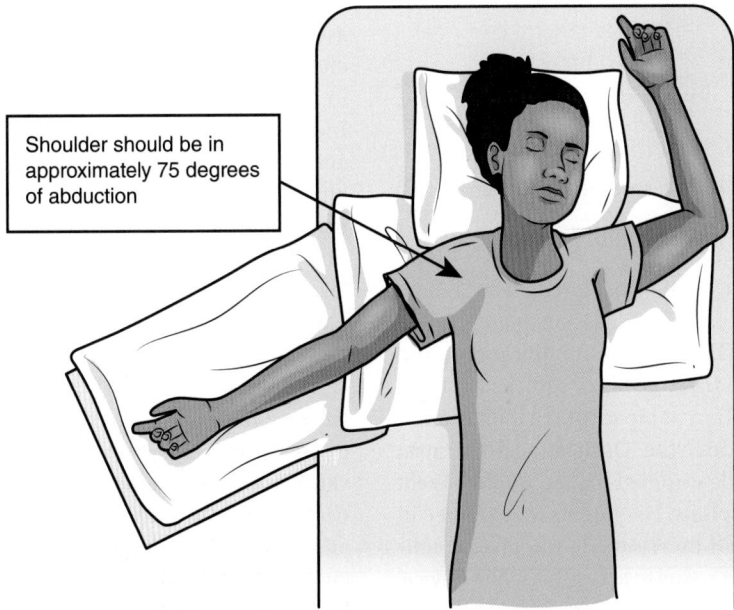

Fig. 37.4 Supine bed positioning for individuals with tetraplegia. Using pillows: *(1)* Position arm out to the side in approximately 75 degrees of abduction. *(2)* Position other arm out to the side, hand back above the head, arm in abduction and external rotation, elbow bent. *(3)* Place pillows on either side of the legs with the railings up to help maintain the legs in a neutral position. *(4)* Place a pillow under the head and shoulders so that the head is not pushed forward.

Shoulder should be in approximately 75 degrees of abduction

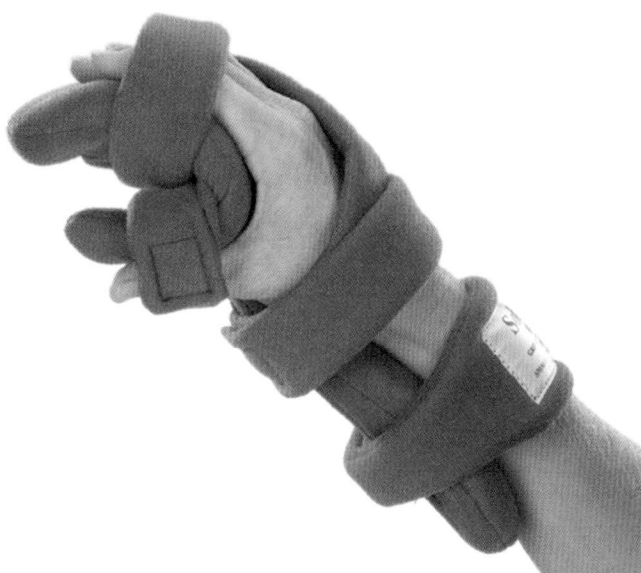

Fig. 37.5 Resting hand splint. (Courtesy AliMed, Dedham, MA.)

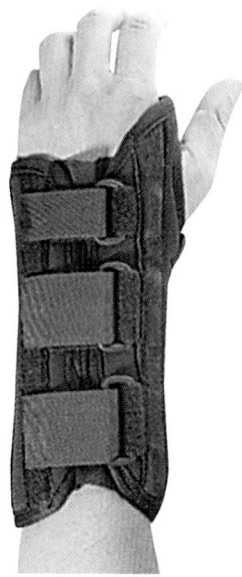

Fig. 37.6 Wrist support. (Courtesy Performance Health, Warrenville, IL.)

tables, and avocational activities, can be explored. Even though the client may be immobilized in bed, discussion of anticipated durable medical equipment (DME), home modifications, and caregiver training should be initiated to allow sufficient time to prepare for discharge or transition to inpatient rehabilitation.

While Jack was in acute care, the Occupational therapist assessed his arm strength and determined that he would benefit from bilateral short opponens splints. His parents were trained in passive and active-assisted ROM exercises. He was given a universal cuff for self-feeding and a stylus to access his tablet device.

Post-Acute Phase: Inpatient Rehabilitation

Some individuals will be transitioned to inpatient rehabilitation within the same facility and will require a quick reassessment of physical status. Others will be transferred from an acute care

setting to a new facility for inpatient rehabilitation and will require a thorough OT evaluation. Still others may be admitted from skilled nursing facilities or from home; these individuals may be several months past their initial injury and are likely to have developed secondary complications, such as pressure injuries and joint contractures. In all cases the beginning of the inpatient rehabilitation program is an opportunity for the Occupational therapist to introduce the importance of self-management and to collaborate with the individual with SCI in setting realistic and attainable goals.

Self-management skills, including being proactive, self-monitoring, problem solving, communicating effectively, staying organized, and managing stress, are emphasized by the rehabilitation team and taught by OT in individual and group sessions.[33] These skills have been found to be effective in increasing self-efficacy and improving health status and behaviors, decreasing pain, increasing compliance with medication programs, and decreasing overall healthcare costs.[33] These skills are essential to independence for all individuals with SCI.

SCI education is integrated into every facet of the rehabilitation program and can be provided in many ways, including individual, small, or large group sessions; written materials, video, and online resources; and through peer mentors. Because individuals learn differently, it is important to identify the client's preferred learning style. Some topics to highlight for the individual with an SCI include transportation and driving resources, emergency preparedness, community resources, nutrition, finance management, how to select and direct caregivers, bladder management, bowel management, skin care and pressure relief, autonomic dysreflexia, pain management, and sexuality.

High tetraplegia/quadriplegia (C1–C4). The intervention and equipment needs of clients with a high-level SCI (C4 and above) are unique and extremely specialized. Individuals with C1–C3 AIS A will be ventilator dependent and require total physical assistance from a caregiver to complete ADLs; however, these clients may be considered independent in living if they are able to direct a personal care assistant to satisfactorily assist them.[4] Individuals with C4 AIS A will initially be ventilator dependent and require total physical assistance from a caregiver to complete ADLs but may progress to breathing on their own and using equipment for self-feeding, such as a hands-free hydration system. Key muscles that may be innervated at the C1–C3 level include the sternocleidomastoid, platysma, and cervical paraspinals; key muscles at the C4 level include the upper trapezius and diaphragm (Table 37.2).

Individuals with high tetraplegia begin to develop upright sitting endurance when medically stable and will require a tilt-in-space or recliner wheelchair with room to accommodate a ventilator. A mechanical lift or dependent transfer technique is used to move the individual between surfaces (e.g., between bed and wheelchair, wheelchair and car), and a pressure-relieving cushion is required. Opportunities for education include teaching the client and family members about dependent pressure relief techniques, orthostatic hypertension, and proper body mechanics.

Upper extremity management for the individual with high tetraplegia includes evaluating neck and arm positioning in bed

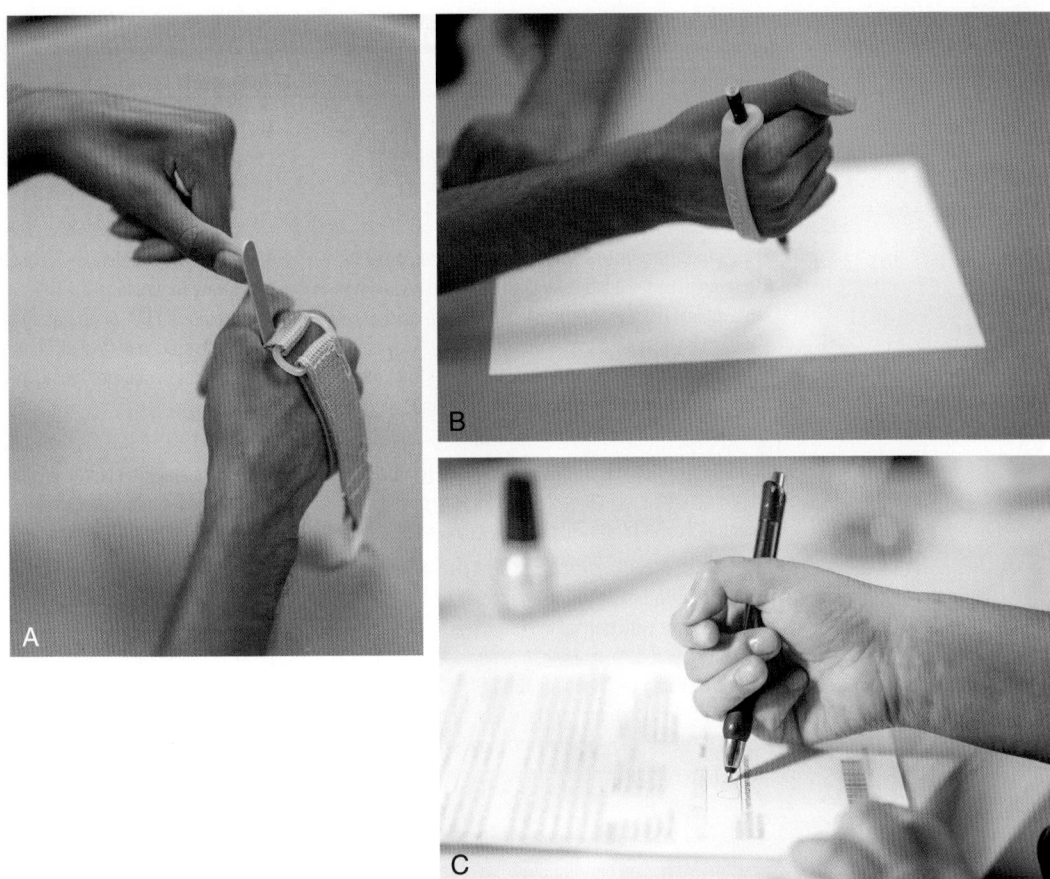

Fig. 37.7 (A) Universal cuff with nail file. (B) Writing with Eazyhold universal cuff. (C) Finger weaving with pen. (Photos courtesy Spencer Toledo, Rancho Los Amigos National Rehabilitation Center, Downey, CA.)

TABLE 37.2	Common Functional Goals for Individuals With a Complete Spinal Cord Injury		
Level of Injury	**Physical Abilities**	**Functional Goals**	**Equipment Used**
C1–C3	C3—Limited movement of head and neck	*Breathing:* Depends on ventilator for breathing.	Suction equipment to clear secretions, two ventilators with backup generator and battery
		Communication: Talking is sometimes difficult, very limited, or impossible. If the ability to talk is limited, communication can be accomplished with adaptive equipment.	Mouth stick and assistive technology (e.g., computer, communication board) for speech or typing
		Daily tasks: Requires full assistance from caregiver for turning in bed, transfers, and all self-care (including bowel and bladder management). Assistive technology can allow for independence in such tasks as reading a book or newspaper, using a telephone, and operating lights and appliances.	Mouth stick, environmental control unit (ECU)
		Mobility: Can operate an electric wheelchair by using a head control, mouth stick, sip and puff, or chin control. Power tilt function on wheelchair allows independence in pressure relief.	Power or manual lift, electric or semi-electric hospital bed, power wheelchair with pressure-relieving cushion

(Continued)

TABLE 37.2   Common Functional Goals for Individuals With a Complete Spinal Cord Injury—cont'd

Level of Injury	Physical Abilities	Functional Goals	Equipment Used
C3–C4	Usually has head and neck control; with injury at C4 level, may shrug shoulders	*Breathing:* May initially require a ventilator for breathing; usually adjusts to breathing full time without a ventilator.	Cough-assist device
		Communication: Normal	
		Daily tasks: Requires full assistance from caregiver for turning in bed, transfers, and all self-care (including bowel and bladder management). May be able to use adaptive equipment to eat independently. May also be able to operate an adjustable bed and perform other tasks, such as painting, writing, typing, and using a telephone with assistive technology.	*Eating:* Sandwich holder on a gooseneck, feeder, long straw for liquids *Other activities:* ECU for operating bed (e.g., head or voice activated, mouth stick controller), hands-free devices, mouth stick for typing
		Mobility: Can operate a power wheelchair by using head control, a mouth stick, sip and puff, or chin control. Power tilt function on wheelchair allows for independence with pressure relief.	Power or manual lift, electric or semi-electric hospital bed, power wheelchair with pressure-relieving cushion
C5	Typically has head and neck control, can shrug shoulders, and has some shoulder control; can bend elbows and turn palms up	*Daily tasks:* With specialized equipment, can be independent with eating and grooming (e.g., face washing, oral care, shaving, makeup application) after setup by caregiver. Requires total assistance from caregiver for bed mobility, transfers, and all other self-care. With adaptive equipment, may be able to assist caregiver with upper body dressing and some bathing.	*Eating:* Universal cuff for attachment of utensils, scoop plate, plate guard, long straw *Grooming:* Universal cuff for attachment of toothbrush, comb, or brush; adapted or electric razor, makeup applicators; wash mitt for face *Bathing:* Roll-in padded shower and commode chair, or padded tub transfer bench; wash mitt; adapted loofah
		Healthcare: Requires assistance from caregiver for cough assist. Can perform pressure relief with power tilt in power wheelchair.	Cough assist
		Mobility: May have strength to push a manual wheelchair for short distances over level surface; however, a power wheelchair with hand controls is required for daily activities. At this level, may be able to drive with specialized hand controls in a modified van with a lift, but still may require attendant to assist with transportation.	*Wheelchair:* Power or manual lift, electric or semi-electric hospital bed, power wheelchair with pressure-relieving cushion *Bed:* Bed ladder, thigh straps, and bed rails for bed mobility
		Bowel and bladder management: Requires total assistance from caregiver for bowel and bladder management. May have indwelling catheter, or caregiver may perform intermittent catheterization for bladder management. Bowel management involves specialized equipment or medication.	*Bowel:* Roll-in padded shower and commode chair, or padded transfer tub bench *Bladder:* Leg bag emptier
C6	Has movement in head, neck, shoulders, arms, and wrists; can shrug shoulders, bend elbows, turn palms up and down, and extend wrists	*Daily tasks:* With some specialized equipment and setup by caregiver, can be independent with most feeding, grooming, and upper body dressing. Still requires some assistance for lower body dressing, and is able to assist with upper body during bathing. With some or total assist from caregiver, can perform sliding board transfers to padded shower commode chair and/or tub bench for toileting and bathing. Can perform some light meal preparation tasks.	*Feeding:* Universal cuff, built-up utensils, scoop plate, long straw, plate guard *Grooming:* Universal cuff, adapted electric razor or toothbrush *Dressing:* Dressing stick, leg lifter, thigh straps, dressing hook splints, adapted or specialized clothing *Bathing:* Adapted loofah, long-handled sponge with universal cuff *Transfers:* Power or manual lift, sliding board, padded drop-arm bedside commode, padded tub bench with cutout, padded shower and commode chair
		Healthcare: Can independently perform pressure relief with power tilt; may require some or no assist for forward or lateral lean pressure relief.	

TABLE 37.2   Common Functional Goals for Individuals With a Complete Spinal Cord Injury—cont'd

Level of Injury	Physical Abilities	Functional Goals	Equipment Used
		Mobility: With use of special equipment, may require some or no assist for turning in bed. With some or no assistance from caregiver, may be able to perform sliding board transfers on level surfaces. Can use a ultralight manual wheelchair for mobility, but some may use a power wheelchair for greater ease over uneven terrain. Can be independent driving a power wheelchair or with manual wheelchair propulsion with specialized equipment.	*Bed:* Bed ladder, thigh straps, bed rails *Wheelchair:* Wheelchair pegs, specialized wheelchair gloves, and rubber tubing on wheels. Also, power-assist wheels can be used for independence with manual wheelchair propulsion *Transportation:* Modified van with lift, specialized hand controls, tie-downs
		Bowel and bladder management: Requires some or total assist with adaptive equipment for management of bowel and bladder.	*Bowel:* Digital stimulation splint device, enema insertion device *Bladder:* Catheter inserter, penis positioner, thigh spreader with mirror
C7–T1	Has movement similar to C6 level, with added ability to straighten elbows With injury at C8–T1 level, has added strength and precision of hands and fingers	*Daily tasks:* With equipment, is independent with all feeding, grooming, and upper body dressing. May require some or no assistance with lower body dressing and bathing with equipment. With some or no assistance, can perform sliding board transfers to padded shower commode chair and/or tub bench for toileting and bathing.	*Feeding:* Universal cuff, built-up handles, curved utensils, long straw, plate guard, adapted techniques for grasp *Grooming:* Universal cuff, splint material to adapt devices *Dressing:* Leg lifter, dressing stick, zipper pull, hooks on shoes *Bathing:* Adapted loofah, long-handled sponge with universal cuff *Transfers:* Sliding board, padded drop-arm bedside commode, padded tub bench with cutout, padded shower and commode chair
		Healthcare: Independent with wheelchair pushup or lateral lean for pressure relief.	
		Mobility: Independent with manual wheelchair propulsion and level surface sliding board transfers. May require some assistance from caregiver for uphill transfers. Can be independent with driving if able to load and unload wheelchair.	*Wheelchair:* Rigid or folding lightweight wheelchair, wheelchair pegs, wheelchair gloves *Transportation:* Hand controls, modified van if unable to perform transfer or load/unload chair
		Bowel and bladder management: Depending on hand function, requires some or total assist for bowel management, with use of adaptive equipment or medication. Can be independent or need some assist for bladder management with ICP or condom catheter.	*Bowel:* Digital stimulation splint device, enema insertion device, toileting aid *Bladder:* Catheter inserter penis holder/positioner (for men), thigh spreader with mirror (for women)
T2–T12	Has normal function in head, neck, shoulders, arms, hands, and fingers Has increased use of rib and chest muscles, or trunk control At the T10–T12 level, more improvements in trunk control because of an increase in abdominal strength	*Daily tasks:* Independent with self-care, including bowel and bladder management, with adaptive equipment if necessary.	*Dressing:* Thigh straps, reacher, dressing stick, sock aid *Bathing:* Long-handled sponge *Transfers:* Sliding board, padded drop-arm bedside commode, padded tub bench with cutout, padded shower/commode chair *Bowel/bladder:* Mirror
		Healthcare: Independent with wheelchair pushup for pressure relief.	
		Mobility: Independent with all bed mobility and transfers, with or without use of equipment. Independent with wheelchair propulsion on uneven and even surfaces and up and down curbs. Able to load and unload wheelchair independently for driving with hand controls.	*Wheelchair:* Ultra-lightweight wheelchair *Transfers:* Sliding board, leg straps *Transportation:* Hand controls

(Continued)

TABLE 37.2	Common Functional Goals for Individuals With a Complete Spinal Cord Injury — cont'd		
Level of Injury	**Physical Abilities**	**Functional Goals**	**Equipment Used**
L1–L5	Has additional return of motor movement in hips and knees	*Mobility:* Independent with all bed mobility and transfers, with or without use of equipment. Independent with wheelchair propulsion on uneven and even surfaces and up and down curbs. Can ambulate with specialized leg braces and walking devices. Functionality of ambulation depends on strength and movement in legs. Ability to ambulate depends primarily on individual's level household distances. May use a wheelchair for community mobility. Able to load and unload wheelchair independently for driving with hand controls.	*Wheelchair:* Ultra-lightweight wheelchair if necessary *Walking:* Leg braces that extend to the hip, the knee, or just the ankle/foot and varying assistive devices *Transportation:* Hand controls
S1–S5	Depending on level of injury, various degrees of return of voluntary bladder, bowel, and sexual function	*Mobility:* Increased ability to walk with fewer or no bracing or assistive devices.	*Walking:* Braces that support ankle/foot

Adapted from the Model Systems Knowledge Translation Center (MSKTC): Understanding spinal cord injury. II. Recovery and rehabilitation. https://www.msktc.org.

and in the wheelchair. As in the acute rehabilitation phase, while the client is in bed, the arms should be intermittently positioned in 80 degrees of shoulder abduction, external rotation with scapular depression, and full elbow extension to assist in preventing the development of ROM limitations and shoulder pain. A lap tray, bilateral arm troughs, or pillows can be used to support the arms with the elbow at 90 degrees while the client is in the wheelchair; remember to consider what will happen to arm position when the individual is reclined or tilted back for a pressure relief. The use of hand splints is continued to maintain available ROM.

Passive and active-assisted/active ROM is started for both the neck and arms to maximize strength in available musculature in preparation for participation in functional activities and to prevent undesirable contractures. Mouth stick training is started, and activities are chosen to reflect each client's functional goals. Card games, drawing, painting, page turning, and typing are some activities that may be used to improve neck ROM and endurance (Fig. 37.8).

Paul, a 25-year-old with a C4 AIS A injury secondary to a gunshot wound, had expressed a goal of being able to use his iPad to communicate with friends and family. At the beginning of his rehabilitation program, he was only able to shrug his shoulders and slightly turn his head. To strengthen these muscles, mouth stick training was initiated. His iPad was placed on a mounting device, and he was given a mouth stick stylus to interact with the touch screen surface. A mouth stick docking station was positioned so that he could independently set the stylus down when he needed to rest. As his neck strength and active ROM increased, his therapist challenged him by changing the position of the iPad and docking station and providing more challenging activities, such as typing emails and navigating the Internet.

Paul had also expressed a goal of being able to attend his daughter's first birthday party. The occupational therapist used

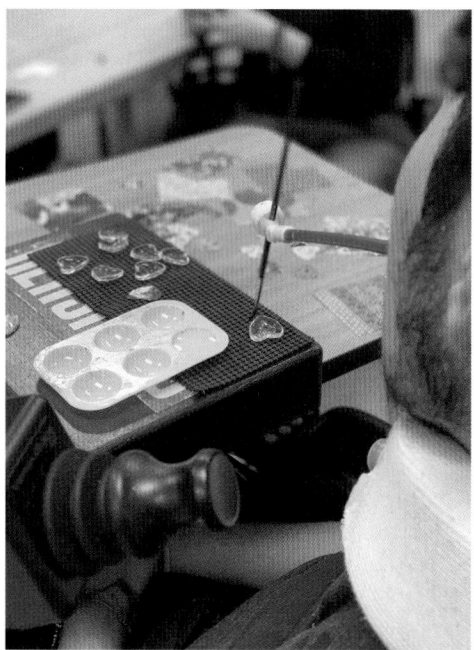

Fig. 37.8 Individual with C2 AIS A tetraplegia painting with mouth stick (Courtesy Rancho Los Amigos National Rehabilitation Center, Downey, CA).

this goal as a springboard to motivate Paul to learn to direct his care needs, including bladder and bowel management, charging his ventilator and wheelchair batteries, organizing accessible transportation, and understanding the purpose and timing of medications.

Assistive technology can be used to enhance performance skills (e.g., typing with a mouth stick to increase neck ROM and endurance) or as preparatory methods and tasks used concurrently with occupations and activities (e.g., using a laptop with voice recognition software to complete a homework assignment

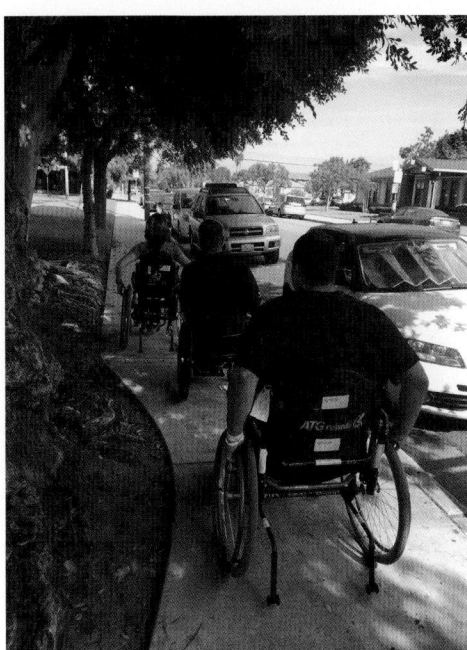

Fig. 37.9 Wheelchair skills, including navigating curb cuts and uneven surfaces, are practiced during an OT-led community outing.

TABLE 37.3 Levels of Spinal Cord Injury and Key Muscles Affected

Level of Injury	Key Muscles Affected
C1–C3	Sternocleidomastoid, cervical paraspinal, neck accessories
C3–C4	Upper trapezius, diaphragm, cervical paraspinal muscles
C5	Deltoid, biceps, brachialis, brachioradialis, rhomboids, serratus anterior (partially innervated)
C6	Clavicular pectoralis supinator, extensor carpi radialis longus and brevis, serratus anterior, latissimus dorsi
C7–T1	Latissimus dorsi; sternal pectoralis; triceps; pronator quadratus; extensor carpi ulnaris; flexor carpi radialis; flexor digitorum profundus and superficialis; extensor communis; pronator/flexor/extensor/abductor pollicis; lumbricals (partially innervated); intrinsics of the hand, including thumbs and lumbricals; flexor/extensor/abductor pollicis
T2–T12	Internal and external intercostals, erector spinae
L1–S5	Fully intact abdominals and all other trunk muscles; depending on level, some degree of hip flexors, extensors, abductors, adductors; knee flexors, extensors; ankle dorsi, flexors, plantar flexors

for school).[3] Commercially available products, such as smart phones, electronic readers, and laptop computers, many with built-in accessibility options, have greatly enhanced the options available to high-level tetraplegics, as have resources such as free adaptive telephone programs and technology lending libraries. If available, an assistive technology specialist can help determine the appropriate equipment to assist the client in reaching both short- and long-term occupational goals.

Specialized equipment, such as turning mattresses, bathing equipment (e.g., inflatable bed bath or padded tilt-in-space and reclining commode chair), and power wheelchairs should be used on a trial basis during the rehabilitation phase. Individuals with C1–C4 SCI can be independent with operating a power wheelchair using a head control, sip-and-puff, or chin control and can be independent with pressure relief when using a power tilt-in-space wheelchair (Fig. 37.9). Accessible transportation options (e.g., a van with a lift) and community transportation services are introduced. Funding resources and grant opportunities should be explored to assist the clients in obtaining this equipment. A home visit with the client as early as possible in the rehabilitation phase helps identify architectural barriers and helps the client and family prepare for discharge.

Tetraplegia (quadriplegia)/high paraplegia (C5–T1). Individuals with C5–T1 tetraplegia will require varying degrees of caregiver assistance (Table 37.3). Key muscles at the C5 level include deltoids and biceps. Individuals with C5 AIS A will be dependent on caregivers for bed mobility. Bed and wheelchair positioning is similar to that of individuals with C1–C4 injuries with one exception: these individuals are at high risk for elbow flexion and supination contractures and their forearms should be positioned in pronation. Elbow extension splints and/or pronation splints may be necessary to maintain ROM as spasticity increases. Splinting or casting of the elbows may be indicated to correct contractures that are developing. Support also should be provided for the wrist and hand; a wrist support can be used during the day and a resting hand splint at night (see Fig. 37.5).

Upper extremity management will include daily passive and active-assisted ROM and activities to maximize strength. Progressive resistive exercise can be introduced through the use of upper extremity skateboard tables. Mobile arm supports are used both to strengthen weak shoulders and elbow flexors and to increase independence in desired tasks. (See the case study for Matt in Chapter 31 to learn about an individual with C4 AIS A with C5 return who uses mobile arm supports and adaptive equipment to engage in his desired occupations, including feeding, computer use, and environmental control.)

The use of adaptive equipment will allow an individual with C5 AIS A to be independent with self-care tasks such as self-feeding and grooming after setup by the caregiver. Key adaptive equipment introduced at the C5 AIS A level includes wrist support used in conjunction with a universal cuff, scoop dish, long straw, swivel spork, long-handled utensils, long-handled comb/brush, Wanchik writer, wrist support, and mobile arm support. Independence in power wheelchair mobility can be achieved using hand controls; adequate trunk support must be provided, and a mobile arm support may initially be used to facilitate driving with a joystick control.

Individuals with C6 AIS A tetraplegia, such as Jack, will have expected functional outcomes that reflect greater independence from caregivers. Key muscles at the C6 level include the extensor carpi radialis brevis, extensor carpi radialis longus, clavicular pectoralis, and serratus anterior. The serratus anterior stabilizes and assists with rotating the scapula, allowing for better control and endurance when flexing the glenohumeral joint, as in

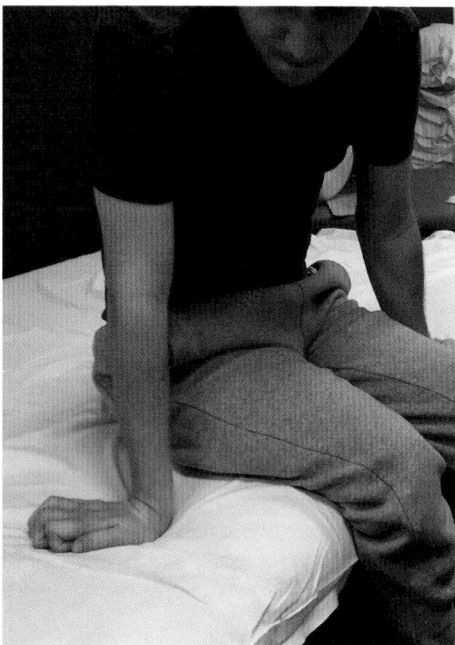

Fig. 37.10 Individual with C6 AIS A preserving tenodesis grasp during sitting balance activities. (Courtesy Rancho Los Amigos National Rehabilitation Center, Downey, CA.)

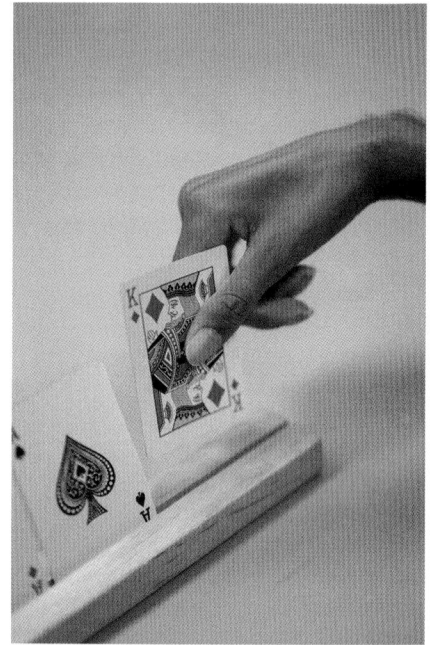

Fig. 37.11 Tenodesis grasp. (Photo courtesy Spencer Toledo, Rancho Los Amigos National Rehabilitation Center, Downey, CA.)

putting a T-shirt over one's head. The clavicular pectoralis allows for horizontal adduction, enabling crossing of the midline and assisting with rolling in bed, turning a steering wheel, and participating in some bimanual activities. Elbow contractures should never be allowed to develop. Full elbow extension is essential for allowing propping to maintain balance during static sitting and for assisting in transfers. With zero triceps strength, an individual with C6 AIS A tetraplegia can maintain forward sitting balance by shoulder depression and protraction, external rotation, full elbow extension ("locked elbows"), and full wrist extension. Special care should be taken to preserve tenodesis during sliding board transfers and sitting balance activities (Fig. 37.10).

The presence of wrist extension allows a functional tenodesis grasp: when the wrist is extended, the fingers automatically flex and allow the individual to grasp objects (Fig. 37.11). It is desirable to develop some tightness in the long finger flexor tendons to give some additional tension to the tenodesis grasp and to maintain the thumb interphalangeal (IP) joint in extension in order to attain alignment of the thumb to the index finger. Tenodesis is maintained by ranging finger flexion with the wrist fully extended and finger extension with the wrist flexed, thus never allowing the flexors or extensors to be in full stretch over all of the joints that they cross (Fig. 37.12).[31] Wrist extensors should be strengthened to maximize natural tenodesis function. Those who have weak wrist movement may use a wrist-driven wrist/hand orthosis, sometimes referred to as a tenodesis hand splint, to properly position their fingers for palmar prehension or a three-jaw chuck pinch (thumb with index and middle fingers). Neuromuscular electrical stimulation also can be used to strengthen weak wrist extensors.[8]

Functional goals for the individual with C6 AIS A range from setup with adaptive equipment to independent for self-feeding, grooming, and upper body dressing (Fig. 37.13). Adaptive equipment to be considered includes a universal cuff, scoop dish, built-up utensils, and a buttonhook. Some to total assistance will likely be required for lower body dressing, toileting, and bathing. Adaptive equipment such as a dressing stick, leg lifter, adapted long-handled sponge, wash mitt, padded tub bench, or padded rolling commode chair may be considered. Simple adaptations can be made to clothing, including widening the button hole, adding loops at the waistband, and using zip ties as zipper pulls to limit the use of adaptive equipment.

During Jack's inpatient rehabilitation stay he was introduced to the peer-mentoring program on the SCI unit. The peer mentors, individuals with SCI who have completed their own rehabilitation programs and received specialized training, were instrumental in facilitating Jack's adjustment to his SCI. The peer mentors offered Jack motivation and emotional support, demonstrated self-care and body handling skills during therapy sessions, and shared valuable resources and experiences. After watching a peer mentor with a similar level of SCI demonstrate independence in lower body dressing on a standard bed and independence with depression transfers, Jack became more motivated and confident during therapy sessions, pushing himself outside of his comfort zone and challenging his problem-solving and body-handling skills.

Individuals with C7–T1 AIS A injuries will show greater independence with self-care tasks and mobility (see Table 37.3). Key muscles at the C7 level include triceps and latissimus dorsi. The triceps muscle gives individuals the ability to extend their elbows and reach overhead; the combination of triceps and latissimus dorsi allows shoulder depression, which assists with sitting balance, transfers, pressure relief, and bed mobility. Key muscles at the C8–T1 level include the flexor carpi radialis,

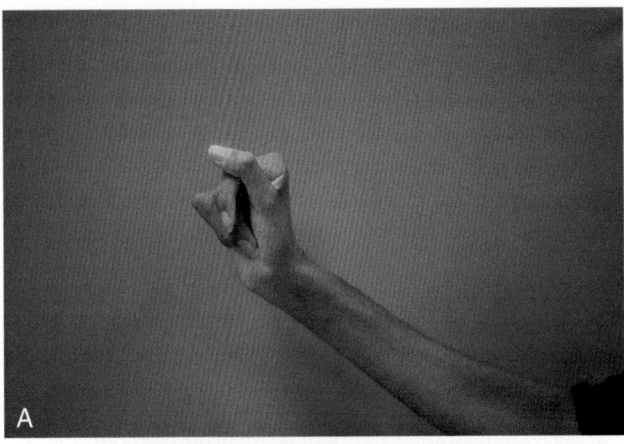 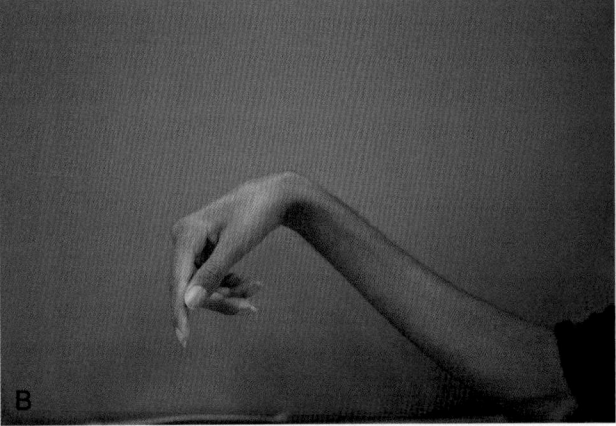

Fig. 37.12 Tenodesis movement. (Photo courtesy Spencer Toledo, Rancho Los Amigos National Rehabilitation Center, Downey, CA.)

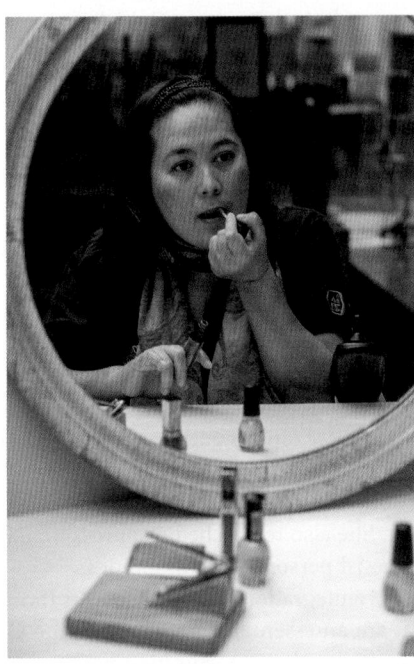

Fig. 37.13 Individual with C5/C6 incomplete tetraplegia applying makeup. (Photo courtesy Spencer Toledo, Rancho Los Amigos National Rehabilitation Center, Downey, CA.)

extrinsic thumb and finger musculature, and intrinsic thumb and finger musculature. The addition of these muscles gives greater strength, control, and precision to the hands and fingers.

Upper extremity management for individuals with a C6–T1 level of injury includes strengthening through a variety of interventions, including the use of occupations (e.g., completing a morning routine, including feeding and dressing oneself), activities (e.g., playing a game of dominoes with a friend, preparing fruit smoothies), preparatory methods (e.g., daily ROM, the use of physical agent modalities such as neuromuscular electrical stimulation), and preparatory tasks (e.g., therapy putty, resisted clothespins, exercise bands). Progressive resistive exercise and resistive activities can be applied to both innervated and partially innervated muscles. Shoulder musculature is strengthened so as to promote proximal stability, with emphasis on the

serratus anterior, latissimus dorsi (shoulder depressors), deltoids (shoulder flexors, abductors, and extensors), and the remainder of the shoulder girdle and scapular muscles. The triceps, pectoralis, and latissimus dorsi muscles are strengthened to increase independence with transfers and pressure relief when the client is in the wheelchair. Strengthening the intrinsic and extrinsic hand musculature is emphasized to create a stronger grasp and pinch. The intervention program should be graded to increase the amount of resistance that can be tolerated during activity. As muscle power and endurance improve, increasing the amount of time in wheelchair activities will help the individual participate in activities and occupations throughout the day.

Principles of energy conservation, in addition to self-management techniques, are important to introduce to individuals with C5–T1 tetraplegia. Jack, for example, can become capable of performing the majority of his self-care, including dressing and bathing, but these tasks require a considerable amount of time and energy for him to complete. On days when he will need to be at work or attend classes, he may choose to have a caregiver come early to help him complete his self-care routine.

Individuals with a C6–T1 level of injury are expected to be independent with pressure relief over time. If the individual with a C6 level of injury has at least 3+/5 shoulder and elbow flexor strength bilaterally, pressure can be relieved on the buttocks by leaning the client forward over the feet. Simple cotton webbing loops are secured to the back frame of the wheelchair. A person who has low tetraplegia (C7 with 3+/5 or better triceps) or paraplegia with intact upper extremity musculature can perform a full depression weight shift off the arms or wheels of the wheelchair. Some clients with C6 tetraplegia can also perform this type of weight shift by mechanically locking the elbows in extension while simultaneously externally rotating the shoulders and using their strong shoulder muscles to support their weight. Pressure relief should be performed every 30 to 60 minutes until skin tolerance is determined.

Paraplegia (T2–T12, L1–L5). Individuals with paraplegia have normal function of the head, neck, and upper extremities and in general have functional goals of independence for all self-care tasks, wheelchair mobility, and health management (see Table 37.2). Factors that may influence goal setting during inpatient rehabilitation include obesity, length of limbs, body handling, spasticity, age, flexibility/ROM, endurance, and psychosocial adjustment. The rate at which these individuals achieve their goals may also vary. For example, individuals with T2–T9 paraplegia have weak or no trunk control, which directly affects their sitting balance, reach, and ability to complete bimanual activities. Individuals with T10–T12 and L1–L5 paraplegia have intact trunk control and will have a reduced fear of falling, a better base of support with increased stability, and an increased ability to perform bimanual activities.

Self-care interventions typically begin at the bed level and progress to the wheelchair level. Modified techniques are introduced to enable an individual to perform tasks efficiently. Adaptive equipment such as a reacher, dressing stick, sock aid, or leg lifter may initially be necessary to accomplish tasks; however, every attempt should be made to have the client perform the task with no equipment or with as little equipment as possible. Some common progressions for self-care include:

- *Lower body dressing:* Begin in the hospital bed with the head of the bed elevated. As sitting balance and bed mobility improve, progress to using a flat bed with the bed rails up and then with the rails down (Fig. 37.14). If possible, practice on a regular bed (similar to the bed the client will have at home). Once bed-level dressing has been mastered, have the individual try from the wheelchair. Note that skin inspection using a mirror must be integrated into the client's daily self-care routine.
- *Bathing:* Initially bathing will be performed at bed level. Once the individual has adjusted to upright sitting, have him or her shower using a padded rolling commode chair. As dynamic sitting balance and transfer skills improve, progress to using a padded tub bench. If a sliding board is used for wet tub/shower transfers, the sliding board should be covered with a pillowcase and the client should be instructed to complete a series of depression lifts across the board. Equipment needs may include grab bars, a handheld shower hose, and a long-handled sponge. The discharge bathroom setup will guide the selection of bathing equipment.

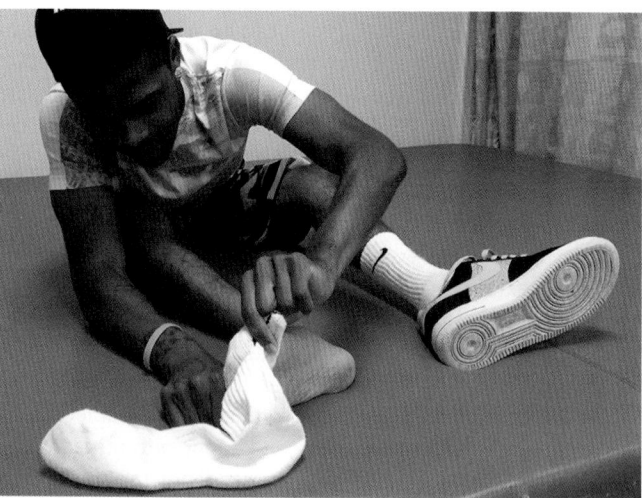

Fig. 37.14 Paraplegic lower body dressing on a flat surface. (Courtesy Rancho Los Amigos National Rehabilitation Center, Downey, CA.)

- *Bowel management:* Initially the bowel program will be performed at bed level for suppository insertion, perineal care, and clothing adjustment. As dynamic sitting balance and transfer skills improve, progress to using a padded rolling commode chair or a padded, height-adjustable commode chair placed over the toilet. Equipment needs may include a mirror, suppository inserter, digital stimulator, and toilet paper aid (see Chapter 10 for additional methods).

Upper extremity management for individuals with paraplegia will focus on strengthening and endurance to achieve clients' functional goals of independence. As with individuals with tetraplegia, occupations, activities, preparatory methods, and tasks will be used and will be specific to each individual. Shoulder preservation strategies should be incorporated into therapy sessions and home exercise programs. The clinical practice guideline established by the Consortium for Spinal Cord Medicine, "Preservation of Upper Limb Function Following Spinal Cord Injury: A Clinical Practice Guideline for Health-Care Professionals," is a comprehensive resource for this purpose.[13]

Vanessa, another client undergoing rehabilitation with Jack and Paul, is a 19-year-old college student who was injured in a motor vehicle accident and has a T10 AIS A SCI. Her goals for inpatient rehabilitation were established with her OT using the COPM. They include being able to get dressed by herself, meet friends for coffee, and return to college. Early in her inpatient stay, Vanessa and her occupational therapist went on a community outing to a nearby coffee shop. During the outing Vanessa worked on endurance training, community safety, and wheelchair skills. One week prior to discharge, Vanessa, her occupational therapist, and her physical therapist went on an outing to her college. To prepare for this outing, Vanessa focused on being independent with bladder management from the wheelchair in a public restroom and being able to place items in a backpack on her wheelchair. She also researched resources available through her college to assist persons with disabilities.

Community reintegration activities, such as those completed with Vanessa, are an essential component of the OT program. These activities provide opportunities not only for practicing skills learned in therapy sessions, but also for psychosocial adjustment, client/caregiver training, and collaboration with interdisciplinary team members. Restaurant outings, work site visits, school visits, grocery store outings, and leisure activities, such as going to the movies, fishing, and going to the park, are just some of the possibilities (Fig. 37.15). These outings also provide opportunities for Jack, Paul, and Vanessa to support each other's accomplishments and to share ideas for solutions, in addition to their feelings about reintegration into the community. The OT leading the outing is in a perfect position to facilitate discussions as they arise.

A home evaluation should be completed for all individuals with SCI before discharge home; this also is an excellent opportunity for hands-on individual and family training. The individual with SCI should accompany the therapy team whenever possible. Consider completing a home evaluation early during the inpatient rehabilitation stay so that the family has sufficient time to make any necessary modifications and then again closer to discharge so that the individual can practice skills learned at

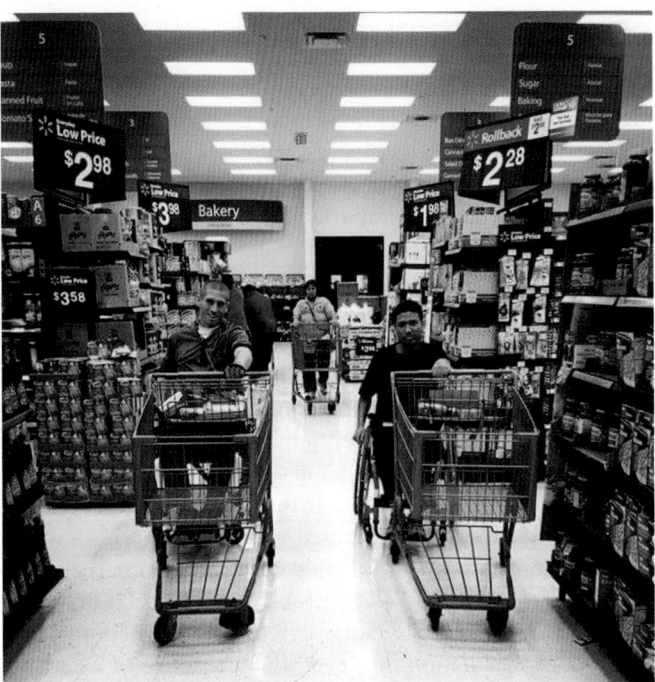

Fig. 37.15 Individuals with SCI practice grocery shopping skills during a community outing with an occupational therapist.

home and with the equipment he or she will have at discharge. The results of the home evaluation should be well documented, and recommendations should be shared with the individual, his or her caregiver, the interdisciplinary team, and third-party payer sources (particularly when specific equipment is recommended).

Jack went on a home visit with his therapists and parents to his two-story home. Together they assessed the safety and accessibility of his home. Jack practiced propelling an ultralightweight manual wheelchair throughout the first floor to make sure all the doorways were wide enough. He practiced tasks such as transferring to a padded tub bench, opening the refrigerator and kitchen cabinets to retrieve a snack, and turning on lights. Some of the immediate recommendations for Jack and his parents included building ramps to access both the front and back entrances of the home, relocating his bedroom from the second floor to the first floor, using furniture risers to raise the height of his bed to facilitate transfers, removing the glass sliding doors in the bathtub and replacing them with a curtain, and placing grab bars in the bathtub. Other options for home accessibility that are more costly involve extensive structural modification and require the services of a contractor well versed in the provisions of the Americans with Disabilities Act of 1990 (ADA; see Chapter 15), including modifying the bathroom to have a roll-in shower and accessible sink and installing a stair lift or elevator for Jack to access the second floor independently.

Incomplete SCI/clinical syndromes. For individuals with an incomplete SCI, functional outcomes are harder to predict. Therapy interventions will be guided by the clinical presentation and will rely on a thorough OT evaluation. Motor return will be greater and occur over a longer period of time, and the potential for ambulation must be considered. Upper extremity management may have the added complexity of protecting a

weak shoulder girdle and preventing shoulder subluxation when the client is standing or ambulating. Supportive devices such as slings and waist/fanny packs can be used to support the shoulder but may require caregiver assistance to put on. Treatment interventions such as neuromuscular electrical stimulation can be used to strengthen partially innervated muscles and can be used in conjunction with taping to provide support.[43]

Equipment

The assessment, ordering, and fitting of DME (e.g., wheelchairs, seating and positioning equipment, mechanical lifts, beds, and bathing equipment) are extremely important parts of the rehabilitation program. This equipment should be specifically evaluated and should be ordered only when definite goals and expectations are known. Inappropriate equipment can impair function and cause further medical problems, such as skin breakdown or trunk deformity. The therapist must take into account all functional, positioning, environmental, psychological, and financial considerations in evaluating the client's equipment needs. The desired equipment—especially wheelchairs, seat cushions, back supports, positioning devices, and bathing equipment—should be available for demonstration and trial by the client before final ordering. The therapist involved in the evaluation and ordering of this costly and highly individualized equipment should be familiar with and have considerable experience with currently available products and also should be knowledgeable about ordering equipment that will provide the client with optimal function and body positioning on a short- and long-term basis. A good working relationship with an experienced and certified assistive technology provider (ATP) (i.e., a durable medical equipment provider who assists in the selection of custom assistive technology for the consumer's needs and provides training in the use of the selected devices) is preferable. Advances in technology and design have provided a wide variety of equipment from which to choose, and working with another professional specializing in such equipment will help ensure correct selection and fit (see Chapter 11 for a more detailed discussion of wheelchairs, seating, and positioning equipment).

In addition to enhancing respiratory function by supporting the client in an erect, well-aligned position that maximizes sitting tolerance and optimizes upper extremity function, wheelchair seating must assist in the prevention of deformity and pressure injuries. An appropriate and adequate wheelchair cushion helps distribute sitting pressure, assists in the prevention of pressure injuries, stabilizes the pelvis as necessary for proper trunk alignment, and provides comfort. Whether it is the occupational therapist's or physical therapist's role to evaluate and order the wheelchair and cushion, the two should work closely together to ensure consistent training and use for the individual needs of each client.

Outpatient Rehabilitation

Decreases in the amount of time devoted to inpatient rehabilitation have moved the extended phase of intervention to an outpatient basis or home therapy context. Adaptive driving, home management, leisure activities (Fig. 37.16), and work skill assessments are feasible and appropriate intervention modalities for evaluating and

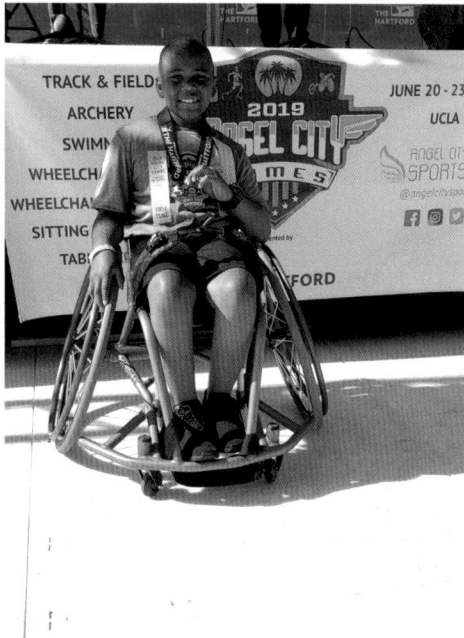

Fig. 37.16 Child with T4 paraplegia participates in wheelchair basketball tournament. (Photo courtesy Eureka Young).

increasing upper extremity strength, coordination, and trunk balance; however, they may not have been a priority during inpatient hospitalization. OT training in such activities can improve the client's socialization skills and can also assess and improve problem-solving skills and potential work habits. (See Chapters 11, 14, 16, and 17 for additional information on these topics.)

OT services can offer valuable evaluation and exploration of the vocational potential of individuals with SCI. The occupational therapist can assess the client's level of motivation, functional aptitudes, attitudes, interests, and personal vocational aspirations during the process of the intervention program and through the use of ADLs, IADLs, mobility, and work simulation occupations. The therapist can observe the client's attention span, concentration, problem-solving ability, judgment, and other high-level cognitive functions, in addition to his or her manual ability with splints and devices, accuracy, speed, perseverance, work habits, and work tolerance level. The therapist can serve as a liaison between the client and the vocational rehabilitation counselor by offering valuable information gleaned from observation during the client's performance of activities and occupations. When suitable vocational objectives have been selected, they may be pursued in an educational setting or in a work setting, usually out of the realm of OT.

Throughout the inpatient and outpatient rehabilitation phases, the occupational therapist should provide psychosocial support by allowing and encouraging clients to express frustration, anger, fears, and concerns. The OT clinic in an SCI center can provide an atmosphere in which clients can establish support groups with other inpatients and outpatients, who can share their experiences and problem-solving advice with those in earlier phases of rehabilitation. Direct OT intervention to address psychosocial issues of SCI can include training in stress management; coping skills training; and education regarding social connectedness, sexuality, relationship-building strategies, and the connection between occupation and emotional health.

SEXUAL FUNCTION

Sexual drive and the need for physical and emotional intimacy are not altered by SCI. However, the ability of the individual with an SCI to engage, develop, and explore sexuality is affected. Education is essential for the individual with SCI and all clinicians. In addition, as an important area of occupation (both in ADLs and social participation), it is a critical part of the rehabilitation process.

In males with SCI, the two most common issues affecting sexual function are the ability to have and maintain erections and ejaculation. These problems vary, depending on the location of and type of SCI and should be evaluated individually. Pharmacological interventions (oral medications, penile injection therapy), vacuum pumps, and penile prostheses are some options that may assist with erections. The decreased ability to ejaculate and decreased motility of sperm in males with SCI can affect fertility. Penile vibrostimulation (inexpensive, used at home) and rectal probe electroejaculation (more costly, done at a fertility clinic) are two of the methods used to produce ejaculation; however, the assistance of a fertility clinic is often needed to fertilize the egg, and these methods can be costly.[2,9,22]

Females with SCI will usually experience changes in lubrication of the vagina during sexual activity and an interruption of menses for weeks to months after injury. In contrast to males, there is no change in female fertility. Females with SCI can conceive and give birth. Special attention must be given to the interaction of pregnancy and childbirth with the SCI, especially with regard to blood clots, respiratory function, bladder infections, autonomic dysreflexia, and the use of medications during pregnancy and breast-feeding.[2,16,44]

The occupational therapist can address sexuality across all phases of SCI recovery. The type of intervention will be guided by the individual with the SCI and influenced by the developmental and life stages of the individual, the nature of the physical impairment, and the client's psychosocial adjustment to the SCI, readiness to learn, and sociocultural influences and expectations. OT interventions may include health promotion (e.g., education on changes in sexual function after SCI, leading support group discussions on body image), remediation (e.g., introduce gentle stretching techniques for spastic muscles as part of foreplay, develop social interaction skills), and modification (e.g., adapt a sexual device for an individual with limited hand function, teach optimal bed positioning using pillows).[2] Recent discussions in the literature emphasize the need for more timely discussions regarding the effects of SCI on sexual intimacy, family planning and parenthood, and developing sexual self-confidence and relationship skills.[20,22] The clinical practice guideline from the Consortium for Spinal Cord Medicine, "Sexuality and Reproductive Health in Adults with Spinal Cord Injury: A Clinical Practice Guideline for Health-Care Providers," is a comprehensive and valuable resource on the impact of SCI on sexuality.[13] There are also many consumer-driven resources available regarding SCI and sexuality (see Resources at the end of this chapter; also see Chapter 12).

SLEEP AND REST

Sleep disturbances for individuals with SCI can be attributed to physiological, psychological, and/or environmental factors. Physiological factors that influence the quality of sleep may include respiratory compromise from muscle weakness (diaphragm, abdominals), spasticity, and pain. Psychological factors include anxiety and depression. Environmental factors include the need for frequent turning in bed to prevent pressure injuries, the need for intermittent catheterization, side effects of medications to control pain and spasticity, and poor sleep hygiene (e.g., frequent napping throughout the day). Promoting optimal sleep and rest patterns and quality is essential to enhancing the quality of life for individuals with SCI. The occupational therapist can help the individual with SCI establish a predictable sleep hygiene routine; identify ideal positioning in bed to decrease pain, prevent pressure injuries, and prevent ROM limitations; promote self-management and caregiver management skills; and explore equipment options (e.g., turning mattresses) that will limit sleep disturbances (see Chapter 13 for more on the OT's role in promoting sleep and rest).

CHILDREN AND ADOLESCENTS WITH A SPINAL CORD INJURY

Of the 12,500 new cases of SCI each year, approximately 3% to 5% affect children and adolescents under the age of 16.[47] Unique manifestations of SCI in children include birth injuries, lap belt injuries, and SCI without radiographic abnormality (SCIWORA), in addition to an increased incidence of higher cervical injuries (C1–C3) versus lower cervical injuries (C4–C8) in younger children.[47] Motor vehicle accidents and sports injuries are the leading cause of injury in teenagers, and violence is the leading cause of injury in African American and Hispanic teenagers.[6,47] Special considerations are required during the ISNCSCI examination for the pediatric population; these guidelines are available at the website https://asia-spinalinjury.org/learning/. Equipment ordered for children and adolescents with SCI must allow for growth; measures should be taken to prevent the formation of scoliosis and hip deformities. Power wheelchair mobility may be appropriate for children with SCI as young as 20 months old; readiness can be assessed via developmental screening tools such as the Pediatric Powered Wheelchair Screening Test.[46]

OT intervention for the pediatric SCI population needs to be developmentally appropriate and family centered. Participation in age-appropriate play, school, leisure, and social activities is integrated into the rehabilitation program. Mouth stick activities could include playing board games and making invitations to a tea party. Upper extremity ROM and strengthening could include word games played on an incline table. Balance and postural retraining activities could be done on a mat or the floor while the child plays with siblings. For children and adolescents with SCI, an area of focus must be the transition to adulthood and the development of independent living skills, vocational exploration, social skill development, and a healthy lifestyle.

Consider the story of Julia, who sustained a T10 AIS A SCI as a result of a gunshot wound from a drive-by shooting when she was 9 years old. During her inpatient rehabilitation program she participated in self-care activities such as dressing and bathing, and her mother was trained in bladder and bowel management. Her mother worked full-time and wanted Julia to be independent with bladder management at school. The occupational therapist first introduced self-intermittent catheterization techniques to Julia using a doll, and over time she was able to learn how to complete her own catheterization.

Julia was a fourth-grade student at the time of her injury, and she was eager to go back to school and be with her friends. A school site visit was completed with Julia and her mother; during this visit the occupational therapist was able to assess the accessibility of the school and make recommendations to school administrators, speak to Julia's teacher about modifications she may need in the classroom (e.g., wheelchair-accessible desk), and allow Julia the opportunity to interact with her classmates for the first time since her injury while having the support of her mother and the occupational therapist.

As the years passed, Julia became involved in a local wheelchair sports program for children and returned to the SCI clinic to participate in a support group for adolescents with SCI. She graduated from high school, and with the encouragement of her support system, pursued a college degree, learned how to drive, and became a peer mentor for newly injured individuals with SCI.

AGING WITH A SPINAL CORD INJURY

Aging with SCI is a multifaceted topic, and several distinct themes must be considered: the onset of SCI at an advanced age, the changing definition of independence as one adjusts to life with SCI, and the consequences of aging with SCI.

There are increasing numbers of individuals aged 65 or older who are diagnosed with SCI; they account for 11.5% to 22.2% of new injuries each year.[48] As mentioned earlier, there has also been a rise in the average age at onset, from 29 years old in the 1970s to 42 years old since 2011.[41] The primary cause of injury for individuals over age 65 is falls, followed closely by motor vehicle accidents. These injuries result predominantly in incomplete tetraplegia, typically CCS. There is also an increased likelihood that these individuals will present with comorbidities that may negatively influence their long-term prognosis for recovery.[48] OT interventions for these individuals may include integration of chronic disease management strategies (e.g., consistently monitoring blood pressure or glucose levels and administering insulin) into daily self-care routines (see Chapter 47 for additional ideas for meeting the needs of the older adult who has a physical disability).

The primary goals of the individual with SCI and the clinician are to maximize independence in all areas of occupation during the initial phases of rehabilitation. The role of the occupational therapist during these initial phases is to introduce the possibilities and mechanisms for independence while simultaneously teaching concepts of directing caregivers, energy conservation, and work simplification. It is ultimately up to the individual with SCI to determine his or her own definition of independence, with the understanding that this definition is fluid and will change throughout the lifespan. For example, after several months at home Jack became physically independent with his morning routine; however, he required 3 hours to complete this routine and was exhausted after doing so. He decided to hire a caregiver to complete the tasks in a fraction of the time so he could focus his energy on other activities, such as school. Jack is still considered independent with his morning routine because he is in control and directing the actions of the caregiver.

Physical aging is a natural, inevitable process. The signs of the process can occur at varying rates for each individual, and aging affects most systems of the body (see Chapter 47). Individuals with SCI are susceptible to an increased rate of changes in their health and abilities as they age. The aging process is accompanied by enhanced secondary effects of the disability, including pressure injuries, infections (urinary and respiratory), muscular imbalance, pain, and joint degeneration secondary to overuse.[17] Regular screening should be performed for chronic health conditions such as diabetes, cardiovascular disease, high cholesterol, and cancer and appropriate maintenance therapies provided.[45]

When SCI is compounded by the increased fatigue and weakness often associated with normal aging, the functional status of the individual with SCI may decline. Occupational therapists may cite this change to justify additional services or equipment. Many considerations must be weighed to make appropriate short- and long-term decisions. Consulting experienced experts who have a perspective on both acute and long-term injuries and issues can provide valuable insight into intervention decisions. Approximately 20 years after injury appears to be a point at which some of the aging problems begin to increase. Thus, an individual with SCI who was independent during transfers at home and with loading a wheelchair into and out of the car may now require assistance getting into and out of bed because his or her shoulders have deteriorated. The client may have to trade the car for a van that requires costly modifications. Similarly, someone who is at a level normally associated with functional independence (e.g., T10-level paraplegia) may now need personal care assistance and possibly a power assist or power wheelchair because of degenerative changes in the shoulders, elbows, and wrists. The occupational therapist should incorporate shoulder preservation strategies (e.g., the Strengthening and Optimal Movements for Painful Shoulders [STOMPS] protocol) into the earliest stages of the rehabilitation program.[39]

RESEARCH

Current research conducted in clinical settings and scientific laboratories around the world focuses on understanding the nature

THREADED CASE STUDY

Jack, Part 2

Upon discharge from acute inpatient rehabilitation, Jack returned to his two-story home, and his mother moved in as his caregiver. Jack's father and friends built ramps for the front and back entrances and moved his bed and clothing to a room on the first floor. Bathroom modifications, including removing the glass doors and installing grab bars, were also completed. Initially his mother assisted him with lower body dressing, bathing, bladder and bowel management, sliding board transfers, and other home-making tasks, such as meal preparation. He required a padded transfer tub bench for bathing and a padded rolling commode for his bowel program, which his mother performed for him.

He was evaluated for an ultra-lightweight manual wheelchair to offer him independent manual wheelchair mobility at home and in his community. He did not wish to use a power wheelchair at this time; however, he is aware that he may require one in the future. He was educated on the premature degenerative changes that will likely occur in his shoulders from pushing a manual wheelchair and transferring himself to many necessary surfaces. He was also educated on skin care and the need for a maximal pressure-relieving wheelchair cushion. He was specifically evaluated for the optimal wheelchair sitting position that will offer him good trunk and pelvic alignment and pressure relief.

Over time Jack's need for caregiver assistance decreased, and he decided to hire a caregiver to assist him in the morning as he prepared for his day and in the evening as he prepared for bed. He regularly visits a neighborhood gym to maintain upper extremity strength and endurance, and he will soon be driving a modified van. He and his occupational therapist had many discussions regarding how he could return to college. Jack decided to return to school with a reduced class schedule and used services available at his school for note taking.

Jack has continued his involvement with the peer-mentoring program at the SCI clinic and loves to interact with clients who have been recently injured, sharing his own tricks and techniques that he has learned since leaving the hospital. He continues to set goals and challenge himself; currently he is learning to play quad rugby and hopes to one day travel to tournaments with his team and without his caregiver.

of SCI and defining the nervous system's response to this injury. There is now a sense of optimism in the scientific community that it will be possible to restore function after SCI. This optimism is based on the combined research efforts of scientists in many disciplines. It is important for occupational therapists treating clients with SCI to be aware of the scientific and technological advances so as to better educate their clients, while at the same time providing them with the most realistic and comprehensive rehabilitation interventions for their immediate and long-term needs. There are many trusted resources, such as the American Spinal Injury Association (https://scitrialsfinder.net/Home) and the U.S. National Institutes of Health (http://www.clinicaltrials.gov), that can provide clinical trials advice to consumers.

SUMMARY

SCI can result in substantial paralysis of the limbs and trunk. The degree of residual motor and sensory dysfunction depends on the level of the lesion, whether the lesion was complete or incomplete, and the area of the spinal cord that was damaged. The goal of OT is to aid the individual with SCI in achieving optimal independence and functioning by exposing the client to what is possible and prioritizing what is important. Areas

of focus are physical restoration of available musculature; self-care; independent living skills; short- and long-term equipment needs; environmental accessibility; and educational, work, and leisure activities. The psychosocial adjustment of the client is instrumental, and the OT offers emotional support and intervention toward this end in every phase of the rehabilitation program.

REVIEW QUESTIONS

1. List three causes of SCI. Which is the most common?
2. What is the difference between tetraplegia and paraplegia?
3. What testing is completed for an accurate diagnosis of neurological level?
4. Describe the difference between complete and incomplete lesions.
5. What is the prognosis for recovery of motor function in complete lesions and incomplete lesions?
6. What are some methods used to manage orthostatic hypotension during therapy sessions?
7. What are the most common causes of autonomic dysreflexia?
8. What is the role of the occupational therapist in the prevention of pressure injuries?
9. Why is vital capacity affected in individuals with SCI, and how does it affect participation in the rehabilitation program?
10. Which level of injury features full innervation of the rotator cuff musculature, biceps, and extensor carpi radialis and partial innervation of the serratus anterior, latissimus dorsi, and pectoralis major?
11. What additional muscle power does the client with C6-level tetraplegia have over the client with C5-level tetraplegia?

What is the major functional advantage of this additional muscle power?
12. What are the additional critical muscles that the client with C7-level quadriplegia has, as compared with the client with C6-level tetraplegia? What additional functional independence can be achieved because of this additional muscle power?
13. What is the first spinal cord lesion level that features full innervation of the upper extremity musculature?
14. Which assessments do OTs use to evaluate the client with SCI? What is the purpose of each?
15. List five goals of OT for the client with SCI.
16. How is wrist extension used to affect grasp by the individual with tetraplegia?
17. What are some self-care activities that the client with a C6-level SCI can accomplish independently?
18. What assistive devices can promote increased independence for an individual with C6 tetraplegia?
19. What considerations must be made when ordering a wheelchair in order to prevent secondary complications?
20. Describe the role of OT in the vocational evaluation of a client with SCI.

REFERENCES

1. American Chronic Pain Association: Neuropathic pain. 2015. www.acpa.org.
2. American Occupational Therapy Association: Sexuality and the role of occupational therapy. 2013. http://www.aota.org/-/media/corporate/files/aboutot/professionals/whatisot/rdp/facts/sexuality.pdf.
3. American Occupational Therapy Association: Occupational therapys' role in acute care. 2017. http://www.aota.org/-/media/corporate/files/aboutot/professionals/whatisot/rdp/facts/acute-care.pdf.
4. American Occupational Therapy Association. (in press): Occupational therapy practice framework: Domain and process (4th ed.), American Journal of Occupational Therapy 74(Supplement 2):1–87, 2020.
5. American Spinal Injury Association (ASIA): ASIA consumer guidelines for SCI rehabilitation. nd. https://asia-spinalinjury.org/wp-content/uploads/2016/02/Consumer_Guidelines_SCI_Rehab.pdf.
6. American Spinal Injury Association (ASIA): WeeStep: pediatric standards training e-program—pediatric considerations for the neurological classification of spinal cord injury. 2009. https://asia-spinalinjury.org/learning/.
7. American Spinal Injury Association (ASIA): International standards for neurological classification of spinal cord injury (ISNCSCI). 2019. https://asia-spinalinjury.org/wp-content/uploads/2019/10/ASIA-ISCOS-Worksheet_10.2019_PRINT-Page-1-2.pdf.
8. Baker LL, et al: Neuro muscular electrical stimulation: a practical guide, ed 4, Downey, CA, 2000, Los Amigos Research & Education Institute.
9. Christopher Reeve Foundation: Sexual health for men. nd. https://www.christopherreeve.org/living-with-paralysis/health/sexual-health/sexual-health-for-men.
10. Cleveland Clinic: Acute vs chronic pain. 2014. http://my.clevelandclinic.org/services/anesthesiology/pain-management/diseases-conditions/hic-acute-vs-chronic-pain.
11. Consortium for Spinal Cord Injury: Autonomic dysreflexia: what you should know – a guide for people with spinal cord injury. 2022. https://pva.org/wp-content/uploads/2022/05/Autonomic-Dysreflexia-Consumer-Guide-2022.pdf .
12. Consortium for Spinal Cord Medicine: Neurogenic bowel management in adults with spinal cord injury. 1999. https://pva.org/wp-content/uploads/2021/09/consumer-guide_neurogenic-bowel.pdf .
13. Consortium for Spinal Cord Medicine: Preservation of upper limb function following spinal cord injury: a clinical practice guideline for health-care professionals. 2005. https://pva.org/wp-content/uploads/2021/09/consumer-guide_upper_limb.pdf.
14. Consortium for Spinal Cord Medicine: Bladder management guidelines for adults with spinal cord injury: a clinical practice guideline for health-care providers. 2006. https://pva.org/wp-content/uploads/2021/09/consumer_guide_bladder_071410.pdf.
15. Consortium for Spinal Cord Medicine: Early acute management in adults with spinal cord injury: a clinical practice guideline for health-care professionals, J Spinal Cord Med 31:403–479, 2008. https://pva.org/research-resources/publications/clinical-practice-guidelines/.
16. Consortium for Spinal Cord Medicine: Sexuality and reproductive health in adults with spinal cord injury: a clinical practice guideline for health-care professionals. 2010. https://pva.org/research-resources/publications/clinical-practice-guidelines/.

17. Craig Hospital: Aging and spinal cord injury. 2015. https://craighospital.org/resources/aging-and-spinal-cord-injury.
18. Curtin M: An analysis of tetraplegic hand grips, *Br J Occup Ther* 62:444–450, 1999.
19. Ditunno J, Cardenas D, Formal C, Dalal K: Advances in the rehabilitation management of acute spinal cord injury, *Handb Clin Neurol* 109:181–195, 2012.
20. Fritz H, Dillaway H, Lysack C: Don't think paralysis takes away your womanhood: sexual intimacy after spinal cord injury, *Am J Occup Ther* 69:1–10, 2015.
21. Grant R, Quon J, Abbed K: Management of acute traumatic spinal cord injury, *Curr Treat Options Neurol* 17:1–13, 2015. https://doi.org/10.1007/s11940-014-0334-1.
22. Hess M, Hough S: Impact of spinal cord injury on sexuality: broad-based clinical practice intervention and practical application, *J Spinal Cord Med* 35:211–218, 2012. https://doi.org/10.1179/2045772312Y.0000000025.
23. Ho C, Wuermser L-A, Priebe MM, et al: Spinal cord injury medicine. Part 1. Epidemiology and classification, *Arch Phys Med Rehabil* 88:S49–S54, 2007. https://doi.org/10.1016/j.apmr.2006.12.001.
24. Juknis N, Cooper J, Volshteyn O: The changing landscape of spinal cord injury, *Handb Clin Neurol* 109:149–166, 2012.
25. Kanwar R, Delasobera B, Hudson K, Frohna W: Emergency Department evaluation and treatment of cervical spine injuries, *Emerg Med Clin North Am* 33:241–282, 2015.
26. Kedlaya D: Heterotopic ossification in spinal cord injury. *Medscape*, 2015. http://emedicine.medscape.com/article/322003-overview#a1.
27. Kirshblum S, Botticello A, Lammertse DP, et al: The impact of sacral sensory sparing in motor complete spinal cord injury, *Arch Phys Med Rehabil* 92:376–383, 2011.
28. Kirshblum S, Priebe MM, Ho CH, et al: Spinal cord injury medicine. Part 3. Rehabilitation phase after acute spinal cord injury, *Arch Phys Med Rehabil* 88:S62–S70, 2007. https://doi.org/10.1016/j.apmr.2006.12.003.
29. Law M, Baptiste S, Carswell A, et al: *Canadian Occupational Performance Measure*, ed 4, Ottawa, ON, 2005, CAOT Publications ACE.
30. Marino R, Burns S, Graves DE, et al: Upper- and lower-extremity motor recovery after traumatic cervical spinal cord injury: an update from the National Spinal Cord Injury Database, *Arch Phys Med Rehabil* 92:369–375, 2011.
31. Mateo S, Roby-Brami A, Reilly KT, et al: Upper limb kinematics after cervical spinal cord injury: a review, *J Neuroeng Rehabil* 12:1–12, 2015. https://doi.org/10.1186/1743-0003-12-9.
32. McKinley W, Santos K, Meade M, Brooke K: Incidence and outcomes of spinal cord injury clinical syndromes, *J Spinal Cord Med* 30:215–224, 2007.
33. Meade M: Facilitating health mechanics: a guide for care providers of individuals with spinal cord injury and disease. 2009. http://www.researchgate.net/publication/242564099_facilitating_health_mechanics_a_guide_for_care_providers_of_individuals_with_spinal_cord_injury_and_disease.
34. Menorca R, Fussell T, Elfar J: Peripheral nerve trauma: mechanisms of injury and recovery, *Hand Clin* 29:317–330, 2013. https://doi.org/10.1016/j.hcl.2013.04.002.
35. Model Systems Knowledge Translation Center: Pain after spinal cord injury. 2009. http://www.msktc.org/sci/factsheets/pain.
36. Model Systems Knowledge Translation Center: Spasticity and spinal cord injury. 2011. https://msktc.org/sci/factsheets/Spasticity.
37. Model Systems Knowledge Translation Center: Understanding spinal cord injury. Part 1. The Body before and after injury. 2015. http://www.msktc.org/sci/factsheets/understanding_sci_part_1.
38. Model Systems Knowledge Translation Center: Understanding spinal cord injury. Part 2. Recovery and rehabilitation. 2015. http://www.msktc.org/lib/docs/Factsheets/Understand_Spin_Crd_Inj_Prt2_508.pdf.
39. Mulroy S, Thompson L, Hatchett PP, et al: Strengthening and Optimal Movements for Painful Shoulders (STOMPS) in chronic spinal cord injury: a randomized control trial, *Phys Ther* 91:305–324, 2011. https://doi.org/10.2522/ptj.20100182.
40. National Institute of Neurological Disorders and Stroke (NINDS): NINDS central cord information page. 2014. https://www.ninds.nih.gov/disorders/all-disorders/central-cord-syndrome-information-page.
41. National Spinal Cord Injury Statistical Center: *Facts and figures at a glance*, Birmingham, AL, 2020, University of Alabama. https://www.nscisc.uab.edu/Public/Facts%20and%20Figures%202020.pdf.
42. Paulson S, editor: *Santa Clara Valley Medical Center spinal cord injury home care manual*, San Jose, CA, 1994, Santa Clara Valley Medical Center.
43. Peterson C: The use of electrical stimulation and taping to address shoulder subluxation for a patient with central cord syndrome, *Phys Ther* 84:634–643, 2004.
44. Pregnancy and spinal cord injury. 2015. https://scisexualhealth.ca/wp-content/uploads/2015/05/Pregnancy-and-SCI-booklet-V7.pdf.
45. Saunders L, Clark A, Tate DG, et al: Lifetime prevalence of chronic health conditions among persons with spinal cord injury, *Arch Phys Med Rehabil* 96:673–679, 2015.
46. Tefft D, Guerette P, Furumasu J: Cognitive predictors of young children's readiness for powered mobility, *Dev Med Child Neurol* 41:665–670, 1999.
47. Vogel L, Betz R, Mulcahey M: Spinal cord injuries in children and adolescents, *Handb Clin Neurol* 109:131–148, 2012.
48. Wirz M, Dietz V: Concepts of aging with paralysis: implications for recovery and research, *Handb Clin Neurol* 109:77–84, 2012.
49. Witiw C, Fehlings M: Acute spinal cord injury, *J Spinal Disord Tech* 28:202–210, 2015.

RESOURCES

American Spinal Injury Association: http://www.asia-spinalinjury.org.
Christopher and Dana Reeve Foundation: http://www.christopherreeve.org.
Innovative products for seniors and people with disabilities: http://www.nuprodx.com.
Life coaching and peer mentoring services for individuals with SCI: http://www.knowbarriers.org.
Model System Knowledge Translation Center: http://www.msktc.org.
National Spinal Cord Injury Statistical Center (NSCISC): https://www.nscisc.uab.edu/.
New Mobility (magazine for active wheelchair users): http://www.newmobility.com.
Paralyzed Veterans of America: http://www.pva.org.
Peer support website run by individuals with spinal cord injuries: http://main.nsic-online.org.uk/useful-information/counselling-and-support/apparelyzed/.
Reachers and grabbers for tetraplegics: http://www.quadtools.com.
Spinal Cord Injury Research Evidence Project: http://www.scireproject.com.
United Spinal Injury Association/NSCIA: https://unitedspinal.org.

38

Disorders of the Motor Unit

Alison Hewitt George and Winifred Schultz-Krohn

KEY TERMS

Brachial plexus	Motor unit	Peripheral neuropathies
Guillain-Barré syndrome	Muscular dystrophy	Post-COVID syndrome (PCS)
Long COVID	Myasthenia gravis	
Lower motor neuron system	Peripheral nerve injuries	

THREADED CASE STUDY

Edith, Part 1

Although this case study is specific to Guillain-Barré syndrome (GBS), many of the aspects of Edith's occupational profile and occupational performance needs apply to the other diagnoses in this chapter.

At age 67, Edith, who identifies as female (prefers the use of the pronouns she/her/hers), had been enjoying her retirement, primarily spending time with her husband, three children, and five grandchildren. She had recently recovered from the flu and was looking forward to a day at the park with her family. While showering, she suddenly lost strength in her legs and collapsed. While lying on the shower floor, she noticed that her arms also felt weak. Her cognition was intact, but she was physically helpless. Her husband called 9-1-1. It was

fortunate that she received immediate medical care because she later required mechanical assistance to breathe. After extensive neurologic testing, Edith was diagnosed with GBS. Neither she nor her family had ever heard of GBS.

Edith suddenly found herself dependent in all of her life roles and occupations. She was hospitalized in the intensive care unit (ICU) for several weeks, was dependent on a ventilator to breathe, and needed complete physical assistance because of her total body paralysis. Her muscles were painful, sore, and tender, and pain medications helped to manage the discomfort.

Jen, the occupational therapist (OT) assigned to the ICU, interviewed Edith, and together they identified the occupational needs and client factors that should be

Continued

THREADED CASE STUDY—cont'd

Edith, Part 1

addressed. Jen performed passive range of motion (ROM) exercises, fabricated static hand orthoses to maintain a functional resting position and to prevent contractures, provided proper bed positioning, and instructed the family about GBS. Jen also provided support, encouragement, and active listening, employing therapeutic use of self during the intervention. Edith often spoke about her spiritual beliefs and reported that she found hope and strength with prayer and meditation. She spoke of her favorite previous performance pattern of reading her Bible every morning, and said she felt depressed because she was now unable to physically hold a book or turn pages. After receiving training and modifications from Jen, Edith was able to listen to the Bible on her tablet or cellular phone, using a mouth switch to turn it on and off; this modification allowed her to resume her previous valued morning routine.

Edith made slow but steady gains in physical abilities and was transferred to an acute rehabilitation hospital to actively participate in an intensive interdisciplinary therapy program. Lara, the occupational therapist on the rehabilitation unit, evaluated Edith's specific functions as they related to supporting performance and engagement in occupations and activities targeted for intervention. The goals for Edith as determined by the Canadian Occupational Performance Measure[34,36] included the following: (1) to be able to feed herself, brush her teeth, and shower, (2) to cook for her family, (3) to go shopping at the mall with her granddaughter, and (4) to drive to her friend's house to play cards. Detailed upper extremity manual muscle testing, muscle belly tenderness screening, ROM measurements, and sensation testing were completed during the evaluation phase.

Intervention strategies focused on using compensatory methods and improving strength and endurance. Lara taught Edith adaptive strategies to eat, groom,

and bathe. The use of adaptive equipment, work simplification, and energy conservation techniques were encouraged while Edith engaged in activities such as cooking and light cleaning. Lara supported Edith's community mobility and accompanied Edith to the mall with her granddaughter. After the brief outing, Edith expressed a sense of increased self-confidence and accomplishment. She practiced playing cards with other clients in a group environment. She also participated in a daily individualized strengthening program.

Lara provided Edith with community resources to aid in her independence. For example, the Guillain-Barré Syndrome/Chronic Inflammatory Demyelinating Polyneuropathy (GBS/CIDP) Foundation International offers local support groups, literature, and conferences to GBS survivors and caregivers.[25,28] In addition, her family received extensive training from the interdisciplinary team members to help Edith apply the learned strategies and equipment in the home and community. Driving was not addressed at an inpatient level, but Edith was referred to an outpatient driving training program.

Critical Thinking Questions

1. What are the phases of Guillain-Barré syndrome, and what occupational therapy interventions might be used in each phase?
2. In what ways were the client's psychosocial needs addressed during recovery?
3. Describe energy conservation techniques that you think would be appropriate for Edith while engaging in her valued occupation of cooking.

This chapter examines the symptoms, course, medical treatment, and occupational therapy (OT) assessment and intervention for clients who have motor unit disorders most often seen in OT practice. The **motor unit** is the basic functional unit of the peripheral nervous system and consists of four elements: the cell body of the motor neuron located in the anterior horn of the spinal cord; the axon of the motor neuron, which travels via spinal nerves and peripheral nerves to muscle; the neuromuscular junction; and the muscle fibers innervated by the neuron (Fig. 38.1). Disorders of the motor unit may be of neurogenic, neuromuscular, or myopathic origin and generally cause muscle weakness and atrophy of skeletal muscle. Those with a neurogenic basis are referred to as lower motor neuron (LMN) disorders, affecting the cell bodies and peripheral nerves of the motor unit. Those with a neuromuscular or myopathic origin affect the neuromuscular junction or the muscle itself.[10,12]

This chapter also discusses the physical, psychosocial, and emotional factors that occupational therapists (OTs) address when assessing and providing interventions for people with motor unit disorders. Occupational performance considers the context, both environmental and personal factors, to support clients with motor unit disorders to participate in desired occupations. Support of occupational performance addresses the client's engagement in the home, school, work environment, and community. Community engagement can range from a quick trip to the grocery store to participating in a community orchestra.

Although long COVID is not a motor unit disorder, this chapter includes a discussion of the role of occupational therapy with those individuals who experience the effects of long

COVID. Literature still uses a variety of terms to describe the residual impact of a COVID 19 infection but the more common term now used is post-COVID syndrome (PCS).[56] This topic is included here since many OT strategies used to support those individuals who experience the effects of long COVID are similar to those used to support individuals who have motor unit disorders.

Occupational therapists, with their holistic view of persons with physical disabilities, are uniquely positioned to recognize and include interventions that address mental health concerns for persons with disorders of the motor unit. The sudden onset of severely disabling peripheral neuropathies, such as Guillain-Barré syndrome (GBS), or the chronic aspects of living with fatigue and experiencing role alterations will have ramifications for the client, the family, and their social network as described in Edith's case study.[35,64]

NEUROGENIC DISORDERS

PERIPHERAL NEUROPATHIES

The motor neurons in the anterior horn of the spinal cord mediate voluntary movement and reflexes that produce motor behavior. Muscle strength and endurance contribute to coordinated and skilled movement and the ability to move through available range of motion (ROM). The characteristics of movement are determined by the pattern and firing frequency of specific motor units. Muscle contraction is the output of the motor system.[10]

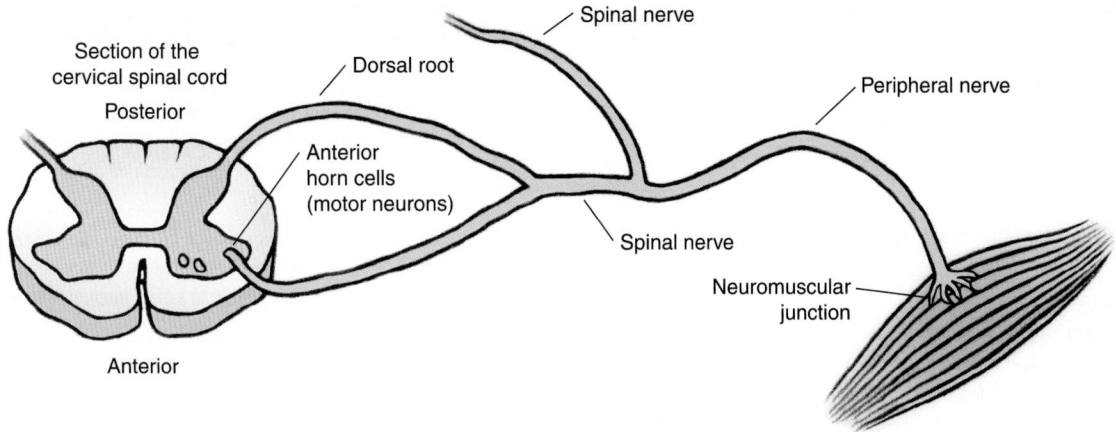

Fig. 38.1 Motor unit consisting of motor neuron cell body in the anterior horn of the spinal cord, the axon of the motor neuron (which travels via spinal nerves and peripheral nerves to muscle), the neuromuscular junction, and the muscle fibers innervated by the neuron.[49]

The lower motor neuron system includes the cell bodies in the anterior horn of the spinal cord and their axons (which pass by way of the spinal nerves and peripheral nerves to the neuromuscular junction) and the nuclei of cranial nerves III through X (located in the brainstem) and their axons. The motor fibers of the lower motor neurons contain somatic motor components, including the alpha motor neurons, which innervate skeletal muscles (extrafusal fibers), and gamma motor neurons, which innervate muscle spindles (intrafusal fibers). A lesion in any of these neurologic structures results in peripheral neuropathy or an a lower motor neuron dysfunction.[10]

Peripheral neuropathies involve lesions of the lower motor neuron system and may be located in the anterior horn cells of the spinal cord, spinal nerves, peripheral nerves, and cranial nerves or their nuclei in the brainstem. Lesions can occur from nerve root compression, physical injury (e.g., bone fractures and dislocations, lacerations, traction, prolonged pressure, compression, or penetrating wounds and friction), nutritional imbalances, exposure to toxins (e.g., lead, mercury, alcohol), infections (e.g., Lyme disease, human immunodeficiency virus, herpes simplex, or varicella zoster), neoplasms (e.g., neuromas and multiple neurofibromatosis), vascular disorders (e.g., atherosclerosis, diabetes mellitus, or peripheral vascular anomalies), autoimmune diseases (e.g., Sjögren's, rheumatoid arthritis, lupus), and congenital malformations.[47] "The peripheral nerves are like the cables that connect the different parts of a computer or connect the Internet. When they malfunction, complex functions can slowly halt."[47]

OT assessments for motor unit disorders follow a similar sequence and are described in Table 38.1. An occupational profile is developed during an interview with the client and caregivers. The Canadian Occupational Performance Measure[36] is an excellent instrument for establishing meaningful goals and measuring intervention outcomes. Performance skills, performance patterns, client factors, and activity demands in context must also be clinically assessed. Specific assessments such as range of motion, manual muscle testing, scales designed to measure coping and depression, and activities of daily living (ADLs) assessments are appropriate for each of the motor unit disorders described in this chapter.

Guillain-Barré syndrome is discussed in detail in the following section. The concepts are applicable to the other motor unit disorders described later in the chapter.

Guillain-Barré Syndrome

Guillain-Barré (ghee-YAN bah-RAY) syndrome (GBS) (also known as acute inflammatory demyelinating polyneuropathy, acute immune-mediated polyneuropathy, or Landry's ascending paralysis) is an acute inflammatory disorder in which the body's own immune system attacks part of the peripheral nervous system. The immune system destroys the myelin sheath that surrounds the axons of many peripheral nerves or even the axons themselves, damaging the nerves' ability to transmit signals to the muscles. GBS has no known cause or cure, and no one knows why this disorder strikes some people and not others.[40,46] The onset of GBS often occurs after an upper respiratory or gastrointestinal viral infection, usually within a few days or weeks. The syndrome also occasionally occurs after surgery, injury, or vaccinations and occasionally occurs with no known precipitating event.[40]

This acute and complex disorder is seen in thousands of new individuals each year. Although anyone can develop GBS, it is more common among adults than children. The incidence of GBS increases with age, and people over age 50 are at greatest risk for developing GBS. On average, each year about 3000 to 6000 people in the United States develop GBS whether or not they received a vaccination. Affecting males slightly more often than females, the incidence of GBS in the United States is approximately 1 to 2 persons in 100,000.[14] The initial symptoms of GBS most often include varying degrees of weakness and sensory changes in the legs. GBS is characterized by rapidly progressive ascending symmetric weakness of bilateral extremities, usually proceeding from distal to proximal (feet to trunk). Descending paralysis with predominant proximal muscle weakness rarely appears.[4,40] Because the myelin sheaths of the peripheral nerves are injured or degraded, the nerves cannot transmit signals efficiently. The muscles begin to lose their ability to respond to the brain's commands. The brain also receives fewer sensory signals from the rest of the body, resulting in an inability to feel textures,

TABLE 38.1   Occupational Therapy Assessments and Descriptions

Assessments	Descriptions
Occupational profile	Interview client (and family members and caregivers, if appropriate) to gain information about problems and concerns, successful and unsuccessful strategies when engaging in occupations, ways in which contexts influence functional abilities, activity demands, and priorities of meaningful occupations.
Canadian Occupational Performance Measure[36]	The interview is conducted before and after intervention to describe problems, level of satisfaction with performing activities, and level of perceived performance abilities in areas of self-care, productivity, and leisure. Testing methods must be measurable to assess intervention results.
Performance skills in areas of occupation: activities of daily living, instrumental activities of daily living, health management, rest and sleep, education, work, play, leisure, social participation	Following the occupations that the client prioritizes in the occupational profile, the therapist can perform formal assessments and observation of the client's performance during activity engagement in the appropriate context, with attention paid to motor, process, and communication/interaction skills. (See Chapter 18 for additional assessment details and Chapter 16 for a description of specific leisure assessments.)
Performance patterns	Client (independently or with assistance from caregivers or occupational therapist) maintains a log of activities and symptoms to analyze. In collaboration with the occupational therapist, the client uses this information to discover habits, routines, roles and rituals that support or inhibit occupational performance. Reestablishment or adjustment of roles should be discussed and implemented.
Client factors: manual muscle testing, range of motion testing, eating and swallowing assessments, pain scale, sensory testing, depression scale, Ways of Coping Scale, clinical observations during activities of daily living	The therapist should perform specific assessments of the client's bodily function, including systems that support participation in meaningful occupations (e.g., neuromusculoskeletal, pain, joint range of motion, sensation, cardiovascular, respiratory, swallowing, skin). Because fatigability is so prevalent in these disorders, assessments should be adequately spaced and preferably performed when clients are feeling their best (often in the morning). Assessment of emotional stability, motivation, sexual activity, depression, ways of coping, and so forth is critical to forming an overall picture of the client's strengths and weaknesses.
Occupation and activity demands	Analysis of the required sequence, performance skills, body functions, and body structures to complete the activity is necessary; as well as considering what is required by the specific client to carry out an occupation. Analysis must include assessment of space demands, social demands, the tools or equipment used to perform the activity, and any adaptations that could be made to ensure success.
Contexts	The therapist should always consider context, including the client's personal factors (e.g., age, gender identity, cultural identification, socioeconomic status, education, professional identity) and environmental factors (e.g., physical, social, and attitudinal).

Data from American Occupational Therapy Association. Occupational therapy practice framework: domain and process, 4th edition, *Am J Occup Ther.* 2020;74(suppl. 2):S1–S87.

heat, pain, and other sensations. Clients often report initial sensations such as tingling, "crawling skin," or painful sensations. The signals to and from the arms and legs must travel the longest distances, so they are most vulnerable to interruption. Therefore, muscle weakness and tingling sensations usually first appear distally in the hands and feet and progress proximally.[42]

Typically, the weakness and abnormal sensations first noticed in the legs progress to the arms and upper body, and some muscles are almost totally paralyzed. As the demyelination continues, the client may experience problems with breathing, speaking, swallowing, blood pressure, or heart rate. The client may require use of a respirator to assist with breathing and is monitored closely for an abnormal heart rhythm, infections, blood clots, and high or low blood pressure. After the initial clinical manifestations of the disease, the symptoms can progress over the course of days or weeks. By the third week of the illness, 90% of all clients are at their weakest. Some may be completely paralyzed and dependent on a respirator for breathing.[40]

The typical progression of GBS occurs in three phases. The *initial*, or *acute, phase* begins with the client's first conclusive

symptoms and lasts until there is no further decline in physical status. This phase may last for up to 4 weeks. The *plateau phase* begins when the client's physical state stabilizes, with no further deterioration of physical status and no evidence of physical recovery. The plateau phase generally lasts a few weeks, during which the physical status of the client remains unchanged. The *recovery phase* is that period when the client slowly begins to recover physical abilities and symptoms gradually decrease (usually 2–4 weeks after disease progression ceases). Recovery can occur over 6 months up to 2 years, depending on the extent of paralysis. Although complete recovery is possible, many individuals (20%–30% of those diagnosed with GBS) will experience long-term residual deficits.[4,64]

Being paralyzed is a frightening experience for people with GBS, their family members, and friends. Clients can be expected to proceed through varying stages of adapting to the acute and residual effects of this physical disability.[51] However, the prognosis is generally good for the majority of clients; therefore, it is appropriate to be optimistic during intervention sessions and encourage clients and families to look forward to recovery (Table 38.2).

TABLE 38.2   Guillain-Barré Syndrome Prognosis and Outcomes

Recovery Status	Percentage of Clients (%)	Description
Recover well spontaneously	80–85	15%–20% of those who recover well have some residual deficits such as distal numbness, weakness, fatigue; these may interfere with some daily functions but usually are not severe; 3% experience a relapse of muscle weakness and tingling sensation years after initial attack.
Significant impairments	10–15	Fatigue and severe weakness in specific muscle groups significantly impair daily function.
Death	5	Death is usually the result of pneumonia, sepsis, adult respiratory distress syndrome, cardiac arrest, autonomic instability, or pulmonary embolism. Mortality rate increases with age.

Data from Centers for Disease Control and Prevention. Guillain-Barré syndrome. 2019. Available at https://www.cdc.gov/campylobacter/guillain-barre.html.

There is no known cure for GBS. However, there are interventions that lessen the severity of the illness and accelerate the recovery in most individuals. Immunomodulatory therapy (plasmapheresis or intravenous immunoglobulin IVIg) is the recommended medical treatment at the onset of GBS. Plasmapheresis has shown clinical improvements, reducing the time required for ventilation and critical care, time to achieve ambulation, and hospital length of stay.[4,64] This process is used to separate the whole blood from the plasma and then return the whole blood to the client without the plasma to reduce the length of the acute phase. IVIg therapy involves the injection of proteins that the immune system uses naturally to fight invading organisms. High doses of these immunoglobulin proteins can lessen the immune attack on the nervous system and hasten recovery.[44,64] There are also a number of ways to treat the complications of this syndrome that pose the greatest risk of death. These interventions include respiratory therapy (such as ventilator support), cardiac monitoring, nutritional supplementation, and monitoring for infectious complications (e.g., pneumonia, sepsis, or urinary tract infection).[44]

Role of the Occupational Therapist

The client with GBS may be referred to OT when medically stable.[11] An occupational profile of the client will be developed through OT assessments related to the level of dysfunction that the client is experiencing. For example, physical abilities are assessed using range of motion (ROM) and manual muscle testing (MMT), sensation testing, and a swallowing assessment. Functional assessments of quality of movement, coordination, and self-care also may be performed. It is critical to assess emotional and psychosocial factors of the client and family. (See Table 38.1 for OT assessments.)

After the initial OT evaluation, an intervention plan is developed to meet the client's needs throughout the disease process. Frequent revisions may be necessary, depending on the client's recovery status. During the initial phases of intervention (the acute phase and plateau phase of the disease), problematic client factors are addressed in conjunction with the healthcare team. These may include providing daily passive ROM, positioning, and splinting to prevent contracture and deformity and to protect weak muscles. Passive ROM should begin with gentle movement of the joints and should not exceed the point of pain. Particular attention should be paid to determining residual weakness in the intrinsic muscles of the hands. Passive activities (e.g., watching television) and nonstrenuous social visits from family and friends are encouraged. Muscle belly tenderness (a flu-type muscle soreness) is closely monitored, and activities are modified as needed.[9] Many clients may benefit from the use of electronic aids for daily living (EADLs). EADLs increase the level of independence in the client's control of the environment through the use of technology. For example, a client with GBS might lack the strength and motor skills to operate the television, lights, telephone, and radio in the environment. With the use of EADLs, the client may be able to use the head, mouth, or other parts of the body to operate switches and successfully control the environment.

An intensive interdisciplinary rehabilitation program is typically implemented during the recovery phase as the client begins to regain physical movement. After the evaluation process, the OT intervention plan, developed in collaboration with the client, must be carefully designed to respect muscle belly tenderness and to prevent fatigue and further damage to the nerves. Because muscle belly tenderness usually decreases in the proximal musculature before it decreases distally, proximal musculature movements can be facilitated first while distal joints continue to be supported (e.g., using mobile arm supports).[9] Activity is gradually increased with close monitoring of pain or fatigue after each intervention session.[58] The therapist should continue to monitor for increased muscle belly tenderness, muscle imbalance, and substitution patterns. Progressive resistive exercises should be used conservatively, with attention to joint protection and fatigue. Throughout the course of recovery, the therapist should guard against fatigue and irritation of the inflamed nerves. Instruction to the client and family in key concepts such as energy conservation, work simplification, avoidance of overstretching, and overuse of muscles is critical to recovery.[54]

As the client's strength increases, activities promoting more resistance can be incorporated into the intervention program. Self-care (grooming, eating, dressing, bathing, and toileting) and other activities of daily living (ADLs), instrumental activities of daily living (IADLs), and leisure occupations should be included as soon as the client is capable of participating in them. Activities should be graded for success as strength and endurance improve. Adaptive equipment, frequent rest breaks, and creative strategies are typically necessary during this phase. Mobile arm supports may be used to alleviate muscle fatigue, promote active assistive use of upper extremities, and encourage independence with occupations. Activities and occupations should be varied among gross motor, fine motor, resistive, and nonresistive exercises to prevent undue fatigue.[54]

OT PRACTICE NOTES

Engagement in light occupations that are meaningful to the client is essential for building the self-confidence necessary to resume previous life roles and interests. For example, a client may be able to participate in enjoyable leisure occupations such as scrapbooking, surfing the web, planning a family gathering, and reading books to grandchildren (see Chapter 16).

People with GBS face not only physical difficulties but emotionally painful periods as well.[40] It is often extremely difficult for clients to adjust to sudden paralysis and dependence on others for help with routine daily activities.[51] Eisendrath et al. found that clients experienced severe anxiety, fear, and panic during the acute progressive phase.[17] When clients reached the plateau phase, they often expressed anger and depression. When improvement began during the recovery phase, severe depression occurred as clients contemplated the long, slow convalescence and the possibility of permanent neurologic deficits. An occupational therapist can support the client by facilitating feelings of self-worth, a positive attitude, and encouragement through the engagement in valued occupations.[51,60] A psychologist or physician should also closely monitor the client's mood and provide necessary interventions as a member of the intervention team.

After becoming medically stable and being discharged from the hospital, many GBS survivors find themselves living at home without proper medical follow-up and therapy. Families are left to their own devices to successfully create real-life solutions to functional limitations and to locate and use resources. Schmidt conducted a survey of 90 voluntary participants from the Guillain-Barré Syndrome Foundation International to explore the extent of functional limitations within home, work, community, and leisure roles after hospitalization.[54] The majority of the participants stated that they had to independently research information about GBS because their doctors and team members either lacked the knowledge or did not provide them with any verbal or written information. One participant noted, "My family had to learn everything about GBS on the Internet. My doctors and nurses didn't know anything about it. We had to educate them (doctors, nurses, therapists, etc.)." These families reported feeling most frustrated about the fact that healthcare professionals did not address significant psychosocial issues such as depression, anxiety, fear, and hopelessness. Physically demanding tasks that required fair to good strength and endurance were scored the lowest in satisfaction and ability by participants. The great majority of respondents (98%) reported that they were living with factors that limited their ability to participate in life, such as fatigue, weakness,

pain, sensation disturbances, coordination problems, and psychosocial changes. Nearly half of the participants agreed that they would benefit from OT services to improve the use of their upper extremities and to learn ways to manage daily fatigue and maintain their current health status. This study indicates the need for continued OT services to optimize occupational performance and occupational roles many years after the onset of the syndrome and apparent recovery.

The complex process of adjusting to the disabling condition, problem solving, learning, and redesigning a life for a GBS survivor is a long-term, therapeutic experience. The lifestyle redesign process can be initiated by the occupational therapist during the inpatient rehabilitation phase; however, there must be a continuum of care established for follow-up treatment. Tomita et al.[62] identified several factors related to successful community reintegration for a woman with GBS. These factors include a holistic approach, short-term achievable goals, accessible home environment, referral to community resources, and social participation and supports, including consideration of spiritual support.[15] An occupational therapist working in an outpatient or home setting can skillfully guide clients back to the resumption of their previous life roles, assist clients in returning to productive community involvement and leisure occupations (see Chapter 16), and teach engagement and participation in meaningful occupations.[38,40,54,62]

GBS is one disorder that requires OT services; it was presented in detail to outline the process used for individuals with this disorder. The remaining portion of this chapter describes other disorders related to the motor unit that result in compromised occupational performance. The principles behind the interventions described for GBS apply to the following disorders as well.

PERIPHERAL NERVE INJURIES

This section covers three specific upper extremity peripheral nerve injuries: axillary nerve, brachial plexus, and long thoracic nerve injury. The brachial plexus includes the nerves from C5 through T1.[7] These nerve fibers, both sensory and motor, intertwine closely to the vertebral column. The fibers join to form trunks of the brachial plexus, and from the trunks arise the divisions at which further interweaving of fibers occurs. The divisions give rise to the cords of the brachial plexus, and from the cords the terminal branches or named peripheral nerves arise. From an anatomic presentation, this complexity has the potential to preserve function if one root is compressed. For example, the radial nerve is composed of fibers originating from C6, C7, C8, and T1. For a list of nerves, muscles innervated, and actions performed, see Table 38.3. (See Chapter 39 for additional information on peripheral nerve injuries, peripheral pain syndromes, and the management of these disorders.)

Many people are injured every year by car accidents, falls, sports mishaps, gunshots, and violent acts (e.g., blunt and sharp wounds) that result in severed, crushed, compressed, or stretched peripheral nerves.[47] The most obvious manifestation of peripheral nerve injury is muscle weakness or flaccid paralysis, with symptoms depending on the extent of the nerve damage. Deep tendon reflexes are depressed or absent. Altered sensation along the cutaneous distribution of the nerve can also be experienced. The individual might experience pain, burning sensation, tingling or a total loss of sensation in the part of the body affected by the damaged nerve. Trophic changes, such as dry skin, hair loss, cyanosis, painless skin ulcerations, and slow wound healing in the area of involvement also may be present.

Extensive peripheral nerve damage may produce deformity if contractures, joint stiffness, and poor positioning are allowed to occur. Disfigurement of the hands is particularly noticeable and may produce psychological distress. Other complications may include osteoporosis of bone and epidermal fibrosis of the joints. See Table 38.3 for descriptions of clinical manifestations of peripheral nerve lesions of the brachial plexus.

Axillary Nerve Injury

The axillary nerve is composed of the C5-C6 spinal nerves and arises from the posterior cord of the brachial plexus. The motor branches of the axillary nerve innervate the deltoid muscle and the teres minor muscle. The sensory branch innervates the lateral aspect of the upper arm (see Table 38.3).[27,30]

The axillary nerve is the most commonly injured nerve in the shoulder, most commonly because of anterior dislocation of the shoulder or fracture of the neck of the humerus.[7,27] Nerve damage may occur as a result of the actual dislocation or of the reduction; other causes include compression (e.g., crutches) or trauma (e.g., blunt or lacerating wounds). As a result, the client has weakness or paralysis of the deltoid muscle, which causes limitations in shoulder flexion, abduction, extension, and weakness in lateral rotation of the arm. In addition to the loss of muscle power, atrophy of the deltoid muscle produces asymmetry of the shoulders, which may cause issues with body image.[37]

See Table 38.1 for OT assessments. ROM assessment and MMT, as well as clinical observation of the client's ability to use the arm functionally, are critical.

Interventions for axillary nerve injury require that the shoulder dislocation be reduced and that the arm be supported for a brief time in a sling. When the physician prescribes OT for rehabilitation of shoulder function, interventions include passive and active ROM of shoulder flexion and extension and shoulder abduction and adduction exercises while the client is supine or lying on the noninjured side to minimize gravity for muscles below a grade of Fair/3 (Table 38.4). Functional movements against gravity are graded as the muscles become stronger (3 and above).

Brachial Plexus Injuries

The nerve roots that innervate the shoulder, arm, and hand originate in the anterior rami between the C5, C6, C7, C8, and T1 spinal segments. This network of peripheral nerves is collectively called the brachial plexus. This important nerve complex can be palpated just behind the posterior border of the sternocleidomastoid as the head and neck are tilted to the opposite side.[26]

Brachial plexus injuries are caused by damage to the nerves and are typically unilateral. The most common cause, obstetric brachial plexus injury, occurs if the baby's shoulders become impacted during delivery, which causes the brachial plexus nerves

TABLE 38.3 Clinical Manifestations of Peripheral Nerve Lesions of the Brachial Plexus

Spinal Nerves	Nerve	Motor Distribution	Clinical Manifestations
C5	Dorsal scapular	Rhomboid major and minor, levator scapulae	Loss of scapular elevation, adduction, downward rotation
C5-6	Suprascapular	Supraspinatus, infraspinatus	Weakened lateral rotation of humerus
C5-6	Subscapular	Subscapularis, teres major	Weakened internal rotation of humerus
C5-6	Axillary	Deltoid, teres minor	Loss of shoulder abduction, flexion, and external rotation and extension
C5-7	Musculocutaneous	Biceps brachii, brachialis, coracobrachialis	Loss of forearm flexion and supination
C5-7	Long thoracic	Serratus anterior	Winging of the scapula
C6-8	Thoracodorsal	Latissimus dorsi	Loss of arm adduction and shoulder extension
C6-8, T1	Radial	All extensors of arm, wrist, fingers, thumb, abductor pollicis longus, supinator, brachioradialis	Wrist drop, extensor paralysis, inability to supinate
C6-8, T1	Median	Flexors of wrist, hand, and digits; forearm pronators; opponens pollicis; abductor pollicis brevis; flexor pollicis brevis; first and second lumbricales	"Ape-hand" deformity, weakened grip, thenar atrophy, unopposed thumb
C8-T1	Ulnar	Supplies muscles on ulnar side of forearm and hand; adductor pollicis, abductor digiti minimi, opponens digiti minimi, flexor digiti minimi brevis, flexor digitorum profundus (digits 4, 5), third and fourth lumbricales, flexor carpi ulnaris, palmaris brevis, dorsal and palmar interossei, flexor pollicis brevis (deep head)	"Claw-hand" deformity, also known as an intrinsic minus hand deformity; interosseus atrophy, loss of thumb adduction

From Hislop HJ, Avers D, Brown M. *Daniels and Worthingham's muscle testing: techniques of manual examination,* ed 9, Philadelphia, 2013, WB Saunders.

TABLE 38.4	Occupational Therapy Interventions for Peripheral Nerve Injuries	
Nerve Injury	**Intervention**	**Example of Activities**
Axillary nerve	Passive ROM to prevent deformity and improve circulation; necessary to protect teres minor and deltoid muscles from stretch during the passive ROM activities	Passive ROM performed two or three times daily while client is supine or lying on uninjured side to minimize effects of gravity; family or caregiver instructed in techniques; client instructed in self-ranging techniques performed on a daily basis
	Adaptive equipment	Instruction in use of long-handled assistive devices to compensate for upper extremity flexion and abduction deficit
	Joint protection	Instruction in joint protection to allow nerve time to heal and to prevent further injury; instruction in adaptive equipment, as needed for activities of daily living and leisure, work, and play occupations
	EMG biofeedback	Biofeedback potentially beneficial in providing the client with visual and auditory incentives during muscle reeducation sessions
	Retrograde massage	Use of retrograde massage if edema occurs in hand or arm; client, family, or caregivers instructed in technique to be performed several times per day
	Graded activities	Shoulder movement critical to recovery; incorporation of long, sweeping shoulder movements in the client's meaningful activities; graded from horizontal to vertical
Brachial plexus	Passive ROM to maintain joint flexibility	Passive ROM performed while supine twice daily, with emphasis on shoulder flexion, abduction, and external rotation; family or caregiver instructed in techniques
	Tactile stimulation to upper extremity to increase awareness	Massage, vibration, application of various textures to the arm
	Proprioceptive stimulation to upper extremity	Joint approximation through progressive weight bearing to increase awareness; always necessary to ensure proper alignment of joints
	Bilateral integration to improve body scheme	Use of developmentally appropriate bilateral activities (e.g., toys, crafts, or activity that requires two hands)
	Pool therapy	Therapeutic exercises with gravity minimized in water; swimming or weight lifting possible as client's strength improves
	Electrical stimulation	As prescribed by physician after EMG
	Slings	For damage to C5 and C6, sling fabricated to fit around humerus to support arm and allow hand to engage in occupations; especially important if arm is flaccid and the individual is able to walk—prevents further traction injury to nerves
	Splints	Resting splint for flaccid hand/wrist seen with damage to C8 and T1 to maintain part in functional position and prevent contractures; other splints available or fabricated for specific joints; air splints sometimes used to provide stability in elbow extension to bear weight with damage to C7
	Retrograde massage	For edema in hand or arm; client, family, or caregivers instructed in technique to be performed several times per day
Long thoracic nerve	Shoulder stabilized to limit scapular motion while nerve heals	After medical treatment, encouragement of maximal functional independence during activities and education in use of long-handled devices to compensate for shoulder limitations
	If nerve regeneration is not complete, possible consideration of surgery to relieve the excessive mobility of the scapula	
	Retrograde massage	For edema in hand or arm; client, family, or caregivers instructed in technique to be performed several times per day

EMG, Electromyography; *ROM*, range of motion.
Data from Storment M. Guidelines for therapists: treating children with brachial plexus injuries, United Brachial Plexus Network, 2022.
https://ubpn.org/resources/medical/pros/therapists/122-therapyguidelins.

CASE STUDY

William

William, who identifies as a man (prefers use of the pronouns he/him/his) and is a 60-year-old husband and teacher, was in a car accident that dislocated his right dominant shoulder. He was taken to the emergency room, given a sling, and sent home. Over the next few days, he noticed that he could neither flex nor abduct his humerus more than approximately 45 degrees. His physician reviewed his radiographs, repositioned the humerus, and diagnosed axillary nerve injury. Once the glenohumeral joint was stable, the physician prescribed occupational therapy to recover arm function.

During his therapy sessions, Marla, his occupational therapist, instructed William and his wife about joint protection, ROM exercises, and use of a reacher. As William's strength improved, Marla explored meaningful activities with him. After he enthusiastically mentioned a map project illustrating the places where he and his family had traveled, the two of them worked together to mount the map on poster board. Marla graded the activity and encouraged William to use long, sweeping movements of his right shoulder in flexion and extension and abduction and adduction when spreading the glue. William then sanded the frame and painted it, again using gliding shoulder movements. His home program also included smooth, gliding shoulder movements (e.g., wiping the counters, which his wife happily endorsed).

Analysis

Injury to the axillary nerve is one of the most common peripheral nerve injuries. Once the dislocation of the humerus has been reduced and the nerve begins to regenerate, rehabilitation of function may be possible. In this case, the occupational therapist was able to identify an activity that related to William's role as husband and home project enthusiast. This meaningful occupation caught his attention and engaged him in participation to accomplish the task.

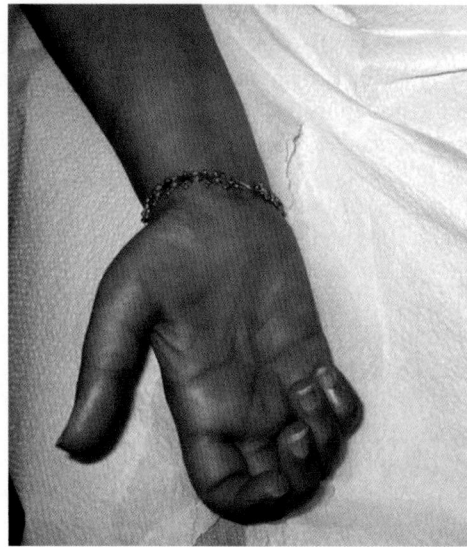

Fig. 38.2 Klumpke's syndrome: paralysis to the distal musculature of the wrist flexors and the intrinsic muscles of the hand that results in a "claw-hand deformity" or intrinsic minus hand. (From Chung KC, Yang LJS, McGillicuddy JE. Practical management of pediatric and adult brachial plexus palsies, Edinburgh, 2012, Saunders.)

to stretch or tear. For example, if the infant's shoulder is stuck in the birth canal during delivery and the head is pulled, the neck is stretched, which can subsequently stretch or tear the peripheral nerves in the brachial plexus.[42] In adults, traumatic brachial plexus injuries are caused by damage to the nerve roots from a variety of causes (e.g., car or motorcycle accidents, sports misadventures, falls, blows to the neck with blunt or sharp objects, tumors).[41] The two types of brachial plexus lesions are Erb-Duchenne syndrome and Klumpke's (Dejerine-Klumpke) syndrome.[26,41] These disorders are also referred to as Erb's palsy and Klumpke's palsy.

Erb-Duchenne syndrome is seen with lesions to the upper trunk of the brachial plexus, which consists of C5 and C6 nerve fibers. It causes significant arm weakness that affects 0.4 to 5 in 10,000 births. The incidence among newborns is 0.9 to 2.6 per 1000 live births with 80% to 96% recovery within 3 to 24 months.[5,59] The incidence among adults is not known because of underreporting. Typically, the muscles of the shoulder and elbow are affected with Erb-Duchenne syndrome, whereas hand movement is retained. Loss of sensation in the arm occurs with paralysis and atrophy in the deltoid, brachialis, biceps, and brachioradialis muscles (see Table 38.3). On observation, the arm hangs limp in internal rotation and adduction of the shoulder. The elbow is extended, forearm pronated, and wrist flexed, resulting in the "waiter's tip position." Even though hand muscles are unaffected, functional movement of the upper extremity is extremely limited.[5,26,59]

Klumpke's syndrome results from compression or traction to the lower trunk of the brachial plexus (comprising nerves arising from C8 and T1) and is seen less often than Erb-Duchenne syndrome. Traction during birth or later in life that is caused by a strong upward pull on the upper extremity when it is in an abducted position can result in this disorder. The involved nerves provide sensation to the medial aspect of the distal upper extremity and innervate muscles whose actions are wrist and finger flexion and abduction and adduction of the fingers (see Table 38.3). Consequently, paralysis of the distal musculature of the wrist flexors and the intrinsic muscles of the hand results in a "claw-hand deformity," also referred to as an intrinsic minus hand deformity (Fig. 38.2).[39,59] (See Table 38.1 for OT assessments.)

OT interventions initially involve partial immobilization and positioning with damage to either the upper or lower trunk of the brachial plexus. Passive ROM is critical for maintaining joint flexibility, and the client's family or caregiver should be taught to perform these exercises with the client two or three times daily. Intervention includes a variety of tactile and proprioceptive sensory input exercises to increase sensory awareness. Preventing contractures is critical to a functional outcome. For individuals with Erb-Duchenne syndrome, performance of passive and active assistive exercises and fabrication of a sling that fits around the humerus to support the arm are important. If strength improves, resistive exercises and activities can be implemented, and the sling may be removed or used intermittently during walking to support the shoulder.[53,59] For those with Klumpke's syndrome, a short opponens hand splint that supports the thumb in opposition is often used. It is important to provide occupations that are appropriate to developmental ages and stages and that appeal to the client and encourage active use of the extremity in bilateral activities. Surgery to improve nerve growth and upper extremity function may be recommended if improvement is not spontaneously observed within a few months.[53,59] Other interventions are described in Table 38.4.

Long Thoracic Nerve Injury

The long thoracic nerve, arising from C5-C7 nerve roots, innervates the serratus anterior muscle, which anchors the apex of the scapula to the posterior of the rib cage. The action of the serratus anterior is scapular abduction and protraction and upward rotation (see Table 38.3).[30] Although injury to this nerve is not common, the nerve can be injured in a number of ways: carrying heavy weights on the shoulder (e.g., backpacks), blows to the neck, compression caused by prolonged lying on the lateral trunk, and wounds. The resulting clinical picture involves "winging" of the scapula where the inferior angle and lower portion of the medial border of the scapula is protruding off the thoracic rib cage. The individual experiences difficulty flexing the glenohumeral joint above shoulder level and performing scapula abduction and protraction.[26,37] Asking the client to perform a wall push-up is a commonly used screening assessment technique. The wall push-up is performed by asking the client to stand facing a wall an arm's distance from the wall, the client places both hands on the wall and then flexes and then extends the elbows for the "push-up." If the long thoracic nerve is impaired, the scapula on that side will elevate and move medially, with the inferior angle rotating medially to produce a winging of the scapula.[37] Other OT assessments are described in Table 38.1.

Lesions of the radial, median, and ulnar nerves and cumulative trauma disorders affecting the hand are discussed in Chapter 40.

Psychosocial Interventions for Peripheral Nerve Injuries

Brachial plexus, thoracic, and axillary nerve injuries are life changing, affecting the psychological and emotional states of clients, their families, and friends. Clients often experience depression, which may be a reaction to the traumatic event that caused the injury. Depression may be short lived or may become chronic and serious. Occupational therapists can be helpful in this regard by discovering activities that are meaningful to the client and adapting them for success. The client's self-image is challenged and may require revision to accommodate the client's changed health status. For example, if the deltoid muscle has atrophied, the client can wear a foam or thermoplastic pad under clothing to round out the shoulders. Use of these aesthetic pads may increase the client's willingness to venture out into society. Referrals to support groups or a psychologist also may help clients adjust to a changed appearance.[51]

Participation in leisure occupations has been found to help people with physical disabilities redefine themselves (see Chapter 16), and occupational therapists should consider leisure as an important area of occupation to include in an intervention plan.[3]

NEUROMUSCULAR DISORDERS

NEUROMUSCULAR JUNCTION: MYASTHENIA GRAVIS

Myasthenia gravis (MG) is the most common chronic disease involving a disorder of chemical transmission at the nerve-muscle synapse, or neuromuscular junction.[10,31] The term myasthenia gravis is derived from Greek and Latin and means "grave muscle weakness."[32,46] It is most commonly caused by an acquired autoimmunological abnormality in which antibodies are produced that block, alter, or destroy the acetylcholine receptors on the postsynaptic membrane and interfere with synaptic transmission at the neuromuscular junction. Because neurotransmission is defective, skeletal (voluntary) muscles, typically the cranial muscles, become weak and easily fatigued with activity. The incidence of MG in the United States is approximately 14 to 20 in 100,000. However, it is underdiagnosed, especially among the elderly, so prevalence is likely higher. The latest statistics show that with the aging of the population, men are diagnosed more often than women, with symptoms typically beginning after 50 years of age.[10,32]

Most clients diagnosed with MG initially experience symptoms in the oculomotor muscles that cause eyelid drooping, referred to as ptosis, and double vision, referred to as diplopia. Oropharyngeal muscle weakness, which results in difficulty in chewing, swallowing, and speaking, is seen in some clients. Weakness of limb musculature is not typically an initial symptom, occurring in about 10% of individuals diagnosed.[32] The severity of muscle weakness fluctuates. People with MG tend to be stronger in the morning, but their strength and endurance decrease as the day progresses and muscles fatigue. Therefore, the client may experience increased double vision, severe drooping of the eyelids, difficulty with speech or swallowing, and fatigue with repetitive activity as muscles tire (Table 38.5).

Most clients with MG have abnormalities of the thymus glands (which is the central organ for immunological self-tolerance), and some have thymic tumors. Removal of the thymus gland (thymectomy) is standard therapy for most clients, but response time for symptom reduction varies with individuals and may take as long as 2 to 5 years after surgery. Clients without thymomas have a better response to surgery than those with a tumor. Clients are also treated with corticosteroids (prednisone) and immunosuppressive and cholinesterase-inhibiting drugs.[10,32] High-dose intravenous immunoglobulin has been reported to decrease symptoms in 50% to 100% of clients for a period of weeks to months. For clients with symptoms that suddenly worsen, those about to have surgery, or those who have not responded well to other interventions, plasma exchange is used as a short-term treatment. Nearly all people with MG improve for weeks to months after plasma exchange.[32]

Most people with MG usually experience maximal weakness during the first year after diagnosis. In 10% to 40% of cases, weakness is restricted to ocular muscles. The rest of cases experience progressive weakness in the first 2 years involving oropharyngeal and limb muscles. The course of the disease fluctuates but is usually progressive according to the Myasthenia Gravis Foundation of America (https://myasthenia.org/). However, with current treatment options, most individuals with MG lead normal or nearly normal lives.[35] Remissions or a decrease in symptoms and an improvement in strength and function can last for years. However, emotional upset, extended exertion, infections, medications, thyroid conditions, elevated

TABLE 38.5 Myasthenia Gravis Initial Symptoms, Description, and Percentage of Clients With Symptoms

Initial Symptoms	Description	Approximate Percentage of Clients With Initial Symptoms (%)
Oculomotor dysfunction	Severe drooping of eyelids (ptosis), double vision (diplopia), inability to move eyes in certain directions	70
Otopharyngeal muscle weakness	Difficulty chewing, swallowing, speaking; in severe cases, problems breathing and coughing resulting in aspiration	20
Limb weakness	May be limited to specific muscles or may progress to generalized fatigue	10

Data from Howard JF. *Myasthenia gravis: a summary.* https://emedicine.medscape.com/article/1171206-clinical?form=fpf; Brown RH, Cannon SC, Rowland LP. Diseases of the nerve and motor unit. In Kandel ER, et al, editors: *Principles of neural science*, ed 6, New York, 2021, McGraw-Hill.

body temperature, or childbirth may induce exacerbations of unpredictable severity.[32]

Role of the Occupational Therapist

Because similarities exist among the diagnoses of motor unit disorders, OT evaluation follows the same pattern, with specific assessments selected according to the disorder (see Table 38.1). A significant area for assessment in MG is eating and swallowing because of the dangers of aspiration. Because some clients may experience difficulty with diaphragmatic and intercostal muscle strength, they may have trouble coughing to clear secretions. An occupational therapist with advanced training in dysphagia should assess and treat clients with severe eating and swallowing dysfunction (see Chapter 27).

CASE STUDY

Jan

For several months, Jan, a 45-year-old photographer, who identifies as female (prefers use of the pronouns she/her/hers), had noticed unusual changes in her body. Her eyelids felt heavy, and her vision would blur after she was reading for a short time; it felt as if she were cross-eyed. Jan's speech became slurred if she was in a lengthy conversation. More recently, she had become aware that when she was drinking thin liquids, such as coffee, she would frequently choke. When she visited her doctor and received the results of medical tests, she was shocked to hear that she had an autoimmune disorder called myasthenia gravis (MG). Jan's physician referred her to a surgeon for removal of her thymus gland, and she was given a prescription for prednisone.

Jeri, an occupational therapist trained in dysphagia, assessed Jan's swallowing abilities and recommended that thickening agents be added to liquids to decrease choking. As Jan improved, Jeri performed ongoing swallowing assessments and was able to gradually add thinner liquids so that Jan could again enjoy coffee. Jan reports that the most important thing that anyone did for her was when Jeri helped her enroll in a myasthenia gravis support group, in which she experienced empathy, was given resources, and, to her surprise, found herself laughing again.

Analysis

People with MG can be helped through a variety of therapies to lead a near normal life. When a swallowing disorder is present, an occupational therapist with advanced training must perform a dysphagia assessment and make recommendations to prevent aspiration and pneumonia. A social support system is critical to the well-being and recovery of people with this disease.

Interventions for clients with MG depend on the results of the OT evaluation, which includes client and caregiver goals. The therapeutic program should focus on how the effects of fatigue impact a person's daily living performance. Interventions should not cause undue fatigue; therefore, the therapist must be aware of the client's medication regimen and ability to tolerate activity and the time of day that the client has the most energy. The client's muscle strength must be monitored on a regular basis, and the occupational therapist keeps an ongoing and updated record to document any important changes that must be reported to the medical team.

An important aspect of treatment is to educate the client and family members on the use of energy conservation and work simplification strategies to employ that can potentially reduce exertion and fatigue when engaging in ADLs, IADLs, and leisure occupations (see Chapters 10, 14, and 16). Adaptive and assistive devices may be introduced to decrease effort during daily activities. Because vision may be impaired, the occupational therapist should visit the client's home to assess architectural barriers, bathroom safety, and furniture arrangements to reduce fall risk and promote safety, thereby reducing the risk for a fall. If chewing and swallowing are problems, a dysphagia program should be designed and monitored by an experienced occupational therapist (see Chapter 27).

Because of the client's facial appearance (e.g., drooping eyelids), fear of choking, or steroid-related changes in appearance, the psychosocial effects of MG may be distressing to clients and their family and friends. The therapist should always treat the client with empathy and encourage honest discussion. For general well-being, the client must be able to express his or her feelings about these physical changes.[51] The client and family members also may be referred to an MG support group, a psychologist, or both.

MYOPATHIC DISORDERS

MUSCULAR DYSTROPHIES

The muscular dystrophies are a group of more than 30 genetic diseases. The dystrophies have in common the progressive degeneration of muscle fibers while the neuronal innervation to muscle and sensation remains intact. As the number of muscle fibers declines, each axon innervates fewer and fewer of

TABLE 38.6   Major Types of Muscular Dystrophy

Type	Description	Age of Onset and Progression
Duchenne	Affects boys only because it is inherited as an X-linked recessive trait	Onset age: 3–5 years—begins in muscles of pelvic girdle and legs
	Results from gene mutation that regulates the protein involved in maintenance of muscle integrity	By 12 years unable to walk; uses wheelchair
		Weakness spreads upward to shoulder girdle and trunk
		By 20 most need respirator to breathe, with death usually occurring by age 30
Becker	Similar to Duchenne, with milder symptoms	Onset age: 2–16 years
	X-linked recessive, affects boys	Slower progression of weakness
		Survival into middle age
Fascioscapulohumeral	Affects both sexes	Onset age: adolescence
	Autosomal dominant	Slow progression of weakness resulting in a near normal lifespan
	Affects primarily the muscles of the face and shoulder girdle (hence its name)	
Myotonic	Affects both sexes	Onset age: varies, often adult
	Causes weakness but also myotonia—prolonged muscle spasm or delayed muscle relaxation after vigorous contraction—especially in fingers and face; floppy, high-stepping gait; appearance of long face and drooping eyelids	Involves cranial muscle and distal limb weakness rather than proximal
		May be mild or severe
		Associated symptoms progress to involve cardiac abnormalities, endocrine disturbances, cataracts, and, in men, testicular atrophy and baldness
Limb girdle	Affects both sexes	Onset age: teens to early adulthood
	Progressive weakness affecting pelvic girdle and shoulder girdle first	Weakness leads to loss of ability to walk within 20 years
		Relatively slow progression
		Death in mid to late adulthood

Data from the National Institute of Neurological Disorder and Stroke: *Muscular dystrophy: hope through research.* Available at https://catalog.ninds.nih.gov/publications/muscular-dystrophy-hope-through-research. Brown RH, Cannon SC, Rowland LP. Diseases of the nerve and motor unit. In Kandel ER, Koester JD, Mack SH, Siegelbaum SA, editors. *Principles of neural science,* ed 6, New York, 2021, McGraw-Hill.

them, resulting in progressive muscle weakness. Some forms of muscular dystrophy (MD) have an onset in childhood, whereas others may not appear until middle age or later. The disorders also differ in terms of the distribution and extent of muscle weakness, rate of progression, and pattern of inheritance.[45] The major types of MD—Duchenne, Becker, facioscapulohumeral, myotonic, and limb girdle—are described in Table 38.6.

Because this group of diseases is degenerative, the decline of muscle function cannot be prevented. As yet, there is no cure. Medical management is largely supportive and designed to slow disease progression and prevent complications that arise from weakness, reduced mobility, and cardiac and respiratory difficulties. Drug therapy includes corticosteroids to slow the rate of muscle degeneration, immunosuppressants to delay some damage to dying muscle cells, drugs to provide short-term relief from muscle spasms and weakness, anticonvulsants to control seizures and some muscle activity, and antibiotics to fight respiratory infections. Various treatment therapies are currently being investigated but are not yet available. These include gene replacement, gene modification, and cell-based and drug-based therapy.[45]

Rehabilitation measures are vital in delaying deformity and achieving maximal function within the limits of the disease and its debilitating effects. In addition to occupational therapy, rehabilitation may include physical therapy, speech therapy, and respiratory therapy services.[45]

Role of the Occupational Therapist

The primary goal of occupational therapy is to help the client with MD maintain maximal independence as long as possible. Self-care activities and assistive devices that promote independence during home, school, leisure, and work activities are a vital part of the treatment program.[53] Leisure occupations need to be considered in a comprehensive OT intervention plan to ensure balance in all areas of the client's life. Social participation, play, and laughter are particularly important to the health, well-being, and social adjustment of the growing youth (see Chapters 6 and 16).

A comprehensive team evaluation of the client's abilities and disabilities should be administered. The team includes the physician, occupational therapist, physical therapist, and psychologist. A social worker may advise the family on community resources. The occupational therapist assesses the client's functional status in ADLs and IADLs and gathers information on client factors such as muscle strength and joint range of motion. After the evaluation process is complete, an OT intervention plan is developed to address specific concerns. Interventions are designed to provide ways for the client to maintain better health and function as independently as possible in self-care, work, and play-related activities. The occupational therapist can recommend and provide training in the use of assistive devices and mobility aids that might be required to foster greater independence. Recommendations for modifications for easy and safe access at home, school, or work, especially when using a wheelchair or a walker, can be made. Interventions should identify ways to engage in leisure and social activities as identified by the client. (See Table 38.1 for assessments.)

Active exercise may help the client maintain strength, but overexertion and fatigue must be prevented. Because people with MD may experience cardiac complications, occupational therapists must be aware of the client's medical history and use exercise judiciously, observing cardiac precautions when necessary. Incorporating exercise into meaningful, age-related activities that are monitored by a therapist can promote engagement in participation.

Two pilot studies involving clients with MD and exercise show that improvements are possible; investigators recommend further research. Clients with myotonic dystrophy showed significant improvement in hand function and self-rated occupational performance on the Canadian Occupational Performance Measure after a 3-month hand training OT intervention.[2] An experimental pilot study quantitatively evaluated qigong and determined that it may be beneficial used as an adjunct therapy program. Subjects with MD who participated in qigong reported perceived maintenance of general health and positive coping when compared to the control group. The treatment group tended to "maintain balance function during training and performance of qigong whilst there was a decline when not training." The researchers concluded that qigong decreased the rate of decline and is worthy of further study.[66]

Adaptive equipment and environmental modifications are often used as OT interventions. Instruction in work simplification and energy conservation—as well as in creative and effective strategies to perform ADLs, IADLs, and various other occupations—is important in the OT program.[53] A powered wheelchair, a wheelchair lap board, suspension slings, or mobile arm supports may facilitate greater independence in self-feeding, writing, reading, computer use, and tabletop leisure activities when there is substantial shoulder girdle and upper limb weakness. Built-up utensils are helpful when grip strength declines. Home and workplace modifications will be necessary for most clients. Client and family education is an important part of a team rehabilitation program.[53] A supportive approach to the client and family is helpful as function declines and new mobility aids, assistive devices, and community resources become necessary. Wheelchair prescription and mobility training in either a manual or powered wheelchair are included in the OT intervention program. The wheelchair may require a special seating system or supports to minimize the development of scoliosis, hip and knee flexion contractures, and ankle plantar flexion deformity.[53] Powered wheelchairs are often recommended to conserve energy and decrease strain on shoulders and trunk. Instruction in methods to maneuver power chairs can cause overexertion, and this activity, like any other, must be graded for difficulty. One study found that young people (i.e., those between 7 and 22 years of age) diagnosed with either MD or cerebral palsy who were inexperienced powered wheelchair drivers significantly improved their wheelchair driving performance through the use of simulator training. The researchers concluded that this method of instruction conserved energy and was effective.[29]

Chronic pain in children, adolescents, and young adults (i.e., persons between 8 and 20 years of age) with physical disabilities has not been widely studied, but research indicates that chronic pain interferes with ADLs and IADLs in young people with MD, cerebral palsy, spinal cord injury, acquired and congenital limb deficiency, and spina bifida.[39] Pain appears to be more prevalent in female subjects than male subjects during the performance of daily routines; it interfered most often with physical activities, and it negatively affected mood. McKearnan noted that the young people in this study frequently reported pain associated with physical therapy, OT, and therapeutic home programs.[38] They also complained that the use of splints, orthotics, and prosthetics was sometimes painful. Therapists must be aware of their client's pain levels and modify activities and orthotics as needed. Helping clients with MD to manage pain will most likely lead to improved quality of life.

The sense of self is challenged as clients with MD realize that they will experience a progressive loss of bodily function. Occupational therapists must realize that these clients are constantly forced to redefine themselves as they go through life, making "continuous trade-offs as function is lost."[51] A critical element in OT intervention is to help the client and family members find meaningful activities in which to participate either as individuals or as a family. For example, connecting with spiritual activities that engage clients and families on the deepest level could be critical to a sense of hope and well-being.[13] Alternatively, encouraging families to use humor and to play and laugh together can promote bonding, reduce fear and anxiety, and produce positive physical and emotional feelings.[8]

Psychosocial issues related to MD involve the whole family. Parents go through phases of shock, fear, and despair when the diagnosis is made and as the child ages and function decreases (e.g., when the wheelchair is prescribed). Encouraging parents not to be overprotective and to continue to promote their child's independence is an important aspect of therapy. Further, therapists can anticipate times in the growing child's life when psychosocial support will be most essential and can offer education and support during intervention sessions. Some potentially disturbing developmental milestones for the client and family occur when the child starts school (at approximately age 5), when the child loses the capacity for independent ambulation (at 8 to 12 years), when adolescent social life is limited, and, of course, when young adulthood arrives with the expectation that death is imminent.[53] Referral to a psychologist, family counselor, or spiritual adviser during these times should be considered.

Edith, Part 2

Return to the case study presented at the beginning of this chapter and compare your answers with the ones given here.

1. What are the phases of Guillain-Barré, and what occupational therapy interventions might be used in each phase?

The typical progression of GBS occurs in three phases. The initial, or acute, phase begins with the client's first conclusive symptoms and lasts until there is no further decline in physical status. This phase may last from 1 to 4 weeks.[43] During this phase, Edith's condition progressed from generalized weakness to paralysis of her extremities and muscles of the trunk and diaphragm. She was completely dependent in activities of daily living (ADLs) and required a ventilator to breathe. Jen, the occupational therapist assigned to the intensive care unit, established four goals with Edith and her family.

Goal	Intervention
Maintain full ROM in all joints.	Perform passive ROM two times per day to all joints.
Prevent contractures.	Fabricate resting hand splints, and educate client, family, and nursing aides in proper ways to position Edith in bed.
Teach Edith and family about GBS.	Provide and discuss handouts, reading materials, and GBS websites.
Provide a strategy for Edith to listen to the Bible.	Instruct Edith in ways to use a mouth stick to control her tablet and phone.

Phase 2, the plateau phase, began when Edith's physical status stabilized, with no further deterioration. She was transferred to a regular hospital unit. She was able to breathe on her own, speak softly, and sit up in bed in a semi-reclining position with pillows positioned for support. Some strength had returned to her proximal musculature, but her hands remained paralyzed and she fatigued easily. The plateau phase lasted a few weeks during which Edith's physical status remained unchanged. The goals for this phase were essentially the same as for the acute phase except that now Edith could choose to either read the Bible by turning the pages with a mouth stick or listen to the e-book using the mouth stick to control the tablet. She could also control the television set with the mouth stick and was able to view her favorite shows. Family and friends were encouraged to visit but were cautioned not to fatigue her.

The recovery phase began when Edith's strength and sensation began to return to her distal extremities. She was transferred to the rehabilitation unit. The occupational therapist, Lara, and Edith came up with four goals during the recovery

phase. The use of adaptive equipment such as built-up handles, work simplification, and energy conservation techniques (e.g., breaking the task down into steps and resting between steps), and the use of electric appliances was encouraged during activities. Edith practiced playing cards with other clients in a group environment. Lara set her up with a cardholder and a battery-powered card shuffler when her hands were too weak to hold the cards, but Edith eventually was able to play independently. Edith went to the mall with her granddaughter and Lara. During the outing, Lara taught them, in the context of shopping, how to gauge fatigue and to rest for 5 or 10 minutes when feeling tired. She also served as a role model, pacing the activity by limiting the initial shopping trip to 30 minutes and encouraging gradual lengthening of the experience over time. Lara provided Edith with community resources to aid in her independence. For example, the Guillain-Barré Syndrome Foundation International (GBSFI) offers local support groups, literature, and conferences to all GBS survivors and caregivers. In addition, Edith's family received extensive training from the interdisciplinary team members on how to continue the learned strategies and use the equipment in the home and community. Driving was not addressed at an inpatient level, but Edith was referred to the OT driver training program, where she would be assessed when her strength returned.

2. In what ways were Edith's psychosocial needs addressed during recovery?

Edith's fears about being paralyzed were addressed in several ways. Edith and her family were taught about the disease and encouraged to have hope because most people with GBS recover well. Edith's spiritual needs were met by making it possible for her to continue her morning Bible routine; she initially used a mouth switch to control page turning, etc., on her tablet and then was able to use a mouth stick to turn pages until her hands recovered strength. Edith expressed a desire to be as independent as possible in activities of daily living (ADLS), to cook for her family, and to enjoy family outings and card playing. These activities were all made possible through occupational therapy adaptive interventions. Her family members and friends were encouraged to visit, gradually increasing the length of time that they stayed.

3. Describe energy conservation techniques that you think would be appropriate for Edith while engaging in her valued occupation of cooking.

First, Edith and Lara reviewed the recipe and listed the necessary items while seated at the kitchen table. Edith used a wheeled kitchen cart to gather items and carry them to the counter. Lara provided her with a reacher to obtain items on high shelves. When the items were assembled, Edith sat and rested on a bar stool near the counter while she and Lara reviewed the next step. Electric appliances were used to chop and stir the ingredients. Edith rested after this step. Lara showed Edith how to slide containers along the counter to the stove without lifting them. They walked back to the table to play a game of cards while the meal cooked. When the food was cooked, Edith placed plates and utensils on the kitchen cart with the one-dish meal and wheeled the cart to the table to enjoy her meal.

OCCUPATIONAL THERAPY AND POST–COVID-19 SYNDROME (LONG COVID)

Winifred Schultz-Krohn

The emergence of the COVID-19 pandemic ushered in substantial unknowns about potential long-term sequelae to those infected.[1,20] Those initially requiring hospitalization for severe respiratory problems recovered and were discharged but then reported persistent problems, post-COVID symptoms, that affected daily life. Those hospitalized for COVID-19 infections

experienced a higher number of post-COVID symptoms (PCS), also referred to as long-haul COVID (long COVID), compared to those infected but not needing hospitalization. Although demographic data continues to be updated, approximately 50% to 75% of those hospitalized for COVID-19 experience continued symptoms 3 to 6 months after discharge from the hospital.[20] The symptoms vary considerably but can be grouped as follows: neurocognitive issues ("brain-fog," decreased attention, confusion), autonomic issues (tachycardia, palpitations), gastrointestinal, respiratory, musculoskeletal, and psychological (anxiety, depression, insomnia).[19]

Individuals with confirmed infection of COVID-19, whether hospitalized or not, are at risk for post-COVID syndrome (PCS). The most common problems noted include fatigue, shortness of breath, cognitive problems, and sleep disorders.[6,24,48,63] Given these problems often persist 3 to 6 months or longer after initial COVID-19 infection, this is an area for occupational therapy intervention. The discussion of PCS in this chapter is appropriate given the need for occupational therapy strategies of fatigue management and energy conservation to support clients with PCS.[57] Over a third of individuals with PCS reported problems completing basic activities of daily living.[63] An instrument designed specifically to record and monitor PCS has been developed and validated using classic psychometric methods for reliability and validity.[48] The COVID-19 Yorkshire Rehabilitation Scale (C19-YRS) provides a tool for initial assessment and also can be used as an outcome measure to record changes in PCS after intervention.[48,56] Various multidisciplinary programs have been developed to meet the persistent needs of those experiencing PCS.[50,63] These programs include occupational therapy services that often provide fatigue management and work simplification strategies along with energy conservation methods.

The persistent cognitive issues of "brain-fog" and fatigue contribute to problems in returning to previous levels of occupational engagement. The Occupational Therapy Practice Framework provides an organizational approach to address the symptoms associated with PCS.[65] Wilcox and Frank[67] illustrated how a systematic approach to address a client's needs resulted in significant improvements in PCS and reduced the impact of the persistent symptoms on occupational engagement. The occupational therapist used strategies of energy conservation and fatigue management along with addressing functional cognitive skills using a multicontext approach. This included analysis of the worksite responsibilities to support the client in returning to a position as a nurse with complex demands. Specific metacognitive strategies were included in the occupational therapy program. Metacognition is the ability to think about your thinking processes.[12,21,22] This includes self-assessment of process and outcomes for a task and reflection of potential changes for future task performance. Metacognitive strategies can focus on the person, task, or approach used for task completion.[55] During services provided for clients with cognitive issues because of PCS, the occupational therapist can prompt the client to engage in assessment of performance and options to continue or consider other options. This model of questioning in the moment is designed to support real-time (in the moment) analysis of how the task is progressing and if the course of action should be continued.

Clients with PCS present with a variety of symptoms, but fatigue management and energy conservation techniques, as described elsewhere in this chapter, will be important supports provided by the occupational therapist.[50] Additionally, functional cognitive strategies (see Chapter 26) and promotion of sleep habits and routines (see Chapter 13) should be included in the occupational therapy services offered to clients with PCS.[67]

SUMMARY

The motor unit consists of the lower motor neuron, neuromuscular junction, and muscle. Some motor unit dysfunctions are reversible, and others are degenerative. In addition, PCS often presents with severe fatigue and shortness of breath, requiring occupational therapy services to support the client's occupational engagement. The role of the occupational therapist is to assess functional capabilities in all occupational performance areas and contexts. ADLs and IADLs (including self-care, home management, mobility, and work-related tasks), energy conservation, work simplification, joint protection, spiritual approaches, and appropriate humor may be used to restore or maintain function. Proper positioning, exercise programs, and pain management techniques are used as indicated to facilitate recovery and increase functional capacity. Orthoses, assistive devices, communication aids, and mobility equipment and training in their use may be necessary. Psychosocial considerations and client and family education are important aspects of the OT program.

REVIEW QUESTIONS

1. Name the components of the motor unit and one disorder that may result in dysfunction for each component.
2. Describe Guillain-Barré syndrome and the occupational therapy interventions used for clients with this disorder.
3. List at least six clinical manifestations of peripheral nerve injury.
4. Describe the occupational therapy treatment strategies, including any contraindications, for peripheral nerve injuries.
5. Describe a method of managing pain that an occupational therapist may use.
6. Discuss the clinical signs of myasthenia gravis.
7. Describe the role of occupational therapy for clients who have myasthenia gravis.
8. What is the primary treatment precaution in myasthenia gravis?
9. Name and differentiate the four types of muscular dystrophy.
10. What are the treatment goals for muscular dystrophy?
11. Discuss ways that occupational therapists address the psychosocial needs of clients with each of the motor unit disorders.
12. Describe how an occupational therapist can support a client with post-COVID syndrome (PCS).

For additional practice questions for this chapter, please visit eBooks.Health.Elsevier.com.

REFERENCES

1. Albu S, Zozaya NR, Murillo N, Garcia-Molina A, Chacón CAF, Kumru H: What's going on following acute COVID-19? Clinical characteristics of patients in an out-patient rehabilitation program, *NeuroRehabilitation* 48:469–480, 2021. https://doi.org/10.3233/NRE-210025.

2. Aldehag AS, Jonsson H, Ansved T: Effects of a hand training programme in five patients with myotonic dystrophy type 1, *Occup Ther Int* 12:14, 2005.

3. American Occupational Therapy Association: Occupational therapy practice framework: domain and process, 4th edition, *Am J Occup Ther* 74 (Suppl. 2):1–87. https://doi.org/10.5014/ajot.2020.74S2001.

4. Andary, M. (2021). Guillain-Barre syndrome clinical presentation. *Medscape*. https://emedicine.medscape.com/article/315632-clinical.

5. Aragonès JM, Bolíbar I, Bonfill X, et al: Myasthenia gravis: a higher than expected incidence in the elderly, *Neurology* 60:1024, 2003.

6. Augustin, M, Schommers, P, Stecher, M, Dewald, F, Gieselmann, L, Gruell, H, et al: Post-COVID syndrome in non-hospitalised patients with COVID-19: a longitudinal prospective cohort study. *The Lancet Regional Health – Europe, 100122, 2021.* https://doi.org/10.1016/j.lanepe.2021.100122.

7. Avers D, Brown M: *Daniels and Worthingham's muscle testing: techniques of manual examination*, ed 10, Philadelphia, 2018, WB Saunders.

8. Basit H, Dewi C, Ali CDM, Madhani N: Erb Palsy, *National Library of Medicine* (2022): https://www.ncbi.nlm.nih.gov/books/NBK513260/.

9. Bayot M, Nassereddin A, Varacallo M: Anatomy, shoulder and upper limb, brachial plexus, *National Library of Medicine* (2021): https://www.ncbi.nlm.nih.gov/books/NBK500016/.

10. Berk L, Tan S, Fry W: Eustress of humor associated laughter modulates specific immune system components, *Ann Behav Med* 15:111, 1993.

11. Blaskey J, et al: *Therapeutic management of patients with Guillain-Barré syndrome*, Downey, CA, 1989, Rancho Los Amigos National Rehabilitation Center.

12. Brown AL: Metacognition, executive control, self-regulation, and other more mysterious mechanisms. In Weinert FE, Kluwe RH, editors: *Metacognition, motivation, and understanding*, Hillsdale, New Jersey, 1987, Lawrence Erlbaum Associates, pp 65–116.

13. Brown RH, Cannon SC, Rowland LP: Diseases of the peripheral nerve and motor unit. In Kandel ER, editor: *Principles of neural science* ed 6, New York, 2021, McGraw-Hill.

14. Centers for Disease Control and Prevention (2019). Guillain-Barré syndrome. https://www.cdc.gov/campylobacter/guillain-barre.html.

15. Christiansen C: Acknowledging a spiritual dimension in occupational therapy practice, *Am J Occup Ther* 51:169, 1997.

16. Reference deleted in proofs.

17. Eisendrath S, Matthay M, Dunkel J: Guillain-Barré syndrome: psychosocial aspects of management, *Psychosomatics* 24:465, 1983.

18. Reference deleted in proofs.

19. Fernández-de-las-Peñas C, Florencio LL, Gómez-Mayordomo V, Cuadrado ML, Palacios-Ceña D, Raveendran AV: Proposed integrative model for post-COVID symptoms, *Diabetes & Metabolic Syndrome: Clinical Research & Reviews* 15(4):102159, 2021. https://doi.org/10.1016/j.dsx.2021.05.032.

20. Fernández-de-las-Peñas C, Palacios-Ceña D, Gómez-Mayordomo V, Cuadrado ML, Florencio LL: Defining Post-COVID symptoms (Post-Acute COVID, Long COVID, Persistent Post-COVID): an integrative classification, *Int. J. Environ. Res. Public Health* 2021(18):2621, 2021. https://doi.org/10.3390/ijerph18052621.

21. Flavell JH: Metacognition and cognitive monitoring: A new area of cognitive-developmental inquiry, *American Psychologist* 34:906–911, 1979.

22. Flavell JH: Speculations about the nature and development of metacognition. In Weinert FE, Kluwe RH, editors: *Metacognition, motivation and understanding*, Hillside, New Jersey, 1987, Lawrence Erlbaum Associates, pp 21–29.

23. Reference deleted in proofs.

24. Graham EL, Clark JR, Orban ZS, Lim PH, Szymanski AL, Taylor C, DiBiase RM, Jia DT, Balabanov R, Ho SU, Batra A, Liotta EM, Koralnik IJ: Persistent neurologic symptoms and cognitive dysfunction in non-hospitalized Covid-19 "long haulers", *Annals of Clinical and Translational Neurology* 8(5):1073–1085, 2021.

25. Grohar-Murray ME, Becker A, Reilly S, Ricci M: Self-care actions to manage fatigue among myasthenia gravis clients, *J Neurosci Nurs* 30:191, 1998.

26. Guillain-Barré Syndrome/Chronic Inflammatory Demyelinating Polyneuropathy Foundation International: GBS. https://www.gbs-cidp.org/gbs/.

27. Gurushantappa P, Kuppasad S: Anatomy of axillary nerve and its clinical importance: a cadaveric study, *J Clin Diagn Res.* 9(3):AC13, 2015.

28. Gutman SA, Schonfeld AB: *Screening adult neurologic populations: a step-by-step instruction manual*, ed 3, Bethesda, MD, 2019, American Occupational Therapy Association.

29. Hasdai A, Jessel AS, Weiss PL: Use of a computer simulator for training children with disabilities in the operation of a powered wheelchair, *Am J Occup Ther* 52:215, 1998.

30. Holmes T: Occupational therapy issues. In Howard, J (Ed.): Myasthenia Gravis: A manual for the healthcare provider. Myasthenia Gravis Foundation of America (2009) https://myasthenia.org/Portals/0/Provider%20Manual_ibook%20version.pdf.

31. Howard JF: Myasthenia Gravis Foundation of America: clinical overview of M, http://www.myasthenia.org/HealthProfessionals/ClinicalOverviewofMG.aspx. https://myasthenia.org/Professionals/Clinical-Overview-of-MG 2015.

32. Keefe FJ: Cognitive behavioral therapy for managing pain, *Clin Psychologist* 49:4, 1996.

33. Reference deleted in proofs.

34. Law M, et al: *Canadian occupational performance measure*, ed 5, Toronto, Canada, 2014, Canadian Association of Occupational Therapy Publications.

35. Leonhard SE, Mandarakas MR, Gondim FAA, et al: Diagnosis and management of Guillain-Barré syndrome in ten steps, *Natures Review Neurology* 15(11):671–683, 2019.

36. Magee DJ, Manske RC, editors: *Orthopedic physical assessment* ed 7, St. Louis, 2020, Elsevier.

37. Mandel DR, Jackson JM, Zemke R, et al: *Lifestyle redesign: implementing the well elderly program*, Bethesda, MD, 2000, American Occupational Therapy Association.

38. McKearnan KA: *Chronic pain in youths with physical disabilities (unpublished doctoral dissertation)*, Seattle, 2004, University of Washington.

39. Merryman J, Varacallo M, Klumpke Palsy. *National Library of Medicine* (2022): https://www.ncbi.nlm.nih.gov/books/NBK531500/.

40. Meythaler J, DeVivo M, Braswell W: Rehabilitation outcomes of patients who have developed Guillain-Barré syndrome, *Am J Phys Med Rehabil* 14:411, 1997.

41. National Institute of Neurological Disorders and Stroke: Brachial plexus injuries information page, p. 1. https://www.ninds.nih.gov/health-information/disorders/brachial-plexus-injuries#.

42. National Institute of Neurological Disorders and Stroke: Erb-Duchenne and Dejerine-Klumpke palsies information page. https://www.ninds.nih.gov/health-information/disorders/erb-duchenne-and-dejerine-klumpke-palsies.

43. National Institute of Neurological Disorders and Stroke: Guillain-Barre. https://www.ninds.nih.gov/health-information/disorders/guillain-barre-syndrome?search-term=Guillian%20Barre.

44. National Institute of Neurological Disorders and Stroke: Guillain-Barré syndrome fact sheet. https://www.ninds.nih.gov/health-information/disorders/guillain-barre-syndrome?search-term=Guillian%20Barre.

45. National Institute of Neurological Disorders and Stroke: Muscular dystrophy: hope through research. https://www.ninds.nih.gov/health-information/disorders/muscular-dystrophy?search-term=muscular%20dy.

46. National Institute of Neurological Disorders and Stroke: Myasthenia gravis fact sheet. https://www.ninds.nih.gov/health-information/disorders/myasthenia-gravis?search-term=myasthenia%20gravis.

47. National Institute of Neurological Disorders and Stroke: Peripheral neuropathy fact sheet. https://www.ninds.nih.gov/health-information/disorders/peripheral-neuropathy?search-term=peripheral%20neuropath.

48. O'Connor RJ, Preston N, Parkin A, Makower S, Ross D, Gee J, Halpin SJ, Horton M, Sivan M: The COVID-19 Yorkshire Rehabilitation Scale (C19-YRS): application and psychometric analysis in a post-COVID-19 syndrome cohort, *J Med Virol.* 94(3):1027–1034, 2022. https://doi.org/10.1002/jmv.27415. PMID: 34676578; PMCID: PMC8662016

49. Netter FH: *The CIBA collection of medical illustrations (vol 1): nervous system*, West Caldwell, NJ, 1986, CIBA.

50. Parkin A, Davison J, Tarrant R, Ross D, Halpin S, Simms A, Salman R, Sivan M: A multidisciplinary NHS COVID-19 service to manage post-COVID-19 syndrome in the community, *Journal of Primary Care & Community Health* 12, 2021. https://doi.org/10.1177/21501327211010994. 21501327211010994.

51. Pendleton HM, Schultz-Krohn W: Psychosocial issues in physical disability. In Cara E, MacRae A, editors: *Psychosocial occupational therapy: a clinical practice* ed 3, Clifton Park, NY, 2013, Delmar Cengage Learning.

52. Reference deleted in proofs.

53. Rogers SL: Common conditions that influence children's participation. In Case-Smith J, editor: *Occupational therapy for children* ed 5, St. Louis, 2005, Mosby.

54. Schmidt A: *How do people with Guillain-Barré syndrome (GBS) participate in daily life? A pilot study (unpublished master's thesis project)*, San Jose, CA, 2004, San Jose State University.

55. Schultz-Krohn W: Best practices in cognition and executive functioning to enhance participation. In Frolek Clark G, Rioux JE, Chandler BE, editors: *Best Practices for Occupational Therapy in Schools* 2nd Ed, Bethesda, MD, 2019, American Occupational Therapy Association, pp 457–464.

56. Sivan M, Parkin A, Makower S, Greenwood DC: Post-COVID syndrome symptoms, functional disability, and clinical severity phenotypes in hospitalized and nonhospitalized individuals: a cross-sectional evaluation from a community COVID rehabilitation service, *J Med Virol* 94(4):1419–1427, 2022. https://doi.org/10.1002/jmv.27456.

57. Sivan M, Halpin S, Hollingworth L, Snook N, Hickman K, Clifton IJ: Development of an integrated rehabilitation pathway for individuals recovering from COVID-19 in the community, *J Rehabil Med* 52(8):1–5, 2020. https://doi.org/10.2340/16501977-2727.

58. Stewart D, et al: The effectiveness of cognitive-behavioral interventions with people with chronic pain: an example of a critical review of the literature. In Law M, editor: *Evidence-based rehabilitation: a guide to practice*, Thorofare, NJ, 2002, Slack.

59. Storment M: Guidelines for therapists: treating children with brachial plexus injuries, *United Brachial Plexus Network*, 2022, https://ubpn.org/resources/medical/pros/therapists/122-therapyguidelins.

60. Taylor RR, Fan C-W: Managing pain in occupational therapy: integrating the Model of Human Occupation and the intentional relationship. In Cara E, MacRae A, editors: *Psychosocial occupational therapy: a clinical practice* ed 3, Clifton Park, NY, 2013, Delmar Cengage Learning.

61. Thanvi BR, Lo TC: Update on myasthenia gravis, *Postgrad Med J* 80:690, 2004.

62. Tomita M, Buckner K, Saharan S, Persons K, Liao S: Extended occupational therapy reintegration strategies for a woman with Guillain-Barré syndrome: case report, *American Journal of Occupational Therapy* 70(4):1–7, 2016.

63. Vanichkachorn G, Newcomb R, Cowl CT, Murad MH, Breeher L, Miller S, Trenar M, Neveau D, Higgins S: (2021) Post-COVID-19 syndrome (long haul syndrome): description of a multidisciplinary clinic at Mayo Clinic and characteristics of the initial patient cohort. *Mayo Clinic Proceedings*, 96(7): 1782–1791, 2021. https://doi.org/10.1016/j.mayocp.2021.04.024 www.mayoclinicproceedings.org.

64. Walling AD, Dickson G: Guillain-Barré syndrome, *Am Fam Physician* 87:191–197, 2013.

65. Watters K, Marks TS, Edwards DF, Skidmore ER, Giles GM: A framework for addressing clients' functional cognitive deficits after COVID-19, *American Journal of Occupational Therapy* 75(Suppl. 1):7511347010, 2021. https://doi.org/10.5014/ajot.2021.049308.

66. Wenneberg S, Gunnarsson LG, Ahlström G: Using a novel exercise programme for patients with muscular dystrophy. Part II: a quantitative study, *Disabil Rehabil* 26:595, 2004.

67. Wilcox J, Frank E: Occupational therapy for the long haul of post-COVID syndrome: a case report, *American Journal of Occupational Therapy* 75(Suppl. 1):7511210060, 2021. https://doi.org/10.5014/ajot.2021.049223.

SUGGESTED READING

Ways of Coping Scale. Available at Mind Garden Inc., 1690 Woodside Road, Suite 202, Redwood City, CA 94961; https://www.mindgarden.com.

39

Arthritis

Lisa Deshaies, Monica Godinez-Becerril, and Honor Duderstadt-Galloway

LEARNING OBJECTIVES

After studying this chapter, the student or practitioner will be able to do the following:

1. Understand the distinct disease processes of osteoarthritis and rheumatoid arthritis.
2. Describe common similarities and differences in the symptoms of osteoarthritis and rheumatoid arthritis.
3. Identify joint changes and hand deformities commonly seen with osteoarthritis and rheumatoid arthritis.
4. Recognize medications commonly used in the treatment of arthritis and their side effects.
5. Understand the physical and psychosocial effects of arthritis and their impact on occupational performance.
6. Identify important areas to evaluate in clients with arthritis.
7. Identify the intervention objectives of occupational therapy for clients with arthritis.
8. Design an appropriate individualized intervention plan based on diagnosis, stage of disease, limitations in functional activity, and client goals and lifestyle.
9. Identify key resources helpful to persons with arthritis and to healthcare providers.
10. Identify evaluation and treatment precautions related to arthritis.

CHAPTER OUTLINE

KEY TERMS

Arthritis
Crepitus
Gelling
Joint laxity

Nodes
Nodules
Osteoarthritis
Rheumatoid arthritis

Subluxation
Synovitis
Systemic
Tenosynovitis

THREADED CASE STUDY

Camilla, Part 1

Camilla is a 65-year-old woman (prefers use of the pronouns she/her/hers) with a 20-year history of rheumatoid arthritis. She lives with her sister, nephew, daughter, and two grandchildren in a one-story home with two steps at the entry. She assists her sister with preparing meals and select light home chores such as folding clothes. Her nephew performs any heavy tasks around the home. Her primary roles include volunteering at the elementary school and taking care of her grandchildren Ava (age 9) and Peter (age 11). She enjoys knitting, gardening, traveling, taking care of her cats, attending church and going to her grandchildren's soccer games. Her duties at school include making photocopies, assembling homework packets, grading papers, and monitoring students on the playground at recess. Her sister provides transportation to medical appointments and to the school.

Camilla was referred to outpatient occupational therapy after an exacerbation of her arthritis that resulted in increasing pain, fatigue, and difficulty engaging in many important daily occupations. On her initial evaluation, Camilla identifies her primary concerns as maximizing her functional level and reducing her pain so that she can resume full participation in her volunteering at school, being active at church, knitting, gardening, pet care, traveling, and attending functions with her grandchildren.

Clinical examination reveals pain and limitations in active range of motion in all of her upper extremity joints (shoulders, elbows, wrists, fingers) and her knees. Synovitis (inflammation of the synovial fluids), subluxation, and mild deviation is present at her wrists. Subluxation and ulnar deviation is noted at her metacarpophalangeal joints with mutilans deformity at her right fifth finger and boutonnière deformity at left fifth finger, with flexible swan neck deformities of digits 2 to 4 bilaterally. She also has laxity and hyperextension of her left thumb interphalangeal (IP) joint. No other significant joint changes are noted.

Pain and stiffness are interfering with daytime activities and are also making sleep difficult. Her energy level has significantly decreased, and she reports feeling tired all the time. Although she still manages to assist her sister with home chores, it is not as much as she would like. She is also having increased difficulty attending her grandchildren's sporting events and performing her volunteer work at school.

Critical Thinking Questions
1. What components of evaluation would you choose to assess regarding Camilla's prior and current clinical and functional status?
2. Which aspects of the disease process are most problematic, and what are the major performance skills, performance patterns, contexts, activity demands, and client factors influencing Camilla's ability to engage in her volunteer work and other areas of occupation?
3. What interventions would you use to help Camilla reach her goal of being able to continue volunteering?

OVERVIEW OF RHEUMATIC DISEASES

The term arthritis is of Greek derivation and literally means "joint inflammation." It is used to describe different conditions that fall under the larger umbrella of rheumatic diseases. Rheumatic diseases encompass more than 100 conditions characterized by chronic pain and progressive physical impairment of joints and soft tissues (e.g., skin, muscles, ligaments, tendons). These conditions include osteoarthritis (OA), rheumatoid arthritis (RA), systemic lupus erythematosus, ankylosing spondylitis, scleroderma, gout, and fibromyalgia. Arthritis continues to be the leading cause of disability in adults. One in every four adults in the United States has signs and symptoms of arthritis, increasing to nearly 50% in persons over the age of 65.[9,16,34] Arthritis is a major public health problem that costs the U.S. economy nearly $304 billion in medical costs and earning losses annually.[9,13,32] Rheumatic diseases are a leading cause of disability with significant economic, social, and psychological impact,[33] resulting in worse health-related quality of life for those affected than for those without arthritis.[50] Between 2013 and 2015, approximately 54.4 million Americans had doctor-diagnosed arthritis and were affected by arthritis and other rheumatic conditions, with an estimated 49.7% experiencing limitations in their ability to participate in daily activities and 31% limited in their ability to work.[12,13,16,34,94,136] As the population continues to age, the prevalence of arthritis-related conditions is expected to increase to an estimated 78.4 million by the year 2040; however, adjusted estimates indicate that there are potentially more than 91 million adults in the United States living with arthritis with disability occurring at a rate of 43.5%.[9,16,34]

Occupational therapists (OTs) are likely to encounter clients with rheumatic diseases in their practice settings, whether the condition is manifested as a primary or secondary type. To recognize problem areas and plan effective intervention strategies, the occupational therapist should know the unique features of each disease, its underlying pathology, and its typical clinical findings; the therapist also should be familiar with commonly prescribed medications and their adverse reactions. Given the scope and intended purpose of this book, it is neither appropriate nor possible to adequately describe every rheumatic disease. Therefore, this chapter focuses on two of the most prevalent diseases: OA and RA. Armed with an understanding of the noninflammatory and inflammatory disease processes that they represent, the therapist can apply many of the evaluation and intervention principles to other rheumatic conditions. Table 39.1 provides a quick summary of the contrasting features of OA and RA.[a]

OSTEOARTHRITIS

Osteoarthritis (OA), also referred to as degenerative joint disease, is the most common rheumatic disease and affects approximately 32.5 million people in the United States.[73,94,107] It ranks third among health problems in the developed world.[23] Its prevalence strongly correlates with age. In fact, evidence of characteristic cartilage damage is almost universal in persons older than 65 years.[23] Before the age of 45, men are more likely to have OA; past the age of 45, women predominate.[9,19,94] In addition to age and gender, risk factors include heredity, obesity, anatomic joint abnormality, injury, and occupation leading to overuse of joints.[19] It is interesting to note that because RA may cause malalignment or instability of joints, it often results in premature OA.[35]

OA is classified as primary or secondary. Primary OA has no known cause and may be localized (i.e., involvement of one or two joints) or generalized (i.e., diffuse involvement generally including three or more joints). Secondary OA can be related to an identifiable cause, such as trauma, anatomic abnormalities, infection, or aseptic necrosis.[23,41]

---

[a] References 3, 19, 34, 41, 73, 107, 126, 128, 131.

TABLE 39.1   Primary Features of Osteoarthritis and Rheumatoid Arthritis

	Osteoarthritis	Rheumatoid Arthritis
Prevalence	Affects 32.5 million Americans	Affects 1.5 million Americans
Peak incidence	Increases with age, <45 years old more common in males and >45 years old more common in females	Ages 40–60, 3:1 female-to-male ratio
Onset	Usually develops slowly over period of years	Usually develops suddenly, within weeks or months
Systemic features	None	Fever, fatigue, malaise, extraarticular manifestations
Disease process	Noninflammatory, characterized by cartilage destruction	Inflammatory, characterized by synovitis
Joint involvement	Individual	Polyarticular, symmetric
Joints commonly affected	Neck, spine, hips, knees, MTPs, DIPs, PIPs, thumb CMCs	Neck, jaw, hips, knees, ankles, MTPs, shoulders, elbows, wrists, PIPs, MCPs, thumb joints
Morning stiffness	<30 minutes	At least 1 hour, often >2 hours

CMC, Carpometacarpal; *DIP,* distal interphalangeal; *MCP,* metacarpophalangeal; *MTP,* metatarsophalangeal; *PIP,* proximal interphalangeal.

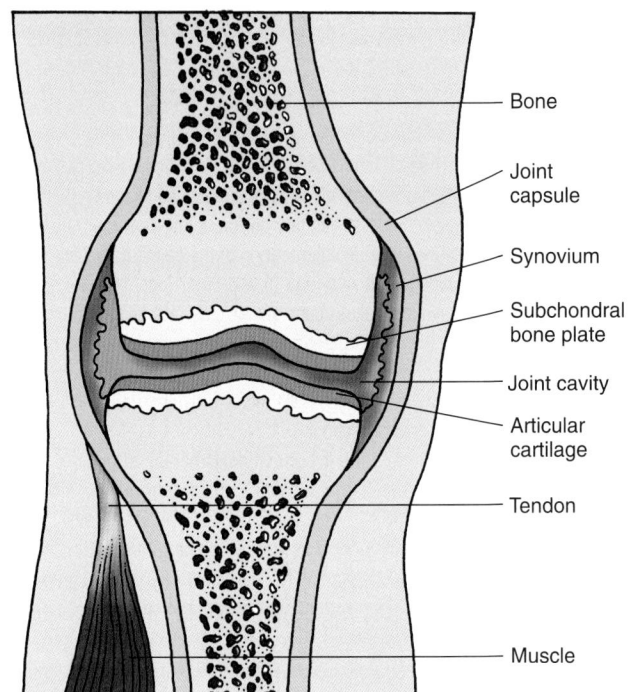

Fig. 39.1 Normal joint structures. (From Ignatavicius DD, et al: *Medical-surgical nursing: concepts for interprofessional collaborative care,* ed 10, St. Louis, 2021, Elsevier.)

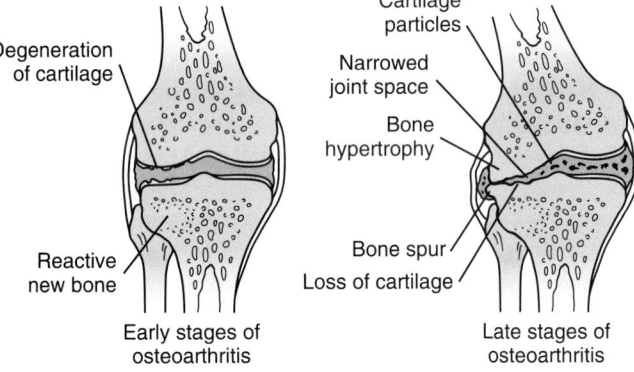

Fig. 39.2 Joint changes in osteoarthritis. (From Magee DJ, et al, editors: *Pathology and intervention in musculoskeletal rehabilitation,* ed 2, St. Louis, 2016, Elsevier.)

OA is a disease that causes the cartilage in joints to break down, with resultant joint pain and stiffness. Unlike RA, which is **systemic** (affecting the entire body), OA limits its attack to individual joints. Also in contrast to RA, the basic process of OA is noninflammatory, although secondary inflammation caused by joint damage is common. Once considered simply "wear and tear" arthritis, OA is now thought to involve more than just the passive deterioration of cartilage. The agent that initiates OA is not well understood, but it is known to involve a complex dynamic process of biomechanical, biochemical, and cellular events.[73] These are affected by local, systemic, genetic, environmental, and mechanical factors, which directly or indirectly influence the vulnerability of cartilage.[19] It is, in essence, the "final common pathway" for a variety of conditions.[23]

A healthy joint is lined by articular cartilage that is relatively thin, highly durable, and designed to distribute loads and limit stress on subchondral bone (Fig. 39.1).[23] OA destabilizes the normal balance of degradation and synthesis of articular cartilage and subchondral bone and involves all of the tissues of a diarthrodial (i.e., synovial-lined) joint.[19,23] OA is basically a two-part process: deterioration of articular cartilage and reactive new bone formation.[87] This breakdown of joint tissue occurs in several stages. First, the smooth cartilage softens and loses its elasticity, which makes it more susceptible to further damage. Eventually, large sections of the cartilage wear away completely and result in reduced joint space and painful bone-on-bone contact. The ends of the bone thicken, osteophytes (bony growths) are formed where ligaments and capsule attach to bone, and the joint may lose its normal shape (Fig. 39.2). Fluid-filled cysts may form in the bone near the joint, and bone or cartilage particles may float loose in the joint space.[3,85]

Clinical Features

OA is characterized by joint pain, stiffness, tenderness, limited movement, variable degrees of local inflammation, and **crepitus** (an audible or palpable crunching or popping in the joint caused by the irregularity of opposing cartilage surfaces).[41,64]

TABLE 39.2 Common Arthritis Medications and Side Effects

Class	Medication	Possible Side Effects
Analgesics		
Nonopioid	Excedrin, Tylenol	Usually none if taken as prescribed
Opioid	Norco, Tylenol with codeine, Vicodin	Constipation, dizziness or lightheadedness, drowsiness, mood changes, nausea, vomiting, drug tolerance, and physical dependence with long-term use
Nonsteroidal Antiinflammatory Drugs (NSAIDs)		
Traditional	Advil, Aleve, Feldene, Indocin, Motrin, Naprosyn, Voltaren	Abdominal pain, dizziness, drowsiness, gastric ulcers and bleeding, greater susceptibility to bruising or bleeding, heartburn, indigestion, lightheadedness, nausea, tinnitus, kidney and liver effects
COX-2 inhibitors	Celebrex	Same as traditional NSAIDs, except less likely to cause gastric ulcers and susceptibility to bruising or bleeding; black box warning for increased risk for heart attack and stroke
Salicylates	Anacin, Bayer, Bufferin, Ecotrin	Abdominal cramps, diarrhea, gastric ulcers, headache, heartburn, increased bleeding tendency, confusion, dizziness, tinnitus, nausea, vomiting, deafness
Corticosteroids	Cortisone, methylprednisolone, prednisone	Cushing's syndrome (weight gain, moon face, thin skin, muscle weakness, osteoporosis), bruising, cataracts, hypertension, elevated blood glucose, insomnia, mood changes, nervousness or restlessness; black box warning for increased risk for cardiovascular problems and gastric bleeding
Disease-Modifying Antirheumatic Drugs (DMARDs)	Imuran	Immunosuppression
	Methotrexate	Liver and blood effects, decreased fertility
	Plaquenil	Visual damage with long-term use
Biological Response Modifiers (Subset of DMARDs)	Enbrel	Dizziness, fatigue, headache, injection site irritation, nausea; black box warning for increased risk for serious infection
	Humira	Injection site irritation; black box warning for increased risk for serious infection
	Remicade	Infusion reaction, injection site irritation; black box warning for increased risk for serious infection

COX, Cyclooxygenase.

It can affect both axial and peripheral joints. The most common joints are the distal interphalangeal (DIP), proximal interphalangeal (PIP) joints, and first carpometacarpal (CMC) joints of the hand; the cervical and lumbar apophyseal joints; the first metatarsophalangeal (MTP) joints of the feet; and the knee and hip joints.[41,73] Symptoms are usually gradual and may begin as a minor ache with motion. Pain and stiffness typically occur with activity and are relieved by rest, but eventually they become present at rest and at night. Morning stiffness (lasting less than 30 minutes) and stiffness after periods of inactivity (known as gelling) may develop. With advanced disease, patients may complain of the "bony" appearance of their joint, which is a result of osteophyte formation and possibly muscle atrophy.[41,73]

Diagnostic Criteria

The diagnosis of OA is initially made on the basis of the patient's history and physical examination, with a lack of systemic symptoms ruling out inflammatory disorders such as RA. The cardinal symptoms are use-related pain and stiffness or gelling after inactivity. The clinical diagnosis is typically confirmed with radiographs of the affected joint, which will show osteophyte formation at the joint margin, asymmetric joint space narrowing, and subchondral bone sclerosis.[41] Magnetic resonance imaging (MRI) may be used to improve diagnostic imaging; MRI is able to detect loss of cartilage, osteophytes, and subchondral cysts more sensitively.

Medical Management

OA currently has no cure. Goals in the treatment of OA are to relieve symptoms, improve function, limit disability, and avoid drug toxicity.[73,110] Pharmacological treatment may be systemic or local. Commonly prescribed systemic medications include analgesic agents and antiinflammatory agents (Table 39.2).[6] Analgesic agents provide relief to painful joints and may be nonnarcotic (nonopioid) or narcotic (opioid) for advanced and severe OA that fails to respond to other measures. Antiinflammatory agents relieve pain, with the added benefit of decreasing local joint inflammation. Because of the risk for gastrointestinal and renal toxicity, these drugs are typically used when analgesics are ineffective. Nonsteroidal antiinflammatory drugs (NSAIDs) and cyclooxygenase-2 (COX-2) inhibitors fall into this category. Although proved effective in treating OA, NSAIDs must be chosen and monitored carefully to minimize potentially serious side effects. COX-2 inhibitors provide clinical benefits similar to NSAIDs but with a lower incidence of gastric problems; however, they carry a black box warning because of links with an increased risk for heart attack and stroke.[6] Local pharmacological treatment of OA includes topical agents and intraarticular corticosteroid injections, alone or as an adjunct to systemic medications. Among topical agents are aspirin and capsaicin creams, as well as the first topical NSAID approved for treating OA pain (Voltaren gel).[6] Cortisone injections in a joint are often limited to fewer than three per year because of the possible risk for progressive cartilage damage.[28]

Use of nonpharmacological agents, also known as nutraceuticals, is extremely common in persons with OA as alternative or complementary treatments and continues to gain favor in the general public.[7,71,73,110] These agents include nutritional supplements such as glucosamine sulfate and chondroitin sulfate. Although they may have some effect in improving symptoms or slowing the progression of OA, studies citing their efficacy have not yet been of optimal quality.[73] However, even if their benefits have not been proved convincingly, use of nutraceuticals typically carries little risk. Even so, patients should be aware that supplements are not regulated like prescription medications. Use of complementary and alternative treatments should be discussed with one's physician to minimize potential negative effects.[71]

Surgical Management

Operative intervention may be performed to slow joint deterioration, improve joint integrity, restore joint stability, or reduce pain, with the overarching goal of improving the patient's overall function. Common surgical procedures for OA include arthroscopic joint debridement, resection or perforation of subchondral bone to stimulate the formation of cartilaginous tissue, use of grafts to replace damaged cartilage, joint fusion, and joint replacement.[28,73]

RHEUMATOID ARTHRITIS

Rheumatoid arthritis (RA) is a chronic, systemic inflammatory condition that affects approximately 1.5 million Americans.[16,107] The cause of RA is not well understood, other than that a yet-unknown trigger causes an autoimmune inflammatory response in the joint lining of a genetically predisposed host.[128,131] Onset can take place at any age, but prevalence does increase with age. The peak incidence occurs between 40 and 60 years of age, with the rate of disease two to three times higher in females.[4,126,131] Its onset is commonly insidious, with symptoms developing over a period of several weeks to several months.

The disease manifests itself as synovitis, which is inflammation of the synovial membrane that lines the joint capsule of diarthrodial joints. The function of normal synovial tissue is to secrete a clear fluid into the joint for the purpose of lubrication.[2,35,36] In RA, synovial cells produce matrix-degrading enzymes that destroy cartilage and bone. Joint swelling results from excessive production of synovial fluid, enlargement of the synovium, and thickening of the joint capsule. This weakens the joint capsule and distends tendons and ligaments. As the inflammatory process continues, the diseased synovial membrane forms a pannus that actively invades and destroys cartilage, bone, tendon, and ligament[36] (Fig. 39.3). Scar tissue can form between the bone ends and cause the joint to become permanently rigid and immovable.

Articular manifestations of RA fall into two categories: (1) reversible signs and symptoms related to acute inflammatory synovitis and (2) irreversible cumulative structural damage caused by recurrent synovitis over the course of the disease. Structural damage typically begins between the first and second years of the disease and progresses as a linear function of the amount of prior synovitis.[49,126] Almost 90% of joints ultimately affected by RA become involved during the first year.[104,126] Progressive joint damage in the majority of patients results in significant disability within 10 to 20 years.[128]

The course of RA is variable from person to person. Approximately 20% of those affected have a single episode of inflammation with a long-lasting remission. The majority of people with RA experience a series of exacerbations and remissions, with periodic flares of inflammation followed by complete or incomplete remissions.[126,131] Outcomes are similarly variable. Patients' functional abilities vary according to the course of the disease, the severity of the symptoms, and the amount of joint damage. Because RA is a systemic disease, certain extraarticular features occur in about half of patients.[126,131] These features include fatigue, rheumatoid nodules, and vasculitis. Ocular, respiratory, cardiac, gastrointestinal, renal, and neurological manifestations are also seen as secondary complications. Patients with severe forms of RA may die between 10 and 15 years earlier than expected as a result of accompanying infection, pulmonary and renal disease, gastrointestinal bleeding, and especially cardiovascular disease.[92]

Clinical Features

RA is characterized by symmetric polyarticular pain and swelling, prolonged morning stiffness, malaise, fatigue, and low-grade fever. Joints most commonly affected are the PIP, MCP, and thumb joints of the hands, as well as the wrist, elbow, ankle, MTP, and temporomandibular joints; the hips, knees, shoulders, and cervical spine are also frequently involved.[126,128] Even though joint involvement is bilateral, disease progression may not be equal on both sides. For instance, a patient's dominant hand may show more severe involvement and different joint changes or deformities than the other hand. Clinical features vary from patient to patient and also in individual patients over the course of their disease. Pain can be acute or chronic. Acute pain occurs during disease exacerbations, or flare-ups. Chronic pain results from progressive joint damage. Synovial inflammation is manifested as warm, spongy, and sometimes erythematous, or red, joints. This is seen in active phases of the disease process. Rheumatoid nodules, a cutaneous manifestation of RA, develop in 25% to 30% of persons with RA during periods

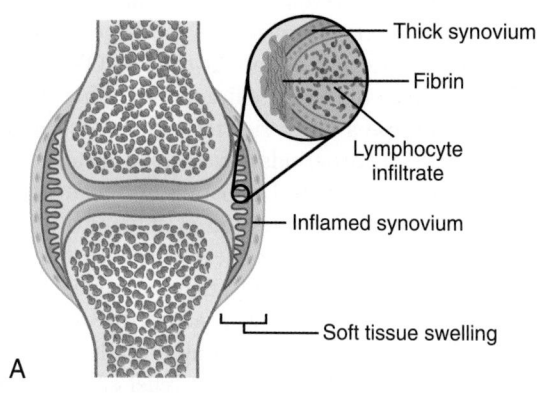

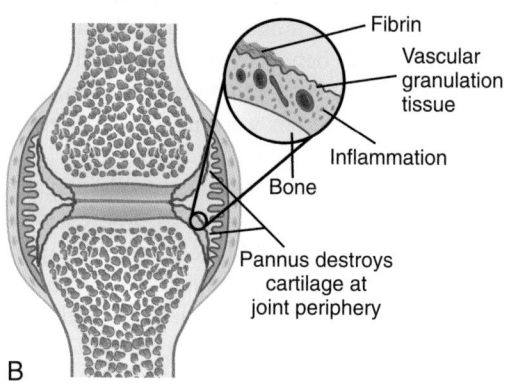

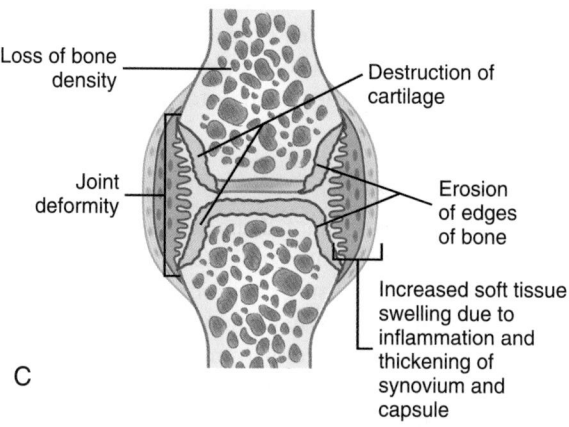

Fig. 39.3 Joint changes in patients with rheumatoid arthritis. A, Early pathological change is rheumatoid synovitis. Synovium becomes inflamed. Lymphocytes and plasma cells increase. B, Over time, articular cartilage destruction occurs, and vascular granulation tissue grows across the cartilage surface (pannus) from the edges of the joint. Joint surface shows loss of cartilage beneath the extending pannus, most marked at joint margins. C, Inflammatory pannus causes focal destruction of bone. Osteolytic destruction of bone occurs at joint edges, causing erosions seen on x-ray films. This phase is associated with joint deformity. (From Harding MM, Kwong J, Hagler D, et al: *Lewis's medical-surgical nursing*, ed 12, St. Louis, 2023, Elsevier.)

of increased disease activity. These soft tissue masses are commonly found over the extensor surface of the proximal end of the ulna or at the olecranon.[126,128] Morning stiffness is an almost universal feature of RA. Unlike the shorter-duration stiffness

seen with OA, RA morning stiffness can last 1 or 2 hours. It frequently disappears during periods of disease remission. The duration of morning stiffness tends to correlate with the degree of synovial inflammation, and its presence and length are useful measures for monitoring the course of RA.[92] Feelings of malaise, fatigue, and depression also fluctuate, with many patients experiencing worse symptoms in the afternoon. These nonspecific symptoms may precede other typical signs of RA by weeks or months.[126]

The inflammatory process has been described as having four stages: acute, subacute, chronic active, and chronic inactive.[85] Stages may overlap, and patients may move back or forward through them, depending on the course of their disease. Clinical symptoms seen in the acute stage include limited movement; pain and tenderness at rest that increase with movement; overall stiffness, weakness, tingling, or numbness; and hot, red joints. In the subacute stage, the limited movement and tingling remain. A decrease in pain and tenderness indicates that the inflammation is subsiding. Stiffness is limited to the morning, and the joints appear pink and warm. The chronic active stage is characterized by less tingling, pain, and tenderness and increased tolerance of activity, although endurance remains low. No signs of inflammation are present in the chronic inactive stage. The patient's low endurance and pain and stiffness at this stage result from disuse. Overall functioning may be decreased as a result of fear of pain, limited range of motion (ROM), muscle atrophy, and contractures.[85]

The characteristic joint deformities will develop as late manifestations of the disease in more than 33% of patients with RA. Deformity of the small joints of the hand will develop within the first 2 years in more than 10%.[128] Wrist radial deviation, MCP ulnar deviation, and swan neck and boutonnière deformities of the digits are the joint changes most often seen. Joint changes, or deformities, can result from a variety of mechanisms, including joint immobility, destruction of cartilage and bone, and alterations in muscles, tendons, and ligaments.[113] Tenosynovitis (inflammation of the tendon sheath) and the presence of nodules within the flexor tendon sheaths can cause trigger finger. Patients may also exhibit symptoms of nerve compression of the median or ulnar nerves at the wrist. Tendon rupture also may be seen, usually in the extensor tendons of the fifth, fourth, and third digits.[10] Stages of the disease based on joint deformity and radiographic changes are defined in Box 39.1.

Diagnostic Criteria

No single test leads to a definitive diagnosis of RA. Diagnosis is based on clinical evaluation of characteristic signs and symptoms, laboratory findings, and radiological findings.[92,126,128] A positive laboratory test is not necessary to establish a diagnosis of RA, but such tests may help confirm the clinical impression. Rheumatoid factor is an antibody found in the blood serum of approximately 85% of persons with RA, but it can also be found in other inflammatory diseases associated with synovitis. The presence of rheumatoid factor correlates with increased severity of symptoms and increased systemic manifestations. The erythrocyte sedimentation rate correlates with the degree of synovial inflammation and is useful in ruling out noninflammatory

BOX 39.1   American College of Rheumatology Classification of Progression of Rheumatoid Arthritis

Stage I: Early
No destructive changes on radiographic examination*
Possible presence of radiographic evidence of osteoporosis

Stage II: Moderate
Radiographic evidence of osteoporosis, with or without slight subchondral bone destruction; possible presence of slight cartilage destruction*
No joint deformities, although possible limitation of joint mobility*
Adjacent muscle atrophy
Possible presence of extraarticular soft tissue lesions, such as nodules and tenosynovitis

Stage III: Severe
Radiographic evidence of cartilage and bone destruction, in addition to osteoporosis*
Joint deformity, such as subluxation, ulnar deviation, or hyperextension, without fibrous or bony ankylosis*
Extensive muscle atrophy
Possible presence of extraarticular soft tissue lesions, such as nodules and tenosynovitis

Stage IV: Terminal
Fibrous or bony ankylosis*
Criteria for stage III

*These criteria must be present to permit classification in any particular stage or grade.
Data from Steinbrocker O, Traeger CH, Batterman RC: Therapeutic criteria in rheumatoid arthritis, *JAMA* 140:659, 1949.

conditions such as OA and tracking the course of inflammatory activity.[126,128] Radiographs (x-rays) may show nothing other than soft tissue swelling early in RA, but in more than half of patients radiographic changes will develop within the first 2 years after onset of the disease.[92,126,128]

Medical Management

RA currently has no known cure. The major goals in the treatment of RA are (1) reducing pain, swelling, and fatigue; (2) improving joint function and minimizing joint damage and deformity; (3) preventing disability and disease-related morbidity; and (4) maintaining physical, social, and emotional function while minimizing long-term toxicity from medications.[93,128] Maintaining normal joint anatomy can be accomplished only by controlling the disease before irreversible damage occurs. Major advances in the treatment of RA have occurred as a result of improved understanding of the pathogenetic mechanisms of the disease, development of therapies that more specifically target the pathophysiological processes, and recognition that early initiation of aggressive drug therapies can alter the outcome and reduce the severity of physical disability and psychological distress of RA.[93,95,128]

Drug categories used for RA include NSAIDs, corticosteroids, and disease-modifying antirheumatic drugs (DMARDs; see Table 39.2).[6] Because the fast-acting NSAIDs can decrease joint pain and swelling but cannot alter progression of the

disease, they are rarely, if ever, used alone for the treatment of RA. The antiinflammatory effects of the large number of medications in this category are about equal. COX-2 inhibitors show no evidence of greater efficacy than other NSAIDs but are thought to pose a lower risk for serious gastrointestinal side effects.[126] Corticosteroids have a long history in the medical management of RA and remain a key element. They produce rapid and potent suppression of inflammation with improvement in joint pain and fatigue. Because of the significant adverse effects of corticosteroids, they are frequently used on a temporary basis in patients with active disease and significant functional decline while awaiting the full therapeutic effect of DMARDs. DMARDs lack a pain relief effect, but they may actually affect the course of the disease. Because of their slow-acting nature, weeks or months of drug therapy may be necessary before a clinical benefit is recognized. The potency of these drugs requires that patients be closely monitored for side effects; they carry a black box warning for increased risk of serious infection.

Traditionally, the approach to treatment of RA began with less toxic medications such as NSAIDs and progressed to the stronger drugs needed later in the disease course. The approach is now more aggressive, with early use of DMARDs to control the disease process as soon as possible, as completely as possible, and for as long as possible.[92,138] Drug therapy constantly changes, depending on the patient's needs and response to treatment, as well as the physician's treatment philosophy. This uncertainty can be frustrating for the patient, who may have to experiment with myriad new medications when current drugs become ineffective or side effects too severe. It is important for the occupational therapist and other team members to know the specific medications that the patient is taking and what adverse reactions may arise.

Surgical Management

Because of the extensive joint damage caused by RA, surgical intervention is frequently indicated to relieve pain and improve function. Several surgical procedures may be of benefit to patients with RA. Synovectomy (excision of diseased synovium) and tenosynovectomy (removal of diseased tendon sheaths) are performed to relieve symptoms and slow the process of joint destruction, but they do not prevent progression of the disease. These procedures are most commonly performed in the wrist and hand. Tendon surgery, including relocation of displaced tendons, repair of ruptured tendons, and release of shortened tendons may be performed to correct hand impairments. Tendon surgery occurs most frequently on the extensor tendons of the wrist and hand. Tendon transfers and peripheral nerve decompression (e.g., carpal tunnel release) are also performed to optimize function. Arthroplasty (joint reconstruction) and arthrodesis (joint fusion) are options when joint restoration is not possible. These procedures may be performed to relieve pain, provide stability, correct deformity, and improve function. Common sites for arthroplasty include the hip, knee, and MCP joints. Common sites for arthrodesis include the wrist, thumb, MCP, and IP joints and cervical spine.[28,85]

OCCUPATIONAL THERAPY EVALUATION

It is important to recognize that every client with arthritis has a unique manifestation of clinical problems and functional impairment. A strong client-centered and occupation-based approach is helpful in determining each client's specific needs. The evaluation process for clients with arthritis includes many of the same elements as for any physical disability. Special considerations related to arthritis include closer attention to pain, joint stiffness, joint changes/deformity, fatigue, and coping strategies, especially as they relate to limitations in activity. Because clients with arthritis typically experience good days and bad days, many symptoms and problems are unpredictable. Thorough systematic assessment of the client's functional, clinical, and psychosocial status is key to prioritizing problems and planning effective intervention.

The extent of specific components of the evaluation often will be driven by the main reason for referral. For example, clients seen for preoperative hand assessment, postoperative hip replacement, education after diagnosis, splinting while in a flare-up, or a decline in functional status will all require the therapist to customize evaluation priorities.

Because of the chronic nature of rheumatic diseases, some clients are able to clearly state their specific needs and should be afforded the opportunity to do so. Other clients may be overwhelmed by multiple problems or a newly made diagnosis and will look to the therapist to guide the intervention process. Regardless of the client's status, close collaboration and partnership among the client, family, therapist, and other team members is crucial in helping deliver the best treatment possible.

The occupational therapy (OT) evaluation process consists of (1) a client history; (2) occupational profile; (3) occupational performance status; (4) cognitive, psychological, and social status; and (5) clinical status.

Client History

A thorough history should be obtained through review of the client's report and medical record. Important details include diagnosis, dates of onset and diagnosis, secondary medical conditions, current medications and medication schedule, alternative or complementary therapies, and surgical history.[115] Asking the client questions such as—"What type of arthritis do you have?" "How long have you had it?" "What medications are you currently taking?" "What other things are you doing to manage your arthritis?" "Are you experiencing pain?" "How are you managing pain and what is a tolerable level of pain for you?"—can provide insight regarding the client's level of understanding about his or her condition, medical treatment, and health habits. Therapists should also ascertain if patients have had previous OT and/or physical therapy (PT) programs to build on those experiences. The therapist must ask and actively listen to the client's current primary complaints through questions: "What is bothering you most about your arthritis?" "How is your arthritis limiting your ability to do things right now?" "What are you hoping therapy can help you with?"

Camilla has some experience with OT from her previous total knee arthroplasty; however, she has limited knowledge about her diagnosis and medications. She is uncertain about the potential benefits of therapy. Through her responses to key questions, Camilla was able to clearly state that addressing her pain and difficulty performing her volunteer, family, and social activities were her main priorities.

Occupational Profile

It is helpful to begin the process of assessing occupational performance with an occupational profile. Obtained through an open-ended interview, the profile yields important details about the client's previous and current roles, occupations, overall activity level, and ability to participate in meaningful activities. It can also provide insight into clients' sense of self-efficacy, adjustment to disability, and themes of meaning in their life.[74,82] An effective method to obtain clients' occupational profile is to have them describe how they spend a typical day. For example, have them describe a typical day(s) from the time they wake up until the time they go to sleep, including their ability to sleep through the night and any physical assistance they may need. This typical-day assessment allows the therapist to become familiar with the client's routines, use of time, sleep/wake habits, energy and fatigue patterns, important people and environments, activity contexts, and other details that may not otherwise come up in conversation. Because arthritis involves fluctuant symptoms, the client should be asked to describe how time is spent on a good day and a bad day so that the therapist can compare the two and understand how arthritis affects the client's daily life and how effectively the client is able to balance activity and rest. It is helpful to ask the client to estimate the percentage of good versus bad days per week or month. It may also be advantageous to explore time spent on weekend days versus weekdays; the client may reveal other occupations, such as those involving spirituality, social participation, and leisure. This fluid dialogue also develops rapport, establishes the client as the valued expert in his or her occupations and lifestyle, and identifies the client's meaningful occupations, thus framing the role of OT in the client's rehabilitation.

Occupational Performance Status

Once the client's typical and preferred occupations are identified, his or her level of independence engaging in these functional activities can be assessed by interview and/or by observation. If observation is used, ideally, the activity should occur as close as possible to the time that it is normally performed because the client's abilities may fluctuate at different times of the day. For instance, stiffness and pain may make dressing very difficult in the early morning, but if this task is assessed in the afternoon, the client's status may appear much better. Ideally, the activity also should be done in the client's own home, community, or work contexts.[11] In addition to assessing the client's level of independence during activities of daily living (ADLs) and instrumental activities of daily living (IADLs) (e.g., school, work, sleep and rest, play, leisure, and social engagements), it is important to note any assistive devices (e.g., mobility aids or adaptive equipment) and compensatory techniques that the client may use. The activity demands of the occupation performed (e.g., tools, equipment, and skills required), as well as the specific contexts in which it is performed (e.g., the client's living situation, others in the home, and architectural set-up relative to occupational performance), should be detailed in tandem with existing physical, environmental, or social barriers. Finally, the amount of time required to complete certain activities should be explored. A client who experiences significant morning stiffness or limited endurance often chooses to accept assistance in an activity such as dressing to save time or conserve energy to participate in a more meaningful occupation later in the day. This strategy may contribute to the client's overall satisfaction with and participation in life, and it should be respected as such.

In RA, functional status may be classified according to the American College of Rheumatology's revised criteria for the classification of functional status in clients with RA (Table 39.3). This system was devised for rapid global assessment of functional status by health professionals.[64] The therapist should be familiar with this system because it is often used in clinical research and can provide a general framework for defining advancing disability.[61,140]

Camilla's status would be considered class III because of limitations in her volunteering and avocational activities.

A decrease in occupational performance in clients with arthritis may be due to pain, joint changes or instability, loss of motion, weakness, fatigue, change in the living environment, or change in social support, among other contributing circumstances. The effects of medication can also limit performance. The challenge for the therapist is not only to identify deficits in occupational performance but also to determine the factors that are causing them. Asking the client why an activity cannot be done yields the important client perspective.[11] Camilla was having difficulty with performing meaningful occupations, including sleeping, attending events (e.g., church and soccer games), caring for her grandchildren, performing volunteer duties and other leisure activities to her level of satisfaction. She reported having to give up or cut back on activities because of increased pain, stiffness, and fatigue from her recent flare-up.

TABLE 39.3　American College of Rheumatology Classification of Global Functional Status in Patients With Rheumatoid Arthritis

Classification	Description
Class I	Completely able to perform usual activities of daily living (self-care,* vocational, and avocational)
Class II	Able to perform usual self-care and vocational activities, but limited in avocational activities
Class III	Able to perform usual self-care activities, but limited in vocational and avocational activities
Class IV	Limited in ability to perform usual self-care, vocational, and avocational activities

*Usual self-care activities include dressing, feeding, bathing, grooming, and toileting. Avocational (recreational or leisure) and vocational (work, school, homemaking) activities are client desired and age and sex specific.
Courtesy American College of Rheumatology ©2004.[52]

Cognitive, Psychological, and Social Status

The effects of arthritis are not merely physical and functional. Clients with arthritis should be screened for cognitive and psychosocial deficits. Although arthritis does not directly affect cognition, pain, sleep disturbances, depression, and medication can all have profound effects on attention span, short-term memory, and problem-solving skills.[85,98] People with a chronic illness must develop coping strategies to deal with the disability. Coping strategies are particularly crucial for persons with arthritis, who may face serious changes in physical function, life roles, and appearance because of deformity and pharmacological side effects. Because arthritis is both unpredictable and painful, normal responses to the disability include depression, denial, need to control the environment, and dependence. Psychosocial adaptation is affected by the complex interplay of physical, psychological, and situational factors.[74,97] Approximately 20% of persons with RA are estimated to suffer from a major depressive disorder, with as high as 48% having significant depression symptoms.[84] A developing theory is that inflammation also plays a role in depression. Those with symptoms of depression had levels of C-reactive protein, a marker of inflammation, that were 31% higher than those with no depressive symptoms.[8]

About half of individuals with RA or OA may experience loss of social relationships.[139] Constant pain and fear of pain, changed body image, perception of self as a sick person, continuous uncertainty about the course and progression of the disease, sexual dysfunction, altered roles, and loss of income resulting from inability to work can lead to significant psychological stress.[74,97] Evidence has shown that the disability associated with RA relates to psychosocial factors almost to the same extent as to biomedical factors.[46] Occupational therapists must understand the ways in which their clients manage stress in their lives because these stressors may exacerbate the disease.[74] Family relationships and cultural backgrounds also affect the client's healthcare behavior and response to disability.[103] The therapist should be sensitive to all factors that will influence rehabilitation. Referral to other health professionals (e.g., psychiatrists, psychologists, and social workers) should be made if needed.[97]

Camilla reported that at times she had difficulty concentrating on tasks because she was unable to get adequate restful sleep. She expressed frustration about her inability to fully participate in the activities that she enjoys, as well as anxiety about losing function, social interactions, and a sense of belonging and feeling needed. She was also fearful about her health because her arthritis had been adequately controlled for the past few years and she had not experienced any flares.

Clinical Status

For clients with arthritis, the elements of inflammation, ROM, strength, hand function, stiffness, pain, sensation, joint instability and deformity, physical endurance, and functional mobility should be included through either brief screening or detailed evaluation. As with assessment of function, the time of day and antiinflammatory or analgesic medications taken should be noted because these factors may influence the results. In addition, future reevaluations should be performed under the same conditions.[85] When the client's functional deficits are identified first, assessment of client factors can be much more focused. Additionally, asking the client a question such as "What joints are you having the most problems with?" can help prioritize assessment needs. Given Camilla's initial findings, the detailed evaluation focused primarily on synovitis, pain, stiffness, ROM, strength, physical endurance, and functional mobility. Because Camilla already has significant joint deformities, the focus was on protecting her joints and slowing the progression of deformity. The therapist was careful to search for signs of joint instability that would place Camilla at risk for additional deformity. The clinical evaluation may take considerable time and should be approached in a systematic manner with the results clearly documented. The occupational therapist may need to perform assessments over several sessions, especially if the client is experiencing significant pain or fatigue. Intervention can begin immediately and does not necessarily depend on completion of the evaluation. The evaluation actually begins with a general observation of the client's posture, willingness to move, and pain behavior during the initial interview.

The presence and location of inflammation or synovitis should be noted because these signs indicate an active disease process. Several types of swelling may be present and should be described. An effusion (excess fluid in the joint capsule) is seen as fusiform swelling that is spindle shaped and conforms to the shape of the joint. Boggy swelling is thin and full of fluid. Puffy, spongy, and soft to the touch, boggy swelling is seen in the early active stages of synovitis. Chronic synovitis feels firm because the joint fills with synovial tissue.[85]

Active and passive ROM can be measured. Depending on the reason for referral and the client's complaints, the therapist may not find it necessary to obtain goniometric measurements of all joints but instead focus only on the joints of most concern. Active motion will allow the therapist to see the amount of mobility that the client has available for function, whereas passive motion will elicit the joint's capacity to move. The client's range of active motion may be significantly less than the range of passive motion; this is known as lag and is caused by pain, weakness, or the mechanical inefficiencies attributable to joint damage. Goniometric measurement of hand joints may be difficult in the presence of deformity. Assessment of composite (combined motion of all joints) flexion, composite extension, and thumb opposition can provide more functional information.[15] Active opening and closing of the hand can be measured by the distance from the fingertips to the tabletop in maximal extension (opening) when the dorsal side of the hand is resting on the table and by the distance from the fingertips to the distal palmar crease (closing). While performing the ROM assessment, the therapist should note whether the client's joints feel stiff or unstable. A hard end-feel in the presence of contracture indicates bony blockage.[87] A firm end-feel that still has some give indicates that the joint capsule or ligaments are limiting motion.[63] The presence and location of crepitus, along with the motions that cause it, should also be noted because crepitus often indicates extensive joint damage. The source of crepitation may be bony, synovial, bursal, or tendinous (see Chapters 20, 21, and 22 for additional information on evaluating clinical status).[15,85]

Gross strength should be assessed with more specific manual muscle testing as indicated. One important detail to understand is that strength testing in clients with arthritis differs from normal testing procedures. Resistance is applied at the end range of pain-free motion rather than at the true end of the ROM. It is not unusual for clients with arthritis to have pain in the last 30 to 40 degrees of joint motion. When resistance is applied within the pain-free range, inhibition of muscle strength by pain will be avoided. It is also important to consider joint protection principles when applying resistance and to discontinue resistance if the client experiences pain. If use of resistance is contraindicated (as may be the case in an acute or active phase of arthritis, in which resistance may be harmful to inflamed tissue and joints), functional muscle or motion testing may be substituted.[85]

Hand strength and function are important to test, but care must be taken to not stress painful or vulnerable joints during assessment. Grip and pinch may be measured by standard meters, but in the presence of severe weakness or hand deformity, adapted methods, such as use of a blood pressure cuff to measure force in millimeters of mercury, may be indicated.[15,85] Although it is more comfortable for the client, the results of strength testing in this manner are less reliable, with no established norms. Other specific devices for measuring grip strength in hands with arthritis, including pneumatic bulb dynamometers, are commercially available. As a result of joint deformity, the client may not be able to assume the standard testing positions for lateral and palmar pinch. Because it is important to assess pinch strength relative to function, pinch should still be tested, with notation made of the client's prehensile pattern (e.g., "4 pounds of pinch with the meter placed in web space between thumb and second metacarpal"). The presence and location of muscle atrophy should be recorded because it indicates severe weakness and possible nerve compression that may require further investigation. Intrinsic atrophy can be seen as flattening of the thenar and hypothenar eminences and as hollowing between the metacarpals on the dorsal aspect of the hand.

Hand function can be assessed through standardized tests (e.g., the Jebsen-Taylor Hand Function Test)[68] or observation of the client performing common functional tasks that involve various grasp and prehensile patterns. These tasks can include opening a medication bottle, writing, holding a glass, using a cell phone, picking up small pins, turning a doorknob and key, cutting with a knife, and fastening buttons. In addition to noting whether the client is able to perform each task, the value of this testing lies in observation of how the client uses his or her hands and determination of which factors interfere most with activity: instability, lack of motion, deformity, pain, weakness, or something else. The therapist cannot predict function solely on the basis of the hand's appearance. Deformities, or joint changes,[b]

---

[b] *Thirty years ago the first editor encountered a client who voiced "horror" and concern when the term "deformities" was used to describe why we were making preventive hand splints. The sadness in his young face convinced his OT that a different term, a less caustic term that was suggested and used by other OTs—joint changes—might be used in its place, which was acceptable to the client. He expressed that hearing the term deformities associated with him was depressing and shocking. The OT has since then tried with some success to draw attention to this issue and uses joint changes whenever possible.*

caused by arthritis often develop slowly, and many clients learn how to adapt their hand function gradually over time. It may be surprising to see significantly deformed hands performing tasks with relatively good function. The therapist should remember this when planning an intervention because it might eliminate a problem that is actually functional for the client.

Joint stiffness is a distinct feeling of excessive stiffness that eventually wears off.[85] It can occur as a result of low-grade inflammation, effusion, synovial thickening, muscle shortening, or spasm.[20,87] The stiffness experience, its impact on daily life, and the adaptations clients need to make greatly vary.[93] The therapist can determine the extent of joint stiffness by asking the client which joints experience stiffness, under what conditions, and for how long. Morning stiffness and gelling should be considered separately and can be measured in hours or minutes. The duration of morning stiffness is often used as an objective indicator of the degree of disease activity present. The gelling phenomenon, that is stiffness after prolonged periods of inactivity, is so named because fluid in the joint and surrounding tissues sets up like gelatin.[87]

Because pain is often the primary clinical manifestation of arthritis, it should be closely evaluated. Pain that interferes with the client's ability to engage in occupations should be of primary concern. The presence and location of joint pain should be noted. The therapist should ask questions to elicit important details ("When does the pain occur?" "What tends to make the pain worse?" "What seems to make the pain better?"). An attempt should be made to distinguish between articular (joint) pain and periarticular (soft tissues surrounding the joint) pain. Secondary conditions such as tendinitis and bursitis are frequent causes of pain. Pain has different meanings for individuals and is often difficult to describe.[116] There are multiple pain scales available that use face, numerical, or other rating methods. For example, a numerical scale enables the therapist to obtain measurements of pain intensity by asking the client to rate the pain on a numeric scale of "1" (no pain) to "10" (greatest pain) or on a visual analogue scale in which the client places a mark along a 10-cm line.[66] These scales can also be used to measure other subjective symptoms, including fatigue and degree of stiffness.[60] Because pain related to arthritis is fluctuant, the client may be asked to rate pain at its current level, at its best, at its worst, and at various times of the day or to compare pain at rest versus pain with motion or activity. Clients may be encouraged to use a pain scale to self-monitor their routine activities. This will allow them to provide more accurate feedback to their primary care provider and take an active role in the management of their pain and arthritis symptoms. Interestingly, pain caused by acute inflammation in the early stages of RA tends to be greater than pain at the end stages, when severe deformities are present.[14] The presence and location of joint tenderness should also be noted. Tenderness is assessed by applying manual compression to the medial/lateral aspects of the joint (see Chapter 28 for additional information).[85]

Sensation should be evaluated if the potential for peripheral nerve damage or compression caused by swelling exists. The therapist should obtain a subjective report from the client with regard to the presence of numbness or tingling. This report can be followed by screening of the touch/pressure threshold of the fingertips with monofilaments.[17] If sensory impairment is noted, further assessment may be indicated. This may include provocative tests to replicate or aggravate symptoms so that areas of compression can be localized. Examples of these tests are the Phalen and Tinel tests in individuals with suspected median nerve compression at the carpal tunnel.[108] When cervical spine involvement is known or suspected, dermatomal light touch, sharp-dull sensation, and proprioception should be evaluated (see Chapters 23 and 40 for additional information).

The examiner assesses joint laxity (instability) by applying stress to individual joints in the medial/lateral and anterior/posterior directions. When testing medial/lateral stability of the MCP joints, the examiner must first place the MCP joints in flexion to tighten the collateral ligaments, which are naturally loose during MCP extension. Unstable joints should be noted. Ligamentous laxity can be described as slight (5–10 degrees in excess of normal), moderate (10–20 degrees in excess), or severe (20 degrees or more in excess).[85] In the hand joints, instability with medial/lateral motion indicates laxity of the collateral ligaments, whereas excessive anterior/posterior motion is caused by laxity of the joint capsule and volar plate. Normal joint stability is highly variable, and whenever possible, it is helpful to compare it to the client's uninvolved joints.[85]

Evaluation of joint deformities is done primarily by observation and palpation. The location and type of deformity should be noted. Comparison with previous evaluations, if available, allows the therapist to see how the deformities have progressed over the course of the disease. If a deformity is correctable, either actively or passively, it is considered flexible; if the deformity cannot be reduced, it is considered fixed. Patterns of deformity can be different in a client's two hands, and a person with RA can also exhibit deformities caused by osteoarthritic joint damage.

Common hand deformities in persons with arthritis include the following:

- A boutonnière deformity is characterized by flexion of the PIP joint and hyperextension of the DIP joint (Fig. 39.4). This zigzag collapse represents an alteration in muscle-tendon balance. Pathological processes begin at the PIP joint with secondary changes in the DIP joint. It occurs when synovitis weakens, lengthens, or disrupts the dorsal capsule and central slip of the extensor mechanism and consequently causes incomplete or weak to absent extension at the PIP joint. The lateral bands of the extensor mechanism displace volarly below the axis of the PIP joint and become flexors of that joint. Increased force on the lateral bands at the DIP joint, where they insert, causes hyperextension. Function of the finger is compromised by the inability to straighten the finger and the loss of flexion at the fingertip for pinching.[2,14,15,85]
- A swan neck deformity is characterized by hyperextension of the PIP joint and flexion of the DIP joint, with possible flexion of the MCP joint (Figs. 39.4 and 39.5). This zigzag collapse is also a result of muscle-tendon imbalance and joint

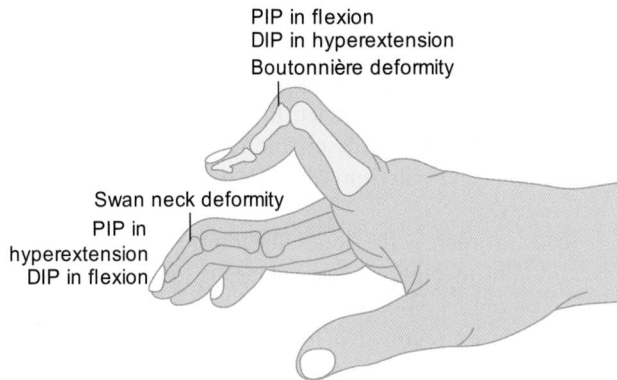

Fig. 39.4 Boutonnière deformity and Swan neck deformity. (From Sud A, Ranjan R: *Textbook of orthopaedics*, ed 2, India, 2022, Elsevier.)

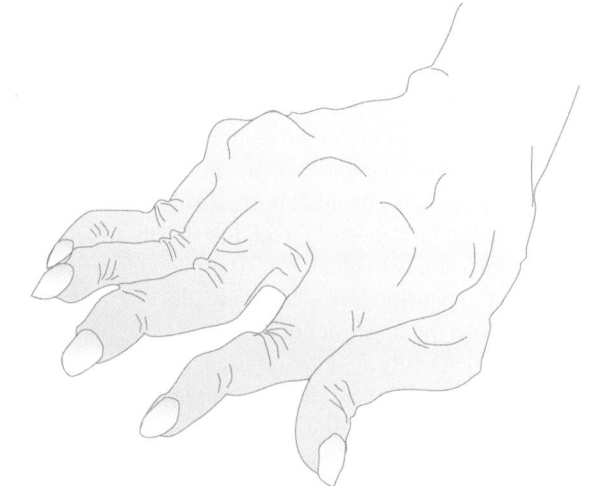

A

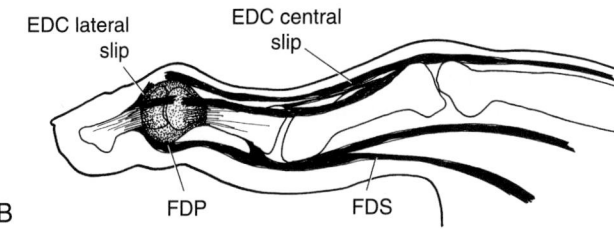

B

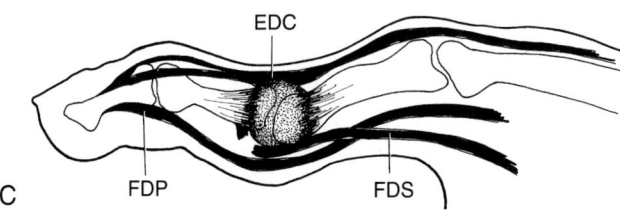

C

Fig. 39.5 (A) Hand displaying swan neck deformity with flexion of the MP joints. (B) Swan neck deformity resulting from rupture of the lateral slips of the extensor digitorum communis tendon. (C) Swan neck deformity as a result of rupture of the flexor digitorum superficialis tendon. (A from Black JM, Hawks JH: *Medical-surgical nursing, clinical management for positive outcomes*, ed 8, Philadelphia, 2009, Saunders.)

laxity. It can originate from abnormalities at any finger joint. Causes of this deformity include intrinsic muscle tightness, stretching or rupture of the terminal extensor tendon at the

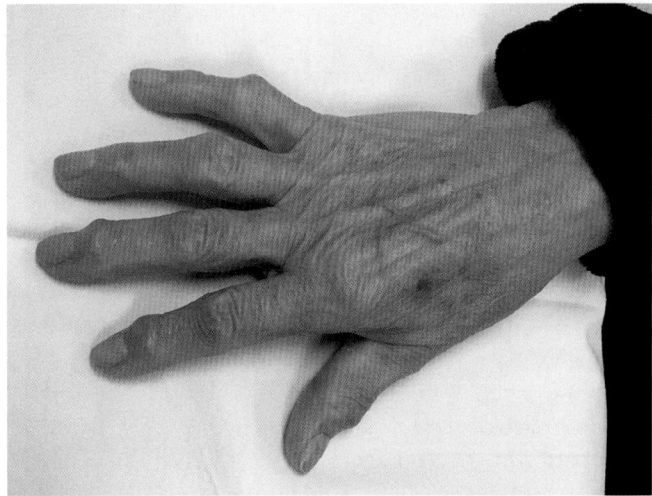

Fig. 39.6 Osteophyte formation in the proximal interphalangeal joints (Bouchard's nodes) and the distal interphalangeal joints (Heberden's nodes) is a common finding with osteoarthritis.

DIP joint, and chronic synovitis that leads to stretching of the volar capsular supporting structures at the PIP joint. Here, the lateral bands of the extensor mechanism slip above the axis of the PIP joint, thereby hyperextending the PIP joint and flexing the DIP joint. Function of the finger is compromised by an inability to flex the PIP joint, with loss of the ability to make a fist or hold small objects.[2,14,15]

- A mallet finger is characterized by flexion of the DIP joint. This is caused by rupture of the terminal extensor tendon as it crosses the DIP joint. The finger loses the ability to extend the distal phalanx.
- **Nodes** are bony enlargements that indicate cartilage damage caused by OA. Joints affected by RA can also have degenerative joint disease, so nodes may be seen in clients with RA as well. These osteophytes are hard to the touch and are typically not painful. They are most commonly seen at the DIP joint (Heberden's nodes) and the PIP joint (Bouchard's nodes; Fig. 39.6).[14,23,85,87]
- Nodules are granulomatous and fibrous soft tissue masses that are sometimes painful. They usually occur along weight-bearing surfaces such as the ulna or at the olecranon (Fig. 39.7) and can be prognostic of the severity of RA.[14]
- Deviation is characterized by a change in the normal joint position. It is typically described as radial or ulnar. In RA the most common pattern of deviation is radial deviation of the wrist and ulnar deviation (commonly referred to as ulnar drift) of the MCP joints (Fig. 39.8). Deviation is caused by ligament weakening or disruption. Small joints are especially vulnerable because daily activities involving gripping and pinching apply strong forces to them.[14,85]
- **Subluxation** is characterized by volar or dorsal displacement of joints. It is any degree of malalignment in which the articular structures are only in partial contact. In RA the most common sites of subluxation are the wrist and MCP joints.[85] Volar subluxation of the wrist occurs as the carpal bones slip relative to the distal end of the radius as a result of weakening of the supporting ligaments by chronic synovitis. Because of

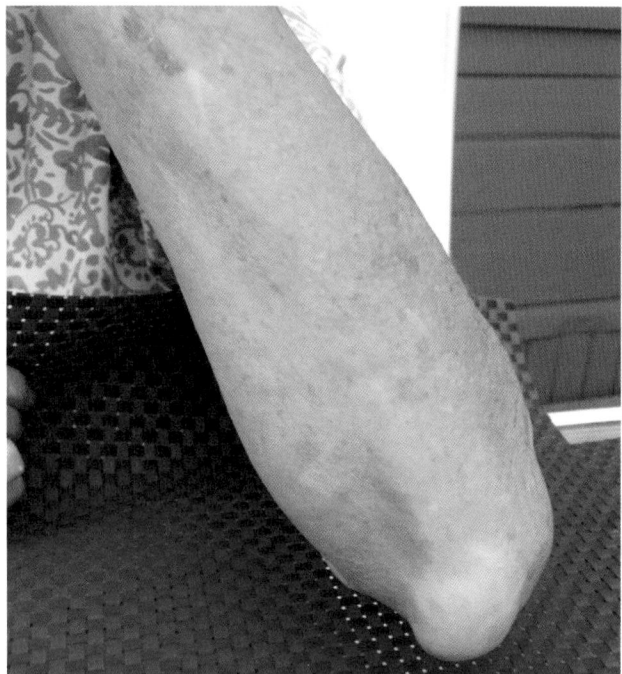

Fig. 39.7 Rheumatoid nodules near the elbow joint. (From Skirven TM, Osterman L, Fedorczyk J, et al: *Rehabilitation of the hand and upper extremity*, ed 7, St. Louis, 2021, Elsevier.)

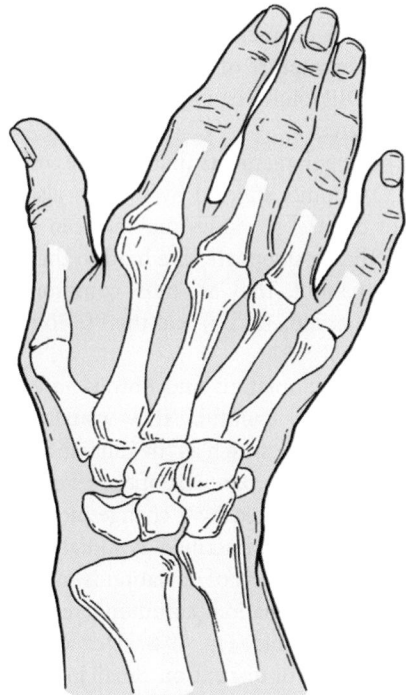

Fig. 39.8 Ulnar drift of the metacarpophalangeal joint. (From Schlenker E, Roth SL: *Williams' essentials of nutrition and diet therapy*, ed 7, St. Louis, 2007, Mosby.)

their condyloid nature, the MCP joints have more planes of movement and are inherently less stable than the IP joints. Volar subluxation of the MCP joints occurs frequently and is often accompanied by ulnar drift and lateral displacement

of the extensor tendons into the ulnar valleys between the metacarpal heads (Fig. 39.9).[2,14,15,85]

- Dislocation is characterized by joints whose articulating surfaces are no longer in contact. In severe cases of RA, volar dislocation of the carpals on the radius or dislocation of other joints can result from complete destruction of ligamentous integrity.[2,85]

- Ankylosis (fusion of the bones of a joint) is characterized by lack of joint mobility. This spontaneous joint fusion can be bony (caused by ossification within or around the joint) or fibrous (caused by growth of fibrous tissue around the joint).[85]

- Extensor tendon rupture is characterized by the inability to actively extend a joint in the absence of muscle weakness (Fig. 39.10). The extensor digiti minimi is often the first to rupture. The extensor pollicis longus and extensor digitorum communis of the third, fourth, and fifth digits are also vulnerable.[2,14] Tendon rupture can occur as a result of rubbing of the tendon over rough bony surfaces or tendon damage caused by direct synovial invasion or increased pressure that decreases blood supply to the tendon.

- Trigger finger is characterized by inconsistent limitation of finger flexion or extension. It is often caused by a nodule on a flexor tendon or stenosis of a tendon sheath, which impedes the tendon's ability to glide.[14,15,85] The client often experiences "catching" or "locking" of a finger into flexion and has to passively extend the finger out of the flexed position.

- Mutilans deformity is characterized by floppy joints with redundant skin (Fig. 39.11). The cause is unknown, but the result is resorption of the bone ends, which shortens the bones and renders the joints completely unstable. This is most commonly seen at the MCP and PIP joints of the hands and the radiocarpal and radioulnar joints of the wrist.[85]

- Thumb deformities can be manifested as any of the deformities previously described. Nalebuff has classified six patterns of thumb deformity (Table 39.4).[127] Type I is the most common in RA, followed by type III, seen in both OA and RA.[85,127] A boutonnière deformity (type I) is characterized by MCP joint flexion and IP joint hyperextension. A swan neck deformity (type III) is characterized by CMC joint subluxation, adduction, and flexion; MCP joint hyperextension; and IP joint flexion. Also common in RA and OA is an adduction contracture of the thumb CMC joint caused by subluxation of the first metacarpal, radial deviation of the MCP joint, or shortening or weakness of intrinsic muscles.[85,127] Subluxation causes a characteristic squared appearance of the CMC joint (Fig. 39.12). Disruption of thumb biomechanics often leads to significant loss of hand function, especially given the fact that the thumb is thought to account for as much as 60% of hand function.[58]

Physical endurance can be evaluated by observation during the assessment process and by client report. Pain, weakness, deconditioning, lack of sleep, and emotional stress can all lead to decreased stamina. The pattern and severity of fatigue should be noted.[115] Functional mobility, including ambulation, sitting and standing tolerances, and ability to transfer, should be assessed relative to occupational performance. It is also important to assess for fall risk, as increased likelihood of falling has been reported in clients with lower extremity arthritis.[42]

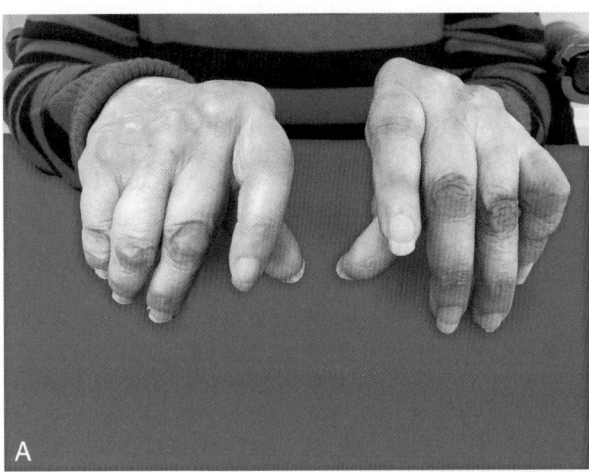 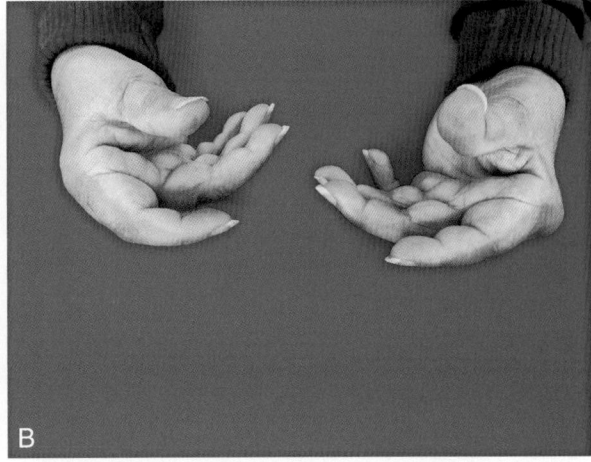

Fig. 39.9 A, Volar subluxation and ulnar deviation of the metacarpophalangeal joints with lateral displacement of the extensor tendons characteristic of rheumatoid arthritis (dorsal view). B, Volar subluxation and ulnar deviation of the metacarpophalangeal joints with lateral displacement of the extensor tendons characteristic of rheumatoid arthritis (volar view). (Courtesy Occupational Therapy Department, Rancho Los Amigos National Rehabilitation Center, Downey California.)

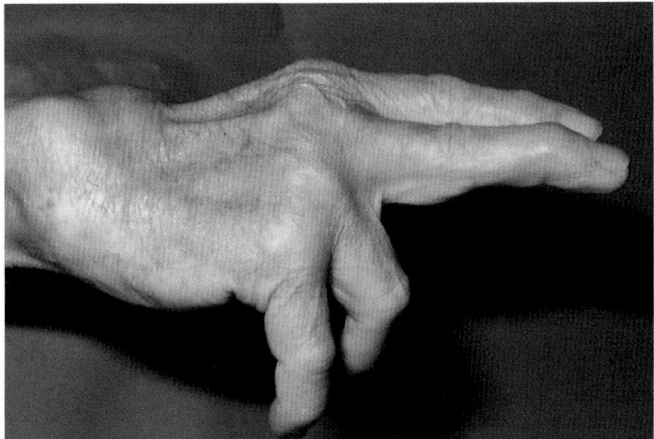

Fig. 39.10 Extensor tendon rupture of the fourth and fifth digits resulting in loss of active extension. Tenosynovitis of the extensor tendons and volar subluxation of the wrist caused by rheumatoid arthritis are contributing factors. (From Evans RC: *Illustrated orthopedic physical assessment,* ed 3, St. Louis, 2009, Mosby.)

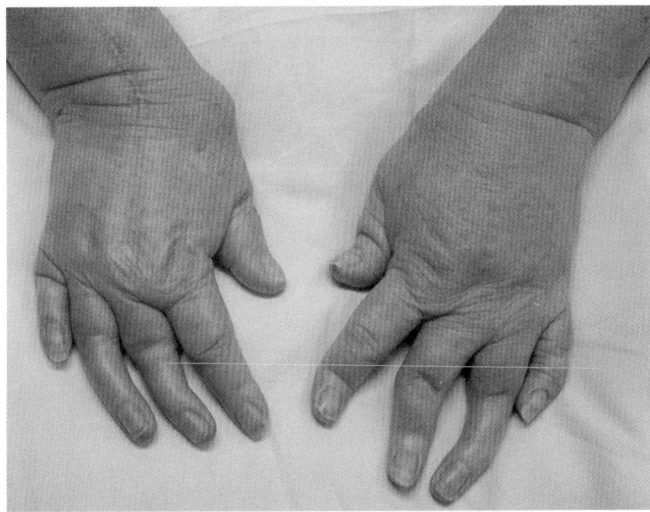

Fig. 39.11 Mutilans deformity. (From Weisman MH, Weinblatt ME, Louie JS: *Targeted treatment of the rheumatic diseases,* Philadelphia, 2010, Saunders.)

GOAL SETTING

The goals of therapy should be determined by careful consideration of the client's stated goals, the client's individual needs, and the stage of the disease process. The Canadian Occupational Performance Measure (COPM) is a useful client-centered tool that can be used for setting goals, planning treatment, and measuring outcomes.[72] It is designed to detect change in a client's self-perception of occupational performance over time. It engages the client in defining problems in activity and helps the client more clearly understand the purpose of OT. The COPM involves a semi-structured interview in which the client is asked to identify occupations that the client needs to, wants to, or is expected to perform but are not done satisfactorily. Occupational goals in the areas of self-care, productivity, and leisure (based on the Canadian Model of Occupational Performance [CMOP]) are listed, and the client is then asked

to rate his or her self-perception of the importance of, current performance of, and satisfaction with performance of each occupation. Through this process of collaboration with the client, occupation-based therapy goals can be identified, priorities determined, and a treatment plan designed to facilitate optimal outcome. The rating process is repeated at time of discharge for outcome purposes. The COPM has been used with people who have arthritis in both inpatient and outpatient settings.[11] COPM goals for Camilla were to return to volunteering, attend church, garden, to take care of her pets, and to attend functions with her grandchildren.

INTERVENTION OBJECTIVES AND PLANNING

Treatment of clients with arthritis must consider the progressive nature of the disease.[35] The overarching goal of therapy is to decrease pain, protect joints, and increase function. General

TABLE 39.4 Rheumatoid Thumb Deformities

Type	CMC Joint	MCP Joint	IP Joint
I (boutonnière)	Not involved	Flexed	Hyperextended
II (uncommon)	CMC flexed and adducted	Flexed	Hyperextended
III (swan neck)	CMC subluxed, flexed, and adducted	Hyperextended	Flexed
IV (gamekeeper's)	CMC not subluxed; flexed and adducted	Hyperextended, ulnar collateral ligament unstable	Not involved
V	May or may not be involved	Volar plate unstable	Not involved
VI (arthritis mutilans)	Bone loss at any level	Bone loss at any level	Bone loss at any level

CMC, Carpometacarpal; *IP,* interphalangeal; *MCP,* metacarpophalangeal.
From Terrono AL, Nalebuff EA, Philips CA: The rheumatoid thumb. In Skirven M, et al, editors: *Rehabilitation of the hand and upper extremity,* ed 6, St. Louis, 2011, Mosby, p 1345.

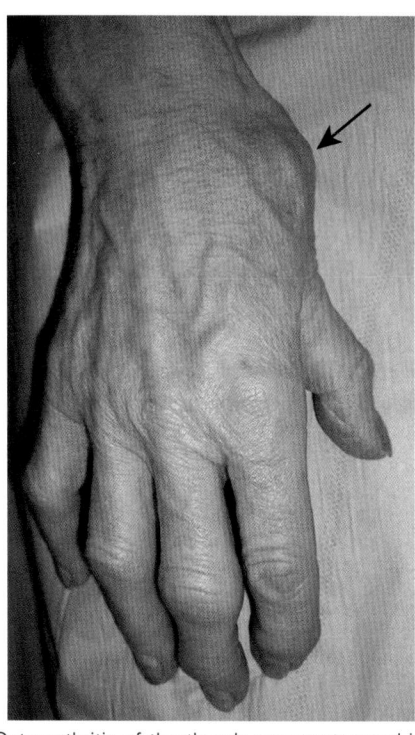

Fig. 39.12 Osteoarthritis of the thumb carpometacarpal joint resulting in squaring and subluxation of the base of the thumb. (From Abhishek A, Doherty M: Diagnosis and clinical presentation of osteoarthritis, *Rheum Dis Clin North Am* 39:45–66, 2013.)

objectives of OT are to (1) maintain or increase the ability to engage in meaningful occupations; (2) maintain or increase joint mobility and strength; (3) maximize physical endurance; (4) protect against or minimize the effect of deformities; (5) increase understanding of the disease and the best methods of dealing with its physical, functional, and psychosocial effects; and (6) assist with adjustment to disability.[85]

The intervention plan should be designed for the individual client and based on the stage of disease, the severity of symptoms, general health status, lifestyle, and mutually agreed goals. Given the limited time for therapy, prioritizing treatment is essential. The therapist should focus on addressing the most important factors by answering the following question: "What are the essential interventions necessary to enable the client to function at an optimal level?" It is important for the client and significant others to be active participants throughout therapy. Everyone involved must understand the disease process and the rationale for the intervention methods. Because therapy intervention will most likely be intermittent throughout the client's course of disease, the client's ability to follow through with and self-manage interventions at home will greatly influence the ultimate success of treatment.

Table 39.5 outlines some common symptoms, general objectives, and OT interventions typically appropriate for each stage of inflammatory disease; it can be used as a starting point for planning treatment.[14,85] Camilla was in the subacute stage of her RA flare-up. All six general objectives listed previously were important to address in her OT program.

OT PRACTICE NOTES

As always, the occupational therapist's clinical judgment of each client's unique status is crucial for tailoring programs appropriately.

TREATMENT METHODS

Treatment methods useful in the remediation of clinical or functional problems include rest, physical agent modalities (PAMs), therapeutic exercise and activity, splinting, occupational performance training, and client education. It is important to foster clients' self-efficacy in their ability to follow through with treatment at home, given the influences of the home contexts, because building the client's confidence will probably lead to the desired behavior. Asking the client a question such as "How certain are you that you can perform this activity at home as well as you did in the clinic?" can provide feedback on the need for further training and practice.[77] The interventions chosen should reflect the individual client's needs and choices whenever appropriate. General treatment precautions related to arthritis are listed in Box 39.2.

Sleep and Rest

Rest should be considered an active means of reducing inflammation and pain. Rest and relaxation can effectively break the vicious cycle of pain, stress, and depression by allowing the body time to heal itself. Rest can be either systemic (whole body sleep) or local (resting individual affected joints). Whole-body general rest, including recuperative sleep, is necessary for health. However, individuals with arthritis are at risk for sleep problems because of pain and depression.[53,67,113] During periods of active systemic inflammatory disease, at least 8 to 10 hours of sleep at night and half-hour to 1-hour morning and

TABLE 39.5   Treatment Objectives by Stage of Inflammatory Disease

Stage	Symptoms	Objectives	Treatment Considerations
I. Acute	Pain; inflammation; hot, red joints; tenderness; overall stiffness; limited motion	Decrease pain and inflammation	Splinting for localized rest day and night, increased bedrest, joint protection, assistive devices, physical agent modalities
		Maintain ROM	Gentle active ROM or passive ROM to point of pain (no stretch), proper positioning
		Maintain strength and endurance	Functional activities to tolerance, isometric exercises
II. Subacute	Inflammation subsiding; warm, pink joints; decreased pain and tenderness; stiffness limited to the morning	Decrease pain and inflammation	Less restrictive splinting during the day, splinting continued at night, joint protection, assistive devices, physical agent modalities
		Maintain ROM	Active ROM or passive ROM with gentle stretch, proper positioning
		Maintain strength and endurance	Increased functional activities to tolerance, isometric exercises
III. Chronic active	Minimal inflammation, less pain and tenderness, increased activity tolerance, low endurance	Decrease pain and inflammation	Joint protection, splinting as needed, assistive devices as needed, physical agent modalities as needed
		Increase ROM	Active ROM or passive ROM with stretch at end range
		Increase strength and endurance	Resistive exercises (isometric or isotonic if no risk of overstressing joints), cardiovascular exercises, increased functional activities
IV. Chronic inactive	No inflammation, pain and stiffness from disuse, low endurance	Decrease pain	Joint protection, splinting as needed, assistive devices as needed, physical agent modalities as needed
		Increase or maintain ROM	Active ROM or passive ROM with stretch at end range
		Increase strength and endurance	Resistive exercises (isometric or isotonic if no risk of overstressing joints), cardiovascular exercises, increased functional activities

---

BOX 39.2   Treatment Precautions Related to Arthritis

Respect pain.
Avoid fatigue.
Avoid placing stress on inflamed or unstable joints.
Use resistive exercise or activity with caution.
Be aware of sensory impairments.
Be cautious with fragile skin resulting from systemic disease or pharmacological side effects.

---

afternoon rest periods are recommended.[18,115] The amount of systemic rest needed varies by individual, from complete bedrest to an extra nap during the day. Localized rest of joints with symptoms of RA and OA may include wearing a splint, avoiding or modifying activity, or positioning during the day or at night to prevent joint stress.[35] Repetitive joint loading or motion with activity should be alternated with rest. The effectiveness of rest will be seen as an improved energy level with less joint swelling, pain, and fatigue.

Camilla required both general rest for her body and localized rest for her inflamed wrists and hands. It was important to help

her realize the physiological need for rest during recovery from her flare-up. In helping to evaluate her sleep and rest needs, it was important to go over her sleep hygiene, that is, her habits and routines around bedtime and other times throughout the day. This assurance permitted her to feel less guilty about tasks left undone and enabled her to understand that taking care of herself in the short term would allow her to return to activity in the long term (see Chapter 13 for more information on sleep and rest).

Physical Agent Modalities

Physical agent modalities (PAMs) may help to relieve pain or to maintain or improve ROM. Although modality use alone has not been shown to provide sustained benefits in rheumatic disease, clients do report less pain and stiffness from a clinical standpoint.[115,129,134] The most commonly used PAMs are superficial heat and cold agents. Benefits of heat in clients with arthritis include increased blood flow, pain relief, and increased tissue elasticity, with a negative effect of increasing inflammation also possible.[24,62] Benefits of cold include reduced inflammation and decreased pain threshold, with possible negative effects of increased tissue viscosity and decreased tissue elasticity causing more joint stiffness.[24,62] Heat can be delivered through hot packs, paraffin, fluid therapy, hydrotherapy in a heated pool, and even a warm shower or bath; cold can be delivered through ice packs or gel packs. When selecting the proper modality, the therapist must consider the activity and stage of the disease process. Acutely inflamed joints may be exacerbated by heat, whereas ice may be more helpful in reducing pain and inflammation. In the subacute or chronic stages, heat or cold may be equally effective.[24] Camilla preferred the use of heat and found it helpful in loosening her joints and lessening her pain. Even though she was in the subacute phase, some inflammation was still present; therefore, her response to heat was closely monitored so that it did not worsen her inflammation. She was educated in the safe use of warm baths and microwave packs at home.

Some medical conditions associated with rheumatic disease contraindicate the use of thermal agents. For example, use of cold is contraindicated in clients with Raynaud's phenomenon, a vasospastic disorder of the digits.[24,62] Clients with RA often have unstable vascular reactions to heat and cold that cause greater than normal heat retention with heat agents or increased coldness and stiffness with cold exposure.[62] Careful monitoring of client responses to PAMs is crucial. Client preference and ease of home application should also be considered before choosing an agent to use. Home paraffin units, microwave packs, and continuous low-level heat wraps are increasingly accessible and affordable in community stores and thus provide clients with more options.[88] Safety should always be a primary concern. Clients and significant others should be carefully instructed in proper application techniques to prevent burns or other tissue damage. Before using any modality, the therapist must fully understand tissue responses and related precautions and be competent in safe delivery of the agent. This typically requires specific education beyond entry-level preparation. Therapists must also adhere to any state licensure or training requirements.

Therapeutic Exercise

The purpose of exercise in the treatment of arthritis is to keep muscles and joints functioning as normally as possible by maintaining muscle strength, preventing disuse atrophy, and maintaining or improving ROM.[137] There is evidence that hand exercise can increase strength, reduce pain, and improve ROM and hand function in OA[129] and that ROM and dynamic and aerobic exercise can have positive effects in RA.[45,81] Regular physical activity can also alleviate depression.[135] It is helpful to find out what exercises the client may already be performing and whether these exercises were suggested by a professional or a well-meaning family member or friend; many self-initiated exercises can be harmful to a person with arthritis. There is no universal exercise program suitable for all clients with arthritis. Exercise programs should be designed with regard to individual client needs and tolerances. As a good rule of thumb, pain lasting greater than 1 or 2 hours after completion of exercise signals a need to modify or decrease an exercise.[85,137] General guidelines for exercise in clients with arthritis are to avoid undue joint stress, avoid pain and joint swelling, and work within the client's comfortable ROM.[14,75,137] The client should be taught to perform

exercises slowly, smoothly, and with proper technique. The client must also understand the rationale behind the prescribed exercises.[137] Exercises to maintain ROM should be performed at least once daily, even during a flare. For RA, each major joint should be taken through its full comfortable ROM. This includes the neck and possibly the jaw if symptomatic. The stiffest joints require the most attention. The type of ROM exercise selected depends on the disease activity and location of the joint. Active ROM is typically preferred, with assisted or passive ROM if pain or weakness precludes it. In cases of active synovitis, active ROM can exert more stress on a joint than gentle passive ROM, so passive ROM exercises may be safer.[85] Performing shoulder exercises is often easier in a supine position, which eliminates the effects of gravity. The number of repetitions should be weighed against the potential inflammatory response. On good days, 10 repetitions may be appropriate; on bad days, 3 or 4 repetitions within a smaller arc of motion may be indicated.[137] If the goal of exercise is to increase joint mobility, active or passive stretch can be incorporated. This is appropriate for the subacute or chronic phases of disease but never for the acute phase.[85] Box 39.3 presents general active ROM exercises for RA.

Exercises for strengthening can be dynamic (isotonic) or static (isometric) and should be aimed toward recovery of function.[39,85,135] Strengthening must be approached cautiously so that pain is not increased, deforming forces are not created, and joint stability is not compromised. Grip-strengthening exercises, even those using TheraPutty with light resistance, can impart large forces to unstable hand joints.[26] Additionally, this type of dynamic exercise may aggravate joints or pose a risk for potential deformity and in general should be avoided in clients with rheumatoid hand involvement.[15] Resistive exercise of any kind should never be performed during periods of acute flare or inflammation but may be used at other stages. Isometric exercises are usually the least painful for clients with RA because they eliminate joint motion and can be as effective or more effective in improving muscle strength and endurance.[85] Isometric contractions are generally held for 6 to 12 seconds.[39] Programs to maintain strength vary depending on the client's overall activity level. Clients who are sedentary may require a daily program, whereas clients who are active may need to perform only specific exercises once a week.[85] Gradual progression of repetitions or resistance is recommended.[135]

Exercises to promote general health and fitness are recommended for all adults as part of a healthy lifestyle and should be encouraged in clients with arthritis. Current evidence supports the benefits of well-designed aerobic and conditioning exercise for people with hip and knee OA, as well as aerobic and strength training in adults with stable RA.[45,65,81,135] Stationary bicycling, walking, and low-impact aerobic dancing, once thought to cause joint damage, have been found to increase flexibility, strength, endurance, and cardiovascular fitness without aggravation of symptoms. Traditional Chinese medicine (TCM) use, such as tai chi, which is a form of complementary and alternative medicine (CAM), appears to represent an approach with increasing interest and benefits.[123] Tai chi has been reported to have positive effects on self-efficacy, quality of life, general health status, pain, stiffness, and physical functioning in older

BOX 39.3 Range-of-Motion Exercises for Rheumatoid Arthritis

Instructions

1. Start with 5 of each exercise, 1 or 2 times each day.
2. Progress to 10 of each exercise, 1 or 2 times each day.
3. Do all exercises slowly, smoothly, and gently.
4. If in a flare, cut down on exercise repetitions. If possible, do not discontinue them entirely.
5. Listen to your body.

Jaw

6. Gently open your mouth as wide as you can and then close it.
7. With your mouth slightly open, move your jaw from side to side.
8. Slide your lower jaw forward and then relax to bring it back.

Neck

9. Look up toward ceiling and then look down to the floor.
10. Looking forward, lean your head toward one shoulder, and then toward the other shoulder.
11. With your mouth closed, slide your chin forward and then relax.
12. With your mouth closed, slide your chin toward the back of your neck and then relax.

Shoulders and Elbows

13. Shrug your shoulders up and down.
14. With your hands on your shoulders, make circles with your elbows.
15. With your hands behind your head (or if unable, on your shoulders), bring your elbows together in front of you and then spread your elbows apart.
16. Touch your shoulders with your hands and then straighten your elbows.

Forearms and Wrists

17. With your elbows partially bent and kept at your sides, turn your palms up and then down.
18. With your fingers and thumbs relaxed, raise your wrists up as far as you can, and then lower them down.

Fingers

19. Make fists and then open your hands and straighten your fingers.
20. Touch your thumb tips to the tips of each finger.
21. With your palms on your thigh or a table, move your thumbs away from your fingers, then gently slide each finger back toward your thumbs.

Courtesy Occupational Therapy Department, Rancho Los Amigos National Rehabilitation Center, Downey, California.

adults with lower extremity OA[59,114] and is being used for clients with RA as well.[55]

Whether the client is exercising to address ROM, strengthening, or overall conditioning, the OT should work closely with the client to help ensure that any exercise program can be successfully integrated into the client's typical daily routine with a proper balance of rest and activity. Exercises ideally should be done when the client feels most limber and has the least pain. Community land- and water-based exercise classes specifically designed for people with arthritis are available through the Arthritis Foundation. They offer the added benefits of social interaction and peer support and have been shown to be safe and effective in increasing fitness and strength and decreasing pain and difficulty in daily functioning.[21,45,65,118,124]

Daily upper body active ROM exercises with gentle stretch and isometric exercises for the shoulders and elbows were prescribed to improve Camilla's motion and strength. It was decided that the best time to perform these exercises was after her morning shower, when she felt less stiff and least fatigued. The therapist initiated simple tai chi exercises in sitting that Camilla could do at home to help with her flexibility, balance, and stress reduction. The therapist also recommended that Camilla become involved in one of the Arthritis Foundation exercise classes once her flare subsided, to build her endurance and cardiovascular conditioning. She was interested in joining and planned to attend classes on the days that she volunteered fewer hours.

Therapeutic Activity

Performance of therapeutic activities offers many benefits, both physical and psychological. Discussing current and past hobbies or having the client complete an interest survey can help the therapist determine activities that may be most appropriate for the client. New activities may be suggested or previously enjoyed activities reintroduced. There is a growing interest in virtual reality-based therapy in rehabilitation that has shown positive effects in ROM, strength, and functional endurance for people with arthritis.[5] A carefully chosen and graded activity can be an effective means of encouraging ROM and strength. When selecting therapeutic activities, the therapist should apply the same principles as with exercise.[85] Activities should be nonresistive, avoid patterns of deformity, and not overstress joints; instead, they should offer enough repetition of movement to help improve ROM and strength. The effect of the activity on all joints should be considered.

It is typically recommended that clients with RA not engage in activities that require use of the hand in prolonged static positions. However, sometimes the psychological benefits of doing activities that one enjoys outweigh the risks involved, especially if the risks can be minimized. Examples of activities that are often frowned on include knitting and crocheting. These activities are truly contraindicated only if there is active MCP synovitis, a developing swan neck deformity, or thumb CMC joint involvement.[85] Potential problems may be averted by having the client wear a hand or thumb splint to support the vulnerable joints while performing the activity or modifying the activity using assistive devices (Figs. 39.13 and 39.14). Additionally, educating the client to incorporate frequent rest breaks and stretching exercises for the intrinsic muscles will help limit risks (see Chapter 29 for additional information regarding therapeutic exercise and activity).[40,85]

Splinting

Indications

Splinting is often an integral component of the treatment of arthritis. Splints can be used for numerous reasons, with the fundamental goal of maximizing function. It is important for the therapist to understand the pathomechanics of the disease process when prescribing an appropriate and feasible splinting plan. Inappropriate use of splints can be harmful. Indications for splinting in clients with arthritis include reducing inflammation,

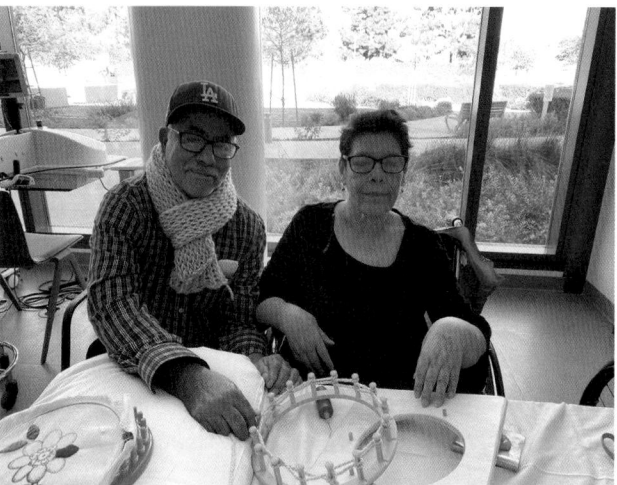

Fig. 39.13 Knitting group using assistive tools.

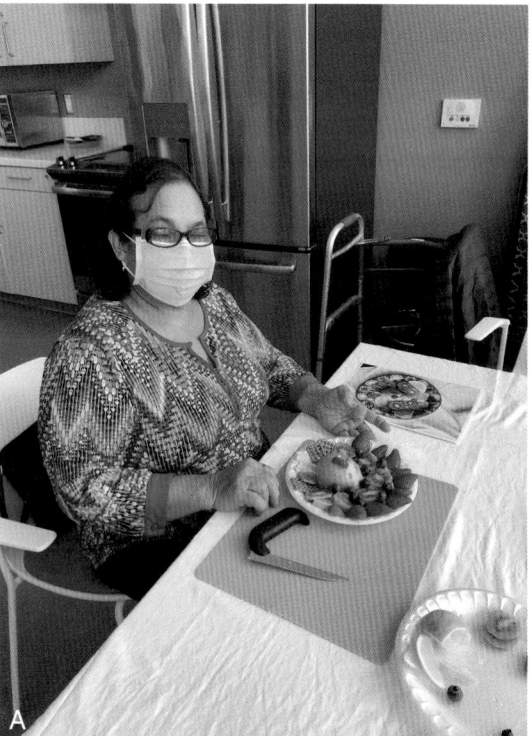

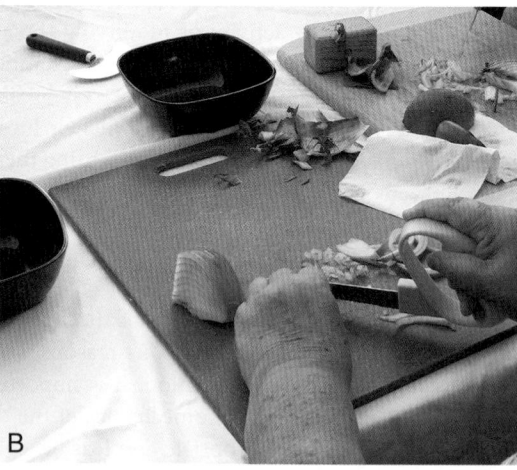

Fig 39.14 Use of modified devices during (A) eating and (B) meal preparation.

TABLE 39.6   Splinting Indications by Classification of Progression of Rheumatoid Arthritis

Stage	Symptoms/ Radiographic Changes	Splinting Indications
Stage I: Early	No destructive changes; possible osteoporosis	Resting splints to decrease acute inflammation, decrease pain, protect joints
Stage II: Moderate	Osteoporosis with or without slight subchondral bone destruction, slight cartilage destruction, no joint deformities, limited joint mobility possible, muscle atrophy, extraarticular soft tissue lesions possible	Day splints to provide comfort Night splints to relieve pain or protect joints against potential deformity Splints to increase ROM
Stage III: Severe	Cartilage and bone destruction, joint deformity, extensive muscle atrophy, extraarticular soft tissue lesions possible	Day splints to improve function (decrease pain, provide stability, limit undesired motion, properly position joints) Night splints to provide positioning and comfort
Stage IV: Terminal	Criteria for stage III, with fibrous and bony ankylosis	Day splints to improve function (decrease pain, provide stability, limit undesired motion, properly position joints) Night splints to provide positioning and comfort

decreasing pain, supporting unstable joints, properly positioning joints, limiting undesired motion, and increasing ROM. Although it is generally agreed that splinting has a place in the acute phase of RA,[45] there are few documented or well-established protocols for splinting in later stages.[48] Table 39.6 summarizes the potential splinting indications on the basis of progression of the joint destruction in RA.[14,85]

Ultimately, the individual needs of each client must be determined carefully. What are the primary goals for splinting? What benefits will a splint provide? What limitations will a splint impose? Which joints are involved and should be incorporated into a splint design? What effect will splinting have on unsplinted joints? Is the client receptive to splinting? What splints has the client tried or worn before? When should the splint be worn? These factors should be considered when deciding on an appropriate splinting plan.

Considerations

There are some special considerations for splinting in clients with RA. Because the added weight of a splint puts additional stress on the upper extremity and may cause problems with pain and fatigue, a splint should be as lightweight as possible. Forces are also transferred from splinted to adjacent unsplinted joints. For example, a thumb splint leaving the wrist and IP joints free may cause these joints to become more symptomatic. Skin tolerance can be an issue because skin is often more fragile as a result of the RA disease process and effects of medication. The presence of sensory impairments may also require closer monitoring for signs of pressure. Finally, splint straps may need to be modified to allow increased ease and decreased joint stress during donning and doffing of splints.

Options

If splinting is indicated, the therapist must then determine which type of splint will work best. The growing array of commercial products has led to a greater number of choices. Should the splint be rigid, semirigid, or soft? This will often be decided by the splint's proposed purpose and the client's preference. Rigid splints provide maximal immobilization or stability, soft splints allow more freedom of motion, and semirigid splints combine elements of both. Should the splint be prefabricated or custom made? This decision is based on many splint- and client-related factors, including splint availability, cost to purchase or fabricate, durability, weight, ease of care, ease of donning and doffing, cosmetic appearance, and extent of the client's existing deformity.

Providing the client with choices will enhance splint use and client satisfaction. Studies have shown that the following additional factors may encourage splint wear: flexibility of the splinting regimen and vigorous client education regarding the splint's purpose and wearing schedule, individualized splint prescriptions based on the client's comfort and preference, strong family support, positive attitudes and behaviors exhibited by healthcare providers, and benefits that are immediately obvious to the client.[30,47,54,91,96,119] Rapport, trust, sensitivity to clients' learning styles, splint trial evaluations, and providing clients with the opportunity to voice their concerns and frustrations can also enhance the collaborative process and splinting outcome.[37] The therapist can recommend splinting, but ultimately the client will decide whether the splint's benefits outweigh the limitations that it imposes.

Commonly Used Splints for Arthritis

A resting hand splint is useful for the treatment of acute synovitis of the wrist and hand. Its primary function is to provide localized rest to the involved joints. It can also relieve pain, decrease muscle spasm, and protect joints vulnerable to contracture or deformity from synovitis. Joints are rested in positions that place the least internal pressure on them and are opposite that of potential deformity.[14] The recommended joint positions during rest are slight wrist extension (0–20 degrees) and ulnar deviation (10–20 degrees), MCP flexion (20–30 degrees), slight PIP and DIP flexion (10–degrees), and slight thumb extension and abduction at the CMC joint with slight flexion of the MCP and IP joints.[48,85] However, the client's comfort should always take precedence and joints should never be forced into the ideal position. The splint is worn continually for the duration of the flare-up and removed at least once a day for skin hygiene and gentle ROM exercises. Splint use should continue full-time for at least 2 weeks after the flare subsides, with a gradual decrease in wearing time to allow the joints to recover.[48,85] In the later

stages of disease, the splint is often used at night only to increase comfort and protect against deforming positions. If bilateral splints are needed, clients may alternate splints or wear the splint on the most symptomatic hand.

Commercial splints, such as those made from wire-foam or a malleable metal frame covered by soft padding (Fig. 39.15), may be used if the limited adjustments that they allow can provide the client with a proper fit. This is often not possible in clients with established joint deformities. A custom-fabricated thermoplastic splint will allow a precise individualized fit. Joints that are asymptomatic may not need to be included in the splint. Modified resting splints with the uninvolved joints left free (Fig. 39.16) may lessen joint stiffness related to splint wear, allow some degree of hand function while the splint is worn, and improve splint wear and comfort.

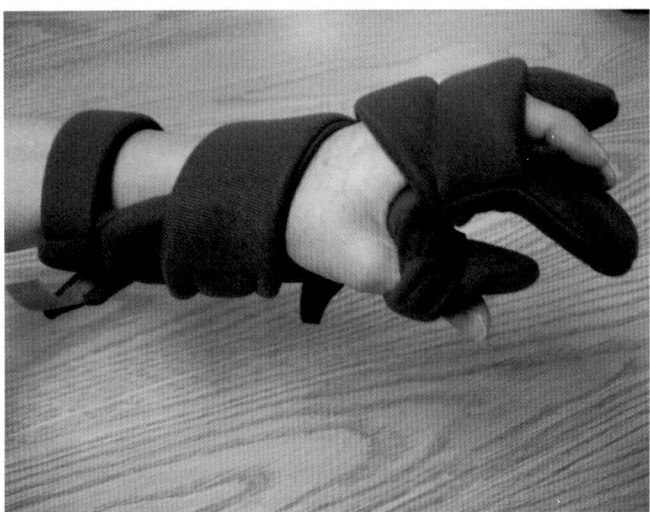

Fig. 39.15 Prefabricated resting hand splint. (Courtesy Occupational Therapy Department, Rancho Los Amigos National Rehabilitation Center, Downey, California.)

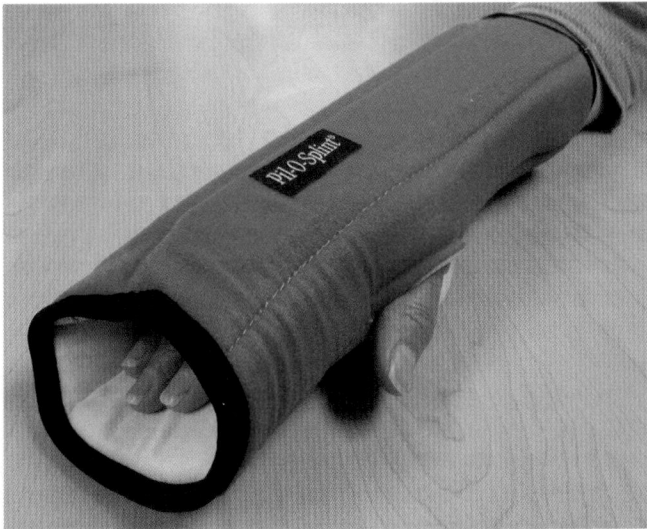

Fig 39.16 Prefabricated wrist-hand splint with thumb left free. (Courtesy Occupational Therapy Department, Rancho Los Amigos National Rehabilitation Center, Downey, California.)

Although the benefits of resting hand splints are recognized by healthcare professionals, studies have shown that client adherence to splint wear is moderate at best.[1,47] In a study comparing the use of soft and hard resting splints in clients with RA, pain was significantly decreased with splint wear, with 57% preferring the soft splint, 33% the hard splint, and 10% no splint at all. The rate of compliance was greater for the soft splint than for the hard splint.[27]

A wrist splint is often used to provide wrist stability, decrease pain, and improve function. Supports may be custom-fabricated (Fig. 39.17) or prefabricated. Because they are intended to provide support while allowing functional use of the hand, fit and comfort are crucial.[122] A variety of commercial splints made from many materials that offer a full range of soft to rigid support are available. Aside from support, clients with arthritis frequently report a benefit from the neutral warmth that many fabrics provide. A systematic review did conclude that wrist splints were effective in reducing pain in clients with RA.[101] When the MCP joints are symptomatic, a splint can be used to support them along with the wrist (Fig. 39.18).

Studies have shown conflicting results of different splint styles in grip strength, dexterity, pain reduction, hand function, comfort, security during performance of tasks, effects of stiffness, or muscle atrophy related to wearing of wrist splints in clients with RA.[93,101,119] In a study of splint preference, most clients were able to identify their preferred splint within only a few minutes of wear when given three styles to try.[120] These studies illustrate the importance of offering a wide variety of splints for each client to try.

MCP ulnar deviation splints may be beneficial in providing relief of pain, stability, alignment, and reduced stress on painful, subluxed, or deviated joints. They may slow the progression of deformity, but they will not prevent or correct it.[14,86,100] Splints can be fabricated or obtained commercially, with support ranging from soft to rigid (Fig. 39.19). Despite the variety of splint designs and materials, MCP ulnar deviation splints are reported to be infrequently prescribed and used by clients.[89] Immobilization of the MCP joints can impede functional use of the hand or increase pain and stress on adjacent PIP joints.[58,86,98] Bulky or volar-based splints can also interfere with palmar sensation or impair the ability to grasp objects. However, some clients benefit from the pain relief and improved digital alignment. High client satisfaction rates have been reported for a custom dorsal-based design.[102] Soft splints are commercially available or can be custom-fabricated.[51] The client's preference for use and selection of an MCP ulnar deviation support should be the primary factor in decision making.[58,86]

A swan neck splint, also known as a PIP hyperextension block, is used to restrict unwanted PIP hyperextension motion. Swan neck deformities often cause difficulty in hand closure because the PIP tendons and ligaments can catch during motion and the finger flexors have less of a mechanical advantage to initiate flexion when the PIP joint is in a hyperextended position. By blocking the PIP joint in slight flexion, the client can flex the PIP joint more efficiently, thus improving hand function. Swan neck splints can be custom-fabricated from thermoplastics for short-term or trial use. For long-term use or for use on adjacent

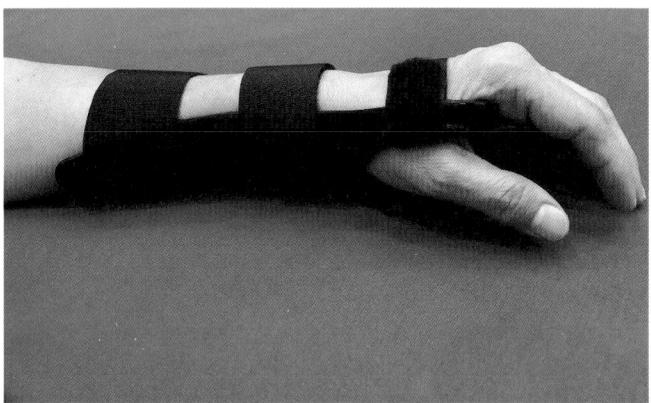

Fig. 39.17 Custom-fabricated thermoplastic wrist splint. (Courtesy Occupational Therapy Department, Rancho Los Amigos National Rehabilitation Center, Downey, California.)

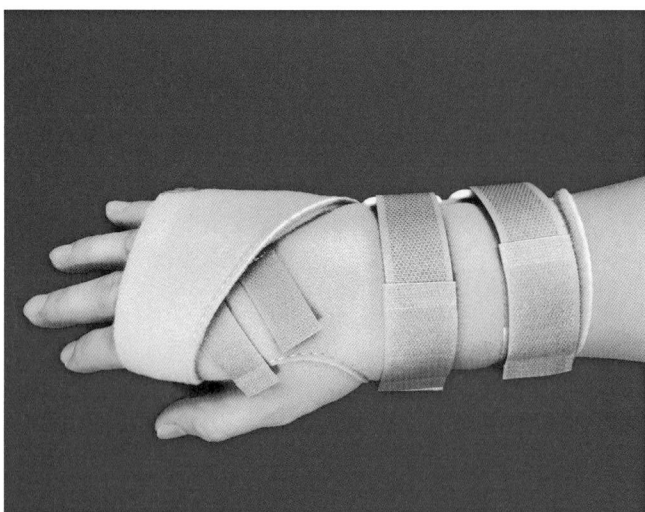

Fig. 39.18 Prefabricated wrist and metacarpophalangeal joint soft support. (Courtesy Occupational Therapy Department, Rancho Los Amigos National Rehabilitation Center, Downey, California.)

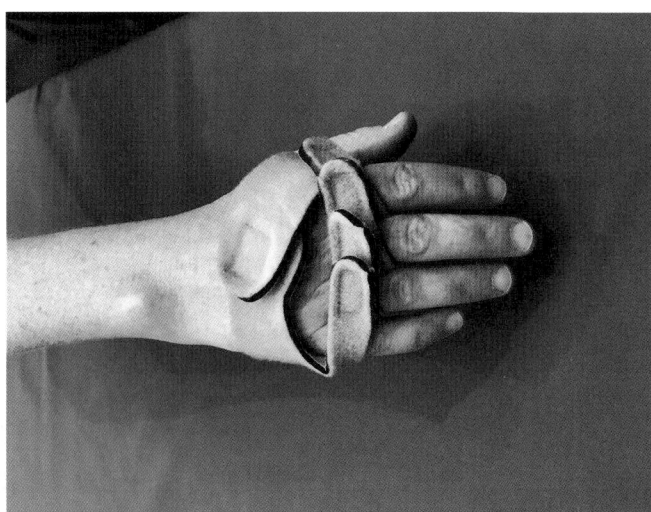

Fig. 39.19 Soft Neoprene metacarpophalangeal joint ulnar deviation splint. (Courtesy Occupational Therapy Department, Rancho Los Amigos National Rehabilitation Center, Downey, California.)

fingers, commercial products made of metal or polypropylene are preferable because they are more durable, less bulky, more easily cleaned, and more cosmetically appealing[130] (Fig. 39.20). Swan neck splints or splints of similar design also can be used to provide lateral stability to unstable IP joints of the fingers or thumb.[14,58]

Flexible boutonnière deformities may benefit from boutonnière splints to block the PIP joint in extension and leave the DIP joint free to flex. These can be fabricated by the therapist or custom-ordered from the same companies that manufacture swan neck splints. As a result of the direct pressure that they exert over the dorsum of the PIP joint, the skin must be monitored closely. Clients may reject wearing these splints during

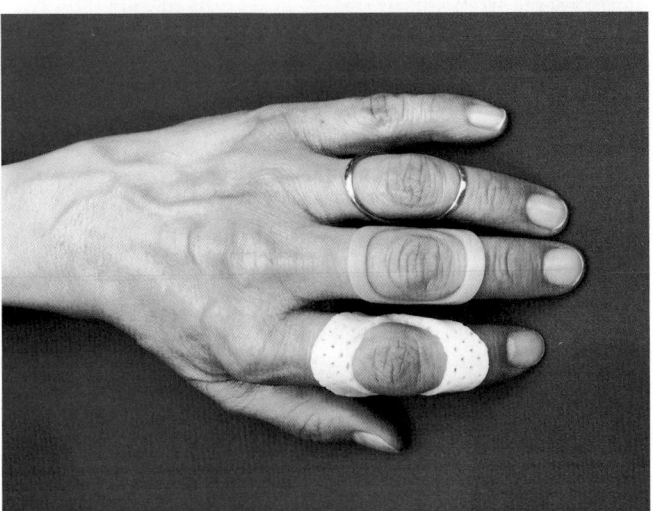

Fig. 39.20 Splints for swan neck deformity: custom-fabricated thermoplastic, commercial custom-sized metal, and prefabricated polypropylene. (Courtesy Occupational Therapy Department, Rancho Los Amigos National Rehabilitation Center, Downey, California.)

the day if limiting PIP flexion impedes function. Night splinting with the PIP joint in maximal extension can be used in an attempt to maintain ROM.[14]

Thumb splinting can provide positioning opposite that of the developing deformity in early stages of disease and a more stable and pain-free pinch for function in later stages.[14] Hand-based short thumb spica splints or opponens splints leave the wrist and IP joints free and can be used for problems at the MCP or CMC joints. Splinting for the CMC joint may sometimes necessitate inclusion of the wrist or MCP joints, but both hand-based and forearm-based (long thumb spica) types have been found to be effective.[58,125,132] Several thermoplastic splint designs exist, as do numerous prefabricated splints made from a variety of materials. Depending on the client's symptoms and stage of disease, a soft support (Fig. 39.21, A) may suffice, or the client may require a rigid support (see Fig. 39.21, B) to counteract the stressors applied to joints during functional use.[52] In studies comparing a short polychloroprene (Neoprene) thumb spica splint and a custom thermoplastic hand-based splint for OA of the CMC joint, both splints improved pain and function and reduced subluxation.[29] The thermoplastic splint reduced subluxation more, but the Neoprene splint provided better pain relief and was preferred by clients.[112,133] Systematic reviews found fair evidence of the effectiveness of splinting in relieving pain and improving function in OA of the CMC joint. Although no evidence was found of a particular splint superiority, patient preferences in splint designs were varied.[44,70]

Dynamic splints and serial static splints may be used to regain ROM lost by shortening of periarticular structures or to maximize motion after surgical procedures such as joint arthroplasty. If the joint space is preserved (as determined by radiographs), there is a soft end-feel, and no more than minimal inflammation is present, gentle splinting may be indicated. The program should be monitored closely for adverse signs of

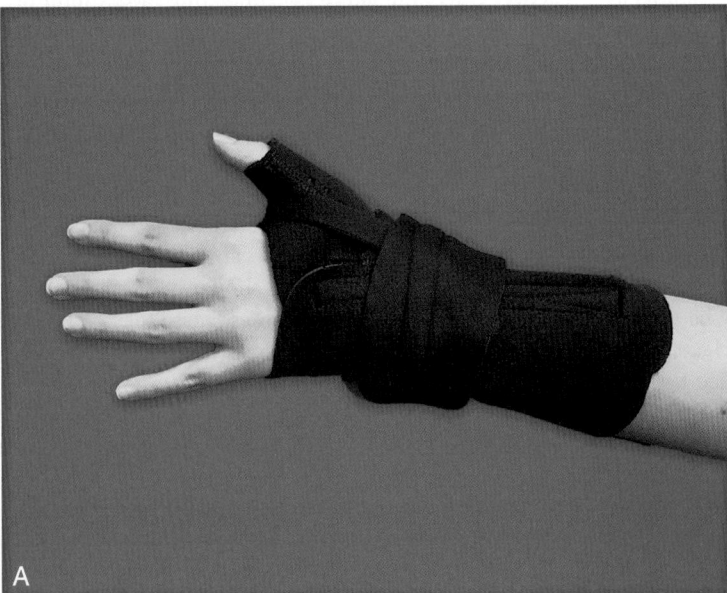
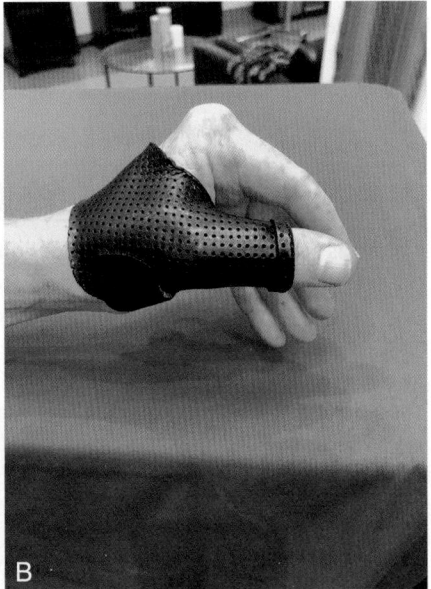

Fig. 39.21 A, Soft prefabricated long thumb and wrist support. B, Custom-fabricated thermoplastic short thumb spica splint. (Courtesy Occupational Therapy Department, Rancho Los Amigos National Rehabilitation Center, Downey, California.)

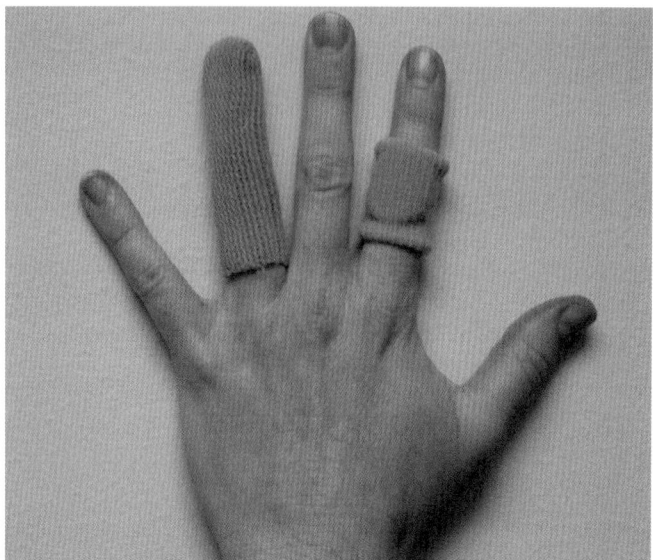

Fig. 39.22 Silicone-lined digital sleeve and pad. (Courtesy Occupational Therapy Department, Rancho Los Amigos National Rehabilitation Center, Downey, California.)

increased pain and swelling. Static splints are often better tolerated than dynamic ones because they apply lesser amounts of force on the joint.[58]

Finally, silicone-lined digital sleeves and pads (Fig. 39.22) may be helpful in protecting painful nodes or nodules from external trauma.

The splinting program for Camilla focused on decreasing her inflammation and pain and protecting her vulnerable joints. Because she had established deformity, most prefabricated splints were not viable options. She preferred soft, lightweight arthritis wrist splints that also provided support and alignment of her MCP joints and were her splints of choice for both day and night use. To afford her some ability to function, she was taught to monitor her symptoms and intermittently use the splints as needed if daytime activity led to increased pain or inflammation. Splint straps were modified by attaching loops to one end so that she could more easily manage them (see Chapter 30 for additional information).

OCCUPATIONAL PERFORMANCE TRAINING

An effective means of maintaining functional motion and strength with arthritis is to have clients perform daily occupations.[85] During active stages of the disease, occupations may be limited to just a few, such as feeding and hygiene. As the client's condition improves, usual life activities should be resumed because this will promote physical status and psychological well-being. An important but sometimes neglected aspect of ADL training is sexual counseling. Given the pain, fatigue, and ROM limitations resulting from arthritis or movement restrictions imposed postoperatively after joint replacement, an open discussion of issues and illustrations of more comfortable and safe positions for intercourse may prove helpful for clients and their partners. Excellent resources for sexual functioning with disabilities are available (see Chapter 12 for additional information).[38,106,111]

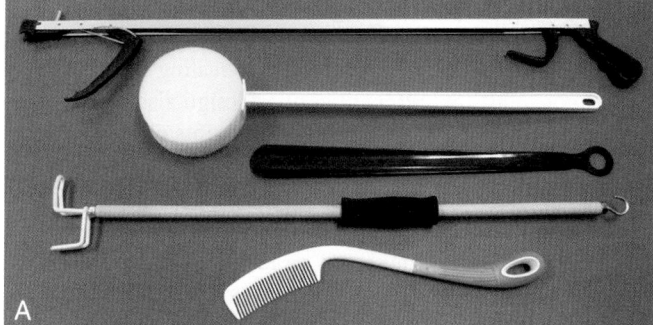

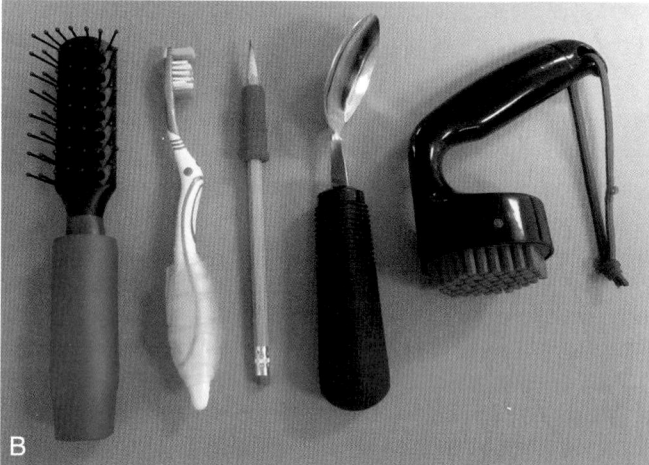

Fig. 39.23 A, Extended-handle devices. B, Built-up handle devices. (Courtesy Occupational Therapy Department, Rancho Los Amigos National Rehabilitation Center, Downey, California.)

Analysis of activity demands and activity contexts is a critical component in helping clients maintain, restore, or enhance their engagement in desired activities and occupations. Environmental modifications, alternative methods, or assistive devices often make a difference by increasing clients' independence, ease, and safety in completing meaningful occupations with less pain and stress on their joints. Creative problem solving with the client as an active participant can lead to solutions for unique challenges. Understanding the client's perspective, the meaning of roles, and the cultural and physical environment will allow the therapist to propose a more effective intervention.[11]

Assistive Devices

Numerous assistive devices can be fabricated or purchased commercially. The therapist should be familiar with the types of devices available and sources where they can be obtained at minimal expense. Many devices that were previously available exclusively from medical suppliers can now be found in retail stores at a much lower cost. Commonly used in arthritis interventions are extended-handle devices (e.g., reacher, bath sponge, shoe horn, dressing stick, comb; Fig. 39.23, A), to compensate for loss of proximal ROM and strength, and devices with built-up handles (e.g., hairbrush, toothbrush, writing implement, eating utensil, knob turner; see Fig. 39.23, B), to compensate for limited hand function (Table 39.7). The therapist should carefully consider the client's goals, factors, activity demands, and contexts when suggesting assistive devices.[85] Most relevant to

TABLE 39.7 Commonly Used Assistive Devices for Arthritis	
Activity	**Assistive Devices**
Dressing	Dressing stick, reacher, shoe horn, sock aid, button hook, zipper pull, elastic shoelaces
Bathing	Handheld shower hose, bath bench, grab bars, long-handled sponge
Toileting	Raised toilet seat, grab bars, extended perineal hygiene aid
Hygiene and grooming	Built-up or extended-handle toothbrush, suction denture brush, extended-handle hairbrush or comb, suction nail brush, mounted nail clipper
Feeding	Built-up or extended-handle utensils, lightweight T-handled mug
Meal preparation	Electric can and jar openers, food processors, adapted cutting board, utensils with built-up handles, lightweight dishes, ergonomic right-angled knives, rolling utility cart, knob turner for stove, reacher
Miscellaneous	Doorknob levers, built-up or extended key holders, extended-handle dust pans, built-up pens, loop or spring-loaded scissors, speaker phones, electronic activities of daily living (EADLs) and other smart home devices, technologies, and applications

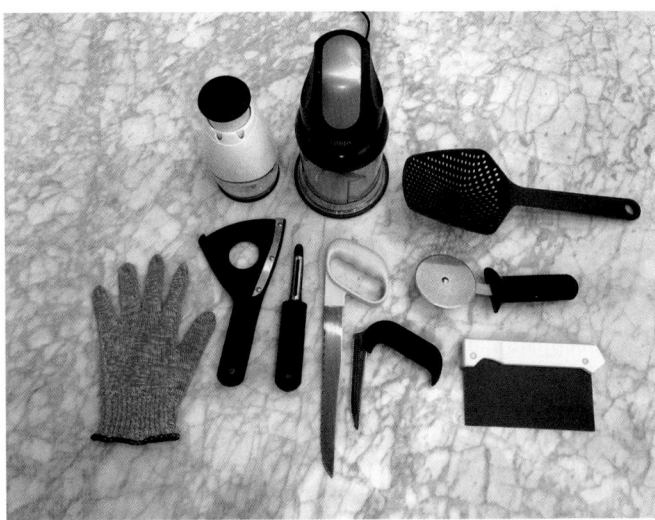

Fig. 39.24 Meal preparation devices to assist with joint protection and energy conservation.

clients with arthritis are the following: Is the client receptive to using a device? Will the device successfully reduce pain, joint stress, energy demands, or time expenditure? Is the device easy to use? Is the device acceptable to the client in terms of appearance, cost, and maintenance needs? Is the device compatible with the physical environment and others in the environment? Is the device likely to cause any negative effects?

Having sample equipment on hand for the client to try can be helpful in finding the best device for each client. For example, having devices available for trial during a meal preparation activity may improve the likelihood of their use of the devices at home (Fig. 39.24). In some cases, it may be necessary to modify existing devices before the client can use them successfully. For example, the handle of a dressing stick may be built up for a client with limited grasp. Surprisingly little research has been done on assistive devices for clients with arthritis and on the characteristics of device users and nonusers, but clinical experience shows that clients are less likely to use devices that they perceive as not helpful, too complicated, too expensive, or too bothersome to others sharing the environment.[105,121] A study of device use in frail elderly clients, including some with arthritis, demonstrated that they were willing to use the devices but required assistance in identifying sources for obtaining them.[79,80] Therapists may need to provide guidance for locating appropriate devices. For example, the therapist may offer specific device names or key words to assist the client with performing online searches independently. Some clients may need to use assistive devices only during a flare or on more symptomatic days. On good days, it may be appropriate to encourage clients to perform tasks without them to promote strength and mobility.

Client and Family Education

Providing clients with as much information as possible regarding their conditions and treatment is a crucial component of OT and should be integrated throughout all phases of the program. Whether it is the client's first visit or one of many therapy encounters, educational needs should always be explored. HEALTH literacy must be considered and fostered because it has been found to be strongly associated with functional status.[31] The use of technology has also played an increasing role in client education. The client's estimation of the therapist's credibility, the quality of the therapeutic relationship, and whether the client's experience confirms the therapist's statements are important factors tied to success in changing the client's knowledge and beliefs.[77] Client education has been shown to empower clients and lead to positive changes in pain reduction, psychological status, disease management, self-efficacy, and overall health promotion.[25,27,45,57,76,78,81–83]

Rather than focusing exclusively on providing basic information and generic skills, encouraging client self-reflection and transformation of client perspectives has been suggested as a helpful part of rehabilitation.[43] Repetition, reinforcement, and real-life application to the client's situation are other keys to education. By focusing on the client's symptoms and concerns, the therapist can capitalize on teachable moments to provide present-oriented and problem-focused learning activities.[22] It may be helpful to provide both verbal and written instructions. The following are some important educational aspects to cover: disease process, symptom management, joint protection and fatigue management, and community resources.

Disease Process

Does the client understand the type of arthritis, basic underlying pathology, medications, and medication side effects? Does the client understand that prolonged synovitis in RA can lead to irreversible joint damage and potential disability? Does the client feel comfortable discussing questions with the physician, nurse, or other treating clinicians? Does the client know of available resources to learn more?

Symptom Management

The occupational therapist determines whether the client knows how to monitor for signs and symptoms of inflammation. Does the client understand that pain lasting for more than 1 or 2 hours after an activity signals a need to modify or cease doing that task? Does the client understand the rationale behind, demonstrate appropriate use of, and appropriately integrate rest, exercise, splinting, and PAMs into a daily routine? Do family members understand the client's abilities and when they should or should not assist the client with activities? Does the client know to take a cautious approach to nontraditional arthritis remedies to avoid falling prey to unethical medical practices?

Joint Protection and Fatigue Management

Also of vital importance is whether the client understands the rationale and general principles of joint protection and fatigue management. More importantly, does the client successfully integrate them into daily activities? It can be challenging not just to help the client understand the potential implications but also to translate learning into action. The purpose of joint protection is to reduce internal and external joint stress, pain, and inflammation in the involved joints and preserve the integrity of joint structures during the performance of daily activities.[85] Although it has not been proved that use of joint protection techniques prevents deterioration, knowledge of the disease process and pathomechanics of deformity and clinical experience suggest that joint protection is a sound idea.[35,81] Studies have shown that clients who experience pain relief or improved function may be more receptive to changing their behavior.[40,56,90,93] Fatigue management, a more contemporary term for energy conservation, is aimed toward saving and expending energy wisely (Box 39.4). Fatigue can have a significant impact on quality of life and functioning of people with RA.[69] Organizing the environment, pacing activity, and resting can successfully moderate fatigue.[40] Instruction of principles should be based on teaching key concepts rather than general rules and should be specifically applied to each client's lifestyle and pattern of occupation with the aim of achieving occupational balance.[85,109,117] Practice in the therapy setting can help with carryover because following these principles often necessitates a change in lifelong habits. General principles for joint protection and fatigue management are especially helpful for clients with RA or clients with OA involving the hands, hips, or knees.[35,40,85]

Joint protection and fatigue management principles are as follows:

- *Respect pain.* Pain is a signal from the body that something is wrong. Clients often feel that they can ignore and work through pain, but the result is often more pain. If pain is present from an acute episode of inflammation, rest and avoidance of activity are indicated so that the pain and inflammation are not worsened. In chronic stages, pain that lasts for more than 1 or 2 hours after completion of an activity indicates that the activity should be modified or avoided. Clients should be encouraged to be aware of their limits and stop activities before pain occurs. Disregarding pain can lead to joint damage.

- *Maintain muscle strength and joint ROM.* Joints that are less stiff and have balanced strength will be less susceptible to further injury. Limited motion at one joint transmits force to another and may require exaggerated motions at other joints to accomplish a task. For example, loss of MCP motion will affect the PIP joint. Daily functioning and exercise programs should be done with all joint protection principles in mind to ensure that they are as least stressful as possible.

- *Use each joint in its most stable anatomic and functional plane.* This plane is the point at which resistance to motion is provided by muscle rather than ligament. Following this principle minimizes excessive stress on ligaments and allows muscle power to be used with the greatest mechanical advantage. Examples include not leaning to either side when rising from a seated position to lessen rotational forces on the knees and pinching with the pad of the thumb and the IP joint in a flexed position to minimize force on the ulnar collateral ligament.

- *Avoid positions of deformity.* The customary way of performing tasks may cause forces to be applied in directions of deformity. Tasks involving tight squeezing, pinching, or twisting motions are especially stressful. Opening a jar lid, turning a doorknob, cutting food with a knife, and lifting a coffee cup are all activities promoting MCP ulnar deviation. Instead, clients with hand involvement can be encouraged to open lids with the palm of their hand and shoulder motion or with a jar opener; to turn a doorknob with an adapted lever; to cut food with a dagger-type grip, rolling pizza cutter, or adapted knife; and to lift coffee mugs with two hands. Static positioning also should be considered. For example, clients should be discouraged from leaning their chin on the back of the fingers because this applies considerable force to the flexed MCP joints.

- *Use the strongest joints available.* Using larger, inherently stronger joints reduces the stress on smaller joints. Carrying bags and purses on the shoulder, elbow, or across the body lessens strain on the wrist and hand. Properly fitting backpacks or waist packs are other good alternatives, as is pushing or pulling a rolling cart instead of carrying items on the body. The palms rather than the fingers should be used to lift, push, or take weight to better distribute the forces.

- *Ensure correct patterns of movement.* The client may adopt incorrect patterns because of pain, deformity, muscle imbalance, or habit. For example, the client may use the dorsum of the fingers to push up from a seated position. This movement places deforming forces toward MCP flexion. A more suitable pattern is to use the flat surface of the palm (Fig. 39.25). In the hand, use of the long extensors during finger movement should be maintained. Finger flexion should be

BOX 39.4   Principles of Fatigue Management

Attitudes and Emotions
Remove yourself from stressful situations.
Refrain from concentrating on things that make you tense.
Close your eyes and visualize pleasant places and thoughts.

Body Mechanics
When lifting something that is low, bend your knees and lift by straightening your legs. Try to keep your back straight.
Avoid reaching (use reachers). Avoid stretching, bending, carrying, and climbing. If you have to bend, keep your back straight.
Incorporate good posture into your activities.
Whenever possible, sit when working.
To get up from a chair, slide forward to the edge of the chair. With your feet flat on the floor, lean forward and push with your palms on the arms or seat of the chair. Stand by straightening your legs.
Before you get tired, stop and rest.

Work Pace
Plan to get 10 to 12 hours of rest daily (naps and nights).
Work at your own pace.
Spread tedious tasks throughout the week.
Do the tasks that require the most energy at the times when you have the most energy.
Alternate easy and difficult activities, and take a 10- to 15-minute rest break each hour.

Leisure Time
Devote a portion of your day to an activity that you enjoy and find relaxing.
Check out what is available in the community.

Work Methods
Keep items within easy reach.
Use good light and proper ventilation and room temperature.
Use joint protection techniques.
Work surfaces should be at a correct height.

Organization
Plan ahead; do not rush or push yourself.
Decide which jobs are absolutely necessary.
Share the workload with family and friends.

How to Begin
Plan ahead by charting your daily routine.
Make a list of tasks, and spread them out in your schedule.
Include daily rest periods and rest breaks during energy-consuming times.
Check your schedule for the following factors:
- Is there 1 day in the week that is longer than the others?
- Are heavier tasks distributed through the week?
- Is there a long task that could be done in several steps?
- Will your plan allow flexibility?
- Have you devoted part of your day to a relaxing activity?
- Does your plan use the principles of energy conservation?

Weekly Schedule

Time	Sun	Mon	Tues	Wed	Thurs	Fri	Sat
7:00							
8:00							
9:00							
10:00							
11:00							
12:00							
1:00							
2:00							
3:00							
4:00							
5:00							
6:00							
7:00							
8:00							
9:00							
10:00							

initiated at the DIP joints while maintaining extension at the MCP joints versus leading motion with the intrinsic muscles.
- *Avoid staying in one position for long periods.* Prolonged static positions can lead to joint stiffness and muscle fatigue. Positional stress is then transmitted to the joint ligaments, which may already be in a weakened state. Changing body positions and gripping postures, taking frequent breaks, and integrating active motion exercises during activities such as computer keyboarding, writing, gardening, and knitting can prevent fatigue, soreness, stiffness, and resulting poor movement patterns.
- *Avoid starting an activity that cannot be stopped immediately if it becomes too stressful.* This will prevent the load from going to the joint capsule and ligaments if muscles tire. Continuing a task that causes sudden or severe pain is likely to cause joint damage, and severe fatigue can cause poor movement

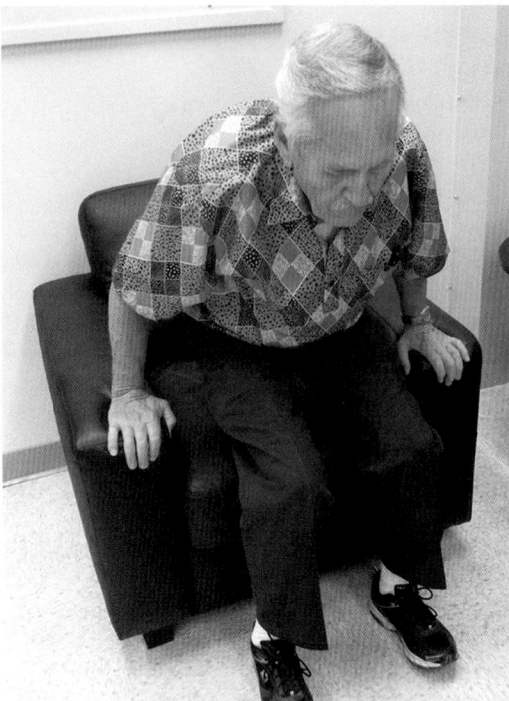

Fig. 39.25 Use of palms to push off a chair helps protect finger joints. (Courtesy Occupational Therapy Department, Rancho Los Amigos National Rehabilitation Center, Downey, California.)

<table>
</table>

BOX 39.5   Selected Arthritis Foundation Resources

Exercise Programs
Walk With Ease
    Online tools
    Mobile applications
Arthritis-friendly exercise videos
    Core exercises
    Strengthening exercises
    Upper body exercises
    Lower body exercises
    Weight-bearing exercises
    Tai chi exercises
    Yoga exercises

Written Materials
Arthritis Answers
Arthritis Today magazine
Arthritis Today Drug Guide
Arthritis Today Supplement and Vitamin Guide
Coping with Arthritis
Living with Osteoarthritis
Living with Rheumatoid Arthritis
Managing Your Pain
Tips for Good Living with Arthritis

Support
Arthritis Foundation Community at Inspire (https://www.inspire.com/groups/arthritis-foundation)

---

patterns and safety risks. Realistic planning of options can help prevent these situations. For example, clients can keep a bath bench available in case they need to rest while standing in the shower. Clients also can note the location of benches in a mall in relation to the stores where they plan to shop.

- *Balance rest and activity.* Chronic pain and a systemic disease such as RA can drain both physical and psychological resources. Helping the client understand the physiological need for proper rest can facilitate this often difficult lifestyle change. The key to increasing functional endurance is to rest before becoming overfatigued, which could mean napping or taking breaks during or between activities. Clients with arthritis often relate similar stories of feeling a need to take advantage of good days by trying to complete as many tasks as possible. These good days are more than likely followed by several bad days as their bodies try to recover. Balancing activities during the day and longer term across the week or month can be accomplished through planning and establishing priorities. The Spoon Theory is another useful means of quantifying the depletion of a person's energy, stamina, and fatigue level.[99]

- The spoon theory is a self-pacing strategy that emphasizes the need for chronic pain patients to work to a certain quota with spoons representing units of measurement of available energy. The metaphor of the spoon theory is that as the client engages in various occupations, a number of spoons of energy are used until all of the spoons for that client per day are depleted.

- *Reduce force and effort.* Less force and effort equate to less joint stress, less pain, and less fatigue. Using built-up handles, levers, more even distribution of loads, alternative methods,

and other aforementioned joint protection and fatigue management techniques can help toward this end. For example, rearranging the kitchen environment to have everything within easy reach, planning tasks and gathering all needed items, sitting down while at the sink or stove, and using assistive devices all contribute to easier meal preparation.

Community Resources

The OT determines whether the client knows of and uses available resources. Clients should be made aware and encouraged to take advantage of them. Reading materials, exercise and educational programs, and support groups can supplement medical and therapy intervention and promote lasting positive self-management behavior. The internet, libraries, YMCA/YWCAs, and senior centers are sources of information and activity or exercise programs. The Arthritis Foundation, a national organization with many local chapters throughout the country, is an excellent resource for clients, families, and clinicians. Among other services, the Arthritis Foundation offers educational pamphlets, exercise programs, self-help tips, and support designed exclusively for persons with arthritis. Box 39.5 highlights some programs and materials of special relevance to persons with RA and OA.

Occupational performance training was an important component of Camilla's OT intervention. Her ability to continue volunteering was addressed through a combination of modification of activities, use of assistive devices, and client education. Client education focused on her ability to better understand her disease process, manage her symptoms, and integrate joint protection and fatigue management principles into her life. Camilla and the therapist reviewed her typical weekly schedule and together planned one that allowed a more suitable balance of rest and activity given her patterns of fatigue and peak energy. The therapist recommended ways to improve Camilla's workstation at school, including adjusting the position of her chair and the height of her table for optimal body positioning, using adaptive devices to reduce the physical demands on her hands such as spring-loaded scissors for cutting papers and built-up handles on her pens and markers when grading papers. Assistive devices were recommended for other occupations she performed, such as gardening, knitting, and pet care. Mutual problem solving identified solutions that allowed Camilla to gradually return to her previous number of volunteer hours. Among these solutions were encouraging Camilla to respect her pain and address her fatigue through more frequent rest breaks and spreading her volunteer hours over the course of the week. Planning and taking an afternoon rest allowed her to go to her grandchildren's soccer games more frequently.

THREADED CASE STUDY

Camilla, Part 2

Critical evaluation components in assessing Camilla's previous and current functional status were the occupational profile and typical-day assessment; assessment of clinical status included pain, inflammation, stiffness, range of motion, strength, endurance, and functional mobility. The aspects of the disease process most problematic to Camilla were inflammation, pain, and fatigue from a flare of her rheumatoid arthritis. Her ability to engage in her occupation of volunteer work was affected by motor and process performance skills; habits, roles, and routine performance patterns; personal and environmental contexts; and client factors, including body functions and body structures.

Camilla benefited from splinting, exercise, heat, and occupational performance training with activity modification, assistive devices, and client education in symptom management, joint protection, fatigue management, and available resources. A collaborative approach throughout the therapy process was essential in promoting lasting benefits and engagement in meaningful occupations.

SUMMARY

Arthritis is a chronic condition that can impose devastating limitations on a person's ability to engage in meaningful occupations. It is important for the therapist to understand the different disease processes and pathomechanics of the joint destruction found in OA and RA. Through a carefully crafted program based on a thorough evaluation of the physical, psychosocial, and functional barriers, OT can decrease pain, protect joints, foster self-management, and enable increased participation in life skills and meaningful occupations.

REVIEW QUESTIONS

1. What are the major differences between osteoarthritis and rheumatoid arthritis?
2. What are three systemic signs of rheumatoid arthritis?
3. What are the clinical signs of joint inflammation?
4. When is resistive exercise appropriate for persons with rheumatoid arthritis?
5. What are the typical indications for splinting in arthritis?
6. What are the purposes and major principles of joint protection and fatigue management?
7. What assistive devices are commonly helpful for clients with arthritis?
8. What are the general treatment precautions related to arthritis?

REFERENCES

1. Adams J, Burridge J, Mullee M, et al: The clinical effectiveness of static resting splints in early rheumatoid arthritis: a randomized controlled trial, *Rheumatology* 47:1548–1553, 2008.
2. Alter S, Feldon P, Terrono AL: Pathomechanics of deformities in the arthritic hand and wrist. In Skirven TM, Osterman AL, Fedorczyk JM, Amadio PC, editors: *Rehabilitation of the hand and upper extremity*, St Louis, 2011, Mosby.
3. American College of Rheumatology: *Osteoarthritis fact sheet*, Atlanta, GA, 2013, American College of Rheumatology.
4. American College of Rheumatology: *Rheumatoid arthritis fact sheet*, Atlanta, GA, 2013, American College of Rheumatology.
5. Arman N, Tarakci E, Tarakci D, Kasapcopur O: Effects of video games-based task-oriented activity training (Xbox 360 Kinect) on activity performance and participation in patients with juvenile idiopathic arthritis: a randomized clinical trial, *American Journal of Physical Medicine and Rehabilitation* 98(3):174–181, 2019.
6. Arthritis Foundation: *Arthritis Today 2015 drug guide*, Atlanta, GA, 2015, Arthritis Foundation.
7. Arthritis Foundation: *Arthritis Today 2015 supplement and herb guide*, Atlanta, GA, 2015, Arthritis Foundation.
8. Arthritis Foundation: *Arthritis and Mental Health*, Atlanta, GA, 2019, Arthritis Foundation.
9. Arthritis Foundation: *Arthritis by the numbers: book of trusted facts and figures*, Atlanta, GA, 2019, Arthritis Foundation.
10. Bachoura A, Pisano K, Wolfe T, Lubahn J: Surgery and therapy for the rheumatoid hand and wrist. In Skirven TM, Osterman AL, Fedorczyk JM, Amadio PC, Feldscher SB, Shin EK, editors: *Rehabilitation of the hand and upper extremity*, Philadelphia, PA, 2021, Elsevier.

11. Backman C: Functional assessment. In Melvin J, Jensen G, editors: *Rheumatologic rehabilitation series, vol 1: assessment and management*, Bethesda, MD, 1998, American Occupational Therapy Association.

12. Barbour KE, Helmick CG, Boring M, Brady TJ: Vital signs: prevalence of doctor-diagnosed arthritis and arthritis-attributable activity limitation – United States, 2013-2015 *MMWR Morb Mortal Wkly Rep*, 66:246–253, 2017.

13. Barbour KE, Moss S, Croft JB, et al: Geographic variations in arthritis prevalence, health-related characteristics, and management – United States, 2015, *MMWR Surveill Summ* 67(4):1–28, 2018.

14. Beasley J: Therapist's examination and conservative management of arthritis of the upper extremity. In Skirven TM, Osterman AL, Fedorczyk JM, Amadio PC, editors: *Rehabilitation of the hand and upper extremity*, St Louis, 2011, Mosby.

15. Beasley J: Arthritis. In Cooper C, editor: *Fundamentals of hand therapy*, St Louis, 2014, Elsevier.

16. Beasley J, Lunsford D: The arthritic hand: conservative management. In Skirven TM, Osterman AL, Fedorczyk JM, Amadio PC, Feldscher SB, Shin EK, editors: *Rehabilitation of the hand and upper extremity*, Philadelphia, PA, 2021, Elsevier.

17. Bell-Krotoski JA: Sensibility testing with the Semmes-Weinstein monofilaments. In Skirven TM, Osterman AL, Fedorczyk JM, Amadio PC, editors: *Rehabilitation of the hand and upper extremity*, St Louis, 2011, Mosby.

18. Belza B, Dewing K: Clinical care in the rheumatic diseases. In Bartlett SJ, editor: *Fatigue*, Atlanta, GA, 2006, Association of Rheumatology Health Professionals.

19. Berenbaum F: Osteoarthritis pathology and pathogenesis. In Klippel JH, Stone JH, Crofford LJ, White PH, editors: *Primer of the rheumatic diseases*, New York, 2008, Springer.

20. Bland JH, Melvin JL, Hasson S: Osteoarthritis. In Melvin J, Jensen G, editors: *Rheumatologic rehabilitation series, vol 1: assessment and management*, Bethesda, MD, 1998, American Occupational Therapy Association.

21. Boutaugh ML: Arthritis Foundation community-based physical activity programs: effectiveness and implementation issues, *Arthritis Rheum* 49:463, 2003.

22. Boutaugh ML, Brady TJ: Patient education for self-management. In Melvin J, Jensen G, editors: *Rheumatologic rehabilitation series, vol 1: assessment and management*, Bethesda, MD, 1998, American Occupational Therapy Association.

23. Bozentka DJ: Pathogenesis of osteoarthritis. In Mackin EJ, editor: *Rehabilitation of the hand and upper extremity* ed 5, St Louis, 2002, Mosby.

24. Bracciano AG: *Physical agent modalities: theory and application for the occupational therapist*, ed 2, Thorofare, NJ, 2008, Slack.

25. Brady TJ, Boutaugh ML: Self-management education and support. In Bartlett SJ, editor: *Clinical care in the rheumatic diseases* ed 3, Atlanta, GA, 2006, Association of Rheumatology Health Professionals.

26. Brand PW, Hollister A: *Clinical mechanics of the hand*, ed 3, St Louis, 1999, Mosby.

27. Brekke M, Hjortdahl P, Kvien TK: Changes in self-efficacy and health status over 5 years: a longitudinal observational study of 306 patients with rheumatoid arthritis, *Arthritis Rheum* 49:342, 2003.

28. Buckwalter JA, Ballard WT: Operative treatment of arthritis. In Klippel JH, Stone JH, Crofford LJ, White PH, editors: *Primer of the rheumatic diseases* ed 13, New York, 2008, Springer.

29. Buhler M, Chapple C, Stebbings S, Sangelaji B, Baxter G: Effectiveness of splinting for pain and function in people with thumb carpometacarpal osteoarthritis: a systematic review with meta-analysis, *Osteoarthritis and Cartilage* 27:547–559, 2019.

30. Callinan NJ, Mathiowetz V: Soft versus hard resting splints in rheumatoid arthritis: pain relief, preference, and compliance, *Am J Occup Ther* 50:347, 1996.

31. Caplan L, Wolfe F, Michaud C, et al: Strong association of health literacy with functional status among rheumatoid arthritis patients: a cross-sectional study, *Arthritis Care Res* 66:508, 2014.

32. Centers for Disease Control and Prevention (CDC): National and state medical expenditures and lost earnings attributable to arthritis and other rheumatic conditions—United States, 2003, *MMWR Morb Mortal Weekly Rep* 56:4, 2007.

33. Centers for Disease Control and Prevention (CDC): Prevalence and most common causes of disability among adults, *MMWR Morb Mortal Weekly Rep* 58:421, 2009.

34. Centers for Disease Control and Prevention (CDC): Prevalence of doctor-diagnosed arthritis and arthritis-attributable activity limitation—United States, 2010-2012, *MMWR Morb Mortal Weekly Rep* 62:869, 2013.

35. Chang RW: *Rehabilitation of persons with rheumatoid arthritis*, Gaithersburg, MD, 1996, Aspen.

36. Chung K, Ross P: Pathomechanics of deformities of the arthritic hand and wrist. In Skirven TM, Osterman AL, Fedorczyk JM, Amadio PC, Feldscher SB, Shin EK, editors: *Rehabilitation of the Hand and Upper Extremity* ed 7, Philadelphia, PA, 2021, Elsevier.

37. Collins L: Helping patients help themselves: improving orthotic use, *OT Pract* 4:30, 1999.

38. Comfort A: *Sexual consequences of disability*, Philadelphia, 1978, George F Stickley.

39. Coppard BM, Gale JR: Therapeutic exercise. In Melvin J, Jensen G, editors: *Rheumatologic rehabilitation series, vol 1: Assessment and management*, Bethesda, MD, 1998, American Occupational Therapy Association.

40. Cordery J, Rocchi M: Joint protection and fatigue management. In Melvin J, Jensen G, editors: *Rheumatologic rehabilitation series, vol 1: Assessment and management*, Bethesda, MD, 1998, American Occupational Therapy Association.

41. Dieppe P: Osteoarthritis clinical features. In Klippel JH, Stone JH, Crofford LJ, White PH, editors: *Primer of the rheumatic diseases* ed 13, New York, 2008, Springer.

42. Doré AL, Golightly YM, Mercer VS, et al: Lower extremity osteoarthritis and the risk of falls in a community-based longitudinal study of adults with and without osteoarthritis, *Arthritis Care Res* 67:633, 2015.

43. Dubouloz CJ, Laporte D, Hall M, et al: Transformation of meaning perspectives in clients with rheumatoid arthritis, *Am J Occup Ther* 58:398, 2004.

44. Egan MY, Brousseau L: Splinting for osteoarthritis of the carpometacarpal joint: a review of the evidence, *Am J Occup Ther* 61:70, 2007.

45. Ekelman BA, Hooker L, Davis A, et al: Occupational therapy interventions for adults with rheumatoid arthritis: an appraisal of the evidence, *Occup Ther Health Care* 28:347, 2014.

46. Escalante A, Rincón I: The disablement process in rheumatoid arthritis, *Arthritis Rheum* 47:333, 2002.

47. Feinberg J: Effects of the arthritis health professional on compliance with use of resting hand splints by patients with rheumatoid arthritis, *Arthritis Care Res* 5:17, 1992.

48. Fess EE, Gettle KS, Philips CA, Janson JR: *Hand and upper extremity splinting: principles and methods*, St Louis, 2005, Mosby.

49. Fleming A, Benn RT, Corbett M, Wood PH: Early rheumatoid disease. II. Patterns of joint involvement, *Ann Rheum Dis* 35:361, 1976.

50. Furner SE, Hootman JM, Helmick CG, et al: Health-related quality of life of US adults with arthritis: analysis of data from the Behavioral Risk Factor Surveillance System, 2003, 2005, and 2007, *Arthritis Care Res* 63:788, 2011.

51. Gilbert-Lenef L: Soft ulnar deviation splint, *J Hand Ther* 7:29–30, 1994.

52. Gottschalk M, Kakar S: Surgery management of the osteoarthritic thumb carpometacarpal joint. In Skirven TM, Osterman AL, Fedorczyk JM, Amadio PC, Feldscher SB, Shin EK, editors: *Rehabilitation of the Hand and Upper Extremity* ed 7, Philadelphia, PA, 2021, Elsevier.

53. Grabovac I, Haider S, Berner C, Lamprecht T, Fenzl K, Erlacher L, Quittan M, Dorner T: Sleep quality in patients with rheumatoid arthritis and associations with pain, disability, disease duration, and activity, *Journal of Clinical Medicine* 7(336), 2018.

54. Groth GN, Wulf MB: Compliance with hand rehabilitation: health beliefs and strategies, *J Hand Ther* 8:18, 1995.

55. Hall A, Maher C, Latimer J, Ferreira M: The effectiveness of tai chi for chronic musculoskeletal pain conditions: a systemic review and meta-analysis, *Arthritis Care and Research* 61(6):717–724, 2009.

56. Hammond A: Joint protection behavior in patients with rheumatoid arthritis following an education program, *Arthritis Care Res* 7:5, 1994.

57. Hammond A, Bryan J, Hardy A: Effects of a modular behavioural arthritis education programme: a pragmatic parallel-group randomized control trial, *Rheumatology* 47: 1712, 2008.

58. Harrell PB: Splinting of the hand. In Bartlett SJ, editor: *Clinical care in the rheumatic diseases*, Atlanta, GA, 2006, Association of Rheumatology Health Professionals.

59. Hartman CA, Manos TM, Winter C, et al: Effects of T'ai Chi training on function and quality of life indicators in older adults with osteoarthritis *J Am Geriatr Soc*, 48:1553–1559, 2000.

60. Hawley DJ: Clinical outcomes: issues and measurement. In Melvin J, Jensen G, editors: *Rheumatologic rehabilitation series, vol 1: Assessment and management*, Bethesda, MD, 1998, American Occupational Therapy Association.

61. Hawley DJ, Fontaine KR: Functional ability, health status, and quality of life. In Bartlett SJ, editor: *Clinical care in the rheumatic diseases* ed 3, Atlanta, GA, 2006, Association of Rheumatology Health Professionals.

62. Hayes KW: Thermal and electrical agents used to manage arthritis symptoms. In Bartlett SJ, editor: *Clinical care in the rheumatic diseases* ed 3, Atlanta, GA, 2006, Association of Rheumatology Health Professionals.

63. Hayes KW, Petersen CM: Joint and soft tissue pain. In Melvin J, Jensen G, editors: *Rheumatologic rehabilitation series, vol 1: Assessment and management*, Bethesda, MD, 1998, American Occupational Therapy Association.

64. Hochberg MC, Chang RW, Dwosh I, et al: The American College of Rheumatology 1991 revised criteria for the classification of global functional status in rheumatoid arthritis, *Arthritis Rheum* 35:498, 1992.

65. Hurkmans E, van der Giesen FJ, Vliet Vlieland TP, et al: Dynamic exercise programs (aerobic capacity and/or muscle strength training) in patients with rheumatoid arthritis, *Cochrane Database Syst Rev*, 2009:CD006853, 2009.

66. Huskisson EC: Measurement of pain, *Lancet* 2:1127, 1974.

67. Janiszewski Goes AC, Busatto Reis LA, Barreto G Silva M, Stadler Kahlow B, Skare TL: Rheumatoid arthritis and sleep quality, *Revista Brasileira De Reumatologia* 57(4):294–298, 2017.

68. Jebsen RH, Taylor N, Trieschmann RB, et al: An objective and standardized test of hand function, *Arch Phys Med Rehabil* 50:311, 1969.

69. Katz P, Margaretten M, Gregorich S, Trupin L: Physical activity to reduce fatigue in rheumatoid arthritis: randomized controlled trial, *Arthritis Care and Research* 70(1):1–10, 2018.

70. Kjeken I, Smedslund G, Moe RH, et al: Systematic review of design and effects of splints and exercise programs in hand osteoarthritis, *Arthritis Care Res* 63:834, 2011.

71. Kolasinski SL: Therapies from complementary and alternative medicine. In Bartlett SJ, editor: *Clinical care in the rheumatic diseases* ed 3, Atlanta, GA, 2006, Association of Rheumatology Health Professionals.

72. Law M, Baptiste S, McColl MA, et al: *The Canadian Occupational Performance Measure manual*, ed 5, Ottawa, Canada, 2014, CAOT Publications ACE.

73. Ling SM, Rudolph K: Osteoarthritis. In Bartlett SJ, editor: *Clinical care in the rheumatic diseases*, Atlanta, GA, 2006, Association of Rheumatology Health Professionals.

74. Livneh H, Antonak RF: *Psychosocial adaptation to chronic illness and disability*, Gaithersburg, MD, 1997, Aspen.

75. Lockard MA: Exercise for the patient with upper quadrant osteoarthritis, *J Hand Ther* 13:175, 2000.

76. Lorig KR, Holman HR: Arthritis self-management studies: a twelve-year review, *Health Educ Q* 20:17, 1993.

77. Lorish C: Psychological factors related to treatment and adherence. In Melvin J, Jensen G, editors: *Rheumatologic rehabilitation series, vol 1: Assessment and management*, Bethesda, MD, 1998, American Occupational Therapy Association.

78. Mallinson T, Fischer H, Rogers JC, et al: Human occupation for public health promotion: new directions for occupational therapy practice with persons with arthritis, *Am J Occup Ther* 63:220–226, 2009.

79. Mann W: Assistive technology for persons with arthritis. In Melvin J, Jensen G, editors: *Rheumatologic rehabilitation series, vol 1: Assessment and management*, Bethesda, MD, 1998, American Occupational Therapy Association.

80. Mann WC, Tomita M, Packard S, et al: The need for information on assistive devices by older persons, *Assist Technol* 6:134–139, 1994.

81. Manning VL, Hurley MV, Scott DL, et al: Education, self-management, and upper extremity exercise training in people with rheumatoid arthritis: a randomized controlled trial, *Arthritis Care Res* 66:217, 2014.

82. Marks R: Efficacy theory and its utility in arthritis rehabilitation: review and recommendations, *Disabil Rehabil* 23:271, 2001.

83. Masiero S, Boniolo A, Wasserman L, et al: Effects of an educational-behavioural joint protection program on people with moderate to severe rheumatoid arthritis: a randomized controlled trial, *Clin Rheumatol* 26:2043, 2007.

84. Matcham F, Rayner L, Steer S, Hotopf M: The prevalence of depression in rheumatoid arthritis: a systematic review and meta-analysis, *Rheumatology* 52:2136, 2013.

85. Melvin JL: *Rheumatic disease in the adult and child: occupational therapy and rehabilitation*, ed 3, Philadelphia, 1989, FA Davis.

86. Melvin JL: Orthotic treatment of the hand: what's new? *Bull Rheum Dis* 44:5, 1995.

87. Melvin JL: Therapist's management of osteoarthritis in the hand. In Mackin EJ, editor: *Rehabilitation of the hand and upper extremity* ed 5, St Louis, 2002, Mosby.

88. Michlovitz SM, Hun L, Erasala GN, et al: Continuous low-level heat wrap therapy is effective for treating wrist pain, *Arch Phys Med Rehabil* 85:1409, 2004.

89. Murphy SL, Smith DM, Alexander NB: Measuring activity pacing in women with lower-extremity osteoarthritis: a pilot study, *Am J Occup Ther* 62:329, 2008.

90. Nordenskiöld U: Evaluation of assistive devices after a course in joint protection, *Int J Technol Assess Heath Care* 10:283, 1994.

91. Oakes TW, Ward JR, Gray RM, et al: Family expectations and arthritis patient compliance to a hand resting splint regimen, *J Chronic Dis* 22:757, 1970.

92. Oliver AM St., Clair EW: Rheumatoid arthritis treatment and assessment. In Klippel JH, Stone JH, Crofford LJ, White PH, editors: *Primer on the rheumatic diseases* ed 13, New York, 2008, Springer.

93. Orbai AM, Smith KC, Bartlett SJ, et al: "Stiffness has different meanings, I think to everyone": examining stiffness from the perspective of people living with rheumatoid arthritis, *Arthritis Care Res* 66:1662–1672, 2014.

94. Osteoarthritis (O.A.) Action Alliance, Thurston Arthritis Research Center. Osteoarthritis Prevention and Management in Primary Care: OA Prevalence and Burden – The University of North Carolina at Chapel Hill, 2020.

95. Overman CL, Jurgens MS, Bossema ER, et al: Change of psychological distress and physical disability in patients with rheumatoid arthritis over the last two decades, *Arthritis Care Res* 66:671, 2014.

96. Pagnotta A, Baron M, Korner-Bitensky N: The effect of a static wrist orthosis on hand function in individuals with rheumatoid arthritis, *J Rheumatol* 25:879, 1998.

97. Parker JC, Smarr KL: Psychological assessment. In Bartlett SJ, editor: *Clinical care in the rheumatic diseases* ed 3, Atlanta, GA, 2006, Association of Rheumatology Health Professionals.

98. Parmelee PA, Tighe CA, Dautovich ND: Sleep disturbance in osteoarthritis: linkages with pain, disability, and depressive symptoms, *Arthritis Care Res* 67:358–365, 2015.

99. Pashby K: "Today is a Four": how students talk about their chronic pain, *The Journal for Undergraduate Ethnography* 8(1):69–83, 2018.

100. Philips CA: Management of the patient with rheumatoid arthritis: the role of the hand therapist, *Hand Clin* 5:291, 1989.

101. Ramsey L, Winder RJ, McVeigh JG: The effectiveness of working wrist splints in adults with rheumatoid arthritis: a mixed methods systematic review, *J Rehabil Med* 46:481, 2014.

102. Rennie HJ: Evaluation of the effectiveness of a metacarpophalangeal ulnar deviation orthosis, *J Hand Ther* 9:371, 1996.

103. Robbins L: Social and cultural assessment. In Bartlett SJ, editor: *Clinical care in the rheumatic diseases* ed 3, Atlanta, GA, 2006, Association of Rheumatology Health Professionals.

104. Roberts WN, Daltroy LH, Anderson RJ: Stability of normal joint findings in persistent classical rheumatoid arthritis, *Arthritis Rheum* 31:267–271, 1988.

105. Rogers JC, Holm MB, Perkins L: Trajectory of assistive device usage and user and non-user characteristics: long-handled bath sponge, *Arthritis Rheum* 47:645, 2002.

106. Ruffing V: Sexual intimacy. In Bartlett SJ, editor: *Clinical care in the rheumatic diseases* ed 3, Atlanta, GA, 2006, Association of Rheumatology Health Professionals.

107. Sacks JJ, Luo YH, Helmick CG: Prevalence of specific types of arthritis and other rheumatic conditions in the ambulatory health care system in the United States, 2001–2005, *Arthritis Care Res*, 62:460–464, 2010.

108. Seftchick JL, Detullio LM, Fedorczyk JM, Aulicino PL: Clinical examination of the hand. In Skirven TM, Osterman AL, Fedorczyk JM, Amadio PC, editors: *Rehabilitation of the hand and upper extremity* ed 6, St Louis, 2011, Mosby.

109. Shapiro-Slonaker DM: Joint protection and energy conservation. In Riggs MA, Gall EP, editors: *Rheumatic diseases: rehabilitation and management*, Boston, 1984, Butterworth.

110. Sharma L: Osteoarthritis treatment. In Klippel JH, Stone JH, Crofford LJ, White PH, editors: *Primer on the rheumatic diseases* ed 13, New York, 2008, Springer.

111. Sidman JM: Sexual functioning and the physically disabled adult, *Am J Occup Ther* 31:81, 1977.

112. Sillem H, Backman CL, Miller WC, Li LC: Comparison of two carpometacarpal stabilizing splints for individuals with thumb osteoarthritis, *J Hand Ther* 24:216, 2011.

113. Smith MT, Wegener ST: Sleep disturbances in rheumatic diseases. In Bartlett SJ, editor: *Clinical care in the rheumatic diseases* ed 3, Atlanta, GA, 2006, Association of Rheumatology Health Professionals.

114. Song R, Lee EO, Lam P, Bae SC: Effects of tai chi exercise on pain, balance, muscle strength, and perceived difficulties in physical functioning in older women with osteoarthritis: a randomized clinical trial, *J Rheumatol* 30:2039–2044, 2003.

115. Sotosky JR, Melvin JM: Initial interview: a client-centered approach. In Melvin J, Jensen G, editors: *Rheumatologic rehabilitation series, vol 1: Assessment and management*, Bethesda, MD, 1998, American Occupational Therapy Association.

116. Spiegel TM, Forouzesh SN: Musculoskeletal examination. In Riggs MA, Gall EP, editors: *Rheumatic diseases: rehabilitation and management*, Boston, 1984, Butterworth.

117. Stamm T, Lovelock L, Stew G, Nell V, el al.: I have a disease but I am not ill: a narrative study of occupational balance in people with rheumatoid arthritis, *Occup Ther J Res* 29:32, 2009.

118. Stenström CH, Minor MA: Evidence for the benefit of aerobic and strengthening exercise in rheumatoid arthritis, *Arthritis Rheum* 49:428, 2003.

119. Stern EB, Ytterberg SR, Krug HE, Mahowald ML: Finger dexterity and hand function: effect of three commercial wrist extensor orthoses on patients with rheumatoid arthritis, *Arthritis Care Res* 9:197, 1996.

120. Stern EB, Ytterberg SR, Krug HE, et al: Commercial wrist extensor orthoses: a descriptive study of use and preference in patients with rheumatoid arthritis, *Arthritis Care Res* 10:27, 1997.

121. Steultjens EM, Dekker J, Bouter LM, et al: Occupational therapy for rheumatoid arthritis: a systematic review, *Arthritis Rheum* 47:672, 2002.

122. Stofer V, McLean S, Smith J: Do wrist orthoses cause compensatory elbow and shoulder movements when performing drinking and hammering tasks? *Irish Journal of Occupational Therapy* 46(1):24–30, 2018.

123. Sun K, Szymonifka J, Tian H, Chang Y, Leng J, Mandl L: Association of traditional Chinese medicine use with adherence to prescribed rheumatic medications among Chinese American patients: a cross-sectional survey, *Arthritis Care and Research* 72(10):1474–1480, 2020.

124. Suomi R, Collier D: Effects of arthritis exercise programs on functional fitness and perceived activities of daily living

measures in older adults with arthritis, *Arch Phys Med Rehabil* 84:1589, 2003.

125. Swigart CR, Eaton RG, Glickel SZ, Johnson C: Splinting in the treatment of arthritis of the first carpometacarpal joint, *J Hand Surg Am* 24:86, 1999.

126. Tehlirian CV, Bathon JM: Rheumatoid arthritis clinical and laboratory manifestations. In Klippel JH, Stone JH, Crofford LJ, White PH, editors: *Primer on the rheumatic diseases*, New York, 2008, Springer.

127. Terrono AL, Nalebuff EA, Philips CA: The rheumatoid thumb. In Skirven TM, Osterman AL, Fedorczyk JM, Amadio PC, editors: *Rehabilitation of the hand and upper extremity*, St Louis, 2011, Mosby.

128. Turkiewicz AM, Moreland LW: Rheumatoid arthritis. In Bartlett SJ, editor: *Clinical care in the rheumatic diseases*, Atlanta, GA, 2006, Association of Rheumatology Health Professionals.

129. Valdes K, Marik T: A systematic review of conservative interventions for osteoarthritis of the hand, *J Hand Ther* 23: 334–351, 2010.

130. Van der Giesen FJ, van Lankveld WJ, Kremers-Selten C, et al: Effectiveness of two finger splints for swan neck deformity in patients with rheumatoid arthritis: a randomized crossover trial, *Arthritis Care Res* 61:1025, 2009.

131. Waldburger JM, Firestein GS: Rheumatoid arthritis epidemiology, pathology, and pathogenesis. In Klippel JH, Stone JH, Crofford LJ, White PH, editors: *Primer on the rheumatic diseases* ed 13, New York, 2008, Springer.

132. Weiss S, LaStayo P, Mills A, Bramlet D: Prospective analysis of splinting the carpometacarpal joint: an objective, subjective, and radiographic assessment, *J Hand Ther* 13:218, 2000.

133. Weiss S, Lastayo P, Mills A, Bramlet D: Splinting the degenerative basal joint: custom-made or prefabricated neoprene? *J Hand Ther* 17:401, 2004.

134. Welch V, et al: Thermotherapy for treating rheumatoid arthritis, *Cochrane Database Syst Rev*, 2002:CD002826, 2002.

135. Westby MD, Minor MA: Exercise and physical activity. In Bartlett SJ, editor: *Clinical care in the rheumatic diseases* ed 3,

Atlanta, GA, 2006, Association of Rheumatology Health Professionals.

136. White PH, Chang RW: Public health and arthritis: a growing imperative. In Klippel JH, Stone JH, Crofford LJ, White PH, editors: *Primer on the rheumatic diseases* ed 13, New York, 2008, Springer.

137. Wickersham BA: The exercise program. In Riggs MA, Gall EP, editors: *Rheumatic diseases: rehabilitation and management, Boston*, 1984, Butterworth.

138. Wilske KR, Healey LA: Remodeling the pyramid: a concept whose time has come, *J Rheumatol* 16:565, 1989.

139. Wright GE, Parker JC, Smarr KL, et al: Risk factors for depression in rheumatoid arthritis, *Arthritis Care Res* 9:264, 1996.

140. Yasuda YL: *Occupational therapy practice guidelines for adults with rheumatoid arthritis*, ed 2, Bethesda, MD, 2001, American Occupational Therapy Association.

SUGGESTED READINGS

Lorig K, Fries JF, editors: *The arthritis helpbook* ed 6, Cambridge, MA, 2006, Da Capo Press.

Melvin JL: *Osteoarthritis: caring for your hands*, Bethesda, MD, 1995, American Occupational Therapy Association.

Melvin JL: *Rheumatoid arthritis: caring for your hands*, Bethesda, MD, 1995, American Occupational Therapy Association.

RESOURCES

American College of Rheumatology and Association of Rheumatology Health Professionals: https://www.rheumatology.org.

Arthritis Foundation: https://www.arthritis.org.

National Institute of Arthritis and Musculoskeletal and Skin Diseases: https://www.niams.nih.gov.

40

Hand and Upper Extremity Injuries

J. Martin Walsh and Nancy Chee[a]

LEARNING OBJECTIVES

After studying this chapter, the student or practitioner will be able to do the following:

1. Discuss the incidence and effect of upper extremity injuries and their effects on occupational performance.
2. Identify three upper quarter screening tests and explain their significance in developing an intervention plan.
3. Discuss the importance of joint mobility in regaining the motor performance skill of hand function.
4. Describe the four categories of tests used to evaluate peripheral nerve function and explain how the results would be used in developing an intervention plan.
5. Compare the standardized tests used to assess the motor performance skill of hand function.
6. Describe the sensory and motor innervation patterns of the three major nerves and differentiate between the effects of proximal and distal lesions in each of the nerves and how they might affect occupational performance.
7. Discuss complex regional pain syndrome and the intervention approaches that should be included in the occupational therapy intervention plan for that disorder.
8. Compare techniques used in the rehabilitation of tendon injuries.
9. Describe the significance of edema with regard to wound healing and joint mobility.
10. Discuss the role of the occupational therapist in the evaluation and rehabilitation of injured workers.

CHAPTER OUTLINE

KEY TERMS

Complex regional pain syndrome
Cumulative trauma disorders
Edema
Ergonomic
Functional capacity evaluation

Orthotics
Peripheral nerve injuries
Provocative tests
Tendon injuries
Upper quadrant

[a] The authors wish to acknowledge the late Mary C. Kasch, OTR/L, CHT, FAOTA, Occupational Therapist, and former Executive Director of the Hand Therapy Certification Commission, whose personal encouragement and foundation work were essential to the original version of this chapter and throughout all subsequent editions of this publication.

Gerry, Part 1

Gerry, 32 years old (prefers use of the pronouns he/him/his), is self-employed as a cabinetmaker. He sustained a table saw injury to his nondominant left hand while working. The thumb, index, and middle fingers of Gerry's left hand were amputated at the level of the proximal phalanges as a result of the saw injury and were subsequently replanted by a hand surgeon using microsurgical techniques. Gerry is single, lives with a roommate, and is in business with his father in a small but busy cabinet shop. Gerry is extremely active at work and during his free time. He is very social and has an extensive network of supportive friends and family.

Gerry was referred to hand therapy as an inpatient 5 days after the replantation surgeries as soon as he was discontinued from the anticoagulation medications. The initial interview between Gerry and his occupational therapist/certified hand therapist (OT/CHT) was performed at bedside. He was to be discharged from the hospital the following day with instructions to return for outpatient hand therapy. A protective orthosis was fabricated on the first therapy session, and Gerry was instructed on his postsurgical precautions, wound care, and dressing changes. During the initial evaluation, Gerry stated that he was very distressed about the potential loss of function of his left hand and that he wanted to accomplish three of his most valued occupations in the months to come. The first occupation was to return to work with his father making cabinets in the family business, the second was to resume playing golf, and the third was to be able to prepare his own meals so that he would not have to rely on family and friends to do this for him. The first occupation was one he valued as a source of livelihood and as a profession in which he demonstrated great skill and derived joy. The second occupation was important to him not only as a source of relaxation but, more importantly, as a primary venue for social interaction with friends and family. The third occupation was something that he also enjoyed and would allow him to be more independent.

Gerry initiated hand therapy in the hospital during the acute phase of his recovery. He was followed in hand therapy for 15 months from the date of his injury, and through several additional surgeries and throughout all phases of his rehabilitative process: the acute or immobilization phase, the intermediate or mobilization phase, and the late or strengthening phase. During the initial evaluation, Gerry clearly expressed a desire to return to three specific occupations of value to him: working as a cabinetmaker, playing golf, and preparing his own meals.

Critical Thinking Questions

1. How will the intervention plan change over the course of Gerry's recovery? What specific intervention approaches will be used during the three phases of his recovery?
2. What specific tools or instruments will be used to assess Gerry's performance skills during the different phases of his recovery?
3. What are some of the specific preparatory methods and purposeful activities that may be used in preparation for Gerry's occupation-based performance activity of cabinetmaker?

training in physical and psychological assessment, prosthetic evaluation, fabrication of orthoses, assessment and training in the activities of daily living (ADLs), and functional restoration is uniquely qualified to treat upper extremity (UE) disorders.

Hand rehabilitation, or hand therapy, has grown as a specialty area of occupational therapy (OT) and physical therapy (PT). Many of the intervention techniques used with hand-injured clients have evolved from the application of therapy and knowledge of both specialties to be used by the hand therapist. It is not the purpose of this chapter to instruct the OT student in physical agent modalities. Rather, intervention techniques that have been found to be beneficial to clients with hand injuries are presented. It is assumed that therapists best trained to provide them will provide these techniques.

As used in this chapter, *hand therapy* is a term that includes intervention of the entire upper quadrant, which includes the scapula, shoulder, and arm. **Upper quadrant** and UE are used interchangeably. UE rehabilitation requires advanced and specialized training by both occupational therapists (OTs) and physical therapists (PTs). A practice analysis study of the theory and knowledge that serves as the underpinning for hand therapy has been reported.[60] Intervention techniques, whether thermal modalities or specifically designed exercises, are used as a bridge to reach a further goal of restoring functional performance. Thus, some modalities may be used as adjunctive or enabling modalities in preparation for functional use. It is within this context that intervention techniques are presented in this chapter.

Intervention for the injured UE is a matter of timing and judgment. After trauma or surgery, a healing phase must occur in which the body performs its physiologic function of wound healing. After the initial healing phase, when cellular restoration has been accomplished, the wound enters its restorative phase. It is in this phase that hand therapy is most beneficial. Early intervention that occurs in this restorative phase is ideal and, in some cases, essential for optimal results.

Although sample timetables may be presented, the therapist should always coordinate the application of any intervention with the referring physician. Surgical techniques may vary, and inappropriate treatment of the client with hand injury can result in failure of a surgical procedure.

Communication among the surgeon, therapist, and client is especially vital in this setting. A comfortable environment that allows group interaction may increase client motivation and cooperation. The presence of the therapist as an instructor and evaluator is essential, but without the client's cooperation,

The hand is vital to human function and appearance. It flexes, extends, opposes, and grasps thousands of times daily, allowing the performance of necessary daily activities. The hand's sensibility allows feeling without looking and provides protection from injury. The hand touches, gives comfort, and expresses emotions. Loss of hand function through injury or disease thus affects much more than the mechanical tasks that the hand performs. Hand injury may jeopardize a family's livelihood and, at the least, affects every daily activity. The occupational therapist (OT) with

OT PRACTICE NOTES

Hand therapy is provided in a number of intervention settings, ranging from private therapy offices to outpatient rehabilitation clinics and hospitals or even in the workplace. Reimbursement for services may come directly from the client or through private medical insurance, workers' compensation insurance, or a variety of managed care programs. Changes in reimbursement have driven changes in the marketplace and employment patterns. In the future, OT will be provided in a variety of new settings and OT intervention will continue to evolve.

limited gains will be achieved. Treating the psychological loss suffered by the client with a hand injury is also an integral part of the rehabilitative therapy.

In UE rehabilitation, changes have included changes in delivery of services. In some cases, therapists are not members of the approved provider panel and are no longer able to treat clients who are members of a health maintenance organization. Reimbursement patterns have altered the provision of services by limiting the number of visits authorized. Therapists are also being asked to provide functional outcome data that support the need for services. They also need high-quality information on which to base clinical decisions, which points to the need for evidence-based practice.

Evidence-based practice uses the best evidence in conjunction with clinical expertise and patient values to make clinical decisions.[65] It is likely that outcome-based or evidence-based intervention plans with functional goals and analysis of goal achievement will become the standard for the reimbursement of OT services. In addition, client satisfaction and perception of health status have become crucial in the delivery of medical care in a consumer-based economy. Continuous quality improvement documentation is often required for participation in managed care programs. With fewer authorized visits, the therapist must be more adept in instructing the client in self-management of the condition being treated. Hand therapists and rehabilitation providers are also subject to intense scrutiny and review by multiple regulatory agencies. Insurance companies and government agencies also review patient records and billing documentation. In addition, reimbursement for therapy services relies on detailed documentation of services provided and reassessments on need for ongoing services. The best way to ensure compliance with all of these agencies is to perform frequent reviews of patients' medical records in the form of chart reviews. Presently and continuing into the future, occupational therapists should anticipate a greater need to justify intervention as part of the national challenge to control medical costs. Aides, certified assistants, and other support personnel are being used increasingly, but the quality of services provided must continue to meet all professional and ethical standards. This climate of change also presents unique opportunities for the occupational therapist. Clinical specialists are finding new roles as consultants and trainers. Just as the OT teaches the client to adapt to changes in health status, the OT profession will need to continue to adapt to social and economic changes to remain a leader in health management.

EXAMINATION AND EVALUATION

Using a client-centered approach, the occupational therapist must gather information about the client's occupational history, including a detailed description from the client's perspective of how the hand injury may interfere with the resumption of daily life activities that are most important to them. Developing this occupational profile includes considerations of a client's performance of daily tasks and their interests, values, and needs.[3] Armed with this occupational profile, the therapist and client continue the evaluation process. The therapist must be able to

evaluate the nature of the injury and the limitations it has produced. First, the injured structures must be identified by consulting with the hand surgeon, reviewing operative reports and x-ray films, and discussing the injury with the client. Assessment of the wound, bone, tendon, and nerve function must be ascertained, using standardized assessment techniques whenever possible.

The client's age, occupation, and hand dominance should be considered in the initial evaluation. The type and extent of medical and surgical treatment that has been received and the length of time since such interventions are important in determining an intervention plan. Any further surgery or conservative intervention that is planned should also be noted. A written intervention plan should have the approval of the referring physician. Most physicians welcome observations and evaluation-based recommendations from the therapist regarding the client's care.

The purposes of hand evaluation are to identify physical limitations, such as loss of range of motion (ROM); functional limitations, such as an inability to perform daily tasks[5]; substitution patterns to compensate for loss of sensibility or motor function; and abnormalities, such as joint contracture.

The movement of the arm and hand must be coordinated for maximal function. Shoulder motion is essential for positioning the hand and elbow for daily activities.[25,29,71] The wrist is the key joint in the position of function.[29,96] Skilled hand performance depends on wrist stability. Although a mobile wrist is preferable, function is possible as long as the wrist is positioned to maximize movement of the fingers. Function also depends on arm and shoulder stability and mobility for fixing or positioning the hand for activity. The thumb is of greater importance than any other digit. Effective pinch is almost impossible without a thumb, and attempts will be made to salvage or reconstruct an injured thumb whenever possible. Within the hand the proximal interphalangeal (PIP) joint is critical for grasp and is considered to be the most important small joint. Limitations in flexion or extension will result in significant functional impairment.

The hand therapy evaluation should, therefore, consist of two concurrent stages. One stage consists of assessing the client's occupational profile to help the therapist select an effective intervention that addresses the client's occupational priorities. The other stage of the hand therapy evaluation consists of assessing specific performance skills, such as coordination and strength, and client factors, such as sensory functions, neuromusculoskeletal and movement-related functions, and the functions of the hand and related structures. Evaluating both the client's occupational profile and the client's performance skills ensures that the client's priorities are addressed and makes the intervention more meaningful.

Observation and Topographic Assessment

The occupational therapist should observe the appearance of the entire UE. The position of the hand and arm at rest and in the carrying posture can yield valuable information about the dysfunction. The therapist should observe the way that the client treats the disease or injury. The therapist should note if the hand and arm are overprotected, carefully guarded, or ignored and if the client carries the arm close to the body in an awkward posture or even covered.

The cervical and shoulder area posture should be observed for evidence of abnormalities in cervical and thoracic curvature that may reduce the potential for shoulder movement. Muscle atrophy may be evident in the scapular area if there has been significant long-term weakness or if the rotator cuff is torn. The scapula may appear asymmetric or altered if muscle imbalances of length or strength are present.

The skin condition of the hand and arm should be noted. In particular, the therapist should note any lacerations, sutures, or evidence of recent surgery; whether the skin is dry or moist; whether scales or crusts are present; and whether the hand appears swollen or has an odor. Palmar skin is less mobile than dorsal skin normally. The therapist should determine the degree of mobility and elasticity and the adherence of scars. The therapist should also observe trophic changes in the skin. To assess the vascular system, the therapist should observe the skin color and temperature of the hand and evaluate for the presence of edema (swelling). Any contractures of the web spaces should be noted. The therapist should observe the relationship between hand and arm function as the client moves about and performs test items or tasks.

The therapist should ask the client to perform some simple bilateral ADLs, such as buttoning a button, putting on a shirt, opening a jar, and threading a needle, and observe the amount of spontaneous movement and use of the affected hand and arm. Similar screening tests can be used to determine shoulder mobility, such as reaching overhead, as well as placing the hand behind the back and behind the head simulating self-care and hygiene activities.

Assessment of Performance Skills and Client Factors

A number of standardized tests can be used to determine physical limitations in the UE. Joint measurement and manual muscle testing are crucial and are described in other chapters (see Chapters 21 and 22). Special tests used by the hand therapist are described here in a general sense, but the student should consult other textbooks for detailed instructions in such areas as assessment of adverse neural tension.[19]

Screening the Cervical Neck and Shoulder

Screening examination of the cervical neck and shoulder regions should be included in evaluation of hand conditions to determine whether these areas are contributing to the client's symptoms or limitations in function.

Active movements of the neck should be conducted, with attention paid to complaints of UE symptoms during cervical extension or lateral flexion to the same side. Complaints during these movements may suggest nerve root irritation. Hand symptoms with opposite side bending may be a sign of adverse neural tension. Few occupational therapists are knowledgeable in the intervention of cervical conditions, and care must be taken not to aggravate an existing condition. The therapist should return the client to the referring physician with recommendations for referral to an appropriate practitioner if the results of this testing are positive.

Assessment of Movement

The effect of trauma or dysfunction on anatomic structures is the first consideration in evaluating hand function. The joints must be assessed for active and passive mobility, fixed deformities, and any tendency to assume a position of deformity. The ligaments must be assessed for laxity or contracture and their ability to maintain joint stability. Tendons must be examined for integrity, contracture, or overstretching; muscles are tested for strength and function.[36]

Limited Movement in the Shoulder

Examples of conditions in the shoulder region leading to reduced strength, reduced ROM, or pain in the shoulder are outlined in Table 40.1. Comparing initial responses with the results of follow-up evaluation will help document a positive response to intervention. Patterns of impairments in UE ROM and strength, as well as a positive response to provocative testing, should be reported to the referring physician if they would affect the client's planned intervention or outcome. Therapists must not attempt to treat conditions that are beyond their scope of knowledge. Referral to an appropriate practitioner should be discussed with the physician if indicated.

Impingement tests. Shoulder impingement syndrome is a common shoulder injury in which tendons of the rotator cuff are pinched or impinged as they pass between the humerus and the acromion. To test for shoulder impingement, the examiner

TABLE 40.1 Clinical Tests for Specific Dysfunction in the Shoulder		
Condition	**Pattern of Impairment**	**Characteristic Findings/Special Tests**
Adhesive capsulitis	Loss of active and passive shoulder motion with the most pronounced loss in external rotation and, to a lesser degree, abduction and internal rotation	• Capsular end feel to passive motions in restricted planes of movement
Subacromial impingement	Painful arc of motion between approximately 80 and 100 degrees elevation or at end range of active elevation	• In early stages, muscle tests may be strong and painless despite positive impingement test
Rotator cuff tendinitis	Painful active or resistive rotator cuff muscle use	• Painful manual muscle test of scapular plane abduction or external rotation • Nonpainful passive motion end ranges • Tenderness at tendons of supraspinatus or infraspinatus
Rotator cuff tear	Significant substitution of scapula with attempted arm elevation	• Positive drop arm test • Very weak, less than three-fifths abduction or external rotation

passively overpressures the client's arm into end-range elevation. This movement causes a jamming of the greater tuberosity against the anterior inferior acromial surface.[43] The test is positive if the client's facial expression shows pain. An alternative test is described by Hawkins and Kennedy.[52] The examiner forward flexes the arm to 90 degrees then forcibly internally rotates the arm. Pain indicates a positive test result.

Drop arm test. To assess a suspected rotator cuff injury or tear, particularly of the supraspinatus tendon, the client's arm is passively abducted by the examiner to 90 degrees with the client's palm down. The client is then asked to lower the arm actively. Pain or inability to lower the arm smoothly with good motor control is considered a positive test result.[43]

Soft-Tissue Tightness

Joints may develop dysfunction after trauma, immobilization, or disuse. Joint play or accessory motions are described as movements that are abnormal and physiological and can only be made with help from someone else.[53] Examples of accessory motions are joint rotation and joint distraction. If accessory motions are limited and painful, the active motions of that joint cannot be normal. Therefore, it is necessary to restore joint play through the use of joint mobilization techniques before attempting passive or active ROM.[53]

Joint mobilization may date back to the fourth century BC, when Hippocrates first described the use of spinal traction. In the 1930s, an English physician, James Mennell, encouraged physicians to perform manipulation without anesthesia. Current theorists include Cyriax, Robert Maigne, F.M. Kaltenborn, G.D. Maitland, Stanley Paris, and John Mennell, son of the late James Mennell. Although physicians originally practiced manipulation, therapists have adapted the techniques, which are now called joint mobilization.[42]

The techniques used to assess joint play are also used in the treatment of joint dysfunction. During assessment the evaluator determines the range of accessory motion and the presence of pain by taking up the slack only in the joint. Some practitioners advocate use of a high-velocity, low-amplitude thrust or graded oscillation to regain motion and relieve pain.[62]

Guidelines must be followed in applying joint mobilization techniques, and the untrained or inexperienced practitioner should not attempt to use the techniques. Postgraduate courses are offered in joint mobilization of the extremities, and the therapist must be familiar with the osteokinematics of each joint and the techniques used.

Joint mobilization is generally indicated with restriction of accessory motions or the presence of pain caused by tightness of the joint capsule, meniscus displacement, muscle guarding, ligamentous tightness, or adherence. It is contraindicated in the presence of infection, recent fracture, neoplasm, joint inflammation, rheumatoid arthritis, osteoporosis, degenerative joint disease, and many chronic diseases.

Limitations in joint motion also may be caused by tightness of the extrinsic or intrinsic muscles and tendons. If the joint capsule is not tight and accessory motions are normal, the therapist should test for extrinsic and intrinsic tightness.

To test for extrinsic extensor tightness, the metacarpophalangeal (MP) joint is passively held in extension and the PIP joint is moved passively into flexion. Then the MP joint is flexed, and the PIP joint is again passively flexed. If the PIP joint can be flexed easily when the MP joint is extended but not when the MP joint is flexed, the extrinsic extensors are adherent.[36]

If there is extrinsic flexor tightness, the PIP and distal interphalangeal (DIP) joints will be positioned in flexion, with the MP joints held in extension. It will not be possible to pull the fingers into complete extension. If the wrist is then held in flexion, the IP joints will extend more easily because slack is placed on the flexor tendons.

Tightness of the intrinsic musculature is tested by passively holding the MP joint in extension and applying pressure just distal to the PIP joint. This action is repeated with the MP joint in flexion. If there is more resistance when the MP joint is extended, intrinsic tightness is indicated.[36]

If passive motion of the PIP joint remains the same whether the MP joint is held in extension or flexion and there is limitation of PIP joint flexion in any position, tightness of the joint capsule is indicated. The therapist should assess the joint for capsular tightness if this has not already been done.

Provocative tests used to assess ligament, capsule, and joint instability are summarized in Table 40.2. For more detailed and comprehensive information regarding administration of these tests, the reader is referred to textbooks dedicated solely to hand therapy or to the specific topic.[15,36]

Assessment of Peripheral Nerve Status

Nerve dysfunction can occur at any point from the nerve roots through the digital nerves in the fingers. A good understanding of the peripheral nervous system is essential for appropriate treatment of the UE. Determining the approximate location of nerve dysfunction can assist in intervention planning.

Categories of tests. A variety of tests may be required to assess nerve function adequately. These tests can be divided into four categories: (1) modality tests for pain, heat, cold, and touch pressure; (2) functional tests to assess the quality of sensibility, or what Moberg[77] described as "tactile gnosis"; (3) objective tests that do not require active participation by the client; (4) and provocative tests that reproduce symptoms.

Examples of functional tests are stationary and moving two-point discrimination and the Moberg pick-up test; objective tests include the wrinkle test, the ninhydrin sweat test, and nerve-conduction studies.[34] Electrodiagnostic testing is the most conclusive and widely accepted method of determining nerve dysfunction.

Provocative tests are highly suggestive of a nerve lesion if results are positive but do not rule out a problem if results are negative. Tests of nerve dysfunction are summarized in Table 40.3. Instructions for administration of the most common tests are described in the following paragraphs.

Adson maneuver. The examiner palpates the radial pulse on the arm to be tested. The client then rotates the head toward the arm being tested. The client then extends the head and holds a deep breath while the arm is being laterally rotated and extended. Disappearance or slowing of pulse rate is considered a positive test result suggesting presence of thoracic outlet syndrome.[1,21,71]

TABLE 40.2   Clinical Tests for Specific Dysfunction in the Wrist

Condition	Pattern of Impairment	Special Tests
Thumb ulnar collateral ligament (gamekeeper's or skier's thumb)	Pain and instability of the thumb MP joint	• Movement greater than 35 degrees when valgus instability stress is applied to the thumb MP joint
Instability of the scaphoid	Pain in the area of the scaphoid bone (anatomic snuffbox) or "clunking" with movement of the wrist	• Watson test • Pain or sound associated with subluxation of the dorsal pole of the scaphoid while performing test
Instability of the distal radioulnar joint	Pain and tenderness in the wrist	• "Piano keys" test • Hypermobility and pain associated with pressure on the distal ulna
Lunate dislocation	Pain or instability in the central wrist	• Murphy's sign • Head of the third metacarpal level with the second and fourth metacarpals while making a fist
Lunotriquetral instability	Pain or instability in the central or ulnar wrist	• Lunotriquetral ballottement test • Crepitus; laxity or pain with isolated movement of the lunate
TFCC tear	Pain and instability in the ulnar wrist	• Wrist arthrogram or MRI • Piano key sign test • Press test • Ulna fovea test

MP, Metacarpophalangeal; *MRI*, magnetic resonance imaging; *TFCC*, triangular fibrocartilage complex tear.

TABLE 40.3   Clinical Tests for Specific Nerve Dysfunction in the Upper Extremity

Condition	Pattern of Impairment	Characteristic Findings/Special Tests
Thoracic outlet syndrome	Nonspecific paresthesias or heaviness with sustained positioning or activity above shoulder level or behind the plane of the body	• Adson test • Roos test
Adverse neural tension	Nonspecific pain or paresthesias with reaching in positions that place tension on brachial plexus nerves	• Positive upper limb screening test
Carpal tunnel syndrome	Pain and numbness, primarily in the thumb, index, and middle fingers Usually worse at night and may be associated with activity	• Tinel's sign at the wrist • Phalen's test • Reverse Phalen's test • Carpal compression test
Cubital tunnel syndrome	Compression of ulnar nerve at elbow	• Elbow flexion test
Ulnar nerve paralysis	Paralysis of the adductor pollicis muscle	• Froment's sign • Jeanne's sign • Wartenberg's sign

authors. The occupational therapist should use this screening process to rule out or confirm the involvement of more proximal structures.

The client is positioned supine, and the examiner takes the client's arm into abduction and external rotation behind the coronal plane at the shoulder. The shoulder girdle is fixed in depression. The elbow is then passively extended with the wrist in extension and the forearm in supination. Symptoms of stretch or ache in the cubital fossa or tingling in the thumb and first three fingers indicate tension on the median nerve. Lateral flexion of the neck to the opposite side will amplify symptoms by increasing tension on the dura mater. Elbow extension ROM should be compared with the uninvolved side to indicate the degree of restriction.[18,71]

Tinel's sign.   The test is performed by tapping gently along the course of a peripheral nerve, starting distally and moving proximally to elicit a tingling sensation in the fingertip. The point at which tapping begins to elicit a tingling sensation is noted and indicates the approximate location of nerve compression. This test is also used after nerve repair to determine the extent of sensory axon growth.[80]

Phalen's test and reverse Phalen's test.   Phalen's test is performed by fully flexing the wrists with the dorsum of the hands pressing against each other. Reverse Phalen's is performed by holding the hands in the "prayer" position for 1 minute. The test results are positive for median nerve irritation or compression at the wrist if the client reports tingling in the median nerve

Roos test.   In this test the client maintains a position of bilateral arm abduction to 90 degrees, shoulder external rotation, and elbow flexion to 90 degrees for 3 minutes while slowly alternating between an open hand and a clenched fist. Inability to maintain this position for the full 3 minutes or onset of symptoms is considered a positive test result for thoracic outlet syndrome.[80]

Upper limb tension test (brachial plexus tension test).   This test is designed to screen for symptoms that are produced when tension stress is placed on the brachial plexus. The maneuver described primarily stresses the median nerve and C5-C7 nerve roots. Adverse neural tension in the ulnar or radial nerves also may be tested. However, we have found that using the median nerve test as a screening device establishes a marker against which to gauge the success of intervention. Although some authors recommend using the neural tension tests for intervention as well as assessment, this has not been the practice of the

distribution (thumb, index, middle and radial aspect of ring finger) within 1 minute.[80]

Carpal compression test. The examiner places pressure over the median nerve in the carpal tunnel for up to 30 seconds. The test result is positive for possible carpal tunnel syndrome if tingling occurs in the median nerve distribution. The combination of wrist flexion and compression of the median nerve for 20 seconds has been found to be more sensitive than other provocative tests used alone.[47,80,90]

Elbow flexion test. The elbow flexion test is used to screen for cubital tunnel syndrome (compression of the ulnar nerve in the cubital tunnel). The client is asked to fully flex the elbows with the wrists fully extended for a period of 3 to 5 minutes. The test result is positive if tingling is reported in the ulnar nerve distribution of the forearm and hand (ulnar ring finger and small finger).[34]

Quick tests for motor function in the peripheral nerves. The ulnar nerve may be tested by asking the client to pinch with the thumb and index finger and palpating the first dorsal interosseous muscle. Another test for ulnar nerve paralysis involves asking a client to grasp a piece of paper between the thumb and index finger. When the examiner pulls away the paper, the tip of the thumb flexes because of absence of the adductor pollicis muscle (Froment's sign). If the MP joint of the thumb also extends at the same time, it is known as Jeanne's sign. Wartenberg's sign for ulnar nerve compression is positive if the client is unable to adduct the small finger when the hand is placed palm down on the table with the fingers passively abducted.

The radial nerve may be tested by asking the client to extend the wrist and fingers. Median nerve function is tested by asking the client to oppose the thumb to the fingers and flex the fingers.[72]

Sensory mapping. Detailed sensibility testing can begin with sensory mapping of the entire volar surface of the hand.[10,70] The hand must be supported by the examiner's hand or be resting in a medium such as therapy putty to stabilize the hand during testing. The examiner draws a probe, usually the eraser end of a pencil, lightly over the skin from the area of normal sensibility to the area of abnormal sensibility. The client must immediately report the exact location where the sensation changes. This is done from proximal to distal and radial and ulnar to medial directions. The areas are carefully marked and transferred to a permanent record. Mapping should be repeated at monthly intervals during nerve regeneration.

Sympathetic function. Recovery of sympathetic response such as sudomotor (sweating), vasomotor (temperature discrimination), pilomotor (gooseflesh), and trophic (skin texture, nail, and hair growth) may occur early but does not correlate with functional recovery.[40] O'Riain observed that denervated skin does not wrinkle. Therefore, nerve function may be tested by immersing the hand in water for 5 minutes and noting the presence or absence of skin wrinkling. This test may be especially helpful in diagnosing a nerve lesion in young children. The ability to sweat is also lost with a nerve lesion. A Ninhydrin test evaluates sweating of the finger.[80]

The wrinkle test and the Ninhydrin test are objective tests of sympathetic function. Recovery of sweating has not been shown to correlate with the recovery of sensation, but the absence of sweating correlates with the lack of discriminatory sensation. Other signs of sympathetic dysfunction are smooth, shiny skin; nail changes; and "pencil-pointing" or tapering of the fingers.[40]

Nerve compression and nerve regeneration. Sensibility testing is performed to assess the recovery of a nerve after laceration and repair, as well as to determine the presence of a nerve compression syndrome and the return of nerve function after surgical decompression or the efficacy of conservative intervention to reduce compression. Therefore, tests such as vibratory tests may be interpreted differently, depending on the mechanism of nerve dysfunction. In the following section, tests are described, and differences drawn as appropriate to assist the therapist in selecting the correct assessment technique and in planning treatment based on the evaluative measures.

During the first 2 to 4 months after nerve suture, axons regenerate and travel through the hand at a rate of about 1 mm/day, or 1 inch (2.54 cm) per month. Tinel's sign may be used to follow this regeneration. As regeneration occurs, hypoesthesia develops. Although this hypersensitivity may be uncomfortable for the client, it is a positive sign of nerve growth. An intervention program for desensitization of hypersensitive areas can be initiated as soon as the skin is healed and can tolerate gentle rubbing and immersion in textures. Desensitization is discussed further in the intervention section.

Vibration. Dellon was an early advocate of the use of 30-cycles-per-second (30-cps) and 256-cps tuning forks for assessing the return of vibratory sensation after nerve repair, as regeneration occurs, and as a guideline for initiating a sensory reeducation program.[32,33,35] However, many clinicians found that use of a tuning fork was not discrete enough to detect sensory abnormalities.

Lundborg et al. have described the use of commercial vibrometers to detect abnormal sensation.[69] This method was less subjective and thought to be more reliable. In a study of induced median nerve compression, Gelberman et al. found that vibration and touch perception as measured by the Semmes-Weinstein monofilaments are altered before two-point discrimination because they measure a single nerve fiber innervating a group of receptor cells.[46,47] Two-point discrimination is a test of innervation density that requires overlapping sensory units and cortical integration. Thus, two-point discrimination is altered after nerve laceration and repair but remains normal if the nerve is compressed, as long as there are links to the cortex. Bell-Krotoski et al. have also found normal two-point values in the presence of decreased sensory function.[9,10]

Vibration and the Semmes-Weinstein test are more sensitive in picking up a gradual decrease in nerve function in the presence of nerve compression where the nerve circuitry is intact. They also correlate with decreases in the potential amplitude of sensory nerve action as measured by nerve conduction studies.[9,10,89] Therefore, Semmes-Weinstein and electrical testing are reliable and sensitive tests for early detection of carpal tunnel syndrome and other nerve compression syndromes. Semmes-Weinstein can be performed in the clinic with no discomfort to the client and is an excellent screening tool when nerve compression is suspected.

Touch pressure. Moving touch is tested using the eraser end of a pencil. The eraser is placed in an area of normal sensibility and, with application of light pressure, is moved to the distal fingertip. The client notes when the perception of the stimulus changes. Light and heavy stimuli may be applied and noted.[34] Constant touch is tested by pressing with the eraser end of a pencil, first in an area with normal sensibility and then placing the eraser distally by lifting up the pencil before placement. The client responds when the stimulus is altered; again, light and heavy stimuli may be applied.[34]

The Semmes-Weinstein monofilaments are the most accurate instruments for assessing cutaneous pressure thresholds.[10,55] The original testing equipment consisted of 20 nylon monofilaments housed in plastic handheld rods. Many therapists today use the smaller five-pack filaments. These five monofilaments correspond to the categories of light touch sensation described later. The diameter of the monofilaments increases, and when applied correctly, they exert a force ranging from 4.5 mg to 447 g. Markings on the probes range from 1.65 to 6.65 but do not correspond to the grams of force of each rod. Normal fingertip sensibility has been found to correspond to the 2.44 and 2.83 probes.

The monofilaments must be applied perpendicularly to the skin and are applied just until the monofilament bends. The skin should not blanch when the monofilament is applied. Probes 1.65 through 2.83 are bounced three times. Probes marked 3.22 to 4.08 are applied three times with a bend in the filament, and probes marked 4.17 to 6.65 are applied once. The larger monofilaments do not bend; therefore, skin color must be observed to determine how firmly to apply the probe.

The examiner should begin with a probe in the normal range and progress through the rods in increasing diameters to find the client's threshold for touch throughout the volar surface.[9,10,55] A grid should be used to record the responses so that varying areas of touch perception can be demonstrated. Two correct responses in three applications are necessary for an area to be considered to have intact sensibility. It is preferable to place the monofilaments randomly rather than to concentrate on an area, to allow the nerves recovery time. When a filament is placed three times, it should be held for a second, rested for a second, and reapplied. Results can be graded from normal light touch (probes 2.83 and above) to loss of protective sensation (probes 4.56 and below). Diminished light touch and diminished protective sensation are in the range reflected by the central probes (probes 3.22 to 4.31).[10,55]

Two-point and moving two-point discrimination. Discrimination, the second level of sensibility assessment, requires the subject to distinguish between two direct stimuli. Static or stationary two-point discrimination measures the slowly adapting fibers. The two-point discrimination test, first described by Weber in 1853, was modified and popularized by Moberg,[77] who was interested in a tool that would assess the functional level of sensation. A variety of devices have been proposed to use in measuring two-point discrimination. The bent paper clip is inexpensive but often has burrs on the metal tip. Other devices include industrial calipers and/or devices with parallel prongs of variable distance and blunted ends

that should produce replicable results. The test is performed as follows[34,68]:

1. The client's vision is occluded.
2. An area of normal sensation is tested as a reference, using blunt calipers or a bent paper clip.
3. The calipers are set 10 mm apart and are randomly applied, starting at the fingertip and moving proximally and longitudinally in line with the digital nerves, with one or two points touching. The caliper should not blanch the skin.
4. The distance is decreased until the client no longer feels two distinct points, and that distance is measured.

Between 3 and 4 seconds should be allowed between applications, and the client should have four correct responses in five administrations. Because this test indicates sensory function, it is usually administered at the tips of the fingers. It may be used proximally to test nerve regeneration. Normal two-point discrimination at the fingertip is 6 mm or less.

Moving two-point discrimination measures the innervation density of the quickly adapting nerve fibers for touch. It is slightly more sensitive than stationary two-point discrimination. The test is performed as follows[34]:

1. The client's vision is occluded.
2. An area of normal sensation is tested as a reference, using blunt calipers or a bent paper clip.
3. The fingertip is supported by the examining table or the examiner's hand.
4. The caliper, separated 5 to 8 mm, is moved longitudinally from proximal to distal in a linear fashion along the surface of the fingertip. One and two points are randomly alternated. The client must correctly identify the stimulus in seven of eight responses before proceeding to a smaller value. The test is repeated down to a separation of 2 mm.

Two-point values increase with age in both sexes, with the smallest values occurring between the ages of 10 and 30 years. Women tend to have smaller values than men, and there is no significant difference between dominant and nondominant hands.[35] (See Chapter 23 for further information on the evaluation of sensation.)

Modified Moberg pickup test. Recognition of common objects is the final level of sensory function. Moberg used the phrase tactile gnosis to describe the ability of the hand to perform complex functions by feel. Moberg described the pick-up test in 1958, and it was later modified by Dellon.[35,77] This test is used with either a median nerve injury or an injury to a combination of median and ulnar nerves. It takes twice as long to perform the tests with vision occluded as with vision unimpaired. The test is performed as follows:

1. Nine or ten small objects (e.g., coins or paper clips) are placed on a table, and the client is asked to place them, one at a time, in a small container as quickly as possible, while looking at them. The client is timed.
2. The test is repeated for the opposite hand with vision.
3. The test is repeated for each hand with vision occluded.
4. The client is asked to identify each object one at a time, with and then without vision.

It is important to observe any substitution patterns that may be used when the client cannot see the objects.

Edema assessment. Hand volume is measured to assess the presence of extracellular or intracellular edema. Volume measurement is generally used to determine the effect of intervention and activities. By measuring volume at different times of the day, the therapist can measure the effects of rest versus activity, as well as the effects of orthotics or intervention designed to reduce edema.

A commercial volumeter may be used to assess hand edema.[30] The volumeter has been shown to be accurate to 10 mL when used in the prescribed manner.[4] Variables that have been shown to decrease the accuracy of the volumeter include the use of a faucet or hose that introduces air into the tank during filling, movement of the arm within the tank, inconsistent pressure on the stop rod, and the use of a volumeter in a variety of places. The same level surface should always be used.[4] The evaluation is performed as follows (Fig. 40.1):

1. A plastic volumeter is filled and allowed to empty into a large beaker until the water reaches spout level. The beaker is then emptied and dried thoroughly.
2. The client is instructed to immerse the hand in the plastic volumeter, being careful to keep the hand in the mid-position.
3. The hand is lowered until it rests gently between the middle and ring fingers on the dowel rod. It is important that the hand not press onto the rod.
4. The hand remains still until no more water drips into the beaker.
5. The water is poured into a graduated cylinder. The cylinder is placed on a level surface, and a reading is made.

A method of assessing edema of an individual finger or joint is circumferential measurement using either a circumference tape or jeweler's ring-size standards. For combined wrist and hand edema, a tape measure may be wrapped in a figure-of-eight pattern to measure hand size.[83] Measurements should be made before and after intervention and especially after the application of thermal modalities or orthoses. Although clients often have subjective complaints relating to swelling, objective data of circumference or volume will help the therapist to assess the response of the tissues to intervention and activity. Edema control techniques are discussed later in this chapter.

Grip and Pinch Strength

UE strength is usually assessed after the healing phase of trauma. Strength testing is not indicated after recent trauma or surgery. Testing should not be performed until the client has been cleared for full-resistive activities, usually 8 to 12 weeks after injury.

A standard adjustable-handle dynamometer is recommended for assessing grip strength (Fig. 40.2). The client should be seated with the shoulder adducted and neutrally rotated, the elbow flexed at 90 degrees, forearm in the neutral position, and wrist between 0 and 30 degrees extension and between 0 and 15 degrees of ulnar deviation. Three trials are taken of each hand, with the dynamometer handle set at the second position. The examiner should hold the dynamometer lightly to prevent accidental dropping of the instrument. A mean of the three trials should be reported.[74] The noninjured hand is used for comparison. Normative data may be used to compare strength scores.[13,61,74] Variables such as age will affect the strength measurements.[4,13]

Pinch strength should also be tested, using a pinch gauge. Two-point pinch (thumb tip to index fingertip), lateral or key pinch (thumb pulp to lateral aspect of the middle phalanx of

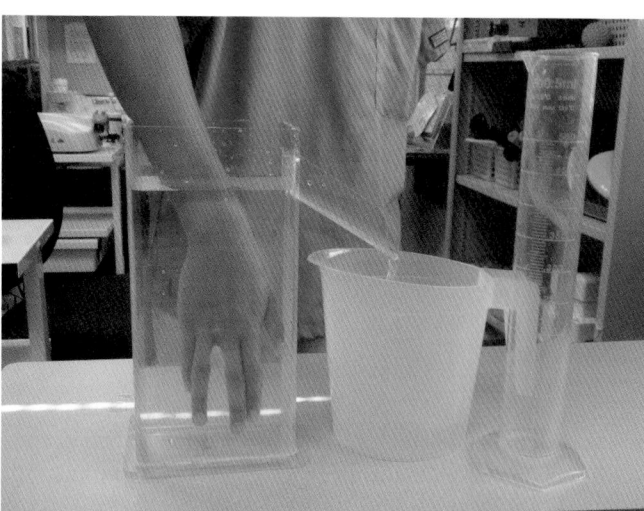

Fig. 40.1 A volumeter is used to measure the volume of both hands for comparison. Increased volume indicates the presence of edema.

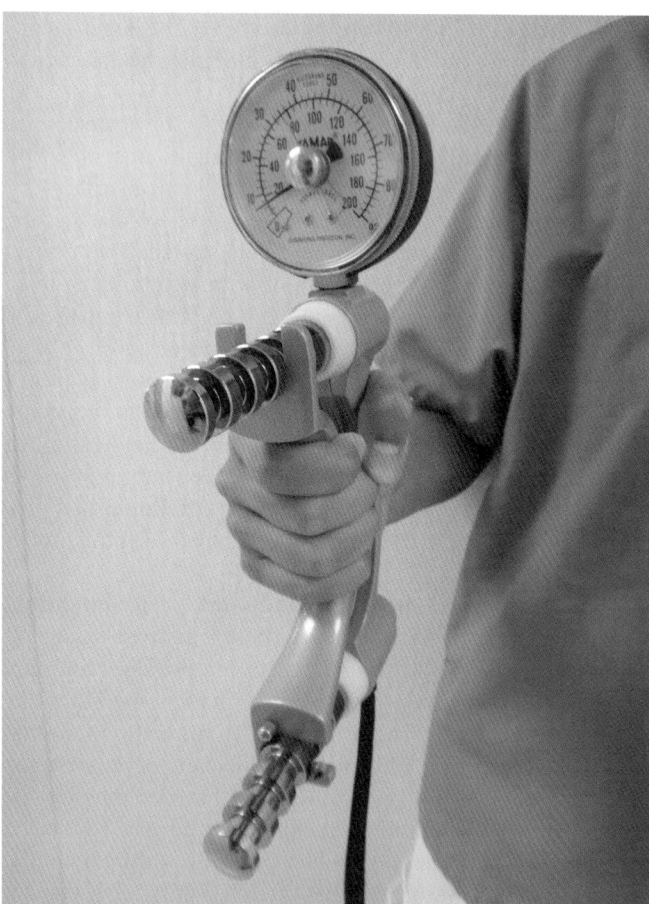

Fig. 40.2 The Jamar dynamometer is used to evaluate grip strength in both hands.

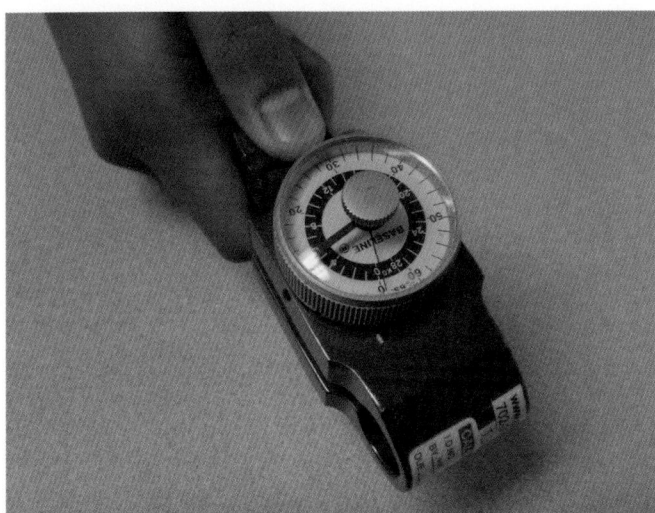

Fig. 40.3 A pinch gauge is used to evaluate pinch strength to a variety of prehension patterns of pinch.

the index finger), and three-point pinch (thumb tip to tips of index and middle fingers) should be evaluated. As with the grip dynamometer, three successive trials should be obtained and compared bilaterally (Fig. 40.3).[4]

Manual muscle testing is also used to test UE strength. Accurate assessment is especially important when the client is being prepared for tendon transfers or other reconstructive surgery. The student who wishes to study kinesiology of the UE is referred especially to Brand's work.[15] In addition, muscle testing is addressed in Chapter 22.

Maximal voluntary effort during grip, pinch, or muscle testing will be affected by pain in the hand or extremity, and the therapist should note if the client's ability to exert full force is limited by subjective complaints. Localization of the pain symptoms and consistency in noting pain will help the therapist evaluate the role that pain is playing in the recovery from injury. Pain problems are discussed in more detail later in this chapter.

Functional Assessment

Assessment of hand function or performance is important because the physical assessment does not measure the client's ingenuity and ability to compensate for loss of strength, ROM, sensation, or the presence of abnormalities.

The physical assessment should precede the functional assessment because awareness of physical dysfunction can result in a critical analysis of functional impairment and an understanding of the reasons for the hand and upper extremity dysfunction.

The occupational therapist should observe the effect of the hand dysfunction on the use of the hand during ADLs. In addition, some type of a standardized performance test, such as the Jebsen Test of Hand Function or the Quantitative Test of Upper Extremity Function,[25] should be administered. The Jebsen Test of Hand Function was developed to provide objective measurements of standardized tasks with norms for client comparison. It is a short test that is assembled by the administrator. It is easy to administer and inexpensive. The test consists of seven subtests, which test writing a short sentence, turning over 3- × 5-inch

cards, picking up small objects and placing them in a container, stacking checkers, simulated eating, moving empty large cans, and moving weighted large cans. Norms are provided for dominant and nondominant hands for each subtest and further categorized by gender and age. Instructions for assembling the test, as well as specific instructions for administering it, are provided by the authors. This has been found to be a good test for overall hand function.[7]

The Quantitative Test of Upper Extremity Function described by Carroll[25] was designed to measure ability to perform general arm and hand activities used in daily living.[7] It is based on the assumption that complex UE movements used to perform ordinary ADLs can be reduced to specific patterns of grasp and prehension of the hand, supination and pronation of the forearm, flexion and extension of the elbow, and elevation of the arm.

The test consists of six parts: grasping and lifting four blocks of graduated sizes to assess grasp; grasping and lifting two pipes of graduated sizes to test cylindrical grip; grasping and placing a ball to test spherical grasp; picking up and placing four marbles of graduated sizes to test fingertip prehension or pinch; putting a small washer over a nail and putting an iron on a shelf to test placing; and pouring water from pitcher to glass and glass to glass. In addition, to assess pronation, supination, and elevation of the arm, the therapist instructs the subject to place his or her hand on top of the head, behind the head, and to the mouth and write his or her name. The test uses simple, inexpensive, and easily acquired materials. Details of materials and their arrangement, test procedures, and scoring can be found in the original source.[7]

Other tests that are useful in the assessment of hand dexterity are the Crawford Small Parts Dexterity Test, Bennett Hand Tool Dexterity Test, the Purdue Pegboard Test, and the Minnesota Manual Dexterity Test.[7,11] The VALPAR Corporation[b] has developed a number of standardized tests that measure an individual's ability to perform work-related tasks. They provide information about the test taker's results, compared with industry performance standards. All of these tests include comparison with normal subjects working in a variety of industrial settings.

This information can be used in predicting the likelihood of successful return to a specific job. The tests are especially useful when administering a work capacity evaluation. Tests may be purchased and come with instructions for administration of the test and the standardized norms.[48] Further discussion of related assessments for vocational evaluation can be found in Chapter 14.

INTERVENTION

Fractures

In treating a hand or wrist fracture, the surgeon attempts to achieve good anatomic position through either a closed (nonoperative) or open (operative) reduction. Internal fixation with Kirschner wires, metallic plates, or screws may be used to maintain the desired position. External fixation also may be

---

[b]VALPAR Assessment Systems (available from VALPAR International, Tucson, AZ, www.valparint.com).

used with internal fixation. The hand is usually immobilized in a position of protection with wrist extension, MP joint flexion, and extension of the distal joints whenever the injury allows this position. Trauma to bone may also involve trauma to tendons and nerves in the adjacent area. Intervention must be geared toward the recovery of all injured structures, and this fact may influence treatment of the fracture.

OT may be initiated during the period of immobilization, which can begin as early as 2 to 3 weeks once cleared by the surgeon. Uninvolved fingers of the hand must be kept mobile, preventing stiffness through the use of active and passive motion. Edema should be carefully monitored and may be treated with elevation and gentle manual edema mobilization.

As soon as there is sufficient bone stability, the surgeon allows mobilization of the injured part. The surgeon should provide guidelines for the amount of resistance or force that may be applied to the fracture site. Activities that correct poor motor patterns and encourage use of the injured hand should be started as soon as the hand is pain free. Early motion will prevent the adherence of tendons and reduce edema through stimulation of the lymphatic and blood vessels.

As soon as the brace or cast is removed, the client's hand must be evaluated. If edema remains present, edema control techniques can be initiated using techniques described later in this chapter. A baseline ROM should be established, and the application of an appropriate orthosis may begin. An orthosis may be used to correct abnormal joint changes that have resulted from immobilization, or it may be used to protect the finger from additional trauma to the fracture site. An example of this type of orthotic would be the application of a Velcro "buddy" orthosis (Fig. 40.4). A dorsal block orthosis that limits full extension of the finger may be used after a fracture or dislocation of the PIP joint. A dynamic orthosis may be used to achieve full ROM or to prevent the development of further abnormal joint changes at 6 to 8 weeks after fracture.

Intraarticular fractures may result in injury to the cartilage of the joint, causing additional pain and stiffness. An x-ray examination will indicate whether the joint surface has been damaged, which might limit the treatment of the joint. Joint pain and stiffness after fracture without the presence of joint damage should be alleviated by a combination of thermal modalities, restoration of joint play, or joint mobilization and a corrective and dynamic orthosis followed by active use. Resistive exercise can be started when bony healing has been achieved.

Wrist fractures are common and may present special problems for the surgeon and therapist. Colles' fractures (dorsal displacement and angulation of the distal radius) are the most common injury to the wrist sustained from a fall on an outstretched hand (FOOSH). This may result in limitations in wrist flexion and extension, as well as pronation and supination resulting from the involvement of the distal radioulnar joint.

Conservative management of closed reduction and cast immobilization may be used if stability of the fracture can be achieved and maintained. A long arm cast extending past the elbow is applied for 2 to 3 weeks to prevent mobility of forearm rotation and wrist. A change to a shorter cast with the elbow free is then made and worn for an additional 4 to 6

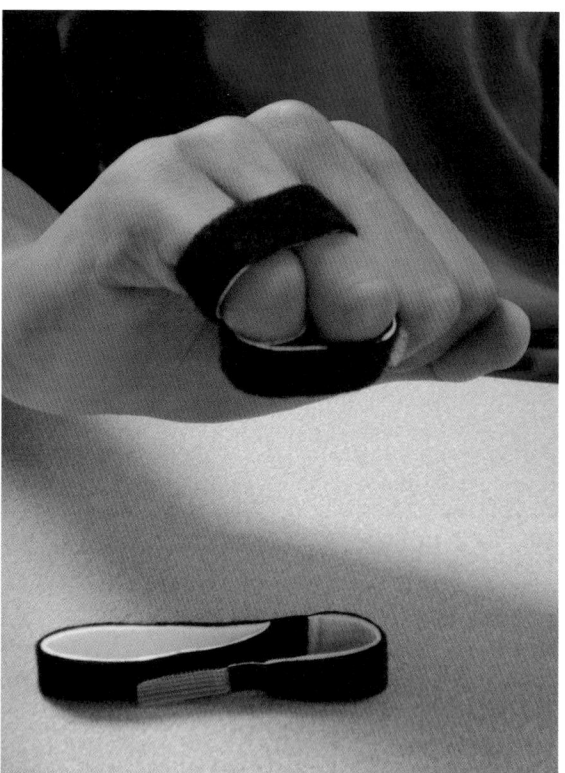

Fig. 40.4 A Velcro "buddy" orthosis may be used to protect the finger after a fracture or to encourage movement of a stiff finger.

weeks depending on fracture healing as shown on x-ray.[27] This is often considered in management of wrist fractures in young children or when surgery is not an option because of a client's medical status.

If a fracture is not reducible or is unstable, surgical strategies for repair of fractures may include internal or external fixations. With recent improvements in volar plating systems, open reduction and internal fixation (ORIF) of distal radius fractures are more commonly used to help restore the bone alignment and joint anatomy and allow for earlier motion of the wrist once cleared by the surgeon.[27,56] A wrist orthosis is applied on referral from the surgeon, and active ROM (AROM) is initiated for forearm rotation and wrist in all planes and to the unaffected fingers to prevent joint stiffness. Wear of the orthosis is gradually decreased at 3 to 6 weeks depending on bone healing on x-ray and on a client's progress with motion, strength, and return to ADLs.[27,56]

Less commonly used, external fixation may still be applied with more comminuted fractures to assist with attaining proper alignment and length of the distal radius. External fixation is drilled into both the distal radius proximally and the index metacarpal distally. Traction is then applied across the wrist to correct length and angulation and/or to reduce any other bony fragments.[86] The therapist should instruct the client in proper care of the pin sites while the fixator is in place and to perform exercise AROM of the unaffected proximal elbow, distal thumb, and fingers to prevent joint stiffness and contractures. Once the fixation is removed, an orthosis may be fabricated to further support the wrist but gradually weaned from as the client improves in ROM and strength and returns safely to ADLs.[27]

Within the eight-bone complex of the wrist itself, the scaphoid bone is the most commonly injured and is often fractured when the hand is dorsiflexed at the time of injury. Fractures to the proximal pole of the scaphoid may result in nonunion because of poor blood supply to this area. Scaphoid fractures require a prolonged period of immobilization, sometimes up to several months in a cast until osseous healing is confirmed, with resulting stiffness and pain. Care should be taken to mobilize uninvolved joints early.

Trauma to the lunate bone of the wrist may result in avascular necrosis of the lunate or Kienböck's disease, which may result from a one-time accident or repetitive trauma. Lunate fractures are usually immobilized for 6 weeks. If the fracture is unstable with loss of joint continuity, surgical intervention may be required with a bone graft, or in salvage procedures with removal of the proximal carpal row, or wrist fusion.

Stiffness and pain are common complications of fractures. The control of edema coupled with early motion and good client instruction and support will minimize these complications.

Nerve Injuries

Nerve injury may be classified into the following three categories:
1. Neurapraxia is contusion of the nerve without wallerian degeneration. The nerve recovers function without intervention within a few days or weeks.
2. Axonotmesis is an injury in which nerve fibers distal to the site of injury degenerate, but the internal organization of the nerve remains intact. No surgical intervention is necessary, and recovery usually occurs within 6 months. The length of time may vary, depending on the level of injury.
3. Neurotmesis is a complete laceration of both nerve and fibrous tissues. Surgical intervention is required. Microsurgical repair of the fascicles is common. Nerve grafting may be necessary in situations in which there is a gap between nerve endings.

Peripheral nerve injuries may occur as a result of disruption of the nerve by a fractured bone, laceration, or crush injury. Symptoms of nerve injuries include weakness or paralysis of muscles that are innervated by motor branches of the injured nerve and sensory loss to areas that are innervated by sensory branches of the injured nerve. Before evaluating the client for nerve loss, the therapist must be familiar with the muscles and areas that are innervated by the three major forearm nerves. A summary of UE peripheral neuropathic conditions can be found in Table 40.4.

Radial Nerve

The radial nerve innervates the extensor-supinator group of muscles of the forearm, including the brachioradialis, extensor carpi radialis longus, extensor carpi radialis brevis, supinator, extensor digitorum communis, extensor carpi ulnaris, extensor digiti minimi, abductor pollicis longus, extensor pollicis brevis, extensor pollicis longus, and extensor indicis proprius. The sensory distribution of the radial nerve is a strip of the posterior

upper arm and the forearm, dorsum of the thumb, index and middle fingers, and radial half of the ring finger to the PIP joints. Sensory loss of the radial nerve does not usually result in dysfunction.

Clinical signs of a high-level radial nerve injury (above the supinator) are pronation of the forearm, wrist flexion, and the thumb held in palmar abduction resulting from the unopposed action of the flexor pollicis brevis and the abductor pollicis brevis. Injury to the posterior interosseous nerve spares the extensor carpi radialis longus and brevis. Posterior interosseous nerve syndrome includes normal sensation and wrist extension with loss of finger and thumb extension. Clinical signs of low-level radial nerve injury include incomplete extension of the MP joints of the fingers and thumb. The interossei extend the interphalangeal (IP) joints of the fingers, but the MP joints rest in about 30 degrees of flexion.

A dynamic or static orthosis, applied to the dorsum of the hand, that provides wrist extension, MP extension, and thumb extension should be provided to protect the extensor tendons from overstretching during the healing phase and to position the hand for functional use (Fig. 40.5).

Median Nerve

The median nerve innervates the flexors of the forearm and hand and is often called the "eyes" of the hands because of its importance in sensory innervation of the volar surface of the thumb, index, and middle fingers. Median nerve loss may result from lacerations, as well as from compression syndromes of the wrist such as carpal tunnel syndrome.

Motor distribution of the median nerve is to the pronator teres, flexor carpi radialis, flexor pollicis longus, flexor digitorum profundus of the index and middle fingers, pronator quadratus, flexor digitorum superficialis, palmaris longus, abductor pollicis brevis, opponens pollicis, superficial head of the flexor pollicis brevis, and first and second lumbricals.

Sensory distribution of the median nerve is to the volar surface of the thumb, index, and middle fingers; radial half of the ring finger and dorsal surface of the index and middle fingers; and radial half of the ring finger distal to the PIP joints.

Clinical signs of a high-level median nerve injury are ulnar flexion of the wrist caused by loss of the flexor carpi radialis, loss of palmar abduction, and opposition of the thumb. Active pronation is absent, but the client may appear to pronate with the assistance of gravity. In a wrist-level median nerve injury, the thenar eminence appears flat and there is a loss of thumb flexion, palmar abduction, and opposition.

The sensory loss associated with median nerve injury is particularly disabling because there is no sensation to the volar aspects of the thumb and index and middle fingers and the radial side of the ring finger. When blindfolded, the client substitutes pinch to the ring and small fingers to compensate for this loss. An injury in the forearm that involves the anterior interosseous nerve does not result in sensory loss. Motor loss includes paralysis of the flexor pollicis longus, the flexor digitorum profundus of the index and middle fingers, and the pronator quadratus. The pronator teres is not affected. Pinch is affected.

TABLE 40.4   Nerve Injuries of the Upper Extremity

Nerve	Location	Affected	Test
Radial nerve (posterior cord, fibers from C5, C6, C7, C8)	Upper arm	Triceps and all distal motors	• MMT
		Sensory to SRN	• Sensory test
Radial nerve	Above elbow	Brachioradialis and all distal motors	• MMT
		Sensory to SRN	• Sensory test
Radial nerve	At elbow	Supinator, ECRL, ECRB, and all distal motors	• MMT
		Sensory to SRN	• Sensory test
Posterior interosseous nerve	Forearm	ECU, EDC, EDM, APL, EPL, EPB, EIP	• Wrist extension—if present, indicates PIN rather than high radial nerve
		No sensory loss	
Radial nerve at ECRB, radial artery, arcade of Frohse, origin of supinator	Radial tunnel syndrome	Weakness of muscles innervated by PIN	• Palpate for pain over extensor mass
			• Pain with wrist flexion and pronation
		No sensory loss	• Pain with wrist extension and supination
			• Pain with resisted middle finger extension
Median nerve (lateral from C5, C6, C7, medial cord from C8, T1)	High lesions (elbow and above)	Paralysis/weakness of FCR, PL, all FDS, FDP I and II	• MMT
		FPL, pronator teres and quad, opponens pollicis, APB, FPB (radial head), lumbricals I and II	• Sensory test
		Sensory cutaneous branch of median nerve	
Median nerve	Low (at wrist)	Weakness of thenars only	• Inability to flex thumb tip and index fingertip to palm
			• Inability to oppose thumb
			• Poor dexterity
Median nerve under fibrous band in PT, beneath heads of pronator, arch of FDS, origin of FCR	Pronator syndrome	Weakness in thenars, but not muscles innervated by AIN	• Provocative tests to isolate compression site
		Sensory in median nerve distribution in hand	
Median nerve under origin of PT, FDS to middle	Anterior interosseous nerve syndrome	Pure motor, no sensory loss	• Inability to flex IP joint of thumb and DIP of index
		Forearm pain precedes paralysis	• Increased pain with resisted pronation
		Weakness of FPL, FDP I and II, PQ	• Pain with forearm pressure
Median nerve at wrist	Carpal tunnel syndrome	Weakness of medial intrinsics	• Provocative tests
		Sensory loss	• Tinel's sign
			• Sensory test
Ulnar nerve at elbow (branch of medial cord from C7, C8, T1)	Cubital tunnel syndrome	Weakness/paralysis of FCU, FDP III and IV, ulnar intrinsics	• Pain with elbow flexion and extension
		Numbness in palmar cutaneous and dorsal cutaneous distribution	
		Loss of grip and pinch strength	
Ulnar nerve at wrist	Compression at canal of Guyon	Weakness and pain in ulnar intrinsics	• Reproduced by pressure at site

AIN, Anterior interosseus nerve; *APB*, abductor pollicis brevis; *APL*, abductor pollicis longus; *DIP*, distal interphalangeal; *ECRB*, extensor carpi radialis brevis; *ECRL*, extensor carpi radialis longus; *ECU*, extensor carpi ulnaris; *ED*, extensor digitorum; *EDC*, extensor digitorum communis; *EDM*, extensor digitorum minimus; *EIP*, extensor indicis proprius; *FDS*, flexor digitorum superficialis; *EPB*, extensor pollicis brevis; *EPL*, extensor pollicis longus; *FCR*, flexor carpi radialis; *FCU*, flexor carpi ulnaris; *FDP*, flexor digitorum profundus; *FPB*, flexor pollicis brevis; *FPL*, flexor pollicis longus; *IP*, interphalangeal; *MMT*, manual muscle test; *PIN*, posterior interosseus nerve; *PL*, palmaris longus; *PQ*, pronator quadratus; *PT*, pronator teres; *SRN*, superficial radial nerve.

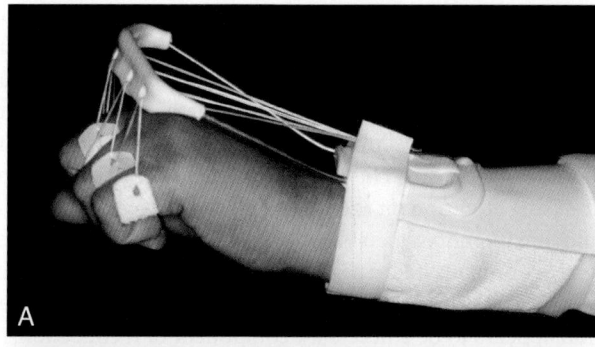

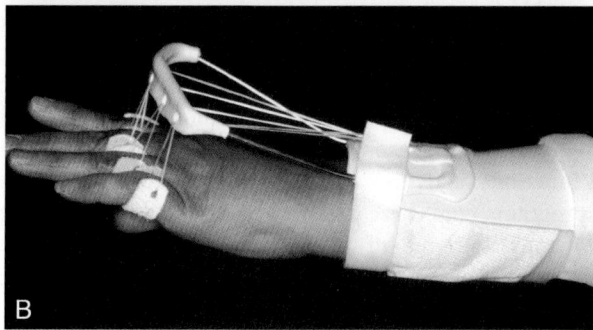

Fig. 40.5 A low-profile radial nerve orthosis is carefully balanced to pull metacarpophalangeal (MP) joints into extension when the wrist is flexed and allows the MP joints to fall into slight flexion when the wrist is extended; it thus preserves the normal balance between two joints and also joint contracture. (Courtesy Judy C. Colditz, HandLab.)

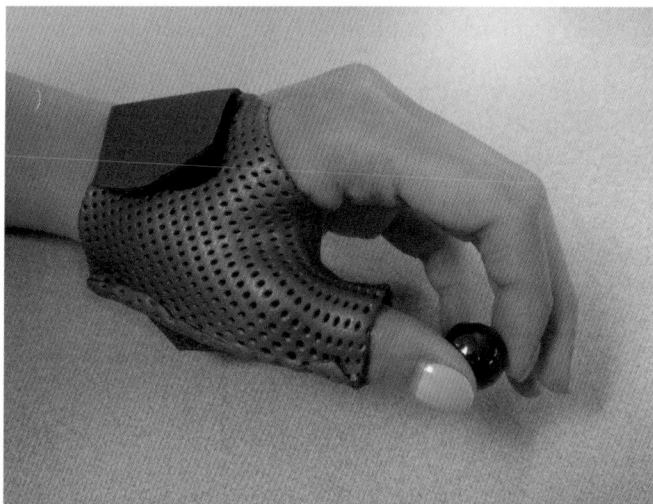

Fig. 40.6 A thumb stabilization orthosis may be used with median nerve injury to protect the thumb and to improve functioning by placing the thumb in a position of pinch. Normal pinch cannot be achieved with a median nerve injury because of paralysis of thumb musculature.

Orthoses that position the thumb in palmar abduction and slight opposition increase functional use of the hand (Fig. 40.6). If clawing of the index and middle fingers is present, an orthosis should be fabricated to prevent hyperextension of the MP joints. Clients report that they avoid use of the hand with a median nerve injury because of lack of sensation rather than because of muscle paralysis. Nevertheless, the weakened or paralyzed muscles should be protected.

Ulnar Nerve

The ulnar nerve in the forearm innervates only the flexor carpi ulnaris and the medial half of the flexor digitorum profundus. It travels down the volar forearm through the canal of Guyon, innervating the intrinsic muscles of the hand, including the palmaris brevis, abductor digiti minimi, flexor digiti minimi, opponens digiti minimi, dorsal and volar interossei, third and fourth lumbricals, and medial head of the flexor pollicis brevis. The sensory distribution of the ulnar nerve is the dorsal and volar surfaces of the small finger ray and the ulnar half of the dorsal and volar surface of the ring finger ray.

A high-level ulnar nerve injury results in hyperextension of the MP joints of the ring and small fingers (also called clawing) as a response to overaction of the extensor digitorum communis that is not held in check by the third and fourth lumbricals. The IP joints of the ring and small fingers do not demonstrate a great flexion deformity because of the paralysis of the flexor digitorum profundus. The hypothenar muscles and interossei are absent. The wrist assumes a position of radial extension caused by the loss of the flexor carpi ulnaris. In a low-level ulnar nerve injury, the ring and small fingers claw at the MP joints and the IP joints exhibit a greater tendency toward flexion because the flexor digitorum profundus is present. Wrist extension is normal.

Clinical signs of a high-level ulnar nerve injury may include claw hand deformity (as described above) with a loss of the hypothenar and the interosseous muscles. In a low-level ulnar nerve injury, the flexor digitorum profundus and flexor carpi ulnaris are present and unopposed by the intrinsic muscles. There is a positive Froment's sign. Long-standing compression of the ulnar nerve in the canal of Guyon results in a flattening of the hypothenar area and conspicuous atrophy of the first dorsal interosseous muscle.

With a low-level ulnar nerve injury a small orthosis may be provided to prevent hyperextension of the small and ring fingers without limiting full flexion at the MP joints. Stabilization of the MP joints will allow the extensor digitorum communis to extend the IP joints fully (Fig. 40.7).

Sensory loss of the ulnar nerve results in frequent injury, especially burns, to the ulnar side of the hand. Clients must be instructed in visual protection of the anesthetic area.

Postoperative Management After Nerve Repair

After nerve repair, the wrist and hand are placed in a position that minimizes tension on the nerve.[49] For example, after repair of the median nerve, the wrist is immobilized in a flexed position. Immobilization usually lasts for 2 to 3 weeks, after which protective stretching of the joints may begin. The therapist must exercise great care not to put excessive traction on the newly repaired nerve.[49] A repaired digital nerve also will be protected with flexion of the MP and PIP joints.[40]

Early intervention is initially directed toward the prevention of deformity and correction of poor positioning during the acute and regenerative stages.[40,49] Correction of a contracture may take 4 to 6 weeks. Active exercise is the preferred method initially of gaining full extension, although a light dynamic orthosis may be applied with the surgeon's supervision. The

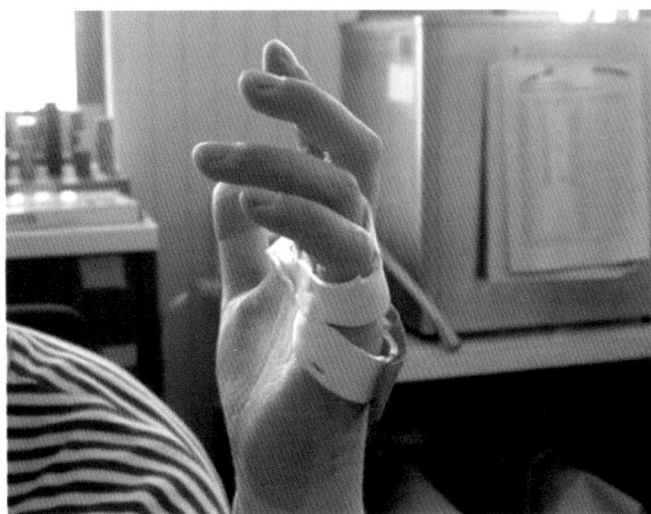

Fig. 40.7 A static ulnar nerve orthosis blocks the hyperextension of metacarpophalangeal (MP) joints that occurs with paralysis of ulnar intrinsic muscles; it also allows MP flexion, which maintains a normal range of motion for the MP joints.

use of orthotics to assist or substitute for weakened musculature may be necessary for an extended period during nerve regeneration. Orthoses should be removed as soon as possible to allow active exercise of the weakened muscles. It is important to instruct the client in correct patterns of motion, however, so that substitution is minimized.

Clients must be instructed in visual protection of the anesthetic area during hand function. ADLs should be assessed, and new methods or devices may be needed for safety and independence. Use of the hand in the client's work should be assessed, and the client should be returned to employment with any necessary job modifications or adaptations of equipment.

Careful muscle, sensory, and functional testing should be done frequently. As the nerve regenerates, orthoses may be changed or eliminated.[40] Exercises and activities should be revised to reflect the client's new gains, and adapted equipment should be discarded as soon as possible.

As motor function begins to return to the paralyzed muscles, a careful program of specific exercises should be devised to facilitate the return. Proprioceptive neuromuscular facilitation (PNF) techniques—such as hold-relax, contract-relax, quick stretch, and icing—may assist a fair-strength muscle and increase ROM. Neuromuscular electrical stimulation (NMES) can also provide an external stimulus to help strengthen the newly innervated muscle. When the muscle has reached a good rating, functional activities should be used to complete the return to normal strength.

Sensory Reeducation. Assessment of sensibility is described in some detail earlier in this chapter. This information should be used to prepare a program of sensory reeducation after nerve repair.

When a nerve is repaired, regeneration is not perfect and results in fewer and smaller nerve fibers and receptors distal to the repair. The goal of sensory reeducation is to maximize the functional level of sensation or tactile gnosis.

Dellon reported a highly structured sensory reeducation program in 1974.[32] Dellon divided his program into early and late-phase training, based on vibratory sensation for early phase and perception of moving and constant touch sensation for late-phase reeducation. Dellon used the localization of stimuli and recognition of objects. Higher cortical integration was achieved by focusing attention on the stimuli through visual clues and by employing memory when vision was occluded. The clients were taught to compensate for sensory deficits by improving specific skills and generalizing them to other sensory stimuli. Daily repetition appears to be a necessary component of reeducation.

As cited in Dellon,[34] Callahan outlined a program of protective sensory reeducation and discriminative sensory reeducation if protective sensation is present and touch sensation has returned to the fingertips. As cited in Dellon,[34] Waylett-Rendall also described a sensory reeducation program using crafts and functional activities, as well as desensitization techniques. All programs emphasize a variety of stimuli used in a repetitive manner to bombard the sensory receptors. A sequence of eyes-closed, eyes-open, eyes-closed is used to provide feedback during the training process. Sessions are limited in length to prevent fatigue and frustration. To prevent further trauma, objects must not be potentially harmful to the insensate areas. A home program should be provided to reinforce learning that occurs in the clinical setting.

Researchers have found that sensory reeducation can result in improved functional sensibility in motivated clients.[34] Objective measurement of sensation after reeducation must be performed and then accurately compared with initial testing to assess the success of the program.

Graded Motor Imagery as described by Butler[19] consists of three sequential exercise phases used to retrain the brain for patients having pain, difficulty moving or initiating movement or a fear of moving. The three stages involve left/right discrimination (also called laterality recognition), motor imagery, and mirror therapy.[84] The clinical approach of Graded Motor Imagery reduces the threatening input, reduces or decreases the pain neuromatrix, targets activation of specific components of the neuromatrix without activating the unwanted parts and upgrades physical and functional tolerance by graded exposure to threatening inputs across sensory and nonsensory domains.[19]

The exercises in Stage I, Left/Right discrimination consist of identifying right and left positions by showing the individual pictures of hands in various positions either with flashcards or photographs. Research has shown that people in pain often lose the ability to identify left or right images of their painful body parts. This ability appears to be important for normal recovery from pain.[19,78] In Stage II, Explicit Motor Imagery involves thinking about movement without actually moving. It is thought that these imagined movements start firing the "mirror neurons" in the brain, which can be affected by pain. In Stage III, Mirror Therapy involves looking into a mirror and viewing the reflection of the uninvolved extremity in the mirror, which gives the appearance of being the involved hand[84] and creates the allusion that the injured extremity is moving without pain. Mirror therapy is thought to work by providing false, but congruent, visual feedback for the unaffected limb, restoring the normal pain-free relationship between sensory feedback and motor intention.[19] The three treatment techniques are delivered sequentially, starting with the activation of cortical areas involved in thinking about movement and then progressing to movement.

Tendon transfers. If a motor nerve has not reinnervated its muscle after a minimum period of 1 year after nerve repair, the surgeon may consider tendon transfers to restore a needed motion. The rules of tendon transfer are to evaluate what is absent, what is needed for function, and what is available to transfer.[31]

Some muscles, such as the extensor carpi radialis longus and the flexor digitorum sublimis to the ring finger, are commonly used for transfers because their motions are easily substituted by the extensor carpi radialis brevis (ECRB) and flexor digitorum profundus (FDP), respectively, to the ring finger. An example in a high radial nerve injury, multiple tendon transfers may be needed to substitute for lost motor function. As median and ulnar nerve innervated muscles are intact, common transfers may include pronator teres (PT) for wrist extension (extensor carpi radialis brevis [ECRB]), palmaris longus (PL) to extensor pollicis longus (EPL) for thumb extension, and flexor carpi radialis (FCR) to extensor digitorum communis (EDC) for finger extension.[45] Choices for transfers are variable, and a surgeon may request assistance from the therapist in evaluating motor status to determine the best motor transfer. Therapy before tendon transfer is essential if the motor being used is not of normal strength. A muscle loses a grade of strength when transferred, and a strengthening program of progressive resistive exercises, NMES, and isolated motion will help ensure success of the transfer. There must be full passive ROM (PROM) of all joints before tendon transfer can be attempted.

After transfer, an initial period of immobilization of 4 to 6 weeks is required to protect the surgical repairs. This may be achieved with casting for those who are not reliable in protecting these repairs or with fabrication of a thermoplastic orthosis. Once cleared by the surgeon, clients begin activation of the tendon transfers through instruction to perceive the correct muscle during active use. Use of surface electromyography, biofeedback, muscle reeducation, and supervised activity to note any substitution patterns during active use can help the client to use the transfer correctly. Therapy must be initiated before the client has time to develop incorrect use patterns. NMES may be used to isolate the muscle and strengthen it postoperatively.

Tendon Injuries
Flexor Tendons

Tendon injuries may be isolated or may occur in conjunction with other injuries, especially fractures or crushes. Flexor tendons injured in the area between the distal palmar crease and the insertion of the flexor digitorum superficialis are considered the most difficult to treat because the tendons lie in their sheaths in this area beneath the fibrous pulley system and any scarring causes adhesions. This area is often referred to as Zone 2 or "no-man's-land."[17,23]

Primary repair of the flexor tendons within Zone 2 is most frequently performed after a clean laceration.[41] With improvements in surgical techniques, advances also have been made

in postoperative management of tendon repairs.[37] Choices for treatment will vary based on surgical repair strength, quality of the tendon, tension of the repair or whether the tendon sheath or pulleys were also restored.[37] Working closely with the surgeon is vital in understanding the delicacy of these repairs.

Other factors to consider are the client's age, cognition level in being able to follow instructions, financial or family supports, and motivation and compliance to the therapy program.

With the ongoing research and improvements in flexor tendon surgeries, postoperative management also continues to evolve,[88] with common goals of protecting the repaired structures, restoring strength, promoting gliding of the tendons, and minimizing the formation of scar adhesions.[2,23,24,67]

Immobilization. Although early mobilization is preferred, immobilization after tendon repairs may be necessary if conditions and circumstances are not optimal to allow for safe early controlled movement.[67] Young children, noncompliant clients, and those with cognitive dysfunction may require cast immobilization or a thermoplastic orthosis initially for 3 to 4 weeks. Wrist is positioned at 10 to 30 degrees of flexion, MP joints at 40 to 60 degrees of flexion, and PIP/DIP joints in extension. No exercises to the fingers are done by the client alone. PROM and protected active extension may be done in therapy. AROM and tendon gliding exercises may then begin after the immobilization period.[23]

Good results have not been consistently achieved with immobilization, and this technique may increase the risk of tendon rupture after repair because a tendon gains tensile strength when submitted to gentle tension at the repair site.[23]

Early passive motion. Early passive motion may be considered when conditions of a tendon repair are not optimal.[41] An injury may involve other structures requiring additional surgical repairs as in fractures or soft tissue injuries. This may prolong the inflammation and edema during this phase of healing. Other factors may include a delay in repair, frayed or repair under tension, or a client who is unable to begin treatment early and is thus delayed after 1 week. Tensile strength of the tendon is diminished between 5 and 21 days during the fibroblastic-collagen producing phase and may be at risk with tension or rupture from early motion.

Early active mobilization. As methods of tendon suturing and the suture materials themselves have evolved, many clinicians have begun to initiate active movement of the repaired tendon within days of surgery.[12] These techniques should be used only when an experienced surgeon and therapist work closely together. The condition of the tendon and the technique of repair must be communicated to the therapist, and the client must be closely monitored. With stronger and more sophisticated repairs, the rate of tendon rupture decreases and improved results are noted after tendon injury. There are several well-documented early active motion protocols, but all of the protocols share important common factors. First, the tendon repair strength must be sufficient to be able to withstand the forces of active mobilization. A strong core suture repair should be performed with a minimum of four strands crossing the repair and with addition of a peripheral suture.[12] Second, the timing and the initiation of therapy must be considered. It has been suggested that early active motion be initiated 2 to 5 days after repair to allow inflammation to subside and to reduce the amount of force on the tendon during active flexion. Third, the client must be able to comprehend and be compliant with the exercise program for the tendon rehabilitation to be successful and to prevent rupture of the tendon by overstressing the repair site.

An early passive place and active hold approach is described by Cannon[23] using two orthoses. A dorsal based blocking orthosis is made and worn at all times except during exercises (Fig. 40.8). An exercise orthosis is fabricated with a hinged wrist and MP joints blocked at 50 degrees. Exercises within this orthosis allow for full flexion of the wrist with simultaneous extension of the IP joints followed by protected wrist extension limited by a dorsal block to 30 degrees (a tenodesis movement). As the wrist is moved into extension, the fingers are passively placed into flexion and the client is asked to actively hold this flexed position by contracting his or her muscles gently. Silfverskiöld and May (as cited in Cannon[23]) adapted this approach by changing the wrist position to neutral.

An active mobilization approach by Gratton applies a dorsal blocking orthosis with the wrist at 20 degrees flexion and the MP joints in more extreme flexion between 80 and 90 degrees. In this protective orthosis, clients perform exercises every 4 hours, two repetitions each of (1) full passive flexion of IP joints, (2) full active extension within the blocking orthosis, and (3) active flexion of the PIP joint to 30 degrees and DIP flexion to 5 to 10 degrees in the first week. Active flexion in this protective position is then gradually increased in subsequent weeks to optimally achieve flexion of the PIP joint to 80 to 90 degrees and DIP to 50 to 60 degrees. For ease of instruction in a home program, the patient is instructed to use the width of four fingers of the opposite hand, placing it across the palm of the affected hand as a guide. The patient then actively touches the affected fingertips to the edge of the index finger on the contralateral side. The active movement is progressed weekly by decreasing

the number of fingers' width and thus increasing active flexion into the palm.[23]

The wide-awake local anesthesia no tourniquet (WALANT) open surgical techniques used by some hand surgeons allows the surgeon to visualize the repair and any gaps to minimize the risk of rupture.[12] While the patient is awake, he or she is asked to actively move the repaired tendon through flexion and extension to ensure an optimal repair. A dorsal blocking orthosis is made initially to protect from bleeding into the wound and for edema to decrease. True active movement can begin at 3 to 5 days postoperatively, with partial flexion of one-third to a half fist for the first several weeks and gradually increased to a full active fist. The patient is encouraged to move the digits but not to use them during this period.

Because early active mobilization of newly repaired flexor tendons involves a higher risk of rupture, close monitoring, and practice with the client, especially those with poor compliance, is required. It is strongly recommended that any of these early mobilization approaches be used with the close collaboration of the surgeon and with caution by less experienced therapists.

Postacute flexor tendon rehabilitation. When active flexion is begun out of the orthosis, after any of the postoperative management techniques described previously, the client should be instructed in exercises to facilitate differential tendon gliding.[92] Wehbé has recommended three positions—hook, straight fist, and fist—to maximize isolated gliding of the flexor digitorum superficialis and the flexor digitorum profundus tendons, in addition to stretching of the intrinsic musculature and gliding of the extensor mechanism.[93] Tendon gliding exercises should be done for 10 repetitions of each position, two or three times a day.

Isolated exercises to assist tendon gliding also may be performed using a blocking orthosis (Fig. 40.9) or the opposite hand (Fig. 40.10). The MP joints should be held in extension during blocking so that the intrinsic muscles that act on it cannot overcome the power of the repaired flexor tendons. Care should be taken not to hyperextend the PIP joints and overstretch the repaired tendons.

After 6 to 8 weeks, passive extension may be started, and the use of orthoses may be necessary to correct limitations in PIP passive and active joint motion.[23] A cylindrical plaster cast may be fabricated to apply constant static pressure into PIP joint extension to decrease a flexion contracture, as described by Bell-Krotoski (Fig. 40.11A).[8] Serially casting into extension requires that the client be able to attend treatment every 2 to 3 days initially so that skin tolerance to casting can be checked and the cast changed as the client makes gains in passive motion. A serial static PIP extension orthosis may be fabricated. When used according to the proper instructions, this orthosis allows the client to make adjustments gradually and independently (see Fig. 40.11B).[28] A finger gutter extension orthosis may be made using {1/16}-inch (0.16 cm) thermoplastic material and worn at night to decrease PIP joint stiffness and to maintain gains in PIP joint passive extension.

At 6 weeks after surgery the hand may be used for light ADLs, such as hygiene, grooming, feeding, and tabletop activities such as writing and using a computer. The client should continue to

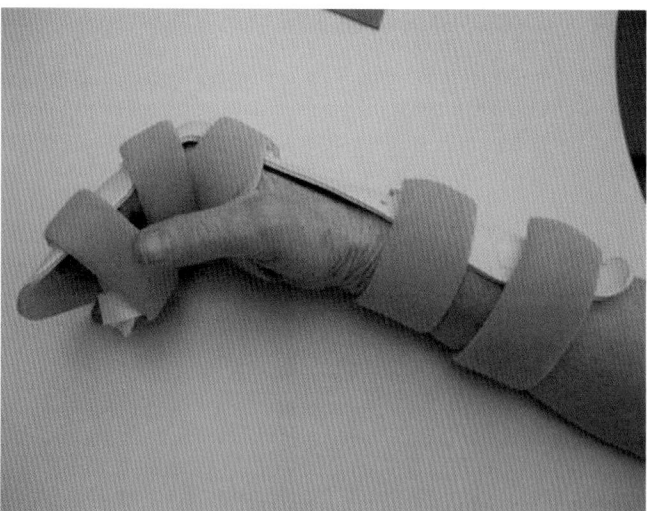

Fig. 40.8 A dorsal blocking orthosis is used after flexor tendon repair. The position of the wrist and fingers in the orthosis is determined by the postoperative approach chosen by the surgeon and therapist.

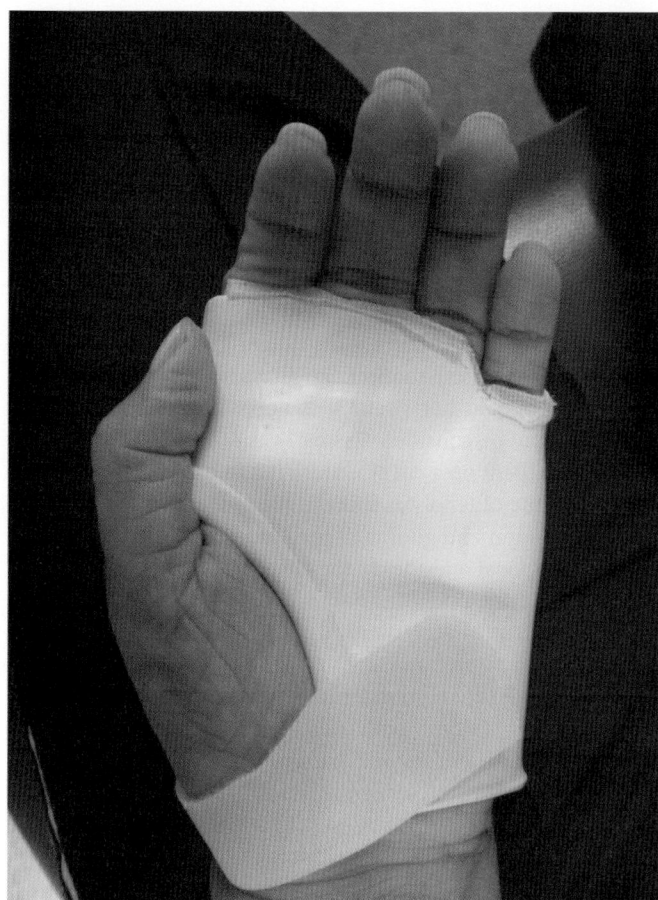

Fig. 40.9 A blocking orthosis can be used to isolate tendon pull-through and joint range of motion by blocking out proximal joints. This orthosis is being used to facilitate motion at the distal interphalangeal joint after repair of the flexor digitorum profundus tendon.

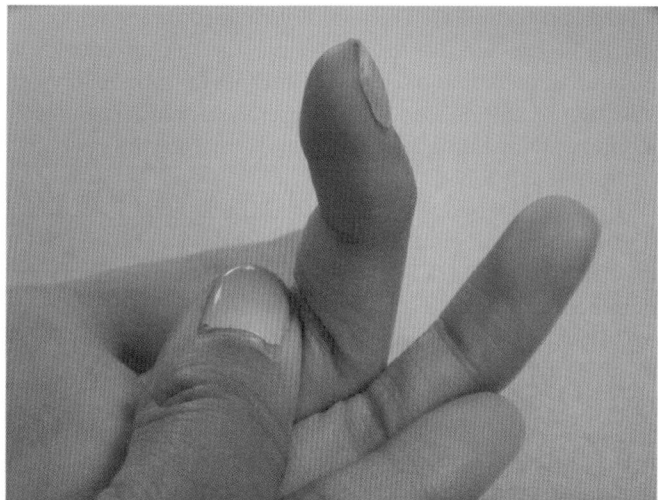

Fig. 40.10 Manual blocking of metacarpophalangeal joint during flexion of the proximal interphalangeal joint.

avoid heavy lifting with the affected hand or excessive resistance. At approximately 8 weeks the client may begin light resistive exercises and progress toward normal activities. Activities such as clay work, woodworking, and macramé are excellent for encouraging return of motion, strength, and coordination, as

are light functional activities such as folding laundry and washing lighter dishes. Full resistance and normal work activities can be started 3 months after surgery. Sports activities should be discouraged until cleared with the surgeon.

After a hand has sustained a tendon injury, passive versus active limitations of joint motion must be evaluated. Limitations in active motion may indicate joint stiffness, muscle weakness, or scar adhesions. If passive motion is greater than active motion, the therapist should consider that tendons may be caught in the scar tissue. The therapist should be able to determine whether a tendon is adhering and causing a flexion contracture or the tendon is free but the joint itself is stiff. Intervention should be based on this type of evaluation. To improve PIP joint active motion, a motion orthosis (relative motion orthosis [RMO]) may be used during the day while the patient is performing functional activities (Fig. 40.12). An RMO can be used to gain PIP joint active extension or flexion. To gain PIP joint active extension, the MCP joint of the affected finger is held in relative flexion compared to the adjacent digits. This increase in MCP joint flexion will block the force of the extensor digitorum communis (EDC) and thus aid the interosseous and lumbrical muscles in transmitting extension to the PIP joint. To gain PIP joint active flexion, the MCP joint of the affected finger is held in relative extension compared to the adjacent digits. This increase in MCP joint extension allows the power of the extrinsic flexors to aid in flexion at the PIP joint.[12] The pencil test is a simple way to simulate relative motion to determine if an RMO would be beneficial for improving active motion at the PIP joint.[75]

ROM, strength, function, and sensibility testing (if digital nerves were also injured) should be performed frequently, with orthoses and activities geared toward progressing the client. Performance of ADLs should continually be assessed and addressed to help maximize a client's return to his or her occupations. Assessments may include use of an ADL checklist or through simulations and observations during treatment. An example of disuse or neglect of an index finger may occur as a client becomes protective of the injured finger. This should be addressed early and prevented.

Gains in flexion and extension may continue to be recorded for 6 months postoperatively. A finger with limber joints and minimal scarring preoperatively will function better after repair than one that is stiff and scarred and has trophic skin changes.[14] Therefore, it is important that all joints, skin, and scars be supple and movable before reconstructive surgery is attempted. A functional to excellent result is obtained if the combined loss of extension is less than 40 degrees in the PIP and DIP joints of the index and middle fingers and less than 60 degrees in the ring and small fingers and if the finger can flex to the palm.[14,87]

Flexor tendon reconstruction. If the tendon is damaged as a result of a crush injury or if the laceration cannot be cleaned up enough to allow for a primary repair, a delayed or staged reconstruction may be needed to provide return of tendon function. Repairs by the surgeon may include tendon transfers, lengthening, or grafting.[31] In severe tendon loss, a staged flexor tendon reconstruction may be performed. At the first operation, a Silastic rod is inserted beneath the pulley system and attached to the distal phalanx. Other reconstructive procedures,

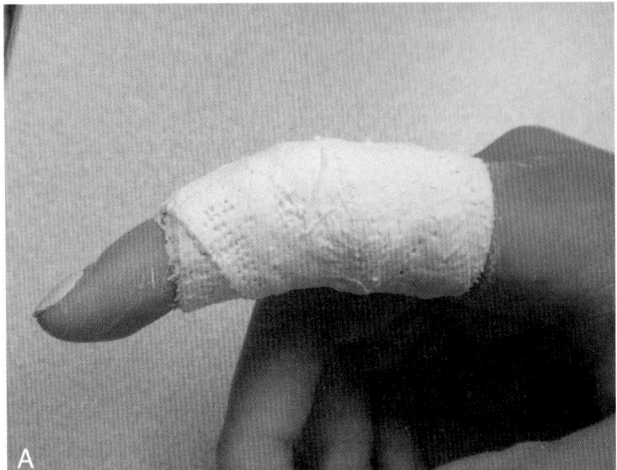

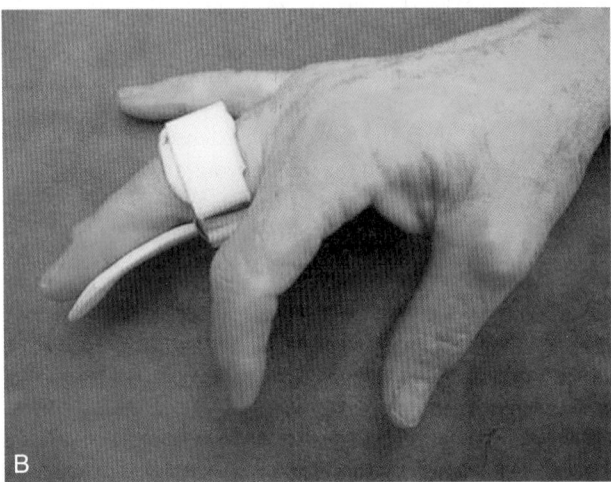

Fig. 40.11 (A) A plaster cylindrical orthosis is used to apply static stretch to a proximal interphalangeal (PIP) joint contracture. It is not removed by the client and must be replaced frequently by the therapist, with careful monitoring of the skin's condition. (B) A static progressive extension orthosis may be fabricated to correct a flexion contracture, allowing the client to make gradual adjustments into PIP joint extension.

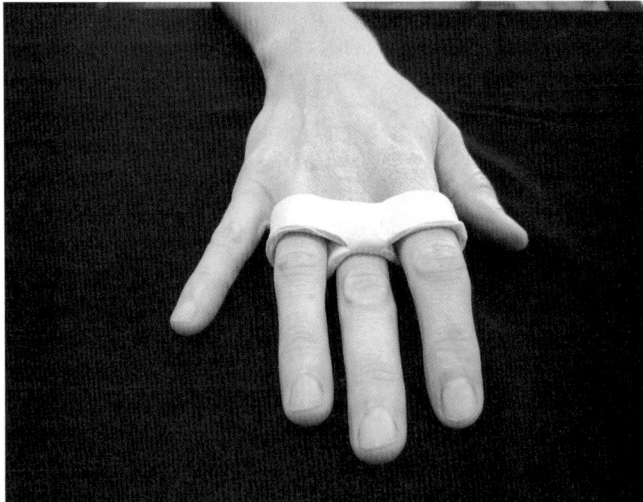

Fig. 40.12 A relative motion orthosis (RMO) is used to position the MCP joint in more extension or more flexion than adjacent digits. The RMO can be used to gain PIP joint active extension or flexion.

such as pulley reconstruction, are performed at the same time. A mesothelial cell-lined pseudosheath is formed about the rod, and a fluid similar to synovial fluid is formed in the postoperative recovery phase.[31,64] The second stage is performed about 4 months later, when the digit can be moved passively to the palm. A tendon graft is inserted and the Silastic rod removed. The postoperative program is carried out in the same manner as for a primary tendon repair.[31]

After a two-stage tendon reconstruction or primary repair, a tenolysis may be performed if the client's progress appears to have plateaued and if there is a substantial difference between the active and passive motion. Surgery also may be considered if motion is equal but strength is not sufficient for function. Tenolysis may be considered as early as 3 months after tendon repair dependent on a client's limitation in progress.

At the time of tenolysis surgery, scar adhesions are removed from the tendon and gliding of the tendons is assessed. If a client is under local anesthesia, the client is asked to move his or her fingers in the operating room at the time of lysis to determine the extent of scar removal. If a client is put under general anesthesia, a proximal incision at the wrist is made and the tendon is pulled there to determine mobility from adhesions.[31] Active motion is begun within the first 24 to 48 hours through tendon gliding exercises and passive flexion of the finger followed with active holds. Gentle blocking exercises of specific joints also may be performed to help improve excursion of the tendon. Transcutaneous electrical nerve stimulation (TENS) and medications may be used to control pain.[24]

Extensor Tendons

Treatment of extensor tendon injuries requires a thorough knowledge of the extensor anatomy and biomechanics of the hand. The extensor mechanism of the hand is a highly sophisticated and complicated system. It is divided into seven zones for the fingers and five for the thumb. The level of injury will dictate the intervention regimen. Timelines for immobilization, initiation of motion, and resistive exercise depend on the level of injury and the unique healing time frames for the structures in the different zones.

There are four zones distal to the MP joint and three zones starting at the MP joint and proximal. Zones I and II consist of the structures at the DIP joint and middle phalanx, and injuries to this area are treated similarly. Zones III and IV are the areas over the PIP joint and proximal phalanx; again, these zones are treated similarly depending on the structures repaired. Zone V consists of the area over the MP joint, whereas zone VI is the area over the dorsal hand and zone VII the area over the wrist. In the thumb, zone T1 consists of the area over the DIP joint, T2 the middle phalanx, T3 the MP joint, T4 the proximal phalanx, and T5 the area over the CMC joint and wrist.

Dorsal scar adherence is the most difficult problem after injury to the extensor tendons because of the tendency of the dorsal extensor hood to adhere to the underlying structures and thus limit its normal excursion during flexion and extension. Overstretching the extensor tendon is another common occurrence and can result in an extensor lag, or lack of full active extension.

Extensor tendon injuries distal to the MP joint (zones I to IV) generally require a longer period of immobilization, usually 6 weeks. As with flexor tendon injuries, controlled mobilization is being used with increasing frequency for zones III and IV. A protocol developed by Evans called the short arc motion protocol, or SAM protocol, allows for immediate active flexion of the PIP joint to 30 degrees followed by full passive extension. Complete immobilization for 6 weeks or longer is necessary for injuries in zones I and II.[44]

Several abnormal finger joint changes are associated with injuries distal to the MP joints. An injury to zones I or II, when there is a traumatic disruption of the terminal extensor tendon, is called a mallet finger. This joint change is characterized by flexion of the DIP joint and the inability to actively extend this joint. A swan-neck posture is a result of the dorsal displacement of the lateral bands (part of the extensor mechanism) in zone III and results in hyperextension of the PIP joint and flexion of the DIP joint. Another abnormal joint position originating from zone III is known as the boutonnière deformity. A boutonnière deformity results when the common extensor tendon is ruptured and the lateral bands sublux volarly. This volar subluxation of the lateral bands results in flexion of the PIP joint and hyperextension of the DIP joint.

Extensor tendons in zones V, VI, and VII (proximal to the MP joints) become adherent because they are encased in paratenon and synovial sheaths and respond to injury in a way similar to that of flexor tendons, resulting in either incomplete extension, also known as extensor lag, or incomplete flexion caused by loss of gliding of the extensor tendon.

Evans studied the normal excursion of the extensor digitorum communis in zones V, VI, and VII to suggest guidelines for early passive motion of extensor tendons.[44] She concluded that 5 mm of tendon glide after repair was safe and effective in limiting tendon adhesions and designed a postoperative orthosis that allows slight active flexion while providing passive extension.[44] The orthosis is worn for 3 weeks, with the initiation of active motion between the third and fourth weeks. A removable volar orthosis is used between exercise periods to protect the tendon for 2 additional weeks. The use of dynamic flexion orthoses may be started at 6 weeks after surgery to regain flexion if needed.

Injuries to extensor tendons proximal to the MP joint may be immobilized for 3 weeks. After this period, the finger may be placed in a removable volar orthosis that is worn between exercise periods for an additional 2 weeks. Progressive ROM is begun at 3 weeks, and if full flexion is not regained rapidly, dynamic flexion may be started at 6 weeks.

Dynamic flexion orthoses may include an orthosis with rubber band traction individualized for affected fingers or a traction glove providing tension to all fingers. For isolated fingers, a PIP-DIP strapping may be used (Fig. 40.13) made of 1-inch-wide pajama elastic with tension applied by adjusting a safety pin.

Early motion also may be employed through an immediate controlled active mobilization (ICAM) program for Zone IV to VII. This requires that at least one extensor tendon is not injured to allow support to other injured tendons. A "yoke," or relative motion orthosis (RMO) is fabricated with the repaired

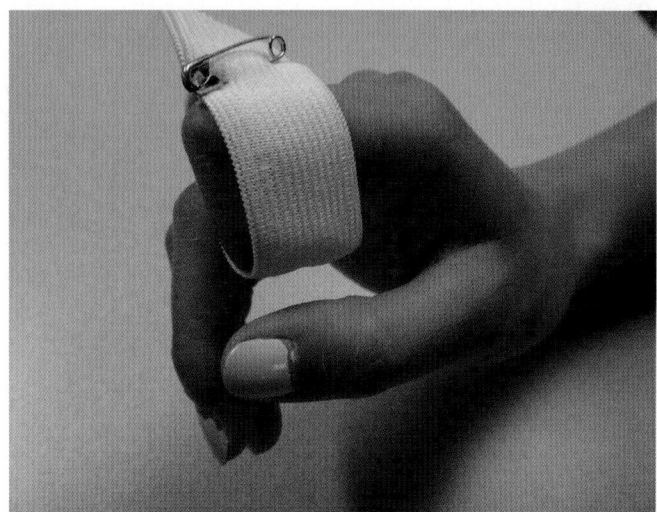

Fig. 40.13 A proximal interphalangeal (PIP)–distal interphalangeal (DIP) orthosis may be used to increase flexion of both PIP and DIP joints. Made with pajama elastic tension, the orthosis can be adjusted by changing position of a safety pin. The therapist should determine tension and wearing time.

digit placed in 15 to 20 degrees more extension than adjacent fingers, thus taking tension off of the repair. An additional wrist orthosis is fabricated holding the wrist at 20 to 25 degrees of extension. In phase 1 after surgery (between 1 to 21 days), passive and active motion is performed after fabrication and wearing of these orthoses. The client is encouraged to perform light activities using his or her hand. In phase 2 (between 22 and 35 days) the client continues to wear the yoke orthosis at all times and can take the wrist orthosis off for light hand function. However, both orthoses must be worn for heavier gripping and lifting activities. At phase 3 (36–49 days after repair), the client may be discharged from the wrist orthosis. The yoke orthosis may be gradually weaned or replaced with a less restrictive buddy strap as the client returns to increasing normal hand function.[54,75]

Total Active Motion and Total Passive Motion

Total active motion (TAM) and total passive motion (TPM) are methods of recording joint ROM that are used to compare tendon excursion (active) and joint mobility (passive). They represent the measure of flexion minus extensor lag of three joints. The American Society for Surgery of the Hand has recommended TAM and TPM for use in reporting joint motion.[4]

TAM is computed by adding the sum of the angles formed by the MP, PIP, and DIP joints in flexion, minus incomplete active extension at each of the three joints. For example, MP joint flexion is 85 degrees with full extension, PIP is 100 degrees and lacks 15 degrees extension, and DIP is 65 degrees with full extension; therefore, the TAM for the digit is 235 degrees.

TAM should be measured while the client makes a fist. It is used for a single digit and should be compared with the same digit of the opposite hand or subsequent measurements of the same digit. It should not be used to compute a percentage of loss of impairment. TPM is calculated in the same manner but measures only passive motion.

Complex Injuries

Complex injuries to the hand or injuries to multiple anatomic structures of the hand are some of the most challenging injuries for the therapist to treat. Complex injuries to the hand differ from other types of hand injuries because they involve trauma to multiple anatomic systems of the hand, resulting in a varied clinical picture. Injuries to these anatomic systems include skin, nerve, tendon, skeletal, and vascular injuries. Because of the complexity of these injuries and because each injured structure has a unique healing time frame, precautions, and treatment approach, there is no set protocol to follow in treating these injuries.

Many of the treatment precautions established for any one of the injuries mentioned earlier contradict one another. Therefore, the therapist's challenge is to determine when it is safe for the client to move forward with treatment without risking injury to healing structures. "The therapist must have a thorough knowledge of anatomy, wound healing, biomechanics, and treatment guidelines of various traumatic injuries"[26] as well as a "thorough understanding of the injuries and types of repairs performed. That understanding should include location and quality of repair, types of sutures used, associated injuries, and any structures that were injured but not repaired."[26] Consequently, the therapist must maintain close communication with the treating surgeon. Types of complex hand injuries include crush injuries, amputations with or without replantation, and avulsion injuries and may be caused by motor vehicle accidents, explosions, gunshots, and machinery accidents. Gerry, the client discussed in the case study at the beginning of this chapter, sustained a complex injury to his hand. All of the anatomic structures of his hand were affected by the saw injury; his intervention plan needed to take into account the unique healing time frames and precautions for each of these anatomic structures.

Generally, and in the case of Gerry, the rehabilitation process for these types of injuries is divided into three stages: early or protective stage (first 5–10 days), intermediate or mobilization stage (1–6 weeks after surgery), and late or strengthening stage (6–8 weeks after surgery). The therapist and surgeon must be skilled and experienced in the rehabilitation of these injuries.

Edema

Although edema is a normal consequence of trauma, it must be quickly and aggressively treated to prevent permanent stiffness and disability. Within hours of trauma, vasodilatation and local edema occur, with an increase in white blood cells in the damaged area. The inflammatory response to the injury results in a decrease in bacteria to control infection.

ETHICAL CONSIDERATIONS

Inexperienced therapists should not treat these clients without the supervision of a more experienced therapist or without additional training in and familiarization with treatment protocols for the various injured structures. Explore further reading for treating these types of injuries.

Edema should be controlled early on through elevation, massage, compression, and AROM. The client is instructed at the time of injury to keep the hand elevated, and a compressive dressing is used to reduce early swelling. Pitting edema appears early and can be recognized as a bloated swelling that creates a pitted appearance when pressed. Pitting may be more pronounced on the dorsal surface, where the venous and lymphatic systems provide return of fluid to the heart. Active motion is especially important to produce retrograde venous and lymphatic flow.

If the swelling continues, a serofibrinous exudate invades the area. Fibrin is deposited in the spaces surrounding the joints, tendons, and ligaments, resulting in reduced mobility, flattening of the arches of the hand, tissue atrophy, and further disuse.[6,38] Normal gliding of the tissues is eliminated, and a stiff, often painful hand is the result. Scar adhesions form and further limit tissue mobility. If untreated, these losses may become permanent.

Early recognition of persistent edema through observation and volume and circumference measurement is important. It may be necessary to use several of the suggested edema control techniques.

Elevation

Early elevation with the hand above the heart is essential. Slings tend to position the hand below the heart and may reduce blood flow. Resting the hand on pillows while seated or lying down is effective. Resting the hand on top of the head or using devices that elevate the hand with the elbow in extension have been suggested.

The client should use the hand for ADLs, within the limitations of resistance prescribed by the physician. Light ADLs that can be accomplished while the hand is in a dressing are permitted.

Manual Edema Mobilization

Manual edema mobilization (MEM) is a method of edema reduction based on ways to activate the lymphatic system. These methods include the principles of manual lymphedema treatment (MLT) massage, medical compression bandaging, exercise, and external compression adapted to meet the specific needs of subacute and chronic postsurgical and poststroke UE edema. The goals are to stimulate the initial lymphatics to absorb excessive fluid and large molecules from the interstitium and to move this lymph centrally. "MEM is not indicated for all hand clients but can be highly effective in cases of recalcitrant subacute or chronic edema. MEM is used to prevent or reduce subacute or chronic high-protein edema as seen in postsurgical, trauma, or post–cerebrovascular accident (CVA) hand edema."[6]

MEM is an advanced skill that requires specialized training of the practitioner. The following overview will acquaint the reader with the techniques involved in MEM[6]:

- Provide light, stroking massage of the involved area. It has been shown that more than 40 mm Hg pressure will cause collapse of the lymphatic pathways.
- Incorporate exercise before and after massage in a specific sequence, following the recommended guidelines.

- Massage, done in segments, is proximal to distal, then distal to proximal, always following movement of the therapist's hand in the proximal direction.
- Massage follows the flow of lymphatic pathways.
- Massage reroutes around the incision area.
- Recognize that this method does not cause additional inflammation.
- Include a client home self-massage program.
- Guide intervention to avoid increased edema from other intervention techniques.
- Incorporate low stretch compression bandaging and warmth to soften hardened tissues, especially at night.

Active Range of Motion

Normal blood flow depends on muscle activity. Active motion does not mean wiggling the fingers; instead, it means maximal available ROM, performed firmly. Casts and orthoses must allow mobility of uninjured parts while protecting newly injured structures. The shoulder and elbow should be moved through full available ROM several times a day. The importance of active ROM for edema control, tendon gliding, and tissue nutrition cannot be overemphasized.

Compression

Compression may be applied through use of various elastic wrap, compression sleeves, and garments. Caution should be observed when applying compression to avoid changes in color or vascularity of the hand or fingers. In cases of vascular repairs, compression is avoided and may be applied with caution after 6 weeks. When first applied, patients should be monitored for any increase in edema, pain, or changes in sensation. Compression may be applied continuously during the night and throughout the day but should not limit a patient's ability to perform exercises and ADLs. Examples of light compression include Coban wraps[b] of the affected area (Fig. 40.14) or light compressive garments such as Isotoner[c] or Jobst[57] (Fig. 40.15).

Wound Healing and Scar Remodeling

The basis of hand therapy is the histology of wound healing. Acute intervention must be planned using the foundation of tissue healing as a guide. Bones, tendons, nerves, and skin follow a progression of healing phases. Intervention must respect healing tissue to promote recovery and prevent further damage. The therapist must take care to do no harm, and that can be accomplished only with a thorough understanding of the physiology of healing.

The first phase of wound healing, the acute inflammatory phase, is initiated within hours, when the tissues are disrupted through injury or surgery, causing vasodilatation, local edema, and migration of white blood cells and phagocytic cells to the area. The phagocytes remove tissue fragments and foreign bodies and are critical to healing. The inflammatory process can subside or persist indefinitely, depending on the degree of bacterial contamination.[82]

---

[b]Coban (available from North Coast Medical, Gilroy, CA).

[c]Isotoner gloves (available from North Coast Medical, Gilroy, CA).

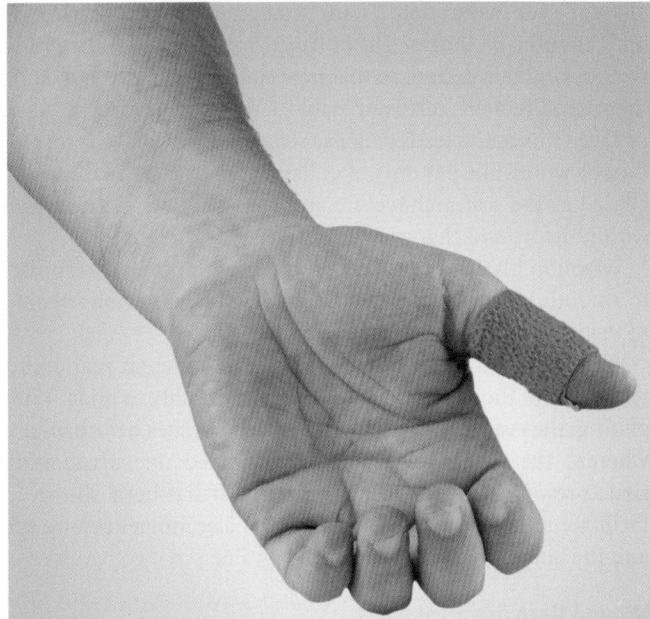

Fig. 40.14 One-inch Coban LF Latex Free Self-Adherent Wrap with Hand Tear is wrapped with minimal stretch. The client is instructed to be alert for the development of swelling, discoloration, pain, numbness, tingling, or other changes in sensation. Coban LF Latex Free Self-Adherent Wrap with Hand Tear may be worn several hours a day to provide compression to reduce edema. (Copyright iStock/melodija. ID: 181832360.)

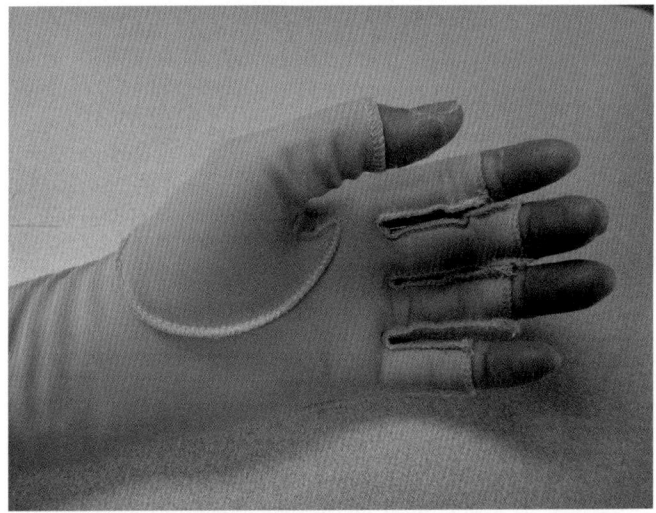

Fig. 40.15 A custom-fit Jobst garment may be used to reduce edema and to decrease and prevent hypertrophic scar formation after burns or trauma. Inserts may be used with the garment to increase pressure over natural curves, such as the dorsum of the wrist.

Fibroblasts, in combination with associated capillaries, begin to invade the wound within the first 72 hours and gradually replace the phagocytes, leading to the second phase: the collagen or granulation phase, between the 5th and 14th days. Collagen fiber formation follows the invasion by fibroblasts, so that by the end of the second week the wound is rich with fibroblasts, a capillary network, and early collagen fibers. This increased vascularization results in the erythema (redness) of the new scar.

During the third to sixth weeks, fibroblasts are slowly replaced with scar collagen fibers, and the wound becomes stronger and more able to withstand progressive stresses, leading to the last phase of scar maturation. Tissue strength continues to increase for 3 months or longer. The collagen metabolizes and synthesizes during this period, so that new collagen replaces old while the wound remains relatively stable. Covalent bonding between collagen molecules leads to dense scar adhesions and the formation of whorl-like patterns of collagen deposits, which may be altered as the scar architecture and collagen fiber organization within the wound change over time.[82]

Myofibroblasts, which are fibroblasts with properties similar to smooth muscle cells, are contractile and cause a shortening of the wound.

Tissues that have restored gliding have different scar architecture from those that do not develop the ability to glide. With gliding, the scar resembles the state of the tissues before injury, whereas the nongliding scar remains fixed on surrounding structures. Controlled tension on the scar has been shown to facilitate remodeling. Scar formation is also influenced by age and the quantity of scar deposited.

Wound Care and Dressings

Wounds may be described using a "three-color concept" (developed in the late 1980s by Marion laboratories) of red, yellow, or black wounds.[82] This system simplifies wound description and intervention. Guidelines for treating the three wound types help the therapist choose the proper method of cleansing and dressing wounds. The reader is encouraged to review this material and obtain advanced education before treating wounds.

A red wound is an uninfected properly healing wound and may be pink or beefy red and consists mainly of granulation and epithelial tissue. A yellow wound indicates the presence of exudate and the need for cleaning. The exudate looks creamy yellow and may contain pus. A black wound is covered with thick necrotic tissue or eschar and indicates the need for debriding or softening of the eschar. Necrotic tissue slows healing and provides an environment for microorganisms to proliferate.[82]

Topical intervention such as antimicrobials may be used to control bacteria. There are a variety of dressings that can be placed on a wound, including gauze that has been impregnated with petroleum, such as Xeroform gauze or Adaptic. Ointments such as Polysporin or Neosporin are also commonly applied. N-Terface[d] is a dry mesh fabric that looks and feels like the interfacing used in sewing. Because it is nonadherent, it can be used directly over wounds. Sterile dressings can be applied directly over the N-Terface without ointments or gels. The selection of materials depends on the amount of exudate and the goal of the dressing (which may include removing debris, absorbing exudate, or protecting new cells).

The wound can be cleaned with sterile saline, with dead tissue then being gently removed with sterile swabs. Sterile saline solution can be used to soak off adherent bandages rather than pulling them off the client. The therapist should pour a small amount of saline on the area that is sticking, wait a few moments,

and gently pry the dressing off. Dead skin can be debrided using iris scissors and pickups. Soft surgical scrub sponges may be used for cleaning and desensitization of the wound once it is healed and the stitches have been removed. Normal handwashing with running water with soap also may be done once cleared by a physician.

Pressure

A hypertrophic scar or a scar that is randomly laid down and thickened is reduced by the application of pressure, often by means of pressure garments.[82] Use of an insert of neoprene[e] fabric or silicone gel sheets or molds made from elastomer under the pressure garment increases the conformity of the garment. Pressure should be applied for most of the 24-hour period, and with a hypertrophic burn scar this intervention should continue for 6 months to 1 year after the injury. Silicone Gel Sheets[f] have been found to reduce hypertrophic scarring when worn on a regular basis for 12 to 24 hours a day.

Massage

Gentle to firm massage of the scarred area using a thick ointment rapidly softens scar tissue and should be followed immediately with active hand use so that tendons glide against the softened scar.[58] Vibration to the area with a small, low-intensity vibrator will have a similar effect.[58,82] Active exercise, using facilitation techniques and against resistance, or functional activity, should follow vibration. Massage and vibration may be started 4 weeks after injury.

Thermal heat in the form of paraffin dips, heat packs, fluidotherapy, or continuous pulse ultrasound may be used as preparatory techniques followed immediately by massage and stretching of scar tissue. Wrapping the scarred or stiff digit into flexion with Coban during the application of heat often increases mobility in the area. Heat should not be used on insensate areas or if swelling persists.

Active Range of Motion and Electrical Stimulation

Active ROM provides an internal stretch against resistant scar, and its use cannot be overemphasized. If the client is unable to achieve active motion because of scar adhesions or weakness, the use of a battery-operated NMES may augment the motion.[22] Stimulation may be performed by the client for several hours at home and has been shown to increase ROM and tendon excursion.[79]

Pain Syndromes

Pain, the subjective manifestation of trauma transmitted by the sympathetic nervous system, may interfere with normal functioning. Because pain leads to overprotection of the affected part and disuse of the extremity, it should be treated early. Limiting the period of immobilization after injury and providing sensory and proprioceptive input to the involved extremity may help in

---

[d]N-Terface, made by Winfield Laboratories (available from North Coast Medical, Morgan Hill, CA).

[e]Neoprene (available from Benik Corp, Silverdale, WA).
[f]Bio-Concepts, Phoenix, AZ. Cica-Care Silicone Gel Sheets (available from Smith & Nephew, Milwaukee, WI).

decreasing maladaptive movement patterns and the response to pain stimuli in the central nervous system.[82]

Desensitization

Stimulation of the large afferent A nerve fibers leads to a reduction of pain by decreasing summation in the slowly adapting, small, unmyelinated C fibers, which carry pain sensation. The A-axons can be stimulated mechanically with pressure, rubbing, vibration, TENS, percussion, and active motion. Desensitization techniques are based on the amplification of inhibitory mechanisms.

Yerxa has described a desensitization program that "employs short periods of contact with three sensory modalities: dowel textures, immersion or contact particles, and vibration."[95] This program allows the client to rank 10 dowel textures and 10 immersion textures on the degree of irritation produced by the stimulus. Intervention begins with a stimulus that is irritating but tolerable. The stimulus is applied for 10 minutes, three or four times a day. The vibration hierarchy is predetermined and based on cycles per second of vibration, the placement of the vibrator, and the duration of the intervention. Complete instructions for assembling the Downey Hand Center desensitization kit can be found in the literature in the references. The Downey Hand Center Hand Sensitivity Test can be used to establish a desensitization intervention program and measure progress in decreasing hypersensitivity.[95]

Neuromas

Neuromas are a complication of nerve suture or amputation. A traumatic neuroma is an unorganized mass of nerve fibers that results from accidental or surgical cutting of the nerve. A neuroma in continuity occurs on a nerve that is intact. Neuromas may be clinically identified by a specific, sharp pain. Stimulation of a neuroma usually causes the client to pull the hand away quickly; many clients report a burning pain that radiates up the forearm. Neuromas are disabling because any stimulation causes intense pain and the client avoids the sensitive area.

A generalized desensitization program may not work because the client never develops a tolerance for stimulation of the neuroma. Injection of cortisone acetate may help break up the neuroma, making desensitization techniques more effective. Surgically excising the neuroma or burying the nerve endings deeper may be necessary.

Complex Regional Pain Syndrome

Complex regional pain syndrome (CRPS) is the term that replaced "reflex sympathetic dystrophy (RSD)" to describe a group of disorders that "involve pain and dysfunction of severity or duration out of proportion to those expected from the initiating event."[63]

Complex denotes the complex nature of the pain response, which may include inflammation and autonomic, cutaneous, motor, and dystrophic changes. Regional refers to the wide distribution of symptoms beyond the area of the original lesion. Pain is the primary characteristic of this syndrome. It includes spontaneous pain, thermal changes, and at times burning pain. CRPS, type I, corresponds to RSD. Type II corresponds to

causalgia, a severe, burning pain first described during the Civil War.[63]

Diagnostic criteria for CRPS must include spontaneous pain beyond the territory of a single peripheral nerve and disproportionate to the inciting event. There is generally edema, skin blood-flow abnormality, or abnormal sudomotor activity in the area of the pain. The diagnosis is excluded by the existence of conditions that would otherwise account for the pain. The hallmarks of CRPS are pain; edema; blotchy-looking, shiny skin; and coolness of the extremity. Sensory changes may occur. Excessive sweating or dryness may occur if there is associated sympathetic dysfunction. The degree of trauma does not correlate with the severity of the pain and may occur after any injury. CRPS, type I may be triggered by a cycle of vasospasm and vasodilatation after an injury. Abnormal edema and constrictive dressings or casts may be a factor in initiating the vasospasm. A vasospasm causes tissue anoxia and edema and therefore more pain, which continues the abnormal cycle.[63] Circulation is decreased, which causes the extremity to become cool and pale.

Fibrosis after tissue anoxia and the presence of protein-rich exudates result in joint stiffness. The client may cradle the hand and prefer to keep it wrapped. There may be an exaggerated reaction to touch, especially light touch. Osteoporosis may be apparent on x-ray films by 8 weeks after trauma after active use of the hand. Burning pain associated with causalgia (CRPS, type II) is a symptom that may be alleviated by interruption of the sympathetic nerve pathways.

There are three stages of CRPS. Stage I (traumatic stage) may last up to 3 months; it is characterized by pain, pitting edema, and discoloration. Stage II (dystrophic stage) may last an additional 6 to 9 months. Pain, brawny edema, stiffness, redness, heat, and bony demineralization are usually found in this stage. The hand usually has a glossy appearance. Stage III (atrophic stage) may last several years or indefinitely. Pain usually peaks in Stage II and decreases in Stage III. Thickening around the joints occurs, and fixed contractures may be present. If swelling is present, it is hard and not responsive to techniques such as elevation. The hand may be pale, dry, and cool. There may be substantial dysfunction of the limb.

CRPS is treated by decreasing sympathetic stimulation. It is most responsive in Stage I. The first goal of intervention is reduction of the pain and hypersensitivity to light touch. This goal may be accomplished with application of warm (not hot), moist heat; fluidotherapy; gentle handling of the hand; acupressure; desensitization; and TENS before active ROM. Intervention that increases pain (e.g., passive ROM) should be avoided. Graded motor imagery is often used to decrease the pain and improve functional use of the involved extremity.[83] Many clients respond well to gentle manual edema mobilization,[6] which reduces the edema and reintroduces touching of the hand. Stellate ganglion blocks to eliminate the pain are effective early. They should be coordinated with therapy so that the client can perform active ROM and functional activities during the pain-free period after the blocks. Active ROM is crucial. Gravity-eliminated exercise, either in water or on a tabletop, may be more easily tolerated.

A variety of drugs may be used, including sympatholytic drugs that reduce the vasoconstrictive action of the peripheral vessels. Neurontin is often effective in reducing pain and increasing temperature in the extremity. Calcium channel blockers are also effective. Carefully monitored use of opioids may interrupt the pain cycle and allow active use of the hand.

Edema control techniques should be started immediately. Elevation, manual edema mobilization, contrast baths, and high-voltage direct current in water have been found to be effective. Surface electromyography-biofeedback training for relaxation may help muscle spasms and increase blood flow, in addition to reducing anxiety.

CRPS frequently triggers shoulder pain and stiffness, resulting in shoulder-hand syndrome or adhesive capsulitis of the shoulder. Therefore, active ROM and functional activities should include the entire upper quadrant. Skateboard exercises are helpful in the early stages for active-assisted exercise of the shoulder. Orthoses that reduce joint stiffness should be used as tolerated. Orthoses must not cause pain or increase swelling. Reliance on immobilization orthoses should be avoided because clients with CRPS prefer not to move the affected part, which ultimately makes their symptoms worse. If progress is not made with the use of traditional treatment interventions, the patient may benefit from casting motion to mobilize stiffness (CMMS). The benefits of CMMS include edema reduction through the circumferential use of a plaster cast that allows specific active motion, while limiting pain and maladaptive movement patterns in the affected wrist and hand.[76]

A tendency to develop CRPS should be suspected in any client who seems to complain excessively about pain, appears anxious, and complains of profuse sweating and temperature changes in the hand. Some clients report nausea associated with touching the hand. Clients tend to overprotect the hand. Early intervention with a structured therapy program of functional activities, group interaction, and exercises that include the hand and shoulder may prevent the occurrence of a fully developed CRPS. This problem is best recognized early and treated with tempered aggressiveness and empathy.

Transcutaneous Electrical Nerve Stimulation

TENS is an intervention technique that is thought to stimulate the afferent A nerve fibers in the high-frequency mode and stimulate the release of morphine-like neural hormones, the enkephalins, in the low-frequency mode. Its efficacy as an intervention for pain control is well documented in medical literature. As with other electrical modalities that may be used by occupational therapists, TENS should be correlated with functional use of the hand.

TENS should be used for intervention periods not to exceed 60 minutes at a time to achieve pain control. A TENS diary should be used to record the level of pain on a scale of 1 to 10 before and after intervention, as well as activities that exacerbate the pain. To prevent overuse, TENS may be tapered as the pain-free periods increase. Intervention can be continued as long as necessary to provide pain control.[22,81]

Joint Stiffness

Joint stiffness has been discussed in other sections of this chapter because it is seen after almost any hand trauma or disease. In

the acute phase it may also result from "internal splinting" done unconsciously by the client to avoid pain. It may be prevented by early mobilization, pain control, reduction of edema, active and passive ROM, use of a continuous passive motion (CPM) device, and appropriate orthotic techniques. Grades I and II joint mobilization are especially helpful in preparing for passive and active motion and providing pain relief.

Treatment of established joint stiffness is more difficult. Thermal modalities, joint mobilization, ultrasound and electrical stimulation, dynamic orthoses, serial casting, static progressive orthoses, relative motion orthoses, casting motion to mobilize stiffness, and active and passive motion in preparation for functional use should all be considered in the intervention regimen.[75,76]

Cumulative Trauma Disorders

A number of terms are used to describe injuries to the musculoskeletal system, including overuse syndromes, repetitive strain injuries, cervical-brachial disorders, repetitive motion injuries, and cumulative trauma disorders (CTDs). The term *cumulative trauma disorder* should be viewed as a description of the mechanism of injury and not a diagnosis. Even when the presenting symptoms are confusing, attempts to define a specific diagnosis are necessary because "each disorder has a different cause, intervention, and prognosis."[85] Diagnoses associated with cumulative trauma usually fall into one of three categories: tendinitis (e.g., lateral epicondylitis—tennis elbow or de Quervain's tenosynovitis), nerve compression syndromes (e.g., carpal tunnel syndrome or cubital tunnel syndrome), or myofascial pain.

Cumulative trauma occurs when force is applied to the same muscle or muscle group, causing an inflammatory response in the tendon or muscle.[85] Muscle fatigue is an important aspect of cumulative trauma. Excessive use of the muscle or body system (overuse or overexertion) is experienced as a muscle cramp. Acute overuse is relieved by rest, but chronic fatigue is not relieved by rest. The amount of fatigue is related to the amount of force and the duration of force application.

Fatigue occurs more quickly with high force. If force is maintained, repetitions must be reduced to allow recovery. Therefore, if the force is decreased while repetitions are maintained and recovery time is adequate, harm is less likely to occur. The combination of repetitions without adequate recovery time and high force establishes an environment that is likely to lead to injury. Brown[16] and Byl et al.[20] found that repetitive hand opening and closing may lead to motor control problems and the development of focal hand dystonia through a degradation of the cortical representation. Applying this research may help therapists develop more effective intervention programs for cumulative trauma and chronic pain.

Intervention may be divided into phases. Acute-phase intervention is geared toward decreasing the inflammation through dynamic rest. Orthoses are used for immobilization to relieve symptoms and may be combined with cortisone injections to reduce symptoms. Icing, ultrasound, iontophoresis (the movement of ions through biological material under the influence of an electric current), and interferential and high-voltage electrical stimulation have all been found to be effective in reducing pain and decreasing inflammation. Nonsteroidal anti-inflammatory drugs are also frequently used. When orthoses are used, they should be removed frequently during the day for stretching of the affected musculature (e.g., the extensor group with lateral epicondylitis) to maintain or increase muscle length and to prevent joint stiffness. Painful activities should be avoided during the dynamic rest phase. Vibration is contraindicated because vibration may contribute to inflammatory problems.

As the acute symptoms decrease, the client begins the exercise phase of intervention. After slow stretching warms up the muscles, the client begins controlled progressive exercise. Resistance should be increased slowly, and the frequency, intensity, and duration of exercises should be monitored and adjusted in response to pain and fatigue levels.

Clients are instructed to continue stretching three times a day, especially before activity, for an indefinite time. Proper body mechanics are critical in the long-term control of inflammatory problems, so clients must become aware of what triggers their symptoms and learn early intervention if symptoms reappear. Icing, orthoses, stretching, and modified activities combined with correct body mechanics are usually effective. The key is that the clients learn self-management techniques and take an active role in their intervention.

Work-related risk factors for CTDs include the following:
- Repetition
- High force
- Awkward joint posture
- Direct pressure
- Vibration
- Prolonged static positioning

An assessment of the job site, tools used, and hand position during work activities may be indicated with the client whose symptoms are related to job demands. Modification of the equipment used and strengthening of the dominant muscle groups and their antagonist muscles may permit continued employment and control the inflammatory problem.

Tendinitis (inflammation of the tendon), tenosynovitis (inflammation of the tendon sheath), and tendinosis (chronic tendon injury with damage to the tendon on a cellular level) are frequently seen in cumulative trauma. The cycle of overuse leading to microtrauma, swelling, pain, and limitations in movement is followed by rest, disuse, and weakness. Normal activity is resumed, and the cycle begins again.[66]

Clients usually have a combination of localized pain, swelling, pain with resisted motion of the affected musculotendinous unit, limitations in motion, weakness, and crepitation of the tendons. Symptoms are reproduced with activity or work simulation. Using functional grades to describe the associated symptoms assists in evaluation and in monitoring of improvement (Table 40.5). Although isometric grip strength may be normal, wrist and forearm strength are often decreased and out of balance. Dynamic grip strength may be more limited because tendon gliding is more likely to increase inflammation and pain. Muscle imbalance leads to positioning and substitution patterns that may result in worsening or spreading of symptoms.

Nerve compression syndromes, especially carpal tunnel syndrome, are frequently seen. Carpal tunnel syndrome is caused by pressure on the median nerve as it travels beneath the transverse carpal ligament at the volar surface of the wrist. The syndrome is associated with increased pressure in the carpal canal because of trauma, edema, retention of fluids as a result of pregnancy, flexor tenosynovitis, repetitive wrist motions, or static loading of the wrist.[47]

Symptoms are night pain that is severe enough to waken the client; tingling in the thumb and index and middle fingers; and, if advanced, wasting of the thenar musculature caused by pressure on the motor branch of the nerve. Early carpal tunnel syndrome may be recognized during a thorough nerve evaluation.

Conservative intervention is usually attempted first and includes orthotics of the wrist in no more than 20 degrees of extension, contrast baths to reduce edema, wearing of compression gloves to reduce edema, and activity analysis. A semiflexible or neoprene orthosis rather than a completely rigid orthosis may be used to provide support while allowing a small amount of flexion and extension for greater functional use in carpal tunnel syndrome.

TABLE 40.5 Functional Grading of Cumulative Trauma Disorders

Grade	Description
Grade I	• Pain after activity; resolves quickly with rest • No decrease in amount or speed of work • Objective findings usually absent
Grade II	• Pain in one site while working • Pain consistent while working but resolves when activity stops • Productivity sometimes mildly affected • May have objective findings
Grade III	• Pain in one or more sites while working • Persistent pain after cessation of activity • Productivity affected and multiple breaks sometimes necessary to continue working • May affect other activities away from work • May have weakness, loss of control and dexterity, tingling, numbness, and other objective findings • May have latent or active trigger points
Grade IV	• All common uses of hand and upper extremity resulting in pain, which is present 50% to 75% of the time • May be unable to work or works in limited capacity • May have weakness, loss of control and dexterity, tingling, numbness, trigger points, and other objective findings
Grade V	• Loss of capacity to use upper extremities because of chronic, unrelenting pain • Usually unable to work • Symptoms sometimes of indefinite duration

From Kasch MC: Therapist's evaluation and treatment of upper extremity trauma disorders. In Mackin EJ, Callahan AD, Skirven TM, et al, editors: *Rehabilitation of the hand and upper extremity*, ed 5, St. Louis, 2002, Mosby.

Ultrasound and iontophoresis may be used to reduce inflammation, and icing techniques are beneficial. Specific strengthening exercises of the wrist, fingers, and thumb should be given when the pain and inflammation have been controlled.

Myofascial pain and fibrositis are also conditions of pain elicited by activation of trigger points within the muscles and resulting in pain referred to a distal area; these are frequently encountered conditions. Travell studied myofascial pain and mapped out the traditional trigger points and their referral patterns.[39] Poor posture and positioning of the body out of normal alignment are often the mechanisms of injury in myofascial pain, so careful examination of the client and his or her normal daily activities is indicated. The therapist should observe the client performing the activity rather than rely on a verbal description.

Myofascial pain should be considered if direct intervention of the painful area does not relieve the pain. Evaluation for trigger points must be done meticulously, and mapping of the trigger points and the referral areas must be documented. Because the pain is referred, the trigger point must be treated, not the referral area. The interventions used for other inflammatory problems, such as ice and ultrasound, can be used. In addition, specific interventions for the trigger points, such as friction massage and TENS, may relieve the pain. Activity analysis is an essential part of intervention to relieve the stresses of functional activities on the affected tissues.

Elastic Therapeutic Taping

Kinesio Tape[g] was developed in Japan in the 1970s. Since its introduction in the United States in 1994, it has become increasingly popular with therapists for use in CTD interventions.[72] The technique of elastic or kinesiology taping uses tapes such as Kinesio Tape, RockTape, and KT Tape. Unlike athletic taping, which is restrictive and is used to provide stability and restrict joint motion, elastic therapeutic tape is designed to "mimic the elastic properties of muscle, skin, and fascia."[59] When properly applied, the elasticity of the elastic tape does not restrict the movement of soft tissue but supports weakened muscles and allows for full movement of the joints by reducing abnormal muscle tension or spasms.

A variety of clinical applications for elastic taping techniques have been described. Depending on the problem, the tape is anchored at either the origin or the insertion of a muscle and then gently stretched and taped over or around either a shortened or an elongated muscle; this puts the muscle back into a neutral position. The tape is believed to affect the peripheral somatosensory receptors in the superficial skin, which in turn affect the skin and lymphatic systems (in addition to muscle and joint function) as they relate to pain, proprioception, and motor control. The goals and concepts of elastic taping include the following[59,72]:

- Decrease pain by increasing the somatosensory system.
- Reduce inflammation and edema by stimulating the lymphatic system.
- Normalize muscle tone by reducing overstretching and overcontraction of muscles.

- Reduce muscle fatigue by supporting and enhancing the contraction of weakened muscles.
- Improve ROM by relieving pain.
- Provide support and alignment to joints by supporting weakened ligaments.
- Prevent injuries during ADLs by providing support to muscles and ligaments.

Strengthening Activities

Acute care is followed by a gradual return of motion, sensibility, and preparation to return to normal ADL and IADL routines.

In addition to the strengthening exercises implemented in the clinic, the therapist and client should work together to discuss which home activities will encourage beginning strengthening, and how to safely return to their gym exercises. Because every hand clinic has its own armamentarium of strengthening exercises and media, only a few suggestions are provided here.

Computerized Evaluation and Exercise Equipment

Baltimore Therapeutic Equipment (BTE) has made available the BTE Work Simulator (https://www.BTEtech.com) (Fig. 40.16), an electromechanical device that has more than

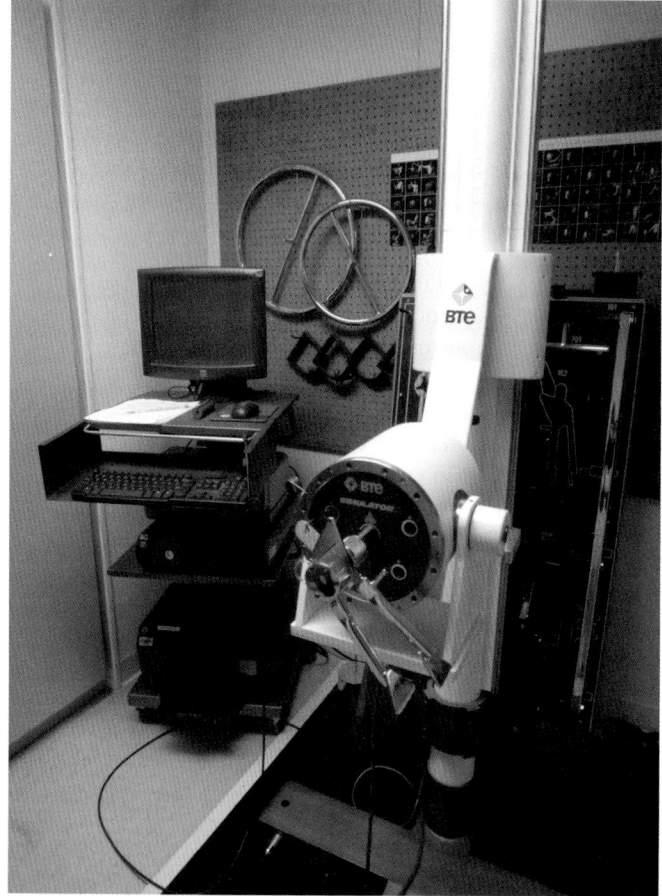

Fig. 40.16 The BTE Work Simulator is an electromechanical device used to simulate real-life tasks, thereby allowing evaluation and strengthening of the upper extremity. The client's progress is monitored through a computerized printout, and the program can be modified to increase resistance and endurance.

---

[g]KinesioTape (available from North Coast Medical, Morgan Hill, CA).

20 interchangeable tool handles and can be used for both work evaluation and UE strengthening. Resistance can vary from no resistance to complete static resistance, with tool height and angle also adjustable. When the device is used for strengthening, the resistance is usually set low and gradually increased. Length of exercise is increased when a base level of strength has been achieved. The BTE Work Simulator allows for close simulation of real-world tasks that are easily translatable into physical demands common to manual work.

Other computerized evaluation equipment allows the therapist to record the results of assessment and print a report. The percentage of impairment also can be determined electronically. Portable systems are being developed that allow the therapist to record daily intervention and download the information into a computerized network. Outcome data from many sources can then be compared. The advancement of technology in rehabilitation will allow the therapist to be more efficient and also capture important information that is not available through traditional means.

Many practitioners use occupation-based interventions that simulate the actual work done, either in the clinic or at the work site. These methods assist the client toward return to their occupations and are in keeping with the Occupational Therapy Practice Framework.

Weight Well

The Weight Well[h] (Fig. 40.17) was developed at the Downey Community Hospital Hand Center in Downey, California, and is available commercially. Rods with a variety of handle shapes are inserted through holes in a box, and weights are suspended from them. The rods are turned against resistance throughout the ROM to encourage full grasp and release of the injured hand, wrist flexion and extension, pinch, and pronation and supination patterns. The Weight Well can be graded for resistance and repetitions and is an excellent tool for progressive resistive exercise.

Theraband

TheraBand[i] is a 6-inch (15.2-cm) wide rubber sheet that is available by the yard and is color coded according to degrees of resistance. It can be cut into any length required and used for resistive exercise for the UE. The uses for TheraBand are limited only by the therapist's imagination; it can be adapted to diagonal patterns of motion, wrist exercises, follow-up intervention of tennis elbow, and other uses. TheraBand can be combined with dowel rods and other equipment to provide resistance throughout the ROM. It is inexpensive and easy to incorporate into a home intervention program.

Hand-Strengthening Equipment

Handgrips of graded resistance are available from rehabilitation supply companies and sporting goods stores. They can be

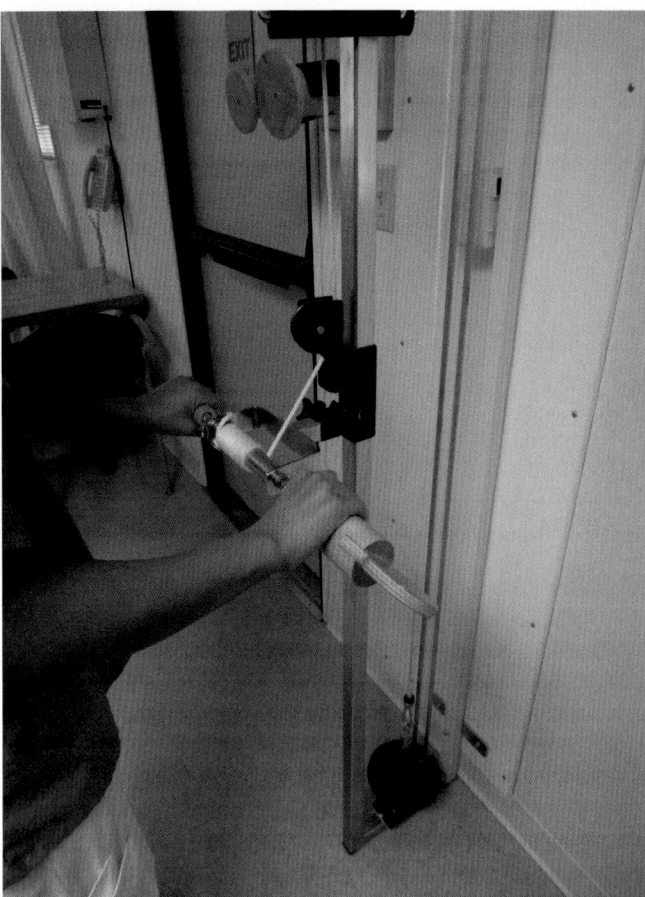

Fig. 40.17 The Weight Well is used to strengthen the upper extremity by applying progressive resistance to weakened musculature. It also is useful in retraining prehension of pinch and grip.

purchased with various resistance levels and can be used for progressive resistive hand exercises.

Therapists must be especially careful not to use the overly resistive, spring-loaded grippers often sold in sporting goods stores. These devices may be beneficial to the seasoned athlete but are usually too resistive for the recently injured.

Therapy putty can be purchased in bulk; the amount given to the client depends on his or her hand size and strength. This medium also is available in grades of resistance, and some types provide chips that can be added to progressively increase resistance. Therapy putty can be adapted to most finger motions, and it is easily incorporated into a home program.

Household items (e.g., spring-type clothespins) have been used to increase the strength of grasp and pinch. Imaginative use of common objects should present a challenge to the hand therapist.

Purposeful and Occupation-Based Activity

Purposeful and occupation-based activities are an integral part of rehabilitation of the hand. Purposeful and occupation-based activities include crafts, games, dexterity activities, ADLs, and work samples. Several studies have shown that clients are more likely to choose occupationally embedded exercise and performed better using this type of exercise over rote exercise.[94]

---

[h] Upper Extremity Technology Weight Well (available from North Coast Medical, Gilroy CA).

[i] TheraBand (available from Patterson Medical, https://www.patterson-medical.com).

With activities that the client has performed multiple times, the brain has a neurological pathway for that activity which assists the client in maneuvering through that task. Many of the intervention techniques described previously are used as preparatory methods for the hand in preparation for purposeful activity.

Activities should be started as soon as possible at whatever level the client can perform them with adaptations to compensate for limited ROM and strength. They should be used in conjunction with other interventions. The occupational therapist must continually assess the client's functional capacities and initiate changes in the intervention plan to incorporate activities as soon as possible in the restorative phase.

Vocational and leisure goals should be established at the time of initial evaluation and taken into account when devising the intervention plan. The needs of a brick mason may be quite different from those of a mother with small children, and the environmental needs of the client must not be neglected.

Crafts should be graded from light resistance to heavy resistance and from gross dexterity to fine dexterity. Crafts that have been found to work extremely well with hand injuries include macramé, Turkish knot weaving, clay molding, leather tooling, and woodworking. All of these crafts can be adapted and graded to the client's capabilities and have been found to have a high level of client acceptance. When integrated into a program of total hand rehabilitation, they are viewed as another milestone of achievement and not as a diversion to fill up empty hours. For example, the pride of accomplishment for Gerry, who was able to complete his first simple woodworking project, is evidence that the purposeful activity of crafts belongs in hand rehabilitation.

Activities that do not have an end product but provide practice in dexterity and ADL skills also fit into the category of purposeful activities. Developmental games and activities that require pinch or grasp and release may be graded and timed to increase difficulty. ADL boards that have a variety of opening and closing devices provide practice for use of the hand at home and increase self-confidence. String and finger games are challenging coordination activities that can be done in pairs and are fun to do. Newer computer games and virtual reality games help to increase speed and coordination.

A hobby often can be adapted for use in the clinic. Fly-tying is a difficult dexterity activity but one that is frequently enjoyed by an avid fisherman. Golf clubs and fishing poles can be adapted in the clinic; in the case of Gerry, therapy with these tools allowed early return to a favorite form of relaxation.

Humor and interaction with the therapists and the other clients are vital but intangible benefits of hand therapy intervention. The intervention should be planned to promote both.

FUNCTIONAL CAPACITY EVALUATION AND WORK HARDENING

The ultimate goal of therapy for an injured worker is to return to full employment. Many weeks or months may have elapsed between the time of the injury and the point at which the

physician thinks that a return to work is appropriate from a medical standpoint. Despite the fact that x-ray examinations may show full healing and restored ROM, many clients do not feel that they have the strength, dexterity, or endurance to return to their former jobs. Pain may continue to be a limiting factor, especially with heavy activities. Light duty or part-time positions may not be available, and the physician, therapist, industrial insurance carrier, and especially the client are frustrated by the lack of an objective method of evaluating an individual's physical capacity for work. Occupational therapists with training in evaluation, kinesiology, and adaptation of environmental factors coupled with a functional approach to the client may play a key role in a functional capacity evaluation.

The terms functional capacity evaluation (FCE) and work tolerance screening (WTS) describe the process of measuring an individual's ability to perform the physical demands of work.[73] The results of the FCE allow the therapist, worker, physician, and vocational counselor to establish a specific, attainable employment goal using reliable data. This approach relieves the physician of the responsibility of returning the client to work without objective information about the client's ability to do a job. It also allows the client to test his or her own abilities and may result in increased self-confidence about returning to work.[48,73] The therapist should consult the Dictionary of Occupational Titles (DOT) to obtain information about the worker traits required for the expected job. Once the physical demand characteristics of work have been documented, it is possible to evaluate the client's ability to perform them.[48,91]

Work hardening is the progressive use of simulated work samples to increase endurance, strength, productivity, and often feasibility. Work hardening may be performed for a period of weeks, and the progressive ongoing nature of the work usually improves physical capacity. It is an important contribution to return to work.

FCE and work hardening are adjuncts to the vocational rehabilitation process. Occupational therapists are trained to observe behavior and have the skills necessary to translate that observation into useful data. FCE and work hardening should not compete with the work of rehabilitation or vocational counselors; instead, they should provide critical information about a worker's physical functioning and foster reentry into the job market. Refer to Chapter 14 for more detailed information regarding work evaluation and work programs.

CONSULTATION WITH INDUSTRY

Occupational therapists may be asked to visit the job site to make recommendations for ergonomic adaptations, including tool modification, ergonomic furniture and accessories, and training of workers in proper positioning to reduce the incidence of CTDs. Because prevention substantially reduces the costs to industry, occupational therapists have a unique opportunity to apply their training in activity analysis and adaptation of the environment in a new setting. The Americans with Disabilities Act (ADA) mandates reasonable accommodations for workers with disabilities. Many occupational therapists have become active in helping companies comply with the requirements of the ADA. The American Occupational Therapy Association is an excellent resource for information about the ways in which therapists can be involved in these efforts in their communities (see Chapter 15).

PSYCHOSOCIAL EFFECTS OF HAND INJURIES

After a hand injury, a number of psychosocial reactions may occur, including changed body image and self-image, depression, anxiety, and decreased self-worth (as experienced by Gerry, the cabinetmaker in the case study with the amputated fingers and surgical replantation. For traumatic hand injuries, acute stress disorder and posttraumatic stress disorder are not

uncommon and can be problematic for the client, especially if they are not addressed promptly.[51] The hand therapist is often the primary contact for the client after injury and may see the client several times per week on a one on one basis. The hand therapist, therefore, plays a very important role in helping the client return to preinjury physical and emotional functioning. Not only do occupational therapists who specialize in hand therapy provide the client with emotional support, but they are also critical in recognizing psychosocial issues that the client may be having; are educated in evaluating and providing intervention for these; and, when necessary, because of the severity of the problem, are capable of facilitating referral to an appropriate mental health professional.

THREADED CASE STUDY

Gerry, Part 2

The case study presented at the beginning of this chapter described Gerry, a 32-year-old cabinetmaker with an acute, complex hand injury involving amputation and surgical replantation of three digits. Gerry progressed through all phases of rehabilitation over the course of 15 months, from the acute hospital stay to return to work and play activities. Based on the case presented, how would the intervention plan change over the course of Gerry's recovery, and what specific intervention approaches could his occupational therapist use?

During the acute phase, one of the therapist's goals was to promote and maintain the health of the client's unaffected joints that were vulnerable to becoming stiff from protective posturing. Another goal during the acute phase was to prevent further injury or abnormal joint changes to the left injured hand. ROM exercises were administered to maintain the healthy function of the client's unaffected joints, such as the shoulder and elbow, and a protective orthosis was fabricated, placing Gerry in a protective and functional position of mild wrist flexion, MP flexion, and IP extension. During this phase of recovery, education was an important component of the client's intervention plan. Gerry was taught appropriate postoperative precautions and orthosis wear and care; his family received education on wound care, dressing changes, and signs of infection. Gerry was given written material regarding this home program.

During the intermediate phase of his recovery, the intervention approach was to restore active and passive ROM, strength, and coordination to Gerry's hand so that he could return to his previous occupations (specifically, cabinetry, golf, and meal preparation). The ROM activities were graded, and motion was progressively added as the tendons, nerves, and vessels healed. Strengthening exercises were added during the late phase of recovery, and at this point Gerry could safely attempt to return to his previous activities. It was at this time that purposeful and occupation-based activities were added to Gerry's therapy regimen. In addition, Gerry's areas of occupation had to be modified for the loss of mobility, strength, and coordination of the hand. Gerry was taught one-handed ADLs during the acute phase of recovery so that he could be self-sufficient until he regained the use of his left hand. Modifications to his activity demands were also implemented, such as enlarging the handles of his golf clubs to compensate for the lack of full finger ROM during the intermediate to late phases of recovery. Finally, Gerry was taught to prevent further injury to his hand through visual compensation techniques for loss of sensation, to monitor for signs of infection, and to undertake postsurgical precautions during the acute phase of his injury.

Throughout Gerry's intervention, his performance skills were reviewed to identify barriers to performance using a variety of assessment tools. A grip dynamometer, pinch meter, and manual muscle tests were used to assess grip, pinch, and muscle strength. A goniometer was used to assess ROM, and Semmes-Weinstein monofilaments were used to assess sensation. A volumeter and circumferential measurements were used to assess edema, and the Jebson Test of Hand Function was used to assess the functional use of Gerry's hand in a standardized format. The evaluation data were then interpreted and the intervention plan modified to achieve the targeted outcomes.

Once the intervention plan was established, various preparatory methods and purposeful activities were chosen to achieve Gerry's occupational goals. For the occupational performance goal of golfing, orthoses were used as a preparatory method during the intermediate phase of recovery to help Gerry gain passive ROM of stiff joints and increase overall flexion of the replanted digits so that he could eventually hold a golf club. Physical agent modalities such as paraffin and ultrasound were applied before performance of purposeful activity during the intermediate and late phases of recovery. Purposeful activities such as swinging a golf club in the clinic, simulating a golf swing on the BTE work simulator, and gradually increasing the physical resistive demands of this golf swing were performed. Gerry also practiced putting in the clinic with special "flexion gloves" early on so that he could hold the golf club; later, he progressed to wearing no glove but instead enlarging the handle of the golf club to facilitate a secure grip.

To address Gerry's occupational goal of returning to work as a cabinetmaker, a volunteer opportunity was arranged for him to participate in the purposeful activity of making "wooden sliding/transfer boards" and other assistive devices for the acute rehabilitation clients. Not only was this activity goal directed and directly related to his work occupation, but it also fulfilled Gerry's desire to use his talents in carpentry to help other clients in the hospital; this contributed to improving his feelings of self-worth. During the late phase of Gerry's recovery, additional occupation-based activity was initiated to address his avocational interests. During the actual performance of golfing and softball outside of the clinic, it was found that Gerry was hypersensitive in the palm over the scars. Desensitization techniques were performed as part of his home program, and he purchased gloves with gel inserts to absorb the shock of hitting the ball.[3]

SUMMARY

This chapter provides an overview of interventions of the UE. Evaluation procedures are discussed, as are as the basic intervention techniques. Management of both acute injuries and cumulative trauma is included, as well as information on strengthening and programs for industrial injuries. Most occupational therapists working in physical disabilities should be familiar with the basic intervention approaches described for the UE because they work with clients who have some limitation in the UEs. Specialization in hand therapy requires both advanced academic study and clinical experience. A therapist who specializes in this area of practice and who meets minimum requirements may choose to take the Hand Therapy Certification Examination and become a certified hand therapist (CHT). For more information on becoming a CHT, contact the Hand Therapy Certification Commission (https://www.

htcc.org).[50] Links to educational resources are also available on this website. Another valuable resource is membership in the American Society of Hand Therapists (https://www.asht.org).

Although much of UE rehabilitation involves the use of preparatory methods such as exercise, orthotics, and physical agent modalities, these interventions should be used in preparation for purposeful or occupation-based activities. The goal is always for the client to be as independent as possible and to use these preparatory methods to achieve the client's occupation-based performance goals. Purposeful activity or occupation is used whenever feasible in the hand clinic according to space and time constraints, and clients are encouraged to use their new skills in their own home or work contexts and bring back to the clinic information about the obstacles that they experience in achieving their performance goals.

REVIEW QUESTIONS

1. A client is seen for a hand problem and found to have limited or painful ROM of the shoulder. List three tests that should be performed.
2. Discuss three approaches to postoperative care of flexor tendon injuries, and describe how the differences among the methods would influence the initiation of OT.
3. What does joint dysfunction refer to? What are its causes?
4. Discuss the three classifications of nerve injury.
5. Define the area referred to as "no-man's land." What distinguishes injury to this area?
6. What techniques are used to evaluate the physical demand characteristics of work?
7. List three methods of applying pressure to a hypertrophic scar.
8. Which functional activities could be used for restoration of hand function following laceration and repair of the extrinsic finger flexors?
9. What are two or three examples of purposeful and occupational-based activities that could be incorporated into Gerry's hand rehabilitation program?
10. List five tests used to assess joint integrity in the hand.
11. List three objectives of the use of orthotics as they relate to injury of the radial, median, and ulnar nerves.
12. What are the characteristics of complex regional pain syndrome, type I? What are the intervention goals?
13. How is the presence of edema evaluated? List three methods used to reduce edema.
14. What are the primary work-related risk factors associated with cumulative trauma?

For additional practice questions for this chapter, please visit eBooks.Health.Elsevier.com.

REFERENCES

1. Adson A, Coffey J: Cervical rib: a method of anterior approach for relief of symptoms by division of scalenus anticus, *Ann Surg* 85:834, 1927.
2. Amadio P: Advances in understanding of tendon healing and repairs and impact on postoperative management. In Skirven T, Osterman L, Fedorczyk J, Amadio P, Feldsher SB, Shin EK, editors: *Rehabilitation of the hand and upper extremity* 7th ed., St. Louis, 2021, Mosby.
3. American Occupational Therapy Association. (2020). Occupational therapy practice framework: Domain and process, 4th edition.
4. American Society of Hand Therapists: *Clinical assessment recommendations*, 3rd ed., Mount Laurel NJ, 2001, American Society of Hand Therapists.
5. American Society for Surgery of the Hand: *The hand: anatomy, examination, and diagnosis*, ed 4, Philadelphia, 2011, Lippincott Williams & Wilkins.
6. Artzberger S: Edema reduction techniques: A biologic rationale for selection. In Cooper C, editor: *Fundamentals of hand therapy: clinical reasoning and treatment guidelines for common diagnoses of the upper extremity* 2nd ed., St. Louis, 2014, Elsevier.
7. Baker K: Functional tests for dexterity. In Skirven T, Osterman L, Fedorczyk J, Amadio P, Feldsher SB, Shin EK, editors: *Rehabilitation of the hand and upper extremity* 7th ed., St. Louis, 2021, Mosby.
8. Bell-Krotoski JA: Plaster cylinder casting for contractures of the interphalangeal joints. In Mackin EJ, editor: *Rehabilitation of the hand and upper extremity* ed 5, St. Louis, 2002, Mosby.
9. Bell-Krotoski JA: Sensibility testing with the Semmes-Weinstein monofilaments. In Skirven TM, editor: *Rehabilitation of the hand and upper extremity* ed 6, Philadelphia, 2011, Elsevier Mosby.
10. Bell-Krotoski J, Weinstein S, Weinstein C: Testing sensibility, including touch-pressure, two-point discrimination, point localization, and vibration, *Journal of Hand Therapy* 6:114–123, 1993.
11. Bennett G: *Hand-tool dexterity test*, Toronto, Pearson.

12. Bo Tang J, Lalonde D: Surgical management of flexor tendon injuries. In Skirven T, Osterman L, Fedorczyk J, Amadio P, Feldsher SB, Shin EK, editors: *Rehabilitation of the hand and upper extremity* 7th ed., St. Louis, 2021, Mosby.

13. Bohannon RW, Peolsson A, Massy-Westropp N, Desrosiers J, Bear-Lehman J: Reference values for adult grip strength measured with a Jamar dynamometer: a descriptive meta-analysis, *Physiotherapy* 92(1):11–15, 2006. https://doi.org/10.1016/j.physio.2005.05.003.

14. Boyes JH, Stark HH: Flexor-tendon grafts in the fingers and thumb, *J Bone Joint Surg Am* 53(7):1332, 1971.

15. Brand PW, Hollister A: *Clinical mechanics of the hand*, ed 3, St. Louis, 1999, Mosby.

16. Brown PW: Psychologically based hand disorders. In Mackin EJ, editor: *Rehabilitation of the hand and upper extremity* ed 5, St. Louis, 2002, Mosby.

17. Bunnell S: Repair of tendons in the fingers and description of two new instruments, *Surg Gynecol Obstet* 26:103–110, 1918.

18. Butler D: *Sensitive nervous system*, Adelaide, 2006, Noigroup.

19. Butler DS: *The graded motor imagery handbook*, Australia, 2012, NOI Group.

20. Byl NN, Kretschmer J, McKenzie A: Focal hand dystonia. In Skirven T, Osterman L, Fedorczyk J, Amadio P, Feldsher SB, Shin EK, editors: *Rehabilitation of the hand and upper extremity* 7th ed., St. Louis, 2021, Mosby.

21. Cameron M, Monroe L: *Physical rehabilitation: evidence-based examination, evaluation, and intervention*, St. Louis, 2007, Saunders.

22. Cameron MH: *Physical agents in rehabilitation: An evidence-based approach to practice* 6th ed., St Louis, 2022, Saunders.

23. Cannon N: Therapist's management of flexor tendon repairs. In Skirven T, Osterman L, Fedorczyk J, Amadio P, Feldsher SB, Shin EK, editors: *Rehabilitation of the hand and upper extremity* 7th ed., St. Louis, 2021, Mosby.

24. Cannon N, et al: Control of immediate postoperative pain following tenolysis and capsulectomies of the hand with TENS, *J Hand Surg Am* 8:625, 1983.

25. Carroll D: A quantitative test of upper extremity function, *J Chronic Dis* 18:479, 1965.

26. Chan SW, LaStayo P: Hand therapy management following mutilating hand injuries, *Hand Clin* 19(1):133, 2003.

27. Chisar J, Chee N: Fractures. In Jacobs M, Austin NM, editors: *Orthotic intervention for the hand and upper extremity* 3rd ed, Philadelphia, PA, 2014, Lippincott Williams & Wilkins.

28. Cifaldi Collins D, Schwarze L: Early progressive resistance following immobilization of flexor tendon repairs, *J Hand Ther* 4(3):111–116, 1991.

29. Commission on Accreditation of Rehabilitation Facilities (CARF): *Guidelines for accreditation*. CARF.org.

30. Creelman G.: Volumeters Unlimited, Phoenix, AZ, 1989.

31. Culp RW, Sirmon B, Feldsher SB: Secondary and reconstructive tendon procedures. In Skirven T, Osterman L, Fedorczyk J, Amadio P, Feldsher SB, Shin EK, editors: *Rehabilitation of the hand and upper extremity* 7th ed., St. Louis, 2021, Mosby.

32. Dellon AL: Clinical use of vibratory stimuli to evaluate peripheral nerve injury and compression neuropathy, *Plast Reconstr Surg* 65(4):466, 1980.

33. Dellon AL: The vibrometer, *Plast Reconstr Surg* 71(3):427, 1980.

34. Dellon AL: *Evaluation of sensibility and reeducation of sensation in the hand*, Baltimore, 2014, Dellon Institutes.

35. Dellon AL, Curtis RM, Edgerton MT: Reeducation of sensation in the hand after nerve injury and repair, *Plast Reconstr Surg* 53(3):297, 1974.

36. DeTullio LM, Wolfe DM, Strohl AB: Clinical examination of the hand. In Skirven T, Osterman L, Fedorczyk J, Amadio P, Feldsher SB, Shin EK, editors: *Rehabilitation of the hand and upper extremity* 7th ed., St. Louis, 2021, Mosby.

37. Diao E, Hariharan JS, Soejima O, Lotz JC: Effect of peripheral suture depth on strength of tendon repairs, *J Hand Surg Am* 21(2):234–239, 1996.

38. Donatelli R, Owens-Burkhart H: Effects of immobilization on the extensibility of periarticular connective tissue, *J Orthop Sports Phys Ther* 3:67, 1981.

39. Donnelly JM, Fernández-de-las-Peñas C, Finnegan M, Freeman JL: *Myofascial pain and dysfunction: the trigger point manual*, 3rd ed., Baltimore, 2018, Williams & Wilkins.

40. Duff SV, Estilow T, Novak CB: Therapy management of peripheral nerve injuries and repairs. In Skirven T, Osterman L, Fedorczyk J, Amadio P, Feldsher SB, Shin EK, editors: *Rehabilitation of the hand and upper extremity* 7th ed., St. Louis, 2021, Mosby.

41. Duran R, et al: Management of flexor tendon lacerations in zone 2 using controlled passive motion postoperatively. In Hunter JM, editor: *Rehabilitation of the hand* ed 3, St. Louis, 1990, Mosby.

42. Edmond SL: *Joint mobilization/manipulation: extremity and spinal techniques*, 3rd ed., Philadelphia, 2017, Elsevier Mosby.

43. Ellenbecker T: *Clinical examination of the shoulder*, St. Louis, 2004, Elsevier Saunders.

44. Evans RB: Rehabilitation following extensor tendon injury and repair. In Skirven T, Osterman L, Fedorczyk J, Amadio P, Feldsher SB, Shin EK, editors: *Rehabilitation of the hand and upper extremity* 7th ed., St. Louis, 2021, Mosby.

45. Feldsher S: Therapist's management of tendon transfers. In Skirven T, Osterman L, Fedorczyk J, Amadio P, Feldsher SB, Shin EK, editors: *Rehabilitation of the hand and upper extremity* 7th ed., St. Louis, 2021, Mosby.

46. Gelberman RH, Szabo RM, Williamson RV, Dimick MP: Sensibility testing in peripheral-nerve compression syndromes: an experimental study in humans, *J Bone Joint Surg* 65(5):632, 1983.

47. Gelberman RH, Hergenroeder PT, Hargens AR, et al: The carpal tunnel syndrome: a study of carpal canal pressures, *J Bone Joint Surg* 63(3):380, 1981.

48. Gerg MJ, Kaskutas K: Work performance. In Skirven T, Osterman L, Fedorczyk J, Amadio P, Feldsher SB, Shin EK, editors: *Rehabilitation of the hand and upper extremity* 7th ed., St. Louis, 2021, Mosby.

49. Goloborod'ko SA: Postoperative management of flexor tenolysis, *J Hand Ther* 12:330–332, 1999.

50. Hand Therapy Certification Commission: *Guidelines for certification*. https://www.htcc.org.

51. Hannah SD, Cheng MK: Psychosocial issues after a traumatic upper extremity injury. In Skirven T, Osterman L, Fedorczyk J, Amadio P, Feldsher SB, Shin EK, editors: *Rehabilitation of the hand and upper extremity* 7th ed., St. Louis, 2021, Mosby.

52. Hawkins R, Kennedy J: Impingement syndrome in athletes, *Am J Sports Med* 8(3):151, 1980.

53. Hengeveld E, Banks K, editors: *Maitland's Peripheral Manipulation* ed 4, London, 2005, Butterworth-Heinemann.

54. Howell JW, Merritt WH, Robinson SJ: Immediate controlled active motion following zone 4–7 extensor tendon repair, *J Hand Ther* 18:182–190, 2005.

55. Jerosch-Herold C: Sensibility testing. In Skirven T, Osterman L, Fedorczyk J, Amadio P, Feldsher SB, Shin EK, editors: *Rehabilitation of the hand and upper extremity* 7th ed., St. Louis, 2021, Mosby.

56. Jiuliano JA, Jupiter J: Distal radius fractures. In Trumble TE, Budoff JE, Cornwall R, editors: *Hand, Elbow & Shoulder: Core Knowledge in Orthopaedics*, Philadelphia, 2006, Mosby, pp 84–101.

57. Jobst Institute https://www.promedica.org/services-and-conditions/institute/jobst-vascular-institute.

58. Kamenetz H: Mechanical devices of massage. In Basmajian JV, editor: *Manipulation, traction and massage* ed 3, Baltimore, 1985, Williams & Wilkins.

59. Kase K, Wallis J, Kase T: *Clinical therapeutic applications of Kinesio taping method*, 3rd edition, Tokyo, 2013, Kinesio Taping Association.

60. Keller JL, Henderson JP, Landrieu KW, Dimick MP, Walsh JM: The 2019 practice analysis of hand therapy and the use of orthoses by certified hand therapists, *Journal of Hand Therapy* 35:628–640, 2022. https://doi.org/10.1016/j.jht.2021.04.008.

61. Kellor M, Frost J, Silberberg N, et al: *Technical manual of hand strength and dexterity test*, Minneapolis, 1971, Sister Kenney Rehabilitation Institute.

62. Kessler RM, Hertling D: Joint mobilization techniques. In Kessler RM, Hertling D, editors: *In Management of common musculoskeletal disorders*, 1983, Harper & Row.

63. Koman LA, Smith BP, Smith TL: Complex Regional Pain Syndrome: In Skirven T, Osterman L, Fedorczyk JM, Amadio P, Feldsher SB, Shin EK, editors: *Rehabilitation of the hand and upper extremity* 7th ed., St. Louis, 2021, Mosby.

64. LaSalle WB, Strickland JW: An evaluation of the two-stage flexor tendon reconstruction technique, *J Hand Surg* 8(3):263, 1983.

65. Law M, MacDermid J: *Evidence-based rehabilitation: a guide to practice*, 3rd ed., 2013, Thorofare: SLACK Incorporated.

66. Lee MP, Biafora SJ, Xelouf DS: Management of hand and wrist tendinopathies. In Skirven T, Osterman L, Fedorczyk J, Amadio P, Feldsher SB, Shin EK, editors: *Rehabilitation of the hand and upper extremity* 7th ed., St. Louis, 2021, Mosby.

67. Lister GD, Kleinert HE, Kutz JE, Atasoy E: Primary flexor tendon repair followed by immediate controlled mobilization, *J Hand Surg (Am)* 2:441–451, 1977.

68. Louis DS, Greene TL, Jacobson KE, et al: Evaluation of normal values for stationary and moving two-point discrimination in the hand, *J Hand Surg* 9(4):552, 1984.

69. Lundborg G, Lie-Stenström AK, Sollerman C, et al: Digital vibrogram: a new diagnostic tool for sensory testing in compression neuropathy, *J Hand Surg* 11(5):693, 1986.

70. Mackinnon SE, Dellon AL: Two-point discrimination tester, *J Hand Surg* 10(6 pt 1):906, 1985.

71. Magee DJ, Manske RC: *Orthopedic physical assessment*, 7th ed., St Louis, 2020, WB Saunders.

72. Marik T: Taping Techniques. In Skirven T, Osterman L, Fedorczyk J, Amadio P, Feldsher SB, Shin EK, editors: *Rehabilitation of the hand and upper extremity* 7th ed., St. Louis, 2021, Mosby.

73. Matheson Education and Training Solutions, LLC. Learn from the leaders. https://www.roymatheson.com/.

74. Mathiowetz V, Weber K, Volland G, Kashman N: Reliability and validity of grip and pinch strength evaluations, *The Journal of Hand Surgery* 9(2):222–226, 1984. https://doi.org/10.1016/s0363-5023(84)80146-x.

75. Merritt WH, Howell JW: Relative motion orthoses the concepts and application to hand therapy management of finger extensor tendon zone III and VII repairs, acute and chronic boutonnière deformity, and sagittal band injury. In Skirven T, Osterman L, Fedorczyk J, Amadio P, Feldsher SB, Shin EK, editors: *Rehabilitation of the hand and upper extremity* 7th ed., St. Louis, 2021, Mosby.

76. Midlgley R, Pisano K: Therapist's management of the stiff hand. In Skirven T, Osterman L, Fedorczyk J, Amadio P, Feldsher SB, Shin EK, editors: *Rehabilitation of the hand and upper extremity* 7th ed., St. Louis, 2021, Mosby.

77. Moberg E: Objective methods of determining functional value of sensibility in the hand, *J Bone Joint Surg* 40B:454–476, 1958.

78. Neuro Orthopaedic Institute. New manual for all healthcare providers and movement specialists. https://www.noigroup.com.

79. Nolan JW, Ballew TP: *Michlovitz's modalities for therapeutic intervention*, 7th ed., Philadelphia, 2022, F.A. Davis Company.

80. O'Riain S: New and simple test of nerve function in hand, *British Medical Journal* 3(5881):615–616, 1973. https://doi.org/10.1136/bmj.3.5881.615.

81. Packham TL, Holly J: Therapist's management of complex regional pain syndrome. In Skirven T, Osterman L, Fedorczyk J, Amadio P, Feldsher SB, Shin EK, editors: *Rehabilitation of the hand and upper extremity* 7th ed., St. Louis, 2021, Mosby.

82. Parrish K, Barret N: Wound classification and management. In Skirven T, Osterman L, Fedorczyk J, Amadio P, Feldsher SB, Shin EK, editors: *Rehabilitation of the hand and upper extremity* 7th ed., St. Louis, 2021, Mosby.

83. Pellecchia GL: Figure-of-eight method of measuring hand size: reliability and concurrent validity, *Journal of Hand Therapy* 16(4):300–304, 2003. https://doi.org/10.1197/S0894-1130(03)00154-6.

84. Priganc V, Stralka S: Graded motor imagery, *Journal of Hand Therapy* 24:164–169, 2011.

85. Rempel DM, Harrison RJ, Barnhart S: Work-related cumulative trauma disorders of the upper extremity, *JAMA* 267(6):838, 1992.

86. Ruch DS, McQueen MM: Distal radius and ulna fractures. In Bucholz RW, Heckman JD, Court-Brown CM, Tornetta Paul III: *Rockwood and Green's Fractures in Adults* 7th ed, Philadelphia, 2010, Lippincott Williams & Wilkins.

87. Strickland JW, Glogovac SV: Digital function following flexor tendon repair in zone II: a comparison of immobilization and controlled passive motion techniques, *J Hand Surg* 5(6):537, 1980.

88. Strickland JW: Development of flexor tendon surgery: twenty-five years of progress, *J Hand Surg [Am]* 25:214–235, 2000.

89. Szabo RM, Gelberman RH, Williamson RV, et al: Vibratory sensory testing in acute peripheral nerve compression, *J Hand Surg* 9A(1):104, 1984.

90. Tetro A, Evanoff BA, Hollstien SB, Gelberman RH: A new provocative test for carpal tunnel syndrome: assessment of wrist flexion and nerve compression, *J Bone Joint Surg Br* 80(3):493, 1998.

91. U.S. Department of Labor Employment and Training Administration: Dictionary of occupational titles, ed 4, Washington, D.C., 1991, U.S. Government Printing Office. Also online at https://www.occupationalinfo.org.

92. Wehbé MA, Hunter JM: Flexor tendon gliding in the hand. Part II: Differential gliding, *J Hand Surg* 10(4):575, 1985.

93. Wehbé MA: Tendon gliding exercises, *Am J Occup Ther* 41:164–167, 1987.

94. Weinstock-Zlotnick G, Mehta SP: A systematic review of the benefits of occupation-based intervention for patients with upper extremity musculoskeletal disorders, *Journal of Hand Therapy* 32:141–152, 2019. https://doi.org/10.1016/j.jht.2018.04.001.

95. Yerxa EJ, Barber LM, Diaz O, et al: Development of a hand sensitivity test for the hypersensitive hand, *Am J Occup Ther* 37(3):176, 1983.

96. Zelouf, David S, Wilson Mathew S, Hussain Haroon: Anatomy and kinesiology of the wrist. In Skirven T, Osterman L, Fedorczyk J, Amadio P, Feldsher SB, Shin EK, editors: *Rehabilitation of the hand and upper extremity* 7th ed., St. Louis, 2021, Mosby.

41

Orthopedic Conditions: Hip Fractures and Hip, Knee, and Shoulder Replacements

Sonia Lawson and Lynne F. Murphy

LEARNING OBJECTIVES

After studying this chapter, the student or practitioner will be able to do the following:

1. Describe the cause and medical management of hip fractures and hip, knee, and shoulder joint replacements and their effect on participation in occupations.
2. Identify precautions associated with hip fractures and joint replacements and their effects on intervention plans and occupational performance.
3. Outline contexts, performance patterns, performance skills, and client factors that are appropriate to include in the occupational therapy evaluation.
4. Develop occupational therapy goals that promote occupational engagement, using information gained from the occupational profile and evaluation results.
5. Explain intervention procedures that incorporate precautions, ensure safety, and promote occupational performance in daily tasks.
6. Discuss the emotional and social impact of hip fractures and joint replacements on occupational performance and performance patterns.

CHAPTER OUTLINE

KEY TERMS

Anterolateral approach
Arthroplasty
Closed reduction
Codman's pendulum exercises

Degenerative joint disease
Direct anterior approach
Hip precautions
Knee immobilizer

Minimally invasive technique
Open reduction and internal fixation
Osteoarthritis
Osteoporosis

Posterolateral approach
Shoulder sling
Shoulder swathe
Weight-bearing restrictions

INTRODUCTION TO ORTHOPEDIC CONDITIONS

Hip fractures and lower extremity (LE) joint replacements are two orthopedic conditions that occur with a relatively high frequency. The Centers for Disease Control and Prevention (CDC) reported that "at least 300,000 older people are hospitalized for hip fractures each year" in the United States.[21] According to the American Academy of Orthopaedic Surgeons (2020), approximately 790,000 knee replacements and 450,000 hip replacements are undertaken in the United States annually.[58,59] As of 2014, the number of shoulder replacements totaled approximately 79,000 per year in the United States.[61] Age-related changes in older adults contribute most to falls resulting in hip fractures or the need to have a joint replaced. Persons who have been involved in activities or occupations that put great amounts of stress on their joints, over time, may experience pain and degeneration as they get older. In addition, older individuals are more likely to have orthopedic problems such as osteoporosis and arthritic joint changes as a part of the aging process. When joint problems occur at the hip, knee, or shoulder, temporary or more long-lasting disability may result. When individuals need to have these joints repaired, there is a period in which the joint is unstable, which limits an individual's participation in meaningful daily occupations. However, medical and rehabilitative advances continue to make orthopedic conditions easier to manage with less of an impact on occupational performance.

The elderly population is most at risk for hip fractures, primarily as a result of age-related changes in muscle strength, bone density, postural alignment, sensory function (e.g., vision impairment, decreased proprioceptive awareness), and nervous system function.[38] Reduced balance, coordination, and mobility are potential risk factors for falls.[5] Postmenopausal women, in particular, develop osteoporosis to a greater degree than men and thus tend to have more hip fractures when they fall.[27]

Mobility is compromised in the elderly population because of decreased flexibility, diminished strength, reduced vision, decreased proprioceptive awareness, slowed reaction time, and the use of assistive ambulatory aids such as canes and walkers. Many elderly people become more cautious when moving about and are fearful of falling. This fear may contribute to more sedentary behavior, which can lead to further declines in strength and mobility. In some cases, individuals use a cane or walker improperly, which contributes to a fall. Not seeing a step or threshold also may cause a fall, as does tripping over items in the home (e.g., throw rugs, cords).[79]

Individuals with a history of osteoarthritis, degenerative joint disease, or other rheumatic disease that limits occupational performance are primary candidates for joint replacement. Individuals who elect to undergo these surgical procedures usually have been living with increasing pain in their joints for many months or years, and their ability to perform daily tasks is limited. By having the painful joint replaced, they hope to return to a more active and satisfying lifestyle. Occupational therapy (OT) plays a key role in identifying the many functional problems imposed by these acute and chronic orthopedic conditions and promoting compensatory or remediation approaches to facilitate the return of the orthopedic client to optimal performance of safe, independent, and meaningful occupations.

This chapter is divided into sections that include a discussion of hip fractures; hip, knee, and shoulder joint replacements; the associated medical and surgical management; and occupational therapy evaluation and intervention for these conditions. The *Occupational Therapy Practice Framework*, Fourth Edition is used to discuss the role of occupational therapy for persons with these conditions.[1] Specific areas addressed in the chapter are occupational therapy evaluation of performance skills in consideration of client context variables, occupational therapy interventions addressing specified occupations, the social and emotional implications of hospitalization and decreased functional abilities, and the interprofessional healthcare team approach in both the acute hospital and rehabilitation settings.

Emotional and Social Factors for the Orthopedic Patient

Attention to emotional and social issues is critical in the overall rehabilitation for the orthopedic client. Many clients in this population are faced with a chronic disability (e.g., rheumatoid arthritis [RA]), a life-threatening disease (e.g., cancer), chronic pain, or consequences of the aging process. The loss or potential loss of mobility and physical ability that limits participation in areas of occupation is a major concern for most of these clients. Adjusting to loss is stressful and requires an enormous amount of physical and emotional energy.[44] An awareness of and a sensitivity toward the psychosocial challenges of the person with an orthopedic problem are critical for the delivery of optimal client care.[64]

Clients with a chronic orthopedic disability often experience one or all of the following challenges: disease of a body part, fear, anxiety, change in body image, decreased functional ability, joint deformity, and pain. Interventions for a client with a chronic orthopedic condition must address these issues, especially in a preoperative phase or if a person chooses to decline surgery. The occupational therapy practitioner should be alert for signs of depression, guilt, anxiety, or fear that may impede participation in valued occupations. These signs may appear differently for each client based on particular context factors within the person (e.g., temperament) and environment (e.g., available social support) and may inhibit the client's progress. In the postoperative phase, clients may also experience pain, fear of operated extremity use, fear of falling, or unexpected delays in recovery that also can have detrimental effects on emotional health.[64]

Occupational therapists can help clients acknowledge and express emotional factors related to their condition, which can ultimately enhance the intervention process. One way to ease anxiety and fear is to make sure the client understands

OT PRACTICE NOTES

It is important for the occupational therapist working with clients who have orthopedic impairments or conditions to have a good understanding of the site, type, cause of the condition, any surgical procedures performed, and treatment precautions before starting the evaluation and intervention processes. A basic understanding of fracture healing and medical management procedures or protocols is also necessary to appreciate the risks, cautions, and implications to occupational performance. The occupational therapist is advised to review additional medical resources if more specific information is needed regarding surgical techniques and healing concerns.

procedures and interventions, as well as the likelihood of a positive outcome. Taking time to answer questions and provide additional information can be crucial for successful adjustment. In addition, communication with the entire healthcare team is important to ensure that these emotional needs are considered in all aspects of healthcare management.

The elderly client experiencing disability deals with additional issues specific to the aging process, such as fear of dependence and relocation trauma. With the onset of a disability late in life, the client may be forced to let go of independence and self-sufficiency.[44] This can be a devastating experience for some clients, and prolonged grieving may be necessary before adjustment. Others may use dependence for secondary gain by manipulating their support systems to avoid taking responsibility for themselves and others. When individuals are removed from their familiar environment, confusion, disorientation, and emotional lability may result. Practitioners must take these factors into consideration when implementing an intervention plan and provide supports as needed.

Learning to cope and adjust to the changes resulting from chronic disability or the aging process is a critical aspect of recovery. Practitioners must realize that the client has relinquished a great deal of functional independence as a result of disease or disability. The occupational therapist must address the emotional and social issues resulting from this loss while focusing on maximizing the client's ability to participate in occupations that are meaningful.[44]

Rehabilitation Team

Optimal rehabilitation for the orthopedic conditions discussed in this chapter requires coordination among the interprofessional team. Collaboration, communication, and clear role delineation among members of the interprofessional team are essential for an effective and efficient therapy program. In addition to the client, the team usually consists of a primary physician/surgeon or physician assistant, nursing staff, an occupational therapist or assistant, a physical therapist (PT) or assistant, a dietitian, a pharmacist, caregiver, and a social worker or case coordinator. Many facilities have a protocol or critical pathway that outlines each team member's responsibilities and a time frame for accomplishing assigned tasks and goals related to the client's rehabilitation. Regular team meetings to discuss each client's ongoing progress and discharge plans are necessary for coordinating individual intervention programs. Members from each service attend meetings to provide information and consultation. Clients are the most important members of the team.

They are involved in goal setting and establishing a plan of care, and they must be able to engage in the interventions specified by other team members. Informal caregivers (e.g., spouses, partners, significant others) are important members of the healthcare team because they provide a good deal of care at home once the patient is discharged. Often, restrictions and protocols must be followed weeks after joint repair, and the caregiver is responsible for ensuring those directions are followed in the home setting.

The role of the physician/surgeon or physician assistant is to manage medical needs and inform the team of the client's medical status. This includes information regarding medical history, diagnosis and treatment of the present problem, and information regarding the surgical procedure performed. The physician specifies any precautions or contraindications that all members of the team must enforce. Information provided may include the type of fixation or prosthesis inserted, the anatomic approach used in the surgery, weight bearing or other types of precautions, and contraindications such as movements that could endanger the client or impede healing. The physician is also responsible for ordering specific medications, overseeing the client's medication regimen, and directing pain-management approaches. The physician orders specific therapies and approves any change in the therapy program resulting from a change in the client's medical status.

The nursing staff is responsible for the physical care of the client during hospitalization, including care and monitoring of the surgical incision and administering prescribed pain medication according to the established pain management protocol. The orthopedic nurse must have a thorough understanding of the surgical procedures and movement precautions for each client. The nurse takes care of proper positioning using pillows and wedges, especially in the first few days after surgery. As the client's therapy program progresses, the client starts to take more responsibility for proper positioning and physical care. The nurse works closely with occupational and physical therapists and caregivers to carry through self-care and mobility skills that the client is learning in therapy and must use at home.

The physical therapist is responsible for evaluation and intervention in the areas of musculoskeletal status, sensation, pain, skin integrity, and mobility (especially gait and bed mobility). In most cases involving joint replacement and surgical repair of a hip fracture, physical therapy is initiated on the first day after surgery along with occupational therapy. Adhering to the prescribed precautions of the protocol, the physical therapist obtains baseline information, including range of motion (ROM), strength of all extremities, muscle tone, and mobility. A treatment program that includes therapeutic exercises, ROM activities, transfer training, and progressive gait activities is established. The physical therapist is responsible for recommending the appropriate assistive device to be used during ambulation. As the client's ambulation status advances, instruction in stair climbing, managing curbs, and outside ambulation is given.[31,51] In the case of shoulder replacements, the physical therapist implements mobility training that allows the client to protect the shoulder, works with occupational therapy to educate the client on strategies to prevent movement that is not permitted, and may progress the client through the postsurgery protocol, gradually increasing ROM and strength of the shoulder.

The dietitian consults with each client to ensure that adequate and appropriate nutrition is received to aid the healing process. The pharmacist monitors the client's pain management and medication routine and provides information and assistance to clients and their caregivers regarding any medications to be continued at home after discharge.

The role of the case coordinator is to ensure that each client is being discharged to the appropriate living situation or facility and the availability of durable medical equipment as recommended by physical and occupational therapy practitioners. The case coordinator is usually a registered nurse or social worker with a thorough knowledge of available community resources, home care agencies, and nursing care facilities. With input from the healthcare team, the case coordinator works with caregivers to arrange ongoing therapy after acute hospitalization, admission to a rehabilitation facility or skilled nursing facility for further intensive therapy if needed, or home healthcare as appropriate. The case coordinator works closely with the interprofessional team and is instrumental in coordinating discharge plans.

The occupational therapist is concerned primarily with improving performance in daily activities and meaningful occupations but may also create exercise programs to address limitations in specific neuromusculoskeletal and movement-related body functions/client factors as a basis for occupational performance. Focus is placed on safe execution of functional mobility, performance of activities of daily living (ADLs), and performance of instrumental activities of daily living (IADLs). The specific role of the occupational therapist will be discussed in detail in each of the following sections.

SECTION 1: HIP FRACTURES AND REPLACEMENT

GENERAL MEDICAL MANAGEMENT OF FRACTURES

In general, a fracture occurs when the bone's ability to absorb tension, compression, or shearing forces is exceeded.[29] The healing process begins after the fracture. Osteoblasts, cells that form bone, multiply to mend the fractured area. Adequate blood supply is necessary to supply the cells with oxygen for proper healing. The fracture site may be protected during the postsurgical healing process by internal fixation, such as pins, plates, screws, or wires. In rare cases in which extra protection is needed, an external abduction brace may be used for the hip. This metal brace extends around the pelvis and down the thigh of the fractured hip and prevents movement, especially hip abduction, according to settings determined by the orthopedic surgeon. Other types of braces or casts may be used for fractures of other parts of the LE (e.g., a knee immobilizer). It may take several months for a bone fracture to heal completely. The time needed varies with the age, health, and nutrition of the client; the site and configuration of the fracture; the initial displacement of the bone; and the blood supply to the fragments.

Etiology of Fractures

Trauma is the major cause of fractures. In most cases, the trauma occurs as a result of falling. Poor lighting, throw rugs,

---

THREADED CASE STUDY

Mrs. Hernandez, Part 1

Mrs. Hernandez (prefers use of the pronouns she/her/hers), a 70-year-old grandmother to three small children, fell outside of the senior center that she attends three times a week for exercise. She sustained a femoral neck fracture of her right hip. Before the fall, she had been experiencing increasing right hip pain because of osteoarthritis and degenerative joint disease, and she was concerned about increasing weakness in the right leg. She remembers not lifting her right leg high enough to clear the entrance step to the center where she tripped up the steps, was not able to catch herself, and fell on her right hip. The fracture was repaired with a total hip replacement that was performed using a direct anterior approach, minimally invasive procedure. Movement precautions include no hip extension or crossing the legs and weight bearing as tolerated on the right lower extremity. Mrs. Hernandez is usually very active; she attends swimming classes twice a week, helps her daughter care for her three children, and heads two committees at her church. These activities became very important to her after her husband died 5 years ago. They give her a sense of purpose and help her feel connected with others. Mrs. Hernandez lives alone in a condominium with elevator access. Her daughter and grandchildren live 15 minutes away and often visit and involve her in many of their family activities.

Mrs. Hernandez was referred for occupational therapy because of her difficulty with functional mobility and completing her daily activities. When asked about what bothered her most about her fall and subsequent hip replacement, she said that she was worried that she would no longer be able to participate in the swimming classes she enjoys so much, nor would she be able to drive herself to all of her appointments and church-related activities. This would make her dependent on her children and church friends. She was afraid of losing her independence, which she valued greatly. She is hoping that the occupational therapy she receives will help her drive again as soon as possible and allow her to remain as independent as possible so that she is not a burden to anyone.

Critical Thinking Questions

1. When completing the occupational profile, what additional information would the occupational therapist need to gather during the evaluation to supplement the information already provided in the case scenario?
2. Identify important occupations and performance skills to address first when educating Mrs. Hernandez to safely resume occupational performance patterns.
3. What prerequisite performance skills and client factors/body functions should be addressed with Mrs. Hernandez before the occupational therapist directly addresses her ability to drive again?

---

and unmarked steps are environmental hazards that can lead to a fall. Osteoporosis is a bone disease that typically results in decreased bone density, most commonly in the vertebral bodies, the neck of the femur, the humerus, and the distal end of the radius. Because the bone becomes porous and therefore fragile, the affected bones are prone to fracture as a result of a fall or other traumatic event. A pathologic fracture can occur in a bone weakened by disease or tumor, as with osteomyelitis and cancers that have metastasized to the bone.[29]

Medical and Surgical Management

The goals of fracture management are to relieve pain, maintain good position of the bone, allow fracture healing, and restore optimal function to the client. Reduction of a fracture refers to restoring the bone fragments to normal alignment.[29] This can be done by a closed procedure called a **closed reduction** (manipulation) or by an open procedure called an open reduction and internal fixation (ORIF) (surgery). The physician performs a closed reduction by applying force to the displaced bone to realign the bone. Depending on the nature of the fracture, the reduction or realignment is maintained by a cast, brace, traction, or skeletal fixation. With open reduction, the fracture site is exposed surgically so that the bone fragments can be aligned. The fragments are held in place with internal fixation such as pins, screws, a plate, nails, or a rod. Further immobilization by a cast or a brace may be deemed necessary by the orthopedic surgeon. Closed reductions and ORIF procedures must be protected from excessive forces during bone healing. Therefore, **weight-bearing restrictions** may be indicated.[29]

There are several levels of weight-bearing restrictions. The physician indicates at which level the client should be placed based on the surgical technique selected and the stability of the surgical repair. Elderly clients may not have the upper extremity (UE) strength to support their body during non–weight-bearing precautions. The surgeon may take this into account and use a more stable procedure to allow the client to bear weight at tolerance through the operated leg, thereby sparing overexertion of the UEs. Restrictions are reduced as the fracture site heals and becomes stronger.[20] The levels of weight-bearing restrictions are listed in Box 41.1.

TYPES OF HIP FRACTURES AND MEDICAL MANAGEMENT

Knowledge of hip anatomy is necessary for understanding the medical management of hip fractures. An anatomy and physiology reference text should be consulted for details. Figs. 41.1 and 41.2 illustrate a normal hip joint and the common locations and directions of fractures (fracture lines). The names of the fractures generally reflect the site and severity of injury and

may signal the form of medical treatment that will be used. For example, a femoral neck fracture will typically be treated with femoral neck stabilization.[68]

Femoral Neck Fractures

Femoral neck fractures, which include subcapital, transcervical, and basilar fractures, are common in adults over 60 years old and occur more frequently in women. If the bone is osteoporotic, fracture may result from even a slight trauma or rotational force.[44] Treatment of a displaced fracture in this area is complicated by poor blood supply, osteoporotic bone that is not suited to hold metallic fixation, and a thin periosteum covering the bone. The type of surgical treatment used is based on the amount of displacement and the vascular supply in the femoral head, as well as the age, health, and activity level of the client.

BOX 41.1   Weight-Bearing Restrictions

- *NWB* (non–weight bearing) indicates that no weight at all can be placed on the extremity involved.
- *TTWB* (toe-touch weight bearing) indicates that only the toe can be placed on the ground to provide some balance while standing—90% of the weight is still on the unaffected leg. In toe-touch weight bearing, clients may be instructed to imagine that an egg is under their foot.
- *PWB* (partial weight bearing) indicates that only 50% of the person's body weight can be placed on the affected leg.
- *WBAT* (weight bearing at tolerance) indicates that clients are allowed to judge how much weight they are able to put on the affected leg without causing pain that may limit function.
- *FWB* (full weight bearing) indicates that clients are able to put 100% of their weight on the affected leg.[71]

From Early MB: Physical dysfunction: practical skills for the occupational therapy assistant, St. Louis, 1998, Mosby.

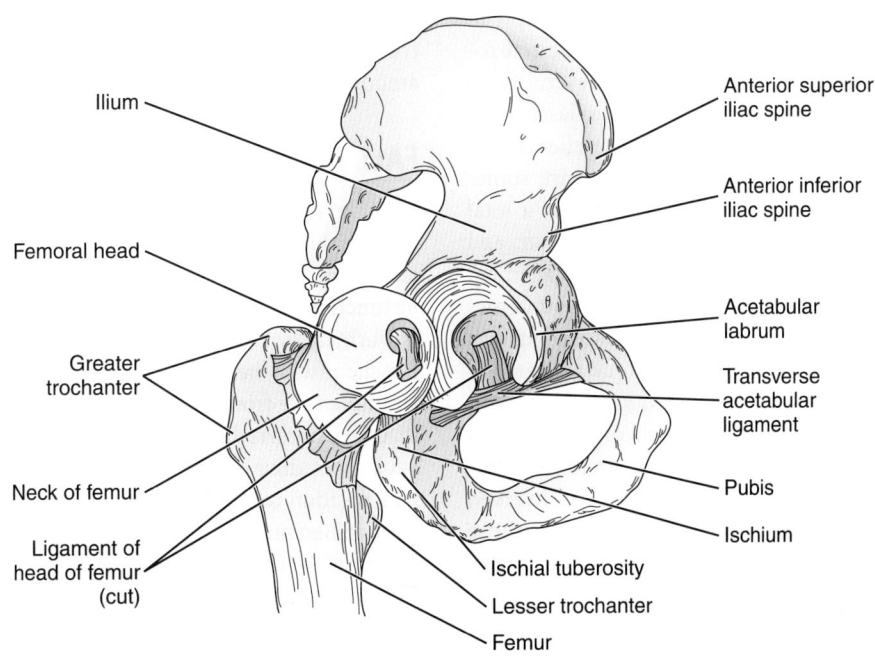

Fig. 41.1 Normal hip anatomy. (From Reese NB, Bandy WD: *Joint range of motion and muscle length testing*, ed 3, St. Louis, 2017, Elsevier.)

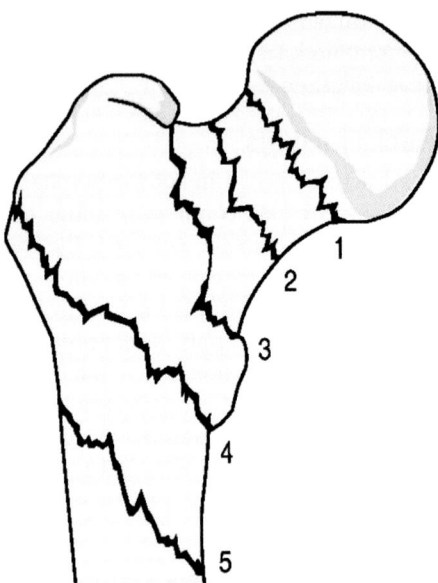

Fig. 41.2 Levels of femoral fracture. *1*, Subcapital. *2*, Transcervical. *3*, Basilar. *4*, Intertrochanteric. *5*, Subtrochanteric. (From Porter S, editor: *Tidy's physiotherapy*, ed 15, Churchill Livingstone, 2013, Elsevier.)

Internal fixation or hip pinning (application of a compression screw and plate) is generally used when displacement is minimal to moderate and blood supply is intact. With a physician's approval, a client is usually able to begin limited out-of-bed activities 1 day after surgery. Per physician's orders, weight-bearing restrictions may be necessary, with the aid of a walker or crutches for at least 6 to 8 weeks while the fracture is healing. Weight bearing may be limited beyond this time if precautions are not observed or if delayed union (slow formation of new bone at the fracture site) occurs.[68]

With severe displacement or in the case of a femoral head with poor blood supply (avascular), nonunion (a poorly healing fracture site where new bone does not form), and degenerative joint disease, the femoral head is surgically removed and replaced by an endoprosthesis (referred to more simply as prosthesis). This joint replacement is called a hemipolar **arthroplasty**, often referred to as a hemiarthroplasty.[51,68] Several types of metal prostheses can be used for a hemiarthroplasty; each has its own shape and advantages to best fit the client's size and hip joint structure. Weight-bearing restrictions are sometimes indicated. Surgeons also may choose to perform a total joint replacement depending on the integrity of the joint and anticipated activity level of the client. A total hip replacement may offer better patient satisfaction and functional outcomes for people who are very active.[17] A total hip replacement may also result in better outcomes for frail older people as there are fewer associated complications for this age group who have suffered a hip fracture.[12] Depending on the surgical procedure used with a hemiarthroplasty or total hip arthroplasty (replacement), specific precautions for positioning the hip must be observed to prevent dislocation. These precautions are the same as those advised for a total hip replacement, which will be outlined later in this chapter. Clients with a hemiarthroplasty or total hip replacement can usually begin limited out-of-bed activity, with a physician's approval, about 1 day after surgery.[50,68,75]

Intertrochanteric Fractures

Fractures between the greater and lesser trochanter are extracapsular, or outside the articular capsule of the hip joint, and the blood supply is not affected. Like femoral neck fractures, intertrochanteric fractures occur mostly in women but in a slightly older age group. The fracture is usually caused by direct trauma or force over the trochanter, as in a fall. The preferred treatment for these fractures is an ORIF. A nail or compression screw with a side plate is used. Weight-bearing restrictions must be observed according to the surgeon's orders for up to 6 to 8 weeks during ambulation, with gradual increases in the amount of weight taken through the affected leg over this time.[50] The client is allowed out of bed 1 day after surgery, pending the physician's approval.[68]

Subtrochanteric Fractures

Subtrochanteric fractures 1 to 2 inches below the lesser trochanter usually occur because of direct trauma, as in falls, motor vehicle accidents, or any other situation in which there is a direct blow to the hip area. These fractures make up 10% to 30% of hip fractures and are most often seen in persons younger than 60 years old or in older clients with severe osteopenia (significant bone loss) who have a low-velocity fall.[20,54] These fractures can be the most challenging to repair because of the muscle attachments in this area that can generate forces to the fracture site, impairing proper fracture healing.[23] An ORIF is the usual surgical method. A nail with a long side plate or an intramedullary rod is used. An intramedullary rod is inserted through the central part of the shaft of bone to help maintain proper alignment for bone healing.[29]

In all types of hip fractures, the practitioner should observe for and address any subsequent issues from the hip fracture that can have an impact on the rehabilitation process and the client's ability to regain the skills needed to complete daily activities. Such issues can be reactions of the body to the surgery such as soft-tissue trauma, edema, and bruising that occur around the fracture or surgical site.[28,50,68] These issues can greatly affect the amount of pain and discomfort a client may experience.

FALL PREVENTION

Another issue that frequently occurs for older adults after hip fracture due to a fall is fear of falling. Frequent falls in older adults can signal to the client and family members that there is a decline in function, which could lead to changes in independence and performance of desired and valued occupations. Psychologically, the client with frequent falls may fear the loss of independence and hide falls from others or under-report the number of falls that have occurred over time. A fear of falling may also lead older adults to reduce their activity level so as not to put themselves in a position to fall in the community. They stay in places that are familiar, putting them at risk for social isolation and further decreases in strength and mobility. These functional decreases can lead to more falls.[79] It is important for the interprofessional team to be attuned to clues related to fall history for the client and potential negative psychosocial reactions to the fall.

Occupational therapists can work with other team members to provide fall prevention education and training. Occupational therapists can teach adaptive strategies, make environmental recommendations, explore community resources, and teach exercises that address strength, mobility, and balance. Physical therapists can also address fall prevention through therapeutic exercise and teaching correct use of an appropriate assistive device for ambulation. Information regarding local community-based fall prevention programs can be provided to the client and family. These programs, typically held at area senior centers, include education and exercise classes specifically geared to improving the body structures and functions that help reduce the risk of falling.[22] The Stopping Elderly Accidents, Deaths and Injuries (STEADI) Program obtained through the CDC is one example of a comprehensive fall prevention program. Materials and resources for professionals and the community can be accessed from the CDC website.[22]

HIP JOINT REPLACEMENT

Etiology and Medical Management

Restoration of joint motion and management of pain by total hip replacement, also called arthroplasty or bipolar arthroplasty, is sometimes indicated when a person experiences decreased occupational performance, often as a result of chronic disease processes involving the hip joint or from congenital hip dysplasia (the hip socket does not fit properly around the head of the femur).[48] Common chronic diseases are osteoarthritis, degenerative joint disease, or rheumatoid arthritis, although other rheumatic and systemic diseases also may be present. Osteoarthritis and degenerative joint disease may develop spontaneously in middle age and progress as the normal aging process of joints accelerates. Degenerative changes may also develop as the result of trauma, congenital deformity, or a disease that damages articular cartilage. Weight-bearing joints such as the hip, knee, and lumbar spine are usually affected. In the hip, there is a loss of cartilage centrally on the joint surface and formation of osteophytes on the periphery of the acetabulum, producing joint incongruity. Pain originates from the bone, synovial membrane, or fibrous capsule and from muscle spasm. When movement of the hip causes pain and limited mobility, the muscles shorten, which can result in a hip position of flexion, adduction, and internal rotation that causes a painful limp.[57]

Rheumatoid arthritis (RA) may involve the hip joint, but because RA affects smaller joints before larger joints in the body, the hip is typically not affected until later stages of RA (see Chapter 39). Arthroscopic surgery can be performed early in the disease process to limit fibrotic damage to the joint and tendon structures.[29] However, once there is significant joint damage, a hip replacement may be the only alternative. Other disease processes (e.g., lupus and cancer) and some medications (e.g., corticosteroids such as prednisone) can compromise the blood flow to the hip joint and lead to avascular necrosis (AVN, a condition in which bone cells die because of poor blood supply) or osteoporosis; either condition results in a painful hip.[57]

When conservative forms of management for the pain and decreased mobility (e.g., cortisone injections, modified activity,

pain medication) are no longer successful, a total joint replacement is considered to restore an individual's ability to more fully participate in daily occupations. Consideration of a total joint replacement relies on a client's ability to comply with a rehabilitation program, the probability of a positive outcome given other medical issues the client may be facing, and the probability of a significant improvement in functional ability.[48,50] There are two mechanical components to the type of prosthesis used for a total hip replacement. Most often, a high-density polyethylene socket is fitted into the acetabulum, and a metallic or ceramic prosthesis replaces the femoral head and neck. Methyl methacrylate or acrylic cement fixes the components to the bone (Fig. 41.3). Hip replacements can last for 15 to 20 years or more before a revision is needed to insert a new prosthesis. Wear and tear on the hip prosthesis are greater for more active people, who may require a revision sooner than for those who are more sedentary. Those who have their hip replaced at a young age will likely have to undergo a revision in later years.[49]

Various surgical approaches are used with the goal of choosing a technique that will provide the best stability for the client and reduces the occurrence of complications. The specific approach is selected based on the surgical skill or technique of the orthopedic surgeon, severity of the joint involvement, anatomic and biomechanical structure of the client's hip, and history of surgery to the hip.[18,68] Three main approaches are used: posterolateral, anterolateral, and direct anterior, which indicate from which direction the surgeon opens the hip for the replacement.[35] All three techniques have variations that involve the surrounding muscles of the hip to a greater or lesser degree. Muscles that must be displaced during the surgery are not able to support the joint after surgery. This results in joint instability in certain directions of movement. With **anterolateral** and **direct anterior approaches**, the client will be unstable in external rotation, adduction, and extension of the operated hip and usually

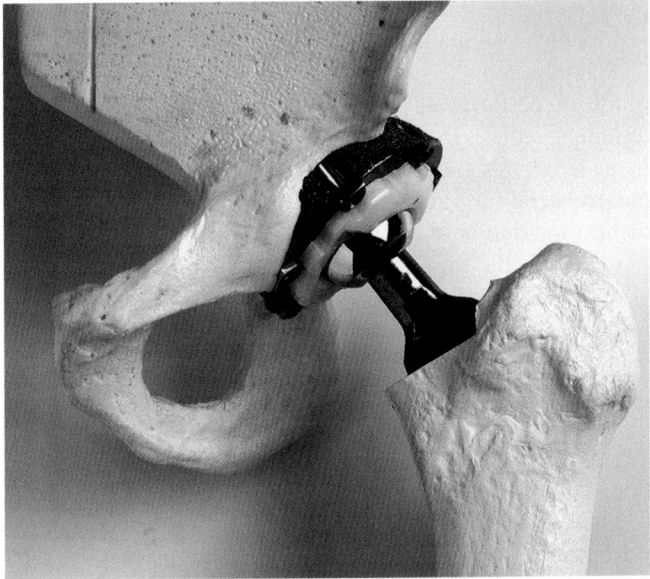

Fig. 41.3 Hip prosthesis. (From Black J, Hawks J: *Medical surgical nursing: clinical management for positive outcomes,* ed 8, St. Louis, 2009, Elsevier.)

BOX 41.2 Hip Precautions

Posterolateral Approach
- No hip flexion greater than 90 degrees
- No internal rotation
- No adduction (crossing legs or feet)

Anterolateral Approach
- No external rotation
- No adduction (crossing legs or feet)
- No extension

must observe precautions to prevent these movements for 6 to 8 weeks. Hip abduction may be prohibited as well with this surgical approach. It is important for the occupational therapist to carefully read the surgeon's postoperative orders. If a posterolateral approach is used, the client will be unstable primarily with hip flexion and must be cautioned not to move the operated hip past specific ranges of flexion (usually 90 degrees) and not to internally rotate or adduct the leg for 6 to 8 weeks. Failure to maintain these hip precautions during muscle and soft-tissue healing may result in hip dislocation and additional surgery (Box 41.2).

In younger people, some surgeons may choose to replace the hip using a hybrid technique in which the acetabular socket is not cemented but the femoral component is cemented. In this case the use of biologic fixation (bony in-growth instead of cement) secures the prosthesis.[23] This can increase the strength of the fixation at the prosthesis interface and can also decrease the possibility of loosening of the prosthesis. In other words, new bone grows into openings in the prosthesis, and this secures the prosthesis to the bone. This noncemented approach can be used for both components of the prosthesis. The precautions after the surgery are identical to those of the anterior or posterior hip replacements, but they may involve an additional restriction on weight bearing.[50]

Many orthopedic surgeons use a minimally invasive technique to perform all approaches for hip replacement. This technique reduces the amount of trauma to the muscle and soft tissue structures and allows for faster recovery. The traditional posterolateral surgical technique requires that a long (about 10 inches) incision be made, and muscles detached to get to the hip joint. In the minimally invasive technique, two incisions of approximately 2 inches are needed and no detachment of muscles is required. Because no muscles are detached, the hip is more likely to remain in a stable position during the healing process. Similarly, for a direct anterior approach, a small vertical incision is made on the anterior surface of the hip joint with the hip placed in hyperextension. In addition to a faster recovery, this technique minimizes the risk of dislocation and postoperative limp.[60,68] The minimally invasive techniques are not appropriate for all total hip replacements or arthroplasties. Persons with severe damage to the hip joint or who have anatomic or biomechanical contraindications will require the traditional surgical method. Hip precautions that are identified for the

posterolateral and anterolateral approaches are also indicated for persons receiving a minimally invasive technique.[74]

To reinforce use of proper hip precautions during occupational performance and to guide intervention and discharge planning, the occupational therapist must know the type of surgical procedure that was performed. For example, someone with a hip replacement in which the minimally invasive technique was used may tolerate more activity after surgery than someone who underwent the traditional surgical technique. Clients with total hip replacements usually begin out-of-bed activity the same day of the surgery or the day after.

Hip resurfacing is another method of repairing a damaged and painful hip. This technique, less commonly used and with mixed evidence for efficacy over a total hip replacement, is a variation of the total hip replacement.[57] Designed for younger clients, the resurfacing technique preserves more of the bone of the femur should a total hip replacement be needed in later years. The surface of the femoral head is reshaped and then capped by a metallic shell. The acetabular cavity also receives a metallic cup or socket. Both are held in place by methyl methacrylate (acrylic cement). This technique preserves the femoral head and neck. With this technique, no weight-bearing restrictions apply.[26,57]

In summary, the occupational therapist must be informed of the surgical technique, movement precautions, and weight-bearing restrictions before beginning the evaluation and intervention of clients recovering from hip replacement surgery. Restrictions on weight bearing for any of the techniques is specified by the orthopedic surgeon and vary in terms of amount of pressure and length of time weight can be placed on the operated leg. A walking aid, usually a walker or crutches, is necessary for at least the first month while the hip is healing and muscles are becoming stronger.[50] The occupational therapist has the responsibility of working with the interprofessional team to educate clients about their hip precautions and restrictions to allow the surgery to heal optimally without adverse effects such as dislocation. A joint that becomes dislocated may need additional surgery for repair. Strategies for completing daily tasks during the recovery process are implemented that allow the client to retain as much independence as possible while maintaining hip precautions and weight-bearing restrictions.

Special Considerations for Hip Replacements

Individuals with joint changes that increase pain may have multiple joint involvement (i.e., both knees, hips, and shoulders). With less frequency than for knee replacements, some clients opt to have two hip joints replaced during the same hospitalization, with procedures spaced apart by a few days.[65] This can complicate the rehabilitation process because the client will not be able to rely on the nonoperated leg when walking, transitioning between seated and standing positions, and performing daily occupations.

It is important for the occupational therapy practitioner to be aware of complications or special procedures that occurred during a client's surgery and to verify precautions or risks with the physician. Surgeons will make specific recommendations based on the client's particular situation, surgical procedures used, or postoperative concerns. Common complications that can occur days, months, or years after the surgery include dislocation of the hip joint, degeneration of the components of the prosthesis, fracture of bone next to implanted parts, loosening of prosthetic parts, and infection of the joint after surgery. A special procedure for individuals at high risk for a hip dislocation after surgery involves using an abduction brace to immobilize the hip joint.[29] This brace adds extra movement restrictions to the performance of daily tasks. Worn component parts, bone fractures, and sometimes dislocations must be repaired surgically. Additionally, clients with hip replacements are required to take prophylactic antibiotics for any future dental work or surgery to prevent infection at the joint replacement site.[63] The implantation of metal and plastic parts makes that area more susceptible to infection. Individuals living with a hip replacement must manage this chronic situation for the rest of their lives.

Postsurgical pain is often managed with a regimen of medications, such as epidural or periarticular anesthetics, patient-controlled analgesia (PCA), oral analgesics or opioids, or peripheral nerve blocks, although side effects and effectiveness are variable with individual clients. The pain may be caused by trauma to soft tissues, edema surrounding the hip joint that places pressure on the incision, or improper positioning. Many hospitals that have a coordinated joint replacement program implement a pain management program in which clients receive regular and timely pain medication to allow optimum recovery and participation in their rehabilitation program. Other methods of pain control amenable to use by rehabilitation professionals include the use of superficial cold modalities, proper positioning during transitional movements, and a balance of rest and activity.

Occupational therapy evaluation and interventions for those following hip surgery increasingly occur in the client's home with very little, if any, time spent in the hospital after the surgery. Outpatient total hip replacements using an anterolateral or direct anterior approach is becoming more frequent for those people who do not have a complicated medical history.[24] For these individuals, preoperative education is even more important, and the occupational therapy practitioner will need to address more of the medical management aspects in the home setting such as medication management, training in hip precautions, and wound management along with ADL and IADL training.

Medical Equipment

The OT practitioner should be familiar with the following equipment that is commonly used in the treatment of hip fracture and total hip replacement:

Hemovac. During surgery, a plastic drainage tube is inserted at the surgical site to assist with postoperative drainage of blood. It has an area for collection of drainage and may be connected to a portable suction machine. The unit should not be disconnected for any activity because this may create a blockage in the system. The Hemovac is usually left in place for 1 to 2 days after surgery.

Abduction wedge. Large and small triangular foam wedges (Fig. 41.4) are used when the client is supine to maintain the lower extremities in the abducted position.

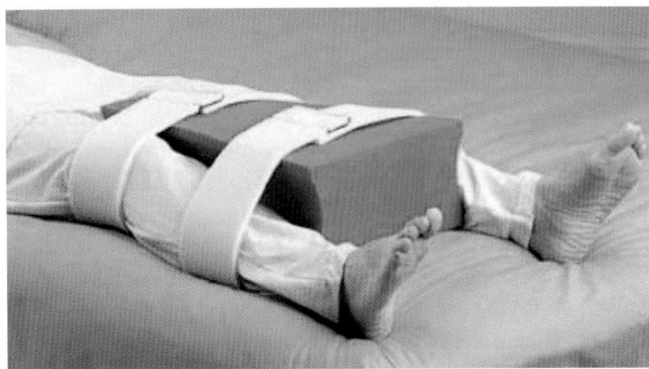

Fig. 41.4 Abduction wedge. (Courtesy Performance Health, Warrenville, IL.)

Balanced suspension. This is fabricated and set up by an orthopedic technician and can be used for about 3 days after surgery. It balances the weight of the elevated leg by weights placed at the opposite end of the pulley system. Its purpose is to support the affected lower extremity in the first few postoperative days. The client's leg can be taken out of the device for exercise only.[68]

Reclining wheelchair. A wheelchair with an adjustable backrest that allows a reclining position is used for clients who have hip flexion precautions while sitting.

Commode chairs. The use of a commode chair that can be adjusted for height instead of the regular toilet aids in safe transfers and allows the client to observe necessary hip flexion precautions.

Sequential compression devices (SCDs). SCDs are used postoperatively to reduce the risk of deep vein thrombosis. They are inflatable pads covering the circumference of the lower leg and provide intermittent pneumatic compression of the legs.[29]

Antiembolus hose. These are thigh-high elastic hosiery that are worn 24 hours a day and removed only during bathing. Their purpose is to assist circulation, prevent edema, and thus reduce the risk of deep-vein thrombosis.[29]

Patient-controlled administration intravenous line. Patient-controlled analgesia (PCA) is delivered through an IV line; patient-controlled epidural analgesia (PCEA) is delivered through an epidural line. A prescribed amount of medication is programmed by the physician and nursing staff to allow the client to self-administer pain medication by pushing a button to inject a safe amount. When dosages have reached a limit, the machine will not administer medication even if the button is pushed.

Incentive spirometer. This portable breathing apparatus is used to encourage deep breathing and prevent the development of postoperative pneumonia.

ROLE OF OCCUPATIONAL THERAPY FOR CLIENTS WITH HIP FRACTURE OR HIP REPLACEMENT

After a hip replacement or surgical repair of a fractured hip, occupational therapy typically begins when the client is ready to start getting out of bed, usually the day of surgery or the following day. The actual time varies, depending on the age and general health of the client, surgical events, or medical complications involved. Before any physical assessment, it is important to introduce and explain the role of occupational therapy and complete an occupational profile. This profile involves gathering information regarding the client's occupational history, prior functional status in activities of daily living (ADLs) and instrumental activities of daily living (IADLs), descriptions of performance contexts (e.g., home environment and social support available), and the client's goals. The goal of occupational therapy is for the client to maximize performance skills in daily occupations, with all movement precautions observed during activities. The role of the occupational therapist and assistant is to teach the client ways and means of performing daily occupations safely.[44]

Evaluation and Intervention

The occupational therapist's role is to assume responsibility for performing any assessments necessary for a complete evaluation. In addition to an occupational profile, an assessment of the psychosocial issues related to the surgery and the surgery's impact on the client's lifestyle is completed via interview. A baseline physical evaluation is necessary for determining whether any physical limitations not related to surgery might prevent functional independence. Client factors/body functions such as upper extremity ROM, muscle strength, sensation, and coordination and status of mental functions such as executive functions are assessed before a functional evaluation is made, because these can affect the client's ability to fully participate in the rehabilitation program. (See Chapters 21, 22, 23, 25, and 26 for more information on these topics.) Evaluation of ADLs, IADLs, and functional mobility is necessary for clinical and professional reasoning and holistic intervention planning (see Chapter 20 for occupation-based functional motion evaluation). During evaluation, it is important to observe and document any signs of pain and fear at rest or during movement. For older adult clients, Chapter 47 offers many ideas helpful for meeting the needs of this population.

Based on evaluation results and a thorough clinical and professional reasoning process, the occupational therapist creates an intervention program of functional activities that gradually enables the client to regain the abilities and skills necessary to participate in identified occupations. The therapist introduces and trains clients in the use of assistive devices, proper transfer techniques, and ADL and IADL techniques while maintaining hip and weight-bearing precautions. An occupational therapy assistant may play a large role in this training. Both the occupational therapist and the occupational therapy assistant are involved in treatment planning, documentation, and discharge planning (including the recommendation of equipment and home exercise programs).

Client Education

Although hip fractures are never a planned occurrence, hip replacements are usually planned and scheduled to be performed on a specific date. Occupational therapists often provide education classes for individuals at risk for fractures and those planning joint replacement. As mentioned earlier in the chapter,

for the person who may be at risk for falling, attending a class on fall prevention is a wise recommendation. Topics may include home modifications (e.g., removal of throw rugs, telephone cords, and clutter), safe transfer techniques, use of public transportation, and community mobility tips. The person who is having an elective total joint replacement may benefit from a class offered before surgery that explains the surgical procedures and precautions, introduces assistive devices, describes the therapy process, and describes the typical recovery period so that the client can be best prepared.

Specific Training Techniques for Participation in Occupations

Some common assistive devices are useful for many people with hip fractures or hip replacements (Fig. 41.5). Helpful assistive devices or adaptive aids include a dressing stick, sock aid, long-handled sponge, long-handled shoehorn, reacher, elastic shoelaces, leg lifter, elevated toilet or commode seat, three-in-one commode, and shower chair or bench. Walker bags are helpful for people using walkers who need to carry small items from one place to another. The OT clinic should have samples of these devices that are available for client use during the intervention process.

The training procedures outlined in the following sections apply to hip fractures and the different types of hip joint replacement. The positions of hip instability for the specific types of surgical procedures for hip replacement are important to remember. For the posterolateral approach (traditional or minimally invasive), positions of instability include adduction, internal rotation, and flexion greater than 90 degrees. For the anterolateral and direct anterior approaches (traditional or minimally invasive), positions of instability include adduction, external rotation, and excessive hyperextension.

Bed Mobility

The supine position with an abduction wedge (see Fig. 41.4) or pillow in place is recommended in bed. If a client sleeps in

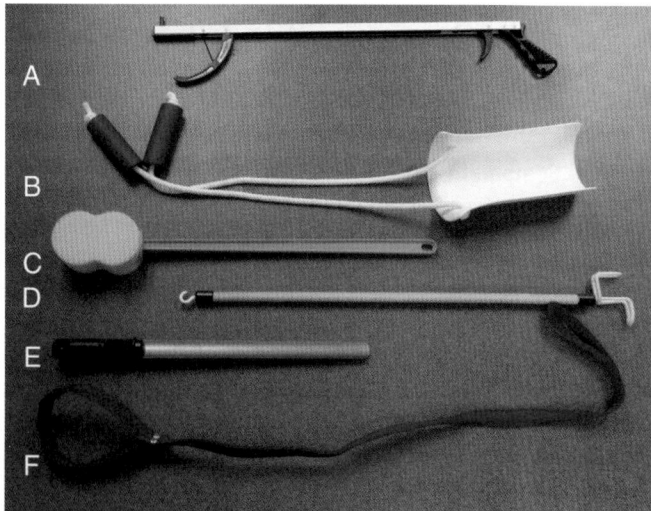

Fig. 41.5 Assistive devices for activities of daily living. (A) Reacher. (B) Sock aid. (C) Long-handled sponge. (D) Dressing stick. (E) Long-handled shoehorn. (F) Leg lifter.

the side-lying position, sleeping on the operated side is recommended if tolerable. When sleeping on the nonoperated side, the client must keep the legs abducted with the abduction wedge or large pillows supporting the operated leg to prevent hip adduction and rotation. The client is instructed in getting out of bed on both sides, although initially it may be easier to observe precautions by moving toward the nonoperated leg. Careful instruction is given to avoid adduction past midline. It is important to determine the type and height of the client's bed at home to determine if other sleeping arrangements are needed. When getting in and out of bed initially, the client may use a leg lifter to help the operated leg move from one position to another. Some clients have an overhead trapeze bar placed on the bed to assist with bed mobility. It is important to wean the clients away from using this device because they will most likely not have one at home.

The best procedure for moving from the supine position to sitting on the edge of the bed is to have clients support the upper body by propping up on their elbows, then moving the lower extremities toward the side of the bed in small increments and following with the trunk and UEs (Fig. 41.6). The client should gradually turn in this manner until he or she can lower the legs out of the bed and push the trunk into the sitting position. Following a posterior approach hip replacement, the occupational therapist should observe the client when sitting to ensure that the client is not flexing the hip more than 90 degrees. If so, the client can extend the knee, which will cause the hip to be less flexed and widen the hip angle so that precautions are maintained.

Transfers

It is always helpful for the client to observe the proper technique for transfers before attempting the movement.

OT PRACTICE NOTES

One way to help therapists understand the impact of maintaining the proper hip position during the healing process is for therapists to tape a goniometer to their own hip when positioned at 90 degrees and attempt to do the transfers listed next. Therapists will soon discover the difficulty of maintaining the proper hip position during functional activities!

Chair. A firmly based chair with armrests is recommended. To move from standing to sitting, the client is instructed to back up to the chair, extend the operated leg forward, reach back for the armrests, and slowly lower to the sitting position. For the person with a posterolateral approach, care should be taken not to lean forward when sitting down (Fig. 41.7). To stand, the client extends the operated leg and pushes up from the armrests. Once standing, the client can reach for an ambulatory aid, such as a walker if it is being used. Because of the hip flexion precaution for the posterolateral approach, the client should sit on the front part of the chair and lean back (see Fig. 41.7). Firm cushions or blankets may be used to increase the height of chair seats and may be especially helpful if the client is tall. Low chairs, soft chairs, reclining chairs, and rocking chairs should be avoided.[2]

Commode chair. Three-in-one commode chairs with armrests can be used in the hospital and at home (see Fig. 41.7). For the person with a posterolateral approach, the height and angle can be adjusted so that the front legs are one notch lower than the back legs; thus, with the client seated, the precautionary hip angle of flexion is not exceeded. A person with an anterolateral or direct anterior approach may have enough hip mobility to use a standard toilet seat safely at the time of discharge. All clients should wipe between the legs in a sitting position or from behind in a standing position and use caution to avoid forward flexion of the hip greater than 90 degrees, or rotation of the hip. The client is to stand up and step to turn to face the toilet when flushing to avoid hip rotation.[2] Comfort height toilets (17-inch seat height) can be considered for installation at home as a permanent modification that eases transfers to the toilet.

Shower stall. Nonskid strips or stickers are recommended in all shower stalls and tubs. When the client is entering the shower stall, the walker or crutches go first, then the operated leg (taking care to avoid active hip abduction if the client is not allowed to perform this motion), and then the nonoperated leg. Installation of a shower chair with adjustable legs or a stool and grab bars is strongly encouraged to prevent the client from losing balance and to maintain weight-bearing precautions. An alternative method to enter the shower stall is to back up to the edge or rim of the shower while using the walker for balance, then stepping into the shower while looking down at the feet and shower rim for safety.

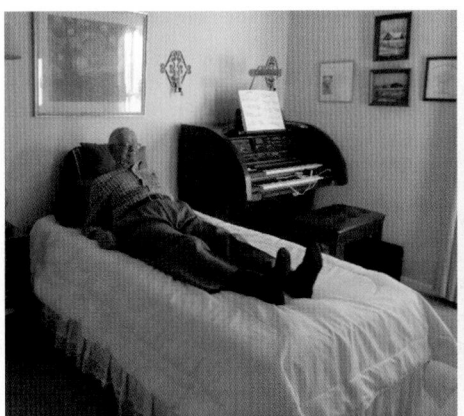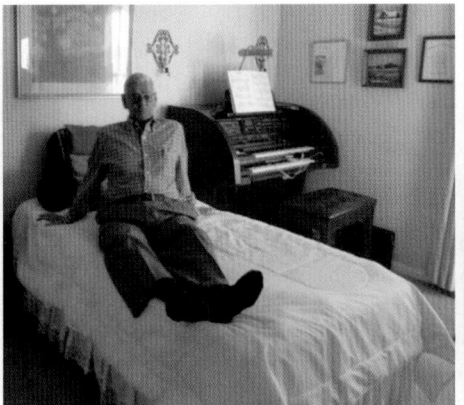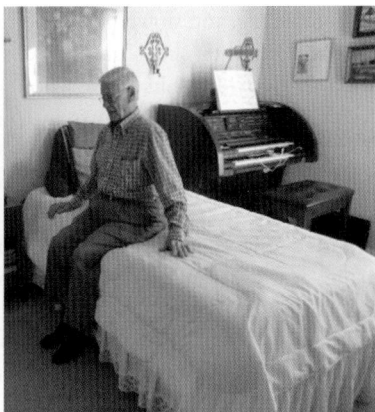

Fig. 41.6 Bed mobility.

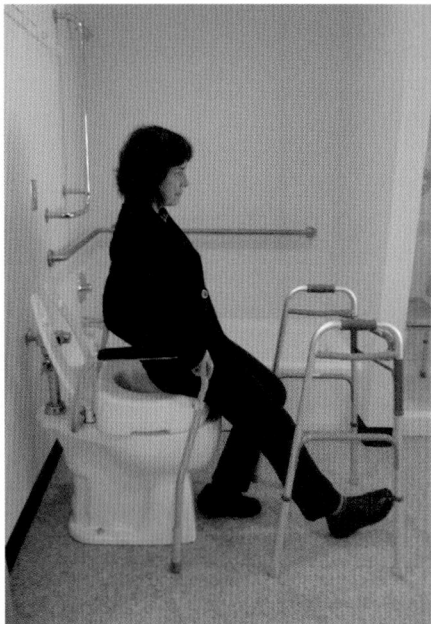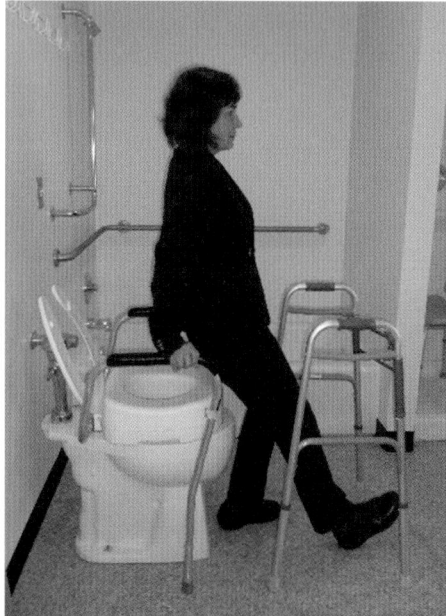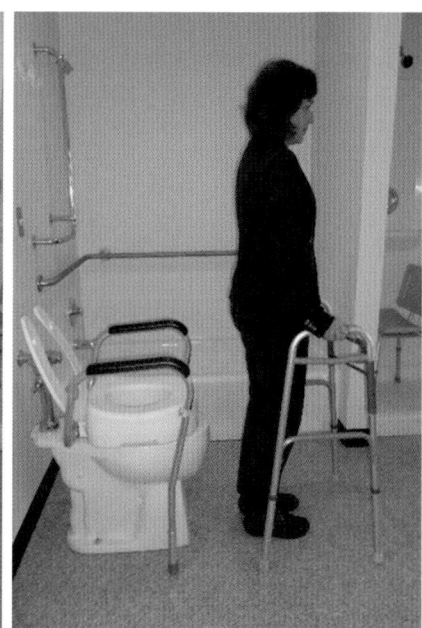

Fig. 41.7 Chair/commode transfer technique. Client's right hip has the hip replacement. The nonoperated leg is used for weight bearing during sitting and standing from the chair/commode.

Tub shower (without shower doors). The client is prohibited from taking a bath sitting on the floor of the tub. This action puts the client at severe risk of causing damage to the impaired joint and other types of injuries. A tub chair or tub transfer bench is strongly recommended to preserve hip precautions. The client is instructed to back up to the tub chair or bench using the walker or crutches for support. Then the client should reach for the backrest, extend the operated leg, and slowly lower to a seated position. The legs can then be lifted into the tub as the client leans back, using a leg lifter or bath towel if needed to support the operated leg. A handheld shower is helpful in directing the water for an effective and comfortable bath. Sponge bathing at the sink is an alternative activity,[2] although use of a long-handled sponge or reacher is recommended to avoid hip flexion when bathing the LEs.

Car. Bucket seats in small cars should be avoided. The client is instructed to have a helper move the front passenger seat back as far as it will go and recline the back of the seat in order to observe the hip flexion precaution. Then the client is instructed to back up to the seat, hold onto a stable part of the car, extend the operated leg, and slowly sit in the car. Remembering to lean back, the client then slides the buttocks toward the driver's seat. The upper body and LEs move as one unit to turn to face the forward direction. Firm pillows in the seat may be necessary to increase the height of the seat. Prolonged sitting in the car should be avoided. If transferring to the front passenger seat is a problem, transferring to the back seat of a four-door car is an alternative. The client backs to the seat, extends the operated leg, and slowly sits in the car. Then he or she slides back so that the operated leg is resting on the seat fully supported. Clients should not return to driving until given permission by their surgeon, even if the operated leg is not the leg used for operating the controls. Certain pain medications may cause driving to be unsafe.

Lower-Body Dressing

The client is instructed to sit in a chair with arms or on the edge of the bed for dressing activities. The client is instructed to avoid hip flexion, adduction and rotation, or crossing the legs to dress. The client must refrain from crossing the operated extremity over the nonoperated extremity at either the ankles or the knees. Assistive devices may be necessary for observing precautions (see Fig. 41.5). To maintain hip precautions, the client uses a reacher or dressing stick to put on and remove pants and shoes. For pants and underwear, the operated leg is dressed first by using the reacher or dressing stick to bring the pants over the foot and up to the knee. A sock aid is used to don socks or knee-high stockings, and a reacher or dressing stick is used to doff them. A reacher, elastic laces, and a long-handled shoehorn can also be provided.[2] It is also prudent for the occupational therapist or occupational therapy assistant to discuss clothing choices with the client for ease of dressing. Slip-on shoes with a nonslip sole, for example, may be easier to put on with appropriate adaptive equipment than sneakers with elastic laces.

Lower-Body Bathing

The section on transfers describes the proper method of getting in and out of the shower or tub. Sponge bathing at the sink is indicated until the physician designates that it is safe for the client to shower. Many surgeons use a waterproof bandage over the incision, which protects the site from infection, thereby allowing the client to shower before the incision is healed. Care must be taken for clients who are given permission to shower early in the recovery process. Pain medication and effects from anesthesia may make the client dizzy when standing or sitting for long periods and requires close monitoring. A sponge bath may still be the safest alternative. A long-handled bath sponge or back brush is used to reach the lower legs and feet safely. Soap-on-a-rope is used to prevent the soap from dropping, and a towel is wrapped on a reacher to dry the lower legs.[2] A handheld shower head is recommended to direct the water and provide a more comfortable shower.

Hair Shampoo

Until able to shower, the client is instructed to obtain assistance for shampooing hair. The client can have a helper wash the hair while the client is supine, using pillows for back support and a bucket or bowl to catch the water poured from a pitcher to rinse the hair. Another method involves having the client sit in a chair with the back to the sink. The client leans backward to position the head over the sink while the helper washes the hair. The client can also visit a hair salon until able to perform hair washing independently. If unable to obtain any assistance, the client may shampoo the hair while standing at the kitchen sink with a handheld sprayer, observing hip precautions at all times. Because bending forward at the kitchen sink can be performed with less than 90 degrees of hip flexion, most clients can observe the proper hip precautions using this method.

Homemaking

The client should initially refrain from heavy housework, such as vacuuming, lifting, and bed making. Kitchen activities can be initiated in therapy, with suggestions made to keep commonly used items at countertop level or within easy reach. The client can carry items by using an apron with large pockets, sliding items along the countertop, using a utility cart, attaching a small basket or bag to a walker, or wearing a fanny pack around the waist. Reachers are provided to grasp items in low cupboards or retrieve items from the floor (Fig. 41.8). Items in the refrigerator should be kept on the higher shelves, with only light items that can be obtained with the reacher on lower shelves. For cooking activities, it is recommended that the client use the stovetop or microwave oven rather than placing items in the oven, because it is difficult to maintain hip precautions when reaching in or out of the oven. Washing dishes should be done at the sink or using the top level only of an automatic dishwasher. The occupational therapy practitioner should also instruct the client in relevant energy conservation techniques for ADLs.

Sexual Activity

Persons with a hip fracture or hip replacement will have difficulty performing sexual activities in their usual manner. It is recommended that such persons refrain from sexual activity for a few weeks as specified by their physician so that they maintain the movement precautions applicable to their condition.[51] However, the occupational therapist must create an environment in which the client feels comfortable enough to ask personal questions. The therapist can do this by being open-minded and realizing that sexual activity is an important and meaningful activity of daily living. For clients with a hip replacement, the therapist can suggest participating in sexual activity while side-lying on the non-operated side when they can resume this activity. Hip abduction precautions can be maintained by placing pillows between the knees. To prevent excessive external rotation at the hips while in the supine position, the client can place pillows under the knees.[51] Written information with diagrams can be helpful when addressing such a personal issue. Clients can read this information privately or with their partners.

Caregiver Training

A family member, friend, or caregiver should be present for OT intervention sessions so that any questions may be answered. Appropriate supervision recommendations and instruction regarding activity precautions are given at this time. So that they fully understand the impact of following the hip precautions, caregivers should be encouraged to practice doing the adapted activities as well. Several online and print resources on hip fractures and total hip surgery can be compiled to provide to the client and caregivers.

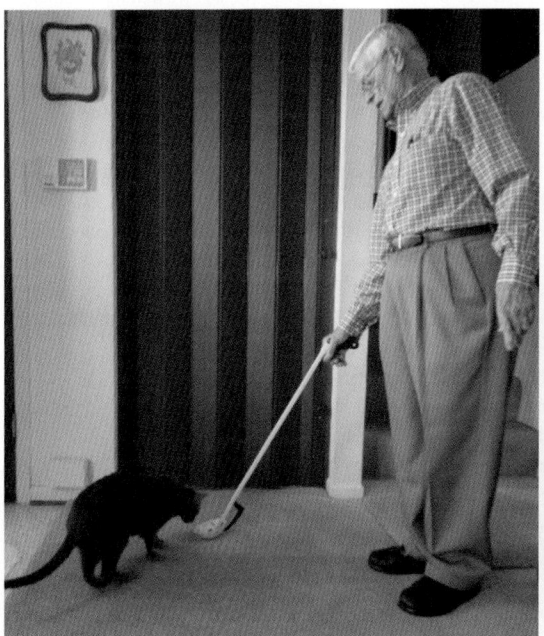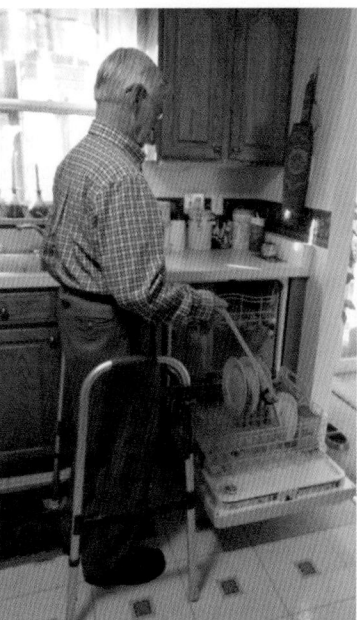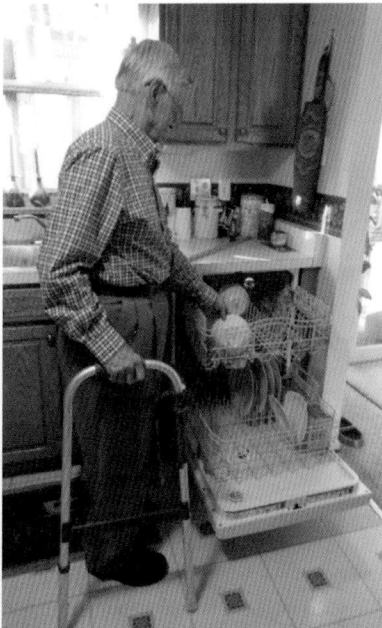

Fig. 41.8 Functional activities.

Evidence Regarding Occupational Therapy Intervention

A limited number of studies have examined OT intervention for hip joint replacements and hip fractures. Mikkelsen and colleagues examined the effects of reduced (less strict) posterior hip precautions along with the use of assistive devices on patient outcomes versus outcomes for patients who followed strict movement precautions but also used assistive devices.[52] They found that initially there were better outcomes for those patients following the strict movement precautions, but after 6 weeks there was no difference. However, patients with the reduced restrictions returned to work at a higher rate than those who followed the strict movement precautions. It was important for both groups in this study to have been trained properly to use assistive devices for daily activities. Therapists should still be sure to follow the surgeon's directions regarding hip precautions.[52]

Sirkka and Branholm[76] examined life satisfaction in 29 Swedish older adults who suffered a hip fracture. Participants reported a significant decline in their ability to perform hobbies and social activities after their hip fracture and that these activities were more important than self-care activities. Elinge and colleagues[32] also found that social interaction was affected more than other occupations for older adults who have had a hip fracture. Therapists can use the results of these studies to support addressing all areas of occupation and not just ADLs. By designing an intervention that targets the client's prior performance patterns and emotional and social needs, the occupational therapist can play a key role in the client's psychosocial adjustment to physical limitations and in maximizing the client's return to participation in meaningful activities.[47]

SECTION 2: KNEE JOINT REPLACEMENTS

Etiology and Medical Management

Knee pain affects the mobility and functional performance of many adults, often due to osteoarthritis in people aged 50 and older. In fact, this knee pain and loss of function are the primary reasons that some people elect to have knee joint replacements.[53] Knee pain is often due to osteoarthritis or degenerative joint disease, trauma or injury to the knee, or other rheumatic conditions and may be compounded by obesity or aging. Surgical knee replacement may be chosen by individuals to alleviate pain, increase motion, and maintain alignment and stability of the knee joint when conservative treatment has failed.

The process of knee replacement involves cutting away the damaged bone (as little bone as possible) and attaching prosthetic components of a new joint.[80] Various types of prostheses are used, depending on the severity and region of knee damage (Figs. 41.9 and 41.10). A partial or unicompartmental knee arthroplasty (UKA) is indicated if there is medial or lateral compartmental damage between the femur and tibia. The UKA is often placed with a minimally invasive technique, which allows greater knee flexion (up to 90 degrees) more quickly after

---

THREADED CASE STUDY

Mrs. Hernandez, Part 2

1. When completing the occupational profile, what additional information would the occupational therapist need to gather during the evaluation to supplement the information already provided in the case scenario?

Mrs. Hernandez's occupational profile revealed that she has many roles that she finds meaningful: grandmother, church member, and swimmer. She also seems to value being independent. She not only does things with her daughter and her family but also has interests and activities in which she participates on her own. Supporting contextual factors include an accessible home, a daughter nearby who involves her in many activities with her children, and church friends who can offer some assistance. Nonsupportive contextual factors include an inaccessible swimming pool and the fact that she lives alone. Additional information that would be useful to obtain from Mrs. Hernandez for the occupational profile includes but is not limited to specific information about the arrangement of furniture and other items in her home, how willing her daughter is to assist Mrs. Hernandez with her needs or whether the daughter is already assisting with some IADLs, prior surgeries or conditions that would have an impact on the current plan of care or lead to additional falls, history of falls, and equipment or home modifications already established. This information will aid the occupational therapist in planning for discharge and specific equipment recommendations.

2. Identify important occupations and performance skills to address first when educating Mrs. Hernandez to safely resume occupational performance patterns.

Motor and process skills that must be assessed before training Mrs. Hernandez to perform her daily activities safely, including driving, are moving herself from one place to another and heeding hip precautions. These skills will affect the extent to which she will be able to engage in and learn the prerequisite performance skills needed to optimize her independence in ADLs and IADLs. The occupational therapist must first be sure that Mrs. Hernandez understands the hip precautions and is able to recall them. Then the occupational therapist must address her ability to move herself in and out of bed and perform toileting functions while observing the hip precautions. These prerequisite skills will prepare her for more advanced skills such as dressing, bathing, driving, and home management activities. Because she lives alone, she needs to be able to complete all her ADLs and IADLs independently. The therapist should be sure to address the prerequisite skills first and progress Mrs. Hernandez to more complex ADL tasks that increase her confidence to return home and resume her typical occupations and performance patterns.

3. What prerequisite performance skills and client factors/body functions should be addressed with Mrs. Hernandez before the occupational therapist directly addresses her ability to drive again?

Because driving allows Mrs. Hernandez to get to her swimming classes, church meetings, and daughter's home, this is placed as a priority in the list of problems, and she verbalizes that this issue is most important. Mrs. Hernandez should have demonstrated strength and coordination to achieve relative independence in different types of transfers, especially car transfers, before she considers driving again. It is important that she obtain medical clearance from her physician or surgeon before resuming driving activities. The occupational therapist can assist her in identifying other community mobility resources available to her until she resumes driving and can complete other assessments directly related to driving, such as an off-road driving assessment.

surgery, fewer postoperative complications, and comparable long-term results with total knee replacements.[40,69] Because limited ligaments and structures of the joint are disrupted, increased stability is obtained immediately.[55]

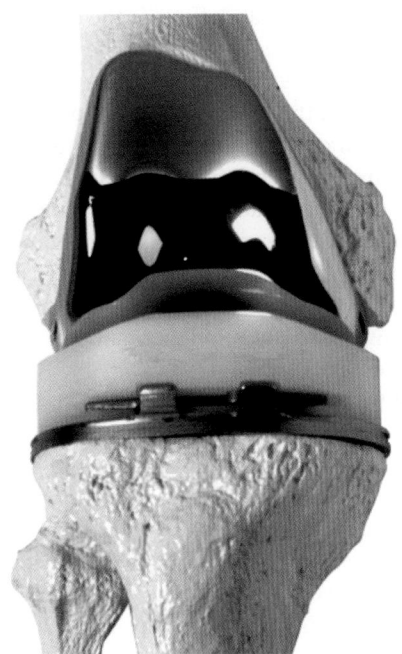

Fig. 41.9 Knee prosthesis. (From Black J, Hawks J: *Medical surgical nursing: clinical management for positive outcomes*, ed 8, St. Louis, 2009, Elsevier.)

Total knee replacement (TKR), or total knee arthroplasty (TKA), is indicated when two or more compartments of the knee are damaged. Various prosthetic devices are chosen based on the medical condition and activities performed by the client.[46] A fixed weight-bearing prosthesis allows only flexion and extension of the knee, as the polyethylene tibia insert is locked into the tibial tray.[73] A rotating platform prosthesis, or mobile weight-bearing prosthesis, allows the slight rotation normally available at the knee, as the tibial component is not locked. This allows for more normal function at the knee, but it has a slightly higher risk of mechanical failure.[73] The rotating platform is typically used for younger, more active people, or for women, because they typically have more rotation available at the knee than men.[37] Both types of prostheses typically decrease pain, improve functional mobility, and enhance quality of life for individuals with degenerative knee conditions. They can be put in place with various surgical techniques, including minimally invasive approaches, in which there is less damage to the quadriceps tendon and the medial collateral ligament, which may improve range of motion at the knee and lead to faster postoperative recovery.[78] However, the minimally invasive approaches are not appropriate for clients who are obese, have comorbidities that influence muscle and bone structure, or have fixed bony deformities before surgery.[66]

The prosthesis can be cemented to the bone with acrylic cement or not cemented. With a cemented prosthesis, clients are usually able to bear weight as tolerated on the operated leg. With a noncemented prosthesis, initial weight bearing is often avoided or restricted. The choice to use cement to hold the

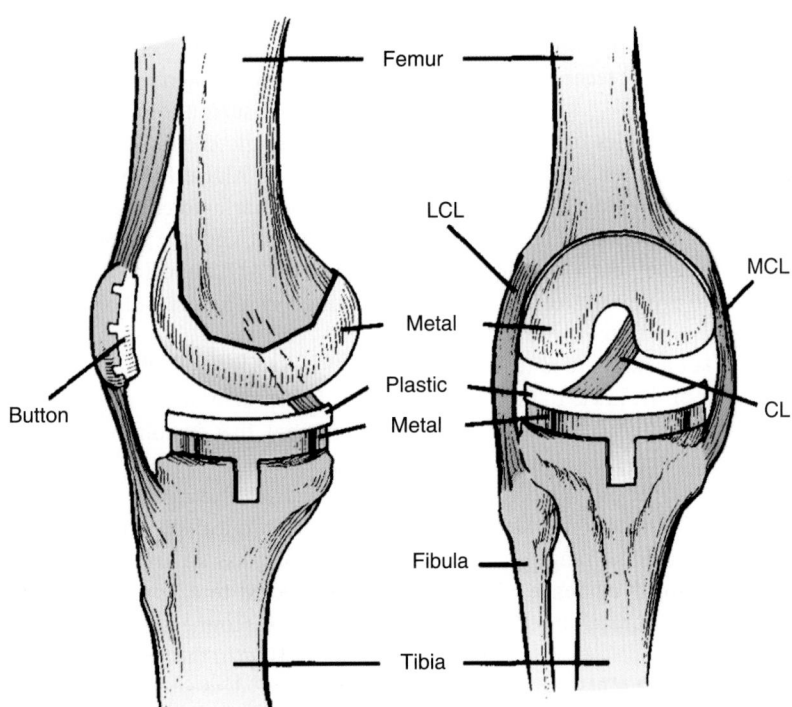

Fig. 41.10 Total knee replacement. The metal aspects of the prosthesis cover the distal portion of the femur and the end of the tibia. There is a polyethylene plastic-bearing surface (plastic) between the metallic aspects of the two surfaces. The patella is replaced by a polyethylene button. The medial collateral ligament *(MCL)*, lateral collateral ligament *(LCL)*, and cruciate ligaments *(CL)* are retained. (From Early MB: *Physical dysfunction: practical skills for the occupational therapy assistant*, ed 3, St. Louis, 2013, Mosby; modified from Calliet R: *Knee pain and instability*, ed 3, Philadelphia, 1992, FA Davis.)

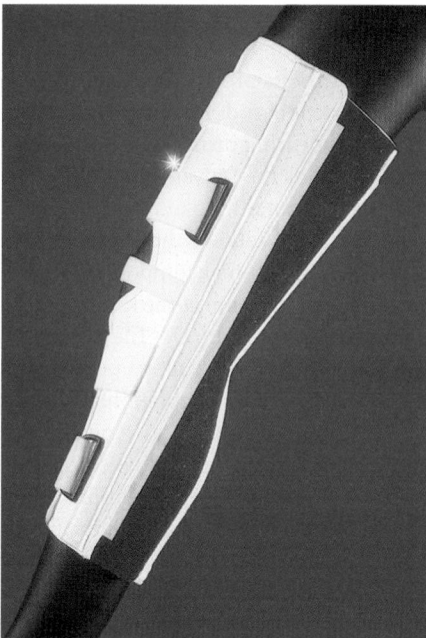

Fig. 41.11 A knee immobilizer is used to support and stabilize the knee joint during mobility. (From Ignatavicius D, Workman ML: *Medical-surgical nursing: patient-centered collaborative care*, ed 8, St. Louis, 2016, Elsevier.)

prosthesis in place is made by the surgeon and considers the medical condition of the client. The noncemented procedure, for example, requires that the client does not have any other health issues that would slow bone growth, thus extending the time frame for restricted weight bearing. There is no evidence indicating that any surgical technique has superior results influencing discharge; therefore, it is up to the orthopedic medical team to make the determination of surgical technique that will be performed for every individual client.[81]

Clients typically start out-of-bed activities on the first day after surgery, with appropriate assistance or supervision. An ambulatory device, such as a walker or crutches, also may be used for greater stability. If the knee joint is unstable after surgery for any reason, the physician may indicate that a knee immobilizer or other brace should be used to preserve knee joint alignment (Fig. 41.11). The client should avoid excessive rotation at the knee for up to 12 weeks after surgery. There is usually no restriction on flexion and extension of the knee. In fact, maintaining the mobility of the knee is important to ensure adequate mobility during healing and to regain normal motion and function.[19,31,50,68] Some surgeons recommend the use of a continuous passive motion (CPM) device to provide slow, controlled movement with the intent of improving functional range of motion and reducing postsurgical edema, although evidence is limited on the long-term effectiveness of the CPM machines.[10,14,31]

SPECIAL CONSIDERATIONS FOR KNEE REPLACEMENTS

As with hip replacements, individuals with joint changes that result in increasing pain may have multiple joint involvement (i.e., both knees). Some clients opt to have two joints replaced during the same hospitalization, either during the same surgery or with procedures 3 to 7 days apart. This can complicate the rehabilitation process because the client will not be able to rely on the nonoperated leg when walking, transitioning between seated and standing positions, and performing daily occupations. However, it eliminates the need for an additional hospitalization if both knees are affected. The orthopedic surgeon should discuss these options with the client to determine the most appropriate course of action.

It is important for the occupational therapy practitioner to be aware of complications or special procedures that occurred during a client's surgery and to verify precautions or risks with the physician. Surgeons will make specific recommendations based on the client's particular situation, surgical procedures used, or postoperative concerns. Common complications include dislocation of the prosthesis, degeneration of parts, fracture of bone next to implanted parts, loosening of prosthetic parts, and infection of the joint after surgery.[29]

Some clients describe postsurgical pain as more significant after TKR compared to total hip replacement. This is often managed with medications, such as epidural or periarticular anesthetics, patient-controlled analgesia, oral analgesics, and NSAIDs, or peripheral nerve blocks; opioids are recommended only when used as part of a full pain management program and only in the immediate postoperative period.[33,81] Side effects and effectiveness of pain management medications vary with individual clients. Other methods of pain control amenable to use by rehabilitation professionals include the superficial cold modalities, proper positioning during transitional movements, CPM machines after therapy if approved by the physician, and balance of rest and activity.

As with hip replacement, the emphasis in rehabilitation is on maintaining or increasing joint motion, slowly increasing the strength of surrounding musculature, decreasing swelling, and increasing the client's functional performance of occupations, particularly ADLs. The occupational therapist's role in this process is primarily to educate the client who has undergone joint replacement and any caregivers about applying adaptive techniques for ADLs and IADLs with limited mobility while maintaining any joint precautions for movement or weight bearing.

Medical Equipment

The OT practitioner should be familiar with the following equipment that is commonly used in the treatment of knee replacement:

- *Hemovac.* During surgery, a plastic drainage tube is inserted at the surgical site to assist with postoperative drainage of blood. It has an area for collection of drainage and may be connected to a portable suction machine. The unit should not be disconnected for any activity because this may create a blockage in the system. The Hemovac is usually left in place for 1 to 2 days after surgery.
- *Commode chairs.* The use of a height-adjustable commode chair instead of a regular toilet facilitates safe transfers and allows the client to limit flexion of the knee during toileting.
- *Sequential compression devices (SCDs).* SCDs are used postoperatively to reduce the risk of deep vein thrombosis. They

are inflatable pads covering the circumference of the lower leg and that provide intermittent pneumatic compression of the legs.[29]

- *Antiembolus hose.* This elastic hosiery may be extended up to the knee or over the knee and on the thigh, depending on physician preference. They are worn 24 hours a day and removed only during bathing. Their purpose is to assist circulation, prevent edema, and thus reduce the risk of deep-vein thrombosis.[29]
- *Patient-controlled intravenous administration.* PCA is delivered through an intravenous line; PCEA is delivered through an epidural line. A prescribed amount of medication is programmed by the physician and nursing staff to allow the client to self-administer pain medication by pushing a button to inject a safe amount. When dosages have reached a limit, the machine will not administer medication even if the button is pushed.
- *Incentive spirometer.* This portable breathing apparatus is used to encourage deep breathing and prevent the development of postoperative pneumonia.
- *Continuous passive motion (CPM) machine.* This mechanical device supports a joint and can be set to move slowly through a designated range of motion to promote controlled movement in the operated joint.

ROLE OF OCCUPATIONAL THERAPY FOR CLIENTS WITH KNEE JOINT REPLACEMENT

After a knee replacement, occupational therapy typically begins on either the day of surgery or the first postoperative day, and this decision is made considering the general health of the client and the physiological response to surgery. Before any physical assessment, it is important to introduce and explain the role of occupational therapy and complete an occupational profile. This profile involves gathering information regarding the client's occupational history, prior functional status in ADLs and IADLs, descriptions of performance contexts (e.g., home environment and social support available), and the client's goals. The goal of occupational therapy is for the client to maximize performance of daily occupations, with all movement precautions observed during activities. This often involves improving activity tolerance, addressing functional mobility, and providing education in the use of adaptive equipment.[28] The role of the occupational therapist and assistant is to teach the client ways and means of performing daily occupations safely and problem-solving any barriers to occupational performance.[44]

Evaluation and Intervention

After the occupational profile, an assessment of the motor, cognitive, social, and emotional factors is recommended, specifically as they relate to occupational performance. Body functions such as UE ROM, muscle strength, sensation, and coordination must be assessed to determine if any adaptations should be made to functional mobility or use of adaptive equipment. Mental functions such as memory, problem solving, and sequencing must be considered when addressing potential precautions, safety awareness, and performance of occupations. ADLs and other relevant occupations should be evaluated through standardized assessments, direct observation, or interview as the context and client conditions allow. The skilled occupational therapist should be able to identify if social or emotional concerns are present, including pain, fear of falling, hesitation to resume normal activities, or concerns about surgical healing.

OT intervention planning requires careful consideration of evaluation data and clinical reasoning skills to determine how the specific client's needs and concerns can be addressed through a program of functional activities that gradually enables a person to resume meaningful occupations. The therapist introduces and trains clients in the use of assistive devices, proper transfer techniques, and ADL and IADL techniques while ensuring safe positioning of the knee and prosthetic components. Discharge planning should be considered early, as many clients are able to return home within a few days if functional mobility and ADL and IADL function can be restored. Clients who need additional rehabilitation to regain occupational performance, who have limited community support, and with inhibitory contexts may be recommended for inpatient rehabilitation after the acute hospital stay.

Specific Training Techniques for Participation in Occupations

Following any type of knee replacement, the occupational therapist should encourage weight bearing as specified by the surgeon, and knee flexion and extension as allowed by pain level and surgical outcomes. It is encouraged that the leg be supported by the occupational therapist when a client is moved from sitting with the legs elevated—for example, in a recliner or geri-chair—to seated with feet on the floor in preparation for transfers or standing. Clients also may be encouraged to participate in deep breathing and relaxation as methods of pain control.

Bed Mobility

The supine position is recommended when the client is resting in bed, with the knee fully extended. Although it is acceptable for a small towel or bolster to be placed under the knee to allow slight flexion for pain control periodically, the client is encouraged to keep the knee extended and the hip in a neutral position when sleeping. This encourages full extension that will be needed for ambulation. A knee immobilizer or other supportive brace can be used if indicated by the physician. As in hip replacement, a pillow or wedge can be placed between the legs if this is necessary for side-lying and if the person lies on the nonoperated side. A CPM machine, used in the supine position, may be used for several hours a day after surgery to facilitate recovery and increased range of motion.[39] However, use of the CPM machine is often discontinued before returning home, when more activities are resumed. To enter or exit the bed, clients can move freely, and specific techniques can be identified according to client preferences. There are no restrictions that dictate bed mobility procedures.

Transfers

Typically, the client can bend freely at the hips if only the knee has been replaced, and this motion may compensate for the more painful knee ROM, often in flexion. Armrests are generally helpful and allow better UE support for the transitions between sitting and standing on a postoperative knee.

Chair or commode chair. To move from standing to sitting, the client is instructed to back up to the chair, extend the operated leg forward, reach back for the armrests, and slowly lower to the sitting position. To stand, the client extends the operated leg and pushes up from the armrests. Once standing, the client can reach for an ambulatory aid, such as a walker if it is being used. As in hip replacement procedures, low chairs, soft chairs, reclining chairs, and rocking chairs should be avoided.[2] If a client has bilateral knee replacements, it may be uncomfortable to flex either knee to promote the sit-to-stand transitions. In this case, to move from standing to sitting, the client again backs up until he or she feels the back of the chair, then takes a small step forward with both feet. Then the client reaches back for the armrests and gently lowers the body onto the chair, slowly advancing the feet forward if necessary, until a seated position is achieved. To move from seated to standing, both feet are placed slightly forward and the arms are used to raise the buttocks off the chair. Then the client can flex forward at the hips and slowly move the feet back toward the chair until the lower extremities are fully supporting the body. Only then should the client release the armrests and reach for a walker or other ambulatory device placed in front of him or her. Three-in-one commode chairs are often recommended because they can be placed over a toilet to raise the height and provide armrests, thereby improving safety during transfers. In addition, the three-in-one can be used as a stand-alone bedside commode if necessary when the home environment does not support easy access to a bathroom on all levels of the home. Comfort height toilets (17-inch seat height) can be considered for a permanent modification at home that can allow for easier transfers to the toilet.

Shower stall. Nonskid strips or stickers are recommended in all shower stalls and tubs. Several methods are possible for movement in shower stalls, and the occupational therapist should problem-solve with the client to determine which method is safest. As in the hip replacement methods, the walker or crutches may go first, then the operated leg, and then the nonoperated leg. An alternative method to enter the shower stall is to back up to the edge or rim of the shower while using the walker for balance, then stepping into the shower while looking down at the feet and shower rim for safety. Installation of a shower chair with adjustable legs or a stool and grab bars is strongly encouraged to help the client maintain balance and preserve endurance.

Tub shower (without shower doors). As in the method for hip replacements, the client is prohibited from taking a bath sitting on the floor of the tub, because this action puts the client at severe risk of causing damage to the knee when transitioning to or from the tub floor. Although a tub seat can be used as in the hip replacement techniques, it is not necessary, as hip flexion is permitted after a knee replacement. To maintain balance during the transfer, it is recommended that the client stand next to the tub, with the hands placed on the short wall of the head or foot of the tub. Then, by flexing the hip and knee, or alternatively by extending the hip and knee, the client can side-step into the tub while using the UEs to maintain balance (Fig. 41.12). A grab bar may be added for safety as needed.

Car. Bucket seats in small cars should be avoided. Bench-type seats are recommended. The client is instructed to have a helper move the front passenger seat back as far as it will go. Then the client is instructed to back up to the seat, hold on to a stable part of the car, extend the operated leg, and slowly sit in the car. The client can lean forward at the hip for clearance of the upper body and head as they move into the car. The upper body and LEs move as one unit to turn to face the forward direction. Prolonged sitting in the car should be avoided. If transferring to the front passenger seat is a problem, transferring to the back seat of a four-door car is an alternative. The client backs to the seat, extends the operated leg, and slowly sits in the car. Then he or she slides back so the operated leg is resting on the seat,

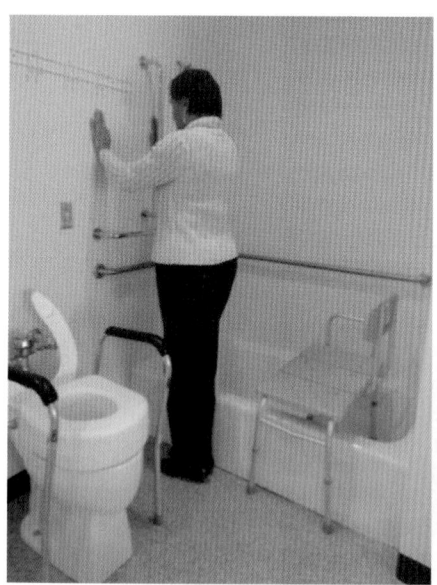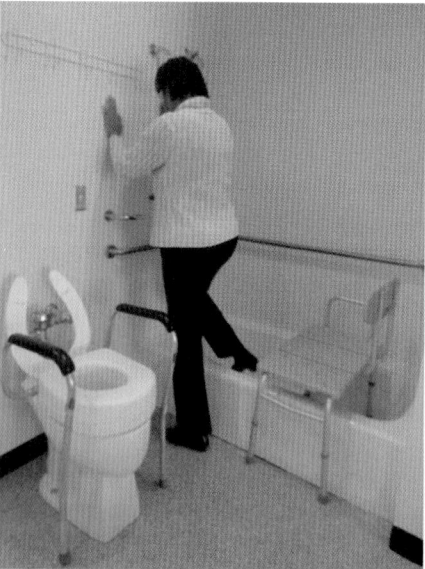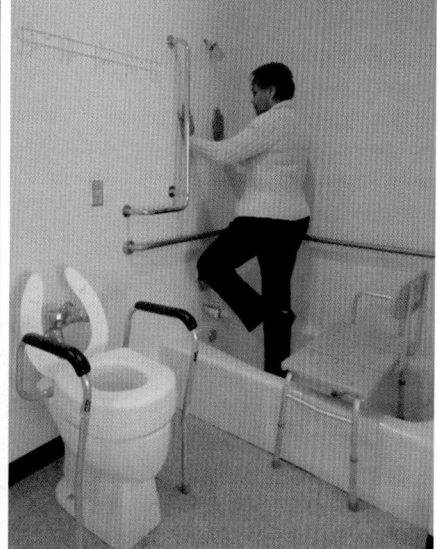

Fig. 41.12 Tub transfers following knee replacement.

fully supported. Clients should not return to driving until given permission by their surgeon, even if the operated leg is not the leg used for operating the controls. Sports utility vehicles, vans, or trucks typically have higher seats and may make the transfers easier for some clients.

Lower-Body Dressing and Bathing

The dressing of lower extremities presents a problem only if the clients are unable to reach their toes, which is usually done by leaning forward at the hips or raising the feet onto a footstool. If necessary, the techniques described for hip replacement can be used, including the use of adaptive equipment. The client also should be instructed in donning and doffing the knee immobilizer or other brace, if used. The client should be cautioned to prevent torque or rotation at the knee joint when dressing by not twisting the body or leg while bearing weight on the operated leg. Clients can take a sponge bath in the initial stages of recovery and typically are not approved to shower until the margins of the incision have healed,[3] approximately 7 to 10 days after the surgery. Showering may be permitted if a waterproof dressing covers the incision.

Homemaking

Homemaking and caregiver training follow the same procedures as for hip replacement techniques, although hip movement is not restricted. Care should be taken when standing or sitting for extended periods, to avoid prolonged static positioning of the knee and for pain management.

Sexual Activity

Much like those with hip replacements, persons with a knee replacement will have difficulty performing sexual activities in their usual manner. It is recommended that they refrain from sexual activity for a few weeks so that they maintain the movement precautions applicable to their condition.[50] For clients who have questions about the level of sexual activity allowed during the healing process, the therapist may need to suggest ways for the client to position the operated leg during sexual activity to maintain precautions or to minimize discomfort. Side-lying on the nonoperated side is one option. Clients with knee replacements or weight-bearing precautions should refrain from kneeling.[50] Written information with diagrams can be helpful when addressing such a personal issue.

Evidence Regarding Occupational Therapy Intervention

Occupational and physical therapies are typically initiated as soon as permitted by surgeons after knee replacements. In fact, a small percentage (13%–15%) of these surgeries are completed as outpatient procedures or considered fast-track surgeries with discharge in 1 to 2 days.[81] When paired with preoperative patient education, early mobilization may reduce potential complications, such as deep vein thrombosis, while offering shorter hospital stays and increased patient satisfaction.[70] Therefore, early evaluation and intervention by the rehabilitation team is important to ensure that clients can return home safely.

Intense postoperative rehabilitation has been proven to enhance patient outcomes, including improved scores on standardized ADL assessments in the areas of self-care, transfers, locomotion, and cognition.[7] Home care and outpatient rehabilitation are also important for the client who needs continued support during recovery. Fewer days between discharge from the inpatient setting and the initiation of outpatient services are associated with greater return of function and lower pain levels.[14]

When rehabilitation is delivered through an interprofessional team that includes occupational therapy, clients experience decreased pain and long-term disability, while achieving improved physical and emotional outcomes and health management.[30]

One occupation that is often overlooked is work, as most patients may be told simply to wait 6 to 12 weeks before returning to work without sufficient guidance about how to make that happen.[56] Occupational therapists are ideally suited to analyze the demands of the job and assess client performance patterns to contribute to the accuracy of those decisions. In fact, occupational therapy can also facilitate improved community-based occupational performance after hip and knee replacements.[30]

SECTION 3: SHOULDER JOINT REPLACEMENTS

The shoulder complex is not a single joint, as functional UE use relies on consideration of the glenohumeral, acromioclavicular, sternoclavicular, and scapulothoracic joints (Fig. 41.13). Musculature acts on the joints to allow complex movements of the shoulder in elevation and depression, retraction and protraction, and rotation of the scapula, as well as flexion, extension, rotation, and horizontal movements typically measured at the glenohumeral joint. The occupational therapist must carefully analyze shoulder dysfunction to determine the potential deficits, to develop interventions, to protect the joints, and ultimately to promote and facilitate UE function during occupations.

Just as osteoarthritis has been described as a contributor to pain that often leads to hip or knee replacement, this orthopedic condition can also contribute to shoulder pain and dysfunction. Other inflammatory or anatomic conditions, biomechanical forces that may cause damage to the shoulder complex, and proximal humerus fractures are often sources of shoulder pain and dysfunction.[15,34] Conservative medical treatments often include oral or injected medication designed to decrease pain and inflammation.[42] In addition, therapeutic exercise and activity modifications may be used to control pain and promote function. In this chapter, only conditions that may result in various types of shoulder replacements will be considered because of the specific rehabilitation needs of this surgical intervention.

ETIOLOGY AND MEDICAL MANAGEMENT

The type of damage to the shoulder complex typically directs the medical intervention undertaken by the orthopedic physician. People who suffer a humeral fracture typically undergo a humeral head replacement or hemiarthroplasty. In this procedure, the humeral head and fractured area are removed and

THREADED CASE STUDY

Mrs. Green, Part 1

Mrs. Green is an 80-year-old (prefers use of the pronouns she/hers/her) with degenerative joint disease that affects many of the joints in her body. She has already had bilateral knee replacements, and her orthopedic surgeon recommended a reverse shoulder replacement of her dominant right arm to improve functional UE use. Mrs. Green lives alone and manages her self-care independently, using a reacher and long shoehorn for dressing. She also completes most housekeeping tasks independently, with a hired housekeeper who assists with the heavy cleaning once a month. She has made some modifications to her home so that she does not need to reach very far. For example, she has moved the microwave oven and most frequently used dishes and glasses to the countertop. Additionally, she moved her hanging clothes to the doorknobs in her bedroom and uses a handheld showerhead when bathing. Mrs. Green drives and just recently stopped working part-time. Her leisure pursuits include visiting with friends and knitting. She is an avid knitter, known to make beautiful scarves and Christmas stockings for family members. This is the activity that is most meaningful to her and the reason she has decided to go ahead with the surgery.

The reverse shoulder replacement technique was chosen because the muscles supporting the shoulder girdle were weak due to prior rotator cuff injuries. Mrs. Green received home-based therapy 2 days after the surgery when she was discharged home. She had to rely on her adult children to help care for her as well as her sister who came to live with her for 2 weeks. Because of the postsurgical pain and movement precautions, Mrs. Green had difficulty completing self-care tasks, bed mobility, and transfers. This frustrated her greatly, especially her inability to perform toilet hygiene with her nondominant hand and difficulty fastening a bra. Most of the therapy sessions focused on developing effective compensatory strategies with Mrs. Green.

After 6 weeks, the movement precautions were lifted, and Mrs. Green progressed faster in her physical rehabilitation, advancing some range of motion and strength. After about 4 months Mrs. Green was able to resume all her prior occupations, including knitting and driving. She reports less pain during activity but still has some range of motion limitation, which she had been informed before surgery might not improve to normal limits.

Critical Thinking Questions

1. What could Mrs. Green have done to better prepare for the surgery knowing that her dominant hand/arm would be restricted for 6 weeks?
2. How could the therapist use caregiver training in this case?
3. Identify self-care tasks that would pose a particular problem due to her movement and weight-bearing precautions (no passive or active shoulder extension or external rotation; no active movement in any direction; only passive shoulder flexion and abduction to about 80 degrees allowed, non–weight bearing).
4. Mrs. Green did not have any movement precautions with her right hand, wrist, or forearm. How could you enable Mrs. Green to use her right hand as an assist (while it was still in the sling) during daily activities without breaking her movement precautions at the shoulder?

---

replaced with an endoprosthesis. In some cases, this procedure includes glenoid resurfacing. The hemiarthroplasty is appropriate for individuals who have rheumatoid or osteoarthritis or have avascular necrosis; it is less effective for individuals being treated for fractures or rotator cuff injury.[62]

A total shoulder arthroplasty (TSA), also referred to as a total shoulder replacement (TSR), is more often performed for a person with degenerative or inflammatory conditions such as osteoarthritis (Fig. 41.14). In this procedure, the humeral head is replaced by a ball-shaped prosthesis and the glenoid is resurfaced or replaced with a prosthetic component.[42] This procedure requires adequate bony support at the glenoid and an intact rotator cuff to maintain the stability of the joint and to facilitate appropriate biomechanical function of the shoulder.[62] This procedure yields good results for patients, including pain relief, return of adequate range of motion, and performance of functional activities, with patient satisfaction rates of up to 95%.[62]

A reverse total shoulder arthroplasty (RTSA), also referred to as a reverse total shoulder replacement (RTSR), is indicated for patients with a degenerative or inflammatory condition present in the shoulder complex, but also with some deficiency of the rotator cuff. In some cases, this procedure is also used when a revision of a traditional TSA is required. When the rotator cuff is extremely weak) or damaged, the muscles are unable to effectively support the newly repaired joint, so a reverse technique is indicated. In the RTSA, the ball and socket of the glenohumeral joint are reversed; the semicircular ball is placed in the glenoid and a polyethylene cap is implanted into the humerus. In this procedure, good deltoid function is needed to stabilize the joint without as much reliance on rotator cuff muscles for support.[8,42,62,72]

All of these procedures are expected to eventually decrease the patient's pain, improve functional use of the shoulder over time, and enhance quality of life.[42] However, when compared with the hemiarthroplasty or replacement of the humeral head, the TSA typically has greater range of motion results and higher patient satisfaction ratings as well as a decreased need for revisions, because further glenoid wear is not a factor.[41,67] The most common postoperative complications for any of the shoulder surgeries is loosening of the glenoid component, loosening of the humeral component, glenohumeral joint instability, or rotator cuff tears. These complications have an incidence of only about 10% to 16% in the 3 to 5 years after surgery and approximately 22% in the 10 to 15 years after surgery.[36,77] Full shoulder ROM may or may not be achieved with shoulder replacements, but the pain relief and functional improvements make the surgery worthwhile for many individuals. Evidence suggests that while range of motion does not match healthy individuals, performance of ADLs and motion gained after the surgery is significantly improved when compared to non-operative individuals with osteoarthritis.[16] A typical prosthesis will last 15 to 20 years for most patients, depending on the conditions of the patient and how the joint is used or protected.[42]

SPECIAL CONSIDERATIONS FOR SHOULDER JOINT REPLACEMENTS

Because orthopedic concerns and surgical techniques may vary among surgeons, so also will the postoperative precautions. The occupational therapist should be familiar with the procedures

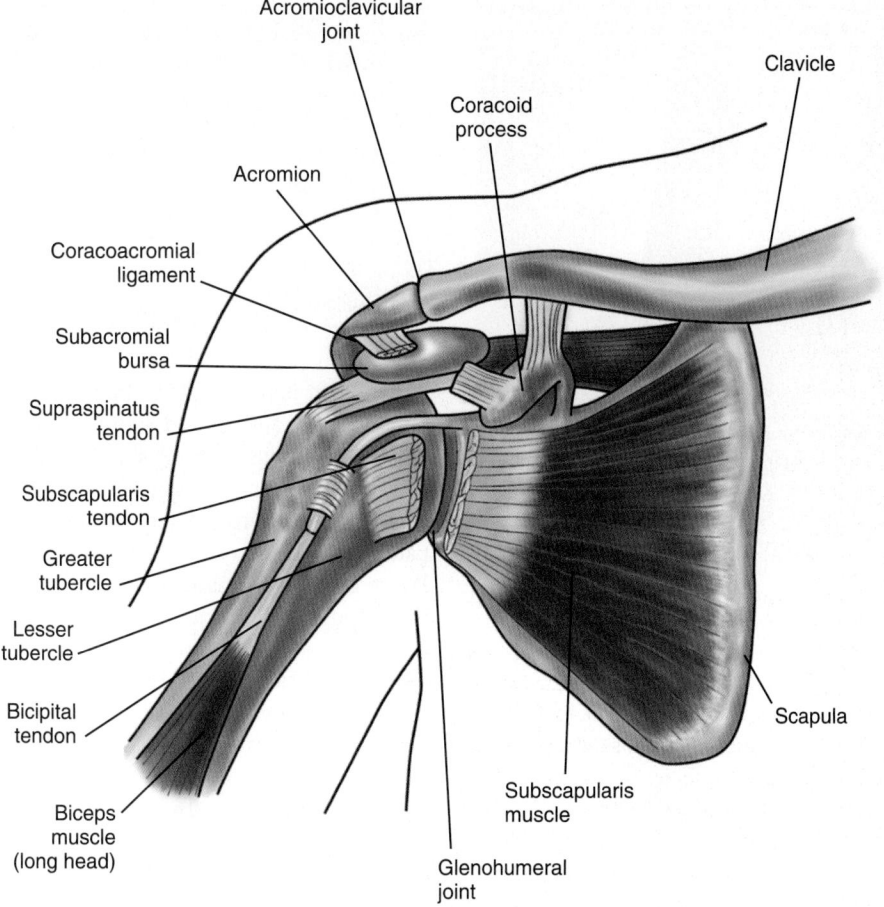

Fig. 41.13 Shoulder complex. (From Miller MD, Hart J, MacKnight JM: *Essential orthopaedics.* Philadelphia, 2010, Saunders. Adapted with permission from Anna Francesca Valerio, MD.)

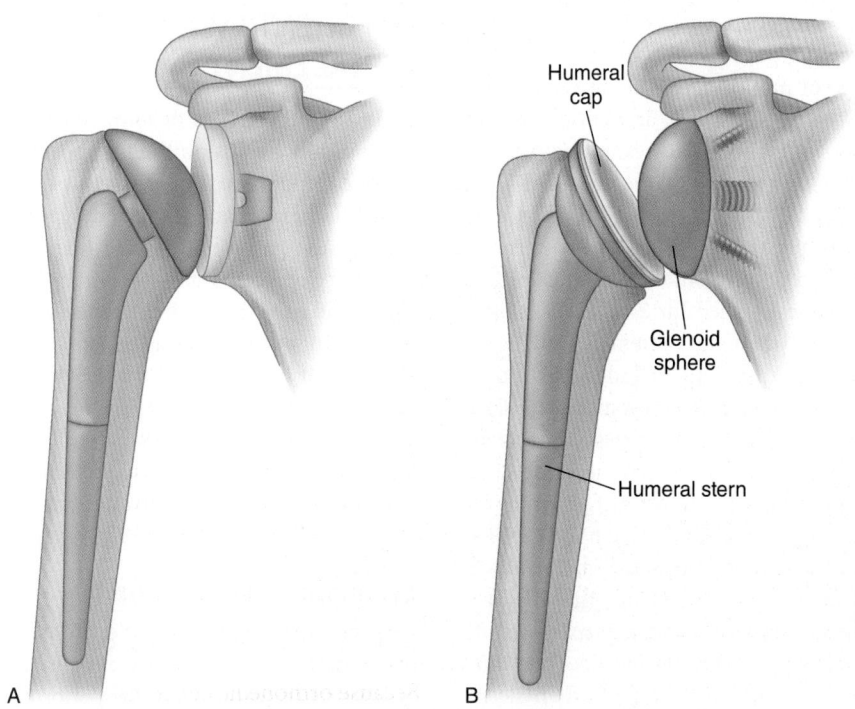

Fig. 41.14 (A) Total shoulder arthroplasty. (B) Reverse shoulder arthroplasty.

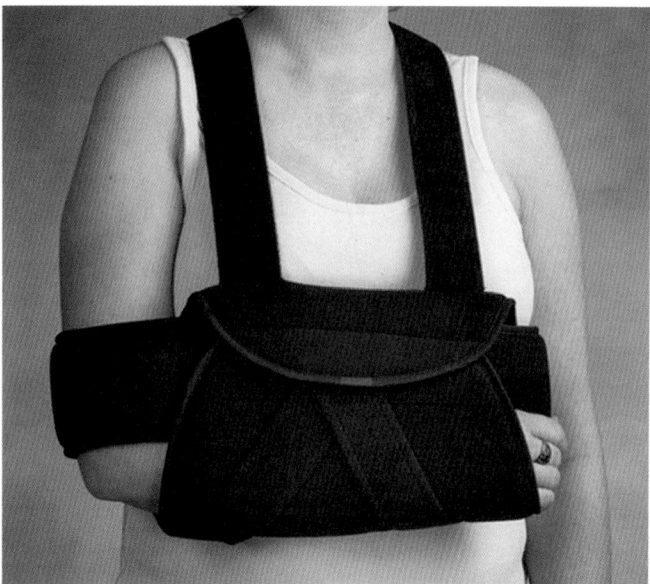

Fig. 41.15 Sling with the swathe. (Courtesy North Coast Medical, Inc., Gilroy, CA.)

and should communicate openly with the surgeon to ensure movements of the shoulder that promote patient safety, prevent complications, and progress function as efficiently as possible.

In the initial postoperative phase, soft tissues that surround and support the joint must be preserved for healing, glenohumeral joint must be maintained in the appropriate anatomic position, and surgical release and repair of supportive musculature must be protected for healing. Edema is managed with modalities or positioning as appropriate. Pain and inflammation are controlled as prescribed by the physician. As with those who have had total hip and knee replacements, the client is provided with a pain medication regimen that provides a consistent level of pain relief to allow full participation in the rehabilitation program. Active range of motion (AROM) is encouraged in the joints of the elbow, wrist, and hand, and contributes to continued participation in occupations. However, only passive range of motion (PROM) is permitted in the shoulder joint and only for motions specified by the surgeon. ADLs should be restored, but typically in compensatory or adaptive patterns as the operative shoulder should not have undue resistance placed on it. A shoulder sling is typically used for 3 to 4 weeks after shoulder surgery and is worn when the patient is moving or sleeping (Fig. 41.15). Options for this sling include a traditional sling with the glenohumeral joint in internal rotation, or a sling with a small abduction pillow wedge that supports a more neutral shoulder position.[41] A shoulder swathe (a long, wide strap that encircles the arm in the sling and the trunk) also may be prescribed to provide extra support and protection for the arm and to prevent prohibited movement. These may be removed for therapeutic activities and when seated with the UE in a supported position (with the humeral head approximated in the glenoid fossa). The sling (or swathe) should be worn during functional activities, during ambulation, and when sleeping to preserve the shoulder joint position. For approximately 6 to 8 weeks, patients may not bear weight on the operated UE,

may not lift items weighing more than 1 to 2 pounds with the operated UE, and should avoid the following motions: shoulder extension past neutral, shoulder abduction past 45 degrees, external rotation past approximately 30 degrees, and internal rotation past approximately 60 degrees. They may not participate in any resistive activities in internal or external rotation. When sleeping, a pillow or towel roll should be placed under the scapula or elbow as needed for comfort to ensure that the shoulder is supported in the front of the body and in adherence to the precautions (Box 41.3).

Pain management is usually achieved in the postoperative phase with patient-controlled anesthesia, which can be administered through an epidural line or a pump with a line inserted into the surgical site. This can be supplemented with superficial cold therapies, movement restrictions and sling wear, and activity modification. After a few days, the anesthesia lines are replaced with oral analgesics or antiinflammatory medications as prescribed by the physician.

ROLE OF OCCUPATIONAL THERAPY FOR CLIENTS WITH SHOULDER JOINT REPLACEMENT

As in the other types of joint replacement, occupational therapy typically begins on the first postoperative day if there is no adverse response to the surgery. Introduction of the role of occupational therapy and expected types of interventions should precede the gathering of data for the occupational profile. In shoulder replacements, it is vital to understand hand dominance and how this may influence occupational performance if the dominant hand is on the side of the surgical intervention. The goal of occupational therapy is for the client to maximize performance of daily occupations, but therapeutic exercise and activities must be advanced carefully in consideration of movement precautions and typical patterns of UE use in occupations. Shoulder use is carefully advanced in the 12 weeks following surgery, but full recovery of function may take up to 9 months.[25,73–76]

Evaluation and Intervention

After the occupational profile, an assessment of motor, cognitive, social, and emotional factors is recommended, specifically as they relate to occupational performance. UE active range of motion (AROM) and muscle strength can be tested in joints of the elbow, wrist, and hand. However, movement, weight bearing, and resistance precautions must be observed in the shoulder in the postoperative phase. Only gentle, controlled passive range of motion (PROM) should be conducted in all shoulder movements. Sensory function and coordination are assessed distally as well, although analgesics inserted through joint or epidural catheters may mask sensory abilities for a few days after surgery. Mental functions such as memory, problem solving, judgment and sequencing must be considered in light of precautions, safety awareness, and performance of occupations. ADLs and other relevant occupations should be evaluated through standardized assessments, direct observation, or interview as the context and client condition allow. Social or emotional concerns may include fear of participation in appropriate therapeutic exercise, hesitation to resume normal activities, or concerns about surgical healing.

OT intervention planning will focus on the primary areas of (1) appropriate health management and therapeutic exercise and (2) resuming normal occupations, primarily routines involving ADLs and IADLs. Therapeutic exercise must be designed to promote controlled movement within precautions to facilitate eventual return of full UE function and to avoid long-term complications of adhesive capsulitis, soft tissue contractures, or bony abnormalities such as heterotopic ossification. Occupations may need to be modified during healing to promote the client's active participation while advancing shoulder use appropriately. Performance in ADLs and IADLs will be used to determine discharge planning and consideration of inpatient rehabilitation or home and outpatient care.

Therapeutic Exercise Considerations
Total Shoulder Replacement

In the immediate postoperative phase, protocols may be adapted so the rehabilitation team should communicate clearly to implement the appropriate and specific surgical precautions for each client. This is based on the musculoskeletal status of the client

and surgical techniques to access the glenohumeral joint.[69] Generally, however, patients are permitted to perform active-assistive range of motion (AAROM) and PROM only of the shoulder in protected ranges. This limited movement can prevent joint stiffening and adhesions while reducing edema and protecting the repair of the subscapularis and muscles released and repaired during the surgical process.[77] PROM is typically limited to 90 to 100 degrees of shoulder flexion, 45 degrees of shoulder abduction, and extension only to neutral. Specific surgical precautions should be followed related to internal and external rotation, but clients are typically permitted to lay the hand across the abdomen in internal rotation and may move to about 30 degrees of external rotation (see Box 41.3). Codman's pendulum exercises may be initiated on the first postoperative day. After removal of the sling, the client is instructed to bend forward by flexing at the hips, allowing up to 90 degrees of passive shoulder flexion, with the arm hanging perpendicular to the floor. The nonoperated UE should rest on a counter or tabletop surface, and a wide base of support with the feet should be maintained to avoid a risk of falls. By shifting the body weight, the arm may passively move in anterior-posterior motions, lateral motions, small clockwise circles, and small counter-clockwise circles (Fig. 41.16).[77,78] Depending on the surgeon's preference, AROM of all distal joints also should be performed several times daily to avoid edema and to promote functional hand use. Over the next 2 to 4 weeks, larger PROM ranges may be initiated at the shoulder. These may include table slides, in which the client sits next to a table with the operated arm supported on the table, and he or she slowly leans forward and allows the shoulder to passively flex. Some physicians allow dowel exercises (the client holds a wooden dowel with both hands) so that the nonoperated arm can be used to assist movement of the operated arm. Isometric exercises can be performed against a wall toward scapular retraction.

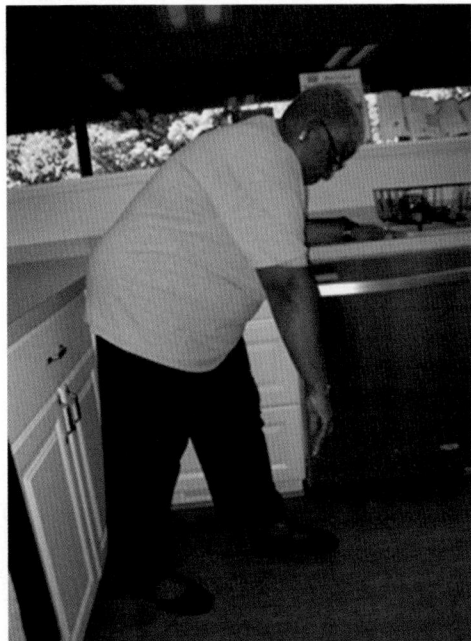 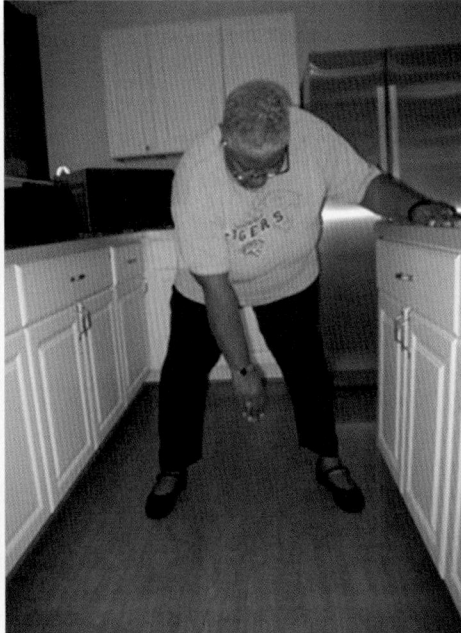

Fig 41.16 Codman's (pendulum) exercises.

Approximately 4 to 6 weeks after the surgery, and if normal movement patterns are observed and healing is progressing as expected, precautions related to movement may be relaxed. Passive shoulder flexion can typically be increased to tolerance, internal rotation to approximately 70 degrees, and external rotation to 60 degrees. Although weight-bearing, closed chain activities and lifting are usually still restricted, active-assisted therapeutic exercise may be initiated. This may include carefully executed overhead pulley exercises, supine dowel exercises, or wall slides.[77] The therapist should assess glenohumeral and scapular-thoracic mobility to ensure normal movement patterns. Light strengthening can be initiated in the elbow, wrist, and hand joints in preparation for greater functional use. Some physicians will allow for a light weight to be added to Codman's pendulum exercises.

In weeks 6 to 12, full movement through all planes is typically initiated and light strengthening begins. This includes shoulder adduction and rotation and flexion in supine, as well as scapular elevation, depression, and retraction in standing with light weights. In addition, light closed-chain activities such as prone-on-elbows and wall push-ups can provide opportunities for controlled strengthening.

By 12 weeks after surgery, full motion may be restored and additional weight training or strengthening exercises may be added. The emphasis of therapy shifts to functional performance of occupations without significant adaptations or compensatory techniques. Impact loading activities, such as bench pressing or use of a sledgehammer, are avoided over the long term to preserve the integrity of the endoprosthesis.[6,13,81,82]

Reverse Total Shoulder Replacement

As for patients with a traditional total shoulder replacement, these patients are permitted to perform AAROM and PROM only of the shoulder in protected ranges in the immediate postoperative period. PROM is typically limited to 90 degrees of shoulder flexion, 45 degrees of shoulder abduction, and extension only to neutral. Because there is limited support of the rotator cuff, there should be no actions that require reaching behind the back, which consists of combined shoulder adduction, extension, and internal rotation. Specific surgical precautions should be followed related to internal and external rotation, but it is typically permitted for the client to lay the hand across the abdomen in internal rotation, to about 30 degrees of external rotation if the shoulder is slightly flexed. Although therapy begins postoperative day 1, Codman's pendulum exercises (see Fig. 41.16) may be performed only with the permission of the surgeon due to rotator cuff instability. PROM may be performed only for the first 5 to 7 days after surgery. Active movement of the distal extremity should be delayed until all anesthesia or nerve blocks that may have been used during surgery for pain control have cleared the patient's system and good motor control returns. Approximately 5 to 7 days after surgery, the patient may begin isometric exercise in the scapula and shoulder and AAROM, up to 90 degrees of flexion and abduction and up to 30 degrees of external rotation. AROM may be initiated approximately 2 weeks after surgery if the glenohumeral joint remains stable and pain is managed.

Table slides, dowel exercises, and pushing items up an incline board may assist in transitioning from AAROM to AROM. From weeks 2 to 6, gains are expected in AROM, isometric control, and shoulder stability. Light strengthening may begin around week 6, although the occupational therapist should carefully monitor progression, and moderate strengthening may begin around week 12.[11]

Specific Training Techniques for Participation in Occupations

Regardless of the type of surgical procedure performed, the occupational therapist must ensure that the client is able to safely and effectively participate in their chosen occupations. Basic ADLs are typically addressed first within the parameters of precautions and allowed movements. Ambulation is generally not affected by the shoulder replacement if balance is functional and there are no other lower extremity problems; however, significant adaptations may be needed for bed mobility, ADLs, and other occupations. The occupational therapist can encourage the patient to use the hand on the side of the operated shoulder as a stabilizer or assist for light activities that do not require weight bearing or strength (e.g., holding toothpaste, buttoning lower buttons, stabilizing paper for writing, or holding a washcloth while soaping it up with the other hand).

Sleeping Positions and Bed Mobility

The sling (and swathe) is worn during sleeping, usually for the first 4 to 6 weeks following the shoulder replacement. A pillow or towel roll should be placed under the scapula or elbow as needed for comfort to ensure that the shoulder is supported in slight flexion with a neutral scapula, and in adherence to the precautions. When entering or exiting the bed or when changing positions in bed, the client may roll over the non-operated shoulder only. The client may need to adjust sleep arrangements to allow for optimal bed mobility that protects the operated shoulder. Core and lower extremity strength and positioning may support movement to and from the bed, but for clients who do not have the necessary core strength, care must be taken that clients do not use the operated arm to push themselves up. Bed ladders or pulls, bed rails, or leg lifters may be needed to assist with bed mobility. Bed mobility routines, including those associated with going to the bathroom at night, should be addressed to anticipate problems that might arise around providing a safe path to the bathroom, managing clothing and hygiene at the toilet, getting back into bed, and adjusting the pillows or towel rolls. (See Chapter 10 for additional ADL and IADL suggestions.)

Functional Mobility

If a cane was required before the surgery, it should be used with the nonoperated arm only. Physical therapy practitioners typically address balance, ambulation, and gait with the client. If a cane is needed, the occupational therapist should ensure its safe use during homemaking tasks or other instrumental ADLs. Use of the operated arm also should be avoided during transfers to prevent weight bearing.

Upper-Body Dressing and Bathing

Clothing should be chosen for ease of dressing and with consideration of sling wear. Button front shirts will be easiest to use for dressing, though stretchy or oversized tops also may be suitable. The client should sit while dressing and bend forward at the waist to promote passive flexion of the shoulder while extending the elbow to put the operated arm in the sleeve first. Once this sleeve is pulled onto the UE and the client returns to sitting upright, he or she can reach around the back to pull the shirt to the other side and to slide the nonoperated arm into the other sleeve. The client can use the hand of the operated shoulder to stabilize and assist in buttoning the shirt. Women should use a bra with the closure in the front so it can be managed like the button-front shirt. The occupational therapist also should ensure that the client is aware of how to put the sling on and off over the clothing. Additional adaptations to clothing or technique may be needed for the client who also has limited shoulder motion on the nonoperated side, as bilateral joint involvement is typical with osteoarthritis.

For bathing, the sling is removed, and a sponge bath can be completed when the client is seated. A rolled towel can be used to support the arm when bathing while seated. A waterproof dressing should be placed over the surgical site if the client will shower during the first week after the surgery. Once sutures or staples are removed, the client can shower normally. Precautions should be maintained during bathing, no matter what method is used. A long-handled sponge may help the client reach the back using the nonoperated arm.

Lower-Body Dressing and Bathing

It is recommended that the client sit to pull on pants and underclothes, to maintain balance and avoid the need to use the operated arm to brace the body during a potential fall. Leaning forward in the seated position will also ensure that precautions are maintained. Again, clothes should be chosen for ease of dressing; for example, slip-on shoes will prevent the necessity of tying shoes.

Homemaking

After shoulder replacements, ambulation is typically unaffected. However, homemaking will need to be done with the shoulder in the sling for the first few weeks. The nonoperated arm can be used primarily for cooking and homemaking, and lifting should be limited in accordance with precautions. A few pieces of adaptive equipment may be helpful, such as a rocker knife or pan stabilizer. The occupational therapist should analyze how the client typically performs household activities to determine if adaptive equipment or compensatory techniques should be used to protect the operated shoulder.

Evidence Regarding Occupational Therapy Intervention

Limited evidence exists that examines specific occupational therapy interventions for people with a shoulder replacement. However, researchers have examined the quality-of-life and return-to-prior-activity levels for this population. Zarkadas

and colleagues[83] collected data from patients on their activity levels after having their shoulder replaced with a total replacement technique or a hemiarthroplasty. Patients reported having continued postrehabilitation difficulty with overhead activities, combing/curling their own hair, washing/drying the back, sleeping on the operated side, and dressing/undressing, as well as other leisure activities.[83]

Boardman and colleagues evaluated the effectiveness of a home-based exercise program for 77 individuals after shoulder

---

THREADED CASE STUDY

Mrs. Green, Part 2

1. What could Mrs. Green have done to better prepare for the surgery knowing that her dominant hand/arm would be immobilized for 6 weeks?

   It is likely that Mrs. Green was seeing either an occupational therapist or a physical therapist before deciding to have her shoulder replaced. The therapist was aware of her prior knee replacements and the assistive devices she already used. Mrs. Green could be directed to practice using the assistive devices she already had with her nondominant arm for completing ADL and IADL tasks. Additionally, the therapist could have provided her with information or suggested she attend a preoperative class to learn tips for postsurgery activity.

2. How could the therapist utilize caregiver training in this case?

   Unlike lower extremity joint replacements, when an individual's arm is immobilized, especially the dominant arm, the ability to perform daily activities can become extremely difficult and a caregiver is needed. It is important to prepare clients for shoulder replacement surgery so that a caregiver can be identified before the surgical procedure to best prepare him or her for assisting the client. Caregivers can be taught the movement and weight-bearing precautions, as well as any home exercises that should be performed daily. Caregivers need to learn ways to assist the client during mobility (e.g., bed mobility, transfers, and ambulation) so that he or she uses proper body mechanics and ensures movement precautions are maintained. If the caregiver cannot be trained before the surgery, it is important to incorporate this training during postoperative rehabilitation.

3. Identify self-care tasks that would pose a particular problem due to her movement and weight-bearing precautions (no passive or active shoulder extension or external rotation; no active movement in any direction; only passive shoulder flexion and abduction to about 80 degrees allowed, non–weight bearing).

   Mrs. Green would have problems with upper body dressing/bathing because she might be tempted to actively move her arm to manage clothing or to wash under her arms. Pulling up her pants/underwear might be difficult if she is unable to pull up both sides evenly without rotating her trunk and potentially extending her operated shoulder. Because Mrs. Green is unable to use her dominant arm for self-care tasks, she would likely use many compensatory movements with her nondominant arm in her efforts to complete tasks that she did in a more coordinated way with her dominant arm. This increases the potential of performing active movement or passively moving the shoulder in directions that are not permitted.

4. Mrs. Green did not have any movement precautions with her right hand, wrist, or forearm. How could you enable Mrs. Green to use her right hand as an assist (while it was still in the sling) during daily activities without breaking her movement precautions at the shoulder?

   Mrs. Green could use her right hand to stabilize objects (e.g., small food packages) while using her left hand to open the package and perform some fine motor tasks (e.g., screwing on the toothpaste top, buttoning lower buttons). She could hold very lightweight objects (e.g., pen, paper, toothbrush) during transport.

replacement.[9] Because most patients return to the home setting within a few days of the surgery, much of the rehabilitation occurs either at home or in an outpatient therapy program. The researchers found that a sequence of exercises, progressing from active hand, forearm, elbow motion, and passive shoulder motion to using a pulley, then a wand or cane exercises, isometric exercises, and ending with Thera-Band exercises, produced good outcomes, with 70% of patients maintaining motion gained during the surgical procedure without causing soft-tissue healing complications.[9]

The primary challenge that continues to face clients after an RTSA remains internal rotation and the ADLs that are associated with this motion, such as washing the back and fastening a bra. Overhead reach and feeding and hygiene activities improve significantly after the procedure. In addition, reaching a high shelf and performing occupations requiring flexion improve

dramatically.[81] However, as both endoprosthetic devices and surgical procedures continue to be refined, and after full rehabilitation and extended recovery time, patients with an RTSA may demonstrate functional skills related to internal rotation, such as toileting, tucking a shirt in at the back, or reaching a back pocket.[4,43,45] In addition, up to 74% of these former patients are able to perform low-demand activities effectively (e.g., cooking and baking), up to 48% performed medium-demand activities (e.g., gardening), and up to 32% performed high-demand activities (e.g., shoveling snow).[4] These studies support intervention priorities that address participation in daily activities, especially self-care tasks, and provide thorough training in home exercises that will help the patient maintain movement precautions and prevent soft-tissue complications while allowing for the maximum functional ability during the healing process.

SUMMARY

Hip fractures and hip, knee, and shoulder replacements are orthopedic conditions in which occupational therapy intervention may speed the client's return to optimal participation in daily activities safely and comfortably. OT evaluation and intervention begin with obtaining the client's occupational profile and an assessment of the emotional and social issues related to the surgery and the surgery's potential impact on the client's lifestyle. Awareness of and a sensitivity to the psychosocial challenges of the person with an orthopedic problem are critical for the delivery of optimal occupational therapy.

The protocol for other areas of OT intervention is determined by the surgical procedure performed and by the precautions prescribed by the physician. Clients who have weight-bearing precautions must be trained to observe these safety measures during all ADL and IADL routines. A simulation of the home environment or a home assessment will prepare the client for potential problems that may arise after discharge. Areas to assess include the entry, stairs, bathroom, bedroom, sitting surfaces, and kitchen. Recommendations to remove throw rugs and slippery floor coverings and obstacles are made because the client will most likely be using an assistive device for ambulation. A kitchen stool or utility cart may be indicated. It is important to assess and instruct the client and caregiver regarding ADLs and IADLs with adaptive equipment, as well as any movement

precautions. Home therapy may be indicated after a hospital stay to ensure safety and independence in daily occupations if these goals were not met during hospitalization.

In addition to the ADL and IADL strategies previously specified, the occupational therapist should address all occupations that may be difficult for the client, as well as those that may pose a safety risk. Occupations such as caring for a pet, navigating through a cafeteria for meals, traveling in vehicles other than cars, and attending religious or other community activities that require specific transfers (e.g., to a church pew) are all examples of activities that may be part of a client's typical performance pattern and should be addressed by occupational therapy. The occupational therapist can assist the client in approaching meaningful occupations safely, observing any movement precautions that are required, and suggesting and demonstrating alternative methods and assistive devices.

Preoperative teaching programs are invaluable in aiding client adjustment. These classes familiarize clients with the hospital, nursing, physical therapy, occupational therapy, and discharge planning. Procedures, equipment, and concerns regarding hospitalization, discharge, and therapy are addressed. Participation in this type of class has been shown to relieve anxiety and fear, empower the client during the hospitalization, and decrease the hospital length of stay.

REVIEW QUESTIONS

1. Explain the difference in precautions for the anterolateral and posterolateral approaches for a hip replacement.
2. When a client is transferring from one surface to another, what is the general procedure to follow to ensure the safety and protection of the involved side?
3. List the most common types of adaptive equipment used during rehabilitation of hip fractures and lower extremity joint replacements and describe their purpose.
4. Describe how the case coordinator and occupational therapist can work together to ensure a safe discharge for the client.
5. List two specific suggestions for performing sexual activities for someone with a hip replacement.
6. What information should be obtained when completing the occupational profile?
7. Identify two factors that affect fracture healing.

8. Identify two ways an occupational therapist can address the psychosocial adjustment to lower extremity joint replacement and hip fracture.
9. Why are weight-bearing precautions observed with an ORIF?
10. Compare the rehabilitation techniques of clients with a hip replacement to those of clients with a knee replacement.
11. What are the benefits of conducting client education pre-operative classes for persons who are at risk for falls or who are planning a joint replacement?
12. How might a person's rehabilitation program be affected by bilateral joint replacements?

13. How do shoulder precautions limit daily activities?
14. During what activities would the occupational therapist suggest that a client wear a sling or swathe after a shoulder replacement?
15. During what activities would the occupational therapist suggest that a client opt not to use a sling after a shoulder replacement?
16. Identify one key exercise that a person should perform multiple times daily after a shoulder replacement. How will you ensure client safety during this exercise?

REFERENCES

1. American Occupational Therapy Association: Occupational therapy practice framework: domain and process, *American Journal of Occupational Therapy* 74(Suppl 2):1–87, 2020. https://doi.org/10.5014/ajot.2020.74s2001.
2. American Occupational Therapy Association: *After your hip surgery: a guide to daily activities*, Rev ed., Rockville, MD, 2001, American Occupational Therapy Association.
3. American Occupational Therapy Association: *After your knee surgery: a guide to daily activities*, Rev ed., Rockville, MD, 2001, American Occupational Therapy Association.
4. Assenmacher AT, Alentorn-Geli E, Aronowitz J, et al: Patient-reported activities after bilateral reverse total shoulder arthroplasties, *Journal of Orthopedic Surgery* 27(1), 2019. https://doi.org/10.1177/2309499018816771.
5. Bello-Haas VD: Neuromusculoskeletal and movement function. In Bonder BR, Bello-Haas VD, editors: *Functional performance in older adults* 3rd ed., Philadelphia, PA, 2009, FA Davis, pp 130–1176.
6. Beth Israel Deaconess Medical Center (BIDMC). Total shoulder arthroplasty rehabilitation protocol, n.d., https://www.bidmc.org/centers-and-departments/orthopaedic-surgery/services-and-programs/sports-med/for-patients/rehab.
7. Bindawas SM, Graham JE, Karmarkar AM, et al: Trajectories in functional recovery for patients receiving inpatient rehabilitation for unilateral hip or knee replacement, *Arch Gerontol Geriatr* 58:344–349, 2014. https://doi.org/10.1016/j.archger.2013.12.009.
8. Blacknall J, Neumann L: Rehabilitation following reverse total shoulder replacement, *Shoulder Elbow* 3:232–240, 2011. https://doi.org/10.1111/j.1758-5740.2011.00138.x.
9. Boardman ND, Cofield RH, Bengston KA, et al: Rehabilitation after total shoulder arthroplasty, *J Arthroplasty* 16:483–486, 2001.
10. Boese CK, Weis M, Phillips T, et al: The efficacy of continuous passive motion after total knee arthroplasty: a comparison of three protocols, *J Arthroplasty* 29:1158–1162, 2014. https://doi.org/10.1016/j.arth.2013.12.005.
11. Boudreau S. Reverse total shoulder arthroplasty protocol. Brigham & Women's Hospital, 2016, https://www.brighamandwomens.org/assets/bwh/patients-and-families/pdfs/shoulder--reverse-total-shoulder-arthroplasty-protocol.pdf.
12. Boukebous B, Boutroux P, Zahi R, Azmy C, Guillon P: Comparison of dual mobility total hip arthroplasty and bipolar arthroplasty for femoral neck fractures: a retrospective case-control study of 199 hips, *Orthopaedics & Traumatology: Surgery & Research* 104(3):369–375, 2018. https://doi.org/10.1016/j.otsr.2018.01.006.

13. Brameier DT, Hirscht A, Kowalsky MS, Sethi PM: Rehabilitation strategies after shoulder arthroplasty in young and active patients, *Clinical Sports Medicine* 37(4):569–583, 2018. https://doi.org/10.1016/j.csm.2018.05.007.
14. Brennan GP, Fritz JM, Houck KM, Hunter SJ: Outpatient rehabilitation care process factors and clinical outcomes among patients discharged home following unilateral total knee arthroplasty, *J Arthroplasty* 30:885–890, 2015. https://doi.org/10.1016/j.arth.2014.12.013.
15. Brox JI: Shoulder pain, *Best Pract Res Clin Rheumatol* 17:33–56, 2003. https://doi.org/10.1016/s1521-6942(02)00101-8.
16. Bruttel H, Spranz DM, Bülhoff M, Aljohani N, Wolf SI, Maier MW: Comparison of glenohumeral and humerothoracical range of motion in healthy controls, osteoarthritic patients and patients after total shoulder arthroplasty performing different activities of daily living, *Gait & Posture* 71:20–25, 2019. https://doi.org/10.1016/j.gaitpost.2019.04.001.
17. Burgers PTPW, Van Geene AR, Van den Bekerom MPJ, et al: Total hip arthroplasty versus hemiarthroplasty for displaced femoral neck fractures in the healthy elderly: a meta-analysis and systematic review of randomized trials, *Int Orthop* 36:1549–1560, 2012. https://doi.org/10.1007/s00264-012-1569-7.
18. Burstein AH, Wright TM: *Fundamentals of orthopaedic biomechanics*, Philadelphia, PA, 1994, Williams & Wilkins.
19. Calliet R: *Knee pain and disability*, 3rd ed., Philadelphia, PA, 1992, FA Davis.
20. Canale ST, Beaty JH: *Campbell's operative orthopedics*, 11th ed., New York, NY, 2007, Mosby.
21. Center for Disease Control and Prevention. Important facts about falls. Centers for Disease Control and Prevention. https://www.cdc.gov/falls/facts.html.
22. Center for Disease Control and Prevention. STEADI—Older adult fall prevention. CDC. https://www.cdc.gov/steadi/index.html.
23. Chapman MW, Campbell WC: *Chapman's orthopaedic surgery*, 3rd ed., Philadelphia, PA, 2001, Lippincott Williams & Wilkins.
24. Coenders MJ, Mathijssen NM, Vehmeijer SBW: Three and a half years experience with outpatient total hip arthroplasty, *Bone Joint J* 102-B(1):82–89, 2020. https://doi.org/10.1302/0301-620x.102b1.bjj-2019-0045.r2.
25. COSM Rehabilitation. Total shoulder arthroplasty/hemiarthroplasty protocol. http://pacosm.com/wp/wp-content/uploads/2015/11/TOTAL-SHOULDER-PROTOCOL-1.pdf. Published 2006.
26. Costa ML, Achten J, Parsons NR, et al: Total hip arthroplasty versus resurfacing arthroplasty in the treatment of patients with

arthritis of the hip joint: single centre, parallel group, assessor blinded, randomised controlled trial, *BMJ* 344:e2147, 2012. https://doi.org/10.1136/bmj.e2147.

27. Crandell T, Crandell C, editors: *Human development* 10th ed., Boston, MA, 2011, McGraw-Hill.

28. DeJong G, Hsieh C-H, Gassaway J, et al: Characterizing rehabilitation services for patients with knee and hip replacement in skilled nursing facilities and inpatient rehabilitation facilities, *Arch Phys Med Rehabil* 90:1269–1283, 2009. https://doi.org/10.1016/j.apmr.2008.11.021.

29. Delisa J, Gans B: *Rehabilitation medicine: principles and practice*, 5th ed., Philadelphia, PA, 2010, JB Lippincott.

30. Dorsey J, Bradshaw M: Effectiveness of occupational therapy interventions for lower-extremity musculoskeletal disorders: a systematic review, *American Journal of Occupational Therapy* 71(1):1–11, 2017. https://doi.org/10.5014/ajot.2017.023028.

31. Ebert JR, Munsie C, Joss B: Guidelines for the early restoration of active knee flexion after total knee arthroplasty: implications for rehabilitation and early intervention, *Arch Phys Med Rehabil* 95:1135–1140, 2014. https://doi.org/10.1016/j.apmr.2014.02.015.

32. Elinge E, et al: A group learning programme for old people with hip fracture: a randomized study, *Scand J Occup Ther* 10:27–33, 2003. https://doi.org/10.1080/11038120310004475.

33. Elmallah RK, Cherian JJ, Pierce TP, et al: New and common perioperative pain management techniques in total knee arthroplasty, *J Knee Surg* 29:169–178, 2016. https://doi.org/10.1055/s-0035-1549027.

34. Farng E, Zingmond D, Krenek L, SooHoo NF: Factors predicting complication rates after primary shoulder arthroplasty, *J Shoulder Elbow Surg* 20:557–563, 2011. https://doi.org/10.1016/j.jse.2010.11.005.

35. Galakatos GR: Direct anterior total hip arthroplasty, *Mo Med* 115(6):537–541, 2018.

36. Gonzalez JF, Alami GB, Baque F, et al: Complications of unconstrained shoulder prostheses, *J Shoulder Elbow Surg* 20:666–682, 2011. https://doi.org/10.1016/j.jse.2010.11.017.

37. Hanusch B, Luo TN, Warriner G, et al: Functional outcome of PFC Sigma fixed and rotating-platform total knee arthroplasty: a prospective randomised controlled trial, *Int Orthop* 34:349–354, 2010. https://doi.org/10.1007/s00264-009-0901-3.

38. Hooper CR, Bello-Haas VD: Sensory function. In Bonder BR, Bello-Haas VD, editors: *Functional performance in older adults* 3rd ed., Philadelphia, PA, 2009, FA Davis, pp 101–129.

39. Kane RL, Saleh KJ, Wilt TJ, et al: *Total knee replacement. Evidence Report/Technology Assessment No. 86, AHRQ Publication No. 04-E006-1*, Rockville, MD, 2003, Agency for Healthcare Research and Quality;.

40. Karson T, Qun-Jid L, Yiu-Chung W: Unicompartmental knee replacement: an underrated alternative of total knee replacement: a matched comparative study analysing their benefits and risks in local population, *Journal of Orthopaedics, Trauma and Rehabilitation* 25(1):58–61, 2018. https://doi.org/10.1016/j.jotr.2017.07.001.

41. Kennedy JS, Garrigues GE, Pozzi F, et al: The American Society of Shoulder and Elbow Therapists' consensus statement on rehabilitation for anatomic total shoulder arthroplasty, *Journal of Shoulder and Elbow Surgery* 29(10):2149–2162, 2020. https://doi.org/10.1016/j.jse.2020.05.019.

42. Killian ML, Cavinatto L, Galatz LM, Thomopoulos S: Recent advances in shoulder research, *Arthritis Res Ther* 14:214–224, 2012. https://doi.org/10.1186/ar3846.

43. Kim MS, Jeong HY, Kim JD, Ro KH, Rhee S-M, Rhee YG: Difficulty in performing activities of daily living associated with internal rotation after reverse total shoulder arthroplasty, *Journal of Shoulder and Elbow Surgery* 29(1):86–94, 2020. https://doi.org/10.1016/j.jse.2019.05.031.

44. Larson KO: *ROTE: the role of occupational therapy with the elderly*, Bethesda, MD, 1996, American Occupational Therapy Association.

45. Levy O, Walecka J, Arealis G, et al: Bilateral reverse total shoulder arthroplasty—functional outcome and activities of daily living, *Journal of Shoulder and Elbow Surgery* 26(4):E85–E96, 2017. https://doi.org/10.1016/j.jse.2016.09.010.

46. Luo S, Zhao J, Su W: Advancement in total knee prosthesis selection, *Zhongguo Xiu Fu Chong Jian Wai Ke Za Zhi* 24:301–303, 2010.

47. Martín-Martín LM, Valenza-Demet G, Jiménez-Moleón JJ, Cabrera-Martos I, Revelles-Moyano FJ, Valenza MC: Effect of occupational therapy on functional and emotional outcomes after hip fracture treatment: a randomized controlled trial, *Clinical Rehabilitation* 28(6):541–551, 2013. https://doi.org/10.1177/0269215513511472.

48. Mayo Clinic. Hip dysplasia. Mayo Clinic. https://www.mayoclinic.org/diseases-conditions/hip-dysplasia/symptoms-causes/syc-20350209. Updated March 20, 2020.

49. McAuley JP, Szuszczewicz ES, Young A, Engh CA Sr: Total hip arthroplasty in patients 50 years and younger, *Clin Orthop Relat Res* 418:119–125, 2004. https://doi.org/10.1097/00003086-200401000-00019.

50. Melvin J, Gall V: *Rheumatic rehabilitation series: Surgical rehabilitation*, Vol 5, Bethesda, MD, 1999, American Occupational Therapy Association.

51. Melvin J, Jensen G: *Rheumatic Rehabilitation Series: Assessment and management*, Vol 1, Bethesda, MD, 1998, American Occupational Therapy Association.

52. Mikkelsen LR, Peterson MK, Søballe K, Mechlenburg I: Does reduced movement restrictions and use of assistive devices affect rehabilitation outcome after total hip replacement? A non-randomized, controlled study, *Eur J Phys Rehabil Med* 50:383–393, 2014.

53. Nguyen US, Zhang Y, Zhu Y, et al: Increasing prevalence of knee pain and symptomatic knee osteoarthritis: survey and cohort data, *Ann Intern Med* 155:725–732, 2011.

54. Nieves JW, Bilezikian JP, Lane JM, et al: Fragility fractures of the hip and femur: incidence and patient characteristics, *Osteoporos Int* 21:399–408, 2010. https://doi.org/10.1007/s00198-009-0962-6.

55. Noble J, Goodall JR, Noble DJ: Simultaneous bilateral knee replacement: a persistent controversy, *Knee*. 16:420–426, 2009. https://doi.org/10.1016/j.knee.2009.04.009.

56. Nouri F, Coole C, Baker P, Drummond A: Return to work advice after total hip and knee replacement, *Occupational Medicine* 70(2):113–118, 2020. https://doi.org/10.1093/occmed/kqaa014.

57. Opitz J: Reconstructive surgery of the extremities. In Kottle F, Lehmann J, editors: *Krusen's handbook of physical medicine and rehabilitation* 4th ed., Philadelphia, PA, 1990, WB Saunders.

58. OrthoInfo: Total Hip Replacement. OrthoInfo. https://orthoinfo.aaos.org/en/treatment/total-hip-replacement/.

59. OrthoInfo: Total knee replacement. https://orthoinfo.aaos.org/en/treatment/total-knee-replacement.

60. Paillard P: Hip replacement by a minimal anterior approach, *Int Orthop* 31(Suppl 1):S13–S15, 2007. https://doi.org/10.1007/s00264-007-0433-7.

61. Palsis JA, Simpson KN, Matthews JH, Traven S, Eichinger JK, Friedman RJ: Current trends in the use of shoulder arthroplasty in the United States, *Orthopedics* 41(3):e416–423, 2018. https://doi.org/10.3928/01477447-20180409-05.

62. Pandya J, Johnson T, Low AK: Shoulder replacement for osteoarthritis: a review of surgical management, *Maturitas* 108:71–76, 2018. https://doi.org/10.1016/j.maturitas.2017.11.013.

63. Peace WJ: Joint replacement infection. OrthoInfo. http://orthoinfo.aaos.org/topic.cfm?topic=A00629. Updated January 2018.

64. Perry M, Hudson HS, Meys S, et al: Older adults' experiences regarding discharge from hospital following orthopaedic intervention: a metasynthesis, *Disabil Rehabil* 34(4):267–278, 2012. https://doi.org/10.3109/09638288.2011.603016.

65. Petridis G, Nolde M: Sequential bilateral total hip arthroplasty through a minimally invasive anterior approach is safe to perform, *The Open Orthopaedics Journal* 11(1):1417–1422, 2017. https://doi.org/10.2174/1874325001711011417.

66. Picard F, Deakin A, Balasubramanian N, Gregori A: Minimally invasive total knee replacement: techniques and results, *European Journal of Orthopaedic Surgery & Traumatology* 28(5):781–791, 2018. https://doi.org/10.1007/s00590-018-2164-4.

67. Radnay C, Setter KJ, Chambers L, et al: Total shoulder replacement compared with humeral head replacement for the treatment of primary glenohumeral osteoarthritis: a systematic review, *J Shoulder Elbow Surg* 16:396–402, 2007. https://doi.org/10.1016/j.jse.2006.10.017.

68. Richardson JK, Iglarsh ZA: *Clinical orthopaedic physical therapy*, Philadelphia, PA, 1994, WB Saunders.

69. Saccomanni B: Unicompartmental knee arthroplasty: a review of literature, *Clin Rheumatol* 29:339–346, 2010 (Retracted article.) See similar article: Kyung TK: Unicompartmental knee arthroplasty. Published online March 1, 2016. https://doi.10.5792/ksrr.18.014.

70. Sattler L, Hing W, Vertullo C: Changes to rehabilitation after total knee replacement, *Australian Journal of General Practice* 49(9):587–591, 2020. https://doi.org/10.31128/ajgp-03-20-5297.

71. Seitz WH, Michaud EJ: Rehabilitation after shoulder replacement: be all you can be, *Semin Arthroplasty* 23:106–113, 2012. https://doi.org/10.1053/j.sart.2012.03.009.

72. Sershon RA, Van Thiel GS, Lin EC, et al: Clinical outcomes of reverse total shoulder arthroplasty in patients aged younger than 60 years, *J Shoulder Elbow Surg* 23:395–400, 2014. https://doi.org/10.1016/j.jse.2013.07.047.

73. Shemshaki H, Dehghani M, Eshaghi MA, Esfahani MF: Fixed versus mobile weight-bearing prosthesis in total knee arthroplasty, *Knee Surg Sports Traumatol Arthrosc* 20:2519–2527, 2012. https://doi.org/10.1007/s00167-012-1946-1.

74. Sherry E, Egan M, Warnke PH, et al: Minimal invasive surgery for hip replacement: a new technique using the NILNAV hip system, *ANZ J Surg* 73:157, 2003. https://doi.org/10.1046/j.1445-2197.2002.02597.x.

75. Singh J, Sloan J, Johanson N: Challenges with health-related quality of life assessment in arthroplasty patients: problems and solutions, *J Am Acad Orthop Surg* 18:72–82, 2010.

76. Sirkka M, Brănholm I: Consequences of a hip fracture in activity performance and life satisfaction in an elderly Swedish clientele, *Scand J Occup Ther* 10:34, 2003. https://doi.org/10.1080/11038120310004501.

77. Strauss EJ, Roche C, Flurin P-H, et al: The glenoid in shoulder arthroplasty, *J Shoulder Elbow Surg* 18:819–833, 2009. https://doi.org/10.1016/j.jse.2009.05.008.

78. Thienpont E: Faster recovery after minimally invasive surgery in total knee arthroplasty, *Knee Surg Sports Traumatol Arthrosc* 21:2412–2417, 2013. https://doi.org/10.1007/s00167-012-1978-6.

79. Tideiksaar R: Falls. In Bonder BR, Bello-Haas VD, editors: *Functional performance in older adults* 3rd ed., Philadelphia, PA, 2009, FA Davis, pp 193–214.

80. Tsai C, Chen C, Liu T: Lateral approach without ligament release in total knee arthroplasty: new concepts in the surgical technique, *Artif Organs* 25:638, 2001. https://doi.org/10.1046/j.1525-1594.2001.025008638.x.

81. Wainwright TW, Gill M, Mcdonald DA, et al: Consensus statement for perioperative care in total hip replacement and total knee replacement surgery: Enhanced Recovery After Surgery (ERAS®) Society recommendations, *Acta Orthopaedica* 91(1):3–19, 2020. https://doi.org/10.1080/17453674.2019.1683790.

82. Wilcox R., Arslanian LE, Millett PJ: Total shoulder arthroplasty/hemiarthroplasty protocol. Brigham & Women's Hospital. https://www.brighamandwomens.org/assets/BWH/patients-and-families/rehabilitation-services/pdfs/shoulder-total-shoulder-arthroplasty-protocol.pdf. Published 2007.

83. Zarkadas PC, Throckmorton TQ, Dahm DL, et al: Patient reported activities after shoulder replacement: total and hemiarthroplasty, *J Shoulder Elbow Surg* 20:273–280, 2011. https://doi.org/10.1016/j.jse.2010.06.007.

42

Low Back Pain[a]

Ashley Uyeshiro Simon

LEARNING OBJECTIVES

After studying this chapter, the student or practitioner will be able to do the following:

1. Identify how low back pain can affect occupational engagement and daily life, physically, psychosocially, and emotionally.
2. Identify the most common causes of low back pain.
3. Define neutral spine.
4. Identify the basic concepts of body mechanics and how this relates to anatomy.
5. Apply general pain intervention strategies to common daily occupations.
6. Identify the occupational therapist's role in evaluation and intervention.
7. Recognize the psychosocial effect of low back pain. Identify adaptive equipment that may improve function.
8. Identify other multidisciplinary pain team members.

CHAPTER OUTLINE

---

[a] The author would like to acknowledge the significant and outstanding contributions of Luella Grangaard to previous editions of this chapter.

KEY TERMS

Activity pacing
Body mechanics
Energy conservation
Ergonomics

Lifestyle modifications
Neutral spine
Self-regulation

THREADED CASE STUDY

Maria, Part 1 (Evaluation)

Maria, a 47-year-old homemaker (prefers use of the pronouns she/her/hers), lives with her husband and adult son in their one-story home. She worked in a retail store before her low back injury, which was caused by a motor vehicle accident (MVA) 3 years ago. Maria has bilateral myofascial (muscular) low back pain and also has herniated disks at L4 and L5. She primarily complains of intense muscle soreness and often compares this to how muscles feel after rigorous exercise. Maria also reports sometimes feeling a sharp shooting pain down the buttock and back of the thigh when she bends over, which only lasts for short periods. She is currently also receiving physical therapy (PT).

Maria has been referred to occupational therapy because she is having difficulty completing activities of daily living (ADLs) (dressing, getting in and out of bed, and meal preparation), difficulty doing home management tasks (laundry, dishes), and was diagnosed with depression. Maria's goals are to decrease her pain, to improve her ability to complete home tasks independently, and to be able to go to a movie with friends.

During the evaluation, the Canadian Occupational Performance Measure (COPM) is used to assess functional limitations and occupational engagement difficulties.[9] Maria reports any activities involving bending or twisting are difficult and painful, including doing laundry, picking items up off the floor, making the bed, and completing her morning hygiene routine. She also reports she is not going out of the house (except for doctor's appointments), has significantly decreased her social activities, and has low energy levels. Maria's baseline level of pain is 5/10 on the Numeric Rating Scale. During self-care and home

management activities, her pain increases to 8/10, and after staying in one position for too long, her pain increases to 7/10, which makes it difficult for her to sleep well. Because of difficulty with meal prep and because her husband and son are at work during the day, Maria also has been eating only one morning snack and one large meal per day.

Maria experiences a lot of guilt about not being a good mother and wife, and she often pushes herself to do tasks despite significant pain increases. She demonstrates little awareness of how her mood affects her pain levels, and vice versa.

Maria's occupational therapy intervention plan will involve education about body mechanics, positioning techniques, and depression management strategies. Problem-solving with Maria and her family about how she can incorporate this education into her daily life to decrease pain and increase engagement in occupations will be a large part of treatment. She will also receive training in relaxation techniques and use of adaptive equipment if necessary.

Critical Thinking Questions

1. What other occupations (not listed in the case study) do you think would be affected by Maria's low back pain?
2. How do you think Maria's depression contributes or relates to her low back pain?
3. What barriers and supports to occupational engagement exist for Maria?
4. What is anatomically happening to the spinal column as Maria bends or twists that is causing pain?

Low back pain (LBP) can have an impact on almost every area of functioning, from self-care activities, to childcare and relationships, to emotional functioning. Low back pain is the number one cause of years lived with disability in the United States and in the world, with a prevalence of 577 million people living with low back pain globally.[14,20]

In the United States, nearly 34% of adults experienced back pain in the past 3 months, making it the most common type of pain experienced among adults (29.1%).[21] Prevalence of LBP was higher for women, generally increased in prevalence by age, and was higher for those with lower socioeconomic standing, less education, or who had Medicaid insurance.[10] For some, this pain will resolve on its own; for others, it can be minimized or eliminated with exercise, core strengthening, and rehabilitation. But for many, back pain is chronic (lasting more than 3 months), and some people will have to function with back pain for the rest of their lives. Chronic pain in particular has become its own emerging health concern, and is listed as one of 20 health condition topics of the *Healthy People 2030* plan.[34,35] This undoubtedly means that an occupational therapist will likely encounter clients with LBP in any adult setting (and some

OT PRACTICE NOTES

It is important that the occupational therapist consider the following personal questions before providing intervention to clients with the LPB diagnosis. Have you ever thrown out your back, had a low back injury, sat in an uncomfortable chair for too long, or just lifted something in the wrong way that caused LBP or muscle strain? Even if you have never personally experienced LBP, perhaps you know someone who has, or you can imagine what it is like. Think of the daily occupations this pain may affect. If prolonged sitting is painful, driving, working at a desk job, studying, or even eating a meal can be difficult. If standing still or leaning forward is painful, cooking a meal, washing your face, showering, or applying makeup can be affected. For many people with low back pain, even lying down can be painful, which can limit restorative sleep routines.

Mentally walk through your day from beginning to end, and think about all of the activities *you* do that involve movement, strength, and flexibility from the low back. Think of how having LBP may influence these activities. What if you want to pick up your child? How will you exercise so you do not gain weight? Would you be able to concentrate to study? How will you do the laundry if you live alone? Would you be as social if you were in pain? Even something as simple as picking up a dropped pen can be difficult, depending on the severity of low back pain. Thinking about the breadth of the impact of LBP will help you to better understand how to help your patients.

pediatric settings), even if the LBP is not the primary reason the client is seeking services. Knowledge of how LBP affects functioning in all aspects of life, as well as how to treat it, will be beneficial for both practitioner and clients.

CLASSIFICATION

LBP can be classified or described in many ways, the most basic of which are by how long it lasts, impact on daily functioning, intensity, and by quality. According to the National Institute of Arthritis and Musculoskeletal and Skin Diseases, acute back pain happens suddenly and typically lasts up to a few weeks. Subacute back pain may have either a sudden onset or an onset over time and lasts 4 to 12 weeks. In addition, the onset of chronic back pain can be sudden or slow but lasts longer than 12 weeks.[26]

Pain also can be described in terms of impact on daily functioning. In 2016, the National Health Interview Survey found about 20.4% of adults in the United States experienced chronic pain (not specific to LBP), which they defined as "pain on most days or every day in the past 6 months." The survey also found that about 8.0% of adults experienced "high-impact" chronic pain, which was defined as "chronic pain that limited life or work activities on most days or every day during the past 6 months" in accordance with the National Pain Strategy.[11]

Intensity and quality of pain are not unique to LBP, but are used to describe how much pain the person is experiencing (often a Numeric Rating Scale from 0–10),[15] and a description of what the pain feels like, respectively. Quality descriptors such as burning, stabbing, shooting, or aching can be offered to the client if they are having difficulty describing the pain independently.

COMMON CAUSES OF LOW BACK PAIN

Understanding the anatomy of the back is essential to help a client with LBP. The occupational therapist must understand both normal anatomy and the pathologic processes underlying numerous back problems and must be able to convey this information in relatable terms to patients of varying backgrounds and levels of understanding. To educate the patient regarding the rationale for proper body mechanics, the occupational therapist must also understand how the anatomy and pathology are related to movement and daily occupations. Patients who understand the causes of their pain are often capable of applying strategies to varying contexts, and are often more intrinsically motivated to make changes to manage their pain.

VERTEBRAL COLUMN AND MUSCULATURE REVIEW

The vertebral column is composed of the vertebrae and intervertebral disks. Each vertebra contains the vertebral body, which is the weight-bearing component, and the vertebral arch, which arises from the back of the vertebral body (Fig. 42.1). The vertebral arch is composed of two pedicles (one on each side) that extend into the lamina. The laminae join to form the vertebral foramina, which make up the vertebral canal in which the spinal cord resides. From the pedicle and joining of laminae are three bony projections called processes. These lateral processes join to form joints with adjacent vertebrae superiorly and inferiorly (Fig. 42.2). Between the joint of these adjacent vertebrae is the intervertebral foramen, from which the spinal nerves enter and exit. At the back of the spinal arch is the spinous process, where muscles attach. The low back region is composed of five lumbar vertebrae.

Between the vertebrae are intervertebral disks, which are composed of fibrocartilage, a harder outer shell, and the nucleus pulposus, a softer gelatinous tissue (Fig. 42.3). The disks work as shock absorbers and are relieved of pressure only when the body is supine. As the nonrigid parts of the vertebral column, they provide spinal flexibility for movement. When a person is standing with a neutral spine—the most comfortable spinal posture and pelvic tilt, yielding equal pressure on all the vertebrae and

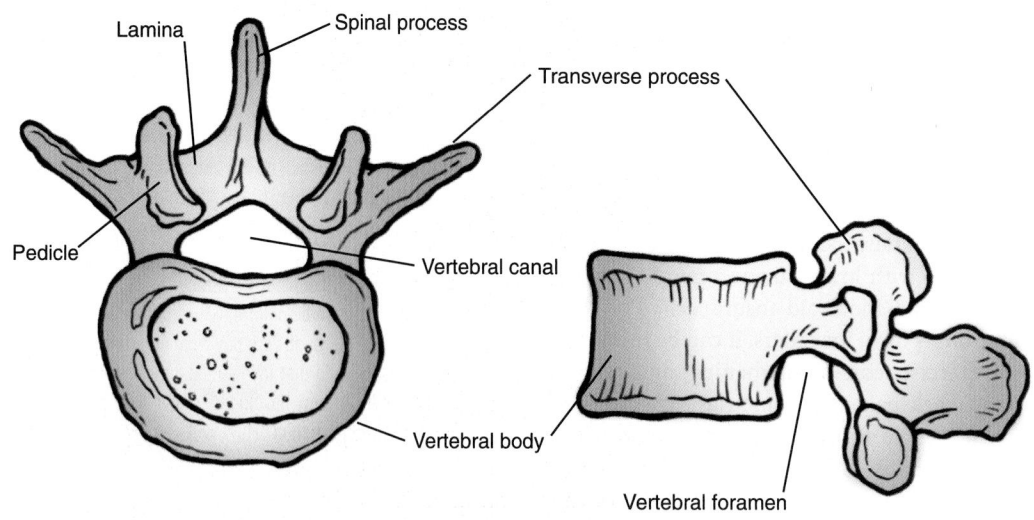

Fig. 42.1 Vertebra from above and side view.

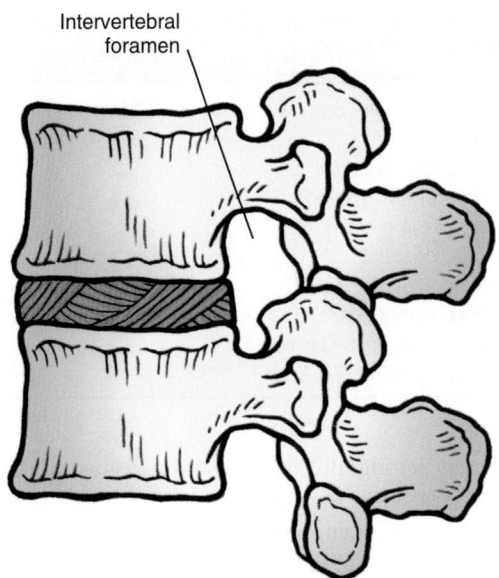

Fig. 42.2 Two vertebrae in articulation. The spinal nerve exits via the intervertebral foramen.

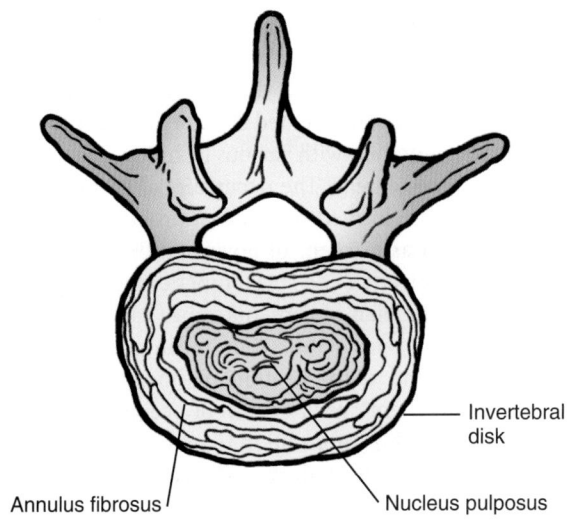

Fig. 42.3 Cut surface of the disk.

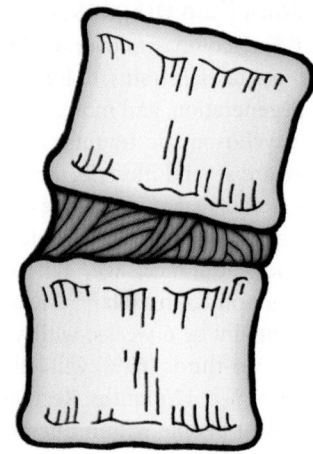

Fig. 42.4 The same disk may be under compression and extension at the same time.

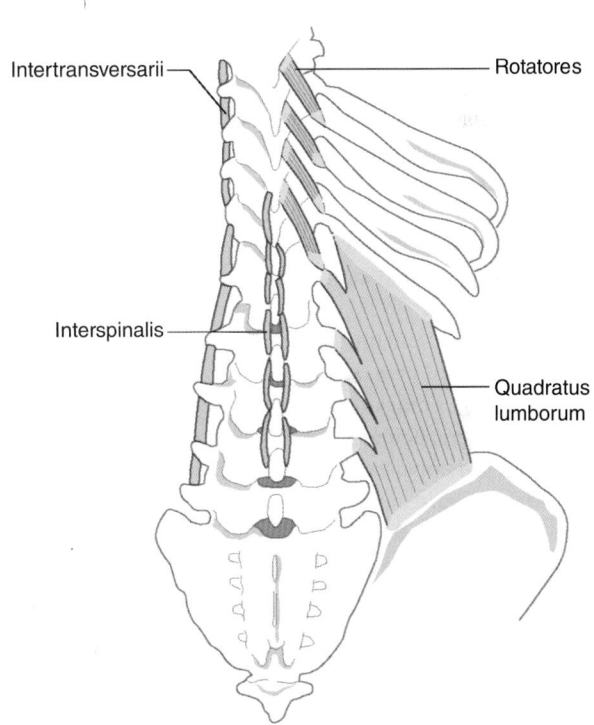

Fig. 42.5 Intertransversarii and interspinales muscles. (From Palastanga N, Soames RW: *Anatomy and human movement: structure and function*, ed 6, Edinburgh, 2012, Churchill Livingstone.)

disks—the pressure on all sides of the disk is equal. Movements such as bending, leaning, and reaching result in disk pressure and bulging on the side that the person is bending toward and stretching of the disk on the opposite side (Fig. 42.4).

Anterior and posterior longitudinal ligaments extend the length of the vertebral column and are attached to the vertebral bodies and intervertebral disks. These ligaments prevent excessive movement of the column. The sacrum is the lower fused portion of the vertebral column and is attached to the pelvis. Movement of the pelvis changes the lordosis, or amount of curve of the lumbar spine: anterior tilt of the pelvis results in more lordosis (arching of the low back), and posterior tilt of the pelvis results in less lordosis (flattening of the low back).

Muscles of the lumbar spine include the intertransversarii and interspinales, which are small intersegmental muscles that connect the transverse process to the spinous process of adjacent vertebrae (Fig. 42.5). The lumbar multifidus, lumbar longissimus, and iliocostalis make up the lumbar muscles. These muscles are primarily extensors for the spine, but the lumbar longissimus and iliocostalis can also assist in lateral flexion. In addition, muscles of the abdominal wall, including the transversus abdominis and obliquus internus abdominis, help to stabilize the spine by providing a corseting effect. For further information on interaction of the back and abdominal muscles during specific movements, the reader is advised to do additional reading in this area.

Common Low Back Pain Diagnoses

Low back pain (LBP) encompasses over 60 differential diagnoses that span from myofascial strains, to inflammatory diseases, to localized joint degeneration, and more.[8] Sometimes LBP can even result from psychosomatic trauma. Anyone can experience LBP, but there are several lifestyle, job-related, psychosocial, and biological factors that may increase a person's risk, such as poor physical fitness, obesity, comorbid depression, reduced muscle strength and endurance, age, genetics, and physical demands or poor ergonomics in a job.[23,26] Most people with LBP will improve substantially by 6 weeks, with very little pain 12 months later. About two-thirds (67%) will still have some pain at three months, and 65% at 12 months. Recurrence of LBP may occur for about 33% of people within one year of recovering from a previous episode.[23]

In 90% of LBP cases seen in primary care, LBP is nonspecific or without a known pathoanatomic cause.[21] Common diagnosable causes of LBP are often due to changes in the structure or mechanics of the lower part of the back, or LBP may be secondary to other diagnoses such as tumors or visceral disease. Some common identifiable causes of LBP include:

- *Degenerative disc disease:* water content of discs decreases with age, the outer annulus fibrosus weakens, and the disc's ability to cushion the vertebrae is impaired causing additional load on the facet joints.[17]
- *Spinal stenosis:* narrowing of the intervertebral foramen decreases the spinal canal where the spinal nerve exits or enters the spine.[3]
- *Facet joint pain:* inflammation or changes in the spinal joints cause facet joint pain.
- *Spondylolysis:* a crack or stress fracture that develops through the pars interarticularis, a thin portion of the vertebra that connects the upper and lower facet joints.[5]
- *Spondylolisthesis:* anterior slipping of one vertebra on the vertebra directly below, often because of untreated spondylolysis.[5]
- *Herniated nucleus pulposus (also known as a herniated disk):* stress may tear fibers of the disk and result in an outward bulge of the enclosed nucleus pulposus. This bulge may press on spinal nerves and cause various symptoms, including nerve entrapment.[2]
- *Sciatic (nerve root) pain:* the nerve is entrapped by a herniated disk.[4]
- Compression/stress fractures: these fractures are usually a result of osteoporosis and occur in the vertebrae.[17]

As noted later in the chapter, behavioral health has a significant impact on pain, and a mental health diagnosis such as anxiety or depression can often worsen, or in some cases cause, LBP as well.

OCCUPATIONAL THERAPY EVALUATION

The occupational therapist's primary goals during the evaluation are to determine which occupations are affected by LBP and how the person's actions influence pain. This can be done by using self-report questionnaires, assessment tools, patient-caregiver interviews, or patient demonstration, depending on

---

BOX 42.1   Common Low Back Pain Assessment Tools

- Canadian Occupational Performance Measure (COPM)[9]
- Brief Pain Inventory[31]
- Pain Self-Efficacy Questionnaire[27]
- Activity of daily living checklists
- Beck Depression Inventory-II[36]
- Numeric rating scale[15]
- Wong-Baker Faces[38]
- Oswestry Disability Index[12,33]
- Roland-Morris Disability Questionnaire[3,33]
- Quebec Back Pain Disability Scale[18]

---

the treatment setting. Box 42.1 lists some common LBP assessment tools. Educating the patient about the role of occupational therapy and how occupational therapists can help improve function and quality of life is vital in the evaluation process, so the patient can correctly identify areas of functional difficulty. Clients should understand the use of occupations as both ends and means of engagement[22] and how these relate to their treatment goals.

The patient's current understanding and knowledge of LBP and pain-relieving strategies can be assessed by asking if patients know any activities that decrease or increase their pain or by listening for action-oriented statements that describe the patient's experimentation with various techniques to find strategies for pain management. The occupational therapist's evaluation should not be limited to physical problematic areas but should include an assessment of how the LBP affects the person's emotional, spiritual, and social functioning.

When creating a plan of care, outcomes can include reduction of pain, use of back stabilization techniques, use of adaptive equipment, and incorporation of body mechanics and ergonomics into client-specific areas of occupation, as well as the ability to adapt this information to new occupations to prevent future problems. Depending on the payer, goals also can be written about stress and mood management, lifestyle and habit changes such as losing weight or managing blood glucose levels, work/school abilities, and socialization.

Postoperative Occupational Therapy Evaluation

Surgical treatment of back problems has undergone many advances. Interventions include laminectomy, spinal fusion, nerve decompression, discectomy, vertebroplasty, and kyphoplasty. Surgical interventions are divided into two basic types: surgery that decompresses the nerve and surgery that stabilizes the spine to reduce pain. Surgeries that decompress the nerve open the transverse foramen and increase the space for exit of the spinal nerve and entrance to the spinal cord. Some surgeries may remove a structure, such as part of a disk or an osteophyte that is putting pressure on the nerve root. Stabilization can include the use of various pieces of hardware, such as screws, wires, rods, and bone grafts, to stabilize the bony structures of the spine. In addition, both vertebroplasty and kyphoplasty use a cement-like substance to stabilize compression/stress fractures. Kyphoplasty involves the use of a balloon that is placed in the fracture and, when inflated, helps restore height and reduce deformity before the cement is injected.[26]

Client precautions must be identified. Therapists should work with the physician to develop protocols or standards of care for specific surgeries. It is also important to identify the types of braces and other equipment that may be used for a specific surgery by a specific physician so that the occupational therapist can provide the expected instructions and precautions for use of the equipment in daily occupations. For example, one physician may allow a client to put a brace on while sitting at the bedside, whereas another physician may require the client to logroll into the brace and completely don it before coming to a seated position. Frequently, braces are ordered and fitted before surgery so that they are available to patients on admission.

When seeing a client for the first time postoperatively, the occupational therapist should obtain the client's history and occupational profile, as well as a description of his or her home environment to ascertain the types of modifications required for safety. During the occupational profile, activities of daily living (ADLs) and instrumental activity of daily living (IADLs) issues should be identified. As part of the home assessment, education in work simplification techniques, in conjunction with directive questions, helps the client identify further needs. For example, when explaining how storing frequently used items within easy reach and infrequently used items in lower or higher places can save energy, the therapist can then ask the client how meal prep and eating items are stored in the home. This return demonstration helps clients to process the training and to independently identify other areas of the home where this concept may apply. Home modifications may include picking up rugs to prevent falls, increasing awareness of pets, and selecting a type of chair that is easy to get in and out of and that provides good support and fits the client well. The therapist should also determine whether the home contains a standard toilet and shower and whether modifications for safety and comfort are required.

Postoperative guidelines, about which occupational therapists should educate and train the patient and their families, are generally as follows, with confirmation needed from the physician[17]:

- Avoid bending and twisting of the spine; try to maintain a neutral spine as much as possible.
- Avoid picking up or carrying anything over 10 lb.
- Avoid sitting or standing in the same position for longer than 30 minutes, with the exception of sleep.
- Do not drive until cleared by the physician.
- Adhere to the physician-prescribed wearing schedule for any orthotic braces. Typical prescription for a rigid thoracolumbosacral orthosis (TLSO) is to wear at all times when the client is out of bed, but consult with the physician to determine if it can be removed for sponge bathing or showering. Flexible orthoses may have less stringent wearing schedules.

OCCUPATIONAL THERAPY INTERVENTIONS

Based on the occupational therapy evaluation, the therapist may implement any of the following intervention areas, depending on the needs and personal goals of the client. Factors to consider when implementing interventions include the client's willingness to change old behaviors, educational level, financial abilities, social support, cognition, and self-awareness.

Client Education

Education is the key to success for a client with LBP. Knowledge of basic anatomy and physiology helps the client understand what is occurring in the body while engaging in an occupation. Understanding how lifestyle factors and stress levels can affect pain helps motivate the client to make behavior changes. Having nonpharmacological tools for pain management and knowing when to use them, which ones to use, and when to combine medication with nonpharmacological strategies can help clients increase their own self-efficacy and decision-making. This knowledge is the foundation on which to build the rest of the intervention plan and ultimately select the appropriate interventions.

Information individualized to each client's needs is ideal. Many books, videos, card systems, and computerized educational systems are available. In addition, charts and models of anatomy can help the client to understand anatomy and physiology. Education can be provided in both group and individual settings.

Body Mechanics

To incorporate body mechanics, the person must first find his or her own "neutral" spinal position by standing with the knees slightly bent and the weight distributed evenly. Using the abdominal muscles to tilt the pelvis, the client should flex and extend the lumbar spine until he or she attains the balanced position of optimal function and stability (Fig. 42.6). The abdominal muscles should be contracted to maintain this position, much as a corset would. This position or stabilization should be maintained and integrated into performance of the client's occupations. Some individuals experience no pain while in a greater degree of extension or with a greater curve in the lower back region, whereas others prefer a neutral position of flexion and have more of a flattened abdomen.

In addition to developing a neutral spine, the client will need to learn and integrate different techniques into activities to help in lifting and movement. These positions include the squat, diagonal lift, and golfer's lift. Performing a squat requires the absence of any knee or hip pathological conditions; the client keeps the back straight while maintaining a neutral spine (Fig. 42.7, A). A diagonal lift requires the lift to be performed with one foot in front of the other and the legs shoulder length apart (see Fig. 42.7, B). A golfer's lift requires bending at the hips while raising one leg behind (see Fig. 42.7, C).

It is important that clients thoroughly understand how to use body mechanics to stabilize their back. This includes maintaining a straight back, bending from the hip, avoiding twisting, maintaining good posture, carrying objects close to the body, lifting with the legs to promote safe performance, and using a wide base of support. To reduce back stress for activities done while standing, the client can use a small stool or open a cabinet door and rest the foot inside the cabinet base. Instruction in avoiding any twisting of the back during activities is also essential, as will

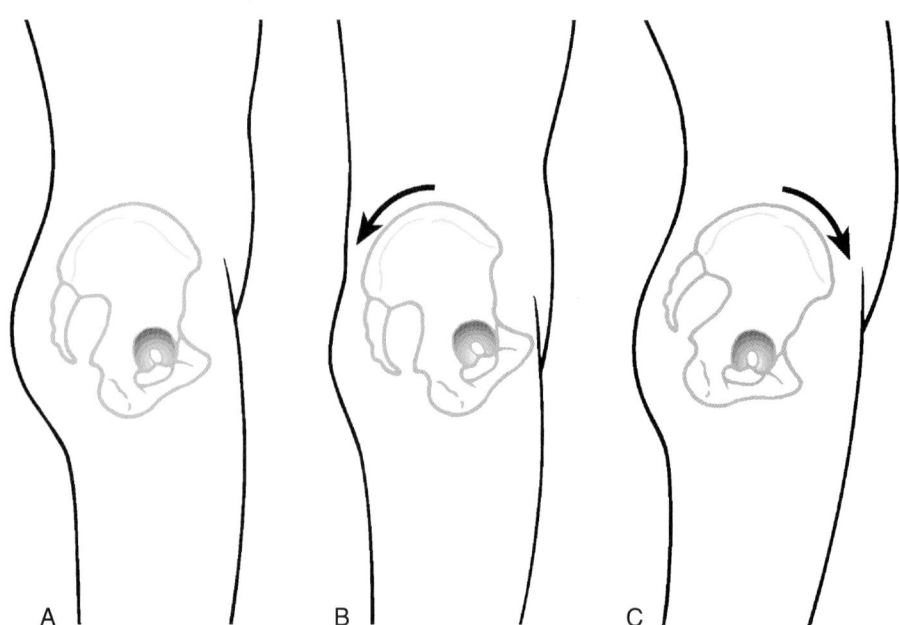

Fig. 42.6 Sagittal plane movements of the pelvis. (A) A pelvis in neutral position. (B) A posteriorly tilted pelvis (pelvis tilted to a flattened back). (C) An anteriorly tilted pelvis (pelvis tilted to an arched back). To obtain a neutral spinal position, a person must find a comfortable position between arched and flattened. (From Muscolino JE, Cipriana S: Pilates and the "powerhouse," *J Body Work Movement Ther* 8:15–24, 2004, Fig. 6, p. 20.)

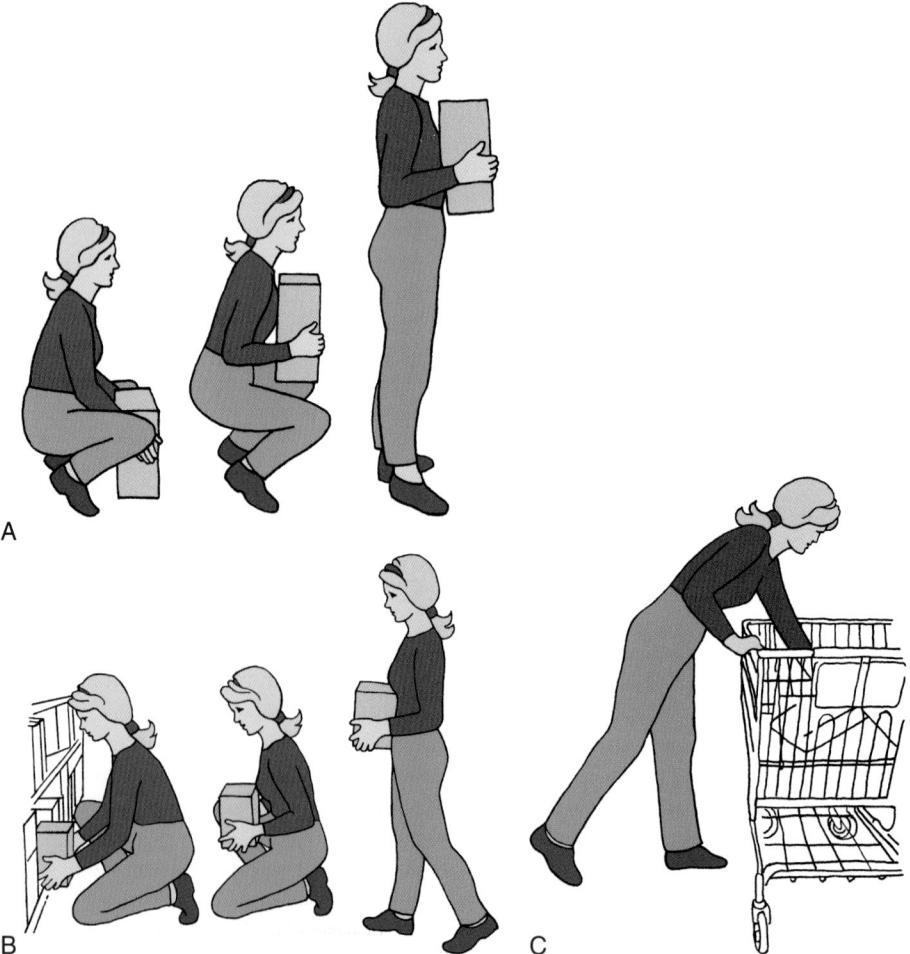

Fig. 42.7 (A) Squat. Squat and lift with both arms held against the upper part of the trunk. Tighten the stomach muscles without holding your breath. Use smooth movements to avoid jerking. (B) Diagonal lift. Squat down and bring the item close for lifting. (C) Golfer's lift. When reaching into the cart, lift the opposite leg to keep the back straight.

be noted in many habitual activities such as flushing the toilet. In these instances the client must be instructed to turn the body as a unit while maintaining a neutral spine.

Ergonomics at Work

Many LBP injuries are caused or exacerbated by working. Whether the person sits at a computer all day or works on an assembly line, the spine is involved with every movement. For labor-intensive jobs, principles of body mechanics are applied to encourage posture and limit strain on the back. For desk jobs, ergonomic principles are applied to ensure a neutrally positioned spine and to minimize muscle strain during periods of extended sitting.

Equipment that allows employees to work while both sitting and standing (Fig. 42.8) can benefit those with LBP, because frequently changing positions reduces muscle strain and promotes more neutral alignment of the spine. Ideally, the person should change positions at least every 30 minutes to alleviate prolonged pressure on disks, pressing of nerves, and muscle strain.

Ergonomic task chairs that permit seat height, seat depth, back angle, and back height or lumbar placement adjustments allow users to fit the chair to their bodies. A chair for desktop work must provide back support (ideally all the way up to the shoulders) and maintain the hips and knees at 90 degrees with the feet flat on the floor or a footrest. Tilt on a chair can also provide desk decompression periodically throughout the day. Often clients place their chairs too high, resulting in pelvic anterior tilt and putting strain on the lower back.

The occupational therapist assesses the client's work tasks and helps the client to modify his or her workspace, equipment, and behaviors. The client is taught to take frequent breaks (again once every 30 minutes), change positions and tasks frequently, and move objects closer to prevent repetitive reaching or leaning. Apps, phone and calendar reminders, and computer software programs can be used to cue clients to take more frequent breaks at work.

Occupational therapists are prime candidates for ergonomic consulting given their anatomic training, occupational analysis, and creative problem-solving skills. Ergonomic equipment manufacturers can help a therapist identify specific products that fit a client's needs, and therapists should make contacts with these vendors.

Chapter 14 discusses ergonomic principles in more detail.

Energy Conservation

Clients may not realize the toll that normal daily activities can take when they have back pain. For instance, a man who usually runs all of his errands in one day may not be aware of how taxing this is on his back and how this pattern is contributing to a pain increase, as opposed to doing one or two errands each day. Teaching clients the principles of energy conservation can alleviate or minimize problems in this area. These principles include planning ahead, setting priorities, learning one's activity tolerance, eliminating or delegating unnecessary tasks, and expending less energy for tasks that are performed (Box 42.2).

Energy conservation analogies are helpful when educating clients about how this concept can be applied to their lives. One analogy is that of a pitcher of water. Imagine the pitcher represents how much *potential* energy a person has, and the amount of water in it is the *actual* amount of energy the person wakes up with at the beginning of the day. Energy levels may differ based on sleep quality, pain levels, or general fatigue.

Now imagine each occupation is a cup, and depending on the activity, the cups may be of varying sizes. The person must prioritize and plan ahead for which cups he or she is going to pour water into, because sometimes the most important tasks come toward the end of the day when energy has already been expended (meal preparation, time with family, sex, etc.). The person must also choose how much water is going to be poured into each glass, because some glasses do not have to be filled completely (instead of cleaning the whole house, a person can choose to dust, decreasing the amount of required energy).

This analogy often helps clients visualize the concepts of energy conservation as well as convey the idea that energy is

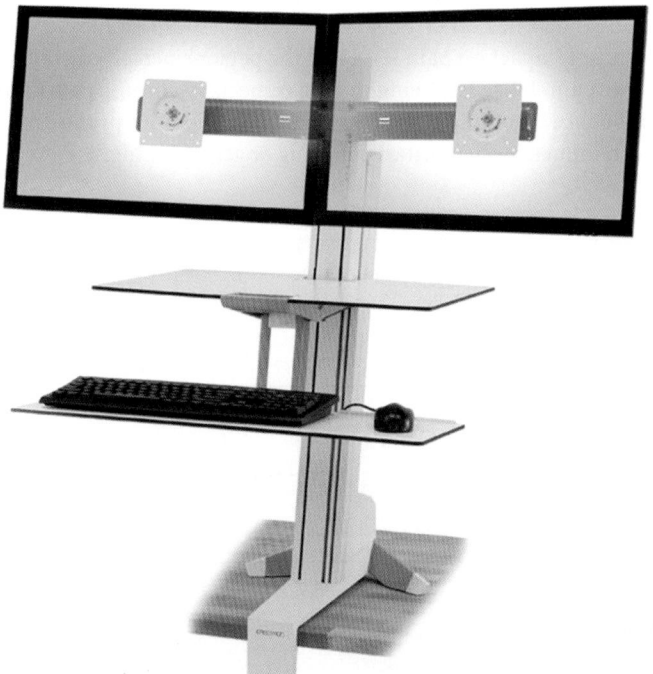

Fig. 42.8 Sit/stand equipment example. (Courtesy Ergotron, Inc., St. Paul, MN.)

BOX 42.2   Energy Conservation Strategies for Hosting Dinner With Friends

- *Plan ahead:* Shop for food 2 days prior; do all chopping and food preparation one day prior.
- *Prioritize:* Do not schedule other events that day to save energy for dinner that night.
- *Eliminate tasks:* Go out to eat to eliminate the need for cooking, cleaning before, and cleaning after the dinner.
- *Delegate:* Make the signature dish, and let others bring side dishes.
- *Learn activity tolerance:* Limit the dinner to a certain amount of time.
- *Decrease required energy for a task:* Sit while preparing food instead of standing; use a fan in the kitchen to decrease heat exhaustion.

finite and must be spent wisely. A person can dig into his or her "reserves" for more energy if needed, but this will result in less energy to start with the next day and often can cause a pain flare-up, decreasing that person's level of functioning. The key to success in incorporating energy conservation into one's daily occupational life is for the client to be aware of his or her individual activity tolerance, including specific knowledge regarding triggers of fatigue and the amount of rest necessary for recovery.

For Maria, implementing energy conservation techniques during laundry tasks may be as simple as sitting while she folds laundry or using an ironing board as a raised table if folding laundry when standing. This technique would decrease the size of the "cup," or required energy, and thus would require less "water" or energy to complete the task, leaving more water for other activities.

Activity Pacing

Activity pacing is a simple concept in theory, but it can be one of the most difficult concepts to help a person implement into daily life. Activity pacing is applied both on a large scale (daily or weekly) and on a small scale (moment to moment). In its simplest form, activity pacing calls for always alternating between periods of activity and periods of rest to prevent overexertion.

On a large scale, people can use time management skills and good planning to make sure they pace themselves with activity. For example, if Maria wants to have her friends over to her home, she may choose to cook foods that can be prepped the day before, go food shopping several days beforehand, and schedule a period of rest just before the event. This would help her to avoid overexertion, which would minimize fatigue and limit pain exacerbation.

On a smaller scale, activity pacing can also happen from moment to moment, as people listen and respond to their changing pain and fatigue levels (Fig. 42.9). Often people with pain will push themselves to finish tasks despite significantly increased pain, as they fear the unpredictability of pain may prevent them from being functional later. However, when people push themselves to their body's limit, they are further

sensitizing and damaging the painful area, as well as putting themselves at risk for a subsequent period of decreased function (usually people report this as being "out of commission" for a few hours to a few days) while their bodies recover. This becomes a vicious cycle, as people push themselves, have a pain flare, then have an abnormally long period of decreased function, causing them to believe they only have small windows of opportunity in which to accomplish tasks. This then leads back to overexertion.

Poor activity pacing can include scheduling too many activities in one day (or one week) without enough rest breaks, having unrealistic expectations of what can be accomplished in a given amount of time, or periods of overexertion followed by a pain flare that lasts for an abnormal period of time.[28]

Occupational Strength and Endurance Building

Once the principles of energy conservation have been taught and incorporated into several of the client's occupations, it is important to build on that knowledge and enable the client to increase strength and endurance for more occupational engagement. Gentle and slow-paced activity grading is the primary strategy for building tolerance when treating someone with pain, because the body's response to increased activity can vary. For example, given the opportunity to prepare a meal nightly, the client can soon develop the endurance to prepare a meal for guests. Likewise, sitting at a computer to write a letter while maintaining a neutral spine strengthens the abdominal muscles and sitting tolerance, which can increase the ability to sit in the car for a moderate to long car ride.

Self-Regulation Training and Coping Skills

LBP can influence, and be influenced by, a person's nervous system regulation. Back pain is associated with a higher risk of depression, anxiety, and stress.[32] Stress, anxiety, depression, and sometimes other behavioral health issues can have a significant impact on pain level and the person's perceived control over pain. Likewise, being in pain (especially chronic pain) can influence emotions and mood (Fig. 42.10). Sensory profiles may also influence client catastrophizing or active coping.[24]

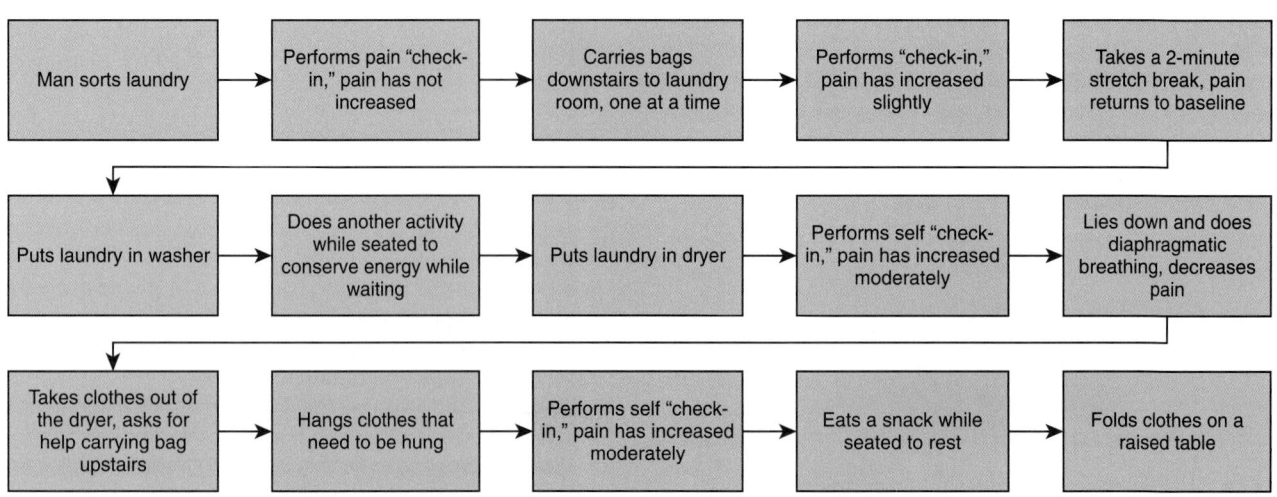

Fig. 42.9 Example of activity pacing while doing laundry.

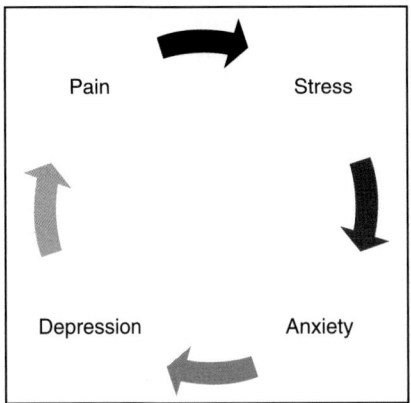

Fig. 42.10 Behavioral health status and the relation to pain.

Stress and Anxiety

Pain causes stress on the body, simply because pain is a signal to the body that something is wrong, and this triggers automatic responses to encourage the body to remove or address the painful stimulus (e.g., moving your foot away from a fire). In addition, feeling stress or anxiety stimulates the sympathetic nervous system, which adds to an already overly excited nervous system, causing a cycle of stress, anxiety, and pain that is difficult to control, as one usually feeds the other. Stress and pain may also reinforce each other via shared pathophysiology,[1] and chronic pain may affect emotional circuitry.[16]

Inversely, psychological stress can also worsen pain, especially in regard to catastrophic thinking, health beliefs about pain and recovery, and coping abilities.

Electromyography (EMG) biofeedback is a noninvasive tool that is useful when training a client in self-regulation strategies, because it provides visual feedback on muscle tension in given area(s).[29] Other forms of biofeedback include heart rate variability, respiratory feedback, thermal feedback, and neurofeedback or electroencephalography (EEG).

Depression

Depression and LBP are often comorbid and are two of the three leading causes of years lived with disability globally.[14] Depression and pain are frequently correlated, with estimates of 5% to 85% of patients with pain conditions experiencing depression, depending on the clinical setting.[7] Theories of pain-depression interactions involve the role of neuroplasticity as well as neurobiological changes.[30] For Maria, her pain and depression influence one another, and she also reports feelings of guilt due to not being able to accomplish the tasks that she feels contribute to her family's needs. She also is dealing with the loss and change of former occupations, which she is both grieving and learning to accept.

Behavioral Health Interventions

Box 42.3 provides basic strategies to encourage patients to self-manage their stress and mood. Occupational therapists in any setting should be certain to assess and treat behavioral and emotional health influences on pain, as client perceived satisfaction of treatment outcomes may be higher when these factors are addressed.[19] Some of these interventions are intended to elicit improved daily routines through biological markers of time (e.g., circadian rhythm). Several interventions listed encourage parasympathetic nervous system activation, thereby decreasing the sympathetic nervous system response, and are deemed **self-regulation** techniques as they promote the client's own ability to regulate and calm an overstimulated nervous system. These strategies not only target the behavioral health of the patient, but often they can directly decrease pain levels and improve functional capacity.[29] Also see the section in Chapter 51 on mindfulness strategies.

Lifestyle Modifications

Lifestyle factors can greatly influence the prognosis, management, and recovery of someone with LBP, yet lifestyle management is not an area of practice most occupational therapists feel readily comfortable addressing. Established programs such as Lifestyle Redesign can be used to inform site- and client-specific lifestyle management plans (see Chapter 53).[35]

Eating

Making **lifestyle modifications** and behavioral changes to keep blood sugar stable, so as to prevent episodes of very low blood sugar, can help people avoid episodes of increased achiness and low energy. Identifying an eating schedule, educating a person about general blood sugar management strategies, and problem-solving when the person is going to go food shopping and how he or she is going to prepare meals without increasing pain are all areas occupational therapists can address.

Sleep

Lack of quality and amount of sleep can cause dysregulation in the body and hypersensitivity of the nervous system and thereby increase pain levels. However, pain can often limit a person's ability to get enough quality sleep because of difficulty falling asleep, frequent waking, anxiety, or discomfort. This creates a problematic cycle for some people with LBP, because pain interferes with restorative sleep, leading to more pain the following day. See Chapter 13 for more information.

Occupational therapists can educate clients about sleep hygiene strategies to help people fall asleep and stay asleep or fall back asleep if frequent waking at night is an issue. Activities performed before bedtime can greatly affect one's ability to fall asleep and the quality of that sleep. Avoiding stimulating activities that will alert the mind or body for at least 30 minutes (ideally 60 minutes) before bed is important. This includes using electronic devices with bright screens, strenuous exercise, house work, answering emails, and sometimes looking at social media. Alcohol and nicotine should also be avoided, because they can interfere with sleep cycles.

Instead, people should be encouraged to engage in calming and relaxing activities before they plan to fall asleep. Reading, listening to music, light stretching, aromatherapy, and hot showers are often used to relax the body and mind before bed. Refocusing thoughts on breathing exercises, guided muscle relaxation, meditation, or even just using white noise can often help people fall asleep more easily by taking their minds off stressful thoughts. Sleep hygiene plans should be individualized to fit the client's preferences and opinions to optimize relaxation before bed (Fig. 42.11).

Exercise

Maintaining muscle tone quality and conditioning is important for those with LBP. Improving muscle strength in the areas surrounding the damaged site can reduce painful symptoms for conditions such as herniated disks or arthritis. For older adults with LBP, trunk muscle integrity is a "key modifiable factor" in reducing pain.[13] Yoga, Pilates, tai chi, swimming, and other strength-building activities that focus on form can be helpful in these situations and can be slow, controlled, and easily graded. This is especially helpful if the person is exhibiting exercise fear-avoidance behaviors.[29] Pool exercises have the added benefit of decreasing strain on muscles and lessening the compression of vertebral disks. Water also provides resistance and fluid movement, which is helpful when trying to gently build strength over time. People with LBP who find the right forms of exercise can often alleviate pain because of the release of synovial fluid in synovial joints, increased blood flow, better muscle tone, released neurotransmitters, and improved endurance and strength.

For clients with acute pain, exercise combined with superficial heat, spinal manipulation, or massage may improve function for occupational therapists with a Physical Agent Modality certification.[29] For those with chronic pain, exercise can result

in some pain relief and functional improvement; however, these results last only as long as the client continues to engage in exercise, which speaks to the need for development of a sustainable exercise routine that it built to fit the lifestyle of the client.[29]

Medication Management and Cognition

Some patients may have difficulty managing their medications, possibly because of cognitive deficits, medication side effects, or being overwhelmed. These difficulties can include the following:
- Frequently forgetting to take medications
- Not taking medications on time
- Not using medication appropriately (addressed with the guidance of a physician)
- Difficulty remembering body mechanic techniques
- Forgetting where adaptive equipment is placed
- Poor attendance at healthcare appointments

Occupational therapists can help people improve medication management skills by providing organization, tracking, and cueing strategies to increase the accuracy of dosages and promote patient safety.

Religious and Spiritual Expression

Spiritual practices can be cognitive-behavioral or social, and spiritual beliefs can shape how a person views or experiences pain. Participation in occupations of spirituality can have an impact on pain intensity and increase social support, and many clients wish to include spiritual issues in their medical care.[37] Occupational therapists should regularly ask clients about the effect that their spiritual or religious occupations have on pain, and vice versa, and also whether the client would like to incorporate spirituality into the plan of care.

Adaptive Equipment

Adaptive equipment is often useful for patients with LBP. The most frequently recommended pieces of equipment for persons with LBP are used primarily to prevent the client making excessive spinal movement and include long-handled sponges or brushes, reachers, long-handled shoehorns, sock aids, elevated commodes or toilet seats, wiping wands for toileting, handheld shower sprayers, footstools, and car door latch grab bars.

Postoperative and Acute Interventions

After surgery, it is the therapist's responsibility to educate the client in the required performance precautions for daily occupations. This should take place before even attempting to have the

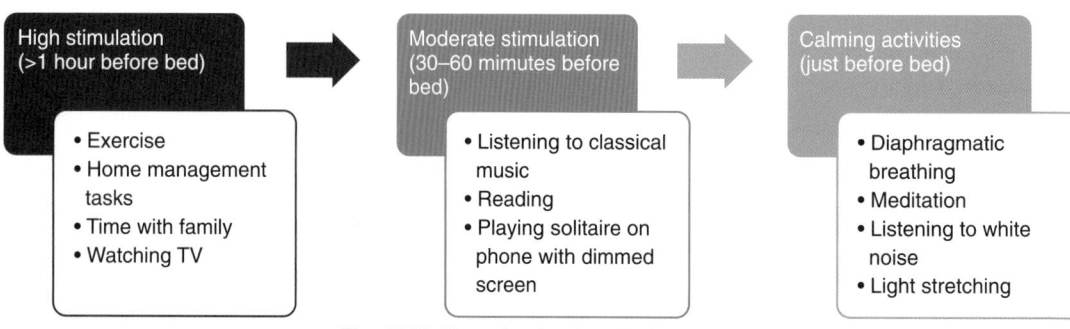

Fig. 42.11 Example of a sleep hygiene plan.

client get out of bed. Contrary to customary practice in occupational therapy in which the therapist observes occupations and makes corrections afterward, in this situation the therapist does not want to observe performance before the intervention. Instead, the primary focus is to educate then cue the client through the process to avoid any improper positions or posture that creates stress on the surgical area. The goal of occupational therapy intervention is to train the patient to perform necessary ADLs while maintaining a straight back, avoiding twisting, incorporating back safety techniques, and using adaptive equipment. Additional goals around self-regulation may be helpful as well, if the person is experiencing stress or anxiety.

The most basic ADLs must be addressed initially while the client is in the hospital. It is important to educate clients on proper positions for sleeping and have them return-demonstrate the positions correctly. The client will need to use the logroll technique for functional mobility in the bed. Proper methods are also taught for getting in and out of bed, in and out of a chair, and on and off a toilet; brushing teeth; washing the face; shaving; and dressing using the back protection techniques discussed previously. Clients are instructed to use adaptive equipment to prevent back stress during daily activities, including getting in and out of an automobile.

Therapists in acute settings may also choose to use superficial heat (if certified to administer physical agent modalities), lumbar supports (if there is no guidance for or against this from the physician), or exercise.[29]

Because hospital stays are often short and because most people will be discharged home, it is good to provide clients with resources (including pictures) should specific occupations not be specifically addressed during the institutional stay. Some facilities develop educational materials that include basic body mechanics information, hints on ADLs, and anatomic and surgical information. Various publications include postsurgical back dos and don'ts. Many hospitals have computerized education programs that allow the provider to issue information on the surgical procedure and the resulting back precautions. Although most insurance plans do not cover adaptive equipment such as reachers, raised commodes, shower chairs, and long-handled sponges, this equipment is necessary to ensure a successful home discharge outcome, and many clients purchase these items and have them delivered to their homes before they leave the care facility. To prepare the client for home and occupation modifications, many hospitals provide preoperative classes.

CLIENT-CENTERED OCCUPATIONAL THERAPY ANALYSIS

Consider the following questions when providing occupational therapy services for a client with LBP:

Evaluation

- What are the client's occupational goals?
- What was the client's functional baseline before injury/surgery, or if the pain is chronic, before exacerbation of symptoms?

- What skills, personal factors, and client factors does the client possess, and which are modifiable?
- What performance patterns are already in place?
- What are the environmental and social contexts in which the occupation is performed?
- What supports and barriers to engagement exist?
- How does the patient perform the necessary occupations currently?

Intervention

- What movements and activities increase pain? Are any specific movements or postures identifiable as the cause for increased pain?
- What anatomic structures are involved during occupational performance?
- Which skills, personal factors, and client factors will be addressed?
- What can the patient do or use to decrease pain?
- How can the environment or task be modified to fit the patient's needs?

Reassessment

- Did the intervention improve the patient's function and/or pains?
- Is the patient able to manage pain during and after activity?
- Does the patient have the education needed to problem-solve through occupational engagement barriers independently after discharge?

In addition, it is important to always consider how the person, occupation, and environment interact when deciding on treatment interventions (Fig. 42.12). Thinking of the complex way in which these three areas support and contradict each other (especially with the help of the patients themselves) is what leads to effective, individualized care plans.

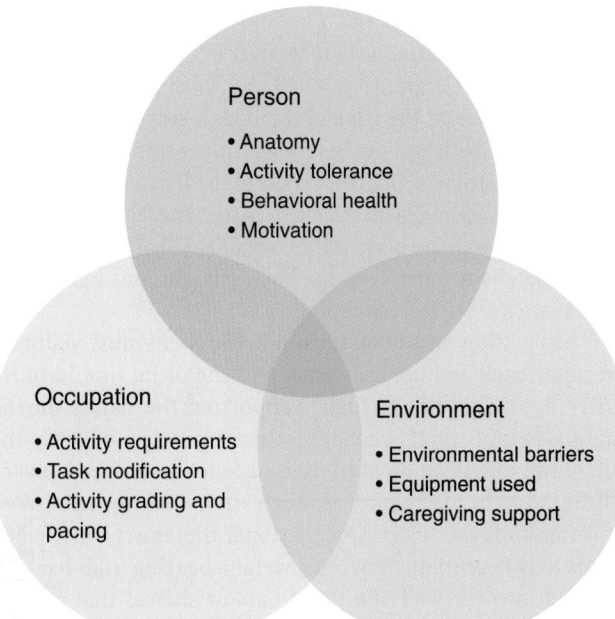

Fig. 42.12 Person, environment, and occupation influences.

THREADED CASE STUDY

Maria, Part 2 (Occupational Analysis)

Maria states her primary goal is to do the family's laundry independently, as this would give her a sense of productivity and fulfillment. The occupational therapist observes Maria attempt to load and unload the top-load washer and observes that Maria often bends at the hips and uses her back to lift the basket of clothing, reporting increased pain. When Maria is unloading the washer and placing clothes in the front-load dryer, the therapist also notes Maria bends forward again to retrieve the clothes, then twists and leans back and to the right to toss the clothing into the dryer.

Person

Maria states laundry is very important for her to do independently, as this will give her a sense of fulfillment. This means delegating part or all of the activity may not be the first option for her. Maria is willing to make changes to the way she goes about doing the laundry, but sometimes her depression makes it difficult to initiate tasks. Maria also states she tends to push herself despite pain increases during activity, because she thinks her pain flare-ups are unpredictable and wants to finish things "while she still can."

To increase motivation, the occupational therapist uses a motivational interviewing approach to help Maria identify why it is important to her that she be able to do the family's laundry. The therapist also has Maria place cue cards around the home to remind her that even small accomplishments are victories (e.g., placing clothes in the hamper instead of in a pile).

The anatomic causes of Maria's LBP (herniated disks, myofascial pain) are mostly fixed, so treatment will focus on managing and minimizing her pain, not necessarily eliminating pain.

Occupation

As Maria bends forward, she is straining the posterior portion of the lumbar disks and causing the anterior portion of the disk to bulge outward. She is also placing strain on the spinal musculature in the lumbar area, especially when she picks up the basket of laundry and when bending to retrieve items from the washer.

These tasks may be modified using good body mechanics to lift a heavy laundry basket, such as using a golf lift for item retrieval and to ensure the hips and shoulders are always facing the same way to prevent twisting. The speed and intensity of the task can also be modified because Maria tends to push herself; if unloading the washer is the most painful part of this activity, Maria can do it in two parts with a break in between to prevent her pain from increasing significantly.

Environment

Barriers to Maria doing laundry independently are lack of assistance during the day, not owning any adaptive equipment, and having laundry equipment that encourages bending forward (top-load washer).

Maria can change to a front-load machine, then put the washer and dryer (also front-loading) on risers to limit the amount of bending she has to do. This will allow her to squat or kneel with a neutral spine next to the open machine door and reach in without twisting or leaning. If this is not possible, Maria can use a long-handled reacher or dressing stick to retrieve the clothes from the washer. If Maria spends a lot of time doing laundry, she can acquire an antifatigue mat to limit disk compression when standing. Maria can also place a small table near her laundry machines, so she can prevent bending and never has to place the laundry basket on the floor. She also may be able to use this table to fold clothing afterward.

If Maria is willing, she can ask her son and husband to carry the laundry baskets to the laundry room before they leave for work, then carry them back when the clothes are washed. This will help her to conserve energy. If Maria is unsure about asking for help, the occupational therapist can suggest this task modification be a temporary solution until Maria is able to tolerate more activity.

INTERVENTION STRATEGIES FOR FREQUENTLY AFFECTED OCCUPATIONS

Functional Mobility

Use of the *logroll* technique to maneuver in bed requires moving the body as a whole unit (Fig. 42.13, A). To sit up, the client lies on one side close to the edge of the bed, bends the knees over the side of the bed, and pushes up with the arms while coming to a sitting position, using the weight of the legs as leverage (see Fig. 42.13, B). To lie down, the client brings the legs up and uses the arms to lower the body to the bedside. During both movements, the client must keep the back straight and tighten the core muscles to support the spine.

When getting on and off the toilet, the client must maintain a straight back and neutral spine, and she or he should move slowly if pain levels are high. Supporting the hands on the thighs is helpful, or, if needed, a toilet frame or grab bars at the side of the toilet can be used. Raised toilet seats are also very helpful, so as to not require as much strain or torque to transfer on and off the toilet. Occupational therapists must teach clients to differentiate between a weight-bearing grab bar that is bolted into the wall and towel bars or shelves that are not meant to bear weight. Clients also need to receive education regarding the safe use of other surfaces for stability, because people often use countertops, tubs, and walls for bracing during transfer, which can jeopardize safety and cause twisting.

It is recommended that clients use an arm chair with a hard seat or firm cushions that is supportive and not too low, compared to an oversized plush couch. The client can use the chair arms to push up to a standing position (Fig. 42.14), and the firm pillows will better support the back while seated. To reduce stiffness, the client should stand and walk or stretch frequently (about every 20–30 minutes). Clients should be trained to activate their hip flexors, extensors, and gluteal muscles to assist as they come into a standing or seated position, while still activating their core muscles for stability but not using them as a primary source of movement.[17]

Therapists should encourage their clients to walk as tolerated and prescribed, as this will promote blood flow to the affected area and improve strength, endurance, and flexibility to support function.[29]

Showering

To promote energy conservation and limit bending, clients can keep all items on a shower rack or ledge that stands between chest and eye height. Use of grab bars, a shower chair, or bench can help if balance and bending when washing lower extremities is difficult or contraindicated while standing. Use of

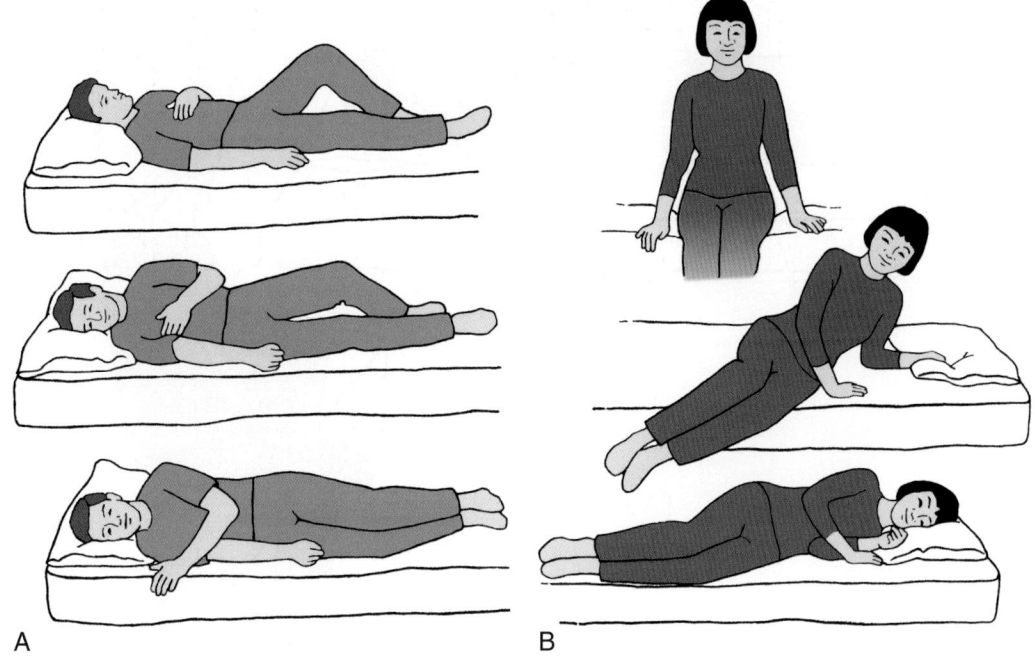

Fig. 42.13 (A) Logroll. Lying on your back, bend your left knee and place your left arm across your chest. Roll all in one movement to the right, using the left leg to assist with starting the roll, and keeping shoulders and hips aligned. Reverse for rolling to the left. Always move as one unit. (B) Movement in and out of bed. Lower your body to lie down on one side by raising your legs and lowering your head at the same time. Use your arms to assist in moving without twisting. Bend both knees to roll onto your back if desired. To sit up, start by lying on your side, and use the same movements in reverse. Keep your trunk aligned with your legs.

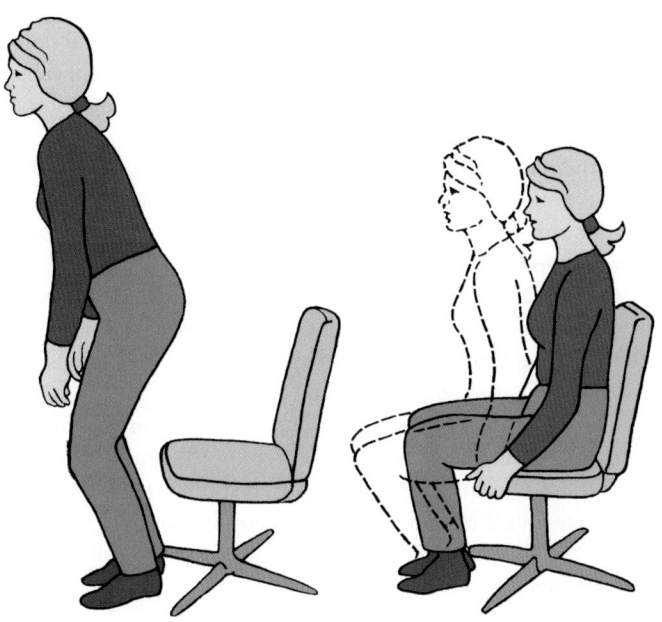

Fig. 42.14 Stand to sit and sit to stand. To sit, bend your knees to lower your body onto the front edge of the chair and then scoot back on the seat. To stand, reverse the sequence by placing one foot forward and scoot to the front of the seat. Use a rocking motion to stand up.

long-handled scrub brushes or sponges allows clients to wash their back, legs, and feet without bending and twisting, especially when used in conjunction with a shower bench or chair. A handheld shower attachment controls water flow and decreases unnecessary movements. For safety, the client should always use a bath mat at home to reduce the chance of slipping, and drain the water from the tub completely before attempting to get out.

Should a client in an acute or subacute care setting not yet be cleared to shower without a prescribed orthosis, most of the bathing can be accomplished in the shower, and a towel bath may be appropriate to clean the skin under the orthosis while supine in bed.

Dressing

Keeping the spine in a neutral position is the main goal when dressing. The client can sit in a chair or at the edge of the bed or lie flat on the bed while using mostly hip flexion to get clothing onto the lower extremities, as opposed to spinal flexion (Fig. 42.15). If the client's balance and strength allow, dressing in a standing position is also possible with use of a walker for stability.

To don and doff socks and shoes, the client should sit and bring the foot to rest on the knee using external rotation and flexion at the hip, or place the foot on a stool while maintaining a neutral back to bring the foot closer. Maria preferred to use slip-on no-tie shoes as a compensatory strategy to minimize and avoid prolonged bending. A long-handled shoehorn and elastic shoelaces are useful for donning shoes that require tying.

To don underwear, pants, or other lower body clothes, clients can begin in a chair or at the edge of the bed to get the clothing over their feet; then they can stand up with a walker for balance if needed to pull the clothing into a fitted position. Dressing hooks, pant clips, and reachers can be useful tools if needed. Back protection techniques should be used for both dressing and undressing, and equipment such as dressing hooks, reachers, sock aids, and long-handled shoe horns can be useful to

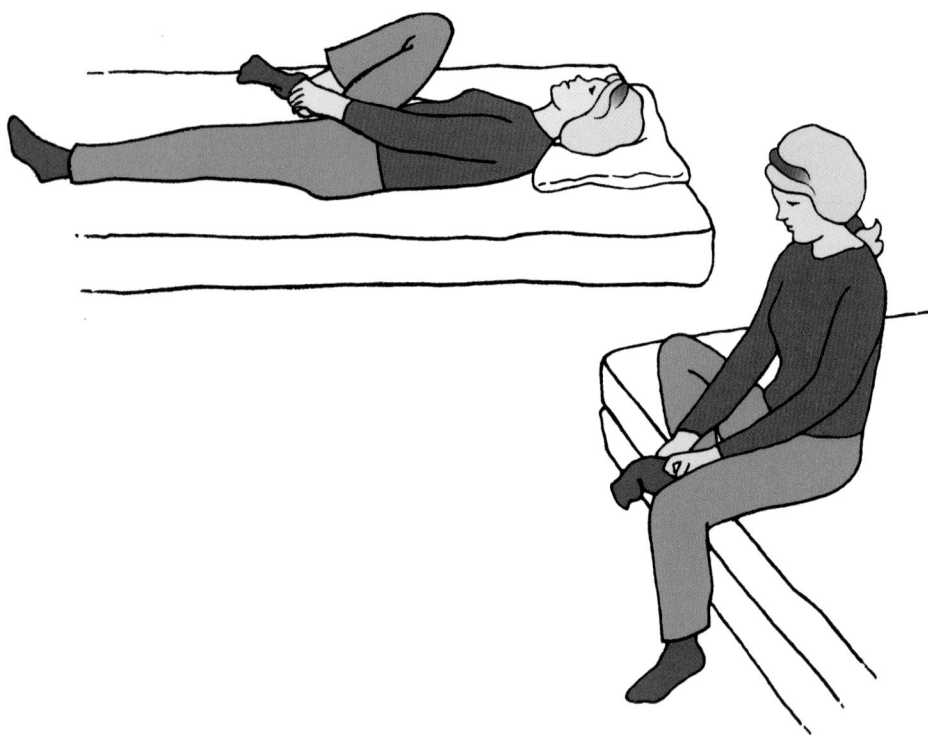

Fig. 42.15 Dressing. Lie on your back to place socks or slacks over your feet, or bend your leg up while keeping your back straight.

assist in donning and doffing lower extremity clothes, and picking them up off the floor.

In addition to the previous discussion about clothing, clients who have undergone back surgery can benefit from clothing choices that are easy to don and doff and can be comfortably worn with any prescribed orthoses.

Donning and Doffing a Thoracolumbosacral Orthosis

To don a TLSO, instruct the patient to log roll to one side, assisting as needed, and with a pillow between the knees if desired. Don the posterior part of the brace first by finding the waist landmarks of the orthosis and match them with the patient's waist (the soft indentation between the hip and the ribs) to ensure the brace is properly aligned with the client's body. It is recommended you first match the side of the orthosis that is furthest from the bed, as the side of the orthosis that is closest to the bed will need to be sufficiently tucked under the patient's body to ensure the orthosis is fitted to the body with no gaps. Hold the orthosis in place, and instruct the client to roll onto the back with the brace in place. Once the client is on the back, ensure the brace is evenly superiorly/inferiorly and laterally on each side and adjust the TLSO as needed. If needed, the client can also roll onto the other side to allow for more significant adjustment.

Don the anterior part of the brace next by again using the waist of the brace and the waist of the client as landmarks to match. Pull the brace open as you place it on the client, because the front piece of the TLSO sits on top of the back piece of the brace, under each arm.

Once the front and back parts of the brace are aligned and fitted, loop the abdominal straps through the buckles, tightening the bottom straps first. The fit should be as snug as possible, while still allowing the patient to breathe comfortably (have the client test this before moving to the next step). After the abdominal straps are secured, loop the shoulder straps (if applicable) through the buckles and tighten, although these straps do not have to be as snug as the abdominal ones.

If there is a chest piece, it should be attached just below the sternal notch, so that it sits directly on the sternum. The straps for this can be under or over the shoulders, so confirm the fit before donning.

Once the brace is secure, have the patient come into a seated position at the edge of the bed. Check to ensure the brace has not moved upward or twisted, because these are indications that it is not tight enough or not fitted properly.

To doff a TLSO brace, the client should lie supine in bed. Undo all of the straps, remove the front of the brace, and assist the patient in rolling toward the therapist onto their side. Push the brace into the bed while simultaneously pulling it out from under the client's body. Finally, assist the client in rolling back into supine.

Personal Hygiene

Activities at the bathroom sink can be difficult, as most sinks are hip or waist height, requiring most adults to bend forward, increasing stress and strain on the low back. While brushing the teeth, shaving, or washing the face, the client should place one foot inside the base cabinet (or on a small stool) to reduce strain on the lower part of the back and bend from the hips while keeping the back as straight as possible (Fig. 42.16). Alternatively, the client may bend forward and bear weight through one knee while extending a straight leg back for balance and support

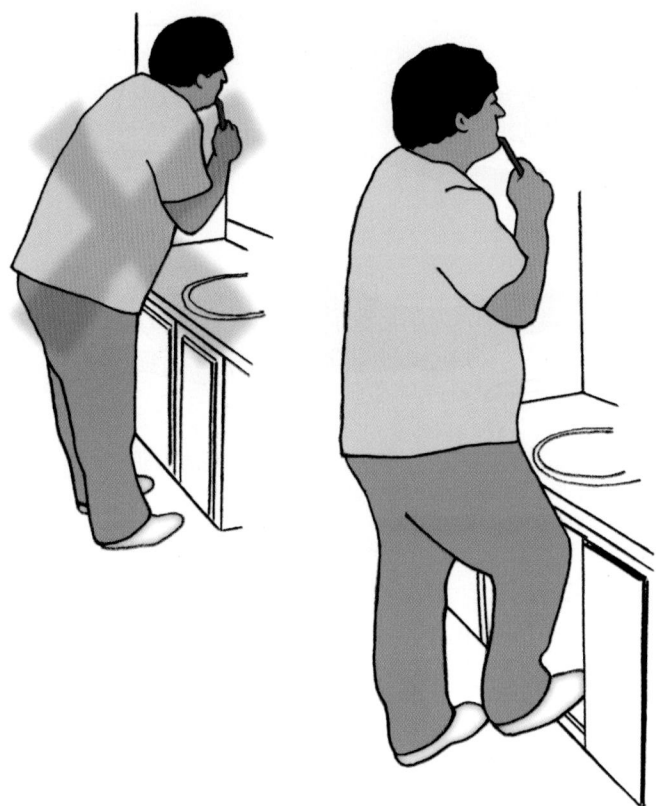

Fig. 42.16 Shaving. Stay upright with one foot on the ledge of the cabinet under the sink. (Courtesy Visual Health Information, Tacoma, WA.)

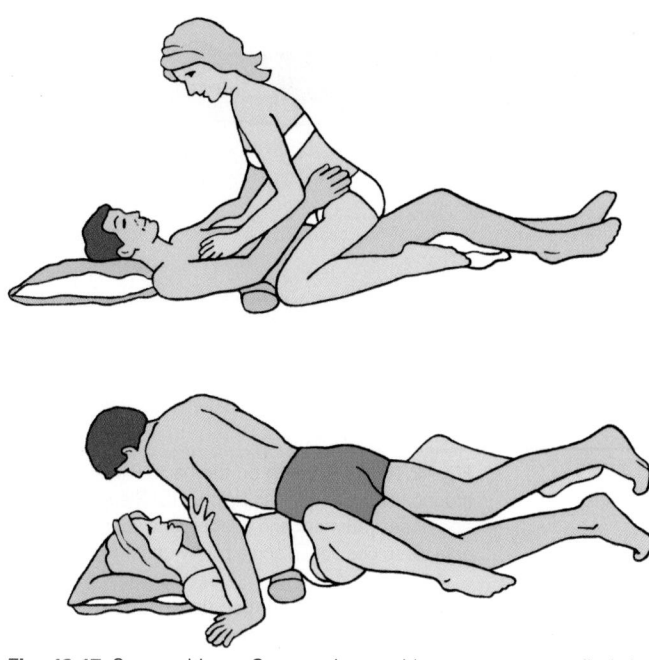

Fig. 42.17 Sex positions. Communicate with your partner to find the position that is most comfortable for you. Plan ahead, and use pillows and rolls for support as needed.

and maintaining a neutral spine position. Maria prefers to lean against the countertop with one hand to relieve some of the compression on her low back when rinsing after brushing her teeth, or she uses a cup to rinse her mouth instead of leaning over the sink to bring water to her mouth. To apply her cosmetics, Maria uses a handheld mirror or a mirror on the wall at face height to limit bending.

Sexual Activity

Sexual activities require positions and movements that keep the lower back in the neutral position and prevent excessive twisting, flexion, or extension of the spine. Clients whose pain increases with spinal extension may be most comfortable lying on their back with pillows under the buttocks or upper part of the back to minimize extension. For those whose pain increases with spinal flexion, a rolled towel under the low back also may help maintain a neutral back position (Fig. 42.17). If the client prefers positions that require being on hands and knees, large wedge pillows can assist the client in keeping a neutral spine. For men, standing during sexual activity and placing one foot in front of the other, or leaning forward on a surface with one or both hands, can promote good alignment.

Activity grading and pacing are especially important with sexual activity, and the client is advised to start slowly and gradually work up to more vigorous movements depending on tolerance. Before sexual activity, stretching and warming up muscles or taking a warm shower may enable greater activity through muscle relaxation.

Communication with a partner is also a key component of engaging in sexual activity. Often clients are too embarrassed, shy, or excited to talk about tolerance levels and speak up during activity when a movement becomes painful. Teaching clients about assertive communication strategies and helping them create an individualized plan for sexual activity can prevent injury and increase a patient's confidence.

Sleep

We spend almost a third of our lives in bed, so it is important to consider the effects that sleep and LBP have on one another. In acute or subacute care settings, medical-grade beds are not often the most comfortable mattresses, but clients can still use the positioning techniques below. If the patient is post-operative and has any positioning or repositioning guidelines from the surgeon, those should be incorporated into the plan. Extra emphasis may need to be placed on self-regulation strategies to promote relaxation for those whose sleep is affected by a care-facility environment.

At home, a firm, supportive mattress is important because mattresses that are too soft or plush will not maintain neutral alignment. The pillow should support the neck and head in neutral alignment, without causing the neck to flex forward or laterally. Many types of contoured cervical pillows are helpful for this purpose.

While sleeping on the back, the client should place a pillow under the knees to reduce strain on the lower part of the back and help maintain a balanced lower back position (Fig. 42.18, A).

While lying on the side, the client should place a pillow between the knees to prevent the hips from collapsing in toward the bed and twisting the lower part of the back (see Fig. 42.18, B). It is also sometimes helpful for people to hold a pillow at chest height when side-lying to minimize rotation of the spine,

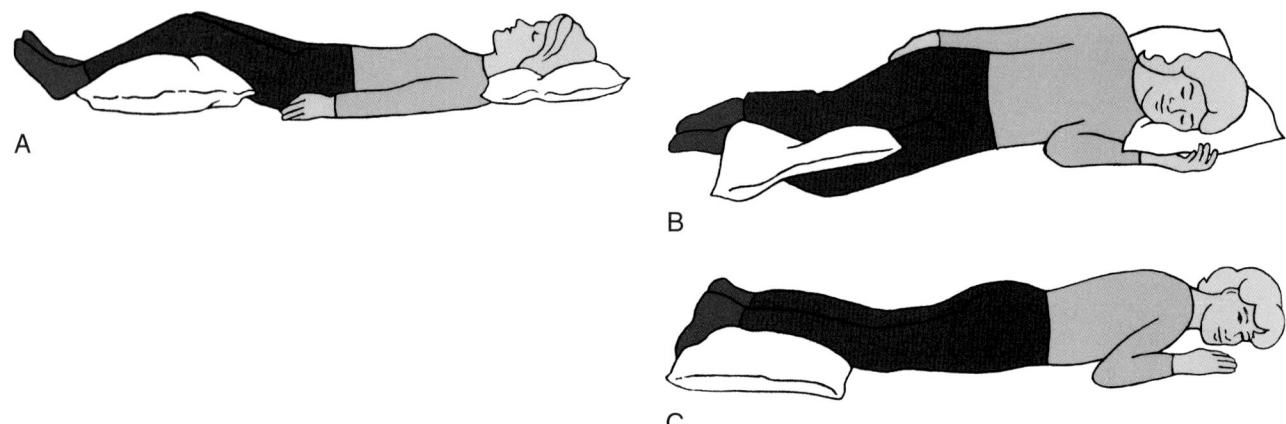

Fig. 42.18 (A) Sleeping on the back. Place a pillow under your knees. A pillow with cervical support and a roll around the waist are also helpful. (B) Sleeping on the side. Place a pillow between your knees. Use cervical support under your neck and a roll around your waist as needed. (C) Sleeping on the stomach. If this is your only desirable sleep position, place a pillow under the lower part of your legs and under your stomach or chest as needed.

because sometimes the shoulders collapse in toward the bed as well. In addition, people who change positions frequently during sleep may find it beneficial to also tuck a pillow behind their back, to prevent rolling onto the back without proper positioning. A long body pillow, or sometimes even very large pregnancy, or bolster, pillows can be used instead of multiple smaller pillows if desired.

It is not recommended that individuals sleep on their stomachs, but individuals who prefer this position should place a small pillow under the ankles to bend the knees and take stress off the lower back region (see Fig. 42.18, C). If back extension is painful, a flat pillow can be placed under the hips.

Many clients with LBP may wake during the night and want to shift positions. This can be helpful, because maintaining one position for a prolonged time can lead to muscle stiffness and reduced synovial fluid in joints. If this is the case, encourage the person to correctly reposition before falling back asleep, to minimize pain on waking and reduce the chance of pain exacerbation.

In addition, providing clients with a gentle morning stretching routine on waking can be helpful, because joints and muscles are often stiff on waking. Breathing exercises, bringing the knees to the chest and gently rocking, small spinal twists (if permitted), and even "cat-cow" movements can be help to warm-up the back before getting out of bed. For additional information on sleep and rest, please refer to Chapter 13.

Toileting

See the previous functional mobility occupation section for guidance on sitting and standing from the toilet. When cleaning after toileting, the client should reach between the legs to avoid twisting the back, using a long-handled tissue holder if needed. When turning to flush the toilet, the client should stand first, then turn all the way around and face the toilet rather than twisting and reaching. If the back pain is acute, the client can straddle the toilet seat, facing the back of the toilet. This affords a wider base of support and allows one to use the toilet tank when coming to a standing position.

Child Care

Handling children requires special precautions for individuals with back pain. Sudden movements can increase the client's pain and interfere with the ability to handle the child safely. Clients should use a changing table or elevated surface when dressing the child. Bathing can be performed in a kitchen sink or in a portable tub on an elevated surface. Many contemporary cribs have drop-down rails so that the client does not need to extend his or her arms to lift the child over the crib.

Always remind the client to bend at the hips and knees while keeping the back straight during these tasks. To lift a child from the ground, the client should squat down and bring the child close before using the legs and buttock muscles to stand up, all while engaging the abdominals. To place a child in a car seat, the client should stand close to the car seat and keep the back straight, minimizing any twisting movements (Fig. 42.19). Therapists should also encourage their clients to think of bonding activities that require less strain on the back, such as reading, doing tabletop puzzles, or snuggling in bed.

Pet Care

Depending on the size and type of the pet, a client may need different strategies to protect the low back. Use of proper body mechanics strategies such as squatting or kneeling with a neutral spine to serve food or water or to pick up the pet itself is advised. Long-handled pet waste scoopers and self-cleaning litter boxes can minimize bending as well. Self-dispensing food and water containers can eliminate the need to bend multiple times per day. Clients with larger dogs need to be cautious when walking or playing with the pet to avoid any sudden twists or jerks.

Computer Use

It is important to remind people to fit the environment and equipment to the body, instead of using the body to compensate for environmental shortcomings. Clients should first position themselves in a seated neutral position by adjusting the chair and their own posture, then place items in close proximity to prevent reaching, bending, or twisting. The

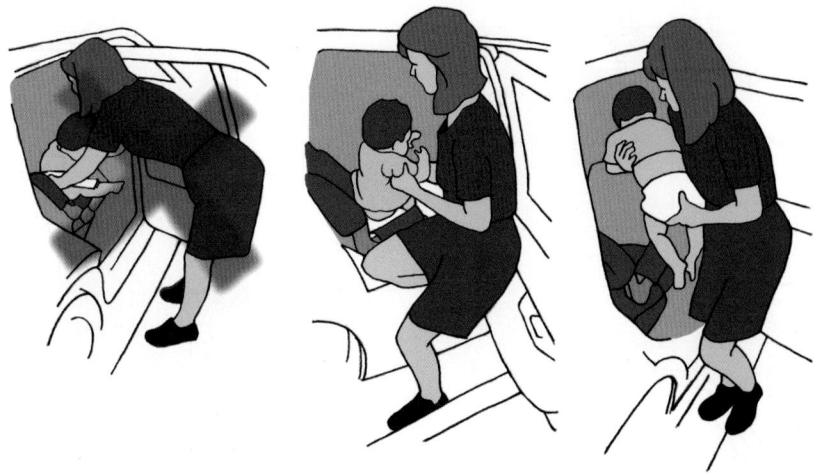

Fig. 42.19 Child care, in and out of a car. Stand close and keep your back straight. Bend your knees to put the baby in or take the baby out of the car seat.

keyboard and mouse should be easily reached without the elbows leaving the sides of the body, which allows the chair to support the back from sacrum to scapulae. Frequently used items should be within arm's length, accessible without the scapulae coming off the back of the chair to prevent repetitive reaching.

The monitor should be placed at a height that encourages sitting up in the chair, rather than slouching. Clients should be taught to use their eyes to look down at the screen, as opposed to using neck and spinal flexion. Document holders can assist in proper placement of papers and books to prevent the need for repetitive or sustained twisting or bending. Tall users may need a different desk height compared to shorter users, and the keyboard (usually placed below the elbows) may need to be a different height than a writing surface (usually above the elbows).

Maria used a laptop computer while seated on the couch, which created much discomfort. To limit spinal flexion, Maria now uses an external keyboard, external mouse, and a laptop stand (or a stack of books) to prevent reaching or slouching. She also now uses the laptop at a desk instead of on the couch to provide herself with more back support. Most important, clients such as Maria are encouraged to stretch, take breaks, and change positions at least every 20 to 30 minutes. (See Chapter 14 for additional information on ergonomics and seating.)

Driving

For postoperative clients, clearance from the surgeon may be necessary to resume driving because of limited range of motion, potential changes to sensory or motor function, and/or use of narcotic/opioid pain medications.[17]

When transferring into a car, the client should slowly sit on the seat while facing the door, then turn the body as a unit until facing forwards to keep from bending and twisting the spine. To transfer out of a car, this procedure can be done in reverse. In some cars, and depending on the person's height, this may require moving the seat forward and backward to get in and out.

If the car is low, the client should also increase the height of the seat to decrease the effort needed to sit and stand, as well as sit with the knees no higher than the hips to reduce strain on the low back. Most cars now allow adjustments in seat height, seat angle, seat position, and steering wheel angle, and some even come with adjustable lumbar support. A small, rolled-up towel positioned in the lumbar area will suffice as well. When riding for extended periods, the client should schedule rest breaks to change positions and use the recline feature of the seat to alleviate any spinal compression from sitting upright for prolonged periods. For drivers with back pain, use of cruise control allows more frequent changes in position, and taking frequent rest stops to stand, walk, and stretch is vital.

Home Management
Organization

The client should organize all work spaces so the equipment and materials needed for specific tasks are within easy reach and the work area is at an optimal height (usually around elbow height). For example, if the client is planning to bake cookies, flour, sugar, baking spices, bowls, measuring cups, and maybe a mixer should all be within reach. Routinely used items should be stored on the countertop, in the lowest cabinets, or in the highest drawers to limit back extension, reaching, and bending. Items in lower cabinets can be accessed with a partial or full squat. This same technique is used to reach items on the lower shelf of the refrigerator (Fig. 41.20), and items above the head can be accessed using a footstool. Cabinets can be modified with slide-out shelves/drawers that eliminate the need to reach far back into the cabinet. Items that are used less frequently can be stored in less accessible cabinets.

Laundry

To remove clothing from a top-load washer, the client should use a golfer's lift to reach inside the machine (Fig. 42.21). To place clothes in a front-load washer or dryer, the client is instructed to use a squat or to use an underhand toss without

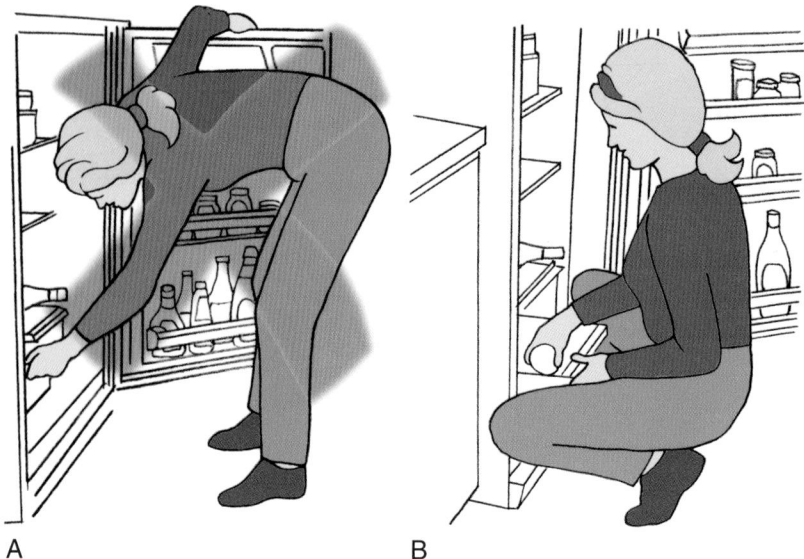

Fig. 42.20 (A) Incorrect way to reach into a refrigerator. (B) Squat with the knees apart to reach the lower shelves and drawers.

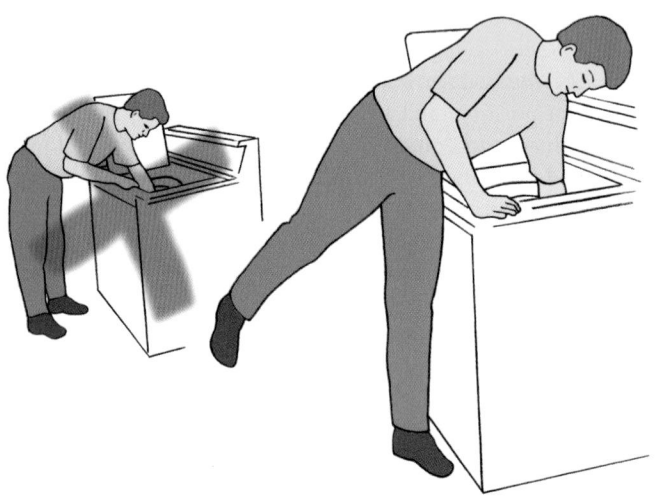

Fig. 42.21 Laundry: unloading the wash. To unload small items at the bottom of the washer, lift your leg opposite the arm used for reaching.

any spinal twisting or bending. To retrieve clothes from a front-load machine, the client repeats the squat, removes the clothes, and places them in a basket that is positioned nearby. When carrying the basket, the client should hold it close to the body and use the body mechanics for lifting that were discussed earlier in this chapter. It is highly recommended that the client fold clothes on an appropriate elbow-height table while standing or seated, to minimize the need for prolonged bending.

For ironing, it is recommended that the client raise the ironing board to elbow height, and to use mostly shoulder flexion and elbow extension to maneuver the iron instead of twisting the lower back. While ironing, the client is instructed to rest one foot on a low stool to help reduce low back strain. Ironing can also be completed while sitting if the ironing board is lowered beforehand. Because of the adjustability of an ironing board, this surface can be used for many other activities, such as folding clothes and wrapping packages.

Dishes

Similar to standing at the sink for bathroom activities, washing dishes sometimes causes people to stand for prolonged periods of time in spinal flexion. Clients should open the cabinets below the sink and use the lowest shelf as a footrest, alternating one foot at a time. In addition, over-the-sink dish racks or countertop tubs can be used to elevate dishes while washing and avoid the need to bend forward to retrieve items repetitively.

Cleaning

A long-handled brush, sponge, or Swiffer mop is recommended to clean low surfaces such as the floor or bottom of a tub. Using a handheld spray cleaner is easier than scrubbing and rinsing the surfaces. While vacuuming, clients should move their feet and legs rather than reach or bend forward. They are also cautioned to avoid twisting; when vacuuming under a table or chair, they should bend at the hips and knees to keep the back in a balanced position.

Yard Work

When mowing the lawn, the client should face forward and align the hips with the mower. The client should keep the back straight, the spine in a neutral position, and the abdominal muscles tight; take frequent breaks; and refrain from twisting or using the back to move the mower. When using a shovel, the client should bend at the hips and knees rather than at the waist and keep the shovel and its load close to the body. The preferred method for emptying the shovel is to turn the entire body and keep the hips and shoulders in alignment while maintaining the load close to the body and facing the location to unload the shovel. None of these yard activities should be attempted when the client is in an unstable condition with acute pain.

Gardening can be challenging for clients with back problems. Raised garden beds, potted plants on windowsills, and light-weight hoses are good options to reduce back strain. Many carts or moving seats can be purchased that allow safer back positioning when working at ground level. Knee pads make gardening in a kneeling position more comfortable. The gardener is cautioned to work only within his or her immediate reach to avoid bending forward or twisting.

Shopping

When retrieving items from a lower shelf, the client should squat or kneel while keeping the back straight. The thigh can be used as support when returning to a standing position; clients are not advised to use the shelf for support, because these are not meant to be weight bearing and may tip. To use a shopping cart, the client should find his or her neutral spine position, keep the abdominals activated, stand up straight, and push the cart with the elbows at the side, using the legs and gluteals for pushing force instead of the back. Use of a cart is preferable to carrying a basket even for small loads, because baskets cause uneven strain on the back. Clients can also place items in the upper portion of the cart, decreasing the need for bending. When unloading the cart, the client should use the golfer's lift to retrieve items. Heavier items should be placed in the tray below the cart if possible, because a squat or kneel can be used to get the item closer to the body.

Work

Job demands vary considerably in the physical demands placed on the spine. Jobs with heavy lifting, repetitive movements, and long periods of standing without breaks place more strain on the back. Seated jobs also have a risk of strain on the low-back, mostly from poor posture and ergonomics, or from prolonged periods of sitting without breaks and movement. Many employers now have health and safety staff to assess workstations, educate employees about body mechanics, and determine whether modifications can be made (see Chapter 14). In many cases, however, it is up to the individual to modify his or her work situation and to implement recommended body mechanic techniques. Many improvements can be made by simply using correct lifting techniques, using the proper equipment for the job, pacing the activity, taking frequent breaks or changing tasks, and asking for help.

Health Management and Maintenance

Establishing good health-promoting habits and routines throughout the day and week that support client goals, increase occupational self-awareness, and infuse pain management precautions and practices into everyday life is an essential part of any pain management intervention. In the Fourth Edition of the Occupational Therapy Practice Framework,[6] Health Management and Maintenance was added as a general occupation category, highlighting the importance of occupational therapists addressing habits and routines, in addition to standalone occupations. Healthy eating, physical activity, managing stress, managing time, and numerous other habits and routines can promote or degrade progress toward LBP recovery and management at any stage of care, but may be particularly helpful for clients with chronic LBP.[25] As always, personal, environmental, and occupational factors should be considered when helping a client build health-promoting routines. For example, Maria did not have ready access to healthy, affordable foods, so much of her healthy eating routine was built around foods which she could freeze or store for longer periods. Her physical activity routines consisted primarily of exercises, stretches, and activities that she could accomplish inside her home, in the event that weather, safety, or pain limited her participation.

Leisure

When reading, clients should sit in a supported chair, not curl up on a sofa. Tabletop hobbies such as sewing and building models require attention to table height, chair comfort, and positioning of the work items. These positioning recommendations resemble those for computer use and will reduce uneven pulling and twisting of the body.

When traveling, the client should use a wheeled suitcase that can be pushed or pulled, which is easier on the back. When wheeling the suitcase, clients should be mindful of pulling the suitcase without twisting at the shoulders or waist. Backpacks and fanny packs with light loads also can be used. Travelers are encouraged to pack lightly and take only what is needed for the trip. Checking luggage and asking for help with placing luggage in overhead bins is also recommended. If needed, the client can also bring a seat or back cushion to promote proper positioning during longer flights. Similar to working at a computer, the person is encouraged to take frequent breaks from sitting (see Chapter 16).

Many clients, male or female, carry briefcases, purses, or bags throughout their daily routines. Decreasing the weight of the bag and frequently switching shoulders can decrease the uneven strain on the back, but using a rolling laptop case or purse is optimal for alleviating back strain.

When using a cell phone, tablet, or other small electronic device, it is important to remember the positioning principles discussed throughout this chapter. Instead of holding a cell phone at a low level and using extreme neck and back flexion to look down, clients should be instructed to hold the device just below eye height, similar to that of a computer monitor. If using the device for prolonged periods, the client can use pillows (if seated) to prop the elbows up without tensing the shoulders. Again, frequent breaks are recommended to avoid prolonged spinal column discomfort.

For Maria, socializing is very important to her well-being. She requires help with problem-solving different social situations, including how to best communicate her health needs to her friends and family. Analyzing different types of social gatherings to identify factors that may influence successful pain management (e.g., ability to sit, stand, or stretch when needed; the ability to bring a lumbar cushion for use when seated) is key in Maria's successful social engagement.

Only a few of the many possible interventions have been described here. Each occupation must be analyzed, and an individualized intervention should be developed for each client. ADL body mechanics cards from Visual Health Information can be used to customize recommendations. This is a card file system from which cards can be selected and copied to develop interventions for each client according to his or her individual needs. Also available are many preprinted booklets and computer programs that may assist in client instruction. It is important to remember that most insurance companies do not cover adaptive equipment, and hospitals typically have large markups on vended equipment. Consequently, many clinics offer sample equipment for clients to try and provide community resources for equipment or consumer catalogs from vendors such as Sammons/Preston and North Coast Medical. Consumers should be made aware that many products once considered adaptive therapy equipment or ergonomic items are frequently available at a lower cost in discount stores.

OTHER MULTIDISCIPLINARY PAIN TEAM MEMBERS

The best intervention strategy for managing LBP is a team approach with the patient as the central and most important team member. Occupational therapists should validate their patients' opinions and goals and remind patients to advocate for themselves. It is important for all team members to remember that the client is the expert on his or her own life, and despite what healthcare providers objectively think and observe, in the end the person's subjective experience is what is real to himself or herself.

Box 42.4 lists common multidisciplinary team members who can play a role in LBP management for patients. Complementary and alternative therapists, although not always part of the immediate medical team, can contribute to the pain management plan for certain patients and should be considered referral resources for the appropriate clients.

BOX 42.4   Multidisciplinary and Complementary Pain Team Members

Multidisciplinary
- Physician
- Occupational therapist
- Physical therapist
- Pain psychologist
- Psychiatrist
- Case worker
- Nurse

Other Pain Team Members
- Surgeon (if needed)
- Pharmacist
- Nutritionist
- Vocational counselor
- Discharge planner
- Social worker

Complementary and Alternative Therapies
- Acupuncture
- Chiropractic
- Reiki
- Animal-assisted therapy
- Gentle yoga
- Massage

THREADED CASE STUDY

Maria, Part 3 (Multidisciplinary Care)

The occupational therapist communicates with the other members of the pain team to create the best possible collective healthcare plan for Maria. The physical therapist plans to work on massaging the low back, as well as core exercises to strengthen the spinal column muscles, in the hope that this will lessen the herniated disk pain.

Because of the lack of motivation to initiate daily activities as a result of depression, the occupational therapist refers Maria to a pain psychologist to help Maria manage her depression. The pain psychologist uses cognitive-behavioral therapy to help Maria change her thought patterns and learn how to use positive self-talk and objective reasoning to feel less guilty about not being able to do certain tasks that she previously performed for her family.

As Maria progresses through her therapies, she shows improvement in strength and motivation, and the occupational therapist uses these improvements to gradually grade and increase Maria's occupational goals.

Physician

The physician is responsible for the client's initial evaluation, usually including a thorough medical history, current symptoms and complaints, functional limitations, posture, gait, strength, reflexes and sensation, and past interventions for this problem. A diagnosis is usually made at this time, or the physician may order additional tests, such as nerve conduction tests, computed tomography scans, magnetic resonance imaging, and blood work. After arriving at a diagnosis, the physician often prescribes medication, determines restrictions in activity and exercise guidelines, and may refer the patient to other physicians for differential diagnoses, a surgeon for surgical consult, physical therapy, occupational therapy, or counseling. To reevaluate progress or lack thereof, the physician will see the patient for follow-up visits at whatever frequency is deemed necessary.

In both acute and chronic LBP, pain medication may be necessary to lower pain levels to allow for client participation in rehabilitation, especially for acute pain or for chronic pain exacerbations. However, it is also important that physicians know occupational therapists can provide vital pain management interventions that supplement, or sometimes replace, pain medications, because opioid prescriptions for acute and chronic LBP are often too frequent given the lack of supporting evidence.[25,29] The American College of Physicians 2017 Guidelines stated strong recommendations that clinicians and patients initially select nonpharmaceutical treatments first before using pharmacological strategies.[29] Physicians, occupational therapists, and other team members must be in frequent communication and coordination about balancing medications with therapies to allow for optimal health outcomes for the client.

Physical Therapist

The client is usually referred to PT to address pain, spasms, limited flexibility, limited strength, and posture. The PT evaluation generally includes a review of the mechanism of injury, date of injury, progression of symptoms, medical history, recent tests and procedures, medications, past treatment history, previous level of functioning, and the client's goal for therapy.

A subjective history of ADLs is reviewed. An objective examination will include analysis of posture, gait, active range of motion (ROM) of the spine, active ROM of the extremities, pelvic symmetry, signs of nerve tension, strength, reflexes and sensation, leg length, and palpation of soft tissue. On the basis of the data collected, the physical therapist develops a treatment plan that includes pain and spasm control, increased core stability and strength, exercises, improved joint mobility, and patient education. The goals of PT are to reduce symptoms and increase strength and flexibility to achieve a functional pain-free outcome for the client.

Physical therapists use dynamic lumbar stabilization (DLS) as a treatment technique that involves integration of the muscle groups that control movement of the spine and the abdominal muscles that support the back. The abdominal muscles act as a corset to support the lumbar area, and the client must learn to balance muscular function and flexibility to control the stresses that are placed on the spinal column during movement.

Pain Psychologist

We have addressed how pain and emotional health are integrally connected. Some clients, especially those with chronic pain, may require the support of a pain psychologist who can assess the person's coping skills and mental health status. Psychologists use cognitive behavioral therapy to help the patient cope with unhelpful thought processes, teach the client self-regulation techniques similar to those discussed earlier, and help the person process any anger, disbelief, or sadness surrounding pain. Psychologists can also help people better manage anxiety, depression, and other behavioral health diagnoses that may be affecting the client's pain levels and self-management capabilities.

SUMMARY

Providing effective occupational therapy for a client with LBP requires a good understanding of how anatomy, physiology, behavioral health, and lifestyle can affect pain. The ability to analyze daily occupations and keep the client at the center of treatment is crucial to attain successful outcomes. Good communication between the patient and the team and among all team members is important for reducing symptoms, integrating knowledge, and supporting the performance of meaningful occupations for a person living with LBP.

REVIEW QUESTIONS

1. Identify five ways low back pain can affect occupational engagement and daily life, physically and emotionally.
2. Identify three common causes of low back pain.
3. Define neutral spine.
4. Identify three body mechanic techniques and how they relate to anatomy.
5. Identify the occupational therapist's role in evaluation and intervention.
6. Identify five occupational therapy interventions used for patients with LBP.
7. Identify other multidisciplinary pain team members.
8. Identify the interventions used for postsurgical patients.

For additional practice questions for this chapter, please visit eBooks.Health.Elsevier.com.

REFERENCES

1. Abdallah CG, Geha P: Chronic pain and chronic stress: Two sides of the same coin? *Chronic Stress*, 2017. https://doi.org/10.1177/2470547017704763.
2. American Academy of Orthopaedic Surgeons: *Herniated disk in the lower back*, 2020, October 9, OrthoInfo. https://orthoinfo.aaos.org/en/diseases-conditions/herniated-disk-in-the-lower-back/.
3. American Academy of Orthopaedic Surgeons: *Lumbar spinal stenosis*, 2020, October 9, OrthoInfo. https://orthoinfo.aaos.org/en/diseases-conditions/lumbar-spinal-stenosis/.
4. American Academy of Orthopaedic Surgeons: *Sciatica*, 2020, October 9, OrthoInfo. https://orthoinfo.aaos.org/en/diseases-conditions/sciatica/.
5. American Academy of Orthopaedic Surgeons: *Spondylolysis and spondylolisthesis*, 2020, October 9, OrthoInfo. https://orthoinfo.aaos.org/en/diseases-conditions/spondylolysis-and-spondylolisthesis/.
6. American Occupational Therapy Association: Occupational Therapy Practice Framework: domain and Process (4th ed.), *American Journal of Occupational Therapy*, 74, 7412410010, 2020. https://doi.org/10.5014/ajot.2020.74S2001.
7. Bair MJ, Robinson RL, Katon W, Kroenke K: Depression and pain comorbidity: a literature review, *Archives of Internal Medicine* 163(20):2433–2445, 2003. https://doi.org/10.1001/archinte.163.20.2433.
8. Borenstein DG, Calin A: *Fast facts: low back pain*, ed 2, Oxford, UK, 2012, Health Press Ltd.
9. Carpenter L, Baker GA, Tyldesley B: The use of the Canadian Occupational Performance Measure as an outcome of a pain management program, *Can J Occup Ther* 68:16–22, 2001.
10. Centers for Disease Control and Prevention: *Summary health statistics: National Health Interview Survey, 2018*, 2020, October 9, National Center for Health Statistics. https://ftp.cdc.gov/pub/Health_Statistics/NCHS/NHIS/SHS/2018_SHS_Table_A-5.pdf.
11. Dahlhamer J, Lucas J, Zelaya C, Nahin R, Mackey S, DeBar L, Kerns R, Von Korff M, Porter L, Helmick C: Prevalence of chronic

pain and high-impact chronic pain among adults—United States, 2016, *MMWR Morbidity and Mortality Weekly Report (CDC)* 67(36):1001–1006, 2018. https://doi.org/10.15585/mmwr.mm6736a2.

12. Fairbank JCT, Pynsent PB: The Oswestry Disability Index, *Spine* 25(22):2940–2953, 2000.

13. Frontera WR, Bean JF, Damiano D, Ehrlich-Jones L, Fried-Oken M, Jette A, Jung R, Lieber RL, Malec JF, Mueller MJ, Ottenbacher KJ, Tansey KE, Thompson A: Rehabilitation research at the National Institutes of Health: Moving the field forward (executive summary), *American Journal of Occupational Therapy* 71(3):7103320010, 2017. https://doi.org/10.5014/ajot.2017.713003.

14. GBD 2017 Disease and Injury Incidence and Prevalence Collaborators: Global, regional, and national incidence, prevalence, and years lived with disability for 354 diseases and injuries for 195 countries and territories, 1990–2017: A systematic analysis for the Global Burden of Disease Study 2017, *Lancet* 392:1789–1858, 2018.

15. Haefeli M, Elfering A. (2006). Pain assessment. *European Spine Journal* 15 Suppl 1(Suppl 1), S17–S24. https://doi.org/10.1007/s00586-005-1044-x.

16. Hashmi JA, Baliki MN, Huang L, Baria AT, Torbey S, Hermann KM, Schnitzer TJ, Apkarian AV: Shape shifting pain: chronification of back pain shifts brain representation from nociceptive to emotional circuits, *Brain: a Journal of Neurology* 136(Pt 9):2751–2768, 2013. https://doi.org/10.1093/brain/awt211.

17. Kerrigan DA, Saltzman KN: Chapter 22: Orthopedics and musculoskeletal disorders. In Smith-Gabai H, Holm SE, editors: *Occupational Therapy in Acute Care*, ed 2. 2017, AOTA Press, 443–469. https://doi.org/10.7139/2017.978-1-56900-415-9.022.

18. Kopec JA, Esdaile JM, Abrahamowicz M, Abenhaim L, Wood-Dauphinee S, Lamping DL, Williams JI: The Quebec Back Pain Disability Scale, *Spine* 20(3):341–352, 1995.

19. Lehman L, Tetzke M, Wanniarachchi G, Wang Y, Sindhu B: Psychological factors' influence on patient-reported outcomes of outpatient rehabilitation in people with lumbar spine impairments, *American Journal of Occupational Therapy* 72(4_Supplment_1):7211515286, 2018. https://doi.org/10.5014/ajot.2018.72S1-PO7030.

20. Lo J, Chan L, Flynn S: A systematic review of the incidence, prevalence, costs, and activity and work limitations of amputation, osteoarthritis, rheumatoid arthritis, back pain, multiple sclerosis, spinal cord injury, stroke, and traumatic brain injury in the United States: A 2019 update, *Archives of Physical Medicine and Rehabilitation* 102(1):115–131, 2021, 2020. https://doi.org/10.1016/j.apmr.2020.04.001.

21. Maher C, Underwood M, Buchbinder R: Non-specific low back pain, *The Lancet* 389(10070):736–747, 2017. https://doi.org/10.1016/S0140-6736(16)30970-9.

22. McLaughlin Gray J: Putting occupation into practice: Occupation as ends, occupation as means, *American Journal of Occupational Therapy* 52:354–364, 1998. https://doi.org/10.5014/ajot.52.5.354.

23. Menezes Costa L da C, Maher CG, Hancock MJ, McAuley JH, Herbert RD, Costa LOP. The prognosis of acute and persistent low-back pain: A meta-analysis. *CMAJ*, 184(11), E613-E624. https://doi.org/10.1503/cmaj.111271.

24. Meredith PJ, Rappel G, Strong J, Bailey KJ: Sensory sensitivity and strategies for coping with pain, *American Journal of Occupational Therapy* 69(4):1–10, 6904240010, 2015. https://doi.org/10.5014/ajot.2015.014621.

25. Mikosz CA, Zhang K, Haegerich T, Xu L, Losby JL, Greenspan A, Baldwin G, Dowell D: Indication-specific opioid prescribing for US patients with Medicaid or private insurance, 2017, *JAMA Network Open* 3(5):e204514, 2020. https://doi.org/10.1001/jamanetworkopen.2020.4514.

26. National Institutes of Health, National Institute of Arthritis and Musculoskeletal and Skin Diseases. *Back Pain*, 2023. https://www.niams.nih.gov/health-topics/back-pain.

27. Nicholas MK: The pain self-efficacy questionnaire: taking pain into account, *Eur J Pain* 11:153–163, 2007.

28. Nielson WR, Jensen MP, Karsdorp PA, Vlaeyen JW: Activity pacing in chronic pain: concepts, evidence, and future directions, *The Clinical Journal of Pain* 29(5):461–468, 2013. https://doi.org/10.1097/AJP.0b013e3182608561.

29. Qaseem A, Wilt TJ, McLean RM, Forciea MA, Clinical Guidelines Committee of the American College of Physicians: Noninvasive treatments for acute, subacute, and chronic low back pain: A clinical practice guideline from the American College of Physicians, *Annals of Internal Medicine* 166(7):514–530, 2017. https://doi.org/10.7326/M16-2367.

30. Sheng J, Liu S, Wang Y, Cui R, Zhang X: The link between depression and chronic pain: Neural mechanisms in the brain, *Neural Plasticity 2017*, 9724371. 2017. https://doi.org/10.1155/2017/9724371.

31. Song CY, et al: Validation of the Brief Pain Inventory in patients with low back pain, *Spine* 41:E937–E942, 2016.

32. Stubbs B, Koyanagi A, Thompson T, Veronses N, Carvalho AF, Solomi M, Mugisha J, Schofield P, Cosco T, Wilson N, Vancampfort D: The epidemiology of back pain and its relationship with depression, psychosis, anxiety, sleep disturbances, and stress sensitivity: Data from 43 low- and middle-income countries, *General Hospital Psychiatry* 43:63–70, 2016. https://doi.org/10.1016/j.genhosppsych.2016.09.008.

33. The Roland-Morris Disability Questionnaire and the Oswestry Disability Questionnaire, *Spine*, 25:3115–3124.

34. U.S. Department of Health and Human Services Office of Disease Prevention and Health Promotion: Chronic pain, *Healthy People 2030*, 2020. https://health.gov/healthypeople/objectives-and-data/browse-objectives/chronic-pain

35. Uyeshiro Simon A, Collins CER: Lifestyle Redesign® for chronic pain management: A retrospective clinical efficacy study, *American Journal of Occupational Therapy* 71(4):7104190040, 2017. https://doi.org/10.5014/ajot.2017.025502.

36. Wang YP, Gorenstein C: Assessment of depression in medical patients: a systematic review of the utility of the Beck Depression Inventory-II, *Clinics* 68:1274–1287, 2013.

37. Weinstein F, Bernstein A, Kapenstein T, Penn E, Richeimer SH: Spirituality assessments and interventions in pain medicine, *Practical Pain Management* 14(5), 2014. https://www.practicalpainmanagement.com/treatments/psychological/spirituality-assessments-interventions-pain-medicine.

38. Wong-Baker Faces Foundation: *Wong-Baker FACES® Pain Rating Scale*, 2016. http://www.WongBakerFACES.org.

43

Burns and Burn Rehabilitation[a,b]

Dawn Kurakazu and Agnes Haruko Hirai

After studying this chapter, the student or practitioner will be able to do the following:

1. Define and identify the characteristics of the different burn depths.
2. Identify the anatomy of skin and its importance to individuals' health and well-being.
3. Understand and describe the different phases of recovery and the role of occupational therapy in each phase.
4. Understand implications of scar formation on the client's occupational roles and identity.
5. Understand the importance of early mobilization with therapy and its implications on recovery of the client's ability to perform activities of daily living.

6. Understand the complications of a severe burn injury and its implications on function in occupational roles.
7. Describe the psychological impact of burn trauma on the individual and the development of adjustment disorder and post-trauma stress disorder.
8. Describe the role of occupational therapy in a multidisciplinary team and support groups.
9. Describe the client context and its effect on occupational performance.

CHAPTER OUTLINE

---

[a] In this chapter, the terms *patient* and *client* are both used, with *client* being used in occupational therapy contexts.

[b] It is important for the reader to recognize that although the American Occupational Therapy Association, to date, does not have an official burn specialization, the American Burn Association (for the burn center verification-type of accreditation) has indicated recommendations for occupational therapists to have the following experiences to work with burn patients: extensive experience in (1) intensive care unit and acute care, (2) hand therapy, (3) pediatrics, and (4) upper and lower extremity splinting.

KEY TERMS

Allograft
Autograft
Compartment syndrome
Deep partial-thickness burn
Dermis
Epidermis
Eschar
Escharotomy
Full-thickness burn
Fasciotomy
Heterotopic ossification

Hypertrophic scar
Ischemia
Keloid scar
Scar maturation
Subdermal burn
Superficial burn
Superficial partial-thickness burn
Total body surface area
Xenograft

THREADED CASE STUDY

Ben, Part 1

Ben is a 27-year-old man (prefers use of the pronouns he/him/his) who suffered a flame burn injury to both hands, both upper extremities (UEs), face, and both lower extremities (LEs). Ben was injured when the car he was a passenger in collided with another car. The car ignited, and Ben was injured as he extricated himself from the car. The driver of the car unfortunately succumbed to her injuries. He was initially taken to a local hospital where his wounds were assessed by their emergency department (ED) physicians. He was placed on resuscitative fluids and transported to a large regional burn center for the area. On arrival, Ben was admitted to the intensive care unit (ICU) because of the suspected size of the injury. His wounds were cleaned by experienced wound care nurses and the size of the burn was determined to be 22% total body surface area (TBSA). Ben was placed on telemetry to monitor his heart rate, oxygen levels, blood pressure, and temperature for signs of hemodynamic instability. His wounds were dressed in an enzymatic debrider and antimicrobial solution to his extremities and antibiotic ointment to his face. His pain was managed initially with intravenous morphine. He received several peripheral intravenous lines, nasogastric feeding tube, and a Foley catheter.

Occupational therapy and physical therapy were ordered on admission. On initial presentation he was very quiet with a flat affect. His initial evaluation consisted of an interview, physical assessment, and medical chart review. Ben's primary occupations were identified as follows: he was employed by the Department of Veterans Affairs in logistics, and he was training to be a firefighter. He had a supportive immediate and extended family. Ben worked out regularly at home in preparation for his firefighter training. He expressed wanting to return to firefighter training as soon as he was able. Ben identified becoming a firefighter as his career goal that he has been working hard to accomplish. He had no previous medical conditions.

Ben had a cousin who was a physical therapy student. His cousin's girlfriend was an occupational therapy student, so Ben had a general idea of the role of occupational therapy in rehabilitation. The confounding factor was the acute nature of his burn injury and the pain associated with the injury. In addition to his burn injury, Ben had also lost his friend in the accident and he expressed feelings of shock and guilt during his hospitalization. The context of Ben's hospitalization was also a factor. Families and loved ones were restricted from visiting him because of the COVID-19 pandemic crisis. Therefore, Ben did not have as much social-emotional support from his family during his hospitalization.

Critical Thinking Questions

1. When should occupational therapy be initiated for optimal patient results?
2. How was the occupational role of the patient affected by his burn injuries?
3. How will the burn injury affect Ben's occupational roles and identity in the future?

As you read and learn more about burn injuries and the role of occupational therapy, consider the effect of OT intervention on this client's life. Consider both the physical and psychological effects of traumatic injuries.

Increasing numbers of individuals are surviving burn injuries that in the past would have proved fatal. Since the 1970s, advances in burn management, such as in resuscitation, early excision and grafting, and surgical critical care, have dramatically improved the percentage of survivors of severe burn injuries. With this improvement in survival comes an increased need for comprehensive burn rehabilitation. A multidisciplinary approach to burn care and rehabilitation is essential for the optimal outcome of a burn survivor.[17]

INCIDENCE OF BURN INJURIES AND BURN-RELATED DEATHS

According to the American Burn Association (ABA) it is estimated that more than 0.5 million burn injuries requiring medical treatment occur each year in the United States.[5] This represents a significant decline in the incidence of burn injuries since the early 1960s, when an estimated 2 million injuries occurred annually.[4] Total fire- and burn-related deaths are currently estimated at 4000 per year. This total includes an estimated 3500 deaths from residential fires and 500 from motor vehicle and aircraft crashes; contact with electricity, chemicals, and hot liquids or objects; and other sources of burn injury.[3] Fire- and burn-related deaths in the United States continue to decline. Burn prevention and fire safety measures have reduced the incidence of severe burn injury to the extent that burn centers are now admitting greater numbers of patients with less severe burns and fewer large, deep burns.[3,6,22]

Since the early 1970s, advances in the medical, surgical, and rehabilitative management of individuals who sustain burns have expanded the focus of burn care professionals from simply ensuring patient survival to include regaining quality of life and the previous life context after a burn injury. Functional recovery can be a long and arduous process, but burn survivors can resume their meaningful occupations and roles with the right interventions. From the date of injury through the outpatient phase of care, a multidisciplinary team approach is necessary to effectively manage the medical, functional, and psychosocial problems encountered during recovery.[2,17,97]

SKIN ANATOMY

The skin is the largest organ of the body. It varies greatly in thickness, flexibility, presence and amount of hair, degree of

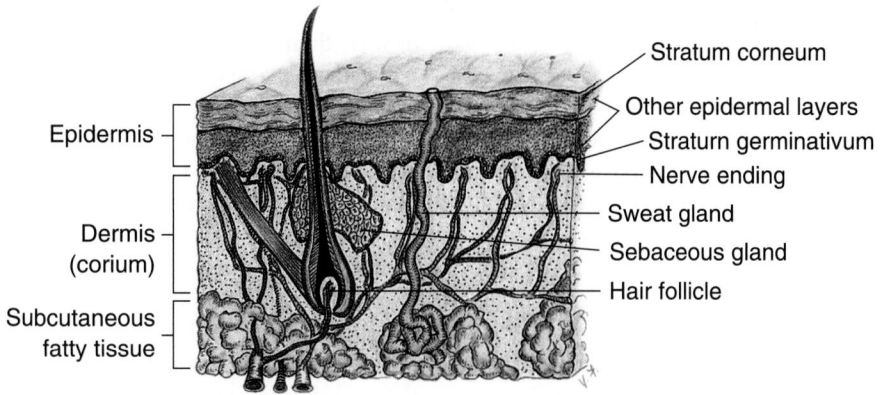

Fig. 43.1 Cross section of the skin. (From Potter PA, et al: *Fundamentals of nursing*, ed 11, St. Louis, 2023, Elsevier.)

pigmentation, vascularity, nerve supply and sensitivity, amount of keratin, and types of glands present in different locations. Keratin is the tough protein substance present in skin and also forms the primary elements of hair, nails, and callused areas of the skin on the hands and feet. Most of the body is covered with thin, hairy skin. However, thicker, tougher, hairless skin, known as glabrous skin, covers the soles of the feet and the palmar surfaces of the hand and fingers.

Anatomically, the skin consists primarily of two layers: the dermis and the epidermis (Fig. 43.1). The **dermis**, or corium, is composed of fibrous connective tissue made of collagen and elastin and contains numerous capillaries, lymphatics, and nerve endings. In it are the hair follicles and their smooth muscle fibers, sebaceous glands, and sweat glands and their ducts.

The **epidermis** is the outermost layer of epithelium, and it also lines the nail beds and the skin appendages, which are pockets of epithelium that extend down into the dermis and contain the hair follicles, sweat glands, and sebaceous glands. The epidermis consists of four or five layers, depending on the location and type of skin. The innermost layer of the epidermis is the stratum germinativum, where the keratinocytes that synthesize keratin are formed. Above this layer lies the stratum spinosum, in which the progressive stages of keratinization occur. The keratinocytes in this layer have a well-developed capacity for phagocytosis, which helps control infection by ingesting and breaking down bacteria and particulate debris. Melanin granules, which give the skin and hair their color, are present in the cytoplasm of certain cells in the stratum spinosum. In the next layer, the stratum granulosum, the cells making their way toward the surface become flattened and accumulate many large keratin granules, termed keratohyalin. In this layer, cells lose their nucleus, change from viable to nonviable, and become a cornified layer composed chiefly of keratin filaments. Above this layer is the stratum lucidum, seen best in glabrous skin, which is thicker. The outermost layer, the stratum corneum, is composed of tightly packed dead keratinocytes known as squames that become the cornified, flattened skin cells that eventually separate from one another and detach from the surface of the epidermis. The time taken by a newly formed keratinocyte to pass from the deepest layer to the surface to be shed is estimated to be 45 to 75 days. This is the natural manner in which the epidermis continually renews itself.[80]

SKIN FUNCTION

The skin serves as an environmental barrier that protects against ultraviolet rays, chemical contamination, and bacterial invasion. It also serves as a moisture barrier to prevent excessive absorption of moisture or evaporative loss. Temperature regulation is also a function of the skin, with hair to insulate and perspiration to cool the body. The skin perceives injury or infection through tactile sensory receptors located in the dermis layer of the skin. These receptors heighten environmental awareness through perceived touch, pressure, pain, and temperature. When the skin is damaged, various systemic, physiological, and functional problems can occur. A burn injury causes destruction of the protective environmental barrier, which results in exposed nerve endings, loss of body heat, seepage of body fluids, and exposure to bacterial invasion.

The skin also influences the development of an individual's body image and personal identity and enhances nonverbal social interaction.[33] Along with age, gender, body type, and voice, the skin's scent, texture, and coloration and the appearance of facial features contribute strongly to a person's external context (physical) and self-concept–related internal contexts (e.g., body image, self-regard, and sense of social and cultural acceptance). Because of all these factors, a large burn injury is considered to be one of the most physically and psychologically painful forms of trauma.

After a burn injury, many factors are taken into consideration in determining the severity of injury, potential for functional recovery, and treatment needs. Primary considerations in evaluating burn wounds are the mechanism of injury, the depth and extent of the burn, specific body areas burned, and associated or concurrent injuries such as inhalation injury and fractures. The individual's age, medical history, preinjury health, and previous life contexts are of equal importance in determining the impact of a serious burn injury on future occupational performance and occupational roles.

MECHANISM OF INJURY AND BURN DEPTH

Burns can be thermal, chemical, or electrical and can be caused by flame, steam, hot liquids, hot surfaces, and radiation.[100] The severity of the injury depends on the area of the body exposed and the duration and intensity of thermal exposure. Thermal burns can be caused by heat in the form of flame, steam, hot liquids, or hot objects. The type of fluid or type of object is important to assess; for example, hot oil boils at a higher temperature than water and retains heat for a longer time, resulting in a deeper burn injury, and objects heated for construction or industrial purposes are often hotter than household items. Thermal burns also can be caused by excessive cold such as in dry ice. Electrical burns often have the appearance of being a small burn with an entrance and exit wound, but this burn injury can be deceptive as the electrical current can cause damage beneath the skin through soft tissue, burning the patient from within. Electrical burns can also affect the heart, and these patients require monitoring for 24 hours with an electrocardiogram to determine that the current did not damage their heart. Chemical burns can often be deep, requiring that the patient be washed with a neutralizing agent. Patients suffering from chemical burns are often asked for the name or type of substance they were using. This information assists the burn team, especially the pharmacist, in identifying the correct neutralizing agent.

Approximately 10 years ago, the American Burn Association made a change to the classification of burn injuries to reflect a description of the burn depth. In the literature, a therapist may see both types of classifications used so it is important to be familiar with both systems. Burn wounds are classified by depth, which is determined by clinical assessment of the appearance, sensitivity, and pliability of the wound.[6]

Burn injuries were traditionally classified as first, second, third, and fourth degree. They are now classified as superficial, superficial partial thickness, deep partial thickness, full thickness, and subdermal.[42] The depth of injury is established by clinical determination of which anatomic layers of the skin are involved.[84]

A superficial burn, previously referred to as a first-degree burn, involves only the upper layers of the epidermis. Damage through the epidermis and upper third of the dermis is referred to as a superficial partial-thickness burn. The term deep partial-thickness burn describes damage to the epidermis and upper two thirds of the dermis, and a full-thickness burn describes an injury that extends down through the entire dermis. A subdermal burn involves the fatty layer, fascia, muscle, tendon, bone, or other subdermal tissues (e.g., those seen in electrical injuries; Table 43.1).

Superficial burns are usually caused by sun exposure or brief contact with rapidly cooling hot fluids or surfaces (e.g., spilled coffee or a hot pan). Superficial partial-thickness burns are typically caused by prolonged sun exposure, contact with flames, or brief contact with hot viscous liquids (Fig. 43.2, A). Deep partial-thickness burns (see Fig. 43.2, B) are caused by longer exposure to intense heat, such as immersion in hot water or contact of the skin with flaming material. Full-thickness burns usually result from prolonged immersion scalding, contact with flaming or high-temperature viscous material such as hot grease or melted tar, extended exposure to chemical agents, and contact with electrical current (see Fig. 43.2, C).

Superficial partial-thickness and deep partial-thickness burns generally heal without surgical intervention. However, once healed, they tend to be excessively dry, itchy, and subsequently susceptible to excoriation (i.e., abrasion or tearing of the skin surface) secondary to shear forces caused by rubbing, scratching, and other trauma. These shear forces can give rise to blisters and compromise long-term skin integrity as a result of repetitious reopening of the wound. Partial-thickness and full-thickness burns usually lead to uneven pigmentation of the healed scar. Deep partial- and full-thickness burns have a greater potential for thick, hypertrophic scar and contracture formation because of the prolonged healing period. This is especially true if a burn converts from partial thickness to full thickness because of infection or repeated trauma. Most full-thickness wounds require surgical intervention or skin grafting for wound closure. Skin graft donor sites generally heal in the same manner that superficial partial-thickness burns do, with less scarring but uneven pigmentation.

In the case study, Ben's burn injuries were a mix of superficial-partial thickness, deep partial, and full-thickness injuries. A large surface area of Ben's injuries required surgical management with skin grafting. This placed him at risk for hypertrophic scar development.[41]

PERCENTAGE OF TOTAL BODY SURFACE AREA INVOLVED

The extent of a burn is classified as a percentage of the total body surface area (%TBSA) burned. The two most common methods for estimating %TBSA are the "rule of nines" and the Lund and Browder chart.[22,54] The rule of nines divides the body surface into areas consisting of 9%, or multiples of 9%, with the perineum making up the final 1%. The head and neck area are 9%, each upper extremity (UE) is 9%, each lower extremity is 18%, and the front and back of the trunk are each 18%. Body proportions vary in children, depending on their age, especially in the head and legs (Fig. 43.3). The Lund and Browder chart[50] provides a more accurate estimate of TBSA and is used in most burn centers. This chart assigns a percentage of surface area to body segments (Fig. 43.4), with the calculations adjusted for different age groups.[68] Computer programs now exist to help clinicians calculate TBSA for a patient. For smaller %TBSA injuries, the therapist can obtain a quick, rough estimate by using the size of the patient's palm (the hand excluding the fingers) to equal approximately 1% of the individual's TBSA.[22]

Ben's burn injury that was initially determined at the outside ED was deemed smaller than it was when measured by the experienced burn physician. This is not uncommon because burn wounds are often larger after the patient's wounds have been debrided of the dead tissue. Calculation of the correct TBSA for a burn patient is an essential lifesaving measure that allows the patient to receive the correct amount of resuscitative fluids, medications, and monitoring to prevent further tissue damage, sepsis, and possible death.

TABLE 43.1   Burn Wound Characteristics

Burn Depth	Common Causes	Tissue Depth	Clinical Findings	Healing Time	Scar Potential
Superficial	Sunburn, brief flash burns, brief exposure to hot liquids or chemicals	Superficial epidermis	Erythema, dry, no blisters, short-term moderate pain	3–7 days	No potential for hypertrophic scar or contractures
Superficial partial thickness and donor sites	Severe sunburn or radiation burn, flash, prolonged exposure to hot liquids, brief contact with hot metal objects	Epidermis, upper dermis	Erythema, wet, blisters; significant pain	Less than 2 weeks	Minimal potential for hypertrophy or contractures if healing is not delayed by secondary infection or further trauma
Deep partial thickness	Flames; firm or prolonged contact with hot metal objects; prolonged contact with hot, viscous liquids	Epidermis and much of the dermis nonviable, but survival of skin appendages from which skin may regenerate	Erythema; larger, usually broken blisters on skin with hair; on glabrous skin of the palms and soles of the feet; large, possibly intact blisters over beefy red dermis; severe pain to even light touch	Longer than 2 weeks, may convert to full thickness with onset of infection	High potential for hypertrophic scarring and contractures across joints, web spaces, and facial contours; high risk for boutonnière deformities if the dorsal surface of fingers involved
Full thickness	Extreme heat or prolonged exposure to heat, hot objects, or chemicals for extended periods	Epidermis and dermis: nonviable skin appendages and nerve endings	Pale, nonblanching, dry, coagulated capillaries possible; no sensation to light touch except at deep partial-thickness borders	Surgical intervention required for wound closure in larger areas; possible for smaller areas to heal inward from borders over extended period	Extremely high potential for hypertrophic scarring or contractures, depending on the method used for wound closure
Full thickness with complications	Electrical burns and severe long-duration burns (e.g., house fires, entrapment in or under a burning motor vehicle or hot exhaust system, smoking in bed or alcohol-related burns)	Full thickness burns with damage to underlying tissue	Possible charring of nonviable surface or, with exposed fat, possible presence of small external wounds on tendons, muscles; with electrical injuries, possibility for small external wounds with significant secondary loss of subdermal tissue and peripheral nerve damage	Requires surgical intervention for wound closure; may require amputation or significant reconstruction	Similar to full thickness burns except when amputation removes the burn site

It is also important as a clinician to understand that the %TBSA of the burn injury will change as the burn injury evolves and fully declares itself in the first 24 to 48 hours.[41] Also to be considered in the case of burn patients that require surgical interventions is that the donor site for surgery adds to the percentage of open wound even though it is not a part of the actual burn injury. This is important for nutritional optimization, wound dressings, functional outcomes, and discharge planning.

In severe cases with large surface area burn injuries, such as Ben's, the donor site must come from whatever intact skin is available. With smaller burn injuries, careful selection of the donor site can help to match the skin to the recipient area better, allowing the donor site scar to be hidden by clothing. This careful selection can be aided by the occupational history provided by the OT to provide more individualized care and greater patient satisfaction.

SEVERITY OF INJURY

The severity of a burn injury is determined by many factors. The size, depth, and location of the injury are of primary concern in a burn-injured patient, but other factors such as a patient's age, previous medical history, social support and resources, functional ability, and pain are also important for determination of admission to a burn center as well as the individual's ability to recover. Usually a burn of 10% or greater with a superficial partial- to full-thickness injury is cause for admission because it will require monitoring by the medical team.[3,22] However, burn centers will at times admit patients with smaller burns if the patient has premorbid conditions that increase the risk of complications, risk of an associated injury or infection, or, the patient's functional ability is severely impaired (i.e., the patient is unable to dress or feed oneself due to an UE burn injury).[3,22]

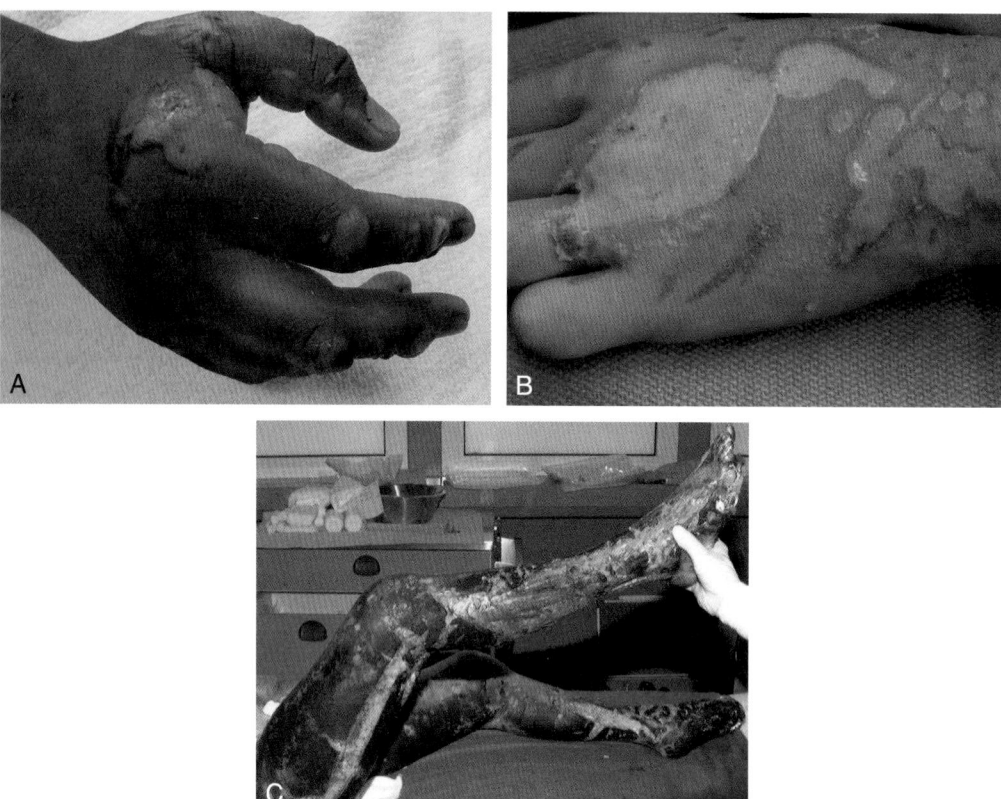

Fig. 43.2 (A) Superficial partial-thickness burns are wet and painful with characteristic fluid-filled blisters. (B) Deep partial-thickness injury. Note the moist open wound. (C) Full-thickness injury with thick adherent eschar. (C, From Song DH, Neligan PC, editors: *Plastic surgery*, ed 3, London, 2013, Saunders.)

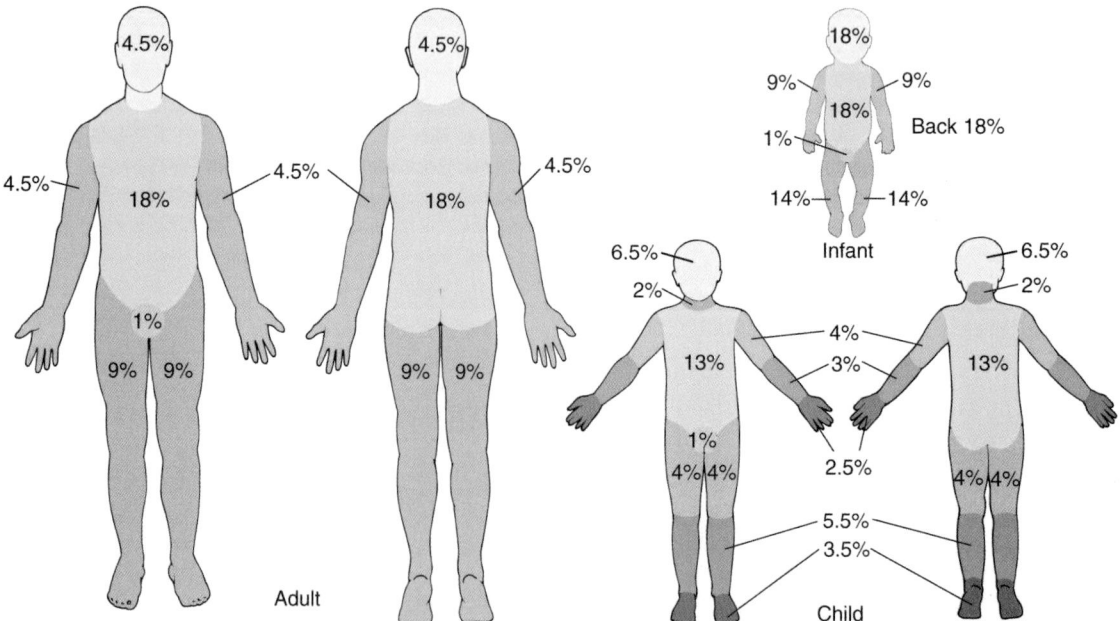

Fig. 43.3 Rule of nines. Proportions for adults/adolescents, children, and infants are shown. Note the relatively greater surface area of the head and slightly lesser surface area of the lower extremities in young children than in adults. (From Lovaasen KR: *ICD-10-CM/PCS coding: theory and practice*, St. Louis, 2016, Elsevier.)

Burns that are partial-thickness, deep partial-thickness, or full-thickness injuries that are larger than 15% to 20% usually require a period of hospitalization that includes complex wound care, fluid resuscitation, medical monitoring, pain management, nutritional optimization, and rehabilitation.[100] The burn injury becomes more severe if the person sustains an inhalational injury in addition to the cutaneous burn injury.

Modified Lund and Browder Chart						% Partial-thickness	% Full-thickness	% Total
Area	Age (Years)							
	0-1	1-4	5-9	10-15	Adult			
Head	19	17	13	10	7			
Neck	2	2	2	2	2			
Ant. trunk	13	13	13	13	13			
Post. trunk	13	13	13	13	13			
R. buttock	2.5	2.5	2.5	2.5	2.5			
L. buttock	2.5	2.5	2.5	2.5	2.5			
Genitalia	1	1	1	1	1			
R. U. arm	4	4	4	4	4			
L. U. arm	4	4	4	4	4			
R. L. arm	3	3	3	3	3			
L. L. arm	3	3	3	3	3			
R. hand	2.5	2.5	2.5	2.5	2.5			
L. hand	2.5	2.5	2.5	2.5	2.5			
R. thigh	5.5	6.5	8.5	8.5	9.5			
L. thigh	5.5	6.5	8.5	8.5	9.5			
R. leg	5	5	5.5	6	7			
L. leg	5	5	5.5	6	7			
R. foot	3.5	3.5	3.5	3.5	3.5			
L. foot	3.5	3.5	3.5	3.5	3.5			
					Total			

Fig. 43.4 Modified Lund and Browder chart. Burn size can be determined most accurately in children by using the Lund and Browder chart, which accounts for changes in the size of body parts that occur with growth. (Modified from Lund CC, Browder NC: The estimation of areas of burns, *Surg Gynecol Obstet* 79:352, 1944.)

Ben's injuries to his arms and legs were full thickness that required surgery. Ben was provided daily evaluations of his wounds and complex wound care to determine his need for surgery and level of surgical intervention. Once surgery was decided upon, the multidisciplinary team, including the OT discussed the surgical plan and intraoperative and postoperative therapy needs.

Burns of less than 15% TBSA that are partial-thickness injuries not requiring surgery can be treated on an outpatient basis as long as the patient has adequate resources, social supports to provide optimal wound care, pain management, nutritional support and functional mobility, and participation in activities of daily living (ADLs) at home.

A patient's medical history will also affect his or her ability to recover from a burn injury, even one that is relatively small. A patient's comorbidities will increase mortality in burn-injured patients. Chronic conditions that are cardiovascular, neurological, renal, endocrine, or pulmonary will increase the likelihood of poor outcomes and or death, especially in the presence of a cutaneous injury or inhalation injury.[58,87]

Because Ben had no previous medical history and was a healthy young individual, his healing progressed without complications. Importantly, he was able to avoid life-threatening complications such as sepsis.[61]

PHASES OF WOUND HEALING

Wound healing takes place in four overlapping phases: hemostasis, the inflammatory phase, the proliferation phase, and the maturation/remodeling phase.

Hemostasis

Hemostasis occurs immediately after the burn. It is characterized by vasocontriction, platelet aggregation and the release of clotting factors. This is the body's response to stop the bleeding at the injury site. This phase lasts approximately 24 hours.[16]

Inflammatory Phase

The inflammatory phase usually lasts 24 hours and can last for days to weeks depending on the severity of the injury. This phase is characterized by a vascular and cellular response, with neutrophils and monocytes migrating to the wound to attack bacteria, debride the wound, and initiate the healing process. The wound is typically painful, warm, and erythematous (red), and edema develops.[16]

During the inflammatory phase, Ben's ability to move and function normally was impaired by severe pain, moderate edema, and bulky dressings to his injuries. The focus of therapy was on edema control, mobility, and reengagement in basic ADLs to mitigate pain and adapt to a new context of functioning.

Proliferation Phase

The proliferation phase begins by the third day after the injury and lasts until the wound heals. It is during this phase that revascularization, reepithelization, and contraction of the burn wound take place. Endothelial cells bud at the end of capillaries, and they grow and create a vascular bed for new skin growth. Epithelial cells migrate over the vascular bed to form a new skin layer. Fibroblasts deposit collagen fibers, which contract to reduce wound size. During this phase the wound remains erythemic, and raised, rigid scars may develop. The tensile strength of the newly healed scars is poor, and they are easily excoriated or injured.[16]

Maturation/Remodeling Phase

The maturation/remodeling phase generally begins by the third week after initial healing and may last from 6 months to 2 or more years after the initial burn injury or the date of the last reconstructive surgical procedure.[16] During this phase, the fibroblasts leave, and collagen remodeling takes place. The erythema fades, and the scar softens and flattens. The tensile strength of the scars increases but never recovers to more than 80% of the original tensile strength of the unburned skin.

Scar Formation

After initial healing, most burn wounds have an erythematous, flat appearance. As the healing process continues, the wound's appearance may change as a result of scar hypertrophy and contraction. The long-term quality of a mature burn scar can be affected by numerous factors, some of which occur during the early phases of burn care.[83] The amount of time needed to achieve wound closure is a strong determinant. Any factor such as patient age, race, burn depth, infection, or any other condition that could delay healing will increase the potential for scarring.

Hypertrophic scars are thick, rigid, erythematous scars that become apparent 6 to 8 weeks after wound closure.[93] Histologically, these immature scars have increased vascularity, fibroblasts, myofibroblasts, mast cells, and collagen fibers arranged in whorls or nodules that make the scar appear raised and rigid.[93] Biochemical investigations have discovered increased synthesis of collagen fibers and connective tissue in hypertrophic scars. As a hypertrophic scar matures, capillaries, fibroblasts, and myofibroblasts decrease significantly, collagen fibers relax into parallel bands, and the scar becomes flatter and more pliable.[16] The time needed for scars to mature differs markedly among individuals and depends on genetics, the age of the patient, the location and depth of the original burn wound, the presence of chronic inflammation, wound contamination, and other factors that have been reported to influence hypertrophic scarring.[16] Superficial burns that heal in less than 2 weeks will not generally form a hypertrophic scar. Deeper burns that take longer than 2 weeks to heal have a greater potential to form hypertrophic scars. Although most hypertrophic scars mature in 6 to 24 months,[16] excessive scar formation, including keloid scars, may take up to 3 years to mature (Fig. 43.5). All three subjects in the case studies were of different age groups and ethnic/genetic backgrounds and had different OT interventions.

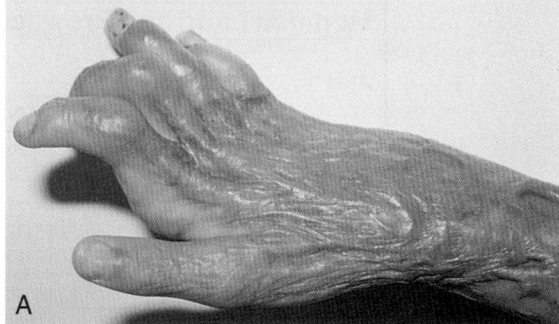
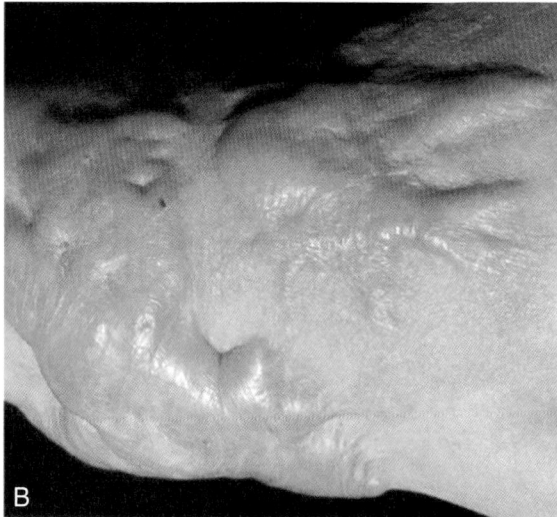

Fig. 43.5 (A) Hypertrophic scars to the dorsum of the hand and in the web spaces of the hand result in a limited ability to grasp objects and impair fine motor function. (B) Severe keloid scars usually require surgical removal and aggressive compression therapy to help prevent recurrence. (A, Courtesy Michael Peck, MD, University of North Carolina Burn Center, Chapel Hill; in Banasik JL: *Pathophysiology*, ed 7, St. Louis, 2022, Elsevier. B, From Lafleur Brooks M, LaFleur Brooks D: *Exploring medical language: a student-directed approach*, ed 11, St. Louis, 2022, Elsevier.)

Nevertheless, they all experienced serious scarring as a result of their burns.

All scars initially have increased vascularity and a red appearance. Scars that remain erythematous for longer than 2 months are more likely to develop into hypertrophic scars. They become progressively firmer and thicker and rise above the original surface level of the skin. There is a marked increase in the production of fibroblasts, myofibroblasts, collagen, and interstitial material, all with contractile properties that help draw together the borders of a wound but can also result in scar tightness. Pain and skin tightness cause most patients to become less active. These patients prefer to rest in a flexed, adducted position for comfort. This allows the new collagen fibers in the wound to link and fuse together in the contracted position. The fibers become progressively more compact and coil up into the whorls and nodules that give the scar surface the textured appearance that often leads to disfigurement.[93] If the scar extends over one or more joints, the progressive tightness leads to a scar contracture and loss of motion. Fortunately, collagen linkage is less stable in new scars, and restructuring of an immature hypertrophic scar contracture can be influenced by sustained mechanical forces such as proper positioning, exercise, splinting, and compression. Scar hypertrophy and contracture are most active for the initial 4 to 6 months after healing.

Keloid scars are thick and raised scars that extend outside of the boundary of the initial injury.[89] They can be unsightly and may take longer than a hypertrophic scar to mature fully. Some races are more likely to form both keloid and hypertrophic scars.[89] If the patient tends to form keloid-type scars, it is important for the treating therapist to be aware of this possibility, because the scars may disrupt daily functional movement more quickly than non–keloid-forming individuals.

At the time of Ben's discharge from the hospital he had a wound burden of less than 5%. It was too early in the healing and scar maturation process to determine the development of hypertrophic scars. Ben will continue to be followed by a qualified burn center or at an experienced private plastic surgeon's office to monitor his healing skin for scar formation and treatment as necessary. In the meantime, he received education by the occupational therapist on the importance of caring for his newly healed skin. In addition to an extensive home exercise program to stretch his skin and maintain normal range of motion (ROM), he was provided instruction on moisturizing his healed skin/scar and protecting his skin/scar from the sun. These education points will allow Ben to protect his skin and allow for its natural improvement in color, texture, and elasticity. Optimizing the appearance of newly healed skin can be important for clients of all ages and cultural backgrounds and should be considered when forming a treatment plan.

Many burn survivors express apprehension about leaving the house to reintegrate into normal social, avocational, and occupational tasks.[11] Consequently, they can be housebound because they want to avoid being seen in public. A significant number of burn survivors describe their regular burn clinic visit as the only time they leave their home during the day. This can foster feelings of isolation and create a barrier to the burn survivor's inclination to reengage in social activities and occupational roles.[11]

The psychological impact of scar formation can be long-lasting.[51] The patient will bear the scars of the burn for his or her whole life. They are very evident and unmistakable, especially in highly visible areas such as the hands, face, and neck. Occupational therapists working in burn care are uniquely qualified to address these issues because of their background in psychology as well as their understanding of physical disabilities. With care and support the burn survivor can find a sense of self-efficacy, self-worth, and self-sufficiency by reengaging in normal daily occupations. By reconnecting them with their occupational roles and identities, occupational therapists help burn survivors to adjust to their environment and reintegration into society.

INITIAL MEDICAL MANAGEMENT (EMERGENT PHASE)

Fluid Resuscitation and Edema

Immediately after a burn injury, during the inflammatory phase, the permeability of blood vessels increases. This causes rapid leakage of protein-rich intravascular fluid into the surrounding extravascular tissues.[59,92] In larger burns, extensive loss of intravascular fluid can result in hypovolemia or burn shock because of decreased plasma and blood volumes and reduced cardiac output.[22] Fluid resuscitation with an intravenous fluid such as lactated Ringer solution is essential for promptly replacing venous fluid and electrolytes. The fluid volume required is determined by various formulas, such as the Parkland and modified Brook formulas,[22] and is based on the extent of the burn and weight of the patient.

The lymphatic system, which normally carries excess tissue fluid away, often becomes overloaded, and subcutaneous edema develops. With circumferential full-thickness burns, loss of elasticity of the burned skin combined with increased edema can cause compartment syndrome, a condition in which interstitial pressure becomes severe enough to compress blood vessels, tendons, or nerves, which could result in secondary tissue damage.[22] When blood vessels are compressed, ischemia, or restriction of circulation, could lead to tissue death in the areas of compromised circulation or even the entire distal end of the extremity. Tight burned tissue can also restrict chest expansion during respiration. Escharotomy, or incision through the necrotic burned tissue, is performed to release the binding effect of the tight eschar (adherent dead tissue that forms on skin with deep partial-thickness or full-thickness burns), relieve the interstitial pressure, and restore the distal circulation (Fig. 43.6, A). In deeper wounds, an incision down to and through the muscle fascia, or fasciotomy, may be required to achieve adequate relief of pressure (see Fig. 43.6, B).

Respiratory Management

A smoke inhalation injury is a common secondary diagnosis with a thermal injury and can significantly increase mortality. When the face is burned, and the burn was caused by a fire in an enclosed space, or when other objective evidence of a possible inhalation injury is present, bronchoscopy, arterial blood gas readings, and chest x-ray examinations are used to confirm the diagnosis.[100] Intubation and mechanical ventilatory support may be required in addition to vigorous respiratory therapy. A tracheostomy is performed if the airway is difficult to maintain or if ventilatory support is prolonged.[41] This procedure, which involves surgical incision through the trachea and relocation of the ventilation tube to the neck, is more comfortable for the patient, allows oral care, and helps prevent permanent damage to the larynx or vocal cords, which may occur with extended oral intubation.

Wound Care and Infection Control (Emergent to Acute Phases)

After a patent airway and fluid resuscitation have been established, attention is directed to wound care.[41] The burn injury itself can be a complex and dynamic injury that requires specialized wound care. The burn injury will often convert or change over time revealing a wound that may be deeper or larger than initially thought. The initial burn injury is thought to declare itself in the first 48 hours if the patient is a healthy, well-nourished individual and received adequate resuscitation at the time of the initial injury.[41] If the patient was not resuscitated properly,

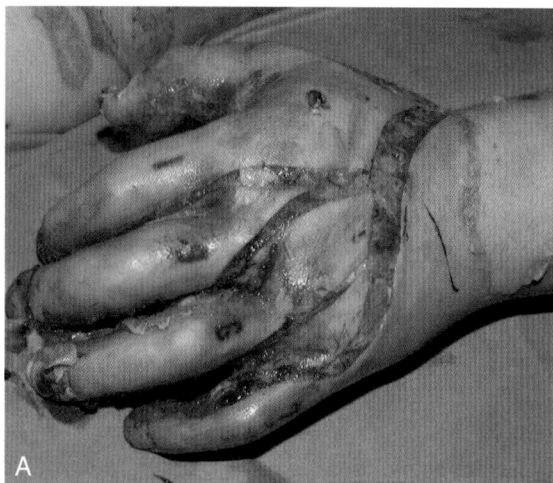

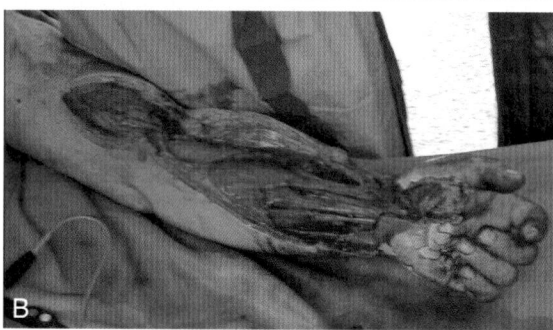

Fig. 43.6 (A) Escharotomies performed on the dorsal surface of a hand with full-thickness burns. (B) Electrical injury requiring fasciotomy, which will allow the muscle belly of the forearm to expand and prevent loss of blood flow to the hand. Note the distances between the edges of the incisions. (A, From Song DH, Neligan PC, editors: *Plastic surgery*, ed 3, London, 2013, Saunders. B, From Herndon DN: *Total burn care*, ed 4, Edinburgh, 2012, Saunders.)

experienced delayed treatment of the burn injury, received inappropriate wound care, or was malnourished, the wounds may continue to worsen and may fail to heal. This leaves the patient at increased risk of infection, hypertrophic scar formation, and requiring surgery for wound closure.

Wound treatment may involve a combination of surgical and nonsurgical therapy.[41] Nonsurgical treatment involves the use of products to promote healing in a partial thickness wound. These products are usually in the form of topical antibiotics, biological dressings, and nonbiological skin substitute dressings.

Daily wound care was a main component of Ben's care in the burn unit. Wound care consisted of hydrotherapy once daily by manual debridement and application of antimicrobial wound care products with occlusive dressings. Wound care is a great source of pain and anxiety for most all burn injured patients. Inadequate pain management combined with the shock and uncertainty of an acute injury can create additional psychosocial stressors on the burn patient.[11,85] These additional stressors can lead to exacerbations of psychiatric issues in patients with a history of psychiatric vulnerabilities. Psychological support is essential and required for comprehensive care of a burn patient.

Topical Antimicrobial Agents

Topical antimicrobials are an integral part of wound care for burn injured clients.[60] There are a variety of different topical antimicrobials that are in use in burn centers throughout the world. It is essential for OTs treating in a burn center to be familiar with the different products used in their facility. There are many different antimicrobial products, and each burn center will decide on the products that are used in their unit based on the collective experience and availability of products.[60] Different antimicrobial products have different properties that may have an impact on functional movement. This knowledge enables the OT to assist the multidisciplinary team to select the appropriate antimicrobial dressing for a client. For example, a client who is living in temporary housing with limited resources may benefit from an antimicrobial dressing that does not require changing for several days.

In Ben's case, his acute injury was initially indeterminate. He required daily dressing changes to debride the wound to try to allow for optimal cell migration while providing antimicrobial protection to prevent infection and sepsis. After approximately 3 to 5 days, Ben's wound was observed to be deep partial to full thickness and requiring surgery. He continued to require antimicrobial dressings before and after surgery to continue to protect him from infection to ensure the optimal healing environment.

Topical antimicrobial agents have been shown to decrease wound-related infections and morbidity in burn wounds when used appropriately.[60] The goal of topical antimicrobial therapy is to control microbial colonization, thereby preventing the development of invasive infections.

An ever-increasing variety of topical antimicrobials are used for burn wound care.[19] The following are several classes of topical antimicrobials used.

Antibiotic ointments.   Neomycin/polymyxin B/bacitracin antibiotic ointments are often used for facial and superficial burns. The ointment is applied, and the burn wound is left open. Mupirocin (Bactroban, GlaxoSmithKline) is an agent used to treat wounds infected with methicillin-resistant *Staphylococcus aureus* and *Staphylococcus pyogenes*.[19,85] Both of these are used in daily wound care/dressing changes.

Antimicrobial solutions.   Mafenide acetate (Sulfamylon, UDL Laboratories, Inc.) is a topical solution and creams that are used to prevent infection.[19] Mafenide hydrochloride cream is hyperosmolar and can be painful when applied to larger areas. However, it is often used on the ears, where it can penetrate eschar to prevent chondritis, or inflammation of the ear cartilage. Vashe irrigation or hypocholorus acid solution is a product that inhibits the growth of bacteria. It is noncytotoxic, removes microorganisms, aids in removal of pseudo-eschar, and assists in wound debridement.[91]

Antifungals.   Nystatin (Nilstat, Lederle Laboratories) may be used in combination with other topical agents for fungal infections caused by secondary immunosuppression. These fungal infections are often caused by long-term antibacterial use, usually originate in the gastrointestinal tract, and can be life threatening if they infect burns covering a large surface area or invade the bloodstream.

Silver solutions. With the improved resuscitation measures developed for burns in the 1960s, infection became the predominant cause of morbidity and mortality. Silver salts and other chemically active silver compounds have been used in various forms because of their potent antimicrobial properties and ability to reduce burn wound infection. These substances have included silver colloidal solution, which was later replaced by silver nitrate solution, and silver sulfadiazine. Silver sulfadiazine is a water-soluble cream that is usually applied one or two times a day to the wound surface, as opposed to the continuous soaking required with silver nitrate.[19,24]

Enzymatic wound debriders. Enzymatic wound debriders are substances that use enzymes to aid in debridement. These products assist in removing dead tissue from a burn wound by affecting the denatured collagen bonds. Removal of dead tissue decreases the likelihood of infection and can speed up the healing process.[78]

Major technological advances have resulted in the ability to crystallize silver in a nanocrystal form, which can release pure silver onto a wound surface in large quantities. This silver nanocrystalline delivery system is a three-ply dressing that may consist of an inner rayon/polyester core between two layers of silver-coated mesh.[12,19] Silver-infused dressings are also available in fabric-mesh or foam form. The ionic silver and silver radicals are released in high concentration when exposed to water. A layer between the wound and silver membrane maintains moisture for healing and decreases the formation of exudate.[19] The dressings, applied directly to the wound surface, promote healing by stimulating cellular dedifferentiation, followed by cellular proliferation. The dressings also have antibacterial, antifungal, and analgesic properties. These dressings have been found to be highly microbicidal against aerobic and anaerobic bacteria (including antibiotic-resistant strains), yeasts, and filamentous fungi,[19] and can remain active and in place for up to 7 days instead of having to be changed every 12 to 24 hours.

Mepilex (Mölnlycke Health Care, Norcross, Georgia) is a silver-infused foam dressing that adheres to the area of the burn injury by a light adhesive. It can stay in place for 7 to 10 days. It provides antimicrobial coverage, and the foam is light and allows for movement of extremities. It is an expensive product, which can affect a burn unit's decision to use it. It is a very good product for children because it is comfortable and does not require a painful dressing change to be done at home. Additional support is provided by using Kerlix wrapping to secure it to the patient and then burn netting to hold the dressing together. It is most effective with superficial partial-thickness injuries (https://www.Molnlycke.us).[55]

Another silver-infused dressing is Acticote[82] (Smith & Nephew, Andover, Maryland) and KerraContact Ag (3M-KCI, St. Paul, Minnesota) dressing. This product is a silver-infused mesh that can be secured to the patient with Kerlix wrap and burn net. Because it is a fabric, it is moldable and able to be secured over joints easily. It requires a light irrigation with water to release the silver into the wound and also to prevent the dressing from adhering to the wound bed and causing pain during movement. These products can be used in preoperative and postoperative periods as burn dressing. These can be effective for up to 5 to 7 days between dressing changes.[82]

Biologic Dressings and Biosynthetic Products

Biologic dressings serve as temporary coverings to close a wound, prevent contamination, reduce fluid loss, and alleviate pain.[23] Theoretically, biological products may deliver growth factors to a wound as well. Traditional biological dressings, such as xenografts (porcine skin) and allografts (human cadaver skin), are still widely used in burn care. Xenografts may adhere to the superficial surface film of partial thickness burns and facilitate debridement of eschar.

Closure of wounds with these dressings mitigates the inflammatory process leading to less pain, faster skin regrowth, and therefore less scarring. They are used until the wound is clean and the wound bed is well vascularized and ready for a skin graft. Typically, biosynthetic dressings are left on from several days to weeks, thereby limiting painful wound care procedures while providing an antimicrobial barrier. Biobrane, a biosynthetic skin substitute wound-dressing sheet, has been used extensively. It is constructed of an outer silicone film (the epidermal analogue) with a nylon fabric partially embedded into the film collagen (https://www.smith-nephew.com).[82] The nylon components bind to the wound surface fibrin and collagen, which results in initial adherence (dermal analogue). Small pores are present in the structure to allow drainage of exudate and increase the permeability to topical antibiotics.[82]

Integra (Integra LifeSciences Corporation, Princeton, New Jersey) is a biosynthetic wound dressing that is made up of an outer semipermeable silicone layer and an inner matrix of bovine collagen and glycosaminoglycan. According to Integra, "the collagen-glycosaminoglycan matrix provides a scaffold for cellular migration and capillary integration." This product is used for partial-thickness and full-thickness burn injuries. Because it facilitates capillary growth into the wound area of coverage, it is often used for areas of tendon exposure, because the exposed tendon will have no blood supply of its own. This can allow for protection of the exposed tendon, maintaining the health and integrity of the tendon and allowing for eventual autograft placement over the area of exposed tendon, thereby preserving the overall function of the joint. In full-thickness injuries where the entire dermis is lost, Integra can facilitate the creation of a fertile wound bed in preparation for skin grafting, thereby creating the optimal environment for the skin graft to adhere and survive.[23]

NovoSorb Biodegradeable Temporizing Matrix (BTM; PolyNovo, Carlsbad, California) is a dermal replacement product that is completely synthetic and used as a temporary skin substitute (https://www.polynovo.com). It is used for full-thickness injuries or over critical structures such as joints. Like other dermal substitutes it helps to create a wound bed that will support a skin graft once the dermal substitute matrix has matured. Unlike other dermal substitutes it contains no biological material (https://www.polynovo.com). It can also require a prolonged period of immobilization to facilitate maturity.[49]

Biosynthetic products change as a result of new technological advances in dermal cell manufacturing.[23] New products are introduced on a yearly basis. New products are usually introduced to burn centers in a systematic fashion through a committee of health professionals that screens new products for use.

It is important for an OT working in a burn center to be aware of new products being introduced in the unit and their specific precautions. Some research indicates that use of these dermal substitutes can improve the appearance of the scar. However, there is no biosynthetic product that can substitute and provide all of the functions of real skin. It appears that biosynthetic products are emerging as a necessary part of burn care; however, most researchers agree that more research is needed on the functional outcomes of these products.[23,43] Additionally, for a burn center, careful consideration for the following must be made when using biosynthetic products: cost of the product (some products can be very expensive), its availability, and the skill required (surgical and wound care) for the product to be effective and safe.[35,79]

Hydrotherapy

Once the patient's condition is sufficiently stable, hydrotherapy is usually performed at least once a day to remove loose debris and "stale" topical antibiotics. It provides thorough cleansing of both the wound and the uninvolved areas. Hydrotherapy is generally accomplished by placing the patient horizontally on a "shower trolley" covered with a sterile plastic sheet and washing and showering the wound for 20 to 30 minutes. This non-submersive showering method of hydrotherapy has become the preferred technique of cleansing burn wounds to prevent cross-contamination of wounds among patients. This method, which has the added benefit of encouraging better body mechanics among care providers, has replaced the traditional whirlpool form of hydrotherapy.[28]

In hydrotherapy, the burn injury is cleaned, often with just a plain white soap (Ivory or Dove) and water. The wound bed is cleaned with soft washcloths. Dead skin, eschar, and pseudoeschar are removed from the wound, sometimes on a daily basis, and a new antimicrobial dressing can be placed. Fresh topical agents are then reapplied to delay colonization of organisms and reduce bacterial counts in the burn wounds. During hydrotherapy the patient has usually received some form of analgesics as well as antianxiety medications, as patients are often afraid or feeling anxious surrounding the anticipated pain of a dressing change. Therefore, the reduced pain and freedom-of-motion characteristic of the hydrotherapy intervention provides an excellent opportunity for the therapist to perform assessments and range-of-motion (ROM) exercises.

Hydrotherapy was a part of Ben's daily wound care routine. It was also an area of great anxiety. Pain management around wound care is often difficult to achieve and can cause great stress to the patient. OT can provide the patient with non-narcotic (non-opiate) pain management through guided meditation, breathing techniques, etc. OTs can also advocate for their patients by informing the multidisciplinary team of issues with inadequate pain management and its impact on the patient's psychological state and functional ability.[7,10,34]

Sepsis

Sepsis is defined as "a life threatening organ dysfunction caused by dysregulated host response to infection."[61,67] Burn wound colonization begins at the moment of injury, with microorganisms invading the wound bed. Once the organism infiltrates the wound, it begins to form a biofilm that will protect the organism from the client's immune system. Wound cultures and biopsies are performed to monitor such growth when signs of possible serious infection are present.[61,67] A severe infection can result in sepsis, in which the infection spreads from the original site through the bloodstream, a condition known as septicemia. Septicemia initiates a systemic response that affects the flow of blood to vital organs. Bacterial infections are the most common source of sepsis, but it can also result from fungal, parasitic, and mycobacterial infections, especially if the patient is immunocompromised.[61,67] Antibiotic therapy is initiated usually with a broad-spectrum antibiotic that affects the organism most likely to be the cause of infection. However, if host defenses continue to be overwhelmed, the bacterial by-products or endotoxins accumulate in the bloodstream, a condition known as toxemia, which eventually leads to septic shock, a cardiovascular response that impedes blood flow to the organ systems, and to generalized circulatory collapse. Septic shock may be characterized by ischemia, diminished urine output, tachycardia, hypotension, tachypnea, hypothermia, disorientation, and coma.[61,67] The patient will require fluid resuscitation and hemodynamic stabilization in addition to antibiotic treatment. Septicemia and septic shock often require multisystem supportive measures for recovery, such as the use of cardiovascular medications, hemodialysis, and mechanical ventilation.[41]

Surgical Intervention

Ben was taken to the operating room for debridement of his burn wounds and skin graft placement to both UEs and both LEs 5 days after admission. This was a large surgical procedure that resulted in all four extremities being immobilized in splints to protect the grafts for 5 days. The impact of surgery on Ben's functional ability was to go from being nearly independent to completely dependent. Because of the pandemic, Ben had little support from family and friends as visitors were restricted from the hospital. Ben relied completely on medical staff, television, and technology to relieve the stress and boredom of confinement. OT provided the patient with daily splint checks, social interaction, and education on distraction techniques that could be implemented. Ben was receptive to all OT recommendations and was able to maintain a positive outlook for the future. Immobilization in splints can be difficult for patients, especially if they are confined to their beds. Some clients with multiple psychosocial stressors in addition to the burn injury and surgery can result in diminished coping skills, which can affect their ability to successfully rehabilitate.[11]

There are a variety of surgical interventions for a burn-injured patient. If a patient is unable to tolerate dressing changes or if the nursing staff is unable to clean the wound sufficiently in hydrotherapy, the burn unit team may decide to take a patient to the operating room for debridement. Some surgeons are certified or have access to conscious sedation in their burn units. In both cases, a surgeon will sedate a patient and then debride the wound down to a clean wound bed. This allows the surgeon to assess the clean wound and determine if the wound will heal on its own or if the patient will require a skin graft.

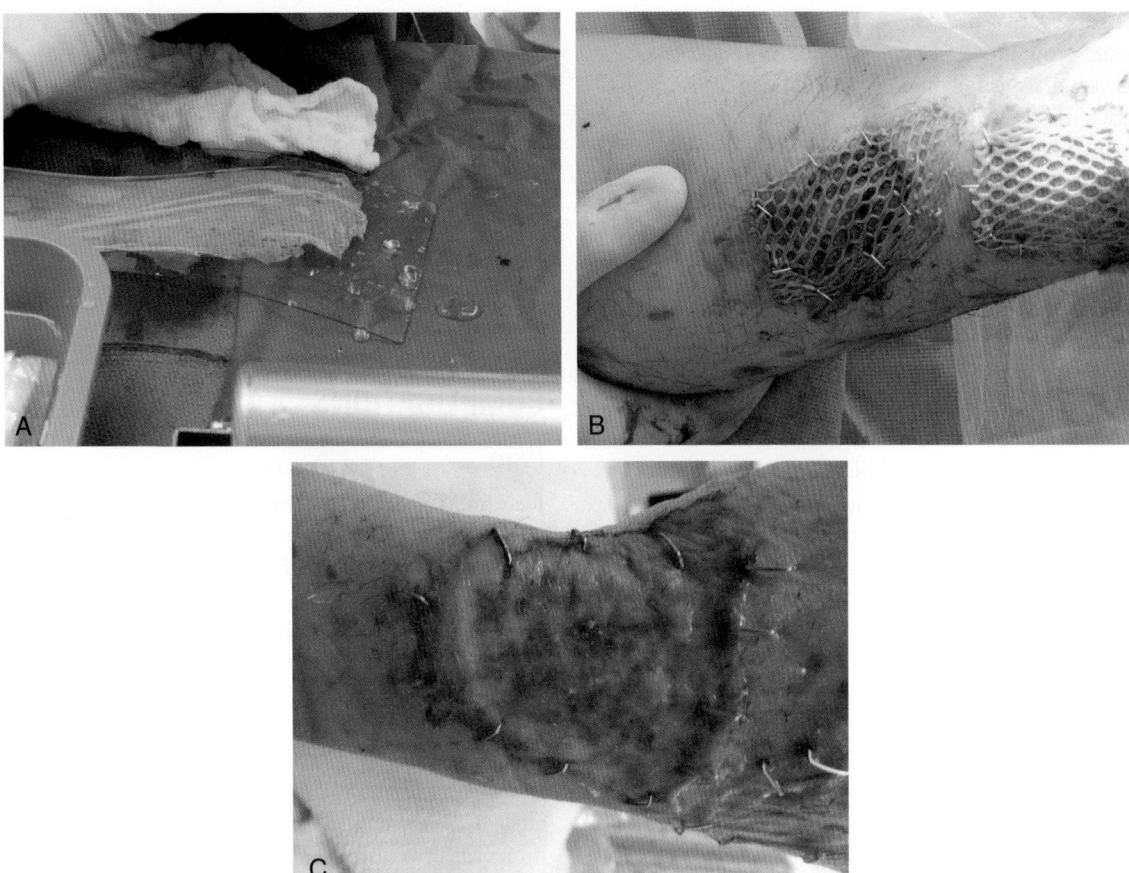

Fig. 43.7 (A and B) Meshed skin grafts can be expanded to cover a larger surface area but have a higher risk of developing hypertrophic scars as they heal. The skin will also heal with the characteristic mesh pattern. (C) Sheet grafts cover a smaller surface area but have a lower risk of developing hypertrophic scars as they heal.

Although all burn wounds are treated with some type of topical antimicrobial agent, when the depth and extent of the wound requires more than 1 week for healing, surgical intervention is indicated to decrease burn morbidity and mortality. Early excision and skin grafting remains the gold standard treatment for deep burn injuries.[23] Surgical treatment of burns usually consists of excision of the nonviable burned tissue, or eschar, and placement of biological or synthetic skin grafts.

Essentially three types of biological grafts are available. A xenograft, or heterograft, is processed pigskin. A homograft, or allograft, is processed human cadaver skin. These grafts are used as biological dressings to provide temporary wound coverage and pain relief. An autograft consists of permanent surgical transplantation of the upper layers or a split-thickness skin graft (STSG) of the person's own skin taken from an unburned donor site.[13] The STSG is applied to the clean, excised tissues of the burn wound graft site. Skin grafts placed as a sheet have superior appearance and quality. These are often used to cover burn wounds to the face, chest, and hands or small wounds and for cosmesis. To cover larger surface areas rapidly, the graft may be "meshed" to allow a single sheet of skin to be expanded for coverage of a larger surface area (Fig. 43.7). The meshed graft attaches to the burn surface in the same manner as a sheet graft, but the interstices, or openings in the meshed skin, must heal by reepithelializing over granulation tissue. This leads to more scarring and a permanent mesh pattern on the skin.

For deeper wounds, a full-thickness skin graft (FTSG) may be used by the surgeon. A FTSG includes the epidermal and dermal layers of the skin and the fat layer.[13] This type of graft is used to cover deeper areas over critical structures such as a joint or where cosmesis is a factor.[13] These types of grafts leave a deep donor site that requires closure by a soft tissue flap or primary closure of the wound.[13]

Now that the size of a survivable burn has increased, the amount of available donor sites for autografting has conversely decreased. For this reason, alternatives to autografts have been developed. Examples of such alternatives are epidermal cultured skin substitutes, cultured epidermal autografts,[13,18,39] and dermal analogues such as Integra (Integra LifeSciences Corporation) and AlloDerm (Lifecell Corporation, Branchburg, New Jersey).[13] A wound may be limited in size, but the defect may be so deep that survival of bone or tendon is at risk. In these instances, STSG adherence is difficult to achieve, and a full-thickness skin graft or microvascular skin flap may be indicated.[13]

Vacuum-Assisted Closure

Negative pressure wound therapy, also known as vacuum-assisted closure (VAC), is a treatment in which a sealed dressing and controlled negative pressure are used to evacuate wound fluid, stimulate growth of granulation tissue, and decrease bacterial colonization, especially in deeper wounds.[53,101] Since their introduction, VAC (VAC Therapy; KCI Concepts, San Antonio, Texas) dressings have been used in a number of surgical specialties, including burn care. By assisting in the debridement of necrotic tissue and removal of soluble inflammatory substances, VAC therapy reduces the number of dressing changes required and shortens the time interval between debridement and wound closure. This has been shown to facilitate the growth of granulation tissue even in deep wounds and thus make graft adherence more successful.[101]

Using a VAC device to secure a skin graft prevents fluid collection beneath the graft, ensures full contact between the wound bed and the transplanted skin, and distributes an even amount of pressure over the entire surface, regardless of the irregularity of the recipient bed. However, the graft could be compromised if the negative pressure is not maintained.[1,101] During treatment the therapist must be attentive to the VAC dressings and avoid activities with the patient that could disrupt the seal around the dressing and cause an air leak.

Nutrition

As part of his multidisciplinary care in the burn unit, Ben worked with a registered dietitian to ensure adequate intake of calories and nutrients. Occupational therapists and dietitians work closely together to promote nutrition, healthy habits, and independence with self-care. Food can be a strong motivating factor for patients and can help them to engage in a rewarding, self-care activity. Self-feeding is an important step toward independence in patients with burn injuries to their hands.[3,7] (See Chapter 10 for more information.)

Adequate nutrition is essential during wound healing because the metabolic rate of a patient with a burn injury greatly increases with corresponding increases in protein, vitamin, mineral, and calorie needs. Protein is especially important for wound healing and must be provided in substantial amounts. Nutritional requirements are calculated on the basis of the %TBSA, the patient's age and weight on admission. Calorie counts and the patient's weight are closely monitored to ensure adequate nutrition. If the patient is unable to meet individual requirements through the diet, high-protein and high-calorie supplements are given either orally or through a nasogastric or gastric tube.[81,100]

Enteral feeding is the preferred method of providing nutrition in burn patients because it is associated with a lower risk of complications. However, if the gastrointestinal tract is compromised, parenteral nutrition becomes necessary, especially in cases with severe burns and extensive %TBSA.[100] There are also some micronutrients such as vitamin C or the trace elements copper, selenium, and zinc that are better absorbed when they are given intravenously.[9,81]

Later, as the wound closes and normal feeding resumes, nutritional demands decrease and the individual's eating habits must be normalized to prevent excessive weight gain. The occupational therapist and dietitian often work together when self-feeding is an issue. The occupational therapist can assist the dietitian in understanding a patient's physical ability in the context of self-feeding so that food choices can be better tailored to suit the patient. For example, patients with mouth (including oral cavity burns) and face burns may find it painful to eat solid foods but may be willing to drink nutritional shakes or softer diets to meet their needs as they are waiting to heal. It is important for occupational therapists to use the activity of feeding to encourage normal hand to mouth and grasping of utensil for self-feeding as well as reinforcing the need for proper nutrition[7] (see Chapter 27).

ASSOCIATED PROBLEMS AND COMPLICATIONS

Pain

Research indicates that pain is a main issue that affects movement and function in burn patients.[10,34,40,63] Pain control was a major issue for Ben. In the acute phase of his injury, he had a large surface area of open wound that required daily wound care. Hydrotherapy and the pain associated with it resulted in anxiety during his hospital stay. Ben required intense pharmacological management of his pain and anxiety through the use of opiates and benzodiazepine. Occupational therapy provided Ben with education on how to move to reduce pain, deep breathing, and meditation to reduce anxiety. Ben was also encouraged to engage in normal daily activities to reduce his anxiety and give him a sense of purpose during his day.

Pain Assessment

Some of the most commonly used pain assessment tools include visual scales, color scales, word and faces scales, and adjective scales. A 1998 study indicated that patients prefer the faces and color scales over commonly used visual analogue and adjective scales.[32] Pain levels should be assessed during a quiet time and again immediately after any painful activity.

Pain Management

Because pain has adverse physiological and emotional effects, pain management is an important factor to achieve better outcomes.[36] Developmentally appropriate and culturally sensitive pain assessment, pain relief, and reevaluation are essential in treatment. Pain control guidelines should address both background and procedural pain and associated anxiety. The occupational therapist should assist nursing staff in focused surveillance of burn pain and its successful treatment because adequate pain management will result in better participation in rehabilitation.[36] Pain management is a main goal of burn care. Multimodal pain management, opioids, and nonpharmacological treatments are a part of burn care. Opiates remain the most common form of analgesic therapy for patients with burns, but due to individual differences, optimal relief of burn pain can be difficult. Alternative pain control methods include the use of nonsteroidal antiinflammatory drugs, benzodiazepines, antiepileptics, antidepressants, and ketamine, each of which can be combined with opiates to provide more effective pain management. Antidepressants appear to enhance opiate-induced analgesia, whereas anticonvulsants are useful in the treatment of sympathetically maintained pain following burns. Ketamine has been used extensively during burn dressing changes causing a dissociative state for the patient.[34]

Nerve blocks are anesthetics that are administered directly to the nerve root. They are effective in relieving pain in the affected limb. They are used when pain is confined to one extremity and the use of pain management drugs has not been effective.[34] Blocks are monitored by the administering physician for side effects and to maintain the medication pump. This treatment can be effective for pain management and improve patient satisfaction.[34] However, nonpharmacological pain management techniques must be explored as well. OTs in burn care are uniquely qualified to distinguish between physical pain and psychological pain. It is important to distinguish between the two and treat them appropriately to prevent long-term psychological distress.[36]

Nonpharmacological intervention using various hypnotic, cognitive, behavioral, and sensory treatment methods is becoming more accepted. Transcutaneous electrical nerve stimulation, topical and systemic local anesthetics, and psychological techniques are also useful adjuncts.[34] Hypnosis may be a very useful alternative when opioid pain medication proves to be dangerous or ineffective; it has received strong anecdotal support from case reports.[34] The mechanisms behind hypnotic analgesia for burn pain are poorly understood; however, patients with burn injuries are more receptive to hypnosis than the general population, possibly because of increased motivation, dissociation, and regressive behavior.[66] Transcutaneous electrical nerve stimulation, topical and systemic local anesthetics, and psychological techniques are also useful adjuncts.[34] Other methods of nonpharmaceutical pain reduction may be helpful. Relaxation techniques such as progressive relaxation, breathing exercises, guided imagery, aromatherapy, music therapy, and teaching individualized coping strategies may be helpful.[73] (See Chapter 51 for additional information.) The occupational therapist can and should use these tools to guide the patient/client through often painful therapeutic exercises and activities. Patients with a severe burn injury naturally respond to pain by resisting painful motions or activities. Adjustment disorder is a common occurrence among burn survivors.[21,95,98] Patients with poor coping skills are at risk for adjustment disorder, which is associated with poorer long-term outcome.[11] Occupational therapists working in burn care and rehabilitation can assist their clients by identifying their occupational roles or identities that encourage more positive coping.[7]

Most patients are usually more interested in whether the procedure will hurt and how long it will last than in lengthy explanations or technical information. Coordinating treatments with scheduled pain medications is often helpful and highly recommended, especially if active participation is necessary. The therapist should be aware of and use techniques to minimize preventable pain (e.g., applying adequate vascular support to the LEs before standing or ambulation). The therapist must also inform the nursing staff about any noted side effects from pain medication, as well as the observed effectiveness of the currently used pain management regimen. The need for short-term breakthrough pain relief should be coordinated with the

nursing staff to reduce discomfort and stress during intensive therapy procedures. If a patient's anxiety or pain is disproportionate to the treatment, antianxiety medication may be indicated both to relieve anxiety and to increase the effectiveness of pain medication. Time limits on painful treatment sessions should be predetermined with all patients who are cognizant and capable of participation. The therapist should consistently adhere to these time limits to foster trust and a sense of control for the patient. By reducing the patient's anxiety, the therapist reduces the fear factor that can exacerbate perceived pain.[34,72] As the wound heals, the amount of opiate/narcotic analgesia is gradually decreased, and patients usually require minimal pain medication by discharge (see Chapter 28).

Psychosocial Factors

Immobilization of affected extremities and social distancing/isolation took its toll on Ben during his hospitalization. Medical staff, especially therapy staff, helped to relieve his sense of isolation and dependence by daily therapy sessions. Occupational therapy was essential in helping him to adapt in the short term to being dependent for most ADLs. OT was able to adapt his nursing call button and television remote control to give him some independence during the period of immobilization.

After a burn injury there is a potential for psychological reactions, including depression; withdrawal reactions caused by disfigurement; adjustment disorder; and anxiety over the uncertain ability to resume work, family, community, and leisure roles.[51] The way in which a person copes with burn trauma is strongly influenced by his or her psychological status before the injury and whether the injury was a result of accident, arson, assault, or suicide attempt. The psychological ramifications can include guilt, anxiety, depression, regression, increased hostility, and existential crisis.[11,51] In the case of permanent loss of function and deformity, the patient may experience severe grief as a result of decreased physical abilities, changes in personal appearance and identity, loss of vocation, or loss of loved ones who were killed in the same accident. In the case of facial disfigurement and amputations, the patient's previous support system also may be reduced or lost as a result of abandonment by friends or significant others who cannot adjust to the physical changes in the patient.

Whether the permanent loss is social or physical, the patient may need to move through stages of grief similar to the five stages of grief in patients with a terminal diagnosis as described by Dr. Kübler-Ross in her book *On Death and Dying*.[47] The stages include the following:

- *Denial*. In this phase a burn-injured patient may express, "Why is this happening to me?" or "The doctor said I'm going to have surgery to fix my burn." In this phase, burn patients may have the belief that their problems will be over once they heal the burn injury or have their surgery. They often do not take into consideration the need for ongoing wound care, scar management, and therapeutic interventions to return to normal function.
- *Anger*. "Leave me alone!" Or "Stop hurting me!" Patients may express anger at medical staff, themselves, or at family or friends. They may refuse treatments or therapeutic interventions in their state of anger.

- *Bargaining.* In this phase, most burn-injured patients do not understand the length of time required for the burn injury to heal and to return to normal functioning. They may make statements such as, "I'll do therapy later."
- *Depression.* When burn-injured patients realize that they are forever altered by their burn injury and that they must endure some amount of pain during their recovery, they will often experience sadness.
- *Acceptance.* The patient accepts the burn injury as part of himself or herself. Patients learn to manage their pain without trying to avoid it. They acclimate to the new sensations of movement and touch. In this phase, patients will adapt to the bodily changes and return to work with modifications as needed; they will learn new physical and coping skills to deal with the burn injury and resume their place within their social/family circle, often creating new additional social supports.

If the patient does not reach the stage of acceptance, the reintegration process can be delayed. It is important to note that there are many rehabilitation professionals who question the stage method and even the concept of acceptance for those with chronic disabilities, seeing it more as a fluid process wherein the individual proceeds and recedes from stage to stage as one encounters problems along the road to coping with a disability. Providing emotional support and education and helping the patient develop coping mechanisms and self-direction can promote the psychological adjustment of patients with burn injuries. An OT should also work together with the burn unit psychologist to provide patients with optimal support to facilitate the reclamation of their life. Severe burn injury can result in a reassessment of personal values and relationships or a renewed appreciation of life. The complex interactions among premorbid personality style, extent of injury, and social and environmental contexts should be considered when determining how patients will adjust psychologically to a severe burn injury.[11]

Stress

Traumatic events associated with severe burns include natural and intentional disasters such as tornadoes, lightning, house fires, motor vehicle accidents, acts of war or terrorism, physical or sexual assault, and the sudden death of loved ones or friends. Burn treatment further traumatizes the patient because of associated painful medical procedures (e.g., wound care, limb amputations, multiple surgeries, and therapies). Mental health professionals are increasing their understanding of the factors associated with increased psychiatric risk and the ways in which burn patients, especially children, cope with the stress and pain triggered by traumatic events. Responses to major stress often include reliving the event, avoidance, and hypervigilance; these responses may continue long after the precipitating event. Posttraumatic stress disorder (PTSD) is a common psychiatric condition after traumatic experiences, including physical injuries such as burns.[21,27] Mood, anxiety, sleep, conduct, learning, and attention problems are often comorbid conditions, especially in children. Treatment involves pain assessment followed by specific interventions such as pain management, psychiatric consultation, and crisis intervention initiated promptly after the traumatic event. Intervention should also involve the burn survivor's family.[17]

OTs working in burn care and rehabilitation should be mindful of the importance of coping self-efficacy. Coping strategies, both negative and positive, will have an impact on the rehabilitation process of burn-injured clients and can affect their quality of life.[11]

Throughout his hospitalization, Ben was encouraged to discuss his thoughts and feelings about his injury. He was offered services from social work and pastoral services. He was able to open up to and express his feelings to an experienced burn nurse with whom he developed good rapport. Providing clients with a safe environment to express their feelings is important for the psychological recovery of clients after traumatic events.

OT PRACTICE NOTES

Occupational therapy intervention must address the psychological aspects from the initial assessment and onset of OT intervention and continue through discharge from OT services at the end of the rehabilitation phase. Even after discharge from rehabilitation, the client may continue to need psychosocial OT intervention as he or she attempts to become actively involved in the community, resume social activities and relationships, and return to or enter the paid workforce.

BURN REHABILITATION

The Team

Successful care and rehabilitation of burn survivors require a multidisciplinary team approach that begins immediately after the patient's admission to the hospital and continues through and beyond hospitalization.[17] Ideally, the burn care team includes physicians, nurses, physical and occupational therapists, respiratory therapists, nutritionists, social workers, psychiatrists and psychologists, speech and language pathologists, orthotists and prosthetists, child care and recreational therapists, pastoral caregivers or clergy, interpreters or cultural support personnel, and vocational counselors. The most important members of the team, however, are the client and the client's family or support system.[17]

OT PRACTICE NOTES

All healthcare professionals must continue to update their knowledge and professional competencies and keep abreast of the rapidly changing treatments and therapies available for treating burned patients.[7] Recommended ways to continue professional development include the following:

- Review professional journals such as the *Journal of Burn Care and Rehabilitation, Burns, Journal of Wound Care, Journal of Trauma, and Journal of Burns.*
- Obtain membership in burn care associations such as the ABA and the International Society of Burn Injuries. Membership includes a subscription to the *Journal of Burn Care and Rehabilitation*, special interest group webinars, literature on established guidelines for burn care and rehabilitation, and access to a database of past publications (ABA website).
- Attend local, regional, and national association meetings. Visit regional burn centers to confer with other burn therapists.
- Visit online websites of professional burn associations and participate in online discussions with other burn care professionals.

Goals of Rehabilitation

The entire burn team is involved in some aspect of burn rehabilitation, whether it is providing verbal support, preparing the patient for self-care tasks, reinforcing the importance of active motion, or providing patient education. The long-term goals of occupational therapy are quite similar to the long-term goals of the entire burn team. Although specific goals may be the responsibility of various team members, everyone's efforts are focused on the same outcome. Occupational therapy treatment goals, therefore, should be compatible with all other treatments and be established in collaboration with the client/patient, family, and entire rehabilitation team. Inherent in this concept is the need for close communication and cooperation of all burn team members. Occupational therapists should take the lead in helping all team members understand the client as a unique occupational being, along with all the relevant factors and contexts that will come into play. Role delineation between different disciplines, especially occupational therapy and physical therapy, differs among burn care facilities and may be determined by insurance reimbursement rather than by traditional roles or the specialized skills of the individual therapist. Therefore, it is especially important that all disciplines work closely together with ongoing communication so that patients benefit from the skills and viewpoints of all areas of specialization. Occupational, physical, and speech therapists who specialize in burn rehabilitation increasingly use co-treatments that promote independence in both mobility and ADLs.

Phases of Recovery

Rehabilitation management of burn survivors can be divided into four overlapping phases to aid in categorizing and determining effective intervention goals. These phases of recovery are the emergent, acute care (both the surgical and postoperative), the inpatient and outpatient rehabilitation, and the reconstructive phases.

The emergent phase is usually the first 72 hours after a major burn injury. However, if it is a superficial partial-thickness burn and heals spontaneously in less than 1 to 2 weeks without surgical intervention, the time from injury until epithelial healing is also considered an acute care phase.[22]

The acute phase follows the emergent phase and continues for varying lengths of time, depending on the size of the burn injury and the presence of associated medical complications. During this period, vulnerability to wound infection, sepsis, and septic shock is especially great, and medical treatment is focused on promoting healing and minimizing infection.

The rehabilitation phase covers both inpatient and outpatient care and can extend for an indeterminate length of time. This phase follows the post-grafting period when the patient is medically stable and most open wounds have healed. The quality of wound healing, scar formation, and need for aggressive rehabilitation make this the most challenging phase for burn patients, their families, and their occupational therapists.

Emergent Phase

During the emergent phase, medical management is of utmost importance for survival of the patient, and the goal of occupational therapy is primarily preventive. As the patient recovers and

wound closure progresses, the nature of occupational therapy also changes, with treatment directed at restoring function. Initially, however, when the wounds are deep partial or full thickness, the emergent phase occupational therapy goals are as follows:

- Provide cognitive reorientation and psychological support.
- Reduce moderate to severe edema.
- Prevent loss of joint and skin mobility through ROM and positioning.
- Prevent loss of strength and activity tolerance.
- Promote occupational performance, such as independence in self-care skills.
- Provide patient and caregiver education.

Acute Phase

The acute phase follows the emergent phase and continues until the wound is closed either by primary wound healing or by skin grafting. It is characterized by continued monitoring of and treatment of the burn wounds. If and when the wounds are too big or deep, surgical intervention is required. Excision and grafting procedures usually require periods of immobilization of the areas treated to allow graft adherence. Occupational therapy goals during the acute phase are focused on preserving or enhancing performance skills and patterns while supporting surgical objectives. The preferred position and length of immobilization will vary by physician prerogative and burn center protocol, with the average period of immobilization being between 2 and 7 days.[56,65,99] Full-thickness skin grafts are immobilized for up to 10 days. When the patient requires biosynthetic grafting, the affected areas are immobilized from 10 to 14 days. The most advantageous postoperative position usually maintains the grafted area in the position that maximizes the surface area of the grafted site. For example, a hand with a dorsal burn should be splinted in the intrinsic plus position where the wrist is in a neutral or slightly extended position, the metacarpophalangeal (MP) joints flexed, and the thumb radially abducted to protect the first web space.

During this phase, the goals of therapy include the following:
- Promote cognitive awareness by providing orientation activities when necessary and continue psychological support.
- Protect and preserve graft and donor sites through splinting and wrapping and establishing positioning techniques that support the surgeon's postoperative care orders while allowing for as much freedom of movement as possible.[3]
- Prevent muscular atrophy and loss of activity tolerance and reduce the risk for thrombophlebitis by providing exercise for areas that are not immobilized.
- Increase independence in self-care by teaching alternative techniques; educate, instruct, and reassure the patient and family members regarding this phase of recovery.

Rehabilitation Phase

The third phase of recovery is the rehabilitation phase, which begins as wound closure occurs. Individuals with large %TBSA burns frequently enter this phase needing further surgeries. However, the majority of their wounds are closed, and scar maturation is commencing. The focus of intervention during this phase is on maximizing function and participation in occupations, promoting physical and emotional independence, and managing scar formation to prevent or correct deformity and contracture formation. Patient and family education is especially important for developing competence in wound/scar care and therapy programs in preparation for discharge.

The rehabilitation phase extends past hospital discharge and continues until maturation of all burn wounds and surgical sites is complete. Before discharge from the hospital, emphasis is placed on independence, self-management, and education. Once the client is home, emotional support and intervention must continue to help sustain the client's confidence, self-esteem, and motivation, qualities that the client needs to cope with the physical, social, and emotional consequences of a severe burn injury.[11]

Intervention goals for this phase can be exhaustive given the potentially disabling effects of burn scars. Therefore, it is important for the therapist to incorporate the patient's personal goals from the beginning of the rehabilitation process.

Treatment goals for the rehabilitation phase are expanded to include the following:

- Continue to provide psychological support as the patient progresses toward physical and emotional independence and faces new challenges.
- Improve joint mobility and reduce contractures by using correct positioning, sustained passive stretching exercises, and splinting as needed.
- Restore muscle strength, coordination, and activity tolerance.
- Initiate a compression therapy and scar management program with the use of vascular support garments, custom scar compression garments, and pressure adapters to minimize scar hypertrophy, contractures, and disfigurement.
- Promote independent self-care skills or the ability to direct others to assist when needed, including appropriate positioning, exercise, and skin care. Provide instruction and opportunities to practice instrumental activities of daily living (IADLs), including vocational and home-care activities.
- Continue to provide instruction on scar development, including potential sensory and cosmetic changes, scar management techniques, and related safety precautions such as sun protection and skin care.
- Guide the implementation of a post-discharge plan that supports resumption of school, work, social, and leisure occupations.

Also important is for the occupational therapist to provide education on support groups or networks to assist the client with the emotional trauma of the burn injury and to be aware of the signs of post-traumatic stress disorder and facilitate referrals to appropriate counseling sources.

Reconstructive Phase

In this phase of burn survivors' recovery, they have often reintegrated into their daily life and have assumed their occupational roles. They have effectively entered the acceptance phase of the grief process and are able to demonstrate hope for the future by learning new occupational skills and acquiring new occupational roles. These patients often return to the outpatient burn clinic for follow-up once or twice a year to assess their scars and functional

ability. These patients are ready to discuss surgery to improve the appearance of scars. In this phase, the patients psychologically understand the limitations of surgery and scar management interventions to improve the burn scar appearance. They are able to have a conversation with the physicians about how they look and the concerns they have. They typically become active participants in the decisions on elective surgeries to improve the appearance of their scars. Though occupational therapy's role during this phase may be limited, occupational therapists can empower the patient to initiate the conversation with the surgeon to discuss options for scar management and reconstruction.

OCCUPATIONAL THERAPY EVALUATION

The initial evaluation is usually a client's first introduction to occupational therapy. In Ben's case, he had an extended family member who was an OT student and so had some knowledge of the profession. A thorough history taken during Ben's initial OT evaluation provided the following information: his occupational history, his values, support system, personal goals, personal strengths, medical history, and current functional status. This information was necessary to create functional and measurable goals for OT. It also allowed OT to provide the multidisciplinary team with a picture of Ben, his life, and his motivations. This enabled the team to provide personalized and relevant care.[7]

At the initial evaluation, Ben was found to have limited ROM of both hands, wrists, elbows, and shoulders due to pain, and bulky dressings. His functional mobility was limited by burn injuries to his LE's. His large surface area burns required fluid resuscitation that resulted in edema of all four extremities and his face that further impaired his ROM. He required maximal assistance for all ADLs due to pain, limited ROM, and decreased functional mobility. He expressed his main goal to be to resume his training in the firefighter program.

Although medical status issues are a primary concern during acute care, whenever possible the occupational therapist should complete an initial evaluation within the first 24 to 48 hours after hospital admission. Burn etiology, medical history, and any secondary diagnoses are obtained from the medical record and team. The wounds are then visually assessed to determine the extent and depth of injury. Any areas affecting future occupational performance and context are noted and documented.

Whenever possible, both the client and family are interviewed to establish rapport and to obtain a history of the client's previous occupational performance. Ben was able to provide his occupational history. His family was not available to interview because of visitor restrictions during the COVID-19 pandemic. Ben was a young man in his 20s who worked full-time during the week in logistics for the local VA hospital. His dream was to become a firefighter and he was currently enrolled in the firefighter's academy. His hobbies included exercising. He had a supportive immediate and extended family who called and provided food and other items for comfort for Ben. He lived in a stable home and had both financial and monetary resources. His primary concern was how his injury would impact his ability to complete the firefighter program in which he was enrolled.

His history included preinjury body structures and body functions (i.e., hand dominance, previous injuries, and performance-limiting illnesses or conditions) and specific information on past performance skills and patterns, daily routines, and activities (including professional, educational, and domestic responsibilities). Obtaining data concerning preinjury personality traits and psychological status is equally important. With this information, the therapist can monitor for changes in the client's behavior and cognitive functioning and choose the most appropriate interactive approach to encourage the client's involvement in goal setting and the therapy process. In the case of a severe burn requiring intubation and mechanical ventilation, this information must be obtained from family members and significant others to verify and supplement what the patient may relay nonverbally.

OT PRACTICE NOTES

Ideally, the client's history of occupational performance would be obtained before assessment of current client factors. However, the acuity of the injury, time constraints, and the need to coordinate physical assessment with pain medications, wound dressing changes, and other medical procedures may supersede completion of a detailed performance history.

Involved and uninvolved areas should be evaluated for joint mobility, strength, sensation, and functional use. However, before beginning this evaluation, the therapist should explain the purpose of occupational therapy and what the client should expect during the assessment, including the potential for discomfort. Preassessment instruction and ongoing encouragement help reassure clients and decrease anxiety so that they can perform at their best. Emphasis is placed on the ultimate long-term goal of resuming engagement in meaningful occupations and participation in life contexts.

The initial clinical evaluation should address all areas of potential occupational therapy intervention, including assessment of wound location and severity, presence and severity of edema, passive range of motion (PROM) and active range of motion (AROM), muscle strength, gross and fine motor coordination, changes in sensation, and level of cognitive awareness. Ideally, these assessments take place during a dressing change or hydrotherapy, when the involved areas are exposed and unencumbered.

During the initial evaluation, distinctions are made among superficial, superficial partial, and deep partial-thickness burns, as well as full-thickness burns, on the basis of appearance and presence of sensation. The therapist must view the wounds as soon as possible after the injury, before the development of burn eschar. Eschar causes deep partial-thickness burns to closely resemble full-thickness burns and makes an accurate evaluation of depth difficult. Attention also should be directed to burned joint surface areas and the presence of any circumferential burns. ROM assessment should be performed to evaluate joint mobility, and general strength should be tested before significant edema develops or restrictive dressings are applied.

Instructing the client regarding the types of movements and the number of repetitions expected while gently guiding the individual through the specific motion can help ensure achievement of full range. When possible, a goniometer should be used for assessing ROM to accurately document baseline deficits and future changes in recorded measurements. If pain, edema, tight eschar, or bulky dressings limit full ROM, such information also should be documented. Preexisting conditions that may alter expected AROM should be investigated during the patient and family interview. Although AROM is preferred, PROM should be measured if a client is unresponsive or unable to move the extremity sufficiently. When using PROM, care must be taken to not apply excessive force, especially with older clients who have degenerative joint disease or small children with hypermobile joints.

With deeper partial- or full-thickness dorsal hand burns, boutonnière precautions should be initiated until the integrity of the hand's extensor hood mechanisms can be verified. Boutonnière precautions involve avoidance of composite active or passive flexion of the fingers. Instead, isolated MP flexion is combined with interphalangeal (IP) joint extension to prevent stress and possible damage to a compromised extensor tendon mechanism. All passive proximal interphalangeal (PIP) flexion is avoided, and protective splinting is promptly initiated to maintain the PIP joints in extension.

A gross sensory screening that includes all sensory distribution areas should be performed. Such screening is especially important in individuals with electrical injury or a history of long-standing diabetes, in whom peripheral neuropathies may be present.

If the client possessed normal functional muscle strength before the injury, an initial test of gross muscle strength may not be needed if the AROM assessment reveals adequate strength to work against gravity. Manual muscle testing of major muscle groups is indicated if the burn resulted from an electrical contact injury, if the presence of severe edema might cause compartment syndrome, or if other musculoskeletal or neurological injuries are suspected.[41] If the hand is unburned or if it is a superficial partial-thickness burn, a dynamometer and pinch gauge provide objective baseline measurements of grip and pinch strength. (See Chapters 21 and 22 for ROM and muscle testing guidance.)

ADL assessment begins by interviewing the client or the family to obtain the client's preinjury level of physical, cognitive, and social performance skills and patterns. When the burn injury is severe, the ADL assessment is postponed until the client is medically stable and able to participate in the pursuit of more advanced occupational goals. Clients with less severe burns and those who are not mechanically ventilated should be assessed for basic ADL skills, such as feeding, basic grooming, and donning and doffing of hospital gowns. Any compensatory actions or awkward movements used to complete the activity should be noted. Any abnormal patterns should be investigated and discussed to determine whether they were present before the burn injury. (See Chapter 10 for more information on ADL assessment.)

After completion of the initial evaluation (Table 43.2), short- and long-term goals should be established with the client's collaboration. The client's previous context and lifestyle, personal long-term goals, and current priorities should be primarily

TABLE 43.2 **Components of Evaluation for Burn Rehabilitation**

Initial Evaluation	Inpatient Rehabilitation	Outpatient Rehabilitation
Cause of the burn	Graft adherence	Skin or scar condition
%TBSA	Skin or scar condition	Compression garment fit
Depth of the burn	Contracture concerns	Volumetrics if needed
Area(s) involved	Edema (if present)	ADL performance level
Age, hand dominance	ADL performance level	Work skills
Functional status	Work skills	Active and passive ROM, TAM
Occupation	Active and passive ROM, TAM	Strength and activity tolerance
ROM and strength	Strength and activity tolerance	Developmental level (child)
Mobility and activity tolerance	Developmental level (child)	Psychological status
Developmental level (child)	Psychological status	Social support
Psychological status	Social support	Leisure activities
Social support	Leisure activities	Compression garment needs
Leisure activities	Compression garment needs	Home management
	Home management	Home care understanding
		Return-to-work capacity
		Return-to-school potential and need for reentry program

ADL, Activity of daily living; *ROM,* range of motion; *TAM,* total active motion; *TBSA,* total body surface area.

considered when establishing occupational therapy intervention goals. All short-term goals should be specific and realistic and have an established time frame for completion. After goals are agreed on, the intervention plan can be formulated. The occupational therapy intervention plan should be practical and should complement and support the goals of the other team members.

Two fundamental principles must be kept in mind when working in burn rehabilitation: (1) the main factor hindering post-burn functional recovery is the formation of scar contractures and hypertrophic scarring, and (2) severe scars and contractures are often preventable with prompt therapeutic intervention.[74] Therefore most burn rehabilitation intervention techniques and objectives are directed at prevention, as well as restoration.

OCCUPATIONAL THERAPY INTERVENTION

Acute Phase

Preventive Positioning

The purpose of preventive positioning is to reduce edema and maintain the involved extremities in an antideformity position (Table 43.3).[25,70] Proper positioning is critical because the position of greatest comfort for the patient is usually the position of contracture. The typical position of comfort consists of adduction and flexion of the UEs, flexion of the hips and knees, and plantar flexion of the ankles. The toes are generally pulled dorsally. Acutely burned hands are held by edema in a dysfunctional position consisting of wrist flexion, MP extension, IP flexion, and thumb adduction.[26] This position, often called

TABLE 43.3 **Antideformity Positioning for Specific Areas of the Body Following Burn Injury**

Body Area	Antideformity Position	Equipment and Technique
Neck	Neutral to slight extension	No pillow; soft collar, neck conformer, or triple-component neck splint, Watusi collar (multi-tubing neck conformer)
Chest and abdomen	Trunk extension, shoulder retraction	Lower the top of the bed, towel roll beneath the thoracic spine, clavicle straps
Axilla	Shoulder abduction of 90 to 100 degrees	Arm boards, airplane splint, modified hip abduction pillow, clavicle straps, overhead traction
Elbow and forearm	Elbow extension, forearm neutral	Pillows, conformer splints, dynamic splints (when wounds healed/closed)
Wrist and hand	Wrist extension to 30 degrees, thumb radial abducted and extended, MP flexion of 50 to 70 degrees, IP extension	Elevate with pillows, volar burn hand splint: may consider a dorsal blocking splint for MP flexion and permit IP ROM
Digits	IP extension; abduction	Gutter splint; webspacers
Thumb	Radial abduction; IP extension	Thumb spica, CMC splint, first web spacer
Hip and thigh	Neutral extension, hips in 10 to 15 degrees of abduction	Trochanter rolls, pillow between the knees, wedges
Knee and lower leg	Knee extension; anterior burn: slight flexion	Knee conformer, casts, elevation when sitting, dynamic splints
Ankle and foot	Neutral to 0 to 5 degrees of dorsiflexion	Custom splint, cast, AFO
Ears, face, nose, mouth, eyes	Prevent pressure; maintain mouth opening, ability to close eyelids	No pillows; headgear, mouth splint; layered tongue depressors; nostril openers

AFO, Ankle-foot orthosis; *CMC,* carpometacarpal; *IP,* interphalangeal; *MP,* metacarpophalangeal.

the "claw hand" or "intrinsic minus" position, can lead to severe dysfunction if not prevented during active scar formation.[26]

Positioning needs are determined during the initial wound assessment by evaluating the surface areas burned and the presence of edema, considering the posture that the individual tends to assume, and assessing whether that posture would limit function if allowed. For example, if the burn injury involves the shoulder, chest, and axillae, the client's UEs should be elevated and positioned in approximately 90 degrees of shoulder abduction, 45 degrees of external rotation, and 60 degrees of horizontal adduction by using pillow inclines and arm boards or supporting the arms with sheepskin slings suspended from an overhead traction rig (Fig. 43.8). Achieving full shoulder flexion and abduction with frequent exercise and activity is critical to prevent axillary contractures and subsequent loss of overhead reach as wound healing progresses. Once positioning needs are determined, illustrated guidelines should be posted at the bedside so that the nursing staff and team can assist in ongoing correct positioning (Fig. 43.9).

After admission, positioning is initiated primarily to reduce edema formation.[70] Elevation of the entire extremity above heart level can reduce the severity of distal edema formation, especially when paired with AROM exercises. As edema decreases and wound closure progresses, positioning goals should be directed toward prevention of skin tightness over joint surfaces (see Table 43.3).

Splinting

Intraoperatively, the OT applied bilateral intrinsic plus hand splints and both elbow extension splints to prevent shearing of the skin grafts. Ben's UEs and hands were immobilized with these splints for 5 days. The OT provided daily splint checks to ensure proper fit and placement and to monitor for areas of pressure from the splints.

Splinting is initiated to maintain correct positioning and protect compromised tissues. It is not necessary for splints to be worn at all times to prevent contractures. When a splint is used during the acute phase, it is generally static in design and applied when at rest, with activity and exercise being emphasized during waking hours. Volar hand splints are indicated if a burned hand has chronic edema, active motion is limited, or unsupervised movement is contraindicated because of deep dorsal burns or other traumatic injury. The typical volar hand splint provides approximately 15 to 30 degrees of wrist extension, 50 to 70 degrees of MP joint flexion, full IP joint extension, and combined thumb abduction and extension (Fig. 43.10).[25] Elbows or knees should be splinted at neutral position and secured with elastic wraps and taped on versus applying metal clips to prevent tears in grafts or surrounding intact skin.

When checking the fit of any splint, the therapist should consider potential pressure points and ensure correct placement. Splints fabricated shortly after injury require daily assessment and may require alterations to accommodate any significant changes in edema. Hand splints are secured in place with a figure-of-eight wrap of gauze bandage or elastic wraps, with the fingertips being exposed so that circulation can be monitored. Folded 4- × 4-inch gauze sponges are used over the proximal phalanges and under the wrap to keep the fingers extended and secured in the splint. Detachable straps, though convenient for later use, may be inappropriate for use with acute burn splints because of infection control concerns and the potential for constriction during fluctuations in distal edema.

The ABA has recommended practices for splinting burn patients. It is essential that the splints applied to the burn patient be applied by a therapist (including OT) and assessed

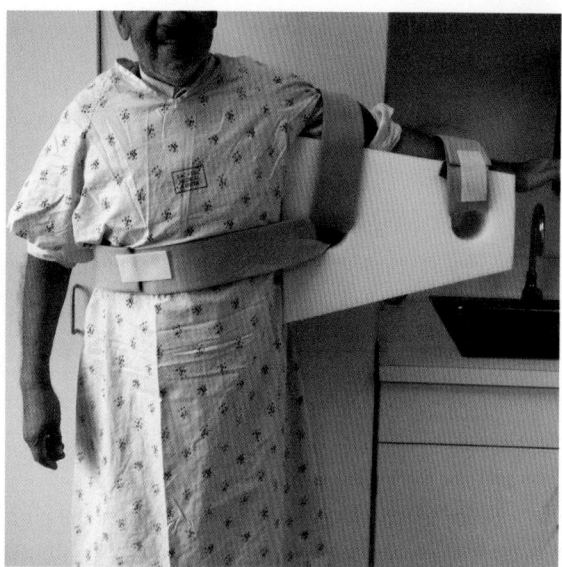

Fig. 43.8 Shoulder positioning postsurgery using a small hip abduction pillow.

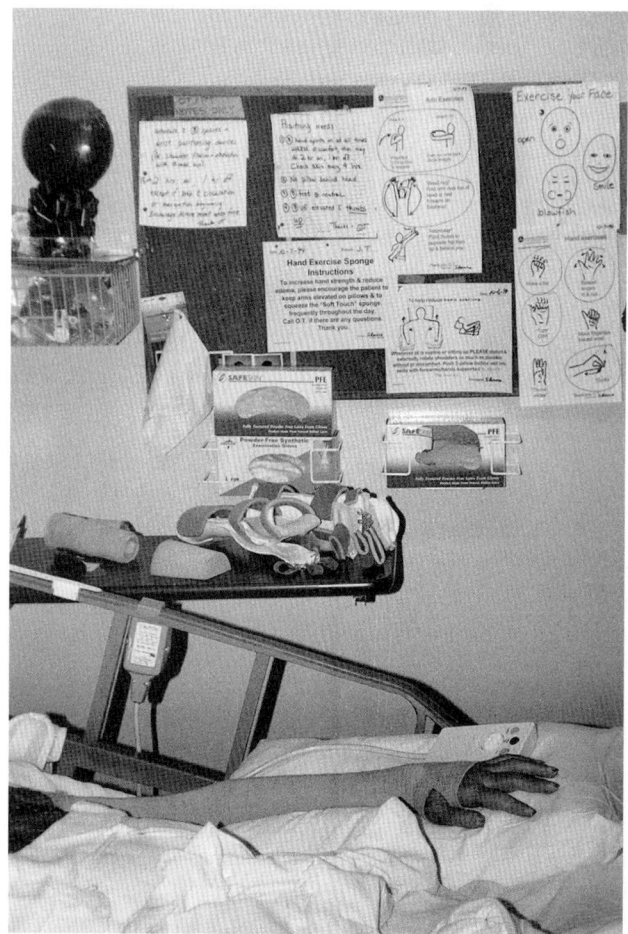

Fig. 43.9 Highly visible bedside posters are beneficial as reminders to the client, staff, and visitors regarding positioning, exercises, and splinting instructions.

for proper fit, especially when being used over wound dressings. The splint also should be applied with consideration toward the patient's tolerance and lifestyle. All splints should be accompanied by patient and caregiver education on application and wear

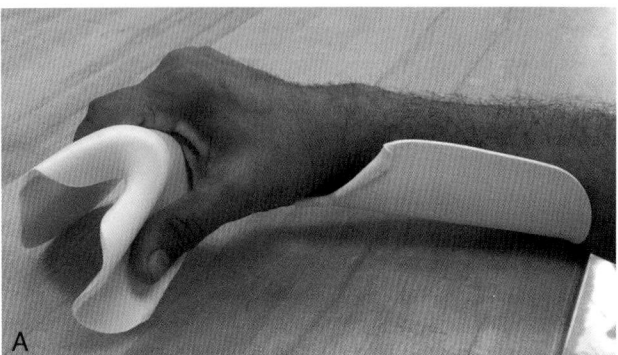
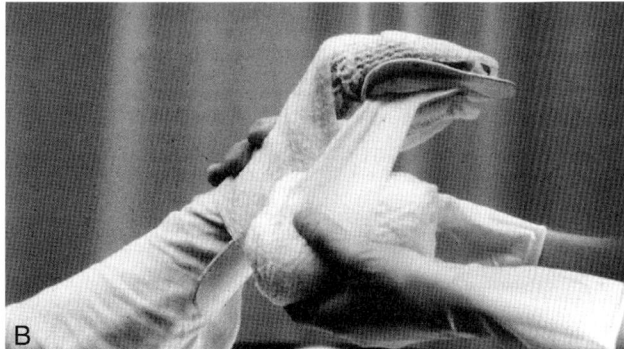

Fig. 43.10 (A) Positioning a hand in a hand splint. (B) Postsurgical placement of a hand in a burn hand splint secured with elastic bandages.

schedule. Splints should be considered whenever the patient is high risk for developing contractures. Splinting of the patient should be based on the patient's need, and the need should outweigh the risk of injury caused by the splint.[44,45,65]

Activities of Daily Living

A client's ability to perform self-care is often limited during the acute care phase because of his or her current medical condition. The need for artificial ventilation, multiple lines, catheters, and other supportive equipment interferes with independence in ADLs, and clients depend on nursing staff for self-care.

While the client is maintained on the ventilator and orally intubated, ADL activity may be limited to self-suctioning of the oral cavity and, if no facial burns have occurred, basic facial hygiene. After extubation, oral care is often the next ADL attempted. When the client is medically cleared to take fluid or food by mouth, the occupational therapist should assess self-feeding abilities. Airway damage, accompanied by compromised speech and swallowing ability, often results from an extended period of intubation or direct damage during the burn injury. In these cases, the occupational therapist works in concert with the speech pathologist on common goals that promote effective communication skills and independent self-feeding. Burns involving the UEs and associated pain, dressings, and edema may interfere with self-feeding, hygiene/grooming, and writing motions and make temporary use of adaptive equipment necessary. This equipment may include built-up or extended handles on utensils, a plate guard, or an insulated travel mug with a lid and straw. Hair grooming and shaving are other self-care activities to initiate early, depending on the client's strength and activity tolerance. Adaptive equipment is sparingly used as the ultimate goal is for the patient to have and use the full range of motion of the upper extremities (UEs) and hands.

In the acute phase, ADL tasks should be selected that are valued by the client and have a high probability of success even though temporary adaptations may be necessary. Modifications in the client's environment, equipment, or previous performance patterns may be necessary to support independence. However, eventual discontinuation of adaptive techniques and devices is a long-term goal of therapy and should be presented to the client as a sign of progress during the course of therapy. A goal shared by both the client and therapist alike should be

independence in all ADLs using previous performance patterns, completed within an appropriate length of time and with minimal adaptations.

Therapeutic Exercise and Activity Tolerance

Sitting tolerance, transfers, and ambulation activities are initiated as soon as the client is medically cleared to get out of bed and bear weight on his or her LEs. If the client has burns on the LEs, elastic wraps should be applied before the client sits up and the feet become dependent. A figure-of-eight pattern should be used from the base of the toes, over and including the heel, to at least the knees, and up to the groin as needed. When the client is sitting in a chair, the LEs should be kept elevated. Any time spent dangling the feet or standing statically should be limited to prevent distal venous congestion and unnecessary discomfort. Donor sites should be considered as new areas of superficial-partial thickness injury and treated as such.

In addition to functional activities, active exercise is a primary component in every burn treatment plan. The exercise techniques used during acute care are not unique to the injury. Active, active-assisted, or passive exercises are used, depending on the client's condition. The focus of exercise in acute care is to preserve ROM and functional strength, build cardiopulmonary endurance, and decrease edema.[31,57]

Strengthening activities are introduced into the acute care intervention program as soon as the patient's condition allows. Such activities range from simple active movement to resistive activities, as tolerated, to counteract the deconditioning effects of hospitalization. Exercise after a severe burn injury was once thought to overstress an already hypermetabolic client. However, research and experience have shown that graded, progressive exercise is beneficial when recovering from acute burns.[31,57]

Client Education

Client education should be thought of as ongoing. Newly injured patients are often in a state of shock from the initial trauma. They can feel overwhelmed and have difficulty processing information. Cognitive studies show that stress can negatively affect the patient's frontal lobe, or thinking brain. This can make providing education more challenging. The patient should be given multiple opportunities to learn information. Ward and home programs are good ways to begin educating a patient on his or her burn injury, expected ROM exercises, safety precautions, and contracture preventions. When the patient is given an array of modalities and opportunities to learn information in multiple ways such as handouts, verbal instruction, video presentations, and return demonstration, outcomes improve significantly. Exercise programs should be a part of the regular treatment session, because this is how patients learn to make stretching and movement a part of their daily routine on returning home. Information should be given to patients as they can tolerate to prevent the patient feeling overwhelmed. The therapist should assess the exercise program on a daily basis to continue to provide the patient with an adequate challenge toward progression in his or her goals.

Although client education is the responsibility of all burn team members, success of the occupational therapy intervention program depends on the client's recognition of long-term activity demands, contextual needs, and role responsibilities. Initial educational objectives should focus on developing an understanding of the stages of burn recovery, the need for and importance of independent activity and motion, and pain and stress management techniques. Meeting these goals promotes motivation, active participation, and engagement in occupation, which are essential for successful treatment outcomes.[7]

Surgical and Postoperative Phase

Positioning and Postoperative Splinting

Excision and grafting procedures usually require a period of postoperative immobilization to allow adherence and vascularization of the grafted skin.[99] It is beneficial for the occupational therapist to discuss postoperative positioning needs with the surgeon before surgery so that splints and positioning devices can be prefabricated and applied in the operating room immediately after the surgical procedure. Various materials and protocols are available. All have the common purposes of immobilizing the grafted area, preventing edema, and assisting in wound healing.[25]

Postoperative positioning may follow standard positioning techniques or may be unique and designed exclusively for the specific surgical procedure. Although standard burn splints position the extremity in the antideformity position, preoperative or postoperative splints should hold the extremity in the position that promotes the greatest surface area for graft placement.

For dorsal hand grafts, the wrist is positioned in neutral or 20 degrees of extension, the MP joints in flexion in the intrinsic plus position, and the thumb in radial abduction to maximize the dorsal grafted surface area. Another example is that in which an axillary skin graft is performed; the shoulder is placed in 90 degrees of horizontal abduction. Gaining prior knowledge of the surgical procedure and determining potential postoperative complications enable the occupational therapist to establish effective positioning and splinting procedures for maximal functional outcomes and minimal scar contractures.

Although postoperative immobilization is often achieved through the use of bulky restrictive dressings and standard positioning equipment, splints are frequently needed to maintain the position. Most splints are typically made with plaster

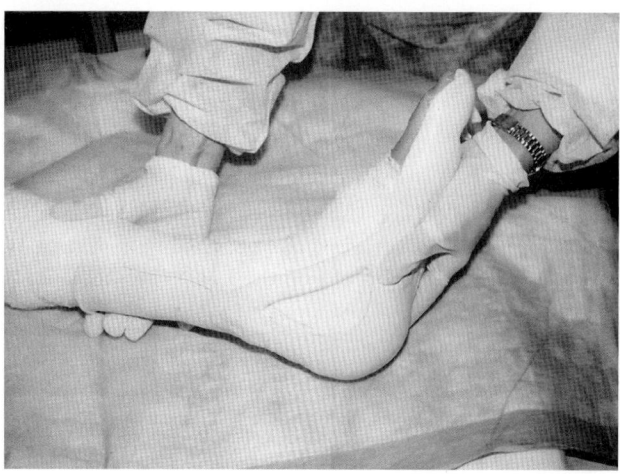

Fig 43.11 Thermoplastic total-contact ankle dorsiflexion splint to prevent plantar flexion contracture.

bandages or thermoplastic material (Fig. 43.11). If a wet dressing will cover the graft site, a perforated or open-weave splinting material may be preferred to permit continuous drainage and prevent graft maceration.[25] In some instances, movement of adjacent joints may disrupt graft adherence even though the graft does not cover the joint surface. In these cases, the splint design should incorporate immobilization of those joints in a functional position. A postoperative thermoplastic splint can generally be made by using a drape-and-trim technique.[25] Most postoperative splints are molded into position for temporary use and are discontinued once graft adherence is ensured. However, if the splints are made of thermoplastic material, they can later be remolded into the antideformity position. These splints/orthoses are valuable as an adjunct to therapeutic activities and exercises to maintain functional positions during a patient's hospital course or as part of their home program.

Therapeutic Exercise and Activity

Throughout the postoperative phase of care, active and resistive exercise of the uninvolved extremities should be continued when possible to prevent loss of ROM and strength. Immediately after excision and grafting procedures, exercises for adjacent body areas are usually discontinued for a short time. Although the time varies among burn centers, the average period of immobilization is 3 to 5 days for most STSGs and 7 to 10 days for cultured epithelial grafts.[65] Exercises can be resumed as soon as graft adherence is confirmed. Before resuming exercises, the occupational therapist should view the grafts and adjacent areas to determine graft integrity and whether any tendons are exposed or subcutaneous tissues are compromised.

Gentle AROM is the treatment of choice to avoid shearing of the new grafts. If the client exhibited normal ROM before surgery and was immobilized for only 3 to 5 days, baseline ROM should be expected within 3 days after resumption of activity. Active exercise of a body area with a donor site is generally permitted after 2 to 3 days if no active bleeding is present. Donor sites on the LEs are treated similar to burns on the LEs; therefore standard treatment involves elevation and wrapping with elastic bandage.

Ambulation after excision and grafting of the LEs is not usually resumed until 5 to 7 days after surgery. With the physician's written consent, the client is encouraged and assisted to ambulate for short distances and then slowly increase the distance. Before ambulation, double elastic bandage wraps should be applied over a fluff gauze dressing to prevent shearing of the graft or vascular pooling. Use of an elastic bandage, elevation, and a stance that discourages static positioning is particularly important for protecting grafts on the LEs. When the client is able to walk, exercise on a stationary cycle ergometer is beneficial for increasing activity tolerance. Additionally, when patients are participating in out of bed (OOB) activities, they are instructed to elevate their UEs at the level of the heart as part of edema management.

Activities of Daily Living and Client Education

Self-care and leisure-promoting activities should be continued and increased in a way that is commensurate with the demands of the activity, the client's physical abilities, and the client's tolerance of activity. Self-care is often difficult during this phase because of the immobilization positions necessary to ensure graft adherence. If a UE is immobilized, creative ADL adaptations may be needed to allow clients continued involvement in their care and control over their environment. Though only temporary, simple techniques such as universal cuffs strapped over splints or extended-handle utensils help preserve newly reacquired independence and foster confidence and feelings of self-actualization. Continued psychosocial support and burn care education are also essential to ensure understanding of postsurgical precautions and procedures.

Rehabilitation Phase: Inpatient

The rehabilitation phase generally begins when a severely burned patient no longer needs the intensive wound care provided by the burn unit. Most of the wounds are now closed, and the patient may move to a step-down unit or transfer to a rehabilitation setting. Here, patients are expected to assume a more active role in establishing treatment goals, demonstrate more independence in their care, and fully participate in their therapy. An upgraded exercise program, a variety of self-help and rehabilitation equipment, and new techniques are introduced to help increase ROM, strength, activity tolerance, and independence in higher-level ADLs and IADLs. Intervention and patient education focus on work, recreation, and the self-care skills necessary to help prepare clients for returning to normal daily activity routines, including resumption of previous performance patterns and roles. Potential roadblocks to resuming participation in occupation in previous personal contexts, including community reentry concerns and psychological adjustments, are anticipated and addressed during this phase. Physical/physiological roadblocks can impede return to occupational role participation. This is especially evident as scar maturation is the hallmark of this recovery/healing phase. Support groups and rehabilitation programs (acute rehabilitation or outpatient) can assist to facilitate a client's reintegration into their social roles and occupational roles. OTs in burn care and rehabilitation should familiarize themselves with resources in their area to help burn survivors find support within the community.

As the wound closes, scar formation develops, and clients frequently report increased skin tightness that restricts certain functional movements and inhibits completion of ADLs. Intervention techniques to counteract the effects of scar development include skin conditioning, scar massage, compression therapy, therapeutic exercise preceded by slow, gentle sustained stretching, and splinting.

During the inpatient rehabilitation phase, the occupational therapy evaluation should emphasize a thorough ongoing assessment of performance skills. Active and passive goniometric measurements should be taken to document any limitations caused by joint restrictions or scar tightness. Joint-specific measurements can be used to document individual joint restriction, but if skin tightness affects several joints in the same extremity, the total active motion measurements or total passive motion measurements of all the joints in a combined movement pattern should be documented. If the injury is unilateral, measurements taken from the unaffected side can be used to establish normal values for the injured extremity. Muscle strength can be measured by manual muscle testing (MMT). However, if MMT is used, caution is required when the therapist applies resistance to avoid shearing of newly healed skin. Other components of the evaluation should include muscular and cardiopulmonary endurance, performance of self-care and home management activities, skin integrity, presence of edema, and scar development indicating the need for scar compression garments (see Table 43.2).

Treatment goals during inpatient rehabilitation are to increase ROM, strength, and activity tolerance to achieve independence in self-care; begin skin conditioning; aid in psychological adjustment; and provide patient and caregiver education, including familiarizing the client with the care necessary for discharge from the hospital. Although these goals are continued and progressively increased during the outpatient rehabilitation phase, other goals are added as the client prepares for reintegration into the home and community.

Skin Conditioning and Scar Massage

Skin-conditioning techniques are used to improve scar integrity and durability against minor trauma caused by pressure or shearing forces, decrease hypersensitivity, and moisturize dry, newly healed skin. These techniques should be used for any burned areas or surgical sites that took longer than 2 weeks to heal. Lubrication and massage with a water-based cream or lotion should be performed three to four times a day or whenever the skin feels excessively dry, tight, or itchy. This action provides needed lubrication for skin that is dry because of damaged sweat and sebaceous glands. Massage is beneficial for desensitizing well-healed but hypersensitive grafted areas or burn scars and for softening tight scar bands during sustained stretching exercises. When massaging a scar band, the therapist should be sure that the scar is fully stretched and pre-moisturized to reduce shearing forces and prevent splitting of immature or unstable, problematic scar tissue. Massage should be performed in a circular motion, with more pressure applied gradually as tolerated over time. Because of damaged or lost skin pigment, burn survivors are at a greater risk for sunburn. Precautions, including the use of sun block and avoidance of prolonged sun exposure, are taught before the client is discharged.

Compression Therapy

Compression therapy should be initiated early in the inpatient rehabilitation phase, as soon as most of the larger wounds are closed. Temporary interim pressure bandages or garments assist in general skin desensitization, edema control, and early scar compression. The type of compression chosen and the degree of compression gradient applied depend on how much pressure and shear force that the client's newly healed skin can initially tolerate; both are upgraded as the integrity of the skin improves. Selection of an interim compression bandage or garment is based on the degree and consistency of pressure that it applies, the ease of application, and the potential for damage from shear forces during application.[15,88] Elastic bandage wraps, self-adherent elastic wraps, tubular elastic support bandages, presized elastic pressure garments, and commercial or custom-made elastic garments are all commonly used (Fig. 43.12).[88] Approximately 5 to 7 days after removal of the postoperative dressings, temporary compression dressings or garments can usually be applied. Tubular elastic bandages, presized or ready-made temporary elastic garments, Spandex "bicycle pants," and Isotoner-style gloves can be worn over light dressings. When patients have small open areas requiring minimal gauze dressings, a standard knee- or thigh-high nylon stocking can be applied over the

dressings before the donning of tubular bandages or garments to reduce shearing forces and prevent displacement of the dressings. Temporary compression dressings and garments are taken off only for bathing, dressing changes, skin care, and garment laundering. Independent donning and doffing of interim garments are incorporated into the client's ADL training.

Therapeutic Exercise and Activity

Newly healed skin tends to blister as a result of shearing forces or to split as a result of overstretching, especially when the skin is dry. Every therapy session should therefore begin with massage of the scars with a moisturizing lotion to prepare the dry or tight skin for increased motion. Whenever possible, clients should learn to perform their own skin care independently before their scheduled therapy. Once the scars are moisturized and lubricated, stretching is performed to increase the flexibility and fluidity of movement. Stretches should be slow and sustained, and forceful dynamic stretching should be avoided, with attention given to the position of adjacent joints during the stretching motion.

Massage with additional moisturizers during stretching exercises helps relieve itching and discomfort. Stretching in front of a mirror provides positive visual feedback for the patient and is helpful in correcting abnormal posturing. The therapist and client should see blanching of the scar as confirmation of an effective stretch.

AROM exercises, strengthening, and tasks to increase activity tolerance should follow stretching exercises. During the

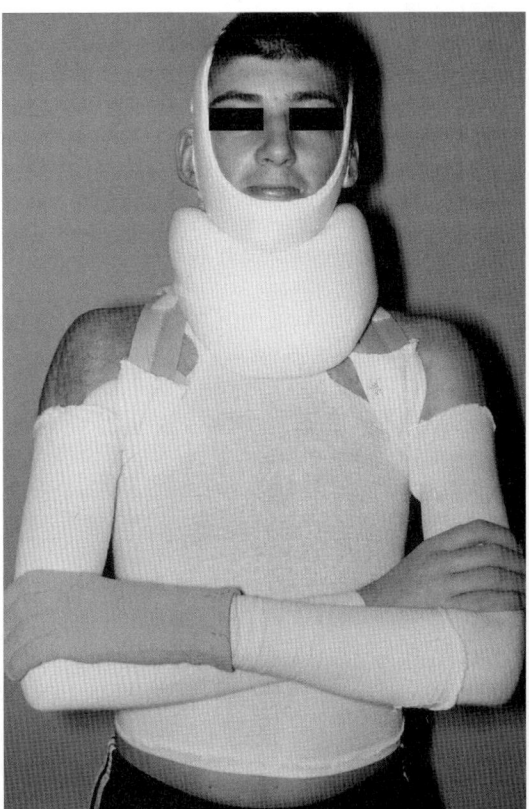
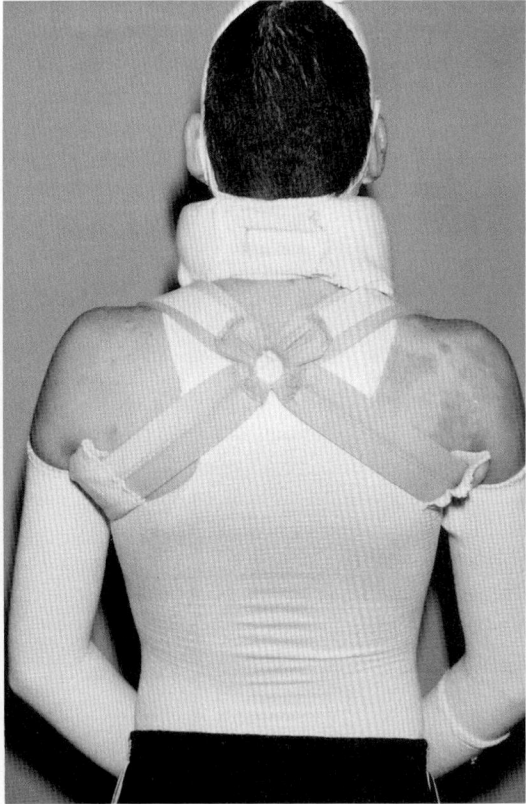

Fig. 43.12 Early compression techniques: tubular elastic dressings, ready-made gloves and chin strap, custom-fabricated foam collar, and padded clavicular strap to preserve the neck and axillary contours.

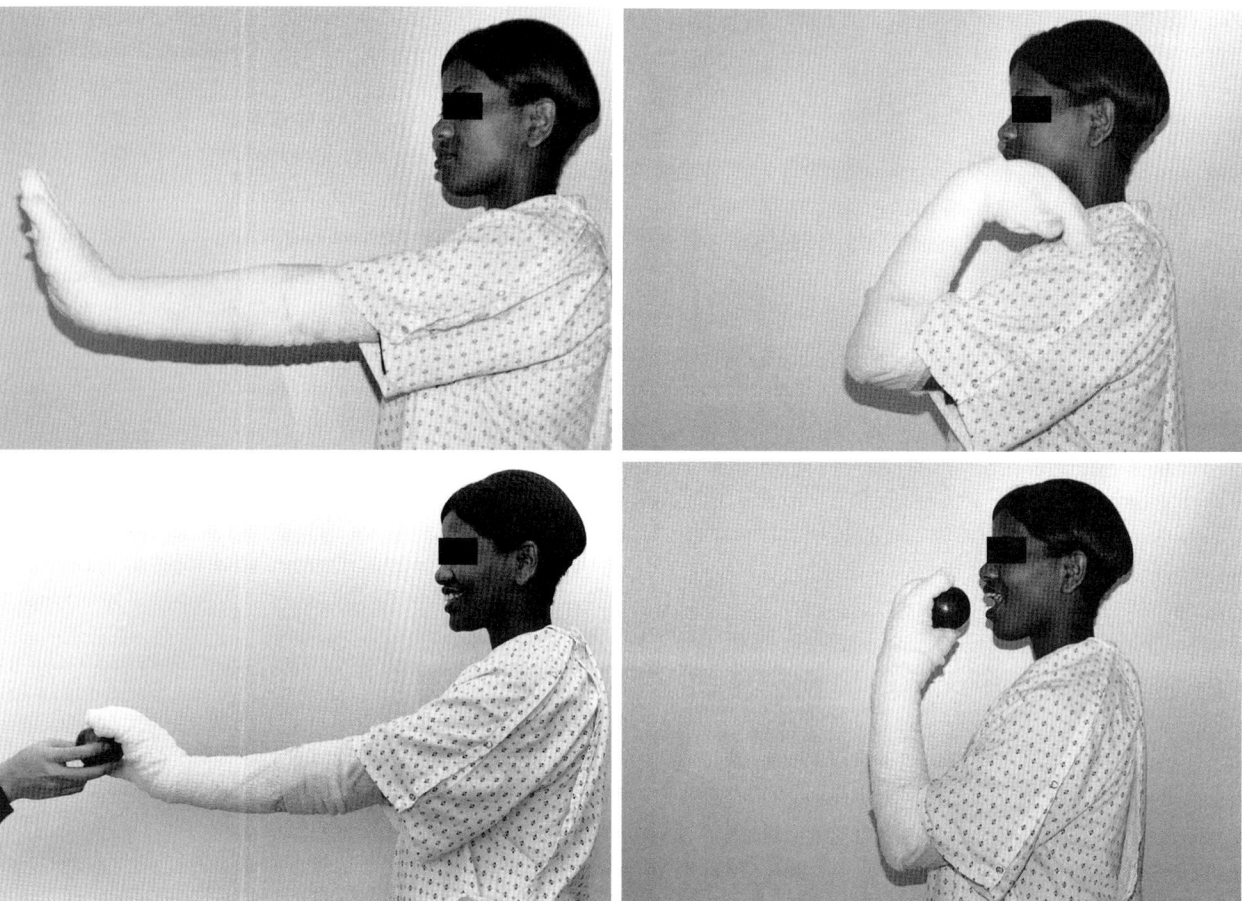

Fig. 43.13 Combined joint motions to obtain the greatest total active motion are often the same functional patterns of movement used when performing activities of daily living.

rehabilitation phase, emphasis is placed on flexibility exercises using complex motions that require the movement of several joints simultaneously. An activity that requires hand manipulation skills while reaching overhead is an example of a complex motion for a burn injury that involves the shoulder, elbow, and hand. Most ADLs require complex motions, and exercise programs should emphasize not just individual joint ROM but also combined joint mobility in functional patterns of movement (Fig. 43.13).

For clients recovering from severe hand and UE burns, intervention activities may include a variety of exercise and activity treatment media. Strengthening activities may involve the use of cuff weights, dumbbells, resistive exercise bands, or work simulation equipment. Activities for hand strengthening and coordination may include using exercise putty, hand manipulation boards, work simulators and work samples, crafts, and meaningful activities such as typing on a computer, dialing a cell phone, and playing cards or board games with visitors.

Edema Management

During the rehabilitation phase, edema often continues because of decreased function, dependent positioning without adequate external compression, or circumferential scarring of the extremity with associated lymphatic damage. When edema is present,

motion is limited and painful; if the edema becomes chronic, it may lead to fibrosis.[92] To treat edema of an extremity, elevation, progressive compression, and activity are recommended.

Self-adherent elastic bandage material (e.g., Coban or Coflex) is often used as an early form of compression for the digits, hands, and feet. It is applied in a spiral fashion, from distal to proximal, with the previous lap overlapped by a half overlap starting on each digit and continuing in this manner across the hand or foot and onto the wrist or ankle. Strips are also applied to each web space (Fig. 43.14). The distal tips of digits are left open to monitor color, which should be rosy and not blanched or bluish. The rest of the extremity is wrapped with an elastic bandage or other form of temporary compression garment. The wrapped hand should be used during ADLs and other functional motions and elevated just above heart level when the client is resting. For edema of the LEs, use of a double layer of elastic wrap when ambulating, elevation when resting, active ankle exercises, and avoidance of static standing are recommended. Intermittent compression pump therapy is often used to treat chronic edema of the distal ends of extremities. Whenever compression therapy is used to treat edema of the hands or feet, before and after circumferential or volumetric measurements are recommended to monitor the effectiveness of the treatment (Fig. 43.15).

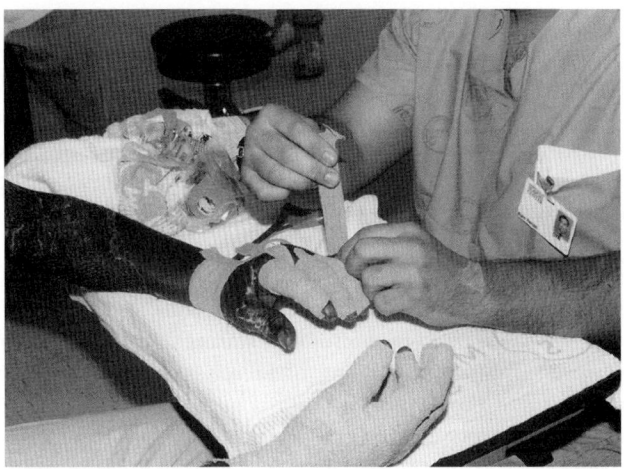

Fig. 43.14 Application of self-adherent elastic wrap to newly healed hands and feet provides external compression for the treatment of edema and early scarring.

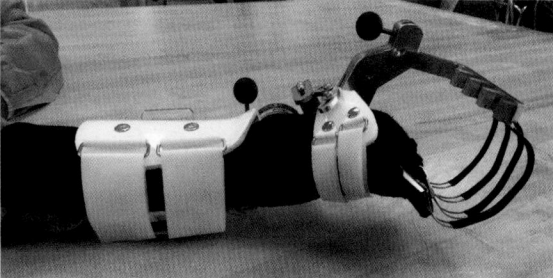

Fig. 43.16 Static-progressive dynamic hand splints allow for a gradual progression of range of motion of the joints of the fingers and wrist during an individual treatment session. Family members or patients can be instructed on how to apply these splints, and they can be incorporated into home exercise programs.

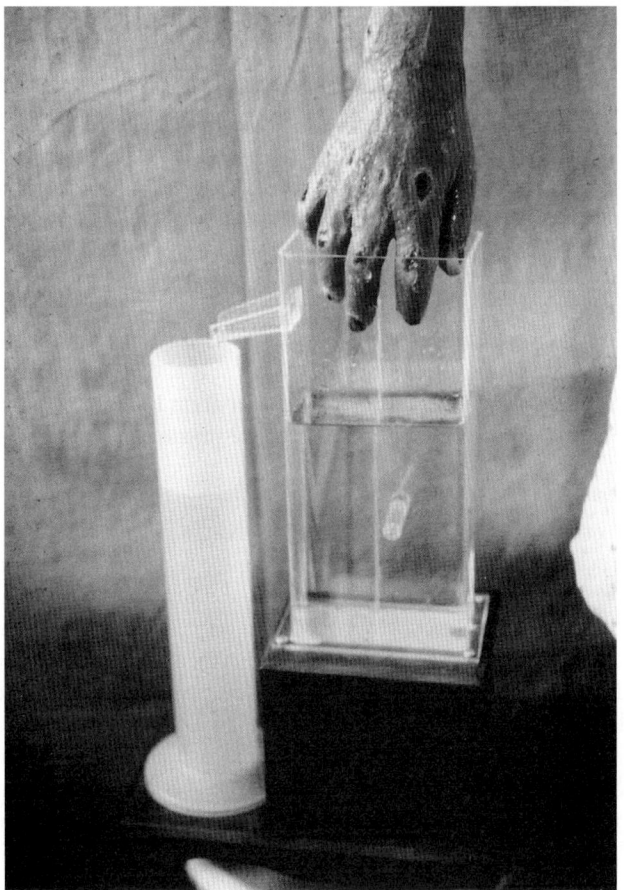

Fig. 43.15 In the treatment of extremity edema, sequential circumferences and volumetric measurements are methods to monitor and document treatment efficacy.

Activities of Daily Living

As patients approach discharge from the hospital, the therapist must stress the importance of independent self-care. Eating, dressing, grooming, and bathing skills should be emphasized as part of the normal daily routine to increase independence

and activity tolerance. When problems occur, the therapist must determine whether the dysfunction originates from a physical limitation, scar contracture, pain, edema, or an assumed abnormal postural reaction. Early identification of abnormal movements helps patients understand and relearn normal movement patterns before the abnormal patterns become habitual.

Practicing ADLs with personal care items and supplies from home fosters self-confidence in functional performance skills before hospital discharge. Clients with major burn injuries may initially require adaptations to support independence. However, when assessing the need for adaptive self-care, the therapist should differentiate between a physical limitation that can be rehabilitated and permanent loss of function.

In addition to basic ADLs and self-care tasks, IADL tasks such as home management responsibilities should be practiced before discharge. Fear of items associated with the injury, such as hot water, the stove, or an electric iron, can hinder functional recovery. For clients injured during a home activity, the therapist should arrange counseling, support, and practice of the skills or activity in the clinic. Prevention techniques taught as part of the inpatient treatment program also should be part of the home program.[102]

Splinting

Splinting in the rehabilitation stage is used to limit or reverse potentially disabling or disfiguring contracture formations, increase ROM, distribute pressure over problem areas, or assist in function (Fig. 43.16). Static splints, dynamic splints, and casting may be used,[25,70,75] depending on the location and severity of the contracture. Regardless of the purpose of the splint, every effort should be made to ensure that its purpose and method of application are fully understood. Splinting at nighttime and during rest periods is preferred because it allows functional use of the extremity during waking hours and provides treatment of contractures while the client is unoccupied. However, splints must fit comfortably, and corrective splinting should not cause discomfort that interferes with the client's rest. Although most clinicians agree about the value of splinting based on the strong rationale for splint use to provide counterforce to contracting scars or to lengthen scars when they limit joint motion, decision making on specifically when and how to splint remains controversial because of lack of strong clinical evidence.[75] The therapist must continually weigh the risk-to-benefit ratio and consider timing, design, and duration of splinting relative to each client's functional needs.

Client Education

Client and caregiver education becomes increasingly important during the predischarge phase to aid the transition from hospital to home. Increased understanding is needed in the areas of wound healing, the importance of preserving independence in ADLs and IADLs, the need for continued activity and exercise, the causes and effects of scar contracture, and scar management techniques and principles. Before discharge from the hospital or transfer to an inpatient rehabilitation facility, the client and family should receive a comprehensive home care education review (Table 43.4).[102] To reinforce learning, information should be presented through a variety of methods, such as verbal instruction, printed handouts, demonstrations, and educational videos. Most important, opportunities should be provided for the client and caregivers to practice wound care, garment and splint application, and all exercises under staff supervision in the weeks preceding discharge. Only with a detailed understanding of home care techniques and potential outcomes can clients be expected to assume responsibility for their own care and recovery.[102]

Rehabilitation Phase: Outpatient

Reassessment

Reassessment procedures take on greater significance after discharge. ROM, strength, activity tolerance, ADLs and IADLs, and skin and scar status must be assessed frequently to ensure early identification of specific problem areas. In addition to these rehabilitation components, the effectiveness of compression garments, the fit and need for continuation of certain splints, home care activities, emotional coping skills, and resumption of engagement in pre-burn occupations to support participation in contexts or life situations should also be closely monitored.

Reassessment of activity tolerance and work skills is indicated to help determine whether clients are ready to return

TABLE 43.4	Home Program Outline
Item	**Information Needed**
Wound care, positioning	Dressing change technique, precautions, elevation
Skin and scar care	Lubricant frequency, sun protection, trauma precautions such as no scratching
Self-care	Techniques and minimizing use of equipment
Splints and orthotics	Donning techniques, schedule, precautions
Pressure garments*	Purpose, washing, reordering, donning techniques, wearing schedule
Exercises	Frequency, techniques for specific areas, contracture prevention

*Custom-made garments are available from Jobst Institute, http://www.jobstcompressioninstitute.com; Barton-Carey, http://www.bartoncarey.com/images/GarmentChart-3.pdf; Bio-Concepts, Inc., http://www.bio-con.com; Medical-Z, http://www.medicalz.com.

to school or work or be referred for vocational rehabilitation. Driving evaluation and prevocational assessment by using simulated work activities or work sample testing also may be indicated for the more severely injured burn survivor. Vocational counseling and exploration should be undertaken in the later stages of recovery if residual dysfunction necessitates a change in the work environment or vocational role.

Therapeutic Exercise and Activity

Inpatient rehabilitation techniques, equipment, and therapeutic activities continue to be appropriate during outpatient therapy. However, progressive grading of exercise and the frequency, intensity, and duration of activity is necessary to successfully regain or improve the client's strength, activity tolerance, and performance skills and patterns, as well as abilities in performance in areas of occupation. Sequencing the order of intervention activities is necessary to prevent injury, minimize client discomfort, and prevent excessive fatigue. Skin lubrication, massage, and stretching should precede progressive strengthening exercises and activities.[52] Before being discharged, clients should learn how to prepare for exercise and activity by performing their own skin lubrication, massage, and stretching. Doing their own pretreatment skin care and stretching will allow outpatients to maximize actual therapy time and develop habits that promote consistent follow-through with their home activities and independent exercise program.

The ABA established guidelines for practice in implementing cardiovascular exercises. The guidelines state that cardiovascular fitness should be assessed in burn patients 7 years or older. Exercise programs can begin as early as discharged from the acute care setting and as late as 14 years after the burn injury. The ABA recommends that the exercise program last 6 to 12 weeks for adults and 12 weeks for children for maximal benefit.[56,58]

Scar Management

A primary objective of most burn rehabilitation techniques is prevention or treatment of hypertrophic scars and scar contractures. For effective treatment of scar problems, scar characteristics must be monitored so that one can recognize when maturation occurs. Active scars are erythematous, raised, and rigid. As they mature, scars become less vascular in color, with flatter and more pliable contours and a smoother texture. Scar maturation usually takes 12 to 18 months after injury, depending on the length of time that the original burn takes to heal. However, it is important to remember that each patient heals differently. Some scars mature in less than 1 year, whereas others may take more than 2 years.[88]

A rating scale has been designed that allows serial assessment of scar pigment, vascularity, pliability, and height.[14] Although the ratings are somewhat subjective and time-consuming, the scale is a useful clinical tool. However, use of digital photography is a time-efficient and objective method of documenting changes in scar appearance; copies of the images can be easily inserted into the medical record.

Wearing intermediate-pressure garments prepares the skin for the later fitting of custom-made compression garments. Use of compression garments is indicated for all donor sites, graft sites, and burn wounds that take more than 2 weeks to heal spontaneously.[88] The occupational therapist is often responsible for measuring, ordering, and fitting of these garments. The occupational therapist must frequently make special on-the-spot modifications during a clinic visit or fabricate underlying conformers to ensure uniform pressure. All custom-made garments are measured and ordered according to the specific instructions of the manufacturer. Most compression garment manufacturers offer a variety of design options, including special zippers or Velcro closures, silicone lining, custom inserts, and assorted colors.

Ideally, clients should be fitted with custom-made compression garments no later than 3 weeks after wound healing; otherwise, interim garments are worn until custom garments can be applied. It may be necessary to order garments on a piecemeal basis because different areas of the client may be ready for compression treatment at different points in time. Custom-made compression garments are constructed to provide gradient pressure, starting at 35 mm Hg distally (Fig. 43.17). They should be worn 23 hours a day and be removed only for bathing, massage, skin care, or sexual activity. Face masks and gloves also may be removed for meals. Compression therapy should be applied to the burned area for approximately 12 to 18 months or until scar maturation is complete. Donor sites may also require compression garments, depending on the thickness of the donor skin taken and whether healing occurred in less than 2 weeks.

Once proper fit is established, it is recommended that the client possess a minimum of two sets of garments at any time to allow both around-the-clock compression therapy and laundering. Because of the elastic construction of the fabric, clients should hand-wash the garments with mild soap and allow them to air-dry unless otherwise advised by the manufacturer. To prolong the life of the garments, washing machines, dryers, direct heat, strong detergents, or bleach should not be used. If they are properly cared for, most garments will last approximately 2 to 3 months before replacements are needed. Children may need replacements more frequently as a result of their growth and active lifestyle. Toddlers undergoing toilet training and incontinent adults may need extra garments and design options that make independent toileting easier. Adults employed indoors are usually able to return to work and previous activities without interference from the garments. However, some individuals who work outside in warmer climates may find compression garments to be too hot in the summer months and may need to change their work setting until compression therapy is no longer required.

To be effective, compression garments must exert equal pressure over the entire burned surface area. Because of body contours, bony prominences, and postural adjustments, flexible inserts or pressure-adapting conformers are often needed under the garments to distribute the pressure more evenly. Areas commonly requiring pressure adapters are the supraclavicular region of the upper part of the chest, the areas between and under the breasts of women or obese men, the nasolabial folds, the midface and chin, the areas between the scapulae and over the axillary folds, the gluteal fold, the perineum, and the web spaces of the hands and feet.

Pressure inserts and conformers are now made from a variety of materials; the choice is based on the area to be treated and the need for flexibility when applied. As with compression garments, the fit of a conformer should be monitored at regular intervals for effectiveness and signs of deterioration and be replaced as needed to maintain exact contouring. Silicone gel pads, Silastic elastomer, Otoform-K (Dreve-Otoplastik GmbH, Unna, Germany), Plastazote (Zotefoams Inc., Croydon, United Kingdom), and Velfoam (North Coast Medical, Inc., Morgan Hill, California) are useful for hand scars. One-sixteenth inch Aquaplast and Silastic (Qfix) elastomer work well on face scars; closed-cell foams, prosthetic foam elastomer, silicone gel pads, Plastazote, Otoform-K, and Velfoam are also useful for other body areas. In addition, Velfoam and silicone gel pads are effective at the flexion creases of the knees, elbows, and anterior aspect of the ankle to equalize pressure and prevent discomfort during activities.

It is important to note that although the use of pressure garments and silicone gel is commonplace, their effectiveness is not well established. A 2009 meta-analysis examining the effectiveness of pressure-garment therapy for the prevention of abnormal scarring after burn injury found sparse evidence to support its widespread use.[8,88] A systematic review of silicone gel sheeting reported inconclusive evidence of its benefits in preventing or treating abnormal scarring.[62,88]

The ABA established practice guidelines for practitioners regarding the use of silicone gel sheets. The ABA recommends that silicone gel sheets be applied whenever hypertrophic scars are likely to develop and as soon as the skin has reepithelialized. Keloid scars may also benefit from silicone gel, and it should be considered as a potential treatment. Silicone gel sheets have been shown to demonstrate less adverse reactions than gel sheets when used for scar management. Only active scars that have not matured yet should be treated with silicone.

The use of lasers is also an effective treatment for hypertrophic scars. The most commonly used types of lasers are the fractional laser and pulsed dye laser. The fractional laser can be ablative or nonablative. Both ablative and nonablative fractional laser treatments will result in decreased inflammation, increased

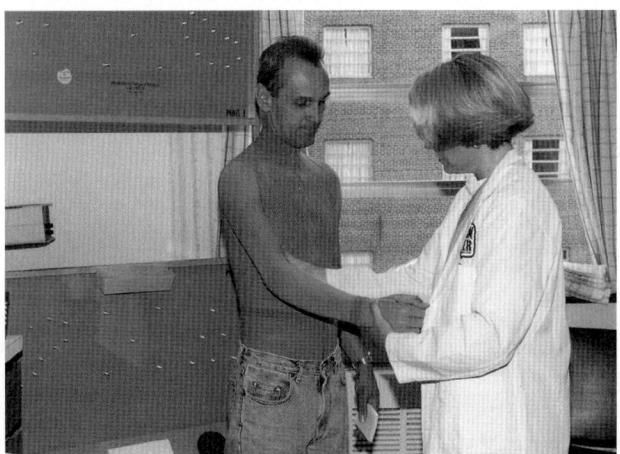

Fig. 43.17 The fit of custom-made compression garments must be regularly reassessed to ensure adequate compression for effective scar management.

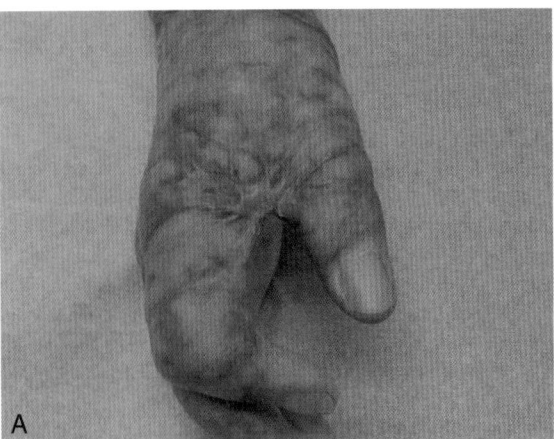
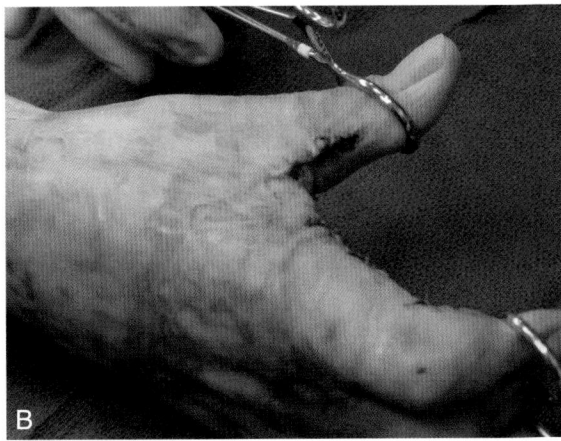

Fig. 43.18 (A) A scar contracture occurs when tight scars limit free motion of a joint. This can be very limiting when the contractures are present in the hand. (B) Surgical scar revisions can be done to reconstruct the hand and improve hand function.

vascularity, and improved collagen remodeling.[96] However, the ablative laser will penetrate deeper into the scar and is more invasive and may be more effective in the treatment of thicker scars. The pulsed dye laser uses pulsed light to treat dyschromia. It is effective for the treatment of erythema and edema.[96]

Activities of Daily Living

In addition to continued exercise, skin care, and scar management, the outpatient intervention plan should be directed at increasing independence in home care while also emphasizing resumption of prior life roles and context, including returning to previous work, school, social, and leisure activities. Scar contracture is often the primary cause of dysfunction (Fig. 43.18). Therefore activities performed during therapy should not only promote strength, activity tolerance, and functional ROM and stretching to counteract the effects of scarring but also preserve independence in performance of occupations related to clients' personal contexts and interests.

Community Reentry

Returning to school or work becomes a primary objective during outpatient rehabilitation. However, most recovering burn survivors are capable of resuming normal daily routines and performance patterns long before their scars completely mature.

Returning to previous community settings (e.g., school, work, and social settings) and becoming reacquainted with friends and co-workers can be a difficult process for burn survivors who have cosmetic disfigurement, loss of functional performance, or restrictions in activity. A community reentry program should be implemented before the client returns to school or work. Correspondence sent to the community setting before the client's return helps educate employers, teachers, and peers about burn injuries and what the client has experienced. This correspondence should explain the purpose of compression garments, splints, exercise, and skin care precautions; digital photos are helpful. The goal of a reentry program is to reduce restrictions in the client's activities and ease the transition of returning to previous areas of occupation.[41,48]

Preparing a burn patient for return to work does not have to be a long-term process. Burn rehabilitation and work skills training have many similarities; therefore, it is possible to design treatment activities that simulate not only functional activities but also various work skills. Strength, activity tolerance, and flexibility, often identified as work tolerances, are obvious goals of burn rehabilitation. Physical demands of jobs, as described in the *Dictionary of Occupational Titles*,[90] are also components of functional skills; lifting, stooping, pushing, pulling, handling, and manipulating are a few examples. A job analysis interview, performed as part of the activity needs analysis, provides the type of information needed to integrate activities into the intervention plan, which should not only improve functional ability but also provide reconditioning for returning to work.

Preparing the client for community reentry after a burn injury also requires attention to two other types of tolerance: skin and temperature. Most clients will still need to wear compression garments and inserts, avoid prolonged sun exposure, and perform skin care while they are at school or work. Skin-conditioning activities and exercises performed while wearing garments will improve skin tolerance for friction and shear force demands (Fig. 43.19). Education regarding the body's response to variations in temperature and precautions for dealing with extremes of temperature are necessary for the patient to plan for anticipated temperature tolerance problems. A systematic review of the literature reported that an average of 66% of patients returned to work after their burn, with the time taken to return to work ranging from 4.7 to 24 months. The extent and severity of the burn were the most significant barriers; others were longer hospital stays and the number of operative procedures.[71] (See Chapters 14 and 15 for further information.)

Children may have a more difficult time reintegrating into their previous roles as students and playmates. Many burn centers offer school reentry programs to assist children in the emotional and physical challenges of returning to their school environment.[41,48] With prior parental permission, predischarge plans are made to send written information to the child's teacher, classmates, and (when available) a community-based therapist

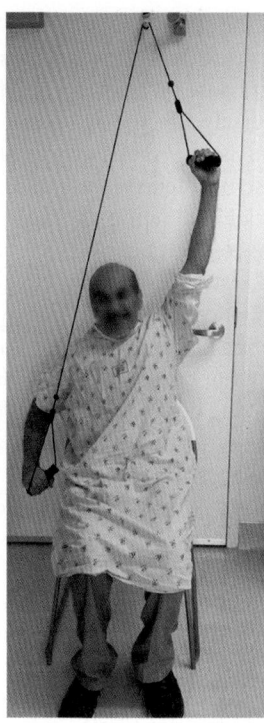

Fig. 43.19 Overhead pulleys are useful to increase range of motion of the upper extremities. They are also easily issued to patients for setup and use at home as a part of their home exercise program.

working in the school system to acquaint them with the child's changed appearance and special needs. A videotaped message recorded by the child to his or her classmates explaining what happened can be very effective, especially when delivered by a family member or healthcare professional, who can then answer the children's questions. The tape can show the child both with and, if appropriate, without compression garments to help satisfy classmates' curiosity and concerns before the burned child returns to the classroom. Such preparations ease resumption of the student role for the child and can help improve acceptance by other children, who may misunderstand the cause of the disfigurement and the need for splints, adapted equipment, and scar compression garments. Informed classmates often serve as advocates for the burned child by passing information to students in other grades or on the bus and providing support when misinformed students reveal their ignorance or fear by teasing or taunting the burned child. Regional burn summer camps, often sponsored by local firefighter organizations or burn centers, also help children adjust by placing them in settings where they can socialize with peers who also have been burned.

For burn survivors of all ages, compression garments should fit the lifestyle of the survivor. Some survivors cannot tolerate compression garments and choose not to have them. Some cannot afford them, and insurance will not cover the expense. In each individual case, the patient's wishes should be respected. It is important that OTs working in burn care and rehabilitation understand that compression garments are one way to treat hypertrophic scars but that all aspects of the client's life need to be considered when determining the right scar management technique.

Psychological Adjustment

During outpatient rehabilitation, clients may undergo numerous physical and emotional changes. Once discharged from the hospital, they must face the overwhelming task of becoming responsible and self-reliant while dealing with the stress associated with developing scars and a changing self-image. They may not participate fully in therapy or adequately follow through with home care activities because of the physical and emotional effects of the injury. Apathy, avoidance of pain, scar tightness, and hypersensitivity all contribute to noncompliance and subsequent dysfunction after injury. Clients may experience symptoms of post-traumatic stress disorder, nightmares, and changes in appetite with subsequent weight gain or loss. They may become reclusive or disengage from previous relationships. Depression may occur even before discharge and some burn-injured clients have preexisting psychiatric issues that are exacerbated by the additional stress of the burn injury.[51,69,74]

In addition to established treatments such as counseling, support, and training in pain management and relaxation techniques, visits from a recovered burn survivor to a new patient are often of great benefit. Attending a burn support group can also help the burn survivor and family members in psychological adjustment. Research has shown that burn survivors at different stages of recovery tend to provide positive support to one another. Group discussions among burn survivors promote acceptance of what they have already experienced and realistic expectations of what they still need to accomplish.[41]

Discharge From Treatment

The outpatient therapy program should be reevaluated periodically to determine whether the frequency of treatment, program progression, or professional or educational status should be changed (e.g., return to work or school).[48] When clients have resumed their preinjury activities, outpatient therapy may be discontinued. Because burn scar maturation may take more than 18 months, a schedule of follow-up care, with appointments every 2 to 3 months, is needed until wearing of compression garments is discontinued. However, for children, annual burn clinic visits are recommended, even after discontinuation of compression garments, until full physical maturity is reached to ensure that growth is not impeded by scar inflexibility.

BURN-RELATED COMPLICATIONS

Heterotopic Ossification

Heterotopic ossification (HO) is formation of bone in locations that normally do not contain bone tissue.[29,30,88] The underlying cause of HO is not yet fully understood. It typically develops either in the soft tissue around the joint or in the joint capsule and ligaments, and it often forms a bony bridge across the joint, resulting in a fused joint.[38,46] Although HO is frequently found in the posterior aspect of the elbow, it may occur in other joint areas such as the shoulder, wrist, hand, hip, knee, and ankle. It may occur in either extremity or bilaterally, even if the extremities were not burned. Signs that HO may be present usually appear during the latter stages of hospitalization, with the patient experiencing increased pain at a certain point in the joint's ROM.

The pain is fairly localized and severe, and loss of ROM is usually rapid, with development of a hard, unyielding feel at the joint's end of available ROM. Inflammatory signs, such as redness or swelling, are not easily discernible within healing burn wounds. Once HO has been detected, frequent AROM exercise of the joint should be carried out within the pain-free range to preserve as much joint motion as possible.[20,46] Use of dynamic splints or forceful passive stretching of the involved joint should be discontinued. If the condition does not resolve with time, surgical intervention may be necessary to resect the limiting bony tissue, followed by therapy to preserve the regained ROM.

Neuromuscular Complications

Peripheral neuropathic conditions are the most common neurological disorder observed in burn patients.[30] They usually occur with high-voltage electrical burns or burns involving greater than 20% TBSA.[37] Peripheral nerve damage may be caused by infections, metabolic abnormalities, or neurotoxicities. A peripheral neuropathic condition is generally manifested as symmetric distal weakness, with or without sensory symptoms. Most conditions improve with time; however, patients often complain of fatigue and decreased activity tolerance that may last for months.[37]

In addition to peripheral neuropathic conditions, localized compression or stretch injuries of nerves are encountered during burn recovery.[30] Causes of localized nerve injury include improper or prolonged positioning in bed or on the operating room table, tourniquet injury, and extreme edema. Common injury sites are the brachial plexus and ulnar and peroneal nerves. Prolonged frog-leg positioning can cause a stretch injury, whereas prolonged side lying can cause a compression injury of the peroneal nerve.[37] The ulnar nerve is subject to a compression injury if the client rests on a firm surface with the elbows flexed and the forearms pronated. The brachial plexus is susceptible to stretch or compression injury if inappropriate shoulder-positioning techniques are used. To implement more effective prevention and intervention techniques, therapists should be aware of the causes and symptoms of various nerve injuries.[30]

Contact with high-voltage electrical current often produces permanent damage to peripheral nerves as a result of thermal damage at the entrance and exit sites of the electrical current.[30] Damage also occurs to peripheral nerves as a result of secondary compression of the blood supply caused by swelling of surrounding tissues. Delayed neurological complications are caused by direct thermal damage, which results in demyelination and subsequent nerve cell death, or by vascular compromise of the brain or spinal cord. This generalized damage may be manifested as paralysis, cognitive impairment, aphasia, seizures, balance problems, or other neurological symptoms. The therapist should be attentive to any developing symptoms of sensory or motor dysfunction in a client who was initially neurologically intact.[30]

Facial Disfigurement

Facial scars can be devastating, both functionally and psychologically.[30] Tight or hypertrophic scars not only distort the smooth contours of the cheeks and forehead but can also flatten the nasal contours, evert the eyelids and lips, and constrict the optic and oral commissures. Vision, speech, feeding, and dental hygiene can be adversely affected by oral and eye contractures. Facial disfigurement is also damaging to an individual's self-image and inhibits social reentry. A significant amount of communication and social interaction depends on nonverbal facial expressions and eye contact. Severe facial burn scars not only distort the face and restrict expression but also undermine the patient's self-esteem when he or she is met by social rejection.

Two main compression therapy methods are used to prevent or manage hypertrophic facial scars. An elastic face mask can be worn with underlying flexible thermoplastic conformers. The other option is a rigid, total-contact transparent facial orthosis.[76] Each has advantages and disadvantages.

Because face masks are made of elastic fabric, generally enclose the entire head and neck, and use flexible conformers, they provide uniform multidirectional compression during movement or changes in position. However, because they occlude the face, they are cosmetically and socially less acceptable. The effectiveness of the compression is based on subjective feedback from the patient and observations made by the therapist during outpatient clinic visits. Most underlying conformers are easy to modify or replace to provide effective distribution of pressure over facial concavities and contours.

Conventional fabrication of a transparent, rigid facial orthosis is an involved and often expensive process. First, a cast is made with dental alginate over the surface of the face, and then the alginate is reinforced with a layer of fast-setting plaster strips. The patient must lie still and breathe through straws or small openings left in the alginate, which can be difficult for claustrophobic adults or small children. For this reason, some patients are unable to cooperate with this procedure unless they are under anesthesia. After the cast is removed from the patient, the breathing and neck openings are closed with more plaster strips and the facial cast filled with plaster of Paris. The resulting exact duplicate plaster model is polished smooth of scars and defects by hand. Additional plaster is carved off as needed to increase pressure on specific scarred areas of the face. Clear, high-temperature thermoplastic is then heated, stretched over the model, and either vacuum-molded to the model or manually stretched and molded by hand. The edges are finished, elastic straps are applied, and the orthosis is fitted to the patient. Because the material is clear, the rigid face mask has the advantage of allowing the therapist to view the face and objectively evaluate the amount of pressure exerted on the scars. By noting the presence of scar blanching under the clear mask, precise adjustments can be made as needed. The clear mask allows the face to be seen but has the disadvantage of exerting primarily unilateral compression, which may be compromised by speech, facial expressions, or side-lying positions. The mask does not allow perspiration to evaporate and must be removed and wiped clean regularly, especially in warmer climates.

Computer-aided design and manufacturing systems have been developed to fabricate transparent face masks efficiently and economically.[77] Three-dimensional (3D) scanning and 3D printers have become more widely available and can be used to fabricate face masks for scar management.[94] A software system integrates shape capture, mask design, and model fabrication with a linear scan noncontact laser imager for the acquisition of facial topography. The computer then integrates with a milling machine to fabricate a positive model out of urethane foam. The foam model is modified through use of the computer program and lined with a layer of polypropylene to smooth the foam texture. The model is then sprayed with silicone and the mold released and used basically in the same manner as the plaster model described previously. The rest of the fabrication process also works in a similar way. The advantage of computerized imaging and model fabrication is the speed of fabrication of the

model and the ability to obtain a model without having to take a direct cast of the patient's face.

With either method, frequent alterations are necessary to achieve and maintain adequate compression of all facial scars (Fig. 43.20). The choice of method is based on the preferences of the patient and physician. However, a combination of both types may be advantageous: the patient wears a clear, rigid face mask in social settings and a fabric mask with conformers at home. Appropriate skin care education is also important. Massage with lotion twice a day will aid in scar desensitization and provide the necessary lubrication. Facial massage and exercises are performed at least four times a day to help stretch tight

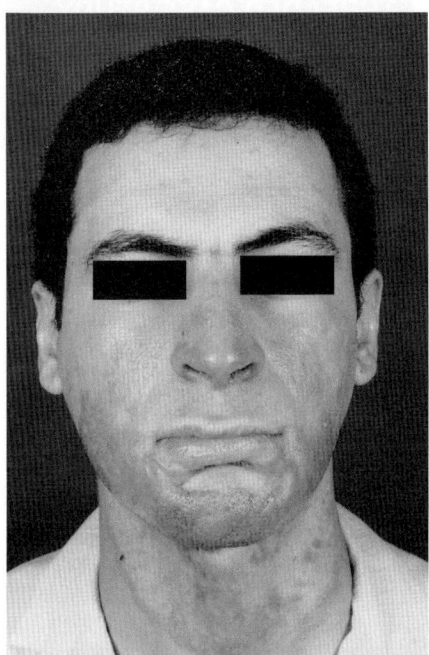
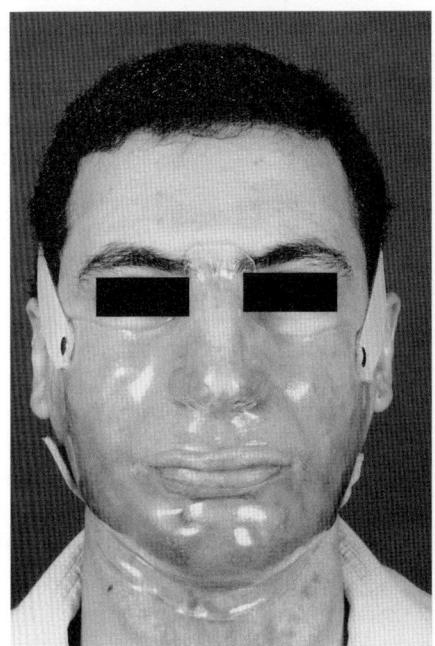
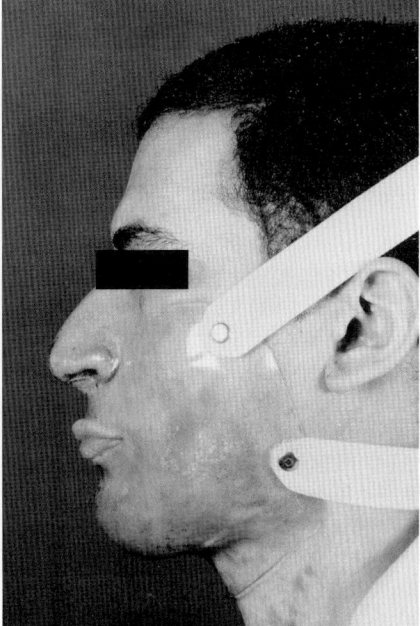

Fig. 43.20 Close-up view of a transparent rigid facial orthosis. The mask contours and strap system are modified to adjust the amount of pressure over specific scarred areas (note the blanching of the scars on the lower lip and lateral aspect of the chin).

facial skin, maintain eyelid and mouth flexibility, and preserve the nostril openings.

Just as with any compression therapy technique, patient compliance is essential for effectiveness of the treatment. The patient is instructed to wear the face mask at all times except while eating, bathing, or engaging in sexual activity. The patient should carry written verification from the burn physician verifying the medical necessity for the mask. Regardless, patients should always consider removing their masks before entering any public facility to avoid provoking suspicion that they are prepared to commit robbery or violence. This is especially important when entering banks, convenience stores, or government facilities, even if the patient is well known to the employees.

Individuals wearing either type of mask initially experience acute feelings of self-consciousness and may avoid going out in public. Parents may have difficulty putting the mask on their children and may experience feelings of guilt if the child rebels. Supportive intervention from family members and therapists is an important way to successfully manage these social and personal issues. Masks are very visible pieces of equipment that can provoke ridicule and bullying from community members for any burn patient. It is important that an OT follow up with a client as to their experiences, thoughts, and feelings about having to wear any compression garment but especially a mask. If the result is negative, then it is the responsibility of the OT to advocate for the client to other members of the multidisciplinary team to provide alternative options for scar management or flexibility with client compliance.

Consistent follow-through is especially critical in preventing or correcting facial scarring and disfigurement. Before applying the mask, the therapist must provide early education, ongoing encouragement, and continual support to ensure that the client wears the facial orthosis. Once the scars are mature and compression therapy is no longer needed, the client should be instructed in the use of special camouflaging cosmetics such as Covermark by Lydia O'Leary, which will cover minor flaws in texture and correct uneven pigmentation.

THREADED CASE STUDY

Ben, Part 2

Ben will continue his process of recovery in an outpatient setting. Because of the nature of his work and career goals, it was recommended that he continue to work with OT in an outpatient setting to progress his UE strength, coordination, and function. It will be essential for the outpatient OT to work with Ben toward improvements in UE function, cosmesis of the scars, and his psychosocial well-being to help him move toward understanding and acceptance of his injury. Because the burn has permanently altered the appearance and texture of his skin, Ben will always be reminded of the incident that resulted in his scars. Once again, rehabilitation for burn injured patients includes psychological recovery as well as the physical one.

SUMMARY

Burn injury is one of the most painful and devastating injuries that can be sustained. Advancements in trauma care and in surgical techniques have significantly improved the survival rate of patients with large burn injuries and those with accompanying multiple medical problems. Treatment of the burn injury is as traumatic as the injury itself at times and can lead to a negative psychological impact on the patient. The occupational therapist treating in a burn center is a valuable member of the team, not just for the patient's physical rehabilitation but also for his or her psychological rehabilitation. Reengaging in normal, valued daily occupations can improve not only a patient's functional ability and movement but also the feelings of competence in occupational performance. Burn survivors often endure more pain than they previously thought they could and must push themselves past what they believed their strength and ability could tolerate to accomplish their goals. As these patients engage in the therapeutic process and recover their functional abilities, they learn new skills to adapt and problem solve. This gives them a tremendous amount of self-esteem and self-efficacy. The word *survivor* then takes on a new meaning of having not only survived traumatic injuries but having learned new skills and created new occupational roles.

REVIEW QUESTIONS

1. Name the two layers of the skin. In which layer are the nerves and sebaceous glands located?
2. Which factors are considered in determining burn severity?
3. What is an escharotomy, and why is it performed? How does it differ from a fasciotomy?
4. Describe two factors that affect the quality of burn wound healing and promote excessive scar formation.
5. During the acute care phase, which factors may limit full ROM?
6. What is a boutonnière deformity, and what are boutonnière precautions?
7. What are the two basic principles underlying most burn rehabilitation treatment techniques?
8. What is the primary objective for positioning during acute care?
9. What are the indications for initiating splints during the acute care phase?
10. When a splint is indicated in the acute phase, what is the preferred wearing schedule and why?
11. When should client education about burn injury and rehabilitation begin?
12. What would cause a patient to require temporary adaptations for self-care during the acute phase?
13. Why are patients immobilized postoperatively? On average, how soon after grafting can gentle AROM exercises be resumed?

14. How soon postoperatively can an intermediate compression dressing or garment be applied?
15. What are the two main compression therapy options for the treatment of facial scars?
16. Why are skin-conditioning activities used in burn rehabilitation? What are examples of skin-conditioning techniques?
17. What is the average length of time required for scar maturation?
18. What are possible causes of limitations in ADLs during the rehabilitation phase?
19. What information should be included in predischarge education and a home program review?
20. What is the primary cause of dysfunction after a burn injury?

REFERENCES

1. Achora S, Muliira JK, Thanka AN: Strategies to promote healing of split thickness skin grafts: an integrative review, *Journal of Wound Ostomy & Continence Nursing* 41(4):335–339, 2014.
2. Al-Mousawi AM, Suman OE, Herndon DN: Teamwork for total burn care: burn centers and multidisciplinary burn teams, *Total Burn Care* 4:9–13, 2012.
3. American Burn Association. (n.d.) https://www.ameriburn.org.
4. American Burn Association: Burn incidence and treatment in the US: 2000 fact sheet. http://www.ameriburn.org.
5. American Burn Association: Burn incidence and treatment in the US: 2016 fact sheet. http://www.ameriburn.org/resources_factsheet.php.
6. American Burn Association: *Relationship between patient characteristics and number of procedures as well as length of stay for patients surviving severe burn injuries: analysis of the American Burn Association National Burn Repository*, 2009. Version 5.0. http://www.ameriburn.org.
7. American Occupational Therapy Association: Occupational therapy practice framework: domain and process (4th ed.), *American Journal of Occupational Therapy*, 74(Supplement 2):1–87, 2020. https://doi.org/10.5014/ajot.2020.74S2001.
8. Anzarut A, Olson J, Singh P, et al: The effectiveness of pressure garment therapy for prevention of abnormal scarring after burn injury: a meta-analysis, *J Plast Reconstr Aesthet Surg* 62:77, 2009.
9. Berger MM, Pantet O: Nutrition in burn injury: any recent changes? *Current Opinion in Critical Care* Volume 22(4):285–291, 2016. https://doi.org/10.1097/MCC.0000000000000323.
10. Bishop S, Maguire S: Anaesthesia and intensive care for major burns. *Continuing Education in Anaesthesia, Critical Care and Pain* 12(3):118–122, 2012.
11. Bosmans MW, Hofland HW, De Jong AE, Van Loey NE: Coping with burns: the role of coping self-efficacy in the recovery from traumatic stress following burn injuries, *Journal of Behavioral Medicine* 38(4):642–651, 2015.
12. Bowler PG, Jones SA, Walker M, Parsons D: Microbicidal properties of a silver-containing hydrofiber dressing against a variety of burn wound pathogens, *J Burn Care Rehabil* 25:192, 2004.
13. Browning JA, Cindass R: *Burn debridement, grafting, and reconstruction*, 2019, https://europepmc.org/article/nbk/nbk551717.
14. Brusselaers N, Pirayesh A, Hoeksema H, Verbelen J, Blot S, Monstrey S: Burn scar assessment: a systematic review of different scar scales, *Journal of Surgical Research* 164(1):e115–e123, 2010.
15. Bruster J, Pullium G: Gradient pressure, *Am J Occup Ther* 37:485, 1983.
16. Bunman S, Dumavibhat N, Chatthanawaree W, Intalapaporn S, Thuwachaosuan T, Thongchuan C: Burn Wound Healing: Pathophysiology and Current Management of Burn Injury, *The Bangkok Medical Journal* 13(2):91–98, 2017.
17. Butler DP: The 21st century burn care team, *Burns* 39(3):375–379, 2013.
18. Capo JT, Kokko KP, Rizzo M, et al: The use of skin substitutes in the treatment of the hand and upper extremity, *Hand (N Y)* 9:156–165, 2014.
19. Cartotto R: Topical antimicrobial agents for pediatric burns, *Burns & Trauma* 5:33, 2017.
20. Crawford CM, Varghese G, Mani MM, Neff JR: Heterotopic ossification: are range of motion exercises contraindicated? *J Burn Care Rehabil* 7:323, 1986.
21. Cukor J, Wyka K, Leahy N, et al: The treatment of posttraumatic stress disorder and related psychosocial consequences of burn injury: a pilot study, *J Burn Care Res* 36:184–192, 2015.
22. Culleiton AL, Simko LM: Caring for patients with burn injuries, *Nursing2020 Critical Care* 43(8):26–34, 2013.
23. Debels H, Hamdi M, Abberton K, Morrison W: Dermal matrices and bioengineered skin substitutes: a critical review of current options, *Reconstructive Surgery: Global Open* 3(1):e284, 2015.
24. Demling RH, DeSanti L: How can silver be delivered to the burn wound? In *The beneficial effects of a nanocrystalline silver delivery system for management of wounds:* part II section III. Copyright 2002, Burnsurgery.org.
25. Dewey WS, Richard RL, Parry IS: Positioning, Splinting and Contracture Management, *Phys Med Rehabil Clin N Am* 22(2):229–247, 2011.
26. Dunpath T, Chetty V, Van Der Reyden D: Acute burns of the hands: physiotherapy perspective, *African Health Sciences* 16(1):266–275, 2016.
27. El hamaoui Y, Yaalaoui Y, Chihabeddine K, et al: Post-traumatic stress disorder in burned patients, *Burns* 28:647, 2002.
28. Embil JM, McLeod JA, Al-Barrack AM, et al: An outbreak of methicillin resistant *Staphylococcus aureus* on a burn unit: potential role of contaminated hydrotherapy equipment, *Burns* 27:681, 2001.
29. Evans EB: Heterotopic bone formation in thermal burns, *Clin Orthop Relat Res* 263:94, 1991.
30. Gauglitz GG, Williams FN: Overview of complications of severe burn injury, *UpToDate. Published March:*5, 2020.
31. Godleski M, Oeffling A, Bruflat AK, Craig E, Weitzenkamp D, Lindberg G: Treating burn-associated joint contracture: results of an inpatient rehabilitation stretching protocol, *Journal of Burn Care & Research* 34(4):420–426, 2013.
32. Gordon M, Greenfield E, Marvin J, et al: Use of pain assessment tools: is there a preference? *J Burn Care Rehabil* 19:451, 1998.
33. Gowland R, Thompson T: *Human identity and identification*, 2013, Cambridge University Press.

34. Griggs C, Goverman J, Bittner EA, Levi B: Sedation and pain management in burn patients, *Clin Plast Surg* 44(3):535–540, 2017. https://doi.org/10.1016/j.cps.2017.02.026.

35. Halim AS, et al: The use of dermal substitutes in burn surgery: acute phase, *Indian J Plast Surg* 43(Suppl):S23–S28, 2010.

36. Hall B: Care for the patient with burns in the trauma rehabilitation setting, *Critical care nursing quarterly* 35(3):272–280, 2012.

37. Helm PA, Fisher SV: Rehabilitation of the patient with burns. In Delisa J, Currie D, Gans B, editors: *Rehabilitation medicine: principles and practice*, Philadelphia, 1988, Lippincott.

38. Hoffer MM, Brody G, Ferlic F: Excision of heterotopic ossification about elbows in patients with thermal injury, *J Trauma* 18:667, 1978.

39. Holmes JH IV, Molnar JA, Carter JE, Hwang J, Cairns BA, King BT, Hickerson WL: A comparative study of the ReCell® device and autologous split-thickness meshed skin graft in the treatment of acute burn injuries, *Journal of Burn Care & Research* 39(5):694–702, 2018.

40. James DL, Jowza M: Principles of burn pain management, *Clinics in plastic surgery* 44(4):737–747, 2017.

41. Jeschke MG, van Baar ME, Choudhry MA, Chung KK, Gibran NS, Logsetty S: Burn injury, *Nature Reviews Disease Primers* 6(1):1–25, 2020.

42. Johnson C: Pathologic manifestation of burn injury. In Richard RL, Staley MJ, editors: *Burn care and rehabilitation: principles and practice*, Philadelphia, 1994, Davis.

43. Jones I, Currie L, Martin R: A guide to biological skin substitutes, *British Journal of Plastic Surgery* 55(3):185–193, 2002.

44. Jordan MH, Gallagher JM, Allely RR, Leman CJ: A pressure prevention device for burned ears, *J Burn Care Rehabil* 13:673, 1992.

45. Jordan MH, Lewis MS, Wiegand LT, Leman CJ: Dynamic plaster casting for burn scar contracture—an alternative to surgery [abstract], *Proc Am Burn Assoc* 16:17, 1984.

46. Kornhaber R, Foster N, Edgar D, Visentin D, Ofir E, Haik J, Harats M: The development and impact of heterotopic ossification in burns: a review of four decades of research, *Scars, Burns & Healing* 3:2059513117695659, 2017.

47. Kübler-Ross E: *On death and dying*, New York, 1997, Simon & Schuster.

48. Leman CJ, Ricks N: Discharge planning and follow-up burn care. In Richard RL, Staley MJ, editors: *Burn care and rehabilitation: principles and practice*, Philadelphia, 1994, Davis.

49. Lo CH, Brown JN, Dantzer EJ, Maitz PK, Vandervord JG, Wagstaff MJ, Barker TM, Cleland H: Wound healing and dermal regeneration in severe burn patients treated with NovoSorb® Biodegradable Temporising Matrix: a prospective clinical study, *Burns* 48(3):529–538, 2022.

50. Lund C, Browder N: The estimation of area of burns, *Surg Gynecol Obstet* 79:352, 1944.

51. Mahendraraj K, Durgan DM, Chamberlain RS: Acute mental disorders and short and long term morbidity in patients with third degree flame burn: A population-based outcome study of 96,451 patients from the Nationwide Inpatient Sample (NIS) database (2001–2011), *Burns* 42(8):1766–1773, 2016.

52. May SR: The effects of biological wound dressings on the healing process, *Clin Mater* 8:243, 1991.

53. Mendez-Eastman S: Negative pressure wound therapy, *Plast Surg Nurs* 18:27,1998.

54. Mlcak R, Buffalo MC: Pre-hospital management, transportation, and emergency care. In Herndon D, editor: *Total burn care* ed 2, New York, 2002, Saunders.

55. Mölnlycke. Introducing Mepilex® Up: An innovative foam dressing for exudating wounds. https://www.molnlycke.us.

56. Nedelec B, Serghiou MA, Niszczak J, McMahon M, Healey T: Practice guidelines for early ambulation of burn survivors after lower extremity grafts, *Journal of Burn Care & Research* 33(3):319–329, 2012.

57. Nedelec B, Carter A, Forbes L, Hsu SCC, McMahon M, Parry I, Boruff J, et al: Practice guidelines for the application of nonsilicone or silicone gels and gel sheets after burn injury, *Journal of Burn Care & Research* 36(3):345–374, 2015.

58. Nedelec B, Parry I, Acharya H, Benavides L, Bills S, Bucher JL, Kloda LA, et al: Practice guidelines for cardiovascular fitness and strengthening exercise prescription after burn injury, *Journal of Burn Care & Research* 37(6):e539–e558, 2016.

59. Nolan WB: Acute management of thermal injury, *Ann Plast Surg* 7:243, 1981.

60. Noronha C, Almeida A: Local burn treatment: topical antimicrobial agents, *Annals of Burns and Fire Disasters* 13(4):216–219, 2000.

61. Nunez Lopez O, Cambiaso-Daniel J, Branski LK, Norbury WB, Herndon DN: Predicting and managing sepsis in burn patients: current perspectives, *Ther Clin Risk Manag* 13:1107–1117, 2017. https://doi.org/10.2147/TCRM.S119938.

62. O'Brien L, Pandit A: Silicone gel sheeting for preventing and treating hypertrophic and keloid scars, *Cochrane Database Syst Rev* (1):CD003826, 2006.

63. Ohrbach R, Patterson DR, Carrougher G, Gibran N: Hypnosis after an adverse response to opioids in an ICU burn patient, *Clin J Pain* 14:167, 1998.

64. Palmieri TL, Greenhalgh DG: Topical treatment of pediatric patients with burns: a practical guide, *Am J Clin Dermatol* 3:529, 2002.

65. Parry IS, Schneider JC, Yelvington M, Sharp P, Serghiou M, Ryan CM, Nedelec B, et al: Systematic review and expert consensus on the use of orthoses (splints and casts) with adults and children after burn injury to determine practice guidelines, *Journal of Burn Care & Research* 41(3):503–534, 2020.

66. Patterson DR, Adcock RJ, Bombardier CH: Factors predicting hypnotic analgesia in clinical burn pain, *Int J Clin Exp Hypn* 45:377, 1997.

67. Zhang P, Zou B, Liou Y-C, Huang C: The pathogenesis and diagnosis of sepsis post burn injury, *Burns & Trauma* 9:tkaa047, 2021. https://doi.org/10.1093/burnst/tkaa047.

68. Pietsch J: Care of the child with burns. In Hazinski MF, editor: *Manual of pediatric critical care,* St Louis, 1999, Mosby.

69. Ptacek JT, Patterson DR, Heimbach DM: Inpatient depression in persons with burns, *J Burn Care Rehabil* 23:1, 2002.

70. Pullium G: Splinting and positioning. In Fisher SV, Helm PA, editors: *Comprehensive rehabilitation of burns*, Baltimore, MD, 1984, Williams & Wilkins.

71. Quinn T, Wasiak J, Cleland H: An examination of factors that affect return to work following burns: a systematic review of the literature, *Burns* 36:1021, 2010.

72. Reeves SU: Adaptive strategies after severe burns. In Christiansen CH, Matuska KM, editors: *Ways of living: adaptive strategies for special needs* ed 3, Bethesda, MD, 2004, American Occupations Therapy Association.

73. Retrouvey H, Shahrokhi S: Pain and the thermally injured patient: a review of current therapies, *J Burn Care Res* 36:315–323, 2015.

74. Richard RL, Staley MJ: Burn patient evaluation and treatment planning. In Richard RL, Staley MJ, editors: *Burn care and rehabilitation: principles and practice*, Philadelphia, 1994, Davis.

75. Richard RL, Ward RS: Splinting strategies and controversies, *J Burn Care Rehabil* 26:392, 2005.

76. Rivers EA, Strate R, Solem L: The transparent face mask, *Am J Occup Ther* 33:108, 1979.

77. Rogers B, Chapman T, Rettele J, et al: Computerized manufacturing of transparent face masks for the treatment of facial scarring, *J Burn Care Rehabil* 24:91, 2003.

78. Rosenberg L, Krieger Y, Bogdanov-Berezovski A, Silberstein E, Shoham Y, Singer AJ: A novel rapid and selective enzymatic debridement agent for burn wound management: a multi-center RCT, *Burns* 40(3):466–474, 2014.

79. Shahrokhi S, Arno A, Jeschke MG: The use of dermal substitutes in burn surgery: acute phase, *Wound Repair Regen* 22(1):14–22, 2014. https://doi.org/10.1111/wrr.12119.

80. Simons M, King S, Edgar D: Occupational therapy and physiotherapy for the patient with burns: principles and management guidelines, *J Burn Care Rehabil* 24:323, 2003.

81. Sinwar PD: Nutrition in burn patient, *Journal of Mahatma Gandhi Institute of Medical Sciences* 21(1):8, 2016.

82. Smith+Nephew. https://www.smith-nephew.com.

83. Sorkin M, Cholok D, Levi B: Scar management of the burned hand, *Hand Clinics* 33(2):305–315, 2017.

84. Staley MJ, Richard RL, Falkel JE: Burns. In O'Sullivan SB, Schmitz TJ, editors: *Physical rehabilitation: assessment and treatment* ed 3, Philadelphia, 1994, Davis.

85. Strock LL, Lee MM, Rutan RL, et al: Topical Bactroban (mupirocin): efficacy in treating burn wounds infected with methicillin-resistant staphylococci, *J Burn Care Rehabil* 11:454, 1990.

86. Tengvall O, Wickman M, Wengström Y: Memories of pain after burn injury—the patient's experience, *Journal of Burn Care & Research* 31(2):319–327, 2010.

87. Travis T, Moffatt L, Jordan M, Shupp J: Factors impacting the likelihood of death in patients with small TBSA burns, *J Burn Care Res* 36:203–212, 2015.

88. Tredget EE, Levi B, Donelan MB: Biology and principles of scar management and burn reconstruction, *Surg Clin North Am* 94(4):793–815, 2014. https://doi.org/10.1016/j.suc.2014.05.005.

89. Tsai CH, Ogawa R: Keloid research: current status and future directions, *Scars, Burns & Healing* 5:1–8, 2019.

90. United States Department of Labor: *Dictionary of occupational titles*, ed 4, Washington, D.C., 1977, US Government Printing Office.

91. Urgo Medical. https://www.urgomedical.us.

92. Villeco JP: Edema: a silent but important factor, *Journal of Hand Therapy* 25(2):153–162, 2012.

93. Walsh K, Nikkhah D, Dheansa B: Burn scar contractures and their management, *Plastic and Reconstructive Surgery*, 2018.

94. Wei Y, Wang Y, Zhang M, Yan G, Wu S, Liu W, Ji G, Li-Tsang CW: The application of 3D-printed transparent facemask for facial scar management and its biomechanical rationale, *Burns* 44(2):453–461, 2018.

95. Wiechman S, Hoyt MA, Patterson DR: Using a biopsychosocial model to understand long-term outcomes in persons with burn injuries, *Archives of Physical Medicine and Rehabilitation* 101(1S):S55–S62, 2020.

96. Willows BM, Ilyas M, Sharma A: Laser in the management of burn scars, *Burns* 43(7):1379–1389, 2017.

97. Win TS, Nizamoglu M, Maharaj R, Smailes S, El-Muttardi N, Dziewulski P: Relationship between multidisciplinary critical care and burn patients survival: a propensity-matched national cohort analysis, *Burns* 44(1):57–64, 2018.

98. Wisely JA, Wilson E, Duncan RT, Tarrier N: Pre-existing psychiatric disorders, psychological reactions to stress and the recovery of burn survivors, *Burns* 36(2):183–191, 2010.

99. Yalagachin G, Hiregoudar AD, Mashal SB, Bagur A, Shivaramu NG: A comparative study of graft uptake in split skin grafting between the first postoperative dressing done on day 3 versus day 5, *International Surgery Journal* 8(12):3615–3621, 2021.

100. Yasti AÇ, Şenel E, Saydam M, Özok G, Çoruh A, Yorganci K: Guideline and treatment algorithm for burn injuries, *Ulus Travma Acil Cerrahi Derg* 21(2):79–89, 2015.

101. Yin Y, Zhang R, Li S, Guo J, Hou Z, Zhang Y: Negative-pressure therapy versus conventional therapy on split-thickness skin graft: a systematic review and meta-analysis, *International Journal of Surgery* 50:43–48, 2018.

102. Yurko L, Fratianne R: Evaluation of burn discharge teaching, *J Burn Care Rehabil* 9:643, 1988.

RESOURCES

American Burn Association: https://www.ameriburn.org

Burn Therapist: www.burntherapist.com

Consumer Review: https://www.consumereview.org/reviews/scars/

Covermark Cosmetics: A vender of special camouflaging cosmetics for burn patients. 157 Veterans Drive, Northvale, NJ 07647, 800-524-1120, https://www.covermark.com

International Burn Foundation: InternationalBurnFoundation.org

Model Systems Knowledge Translation Center: https://www.msktc.org/burn/model-system-centers

Phoenix Society for Burn Survivors: https://phoenix-society.org

44

Amputations and Prosthetics

Annemarie E. Orr and Kelly McGaughey Roseberry[a]

LEARNING OBJECTIVES

After studying this chapter, the student or practitioner will be able to do the following:

Sections 1 and 2

1. Understand the role of the occupational therapist in the evaluation and treatment of upper limb amputations.
2. Identify the upper limb amputation levels and describe the prosthetic systems and componentry associated with each level of amputation.
3. Identify the phases of upper limb prosthetic training and describe key characteristics of each phase of intervention.
4. Name the five types of prosthetic systems and explain the advantages and disadvantages of each type of system.
5. Identify the outcome measures that are used specifically with upper limb amputations.
6. Recognize the emerging technologies and advances in the area of prosthetics and analyze how these may affect functional outcomes for individuals with upper limb loss.
7. Analyze how upper limb amputation affects an individual's performance skills and patterns as they relate to occupational performance.

Section 3

1. List the types and causes of lower extremity amputation (also known as lower limb amputation).
2. Describe the types of equipment that may be used by a person who has had a lower limb amputation.
3. Describe how lower limb amputation may affect a person's occupational performance.
4. Identify the effects that lower limb amputation may have on client factors, performance skills, and performance patterns.
5. Discuss the potential psychosocial repercussions of lower limb amputation.
6. Describe the role of the occupational therapist in working with a person who has had a lower limb amputation.
7. Explain how context and activity demands can be altered to improve a client's ability to participate in a given occupation.
8. Discuss possible additional concerns for an older person who has had a lower limb amputation.

CHAPTER OUTLINE

[a] Annemarie E. Orr and the editors of this text would like to acknowledge the contributions of the late Kelly McGaughey Roseberry, DPT. Kelly brought her kindness, optimistic personality, wealth of knowledge, and experience working with people with amputations to prospective occupational therapy practitioners. Her words and treatment suggestions will be incorporated into untold numbers of treatment sessions and clinical interactions with clients for years to come. Kelly valued occupational therapy, understood our different contributions, and embraced the importance of team effort. We are saddened by our great loss but, in tribute to Kelly and her family, will remember her influence on our everyday practices.

KEY TERMS

Above-knee amputation	Interscapular thoracic	Preprosthetic phase	Syme's amputation
Acquired amputation	Myoelectric prosthesis	Prosthetic training	Terminal device
Below-knee amputation	Myosite	Pylon	Transhumeral
Body-powered prosthesis	Neuroma	Residual limb	Transradial
Disarticulation	Phantom limb pain	Residual limb support	
Hybrid prosthesis	Phantom limb sensation	Separation of controls	

SECTION 1: GENERAL CONSIDERATIONS IN UPPER LIMB AMPUTATIONS[b]

Annemarie E. Orr

Amputation can result from several causes, including disease, trauma, infection, tumor, or congenital limb deficiency. Individuals with congenital limb deficiencies and those whose amputations occur early in life usually develop sensorimotor skills and a self-image without the limb; therefore, these two populations present different problems for the rehabilitation worker.[16,106,107] This chapter discusses adults with acquired amputations; that is, surgical removal of a limb as a result of disease or trauma.

CAUSES AND INCIDENCE OF AMPUTATION

Approximately 1.6 million persons live with limb loss in the United States.[130] This number is projected to more than double to 3.6 million by 2050.[130] Annually, more than 185,000 persons in the United States undergo an amputation. Dysvascular disease and diabetes are the primary reasons for amputation of the lower limb, and trauma is the primary cause of upper limb amputation in adults.[26] Approximately 75% of upper limb amputations are the result of trauma caused by work-related accidents, gunshot wounds, and burns.[61] The ratio of upper limb to lower limb amputation is estimated to be 1:3.[37] Limb loss as a result of trauma is increased during times of active warfare.[78] As of June 1, 2015, more than 1600 U.S. military service members had undergone an amputation as a result of the wars in Iraq and Afghanistan[28]; this was the case for Daniel, described in the case study in Section 2.[28]

CLASSIFICATION OF AMPUTATION LEVELS

The classifications for levels of upper extremity amputation are illustrated in Fig. 44.1. The term interscapular thoracic

(forequarter) describes an amputation of the entire upper extremity, scapula, and clavicle; transhumeral describes an amputation through the humerus; and transradial describes an amputation through the radius and ulna. These levels of amputation are also

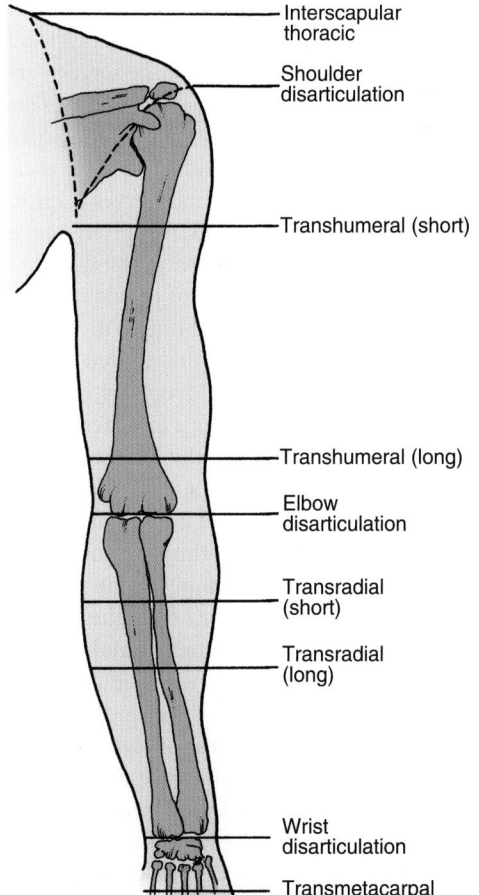

Fig. 44.1 Classification levels of upper limb amputation. (From Saunders R, Astifidis R, Burke SL, et al., editors: *Hand and upper extremity rehabilitation: a practical guide*, ed 4, St Louis, 2016, Elsevier.)

Labels on figure:
- Interscapular thoracic
- Shoulder disarticulation
- Transhumeral (short)
- Transhumeral (long)
- Elbow disarticulation
- Transradial (short)
- Transradial (long)
- Wrist disarticulation
- Transmetacarpal

---

[b] The authors wish to acknowledge the outstanding work of Denise D. Keenan in previous editions of this text. The present chapter Sections 1 and 2 are built on her foundational work.

commonly referred to by their relationship to the elbow joint: above elbow (AE) and below elbow (BE). The term disarticulation, at the shoulder, elbow, or wrist level, describes an amputation through the joint. The higher the level of amputation, the more difficult it may be for a person to use a prosthesis because fewer joints and muscles are available to control the prosthesis.

REHABILITATION AS A TEAM APPROACH

Rehabilitation after amputation requires a team approach. Members of the interdisciplinary team include the physician, nurse, occupational therapist, physical therapist, prosthetist, social worker, and psychologist. The client is the primary member of this team and should be encouraged to be an active participant in the rehabilitation plan of care. The primary role of the occupational therapist in the rehabilitation of amputations is to facilitate an individual's return to maximum performance of daily occupations and roles that lead to a meaningful life.[52,103,104,113]

SURGICAL MANAGEMENT

Although the mechanism of injury may vary, the primary goal of surgical management of upper limb amputations is the same—to maintain limb length and provide an opportunity for an optimal prosthetic fit that allows for maximal use of the prosthesis.[103,113] A longer residual limb typically leads to improved functional outcomes. Increased limb length and preservation of each progressive joint allows for greater opportunities for clients to position the residual limb in space and to feel, grasp, and manipulate objects in their own environment. It is important for the surgeon and interdisciplinary team to understand the capabilities of each prosthetic device as they correspond to the amputation level, so as to maximize the functional outcomes and overall satisfaction of the client.[113]

Surgical management of muscles and nerves is critical with upper extremity amputation. Myodesis, myoplasty, and myofascial closure are surgical techniques used to stabilize the muscle and tendons of the residual limb and to provide adequate soft tissue padding to the distal end of the bone. With myodesis, the muscle and fascia of the residual limb are sutured directly to the bone, making it structurally stable. Myoplasty involves suturing the residual opposing muscle groups together over the transected bone end. Myofascial closure, the least stable technique, involves suturing the residual muscle and its fascia together.

Nerve management in the residual limb is also important to limit neuroma development and optimize myosite signals for myoelectric control. Traction neurectomy is a surgical technique that moves the eventual neuroma away from the skin and muscle closure by isolating all the major nerves and allowing them to retract proximal to the closure into the residual muscle.[103,113]

Surgical techniques vary with the level and cause of amputation.[105,107] A closed or open surgical procedure may be performed. The open method allows drainage as the surgical site heals and minimizes the possibility of infection. The closed method reduces the period of hospitalization but also reduces free drainage and increases the risk of infection.[107] The specific type of amputation performed is left to the discretion of the surgeon and is often determined by the status of the limb at the time of amputation. The surgery may be ablative only (removal of devitalized tissues) or reconstructive. In either case the surgeon must remove the part of the limb that has to be eliminated and allow for primary or secondary wound healing. The surgeon reconstructs a residual limb (sometimes referred to as a stump) to achieve the optimal prosthetic fit and function.[107]

SECTION 2: UPPER LIMB AMPUTATIONS

Annemarie E. Orr

THREADED CASE STUDY

Daniel, Part 1

Daniel is a 19-year-old combat engineer (prefers use of the pronouns he/him/his) in the U.S. Army. While on patrol in Afghanistan, his vehicle came under attack by enemy fire. Seated in the passenger side of the vehicle, Daniel was hit by a rocket-propelled grenade, resulting in the traumatic amputation of his nondominant left upper extremity below the elbow. Daniel was medically stabilized in theater and medevaced to a military hospital in the United States for continued medical treatment and rehabilitation. Daniel underwent multiple surgeries, including a myoplasty, to optimize limb closure and healing. He had no postoperative complications. Occupational therapy was consulted for an evaluation after closure of his residual limb.

Daniel is originally from California, where he enlisted in the Army directly after high school. He is engaged to his high school sweetheart and had planned to be married after his deployment. Daniel and his family lived in the desert of California, where he and his father would work together on restoring cars and riding dirt bikes. Before this deployment Daniel was stationed at Fort Stewart in Georgia. He was living in the barracks on base, and his fiancée remained in California. Before his injury, Daniel was independent with all activities of daily living (ADLs) and instrumental activities of daily living (IADLs). He has a passion for motocross and expressed concern about his ability to participate in the sport he loves after the amputation. He identifies primarily with his role as a soldier and is unsure whether he will be able to stay on active duty as a combat engineer in the Army after the amputation.

Daniel's parents and fiancée are present for the initial evaluation. A comprehensive occupational therapy evaluation is performed at Daniel's bedside on the inpatient unit. On arrival the occupational therapist notes that a compressive elastic bandage wrap has been applied to Daniel's left residual limb. Range-of-motion, strength, and sensory assessments are performed for both upper extremities. Daniel has full range of motion throughout all joints except his left elbow. His left elbow is limited in both flexion and extension as a result of postoperative edema and pain. Daniel is educated on the various forms of pain that occur after amputation. He is able to describe his pain as phantom pain; he reports that his hand feels as if it is in a tight fist position, and he is unable to move it. Daniel has sutures in place along the distal end of the residual limb and no other open wounds. Daniel and his family are educated on the use and application of an elastic shrinker to assist with residual limb volume reduction and shaping.

During the evaluation Daniel reports that he is initiating basic ADLs performance (e.g., feeding, hygiene and grooming, and dressing) with his right arm using one-handed techniques. Overall he shows a positive affect throughout the initial meeting with the occupational therapist, and he is motivated to begin his therapy and preprosthetic training.

Critical Thinking Questions

1. For Daniel, how will each area of occupational performance (ADLs, IADLs, work, education, leisure, play, and social participation) be affected as a result of the loss of his left arm?
2. How will Daniel's occupational profile and contexts influence and guide occupational therapy treatment interventions?
3. What is the therapeutic role of the occupational therapist in Daniel's psychological and psychosocial adjustment to life after amputation?

PREPROSTHETIC TRAINING

The **preprosthetic phase** of training begins immediately after amputation and continues through prosthetic fitting. During the period between amputation and fitting of the prosthesis, the client participates in a program designed to prepare the residual limb for a prosthesis, facilitate adjustment to his or her loss, and achieve maximal independence in self-care.[82,122] The primary goals of this phase of rehabilitation are to promote wound healing and closure, pain management, initiation of basic activities of daily living (ADL) retraining, and client and family education.[102,103]

Evaluation

A comprehensive evaluation is administered to determine baseline information about the client's past medical history, functional status, and rehabilitation goals. An interview with the client and family members is performed to identify occupational roles, the home and work environments, and premorbid interests. The occupational therapist evaluates the client's medical history, upper quadrant range of motion and strength, sensation in the residual and intact limb, wound and skin healing, edema and limb volume measurement, residual limb and phantom limb pain, and psychological and emotional adjustment after amputation.[104] A baseline functional assessment is performed to evaluate the client's level of independence with basic ADLs performance in such tasks as self-feeding, dressing, toileting, and bathing, and with instrumental activities of daily living (IADLs), such as work and leisure.[1] The findings from the initial perioperative evaluation and a statement of the client's goals are important for guiding the rehabilitation program toward meeting these functional goals.[6]

Activities of Daily Living

One of the primary goals of occupational therapy is independence in basic self-care after amputation. During this acute phase of recovery, feelings of helplessness for the client are typical. It is important for the occupational therapist to provide the clients with control over their environment and a sense of independence in basic ADLs. Modifications to the environment, such as adaptive call bells and pain-controlled analgesia (PCA), are a simple first step toward independence. Adaptive equipment, such as universal cuffs, bidets, and hook-and-loop-adapted clothing, can provide initial independence in basic ADLs (Fig. 44.2). The ADLs that should be addressed immediately after amputation are (1) self-feeding, (2) toileting, and (3) oral hygiene.[104] If the client is medically stable and the wounds have healed, training in additional ADLs (e.g., dressing and bathing) may be initiated. It is the role of the occupational therapist to creatively adapt and modify the client's environment to achieve maximum independence.

The change in hand dominance is introduced during this phase of recovery for persons with amputation of the dominant limb. Because a prosthesis has limited fine motor prehension and dexterity, it is important to transfer hand dominance in handwriting to maintain independence with written

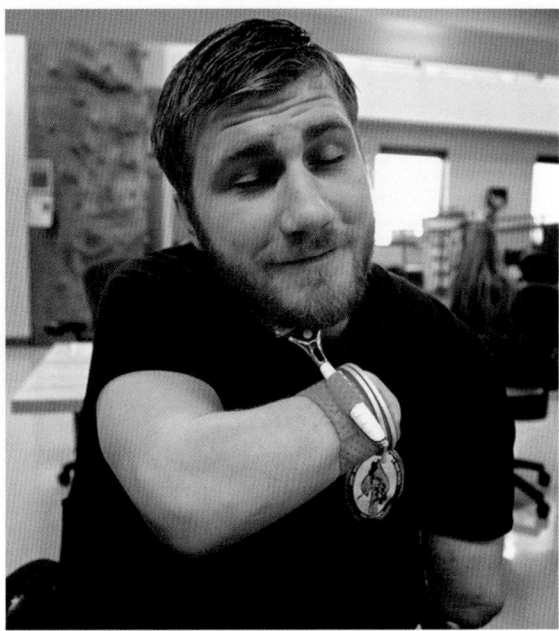

Fig. 44.2 Adaptive cuff fabricated for shaving using the residual limb.

communication.[128,129] Clients learn and adapt quickly to limb loss and often begin to perform ADLs on their own with the nondominant hand. The occupational therapist will also educate the client on one-handed techniques for performing ADLs and will make recommendations for adaptive equipment as necessary. The occupational therapist educated Daniel in the use of adaptive equipment, such as a pump soap dispenser and a rocker knife, to increase his independence in bathing and self-feeding.

Wound Healing and Limb Shaping

During the initial wound healing phase, the occupational therapist performs wound care and dressing changes according to the physician's guidelines. Immediately after surgery, limb wrapping is initiated to decrease edema and promote optimal limb shaping for the prosthesis. Figure-8 limb wrapping with an elastic bandage is performed for distal to proximal compression and shaping of the residual limb. The limb must never be wrapped in a circular manner because this restricts circulation and causes a tourniquet effect. Once the wound has stopped draining and clearance has been obtained from a physician, progression to use of an elastic shrinker or a compression garment can be initiated. Shrinkers come in a range of measurements; therefore, progression of residual limb volume change can be documented accordingly. Use of a cylindrical tube, or donner, is recommended for ease of application of the shrinker on the residual limb (Fig. 44.3). If the shrinker loosens, a smaller size is indicated. A shrinker should be worn whenever the client is not in a prosthesis to maintain residual limb volume and shaping. The client is educated to remove the shrinker two or three times daily to examine the skin for any redness or pressure. The client and family are instructed in donning and doffing the compression garment with the goal of independence for the client in this technique.

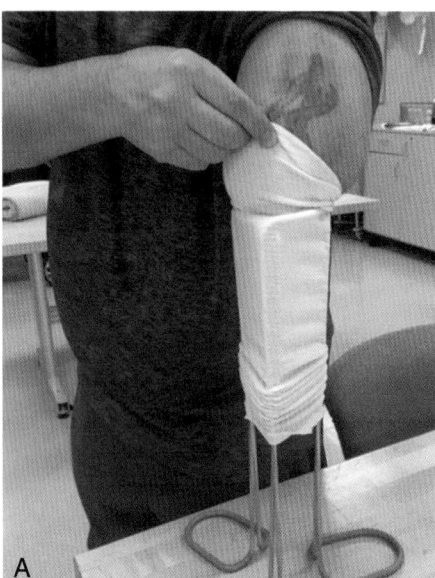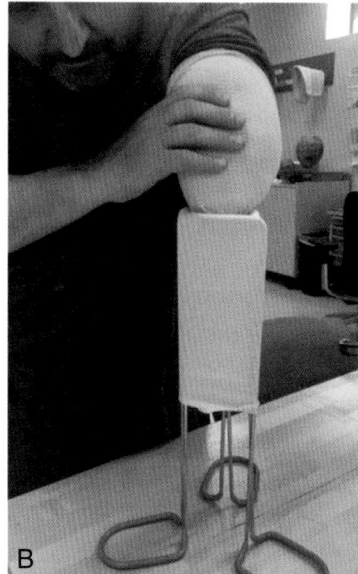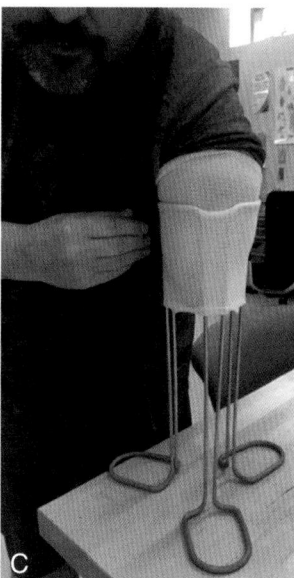

Fig. 44.3 A and C, The process of donning an elastic shrinker.

Pain Management

Residual limb hyperesthesia, phantom limb pain, phantom limb sensation, and neuroma are common problems after amputation that can interfere with functional use of the limb with or without the prosthesis.

Desensitization

A residual limb may be hypersensitive after surgery, requiring a technique known as desensitization. Overstimulating a hypersensitive peripheral area with nonharmful stimuli teaches the central nervous system to accept these stimuli as nonharmful and to minimize aversive responses to them. Residual limb hyperesthesia, or an overly sensitive limb, limits functional use and causes discomfort. Reduction in hypersensitivity of the residual limb improves the client's tolerance to wearing of the prosthesis. Desensitization techniques are implemented after wound closure. Methods include tapping, vibration, constant pressure, and rubbing of various textures on the limb. The therapist introduces the tissue to soft, lightweight, smooth textures and progresses to rough, hard, uneven, heavier textures as the client is able to tolerate them. As the techniques are performed, the therapist teaches them to the client, family members, or caregivers to facilitate use of the techniques at home.[6,91] Desensitization is used to prepare the residual limb to tolerate the initial socket.

Phantom Limb Pain

Approximately 90% of individuals who have had an amputation experience phantom limb pain.[15-17] Phantom limb pain can have a number of varying characteristics, such as stabbing, cramping, burning, or throbbing.[30] Changes in the central nervous system and peripheral nerve damage are thought to be the cause of phantom limb pain.[30,31] Oftentimes psychological factors, such as stress, are the triggers for phantom limb pain.[21,22]

Phantom limb pain and its causes and treatment are highly debated topics. Research in this area continues to make progress,

but no evidence strongly supports any one approach as clearly successful in the management of phantom limb pain. A team approach should be used to address phantom limb pain and to find the best method for the client in the management of this pain.

Treatment methods for those with phantom limb pain may include analgesics, acupuncture, electrical nerve stimulation, and mirror therapy, among others. Isometric exercises of the phantom and residual limb initiated 5 to 7 days after the amputation and performed several times throughout the day may help to minimize pain. Active movement of muscles associated with the phantom limb can be beneficial, especially when the sensations are described as stuck, cramped, or tight. Daniel experienced this kind of phantom pain, describing his phantom hand as stuck in a fist position. He had positive results from active movement and visualization exercises with the phantom limb. Mirror therapy has elicited some positive results in decreasing the pain of phantom limbs.[31,89] The use of mirror therapy in the management of phantom limb pain is now widely accepted as standard therapy after amputation.[89,121] Biofeedback, transcutaneous electrical nerve stimulation (TENS), ultrasound, progressive relaxation exercises, and controlled breathing exercises also have been used.[102,103] Activities such as massaging, tapping, and applying pressure to the residual limb may be beneficial. A physician may treat the pain by prescribing oral medications, injecting anesthetics into a specific soft tissue area, or performing sympathetic nerve blocks. Surgical revision of the residual limb is sometimes necessary to alleviate the pain.[7,22,119] An individual also may take nonpharmaceutical oral supplements to decrease the pain. Management of phantom limb pain requires an interdisciplinary team approach.

Phantom Limb Sensation

Phantom limb sensations are sensations of the amputated limb. In its simplest form, the phantom limb sensation is the sensation of the limb that is no longer there. The phantom limb sensation is present because the neural system in the brain still exists, even when the input to the body is interrupted by an amputation.[68] Almost all individuals who have undergone amputation report this painless sensation.[67] Although phantom limb sensation is more common after traumatic amputation, it also has been known to occur in persons with congenital limb absence.[88] The distal part of the limb is most frequently felt, although sometimes the person feels the whole extremity. The sensation may dissipate over time, or the person may experience it throughout life. The individual may feel that the distal portion of the phantom hand has retracted closer to the end of the residual limb in a phenomenon called telescoping. Research has recently begun to focus on the use of phantom limb sensation and its potential to improve control with a myoelectric prosthesis.[79]

Neuroma

Severed peripheral nerves may form neuromas in the residual limb.[64,70] A neuroma is a small ball of nerve tissue that develops when growing axons attempt to reach the distal end of the residual limb. As the axons grow, they turn back on themselves, producing a ball of nerve tissue. If the neuroma adheres to scar tissue or to skin subjected to repetitive pressure, it can be painful when pressed. The diagnosis is made by palpating the neuroma and is confirmed with ultrasound.[9] Most neuromas occur 1 to 2 inches (2.5 to 5 cm) proximal to the end of the residual limb and are not troublesome.[6] To minimize negative effects of a neuroma, surgeons perform a traction neurectomy to move the eventual neuroma away from the skin closure.[64,70]

One treatment option for a painful neuroma is local steroid injections. If surgical intervention is indicated, the options are to (1) redirect the nerve more proximally into a padded area, (2) tie the nerve ending into a proximal wound bed to protect it, or (3) tie two nerve ends to each other to prevent the development of a neuroma. In addition, the residual limb socket may be fabricated or modified to accommodate the neuroma.[6,119,122]

Upper Extremity Range of Motion, Strength, and Endurance

The days and weeks immediately after amputation are the most critical for implementation of a comprehensive exercise program. Once medical approval has been provided, the client begins exercises designed to maintain and increase range of motion (ROM) and to strengthen the upper quadrant and trunk muscles. Daily upper extremity flexibility training and strengthening are critical to preparing the residual limb for prosthetic use. Depending on the level of amputation, the client may perform specific exercises that mimic the movements required to operate the prosthesis. Of utmost importance is the maintenance of ROM and strength to the shoulder flexors, abductors, and rotators, as well as the scapular protractors and retractors, because limitations in these motions may result in an increased risk of rejection of the prosthesis.[26] The therapist manually positions and holds the residual limb in the desired posture and asks the client to resist the hold, facilitating increased strength of the appropriate muscles. Isometric exercises enable the client to engage in a strengthening program without equipment. Exercises also may be performed with rubber tubing, elastic

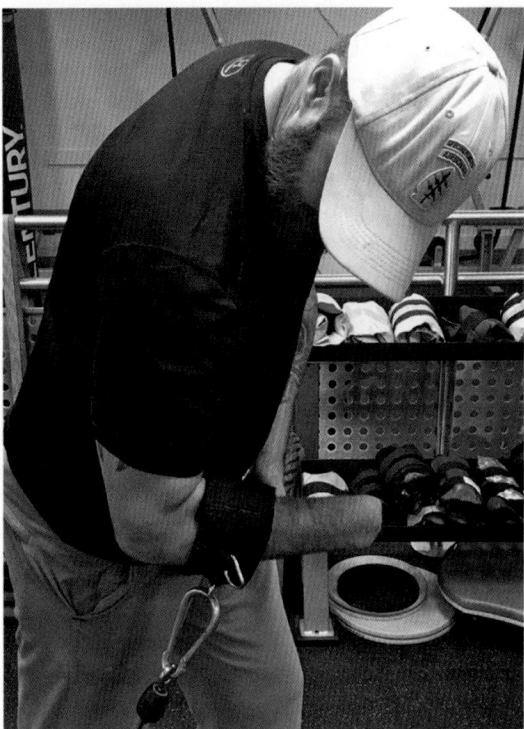

Fig. 44.4 Weight-lifting cuff with D-ring used on a cable machine to perform upper extremity strengthening exercises.

bands, or strap-on weights. As the client progresses, adaptive cuffs with D-rings can be used on cable machines (Fig. 44.4). It is appropriate for the occupational therapist to guide the client through a home exercise program for self-stretching and use of modified home or gym equipment to perform exercises.

Body symmetry and proper trunk alignment can limit the possibility of cumulative trauma or overuse injuries of the upper limbs, neck, or back.[103] Therapeutic activities are facilitated in front of a mirror to increase visual feedback and the client's body awareness. Verbal and tactile cues are provided as necessary to promote proper body mechanics and alignment during therapeutic activities. The client will participate in physical therapy, along with occupational therapy, to address core strengthening and cardiovascular fitness. After amputation the use of a prosthesis increases cardiovascular demands; therefore, it is important for the client to maintain an active lifestyle and engage in regular aerobic activities.

Myosite Testing and Training

When early prosthetic fitting is not possible, preprosthetic training for a myoelectric prosthesis can be initiated. A myoelectric prosthesis functions by detecting electromyographic (EMG) signals produced by muscles in the residual limb. Locating appropriate superficial muscle sites (i.e., myosites) is the most important aspect of the successful operation of a myoelectric prosthesis. Physical examination of a person's arm often reveals sufficient strength in natural agonist-antagonist pairs, such as the wrist extensor and wrist flexor muscles in the person with a transradial amputation, and the biceps and triceps muscles in the person with a transhumeral amputation. Individuals with a short transhumeral amputation often have an effective myosite in the pectoralis or deltoid anteriorly and in the infraspinatus or trapezius posteriorly. Use of an agonist-antagonist pairing for control of the prosthesis is called two-site control. Preference is given to distal myosites that are adequate in signal to allow the prosthetist room to position the electrodes within a well-suspended socket. In some cases trauma or nerve injuries do not allow the choice of a natural pair. In such cases a single muscle site can be used to control two functions. A strong contraction controls one operation, a weaker contraction controls another, and relaxing the muscle turns the system off.[73] Alternative methods for control also have been developed (these are discussed briefly later in the chapter).

Both the therapist and the prosthetist can perform myosite testing. A biofeedback system or myotester is used to identify the amount of signal generated by the muscle. Surface electrodes are positioned on the residual limb and connected to the myotester or biofeedback system. Examples of commonly used systems are the Myolab II (Motion Control), MyoBoy (Ottobock), and a biofeedback computer program or electric demonstration hand (Fig. 44.5). It is important that all electrodes have good contact with the skin and are aligned along the general direction of muscle fibers. Moistening the skin slightly with water may improve the EMG signal by lowering skin resistance.

The goal of myosite testing is to identify two muscle sites that would fit appropriately within the socket with the greatest microvolt difference between them, not necessarily the two muscle sites with the strongest signals. Selection is complete when the client is consistently generating sufficient signals to operate the prosthesis in its basic functions, such as opening and closing the terminal device (TD). The therapist should check with the prosthetist to determine the minimum signal required to operate the myoelectric system chosen for the client.[80]

The more proximal the level of the client's amputation, the more challenging it is for the prosthetist to fit the prosthesis and

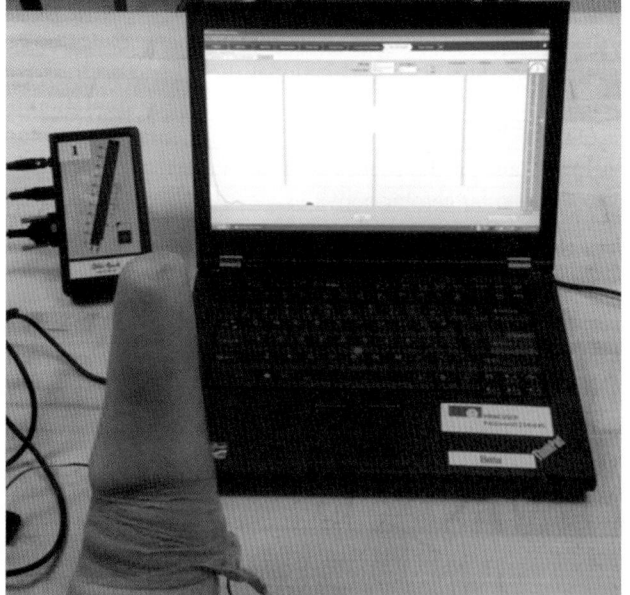

Fig. 44.5 MyoBoy system (Ottobock) with myosimulator used for myosite testing and training.

for the therapist to train the person to control the prosthesis. To help the client understand a desired muscle contraction, the therapist instructs the client to imitate the desired contraction or movement with both arms. For instance, the therapist can ask the client to raise the sound hand at the wrist (wrist extension) and imagine this motion with the phantom hand on the amputated side. Muscle groups are most frequently used according to their physiological function. For example, the wrist extensors are used for hand opening and the wrist flexors for hand closing. The therapist often can palpate the wrist flexors and extensors on the residual limb during this exercise. The client is instructed to contract and relax each muscle group separately and on command. For this step a myotester is particularly useful because it indicates the magnitude of the EMG signal as the client contracts the muscle, in addition to the decrease in signal as the client relaxes the muscle. Many clients have difficulty relaxing a muscle completely; this causes a decrease in muscle signal separation.

The myotester can be used to train the muscles with both visual and auditory feedback. Various models are available to therapists. The goals of training at this point are to increase muscle strength and to isolate muscle contractions. As the client's confidence and accuracy improve, visual or auditory feedback should be removed. Practicing muscle contractions without feedback teaches the client to internalize the feeling of each control movement. The advantage of creating this internalized awareness of proper muscle control is that control and strengthening practice can be continued between treatment sessions without feedback equipment.[108] The therapist must learn to recognize muscle fatigue, which is frequently a side effect in this process, and should allow sufficient time for that muscle to recover during the treatment session.

Ideally the client with an amputation receives adequate training and practice in initiating these muscle contractions before receiving the completed myoelectric prosthesis from the prosthetist. Prosthetists commonly engage a client in muscle site training with the preparatory socket and prosthesis fitting. This training, which usually occurs when the prosthetist looks for optimal electrode placement and socket fit, is not adequate for most clients to operate a prosthesis immediately and successfully. Anxiety and frustration are common for clients during preprosthetic training in the use of a myoelectric prosthesis. A team approach during training with the therapist and prosthetist can minimize these responses. The client's success and effectiveness in using the prosthesis are closely related to the quality of the preprosthetic training.

Psychological Support

Psychosocial adjustment depends on various factors: the individual's character and essence, the quality of the social support systems available, sociocultural reactions to amputation, and the team's management of rehabilitation.[32] Social, personal, and spiritual contexts may be significantly altered for those who have experienced amputation. Through the interview with Daniel, the therapist identified successful adaptation and coping strategies already in place.

The process of adjustment to amputation is analogous to the grieving process. The client experiences identifiable stages of denial, anger, depression, coping, and acceptance.[32] Most clients move through these stages and ultimately adapt to the loss. It is important to note that depression rates in amputees are higher than general population rates for up to 2 years after amputation.[48] During any phase, clients may react with anger toward themselves, family members, and the medical team. The therapist should build a relationship of trust and respect with the client, one that encourages open discussion about the person's psychological adjustment to the amputation and loss of the limb. Positive reinforcement through involvement in the rehabilitation process and contact with people who have experienced similar amputations may help the client in returning to former life roles.[32] Meetings with a peer mentor or visitor are encouraged to facilitate a discussion about the rehabilitation process and the phases of recovery and psychological adjustment and also to provide problem-solving strategies. The client may be afraid to return to family, social, vocational, or sexual roles. Frequent discussions of fears and solutions to real or imagined problems are important for facilitating adjustment.[32] The therapist is encouraged to build a collaborative relationship with the client, to listen and understand the client's life roles, and to facilitate the rehabilitation to meet the individual's future goals.

Reactions after amputation are complex and unique to each individual. Although occupational therapists play a vital role in the psychological adjustment of the client, it is important that they communicate with and refer the client to a psychologist, spiritual counselor, or other behavioral health specialist as indicated.[118]

> ### OT PRACTICE NOTES
>
> The entire rehabilitation team is responsible for providing the client with the reassurance and motivation he or she needs. The team should focus on occupational therapy intervention and facilitation of participation and engagement in meaningful occupations.[81]

CHOOSING THE PROSTHESIS

The occupational therapist and prosthetist begin by educating the client about the various upper extremity prosthetic systems available for and appropriate to each level of amputation. The client's age, medical status, amputation level, cognitive status, functional goals, and desire for a prosthesis are important factors in choosing the prosthesis. A discussion about the advantages and disadvantages of each prosthetic system and terminal device allows the team to make the appropriate recommendation. The prosthetist generally provides information about specific prosthetic options, and the therapist helps the client understand the options as they relate to the client's performance in areas of occupation. This discussion allows the client to stay informed throughout the entire prosthetic fitting and training process and establishes realistic expectations for the functional outcomes of the prosthesis.

Early fitting of a prosthesis has been shown to significantly enhance functional prosthetic use and acceptance.[3,86] Studies suggest that fitting an individual with a prosthesis within 30 days of amputation significantly increases the chances of acceptance of the prosthetic limb. This 30-day period is known as the "golden window."[13,65] Early fitting programs have been very successful in helping the clients who have had an amputation incorporate the new extremity more rapidly into their daily activities.[3,4]

The importance of early fitting of a prosthesis cannot be overemphasized; it may be one of the most important factors in client acceptance and use of a prosthesis.

TYPES OF PROSTHETIC SYSTEMS

The five most common upper extremity prosthetic systems are body-powered, electrically powered, hybrid, activity-specific, and passive prostheses. As discussed, the type of prosthesis recommended is based on many factors. Each type has its advantages and disadvantages; therefore, more than one option is often required to maximize occupational performance.

Body-Powered Prosthesis

A body-powered prosthesis is cable driven and controlled by gross body movements. This type of prosthesis uses body motions proximal to the amputation to pull tension on a cable operating the terminal device. The client must have sufficient musculature and ROM in the upper quadrant to operate a body-powered prosthesis. The client must be able to perform one of the following movements to control this prosthesis: (1) glenohumeral flexion, (2) scapular abduction or adduction, (3) shoulder depression or elevation, (4) chest expansion, or (5) elbow flexion.[71] Because of its simple design, the body-powered prosthesis is durable, lightweight, and has low maintenance costs. The harness and cable system on the prosthesis also gives good proprioceptive feedback to the wearer on the position of the terminal device in space.[71] However, a body-powered prosthesis harness may restrict ROM and limit the functional envelope for operation of the terminal device. This design also limits the potential grip force of the terminal device, and for some users the hook may create an undesirable appearance (Box 44.1).

> ### BOX 44.1   Advantages and Disadvantages of a Body-Powered Prosthesis
>
> **Advantages**
> - Durable and can be exposed to environmental conditions (e.g., water and dirt)
> - Provides proprioceptive feedback
> - Lower maintenance costs than myoelectric prostheses
>
> **Disadvantages**
> - Restrictive harness
> - Decreased grip force compared to myoelectric options
> - Force is exerted on the residual limb
> - Can be difficult to control for high levels of amputation

Electrically Powered Prosthesis

An electrically powered prosthesis, also known as a myoelectric prosthesis (mentioned earlier), uses muscle surface electricity to control the operations of the terminal device. The muscle generates an electric potential at the time of contraction. The myoelectric signal is sensed, amplified, and processed by a control unit that generates a motor, which in turn drives the terminal device.[19] Surface electrodes are embedded in the prosthetic socket, eliminating the need for harnessing or cable systems.

Myoelectric upper limb prostheses have opened a new world of freedom and function for persons who have had upper limb amputations. The advent of electronic microminiaturization has allowed the development of prosthetic devices with totally self-contained services of power, motor units, and electrodes.[47,49] Powered prostheses have existed for decades, but not until the 1960s were electrically powered prostheses introduced clinically. Ottobock, a firm based in Duderstadt, Germany, began this process by aiming for the development of an electromechanically driven prosthetic hand that would match the technical and cosmetic demands of a human hand.[77]

The electric motors used to operate the terminal device give myoelectric prostheses significantly increased grip force, upward of 20 to 32 lb per square inch.[71] These types of prostheses provide a more natural appearance and increase the functional envelope of operation without the restriction of a harness or cable. Myoelectric prostheses are battery operated and therefore require regular maintenance for charging, repairs, and component replacement. The electrical components that drive the prosthesis also add to the overall weight of the device (Box 44.2).

Daniel was first considered for a myoelectric prosthesis. He received myosite testing and training during the preprosthetic phase and demonstrated good strength and control. After discussions that included the prosthetist, occupational therapist, and Daniel, in which Daniel's age, level of amputation, and functional goals also were considered, a myoelectric prosthesis was recommended for him.

Hybrid Prostheses

A hybrid prosthesis combines body-powered and electrically powered components in one design. These prostheses are most commonly used with a transhumeral amputation. The components can be combined to create a variety of options. Often a body-powered elbow is used with an electrically powered terminal device, or an electrically powered elbow can be combined with a body-powered hook or hand.[11,12,71] All excursion of the existing cable is dedicated to one component, rather than to multiple components; this feature requires less overall force on the part of the wearer for operating the prosthesis. Advantages of hybrid prostheses include simultaneous control of the elbow and terminal device, decreased overall weight of the prosthesis, and decreased cost (Box 44.3).

Passive Prosthesis

A passive prosthesis can serve in both cosmetic and functional restoration of the hand after amputation. A passive prosthesis is static and does not have an active grasp. Often the digits can be passively positioned to assist with stabilizing, carrying, or grasping objects. For example, for an individual who has undergone a thumb amputation, a static thumb post with a friction joint can be passively prepositioned to allow for opposition. Cosmetic restoration can be achieved with a rubberized glove or a custom-sculpted, painted covering that replicates the individual's remaining hand or fingers (Fig. 44.6). Typically these prostheses are made from flexible latex, rigid polyvinyl chloride (PVC), or silicone.[71] They are lightweight, require less maintenance, and can help promote a positive self-image for the user (Box 44.4).

Activity-Specific Prosthesis

Activity-specific prostheses are designed for a particular activity or task (Fig. 44.7). They are often used when body-powered or electrically powered prostheses cannot perform the needed function or provide the required durability for a specific activity. These prostheses are typically used for recreational or work activities, such as sports, hobbies, and tool use. The design is typically a lightweight socket with limited or no harness or control cable. Terminal devices specific to the activity can be easily interchanged using a Hosmer Dorrance quick disconnect wrist unit. Advantages of activity-specific prostheses are durability, decreased burden on the primary prosthesis, and increased independence and function in a particular activity (Box 44.5).[71]

Upper Limb Prosthetic Componentry

Various prosthetic components are available for each level of amputation. The higher the level of amputation, the greater

---

BOX 44.2   Advantages and Disadvantages of a Myoelectric Prosthesis

Advantages
- Improved cosmesis
- Increased and proportional grip force
- Minimal or no harnessing
- Provides a larger functional work envelope for use
- Minimal effort needed to control
- Can be fitted early in rehabilitation phase

Disadvantages
- Increased cost
- Frequency of maintenance and repair for battery
- Lack of sensory feedback
- Susceptible to interference from moisture or other environmental factors
- Increased overall weight

BOX 44.3   Advantages and Disadvantages of a Hybrid Prosthesis

Advantages
- Simultaneous control of elbow and wrist or terminal device
- Less weight than an entirely electrically powered prosthesis
- Increased grip force

Disadvantages
- Harness is required for operation of elbow
- May be difficult to operate with a short transhumeral or higher amputation because of the force required to operate the elbow

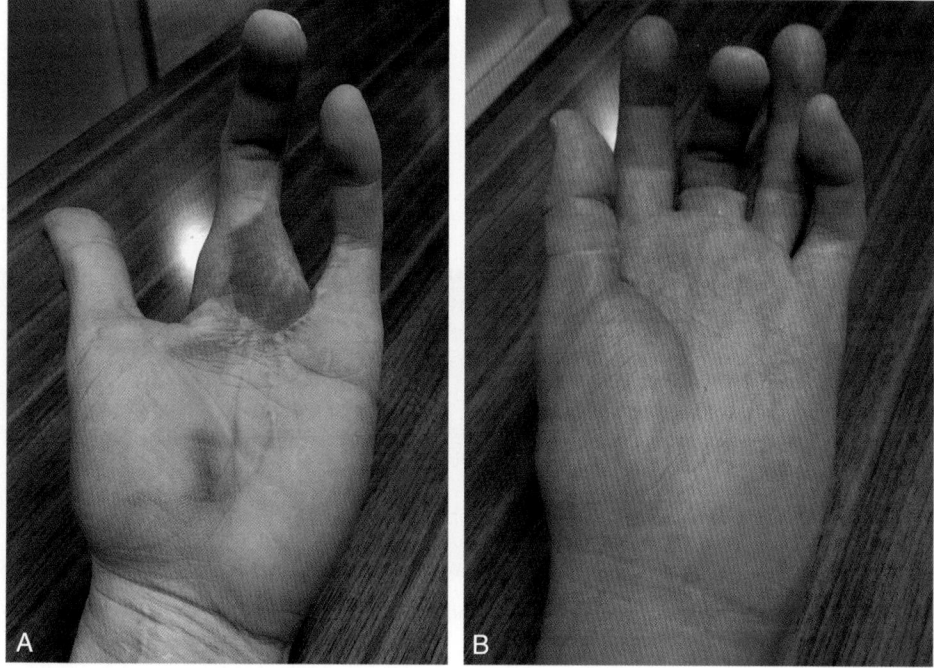

Fig. 44.6 Example of a passive cosmetic glove on a partial hand amputation. (A) Without cosmetic glove. (B) With cosmetic glove.

BOX 44.4   Advantages and Disadvantages of a Passive Prosthesis

Advantages
- No harnessing or control cables
- Provides cosmetic restoration and positive body image
- Low maintenance
- Lightweight
- Digits can be positioned for static grasp or opposition

Disadvantages
- Does not provide active grasping function
- Cosmetic covers made of latex or polyvinyl chloride can stain easily

---

the functional loss of the limb. Greater functional loss often necessitates a more complex prosthetic system. Each prosthetic system is custom made, individually fitted, and prescribed, according to the client's level of amputation, lifestyle, and goals.

Body-Powered Components

The first five components described in the following sections are common to all body-powered prostheses prescribed for the wrist disarticulation level and higher (Fig. 44.8). These components are the prosthetic sock, socket, harness and control system, terminal device, and wrist unit. (Components specific to each level of amputation are also discussed.)

Prosthetic sock. A prosthetic sock of knit wool, cotton, or Orlon Lycra is worn between the prosthesis and the residual limb. The function of the prosthetic sock is to absorb perspiration and protect against irritation that can result from direct contact of the skin with the socket. The sock compensates for volume change in the residual limb and contributes to fit and comfort in the socket.[105,125]

Socket. The socket is the fundamental component, to which the remaining components are attached. A cast molding of the residual limb is used to construct the socket so as to optimize fit, comfort, and function. The original socket is made of a transparent, thermoform plastic material, which allows quick modification to accommodate changes in limb volume and to optimize fit. Once the limb volume has stabilized and a good fit has been found, the socket is made in its definitive form of carbon fiber. The socket should cover enough of the residual limb to be stable and provide suspension, but not so much that it unnecessarily restricts ROM of the residual limb.[105,122]

The socket is typically made of an inner flexible socket and an external rigid frame. The outer wall provides a structurally cosmetic surface and houses the hardware for the prosthesis. The inner wall maintains total contact with the skin surface of the residual limb to distribute socket pressure evenly. Flexible-frame sockets have been favored because they allow for volume and contour changes that occur when muscles contract and relax. In addition, wearers report that this type of socket is cooler than conventional alternatives.[5]

Harness and control system. In a body-powered prosthesis the control system functions through the interaction of a Dacron harness and stainless steel cable. The harness is composed of a system of nonelastic straps, which provide suspension for the socket and house the cable system. Several types of harnesses are available, including the standard figure-8, figure-9, and chest strap models. The higher the level of amputation, the more complex the harness design system. Loss of muscle power and ROM may necessitate variations in the harness design. A properly fitted harness is important for both comfort and function.[96,105,122]

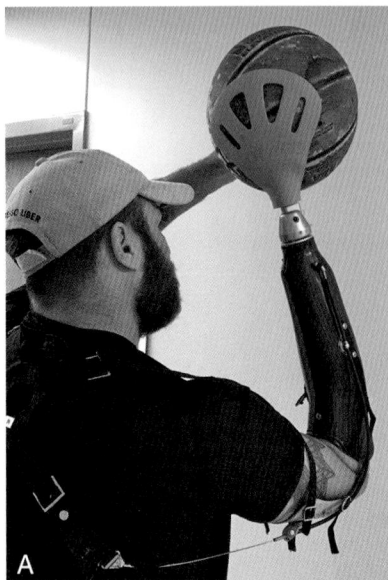
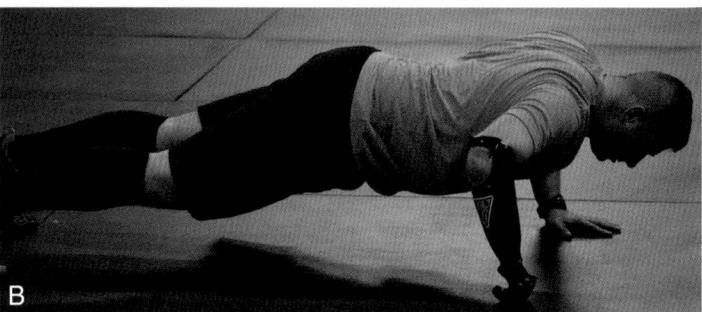

Fig. 44.7 Activity-specific prostheses. (A) Mill's Rebound Pro Basketball Hand (TRS Prosthetics). (B) Shroom Tumbler for push-ups (TRS Prosthetics).

BOX 44.5 Advantages and Disadvantages of an Activity-Specific Prosthesis

Advantages
- Allows enhanced function and task-specific participation in a variety of activities
- Minimal harness or cabling
- Durable and low maintenance
- Reduces wear and tear on primary prosthesis

Disadvantages
- Does not provide active grasp
- Appropriate for specific tasks only, not for a broad range of functions

---

A transradial control system is a one-cable design (Fig. 44.9). A flexible, stainless steel cable, contained in Teflon housing, attaches to the harness proximally with a T-bar or hanger fitting and attaches distally to a prehension device or terminal device.[33] Recently, Spectra fiber, an extremely strong material, has come into use in place of the stainless steel cable because it glides through the housing with less friction. The axilla loop is placed around the nonamputated side and serves as the primary anchor from which the other components originate.

A transhumeral prosthesis uses a two-cable design. One cable operates open and close of the terminal device, and the other cable allows the elbow unit to lock and unlock. Specific upper body movements create tension on the cables, thereby operating the various components of the prosthesis. A properly fitted control system maximizes prosthetic control while minimizing body movement and exertion.[4,96,122]

Terminal device. The terminal device (TD) (or prehensors) is the most distal component of the prosthesis. Body-powered TDs are classified as either a voluntary open (VO) mechanism or a voluntary close (VC) mechanism.[76] The VO TD is held closed

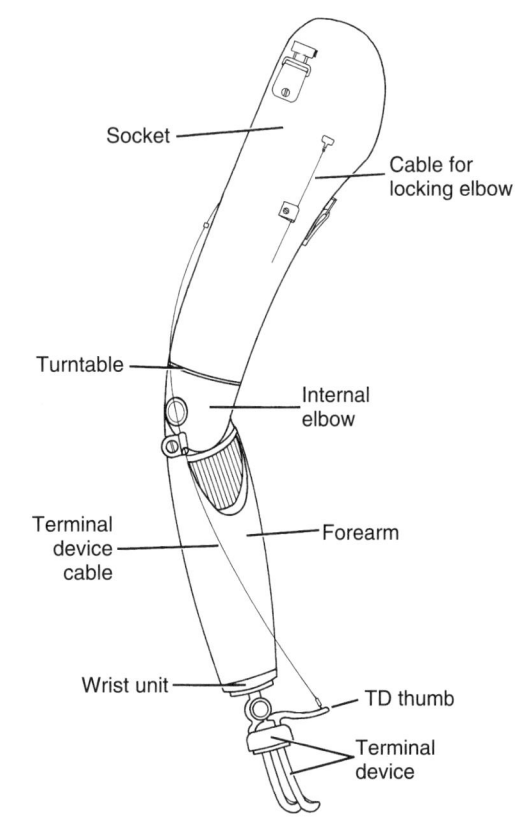

Fig. 44.8 Components of a standard transhumeral prosthesis. *TD,* Terminal device.

in a relaxed position, and it opens when the wearer exerts tension on the control cable that connects to the "thumb" of the TD. When the tension is released, rubber bands or springs close the fingers of the TD. The number of rubber bands or springs determines the holding force of the TD. The force of the pinch can

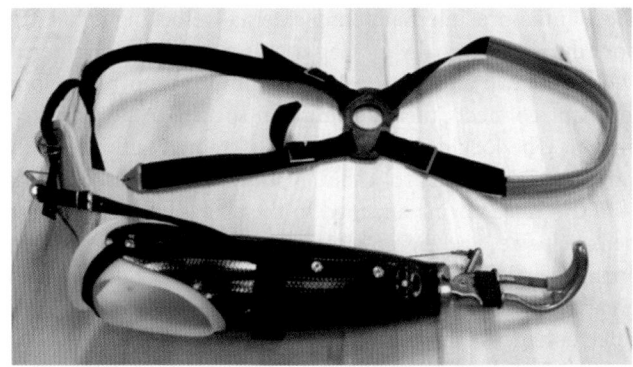

Fig. 44.9 Transradial body-powered prosthesis with a one-cable design and figure-8 harness.

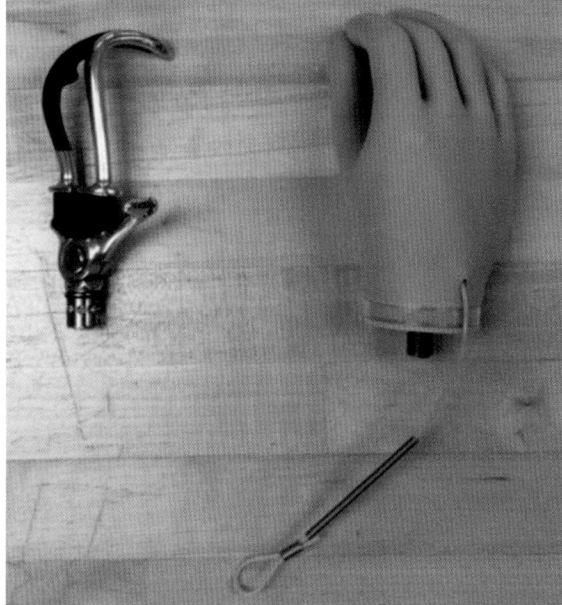

Fig. 44.10 Examples of body-powered terminal devices. *Left*, Model 5X Hook, adult size (Hosmer Dorrance Corp.). *Right*, Voluntary opening hand (Ottobock).

be adjusted by changing the number of rubber bands (approximately 1 lb per rubber band). The VC TD is open in a relaxed position; it closes when tension is applied to the control cable, and it is automatically opened by a spring mechanism when the cable is relaxed. The amount of pinch force in a VC TD is determined by the amount of tension applied on the cable.[4,5,11,33,73]

Two styles of body-powered TDs are commonly prescribed, the hook and the hand (Fig. 44.10). The VO split hook is the most prescribed terminal device in the United States.[33] Hooks have two basic designs, canted or lyre shaped. Canted describes the slanted design of the hook fingertips, which provides visual feedback to the client during functional use. Lyre-shaped TDs provide symmetry for grasp (e.g., of cylindrical items). Because TDs do not provide sensory feedback, the client must rely on visual feedback during object manipulation.

The hook design is made in a variety of materials, such as stainless steel or aluminum. Stainless steel TDs are prescribed

for activities requiring a durable TD, such as yard work or construction. Aluminum TDs are recommended for lighter work and to reduce the total weight of the prosthesis for a person with a higher level amputation. Most TDs have a rubber lining or a serrated grid between the fingers. The rubber lining increases the holding friction and minimizes damage when the client holds objects.

A prosthetic hand is also available as a TD. It attaches to the wrist unit and is either passively operated or cable operated. The same control cable that operates the hook activates the prosthetic hand in either a VO or VC mechanism. As with the hook TD, the VO hand is preferred and prescribed more often than the VC hand. A flesh-colored rubber glove fits over the prosthetic hand for protection and cosmesis.[105] Body-powered hands offer limited pinch force. Additionally, the fingers that improve the cosmesis of the TD often block visual feedback during fine motor tasks.[33]

The client's lifestyle and activity demands determine the most appropriate TDs. It is important to provide the wearer with information about the advantages and disadvantages of each TD style. Many individuals who have undergone amputation choose interchangeable TDs, using a hand TD for social occasions and a hook TD for daily activities.[33]

Wrist unit. The wrist unit connects the TD to the prosthesis. It serves as the unit for interchange and provides pronation and supination of the TD for prepositioning purposes. The wearer can passively or actively rotate the TD by turning it with the sound hand, by pushing the TD against an object or a surface, or by stabilizing the TD between the knees and using the arm to rotate it. The wrist unit for a particular client must be chosen according to its ability to meet the individual's needs in daily living and vocational activities.

Friction-held wrist units hold the TD in place by friction, which is provided by a rubber washer or setscrews. Tightening the washer or screws increases friction. The wrist is passively rotated and positioned by the other hand. Friction is sufficient to hold the TD against moderate loads while still allowing manual rotation of the terminal device. Friction-held units are mechanically simple but are not as strong as locking units.

The locking wrist unit allows the TD to be manually positioned and locked into place. In the unlocked position the TD can be prepositioned in almost any degree of rotation throughout a 360-degree range. In the locked position the locking wrist provides greater resistance under load than do the friction units.[33] The quick disconnect locking wrist unit is most common. The quick disconnect function allows the wearer to easily interchange TDs based on the needs of the activities performed.

The wrist flexion unit allows the TD to be manually flexed and locked into position. The wrist unit can be manually positioned into neutral, 30 degrees of flexion, or 50 degrees of flexion.[73] This unit is generally used on the dominant side of a person who has undergone bilateral amputation to facilitate midline activities close to the body, such as dressing and toileting.[4,76,105,122,125]

The N-Abler V Five-Function Wrist (Texas Assistive Devices) combines a rotational wrist with a flexion unit. It also allows quick disconnect of the TD.[111] This wrist unit provides the prosthetic user with flexibility in performing ADLs.

A ball-and-socket wrist unit is also available. This unit is unique in that it allows prepositioning in multiple wrist positions. It has constant friction, and the magnitude of loading is adjustable.[33] They do not lock, which can present a problem for clients engaging in activities that are heavy duty in nature.[45] As mentioned, the sock, socket, harness and control system, TD, and wrist unit are components common to all body-powered prostheses. The remaining body-powered prosthetic components—transradial hinges, elbow units, and shoulder units—maximize function at specific levels of amputation.

Transradial hinges. A transradial prosthesis uses two hinges, one on each side of the elbow, that attach to the socket below the elbow and to a pad or cuff above the elbow. These hinges stabilize and align the transradial prosthesis on the residual limb. When properly aligned, the hinges help distribute the stress of the prosthesis on the limb.

Two hinge styles, flexible and rigid, are available for use with transradial amputations. Flexible hinges are used with amputations of the distal third of the forearm. They usually are made of Dacron and connect the socket to a triceps pad positioned over the triceps muscle. Their flexibility permits at least 50% of the anatomic residual forearm rotation, reducing the need to rotate the TD manually in the wrist.[33] Rigid hinges are used with amputations at or above the midforearm to protect the residual limb against torque load.[33] Rigid hinges usually are made of steel and are attached to a laminated Dacron biceps half-cuff positioned behind the arm, which is sturdier and provides more support than the triceps pad. They are now used less frequently, having largely been replaced by a design using a self-suspending socket, in which supercondylar flares mimic some of the function of the hinges and triceps pad. Team members consider the amount of residual function and the length of the limb when choosing the appropriate hinge style for the transradial prosthesis.[76]

Elbow units. A prosthetic elbow unit is prescribed for the person who has had an amputation through the level of the elbow or higher. The elbow unit allows 5 to 135 degrees of elbow flexion and locks in various positions. The two main types of elbow units are internally and externally locking units. The more durable internally locking unit is prescribed for a person who has had an amputation 2 inches or more above the elbow. This unit connects the transhumeral socket to the prosthetic forearm. The locking mechanism is contained within the unit and attaches to a control cable. A lift assist, which consists of a tightly coiled spring attached to the elbow unit and forearm shell, helps reduce the amount of energy required to lift the forearm shell. The lift assist also allows a slight bounce in the forearm when the person is walking with the elbow unlocked, which enhances the appearance of a natural arm swing.

A friction-held turntable positioned on top of the elbow unit allows the prosthetic forearm to be rotated manually toward or away from the body. Lateral and medial aspects of a transhumeral prosthesis are shown in Fig. 44.11. The internally locking unit is 2 inches long and therefore not appropriate for an individual who has had an amputation proximal to the elbow.

The externally locking elbow unit is prescribed for a person who has an elbow disarticulation or an amputation within 2 inches above the elbow. This unit, which consists of a pair of hinges positioned on either side of the prosthesis, attaches the socket to the forearm. The cable attaches to one of the hinges, which locks and unlocks the unit.

Shoulder units

With a high-level amputation, shoulder and back movements typically are not sufficient to allow use of a cable-operated shoulder unit. Therefore, most shoulder units are manually operated and friction held. Two shoulder unit mechanisms that are often prescribed are the moveable friction-loaded shoulder unit and the locking shoulder unit. Shoulder units are classified by the degree of motion allowed in the prosthesis. A single-axis joint provides abduction; a double-axis joint provides positioning in abduction and flexion; and a triple axis and ball and socket joint allows for universal motion. A locking shoulder unit allows the prosthesis to be locked in various degrees of shoulder flexion.

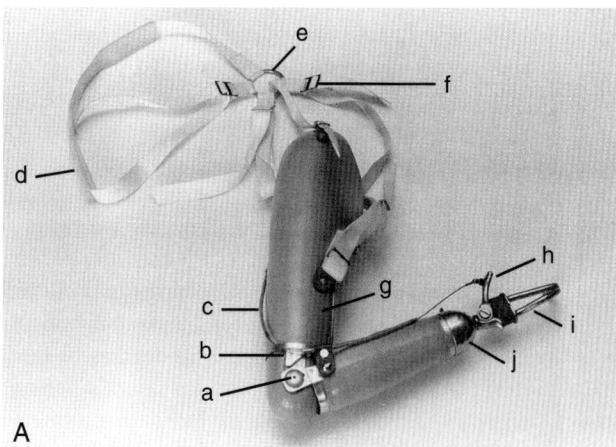
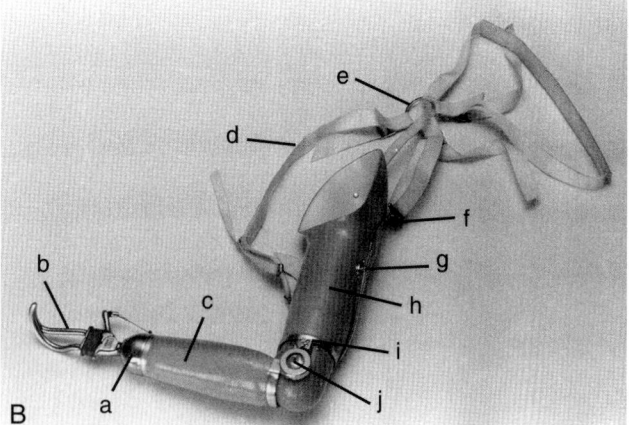

Fig. 44.11 (A) Lateral side of a transhumeral prosthesis: *a*, elbow unit; *b*, turntable; *c*, control cable; *d*, adjustable axilla loop; *e*, harness ring; *f*, figure-eight harness; *g*, elbow lock cable; *h*, terminal device (TD) thumb; *i*, hook TD; *j*, wrist flexion unit. (B) Medial side of a transhumeral prosthesis: *a*, wrist unit; *b*, hook TD; *c*, forearm; *d*, harness; *e*, harness ring; *f*, control cable; *g*, baseplate and retainer; *h*, socket; *i*, turntable; *j*, spring-loading device.

This shoulder unit allows for activities such as reaching for items in a cabinet or overhead.

With an interscapular thoracic amputation, all or a portion of the scapula and clavicle is removed with the arm. In these cases, standard prosthetic components may make the prosthesis too heavy for practical use. An endoskeletal prosthesis, made from lightweight materials such as a single aluminum alloy surrounded by a soft foam shape, is often prescribed to decrease the weight. The system provides its own style of prosthetic joints, which will not withstand heavy-duty usage. An endoskeletal prosthesis with a lightweight cosmetic cover is commonly prescribed as a cosmetic prosthesis with limited functional value.

Electrically Powered Components

The two prosthetic components common to all powered prostheses are the terminal device and the wrist unit. (Elbow and shoulder units specific to each level of amputation are also discussed later.) Research and technological advances in myoelectric componentry are proceeding at a rapid pace. This section provides an overview of the components that are commercially available and readily used (Fig. 44.12).

Terminal devices. Electrically powered terminal devices or prehensors are available in two speed systems: digital control and proportional control.[5] Digital control systems operate at a constant speed. In a proportional control system the myoelectric signal (power) to the hand is proportionate with the level of muscle signal the wearer generates; therefore, the intensity of the muscle contraction directly controls the speed and pinch force of the hand.[5]

Myoelectric terminal devices come in two designs, the hook or the hand (Fig. 44.13). The electric hook has two prehensors to provide precision pinch. Myoelectric TDs combine powered pinch force with a tip pinch for manipulation of small objects. The Electric Terminal Device (Motion Control) is designed with one nonmoving prehensor and a second, which opposes it. The System Electric Greifer (Ottobock) has two prehensors, which have a parallel opening and closing mechanism.[9,84]

The development of the electric hand has served to preserve the anthropomorphic nature of the human hand. The belief is that our environment is made up of objects designed to be handled by the human hand. Therefore, it would follow that a device designed with the same qualities as the human hand would offer the most function.[101] Electric hand terminal devices also provide an aesthetic quality and appeal. The cosmesis of a hand prehension mechanism has been shown to be a strong determinant for acceptance of the prosthesis.[11,12,17,72,79] An example of an electric hand is the SensorHand Speed (Ottobock).[84] This hand has a mechanism that drives the hand to open and close into a three-point prehension pinch. The motor also has a feature in the thumb that automatically increases pressure applied to an object being held if the device detects slippage.[73]

Advances in technology and myoelectric control have brought about the advent of multiarticulating prosthetic hands. Multiarticulating hands are defined by the multiple degrees of freedom they provide to assume a variety of grasp patterns. These TDs, which have powered articulating digits, offer prosthesis users increased functional grasp patterns that are unavailable with previous myoelectric hands designed with a single degree of freedom.[120] Individual motors in each digit drive the movement of the hand into a variety of preset pinch and grasp patterns. Multiarticulating hands provide the opportunity for advanced functionality combined with the natural appearance of the human hand. There are multiple ways the prosthesis user can access the preset grasps associated with each TD. Triggers such as co-contraction, single impulse, or double impulse allow the client to switch grasps from tip pinch to mouse grip, for example. The Bebionic hand (Ottobock) has 14 selectable grip patterns and hand positions, accessed by input triggers and/or an external switch on the back of the hand.[7,84]

The i-Limb Quantum (Össur) offers 36 preset grasp patterns and a powered thumb that switches between lateral pinch and opposition. The grasps for this hand can be accessed with input triggers and/or mobile app control.[83]

Education by the occupational therapist and prosthetist on the benefits and limitations of these advanced terminal devices should be provided to the client before a device is recommended and prescribed.

Wrist units. Electric wrist rotators are used to provide an attachment point for the TD to the forearm. The rotator also

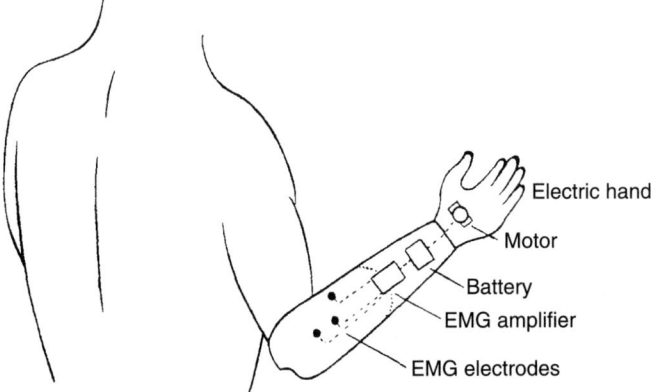

Fig. 44.12 Typical electrically powered, myoelectrically controlled, transradial prosthesis with an electromechanical hand terminal device that is activated by electromyographic *(EMG)* potentials. (From Billock JN: Upper limb prosthetic terminal devices: hands versus hooks, *Clin Prosthet Orthot* 10:59, 1986.)

Labels on Fig. 44.12: Electric hand, Motor, Battery, EMG amplifier, EMG electrodes

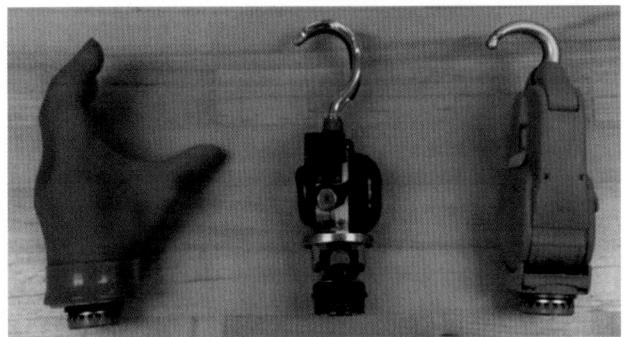

Fig. 44.13 Examples of electrically powered prehensor terminal devices. *Left,* System Electric Hand (Ottobock). *Center,* Electric Terminal Device (Motion Control, Inc.). *Right,* System Electric Greifer (Ottobock).

provides the important function of forearm supination and pronation for prepositioning of the TD for functional use.[5,41] The rotator is not recommended for work that generates high torque[41]; it should be used only for TD orientation and prepositioning. Currently, no electrically powered wrist flexion units are available. Wrist flexion is an important function for individuals who have undergone bilateral upper extremity amputation. It allows the user to reach midline for tasks such as dressing and eating. The Motion Control Powered Flexion Wrist (Fillauer) provides a previously unavailable degree of freedom with powered wrist flexion and extension.[27]

The need for wrist motion that replicates the requirements for prepositioning of the human hand will continue to drive development efforts with electrically controlled wrist units.[41]

Elbow units. Electrically powered elbows reduce the need for the glenohumeral ROM or strength that typically is needed to operate body-powered prostheses.[71] Myoelectric elbows position the forearm and TD in space for activity performance. For manual humeral rotation a friction joint or turntable is used in addition to the elbow unit.[41] The functional advantage of a myoelectric elbow comes with the cost of increased weight. Locking of the elbow unit is performed in two ways: when the elbow is held for a stationary set of time or when a momentary switch is activated. Unlocking the elbow is controlled by the following: rapid contraction of the controlling muscle known as rate control, slow contraction of the controlling muscle known as threshold control, or by actuation of the momentary switch. When the elbow is locked in position, the myosites used to control the elbow are transmitted to control the TD.[41] Although advances have been made in the design and performance of electrically powered elbow units, functional performance still needs improvement.

Shoulder units

Shoulder disarticulation and other higher level amputations are uncommon; therefore, there are few commercially available shoulder component options. Prosthetic shoulder components offer two degrees of freedom: flexion/extension and adduction/abduction. A shoulder component with an electric lock actuator is used to provide increased function for clients with shoulder amputations. Manual operation of flexion and extension involves actuating a nudge control that disengages the lock on the joint, allowing it to swing freely. Releasing the nudge control engages the lock to hold the shoulder in a fixed degree of flexion. If the wearer cannot operate a manual nudge control, a myoelectrode or force-sensitive resistor can control the actuator.[41]

The Luke Arm (Mobius Bionics) offers a commercially available option for powered humeral rotation, shoulder flexion and extension, and/or shoulder abduction. The Luke Arm provides a flexible control system that allows the prosthesis to be controlled by a variety of input devices to include EMG, inertial measurement unit foot controls, and/or a linear transducer.[74]

PROSTHETIC TRAINING

Upper extremity prosthetic training begins after the final fitting of the prosthesis. The final fitting may be done with a preparatory prosthesis rather than a definitive prosthesis. The occupational therapy intervention is occupation based and includes purposeful activity and preparatory methods to facilitate therapeutic goals.

Evaluation of the Prosthesis

When the prosthesis is received, team members check to ensure that it meets the prescription's requirements, functions efficiently, and is mechanically sound. The prosthesis is checked for fit and function against specific mechanical standards developed from actual tests on prostheses worn by individuals. The tests performed are comparative ROM with the prosthesis on and off; control system function and efficiency; TD opening in various arm positions; amount of socket slippage on the residual limb under various degrees of load or tension; compression fit and comfort; and force required to flex the forearm or open and close the TD.[4,96,122] Ideally the prosthetist and the therapist coordinate fitting of the prosthesis and initiation of therapy. Communication among the client, therapist, and prosthetist is essential to ensure that the prosthesis fits and functions optimally.

Donning and Doffing the Prosthesis

Donning and doffing the full prosthetic system is a critical first step in training for the user. It is important for the client to be able to don and doff the prosthesis as independently as possible. The full prosthetic system includes the residual limb sock, prosthetic donning liner, prosthetic socket, and/or harnessing.[102]

The two most common methods of donning and doffing the body-powered prosthesis are the coat method and the pullover (or sweater) method. Either method can be used for unilateral or bilateral amputations. The method used depends on the client's choice and ease of use. The coat method is similar to placing one arm in a coat sleeve and manipulating the coat to a position where the other arm can reach the other sleeve. The residual limb is inserted into the socket while the harness and axilla loop dangle behind the back. The sound hand reaches around the back and slips into the axilla loop. The person then slips into the harness as if putting on a coat. The shoulders are shrugged to shift the harness forward and into the correct position. To remove the prosthesis, the person uses the TD to slip the axilla loop off the sound side and then slips the shoulder strap off the amputated side. The harness is slipped off like a coat.[4,96,122]

The person who has had bilateral amputations can use the coat method by placing the prostheses face up on a surface, placing the longer residual limb in the socket, and elevating the prosthesis, allowing the other prosthesis to hang across the back. The person then leans to the side and places the shorter limb in the prosthesis.[96,125] To remove the prosthesis, the person shrugs the harness off the shoulders and removes the prosthesis from the shorter side first. Before removing the prosthesis on the longer side, the person should position the prostheses somewhere convenient for the next donning.

For the pullover method, the client positions the prosthesis face up, places the residual limb in the socket, and threads the opposite arm through the harness. The person then raises both arms above the head, allowing the axilla loop to slide down to

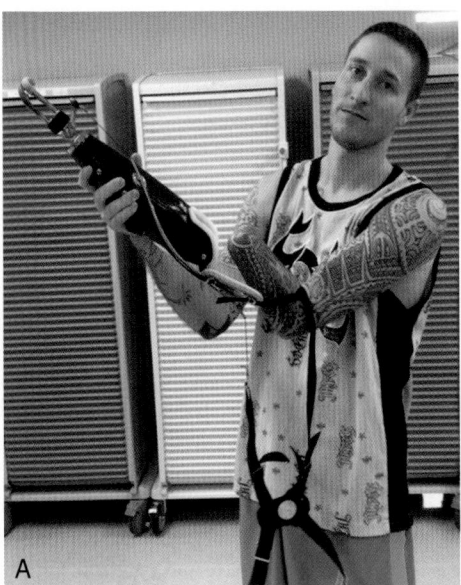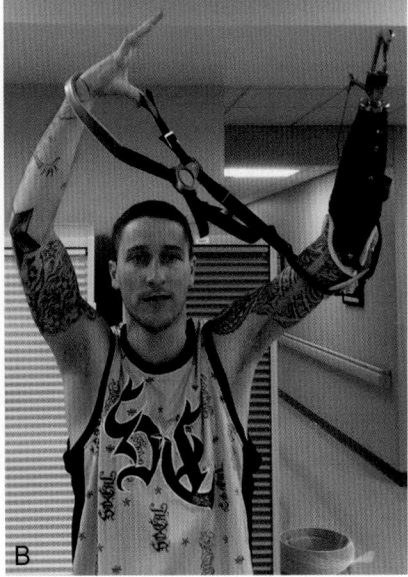

Fig. 44.14 (A–B) Pullover (or sweater) method for donning a transradial body-powered prosthesis.

the axilla and the harness to be properly positioned across the back and on the shoulders (Fig. 44.14). To remove the prosthesis, the person raises both arms above the head and grasps and removes the prosthesis with the sound arm while allowing the axilla loop to slide off the arm.[96]

A person who has had bilateral amputations dons the prostheses using the pullover method by placing the prostheses on a surface, face up. With the longer limb stabilizing the socket, the shorter residual limb is positioned under the harness and in the socket. The longer limb is positioned similarly under the harness in the socket, and the arms are raised, allowing the harness to flip over the head and across the back and shoulders. The person removes the prostheses by shrugging the shoulders to bring the harness up, grasping it with one TD, and pulling it over the head while allowing the residual limbs to come out of their sockets.

In the case of donning an electrically powered prosthesis, the client may use a pull sock to facilitate an intimate interface between the skin and socket. For this method a pull sock is placed over the residual limb, and a weighted cord from the pull sock is guided through a hole in the bottom of the socket. The client then pulls the sock off the arm and through the hole in the socket, creating optimal contact with the surface electrodes. Daniel preferred the pull sock method to don and doff his prosthesis because it provided a tight fit and good suction in his myoelectric socket.

Donning of the prosthesis should be performed with the electronic components in the OFF position to prevent any uncontrolled movements. Applying a silicone-based skin lotion to the skin before donning the pull sock enables the person to remove the pull sock with less effort. It may be necessary to experiment with different sock materials, powder on the skin, and various donning techniques until the most successful materials and techniques are identified. Good electrical contact is achieved after approximately 1 minute of donning. A wearer can moisten the skin at the electrode sites to eliminate the waiting

period for skin warmth to occur. The prosthetic arm should be stored in the OFF position with the batteries removed. The hand should be fully opened when stored to keep the thumb web space stretched.

Wearing Schedule

A wearing schedule for the prosthesis is established and reviewed during the first training session. The client increases the wearing time gradually to develop a tolerance and decrease the likelihood of skin breakdown. The prosthesis initially is worn 15 to 30 minutes 3 times a day. Each time the prosthesis is removed, the skin must be inspected for redness or irritation. The skin must be closely monitored, and the wearing time is increased only if the skin remains in good condition. If no skin problems develop, the three scheduled wearing periods may be increased by 30-minute increments until the prosthesis can be worn all day. If skin problems occur, the therapist, prosthetist, or physician must be notified, and the prosthesis should not be worn until the problem has cleared. Restarting the initial wearing schedule may be necessary to decrease the risk of additional skin problems.[6]

Residual Limb Hygiene

The client is instructed in residual limb hygiene in the early phase of prosthetic training. Perspiration is common when a prosthesis is worn because the residual limb is enclosed in a rigid socket. Excessive perspiration can cause irritation or maceration of the skin; therefore, it is important to teach the client to inspect the skin of the residual limb, each time the prosthesis is removed, to look for areas of redness or breakdown. The client is also instructed to wash the residual limb daily with mild soap and water and to pat it dry. To minimize sweating, education is provided to the client in the application of antiperspirants, socks, or liners that will not compromise the fit of the prosthesis or interfere with myoelectric surface electrodes.

Operational Prosthetic Knowledge

The wearer should learn and demonstrate knowledge of the terminology and function of each prosthetic component. A basic knowledge of the following terminology is recommended: socket and harness design and use; types of control systems; and basic mechanics of the prosthesis. This allows the client to communicate with the rehabilitation team, using terminology understood by all, about the operation of the prosthesis and any difficulties with or repairs needed for the device.[6,122,125]

Care of the Prosthesis

Instructions regarding care of the prosthesis are provided and reviewed. In general, the prosthetist educates the person in this area, and the therapist reviews and reinforces the information with the wearer. The socket should be cleaned daily with mild soap and water or weekly with rubbing alcohol. Cleaning at night is recommended to allow the prosthesis to dry completely. Wearing the prosthesis when the socket is wet may lead to skin problems. The components should be cleaned and maintained according to the manufacturer's specifications. Daily inspection of the prosthesis helps prevent problems.[6] The client should be proficient in basic maintenance procedures, including daily socket cleaning and inspection, battery charging procedures for the prosthesis, component maintenance, harness adjustment, and cable system changes and rubber band replacement.[73,102] It is the role of the occupational therapist to ensure that the client is trained and independent in the maintenance and care of the prosthesis.

INTERMEDIATE PROSTHETIC TRAINING

Controls Training

Therapy progresses through two phases of training: (1) prosthetic controls training and (2) use training. The goal of prosthetic controls training is to achieve smooth movement of the prosthesis with minimal delay or awkward movements with task performance.[6] Functional use training is designed to apply the skills learned during controls training and apply them to functional use of the prosthesis. Acquiring skill in the operation of the prosthesis is emphasized in controls training. The therapist educates the wearer on the importance of the practice drills that will ensure more successful function with the prosthesis in daily activities. Joint protection, energy conservation, and work simplification principles and techniques should be stressed during this phase of training. Each prosthetic component should be reviewed separately and understood before the components are combined into functional activities.

Body-Powered Prosthesis

Controls training for a body-powered prosthesis begins with the operation of each component, starting with the TD. For a transradial prosthesis there is a single control system to activate the TD. Scapula abduction and glenohumeral flexion are the motions used to open and close the TD. The client is instructed to activate the TD with the arm in various positions in space, such as overhead and leaning over toward the floor.[125] The client is instructed in how to exchange the TD if more than one

is prescribed. To complete controls training with a transradial prosthesis, the client demonstrates the motions required to position and operate the TD until they are performed in one continuous, smooth, and natural sequence in both sitting and standing positions.[122]

Transhumeral prostheses operate through the use of a dual-control cable system. When tension is applied on the cable attached to the elbow unit, the unit locks and unlocks. The motions necessary to lock and unlock the elbow are a combination of scapular depression, humeral extension, and abduction. This movement places tension on the cable that attaches the harness to the elbow unit. The reminder "down, out, and away" may be repeated until the client develops a proprioceptive memory. The client is then asked to practice locking and unlocking the elbow in various ranges of elbow flexion and extension.[4,6,125] The client may also learn to operate the turntable that manually rotates the arm medially and laterally, allowing for internal and external rotation. The same motions of shoulder flexion and scapula abduction that flex the forearm with the elbow unlocked control the TD when the elbow is locked. The person is instructed to lock the elbow, first at 90 degrees, and to perform the motions to operate the TD. The sequence of elbow positioning, elbow locking, TD operation, elbow unlocking, elbow repositioning, and locking is repeated at various points in elbow ROM from full extension to full flexion.[4,125]

A prosthesis used for a shoulder disarticulation may have a manually operated, friction-held shoulder unit that the client pre-positions using the sound arm. A chin-operated nudge control may be used to operate the elbow unit if the client does not have the shoulder movements necessary to lock and unlock the elbow. The client still is instructed in the dual-control cable system of operation, as described for a transhumeral prosthesis. For clients with higher levels of amputation, such as shoulder disarticulation, chest expansion is used to assist with TD operation.

The progression of controls training for body-powered prostheses at each level of upper limb amputation is described in Fig. 44.15.

Electrically Powered Prosthesis

Each myoelectric prosthesis has a unique control system based on the manufactured componentry and/or the person's musculoskeletal integrity. Typically a two-site system is used, in which two separate muscle groups operate the TD. For transradial prostheses, wrist flexors and extensors are commonly used to open and close the TD; the biceps and triceps are often used with a transhumeral prosthesis. With higher level amputations (e.g., shoulder disarticulation), the muscles used for control are typically the pectoralis or infraspinatus.

Controls training typically begins with opening and closing of the TD. Simple opening and closing of the terminal device is practiced in various arm positions to ensure that the electrodes maintain contact with the skin in each position. Next, the client practices opening the TD through one-third, one-half, and three-fourths of range. If a proportional control system is used, the client may also practice opening and closing quickly and slowly. Daniel demonstrated difficulty with proportional

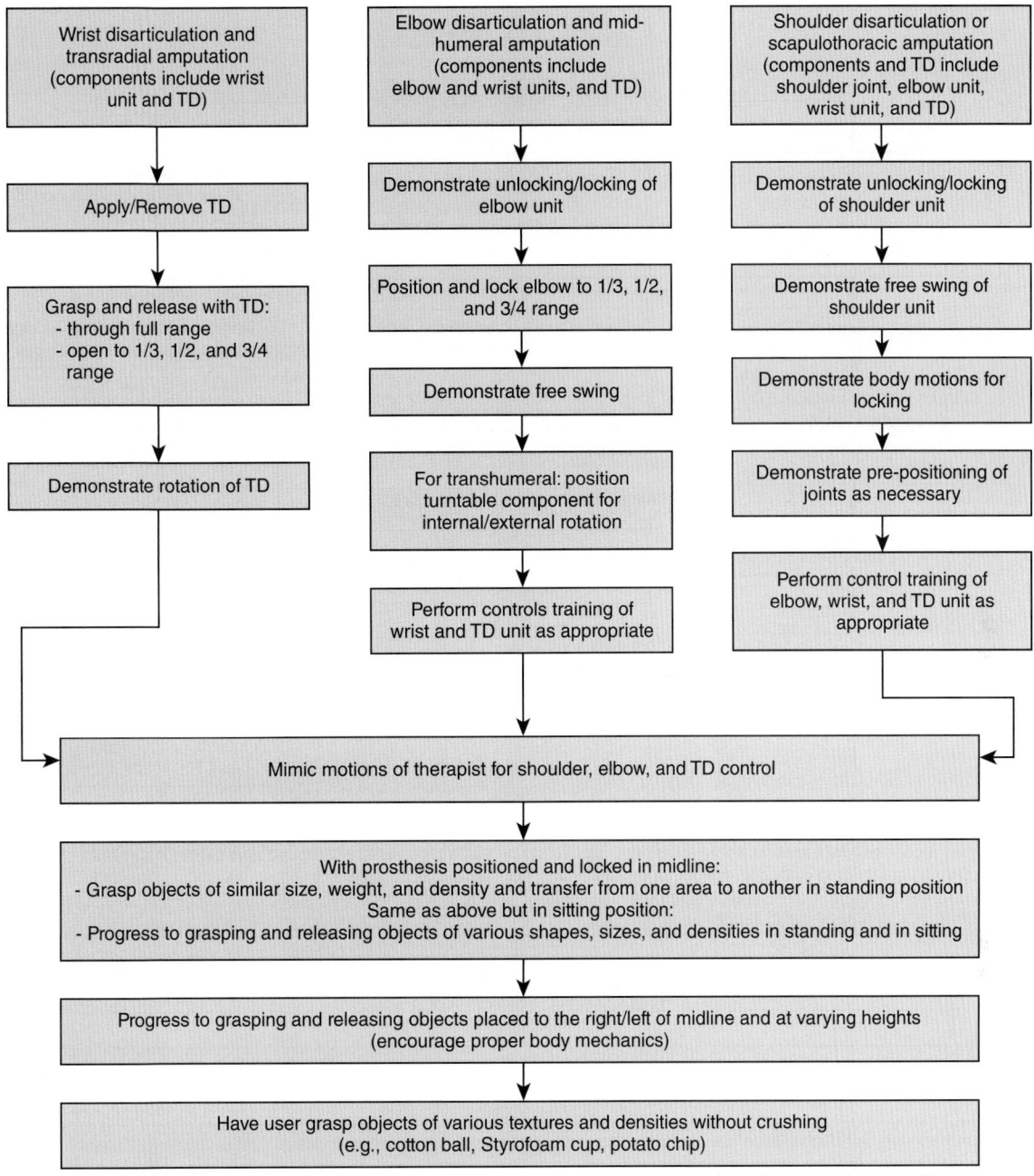

Fig. 44.15 Controls training for body-powered prostheses by level of amputation. *TD,* Terminal device. (From Smurr LM, Yancosek K, Gulick K, et al: Occupational therapy for the polytrauma casualty with limb loss. In Pasquina PF, Cooper RA, editors: *Care of the combat amputee,* Washington, DC, 2009, Department of the Army, the Borden Institute.)

control initially during training. To offer more practice, the therapist often will design a home program of specific patterns of terminal device action that the person performs. Control of the TD improves in accuracy and speed with practice and use throughout the other phases of training. The progression of controls training for myoelectric prostheses at each level of upper limb amputation is described in Fig. 44.16.

Use Training

Once the client understands how to operate and control the pros-thetic components, he or she can begin to apply the mechanics of

operation to activities. Instruction on pre-positioning the pros-thesis is important because this involves moving the prosthetic units in their optimal position to grasp an object or perform a given activity in the most efficient manner, thereby avoiding awkward body movements used to compensate for poor pre-positioning.[96] The client is instructed in control drills in patterns of reach, grasp, and release of objects of various sizes, weights, densities, and shapes. The sequence (and progression) typically is from large, hard objects to smaller, softer ones. These objects should be placed in positions that require elbow and TD pre-positioning and TD operation, both for prehension practice

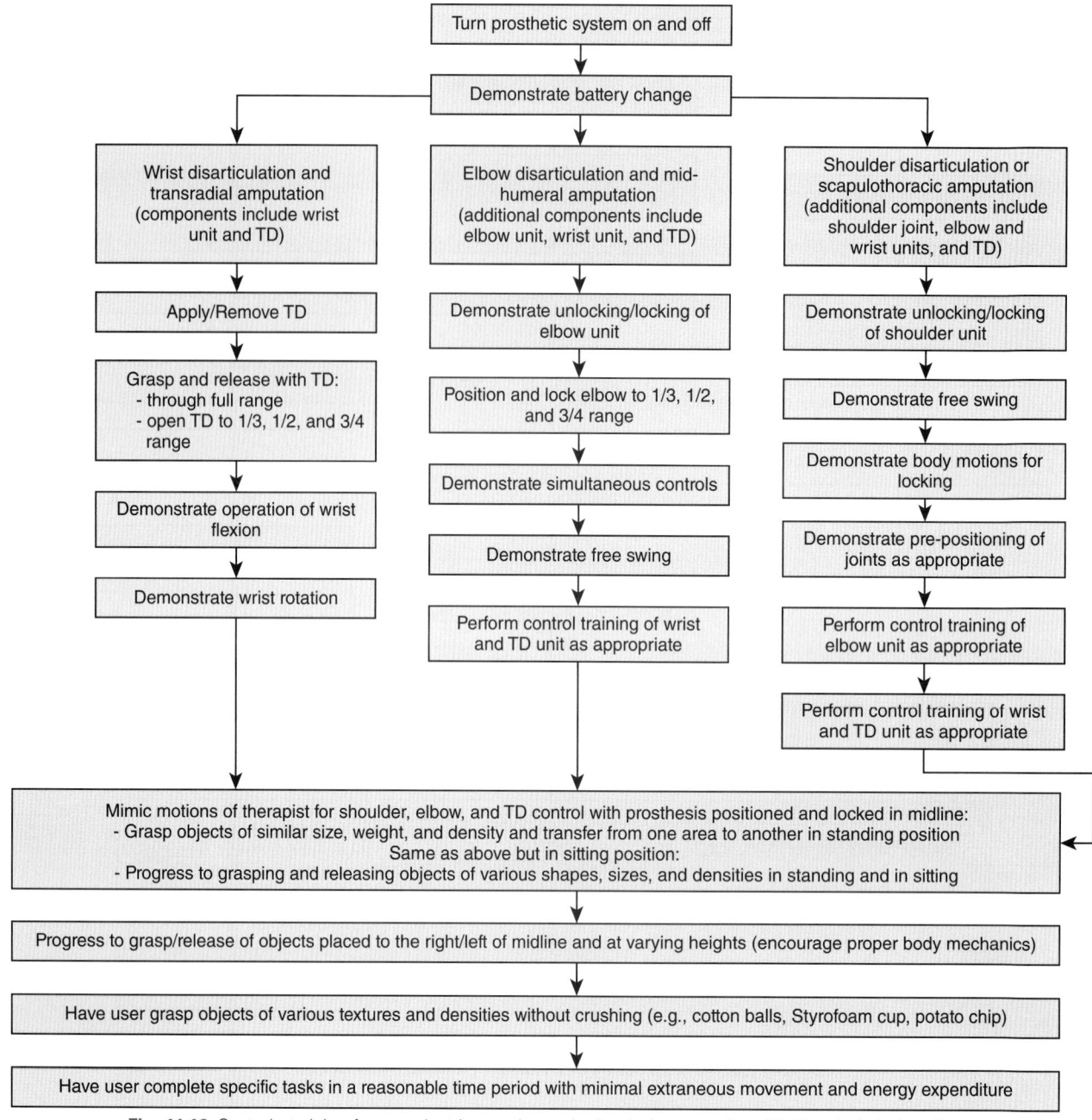

Fig. 44.16 Controls training for myoelectric prostheses by level of amputation. *TD*, Terminal device. (From Smurr LM, Yancosek K, Gulick K, et al: Occupational therapy for the polytrauma casualty with limb loss. In Pasquina PF, Cooper RA, editors: *Care of the combat amputee*, Washington, DC, 2009, Department of the Army, the Borden Institute.)

at tabletop or at various heights around the room. Working on reach, grasp, and release in multiple arm positions then follows. The client will attempt to grasp objects at counter height, at table height, overhead, on the floor, at cupboard height, alongside the body, and behind the body. This area of space in which the client can operate the prosthesis is referred to as the functional envelope.

Another goal of use training is mastering pressure control, or the gripping force of the TD. Particularly with myoelectric control, this skill involves close visual attention to appropriately grade the muscle contraction for a specific result in the TD. The

client must learn how to pick up the object without applying too much force and crushing it. Good grasp control through training with foam, cotton balls, or wet sponges will help the client develop the control necessary to handle paper cups, vegetables, boxes, lotion bottles, and sandwiches or even to hold someone's hand.[108]

The client with a transhumeral amputation who uses a body-powered or myoelectric elbow should ensure that the position of the terminal hand and the angle of elbow flexion are appropriate to complete the grasp in a natural manner. Often the client automatically adjusts the body using compensatory body motions (e.g., bending forward rather than adjusting the elbow position or pre-positioning the hand). It is important to discourage this adjustment because it looks unnatural, becomes habitual, and may lead to secondary musculoskeletal problems in the neck, shoulder, or trunk. The ability to perform specific movements will eventually take less conscious effort, and movements will become automatic.

The wearer now has increased muscle endurance and prosthetic tolerance. Next, functional activities are introduced into the therapy program.

ADVANCED PROSTHETIC TRAINING

Functional Training

Functional training applies the concepts of control and use of the prosthesis for completion of functional and meaningful activities. The goal is to perform functional tasks with automatic, spontaneous, smooth movements. Five characteristics of advanced prosthetic training can help guide therapy. First, a person's rehabilitation is individualized, and each client has a unique set of goals. Second, the client uses tools or interacts with an object such as a cooking utensil or a piece of sports equipment (Fig. 44.17). The third characteristic of advanced prosthetic training is that it involves complex, multistep tasks that are typically bimanual (Fig. 44.18). The fourth characteristic is that the training involves the prosthesis of choice for the client. Training should focus on advancing and refining the control of the preferred prosthesis for functional use. The final characteristic is that the training and activity selection are meaningful to the client.[102] The key to successful functional training is to teach the client problem-solving techniques and ways to

analyze each activity with respect to the environment in which it is performed. The client recognizes the altered environment and learns to successfully complete activities within it.

Although there is no specific technique to accomplish most tasks, the therapist will offer guidance to enable completion of activities in an efficient way. A client with a unilateral amputation quickly learns to perform activities with one hand. Therefore, when incorporating a prosthesis into bimanual tasks, the prosthesis is primarily used for stabilization or support.[122] Table 44.1 offers suggestions for ways some activities can be accomplished with a prosthesis.[128]

During advanced prosthetic training, therapy will focus on incorporation of the prosthesis into ADL and IADL performance. Practice in handwriting and activities requiring dexterity and fine motor coordination may be useful in this phase of the training process.[82,105,122] A rating guide developed by Atkins, the Unilateral Upper Extremity Amputation: Activities of Daily Living Assessment, provides a comprehensive checklist of functional activities that can be used as a reference to show progression with advanced prosthetic training (Fig. 44.19).[6] Vocational and recreational activities, including driving, community reintegration, and adaptive sports, are introduced during this phase. The occupational therapist should bring the client into the actual environment, when possible, to encourage realistic, deliberate training with the prosthesis (Fig. 44.20). By the end of this phase of training, the client will have learned to perform functional tasks and meaningful occupations in the most efficient way. This would result in saved energy for the body and decreased biomechanical stress on the sound limb.[102]

Adaptive Sports and Recreation

Adaptive sports and recreational activities are an important part of rehabilitation after limb loss. Various levels of recreational activity and adaptive sports options are available, from low to high intensity, and a number of activity-specific and customized prostheses are available to facilitate participation in these activities (Fig. 44.21). It is the role of the occupational therapist and interdisciplinary clinical team to encourage participation

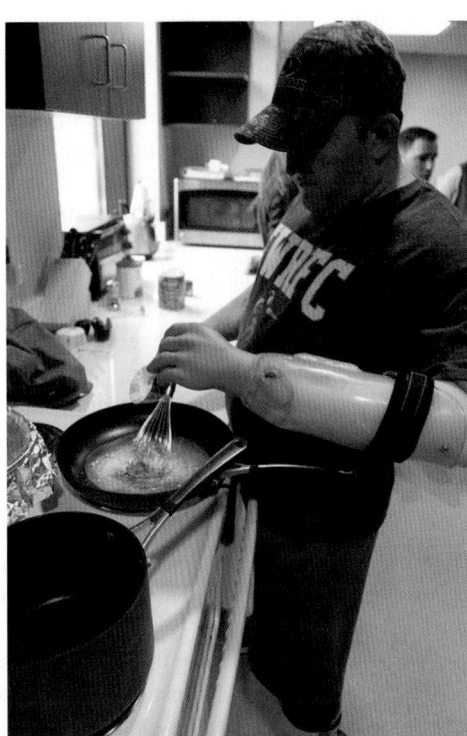

Fig. 44.17 Example of functional training: interacting with an object such as a cooking utensil.

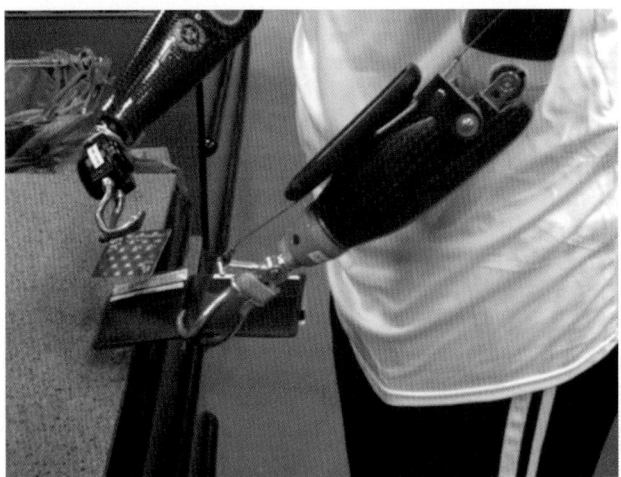

Fig. 44.18 Individual with bilateral upper limb loss removing credit cards from a wallet. This is an example of a multistep, bimanual task that is taught during advanced prosthetic training.

TABLE 44.1   Roles of Prosthetic Terminal Device and Sound Hand in Bilateral Activities of Daily Living

Activity	Prosthetic Terminal Device	Sound Hand
Cutting meat	Hold the fork with prongs facing downward; hold the knife as grip strength increases.	Hold knife. Hold fork.
Opening a jar	Hold the jar.	Turn the lid.
Opening a tube of toothpaste	Hold the tube.	Turn the cap.
Stirring something in a bowl	Hold the bowl with a strong grip.	Hold the mixing spoon or fork.
Cutting fruit or vegetables	Hold the fruit or vegetable firmly.	Hold the knife to cut.
Using scissors to cut paper	Hold the paper to be cut.	Use scissors in normal fashion.
Buckling a belt	Hold buckle end of belt to keep it stable.	Manipulate long end of belt into buckle.
Zipping a jacket from the bottom up	Hold anchor tab.	Manipulate pull tab at base, and pull upward.
Applying socks	Hold one side of sock.	Hold other side of sock, and pull upward.
Opening an umbrella	Hold base knob of umbrella.	Open as normal.

in adaptive sports and to train the client in the use of activity-specific prostheses. Modifications can be made to all types of sporting and recreational equipment. Additionally, a number of nonprofit organizations have been established to support individuals with amputations in their participation in adaptive sports and recreation. Participation in adaptive sports has been shown to promote social and psychological health and also helps individuals with a disability focus on their abilities rather than their functional limitations.[100,123] Studies have shown that adaptive sports participation for persons with disabilities improves overall quality of life and satisfaction across physical, social, and psychological domains.[127] The interdisciplinary team of healthcare providers should educate the client on the benefits of participation in adaptive sports and recreation, assist with modifications to equipment, and provide information on available resources to support reintegration into meaningful activities.

OT PRACTICE NOTES

Encourage clients to try new sports or activities that may be outside their comfort zone. Reinforce the positive idea of finding a "new norm" in the context of occupational performance after amputation.

Driver Training

The ability to drive is a valued occupation in today's society. For many clients, returning to driving after amputation is a primary goal. Driving is a complex process, involving an individual's physical, cognitive, visual, and behavioral abilities. The occupational therapist will make a referral for a comprehensive driving evaluation when appropriate. A driving rehabilitation specialist will do a clinical assessment and will make recommendations for adaptive equipment or vehicle modifications. The driving rehabilitation specialist may also provide behind the wheel training with the client as necessary. Modifications can be made to improve safety and comfort. For example, a person with a unilateral upper extremity amputation can have a spinner knob or driving ring installed (Fig. 44.22). Clients are

always encouraged to contact their state's Department of Motor Vehicles or driver's licensing agency to determine whether any driving restrictions apply to persons with amputations.

CONSIDERATIONS FOR BILATERAL AMPUTATIONS

In the case of bilateral amputations, adaptive equipment should be introduced as soon as possible to increase the client's level of independence. The equipment may include a universal cuff secured by elastic or Velcro to the residual limb to aid in eating, writing, and hygiene; a dressing tree with hooks to hold articles of clothing in a position conducive to donning them, to improve dressing independence; and loops added to items such as socks and towels. Individuals with bilateral amputations can learn to complete activities using foot skills, such as holding items between the toes in a functional pinch for dressing, eating, and reaching items. The therapist can also encourage the use of the chin, knees, and teeth for activity performance.[24] The therapist and client will problem-solve and analyze activities together, with emphasis placed on how to maximize the individual's environment to accomplish a particular task.

The use of an immediate or early postoperative prosthesis (IPOP or EPOP, respectively) is strongly recommended in bilateral upper extremity amputations.[116] Fitting an individual with an early temporary prosthesis not only promotes immediate participation and independence in ADLs, but also may facilitate acceptance and use of the permanent prosthesis.[29,51,58,61]

Bilateral upper extremity amputations present unique challenges for prosthetic selection, fitting, and training. A person with bilateral upper extremity amputations commonly is fitted with a combination of systems (Fig. 44.23). For example, an individual may be fitted with a body-powered system for one side and a myoelectric system for the other. It is important to include the client in this decision-making process and to include the individual's goals when discussing prosthesis selection with the rehabilitation team. The progression and phases of training for bilateral upper extremity amputations are the same

Name:	Age:	Occupation:	Date(s) of Test:
Therapist:	Sex:	Type of terminal device:	

RATING GUIDE KEY:

0 Impossible	1 Accomplished with much strain, or many awkward motions	2 Somewhat labored, or few awkward motions	3 Smooth, minimal amount of delays and awkward motions

ACTIVITIES OF DAILY LIVING	0	1	2	3	ACTIVITIES OF DAILY LIVING	0	1	2	3
PERSONAL NEEDS:					**GENERAL PROCEDURES:**				
Don/doff pull-over shirt					Turn key in lock				
Dress button-down shirt: cuffs and front					Operate door knob				
Manage zippers and snaps					Place chain on chain lock				
Don/doff pants					Plug cord into wall outlet				
Don/doff belt					Set time on watch				
Lace and tie shoes					**HOUSEKEEPING PROCEDURES:**				
Don/doff pantyhose					Perform laundry				
Tie a tie					Fold clothes				
Don/doff brassiere					Set up ironing board				
Don/doff glove					Iron clothes				
Cut and file finger nails					Hand-wash dishes				
Polish finger nails					Dry dishes with a towel				
Screw/unscrew cap of toothpaste tube					Load and unload dishwasher				
Squeeze toothpaste					Use broom and dustpan				
Open top of pill bottle					Operate vacuum cleaner				
Set hair					Use wet and dry mops				
Take bill from wallet					Make bed				
Open pack of cigarettes					Change garbage bag				
Light a match					Open/close jar				
Don/doff prosthesis					Open lid of can				
Perform residual limb care					Cut vegetables				
EATING PROCEDURES:					Peel vegetables				
Carry a tray					Manipulate hot pots				
Cut meat					Thread a needle				
Butter bread					Sew a button				
Open milk carton					**USE OF TOOLS:**				
DESK PROCEDURES:					Saw				
Use phone and take notes					Hammer				
Use pay phone					Screwdrivers				
Sharpen pencil					Tape measure				
Use scissors					Wrenches				
Use ruler					Power tools: drill, sander				
Remove and replace ink pen cap					Plane				
Fold and seal letter					Shovel				
Use paper clip					Rake				
Use stapler					Wheelbarrow				
Wrap package					**CAR PROCEDURES:**				
Use computer: typing, access Internet					Open and close doors, trunk and hood				
Demonstrate handwriting					Perform steps required to operate vehicle				

COMMENTS:	COMMENTS:

Fig. 44.19 Assessment of activities of daily living for a client with unilateral upper extremity amputation. (From Atkins DJ. In Atkins DJ, Meier RH, editors: *Comprehensive management of the upper-limb amputee*, New York, 1989, Springer-Verlag.)

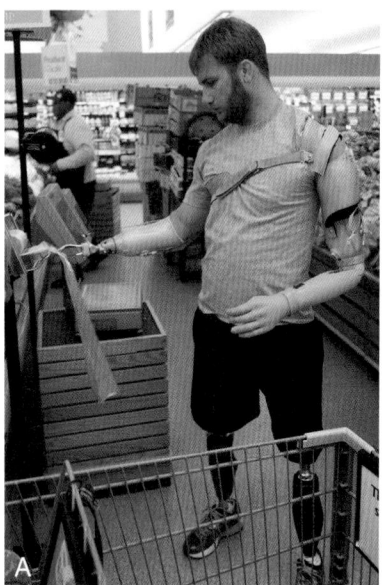
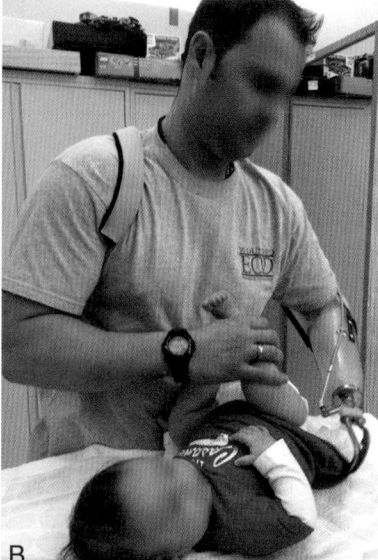
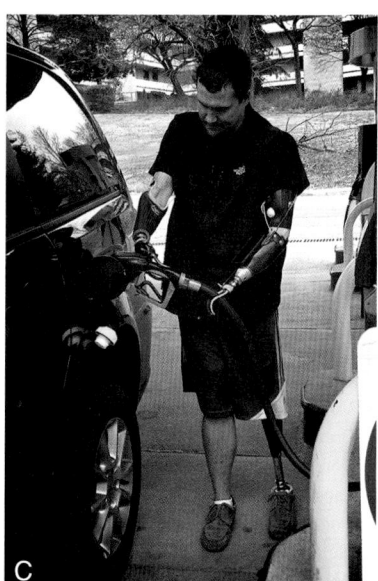
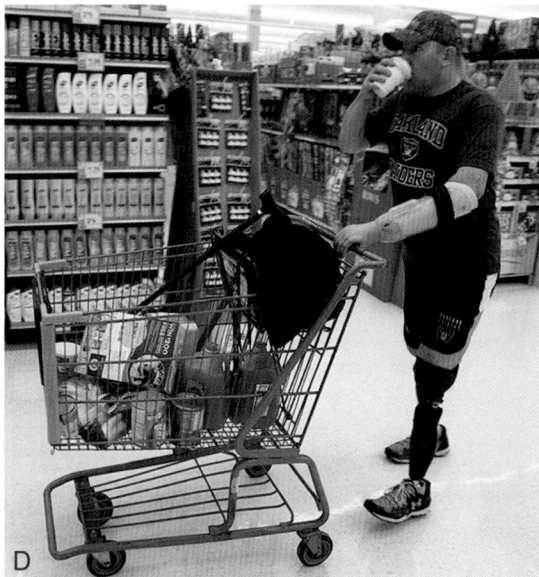

Fig. 44.20 Instrumental activities of daily living. (A) Individual with bilateral upper limb amputation and bilateral lower limb amputation grasps a plastic bag for produce while grocery shopping. (B) Father dresses his son using a body-powered prosthesis. (C) Individual putting gas in a car using bilateral upper limb prostheses. (D) Individual uses a myoelectric prosthesis to push a grocery cart while sipping a cup of coffee.

as for unilateral amputation. Techniques for donning and doffing, componentry, and controls training vary slightly to accommodate variations in the designs of the two prosthetic systems. Refer to donning and doffing techniques for bilateral upper extremity amputations presented earlier in this chapter under Prosthetic Training.

A client with bilateral amputations typically receives two prostheses that are attached to one harness. Operating one of the prostheses may transmit tension through the harness to the other prosthesis, causing it to operate. The client must learn to operate each prosthetic component without affecting the components on either side. This skill is called separation of controls, and the client may need extensive practice to master it. Each prosthesis operates according to the level of amputation, as described in the previous sections.

OUTCOME MEASURES

Outcome measures for upper limb amputations are used to assess progress and analyze the effectiveness of a prosthetic device.[93,126] Evaluation of upper extremity prosthetic use presents a unique challenge because only a limited number of measures have been validated for adults.[93] Traditional dexterity assessments, such as the 9-Hole Peg Test and the Purdue Pegboard, provide occupational therapists with a measure of progress in performance over time but are not validated as true determinants of the effectiveness of prosthetic use. Efforts are ongoing for the development and validation of outcome measures for prosthetic use and upper limb amputation.[46,93]

For the purpose of this chapter, five assessments that have been recommended for use will be discussed. The Assessment of Capacity for Myoelectric Control (ACMC) is a measurement

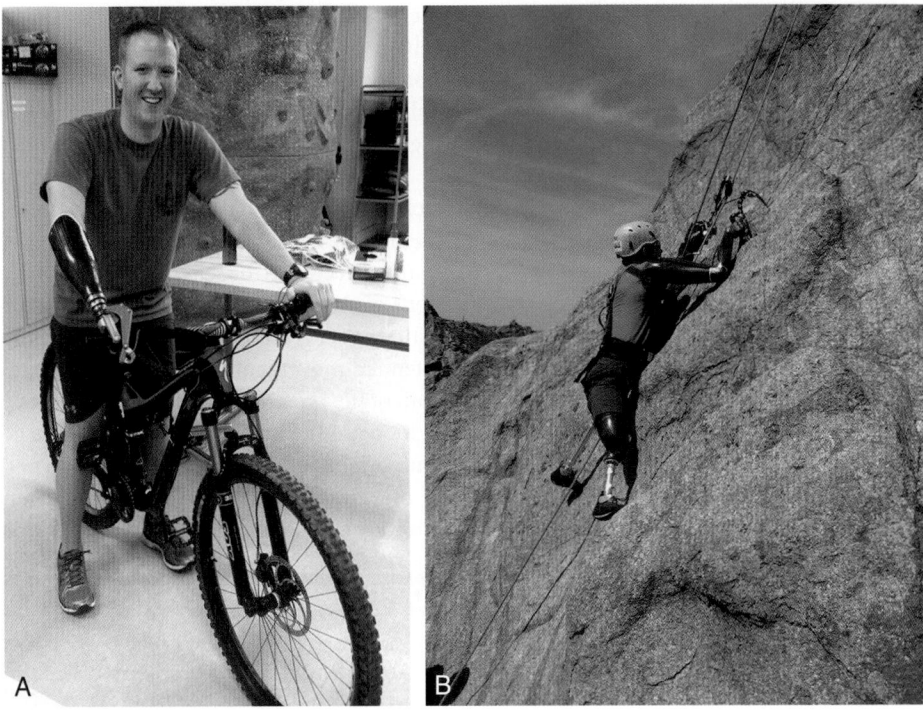

Fig. 44.21 (A) Mountain biking using an activity-specific terminal device. (B) Individual with multiple limb loss rock climbing using activity-specific terminal devices.

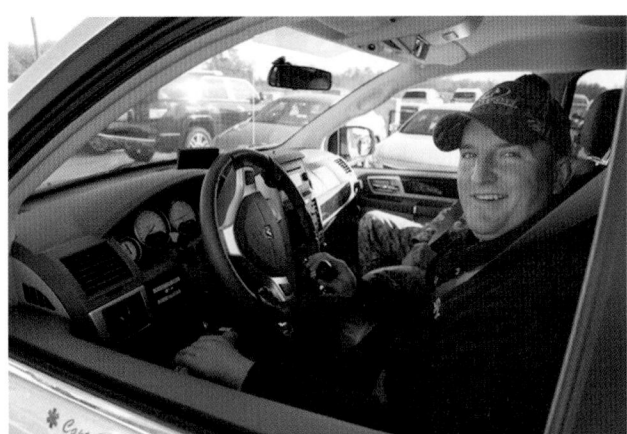

Fig. 44.22 Individual with left upper extremity amputation and bilateral lower extremity amputations uses hand controls and spinner knob for driving.

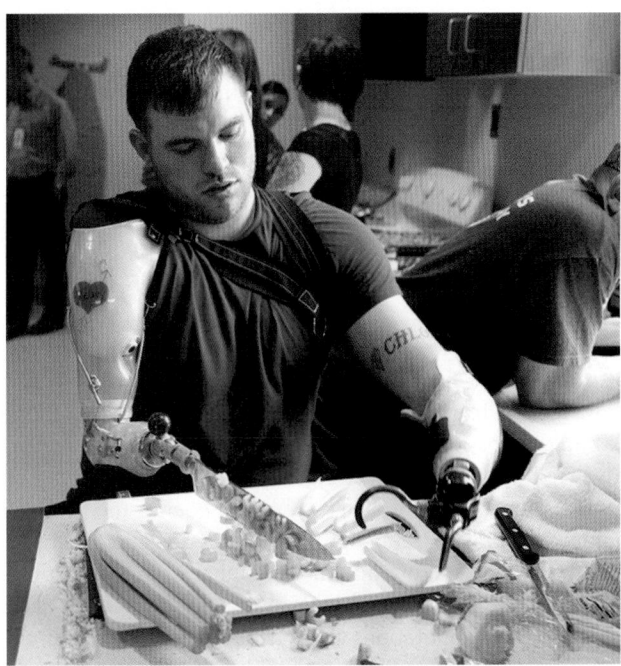

Fig. 44.23 Individual with bilateral upper limb loss using a combination of prosthetic systems. On the right side he is using a transhumeral body-powered system with an activity-specific terminal device. On the left side he is using a transradial myoelectric system with an electric hook.

of an electrically controlled prosthesis in the performance of bimanual tasks. The assessment evaluates performance with the prosthesis in the areas of gripping, holding, releasing, and bimanual manipulation.[43,44] The Trinity Amputation and Prosthesis Experience Scales–Revised (TAPES-R) is a self-report measure that evaluates psychosocial adjustment, activity restriction, and satisfaction with the prosthetic device.[35] The Southampton Hand Assessment Procedure (SHAP) examines upper limb prosthetic use during manipulation of 8 objects and 14 ADLs tasks (Fig. 44.24).[63] The Orthotics and Prosthetics User Survey (OPUS) is a self-report instrument that assesses for functional status, quality of life, and client satisfaction with the prosthetic devices and services. The survey is used to examine both upper and lower extremity function.[42] The final outcome measure that will be addressed is the Activities Measure for Upper Limb Amputees (AM-ULA); this

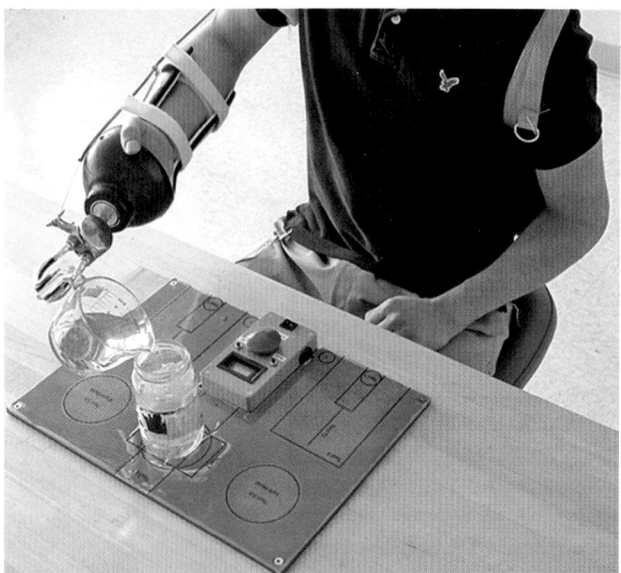

Fig. 44.24 Southampton Hand Assessment Procedure (SHAP). (From Berning K, Cohick S, Johnson R, et al: Comparison of body-powered voluntary opening and voluntary closing prehensor for activities of daily life, *J Rehabil Res Dev* 51:253–261, 2014.)

is an observational measure of activity performance for adults with upper limb amputation that evaluates task completion, speed, movement quality, skillfulness of prosthetic use, and independence.[93]

Work is still needed in the development of normative data and outcome measures for upper extremity prosthetic use. Continued development of standardized assessments for this population would serve to identify standards of performance and provide an evidence base for intervention and practice.[14,15]

CURRENT RESEARCH AND EMERGING TECHNOLOGIES

Research in the field of upper limb prosthetics continues to grow, thanks in part to the program Revolutionizing Upper Extremity Prosthetics, which was established by the Defense Advanced Research Project Agency (DARPA), an agency of the U.S. Department of Defense.[20,92] The goal of the project is to improve upper extremity prosthetic function and "to create a fully functional (motor and sensory) upper limb that responds to direct neural control, within this decade."[20] As a result of this program and collaborations with various institutions, a number of advances have been made in signal control schemes, socket design, and prosthetic components.[14,51]

Targeted muscle reinnervation (TMR) is a surgical technique used to increase the number of myosites (control signals) available for use, thereby increasing the potential for improved prosthetic function. This procedure maximizes the function of the intact residual nerves by transferring them to unused muscle in the residual limb. The goal is reinnervation of the "target" muscle so that the myosites physiologically correlate with the prosthetic movements.[55,109] TMR has also elicited a targeted sensory reinnervation response in which sensory nerves from

the residual limb can be directed to the chest, resulting in perceived touch of the phantom limb. Targeted sensory reinnervation can provide sensory feedback while a prosthesis is used for enhanced control.[56] TMR has also been shown to have a promising effect in pain and neuroma management.[54]

Pattern recognition, a new development in myoelectric control, offers individuals with upper limb loss a natural, intuitive method of control with a myoelectric prosthesis.[87] In contrast to the direct control scheme in which isolated muscle contractions control discrete movement at each prosthetic component, pattern recognition uses multiple electrodes to map a user's intended movement patterns to control several degrees of freedom of the prosthetic device.[57] The goal of pattern recognition is to increase the overall picture of muscle activity in the residual limb by allowing the prosthetic user to perform a large number of movements with the prosthesis by simply reproducing the intuitive movements of the amputated limb.[40,55,87,97,99]

> ### OT PRACTICE NOTES
>
> An occupational therapy protocol for clients who have undergone targeted muscle reinnervation (TMR) has been developed and should be used throughout their rehabilitation.

Surface electrodes provide a challenge for maintaining consistent contact over the targeted muscle belly (myosite). Internal electrodes as a control scheme is being researched to combat the challenges that surface electrodes can present. The Alfred Mann Foundation, for example, has worked on the use of implantable myoelectric sensors which are surgically implanted into various muscles in the residual limb. The goal is to improve the accuracy of signal reception, provide intuitive control, and enhance simultaneous control of multiple degrees of freedom of the prosthetic hand.[69]

Osseointegration is a surgical procedure in which an implanted device is fixed to the bone of the residual limb. A component of the implant protrudes from the skin and anchors the prosthesis directly to the residual limb, eliminating the need for suspension.[39] The procedure was developed as an alternative for individuals who cannot tolerate a conventional socket-based prosthesis because of skin breakdown, residual limb length, shape and volume fluctuation of the residual limb, or poor maintenance of suspension as a result of perspiration. Osseointegration is best viewed as a combined surgical and rehabilitation technique which requires integrated coordination and care among the orthopedic surgeons, occupational therapists, physical therapists, and prosthetists to achieve long-term success for the client.[10,34,94]

Loss of any part of the upper extremity significantly affects participation in every activity of daily living. Despite promising technological advances in upper limb prosthetics, prostheses cannot replicate the complex prehensile and sensory function of the native hand.[110,113] Vascularized composite allotransplantation (VCA) provides a valuable restorative option for upper extremity amputations. VCA is defined as "transplantation of multiple tissues such as muscle, bone, nerve and skin, as a functional unit (e.g., a hand or face) from a deceased donor to a recipient with a severe injury."[2] Hand transplantations are performed with the aim of achieving improved functionality, cosmesis, and psychological recovery, compared to prostheses.[25,112] Although this is a feasible therapeutic option, the risks of this surgical procedure also must be considered. Hand transplantation carries a risk of rejection, necessitates the lifetime use of immunosuppressive therapies, and requires dedicated time in intensive rehabilitative therapies.[23,25]

SECTION 2 SUMMARY

At the beginning of the chapter, three critical thinking questions are posed for you to consider and refer to as you read through. Examples from Daniel's case study are used to answer each of the critical thinking questions and are integrated throughout the chapter for reference. Daniel is a single case example that serves as a guide when working with all clients with upper limb amputation.

Loss of a limb had a significant impact on an individual's ability to participate in meaningful occupation. For Daniel, it affected his ability to effectively and safely work as a combat engineer, a career he identified as part of his occupational profile. In addition, Daniel was initially unable to prepare his own food or participate in his favorite sport of motocross. While Daniel adapted well to his amputation, the lack of participation in activities that he loved was difficult for him to process. The occupational therapist listened to Daniel, thus building a collaborative relationship in order to design Daniel's rehabilitation to include facilitating his return to his favorite sport of motocross. Prosthetic training was focused on functional use of a prosthesis for daily activities as well as adaptive sports. Not only is this an example of the therapeutic role of the occupational therapist in Daniel's psychological adjustment, it also demonstrates how Daniel's occupational profile guided the therapeutic process and interventions for prosthetic rehabilitation.

The rehabilitation process for individuals with upper limb loss can be challenging and rewarding. In the case of upper extremity prosthetic training, expertise on the part of the therapist and interdisciplinary rehabilitation team is essential. Occupational therapists play a vital role in the rehabilitation process by addressing residual limb management and care, in addition to preprosthetic and prosthetic training. Desired outcomes of occupational therapy include a positive self-image after limb loss, independent management of ADLs; and resumption of work, social, and leisure roles that support the client's health and occupational performance.

THREADED CASE STUDY

Daniel, Part 2

After the initial evaluation, regular occupational therapy treatment sessions were initiated on an outpatient basis. Daniel was educated on the use of adaptive equipment, such as a rocker knife and buttonhook, and one-handed techniques to perform basic ADLs. He was a quick learner and adapted well to his loss, physically and psychologically. His family members were present throughout each treatment session and were active participants in his rehabilitation. His fiancée encouraged him to maximize his functional independence. The social support network that he had was critical in his rehabilitation success.

The occupational therapist educated Daniel and his family on the various prosthetic options available, and the advantages and disadvantages of each prosthetic system. Preprosthetic training was initiated while Daniel was still in the perioperative phase and sutures were intact. His residual limb was tested for possible myosites to use to control a myoelectric prosthesis. The occupational therapist, along with the prosthetist, was able to identify strong myosites for the flexors and extensors in the forearm. Preprosthetic controls training began with the use of a myotester and simulator. Daniel was educated in strengthening the muscles in his residual limb and performing isolated contractions for increased control. Daniel had good muscle tone and strength in his residual limb but had difficulty isolating the muscle contractions that control the terminal device. With practice and repetitive training and cueing, Daniel was able to accurately control the signals for hand open and close and wrist rotation on the myosimulator.

Once the sutures were removed, Daniel was casted and fitted with his initial myoelectric prosthesis. Because Daniel's arm was amputated through the forearm (transradial), he was fitted with a two-site myoelectric control system with a wrist rotator, a wrist flexion unit, and an electric hand terminal device. Daniel used the pull sock method to don his prosthesis to ensure a tight prosthetic fit and good skin contact with the surface electrodes. The names and operations of all of the component parts of the prosthesis were reviewed. Daniel's mechanical history of working on cars helped him to quickly learn and understand the operations of the prosthesis.

The next phase of therapy for Daniel was controls training with the prosthesis. This included practice in open and close of the terminal device in various arm positions, wrist rotation in both supination and pronation, and pre-positioning of the terminal device in various degrees of wrist flexion and extension. Training in grasp and release of objects of various sizes, shapes, and densities was completed with good performance. Daniel had difficulty performing proportional control during training but was able to improve with continued practice.

Once Daniel had mastered the basics of controls training, ADL training was initiated. This included tasks such as cutting food, buttoning a shirt, using a computer, and manipulating a wallet and credit cards. Daniel was encouraged to use his prosthesis as a stabilizer and functional assist during bimanual tasks. IADLs training specific to Daniel's vocational and recreational interests included weapon manipulation, working on cars, woodworking, and driving.

One of Daniel's goals for occupational therapy was to continue to participate in the various sports that he loved, such as mountain biking and motocross. To maximize his functional independence in adaptive sports, Daniel was prescribed an activity-specific prosthesis. The activity-specific prosthesis had a quick disconnect wrist unit to allow easy interchange of terminal devices. Daniel brought his mountain bike into the clinic during therapy, and the occupational therapist and prosthetist educated him on the various sport-specific terminal devices available for this activity. Daniel's understanding and use of the terminal device was assessed in the clinic to ensure his safety with this high-level activity.

Throughout his time in occupational therapy, Daniel was able to reach his goals of functional independence with ADLs and IADLs performance with a prosthesis. During his rehabilitation, Daniel reevaluated his goals for his career. He reported that he would always identify as a soldier, but realized that he had the opportunity to pursue other occupational roles and opportunities through participation in adaptive sports. Daniel was connected with a nonprofit organization during his rehabilitation that specialized in motocross sports for disabled veterans. Through this peer mentorship and participation in various adaptive sports activities during his rehabilitation, Daniel was able to pursue his dream and began competitively racing in motocross events around the country. He medically retired from the army, married his high school sweetheart, and moved back to California to begin life after the military.

Careful assessment of the client's needs, a creative approach to therapeutic intervention, an emphasis on problem solving, and close communication with the rehabilitation team can make the challenge rewarding and the outcome successful.

SECTION 3: LOWER LIMB AMPUTATIONS[c]

Kelly McGaughey Roseberry

THREADED CASE STUDY

Lena, Part 1

Lena is a 72-year-old woman (prefers pronouns she/her/hers) who lives by herself in a one-story house near downtown. She was widowed 5 years ago and has two adult children who also live in town. Lena has adult-onset diabetes and chronic obstructive pulmonary disease (COPD). She worked part-time as a clerk at a department store until her 50s, when she retired because she could no longer stand comfortably for long periods. After retirement, Lena would drive for shopping and appointments and would walk the short distance to church. The circulation in Lena's legs got progressively worse over the years, and she began to spend increasing amounts of time at home. Lena's day usually involved watching television, bird watching through the window, and occasionally painting ceramic figurines.

At age 62 Lena stubbed the toe on her left foot, cutting the toe. The circulation in her foot was not sufficient for it to heal, and the toe was amputated. She had another toe amputated 2 years later, and 2 weeks ago she had a below-knee amputation (transtibial) of her left leg because of wounds that would not heal.

Lena has just been transferred to a skilled nursing facility in her hometown. The occupational therapist met with Lena for her initial evaluation today, after which the two set goals for Lena's course of treatment.

Critical Thinking Questions

1. What is an occupation that will make Lena feel like herself again?
2. What treatment activities can be used to best address challenges presented by Lena's amputation and help her return to participation in her chosen occupations?
3. How can the occupational therapist help Lena prepare not only to return home but also to reduce her risk of rehospitalization?

LEVELS OF LOWER LIMB AMPUTATION

Lower limb (LL) amputations are typically discussed as above-knee or below-knee; however, variability exists even within these categories (Fig. 44.25).[9] Generally, the more proximal an amputation, the more energy expenditure required to use a prosthesis. Proximal LL amputations include hip disarticulation and hemipelvectomy amputations, resulting in loss of the entire lower limb and part of the pelvis; such severe amputations are typically a result of trauma or malignancy. Wound healing from such proximal amputations is often slow, and skin grafting may be required for full healing. In cases of hemipelvectomy, a muscle flap covers and helps to stabilize the internal organs. Prosthetic limbs or prostheses can still be used but require creativity by the prosthetist for comfort and functional capacity for the client.

[c] The authors wish to acknowledge Jennifer Glover and Chelsey E. Cook for their excellent contributions to earlier editions of Section 3 addressing lower limb amputations and rehabilitation.

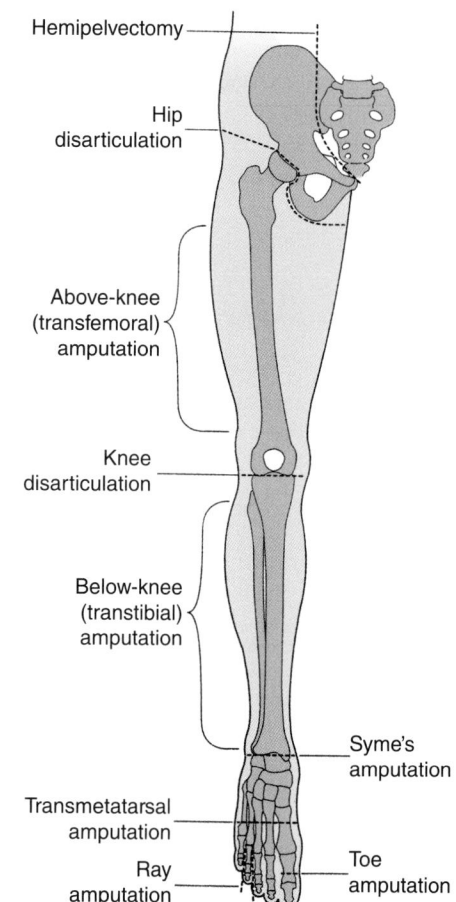

Fig. 44.25 Levels of lower extremity amputation. (From Cameron MH, Monroe LG: *Physical rehabilitation: evidence-based examination, evaluation, and intervention,* St Louis, 2007, Saunders.)

A transfemoral amputation, or above-knee amputation (AKA), results in loss of the knee joint and everything distal to it.[8,9] Residual limb length from an AKA typically varies greatly and can be classified as upper, middle, or lower third, indicating the amputation distance from the ischium. The longer the residual limb, the more surface area available for socket fit and the faster self-selected walking speeds of clients.[8,9] A through-the-knee amputation, or knee disarticulation, results in loss of knee joint function but maintains full length of the femur, allowing a high level of prosthetic control and mobility. Maintaining length of the femur and condyles allows for weight bearing on the distal end of the residual limb itself as well.

A transtibial amputation, or below-knee amputation (BKA), preserves the knee and thigh musculature attachments, thus eliminating the necessity for a mechanical knee joint in the prosthesis. The ideal residual limb length of a BKA is typically 12.5 to 17.5 cm from the tibial tuberosity.[114] A Syme's amputation, or ankle disarticulation, results in loss of both ankle and foot function, but maintains length of the tibia and fibula and their condyles, and is typically performed in cases of trauma or infection. Prosthetic options can be limited based on long length of the limb and build height of prostheses for this type of amputation. A transmetatarsal amputation results in severing of the foot through the metatarsal bones, but the ankle remains intact. Clients may also experience amputation of individual toes. Ambulation is most effected by amputation of the first toe, as it prevents proper toe-off in terminal stance.[75] The loss of the small toes does not usually result in impaired ambulation and often can be compensated for with proper footwear. In Lena's case, the amputation is considered a BKA because her left leg was amputated approximately 5 inches below the tibial tuberosity, resulting in the loss of her foot and ankle joint completely.

CAUSES OF LOWER LIMB AMPUTATION

In the United States, 95% of LL amputations are performed as a result of complications of peripheral vascular disease (PVD)[50]; ultimately, 25% to 50% of these cases are caused by diabetes mellitus.[90] Trauma is the second most common cause of amputation in the United States, but it is the leading cause in developing countries because of land mines and other environmental hazards.[90] Amputation also may be performed in cases of malignancy in an effort to prevent it from spreading to other sites or systems in the body.

In Lena's case, both diabetes mellitus and PVD resulted in poor circulation in her lower limbs. Because of this complication, blood flow to her left foot and leg was not adequate for her limb to heal, even from what initially appeared to be a small wound. Therefore, she was forced to undergo progressive amputations of her left lower limb, eventually leading to the recent BKA.

POSTSURGICAL RESIDUAL LIMB CARE

Skin care and positioning are extremely important throughout the course of rehabilitation, especially immediately after surgery, regardless of the procedure that was done. Once the surgical wound has begun to heal, some form of specialized postsurgical dressing will be used to help prevent swelling and to shape the residual limb for ease of future prosthesis use. Figure-8 wrapping with an elastic bandage (e.g., an elastic wrap) is a common method to control edema after surgery. The advantage to wrapping with an elastic bandage is that it can be applied around drains and tubes the residual limb may still have in the immediate postoperative period. However, smooth wrapping does require a skilled and consistent technique, which is necessary to prevent poor shaping of the residual limb. A series of gradually smaller residual limb shrinkers can be worn as an alternative to elastic bandage wrapping to encourage constant, uniform shrinkage of the residual limb to facilitate fitting with a final prosthesis. Both elastic bandages and shrinkers can be used early after surgery, even if the client's surgical wound still has a dressing on it. The client should be encouraged to continue to wear the shrinker even once the final prosthesis has been built. Shrinkers should be worn anytime the prosthesis is not worn, for up to 1 year after amputation, to continue to help with shaping and shrinking the residual limb.

If the client (or one's caregiver) is unable to demonstrate proper technique with wrapping or shrinker use, a Jobst compression pump may be used. The pump is an air-filled sleeve that surrounds the residual limb, placing constant, equal pressure on all sides, quickly shrinking and shaping the residual limb. A rigid dressing or cast, commonly called an IPOP, can be used for active clients after surgery. The end of the cast is made to work with a simple training prosthesis, so the client can begin training for standing with minimum weight (typically about 20 lb) and walking immediately. However, this requires immediate postoperative prosthetist intervention and may not be covered by insurance. Scar massage is often necessary later in the healing process to prevent adhesions and enhance comfort and mobility around the surgical site; this massage technique can be taught to the client or caregiver.

The elastic wrap bandaging of Lena's residual limb was performed by nurses in the hospital. After Lena's arrival at the skilled nursing facility, the nursing staff consulted the occupational therapist to determine whether Lena had the cognitive and visual function and the necessary motor skills to learn how to apply her own wrap or shrinker and to perform her own scar massage.

LOWER LIMB EQUIPMENT AND PROSTHESES

Movement and time out of bed are typically reduced immediately after LL amputation. The surgery itself can make movement uncomfortable, and many persons who have undergone amputation surgery have preexisting conditions that may further reduce mobility. For these reasons, clients may require the use of bed rails or a metal trapeze bar hanging over the bed to help reposition themselves in bed and to transition between supine and sitting. Wheelchairs also present a challenge because the client is no longer able to support the affected limb by resting the now absent foot on the floor or on the footrest of the wheelchair. A residual limb support is a padded board that is attached to the frame of the wheelchair and extends from the seat on the side of the affected limb to support the residual limb in an extended position (Fig. 44.26). This extension provides a surface for the residual limb to rest on, thus placing the limb in a nondependent position and reducing stresses on the hip joint. A person with a BKA is often at risk for developing a flexion contracture of the knee joint, and a residual limb support facilitates extension of the knee in sitting, thus helping to prevent both edema in the residual limb and flexion contracture of the knee joint.[124] A residual limb support is sometimes still referred

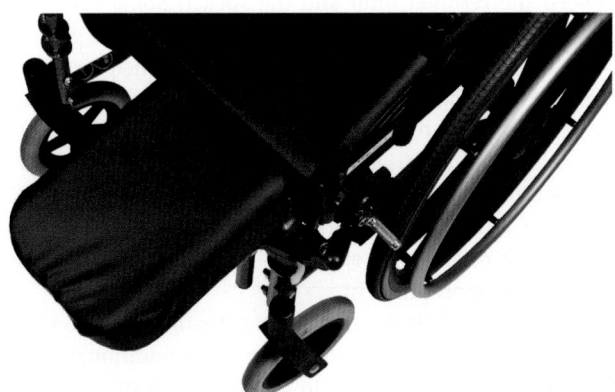

Fig. 44.26 Wheelchair with support for residual limb. (Courtesy Comfort Company, Bozeman, MT.)

to, in less acceptable terminology, as a stump support. For a person with bilateral LL amputations, the large wheels on the wheelchair must be placed farther back to accommodate the change in body weight distribution. Anti-tip bars, which are commercially available wheelchair accessories, also can be used on the back of the chair to reduce the likelihood of tipping backward during weight shifting. These are often used initially for safety, but removed later to allow the client to perform wheelies and functional tasks such as getting up or down a curb.

Most clients will use a walker or other assistive device during at least the initial phases of their rehabilitation. Some clients with LL amputations will go on to use a walker at all times for ambulation. Both four-footed (standard) and two-wheeled (rolling) walkers may be used, depending on the client's individual characteristics and needs. It has been suggested that using a two-wheeled walker may allow those with prosthetic limbs to ambulate more quickly and effeciently,[115] but assistive device choice should always be made on the basis of a total assessment of the client's abilities and needs.

Many types of prostheses are available for the lower limbs, and technology is improving daily. For all prostheses, comfort, ease of application, appearance, and functioning of the prosthesis, including the client's ability to perform ADLs and IADLs with use of the affected limb, all go into deciding the proper prosthetic components. These factors correlate significantly with the client's walking distance and with the client's perceived quality of life after an LL amputation.[66] It is very important for the rehabilitation team to keep this in mind during a client's fitting for and training with a prosthesis.

The main components of an LL prosthesis are a liner or other interface, socks, the socket, a suspension system, a pylon, and a terminal device. For most prostheses, an articulating joint is also necessary. The socket is the direct connection between the residual limb and the prosthesis.[53,122] The order of properly donning a LL prosthetic is a liner, socks if needed, and socket/suspension system. A person's residual limb may change in volume during the day and over the course of time, presenting challenges for maintaining an adequate fit within the socket. This challenge is frequently addressed by adding or removing socks to adapt to these volume changes in the limb. Socks come in different thicknesses, called ply, and can be combined to accommodate volume changes to maintain total contact between the residual limb and the socket. Some sockets are specially designed using either fluid (Smart variable geometry socket technology) or air (vacuum socket) to help accommodate volume changes in the residual limb as well.[38] Static elastomeric liners are also used for the prosthesis socket; the choice of liner is based on variables such as fit, comfort, friction tolerance, and price.[95] Various suspension mechanisms are used to attach the socket to the residual limb, including belts, straps, pins, sleeves, or suction; sometimes mechanisms are combined to ensure the appropriate fit.

The **pylon** is the structure that attaches the socket to the TD (Fig. 44.27). Some LL prostheses can have additional vertical shock absorber components to assist with absorbing ground forces. Many clients who have had an LL amputation express a preference for walking with these devices.[36] Such shock

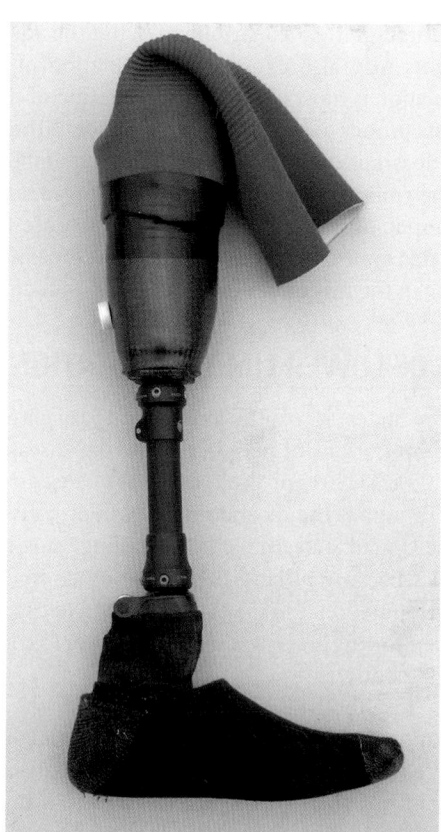

Fig. 44.27 Typical pylon, the internal frame or skeleton of the prosthetic limb.

absorption is especially beneficial during high-impact activities, such as running, and for other activities that are part of daily life for many clients, such as descending curbs and stairs. A pylon can be a basic, static device that provides minimal cosmetic benefits; it also can be a dynamic device, such as that outlined in the preceding paragraph. The pylon also can have a cosmetic cover added over it to mimic the shape of the unaffected limb.

The TD is the prosthetic foot/ankle, which provides a stable, weight-bearing surface and can itself function as a shock absorber. There are many types of available TDs that provide varying degrees of mechanical ankle movement and dynamic response, according to the needs and abilities of the client. Specialized TDs, such as a running or swimming foot, are designed to accommodate the challenges presented by various sports and activities (Fig. 44.28). To help select the best prosthesis, Lena's prosthetist consulted with her occupational therapist to explore the activities and lifestyle to which Lena wished to return.

PARTICIPATION IN OCCUPATIONS

OT PRACTICE NOTE

A thorough occupational profile obtained during the initial evaluation, along with evaluation and analysis of occupational performance, will help the occupational therapist identify areas of strength and of challenge for the client who has undergone a limb amputation.

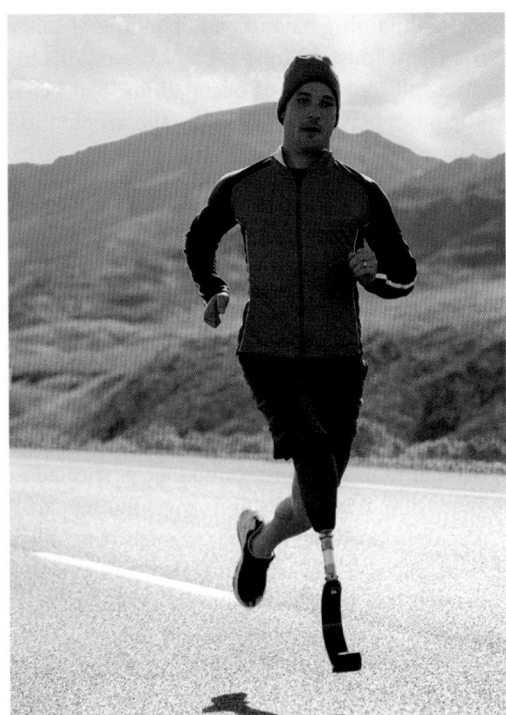

Fig. 44.28 Athlete with a specialized running prosthesis competing in a marathon. (From GettyImages.com.)

For some clients, particularly those who have undergone a traumatic amputation, the activities to which they wish to return are ones they engaged in right up to the point of injury or illness. However, given the nature of PVD and diabetes, many clients with LL amputations experience a progressive decline in function over the course of several years leading up to amputation. For these clients, amputation and subsequent rehabilitation, although difficult, may allow a return to fulfilling occupations that had been absent from the clients' repertoire for quite some time.

Participation in most ADLs will be affected by LL amputation, at least initially. Although a client with an LL amputation will be learning new mobility techniques in physical therapy, he or she must also participate in occupational therapy to learn new functional mobility techniques with which to accomplish familiar tasks. Comprehensive client-centered care requires a close working relationship between physical and occupational therapists to provide the best care for the client. The level of adaptation and modification largely depends on level of amputation and existing comorbidities. Bathing, dressing, personal hygiene, grooming, and toilet hygiene will likely need to be addressed as part of an occupational therapy intervention program. Personal device care must be addressed if the client is using an LL prosthesis. Participation in IADLs also will be affected. Particular attention should be paid to care of others, care of pets, childrearing, community mobility, health management and maintenance, home establishment and management, meal preparation and cleanup, safety and emergency maintenance, and shopping. As an occupational therapist you always have to consider quality of life of the client and make sure goals match the desired functional outcome of the client. The areas of rest and sleep may also

present challenges to a person with a new LL amputation. For example, a client's evening routine may be disrupted by having to perform it from a wheelchair instead of at an ambulatory level (sleep preparation). A client may experience difficulties interacting with a partner in the sleeping space as they both adjust to a new amputation (sleep participation). This may be affected by both pain and general mobility limitations. The occupational therapist should assess how these occupations may be affected by the amputation and should help the client develop adaptations that facilitate improved rest and sleep. Treatments addressing phantom sensations may also benefit the client's rest and sleep (see Chapter 13 for further information).

Participation in educational, work, play, and leisure activities are usually affected by LL amputation and should be addressed during occupational therapy, as should social participation. Although intervention often assumes a greater role with these occupations later in the rehabilitation process, they still can be addressed even during the acute rehabilitation phase, thus reinforcing to the client that these are occupations in which a return to active participation is indeed possible and encouraged. Time should be spent to educate patients about defining their "new normal" after amputation. It is essential that the occupational therapist help clients to explore all avenues of an occupation in which they may wish to participate, ensuring that even activities that had been abandoned in the past are possible again.[60] As a result of changes in function after amputation, clients may not be able to return to participation in prior work or leisure activities or to participation at the level to which they were accustomed. In such cases the occupational therapist should help clients explore modifications or other opportunities that they might find fulfilling through identification of interests, skills, and opportunities.

Early in her course of occupational therapy at the skilled nursing facility, Lena spoke with her therapist about how much she missed walking to her church and helping to bake pies for its annual autumn festival. Lena said that she stopped doing this about 10 years ago because it became so difficult; she then discussed feelings of isolation and uselessness. Lena said that she had been known throughout her town for her pies, and she proudly recounted how each year people would tell her that she should open her own restaurant. Although Lena and her occupational therapist had initially set her long-term goals for independence with self-care and basic home management, they decided to add a goal for community reentry that focused on being able to reengage in this occupation.

CLIENT FACTORS

Structures affecting movement, in addition to skin and related structures, are always altered by LL amputation. However, the status of other body structures also must be assessed to determine the level of support or challenge these structures might present during the rehabilitation process.

Neuromuscular and movement-related functions will be altered by LL amputation, and this will affect occupational performance after amputation. This alteration of function may occur not only in the affected limb, but also in other parts of the body. Because of changes in the affected limb, greater stresses will be placed on the rest of the body; a person's unaffected leg and arms will experience increased weight bearing during many functional activities, and both surgical wound healing and increased time in bed will place greater demands on skin functions. All of these additional stresses can be combated with physical and occupational therapies to adapt activity and strengthen other structures.

Of particular importance is attention to sensations of pain. Up to 84% of persons who have had an LL amputation have experienced phantom limb pain.[18] In such an instance the client may experience painful sensations in the part of the limb that has been removed, such as feelings of cramping, squeezing, shooting, or burning pain. In these cases, the therapist can use desensitization techniques (e.g., deep pressure or massage of the residual limb), exercise, hot and cold therapy, or electrical stimulation[90] to help decrease these sensations and allow the client to more easily and comfortably participate in chosen occupations.

Clients with PVD already have compromised cardiovascular function, and care must be taken to determine how much activity can safely be tolerated during therapy. It is important to check a client's skin integrity at the start and end of each session to determine skin tolerance to activity. A client's mental and sensory functions will affect the way therapy, including education, is delivered and what types of prosthesis and equipment are used.[59] Some clients may be able to incorporate new techniques quickly, recalling information from one session or even from reading material, and may be able to independently apply this learning to new situations. However, other clients will require adaptation of training and may require prolonged treatment to turn the new techniques they have learned into habits. Understanding a client's values, beliefs, and spirituality will further help the therapist to develop an individualized treatment program and to choose interventions that are tailored to that client and best meet one's needs.

The occupational therapist found that Lena would need to increase her upper body strength to help support herself during transfers and ambulation with the walker. She also needed to improve her postsurgical postural alignment and gait patterns to participate in her chosen occupations. Lena was experiencing pain and sensitivity in her residual limb. However, Lena's mental functions were found to be strengths, and her vision and the sensation in her hands, although slightly diminished, were functioning at a level sufficient to support her desired functional activities. Additionally, Lena's belief that good efforts yield results, in addition to her commitment to her spiritual and social communities, would facilitate her engagement in her occupational therapy program. Her treatment plan was devised around these specific needs to meet her occupation goals. She would not have benefited from interventions focused on running, or jumping.

PERFORMANCE SKILLS

The most overt effects of LL amputation will be evident in the area of motor skills. Adjusting posture, coordinating movements, maintaining balance, and bending are altered after surgery. The client must address each of these skills in therapy to return to a full repertoire of occupations. Sensory and perceptual skills also may be affected by the amputation, and a client may have had prior difficulty with these skills caused by impaired sensory function. Clients' processing skills (e.g., judging, sequencing, and multitasking) and communication and social interaction skills will affect their participation in treatment and the therapist's choice of treatment methods. Overall function is affected by many factors, including length of residual limb, cause of amputation, additional comorbidities, living environment, prior level of function, support, insurance access to rehab and prosthetics, etc. All of these factors are considered when formulating treatment methods.

Lena's occupational therapist found that, as she had expected, Lena exhibited impairment in stabilizing, aligning, positioning, walking, reaching, bending, moving, transporting, lifting while standing, and pacing. The therapist also found that processing skills were at functional levels for Lena. However, Lena did exhibit difficulty with adaptation as she began attempting to perform activities with a changed body structure and in different positions. The therapist also noticed that Lena was having difficulty with social interaction skills, exhibiting trouble focusing and collaborating during many occupations. The therapist would need to address these areas in therapy to help Lena return to her optimal level of participation in occupations.

PERFORMANCE PATTERNS

Whatever clients' performance patterns were before their amputation, they are likely to be altered after amputation. The client may already have useful habits, routines, rituals, and roles that can be drawn upon in therapy to facilitate return to prior levels of occupational performance. However, for many clients, the occupational history will reveal prior impoverished habits and lack of or maladaptive routines that may present challenges to the rehabilitative process. Although Lena's diabetes and PVD placed her at increased risk for poor wound healing, she had also never developed the habit of routinely checking her feet and legs for cuts or infections, which further increases her risk of poor outcomes. For Lena, this impoverished habit led to three amputations on her left leg. Lena's morning routine in her kitchen involved crossing the room many times and carrying multiple items in her hands at once. In conversations with her occupational therapist, Lena did indicate that she had already begun to drop things during this routine, that she had nearly fallen a few times, and that she worried about being able to safely make her own breakfast at home. All of these concerns are consistent with her deficits and can be addressed with a comprehensive plan of care.

PSYCHOSOCIAL REPERCUSSIONS

Amputation of a limb represents a loss, and processing this loss is often related to going through a grief process. This process involves dealing with one's feelings regarding change in body structure, functional abilities, and participation in occupations.

It can also involve anger, acknowledgment of unpleasant realities regarding one's health status, and fears about one's functional and financial future. Social acceptance and community function are also significant concerns for a person who has undergone an amputation. Areas of body image and sexual health are also affected and should be acknowledged. These are all areas that can be addressed by an interdisciplinary rehabilitation team in an effort to help the client adapt and should address all aspects of occupational therapy intervention.

The occupational therapist may use several techniques to help a person adapt to the amputation and create a new sense of self. The therapeutic relationship and the therapeutic use of self can provide a safe environment and catalyst for the client to discuss feelings of loss, thoughts regarding body changes, and fears for the future. The therapist can teach the client coping skills for dealing with anxiety and depression, in addition to techniques for improving one's postsurgical body image.[85] The consultation process can include recommendations for workplace adaptations and suggestions for how to make the home more accessible to a client with a new amputation. The therapeutic use of occupations that have been graded to the client's current abilities provides opportunities to master skills and experience success. The therapist's encouragement during such sessions not only fosters development and provides support, but also provides evidence to the client that recovery of function and return to participation in chosen occupations are indeed possible[85]; this knowledge fosters hope and a vision of the future. Success can also help the client to believe in the rehabilitation process and plan and be more motivated and willing to continue to work hard in the future.

It is important to recognize that an outside observer's rating of a person's adaptation to an LL amputation may not be the same as that person's self-rating. A surgeon may rate success on the basis of healing of the surgical wound, a prosthetist on the fit between residual limb and prosthesis, a physical therapist on the client's ability to ambulate, and an occupational therapist on the client's ability to participate in occupations. However, clients may place greater emphasis on other criteria in their determination of successful adaptation to an LL amputation. Some related variables that appear to be of primary concern to clients include feeling comfortable while being active in the presence of strangers, not feeling like a burden to one's family, being able to care for others, and being able to exercise recreationally.[66]

CONTEXT, ENVIRONMENT, AND ACTIVITY DEMANDS

An understanding of the client's contexts, environments, and demands of daily activities will help the therapist design a treatment program that will best help the client reengage in chosen occupations within the everyday environment. It will also help the therapist adapt the activity demands of the client's chosen occupations to facilitate greater independence and development of proficiency. Lena's occupational therapist took a detailed floor plan of Lena's bedroom and was able to move the furniture in her room in the skilled nursing facility so it closely approximated her bedroom setup at home. When Lena performed her

morning and evening ADLs in the room, she was then doing so in a more natural environment, making it easier to transition those skills to her home. Lena's therapist initially made significant adaptations to Lena's morning routine demands, wheeling Lena up to the sink in the bathroom for sponge bathing and bringing her clothes to her in the bathroom, where she would stand with the help of a grab bar so the therapist could pull Lena's pants up. Over the course of time, as Lena improved her performance skills and her performance patterns and incorporated her new ADLs techniques taught during therapy into her routine, her occupational therapist was able to decrease the adaptation of activity demands. Lena was able to progress to independence with routines that she would be able to sustain at home.

ADDITIONAL CONSIDERATIONS WITH ELDERLY CLIENTS

Although LL amputation may be performed to preserve function or to save the client's life, it does carry an increased mortality risk as the age of the client increases. One study of older persons who underwent a BKA found the survival probability after BKA to be 77% at 1 year, 57% at 3 years, and 28% at 7{1/2} years.[62] Because this increased mortality risk is related not only to the amputation surgery but also to preexisting health and environmental factors, attention to the overall health status of the client is of utmost importance. Education, skin checks of remaining limbs, and controlling blood sugar levels become very important in decreasing mortality risk.

Many body structures and functions are already compromised in elderly clients, making the rehabilitation process longer and more delicate. An elderly person may take more time to recover from the effects of anesthesia after surgery, including effects on cognition and the respiratory system. For unilateral amputees, leg balance on the unaffected limb is a significant predictor for prosthetic use.[98] Because balance may already be decreased and cognitive skills may have declined, elderly clients learning to use a prosthetic limb may experience greater challenges. There are changes in skin integrity and elasticity that also influence prosthetic fit, function, and comfort. Elderly clients have already experienced many losses, which may include family and friends, home, health, and function; the psychological sequelae of amputation can be all the more traumatic when layered over these previous losses.

SECTION 3 SUMMARY

Three critical thinking questions were posed at the beginning of the chapter to think about as you read. Lena's case study is threaded throughout the chapter to help you apply what you are learning. The most important part of understanding information is being able to think critically about how it would apply to a real-life client. Lena's case is very indicative of a client you may see in the clinic, with multiple lower limb amputations and complications that have resulted in further amputations and altered function.

Lena, Part 2

Amputation of a lower limb has a significant functional impact on a person, but returning to an active and fulfilling life is still possible. Lena required extensive assistance to take care of herself when she entered the skilled nursing facility, but her goal was to return home and independently take care of herself and her home. During the course of occupational therapy, Lena realized that she had been slowly decreasing her participation in the very activities that helped her feel active and vital and helped her define who she was. She then decided to work with her therapist toward being able to reclaim these activities, particularly going back to her church and helping to bake pies for its upcoming autumn festival.

During the course of her occupational therapy, Lena's therapist presented her with activities that addressed the areas that Lena needed to improve to reach her goals. These goals, which Lena had identified as of interest to her, were adapted to provide an appropriate level of challenge. Because Lena liked to watch birds and had enjoyed decorative painting in the past, her occupational therapy sessions included building and painting birdhouses. This increased Lena's upper body strength and provided progressive challenges to her sitting and eventually standing balance, facilitating her return to independence with ambulatory tasks and providing an activity that Lena could perform at home and a product that she could donate to her church's fall festival.

As Lena's stay at the skilled nursing facility neared its end, she participated in community reentry sessions with her occupational therapist. Because Lena had mentioned her desire to help bake pies with the congregation for the fall festival, she and her occupational therapist visited the church together during a community reentry session. This visit gave Lena a chance to interact with some of the members of the baking committee so that they could see Lena's capable self, allaying their fears about interacting with a person with a disability and setting the expectation that Lena would be involved. Through supported engagement in this social community occupation, Lena gained confidence that she was still an accepted and desired member of her community. Together, Lena and her occupational therapist identified potential challenges presented by the layout of the kitchen and access to the building. Lena engaged in trials and problem-solving strategies with her therapist to determine methods to allow safe participation in baking. In preparation for her return to the church as a member of the baking team, Lena then perfected these techniques in the occupational therapy kitchen back at the facility.

Lena's occupational therapist also worked with Lena to discuss the ways in which some of her prehospitalization habits and routines had contributed to high-risk situations and to identify strategies to help reduce her risks of rehospitalization. Lena learned how to perform her own lower body skin checks, and she was performing them regularly by the end of her stay. She went home with a daily routine that would help her stay active throughout the day, but also incorporated techniques that minimized periods of prolonged standing and reduced the amount of energy required to accomplish tasks. Lena's family then reorganized items in her kitchen, according to recommendations determined by Lena in collaboration with her occupational therapist, so that her environment placed less strain on her during daily activities. Lena went home independent in her daily activities, able to engage in individual and social occupations that made her feel happy and vital, and reclaimed a role that had long been abandoned.

Lena had many occupations that have been affected over the years by her LL amputations—her job as a clerk, her ability to participate in and attend church, and paint. At the top of Lena's list of occupations she would like to return to is her role with the church and baking pies. Her occupational therapist was able to tailor her treatments to address these specific areas. She was able to focus on balance, increasing strength and endurance, and functional activities such as painting birdhouses to address multiple hobbies Lena had. Each task Lena wanted to return to had to be broken down into elements that could be practiced: balance, strength, endurance, etc. Education on proper skin checks and wound care are extremely important for clients such as Lena to help prevent rehospitalization and further amputation in the future. Lena worked on setting up a safe home environment to minimize tripping hazards and make mobility around her home easier, as well as learning how to properly care for her skin to prevent breakdown and additional wounds in the future.

REVIEW QUESTIONS

1. List the common causes of acquired amputation.
2. Describe the role of the occupational therapist, as a team member, in the rehabilitation of an individual with an upper limb amputation.
3. What are the goals of amputation surgery?
4. Name three types of surgical techniques performed for amputations.
5. Name three ADLs that should be addressed immediately after amputation.
6. What is the purpose of a shrinker?
7. Name at least four postsurgical factors that can interfere with prosthetic training and rehabilitation. How is each factor managed?
8. What is the difference between phantom limb pain and phantom limb sensation?
9. Discuss the impact of the residual limb status on successful fitting and operation of an upper limb prosthesis.
10. Describe the goal of myosite testing for an electrically powered prosthesis.
11. Describe the typical psychological consequences of amputation surgery, and discuss how the occupational therapist facilitates adjustment to limb loss.
12. Define the "golden window" and identify its importance in upper extremity amputation rehabilitation.
13. What are the five most common types of upper limb prostheses?
14. List the motions used to operate the body-powered prosthesis.
15. Name at least two techniques for donning the body-powered prosthesis and describe them.

16. What is the importance of pre-positioning the terminal device?
17. Name three types of electric terminal devices. What are the advantages of each?
18. What components are specific to body-powered prostheses? To electrically powered prostheses?
19. List the five characteristics of advanced prosthetic training in the use of upper limb prostheses.
20. Discuss the primary function of a prosthesis in the functional performance of various ADL and IADL tasks.
21. What are the special considerations discussed in this chapter for treating persons with bilateral upper extremity amputations?
22. Identify and describe three outcome measures used with upper limb amputations.
23. How will advances in prosthetic technology and surgical techniques affect the outcomes for persons with upper limb loss?
24. Name two significant concerns for the residual limb immediately after surgery.

25. What is the purpose of a shrinker?
26. What should be done with the wheelchair to accommodate the residual limb? To accommodate a person with bilateral AKA?
27. Name the main components of an LL prosthesis.
28. What is the purpose of using a sock on the residual limb?
29. How will LL amputation affect other parts of the body?
30. How might LL amputation affect an individual's participation in occupations?
31. Which performance skills are most likely to be affected after LL amputation?
32. How can preexisting performance patterns affect a client's participation in occupations after an amputation?
33. What are the potential psychosocial repercussions of LL amputation?
34. How can the demands of ADLs be adapted to foster greater independence after LL amputation?
35. What additional considerations does LL amputation present for elderly clients?

For additional practice questions for this chapter, please visit eBooks.Health.Elsevier.com.

REFERENCES

1. American Occupational Therapy Association: Occupational therapy practice framework: domain and process, ed 4, *Am J Occup Ther* 74(Suppl 2):1–87, 2020.
2. American Society of Transplantation: Vascularized composite allotransplantation (VCA) research. http://www.myast.org/public-policy/vascularized-composite-allotransplantation-vca-research.
3. Anderson MH, Bechtol CO, Sollars RE: *Clinical prosthetics for physicians and therapists*, Springfield, IL, 1959, Charles C Thomas.
4. Andrew JT: Prosthetic principles. In Bowker JH, Michael JW, editors: *Atlas of limb prosthetics: surgical, prosthetic, and rehabilitation principles*, ed 2, St Louis, 1992, Mosby.
5. Atkins DJ: Adult upper limb prosthetic training. In Atkins DJ, Meier RH, editors: *Comprehensive management of the upper-limb amputee*, New York, 1989, Springer-Verlag.
6. Atkins DJ: Postoperative and preprosthetic therapy programs. In Atkins DJ, Meier RH, editors: *Comprehensive management of the upper-limb amputee*, New York, 1989, Springer-Verlag.
7. Beachler DM, Oddie LH: Upper limb externally powered components. In Krajbich JI, Pinzur MS, Potter BK, Stevens PM, editors: *Atlas of amputations and limb deficiencies*, ed 4, Rosemont, IL, 2016, American Academy of Orthopedic Surgeons.
8. Bell JC, Wolf EJ, Schnall BL, et al: Transfemoral amputation: is there an effect of residual limb length and orientation on energy expenditure? *Clin Orthop Relat Res* 472(10):3055–3061, 2014.
9. Bennett JB, Alexander CB: Amputation levels and surgical techniques. In Atkins DJ, Meier RH, editors: *Comprehensive management of the upper-limb amputee*, New York, 1989, Springer-Verlag.
10. Berlin O., et al: Osseointegrated prosthesis for the rehabilitation of amputees: two-year results of the prospective OPRA study. In syllabus abstracts of the 2012 Orthopedic Surgical Osseointegration Society, Fourth International Advances in Orthopedic Osseointegration Conference, Orthopedic Surgical Osseointegration Society, San Francisco, 2012.
11. Billock JN: Upper limb prosthetic terminal devices: hands versus hooks, *Clin Prosthet Orthot* 10:57–65, 1986.
12. Billock JN: Prosthetic management of complete hand and arm deficiencies. In Hunter JM, Mackin EJ, Callahan AD, editors: *Rehabilitation of the hand: surgery and therapy*, ed 4, St Louis, 1995, Mosby.
13. Bowker JH: The art of prosthesis prescription. In Smith DG, Michael JW, Bowker JH, editors: *Atlas of amputations and limb deficiencies*, Rosemont, IL, 2004, American Academy of Orthopedic Surgeons.
14. Bridges M, Para M, Mashner M: Control system architecture for the modular prosthetic limb, *Johns Hopkins APL Tech Dig* 30:217–222, 2011.
15. Butkus J, Dennison C, Orr A, St. Laurent M: Occupational therapy with the military upper extremity amputee: advances and research implications, *Curr Phys Med Rehabil Rep* 2:255–262, 2014.
16. Chan BL, Witt R, Charrow AP, et al: Mirror therapy for phantom limb pain, *N Engl J Med* 357:2206–2207, 2007.
17. Chan KM, Lee SY, Leung KK, Leung PC: A medical-school study of upper limb amputees in Hong Kong: a preliminary report, *Orthot Prosthet* 37:43–48, 1984.
18. Czerniecki JM, Ehde DM: Chronic pain after lower extremity amputation, *Crit Rev Phys Med Rehabil* 15:309, 2003.
19. Dalsey R, Gomez W, Seitz WH Jr, et al: Myoelectric prosthetic replacement in the upper extremity amputee, *Orthop Rev* 18:697, 1989.
20. Defense Advanced Research Project Agency. Revolutionizing upper extremity prosthetics, nd, https://www.jhuapl.edu/work/projects/revolutionizing-prosthetics#:~:text=Revolutionizing%20Prosthetics%20is%20an%20ambitious,to%20upper%20Extremity%20amputee%20patients.
21. Desmond DM, Maclachlan M: Affective distress and amputation-related pain among older men with long-term,

traumatic limb amputations, *J Pain Symptom Manage* 31: 362–368, 2006.

22. DiMartine C: Capturing the phantom, *inMotion* 10:7, 2000.

23. Dubernard JM, Petruzzo P, Lanzetta M, et al: Functional results of the first human double-hand transplantation, *Ann Surg* 238:128–136, 2003.

24. Edelstein JE: Rehabilitation without prosthesis. In Smith DG, Bowker JH, editors: *Atlas of amputations and limb deficiencies: surgical and prosthetic rehabilitation principles*, ed 3, Rosemont, IL, 2004, American Academy of Orthopedic Surgeons.

25. Errico M, Metcalfe NH, Platt A: History and ethics of hand transplants, *JRSM Short Rep* 3:74, 2012.

26. Esquenazi A, Wikoff E, Lucas M: Amputation rehabilitation. In Grabois M, Garrison SJ, editors: *Physical medicine and rehabilitation: the complete approach*, Ames, IA, 2000, Blackwell Science.

27. Fillauer: MC Powered Flexion Wrist: https://fillauer.com/products/mc-powered-flexion-wrist/.

28. Fischer H, Congressional Research Service, Federation of American Scientists: A guide to U.S. military casualty statistics: Operation Freedom's Sentinel, Operation Inherent Resolve, Operation New Dawn, Operation Iraqi Freedom, and Operation Enduring Freedom. https://www.fas.org/sgp/crs/natsec/RS22452.pdf.

29. Fletchall S: Returning upper-extremity amputees to work, *O&P Edge* 4:28–33, 2005.

30. Flor H, Nikolajsen L, Jensen TS: Phantom limb pain: a case of maladaptive CNS plasticity? *Nat Rev Neurosci* 7:873–881, 2006.

31. Franz EA, Ramachandran VS: Bimanual coupling in amputees with phantom limbs, *Nat Neurosci* 1:443–444, 1998.

32. Friedman LW: *The psychological rehabilitation of the amputee*, Springfield, IL, 1978, Charles C Thomas.

33. Fryer CM, Stark GE, Michael JW: Body-powered components. In Smith DG, Bowker JH, editors: *Atlas of amputations and limb deficiencies: surgical and prosthetic rehabilitation principles*, ed 3, Rosemont, IL, 2004, American Academy of Orthopedic Surgeons.

34. Forsberg JA, Branemark R: Osseointegration: surgical management. In Krajbich JI, Pinzur MS, Potter BK, Stevens PM, editors: *Atlas of amputations and limb deficiencies*, ed 4, Rosemont, IL, 2016, American Academy of Orthopedic Surgeons.

35. Gallagher P, MacLachlan M: Development and psychometric evaluation of the Trinity Amputation and Prosthesis Experience Scales (TAPES), *Rehabil Psychol* 45:130–154, 2000.

36. Gard SA, Childress DS: A study to determine the biomechanical effects of shock-absorbing pylons, *Rehabil R&D Progr Rep* 35:18, 1998.

37. Goodney PP, Beck AW, Nagle J, et al: National trends in lower extremity bypass surgery, endovascular interventions, and major amputations, *J Vasc Surg* 50:54–60, 2009.

38. Greenwald RM, Dean RC, Board WJ: Volume management: smart variable geometry socket (SVGS) technology for lower-limb prostheses, *J Prosthet Orthot* 15:107, 2003.

39. Hagberg K, Branemark R: One hundred clients treated with osseointegrated transfemoral amputation prostheses—rehabilitation perspective, *J Rehabil Res Dev* 46:331–344, 2009.

40. Hargrove LJ, Li G, Englehart KB, Hudgins BS: Principal components analysis preprocessing for improved classification accuracies in pattern recognition-based myoelectric control, *IEEE Trans Biomed Eng* 56:1407–1414, 2009.

41. Heckathorne CW: Components for electric-powered systems. In Smith DG, Michael JW, Bowker JH, editors: *Atlas of amputations and limb deficiencies: surgical, prosthetic and rehabilitation principles*, ed 3, Rosemont IL, 2004, American Academy of Orthopedic Surgeons.

42. Heinemann AW, Bode RK, O'Reilly C: Development and measurement properties of the orthotics and prosthetic user survey (OPUS): a comprehensive set of clinical outcome instruments, *Prosthet Orthot Int* 27:191–206, 2003.

43. Hermansson LM, Bodin L, Eliasson AC: Intra- and inter-rater reliability of the assessment of capacity for myoelectric control, *J Rehabil Med* 38:118–123, 2005.

44. Hermansson LM, Fisher AG, Bernspång B, Eliasson A-C: Assessment of capacity for myoelectric control: a new Rasch-built measure of prosthetic hand control, *J Rehabil Med* 37:166–171, 2005.

45. Hess A: Upper limb body-powered components. In Krajbich JI, Pinzur MS, Potter BK, Stevens PM, editors: *Atlas of amputations and limb deficiencies*, ed 4, Rosemont, IL, 2016, American Academy of Orthopedic Surgeons.

46. Hill W, et al: Limb Prosthetic Outcome Measures (ULPOM): a working group and their findings, *J Prosthet Orthot* 21:69–82, 2009.

47. Hirschberg G, Lewis L, Thomas D: *Rehabilitation*, Philadelphia, 1964, JB Lippincott.

48. Horgan O, MacLachlan M: Psychological adjustment to lower-limb amputation: a review, *Disabil Rehabil* 26:837–850, 2004.

49. Jacobsen SC, Knutti DF, Johnson RT, Sears HH: Development of the Utah artificial arm, *IEEE Trans Biomed Eng* 29:249–269, 1982.

50. Jelic M, Eldar R: Rehabilitation following major traumatic amputation of lower limbs: a review, *Crit Rev Phys Rehabil Med* 15:235–252, 2003.

51. Johns Hopkins Applied Physics Laboratory: Modular prosthetic limb. http://www.jhuapl.edu/prosthetics/scientists/mpl.asp.

52. Johnson SS, Mansfield E: Prosthetic training: upper limb, *Phys Med Rehabil Clin North Am* 25:133–151, 2014.

53. Kapp S, Miller J: Lower limb prosthetics. In Pasquina PF, Cooper RA, editors: *Care of the combat amputee*, Washington, DC, 2009, Department of the Army, the Borden Institute.

54. Kuiken TA, Schultz Feuser AE, Barlow AK: *Targeted muscle reinnervation: a neural interface for artificial limbs*, Boca Raton, FL, 2014, Taylor & Francis Group.

55. Kuiken TA, Li G, Lock BA, et al: Targeted muscle reinnervation for real-time myoelectric control of multifunction artificial arms, *JAMA* 301:619–628, 2009.

56. Kuiken TA, Marasco PD, Lock BA, et al: Redirection of cutaneous sensation from the hand to the chest skin of human amputees with targeted reinnervation, *Proc Natl Acad Sci U S A* 104:20061–20066, 2007.

57. Kyberd P, Bush G, Hussaini A: Control options for upper limb externally powered components. In Krajbich JI, Pinzur MS, Potter BK, Stevens PM, editors: *Atlas of amputations and limb deficiencies*, ed 4, Rosemont, IL, 2016, American Academy of Orthopedic Surgeons.

58. Lake C, Dodson R: Progressive upper limb prosthetics, *Phys Med Rehabil Clin North Am* 17:49–72, 2006.

59. Larner S, van Ross E, Hale C: Do psychological measures predict the ability of lower limb amputees to learn to use a prosthesis? *Clin Rehabil* 17:493–498, 2003.

60. Legro MW, Reiber GE, Czerniecki JM, Sangeorzan BJ: Recreational activities of lower-limb amputees with prostheses, *J Rehabil Res Dev* 38:319–325, 2001.

61. Leonard JA, Meier RH: Prosthetics. In DeLisa JA, editor: *Rehabilitation medicine: principles and practice*, Philadelphia, 1988, JB Lippincott.
62. Levin AZ: Functional outcome following amputation, *Top Geriatr Rehabil* 20:253–261, 2004.
63. Light CM, Chappell PH, Kyberd PJ: Establishing a standardized clinical assessment tool of pathologic and prosthetic hand function: normative data, reliability and validity, *Arch Phys Med Rehabil* 83:776–783, 2002.
64. Malone JM, Goldstone J: Lower extremity amputation. In Moore WS, editor: *Vascular surgery: a comprehensive review*, New York, 1984, Grune & Stratton.
65. Malone JM, Fleming LL, Roberson J, et al: Immediate, early, and late postsurgical management of upper-limb amputation, *J Rehabil Res Dev* 21:33–41, 1984.
66. Matsen SL, Malchow D, Matsen FA III: Correlations with clients' perspectives of the result of lower-extremity amputation, *J Bone Joint Surg Am* 82:1089–1095, 2000.
67. McMahon SB, et al: *Wall and Melzack's textbook of pain*, ed 6, Philadelphia, 2013, Elsevier/Saunders.
68. Melzack R: Phantom limbs, the self and the brain, *Can J Psychol* 30:1–16, 1989.
69. Merrill DR, Lockhart J, Troyk PR, Weir RF, Hankin DL: Development of an implantable myoelectric sensor for advanced prosthesis control, *Artif Organs* 35(3):249–252, 2011.
70. Michaels JA: The selection of amputation level: an approach using decision analysis, *Eur J Vasc Surg* 5:451–457, 1991.
71. Miguelez J, et al: Upper extremity prosthetics. In Pasquina PF, Cooper RA, editors: *Care of combat amputee*, Washington, DC, 2009, Department of the Army, Borden Institute.
72. Millstein SG, Heger H, Hunter GA: Prosthetic use in adult upper limb amputees: a comparison of the body powered and electrically powered prostheses, *Prosthet Orthot Int* 10:27–34, 1986.
73. Mitsch S, Walters LS, Yancosek K: Amputations and prosthetics. In Radomski MV, Latham CAT, editors: *Occupational therapy for physical dysfunction*, ed 7, Philadelphia, 2014, Wolters Kluwer Health/Lippincott Williams & Wilkins.
74. Mobius Bionics: Luke Arm system product specifications: https://www.mobiusbionics.com/luke-arm/#section-five.
75. Motawea M, Kryillos F, Hanafy A, et al: Impact of big toe amputation on foot biomechanics, *Int J Adv Res* 3(12): 1224–1228, 2015.
76. Muilenburg AL, LeBlanc MA: Body-powered upper-limb components. In Atkins DJ, Meier RH, editors: *Comprehensive management of the upper-limb amputee*, New York, 1989, Springer-Verlag.
77. Näder M: The artificial substitution of missing hands with myoelectric prostheses, *Clin Orthop Relat Res* 258:9–17, 1990.
78. National Limb Loss Information Center: Fact sheet: limb loss in the United States. (2007). Amputee Coalition of America. http://www.amputee-coalition.org/fact_sheets/limbloss_us.html.
79. Northmore-Ball MD, Heger H, Hunter GA: The below-elbow myo-electric prosthesis: a comparison of the Otto Bock myo-electric prosthesis with the hook and functional hand, *J Bone Joint Surg Br* 62:363–367, 1980.
80. NovaCare: Motion control: training the client with an electric arm prosthesis (videotape), King of Prussia, PA, 1997, NovaCare. http://utaharm.com/.
81. Novotny MP: Psychosocial issues affecting rehabilitation, *Phys Med Rehabil Clin North Am* 2:373–393, 1991.
82. Olivett BL: Management and prosthetic training of the adult amputee. In Hunter JM, editor: *Rehabilitation of the hand*, St Louis, 1984, Mosby.
83. Össur. i-Limb Quantum. https://www.ossur.com/en-us/prosthetics/arms/i-limb-quantum.
84. Ottobock. Bebionic hand: https://www.ottobockus.com/prosthetics/upper-limb-prosthetics/solution-overview/bebionic-hand/.
85. Pendleton HM, Schultz-Krohn W: Psychosocial issues in physical disability. In Cara E, MacRae A, editors: *Psychosocial occupational therapy: a clinical practice,*, Clifton Park, NY, 2005, Thomson Delmar Learning.
86. Pinzur MS, Angelats J, Light TR, et al: Functional outcome following traumatic upper limb amputation and prosthetic limb fitting, *J Hand Surg Am* 19:836–839, 1994.
87. Powell MA, Thakor NV: A training strategy for learning pattern recognition control for myoelectric prostheses, *J Prosthet Orthot* 25:30–41, 2013.
88. Price EH: A critical review of congenital phantom limb cases and a developmental theory for the basis of body image, *Conscious Cogn* 15:320–322, 2006.
89. Ramachandran VS, Brang D, McGeoch PD: Size reduction using mirror visual feedback (MVF) reduces phantom pain, *Neurocase* 15:357–360, 2009.
90. Rand JD, Paz JC: Amputation. In Paz JC, West MP, editors: *Acute care handbook for physical therapists*, Woburn, MA, 2002, Butterworth-Heinemann.
91. Raney R, Brashear H: Shands' handbook of orthopaedic surgery, ed 8, St Louis, 1971, Mosby.
92. Resnick L, Klinger SL, Etter K: User and clinical perspectives on DEKA arm: results of VA study to optimize DEKA arm, *J Rehabil Res Dev* 51:27–38, 2014.
93. Resnick L, Adams L, Borgia M, et al: Development and evaluation of the Activities Measure for Upper Limb Amputees (AM-ULA), *Arch Phys Med Rehabil* 94:488–494, 2013.
94. Rosenbaum-Chou T: Update on osseointegration for prosthetic attachment, *Acad Today* 9(2):A9–A11, 2013.
95. Sanders JE, Nicholson BS, Zachariah SG, et al: Testing of elastomeric liners used in limb prosthetics: classification of 15 products by mechanical performance, *J Rehabil Res Dev* 41:175–186, 2004.
96. Santschi WR, editor: Manual of upper extremity prosthetics, ed 2, Los Angeles, 1958, University of California Press.
97. Scheme EJ, Englehart KB, Hudgins BS: Selective classification for improved robustness of myoelectric control under nonideal conditions, *IEEE Trans Biomed Eng* 58:1698–1705, 2011.
98. Schoppen T, Boonstra A, Groothoff JW, et al: Physical, mental and social predictors of functional outcome in unilateral lower-limb amputees, *Arch Phys Med Rehabil* 84:803–811, 2003.
99. Sensinger JW, Lock BA, Kuiken TA: Adaptive pattern recognition of myoelectric signals: exploration of conceptual framework and practical algorithms, *IEEE Trans Neural Syst Rehabil Eng* 17:270–278, 2009.
100. Sherril C: Social and psychological dimensions of sports for disabled athletes. In Sherril C, editor: *Sport and disabled athletes*, Champaign, IL, 1986, Human Kinetics.
101. Simpson DC: Functional requirements and system of control for powered prostheses, *Biomed Eng* 1:250–256, 1966.
102. Smurr LM, Gulick K, Yancosek K, Ganz O: Managing the upper extremity amputee: a protocol for success, *J Hand Ther* 21: 160–176, 2008.

103. Smurr LM, Yancosek K, Gulick K, et al: Occupational therapy for the polytrauma casualty with limb loss. In Pasquina PF, Cooper RA, editors: *Care of the combat amputee*, Washington, DC, 2009, Department of the Army, Borden Institute.

104. Spencer EA: Amputations. In Hopkins HL, Smith HD, editors: *Willard & Spackman's occupational therapy*, ed 5, Philadelphia, 1978, JB Lippincott.

105. Spencer EA: Amputation and prosthetic replacement. In Hopkins HL, Smith HD, editors: *Willard & Spackman's occupational therapy*, ed 8, Philadelphia, 1993, JB Lippincott.

106. Spencer EA: Functional restoration. III. Amputation and prosthetic replacement. In Hopkins HL, Smith HD, editors: *Willard & Spackman's occupational therapy*, ed 8, Philadelphia, 1993, JB Lippincott.

107. Spencer EA: Musculoskeletal dysfunction in adults. In Neistadt ME, Crepeau EB, editors: *Willard & Spackman's occupational therapy*, ed 9, Philadelphia, 1998, JB Lippincott.

108. Spiegal SR: Adult myoelectric upper-limb prosthetic training. In Atkins DJ, Meier RH, editors: *Comprehensive management of the upper-limb amputee*, New York, 1989, Springer-Verlag.

109. Stubblefield KA, Miller LA, Lipschutz RD, Kuiken TA: Occupational therapy protocol for amputees with targeted muscle reinnervation, *J Rehabil Res Dev* 46:481–488, 2009.

110. Sullivan J, Uden M, Robinson KP, Sooriakumaran S: Rehabilitation of the trans-femoral amputee with an osseointegrated prosthesis: the United Kingdom experience, *Prosthet Orthot Int* 27:114–120, 2003.

111. TAD reveals N-Abler V five-function wrist. O&P Edge (serial online). http://www.oandp.com/articles/news_2003-10-02_02.asp.

112. Tintle SM, Shores JT, Levin SL: Hand transplantation. In Krajbich JI, Pinzur MS, Potter BK, Stevens PM, editors: *Atlas of amputations and limb deficiencies*, ed 4, Rosemont, IL, 2016, American Academy of Orthopedic Surgeons.

113. Tintle SM, Baechler MF, Nanos GP III, et al: Traumatic and trauma-related amputations. part II: upper extremity and future directions, *J Bone Joint Surg Am* 92:2934–2945, 2010.

114. Tooms RE: Amputations of lower extremity. In Crenshaw AH, editor: *Campbell's operative orthopaedics. 8*, St. Louis, 1992, Mosby-Year Book, Inc, pp 689–702.

115. Tsai HA, Kirby RL, MacLeod DA, Graham MM: Aided gait of people with lower-limb amputations: comparison of 4-footed and 2-wheeled walkers, *Arch Phys Med Rehabil* 84:584–591, 2003.

116. Uellendahl JE: Bilateral upper limb prostheses. In Smith DG, Bowker JH, editors: *Atlas of amputations and limb deficiencies: surgical and prosthetic rehabilitation principles*, ed 3, Rosemont, IL, 2004, American Academy of Orthopedic Surgeons.

117. Reference deleted in proofs.

118. Van Dorsten B: Common emotional concerns following limb loss. In Atkins DJ, Meier RH, editors: *Functional restoration of adults and children with upper extremity amputation*, New York, 2004, Demos Medical Publishing.

119. Walsh NE, et al: Treatment of the client with chronic pain. In DeLisa JA, editor: *Rehabilitation medicine: principles and practice*, Philadelphia, 1988, JB Lippincott.

120. Waryck B: Comparison of two myoelectric multi-articulating prosthetic hands, Proceedings of the MEC '11 Conference, UNB, 2011.

121. Weeks SR, Anderson-Barnes VC, Tsao JW: Phantom limb pain: theories and therapies, *Neurologist* 16:277–286, 2010.

122. Wellerson TL: *A manual for occupational therapists on the rehabilitation of upper extremity amputees*, Dubuque, IA, 1958, William C Brown.

123. Wetterman KA, Hanson C, Levy CE: Effect of participation in physical activity on body image of amputees, *Am J Phys Med Rehabil* 81:194–201, 2002.

124. White EA: Wheelchair stump boards and their use with lower limb amputees, *Br J Occup Ther* 55:174–178, 1992.

125. Wright G: Controls training for the upper extremity amputee (film), San Jose, CA, Instructional Resources Center, San Jose State University.

126. Wright V: Measurement of functional outcome with individuals who use upper extremity prosthetic devices: current and future directions, *J Prosthet Orthot* 18:46–56, 2006.

127. Yazicioglu K, Yavuz F, Goktepe AS, Tan AK: Influence of adapted sports on quality of life and life satisfaction in sport participants and non-sport participants with physical disabilities, *Disabil Health J* 5:249–253, 2012.

128. Yancosek KE: Amputations and prosthetics. In Skirvin T, editor: *Rehabilitation of the hand*, ed 6, Philadelphia, 2011, Mosby.

129. Yancosek KE, Howell D: Systematic review of interventions to improve or augment handwriting ability in adult clients, *Occup Ther J Res* 31:55–63, 2011.

130. Ziegler-Graham K, MacKenzie EJ, Ephraim PL, et al: Estimating the prevalence of limb loss in the United States: 2005 to 2050, *Arch Phys Med Rehabil* 89:422–429, 2008.

RESOURCES

Amputee Coalition

601 Pennsylvania Avenue NW, South Building, Suite 420
Washington DC, 20004
Telephone: 888-267-5669
Website: http://www.amputee-coalition.org

Challenged Athletes Foundation

9591 Waples Street
San Diego, CA 92121
Telephone: 858-866-0959
Website: http://www.challengedathletes.org

Move United

451 Hungerford Drive, Suite 608
Rockville, MD 20850
Telephone: 301-217-0960
Website: http://www.disabledsportsusa.org

45

Cardiac and Pulmonary Disease

Shohei Takatani[a]

LEARNING OBJECTIVES

After studying this chapter, the student or practitioner will be able to do the following:

1. Demonstrate a beginning understanding of the cardiovascular function and how heart rate and rhythm and blood pressure affect engagement in occupation.
2. Identify the significance of ischemic heart disease and valvular diseases of the heart and the potential impact of these conditions on occupational performance.
3. Differentiate between modifiable and nonmodifiable risk factors and discuss how these risk factors might be affected by context and environment.
4. Identify signs and symptoms of cardiac distress.
5. Describe the course of action that should be taken if signs and symptoms of cardiac distress are present.
6. Define sternal precautions and identify three modifications of activities of daily living (ADLs) for these precautions.
7. Identify how performance patterns are affected for persons with cardiovascular or pulmonary disease.
8. Describe methods for determining the heart rate and blood pressure and calculate the rate-pressure product given the heart rate and blood pressure.
9. Give a brief overview of the respiratory system and identify its primary function.
10. Define chronic obstructive pulmonary disease (COPD) and identify how occupational performance might be affected by COPD.
11. Identify pulmonary risk factors and psychosocial considerations within the context of social justice.
12. Describe dyspnea control postures, pursed-lip breathing, and diaphragmatic breathing.
13. Describe a relaxation technique and explain the benefits of relaxation from an occupational perspective.
14. List interview questions that will help the clinician know what the patient understands about intervention.
15. List the principles of energy conservation and identify how you might focus patient education based on the environment of a patient in an assisted living facility.
16. Explain the significance of a metabolic equivalent chart in the progression of ADL and instrumental ADLs (IADL) and describe how to use it.

CHAPTER OUTLINE

[a]The author wishes to acknowledge the outstanding work of Maureen Michele Matthews in previous editions of this text. The present chapter is built on her foundational work.

KEY TERMS

Atrial fibrillation

Blood pressure

Cardiac ablation

Chronic obstructive pulmonary
  disease

Diaphragmatic breathing

Energy conservation

Heart rate

Ischemic heart disease

Mechanical circulatory support

Metabolic equivalent

Myocardial infarction

Pack-year history

Pulmonary rehabilitation

Pursed-lip breathing

Rate-pressure product

Sternal precautions

Ventricular assist device

THREADED CASE STUDY

Joe, Part 1

Joe, a 64-year-old married man (prefers the pronouns he/his/him) with diabetes, was enjoying his daily exercise of running 3 miles when he suddenly experienced significant fatigue and difficulty breathing. In the emergency room his heart rate (HR) was 140 beats per minute, his blood pressure was 128/70 mm Hg, and his respiratory rate was 20 breaths per minute with oxygen saturation of 93% on room air. He was diagnosed with atrial fibrillation, and his previously diagnosed defective heart valve was failing. He was admitted to the hospital and underwent an aortic valve replacement and cardiac ablation.

Joe's surgeon had accessed his heart through a large incision made through the sternum. This approach is referred to as a median sternotomy. At the end of the procedure, Joe's sternum was closed and stabilized with wire, and his physician placed activity orders with sternal precautions to maintain the integrity of the healing bone. During the occupational therapy (OT) evaluation, Joe got out of bed, ambulated to the bathroom with a front wheel walker, and transferred on and off the toilet with minimal assist. He then washed his hands standing at the sink with contact guard assist for balance and then ambulated to the bedside chair with the front wheel walker and sat up in the bedside chair for lunch. He rated his pain as 3 on a scale of 0 to 10 at the chest incision and was premedicated by his nurse. Of note, Joe moved impulsively and demonstrated significant difficulty adhering to his sternal precautions, requiring multiple verbal and tactile cues. Joe and his wife live in a three-story townhouse with 15 steps to enter and

with the bedroom and bathroom on the third floor. Joe's wife works during the day, and so Joe would be home alone for the greater part of the day if he were to go home after discharge from the hospital.

Joe has an executive desk job and plans to return to work in 3 weeks. He added that his goal is to resume everything he did before his recent decline. Joe and his wife were anxious and asked lots of questions. Joe stated, "I need to go to the bathroom and dress by myself." Joe's wife, who works outside the home, said she was afraid of potentially harming Joe by expecting too much of him and also afraid that he would potentially harm himself by not limiting his activity level. Joe expressed concern that his wife was avoiding intimacy based on her fears of hurting him. A barrier to recovery revealed by Joe was his regular alcohol consumption. This was not in evidence as a problem in the medical record.

Critical Thinking Questions

1. What probative questions might the occupational therapist ask to clarify what Joe means by "everything he did"?
2. What skills must Joe acquire to protect his healing sternum and resume safe participation in his daily activities?
3. What areas of occupation might the therapist choose for the next intervention session, and based on Joe's occupational profile, what goals might be included in his occupational therapy intervention plan?[3]

In this chapter the term *patient* is used instead of *client* to reflect the practice setting and the acute nature of the diagnoses in the individuals described in the case studies.

Individuals with disorders of the cardiovascular or pulmonary system may be severely limited in endurance and performance in areas of occupation, including activities of daily living (ADLs) and instrumental activities of daily living (IADLs). Occupational therapy (OT) services may benefit such individuals and are available throughout the continuum of healthcare. An understanding of the normal function of the cardiopulmonary system, the pathology of cardiopulmonary disease, common risk factors, clinical terminology, medical interventions, precautions, and standard treatment techniques will guide the occupational therapist (OT) in providing effective care and promoting recovery of function in patients with compromised cardiovascular or pulmonary systems.

ANATOMY AND CIRCULATION

The heart and blood vessels work together to maintain a constant flow of blood throughout the body. The heart, located between the lungs, is pear shaped and about the size of a fist.

It functions as a two-sided pump. The right side pumps blood from the body to the lungs; the left side simultaneously pumps blood from the lungs to the body. Each side of the heart has two chambers: an upper atrium and a lower ventricle.

Blood flows to the heart from the venous system. Blood enters the right atrium, which contracts and squeezes the blood into the right ventricle. Next, the right ventricle contracts and ejects the blood into the lungs, where carbon dioxide is exchanged for oxygen. Oxygen-rich blood flows from the lungs to the left atrium. As the left atrium contracts, it forces blood into the left ventricle, which then contracts and ejects its contents into the aorta for systemic circulation (Fig. 45.1). Blood travels from the aorta to the arteries and through progressively smaller blood vessels to networks of very tiny capillaries. In the capillaries, blood cells exchange their oxygen for carbon dioxide.

Each of the ventricles has two valves: an input valve and an output valve. The valves open and close as the heart muscle (myocardium) contracts and relaxes. These valves control the direction and flow of blood. The input valves are the mitral, or bicuspid, valve (between the left atrium and ventricle) and the tricuspid valve (between the right atrium and ventricle). The output valves comprise the aortic and pulmonary valves.

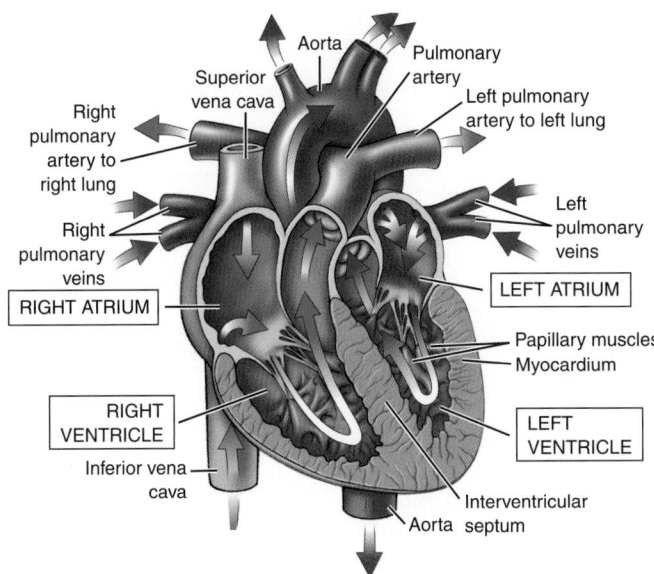

Fig. 45.1 Anatomy of the heart. (From Herlihy B: *The human body in health and illness,* ed 7, St. Louis, 2022, Elsevier.)

The heart is living tissue and requires a blood supply (through an arterial and venous system of its own), or it will die. Coronary arteries cross over the myocardium to supply it with oxygen-rich blood. The coronary arteries are named for their location on the myocardium (Fig. 45.2). Cardiologists generally refer to these arteries by abbreviations, such as "LAD" for "left anterior descending" and "RCA" for "right coronary artery." The LAD artery is on the left, anterior portion of the heart and runs in a downward direction; it supplies part of the left ventricle. Blockage of this coronary artery will interrupt the blood supply to the left ventricle. Because the left ventricle supplies the body and brain with blood, a heart attack caused by blockage of the LAD artery can have serious consequences.

WHAT CAUSES THE HEART TO CONTRACT?

In addition to the ordinary muscle tissue of the heart, the myocardium is composed of two other types of tissue: nodal and Purkinje. These tissues are part of a specialized electrical conduction system that causes the heart to contract and relax (Fig. 45.3). An electrical impulse usually originates in the right atrium at a site called the sinoatrial node. The impulse travels along internodal pathways to the atrioventricular node, through the bundle of His, to the left and right bundle branches, and then to the Purkinje fibers. Nerve impulses normally travel this pathway 60 to 100 times every minute, first causing both atria to contract, pushing blood into the ventricles, and then provoking the ventricles to contract. The electrical impulse created by the heart's conduction system can easily be studied. Electrodes placed on a person's limbs and chest can pick up the heart's electrical impulse, which can be translated to paper as an electrocardiogram (ECG). The resulting ECG tracing is frequently used to help diagnose cardiac disease.

The sinoatrial node responds to vagal and sympathetic nervous system input.[34] This is why the heart rate (HR) increases in response to exercise and anxiety and decreases in response to relaxation techniques, such as deep breathing and meditation. Each cell within the electrical conduction system of the heart can respond to, conduct, resist for a brief period, and generate an electrical impulse. Because of this capacity, electrical impulses causing the heart muscle to contract can be generated from anywhere along the electrical conduction system. This is desirable when part of the conduction system has been damaged and is unable do its job, but it is undesirable when life-threatening conduction irregularities develop.

CARDIAC CYCLE

HR and **blood pressure** (BP) determine cardiac output, the amount of blood ejected by the heart each minute. The cardiac cycle occurs in two phases: input (diastole) and output (systole).

During the input phase, blood flows through the atria and into the ventricles. The atria contract and push more blood into the ventricles. Once the pressure inside the ventricles is equal to the pressure in the atria, the input valves (tricuspid in the right ventricle and mitral [or bicuspid] in the left ventricle) close. The ventricles then contract, which results in rapidly increasing ventricular pressure. When the pressure inside the ventricles exceeds the pressure in the blood vessels beyond, the output valves (pulmonary in the right and aortic in the left) open, and diastolic BP (DBP) is attained.

The ventricles continue to contract and squeeze blood under increasingly greater pressure into the pulmonary and body circulation. Systolic BP (SBP) is attained when pressure in the emptying ventricles falls below pressure in the blood vessels beyond, which causes the output valves to close.

ISCHEMIC HEART DISEASE

Ischemic heart disease (ischemia) occurs when a part of the heart is temporarily deprived of sufficient oxygen to meet its demand. The most common cause of cardiac ischemia is coronary artery disease (CAD). CAD is the most common form of heart disease in the United States.[48,74]

CAD usually develops over a period of many years without causing symptoms. The internal wall of an artery can become injured. Once the wall is damaged, it becomes irregular in shape and more prone to collect plaque (fatty deposits such as cholesterol). Platelets also gather along the arterial wall and clog the artery, thereby creating a lesion in the same manner in which rust can clog a pipe. The artery gradually narrows and thus allows a smaller volume of blood to pass through it. This disease process is called atherosclerosis.[13]

If a coronary artery is partially or completely blocked, the part of the heart supplied by that artery may not receive sufficient oxygen to meet its needs. Persons with partial blockage of a coronary artery may be free of symptoms at rest but have angina, a type of chest pain, with eating, exercise, exertion, or exposure to cold. Angina varies from individual to individual and has been described as squeezing, tightness, fullness, pressure, or a sharp pain in the chest. The pain may also radiate to other parts of the body, usually the arm, back, neck, or jaw.

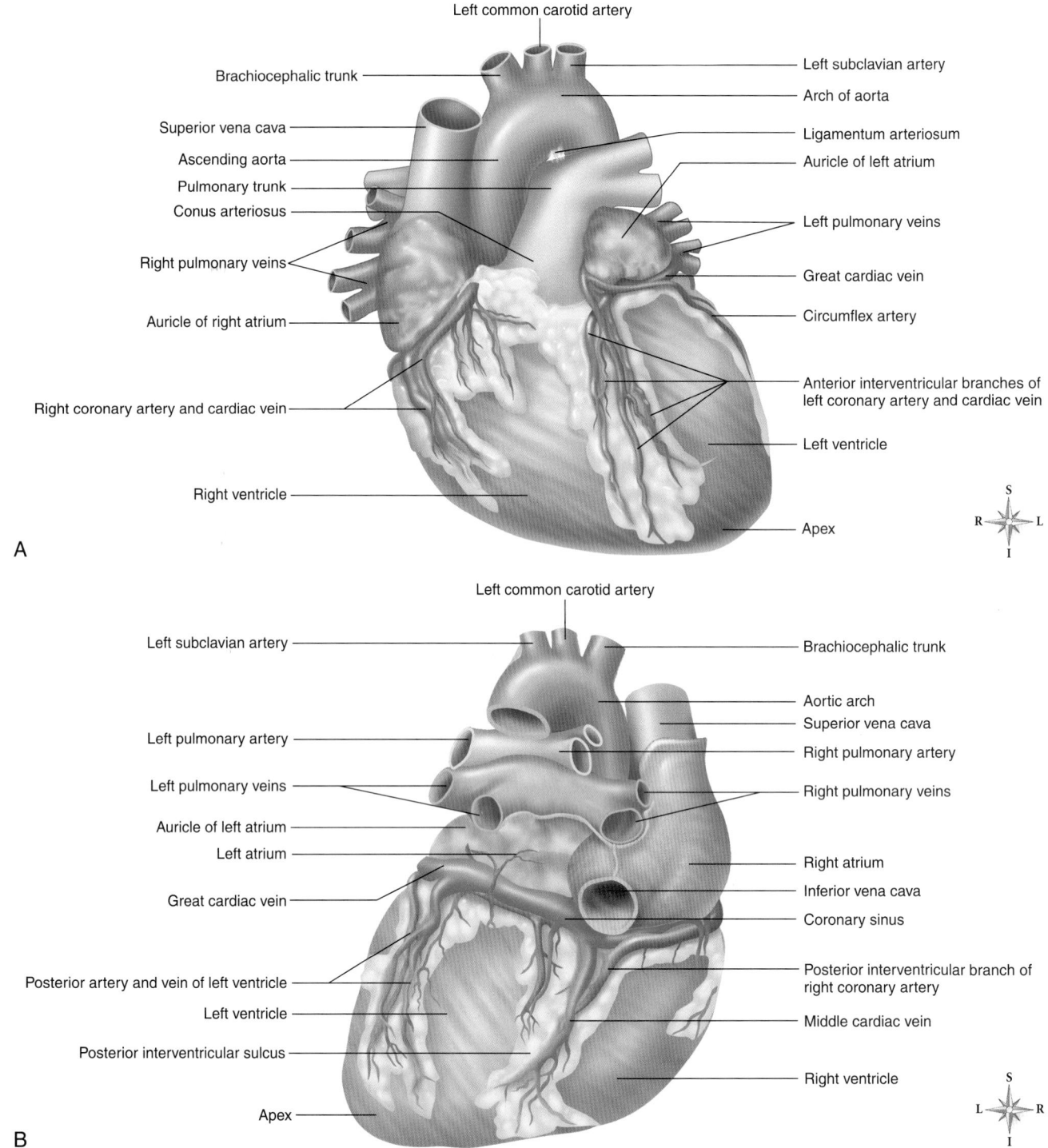

Fig. 45.2 Coronary circulation. (From Patton KT, Thibodeau GA: *Anatomy & physiology*, ed 11, St Louis, 2022, Elsevier.)

Angina also has been confused with indigestion. Rest or medication (or both) will frequently relieve angina. Usually, no permanent heart damage results. Angina is a warning sign that should not be ignored.

Chest pain that is not relieved by rest or nitroglycerin likely indicates a myocardial infarction (MI), or heart attack. A patient who has this type of pain should seek emergency medical help immediately. Individuals who attribute their symptoms to anxiety and stress are more likely to delay emergency care.[60]

Substernal chest pain can be a warning sign that one or more of one's coronary arteries are blocked. If the blood flow to the heart muscle is interrupted and starved of the necessary oxygen, the heart will begin to die. This is an MI. If a substantial section of the heart is damaged, it will stop pumping (cardiac arrest).

Restrictions in activity are prescribed for the first 6 weeks after a heart attack because newly damaged heart muscle, like any injured body tissue, is easily reinjured.[20] During a heart attack, metabolic waste products accumulate in the damaged myocardium and make

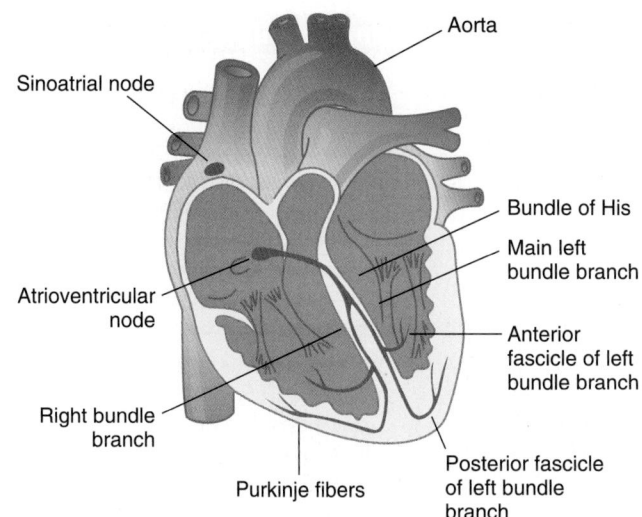

Aorta

Sinoatrial node

Bundle of His

Main left
bundle branch

Atrioventricular
node

Anterior
fascicle of left
bundle branch

Right bundle
branch

Posterior fascicle
of left bundle
branch

Purkinje fibers

Fig. 45.3 Cardiac conduction. (From Benjamin IJ, Griggs RC, Wing EJ, Fitz JG: *Andreoli and Carpenter's Cecil essentials of medicine*, ed 9, Philadelphia, 2016, Saunders.)

it irritable and prone to electrical irregularities such as premature ventricular contractions. A delicate balance of rest and activity must be maintained to allow the damaged area of myocardium to heal while also sustaining the strength of the healthy part of the heart. Occupational therapy is often ordered by the physician to guide the patient toward a safe level of activity or participation in occupation during this acute period of recovery. Therapists teach persons with cardiac compromise the signs of fatigue, applied energy conservation strategies to daily activities and other occupation, including but not limited to work simplification concepts and pacing to help facilitate safer resumption of occupation.

At approximately 6 weeks after an MI, scar tissue forms and the risk of extending the MI decreases. The scarred part of the heart muscle is not elastic and does not contract with each heartbeat. Therefore, the heart does not pump as well. A graded exercise program will help strengthen the healthy part of the myocardium and improve cardiac output.[11,28,75] Cardiac rehabilitation is generally prescribed for persons recovering from heart attacks and for those recovering from cardiac surgery.

CAD can also lead to congestive heart failure (CHF). Similarly, infections can lead to CHF. This disease process develops over time, with the heart becoming progressively weaker. CHF occurs when the heart is unable to pump effectively enough to meet the demand and fluid backs up into the lungs or the body. The fluid buildup in the lungs causes shortness of breath. Fluid overload is problematic because it puts a greater workload on the heart as the heart strains while attempting to clear the excess fluid, which may result in further congestion. Heart size is often enlarged in persons with CHF because the heart muscle thickens (hypertrophy) from working so hard. Diuretics can be prescribed for persons with CHF to promote diuresis or fluid loss through the urinary system. Low-sodium diets and fluid restrictions reduce the overall amount of fluid in the body. CHF cannot be cured, but with medication, diet modification, and applied energy conservation strategy, people with this condition can live longer and participate more fully in life.

Once an acute exacerbation of CHF is controlled, gradual resumption of activity will promote improved function. If activity is resumed too quickly, another acute episode may follow. Patients who have difficulty resuming their former level of activity may self-limit their recovery. Occupational therapy can guide patients with acute CHF toward an optimal level of function via graded self-care tasks, thus facilitating the goal of "Achieving Health, Well-being and Participation in Life through Engagement in Occupation" (p. 5).[3] "About 5.7 million people in the United States have heart failure"[24] and "about half of the people diagnosed with heart failure die within 5 years of the diagnosis."[24] Table 45.1 delineates the four functional classifications of heart disease. Occupational therapy can be of great benefit to persons with stage III and IV heart disease and can provide preventive programs for persons with stages I and II.

VALVULAR DISEASE

The heart valves, which are responsible for controlling the direction and flow of blood through the heart, may become damaged by disease or infection. Two complications result from valvular disease: volume overload and pressure overload. A fibrous mitral valve will fail to close properly, and blood will be regurgitated back to the atria when the left ventricle contracts. Volume overload results when fluid accumulates in the lungs, thereby causing shortness of breath. Volume overload increases the potential for atrial fibrillation, which results in irregular and ineffective contractions in both atria. Blood flow through the heart slows, and blood clots (emboli) may develop in the ventricles. Many cerebrovascular accidents are caused when emboli ejected from the left ventricle enter the circulatory system of the brain. Volume overload caused Joe's shortness of breath and rapid HR and also can manifest with swelling of the ankles.

If the aortic valve fails to close properly (aortic insufficiency), CHF or ischemia may result. Another disorder of the aortic valve is aortic stenosis (narrowing), which results in pressure overload. The left ventricle, which must work harder to open the sticky valve, becomes enlarged, and cardiac output decreases. Ventricular arrhythmia (irregular rhythm of heartbeats), cerebral insufficiency, confusion, syncope (fainting), and even sudden death may result from aortic stenosis. Surgery to repair or replace the damaged valves is frequently recommended.

CARDIAC RISK FACTORS

Many scientific studies have been conducted to determine the causes of heart disease. The most famous of these, the Framingham study,[14] helped identify many factors that put an individual at risk for atherosclerosis. Risk factors are divided into three major categories: those that cannot be changed (heredity, male sex, and age), those that can be changed (high BP, cigarette smoking, cholesterol levels, and an inactive lifestyle), and contributing factors (diabetes, stress, and obesity). The Framington Heart Study continues with research milestones in identifying specific genetic and social factors associated with heart disease, dementia, and stroke.[19] Other factors that contribute to CAD include sleep apnea, alcohol, and preeclampsia.[52] There is a

TABLE 45.1   Comparison of Three Methods of Assessing Cardiovascular Disability

Class	New York Association Functional Classification[69]	Canadian Cardiovascular Society Functional Classification Severity of Unstable Angina[44]	Specific Activity Scale[23]
I	This category includes patients with cardiac disease but without resulting limitations in physical activity. Ordinary physical activity does not cause undue fatigue, palpitations, dyspnea, or anginal pain.	Ordinary physical activity, such as walking and climbing stairs, does not cause angina. Angina occurs with strenuous, rapid, or prolonged exertion during work or recreation.	Patients can perform to completion any activity requiring ≤ 7 METs (e.g., can carry objects that weigh 80 lb, do outdoor work [shovel snow, spade soil], and do recreational activities [skiing, basketball, squash, handball, jog/walk 5 mph]).
II	This category includes patients with cardiac disease resulting in slight limitations in physical activity. They are comfortable at rest. Less than ordinary physical activity causes fatigue, palpitations, dyspnea, or anginal pain.	Ordinary activity is somewhat limited. This includes walking or climbing stairs rapidly; walking uphill; and walking or climbing stairs after meals, in cold, in wind, when under emotional stress, or only during the few hours after waking. This also includes walking more than two blocks on a level surface and climbing more than one flight of stairs at a normal pace and in normal conditions.	Patients can perform to completion any activity requiring ≤ 5 METs (e.g., have sexual intercourse without stopping, garden, rake, weed, roller skate, dance the fox-trot, walk at 4 mph on level ground) but cannot and do not perform to completion activities requiring ≥ 7 METs.
III	This category includes patients with cardiac disease resulting in marked limitation in physical activity. They are comfortable at rest. Less than ordinary physical activity causes fatigue, palpitation, dyspnea, or anginal pain.	Ordinary physical activity is significantly limited. This includes walking one to two blocks on a level surface and climbing more than one flight in normal conditions.	Patients can perform to completion any activity requiring ≤ 2 METs (e.g., shower without stopping, strip and make the bed, clean windows, walk 2.5 miles, bowl, play golf, dress without stopping) but cannot and do not perform to completion activities requiring ≥ 5 METs.
IV	This category includes patients with cardiac disease resulting in an inability to carry out any physical activity without discomfort. Symptoms of cardiac insufficiency or angina syndrome may be present even at rest. If any physical activity is undertaken, discomfort is increased.	Patients are unable to carry out any physical activity without discomfort; angina syndrome may be present at rest.	Patients cannot perform to completion any activity requiring ≥ 2 METs and cannot carry out activities listed previously (Specific Activity Scale, class III).

METs, Metabolic equivalents.

From Goldman L, Hashimoto B, Cook EF, et al: Comparative reproducibility and validity of systems for assessing cardiovascular functional class: advantages of a new specific activity scale, *Circulation* 64:1227, 1981.

bidirectional link between CAD and depression. Persons with CAD are more likely to develop depression, and persons with depression are more likely to develop CAD than others.[25]

The more risk factors that an individual has, the greater is the individual's risk for CAD. All team members—the physician, nurse, physical therapist (PT), case manager, social worker, nutritionist, and OT—should support the patient's attempts to reduce risk factors. In reviewing Joe's case study, several risk factors are clearly present, whereas others appear to be absent.

MEDICAL MANAGEMENT

A heart attack is a medical emergency, and treatment with aspirin and oxygen is usually initiated before diagnosis. Early treatment is usually started before confirmation of the diagnosis and includes aspirin, nitroglycerin, oxygen, and treatment of chest pain.[49] After emergency treatment, heart attack survivors are typically managed in a coronary care unit, where they are closely observed for complications. Approximately 90% of persons who have suffered an MI will have arrhythmia.[6] Heart failure, the

development of blood clots (thrombosis and embolism), aneurysms, rupture of part of the heart muscle, inflammation of the sac around the heart (pericarditis), and even death are potential outcomes of MI. Close medical management is imperative.

Generally, patients are managed for 1 to 3 days after MI in an intensive care unit (ICU). Once their condition has stabilized, they are transferred from the ICU to a less acute step-down telemetry unit (determined by nursing to patient ratio) with ongoing cardiac monitoring. Patients typically stay 5 to 10 days in the hospital after an acute MI. Vital signs are monitored closely while activity is gradually increased. Occupational therapists may be consulted to monitor the patient's response to activity and educate the patient about the disease process, risk factors, and lifestyle modification to help facilitate safe and successful resumption of occupation.

Various surgical procedures can correct the circulatory problems associated with CAD. Balloon angioplasty, also called percutaneous transluminal coronary angioplasty (PTCA), and coronary artery bypass grafting (CABG) are most common.

In PTCA, a catheter is inserted into the femoral artery and guided through the circulatory system into the coronary arteries.

Radioactive dye is injected into the arteries, and the site of the lesion is pinpointed. A balloon is then inflated at the site of the lesion to push the plaque against the arterial wall. When the balloon is deflated and the catheter removed, improved circulation to the myocardium usually results. During PTCA, a wire mesh tube, called a stent, may be implanted into the coronary artery to keep the artery open.[42]

If a lesion is too diffuse or if an artery reoccludes after PTCA, CABG may be performed. The diseased section of the coronary arteries is bypassed with healthy blood vessels (taken from other parts of the body), thus improving the coronary circulation. In performing CABG, the surgeon usually opens the chest wall by cutting through the sternum (sternotomy) and spreading the ribs to gain access to the heart. Sternal precautions to prevent trauma to the compromised chest are generally in place for 6 to 8 weeks after a sternotomy. Survival rates at 10 years after a CABG vary between 70% and 93% depending on the number of grafts, the sex of the patient, and the vein or artery recruited for the bypass.[9,10]

When heart rhythms are abnormal—too fast, too slow, or too irregular to support normal activity—medical intervention is indicated. Arrhythmias that cannot be controlled with medication may be managed by the insertion of a pacemaker in the chest. Wires are run from the pacemaker to specific spots on the heart. The pacemaker delivers a small electrical impulse to the heart muscle and sets the pace of the heart's electrical conduction. The impulse may be set to deliver a regular impulse or to send an impulse only if the HR drops below a certain number of beats per minute (demand). Modern pacemakers can monitor physiologic responses such as BP and temperature. Implantable cardioverter-defibrillators (ICDs) also may be used to treat cardiac arrhythmias. An ICD can both pace the heart muscle and deliver a high-energy impulse to reset the heart muscle if certain dangerous arrhythmias develop.

Cardiac ablation is a medical procedure used to destroy small areas of the heart that are emitting dangerous signals that cause the heart to contract abnormally. Small catheters are threaded through a vein to the heart. The dysfunctional cardiac tissue is reached, and an electrical impulse is sent to the site, destroying the abnormal tissue.[50]

When the heart's pumping ability has become too compromised by CHF or cardiomyopathy, a heart transplant or heart-lung transplant may be considered. After the healthy tissue of a recently deceased person is harvested, the patient's diseased organ (or organs) is removed, and the harvested tissue is transplanted into the patient's body. Transplant patients are typically maintained on special medication to decrease the risk for organ rejection. Median survival after heart transplant is about 12 years.[26] Most recipients resume normal lifestyles, but only about 40% return to work.[53]

Ventricular assist devices (VADs), total artificial hearts (TAHs), and extracorporeal membrane oxygenation (ECMO) are some life-sustaining therapy options for individuals with end-stage heart failure or for extremely sick persons awaiting heart transplant. ECMO is only used in the ICU and is for patients recovering from heart failure, lung failure, or heart surgery. ECMO is a life support machine that uses a pump to circulate blood outside of the body, through an artificial lung to remove carbon dioxide and oxygenate the blood, before the blood is warmed and returned back to the body.[58] Sometimes it is used as a bridge option to further surgical treatment when doctors want to assess the state of other organs such as the kidneys or the brain before performing heart or lung surgery. ECMO is often used as a short-term bridge to implantation of a left ventricular assist device (LVAD) or as a bridge for patients awaiting heart, lung, or heart and lung transplant. There are two types of ECMO: venoartirial (VA) and venovenous (VV) ECMO. VV ECMO is typically used for respiratory failure, and VA ECMO is typically used for cardiac failure.[4,32]

VADs and TAHs are surgically implanted pumps, with a battery pack worn externally. These devices, referred to as mechanical circulatory supports, allow patients to return home to a more active occupational level while they await a transplant. Nearly 80% of persons using these devices in clinical trials have survived the wait for a new heart.[30] Although many patients undergo VAD implantation as a "bridge to transplant," there are two other treatment pathways for VAD candidates. Patients who do not meet the strict criteria for solid organ transplantation but require advanced therapies for end-stage heart failure may have a LVAD implanted for what is often referred to as "destination therapy." These patients will live out the rest of their lives with the LVAD and will not pursue heart transplantation. If a patient is not eligible for heart transplant at present but may be able to undergo transplantation in the future after demonstrating favorable changes in risk factors such as hypertension, obesity, and or social situation, there is an LVAD pathway referred to as "bridge to decision."[26] In cases that present with significant right ventricular dysfunction and arrythmias, implantation of a total artificial heart as a bridge to transplant may be considered. There are more hospitalizations after LVAD placement than after heart transplantation because patients with LVAD are at high risk for complications, including but not limited to arrythmias, bleeding, stroke, and infection.[18,21,26]

OT intervention often focuses on self-care and leisure activities, providing education and training on adaptive strategies in daily routines and modification of environmental obstacle, facilitating maximal functional independence and quality of life while managing the LVAD. Shower training LVAD patients at some medical centers is a role primarily led by occupational therapists. The median survival after LVAD support is about 7 years.[26]

Valvular stenosis may be managed surgically with valvuloplasty, in which a balloon is inflated in the damaged valve, stretching and breaking up scar tissue, thus opening and restoring blood flow within the heart. Damaged valves may need to be replaced to restore optimal blood flow. A valve replacement may require a sternotomy (opening of the breast bone) or only a small incision, in the case of a transcatheter valve replacement.[2] A sternotomy was performed to replace Joe's valve.

Cardiac Medications

Knowledge of the purpose and side effects of cardiac medication promotes understanding of the patient's response to activity. Table 45.2 lists common cardiac medications.

TABLE 45.2   Common Cardiac Medications

Category	Common Names	Purpose and Uses	Reason Prescribed
Anticoagulants (blood thinners)	Warfarin (Coumadin) Heparin	Decrease the blood's ability to clot	Prevent clot formation or enlargement; prevent stroke
Antiplatelet agents	Aspirin Clopidogrel (Plavix)	Prevent clots by preventing platelets from sticking together	Prevent clots after MI; with unstable angina, ischemic stroke, plaque
Angiotensin-converting enzyme (ACE) inhibitors	Fosinopril (Monopril) Catopril (Capoten) Quinapril (Accupril)	Expand blood vessels, lower levels of angiotensin II; make the heart work more easily	Treatment of: <ul><li>Hypertension</li><li>Heart failure</li></ul>
Angiotensin II receptor blockers (or inhibitors)	Losartan (Cozaar) Irbesartan (Avapro)	Keeps blood pressure from rising by preventing angiotensin II from having an effect on the heart	Treatment of: <ul><li>Hypertension</li><li>Heart failure</li></ul>
Angiotensin-receptor neprilysin inhibitors (ARNIs)	Sacubitril/valsartan (Entresto)	Opens narrow arteries, improves artery opening Improves blood flow Reduces sodium retention Decreases the work of the heart	Treatment of heart failure
β-Blockers	Atenolol (Tenormin) Propranolol (Inderal)	Decreases heart rate and cardiac output, lowers blood pressure, and makes the heart beat more slowly and with less force	Treatment of: <ul><li>Abnormal cardiac rhythms</li><li>Chest pain</li><li>Prevention of recurrent heart attacks</li><li>Lowers blood pressure</li></ul>
Calcium channel blockers	Amlodipine (Norvasc, Lotrel) Diltiazem (Cardizem, Tiazac)	Interrupt movement of calcium into cells of the heart and blood vessels	Used to treat high blood pressure, angina, and some arrhythmias
Cholesterol lowering medications	Statins (Lipitor) (Crestor) Nicotinic Acids: (Advicor) Cholestero Absorption Inhibitors: (Vytorin)	Lower blood cholostrol levels	Lowers LDL
Digitalis preparations	Digoxin (Lanoxin)	Increase the force of cardiac contractions	Treatment of: <ul><li>Heart failure</li><li>Arrhythmias</li><li>Atrial fibrillation</li></ul>
Diuretics (water pills)	Furosemide (Lasix) Hydroclorothiazide (Esidrix, HydroDIURIL)	Cause loss of excess water and sodium by urination, thus relieving heart workload and buildup of fluid in lungs and body tissues	Lower blood pressure; reduce edema in lungs, stomach, and extremities
Vasodilators	Nitroglycerin Minoxidil	Relax blood vessels; increase supply of blood and oxygen to the heart while reducing its workload	Ease chest pain

HDL, High-density lipoprotein; *LDL,* low-density lipoprotein; *MI,* myocardial infarction.
Data from Kizior RJ, Hodgson KJ: *Saunders nursing drug handbook 2025,* St Louis, 2025, Elsevier; Benisek A: *Common heart disease medications,* 2023, https://www.webmd.com/heart-disease/heart-disease-medications; Mandal A: *Cardiovascular drugs,* 2023, https://www.news-medical.net/health/Cardiovascular-Drugs.aspx.

Psychosocial Considerations

Depression, anger, anxiety disorders, and social isolation are common in individuals receiving cardiac rehabilitation. Improvement in event-free survival for persons receiving treatment for these problems was not found to have improved survival versus an untreated control group. However, the treated individual in a large randomized multicenter trial improved in socialization and mood compared with the control group.[5] "Nevertheless, even if psychosocial interventions ultimately are shown not to alter the prognosis of CHF patients, they remain an integral part of cardiac rehabilitation services to improve the psychological well-being and quality of life of cardiac patients."[37]

As patients begin to resume more normal activities, such as self-care and walking around the ward, feelings of helplessness may begin to subside. Patients feel more secure when familiar coping mechanisms allow them to respond to the stress, but some former coping mechanisms (e.g., smoking, drinking, consuming fatty foods) are harmful and should be discouraged and replaced by newly learned coping strategies, often those taught by the occupational therapist and other members of the intervention team. Typically, the nutritionist directs the patient toward healthy food choices, the physical therapist provides guidance toward exercise, and the nurse oversees management of medications.

Denial is common in patients with cardiac disease. Patients in denial must be closely monitored during the acute phase of recovery. Persons in denial may ignore all precautions and could stress and further damage their cardiovascular systems. Clinical evidence supports psychosocial counseling after MI that focuses on improving self health appraisal, improving social support, and establishing an effective means of coping to improve quality of life.[67] The patient's family must be included in the education so that their misconceptions and anxieties do not compound the patient's fears. In Joe's case, his wife's anxiety that she might accidentally harm him or that he might harm himself and Joe's concern that his wife is avoiding intimacy and self-identified barrier of alcohol consumption should be addressed in his intervention plan.

Depression and lack of social support adversely affect persons with CHF and need to be addressed.[62] Quality of life is affected by sense of control and perception of symptoms at hospital discharge in persons with heart disease as much as 3 years after a cardiac event.[36] Patients' perceptions of their illness can have an impact on their ability to make the changes in lifestyle necessary for healthy living after an acute coronary event. Occupational therapists' understanding of patient factors, specifically values, beliefs, and spirituality, can help the healthcare team better understand the uniqueness of each individual and positively affect recovery.

Cardiac Rehabilitation

During the first 1 to 3 days after MI, stabilization of the patient's medical condition is usually attained. This acute phase is followed by a period of early mobilization. Phase 1 of treatment, inpatient cardiac rehabilitation, includes monitored low-level physical activity, including self-care; reinforcement of cardiac and postsurgical precautions; instruction in energy conservation and graded activity; and establishment of guidelines for appropriate activity levels at discharge. Through monitored activity, the ill effects of prolonged inactivity can be averted while medical problems, poor responses to medications, and atypical chest pain can be addressed (Table 45.3).

Phase 2 of treatment, outpatient cardiac rehabilitation, usually begins at discharge. During this phase, exercise can be advanced while the patient is closely monitored on an outpatient basis. Community-based exercise programs follow in phase 3. Some individuals require treatment in their place of residence because they are not strong enough to tolerate outpatient therapy.

There is a strong base of clinical evidence that cardiac rehabilitation improves survival and quality of life and reduces the cost of medical care in the long run.[28] This has led the Center for Medicare and Medicaid Services to expand the indications for cardiac rehabilitation programs.[75] These physician-directed, exercise-based programs include regular monitored exercise, lifestyle modification, and medical therapy. Individuals are taught how to monitor their response to activity and what to do in the event of an adverse response.

The Borg Rate of Perceived Exertion Scale (Box 45.1) is a tool used to measure perceived exertion. The patient is shown the scale before an activity and instructed that a rating of 6 means no exertion at all and a rating of 19 indicates extremely strenuous activity, equal to the most strenuous activity that the patient has ever performed. After the activity has been completed, the patient is asked to appraise his or her feelings of exertion as accurately as possible and give the activity a rating.

TABLE 45.3 Signs and Symptoms of Cardiac Distress

Sign/Symptom	What to Look For
Angina	Look for chest pain that may be described as squeezing, tightness, aching, burning, or choking. Pain is generally substernal and may radiate to the arms, jaw, neck, or back. More intense or longer-lasting pain forewarns of greater ischemia.
Dyspnea	Look for shortness of breath with activity or at rest. Note the activity that brought on the dyspnea and the amount of time that it takes to resolve. Dyspnea at rest with a resting respiratory rate of greater than 30 breaths per minute is a sign of acute congestive heart failure. The patient may require emergency medical help.
Orthopnea	Look for dyspnea brought on by lying supine. Count the number of pillows that the patient needs to breathe comfortably during sleep (1, 2, 3, or 4 pillows needed to relieve orthopnea).
Nausea/emesis	Look for vomiting or signs that the patient feels sick to the stomach.
Diaphoresis	Look for cold, clammy sweat.
Fatigue	Look for a generalized feeling of exhaustion. The Borg Rate of Perceived Exertion Scale is a tool used to grade fatigue (see Box 45.1). Cerebral signs—ataxia, dizziness, confusion, and fainting (syncope)—are all signs that the brain is not getting enough oxygen.
Orthostatic	Look for a drop in systolic blood pressure and hypotension of greater than 10 mm Hg with a change in position from supine to sitting or sitting to standing.

Sternal Precautions

Sternal precautions vary widely among hospitals, surgeons, and therapy departments. This is likely because they were developed on anecdotal and indirect evidence. Commonly observed sternal precautions often include the following criteria: do not lift, push, or pull more than 5 to 10 lb; do not push or pull with arms when getting in and out of bed or up from a chair; do not bring elbows above shoulders; do not twist the trunk or do deep bending; hug a pillow to splint the chest when coughing or sneezing; and do not drive for 4 weeks or until cleared by surgeon. Concern has been expressed in the literature that sternal precautions that are too restrictive might interfere with long-term functional outcomes and that individualized precautions based on surgical closure techniques and individual patient profiles would yield an improved functional outcome.[11]

Studies have investigated less restrictive approaches that allow any unrestricted, unweighted arm movement provided there is no increase in pain or instability of the sternum (popping, cracking sounds or sensations of a moving sternum).[1,7] Load-bearing activities are allowed through the arms as long as the patient keeps the elbows against the body. Patients are encouraged to

BOX 45.1   Instructions for Using the Borg Rate of Perceived Exertion Scale

During the work we want you to rate your perception of exertion (i.e., how heavy and strenuous the exercise feels to you and how tired you are). The perception of exertion is felt mainly as strain and fatigue in your muscles and as breathlessness or aches in the chest. All work requires some effort, even if only minimal. This is also true if you move only a little (e.g., walking slowly).

Use this scale from 6 to 20, with 6 meaning "no exertion at all" and 20 meaning "maximal exertion."

6—"No exertion at all" means that you don't feel any exertion whatsoever (e.g., no muscle fatigue, breathlessness, or difficulty breathing).

9—"Very light" exertion, such as taking a shorter walk at your own pace.

13—A "somewhat hard" work, but it still feels okay to continue.

15—It is "hard" and tiring, but continuing isn't terribly difficult.

17—"Very hard." This is very strenuous work. You can still go on, but you really have to push yourself and you are very tired.

19—An "extremely" strenuous level. For most people this is the most strenuous work that they have ever experienced.

Try to appraise your feeling of exertion and fatigue as spontaneously and as honestly as possible without thinking about what the actual physical load is. Try to not underestimate and to not overestimate your exertion. It's your own feeling of effort and exertion that is important, not how this compares with other people. Look at the scale and the expressions and then give a number. Use any number you like on the scale, not just one of those with an explanation behind it.

---

continue to protect the sternum by splinting it with a pillow during coughing or sneezing.[31] Studies have found that there were no statistically significant differences in wound healing problems, use of pain medications, or antibiotic between the commonly used sternal precautions and the less restrictive version.[1,7,31,56]

Occupational therapists play a key role in assessing and educating individuals on sternal precautions. Engagement of patients in functional activity frequently will challenge individuals to maintain precautions while engaged in an ADL. Therapists need to assess factors that interfere with the individual's ability to adhere to the precautions and subsequently make suggestions for modification to education and recommendations for discharge. Cognitive impairments can limit one's ability to comply and may be temporary if influenced by medication or, of more long-term concern, if underlying conditions such as dementia are present. Given the potential for neurological events such as cerebrovascular accident (CVA) or transient ischemic attack (TIA) after surgery, the therapist may be the first to observe deficits from such events, which may appear as a lack of ability to comply with precautions.[76]

Monitoring Response to Activity

When the patient's response to an activity is being assessed, symptoms provide one indication that the patient is or is not tolerating the activity. HR, BP, rate-pressure product (RPP), and ECG readings are other measures that may be used to evaluate the cardiovascular system's response to work.

Heart Rate

Heart rate (HR), or the number of beats per minute, can be monitored by feeling the patient's pulse at the radial, brachial,

or carotid sites. The radial pulse is located on the volar surface of the wrist, just lateral to the head of the radius. The brachial pulse is found in the antecubital fossa, slightly medial to the midline of the forearm. The carotid pulse, located on the neck lateral to the Adam's apple, should be palpated gently; if overstimulated, it can cause the HR to drop below 60 beats per minute (bradycardia). To determine HR, the clinician applies the second and third fingers (flat, not with the tips) to the pulse site. If the pulse is even (regular), the clinician counts the number of beats in 10 seconds and multiplies the finding by 6. The thumb should never be used to take a pulse because it has its own pulse.

All clinicians who assess HR, as well as the patient, should be able to note the evenness (regularity) of the heartbeat. HR can be regular or irregular. An irregular heartbeat may be described as regularly irregular, which means that there is a consistent irregular pattern (e.g., every third beat is premature), or it may be described as irregularly irregular, which means that there is no pattern to the premature or skipped beats. HR irregularities include skipped beats, delayed beats, premature beats, and beats originating from outside the normal conduction pathway in the heart. Although an irregular HR is not normal, many individuals function quite well with an irregular rate. Clinicians should note the patient's normal rate pattern, as well as any variations. The therapist evaluating a patient for the first time should compare his or her observations about HR and regularity with the patient's record. A sudden change in HR from regular to irregular should be reported to the physician. An ECG or other diagnostic test may be ordered on the basis of such findings. When the HR is irregular, the number of beats should be counted for a full minute. Patients can be taught to take their own pulse and monitor the response of HR to activity. As a general rule, HR should rise in response to activity.

Blood Pressure

BP is the pressure that the blood exerts against the walls of any vessel as the heart beats. It is highest in the left ventricle during systole and decreases in the arterial system with distance from the heart.[73] A stethoscope and BP cuff (sphygmomanometer) are used to indirectly determine BP. The BP cuff is placed snugly (but not tightly) around the upper part of the patient's arm just above the elbow, with the bladder of the cuff centered above the brachial artery. The examiner inflates the cuff while palpating the brachial artery to 20 mm Hg above the point at which the brachial pulse is last felt. With the earpieces of the stethoscope angled forward in the examiner's ears, the dome of the stethoscope is placed over the patient's brachial artery. Supporting the patient's arm in extension with the pulse point of the brachial artery and the gauge of the stethoscope at the patient's heart level, the examiner deflates the cuff at a rate of approximately 2 mm Hg per second. Listening is imperative when recording BP. The first two sounds heard correspond to SBP. The examiner continues to listen until the last pulse is heard and DBP is attained.

Physicians usually indicate treatment parameters for the HR and BP of patients in medical facilities. Parameters are frequently written in abbreviations, such as "Call HO if SBP > 150

< 90; DBP > 90 < 60; HR > 120 < 60." (In other words, "Call the house officer or physician on call if SBP is greater than 150 or less than 90, if DBP is greater than 90 or less than 60, and if HR is greater than 120 or less than 60.").

HR and BP will fluctuate in response to activity, and cardiac output is affected by both HR and BP. Measurement of the RPP (measurement of the workload or oxygen demand) can give a more accurate indication of how well the heart is pumping. The RPP is the product of HR and SBP (RPP = HR × SBP). It is usually a 5-digit number but is reported in 3 digits by dropping the last 2 (e.g., HR 100 × SBP 120 = 12,000 = RPP 120). During any activity, the RPP should rise at peak and return to baseline in recovery (after 5 to 10 minutes of rest).

Correctly reading and interpreting an ECG is a skill that requires hours of learning and practice for proficiency. Electrocardiography is not available in most nonacute settings. The reader is referred to Dubin's *Rapid Interpretation of EKGs*,[16] which is an excellent resource for persons unfamiliar with the subject.

There are many similarities in the evaluation and treatment of persons with cardiac disease and those with pulmonary dysfunction. A review of the pulmonary system and its disease processes follows.

THREADED CASE STUDY

Harriet, Part 1

Harriet is a 64-year-old widow and mother of an adult daughter. She retired 3 years ago from her housekeeping job because of fatigue and shortness of breath. Chronic obstructive pulmonary disease (COPD) was diagnosed at that time. She has been smoking cigarettes since the age of 20 and currently smokes one pack per day. She shares a small one-bedroom apartment with her terrier Sir Filo. There is a first-floor laundry room in her building. Harriet's daughter lives three blocks away and checks on her mother daily. Harriet's baseline level of function 4 weeks ago consisted of walking the dog around the block slowly, fixing meals, doing laundry, and performing ADLs independently. She also enjoys playing bingo on Tuesday nights at her local church and cards with her widowers and widows group. Her daughter assists her in grocery shopping and cleaning.

Harriet was released from the acute care hospital 3 days ago, with her condition having stabilized after an acute exacerbation of her COPD. Since her recent discharge, her daughter empties Harriet's bedside commode, shops for groceries, and fixes dinner for Harriet and Sir Filo. Results of the occupational therapy evaluation indicated that Harriet became short of breath when combing her hair. She was unable to pace her activity, to coordinate pursed-lip breathing with activity, or to assume dyspnea control postures when needed. She was receiving 2 L of oxygen by nasal cannula at all times. Harriet wants to be able to feed Sir Filo herself, stating that dogs become attached to people who feed them. She does not want her daughter to empty her commode and wants to be able to prepare dinner for herself. She does not want to be a burden to her daughter but rather to enjoy visiting with her.

Critical Thinking Questions
1. What goals may Harriet find relevant in her therapy?
2. What safety concerns might arise?
3. Do Harriet's goals appear realistic given her baseline level of function?

ANATOMY AND PHYSIOLOGY OF RESPIRATION[6,45,47,59]

The heart provides oxygen-rich blood to the body and transports carbon dioxide and other waste products to the lungs, and the respiratory system exchanges oxygen for carbon dioxide. The cardiac and pulmonary systems are interdependent. If no oxygen were delivered to the bloodstream, the heart would soon stop functioning for lack of oxygen; conversely, if the heart were to stop pumping, the lungs would cease functioning for lack of a blood supply. All body tissues depend on the cardiopulmonary system for their nutrients.

The respiratory system supplies oxygen to the blood and removes waste products, primarily carbon dioxide, from the blood. Air enters the body via the nose and mouth and travels through the nasopharynx to the larynx or voice box. From there, the air continues downward into the lungs by way of the trachea or windpipe. The trachea consists of ribbed cartilage approximately 10 cm long. When the trachea or pharynx becomes blocked, a small incision may be made in the trachea to allow air to pass freely into the lungs. This procedure is called a tracheotomy.

The trachea divides into two main bronchi that carry air into the left and right lungs. The bronchi continue to branch off into smaller tubes, called bronchioles. Bronchioles are segmented into smaller passages called the alveolar ducts. Each alveolar duct is divided and leads into three or more alveolar sacs. The entire respiratory passageway from bronchi to alveolar sacs is often referred to as "the pulmonary tree" because its structure is much like that of an upside-down tree, with the alveolar sacs representing the leaves.

Each alveolar sac contains more than 10 alveoli. A very fine, semipermeable membrane separates the alveolus from the capillary network. Across this membrane, oxygen is transported and exchanged for carbon dioxide. Carbon dioxide is exhaled into the air after traveling upward through the "pulmonary tree" (Fig. 45.4).

With the exception of the nose and mouth, all the airways are lined with cilia and coated with mucus. Mucus and cilia provide a filtering shield that protects the fragile airway respiratory structures from dust and germs.

The musculature of the thorax helps in inspiration and expiration. During inspiration, the muscle power for breathing air into the lungs is provided primarily by the diaphragm.[59] Originating from the sternum, ribs, lumbar vertebrae, and lumbocostal arches, the diaphragm forms the inferior border of the thorax. The muscle fibers of the diaphragm insert into a central tendon. Innervated by the left and right phrenic nerves, the diaphragm contracts and domes downward when stimulated. This downward doming of the diaphragm enlarges the volume of the thorax and causes a drop in pressure in the lungs relative to the air in the environment. Air then enters the lungs to equalize inside and outside pressure.[59] Accessory muscles, the intercostals and scalenes, are also active during inspiration. The intercostals maintain alignment of the ribs, and the scalene helps elevate the rib cage.[45]

At rest, expiration is primarily a passive relaxation of the inspiratory musculature. The lungs help draw the thorax inward

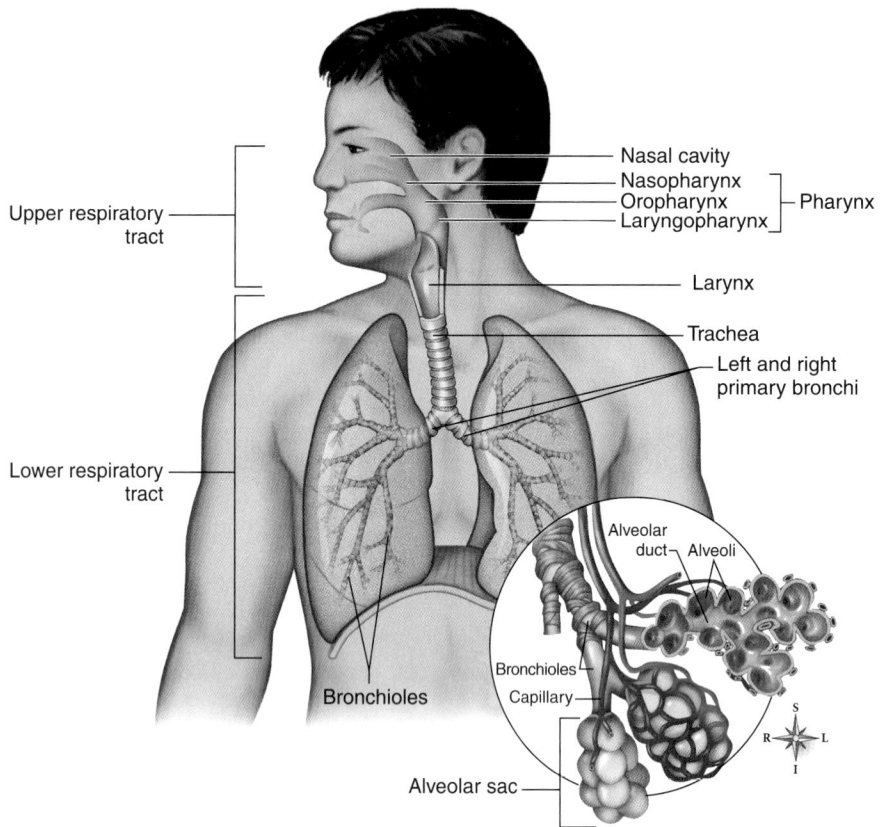

Fig. 45.4 Major structures of the respiratory system. (From Patton KT, Thibodeau GA: *The human body in health and disease,* ed 7, St Louis, 2018, Elsevier.)

as the inspiratory muscles relax. Forced expiration requires active contraction of the abdominal muscles to compress the viscera and squeeze the diaphragm upward in the thorax. Expiration can be further forced by flexing the torso forward and pressing with the arms on the chest or abdomen. As the volume of the thorax decreases, air is forced out of the lungs. Accessory muscles in the neck and collarbone region can be recruited to assist in respiration when lung disease is active or other respiratory musculature is impaired.

INNERVATION OF THE RESPIRATORY SYSTEM

Breathing is mostly involuntary. A person does not have to think to take a breath. The autonomic nervous system has control over breathing. With anxiety and increased activity, the sympathetic nervous system will automatically increase the depth and rate of inspiration.

Inspiration and expiration have a volitional component. Volitional control allows us to control our breathing as we swim and to play the harmonica. Additionally, receptors within and outside the lungs can, when stimulated, cause changes in the depth and rate of breathing. Although the pons, medulla, and other parts of the brain provide the central control for breathing, they adjust their response to input from receptors in the lungs, the aorta, and the carotid artery.

CHRONIC LUNG DISEASE

Occupational therapy is frequently prescribed for individuals with chronic lung conditions that functionally affect their ability to participate in their usual occupations. Persons with chronic obstructive pulmonary disease (COPD), sarcoidosis, asthma, idiopathic pulmonary fibrosis, or cystic fibrosis may benefit from learning better ways to breathe and to conserve their energy. COPD includes two primary medical conditions: emphysema and chronic bronchitis. The air sacs of the lungs (alveoli) are damaged, lose their elasticity, and may become clogged with mucus.[34a,41,43,51,57] It becomes harder to breathe, and as the disease progresses individuals experience a decrease in their IADL and ADL abilities. COPD is not curable, and the damage caused by the disease is irreversible. With medical management and lifestyle changes, the disease progression can be slowed and ability to participate in occupations can improve.

Emphysema is a medical condition in which the alveoli are gradually damaged. Although cigarette smoking is the leading cause of emphysema,[43] airborne irritants such as air pollution, marijuana smoke, and particles produced in manufacturing are contributing causes. Persons with chronic bronchitis experience shortness of breath (dyspnea) on exertion, and as the disease progresses, dyspnea occurs at rest.

In bronchitis the bronchial airway becomes inflamed, leading to increased mucus production, cough, and airway obstructions. When the airway is constantly irritated a chronic cough with mucus results. Smoking is the major contributing cause of chronic bronchitis. Persons with chronic bronchitis are prone to upper respiratory tract infections causing a worsening of their disease process. Persons with severe chronic bronchitis are unlikely to recover fully.

Inflammation, fibrosis (thickening of the connective tissue), and narrowing of the terminal airways of the lungs are physiological changes that occur with peripheral airway disease. Smoking and other environmental pollutants irritate the airways, which leads to the development of abnormal terminal airways. Coughing and spitting up mucus from the lungs are common clinical manifestations of this disorder. The disease process may never progress beyond this initial phase, or it may evolve into emphysema and full-fledged COPD.[34a,41,43,51]

Asthma is characterized by irritability of the bronchotracheal tree and is typically episodic in onset.[49] Persons with asthma experience wheezing and shortness of breath that may resolve spontaneously or necessitate the use of medication for calming the airway. Persons with asthma may be free of symptoms for periods between the episodes of wheezing and dyspnea. Some individuals appear to have a genetic predisposition to asthma. Allergenic causes of asthma may include pollen and respiratory irritants such as perfume, dust, and cleaning agents. Bronchospasm occurring with exposure to cold air or induced by exercise is sometimes the first clinical manifestations of asthma. Irritation of the airway leads to narrowing of the air passages and interferes with ventilation of the alveolar sacs. If left untreated, a severe asthmatic episode may result in death. Persons with severe asthma may be referred to occupational therapy to address declining ADL function.

Idiopathic pulmonary fibrosis (IPF) is the most common type of idiopathic interstitial pneumonia and is defined as a spontaneously occurring (idiopathic) specific form of chronic fibrosing interstitial pneumonia. Most cases of IPF are sporadic; familial cases have been found but tend to present at a younger age then typical IPF.[70] Patients with IPF typically present at age 60 and older, men appear to be affected more often than women, and the majority of patients have a history of cigarette smoking, gastroesophageal reflux, occupational and/or environmental exposure to specific agents. Patients commonly report a gradual onset of dyspnea on exertion and nonproductive cough over several months that may precede diagnosis by 1 to 2 years. During this time IPF is frequently misdiagnosed, often leading to late access to treatment.[71] The natural course of IPF is highly variable and unpredictable, with some patients demonstrating a slow functional decline and others demonstrating a rapid decline leading to death.[33] The diagnostic process of interstitial lung disease is complex; therefore, patients are evaluated together with experts in a multidisciplinary approach with pulmonologists, radiologists, and pathologists. In addition to pharmacological treatment, nonpharmacological treatment may include pulmonary rehabilitation, lung transplantation, and palliative intervention.[71] Unfortunately, the progressive lung function impairment associated with IPF is fatal without lung transplantation, because no curative pharmacological treatment exists at this time.[38] Occupational therapists may be consulted at any stage in a patient's course of the disease to assess and help facilitate safe resumption of participation in ADLs and other occupations with applied energy conservation and effective adaptive strategies.

Lung transplantation has become a viable treatment option for patients with a variety of end-stage lung diseases.[27] The most common diseases that lead to lung transplant are interstitial lung disease, including IPF, COPD, and cystic fibrosis.[27] Since 2005 the order of patients on a waiting list for lung transplantation has been based on a Lung Allocation Score that was developed to address high waiting list mortality and progressively earlier placement of patients on the waiting list.[24] Patients with untreatable, advanced-stage lung disease are referred to a regional transplant center for evaluation.

The transplant centers thoroughly evaluate patients to determine the appropriateness of placing them on a transplant waiting list and to collect the information from which lung allocation score is derived.[29] A single lung transplant is a faster and easier to perform surgical procedure than double lung transplant and is associated with lower perioperative mortality and morbidity. However, better long-term survival and less chronic lung allograft dysfunction have been reported with double lung transplant.[38] Surgical approaches to single lung transplant and double lung transplant may vary according to surgeon preference and clinical judgment, but the standard approach many surgeons will employ is through a transverse thoracosternotomy (clamshell incision), typically through the fourth intercostal space. Two alternative surgical approaches to bilateral lung transplant are median sternotomy and bilateral anterior thoracotomies.[29] Both clamshell and median sternotomy patients will have sternal precautions postoperatively. All patients who have undergone lung transplantation require immunosuppressive therapy to prevent allograft dysfunction. This subsequently puts this patient population at high risk for developing infection and in addition to the pharmacological prophylactic therapies. A common practice found in the hospital is for transplant patients to wear masks (N99, P100 rated) in shared areas and common spaces.

Patients with advanced lung disease often show cognitive impairment possibly due to hypoxia and hypercapnia associated with lung disease.[76] An observational cohort study conducted in Germany found that most lung transplant recipients have a cognitive impairment in visual memory, concentration, speed of processing/attention, and or executive functioning. Verbal memory and executive functioning were the two most commonly affected domains. In the patients with two domains impaired, all patients had impairment in executive functioning. When three domains showed impairments, lung transplant recipients most often showed impairment in concentration, speed of processing/attention followed by verbal memory and then executive functioning. Less than a quarter of participants performed within their age range on these tests.[68]

OT PRACTICE NOTE

The OT practitioner may use various assessment tools to further assess the patient factor of cognition and provide appropriate and effective interventions to help facilitate successful engagement in occupation.

PULMONARY RISK FACTORS

Smokers are 12 times more likely to die from COPD than non-smokers.[72] Cigarette smoking also causes emphysema and chronic bronchitis.[43] Clinical manifestations of the respiratory disease increase as the pack-year history increases. Pack-year history is calculated by multiplying the number of packs of cigarettes consumed per day by the number of years of smoking. A person who started smoking at the age of 20 and is now 64 has a pack-year history of 44 (64 − 20 = 44 × 1 pack/yr = 44 pack-years). Because cigarette smoke is a pulmonary irritant, it can also be a causative agent in asthmatic episodes.[72] Other environmental irritants, such as air pollution, chemical exposure, and dust, are contributory risk factors in the development of COPD and asthma.

MEDICAL MANAGEMENT

COPD is a progressive, chronic disease. The onset of the disease is insidious. When patients initially seek medical attention, they are frequently seen in a physician's clinic rather than at a medical center. Besides evaluating the patient's medical history and symptoms and performing a physical examination, the physician will assess the patient's history of smoking and occupational exposure to respiratory irritants. Blood work and an x-ray examination will be performed to further assess the patient's clinical status. Most people with COPD take medication every day. Medications prescribed include antiinflammatory agents (e.g., steroids and cromolyn sodium), bronchodilators (e.g., albuterol and theophylline) to help open the airway, and expectorants (e.g., iodides and guaifenesin) to help loosen and clear mucus. Flu shots and pneumonococcal vaccines are recommended. Oxygen therapy also may be prescribed at a specific flow rate. Occasionally, persons receiving oxygen therapy may be tempted to increase the liter-per-minute flow in the erroneous thinking that more is better. This can result in retention of carbon dioxide and lead to failure of the right side of the heart.

Persons in acute respiratory distress may initially be managed with a ventilator before being weaned to oxygen. Ventilators provide mechanical assistance to the process of inspiration and do not increase the number of healthy alveolar sacs. Ventilators will not slow the end-stage disease process of COPD, but mechanical ventilation is recommended for patients with acute exacerbation of COPD because mortality from respiratory failure is much lower than mortality from other causes in patients with COPD.[55]

Pulmonary rehabilitation is a multidisciplinary, comprehensive program tailored to the individual needs of each recipient. Psychological, emotional, physical, and emotional problems are addressed. The physician-directed team may include nurses, respiratory therapists, physical therapists, occupational therapists, psychologists, and others with relevant skill sets. Pulmonary rehabilitation improves dyspnea symptoms in persons with COPD, reduces the number of hospital days, and results in efficacious use of medical services.[63]

OT PRACTICE NOTES

Frequently, the occupational therapist's role in treating patients with COPD involves salvage rather than prevention of the disease process. Earlier intervention by an occupational therapist is critical for prevention of disease.

Signs and Symptoms of Respiratory Distress

Dyspnea is probably the most obvious sign of breathing difficulty. In the most severe form of dyspnea, the patient is short of breath even at rest. Patients with this level of dyspnea are unable to utter a short phrase without gasping for air. When reporting that a patient has dyspnea, the practitioner should note the precipitating factors and associated circumstances; for example, "Harriet becomes short of breath when washing her face while seated in front of the sink."

Other signs that the body is not getting enough oxygen include extreme fatigue, a nonproductive cough, confusion, impaired judgment, and cyanosis (bluish skin color caused by insufficient oxygen in the blood).

Psychosocial Considerations

Because COPD is a progressive, debilitating physical illness, it is not surprising that the psychosocial effects of the disease are considerable. Chan identified five themes related to barriers preventing engagement in occupation for people with COPD: uncertainty about progression of the disease, attributing the cause of the disease to external factors, progressing restriction in activity and isolation, anxiety and depression, and passive acceptance.[8,12] For persons with COPD, anxiety and depression are most strongly linked to decreased exercise capacity and shortness of breath.[64] Training in progressive muscle relaxation can be a successful tool for controlling the dyspnea and anxiety and for lowering the HR.[12,61]

Most cardiac and respiratory disease processes are preventable. Individuals with these diseases may lack basic skills in coping and setting limits with themselves or with others. The therapist's role includes encouraging the patient to engage in activities that will develop his or her skills and promoting resumption of occupations that bring value, meaning, and participation back into the patient's life. With these skills, the patient begins to see himself or herself as a person actively making choices to get better. By working with Harriet on ways to engage with her dog when she does not have the endurance to take a walk, the OT not only teaches energy conservation but also conveys this information in a meaningful manner to the patient.

Pulmonary Rehabilitation

The goal of pulmonary rehabilitation is to stabilize or reverse the disease process and return the patient's function and participation in activity/occupation to the highest capacity. A multidisciplinary rehabilitation team working with the patient can design an individualized intervention program to meet this end. Accurate diagnosis, medical management, therapy, education, and emotional support are components of a pulmonary rehabilitation program. Occupational therapy personnel are frequently part of the patient's team, which is headed by the patient and also includes the physician, nurse, and the patient's family and social supports. Respiratory therapists, dietitians, PTs, social workers, and psychologists also may be team members. Roles of team members vary slightly among facilities. Knowledge of specialized pulmonary treatment techniques is imperative for each team member when treating persons with pulmonary disease.

Recognized pulmonary rehabilitation guidelines state that both low- and high-intensity exercises are beneficial, although higher intensity is better. Arm exercises should be unsupported (active motion with no outside assistance), against gravity and with and without resistance; leg exercise should be included. Supplemental oxygen is helpful during rehabilitation exercise.[63] The occupational therapist should apply these guidelines during ADLs training. By continuing to maintain the higher level of activity gained in a pulmonary rehabilitation program, individuals can have sustained benefit from the program for years.

Intervention Techniques

Dyspnea control postures. Adopting certain postures can improve dyspnea. Body positions that increase abdominal pressure may improve the condition of the respiratory muscles and their function. Leaning forward has been reported to reduce recruitment of accessory muscles, improve diaphragm participation, improve overall inspiratory muscle strength, and reduce dyspnea in COPD.[15,17,59] In a seated position, the patient bends forward slightly at the waist while supporting the upper part of the body by leaning the forearms on a table or the thighs. In a standing position, relief may be obtained by leaning forward and propping oneself on a counter or shopping cart.[15]

Pursed-lip breathing. Pursed-lip breathing (PLB) is thought to prevent tightness in the airway by providing resistance to expiration. PLB improves air movement, releasing trapped air in the lungs and helps to keep the airways open. Persons with COPD sometimes instinctively adopt this technique, whereas others may need to be taught it. Instructions for PLB are as follows:

1. Relax your neck and shoulder muscles.
2. Inhale slowly through the nose for a count of two.
3. Purse the lips as if to whistle.
4. Exhale—slowly, to a count of 4—through pursed lips as if trying to make a candle flicker without blowing it out.

Pursed lip breathing should be used when bending, lifting, or stair climbing.[6]

Diaphragmatic breathing. Another breathing pattern, which calls for increased use of the diaphragm to improve chest volume, is diaphragmatic breathing. Many persons learn this technique by placing a small paperback novel on the abdomen just below the xiphoid process (base of the sternum or breastbone). The novel provides a visual cue for diaphragmatic movement. The patient lies supine and is instructed to inhale slowly and make the book rise. Exhalation through pursed lips should cause the book to fall.[15]

Relaxation. Progressive muscle relaxation in conjunction with breathing exercises can be effective in decreasing anxiety and controlling shortness of breath. One technique involves tensing muscle groups while slowly inhaling and then relaxing the muscle groups while exhaling twice as slowly through pursed lips. It is helpful to teach the patient a sequence of muscle groups to tense and relax. One common sequence involves tensing and relaxing first the face; followed by the face and the neck; then the face, neck, and shoulders; and so on, down the body to the toes. A calm, quiet, and comfortable environment is important for the novice in learning any relaxation technique.

Other treatments and considerations. PTs are generally called on to instruct patients in chest expansion exercises, a series of exercises intended to increase the flexibility of the chest. Percussion and postural drainage use gravity and gentle drumming on the patient's back to loosen secretions and help drain the secretions from the lungs. By isometrically contracting the arms and hands while they are placed on the patient's thorax, the therapist may transmit vibration to the patient. Vibration is performed during the expiratory phase of breathing and helps loosen secretions. Percussion and postural drainage may, however, be contraindicated in acutely ill patients and those who are medically unstable.

Humidity, pollution, extremes of temperature, and stagnant air have deleterious effects on persons with respiratory ailments. The therapist and patient should take these factors into consideration when planning activity.

Migliore's guidelines for the management of dyspnea provide a clinical progression and direction for the integration of dyspnea control techniques with progression of activity.[46]

Individuals with chronic respiratory or cardiovascular limitations are frequently restricted in their ability to perform ADLs. Occupational therapy intervention can promote improvements in the patient's life management skills and quality of life.

EVALUATION

Review of the Medical Record

A review of the medical record will identify the patient's medical history (diagnosis, severity, associated conditions, and secondary diagnoses), social history, test results, medications, and precautions.

Patient Interview

It is common courtesy and good medical practice to begin every encounter with a patient by introducing oneself and explaining the purpose of the evaluation or intervention. Good interviewing skills, including asking the right questions, listening to the patient's response, and observing the patient while responding, are considered integral aspects of the therapeutic use of self. Thoughtful, probing questions will help the patient and therapist identify areas of concern and lay the groundwork for establishing mutually agreeable goals. The therapist should observe the patient for signs of anxiety, shortness of breath, confusion, difficulty comprehending, fatigue, abnormal posture, reduced endurance, reduced ability to move, and stressful family dynamics. Interview questions should not only seek clarification of information that was unclear in the medical record but also clarify the patient's understanding of his or her condition and treatment.

A patient with a history of angina should be asked to describe what the angina feels like. If the patient has also had an MI, the patient should be asked whether he or she can differentiate between the angina and the MI chest pain. Clarification of symptoms before treatment can prove invaluable should symptoms arise. What clarifying questions might the therapist ask in the evaluation of Joe or Harriet?

Asking patients to describe a typical day, to identify activities that bring on shortness of breath or angina, and to tell how their physical limitations interfere with the activities or occupations that they need to do or most enjoy doing will reveal problems that are meaningful and relevant to the patient.

Clinical Evaluation

The purpose of clinical assessment is to establish the patient's present functional ability and limitations. The content of an occupational therapist's clinical evaluation will vary from patient to patient and from setting to setting. Patients with impairments in the cardiovascular system will require monitoring of HR, BP, signs and symptoms of cardiac distress, and possibly ECG readings during an assessment of tolerance to postural changes and during a functional task. Table 45.4 provides a summary of appropriate versus inappropriate responses to activity. Individuals with disorders involving the respiratory system should be monitored closely for signs and symptoms of respiratory distress. If an oxygen saturation monitor is available, the patient's range of motion, strength, and sensation may be grossly assessed within the context of the ADL assessment. The patient's cognitive and psychosocial status will become apparent to a skilled clinician via interview and observation.

After completing the evaluation, the clinician has sufficient information to formulate an intervention plan. In establishing the intervention goals and objectives, the clinician verifies that the patient agrees with the intervention plans and projected outcome. At this point it is helpful to assess the patient's perspective on barriers to attaining the goals identified. Asking "what might prevent you from being successful in . . . ?" can yield unexpected information and identify other areas of concern. The occupational therapist discovered Joe's possible alcohol dependence by using such a probative question.

INTERVENTION

Patient goals, present clinical status, recent occupational performance history, response to current activities and occupations, and prognosis all help guide the progression of intervention for persons with cardiovascular or respiratory impairment. Patients with significant cardiac or pulmonary impairment, limited recent ability to participate in occupation, inappropriate responses to activities and occupations or orthostatic change, and a poor prognosis will progress very slowly. Individuals with little impairment of the heart or lungs, a recent history of normal occupational performance, appropriate responses to orthostatic change and activities and occupations, and a good prognosis will progress rapidly by comparison.

Progression and Energy Costs

The energy costs of an activity or occupation and the factors that influence energy costs can further guide the clinician in the safe progression of activity or participation in occupation. Oxygen consumption suggests how hard the heart and lungs are working and is indicative of the amount of energy needed to complete a task. Resting quietly in bed requires the lowest amount of oxygen per kilogram of body weight, roughly 3.5 mL O_2/kg body weight. This also can be expressed as 1 basal metabolic equivalent (MET). As activity increases, more oxygen is needed to meet the demands of the task. For instance, dressing requires 2.5 METs, or roughly twice the amount of energy that lying in bed requires (Table 45.5). Guided by a MET table,

TABLE 45.4	**Cardiovascular Response to Activity**	
	Appropriate	**Inappropriate**
Heart rate (HR)	Increases with activity to no more than 20 beats/min above the resting heart rate	HR more than 20 beats/min above the resting heart rate (RHR) with activity, RHR ≥120, HR drops or does not rise with activity
Blood pressure (BP)	Systolic blood pressure (SBP) rises with activity	SBP ≥220 mm Hg postural hypotension (drop in SBP ≥10 to 20 mm Hg), decrease in SBP with activity
Signs and symptoms	Absence of adverse symptoms	Excessive shortness of breath, angina, nausea and vomiting, excessive sweating, extreme fatigue (RPE ≥15), cerebral symptoms

RPE, Rate of perceived exertion.

TABLE 45.5	**Basal Metabolic Equivalent Table of Self-Care and Homemaking Tasks**	
MET Level	**Activities of Daily Living**	**Instrumental Activities of Daily Living, Work, Play, and Leisure**
1-2	Eating, seated[40]; transfers, bed to chair; washing face and hands; brushing hair[40]; walking 1 mph	Hand sewing[11]; machine sewing; sweeping floors[8]; driving automatic car, drawing, knitting[65]
2-3	Seated sponge bath,[65] standing sponge bath,[65] dressing and undressing,[22] seated warm shower,[65] walking 2–3 mph, wheelchair propulsion 1.2 mph	Dusting,[40] kneading dough,[11] hand-washing small items,[11] using electric vacuum,[40] preparing a meal,[35] washing dishes,[65] golfing[65]
3-4	Standing shower, warm[35]; bowel movement on toilet[11]; climbing stairs at 24 ft/min[65]	Making a bed[35]; sweeping, mopping, gardening[65]
4-5	Hot shower,[35] bowel movement on bedpan,[35] sexual intercourse[65]	Changing bed linen[40]; gardening, raking, weeding; rollerskating[23] swimming 20 yards/min[65]
5-6	Sexual intercourse,[65] walking up stairs at 30 feet/min[65]	Biking 10 mph on level ground[65]
6-7	Walking with braces and crutches	Swimming breaststroke[65]; skiing, playing basketball, walking 5 mph, shoveling snow, spading soil[65]

the patient's response to activity or occupation, the prognosis, and the patient's goals, the occupational therapist will be able to determine a logical intervention progression. As a general rule, once a patient tolerates an activity (e.g., seated sponge bathing) with appropriate responses, the patient may progress to the next higher MET-level activity (e.g., standing sponge bath).

The duration of sustained physical activity must be taken into account when activity guidelines are being determined. Obviously, persons who have difficulty performing a 2-MET activity must still use a commode (3.6 METs) or bedpan (4.7 METs) for their bowel management. This is possible because a person can perform at a higher than usual MET level for brief periods without adverse effects.

At 5 METs, sexual activity is frequently a grave concern to persons with impaired cardiovascular function and to their partners. Sexual intercourse is intermittent in its peak demands for energy. Very few patients recall receiving counseling about sexual activity after a heart attack.[39] Bringing up the topic of sexual intimacy with both partners present is one technique that can put both the patient and therapist in an open frame of mind. Patients are frequently able to return to sexual intercourse once they can climb up and down two flights of steps in 1 minute with appropriate cardiovascular responses.[66] Providing the patient with information about when it is safe to resume sexual activity can reduce anxiety surrounding the resumption of sexual intercourse.[39] Anxiety may be further decreased through discussion of sexual activity guidelines with the patient and partner and identification of various forms of romantic intimacy, such as hand-holding and kissing, when intercourse is not feasible. Besides instructing the patient to monitor HR and symptoms of cardiac distress before and after intercourse, the therapist should inform the patient and partner that cardiac medications might affect the patient's libido. The patient should be encouraged to inform the physician of problems related to sexual activity. In many cases the physician can adjust the patient's medications to control symptoms.

Energy Conservation

When patients are taught methods to conserve their energy resources, they will be able to perform at a higher functional level without expending more energy. The principles of energy conservation and work simplification are based on knowledge of the ways in which specific factors cause various cardiovascular responses. Ogden identified six variables that increase oxygen demand: increased rate, increased resistance, increased use of large muscles, increased involvement of the trunk musculature, raising one's arms, and isometric work (straining).[54] Upper extremity activity also has been shown to require greater cardiovascular output than lower extremity activity, and standing activity requires more energy than seated activity. Extremes of temperature, high humidity, and pollution make the heart work harder. By applying this information, a skilled clinician can suggest modifications in activity that will decrease the amount of energy needed for the task.

Energy conservation training should be individualized for each patient. Time management is an invaluable tool for energy conservation. Time management involves learning to plan one's activity or participation in occupation so that tasks requiring high energy expenditure are interspersed with lighter tasks and rest breaks are scheduled throughout the day, especially after meals. The most important part of educating the patient is incorporating his or her active involvement in planning the day. Patient involvement increases the likelihood of realistic goal attainment. Rather than prescribing how Harriet might sequence her ADLs, IADLs, and rest breaks throughout her typical day, the therapist might engage her in a conversation about what works or does not work well for her in her current performance patterns. The therapist would then ask probing questions, such as "Have you tried taking your shower at a different time of day?" and "Would laying your clothes out the night before help your morning go more smoothly?" Such a patient-centered approach engages the patient in the process of designing realistic performance patterns that incorporate principles of energy conservation according to his or her own circumstances and values. Through such collaboration, the therapist demonstrates respect for the patient's needs and increases the likelihood that changes will be implemented successfully.

Written material may augment energy conservation instruction. However, until the patient has successfully applied energy conservation principles to activity, the therapist should expect little follow-through with energy conservation recommendations. Practice and practical application of skills are critical to changing behavior.

The specific pulmonary rehabilitation intervention techniques of PLB, diaphragmatic breathing, dyspnea control postures, and relaxation techniques were discussed earlier in this chapter. Exhaling with exertion is another breathing principle for persons with compromised cardiac or pulmonary function. Franklin might be taught to exhale when having a bowel movement rather than holding his breath and straining. Harriet might be taught to exhale when lifting or lowering her pet's water bowl. This technique is more energy efficient and helps control SBP responses to activity. It is important for the patient to practice these skills during treatment. Therapeutic support is often critical in learning.

Lifestyle Modification

Modification of lifestyle is a key component in improving cardiovascular health. Exercise education should include the benefits of exercise; a graded program of increased activity and participation in occupation; stretching, strengthening, and aerobic activity; guidelines for monitoring HR, BP, and rate of perceived exertion; cool down; safety issues related to clothing, environmental factors, and warning signs; a plan for resuming exercise if it is skipped for a period; and emergency guidelines. Although the PT typically designs and oversees the exercise program, the occupational therapist can provide valuable insight into forms of exercise that might be meaningful to the patient. Modification of diet may be addressed by the dietitian but can readily be reinforced during meal preparation activities. To stop smoking, refrain from excessive alcohol consumption, and stop abusing drugs are challenging goals for patients who have developed these habits. Support groups, counseling, and medical management play key roles in successful cessation or modification of these risk factors. Occupational therapists think that enabling the patient's participation in rounds of personally meaningful and healthy occupations can also play a key role in supporting health and controlling such risk factors (see Chapter 53). The therapist worked with Joe's treatment team to address his alcohol use concerns and helped him identify healthy occupational patterns (regular yoga) he had previously abandoned that would support sobriety.

Patient and Family Education

As members of the healthcare team, Occupational therapists share the responsibility for patient and family education. The team must instruct the patient and family members in cardiac or pulmonary anatomy, the disease process, management of symptoms, risk factors, diet, exercise, and energy conservation and must reinforce the teaching. Inclusion of family members in an education program provides support indirectly to the patient through the family unit. Such support is critical when the patient depends on the assistance of a family member to accomplish everyday tasks.

THREADED CASE STUDY

Joe, Part 2

Reflecting on the case of Joe (who had undergone a valve replacement after a cardiac episode), the reader should consider the importance of really listening to the patient and following up with probative questions to develop more patient-centered and thus more relevant goals. The first question the reader was asked to consider while reading the chapter was "What probative questions might the occupational therapist ask to clarify what Joe means by "everything he used to do"? Joe provided some clues in his occupational profile that yield themselves to further exploration. Besides returning to work, being able to dress himself and managing his toileting, a therapist might further inquire as to (1) the role Joe normally has in management of the home, how he previously showered, and in what other avocational activities he participates; (2) whether he and his wife would like to discuss safe resumption of sexual activities; and (3) the job-specific tasks that are most relevant for him to return to work.

With regard to the second question involving resumption of sexual activity, the therapist must first assess Joe's understanding of his precautions and any factors that are interfering with his ability to apply those precautions. Besides asking Joe to list his precautions and providing a written list of precautions, the therapist can better support Joe's compliance by reviewing the at-risk postures before an activity as well as pacing the activity according to Joe's ability to

comply. The occupational therapist should consider if Joe's memory and ability to apply precautions might be affected by his pain medications, his premorbid personality, any neurological condition associated with alcohol abuse, or perhaps even portend an impending CVA.

Finally, the reader was asked to consider what areas of occupation the therapist might choose for the next intervention session and, depending on Joe's occupational profile, what goals might be included in his occupational therapy intervention plan. Performing the seated sponge bathing task and repeating bed mobility training while reinforcing sternal precautions would be a good choice of activities for the next therapy session. Joe required frequent cuing and therapeutic intervention to keep him safe. By incorporating practice in safely pacing the activity and self-monitoring his HR and application of sternal precautions, his therapist will begin practical application of the skills essential to safe management of his cardiac condition. Occupational therapy intervention will most likely end before Joe returns to work. It is critical for him to understand how he might apply his sternal precautions at home and at work. The occupational therapist intervenes by using education to engage Joe in a conversation about ways that he might adapt these principles to his work. Thus, the therapist sets the groundwork for carryover of principles into that setting.

THREADED CASE STUDY

Harriet, Part 2

When considering the case of Harriet, the reader was asked what goals she might find relevant in her therapy. Harriet identified several meaningful goals during the initial occupational therapy evaluation, including feeding her dog Sir Filo, preparing her own dinner, and being able to empty her bedside commode herself. Another question involved the safety concerns that might arise in treating Harriet. Additional goals relevant to her safety include learning to pace her activity, coordinating her breathing with function, increasing her ability to

assume dyspnea control postures when needed, and increasing her safety with oxygen. The oxygen line not only poses a potential trip hazard but also presents a fire hazard given her meal preparation goals and smoking habit. Smoking cessation is a goal that can be explored but will be meaningful only if Harriet wants to quit. Finally, the reader was asked to determine what goals appear realistic given Harriet's baseline level of function. Given her baseline level of function, all the goals she identified appear to be realistic.

SUMMARY

Healthy persons are able to meet the varying demands of their bodies for oxygen because their heart and respiratory rates adjust to meet oxygen demand. When either the cardiovascular or the pulmonary system (or both) is compromised, the ability to perform normal activities or occupations declines. This chapter is intended to guide the occupational therapist in the treatment of patients with impairment of the heart or lungs and in designing programs to maximize patients' independent performance in areas of occupation to support participation in context. The two case studies presented in this chapter and related information portray the range of problems involving patient factors, contextual issues, performance skills, and performance patterns that typically interfere with the patient's ability to perform customary activities and occupations.

REVIEW QUESTIONS

1. Describe the heart, including its size, anatomy, and functional parts.
2. Name the heart valves and give their locations and functions.
3. Discuss the relationship between the coronary arteries and health of the heart.
4. List and describe the symptoms of cardiac distress.
5. What are the typical psychosocial responses to a diagnosis of heart disease?
6. How is cardiac response to activity monitored? How does the therapist know that a change in level of activity is warranted?
7. Describe the functional parts of the pulmonary system.
8. What is COPD, and what is its significance for occupational performance?
9. What can the OT practitioner do to help prevent or reduce the incidence of COPD?
10. Demonstrate the recommended dyspnea control postures.
11. Compare pursed-lip breathing with diaphragmatic breathing. When should one be used rather than the other?
12. Describe the appropriate evaluation content and approach for patients with cardiac and pulmonary problems.
13. What is a MET, and what is the clinical value of a MET table for occupational therapists?
14. How would you teach energy conservation techniques to the following individuals, all of whom have cardiac or pulmonary disease?

- A 40-year-old female marathon runner
- A 50-year-old homemaker and adoptive mother of eight (including three children younger than 6 years)
- A 60-year-old air conditioner repairman
- A 72-year-old man who says his main pleasures are riding thoroughbreds, drinking good Kentucky bourbon, smoking cigars, and enjoying the company of lovely women

For additional practice questions for this chapter, please visit eBooks.Health.Elsevier.com.

REFERENCES

1. Adams, J., Lotshaw, A., Exum, E., Campbell, M., Spranger, C.B., Beveridge, J., . . . Schussler, J.M. (2016). An alternative approach to prescribing sternal precautions after median sternotomy, "Keep your move in the tube," *Proc (Bayl Univ Med Cent)* 2016;29(1), 97–100. https://doi.10.1080/08998280.2016.11929379.
2. American Heart Association. Options for Heart Valve Replacement, Available at http://www.heart.org/HEARTORG/Conditions/More/HeartValveProblemsandDisease/Options-for-Heart-Valve-Replacement_UCM_450816_Article.jsp#.VqR9fDbAeCc. Visited January 23, 2016.
3. American Occupational Therapy Association: Occupational therapy practice framework: domain and process, fourth edition, *Am J Occup Ther* 74(Suppl_2), 2020. 7412410010p1-7412410010p87.
4. Bartlett, R., (2020). Extracorporeal membrane oxygenation (ECMO) in adults. *UpToDate.* Retrieved November 2, 2020, from https://www-uptodate-com.laneproxy.stanford.edu/contents/extracorporeal-membrane-oxygenation-ecmo-in-adults.
5. Berkman LF, Blumenthal J, Burg M, et al: Enhancing Recovery in Coronary Heart Disease Patients Investigators (ENRICHD). Effects of treating depression and low perceived social support on clinical events after myocardial infarction: the Enhancing Recovery in Coronary Heart Disease Patients (ENRICHD) randomized trial, *JAMA.* 289:3106–3116, 2003.
6. Brannon FJ, Foley MW, Starr JA, Saul LM: *Cardiopulmonary rehabilitation: basic theory and application,* ed 3, Philadelphia, Pa, 1997, Davis.
7. Cahalin LP, Lapier TK, Shaw DK: Sternal precautions: is it time for change? precautions versus restrictions – a review of literature and recommendations for revision, *Cardiopulm Phys Ther J.* 22(1):5–15, 2011 Mar.
8. Chan SCC: Chronic obstructive pulmonary disease and engagement in occupation, *Am J Occup Ther* 58:408–415, 2004.
9. Cleveland Clinic: Treatments and procedures: CABG 10-year survival. Available at: http://my.clevelandclinic.org/services/heart/lytle_imagraft10yrsurvival.
10. Cleveland Clinic. Diseases and conditions:- COPD –treatment. Available at http://my.clevelandclinic.org/health/diseases_conditions/hic_Understanding_COPD/hic_Pulmonary_Rehabilitation_Is_it_for_You/hic_Pursed_Lip_Breathing. Accessed Jan 12, 2016.
11. Colorado Heart Association: Exercise equivalent (pamphlet), Boston, Mass, 1970, Cardiac Reconditioning & Work Evaluation Unit, Spaulding Rehabilitation Center.
12. Dahlén I, Janson C: Anxiety and depression are related to the outcome of emergency treatment in patients with obstructive pulmonary disease, *Chest* 122:1933, 2002.
13. Dangas G, Kuepper F: Cardiology patient age, restenosis: repeat narrowing of a coronary artery: prevention and treatment, *Circulation* 105(22):2586, 2002.
14. Dawber TR: The Framingham study, the epidemiology of atherosclerotic disease, Cambridge. MA, 1980, Harvard University Press.
15. De Troyer, A., & Moxham, J. (2020). Chest wall and respiratory muscles. https://doi-org.laneproxy.stanford.edu/10.1002/9781118597309.ch10.
16. Dubin D: 2000, updated *Rapid interpretation of EKGs,* ed 6, Tampa, Fla, 2007, Cover Publishing.
17. Dyspnea. Mechanisms, assessment, and management: a consensus statement. American Thoracic Society. (1999). *American Journal of Respiratory and Critical Care Medicine,* 159(1), 321–340. https://doi.org/10.1164/ajrccm.159.1.ats898.
18. Fishman, J.A., Alexander, B.D., (2020). Prophylaxis of infections in solid organ transplantation. *UpToDate.* Retrieved October 27, 2020 from https://www-uptodate-com.laneproxy.stanford.edu/contents/prophylaxis-of-infections-in-solid-organ-transplantation.
19. Framingham Heart Study, A Project of the National Heart, Lung, and Blood Institute and Boston University. Available at https://www.framinghamheartstudy.org/.
20. Froom P, Gofer D, Boyko V, Goldbourt U: Risk for early ischaemic event after acute myocardial infarction in working males, *Int J Occup Med Environ Health* 15:43–48, 2002.

21. Gazda AJ, Kwak MJ, Akkanti B, Nathan S, Kumar S, de Armas IS, et al: Complications of LVAD utilization in older adults. *Heart & Lung* 50(1):75–79, 2021. https://doi.org/10.1016/j.hrtlng.2020.07.009.

22. Go AS, Mozaffarian D, Roger VL, Benjamin EJ, Berry JD, et al: Heart disease and stroke statistics—2013 update: a report from the American Heart Association, *Circulation* 127:e6–e245, 2013.

23. Goldman L, Hashimoto B, Cook EF, Loscalzo A: Comparative reproducibility and validity of systems for assessing cardiovascular functional class: advantages of a new specific activity scale, *Circulation* 64:1227–1234, 1981.

24. Gottlieb J: Lung allocation, *Journal of thoracic disease* 9(8):2670–2674, 2017. https://doi.org/10.21037/jtd.2017.07.83.

25. Grippo AJ, Johnson AK: Biological mechanisms in the relationship between depression and heart disease. *Neurosci Biobehav Rev* 26:941–962, 2022.

26. Guglin M, Zucker MJ, Borlaug BA, Breen E, Cleveland J, Johnson MR, Bozkurt B, et al: Evaluation for heart transplantation and LVAD implantation: JACC council perspectives, *Journal of the American College of Cardiology* 75(12):1471–1487, 2020. https://doi.org/10.1016/j.jacc.2020.01.034.

27. Hachem, RR: Lung transplantation: an overview. *UpToDate*. Retrieved October 26, 2020, from https://www.uptodate.com/contents/lung-transplantation-an-overview.

28. Hambrecht R, Gielen S, Linke A, et al: Effects of exercise training on left ventricular function and peripheral resistance in patients with chronic heart failure: a randomized trial, *JAMA* 283(23):3095–3101, 2000.

29. Hartwig, MG, Klapper, JA: Lung transplantation: procedure and postoperative management. *UpToDate*. Retrieved October 10, 2020, from https://www-uptodate-com/contents/lung-transplantation-procedure-and-postoperative-management.

30. Heart & Vascular Institute – Temple Health – Mechanical Circulatory Support Devices. Available at: http://heartsurgery.templehealth.org/content/mechanical_circulatory_support.htm. Visited January 23, 2016.

31. Holloway C, Pathare N, Huta J, Grady D, Landry A, Christie C, Pierce P, Bopp C: The impact of a less restrictive poststernotomy activity protocol compared with standard sternal precautions in patients following cardiac surgery, *Physical Therapy & Rehabilitation Journal* 100(7):1074–1083, 2020. https://doi.org/10.1093/ptj/pzaa067.

32. Javidfar J: The challenges faced with early mobilization of patients on extracorporeal membrane oxygenation, *Critical Care Medicine* 46(1):161–163, 2018. https://doi.org/10.1097/CCM.0000000000002822.

32a. King TE Jr: Clinical manifestations and diagnosis of idiopathic pulmonary fibrosis. *UpToDate*. Retrieved October 26, 2020, from https://www.uptodate.com/contents/clinical-manifestations-and-diagnosis-of-idiopathic-pulmonary-fibrosis.

33. King TE, Pardo A, Selman M: Idiopathic pulmonary fibrosis, *The Lancet* 378(9807):1949–1961, 2011. https://doi.org/10.1016/S0140-6736(11)60052-4.

34. Kinney M: *Andreoli's comprehensive cardiac care*, ed 8, St. Louis, 1995, Mosby.

34a. Kon OM, Hansel TT, Barnes, PJ: *Chronic Obstructive Pulmonary Disease (COPD)*, Oxford, 2008, OUP.

35. Kottke FJ: Common cardiovascular problems in rehabilitation. In Krusen FH, Kottke FJ, Elwood PM, editors: *Handbook of physical medicine and rehabilitation*, Philadelphia, Pa, 1971, Saunders.

36. Lau-Walker MO, Cowie MR, Roughton M: Coronary heart disease patients' perception of their symptoms and sense of control are associated with their quality of life three years following hospital discharge, *J Clin Nurs* 18(1):63–71, 2009. https://doi.org/10.1111/j.1365-2702.2008.02386.x.

37. Leon AS, Franklin BA, Costa F, et al: Cardiac rehabilitation and secondary prevention of coronary heart disease, *Circulation* 111(3):369–376, 2005.

38. Le Pavec J, Dauriat G, Gazengel P, Dolidon S, Hanna A, Feuillet S, Fadel E, et al: Lung transplantation for idiopathic pulmonary fibrosis, *La Presse Médicale* 49(2):104026, 2020. https://doi.org/10.1016/j.lpm.2020.104026.

39. Lindau ST, Abramsohn EM, Bueno H, et al: Sexual activity and counseling in the first month after acute myocardial infarction among younger adults in the United States and Spain: a prospective, observational study, *Circulation* 130(25):2302–2309, 2014.

40. Maloney FP, Moss K: Energy requirements for selected activities, Denver, Colo, 1974, Department of Physical Medicine, National Jewish Hospital (unpublished).

41. Mason RJ, Broaddas VC, Martin TR, et al: *Murray and Nadel's Textbook of Respiratory Medicine*, 5th ed., Philadelphia, Pa, 2010, Saunders Elsevier. http://www.clinicalkey.com. Accessed Nov. 18, 2013.

42. Mayo Clinic: Tests & procedures: coronary angioplasty and stents. Available at: http://www.mayoclinic.org/tests-procedures/angioplasty/basics/definition/prc-20014401. Last updated February 13, 2014, visited January 25, 2016.

43. Mayo Clinic: Diseases and conditions: emphysema. http://www.mayoclinic.org/diseases-conditions/emphysema/basics/definition/CON-20014218. Visited January 20, 2016.

44. *McGraw-Hill concise dictionary of modern medicine,* 2002. New York: McGraw-Hill.

45. Medline Plus: Lungs and breathing. Available at https://www.nlm.nih.gov/medlineplus/lungsandbreathing.html. Visited January 30, 2016.

46. Migliore A: Management of dyspnea guidelines for practice for adults with chronic obstructive pulmonary disease. In *Occupational therapy in health care*, Binghamton, NY, 2004, Haworth Press.

47. Mythos for SoftKey: BodyWorks 4.0: human anatomy leaps to life, Cambridge, Mass, 1993–1995, SoftKey International.

48. National Center for Chronic Disease Prevention and Health Promotion, Division for Heart Disease and Stroke Prevention: What is coronary artery disease? 2021. Available at: http://www.cdc.gov/heartdisease/coronary_ad.htm.

49. National Heart, Lung, and Blood Institute: How is a heart attack treated? and What Is Asthma? https://www.nhlbi.nih.gov/health/heart-attack/treatment and https://www.nhlbi.nih.gov/health/asthma.

50. National Heart, Lung, and Blood Institute: What is cardiac ablation? Available at: http://www.nhlbi.nih.gov.

51. National Heart, Lung, and Blood Institute – What is COPD? http://www.nhlbi.nih.gov/health/health-topics/topics/copd.

52. National Heart, Lung and Blood Institute: Who is at risk for coronary heart disease? Available at: http://www.nhlbi.nih.gov.

53. National Institutes of Health: What is a heart transplant? https://www.nhlbi.nih.gov/health/heart-treatments-procedures.

54. Ogden LD: Guidelines for analysis and testing of activities of daily living with cardiac patients, Downey, Calif, 1981, *Cardiac Rehabilitation Resources*.

55. Reference deleted in proofs.

56. Park L, Coltman C, Agren H, Colwell S, King-Shier K: "In the tube" following sternotomy: A quasi-experimental study,

European Journal of Cardiovascular Nursing, 20(2):160–166, 2021. https://doi.org/10.1177/1474515120951981.

57. Patel A, Chernyak Y: The need for psychological rehabilitation in lung transplant recipients, *Progress in Transplantation (Aliso Viejo, Calif.)* 30(2):140–143, 2020. https://doi.org/10.1177/1526924820913510.

58. Pavlushkov E, Berman M, Valchanov K: Cannulation techniques for extracorporeal life support, *Annals of translational medicine* 5(4):70, 2017. https://doi.org/10.21037/atm.2016.11.47.

59. Pellegrini M, Hedenstierna G, Roneus A, Segelsjö M, Larsson A, Perchiazzi G: The diaphragm acts as a brake during expiration to prevent lung collapse, *American Journal of Respiratory and Critical Care Medicine* 195(12):1608–1616, 2017. https://doi.org/10.1164/rccm.201605-0992OC.

60. Perkins-Porras L, Whitehead D, Strike P, Steptoe A: Causal beliefs, cardiac denial and pre-hospital delays following the onset of acute coronary syndromes, *J Behav Med* 31(6):498–505, 2008.

61. Renfroe KL: Effect of progressive relaxation on dyspnea and state anxiety in patients with chronic obstructive pulmonary disease, *Heart Lung* 17(4):408, 1988.

62. Richardson LG: Psychosocial issues in patients with congestive heart failure, *Prog Cardiovasc Nurs* 18(Issue 1):19–27, 2003.

63. Ries AL, Bauldoff GS, Carlin BW, et al: Pulmonary Rehabilitation: joint ACCP/AACVPR evidence-based clinical practice guidelines, *Chest*(5-suppl):4S–42S, 2007. https://doi.org/10.1378/chest.06-2418.

64. Salerno, FG, Carone M: Anxiety and depression in COPD, *Multidisciplinary Respiratory Medicine*, 6(4):212–213, 2011. http://doi.org/10.1186/2049-6958-6-4-212.

65. Santa Clara Valley Medical Center: Graded activity sheets, San Jose, Calif, 1994, Santa Clara Valley Medical Center.

66. Scalzi C, Burke L: Myocardial infarction: behavioral responses of patient and spouses. In Underhill SL, editor: *Cardiac nursing*, Philadelphia, Pa, 1982, Lippincott.

67. Sheikh A, Marotta S: Best practices for counseling in cardiac rehabilitation settings, *J Counsel Dev* 86(1):111–120, 2008.

68. Sommerwerck U, et al: Cognitive Function After Lung Transplantation. In *Medical research and innovation*, New York, NY, 2020, Springer. https://doi.org/10.1007/5584_2020_590.

69. *Stedman's Medical Dictionary*: 2006, Philadelphia: Lippincott Williams & Wilkins.

70. Reference deleted in proofs.

71. Torrisi SE, Kahn N, Vancheri C, Kreuter M: Evolution and treatment of idiopathic pulmonary fibrosis, *La Presse Médicale* 49(2):104025, 2020. https://doi.org/10.1016/j.lpm.2020.104025.

72. U.S. Department of Health and Human Services: The health consequences of smoking—50 years of progress: a report of the Surgeon General. Atlanta: U.S. Department of Health and Human Services, Centers for Disease Control and Prevention, National Center for Chronic Disease Prevention and Health Promotion, Office on Smoking and Health, Washington, D.C. 2014.

73. Venes D, Thomas CL, Taber CW: *Taber's cyclopedic medical dictionary*, ed 19, Philadelphia, Pa, 2001, Davis.

74. Virani SS, Alonso A, Benjamin EJ, et al: Heart disease and stroke statistics – 2020 update: a report from the American Heart Association, *Circulation*. 141(9):e139–e596, 2020. https://doi.org/10.1161/CIR.0000000000000757.

75. Williams MA, et al: Clinical evidence for a health benefit from cardiac rehabilitation: an update, *Am Heart J* 152(5):835–841, 2006.

76. Yohannes AM, Chen W, Moga AM, Leroi I, Connolly MJ: Cognitive impairment in chronic obstructive pulmonary disease and chronic heart failure: a systematic review and meta-analysis of observational studies, *Journal of the American Medical Directors Association* 18(5):451.e1–451.e11, 2017. https://doi.org/10.1016/j.jamda.2017.01.014.

46

Cancer and Oncology Rehabilitation

Brent Braveman, Jennifer Kaye Hughes, and Jennifer Nicholson

LEARNING OBJECTIVES

After studying this chapter, the student or practitioner will be able to do the following:

1. Identify and describe the range of impacts that cancer and cancer treatments can have on occupational performance.
2. Understand the various types of cancer, which are most common in men and women, and the most common medical and therapeutic interventions.
3. Identify the types of occupational therapy interventions that are used to promote occupational performance in adults with cancer.
4. Explain the side effects of surgery, radiation, and chemotherapy and their impact on occupational performance.
5. State the distinct value that occupational therapy adds to rehabilitation of the person with cancer.

CHAPTER OUTLINE

KEY TERMS

Cancer
Cancer-related cognitive impairment
Cancer-related fatigue
Chemotherapy
Hospice

Lymphedema
Metastasis
Palliative care
Radiation therapy

CASE STUDY

Kay

Kay is a 36-year-old woman (prefers use of the pronouns she/her/hers). She is a mother of two children, resides with her spouse, and works full time. She was diagnosed with invasive ductile breast cancer and underwent surgery followed by radiation and chemotherapy. She received occupational therapy services as an inpatient and was referred for outpatient services after discussing with her treating physician and nurse practitioner the difficulty she is experiencing with performance of her daily occupations.

Kay was evaluated by the outpatient occupational therapist to identify challenges to occupational performance in her various roles (e.g., parent, spouse, worker, homemaker, volunteer, sports enthusiast, religious participant). Kay is functioning independently in many occupations but is feeling stretched to her limits because of fatigue and mild cognitive issues caused by the radiation and chemotherapy. She reports that she is no longer able to consistently perform homemaking tasks independently. She has also taken a leave of absence from her job and is unable to perform her valued work occupations.

Kay is also experiencing psychosocial distress related to her body image and impending reconstructive surgery. Kay told her occupational therapist, "I barely am making it through the day and am trying to hold it together while I care for my kids and take care of our home. I am exhausted all the time and continually make stupid mistakes and feel confused over things that used to be so simple. I had to take a leave of absence from work; I just couldn't handle it anymore. I

can't even imagine getting back to running or my volunteer work at my church. I am at the end of my rope!"

Critical Thinking Questions
1. If Kay is able to bathe and dress herself and get support from her spouse over the short term, why does she need occupational therapy?
2. Kay has identified fatigue and cognitive issues as primary issues but is struggling with performance of all of her daily roles, so where should the occupational therapist begin?
3. In addition to the physical symptoms that Kay is experiencing, what are the psychosocial issues that should be addressed by the occupational therapy practitioners working with Kay?

AN INTRODUCTION TO CANCER AND ONCOLOGY REHABILITATION

In 2022 there were an estimated 1.9 million new cancer cases diagnosed and over 600,000 cancer deaths in the United States.[4] Approximately 38.4% of men and women will be diagnosed with cancer at some point during their lifetimes (based on 2013–2015 data).[37] The most common cancers in men are prostate, lung and bronchus, colon and rectum, urinary and bladder, and melanoma of the skin. The most common cancers in women are breast, lung and bronchus, colon and rectum, uterine corpus, and thyroid.[4] Overall men have a 50% chance of developing some form of cancer in their lifetime and women have a 33% risk of incidence. The number of cancer survivors in the United States is expected to reach 20.3 million by 2026.[37] Cancer is typically described according to where the cancer originates, with the most common forms being melanoma (skin), carcinoma (skin or tissue lining organs), sarcoma (connective tissue), leukemia (bone marrow or blood forming organs), lymphoma (immune system), multiple myeloma (plasma cells and bone marrow), and central nervous system (brain and spine).

Oncology rehabilitation, including occupational therapy, physical therapy, speech and language pathology, and rehabilitation medicine, has grown rapidly in the last decade. Oncology rehabilitation services are provided at large National Cancer Institutes such as the University of Texas MD Anderson Cancer Center in Houston Texas, at smaller cancer centers and community-based hospital, and in the home. Rehabilitative services are provided at all stages of cancer or what is referred to as the *cancer care continuum*. The stages of the cancer care continuum include (1) pretreatment (newly diagnosed but no treatment initiated), (2) active treatment (treatment with a curative goal), (3) maintenance (long-term therapy with a goal of remission), (4) post-treatment or survivorship (medical treatment complete with no sign of disease), and (5) palliative care (treatment when cancer is incurable with a focus on comfort and function). Occupational therapy practitioners also have roles in cancer prevention through lifestyle redesign and occupational performance to support health.

TREATMENT OPTIONS

There are a range of treatments for cancer that are driven by the type of cancer, how early the disease is discovered and how advanced the cancer has become. The length of time that treatment lasts and the impact of treatment on an individual can be wide ranging. The most common forms of treatment include[4]:
- Surgical removal of cancer cells/tumors from the body.
- Radiation therapy focused on killing cancer cells and shrinking tumors.
- Chemotherapy using drugs to kill cancer cells.
- Immunotherapy focused on strengthening and using a person's immune system to fight cancer.
- Targeted therapy, which uses drugs or others substance to precisely identify and attack certain types of cancer cells.
- Hormone therapy, which uses hormones to slow or stop cancer cell growth.
- Stem cell transplants, which restore blood-forming cells destroyed by high-dose chemotherapy or radiation.

Precautions, Contraindications, and Medical Complexity

Providing safe occupational therapy intervention with people with cancer can be complex and requires specialty and sometimes advanced knowledge and understanding of how medications, treatments, and the status of body systems affect the course of evaluation and treatment.[7] Medications and the disease process can influence the body that is attempting to maintain homeostasis. Some areas that could be affected would include changes in heart rate and rhythm, dizziness, blood pressure, changes in vision, changes in cognitive status, appetite, or metabolism. Vital signs (i.e., blood pressure, arterial blood pressure, intracranial pressure, respiration rate, heart rate, and oxygen saturation) and laboratory values are two important measures of body functions to monitor during intervention with cancer survivors. Laboratory values provide the practitioner with information regarding a client's biochemistry that could affect performance.

Common laboratory values that should be reviewed before each occupational therapy intervention session include the following:

- Blood cell counts such as red blood cell count, white blood cell count, hemoglobin, and hematocrit.
- Coagulation panels such as prothrombin time, international normalized ratio, and partial thromboplastin time.
- Basic metabolic panels, including blood sugar, calcium, creatinine, potassium, and blood urea nitrogen.

These laboratory values each have a range within which functional activity and participation in rehabilitation activities is safe and appropriate. Functional activity is contraindicated when laboratory values that are critically outside the normal range. Tests such as a complete blood count can help practitioners determine safe functional activity guidelines, particularly for patients who are undergoing or have just completed chemotherapy, radiation therapy, or bone marrow transplants. Criteria for exercise vary depending on the type of cancer, the treatment that a patient is receiving and the patient's reaction medically and physiologically. Patients who may be able to safely exercise at one point in their course of treatment may be under activity restrictions at other times. Table 46.1 includes examples of three common laboratory values seen in the oncology setting: platelets, hematocrit, and white blood cells. The precautions associated with abnormal values for each are also noted. The ranges provided are reflective of commonly used values. Medical and rehabilitative practice in regard to laboratory values may vary, so practitioners should become familiar with the specific ranges considered "normal" in their setting and consult with the medical team to determine when participation in rehabilitation is contraindicated.

Radiology and Imaging

Occupational therapy practitioners should consult and review imaging reports such as computerized tomography scans (CT or CAT scans), magnetic resonance imaging (MRI) scans, ultrasound, or X-ray films in the event of acute fractures, metastasis (the spread of cancer to another part of the body), or any changes in status that could affect precautions or treatment. These test results may influence the type of testing that the occupational therapy practitioner performs or alter the intervention plan. For example, evidence on an MRI may show new metastatic disease to the brain that would result in more intense cognitive testing. An MRI exhibiting new pathologic fractures could alter activities of daily living (ADLs) that require weight bearing or lifting.

In general, the occupational therapy practitioner should verify blood counts, vital signs, and images before evaluation and treatment. The practitioner should also verify any specific precautions that are associated with the type of cancer before attempting interventions including mobilization, weight bearing, manual muscle testing, or any activities that may have a resistive component.

OCCUPATIONAL THERAPY AND CANCER: DOMAIN AND PROCESS

Because of the variations in types of cancers and the broad-ranging impact of the disease and its treatments, understanding the occupational therapy process and cancer requires consideration of the full domain of occupational therapy and the full scope of the occupational therapy process as represented in the Occupational Therapy Practice Framework: Domain and Process, Fourth Edition.[11] Table 46.2 provides examples applied to Kay, who was introduced at the start of the chapter.

COMMON ASSESSMENTS USED IN ONCOLOGY REHABILITATION BY OCCUPATIONAL THERAPISTS

In addition to routine assessment of ADLs, instrumental ADLs (IADLs) and other areas of occupation through observation of performance, there are specific assessments or categories of

TABLE 46.1   Examples of Common Laboratory Values in the Oncology Rehabilitation Setting and Their Indication for Participation in Rehabilitation Activity

Laboratory Name	Normal Range	Accepted Values for Participation	Rehabilitation Implications	Other Findings
Platelets	150–450 k/µL	140–440 k/µL	• <5 K only active assistive movements/no Valsalva maneuvers • <20 K active movements • >50 K resistive movements • Fall risk assessments are paramount when platelets are low	Check for petechiae: a reddish-purple rash Check for any active signs of bleeding: nosebleeds, excessive bleeding from cuts, blood tinged sputum, swollen joints, etc. Below 20 K (+) increased risk for intracranial bleed
White blood cells (WBC)	3.5–10.5 k/µL	4.0–11.0 k/µL	(+) Risk for infection Neutropenia: absolute neutrophil count <0.5 cells/mm³	Adhere to hand hygiene and infection control policies Patient may present with a fever when neutropenic
Hematocrit	Normal male: 37%–49% Female: 36%–46%	Male: 40%–54% Female: 37.0%–47.0%	<20%: can result in cardiac failure/death <25%: defer therapy 25%–30% ADL and exercise, as tolerated 30%: can add resistive exercise	• Consult with medical team

TABLE 46.2   The Occupational Therapy Domain and Process in Oncology Rehabilitation

Occupational Therapy Domain	Examples Related to Kay
Occupations	Occupations related to Kay's identified roles of parent, spouse, worker, homemaker, volunteer, sports enthusiast, and religious participant. Physical, cognitive, emotional and psychosocial factors can affect all areas of occupation, including ADLs, IADLs, health management, rest/sleep, education, work, play, leisure and social participation
Patient factors	All areas of patient factors must be considered, including values and beliefs about health and illness as Kay confronts the impact of cancer on body functions such as respiration, sensation, cognition, and organ function and body structures such as bone, joints, and muscles.
Performance skills	Depending on the location of the cancer and the effects of treatment performance skills, including cognitive abilities, motor skills, process skills, and social interaction skills.
Performance patterns	Kay's habits, routines, roles, and rituals used in the process of engaging in occupations can be disrupted by surgery or the effects of chemotherapy or radiation on level of energy, endurance, interest in continuing in roles, and interacting with others.
Contexts	Cultural, personal, temporal, and virtual contexts can support or inhibit the occupational performance of persons with cancer. The physical and social environment, including natural and built environments, objects and relationships with family members, friends, co-workers, and others must be considered.
Occupational Therapy Process	
Evaluation	Identification of information about Kay's needs, problems and concerns.
Occupational profile	Summary of Kay's occupational history, patterns of daily life, interests, values and needs.
Analysis of occupational performance	Using assessment tools to identify Kay's assets and problems.
Intervention	The skilled services provided by occupational therapy practitioners to facilitate Kay's engagement in occupational performance.
Intervention plan	Guides the actions of the practitioner and the approaches used to achieve the Kay's goals.
Intervention implementation	Putting the intervention plan into action.
Intervention review	Continuous process of reevaluating the intervention plan to improve outcomes.
Targeting of outcomes	Selecting the end results to be achieved through occupational therapy interventions.

assessments commonly used by the occupational therapist in treating the person with cancer. A few examples include:
- Activities of daily living assessment scales such as the Katz ADL Scale.
- *A-One* is a cognitive assessment that directly links functional performance (basic activities of daily living and mobility) to neurobehavioral deficits, including cognitive-perceptual and motor impairments. The A-ONE is appropriate to use for patients over the age of 16 who present with damage to the central nervous system.
- *Brief Fatigue Inventory (BFI)* is a short assessment of the severity of fatigue experienced over the last 24 hours and its impact on function.
- *Executive Function Performance Test* is a performance-based standardized assessment of cognitive function available for free in the public domain.
- Functional Assessment of Cancer Therapy (FACT) is a general assessment of quality of life.
- Functional Assessment of Cancer Therapy-Cognitive Function (FACT-Cog) is a cognitive assessment tool specific to cancer survivors
- *Kettle Test* is a performance-based assessment of cognitive functional performance.
- *The Multiple Errands Test (MET)* evaluates the effect of executive function deficits on everyday functioning through a number of real-world tasks.

- *Pain scales* such as rating pain from 0 to 10, with 0 indicating no pain and 10 the worst pain imaginable, or the Wong-Baker Faces Pain Rating Scale, which uses pictures to express "no hurt" to "worst hurt."

SIGNIFICANT SECONDARY CONDITIONS RELATED TO CANCER AND TREATMENT

In addition to problems caused directly by cancer, there are several significant secondary conditions that can be caused by the cancer or its treatment (e.g., surgery, radiation, and chemotherapy). The following are examples of such secondary conditions and brief explanations of the significance for occupational performance.

Cancer-Related Fatigue

The National Comprehensive Cancer Network (NCCN) has defined cancer-related fatigue (CRF) as "a distressing, persistent subjective sense of physical, emotional and/or cognitive tiredness or exhaustion related to cancer or cancer treatment that is not proportional to recent activity and interferes with usual functioning."[39] Occupational therapy practitioners empower patients by helping them distinguish between CRF and other types of normal exhaustion or fatigue experienced in the past. This differentiation is important because fatigue related to cancer is not proportional to current activities and prolonged rest or sleep will only worsen the symptoms, which is counterintuitive for most people.[39] Patients further need to comprehend that CRF is multidimensional and comprises much more than the physical realm. Hann et al.[23] describe CRF as having four subcomponents: (1) general fatigue, (2) emotional fatigue, (3) physical fatigue, (4) and mental fatigue. Occupational therapy practitioners play a vital role in helping clients identify how each dimension directly contributes to CRF, as well as strategies for addressing the controllable factors interfering with engagement and participation in daily activity.[24] The incidence of CRF experienced by patients with cancer is difficult to determine because published studies are restricted to prevalence data.[18] However, some studies reveal that CRF is experienced by most patients during the course of treatment, and one third will experience persistent fatigue after treatment is completed.[17,18] In practice, almost 80% of patients report CRF as the most distressing symptom experienced because it can drastically decrease participation and performance of all occupations, roles, and routines.

CRF profoundly affects the quality of life (QOL) of both patients and their families, including mental, physical, psychosocial, and economic aspects.[18] CRF can result in an altered lifestyle, decreased participation, a decline in performance capacity because of inefficient use of energy, loss of control and identity, impaired volition and motivation, reduced ability to work, reduced self-efficacy, poor QOL, lack of social interaction, and loss of important roles.

All patients should be screened for CRF throughout the continuum of care recognizing that the experience of CRF is unique to each individual. There are no accurate objective measures; however, patient-reported outcomes (PROs) are commonly used to identify improved subjective outcomes such as perceived well-being and sustainability of valued occupations. It is also important to recognize that symptom severity is not equivalent to the degree to which symptoms interfere with the performance and participation in meaningful activities; therefore what matters is how occupational performance and participation are directly affected by CRF.[15,33]

Table 46.3 provides examples of each of the types of occupational therapy interventions identified in the Occupational Therapy Practice Framework: Domain and Process that are appropriate to CRF.[11]

Occupational therapy intervention for CRF varies depending on its severity and can include participation in the full range of human occupation. The following are some basic guidelines to follow in interventions for CRF:

- Remain patient-centered, use active listening, and use a holistic approach focusing on therapeutic use of self.
- Assess the patient's motivation and volition for performance of occupations and roles.
- Assess all areas of function (e.g., physical, cognitive, psychosocial/emotional).
- Intervention should include application of skills and include use of occupation rather than remain solely didactic.
- Provide demonstrations and give homework to facilitate carryover of skills and learning.
- Assess response to treatment and indications that treatment or homework is too intense or counterproductive.

Cancer-Related Cognitive Impairment

Up to 75% of patients with cancer experience cancer-related cognitive impairment in memory, executive functioning, and attention span during or after cancer treatment. It is estimated that nearly 4 million cancer survivors have some form of cognitive difficulty. Cancer-related cognitive impairment (CRCI) is characterized as deficits in areas of cognition, including memory, attention, concentration, and executive function.[27] Development of CRCI can impair quality of life and affect treatment decisions. CRCI is highly prevalent; these problems can be detected in up to 30% of patients before chemotherapy, up to 75% of patients report some form of CRCI during treatment, and CRCI is still present in up to 35% of patients many years after completion of treatment.[26]

Cognitive impairments resulting from cancer-related treatment can vary from subtle to dramatic and can be temporary or permanent. Table 46.4 correlates different treatments used in treating cancer with predicted cognitive impairments.[1]

TABLE 46.3	**Examples of Occupational Therapy Interventions Related to Cancer Related Fatigue**
Occupational Therapy Intervention Approach	**Example**
Create and promote	Create educational materials to guide patients in management of cancer-related fatigue (CRF) or cognitive impairment.
Prevent	Screen for early signs of CRF and educate patients and family members on the potential for the onset of CRF with new treatments.
Establish and restore	Examine daily routines and establish habits and patterns that incorporate rest and exercise to minimize CRF.
Modify	Simplify ADL and IADL tasks and add cuing strategies to compensate for cancer-related cognitive impairment such as impaired short-term memory and lowered attention span.
Maintain	Identify occupations and roles important to the patient and prioritize involvement in meaningful occupations that will allow the patient to continue role fulfillment. Use lifestyle redesign approaches to maintain strength, endurance, and mobility during and after treatment.

In approaching intervention for cancer-related cognitive dysfunction the occupational therapy practitioner has several options. These options are presented in Table 46.5. The approach depends on the treatment context and the severity of the impairments experienced by the patient. It is important to note that the approaches are not exclusive and several may be used throughout the episode of care.

Cancer-Induced Peripheral Neuropathy

Cancer-induced peripheral neuropathy (CIPN) is experienced by patients undergoing treatment with certain neurotoxic chemotherapy agents.[12] The platinum drugs cause dysfunction or damage to peripheral nerves, and functional recovery can take months to years depending on many factors.[28] CIPN can manifest as motor, sensory, autonomic, or mixed impairments and typically follows a symmetric stocking-glove distribution with the earliest symptoms developing at the fingertips and toes. Common symptoms that impair occupations include tingling, numbness, paresthesia, temperature sensitivity, pain, feeling

TABLE 46.4 Common Cancer Treatment Methods and Their Predicted Cognitive Impairments

Chemotherapy	• Inattention • Lack of concentration • Decreased working memory • Impaired executive functioning
Radiation therapy	• Inattention • Decreased memory • Impaired executive functioning • Impaired visual/perceptual skills
Steroids	• Behavioral changes • Decreased verbal memory • Inattention
Sedatives	• Decreased level of arousal • Delirium • Confusion/disorientation

TABLE 46.5 Intervention Approaches for Cancer-Related Cognitive Dysfunction

Cognitive-behavioral strategies	• Coping skills/relaxation • Sleep hygiene and education • Self/goal management
Remediation/restoration	• Repeated practice of drills, exercises, or activities • Relevant real-life tasks • Computer-based training
Compensatory skills training	• Environment or task modifications • Adjustment of task features/sensory cues • Involvement of the individual's mental operations; use of imagery
Meaningful functional activity	• Promotes and maintains focus; concentration • Decreases anxiety • Improves psychological well-being

of wearing gloves and stockings, weakness and impaired balance.[34,47] Many patients report the effects of CIPN as painful, disabling, creating significant loss of function, and decreasing quality of life. Overall survival might be affected with dose reductions or discontinuation of treatment when severe symptoms arise.[35]

Standard sensory testing, balance tests, outcome measurements, and functional timed tests to better determine underlying problems related to performance skill deficits are appropriate for the patient with CIPN. Standard sensory tests will help establish a baseline and determine change over time as well as identify which type of sensation is potentially affecting occupational outcomes. It is also beneficial to assess balance and the patient's confidence with activities requiring balance.[16,52]

Intervention for patients with CIPN include compensation strategies for safety, foot care and proper shoes, strategies to reduce ischemic and thermal injuries and management of symptoms of autonomic dysfunction, falls prevention, and use of assistive devices to compensate for loss of sensation or weakness to promote independence and remain active in daily activities.[47,50] Activity pacing and gradation of activity is also beneficial, as are use of energy conservation techniques to manage muscle fatigue. Exposure to different surfaces during functional tasks (i.e., desensitization) can reduce anxiety associated with CIPN.

Cancer-Related Pain

Cancer-related pain (CRP) is a notable and pervasive sequela of cancer and one of the most common reported symptoms in oncology literature.[22,25] As many as 90% of adults with cancer may have some experience of pain.[13] In the pediatric population, 49% of patients in one study reported pain at diagnosis and during early phases of treatment.[2] Pain caused by cancer is a complex symptom that affects a person's life, including physical functioning, the performance of ADLs, psychological and emotional status, and social interactions.[44] The symptom of pain is a mixed mechanism, including both neuropathic and nonneuropathic origins. It involves inflammatory, neuropathic, ischemic, and compression mechanisms at multiple sites. Cancer survivors might experience pain as one discrete symptom or experience several types of pain concurrently. Typical types of pain in cancer might include neuropathic, testing, surgical and procedural, radiation-induced, and metastatic disease and pathological fracture.

Pain can be a devastating consequence of cancer or its treatment at any stage of the life. As a result of advancements in the field of oncology, cancer is considered a chronic rather than fatal condition; therefore, occupational therapy practitioners must consider the impact of pain throughout the lifespan and at any stage of the cancer journey.[40] Occupational therapy practitioners evaluate the symptoms of pain and the impact of pain on a client's desired activities and quality of life. Through skilled and thoughtful intervention, the occupational therapy practitioner must then equip the client with the skills and strategies to manage the pain with the goal of optimizing engagement in valued occupations. Interventions might include, but are not limited to the activity modification, use of orthotics, adaptive techniques, incorporation of physical agent modalities (PAMs) and therapeutic exercise. The literature additionally supports use of guided imagery, deep-breathing techniques, and patient journaling as means to manage pain.[25]

Deconditioning in Oncology

As occupational therapy practitioners working with patients in the oncology setting, an emphasis must be placed on the relationship between deconditioning and occupational performance. Deconditioning, sometimes referred to as debility, is described as complex process of physiological change that can affect multiple systems within the body.[19,30,45] Deconditioning, as associated with disease process and anticancer interventions, can have a dramatic impact on quality of life and can be associated with poor responses to cancer-related treatments. The literature also suggests that the mechanism for fatigue may be related to a "vicious circle between fatigue, physical inactivity, and deconditioning."[51]

Occupational therapy practitioners are primarily concerned with the degree of activity limitation and the reduced capacity for occupational participation, which are negative consequences of deconditioning.[49] Occupational therapy practitioners have a key function of supporting cancer survivors with restoring typical levels of participation or with developing strategies or appropriate modifications to support engagement in valued occupations.

Cardiovascular and Pulmonary Considerations

At the core of occupational performance is the functionality of the cardiovascular and pulmonary systems. In the oncological setting, the occupational therapy practitioner must consider the disease burden and the unfortunate impact of anticancer therapies on these systems. Chemotherapy, radiation therapy, supportive medications such as steroids, and surgical resection may cause damage or risk of complications to the heart, lungs, and larger circulatory system. Specific to radiation therapy, a cornerstone in the treatment of thoracic malignancies, the lungs may develop inflammatory changes and scarring as a side effect of treatment.[14] Comorbid conditions, such as history of myocardial infarction, coronary artery disease, and atrial fibrillation, further complicate the clinical picture and must be considered when evaluating activity tolerance. There are strong implications for the efficacy of skilled occupational therapy intervention in this patient population because support for engagement in occupations, exercise prescription, normalization of routine for activities, as examples, may improve the performance of the cardiovascular and pulmonary systems thereby reducing debility.

Psychosocial Issues (Body Image, Depression, Anxiety)

The patient with cancer is faced with many psychosocial challenges such as distress, anxiety, or depression starting at initial diagnosis and often lasting throughout survivorship.[32] The word *cancer* is often associated with a "life-threatening" disease, although it is more recently used to refer to a chronic illness in the field of medicine. Beyond thoughts of death, patients begin to worry about how the diagnosis and treatment will affect the

occupational performance of not only themselves but also family, and friends. Lyons[31] suggested, "The awareness of mortality and resultant uncertainty can create tension in the lives of those with cancer." There are many effects of psychosocial challenges on everyday occupations, including but not limited to altered or disrupted roles, routines, and habits; changes to social contexts; negative emotions, loss of control and identity; impaired motivation; and decline in quality of life.[31] Still, some cancer patients may experience post-traumatic growth, which occurs when the cancer experience prompts increased resilience and mental health.[32,54]

Body image and self-efficacy is a common psychosocial issue experienced by patients with cancer secondary to unavoidable changes to appearance and decline in function. Body image is a complex concept that goes far beyond one's perceptions of physical appearance and includes the resultant feelings associated with those perceptions.[29] Body image is further defined as a multidimensional construct that involves perceptions, thoughts, feelings, and behaviors related to the entire body and its functioning.[20]

Moreover, Zabora et al.[53] stated that 60% of cancer patients suffer psychological distress. Distress can be defined as multifactorial, unpleasant emotional experience of a psychological, social, or spiritual nature that interferes with effective coping.[38] Some literature, however, estimates that the proportion exceeds 60%, which is often what we see in practice. Although statistics do not exist, we find that many of the patients who are referred for occupational therapy experience a higher incidence of psychosocial challenges, most likely secondary to decline in function and occupation-based activities, than patients who are never referred to occupational therapy.[16]

Occupational therapy practitioners are trained to assess the needs of the whole person in different environments and contexts, which includes any psychosocial issues interfering with occupational performance and participation.[8]

Occupational therapy intervention for psychosocial issues can include adaptations to the physical and social environment to promote occupations.[8] Occupational therapy practitioners can develop programs and interventions that promote health, well-being, and social participation.[10]

The focus of occupational therapy intervention can include:
- Stress management and coping strategies to increase one's sense of control.
- Relaxation techniques, guided imagery, and breathing techniques as part of a personal plan to manage anxiety.
- Lifestyle management and redesign.
- Cognitive behavioral techniques and adaptive solutions to practical problems.
- Facilitate positive lifestyle change and adoption of healthy behaviors.
- Interventions related to disturbance in body image.
- Psychosexual therapy focusing on communication training, sensate focus, and body image exposure.
- Expressive-supportive therapy focusing on expression of thoughts and emotions, receiving and offering support, coping skills.
- Educational interventions including information disseminated in lecture formats to increase knowledge on disease and treatment with the aim of increasing self-efficacy.

Although it is easy to direct the clinical eye to physical changes and manifestations of cancer, the occupational therapy practitioner working in oncology must have a keen awareness of a number of detrimental effects on occupational performance and participation that are not observable, namely anxiety and depression. People with cancer and their families experience a substantial amount of psychological morbidity. Depression and anxiety can have an impact on functioning, quality of life, and survival. Tang et al.[48] discuss that the cancer patients, especially in terminal cases, are predisposed to depressive symptoms as a result of progressive functional decline, accelerating symptom severity, deteriorating social support, and self-perceived burden to others. Pain associated with treatments is also correlated to depression and anxiety. Typical assessments found and used in the oncology setting to detect these include the Hospital Anxiety and Depression Scale, the Beck Depression Inventory, and the Beck Anxiety Inventory.

LYMPHEDEMA

Lymphedema, a condition caused by inadequate drainage of lymphatic fluid, is a common secondary condition associated with some forms of cancer treatment.[3,5] Lymphedema is most commonly associated with breast cancer but can be seen with other forms of cancer, including lymphoma. There are multiple causes of inadequate lymphatic drainage, including blockage of lymphatic flow by a tumor, scarring and inflammation of the lymph nodes and vessels after radiation therapy, and surgical resection of a lymph node or multiple lymph nodes. Lymphedema can occur in the head and neck region but most commonly occurs in the arms or the legs. Scrotal edema also can occur after surgery.

According to the American Cancer Society,[4] lymphedema can begin soon after surgery or radiation but can also appear many years after treatment, and cancer survivors should be educated to the fact that they will remain at risk for lymphedema throughout their life. Several studies have shown that 80% of individuals experience an onset of lymphedema within 3 years of surgery.[42,43] O'Toole and colleagues[41] note that lymphedema can have significant functional implications and increased attention has been given to lymphedema with increased survivorship. Treatment approaches for lymphedema include gentle exercise paired with diaphragmatic breathing, compression garments and lymphedema wrapping techniques, manual lymphatic drainage, pneumatic compression, and complete decongestive therapy (CDT).[3,5,6] Certification in the management of lymphedema is available to both occupational therapy practitioners and physical therapy practitioners.

PALLIATIVE CARE AND HOSPICE

According to the American Occupational Therapy Association (AOTA), hospice and palliative care are closely related. In both instances, practitioners intervene with persons facing life-threatening illnesses.[36] The official document, "The Role of Occupational Therapy in End of Life Care" states, "Palliative care differs from hospice care in that palliative care can be initiated at any point in the client's illness, whereas hospice is reserved for the terminal stage of the client's condition. Curative care interventions may be used within the context of the palliative approach, whereas curative services are not provided when a client is receiving hospice care. A client simultaneously receiving palliative and curative services may transition to a hospice service when curative therapies are no longer appropriate or desired and the end of life is more imminent."[9]

A key element of occupational therapy practice in palliative care and in hospice is remaining patient-centered and providing occupation-based intervention. The occupational therapy practitioner in hospice collaborates with the patient and the patient's family to identify goals and to assist the patient to remain self-determinant. Because persons with cancer may be under hospice care for a short time before death or for many months, and because hospice care is provided on an inpatient basis and at home, patients may wish to continue performance of occupations across the spectrum of occupational roles, including worker, home manager, parent, spouse, religious participant, and others. The occupational therapy process is the same with the patient who is dying as it is with any other occupational therapy patient. Even those who are faced with imminent death typically have goals and wish to remain in control and self-determinant.

SUMMARY

The number of cancer survivors is growing significantly, and persons with cancer have rehabilitation needs, including needs for occupational therapy intervention during active treatment and following. Cancer can result in a range of problems that affect occupational performance, including cancer-related fatigue, cancer-related cognitive dysfunction, pain, cancer-induced neuropathy, lymphedema, depression, and a range of psychosocial issues related to body image, reproduction, and identity.

Although many persons with cancer may be able to physically perform basic ADLs and IADLs, the effects of cancer and its treatment such as surgery, radiation, and chemotherapy can be devastating. Many cancer survivors will require some support and assistance to manage multiple roles and even common occupations. Occupational therapy assessment and intervention should be comprehensive and identify the full range of factors that are influencing occupational performance. Strategies including but not limited to energy conservation, work simplification, compensatory strategies for decreased attention or memory, prevention of edema and lymphedema and to address psychosocial issues including body image and sexuality are appropriate.

Comprehensive oncology rehabilitation by the occupational therapy practitioner begins with evaluation of occupational performance and the development of the occupational therapy profile. Remaining patient-focused, theory-driven, and evidence-based during the intervention planning and implementation phases will help to ensure positive outcomes.

REVIEW QUESTIONS

1. What are the most common forms of cancer in men and women and what is the likelihood of experiencing cancer during one's life?
2. What are common treatment approaches for cancer and how can they affect the occupational performance of persons with cancer?
3. Why is occupational therapy intervention with persons with cancer medically complex?
4. What areas of specialty and advanced knowledge must the occupational therapy practitioner have when working with persons with cancer?
5. What are common approaches to assessment of occupational performance in the person with cancer?

For additional practice questions for this chapter, please visit eBooks.Health.Elsevier.com.

REFERENCES

1. Ahles T, Root J, Ryan E: Cancer and cancer treatment associated cognitive change: An update on the state of the science, *Journal of Clinical Oncology* 30:675–686, 2012.
2. Allen JM, Graef DM, Ehrentraut JH, Tynes BL, Crabtree VM: Sleep and pain in pediatric illness: A conceptual review, *CNS Neuroscience & Therapeutics* 22:880–893, 2016. https://doi.org/10.1111/cns.12583.
3. American Cancer Society. What is lymphedema? 2021. https://www.cancer.org/cancer/managing-cancer/side-effects/swelling/lymphedema/what-is-lymphedema.html.
4. American Cancer Society. Cancer Facts & Figures 2022; 2022. https://www.cancer.org/research/cancer-facts-statistics/all-cancer-facts-figures/cancer-facts-figures-2022.html.
5. American Cancer Society. For people at risk of lymphedema. 2020. Online at: https://www.cancer.org/treatment/treatments-and-side-effects/physical-side-effects/lymphedema/for-people-at-risk-of-lymphedema.html.
6. American Cancer Society. Types of cancer treatment. 2020. Online at: https://www.cancer.org/treatment/treatments-and-side-effects/treatment-types.html.
7. American Occupational Therapy Association. AOTA approves updates to Occupational Therapy Model Practice Act, 2023. https://www.aota.org/advocacy/advocacy-news/2023/occupational-therapy-model-practice-act.
8. American Occupational Therapy Association: Occupational therapy services in the promotion of psychological and social aspects of mental health, *American Journal of Occupational Therapy* 64(Suppl.):S78–S91, 2010.
9. American Occupational Therapy Association: The role of occupational therapy in end-of-life care, *American Journal of Occupational Therapy* 70(Suppl. 2):7012410075, 2016. https://doi.org/10.5014/ajot.2016.706S17
10. American Occupational Therapy Association. Occupational therapy in the promotion of health and well-being. 2020. https://research.aota.org/ajot/article/74/3/7403420010p1/6636/Occupational-Therapy-in-the-Promotion-of-Health.
11. American Occupational Therapy Association. Occupational therapy practice framework: Domain and process (4th ed.). *American Journal of Occupational Therapy* 74 (Supplement 2), 2020. Advance online publication.
12. Argyriou AA, Bruna J, Marmiroli P, Cavaletti G: Chemotherapy-induced peripheral neurotoxicity (CIPN): An update, *Critical Reviews in Oncology/Hematology* 82(21):51–77, 2011.
13. Bao YJ, Hou W, Kong XY, Yang L, Xia J, Hua BJ, Knaggs R: Hydromorphone for cancer pain, *Cochrane Database of Systematic Reviews* 2016:CD011108, 2016. https://doi.org/10.1002/14651858.CD011108.pub2.
14. Benveniste MF, Gomez D, Carter BW, Betancourt Cuellar S, Shroff GS, Benveniste A, Marom E: Recognizing rational therapy-related complications in the chest, *Radiographics* 39:344–366, 2019.
15. Bower JE, Bak K, Berger A, Breitbart W, Escalante CP, Ganz PA, Jacobsen PB: Screening, assessment, and management of fatigue in adult survivors of cancer: an American Society of Clinical oncology clinical practice guideline adaptation, *Journal of Clinical Oncology* 32(17):1840–1850, 2014.
16. Campbell C, Hughes J, Munoz L: *Occupational therapy's unique contributions to cancer rehabilitation*, Bethesda, Maryland, 2012, AOTA Press.
17. Chidinma C, Ebede MD, Yongchang Jang BS, Carmen P, Escalante MD: Cancer-related fatigue in cancer survivorship, *Medical Clinics of North America,* 101:1085–1097, 2017.
18. Escalante CP (2014): Cancer-related fatigue: Prevalence, screening and clinical assessment. http://www.uptodate.com/contents/cancer-related-fatigue-prevalence-screening-and-clinical-assessment.
19. Escalante CP, Kallen MA, Valdres RU, Morrow PK, Manzullo EF: Outcomes of a cancer related fatigue clinic in a comprehensive cancer, *Journal of Pain Symptom Management* 39(4):691–701, 2010.
20. Fingeret MC, Teo I, Epner D: Managing body image difficulties of adult cancer patients: lessons from available research, *Cancer* 120(5):633–641, 2014.
21. Reference deleted in proofs.
22. Goudas LC, Bloch R, Gialeli-Goudas M, Lau J, Carr DB: The epidemiology of cancer pain, *Cancer Investigation* 23(2):182–190, 2005.
23. Hann DM, Jacobson PB, Azzarello LM, Martin SC, Curren SL, Field KK, et al: Measurement of fatigue in cancer patient: Development and validation of the Fatigue Symptom Inventory, *Quality of Life Research* 7:301–310, 1998.
24. Hill AE: Cancer related fatigue. In Braveman B, Newman R, editors: *Cancer and occupational therapy: Enabling performance and participation across the lifespan*, North Bethesda, Maryland, 2020, AOTA Press, pp 187–198.
25. Hunter EG, Gibson RW, Arbesman M, D'Amico M: Systematic review of occupation therapy and adult cancer rehabilitation: Part 1. Impact of physical activity and symptom management interventions, *American Journal of Occupational Therapy* 71:7102100030, 2017. https://doi.org/10.5014/ajot.2017.023564.
26. Janelsins MC, Kesler SR, Ahles TA, Morrow GR: Prevalence, mechanisms, and management of cancer-related cognitive impairment, *International Review of Psychiatry* 26(1):102–113, 2014.

27. Janelsins MC, Kohli S, Mohile SG, Usuki K, Ahles TA, & Morrow GR: An update on cancer-and chemotherapy-related cognitive dysfunction: current status. In *Seminars in Oncology* 38(3):431–438, 2011.

28. Kautio AL, Haanpää M, Kautiainen H, Kalso E, Saarto T: Burden of chemotherapy-induced neuropathy—A cross-sectional study, *Supportive Care in Cancer* 19:1991–1996, 2011. https://doi.org/10.1007/s00520-010-1043-2.

29. Kelly D: Special considerations for adolescents and young adults with cancer. In Braveman B, Newman's R, editors: *Cancer and Occupational Therapy: Enabling Performance and Participation Across the Lifespan*, North Bethesda, Maryland, 2020, AOTA Press, pp 67–77.

30. Kortebein P: Rehabilitation for hospital-associated deconditioning, *American Journal of Physical Medicine and Rehabilitation* 88:66–77, 2009. https://doi.org/10.1097/PHM.0b013e3181838f70.

31. Lyons K: Occupation as a vehicle to surmount the psychosocial challenges of cancer, *Occupational Therapy in HealthCare* 20(2):1–16, 2006.

32. Lyons K: Psychosocial issues. In Braveman B, Newman's R, editors: *Cancer and Occupational Therapy: Enabling Performance and Participation Across the Lifespan*, North Bethesda, Maryland, 2020, AOTA Press, pp 253–266.

33. McColl E: Best practice in symptom assessment: A review, *Gut* 53(4):49–54, 2004.

34. Miaskowski C, Mastick J, Paul SM, Topp K, Smoot B, Abrams G, Chen LM, Kober KM, Conley YP, Chesney M, Bolla K, Mausisa G, Mazor M, Wong M, Schumacher M, Levine JD: Chemotherapy-induced neuropathy in cancer survivors, *Journal of Pain Symptom Management* 54(2):204, 2017.

35. Miltenburg NC, Boogerd W: Chemotherapy-induced neuropathy: A comprehensive survey, *Cancer Treatment Reviews* 40:872–882, 2014.

36. Munoz, L., & Campbell, C. (2010). AOTA Fact Sheet: The role of occupational therapy in palliative and hospice care. American Occupational Therapy Association.

37. National Cancer Institute. Cancer Statistics. 2018. https://www.cancer.gov/about-cancer/understanding/statistics.

38. National Comprehensive Cancer Network. NCCN Clinical Practice Guidelines for Distress Management. 2023. https://www.nccn.org/guidelines/guidelines-detail?category=3&id=1457.

39. National Comprehensive Cancer Network. NCCN Clinical Practice Guidelines in Oncology: Cancer-Related Fatigue. 2020. https://allofmeiowa.org/wp-content/uploads/2020/09/Cancer-Related-Fatigue.pdf.

40. Nicholson J: Cancer-related pain. In Braveman B, Newman R, editors: *Cancer and Occupational Therapy: Enabling Performance and Participation Across the Lifespan*, 199-212, North Bethesda, Maryland, 2020, AOTA Press.

41. Norman SA, Localio AR, Potashnik SL, Torpey HAS, Kallan MJ, Weber AL, Solin LJ: Lymphedema in breast cancer survivors: incidence, degree, time course, treatment, and symptoms, *Journal of Clinical Oncology* 27(3):390, 2009.

42. O'Toole JA, Ferguson CM, Swaroop MN, Horick N, Skolny MN, Brunelle CL, Miller CL, Jammallo LS, Specht MC, Taghian AG: The impact of breast cancer-related lymphedema on the ability to perform upper extremity activities of daily living, *Breast Cancer Research and Treatment* 150:381–388, 2015.

43. Petrek JA, Senie RT, Peters M, Rosen PP: Lymphedema in a cohort of breast carcinoma survivors 20 years after diagnosis, *Cancer* 92(6):1368–1377, 2001.

44. Portenoy, R.K. & Dhingra, L.K. (2015). Assessment of cancer pain. UpToDate. http://www.uptodate.com/contents/assessment-of-cancer-pain.

45. Siebens H, Aronow H, Edwards D, Ghasemi Z: A randomized controlled trial of exercise to improve outcomes of acute hospitalization in older adults, *Journal of the American Geriatrics Society* 48:1545–1552, 2000. https://doi.org/10.1111/j.1532-5415.2000.tb03862.x

46. Reference deleted in proofs.

47. Stubblefield MD, Burstein HJ, Burton AW, Custodio CM, Deng GE, Ho M, et al: NCCN Task Force report: Management of neuropathy in cancer, *Journal of the National Comprehensive Cancer Network* 7(Suppl. 5):S1–S26, 2009; quiz S27–S28.

48. Tang ST, Chen JS, Chou WC, Lin KC, Chang WC, Hsieh CH, Wu CE: Prevalence of severe depressive symptoms increases as death approaches and is associated with disease burden, tangible social support, and high self-perceived burden to others, *Support Care Cancer* 24(2):83–91, 2015.

49. Timmer AJ, Unsworth CA, Browne M: A randomized controlled trial protocol investigating effectiveness of an activity-pacing program for deconditioned older adults, *Canadian Journal of Occupational Therapy* 86(2):136–147, 2019. https://doi.org/10.1177/0008417419830374.

50. Ubrich S, Mohammed A: Chemotherapy-induced peripheral neuropathy. In Braveman B, Newman R, editors: *Cancer and Occupational Therapy: Enabling Performance and Participation Across the Lifespan*, North Bethesda, Maryland, 2020, AOTA Press, pp 241–252.

51. Vermaete N, Wolter P, Verhoef G, Gosselink R: Physical activity and physical fitness in lymphoma patients before, during, and after chemotherapy: a prospective longitudinal study, *Annals of Hematology* 93(3):411–424, 2014.

52. Winters-Stone KM, Horak F, Jacobs PG, Trubowitz P, Dieckmann NF, Stoyles S, Faithfull S: Falls, functioning, and disability among women with persistent symptoms of chemotherapy-induced peripheral neuropathy, *Journal of Clinical Oncology* 35(23):2604, 2017.

53. Zabora J, BrintzenhofeSzoc K, Curbow B, Hooker C, Piantadosi S: The prevalence of psychological distress by cancer site, *Psycho-Oncology* 10(1):19–28, 2001.

54. Zamora ER, Yi J, Akter J, Kim J, Warner EL, Kirchoff AC: "Having cancer was awful but also something good came out": Post-traumatic growth among adult survivors of pediatric and adolescent cancer, *European Journal of Oncology Nursing* 28(Suppl. C):21–27, 2017. https://doi.org/10.1016/j.ejon.2017.02.001.

ADDITIONAL RESOURCES

- National Cancer Institute (NCI): https://www.nci.nih.gov
- American Cancer Society: https://www.cancer.org
- Cancer Hope Network: https://www.cancerhopenetwork.org
- Coping with Cancer Magazine: https://www.copingmag.com

47

Meeting the Needs of the Older Adult[a]

Samia Husam Rafeedie

LEARNING OBJECTIVES

After studying this chapter, the student or practitioner will be able to do the following:

1. Describe the importance of wellness and productive aging for the baby boomer generation.
2. Describe what an occupational therapist can do to help an older adult to age in place.
3. Identify the environmental factors (services, systems, and policies) affecting older adults in the United States and their access to healthcare.
4. Describe how the learning needs and styles of older adults may differ from those of younger persons.
5. Describe the accepted theories of how aging occurs.
6. Describe the therapeutic benefits of using occupations as a primary modality with older adults.
7. Describe how mental functions may change as a person ages.

8. Identify basic age-related changes in sensory functions and body structures.
9. Identify basic age-related changes in neuromusculoskeletal functions.
10. Identify basic age-related changes in cardiovascular, hematological, immunological, and respiratory functions.
11. Identify basic age-related changes in voice and speech functions; digestive, metabolic, and endocrine functions; and genitourinary and reproductive functions.
12. Identify basic age-related changes in skin and related structure functions.
13. Describe the concept of "flipping a nursing facility" and facilitating a paradigm shift with clients and colleagues alike.

CHAPTER OUTLINE

[a] The author would like to acknowledge the outstanding contributions of Joanne Wright and Jennifer Glover to previous editions.

KEY TERMS

Aging in place

Allostatic load

Andropause

Mild cognitive impairment

Old-old

Productive aging

Senescence

Shared governance

THREADED CASE STUDY

Doris, Part 1

Doris (prefers use of the pronouns she/her/hers) has been an assistant to a local certified public accountant for decades and is responsible for the bookkeeping and bills in her home. She enjoys sending e-mails on her personal computer and playing the piano. In fact, Doris was a piano instructor for many years and enjoyed teaching the young people in her neighborhood as a side job. Her husband, Don, says that this was the only thing that kept her going before her most recent fall. Doris is a 79-year-old mother of two, grandmother of four, and great grandmother of two who lives in Indiana with her husband of 55 years.

Doris and Don have recently moved into a senior living community right behind the skilled nursing and rehabilitation facility where she was admitted for 1 month after an incident at home in which she fell and could not be assisted by her husband, who also has medical complications with his heart. Doris' family became concerned after recent falls at the new apartment and Doris showing signs of increased forgetfulness and bouts of confusion. She was recently diagnosed with senile dementia–Alzheimer's type and has a medical history of hypertension, spinal stenosis, diverticulitis, osteoarthritis, laser eye surgery, and a colonoscopy. Her admitting diagnosis is right hip fracture.

Doris' occupational therapy (OT) evaluation took place at bedside with her husband present. She required supervision for feeding and maximum assistance with grooming and bathing activities; she also required maximum verbal cues for thoroughness and attention to detail. Doris required supervision for upper

body dressing and minimal assistance for lower body dressing and toileting. She required stand-by assistance for bed mobility and minimal assistance for functional mobility during performance of everyday tasks with the use of a front-wheeled walker. She was oriented × 2 (to her name and situation) and could follow simple directions. Her long-term memory and short-term memory were impaired. On observation, her oculomotor skills and visual fields appeared intact. However, she had two pairs of glasses; one pair was for reading and one was for distance, but she was uncomfortable with both pairs and said she was waiting for a new pair from her doctor. Range of motion was within normal limits in the bilateral upper extremities. She demonstrated good (4/5) manual muscle grades throughout both upper extremities and is right-hand dominant. No apparent tone impairments were noted, and she had no complaints of pain at the time of evaluation. Fine motor and gross motor coordination appeared within functional limits for both upper extremities. Minimal edema was present in both lower extremities.

Critical Thinking Questions

1. What intervention activities might be used to support engagement in meaningful occupation while Doris is at the rehabilitation facility?
2. What are the areas of concern with Doris' caregiver and home situation?
3. How will Doris' current status and medical history complicate the rehabilitation process?

INTRODUCTION

Occupational therapy (OT) practitioners have a unique opportunity to be at the forefront of healthcare delivery to our society's older adults. Occupational therapy's holistic and client-centered approach highlights strengths and resources and supports the complex and challenging physical, social, cognitive, and emotional changes experienced by this population. These changes may have an impact on occupational independence and participation in meaningful activity; therefore, a careful and thorough approach to evaluation and intervention is required to meet the needs of our aging population.

Americans born between 1946 and 1964 are members of the baby boom generation, and this cohort turned 74 years of age in 2020.[43] Chop estimates that from this time on, "approximately one American will turn 65 years of age every 8 seconds for the next 18 years" (p. 2).[43] In 2019, the United States (U.S.) Census Bureau reported that more than 54 million people residing in the U.S. were 65 years or older (2020).[185] Werner reported that more people were 65 years of age and over in 2010 than in any other census reporting period,[183,200] and this population increased at a faster rate (15.1%) than the total U.S. population (9.7%). By the year 2030, it is estimated that 22% of Americans (70.2 million) will be 65 years of age and older.[43]

Another fast-growing population of interest for occupational therapy in the United States is the group older than 85 years of age.

This cohort is referred to as the old-old and is expected to increase from 5.5 million in 2010 to 6.6 million in 2020 (19% increase) according to Chop.[43] Opportunities for occupational therapy are also presenting themselves on the global scale with an estimated 1 billion people in the 65 years and older bracket worldwide by 2030, which is 12% of the projected total world population. By 2050, 1.6 billion (or 17%) of the total population of 9.4 billion will be 65 and older.[147] For the first time in history, people over 65 years of age will outnumber children under the age of 5, and according to Chop,[43] this will likely happen between 2015 and 2020. These population trends demand special attention as OT practitioners work with older adults in a variety of settings, including, but not limited to, home healthcare, assisted living, skilled nursing, inpatient rehabilitation, outpatient clinics, community health programs, adult day programs, and extended care facilities, as well as in palliative care. Not only will the role of occupational therapy in healthcare support the aging population with physical disabilities, but occupational therapy is also positioned to address aging in place, wellness, and prevention.

This chapter highlights the unique contributions OT practitioners can make when working with older adults who may have physical limitations but who are also getting older and experiencing the many developmental and biopsychosocial (biological, psychological, and sociological) changes that naturally occur from the moment a person is born. The fourth edition of the

Occupational Therapy Practice Framework (OTPF) is used as a foundation to paint a comprehensive picture from a top-down approach, starting with wellness and productive aging, then moving to occupation and participation in meaningful activity and, finally, highlighting body functions and structures that have the potential to physiologically decline as a person ages.[7]

WELLNESS AND PRODUCTIVE AGING

Improvements in healthcare technology and lifestyle have positively affected the lifespan, with people now living longer and healthier lives as a result of productive aging.[28] According to the National Institute on Aging,[130] people are living longer. In 1970, people were expected to live approximately 71 years, but this number has been on the rise. In 2020, the average life expectancy was 78.6 years of age, according to the U.S. Census Bureau (2020).[185] Given this increase in life expectancy, the myths of aging would have society believe that with age comes disability and limitations, but this is not necessarily true.

Important information regarding nutrition, exercise, and health management can be accessed instantly by way of smart phones, computers, and other personal electronic devices. Older adults do experience problems with health if the body is not taken care of over time. The National Institute on Aging[130] reports that problems with health can arise if the body has been subjected to overeating, poor nutrition, and lack of adequate exercise and activity, as well as exposure to toxins (such as drugs and alcohol); therefore, preventive measures are critical for the older adult population.

Healthy People 2020 includes a goal for improving the health of all Americans and strives to encourage collaborations across communities, empower individuals to make informed health decisions, and measure the impact of activities associated with prevention.[78] A gerontological approach is reflected in the work this organization has developed for older adults, including socioeconomic and lifestyle-related influences on health. *Healthy People 2020* highlights the importance of independence and vitality with aging and uses a health-oriented approach rather than a disease-oriented approach.[78] According to *Healthy People 2020*, common complaints experienced frequently by older adults include joint stiffness, weight gain, fatigue, loss of bone density, and loneliness. The research presented by this organization also indicates that these conditions can be prevented, or even eliminated, with activities such as exercise, stress management, nutrition counseling, and substance control.[78,79] Older adults who do not get physical activity are more likely to experience a fall or develop a disability, according to the most recent version of *Healthy People 2030*.[79] For older adults, falls are a major cause of "premature death, physical injury, immobility, psychosocial dysfunction, and nursing home placement" (p. 194).[180] Falls are more prevalent in the adult population who are 65 years and older, with the age-adjusted fall death rate climbing to 64 deaths per 100,000 older adults.[34] Having one fall will increase the risk for an older adult to fall again, and, alarmingly, the psychological consequences such as fear associated with falls, according to Schoene et al., may be just as detrimental as the fall itself over time.[159] They concluded that the importance of fear of falling on quality of life in older adults, "appears

to be more important than actual falls" (p. 716).[159] According these researchers, fear of falling and quality of life can be clinically addressed through increased amounts of physical activity, which can also improve physical and cognitive functioning in older adults.[159]

According to Florence associates, about one third of older adults will fall each year, resulting in more than just the injuries after the fall, but also includes acquired injuries such as head trauma, lacerations, and hip fractures.[65] With a rise in the lifespan of older adults, the burden of cost in the United States for fatal and nonfatal falls in 2018 was approximately $50 billion dollars.[65] As Leland et al. stated, "Falls are a serious public health concern among older adults in the United States" (p. 149)[105]; therefore, OT practitioners should assess and intervene accordingly based on current evidence and practice guidelines. More information can be found through publications by the American Occupational Therapy Association (AOTA),[5] American Geriatrics Society (AGS), and the British Geriatrics Society (BGS) for specific algorithms and intervention approaches for older adults in the community, those living in long-term care facilities, and those with cognitive impairments.[4]

Prevention in the hospital setting is just as critical as prevention in the community. Rogers and colleagues examined the association between hospital spending for specific services and 30-day readmission rates for patients who were diagnosed with heart failure, pneumonia, and acute myocardial infarction.[151] An outcome of their study was that occupational therapy was the only "spending category where additional spending was a statistically significant association with lower readmission rates for all three medical conditions."[151] It was determined that occupational therapy provides "a unique and immediate focus on patients' functional and social needs, which can be important drivers of readmission if left unaddressed."[151] OT interventions that could potentially decrease readmissions described in Roger's study include addressing cognitive abilities; patient education and caregiver training in preparation for discharge; addressing functional needs related to self-care and recommendations for after discharge; prescribing adaptive equipment and durable medical equipment to increase independence in self-care and functional mobility; and performing home safety assessments, which are found to prevent falls—interventions described in a study by Clemson.[49]

OT practitioners work with older adults on all aspects of their lives so that they are ready to face the challenges ahead as they work to age in place and participate fully in life. With the holistic perspective occupational therapy brings to the table, it is essential that the field addresses promotion of health at both the individual and the population level. The basic tenets of occupational therapy have always helped with identification, realization, and change in the person, the occupation, or the environment in an effort to enhance participation and quality of life.[201] Community-based practice will be critical as increasingly more baby boomers require services. OT practitioners have opportunities for employment in senior centers, community centers, and skilled nursing facilities where innovative programs can be designed and implemented.

An example of an innovative program developed by occupational therapists (OTs) includes Farewell to Falls. Farewell to Falls is part of a fall prevention program developed at the Trauma Service of Stanford University Medical Center. According to Corman,[51] best practice in fall prevention should include a multifactorial risk assessment and intervention, with a focus on home safety and modifications,[116] medication management, and regular exercise. The development of this program also included best opportunities for patient compliance with suggestions related to behavior change by way of individualized assessment and home-based intervention.[51]

The Home Safety Council and National Council on Aging named the Farewell to Falls program as one of the 10 best programs nationally with respect to providing "creative programs and practices in home assessment and modifications" (p. 206)[51] in March of 2007. The program is designed to send an occupational therapist to a patient's home for two visits to complete a health and daily living skills interview, as well as a safety checklist and sensory-motor assessment. A basic fall prevention screening is completed, and simple home modifications are recommended. The program will even cover the cost of some modifications, such as grab bars. A pharmacy resident participates in the initial home visit to review medications and provide information on drug interactions and side effects. During the second home visit, the occupational therapist reviews the pharmacy-prepared medication report and prescribes an individualized exercise program for the patient. Patients receive a follow-up phone call once per month to encourage compliance, and after the first year of the implementation an occupational therapist reevaluates the patient during a home visit.[51]

Older adults not only need fall prevention strategies when living on their own or in a care facility, they also require interventions that enable them to "infuse sustainable, personally satisfying, health-promoting activities into daily life."[45] In a groundbreaking study, the USC Well Elderly Study[44–46] demonstrated in a dramatic way that occupational therapy intervention, based on sound occupational science principles, was more effective than other types of group activities and beneficial overall to older adults. During the 9-month study period, participants were randomly assigned to the Lifestyle Redesign intervention, a social activity control group, or a no-treatment control group. Participants who were assigned to the Lifestyle Redesign intervention group maintained or improved their health-related quality of life and life satisfaction.[87] These changes were a direct cause of involvement in the specific occupational therapy intervention, not merely involvement in busy work, or social activity.[45] This study was followed up by the Well Elderly 2 randomized controlled trial that "demonstrated that a 6-month preventative lifestyle-oriented intervention has positive effects for a sample of ethnically diverse older people recruited from a variety of community sites."[46] In the profession's earliest days, occupation was seen as health promoting and necessary for a productive and satisfying life.[136]

AGING IN PLACE

Aging in place is a phrase used in healthcare, among policy makers and advocacy groups, meaning to continue to live in the community, with some level of independence, rather than moving into an institution or care facility.[54] With the rise of healthcare costs and the increase in the number of older adults, the cost of healthcare programs has risen to staggering levels.[28] According to the Centers for Disease Control and Prevention (CDC), the national health expenditures as a percentage of the gross domestic product for national health programs (i.e., Medicare, Medicaid, veterans' medical care) increased from 0.4% in 1962 to approximately 17.9% in 2017.[35,40] Older adults with declining health spend more money on long-term institutionalization care than on any other kind of healthcare.[28]

The cost for long-term care varies by state, but on average, it costs $87,000 per year for a semiprivate room. It is estimated that by 2030, the cost for institutionalized care will grow to $190,600 per year.[28] This is a cost that the majority of older adults will likely not be able to afford and is therefore not a realistic option when extensive medical care is needed. A person's health and well-being is strongly connected to the environment in which that person lives. Older adults who are physically and cognitively able to stay at home prefer to do so; however, those with physical or cognitive limitations, as well as other complex medical conditions, may need assistance or a more supportive environment.[149] The National Conference of State Legislatures and the American Association of Retired Persons (AARP) reported that 90% of seniors wish to stay at home as they age, and even if these older adults require some sort of assistance or ongoing healthcare during retirement, 83% would prefer to stay in their homes.[126] A small number of seniors prefer to move to a care facility (9%), and an even smaller percentage (4%) prefer to move in with a family member.[126] The AARP published an executive report highlighting policies that integrate land use, housing and transportation, efficient delivery of in-home services, provision of transportation options, and improvement of affordable and accessible housing to prevent social isolation.

Wanting to age in place is based on the accumulation of memories, habits, roles, and routines, or what may be described as the context or the environment. A number of helpful web-based resources focus on older adults and aging in place, as well as a number of services that can be used by older adults and OT practitioners working in the community. A growing number of developers and contractors use universal design principles in new construction and have an overall goal of creating aging-friendly communities—places where all areas of a community are accessible and user-friendly for older adults and people with a variety of abilities and disabilities. Many housing alternatives are available for older adults to age in place, with the idea being that aging in place relates to the preferred place of residence. When there is a good person-environment fit, a person is more likely to increase or maintain occupational performance. This environment can be a single-family home, an apartment, an assisted living senior complex, or with family.

The Community Aging in Place, Advancing Better Living for Elders (CAPABLE) intervention is a coordinated effort of an occupational therapist (for up to six visits), nurse (for up to four visits), and handyman (spending $1300 on average for home repairs and modifications) who visit clients in their homes who are waiting for home-based care. It is "funded by the Center for Medicare and Medicaid Innovation, and aims to reduce the impact of disability among low-income older adults by addressing the individual capacities and the home environment."[172] This intervention targeted intrinsic and extrinsic disability factors in a population of older adults who were categorized as low-income and African-American and had higher rates of disability, chronic disease, pain, and depression and less access to primary care services.[173] The findings from the study suggest that occupational therapy, nursing, and a handyman have the potential to improve daily function and well-being while a person ages in place at home.

Until residences are more accessible, evaluations and interventions for home modification will continue to be an important aspect of occupational therapy services. Whether it is an actual onsite evaluation or a review of the home and community by report, assessment of context is important when looking at the whole person. When performing a home evaluation, it is important to look at the fit between the person and the environment and then consider what modifications or services can help a person age in place. It is also critical to look beyond the physical and cognitive to the psychosocial, financial, and support-related change.

There are empowering movements in the community that support older adults who wish to maintain their independence and stay actively engaged in meaningful activity. One such movement is known as the Village to Village Network[192] and was developed to promote aging in place to foster a person's ability to continue to live in his or her home as safely, comfortably, and independently as possible, regardless of age, income, or ability level. The promoters of this network believe that older adults who are empowered can take control over their own lives, and as a cohesive and collective group, they can design and implement the future they desire for themselves.

A similar movement is the Green House Project, which has been growing since the early 2000s. Organizations are running successful Green House homes in a variety of settings, including skilled nursing facilities, assisted living centers, short-term rehabilitation centers, veterans' homes, and memory care facilities. On the Robert Wood Johnson Foundation (RWJF) website, this project is described as "a revolution in long-term care, creating small homes that return control, dignity, and a sense of well-being to elders, while providing high-quality, personalized care."[146] Older adults are living happier and healthier lives, according to the research conducted by the RWJF. This is an alternative to traditional nursing homes and provides opportunities for older adults to contribute to the everyday operational tasks of the home, to engage in purposeful activity, and, most importantly, to age in place.

OT practitioners have an important opportunity when working with older adults in community-based settings or healthcare facilities. The field thrives on empowering clients through meaningful occupations and "engagement in enjoyable and productive activity is paramount to productive aging" (p. 263).[149] Teaching our clients, caregivers, and colleagues about advocacy and empowerment changes perspectives and shifts attitudes in traditional medical settings, like skilled nursing facilities. There is an organizational structure known as shared governance, believed to be a nursing-derived concept or at least introduced first by nursing into the healthcare setting (though it is also used in academia, business, etc.) that can lend a great deal to OT practitioners who

are in leadership positions or seeking leadership opportunities in interprofessional settings. The emphasis is on a nonhierarchical matrix that disseminates accountability and decision-making to front-line staff [48] working directly with residents, patients, clients, or elders in the various healthcare settings. Transforming the leadership style in health facilities with one of shared governance has many benefits, according to Myers and colleagues.[122] Some of these benefits include overall patient satisfaction, improved patient outcomes, improved patient care, increased staff morale, increased job satisfaction (leading to staff retention), personal and professional growth and development, increased staff autonomy and decision-making, and improved communication among interdisciplinary team members. All of these benefits support a culture for aging in place and "flip" the very traditional (and at times, stigmatized) perception of a nursing home into a client-centered and occupation-based program where clients and clinicians equally thrive.

Clinicians are expected to be good stewards of limited resources, promote a positive work culture, and use best evidence when working with patients, caregivers, and colleagues through a lens of shared governance.[122] OT practitioners are the experts of occupational analysis, occupational balance, and wellness. Therefore, incorporating meaningful activity into an intervention should remain at the forefront of what OT practitioners do—provide therapeutic intervention based on everyday activities or occupations.

OCCUPATIONS

Activities of Daily Living

Completion of activities of daily living (ADLs) is a significant component of independent living for older adults and a top priority in the hospital setting. Because OT providers recognize deficits in self-care and function, they may be in a better position than any other healthcare provider in assessing ADLs and preventing a readmission because of complications after discharge from a hospital. Once discharged from a hospital, an older adult may be considered generally vulnerable, which could lead to challenges performing ADLs, the development of new disabilities, decreased independence in functional mobility, and overall weakness.[151] Continued participation in the basic self-care tasks and routines followed by older adults is viewed as critical in avoiding disability.[140] According to Robnett and O'Sullivan, 88% of people age 75 and older are independent with basic ADLs.[149] In a study by Jacobs and colleagues,[89] functional status declined progressively according to age with a trend from independence at age 70 to difficulty in performing ADLs at age 78, to dependence in performance by age 85. The study consisted of following a longitudinal cohort with a representative sample of 1861 people born between 1920 and 1921.[89]

According to Keeler and colleagues,[95] functional status has a dramatic impact on life expectancy, with declines in both ADLs and mobility resulting in decreased life expectancy and the remaining years of survival categorized as living with a disability. In fact, an association was identified between unmet needs for assistance in one to two ADLs and 1-year mortality, revealing a greater risk for mortality among older adults with mild disability.[76]

Of particular interest for the older adult population are the ADLs of feeding and swallowing and the connection between nutrition and chronic conditions. According to Thompson, approximately 15% of the older adult population living in the community and 50% of hospitalized older adults are malnourished, and the incidence of chronic disease in this population is high, "with 80% of older adults having at least one chronic disease and 50% having at least two" (p. 192).[179] An OT practitioner may consider several factors when weight loss or malnourishment has been identified as an issue. An individual who has been losing weight could have difficulty chewing because of poor dentition or ill-fitting dentures.[3] The death of a spouse or friend could affect appetite or a feeling of isolation during mealtime, limiting caloric intake.[82,179] An older adult may also have difficulty sitting comfortably at the table or maintaining safe posture required for feeding and swallowing. Older adults may also be losing weight because of difficulty preparing meals, transporting food within the kitchen, grocery shopping, or getting to the store or restaurant.

An older adult's ability to engage in functional mobility will affect other ADLs, including toileting and issues of continence. The likelihood of incontinence increases with age; Kuchel and DeBeau[102] reported that 23% of people who are 60 to 79 years of age and 32% of people 80 years of age and older are diagnosed with incontinence. Both men and women experience incontinence and may not feel comfortable initiating a discussion upon evaluation; however, the clinician can broach the topic in a sensitive manner. Quality of life, self-esteem, and self-concept may be affected by incontinence.[102] Intervention sessions can address management within the scope of ADLs, in collaboration with nursing and the physician. A referral to a specialist may also be warranted. It should be noted that side effects to medications impacting balance or cognition, access to toilets, and functional impairments (including the ability to transfer independently) are of concern for older adults living with this condition.

Incontinence and functional mobility impairments are also essential when addressing sexuality with the older adult population. Not only are physical abilities and limitations taken into consideration, but a number of chronic mental and psychological disorders, chronic illnesses and medication side effects, gender-specific health concerns, and lifestyle changes experienced over the lifespan should be taken into account.[83] According to Hillman,[83] only recently has society viewed aging and sexuality as an important topic that deserves attention from a clinical perspective. In her work, Hillman highlighted what clinicians can expect when working with baby boomers regarding sexuality and aging. Older adults may seek support for sexual dissatisfaction through medical and psychological treatment. Sexual disturbances may be a result of underlying interpersonal problems, which reflect changes in family structure over the course of time, such as divorce, stepfamily members, and multiple marriages. Eating disorders, institutionalization, openness to diversity, less traditional gender roles, and the influence of the internet and related technologies also will have an impact on the aging population seeking professional services.[83] This is an important area of human interaction and life satisfaction and also a sensitive discussion to have with an older client. Should the client wish

to engage in discussion, open-ended questions and a comprehensive occupational therapy intervention are encouraged. The extended PLISSIT model (Permission, Limited Information, Specific Suggestions, Intensive Therapy), or Ex-PLISSIT, extends the original model developed by Annon,[11] which was a conceptual scheme for the behavioral treatment of sexual problems. By emphasizing the importance of explicitly obtaining permission during every phase of an intervention geared toward sexuality and rehabilitation, the Ex-PLISSIT model is a more contemporary approach available to practitioners.[177] The reader is referred to Chapter 12 on sexuality and physical dysfunction as well as the work of Kontula and Haavio-Mannila,[101] Bauer and colleagues,[18] and Hinchliff and Gott[84] for more research, clinical relevance, and adaptive approaches related to this topic.

Adaptive approaches with functional mobility should always be assessed carefully because many older adults experience changes in this area. An older adult may use an assistive device for mobility, although it may not be used all of the time. Sometimes individuals are self-conscious in public and may use a cane or walker only at home.[143] Others feel comfortable walking in their home environment or using the furniture to help maintain their balance but will use a device when walking long distances. It is important to ask each client about a variety of situations to ensure an understanding of how the client maneuvers in different settings, because functional mobility is a critical aspect of the completion of instrumental activities of daily living (IADLs). See Chapter 11 for information on individual and community mobility.

Instrumental Activities of Daily Living

According to Depp and Jeste, autonomy in IADLs completion plays an important role in successful aging.[55] Contrary to common belief, over 80% of people 75 years of age (and older) are free of functional limitations requiring assistance for IADLs, according to Robnett and O'Sullivan.[149] Performance of IADLs is a factor in determining whether a person can continue living at home independently and should therefore be addressed when working with an older adult client. The use of tailored, interdisciplinary, home-based interventions combined with the use of cognitive intervention are reported as strong evidence to maintain IADL improvements over time.[85] Cognitive interventions should be used for improving executive function, functional status, everyday problem-solving, and memory in support of IADL completion. There is also strong evidence that individualized and client-based interventions in the home are beneficial to mediate functional disability and satisfaction with performance.[85] Difficulty in performing IADLs is associated with poor self-efficacy and decreased quality of life.[135,165] A change in performance of home management skills is sometimes the first sign that a person needs assistance in the home, and this may trigger considerations for moving into a family member's home or another community-based setting such as assisted living.[70]

Living in the community requires a means of transportation, whether it is driving or using public transportation. Maintaining the ability to drive is critical for older adults in that it allows the freedom they desire, and it promotes healthy aging and access to community resources, including shopping centers, medical

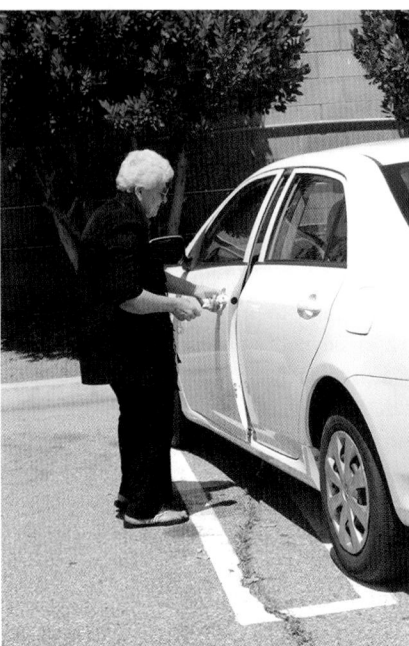

Fig. 47.1 An older adult driver accessing the community to complete daily tasks. (Photo courtesy Ramez Ethnasios.)

appointments, and visiting friends and family.[71] According to the CDC, there were nearly 44 million licensed drivers in the United States who were 65 years of age or older in 2017, which is a 63% increase from 1999.[36] The risk for accidents and injuries while driving increases with age, making the need for OT practitioners greater with this population.[128] OT practitioners can intervene at many levels, including in the areas of vision, cognition, functional mobility, and upper extremity strength, among others (Fig. 47.1).[128]

According to Rosenbloom,[153] older adults are not likely to use public transportation when they turn 65 years of age; they prefer to continue to drive or use private cars. Public transportation has traditionally been used by those who are commuting to work and underused by this population for many reasons, including cost, accessibility, and a fear of being stigmatized.[153] In fact, the National Council on Disability (NCD) stated that some people with disabilities cannot work, even though they would like to, and completing basic IADLs such as shopping or visiting friends becomes a challenge as a result of a lack of safe and reliable transportation options.[127] Safety is paramount in the area of transportation and driving, as well as in the home.

Safety when functioning in the home is a primary concern and should be addressed on multiple levels. Common factors to assess include vision (particularly in the areas of visual acuity, contrast sensitivity, glare sensitivity, adaptation to the dark, and visual field cuts), whether sufficient lighting and contrast are available for the older adult to be able to see, whether the home is in good condition or in need of repair, whether the person can move around the environment successfully, whether the neighborhood is safe, and whether the older adult is cognitively intact to understand whether risks are present. Doris and Don recently moved into a new home and although they continue to unpack and organize personal items, the living space is cluttered

with boxes and stacks of books, magazines, and clothing. This is creating a fall risk for Doris and limits the space in the hallways and rooms for safely using her walker. Doris has been diagnosed with Alzheimer's disease, so she is disoriented at baseline and the new living space further confuses her when she tries to use the bathroom in the middle of the night. Clearing a pathway in the hallway and removing items from the floors will decrease Doris' fall risk and promote functional mobility. The possibility of using a bedside commode also should be discussed with both Don and Doris.

Other factors affecting a person's ability to safely remain in the home is pain. Pain can decrease mental flexibility, which includes immediate and delayed memory, as well as language; and it can also decrease physical functioning.[93,198] Depression can influence cognitive processing and has been associated with cognitive decline,[203] and older adults should be screened upon evaluation when assessing safety in the home. Once the physical portion of the home evaluation is completed with the particular client in mind—including abilities and inabilities—it is time to address components that are important to aging in place that can be considered part of the extended context or the environment. What services are available in the community? How can the person access these services? Is the person willing and able to access them? Is the person socially isolated? Does the person drive despite not being able to see well enough or not being cognitively intact? Can modifications be made to the routine that will keep the client safe and socially connected? What are the client's social supports? These are just a few of the many questions that a clinician needs to start asking when evaluating a client regarding aging in place and safety in the home.

An OT practitioner may consider any of a number of home evaluations. Some of the home evaluations are based on performance and some are based on the physical characteristics of a home only. Psychometrically sound evaluations include the Safety Assessment of Function and the Environment for Rehabilitation (SAFER),[106] the In-Home Occupational Performance Evaluation (I-HOPE),[167] and the Home and Community Environment Assessment (HACE).[96] See Chapter 10 for an example of a home evaluation. A home evaluation was completed at Don and Doris' home using the facility's home assessment form to capture information and make recommendations. It was decided that Doris would benefit greatly from a bedside commode for use during the middle of the night, to avoid walking to the bathroom. A shower chair was also recommended, as well as a long-handled bath sponge. Doris did not like using the long-handled reacher and decided she did not need that "gadget." Don was tasked with asking their oldest daughter for help unpacking and clearing the hallways and floors, and Doris agreed to allow their oldest daughter to help with finances until Doris and Don were "back on their feet."

Community-based occupations, such as going to the pharmacy, shopping at a department store, or taking a grandchild to school can be intimidating to an older adult who has experienced a change in health status. Older adults have the same responsibilities younger adults have, such as caring for pets, caring for a spouse or loved one, or child rearing. According to Brossoie and Chop,[28] there is a recent trend in grandparents raising their grandchildren. In 2015, the U.S. Census Bureau reported approximately 2.6 million grandparents claiming responsibility and providing basic needs for their grandchildren.[184] This can become an enjoyable, rewarding, yet challenging responsibility, with financial restrictions, taking on new social roles, and coping with any social stigmas attached to the grandchild's parents, who are unable to care for their children.[28] Financial management is an area for occupational therapy assessment if an older adult client is a caregiver for a grandchild, particularly if the person is retired and has a limited income. Safety and emergency maintenance and preparedness also should be considered, such as having a list of emergency contacts and knowing what to do in case of a natural disaster.

Becoming a caregiver for an adult family member or friend is also a reality with the older adult population. The responsibilities often occur in a slow and progressive manner, and the full extent of functional decline is not realized by the caregiver or the person receiving the care.[124] For many caregivers, the initiation of services is subtle and not many other family members will recognize how much support the caregiver is providing to a spouse until it becomes a full-time job. Care recipients wish to stay as independent as possible and try to decline this care from loved ones and family members, until they reach a point where they simply cannot function without the support. In the United States, the trend is for the oldest daughter (or daughter-in-law) to provide assistance with basic ADLs and IADLs, whereas the son typically manages the finances and estate affairs. Other family members are also called upon for help, and certainly many offer to help.[28]

In many families, a child is not aware of the habits, roles, and routines of an aging parent until a health issue arises and a parent needs physical assistance in the home. Aging parents do not wish to move in with a child, because maintaining independence and control over their lives is important; however, approximately 83% of caregiving support is provided by family.[28]

According to the National Alliance for Caregiving and the AARP, the number of Americans providing unpaid care has increased from 43.5 million in 2015 to 53 million in 2020 with the health of the caregivers worsening compared with the number in 2015.[124] It is important to keep in mind the health and well-being of the caregiver, as the needs of an older adult client are being evaluated. Caregivers primarily support care recipients by assisting with ADLs, IADLs, and a variety of health management tasks such as taking their loved one to a medical appointment. Caregiver burden can be defined in terms of emotional, physical, and financial difficulties associated with caregiving, in addition to decreased participation in social events and activities.[144] A study by Riffin and colleagues revealed that caregivers for those who are diagnosed with dementia, or who have moderate or substantial disability, experienced the greatest burden.[144] Caregiver burnout and stress are real indicators that the caregiver may need respite care to provide a break, or counseling to learn how to handle a new familial role as a caregiver. Older caregivers also may have their own medical conditions and limitations, which take a backseat to the needs and priorities of the care recipient. This was the case with Don, who also had a medical condition that affected his ability to care for

Doris. Not wanting to draw attention onto himself and away from his spouse, Don simply stated, "I have a heart condition; but I am just fine." It was important to assess Don's ability to care for Doris by asking questions related to his role in Doris' everyday activities, but then to also question if his needs were being met and if he was able to take breaks during the day as he needed. Don was adamant about not "worrying the girls" with their problems and not wanting to rely on their daughters for support, as "they were busy with their own children and families."

In the United States, when adults are in a position of caring for their own children and their parents, they become members of the sandwich generation because they are "caught between two caregiving roles—caring for a child and caring for a parent" (p. 36).[28] The average woman in the United States can expect to spend more time caring for her aging parent than she did caring for her own children.[58] Caregivers also need support and attention from the OT practitioner. It is vital for the clinician to be aware of the context or environment, the requisite occupations the caregiver is responsible for, and to provide resources that address the emerging needs of the caregiver during an intervention. These resources may include referral for counseling, respite services, or assessment of coping skills and intervention to address prioritizing to better meet the needs of the caregiver and person receiving the care. During an intervention session, the OT practitioner discussed respite care with Don and encouraged him to call and learn more about a local support group for spouses who are caring for a loved one with Alzheimer's disease. He said that it sounded interesting but was not sure where Doris would go during the meeting. The OT practitioner and Don researched the support group and found that there was a respite program in the same building as the support group and he and Doris could go together. Doris would be safe and engaged in activity while he attended the meeting. Don also asked the clinician for resources on Alzheimer's disease and how to help a loved one in the home through compensatory strategies and "tricks" to keep them going. Don worried that Doris would stop doing what she loved—playing the piano—and then "things would snowball into bigger problems."

Unfortunately, there is a link between caregiving and elder abuse. Some studies suggest that "family members who provide care for persons with dementia are up to three times more likely to physically abuse the care recipient as those who care for relatives without dementia" (p. 620).[10] Elder abuse is defined as any knowing, intended, or careless act that causes harm or serious risk of harm to an older person, physically, mentally, emotionally, or financially,[125] and includes many different kinds of abuse. Elder abuse can be physical, emotional, or sexual; other forms include exploitation, neglect, abandonment, and self-neglect. Elder abuse can take place in a private home, a healthcare institution, or a senior center and can be inflicted by a family member or a healthcare provider.

There are signs and symptoms to be aware of, and OT practitioners are considered mandated reporters and must contact the appropriate authorities (either directly or by way of a social worker or case manager, depending on the facility, employer, or policy in place). Once adult protective services is contacted, an investigation begins. The various signs or symptoms depend on the type of abuse and can be anything from shouting at an older adult or unexplained bruises, burns, and injuries with the outline of an object or hand, to torn clothing, poor skin condition, and indications that the older adult is withdrawn or frightened. Other signs to be aware of include poor hygiene, pressure ulcers, malnourishment or dehydration, or bruising around the breasts or genitals.[29] Injury, illness, or chronic disease can lead to limitations in participation in IADLs, making it difficult for older adults to remain at home and manage their health.[78]

Health Management

Health management refers to "activities related to developing, managing, and maintaining health and wellness routines, including self-management, with the goal of improving or maintaining health to support participation in occupations."[7] Management of chronic conditions such as diabetes, osteoporosis, and Alzheimer's disease are expected to be priorities in the next decade in addition to continued hospitalization for older adults with infectious diseases such as influenza and pneumonia, which is the leading cause of death for this age group.

According to Berger et al., addressing health management and maintenance is certainly within the scope of occupational therapy practice and "has been shown to improve occupational performance and QOL [quality of life] for older adults.[23] Recommendations published in this systematic review included providing group or individual health promotion, management, and maintenance interventions to older adults to improve their quality of life and occupational performance. The researchers also recommended the inclusion of individualized goal-setting, coping strategies, specific skills in health management, and problem-solving techniques to best meet the needs of older adults.[23]

A systematic review by Arbesman and Mosley revealed that client-centered occupational therapy intervention does improve occupational performance related to health management.[13] They report that health education programs reduce pain and increase physical activity, and individualized health action plans improve ADL performance and participation in physical activity. Additionally, they synthesized that the development of health routines is critical for older adults. According to the OTPF (AOTA, 2020), the goal of engagement in health management and sleep "includes maintaining or improving performance of work, leisure, social participation, and other occupations" (p. 12).[7]

Rest and Sleep

Sleep is an important occupation because of its restorative qualities, as well as its ability to support healthy aging and participation in meaningful activity.[7] According to the OTPF-4 (2020), the occupation of sleep and rest also includes sleep preparation. This can be described as undressing and grooming before going to sleep, listening to music as a form of unwinding, saying goodnight to loved ones, setting an alarm clock, or even locking the house door before retiring to the bedroom.[7]

The National Sleep Foundation (NSF) reports that 39% of people who are 65 years of age or older report having sleep-related problems.[26] The NSF also recommends between 7 and 9 hours of sleep per night for an adult who is 65 years of age or older[132,133]; when this amount of sleep is not achieved, it can have significant effects on how one feels and responds to events during the day. This is particularly important when older adults are hospitalized, because it is challenging to achieve undisturbed sleep in a hospital setting. According to a pilot study with 48 older adults completed by Missledine et al.,[119] noise levels, light, and disturbances prevented a restful night's sleep with an average of 13 awakenings per night. This resulted in an average of 3.5 hours of sleep per night, which falls short of the recommended 7 to 9 hours. OT practitioners can support hospitalized older adults by collaborating with the nursing team to reduce light and sound disturbances and post a "do not disturb" sign on the door to facilitate sleep hygiene and sleep preparation in the hospital setting.

Intervention outside of the hospital setting can include mindfulness meditation, which was described in a study by Black et al., to be effective in remediating sleep problems among older adults in the short-term, but that also could play a role in overall improved quality of life.[25] According to Leland et al., OT practitioners "can help older adults with their sleep problems by ensuring a sleep-conducive environment, address[ing] evening routines that incorporate desired sleep behaviors, and modify[ing] daily routines to include appropriate activity participation."[105] Other effective strategies also include stimulus control, sleep hygiene, cognitive-behavioral therapy, and relaxation techniques.[181] See Chapter 13 for additional information on sleep and rest.

Education

In 2015, approximately 84% of older adults had completed high school and 27% completed a bachelor's degree, with near-equal bachelor degree completion rates between men and women.[197] Educational opportunities can be enriching, engaging, and provide a means for social participation and improved self-efficacy.

There is a program titled "Road Scholar," previously known as Elderhostel, which offers thousands of courses appealing to older adults who are already well educated and focuses on college-level studies and cultural enrichment. The courses most commonly taken are those related to financial planning, health and wellness, and contemporary civic responsibilities. Older adults choose to return to school for a variety of reasons, including transitions in life, to learn a subject area of interest, to meet new people, and to remain occupied and have "something to do."[60] An OT practitioner should inquire about an older adult's educational level and complete an onsite assessment of the campus/classroom, if possible, for any environmental modifications, accommodations, or functional mobility concerns.

Educational attainment has been on the rise over the last six decades and is associated with improved health, lower mortality rates, and reduced poverty. It is also associated with longer work lives and employment opportunities.[197]

Work

Even though the standard for retirement in the United States is at 65 years of age, many older adults choose to continue working full-time or part-time for many reasons, including financial need, social participation, and the desire to maintain productivity in later years.[197] The health of an older adult is associated with the ability to work. According to Adams et al.,[1] adults who are 45 to 69 years of age are approximately three times more likely than their younger counterparts (adults who are 18–44 years of age) to report an inability to work because of health reasons. In workers 50 years of age or older, researchers found that approximately 22% reduced their employment hours, 20% have tried to eliminate demanding physical aspects of the job, and 5% reported trying to accept fewer mentally challenging tasks while in the workplace.[21]

Studies have also pointed to planned or unplanned retirement, with health issues playing a larger role in nonprofessional jobs.[21] According to Goyer, over 50% of retired adults made the transition to retirement before truly wanting to retire, with 32% of these adults blaming a decline in health as the reason.[73] Ewald stated, "The ability to retire was determined primarily on the basis of finances and health, factors working as incentives or disincentives depending on individual circumstances" (p. 345).[60] Many older adults continue to work for the enjoyment and desire to do so; others continue to work because of financial necessity, including repayment of second or third mortgages that were taken out to support children or grandchildren who experienced financial distress during the economic recessions in the 2000s.

Work also positively affects health and well-being. Older adults who are highly engaged in their work have been identified as being less stressed, less dependent on healthcare, and less likely to call in sick or use sick days. These adults also stay on the job longer than their less engaged counterparts.[67] Kim et al. report that older adults who remain in the workforce have decreased risks of physical decline and an increased sense of life purpose.[97] According to Pitt-Catsouphes et al., workplace-based health and wellness programs (HWPs) may be beneficial "for promoting positive health-related behaviors among older workers and for increasing their ability to continue to work" (p. 262).[139] This is an area in which an OT practitioner could thrive while supporting older adults in their quest to maintain health, wellness, and employment.

Volunteer work is also often part of an older adult's repertoire of occupations and is just as important as paid employment. About 25% of adults 65 years of age or older engage in some type of volunteering in the community for many reasons including achievement of higher levels of mastery, life satisfaction, and energy.[52,154] Others participate in volunteering for other reasons, such as making a contribution to society, meeting others, gaining career-related opportunities, enhancing self-esteem, reducing negative feelings, and strengthening social relationships.[47,194] Crittenden et al., report that volunteering increases physical and mental wellness through increased physical activity; all of these benefits have the potential to contribute to a longer and healthier life.[52] Paid and volunteer work may present the need to do an onsite community evaluation so that the client can prepare for engaging or reengaging in these occupations (Fig. 47.2).

Play

The fourth edition of the OTPF (2020) defines play as "activities which are intrinsically motivated, intrinsically controlled,

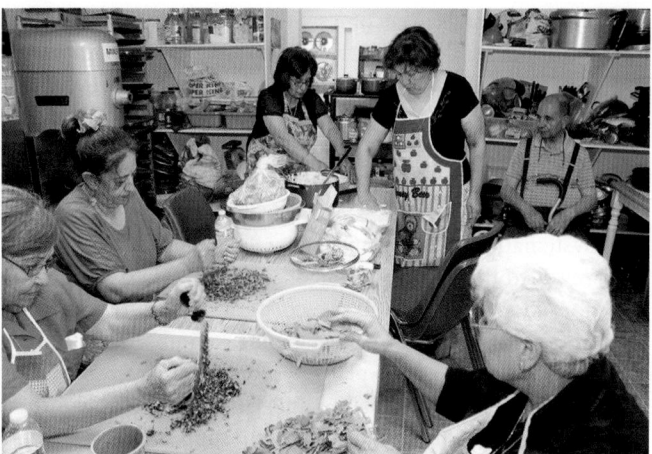

Fig. 47.2 Volunteers preparing food to sell at a Coptic Orthodox church for fundraising efforts in their community. (Photo courtesy Ramez Ethnasios.)

and freely chosen and that may include suspension of reality" (p. 34).[7] Play, in the OTPF (4th edition) is also described as engagement in exploration, humor, risk-taking, contests, and celebrations, and which is shaped by sociocultural factors.[7] The phenomenon of play was studied by Burr et al. in older adults, something that is not commonly done.[32] Typically, the benefits of play are described in the development of children; however, these researchers report that theoretical ideas help frame play as not simply a childhood experience but one that connects to later experiences across the lifespan. The planning and implementation of meaningful intervention, they proffer, can be associated with memories of play and engagement in intergenerational play.[32]

In a study conducted by Dobbins et al., exercise video games for older adults with serious mental illness promoted recovery by increasing social participation, improving self-efficacy, and facilitating physical health through exercise.[57] A study by Waldman-Levi et al. produced evidence that playfulness and play should be considered and implemented into the concept of well-being as adults age because it could help to increase feelings of empowerment, self-efficacy, and a positive self-concept.[193] Play and sport also have been shown to contribute to the overall experience of successful aging, as reported by Stenner et al.[169] Other positive benefits of sports and play include increased opportunities for developing relationships, experiencing competition, and achieving goals.[169] Play can be incorporated into any intervention plan of care, regardless of context or setting in which older adults are receiving occupational therapy services.

Leisure

"Although the aging process is one factor that influences occupational engagement, the older adult's individual perspective affects not only what the older adult is able and may need to do but also what the older adult chooses and wants to do" (p. 302).[168] According to a systematic review completed by Stav et al.,[168] leisure activities have positive health benefits and when incorporated into everyday activities, behaviors such as gardening, visiting friends, participating in clubs, or reading result in a variety of health outcomes. Some activities such as playing board games, taking a trip to a museum, and completing cognitive puzzles play a role in decreasing the risk of dementia and result in higher cognitive levels.[69,157,191] There are also global health benefits that have been identified in the literature, such as increased survival rates and increased coping and well-being strategies for widows.[88,90]

A systematic review completed by Smallfield and Molitor in 2018 revealed the many benefits of supporting leisure occupations for older adults, as well as incorporating leisure education and chronic disease self-management programs into occupational therapy intervention plans.[161] If older adults are at risk for a decline in social participation and leisure engagement, then community-based group intervention to support social participation should be considered, in addition to electronic gaming and assistive device intervention to maximize participation in leisure occupations.[161]

Standardized and nonstandardized assessments of leisure and social participation should be used in clinical settings; however, formal or informal assessments can also capture relevant information to inform the intervention plan of care. It is common for OT practitioners to work in adult physical rehabilitation settings that do not allow for direct billing and reimbursements of leisure activities as part of an intervention due to many third-party payer restrictions regarding treatment goals. However, in implementing occupations as ends and occupations as means, as described by Gray,[74] leisure activities can be used as a complement to ADLs and functional mobility goals established for clients, as well as a therapeutic tool to address performance skills and client factors in the areas of vision, cognition, and motor control. Meaningful activities and creativity in intervention planning are important for success when working with this population. In the skilled nursing environment, it may be possible to design a functional maintenance program for a client that involves recreation activities to address particular performance skills or client factors, or occupation-based goals as well (see Chapter 16 for more information regarding leisure).

Social Participation

Just as leisure activities have been proven to affect health positively, so has social participation. In their systematic review of the literature, Stav et al.[168] synthesized 33 different research articles and concluded that there is strong evidence linking participation in social activities with preventing decreased cognition and physical decline. Social activities identified in the review included attendance in groups outside of the home, regular visits and contact with friends, and participation in social networks. These types of activities also improved physical health and functioning in terms of ADL performance, as well as showed lower mortality rates and improved quality of life.[168]

The OT practitioner can be of particular support in assessing a community environment and making recommendations for adaptation to promote the participation and independence of older adults. Incorporation of family and friends into intervention, although directed by the client, can also ease concerns about what a client can safely do and can often support increased client participation in social activities.

Another approach to social participation is to consider multisocial media use or use of multiple social media platforms for older adults. According to a study by Yu, the use of social media by older adults has increased, and this population has embraced various platforms that offer social participation, including WhatsApp, Facebook, and other social network sites.[205] Messaging applications (apps) are also becoming more popular, with older adults obtaining health benefits from using these apps to stay connected with close family and friends and to develop new relationships with acquaintances. These platforms may support social engagement as older adults try to navigate retirement, bereavement, and changes in health that could limit more traditional in-person social engagements.

The Wellness Program for Older Adults demonstrated that occupational therapy intervention that addresses prevention efforts for older adults living in the community enhances ADLs, IADLs, physical and mental health, occupational functioning, and life satisfaction.[114] OT practitioners play a role in personal aspects of an older adult's life; therefore, they can address modification of components of occupations that are important to an older adult either in a group setting or in individual intervention before it becomes problematic for the older adult. This can be done through a community model and results in an overall increase in participation by older adults and an increase in quality of life.

ENVIRONMENTAL AND PERSONAL FACTORS

The context in which a person, group, or population lives and participates in everyday life activities will certainly influence what is done and how it is done. Not only is access considered but the quality and satisfaction of performance also must be considered by the occupational therapist when addressing environmental and personal factors. Personal factors reflect who a person is and includes "customs, beliefs, activity patterns, behavioral standards, and expectations accepted by the society or cultural group of which a person is a member" (p. 10) and oftentimes described as demographic information.[7] AOTA defines environmental factors as "aspects of the physical, social, and attitudinal surroundings in which people live and conduct their lives. Environmental factors influence functioning and disability and have positive aspects (facilitators) or negative aspects (barriers or hindrances)" (p. 9–10) to occupation, including the natural and human-made environment, products and technology, support and relationships, and attitudes.[7] Services, systems, and policies also must be considered because certain benefits, structured programs, and regulations will also either be a facilitator or barrier to accessing care, particularly healthcare, in the United States.

Policy Affecting Older Adults

To provide the best healthcare, OT practitioners should be aware of the policies affecting older adults in the United States. Policies not only impact the way clinicians document services, but they also impact reimbursement and payment systems in several settings, including inpatient hospital settings, acute rehabilitation settings, skilled nursing facilities, home healthcare, outpatient, or even palliative care.

An overview of important financial and healthcare policies is presented here as a framework for working with this population. Practitioners and students are encouraged to research the specific policies related to their state of employment and, generally speaking, in the facilities of employment. Learning how policies affect practice is also learned on the job. A plethora of resources can be found online, and trusted online resources, such as https://www.cms.gov (Centers for Medicare and Medicaid Services), should be used for more detail and to stay abreast of changes that occur frequently.

A significant change In healthcare policy was the passing of the Patient Protection and Affordable Care Act (ACA) in 2010. This was part of President Barack Obama's healthcare reform legislation, which requires most individuals living in the United States to have health insurance through employer-based insurance, health insurance exchanges, or the optional expansion of state programs (including Medicaid).[81] There are specific provisions of this policy that affect older adults, including Medicare Part D's prescription drug plan (closing the coverage gap in prescription drug coverage through Medicare [also known as "the doughnut hole"]), the creation of a center in each state to provide funds to individuals who are Medicare or Medicaid eligible, as well as expanded services in the home and community for those who receive Medicaid.[186]

The issues and debates surrounding the ACA continue as this chapter is written in 2020, with the Trump Administration's efforts to repeal and replace certain features of the ACA. As described by Conhoto, this is a "fluid and evolving situation" (p. 131), with the latest changes implemented in 2017.[50] Those changes repealed the ACA's individual mandate of requiring most individuals living in the United States to have health insurance through employer-based insurance, health insurance exchanges, or the optional expansion of state programs. Other changes resulting from the Trump Administration provisions may have an impact on drug rebates and discounts for Medicare recipients, annual wellness visits, preventive screenings, and access to home and community-based services.[50]

With the passage of the Social Security Act in 1935, the national government highlighted a realization that older adults required support and assistance, and, since that time, Social Security has helped millions of older adults financially. Specifically, 15 million adults were assisted out of poverty in 2015.[152,158] In 1961, the first White House Conference on Aging was held; these conferences continue to be held once every decade (with the most recent conference in 2015) in Washington, D.C. In 1962, the Commission on Aging was established, and, in 1965, the Older Americans Act was created, which was a catalyst for the creation of the Federal Administration on Aging. In 1965, Medicare was established as a federal healthcare insurance for older adults, and Medicaid was also enacted, providing healthcare assistance programs for individuals with low income, including those with disabilities. In 1990, the Americans with Disabilities Act (ADA) was established, facilitating the integration of people with disabilities into employment, services, and healthcare.[29] Of course, all of these policies are implemented

in a unique way, as the current situations in the United States change by way of politics and demographics.

Social Security is the Old-Age, Survivors, and Disability Insurance (OASDI) program. Current taxpayers pay for this program and the longer one works, the longer one pays into the system. This program is for older adults, retired workers, workers with disabilities, and dependents and survivors of workers who have participated in Social Security. Benefits can be received as young as 62 years of age; however, the benefit is greater for workers who wait until full retirement (which is based on their birth year).[163]

Supplemental Security Income (SSI) provides a monthly monetary payment for eligible individuals who have low income or resources. Criteria for eligibility include being 65 years of age or older, being legally blind, or being disabled. SSI is funded through the U.S. Treasury's general fund and is not recognized as an entitlement, like Social Security. The payment amount varies and depends on each individual's income, resources, and living arrangement.[29]

Medicare is a social insurance that is government-sponsored and covers people 65 years of age and older, certain people under 65 years of age with long-term disabilities, and adults with end-stage renal disease requiring dialysis or kidney transplant. Medicare is divided into four parts: Parts A, B, C, and D. Part A is known as hospital insurance and covers inpatient hospitalizations, limited skilled nursing care (100 days, renewable over the lifespan), hospice, and home healthcare. Part B is also known as Medical Insurance and covers doctors' services, outpatient care, home healthcare, durable medical equipment, and some types of preventive services. Part C is also known as Medicare Advantage plans (and includes Parts A and B) but is run by private insurance companies. Part D is also known as the Medicare Prescription Drug Coverage plan and is also run by private insurance companies.[164] Occupational therapy services (among other rehabilitation services) are covered under Parts A, B, and C, and coverage is specific to the setting in which services are being delivered. Documentation requirements and expectations vary from setting to setting; practitioners are encouraged to learn the details and keep abreast of the Medicare policies specific to the place of employment (see Chapter 8 for additional information on documentation).

Medicaid is a public assistance program that provides healthcare to people of all ages with low income, including those with disabilities. Medicaid is a federal and state partnership, not the responsibility of the federal government (as is Medicare). Eligibility differs by state, and each state has specific income levels and resource amounts for qualification. Medicaid is the largest payer of long-term services and supports in the United States, including nursing facility care and home- and community-based services. Nursing facility care is one of the mandatory services covered by Medicaid in all states; however, Medicaid does not currently mandate home- and community-based services. For all Medicaid services, individuals must meet the eligibility requirements for the state to qualify for long-term services and supports. There are financial requirements that must be met, and if an individual has more financial resources and supports than is considered the minimum requirement, a "spend down" occurs in which the assets and income are depleted to the point at which the individual does qualify for Medicaid services. In-home services, such as personal care services and community-based services, are also provided.[112]

The Aging Network, established under the Older Americans Act of 1965, defines an older adult as being 60 years of age or older. Caregivers of older Americans are also covered, according to this act. Funds are provided to the states and tribal organizations to offer specific services as mandated by the Older Americans Act. These services include nutrition services; congregate services and home-delivered meals (Meals on Wheels); and supportive services, including transportation, in-home care, adult daycare, and preventive health services. One important service is the Long-Term Ombudsman Program and the National Family Caregiver Support Program, which offers counseling, training, and respite care to caregivers.[29]

Finally, some older adults do carry long-term care insurance. These policies are sold by private companies and only fund about 6% of long-term services and supports in the United States.[134] Depending on the policy and coverage, home- and community-based services may be provided, as well as nursing facility care. Policies can be expensive, and premiums typically rise as a person ages. When working with older adult clients, it will be necessary to understand the medical insurance the client carries and what services are covered by the insurance. Healthcare policy and insurance impact occupational therapy services, including evaluation, assessments, and intervention; therefore, collaboration with the client, family members, case manager, and social worker is essential for best practice.

Coronavirus (COVID-19) Pandemic

Aside from environmental factors related to policies that affect older adults, the coronavirus disease (COVID-19) pandemic, as described by the World Health Organization (WHO) in 2020, is a world-wide emergency that has affected the day-to-day living of everyone around the globe. COVID-19 is defined as a "disease caused by a new coronavirus, which has not been previously identified in humans" and is transmitted from person to person through small droplets from the nose or mouth when a person sneezes, coughs, or exhales; it can even be transmitted if the droplets land on objects and surfaces that are then touched by other people who then touch their eyes, nose, or mouth. According to the WHO, older people and people of all ages who have preexisting medical conditions are at higher risk for developing serious illness, whereas most people will recover from the disease without needing specialized intervention. Loneliness and social isolation became a by-product for older adults with adherence to the recommended physical distancing and "safer at home" orders observed in many counties across the United States.

The U.S. Surgeon General Vivek Murthy had already proclaimed loneliness and social isolation as a global epidemic for the world's older adult population, according to Berg-Weger and Morley, with nearly one-third of older adults experiencing loneliness and/or social isolation since 2017.[22] Berg-Weger and Morley reported that loneliness and social isolation are indicative of significant and long-term negative physical and mental health outcomes for older adults who had their exercise and

social activities, in-person interactions, and volunteer responsibilities suspended during the COVID-19 pandemic (2020).[22] Creative solutions for connecting with older adults, reassuring them through telephone visits, and providing workshops and education in a virtual environment became a new "norm" in the summer of 2020.[22] It is critical to assess loneliness and social isolation, develop adaptive evidence-based interventions to work with other healthcare providers when providing services to older adults, and address various needs through client-centered and meaningful occupations that combat ageism.

The COVID-19 pandemic forced millions to prepare for staying indoors and limiting physical interactions with others to prevent community spread of the disease. In March of 2020, people began working from home, using telehealth services for appointments with healthcare providers, using online video communications platforms for meetings and schoolwork (i.e., Zoom), and ordering food and medications for delivery to their homes.

In July of 2020, the U.S. Bureau of Labor Statistics reported that 31.3 million people were unable to work at home because their employer closed or lost business as a result of the pandemic.[182] This statistic was reported in a survey that asked about the previous 4 weeks at the time of completion. Of the 16.9 million people unemployed in July of 2020, 9.6 million were unable to work because their employer closed or lost business because of the pandemic.[182] Employment is not the only area impacted by the pandemic, access to healthcare has also shifted, with more older adults using telehealth services than ever before.

Telehealth is defined by the Health Resources Services Administration as "the use of electronic information and telecommunications technologies to support long-distance clinical healthcare, patient and professional health-related education, public health and health administration."[77] It includes video-conferences, use of the internet, store-and-forward imaging, streaming media, and terrestrial and wireless communications. Ever since the pandemic began, more older Americans have been using telehealth to see their physicians and healthcare providers virtually, and as one report cites, one in four patients over the age of 50 used telehealth between March and June of 2020.[189] In fact, in 2019, only 4% of older adults (50–80 years of age) used telehealth, and in June of 2020, this number increased to 26%. Comfort in using video conferencing technologies rose from 53% in May of 2019 to 64% in June of 2020, as older adults were faced with decisions to use virtual services or not communicate with their providers.[189] Results from the 2020 National Poll on Healthy Aging revealed that older adults have experienced this rapid expansion of telehealth services, with respect to availability, use, and interest, and older adults will likely continue to use this type of communication for years to come.[30]

Global Warming and Climate Change

Just as a global infectious disease pandemic can cause a shift in healthcare delivery models, another environmental factor that must be considered is that of climate change and global warming. According to Li et al., "[a]n aging population could substantially enhance the burden of heat-related health risks in a warming climate because of their higher susceptibility to extreme heat health effects."[110] These researches encourage countries around the globe to develop public health policies that address climate change and the aging population.[110] Another threat to older adults related to global warming is the ability to adapt ambient temperature and maintain a normal core body temperature for physiological function through thermoregulatory mechanisms.[2] Ahima's research points to extreme temperatures driven by global warming disrupting this normal thermoregulation mechanism and warns that it can negatively affect an older adult's health and well-being by putting them at risk for heat cramps, heat exhaustion, or even heat stroke.[2] Assessments and interventions with healthcare providers are critical for health management and health maintenance during these uncertain times of global change; this includes patient and caregiver education regarding safety when temperatures are deemed unsafe to be outdoors.

THREADED CASE STUDY

Doris, Part 2

Several assessment tools were used with Doris as part of her occupational therapy evaluation and intervention plan. The Brief Cognitive Rating Scale (BCRS),[141] which is used with the Global Deterioration Scale (GDS),[142] was used initially to acquire a baseline for cognitive function. Doris scored 4.6 on the GDS, which indicates a moderate cognitive decline/late confusional state. At this level, definite concentration deficits are present, with marked deficit on serial 7s and frequent deficits in subtraction of serial 4s from 40. Doris was unsure of the weather and did not know her current address. There was a clear-cut deficit in long-term memory, and most of Doris' history was obtained from Don. She could not recall childhood friends or teachers but could state the name of her high school. Confusion in chronology of personal history is also found at this stage.

The Cognitive Performance Test[31] was also administered, resulting in findings that were consistent with a moderate stage of Alzheimer's disease and difficulties completing detailed tasks. This score was consistent with Don's report of Doris' need for assistance with most IADLs and ADLs, and the outcomes of this assessment complemented those of the GDS.

The Geriatric Depression Scale[204] was also administered, and the outcome indicated that Doris should meet with her physician for diagnostic testing for possible major depressive disorder. The OT practitioner notified the charge nurse at the facility and asked her to relay this information to the admitting physician so that Doris could be evaluated by the proper healthcare provider. Lastly, the Canadian Occupational Performance Measure (COPM)[104] was used with Doris and Don. This assessment tool was an excellent way to find out what Doris wanted to do, needed to do, or was expected to do through a semi-structured interview with Don and Doris. This tool is used not to assess performance but to assess self-perception of importance, as well as performance and satisfaction with performance in three general areas: self-care, work, and leisure.

ASSESSMENT AND INTERVENTION

Customary assessment and intervention strategies for adults with physical disabilities are recommended for older adults, as presented throughout this textbook. There are, however, many assessments and intervention approaches recommended for older adults specifically. Smallfield et al. published occupational therapy guidelines for productive aging for community-dwelling older adults, which include evidence-based guidelines for this population.[162] For a thorough and detailed table

highlighting examples of standardized screening tools and assessments, please refer to these guidelines, published by the AOTA.[162]

These recommendations are also published in the National Guideline Clearinghouse to clarify the role of occupational therapy in treating community-living older adults and to support productive aging efforts. Areas of intervention specifically named in the guidelines include those that improve ADL, IADLs, fall prevention, home modification, health management, and health maintenance. It is recommended that OT practitioners use standardized assessment tools and outcome measures for evaluating occupational performance consistently and whenever possible. Habits, routines, roles, and rituals should be assessed and addressed; a person's values, beliefs, and spirituality also should be included for the most thorough and comprehensive plan of care. Client-centered and occupation-based intervention plans that are meaningful and individualized show positive benefits to older adult clients. Performing functional and occupation-based activities within the older adults' actual environment will facilitate carryover and generalizing of information learned during intervention. Research shows that gains observed in physical performance (client factors and performance skills) do not always translate to an improvement in ADL and IADL performance.[135]

With changes in reimbursement for occupational therapy services through the Patient-Driven Payment Model (PDPM) in 2019, intervention and documentation demonstrating occupational therapy's distinct value is of utmost importance. Sites where older adults are being treated are held accountable for the quality of care they are providing and according to the Improving Medicare Post-Acute Care Transformation (IMPACT) Act of 2014,[38] which is based on several identified factors, including rates of readmissions, community discharge, skin integrity, medication reconciliation, and major falls.

Clinical decision-making and quality of care priorities are elevated when assessing services provided in post-acute care settings, and occupational therapy can play a pivotal role in identifying risks for falls, readmission, failed community transition, psychosocial factors, lack of social support, and so many other essential areas affecting a person's health and well-being. The AOTA advocates that all practitioners address the following areas with every single interaction they have with an older adult in any clinical setting to ensure best practice and to meet the occupational needs of every client: ADL; IADL; functional cognition; vision; psychosocial or behavioral skills; fear of falling; habits, routines, and roles; patient and caregiver education; and safety.[6]

Intervention activities should always be meaningful and age appropriate. Many older adults enjoy occupations that are fun and playful, including games and crafts. These activities should be considered carefully, however, to be sure that they are meeting the needs of each individual client. A thoughtful interview should be completed, and a thorough occupational profile will support the use of occupation-based and client-centered practice. While searching for activities that present the "just right" challenge for the client, it may be tempting to use tasks that meet most specifications for intervention, but some of those tasks may also be demeaning. During the occupational therapy evaluation, Don mentioned, "I know you therapists mean well when you set up those cones and have Doris walk around them, but they really don't do her a bit of good. She needs to do real things so she can get back to our real home and take care of herself, because I can't do it all anymore."

If an older adult comments that an activity seems childish or questions why an activity is being used as part of therapy, participating will probably not prove to be a significant benefit. Remnants of the reductionist paradigm of the field exist in all practice settings, where clients are given a "restorator" bike for the upper extremities or asked to raise the weighted bar 15 times and repeat. At times, clinicians can function on autopilot and execute more of a cookie cutter approach to therapy, which is not meaningful or even therapeutic for the older adult client, or any client for that matter. It can lead to frustration, dissatisfaction, and confusion of the role occupational therapy plays in a variety of settings, such as skilled nursing facilities, inpatient rehabilitation facilities, and outpatient settings. The match between the client and the intervention task is especially important for members of this age group. Working with the client to problem-solve strategies for therapy and the best approach to meeting established goals will further engage the client in the intervention process, while increasing self-esteem and effectiveness. After completing the OT evaluation, the clinician reviewed the results with Don and Doris and asked about the goal for occupational therapy. Without hesitation Doris said, "Play the piano again"; and without hesitation Don said, "Be able to get around and do some of the things she needs to do to take care of herself." These goals were meaningful to Doris and would be used as a means to an end during her rehabilitation.

It is recommended that OT practitioners incorporate involvement or participation of physical, social, leisure, religious, work-related, or volunteer activities into intervention approaches and use an evidence-based approach to develop healthy routines and habits in this population. Health management approaches, self-management programs, and health education programs are also recommended.[13] The recommendations also encourage clinicians to consult with organizations that focus on aging to develop preventive educational and intervention programs for this population, including the area of driving to support productive aging.[135,168]

Educational programs and teaching aimed at older adult clients and their families or caregivers also must be considered carefully with respect to health literacy. To an older adult, this could mean anything from reading and writing to speaking and listening. In a literacy survey processed by the United States Department of Education, adults 65 years of age and older had the lowest average prose, document, and quantitative literacy.[103] Oftentimes, health professionals communicate at higher levels than older adults understand. According to Stableford,[166] "Many, if not most, older adults have trouble understanding both verbal and written health communication" (p. 324). The cause does not need to be linked to English as a second language, although at times this is a reason.

There are common assumptions that have been made about the learning needs of older adults. In 1984, Knowles[100] identified specific concepts that he thought should be a foundation of adult education and included understanding why something needs to be learned (before learning it), motivating oneself to learn through internal forces (versus external forces), being solution driven and problem based, associating learning with social roles, tapping into the rich experiences of life to enhance learning, and lastly, becoming more self-directed with respect to learning. All of this should occur as one's personality matures. These general assumptions do not always fit the needs and desires of older adult clients in occupational therapy for several reasons. However, older adult learners must have their developmental needs and interests met; therefore, Knowles recommended an environment of mutual trust, respect, and acceptance of differences.[100]

Many obstacles can get in the way of an older adult understanding instructions during patient education, including family members, the healthcare provider's style, or the language being used. The experience of learning will be affected by the assumptions being made about older adults; therefore, it is critical to analyze learning assumptions being made about older adults by clinicians and educators.[41] In a review and critique of the portrayal of older adult learners, it was reported that society views older adult learners as a homogeneous group of people not affected by age-related changes to the mind and body. Clinicians must pay attention to the diversity that exists among the older adult population with respect to age, race, ethnicity, educational levels, and income, as well as physical and cognitive abilities. Not all older adults are capable and motivated learners, as much of the literature would convey in this review.[41] Many older adults do have age-related changes associated with cognition, which have an impact on their learning abilities. Others have decreased motivation to participate in learning opportunities secondary to lower socioeconomic status or residing in an isolated rural community.

Stress, anxiety, decreased vision, and decreased hearing can contribute to misunderstandings or lack of comprehension with written and verbal instructions provided by health professionals. Older adults take a longer amount of time to process information, and hearing information repeatedly helps older adults to make associations and connections to existing knowledge, so hearing information once before discharge will likely not be recalled upon reaching home.[87,89] Medical interpreters and translated brochures are helpful and recommended, as are "teach-back" strategies, in which clients are asked to demonstrate what the healthcare provider just reviewed or taught to prove learning occurred.[134] Levy recommended other strategies,[108,109] such as chunking information in an organized way to promote effective storage of new information, being mindful of internal and external contextual factors during the learning process to facilitate recall in a new environment, and providing cues that offer opportunities for recognition or matching information with previously learned information.

The American Medical Association also recommends that clinicians apply the following verbal communication tips, which contribute to improved patient understanding: slow down, use plain/nonmedical language, show or draw pictures, limit the amount of information and repeat that information, use the teach-back technique, and create a shame-free environment in which clients are encouraged to ask questions.[199] When using plain/nonmedical language, it is important to write down what the patient should do, how to do it, and why the patient should do it; these reminders facilitate communication with loved ones or caregivers who may not be present at the time of teaching. Additional suggestions made by Stableford[166] include framing the conversation first, before diving into the discussion, as well as encouraging the older adult to bring a friend or family member to appointments.

During initial contacts with an older adult, the OT clinician must take the time to listen to and get to know the client. By the time that intervention begins, the clinician will have an understanding of the client's learning style, deficits that may require specific types of teaching, and any cognitive or perceptual deficits that should be considered. The pace and style of the intervention will be individualized to meet the client's learning needs. If increased recovery time is needed for limitations in cardiovascular function, the clinician should plan for this and allow time to assess vital signs and monitoring. The clinician should also incorporate energy conservation or work simplifications into the intervention plan, if the patient needs these strategies. The client is the best judge of what fits within their life and goals, and this should ultimately be respected and interwoven into the intervention plan. Don and Doris were provided with printed information regarding compensatory strategies and durable medical equipment recommendations. Because Doris has Alzheimer's disease, the majority of the patient education was directed at Don, who was serving as the caregiver and would follow through with the strategies at home. Don requested information in the most "straightforward way" and preferred to be hands-on during intervention sessions. He often wanted to try the various hand placements during functional mobility and wrote down when and how to provide verbal cues to Doris during self-care activities. Don mentioned, "Writing things down helps; that way, I will not forget what I learned." Don also requested help making memory books and sequencing cards to help Doris complete tasks on her own. These requests were incorporated into Doris' intervention sessions, and Don attended every one of them.

One of the critical components of processing life changes— especially changes in health or changes in environment—relates to coping style. The emphasis is less on context and more on how the older adult deals with the reality of a situation. Older adults generally have a well-established style of coping, and regardless of whether their style may be effective or ineffective, it should be a personal factor that is taken into account during evaluation or intervention. As a group, older adults have seen wide-sweeping political, social, cultural, economic, and technological changes in their lifetimes. Some of the old support systems such as an extended family have changed for many older adults, whereas others have taken new caregiver roles within the extended family that were not prevalent in previous generations—such as parenting grandchildren.

New support systems have become available for this population through technology and the internet. Computers and personal electronic devices play a large role in keeping older adults connected to family, friends, and grandchildren who live in

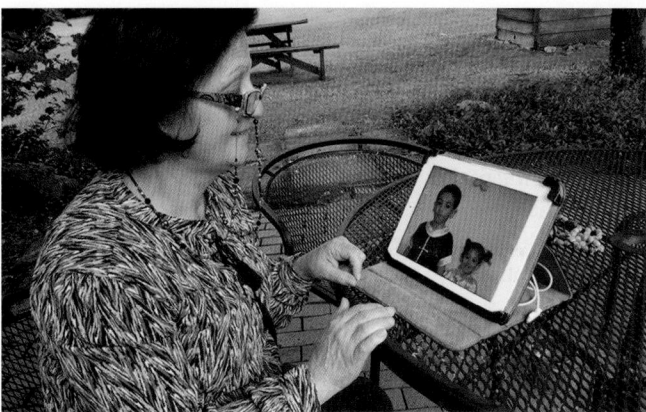

Fig. 47.3 A grandmother using her personal electronic device and the internet to communicate with her grandchildren across the miles. (Photo courtesy Julie Rafeedie Haar.)

other states or countries (Fig. 47.3). This population also uses chat rooms and online dating services to establish relationships or for companionship.[16] Learning to use a computer and the internet can be challenging initially; however, many community centers provide workshops and tutorials on how to send e-mails, surf the internet, or join social media sites such as Facebook.[28] The internet is also a way for older adults to learn more about any given topic, and like their younger counterparts, they can use the internet to learn more about medical conditions and health concerns and to become more informed.

THE AGING PROCESS

The aging process is complex; many theories for why and how people age have been researched and published in the field of gerontology (the study of aging). It is inevitable that people age, and with the aging process comes a change in body structure and function. There is increased prevalence of degenerative diseases and the potential for physiological decline in several body systems. Gregory and Sandmire stated, "From a strictly scientific standpoint, however, the distinction between aging and disease is, at best, a blurry one" (p. 53).[75]

Distinctions between aging and disease include the fact that aging is a universal process, shared by all human beings; it is intrinsic and dependent on genetic factors. We are constantly aging and it is a progressive process, which may ultimately lead to decreased functional capacity. The aging process is not reversible. Disease, on the other hand, is a selective process and varies from person to person; it is categorized as intrinsic and extrinsic with genetic and environmental factors to consider, as well as uncertainty with respect to progression, regression, or termination/cure with treatment. Disease does cause damage but has the potential for being reversible, and disease may be treatable and often has a known cause.[75]

Many of the physiological changes associated with aging can be slowed or prevented with lifestyle choices, such as incorporating a healthy diet and exercise into a daily routine. Many of the chronic conditions seen in older adults also can be prevented by adjusting behaviors and habits; however, these changes should happen in early to middle life so that the maximum effect can be achieved. OT practitioners can play a role in this prevention by working with younger and older clients in wellness, prevention, and primary care.

Most biological theories of aging can be roughly grouped according to two major suppositions: genetic theories on aging and environmental theories on aging.[62,75,118] One genetic theory claims that senescence, or the process of deterioration with age, results from the gradual mutations (alternations in deoxyribonucleic acid [DNA]) in somatic cells of the body. This is known as the somatic mutation theory, and it is thought that over time the radiation and environmental factors people withstand actually mutate and alter critical genetic code, changing the sequence of amino acids found in enzymes and other proteins.[61,174] Two other genetic theories are related to the endocrine and immunological systems in which there is decline over time; however, hormones and "biological clocks" regulate and control the aging process.[75]

The environmental theories on aging branch off into another direction, with one theory known as the *wear-and-tear* theory of aging (sometimes referred to as allostatic load). This theory basically states that it is inevitable that cells, tissues, and organs gradually wear out from continued use over time.[75] There is another theory called the *rate-of-living* theory of aging, which states that each living organism is given the ability to burn up a fixed number of calories within the lifespan, and once that number is reached, the organism dies.[98] The rate-of-living theory led to the *free radical* theory, which is similar to the wear-and-tear theory, "but attributes cellular and organismal aging to random accumulating damage of macromolecules by the highly reactive by-products of oxidative metabolism known as free radicals" (p. 59).[75] What is clear is that the explanation for aging is unclear, given so many theories that are constantly challenged and reevaluated. It is important for OT practitioners to adopt a holistic view of the individual and appreciate that, for example, hypertension, high cholesterol, and diabetes increase health risk exponentially. Such a view also can be taken of other areas in a person's life. Older adults with low vision who also have difficulty hearing and who have diabetic neuropathy with altered sensation in their fingers will have a greater challenge in adapting daily activities to achieve functional independence. Because aging is a process that is generally predictable from infancy through older adulthood, it is helpful to understand and appreciate the body structures and functions by system and how they change, or have the potential to change, as a person ages.

CHANGES IN MENTAL STRUCTURES AND FUNCTIONS

The brain decreases in weight and size with older age, even in those with normal cognitive function.[156,171] Some neurons shrink with age and others are lost. It is estimated that we use only a small percentage of the neurons in our brain, so the effect of these changes could be very small. It is also normal to see neurofibrillary plaques and tangles in older brains,[156,171] although excessive levels can be indicative of Alzheimer's disease (see Chapter 36 for more details). Messages moving through the nervous system may not get through as quickly as they used to,[171]

thereby slowing the speed of some cognitive functions such as memory. This reduction in the efficiency of transmission of signals in the nervous system may contribute to the declines seen in some mental functions.

Changes in cognition often affect the ability to function because information processing and problem-solving are so vital to safety and independence in ADLs. Actual cognitive decline can have a major impact on the quality of life, and this is compounded when physical function, especially sensation, is impaired as well.[108] Many of these cognitive changes are related to treatable, temporary, or manageable medical problems. Many important considerations when working with an older adult include medication side effects, alcohol and nonprescription drug use, vision and hearing deficits, nutritional deficiencies, stress, sleep dysfunction, depression, and medical illnesses such as diabetes, high cholesterol, and high blood pressure. These conditions may also be predictive of functional decline.[56,148] Cognitive decline becomes more substantial with each new medical condition that develops.

OTs find that cognitive capacity greatly affects the client's ability to benefit from rehabilitation. A more detailed discussion of cognitive aging can be found in other sources.[15,107,108,148] Cognition as a mental function is also discussed in Chapter 26. Age-associated differences are seen in almost all aspects of cognition in healthy older adults, but this difference is typically minor, with more time and more extensive processing being required. Age-associated differences in cognition do not generally present serious implications for ADLs and IADLs.[87,122] Researchers have found that cognitive processing efficiency, especially for working memory, information processing, and reaction time, is 1.5 times slower in older adults than in middle-aged or young adults.[94] Generally, older adults can, with effort and training, remember details with the same accuracy as that of younger persons.

Robnett and Bolduc[148] described the cognitive changes of aging, relevant for rehabilitation. In a typically aging adult, orientation, for the most part, remains intact as part of crystallized intelligence (basic knowledge and skills that accumulate over the lifespan). With lifestyle changes, like retirement, difficulty remembering the date or the day can occur in older adults. Attention (to sustain attention or focus on a task, alternate attention between two tasks, or divide attention between two or more tasks), or selective attention (to pay attention to relevant stimuli and ignore noise) generally remains intact if there are no distractions with a typically aging adult. However, as adults grow older, they tend to be less able to ignore distractions while trying to attend to a task (such as driving). Crystallized intelligence remains intact or may continue to improve as one ages, particularly for overlearned material and skills needed for work. Older adults tend to see the "gray areas" and pride themselves on seeing beyond the "black and white." Lastly, fluid intelligence is the ability to problem-solve and find meaning at times of confusion, with the ability to develop inferences and understand relationships of various concepts without acquiring new knowledge. This includes skills such as judgment, awareness, and problem-solving (executive skills). Fluid intelligence shows decline with aging to a degree. Older adults have more challenges with multistep tasks, and because learning requires multiple-step tasks, this process may slow down but does not stop in typically aging adults.[147]

Loss of memory is a concern for many older adults because memory involves the retention, storage, and retrieval of information. Memory requires adequate attention to sensory-perceptual cues at the initial stages of reception and encoding.[15,109,160] Age differences have been found to affect working memory—one component of short-term memory. Older adults exhibit poorer function in complex deliberate processing (i.e., simultaneously performing a cognitive task while trying to remember the information for a later task) than they do in automatic processing (i.e., remembering how to perform an activity).[94,148,160] Older adults also have a decreased ability to inhibit thoughts that are irrelevant to the task.[109,148] Age-related deficits have been found in the recall of information when it is retrieved from secondary (storage) memory levels, and this deficit worsens with advancing age.[107,108] However, the overall effects of age-related differences or changes in memory on daily function are minimal. Most healthy older adults are able to compensate for reduced processing resources by using the relevant context of situations, targeting environmental cues, providing environmental supports, rehearsing with elaboration, and developing new skills built on personal associations.

Intervention for the cognitive changes of aging includes using calendars for orientation and making sure that calendars or dry-erase boards are up-to-date at extended care facilities or nursing homes. To address attention, OT practitioners can eliminate distractions when older adults are attempting to complete a complex task. Repetition for learning is important; however, clinicians should not assume that the client will remember patient education and strategies without writing them down. Providing written instruction or having a client write information down will be more effective for intervention and carryover. Older adults are more likely to use written lists to recall important items, unlike their younger counterparts.[148] Generally speaking, if material to be learned is interesting and the client can draw associations to his or her life, it is more likely that the learning will take place. Multimodal sensory input, such as hearing the information, reading the information, and writing it down, will also increase the likelihood of recall.

When impaired cognition (especially memory) interferes with relationships, diminishes daily function, or affects quality of life, the causes should be explored because many of them are potentially treatable. Problems with memory tasks, whether subjective or objective, are the most commonly acknowledged types of age-related cognitive changes.[17] Displaying decreased memory skills does not, however, indicate that a person has dementia. Mild forgetfulness is experienced by the young and old alike, and it should not cause alarm or lead a person to think about dementia. In fact, decreased memory, or age-associated memory impairment (AAMI), "is widespread and refers to memory skills that are lower than average. AAMI is not as serious and may or may not relate to mild cognitive impairment" (p. 114).[148] AAMI is a part of normal aging, affecting as many as 90% of older adults.[108] This is not a psychiatric disorder. Among the criteria for these cognitive changes is a decline in memory that is sufficient to worry the older adult but not in excess of normal age function, as seen with dementia. The decline must be within normal limits when the client is compared, through psychometric testing, with others who are the same age. Older adults who are tired, under stress, sick, or distracted are more likely to experience slower thinking and recall, experience more difficulty attending to and organizing information, and have difficulty recalling information, especially names, placement of objects, and tasks requiring multiple actions.[108]

According to Petersen et al.,[138] memory loss that falls outside of normal limits by 1 standard deviation on test scores, with more severe memory lapses evident in recent memory that are persistent and begin to interfere with work and social activity (not ADLs), is identified as mild cognitive impairment (MCI). In 50% of individuals with MCI, dementia develops within 3 years, although symptoms may have been evident for up to 7 years previously.[108,138] When cognitive impairment becomes so severe that it affects daily function, particularly a significant decline resulting in dependence in ADLs, a diagnosis of dementia is often made. This was the case with Doris, as Don mentioned that she began needing assistance with everyday tasks that included balancing the checkbook and preparing meals. Don encouraged Doris to stop driving, and months later she needed assistance with simple tasks such as bathing, dressing, and grooming. Don would oftentimes find Doris in layers of clothing sitting on the floor unsure of what she was doing. Doris was no longer able to keep records of the bills or teach piano to the children in the neighborhood, which was difficult for both Don and Doris, personally and financially.

Differentiated from dementia is delirium, a condition that is estimated to affect 30% of hospitalized older adults.[190] The cardinal features of delirium include a transient state of fluctuating cognitive abilities, often characterized by hallucinations, decreased ability to focus, poor memory, and increased confusion.[64] People who are delirious can have difficulty following multistep commands and have disorganized thoughts, as well as an altered level of consciousness. Delirium can fluctuate during the course of the day, even with lucid intervals occurring. Although delirium can resolve, most people with the condition still experience some symptoms 6 months after diagnosis. Treatment is often nonpharmacological and focuses on reorientation strategies such as the use of clocks, calendars, familiar objects from home, and personal contact to reinforce orientation.[86] Also beneficial in communication is frequent eye contact and the use of clear instructions. It is important to maintain a quiet environment as much as possible and to involve the client in both self-care and general decision-making.

Clinicians working with older adult clients will encounter varying degrees of cognitive decline, and it is essential that they screen for cognitive impairments and consider cognition as a major factor when planning the intervention approach and carrying out interventions. Levy has suggested that occupational therapists can make an important contribution in the early detection and monitoring of cognitive decline by regularly assessing mental status on an informal basis during intervention and formally screening both during the initial evaluation and periodically.[108] Assessments such as the Mini-Mental State

Examination,[66] with scoring adjusted for age, culture, and educational level, are helpful as screening tools. Other standardized assessment tools include the Montreal Assessment of Cognition (MoCA),[123] the Saint Louis University Mental Status (SLUMS),[176] and the Executive Function Performance Test (EFPT),[19] which is more occupation-based. An assessment tool such as the Functional Activities Questionnaire[178] has been used to assess functional abilities in IADLs to distinguish older adults who are experiencing more severe cognitive impairment from those who are experiencing MCI.[175]

Approximately 20% of the people ages 55 years or older experience some type of mental health concern,[37] and at times, what seems to be a loss of memory or decline in cognition can actually be another medical condition in disguise. Pathological mental conditions often occur in older adulthood because of physiologically based changes in brain function or brain disorders.[8] Less frequently, the cause is an inability to adapt to changes, losses, and transitions, or these factors may exacerbate an existing condition. Older adults who have adjusted poorly to previous stressors, who are overwhelmed by multiple simultaneous stressors, or who have little social support are particularly vulnerable. Depression, anxiety, and severe cognitive disorders are of concern for the older adult population, as is substance abuse and suicide.[148]

Depression

At least 1 in 20 older adults (65 years of age or older) who live in the community are diagnosed with clinical depression.[148] The percentage of older adults with depression increases among the population living in institutions or in the hospital setting.[92] Depression often does go unnoticed or is mistaken for other ailments, grieving, or health conditions; however, a person can experience impaired cognition and depression simultaneously. There are specific differences between depression and dementia, requiring careful diagnosis from an appropriate healthcare provider based on the patient and family report. Signs and symptoms indicative of dementia include a gradual onset of cognitive impairments (over a period of years), unawareness of memory deficits, impairments on various neuropsychological testing, and progressively worsening impairments over time.[145] Signs and symptoms indicative of depression include a more sudden onset of cognitive limitations that happens near the same time as other depressive symptoms, self-report of memory impairment, impairments that are more limited in scope and severity on various neuropsychological testing, and reports of cognitive impairment not advancing, but resolving with treated depression.[145] Older adults are reluctant to seek care from mental health practitioners; however, intervention is critical as depression can lead to withdrawal from social engagement or the inability to perform self-care. This can spiral, and the older adult could become isolated and experience occupational dysfunction as a result.

It is important for OT practitioners to be aware of the signs and symptoms of clinical depression, screen for the condition, make referrals, and seek out support for clients and their family members if depression is suspected. An OT practitioner can use the Geriatric Depression Scale[204] or the Beck Depression Inventory[20] to assess a client in any clinical setting. In general, a person may have a sad or depressed mood; decreased interest in activities, attention, concentration, or memory; feelings of guilt and worthlessness; apathy or a lack of motivation; changes in sleep, appetite, weight, energy, or sexual desire; as well as suicidal thoughts.[5] Despite the myths of aging, many older adults do not have depression; depression is not an expected outcome of aging. Suicide is "not always a consequence of depression, [however] death is the most definitive outcome of depression" (p. 126).[148]

Suicide is a major risk in late-life depression. Caucasian (now called White) men between the ages of 60 and 85 years have an increased risk for suicide, especially if they are 85 and older, have a medical illness, or live alone. Common indicators of possible impending suicide include a history of suicidal attempts, symptoms of depression or other psychiatric disorders, discharge from a facility against medical advice, spontaneous recovery from a depressed mood, substance abuse; bereavement, or giving very personal items away.[80] Through psychotherapy, electroconvulsive shock treatment, or medication management, depression can be treated, and more than 80% of older adults with clinical depression who are properly diagnosed and treated can recover and return to their previous level of functioning.[129]

Anxiety

Older adults are less likely to report mental health concerns and more likely to emphasize their physical ailments; therefore, anxiety disorder can also go unrecognized or untreated in this population. According to the Anxiety and Depression Association of America (ADAA), older adults with anxiety disorder likely had one when they were younger, and it is just as common among the older population as it is among the younger generation of adults.[12] Recognizing that an older adult has anxiety disorder can present with challenges, because older adults may present with increased numbers of comorbidities and other health concerns. Some symptoms described by the ADAA include headaches, back pain, or a rapid heartbeat. Therefore, it is difficult to separate these symptoms from other medical conditions.

Older adults may not be as open to discussing anxiety or seeking professional help because they were raised during a time when mental illness was more stigmatized and less talked about than in today's society. They also may be concerned about the loss of friends and relatives, decreased mobility, isolation, and increasingly stressful situations and are unaware themselves that this could be a treatable disorder. Anxiety disorders can manifest in various forms, including intense apprehension with shortness of breath and chest pain; fear and the disproportionate avoidance of a perceived danger; as well as chronic, persistent, and excessive anxiety.[68] Occupational therapy practitioners can perform a screen for this disorder with basic questions recommended by the ADAA,[12] inquiring about what triggers the anxiety, if the client has had concern or fretted about a number of things or if there is anything going on in life that is causing concern. Referrals should be made to a physician or psychiatrist as needed.

Substance Abuse

Substance abuse is not as prevalent among older adults as it is with younger adults; however, the problem does exist. In fact, substance abuse is on the rise and the baby boom generation will have an increased need for treatment of illicit drug use, according to the Substance Abuse and Mental Health Services Administration (SAMHSA).[170] Age-related physiological and social changes make this population vulnerable to the harmful effects of illicit drug use.

Opioids are being used increasingly more by older adults to manage short-term and more chronic pain.[121] Of particular concern are those older adults who are prescribed high daily doses of opioids, which could lead to an emergency room visit, cause psychomotor impairments, falls, respiratory depression, sedation, or death secondary to overdose. Older adults are often prescribed opioids for chronic pain associated with arthritis, back pain, chronic obstructive pulmonary disease (COPD), or cardiovascular conditions, and they are proven to be more effective for short-term versus long-term management of these conditions.[121] In addition to making referrals to appropriate care providers, OT practitioners should increase their awareness of substance abuse issues and consider interventions that integrate mental health, sleep management, and pain management into an intervention plan of care.

SAMHSA estimates that 4.3 million adults who are 50 years of age and older have used an illicit drug in the past year.[170] However, the more pressing concern is the abuse of alcohol.[63] Older adults may be taking several prescription medications that would negatively interact with alcohol. Symptoms of alcohol abuse include an increased tolerance of the effects of the substance and increased consumption over time. Older adults are more susceptible to the effects of alcohol, even when they consume less of it, because of age-related changes such as possible decreased liver and kidney function and reduced water content and body mass. Substance abuse can lead to increased accidents, increased risk for falling, poor nutrition, poor hygiene, increased mental health problems, and increased suicide risk, among many other medical conditions. Older adults should be screened by OT practitioners and referrals made to self-help groups such as Alcoholics Anonymous, counseling, psychotherapy, and a primary care physician for intervention.

CHANGES IN SENSORY STRUCTURES AND FUNCTIONS

The sensory systems of the human body are not immune to the changes that occur with aging. Older adults are often more susceptible to a number of diseases and chronic conditions or to the cumulative effect of having a disease for a long period of time, which can take a toll on the visual and hearing systems.

Vision

Normal aging of the visual system takes place at varying degrees, depending on genetic factors and lifestyle choices. These changes in the visual system are related to the eye structure itself and to the mechanisms of visual processing in older adults. (For a full discussion of how the visual system works, please refer to Chapter 24.)

Because vision is such a critical sensory system in humans and plays a significant role in social interactions and safety, any decrease in vision can have an impact on an older adult's ability to engage in occupations. In fact, in a nationally representative sample of older adults in the United States, visual dysfunctions were associated with poor cognitive function, based on self-report.[42] An occupational therapy practitioner may be seeing a client with low vision as a primary diagnosis or as an underlying secondary diagnosis; at times no diagnosis has yet been made. The clinician should encourage the client to see an eye care professional to obtain the best correction if glasses are worn and so that the client's eye health can be evaluated and addressed. Recommendations also should be made to the many professionals serving individuals with blindness and visual impairment.

It is estimated that 33% of adults have some form of vision-reducing eye disease by the age of 65.[59,196] Normal aging in the eye creates a number of changes. As the eye ages, the cornea becomes thicker and more opaque and the lens becomes less elastic, which in turn decreases accommodation, or the ability to make a change from distance to near vision. This condition is called presbyopia. Presbyopia occurs so universally that nearly everyone older than 55 requires some type of corrective lens to be able to read.[75] The lens of the eye may also become more opaque and eventually result in a cataract. Clouding of the lens can be gradual enough that an older adult is not aware of a change in color vision and a decrease in overall vision until the disease is well advanced and occupations have been affected. The iris muscles tend to atrophy, which causes the pupil to constrict. This makes it more difficult for the eye to bring enough light in for the retina to work effectively. The macula (used for central vision), which is part of the retina, has a decreased number of cones and therefore a decrease in effective color discrimination. The rods (peripheral vision) of the retina decrease and are less sensitive. There is also a decrease in the ability to transition between light and dark. Night vision is more difficult for older adults. The need for additional light increases with each decade, and the cones need increased light to effectively discriminate colors. Contrast sensitivity also decreases because of these changes in the eye structures. These changes in the anterior portion of the visual system make it more difficult to adjust for the changing visual requirements of life.[75,158]

In addition to the natural changes in the visual system, the incidence of macular degeneration and diabetic retinopathy, which can destroy central vision, is high. Any neurological disease that affects the brain will more than likely affect the visual system. This can be seen with diseases such as multiple sclerosis and Parkinson's disease. Peripheral vision is affected by various conditions, including glaucoma, retinitis pigmentosa, and field cuts related to acquired brain injuries such as stroke. Vision accounts for a high percentage of the sensory information that we use to participate in occupations. When visual acuity is reduced, as can occur in older adults, self-sufficiency in ADLs and IADLs may decrease, the potential for falls increases, and an increase in depression may be seen. It is an all-encompassing system that has an impact on every other perceptual system in the body.[113,196]

Vision functionally can be divided into central field functioning and peripheral field functioning. Each category tends to have a different impact and different intervention goals. Central visual loss (which is experienced with macular degeneration) takes away part or all of the fine detailed vision that we use for reading, shopping, community mobility, and leisure activities.[137] Something key to remember in any assessment or intervention is that if a client wears glasses, they should be worn to elicit the best performance.

Key areas of intervention to enhance participation are magnification, lighting, contrast, and organization. Magnification helps make the object larger on the retina so that the brain has more sensory input for processing. This may be accomplished by bringing the object closer client, such as with lenses, magnifiers, and electronic magnification. Because of occupational therapy's involvement in assistive technology and with the increase in all areas of technology, electronic visual enhancement may become the most popular adjustment among older adults in the future. There are ways to read, or to be read to, that are now economically feasible for almost every client. Computers come with magnification programs already installed for those with a visual impairment. Other electronic magnification devices can be used in multiple settings to increase the ability to see functionally. Each state has an agency whose mission is to provide low-vision service for individuals who are blind or have a visual impairment. There are also national and local service agencies and vendors for products.[85]

Lighting is an important component of vision and includes not only the type of light but also where it is placed. It should be close to the task and in a position that will eliminate any glare. Glare may be controlled by window dressings or by changing locations in a room. Glare is a component of contrast sensitivity.[85]

Contrast sensitivity is the ability to detect detail when gradation between an object and the background is subtle. An example might be a white banister on a white wall in a hallway that a client is unable to see or a client's inability to distinguish coffee when it is being poured into a black cup. With poor contrast sensitivity, it would be impossible to discriminate between the background and the object. This has a functional impact not only on living tasks but also on mobility. Contrast and contrast sensitivity are important determiners of how well someone sees in order to function. They are strongly associated with reading performance, mobility, driving, and face recognition.[156] Persons with central visual loss may isolate themselves from friends and family because they can no longer recognize those close to them and are embarrassed.

Decluttering spaces, grouping items by function, and further organizing objects can eliminate what has been called "visual static." An older adult with low vision is then able to more easily find and use the tools needed during a task.[85]

With peripheral field loss (such as seen with glaucoma or retinitis pigmentosa), mobility becomes an issue because of loss of part of the visual field. Central vision is often spared during this disease process. With field deficits, older adults can have difficulty using their environmental context effectively and consistently. Other areas of participation that may be affected by visual field loss include driving, shopping, financial management, and meal preparation. Grooming also may be affected by field loss.[195,196] Many older adults with peripheral field loss are able to function independently within their living environment because they rely on the habit of navigation rather than their vision. However, the field loss becomes more apparent and

function decreases when the older adult is in an unfamiliar situation. Intervention would include more effective use of scanning for detection of items. It is within occupational therapy's scope of practice to work on mobility as related to familiar space and ADL training. Teaching of mobility outside of familiar surroundings should be referred to an orientation and mobility specialist.

Hearing

Hearing is a multistep process in which sound waves result in vibration of the eardrum and movement of the ossicles. This movement is transferred to the fluid medium of the cochlea within the inner ear. The hair cells in the cochlea turn these vibrations into nerve impulses. Any impedance such as ear wax, ear infection, or hair cells that have died will have an impact on what is perceived as sound.[75] Generally, with normal aging there is a gradual progressive loss called presbycusis. Environmental factors may contribute to an increase in this loss, as may genetic factors and gender differences. Sound seems muffled to older adults. It becomes more difficult for older adults to be able to separate background and foreground noise.[75] Hearing loss is a common chronic condition seen in older adults. Anywhere from 33% to 87% of the older population in the community have some form of impairment.[137] There is increasing evidence that in addition to the ear and its parts, the central nervous system plays a part in the ability to perceive speech in a naturalistic environment.[202] With hearing loss, participation may be limited in the area of phone use, socialization, safety, and participation. Because the sound is muffled or the older adult has difficulty separating foreground and background noise, it may take longer to process what is being said. This loss is gradual and a person often compensates through lip reading. Older adults affected by hearing loss may isolate themselves from others and stop participating and socializing with family and friends.[85] Research shows that decreased hearing is associated with impaired cognition, which increases the risk for depression in older adults.[155] Screening for hearing and depression should be a consideration for occupational therapy practitioners. Hearing loss should be taken into consideration when planning intervention and recommending adaptive strategies to older adults, as well as making referrals to other healthcare providers who specialize in hearing loss.

Dual Sensory Loss

When one sense is impaired, the other senses are relied on more heavily to interpret social cues, physical cues, and safety cues. With visual and hearing loss, or what is often termed *dual sensory loss*, the impact is that much greater. It is estimated that 23% of people older than 81 years have some degree of dual sensory impairment.[24] Dual sensory loss is typically considered hearing and vision, although a decrease in the tactile system could also make participation and adjustment difficult for an older adult. The combination of loss in more than two sensory systems is considered multisensory loss.

Smell and Taste

The ability to detect smells and correctly identify smells decreases with age. Most people over the age of 80 years have impaired olfaction, or smell,[120] and there is a high prevalence of people ages 65 and older who report decreased smell sensation and complete loss of smell.[148] This is a sensory loss of major concern for OT practitioners who are assessing safety in the home and one's ability to live independently. Compensatory strategies such as natural gas and smoke detectors can be critical, as well as a family member or friend checking for food spoilage.

Because of the fact that the sense of smell is connected so intricately with the sense of taste, a decrease in olfaction can negatively affect eating and nutrition. Olfaction impairments have been associated with depressive symptoms and poorer quality of life, which can also affect the enjoyment of food, drink, and socialization.[72] As people age, the ability to distinguish among salty, sour, and bitter decreases; therefore, older adults may use more salt on foods. The thirst sensation can also decrease, placing an older adult at risk for dehydration.[150] Older adults may purposefully reduce the amount of fluids they drink to avoid frequent and energy-depleting trips to the bathroom. Food and water intake is monitored in hospitals, long-term care, and rehabilitation facilities. It is also critical for caregivers and family members to encourage proper nutrition and hydration in the home.

CHANGES IN NEUROMUSCULOSKELETAL AND MOVEMENT-RELATED STRUCTURES AND FUNCTIONS

Although age-related changes do occur in the musculoskeletal system, older adults also have the capacity to maintain or even increase their strength in later years. Exercise is highly effective in older adults,[28,75] as is a program of functional activity, as long as it is adapted to the client's unique needs.

Early in life the body builds bone mass, with a peak at around 35 years.[47,156] After this age, calcium is gradually lost from the bones, which results in loss of bone strength. This condition is termed *osteopenia* when bone volume reaches below-normal levels because of bone resorption exceeding bone synthesis. This is different from *osteoporosis*, in which the reduction in bone mass is significant enough to cause fractures. Primary osteoporosis occurs when the bones become more porous but no other disease is causing this process. Secondary osteoporosis can be due to a number of different processes, including rheumatoid arthritis, diabetes, and drug use, especially corticosteroids.[156] In the United States it is estimated that 10 million people who are 50 years of age or older have the diagnosis of osteoporosis, whereas another 34 million older adults have bone mass that is lower than normal, putting this population at risk for bone fractures. Risks for osteoporosis include estrogen depletion, testosterone depletion, calcium deficiency, cigarette smoking, alcoholism, or physical inactivity. The loss of bone mass can also contribute to a collapse of spinal vertebrae causing a kyphotic appearance in the back with a possible impact on respiration.[75]

Joints also exhibit normal age-related changes. Over time a reduction in joint range of motion of 20% to 25% can be seen.[111] As people age, the water content in tissues, including cartilage, decreases.[156] Cartilage also becomes stiffer and has less of a cushioning effect for the joint over time.[53] The cartilage surfaces become rougher in areas of each joint with the greatest stress, thereby reducing the smoothness of movement. These changes are more significant in areas of increased wear and tear, but they are even seen in sedentary individuals. At a pathological level, articular cartilage can degenerate to such a point that pain and stiffness result, as well as impaired movement, which can be diagnosed as osteoarthritis (see Chapter 39 for further details). Although pain and decreased joint mobility are often factors limiting a person's function, arthritic changes can be seen radiographically in the joints, even in individuals with no other symptomatology. Changes are seen in tendons and ligaments, which also have reduced water content over time.[111] Increased cross-linking of collagen fibers occurs and can cause stiffness of the collagen. Tendon and ligament strength declines with age,[156] as does the strength of attachment to bone, which results in decreased joint stability and greater risk for injury. Doris was diagnosed with osteoarthritis, and the physical changes in her hip joint placed her at an increased risk for injury, which occurred when she fell in her new home. The hip fracture was stabilized with open reduction and internal fixation. Don was grateful that a total joint replacement was not indicated at the time because, as he reported, he worried about how her therapy would go, because she would not remember any of the restrictions after a replacement. Her orthopedic surgeon cleared her to bear weight as tolerated on her leg. Doris did not have postoperative pain nor did she have any other precautions or restrictions (for further information on hip fractures and lower extremity joint replacements, please see Chapter 41).

In general, older adults exhibit some muscle atrophy.[156] This is due in part to age and in part to disuse, and it is difficult to distinguish the two. Some motor units and muscle fibers are lost over time, with the loss being most pronounced in fast-twitch fibers.[156] Denervation of fast fibers in aging can be followed by reinnervation from slow fibers and result in this conversion. It takes more time for older muscles to recover from use, and the recovery may not be complete, resulting in decreased muscle endurance. The decrease in muscle mass and contractile force is termed *sarcopenia*,[111] which can be a consequence of age or a disease process and results in decreased muscle power. Encouraging older adults to continue exercising or to resume exercise after a hospitalization cannot be overemphasized for its benefits and therapeutic effects. Regular physical training can improve muscle strength and endurance, even in the older adult population.[117] This type of exercise program (completed with caution and under the supervision of a healthcare provider) is also beneficial to the cardiovascular system.

CHANGES IN CARDIOVASCULAR, HEMATOLOGICAL, IMMUNOLOGICAL, AND RESPIRATORY SYSTEM STRUCTURES AND FUNCTIONS

The cardiovascular system is responsible for pumping blood throughout the body, enabling oxygen and nutrients to be delivered to all systems, as well as removing waste products from all parts of the body. Therefore, damage to this system can have a negative impact on the functioning of the entire body. Cardiovascular disease is the most common cause of death around the globe; however, with improved diet, increased exercise, and less smoking, mortality rates are decreasing in the United States.[75]

Although high blood pressure is a pathological function and not part of normal aging, it is normal for systolic blood pressure to increase with age because of increased stiffness of the arteries.[99] Athletic individuals have lower systolic pressure than do sedentary individuals, but systolic pressure is still, on average, higher than that in younger individuals. Veins also dilate and stretch with age, and their valves function less efficiently,[156] so blood return to the heart is slowed. With age the heart requires slightly longer rest periods between beats, or longer recovery, which may have an impact during activities requiring a higher heart rate. The maximum attainable heart rate declines with age, though not as steeply as in those who exercise. Cardiac output is also somewhat decreased, which may explain some of the fatigue felt by older adults during strenuous activities.[156] During exercise, older adults may become short of breath (dyspnea) and fatigue more quickly than younger adults. Older adults are also susceptible to postural, or orthostatic, hypotension, which is a fall in systemic blood pressure upon changing positions (such as rising from supine to sitting at the edge of the bed) too quickly. This can cause a person to feel lightheaded upon standing, increasing yet another risk for a fall.[75] See Chapter 45 for further information on cardiac and pulmonary diseases.

Arteriosclerosis is hardening of the arteries, which can occur in older persons; symptoms may include headache or dizziness.[99] Atherosclerosis is a form of arteriosclerosis in which plaques decrease the diameter of the arteries, and it is the predominant change that occurs in blood vessels with age. These fatty plaques and the proliferation of connective tissue in the walls of the arteries contribute to the slow destruction of the arterial walls and can lead to blockage of the artery, especially when there is a blood clot. There is evidence that this accumulation of plaque in the walls of the arteries begins in the first decade of life, with complications of atherosclerosis beginning as early as the fourth decade of life.[75] Heart attacks are more common in individuals older than 50 years of age, and the coronary artery disease that causes the heart attack is the number one killer of people in the United States.[91] Given the prevalence of atherosclerosis in older adults, it is important that OT practitioners do their part and address diet and exercise, stress and weight management, smoking cessation and lifestyle modification, as well as medication management and adherence to prescription medications.

One important hematological condition in older adults is anemia. Anemia is defined as "a lower than normal oxygen-carrying capacity of blood" (p. 81).[75] It can occur in older adults during a hospitalization or when placed in long-term care settings. There is no single cause for the disease; it is treated more like a syndrome that has many different causes. People with anemia generally have pale skin, fatigue, and shortness of breath. OT clinicians should check with the physician or nurse before treating someone who may have these symptoms in a hospital setting, because the person may require a blood transfusion.

The immune system is important to ensure that our bodies remain free of infections and cancer. The white blood cells in the immune system must be able to recognize healthy cells from invading microorganisms and parasites or abnormal cancerous cells.[75] Immunological function is decreased at multiple levels and typically gives rise to three categories of illness that affect older adults: infections, cancer, and autoimmune disease. The thinner skin of elderly persons provides less of a barrier to infectious agents with increased risk for skin tears and subsequent infection. Fewer cilia are found in the lungs, which reduces the body's ability to keep infectious agents out of the lungs. There is also evidence that immunity is decreased at a cellular level, with a reduction in adaptive immune responses, such as those of T cells.[156]

The function of the respiratory system is to deliver oxygen to and remove carbon dioxide from the bloodstream.[75] Production of mucus in the respiratory system, which helps prevent respiratory infections, is decreased, and thus older adults' susceptibility to these ailments increases. The cough reflex is also less effective.[156] Numerous changes occur and can result in chest wall stiffness, such as kyphosis (appears hunched over), calcification of the costal cartilages, and scoliosis. This limits chest expansion and requires increased use of the diaphragm for breathing. This heightened energy requirement just to breathe can increase older adults' fatigue even when at rest or during light activities. The efficiency of oxygen–carbon dioxide exchange also decreases because of increased residual volume in the lungs, enlarged alveoli, and fewer capillaries.[27]

The normal age-related changes to the respiratory system can be coupled with common diseases that increase in frequency from the fifth decade of life and onward to complicate this picture. These conditions include emphysema, pneumonia, chronic bronchitis, and lung cancer. Emphysema and bronchitis can be grouped together and discussed as COPD, which is primarily caused by cigarette smoking or long-term exposure to unhealthy air (see Chapter 45 for more details). Energy conservation and work simplification techniques should be incorporated into intervention when respiratory dysfunction is limiting engagement in occupations. Pursed lip breathing techniques and diaphragmatic breathing also can be incorporated into a stress management approach.

CHANGES IN VOICE AND SPEECH FUNCTIONS; DIGESTIVE, METABOLIC, AND ENDOCRINE FUNCTIONS; AND GENITOURINARY AND REPRODUCTIVE FUNCTIONS

The vocal mechanism is affected by age and results in weakness, reduced intensity, hoarseness, trembling, and alterations in vocal pitch, which is a common characteristic of the older adult's voice. These changes in the vocal mechanism are in part due to the aging larynx and supporting structures, as well as an increase in calcium and hardening of the cartilage in the larynx. Blood supply to the vocal mechanism may be decreased, and there may be edema of the vocal cords that affects the quality of voice and speech functions. The vocal pitch of older male adults increases, whereas the pitch of older females decreases. The trembling or jittering of the voice is caused by a decrease in neuromuscular control of the muscles that support the larynx. These changes are subtle and usually are recognized only by a trained professional; they may have minimal impact on the daily communication functioning of an older adult.[33]

A major function of the digestive system is to process incoming foods to deliver nutrients to the body. A common problem experienced by older adults in eating and swallowing is due to tooth loss and compromised dentition. Aging causes tissue, glandular, and muscular changes in the jaw, as well as changes in the tongue, salivary glands, and throat with a decrease in the number of salivary glands and reduced taste sensation. These changes may cause an older adult to exert greater effort in swallowing and require more time to swallow food. Some older adults will choose foods that are soft and easier to swallow, whereas others reduce their food intake, affecting nutrition and weight negatively.[9]

Eating also can be challenging when there is not the proper amount of saliva in the mouth to create a bolus. This condition can be caused by decreased saliva production, cigarette smoking, or medication side effects. If a person is having difficulty swallowing, an assessment of swallowing is recommended for dysphagia (difficulty in swallowing). This would be an assessment of a complex coordination of several muscles of the tongue, palate, pharynx, and esophagus and can be administered by an OT practitioner with advanced practice or a speech and language pathologist.[75] See Chapter 27 for more information on the assessment and interventions for eating and swallowing.

In the stomach, food is chemically digested by gastric acid. As people get older, the amount of gastric acid secretions decreases, whereas the incidence of peptic ulcers and gastritis increases. This can be due to drug ingestion, aspirin, caffeine, or alcohol; it also can be caused by a genetic predisposition causing inflammation of the stomach lining. The liver's ability to detoxify many foreign and potentially damaging chemicals that enter (or are produced by) the body also decreases with age.[75]

One common problem with older adults is diverticulosis, which is "the development of small sacs where the large intestinal lining has herniated through the intestinal muscular wall" (p. 87).[75] These pockets can become impacted with feces, resulting in an ulceration and inflammation of the mucosal lining (known as diverticulitis). This can be a painful experience for older adults and can complicate the bowel routine by causing constipation. In extreme cases, it can also lead to an intestinal obstruction.[75] An occupational therapy practitioner can address issues of feeding, digestion, and bowel routine in collaboration with nursing and dietary services, as well as the client and family. Doris had a diagnosis of diverticulitis, and when asked about her experience with it, Don mentioned that it did cause Doris a lot of pain and it was something that he felt was at times more painful than the hip fracture. Don thought a reason why Doris got up and went to the bathroom so much at night was because of the constipation and her attempts to have a bowel movement. Doris stopped taking her medications for diverticulitis; however, Don thought it was something she needed to resume taking to prevent the discomfort experienced before admission. A follow-up appointment with Doris' primary care physician was recommended.

The kidneys filter the blood and help remove wastes and extra fluid from the body. They also help control the chemical balance within the body. The kidneys work with the ureters, bladder, and urethra to excrete urine and waste, and this process can be affected by muscle changes and changes in the reproductive system with respect to bladder control. As a person ages, the kidneys and bladder change because the amount of kidney tissue decreases, the number of filtering units (nephrons) decreases, and the blood vessels supplying the kidneys become hardened, causing the kidneys to filter blood more slowly. The bladder wall changes and the elastic walls become tough and less elastic, limiting how much urine the bladder can hold. The bladder muscles weaken and can cause the bladder or vagina to fall out of position (prolapse) in women. In men, the urethra can become blocked by an enlarged prostate gland. These conditions can place an older adult at risk for urinary incontinence or urinary tract infections. Collaborating with the client and the family, as well as the nursing team, to work on a bladder program is under the scope of practice of an OT practitioner and is a critical component of self-care and independence with ADLs.[187]

Often, OT practitioners work with clients who are undergoing dialysis for chronic (or acute) renal failure. Dialysis is a treatment that replaces the function of the kidneys by removing waste, salt, and extra water to prevent them from building up in the body. It also keeps a safe level of certain chemicals in the blood, such as potassium, sodium, and bicarbonate. One other effect is maintaining control of blood pressure.[131] Clients who are undergoing dialysis treatments can experience exhaustion after a treatment, weakness in the lower extremities, decreased blood pressure, muscle cramps, itching, insomnia, anemia, bone disease, fluid overload, and depression. It is critical to pace any occupational therapy intervention and teach energy conservation and work simplification techniques. Caregivers and family members should also receive the attention of the clinician, as dynamics in family responsibilities and relationships can be altered.[115] Meal planning and grocery shopping can be included in the intervention plan, as patients receiving dialysis must maintain a special diet with supplements and an extensive prescription medication list.

The endocrine system is another regulatory system in the human body and controls many aspects of the body's physiology, such as body temperature; basal metabolic rate; growth rate; carbohydrate, lipid, and protein metabolism; stress response; and reproductive events.[75] Because the endocrine system is responsible for producing and secreting hormones into the body, dysfunction of this system has widespread impact on the health and well-being of an older adult.

Gregory and Sandmire have described a hierarchy of control[75] that starts with the higher brain centers that influence the activity of the hypothalamus. The hypothalamus releases hormones that control the activity of the pituitary gland, which in turn releases hormones that control the activity of lower endocrine glands and other tissues. These lower endocrine glands release hormones that control other body functions related to the thyroid gland, adrenal gland, testes, and ovaries. An overall decline in the production and secretion of hormones and the impact this has on the human body goes beyond the scope of this chapter; however, one condition that is prevalent in the older adult population is diabetes mellitus (DM).

Diabetes is a condition in which the body does not properly process food for use as energy. The pancreas makes a hormone called insulin to help glucose get into the cells of the body. With diabetes, the body either does not make enough insulin or cannot use its own insulin as well as it should. This causes sugars to build up in the blood.[39] Long-term complications such as blindness (resulting from cataracts and retinal damage), renal failure, nerve damage, atherosclerosis, and gangrenous infection often necessitating amputation (below or above the knee) are all factors that will have an impact on participation in occupations. Non–insulin-dependent diabetes mellitus (NIDDM), or type 2, accounts for approximately 90% to 95% of all cases. In the United States, 21 million people have been diagnosed with DM, and 27% of those 65 years of age and older have the disease.[39] This is another area in which OT practitioners can intervene with lifestyle modification programs, weight management, exercise and diet programs, and stress management. The client and family should be working closely together to address the needs of an older adult with DM.

Reproductive function will also change as a person ages. For women, menopause is associated with physiological and psychological changes that can influence sexuality. There is a decrease in estrogen levels, which affects the menstrual cycle and vaginal lubrication. The changes in estrogen levels also affect the vascular and urogenital systems. Women may experience changes in mood, sleep, and cognitive function, which can contribute to lower self-esteem, decreased self-image, and decreased sexual desire. Prescribed medications and current medical status can also affect sexuality and sexual drive.[14] There are medications and hormone replacement therapies that can be used to address these issues medically; therapy and counseling also can be of benefit psychologically.

For men, there is not a major or rapid change in fertility with age as there is with women. The changes are gradual, and the condition is referred to as andropause. The changes for men primarily occur in the testes, with decreased testicular mass and a gradual decline of testosterone; these changes may make it more challenging to achieve an erection. The testes continue to produce sperm; however, the rate of sperm cell production decreases and the tubes that carry the sperm may become less elastic with age. With the enlargement of the prostate gland, urination and ejaculation are negatively affected. Approximately 50% of older men are diagnosed with benign prostatic hypertrophy.[188] Fertility varies among older men; age does not predict male fertility. The volume of fluid ejaculated usually remains the same; however, there may be a decreased number of sperm. Some men experience decreased sex drive, which can be caused by psychological concerns, lack of a willing partner, medication side effects, or other chronic medical conditions.[188]

Erectile dysfunction (ED) also may be a concern for aging men; however, this is not because of the aging process itself but because of other medical conditions or medication side effects. Hypertension and DM are known causes of ED, and medications can be used to treat this condition. Prostate cancer and bladder cancer are more likely to occur with age, and preventive measures and visits to a primary care physician are encouraged

for early detection.[188] OT practitioners can use their interview skills and the EX-PLISSIT model (previously mentioned in this chapter) for sexuality to obtain information and provide information in the area of sexuality. There are also clinicians who have advanced practice in this area and can provide more intensive and comprehensive therapy. Referrals also should be made to sex therapists as needed.

CHANGES IN SKIN AND RELATED STRUCTURE FUNCTIONS

The integumentary system consists of the skin and accessory structures such as the nails, hair, oil glands, and sweat glands. An obvious sign of aging is the change in hair color to gray, as well as the thinning and loss of hair, experienced by many older adults. Because skin covers the entire body, another obvious sign associated with aging is the changing skin. As the aging process progresses, skin becomes more vulnerable to shearing forces, abrasions, and blister formation.[74] It is important for OT practitioners to protect the client's skin during functional mobility and ADL transfers from surface to surface, to avoid any shearing or tearing of the skin. Any open tears or wounds should be covered to protect the client and the clinician.

It is also important for older adults to protect the skin from ultraviolet rays of the sun. The turnover rate of the epidermis shedding and replacing itself every month starts to slow down with aging, slowing the amount of protective melanin pigment produced. This makes the ultraviolet light more dangerous and leaves older adults more prone to developing skin cancer.[58]

The thinning and wrinkling of the skin are results of the decreased amounts of collagen and elastin in the dermis of the skin. With the loss of elastin, the skin loses its resilience as a person ages, and with the loss of collagen, the skin is more susceptible to wear and tear. These changes are accompanied by a decreased flow of dermal blood supply, affecting the typical signs of inflammation in the skin. Older adults may not show initial signs and symptoms of tissue injury such as sunburn, bacterial infection, or even skin cancer. Because the dermal layer of the skin holds sensory receptors, the changes in this layer will also affect tactile sensitivity of the skin while increasing the pain threshold at the fingertips.[58] These changes may make it difficult for older adults to perform fine motor movements, such as turning on a hearing aid, snapping buttons, or putting in earrings. Fine motor movements and dexterity should be assessed, and compensatory strategies should be integrated into intervention for the completion of ADLs such as grooming and other meaningful activities.

Aging is a natural process, and the changes described here are expected and typical. "It is this interdependence of our organ systems that, on the one hand, allows for appropriate compensatory adjustments to homeostatic disturbances in younger, healthy individuals but, on the other hand, can create a chain reaction of dysfunction in older, less healthy persons with decreased physiological functional reserve" (p. 82).[75] When there is a chronic medical condition or injury, the aging process becomes more complicated; therefore, it is important to consider prevention and wellness with the older adult and intervene with our clients when they are younger adults, if possible.

THREADED CASE STUDY

Doris, Part 3

Strengths that were identified for Doris included the fact that she required minimal assistance or less during functional mobility and could feed herself with supervision. These were two areas that did not require much physical assistance from Don. Doris also showed active range of motion and strength in her upper extremities, which were considered within functional limits. Doris had a passion for piano and teaching young children to play piano, which was also a strength, as it was motivating for her and provided her with hope. Supports included her relationship and assistance from Don and their loving family. Don and Doris lived right behind the rehabilitation facility, and Don could visit Doris and learn from the occupational therapy each day for family/patient education.

Areas of potential occupational disruption included resuming instrumental activities of daily living and resuming her roles in the home management tasks of bookkeeping and paying the bills secondary to her cognitive deficits and expected limitations in the future, given her diagnosis of Alzheimer's disease. Barriers included safety in the home (and at the facility) secondary to the cognitive component, which is progressive, requiring increasingly more compensatory measures. There is also concern about Don's health and his abilities to serve as the sole care provider upon discharge to their home.

Priorities included patient and family education, particularly with Don, in preparation for discharge. Don identified two major goals for Doris as being very important: safely performing toileting activities (particularly in the middle of the night) and resuming piano instruction. The OT practitioner recommended that Don also consider a caregiver support group and in-home support services for the physical work that he may not be able to complete with Doris, due to his own physical limitations and heart condition.

Doris' case has several layers, including a new home environment and medical conditions that added to the complexity of the aging process. All of these layers had to be considered when designing an intervention plan that could meet Doris' and Don's needs. Compensatory strategies and environmental adaptations were recommended for Doris, and caregiver education was paramount for the carryover and execution of the strategies in the home. Attention was given to the caregiver and his needs, as Don himself is an older adult with a complicated medical condition who also demonstrated physical limitations in his role as caregiver.

Don brought Doris' keyboard to therapy, and as Doris progressed in OT, she began to play the keyboard again. She was able to complete bathing and dressing activities with minimal verbal cues using sequencing cards designed in therapy and was soon inviting other residents at the facility to the rehabilitation gym to sing along as she played the keyboard. Don said she finally looked like herself again. He attended a support group specifically designed for caregivers who were spouses of loved ones with Alzheimer's disease, and he agreed to in-home support services and respite services so that he could take time for himself. The new apartment was organized, and the hallways and floors were cleared. Don and Doris felt ready for the discharge to their home.

SUMMARY

Older adults are an extremely diverse population with whom OT practitioners work; they provide complex challenges yet offer rewarding experiences and opportunities in both habilitation and rehabilitation settings. Older adults bring a lifetime of experiences, habits, wisdom, and problem-solving strategies to the occupational therapy process, as well as the possibility of functional decline as a result of the aging process. From the stories of "when I was your age" to the excitement experienced while surfing the internet, this population presents opportunities and potential for the field of occupational therapy to truly make a difference with people who deserve comprehensive and holistic care.

Empowering older adults, their families, and their caregivers is a reflection of the respect and dignity the older adult population deserves. Baby boomers must be a priority to society and to healthcare because their needs are growing as they continue to age. Meanwhile, the healthcare policies and systems driving reimbursement and documentation continue to challenge the delivery of services. An occupation-based, client-centered approach makes sense when addressing the needs of an older adult, because like any other client, the desired outcome is to live life to its fullest.

REVIEW QUESTIONS

1. Describe four elements of treatment to enhance participation by an older adult with low vision, impaired hearing, impaired sensation, and low endurance.
2. Name three cognitive changes associated with aging, and provide three strategies to enhance the learning of new information.
3. List five age-related physical changes that a therapist would consider in a client who is 80 years of age.
4. Identify areas of occupation to assess when working with an older client who recently had significant weight loss.
5. Describe three key considerations when assessing an older adult's home for the potential to age in place.
6. What are the benefits to a shared governance structure in facilities providing care to older adults?
7. Describe the paradigm shift that can occur when "flipping a nursing facility."
8. Describe the significance of policies established for older adults in the United States with respect to documentation and reimbursement.

For additional practice questions for this chapter, please visit eBooks.Health.Elsevier.com.

REFERENCES

1. Adams PF, Kirzinger WK, Martinez ME: QuickStats: percentage of adults aged 18-69 years with a limitation in their ability to work because of health problems, by age group—National Health Interview Survey, United States, 2012, *MMWR Morb Mortal Wkly Rep* 63:519, 2014.

2. Ahima RS: Global warming threatens human thermoregulation and survival, *The Journal of Clinical Investigation* 130(2): 559–561, 2020.

3. Ahmed T, Haboubi N: Assessment and management of nutrition in older people and its importance to health, *Clin Interv Aging* 5:207–216, 2010.

4. American Geriatrics Society and British Geriatrics Society: Guideline for the prevention of falls in older persons. https://pubmed.ncbi.nlm.nih.gov/11380764.

5. American Occupational Therapy Association: Falls prevention and home modification. http://www.aota.org/-/media/Corporate/Files/Practice/Aging/Resources/Focus-On-Falls-Prevention-Home-Mod-Booklet.pdf.

6. American Occupational Therapy Association (2019). Specialty conference: PDPM & occupational therapy: navigating from volume to value. Retrieved from https://myaota.aota.org/shop_aota/product/OL5176.

7. American Occupational Therapy Association. Occupational therapy practice framework: Domain and process (4th ed), *American Journal of Occupational Therapy*, 74(2):1–87, 2020.

8. American Psychiatric Association: *Diagnostic and statistical manual of mental disorders*, ed 5, Arlington, VA, 2013, American Psychiatric Association.

9. American Speech and Hearing Association: Let's talk: normal aging changes in speech, language, and swallowing. https://www.asha/siteassets/puplications/0499asham.

10. Anetzberger GJ: Elder abuse. In Bonder BR, Dal Bellow-Haas V, editors: *Functional performance in older adults*, Philadelphia, 2009, FA Davis, pp 609–632.

11. Annon J: The PLISSIT model: a proposed conceptual scheme for the behavioural treatment of sexual problems, *J Sex Educ Ther* 2:1–15, 1976.

12. Anxiety and Depression Association of America: Older adults. http://www.adaa.org/living-with-anxiety/older-adults.

13. Arbesman M, Mosley LJ: Systematic review of occupation- and activity-based health management and maintenance interventions for community-dwelling older adults, *Arch Occup Ther* 66:277–283, 2012.

14. Bachmann GA, Leiblum SR: The impact of hormones on menopausal sexuality: a literature review, *Menopause* 11: 120–130, 2004.

15. Baltes PA, Lindenberger U: Emergence of a powerful connection between sensory and cognitive functions across the adult lifespan: a new window to the study of cognitive aging? *Psychol Aging* 12:12–21, 1997.

16. Bargh JA, McKenna KYA: The Internet and social life, *Annu Rev Psychol* 55:573–590, 2004.

17. Bartrés-Fax D, Junqué C, López-Alomar A: Neuropsychological and genetic differences between age-associated memory impairment and mild cognitive impairment entities, *J Am Geriatr Soc* 49:985–990, 2001.

18. Bauer M, McAuliffe L, Nay R, Chenco C: Sexuality in older adults: effect of an education intervention on attitudes and beliefs of residential aged care staff, *Educ Gerontol* 39:82–91, 2012.

19. Baum CM, Tabor Connor L, Morrison T, et al: Reliability, validity, and clinical utility of the Executive Function Performance Test: a measure of executive function in a sample of people with stroke, *Arch Occup Ther* 62:446–455, 2008.

20. Beck A, Steer R: *Beck Depression Inventory manual*, San Antonio, TX, 1987, The Psychological Corp.

21. Benz J, Sedensky M, Tompson T, Agiesta J: Working longer: older Americans' attitudes on work and retirement, Chicago, 2013, The Association Press–NORC Center for Public Affairs Research. https://apnorc.org/projects/working-longer-older-americans-attitudes-on-work-and-retirement/.

22. Berg-Weger M, Morley JE: Loneliness and social isolation in older adults during the COVID-19 pandemic: implications for gerontological social work, *Journal of Nutrition, Health, and Aging* 24(5):456–458, 2020.

23. Berger S, Escher A, Mengle E, Sullivan N: Effectiveness of health promotion, management, and maintenance interventions within the scope of occupational therapy for community-dwelling older adults: a systematic review, *American Journal of Occupational Therapy* 72:1–10, 2018. https://doi.org/10.5014/ajot.2018.030346.

24. Bergman B, Rosenthal U: Vision and hearing loss in old age, *Scand Audiol* 30:255–264, 2001.

25. Black DS, O'Reilly GA, Olmstead R: Mindfulness meditation and improvement in sleep quality and daytime impairment among older adults with sleep disturbances: a randomized clinical trial, *JAMA Internal Medicine* 175(4):494–501, 2015.

26. Bolduc JJ: Functional performance in later life: basic sensory, perceptual, and physical changes associated with aging. In Robnett RH, Brossoie N, Chop WC, editors: *Gerontology for the health care professional*, Burlington, MA, 2019, Jones & Bartlett Learning, pp 233–256.

27. Brashers VL: Structure and function of the pulmonary system. In McCance KL, Huether SE, Brashers VL, Rote NS, editors: *Pathophysiology: the biologic basis for disease in adults and children*, ed 6, Maryland Heights, MO, 2010, Mosby.

28. Brossoie N, Chop WC: Social gerontology. In Robnett RH, Brossoie N, Chop WC, editors: *Gerontology for the health care professional*, Burlington, MA, 2019, Jones & Bartlett Learning, pp 27–56.

29. Bruner-Canhoto LA: Policy and ethical issues for older adults. In Robnett RH, Chop W, editors: *Gerontology for the health care professional*, Burlington, MA, 2015, Jones & Bartlett Learning, pp 293–321.

30. Buis L, Singer D, Solway E, Kirch M, Kullgren J, Malani P. (2020). Telehealth use among older adults before and during COVID-19. *University of Michigan National Poll on Healthy Aging*. Retrieved from https://www.healthyagingpoll.org/report/telehealth-use-among-older-adults-and-during-covid-19.

31. Burns T, Mortimer JA, Merchak P: Cognitive performance test: a new approach to functional assessment in Alzheimer's disease, *J Geriatr Psychiatry Neurol* 7:46–54, 1994.

32. Burr B, Atkins L, Bertram AG, Sears K, McGinnis AN: "If you stop playing you get old": investigating reflections of play in older adults, *Educational Gerontology* 45(5):353–364, 2019. https://doi.org/10.1080/03601277.2019.1627058.

33. Caruso A, Mueller P: Age-related changes in speech, voice, and swallowing. In Shadden BB, Tone MA, editors: *Aging and communication*, Austin, TX, 1997, Pro-Ed, pp 117–134.

34. Centers for Disease Control and Prevention: Falls among older adults: an overview, 2013. https://www.cdc.gov/falls/index.html.

35. Centers for Disease Control and Prevention: Health expenditures. http://www.cdc.gov/nchs/fastats/health-expenditures.htm.

36. Centers for Disease Control and Prevention: Older adult drivers, 2022. https://www.cdc.gov/transportationsafety/older_adult_drivers/index.html.

37. Centers for Disease Control and Prevention: The state of mental health and aging in America. http://www.cdc.gov/aging/pdf/mental_health.pdf.

38. Centers for Medicare and Medicaid Services. 2014. IMPACT Act of 2014 data standardization and cross setting measures. Retrieved from https://www.cms.gov/Medicare/Quality-Initiatives-Patient-Assessment-Instruments/Post-Acute-Care-Quality-Initiatives/IMPACT-Act-of-2014/IMPACT-Act-of-2014-Data-Standardization-and-Cross-Setting-Measures.

39. Centers for Disease Control and Prevention: 2014 National diabetes statistics report. https://www.cdc.gov/diabetes/data/statistics-report/index.html.

40. Centers for Medicare and Medicaid Services. 2017. National Health Expenditures 2017 Highlights. Retrieved from https://www.cms.gov/research-statistics-data-and-systems/statistics-trends-and-reports/nationalhealthexpenddata/downloads/highlights.pdf.

41. Chen LK, Kim YS, Moon P, Merriam S: A review and critique of the portrayal of older adult learners in adult education journals, 1980–2006, *Adult Educ Q* 59(1):3–21, 2008.

42. Chen SP, Bhattacharya J, Pershing S: Association of vision loss with cognition in older adults, *JAMA Ophthalmology* 135(9):963–970, 2017.

43. Chop WC: Demographic trends of an aging society. In Robnett RH, Chop W, editors: *Gerontology for the health care professional*, Burlington, MA, 2015, Jones & Bartlett Learning, pp 2–15.

44. Clark F, Azen SP, Zemke R, et al: Occupational therapy for independent-living older adults: a randomized controlled trial, *JAMA* 278:1321–1326, 1997.

45. Clark F, et al: *Lifestyle Redesign®: the intervention tested in the USC Well Elderly Studies*, ed 2, Bethesda, MD, 2015, AOTA Press.

46. Clark F, Jackson J, Carlson M, et al: Effectiveness of a lifestyle intervention in promoting the well-being of independently living older people: Results of the Well Elderly 2 randomised controlled trial, *Journal of Epidemiology and Community Health* 66:782–790, 2012. https://doi.org/10.1136/jech.2009.099754.

47. Clary EG, Snyder M: The motivations to volunteer: theoretical and practical considerations, *Curr Dir Psychol Sci* 8:156–159, 1999.

48. Clavelle JT, Porter O'Grady T, Drenkard K: Structural empowerment and the nursing practice environment in Magnet® organizations, *J Nurs Adm* 43:566–573, 2013.

49. Clemson L, Cumming RG, Kendig H, Swann M, Heard R, Taylor K: The effectiveness of a community-based program for reducing the incidence of falls in the elderly: a randomized trial, *Journal of American Geriatric Society* 52:1487–1494, 2004.

50. Conhoto LB: Policy issues for older adults. In Robnett RH, Brossoie N, Chop WC, editors: *Gerontology for the health care professional*, Burlington, MA, 2019, Jones & Bartlett Learning, pp 129–152.

51. Corman E: Including fall prevention for older adults in your trauma injury prevention program: introducing farewell to falls, *J Trauma Nurs* 16:206–207, 2009.

52. Crittenden J, Butler S, Silver N, Hartford A, Coleman R: Juggling multiple roles: an examination of role conflict and its brief report: relationship to older adult volunteer satisfaction and retention, *Maine Center on Aging Research and Evaluation* 43:1–16, 2020.

53. Crowther-Radulewicz CL: Structure and function of the musculoskeletal system. In McCance KL, Huether SE, Brashers VL, Rote NS, editors: *Pathophysiology: the biologic basis for disease in adults and children*, ed 6, Maryland Heights, MO, 2010, Mosby.

54. Davey J, de Joux V, Arcus M: Accommodation options for older people in Aotearoa/New Zealand, Wellington, New Zealand, 2004, NZ Institute for Research on Ageing/Business and Economic Research Ltd, for Centre for Housing Research Aotearoa/New Zealand.

55. Depp C, Jeste D: Definitions and predictors of successful aging: A comprehensive review of larger quantitative studies, *Focus* 7:137–150, 2009. https://focus.psychiatryonline.org/doi/full/10.1176/foc.7.1.foc137.

56. Deeg D, Kardaun J, Fozard J: Health, behavior and aging. In Birren JE, Schaie KW, editors: *Handbook of the psychology of aging*, ed 4, San Diego, CA, 1996, Academic Press.

57. Dobbins S, Hubbard E, Flentje A, Dawson-Rose C, & Leutwyler H: Play provides social connection for older adults with serious mental illness: a grounded theory analysis of a 10-week exergame intervention, *Aging & Mental Health*, 24:4, 596-603, 2020.

58. Dychtwald K: *Age wave*, New York, 1990, Bantam Books.

59. Ellexson MT: Access to participation: occupational therapy and low vision, *Top Geriatr Rehabil* 20:154–172, 2004.

60. Ewald PD: Future concerns in an aging society. In Robnett RH, Chop W, editors: *Gerontology for the health care professional*, Burlington, MA, 2015, Jones & Bartlett Learning, pp 337–371.

61. Failla G: The aging process and cancerogenesis, *Ann N Y Acad Sci* 71:1124–1140, 1958.

62. Ferrini AF, Ferrini RL, editors: *Health in later years*, ed 3, Boston, 2000, McGraw-Hill.

63. Fink A, Elliot MN, Tsai M, Beck JC: An evaluation of an intervention to assist primary care physicians in screening and educating older patients who use alcohol, *J Am Geriatr Soc* 53:1937–1943, 2005.

64. Flinn DR, Diehl KM, Seyfried LS, Malani PN: Prevention, diagnosis, and management of postoperative delirium in older adults, *J Am Coll Surg* 209:261–268, 2009.

65. Florence CS, Bergen G, Atherly A, Burns E, Stevens J, Drake C: The medical costs of fatal falls and fall injuries among older adults, *Journal of American Geriatrics Society* 4(66):693–698, 2018.

66. Folstein MF, Folstein SE, McHugh PR: Mini-mental state: a practical method for grading the cognitive state of patients for the clinician, *J Psychiatr Res* 12:189–198, 1975.

67. Gallup Organization: Gallup study: engaged employees inspire company innovation, 2006. https://www.employment-studies.co.uk/system/files/resources/files/469.pdf.

68. Gatz M, Kasl-Godley J, Karel M: Aging and mental disorders. In Birren JE, Schaie KW, editors: *Handbook of the psychology of aging*, ed 4, San Diego, CA, 1996, Academic Press.

69. Ghisletta P, Bickel J, Lövdén M: Does activity engagement protect against cognitive decline in old age? Methodological and analytical considerations, *J Gerontol B Psychol Sci Soc Sci* 61:253–261, 2006.

70. Gill TM, Kurland BF: Prognostic effect of prior disability episodes among nondisabled community-living older persons, *Am J Epidemiol* 158:1090–1096, 2003.

71. Golisz K: Occupational therapy interventions to improve driving performance in older adults: a systematic review, *Arch Occup Ther* 68:662–669, 2014.

72. Gopinath B, et al: Olfactory impairment in older adults is associated with depressive symptoms and poorer quality of life scores, *Am J Geriatr Psychiatry* 19:830–834, 2011.

73. Goyer A: *The Metlife report on the oldest boomers: healthy, retiring rapidly and collecting social security Business Wire*, 2013, https://www.businesswire.com.

74. Gray JM: Putting occupation into practice: occupation as ends, occupation as means, *Arch Occup Ther* 52:354–364, 1988.

75. Gregory CJ, Sandmire DA: The physiology and pathology of aging. In Robnett RH, Chop W, editors: *Gerontology for the health care professional*, Burlington, MA, 2015, Jones & Bartlett Learning, pp 51–101.

76. He S, Craig BA, Xu H, et al: Unmet need for ADL assistance is associated with mortality among older adults with mild disability, *J Gerontol A Biol Sci Med Sci* 70:1128–1132, 2015.

77. HealthIT.gov (2020). What is telehealth? How is telehealth different from telemedicine? Retrieved from https://www.healthit.gov/faq/what-telehealth-how-telehealth-different-telemedicine.

78. HealthyPeople.gov: Healthy people 2020: older adults. http://www.healthypeople.gov/2020/topics-objectives/topic/older-adults.

79. Healthy People 2030: Older Adults (2020, September 26). Retrieved from https://health.gov/healthypeople/objectives-and-data/browse-objectives/older-adults.

80. Hemphill BJ: Depression among suicidal elderly: a life-threatening illness, *Occup Ther Pract* 4:61–66, 1992.

81. Henry J. Kaiser Family Foundation: Focus on health reform—summary of new health reform law (#8061). http://kff.org/health-reform/fact-sheet/summary-of-the-affordable-care-act/.

82. Heuberger R, Wong H: The association between depression and widowhood and nutritional status in older adults, *Geriatr Nurs* 35:428–433, 2014.

83. Hillman J: An introduction including media, boomer, and cross-cultural perspectives. In *Sexuality and aging: clinical perspectives, Reading*, PA, 2012, Springer, pp 1–27.

84. Hinchcliff S, Gott M: Challenging social myths and stereotypes of women and aging: heterosexual women talk about sex, *J Women Aging* 20:65–81, 2008.

85. Hooper CR, Bello-Haas VD: Sensory function. In Bonder BR, Bello-Haas VD, editors: *Functional performance in older adults*, ed 3, Philadelphia, 2009, FA Davis, pp 101–129.

86. Inouye SK, Fearing MA, Marcantonio ER: Delirium. In Halter JB, editor: *Hazzard's geriatric medicine and gerontology*, New York, 2009, McGraw-Hill.

87. Jackson J, Carlson M, Mandel D, Zemke R, Clark F: Occupation in lifestyle redesign: the Well Elderly Study Occupational Therapy Program, *Arch Occup Ther* 52:326–336, 1998.

88. Jacobs JM, Hammerman-Rozenberg R, Cohen A, Stessman J: Reading daily predicts reduced mortality among men from a cohort of community-dwelling 70-year-olds, *J Gerontol B Psychol Sci Soc Sci* 63:73–80, 2008.

89. Jacobs JM, Maaravi Y, Cohen A, et al: Changing profile of health and function from age 70 to 85 years, *Gerontology* 58:313–321, 2012.

90. Janke MC, Nimrod G, Kleiber DA: Leisure patterns and health among recently widowed adults, *Act Adapt Aging* 32:19–39, 2008.

91. Johnson D, Sandmire D: *Medical tests that can save your life: 21 tests your doctor won't order unless you know to ask*, New York, 2004, Rodale and St. Martin's Press.

92. Johnson JC: Depression and dementia in the elderly: a primary care perspective, *Compr Ther* 22:280–285, 1996.

93. Karpe JF, Reynolds CF 3rd, Butters MA, et al: The relationship between pain and mental flexibility in older adult pain clinic patients, *Pain Med* 7:444–452, 2006.

94. Kausler DH: *Learning and memory in normal aging*, San Diego, CA, 1994, Academic Press.

95. Keeler E, Guralnik JM, Tian H, et al: The impact of functional status on life expectancy in older persons, *J Gerontol A Biol Sci Med Sci* 65:727–733, 2010.

96. Keyser JJ, Kette AM, Haley SM: Development of the Home and Community Environment (HACE) instrument, *J Rehabil Med* 37:37, 2005.

97. Kim ES, Kawachi I, Chen Y, Kubzansky LD: Association between purpose in life and objective measures of physical function in older adults, *JAMA Psychiatry* 74:1039–1045, 2017.

98. Kirkwood TBL: Evolution of aging, *Nature* 270:30–304, 1977.

99. Kitzman DW, Taffet G: Effects of aging on cardiovascular structure and function. In McCance KL, Huether SE, Brashers VL, Rote NS, editors: *Pathophysiology: the biologic basis for disease in adults and children,* ed 6, Maryland Heights, MO, 2009, Mosby.

100. Knowles M: *The adult learner: a neglected species*, Houston, TX, 1984, Gulf Publishing.

101. Kontula O, Haavio-Mannila E: The impact of aging on human sexual activity and sexual desire, *J Sex Res* 46:46–56, 2009.

102. Kuchel GA, DuBeau CE: Chapter 30: Urinary incontinence in the elderly. https://www.asn-online.org/education/distancelearning/curricula/geriatrics/Chapter30.pdf.

103. Kutner M, Greenberg E, Jin Y, et al: Literacy in everyday life: results from the 2003 National Assessment on Adult Literacy. http://nces.ed.gov/Pubs2007/2007480_1.pdf.

104. Law M, Baptiste S, McColl M, et al: The Canadian occupational performance measure: an outcome measure for occupational therapy, *Can J Occup Ther* 57:82–87, 1990.

105. Leland NE, Marcione N, Schepens Niemiec SL, Kelkar K, Fogelberg D: What is occupational therapy's role in addressing sleep problems among older adults? *OTJR: Occupation, Participation, and Health* 34(3):141–149, 2014.

106. Lets L: Assessing safe function at home: the SAFER tool, *AOTA Home Community Health SIS Q* 2:1, 1995.

107. Levy L, editor: *Cognition and the aging adult,* ed 2, Bethesda, MD, 1996, American Occupational Therapy Association.

108. Levy L: Cognitive aging in perspective: implications for occupational therapy practitioners. In Katz N, editor: *Cognition & occupation across the life span: models for intervention in occupational therapy,* ed 2, Bethesda, MD, 2005, American Occupational Therapy Association.

109. Levy L: Cognitive aging in perspective: information processing, cognition and memory. In Katz N, editor: *Cognition & occupation across the life span: models for intervention in occupational therapy,* ed 2, Bethesda, MD, 2005, American Occupational Therapy Association.

110. Li T, Horton RM, Bader DA, Zhou M, Liang X, Ban J, Sun Q, Kinney PL: Aging will amplify the heat-related mortality risk under a changing climate: projection for the elderly in Beijing, China. *Scientific Reports* 6:28161, 2016. https://doi.org/10.1038/srep28161.

111. Loeser RF, Delbono O: Aging of the muscles and joints. In Halter JB, editor: *Hazzard's geriatric medicine and gerontology*, New York, 2009, McGraw-Hill.

112. LongTermCare.gov: Medicaid. https://www.medicaid.gov/medicaid/long-term-services-supports.

113. Lotery AJ, Wiggam MI, Jackson AJ, et al: Correctable visual impairments in stroke rehabilitation patients, *Age Ageing* 29: 221–222, 2000.

114. Matuska K, Giles-Heinz A, Flinn N, et al: Outcomes of a pilot occupational therapy wellness program for older adults, *Am J Occup Ther* 57:220–224, 2003.

115. Mayo Clinic: Hemodialysis: risks. http://www.mayoclinic.org/tests-procedures/hemodialysis/basics/risks/prc-20015015.

116. McNulty MC, Johnson J, Poole JL, Winkle M: Using the transtheoretical model of change to implement home safety modifications with community-dwelling older adults: an exploratory study, *Phys Occup Ther Geriatr* 21:53–66, 2003.

117. Mian OS, Baltzopoulos V, Minetti AE, Narici MV: The impact of physical training on locomotor function in older people, *Sports Med* 37:683–701, 2007.

118. Miller B: Theories of aging. In Lewis CB, editor: *Aging: the health care manager*, ed 4, Philadelphia, 2002, FA Davis.

119. Missildine K, Bergstrom N, Meininger J, Richards K, Foreman MD: Sleep in hospitalized elders: a pilot study, *Geriatr Nurs* 31:263–271, 2010.

120. Murphy C, Shubert CR, Cruickshanks KJ, et al: Prevalence of olfactory impairment in older adults, *JAMA* 288:2307–2312, 2002.

121. Musich S, Wang SS, Slindee L, Kraemer S, Yeh CS: Prevalence and characteristics associated with high dose opioid users among older adults, *Geriatric Nursing* 40:31–36, 2018.

122. Myers M, Parchen D, Geraci M, et al: Using a shared governance structure to evaluate the implementation of a new model of care: the shared experience of a performance improvement committee, *J Nurs Adm* 43:509–516, 2013.

123. Nasreddine ZS, Phillips NA, Bédirian V, et al: The Montreal Cognitive Assessment, MoCA: a brief screening tool for mild cognitive impairment, *J Am Geriatr Soc* 53:695–699, 2005.

124. National Alliance for Caregiving: Caregiving in the U.S. https://www.caregiving.org/wp-content/uploads/2020/06/AARP1316_RPT_CaregivingintheUS_WEB.pdf.

125. National Center on Elder Abuse: Frequently asked questions. https://ncea.acl.gov/home#gsc.tab=0.

126. National Conference of State Legislatures and the American Association of Retired Persons: Aging in place: a state survey of livability policies and practices. http://assets.aarp.org/rgcenter/ppi/liv-com/ib190.pdf.

127. National Council on Disability: Transportation update: where we've gone and what we've learned. https://www.bts.gov/archive/publications/special_reports_and_issue_briefs/issue_briefs/number_03/entire.

128. National Highway Traffic Safety Administration: Older driver program: five-year strategic plan 2012–2017 (Publication No. DOT HS 811 432). https://www.nhtsa.gov/document/older-driver-program-five-year-strategic-plan-2012-2017.

129. National Institute of Health: Depression. http://www.nimh.nih.gov/health/topics/depression/index.shtml.

130. National Institute on Aging: Health and aging: can we prevent aging? https://www.nia.nih.gov/health/publication/can-we-prevent-aging.

131. National Kidney Foundation: Dialysis. https://www.kidney.org/atoz/content/dialysisinfo.

132. National Sleep Foundation: How much sleep do we really need? http://sleepfoundation.org/how-sleep-works/how-much-sleep-do-we-really-need.

133. National Sleep Foundation: Insomnia. Retrieved from https://www.sleepfoundation.org/insomnia.

134. Nguyen V: *Long-term support and services*, Washington, D.C., 2017, AARP Public Policy Institute. Retrieved from https://www.aarp.org/content/dam/aarp/ppi/2017-01/Fact%20Sheet%20Long-Term%20Support%20and%20Services.pdf.

135. Orellano E, Colon WI, Arbesman M: Effect of occupation- and activity-based interventions on instrumental activities of daily living performance among community-dwelling older adults: a systematic review, *Am J Occup Ther* 66:292–300, 2012.

136. Peloquin SM: Occupational therapy service: individual and collective understanding of the founders: part 1, *Am J Occup Ther* 45:352–360, 1991.

137. Perlmutter MS, Bhorade A, Gordon M, et al: Cognitive, visual, auditory, and emotional factors that affect participation in older adults, *Am J Occup Ther* 64:570, 2010.

138. Petersen RC, Smith GE, Waring SC, et al: Mild cognitive impairment: clinical characterization and outcome, *Arch Neurol* 56:303–308, 1999.

139. Pitt-Catsouphes M, James JB, Matz-Costa C: Workplace-based health and wellness programs: the intersection of aging, work, and health, *Gerontologist* 55:262–270, 2015.

140. Raia P: Habilitation therapy: a new starscape. In Volicer L, Bloom-Charette L, editors: *Enhancing the quality of life in advanced dementia*, London, 1999, Churchill Livingstone, pp 61–75.

141. Reisberg B, Ferris SH: Brief cognitive rating scale, *Psychopharmacol Bull* 24:629–636, 1988.

142. Reisberg B, Ferris SH, de Leon MJ, Crook T: The global deterioration scale for assessment of primary degenerative dementia, *Am J Psychiatry* 139:1136–1139, 1982.

143. Resnik C, Allen S, Isenstadt D, et al: Perspectives on use of mobility aids in a diverse population of seniors: implications for intervention, *Disabil Health J* 2:77–85, 2009.

144. Riffin C, Van Ness PH, Wolff JL, Fried T: Family and other unpaid caregivers and older adults with and without dementia and disability, *Journal of the American Geriatric Society* 65: 1821–1828, 2017.

145. Riley KP: Depression. In Bonder B, Bello-Haas VD, editors: *Functional performance in older adults*, ed 3, Philadelphia, 2009, FA Davis.

146. Robert Wood Johnson Foundation: The Green House® Project. https://thegreenhouseproject.org/.

147. Roberts AW, Ogunwole SU, Blakeslee L, Rabe MA. (2018). The population 65 years and older in the United States: 2016. *American Community Survey Reports*. https://www.census.gov/content/dam/Census/library/publications/2018/acs/ACS-38.pdf.

148. Robnett RH, Bolduc JJ: The cognitive and psychological changes associated with aging. In Robnett RH, Chop W, editors: *Gerontology for the health care professional*, Burlington, MA, 2015, Jones & Bartlett Learning, pp 103–145.

149. Robnett RH, O'Sullivan A: Living options and the continuum of care. In Robnett RH, Chop W, editors: *Gerontology for the health care professional*, Burlington, MA, 2015, Jones & Bartlett Learning, pp 259–291.

150. Robnett RH, Bolduc JJ, Murray J: Functional performance in later life: basic sensory, perceptual, and physical changes associated with aging. In Robnett RH, Chop W, editors:

Gerontology for the health care professional, Burlington, MA, 2015, Jones & Bartlett Learning, pp 147–170.

151. Rogers AT, Bai Ge, Lavin RA, Anderson GF: Higher hospital spending on occupational therapy is associated with lower readmission rates, *Medical Care Research and Review* 74(6): 668–686, 2017.

152. Romig K, Sherman A. (2016). Social security keeps 22 million Americans out of poverty: A state by state analysis. *Center on Budget and Policy Priorities*. Retrieved from https://www.cbpp.org/research/social-security/social-security-keeps-22-million-americans-out-of-poverty-a-state-by-state.

153. Rosenbloom R: Meeting transportation needs in an aging-friendly community, *J Am Soc Aging* 33:33–43, 2009.

154. Rozario PA: Volunteering among current cohorts of older adults and baby boomers, *Generations* 30:31–36, 2007.

155. Rutherford BR, Brewster K, Golub JS, Kim AH, Roose SP: Sensation and psychiatry: Linking age-related hearing loss to late-life depression and cognitive decline, *The American Journal of Psychiatry* 175(3):215–224, 2018.

156. Saxon SV, Etten MJ, Perkins EA: *Physical change and aging: a guide for the helping professions*, New York, 2010, Springer.

157. Scarmeas N, et al: Influence of leisure activity on the incidence of Alzheimer's disease, *Neurology* 57:2236–2242, 2001.

158. Scheiman M, Scheiman M, Whittaker SG: *Low vision rehabilitation: a practical guide for occupational therapists*, Thorofare, NJ, 2007, Slack.

159. Schoene D, Heller C, Aung YN, Sieber CC, Kemmler W, Freiberger E: A systematic review on the influence of fear of falling on quality of life in older people: Is there a role for falls? *Clinical Interventions in Aging* 14:701–719, 2019.

160. Smith A, editor: *Memory*, San Diego, CA, 1996, Academic Press.

161. Smallfield S, Molitor WL: Occupational therapy interventions supporting social participation and leisure engagement for community-dwelling older adults: a systematic review, *American Journal of Occupational Therapy* 72:7204190020, 2018. https://doi.org/10.5014/ajot.2018.030627.

162. Smallfield S, Elliott S, Leland NE: *Occupational therapy practice guidelines for productive aging for community-dwelling older adults*, Bethesda, MD, 2019, American Occupational Therapy Association.

163. Social Security Administration: Benefits. http://www.ssa.gov/.

164. Social Security Administration: Medicare. http://www.ssa.gov/pubs/EN-05-10043.pdf.

165. Spillman BC: Changes in elderly disability rates and the implications for health care utilization and cost, *Milbank Q* 82:157–194, 2004.

166. Stableford S: Health literacy and clear health communication: teaching and writing so older adults understand. In Robnett RH, Chop W, editors: *Gerontology for the health care professional*, Burlington, MA, 2015, Jones & Bartlett Learning, pp 323–336.

167. Stark S, Somerville EK, Morris JC: In-home occupational performance evaluation (I-HOPE), *Am J Occup Ther* 64:580, 2010.

168. Stav WB, Hallenen T, Lane J, Arbesman M: Systematic review of occupational engagement and health outcomes among community-dwelling older adults, *Am J Occup Ther* 66:301–310, 2012.

169. Stenner, BJ, Buckley, JD, Mosewich, AD: Reasons why older adults play sport: a systematic review, *J Sport Health Sci* 9(6):530–541, 2020.

170. Substance Abuse and Mental Health Administration: Increasing substance abuse levels among older adults likely to create sharp rise in need for treatment services in next decade, 2010. https://www.samhsa.gov.

171. Sugerman RA: Structure and function of the neurologic system. In McCance KL, Huether SE, Brashers VL, Rote NS, editors: et al, editors: Pathophysiology: the biologic basis for disease in adults and children, ed 6, Maryland Heights, MO, 2009, Mosby.

172. Szanton SL, Leff B, Wolff JL, Roberts L, Gitlin LN: Home-based care program reduces disability and promotes aging in place, *Health Affairs* 35(9):1558–1563, 2016.

173. Szanton SL, Thorpe RJ, Boyd C, Tanner EK, Leff B, Agree E, Xue Q, Allen JK, Seplaki CL, Weiss CO, Guralnik JM, Gitlin LN: Community Aging in Place, Advancing Better Living for Elders (CAPABLE): A bio-behavioral-environmental intervention to improve function and health-related quality of life in disabled, older adults, *Journal of American Geriatrics Society* 59(12): 2314–2320, 2011.

174. Szilard L: On the nature of the aging process, *Proc Natl Acad Sci U S A* 45:30–45, 1959.

175. Tabert MH, Albert SM, Borukhova-Milov L, Camacho Y, et al: Functional deficits in patients with mild cognitive impairment: prediction of AD, *Neurology* 58:758–764, 2002.

176. Tariq SH, Tumosa N, Chibnall JT, et al: Comparison of the Saint Louis University Mental Status Examination and the Mini-Mental State Examination for detecting dementia and mild neurocognitive disorder: a pilot study, *Am J Geriatr Psychiatry* 14:900–910, 2006.

177. Taylor B, Davis S: The extended PLISSIT model for addressing the sexual wellbeing of individuals with an acquired disability or chronic illness, *Sex Disabil* 25:135–139, 2007.

178. Teng E, Becker BW, Woo E, et al: Utility of the Functional Activities Questionnaire for distinguishing mild cognitive impairment from very mild Alzheimer's disease, *Alzheimer Dis Assoc Disord* 24:348–353, 2010.

179. Thompson KH: Nutrition and aging. In Robnett RH, Chop W, editors: *Gerontology for the health care professional*, Burlington, MA, 2015, Jones & Bartlett Learning, pp 191–211.

180. Tideiksaar R: Falls. In Bonder BR, editor: *Functional performance in older adults*, Philadelphia, 2009, FA Davis, pp 193–214.

181. Trauer JM, Qian MY, Doyle JS, Rajaratnam SM, Cunnington D: Cognitive behavioral therapy for chronic insomnia: a systematic review and meta-analysis, *Annals of Internal Medicine* 163(3):191–204, 2015.

182. United States Bureau of Labor Statistics (2020). Labor force statistics from the current population survey: Supplemental data measuring the effects of the coronavirus (COVID-19) pandemic on the labor market. Retrieved from https://www.bls.gov/cps/effects-of-the-coronavirus-covid-19-pandemic.htm.

183. United States Census Bureau: Facts for features: older Americans month: May 2014. http://www.census.gov/newsroom/facts-for-features/2014/cb14-ff07.html.

184. United States Census Bureau: Grandparents and grandchildren. 2016, https://www.census.gov/newsroom/blogs/random-samplings/2016/09/grandparents-and-grandchildren.html.

185. United States Census Bureau (2020). Life expectancy. https://www.cdc.gov/nchs/fastats/life-expectancy.htm.

186. U.S. Department of Health and Human Services: Key features of the Affordable Care Act, by Year. http://www.hhs.gov/healthcare/facts/timeline/timeline-text.html.

187. U.S. National Library of Medicine: Aging changes in the kidneys and bladder. https://www.nlm.nih.gov/medlineplus/ency/article/004010.htm.

188. U.S. National Library of Medicine: Aging changes in the male reproductive system. https://www.nlm.nih.gov/medlineplus/ency/article/004017.htm.

189. U.S. World and News Report. Telehealth skyrocketing among older adults. Retrieved from https://www.usnews.com/news/health-news/articles/2020-08-20/telehealth-skyrocketing-among-older-adults.

190. Vasilevskis EE, Han JH, Hughes CG, Fly EW, et al: Epidemiology and risk factors for delirium across hospital settings, *Best Pract Res Clin Anaesthesiol* 26:277–287, 2012.

191. Verghese J, Lipton RB, Katz MJ, et al: Leisure activities and the risk of dementia in the elderly, *N Engl J Med* 348:2508–2516, 2003.

192. Village to Village Network: About VtV Network. http://www.vtvnetwork.org/content.aspx?page_id=22andclub_id=691012andmodule_id=65139.

193. Waldman-Levi A, Bar-Haim AE, Katz N: Healthy aging is reflected in well-being, participation, playfulness, and cognitive-emotional functioning, *Healthy Aging Research* 4:1–7, 2015. https://doi.org/10.12715/har.2015.4.8.

194. Warburton J, Terry D, Rosenman L, Shapira M: Difference between older volunteers and nonvolunteers: attitudinal, normative, and control beliefs, *Res Aging* 23:586–605, 2001.

195. Warren M: Pilot study on activities of daily living limitations in adults with hemianopsia, *Am J Occup Ther* 63:626, 2009.

196. Watson GR: Low vision in the geriatric population: rehabilitation and management, *J Am Geriatr Soc* 49:317–330, 2001.

197. Weaver RH: Reframing aging issues to ensure a better future. In Robnett RH, Brossoie N, Chop WC, editors: *Gerontology for the health care professional*, Burlington, MA, 2019, Jones & Bartlett Learning, pp 345–372.

198. Weiner DK, Rudy TE, Morrow L, Slaboda J, Lieber S: The relationship between pain, neuropsychological performance, and physical function in community-dwelling older adults with chronic low back pain, *Pain Med* 7:60–70, 2006.

199. Weiss B: *Health literacy and patient safety: help patients understand: a manual for clinicians*, ed 2, Chicago, 2007, American Medical Association.

200. Werner CA: *The older population: 2010. 2010 census briefs*, Washington, DC, 2011, U.S. Census Bureau. https://www.census.gov.

201. Wilcock A: Population health: an occupational rational. In Scaffa ME, Reitz MA, Pizzi M, editors: *Occupational therapy in the promotion of health and wellness*, Philadelphia, 2015, FA Davis.

202. Wong CM, Ettlinger M, Sheppard JP, et al: Neuroanatomical characteristics and speech perception in older adults, *Ear Hear* 31:471–479, 2010.

203. Yaffe K, Blackwell T, Gore R, et al: Depressive symptoms and cognitive decline in nondemented elderly women: a prospective study, *Arch Gen Psychiatry* 56:425–430, 1999.

204. Yesavage JA, Brink TL, Rose TL, et al: Development and validation of a geriatric depression screening scale: a preliminary report, *J Psychiatr Res* 17:37–49, 1983.

205. Yu RP: Use of messaging apps and social network sites among older adults: a mixed-method study, *International Journal of Communication* 14:4453–4473, 2020.

48

HIV Infection and AIDS

Michael A. Pizzi and Graham Teaford

LEARNING OBJECTIVES

After studying this chapter, the student or practitioner will be able to do the following:

1. Understand the stages of HIV and AIDS.
2. Describe the impact of medical interventions on HIV.
3. Describe how to assess a person with HIV or AIDS holistically.
4. Identify occupational therapy interventions directed toward optimizing health as an occupational participation.
5. Understand the importance of a health promotion and prevention perspective in occupational therapy services for people with HIV and AIDS.

CHAPTER OUTLINE

KEY TERMS

AIDS-dementia complex
Antiretroviral therapy
HIV infection

Opportunistic infection
Retrovirus
Seroconversion

THREADED CASE STUDY

Billy, Part 1

Billy is a lawyer and internal medicine physician (prefers use of the pronouns he/his/him). Billy is living with Tom, his partner of 15 years. He has lived for more than 20 years with a diagnosis of HIV infection, and the mode of infection for Billy is unknown. Billy has been practicing medicine successfully, as well as doing pro bono work as a legal advocate for people diagnosed with HIV and with AIDS. He began highly active antiretroviral therapy approximately 15 years earlier. His CD4+ count has remained above 500, and he has not had any opportunistic infections. He continues to be active in his career as a physician and with his pro bono legal work.

He has recently noticed that he has more difficulty with his memory, decreased fine motor coordination, difficulty coordinating his movements, burning sensations in his hands and feet, and lower extremity weakness. These changes have had an impact on his life in a variety of ways, such as difficulty remembering his appointments, taking his medications as scheduled, writing, and awakening at night because of pain.

During the course of developing an occupational profile, he stated that his primary concerns involve how these changes have affected his professional activities. He values his roles as both physician and attorney, as well as his paid employment and his pro bono work. His work has been affected by his diminished writing skills (requiring more time and effort to write legibly) and his pain (limiting his rest and causing him to have difficulty concentrating on work tasks). However, he is most concerned with his changes in memory because it has caused him to forget appointments and miss deadlines, has compromised the quality of his work, and has placed his professional competence and identity at risk. This deficit became his greatest concern because of his pride in having what he calls a "mind like a steel trap." As a health professional, Billy possesses the knowledge required to care for his own health and well-being; however, he does not apply this knowledge to his own daily life. His partner, though supportive, is becoming increasingly angry, irritable, and concerned, and these emotions appear to have impaired his own occupational performance in work, home, and leisure occupations.

ORIGINS AND CURRENT STATUS OF HIV INFECTION

An estimated 37.7 million people globally are infected with human immunodeficiency virus (HIV) or have acquired immunodeficiency syndrome (AIDS), with an estimated 34% of infected persons aware of their HIV status.[53] In 2020, approximately 1.2 million people died of HIV/AIDS, and an estimated 1.5 million persons were newly infected with HIV. An estimated 36.3 million people have died of HIV/AIDS since the virus was first detected.

HIV originated in Africa and has likely been present in humans since the late 19th century.[19] The virus has been present in the United States since the 1970s, possibly decades earlier, and has since spread globally.[26]

AIDS was first clinically identified in the United States in 1981.[7] These initial cases of AIDS in the United States were concentrated in men having sex with men, injection drug users, and persons receiving contaminated blood supplies (from transfusions or clotting factor for persons with hemophilia). By 1983, HIV, the virus that causes AIDS, was identified.[18] It soon became apparent that HIV is spread by contact with specific body fluids (including blood products, semen, and vaginal fluids). The eventual discovery of HIV as a virus made it apparent that AIDS does not discriminate among sex assigned at birth (Table 48.1 and Fig. 48.1), race or ethnicity (Tables 48.2, 48.3, and 48.5), culture, sexual orientation (see Table 48.1), or age (Table 48.4). HIV affects all of humanity. It affects not only the people infected with the virus but also their parents, siblings, friends, lovers, children, and co-workers. After a person's diagnosis of being HIV positive has been confirmed, the person can become immobilized and drastically alter his or her occupational performance and participation in society, or the person can treat the diagnosis as an impetus to act in positive, life-transforming ways.

The majority of global HIV cases are caused by exposure to HIV type 1 (HIV-1), with HIV type 2 (HIV-2) being much less common and primarily found in western Africa. The global patterns of the HIV epidemic are complex and vary greatly by region and within different regions. The 2021 UNAIDS Global AIDS Update[54] identifies a number of trends:

- Global inequalities continue to be a factor in infection prevention and access to treatment for HIV. It is unclear how the long-term effects of COVID-19 will affect persons with HIV, but the majority of persons living with HIV reside in lower income and lower-middle income status nations.[32] These nations have had much more limited access to vaccines for SARS-CoV-2. Preliminary evidence suggests the persons infected with HIV are at greater risk of severe COVID-19 and death than persons not infected with HIV.
- Tremendous progress has been made in saving lives of persons infected with HIV due, in large part, to increasing access to antiviral medications. There has been a 47% decline in AIDS-related mortality, and an estimated 16.6 million deaths have been averted during the past decade.
- Despite the progress made during the past decade, the targets for testing and treatment were not met. The goal has been to reach 90-90-90 (90% of people living with HIV: knowing their status, on treatment, and virally suppressed). An estimated 10.2 million people globally were not on HIV treatment (4.1 million of whom did not know their status and 6.1 million of whom knew their status but could not access treatment).
- In addition, efforts to prevent new HIV infections have fallen short of goals with no significant progress during the past 4 years and only a 31% decline in new infections since 2010.
- The estimated annual number of new HIV infections globally declined to 1.5 million in 2020 from 2.3 million in 2012 and 3.4 million in 2001.
- There were an estimated 680,000 AIDS-related deaths in 2020. A decline from 1.6 million annual deaths in in 2012 and 2.3 million deaths in 2005.
- Inequalities and resource limitations remain barriers to HIV prevention and treatment. These inequalities are found

TABLE 48.1   Distribution of New HIV Diagnoses in 2019

Exposure Category	Male	Female	Total
Gay and bisexual men	25,552	—	25,552
Transgender people	46 (FTM)	625 (MTF)	671
People who inject drugs	1397	1111	2508
Heterosexual contact	2754	5863	8617

In 2019, 36,801 people were diagnosed with HIV infection in the United States. The number of new HIV diagnoses between 2015 and 2019 fell by 9% in the United States and dependent areas. Because HIV testing has remained stable or increased in recent years, this decrease in diagnoses suggests a true decline in new infections. The decrease may be due to targeted HIV prevention efforts. However, progress has been uneven, and diagnoses have increased among a few groups.
From Centers for Disease Control and Prevention. HIV Surveillance Report, 2019; http://www.cdc.gov/hiv/library/reports/hiv-surveillance.html, 2021; and https://www.cdc.gov/hiv/statistics/overview/ataglance.html.

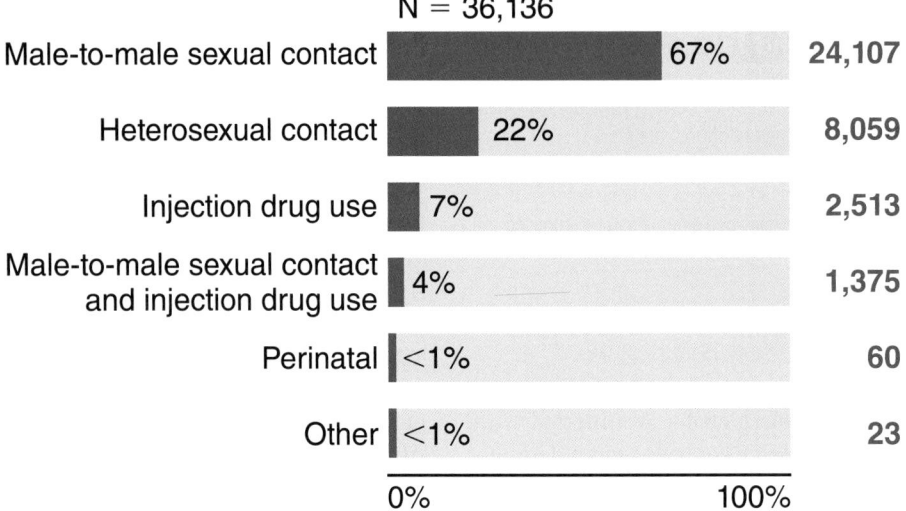

Fig. 48.1 Differences in new HIV diagnoses among people age 13 years and older by transmission category. Transmission category is classified based on a hierarchy of risk factors most likely responsible for HIV transmission. Classification is determined based on the person's assigned sex at birth. Data have been statistically adjusted to account for missing transmission category. (Source: CDC. Diagnoses of HIV Infection in the United States and Dependent Areas, 2021. *HIV Surveillance Report* 34, 2023. https://www.cdc.gov/hiv/library/reports/hiv-surveillance/vol-34/index.html.)

TABLE 48.2 Percentages of Adults and Adolescents Living With Diagnosed HIV Infection, by Sex at Birth and Race/Ethnicity, Year-End 2019—United States and 6 Dependent Areas

In 2019, the percentages of persons living with HIV infection in the United States was as follows:

Race or Ethnicity	Male Percentage (N = 811,640)	Female Percentage (N = 248,144)
American Indian/Alaska Native	<1	<1
Asian	2	1
Black/African American	35	57
Hispanic/Latino*	26	21
Native Hawaiian/Other Pacific Islander	<1	<1
White	32	16
Multiracial†	5	5

*Hispanics/Latinos can be of any race.
†Includes Asian/Pacific Islander legacy cases.
Data from https://www.cdc.gov/hiv/library/reports/hiv-surveillance/vol-32/content/national-profile.html#Prevalence.
For more details on HIV infection and race/ethnicity, see CDC's Populations and Surveillance fact sheets.

TABLE 48.3 New HIV Diagnoses by Race/Ethnicity

Race/Ethnicity	Number of Cases	By Percentage
Black/African American*	15,340	42
Hispanic/Latino†	10,502	29
White	9,018	25
Multiracial	918	2
Asian	743	2
American Indian/Alaska Native	210	1
Native Hawaiian and other Pacific Islander	70	<1

*Black refers to people having origins in any of the Black racial groups of Africa. *African America*n is a term used for people of African descent with ancestry in North America.
†Hispanics/Latinos can be of any race.
Data from https://www.cdc.gov/hiv/images/statistics/overview/ataglance/2021/cdc-hiv-stats-us-race-ethnicity-1200x630.png.

across countries but also within countries. In particular, poverty and lack of schooling are barriers within countries.

- In the United States, HIV burden is disproportionately higher among Black Americans and Hispanic/Latinos. These groups have disparities in outcomes and a host of barriers to access of services.
- People between 13 and 34 years of age accounted for more than half (57%) of the new HIV diagnoses in 2020.[19]
- Key risk populations include gay men and other men who have sex with men (25 times greater risk than heterosexual men), female sex workers (26 times greater risk than women in the general population), transgender women (34 times greater risk than other adults), people who inject drugs (35 times greater risk than those who do not inject drugs).

TABLE 48.4 AIDS Information Tracked by CDC on Various Racial and Ethnic Groups*

In 2015, the number of persons in the United States with diagnosed HIV infection classified as stage 3 (AIDS), by race/ethnicity, was as follows:

American Indian/Alaska Native	96	3,543
Asian†	325	9,932
Black/African American	8,702	506,163
Hispanic/Latino‡	3,870	222,227
Native Hawaiian/Other Pacific Islander	22	845
White	4,668	439,207
Multiple Races	620	35,000

*From the beginning of the epidemic through 2015.
†Includes Asian/Pacific Islander legacy cases.
‡Hispanics/Latinos can be of any race.
For more details on AIDS and race/ethnicity, see CDC's fact sheets.

TABLE 48.5 New HIV Diagnoses by Age

Age in Years	Number of Cases in 2019
13–24	7,648
25–34	13,127
35–44	7,147
45–54	4,931
55 and older	3,887

Data from Centers for Disease Control and Prevention, https://www.cdc.gov/hiv/images/statistics/overview/ataglance/2021/cdc-hiv-stats-us-age-1200x630.png.

- Criminalization of key populations has slowed response to HIV prevention and services. Key populations have seen criminalization for gender identities and expression, sexual orientation, and their livelihood.
- Women, men, and young people face different challenges.
- Discrimination against persons with HIV remains a barrier to treatment and prevention efforts.

Currently, an estimated 1.2 million persons in the United States have diagnosed or undiagnosed HIV/AIDS.[14] As of 2012, 12.8% of persons infected with HIV in the United States are unaware of their HIV-positive status.[20] According to estimates from the Centers for Disease Control and Prevention (CDC), more than 50,000 new cases of HIV infection occur in the United States each year. The number of new infections per year (incidence rate) has remained relatively stable. However, the number of persons living with HIV (prevalence rate) has continued to grow as mortality rates from HIV have decreased, in large measure as a result of available and effective antiviral medications.[13] The demographic trends in the United States have changed since the earliest years of the pandemic.

Although overall rates of new infections have been relatively stable in the United States, certain groups are at greater risk for HIV infection and bear a disproportionate burden of HIV.

Among ethnic groups, African Americans are the most disproportionately affected population in the United States. African Americans represent approximately 13% of the U.S. population but account for 42% of HIV infections and have lower viral suppression rates than the general population.[16]

Hispanics/Latinos are also disproportionately affected by HIV in the United States. In 2020, Hispanic/Latinos accounted for 27% of new HIV infections.[17] They also have lower rates of viral suppression than the general population.

The earliest cases of HIV infection in the United States, though having a broad impact on society, were concentrated in White males.[7] In contrast, current infection patterns in the United States demonstrate changes in the groups currently at risk, as well as underscore the fact that HIV infection is not a concern of only one ethnic group.[19]

Although male-to-male sexual contact remains the most common means of transmission of new infections, heterosexual contact accounts for nearly a quarter of all new HIV infections.

The course of the HIV pandemic has changed significantly with the advent of effective medical treatments. For persons with access to effective medications, management of HIV has, to some extent, changed the focus of medical management to the chronic medical needs of persons with HIV infection rather than more acute management of opportunistic infections. In the earliest years of the pandemic, before effective pharmaceutical treatment, death typically occurred within 10 years of HIV infection and 1 to 2 years after the onset of AIDS.[6] Mortality rates and the frequency of opportunistic infections have decreased significantly. However, this also presents public health concerns. The health delivery model in the United States is not always effective in addressing the increasingly chronic needs of persons infected with HIV rather than the more acute cases that were more common in the earlier years of the pandemic.[11] Occupational therapy (OT) practitioners can potentially play a significant role in the promotion of health and management of chronic medical needs to ensure that persons remain active participants in meaningful occupations.

INFECTION PROCESS

HIV is the virus that causes AIDS[18] and belongs to a class of viruses known as retroviruses. Retroviruses share a unique process of replication characterized by the viral genetic material being encoded by RNA rather than DNA. Retroviruses, including HIV, replicate as viral RNA is transcribed into DNA in the host cell. The cellular process is complex, with many components and processes occurring. The following is a simplified description of the infection process.

The process begins as the virus binds to a cell surface receptor.[38] During the attachment phase, HIV binds with the surface protein receptors on the cell membrane. The receptors operate in a lock-and-key fashion, with CD4 being the primary receptor for HIV (although other receptors and processes are also critical in the process of HIV cellular infection). The initial binding with surface receptors is a necessary stage for cellular infection.

Once the initial binding to cell receptors is completed, the virus passes through the cellular membrane and enters the cytoplasm. On entering the cytoplasm, the retrovirus uses an enzyme called reverse transcriptase to synthesize a proviral DNA copy from the viral RNA template (a process referred to as reverse transcription). During this process, the transcriptase reads the RNA material as it is converted to DNA that can be integrated into the host cells' genetic material. However, errors are frequently made in the replication process. As a result, not all copies of HIV DNA are identical. The modifications or mutations during this process contribute to the resistance of the virus to the body's immune system and to certain antiviral treatments.

The completed proviral DNA migrates to the nucleus of the host cell and is inserted into or integrates with the host cell DNA. Once this integration occurs, the integrated viral DNA (or provirus) is replicated along with normal cellular genes as part of the routine cellular division process. Virions containing HIV RNA and HIV proteins are assembled within the host cell body, and an enzyme called protease is required at this phase to divide the polypeptide chain into discrete functional enzymes. The completed HIV virions (containing HIV, RNA, and HIV proteins or enzymes) are released from the host cell membrane in a process referred to as budding. Once the virions are released and the transcriptase has completed division of the proteins, the mature virus is capable of infecting additional cells. The newly created mature virus resembles the original virus but may also have undergone some variation during the replication process, thus complicating medical treatment.

TRANSMISSION

HIV is transmitted through exchange of certain body fluids (blood, semen, preseminal fluid, rectal fluid, vaginal fluid, and breast milk) from a person with HIV. Sexual behaviors and injection drug use are the most common means of transmission for new infections.[21] Less common means of transmission include mother to child during pregnancy, birth, or breastfeeding, and accidental exposure to infected needles (primarily occupational exposure). HIV is not transmitted through casual (nonsexual) contact with persons.[6]

In the early years of the AIDS pandemic, many people were infected with HIV because of contamination of the blood supply (primarily through transfusions or clotting factor given to persons with hemophilia). However, the blood supply is tested for HIV in the United States.[15] The risk of contracting HIV via blood products, transfusions, or organ/tissue transplants is very low.

The risk of infection to healthcare providers is also very low.[21] The risk for HIV infection following a needle stick is 0.3%, and the risk for infection after exposure of infected blood to the eyes, nose, or mouth is 0.1%.[9] The risk with exposure of nonintact skin to infected blood is less than 0.1%, and exposure of infected blood to intact skin probably poses no risk at all. It is important to remember that healthcare workers, or any other persons, are not at risk for HIV infection through casual, everyday contact with persons infected with HIV. The CDC recommends that healthcare workers practice universal precautions.

Universal precautions in the workplace include assuming that blood and body fluids from all clients are potentially infectious.[12] Healthcare workers should take certain precautions when working with all clients. Such precautions include the routine use of barriers (such as gloves) when anticipating contact with blood or body fluids. Workers should also wash hands and other skin surfaces immediately after contact with blood and body fluids. Finally, although the risk for HIV infection from an accidental needle stick is very low, this route of transmission constitutes the most likely risk for infection in healthcare workers. Workers should practice careful handling and disposal of any needles or potentially infectious sharp objects.

DIAGNOSIS

HIV may be detected by using a variety of tests.[6] In general, three broad categories of tests are available: antibody tests, combination tests, and nucleic acid tests (NATs).[20] Antibody tests detect the presence of HIV antibodies following the initial HIV infection. It is important to note that during the process of seroconversion (the immune response producing detectable antibodies), the person may be infected but not have a positive antibody test result. The process of seroconversion (producing a positive antibody detection test result) may take up to 2 months after the initial infection, and the infected person is capable of transmitting HIV during this time. It is recommended that antibody tests be repeated 3 months after exposure if the initial test failed to detect antibodies. Combination tests detect both the antigen and HIV antibodies. NATs detect the virus itself in the blood rather than the presence of antibodies. It is expensive and is not typically used for standard screening purposes.

HIV infection can be categorized along a continuum ranging from asymptomatic persons with high CD4+ counts to persons with clinical AIDS (representing the most advanced and serious stage of HIV infection). In 1993, the CDC revised the categories that determine HIV or AIDS status.[8] They include the following:

- *Category 1 (C1):* counts of 500 or more CD4+ cells per microliter of blood
- *Category 2 (C2):* counts from 200 to 499 CD4+ cells
- *Category 3 (C3):* counts below 200 CD4+ cells

The second set of categories relates to the expression of HIV from a clinical perspective:

- *Category A:* individuals who have been asymptomatic except for persistent, generalized lymphadenopathy seroconversion syndrome. This includes the initial acute onset of HIV exposure.
- *Category B:* individuals who have never had an AIDS-defining illness but have had some symptoms of HIV infection, such as candidiasis, fever, persistent diarrhea, oral hairy leukoplakia, herpes zoster, idiopathic thrombocytopenic purpura, peripheral neuropathy, cervical dysplasia, or pelvic inflammatory disease.
- *Category C:* individuals who have or have had one or more of the AIDS-defining illnesses.

In 2021 the National Institutes of Health (NIH) identified three stages of HIV infection.[38] The acute infection stage develops within 2 to 4 weeks after infection with HIV. The second stage is chronic HIV infection (sometimes called the asymptomatic stage), and the final stage is AIDS.

THREADED CASE STUDY

Billy, Part 2

Billy appears to have more mental health issues surrounding his illness than physical concerns at this time. He does experience fatigue and slight memory problems. The occupational therapist may ask the following questions:

1. Is the fatigue experienced related to the medical condition or the mental health issues that Billy is experiencing?
   - In this case, the fatigue that Billy reports could certainly be related to both physical and mental health issues. He could be experiencing **AIDS-dementia complex** (ADC), which is manifested, in the context of occupational performance, as altered cognitive processing and impaired memory. ADC appears to be related to the destruction of subcortical structures in the central nervous system (CNS) and is estimated to be present in more than half of individuals in whom AIDS is diagnosed. A peripheral neuropathy also may be developing, among other conditions. Having an awareness of these disease processes could lead to increased anxiety, fear, and possibly depression, especially with regard to the impact on his worker role. Billy should be encouraged to discuss these fears in the context of his daily living occupational performance.
   - Billy's ability to use effective habits and routines in the workplace might reduce his anxiety about his diminished memory. Devices such as electronic organizers and calendars may be helpful to Billy as memory aids. A conversation about these issues would involve Billy's knowledge of his life situation, thus making the OT sessions very client centered.
2. If Billy is preoccupied with his change in health status, how does he function in his work, home, community, and other contexts?
   - Using specifically guided questions, the therapist might examine the contexts in which Billy engages to elicit information that might have been unknown to him before OT interventions. He would benefit from an evaluation such as the Pizzi Holistic Wellness Assessment (discussed later).
3. *Are there mental and physical health issues that can be incorporated into a prevention and health promotion OT program?*
   - Billy could engage in a reality-checking exercise in which he explores the positive aspects and strengths in his life (e.g., good social support, advanced knowledge in the area of healthcare). These strengths can help him maintain a positive sense of self and engage in more health-promoting behavior on a physical level, such as a regular exercise program.

BOX 48.1 Classes of Antiretroviral Drugs Used to Treat HIV Infection

- Multiple classes of antiretrovirals are used in ART. Two classes inhibit HIV entry, and the others inhibit one of the three HIV enzymes needed to replicate inside human cells; three classes inhibit reverse transcriptase by blocking its RNA-dependent and DNA-dependent DNA polymerase activity.
- *Nucleoside reverse transcriptase inhibitors (NRTIs)* are phosphorylated to active metabolites that compete for incorporation into viral DNA. They inhibit the HIV reverse transcriptase enzyme competitively and terminate synthesis of DNA chains.
- *Nucleotide reverse transcriptase inhibitors (nRTIs)* competitively inhibit the HIV reverse transcriptase enzyme, as do NRTIs, but do not require initial phosphorylation.
- Nonnucleoside reverse transcriptase inhibitors (NNRTIs) bind directly to the reverse transcriptase enzyme.
- *Protease inhibitors (PIs)* inhibit the viral protease enzyme that is crucial to maturation of immature HIV virions after they bud from host cells.
- *Entry inhibitors (EIs)*, sometimes called fusion inhibitors, interfere with the binding of HIV to CD4+ receptors and chemokine co-receptors; this binding is required for HIV to enter cells. For example, CCR-5 inhibitors block the CCR-5 receptor.
- *Postattachment inhibitors* bind to the CD4 receptor and prevent HIV (which also binds to the CD4 receptor) from entering the cell.
- *Integrase inhibitors* prevent HIV DNA from being integrated into human DNA.
- *Attachment inhibitors* bind directly to the viral envelope glycoprotein 120 (gp120), close to the CD4+ binding site, which prohibits the conformational change necessary for initial interaction between the virus and the surface receptors on CD4 cells, thereby preventing attachment and subsequent entry into host T cells and other immune cells.

Data from Cachay ER: Drug treatment of HIV infection. In Merck manual professional version online, 2021. https://www.merckmanuals.com/professional/infectious-diseases/human-immunodeficiency-virus-hiv/human-immunodeficiency-virus-hiv-infection.

An individual is determined to have HIV infection if one category from each set applies. For example, AIDS would be diagnosed if the person is designated category 3 (<200 CD4+ cells) and has had at least one AIDS-defining illness. Categories 1 and 2 and A and B are considered HIV positive (a less grave condition), whereas categories 3 and C are defined as AIDS. These categories are used primarily to pinpoint an individual's placement along the continuum of HIV infection.[36]

Occupational therapists and OT assistants have the opportunity to positively affect the daily lives of people with HIV and AIDS in all of these stages of illness. Promoting health, quality of life, and well-being is one focus of OT intervention.[1]

PHARMACOLOGY

Decades after the origins of the HIV epidemic, there is still no cure. Over the years, researchers have made extraordinary progress in the development of medications to alter the course of the disease. The medications used to treat HIV infection have helped promote healthier functioning in people with HIV and AIDS, which facilitates continued occupational participation.[39]

Several classes of antiretroviral drugs are used to treat HIV infection.[6] They can be grouped into different classes of medication based on the mechanism by which the drug limits viral replication. These medications act on specific enzymes required for viral replication. By restricting viral replication, these medications can increase the CD4+ cell count and thus improve immune function and, as a result, limit the individual's susceptibility to opportunistic infections.

The general categories or classes of drugs are listed in Box 48.1, and it is important for the occupational therapist to understand the potential side effects of the medications used by the client.

HIV has considerable variation as a result of the replication process described previously. HIV quickly develops resistance to any of the antiretroviral medications used individually because of these mutations occurring during replication. Antiretroviral treatment is most effective when the medications are used in combination. Current protocols use multiple antiretroviral medications simultaneously to limit the ability of the virus to develop resistance to a single medication. The combination of medications has the benefit of reducing HIV blood levels more than is possible with a single medication, the combination helps prevent drug resistance, and some of the medications used in combination have a synergistic effect (increasing levels of other HIV drugs in blood). Current treatment with antiretroviral medications have been simplified in recent years to reduce pill burden and complexity of medication management. The current medications are more potent and less toxic than in the earlier years of HIV treatment.

These combined antiretroviral medications are referred to as antiretroviral therapy (ART). The introduction of ART has significantly changed the course of the AIDS pandemic.[52] In the United States, more people than ever before are living with HIV. The increased survival rate is most likely due to a combination of an increasing percentage of persons knowing their HIV infection status and persons receiving access to ART. It is particularly important for people to be tested and be aware of their HIV status. This is significant because it increases the likelihood that these persons will receive ART at an appropriate time, but it is also significant that persons who are aware of being HIV positive are less likely to transmit the virus (further reducing the incidence of infection). Successful ART treatment can lower viral load to undetectable levels at which point an infected person can no longer transmit the virus to partners or to infants (for pregnant persons).

The use of ART has significantly extended the life expectancy of persons infected with HIV. Many persons treated with ART live decades after the initial infection.[52] As a result of the effectiveness of this treatment, the overall prevalence rate of HIV infection in the United States has increased despite incidence rates of the infection remaining relatively stable (see the section "Origins and Current Status of HIV Infection"). Overall hospital use has declined since the introduction of ART, as well as morbidity and mortality in persons infected with HIV.[5] For persons able to maintain ART treatment, it is possible to have the same life expectancy as persons without HIV infection and live without opportunistic infections. However, medical management of persons infected with HIV throughout the lifespan is now more complex and includes multiple medical conditions associated with aging or chronic conditions.

The improved survival rates resulting from access to ART have become a significant factor in the management of HIV infection. However, it should be noted that ART is not a panacea. Despite prevention and treatment successes (including ART), people still die of AIDS. The overall survival rate trends are encouraging, but there remain too many persons in whom HIV is not diagnosed until late in the course of the infection process, and this represents a missed opportunity for prevention and treatment.[14,54] ART also has potential complications resulting from medication side effects and other issues.

Adherence to ART is correlated with viral suppression, improved immune function, increased survival from HIV, and improved quality of life.[24] However, maintaining medication compliance is challenging for reasons other than side effects. Persons who begin ART are often young and frequently display minimal symptoms from HIV at the initiation of ART. Because HIV infection is a lifelong condition, it may be a challenge for persons to continue adhering to the medication regimen as

prescribed. Reasons for poor adherence are many and complex, but there are several predictors of poor medication adherence. Low levels of literacy, psychosocial issues (including depression, limited social support, stress, and dementia), active substance use, cognitive impairment, complex regimens, age-related changes, medication fatigue, and medication scheduling issues are all predictors of poor medication adherence independent of side effects of the medications.[24]

Effective use of medications for the treatment of HIV requires consistency in maintaining the schedule of administration of the medications.[24] Failure to maintain consistency with the medications may result in HIV developing resistance to medications and allowing viral replication. ART reduces the viral load and allows the immune system to continue to function and prevent the presence of opportunistic infections. The effectiveness of the ART regimen can be measured by detecting the level of viral load present and by monitoring helper T-cell counts. In many instances, persons taking ART have a nearly undetectable level of virus. However, once a person is infected with HIV, that person is always able to transmit the virus.

Unfortunately, these life-enhancing medical regimens are associated with myriad side effects, many of which clients receiving OT services will experience. Understanding these side effects is important because they affect occupational performance. Side effects include CNS disorders, peripheral polyneuropathy, gastrointestinal disorders, hepatotoxicity, anemia, pancreatitis, osteopenia and osteoarthritis, metabolic effects (including lipodystrophy, hyperlipidemia, diabetes, and hyperglycemia), and immune reconstitution inflammatory syndrome.[6,24] Because of the extensive and varied pharmacological side effects, many people with HIV have great difficulty in deciding the appropriate time to begin a drug regimen.[31] Persons taking ART also may be at risk as a result of being unable to take ART consistently. This can occur because of either side effects or poor medication management (e.g., persons with HIV-related neurocognitive deficits are 2.5 times more likely to be at risk for medication noncompliance than are persons without dementia).[30]

ART has been an effective medical intervention that has significantly altered the landscape of HIV infection by creating improved health and well-being for many infected individuals. Unfortunately, access to affordable healthcare is limited or nonexistent for millions of people worldwide, and improving outreach to persons who do not yet have access to testing and who do not have access to ART remains a public health priority. Recent efforts have made these important medications more accessible.[32] Despite best practice in medicine, a cure for AIDS remains elusive. However, thanks to medical advances, people continue to live full and productive lives while coping with the daily issues of living with HIV.

AGING AND HIV INFECTION

A few issues related to aging in persons infected with HIV are important and require the attention of the OT practitioner. As ART prolongs the life of persons with HIV, the presence of HIV with other age-related conditions is becoming more common. Research has indicated that both hospitalizations and deaths from HIV-related causes have declined. The reduction in opportunistic infections and clinical AIDS has resulted in alternative causes of mortality in aging persons infected with HIV. Elderly persons with HIV are more likely to have additional medical comorbid conditions.[22,55]

Several considerations influence the health outcomes of elderly persons with HIV.[28] The elderly (classified by the CDC as persons older than 50 years) are a growing demographic in the United States for HIV infection. The number of persons older than 50 years infected with HIV has increased because of at least two factors. The first is sometimes referred to as an *aging cohort effect*, which describes a group of persons infected with HIV earlier in life and who age as a result of ART prolonging life expectancy. The other factor involves new infections diagnosed in persons older than 50 years. The incidence and prevalence of HIV infection have both increased in persons older than 50.

Some research suggests that persons in whom HIV infection is diagnosed after 50 years of age have worse outcomes than their younger cohorts do. One important factor appears to be that HIV infection diagnosed in persons older than 50 is at a more advanced stage than in their younger counterparts.

Possible explanations for the more advanced progression at the time of diagnosis in older persons with HIV includes less common routine screening for HIV in this population, poorer awareness of the risks for HIV infection and safer sex practices in this age group, and physicians perhaps being less likely to consider HIV clinically. The symptoms or signs of HIV infection also may be more likely to be attributed to comorbid medical conditions or to other conditions more commonly associated with aging populations.

NEUROLOGICAL SEQUELAE OF HIV/AIDS

Various medical complications are associated with HIV/AIDS, and multiple body functions and body structures can be affected by HIV/AIDS. Neurological disorders related to HIV infection are common and may be potentially debilitating in the performance of activities of daily living (ADLs) and instrumental activities of daily living (IADLs).[34] Estimates of the frequency of neurological disorders vary, but it appears that as many as 66% of persons with HIV may have peripheral neuropathy.[33] It is likely that at least 20% of persons with HIV infection have some type of neurocognitive impairment,[48] and some evidence suggests that more than 50% of persons on ART may have cognitive deficits.[29,51] The estimated prevalence of neurocognitive impairment varies considerably, in part because of the clinical standard used to determine the presence of cognitive impairment. If mild cognitive impairment is used as the criterion, the prevalence of neurocognitive impairment is significantly higher.[47] Despite the effectiveness of ART in improving overall immune function, neurological deficits have persisted, although advanced stages of dementia are less common than before the use of ART.[52]

Neurological disorders are of particular concern to occupational therapists working with persons with HIV/AIDS. HIV is capable of passing the blood-brain barrier and entering the CNS.[35] HIV has been detected in CNS structures, as well as in cerebrospinal fluid, in persons infected with HIV, including those who are asymptomatic and with functioning immune systems. The neurological sequelae of HIV/AIDS can be an indirect result of the virus via opportunistic infections (resulting from compromised immune function) or a direct or primary effect of HIV. The presence of neurological opportunistic infections has been greatly reduced in the United States since the advent of antiretroviral therapies.[48] However, primary effects of HIV on the CNS remain common and should be considered when addressing the needs of this population. Various neurological conditions or clinical manifestations are associated with HIV/AIDS. However, this section focuses on neuropathies (the most common neurological complication of HIV/AIDS) and AIDS-related dementia (which can have a profound impact on occupational performance) (Box 48.2). Not all persons display clinically significant neurological deficits. However, neurological deficits will develop in a significant number of persons as a result of this process.

Some changes in the course of neurological deficits do appear to be a result of ART. Before ART, the more advanced stages of AIDS dementia were commonly found in the advanced stages of clinical AIDS. As ART has improved immune functioning and decreased the number of persons with advanced clinical AIDS, the number of advanced dementia cases appears to have decreased as well. Although HIV dementia is common in advanced AIDS,[46,50] it is also found early in HIV infection and without AIDS or in the presence of opportunistic infections. The prevalence rate is significantly higher when including persons displaying signs of neurological involvement detected by neuroimaging but without clinical changes or when including persons with mild cognitive impairment.

BOX 48.2 Neurological Complications of HIV-1 Infection

HIV-1 Associated
- HIV-1 encephalopathy
- HIV-associated cognitive-motor disorder
- HIV-1 meningitis
- Vacuolar myelopathy
- Peripheral neuropathy
- Distal sensory polyneuropathy
- Antiretroviral toxic neuropathy
- Ascending neuromuscular syndrome
- Mononeuritis multiplex
- Inflammatory demyelinating polyneuropathy
- HIV-associated polymyositis

Opportunistic Infections
- Cerebral toxoplasmosis
- Tuberculosis
- Cryptococcal meningitis
- Cytomegalovirus retinitis/encephalitis/polyradiculitis
- Progressive multifocal leukoencephalopathy
- Other viral/fungal/bacterial/protozoal central nervous system infections
- Neoplasms
- Primary central nervous system lymphoma
- Metastatic systemic lymphoma
- Metastatic Kaposi's sarcoma

Despite the effectiveness of ART in improving overall immune function, neurological deficits have persisted,[52] and prevalence rates for dementia, when including mild cognitive impairment, have increased since the advent of ART, although advanced dementia is less common.[2,3,23,25] Some evidence also suggests that the cognitive deficits may be related to a combination of the aging process, extended period of HIV infection, medication side effects, and the comorbid neurological conditions that are more common in aging persons.[22,30]

NEUROPATHIES

Peripheral neuropathies are the most common neurological complication of HIV. They can occur both as a primary effect of the virus and as a side effect of antiviral medications used to treat HIV.[35] It is often difficult to distinguish clinically between the two causes of neuropathy. Although many peripheral nerve disorders are associated with HIV, distal sensory polyneuropathy is by far the most common disorder. Persons with distal symmetric polyneuropathy frequently have burning, painful sensations on the distal end of the lower extremities, often accompanied by numbness or tingling sensations. Individuals may also have decreased sensation of thermal stimuli. If lower extremity weakness is present, it is more likely to be distal than proximal. Distal sensory polyneuropathy follows a stocking-glove distribution of sensory impairment involving the feet and hands (typically with greater lower extremity involvement initially), and impairment spreads proximally as the condition progresses.

The functional deficits associated with peripheral neuropathy may include numbness or impaired sensation, loss of balance because of diminished proprioception in the lower extremities, and abnormal pain sensations (dysesthesias). Distal sensory polyneuropathy results in damage to both large myelinated and unmyelinated nerve fibers and is clinically similar to diabetic neuropathy (in that small sensory fibers are also involved).

Occupational therapists should assess clients for pain. Chronic pain is a common condition associated with HIV infection in general and with distal symmetric polyneuropathy in particular. The pain may limit occupation performance and is frequently underdiagnosed and undertreated. Current evidence suggests that the pain sensations are probably caused by dysfunctional regulation of pain fibers in both the central and peripheral nervous systems and that it results in severe pain out of proportion to the extent of epidermal nerve fiber loss.

In HIV-associated distal sensory polyneuropathy, it is hypothesized that the abnormal pain may be caused by damage to peripheral nerve fibers as a result of multifocal inflammation and infiltration of activated macrophage into peripheral nerves, with subsequent abnormal activity occurring in uninjured neighboring nociceptive fibers. The abnormal inflammatory response and macrophage infiltration are also found in the dorsal root ganglion. It is possible that this results in changes in neuronal calcium and sodium channels and ectopic impulse generation causing abnormal neuronal hyperexcitability. Finally, it is possible that remodeling occurs in the dorsal horns as a result of A-fiber sprouting and synaptic formation within lamina II of the spinal cord.

DEMENTIA

AIDS dementia complex (ADC) is also referred to as AIDS-related dementia, HIV-associated dementia, AIDS encephalopathy, or HIV encephalitis and is a common neurological condition associated with HIV infection.[45] Dementia associated with HIV infection has been identified since the earliest years of the HIV/AIDS pandemic and has been characterized by the cardinal features of progressive dementia with motor and behavioral deficits.[40] ADC appears to be a result of the presence of HIV in the CNS and is a primary effect of the virus. HIV can enter the CNS shortly after the initial infection. The most likely mechanism for entry appears to be infected monocytes passing through the blood-brain barrier.[51] The precise mechanism by which infected cells within the CNS are activated and cause dementia is not known at this time. It is possible that the brain may act as a sanctuary for HIV replication inasmuch as the blood-brain barrier may prevent ART from passing through the barrier to the CNS and create a viral reservoir.[42] The cells that are most frequently infected are macrophages, microglial cells, and astrocytes (although many other cells also may be infected within the CNS). It appears that neurons are rarely if ever infected by HIV.

ADC remains a complication in persons infected with HIV despite the introduction of ART.[49] ADC is characterized by subcortical involvement and is considered a subcortical dementia. There is evidence of damage to the basal ganglia and caudate nuclei,[27,41] and the clinical manifestations of ADC have some similarities to other subcortical dementias, including Parkinson's disease and Huntington's disease. Persons with ADC frequently display motor disturbances, such as imbalance, unsteady gait, tremors, difficulty performing fine motor tasks (including handwriting), weakness, and motor-processing delays and reduced speed of motor responses (primarily in the more advanced stages of ADC) (Box 48.3).

ADC may cause impairment of visuospatial function, executive function, and recall of information, as well as slowed psychomotor speed. Persons with ADC may have impaired episodic memory (the ability to remember facts, places, and subjective historical information) and deficits in retrieving information. It appears that ADC spares semantic memory (ability to recall facts and information unrelated to personal experience) and the ability to retain information until the relatively advanced late stages of ADC. Unlike Alzheimer-type dementia, persons in the earlier stages of ADC may not have significant deficits in naming objects or other language functions associated with the cerebral cortex but will probably have deficits in retrieving and manipulating retained information, as well as slowing of information processing.[37]

Persons with ADC may also exhibit behavioral changes, potentially including increased agitation, apathy, isolation, or changes in personality. Cognitive deficits are also present in the earliest stages of ADC. The cognitive deficits are most likely to involve executive function (including delays in information processing, limited attention to tasks, and visuospatial deficits). In the early stages of ADC, the manifestation of these deficits in executive functioning is different from dementia of the Alzheimer type, in which the person typically has more

BOX 48.3 Clinical Manifestations of AIDS-Dementia Complex

Affective: Apathy (Depression-Like Feature)
- Irritability
- Mania, new-onset psychosis

Behavioral: Psychomotor Retardation (Slowed Speech or Response Time)
- Change in personality
- Social withdrawal

Cognitive: Lack of Visuospatial Memory (Misplacing Things)
- Lack of visuomotor coordination (eye movement abnormalities)
- Difficulty with complex sequencing
- Impaired concentration and attention
- Impaired verbal memory (word-finding ability)
- Mental slowing

Motor: Unsteady Gait, Loss of Balance
- Dropping things
- Tremors, poor handwriting
- Decline in fine motor skills

pronounced memory deficits, word retrieval deficits, decreased comprehension or other language difficulties, and disorientation. However, as the dementia reaches more advanced stages and the deficits become more global, it may be difficult to differentiate ADC from dementia of the Alzheimer's type.

ADC appears to influence dopamine production, and a subtype of persons with ADC may exhibit mood disorders, including mania, probably as a result of the dopaminergic changes caused by ADC.[37] The likelihood of dopamine involvement is also supported by the movement disorders described previously.

The incidence and prevalence of HIV dementia or ADC have changed in the ART era. It appears that the incidence of ADC has decreased with the use of ART, but prevalence rates are increasing. One hypothesis is that new multiple patterns or progressions of ADC have arisen following the introduction of ART.[35] The first type is a subacute progressive form of dementia that is seen in untreated persons and marked by severe progressive dementia similar to the pattern seen before ART. The second pattern involves a chronic active dementia seen in persons prescribed ART who have poor compliance or exhibit viral resistance. These persons are at risk for progression of the dementia. The final category is chronic inactive dementia, in which persons receiving ART with good adherence and viral suppression remain neurologically stable but have some degree of cognitive impairment or early-stage ADC.

Advanced ADC was most common in the late stages of AIDS before the use of ART. The use of ART appears to have decreased the frequency of advanced stages of dementia in persons infected with HIV. However, the incidence of cognitive impairment and ADC has not abated despite the use of ART. It appears that mild cognitive impairment and early-stage ADC are more common than later stages of ADC as a result of ART,

but the overall incidence of cognitive deficits has remained at higher than 20% for persons infected with HIV.

It is important to be aware of the clinical manifestations of ADC during different stages of the dementia.[40]

Early Stages of AIDS-Dementia Complex

During the early phases of the disorder, it is possible for the deficits to be overlooked or be attributed to other causes. The early stages are consistent with subcortical dementia and are characterized by difficulty concentrating and attending to tasks and delayed processing of information, which may require extended time for completion of ADLs; minor forgetfulness and difficulty with executive functioning tasks are not unusual. Motor deficits also occur frequently and include tremors, gait imbalances, lower extremity weakness, and slowing of motor function. Persons may also display behavioral changes, including increased withdrawal from ADLs or social situations, agitation or irritability, and other changes in personality.

The early stages of ADC can potentially have an impact on a number of ADLs and IADLs. Persons may have particular challenges with IADLs involving executive functioning and may have difficulty managing finances, medications, or scheduling and keeping appointments. In particular, tasks involving multiple steps and sequencing may be problematic and lead to difficulties with related IADLs. Persons with HIV-related neurocognitive deficits are much more likely to be at risk for medication noncompliance than are persons without dementia.[30] Persons also may have difficulty with tasks requiring sustained attention (e.g., the person may have difficulty reading or listening to lengthy conversations). The motor deficits related to ADC may be minimal in the early stages but may be observed by noting difficulty with ADLs involving fine motor coordination, including handwriting, managing clothing fasteners, using utensils during meals, and performing grooming activities (such as shaving or applying makeup). The person also may have difficulty maintaining balance while walking, tremors, and weakness.

Later Stages of AIDS-Dementia Complex

As ADC progresses, the deficits become more generalized or global and may be difficult to distinguish from other types of advanced dementia. It is worth noting that given the use of ART, many persons with ADC or minor cognitive impairment have maintained relatively stable cognitive functioning without significant progression of symptoms over an extended period. In these cases, although deficits are present, the person may not progress to later stages of ADC. Late-stage ADC remains most common in people with significant progression of HIV or AIDS. By the late stages, ADC is characterized by global deterioration involving cognition, motor skills, behavioral deficits, and limited insight into the client's condition and deficits. As ADC progresses, the person will probably exhibit significant cognitive deficits, disorientation, general confusion, and impaired speech and language ability. Motor symptoms also progress at this point, with continued weakness, changes in muscle tone (spasticity in particular), ataxia, and dyskinesia. Some behavioral changes are also common as ADC progresses, including disinhibition of behavior and incontinence of the bowel or

TABLE 48.6 Staging of AIDS-Dementia Complex

Stage/Grading	Manifestation
0	Normal
0.5	Subclinical or equivocal—Minimal or equivocal symptoms • Mild (soft) neurological signs • No impairment in work or activities of daily living
1	Mild—Unequivocal intellectual or motor impairment • Able to do all but the most demanding work
2	Moderate—Cannot work or perform demanding activities of daily living • Capable of self-care • Ambulatory, but may need a single prop • Major intellectual disability or cannot walk unassisted
3	Severe—Major intellectual disability or cannot walk unassisted
4	End-stage—Nearly vegetative • Rudimentary cognition • Paraplegic or quadriplegic

bladder. At this point in the disorder, persons with HIV will probably require assistance in performing all IADLs and most ADLs. Refer to Table 48.6 for a summary of the stages of ADC.

HIV/AIDS PATHOLOGIES: CLIENT FACTORS

People with HIV are living longer and healthier lives as a result of improvements in medications, health education, and behavioral changes. However, medications are costly and often provided only to those who can afford them or have other access to them. Thus, people with HIV who are not privy to information on community resources or whose accessibility is otherwise limited experience numerous opportunistic infections (infections resulting from a compromised immune system), such as *Pneumocystis pneumoniae* infection or Kaposi's sarcoma (the latter being less common).

OT practitioners may see a diverse population of people with AIDS who have numerous occupational deficits. Many physical and psychosocial factors indicate the need for occupational therapy. Factors experienced by people with HIV and AIDS include, but are not limited to, the following:

• Fatigue and shortness of breath
• Impairment of the CNS
• Impairment of the peripheral nervous system
• Visual deficits
• Sensory deficits (including painful neuropathies)
• Cardiac problems
• Muscle atrophy
• Altered ability to cope with and adapt to changes that the illness creates
• Depression
• Anxiety
• Guilt

• Anger
• Preoccupation with illness versus wellness

All of these factors affect clients' occupational performance in meaningful, health-promoting daily occupations. Occupational therapy can benefit all people with HIV and AIDS who experience any of the aforementioned problems.

POSITIVE PREVENTION

Reflecting the changing needs of people with HIV and in consideration of the improved drugs to combat the disease and its secondary conditions, the term *positive prevention* has been developed and used by the CDC.[10] The Serostatus Approach to Fighting the Epidemic (SAFE) helps reduce the risk for transmission to supplement current risk reduction programs. Several action steps are recommended that focus on diagnosing HIV: linking infected persons to appropriate preventive services, helping them adhere to treatment regimens, and providing support to develop healthy habits for sustaining behavior that reduces the risk associated with HIV infection. It is one of the first programs to dovetail traditional infectious disease control with behavioral interventions. Although occupational therapists may primarily intervene with people who have already been infected, prevention can still be integrated into a holistic program of care.

Prevention and health promotion can be a primary area of intervention in OT. In primary prevention, the practitioner may develop and implement health education and risk reduction strategies to help individuals and communities understand the impact of reducing risk in occupational participation. An OT primary prevention strategy could be the establishment of a developmentally appropriate lecture or workshop on abstinence and safe sex for schools, religious groups, and community centers. These workshops could incorporate mental health strategies, culturally relevant information, and interpersonal skill-building exercises, areas in which OT practitioners are well educated.

Secondary prevention, wherein OT services are provided for people who are already infected with the virus, would include activities that create and promote healthy lifestyles and thereby prevent future opportunistic infections and promote balance and well-being. OT intervention focused on providing secondary prevention can significantly affect communities that have large numbers of people who are infected with HIV. An emphasis on establishing and maintaining the habits and routines that support engagement in occupations would be appropriate for secondary prevention programs.

Tertiary prevention is provided when clients suffer from a disability that is secondary to the disease. Tertiary prevention includes a strong emphasis on rehabilitation; health promotion programming also can be included to positively affect a person's lifestyle and provide hope for continued and healthful functioning. Strategies that support continued participation in occupations, even if the occupation has been modified, would be addressed in tertiary prevention programs. An example would be the use of adaptive equipment to support continued engagement in a desired occupation (e.g., woodworking, cooking) when muscular weakness or peripheral nerve damage compromises occupational performance.

ASSESSMENT

Pizzi developed two assessments that focus on enhancing health and well-being (see Chapter 5): one is for general use, and the other is for use in people infected with HIV.[44] The one related to HIV specifically is the Pizzi Assessment of Productive Living for Adults with HIV Infection and AIDS (PAPL; Fig. 48.2).

One of the first assessments in OT specifically designed as a client-centered and subjective health promotion tool is the Pizzi Health and Wellness Assessment (PHWA).[44] An occupational

---

Pizzi Assessment of Productive Living for Adults with HIV Infection and AIDS (PAPL)

Demographics

Name_____Age_____

Sex_____Lives with (relationship)_____

Identified caregiver_____

Race _____Culture_____Religion_____

Practicing?_____How does spirituality play a role in your life, if

any?_____

Primary occupational roles:

_____

Primary diagnosis:

_____

Secondary diagnosis:

_____

Stage of HIV_____

Past Medical History:

_____

Medications:

_____

Activities of Daily Living (use ADL performance assessment)
Are you doing these now?

_____

Do you perform homemaking tasks?

_____

(For areas of difficulty) Would you like to be able to do these again like you did

before?_____ Which ones? _____

Work

Job _____When last worked_____

Describe type of activity_____

Work environment _____

If not working, would you like to be able to?_____

Fig. 48.2 Pizzi Assessment of Productive Living for Adults with HIV and AIDS (PAPL). *LTG*, Long-term goals; *STG*, short-term goals. (Courtesy Michael Pizzi © 1991.)

(Continued)

Do you miss being productive?_____

Types of activity engaged in_____

If not, would you like to?_____Which ones?_____

Would you like to try other things as well?_____

Is it important to be independent in daily living activities?_____

Play/Leisure (interests and current participation)_____

_____

Sleep issues (habits, patterns)_____

Physical Function

Active and passive range of motion:

Strength:

Sensation:

Coordination (gross and fine motor or dexterity):

Visual-perceptual:

Hearing:

Balance (sit and stand):

Ambulation, transfers, and mobility:

Activity tolerance/endurance:

Physical pain:

Location:

_____

Does it interfere with doing important activities?_____

Sexual function:

Cognition

(Attention span, problem solving, memory, orientation, judgment, reasoning, decision making, safety awareness)

Time Organization

Former daily routine (before diagnosis)

Fig. 48.2 cont'd

Has this changed since diagnosis?_____

If so, how? _____

Are there certain times of day that are better for you to carry out daily tasks?

_____

Do you consider yourself regimented in organizing time and activity or pretty

flexible? _____

What would you change, if anything, in how your day is set up?

_____

Body image and self-image

In the last 6 months, has there been a recent change in your physical body and how it

looks?_____How do you feel about this?_____

_____

Social environment (Describe support available and utilized by patient)

Physical environment (Describe environments where patient performs daily tasks and

level of support or impediment for function)

Stressors

What are some things, people, or situations that are/were stressful?_____

_____

What are some current ways you manage stress?_____

_____

Situational Coping

How do you feel you are dealing with:

a) your diagnosis

_____

_____

b) changes in the ability to do things important to you?

_____

_____

c) other psychosocial observations

_____

_____

Fig. 48.2 cont'd

(Continued)

Occupational Questions

What do you feel to be important to you right now?

Do you feel you can do things important to you now? In the future?

Do you deal well with change?

What are your hopes, dreams, aspirations? What are some of your goals?

Have these changed since you were diagnosed? How?

Do you feel in control of your life at this time?

What do you wish to accomplish with the rest of your life?

Plan:

STG:

LTG:

Frequency:

Duration:

Therapist:

Fig. 48.2 cont'd

history format is used. The emphasis of the PHWA is to explore an individual's self-perception of health and strategies for self-responsibility. It is vital that practitioners incorporate the goals, beliefs, values, attitudes, and occupational meanings identified by the client being served. Reductionistic interventions (e.g., range of motion, strengthening, cognitive retraining) are incorporated into meaningful occupations and not addressed separately.

The PHWA is a self-assessment tool that incorporates both a qualitative and a quantitative component. Clients self-assess six areas of health on a scale of 1 through 10. They then address each area with the help of the practitioner in terms of their self-perception of occupational participation in the respective area. This dialogue helps clients become aware of important health issues affecting their daily occupational performance. In each area of health, the client explores strategies to optimize health and determines which strategies could be used to promote health and well-being.

Even when it appears that a specific intervention positively changes occupational performance, the person experiences wellness through self-discovery of how to best manage his or her well-being. After self-discovery, the therapy process unfolds collaboratively between the client and therapist.[44]

Immediate and meaningful occupational areas and self-identified health concerns are identified through this assessment. A holistic view of the client is inherent in the assessment and is guided by the principles of health promotion and the values of occupational therapy.

PAPL (see Fig. 48.2) is a holistic assessment for therapists to gather data on the physical, psychosocial, emotional, and spiritual aspects of the client's life. The resultant data are synthesized by the practitioner's clinical reasoning skills to produce a collaborative intervention that is client centered. All areas of occupational performance are addressed.

Holistic assessments are useful for practitioners because they address the multitude of issues and problem areas experienced by people with HIV and AIDS. The clinical reasoning of practitioners will then be challenged to integrate knowledge and skill in all areas of occupational therapy to best serve the client's needs.

In as many as 10% of persons infected with HIV and experiencing chronic pain, no specific cause is known.

INTERVENTION

The OT intervention process involves both the therapeutic use of self by the practitioner and the therapeutic use of occupations and activities. OT practitioners engage and facilitate engagement in meaningful and productive daily life occupations through a variety of techniques, strategies, and inventive programming. Promotion of healthy lifestyles while living with the disease is crucial for all clients infected with HIV. Interventions are individually tailored to meet the many physical, psychosocial, and contextual issues of people with HIV and AIDS. Because of the diverse features of HIV and AIDS, there are many considerations for practitioners when developing plans and goals. These considerations, listed in the following sections, also incorporate several occupational interventions that can be implemented.[43]

Prevention of Disability

Occupational therapists can play a significant role in primary prevention by participating in occupation-based education for various community groups to reduce the risk for infection and by promoting health. Occupational therapists can address secondary prevention through various health promotion strategies to enhance occupational engagement and performance with an emphasis on maintaining performance patterns, including significant habits, routines, rituals, and roles. OT intervention addressing tertiary prevention can focus on health promotion and rehabilitation to enhance occupational performance.

Education and Health Promotion

Occupational therapists can provide educational opportunities for clients to address multiple concerns, including energy conservation strategies to address fatigue, generalized weakness, and deconditioning, which are primary physical manifestations of HIV. Energy conservation, work simplification, and occupational adaptations are used to enhance productivity and participation. Education can address proper nutrition, which is vital for people with HIV and AIDS. In addition, occupational therapists can provide educational interventions to promote awareness of clients' medical status and medication management, as well as to improve awareness of side effects of the medications.

Maintaining and Restoring Performance

Occupational therapists work with clients with HIV/AIDS to maintain or restore occupational performance in the presence of changes in client factors related to HIV/AIDS. Considerations for OT interventions include the following:

1. Control and choices of daily living options must be provided as much as possible. Frequently people infected with HIV feel a sense of loss of control as the virus slowly invades body systems and manifests itself by further limitations in occupational performance. Providing choices can prove beneficial to clients when the virus compromises control in life.
2. Most clients with symptomatic HIV and AIDS have an altered worker role. Specific interventions regarding alternatives to

work and productive living are necessary if work is a valued role. Physical as well as psychosocial work assessment for holistic work-hardening programming is vital.
3. Habit training and adaptation of the routine of daily living are essential interventions and include performance of favored occupations with respect to physical and cognitive status; the level at which the person feels comfortable adapting routines; and times of day, contexts, and with whom the person chooses to perform the occupations. Whenever possible, clients must be given choices of scheduling within their own personal routines and not those that fit health professionals' schedules.
4. Short- and long-term goals must be readily adapted and changed as needed.

Complementary therapies must be considered as interventions before and during occupational performance. Such therapies can include progressive relaxation, biofeedback, prayer, therapeutic touch, traditional Chinese medicine techniques, myofascial release, craniosacral therapy, imagery, and visualization.

Modifications, Adaptations, and Compensatory Approaches to Intervention

Occupational therapists can provide intervention that includes a variety of modifications, adaptations, and compensatory techniques to promote occupational performance skills and patterns. Such approaches include the following:

1. Adaptive equipment and positioning can be used to assist clients in returning to independent performance of ADLs, work, and leisure occupations. Often people with HIV may reject such equipment even though it can benefit them. This rejection signals a rejection of the sick role and sometimes a denial of diminished abilities. This attitude must be respected until the time when the person chooses, if at all, to use the equipment.
2. Changes can be made in the physical environment or performance patterns to help the client continue important roles despite medical changes, including fatigue. Energy conservation approaches and work simplification can be useful to allow continued participation in ADLs.
3. A variety of strategies can be used to compensate for cognitive changes that may have an impact on occupational performance, including activities that involve executive function (medication management, work responsibilities, financial management) and motor performance. Occupational therapists can adapt tasks to compensate for neurological deficits, including sensory loss related to peripheral neuropathies. Therapists also can be involved in modifications to optimize function in persons with ADC and related cognitive deficits.

Advocacy and Psychosocial Considerations

Occupational therapists can be involved in both advocating for clients with HIV/AIDS and helping support client efforts for personal advocacy. More unique psychosocial aspects of HIV rehabilitation are present than in most other physical or psychosocial cases.

Many people with HIV have lost numerous friends to the same disease for which they are receiving therapy; have undergone loss of work and family as a result of discrimination, rejection, or physical inabilities; and may have lost life partners to the same disease. For many clients, all of these losses can occur before the age of 40. Women with HIV experience the aforementioned losses but must also frequently cope with poverty and homelessness; women are often underrecognized in the epidemic.

There is no known cure or vaccine for HIV to date, although research is promising. This is a major consideration as a stressor of daily living.

The aforementioned considerations are several areas of intervention that can help maintain and restore occupational performance and prevent secondary conditions and impairments from emerging.

THREADED CASE STUDY

Billy, Part 3

Billy required assessment to determine how the changes in client factors and body functions have altered various areas of occupation and life roles. After developing the occupational profile, several types of OT interventions are needed to strengthen the mind, body, and spirit. Promotion of the therapeutic use of self, with a nonjudgmental and caring, compassionate attitude, will help Billy relax during occupational therapy sessions and engage him in discovering the best ways to establish balance and well-being in his life. As a result of his apparent depression and fatigue, he may be experiencing altered occupational role performance. Fatigue and depression can also impair cognition. Understanding exactly how these roles are compromised and the underlying impairments in body function will help the therapy process unfold, with specific interventions

being implemented as appropriate. Billy, as determined through the occupational profile, is a habit-oriented man. Helping him explore his daily habits and routines, understanding the areas in which he senses an impairment (along with OT evaluation data), and encouraging him to adapt to change can help him to restore both his emotional health and his physical well-being.

Using an occupation- and client-centered approach and understanding the disease process afford the occupational therapist unique insight into the best ways to assess and treat people with HIV and AIDS. Promoting health and well-being will also establish a higher quality of life. The focus of occupational therapy is always to enable participation in meaningful life occupations that support life satisfaction and quality of life.

SUMMARY

Many changes have taken place since the earliest days of the HIV/AIDS epidemic. These changes include the demographics of persons infected by the virus, the areas globally in which infections are concentrated, populations infected in the United States, treatments available, survival rates, and medical management of the condition. Fortunately, the development of antiretroviral treatments has extended the life expectancy of many persons with HIV in the United States (and increasingly on a global basis). These encouraging developments also present a number of challenges in managing the chronic health and medical needs of persons infected with HIV.

Occupational therapy has many roles in addressing the needs of persons with HIV/AIDS. It can help address the range of client factors and performance skills that are affected by HIV/AIDS. Prevention is critical in the management of HIV, and occupational therapy can help emphasize prevention and reduce the incidence of HIV infections. Occupational therapy can also address the needs of persons infected with HIV.

OT assessment should focus on developing an occupational profile that includes the individual's previous occupational performance patterns, roles, habits, and routines to better understand how HIV influences function. Specific assessments can identify which client factors are most affected by HIV and provide guidance for OT interventions. Of particular importance in assessing client factors are the common neurological deficits that can greatly influence functional performance and are often present even in the absence of opportunistic infections or AIDS.

Occupational therapists can promote function and independence in ADLs and IADLs by a variety of means and interventions. These approaches include prevention of disability, education/health promotion, maintaining/restoring performance, modifying/adapting environments, compensatory strategies, advocacy, and addressing psychosocial factors. Through the use of these interventions, Occupational therapy can help persons with HIV maintain active participation in individual meaningful daily activities and be active in the community.

REVIEW QUESTIONS

1. What is the difference between HIV infection and AIDS?
2. What are the routes of HIV transmission?
3. Name three side effects of the drug regimen that affect the quality of life of persons who have HIV or AIDS.
4. Differentiate primary, secondary, and tertiary prevention programs.
5. Identify one potential neurological, physical, and psychosocial problem seen in clients who have HIV or AIDS.
6. Why might a client be hesitant to accept the use of adaptive equipment to engage in occupation?
7. What are at least three health promotion and prevention goals for a client with HIV? For a client with AIDS?
8. How might you address caregiver concerns regarding sexuality issues when both partners are in their sexual prime?
9. If a client with AIDS came to you about the perception of prejudice from other healthcare personnel, how might you respond?
10. List and discuss at least four strategies to promote the health and well-being of Billy and his partner, Tom.

REFERENCES

1. American Occupational Therapy Association: Occupational therapy practice framework: domain and process, 4th edition, *Am J Occup Ther* 74:7412410010p1–7412410010p87, 2020.
2. Brew BJ, Crowe SM, Landay A, Cysique L: Neurodegeneration and ageing in the HAART era, *J Neuroimmune Pharmacol* 4:163–174, 2009.
3. Brew B, Halman M, Catalan J, et al: Abacavir in AIDS dementia complex: efficacy and lessons for future trials, *PLoS Clin Trials* 2:e13, 2007.
4. Bruce RD, Kresina TF, McCance-Katz EF: Medication-assisted treatment and HIV/AIDS: aspects in treating HIV-infected drug users, *AIDS* 24:331–340, 2010.
5. Buchacz K, Baker RK, Moorman AC, et al: Rates of hospitalizations and associated diagnoses in a large multisite cohort of HIV patients in the United States, 1994–2005, *AIDS* 22:1345, 2008.
6. Catchay ER: Drug treatment of HIV infection. In Merck manual professional version online, 2021. https://www.merckmanuals.com/professional/infectious-diseases/human-immunodeficiency-virus-hiv/drug-treatment-of-hiv-infection.
7. Centers for Disease Control and Prevention (CDC): *Pneumocystis pneumoniae—Los Angeles, MMWR Morb Mortal Wkly Rep* 30:250–252, 1981.
8. Centers for Disease Control and Prevention: Revised classification system for HIV infection and expanded surveillance case definition for AIDS among adolescents and adults, *MMWR Recomm Rep* 41(RR-17):1–19, 1993.
9. Centers for Disease Control and Prevention: Infection control in healthcare personnel, 2022. https://www.cdc.gov/infectioncontrol/guidelines/healthcare-personnel/index.html.
10. Centers for Disease Control and Prevention: National Prevention Information Network (CDC-NPIN), nd, https://clinicalinfo.hiv.gov/en/glossary/centers-disease-control-and-prevention-national-prevention-information-network-cdc-npin#:~:text=Centers%20for%20Disease%20Control%20and%20Prevention-National%20Prevention%20Information,other%20sexually%20transmitted%20diseases%20%28STDs%29%2C%20and%20tuberculosis%20%28TB%29.
11. Centers for Disease Control and Prevention: Health, United States, 2009 report. http://www.cdc.gov/nchs/data/hus/hus09.pdf.
12. Centers for Disease Control and Prevention: HIV and Occupational Exposure, 2019. https://www.cdc.gov/hiv/workplace/healthcareworkers.html.
13. Centers for Disease Control and Prevention: HIV surveillance report, 2019. https://www.cdc.gov/nchhstp/newsroom/2021/2019-national-hiv-surveillance-system-reports.html.
14. Centers for Disease Control and Prevention: HIV surveillance report: Diagnoses of HIV Infection in the United States and Dependent Areas, 2019. https://www.cdc.gov/hiv/library/reports/hiv-surveillance/vol-32/index.html.
15. Centers for Disease Control and Prevention: Blood safety basics, 2021. http://www.cdc.gov/bloodsafety/basics.html.
16. Centers for Disease Control and Prevention: HIV and African American People, 2021. http://www.cdc.gov/hiv/group/racialethnic/africanamericans/.
17. Centers for Disease Control and Prevention: HIV and Hispanics/Latinos, 2021. http://www.cdc.gov/hiv/group/racialethnic/hispaniclatinos/.
18. Centers for Disease Control and Prevention: HIV basics, 2021. http://www.cdc.gov/hiv/basics/.
19. Centers for Disease Control and Prevention: HIV: Basic statistics, 2021. https://www.cdc.gov/hiv/basics/statistics.html.
20. Centers for Disease Control and Prevention: HIV: HIV testing, 2021. https://www.cdc.gov/hiv/testing/index.html.
21. Centers for Disease Control and Prevention: HIV transmission, 2021. https://www.cdc.gov/hiv/basics/transmission.html.
22. Cooley SA, Paul RH, Ances BM: Medication management abilities are reduced in older persons living with HIV compared with healthy older HIV-controls, *Journal of Neurovirology* 26(2):264–269, 2020.
23. Cysique LA, Brew BJ, Halman M, et al: Undetectable cerebrospinal fluid HIV RNA and beta-2 microglobulin do not indicate inactive AIDS dementia complex in highly active antiretroviral therapy–treated patients, *J Acquir Immune Defic Syndr* 39:426–429, 2005.
24. Department of Health and Human Services: Guidelines for the use of antiretroviral agents in adults and adolescents with HIV, 2022. https://clinicalinfo.hiv.gov/en/guidelines/hiv-clinical-guidelines-adult-and-adolescent-arv/introduction.
25. Dore GJ, McDonald A, Li Y, et al: Marked improvement in survival following AIDS dementia complex in the era of highly active antiretroviral therapy, *AIDS* 17:1539–1545, 2003.
26. Gilbert MTP, Rambaut A, Wlasiuk G, et al: The emergence of HIV/AIDS in the Americas and beyond, *Proc Natl Acad Sci U S A* 104:18566, 2007.
27. Glass JD, Fedor H, Wesselingh SL, McArthur JC: Immunocytochemical quantitation of human immunodeficiency virus in the brain: correlations with dementia, *Ann Neurol* 38:755–762, 1995.
28. Grabar S, Lanoy E, Allavena C, et al: Causes of the first AIDS-defining illness and subsequent survival before and after the advent of combined antiretroviral therapy, *HIV Med* 9:246–256, 2008.
29. Heaton RK, Marcotte TD, Rivera Mindt M, et al: The impact of HIV-associated neuropsychological impairment on everyday functioning, *J Int Neuropsychol Soc* 10:317–331, 2004.
30. Hinkin CH, Hardy DJ, Mason KI, et al: Medication adherence in HIV-infected adults: effect of patient age, cognitive status, and substance abuse, *AIDS* 18:19–25, 2004.
31. Hoffman C, Rockstroh JK, Kamps BS: *HIV medicine* 2007.
32. Joint United Nations Programme on HIV/AIDS (UNAIDS): The path that ends AIDS, 2022. https://www.unaids.org/en.
33. Letendre S, Ellis RJ, Everal I, et al: Neurologic complications of HIV disease and their treatment, *Top HIV Med* 17:46–56, 2009.
34. McArthur JC, Brew BJ, Nath A: Neurological complications of HIV infection, *Lancet Neurol* 4:543–555, 2005.
35. McArthur JC, Haughey N, Gartner S, et al: Human immunodeficiency virus–associated dementia: an evolving disease, *J Neurovirol* 9:205–221, 2003.
36. McGovern T, Smith R: Case definition of AIDS. In McGovern T, Smith R, editors: *Encyclopedia of AIDS: a Social, Political, Cultural and Scientific Record of the HIV Epidemic*, Chicago, 1998, Fitzroy Dearborn.
37. Meehan RA, Brush JA: An overview of AIDS dementia complex, *Am J Alzheimers Dis Other Demen* 16:225–229, 2001.
38. National Institutes of Health: HIV Overview, 2021. https://hivinfo.nih.gov/understanding-hiv/fact-sheets/stages-hiv-infection.
39. National Institutes of Health: Guidelines for the Use of Antiretroviral Agents in Adults and Adolescents Living with HIV, 2021. https://clinicalinfo.hiv.gov/en/guidelines/adult-and-adolescent-arv/whats-new-guidelines.

40. Navia BA, Jordan BD, Price RW: The AIDS dementia complex: I. clinical features, *Ann Neurol* 19:517–524, 1986.

41. Neuen-Jacob E, Arendt G, Wendtland B, et al: Frequency and topographical distribution of CD68–positive macrophages and HIV-1 core proteins in HIV-associated brain lesions, *Clin Neuropathol* 12:315–324, 1993.

42. Nightingale S, Winston A, Letendre S, et al: Controversies in HIV-associated neurocognitive disorders, *Lancet Neurol* 13:1139–1151, 2014.

43. Pizzi M: HIV infection and AIDS. In Hopkins H, Smith H, editors: *Willard and Spackman's Occupational Therapy* ed 8, Philadelphia, 1993, Lippincott Williams & Wilkins.

44. Pizzi M: The Pizzi Holistic Wellness Assessment. In: Velde B.Wittman P, editors: *Occupational Therapy in Health Care (Special Issue on Community Based Practice)*, 13, Binghamton, NY, 2001, Haworth Press.

45. Price RW, Brew B, Sidtis J, et al: The brain in AIDS: central nervous system HIV-1 infection and AIDS dementia complex, *Science* 239:586, 1988.

46. Price RW, Yiannoutsos CT, Clifford DB, et al: Neurological outcomes in late HIV infection: adverse impact of neurological impairment on survival and protective effect of antiviral therapy, *AIDS* 13:1677–1685, 1999.

47. Robertson KR, Smurzynski M, Parsons TD, et al: The prevalence and incidence of neurocognitive impairment in the ART era, *AIDS* 21:1915–1921, 2007.

48. Sacktor N: The epidemiology of human immunodeficiency virus–associated neurological disease in the era of highly active antiretroviral therapy, *J Neurovirol* 8:115–121, 2002.

49. Schifitto G, Deng L, Yeh T: Clinical, laboratory, and neuroimaging characteristics of fatigue in HIV-infected individuals, *J Neurol* 17:17–25, 2011.

50. Selnes OA, Miller E, McArthur J, et al: HIV-1 infection: no evidence of cognitive decline during the asymptomatic stages, *Neurology* 40:204–208, 1990.

51. Simioni S, Cavassini M, Annoni J-M, et al: Cognitive dysfunction in HIV patients despite long-standing suppression of viremia, *AIDS* 24:1243–1250, 2010.

52. Tozzi V, Balestra P, Bellagamba R, Corpolongo A, et al: Persistence of neuropsychologic deficits despite long-term highly active antiretroviral therapy in patients with HIV-related neurocognitive impairment: prevalence and risk factors, *J Acquir Immune Defic Syndr* 45:174–182, 2007.

53. UNAIDS: *Fact sheet - latest global and regional statistics on the status of the aids epidemic*, 2021. https://www.unaids.org/en/resources/documents/2021/UNAIDS_FactSheet.

54. 2021 UNAIDS: Global AIDS Update — Confronting inequalities — Lessons for pandemic responses from 40 years of AIDS. https://www.unaids.org/sites/default/files/media_asset/2021-global-aids-update_en.pdf.

55. Valcour V, Watters MR, Williams AE, et al: Aging exacerbates extrapyramidal motor signs in the era of ART, *J Neurovirol* 14:362, 2008.

SUGGESTED READINGS

Centers for Disease Control and Prevention: Blood safety, 2021. https://www.cdc.gov/nhsn/biovigilance/blood-safety/index.html?CDC_AA_refVal=https%3A%2F%2Fwww.cdc.gov%2Fnhsn%2Facute-care-hospital%2Fbio-hemo%2Findex.html.

Jaffe HW, Valdiserri RO, De Cock KM: The reemerging HIV/AIDS epidemic in men who have sex with men, *JAMA* 298:2412, 2007.

Thompson MA, Horberg MA, Agwu AL, Colasanti JA, Jain MK, Short WR, Aberg JA: Primary care guidance for persons with human immunodeficiency virus: 2020 update by the HIV Medicine Association of the Infectious Diseases Society of America, *Clin Infect Dis* 73(11):e3752–e3605, 2020. https://pubmed.ncbi.nlm.nih.gov/33225349/

University of Arizona: HIV/AIDS pandemic began around 1900, earlier than previously thought; urbanization in Africa marked outbreak, *ScienceDaily*, 2008. http://www.sciencedaily.com/releases/2008/10/081001145024.htm

49

Polytrauma and Occupational Therapy[a]

Sharon Dekelboum and Karen Parecki

LEARNING OBJECTIVES

After studying this chapter, the student or practitioner will be able to do the following:

1. Understand the definition of polytrauma.
2. List several standard occupational therapy assessments used for patients with polytrauma.
3. Identify the areas in which the occupational therapist needs basic knowledge to care for patients with polytrauma.
4. Define the term *emerging consciousness.*
5. Understand the importance of an interdisciplinary approach to polytrauma care.
6. Describe the continuum of care process available within the Veterans Affairs system of care.
7. Describe the multisystem effects of a blast injury.
8. Explain the impact of post-traumatic stress disorder on the recovery process.
9. Identify the use of assistive technology in this population.
10. Provide examples of how return-to-work/return-to-school programs can be included in rehabilitation services.
11. Articulate the importance of treating the client and family as a unit.
12. Understand the implications of sensory loss for the rehabilitation process.

CHAPTER OUTLINE

KEY TERMS

Amputation
Assistive technology
Blast injury
Emerging consciousness
Interdisciplinary
Polytrauma

Post-traumatic stress disorder
Sensory loss
Shrapnel
Skull flap
Traumatic brain injury
Triage

---

[a] The opinions expressed in this chapter do not necessarily represent those of the Department of Veterans Affairs.

THREADED CASE STUDY

Alex, Part 1

Alex, a 25-year-old man (prefers use of the pronouns of he/his/him), was serving in the Marines. Alex sustained a polytraumatic injury from the blast of an improvised explosive device while stationed in Iraq. As a result of the blast, Alex incurred a traumatic head injury (diffuse axonal injury and temporal lobe contusion with subarachnoid hemorrhage), a right arm degloving injury, maxillary and mandibular fractures, and traumatic amputation of his right leg below the knee along with a femoral fracture. Additionally, his injuries included a penetrating eye injury with subsequent surgical excision of the foreign body. He also demonstrated clinical signs of post-traumatic stress disorder. Alex is married, and his wife was 3 months pregnant at the time of his injury. He was living in Hawaii before his deployment to Iraq; the home is a single level with two steps to enter the home. His role in the Marines was as a corpsman (medic).

Alex was referred to occupational therapy 1 month after injury when he arrived, medically stable, at the polytrauma rehabilitation unit. Initially, Alex was evaluated at a Rancho Los Amigos Cognitive Function Scale Level of II or III with an altered level of consciousness and was evaluated with the Coma Recovery Scale–Revised (CRS-R).[15] Additionally, he was assessed for positioning and splinting needs, range of motion (ROM), and gross strength. Because of decreased arousability, restlessness, and an inability to consistently follow commands, much of the psychosocial components, including occupational history and profile, were obtained by interviewing his wife. As Alex was unable to identify occupational goals, his wife assisted in determining rehabilitation goals that related to increased cognitive skills, including alertness and orientation, along with improved self-care skills. Within a week Alex demonstrated improved cognitive abilities as measured by the CRS-R, functional mobility, activities of daily living (ADLs), and cognitive and visual-perceptual screening was initiated. Alex required minimal assistance for bed mobility, maximal assistance for transfers and wheelchair mobility, and moderate to maximal assist for all ADLs. Cognitively, he was able to follow simple one-step commands 80% of the time, easily became overstimulated and distractible in any setting but a quiet environment, had poor endurance, easily became frustrated, and had difficulty with orientation, problem solving, and other executive skill functions. Safety awareness was also impaired. In addition, Alex's visual-perceptual skills were impaired and he demonstrated dysmetria and double vision. Strength and ROM in his left upper extremity were within normal limits; however, his right hand had decreased strength and ROM. Coordination was slightly impaired on the right but normal on the left. Alex also demonstrated signs of hypervigilance and reported difficulty sleeping.

The objectives of occupational therapy intervention included (1) increasing independence in performance of ADLs; (2) achieving increased independence in transfers and wheelchair mobility; (3) achieving optimal ROM in all joints of the right upper extremity for function and maintaining ROM in all other joints for optimal seating and positioning; (4) achieving improved visual-perceptual skills or implementing compensatory strategies to promote safety and ease in ADLs, mobility, and performance of instrumental activities of daily living (IADLs); (5) promoting the highest level of functional cognition, including implementation of compensatory strategies and cognitive prosthetics to increase independence and safety in all functional skills; (6) achieving optimal independence in performing IADLs, including parenting skills; (7) optimizing independent ability to access the community, including transportation; (8) optimizing independence in return-to-school and return-to-work skills; (9) receiving appropriate durable medical equipment to meet both short-term and long-term needs (including wheelchair, cushion, ADL equipment, and prosthetic limb care needs); (10) optimizing self-regulation and promoting good sleep hygiene; and (11) educating the family and patient in all aspects of care needs, compensatory strategies, and safety recommendations.

Because of significant impairment in cognitive skills, an interdisciplinary team approach was implemented to ensure that compensatory strategies were carried over throughout the day. As Alex gained insight into his deficits and how they were currently having an impact on his life (community skills, employment, parenting, independence in self-care, and self-efficacy), he had mood fluctuations that ranged from depressed to feeling hopeful and accepting of his current situation. Additionally, supporting the family members and working with Alex and his wife as a couple, on their roles in the relationship, and how that has been changed was addressed through the psychology service and with a family therapist.

Throughout the chapter, consider the short-term and long-term consequences of Alex's injuries. The many body systems that were affected with this type of polytraumatic brain injury will have effects on client factors, performance skills and patterns, occupational performance, and the relationship of activity demands to selection of optimal equipment and strategies to optimize his performance in all aspects of his life.

Critical Thinking Questions

1. How would you determine what occupations need to be addressed and in what order you would address them?
2. Thinking about client factors, how would you prioritize treatment interventions?
3. How would you integrate your treatment plan and interventions with the needs and goals of the client, family, and whole treatment team?

POLYTRAUMA

The definition of polytrauma stems from the Latin *poly*, meaning many, and *trauma*. The term is generic and has been in use for a long time for any case involving multiple traumas. It has become a common term for U.S. military doctors to describe seriously injured soldiers returning from Operation Iraqi Freedom (OIF, Iraq) and Operation Enduring Freedom (OEF, Afghanistan).[34]

The term *polytrauma* is now consistently used by U.S. military medical personnel and the Veterans Administration (VA) to describe the multiple, extreme, and often totally incapacitating complex of traumatic injuries that individual U.S. service members suffer in the aftermath of war. The severity and complexity of these multiple wounds and injuries would have proved fatal in previous wars. Advances in medicine and especially in battlefield medicine, as well as quick evacuation of these patients to complex trauma centers, have decreased the mortality rate. Many polytrauma injuries include multiple, severe shrapnel injuries leading to multiple amputations, wounds, loss of normal body function and systemic complications, brain damage, sensory impairment, and partial to full paralysis. This type of complex injury is not typically seen, even in the trauma centers of major urban centers. This type of injury needs the rehabilitation plan to address changing needs throughout the recovery process; therefore, the focus and care need to be adjustable–in other words, to for the right rehabilitation care at the right time, throughout the recovery.

Polytrauma centers have been developed throughout the Department of Veterans Affairs to address the complex medical and rehabilitation needs of these patients. The VA defines poly-trauma as "injuries to more than one physical region or organ system, one of which may be life threatening and results in physical, cognitive, psychological, or psychosocial impairments and functional disability."[10] Not only has the VA taken on the challenge of finding best-care practices to optimize the long-term outcome of these clients, but the civilian sector has also begun to adopt the term *polytrauma* and has set out to provide treatment for this population as well.

Types of Blast Injuries

One of the most common causes of polytrauma is exposure to a blast, such as from an improvised explosive device or a rocket-propelled grenade. According to the Defense and Veterans Brain Injury Center (DVBIC),[8] blast injury can have differ-ent effects on the body based on proximity to the blast and the body's reaction to the blast. The DVBIC indicates that "exposure to blast events can affect the body in a number of ways, in addi-tion, these different injury mechanisms can interact and result in more impairments or prolonged periods of recovery."

Primary blast injury is the result of exposure to the overpres-surization wave or the complex pressure wave that is generated by the blast itself. This blast overpressurization wave travels at high velocity and is affected by the surrounding environment; for example, the effects of the blast wave may be increased in a closed environment such as a vehicle. Air-filled organs such as the ear, lung, and gastrointestinal tract and organs surrounded by fluid-filled cavities such as the brain and spinal cord are espe-cially susceptible to primary blast injury.[13,23] The overpressur-ization wave dissipates quickly and causes the greatest risk for injury to those closest to the explosion.

- *Secondary blast injury* is the result of energized fragments flying through the air; these fragments may cause penetrat-ing brain injury.
- *Tertiary blast injury* may occur when the individual is thrown from the blast into a solid object such as an adjacent wall or even a steering wheel. These types of injuries are associated with acceleration/deceleration forces and blunt force trauma to the brain, similar to that observed following high-speed motor vehicle accidents.
- Finally, with severe blast-related trauma, *quaternary blast injury* can occur as a result of significant blood loss associ-ated with traumatic amputations or even the inhalation of toxic gases released by the explosion.[9]

Impairments from a polytraumatic injury are not predict-able, and the outcome for each individual is unique. Some of the common sequelae include brain injury; spinal cord injury; amputation; infections; orthopedic problems such as fractures; wounds; psychological stressors such as post-traumatic stress disorder (PTSD); crush injuries; burns; auditory and vestibular impairments; eye, orbit, and facial injuries; dental complica-tions; renal, respiratory, cardiac, and gastrointestinal compro-mise; peripheral nerve injuries; and pain (Table 49.1).

Although the polytrauma population is defined as a unique population, the principles of treatment and the factors that must be considered when planning treatment are applicable to all rehabilitation populations.[16,28] Some of the factors typically seen

TABLE 49.1	Overview of Explosive-Related Injuries
System	**Injury or Condition**
Auditory or vestibular	Tympanic membrane rupture, ossicular disruption, cochlear damage, foreign body, hearing loss, distorted hearing, tinnitus, earache, dizziness, sensitivity to noise
Eye, orbit, face	Perforated globe, foreign body, air embolism, fractures
Respiratory	Blast lung, hemothorax, pneumothorax, pulmonary contusion and hemorrhage, arteriovenous fistulas (source of air embolism), airway epithelial damage, aspiration pneumonitis, sepsis
Digestive	Bowel perforation, hemorrhage, ruptured liver or spleen, sepsis, mesenteric ischemia from air embolism, sepsis, peritoneal irritation, rectal bleeding
Circulatory	Cardiac contusion, myocardial infarction from air embolism, shock, vasovagal hypotension, peripheral vascular injury, air embolism–induced injury
Central nervous system injury	Concussion, closed and open brain injury, petechial hemorrhage, edema, stroke, small blood vessel rupture, spinal cord injury, air embolism–induced injury, hypoxia or anoxia, diffuse axonal injury
Renal injury	Renal contusion, laceration, acute renal failure from rhabdomyolysis, hypotension, hypovolemia
Extremity injury	Traumatic amputation, fractures, crush injuries, compartment syndrome, burns, cuts, lacerations, infections, acute arterial occlusion, air embolism–induced injury
Soft tissue injury	Crush injuries, burns, infections, slow-healing wounds
Emotional or psychological	Acute stress reactions, post-traumatic stress disorder, survivor guilt, postconcussive syndrome, depression, generalized anxiety disorder
Pain	Acute pain from wounds, crush injuries, or traumatic amputation; chronic pain syndrome

Adapted from Centers for Disease Control and Prevention (CDC): Explosions and blast injuries: a primer for clinicians. https://stacks.cdc.gov/view/cdc/28987. Accessed May 31, 2023.

in the polytrauma population include young age at the time of injury, developmental stage and life role participation, includ-ing work and family role, familiarity with assistive technology, and military culture, as well as ethnic/racial background, PTSD/acute stress reaction, previous or current substance abuse, high incidence of mental health complications and suicide risk, and vocational and community reintegration factors. Additionally, this population may need to be supported by a case manager for an extended period because their life roles and secondary conditions start to have an impact on their function (Fig. 49.1).

Treatment and implementation of treatment triage begin at the acute onset of injury.[12] The priority in the field and once in the hospital is medical stabilization. Once the patient is medically stable, the occupational therapist (OT) may be consulted, even while the patient is in the intensive care unit. As soon as the individual is ready for a rehabilitation program, the client's needs are again triaged to see which type of rehabilitation program will be the best fit. Within the VA system is the Polytrauma System of Care, which is further divided into several levels of rehabilitation programs. Every VA facility has a Polytrauma Point of Contact (PPOC) that connects veterans with polytrauma to the appropriate facility and program. Once connected, the veteran is referred to the Polytrauma Rehabilitation Center (PRC—inpatient rehabilitation), the Polytrauma Transitional Rehabilitation Program (PTRP—residential treatment), the Polytrauma Network Sites (PNSs—outpatient rehabilitation), or the Polytrauma Support Clinic Teams (outpatient rehabilitation).[10] Additionally, the VA offers polytrauma telehealth for those who are not able to come to a local polytrauma site (Fig. 49.2).

Polytrauma Rehabilitation Centers

PRCs provide acute, comprehensive, inpatient rehabilitation and comprehensive interdisciplinary evaluation of patients with varying levels of acuity or severity. A patient at any level on the Rancho Los Amigos Level of Cognitive Function Scale[17] may be admitted. These evaluations help determine the range and types of services needed to manage the full scope of medical, rehabilitation, and psychosocial sequelae resulting from combat injury and the most appropriate setting in which to deliver these services.[10] PRCs maintain a full team of rehabilitation

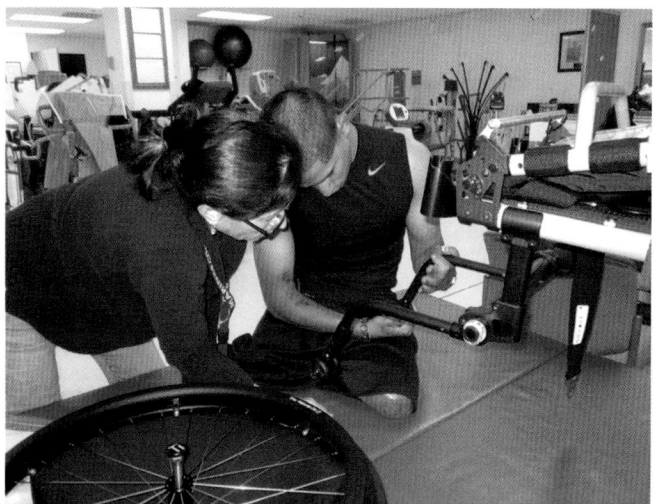

Fig. 49.1 Learning to break down a new wheelchair.

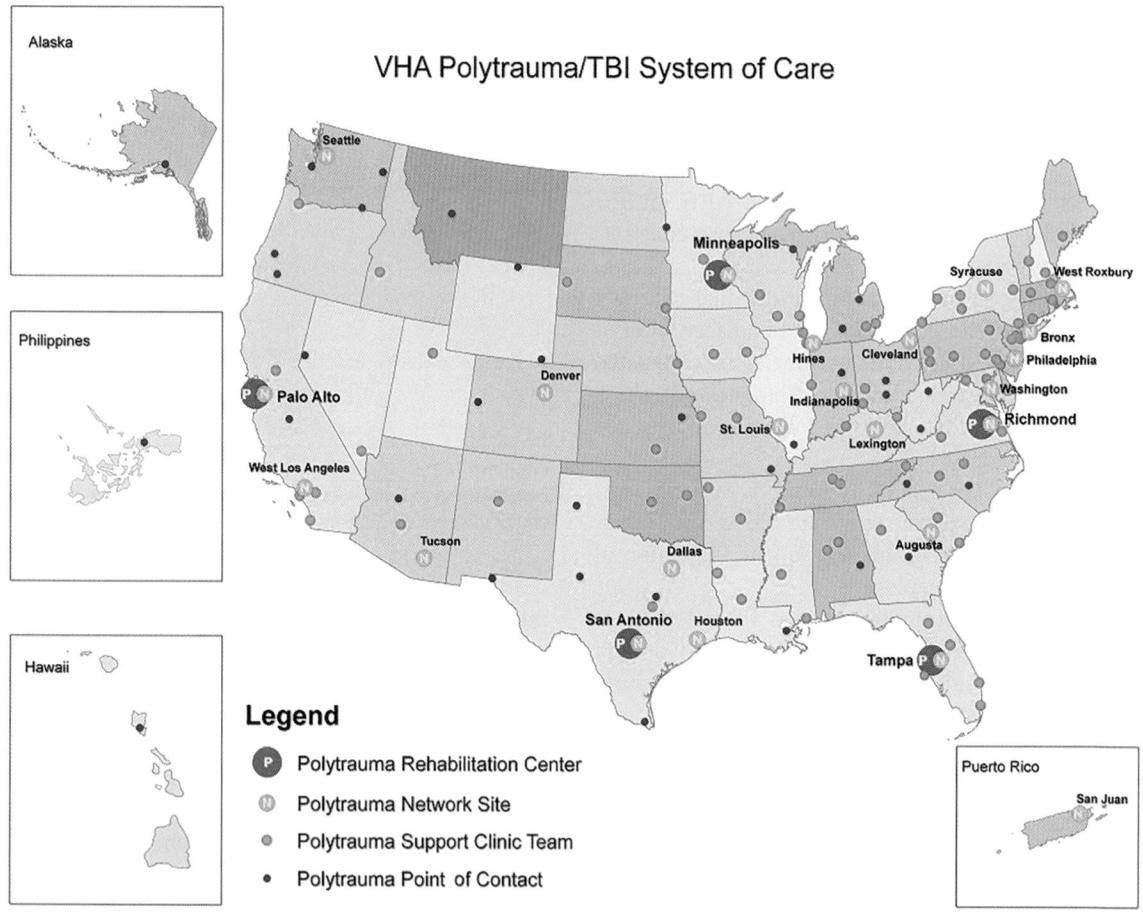

Fig. 49.2 Map of polytrauma system of care facilities. (From U.S. Department of Veterans Affairs. *Polytrauma/TBI System* of Care. VA Polytrauma System of Care. https://www.polytrauma.va.gov/system-of-care/index.asp.)

professionals, as well as consultants from other specialties related to polytrauma. PRCs also serve as consultants to other facilities in the Polytrauma System of Care.

As an occupational therapist serving on a polytrauma team, it is imperative to have knowledge and experience in treating a wide variety of conditions. For example, rehabilitation care is often focused on head/brain injury. Therefore, the therapist must have specialized skill in rehabilitation of **traumatic brain injury** (TBI), including cognitive rehabilitation, visual-perceptual skill training, **sensory loss** training, and behavioral skill training.[16,28] Additionally, occupational therapists need to have a solid understanding of the rehabilitation of physical disabilities, including upper extremity rehabilitation, amputation care, functional mobility, burns, wound prevention, balance, and hand therapy, including splinting. Moreover, the occupational therapist must be skilled in psychosocial rehabilitation, with a focus on family care, as well as how to work with patients with PTSD, anxiety, and pain.[18] Finally, the occupational therapist must be proficient in retraining performance of ADLs and IADLs, as well as community reintegration training.

The occupational therapist is just one member of an interdisciplinary team assigned to the PRC. Some of the other team members include the rehabilitation physician (physiatrist), nurses, social work case managers, speech-language pathologists, physical therapists, recreation therapists, counseling psychologists, and neuropsychologists. Some teams also include family therapists, military liaisons, blind rehabilitation and outpatient specialists, and massage therapists. Consulting services play a large part in the care of these patients. Consultants frequently involved in care include plastic surgeons, orthopedists, pain management specialists, psychiatrists, dentists, audiologists, neurologists, ophthalmologists, and internists. The key component in the treatment of patients with more acute polytrauma is working within and in conjunction with a large team to best serve the patient. The interdisciplinary team meets regularly to ensure that all treating specialists are working as a fluid team to address the primary issues and ensure that the treatment is clinically appropriate and patient centered. Interdisciplinary communication is essential to ensure that all members of the team are reenforcing techniques and compensations that are initiated by the different disciplines or to collaborate on what techniques and compensations may be most effective to implement for that patient. This often requires co-treatment between disciplines to ensure the best care.[7,35,36]

Once a patient is admitted to a PRC, the occupational therapist is consulted. The occupational therapist will always start with a chart review and review the precautions for the client. This population frequently has **skull flaps** removed and must therefore wear helmets when out of bed as a safety and protective measure. Clients with polytrauma often have infections such as methicillin-resistant *Staphylococcus aureus* and *Acinetobacter*, which require contact precautions (gown and glove); they also may be at risk for seizures, have visual deficits, be at risk for falling, and have behavioral difficulties, as well as having PTSD. Once the occupational therapist is aware of the patient's background and precautions, the next step is to communicate with the treatment team to determine whether any

additional information is available and then meet with the client. One of the most important pieces of information to gather is the client's and family's goals and expectations for the rehabilitation program. These goals, as well as the extent of the brain injury, will direct care of the client.

The occupational therapy evaluation is tailored to the needs of the client. For example, clients at Rancho Los Amigos levels I to III will be evaluated with the CRS-R[14] and the Coma–Near Coma Scale.[31] Clients will generally be considered to be at the level of "**emerging consciousness**" if they demonstrate minimal arousal, limited capacity to interact with the environment, significantly impaired ability to follow commands and communicate, and little to no intentional movement.[2] At this level there is no functional use of objects, which limits the client's engagement in ADLs. A client at the level of "emerging consciousness" will then follow a different pathway from an acute rehabilitation patient. Interventions for these clients often include sensory stimulation, maintenance and restoration of neuromuscular and movement-related functions, prevention of secondary disability, and family education and involvement (see Chapter 35 for additional details). The goal of occupational therapy intervention is to increase arousal and alertness, increase functional use of objects, work with a speech-language pathologist to determine the most accurate form of yes/no communication, and be able to follow basic commands. In addition, the occupational therapist is involved in maintaining or restoring ROM to the upper extremities through passive ROM exercises, splinting, and tone management techniques. The occupational therapist will also ensure optimal positioning for seating and maintenance of skin integrity through cushion and wheelchair evaluation. Once a patient emerges from the minimally conscious state, the client will transition out of the emerging consciousness program and become an acute rehabilitation candidate (Fig. 49.3).

Acute rehabilitation begins with an evaluation of the patient that is used in clinical decision making for triage of the client's needs. Goal setting is based on clinical reasoning with direct input from the client and family members. Goals must reflect occupational performance of functional outcomes. Common evaluation tools focused on assessing body functions include basic goniometry for upper extremity ROM; manual muscle testing; and coordination testing, including standardized assessments such as the Moberg Pickup Test, Purdue Pegboard Test, Jebson-Taylor Hand Function Test, and the Minnesota Rate of Manipulation. Sensory testing is performed, and if needed, Semmes-Weinstein filaments can be used for additional detailed sensory assessment. Basic ADLs and IADLs are assessed. Some examples of assessments that are used for ADLs/IADLs are the Kohlman Evaluation of Living Skills, Executive Function Performance Test, Canadian Occupational Performance Measure, and the VALPAR 5 Workstation Analysis. Transfers and functional mobility are assessed, in addition to skin maintenance and seating needs. Visual-perceptual skills are evaluated; some standardized tools that are used include the Motor Free Visual Perceptual Test, the BiVABA, and Dynavision, and nonstandardized assessments for neglect, saccades, acuity, and color perception are also administered. Finally, basic cognitive skills are evaluated with tools such as the Loewenstein Occupational

JFK COMA RECOVERY SCALE - REVISED ©2004
Record Form

This form should only be used in association with the "CRS-R ADMINISTRATION AND SCORING GUIDELINES" which provide instructions for standardized administration of the scale.

| Patient: | | Diagnosis: | | Etiology: |
| Date of Onset: | | Date of Admission: | | |

Date																
Week	ADM	2	3	4	5	6	7	8	9	10	11	12	13	14	15	16
AUDITORY FUNCTION SCALE																
4 - Consistent movement to command*																
3 - Reproducible movement to command*																
2 - Localization to sound																
1 - Auditory startle																
0 - None																
VISUAL FUNCTION SCALE																
5 - Object recognition*																
4 - Object localization: Reaching*																
3 - Visual pursuit*																
2 - Fixation*																
1 - Visual startle																
0 - None																
MOTOR FUNCTION SCALE																
6 - Functional object use†																
5 - Automatic motor response*																
4 - Object manipulation*																
3 - Localization to noxious stimulation*																
2 - Flexion withdrawal																
1 - Abnormal posturing																
0 - None/flaccid																
OROMOTOR/VERBAL FUNCTION SCALE																
3 - Intelligible verbalization*																
2 - Vocalization/oral movement																
1 - Oral reflexive movement																
0 - None																
COMMUNICATION SCALE																
2 - Functional: Accurate†																
1 - Non-functional: Intentional*																
0 - None																
AROUSAL SCALE																
3 - Attention																
2 - Eye opening w/o stimulation																
1 - Eye opening with stimulation																
0 - Unarousable																
TOTAL SCORE																

Denotes emergence from MCS†

Denotes MCS*

Fig. 49.3 JFK Coma Recovery Scale. (Data from Giacino JT, Kalmar K, Whyte J: The JFK Coma Recovery Scale—Revised: measurement characteristics and diagnostic utility, *Arch Phys Med Rehabil* 85:2020–2029, 2004.)

Therapy Cognitive Assessment, Test of Everyday Attention, Contextual Memory Test, and informal assessments such as components of functional task performance.

Once the evaluation is complete, it is the occupational therapist's role to ensure that the client engages in functional activities that promote and maintain optimal upper extremity ROM for later functional tasks. This includes basic self-care tasks along with tone management, splinting, and ROM exercises. Additionally, maintenance of skin integrity is a priority. Many clients with polytrauma have shrapnel wounds, burns, and pressure wounds from bed surfaces, seating surfaces, and splints. It is critical that the occupational therapist work with the medical provider, nursing, and physical therapy to ensure that client has optimal skin integrity and contact surfaces that provide pressure relief.

If sensory impairments are present, they must be addressed for the client to function within the environment. With decreased sensation in areas such as pain, touch, and temperature, the occupational therapist must make sure that the client has training in the use of compensatory strategies for safety. If the patient has hearing loss, it is critical that the therapist face the patient when speaking, speak at a louder volume, or ensure that the client uses appropriate devices to compensate for the hearing loss. Finally, with visual loss, it is important to maintain a clutter-free environment for the client, keep all necessary items and furnishings in the same place at all times, and orient the client for safe functional mobility within the room. The occupational therapist also works closely with the blind rehabilitation outpatient specialist to ensure that client can perform basic ADLs and IADLs by using low-vision or blind rehabilitation techniques and devices.

After these performance components are evaluated, the occupational therapist can focus on basic ADLs. This includes issuance of and training on any assistive devices or durable medical equipment needed to optimize independence. For example, a client may need a long-handled mirror to inspect the skin for wounds or observe a healing amputation site. A client may also require specialized feeding tools such as plate guards or rocker knives for one-handed feeding. In addition, clients may require shower benches or grab bars if balance or mobility issues are present. Part of basic ADL performance includes the ability to get to places safely, such as the toilet or shower. Therefore, the occupational therapist must address any seating and mobility needs for a client who is nonambulatory. A seating evaluation can be performed as part of the wheelchair assessment for a client who is nonambulatory. Wheelchair issuance includes training on safety, training on mobility, and evaluation of visual-perceptual skills for safe propulsion of the chair. Ambulatory clients who have deficits that affect toileting or shower safety because of balance issues or motor planning would also need occupational therapy services. Caregiver training is also initiated with ADL and functional mobility training, and as a client progresses, the training needs to be revised and readdressed.

IADLs are also addressed for this population. It may start with simple meal preparation, basic money management, or simple homemaking skills and progress to higher-level money

management skills; work-, school-, and family care–related skills; time management; and community living skills. It is important to incorporate cognitive retraining and compensatory strategies to optimize independence in these skills. Clients are often issued and trained on the use of cognitive prosthetic tools such as electronic cognitive devices (ECDs), alarm watches, cell phone, and global positioning system (GPS) devices. Use of these tools and the strategies provided for executive skill functions such as pathfinding, problem solving, organization, and planning is then integrated into community reintegration sessions. Community reintegration also includes training on use of public transit, as well as driving rehabilitation.

Many clients who have sustained polytrauma experience PTSD, anxiety, and pain. A polytrauma occupational therapist may initiate training in the use of biofeedback for management of stress, relaxation, and management of pain. Additionally, sleep hygiene is addressed by the occupational therapist in conjunction with psychology services, medical service, and nursing. The client is able to learn and practice these sleep hygiene techniques while in the PRC to support the use of these skills after discharge. Techniques such as deep regular breathing with attention drawn to both inhaling and exhaling can support transition to sleep.

Throughout the inpatient stay, a client with polytrauma may have many medical procedures and additional medical appointments that interrupt the scheduled occupational therapy sessions. These procedures may result in a change in status and thereby necessitate reevaluation and reassessment of the client's

THREADED CASE STUDY

Alex, Part 2

On completion of his inpatient PRC stay, Alex was independent in basic ADLs, transfers, and manual wheelchair mobility on indoor and outdoor surfaces. He was fitted for a prosthetic limb and had achieved functional grip strength in his right hand and sufficient coordination to don and doff the prosthesis. Alex was issued an electronic cognitive device (ECD) to assist in his memory deficits, performance of IADLs, and organizational skills. He still required minimal assistance to perform basic IADLs such as meal preparation, household management, and financial management. With visual-perceptual skill retraining, Alex no longer complained of double vision and was able to identify and reach for targets accurately. With the use of compensatory strategies, such as deep breathing, biofeedback, and sleep hygiene skills, Alex was sleeping well and less anxious, and his tolerance of frustration had improved. Distractibility continued to have a negative impact on his time management skills and ability to follow through with assignments; however, he was able to create a less distracting environment for himself with cueing. His safety awareness improved, although supervision was still required for higher-level judgment and safety. As Alex moved to the Polytrauma Transitional Rehabilitation Program (PTRP), his occupational therapy program continued and progressed in accordance with his stated goals and the inpatient team recommendations. Occupational therapy objectives for the PTRP included (1) promoting the highest level of functional cognition, including implementation of compensatory strategies and cognitive prosthetics to increase independence and safety in all functional skills; (2) achieving optimal independence in IADLs, including parenting skills; (3) optimizing independent ability to access the community, including transportation; (4) optimizing independence in return-to-school and return-to-work skills; and (5) receiving appropriate durable medical equipment to meet both short- and long-term needs.

functional and cognitive status. Updating of goals and priorities must continually be on the forefront as the client's status or the client and family goals change. The families are generally very involved in all aspects of the client's care and are incorporated into the treatment-planning process.

Polytrauma Transitional Rehabilitation Program

The PTRP provides comprehensive, postacute cognitive retraining and community reentry rehabilitation to patients with TBI who have progressed beyond the needs of basic rehabilitation interventions. The goals of this program are to integrate clients back into their community, assist them in achieving independent living, and help them return to their life roles. Not all clients who enter the PTRP have been through a PRC; many are direct referrals from other VA facilities, from Polytrauma Network Sites (PNSs), and from outside private facilities or military treatment facilities. Because these clients have already achieved the goal of basic inpatient rehabilitation, that is, independence in ADLs and basic functional mobility, the focus while involved in the PTRP is on the higher-level skills needed to return to the community. There is more of a cognitive retraining focus with an emphasis on group work and community reentry. The majority of clients reside within the PTRP facility; however, some clients have already transitioned back to the community and come to the facility for the day program.[20]

As is similar with all rehabilitation settings, the occupational therapy program begins with an evaluation of the patient and leads to clinical decision making. Goal setting is based on clinical reasoning, input from the patient and family, and the interdisciplinary team goals. Occupational therapists in the PTRP use many functional nonstandardized evaluation tools, but they also use standardized TBI evaluation tools such as the Mayo-Portland Adaptability Inventory (MPAI-4).[21] The MPAI-4 focuses specifically on the most frequent sequelae to be considered during rehabilitation planning or other clinical interventions, such as physical, cognitive, emotional, behavioral, and social problems. MPAI-4 items also provide an assessment of major obstacles to community integration that may result directly from a brain injury, as well as the environment and context of the activity. With input from other team members, including psychology and neuropsychology, speech-language pathology, and physical therapy personnel, realistic goals and community reintegration training can be initiated.

The occupational therapist addresses a client's ability to participate in basic IADLs such as money management, including establishing banking accounts, budgeting, financial planning, and paying bills. Additional areas addressed include cooking skills, home management and organization, health management and maintenance, child rearing, pet care, safety awareness and emergency responses, and shopping. The use of compensatory strategies and cognitive prosthetics is integral for IADL retraining, especially for clients with disorders in memory and executive functions. Many of these clients are issued and trained on use of an ECD, which is then reinforced throughout all therapies within the program.

Community reintegration training facilitates the client's ability to access the community. This includes training a client on the use of public transit, addressing driving needs, or addressing the client's ability to procure transportation in the community. It also requires the client to learn pathfinding skills, often with the use of a GPS device on a cell phone, and executive skill functions such as trip planning, budgeting, time management, and problem solving. The occupational therapist provides opportunities for practice in using strategies and cognitive prosthetics (such as ECDs, smart phones, or GPSs) to aid the client in becoming successful in this occupational performance area.

Another key component of this rehabilitation program is training and interventions to assist the client in meeting the goals of returning to school and learning. This includes training in basic academic skills such as math, note taking, and general study habits. It also includes exploration of educational needs and interests, some of which may lead to prevocational or vocational participation. The occupational therapist must also address any assistive technology needs such as computer access, ECDs, and specialized software designed to increase ability to succeed in school-based programs.

If return to work is the primary goal for the client, the occupational therapist must assist him or her in gaining the skills needed to return to productive employment or volunteer activities. The occupational therapist may work on goals to identify and select work opportunities based on the client's level of function, as well as likes and dislikes. Occupational therapy services are often provided to retrain the client in how to identify job opportunities, complete and submit appropriate application materials, and prepare for interviewing. Work habits, such as attendance, punctuality, appropriate relationships with co-workers, appropriate dress, completion of assignments, timeliness, and compliance, also must be addressed. The use of cognitive prosthetics is incorporated to assist the client in succeeding in these areas. Finally, the client may not be ready to engage in full-time or even part-time paid employment, and thus volunteer exploration and participation may be the first step in returning to the workforce. The occupational therapist may provide job coaching at the work or volunteer site to identify adaptive or compensatory strategies for successful performance.

Leisure exploration, participation, and social skills also need to be addressed by the occupational therapist to improve a clients' reintegration into the community. Key elements in addressing these skills include social skills groups, practice on appropriate interactions within the milieu or environment, and role-playing with feedback. Peer interaction, both within the program and within the community, as well as family and community interactions, allows greater practice and skill training. Leisure exploration may include administering interest checklists and assessing abilities and opportunities available. It also includes training in the ability to plan for leisure, obtaining and maintaining equipment and supplies, and balancing leisure participation with work and self-care needs. The occupational therapist may work in conjunction with the physical therapist and the recreation therapist to ensure that adaptive sporting equipment and assistive technology are available as needed to best meet the leisure needs of the client.

Stress management also needs to be addressed. Many clients experience stress related to adjusting to their limitations, changes in their life roles and patterns, pain or sleep issues, and PTSD. Biofeedback may be used to aid these clients in learning techniques to decrease overall stress reactions, manage pain, and improve sleep. Sleep hygiene education, as well as various mind-body techniques, can also be introduced and incorporated into this program.

Overall, occupational therapists working in the PTRP have to address all the aforementioned areas in the context of clients' current physical and cognitive abilities while also addressing how to improve their current functional abilities. Any physical limitations such as in ROM, strength, and coordination are addressed to improve functional performance. A client's sensory issues, such as low vision or visual-perceptual skill deficits, must be addressed and compensations incorporated into treatment planning for all the previously mentioned areas of function. Finally, cognitive skills, remediation, and compensation must be addressed to ensure that the patient has an optimal outcome in these areas of function.

As the patient transitions out of the PTRP, the occupational therapist plays a role in helping the patient relocate to appropriate housing, makes recommendations for levels of assistance still needed, addresses caregiver training if required, and ensures that prerequisite skills for the housing option are in place. Any durable medical equipment and environmental modifications needed will be addressed by the occupational therapist.

THREADED CASE STUDY

Alex, Part 3

After 3 months in the PTRP, Alex demonstrated improved integration of his ECD into performance of IADLs. He is now using it for appointment reminders, direction finding, list making, note taking, and medication management, with occasional cueing from the therapist. Although Alex is still unable to drive, he has learned to use the local public transportation system of buses and is able to access restaurants, malls, grocery stores, and specialty stores in the local area. Pathfinding with use of the ECD and GPS on cell phone maps is adequate for familiar areas. Safety awareness has improved, and Alex is now safe to be left alone for long periods, is able to independently access his local community, and demonstrates improved reasoning and insight in decision making/problem solving. Alex is now independent in light hot meal preparation and basic home management tasks such as laundry and cleaning. He began to volunteer part-time in the local preschool program to address work skills and child care skills. Training in the use of biofeedback has continued, and Alex has become more skilled at self-regulation.

As Alex completed the PTRP, he moved home with his pregnant wife and was referred to a Polytrauma Network Site (PNS) for further occupational therapy intervention. The objectives of occupational therapists in the PNS, which were determined by client and family input, as well as the PTRP team recommendations, included (1) promoting the highest level of functional cognition, including implementation of compensatory strategies and cognitive prosthetics to increase independence and safety in all functional skills; (2) achieving optimal independence in IADLs, including parenting skills; (3) maximizing his ability to independently access the community, including transportation; (4) optimizing independence in return-to-school and return-to-work skills; (5) receiving and training on appropriate durable medical equipment to meet both short- and long-term needs; and (6) optimizing independence in the use of stress management and coping skill strategies, including mind-body techniques. At this level of care, the focus shifts to community reentry and return to prior or desired occupations.

Polytrauma Network Sites

PNSs are outpatient clinics that serve two roles. The first is to provide specialized, postacute rehabilitation in consultation with rehabilitation centers. The occupational therapist consults with and provides follow-up based on recommendations made by the inpatient therapists. Depending on the client's current status and outcomes, the client's occupational needs can range from reeducation of caregivers in skilled nursing facilities to seating and mobility needs for returning to school or the workplace. Ambulatory clients who have deficits that affect getting to the toilet or shower safely because of balance issues or motor planning would also need occupational therapy services. Another focus may be on reinforcing the integration of assistive technology and other compensatory techniques for optimal independence in performance skills and patterns. The occupational therapist creates a treatment plan based on the client's needs (environment, client factors, client and family goals, activity demands, and current performance skills), not one that is based on the particular diagnosis. Treatment is provided in the context and environment most appropriate to meet the needs of the client.

A significant increase in the incidence of mild traumatic brain injury (mTBI) has been seen in service members as a result of serving in the OIF/OEF conflicts.[11] There is no standard, agreed-on definition of mTBI. The Department of Veterans Affairs uses the following definition of mTBI in all its TBI screening evaluations: a patient with mTBI is one who has experienced a traumatically induced, physiological disruption of brain function as manifested by at least one of the following[8,22,24,30]:

1. Any period of loss of consciousness
2. Any loss of memory of events immediately before or after the accident
3. Any alteration in mental state at the time of the accident (e.g., feeling dazed, disoriented, or confused)
4. Focal neurological deficit or deficits that may or may not be transient but in which the severity of the injury does not exceed the following:
   a. Loss of consciousness of approximately 30 minutes or less
   b. After 30 minutes, an initial Glasgow Coma Scale score of 13 to 15
   c. Post-traumatic amnesia not longer than 24 hours

Common symptoms of mTBI include headache, dizziness, nausea and vomiting, sleep disturbances, sensitivity to light, sensitivity to noise, slowed processing, memory difficulties, irritability, depression, and visual changes. An individual may experience symptoms at the time of the event or weeks later after the mTBI. The majority of the population who sustain mTBI experience a resolution of symptoms within 3 months.[32] However, 15% to 30% of individuals have ongoing symptoms and are at risk for the development of postconcussive syndrome.[1,29] In postconcussive syndrome, the aforementioned symptoms or clusters of symptoms persist for longer than 3 months.[5]

Postconcussive syndrome can have an impact on outcomes at any stage of polytrauma rehabilitation. Sometimes postconcussive syndrome does not become apparent until many of the life-threatening injuries have been stabilized.[19,30] While in the acute phase of rehabilitation, the symptoms may have an impact on function; however, the focus may be more on the acute injury, not on the persistent postconcussive symptoms. While in the postacute phase, postconcussive symptoms are identified during higher-level functional activities. Patients also can be treated for PTSD when mTBI and postconcussive symptoms are recognized.

Clients who experience multiple blast exposures are at higher risk for more complicated mTBI. This, in conjunction with exposure to stressful environments, increases the risk for mTBI and acute stress reaction/PTSD. This is true for mTBI sustained in automobile accidents in the private sector as well.[4] The stressful environment, multiple exposures, and acute stress reaction/PTSD can have a significant impact on natural recovery from mTBI.

The symptoms of acute stress reaction, depression, and PTSD are very similar to those of mTBI/postconcussive syndrome and can include difficulties in memory and concentration, sleep problems, impaired attention, irritability, and headache. The best approach for identifying the cause of the various symptoms is to incorporate the treatment team. The PNS uses an interdisciplinary team model to determine the most likely cause of the deficits and the most appropriate treatment to address the symptoms (Fig. 49.4).

When the PNS system was developed in 2007, there were no standards for rehabilitative treatment of mTBI. As this diagnosis became so prevalent from the OIF/OEF conflict, the Department of Defense and the Department of Veterans Affairs developed best-practice guidelines.[11] Additionally, an occupational therapy– and physical therapy–specific guideline was developed by the Propenency Office for Rehabilitation and Reintegration (OT/PT: Clinical Practice Guidance: Occupational Therapy and Physical Therapy for Mild Traumatic Brain Injury). The clinical guidance document recommended treatments focused on client education, visual dysfunction, headache, cognition, resumption of roles, and emotional well-being.

Studies show that mTBI needs to be approached and treated differently from moderate or severe TBI. The goal is to increase awareness of deficits in those with more severe TBI, whereas with mTBI, studies have shown that focusing on abilities, stress management/coping skills, and compensatory strategies improves outcomes.[b] Clients with mTBI tend to be overly sensitive to errors and have decreased perceived self-efficacy, which can lead to decreased self-esteem, depression, and isolation. These factors can affect return to life roles and community reintegration. Clients may be able to follow through with routine and familiar tasks yet may demonstrate difficulty in problem solving, insight, and self-control.[26]

Occupational therapists working in the PNS system start the initial interaction with the client during the evaluation. This includes the use of standardized assessments, self-report tools, and observation of performance of functional tasks. The therapist also provides visual-perceptual screening because visual deficits are frequently seen in clients exposed to multiple blasts. From that screening, the therapist can then refer the client for further assessments as needed. The evaluation also includes screening for ADL needs, cognitive deficits, current use of assistive technologies, home modification needs, home management skills, organizational skills, predriving skills, physical rehabilitation needs, emotional regulation, sleep hygiene, pain, headache, and relaxation skills. Additionally, the occupational therapist will address current needs in relation to study skills, vocational needs, community reentry skills, return and transition to life roles (including follow-through with entering school, the workforce, or both), managing a household for the first time, higher-level money management, and parenting skills.

The therapist focuses on client goals in relation to activity demands and any deficits identified. The therapist will address the aforementioned areas by intervention consisting of remediation techniques and training in compensatory strategies, assistive technology, and biofeedback/mind-body techniques. This may include removing distractions, creating routines, and integrating self-awareness training tools. Client education is also an integral part of treatment. Client education may consist of discussing the effects of mTBI, expected outcomes, and how typical stressful situations and sleep problems can have an impact on function. Within the context of this education, the therapist must provide guidance on strategies for increasing insight, using compensatory mechanisms, and achieving effectiveness in participation in desired occupations. Overall, it has been documented that outcomes are better for mTBI when clients receive adequate education.[25,28]

Because the PNS works with many returning service members who bring combat driving skills to the civilian environment, their safety in driving skills must be assessed. Such driving skills include attention, multitasking ability, reaction speed, and visual-perceptual skills, as well as addressing stress reactions and hypervigilance. Many soldiers avoid driving or rely on others for assistance. Occupational therapists address predriving skills by assessing and remediating performance components. The VA has therapists who are driving rehabilitation specialists. These specialists are trained to evaluate this population by working both with driving simulators and behind the wheel. They also can provide driver's training and adaptive controls or vehicles as indicated.

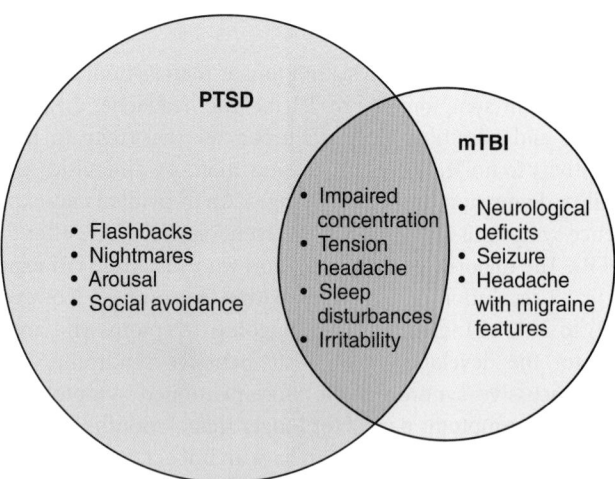

Fig. 49.4 Common symptoms of mTBI and PTSD. (From Ruff RL, Riechers RG, Ruff SS: Relationships between mild traumatic brain injury sustained in combat and post-traumatic stress disorder. *F1000 Med Rep* 2:64, 2010 [government publication].)

[b] References 3, 6, 8, 27, 33, 37.

Alex, Part 4

Alex was initially evaluated by the occupational therapist at the PNS on a weekly basis and then once a month. Alex's primary concern on initial PNS evaluation was the upcoming arrival of his baby. Although some child care skills were addressed during his volunteer experience, he was unsure of how to care for a newborn, combined with the stressors of lack of sleep, poor tolerance of frustration, and distractibility. Trial and training with a programmable infant simulator were successful in the integration of self-regulating strategies and ECD use and increased his confidence in his abilities. After training on the use of GPS, a feature on his cell phone, Alex is able to navigate in unfamiliar areas with confidence. He also completed a driver's rehabilitation program and has been cleared to drive independently. Alex has enjoyed his volunteer experience and has identified teaching as a vocational goal. He is now taking one course per semester at the local community college and is implementing the study skills taught during his PNS sessions.

Monthly, Alex brings in a list of difficulties identified (tracked in his ECD) in work, home care, and child care, and he works with the occupational therapist to further address these needs. At the 1-year postinjury mark, Alex reports that he has a well-balanced life with volunteering, school, family, and social/leisure activities.

The PNS as a team is tasked to monitor and follow clients' needs for their lifetime. These network sites provide proactive case management for existing and emerging conditions and identify local resources for both VA and non-VA care.

Long-Term Management/Polytrauma Support Clinic Teams

Long-term polytrauma management is accomplished in clients' home community, where they are monitored by either the PNS or Polytrauma Support Clinic Teams. These teams are groups of rehabilitation providers who deliver follow-up services in consultation with regional and network specialists. They assist in managing the long-term effects of polytrauma through direct care, consultation, and the use of tele-rehabilitation technologies, as needed. Polytrauma telehealth is a burgeoning field in rehabilitation. Telehealth is the use of electronic information and telecommunications technologies to support long-distance clinical healthcare, client and professional health-related education, public health, and health administration.

Technologies used in telehealth typically consist of videoconferencing, internet-based video applications, store-and-forward imaging, streaming media, and wireless communications. As technology and telehealth use become an integral part of daily healthcare practice, there still remain barriers for some clients. The occupational therapist's role in telehealth is either as a presenter, consultant, or direct care provider.

The Polytrauma System of Care encompasses all the programs described earlier and ensures that there is a smooth, seamless continuum of care for these clients, including case management for life.

SUMMARY

Polytrauma can result in substantial impairments that affect all areas of occupation. The injuries can vary from mild to severe and can include multiple body systems and affect performance skills and patterns. When treating these clients a therapist must take into consideration the specific client factors and the context and environment in which activities will occur. The goal of occupational therapy is to facilitate the client's achievement of optimal independence and functioning at each stage of recovery. Polytrauma affects the entire family unit, and thus rehabilitation goals must be client and family centered and coordinated and reinforced by all those working with the client.

REVIEW QUESTIONS

1. What is the definition of polytrauma?
2. Differentiate among primary, secondary, tertiary, and quaternary blast injury?
3. What are some common sequelae of polytrauma?
4. What makes a polytrauma patient from the OIF/OEF conflict unique in today's rehabilitation population?
5. In the inpatient/acute unit, what primarily drives the rehabilitation course?
6. Why is an interdisciplinary team more effective than siloed care in treating polytrauma patients?
7. What are the common symptoms of and interventions for mTBI and PTSD?
8. What are the roles and treatment interventions for occupational therapists in treating an emerging consciousness patient?
9. How does the focus of treatment change as the patient progresses through the Polytrauma System of Care?
10. How does PTSD affect the recovery process for a patient with polytrauma?

For additional practice questions for this chapter, please visit eBooks.Health.Elsevier.com.

REFERENCES

1. Alves WC, Colohan A, O'Leary T, et al: Understanding posttraumatic symptoms after minor head injury, *J Head Trauma Rehabil* 1(2):1–12, 1986.
2. American Congress of Rehabilitation Medicine: Recommendations for the use of uniform nomenclature pertinent to patients with severe alterations of consciousness, *Arch Phys Med Rehabil* 76:205–209, 1995.
3. American Occupational Therapy Association: Occupational therapy practice framework: domain and process, 4th Edition edition, Am J Occup Ther 2020;74 (Suppl 2): 7412410010 p1–7412410010p87. https://doi.org/10.5014/ajot.2020.74S2001
4. Bryant RA, Harvey AG: Post-concussive symptoms and post-traumatic stress disorder after mild traumatic brain injury, *J Nerv Mental Dis* 187(5):302–305, 1999.
5. Carroll LJ, Cassidy JD, Peloso PM, et al: Prognosis for mild traumatic brain injury: results of the WHO Collaborating Central Task Force on Mild Traumatic Brain Injury, *J Rehabil Med* 43:84–105, 2004.
6. Cicerone KD, Kalmar K: Persistent postconcussion syndrome: the structure of subjective complaints after mild traumatic brain injury, *J Head Trauma Rehabil* 11:1–17, 1995.
7. Darkins A, Cruise C, Armstrong M, et al: Enhancing access of combat wounded veterans to specialist rehabilitation services: the VA Polytrauma Telehealth Network, *Arch Phys Med Rehabil* 89:182–187, 2008.
8. Defense and Veterans Brain Injury Center: *DVBIC Working Group on the Acute Management of Mild Traumatic Brain Injury in the Military Operational Settings: Clinical Guideline and Recommendations*, Silver Spring, Md., 2006, DVBIC.
9. DePalma RG, Burris DG, Champion HR, Hodgson MJ: Blast injuries, *N Engl J Med* 352:1335–1342, 2005.
10. Department of Veterans Affairs: *Polytrauma Rehabilitation Procedures*, Washington DC, 2005, Department of Veterans Affairs.
11. Department of Veterans Affairs and Department of Defense: VA/DoD clinical practice guideline for management of concussion/mild traumatic brain injury, Washington, DC, 2009, VA/DoD Evidenced Based Practice.
12. Directive from Department of Defense: (2009). *Screening and Evaluation of Possible Traumatic Brain Injury in Operation Enduring Freedom (OEF) and Operation Iraqi Freedom (OIF) Veterans*, Washington, DC, 2009.
13. Elsayed NM: Toxicology of blast overpressure, *Toxicology* 121:1–15, 1997.
14. Giacino J, Kalma K: *Coma Recovery Scale–Revised*, 2006, The Center for Outcome Measurement in Brain Injury. Retrieved April 28, 2010. Available at: http://www.tbims.org/combi/crs.
15. Giacino JT, Kezmarsky MA, DeLuca J, Cicerone KD: Monitoring rate of recovery to predict outcome in minimally responsive patients, *Arch Phys Med Rehabil* 72:897–901, 1991.
16. Golisz K: *Neurorehabilitation in Traumatic Brain Injury. Self-Paced Clinical Course Series, American Occupational Therapy Association*, Bethesda, Md., 2009, AOTA.
17. Hagan CM: *The Rancho Level of Cognitive Functioning: the Revised Levels*, ed 3, Downey, Calif, 1998, Los Amigos Research and Educational Institute.
18. Harvey AG, Bryant RA: The relationship between acute stress disorder and post traumatic stress disorder following motor vehicle accidents, *J Consult Clin Psychol* 66:507–512, 1998.
19. Helmick K: Cognitive rehabilitation for military personnel with mild traumatic brain injury and chronic post-concussive disorder: results of April 2009 consensus conference, *NeuroRehabilitation* 26:239–255, 2010.
20. Klonoff PS, Lamb DG, Henderson SW: Milieu-based neurorehabilitation in patients with traumatic brain injury: outcome at up to 11 years postdischarge, *Arch Phys Med Rehabil* 81:1535–1537, 2000.
21. Malec J: The Mayo-Portland Adaptability Inventory, 2005, The Center for Outcome Measurement in Brain Injury. Available at: http://www.tbims.org/combi/mpai.
22. Mateer CA, Sira CS, O'Connell ME: Putting Humpty Dumpty back together again: the importance of integrating cognitive and emotional interventions, *J Head Trauma Rehabil* 20:62–75, 2005.
23. Mayorga MA: The pathology of primary blast overpressure injury, *Toxicology* 121:17–28, 1997.
24. Mild Traumatic Brain Injury Interdisciplinary Special Interest Group of the American Congress of Rehabilitation Medicine: Definition of mild traumatic brain injury, *J Head Trauma Rehabil* 8:86-87, 1993.
25. Mittenberg W, Tremont G, Zielinski RE, et al: Cognitive-behavioral prevention of post-concussive syndrome, *Arch Clin Neuropsychol* 11:139–145, 1996.
26. Montgomery SA: Managing depression in the community, *Professional Nurse* 10(12):805–807, 1995.
27. OT/PT MTBI Work Team; Bolgla RD: Clinical practice guidance: occupational therapy and physical therapy for mild traumatic brain injury, 2007, Office of the Surgeon General, Washington, D.C.
28. Ponsford J: Rehabilitation interventions after mild head injury, *Curr Opin Neurol* 18:692–697, 2005.
29. Ponsford J, Willmott C, Rothwell A, et al: Factors influencing outcome following mild traumatic brain injury in adults, *J Int Neuropsychol Soc* 6:568–579, 2000.
30. Radomski MV, Davidson L, Voydetich D, Erickson MW: Occupational therapy for service members with mild traumatic brain injury, *Am J Occup Ther* 63:646–655, 2009.
31. Rappaport M, Dougherty AM, Kelting DL: Evaluation of coma and vegetative states, *Arch Phys Med Rehabil* 73:628–634, 1992.
32. Ruff R: Two decades of advances in understanding of mild traumatic brain injury, *J Head Trauma Rehabil* 20:5–18, 2005.
33. Ruff RM, Camenzuli L, Mueller J: Miserable minority: emotional risk factors that influence the outcome of a mild traumatic brain injury, *Brain Inj* 10:551–565, 1996.
34. Schnurr PP, Kaloupek D, Sayer N: Understanding the impact of the wars in Iraq and Afghanistan, *Journal of Stress* 23:3–4, 2010.
35. Smits SJ, Falconer JA, Herrin J, et al: Patient-focused rehabilitation team cohesiveness in Veterans Administration hospitals, *Arch Phys Med Rehabil* 84:1332–1338, 2003.
36. Strasser DC, Uomoto JM, Smits SJ: The interdisciplinary team and polytrauma rehabilitation: prescription for partnership, *Arch Phys Med Rehabil* 89:179–181, 2008.
37. Tipton-Burton M: Traumatic brain injury. In Pendleton H, Schultz-Krohn W, editors: *Pedretti's Occupational Therapy Practice Skills for Physical Dysfunction*, St. Louis, 2006, Mosby.

50

Occupational Therapy in Hospice and Palliative Care

Janice Kishi Chow

LEARNING OBJECTIVES

After studying this chapter, the student or practitioner will be able to do the following:

1. Define hospice and palliative care.
2. Explain the therapeutic value of occupational participation while living with a life-threatening illness.
3. Describe the role of occupational therapy in hospice and palliative care within the Occupational Therapy Practice Framework (OTPF-4).[5]
4. Discuss how professional reasoning adjusts to accommodate the dying process.
5. Identify outcome measures for hospice and palliative occupational therapy.
6. Articulate strategies for practitioner self-care.

CHAPTER OUTLINE

KEY TERMS

Actively dying
Chronic disease/Chronic illness
Dying trajectories
Grief/Grieving process
Hospice
Loss

Palliative/Palliative care
Practitioner self-care
Terminal Phase
Terminal/Terminal illness
Transitions/Transitioning

THREADED CASE STUDY

Kay

Kay watched Dr. Kato's lips move. "You have pancreatic cancer. . ." The movement of his mouth didn't seem to match the sounds she heard. "with liver metastasis and biliary duct obstruction. . . ." Kay slowly turned to watch her daughter frantically write down every word. Dr. Kato further explained that surgery was not indicated given the extent of metastasis—the cancer's spread to multiple organs, but palliative chemotherapy may slow the growth of the tumors and a stent in her biliwary duct could reduce her jaundice. These procedures would lessen her symptoms but were not curative. Dr. Kato paused and then said, "You have a **terminal** disease and probably 6 months or less to live." Her daughter's pen froze in place. As they recalibrated their gaze upon Dr. Kato, he suggested hospice to support Kay and her family during this difficult time.

Kay followed through with the recommended treatment plan in disbelief. Divorced at age 50, Kay worked long hours as a housecleaner to support herself and four children until her retirement at age 62. At 82, she highly valued being able to take care of herself and remained fiercely independent. Kay enjoyed spending time with family and friends, attending church on Sundays, participating in a weekly Bible study, traveling, and cooking for others. "I can't be dying," she would say to herself, "I have plans to travel, see the grandkids married, and be a great-grandmother!"

Within 3 months of her diagnosis, Kay began experiencing increased fatigue, weakness, and abdominal discomfort. The hospice nurse and physician adjusted her medications to control her pain, but she became frustrated not being able

Continued

Kay

to maintain her self-care routines. Each day, she was less able to do for herself. An unspoken realization arose within her and her family that she would not get better and now required more help. Her children and grandchildren assisted with homemaking, financial affairs, and transportation, but Kay insisted on attending to her own bathing, dressing, and toileting as much as possible. She compromised by moving in with her eldest daughter to get assistance as needed. Seeing Kay's angst to remain as independent as possible, the hospice team consulted occupational therapy services.

Critical Thinking Questions

1. Is the hospice team appropriately consulting occupational therapy services for someone who is declining and dying?
2. How will the occupational therapist help Kay meet her goals as she continues to decline?
3. How will the occupational therapist know if the intervention is effective?

Kay is one of 1.49 million Medicare beneficiaries who receive hospice, or end-of-life care, annually.[99] In addition, an estimated 133 million Americans live with a chronic disease, or an incurable illness not yet in the end-stages of the disease process.[29,44,97] With our geriatric population tripled in the last 50 years and expected to triple again in the next 50 years,[125] there will foreseeably be more people living longer with chronic conditions[29] but dying with more complex disease processes.[32] The needs of those with incurable illness, chronic or terminal, will increase exponentially.

What is occupational therapy's role in addressing this crisis? Is occupational therapy, a profession known for promoting health and well-being through occupation participation, effective with people who are declining and dying? This chapter will provide a background on hospice and palliative care, present the evidence-base for hospice and palliative care occupational therapy (OT), describe the role of occupational therapy with this population within the parameters of the fourth edition of the Occupational Therapy Practice Framework (OTPF-4), and recommend strategies to support ongoing quality care.[5]

HOSPICE AND PALLIATIVE CARE

Derived from two Latin words—*hospis*, for both host and guest, and *hospitium*, for the dwelling offering hospitality[34,100]—hospice initially referred to monastery-based hostels during the 11th to 15th centuries set up throughout Europe along pilgrim routes to provide shelter for weary travelers, the poor, and the sick as they sojourned to sacred places.[7,34,105,117] When religious orders lost their influence and the monasteries ceased to exist in Britain, the number of hospices waned for three to four centuries.[84,105]

From the 17th century, there was a resurgence of hospice care. In 1633, St. Vincent De Paul founded the Sisters of Charity in Paris to care for the orphaned, sick, and dying in the community.[34] In 1842, Madame Jeanne Garnier further defined hospice by first using the term *hospice* to specifically describe care for the dying.[7,34] In 1879, the Irish Sisters of Charity opened Our Lady's Hospice of Dublin, which expanded to England with the opening of St. Joseph's in 1905 in London.[7,100]

As hospice care developed, the mid-20th century brought advances in modern medicine. The discovery of antibiotics and the development of cardiopulmonary resuscitation brought hope that certain fatal illness could be cured.[19,44] Healthcare shifted from a model of healing to a biomedical culture focused on cure and the elimination of disease.[19,44] Health became defined "as the absence of disease."[122] Those living with an incurable, terminal disease, however, were ignored and marginalized as failures of medical advances within this new model of healthcare.[19,44]

In response to the neglected needs of the terminally ill, Dr. Cicely Saunders opened the first modern hospice, St. Christopher's Hospice, in South London in 1967.[19,44] Radically different from previous hospice centers, Saunders based St. Christopher's Hospice on solid research. Dr. Saunders was a strong opponent of euthanasia and desired to find effective pain management options so patients could live fully until the end of their lives.[56] Defying conventional fears of addiction and practice of using opioids only as a "last resort," she integrated evidence on the effective use of opioids for pain management with a fixed scheduled dosing regimen to promote pain control rather than dosing only as pain occurred.[19] Based on her own research of 340 cases in 1960 and 1100 in 1967, Saunders defined "total pain" as the integral relationship between physical, mental, and spiritual suffering and gathered an interdisciplinary team to provide medical, psychosocial, and spiritual support through the dying process.[19,100]

Soon, the modern hospice movement came to the United States. In 1975, the first U.S. hospices opened in Connecticut and New York, funded by grants and contributions.[44] In 1982, U.S. Congress passed the landmark Medicare Hospice Benefit, providing federally funded home hospice care.[20,98] Today, Medicare-funded hospice care is defined as noncurative comfort care and psychosocial support for those with a life expectancy of 6 months or less.[13] In 2017, there were 4515 Medicare-certified hospices, spanning all 50 U.S. states and the District of Columbia.[97] Approximately 48% of hospice care is provided in the patient's home, 31.8% in a nursing facility (nursing facilities, assisted living facilities, and long-term care facilities), 11.2% in an inpatient hospice facility, and 7% in an acute care hospital.[99]

As the needs of the terminally ill were gradually being addressed, the needs of the chronically ill became more apparent.[44] Palliative care subsequently formed to help alleviate suffering of those with life-limiting illness not yet in the terminal or end-stages of the disease process.[44] Both hospice and palliative care affirm life, see dying as a normal process, seek to provide relief from pain and distressing symptoms, help patients remain as active as possible until death, and provide support to both patient and family.[1,96,131] Palliative care, however, can be used at any stage of the disease process and in conjunction with curative treatments, whereas hospice is a specialty of palliative care, reserved for the last 6 months of life.[1,13,96]

When Kay considered her doctor's recommendations for hospice, she wondered if she would die faster while on hospice care as opposed to pursuing aggressive treatments. Using retrospective statistical analysis of 4993 patients, Conner et al.[21] compared the mean survival rate of hospice patients with non-hospice patients with congestive heart failure as well as colon, lung, pancreatic, prostate, and breast cancers at similar stages of illness. The mean survival rate of the six diagnoses combined revealed that hospice patients lived an average of 29 days longer than nonhospice patients who pursued curative treatments.[21] Ternel et al.[121] found that patients with lung cancer who received palliative care in the early stages of their disease process lived 2.7 months longer and reported lower rates of depression than lung cancer patients who waited until the end stages.[121] Hoerger et al. noted in a meta-analysis of randomized controlled trials comparing outpatient specialty palliative care with usual care of adults with advanced cancer, patients in an outpatient specialty palliative care program lived 4.56 months longer and reported greater quality of life in comparison to controls.[47] Wang et al. found patients who enrolled early in home-based palliative care had fewer hospitalizations and skilled nursing facility stays and more time at home in the last 6 months of life than patients who received only home hospice or no hospice care.[128] Researchers speculate patients at the end of life may live longer because of avoidance of aggressive cure-directed interventions that carry a high mortality risk for debilitated patients (i.e., high-dose chemotherapy), improved treatment monitoring, increased social support amongst the multidisciplinary team, and early symptom management stabilizing the disease process.[21,121]

Based on this current evidence and given the extensiveness of her disease process, Kay may even live longer and have a better quality of life with early symptom management and hospice care. Her doctor exemplifies how health providers need to understand the benefits of hospice and palliative care. Knowing about local services, initiating discussions about end-of-life issues and making timely referrals may promote early symptom management, increase psychosocial support, minimize needless suffering, and support the utmost quality of life at the end of life.

EVIDENCE BASE FOR OCCUPATIONAL THERAPY SERVICES

Kay's daughter wanted to support her mother's independence and ability to do things that mattered to her, but her mother was dying. *Is there evidence that occupational therapy is effective with someone like her mother?*

Occupational participation at the end of life may provide "a means of self-expression and engagement while serving as a vehicle by which the client finds peace with the dying process."[4] Studies by Jacques and Hasselkus,[54] Lala and Kinsella,[73] Lyons et al.,[85] Vrkljian and Miller-Polgar,[127] and Sviden et al.[118] highlight the therapeutic value of occupational participation while living with a life-threatening illness and infer the need for occupational therapy in hospice and palliative care. Based on qualitative design methods, semi-structured interviews, and participant observations, these studies found disengagement in valued occupations led to loss of control, sense of helplessness,

and disruption of self-identity.[73,127] However, with occupational participation, participants experienced a sense of normalcy, restoration, health, well-being, and pleasure.[54,73,85,118,127] This research establishes occupational participation at the end of life is essential to remain engaged in life and have quality of life at the end of life.

Occupational therapy practitioners uniquely support occupational participation at the end of life, supporting both life engagement and preparation for death.[45] Through consideration of meaningful occupations, contexts, performance patterns and skills, and client factors, occupational therapy practitioners affirm life[45] by maximizing occupational performance with available supports and abilities.[4,45,119] Common interventions include collaborative goal setting based on functional changes through the disease process, prioritization of valued activities, activities of daily living retraining,[103] environmental modification,[62] fatigue and stress management,[80,90] caregiver training,[59] leisure activities,[101] creative arts,[71] and introduction of new occupations when the client is unable to satisfactorily participate in established occupations.[85] While affirming life, practitioners also prepare clients and their families for death[45] through facilitation of end-of-life discussions,[4] life review,[111] legacy making and transmission,[52] and closure (e.g., putting affairs into order, reconciling estranged relationships, and saying goodbye).[4] Balancing both life affirmation and preparation for death, occupational therapists play a key role in helping clients experience quality of life at the end of life.

Unfortunately, occupational therapy remains underused in end-of-life care. Decision makers, such as referring physicians and nurses, frequently deem OT services as unnecessary because of their patient's assumed decline.[9,85,113,132] Despite literature showing people with incurable diseases desire rehabilitative services to address their unmet occupational engagement needs,[61,113,132] the terminally ill are not seen as "proactive, occupational beings . . . who engage purposefully in occupations as part of living with a life-threatening illness."[85] Within the Hospice Medicare Benefit, Medicare also narrowly views occupational therapy's role as "providing adaptive equipment training, home safety assessment, and caregiver instruction for safe body mechanics."[14] Many end-of-life care decision makers do not realize their patient's unique occupational needs nor understand the range of services occupational therapists can offer beyond equipment issue and caregiver training. Occupational therapy is not being used to its fullest capacity to support the needs of people living with chronic and terminal illness.

Weakening occupational therapy's cause further, there is a paucity of evidence supporting the efficacy of occupational therapy in hospice and palliative care. There are a limited number of outcome studies with small sample sizes demonstrating the use of occupational therapy to increase participation in self-care tasks,[59,78,101,103] to teach fatigue management,[80] and facilitate life review.[111] However, there is currently no high-level evidence study that generalizes the value of occupational participation and the efficacy of occupational therapy intervention at the end of life.[63] Some researchers speculate the limited body of evidence may be due to the difficulty ascertaining occupational therapy-specific outcomes from the outcomes of the interdisciplinary palliative care team[33,89] and the ethical issues of research as a patient's symptoms worsen.[132,133] Cyclical in nature, lack of evidence results in lack of funding and workforce, further reducing therapeutic efficacy.[43,62]

Despite the lack of evidence supporting the use of occupational therapy in hospice and palliative care, the hospice team had already seen positive occupational therapy outcomes with previous patients. Kay's hospice team knew occupational therapy is effective not only with equipment issues and caregiver training but also with problem-solving innovative ways to help people "do what is important." Regardless of Kay's prognosis, her declining function, and ample help, an occupational therapy consult was highly appropriate to uphold what Kay found meaningful. Upon receiving a doctor's referral, Tess, an occupational therapist, called Kay to arrange an initial visit.

ROLE OF OCCUPATIONAL THERAPY

What would Tess's role be in Kay's care? Similar to other areas of care, hospice and palliative occupational therapy seeks to promote health and well-being through participation in meaningful occupation, yet distinguishes itself with specialized knowledge of the grieving process, dying trajectories, and the terminal phase of life. Integration of these factors with the domain and process of the Occupational Therapy Performance Framework (OTPF-4) shapes the unique role and purpose of occupational therapy in the care of those living with life-threatening disease.[5]

The Grieving Process

Central to working with Kay is understanding how she is responding to the loss of her life. Rando defines two types of loss: physical and symbolic loss.[106] Physical loss is tangible, such as Kay's loss of strength and ability to care for herself. Symbolic loss relates to psychosocial significance such as her consequent loss of independence, self-reliance, and privacy.

Grief is a normal, universal, individualized, and emotional reaction to loss.[69,105] Anticipatory grief can also occur in expectation of eventual loss.[69] Grief responses may be culturally and socially defined and expressed in social, physical, cognitive, spiritual, psychological, and emotional behaviors.[69,107] Expression about loss may be directly articulated ("I am angry that I am dying") or wrapped up in an indirect symbolic language ("I am angry that my wheelchair does not work properly").[70,106] It is essential that Tess identifies Kay's losses, both physical and symbolic, and the meaning Kay assigns to these losses to fully support her grieving process.[70,106]

Kübler-Ross's Five Stages of Grief Model remains the best-known and most frequently cited theory on the grieving process.[70,116] Although research refutes sequential progression through all stages or the generalization of experiencing any of the stages,[48] Kübler-Ross's Five Stages (denial, anger, bargaining, depression, and acceptance) provide a framework for practitioners to understand the dynamic process clients and their loved ones may experience through disease progression and dying.

Tess had yet to meet and assess Kay, but she had experience working with clients at different stages of the grieving process. In **denial** of being in the end-stages of heart disease, Paul, one of Tess's clients, vehemently declined OT services because he "was taking care of himself fine." Unfortunately, it took a collapse at home for him to accept that he indeed was ill and needed help. Simona, another client, readily accepted OT services but constantly lashed out in **anger** at Tess for not fully addressing and "fixing" her functional limitations rather than acknowledging that her cancer was progressing. **Bargaining** for more time, Bob followed all of Tess's recommendations with great fervor. Tess had to gently and repeatedly explain that therapy would help make the most of today but would not cure him. Seeing his situation as futile, Kevin remained tethered by **depression** and refused any of Tess's interventions despite potential for some gains in occupational participation. Realizing her disease was progressing, Joan was in **acceptance** that she was dying. She knew occupational therapy would not cure her but remained open to Tess's visit to maximize her ability to transfer to a wheelchair so she could sit out on her porch. When Joan transitioned toward the end stages of the dying process and became unable to get out of bed, she positively reflected on being able to sit out in the sun for a few days and was at peace ending OT services.

Initially, Kay was in denial of her illness. As symptoms began to affect her daily life, she became angry with God that she was sick and would likely not see her great-grandchildren born. Her anger sapped her energy further. She prayed for God to save her, but as she became more ill, she began to accept she was dying. When Tess contacted her, Kay thought she had nothing to gain, but perhaps nothing to lose, working with an occupational therapist. She agreed to meet Tess later that week.

Dying Trajectories

Although there are uncertainties regarding when people will die, there are some evidence-based patterns, or *dying trajectories*, which describe common changes in functional status as the patient approaches death. Lunney et al. interviewed 4190 U.S. patients and caregivers before death and identified four common trajectories of dying: sudden or unexpected death trajectory, the chronic organ failure trajectory, the dementia/frailty trajectory, and the cancer trajectory.[83] Knowledge of established dying trajectories helps guide and suggest appropriate and timely interventions.

Sudden or unexpected death may be due to trauma, cardiac arrest, or a cerebral vascular accident.[44] Practitioners are unable to provide treatment for the deceased, but they may be able to make referrals or recommendations for bereavement support as indicated for the family and friends. Grief may be complicated by violence, lack of making amends before death, or inability to say a final goodbye. Survivors may have emotional, financial, or psychosocial dependence on the deceased. Caregivers may be lost without their caregiving roles. Bereavement support draws upon the multidisciplinary team and may include counseling services, social services, support groups, and training in life skills for role transitions into a new period of their lives. Occupational therapists may support the bereaved in taking on roles the deceased assumed, developing new skills and routines, and exploring new roles.[4]

The *chronic organ failure trajectory* applies to conditions such as heart failure and chronic obstructive pulmonary disease

(COPD) and is characterized by decline with an oscillating, or sine-wave pattern, between chronic health and acute exacerbations.[44,94,112] The span of decline can be 2 to 5 years, with low health status in the last 6 to 24 months and significant decline in the last three months.[44,94] Morgan et al. more specifically noted patients often have a period of sharp functional decline within the last 14 days before death, similar to cancer patients as described later.[93] With each acute event, patients have a functional dip and a period of recovery; however, patients typically do not return to their previous baseline.[93] Occupational and physical therapists may be consulted to rehabilitate only to have the patient quickly readmitted for another rehabilitation course after a sequential exacerbation. Although patients may have gains after medical intervention and return home, the cumulative effect is an overall functional decline. Each acute event also has a risk of death; despite long-term functional decline, death may still seem "sudden."[94] Patients often struggle to provide a narrative about their disease process,[65] have difficulty speaking about death,[108] and prefer to focus instead on maintaining function.[108] Houben et al. observed that physicians frequently saw exacerbations in the disease process as signs of decline but deferred speaking about dying out of desire to maintain a patient's hope.[50] Consequently, patients with chronic organ failure may highly benefit from a palliative care referral early in the disease process to prepare the patient and family, initiate end-of-life care planning, and provide psychosocial support.[44,82]

People who do not develop organ failure or cancer often develop dementia or generalized frailty of multiple body systems.[44,94] Dementia is typically characterized by gradual cognitive and functional decline, while frailty is defined by weakness, weight loss, fatigue, slowed performance, and low activity.[38] The *dementia/frailty trajectory* is a progressive decline that begins at a low baseline of cognitive or physical function and may be variable and unpredictable over six to eight years.[94] General decline often leads to inability to recover from trivial illnesses.[38,94] Death may soon follow an acute event such as a femoral neck fracture, pneumonia, infections, or an aspiration.[38,91,94,110]

Although the dementia/frailty trajectory may be long and slow, there remains great complexity in end-of-life care needs. In a qualitative, serial interview study, Lloyd et al. observed that people with frailty frequently sustained well-being through maintaining a sense of self but reported greater fear of losing self-identity and being institutionalized than the fear of death.[81] Morgan et al. found patients with dementia were typically at a lower functional status and a slower rate of decline 120 days before death than patients with cancer and chronic organ failure, underscoring patients and caregivers need support sooner and longer.[93] Hoveland and Mallette (2020) found people with dementia in the last weeks of life frequently had a drastic decline in self-care function, were unable to recognize their caregiver, and exhibited behavioral and psychological changes such as fear, paranoia, confusion, verbal and physical aggression, and deathbed visions.[51] Mitchell et al. found that of 323 nursing home residents with dementia, 40% of the residents endured at least one burdensome intervention in the last 3 months of life such as a hospitalization, tube feeding, or parenteral therapy, whereas residents with proxies who understood the resident's poor prognosis and dementia/frailty trajectory were less likely to have burdensome interventions in the last 3 months.[91] Given the lengthy period of decline of these chronic conditions, palliative care is essential to control pain and other negative symptoms, maximize functional status, connect patients and caregivers with social and community supports, educate patients and their families on the disease and dying process, and initiate discussions and care planning to support the patient's autonomy and avoid burdensome interventions at the end of life.[11,30,38,91,110]

The *cancer trajectory* is a more predictable pattern than the chronic organ and dementia/frailty trajectories.[44,94] Many cancer patients may remain quite functional until 5 to 6 months before death.[44] In the last 2 to 3 months, patients may experience weight loss, decline in self-care performance, and need for increased pain management.[44,94] Morgan et al. noted that cancer patients were often at a higher level of function 120 days before death in comparison to patients with neurological conditions or dementia but had a steeper decline in the last 14 to 22 days of life.[93] During the rapid decline phase, patients often become bedfast and typically die within a few months to weeks.[37,44,94] People with cancer frequently balance a hope of being cured with a fear of death[65,95] and often desire to have effective pain management, maximize function to lessen the care burden on their family, prepare loved ones for their death, put affairs into order, leave a legacy, and die at home.[66] They commonly have a clear disease narrative, being able to account for specific details about their disease management and progression.[65,95] Murray et al. observed lung cancer patients had marked psychological and spiritual distress experience at key disease transition points—diagnosis, discharge from treatment, disease progression, and the terminal stage.[95] Given both the physical and psychosocial needs along the entire trajectory, it is important to refer patients with cancer at the beginning of the disease process to provide holistic support for the patient and family.

Because the hospice nurse reported Kay was still getting up and dressed daily and walking household distances, Tess foresaw a meaningful window of time to help Kay develop and work toward her personal goals as well as offer her support.

The Terminal Phase

With experience in hospice care and self-study, Tess has learned much about the dying process, or the **terminal phase**. Understanding what dying "looks like" is an asset not only to educate and allay fears of her clients and families, but also to appropriately direct Tess' interventions. Although there is some variation if the patient has an acute event or sudden death, common patterns typify the terminal phase.

During the months before death, the patient endures changes caused by disease and prepares for death. In the 6 to 12 months before death, patients may be less active, functionally decline, and complain of increased fatigue, weakness, pain, and bowel and bladder problems (incontinence, constipation, or diarrhea).[49] In anticipation of death, they may begin to withdraw from others, experience a range of emotions, and ponder spiritual and existential concerns.[49] In the last 1 to 3 months, the dying may be less communicative, sleep more, and eat less.[58]

There are many salient changes as the patient transitions and begins to actively die. In the final weeks to days, they may be less responsive and disorientated to their surroundings, yet have a surge of energy and be restless.[49] They have minimal to no oral intake, exhibit hemodynamic changes (decreased blood pressure, faster or slower pulse, and tachycardia), and have decreased to no urine output.[46,49,58,92] Patients' extremities may become *mottled* (purplish discoloration of skin) and feel cold to touch.[46,58] They may have hallucinations of deceased relatives and express an urgency to "leave" ("I need to catch the train").[44,49] In the last days to hours, fluid may accumulate in the pharynx causing a crackling sound in the chest, commonly known as a "*death rattle*."[16] Caregivers and family may observe *Cheyne-Stokes breathing*—periods of *agonal breathing* (rapid, shallow breaths) separated by *apneic* periods (no breathing) of 1 to 3 minutes.[46] When breathing stops, the heart will cease to beat several minutes later.[46] Death is confirmed on determination the heart has stopped, breathing has ceased, and pupils are dilated and fixed.[92]

As patients progress from the beginning to final stage, regular communication with the hospice team is imperative to help manage physical symptoms, discontinue unnecessary interventions, and address psychosocial needs to provide the utmost care for patients and their families.

OTPF-4 Domain

The domain describes the body of knowledge and expertise of occupational therapy.[5] Constructs include occupations, context, performance patterns and skills, and client factors.[5] How does the charged nature of life-threatening illness shape the domain of occupational therapy?

Occupations

Occupational participation is critical while living with a life-threatening disease.[73,87,127] Regardless of the level of performance, occupational participation promotes involvement in life[118] and maximizes physical and mental function.[85] Rest and sleep are essential as "a respite from physical discomfort and psychological stressors."[28] Educational and play occupations encourage social engagement with peers, feed a need to learn, encourage discovery of new occupations, build self-esteem and mastery, and promote goal setting.[27,130] Work occupations provide a means to make contributions to one's community.[85] Social and leisure occupations foster social support, a sense of belonging, and enjoyment (Fig. 50.1).[85]

Research has also identified occupations specific to the end of life. Jacques and Hasselkus found hospice patients gravitated toward activities "that matter[ed]" (p. 48).[54] In the context of dying, the most mundane tasks such as playing cards or sharing pie with family transformed into extraordinary events. Precious time focused on preparing for death by putting one's affairs into order, making amends, and saying goodbye to loved ones. Bye noted patients often desired closure, such as going home to die.[9] Bye[9] and Hunter[52] both identified the importance of building a legacy through passing on belongings or instilling one's values.

Although the team requested occupational therapy for Kay primarily to help her with self-care tasks, Tess looked forward

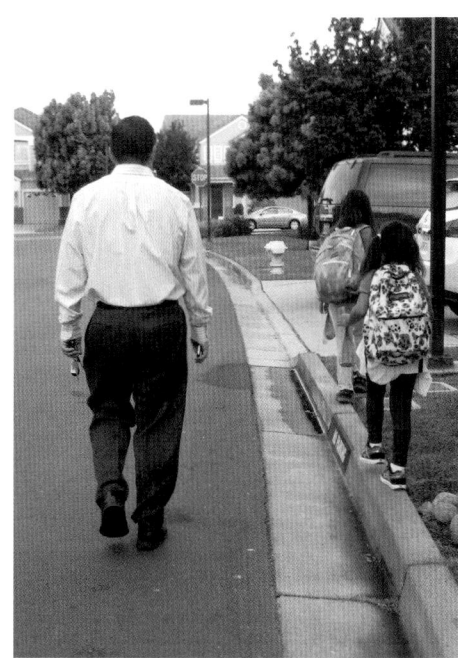

Fig. 50.1 Participating in meaningful occupations, such as a father walking his daughters to school, helps to keep a client with a life-threatening illness engaged in living.

to speaking with Kay further to inquire of other occupations of interest, if able. It is critical that occupational therapy practitioners not dismiss opportunities to engage in occupation, based on a client's prognosis, nor get locked into occupation only being activities of daily living. We need to take the time to identify the client's valued occupations, determine whether client factors, performance skills and patterns, and context support participation in choice occupations, and see if intervention can enable continued participation.

Contexts

As a home hospice occupational therapist, Tess valued being able to visit Kay in her home context. The OTPF-4 states "context is a broad construct defined as the environmental and personal factors specific to each client (person, group, population) that influence engagement and participation in occupations."[5] Environmental factors consist of physical, social, and attitudinal surroundings and include the natural environment and human-made changes, products and technology, support and relationships, attitudes, and service; systems; and policies.[5] Personal factors are "unique features of a person that are not part of a health condition or health state and that constitute the particular background of the person's life and living."[5] Tess was interested in seeing how Kay's environmental factors were affecting her ability to engage in her valued occupations as well as learning how Kay's personal factors were shaping how she viewed this stage of her life.

Environmental Factors

As clients experience disease progress and performance decline, the *natural environment and human-made changes* may limit occupational participation and compromise safety for both client and caregiver in one's home, school, work, community, recreational facilities, and places of worship. Depending on the client's resources, remodeling may be an option; however, there may not be enough time at the end of life to make extensive changes. More accessible and timely options may be to rearrange furniture, move items within reach, or provide *products* such as durable medical equipment (e.g., wheelchair, ramps, shower chair, or raised toilet seat) or install additional supports (e.g., grab bars, handrails, or bedrails).[23,89] Tess looked forward to assessing whether she could help make Kay's physical surroundings more accessible. Given Kay had just moved in with her daughter, perhaps she would need help building a personal and functional space to safely, efficiently, and privately access belongings and attend to her self-care. Tess's experience taught her that simple changes such as clearing hallways to allow passage of a four-wheeled walker, raising the height of a favorite chair with a cushion for greater ease with standing, and moving a bed so that one could turn to a less painful side while getting up could make a significant impact. Other times, Tess had used more involved interventions such as setting up a tilt-in-space recliner wheelchair to enable a client confined to her bed to get outside or training another client to drive a scooter to attend a grandchild's baseball game at the far end of the park. Knowing that decline is inevitable with terminal illness, Tess continuously looked for ways to modify environmental factors to maximize occupational participation.

Technology may also enable the client with limited accessibility to connect with others through texting, email, social media, video conferencing, and phone calls. The hospitalized client may be able to build a virtual shared space for social participation and a sense of being at home while away from home.[114] One of Tess's occupational therapy colleagues taught a client to use video conferencing to maintain his relationship with his grandchildren living out-of-state when he was no longer able to travel. With the coronavirus disease (COVID-19) pandemic, Kay was already feeling isolated from not being able to see all of her family, go to church, or participate in her Bible study group. Could Tess help Kay learn how to connect with her family and community through FaceTime or Zoom? Such interventions may help support ongoing participation in valued roles and continued connection with others when Kay would need her family and friends most.

Support and relationships are critical and an essential for the chronically and terminally ill. However, fearful *attitudes* toward death may hinder positive interactions. Family and friends may unintentionally isolate a loved one by avoiding conversations about dying and death.[24] Clients and caregivers may also feel shunned by lack of medical and social *services and policies* for those with life-limiting illness within our cure-centric healthcare system. As the client physically declines, caregiver needs will increase, causing further stress and strain between the client and the caregiver. Bye found that at the end of life, the work of occupational therapists with caregivers influences occupational therapy outcomes more than addressing the client's functional status.[9] Practitioners may need to educate family, friends, and caregivers on positive communication strategies, the dying and grieving process, and available social and healthcare services

for end-of-life care in the local area. To ease burden of care, practitioners can train caregivers on safe body mechanics, use of equipment, and techniques to enable occupational participation.[23,89] To develop the client's locus of control, practitioners can coach clients in how to direct their care.[9,22,105]

Kay's family seemed to be well connected with medical services and could likely reestablish Kay's community connections through technology, but Tess was not sure how they were coping with Kay's decline and impending death. Tess recalled working with another client, Joe, and his family on new ways to communicate and interact with each other. As Joe's dementia progressed, his family struggled to visit as he repeated himself multiple times within the same conversation. Tess coached Joe's children on facilitating life review conversations, helping Joe recall new details about the past. Tess also drew upon Joe's love of cooking by asking about family recipes and then working with him to make a dish with plenty of leftovers on Fridays. When his children visited on Saturdays, Joe would proudly serve them a meal. As they ate together, Joe and his children would talk about how Joe made the dish, reflect on their favorite dishes, and build new experiences together. For Kay's family, were they able to speak freely about their feelings, fears, grief, and concerns? Did engrained family dynamics support or isolate Kay? Would they benefit from coaching and practice with different communication skills? How could Tess use occupation to keep Kay connected with her family and friends as she continued through the dying process?

Personal Factors

Personal factors are aspects of the person's background and attributes such as age, race and ethnicity, cultural identification, and character traits.[5] These factors can shape how people view and approach the end of life. When Kay celebrated her 82nd birthday earlier in the year, she did not feel that age. She felt and acted much younger than her peers. Perhaps that is why she got divorced, frustrated by cultural expectations to be the typical housewife by her husband or to "act her age." A third-generation Japanese-American and native Californian, she was a small child during World War II when she, her parents, and grandparents were sent to a Japanese-American internment camp in Topaz, Utah. Although many years had passed since "camp," no one spoke about their experiences or feelings about this social injustice. Kay continued throughout her life to negotiate and sometimes fight with how others saw her, how she saw herself, and how she lived her life. She never mastered verbalizing her feelings, but her children knew she loved them by her consistent presence and provision for them. Kay was proud of the life she built for herself and family after her divorce and hoped she could somehow define her death on her own terms. However, cancer was ruining her life plans. Although her peers approached their 80s reflectively saying, "I have lived a good life," Kay would emphatically say, "I still have much to do!" and strongly desired to meet her great-grandchildren one day. How would Tess help Kay reconcile how cancer was disrupting her life plan? Could Tess help Kay define what was important to her, set obtainable goals, and build a legacy for her great-grandchildren through which they could come to know their great-grandmother?

Consideration of the client's context plays a vital part in occupational therapy intervention. Despite decline and loss of functional performance, the client may experience continued occupational participation through modification of the client's environmental factors. Understanding the client's personal factors may help the practitioner understand how the client views and approaches the end of life to then make intervention client-centered and consistent with the client's sense of self.

Performance Patterns and Skills

Our values draw us to what we feel is important. As we gravitate to meaningful occupations, we seek to meet occupational and contextual demands, develop proficiency, shape habits, and blend habits into performance patterns.[5,76] These performance patterns structure our daily lives, define our roles in society, and provide purpose.[76] To maintain these performance patterns, we rely upon body structures and functions to support performance skills.[5]

Incurable disease can impair body functions and structures and limit performance skills. Loss of performance skills disrupts habits, dissolves routines, and collapses one's ability to uphold defining roles.[5,75] Although palliative medical interventions may stabilize symptoms and occupational therapy may help provide a window of improved functional performance, people with incurable illness continue to face decline. Inability to fulfill roles may rob one's self-identity, invalidate social membership, and erode sense of self-worth.[75] A social death occurs long before a biological death.[60]

When addressing performance patterns and skills, consider the client's defining roles, habits, and routines. How has disease disrupted or limited these factors? Can these roles be modified or adapted to allow continued participation? Can the client's expectations of role requirements be reframed? Can the client participate in a role without performing a skill? Can new occupational roles be introduced and tried? Can the client be affirmed of inherent value, regardless of current role performance (Fig. 50.2)?

Client Factors

Client factors are "specific capacities, characteristics, or beliefs that reside within the person and that influence performance in occupation."[5] OTPF-4 further breaks client factors into values, beliefs, spirituality, body functions, and body structures.[5] The disease and dying process can affect each of these constructs.

Values, beliefs, and spirituality. Values, beliefs, and spirituality collectively connect meaning with our occupational experiences. *Values* are principles that personally define "what is good, right, or important."[5] *Beliefs* are "something that is accepted, considered to be true, or held as an opinion."[5] *Spirituality* is the process of finding meaning "by engaging in occupations that involve the enacting of personal values and beliefs, reflection, and intention within a supportive contextual environment."[5] When we satisfactorily participate in valued occupations, we experience coherence with our beliefs, validation of our actions, and sense of purpose in our lives.

Incurable disease may cause angst and struggle with our values, beliefs and spirituality. Although life-limiting illness may help prioritize "what matters" with remaining time and resources,[54] disease may limit the ability to satisfactorily maintain valued and self-defining roles and occupations (Fig. 50.3).[77] Faced with their mortality, clients may question beliefs, the purpose of life, and the reason for suffering and loss.[87] Practitioners need to determine the client's values, supporting beliefs, and what is meaningful in their lives to help them reframe perceptions, accommodate illness, and experience self-worth in the face of decline and functional loss.

Kay highly valued self-sufficiency. As a child, she was frequently sick and unable to help with household duties like her siblings. Her mother often called her "a weak child." Although she regained full health in her adolescence, she continued to see herself as "weak" and overcompensated with self-reliance. Now, unable to fully care for herself, she felt worthless and a burden to her children. Countering these self-labels, however, Kay believed God knows her and has a plan for "good" in her life.

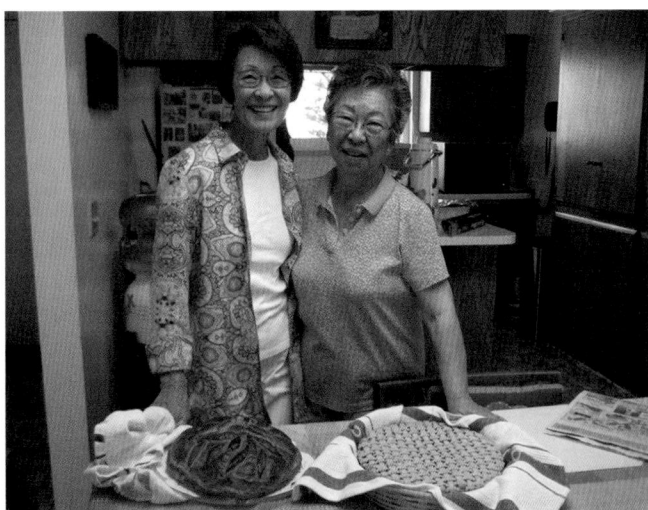

Fig. 50.2 Illness can affect a client's ability to perform defining tasks such as baking for the family.

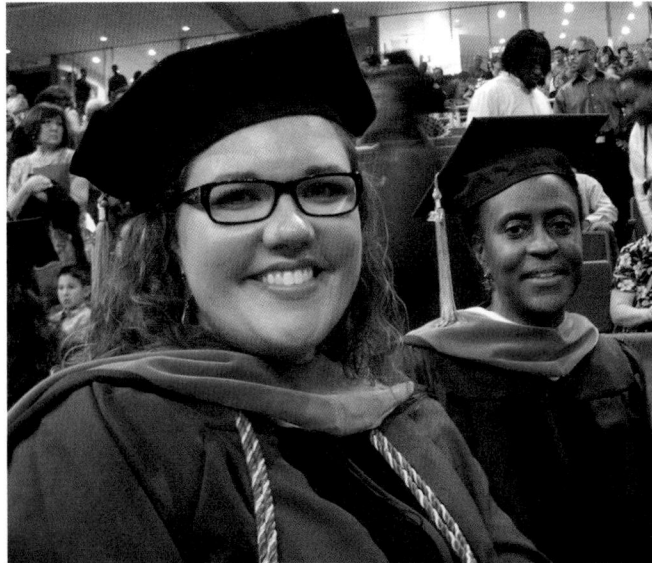

Fig. 50.3 Graduation, as shown here, is an example of an anticipated life moment that can be disrupted by illness.

Could Tess help Kay draw upon her spiritual beliefs to help her find purpose, meaning, and inherent value despite functional dependence on her children?

Body structures and body functions. Hospice and palliative care address an array of illnesses. Common diagnoses include cancer (30.1%), circulatory and heart conditions (17.6%), dementia (15.6%), respiratory diseases (11.0%), stroke (9.2%), and chronic kidney diseases (2.3%).[99] With such a range of illness in hospice and palliative care, this chapter is unable to address the full array of pathological issues; however, four general guidelines may help the practitioner consider how incurable illness affects body structures and function and, consequently, occupational participation.

1. *Learn the pathology of the client's primary diagnosis.* Find out which structures are affected and how disease compromises body function. Be aware of how the disease and symptoms change with disease progression. Consider how these changes will affect occupational participation. In Kay's situation, pancreatic cancer will affect the function of the pancreas, which produces digestive enzymes and hormones to control blood glucose levels.[55] Pancreatic cancer is often undetected at early stages because there are no established routine screening tests and symptoms are vague or nonexistent.[2,3,55] As the tumor grows, symptoms become more apparent. A tumor in the head of the pancreas may obstruct the bile duct and backlog bile into the liver and the bloodstream, causing jaundice in the skin and eyes, darkened urine, and light-colored stool.[55] The tumor may block the digestive system, causing nausea and vomiting.[55] Continued growth may push against surrounding organs, resulting in abdominal pain and distention.[55] As cancer cells rob nutrients from normal cells in the advanced stages of the disease, the client will experience weakness, fatigue, and weight loss (cachexia).[3,55] Each sequential stage will pose increasing difficulties for Kay, as digestive problems, pain, distention, and fatigue will progressively limit her function. (See Chapter 46 for more information.)

2. *Account for a secondary diagnosis or premorbid conditions.* These factors may complicate the primary disease process and have an exponential effect on body structures and function. Kay has a history of COPD and experienced dyspnea with moderate exertion. As her pancreatic cancer progresses, the abdominal pressure may cause shortness of breath and anxiety. Tess will need to address both her COPD and her cancer symptoms in treatment. (See Chapter 45 for more details.)

3. *Consider the body systems as integrated.* Impairment of one body structure can affect multiple body systems. Pancreatic cancer can spread into the lymphatic system, impairing drainage of lymph in the surrounding areas. Severe edema may develop in the abdomen and lower extremities, causing pain, immobility, and poor skin integrity.

4. *Be aware of the mind-body connection.* Practitioners need to consider the psychological implications of disease in order to holistically care for clients. At the early stages of her disease, Kay was dyspneic with moderate exertion. Although her symptoms were more related to her COPD at the time, she assumed her breathlessness was due to her growing tumor pushing onto her diaphragm. Kay would spiral in anxiousness and feel she was about to suffocate and die. The context of living with a life-limiting illness may heighten emotional reactions and existential pain.[44] Somatic pains that seem excessive or not congruent with the identified organic pathological conditions may be of psychogenic origins.[17] Also, physical changes to body structures due to surgical intervention (e.g., amputation, mastectomy, or facial surgery) or disease progression may result in an altered body image, highly affecting self-esteem, emotional well-being, spirituality, socialization, intimacy, sexuality, and function in daily activities.[115] The psychological impact of life-limiting disease can significantly affect occupational participation.

Working with Kay, Tess will need to be aware of how cancer and COPD will affect multiple body functions and systems along the disease trajectory. With such knowledge, Tess will effectively address Kay's limitations and support her occupational participation through the dying process.

OTPF-4 Process

Within context of the grieving and dying process, provision of hospice and palliative occupational therapy services involves evaluation, intervention, and targeting intervention outcomes to support occupational participation throughout the lifespan.[4,5] *Upon Tess knocking on the front door, she heard shuffling steps approached from behind. As the deadbolt clicked and the doorknob turned, Tess looked up to see Kay peering from behind the door. "Hi, I'm Tess . . . Mrs. Shimada?" Kay replied, "It's Kay. Come in."*

Evaluation

The evaluation process seeks to determine the client's goals, needs, functional baseline, and supports and barriers to occupational participation.[5] Through preparation, evaluation analysis, and synthesis, the occupational therapist develops an occupational profile and determines appropriate interventions.[5]

After receiving a consultation to evaluate and treat, *preparation* for the evaluation process begins with gathering data from chart review, staff and caregiver reports, and clinical observation.[105] In addition to areas that may affect occupational participation, special attention is given to the grieving and dying processes. Information may need to be verified by the client and/or family; however, preparation may prevent asking redundant questions, conserve the client's energy, build a foundation for an occupational profile, and provide segues for therapeutic interaction. See Table 50.1 for suggestions in the preparation process.

Building upon the preparation process, *evaluation* begins by identifying the client's needs and goals and developing an occupational profile. Depending on the client's physical, emotional, and cognitive stamina, the evaluation process may vary. A palliative care client at the early stages of the disease process may have a relatively high activity tolerance and occupational performance capacity, despite living with a life-threatening disease. A more formal assessment may be indicated to determine more progressive interventions. For a hospice client with poor activity

TABLE 50.1 Preparation Guide

Areas of Concern	Subtopics	Sources of information	Probing Questions
Medical history	• Primary diagnosis (dx) • Symptoms • Secondary dx • Comorbidities • Prior medical issues • Mental health status	• MD, nursing, & mental health services notes • Staff/family reports	• What are the events leading up to admission for primary dx? • How long since initial dx? • How is the client coping/grieving? • Do comorbidities complicate treatment (tx)? • How do/will medical issues affect occupational participation?
Medical orders	• Precautions • Contact isolation • Advance directive	• Medical orders • MD, nursing notes	• Are there orders that should be in place that are not? (i.e., total hip replacement precautions) • Review advance directive • Will precautions affect treatment?
Social history	• Age • Marital status • Work history • Education • Cultural background	• MD, nursing, social work, and mental health services notes • Staff/family reports	• Do these client factors support or limit occupational participation?
Areas of occupation and performance patterns	• Values • Leisure interests • Roles • Routines • Performance • Goals	• MD, nursing, social work, mental health services, physical therapy, or previous OT notes • Staff/ family reports • Observation	• What is the client's previous level of occupational participation/performance? • How much assistance was needed? • Any discharge needs? • Any end-of-life goals and wishes?
Contexts	• Environmental factors • Personal factors	• Home health services notes, physical therapy, social work, nursing, mental health services, and MD notes • Staff/family reports	• See "Discharge Check List"

tolerance, a formal assessment process may be invasive and burdensome.[9,89,105] In a qualitative study of hospice occupational therapists, Bye (1998) found that practitioners often used a "low-keyed" approach of observation and interview with the client, staff, and caregivers rather than exhausting clients with a formal assessment.[9] Although administering an incomplete assessment may compromise validity and reliability, subsets of assessments may also address the client's particular need while accommodating the client's limited endurance.[6] For example, using only the grooming portion of the Functional Independence Measure (FIM)[39,64] rather than completing all areas of self-care may provide evaluative data and conserve the client's energy to complete the single goal of brushing the teeth that day. Table 50.2 presents more evaluation strategies.

Given the challenges of assessing people with life-threatening illness, are there accepted assessments for hospice and palliative care occupational therapy? Currently, there are no established hospices and palliative care occupational therapy outcome measures or assessment tools.[45,89] However, two occupation-based measures may be appropriate for use with hospice and palliative care clients: the Occupational Case Analysis Interview and Rating Scale (OCAIRS)[35] and the Canadian Occupational Performance Measure (COPM).[75]

The OCAIRS is primarily a descriptive assessment of occupational participation. Based on the Model of Human Occupation (MOHO),[120] the OCAIRS addresses all of the domain areas of the OTPF-4 by evaluating volitional, habitual, and performance components and the influence of context on occupational participation.[5] This 20- to 30-minute, standardized, semi-structured interview is portable and flexible to the client's level of endurance. The OCAIRS has adequate reliability[41,42,57] and excellent to adequate validity.[8,72,123,127,129] The brief, MOHO-based interview format may enable the practitioner to determine the client's goals and assess multiple domains quickly without excessive burden on the client. There are no studies on the use of the OCAIRS in hospice and palliative care. However, an unpublished quality improvement study found the OCAIRS an effective assessment tool for developing a rich narrative with hospice clients.[18]

Based on Canadian Model of Occupational Performance and Engagement (CMOP-E),[10] the Canadian Occupational Performance Measure (COPM)[75] is an extensively researched assessment tool with excellent reliability[25,102] and excellent validity.[12,15,26,88,109] This portable, 15- to 30-minute semi-structured interview is primarily an evaluation assessment that organizes occupational participation under self-care, productivity, and leisure categories, with an emphasis on occupation performance.[75] The client identifies occupational performance issues and self-rates performance and satisfaction on a Likert scale.[75] The COPM was shown to be problematic with the terminally ill, because focus on occupational performance was psychologically distressing for

TABLE 50.2 Evaluation Strategies for OTPF-4 Domains

Domains	Evaluation Strategies

Occupation
• Activities of daily living
• Instrumental activities of daily living
• Health management
• Rest/sleep
• Education
• Work
• Play
• Leisure
• Social participation
	• Use chart review, interview, family reports
	• Focus on areas pertinent to client's goals and interests
	• Administer assessments only if data will support client's goals; client is willing; and client has the emotional, cognitive, and physical stamina to participate
	• Possible occupation-based assessments[a] include:
	  • Occupational Circumstance Assessment and Interview Rating Scale (OCAIRS)[35] (client report)
	  • Canadian Occupational Performance Measure (COPM)[75] (client report)
	  • Functional Independent Measure (FIM)[39,64] (subtests as indicated)

Client Factors • Values, beliefs, spirituality • Body functions • Body structures	• Use chart review, interview, and family reports • Observation • OCAIRS[a] (values, beliefs, and spirituality) • Only assess body structures and functions that support client's goals and interests. For example, instead of doing comprehensive manual muscle testing, assess just hip and knee flexors and extensors to determine if at least grossly 3+/5 and safe to attempt functional transfer.
Performance Patterns • Habits • Routines • Rituals • Roles	• Chart review, interview, staff, and family report • OCAIRS[a] (habits, routines, roles)
Performance Skills • Motor • Process • Social interaction	• Observation • FIM[a] (Subtests as indicated) • OCAIRS[a] (client report) • COPM[a] (client report)
Contexts • Environmental factors • Personal factors	• Chart review, interview, staff, and family report • If client will be going home, see "Discharge Checklist" • OCAIRS[a]

[a]Administer assessments only if data will support client's goals and client is willing and has the emotional, cognitive, and physical stamina to participate.

clients confronting functional decline and disease progression.[102] However, as a client-centered and individualized measure with excellent psychometric strength, the COPM may be a good alternative to measures with preset performance levels[23] and appropriate for higher functioning palliative care clients.[101]

The OCAIRS and COPM are two possible hospice and palliative occupational therapy assessments. Both are brief, semi-structure interviews that can accommodate low endurance. The OCAIRS accounts well for volitional and environmental components, which may be the only modifiable factors as the client loses functional performance.[9,103] Although suited more for higher functioning clients, the COPM offers excellent psychometric strength and clinical utility. Further research is needed to validate the appropriateness of the OCAIRS and COPM in hospice and palliative occupational therapy.

The evaluation process requires the practitioner to assess the client's stamina and apply professional reasoning to ascertain the appropriate approaches and assessment tools to use. After drawing from numerous sources, the practitioner integrates and *analyzes* evaluation findings. Based on identified supports and limitations of occupational participation, the practitioner prepares to develop a treatment plan and implement intervention.

Kay's evaluation. As Tess followed Kay into the living room, she observed Kay occasionally skimming the wall with her hand and leaning onto the console *(movement function/gait pattern)* before sitting down onto the couch *(motor skill-functional transfer)*. Kay pointed to the seat across from her for Tess. Kay's daughter, Liz, came in, introduced herself, and asked if she could join the conversation. Tess said it would be fine with her if it were all right with Kay. Kay nodded in agreement.

Kay asked right away with a smile *(social interaction skills)*, "Are you here to give me a job?" Tess explained that her job was to help Kay be able to "do" what she feels is important, or her occupations. Although Kay's cancer will cause decline, Tess would try to help modify and accommodate everyday tasks, routines, and activities as much as possible. The reason for Tess' first visit is to get to know Kay better and define her goals and needs.

With Kay's permission, Tess initiated the OCAIRS interview. Folding questions from the OCAIRS into a casual conversation, Tess was able to find out that Kay's current *roles* are being a mother, grandmother, and friend. She enjoyed traveling, cooking, and going to church *(interests)*, but her *routines* had slowly changed due to her fatigue, abdominal pain, and occasional shortness of breath *(body structures/function)*. Kay used to attend different events three times a week for church or to meet friends. She had not attended church in the last few months *(routine, performance skills)* mainly because of COVID-19, but Kay speculated she would be too fatigued to go to church anyway. Although she is still able to get to the toilet independently, she needs minimal assistance from her daughters for bathing and dressing.

When asked what Kay *values* most, she said God, her family, and being independent. Liz added that her mother worked hard to send all four kids to college and taught them to be self-sufficient. Kay said she is most proud of *(personal causation)* her children and grandchildren, adding, "They are all good people who get along with each other. I can't ask for more." She reflected that her life had been tough at times, but she felt that "God made me a better person through it all *(spirituality)*." Tess asked how she got through tough times in the past *(interpretation of past experiences)*. Kay explained her *belief* that God had a purpose for her and her kids, and this kept her going *(spirituality)*. Tess asked about how she is doing getting through this challenging time. Kay paused and said, "I regret not being able to see my great-granddaughter, expected in 6 months, but I have to believe that God is somehow using me now *(grieving–acceptance; spirituality)*." Kay added, however, she feels like a burden on her children and grandchildren because they are all taking turns from their jobs and schoolwork to help her out *(social environment, belief)*. Liz tried to reassure Kay that she is not a burden, but Kay just looked down.

Tess then asked, "If there were two things that you could do with greater ease, what would they be *(goals)*?" Kay looked up and said without hesitation, "Be able to get dressed and take a shower by myself without being so tired." Tess asked if doing things differently or having change is hard *(readiness for change)*. Kay said, "Sometimes. Especially if it means that things will never be the same."

Kay began to fatigue from the interview *(motor skill-endurance)*. To allow Kay to rest, Tess asked if it would be OK to have Liz show Kay's bedroom, the bathroom, and places she likes to spend time *(physical environment)*. Kay agreed and remained in the living room. While Liz showed Tess the main living areas and Kay's bedroom and bathroom, Liz mentioned Kay is "still getting around, but she is getting weaker." Tess asked Liz how she is doing. Liz remarked her mom's illness has been so sudden and the whole family is struggling watching their feisty mother and grandmother wither. "She's the glue of our family. I don't know what I am going to do without her. My sister thinks she should get more chemo and go to rehab *(grieving-denial vs. bargaining)*, but I know that is not going to help her *(grieving-acceptance)*." Tess listened intently and then remarked on how Liz and her family seem to be working well together. Liz laughed, "What do you mean? We don't agree on things." Tess replied, "Maybe, but you talk with each other. Many families don't." Liz paused. "I guess we do."

Tess and Liz returned to find Kay asleep on the couch *(motor skill-endurance)*. To allow Kay to rest, Tess asked if it would be OK if she came back tomorrow morning to discuss possible ways to make it safer for Kay to do her self-care and get around the house. Liz thought that would be fine.

Although Tess would have liked to spend more time, Kay was too fatigued. However, based on the OCAIRS and home assessment, Tess was able to find out Kay's goals—to be independent as possible with dressing and bathing. Kay is limited by fatigue, abdominal pain, and shortness of breath, but she continues to have fair motor strength, fair/good balance, resilience, and strong social support. Perhaps with equipment, modification of her routine, and energy conservation principles (also referred to as fatigue management), Kay may be more independent with her self-care and able to get out into the community for a bit longer. Tess also thought about that great-grandchild coming and wondered if Kay would want to somehow share a part of herself with the baby.

Intervention

Using analysis of evaluation data, the practitioner collaborates with the client to develop a plan, implements intervention, and continually reevaluates treatment effectiveness.[5] Like the evaluation process, intervention remains focused on the client's goals and considers the changing needs of the dying and grieving

process. The context of dying shapes the selection of occupations and interventions.

The *intervention plan* is the map to care. Taking the client's goals, the practitioner translates them into treatment goals. In hospice and palliative care, the client's goal may not be realistic, such as "I want to get better." However, the practitioner may have to dig deeper to understand if there are other ways to feel "better," such as participating in a beloved hobby or spending time with family. Together, the practitioner and client collaborate to develop a desired plan and outcomes.

Another frequently heard goal is to "return home." Within the context of dying, the wish to return home may be even stronger. Similar to other areas of care, practitioners need to access the physical and social environments and determine if discharge home is feasible and safe. Table 50.3 presents discharge planning checklists.

Tess discussed with Kay her goals to dress and bathe with less assistance. Kay was open to working with Tess on changing her routine and trying out adaptive equipment. Tess used goal attainment scaling (GAS)[67] to develop treatment goals and later serve as an outcome measure of treatment efficacy. Initially developed for mental health services, GAS asserts goals are best defined by the client's challenges,[53] provides a means to detect meaningful change relevant to the clients and their families that may be difficult to capture on standardized measures,[36,86,124] and can be administered in a time-effective manner.[36] Goals are ranked on a 5-point scale, ranging from −2 to 2, with −2 being much less than expected outcome, 0 being expected outcome, and 2 being much more than expected outcome[67,86] (Table 50.4). Preintervention and postintervention scores can be converted to a standardized score to show outcome changes.[124] Tables are available for easy conversion of outcome scores to T-scores.[68] There is insufficient evidence to determine test-retest reliability.[31,53] Concurrent validity is fair to poor.[31,53] Congruent validity is fair.[53] Despite low to moderate psychometric strength, however, GAS is still widely used based on its clinical utility[31] and provides an individualized, client-centered outcome measure when standardized tests are not available.[84] Box 50.1 lists Kay's GAS goals.

With the intervention plan established, *intervention implementation* begins. Interventions used in hospice and palliative care include pain and symptom control (Table 50.5),[4,23,45] occupational modification,[4,23,61] and training of both the client and caregiver.[9,107] Table 50.6 lists intervention examples. Although these interventions seem similar to other areas of care, qualitative studies of hospice occupational therapists have found practitioners uniquely balance between maximizing occupational participation for today while preparing clients for death through occupations that promote closure during the intervention process.[9,45,54]

To help Kay increase her safety and independence bathing, Tess gave suggestions for equipment in the bathroom such as grab bars, a shower chair, and a nonskid mat. Kay practiced transferring in and out of the shower, using the shower chair. Liz said she would have someone install the grab bars at the shower entrance, in the stall, and by the toilet. Kay felt that she would be more stable getting in and out by herself with the grab bars,

TABLE 50.3 Discharge Planning Checklists

Context	Checklist
Physical Environmental Factors	

Entrances	• Accessible entrances? (primary and secondary entrances)
	  • Door wide enough for wheelchair or scooter?
	  • Accommodation for turning radius?
	  • Ramp or railing needed?
	  • Access to driveway or car drop off?
	• Will client be able to safely access home at current level of function and expected level of function? Will ambulance/gurney services be needed at discharge?

Bathroom	• Accessible entrance with room for turning radius? • Tub/shower accessible? Modifications needed? • Shower chair, grab bars, and shower hose? • Bedside commode, raised toilet seat, or toilet frame needed? • Is it possible to provide safe care in this area at client's current and expected level of function?

Bedroom	• Accessible entrance with room for turning radius?
	• Clear pathways and access to belongings?
	• Bed
	  • Height too high/low for transfers?
	  • Bed rail needed?
	  • Hospital bed needed?
	  • Room for hospital bed?
	• Bedside commode needed? Space available?
	• Room for mechanical lift if needed?
	• Is it possible to provide safe care in this area at client's current and expected level of function?

Living space Outdoor areas Community areas	• Accessible entrance/area for wheelchair or walker? • Accessible sitting areas? • Modifications needed to enable occupational participation?
Caregiver's area	• Living space for caregiver that allows for sleep, self-care, respite, and privacy?
Social and Attitudinal Environmental Factors	

Support and relationships	• Does the caregiver have the emotional, spiritual, and physical stamina to provide the care needed?
	• What are the caregiver's coping strategies?
	• Does the caregiver have a support system?
	• Are there multiple caregivers to allow for respite?
	• Is the caregiver knowledgeable of:
	  • The dying and grieving process?
	  • Proper body mechanics?
	  • Caregiver techniques?
	  • Use of equipment (i.e., lift, hospital bed)?
	  • Community supports?

Attitudes	• Does the client feel supported or isolated? • Does the client have support to speak about dying and death?

Services, systems, and policies	• Client and/or caregiver aware of:
	  • Community resources?
	  • Support groups?
	  • How to contact their healthcare team?

TABLE 50.4 Scaled levels of Goal Attainment Scaling[67,86]

Rating	Level Description
−2	Much less than expected outcome
−1	Somewhat less than expected outcome
0	Expected outcome
+1	Somewhat more than expected outcome
+2	Much more than expected outcome

but reassured Tess she would have her daughters stand by. To decrease her fatigue, Tess instructed Kay in energy conservation principles, coaching Kay on pacing, prioritizing tasks, sitting with activity, and use of long-handled equipment. They discussed situations and thoughts that may trigger Kay's dyspnea and practice pursed-lipped breathing and mindfulness techniques to help center herself. Tess gave Kay permission to not take a shower every day and to delegate other tasks so she could focus on what was important to her. She also showed Kay how to use a four-wheeled walker not only for stability, but to carry her

BOX 50.1   Kay's Treatment Goals

Goal 1: With energy conservation principles and adaptive equipment, Kay will be able to complete her bathing routine independently.

−2: Kay will be able to complete her bathing routine with min A.

−1: Kay will be able to complete her bathing routine with CGA.

0: Kay will be able to complete her bathing routine with SBA/setup.

+1: Kay will be able to complete her bathing routine with setup.

+2: Kay will be able to complete her bathing routine with modified I.

Today's score: −2

Goal 2: With energy conservation principles and adaptive equipment, Kay will be able to dress herself independently.

−2: Kay will be able to dress herself with min A.

−1: Kay will be able to dress herself with CGA.

0: Kay will be able to dress herself with SBA/setup.

+1: Kay will be able to dress herself with setup.

+2: Kay will be able to dress herself with modified I.

Today's score: −2

Cumulative raw score for 2 goals: −4

Standardized score: +25

min A, Minimal assistance; *CGA*, contact guard assist; *SBA*, stand-by assist; *modified I*, modified independence.

TABLE 50.5   Symptom Control Strategies[22,23,89,123]

Symptom(s)	Strategies for Symptom Control

Pain, dyspnea, anxiety	• Work with team on use and timing of medications with daily routines
	• Understand source of symptoms (physical, psychological, or both)
	• Identify triggers of symptoms
	• Identify any positioning that exacerbates symptoms
	• Provide means for better positioning and body mechanics that decrease symptoms:
	  • *Dyspnea:* Side-line sleeping, avoid compressing abdominal/chest area
	  • *Pain:* Good body mechanics with daily tasks
	  • *Anxiety:* Note posturing that may cause muscle tension
	• Assess and address quality of sleep and sleep hygiene
	• Instruct client in relaxation techniques and mindfulness training
	• Integrate stress management principles
	• Instruct client in adaptive breathing techniques (e.g., pursed-lipped breathing)
	• Make referrals as indicated to other disciplines (e.g., massage and physical therapies, psychology, chaplain, social work)

Nausea, vomiting	• Identify triggers • Work with team (speech and physical therapy, nursing) on positioning to avoid dysphagia • Coach on positioning that decreases symptoms while performing daily tasks • Integrate relaxation techniques and mindfulness training as indicated
Fatigue	• Identify and address psychological stressors that may exacerbate fatigue • Assess and address sleep hygiene • Analyze daily tasks. Coach on simplifying and/or modifying tasks • Instruct in energy conservation principles (e.g., pacing, prioritizing, delegating, sitting with tasks)

For additional resources and information, please refer to Chapter 51 (Therapeutic Use of Self: Embodying Mindfulness in Occupational Therapy), Chapter 13 (Rest and Sleep), Chapter 27 (Eating and Swallowing), Chapter 28 (Pain Management), Chapter 34 (Cerebrovascular Accident [Stroke]), Chapter 39 (Arthritis), Chapter 42 (Low Back Pain), and Chapter 45 (Cardiac and Pulmonary Disease).

things and allow her to take a break on the walker seat. At first she seemed hesitant, but when Tess mentioned she would probably be more independent with the walker, she decided to try it.

Although not specifically a part of Kay's treatment plan, Tess integrated a *therapeutic use of self* strategy to connect with Kay and bring out Kay's previous occupational roles. At the end of one session, Tess noticed at a picture of Kay's children by her bedside, and commented, "I have two kids I am raising on my own. Any parental advice?"

Kay paused. "I never thought I would have to raise four kids by myself."

Tess asked, "How did you do it?"

"Forgiveness."

"Forgiveness?"

"I wasted a lot of energy being angry at my ex-husband. When I hit a wall, I realized I needed to make a change for the better. I had to choose to forgive him and not wait until I felt like I could forgive. When I finally did, a big weight lifted, and I was freed up to live my life and be there for my kids."

"Did he ask for forgiveness?"

"Are you kidding? Of course not . . . have you ever tried oregano tea?

Surprised by the sudden change of subject, Tess replied, "No, never heard of it.

"My neighbor told me it's a good household remedy for a nagging cough. I thought it was the strangest idea. When I couldn't get over my cold, I decided to steep some. Terribly bitter but surprisingly soothing. Sometimes you have to try something totally different for a change for the better."[a]

Kay smiled. Tess realized roles were reversed. Kay was the occupational therapist for the day. Although weak and tired, in that moment, Kay was the strong, vibrant, self-reliant mother teaching Tess.

Tess returned the next week. Kay was able to bathe herself after Liz set things up. With Kay using the grab bars and sitting while she completed her bathing routine, Liz felt more comfortable leaving for periods of time and providing Kay privacy. By implementing the energy conservation suggestions of pacing, putting out her clothes the day before, carrying things with the four-wheeled walker, sitting down, using long-handled equipment, she was able to get dressed with modified independence

---

[a]The author does not endorse the use of oregano tea and recommends consulting one's healthcare provider to inquire whether it is appropriate for personal use.

TABLE 50.6 Interventions

Types of Interventions	Examples
Occupations and activities	**Occupations** • Completes a morning routine with adaptive equipment • Prepares own breakfast with energy conservation principles • Does grocery shopping with use of a scooter • Writes a legacy letter expressing hopes, dreams, and values to children • Makes amends with estranged sibling • Gives possessions away to desired loved ones • Sits outside on porch to have a cup of coffee with friend **Activities** • Practices getting in/out of shower while using grab bar • Develops a list of affairs that need to be attended to • Decides who to give belongings to • Participates in life review about raising children • Practices how to ask caregiver for help
Interventions to support occupations	**PAMs and Mechanical Modalities** • Heels floating off pillow to prevent skin breakdown • Retrograde massage to decrease upper extremity edema • Hand-strengthening program with putty or exercise hand ball • Upper extremity range of motion (ROM) program **Orthotics and prosthetics** • Positioning device to foster comfort while in bed **Environmental modifications** • Shower chair and shower hose for bathing tasks • Long-handled equipment for dressing and bathing tasks • Recommendation for equipment installation (i.e., grab bars, ramp, lift) **Wheeled mobility** • Determination of appropriate wheelchair and seat positioning **Self-regulation** • Pursed-lipped breathing to control shortness of breath (SOB)
Education and training	**Client education and training in use of:** • Adaptive equipment with bathing and dressing • Energy conservation strategies • Pursed-lipped breathing to decrease SOB with ADLs • Manual or power wheelchair mobility **Caregiver education and training in use of:** • ROM • Edema control • Positioning • Body mechanics • Mechanical lift • Provided equipment
Advocacy	**Advocacy** • Therapist advocates for the client's interests in team meetings • Therapist explains to family that the client does not want to continue with aggressive rehabilitation anymore **Self-advocacy** • Client practices how to ask caregiver for help • Client directs own care • Client makes a request for palliative treatments
Group interventions	• Day hospice program • Group to discover new occupations such as art making or computer use • Legacy writing group • Support groups • Caregiver support groups
Virtual interventions	**Instruction and support in:** • Using a smart phone to text, email, and/or video call • Blogging experiences and reflections

For additional resources and intervention strategies, please refer to Chapter 10 (Activities of Daily Living), Chapter 11, Section 2 (Functional Ambulation) and Section 3 (Wheelchair Assessment and Transfers), Chapter 13 (Sleep and Rest), Chapter 16 (Leisure Occupations), Chapter 17 (Assistive Technology), Chapter 34 (Cerebrovascular Accident [Stroke]), Chapter 39 (Arthritis), Chapter 42 (Low Back Pain), and Chapter 45 (Cardiac and Pulmonary Disease).

BOX 50.2 Review of Kay's Treatment Goals

Goal 1: With energy conservation principles and adaptive equipment, Kay will be able to complete her bathing routine independently.
−2: Kay will be able to complete her bathing routine with min A.
−1: Kay will be able to complete her bathing routine with CGA.
0: Kay will be able to complete her bathing routine with SBA/setup.
+1: Kay will be able to complete her bathing routine with setup.
+2: Kay will be able to complete her bathing routine with modified I.
    Baseline's score: −2
    Highest score achieved to date: +1

    Goal 2: With energy conservation principles and adaptive equipment, Kay will be able to dress herself independently.
−2: Kay will be able to dress herself with min A.
−1: Kay will be able to dress herself with CGA.
0: Kay will be able to dress herself with SBA/setup.
+1: Kay will be able to dress herself with setup.
+2: Kay will be able to dress herself with modified I.
    Baseline score: −2
    Highest score achieved to date: +2

Cumulative baseline raw score for 2 goals: −4
Cumulative raw score after second session: +3
Baseline standardized score: 25

Second session standardized score: 69
Outcome change: +44
    min A, Minimal assistance; *CGA*, contact guard assist; *SBA*, stand-by assist; *modified I*, modified independence.

BOX 50.3 Kay's Revised Treatment Goals

Goal: Kay will write legacy letters to her family.
−2: Kay will decide whom she will write letters to.
−1: Kay will finish writing 1 or 2 letters.
0: Kay will finish writing 3 or 4 letters.
+1: Kay will finish letters to her children and 1 letter to her grandchildren.
+2: Kay will write letters to her children, grandchildren, and great-grandchild.

Baseline score: -2
Highest score achieved to date: +2
Baseline standardized score: 30
Three-week reevaluation score: 70
Change in outcome score: +40

BOX 50.4 Family Goals

Goal: Family will safely and independently assist Kay with care.
−2: Family will verbalize understanding of good body mechanics.
−1: Family will demonstrate good body mechanics with 3 or 4 verbal cues during care.
0: Family will demonstrate good body mechanics with 1 or 2 verbal cues during care.
+1: Family will demonstrate good body mechanics with 1 verbal cue during care.
+2: Family will demonstrate good body mechanics with no cuing during care.

Baseline score: −2
Highest score after 2 sessions: +2
Baseline standardized score: 30
Standardized score after 2 sessions: 70
Change in outcome scores: +40

---

and without shortness of breath. Kay had a brighter affect than last week and seemed pleased with her progress.

At the end of the session, Tess did an *intervention review* of Kay's plan (Box 50.2). Kay had made great progress over the last week. Although her progress may be momentary, it was evident that having more independence and privacy was priceless to Kay.

With Kay meeting her goals, Tess considered discharging Kay, but then asked her if she would like to work on a legacy project—creating something by which her family could remember her and the things she valued. Kay was taken back a bit. Tess asked, "With your great-granddaughter coming, would you like to leave her a message or tell her something about yourself? Or your children and grandchildren?" Tess went on, "Recently, I read about people writing letters to their children—sometimes just a couple of sentences, expressing their feelings and hopes for their future." Kay replied, "My parents never 'talked.' I guess they just assumed that as long as I was fed, I knew they cared for me." "Did you ever wish they said, 'I love you?'" Kay paused. Tess broke the silence and asked, "How about writing a couple of letters to your family?"

Tess and Kay worked out a goal for the next 3 weeks (Box 50.3). Kay did not know if she would have the time and energy to write everyone a letter. So, she decided to write a letter each to her children first. If able, she would write one letter to all her grandchildren, and then one letter to her great-grandchild. Over the next few weeks, Tess gave Kay prompts like, "How would you describe your son?" or "What do you admire most about your daughter?" to help Kay put her thoughts into words. By the end of 3 weeks, Kay completed her letters and put them in a large envelope to be opened after she passed away.

Upon completion of her letters, Kay felt that she had met her goals. She continued to dress and bathe relatively independently and expressed feeling at peace. Tess also thought that there were no other occupational therapy issues to address at the moment, but she informed Kay and her family to ask for occupational therapy again "when things change." Tess then discharged Kay from OT services.

About a month after Tess discharged Kay, she received another consultation to train the family in body mechanics with caregiving. Tess knew that Kay was declining quickly and that it would be a few weeks to perhaps a month before Kay would pass away. She worked with designated family members who would be providing care and ordered additional equipment such as a bedside commode, so Kay could toilet with assistance bedside instead of using diapers, and a wheelchair with a pressure-relieving cushion to get outside. Kay was sleeping a lot more, but when Tess visited, Kay awoke, smiled, and asked Tess how her daughters were doing.

Tess made one more visit to check in with the family, see if the equipment was sufficient, and offer support. The family was able to safely provide care for Kay without cuing. Given that goals were met with positive outcomes (Box 50.4) and no other occupational therapy issues, Tess discharged Kay from OT services.

Targeting Intervention Outcomes

Outcomes determine whether occupational therapy intervention is effective. What are the recommended occupational therapy outcome measures in hospice and palliative care? What constructs do we measure with a population living with a life-threatening illness? How do we determine if our intervention has been effective with clients who are declining?

There is currently no accepted hospice and palliative care outcome measure that distinguishes OT-specific outcomes.[33,45,89] However, to accommodate probable functional decline of hospice and palliative care clients, the literature suggests using reliable, valid, and individualized measures rather than one with preset performance levels on a traditional standardized measure.[74,89,124] Such client-centered measures may be more sensitive to subtle changes and more effective in capturing personal and meaningful outcomes.[124] For example, upon admission, a hospice client confined to the bed with severe pain and inability to tolerate being transferred to a wheelchair would be rated on the Functional Independent Measure (FIM) scale as 1 or dependent. The client's goal may be just to be able to tolerate being lifted into a chair and escorted outside. On a Goal Attainment Scale (GAS), the client tolerating a lift transfer and getting outside may progress 3 levels from −2 (much less than expected outcome) to 0 (expected outcome). Although the client would accomplish a major personal goal, the FIM is not sensitive to show this progress, because the performance level for functional transfers remains 1–dependent.

In the previous example, the GAS is measuring occupational participation and the FIM is measuring performance. This raises the question of what constructs should we measure to capture positive outcomes with clients who are functionally declining. With Kay, Tess measured occupational performance changes given adaptations and modifications. *Occupational performance* (or functional performance) is often used in healthcare to determine efficacy[33]; however, with life-limiting disease, a focus on occupational performance does not accommodate functional decline and may cause emotional distress over limited functional improvement as the client's disease progresses.[33,101] As Kay became more debilitated, using an occupational performance outcome measure would be less ineffective. *Occupational participation* outcomes strike a balance of detecting change in participation in meaningful occupations without focusing on performance outcomes. Occupational participation is the involvement and interaction in a life situation[5] and does not necessarily require occupational performance.[134]

The purpose of hospice and palliative care is commonly said to increase *quality of life* (QoL). With medical advances, people are living longer but with chronic and incurable diseases.[29] Longevity cannot be assumed to correlate with wellness; consequently, the concept of *quality of life* (QoL) arose to determine if treatments improve life rather than just prolong it.[79] QoL shifts the focus on functional performance to the value of life[79] and is conceptually aligned with the philosophies of occupational therapy.[79,104] Use of QoL as an outcome measure, however, can be problematic with terminally ill clients because there is no universal definition of QoL, outcomes can be affected by subjective experience, and it may be impossible to ascertain QoL outcomes due to occupational therapy intervention versus the cumulative team effect.[33,79,104]

Contextual factors are not specifically cited in the literature as a hospice outcome measure; however, the context can affect occupational therapy outcomes and must be addressed in hospice care.[9,103] In the end stages of life, modification of the physical and social environments may lessen the burden of functional problems, may affect occupational therapy outcomes more than functional status, and may be the only elements that can be varied as the client's status declines.[9,89,105] The context of dying can transform mundane occupations to highly significant life moments,[53] whereas cultural and personal factors may conjure up taboos, fears, and inhibitions that isolate the client.[24] Focus on the physical environment may maximize a client's participation in occupations and the caregiver's ability to provide safe and effective care.[9,105] Focus on the supports and relationships can facilitate social participation, enhance social support, connect the client and family to essential community and medical resources, and help facilitate closure in the end of life.[9,24,54,89,105]

Overall, there is not a consensus on what constructs we should measure with hospice and palliative care clients to capture positive occupational therapy outcomes. Selection of constructs relies on the practitioner's clinical reasoning to discern outcomes appropriate to the client's status and stage in the dying process and whether chosen constructs will effectively distinguish occupational therapy outcomes from other disciplinary interventions.

In the end, a reliable and valid client-centered measure that has an appropriately chosen construct may determine whether occupational therapy intervention has been effective. Practitioners can use client-centered measures such as GAS and the COPM, if conducive to the selected construct. For Kay, Tess was able to quantifiably capture Kay's improved occupational participation and her family's occupational performance in caregiving with GAS. Further research, however, is needed to validate whether these measures effectively and accurately capture occupational therapy outcomes in hospice and palliative care.

In summary, the role of hospice and palliative occupational therapy is to promote occupational participation throughout the lifespan. The practitioner integrates knowledge of the dying and grieving process together with the OTPF-4 domain and process to meet the unique needs of people living with life-threatening illness.[5] While focused on the client's goals, the practitioner draws upon clinical reasoning to adjust and accommodate evaluation, intervention, and selection of outcomes to the changing needs of the dying process. This method serves the needs of the client, but how do practitioners take care of themselves to sustain ongoing quality care?

PRACTITIONER SELF-CARE

Within 2 weeks of her last visit, Tess got a call from the case manager that Kay died peacefully with all her children at her bedside. People often asked Tess how she could work in hospice and palliative care with constant loss, death, and sadness. Hospice and palliative care practitioners are at high risk of burnout given the stress of working with dying clients and being constantly confronted with their own mortality.[126] Other contributing factors may include high workloads, lack of financial compensation, or lack of administrative support of palliative care programs.[40,126] To cope and sustain quality care, practitioner self-care is essential. Research has found that setting strong work-home boundaries, spending time with loved ones, focusing on the satisfying aspects of one's job, maintaining self-awareness and good physical care, practicing a daily spiritual or meditative routine, having a personal philosophy about illness and death, and knowing one's role in life may provide healthy coping strategies and decrease the risk of burnout.[40,126] For Tess, after that call, she took a moment to remember Kay's glow when she was able to "do what was important" and the privilege of working with such a vibrant person. How could she not do this job?

SUMMARY

Regardless of diagnosis or prognosis, people with life-threatening illness need opportunities and support for occupational participation to experience normalcy, purpose, well-being, and connection with others into the end of life. The hospice team appropriately consulted occupational therapy to enable Kay to "do what is important" within her limited life expectancy. Although Kay had ample help, attending to her own self-care was critical to her values and self-identity of self-sufficiency. With modifications, compensatory strategies, and adaptive equipment, Tess helped Kay maximize her occupational participation in self-care for a finite but meaningful period. Tess also helped Kay remain active in her role as mother and grandmother, sharing words of wisdom in letters to her family and in her interactions with Tess. As Kay declined, Tess continued to work with her family and provided additional equipment, modifying Kay's environment to support Kay's occupational participation through the dying process. Using a client-centered outcome measure, Tess was able to quantifiably determine positive occupational therapy outcomes of occupational participation until the end of life. However, seeing the sense of satisfaction on Kay's face truly confirmed to Tess that treatment was effective and worthwhile.

Epilogue

A month after Kay's death, Tess received a card from Liz—"I know you worked with Mom on writing letters to us all. Per her wishes, I opened up mine the night she died. Mom wrote, 'You have become what I always wanted to be. I love you.' She never told me that before. . . . Thank you. The enclosed letter is for you from Mom."

Tess slowly opened the letter and chuckled as she read, "Drink a cup of oregano tea.[b] Thank you for everything.—Kay"

---

[b]The author does not endorse the use of oregano tea and recommends consulting one's healthcare provider to inquire whether it is appropriate for personal use.

ACKNOWLEDGMENTS

The author thanks Ms. Treva Smith and Dr. Noralyn Pickens for their editorial assistance.

REVIEW QUESTIONS

1. How are hospice and palliative care interconnected yet differentiated?
2. What are therapeutic benefits of occupational participation while living with life-threatening illness?
3. What are common grief reactions we may see in clients, families, and ourselves?
4. Identify four dying trajectories.
5. What occupations has research identified as common in the end of life?
6. How does incurable disease and dying affect the domain areas of occupational therapy?
7. How can the evaluation process accommodate a declining and dying client?
8. How can the intervention process foster occupational participation in declining and dying clients?
9. Identify three possible hospice and palliative occupational therapy outcome measures.
10. Identify five coping strategies for preventing burnout.

For additional practice questions for this chapter, please visit eBooks.Health.Elsevier.com.

REFERENCES

1. American Academy of Hospice and Palliative Medicine. (n.d.). *What is hospice and palliative care?* http://aahpm.org/about/about.
2. American Cancer Society. (n.d.) *Can pancreatic cancer be found early?* https://www.cancer.org/cancer/pancreatic-cancer/detection-diagnosis-staging/detection.html.
3. American Cancer Society. (n.d.). *Signs and symptoms of pancreatic cancer.* https://www.cancer.org/search.html?q=Signs+and+symptoms+of+pancreatic+cancer
4. American Occupational Therapy Association: The role of occupational therapy in end-of-life care, *American Journal of Occupational Therapy* 70(Supplement 2):1–16, 2016. https://doi.org/10.5014/ajot.2016.706S17.

5. American Occupational Therapy Association: Occupational therapy practice framework: domain and process (4th ed.). *American Journal of Occupational Therapy* 74(Supplement 2):1–87, 2020. https://doi.org/10.5014/ajot.2020.74S2001.

6. Barrett H, Watterson J: Occupational therapy in neuro-oncology. In Cooper J, editor: *Occupational therapy in oncology and palliative care*, ed 2, 2006, Whurr Publishers Limited, pp 145–160.

7. Bostock A, Ellis S, Mathewson S, Methven L: Occupational therapy in hospices and day care. In Cooper J, editor: *Occupational therapy in oncology and palliative care*, ed 2, 2006, Whurr Publishers Limited, pp 161–173.

8. Broiller CB, Watts JH, Bauer D, Schmidt WA: A concurrent validity study of two occupational therapy evaluation instruments: the AOF and OCAIRS, *Occupational Therapy in Mental Health* 8(4):49–59, 1989. https://doi.org/10.1300/J004v08n04_04.

9. Bye R: When clients are dying: occupational therapists' perspectives, *The Occupational Therapy Journal of Research* 18(1):3–24, 1998. https://doi.org/10.1177/153944929801800101.

10. Canadian Association of Occupational Therapists: *Enabling occupation: an occupational therapy perspective*, 1997, CAOT Publications ACE.

11. Cardona-Morrell M, Lewis E, Suman S, Haywood C, Williams M, Brousseau A, Greenaway S, Hillman K, Dent E: Recognising older frail patients near the end of life: what next? *Eur J Intern Med* 45:84–90, 2017. https://doi.org/10.1016/j.ejim.2017.09.026.

12. Carpenter L, Tyldesley B, Baker GA: The use of the Canadian Occupational Performance Measure as an outcome of a pain management program, *Canadian Occupational Therapy Journal* 68(1):16–22, 2001. https://doi.org/10.1177/000841740106800102.

13. Centers for Medicare and Medicaid Services: *Medicare hospice benefits*. Centers for Medicare & Medicaid Services. 2020. https://www.medicare.gov/Pubs/pdf/02154-medicare-hospice-benefits.pdf.

14. Centers for Medicare and Medicaid Services: *State operations manual: appendix M—Guidance to surveyors: hospice—Rev.200, 02-21-20*. http://www.cms.gov/Regulations-and-Guidance/Guidance/Manuals/downloads/som107ap_m_hospice.pdf.

15. Chan CCH, Lee TMC: Validity of the Canadian occupational performance measure, *Occupational Therapy International* 4(3):231–249, 1997. https://onlinelibrary.wiley.com/doi/pdfdirect/10.1002/oti.58.

16. Chan K, Tse DMW, Sham MMK: Dyspnoea and other respiratory symptoms in palliative care. In Cherny N, Fallon M, Kaasa S, Portenoy RK, Currow DC, editors: *Oxford textbook of palliative medicine*, ed 5, 2015, Oxford University Press, pp 421–434.

17. Cherny N: Pain assessment and cancer pain syndromes. In Hanks G, Cherny NI, Chistakis NA, Fallon M, Kaasa S, Portenoy RK, editors: *Oxford textbook of palliative medicine*, ed 4, 2010, Oxford University Press, pp 599–623.

18. Chow JK: *Is the OCAIRS a suitable hospice occupational therapy outcome measure?* [Unpublished manuscript]. In *Department of Rehabilitation Sciences*, 2014, Temple University.

19. Clark D: International progress in creating palliative medicine as a specialized discipline. In Hanks G, Cherny NI, Chistakis NA, Fallon M, Kaasa S, Portenoy RK, editors: *Oxford textbook of palliative medicine*, ed 4, 2011, Oxford University Press, pp 9–16.

20. Connor SR, Fine PG: Lessons learned from hospice in the United States of America. In Hanks G, Cherny NI, Chistakis NA, Fallon M, Kaasa S, Portenoy RK, editors: *Oxford textbook of palliative medicine*, ed 4, 2010, Oxford University Press, pp 17–22.

21. Connor SR, Pyenson B, Fitch K, Spence C, Iwasaki K: Comparing hospice and nonhospice patient survival among patients who die within a three-year window, *Journal of Pain Symptom Management* 33(3):238–246, 2007. https://doi.org/10.1016/j.jpainsymman.2006.10.010.

22. Cooper J: Occupation therapy approach in symptom control. In Cooper J, editor: *Occupational therapy in oncology and palliative care*, ed 2, 2006, Whurr Publishers Limited, pp 27–39.

23. Cooper J, Kite N: Occupational therapy to palliative care. In Cherny N, Fallon M, Kaasa S, Portenoy RK, Currow DC, editors: *Oxford textbook of palliative medicine*, ed 5, 2015, Oxford University Press, pp 177–183.

24. Costa A, Othero M: Palliative care, terminal illness, and the model of human occupation, *Phys Occup Ther Geriatr* 30(4):316–327, 2012. https://doi.org/10.3109/02703181.2012.743205.

25. Cup EH, Scholte op Reimer WJ, Thijssen MC, Van Kuyk-Minis MA: Reliability and validity of the Canadian occupational performance measure in stroke patients, *Clin Rehabil* 17(4):402–409, 2003. https://doi.org/10.1191/0269215503cr635oa.

26. Cusick A, Lannin NA, Lowe K: Adapting the Canadian Occupational Performance Measure for use in a paediatric clinical trial, *Disability & Rehabilitation* 29(10):761–766, 2007. https://doi.org/10.1080/09638280600929201.

27. Davies B, Siden H: Children in palliative medicine: an overview. In Hanks G, Cherny NI, Chistakis NA, Fallon M, Kaasa S, Portenoy RK, editors: *Oxford textbook of palliative medicine*, ed 2, 2010, Oxford University Press, pp 1301–1317.

28. Delgado Guay MO, Yennurajalingam S: Sleep disturbance. In Yennurajalingam S, Bruera E, editors: *Oxford American handbook of hospice and palliative medicine*, 2011, Oxford University Press, pp 115–126.

29. DeRosa J: Providing self-management support to people living with chronic conditions, *OT Practice* 18(17):CE-1-8, 2013. https://www.aota.org

30. Ding J, Johnson CE, Lee YC, Gazey A, Cook A: Characteristics of people with dementia vs other conditions on admission to inpatient palliative care, *Journal of American Geriatrics Society* 68(8):1825–1833, 2020. https://doi.org/10.1111/jgs.16458.

31. Donnelly C, Carswell A: Individualized outcome measures: a review of the literature, *Canadian Journal of Occupational Therapy* 69(2):84–94, 2002. https://doi.org/10.1177/000841740206900204.

32. Etkind SN, Bone AE, Gomes B, Lovell N, Evans CJ, Higginson IJ, Murtagh FEM: How many people will need palliative care in 2040? Past trends, future projections and implications for services, *BMC Med* 15(1):1–10, 2017. https://doi.org/10.1186/s12916-017-0860-2.

33. Eva G: Measuring occupational therapy outcomes in cancer and palliative care. In Cooper J, editor: *Occupational therapy in oncology and palliative care*, ed 2, 2006, Whurr Publishers Limited, pp 189–199.

34. Faguet G: *The war on cancer: an anatomy of failure, a blueprint for the future*, 2008, Springer Science and Business Media.

35. Forsyth K, Deshpande S, Kielhofner G, Henriksson C, Haglund L, Olson L, Skinner S, Kulkarni S: A user's manual for the Occupational Circumstances Assessment Interview and Rating Scale (OCAIRS), *The MOHO Clearinghouse Department of Occupational Therapy*, 2006.

36. Fuller K: The effectiveness of occupational performance outcome measures within mental health practice, *British Journal of Occupational Therapy* 74(8):399–405, 2011. https://doi.org/10.4276/030802211X13125646371004.

37. Glare P, Sinclair C, Downing M, Stone P: Predicting survival in patients with advanced disease. In Hanks G, Cherny NI,

Chistakis NA, Fallon M, Kaasa S, Portenoy RK, editors. *Oxford textbook of palliative medicine*, ed 4, 2010, pp. 81–110.

38. Goldstein NE, Meier DE: Palliative medicine in older adults. In Hanks G, Cherny NI, Chistakis NA, Fallon M, Kaasa S, Portenoy RK, editors: *Oxford textbook of palliative medicine*, ed 4, 2010, Oxford University, pp 1386–1399.

39. Granger CV, Hamilton BB, Linacre JM, Heinemann AW, Wright BD: Performance profiles of the functional independence measure, *Am J Phys Med Rehab* 72:84–89, 1993. https://doi.org/10.1097/00002060-199304000-00005.

40. Gupta S, Paterson ML, Lysaght RM, von Zweck CM: Experiences of burnout and coping strategies utilized by occupational therapists, *Canadian Journal of Occupational Therapy* 79(2): 86–95, 2012. https://doi.org/10.2182/cjot.2012.79.2.4.

41. Haglund L, Henriksson C: Testing a Swedish version of OCAIRS on two different patient groups, *Scand J Caring Sci* 8(4):223–230, 1994. https://doi.org/10.1111/j.1471-6712.1994.tb00248.x.

42. Haglund L, Thorell L, Walinder J: Assessment of occupational functioning for screening of patients to occupational therapy in general psychiatric care, *Occupational Therapy Journal of Research* 18(4):193–206, 1998. https://doi.org/10.1177/153944929801800405.

43. Halkett G, Ciccarelli M, Keesing S, Aoun S: Occupational therapy in palliative care: is it under-utilised in Western Australia? *Australian Occupational Therapy Journal* 57(5):301–309, 2010. https://doi.org/10.1111/j.1440-1630.2009.00843.x.

44. Hallenbeck J: *Palliative care perspectives*, 2003, Oxford Press.

45. Hammill K, Bye R, Cook C: Occupational therapy for people living with a life-limiting illness: a thematic review, *British Journal of Occupational Therapy* 77(11):582–589, 2014. https://doi.org/10.4276/030802214X14151078348594.

46. Harlos M: The terminal phase. In Hanks G, Cherny NI, Chistakis NA, Fallon M, Kaasa S, Portenoy RK, editors: *Oxford textbook of palliative medicine*, ed 4, 2010, Oxford University Press, pp 1549–1559.

47. Hoerger M, Wayser GR, Schwing G, Suzuki A, Perry LM: Impact of interdisciplinary outpatient specialty palliative care on survival and quality of life in adjust with advanced cancer: a meta-analysis of randomized controlled trials, *Annals of Behavioral Medicine* 53(7):674–685, 2019. https://doi.org/10.1093/abm/kay077.

48. Holland JM, Neimeyer RA: An examination of stage theory of grief among individuals bereaved by natural and violent causes: a meaning-oriented contribution, *OMEGA J Death Dying* 61(2): 103–120, 2010. https://doi.org/10.2190/OM.61.2.b.

49. Hospice Foundation of America (2011). *A caregiver's guide to the dying process*. http://hospicefoundation.org/hfa/media/Files/Hospice_TheDyingProcess_Docutech-READERSPREADS.pdf.

50. Houben CH, Spruit MA, Schols JM, Wouters EF, Janssen DJ: Patient-clinician communication about end-of-life care in patients with advanced chronic organ failure during one year, *J Pain Symptom Manage* 49(6):1109–1115, 2015. https://doi.org/10.1016/j.jpainsymman.2014.12.008.

51. Hovland CA, Mallett CA: Dying with dementia: caregiver observations of their family members' physical decline and behavioral or psychological changes during their last days, *OMEGA J Death Dying* 84(2):653–672, 2021. https://doi.org/10.1177/0030222820906684.

52. Hunter EG: Legacy: The occupational transmission of self through actions and artifacts, *Journal of Occupational Science* 15(1):48–54, 2008. https://doi.org/10.1080/14427591.2008.9686607.

53. Hurn J, Kneebone I, Cropley M: Goal setting as an outcome measure: a systematic review, *Clin Rehabil* 20(9):756–772, 2006. https://doi.org/10.1177/0269215506070793.

54. Jacques ND, Hasselkus BR: The nature of occupation surrounding dying and death, *Occupational Therapy Journal of Research* 24(2):44–53, 2004. https://doi.org/10.1177/153944920402400202.

55. Johns Hopkins Medicine: *Pancreatic cancer*. https://www.hopkinsmedicine.org/health/conditions-and-diseases/pancreatic-cancer#:~:text=This%20cancer%20occurs%20when%20a,at%20age%2065%20or%20older.

56. Johnson, S: *Living fully until we die.* 2009. http://www.christianitytoday.com/ch/thepastinthepresent/storybehind/livingfully.html?start=2.

57. Kaplan K: Short-term assessment: the need and a response, *Occupational Therapy in Mental Health* 4(3):29–45, 1984. https://doi.org/10.1300/J004v04n03_05.

58. Karnes, B: *Gone from my sight: the dying experience.* [Pamphlet]. 2001. Barbara Karnes.

59. Kasven-Gonzalez N, Sourverain R, Miale S: Improving quality of life through rehabilitation in palliative care: case report, *Palliative and Supportive Care* 8(3):359–369, 2010. https://doi.org/10.1017/S1478951510000167.

60. Kaye, P: Notes on symptom control in hospice and palliative care, 2006, Hospice Education Institute.

61. Kealey P, McIntyre I: An evaluation of the domiciliary occupational therapy service in palliative cancer care in a community trust: a patient and carers perspective, *Eur J Cancer Care (Engl.)* 14(3):232–243, 2005. https://doi.org/10.1111/j.1365-2354.2005.00559.x.

62. Keesing S, Rosenwax L: Is occupation missing from occupational therapy in palliative care? *Australian Occupational Therapy Journal* 58(5):329–336, 2011. https://doi.org/10.1111/j.1440-1630.2011.00958.x.

63. Keesing S, Rosenwax L: Establishing a role for occupational therapists in end-of-life care in Western Australia, *Australian Occupational Therapy Journal* 60(5):370–373, 2013. https://doi.org/10.1111/1440-1630.12058.

64. Keith RA, Granger CV, Hamilton BB, Sherwin FS: The functional independence measure: a new tool for rehabilitation. In Eisenberg MG, Grzesiak RC, editors: *Advances in Clinical Rehabilitation*, New York, 1987, Springer Publishing, pp 6–18.

65. Kendall M, Carduff E, Lloyd A, Kimbell B, Cavers D, Buckingham S, Boyd K, Grant L, Worth A, Pinnock H, Sheikh A, Murray SA: Different experiences and goals in different advanced diseases: comparing serial interviews with patients with cancer, organ failure, or frailty and their family and professional carers, *J Pain Symptom Manage* 50(2):216–224, 2015. https://doi.org/10.1016/j.jpainsymman.2015.02.017.

66. Khan SA, Gomes B, Higginson IJ: End-of-life care—what do cancer patients want? *National Review of Clinical Oncology* 11:100–108, 2014. https://doi.org/10.1038/nrclinonc.2013.217.

67. Kiresuk T, Sherman R: Goal attainment scaling: a general method for evaluating comprehensive community mental health programs, *Community Ment Health J* 4:443–453, 1968. https://doi.org/10.1007/BF01530764.

68. Kiresuk TJ, Smith A, Cardillo JE: *Goal attainment scaling: applications, theory, and measurement*, Mahwah, NJ, 1994, Lawrence Erlbaum Associates.

69. Kissane DW, Zaider T: Bereavement. In Cherny N, Fallon M, Kaasa S, Portenoy RK, Currow DC, editors: *Oxford textbook of palliative medicine,* ed 5, 2015, Oxford University Press, pp 1110–1122.

70. Kübler-Ross E: *On death and dying*, 1969, Collier Books.

71. la Cour K, Josephsson S, Tishelman C, Nygård L: Experiences of engagement in creative activity at a palliative care facility, *Palliative and Supportive Care* 5(3):241–250, 2007. https://doi.org/10.1017/S1478951507000405.

72. Lai J, Haglund L, Kielhofner G: Occupational case analysis interview and rating scale: an examination of construct validity, *Scand J Caring Sci* 13(4):267–273, 1999. https://doi.org/10.1111/j.1471-6712.1999.tb00550.x.

73. Lala AP, Kinsella EA: A phenomenological inquiry into the embodied nature of occupation at end of life, *Canadian Journal of Occupational Therapy* 78(4):246–254, 2011. https://doi.org/10.2182/cjot.2011.78.4.6.

74. Laver-Fawcett A: *Principles of assessment and outcome measurement for occupational therapists and physiotherapists: theory, skills and application*, 2007, John Wiley & Sons, Ltd.

75. Law M, Baptiste S, Carswell A, McColl MA, Polatajko H, Pollack N: *Canadian occupational performance measure*, ed 4, 2005, CAOT Publications ACE.

76. Lee SW, Kielhofner G: Habituation: patterns of daily occupation. In Taylor R, editor: *Kielhofner's model of human occupation*, ed 5, 2017, Wolters Kluwer, pp 57–73.

77. Lee SW, Kielhofner G: Volition. In Taylor R, editor: *Kielhofner's model of human occupation*, ed 5, 2017, Wolters Kluwer, pp 38–56.

78. Lee WTK, Chan HF, Wong E: Improvement of feeding independence in end-stage cancer patients under palliative care—a prospective, uncontrolled study, *Support Care Cancer* 13:1051–1056, 2005. https://doi.org/10.1007/s00520-005-0859-7.

79. Liddle J, McKenna K: Quality of life: an overview of issues for use in occupational therapy outcome measurement, *Australian Occupational Therapy Journal* 47(2):77–85, 2000. https://doi.org/10.1046/j.1440-1630.2000.00217.x.

80. Littlechild B: Managing fatigue: A trial of group and individual educational support for hospice outpatients, *European Journal of Palliative Care* 23(4):166–168, 2016. http://www.haywardpublishing.co.uk/_year_search_review.aspx?JID=4&Year=2016&Edition=573.

81. Lloyd A, Kendall M, Starr JM, Murray SA: Physical, social, psychological and existential trajectories of loss and adaptation towards the end of life for older people living with frailty: a serial interview study, *BMC Geriatr* 16(176):1–15, 2016. https://doi.org/10.1186/s12877-016-0350-y.

82. Lowey SE, Norton SA, Quinn JR, Quill TE: Living with advanced heart failure or COPD: experiences and goals of individuals nearing the end of life, *Research in Nursing and Health* 36(4):349–358, 2013. https://doi.org/10.1002/nur.21546.

83. Lunney JR, Lynn J, Foley DJ, et al: Patterns of functional decline at the end of life, *J Am Med Assoc* 289(18):2387–2392, 2003. https://doi.org/10.1001/jama.289.18.2387.

84. Lutz S: The history of hospice and palliative care, *Curr Probl Cancer* 35(6):304–309, 2011. https://doi.org/10.1016/j.currproblcancer.2011.10.004.

85. Lyons M, Orozovic N, Davis J, Newman J: Doing-being-becoming: occupational experiences of persons with life-threatening illnesses, *American Journal of Occupational Therapy* 56(3):285–295, 2002. https://doi.org/10.5014/ajot.56.3.285.

86. Mailloux Z, May-Benson TA, Summers CA, Miller LJ, Brett-Green B, Burke JP, et al: Goal attainment scaling as a measure of meaningful outcomes for children with sensory integration disorders, *American Journal of Occupational Therapy* 61(2):254–259, 2007. https://doi.org/10.5014/ajot.61.2.254.

87. McClement SE, Chochinov HM: Spiritual issues in palliative medicine. In Hanks G, Cherny NI, Chistakis NA, Fallon M, Kaasa S, Portenoy RK, editors: *Oxford textbook of palliative medicine*, ed 4, 2010, Oxford University Press, pp 1403–1409.

88. McColl MA, Paterson M, Davies D, Doubt L, Law M: Validity and community utility of the Canadian Occupational Performance Measure, *Canadian Journal of Occupational Therapy* 67(1):22–30, 2000. https://doi.org/10.1177/000841740006700105.

89. Miller J, Cooper J: The contribution of occupational therapy to palliative medicine. In Hanks G, Cherny NI, Chistakis NA, Fallon M, Kaasa S, Portenoy RK, editors: *Oxford textbook of palliative medicine*, ed 4, 2011, Oxford University Press, pp 206–213.

90. Miller J, Hopkinson C: A retrospective audit exploring the use of relaxation as an intervention in oncology and palliative care, *Eur J Cancer Care (Engl.)* 17(5):488–491, 2008. https://doi.org/10.1111/j.1365-2354.2007.00899.x.

91. Mitchell SL, Teno JM, Kiely DK, Shaffer ML, Jones RN, Prigerson HG, Volicer L, Givens JL, Hamel MB: The clinical course of advanced dementia, *N Engl J Med* 361(16):1529–1538, 2009. https://doi.org/10.1056/NEJMoa0902234.

92. Moneymaker KA: Understanding the dying process: transitions during final days to hours, *J Palliat Med* 8(5):1079, 2005. https://doi.org/10.1089/jpm.2005.8.1079.

93. Morgan DD, Tieman JJ, Allingham SF, Ekström MP, Connolly A, Currow DC: The trajectory of functional decline over the last 4 months of life in a palliative care population: a prospective, consecutive cohort study, *Palliat Med* 33(6):693–703, 2019. https://doi.org/10.1177/0269216319839024.

94. Murray SA, Kendall M, Boyd K, Sheikh A: Illness trajectories and palliative care, *Br Med J* 330(7498):1007–1011, 2005. https://doi.org/10.1136/bmj.330.7498.1007.

95. Murray SA, Kendall M, Grant E, Boyd K, Barclay S, Sheikh A: Patterns of social, psychological, and spiritual decline toward the end of life in lung cancer and heart failure, *J Pain Symptom Manage* 34(4):393–402, 2007. https://doi.org/10.1016/j.jpainsymman.2006.12.009.

96. National Consensus Project for Quality Palliative Care: *Clinical practice guidelines for quality palliative care, 4th edition*, 2018, National Consensus Project for Quality Palliative Care.

97. National Health Council (2013). *About chronic diseases*. https://www.nationalhealthcouncil.org/sites/default/files/NHC_Files/Pdf_Files/AboutChronicDisease.pdf.

98. National Hospice and Palliative Care Organization (NHPCO). *History of hospice*, n.d. https://www.nhpco.org/hospice-care-overview/history-of-hospice/.

99. National Hospice and Palliative Care Organization (NHPCO). Hospice facts and figures, 2020, https://www.nhpco.org/hospice-facts-figures/.

100. Noe K, Smith PC, Younis M: Call for reform to the U.S. hospice system, *Ageing Int* 37:228–237, 2012. https://doi.org/10.1007/s12126-010-9106-8.

101. Norris A: A pilot study of an outcome measure in palliative care, *Int J Palliat Nurs* 5(1):40–45, 1999. https://doi.org/10.12968/ijpn.1999.5.1.9931.

102. Pan A, Chung L, Hsin-Hwei G: Reliability and validity of the Canadian Occupational Performance Measure for clients with psychiatric disorders in Taiwan, *Occup Ther Int* 10(4):269–277, 2003. https://doi.org/10.1002/oti.190.

103. Panchmatia N, Urch C: The feasibility of using goal attainment scaling in an acute oncology setting, *European*

Journal of Palliative Care 21(3):138–143, 2014. http://www.haywardpublishing.co.uk/_year_search_review.aspx?JID=4&Year=2014&Edition=509.

104. Pearson E, Todd JG, Futcher JM: How can occupational therapists measure outcomes in palliative care? *Palliat Med* 21(6):477–485, 2007. https://doi.org/10.1177/0269216307081941.

105. Pizzi M: Environments of care: hospice. In Hopkins HL, Smith H, editors: *Willard and Spackman's occupational therapy*, ed 8, 1993, J.B. Lippincott Company, pp 853–864.

106. Rando TA: *Grief, dying, and death: clinical interventions for caregivers*, Champaign, IL, 1984, Research Press.

107. Reed KS: Grief is more than tears, *Nurs Sci Q* 16(1):77–81, 2003. https://doi.org/10.1177/0894318402239070.

108. Reinke LF, Engelberg RA, Shannon SE, Wenrich MD, Vig EK, Back AL, Curtis R: Transitions regarding palliative and end-of-life care in severe chronic obstructive pulmonary disease or advanced cancer: themes identified by patients, families, and clinicians, *J Palliat Med* 11(4):601–609, 2008. https://doi.org/10.1089/jpm.2007.0236.

109. Rochman D, Ray S, Kulich R, Mehta NR, Driscoll S: Validity and utility of the Canadian Occupational Performance Measure as an outcome measure in a craniofacial pain center, *Occupational Therapy Journal of Research* 28(1):4–11, 2008. https://doi.org/10.3928/15394492-20080101-06.

110. Sachs GA: Dying from dementia, *N Engl J Med* 361(16):1595–1596, 2009. https://doi.org/10.1056/NEJMe0905988.

111. Sakaguchi S, Okamura H: Effectiveness of collage activity based on a life review in elderly cancer patients: a preliminary study, *Palliative and Supportive Care* 13(2):285–293, 2015. https://doi.org/10.1017/S1478951514000194.

112. Sands MB, O'Connell DL, Piza M, Ingram JM: The epidemiology of death and symptoms: planning for population-based palliative care. In Cherny N, Fallon M, Kaasa S, Portenoy RK, Currow DC, editors: *Oxford textbook of palliative medicine*, ed 5, 2015, Oxford University Press, pp 49–77.

113. Schleinich MA, Warren S, Nekolaichuk C, Kaasa T, Watanabe S: Palliative care rehabilitation survey: a pilot study of patients' priorities for rehabilitation goals, *Palliat Med* 22:822–830, 2008. https://doi.org/10.1177/0269216308096526.

114. Seamon D: Physical and virtual environments. In Boyt Schell BA, Gillen G, Scaffa ME, Cohn E, editors: *Willard and Spackman's occupational therapy*, ed 12, 2014, J.B. Lippincott Company, pp 202–214.

115. Shearsmith-Farthing K: The management of altered body image: a role for occupational therapy, *British Journal of Occupational Therapy* 64(8):387–392, 2001. https://doi.org/10.1177/030802260106400803.

116. Steinhauser KE, Tulsky JA: Defining a 'good death.' In Cherny N, Fallon M, Kaasa S, Portenoy RK, Currow DC, editors: *Oxford textbook of palliative medicine*, ed 5, 2015, Oxford University Press, pp 77–83.

117. Stoddard, S: *The hospice movement: a better way of caring for the dying*, 1978, Stein.

118. Svidén GA, Tham K, Borell L: Involvement in everyday life for people with a life threatening illness, *Palliative and Supportive Care* 8(3):345–352, 2010. https://doi.org/10.1017/S1478951510000143.

119. Tavemark S, Hermansson LN, Blomberg K: Enabling activity in palliative care: focus groups among occupational therapists, *BMC Palliat Care* 18(1):17, 2019. https://doi.org/10.1186/s12904-019-0394-9.

120. Taylor R: *Kielhofner's model of human occupation*, 2017, Wolters Kluwer.

121. Temel JS, Greer JA, Muzikansky A, Gallagher ER, Admane S, Jackson VA, Dahlin CM, Blinderman CD, Jacobsen J, Pirl WF, Billings JA, Lynch TJ: Early palliative care for patients with metastatic non-small-cell lung cancer, *New England Journal of Medicine* 363(8):733–742, 2010. https://doi.org/10.1056/NEJMoa1000678.

122. Thew M, Edwards M, Baptiste S, Molineux M: *Role emerging occupational therapy: maximizing occupation-focused practice*, 2011, Wiley-Blackwell. [(Wade & Halligan as cited in Thew et al., 2011, location 346 of 5018).]

123. Thompson, B. Mindfulness-based stress reduction for people with chronic conditions. Br J Occup Ther, 72(9), 405–410, 2009.

124. Turner-Stokes L: Goal attainment scaling (GAS) in rehabilitation: a practical guide, *Clin Rehabil* 23(4):362–370, 2009. https://doi.org/10.1177/0269215508101742.

125. United Nations Department of Economic and Social Affairs: Population Division. *World population ageing 2019. United Nations*, 2019. https://www.un.org/en/development/desa/population/publications/pdf/ageing/WorldPopulationAgeing2019-Report.pdf.

126. Vachon MLS: Burn-out in health care providers. In Yennurajalingam S, Bruera E, editors: *Oxford American handbook of hospice and palliative medicine*, 2011, Oxford University Press, pp 449–464.

127. Vrkljan B, Miller-Polgar J: Meaning of occupational engagement in life-threatening illness: a qualitative pilot project, *Canadian Journal of Occupational Therapy* 68(4):237–246, 2001. https://doi.org/10.1177/000841740106800407.

128. Wang SE, Liu IA, Lee JS, Khang P, Rosen R, Reinke LF, Mularski RA, Nguyen HQ: End-of-life care in patients exposed to home-based palliative care vs hospice only, *J Am Geriatr Soc* 67(6):1226–1233, 2019. https://doi.org/10.1111/jgs.15844.

129. Watts JH, Brollier C, Bauer D, Schmidt W: A comparison of two evaluation instruments used with psychiatric patients in occupational therapy, *Occupational Therapy in Mental Health* 8(4):7–27, 1989. https://doi.org/10.1300/J004v08n04_02.

130. Webb J: Play therapy with hospitalized children, *International Journal of Play therapy* 4(1):51–59, 1995. https://doi.org/10.1037/h0089214.

131. World Health Organization. (2018, February 23). *10 facts on palliative care*. https://www.who.int/news-room/facts-in-pictures/detail/palliative-care.

132. Wu J, Quill T: Geriatric rehabilitation and palliative care: opportunity for collaboration or oxymoron? *Topics in Geriatric Rehabilitation* 27(1):29–35, 2011. https://doi.org/10.1097/TGR.0b013e3181ff6844.

133. Yennurajalingam S, Bruera E: Research in terminally ill patients. In Yennurajalingam S, Bruera E, editors: *Oxford American handbook of hospice and palliative medicine*, 2011, Oxford University Press, pp 439–447.

134. Zhang C, McCarthy C, Craik J: Students as translators for the Canadian Model of Occupational Performance and Engagement, *Occupational Therapy Now* 10(3):3–5, 2008. https://caot.in1touch.org/document/3899/OTNow_May_08.pdf.

51

Therapeutic Use of Self: Embodying Mindfulness in Occupational Therapy

Rochelle McLaughlin

LEARNING OBJECTIVES

After studying this chapter, the student or practitioner will be able to do the following:

1. Define mindfulness and the therapeutic use of self.
2. Explain ways in which the therapeutic use of self can be cultivated and fostered.
3. Describe ways in which the Western medicine medical culture and Western societal and cultural norms in general undermine our capacity to cultivate and foster the therapeutic use of self.
4. Differentiate between mindful occupational participation and automatic-pilot mode occupational participation.
5. Identify ways in which mindfulness is currently embedded within the Western medical system.
6. Examine ways in which the act and practice of embodying mindfulness as an occupational therapist can enhance the cultivation and development of the therapeutic use of self. Assess and justify the efficacy of mindfulness as a skillful way to develop the therapeutic use of self.

CHAPTER OUTLINE

KEY TERMS

Coping
Maladaptive Coping

Mindful Awareness
Mindfulness-based healthcare practitioners

Resilience
Therapeutic Use of Self

KEY PHRASES

Development of the therapeutic use of self
Habitual stress reactivity
Mindfulness-mediated stress response

Quality of the engagement and participation in occupations

Prepared and effective interpersonal interaction

THREADED CASE STUDY

Kay, Part 1

Kay (prefers use of the pronouns she/her/hers), an experienced occupational therapist (OT), works full time in a rehabilitation hospital in her metropolitan area. In the past, Kay has experienced a great deal of gratification from her work as an OT and prided herself in being great at building rapport with her clients. Over the past few years, however, with the intensifying productivity demands in healthcare, the development of the pandemic, and ubiquitous cultural unrest, her stress has increased to a level she's never experienced before. On top of her family responsibilities and challenges, Kay is finding it increasingly difficult to skillfully and effectively meet the needs of the complexity of the patient-family-care demands, the intense productivity standards at work, the overwhelmingly large caseload, the complex needs of her team, and taking care of herself. She has also noticed she has less time and feels less energy for building meaningful connections with her clients.

Kay has identified various signs and symptoms of her challenges in meeting and responding to all that is unfolding. She has been experiencing insomnia, heart palpitations, shallow breathing, muscle tension, headaches, back pain, and digestive issues. Kay also noticed that she has been making increasingly poor food choices, as well as increased media use, and she has noticed a frazzled sense of being "overly busy" with little time to take care of her basic needs. She notes increased feelings of cynicism, hopelessness, and disengagement from routines and occupations that she usually considers restorative and nourishing.

Kay wishes that she could have greater ease and well-being in her work and in her family life despite all that is unfolding. She desires to be more effective at work and in her community, as well as feeling more connected to herself and her family. She feels stuck and thinks that there must be a healthier, more effective way to be in relation to all that is going on.

Critical Thinking Questions

1. How might Kay's access to valuable clinical reasoning and critical thinking skills be compromised as a result of stress reactivity, maladaptive coping, and lack of self-care?
2. In what specific ways might Kay's relationship to the stress in her life affect her capacity to meet the demands of our complex profession of occupational therapy.
3. What are Kay's patterns of occupational engagement? How have they changed and why have they changed? Consider her **quality of engagement and participation in occupations**.
4. What barriers are affecting Kay's capacity to be a thriving person, mother, partner, occupational therapist, community member, and caregiver?
5. Consider Kay's priorities and desired outcomes related to occupational performance, prevention, participation, role competence, health and wellness, quality of life, and well-being, how might mindfulness help enhance Kay's capacity to build meaningful rapport with her clients or foster her capacity to use herself in an effective and therapeutic way?

INTRODUCTION

The development of the therapeutic use of self is a cornerstone of the occupational therapy (OT) process (OTPF-4, 2020)[2] and can be considered the single most important line of intervention we can provide as occupational therapists (OTs) because it is the foundation from which practitioners experience their relationship with clients and their occupations.[1,2,98] However, there remains little focus in the literature or even in OT education on *how* to access, develop, and implement this critical yet elusive skill. Mindfulness, defined as the steady, intentional gathering

of one's attention into the present moment in a nonjudgmental way,[43] has the potential to offer the essential skillset necessary for the development of the therapeutic use of self, particularly in these times of uncertainty and change.

Kay's situation is unfortunately not unique. The current medical environment in which occupational therapists work tends not to foster institutional norms for supporting the development of these skills for their employees.[40] The modern Western medicine environment itself disproportionately values productivity and self-sacrifice over employee health and well-being. Even before the pandemic, the healthcare system has been increasingly overburdened by the chronic public health disease crisis. Industry experts state that hospital admissions have been continuously rising over the past 30 years, to the point at which U.S. hospitals are being stretched to their limits—placing a heavy burden of care on the staff.[3,8] It is not surprising, then, that burnout and chronic disease statistics among healthcare professionals are staggering and growing.[77] The United States reports 25% to 90% burnout rate among healthcare workers,[10,52] depending on the working conditions and setting.[a]

Although these statistics demonstrate dire circumstances for healthcare workers, there is promising and emerging research demonstrating the beneficial and encompassing effects of the psychological characteristics that mindfulness develops and can be a remedy and healing antidote to meet the mental, emotional, physical, contextual, and therapeutic needs of our world's healthcare workers and the individuals they work with.[b] The characteristics of mindfulness-based healthcare practitioners (MBHPs; healthcare workers who embody mindfulness in their lives and work, which includes occupational therapy practitioners) are aligned with the characteristics of providers who demonstrate skillful and effective therapeutic use of self.[c]

The practices, skills, characteristics, and qualities of mindfulness take time to develop in one's life and work, just as the development of the therapeutic use of self does, and yet they are incredibly portable, practical, and useful. Employing mindfulness in occupational therapy practice with the intention to develop one's capacity to use oneself in an effective and therapeutic way is not a quick fix for any of the complex problems an occupational therapist encounters in life and work. According to extensive research, however, the implications of this kind of training are profound and far-reaching.[d] In this chapter, with the assistance of Kay's case example, will take a look at how the embodiment of mindfulness in occupational therapy can elicit the development of the therapeutic use of self and enhance our health, well-being, effectiveness, and sense of purpose and meaning.

THE THERAPEUTIC USE OF SELF

The Commission on Practice of the American Occupational Therapy Association (AOTA) added "the therapeutic use of self" to the OTPF-3 process overview in 2014.[2] The OTPF-4 states, "An integral part of the OT process is therapeutic use of self, which

---

[a] References 9,17,22,23,37,38,48,53,58,59,65,66,75,83,84.
[b] References 7,12,14,18–20,25,31,33,36,41,45,49,69,74.
[c] References 27,29,31,80,86–89,93,96.
[d] References 13,27,29,31,39,80,86–89,92,96.

allows OT practitioners to develop and manage their therapeutic relationship with clients by using professional reasoning, empathy, and a client-centered, collaborative approach to service delivery.[2] The initial change in the OTPF-3 was made to ensure that practitioners understand that use of the self as a therapeutic agent is integral to the occupational therapy process and is used in *all* interactions with *all* clients.[1,2] The commission states that the *therapeutic use of self* allows OT practitioners to develop and manage their therapeutic relationship with clients by using professional reasoning[49,79]; empathy[97]; and a client-centered,[19,69,72] collaborative approach to service delivery.[49,79] Open communication ensures that practitioners connect with clients at an emotional level to assist them with their current life situation.[30,31] The use of the self in a therapeutic way is defined as the capacity and skill to use oneself in such a way that one becomes an *effective* tool in the evaluation and intervention process (as cited by Taylor RR, 2020 in AOTA OTPF-4 document).[1,2]

The following text highlights a few qualities and characteristics of the effective use of the therapeutic use of self to help us begin to articulate the practice and skills. They can be described as being embedded within the Mindfulness Model,[89] which, as described by Shapiro and colleagues,[89] highlights three important aspects of the development of the therapeutic use of self: the level of attention, the attitude, and the intention the occupational therapist brings to therapeutic relationships. As you consider the list below, identify whether the characteristic, quality, or behavior is expressed by a *level of attention, attitude,* or *intention (or all three)* on the part of the therapist. For example, as Kay integrated mindfulness into her life, she engaged in the *intentional* cultivation of *attitudes* of openness, curiosity, gentleness, and compassion toward her internal experiences, thereby enhancing her willingness to *attend to*, honor, and acknowledge her own physical, mental, and emotional experiences as they arose in the field of her awareness. Therefore, for this example (Fig. 51.1), all three of the characteristics defined by Shapiro and colleagues are present.

It is important to recognize that the mindfulness skills the therapist uses in the therapeutic relationship must come from a place of embodied knowing meaning that therapists must be working with mindfulness practices and integrating awareness into their own lives. If, for example, Kay is unable to recognize her own mental, physical, or emotional state or if she tends to numb or subjugate her own feelings and not process, metabolize, or integrate them, her capacity to recognize and be in a skillful relationship to another's pain and suffering will be limited. This could undermine the development of Kay's therapeutic use of self and could contribute to burnout and affect her therapeutic and personal relationships.[73]

Attuning to oneself and another person with awareness of the full dimensionality of the situation with the intention to provide prepared and effective interpersonal interaction is a part of the development of the therapeutic use of self.[90] Prepared and effective interpersonal interaction requires a specific intention, level of attention, attitude, and skill set on the part of the therapist that can be developed via mindfulness training in the therapist's personal and work life over time. Integrating mindfulness thereby becomes a "practice" and a "way of being."

These characteristics and qualities also can be related to occupational therapy's established core values and standards of conduct, illustrating the relationship between characteristics and qualities of mindfulness skills, prepared and effective interpersonal interaction, and the therapeutic use of self with occupational therapy's core values, ethical principles, and standards of conduct. The profession of occupational therapy is grounded in seven long-standing core values: (1) altruism, (2) equality, (3) freedom, (4) justice, (5) dignity, (6) truth, and (7) prudence. It also follows six ethical principles and standards of conduct for determining the most ethical course of action: (1) beneficence, (2) nonmaleficence, (3) autonomy, (4) justice, (5) veracity, and (6) fidelity. These concepts or words are not regularly used in our modern lexicon, but each word benefits from a greater depth of inquiry and engagement so that there is a deeper understanding of its true meaning and potential impact. In-depth study of the original documents wherein these principles are fully defined and discussed is recommended. It is also beyond the scope of this chapter to thoroughly explore the Occupational Therapy Code of Ethics (2020); however, readers are encouraged to do their own investigation into the personal, cultural, societal, and even spiritual meaning they each hold.

This list of characteristics and qualities of prepared and effective interpersonal interaction can easily just become another concept or intellectual understanding that we operationalize without much effort and with mindlessness. The key is to engage with them in the choices we make and the actions we take, thereby tilting our lives in their direction as a kind of life-long process of unfolding, growth, learning, and evolution.

Mindfulness is a powerful practice that can help us learn to turn toward our own human experience no matter what is here for us as a way to help integrate all aspects of ourselves and our experience. Mindfulness can help us cultivate courage to be with and tend to our challenges, habitual stress reactivity, and our human experience as it is and can assist us in reducing the tendency to fall into habitual modes of stress reactivity and maladaptive coping mechanisms such as blocking, numbing over, or checking out from experiences. We can use mindfulness as a way to mitigate reactivity, whereby we might be more able to respond to the situation at hand. This practice would be considered a mindfulness-mediated stress response. This is a way of being that comes with dedicated, intentional and compassionate practice. Although mindfulness is certainly not a quick fix, it is a fruitful journey that is sorely needed during this critical time.

Every single present moment is an opportunity to arrive here fully, to come to terms with the actuality of things as they are, and every moment one embodies these qualities in one's life, they will be deepened and become a part of who one is; they are an essential skill in the development of the therapeutic use of self.[45,104,105]

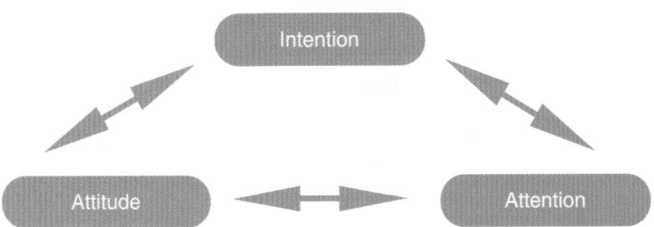

Fig. 51.1 The Mindfulness Model, in which each quality and characteristic affects the others.

ENVIRONMENTAL EFFECTS ON THE DEVELOPMENT OF THE THERAPEUTIC USE OF SELF

Most would agree that the development of the therapeutic use of self is a welcome and necessary component to becoming and being an effective occupational therapist. The challenge lies in the fact that health professionals, including occupational therapists, are working in increasingly fast-paced, production-oriented, resource-driven environments in Western medicine that disproportionately value hard work and self-sacrifice over employee health and well-being. Increased productivity standards, increased client loads, and self-care discrepancy measures among health professionals demonstrate staggering and unfortunate impacts on the health professional's mental, physical, and moral health. Research has demonstrated that the resulting burnout among health professionals significantly affects and reduces client outcomes, the development of the therapeutic use of self, and rapport building.[e]

Burnout refers to a state of emotional exhaustion in health and mental health workers that can manifest in the form of mental health problems, physical ailments, illness, and disease, and it is on the rise—particularly in these times of the pandemic and cultural unrest.[23,57–59,75]

Depression, suicide, substance abuse, and relational problems all can be serious concerns for therapists who do not effectively care for themselves and do not have the skills to effectively engage with the unique and staggering personal and occupational stressors they face.[7] Burnout has been associated with suboptimal patient care.[87,89]

Chronic sympathetic nervous system activation and operating in perpetual modes of fight, flight, freeze takes an enormous toll on interpersonal relationships.[76] In his book, *The Body Keeps the Score: Brain, Mind, and Body in the Healing of Trauma*,[101] Dr. Bessel van der Kolk explains why sympathetic nervous system activation affects concentration and memory and leads to difficulty forming trusting relationships, in addition to difficulty attending to and feeling a sense of safety in one's own body.

Kay's situation articulates these unfortunate realities. Like so many millions of healthcare workers, Kay too was not taught skills to regulate her nervous system; she did not learn how important it is to care for her own mental, physical, and spiritual health. She too was reared to be disconnected from her body. She was not taught skills that would enable her to be in effective and skillful relationship to the suffering in her personal or professional life. She has been relying on maladaptive coping strategies and habitual patterns to cope with her suffering. She is avoiding coming to terms with the actuality of her own suffering, and the habitual patterns of stress reactivity via numbing and subjugating her experience has caught up with her in the form of burnout and disease. Kay's declining mental, emotional, and physical health are compounding the suffering even further and significantly affecting her interpersonal relationships and effectiveness as an OT.[67]

Acknowledging this current healthcare climate reality can make anyone feel hopeless about the situation; however, there is potential for learning and meaningful change in the midst of today's challenges and difficulties. As stated by Elizabeth Lesser in her book *Broken Open: How Difficult Times Can Help Us Grow*,[50] every experience of struggle offers individuals what they need to be born anew. As we turn toward and acknowledge the suffering occurring within the current reality of Western medicine, we can allow the circumstances to become a catalyst for engaged transformation as we learn to integrate the skills of mindfulness in meaningful ways that foster a sense of groundedness, strength, resilience, and clarity. We can do this co-collectively and co-creatively, and there are maps and practices to help guide us on this journey. In this chapter we will be exploring aspects of the development of mindfulness as that guiding compass.

An ever-increasing number of studies demonstrates that the skills of mindfulness appear to be an effective intervention for many of our social, emotional, physical, occupational, contextual, moral, ethical, spiritual, and environmental ills.[f] Research suggests that mindfulness training for healthcare professionals can function as a viable, practical, and useful tool for promoting effective and skillful engagement in one's profession.[36] The development of body awareness in particular has been shown to enhance one's sense of connectedness to our core values.[76,101]

The core values, ethical standards, and principles of care of occupational therapy as demonstrated in the preamble to the Occupational Therapy Code of Ethics states:

Ethical action goes beyond rote compliance with these Principles and is a manifestation of moral character and mindful reflection. It is a commitment to benefit others, to virtuous practice of artistry and science, to genuinely good behaviors, and to noble acts of courage. Recognizing and resolving ethical issues is a systematic process that includes analysis of the complex dynamics of situations, weighing of consequences, making reasoned decisions, taking action, and reflecting on outcomes.

As an example, the code lists Principle 2 as "nonmaleficence," which states that "Occupational Therapy personnel shall intentionally refrain from actions that cause harm." Specifically, subprinciple 2C states that we must recognize and take appropriate action to remedy personal problems and limitations that might cause harm to recipients of service, colleagues, students, research participants, or others.[1]

For Kay, her personal problems and habitual pattern of maladaptive/adaptive coping affected her capacity to build rapport and reduced her capacity to provide the best possible service to her clients. As Kay began engaging in mindfulness training, as she developed awareness in her life and work, and as she began getting support and making lifestyle changes, she became clearer about her values, became more connected to her experience, and began developing mental clarity and flexibility, resilience,

[e]References 9,17,22,23,37,38,48,53,58,59,65,66,75,83,84.

[f]References 27,29,30,80,86–90,96.

stress-hardiness, and self-compassion. All of these enhance the psychological characteristics that support the development of the therapeutic use of self, especially in the midst of challenge and difficulty.

MINDFULNESS AND THE ENHANCEMENT OF THE THERAPEUTIC USE OF SELF

Research has shown mindfulness training enhances health-care professionals' personal self-care and their interpersonal relationships. Such professionals are found to be markedly more fully present with clients and their needs, less resentful, less reactive, and less defensive. Additionally, they demonstrate increased positive affect and self-compassion, more self-awareness and acceptance, improved attention and concentration, enhanced life satisfaction and meaning, and improved morale. Furthermore, they show increased performance and decision-making, improved self-regulation and impulse control, improved empathic responses, enhanced creativity, and improved senses of self-mastery, self-esteem, self-trust, and mental flexibility.[4,6,32,85] These specific qualities of attention, attitude, and intention are foundational components in the development of the therapeutic use of self and can have profound and far-reaching effects.[14,35,79,86,100]

Mindfulness is the skill of being deliberately attentive to one's experience; to encounter what is here in the present, as it unfolds, to come to terms with the actuality of things as they are without the often unacknowledged overlay of judgments, expectations, and conceptualizations.[5] This does not mean that the therapist would suddenly become a perpetually unflustered and calm person. Practicing mindfulness is messy. Turning toward one's experience with courage can initially be more challenging than we might think. However, with steadfast practice and curiosity, the human capacity to be mindful provides a wholesome way to attend to our subjective experiences and helps us learn, grow, and overcome maladaptive habits of mind that cause us to suffer unnecessarily.[100] The practice of nonjudgmental noticing what is here for you in the moment takes courage, and over time this sense of courage can grow and instill a personal sense of strength and empowerment. It is clear that mindfulness appears to help foster states of mind that are conducive to developing and enhancing the therapeutic use of self.[37,92,93,95]

Although it may sound simple to attend to the present moment, the mind's default mode tends to be entropy, and because we live in a society that does not typically appreciate or teach the skills of present moment awareness, nor of being with the actuality of things as they are, we tend to rely on maladaptive coping strategies. In addition, our society offers up a plethora of opportunity to disconnect from our experience—such as, in Kay's example, excessive use of media and technology, excessive busyness, mindless autopilot mode when participating in occupation, mindless eating, and other distractions—in a desperate attempt (albeit adaptive) to avoid the discomfort of unacknowledged thoughts and emotions or body sensations.[12,15]

As we integrate mindfulness in our lives, we are given the opportunity to recognize how familial, societal, and cultural conditioning encourages us to avoid and deny discomfort of

any kind, to cling to pleasant experiences, and begin to appreciate ways in which the formal mindfulness practices can both deepen the awareness of life's challenges and help us recognize our capacity as human beings to be in skillful relationship to them. In her book, *A Mind of Your Own*,[11] Dr. Kelly Brogan encourages the reader to recognize this kind of conditioning as a way to begin to reclaim personal power and innate wisdom to heal one's body and reclaim one's life.

As Kabat-Zinn wrote, "If there was such a thing as a self-distraction index, in the technologically bombarded society we live in today, it would be going through the roof."[41,42] This level of distraction contributes to enormous degrees of stress and anxiety, and it has very real and lasting repercussions for the mind and body. As Dr. Steven Cole, professor of medicine and psychiatry at the University of California–Los Angeles, states, "The experience you have today will influence the molecular composition of your body for the next 80 days, because that's how long the average protein synthesized in your body today will hang around in the future, so plan your day accordingly."[71a]

In response, one might ask: *Okay, so how do we do this?* The key practices necessary for the cultivation of mindful awareness are the formal practices or meditations. The formal practices are a form of mental and physical exercises that are meant to strengthen and deepen the inherent human capacity to bring our awareness to the present moments of our lives.[89,90,92] Because mindfulness is the skill of leaning into the present moments of life without judgment, it is important that we approach the practices in this spirit, relinquishing preconceptions, as much as possible, with no agenda about the practices and cultivating an open and curious state of mind. This offers a greater opportunity to benefit from these practices and deepens these experiences and growth. Of course, a healthy dose of skepticism is valuable; testing out the practices for each individual is important, and reflecting on and acknowledging the experiences throughout the process of developing insight, empathy, compassion, and understanding are crucial.[72] This is a true expression of "evidence-based practice"; when the fruits of practicing these skills are perceived as "self-evident," they become personal, palpable, and recognized by the practitioner for their inherent value.

Therefore, the key to using mindfulness with the intention of developing the therapeutic use of self in the context of occupational therapy is the steadfast personal work with the formal and informal mindfulness practices. Mindfulness practices are highly adaptable for any population and can be applied to participation in any occupation, such as sitting, eating, washing hands, driving, walking, shopping, taking in media, studying, reading, expressing loving kindness, the occupation of sleep, and so on.

Although the practices may seem simple at first, what comes up can actually be quite complex, offering infinite opportunities to bring the foundational qualities of compassion and kindness to the present-moment experiences.[80] Offering compassion (a desire to alleviate suffering) to ourselves throughout the journey is quite possibly the greatest practice of all. It can be challenging at times to offer ourselves compassion, and it is important to be aware of when it is needed most. Mindfulness skills and techniques can help one to open, lean into, and acknowledge challenges, and through that opening deepen the potential for greater freedom, humility, and a deeper connection with humanity. Practitioners, so prepared, are more capable of showing up for another human being's suffering when they can trust that they can be in wise, compassionate relationship to themselves.

The primary formal practices taught in mindfulness-based stress reduction curriculum are the body scan, the breath awareness practice, the sitting awareness practice, mindful lying yoga, mindful standing yoga, walking meditation, and loving kindness. Each of these practices is unique to its intended focus, yet they all share significant commonalities, such as intentionally attuning nonjudgmentally to one's experience in the present moment.[34,61] (See the Apply it Now section of this chapter for examples of formal mindfulness practices.)

Practicing mindfulness over time develops human qualities of connection and compassion; it builds a sense of groundedness and clarity, as well as insight and courage. Wisdom means seeing clearly into the nature of reality. Through mindfulness practices, practitioners can begin to acknowledge the actuality of things as they are without needing to numb over and check out, without needing to resist or subjugate the experience. In fact, one can shift one's relationship to challenge, to anxiety, to all of one's emotions and feelings, to a relationship of curiosity and openness rather than fear and feeling overwhelmed. The practitioner comes to terms with the full dimensionality of the present moment. One builds the capacity to recognize the impermanent nature of all phenomena and all "events" and to separate the event itself from the content of the thoughts we may have about the event or experience. They begin to see the unsatisfactory nature of ordinary human experience that arises from the illusion that the self is an existence separate from the rest of reality.[24,69] Practitioners begin to sense their interconnectedness within the full spectrum of our shared human experience. They have a greater capacity to meet grief and loss without fear or aversion. They are more capable of behaving with wisdom and compassion while staying centered and engaged, regardless of the situation.[103] They begin to recognize what is most essential for one's own well-being and to tune into their experience and the experience of others with greater degrees of insight and understanding (Fig. 51.2).[76,81]

Mindfulness offers an opportunity to realize the arising and passing away of all phenomena and the impermanence of all experience, including our thoughts and emotions, pain and discomfort, and life itself. Through this recognition, which arises out of our own subjective experiences with the practices, we are capable of learning to embrace life's transient nature and to understand the value of capturing each present moment as it arrives as fully as possible, with all our senses. This especially applies to preparing the OT self to work in the moment and value the moment, and to convey this to our clients, regardless of their loss or the severity of their circumstances. The presence of a practitioner can be a palpable anchoring presence in the midst of catastrophic life experiences. It may be imperceptible, but research has shown that these qualities are very much present and can be profoundly effective and healing.[62]

Mindfulness skills offer powerful means to work with pain and physical discomfort—by becoming aware of and experiencing for oneself the distinction between pain and suffering—as

---

OT PRACTICE NOTE

Extended Mindfulness Retreat Training

Participating in extended mindfulness training retreats is one of the best ways to deepen the skills of mindfulness in one's life and to experience the benefits more deeply. It is assistive to cultivate a relationship to mindfulness with an attitude of nonstriving, of not needing anything to be "fixed," of having no agenda other than to be fully present to whatever is unfolding, and to sense that we are already whole and complete just as we are as we engage with the mindfulness practices—to trust as we turn toward our own completeness and humanity while being held in the container of mindfulness that we will open to greater degrees of insight and well-being (see resources for mindfulness-based retreat centers in the United States). In fact, we can consider the shelter-in-place situation as a kind of extended retreat and potentially shift our potential discordant perspective about the shelter-in-place situation a bit from one that is punitive to one that is health-enhancing and begin to open to the possible benefits from the situation. For example, for some the daily commute in traffic was eliminated, and for some they saw their children more often and were able to share more meals together. Of course, this was not true for everyone; for some the pandemic caused family businesses to close, and substance abuse and other mental health challenges are on the rise. Yet, it may be that there are aspects of the difficult situation that may have been a catalyst for necessary and meaningful change that would not have otherwise occurred.

---

it pertains to our own perception of the experience.[42] These qualities are invaluable as we participate in the compelling and complex practice of OT, working on the front lines of incredible human suffering: our own, the world's, and that of the individuals with whom we work.

The shift for Kay was slow but palpable as she began to recognize the difference (perceptual shift) between "pain" and "suffering." Her most valuable experiences at first were those that pertained to her own pain and experience of what it really means "to suffer." As she built mindful awareness into her life, Kay began to recognize that the physical pain she experienced in her back fluctuated, depending on what she was doing, that it was impermanent and not present "all the time," and that it did not spread throughout her whole body, as she had previously "thought." Kay recognized that when she mentally resisted or ruminated about the pain in her back, it would get stronger and intensify. She recognized that the mental and emotional resistance and rumination were the root of her "suffering," and the physical pain was something separate and was to be honored and acknowledged. The physical pain sensations were messages from her body that she could turn toward, tend to, and to which she could actually listen and skillfully respond. She recognized that steadfast personal self-care and self-compassion were particularly healing remedies for her physical pain. As she released the mental and emotional ruminations and resistance, she noticed she had much more energy to devote to her healing and she had greater mental clarity and curiosity, all of which reduced her experience of the mental and emotional "suffering" previously associated with the physical pain.

Kay sensed parallels between her reaction to her physical pain and her mental pain. She noticed that when she was ruminating about an event or situation, her thoughts would spin off and she would lose focus and become agitated, easily frustrated, and mentally unclear. She recognized rather quickly

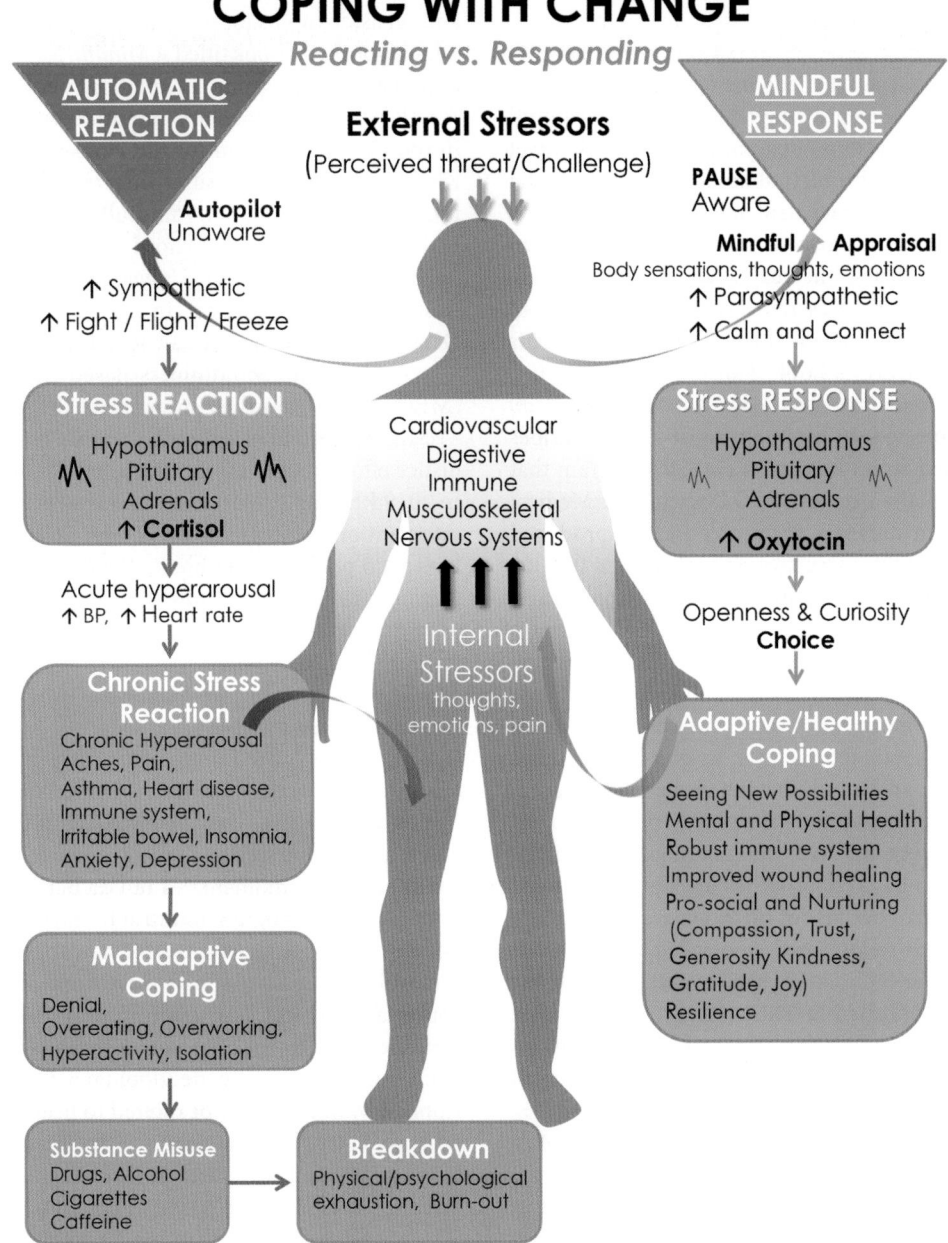

Fig. 51.2 Coping with change. (©2015 Elizabeth Lin MD, MPH, ehblin@uw.edu. Adapted with permission from Kabat-Zinn J: *Full catastrophe living*, 2013, New York: Bantam; and Bardacke N: *Mindful birthing*, 2012, New York: Harper Collins. Graphics courtesy R. Ryan.)

that when she did not feed into or resist the persistent thinking patterns, she could gently observe her thought patterns and emotions, not take them so personally, and actually find humor in her automatic habitual patterns that she could now let go of if she chose to. She sensed greater ease from this mindfulness practice, and each moment became a practice and a choice for how to respond to her physical, mental, or emotional pain. Every moment she was aware, she chose, and each moment she chose to expand her perspective, allow thoughts and emotions to pass if she was able to, she became aware of the sensation of her breath to ground her awareness into the present moment. This brought greater degrees of ease and this empowered her.

She was aligning her present moment experience with her values of self-care, compassion, clarity, and insight.

Kay noticed the difference between the physical pain and the mental and emotional suffering her clients might be experiencing. She realized that mindfulness skills training (if the person chose to engage in it) could reduce suffering and foster greater degrees of clarity and well-being. She also recognized that this is a path persons must choose for themselves, and she was careful not to push mindfulness on her clients. In some situations she knew that the only way she could bring the healing power of mindfulness to the table was through her own therapeutic use of self, through her own presence, clarity, openness, and well-being.

MINDFULNESS IN WESTERN MEDICINE, HEALTHCARE, AND SOCIETY

Complementary and alternative medicine (CAM) and integrative medicine (IM) have been growing rapidly in the psychodynamic and humanistic traditions of psychotherapy to help meet the needs of our growing chronic public physical and mental health disease crisis. The current demand for highly qualified professionals who teach the skills of mindfulness has grown exponentially in recent years. The year 1990 was a watershed, after which "mindfulness" as a discrete term began to take hold in the discourse of academic medicine and psychology.[16] This was the year Jon Kabat-Zinn's book, *Full Catastrophe Living: Using the Wisdom of Your Body and Mind to Face Stress, Pain, and Illness,*[41] was published. In his book Kabat-Zinn describes the Mindfulness-Based Stress Reduction (MBSR) program that he developed in 1979 at the University of Massachusetts Medical Center. The curriculum started at the center and has produced nearly 1000 certified MBSR instructors and taken over 100,000 people through the MBSR course in the United States and in more than 30 countries.[61]

Almost every major medical center in the United States currently has an IM center, and many include mindfulness and/or MBSR as an integral component of their programming. MBSR is now used as a therapeutic intervention in over 700 hospitals worldwide. Meditation and mindfulness have been featured in cover stories in *Scientific American, The New York Times, Time Magazine, The New Yorker*, and *Newsweek*, among others. MBSR and other mindfulness-based approaches are now considered evidence-based treatment because of the extensive amount and quality of research with randomized, controlled clinical trials that have abounded over the past 10 years. In fact, 52 academic journal articles were published in 2003, rising to 1203 by mid 2018.[61] During 2020 alone more than 3000 related publications were released and can be found through the National Library of Medicine (https://bit.ly/3Jklymy).

Clinical trials that are currently under way studying the efficacy of mindfulness-based interventions (MBIs) include the following conditions: asthma, bone marrow transplant, breast cancer, chronic pain, chronic obstructive pulmonary disease, human immunodeficiency virus infection and acquired immunodeficiency syndrome (HIV/AIDS), hypertension, immune response, irritable bowel syndrome, lupus, myocardial ischemia, obesity, cancer, arthritis, organ transplant, diabetes, and other medical conditions, including psychiatric disorders, such as anxiety disorders, eating disorders, personality disorders, post-traumatic stress disorder, burnout, schizophrenia, and suicidality.[26,55] Grossman and associates[28] characterized the current research findings with this statement: "Thus far, the literature seems to clearly slant toward support for basic hypothesis concerning the effects of mindfulness on mental and physical well-being."[21,68]

Mindfulness and MBSR are not just in Western medicine. More than 2000 people from companies such as Google, Facebook, and Instagram met in San Francisco in 2018 for a mindfulness conference called Wisdom 2.0. Google offers its 99,000 employees free lessons in mindfulness. Corporations such as General Mills have made it available to their employees and set aside rooms for meditation. Representative Tim Ryan of Ohio published a book titled *A Mindful Nation*, and he has helped organize regular group meditation periods on Capitol Hill. An all-party parliamentary mindfulness group was developed in the United Kingdom for the House of Lords. In the United Kingdom, three universities offer master's level postgraduate professional training in mindfulness-based approaches: The University of Exeter and Oxford University Mindfulness Centre in England and Bangor University Center for Mindfulness, Research, and Practice in Wales. The Department of Occupational Therapy at San Jose State University has offered a semester-long Mindfulness-Based Occupational Therapy (MBOT) course for their students for the past 10 years.

Mindfulness interventions are also being applied in social justice efforts and to minimize the effects of social identity bias. In 2019 Rhonda V. Magee, facilitator of trauma-sensitive MBSR interventions and professor of law at the University of San Francisco published her book, *The Inner Work of Social Justice: Healing Ourselves and Transforming Our Communities Through Mindfulness*, as a call for courageous political action in support of equitable justice for all.[56]

MBIs are growing in number as well. Mindfulness-Based Cognitive Therapy (MBCT), Dialectical Behavioral Therapy (DBT), Acceptance and Commitment Therapy (ACT), Mindfulness-Based Relapse Prevention (MBRP), and Mindfulness-Based Therapeutic Community (MBTC) treatment are several MBIs that are drawing the most cultural attention at this moment.[61] The UC Berkeley Greater Good in Action (GGIA) program found at http://ggia.berkeley.edu highlights science-based practices for how to build qualities such as mindfulness, compassion, connection, empathy, forgiveness, appreciation, happiness, optimism, and resilience, to name a few. The Department of Occupational Therapy at San Jose State University is currently developing a Certificate Program in Applied Mindfulness to be offered to health and human service professionals all over the world with the intention of continuing to deepen the effectiveness of the emerging mindfulness-based discourse and evidence-based interventions.[64]

Occupational therapists are currently using elements of MBIs in a variety of ways as interventions within their practice, and yet there is a need for more direct training for occupational therapists in applying mindfulness more explicitly into the complexities of occupational therapy practice.[44] A couple of related questions to ponder are, "How might mindfulness affect the quality of participation in daily occupations?" and "What affect does poor quality of participation in occupation play on an individual's health and well-being?" This chapter is meant to begin to explore these questions.

INTEGRATING MINDFULNESS IN OCCUPATIONAL THERAPY PRACTICE

OT promotes health by enabling people to participate in meaningful and purposeful occupations[2]; however, it is often the case that we may not be present or "conscious" while engaging in so-called meaningful and/or purposeful occupations. Not only are

THREADED CASE STUDY

Kay, Part 2

Occupational Therapists Embodying Mindfulness in Their Lives and Work

Kay began to realize that her ethical and moral duty to her work as an occupational therapist was not separate from her duty to her own mental, emotional, spiritual, and physical health and self-care. She realized that she deeply valued the ethical principle of "do no harm." She also knew she wanted to make a meaningful contribution to her clients' lives. With this desire to improve her own well-being, quality of life, occupational participation, and therapeutic use of self, Kay pursued mindfulness practice in her own life, and, over time, this had beneficial effects. The effects of building mindfulness into her life were significant and clear. Kay's life challenges became learning opportunities, she found that she felt more centered, and life's intensities became edges that actually propelled her into greater degrees of understanding and insight. She recognized that cultivating awareness, curiosity, and self-compassion during her most difficult moments transformed those instances into moments of great courage, strength, growth, and learning.

Mindfulness of Self

Body Awareness

With the cultivation of mindful awareness through the formal and informal practices of mindfulness, Kay became more aware of her body and the needs of her body. Initially Kay noticed a great deal of tension, discomfort, and pain in her body. She noticed how she wanted to numb and distract herself from the discomfort, and she recognized that she would fall into habitual stress reactivity of blocking or subjugating her experiencing or distracting herself in a number of ways. As she integrated the mindfulness practice qualities of kindness and self-compassion, she noticed her growing capacity to keep showing up for the discomfort, the pain, and difficulty with no agenda other than to come to terms with the actuality of things as they were. She simply noticed her experience with nonjudgmental, open, curious awareness without needing to alter her experience in any way. She would come back to the formal practices and each time was increasingly more capable of showing up for whatever was there without needing it to go away and without needing to numb over and check out.

As Kay developed greater degrees of body awareness, she moved through her daily routines and daily occupations with greater intention and ease. She slowed her pace. As she slowed during her activities of daily living (ADLs) participation, she was able to recognize which activities exacerbated her pain, and she made adjustments over time that supported the needs of her body. Initially she took frequent mindful breaths, wherever possible, to release any unnecessary tension that she noticed. This increased blood flow and oxygenation to these areas. The attention and expression of kindness toward her body that she developed over time helped her remain in a more parasympathetic nervous system response and helped to regulate her nervous system. At times she noticed herself expressing appreciation and gratitude toward her body, which felt healing and nourishing to her and brought about a greater sense of ease and well-being. Kay noticed that daily activities such as watching television and surfing social media sites increased ruminative thought patterns, which activated her sympathetic stress response. Fig. 51.3 is a visual representation of how Kay became empowered to choose how she was going to respond and to tilt her life in the direction of making more empowered lifestyle choices that aligned with her intention for greater health, effectiveness, and well-being. As stress reactivity mode was reduced, this in turn opened up more time and energy for her to be with and connect with her husband and daughter and for preparing healthy meals for her family, all of which activated her parasympathetic response and nourished her health and well-being.

Kay's digestion improved, allowing her to reap greater nutritional benefits from the foods she was eating. She began to eat foods that she recognized would nourish her body and noticed how her body felt after eating foods that were not nourishing. She made more dietary adjustments that supported the experience of greater health in her body. She became more aware of these health feedback loops, which motivated her further to continue to deepen the practices in her life and continue making healthy dietary adjustments for her family. She could physically sense the difference in her health and well-being with the body awareness practices and with integrating qualities of kindness and self-compassion toward herself. Her insomnia began to lessen, she had fewer headaches, and she felt more in control of her eating habits. She noticed that her daughter's behavior also responded positively to the dietary changes, and this continued to motivate her to make healthier choices over time. Kay was ever more empowered by her and her family's healing journey at the hands of none other than herself.

Breath Awareness

Kay learned to use the awareness of breath practice to anchor her awareness in the present moment when she noticed that her mind was wandering needlessly and exacerbating her stress. She noticed that her thoughts were often ruminating over situations that she had little or no control over, such as the health of her father, the overwhelming workload for which she was responsible, the pandemic, and her husband's lack of income. She would kindly and gently refocus her attention on the occupation at hand, and when she had time in the day, she would sit down and problem-solve with her husband about what adjustments needed to be made in their life to support greater ease, sense of control, and a sense of connectedness. They worked together over time to make necessary adjustments to their lifestyle, simplifying, reducing extraneous expenditures, getting support from community resources, and making small but meaningful problem-focused and emotion-focused shifts that gave them a sense of self-efficacy and hope for a better situation for their family. Kay had a new and embodied sense of the true value of what occupational therapists often teach in their work, and these personal-life adjustments developed a deep sense of trust and self-efficacy in her capacity to help others make meaningful lifestyle changes that might enhance their life satisfaction and well-being.

Although Kay recognized that she could not alter the productivity or billability standards of her work environment, she now realized that she had complete control over how she responded to the work environment demands. She noticed that when she mentally resisted the situation in any way, this would activate her stress response, she would get tension throughout her body, feel a knot in her stomach, and release a storm of stress chemicals that affected every cell of her body. Over time and with practice, Kay noticed how she could allow the work environment to be as it is. She realized she could come to greater degrees of acceptance over the reality of the situation and not need to mentally or physically resist it, but rather to hold it with curiosity and openness—all the while acknowledging and honoring her own experience of the situation and bringing kindness and compassion toward herself, her team, and her clients, all of whom were participating in and managing the system in their own unique ways. She noticed how her usual mode of cynicism melted away over time and was replaced with more moments of clarity and curiosity about the complexities of a rehabilitation environment such as the one in which she worked. She was better able to recognize the simple yet deeply moving details of her workday, such as how a family dealt courageously with the suffering of their loved one. Furthermore, she noted how, day in and day out, the staff members arrived and did the best they could with what they knew, and how society has developed such inspiring emergency medical care for its people. She recognized what a beautiful profession occupational therapy is, with its holistic view of each individual client and the client's unique situation. Kay noticed how there was less tension in her body, and she sensed greater degrees of ease and equanimity even during some of the more intense moments in her day. She observed that she was more capable of responding skillfully to the complexities of patient and

(Continued)

THREADED CASE STUDY—cont'd

Kay, Part 2

family care and was able to be more present and respond with greater clarity to the needs of her team. Similarly, she was less mentally and emotionally affected by the billability and productivity standards and continued to do the best she could to meet them with integrity and ethical behavior without the usual overlay of self-criticism or judgment.

Kay recognized a deepening sense of self-compassion and appreciation for simple experiences in her life that seemed to remotivate her to engage in occupations that she previously found nourishing and rejuvenating but had given up as life and work became more intense and less manageable. She made sure to take frequent "three-breath cycle breaks" while at work, usually while she washed her hands between clients and team meetings. She found this to be particularly grounding and restorative, and it gave her a pause to check in on how she was doing mentally, emotionally, and physically. Based on this self–check-in practice, she would make adjustments to gently bring herself back to the present, to let go of any unnecessary tension if she was able to, and to cultivate a state of greater equanimity and a sense of groundedness before she moved on to her next task of the day. She noticed that she felt more clarity and felt more capable when she needed to have difficult conversations with her team or supervisors. She spoke with greater courage and calm. She was able to stay on point, centered in her own experience, and be an effective leader during difficult situations.

Kay reconnected with her family by planning regular activities that they all enjoyed participating in together, such as being in nature, camping, and going for walks. They incorporated more check-in time/connection during the week and ate at least one meal a day at the kitchen table together, enjoying healthy food and pleasant conversation. The greatest adjustment Kay made was to reduce her level of "busyness." She and her family took a fresh look at their deeply held family values and made adjustments and even removed tasks or activities that did not align with those values; this opened up more spaciousness in their lives. They all felt less hurried and harried. Over time and together, Kay's family developed a greater sense of connectedness, simplicity, and well-being overall for the whole family. This experience and newly practiced behavior opened her up for more authentic and present interactions and relationships with her clients and colleagues. Kay became a source of groundedness for her team and was often approached for guidance about important matters and decisions that needed to be made for her team and her clients.

Awareness of Thoughts and Emotions

Over time, with her deepening experiences with the formal and informal mindfulness practices, increased reflective observation, and open, curious, nonjudgmental investigation, Kay began to gradually notice how her *quality* of participation and engagement in her daily occupations affected the quality of her life and her mental, emotional, and physical well-being. She experienced how before integrating mindfulness into her life, she was frequently on autopilot mode during basic ADLs, often ruminating about unpleasant past events and experiences or fabricated fears about the future, all of which activated her sympathetic nervous system, released a storm of stress chemicals throughout her body, and increased tension in her body and affected her digestion. Kay noticed it was a habit to neglect her body's cues when she participated in her ADLs and would often overdo it and feel exhausted after. With mindfulness practice, however, Kay had greater control over where her mind went and she was able to release ruminative patterns of thinking when she noticed it and she was more capable of keeping her attention and awareness in the present moment. She noticed more often when her mind was not in the present, and she noticed the thoughts and emotions with curiosity and compassion rather than judgment. When she needed to plan for the future, she scheduled time in her day for this and focused her attention on the task at hand. She did her "planning" in the present moment. With the energy that previously had been spent on ruminating and stressful thinking, Kay shifted the focus of her energy on approaching her daily occupations with appreciation. Kay began recognizing things in her life that she was grateful for, such as how wonderful it was to have running water. When she noticed herself getting lost in a stream of ruminative thought patterns about the past or future that used to run her life and sap her energy, she simply paused, turned her awareness to the sensation of her breath and proceeded with what she was doing. With practice she was developing new neural pathways in her brain that supported a sense of connectedness, and it became increasingly easier to stay present over time.

Situational Awareness

As Kay developed a kind attunement to her present moment experience in basic ADLs, she noticed that her senses awakened. She was able to find enjoyment and appreciation for the simplest of daily life experiences, such as the warm sensations of the water while washing her hands, the smooth texture of her favorite pants as she put them on in the morning, the scent of her daughter's clean hair

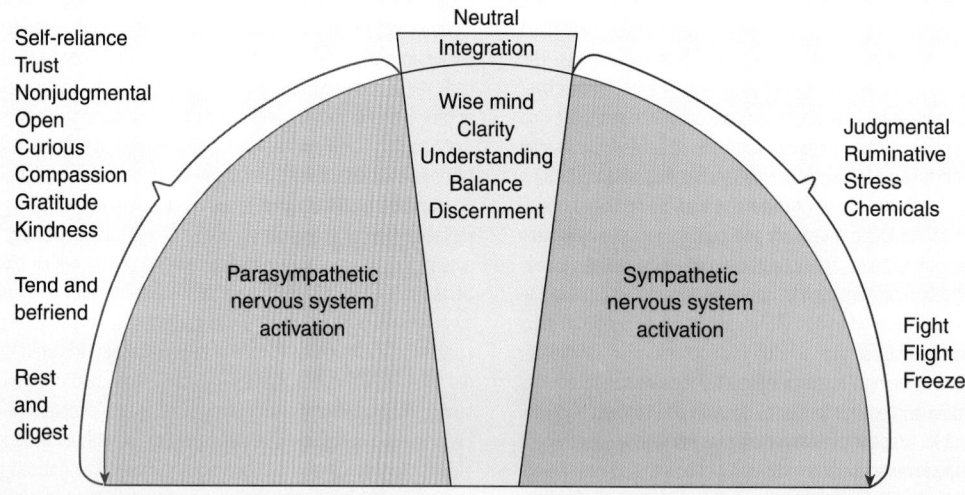

Fig. 51.3 Visual representation of how Kay became empowered to choose how she was going to respond and to make empowered lifestyle choices that aligned with her intention to achieve greater health, effectiveness, and well-being.[99]

THREADED CASE STUDY—cont'd

Kay, Part 2

as she brushed it. She recognized that being present during her basic self-care in this way increased her appreciation for her ability to participate in these occupations. It activated her parasympathetic nervous system, thereby releasing the healing "tend and befriend" hormones (e.g., oxytocin and endorphins), which helped her release tension and regulate her nervous system and reduced her mental, emotional, and physical pain (see Fig. 51.3).

During more instrumental ADLs, such as meal planning, preparation, and cleanup, Kay began to notice how her thoughts and emotions tended toward resentment for having to do housework. She perceived anger and frustration in her body, which increased tension and pain in her body. Once again, she skillfully met these kinds of thoughts with self-compassion and the recognition that she was having to do more than her share of the household work. She began to share her frustration with her family and to express her needs in such a way that she might tilt the dynamic in her family to one that felt more equitable in how the housework was divided. She also used the grounding practices of mindfulness to stabilize herself as she approached difficult conversations in interpersonal situations such as navigating the terrain of enhancing equity in her home life responsibilities. Kay consciously chose thoughts that aligned with her core values of family and connection. She noticed that as she paid attention to the task at hand, such as preparing a healthy meal for her family, she developed appreciation for her strength and capacity to do these complex occupational tasks. She became more vocal in expressing her needs and made the conscious efforts to bring more balance into sharing household contributions. At the same time, as she was more present during her ADLs, she noticed how the level of attention she brought to the occupation could transform it from one of drudgery, resentment, and disconnection to one of appreciation and connectedness for herself and her family. If she noticed her mind wandering into thought, she would anchor herself by becoming aware of the sensations of the breath in her body and then focus on the sensations and experience of the task at hand. As with all the mindfulness awareness practices, she was developing new neural pathways in her brain that supported being present, and it became increasingly easier to stay present over time. She expressed her appreciation to her family more often, and she asked for help more when she thought she needed it. The whole family was developing new routines that supported their engagement with one another, and they all began to contribute, which made for a more equitable share of the household responsibilities. The same daily occupations that were once drudgery and prompted resentment became, over time, filled with appreciation and a sense of connectedness to her family and herself. (See the mindful listening exercise in Box 51.1).

Kay also noticed how much more present she was able to stay when she was with clients. She recognized that she was much more capable of attuning to her client's mental, emotional, and physical states, and she felt more capable of responding to the needs of the moment as it required of her. She also experienced how she was better able to stay grounded in her own experience, not needing to be drawn into the suffering of her client and be taken away by it so readily. She was able to recognize and to be with the suffering and to stay centered in and honor her own experience. She recognized she was more able to acknowledge and validate her feelings with gentleness and to seek support and respite when needed.

As Kay became more aware of how she approached her clients and team members, she was also more aware of her intention, her body language, her communication style, and her energy and presence and how she affected others. She was more likely to identify when she made mistakes, reflect on the experiences, learn from them, make necessary adjustments, and move forward with greater degrees of courage. She noticed how the practice of self-compassion and expression of kindness and gentleness was particularly healing during times when she felt like she could have done better.

BOX 51.1 Mindful Listening/Mindfulness Communication Exercise

To keep the language of this guidance clear and uncomplicated, let's assume that your partner is a young woman. The process is the same, regardless of gender or identity.

Sit about 3 to 4 feet away from your partner with nothing in between you. Lower your gaze or close your eyes. Begin by dropping your awareness into the sensations in your body, acknowledging whatever is here for you with no agenda other than tending to whatever is here, without needing it to be any other way, just noticing and recognizing the condition of your body in this moment. (pause) Bring awareness to what is the condition of your mind in this moment, again not trying to make any thoughts or emotions go away, just noticing them as they are in this moment. (pause)

Draw your awareness gently into the sensations of your body. If you notice any unnecessary tension, see if you can allow those areas to release, and, if not, just allow those sensations to go wherever they need to go . . . . Now anchor your awareness into the sensation of your breath, letting the breath be just as it is, without trying to change or regulate it in any way . . . allowing it to flow easily and naturally, with its own rhythm and pace, knowing you are breathing perfectly well right now, nothing for you to do . . . .

Become aware of what your intention is in communicating with your partner.

Before opening your eyes to share in this communication, see if you can keep some of your awareness anchored in your body and/or your breath sensations. Open your eyes and listen as best you can to your partner without any judgments, with openness, without needing to have thoughts about what you are going to say next or without your own mental dialogue distracting you from your partner's sharing. Just listen as deeply as you are able.

When your partner is done sharing, guide your awareness gently back into your body sensations; notice any unnecessary tension and see if you can allow it to release. You can state as clearly as you can what you heard. Ask your partner if you heard her correctly.

Now take a few moments to formulate and articulate what is true for you/ what it is you would like to share.

Before opening your eyes to share in this communication once again, see if you can keep some of your awareness anchored in your body and/or your breath sensations. Open your eyes and speak what is true for you. Notice any body sensations that may arise as you share. If you ever feel like you are getting off-center, just close your eyes, anchor your awareness back in your body sensations, and see if you can release tension. Connect back in with your truth and begin again when you are ready.

When you both feel that the communication is complete, thank each other for her presence and mindful listening. Being deeply heard and listened to is a practice of compassion and is an incredible gift we can give to ourselves and others.

Interoccupational Awareness

The Quality of Engagement and Participation in Occupations (QPIO)

As we integrate mindful awareness into our daily personal and professional lives, we begin to become aware of our quality of participation in daily occupations. Through engaged participation in meaningful occupations, we gain insight into the significance of the healing nature of being more aware and present with

(Continued)

Kay, Part 2

our unfolding experience in each given moment. Interoccupational awareness is a state in which we intentionally establish an awake, alert, nonjudgmental awareness during occupational participation. Establishing connection to our experience during daily occupations gives us the opportunity to develop deeper levels of understanding of the significance of daily occupations in our lives, of awareness of our own habitual patterns of thought and behavior, and of the effect of these patterns on our health and well-being and on those around us.

As an example, Kay described that as she developed mindful awareness during her daily activities, she noticed that the occupation of washing the dishes was overlaid with her thoughts of resentment toward her family. She questioned why she had to do the dishes, when she had other things to do that were "a better use of her time." She experienced how this thought about the occupation of doing the dishes activated her sympathetic nervous system response, which in turn released stress chemicals that affected her body, shut down her digestion, and reduced her capacity to appreciate the occupation in which she was participating. Over time, once she developed greater awareness and made conscious choices about her relationship (in the form of thoughts, ideas, beliefs, and expectations) to washing the dishes, she was first able to cultivate a quality of neutrality, and eventually she was able to actually enjoy the activity. She noticed that it was her choice as to how she would relate to the activity. She noticed how she began to experience gratitude for having the strength to stand at the sink, to be able to use both of her arms, to have running water and hot water, to be able to afford and prepare healthy food for her family, and to feel the sensory experience of washing the dishes. She noticed how her capacity to appreciate washing the dishes then became an activity that engaged her parasympathetic "rest and digest, tend and befriend" nervous system (see Fig. 51.3). She felt at ease and almost as if the activity of washing dishes was a restorative activity, rather than her previous experience of dismay, resentment, and frustration. She also recognized that the equitable balance of household contributions within her family was off and over time, and with mindful communication, she was able to shift the dynamic so that the share of the work in the home was more equitable.

Kay's example demonstrates that enhanced awareness allows us to notice our relationship to our daily occupations and to the objects we come into contact with in our lives. This awareness offers us information that can empower us and give us the opportunity and freedom to choose and establish wise relationships with our occupations. Parasympathetic nervous system activation can be experienced during *any* occupation in which we participate. Not just the occupations we ascribe meaning to, but *all* of our occupations hold the key to our freedom if we are open to the potential within the power of our choice as to how we relate to them. This is the essence of personal empowerment; choosing to experience all of our interoccupational relationships with a sense of openness, curiosity, and maybe even wonder and gratitude. At the same time, with mindfulness on board, we are more likely to express our needs and we are more able to get our needs met. If we need help for example, with completing housework, we are more likely to ask for help, to stay centered in our experience, and to work toward a meaningful resolution.

we not present, but we can often be lost in a cascade of ruminative thoughts, expectations, and unacknowledged judgments. We can often be lost in thoughts about the past or future, completely disengaged from what we are actually doing in the moment—the only moment in which we ever have to live. Habitual, and at times, ruminative mental events/phenomena, such as plans, worries, anticipations, expectations, fantasies, and so on, can not only disengage us from our present-moment experience and occupational participation, but they also can often be destructive to our emotional, mental, spiritual, and physical health by perpetuating stress reactivity. These thoughts and ruminations are often not even our own. We take on implicit biases, perceptions, and underlying ideas by our culture, family, teachers, communities, societies, religions, popular media, and other sources. We can be significantly limiting our experience of our lives by living only in the unacknowledged, often habitual, cognitive domain of experience. We can be disconnected from our occupational experiences and our bodies for long periods of time and even lifetimes. When we are disconnected from our lives, we are unable to fully experience our daily activities, even those that we might consider "meaningful," and the quality of participation in occupations can suffer greatly, affecting every aspect of our lives.

Our occupations can even lose their "occupation-ness" when we are not engaged, not present, or are even not conscious. If we participate in our occupations in this way out of habit because of familial, cultural, or societal norms, are they really occupations? Are they really meaningful or purposeful? Or do they become an end in and of the means and sheer drudgery? Can occupational participation really be considered a healing agent and skillful tool if we as therapists do not really know what it means to be present for our own occupations? These are questions to be lived, engaged in, embodied, and considered as we integrate mindfulness into the practice of occupational therapy.

Another potential benefit of mindfulness is that is connects us to our body. Becoming aware of one's body can be assistive in mitigating many of the underlying problems of modern diseases. Mindfulness is the practice of purposefully attending to the present moment with an attitude of curiosity and gentleness, with no agenda other than to encounter what is here with open awareness. When we integrate mindfulness into our work as occupational therapists we become facilitators of our client's capacity to become a co-healer in their own journey, using the wisdom of their own body and mind.[46,47,51,54,78]

The AOTA defines occupational therapy as a practice that maximizes health, well-being, and quality of life for all people, populations, and communities through effective solutions that facilitate participation in everyday life.[2] Mindfulness is an effective practice or "antidote" that cultivates deeper levels of personal understanding, insight, and freedom that facilitates empowered and awake participation in everyday life. Mindfulness is "emancipatory education" because it is "really useful knowledge" that is integrated via procedural, "self-evident" learning that empowers us to rise out from under often unacknowledged forces of oppression. These forces may come in the form of our own underlying ideas, judgments, thought patterns, and perception that we've taken on through cultural and familial norms over the course of our lifetimes without our even knowing.

The skills of mindfulness help us come into contact with and engage in close connectivity in each moment with our tattered hearts with compassion and gentleness. Awareness sheds light on our present-moment experience and helps us build trust in our capacity to make effective lifestyle shifts that tilt us in the direction of what we value most.

Occupational therapists, work on the front lines of incredible human suffering. Occupational therapists, who have their own personal mindfulness practice will be more able to remain present to their own internal mental and emotional experience and physical well-being from one moment to the next, thereby reducing potential for burnout and enhancing self-efficacy.[60] Dr. Dan Siegel, researcher, author, and director of The Mindsight Institute at the University of California–Los Angeles, describes this process as neurologic "integration."[90,91,93,94] He invites the reader to "connect rather than correct." This process of integration involves learning to be in wise relationship to our experience in each moment, without needing it to be any other way. Mindfulness helps to build our capacity to come to terms with the actuality of things as they are without trying to alter the experience in any way. In this way we are capable of learning, growing, and cultivating a wiser and more embodied relationship to our work as occupational therapists, capable of expanding our perspective and enhancing our mental flexibility.

MBOT invites us to live the following questions as a journey of inquiry, growth, and learning:

- How do I experience my *quality* of participation and engagement in my daily occupations?
- What is my relationship (underlying ideas, attitudes, expectations, perceptions) of my occupations, and how can I cultivate an effective and meaningful relationship with them?
- How can I assist my client in cultivating and embodying a higher quality of participation, engagement, and relationship to his or her occupations? How might this affect my client's health and well-being?

Integrating mindfulness in our own lives is essential to exploring these questions in a meaningful way. The mindfulness-based occupational therapist (MBOT) practices and develops mindfulness skills in their life that become a part of daily performance patterns (habits, routines, rituals, and roles). Mindful awareness tools and skills become embodied and integrated into the therapist's clinical practice, whether it be addressing interventions for physical conditions or mental health concerns.[70] As an MBOT integrates mindfulness practice as a therapeutic modality, they bring it with the intention that occupational therapists will also benefit and grow themselves from the practice. (See the Additional Resources section at the end of the References for suggested training pathways and a few simple mindfulness exercises with which to begin.)

INTEGRATING OCCUPATIONAL THERAPY AND MINDFULNESS: MINDFULNESS-BASED OCCUPATIONAL THERAPY COMPETENCIES

When occupational therapy and mindfulness are skillfully integrated, mindfulness-based OT competencies have more fertile ground in which to grow and ultimately be embodied by the occupational therapist and shared with the client in meaningful ways. The following list presents the five interrelated sets of cognitive, affective, and behavioral competencies. The definitions of the five competency clusters for therapists are:

- *Competency 1: Self-Awareness:* An occupational therapist's self-awareness deepens when it is enhanced by the mindfulness practices of focusing attention and cultivating self-compassion. It includes the capacity to recognize one's emotions, thoughts, attitudes, underlying ideas, beliefs, and perceptions and their influence on behavior. This includes accurately assessing one's strengths and limitations and possessing a well-grounded sense of confidence and enthusiasm.
- *Competency 2: Self-Management:* Mindfulness increases the occupational therapist's emotion, thought, and behavior regulation skills, which enhances the ability to meet the needs of our complex profession, resolve internal and situational conflict more creatively, recognize and honor how he or she is feeling in an emotionally balanced way, and learn and grow from insights and deepening awareness. This includes managing stress responses skillfully, recognizing impulses that may be unskillful, motivating oneself, finding meaning, and setting and working toward achieving personal and professional goals that are guided by personal values.
- *Competency 3: Social Awareness:* Mindfulness increases the empathic drives of occupational therapists by helping them validate, acknowledge, and regulate their own emotions rather than get emotionally overwhelmed or block emotions when faced with difficult situations. As a result, their capacity to notice and honor both their own suffering and another person's suffering and respond to it is fostered. In addition to this, they are able to take a broader contextual perspective and embrace others from diverse backgrounds and cultures, to respond to the needs of the situation, and offer appropriate resources and support.
- *Competency 4: Relationship Skills:* Mindfulness increases compassion. Thus, when occupational therapists practice mindfulness skills, such as non-striving, they are doing so with more compassionate, open, curious, accepting, and nonjudgmental understanding. This manifests as communicating clearly, listening actively, and seeking and offering help when needed. This also includes recognizing the relationship therapists have with their own occupational participation, in addition to recognizing how their perceptions and underlying ideas about an occupation shape their experience and can make the occupational participation health enhancing or health degrading. The occupational therapist recognizes that the quality of participation is up to them, which is empowering, and can foster life-enhancing adjustments over time.
- *Competency 5: Decision-Making:* Mindfulness increases cognitive flexibility and creativity, which gives occupational therapists a broader contextual perspective and a wider range of potential responses to challenging situations. This includes being able to make constructive and respectful choices about personal behavior and interpersonal interactions based on consideration of cultural norms, including those that oppress marginalized populations, those that bestow privilege to specific groups based on the color of their skin, gender, identity, or socioeconomic status. Mindfulness fosters the realistic evaluation of consequences of various actions, cultural norms, and the well-being of oneself and others.[63,102]

Ultimately, when taught and learned together, mindfulness and occupational therapy have the potential to transform our profession from one focused on what can feel more like encouraging our clients to be occupational "doings" and instead foster and cultivate the qualities of what it means to be occupational "beings."

As mindfulness-based healthcare practitioners, we can help co-create a new paradigm in Western medicine; one that honors our power individually and collectively to come to terms with the actuality of things as they are and one that fosters embodied, courageous, and compassionate engagement with the world. Each of us has the opportunity to participate in this exciting stage of human evolution[35] and the movement toward a new model of care that is so deeply needed. This is a model of care that acknowledges the situation as it is and works to tilt the dynamic in the direction of one that is inclusive, equitable, just, grounded, compassionate, courageous, and reverent. In this way we become empowered mindfulness-based healing agents for the bloodstream of humanity.[71]

APPLY IT NOW: PRACTICE DESCRIPTIONS

This section describes modified versions of the core practices of mindfulness-based stress reduction. The traditional MBSR practices of body scan, sitting meditation, mindful yoga, and walking meditation have been adjusted to better fit the needs of the occupational therapist interested in integrating a practice into a treatment session. The best way to integrate these practices authentically into OT practice is for the therapist to integrate them into his or her own life first. The therapist who has had his or her own embodied experience of what it really means to participate in mindfulness practices will bring the practices into occupational therapy interventions in an authentic way. It is not recommended to integrate these practices into interventions if therapists themselves are not already clear about its usefulness or effectiveness and are not integrating them fully into their lives as well.[61]

Practice 1: Body Awareness Practice in Sitting or Lying Down

Approximate timing: introduction 3 minutes; practice 25 minutes.

Introduction: This is a body awareness practice designed for you (the OT) to use regularly to help assume an active and powerful role in your own health and well-being. It is best to use a guided body scan recording (see Additional Resources for links) and do what it says while in a comfortable place where you feel safe, secure, and free from interruption. Consider this practice time as an opportunity to be both by yourself and fully with yourself . . . an opportunity to nourish yourself, to open to and experience the potential of strength and insight within yourself.

You are choosing to show up for whatever is happening in this moment . . . making the choice to allow yourself to be exactly as you are in this moment. Completely as you are and complete as you are with no agenda other than to fall awake to the full dimensionality of the moment.

Our culture asks us to live so much in the cognitive and intellectual domain of experience. We often forget that the whole body feels and knows and that there is a wisdom beyond words.

The body awareness practice, as with all the others described here, provides ample opportunities to reinforce the powerful practice of cultivating nonjudgment and curiosity, in addition to nonstriving, kindness, and compassion toward oneself.

Mindfulness Practice: The 3-Minute Breathing Space: The following instructions for the 3-minute breathing space are adapted from Segal, Williams, and Teasdale.[82] You may wish to take about 5 minutes right now to read the instructions and use them to guide you through the practice, spending about a minute practicing each step after you read it.

- **Step 1: Becoming aware of present-moment experience.** Begin by taking an intentional posture that is upright but not stiff, eyes gently closed, or holding a soft gaze on the floor or wall a few feet in front of you. Next, begin to bring your attention to your internal experience, perhaps by asking, "What is my experience right now?" "What thoughts are passing through my mind?" Acknowledge thoughts as mental events as best you can, perhaps putting thoughts into words. "What feeling tone is here?" "Is there a sense of pleasant, unpleasant, or neutral feeling present?" In particular, allow any unpleasant feelings to be known. "What body sensations or reactions are noticeable right now?" Acknowledge any sensations in your body, including any areas of tightness or tension. Just letting them be, not needing to alter them in any way.

- **Step 2: Gathering attention on the breath.** In this step, redirect your attention to the physical sensations of the breath in your body. Focus on a particular area of the body where the breath sensations are most accessible, perhaps the abdomen rising and falling, or the air passing in and out through your nostrils. Follow the breath in your chosen area of the body from the very beginning of the in-breath, all the way to the pause when the breath turns and becomes the out-breath and follow the sensations all the way through the out-breath. Letting the breath be just as it is, without trying to change or regulate it in any way...allowing it to flow easily and naturally, with its own rhythm and pace, knowing you are breathing perfectly well right now, nothing for you to do. . . . Continuing in this way, allow your attention to rest on the breath sensations and gently return your attention to these sensations whenever you notice that it has wandered away.

- **Step 3: Expanding attention to whole body.** In the third step expand the spotlight of your attention once again, maintaining awareness of breathing while including a sense of whole body, perhaps a sense of the posture, and the internal sense of your facial expression.

- If any sensations of discomfort, tension, or resistance are present, allow them to be acknowledged and breathe with them. Perhaps on the out-breath, see if any tension can be released.

As best you can, bring this expanded awareness to the next moments of your day.

Exploring the breath and its soothing and anchoring potential. Come to gently notice the breath. It's such a constant feature of life that we often ignore it...so take time with it now...actually feel the sensations as the breath enters the body and leaves the body of its own accord…allow it to move through its cycle of in-breath and out-breath without controlling or needing it to be any other way than it is… if it feels right to you, attend to the belly, the lower abdomen, noticing that it may be rising and falling with the cycle of the breath. If you care to, place your hands on your belly, feeling the movement of breath, the rhythm, the waves of the breath… simply ride the waves of your breath from moment to moment.

Offering a safe haven. As you listen to the body scan, if at any time sensations in the body become too uncomfortable, or emotions arrive that are too difficult, know that it is always possible to return to the breath as a safe place, as a haven, a retreat for you to rest in, until you are ready to venture again and into the body scan…wherever the recording is in its progress.

Body awareness practice—in this practice we are building awareness of sensations and moving away from concepts toward direct experience. If you have placed your hands on your belly, allow your arms and hands to rest by your sides, and move your attention to the top of your head. Notice that sensations may arise when you bring attention to a particular part . . . maybe tingling, maybe pressure, maybe a feeling of breath. Or perhaps there is no sensation . . . that is OK; that is simply your experience at this moment. And when you're ready, move your attention to your forehead . . . observe sensation . . . perhaps sensations of tension, or tingling, or a sense of relaxation. Allow yourself to feel whatever you feel.

Now move your attention from the forehead to the eyes and eyelids . . . notice how you're holding them. How much or how little pressure does it take to keep them closed? Experience the eyes from the inside, from behind the eyelids. Are the eyeballs moving or still? Is there darkness? Light? Color? How does the breath affect this area?

When it feels right, begin to pay attention to the cheeks . . . sense the bones and the muscles coming to the skin of the cheeks . . . the air, sensations of coolness or warmth . . . note perhaps that some sensations stay for a while, whereas others pass quickly . . . and that intensity may change as you bring attention to them. Attend now to the nose, from the bridge to the edges of the nostrils . . . perhaps feeling the breath in the nostrils as it enters and leaves. Notice there are temperature, moisture, and sensations on the upper lip.

Moving the attention to the jaw . . . be aware of tightness or softness . . . allow the lower jaw to drop down slightly, and notice any changes in sensations in the muscles of the face and neck, or in other parts of the body, that this small movement may create. Expand your focus of attention to include the mouth and lips . . . inside the mouth, tongue against the teeth, sense the roof of the mouth, the gums . . . if you care to, breathe in through the nose and out through the lips, observing the sensations of dampness, dryness, warmth, or coolness.

Expanding the attention to encompass the entire face . . . don't just picture your face in your mind, but really feel the sensations in that area we call the face. Where is that for you? Be aware of any thoughts and emotions as well . . . and if thoughts or emotions arise, just allow them to simply come into awareness and then pass, like clouds in the sky.

Shifting the attention to your neck . . . notice how it is right now in the big muscles in the back of the neck, from the base of the skull to the shoulders . . . the throat . . . perhaps be aware of the sensation of air or the touch of clothing . . . be present in this experience.

Now to the shoulders; check into their condition in the moment . . . notice any tightness or softness, recognizing that this is the current condition . . . accept it, know that it does not need to be some other way. And know also that conditions change . . . notice if there is a sense of breath in the shoulders. How much of the body does breathing affect?

Allow attention to travel to the upper and midback . . . sense the muscles, tight or loose . . . perhaps be aware of sensations of the weight of the body here . . . pressure against the chair, feelings of the texture of clothing. Notice how the breath moves in this area.

Bring attention to the lower back…sense the contact or lack of contact with the chair…a sense of yielding to gravity or resisting . . . any tightness or softness. Notice any tendency to move away from or toward any sensations or thoughts, feelings, or judgments that may arise . . . remember this is simply how it is in the lower back at this moment.

Experience the whole back now, from the shoulders to the base of the spine . . . be aware of the subtle and not so subtle motions of the back as you breathe . . . dwell in the sensations in the back, not watching from your head, just knowing what the back knows.

Shift to the arms . . . to the upper arms and forearms . . . be aware of the pull of gravity, the weight of the arms . . . feel the muscles and joints . . . the touch and texture of clothing. Expand the attention to the wrists and hands . . . notice warmth or coolness, tingling, moisture, or dryness. How does the breath affect the arms and hands? Is it possible to feel the pulse here? Just be with what's here now.

And move, as you are ready, to the chest . . . to the lungs and heart in this space . . . maybe sensing inside, as the lungs fill and empty . . . perhaps noticing the heartbeat . . . the rhythm of the heart and the breath together. Be present to the sensations of life . . . what it feels like to be alive . . . and feel the surface, the touch of the clothing and any sense of movement.

Now extend attention to the abdomen, the belly, feeling inside first . . . this is the place where we have our gut feelings . . . there really are nerves here that sense and *know* . . . feel into the motion of the diaphragm, sense the breath in the belly.

When it seems right, move attention to the pelvic region, from hip to hip . . . be aware of the effects of gravity, the weight of the lower body . . . the buttocks pressed into the floor or chair, sensations in the joints . . . the groin, genitals . . . the lower abdomen . . . tune into the sense of the breath, or the pulse here. How far do they reach? And notice thoughts and feelings that may arise . . . be aware of any judgments and, as it's possible for you, let them go.

Shift the focus to the upper legs, the thighs . . . be aware of the sense of gravity, the pressure against the floor or chair, the feeling of clothing against the skin, and sense the quality of the muscles. Are the muscles tight or loose? Is it possible to feel the bone running through?

Extend the attention now to the lower legs, calves, and shins . . . notice points of contact or lack of contact with the floor or chair . . . be aware of gravity . . . be aware also that the legs are alive. How does the breath affect them? How does the pulse? Is there a sense of the blood flowing?

When you are ready, explore the feet . . . feel where they are . . . the floor . . . perhaps feel temperature sensations . . . warmth or coolness. Sense the heartbeat in the feet, perhaps?

Now, expand the attention to include the entire body, from the soles of the feet to the top of the head . . . be fully present to the totality of the experience of sitting or lying in this moment . . . sense perhaps the breath, the pulse, the heartbeat . . . feel a sense of gravity . . . a sense of being held gently, closely, without fail . . . dwell in what the body feels . . . and what it knows.

In the last moments of this body awareness practice, congratulate yourself for spending the time and energy to nourish yourself in this way . . . for continuing to make choices to live a more healthy, satisfying life . . . and know that you can carry this awareness of your body's deep wisdom beyond this practice session into each moment of your day, wherever you may find yourself.

Practice 2: Opening to and Expanding Awareness Practice

Approximate timing: introduction 3 minutes; practice 25 minutes.

Introduction. In your formal practice of sitting meditation, you are taking a seat right in the middle of your life. You are intentionally bringing yourself into a direct and intimate relationship with the present moment and what is arising in it for you—as much as possible, without judgment.

In this practice you have the opportunity to expand your attention to explore body sensations, sounds, thoughts, emotions, and, when you are ready, to open to all of these—to the full range of events and phenomena, within and without as they move and change, appear and disappear in awareness. You're taking time to become more familiar—moment by moment—with who you are, beyond all the wanting and having and doing . . . learning to dwell more in a domain of doing and learning to come to terms with the actuality of things as they are.

In a sense this practice is a perfect expression of your own unique presence in the world. It is helpful to come to this practice with a sense of kindness and care for yourself and bring a dignity and ability that resonates with your special status to the time, place, and posture of your sitting practice. Set aside a regular time when you won't be interrupted and can be in a quiet and comfortable place that can nurture your practice. When sitting, whether in a chair cushion or on the floor, maintain an attitude of confidence and stability—not leaning into or moving away from anything, simply be present with and open to what is happening now.

Opening to and expanding awareness practice. Sit in an upright position with your back straight and belly relaxed. Embody dignity and confidence . . . allow the sense of dignity to be both an expression and a reflection of your own innate integrity and wakefulness. Feel the floor or chair cushion beneath you, supporting you. Sense the pull of gravity holding you, receiving you. Find a point of balance where gravity is holding you comfortably upright, without strain. Allow the body to become still.

Bring your attention now to the sense of the body breathing, orient yourself to the breath entering and leaving the body . . . bring openness and curiosity to this moment. Notice where you feel the sensation of the breath most now . . . center your attention there.

Notice that there is a beginning, middle, and end of the in-breath and a beginning, middle, and end of the out-breath . . . (long pause).

Watch the entirety of the cycle of breath from beginning to the end. Notice the moment when the in-breath shifts to become an out-breath . . . and then notice the out-breath, from its beginning to when it shifts to become an in-breath . . . (long pause).

Realize that no matter how many times the attention leaves the breath, awareness of that does arise and there is an opportunity to choose and to bring the attention back . . . to this in-breath and/or the out-breath, now . . . (long pause).

Allow the breath to be at the center of your attention . . . to be center stage . . . allow any thoughts to come and go like clouds in the sky. If attention has wandered from the breath, gently but firmly escort it back, making the breath the focus of attention again . . . (long pause).

When you are ready, expand your attention beyond the breath to also include the entire body, sitting. Begin where there are distinct sensations in the body . . . perhaps in sensations of contact with the chair cushion . . . perhaps the touch of the clothes on your body or how your hands are feeling in the moment . . . perhaps sensations of temperature. Be present with any sensations as they rise.

Notice how sensations sometimes stay for just a short while, and how other times they linger . . . notice they may change in intensity, shift, and pass away as new sensations arise. Like the breath, they, too, have a beginning, middle, and end . . . (long pause).

Stay in touch with the sensations in the body as you sit . . . when attention wanders, notice you are making a choice to bring it back, with care and kindness, to the awareness of the body in the breath . . . (long pause).

We always have options and permission to explore our experience and notice the impermanence of all phenomena. If sensations arise in the body that are very intense, making it difficult to focus on the body or the breath, there are two ways to address this:

1. You may choose to mindfully change your posture, attending to the sensations of the movement as you shift.
2. You may choose to direct attention right into the intensity and sensation itself. Explore it with a gentle curiosity . . . notice nuances of sensation . . . perhaps notice thoughts and judgments . . . perhaps notice resistance or bracing . . . and, as much as possible, step back to observe, to open space in awareness, perhaps to soften the intensity of the sensation. Attend to duration . . . notice the duration and changes in

sensations . . . notice they have a beginning, middle, and end . . . (long pause).

Now, allow your attention to shift from the breath and body to the sense of hearing . . . not seeking sound, rather, receiving whatever is available from within the body and from the environment near and far. Become particularly aware of hearing . . . notice how the awareness receives sounds without effort . . . (long pause).

Be aware of how sounds have a beginning, middle, and end . . . how some sounds are short and some are long . . . sounds are varied and textured . . . there is space between sounds. Notice how the mind labels sounds . . . has opinions about sounds . . . it likes and dislikes certain sounds. Notice any desire to move away from some sounds and toward others . . . as much as possible, make a space in which sounds can be experienced as they are . . . (long pause).

And when you're ready, allow your attention to shift from hearing and let it expand to thinking—the realm of thought. See thoughts not as distractions but, rather, bring your awareness to the thinking process itself. Notice how thoughts arise, stay briefly, or for a more extended period, and then dissolve . . . they, too, have a beginning, middle, and end. So as not to get lost in the content of the thoughts, allow thoughts to be in the foreground of awareness, with sound, body sensations, and breath in the background . . . (long pause).

Notice thoughts . . . they may be about anything—sleep, obligations, the past, the future . . . if you get carried away in the current of thinking, come back to observing thoughts as separate events that come and go . . . thoughts moving through an open and spacious mind.

Emotions also arise in the body and mind . . . perhaps frustration, restlessness, peacefulness, sadness, joy, or fear . . . observe the emotion . . . bring attention to emotion and to the mood state. What is here for you right now? Notice where in the body certain emotions seem to live . . . (long pause).

Explore emotions . . . notice how what is here may be wanted or unwanted . . . how there may be a tendency to cling to emotion judged as pleasant and to struggle with emotions judged negatively—such as sadness or fear . . . (long pause).

Notice whatever emotions arise in the moment . . . Know that they have a beginning, middle, and end . . . Perhaps simply observing them in the body—letting go of supporting thoughts, narratives, or stories . . . (long pause).

If at any time emotions or sensations become too uncomfortable, remember that you can always return to the breath . . . find a safe harbor and focus there until you are ready to venture out again . . . (long pause).

Move now, if you care to, into a choiceless awareness . . . not choosing to bring your attention to anything in particular. Simply sit, fully aware of whatever is presenting itself to you in each moment. If sound arises, allow sound to be the center of attention. . . . If a body sensation arises, let that be the center of your attention until the next sensation arises, which may be another body sensation . . . or a thought about the body sensation . . . or an emotion . . . (long pause).

In one moment, the breath may be predominant and then, perhaps, sound might be most prominent . . . simply dwell with an open awareness, attending to whatever arises . . . (long pause).

Observe whatever presents itself to you in the moment . . . be spacious with whatever arises . . . (long pause).

Sit in stillness with whatever comes and goes . . . (pause) . . . be present with it all . . . (pause) . . . be here now . . . (pause) . . . open to the totality of your experience . . . (pause) . . . be fully human . . . (long pause).

Now return the attention to the body as you sit . . . feel the breath coming and going . . . stay fully present with body and breath . . . (long pause).

As this meditation practice comes to a close, realize that by practicing mindfulness you are intentionally deepening your ability to be fully present in your daily life. If it feels right, perhaps congratulate yourself for having taken this time and energy to nourish and care for yourself. Remember that practicing in this way helps create access to a wider, deeper, more open way of being in your life, in which you can see more clearly and make more conscious choices for health, well-being, and freedom.

Practice 3: Mindful Movement Practice During Activities of Daily Living

Approximate timing: introduction 3 minutes; practice 20 minutes.

Introduction. This guiding of gentle movement during an ADL is an invitation to enter more deeply into the life of the body . . . experience the mind and body as one, as a unit while moving the body . . . to bring them together. And as with all mindfulness practices, this movement practice is about paying attention, moment to moment, to sensations, thoughts, and feelings that arise in your awareness. The movements in this guided meditation are designed to be done during basic and routine ADLs, such as washing your hands or face or folding the laundry.

As you go through this guided practice, you will be entering into the experience of the body as deeply as you can, without judgment. This is not about performing, about doing the mindful movements in some ideal way for a critical audience . . . rather, it's about doing them to help connect more closely to, and better understand, the body while you move and participate in ADLs. Not forcing any movement but, rather, relaxing into it . . . using discernment and knowledge of your own body and its limits to guide you and to override the instructions, adapting the practice in a way that works for you. Or perhaps imagining yourself doing the movements in a mindful way, feeling them in stillness as you visualize participating in the ADL in a mindful way, which is a valuable practice in itself.

Mindful Movement Practice During ADLs. For this mindful ADL practice let's begin in an alert, dignified, seated posture . . . notice the how the chair or other support accepts you . . . how gravity works so you don't have to . . . sense the areas of your body that touch the seat or chair . . . sense your feet on the floor. Bring your attention to the sensations of the breath in the body . . . be aware of sensations of rising and falling, expanding and contracting, on the in-breath and out-breath . . .

and with each breath, allow the chair or support to receive more of your weight . . . working less, trusting and accepting more . . . breathing in and out.

When you're ready, breathe in and imagine yourself preparing to wash your hands as you stand at your sink . . . notice your body sensations as you stand at your sink, notice any thoughts or emotions that may arise in the moment and let them be, and guide your attention, with kindness and firmness, back to sensations of your body. Then actually walk mindfully to your sink . . . bring a sense of curiosity and freshness to the movement . . . feel the pressure of the soles of the feet as you take each step . . . feel the lifting, swinging, placing phase of each step you take. Stand still with your arms and hands at your side as you reach the sink and just feel the sensations of standing . . . sense the pull of gravity and the support of the surface you are standing on. Notice any unnecessary tension in your muscles and see if you might be able to release any tension . . . and, if not, just allow the sensations to go wherever they need to go.

Notice any thoughts or feelings that may enter your awareness, and as much as possible, allow them to simply come and go like clouds in the sky . . . keeping attention centered on the sensations of the body.

Now, bring your hands to the soap dispenser or bar of soap, hold the soap in your hand and experience the sensations of the force of gravity on the soap in your hand, the weight of the soap, the coolness or warmth, the texture . . . you may notice there is a scent to the soap, just notice it without judgment,

without narrative . . . then slowly, aware of the sensations of movement but without anticipating the next movement, begin to wash your hands. Allow an element of freshness of experience as you move the soap around in your hands. Now sense into the body as you move your hands to turn on the faucet and feel the sensation of the water as you rinse your hands, the warmth or coolness, the weight and texture, the sounds as just sounds. Notice how much of the body is involved in this activity, how the breath may change as you move. Now mindfully reach to dry your hands off with a towel, sensing the texture of the towel on your hands and wrists, and return to standing with your hands at your sides. As you stand still, notice how you feel in your body after having experienced the ADL of washing your hands in this way—with open, curious awareness.

In your own time, mindfully walk and return to a tall, dignified seated position and become aware of how you feel . . . aware of thoughts and emotions, and as much as possible, let them go as you focus on bodily sensations in this moment . . . allowing them to pass as clouds in the sky as you focus on the sensations in the body after experiencing this ADL in this way. If it feels right, perhaps congratulate yourself for having taken this time and energy to nourish and care for yourself . . . remembering that practicing in this way helps create access to a wider, deeper, more open and healthy way of being and doing in your life, in which you can see more clearly and make more conscious choices for your health, well-being, and freedom.

SUMMARY

How fortunate we are as a profession, in these efforts, in this time, to be able to draw upon a body of research that identifies practical and reasonable ways for us as individuals and as a profession to be able to articulate specific skills, qualities, characteristics, and practices that can, like a magic carpet, take us on a journey of compassionate self-exploration and enhanced insight and understanding, and ultimately bring us closer to an embodied experience of what it really means to use ourselves in a therapeutic way and to find for ourselves a meaningful balance

between what it means to "be" and "do." Mindfulness must be embodied, just as the use of the self as a therapeutic modality must be embodied. These practices are inextricably interconnected and inseparable, with an infinite depth. Developing one does not happen without developing the other, and when working on one, we also work on deepening the other. It is a true journey of exploration and one that is just emerging for our beautiful and complex healing profession.

REVIEW QUESTIONS

1. Define mindfulness and the therapeutic use of self. Who is mindfulness appropriate for? What are the major practices of mindfulness? Why is self-compassion such an integral part of developing mindfulness in one's life?

2. Explain ways in which the therapeutic use of self can be cultivated.

3. Describe ways in which the Western medical system and our modern culture might undermine our capacity to develop the therapeutic use of self. What is the potential impact of the current Western medical environment on the development of the therapeutic use of self? How might you mitigate these modern-day challenges?

4. Describe three or four ways in which the art and practice of embodying mindfulness as an occupational therapist can enhance the cultivation and development of the therapeutic use of self.

5. What is the significance of learning to turn toward one's own present-moment experience with openness and curiosity? How might occupational therapists skilled in this particular characteristic be able to benefit their client and/or the therapist-client relationship?

6. What is the distinction between pain and suffering?

7. List a few of the mindfulness-based interventions in which an occupational therapist could be trained.

8. In what ways did developing breath and body awareness empower Kay to make meaningful and lasting lifestyle changes that enhanced her health and well-being?

9. What is the point of cultivating interoccupational awareness?

10. Can occupational participation really be considered a healing agent and skillful tool if we as occupational therapists do not really know what it means to show up fully for our own occupations?

11. What is the significance of the word "being" in the term "occupational being"? What is an MBOT's role in cultivating "being" over "doing" for one's clients?

REFERENCES

1. American Occupational Therapy Association: AOTA 2020 occupational therapy code of ethics, *American Journal of Occupational Therapy* 74(Suppl. 3):7413410005, 2020.

2. American Occupational Therapy Association: Occupational therapy practice framework: domain and process, fourth edition, *Am J Occup Ther* 68(Suppl 1):S1–S48, 2020.

3. American Hospital Association: AHA hospital statistics: 2005, Chicago, 2005, Health Forum.

4. Birnie K, Speca M, Carlson L: Exploring self-compassion and empathy in the context of mindfulness-based stress reduction (MBSR), *Stress Health* 26(5):359–371, 2010.

5. Bishop SR, et al: Mindfulness: a proposed operational definition, *Clin Psychol (New York)* 11:230–241, 2004.

6. Bowen S, et al: Mindfulness-based relapse prevention for substance use disorders: a pilot efficacy trial, *Subst Abuse* 30(4):295–305, 2009.

7. Brady J, Guy J, Norcross J: Managing your own distress: lessons from psychotherapists healing themselves, *Innovations in Clinical Practice: A Source Book* 14:294–306, 1994.

8. Brazzoli GJ, Brewster GL, Kuo S, Does U.S.: hospital capacity need to be expanded? *Milbank Q* 22(6):40–54, 2003.

9. Brice H: Working with adults with enduring mental illness: emotional demands experienced by occupational therapists and the coping strategies they employ, *Br J Occup Ther* 64(4):175–182, 2001.

10. Bridgeman PJ, et al: Burnout syndrome among healthcare professionals, *American Journal of Health-System Pharmacy* 75(3):147–152, 2018.

11. Brogan K: *A mind of your own: the truth about depression and how women can heal their bodies to reclaim their lives*, New York, 2016, Harper Wave.

12. Brown KW, Ryan RM: The benefits of being present: mindfulness and its role in psychological well-being, *J Pers Soc Psychol* 84:822–848, 2003.

13. Chiappetta M. et al: Stress management interventions among healthcare workers using mindfulness: a systematic review, *Senses Sci* 5(2): 517–549.

14. Christopher JC, et al: Teaching self-care through mindfulness practices: the application of yoga, meditation, and qigong to counselor training, *Journal of Humanistic Psychology* 46:494, 2006.

15. Csikszentmihalyi M: *Flow: the psychology of optimal experience*, New York, 2008, Harper Perennial Modern Classics.

16. Dryden W, Still A: Historical aspects of mindfulness and self-acceptance in psychotherapy, *J Ration Emot Cogn Behav Ther* 24(1):3–28, 2006.

17. Embriaco N, et al: Burnout syndrome among critical care healthcare workers, *Curr Opin Crit Care* 13(5):482–488, 2007.

18. Epstein RM: Mindful practice, *JAMA* 282(9):833–839, 1999.

19. Epstein RM: Mindful practice in action, Part 1. Technical competence, evidence-based medicine, and relationship-centered care, *Families, Systems & Health* 21(1):1–9, 2003.

20. Epstein RM, Siegel DJ, Silberman J: Self-monitoring in clinical practice: a challenge for medical educators, *J Contin Educ Health Prof* 28(1):5–13, 2008.

21. Fang CY, et al: Enhanced psychosocial well-being following participation in a mindfulness-based stress reduction program is associated with increased natural killer cell activity, *J Altern Complement Med* 16(5):531–538, 2010.

22. Figley CR, editor: *Treating compassion fatigue*, New York, 2002, Brunner-Routledge.

23. Freudenberger H: Staff burn-out, *J Soc Issues* 30(1):159–165, 1974.

24. Germer CK: *The mindful path to self-compassion: freeing yourself from destructive thoughts and emotions*, New York, 2009, Guilford Press.

25. Goodman MJ, Schorling JB: A mindfulness course decreases burnout and improves well-being among healthcare providers, *The International Journal of Psychiatry in Medicine* 43(2): 119–128, 2012.

26. Greeson JM: Mindfulness research update: 2008, *Complementary health practice review* 14(1):10–18, 2009.

27. Grepmair L, et al: Promoting mindfulness in psychotherapists in training influences the treatment results of their patients: a randomized, double-blind, controlled study, *Psychother Psychosom* 76(6):332–338, 2007.

28. Grossman P, Niemann L, Schmidt S, Walach H: Mindfulness-based stress reduction and health benefits: a meta-analysis, *J Psychosom Res* 57(1):35–43, 2004.

29. Gura ST: Mindfulness in occupational therapy education, *Occup Ther Health Care* 24(3):266–273, 2010.

30. Guy J: Holding the holding environment together: Self-psychology and psychotherapist care, *Prof Psychol Res Pr* 31(3):351–352, 2000.

31. Guy JD, Poelstra P, Stark MJ: Personal distress and therapeutic effectiveness: national survey of psychologists practicing psychotherapy, *Prof Psychol Res Pr* 20(1):48–50, 1989.

32. Hanson R: *Hardwiring happiness: the new brain science of contentment, calm, and confidence*, New York, 2013, Random House.

33. Hashem Z, Zeinoun P: Self-compassion explains less burnout among healthcare professionals, *Mindfulness* 11:2542–2551, 2020.

34. Hazlett-Stevens H: Mindfulness-based stress reduction for health care staff: expanding holistic nursing paradigms to the whole system, *Holistic Nursing Practice* Volume 34(5):301–305, 2020.

35. Hubbard BM: *Conscious evolution: awakening the power of our social potential*, Novato, CA, 2015, New World Library.

36. Irving J, Dobkin P, Park J: Cultivating mindfulness in health care professionals: a review of empirical studies of mindfulness-based stress reduction (MBSR), *Complement Ther Clin Pract* 15:61–66, 2009.

37. Jackson S, Maslach C: After-effects of job-related stress: families as victims, *Journal of Occupational Behavior* 3:63–77, 1982.

38. Jackson SE, Schwab RL, Schuler RS: Toward an understanding of the burnout phenomenon, *J Appl Psychol* 71:630–640, 1986.

39. Janssen M, Heerkens Y, Kuijer W, van der Heijden B, Engels J: Effects of Mindfulness-Based Stress Reduction on employees' mental health: A systematic review, *PLoS ONE* 13(1):e0191332, 2018.

40. Johnson J, et al: Mental healthcare staff well-being and burnout: a narrative review of trends, causes, implications, and recommendations for future interventions, *International Journal of Mental Health Nursing* 27(1):20–32, 2018.

41. Kabat-Zinn J: *Full catastrophe living: using the wisdom of your body and mind to face stress, pain, and illness*, New York, 1990, 2013, Bantam Dell.

42. Kabat-Zinn J: *Coming to our senses: healing ourselves and the world through mindfulness*, London, 2005, Piatkus.

43. Kabat-Zinn J: *The healing power of mindfulness: a new way of being*, New York, 2018, Hachette Group.

44. Katz N, Hartman-Maier A: Metacognition: the relationships of awareness and executive functions to occupational performance. In Katz N, editor: *Cognition and occupation in rehabilitation: cognitive models for intervention in occupational therapy*, Bethesda, MD, 1998, American Occupational Therapy Association.

45. Keng S-L, et al: Mechanisms of change in mindfulness-based stress reduction: self-compassion and mindfulness as mediators of intervention outcomes *J Cogn Psychother*, 26, 2012. pp 270–280.

46. Kramer G, Meleo-Meyer F, Turner ML: Cultivating mindfulness in relationship: insight dialogue and the interpersonal mindfulness program. In Hick SF, Bien T, editors: *Mindfulness and the therapeutic relationship*, New York, 2007, Guilford Press, pp 195–214.

47. Krasner M, Epstein R: *Mindful communication: bringing intention, attention, and reflection to clinical practice (curriculum guide)*, Rochester, NY, 2010, University of Rochester.

48. Krasner M, et al: Association of an educational program in mindful communication with burnout, empathy, and attitudes among primary care physicians, *JAMA* 302:1284–1293, 2009.

49. Leitch SB, Dickerson A: Clinical reasoning, looking back, *Occup Ther Health Care* 14(3/4):105–130, 2001.

50. Lesser E: *Broken open: How difficult times can help us grow*, New York, 2005, Random House.

51. Levin MF, Weiss PL, Keshner EA: Emergence of virtual reality as a tool for upper limb rehabilitation: incorporation of motor control and motor learning principles, *Phys Ther* 95:415–425, 2015.

52. Lin M, et al: High prevalence of burnout among US emergency medicine residents: results from the 2017 national emergency medicine wellness survey, *Annals of Emergency Medicine* 74(5):682–690, 2019.

53. Lloyd C, King R: A survey of burnout among Australian mental health occupational therapists and social workers, *Soc Psychiatry Psychiatr Epidemiol* 39:752–757, 2004.

54. Lloyd C, McKenna K, King R: Is discrepancy between actual and preferred work activities a factor in work-related stress for mental health occupational therapists and social workers? *Br J Occup Ther* 67(8):353–360, 2004.

55. Ludwig DS, Kabat-Zinn J: Mindfulness in medicine, *JAMA* 300(11):1350–1352, 2008.

56. Magee R: *The inner work of social justice: healing ourselves and transforming our communities through mindfulness*, New York, 2019, Penguin Random House.

57. Maslach C: Characteristics of staff burnout in mental health settings, *Hosp Community Psychiatry* 29(4):233–237, 1978.

58. Maslach C: The client role in staff burn-out, *J Soc Issues* 34(4):111–124, 1978.

59. Maslach C: Burnout research in the social services: a critique, *J Soc Serv Res* 10:95–105, 1986.

60. Mate G: *When the body says no: exploring the stress-disease connection*, Hoboken, NJ, 2011, John Wiley & Sons.

61. McCown D, Reibel DC, Micozzi MS: *Teaching mindfulness: a practical guide for clinicians and educators*, New York, 2010, Springer.

62. McCraty R, Childre D, Martin H, Rozman D: *Heart intelligence: connecting with the intuitive guidance of the heart*, Cardiff, Calif., 2016, Waterfront Press.

63. McLaughlin R, Giroux J, Cara L, Chang M: *Proposal and curriculum for mindfulness-based occupational therapy advanced certificate program*, 2015, SJSU.

64. McLaughlin R, Giroux J: In Brown C, Stoffel VC, and Muñoz JP *Occupational therapy in mental health: a vision for participation*, ed 2, Philadelphia, PA: 2019, FA Davis.

65. McLean S, Wade T: The contribution of therapist beliefs to psychological distress in therapists: an investigation of vicarious traumatization, burnout and symptoms of avoidance and intrusion, *J Behav Cogn Psychother* 31:417–428, 2003.

66. Miller KI, Stiff JB, Ellis BH: Communication and empathy as precursors to burnout among human service workers, *Commun Monogr* 55:250–265, 1988.

67. Moore K, Cooper C: Stress in mental health professionals: a theoretical overview, *Int J Soc Psychiatry* 42:82–89, 1996.

68. Morgan N, Irwin MR, Chung M, Wang C: The effects of mind-body therapies on the immune system: meta-analysis, *PLoS ONE* 9(7):e100903, 2014.

69. Morse JM, et al: Beyond empathy: expanding expressions of caring, *J Adv Nurs* 1:809–821, 1992.

70. Nelson DL, et al: The effects of an occupationally embedded exercise on bilaterally assisted supination in persons with hemiplegia, *Am J Occup Ther* 50:639–646, 1996.

71. Nepo M: *The book of awakening: having the life you want by being present to the life you have*, Boston, 2000, Red Wheel/Weiser.

71a. Nerurkar A: What a happy cell looks like. The Altantic, February 10, 2025. https://bit.ly/48s6Sgu.

72. Nugent P, Moss D, Barnes R, Wilks J: Clearing space: mindfulness-based reflective practice, *Reflective Practice* 12(1):1–13, 2010.

73. Panagioti M, Geraghty K, Johnson J, et al: Association between physician burnout and patient safety, professionalism, and patient satisfaction: a systematic review and meta-analysis, *JAMA Intern Med.* 178(10):1317–1331, 2018.

74. Philippot P, Segal Z: Mindfulness based psychological interventions: developing emotional awareness for better being, *J Conscious Stud* 16(10–12):285–306, 2009.

75. Pines AM, Maslach C: Characteristics of staff burnout in mental health settings, *Hosp Community Psychiatry* 29(4):233–237, 1978.

76. Porges S: *The polyvagal theory: neurophysiological foundations of emotion, attachment, communication, and self-regulation*, New York, 2011, WW Norton.

77. Raquepaw J, Miller R: Psychotherapist burnout: a componential analysis, *J Prof Psychol Res Pract* 20:32–36, 1989.
78. Reid D: Capturing presence moments: the art of mindfulness practice in occupational therapy, *Can J Occup Ther* 76(3): 180–188, 2009.
79. Reid D: Mindfulness and flow in occupational engagement: presence in doing, *Can J Occup Ther* 78:50–56, 2011.
80. Santorelli S: *Heal thy self: lessons on mindfulness in medicine,* New York, 1999, Random House.
81. Sapolski R: *Why zebras don't get ulcers: the acclaimed guide to stress, stress-related diseases, and coping,* New York, 2004, St Martin's Press.
82. Segal ZV, Williams JMG, Teasdale JD: *Mindfulness-based cognitive therapy for depression: a new approach to preventing relapse,* New York, 2002, Guilford Press.
83. Seyle H: Stress without distress, *Vie Med Can Fr* 4(8):964–968, 1975.
84. Shanafelt TD, Bradley KA, Wipf JE, Back AL: Burnout and self-reported patient care in an internal medicine residence program, *Fam J Alex Va* 12:396–400, 2002.
85. Shapira LB, Mongrain M: The benefits of self-compassion and optimism exercises for individuals vulnerable to depression, *J Posit Psychol* 5:377–389, 2010.
86. Shapiro S, Brown KW, Biegel GM: Teaching self-care to caregivers: effects of mindfulness-based stress reduction on the mental health of therapists in training, *Train Educ Prof Psychol* 1(2):105–115, 2007.
87. Shapiro S, Astin J, Bishop S, Cordova M: Mindfulness-based stress reduction for health care professionals: results from a randomized trial, *Int J Stress Manag* 12(2):164–176, 2005.
88. Shapiro SL, Schwartz GE, Bonner G: Effects of mindfulness-based stress reduction on medical and premedical students, *J Behav Med* 21(6):581–599, 1998.
89. Shapiro SL, Carlson LE, Astin JE, Freedman B: Mechanisms of mindfulness, *J Clin Psychol* 62:373–386, 2006.
90. Siegel DJ: *The mindful therapist,* New York, 2010, WW Norton.
91. Siegel DJ: *Brainstorm: the power and purpose of the teenage brain,* New York, 2013, Penguin Group.
92. Siegel DJ: *The developing mind: how relationships and the brain interact to shape who we are,* New York, 2015, Guilford Press.
93. Siegel DJ, Bryson TP: *The whole-brain child: 12 revolutionary strategies to nurture your child's developing mind,* New York, 2011, Delacorte Press.
94. Smith BW, et al: Mindfulness is associated with fewer PTSD symptoms, depressive symptoms, physical symptoms, and alcohol problems in urban firefighters, *J Consult Clin Psychol* 79(5):613–617, 2011.
95. Spoorthy MS, Pratapa SK, Mahant S: Mental health problems faced by healthcare workers due to the COVID-19 pandemic: a review, *Asian Journal of Psychiatry* 51:102119, 2020.
96. Stew G: Mindfulness training for occupational therapy students, *Br J Occup Ther* 74(6):269–276, 2011.
97. Szalavitz M, Perry BD: *Born for love: why empathy is essential – and endangered,* New York, 2010, William Morrow.
98. Trombly CA: Occupation: purposefulness and meaningfulness as therapeutic mechanisms: 1995 Eleanor Clark Slagle Lecture, *Am J Occup Ther* 49:960–972, 1995.
99. Urbanowski F, Harrington A, Bonus K, Sheridan J, et al: Alterations in brain and immune function produced by mindfulness meditation, *Psychosom Med* 65(4):564–570, 2003.
100. Valente V, Marotta A: The impact of yoga on the professional and personal life of the psychotherapist, *Contemp Fam Ther* 27(1):65–80, 2005.
101. van der Kolk B: *The body keeps the score: brain, mind, and body in the healing of trauma,* New York, 2014, Viking.
102. Weissberg R, Goren P, Domitrovich C, Dusenbury L: *Collaborative for Academic Social and Emotional Learning (CASEL),* Arlington, VA, KSA-Plus Communications, 2012.
103. Wigglesworth C: SQ21: the twenty one skills of spiritual intelligence, New York, 2014, SelectBooks.
104. Winfrey O, interviewer. Interview with Jon Kabat-Zinn. OWN Network, 2015 (videotape).
105. Yela JR, Crego A, Gómez-Martínez MÁ, Jiménez L: Self-compassion, meaning in life, and experiential avoidance explain the relationship between meditation and positive mental health outcomes, *Journal of Clinical Psychology* 76(9):1631–1652, 2020.

ADDITIONAL RESOURCES

Mindfulness Recording Resources
Kabat-Zinn J: *Mindfulness meditation practices.* http://www.mindfulnesscds.com
Stahl B: Mindful healing recordings. http://www.mindfulnessprograms.com
Sounds True Audio. http://www.Soundstrue.com
Parallax Press: Books and recordings of Thich Nhat Hanh. http://www.parallax.org

Professional Training in MBSR
Brown School of Public Health: An International Learning Center for MBSR Teacher training: Center for Mindfulness in Medicine, Health Care and Society. https://www.brown.edu/public-health/mindfulness/home
El Camino Hospital Mindfulness Stress Reduction Program, Mountain View, CA: http://www.mindfulnessprograms.com/teacher-training.html
Duke Integrative Medicine, Durham, NC: https://dukeintegrative medicine.org/
Academic Education in Teaching Mindfulness-Based Interventions
Center for Mindfulness Research and Practice, School of Psychology, Bangor University, UK: https://www.bangor.ac.uk/mindfulness/
Postgraduate Master of Science in MBCT at Oxford University: http://www.oxfordmindfulness.org
Centre for Mindfulness Studies affiliated with the University of Toronto, in Toronto, ON: Canada, offers a certificate program in MBCT facilitation. http://www.mindfulnessstudies.com/pro-training/
Mindfulness-Based Health and Human Services Certificate (available Fall 2023). San Jose State University, https://catalog.sjsu.edu › preview_program
DBT Training Resource: Marsha Linehan Behavioral Tech Research, Inc: http://www.behavioraltech.org
ACT Training Resource: Steven Hayes Association for Contextual Behavioral Science: http://www.contextualpsychology.org

52

Integrating Telehealth Services Into Occupational Therapy Practice

Michelle Tipton-Burton and Fiona Dunbar

LEARNING OBJECTIVES

After studying this chapter, the reader will be able to do the following:

1. Define telehealth and its application in the delivery of occupational therapy services.
2. Examine the basic skills required for the delivery of telehealth occupational therapy services.
3. Understand regularity, legal, ethical, and supervision considerations in the delivery of telehealth services.
4. Identify special population considerations in telehealth delivery.
5. Understand technical considerations in implementing telehealth services.
6. Describe clinical decision-making strategies.
7. Consider telehealth-specific documentation requirements.

CHAPTER OUTLINE

KEY TERMS

Asynchronous technologies
Legal and regulatory
Privacy and confidentiality
Synchronous technologies

Telehealth
Telemonitoring
Telerehabilitation

Nikolas

The global pandemic of COVID-19 necessitated substantial changes in the method of service delivery for many clients receiving occupational therapy. The following case study is presented to illustrate how the abrupt pivot to telehealth continued to use skilled occupational therapy intervention and benefits were noted in the process of providing telehealth services. Although this case presentation represents the abrupt changes required given the global pandemic, the strategies provided can be used in constructing authentic outpatient occupational therapy intervention services for all clients.

Nikolas (prefers use of the pronouns he/him/his) is 35 years old and sustained a traumatic brain injury (TBI) 3 years ago. Following the TBI, Nikolas returned to live with his mother. His mother additionally serves as Nikolas' primary caregiver following the TBI.

Nikolas returned to an outpatient clinic recently and has been receiving occupational therapy services twice per week for 1 hour. The initial evaluation revealed significant motor planning deficits and spasticity throughout his limbs. Nikolas and his mother's primary goals were to increase independence with transfers and dressing and to safely perform therapeutic exercises. His mother attends all in-person sessions and is safe and independent with assisting Nikolas with mobility and self-care activities.

Because of an emergency mandated shut-down with the pandemic, Nikolas was no longer able to attend the clinic and was transitioned to telehealth sessions. The occupational therapist was able to complete six in-person sessions before transition to telehealth services. The in-person sessions focused on facilitation techniques to advance transfer and dressing skills and on therapeutic exercises to increase range of motion (ROM) and decrease spasticity in both upper and lower extremities.

The use of a telehealth service delivery model enabled Nikolas to continue to receive direct occupational therapy services using videoconferencing technology. The occupational therapy sessions continued at the same schedule initially established. One advantage identified during telehealth sessions was that Nikolas performed and practiced the functional skills in his natural environment. Nikolas' parents were actively involved in the occupational therapy sessions and able to facilitate the use of therapeutic strategies during dressing and transfer training. Initially the treatment sessions were challenging and time consuming, especially when collaboratively problem solving safe techniques during chair to floor transfers. The safety of Nikolas and his mother was a priority; therefore, using additional family members when addressing transfers was a key to success. Another advantage noted during telehealth sessions included assessment of the use of equipment such as bed rails that supported Nikolas with bed mobility and transfers. Advantages for the occupational therapist was not only observation of both parents' body mechanics but also the ability to provide real-time feedback during transfer practice in the natural environment. After the virtual sessions, the occupational therapist was also able to review video recordings with the supervisor, which promoted progression of clinical reasoning as well as professional growth.

Nikolas continued to demonstrate functional improvements in performance of self-care activities as well as instrumental activities of daily living (IADLs) such as simple meal preparation and home management tasks such as washing dishes and folding laundry. Client and parent satisfaction for telehealth sessions exceeded expectations, so when in-person sessions resumed, the family opted for a hybrid approach and continued with intervention sessions provided both virtually and in person.

TELEHEALTH DEFINITION, FORMATS, AND TYPES OF DELIVERY

The American Occupational Therapy Association (AOTA) describes telehealth as the use of telecommunication and electronic information technologies that support and promote remote clinical health services to patients and professional health-related education, public health, and health administration. AOTA also recognizes and uses the term *telehealth* for all nontraditional healthcare provided at long distance.[3,4] In March 2020, the United States underwent the national emergency of the COVID-19 pandemic in which shelter-in-place mandates were instituted throughout the country. The pandemic created a situation in which most nonemergency healthcare came to a sudden halt. In many instances, healthcare professionals had to quickly shift to remote (telehealth) services to continue to provide crucial services to their clients.

AOTA further describes telehealth services as "The application of evaluative, consultative, preventative, and therapeutic services delivered through information and communication technology (ICT)."[1] Telehealth services are provided in real time (live) between the client and healthcare provider. The methods to choose from include communication by telephone call or text, email, and phone- or computer-based video chat technologies. To provide confidential services, the occupational therapist must use Health Insurance Portability and Accountability Act (HIPAA)-compliant videoconferencing software.

Telerehabilitation

Telerehabilitation is described as the larger realm of telehealth and is the application of ICT specifically for the delivery of rehabilitation and habilitation services.[14] However, the term *telehealth* best represents the scope of occupational therapy services.[10,11] and is the prevailing term used in both state and federal policy. *Telehealth* is the recommended term used for all occupational therapy services provided through ICT.

Telemonitoring

Remote patient monitoring (RPM), or telemonitoring, is the monitoring and management of client factors such as vital signs (e.g., heart rate, blood pressure, oxygen levels) and other health data (e.g., blood sugar levels, activities of daily living (ADL) performance and fall events) for ongoing review and intervention by the clinician. This type of monitoring can prevent significant health issues and hospitalizations, promote health and wellness, and optimize independence with ADLs functioning. With the ongoing emergence of technologies, a range of telemonitoring devices have been designed for individuals with varying technology literacy and are available at a variety of cost ranges. Wearable (e.g., Apple watch, Fitbit) and home-based sensor monitoring systems such as artificial intelligence (AI) devices (e.g., Google Home, Alexa, Siri) are available.

Synchronous Technologies

Synchronous technologies such as videoconferencing allow the exchange of health information in real time by interactive video and audio between the healthcare provider and the client. Several options for HIPAA-compliant videoconferencing software are available, and more are being developed. Software features that are commonly used with telehealth include text chat, on-screen annotation (note of explanation added to a text or diagram), and computer screen sharing, which allows practitioners to share content from their own computer screen with the client in real time. Videoconferencing is the most common form of telehealth service delivery and can be provided using a variety of forms of technology. The advantage of synchronous technology using telehealth principles is the provision of services within the context where occupations naturally occur, such as the client's home, work site, or community. There are minimal infrastructure requirements and lower costs for equipment and connectivity (e.g., residential service plan, data plan). Disadvantages may include confidentiality, privacy (difficult to control with the end-user), poor bandwidth for connectivity (slow internet/frozen screen, abrupt disconnection), ongoing expenses (e.g., residential service plan, data plan), diminished sound or image quality, and technological challenges associated with end-user experience and expertise with videoconferencing technology.[9]

Asynchronous Technologies

Asynchronous technologies refers to a communication exchange in which the provider and client are not connected at the same time. Telehealth applications that are asynchronous may include video clips, digital images, and PDF handouts with illustrations and activity ideas. Applications within the practice of occupational therapy may include:

- Home evaluations and modifications
- Ergonomic assessments
- Home programs
- Mobility and ADL techniques and adaptations

GENERAL CONSIDERATIONS FOR OCCUPATIONAL THERAPY PRACTICE

As an occupational therapy practitioner, one must ensure safe and ethical delivery of services. To achieve that outcome, the clinician must consider the unique features of service delivery through the use of telecommunication methods. Although in-person evaluation and treatment procedures are ideal and offer the practitioner the ability to physically assess and observe clients' skills, behaviors, and responses to tactile and physical cues, telehealth services provide opportunities for clients who may not be able to attend in-person sessions because of shelter-in-place mandates, difficulty traveling, or residing in rural locations with limited availability to occupational therapy services. Without telehealth delivery methods, some individuals may not be able to receive services, which could prove detrimental.

Legal and Regulatory

Regulatory agencies such as Centers for Medicare & Medicaid Services (CMS), Department of Health and Human Services (DHHS), and Office of Civil Rights (OCR) enforce rules to ensure privacy and security for individuals receiving healthcare services. During the public health emergency (PHE) of 2020, covered health providers were not subject to penalties for violations of HIPAA privacy, security, and breach notification rules that occurred in good faith. If providers used technology during the public health emergency that was not fully compliant with HIPAA, individuals were not subject to imposed penalties; however, when the PHE restrictions were lifted, providers had to conform to HIPAA-compliant technology. Before implementing telehealth treatment:

- Examine state telehealth laws and regulations that may affect the delivery of services using information and communications technology (ICT).
- Research your state occupational therapy practice act and state occupational therapy board website for additional guidance on the use of telehealth to deliver occupational therapy services in the state in which treatment will occur.

Privacy and Confidentiality

Providers should ensure that clear policies related to services rendered, documentation and transmission, retention, and storage of video, audio, and electronic recordings and records are in place and are in accordance with the Health Insurance Portability and Accountability (HIPAA) privacy rule to protect the confidentiality and privacy of clients' protected health information. Healthcare providers are subject to penalties for violations of HIPAA privacy security and breach notification rules that occur; however, during emergency situations (e.g., mandated shelter-in-place), penalties for violations may be waived. Clients have the right to know that, despite efforts to protect their privacy and confidentiality, breaches may occur. In these instances, clinicians should understand and adhere to appropriate procedures addressing the compromise of the client's privacy and confidentiality of protected health information.[1]

Ethical Practice

Occupational therapy practitioners who provide telehealth services face unique ethical considerations. The Occupational Therapy Code of Ethics (2020) (referred to as the "Code"; AOTA[5]), in conjunction with other AOTA official documents, offers guidance for these considerations.[5] Clients should be informed of risks and benefits, their rights (e.g., right to refuse), and responsibilities and organizational policies for the retention and storage of audio and video recordings and electronic medical records. Practitioners should document and the client should sign the consent-to-treat process and telehealth content. Furthermore, the occupational therapist must respect the clients' right to refuse these telecommunication services.

Supervision

State licensure laws, facility-specific policies and procedures, and the *Guidelines for Supervision, Roles, and Responsibilities During the Delivery of Occupational Therapy Services*[2] and the Occupational Therapy Code of Ethics[5] must be followed, regardless of the method of supervision. Adherence to those guidelines to support both occupational therapy students and practitioners using telecommunication as part or in its entirety during assessment and treatment sessions. Direct supervision can be provided by joining the telehealth session and providing feedback during the interaction or discreetly using the "chat" option. Indirect options can be accomplished by reviewing recorded sessions and documentation. Precautions should be followed as they would be during in-person sessions. For example, use caution and assistance when performing activities that may be a safety risk such as transfers, activities that use appliances or sharps, and balance tests. Involving a caregiver or family member to assist will minimize such risks.

Documentation, Funding, and Reimbursement

Occupational therapy services provided through telehealth should be valued, recognized, and reimbursed in the same manner as in-person occupational therapy services. It is prudent to explore whether telehealth services will be covered by the client's insurance. When billing for occupational therapy services, practitioners may be required to distinguish the service delivery model. When completing documentation it is important to take the following steps[5]:

- Investigate with the payer source reimbursement and coding requirements for telehealth services.
- Ensure malpractice insurance carrier provides similar coverage for services provided through ICT.

BENEFITS AND CHALLENGES IN THE PROVISION OF TELEHEALTH SERVICES

The use of telehealth for the provision of occupational therapy and other healthcare services increased exponentially during the COVID-19 pandemic, and current trends indicate that telehealth will continue to be widely used even after the public health emergency is over. Literature investigating the effects of more widespread use of telehealth is emerging, with both benefits and challenges of this form of healthcare delivery process being examined.

Despite some skepticism at the perceived challenges of telehealth compared to in-person therapeutic interventions, benefits to receiving occupational therapy by telehealth have been recognized by clients and therapists. Telehealth permits occupational therapists to meet with clients within the natural environments and contexts of clients' everyday lives, whether at home, work, or in the community. Therefore, the delivery of occupational therapy services by telehealth promotes rehabilitation and habilitation within the framework of clients' (and their caregivers') normal routines, behaviors, and roles,[6] as well as the comfort of their own familiar environment. Some clients experience an increased sense of autonomy and independence

as they receive occupational therapy in the "hands-off" context of telehealth. Additionally, telehealth may increase access to healthcare services for some populations, including those in underserved or rural areas, those who lack transportation to get to and from traditional clinic-based settings, and those restricted by shelter-in-place regulations associated with a public health emergency. For the medically fragile, for whom traveling to a clinic visit may be strenuous and demanding of time and energy on the part of both the client and the caregiver, telehealth may be an optimal choice for treatment. By eliminating travel time and expenses for clients and offering therapy outside of traditional work hours, access to services may be further improved, making therapy sessions more time-effective and convenient. Access to healthcare at home through telehealth may decrease overall healthcare costs while contributing to positive health outcomes.[12] Finally, this service delivery method allows multidisciplinary team members to collaborate remotely on patient care.

Even while telehealth has proven effective for many clients and caregivers, it can create challenges not typically faced during traditional in-person occupational therapy and may not be appropriate for all individuals or populations. A certain level of technological literacy is required of clients to download, install, and adequately use videoconferencing applications for telehealth sessions. The need for internet connection can be a barrier, either because of issues with connectivity before or during occupational therapy sessions, or for those economically disadvantaged clients who lack broadband in their home.[15] Screen placement for clear visibility on the part of the client and occupational therapist can at times be a challenge, limiting accurate observations.

In addition to challenges presented by technology, the absence of hands-on care (particularly when there is no caregiver present) has been cited as a drawback to virtual visits and may especially limit therapeutic interventions in the case of clients with musculoskeletal conditions who require specialized facilitation and handling.[16] In the virtual setting, physical assistance and cueing are limited to verbal and visual cues. Clients receiving occupational therapy via telehealth may have decreased access to therapeutic equipment and modalities (e.g., pediatric sensorimotor gym, physical agent modalities, driving simulator) otherwise available when seen in person at a clinic. Therapists of pediatric clients expressed challenges faced when children eloped from or had difficulty sustaining attention during telehealth visits, and when intervening during aggressive or other problematic behaviors.[16] Limitations have additionally been observed when conducting assessments and evaluations by telehealth and may require the use of alternative strategies in place of the more standardized tools typically used in clinical settings. Additional drawbacks include challenges with developing therapeutic use of self and relying primarily on verbal communication in service delivery. Occupational therapists must at times use ingenuity and keen observation skills to be able to accurately evaluate and clinically observe clients through this method of healthcare.

In many cases, the involvement of caregivers may be mandatory or strongly advised during telehealth visits to ensure client safety, proper facilitation, positioning, skill development, and understanding of intervention strategies. This added caregiver involvement in therapeutic interventions has been reported as valuable to clients and caregivers, leading to improved outcomes because of carryover of skills and techniques used increasingly outside of therapy sessions. An example is the use of telehealth in school-based practice, in which Rortvedt et al.[15] reported that parents and teachers benefited from increased procedural knowledge of therapeutic interventions used with students.

Despite the challenges posed by telehealth, occupational therapists and clients report positive outcomes in its use. Patients and patient care advocates reported receiving high-quality healthcare across a variety of metrics and overall positive regard for future telehealth visits.[16]

OPTIMAL DELIVERY STRATEGIES

Interventions delivered through telehealth encompass the full scope of occupational therapy practice and must be client-centered and occupation-based.[6] Therapists should engage in up-to-date evidence-based practice as literature on telehealth emerges to ensure optimal treatment and outcomes for clients. Although occupational therapy provided by telehealth employs many of the same strategies and techniques used when treating in-person, distinctive considerations must be addressed.

Special Preparation

To maximize efficacy and efficiency of every telehealth visit, the occupational therapist should contact clients (or their caregivers) in advance by phone call, email, or text message to confirm logistics (e.g., session date and time and, when relevant, send an internet link for accessing the telehealth appointment). The therapist may also choose to instruct clients on the optimal location to set up for the visit within their environment (e.g., kitchen, bedroom, or workplace cubicle) and the materials to have ready for the session to best accomplish interventions as planned. It is incumbent upon the occupational therapist to perform a careful chart review and note any precautions or safety considerations for each client before any therapeutic interventions. For reasons of safety, and in some cases to facilitate functional mobility, fine and gross motor tasks, proper handling, or understanding of task, it may be necessary to ensure that a caregiver or family member will be present and actively engaged in part or all of a client's telehealth session.

The occupational therapist must be prepared for potential technical difficulties (e.g., abrupt internet loss, patchy connection, challenges logging in to a session) and have the capacity to talk a client through trouble-shooting over the phone. Professional flexibility and creativity are required of therapists to swiftly adjust interventions as needed given potential technical challenges, or when clients do not have materials or caregiver assistance, or are not in a prespecified location as anticipated.

Technology and Visibility

Videoconferencing applications used on smartphones, tablets, and computers are the most widely used format for telehealth delivery at this time. Occupational therapy sessions are most effective when both therapist and client are in a quiet, distraction-free location with reliable internet connection. Therapists should be mindful that the type of device each client uses may affect visibility (e.g., screen size) and therefore may influence the selection of evaluations and interventions, or the decision to use screen sharing technologies. The type of device used, the presence of a caregiver during the session, and/or the capacity of the client will also influence whether the device can be repositioned during telehealth interventions. At times, repositioning either the client's or the therapist's screen view, or both, is necessary for optimal observation of engagement in the occupation or activity. If using a smartphone or tablet without a stand, one may need to hold or prop the device throughout the session, thereby limiting some activities. Sometimes the use of two devices simultaneously in the client's or therapist's environment may be optimal in observing an activity to completion—for example, a client preparing a meal in the kitchen and transporting it to the dining room. This allows not only observation of meal preparation but also of mobility and ability to carry the food to the table.

Client Safety, Fatigue, and Frustration

As always, developing rapport with clients is foundational to the successful provision of occupational therapy services and needs to be a foundation for services delivered by telehealth. Open communication and keen clinical observations are critical to anticipating safety precautions and to noting signs of fatigue, frustration, or other client concerns during a session.

Safety is the priority during telehealth sessions. If one anticipates a transfer or functional task to be potentially unsafe for a client, it is best to err on the side of caution and postpone until a later time when conditions are optimal or select another way to achieve the client's treatment goals. In some situations, a competent and willing caregiver may need to be present; in this event, the therapist must take caution that the task is safe for all parties. For example, when caregivers actively assist clients during telehealth, caregivers may require coaching on proper body mechanics for themselves as well as for the client. In contrast to an in-person session, in which the occupational therapist might provide tactile cues and special handling of a client, during telehealth the therapist may need to remind clients/caregivers to wait for instructions and demonstrations before attempting a task to ensure safety.

For clients with physical disabilities, telehealth visits should be designed to minimize unnecessary fatigue. Strategies include modeling actions or tasks to clients and caregivers, so they understand a task before undertaking it; sequence intervention activities and the need to transfer or move around in the environment during the session based on principles of energy conservation; and regularly check in with the client during every session to ascertain energy level. Because telehealth demands a high level of verbal and visual input, therapists must also consider cognitive, auditory, or visual fatigue for some clients and adjust interventions accordingly.

Conducting Evaluations, Assessments, and Interventions

Telehealth evolved rapidly during the beginning of the COVID-19 pandemic; before that little to no research existed on the use of occupational therapy evaluations conducted by telehealth. Evaluations were a perceived barrier to the efficacy of telehealth by some practitioners[15]; however, circumstances related to the public health emergency required that many clients be evaluated, assessed, and reevaluated through videoconferencing and other telehealth mechanisms.

Evaluation is a key and necessary component of the occupational therapy process[6] and can take a variety of formats, including standardized and nonstandardized tools, questionnaires, checklists, client and caregiver interviews, and clinical observations. When selecting assessment tools for telehealth, occupational therapy practitioners should approach this process in a manner similar to evaluating clients in person, with some additional considerations. Clinical reasoning and practitioner competence for administering an evaluation tool should dictate assessment selection to best meet the needs of each client.[4] The practitioner must also consider whether a specific tool or method for evaluation is safe for the client to perform independently or with the assistance of a caregiver or family member. If a caregiver is needed to safely administer an assessment, it is imperative that the caregiver be comfortable and safe in the role of assistant. Additionally, occupational therapy practitioners should appraise the client's environment to determine whether it is an appropriate and safe location for the evaluation, and know if the client will have the necessary materials and camera placement available to properly conduct and view the client's performance during the assessment. Reliability and validity for use of any assessment in a telehealth setting should be noted when selecting tools.

When clients are evaluated remotely by telehealth, this should be noted in the documentation. Also, if modifications are made to standardized testing protocols to facilitate the evaluation of a client, or if alternative materials or the assistance of a caregiver are employed during the evaluation, this must be documented.[4] When using telehealth, practitioners may need to rely more on nonstandardized methods for evaluating than is typical in a clinical setting because some assessments are not designed for application via telehealth. Therefore, observations of functional tasks and clinical assessments such as range of motion (ROM), sensation, strength, and tone are especially important for evaluating clients, which may require a caregiver to assist in facilitating and reporting findings. This will require skilled observations versus the specific measurements ordinarily taken when occupational therapy is delivered in person. An increasing number of standardized assessments can be conducted remotely, and some tools (e.g., the Sensory Processing Measure) can be emailed to clients or caregivers directly from the publishing company (Box 52.1). These will automatically generate scores upon completion for the occupational therapist and multidisciplinary team members to review. Telehealth will continue to evolve, with increased attention given to the appropriateness, reliability, and validity of assessment tools for accurate evaluation of clients' occupational performance. Therefore, practitioners should refer to current

> **BOX 52.1 Assessment Tools With Established Use for Telehealth[5]**
>
> - Montreal Cognitive Assessment (MoCA)
> - Mini-Mental State Examination
> - Kohlman Evaluation of Living Skills
> - Functional Reach Test
> - European Stroke Scale
> - Canadian Occupational Performance Measure (COPM)
> - Timed Up and Go Test
> - Functional Independence Measure (FIM)
> - Jamar Dynamometer
> - Preston Pinch Gauge
> - Nine-Hole Peg Test
> - Unified Parkinson's Disease Rating Scale
> - The Ergonomic Assessment Tool for Arthritis (from https://otpotential.com/blog/guide-to-ot-telehealth-assessments)
> - Beery VMI
> - Berg Balance Test
> - Katz Index of Independence in Activities
> - Lawton Instrumental Activities of Daily Living Scale
> - Manual Ability Measure-16
> - McMaster Handwriting Assessment Protocol
> - Mini-Cog
> - Modified Barthel Index
> - Pediatric Evaluation of Disability Inventory
> - Sensory Processing Measure and Sensory Profile-2
> - Short-Form Everyday Technology Use Questionnaire
> - Visual Symptoms Assessment
> - World Health Organization Disability Assessment Schedule II

research and evidence-based practice when selecting methods to evaluate and reevaluate clients.[4]

SPECIAL POPULATION CONSIDERATIONS

Research on the efficacy of telehealth delivery for specific populations is emerging in the field of occupational therapy and allied health disciplines. It is therefore incumbent upon occupational therapy practitioners to remain current on telehealth best standards and evidence-based practices specific to the client populations they serve.

Pediatrics

The use of telehealth for occupational therapy has become increasingly common and was a primary form of service delivery during the COVID-19 public health emergency among pediatric outpatient clinics, schools, and early intervention settings. Even before the pandemic, the literature indicated satisfaction among parents and therapists with the use of telehealth for pediatric rehabilitation services.[17] A key difference to providing pediatric occupational therapy through telehealth is an increased reliance on parent or caregiver involvement. With practice, some children as young as 3 years old can learn the basic technology skills to engage with a therapist virtually (e.g., muting and unmuting the microphone, observing demonstrations, answering questions, showing their work), but generally, younger children will need assistance for accessing technology and participating fully in therapeutic interventions.

This reliance on adult support can have the beneficial effect of increasing opportunities for direct caregiver involvement in and facilitation of their children's interventions to support occupational performance. By repeatedly and briefly explaining the rationale for interventions, families can learn why certain skills are being addressed and how to facilitate proper performance. This gives families and caregivers the tools to transfer learning and therapeutic techniques into everyday life with their children. However, in some cases, family circumstances may limit or preclude adult participation in their child's therapy sessions and practitioners should grade and adapt interventions to maximize each child's ability to independently attend and participate in therapy.

In school-based practice, occupational therapy practitioners have cited telehealth benefits, including flexible scheduling, the ability to observe children unobtrusively in natural environments, and increased accessibility for providing services to homebound children.[15] Increased capacity for multidisciplinary collaboration and real-time communication with the ability to text messages privately to other practitioners without disturbing a child mid-session have also emerged as beneficial to virtual service delivery.[8] However, evaluating and assessing pediatric clients may be more challenging virtually, so observation, interviews, and questionnaires play a greater role than they might in a clinical setting, in which standardized measurements not calibrated for telehealth are more typically used.

Some practitioners recommend using common, familiar household items during pediatric interventions, because not all families will have or be able to purchase special materials (e.g., dry rice or beans and a kitchen spoon could be used in place of kinetic sand and a spade for tactile exploration and tool manipulation). The use of simple and everyday materials allows families to prepare quickly and easily for teletherapy sessions, and for older children to prepare or gather materials independently. Very young children or clients with decreased attention may benefit from shorter sessions or the inclusion of short breaks during telehealth. Depending on the need for physical or other assistance, many older children and teens may participate in virtual therapy sessions with little to no in-home adult support.

Persons With Dementia

Positive outcomes have been identified with the use of telehealth for persons with dementia (PWDs) and their caregivers.[13] PWDs and their caregivers benefit from receiving health services within the natural home environment and from reducing the challenges associated with leaving home for health-related appointments. Telehealth interventions often focus primarily on caregiver education when cognitive capacity is significantly limited in clients with dementia. Caregiver education may include training in accessing social supports and community resources and in developing effective communication with the PWD, family members, and healthcare providers. Strategies for addressing problematic behaviors displayed by the PWD and for decreasing caregiver burden through self-care and respite opportunities also may be addressed.[14] Outcomes have been particularly effective for caregivers, with observed diminished caregiver burden, stress, and depression; improvements in caregiver ability to manage dementia-related behaviors; increases in accessing social supports and resources; and improvements in caregiver physical and mental health.[13]

Occupational therapy interventions to support clients with dementia have been effective using a variety of delivery methods including synchronous, asynchronous, combined with in-person treatment, and by telephone, video conferencing, and email. A number of assessment tools have been identified for use with this population, although it has been noted that increased time may be required to conduct these evaluations by telehealth. The Montreal Cognitive Assessment (MoCA), Revised Memory and Behaviors Problem Checklist (RMBPC), and Zarit Burden Interview (ZBI) have excellent test-retest reliability, and the Clinical Dementia Rating Scale (CDR) has good reliability.[13]

GROUP THERAPY DELIVERY

Telehealth video conferencing is an effective way to conduct group occupational therapy sessions for a range of client populations, including school-based and outpatient pediatrics and youth and adults with mental health needs and physical disabilities. Occupational therapy practitioners use clinical reasoning to judge whether individuals may benefit from telehealth provided in a group setting. Factors such as the size of the group, therapeutic goals, and optimal setup and format for interventions should be established before initiating group interventions.

Therapeutic interventions in a group telehealth setting create opportunities for social participation. Clients, as well as their family members or caregivers, can benefit from the support network and social outlet that may develop within occupational therapy groups. This may be especially true for clients who face isolation because of limited functional mobility or reduced access to transportation for accessing community resources and social interaction outside of the home. For some clients during the COVID-19 shelter-in-place period, weekly occupational therapy groups were their only social interaction, and therefore an important place to connect with others. Video conferencing platforms facilitate new ways for participants to engage in a group, including anonymously, thanks to the ability to direct public or private text messages to the facilitator or other group members, or to respond to anonymous surveys in real time. By using breakout rooms during the course of a group session, practitioners can facilitate more intimate conversations among smaller groups of participants.

Furthermore, participation is made more convenient because clients can join from home or any other location with internet connection with no additional time commitment for travel to and from a session. Practitioners may have increased flexibility to schedule group sessions at times of day that are most convenient for participants. Telehealth can eliminate or reduce logistical hurdles sometimes encountered in a clinic or healthcare facility, such as the ability to book a conference room at a desired time or having to cap the number of participants because of space limitations.

When delivering occupational therapy to a group by video conferencing technology, occupational therapists must address several special considerations. First, to decrease unanticipated distractions and interruptions, it is best for only one active speaker to have the sound on, with the remainder of the group muted. When participants are performing therapeutic activities and have microphones muted, keen visual observation skills on the part of the practitioner are required, lacking the audio from each client's voice and environment. Second, clarity of communication by the occupational therapist is crucial, with extra effort given to ensure privacy and tactfulness when giving cues to individuals rather than the whole group. Directly addressing people by name can be particularly important in groups. Third, when selecting interventions, practitioners should consider what materials all members of a group have readily available, as well as possible alternatives, and plan for the gradation of activities for individual client needs. Finally, as with running groups in person, practitioners may need to address group dynamics and actively facilitate communication and participation among differing personalities. The focus of group therapy may be wide ranging. Examples are found in Box 52.2.

BOX 52.2 **Focus of Group Therapy**	
Activity Groups/Thematic Groups	**Education/Discussion Groups**
• Seated yoga, tai chi, movement • Arts and crafts • Gardening • Virtual games, trivia • Mindfulness meditation • Stretches and strengthening exercises	• Pain and fatigue management • Healthy habits and routines (sleep, nutrition, etc.) • Energy conservation • Safety and home/environmental modifications • Coping skills

SUMMARY

Telehealth has the potential to increase client access to occupational therapy services. Provision of occupational therapy services, regardless of the mode of delivery, requires the practitioner to adhere to the Occupational Therapy Code of Ethics and maintain client confidentiality. The use of telehealth in occupational therapy offers both advantages and challenges, as outlined in this chapter. The decision to use occupational therapy telehealth services requires careful consideration of the client's needs and abilities along with the advantages and challenges posed by telehealth services. It should be a collaborative decision made by the client and occupational therapy practitioner to meet the client's occupational goals.

REVIEW QUESTIONS

1. Define telehealth.
2. What are some benefits of telehealth services?
3. What is the difference between synchronous technologies and asynchronous technologies?
4. What requirements are specific to telehealth documentation?
5. Identify 3 things the occupational therapy practitioner (OTP) needs to prepare for before the telehealth session.
6. What steps can the OTP take to maximize the use of technology during the telehealth session?
7. What are the HIPAA requirements for telehealth services?
8. Identify special considerations the OTP must make when providing group occupational therapy telehealth services.

REFERENCES

1. American Occupational Therapy Association.: Telehealth, *Am J Occup Ther* 67(Suppl):S69–S90, 2013. https://doi.org/10.5014/ajot.2013.67S69.
2. American Occupational Therapy Association: Guidelines for supervision, roles, and responsibilities during the delivery of occupational therapy services via telehealth technology, *Am J Occup Ther* 68(Suppl 3):S16–S22, 2014. https://doi.org/10.5014/ajot.2014.686S03.
3. American Occupational Therapy Association: Advisory opinion for the ethics commission: Telehealth, (2017). Retrieved March 17, 2020 from http://www.aota.org/-/,edoa/Corporate/Files/Practice/Ethics/Advisory/telehealth-advisory.pdf.
4. American Occupational Therapy Association: Position paper: Telehealth in occupational therapy, *American Journal of Occupational Therapy* 72(2), 7212410059p1-7212410059p18, 2018. https://doi.org/10.5014/ajot.2018.72S219.
5. American Occupational Therapy Association: AOTA 2020 occupational therapy code of ethics, *American Journal of Occupational Therapy* 74(Suppl. 3), 7413410005–7413410005p13, 2020. https://doi.org/10.5014/ajot.2020.74S3006.
6. American Occupational Therapy Association: Occupational therapy practice framework: Domain and process (4th ed.), *American Journal of Occupational Therapy* 74(Suppl. 2): 7412410010–7412410010p87, 2020. https://doi.org/10.5014/ajot.2020.74S2001.
7. Brennan D, Tindall L, Theodoros D, J, et al: A blueprint for telerehabilitation guidelines, *International Journal of Telerehabilitation* 2:31–34, 2010. https://doi.org/10.5195/IJT.2010.6063.
8. Camden C, Silva M: Pediatric telehealth: Opportunities created by the COVID-19 and suggestions to sustain its use to support families of children with disabilities, *Physical & Occupational Therapy in Pediatrics* 41(1):1–17, 2021. https://doi.org/10.1080/01942638.2020.1825032.
9. Cason J: Telerehabilitation: An adjunct service delivery model for early intervention services, *International Journal of Telerehabilitation* 3:19–28, 2011. https://doi.org/10.5195/ijt.2011.6071.
10. Cason J: An introduction to telehealth as a service delivery model within occupational therapy, *OT Practice* 17:CE1–CE8, 2012.
11. Cason J: Telehealth and occupational therapy: Integral to the triple aim of health care reform, *American Journal of Occupational Therapy* 69(2):6902090010 p1–69020900p8, 2015. https://doi.org/10.5014/ajot.2015.692003.
12. Nissen RM, Serwe KM: Occupational therapy telehealth applications for the dementia-caregiver dyad: A scoping review, *Physical & Occupational Therapy in Geriatrics* 36(4):366–379, 2018. https://doi.org/10.1080/02703181.2018.1536095
13. Nissen RM, Hersch G, Tietze M, Chang PFJ: Persons with dementia and their caregivers' perceptions about occupational

therapy and telehealth: A qualitative descriptive study, *Home Healthcare Now* 36(6):369–378, 2018.

14. Richmond, T, Peterson, C, Cason, J, et al. (2017). Principles for delivering telerehabilitation services. Retrieved from https://www.americantelemed.org/main/membership/ata-sigs/telerehabilitation-sig

15. Rortvedt D, Jacobs K: Perspectives on the use of a telehealth service-delivery model as a component of school-based occupational therapy practice: Designing a user-experience, *Work* 62(1):125–131, 2019.

16. Tenforde AS, Borgstrom H, Polich G, Steere: Outpatient physical, occupational, and speech therapy synchronous telemedicine: A survey study of patient satisfaction with virtual visits during the COVID-19 pandemic, *American Journal of Physical Medicine & Rehabilitation* 99(11):977–981, 2020.

17. Zylstra SE: Evidence for the use of telehealth in pediatric occupational therapy, *Journal of Occupational Therapy, Schools, & Early Intervention* 6(4):326–355, 2013. https://doi.org/10.1080/19411243.2013.860765.

53

Lifestyle Redesign®, Other Lifestyle Interventions, and Self-Management

Michal S. Atkins, Monica Godinez-Becerril, Stephanie Yang, and Jane Baumgarten[a]

LEARNING OBJECTIVES

After studying this chapter the student or practitioner will be able to do the following:

1. Identify the key theories and occupational therapy (OT) concepts framing Lifestyle Redesign® (LR).
2. State important criteria for successfully embedding new or renewed healthy daily routines.
3. Describe key intervention modules and related occupations that can empower the client to make a positive behavior change.
4. Describe the benefits and challenges of group vs. individual LR interventions.

CHAPTER OUTLINE

KEY TERMS

Chronic conditions
Healthy living
Lifestyle interventions
Lifestyle Redesign
Occupational engagement

Prevention
Readiness for behavior change
Routines and habits
Self-management
Well-being

THREADED CASE STUDY

Carmen, Part 1

Carmen (prefers use of the pronouns she/her/hers) had a stroke 2 years ago. She begins to cry as she looks in the mirror and barely recognizes herself. Carmen completed an inpatient rehabilitation program and months of outpatient therapy, and yet she feels hopeless about her future. Her right arm feels stiff and painful and she can hardly move it, and her right leg drags a little when she walks. She used to think that this would eventually all go away, but it has not, and the constant pain has become part of her. After the stroke, Carmen's occupational therapy goals and interventions focused on returning function to her right upper extremity and on activities of daily living (ADLs). During outpatient therapy she continued to focus on her right upper extremity (UE) function, and learned ways to cook, clean, and manage laundry with one hand. In addition, she learned to take public transportation independently. Carmen was recently referred to an OT Lifestyle Redesign (LR) program. She is ready to address her current challenges and set some goals that better address her limitations and barriers.

Can Carmen regain a sense of hope, engage in life-affirming activities, and experience less pain and isolation? To do this, Carmen must first feel hopeful. LR offers clients hope through the exploration of new and renewed occupational engagement. The path to a successful outcome lies in the client's willingness to accept and trust that changes to daily routines and habits can make the client feel better.

[a] The authors would like to thank the RLANRC clients who have entrusted occupational therapists to guide them to healthier, more meaningful lives, through the implementation of LR principles. Additionally, we would like to thank Michele Berro for her OT vision and unwavering support in building our LR programs, and to the USC Chan Division of Occupational Science and Occupational Therapy for decades of fruitful collaboration.

Lifestyle Redesign® (referred to as Lifestyle Redesign or LR throughout chapter) enables individuals to integrate health-promoting activities into their daily routines.[5] During therapy, individuals explore and practice healthful activities. This outpatient intervention seeks to embed engagement in new and renewed occupations into the home and community environments. LR is a manualized therapeutic intervention that uses self-analysis, education, and the practice of both new and renewed skills. This occupational therapy intervention framework originated at the University of Southern California (USC) Chan Division of Occupational Science and Occupational Therapy in the late 1990s. We note that although use of the term "Lifestyle Redesign" to describe occupational therapy services is limited to those who have completed rigorous training and certification by USC, the concepts outlined in this chapter may be integrated into occupational therapy interventions that are not referred to as Lifestyle Redesign.

LR is most appropriate when individuals are ready to incorporate new behaviors into their daily routines and improve their health. As clients become aware of their health status, such as acquiring a new diagnosis of diabetes, they may be ready to incorporate behavioral changes to reduce the risk of future complications. After traumas and/or new disabilities (e.g., spinal cord injury or stroke) individuals often require time (months or years) to gain some level acceptance of their permanent residual chronic condition and/or disability before participating in a LR program. Participants in the initial successful Well Elderly Study were healthy older adults, who benefited from the Lifestyle Redesign intervention to optimize their health and well-being through engagement in healthy occupations. As this intervention ultimately seeks to optimize people's health regardless of their medical status and life challenges, it can be offered to all individuals invested in bettering their own lives.

The focus of LR is on the performance patterns of habits, routines, life roles, and rituals. The occupational domains (which reflect the American Occupational Therapy Association [AOTA] Occupational Therapy Practice Framework-4)[1] addressed in LR interventions include activities of daily living (ADLs), instrumental activities of daily living (IADLs), health management, rest and sleep, education, work, play, leisure, and social participation.

As of this writing, LR programs are available for a wide range of conditions and populations, including for metabolic disorders (e.g., diabetes and obesity), for movement and neurological disorders (such as Parkinson's disease, spinal cord injury, post stroke and multiple sclerosis), for the well elderly, for arthritis and chronic pain, for cardiac conditions, and for mental health conditions. The chapter authors have observed that when treating clients with greater than mild cognitive impairments, successful carryover to the home and community environment requires the help of dedicated, consistent caregivers.

The authors of this chapter have been involved in the implementation of Occupational Therapy Lifestyle Redesign (LR) programs at Rancho Los Amigos National Rehabilitation Center (RLANRC), in close collaboration with the USC Chan

Division of Occupational Science and Occupational Therapy (OSOT). One of the authors was an intervening therapist in the USC OT Lifestyle Redesign Pressure Ulcer Prevention Study (PUPS), for people with spinal cord injury. This collaboration has allowed therapists in community settings to have a positive impact on the lives of consumers with a wide variety of challenging life circumstances. Clients are able to improve their health and well-being by implementing innovative strategies designed to prevent disease or more effectively manage existing conditions.

LIFESTYLE REDESIGN FOUNDATION AND CONCEPTS

Answers to questions regarding what motivates people, how to bring about positive behavior change, and how to promote feelings of well-being have been the focus of healthcare professionals for some time. The contribution of occupational science (OS) and occupational therapy to answering these questions lies in our understanding of the centrality of human engagement in occupation. Core occupational therapy concepts that inform LR are the assertion that humans are occupational beings, driven and transformed by doing (Occupational Therapy Practice Framework[1] and LR writings), and that the "just right" balance of productive and restorative behaviors facilitates personal health and well-being.

In addition to occupational science and occupational therapy, Lifestyle Redesign incorporates theories, models, and practical tools from the sciences and the humanities, especially from philosophy, psychology, and sociology. Theories that inform LR include Social Cognitive Theory (self-efficacy),[2] the Transtheoretical Model (Stages of Change),[19] the Patient Activation Model,[10] Self-Determination Theory,[27] Habit Theory,[18] Motivational Interviewing,[26] and Flow Theory.[17]

Each of these theories contributes to the understanding of human emotions, cognition, and behaviors. Individuals are viewed as independent agents, motivated by internal and contextual factors. The authors of LR built on former studies and models that inform healthcare providers of better practices to facilitate desired lifestyle changes. These models depart from the medical model of prescriptive, authoritarian treatment regimens, moving toward a healthcare model that allows the client to experience successful learning and incorporates conducive environmental conditions for improved self-efficacy.[2] Expanding on our professional foundation, Habit Theory, the Transtheoretical Model, and Motivational Interviewing provide the LR occupational therapist with practical tools to assess and treat individuals with a variety of chronic conditions.

LR first received worldwide recognition with the publication of the Well Elderly study.[5,12] This study of 361 independently living elders evaluated a new preventive occupational therapy intervention that led to improved health and well-being. Its innovation was the recognition that providing an individual with insight, autonomy, and control over occupational choices leads to improved health and increased feelings of well-being. In this randomized clinical trial, conducted from 1994 to 1996, participants were assigned to one of three groups: an occupational therapy group (later called LR), a social activity control group, and a nontreatment control group. The LR occupational therapy group was led by occupational therapists, and the therapeutic emphasis centered on self-analysis and the understanding of values, goals, and individual choices. Participants met for 9 months and engaged in lessons, peer exchange, and experiential learning. The social activity group was led by non-OTs and included crafts, games, viewing films, and going on outings. Outcome measures included the participants' perception of their own quality of life, physical capacity, functional capabilities, and emotional health. Results of this study demonstrated the effectiveness of LR in embedding health-promoting behaviors in daily life for independently dwelling seniors.

To test the effectiveness of LR, the Well Elderly study was successfully replicated in more diverse populations and settings, with fewer fidelity measures in place, to more closely approximate real-world clinical practice.[6] It was followed by research examining the potential of LR to address the needs of other populations. The intervention was tested with people with spinal cord injuries who had recurring pressure ulcers[4] and in individuals with chronic pain,[28] such as those with diabetes mellitus,[23] multiple sclerosis, or other chronic medical conditions.

LR is a manualized intervention to ensure standardization of the program, because accurately delivering LR services in varied settings and locations is key to its success.[22,25] The process of manualization involves adhering to the main philosophies of OT, OS, and LR theories, conducting needs assessments of target populations, evaluating expert feedback and reviews, and running feasibility studies. The manuals are dynamic in nature and require content revisions as feedback regarding practical program considerations is received (e.g., the optimal number of group participants or the need to change an activity to better emphasize the educational element of a session).[3,22]

THREADED CASE STUDY

Carmen, Part 2

Motivation and Stage of Change
Motivating clients to change their behavior is challenging, because people's motives are fundamentally internal and significant energy is required to change daily routines. To help clients change their perceptions and ultimately their behavior, occupational therapists use their professional tools, including occupational analysis, occupational exploration (verbal or practiced), and motivational interviewing.

During the initial evaluation and initial intervention sessions, Carmen wore fashionable clothes but poorly applied makeup. It became clear that she was unhappy with her current appearance. The therapist reasoned that with improved appearance and self-image, Carmen would be able to work on other goals. The therapist designated Carmen as the teacher, and she instructed the therapist on makeup application. As Carmen became invested in teaching her therapist how to apply makeup, her appearance improved, as did her mood and her outlook on her future. It was then time to address other goals that were important to her.

LIFESTYLE REDESIGN EVALUATION AND INTERVENTION PROCESS

A client's referring diagnosis guides the focus of the LR intervention. At present, there is no dedicated LR evaluation tool. Pyatak et al.[20] recommend four categories of measures, including the Canadian Occupational Performance Measure (COPM) for occupational goal setting, performance, and satisfaction, a health management capability measure (e.g., a self-efficacy or patient activation measure, or if less formal assessing ADL/IADL performance, overall health status (e.g., SF-36 or WQ-5D) and diagnosis-specific measures[20] (e.g., in the Pain, Enjoyment of Life and General Activity Scale (PEG) for pain or the hemoglobin A_{1C} (Hb A_{1C}) blood sugar test results for diabetes.

LR focuses on developing a healthy, well-balanced day; therefore, assessing the client's typical day and the equilibrium of sleep, self-care, productive activities, and restful activities is an important step in making both client and therapist aware of daily buffers and challenges. This can be accomplished by administering the Balance Wheel activity Fig. 53.1.

Criteria for successful intervention depend on readiness for behavior change and ability to learn and retain new skills and routines. Adjusting to a new chronic condition and accepting new daily habits often requires months or even years; thus, expectations for learning during acute rehabilitation must be realistic.

Insight and short-term memory are also important for successfully embedding new behaviors. Consistent, involved caregivers can assist clients living with cognitive impairment to acquire and retain skills leading to successful LR outcomes.

THREADED CASE STUDY

Michael, Part 1

Michael (prefers use of the pronouns he/him/his) had a right cerebrovascular accident (CVA) 2 years ago. Additionally, he has had poorly controlled type 2 diabetes for the past 12 years, as well as obesity and depression. During his inpatient rehabilitation program and outpatient occupational therapy sessions, his therapists focused on his left upper extremity deficits and activities of daily living. Following his discharge from therapy, Michael stayed at home, lived a sedentary life, and stayed in bed for long hours. Fearful of having another stroke, and perhaps needing to have his foot amputated, he agreed to join the LR Stroke survivors' program. Like Carmen, Michael received several individual sessions before joining the LR Stroke group.

Lifestyle Redesign Intervention

The goal of LR is to embed healthy behaviors in everyday life. Clients may participate in the intervention individually, in a group setting, or a combination of both.

LR Individual Therapy

After clarifying and prioritizing goals, the client selects relevant topics from the manual to begin the work. Sessions typically last 1 to 2 hours. Most sessions include both educational and practice components. For example, stress management (which

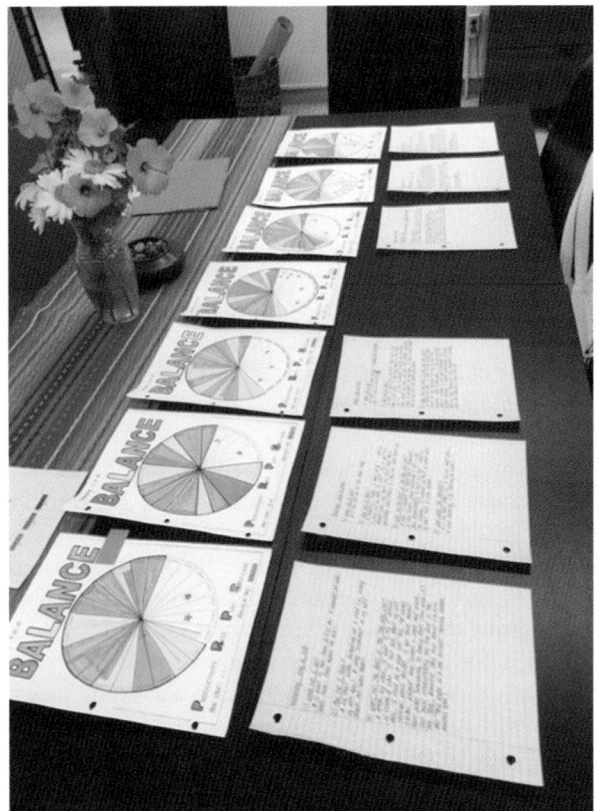

Fig. 53.1 A week of balance wheel home assignment raises clients' awareness of present routines and habits and assists in facilitating a needed change talk toward optimal daily balance.

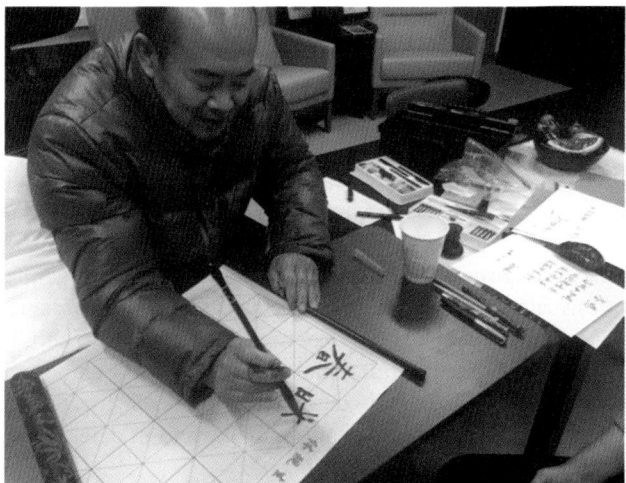

Fig. 53.2 Engaging in a meaningful activity facilitates pain reduction.

is relevant to most clients) may include education about the physiological mechanisms of stress followed by the practice of stress management techniques such as deep breathing and imagery. Another common topic, healthy eating, may involve learning to read and understand nutrition labels, comparing items at the market to make a healthier choice, and identifying healthier ways of cooking. Choice of ingredients will differ for each client, depending on the client's medical conditions and preferences.

To embed new daily routines and habits, clients are encouraged to practice what was learned in the intervention session at home. Subsequent sessions begin with an inquiry and discussion about successes with and barriers to the newly learned behaviors. Frequently, this dialogue involves the use of motivational interviewing techniques to further empower clients to reach their goals. A module (or topic) may require a single or multiple sessions to complete, depending on contextual barriers to behavior change, or the status of individual client factors.

The frequency and duration of sessions varies with the population, setting, diagnoses, and constraints imposed by payors. In the chapter authors' facility, sessions are typically held once a week for 3 to 4 months. These authors/practitioners have found that gradually decreasing the frequency of intervention sessions to once every 2 weeks or once a month may enhance a client's ability to continue with their newly learned behaviors.

Challenging behavioral changes such as weight loss require longer intervention duration.

During each therapy session clients receive home assignments. These assignments serve to ensure clients' ongoing engagement in their attempt to introduce and embed new daily behaviors and to assess the barriers to implementing their desired activity. "Homework" also serves to empower clients to assert self-efficacy in their ability to manage care away from the clinical setting (Fig. 53.2).

Successfully embedded healthy behaviors are celebrated, empowering clients to stay on course. Clients are encouraged to "own" their success and attribute their behavior change to their performance at home, away from the clinic setting. Some clients work on their goals sequentially and others may work on several goals simultaneously.

Working with clients individually has the advantage of tailoring the program specifically to that person, being able to provide undivided attention, and having fewer scheduling conflicts. Individual sessions, however, lack the dynamic nature of group interaction, missing out on learning from and sharing experiences with others encountering similar concerns.

LR Group Therapy

The advantages of group therapy for embedding new behaviors are well documented,[8,9,14] because clients value the relatedness to others. Participants in group therapy learn from one another and share their experiences with individuals who are living with similar conditions and challenges. Using activities as part of group therapy enhances interpersonal learning and group cohesiveness.[14]

In group therapy settings, clients are initially evaluated individually and then matched by diagnosis or shared goals. After the evaluation, the first sessions are dedicated to increasing a client's awareness of group processes and LR. These initial education sessions and discussions include group norms, awareness of daily behavioral choices, and the meaning of healthy living. Most sessions last 2 hours, and larger groups (more than 4 clients) require two therapists. Typical groups consist of 4 to 6 clients. At the beginning of most sessions, clients may meet individually with a therapist to identify and clarify their specific goals, after which all participants meet together to learn, discuss, share, explore, and engage in activities.

To further solidify new routines and habits, clients are encouraged to practice what was learned in the clinic in their own home environment. The next session begins with a discussion of what did and did not work within clients' homes. This allows individuals to reflect, share, and evaluate their behavior in a supportive environment.

Organizational challenges can make group therapy difficult. It takes time to select appropriate clients, coordinate schedules, and complete the necessary preparations for successful outcomes. Additionally, client factors influence the consistency of group attendance, because clients with chronic conditions and disabilities may become ill, experience transportation difficulties, or have conflicting schedules (Fig. 53.3).

THREADED CASE STUDY

Carmen and Michael

Participation in a LR Group

When Carmen felt better and began integrating healthier behaviors, she joined a group of five clients who shared common diagnoses and goals. Michael also joined the group, along with three additional stroke survivors. The group met for 2 hours weekly for 3 months. Because all of the clients were stroke survivors, topics included monitoring vital signs, managing medication, preventing another stroke, being active and exercising, eating healthy, engaging in meaningful occupations, sleeping well, establishing daily routines, engaging socially, and sharing community resources.

Carmen and Michael were active participants in the group and focused on achieving their goals. Like the other group members, they understood the importance of healthy eating but did not know how to achieve that goal. During intervention sessions, discussion topics included food groups, portion control, shopping on a budget, eating out, emotional eating, and food-related smart phone applications. The group members learned to compare products and make informed choices to support their health. Family members were encouraged to participate in these sessions to provide support and foster behavior change that could have an impact on the entire family (Fig. 53.4).

Participation in community activities with her group allowed Carmen's self-confidence to soar, and she returned to engaging in activities out in the community with family and friends, which was a very important goal for her.

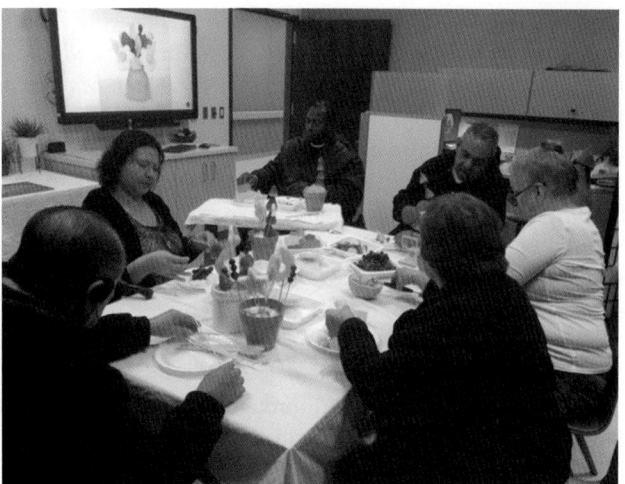

Fig. 53.3 While engaging in a fun group activity, the occupational therapist facilitates a discussion about the importance of increasing daily intake of vegetables and fruits to lose weight.

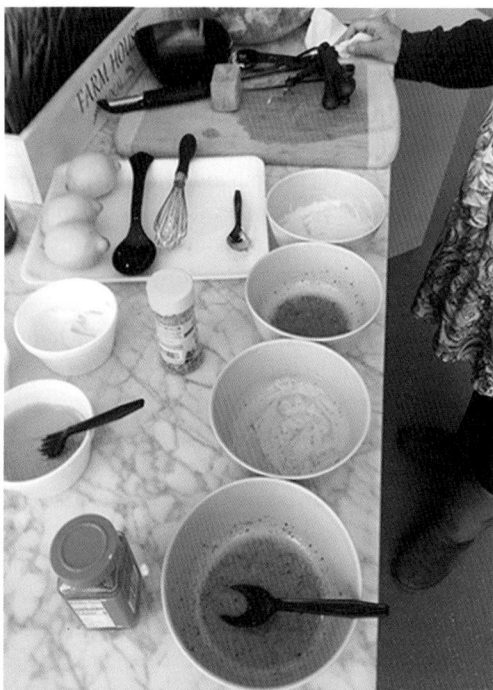

Fig. 53.4 Preparing different salad dressings that offer good taste with no sugar, reduced calories, and fat as an LR Diabetes group activity.

LR Modules

The manuals for LR are an integral part of the program. Topics and content are developed following needs assessment, literature reviews, and expert input. These manuals are created to meet the needs of varied populations in diverse locations and settings. Common topics are discussed and practiced with all participants, and are based on the core principles and values of occupational therapy. These include increased awareness of daily choices that foster good health and well-being, the centrality of the "just right" selection and balance of activities throughout the day, and the importance of sound daily routines and habits.

Common topics for populations with chronic conditions include exploring meaningful occupations, understanding routines and habits, stress management, healthy eating, exercise, and sleep hygiene.

Exploring meaningful occupations. Central to OT, finding activities that add meaning to the client's life is essential for individuals' health and feeling of well-being.

Carmen and Michael's group identified journaling and gardening as activities they would like to try. Carmen and Michael both found that journaling increased their sense of well-being. It also sparked Michael's love of writing, and he later volunteered at the hospital's gift shop, writing greeting card sentiments.

Gardening was explored to relax, exercise, practice mindfulness, meditate, and help manage pain. Both Carmen and Michael found that after being in the garden they felt better. Michael and his wife began to grow herbs for cooking and making his delicious orange and mint-flavored sparkling water (Fig. 53.5).

Understanding routines and habits. Fundamental to LR is becoming aware of the decisions people make in allocating daily "chunks of time" to engage in activities. Maintaining a daily activity log may increase awareness of the choices one makes and of environmental constraints that may interfere with daily plans.

As a result of depression, Michael explained that he did not "feel like doing much at home." He slept until after noon, did not eat breakfast, and snacked throughout the day "to keep my blood glucose levels in a good range." Michael spent the rest of his time watching TV and using his smart phone to play games. During therapy he was encouraged to explore using daily activity tracker phone applications as a means of increasing awareness of his time use. This allowed Michael to improve his routine for monitoring blood pressure and blood glucose level.

Stress management. Educating clients about the potential effects of stress (including triggers and buffers/relievers), as well as practicing stress management techniques is essential to improving feelings of health and well-being. Sessions may include breathing techniques, guided imagery, and body scan meditation, as well as introducing clients to phone apps and internet options for mindfulness practices and other stress management resources (Fig. 53.6). See Chapter 51 for more information on mindfulness.

All group members identified nature walks as enjoyable and relaxing. The group explored places to go for a walk and eat lunch together. After researching food options, the group went to the nearby pier for lunch, followed by a walk on the beach. Both Carmen and Michael have continued to use nature walks to manage stress, help them relax, and practice mindfulness, all of which lead to an increased sense of well-being.

Healthy eating. Following introduction to basic nutritional concepts, the educational component varies, depending on the chronic condition, and the socioeconomic and cultural background of the participants.

After his stroke, Michael understood that he must change his eating habits to manage his diabetes, lose weight, and decrease his risk of another stroke. He learned to read nutrition labels, analyze his food intake, shop on a limited budget, and cook simple meals, paying closer attention to healthier eating choices.

Exercise. The importance of daily exercise is stressed in maintaining clients' health. This may pose a challenge for individuals with mobility impairment, and occupational therapists are challenged to find a safe exercise option for each client. Options may include sitting yoga or tai chi, assessment of community resources that provide group exercise, and exploring online exercise programs.

Both Carmen and Michael identified dancing as a valued occupation. The group was introduced to a dance class, and the therapist modified their "moves" and the environment to provide a safe and enjoyable experience. They were able to resume their love of dancing with the added benefits of exercise.

Sleep hygiene. Many individuals with chronic conditions experience sleep disturbances. Difficulty falling asleep, waking

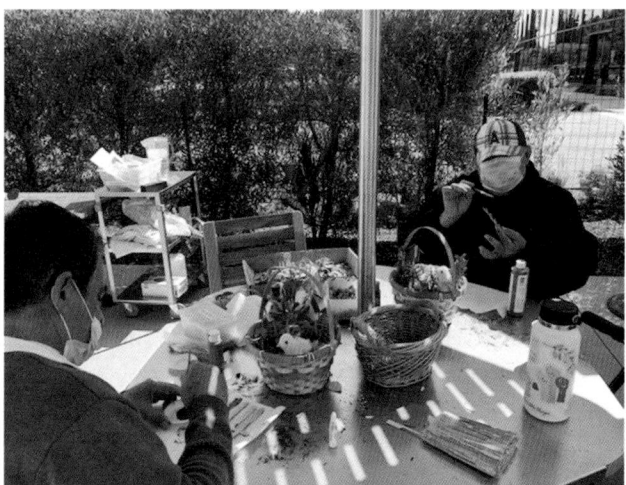

Fig. 53.5 A therapeutic garden is a backdrop to celebrating spring and the power of experiencing nature with its healing powers.

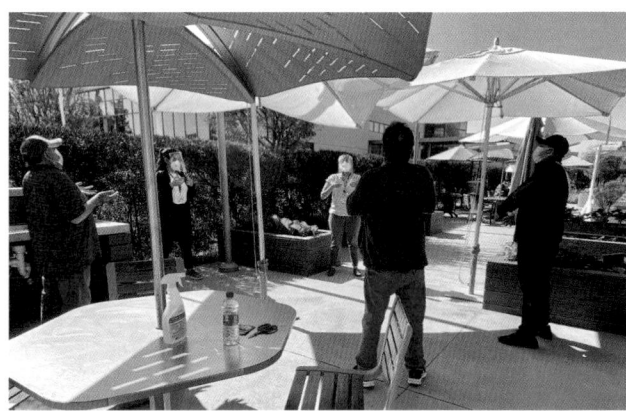

Fig. 53.6 To explore relaxation techniques, tai chi, a meditative and contemplative practice, is introduced to the group and can accommodate people with most physical limitations.

up multiple times without being able to fall back asleep, and not getting enough sleep are common challenges. Understanding and embedding sleep hygiene techniques and developing consistent sleep routines can augment medical solutions offered to the client by the physician. See Chapter 13 for more on sleep and rest.

Both Carmen and Michael identified sleeping better as an important goal. Each developed a sleep hygiene routine that helped them fall and remain asleep during the night.

SELF-MANAGEMENT AND OTHER LIFESTYLE INTERVENTIONS

Healthcare professionals have long understood that an authoritarian medical approach to changing clients' behavior seldom yields the desired results. Instead, providers have begun to seek out ways to engage their clients, to emphasize personal responsibility in disease prevention, and to form a patient-provider partnership that fosters problem solving. Self-care management and lifestyle interventions often focus on managing medical conditions, such as checking blood sugar for individuals with type 2 diabetes or monitoring blood pressure after a stroke.

In the mid-1980s, K. Lorig, a nurse and Stanford researcher, and her colleagues developed The Chronic Disease Self-Management Program (CDSM), which has been adopted nationally.[15] The program trains nonprofessionals to lead groups, educating clients in managing chronic illness effectively, and enhancing health-promoting behaviors using the principles of increased self-efficacy and problem-solving skills.

The model of recruiting nonprofessionals with the same medical condition as the client has been hailed for its success and low cost. It is important to note that the CDSM authors acknowledge that the program is not meant to conflict with existing programs or treatments but rather to augment them.

Occupational therapy has long been involved in healthcare education, health-promoting occupations, and fostering problem-solving skills. An increasing number of occupational therapy programs have expanded their focus on lifestyle interventions. Similar to the LR model, these programs offer individual and group therapy with the focus on healthy daily occupations. They address health and disease prevention with an occupational therapy lens first, analyzing individuals' occupational profile and environmental context to facilitate healthy behaviors. These programs also emphasize "the doing"—practicing skills in the clinic at home and in the community. Intervention is centered around daily occupations. Along with managing aspects of chronic conditions, individuals are guided in embedding meaningful, joyful, and restorative activities throughout the day.[16]

LIFESTYLE RESDESIGN AND TELEHEALTH

Telehealth, long thought of as a good idea for delivery of certain occupational therapy services, has received a substantial boost because of the COVID-19 pandemic.[11] Telehealth has become an important means of delivering services to clients with serious health conditions who have been advised to stay at home to prevent further medical complications.[7] Service delivery by phone or video is now being reimbursed by the Centers for Medicare & Medicaid Services (CMS) and may continue to be covered after the pandemic.

Therapists and clients communicate by secure telephone or video Wi-Fi connection. These authors have found that a blended model of in-person and telehealth sessions works well and is highly compatible with LR. Optimally, the program includes an in-person initial evaluation, followed by a combination of in-person and video intervention sessions. Seeing clients in their home environment promotes a better understanding of challenging circumstances and enhances problem solving. See Chapter 52 for more on Telehealth.

When addressing Carmen's UE pain and quality of sleep, the therapist explored her challenges with optimal bed positioning. During a video session, the therapist was able to assess her in her own bed, and together they problem solved optimal

THREADED CASE STUDY

Carmen and Michael: Follow-Up at 6 Months

Carmen is driving to work at a hospital food kitchen where she works part-time and has made new friends. She now attends her sons' sporting events and goes out regularly with her girlfriends. She routinely cooks for her family, something she had longed to do since her stroke.

Michael is happily married. Because of the lifestyle changes he has made, he no longer takes medication for his diabetes. His blood pressure and diabetes are better controlled by watching what he eats, keeping active, getting good sleep, and managing his pain and stress levels. He is doing stand-up comedy, a prior occupation at a community center near his house for special fund-raising events. He also volunteers at the hospital, helping people who are experiencing challenges managing their conditions, by offering insight, providing support, and sharing his experiences.

pillow placements. After some trial and error, Carmen reported decreased UE pain and improved sleep.

USE OF LIFESTYLE REDESIGN IN PRIMARY CARE

The goal of primary care is to deliver seamless treatment and monitor clients' health throughout the lifespan. This is especially important, considering the number of individuals living longer with multiple chronic conditions. Preliminary studies indicate that LR programs can complement the efforts of the primary care team in the provision of comprehensive health services to clients.[13]

In a preliminary study of clients with diabetes who received 8 hours of LR intervention in a primary care setting, participants (N = 38) who completed the program exhibited positive changes to their Hb_{A1c}, health status, and diabetes self-management.[21,24,25]

It is the hope of the chapter authors that more primary care clinics will routinely include LR programs, although more data needs to be collected and analyzed to demonstrate its efficacy in the primary care setting.

FUTURE DIRECTION FOR LIFESTYLE REDESIGN

USC occupational scientists, in collaboration with the USC OT Faculty Practice, are in the process of developing programs to promote the widespread implementation of LR. At the time of this publication, they are developing a certification program allowing occupational therapists to practice LR in their individual healthcare settings. The *Lifestyle Redesign* certification program is anticipated to launch in Fall 2024. More information about this program will be posted as it is available at https://chan.usc.edu/about-us/lifestyle-redesign.

SUMMARY

LR is an occupational therapy intervention that enables individuals to integrate health-promoting activities into their everyday routines. In therapy, clients explore and practice healthful activities. This outpatient intervention seeks to embed new and renewed occupations in the home and community environment. Manuals assist the therapist to organize, structure, and lead individual and group sessions.

OT Lifestyle interventions and self-management programs such as LR aim to assist individuals with chronic conditions to prevent further complications and live a healthy life. As people live longer and wish to continue to be active and productive in their homes and communities, occupational therapy is there to meet the challenge.

REVIEW QUESTIONS

1. When is Lifestyle Redesign most appropriate?
2. How is the effectiveness of Lifestyle Redesign tested?

3. What is the Chronic Disease Self-Management Program?

For additional practice questions for this chapter, please visit eBooks.Health.Elsevier.com.

REFERENCES

1. American Occupational Therapy Association.: Occupational therapy practice framework: Domain and process (4th ed.), *American Journal of Occupational Therapy* 74(Supplement 2), 7412410010 p1–7412410010p87, 2020. https://doi.org/10.5014/ajot.2020.74S2001.
2. Bandura A: Social cognitive theory: An agentic perspective, *Annual Review of Psychology* 52(1):1–26, 2001.
3. Blanche EI, Fogelberg D, Diaz J, Carlson M, Clark F: Manualization of occupational therapy interventions: Illustrations from the pressure ulcer prevention research program, *American Journal of Occupational Therapy* 65(6):711–719, 2011.
4. Carlson M, Vigen CL, Rubayi S, Blanche EI, Blanchard J, Atkins M, Clark F: Lifestyle intervention for adults with spinal cord injury: Results of the USC–RLANRC Pressure Ulcer Prevention Study, *The Journal of Spinal Cord Medicine* 42(1):2–19, 2019.
5. Clark F, Azen SP, Zemke R, et al: Occupational therapy for independent-living older adults: A randomized controlled trial, *JAMA* 278(16):1321–1326, 1997. https://doi.org/10.1001/jama.1997.03550160041036.
6. Clark F, Jackson J, Carlson M, Chou CP, Cherry BJ, Jordan-Marsh M, Wilcox RR: Effectiveness of a lifestyle intervention in promoting the well-being of independently living older people: Results of the Well Elderly 2 Randomised Controlled Trial, *J Epidemiol Community Health* 66(9):782–790, 2012.
7. Dahl-Popolizio S, Carpenter H, Coronado M, Popolizio NJ, Swanson C: Telehealth for the provision of occupational therapy: Reflections on experiences during the COVID-19 pandemic, *International Journal of Telerehabilitation* 12(2):77, 2020.
8. Edelman D, McDuffie JR, Oddone E, Gierisch JM, Nagi A, Williams JW:Jr, *Shared Medical Appointments for Chronic Medical Conditions: A Systematic Review*, Washington, DC, Department of Veterans Affairs, 2012.
9. Frates EP, Morris EC, Sannidhi D, Dysinger WS: The art and science of group visits in lifestyle medicine, *American Journal of Lifestyle Medicine* 11(5):408–413, 2017.
10. Hibbard JH, Mahoney ER, Stock R, Tusler M: Do increases in patient activation result in improved self-management behaviors? *Health Services Research* 42(4):1443–1463, 2007.
11. Hoel V, von Zweck C, Ledgerd R: Was a global pandemic needed to adopt the use of telehealth in occupational therapy? *Work,* 68(1):13–20, 2021.
12. Jackson J, Carlson M, Mandel D, Zemke R, Clark F: Occupation in lifestyle redesign: The Well Elderly Study occupational therapy program, *American Journal of Occupational Therapy* 52(5):326–336, 1998.
13. Jordan K: Occupational therapy in primary care: Positioned and prepared to be a vital part of the team, *The American Journal of Occupational Therapy* 73(5), 7305170010p1–7305170010p6, 2019.
14. Lloyd C, Maas F: Occupational therapy group work in psychiatric settings, *British Journal of Occupational Therapy* 60(5):226–230, 1997.
15. Lorig KR, Holman HR: Self-management education: History, definition, outcomes, and mechanisms, *Annals of behavioral medicine* 26(1):1–7, 2003.
16. Mountain GA, Craig CL: The lived experience of redesigning lifestyle post retirement in the UK, *Occupational Therapy International* 18(1):48–58, 2011.
17. Nakamura J, Csikszentmihalyi M: The concept of flow. In *Flow and the Foundations of Positive Psychology*, Dordrecht, 2014, Springer, pp 239–263.
18. Neal DT, Wood W, Quinn JM: Habits—A repeat performance, *Current Directions in Psychological Science* 15(4):198–202, 2006.
19. Prochaska JO, Velicer WF: The transtheoretical model of health behavior change, *American Journal of Health Promotion* 12(1):38–48, 1997.
20. Pyatak E, Carandang K, Collins Rice C, Carlson M: Optimizing occupations, habits and routines for health and well-being with Lifestyle Redesign®: A synthesis and scoping review, *American Journal of Occupational Therapy,* 76(5): 7605205050, 2022.
21. Pyatak EA: The role of occupational therapy in diabetes self-management interventions, *OTJR: Occupation, Participation and Health* 31(2):89–96, 2011.

22. Pyatak EA, Carandang K, Davis S: Developing a manualized occupational therapy diabetes management intervention: Resilient, Empowered, Active Living with Diabetes, *OTJR: Occupation, Participation and Health* 35(3):187–194, 2015.

23. Pyatak EA, Carandang K, Vigen CL, Blanchard J, Diaz J, Concha-Chavez A, Peters AL: Occupational therapy intervention improves glycemic control and quality of life among young adults with diabetes: The Resilient, Empowered, Active Living with Diabetes (REAL Diabetes) randomized controlled trial, *Diabetes Care* 41(4):696–704, 2018.

24. Pyatak E, King M, Vigen CL, Salazar E, Diaz J, Niemiec SLS, Shukla J: Addressing diabetes in primary care: Hybrid effectiveness–implementation study of Lifestyle Redesign® occupational therapy, *American Journal of Occupational Therapy* 73(5), 7305185020p1–7305185020p12, 2019.

25. Pyatak B, Diaz J, Linderman M, Niemiec SLS, Lee ES, Mehdiyeva K, Banerjee J: Addressing diabetes in a safety net primary care clinic: Effectiveness of Lifestyle Redesign occupational therapy, *Annals of Behavioral Medicine* 54: s68–s68, 2020.

26. Rollnick S, Allison J: Motivational interviewing. In *The Essential Handbook of Treatment and Prevention of Alcohol Problems*, Hoboken, NJ, 2004, Wiley and Sons, pp 105–116.

27. Ryan RM, Deci EL: Self-determination theory and the facilitation of intrinsic motivation, social development, and well-being, *American Psychologist* 55(1):68, 2000.

28. Uyeshiro Simon A, Collins CE: Lifestyle Redesign® for chronic pain management: A retrospective clinical efficacy study, *The American Journal of Occupational Therapy* 71(4): 7104190040p1–7104190040p7, 2017.

INDEX

Note: Page numbers followed by *f* indicate figures, *t* indicate tables, and *b* indicate boxes.